S0-APQ-001

Current Therapy in Adult Medicine

CURRENT THERAPY SERIES

Bardin:
Current Therapy in Endocrinology and Metabolism

Bayless:
Current Therapy in Gastroenterology and Liver Disease

Brain, Carbone:
Current Therapy in Hematology-Oncology

Callaham:
Current Practice of Emergency Medicine

Cameron:
Current Surgical Therapy

DeFronzo:
Current Therapy of Diabetes Mellitus

Ernst, Stanley:
Current Therapy in Vascular Surgery

Fazio:
Current Therapy in Colon and Rectal Surgery

Gates:
Current Therapy in Otolaryngology–Head and Neck Surgery

Glassock:
Current Therapy in Nephrology and Hypertension

Grillo, Austen, Wilkens, Mathisen, Vlahakes:
Current Therapy in Cardiothoracic Surgery

Hurst:
Current Therapy in Cardiovascular Disease

Johnson, Griffin:
Current Therapy in Neurologic Disease

Kadir:
Current Practice of Interventional Radiology

Kaplan:
Current Therapy in Pediatric Infectious Disease

Kassirer, Greene:
Current Therapy in Adult Medicine

Lichtenstein, Fauci:
Current Therapy in Allergy, Immunology, and Rheumatology

Niederhuber:
Current Therapy in Oncology

Parrillo:
Current Therapy in Critical Care Medicine

Rogers:
Current Practice in Anesthesiology

Schlossberg:
Current Therapy of Infectious Disease

Thrall:
Current Practice of Radiology

Torg, Shephard:
Current Therapy in Sports Medicine

Current Therapy in Adult Medicine

FOURTH EDITION

Jerome P. Kassirer, M.D.

Editor-in-Chief
The New England Journal of Medicine
Boston, Massachusetts

Harry L. Greene II, M.D.

Executive Vice-President
Massachusetts Medical Society
Waltham, Massachusetts

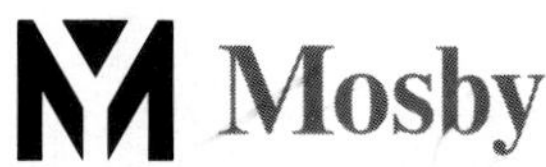

St. Louis Baltimore Boston Carlsbad Chicago Naples New York Philadelphia Portland
London Madrid Mexico City Singapore Sydney Tokyo Toronto Wiesbaden

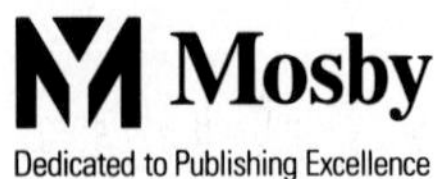

A Times Mirror
Company

Publisher: Anne S. Patterson
Senior Managing Editor: Lynne Gery
Editorial Assistant: Amanda Starr
Project Manager: Chris Baumle
Production Editor: Anthony F. Trioli
Designer: Nancy McDonald
Manufacturing Manager: William A. Winneberger, Jr.

FOURTH EDITION

Printed in the United States of America.
Composition by Graphic World, Inc.
Printing/binding by R.R. Donnelley and Sons Company

Mosby–Year Book, Inc.
11830 Westline Industrial Drive
St. Louis, Missouri 63146

ISBN: 0-8151-5480-1

97 98 99 00 01 / 9 8 7 6 5 4 3 2 1

Section Editors

C. Wayne Bardin, M.D.
Adjunct Professor, Department of Medicine, New York Hospital—Cornell Medical Center, New York, New York

Theodore M. Bayless, M.D.
Professor of Medicine, and Clinical Director, Meyerhoff Digestive Disease and Inflammatory Bowel Disease Center, The Johns Hopkins Medical Institutions, Baltimore, Maryland

Michael C. Brain, D.M., F.R.C.P., F.R.C.P.C.
Honorary Clinical Professor of Medicine, University of Calgary Faculty of Medicine, Calgary, Alberta; Emeritus Professor of Medicine and Pathology, McMaster University Faculty of Medicine, Hamilton, Ontario, Canada

Paul P. Carbone, M.D., D.Sc. (Hon), F.A.C.P.
Wattawa Bascom Professor in Cancer Research, and Professor, Department of Human Oncology and Medicine, University of Wisconsin Medical School; Director, University of Wisconsin Comprehensive Cancer Center, Madison, Wisconsin

Richard J. Glassock, M.D.
Chairman, Department of Internal Medicine, University of Kentucky College of Medicine, Lexington, Kentucky

John W. Griffin, M.D.
Professor of Neurology and Neuroscience, The Johns Hopkins University School of Medicine, Baltimore, Maryland

J. Willis Hurst, M.D.
Consultant to the Division of Cardiology (Professor of Medicine and Chairman of the Department, 1957-1986), Emory University School of Medicine and Hospital, Atlanta, Georgia

Richard T. Johnson, M.D.
Professor and Director of Neurology, and Professor of Microbiology and Neuroscience, The Johns Hopkins University School of Medicine, Baltimore, Maryland

Lawrence M. Lichtenstein, M.D.
Professor of Medicine, The Johns Hopkins University School of Medicine; Director, Johns Hopkins Asthma and Allergy Clinic, Baltimore, Maryland

David Schlossberg, M.D., F.A.C.P.
Professor of Medicine, Jefferson Medical College of Thomas Jefferson University; Director of Medicine, Episcopal Hospital, Philadelphia, Pennsylvania

Contributors

Elias Abrutyn, M.D.
Professor and Vice-Chairman, Department of Medicine, MCP-Hahnemann School of Medicine, and Professor of Public Health, School of Public Health, Allegheny University of the Health Sciences, Philadelphia, Pennsylvania

David W.K. Acheson, M.D.
Assistant Professor of Medicine, Tufts University School of Medicine, Boston, Massachusetts

Adaora A. Adimora, M.D., M.P.H.
Clinical Assistant Professor of Medicine, University of North Carolina at Chapel Hill School of Medicine, Chapel Hill, North Carolina

Gail K. Adler, M.D., Ph.D.
Assistant Professor of Medicine, Harvard Medical School; Associate Physician, Brigham and Women's Hospital, Boston, Massachusetts

Sharon G. Adler, M.D.
Professor of Medicine, UCLA School of Medicine, Los Angeles; Associate Chief, Division of Nephrology, Harbor-UCLA Medical Center, Torrance, California

Sanjay K. Agarwal, M.B., B.S.
Assistant Professor, Department of Obstetrics and Gynecology, UCLA School of Medicine; Director, Reproductive Medicine, Cedars Sinai Medical Center, Los Angeles, California

Gregory W. Albers, M.D.
Associate Professor of Neurology and Neurological Sciences, and Director, Stanford Stroke Center, Stanford University School of Medicine, Stanford, California

Garrett E. Alexander, M.D., Ph.D.
Professor of Neurology, Emory University School of Medicine; Attending Neurologist, Emory University Hospital, Atlanta, Georgia

Juan-Manuel Anaya, M.D.
Postdoctoral Research Fellow, Division of Clinical Immunology, University of Texas Health Science Center at San Antonio, San Antonio, Texas

Robert J. Anderson, M.D.
Professor of Medicine, University of Colorado School of Medicine; Chief, Medical Service, Veterans Affairs Medical Center, Denver, Colorado

Joseph D. Ansley, M.D.
Associate Professor of Surgery, Emory University School of Medicine, Atlanta, Georgia

Elliott M. Antman, M.D.
Associate Professor of Medicine, Harvard Medical School; Director, Samuel A. Levine Coronary Unit, Brigham and Women's Hospital, Boston, Massachusetts

George R. Aronoff, M.D., F.A.C.P.
Professor of Medicine and Pharmacology, and Chief, Division of Nephrology, University of Louisville, Louisville, Kentucky

Aris P. Assimacopoulos, M.D.
St. Paul Infectious Disease Associates, St. Paul, Minnesota

Maria R. Baer, M.D.
Research Associate Professor, Department of Medicine, State University of New York at Buffalo; Associate Professor, Division of Medicine, Departments of Hematologic Oncology and Bone Marrow Transplantation, Roswell Park Cancer Institute, Buffalo, New York

John Baillie, M.B., Ch.B., F.R.C.P.(Glasg.)
Associate Professor of Medicine, Duke University School of Medicine; Director, Duke Biliary Services, Duke University Medical Center, Durham, North Carolina

Laurence H. Baker, D.O.
Professor of Internal Medicine, University of Michigan Medical School; Deputy Director and Director for Clinical Research, University of Michigan Comprehensive Cancer Center, Ann Arbor, Michigan

C. Wayne Bardin, M.D.
Adjunct Professor of Medicine, New York Hospital-Cornell Medical Center, New York, New York

John B. Barlow, M.D., Hon. D.Sc. (Med)., F.R.C.P.
Emeritus Professor and Honorary Research Fellow, University of the Witwatersrand; Part-Time Cardiologist,Department of Cardiology, Johannesburg Hospital, Johannesburg, South Africa

John G. Bartlett, M.D.
Professor of Medicine, and Chief, Division of Infectious Diseases, The Johns Hopkins University School of Medicine, Baltimore, Maryland

Joseph H. Bates, M.D.
Professor of Medicine and Microbiology, University of Arkansas College of Medicine; Chief, Medical Service, Veterans Affairs Medical Center, Little Rock, Arkansas

Roy D. Baynes, M.D., Ph.D., F.C.P.S.A., F.A.C.P.
Professor of Medicine, and Director of Bone Marrow Transplantation, Wayne State University; Professor of Oncology, and Director of Bone Marrow Transplantation, Karmanos Cancer Institute, Detroit, Michigan

Arthur C. Beall, Jr., M.D.
Professor of Surgery, Baylor College of Medicine, Houston, Texas

Ivan T. Beck, M.D., Ph.D., F.R.C.P.C., F.A.C.P., F.A.C.G.
Emeritus Professor of Medicine and of Physiology, Queen's University Faculty of Medicine; Consultant, Hotel Dieu Hospital and the Kingston General Hospital, Kingston, Ontario, Canada

Kyra J. Becker, M.D.
Assistant Professor, Department of Neurology, University of Washington School of Medicine, Seattle, Washington

William R. Bell, M.D.
Edythe Harris Lucas-Clara Lucas Lynn Professor in Hematology, and Professor of Medicine, Radiology and Nuclear Medicine, and Clinical Director, Division of Hematology, The Johns Hopkins University School of Medicine; Physician on Duty, The Johns Hopkins Hospital, Baltimore, Maryland

Snunit Ben-Ozer, M.D.
Former Fellow, Reproductive Endocrinology and Infertility, University of California, San Diego, School of Medicine, La Jolla, California

Al B. Benson III, M.D., F.A.C.P.
Associate Professor of Medicine, Northwestern University Medical School; Director, Clinical Investigations Program and Adult Oncology Program, Robert H. Lurie Cancer Center, Northwestern University, Chicago, Illinois

Steven L. Berk, M.D.
Professor and Chairman, Department of Internal Medicine, East Tennessee State University, James H. Quillen College of Medicine, Johnson City, Tennessee

José Biller, M.D., F.A.C.P.
Professor and Chairman, Department of Neurology, Indiana University School of Medicine; Chief, Neurology Services, Indiana University Medical Center, Indianapolis, Indiana

Victor S. Blanchette, M.B., M.A., B.Chir., M.R.C.P., F.R.C.P.(Lon), F.R.C.P.C.
Professor of Medicine, University of Toronto Faculty of Medicine; Medical Director, Comprehensive Care Hemophilia Program and Pediatric Hemostasis Program, Hospital for Sick Children; Deputy Medical Director, Toronto Center, Canadian Red Cross Society Blood Services, Toronto, Ontario, Canada

Mitchell A. Blass, M.D.
Fellow, Division of Infectious Diseases, Emory University School of Medicine, Atlanta, Georgia

Andres T. Blei, M.D.
Professor of Medicine, Northwestern University School of Medicine; Associate Chief, Clinical Hepatology, and Medical Director, Liver Transplantation, Northwestern Memorial Hospital, Chicago, Illinois

Clara D. Bloomfield, M.D.
Professor of Medicine, and Chief, Division of Medicine, State University of New York at Buffalo; Chair, Division of Medicine, Roswell Park Cancer Center, Buffalo, New York

Charles D. Bluestone, M.D.
Eberly Professor of Pediatric Otolaryngology, University of Pittsburgh School of Medicine; Director, Department of Pediatric Otolaryngology, Children's Hospital of Pittsburgh, Pittsburgh, Pennsylvania

Frank G. Boineau, M.D.
Professor of Pediatrics, Tulane University School of Medicine; Chief, Section of Pediatric Nephrology, Tulane Hospital for Children, New Orleans, Louisiana

W. Kline Bolton, M.D.
Professor of Medicine, University of Virginia Health Sciences Center, Charlottesville, Virginia

Gianni Bonadonna, M.D.
Director, Division of Medical Oncology, Istituto Nazionale Tumori, Milan, Italy

Roger C. Bone, M.D., Ph.D.(Hon.), M.A.C.C.P., M.A.C.P.
Distinguished Professor of Medicine, Rush Medical College, Chicago, Illinois

José O. Bordin, M.D.
Associate Professor of Hematology and Transfusion Medicine, and Blood Bank Director, Escola Paulista De Medicina, Sao Paulo, Brazil

William R. Bowie, M.D., F.R.C.P.C.
Professor of Medicine, Division of Infectious Diseases, University of British Columbia Faculty of Medicine; Acting Staff, Vancouver Hospitals and Health Sciences Center, Vancouver, British Columbia, Canada

Suzanne F. Bradley, M.D.
Associate Professor of Internal Medicine, University of Michigan Medical School; Staff Physician, Veterans Affairs Medical Center, Ann Arbor, Michigan

Michael C. Brain, D.M., F.R.C.P., F.R.C.P.C.
Honorary Clinical Professor of Medicine, University of Calgary, Calgary, Alberta; Emeritus Professor of Medicine and Pathology, McMaster University Faculty of Health Sciences, Hamilton, Ontario, Canada

Nachman Brautbar, M.D.
Clinical Professor of Medicine and Pharmacology, and Director, Center for Toxicology, University of Southern California School of Medicine, Los Angeles, California

James L. Breeling, M.D.
Instructor in Medicine, Harvard Medical School; Associate Chief of Staff, Ambulatory Care, West Roxbury VA Medical Center, Boston, Massachusetts

Michael E. Brier, Ph.D.
Associate Professor of Medicine, University of Louisville School of Medicine, Department of Veterans Affairs, Louisville, Kentucky

Dan W. Brock, Ph.D.
University Professor, Professor of Philosophy and Biomedical Ethics, and Director, Center for Biomedical Ethics, Brown University, Providence, Rhode Island

Staley A. Brod, M.D.
Associate Professor of Neurology, Multiple Sclerosis Research Group, University of Texas Health Science Center, Houston, Texas

Steven L. Brody, M.D.
Assistant Professor of Medicine, Washington University School of Medicine; Attending Physician, Pulmonary and Critical Care Medicine, Barnes-Jewish Hospital, St. Louis, Missouri

Itzhak Brook, M.D., M.Sc.
Professor of Pediatrics, Georgetown University School of Medicine, Washington, DC; Senior Investigator, Naval Medical Research Institute, Bethesda, Maryland

Eduardo Bruera, M.D.
Professor of Oncology, and Alberta Cancer Foundation Chair in Palliative Medicine, University of Alberta, Edmonton, Alberta, Canada

Askiel Bruno, M.D., M.S.
Associate Professor, Department of Neurology, Indiana University School of Medicine; Director, Indiana Stroke Center, Indianapolis, Indiana

David W. Buchholz, M.D.
Associate Professor of Neurology, The Johns Hopkins University School of Medicine; Director, Neurological Consultation Clinic, The Johns Hopkins Outpatient Center, Baltimore, Maryland

M. Andrew Burgess, M.D., B.S., F.R.A.C.P.
Professor of Medicine, University of Texas M.D. Anderson Cancer Center, Houston, Texas

Thomas Butler, M.D.
Professor, Department of Internal Medicine, Texas Tech University Health Sciences Center; Consultant, and Attending Physician, University Medical Center, Lubbock, Texas

Alfred E. Buxton, M.D.
Professor of Medicine and of Cardiology, Temple University School of Medicine; Associate Chief of Cardiology, Temple University Hospital, Philadelphia, Pennsylvania

A. John Camm, M.D.
Professor of Cardiology, St. George's Hospital Medical School, London, United Kingdom

Paolo Caraceni, M.D.
Clinical and Research Fellow, Servizio di Patologie Medica, University of Bologna, Bologna, Italy

Hugh J. Carroll, M.D.
Professor of Medicine, State University of New York Health Science Center, Brooklyn, New York

Richard Casaburi, M.D., Ph.D.
Professor of Medicine, UCLA School of Medicine, Los Angeles; Associate Chief, Division of Respiratory and Critical Care Physiology and Medicine, Harbor-UCLA Medical Center, Torrance, California

Gail H. Cassell, Ph.D.
Charles H. McCauley Professor and Chairman, and Director, Clinical Mycoplasma Laboratory, University of Alabama School of Medicine, University of Alabama at Birmingham, Birmingham, Alabama

Peter A. Cassileth, M.D.
Professor of Medicine, and Chief of Hematology-Oncology Division, University of Miami School of Medicine, Miami, Florida

Daniel C. Cattran, M.D.
Professor of Medicine, University of Toronto Faculty of Medicine, Toronto, Ontario, Canada

Lawrence S. Chan, M.D.
Assistant Professor of Dermatology, and Director of Immunodermatology Division, Northwestern University Medical School; Attending Physician, Veterans Affairs Medical Center—Lakeside, Chicago, Illinois

Richard K.T. Chan, M.B.B.S., M.R.C.P.(UK)
Clinical Fellow, Department of Clinical Neurological Sciences, University of Western Ontario, London Health Sciences Centre, London, Ontario, Canada

Eugene B. Chang, M.D.
Martin Boyer Professor of Medicine, and Director, Inflammatory Bowel Disease Center, University of Chicago Pritzker School of Medicine, Chicago, Illinois

Feng-Yee Chang, M.B., D.M.S.
Associate Professor of Medicine, National Defense Medical Center; Attending Physician, Division of Infectious Diseases and Tropical Medicine, Department of Internal Medicine, Tri-Service General Hospital, Taipei, Taiwan, Republic of China

Gregory Y. Chang, M.D.
Associate Professor of Neurology, University of Southern California School of Medicine, Los Angeles, California

Kanu Chatterjee, M.B., F.R.C.P., F.A.C.C., F.C.C.P. M.A.C.P.
Professor of Medicine, and Lucie Stern Professor of Cardiology, University of California, San Francisco, School of Medicine, San Francisco, California

Lawrence J. Cheskin, M.D.
Associate Professor of Medicine, The Johns Hopkins University School of Medicine; Associate Professor of International Health (Human Nutrition), The Johns Hopkins University School of Public Health; Chief, Division of Gastroenterology, Johns Hopkins Bayview Medical Center; Director, Johns Hopkins Weight Management Center, Baltimore, Maryland

Judy H. Cho, M.D.
Instructor, Department of Medicine, University of Chicago Pritzker School of Medicine, Chicago, Illinois

Sanford Chodosh, M.D.
Associate Professor of Medicine, Boston University School of Medicine; Chief of Staff, and Chief of Pulmonary Medicine, Veterans Affairs Outpatient Clinic, Boston, Massachusetts

Charles S. Cleeland, Ph.D.
Professor of Medicine, University of Texas M.D. Anderson Cancer Center, Houston, Texas

Thomas J. Coates, Ph.D.
Professor of Medicine and Epidemiology, Director, Center for AIDS Prevention Studies, and Director, AIDS Research Institute, University of California at San Francisco, San Francisco, California

Thomas A. Cochran, M.D.
Assistant Professor of Surgery, Baylor College of Medicine, Houston, Texas

Arthur H. Cohen, M.D.
Professor of Pathology and Medicine, UCLA School of Medicine; Attending Pathologist, Cedars-Sinai Medical Center, Los Angeles, California

Zane Cohen, M.D., F.R.C.S.C., F.A.C.S.
Professor of Surgery, University of Toronto Faculty of Medicine; Surgeon-in-Chief, Mount Sinai Hospital, Toronto, Ontario, Canada

Nananda F. Col, M.D., M.P.P., M.P.H.
Assistant Professor, Department of Medicine, Division of Clinical Decision Making, Informatics and Telemedicine, New England Medical Center, Tufts University School of Medicine; Assistant Physician, New England Medical Center, Boston, Massachusetts

James D. Cook, M.D.
Phillips Professor of Medicine, University of Kansas Medical Center, Kansas City, Kansas

Bernard A. Cooper, M.D.
Clinical Professor of Medicine (Hematology), Stanford University, Palo Alto, California

David S. Cooper, M.D., F.A.C.P.
Director, Division of Endocrinology, Sinai Hospital of Baltimore; Director, Thyroid Clinic, The Johns Hopkins Hospital; Professor of Medicine, The Johns Hopkins University School of Medicine, Baltimore, Maryland

Martin G. Cormican, M.D.
Fellow, Division of Microbiology, Department of Pathology, University of Iowa Hospitals and Clinics, Iowa City, Iowa

Andrea M. Corse, M.D.
Assistant Professor of Neurology, The Johns Hopkins University School of Medicine; Attending Physician, The Johns Hopkins Hospital, Baltimore, Maryland

Joseph S. Coselli, M.D.
Professor of Surgery, Baylor College of Medicine; Attending Surgeon, The Methodist Hospital, Houston, Texas

James D. Cox, M.D., F.A.C.R.
Professor of Radiation Oncology, University of Texas M.D. Anderson Cancer Center, Houston, Texas

E. Stanley Crawford, M.D. (Deceased)
Formerly Professor of Surgery, Baylor College of Medicine; Senior Attending Surgeon, The Methodist Hospital, Houston, Texas

I. Sylvia Crawley, M.D.
Former Professor of Medicine (Cardiology), Emory University School of Medicine, Atlanta; Private Practice, Cardiology of Georgia, DeKalb Medical Center, Decatur, Georgia

Peter S. Creticos, M.D.
Associate Professor, Division of Allergy and Clinical Immunology, Department of Medicine, The Johns Hopkins University School of Medicine; Medical Director, Asthma and Allergic Diseases, The Johns Hopkins Asthma and Allergy Center, Baltimore, Maryland

J. Thomas Cross, Jr., M.D., M.P.H.
Assistant Professor, Departments of Internal Medicine and Pediatrics, Louisiana State University School of Medicine in Shreveport, Shreveport, Louisiana

Mark A. Crowther, M.D., F.R.C.P.C.
Clinical Fellow, Thromboembolism Program, McMaster University and Hamilton Civic Hospitals, Hamilton, Ontario, Canada

Steven R. Cummings, M.D.
Professor of Medicine and Epidemiology, University of California at San Francisco; Attending Physician, and Chief of General Internal Medicine, Moffitt-Long Hospital, San Francisco, CA

Burke A. Cunha, M.D.
Professor of Medicine, State University of New York School of Medicine, Stony Brook; Chief, Infectious Disease Division, and Vice Chairman, Department of Medicine, Winthrop-University Hospital, Mineola, New York

Marinos C. Dalakas, M.D.
Professor of Neurology, Georgetown University Medical Center, Washington, D.C.; Chief, Neuromuscular Diseases Section, National Institute of Neurological Disorders and Stroke, National Institutes of Health, Bethesda, Maryland

Vincent A. DeLeo, M.D.
Associate Professor and Vice Chairman, Department of Dermatology, Columbia University College of Physicians and Surgeons; Interim Director of Services, Department of Dermatology, St. Luke's-Roosevelt Hospital Center, New York, New York

Louis J. Dell'Italia, M.D.
Associate Professor and Clinical Director, Cardiology Fellowship Training Program, University of Alabama School of Medicine, Birmingham, Alabama

Samuel J. DeMaio, Jr., M.D.
Attending in Cardiology, Texas Cardiology Consultants, Baylor University Medical Center, Dallas, Texas

Richard D. DeShazo, M.D.
Professor of Medicine and Pediatrics, Director, Division of Allergy and Immunology, and Chair, Department of Internal Medicine, University of South Alabama, Mobile, Alabama

Stephen F. Deutsch, M.D., F.A.C.G.
Attending Physician, West Suburban Hospital Medical Center, Oak Park, Illinois

Lisa L. Dever, M.D.
Assistant Professor of Medicine, University of Medicine and Dentistry of New Jersey-New Jersey Medical School,Newark; Chief, Infectious Diseases Clinic, Department of Veterans Affairs Medical Center, East Orange, New Jersey

Luis A. Diaz, M.D.
Professor and Chairman, Department of Dermatology, Medical College of Wisconsin; Senior Attending Staff, Froedtert Memorial Lutheran Hospital, Staff Physician, Clement J. Zablocki Veterans Affairs Medical Center, and Consulting Staff, Children's Hospital of Wisconsin, Milwaukee; Courtesy Staff, Waukesha Memorial Hospital, Waukesha, Wisconsin

James D. Dick, Ph.D.
Associate Professor of Pathology, Molecular Microbiology, and Immunology, The Johns Hopkins University School of Medicine; Director of Bacteriology, The Johns Hopkins Hospital, Baltimore, Maryland

Wolfgang H. Dillmann, M.D.
Professor of Medicine, University of California, San Diego, School of Medicine, La Jolla, California

Germano DiSciascio, M.D.
Associate Professor of Medicine, Medical College of Virginia, Richmond, Virginia

Bruce H. Dobkin, M.D.
Professor of Neurology, and Director, Neurologic Rehabilitation and Research Unit, UCLA School of Medicine, Los Angeles, California

Thomas F. Dodson, M.D.
Associate Professor of Surgery, Associate Program Director, and Vice-Chairman for Education, Department of Surgery, Emory University School of Medicine, Atlanta, Georgia

John S. Douglas, Jr., M.D., F.A.C.C., F.A.C.P., F.A.C.S.
Associate Professor of Medicine, Emory University School of Medicine, Atlanta, Georgia

Leonard S. Dreifus, M.D.
Clinical Professor of Medicine, University of South Florida College of Medicine, Tampa, Florida

Daniel B. Dubin, M.D.
Instructor in Dermatology, Harvard Medical School; Associate Physician, Brigham and Women's Hospital, Boston, Massachusetts

David C. Dugdale, M.D.
Associate Professor of Medicine, University of Washington School of Medicine, Seattle, Washington

Marshall B. Dunning, III, Ph.D.
Assistant Professor of Medicine, Division of Pulmonary/Critical Care Medicine, Medical College of Wisconsin; Physician, Froedtert Memorial Lutheran Hospital, Milwaukee, Wisconsin

Herbert L. DuPont, M.D.
H. Irving Schweppe, Jr., M.D. Chair in Internal Medicine, and Vice-Chairman, Department of Internal Medicine, Baylor College of Medicine; Mary W. Kelsey Professor of Medical Sciences, University of Texas Health Science Center; Chief, Internal Medicine Service, St. Luke's Episcopal Hospital, Houston, Texas

Asim K. Dutt, M.D., F.C.C.P.
Professor and Vice Chairman, Department of Medicine, Meharry Medical College, Nashville; Chief, Medical Service, Alvin C. York Veterans Affairs Medical Center, Murfreesboro, Tennessee

Sudhir K. Dutta, M.D., F.A.C.P., F.A.C.G., F.A.C.N.
Division of Gastroenterology, Sinai Hospital of Baltimore, Baltimore, Maryland

Mark H. Eckman, M.D.
Associate Professor of Medicine, Tufts University School of Medicine; Physician and Chief, Division of General Medicine, New England Medical Center, Boston, Massachusetts

Steven V. Edelman, M.D.
Associate Professor of Medicine, Division of Endocrinology and Metabolism, University of California, San Diego; Director, Endocrine Fellowship Program, Veterans Affairs Medical Center, San Diego, California

Richard M. Effros, M.D.
Professor and Chief, Pulmonary and Critical Care, Medical College of Wisconsin, Milwaukee, Wisconsin

N. Joel Ehrenkranz, M.D.
Director, Florida Consortium for Infection Control, South Miami, Florida

Bruce Ettinger, M.D.
Clinical Professor of Medicine and Radiology, University of California, San Francisco, School of Medicine, San Francisco; Senior Investigator, Division of Research,Kaiser Permanente Medical Care Program, Los Angeles, California

Douglas B. Evans, M.D.
Associate Professor of Surgery, University of Texas M.D. Anderson Cancer Center, Houston, Texas

Janine Evans, M.D.
Assistant Professor of Medicine, Yale University School of Medicine, New Haven, Connecticut

Stefano Fagiuoli, M.D.
Senior Fellow in Transplant Medicine, Oklahoma Transplantation Institute, Baptist Medical Center of Oklahoma, Oklahoma City, Oklahoma

Richard J. Falk, M.D.
Clinical Professor, Department of Obstetrics/Gynecology, Georgetown University School of Medicine; Director, Division of Reproductive Endocrinology/Infertility, Columbia Hospital for Women, Washington, DC

Eben I. Feinstein, M.D.
Clinical Professor of Medicine, University of Southern California School of Medicine; Chairman, Department of Medicine, Good Samaritan Hospital, Los Angeles, California

M. Brian Fennerty, M.D., F.A.C.P., F.A.C.G.
Associate Professor of Medicine, Oregon Health Sciences University School of Medicine, Portland, Oregon

David W. Ferguson, M.D., F.A.C.C., F.A.C.P., F.C.C.P., Capt., M.C. U.S.N.
Professor of Medicine, Uniformed Services University of the Health Sciences; Director of Cardiology Training Programs, and Associate Chairman of Medicine, National Naval Medical Center,Bethesda, Maryland

James J. Ferguson III, M.D.
Assistant Professor, Baylor College of Medicine; Clinical Assistant Professor, University of Texas Health Science Center at Houston; Associate Director, Cardiology Research, Texas Heart Institute and St. Luke's Episcopal Hospital, Houston, Texas

Charles Fisch, M.D.
Distinguished Professor Emeritus of Medicine, Krannert Institute of Cardiology, Indiana University School of Medicine, Indianapolis, Indiana

Evelyn J. Fisher, M.D.
Associate Professor of Medicine, Division of Infectious Diseases, Medical College of Virginia, Virginia Commonwealth University; Director, Infectious Diseases Clinic, Medical College of Virginia Hospital, Richmond, Virginia

Richard I. Fisher, M.D.
Professor of Medicine, Loyola University of Chicago Stritch School of Medicine; Dorothy W. and J.D. Stetson Coleman Professor of Oncology, Director, Cardinal Bernardin Cancer Center, and Director, Division of Hematology-Oncology, Loyola University Medical Center, Maywood, Illinois

Robert S. Fisher, M.D., Ph.D.
Professor of Clinical Neurology, University of Arizona College of Medicine, Tucson; Chief, Epilepsy Center, Barrow Neurological Institute, Phoenix, Arizona

Neil Fishman, M.D.
Assistant Professor of Medicine, University of Pennsylvania School of Medicine, Philadelphia, Pennsylvania

J. Mark Fitzgerald, M.D., F.R.C.P.I., F.R.C.P.C.
Associate Professor, Respiratory Division, Department of Medicine, University of British Columbia Faculty of Medicine; Staff Physician, Respiratory Division, Vancouver Hospital and Health Sciences Center, Vancouver, British Columbia, Canada

Ronan Foley, M.D., F.R.C.P.C.
Hematologist, McMaster University Medical Center, Hamilton, Ontario, Canada

Noble O. Fowler, M.D.
Professor of Medicine Emeritus, University of Cincinnati College of Medicine; Attending Physician, University of Cincinnati Hospital, Cincinnati, Ohio

Robert H. Franch, M.D.
Professor of Medicine (Cardiology), Emory University School of Medicine; Senior Cardiologist, Emory Clinic, Emory University Hospital, Grady Memorial Hospital and Egleston Children's Hospital, Atlanta, Georgia

Martin J. Frank, M.D.
Formerly Professor of Medicine and Radiology, Medical College of Georgia School of Medicine, Augusta, Georgia

Harvey M. Friedman, M.D.
Professor of Medicine, University of Pennsylvania School of Medicine; Chief, Infectious Diseases, Hospital of the University of Pennsylvania, Philadelphia, Pennsylvania

Lawrence S. Friedman, M.D.
Associate Professor of Medicine, Harvard Medical School; Associate Physician, Gastrointestinal Unit, Massachusetts General Hospital, Boston, Massachusetts

Edward D. Frohlich, M.D., M.A.C.P., F.A.C.C.
Vice President for Academic Affairs, Alton Ochsner Medical Foundation; Professor of Medicine and Physiology, Louisiana State University; Clinical Professor of Medicine, and Adjunct Professor of Pharmacology, Tulane University, New Orleans, Louisiana

J. Pedro Frommer, M.D.
Department of Medicine, Baylor College of Medicine and the Methodist Hospital, Houston, Texas

J. Timothy Fulenwider, M.D., F.A.C.S.
Director, Noninvasive Vascular Laboratory, Northeast Georgia Medical Center, Gainesville, Georgia

Richard K. Fuller, M.D.
Director, Division of Clinical and Prevention Research, National Institute on Alcohol Abuse and Alcoholism, National Institutes of Health, Bethesda, Maryland

Robert F. Gagel, M.D.
Professor of Medicine, University of Texas M.D. Anderson Cancer Center, Houston, Texas

Eduardo Gaitan, M.D., F.A.C.P.
Professor of Medicine, University of Mississippi School of Medicine; Attending Physician and Chief, Endocrinology Section, G.V. (Sonny) Montgomery Veterans Affairs Medical Center, Jackson, Mississippi

John H. Galla, M.D.
Professor of Medicine and of Molecular and Cellular Physiology, and Director, Division of Nephrology and Hypertension, University of Cincinnati, Cincinnati, Ohio

Renee E. Garrick, M.D.
Associate Professor of Medicine, New York Medical College; Director of Dialysis Services, Westchester County Medical Center, Valhalla, New York

Ellen R. Gaynor, M.D.
Associate Professor of Medicine, Division of Hematology-Oncology, Loyola University of Chicago Stritch School of Medicine, Maywood, Illinois

Jack Geller, M.D.
Clinical Professor of Medicine, University of California, San Diego, School of Medicine; Director of Research, Mercy Hospital and Medical Center; Director of Clinical Research, Anti-Cancer Inc., San Diego, California

Saul M. Genuth, M.D.
Professor of Medicine, Case Western Reserve University School of Medicine; Chief, Division of Endocrinology, Mount Sinai Medical Center, Cleveland, Ohio

Hossein Gharib, M.D., F.A.C.P.
Professor of Medicine, Mayo Medical School; Consultant in Endocrinology and Metabolism, Mayo Medical Center, Rochester, Minnesota

Ray W. Gifford, Jr., M.D.
Professor of Internal Medicine, Ohio State University, Columbus; Consultant, Department of Nephrology and Hypertension, Cleveland Clinic Foundation, Cleveland, Ohio

Mark R. Gilbert, M.D.
Associate Professor of Neurology, Emory University School of Medicine, Atlanta, Georgia

Francis J. Giles, M.D.
Associate Professor, Department of Medicine, UCLA Medical School; Director, Stem Cell Transplantation and Myeloma Program, Cedars-Sinai Medical Center, Los Angeles, California

Jens Gille, M.D.
Resident, Department of Dermatology, J.W. Goethe University , Frankfurt, Germany

Gary Gitnick, M.D.
Professor of Medicine, Chief, Division of Digestive Diseases, and Director, Division of Gastroenterology Research Laboratories, UCLA School of Medicine, Los Angeles, California

Aaron E. Glatt, M.D., F.A.C.P., F.C.C.P., F.I.D.S.A.
Chief, Infectious Diseases, Catholic Medical Center of Brooklyn and Queens, Jamaica; Associate Director of Medicine, Albert Einstein College of Medicine of Yeshiva University, Bronx, New York

Helmuth Goepfert, M.D.
Professor and Chair, Department of Head and Neck Surgery, and Head, Division of Surgery, University of Texas M.D. Anderson Cancer Center, Houston, Texas

Stanley Goldfarb, M.D., F.A.C.P.
Professor of Medicine, University of Pennsylvania School of Medicine; Vice Chairman for Network Development, University of Pennsylvania Health System, Philadelphia, Pennsylvania

John M. Goldman, D.M., F.R.C.P., F.R.C.Path.
Professor of Leukemia Biology, Royal Postgraduate Medical School; Consultant Haematologist, Hammersmith Hospital, London, United Kingdom

Ernesto Gonzalez, M.D.
Associate Professor of Dermatology, Harvard Medical School; Dermatologist, Massachusetts General Hospital, Boston, Massachusetts

Enoch Gordis, M.D.
Director, National Institute on Alcohol Abuse and Alcoholism, National Institutes of Health, Bethesda, Maryland

David F. Graft, M.D.
Chairman, Allergy Department, Park Nicollet Clinic, Minneapolis, Minnesota

Richard D. Granstein, M.D.
George W. Hambrick, Jr. Professor, and Chairman, Department of Dermatology, Cornell University Medical College; Dermatologist-in-Chief, The New York Hospital, New York, New York

Malcolm Greaves, M.D., Ph.D., F.R.C.P.
Professor of Dermatology, and Consultant Dermatologist, St. John's Institute of Dermatology, United Medical and Dental Schools, St. Thomas's Hospital, London, England

F. Anthony Greco, M.D.
Director, The Sarah Cannon-Minnie Pearl Cancer Research Center, Nashville, Tennessee

Harry L. Greene II, M.D.
Executive Vice-President, The Massachusetts Medical Society, Waltham, Massachusetts

Peter Greenwald, M.D., Dr.P.H.
Director, Division of Cancer Prevention and Control, National Cancer Institute, Bethesda, Maryland

David W. Gregory, M.D.
Associate Professor of Medicine, Vanderbilt University School of Medicine; Associate Chief of Staff, Veterans Affairs Medical Center, Nashville, Tennessee

John W. Griffin, M.D.
Professor of Neurology and Neuroscience, The Johns Hopkins University School of Medicine, Baltimore, Maryland

James C. Grotta, M.D.
Professor of Neurology, Adjunct Professor of Radiology, and Director of Stroke Program, University of Texas Medical School, Houston, Texas

Anton Grunfeld, M.D., F.R.C.P.C.
Assistant Professor, Division of Emergency Medicine, Department of Surgery, University of British Columbia Faculty of Medicine, Vancouver, British Columbia, Canada

Alan D. Guerci, M.D.
Associate Professor of Clinical Medicine, Columbia University College of Physicians and Surgeons, New York, New York

Arnold W. Gurevitch, M.D.
Professor of Clinical Medicine, UCLA School of Medicine; Chief, Division of Dermatology, Harbor-UCLA Medical Center, Torrance, California

Alejandra C. Gurtman, M.D.
Assistant Professor of Medicine, Mount Sinai School of Medicine; Assistant Medical Director, Jack Martin Fund Clinic,The Mount Sinai Medical Center, New York, New York

Vladimir C. Hachinski, M.D., F.R.C.P.C., M.Sc.(DME), D.Sc.(Med)
Richard and Beryl Ivey Professor and Chair, Department of Clinical Neurological Sciences, University of Western Ontario, London Health Sciences Centre, London, Ontario, Canada

Timothy C. Hain, M.D.
Associate Professor of Neurology and Otolaryngology, Northwestern University Medical School; Director, Vestibular Laboratory, Northwestern Memorial Hospital, Chicago, Illinois

John D. Hainsworth, M.D.
Director, Clinical Research, The Sarah Cannon-Minnie Pearl Cancer Research Center, Nashville, Tennessee

W. Dallas Hall, M.D.
Professor of Medicine, and Director, Division of Hypertension, Emory University School of Medicine, Atlanta, Georgia

Scott M. Hammer, M.D.
Associate Professor of Medicine, Harvard Medical School; Director, Research Virology Laboratory, Beth Israel Deaconess Hospital, Boston, Massachusetts

E. William Hancock, M.D.
Professor of Medicine (Cardiovascular), Stanford University School of Medicine, Stanford, California

Jules Hardy, O.C., M.D., F.R.C.S.C.
Professor of Neurosurgery, Department of Surgery, University of Montreal Faculty of Medicine; Adjunct Professor, Department of Neurosurgery, McGill University Faculty of Medicine, Montreal, Quebec, Canada

William V. Harford, M.D.
Associate Professor of Medicine, University of Texas Southwestern Medical Center at Dallas; Director, GI Endoscopy Laboratory, Veterans Affairs Medical Center, Dallas, Texas

Kiyoshi Hashizume, M.D., Ph.D.
Professor, Department of Geriatrics, Endocrinology, and Metabolism, Shinshu University School of Medicine, Matsumoto, Japan

Eric I. Hassid, M.D.
Associate Clinical Professor, University of Texas Health Science Center, San Antonio; Staff Neurologist, Brooke Army Medical Center, Fort Sam Houston, Texas

Barton F. Haynes, M.D.
Frederic M. Hanes Professor of Medicine, and Chair, Department of Medicine, Duke University Medical Center, Durham, North Carolina

Nancy M. Heddle, M.Sc., A.R.T.
Assistant Professor, Department of Pathology, McMaster University Faculty of Health Sciences; Diagnostic Unit Manager, Hematology, Coagulation and Transfusion Medicine, McMaster University Medical Center, Hamilton, Ontario, Canada

Peter S. Heeger, M.D.
Assistant Professor of Medicine and Pathology, Case Western Reserve University and Cleveland Veterans Affairs Medical Center, Cleveland, Ohio

Robert R. Henry, M.D.
Professor of Medicine, University of California, San Diego, School of Medicine; Director, Endocrine, Diabetes and Metabolism Clinic, Veterans Affairs Medical Center, San Diego, California

Geoffrey P. Herzig, M.D.
Professor of Medicine, State University of New York at Buffalo; Chief, Departments of Hematologic Oncology and Bone Marrow Transplantation, Roswell Park Cancer Institute, Buffalo, New York

Scott E. Hessen, M.D.
Assistant Professor of Medicine, Allegheny University of the Health Sciences; Associate Director, Clinical Cardiac Electrophysiology, Allegheny University Hospitals-Hahnemann Division, Philadelphia, Pennsylvania

Jack Hirsh, M.D., F.R.C.P.C.
Professor Emeritus, Department of Medicine, McMaster University Faculty of Medicine; Director, Hamilton Civic Hospitals Research Center, Hamilton, Ontario, Canada

Tony W. Ho, M.D.
Postdoctoral Fellow in Neurology, The Johns Hopkins Hospital, Baltimore, Maryland

Dieter F. Hoelzer, M.D., Ph.D.
Professor of Medicine, Johann Wolfgang Goethe-Universitat; Head, Medizinische Klinik III, Frankfurt, Germany

Gary P. Holmes, M.D.
Assistant Professor, Division of Infectious Diseases, Texas A&M University Health Science Center, Temple, Texas

James Wm. C. Holmes, M.D., M.S., F.A.C.S.
Professor of Clinical Surgery, Colo-Rectal Surgery, Tulane University School of Medicine; Assistant Dean for MCLANO Affairs, CAO, Charity Hospital, New Orleans, Louisiana

Robert B. Holtzman, M.D.
Clinical Assistant Professor of Surgery, University of Miami School of Medicine, Miami, Florida

Richard Horton, M.D.
Professor of Medicine, University of Southern California School of Medicine, Los Angeles, California

Lyn Howard, M.B., F.R.C.P., F.A.C.P.
Professor of Medicine, and Associate Professor of Pediatrics, Albany Medical College, Albany, New York

Walter T. Hughes, M.D.
Professor of Pediatrics, University of Tennessee College of Medicine; Arthur Ashe Chair for Pediatric AIDS Research, St Jude Children's Research Hospital, Memphis, Tennessee

Robert A. Hyndiuk, M.D.
Professor of Ophthalmology, Medical College of Wisconsin, John L. Doyne Hospital, Froedtert Memorial Lutheran Hospital, and Children's Hospital of Milwaukee, Milwaukee, Wisconsin

Roger T. Inouye, M.D.
Senior Fellow in Infectious Diseases, Harvard Medical School; Research Fellow, Beth Israel Deaconess Medical Center, Boston, Massachusetts

Richard F. Jacobs, M.D., F.A.A.P.
Horace C. Cabe Professor of Pediatrics, University of Arkansas College of Medicine; Chief, Division of Pediatric Infectious Disease, Arkansas Children's Hospital, Little Rock, Arkansas

D. Geraint James, M.D., F.R.C.P., F.A.C.P.(Hon.)
Adjunct Professor of Medicine, Royal Free Hospital of Medicine, London, United Kingdom

Dennis M. Jensen, M.D.
Professor of Medicine, UCLA School of Medicine, Los Angeles, California

Waldemar G. Johanson, Jr., M.D., M.P.H.
Professor and Chairman, Department of Medicine, University of Medicine and Dentistry of New Jersey-New Jersey Medical School; Physician-in-Chief, Department of Medicine, University of Medicine and Dentistry of New Jersey-University Hospital, Newark, New Jersey

Richard Allen Johnson, M.D.
Instructor in Dermatology, Harvard Medical School; Clinical Associate in Dermatology, Massachusetts General Hospital; Attending Physician, Beth Israel Deaconess Medical Center; Consultant in Dermatology, Dana Farber Cancer Institute and New England Baptist Hospital, Boston, Massachusetts

Ronald N. Jones, M.D.
Professor of Pathology, University of Iowa College of Medicine; Director, Medical Microbiology Division, Department of Pathology, University of Iowa Hospitals and Clinics, Iowa City, Iowa

Elaine C. Jong, M.D.
Clinical Professor of Medicine, Director, Hall Health Primary Care Center, and Co-Director, Travel and Tropical Medicine Service, University of Washington School of Medicine, Seattle, Washington

Howard L. Judd, M.D.
Professor and Vice-Chair, Department of Obstetrics and Gynecology, UCLA School of Medicine, Los Angeles; Chair, Department of Obstetrics and Gynecology, Olive View/UCLA Medical Center, Sylmar, California

Bruce A. Julian, M.D.
Professor of Medicine, University of Alabama School of Medicine and University Hospital, Birmingham, Alabama

Jagmohan Kalra, M.D., F.A.C.P.
Associate Clinical Professor of Medicine, Albert Einstein College of Medicine of Yeshiva University, Bronx; Attending Physician, Division of Hematology/Oncology, Long Island Jewish Medical Center, New Hyde Park, New York

Kamel S. Kamel, M.D., F.R.C.P.C.
Associate Professor of Medicine, University of Toronto Faculty of Medicine; Staff Nephrologist, St. Michael's Hospital, Toronto, Ontario, Canada

Allen P. Kaplan, M.D.
Professor of Medicine, Medical University of South Carolina, Charleston, South Carolina

Michael S. Kaplan, M.D.
Clinical Professor of Pediatrics (Voluntary), UCLA School of Medicine; Chief and Training Program Director, Allergy/Immunology, Kaiser Permanente, Los Angeles Medical Center, Los Angeles, California

Judith E. Karp, M.D.
Professor of Medicine and Oncology, Greenebaum Cancer Center, University of Maryland Medical Systems, Baltimore, Maryland

Jerome P. Kassirer, M.D.
Editor-in-Chief, *The New England Journal of Medicine*

William N. Katkov, M.D.
Assistant Clinical Professor of Medicine, UCLA School of Medicine, Los Angeles, California

Takakazu Katoh, M.D.
Katoh Cardiovascular Clinic, Japan

Carol A. Kauffman, M.D.
Professor of Internal Medicine, University of Michigan Medical School; Chief, Infectious Diseases Section, Veterans Affairs Medical Center, Ann Arbor, Michigan

David T. Kawanishi, M.D.
Associate Professor of Medicine, University of Southern California School of Medicine; Director of Cardiac Catheterization Laboratory, LAC+USC Medical Center, and of University of Southern California Pacemaker Center, Los Angeles, California

Claudia Kawas, M.D.
Associate Professor of Neurology, and Clinical Director, Alzheimer's Disease Research Center, The Johns Hopkins University School of Medicine, Baltimore, Maryland

Donald Kaye, M.D.
Klinghoffer Professor of Medicine, and Executive Vice President for Health Affairs, Allegheny University of the Health Sciences; President and CEO, Allegheny University Hospitals, Philadelphia, Pennsylvania

James R. Keane, M.D.
Professor of Neurology, University of Southern California School of Medicine, Los Angeles, California

Clive Kearon, M.B., M.R.C.P.I., F.R.C.P.C., Ph.D.
Assistant Professor of Medicine, McMaster University Faculty of Health Sciences; Physician, Thrombosis and Respiratory Medicine, McMaster Medical Clinic, Henderson General Hospital, Hamilton, Ontario, Canada

Roger G. Keith, M.D., F.R.C.S.C., F.R.C.S., F.A.C.S.
Fred H. Wigmore Professor and Chairman, Department of Surgery, University of Saskatchewan College of Medicine; Chief of Surgery, Royal University Hospital, Saskatoon, Saskatchewan, Canada

Steven M. Keller, M.D.
Associate Professor of Surgery, Albert Einstein College of Medicine of Yeshiva University, Bronx; Chief of Thoracic Surgery, Beth Israel Medical Center, New York, New York

John G. Kelton, M.D.
Professor and Chairman, Department of Medicine, and Professor of Pathology, McMaster University Faculty of Health Sciences; Acting Chief of Medicine, and Director of Transfusion Medicine Laboratories, Hamilton Health Sciences Corporaton, Chedoke-McMaster Campus, Hamilton, Ontario, Canada

John F. Kerrigan, M.D.
Associate Director, Pediatric Epilepsy, Epilepsy Center, Barrow Neurological Institute, Phoenix, Arizona

Kenneth M. Kessler, M.D.
Professor of Medicine, and Associate Director of Cardiology, University of Miami School of Medicine; Chief, Cardiology Section, Department of Veterans Affairs Medical Center, Miami, Florida

Jay S. Keystone, M.D., M.Sc. (C.T.M.)
Professor of Medicine and Microbiology, University of Toronto Faculty of Medicine; Director, Tropical Disease Unit, The Toronto Hospital, Toronto, Ontario, Canada

David W. Kimberlin, M.D.
Assistant Professor, Department of Pediatrics, University of Alabama School of Medicine, Birmingham, Alabama

Kirsten J. Kinsman, M.D.
Fellow, Gastroenterology, Oregon Health Sciences University School of Medicine, Portland, Oregon

Craig S. Kitchens, M.D.
Professor and Vice-Chairman, Department of Medicine, University of Florida College of Medicine; Chief, Medical Service, Veterans Affairs Medical Center, Gainesville, Florida

Saulo Klahr, M.D.
Simon Professor of Medicine, Washington University School of Medicine, St. Louis, Missouri

Natalie C. Klein, M.D., Ph.D.
Assistant Professor of Medicine, State University of New York School of Medicine, Stony Brook; Associate Director, Infectious Disease Division, Winthrop-University Hospital, Mineola, New York

Adrienne N. Knopf, M.D.
Assistant Professor of Medicine, Tufts University School of Medicine, Boston, Massachusetts

Timothy R. Koch, M.D.
Professor of Medicine, and Chief, Section of Gastroenterology, West Virginia University, Morgantown, West Virginia

Ritsuko Komaki, M.D., F.A.C.R.
Professor of Radiation Oncology, University of Texas M.D. Anderson Cancer Center, Houston, Texas

Joel D. Kopple, M.D.
Professor of Medicine and Public Health, UCLA School of Medicine, Los Angeles; Chief, Division of Nephrology and Hypertension, Harbor-UCLA Medical Center, Torrance, California

Joseph H. Korn, M.D.
Professor of Medicine and Biochemistry, Boston University School of Medicine; Director, Arthritis Center, and Chief, Rheumatology Section, Boston University Medical Center and Veterans Affairs Medical Center, Boston, Massachusetts

Phyllis E. Kozarsky, M.D.
Associate Professor of Medicine/Infectious Diseases, and Assistant Professor of International Health, Emory University School of Medicine; Atlanta, GA

Elizabeth Krecker, M.D.
Medical Oncology Fellow, LAC+USC Medical Center, Los Angeles, California

Ralph W. Kuncl, M.D., Ph.D.
Professor of Neurology, The Johns Hopkins University School of Medicine; Attending Physician, The Johns Hopkins Hospital, Baltimore, Maryland

Steven P. Kutalek, M.D.
Associate Professor of Medicine and Pharmacology, and Director of Cardiac Electrophysiology Laboratory and of Pacing, Allegheny University of the Health Sciences-Hahnemann Division, Philadelphia, Pennsylvania

Michael A. Kutcher, M.D.
Associate Professor of Internal Medicine (Cardiology), Bowman Gray School of Medicine of Wake Forest University; Director of Interventional Cardiology, North Carolina Baptist Hospital, Winston-Salem, North Carolina

Timothy M. Kuzel, M.D.
Associate Professor of Medicine, Division of Hematology-Oncology, Northwestern University Medical School,Chicago, Illinois

Robert A. Kyle, M.D.
Professor of Medicine and Laboratory Medicine, Mayo Medical School; Consultant, Division of Hematology and Internal Medicine, Mayo Clinic and Mayo Foundation, Rochester, Minnesota

F. Marc LaForce, M.D.
Professor of Medicine, University of Rochester School of Medicine and Dentistry; Physician-in-Chief, The Genesee Hospital, Rochester, New York

Parviz Lalezari, M.D.
Clinical Professor of Medicine and Pathology, Albert Einstein College of Medicine of Yeshiva University; Attending Physician, Departments of Medicine and Pathology, Montefiore Medical Center, Bronx, New York; President and CEO, Bergen Community Regional Blood Center, Paramus, New Jersey

Frances Lawlor, M.D., F.R.C.P.I., D.C.H.
Honorary Senior Lecturer in Dermatology, United Medical and Dental Schools of Guys and St. Thomas; Honorary Consultant Dermatologist, St. John's Institute of Dermatology, London, United Kingdom

William J. Ledger, M.D.
Given Foundation Professor of Obstetrics and Gynecology, Cornell University Medical College; Obstetrician and Gynecologist-in-Chief, The New York Hospital, New York, New York

Belle L. Lee, Pharm.D.
Associate Professor of Medicine and Pharmacy, Division of Infectious Disease and Clinical Pharmacology, University of California at San Francisco and San Francisco General Hospital, San Francisco, California

David B.N. Lee, M.D.
Professor, UCLA/San Fernando Valley Renal Program, Los Angeles; Chief, Nephrology Division, Veterans Affairs Medical Center, Sepulveda, California

John E. Lennard-Jones, M.D., F.R.C.P., F.R.C.S.
Emeritus Professor of Gastroenterology, University of London; Emeritus Consultant Gastroenterologist, St. Mark's Hospital, London, United Kingdom

A. Martin Lerner, M.D.
Clinical Professor of Medicine, Wayne State University School of Medicine, Detroit; Attending Physician, William Beaumont Hospital, Royal Oak, Michigan

Lucy A. Levandoski, P.A.-C
St. Louis Children's Hospital, St. Louis, Missouri

Daniel P. Lew, M.D.
Professor of Medicine, and Chief, Infectious Diseases Division, Geneva University Hospital, Geneva, Switzerland

Richard P. Lewis, M.D.
Professor of Internal Medicine, Ohio State Univers College of Medicine, Columbus, Ohio

John E. Lewy, M.D.
Professor and Chairman, Department of Pediatrics, Tulane University School of Medicine; Chief of Staff, and Professor of Pediatrics, Tulane Hospital for Children, New Orleans, Louisiana

Darla Liles, M.D.
Research Assistant Professor, University of North Carolina at Chapel Hill School of Medicine; Attending Physician, University of North Carolina Hospitals, Chapel Hill, North Carolina

Joseph Lindsay, Jr., M.D.
Professor of Medicine, The George Washington University School of Medicine; Director, Section of Cardiology, Washington Hospital Center, Washington, D.C.

J. William Lindsey, M.D.
Assistant Professor of Neurology, University of Texas Health Science Center, Houston, Texas

Nicholas J. Linker, M.D.
Senior Registrar in Cardiology, Manchester Royal Infirmary, Manchester, United Kingdom

Richard B. Lipton, M.D.
Professor of Neurology, Epidemiology, and Social Medicine, Albert Einstein College of Medicine of Yeshiva University, and Co-Director, Montefiore Headache Unit, Bronx, New York; CEO, Innovative Medical Research, Stamford, Connecticut

Peter I. Lobo, M.D.
Associate Professor, Department of Internal Medicine, University of Virginia Health Science Center, Charlottesville, Virginia

Patrick J. Loehrer, Sr., M.D.
ofessor of Medicine, Section of Hematology-cology, Indiana University School of Medicine, anapolis, Indiana

n A. LoGiudice, M.D.
tor of Gastroenterology, West Suburban Hospital al Center, Oak Park, Illinois

Long, M.D., Ph.D.
r and Director of Neurosurgery, The Johns University School of Medicine; irgeon-in-Chief, The Johns Hopkins Hospital, e, Maryland

Donald P. Lookingbill, M.D.
Professor of Medicine, and Chief, Division of Dermatology, The Pennsylvania State University College of Medicine, Hershey, Pennsylvania

Robert G. Luke, M.D.
Chairman, Department of Internal Medicine, University of Cincinnati Medical Center, Cincinnati, Ohio

Valerie J. Lund, M.S., F.R.C.S., F.R.C.S.Ed.
Professor of Rhinology, Institute of Laryngology and Otology, University College London; Consultant ENT Surgeon, Royal National Throat, Nose and Ear Hospital and Moorfields Eye Hospital, London, United Kingdom

Rodger D. MacArthur, M.D.
Associate Professor of Medicine, Division of Infectious Diseases, Wayne State University School of Medicine; Director of HIV/AIDS Clinical Research, Wayne Sate University — Detroit Medical Center, Detroit, Michigan

Peter Hugh MacDonald, B.Sc., M.D., F.R.C.S.C.
Assistant Professor of Surgery, Queen's University Faculty of Medicine, Kingston, Ontario, Canada

Stephen E. Malawista, M.D.
Professor of Medicine, Yale University School of Medicine; Consultant in Medicine, Yale-New Haven Medical Center, New Haven, and West Haven Veterans Affairs Medical Center, West Haven, Connecticut

Margaret Malone, Ph.D., M.R.Pharm.S., F.C.C.P.
Professor of Pharmacy Practice, Albany College of Pharmacy, Albany, New York

Pier Mannuccio Mannucci, M.D.
Professor of Medicine, University of Milan; Director, Hemophilia and Thrombosis Center—Institute of Internal Medicine, Milan, Italy

Christina M. Marra, M.D.
Assistant Professor, Departments of Neurology and Medicine (Infectious Diseases), University of Washington School of Medicine, Seattle, Washington

Rebecca Edge Martin, M.D.
Associate Professor of Medicine, Division of Infectious Disease, University of Arkansas College of Medicine and John L. McClellan Veterans Affairs Medical Center, Little Rock, Arkansas

José M. Mascaro, Jr., M.D.
Department of Dermatology, Hospital Clinic, Barcelona, Spain

Carol M. Mason, M.D.
Assistant Professor of Medicine (Pulmonary/Critical Care Medicine), Louisiana State University School of Medicine; Medical Director of Respiratory Therapy, Charity Hospital, New Orleans, Louisiana

Axel C. Matzdorff, M.D.
Fellow of Hematology, Justus-Leibig University, Giessen, Germany

John H. McAnulty, M.D.
Professor of Medicine, and Director, Arrhythmia Service, Oregon Health Sciences University School of Medicine, Portland, Oregon

Rex M. McCallum, M.D.
Assistant Professor of Medicine, Division of Rheumatology, Allergy and Clinical Immunology, and Vice Chair for Clinical Services, Department of Medicine, Duke University Medical Center, Durham, North Carolina

Robin S. McLeod, M.D., F.R.C.S.C., F.A.C.S.
Professor of Surgery, University of Toronto Faculty of Medicine; Head, Division of General Surgery, Mount Sinai Hospital, Toronto, Ontario, Canada

Barbara Menzies, M.D.
Assistant Professor in Medicine, Vanderbilt University School of Medicine and Veterans Affairs Medical Center, Nashville, Tennessee

William G. Merz, Ph.D.
Associate Professor of Pathology, Dermatology, and Epidemiology, The Johns Hopkins University School of Medicine; Acting Director, Microbiology Laboratory, and Director, Mycology Laboratory, The Johns Hopkins Hospital, Baltimore, Maryland

Dean D. Metcalfe, M.D.
Chief, Laboratory of Allergic Diseases, National Institute of Allergy and Infectious Diseases, National Institutes of Health, Bethesda, Maryland

Burt R. Meyers, M.D.
Professor of Medicine, Mount Sinai School of Medicine of the City University of New York; Director, Transplantation Infectious Diseases, Division of Infectious Diseases, The Mount Sinai Medical Center, New York, New York

William M. Miles, M.D.
Professor of Medicine, Indiana University School of Medicine, and Research Associate, Krannert Institute of Cardiology; Director, Cardiac Electrophysiology Laboratory, Indiana University Hospital, and Staff Physician, Richard L. Roudebush Veterans Affairs Medical Center, Indianapolis, Indiana

Paul F. Milner, M.D., F.R.C.Path
Professor Emeritus of Pathology and Medicine, Medical College of Georgia, Augusta, Georgia

Philip B. Miner, Jr., M.D.
Professor of Medicine, and Director, Division of Gastroenterology, University of Kansas, Kansas City, Kansas

Taseer A. Minhas, M.D.
Assistant Professor of Neurology, United Health Services Hospitals, Binghamton, New York

Daniel R. Mishell, Jr., M.D.
The Lyle G. McNeile Professor and Chairman, Department of Obstetrics and Gynecology, University of Southern California School of Medicine; Chief of Professional Services, LAC+USC Medical Center, Women's and Children's Hospital, Los Angeles, California

Herman S. Mogavero, Jr., M.D.
Assistant Clinical Professor of Medicine and Dermatology, State University of New York School of Medicine; Dermatologist, Buffalo Medical Group, Buffalo, New York

Arlene J. Morales, M.D., F.A.C.O.G.
Assistant Professor, Division of Reproductive Endocrinology, University of California San Diego School of Medicine, La Jolla, California

Douglas R. Morgan, M.D., M.P.H.
Clinical Assistant Professor, University of North Carolina; Staff Physician, and Gastroenterology Consultant, Wake Medical Center, Raleigh, North Carolina

Lewis B. Morgenstern, M.D.
Assistant Professor of Neurology, University of Texas Medical School; Attending Neurologist, Hermann Hospital, Houston, Texas

Warwick L. Morison, M.B., B.S., M.R.C.P..
Professor of Dermatology, The Johns Hopkins University School of Medicine, Baltimore, Maryland

Gabriella Moroni, M.D.
Physician, Division of Nephrology and Dialysis, Ospedale Maggiore di Milano, Milan, Italy

Ann Morrison, M.S., R.N., C.S.
Clinical Nurse Specialist, The Johns Hopkins Medical Institutions, Baltimore, Maryland

Monica Morrow, M.D.
Associate Professor of Surgery, Northwestern University Medical School; Director, Lynn Sage Comprehensive Breast Program, Northwestern Memorial Hospital, Chicago, Illinois

Joseph F. Mortola, M.D.
Director, Division of Reproductive Endocrinology, Cook County Hospital, Chicago, Illinois

Maurice A. Mufson, M.D.
Professor and Chairman, Department of Medicine, Marshall University School of Medicine; Active Staff, Cabell Huntington Hospital and St. Mary's Hospital; Staff Physician, Veterans Affairs Medical Center, Huntington, West Virginia

Franco M. Muggia, M.D.
Professor of Medicine, New York University Medical Center, New York, New York

Lutifiye Mulazimoglu, M.D.
Associate Professor of Infectious Disease and Clinical Microbiology, Marmara University School of Medicine, Istanbul, Turkey

Jerry Nadler, M.D.
Adjunct Associate Professor of Medicine, University of Southern California School of Medicine, Los Angeles; Director, Department of Diabetes and Endocrine, City of Hope Medical Center, Duarte, California

Manoochehr Nakhjavani, M.D.
Associate Professor of Medicine, Tehran University School of Medical Sciences, Tehran, Iran; Visiting Clinician, Division of Endocrinology and Metabolism, Mayo Clinic and Foundation, Rochester, Minnesota

Eric G. Neilson, M.D.
C. Mahlon Kline Professor of Medicine and Pediatrics, Chief, Renal Electrolyte and Hypertension Division, and Director, Penn Center for the Molecular Studies of Kidney Diseases, University of Pennsylvania School of Medicine; Attending Physician and Chief, Renal Division, Hospital of the University of Pennsylvania, Philadelphia, Pennsylvania

Bill Nelems, M.D., F.R.C.S.C.
Professor of Surgery, University of British Columbia Faculty of Medicine, Vancouver, British Columbia, Canada

Harold S. Nelson, M.D.
Professor of Medicine, University of Colorado Health Sciences Center; Senior Staff Physician, Department of Medicine, National Jewish Medical and Research Center, Denver, Colorado

Joseph M. Nesta, M.D.
Clinical Instructor, Department of Medicine, University of Connecticut, Hartford, Connecticut

Ronald Lee Nichols, M.D., M.S., F.A.C.S.
William Henderson Professor of Surgery, and Professor of Microbiology and Immunology, Tulane University School of Medicine; Attending Surgeon, Tulane University Hospital and Clinic, New Orleans, Louisiana

John E. Niederhuber, M.D.
Emile Holman Professor of Surgery, Professor of Microbiology and Immunology, and Attending Surgeon, Stanford University, Stanford, California

Masao Nishimura, M.D.
Attending Cardiologist, Department of Medicine, Ageo Central General Hospital, Ageo, Saitama, Japan

Dennis H. Novack, M.D.
Professor of Medicine, and Associate Dean of Clinical Skills, Allegheny University of the Health Sciences, MCP-Hahnemann School of Medicine, Philadelphia, Pennsylvania

Judith A. O'Donnell, M.D.
Assistant Professor of Medicine, Division of Infectious Diseases, Allegheny University of the Health Sciences, Philadelphia, Pennsylvania

Celia M. Oakley, M.D., F.R.C.P., F.A.C.C., F.E.S.C.
Professor of Clinical Cardiology, Royal Postgraduate Medical School, University of London; Honorary Consultant Cardiologist, Hammersmith and St. Mary's Hospitals, London, United Kingdom

Nancy F. Olivieri, M.D., F.R.C.P.C.
Professor of Pediatrics and Medicine, and Director, Hemoglobinopathy Program, University of Toronto Faculty of Medicine, Toronto, Ontario, Canada

Rapin Osathanondh, M.D.
Associate Professor of Obstetrics, Gynecology, and Reproductive Biology, Harvard Medical School; Director, Family Planning Division, Brigham and Women's Hospital, Boston, Massachusetts

David N. Ostrow, M.D., B.Sc.(Med), M.A., F.R.C.P.C., F.C.C.P., F.A.C.P.
Professor of Medicine, University of British Columbia Faculty of Medicine; Vice President, Clinical Services, Vancouver Hospitals and Health Science Center, Vancouver, British Columbia, Canada

Rosemary Ouseph, M.D.
Assistant Professor of Medicine, University of Louisville School of Medicine, Louisville, Kentucky

Robert L. Owen, M.D.
Professor of Medicine, Epidemiology and Biostatistics, University of California at San Francisco; Environmental Health Physician, and Gastroenterologic Infectious Diseases Consultant, Veterans Affairs Medical Center, San Francisco, California

Robert F. Ozols, M.D., Ph.D.
Senior Vice President, Medical Science, Fox Chase Cancer Center, Philadelphia, Pennsylvania

Charles Y.C. Pak, M.D.
Professor of Internal Medicine, and Director, Center for Mineral Metabolism and Clinical Research, University of Texas Southwestern Medical Center at Dallas, Dallas, Texas

Paul M. Palevsky, M.D.
Associate Professor of Medicine, Renal-Electrolyte Division, University of Pittsburgh School of Medicine; Chief, Renal Section, Medical Service, Veterans Affairs Pittsburgh Health Care System, Pittsburgh, Pennsylvania

Amy S. Paller, M.D.
Professor of Pediatrics and Dermatology, Northwestern University Medical School; Head, Division of Dermatology, Children's Memorial Hospital, Chicago, Illinois

Richard H. Parker, M.D.
Associate Professor of Medicine, Howard University College of Medicine; Director, Antimicrobial Agent Research and Education, Section of Infectious Diseases, Providence Hospital, Washington, D.C.

Andrew T. Pavia, M.D.
Assistant Professor of Medicine and Pediatrics, University of Utah School of Medicine; Director for Clinical Research, University AIDS Center, Salt Lake City, Utah

John M. Pellock, M.D.
Professor of Neurology, Pediatrics, and Pharmacy and Pharmaceuticals, Chairman, Division of Child Neurology, and Director, Comprehensive Epilepsy Institute, Medical College of Virginia, Virginia Commonwealth University, Richmond, Virginia

Rosalie Pepe, M.D.
Clinical Associate Professor, Jefferson Medical College of Thomas Jefferson University; Physician, Episcopal Hospital, Philadelphia, Pennsylvania

Mark A. Peppercorn, M.D.
Associate Professor of Medicine, Harvard Medical School; Director, Center for Inflammatory Bowel Disease, Beth Israel Deaconess Medical Center, Boston, Massachusetts

Stephen J. Peroutka, M.D., Ph.D.
Former Assistant Professor of Neurology and Neurological Sciences, Stanford University Medical Center, Stanford, California

Michelle Petri, M.D., M.P.H.
Associate Professor of Medicine, and Director, Lupus Center and Hopkins Lupus Cohort, The Johns Hopkins University School of Medicine, Baltimore, Maryland

Joann Pfundstein, M.D.
Infectious Diseases Physicians, Inc., Annandale,Virginia

John P. Phair, M.D.
Professor of Medicine, Northwestern University Medical School; Chief, Infectious Disease, and Director, Comprehensive AIDS Center, Northwestern Memorial Hospital, Chicago, Illinois

Dominique Q. Pham, M.D.
Former Fellow in Gastroenterology and Hepatology, Veterans Affairs Medical Center, Washington, D.C.

Philip A. Pizzo, M.D.
Thomas Morgan Rotch Professor, and Chair, Department of Medicine, Harvard Medical School; Physician-in-Chief, The Children's Hospital, Boston, Massachusetts

Andrew G. Plaut, M.D.
Professor of Medicine, Tufts University School of Medicine; Staff Physician, New England Medical Center Hospital, Boston, Massachusetts

Peter E. Pochi, M.D.
Professor Emeritus of Dermatology, Boston University School of Medicine, Boston, Massachusetts

Claudio Ponticelli, M.D., F.R.C.P.
Director, Division of Nephrology and Dialysis, Ospedale Maggiore di Milano, Milan, Italy

John H. Powers, M.D.
Clinical Instructor in Medicine, Jefferson Medical College of Thomas Jefferson University, Philadelphia, Pennsylvania; Attending in Infectious Diseases, Department of Medicine, Medical Center of Delaware, Wilmington, Delaware

Craig M. Pratt, M.D.
Professor of Medicine, and Director, Clinical Cardiology Research, Baylor College of Medicine; Director, Coronary Intensive Care Unit, Methodist Hospital, and Director, Outpatient Cardiovascular Services, MacGregor Clinic, Houston, Texas

Daniel H. Present, M.D.
Clinical Professor of Medicine, Mount Sinai School of Medicine, New York, New York

Ahmed S. Rabbat, M.D.
Physician; Attending Physician, Infectious Diseases, Catholic Medical Center of Brooklyn and Queens, Jamaica, New York

Arthur I. Radin, M.D., F.A.C.P.
Clinical Assistant Professor of Medicine, Cornell University Medical College; Assistant Attending Physician, The New York Hospital-Cornell Medical Center and St. Vincent's Hospital and Medical Center, New York, New York

Shahbudin H. Rahimtoola, M.B., F.R.C.P., M.A.C.P.
Distinguished Professor, George C. Griffith Professor of Cardiology, Professor of Medicine, and Chairman, Griffith Center, University of Southern California School of Medicine, Los Angeles, California

Kanti R. Rai, M.D., F.A.C.P.
Professor of Medicine, Albert Einstein College of Medicine of Yeshiva University, Bronx; Chief, Division of Hematology-Oncology, Long Island Jewish Medical Center, New Hyde Park, New York

Albert E. Raizner, M.D.
Professor of Medicine, Baylor College of Medicine; Director, Cardiac Catheterization Laboratories, The Methodist Hospital, Houston, Texas

Paul G. Ramsey, M.D.
Robert G. Petersdorf Professor, and Chair, Department of Medicine, University of Washington School of Medicine; Physician-in-Chief, University of Washington Medical Center, Seattle, Washington

John H.C. Ranson, B.M., B.Ch., M.A . (Deceased)
Formerly S. A. Localio Professor of Surgery, New York University School of Medicine; Director, Division of General Surgery, New York University Medical Center; Associate Director of Surgery, Tisch Hospital; Attending Physician, Bellevue Hospital Center and New York University Medical Center, New York, New York

David P. Rardon, M.D.
Electrophysiologist, Division of Clinical Electrophysiology, St. Vincent's Hospital, Indianapolis, Indiana

Robert W. Rebar, M.D.
Professor and Director, Department of Obstetrics and Gynecology, University of Cincinnati College of Medicine; Chief, Obstetrics and Gynecology, University Hospital, Cincinnati, Ohio

William G. Rector, Jr., M.D.
Associate Clinical Professor of Medicine, University of Colorado Health Sciences Center, Denver, Colorado

S. Frank Redo, M.D.
Emeritus Professor of Surgery, Cornell University Medical College; Attending Surgeon, The New York Hospital-Cornell Medical Center, New York, New York

Andrew J. Rees, M.B., Ch.B., M.Sc., F.R.C.P.
Regius Professor of Medicine, Unversity of Aberdeen; Honorary Consultant Physician, Aberdeen Royal Infirmary, Aberdeen, Scotland

Michael F. Rein, M.D.
Professor of Medicine, Division of Infectious Diseases, University of Virginia School of Medicine; Attending Physician, University of Virginia Health Sciences Center; Medical Director, Sexually Transmitted Diseases Clinic, Thomas Jefferson District Health Department, Charlottesville, Virginia

Joel E. Richter, M.D.
Chairman, Department of Gastroenterology, Cleveland Clinic Foundation, Cleveland; Professor of Medicine, Ohio State University College of Medicine, Columbus, Ohio

Roger S. Rittmaster, M.D.
Professor of Medicine, Dalhousie University; Active Staff, Queen Elizabeth II Health Sciences Center, Halifax, Nova Scotia, Canada

W. Neal Roberts, Jr., M.D.
Charles W. Thomas Associate Professor of Medicine, and Director of Training in Rheumatology, Medical College of Virginia, Virginia Commonwealth University, Richmond, Virginia

Harold R. Roberts, M.D.
Sarah Graham Kenan Professor of Medicine, and Director, Center for Thrombosis and Hemostasis, University of North Carolina at Chapel Hill School of Medicine; Attending Physician, University of North Carolina Hospitals, Chapel Hill, North Carolina

Robert Roberts, M.D.
Don W. Chapman Professor of Medicine, Professor of Cell Biology, and Chief of Cardiology, Baylor College of Medicine, Houston, Texas

Alan G. Robinson, MD
Professor of Medicine (Endocrinology), Vice Provost, Medical Sciences, and Executive Associate Dean, UCLA School of Medicine, Los Angeles, California

Noppomas Rojanasthien, M.D.
Division of Clinical Pharmacology and Experimental Therapeutics, University of California, San Francisco, School of Medicine, San Francisco, California

James A. Ronan, Jr., M.D.
Clinical Professor of Medicine, Georgetown University School of Medicine, Washington, D.C.; Co-Director, Department of Cardiology, Washington Adventist Hospital, Takoma Park, Maryland

Steven T. Rosen, M.D., F.A.C.P.
Director, Robert H. Lurie Cancer Center, Genevieve Teuton Professor of Medicine, Northwestern University Medical School; Director, Cancer Programs, Northwestern Memorial Hospital, Chicago, Illinois

Gayle M. Rosenthal, M.D.
Staff Physician, West Suburban Gastroenterology, Oak Park, Illinois

Bruce S. Rothschild, M.D.
Assistant Clinical Professor, Department of Psychiatry, University of Connecticut School of Medicine, Farmington; Director, Consultation- Liaison Services, St. Francis Hospital and Medical Center, Hartford, Connecticut

Lewis J. Rubin, M.D.
Head, Division of Pulmonary and Critical Care Medicine, and Professor of Medicine and Physiology, University of Maryland School of Medicine, Baltimore, Maryland

Shaun Ruddy, M.D.
Chairman, Division of Rheumatology, Allergy and Immunization, and Attending Surgeon, Medical College of Virginia, Virginia Commonwealth University, Richmond, Virginia

Zaverio M. Ruggeri, M.D.
Professor and Member, Departments of Molecular and Experimental Medicine and Vascular Biology, Head, Division of Experimental Hemostasis and Thrombosis, and Director, Roon Research Center for Arteriosclerosis and Thrombosis, The Scripps Research Institute, La Jolla, California

Anil K. Rustgi, M.D.
Assistant Professor of Medicine, Harvard Medical School; Assistant Physician in Medicine, Massachusetts General Hospital, Boston, Massachusetts

Preston C. Sacks, M.D.
Clinical Instructor, Department of Obstetrics and Gynecology, Georgetown University School of Medicine; Reproductive Endocrinologist, Columbia Hospital for Women, Washington, DC

Merle A. Sande, M.D.
Professor and Chairman, Department of Internal Medicine, University of Utah School of Medicine, Salt Lake City, Utah

Julio V. Santiago, M.D.
Professor of Medicine and Pediatrics, Washington University School of Medicine, St. Louis, Missouri

Thomas J. Savides, M.D.
Assistant Professor of Clinical Medicine, University of California, San Diego, School of Medicine, La Jolla, California

Joan H. Schiller, M.D.
Associate Professor of Medicine, University of Wisconsin Medical School, Madison, Wisconsin

Robert C. Schlant, M.D.
Professor of Medicine (Cardiology), Emory University School of Medicine; Chief of Cardiology, Grady Memorial Hospital, Atlanta, Georgia

Patrick M. Schlievert, Ph.D.
Professor of Microbiology, University of Minnesota Medical School, Minneapolis, Minnesota

David Schlossberg, M.D., F.A.C.P.
Professor of Medicine, Jefferson Medical College of Thomas Jefferson University; Director, Department of Medicine, Episcopal Hospital, Philadelphia, Pennsylvania

Arnd Schulte-Bockholt, M.D.
Director, Gastrointestinal Endoscopy and Motility, Medizinische Klinik II Lab, Klinikum Meiningen, Germany

Marvin M. Schuster, M.D., F.A.C.P., F.A.P.A., F.A.C.G.
Professor of Medicine and Psychiatry, The Johns Hopkins University School of Medicine; Director, Marvin M. Schuster Center for Gastrointestinal Motility and Digestive Diseases, Johns Hopkins Bayview Medical Center, Baltimore, Maryland

Darryl M. See, M.D.
Assistant Professor of Medicine, University of California, Irvine, College of Medicine, Irvine, California

Leonard B. Seeff, M.D.
Professor of Medicine, Georgetown University School of Medicine; Chief of Gastroenterology and Hepatology, Veterans Affairs Medical Center, Washington, D.C.

Edward J. Septimus, M.D., F.A.C.P.
Clinical Professor of Medicine, University of Texas Medical School at Houston; Director, Infectious Diseases Program, Memorial Health Care System, Houston, Texas

Eldon A. Shaffer, M.D., F.R.C.P.C., F.A.C.P.
Professor and Head, Department of Medicine, University of Calgary Faculty of Medicine; Regional Clinical Department Head, Internal Medicine, Calgary Regional Health Authority, Calgary, Alberta, Canada

Peter Shamamian, M.D.
Assistant Professor of Surgery, New York University School of Medicine; Attending Surgeon, Tisch Hospital, New York University Medical Center Bellevue Hospital Center, Manhattan Veterans Affairs Medical Center, Gouverneur Hospital, and New York Downtown Hospital, New York, New York

Andrew M. Shapiro, M.D.
Assistant Professor of Surgery, Milton S. Hershey Medical Center, Hershey, Pennsylvania

Sandor S. Shapiro, M.D.
Thomas Drake Martinez Cardeza Research Professor of Medicine, Professor of Biochemistry, and Director of Cardeza Foundation for Hematologic Research and the Division of Hematology, Jefferson Medical College, Philadelphia, Pennsylvania

Peder M. Shea, M.D.
La Jolla, California

Bhavna P. Sheth, M.D.
Assistant Professor of Ophthalmology, The Eye Institute/Medical College of Wisconsin, Milwaukee, Wisconsin

Craig O. Siegel, M.D.
Clinical Instructor, University of North Carolina at Chapel Hill School of Medicine, Chapel Hill, North Carolina

Mark Siegler, M.D.
Lindy Bergman Professor, and Director, MacLean Center for Clinical Medical Ethics, and Professor, Department of Medicine, University of Chicago, Chicago, Illinois

Stephen D. Silberstein, M.D., F.A.C.P.
Clinical Professor of Neurology, Temple University School of Medicine; Co-Director, Comprehensive Headache Center at the Germantown Hospital and Medical Center, Philadelphia, Pennsylvania

Irwin Singer, M.D.
Clinical Professor of Medicine, University of Miami School of Medicine; Nephrology Section, Medical Services, Veterans Affairs Medical Center, Miami, Florida

Peter A. Singer, M.D., M.P.H., F.R.C.P.C.
Assistant Professor of Medicine, and Associate Director, Center for Bioethics, University of Toronto Faculty of Medicine, Toronto, Ontario, Canada

Régine Sitruk-Ware, M.D.
Senior Consultant in Reproductive Endocrinology, Hospital Saint Antoine, Paris, France

Roland T. Skeel, M.D.
Professor of Medicine, Medical College of Ohio; Attending Physician, Medical College Hospital, Toledo, Ohio

Raymond G. Slavin, M.D.
Professor of Internal Medicine, and Director, Division of Allergy and Immunology, St. Louis University School of Medicine, St. Louis, Missouri

Linda A. Slavoski, M.D.
Former Fellow, Division of Infectious Diseases, Medical College of Pennsylvania, Philadelphia, Pennsylvania

Corey M. Slovis, M.D., F.A.C.P., F.A.C.E.P.
Professor of Emergency Medicine and Medicine, Vanderbilt University School of Medicine; Director of Emergency Services, Vanderbilt University Medical Center, Nashville, Tennessee

Fiona Smaill, M.B., Ch.B.
Associate Professor, Departments of Pathology and Medicine, McMaster University Faculty of Health Sciences; Chief of Service, Microbiology and Infectious Diseases, Hamilton Health Sciences Corporation, Chedoke-McMaster Site, Hamilton, Ontario, Canada

David L. Smith, M.D.
Assistant Professor (Retired), Allergy and Immunology, University of South Alabama, Mobile, Alabama

Robert B. Smith III, M.D.
John E. Skandalakis Professor of Surgery, Emory University School of Medicine; Head, General Vascular Surgery, and Medical Director, Emory University Hospital, Atlanta, Georgia

Thomas W. Smith, M.D. (Deceased)
Formerly Professor of Medicine, Harvard Medical School; Chief, Cardiovascular Division, Brigham and Women's Hospital, Boston, Massachusetts

Dilip L. Solanki, M.D., F.A.C.P.
Partner, Texas Oncology, Dallas, Texas

Andrew H. Soll, M.D.
Professor of Medicine, UCLA School of Medicine; Staff Physician, West Los Angeles VA Medical Center, Los Angeles, California

John G. Stagias, M.D.
Former Gastroenterology Fellow, Yale University School of Medicine, New Haven, and Griffin Hospital, Derby, Connecticut

Deborah J. Statters, B.M., B.Ch., M.A.
Specialist Registrar, Queen Elizabeth Hospital, Birmingham, West Midlands, United Kingdom

William W. Stead, M.D., M.A.C.P.
Professor of Medicine, University of Arkansas College of Medicine; Director, Tuberculosis Control, Arkansas Department of Health, Little Rock, Arkansas

Richard A. Steeves, M.D., Ph.D.
Professor of Human Oncology, University of Wisconsin Medical School, Madison, Wisconsin

James P. Steinberg, M.D.
Associate Professor of Medicine, Division of Infectious Diseases, Emory University School of Medicine; Associate Chief of Medicine, Crawford Long Hospital of Emory University, Atlanta, Georgia

Dennis L. Stevens, M.D., Ph.D.
Professor of Medicine, University of Washington School of Medicine, Seattle, Washington; Chief, Infectious Disease Section, Veterans Affairs Medical Center, Boise, Idaho

James A. Stewart, M.D., F.A.C.P.
Associate Professor of Medicine, and Associate Director for Clinical Affairs, University of Wisconsin Comprehensive Cancer Center; Clinical Director, Medical Oncology, University of Wisconsin, Madison, Wisconsin

Eric H. Stocker, M.D.
Fellow in Cardiology, Baylor University Medical Center, Dallas, Texas

James M. Stone, M.D., F.A.C.S.
Private Practice, Northern California Surgical Group, Redding, California

Harris R. Stutman, M.D.
Formerly Associate Professor of Pediatrics, University of California at Irvine; Director, Pediatric Infectious Disease, Memorial Miller Children's Hospital, Irvine, California

Darryl Y. Sue, M.D.
Professor of Clinical Medicine, UCLA School of Medicine, Los Angeles; Division of Respiratory and Critical Care Physiology and Medicine, and Associate Chair, Department of Medicine, Harbor-UCLA Medical Center, Torrance, California

Wadi N. Suki, M.D.
Professor of Medicine and of Molecular Physiology and Biophysics, and Chief, Renal Section, Baylor College of Medicine, Houston, Texas

Warren R. Summer, M.D.
Howard A. Buechner Professor, and Section Chief, Pulmonary/Critical Care Medicine, Louisiana State University School of Medicine; Director, Pulmonary Services, Medical Center of Louisiana; Section Chief of Pulmonary Services, Ochsner Clinic, New Orleans, Louisiana

Satoru Suzuki, M.D., Ph.D.
Professor, Department of Geriatrics, Endocrinology and Metabolism, Shinshu University School of Medicine, Matsumoto, Japan

Barbara E. Swartz, M.D., Ph.D.
Associate Professor, UCLA School of Medicine; Director, Epilepsy Unit, West Los Angeles Medical Center, Los Angeles, California

Robert A. Swerlick, M.D.
Associate Professor of Dermatology, Emory University-Emory Clinic, Atlanta, Georgia

Norman Talal, M.D.
Professor of Medicine, University of Texas Health Science Center at San Antonio, San Antonio, Texas

Jerome Teitel, M.D., F.R.C.P.C.
Associate Professor, University of Toronto Faculty of Medicine; Director, Toronto and Central Ontario Adult Comprehensive Hemophilia Program; Department of Medicine, Division of Hematology, St. Michael's Hospital, Toronto, Ontario, Canada

Tate Thigpen, M.D.
Professor of Medicine, and Director, Division of Oncology, University of Mississippi Medical Center, Jackson, Mississippi

Michael A. Thomas, M.D.
Assistant Professor, Division of Reproductive Endocrinology and Infertility, Department of Obstetrics and Gynecology, University of Cincinnati College of Medicine, Cincinnati, Ohio

W. Grant Thompson, M.D., F.R.C.P.C.
Professor of Medicine, University of Ottawa Faculty of Medicine; Chief, Division of Gastroenterology, Ottawa Civic Hospital, Ottawa, Ontario, Canada

Paul J. Thuluvath, M.D., M.R.C.P.
Medical Director, Liver Transplantation, Division of Gastroenterology, The Johns Hopkins University, Baltimore, Maryland

Jeremiah G. Tilles, M.D.
Professor of Medicine, Professor of Microbiology and Molecular Genetics, and Associate Dean for Academic Affairs, University of California at Irvine; Principal Investigator, California Collaborative Treatment Group, Irvine, California

James R. Tillotson, M.D.
Formerly Clinical Professor of Medicine, Albany Medical College, Albany, New York

Janelle Tipton, M.S.N., R.N., A.O.C.N.
Adjunct Instructor, School of Nursing, Medical College of Ohio; Oncology Clinical Nurse Specialist, Medical College Hospitals, Toledo, Ohio

Marcia G. Tonnesen, M.D.
Associate Professor of Medicine and Dermatology, State University of New York School of Medicine, Stony Brook; Chief of Dermatology, Veterans Affairs Medical Center, Northport, New York

Vicente E. Torres, M.D.
Professor of Medicine, Mayo Medical School; Consultant, Division of Nephrology and Internal Medicine, Mayo Clinic and Mayo Foundation, Rochester, Minnesota

Edmund C. Tramont, M.D.
Professor and Director, Medical Biotechnology Center, and Professor, Department of Medicine, University of Maryland School of Medicine, Baltimore, Maryland

Morris Traube, M.D.
Associate Professor of Medicine, and Director, Clinical Affairs, Section of Digestive Diseases, Yale University School of Medicine; Director, Gastrointestinal Procedure Center, Yale-New Haven Hospital, New Haven, Connecticut

Charles B. Treasure, M.D.
Formerly Assistant Professor of Medicine, Emory University School of Medicine; Director, Cardiac Catheterization Laboratory, Grady Memorial Hospital; Interventional Cardiologist, The Emory Clinic, Atlanta, Georgia

Allan R. Tunkel, M.D., Ph.D.
Associate Professor of Medicine, Allegheny University of the Health Sciences; Director, Internal Medicine Residency Program, Allegheny University Hospitals, Philadelphia, Pennsylvania

Antonio Ucar, M.D.
Clinical Director, The League Against Cancer, Miami, Florida

John A. Ulatowski, M.D., Ph.D.
Assistant Professor of Anesthesiology/Critical Care Medicine, Neurology and Neurosurgery, and Co-Director, Neuroscience Critical Care Unit, The Johns Hopkins Hospital, Baltimore, Maryland

Mark E. Unis, M.D.
Clinical Instructor, Division of Dermatology, University of Florida College of Medicine, Gainesville; Chief of Dermatology, Holy Cross Hospital and Northridge Hospital, Fort Lauderdale, Florida

Jaime Uribarri, M.D.
Assistant Professor of Medicine, Mount Sinai School of Medicine; Director, Dialysis Services, Mount Sinai Hospital, New York, New York

Luis M. Valdez, M.D.
Fellow, Divison of Infectious Diseases, University of Texas Health Science Center, Houston, Texas

A.W. L. van den Wall Bake, M.D., Ph.D.
Consultant Physician, St. Joseph Hospital, Veldhoven, The Netherlands

David H. Van Thiel, M.D.
Formerly Medical Director of Transplantation, Baptist Medical Center of Oklahoma, Oklahoma City, Oklahoma

Rama P. Venu, M.D., F.A.C.P., F.A.C.G.
Clinical Professor of Medicine, and Director, Therapeutic Endoscopy, Digestive Disease and Liver Center, University of Illinois, Chicago, Illinois

Joseph G. Verbalis, M.D.
Professor of Medicine and Physiology, and Chief of Endocrinology and Metabolism, Georgetown University Medical Center, Washington, D.C.

George W. Vetrovec, M.D.
Professor of Medicine, Interim Chairman of Cardiology, and Director, Adult Catheterization Laboratories, Medical College of Virginia, Virginia Commonwealth University, Richmond, Virginia

Thomas W. Von Dohlen, M.D.
Chief Fellow in Cardiology, Instructor in Medicine, and Assistant Professor of Medicine and Radiology, Medical College of Georgia School of Medicine, Augusta, Georgia; Associate Professor of Medicine, West Virginia University School of Medicine, Charleston, West Virginia

Elaine Lee Wade, M.D.
Assistant Professor of Medicine, Part Time Faculty, Loyola University Medical Center, Maywood; Attending Physician, Hematology-Oncology, West Suburban Hospital Medical Center, Oak Park, Illinois

John F. Wade III, M.D.
Instructor in Medicine, University of Colorado School of Medicine, Denver, Colorado

Ken B. Waites, M.D.
Associate Professor of Pathology and Microbiology, and Director of Clinical Microbiology, University of Alabama School of Medicine, Birmingham, Alabama

Arnold Wald, M.D.
Professor of Medicine, University of Pittsburgh School of Medicine; Associate Chief, Division of Gastroenterology and Hepatology, University of Pittsburgh Medical Center, Pittsburgh, Pennsylvania

Francis A. Waldvogel, M.D.
Professor and Chairman, Department of Medicine, University of Geneva Faculty of Medicine; Physician-in-Chief, Clinique de Medecine II, University Hospital, Geneva, Switzerland

Paul G. Walfish, C.M., M.D., F.R.C.P.C., F.A.C.P., F.R.S.M.
Professor of Medicine and Paediatrics, University of Toronto Faculty of Medicine; Senior Scientist, Samuel Lunenfeld Research Institute of Mount Sinai Hospital and The Isabel Silverman Canada International Scientific Exchange Program; Senior Attending Physician, Division of Endocrinology and Metabolism, and Senior Consultant, Endocrinology and Head and Neck Oncology, Mount Sinai-Toronto Hospital, Toronto, Ontario, Canada

Thomas J. Walsh, M.D.
Senior Investigator, and Chief, Immunocompromised Host Section, National Cancer Institute, Bethesda, Maryland

Theodore E. Warkentin, M.D., F.A.C.P.C., F.A.C.P.
Associate Professor of Pathology and Medicine, McMaster University Faculty of Health Sciences; Head, Transfusion Medicine and Hemostasis, and Hematologist, Service of Clinical Hematology, Hamilton Health Sciences Center, Hamilton General and Henderson Campuses, Hamilton, Ontario, Canada

Steven A. Wartman, M.D., Ph.D.
Professor of Medicine, Albert Einstein College of Medicine of Yeshiva University, Bronx, New York; Physician-in-Chief, and Chairman, Department of Medicine, Long Island Jewish Medical Center, New Hyde Park, New York

Karlman Wasserman, M.D., Ph.D.
Professor of Medicine, UCLA School of Medicine, Los Angeles, and Harbor-UCLA Medical Center, Torrance, California

Yoshio Watanabe, M.D., D.M.Sc.
Professor Emeritus of Medicine, Fujita Health University School of Medicine, Toyoake; Director, Toyota Regional Medical Center, Toyota, Aichi, Japan

Nathan Watemberg, M.D.
Fellow, Neurophysiology, Department of Neurology, Medical College of Virginia, Virginia Commonwealth University, Richmond, Virginia

Jeffrey N. Weiser, M.D.
Assistant Professor, Departments of Pediatrics and Microbiology, University of Pennsylvania School of Medicine; Medical Staff, Children's Hospital of Philadelphia, Philadelphia, Pennsylvania

Jeffrey I. Weitz, M.D., F.R.C.P.C., F.A.C.P.
Professor of Medicine, McMaster University Faculty of Health Sciences; Head, Experimental Thrombosis/ Atherosclerosis Group and Division of Thromboembolism, Hamilton Civic Hospitals, Hamilton, Ontario, Canada

Richard J. Whitley, M.D.
Loeb Eminent Scholar Chair in Pediatrics, and Professor of Pediatrics, Microbiology, and Medicine, University of Alabama School of Medicine, Birmingham, Alabama

James T. Willerson, M.D.
Professor and Chairman, The University of Texas Medical School at Houston; Medical Director, and Chief of Cardiology, Texas Heart Institute; Chief of Medicine, Hermann Hospital; Chief of Cardiology, St. Luke's Episcopal Hospital, Houston, Texas

Elizabeth A. Williams, M.D., Ph.D.
Associate Professor of Medicine, Department of Internal Medicine, East Tennessee State University, James H. Quillen College of Medicine, Johnson City, Tennessee

Gordon H. Williams, M.D.
Professor of Medicine, Harvard Medical School; Chief, Endocrine-Hypertension Division, Brigham and Women's Hospital, Boston, Massachusetts

Richard H. Winterbauer, M.D.
Chief, Section of Pulmonary and Critical Care Medicine,Virginia Mason Clinic, Seattle, Washington

Jerry S. Wolinsky, M.D.
Professor of Neurology, University of Texas Health Science Center; Staff Physician, Hermann Hospital, Houston, Texas

David T. Woodley, M.D.
Walter J. Hamlin Professor, and Chair, Department of Dermatology, Northwestern University Medical School, Chicago, Illinois

Alexandra S. Worobec, M.D.
Clinical Associate, Laboratory of Allergic Diseases, National Institute of Allergy and Infectious Diseases, National Institutes of Health, Bethesda, Maryland

Harlan I. Wright, M.D.
Interim Chief, Abdominal Transplant Medicine, Oklahoma Transplantation Institute, Baptist Medical Center of Oklahoma, Oklahoma City, Oklahoma

Neal S. Young, M.D.
Chief, Hematology Branch, National Heart, Lung and Blood Institute, National Institutes of Health, Bethesda, Maryland

William B. Young, M.D.
Clinical Instructor, Department of Neurology, Temple University School of Medicine; Co-Director, Comprehensive Headache Center, Germantown Hospital and Medical Center, Philadelphia, Pennsylvania

George C.S. Yu, M.D., F.A.C.P., F.C.C.P.
Ventura County Pulmonary Medical Group, Oxnard, California

Victor L. Yu, M.D.
Professor of Medicine, University of Pittsburgh School of Medicine; Chief, Infectious Disease Section, Veterans Affairs Medical Center, Pittsburgh, Pennsylvania

John A. Zaia, M.D.
Professor of Pediatrics, and Director, Department of Virology and Infectious Diseases, Division of Pediatrics, City of Hope National Medical Center, Duarte, California

Mark M. Zalupski, M.D.
Associate Professor of Medicine, Wayne State University School of Medicine, Detroit, Michigan

Jonathan M. Zenilman, M.D.
Associate Professor of Medicine, Division of Infectious Diseases, The Johns Hopkins University School of Medicine; Attending Physician, The Johns Hopkins Hospital, Baltimore, Maryland

Douglas P. Zipes, M.D.
Distinguished Professor of Medicine, Pharmacology and Toxicology, Indiana University School of Medicine; Director, Krannert Institute of Cardiology and Division of Cardiology, Indiana University School of Medicine, Indianapolis, Indiana

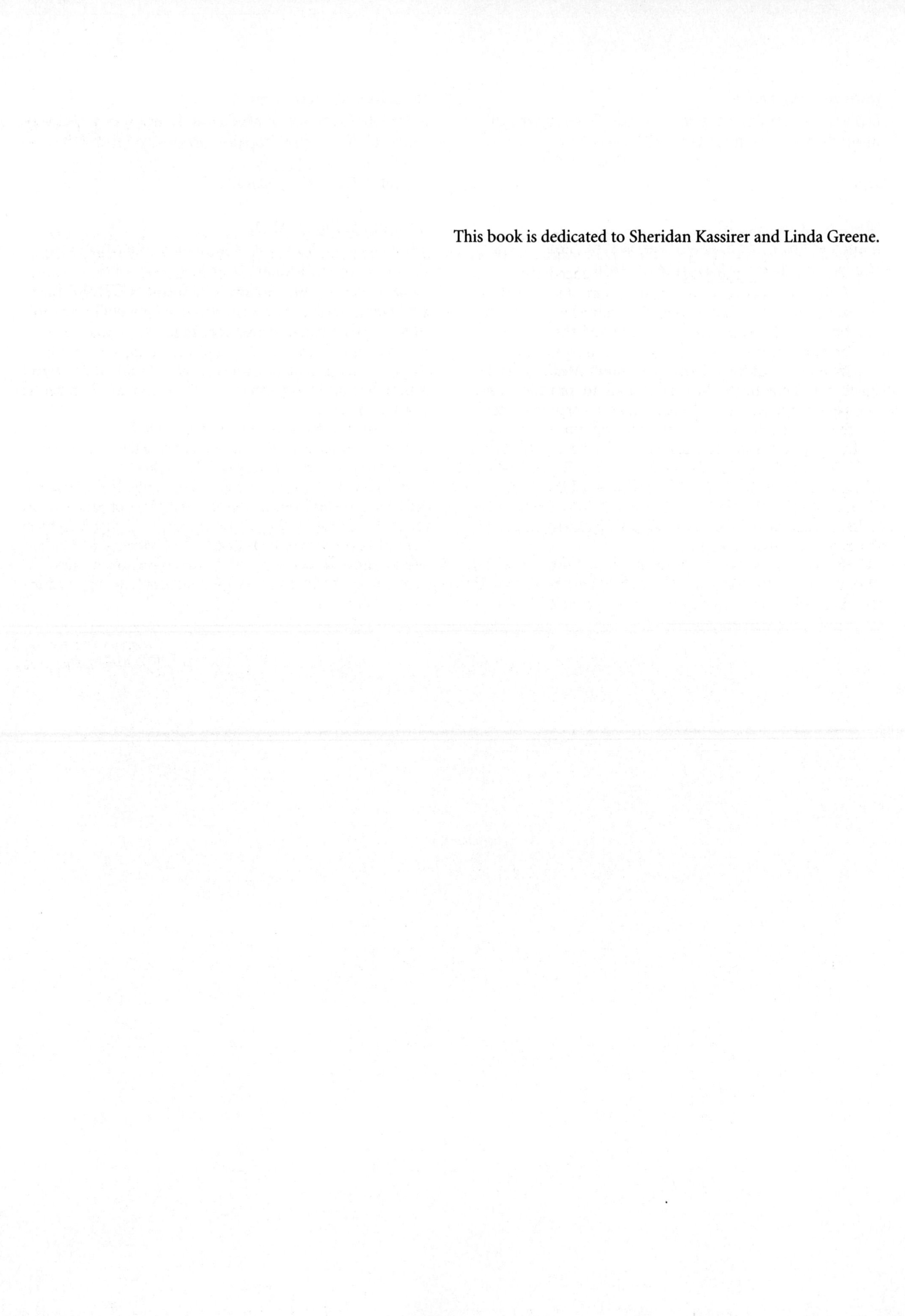

This book is dedicated to Sheridan Kassirer and Linda Greene.

PREFACE

Medicine has moved at an incredible pace since the first publication of *Current Therapy in Internal Medicine* in 1984. Specialists and subspecialists are being challenged to broaden their focus, while primary care physicians must increase their depth. The time for patient visits is diminishing, while the amount of work required is increasing and the margin for error is diminishing. The fourth edition, now more appropriately entitled *Current Therapy in Adult Medicine,* is designed for these times. We have tried to provide broad therapeutic options in a context that incorporates cost-effective choices. We have presented the opinions of some of the best physicians in the world with the work ably edited by C. Wayne Bardin, M.D., Theodore M. Bayless, M.D., Michael C. Brain, D.M., Paul P. Carbone, M.D., Richard J. Glassock, M.D., John W. Griffin, M.D., J. Willis Hurst, M.D., Richard T. Johnson, M.D., Lawrence M. Lichtenstein, M.D., and David Schlossberg, M.D.

This edition contains new chapters in virtually every specialty of internal medicine and should help keep subspecialists and generalist physicians of all stripes at the forefront of therapeutics. A new section on women's health responds to the evolving needs of our patients. *Current Therapy in Adult Medicine* will be at home in all treatment settings: clinical problems ranging from those encountered in the office to the intensive care unit are all addressed. The emphasis of this book is on therapy, but because treatment decisions take place in a context which includes an understanding of pathophysiology, we have included substantial pathophysiology and critical diagnostic issues to provide structure for therapeutic decision making.

We are grateful to many for their help, but especially to Michele Boutin, Marie Chieppo, Linda Healy, and Lesley Traver. We have been encouraged throughout this process by Lynne Gery of Mosby–Year Book. She is a highly professional and effective editor who knows the challenges of practice and understands how to design and deliver books that help busy clinicians provide the best care for their patients. At Mosby–Year Book we are also grateful to Anthony Trioli, production editor; Nancy McDonald, designer; and Amanda Starr, editorial assistant.

Harry L. Greene II
Jerome P. Kassirer

Contents

CARDIOVASCULAR DISEASES

GASTROINTESTINAL DISEASES

ENDOCRINE DISORDERS

IMMUNE, ALLERGIC, AND RHEUMATOLOGIC DISEASES

SKIN DISEASES

NEUROLOGIC DISEASES

EYE DISEASES

APPENDIX

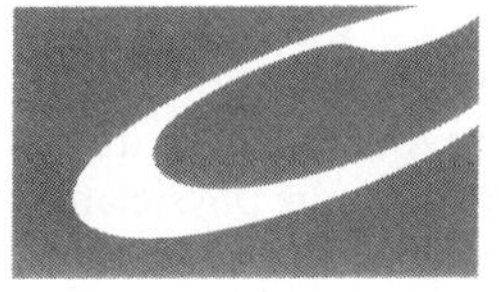

THERAPEUTIC PRINCIPLES AND PROBLEMS

PRINCIPLES OF THERAPEUTIC DECISION MAKING

Mark H. Eckman, M.D.
Nananda F. Col, M.D., M.P.P., M.P.H.
Jerome P. Kassirer, M.D.

Selecting the right treatment at the right time is a prime function of the physician, and a dazzling array of therapeutic approaches is available. Choices lie along a spectrum of dissimilar options: avoidance or cessation of all modalities on the one hand and the use of accepted drugs and operative approaches or radical new, incompletely effective, and high-risk medical and surgical treatments on the other. The penalties for unwise and inappropriate selection of therapy are formidable, including disappointments, disability, and death.

Needless to say, accurate diagnosis is the critical first step in deciding which treatment to choose; however, many therapeutic decisions must be made before all diagnostic information is available and before we are confident of a diagnosis. In many instances selection of therapy is simple and straightforward because long experience has confirmed the value and safety of a given approach. In such instances we develop comfortable and familiar rules that guide our every day decisions. "Treatments of choice," which vary little from year to year, are available for many disease entities.

Not all therapeutic decisions can be based on simple rules or guidelines, however. In many instances we must return to first principles to make such choices—instances in which we are not guaranteed that a given disease is present, instances in which one approach seems only marginally better than another, and instances of newly discovered drugs or novel diseases.

By tradition, we try to select a treatment according to the highest scientific principles. Anecdotal reports of therapeutic efficacy and risk are not sufficient because factors such as placebo effect, spontaneous remissions, and regression toward the mean seriously cloud the interpretation of individual responses. To avert these confounding variables, we rely heavily on randomized controlled trials of therapeutic approaches. We insist that, for a study to qualify as appropriate, patients must be assigned randomly to treatment, neither the patient nor the physician must know which treatment is being administered, outcomes must be measured and defined with precision, and analysis of data must be done using accepted statistical methods. Such trials are laborious, expensive, and subject to flaws, both in design and implementation, but many such studies have been performed well and have provided invaluable therapeutic insights. Even the best of the randomized controlled studies, however, provide only an anchor point or a benchmark when it comes to selecting therapy for an individual patient. To the extent that a patient differs notably from the subjects studied in a randomized trial, that patient's response to the treatment also may differ. Patients may differ in many ways, including their age, sex, race, genetic makeup, and the stage at which their disease is encountered.

Of course, many instances exist in which no randomized controlled trial has been carried out or is likely ever to be carried out. When the patient fails to match a cohort in a controlled study or when no study is available, the physician's good judgment must be relied on. The elements of therapeutic judgment become critical in such circumstances, forming the basis for our ability to return to first principles in making decisions in the face of uncertainty.

In the past two decades, the principles of therapeutic decision making have been organized and codified into a prescriptive method called *decision analysis.* Although decision analysis is a highly useful quantitative approach that applies probability and utility theory to therapeutic decision making under conditions of uncertainty, the principles underlying the application of decision analysis to therapeutic choices can be enunciated and applied even without reverting to numbers and calculations. To explicate these principles, we first describe many of them qualitatively. Then, to demonstrate how these principles translate into therapeutic decision making, we provide a formal decision analysis for a particular therapeutic dilemma.

■ SOME THERAPEUTIC PRINCIPLES

Not surprisingly, the principles of therapy are intertwined inextricably with the principles of diagnosis. Because a diagnosis is only an inference about a patient's illness, we can never be absolutely certain that the disease label we assign to a patient's illness is correct. Even if we have a treatment for a disease that is regularly effective and devoid of risk or cost, we inevitably will give the treatment to some patients who do not have the disease and inevitably will not give the treatment to some who have the disease. Both circumstances deprive patients of appropriate therapy. To the extent that the treatment is effective, patients who have the disease will derive the benefit of therapy. However, this benefit will be offset to some extent by the risks of therapy. The patients who do not have the disease, however, derive no therapeutic benefit but nonetheless are subjected to the risks of treatment.

The interrelations between a diagnosis and the benefits and risks of treatment can be specified in the concept of a therapeutic threshold, a probability of disease above which administering the treatment is optimal and below which withholding the treatment is optimal. The efficacy and risks of a treatment for a given disease determine how confident a physician must be of a given diagnosis before administering therapy. For treatments with a high ratio of benefits to risks, the treatment can be given even when the probability of disease is relatively low (e.g., penicillin for suspected streptococcal pneumonia infections). For these treatments, the therapeutic threshold is quite low. For treatments with a low ratio of benefits to risks, however, the physician must be quite certain that the patient has the disease before administering therapy (e.g., amphotericin B for suspected cryptococcal meningitis). For these treatments, the therapeutic threshold is quite high. Of course, low efficacy of treatment, high risk, or both can contribute to such a low benefit-risk ratio.

Independent of diagnosis, decision analysis makes explicit the tradeoffs between disparate therapeutic choices. Physicians often are compelled to help patients choose between short-term and long-term risks (e.g., in a patient with asymptomatic gallstones, the risk of immediate cholecystectomy must be weighed against the future risk of biliary colic and cholecystitis; and in a patient with significant coronary artery disease, the risk of early surgical mortality from bypass grafting must be compared with the future risk of myocardial infarction). In addition, the greater efficacy of one therapeutic approach over another must sometimes be measured against its adverse effect on the quality of a patient's life (e.g., in a patient with laryngeal carcinoma, the choice between less aggressive, speech-preserving surgery has to be weighed against a more aggressive procedure that might result in loss of speech but might yield a cure or at least longer cancer-free survival).

When comparing treatments, both randomized controlled trials and decision analysis disclose the marginal benefit of one therapy over another. In many instances this benefit is large and the decision is clear. In some instances, however, no clear therapeutic approach emerges. Such decisional "toss-ups" are well known in lay decision making, but physicians have been slow to appreciate their existence in clinical decision making. The principal problem in dealing with therapeutic toss-ups lies in judging the clinical relevance of a small benefit. A difference of several years of life expectancy between two treatments seems like quite a lot, whereas a difference of only several weeks could easily allow the physician to recommend either treatment. However, even a few weeks' difference could be important to a particular patient. Given these features of therapeutic decision making, patients' preferences must always be taken into consideration. Doing so is especially important when marginal differences in the outcomes of two therapeutic approaches are quite small.

Comparing therapeutic choices quantitatively discloses the benefits of these choices clearly. In some instances the principal benefit of one choice over another lies in a small improvement in the quality of an individual's life. In other instances it is apparent that, no matter which therapeutic choice is made (e.g., extensive chemotherapy versus radical surgery in a patient with metastatic cancer), the outcome will be poor. If nothing more, such an assessment may have important prognostic implications.

As noted previously, physicians often conduct their therapeutic reasoning based on experience-proven rules. Given the repetitiveness of our day-to-day patient experiences, this practice generally stands us in good stead. Nonetheless, situations often arise in which the patient or clinical setting is in some way atypical—the operative mortality may be higher than usual because of a patient's other risk factors and illnesses, the diagnosis may be uncertain, or the efficacies of competing therapies may be in doubt. Sometimes we are confronted with innovative techniques for testing new therapies or developments in health technology for which adequate information is not yet available. In these settings a more formal and quantitative approach to therapeutic decision making may be especially useful. The following section discusses how decision analysis can be used to deal with a therapeutic quandary.

■ FORMAL DECISION-MAKING METHODS

Decision analysis prescribes how decisions should be made, rather than describing how they are made in practice. A model of the decision in the form of a decision tree provides a uniform and formal framework around which all of the involved medical caretakers can gather. It makes explicit the questions that are being asked. It provides a common language, so that when either a patient or a physician asks, for example, "How will the high risk of this proposed therapy effect our decision?", we can specify clearly the parameter to be discussed and the range of risk to be considered.

Decision analysis also quantifies the language of uncertainty. Where one physician's use of the qualifying term *likely* may indicate a probability of 90 to 100 percent, another physician's use of the same term in the same clinical setting may mean 50 to 80 percent. Although no one can rightfully say what *likely* actually means in probabilistic terms, the use of a common model and numeric probabilities as focal points of discussion ensures that all parties are speaking the same language.

The steps in performing a decision analysis include (1) framing the question; (2) structuring the problem; (3) determining the probabilities of each outcome; (4) assigning utilities (i.e., numeric values for each possible outcome); (5) calculating and comparing the expected (average) utility for each strategy, thus determining which strategy is best; (6) performing sensitivity analyses to examine the important numeric assumptions used; and (7) interpreting the results. Frequently, this final step leads to an iterative reconsideration of the previous six steps as oversights in assumptions or mistakes in the model are uncovered.

Here the problem is illustrated: A male Jehovah's Witness aged 55 years with stable exertional angina was found to have critical occlusion of two coronary arteries on cardiac catheterization. Based on religious beliefs, he refuses to receive any blood transfusion, although he consents to the use of cardiopulmonary bypass, if necessary. He has normal left ventricular function and is otherwise healthy. What is the optimal approach to his treatment? Should he be treated medically? Should a surgical approach be considered? Are there other options?

Structuring the Problem

We first structure the problem making all of the assumptions, events, and outcomes explicit. This structure usually is provided in the form of a decision tree in which all possible outcomes of each of the choices are laid out and the end branches represent final outcomes. The symbolic notation of a decision tree consists of three basic elements: (1) decision nodes (*square*) describing the choices to be made by the clinician(s) and patients; (2) chance nodes (*round*) representing probabilistic events not under our control; and (3) terminal nodes (*rectangular*) representing outcomes (i.e., summaries of events beyond the time horizon of the decision tree). In Figure 1, the initial decision node at the left delineates four choices: medical management, initial medical management with subsequent cross-over to either coronary artery bypass grafting (CABG) or percutaneous transluminal coronary angioplasty (PTCA) if symptoms worsen, and immediate CABG or PTCA. Prognosis is determined by whether the patient dies or develops an acute myocardial infarction as an immediate consequence of surgery or PTCA, whether or not the procedure is successful in achieving and maintaining patency of the occluded vessels, and by the efficacy of medical management, CABG, or PTCA in decreasing long-term coronary artery disease mortality and symptomatology. We explicitly modeled events that occur within the first year. After this time, long-term prognosis is summarized by a quality-adjusted life expectancy for each outcome, based on the presence and severity of angina and revascularization status.

As shown in Figures 2 through 4, we explicitly model both short-term (i.e., 30 days) and long-term (i.e., within the first year) events. Those patients who are managed medically may die or suffer myocardial infarction during the first 30 days (corresponding to the perioperative period during which they were to have had a revascularization procedure). After this time, some patients may die within the first year from coronary artery disease ('DIE FROM CAD'). At the end of the first year, patients may continue to have symptomatic angina, which can be mild (class I or II) or severe (class III or IV).

Events for patients undergoing CABG are shown in Figure 3. These patients may die or suffer a myocardial infarction ('NONFATAL MI') during the perioperative period. Some patients will die within the first year from nonexplicitly modeled events related to coronary artery disease ('DIE FROM CAD'), and some will develop symptomatic occlusion

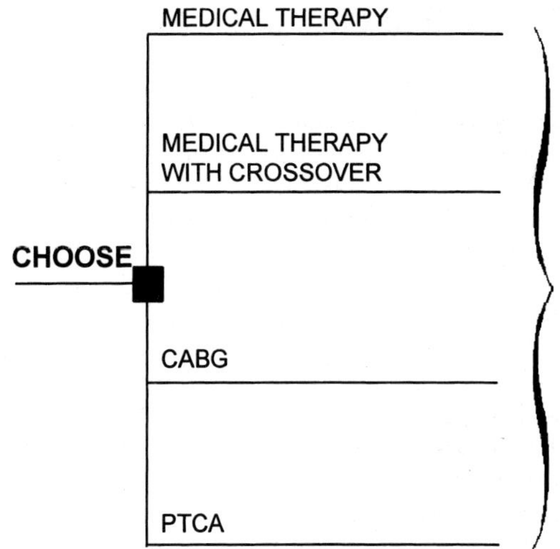

Figure 1
Decision tree analyzing revascularization strategies for a man aged 55 years who is a Jehovah's Witness and who refuses blood products during CABG with stable angina and two-vessel coronary disease. The square on the left represents the decision node between the four strategies: medical therapy, medical therapy with cross-over to revascularization, CABG, and PTCA.

of their grafts that leads to repeat cardiac catheterization ('CARDIAC CATH'). Patients who do not undergo a revascularization procedure may develop recurrent angina, which may be mild or severe ('? ANGINA' subtree).

Patients who receive medical management initially but who may cross-over to a revascularization procedure (either CABG or PTCA) face the same chance events described in Figure 3 for patients who initially undergo CABG.

Finally, Figure 4 details events for patients who initially undergo PTCA. These patients may die or suffer a nonfatal perioperative myocardial infarction, and some may require emergent CABG. A proportion of those patients in whom PTCA is clinically successful ('PTCA SUCCESSFUL') may die from coronary artery disease within the first year ('DIE FROM CAD'). Survivors may reocclude and undergo repeat cardiac catheterization followed by another attempt at revascularization. Patients in whom PTCA is not successful undergo CABG unless they are deemed inoperable (i.e., they already have experienced CABG twice).

We assume that a maximum number of two CABG procedures and three PTCAs will be performed within the first year. If symptomatic reocclusion occurs after this point, medical therapy is continued and no further revascularization procedures are attempted. This therapy is implemented through the use of a Boolean node, which acts like a switch by allowing recursion when equal to 1 and terminating recursion when equal to 0.

Probabilities

After the decision tree is structured, the likelihood of each event being modeled must next be determined. These probabilities should come from the literature, when available, but if not, they may represent the subjective best estimates of

DIE DURING FIRST 30 DAYS
DEATH
NONFATAL MI
DIE FROM CAD
DEATH
MEDICAL
THERAPY
SEVERE ANGINA
LE
ANGINA
MILD ANGINA
LE
WELL
? ANGINA
NO ANGINA
LE

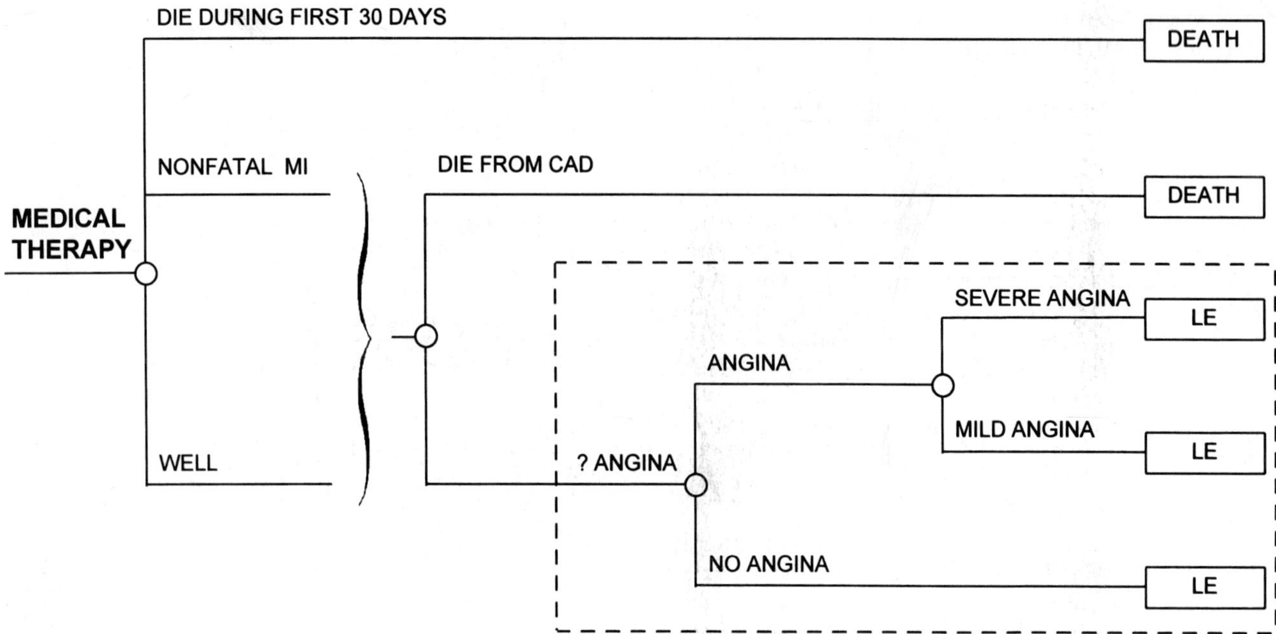

Figure 2
Medical therapy strategy. The brace indicates subtree notation. The open circles represent chance nodes. The rectangles on the right represent terminal nodes. The subtree '? ANGINA' is enclosed by the dashed rectangle.

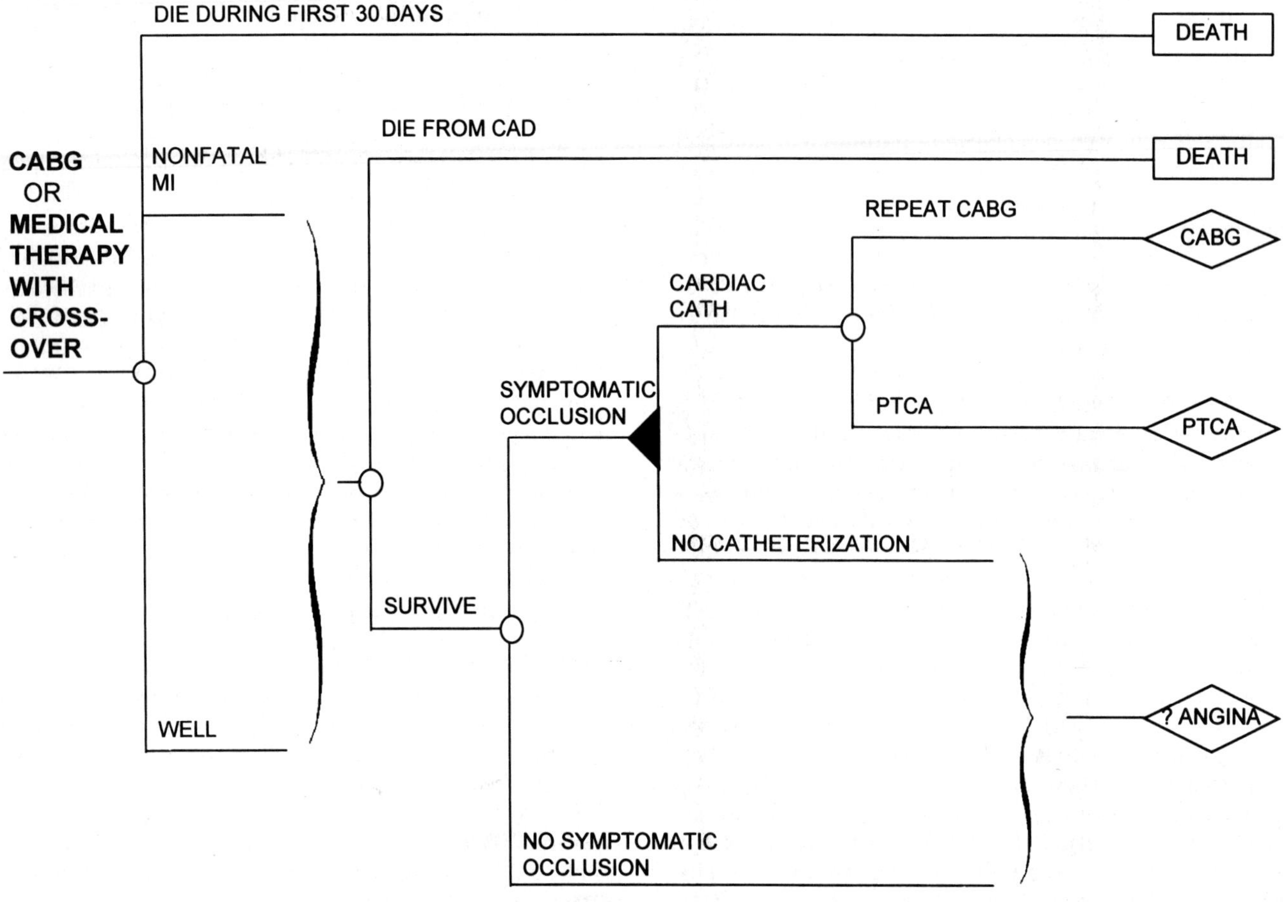

DIE DURING FIRST 30 DAYS
DEATH
DIE FROM CAD
CABG
OR
MEDICAL
THERAPY
WITH
CROSS-
OVER
NONFATAL
MI
DEATH
REPEAT CABG
CABG
CARDIAC
CATH
SYMPTOMATIC
OCCLUSION
PTCA
PTCA
NO CATHETERIZATION
SURVIVE
WELL
? ANGINA
NO SYMPTOMATIC
OCCLUSION

Figure 3
Medical therapy with cross-over to revascularization. The triangle represents a Boolean node. The diamonds at the far right denote subtrees. This figure also models the CABG strategy.

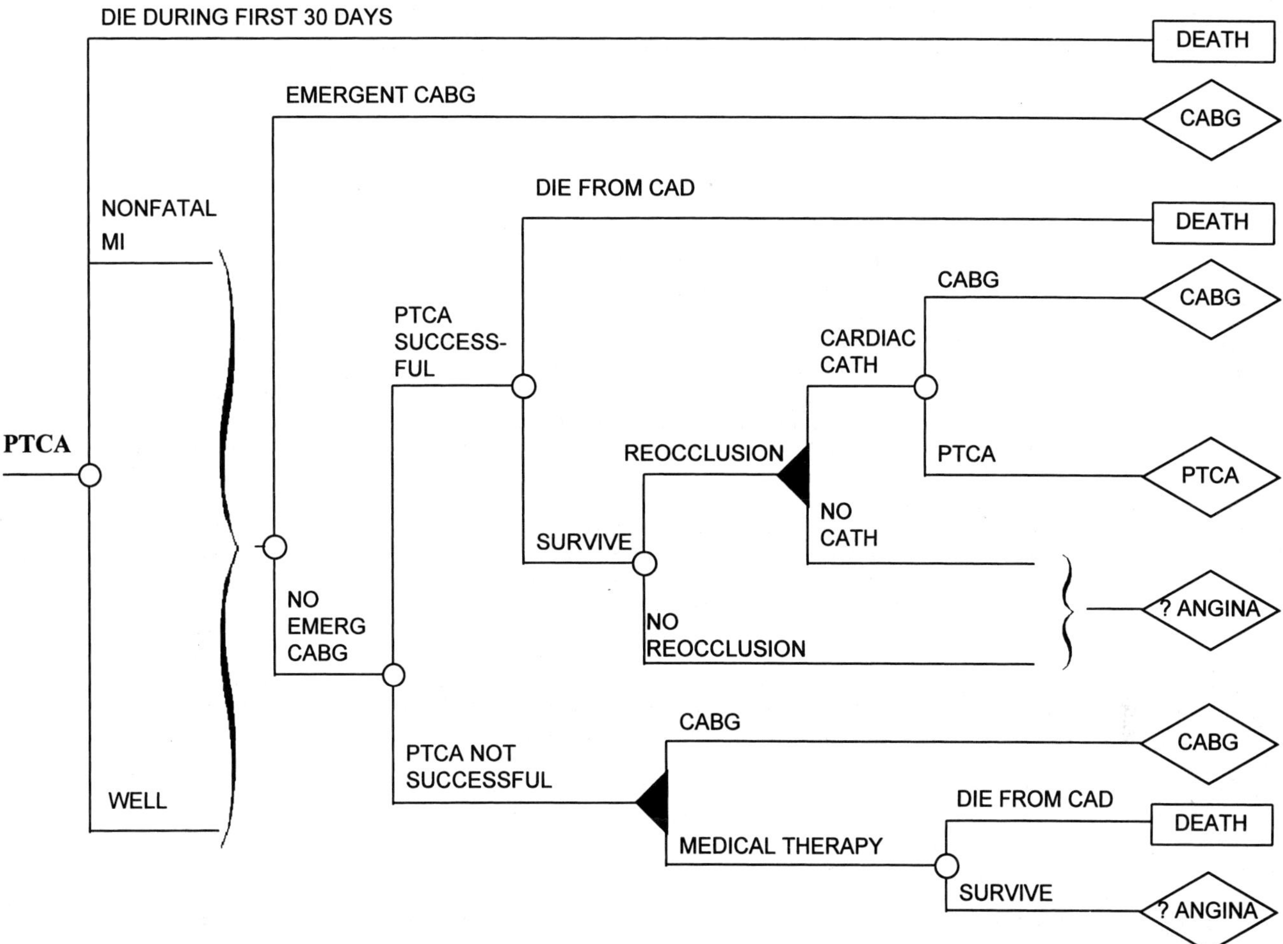

Figure 4
PTCA strategy.

experts. Table 1 describes the probabilities used in this analysis. Whenever possible, we used data on men with two-vessel disease and mild angina.

Medical Management

Because we explicitly modeled the risk of death and nonfatal myocardial infarction occurring during the perioperative period for the revascularization strategies, we also must consider these same short-term events in the medical strategy. Under medical management, 2.2 percent of patients suffer nonfatal myocardial infarction over a 1-year period, corresponding to a monthly probability of 0.2 percent. The yearly probability of dying from coronary artery disease is higher among those patients who have suffered acute myocardial infarction and survived the first 30 days than among those who have not had a myocardial infarction (8 percent versus 1.8 percent, respectively). The probability of developing symptomatic occlusion requiring revascularization is roughly 10 percent, based on the proportion of medical patients in the Coronary Artery Surgery Study (CASS) who crossed over to surgical treatment during the first year of the study. To account for the increased utilization of PTCA since the CASS was performed, we assumed that half of those patients requiring revascularization would undergo PTCA. Although the use of coronary-artery stents is an effective new alternative to angioplasty, we did not consider this therapeutic option because of the high risk of hemorrhagic complications with present protocols.

Medical therapy is less effective than CABG or PTCA in reducing anginal symptoms. Among patients with mild angina, 78 percent of those receiving medical therapy continue to have angina at the end of one year, 27 percent of whom have severe angina. The probability of anginal symptoms increases to 100 percent when patients are deemed inoperable (i.e., they have completed the maximum number of revascularization procedures and reocclude). These patients have a threefold increase in long-term mortality from cardiovascular events.

CABG

We assume that the saphenous vein would be used as the conduit rather than the internal mammary artery because of the lower risk of hemorrhage associated with the former, even though the internal mammary artery approach recently has been shown to confer a survival advantage. To estimate the increased risk of perioperative death among patients who refuse blood transfusion, we developed a ratio of the mortality rates of Jehovah's Witnesses who underwent CABG without transfusion (5.1 percent) to that of the general population (2.3 percent). We used this relative risk of 2.2 as a multiplier to adjust the surgical mortality rate for CABG in our patient.

Table 1 Probabilities and Rates Used in Decision Tree for 55-Year-Old Male Jehovah's Witness with Stable Angina and Two-Vessel Coronary Disease

OUTCOMES	CABG	EMERGENCY CABG	PTCA	MEDICAL THERAPY
PROBABILITIES:				
Procedural complications				
Death				.0015*
First procedure, no previous myocardial infarction	0.055†	0.055†	0.011	—
Repeat procedure	0.086†	—	0.011	—
After myocardial infarction	0.108†	0.095†	0.067	—
Myocardial Infarction	0.20†	0.46†	0.027	0.002*
Emergent CABG				
Previous myocardial infarction	—	—	0.38	—
No previous myocardial infarction	—	—	0.02	—
Procedural efficacy				
Initial clinical success	1.00	1.00	0.90	—
Symptomatic reocclusion over the next year	0.06	0.06	0.44	0.10
Angina 1 year later	0.26	0.26	0.29	0.78
Severe angina††	0.27	0.27	0.27	0.27
First-year mortality (among survivors)				
After myocardial infarction	0.014	0.014	0.021	0.08
No myocardial infarction	0.01	0.01	0.016	0.018
RATES:				
Long-term mortality	0.023	0.023	0.023	0.029

*Events during the first 30 days.
†Probabilities are multiplied by the increased risk of complications for Jehovah's Witnesses.
††Probability of having severe angina among those patients with angina.

Myocardial infarction, the principal nonfatal complication of CABG, occurs in approximately 9 percent of patients. Although there are no data describing the increased risk of perioperative myocardial infarction in Jehovah's Witnesses, we assumed this risk was increased in proportion to their overall increased risk of perioperative death.

Perioperative mortality is higher if the surgery is performed emergently after PTCA in the setting of acute myocardial infarction or if it is a repeat procedure. Patients who have suffered a perioperative myocardial infarction but survived the initial 30 days have an increased mortality rate attributable to coronary artery disease during the first year (1.4 percent per year versus 1.0 percent per year in other CABG survivors). Deaths that occur during the first year are modeled as occurring at mid-year.

Approximately 6 percent of CABG survivors will have occlusion in at least one of their coronary artery grafts and require revascularization within the first year. Most patients (83 percent) undergo angioplasty, whereas the remainder undergo repeat CABG.

We assumed that CABG would be 100 percent effective initially in relieving mild angina. However, by the end of the first year 26 percent of patients develop recurrent angina, 27 percent of whom have severe symptoms.

PTCA

We used the most recent data on patients with multivessel disease to obtain the perioperative risk of death (1.1 percent) and nonfatal myocardial infarction (2.7 percent). Perioperative mortality is higher among those patients who have previously suffered a myocardial infarction, but not after a repeat procedure. Among those patients who survive a myocardial infarction during the initial perioperative period, mortality from coronary artery disease within the first year is increased. Approximately 90 percent of angioplasties are clinically successful, although nearly half of these patients will restenose over the next year. Most patients (57 percent) undergo repeat angioplasty rather than CABG surgery. Nearly 4 percent of patients undergoing angioplasty require emergent CABG. The efficacy of PTCA in relieving angina after the first year is comparable to that of CABG.

Utilities

The fourth step in performing a decision analysis is to assign numeric values (utilities) to all of the outcomes in the tree using a single consistent scale. There are many possible measures of utility, from simple rank ordering schemes using arbitrary scales (i.e., 0 being the worst outcome to 1 being the best), to more sophisticated utilities that capture multiple attributes of patients' outcomes. A particularly useful utility measure is quality-adjusted life expectancy, a measure that takes into account not only the quantity of life but also the quality of life. This measure depreciates the average life expectancy for outcomes that consist of health states with less-than-ideal quality of life. In this way patient preferences for the various outcomes in a model can be taken into account. In this analysis we depreciated the life expectancy of patients suffering from mild angina by 5 percent and that of patients with severe angina was depreciated by 30 percent. As a simplification we assumed that the level of angina experienced at the end of the first year remains unchanged thereafter. We debited a fixed amount of time for patients who suffered adverse events or underwent invasive procedures to account for the short-term disutility of these events, deducting all time spent in the hospital (19 days for a CABG, 5 for a PTCA, 7 for a myocardial infarction, and 1 for a cardiac catheterization).

We used a declining exponential approximation to calculate average life expectancy from survival data. In an otherwise healthy man 55 years of age, the average life expectancy is approximately 22 years. The average yearly mortality rate of such an individual is the inverse of the life expectancy, or approximately 4.7 percent per year. Among men with mild angina enrolled in the CASS, 58 percent of those men randomized to medical treatment were alive at the end of 15 years, compared with 60 percent of those assigned to surgical treatment. The average mortality rate can be calculated by the equation $-1/t \times \ln$ (percent survival), in which percent survival is measured at time (t). Solving this equation for patients assigned to medical management yields an average mortality rate of $[-(\frac{1}{15}) \times \ln (0.58)]$, or 0.0462 deaths per year. Similarly, the average annual mortality rate for those patients randomized to CABG is 0.0436. Because we wish to examine the prognosis of a patient whose age is different from that of the cohort from which these data were derived, we must separate the excess mortality rate attributable to coronary artery disease from the overall mortality rates reported in the trial. Because deaths from all causes were included in these survival data, we must subtract mortality attributable to demographic-related causes (i.e., age-, sex-, and race-related mortality [μASR]) to calculate the excess mortality attributable to coronary artery disease (μCAD). From life tables, we calculate the average annual mortality rates for men 53 and 55 years of age (the average age of men within the medical and surgical treatment arms of the CASS, respectively) over the follow-up period of 15 years, yielding μASRs of 0.0173 and 0.0205, respectively. The excess mortality attributable to coronary artery disease (μCAD) is derived by subtracting μASR from the total observed mortality. For medical management, this yields 0.0289 (0.0462 – 0.0173), and for surgery, 0.0231 (0.0436 – 0.0205). Because no significant difference in long-term survival has been demonstrated following treatment with CABG or PTCA, we used the same excess mortality rate following PTCA as for patients who have had CABG surgery.

Evaluation

In evaluating a decision tree the analyst starts at the distal end of the tree and applies two simple rules. The first rule is that the average or expected value at any chance node is calculated as the utility (i.e., in units of quality-adjusted life years [QALYs]) of the events at that chance node weighted by the probability distribution over those events (i.e., branches). With the aid of a computer program, this process is repeated for each chance node in the decision tree, yielding an average or expected utility for each strategy—11.99 QALYs for 'Medical Therapy', 12.10 QALYs for 'Medical Therapy with Crossover', 13.35 QALYs for 'PTCA', and 13.11 QALYs for 'CABG'.

The second rule is that whenever a choice must be made (i.e., at a decision node), a rational decision maker would select the option with the greatest expected utility. Invoking this rule, we select the 'PTCA' strategy as the preferred strategy, which has a slightly greater expected utility (0.24 QALYs, or 3 months) than the CABG strategy. The small gain afforded by PTCA seems reasonable in light of the small increase in surgical risk associated with performing CABG without the use of blood products and in light of the similar efficacies of PTCA and CABG in decreasing mortality attributable to coronary disease.

Sensitivity Analyses

How convincing is this result? If the relative risk of surgical mortality in patients undergoing CABG without the benefit of transfusion were lower, would PTCA still be the optimal strategy? What if the operative mortality for performing CABG without transfusion were 1.5-fold that of the general population (compared with 2.2 in our base case)? Better yet, we can ask, "Above what increased risk of surgical death among like patients would PTCA be the optimal choice?" Attempting to answer such questions allows us to exploit one of the most powerful aspects of decision analysis, namely, sensitivity analysis.

We can perform sensitivity analyses on any or all of the probabilities and utilities in the model, and we can even vary multiple parameters simultaneously. We typically examine the "softest" data first in what are termed *one-way sensitivity analyses.* Figure 5, for example, demonstrates the impact of changes in the relative risk of surgical mortality among Jehovah's Witnesses undergoing CABG. The relative risk is shown on the horizontal axis in the range 1 to 5 (i.e., no increased risk to fivefold increased risk). A second horizontal axis displays the corresponding absolute surgical mortality rate. The vertical axis displays the expected utility of all four strategies in units of QALYs. In the strategy 'Medical Therapy', the expected utility remains unchanged as the risk of surgical mortality increases. This result is expected, because patients receiving medical therapy are not subject to surgical risk. However, the 'CABG' strategy is markedly affected by changes in this parameter, with expected utility declining as surgical mortality increases. The 'PTCA' strategy also is affected by changes in surgical mortality, although not as profoundly as is the surgical strategy. This result occurs due to the considerable cross-over from PTCA to CABG—many patients initially treated with PTCA will later have CABG surgery. A threshold exists at the point where both strategies have the same expected utility. In Figure 5, this threshold occurs at a surgical risk of 1.19, corresponding to a surgical mortality rate of 0.030 (0.025 × 1.19) for like patients undergoing CABG. Therefore, for all values greater than 1.19, PTCA is preferred, whereas CABG is favored if the relative risk of surgical mortality is less than 1.19. Recall that our assumption for the baseline risk of surgical mortality for like patients was 2.2 times that of the general population, a value that lies in the region in which PTCA is favored.

There is considerable uncertainty concerning the long-term survival benefit associated with CABG or PTCA. Although we assumed that there was no difference in long-term mortality following either PTCA or CABG, this assumption was based on results from a single study that followed patients for only 3 years. It is possible that mortality rates may diverge after this time. By performing a two-way sensitivity analysis, we can examine the effect of changes in these two parameters simultaneously. In Figure 6, the increased surgical risk for like patients is shown on the horizontal axis, whereas the long-term excess annual mortality rate attributable to coronary artery disease (μCAD) following PTCA is shown on the vertical axis. In a two-way analysis, the threshold curve divides

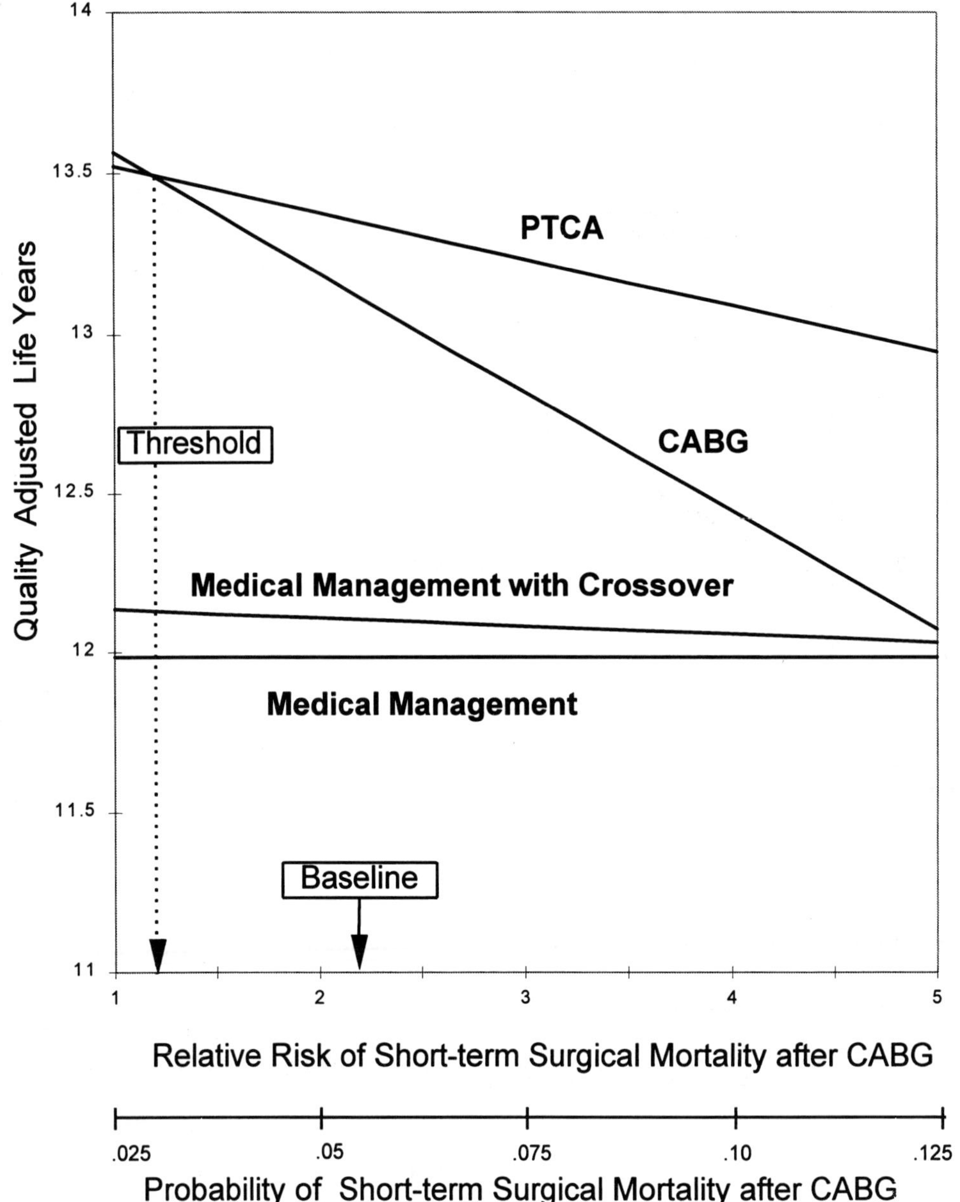

Figure 5
One-way sensitivity analysis examining the effect of changes in the relative risk of surgical mortality among like patients (shown on the upper horizontal axis). The lower horizontal axis displays the corresponding surgical mortality. The baseline relative risk of surgical mortality is 2.21. Below a threshold relative risk of 1.19 the preferred strategy is CABG, whereas above this threshold the preferred strategy is PTCA.

the space into regions in which each strategy is preferred. In the lower right corner, where the surgical risk associated with like patients is high and the long-term cardiovascular mortality following PTCA is low, PTCA is preferred. In the upper left corner, where the surgical risk is low and the long-term cardiovascular mortality following PTCA is high, CABG is preferred. The bold X marking the baseline values for these two parameters falls within the region in which PTCA is favored.

Using the same axes as in Figure 6, Figure 7 demonstrates a three-way sensitivity analysis examining the increased surgical risk for like patients on the horizontal axis and the long-term excess cardiovascular mortality following PTCA on the vertical axis, for a series of values for the probability of developing severe angina within 1 year after PTCA. Whereas in Figure 6 there was only a single curve, there is now a family of curves in Figure 7, each representing a different probability of developing severe angina following PTCA. As in the two-way analysis, the curves separate the graph into regions in which either PTCA or CABG is preferred. As the probability of developing severe angina after PTCA increases, the region in the lower right in which PTCA is preferred becomes smaller, whereas the region in which CABG is preferred becomes larger.

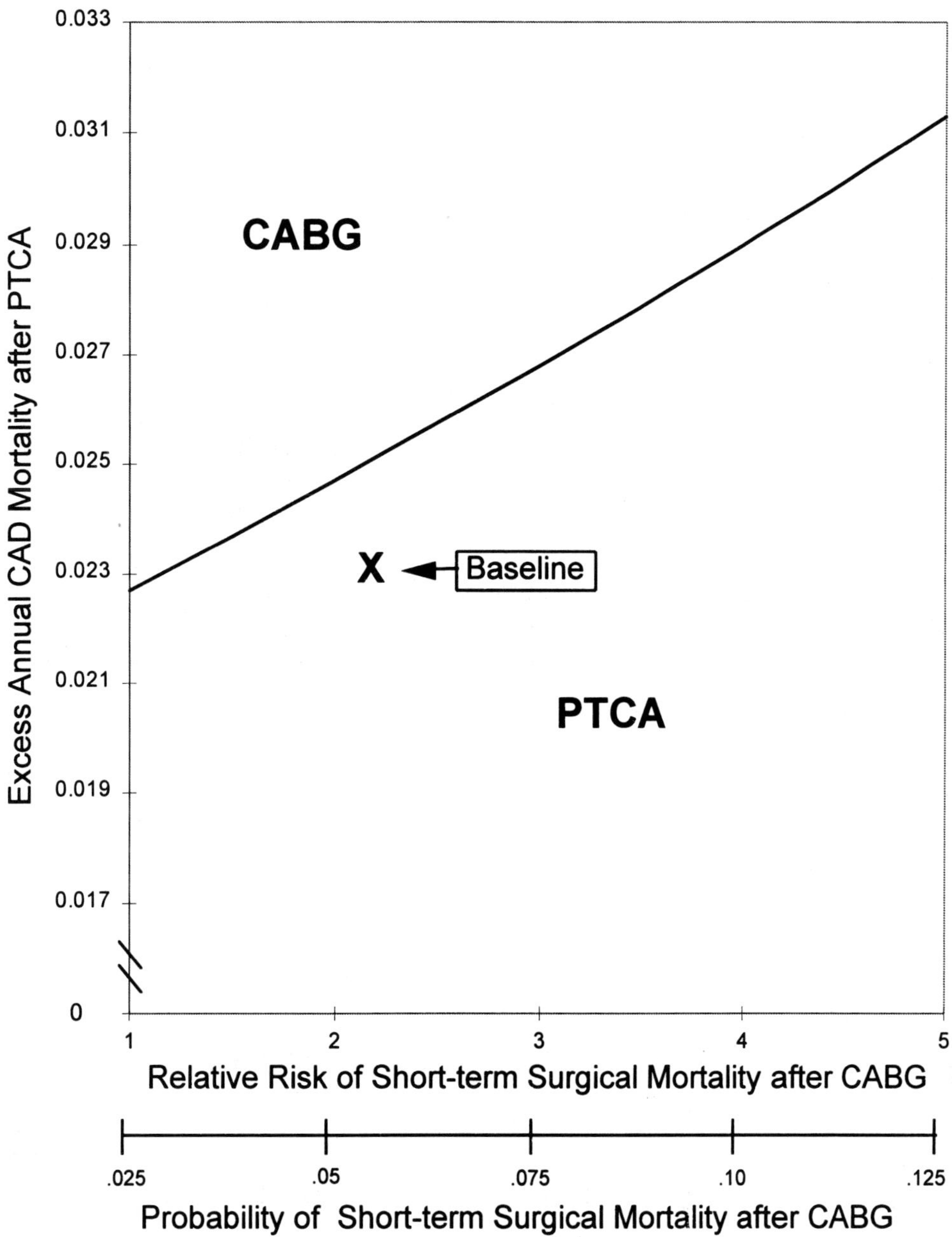

Figure 6
Two-way sensitivity analysis examining both the relative risk of surgical mortality among like patients (shown on the upper horizontal axis with the lower horizontal axis displaying the corresponding surgical mortality) and the long-term excess mortality rate attributable to coronary artery disease (μCAD) following PTCA (shown on the vertical axis). The baseline values for both probabilities are marked by the bold **X,** falling within the region in which PTCA is preferred.

Interpretation of the Results

Although PTCA is favored in this analysis, the amount of quality-adjusted life expectancy gained by PTCA compared with CABG is relatively small. However, the gain in quality-adjusted life expectancy afforded by PTCA compared with medical therapy with cross-over is substantial (1.25 QALYs), although much of this gain is due to the improved quality of life associated with the control of angina. As noted earlier, CABG and PTCA are considerably more effective in decreasing anginal symptoms than medical therapy. Repeating the analyses without adjustments for quality of life (either short- or long-term) results in an expected utility of 13.20 QALYs for the 'Medical Therapy' strategy, 13.24 for the 'Medical Therapy with Cross-over' strategy, 13.84 for the 'PTCA' strategy, and 13.58 for the 'CABG' strategy. Although the difference in quality-adjusted life expectancy between PTCA and medical therapy with cross-over diminishes when quality of life adjustments are not considered (1.25 versus 0.59 QALYs), PTCA remains the preferred strategy, and the gain in quality-adjusted life expectancy afforded by PTCA compared with CABG remains relatively unchanged (0.26 QALYs). Thus, the optimal choice for this patient is PTCA.

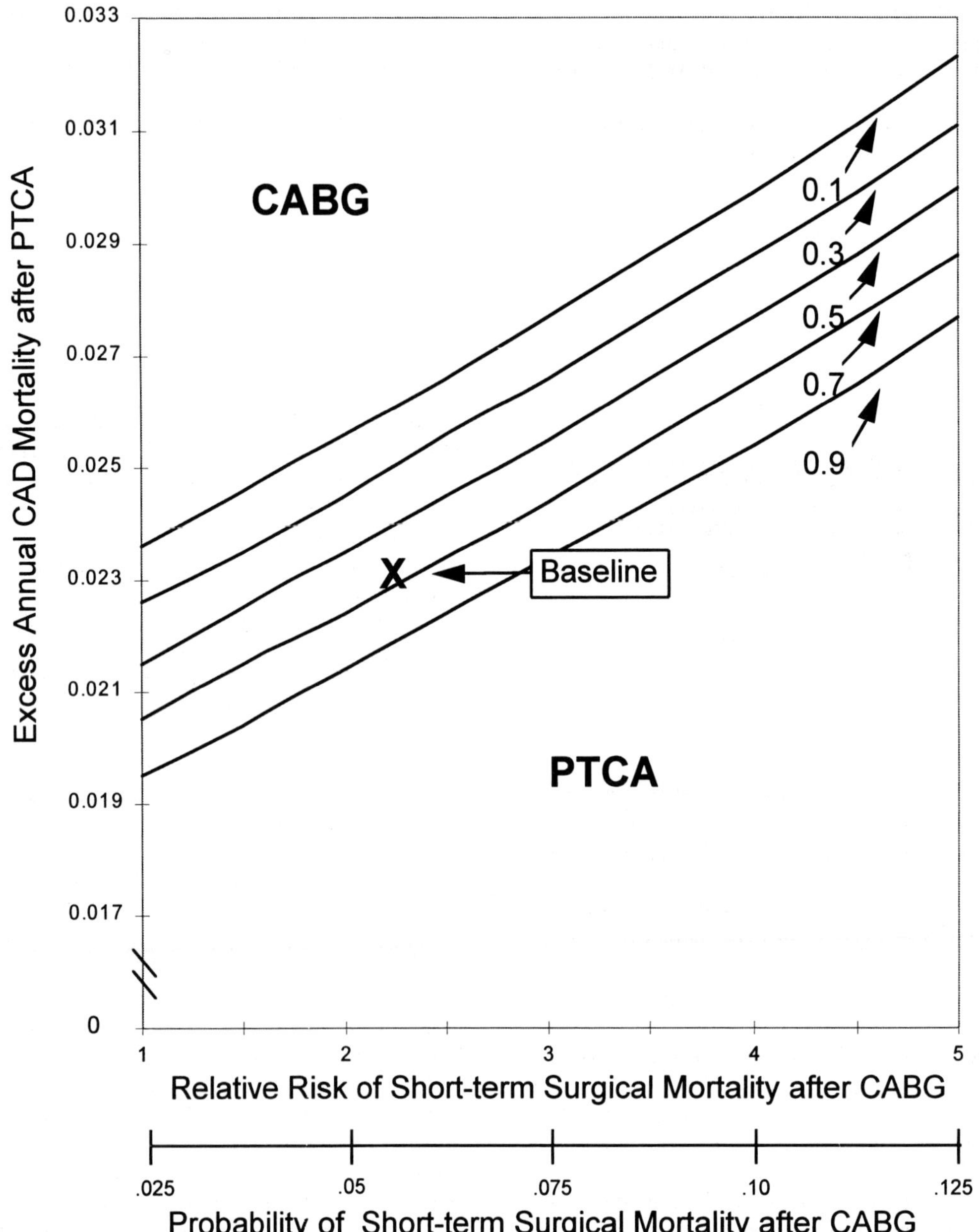

Figure 7
Three-way sensitivity analysis examining both the relative risk of surgical mortality among like patients (shown on the upper horizontal axis with the lower horizontal axis displaying the corresponding surgical mortality) and the long-term excess mortality rate attributable to coronary artery disease (μCAD) following PTCA (shown on the vertical axis). Each of the five curves represents the decision threshold given a different probability of developing severe angina following PTCA (0.1, 0.3, 0.5, 0.7, 0.9). Larger probabilities of developing severe angina after PTCA diminish the region in which PTCA is the preferred strategy. Even if the probability of developing angina after PTCA is twice the baseline value (0.27), PTCA is still the preferred strategy.

■ WHEN TO TURN TO DECISION ANALYSIS

Decision analysis provides a formal quantitative method for considering the tradeoffs between the benefits of therapy and its risks. It is most useful when the patient fails to conform to predetermined rules. Such circumstances include greater than usual uncertainty, poorly established efficacies of treatment, enhanced risks of treatment, unusually expensive treatment, confusion about the optimal timing of a necessary procedure, ambiguity about the optimal sequence of multiple procedures, situations in which patient preferences are critical, or instances in which rare, new, or unique problems are encountered. Analysis can be done, as described here, for individual patients or for complex and controversial choices in classes of patients.

Suggested Reading

Beck JR, Kassirer JP, Pauker SG. A convenient approximation of life expectancy (the "DEALE"): I. Validation of the method. Am J Med 1982; 73: 883–888.

Beck JR, Pauker SG, Gottlieb JE, et al. A convenient approximation of life expectancy (the "DEALE"): II. Use in medical decision making. Am J Med 1982; 73:889–897.

Kassirer JP, Moskowitz AJ, Lau J. Decision analysis: A progress report. Ann Intern Med 1987; 106:275–291.

Pauker SG, Kassirer JP. The threshold approach to clinical decision making. N Engl J Med 1980; 302:1109–1117.

Plante DA, Kassirer JP, Zarin DA, Pauker SG. Clinical decision consultation service. Am J Med 1986; 80:1169–1176.

THERAPEUTIC BENEFITS OF THE PHYSICIAN-PATIENT INTERACTION

Dennis H. Novack, M.D.

Before powerful therapies became available, physicians mainly relied upon the healing power of the physician-patient relationship. Hippocrates observed that "The patient, though conscious that his condition is perilous, may recover his health simply through his contentment with the goodness of the physician." More recently, Balint reaffirmed the importance of doctor-patient interaction, asserting that by far the most frequently used "drug" in medical practice is the physician.

Although physicians use their relationships with patients to enhance therapy, few pause to identify the therapeutic elements of their patient encounters, explaining their effectiveness by their use of the "art of medicine." Yet, if using the healing power of the physician-patient relationship is an art, physicians could become more skillful artists; by identifying the therapeutic elements of their clinical encounters, they might use them more consistently and effectively. Much research has elucidated the therapeutic aspects of clinical encounters. In this chapter, this research is summarized and therapeutic strategies relevant to practicing physicians are discussed.

■ UNDERSTANDING THE THERAPEUTIC EFFICACY OF THE PHYSICIAN-PATIENT RELATIONSHIP

Two concepts are central to understanding the therapeutic efficacy of the physician-patient relationship: the essential unity of mind and body, and the definitions of and relationships between disease and illness.

Although for historical and scientific reasons it has been useful to separate the concepts of mind and body, the many advances of psychosomatic research have demonstrated their essential unity. One way of understanding this unity is by reflecting that thought, feelings, and abstract reasoning are also neurobiologic processes. While you are reading this chapter, neurochemical processes are being stimulated in your brain. Changes in messenger RNA and neurotransmitter metabolism are occurring as new information is being processed. If your feelings are aroused, neuroendocrine mechanisms are affecting other bodily processes, all of which can, in turn, affect your behavior.

Another central concept is the notion of the differences and relationships between disease and illness. Disease and illness are, respectively, objective and subjective phenomena. Disease can be identified by a laboratory test or a microscopic examination. Illness is a sense of disease, a sense of distress, related to a patient's perceptions and feelings. There can be disease without illness (e.g., hypertension), and illness without disease (e.g., hypochondria). Many patients have a disease and a sense of illness determined not only by the severity of disease but also by a host of psychological and social factors. For the most part, patients come to physicians seeking relief from illness. In contrast to curing disease, which may be accomplished with a scalpel or a drug, to heal illness the physician must often attend to psychosocial issues.

A key therapeutic process by which physicians' communication can affect healing of illness is the reduction of patient anxiety and depression. Significant anxiety and depression are found in up to 35 percent of patients visiting clinicians for physical complaints. Anxiety and depression have a number of deleterious effects. At a biologic level, the neural and neuroendocrine factors associated with anxiety can increase blood glucose levels in the diabetic, increase gastric acid in the patient with an ulcer, or increase cardiac work and tip the compromised heart into congestive failure or induce a fatal arrhythmia. Grief and depression are associated with depressed immune function, which could predispose to infection or neoplasia. At a psychological level, the somatic symptoms of anxiety and depression (e.g., tremor, palpitations, loss of appetite, impotence) may prolong illness and confuse assessment of recovery. Depression is associated with self-defeating thoughts and negative self-images (e.g., "I'm no good, I'll never get better"), which may diminish patients' compliance. At a social level, these effects may undermine relationships with physicians, family, and friends and increase patients' isolation and sense of illness. Thus, to the extent that their interventions relieve anxiety and depression, physicians reduce the negative influences of these effects. With less anxiety and depression, patients begin to feel less ill and are more amenable to the physician's efforts to promote positive attitudes and compliance.

■ FACTORS CONDUCIVE TO EFFECTIVE THERAPY

Certain factors are conducive to effective therapy, including the clinical setting and physician attitudes, knowledge, and skills.

Clinical Setting

Before patients enter a physician's examining room, they have already had much contact with the physician's setting. The parking facilities, waiting room, administrative procedures, and waiting times affect patients' initial impressions of the physician. The attitudes and practices of receptionists, nurses, and ancillary personnel can either put patients at ease or heighten their anxieties (e.g., a patient did not want to discuss her personal life because she had seen the receptionist reading another patient's chart). A busy practice setting with multiple interruptions can restrain communication. A setting that is comfortable, unhurried, and puts the patient at ease is conducive to effective communication and therapy.

Physician Attitudes and Personal Qualities

Certain attitudes facilitate effective therapy. Accepting the importance of psychosocial factors in illness enhances the evaluation of the patient because more relevant psychological and social data are included. As another benefit of this approach, the physician's active concern for psychological and social issues may convince patients of his or her caring.

Peabody advised, "... the secret of the care of the patient is in caring for the patient." Patients want their physicians to be warm and caring. Patients' perceptions of these qualities are related to their evaluations of their physicians' general competence and their satisfaction and compliance with medical visits. Rogers identified an attitude of unconditional positive regard toward patients as the most important of the necessary and sufficient conditions for therapeutic personal change. This attitude implies a nonjudgmental approach, respect for a patient's individuality, and the ability to offer warmth and genuineness. Conversely, if a physician dislikes a patient or feels that a patient is untruthful, these attitudes are likely to be communicated and have a detrimental effect on therapy.

Several authors have commented on the necessity for physicians to be tolerant of ambiguity, uncertainty, and stress in the clinical setting. With all the uncertainty in clinical medicine, this tolerance prevents injudicious use of procedures and laboratory tests and physician anxiety that could undermine patient confidence.

Basic Knowledge and Skills

In addition to biotechnical knowledge and skills, the physician needs to master certain psychosocial knowledge and skills. Examples of key knowledge areas are the somatoform disorders, such as psychogenic pain disorder and conversion disorders, the phenomenology and treatment of depression and anxiety, and the importance of stress and life change in the development of illness. Examples of key skills are the ability to perform an effective patient-centered interview, the ability to interpret and use nonverbal behavior, the ability to recognize and use emotional reactions to patients as data, and skills in patient education and behavior modification techniques.

■ THERAPEUTIC STRATEGIES

The therapeutic process begins with the patient's decision to seek help. The physician's personal contributions to this process begin with the first interview: attentive listening in itself imparts great therapeutic value. A comprehensive diagnosis guides selection of appropriate therapeutic strategies. This diagnosis involves understanding the contributions of biologic, psychosocial, and personality factors to the onset and maintenance of the illness.

For people to change, they must change the way they think, feel, or behave in their social contexts. Major changes in any of these spheres change the whole person. Interventions, then, are presented in four categories: cognitive, affective, behavioral, and social. Although these are categorized for explanatory purposes, there is great overlap in these interventions and in their effects (e.g., giving an explanation often changes the way a person thinks, feels, and behaves). Many of these strategies and interventions have proved useful, as evidenced by their common presence in diverse healing disciplines.

Cognitive Therapeutic Strategies

A patient's thoughts, perceptions, and attitudes are involved in the illness process and can be addressed directly.

Negotiation of Priorities and Expectations

There is value in a negotiated approach to patient care. This approach recognizes the critical importance of eliciting and attending to the patient's perspective, which begins by asking: "How do you hope that I can help?" Physician and patient then negotiate some agreements about the nature of the patient's problems, the patient's requests and expectations, and the goals, methods, and conditions of treatment. Although it may seem obvious that the physician and patient must agree on the problems to be addressed, studies show that physician-patient concordance is often low. In a study of more than 400 patient visits to a medical clinic, physician and patient were fully concordant in the identification of the principal problem only about half the time. Patients often have hidden reasons for visiting doctors, and by focusing too early on chief complaints, physicians often do not elicit patients' real major concerns. Patients report better outcomes when there is physician-patient agreement about problems. In addition to improving physician-patient concordance on a variety of therapeutic issues, the negotiated approach helps both physician and patient to share the responsibility for therapy and prevents unrealistic patient expectations of the relationship.

Giving an Explanation

All healing disciplines give explanations to patients about causes of illness. Patients have intense needs for information and explanations about the causes of illness and are dissatisfied when these are not given. Confusion and uncertainty about diagnosis are noxious emotions for patients. Giving a symptom complex a name and an explanation thus has a salutary effect; patients feel comforted that the physician knows what is wrong and can thus begin appropriate therapy. For instance, one of my patients at first was relieved to learn that he had multiple sclerosis because for years he felt that his doctors were implying that his evanescent neurologic symptoms were not real.

When psychosocial factors are a major part of illness, an effective form of explanation is to tell the patient's story back to him or her in a way that makes the development of illness almost a logical progression. This demonstrates to the patient that the physician has listened and has understood and may help the patient to make sense out of confusing feelings and impressions. In sharing an understanding of the diagnosis, the physician can briefly teach the patient how mind and body work together in the promotion of illness and health. The physician uses his or her authority as an expert to legitimize psychosocial explanations when these are appropriate.

It is often difficult to discuss the etiologic role of psychosocial factors with patients whose long-standing symptoms are related to emotional conflicts and whose "secondary gains" have perpetuated symptoms in their lives. These individuals are often called "problem patients," and many are given psychiatric diagnoses. Although they reject a psychiatric explanation, many such patients are willing to accept that stress plays some role in how they feel, and most would agree that their anxiety and depression about their symptoms make them feel worse. These admissions may be the opening the physician can use to begin to help these patients change their psychosocial situations.

Bringing the Patient to a Crossroad

In some patients, denial contributes to their illness. The business executive who denies that he or she has had a heart attack or the alcoholic who denies his or her drinking habit are examples. Sometimes symptoms of illness serve a purpose in a patient's life. In certain dysfunctional families, illness may help maintain family equilibrium. Symptoms may serve to prevent the recognition of an intrapsychic conflict (which is fantasied to be more painful than the symptoms). Patients frequently hint at or relate interpersonal or intrapsychic conflicts to physicians without recognizing the relation to their symptoms. In these instances, it is often effective for physicians to confront their patients.

For example, when symptoms seem to represent an intrapsychic conflict, sometimes it is effective to discuss conflicts with patients, relate the conflicts to symptoms, and then let patients know that they are at a crossroad; they can begin to work on resolving the conflicts or choose to continue to have symptoms. These confrontations can initiate new relationships between the conflicts, the patients, and the illnesses. In essence, illness has been "reframed" from a biologic problem to a biopsychosocial one.

Suggestion

Suggestion is a powerful therapeutic tool that works in part by influencing patients' expectations of therapy. Suggestion via the placebo response can induce a wide variety of physiologic effects in patients, including release of endorphins. Physicians can use suggestion to enhance the effectiveness of any therapy. If a physician honestly communicates optimism in a therapy, it will often be more effective than if prescribed casually. Prescriptions given with hesitation or uncertainty may have diminished effectiveness. One hypnotic technique that may be useful is to make self-reinforcing positive suggestions. That is, patients may respond to positive suggestions such as, "As you recover from this heart attack and begin to be more active, you will feel less anxious and more optimistic." Suggestions such as this can set up a positive feedback loop: patients may respond to positive suggestions with hope and increased well-being. As their physical conditions improve, these positive emotions not only confirm their sense of recovery but also tend to improve confidence in the physician whose predictions have been accurate. Positive suggestions have limited value for patients with somatoform disorders. Although there may be initial benefits, the predictable recurrence of symptoms may then undermine patient confidence.

Patient Education

Patient education has proven benefits in increasing patient satisfaction and compliance and an overall positive effect on patients' coping. Information can reduce patient anxiety, enhance feelings of personal control, improve a patient's attitude toward a painful procedure, and help patients cope with pain. Presurgical educational interventions increase cooperation with treatment and speed of recovery and decrease postoperative pain and post-hospital complications. In general, physicians spend little time giving information to their patients, overestimate the time they have spent, and underestimate the amount of information the patient wants to receive. Explanations about illness or about tests and procedures should be given in clear language without jargon, using concrete familiar examples and frequently testing for understanding. Careful attention to patient education is important because patients forget or misunderstand so much of what physicians tell them.

Patient education includes correcting misconceptions and incorrect illness attributions. A common example is the belief that hypertension is hyper-tension, that is, feeling too nervous, and that antihypertensive medications can be discontinued when the patient is not feeling stressed. Clinical reality may be viewed quite differently by patient and physician; explanatory models of illness, which are often culturally derived, may give rise to misconceptions that can interfere with therapy. Physicians who elicit these explanatory models can then address points of misunderstanding or disagreement.

Giving a Prognosis

Prognoses should be realistic so that patients do not feel deceived if they become more ill than predicted, and they should be optimistic so as to engender hope. For example, in conveying the diagnosis of a malignancy, many physicians emphasize promising new therapies and describe other patients with the same disease who did well. As in learning a diagnosis, knowledge about prognosis can help patients cope with illness by reducing the dysphoria of uncertainty. Patients told what to expect can prepare and adapt. If the physician can correctly predict certain feelings or physical sensations, patients may avoid misinterpreting these sensations. For example, the patient who returns from the hospital after a heart attack may experience marked tiredness. If the physician explains that this is a natural and common occurrence, the patient will not misinterpret this tiredness as symptomatic of a failing heart.

Affective Therapeutic Strategies

Anger, depression, and anxiety are not only common reactions to illness but also can amplify illness. Physicians can diminish these negative emotions and arouse positive emotional states through a variety of interventions.

Empathy

Expression of empathy is one of the most potent therapeutic interventions. Empathy is sharing in another's emotions or feelings as if they are one's own. All people have a need to be understood, a need made more pressing by illness. Empathy involves accurately identifying a patient's feelings and then communicating this to the patient: "I understand how difficult it is for you to be going through this illness," or "It sounds like your mom's illness has been a real burden to you." Empathy also involves eliciting and responding to the meaning of illness for the patient (e.g., "I can understand your worries about this angina, especially since your brother died of a heart attack"). In addition to strengthening the bond between physician and patient, expression of empathy can aid the diagnostic process. After experiencing physicians' empathy, patients are often encouraged to reveal their most difficult problems. Communication of empathy is a skill that can be effectively learned.

Encouraging Emotional Expression

Many physicians, especially physicians in training, feel uncomfortable when patients cry or grow angry in their offices. However, there are good reasons for encouraging emotional expression, without feeling the need to "resolve" negative feelings. "Ventilation" of strong emotions provides immediate relief for some patients. Conversely, being unable to express emotion makes patients feel alone and creates barriers between patients and physicians. Many forms of psychotherapies and healing disciplines arouse the patient's emotions, recognizing these as the motive power for attitude change. Emotional "catharsis" is considered crucial in some psychotherapies and in many religious and magic healing rituals. In some instances, when a patient realizes that a physician is not threatened or appalled by his or her admissions, a "corrective emotional experience" may take place. The physician can encourage emotional expression by making empathic comments, by inquiring about feelings, or by commenting on nonverbal expressions of affect such as, "You looked sad when you mentioned your son."

Praise

Praise is supportive of patients, conveys respect, and helps give them confidence and hope. Physicians may praise patients' personality strengths, attitudes, or actions (e.g., "You are a bright and conscientious man, and I think you will do fine in dealing with this complicated regimen," or "I think your sensitivity to your wife's feelings is laudable and will help her a lot during these difficult times"). Praise as a reinforcer of desired behaviors is discussed further on. When there is a dearth of personality strengths, the physician may need to resort to paradox and redefine weakness as strength. For example, the physician can redefine a patient's masochism into ability to cope with suffering and thus can encourage and praise a patient's coping abilities.

Offering Hope

Hope is a central coping mechanism; it defends against despair, diminishes anxiety, is energizing, and can stimulate patients to undertake health-promoting activities. On the other hand, hopelessness, the most noxious of emotions both psychologically and physiologically, has been linked to disease onset and sudden death. Patients' hopelessness can engender pessimism in their caregivers, which impedes therapy. Mobilizing hope and instilling "expectant faith" that the physician will help the patient recover is a device used by all healing disciplines. Offering hope is appropriate for patients with diverse illnesses, although the manner in which it is offered varies. Most dying patients maintain some hope until the end, feeling nourished by it in difficult times, and appreciate it when hope is offered despite bad news. Physicians can maintain hope in their dying patients without deception by accepting their hopes and sharing with them the hope that they may have a remission or that they will live longer than expected. For patients with long-standing psychosomatic illness in whom symptoms serve an adaptive function, it is best not to raise hopes for recovery; instead one should assert that these patients deserve and have a good chance for some improvement. In these patients, it is helpful to emphasize coping as the goal rather than cure.

Touch

Placing a hand on his or her shoulder when talking to a hospitalized patient or holding a patient's hand during a moment of reassurance is an important therapeutic intervention. Lewis Thomas calls touching "the oldest and most effective act of doctors." From infancy on, touch is associated with comfort and the relief of anxiety. "Laying on hands" is common to most healing disciplines. It is significant that some patients begin to talk about emotional issues only while the physician is examining them. There is probably an optimal "dose" of touching, however. Too much touching or touching too early in the relationship may be associated with untoward consequences.

Facilitation of Self-Forgiveness

Some symptoms are related to feelings of guilt. Guilt has been linked to the symptoms of conversion disorders, pathologic grief, depression, and psychogenic pain disorders. The associated somatic symptoms are conceptualized as forms of self-punishment to expiate guilty feelings. Guilt may be related to the death of someone close toward whom the patient had harbored angry feelings. Much can be accomplished by exploring these feelings in the context of the past relationship and giving support to the patient about the appropriateness of past behavior and feelings. Often by exploring a patient's feelings of guilt and occasionally by merely listening to a patient's confessions, the physician can help patients forgive themselves. Listening to a patient's confession is a part of many psychotherapies, religious practices, and diverse healing ceremonies in primitive cultures in which sickness is often viewed as punishment for sins.

Reassurance
Most physicians have observed the beneficial effects of reassurance in allaying patient anxiety and diminishing the patient's sense of illness. However, reassurance is a complex phenomenon. It is most ineffective when given prematurely, casually, or without conviction. Reassurance is most effective when it accurately addresses the patient's concerns and personal meanings of illness. It usually cannot be given effectively until the patient senses that the physician has listened to and understood his or her problems and has performed the necessary evaluation. There are several categories of reassurance. The physician can reassure patients that their illnesses are not as severe or threatening as they had imagined. Physicians can help remove the sense of isolation that illness imposes by reassuring patients that they have successfully treated other patients with similar illnesses. Physicians can allay specific fears. It is also reassuring to patients to be told that the physician will continue to work with them whatever the course of the illness.

Behavioral Therapeutic Strategies
One of the major contributions of behavioral therapy research has been the demonstration that accomplishing behavioral changes through successful performance leads to lasting cognitive and affective changes. The emphasis of most behavioral therapies is on changing current determinants of behavior. The therapist focuses on changing environmental cues, thoughts and feelings, and consequences of behavior that make the behavior more likely. Physicians can use specific behavioral approaches in treating obesity, smoking, and noncompliance. Relaxation techniques can be useful in the management of anxiety. In addition, some behavioral therapy principles are applicable in general medical practice.

Emphasis on the Patient's Active Role
Many patients take a passive attitude toward their illnesses, often feeling that their illnesses are controlling them. This contributes to demoralization and depression. On the other hand, a sense of control or mastery has been linked to improved health status. Physicians accomplish much by emphasizing that patients have some control in overcoming illness and by encouraging an "active patient orientation." In this approach, patients are viewed as collaborators in their care; they are given information that will help them discuss diagnostic and management decisions with their physicians, and skill training and technical aids are made available to assist self-care activities (e.g., home blood pressure or glucose monitoring). This approach improves satisfaction, compliance, and functional abilities.

Assigning to the patient self-monitoring of behavior also encourages an active patient role. In asking patients to keep diaries in which they record events relevant to their problems, physicians and patients are provided not only with a useful way to monitor progress but also with valuable information on the determinants of behavior. Other strategies that encourage a patient's role include prescribing physical activity, giving assignments such as books to read or courses to take, and working with patients to delineate conflicts that they must actively resolve.

Praising Desired Behaviors
In behavior modification techniques, praise is recognized as a reinforcer of desired behaviors. When patients successfully perform suggested behaviors, praise encourages them to continue their efforts. Praise can be used in this way to shape a patient's behavior; even when patients have made only small improvements in their behavior, the physician praises these improvements and praises successive approximations of the desired behavior until it is achieved. When treating hypertension or promoting dietary compliance for management of diabetes or hypercholesterolemia, for example, physicians' praise of improving parameters reinforces a patient's progress.

Suggesting Alternative Behaviors
Patients may react to intolerable social situations with an exacerbation of symptoms. Sometimes illness may be in large part a reaction to or solution to an intolerable social situation. Because they are enmeshed in the situations, patients may be unable to perceive alternative strategies for coping. There are several types of responses to intolerable situations: changing the situation, changing one's reaction to the situation, or leaving it. It is often helpful to explore these options with patients and to suggest alternatives the patient is unable to see.

In suggesting alternative behaviors, physicians often engage in covert modeling. They suggest behaviors they feel would be appropriate if they were in a similar situation. Overt modeling in the form of a mini role play is often effective (e.g., "I'll be you for a minute and you be your angry son, and I'll demonstrate one technique that might just work").

Occasionally a patient hesitates to carry out a decision he or she has made that is a viable solution to an intolerable situation. The physician's agreement with and support of a difficult decision may enable the patient to begin to do what is adaptive. A key concept is that only by carrying out feared behaviors can patients compare their dire predictions with the actual events and correct their misapprehensions.

Attending to Compliance
Healing is promoted when patients follow an effective therapeutic plan and take their medications as prescribed. Unfortunately, noncompliance has been found to be as high as 20 to 60 percent, depending on the type of regimen. Physicians typically overestimate rates of compliance among their patients and are often inaccurate in identifying noncompliant individuals. At a most basic level, simply checking with patients about their compliance tends to increase it. When physicians ask about compliance, patients are more likely to express complaints or to admit having problems conforming to a regimen. Other strategies for improving patient compliance have proved effective, such as improving patients' levels of information concerning the specifics of their regimens; reinforcing essential points with review, discussion, and written instruction; emphasizing the importance of the therapeutic plan; simplifying and reducing the cost of the regimen; suggesting behavior prompts (e.g., notes on the refrigerator); and creating physician-patient contracts that include a writ-

ten outline of behavioral expectations and specified rewards or reinforcements.

Social Therapeutic Strategies

Use of Family and Social Supports

A noxious social environment and a lack of social and community ties have been associated with an overall increase in morbidity and mortality. Conversely, positive family and social supports ameliorate illness and improve compliance. An essential ingredient of many healing rituals is the active participation of family and friends, which begins the reintegration of the ill person into family and community. This reintegration helps to dispel the social isolation frequently imposed by illness. Many rituals also stress mutual service, which counteracts the patient's morbid self-preoccupation and strengthens self-esteem by demonstrating that he or she can do something for others.

Families should be evaluated to see if they are potential resources. Sometimes disengagement from a dysfunctional family is effective therapy. Often, though, families and friends are helpful. As well as providing support and encouragement for patients, they provide valuable perspectives that can help in designing therapy. Family members often have specific informational needs that must be met in order to participate effectively in therapy.

Use of Community Agencies and Other Health Care Providers

Involvement in community agencies, self-help groups such as Alcoholics Anonymous, and religious, cultural, and social groups can play a major role in a patient's recovery. It is helpful for physicians to have a first-hand knowledge of the make-up or workings of the important community agencies to which they can refer patients (particularly programs such as Alcoholics Anonymous, Al-Anon, Overeaters Anonymous, and cardiac rehabilitation programs). Involvement of other members of the health care team, including office staff and pharmacists, increases the patient's social interaction and helps the therapeutic process. Nurses often play essential roles in monitoring compliance, implementing and clarifying health education and attitude change strategies, enlisting family support, and helping with behavior modification strategies.

■ COMMENT

Although the therapeutic process can be analyzed and studied, medical therapy is also an art. Each physician uniquely synthesizes biopsychosocial knowledge, skills, and attitudes and combines this synthesis with his or her own intuition, natural empathy, and caring for patients. With an organized approach to the therapeutic aspects of the physician-patient relationship, the result is medical care that is both more scientific and more humanistic.

Suggested Reading

DiMatteo MR, DiNicola DD. Achieving patient compliance. New York: Pergamon Press, 1982.

Engel GL. The need for a new medical model: A challenge for biomedicine. Science 1977; 196:129–135.

Frank JD. Persuasion and healing. New York: Schocken Books, 1977:75.

Lipkin M Jr, Lazare A, and Putnam S. The medical interview. New York: Springer-Verlag, 1995.

Novack DH. Therapeutic aspects of the clinical encounter. J Gen Intern Med 1987; 2:346–355.

Portions of this chapter appeared originally in Novack DH. Therapeutic aspects of the clinical encounter. J Gen Intern Med 1987; 2:346–355.

RESPECTING PATIENTS' TREATMENT PREFERENCES

Dan W. Brock, Ph.D.
Steven A. Wartman, M.D., Ph.D.

In recent years, physicians and patients have tended to move toward a model of shared treatment decision making. Although this sounds reasonable on the surface, i.e., that patients and physicians collaborate in the process of making decisions regarding medical care, surprisingly little attention has been given to the complex and troubling issues that can arise within this model. In this chapter, we discuss the rationale for the model of shared physician-patient decision making, followed by what that model implies for physicians' responsibilities when an apparently competent patient's preference appears to be irrational. A discussion of this issue requires the development of a taxonomy of the different forms and sources of irrational decision making. These include the bias toward the present and near future; the belief that "it won't happen to me"; fear of pain or the medical experience; patient values or wants that do not make sense; framing effects; and conflicts between individual and social rationality. Our main aim is to develop this taxonomy and thereby to bring out some of the theoretical and practical obstacles in distinguishing irrational patient choices, which physicians might seek to change or override, from merely unusual choices that should be respected.

■ SHARED DECISION MAKING BETWEEN PHYSICIAN AND PATIENT

Historically, the most common professional ideal of the physician-patient relationship held that the physician directed care and made decisions about treatment, whereas the patient's principal role was to comply with "doctor's orders." Although this paternalistic ideal often did not ignore at least the patient's general preferences and attitudes toward treatment, it nevertheless gave the patient only a minimal role in treatment decision making. This model reflected, on the one hand, the inequality between the medical training, knowledge, and experience of the physician and the average patient, and, on the other, the anxiety, fear, dependency, and regression that can impair or seriously alter sick patients' usual decision-making abilities. When faced with what appeared to be irrational choices or preferences expressed by their patients, this paternalistic model encouraged physicians to overlook or override those choices as not being in the patients' true interests or not what patients would prefer in the absence of their decision-making impairment.

The paternalistic ideal of the physician-patient relation has been challenged by a number of forces from both within and outside of medicine during the last two or three decades and has generally been replaced by an ideal of shared decision making. In this model, health care treatment decisions are a collaborative process in which both physician and patient make active and essential contributions. The physician brings his or her medical training, knowledge, and expertise to the diagnosis and management of the patient's current condition, including available treatment alternatives. The patient brings knowledge of his or her own subjective aims and values through which the risks and benefits of various treatment options can be evaluated. The selection of the best treatment of this particular patient requires the contributions of both parties.

This division of labor oversimplifies, of course, the complexities of the actual roles and contributions of physicians and patients in real instances of treatment decision making, but it does serve to highlight the new, active role of the patient in that process. Some have concluded that in shared decision making, respecting patient autonomy or self-determination requires respecting the patient's treatment preferences no matter how they have been arrived at. However, we believe that such a conclusion is not warranted. It fails to recognize the trade-off between the different, conflicting values involved in the decision to respect or to seek to change or override patients' choices and relies on an inadequate account of the nature and value of self-determination.

Three examples serve to illustrate the kinds of difficulties that can arise when patients are offered the opportunity to participate in the decision-making process and make decisions that appear "irrational" to the physician.

Example No. 1: The Bias Toward the Present or Near Future. A 35-year-old healthy man with a strong family history of heart disease has been found to have hypertension and an elevated cholesterol level. In response to his physician's recommendation of medication to lower blood pressure and a low-cholesterol diet, he responds, "I don't care what happens to me when I'm 65, I know these drugs have side effects, and I want to eat what I like now." This patient seems irrational in caring only about his present situation and disregarding potential future morbidity.

Example No. 2: The Belief That "It Can't Happen to Me." Despite detailed counseling by her physician, an 18-year-old woman with numerous sexual partners continues to practice unsafe sex. When advised again of the risks, she responds by saying that she does not think she will develop any sort of problem. Her seemingly irrational decision appears based on her belief that "It can't happen to me."

Example No. 3: Fear of a Medical Experience. A 44-year-old patient has been admitted to the hospital with a partial bowel obstruction. Despite medical management, his condition steadily worsens. When surgery is repeatedly advised, he refuses because of a fear of "being put to sleep."

How do physicians respect these patients' preferences while trying to offer what they believe is the best medical care? This is especially difficult because, from the physician's point of view, these preferences appear to be "irrational"; that is, they are based on biases, beliefs, or fears that are not necessarily amenable to scientific or medical reasoning. When the physician properly judges the patient's treatment choice to be irrational, attempts to change that choice through persuasion are commonly appropriate. However, it can be difficult to distinguish choices that are truly irrational from those that are merely unusual.

When persuasion fails, the decision to respect or to seek to override a patient's treatment choice is ultimately a question of the patient's competence in making that choice. This is because Anglo-American law holds that a patient's informed and voluntary treatment choice can only be set aside for the patient's own good if that choice is found to be incompetent. Physicians lack both ethical and legal authority unilaterally to override patients' treatment choices. Thus, when we speak of the physician "seeking to override" the patient's choice, we mean initiating the process of determining incompetence and selecting a surrogate, which commonly involves recourse to the courts.

■ WELL-BEING AND SELF-DETERMINATION

Determining what degree of decision-making impairment on a particular occasion warrants a finding of incompetence involves balancing two principal interests or values of patients. The first value is the patients' own well-being, which can require protecting patients from the harmful consequences of their seriously impaired treatment choices. The second value is respecting patients' self-determination in making significant decisions about their lives for themselves when they are able. When patients appear to be making treatment choices contrary to their own well-being and further discussion is unsuccessful in changing their opinion, these two values will be in conflict.

We use the notion of patient well-being to emphasize that medical care, which relieves pain and suffering, prevents disability, restores function, and prevents loss of life, is ultimately of value to the extent that it serves those aims and purposes that give content and meaning to the patient's overall plan of life. For many conditions, there are alternative treatments that are medically acceptable. These treatment options often have different mixes of risks and benefits, such that the "medical facts" alone will not settle which treatment is best for a particular patient. Moreover, treatment choices usually have an impact on other important values of patients, requiring trade-offs between medical and nonmedical values. The ultimate responsibility of physicians is to use their knowledge, skills, and expertise to serve patients' overall well-being and to facilitate patients' pursuit of their own plans of life. Thus, determining what treatment will best serve a particular patient's well-being has both medical components and patient preference or value components. However, as noted in the previous examples, patients can often be mistaken about what best serves their well-being.

Patient self-determination involves patients' making important decisions that shape and affect their lives and having these decisions be respected by others. Self-determination is given great importance throughout American life, and in the field of medicine it has long been the central principle underlying the doctrine of informed consent. Since what serves patients' well-being often depends on their own wishes and values, informed patients are reasonably presumed to be the best judges of how specific treatment choices would contribute to their well-being. In this way, self-determination has instrumental value because respecting patients' self-determination usually serves their well-being. In addition, most persons want to make important decisions about their lives for themselves, even if they believe that others may be able to decide for them better than they themselves can. In this respect, self-determination is valued for its own sake and has noninstrumental value. It is in exercising our capacities to reflect on what kinds of persons we want to be and become and in adopting or affirming our own particular aims and values that we create a unique self and take responsibility for our lives.

It is important to realize that in the physician's decision to respect, attempt to change through persuasion, or seek to override a patient's choice, both the instrumental and noninstrumental values of self-determination vary with different decisions. The more that a patient's decision making is impaired and results in a choice that fails to promote his or her well-being, the less instrumental value self-determination has in promoting well-being; indeed, when the choice is positively harmful, this instrumental value may be thought of as negative. The more far-reaching the effects of the choice for the patient's life and what the patient most cares about, the greater the noninstrumental value of making the choice for oneself. Moreover, the more a choice is based on specific values that have stood some significant test of time in guiding the patient's life, the more weight self-determination deserves in making that choice. The noninstrumental value of self-determination also varies among persons according to how much weight they give to making their own choices, even when those choices are nonoptimal or harmful.

It is common to think that respecting patient self-determination always requires respecting the patient's choice and giving the same weight to all such patient choices. These views, however, are mistaken. First, just because the decision of whether to respect, seek to override, or attempt to change through persuasion a patient's choice sometimes involves weighing patient self-determination against protecting patient well-being, in some cases giving due weight to patient self-determination can be compatible with setting aside patient choices. Second, an assessment is needed in each instance of decision making of how much weight self-determination should properly be given.

Physicians thus have the option of respecting the patient's choice or attempting to override or to change that choice through persuasion, which must reflect both the values of patient well-being and self-determination. It may be the case that these values come into conflict, as in the examples cited previously. In these cases, the patients' preferences appear to be irrational, making the physicians' choice to respect, seek to override, or attempt to persuade a difficult one.

■ THE STANDARD OF RATIONAL DECISION MAKING

Any discussion of irrational decision making must rely on an account of rational decision making. We believe that it is helpful to make that account explicit, even if only in brief outline. Specifically, what is the norm of rational decision making that underlies the ideal of shared decision making between patient and physician? Shared decision making essentially entitles the patient (or surrogate if the patient is incompetent) to weigh the benefits and risks of alternative treatments, including the alternative of no treatment, according to the patient's values and to select the alternative that best promotes those values. In the language of decision theory, the patient's own values determine his or her utility function, and the rational choice is the choice that maximizes expected utility for the patient. Since treatment decisions always involve some degree of uncertainty about both the benefits and harms of alternative treatments, these benefits and harms should be discounted by their probabilities, to the extent that they are known, in calculating the expected utility of different treatment alternatives. When the probabilities are not known, the patient's particular attitude toward risk, including the extent to which the patient is risk-averse or risk-taking, will determine the weight given to uncertain benefits or harms.

Shared decision making requires the physician, in part, to ensure that the patient is well informed. Thus, another aspect of ideal rational decision making is that the patient has and employs correct factual information about relevant alternatives, to the extent that it is available. This sketch of rational decision making ultimately relies on the patient's own aims and values as the ends that guide decision making. Irrational choice then can be conceived instrumentally as a choice that less completely satisfies those aims and values than would some available alternative.

Sometimes physicians employ a second notion of irrational choice that deems a patient's choice irrational if it fails to promote a set of basic aims and values that belong to the physician and/or standard medical practice guidelines. When physicians criticize patient's choice as irrational in this sense, they express their disagreement with the basic aims and values by which the patient defines his or her own good as opposed to the judgment that the patient's choice will fail to promote best the patient's own aims and values. Since this second notion ignores the patient's own aims and values and thereby fails to respect the patient's self-determination adequately, we rely here on the first account of rational and irrational choice.

■ FORMS OF IRRATIONAL DECISION MAKING

We turn now to developing a taxonomy of common forms of irrational decision making by patients or their surrogates (but also sometimes physicians) when making treatment choices. In many actual treatment decisions, more than one form of irrationality affects a single choice, but we separate them here for analytic clarity.

Bias Toward the Present and Near Future

The ideal of rational decision making gives equal weight to a benefit or harm whenever it occurs in a person's life, with differences determined only by the size and probability of the benefit or harm. In the case of money, it is rational to apply a discount rate because a dollar received today can then earn interest and so is worth more than a dollar received 10 years from now. Some effects of health care are similar in that it is rational to prefer a restoration of function now rather than in the far future and to prefer that a loss of function occur as far in the future as possible, so as to minimize the period of disability. Similarly, it is rational to prefer that the loss of one's life be postponed as far as possible into the future. For other effects of medical care, however, especially pain and suffering, rational choice would seem to require indifference to when the experience occurs. In particular, it is a paradigm of prudential *ir*rationality to refuse to undergo a bad experience now, when doing so would avoid a much worse experience in the future. The reason such choices are commonly considered irrational is that the choice amounts to preferring that there be more rather than less bad experience or suffering in one's life.

Yet, as clinicians know, medical practice is replete with such irrational choices by patients. Patients who continue heavy smoking or alcohol use or who fail to comply with relatively simple steps to control moderate hypertension are often most plausibly understood as having given inadequate weight in their present decision making to the harms likely to occur to them in the relatively distant future. We call this a bias to the present and near future, because such persons commonly give disproportionate weight to securing benefits or avoiding harms in their present and near future as opposed to their more distant future. The physician's task in such cases is to help the patient fully appreciate the more distant harm or benefit, commensurate with its size or seriousness, so that it can play an appropriate role in the patient's decision making. A variety of methods for doing so may be useful, depending on the particular patient, such as letting the patient see similar effects that have actually occurred in other patients or the use of especially graphic accounts of the nature of the future benefits or harms.

The Belief That "It Won't Happen To Me"

Patients may have differing views as to the nature of the risk or harm to them of not following medical advice. This is especially true for events that have a low probability of occurring. However, what constitutes low probability may vary considerably from patient to patient. Further, since some patients may be greater risk-takers than others, it is often difficult to determine whether a given patient is just more of a risk-taker than most patients or whether this patient has simply failed to give adequate weight to a low-probability, distant event. This situation becomes more complicated by the difficulty of distinguishing among patients who tend to deny the possibility of an untoward event's happening to them, or who have "magical" or illusory beliefs regarding their vulnerability to harm, or who simply have a different way of viewing the medical problem. Adolescents, for example, are commonly subject to feelings of invulnerability to certain harms that are disproportionate to the real risk of those harms.

The physician often needs to gain some understanding of the patient's general attitude toward risk and the extent to which the patient is risk-averse or a risk-taker, perhaps as evidenced by the patient's past behavior. The physician should attempt to distinguish among the possibilities noted previously. Sometimes the physician can help the patient more vividly appreciate the risk and relate it to the patient's life. However, in the case of the patient who denies the risk or who uses magical thinking, a more detailed medical and scientific explanation is not likely to be helpful. In these cases, formal counseling or psychiatric evaluation may prove more fruitful.

Fear of Pain or of a Medical Experience

Many patients delay or will not even consider a particular form of treatment for fear of the perceived nature of the experience. In many cases they may even acknowledge that the treatment or procedure is clearly in their best interest. Sometimes their decision is coupled with some form of rationalization—"there's no need to do it yet," or "I'm too busy now with other things." In other cases, when a dreaded experience draws near, a patient may become almost paralyzed by fear. Sometimes the fear may be focused not on pain or suffering but on other dreaded experiences, such as "being cut open" or of "being put to sleep" in surgery. In still other cases, fear of a disease such as cancer or acquired immunodeficiency syndrome can disable a person from making informed decisions about its treatment.

Determining when this form of irrational decision making is present is considerably complicated by the fact that there is no single, correct weight to give to pain or a particular medical experience as measured against the beneficial outcomes for which the experience may be necessary. Patients differ, for example, in the degree to which they are prepared to tolerate painful treatments or conditions for the sake of other ends. Adding to this complexity is the inaccessibility to physicians of other persons' pain. Although we can identify and often quantify the physiologic causes of pain in a particular person as well as the person's associated pain behavior, the person's conscious experience of the pain itself is not accessible to anyone else. As a result, it is often difficult to determine whether a patient gives more or less weight or importance to pain than do most others or is experiencing more or less pain than do others in similar circumstances.

More to the point here, however, is the difficulty of distinguishing persons who give undue weight to certain aspects of treatment because of irrational fear. Physicians may have had prior experience of patients who later were grateful that they were pressured or even forced to undergo such painful or dreaded treatments. The physician's responsibility in these cases is a difficult one—to respect the varying importance different persons give to avoiding pain while helping patients to overcome irrational fears that prevent them from pursuing promising treatment plans. This often involves helping patients to distinguish whether they are experiencing fear of a medical experience which they want to overcome or have instead made a choice with which they are comfortable.

What the Patient Wants Does Not Make Sense

When a competent patient prefers a certain form of treatment or wishes to decline a recommended course of treatment because of an obvious and understandable, although unusual, belief, physicians (and the courts) commonly yield to that belief. Examples include the Jehovah's Witness patient who refuses a blood transfusion, or the Asian patient who requests acupuncture or coining. If the patient's refusal of beneficial treatment is clearly incompetent, such as when a grossly psychotic patient reports that voices told him to refuse therapy, there are institutional and legal mechanisms to transfer medical decision making to another person or to the state. The real difficulties arise when what a competent patient wants does not make sense but is not attributable to something clearly recognizable as a religious belief or cultural preference. It can be extremely difficult in these situations for the physician to determine the basis of a patient's preference. However unusual, the more the preference reflects a deeply held enduring value that is important in the patient's life plan, the stronger the case for respecting it.

In other cases it is what the patient does *not* care about that does not make sense. For example, a patient may state that he or she understands but simply does not care that death or serious disability will result from a refusal of treatment. It may be difficult to determine whether this is an authentic, although unusual, choice or instead a result of a distortion of the patient's values caused by a treatable condition such as depression.

Framing Effects—Avoiding a Harm or Gaining a Benefit

It is well known that the way choices are formulated and presented, or framed, can have major effects on these choices. A simple example is the alternative presentation of a surgical treatment as "substantially extending the lives of 70 percent of patients who select it" or as "killing on the operating table up to 30 percent of the patients who select it." Both characterizations may be true, but which is used, or emphasized, may have a substantial impact on the rate of selection of the surgery.

There are a variety of different and more subtle kinds of framing effects. Some parents in the face of publicity about the diphtheria/pertussis/tetanus (DPT) vaccine refused the vaccine for their children because of the vaccine-related risk of neurologic damage or death. They continued to do so even after being told of the substantially greater risk of the negative outcome from the disease itself without vaccination. If the only relevant outcome of the vaccinate/do not vaccinate choice is the risk of harm to the child, parents' choices not to vaccinate their children are irrational and physicians' responsibilities might then arguably be to seek to persuade those parents to accept vaccination. But attempting to understand such choices of parents is often complex and may not always allow the choices to be so easily and quickly dismissed as irrational. For example, in the case of DPT, one factor affecting some parents' thinking may be a feeling on their part of a greater responsibility for the harm to their child if that harm results from a decision they made as opposed to random bad luck in acquiring the naturally occurring disease.

Work in the psychology of choice shows that losses tend to loom larger than gains in most people's decision making. Of course, whether a particular outcome is viewed as a gain or a loss depends on the status quo or reference point against which the outcome is compared. Many choices in medicine can be framed in either way, as obtaining a gain or avoiding a loss. For example, lowering moderate hypertension can be presented to a patient as adding months to his or her expected life span or as avoiding a shortening of life span from untreated hypertension. Neither framing of the patient's choice is obviously correct or mistaken; instead, each simply relies on different characterizations of the patient's present situation. Tversky and Kahneman have compared the framing effects in decision making to perspective changes in visual judgments; for example, which of two mountains appears higher depends on the position from which one views them. In this case, there is an objective standard by which one mountain could be determined to be higher. But there appears to be no objectively correct framing of many medical decisions, such as that of the patient with moderate hypertension. There are simply the two different but both correct ways of framing the choice, and the one that is used will influence whether some patients choose treatment. Sometimes the best that physicians can do is to present choice framed in alternative ways in the hope that doing so will at least minimize framing effects.

Individual Versus Social Rationality: Irrational Use of Resources

Sometimes the circumstances that make individual choices rational also make the outcome of those choices irrational when viewed from a different perspective. One factor fueling the intense pressure to control rapidly rising health care costs is the perception that health care resources are often utilized in circumstances in which their expected benefits do not justify their true costs. In the extreme case of a patient's having full insurance coverage with no copayments or deductibles, the patient has no economic incentive to weigh the true costs of medical care under consideration against its expected benefits. Since using that care has no out-of-pocket costs for the patient, it is rational for the patient to choose to use all care with any expected medical benefit, no matter how small the benefit, and without regard for its costs. If the patient's physician employs the commonly accepted professional norm that his or her obligation to patients is to do whatever may be of benefit to them, without regard to cost, then it is rational for the physician also to ignore the cost of care in recommendations and decisions about the patient's treatment. The result will be overutilization of health care as against other goods and services whose benefits are weighed against their true costs. From the perspective of the group paying insurance premiums (for example, employers or the government), the result is an irrational overallocation of resources to health care.

Very different issues are raised by this form of irrational social choice in the use of resources than by the forms of irrational patient choice discussed previously. It would be misdirected for physicians to seek to convince insured patients that their choices to employ non-cost-worthy care are irrational. On the contrary, the point is that an insured patient's choice to use non-cost-worthy care *is* rational, although it leads to an irrational social overallocation of resources to health care. Since the irrationality is not at the level of the insured patient's choice of treatment, the response to the irrationality should not be principally at that level. This form of social irrationality in the allocation of resources to health care does not justify a physician's failing to respect the insured patient's individual choice to employ non-cost-worthy care on grounds that the choice is irrational. Instead, this irrationality must be addressed where it exists—in the social and economic health care financing system.

Individual Versus Social Rationality: Public Health Versus Individual Benefit

Often physicians are concerned about the public health benefits of medical interventions, whereas their patients are not. For example, national campaigns to reduce serum cholesterol levels will clearly benefit the nation's health as a whole. However, the beneficial effects for a given individual patient may be minimal or nonexistent. Consequently, some individuals may rationally decide that for them the benefits of the intervention do not outweigh its burdens. This distinction between community-wide and individual benefits has been called the "prevention paradox," whereby a treatment that brings large benefits to the community may offer little to each participating individual. There is no true paradox, however. The society-wide benefit constitutes no reason to view as irrational and to not respect an individual's choice to decline the intervention.

For some infectious diseases, preventing the infection through vaccination (or shortening the period of transmissibility through treatment) of one individual lessens the risk of disease for others. A patient's or parent's refusal of immunization might be rational if the patient or parent is not concerned with the risks for others or believes that because enough of the population is immunized, the threat of the disease is minimal and therefore the risks of immunization outweigh the benefits. In this case, society may adopt mandatory immunization programs or the physician may seek to change the patient's refusal, not because the refusal is irrational but rather because of the social benefit for others.

■ WHAT SHOULD PHYSICIANS DO?

The model of shared decision making between patient and physician, while respecting the patient's self-determination, does not always require accepting the patient's preferences, particularly when these preferences are irrational. It is appropriate in some cases for the physician to attempt to persuade the patient to change his or her irrational choice or seek to have the patient's choice overridden as incompetent. However, distinguishing when a patient's preferences are truly irrational from when they simply express different attitudes, values, and beliefs can be difficult both in theory and in practice. Physicians need to be sensitive to the complexity of these judgments in helping patients to make sound treatment choices. More research is needed on the frequency and different forms of irrational treatment choices as well as on how physicians and patients can work together to overcome these decision-making irrationalities.

Suggested Reading

Forrow L, Wartman SA, Brock DW. Science, ethics and the making of clinical decisions. JAMA 1988; 259:3161–3167.

Gillick MR. Talking with patients about risk. J Gen Intern Med 1988; 3:166–170.

Rose G. Strategy of prevention: Lessons from cardiovascular disease. Br J Med 1981; 282:1847–1851.

Tversky A, Kahneman D. The framing of decisions and the psychology of choice. Science 1981; 211:453–459.

HEALTH PROMOTION AND DISEASE PREVENTION

F. Marc LaForce, M.D.

Practicing physicians have become somewhat disappointed with the results of many of the so-called medical miracles. The preponderance of these advances are applied relatively late in the course of a patient's illness and interventions at that stage, irrespective of their drama and intensity, often yield limited dividends. Some physicians have remarked that we seem to be doing more and more to sicker and sicker patients with gains that are at best marginal. A visit to any intensive care unit will attest to at least a partial truth to this assertion. This chapter is aimed at the opposite end of this spectrum and describes primary and secondary preventive maneuvers that are appropriate for the office setting. Primary preventive maneuvers such as immunizations are aimed at asymptomatic persons with no evidence of the condition to be prevented; secondary prevention refers to screening for the early diagnosis of disease in asymptomatic persons. The basic premise is that it is far better, though not necessarily cheaper, to prevent rather than to treat disease.

Most physicians first learn about disease prevention on

Table 1 Leading Causes of Death by Age

AGE, YR	CONDITION	RISK FACTOR OR INTERVENTION
11–24	Motor vehicle crashes	Seatbelt noncompliance, alcohol use
	Homicide	Gun ownership
	Suicide	Depression
	Injuries (nonvehicular)	Alcohol use
25–64	Heart disease	Hypertension, elevated cholesterol, smoking
	Lung cancer	Smoking
	Breast cancer	Clinical examination and mammography
	Colorectal cancer	Stool for occult blood and/or sigmoidoscopy
	Human immunodeficiency virus infection	Avoid high-risk behavior, use condoms
65+	Heart disease	Hypertension, elevated cholesterol, smoking
	Cerebrovascular disease	Hypertension, elevated cholesterol
	Obstructive lung disease	Smoking
	Pneumonia/influenza	Smoking, influenza, and pneumococcal vaccines
	Lung cancer	Smoking
	Colorectal cancer	Stool for occult blood and/or sigmoidoscopy

pediatric services during which the virtues of immunization are emphasized. Until recently, training in internal medicine has largely emphasized the diagnosis and treatment of adult diseases with little emphasis on prevention. This attitude is changing with the realization that treatment can be very expensive and may not necessarily result in increased life expectancy or a better quality of life.

The leading causes of death in the United States by age are presented in Table 1 along with modifiable risk factors or interventions that can prevent or delay development of these diseases. Screening and attempts at risk factor modification are appropriate to the office setting but require a change in how medicine is generally practiced.

Primary prevention requires that patients assume greater responsibility for their own health. The older paradigm in which the physician assumed total responsibility for the patient's illness must give way to a model whereby patients become responsible for acts likely to put them at risk.

Much of the material in this chapter is taken from the 1995 second edition of the U.S. Preventive Services Task Force report entitled "Guide to Clinical Preventive Services." The Task Force was originally asked to produce a series of recommendations on health promotion and disease prevention appropriate for the office setting. The Task Force methodology emphasized a rigorous review of the medical literature with the evaluation of specific maneuvers according to strict rules of evidence. More weight was given to results from properly controlled studies, and recommendations from expert groups in the absence of solid experimental data were downgraded. Population benefits were an important consideration when recommending specific maneuvers. For example, a highly effective intervention for a relatively rare disease was deemed less important, because of the small population benefit, than a maneuver of moderate or even minor effectiveness that could be applied to a common disease associated with significant morbidity and mortality.

Lastly, a special effort was made to present recommendations in age-specific packages that recognized the leading causes of morbidity and mortality in specific age groups. A teenager or a young adult is far more likely to die from an automobile collision than from any other condition. In 1986 50 percent of the approximately 40,000 deaths among persons 15 to 24 years of age were due to injuries, and more than 75 percent of these injuries occurred in motor vehicle collisions. All forms of cancer accounted for only 6 percent of deaths in this age group. To lower mortality rates in teenagers and young adults it is far more productive for the practitioner to promote the use of safety belts and to discourage driving under the influence of drugs or alcohol than to do a comprehensive physical examination.

■ SCREENING

Most physicians vigorously adhere to the dogma that finding disease early is always good. However, when carefully studied, screening has been shown to have its downside. All procedures, no matter how minor, have side effects, ranging from a direct effect such as sigmoid perforation during screening sigmoidoscopy to the psychologic effects of labeling a person ill when identified by a positive screening test. This negative effect of labeling was studied in a group of asymptomatic steelworkers who were screened for hypertension. Some of the workers were told they were ill with hypertension, and, during the next 2 years, these workers had a significant increase in work absenteeism that was not related to any complications of hypertension but represented a new response to minor illnesses.

Screening for a particular disease or condition, particularly in an asymptomatic person, carries with it a special burden. The person is feeling well, and searching for a particular condition implies an improved outcome as a result of identification of that condition. In an important series of papers, Frame and Carlson (1975) defined conditions that had to be met for a screening maneuver to be recommended: (1) the disease must have a significant effect on quality and quantity of life; (2) acceptable methods of treatment must be available; (3) the disease must have an asymptomatic period during which detection and treatment significantly reduces morbidity and mortality; (4) treatment in the asymptomatic phase must yield a therapeutic result that is superior; (5) tests must be available at reasonable cost to detect the condition during the asymptomatic period; and (6) the incidence of the condition must be high enough to justify the cost of screening. These conditions are still valid and serve as a convenient standard against which all proposed screening maneuvers should be measured.

In addition, the benefits of screening tests usually have been overestimated. The phenomenon of lead-time bias is an important confounder because early diagnosis, invariably associated with improved survival, will always lengthen the

Table 2 Recommended Screening Questions in the History (All Ages)

Dietary intake
Physical activity
Tobacco/alcohol/drug use
Sexual practices
Safety use

time period between diagnosis and death without necessarily having improved survival. Thus, early identification of disease may not necessarily improve life expectancy but rather lengthen the time a person is diagnosed as "ill." The effectiveness of screening also can be overestimated due to length-time bias because of the tendency of screening procedures to detect a disproportionately high number of cases of slowly progressive disease. Cases of aggressive disease are less likely to be picked up by a screening maneuver in the population because these diseases are present for a relatively short time. Because these cases will be underrepresented, results from screening tests may be associated with a better-than-average survival.

One final problem is the issue of efficacy and effectiveness. A specific screening maneuver may be shown to be effective under study conditions but may lack effectiveness when applied on a population basis. Poor vaccination levels against influenza in the elderly is one such example. Other factors may limit the beneficial impact of screening services. Screening maneuvers are usually furnished free in a study setting, but in the real world they must be billed for and patients may not be willing to assume this financial burden for a future benefit. Physicians may not be willing to spend the time necessary for counseling because it is considered unreimbursable. Despite all of these limitations, the following screening maneuvers appropriate for the office setting are recommended.

History

Table 2 lists topics that should be reviewed in individuals of all ages. The importance of each of these areas cannot be overemphasized. General information about alcohol and drug consumption can be easily linked to an inquiry, as well as counseling about the need for safety belts to be used at all times. Information in any of these areas may help direct the physical examination. Dietary questions that are appropriate for age and sex help direct counseling and educational strategies. The threat of acquired immunodeficiency syndrome (AIDS) and the increasing prevalence of sexually transmitted diseases make it mandatory for a physician to inquire into a patient's sexual practices. Approximately 25 percent of Americans still smoke, and 390,000 Americans die annually from smoking-related causes. Hence, all smokers need to be identified and counseled to quit. Nutrition questions should be age- and gender-specific but should focus on the need to maintain ideal weight and to limit fat intake in general. Cancer of the colon, breast, and prostate have been epidemiologically linked with increased fat consumption. These questions quite logically lead to an inquiry about a patient's level of physical activity.

The quality of the information gathered depends on the physician's sensitivity to the patient's concerns. Patients are often uncomfortable about answering questions dealing with sexual practices or drug use for fear of being thought of as deviant, with all that the connotation implies. Physicians must be aware of these concerns and in a nonjudgmental manner elicit the patient's trust. Several health risk appraisal aids have been developed for the office setting and can serve as instruments to analyze a patient's lifestyle in order to provide guidance. Some practitioners have favored use of these instruments because they help personalize risk and facilitate the prioritization of behavioral changes necessary to reduce risk.

Table 3 Recommended Screening Maneuvers in the Physical Examination for Individuals at Average Risk

AGE, YR		
11–24	**25–64**	**65+**
Height	Height	Height
Weight	Weight	Weight
Blood pressure	Blood pressure	Blood pressure
	Breast examination*	Breast examination*
		Visual acuity
		Hearing

*In association with mammography.

Physical Examination

One of the rituals of office practice is the annual physical examination. Practitioners expect to do them, and patients have been conditioned to expect them. Nonetheless, a critical review of published studies suggests that the routine physical examination has little screening value in the asymptomatic patient. The Canadian Task Force on the Periodic Examination and the U.S. Preventive Services Task Force have concluded that the annual complete physical examination is unnecessary. Some maneuvers, however, were found to have screening value (Table 3).

Properly conducted randomized or cohort studies have shown that only three screening maneuvers should be routinely performed: blood pressure determination, clinical breast examination for women over 40 years of age, and a Papanicolaou test for all sexually active women.

Hypertension is a common disease, and data show that treating patients with moderate and severe hypertension decreases morbidity and mortality from congestive heart failure, stroke, renal disease, and retinopathy. The Kaiser randomized trial of multiphasic screening determined that there was less mortality from the intervention group subjects who were screened every 2 years when compared with control subjects who were screened every 5 years. Therefore, blood pressure should be measured at least every 2 years.

A randomized controlled trial in the United States has shown that breast examination by a physician along with mammography decreases breast cancer mortality in women 50 to 59 years of age. For women above 60 years of age there are case control data supporting annual physical examination and mammography. Cervical cancer is another ideal disease for screening. The disease can be recognized early and is a relatively slow-growing cancer. Cohort studies have shown that routine screening by Papanicolaou tests reduces the incidence and mortality from invasive cervical cancer. The main screening argument has centered on how frequently the test should be done. The U.S. Preventive Services Task Force has suggested that sexually active women should have a Papanicolaou test every 3 years after two initial negative tests obtained 1 year apart.

Because visual and hearing problems frequently occur with aging, annual examinations are recommended for persons above age 60 years. Data show that annual dental visits are associated with less dental disease, therefore referral for dental care is encouraged. To identify valvular abnormalities requiring antibiotic prophylaxis, cardiac auscultation should be done early in life and again in the patient's mid-sixties. Neither the bimanual pelvic examination nor the rectal examination is recommended. Critical review of published data show that these tests have low sensitivity, specificity, and positive predictive value.

Controversy has surrounded screening recommendations dealing with the physical examination in asymptomatic patients. Some physicians have argued that the bonding that is essential to the physician-patient relationship is facilitated by the touching that is intrinsic to the physical examination. Nonetheless, an unbiased review of the physical examination suggests that much of it is ritualistic and, in the absence of specific complaints, largely unnecessary. On the positive side is the observation that there are relatively few appropriate screening maneuvers that need to be done when a patient presents to the office with symptoms.

These recommendations should not be overinterpreted. They refer to asymptomatic patients and reflect a paucity of properly conducted clinical trials. In addition, certain maneuvers may be done for other reasons, such as a rectal examination to obtain stool for occult blood testing, and in such circumstances a digital search for rectal masses and prostatic nodules would not be discouraged. The point that must be emphasized is that the time-limited patient-physician encounter requires that the most efficacious activities should be done. For example, it makes little sense to do a complete physical examination in an asymptomatic patient 25 years of age without discussing the hazards of AIDS and alcohol use and the importance of using safety belts, counsel that is far more likely to decrease morbidity and increase life expectancy.

Laboratory Procedures

Few laboratory or diagnostic studies are recommended for persons of average risk (Table 4). Periodic measurement of cholesterol level is recommended for middle-aged men because of the large body of epidemiologic, clinical, and animal studies that have linked serum cholesterol levels to coronary atherosclerosis. The ability of cholesterol-lowering drugs to reduce the incidence of coronary atherosclerosis in middle-aged men has been demonstrated in randomized controlled studies. Controversy exists as to whether these results can be generalized to the general population such as premenopausal women or the elderly. The Framingham data show that coronary artery disease risk rises in a graded fashion with a sharp increase after cholesterol levels of 220 to 240 mg/dl. Asymptomatic adults with cholesterol levels above 240 mg/dl should receive dietary counseling and follow-up evaluation. The need for Papanicolaou testing and mammography in women over 50 years of age has been discussed previously. Screening for colorectal cancer is recommended for all persons aged 50 years and older with annual fecal occult blood testing or sigmoidoscopy. These interventions are consistent with the well-documented observation that early-stage diagnosis of colorectal cancer is associated with longer survival than that of persons with advanced disease.

Persons who fall into high-risk groups are another matter, and recommendations for screening are far more aggressive (Table 5). For example, breast cancer in a first-order relative significantly increases the risk of breast cancer in the propositus, and for that reason annual breast examinations and mammography have been recommended for women beginning at 35 years of age. Patients who are sexually active with multiple partners should be screened for sexually transmitted diseases. Laboratory tests and procedures for high-risk groups are beyond the scope of this chapter and readers are referred to the U.S. Task Force report for more details.

There are specific screening tests that are not recommended because of poor sensitivity, specificity, or, if the condition is identified, the absence of good therapy. Although lung cancer is the leading cause of cancer deaths in the United States, screening chest radiographs and sputum cytologic examinations have been studied prospectively in smokers and

Table 4 Recommended Screening Laboratory or Diagnostic Studies for Adults of Average Risk

AGE, YR		
11–24	25–64	65+
Chlamydia screen	Blood cholesterol	Papanicolaou smear
Papanicolaou smear	Papanicolaou smear	Fecal occult blood test and/or sigmoidoscopy
Rubella serology	Mammogram* Fecal occult blood test and/or sigmoidoscopy	Mammogram*

*In association with clinical breast examination.

Table 5 Recommended Screening Laboratory or Diagnostic Studies for Adults Deemed to Be at High Risk

AGE, YR		
11–24	25–64	65+
Fasting glucose level	Fasting glucose level	Fasting glucose level
VDRL test	VDRL test	Tuberculin test
Urinalysis (bacteria)	Chlamydia test	ECG
Culture for gonorrhea	Urinalysis (bacteria)	Colonoscopy
HIV test	Culture for gonorrhea	Papanicolaou smear
Hearing test	HIV test	Fecal occult blood/ sigmoidoscopy
Tuberculin test	Tuberculin test	
ECG	Hearing test	
	ECG	
	Fecal occult blood/ sigmoidoscopy	

ECG, electrocardiogram; HIV, human immunodeficiency virus; VDRL, Venereal Disease Research Laboratories.

found not to be helpful. Pancreatic cancer is the fifth most common cancer in the United States, but there are no appropriate screening tests for this type of cancer. Potential screening tests such as computerized tomography and endoscopic retrograde cholangiopancreatography are expensive, and there is little evidence that early detection lowers morbidity or mortality from the disease. Neither the physical examination nor the Papanicolaou test is accurate enough to be used routinely as a screening test for ovarian carcinoma. Similarly, there are no data to suggest that screening electrocardiograms reduce morbidity or mortality.

■ COUNSELING

As discussed previously, patient education and physician-based efforts at curbing cigarette smoking, lack of exercise, poor nutrition, and alcohol and other drug abuse are more likely to favorably impact life expectancy than more traditional clinically based interventions. However, as any experienced physician will attest, identifying a risk factor is not synonymous with controlling it. Many physicians do not feel comfortable in their counseling roles. Internists have been trained to diagnose and treat illnesses but have had little formal training in counseling. Studies have compared physician-reported compliance with counseling with medical record reviews and data from consumer surveys. For the most part, physicians either overestimate the amount of counseling they do or do it in such a way that patients have little realization that they are being counseled. More research in office-based counseling is urgently needed.

The U.S. Preventive Services Task Force has proposed 12 counseling guidelines for physicians.

1. Frame the teaching to match the patient's perception of the problem. Physicians should not assume that patients understand the relationship between smoking, poor nutrition, alcohol, and lack of exercise to poor health. Simple terms should be used to explain how these factors affect health singly and together. Patient beliefs that are not conducive to healthy behavior should be identified and assessed. Obstacles should be identified and patients helped to overcome them.
2. Fully inform patients of the purposes and expected effects of interventions and when to expect the effects. Patients must know what to expect.
3. Suggest small changes rather than large ones.
4. Be specific. Agree on a time-limited goal to be achieved and note it in the medical record. Assist patients in writing action plans, and stress willingness to continue to be involved.
5. Try to add new behaviors rather than eliminate established behaviors.
6. Link new behaviors to old ones. Recommending that patients exercise before eating lunch is one such example.
7. Use the power of the profession. Patients view physicians as health experts and regard their advice as important.
8. Get explicit commitments from the patient. This is a key step—if patients do not agree that their behaviors are significantly related to health outcomes, attempts at patient education may be irrelevant.
9. Use a combination of strategies that will help integrate the message. Educational efforts that integrate individual counseling, group classes, written materials, and community resources are far more effective than those employing a single technique. However, studies have shown that the practitioner's individual attention and feedback are more important than other communication channels.
10. Involve office staff. Use the team approach to patient education so that patients hear the same message.
11. Monitor progress through follow-up contact. Schedule a follow-up appointment or telephone call within the next few weeks to evaluate progress. Reinforce success, and, if unsuccessful, work with the patient to identify and overcome obstacles.
12. Refer the patient when it is not feasible to provide appropriate counseling.

■ IMMUNIZATIONS AND CHEMOPROPHYLAXIS

Recommended immunizations for adults are presented in Table 6. Influenza continues to be an important public health problem in the United States. At least 10,000 excess deaths have been documented in 19 different epidemics between 1957 and 1986. Influenza vaccine contains antigens that are chosen each year on the basis of predictions of which influenza viruses will circulate. During seasons in which the match has been good, vaccine efficacy levels of about 70 percent have been documented. Because the elderly make up 80 to 90 percent of all deaths from influenza, they are a particularly important target. The vaccine should be given annually to all persons above age 65 years and to those under 65 years who are considered at high risk, predominantly persons with chronic cardiopulmonary disease. To limit spread of the disease, all health care providers with contact with either the elderly or younger high-risk persons should also receive influenza vaccine annually.

More than 70 percent of reported cases of tetanus in the United States occur in the elderly. Serosurveys in the elderly have shown that approximately 50 percent have tetanus antitoxin levels that are not protective. There is universal need for tetanus immunization in adults. Pneumococcal vaccine should be given to all persons above age 65 years and to all others with medical conditions that put them at special risk

Table 6 Immunization by Age Group (Individuals at Average Risk)

AGE, YR	ANTIGENS
19–39	Tetanus-diphtheria booster Measles Hepatitis B
40–64	Tetanus-diphtheria booster
65+	Tetanus-diphtheria booster Influenza vaccine Pneumococcal vaccine

from pneumococcal infection. Case-control studies and studies comparing the distribution of pneumococcal serotypes in the blood of vaccinated and unvaccinated persons have shown an efficacy of about 60 percent.

The introduction of measles vaccine more than 20 years ago has been associated with a dramatic decrease in U.S. cases. In 1989 the Advisory Committee on Immunization Practices adopted a two-dose measles vaccine strategy for all adults born after 1956 who do not have either laboratory evidence of measles immunity or a history of physician-diagnosed measles.

Suggested Reading

Canadian Task Force on the Periodic Health Examination. The periodic health examination. Can Med Assn J 1979; 121:1193–1254.

Frame P, Carlson SJ. A critical review of periodic health screening using specific screening criteria. Parts 1–4. J Fam Prac 1975; 2:29–36, 123–129, 189–194, 283–289.

Morbidity and Mortality Weekly Report: Premature mortality in the United States. MMWR 35(2S):1S–11S.

Oboler SK, LaForce FM. The periodic physical examination in asymptomatic adults. Ann Intern Med 1989; 110:214–226.

U.S. Preventive Services Task Force. Guide to clinical preventive services. 2nd ed. Baltimore: Williams & Wilkins, 1995.

BEHAVIOR MODIFICATION

Thomas J. Coates, Ph.D.
Steven R. Cummings, M.D.

Changing patient behavior is essential to the practice of medicine. The major causes of death and disability in the United States today are chronic diseases (e.g., heart disease, cancers, diabetes) and accidents. Individual behaviors are related strongly to the incidence and course of these causes of death. Tobacco (inhaled, snuffed, or chewed) increases the risk of heart disease, cancers, stroke, accidents (e.g., fires), and influenza. Alcohol is related to heart disease, stroke, some cancers, motor vehicle accidents, cirrhosis, and suicide. Diets high in saturated fats and cholesterol are related to heart disease, cancers, stroke, and arteriosclerosis. High-risk sexual behavior is related to sexually transmitted diseases and pregnancy and increasingly to mortality in diseases such as the acquired immunodeficiency syndrome (AIDS). It is clear that many diseases might be prevented and that the course of disease, once begun, might be altered if individuals were motivated to adopt healthier lifestyles.

In 1974, the Secretary of Health and Human Services of the United States, Joseph Califano, Jr., summarized the challenge as follows:

> We are killing ourselves by our own careless habits. We are killing ourselves by carelessly polluting the environment. We are killing ourselves by permitting harmful social conditions to persist—conditions like poverty, hunger, and ignorance—which destroy health, especially for infants and children. You, the individual, can do more for your own health and well-being than any doctor, any hospital, any drug, any exotic medical device.

Many patients do not feel confident that they can engage in healthful behaviors, and many physicians do not feel confident in their ability to motivate patients to develop and maintain health-promoting behaviors. The task is difficult, the results are not immediate, and formal and systematic training in this aspect of medicine has been lacking. Our objective is to present a guide to the theory and the specific techniques for helping patients to change.

■ BEHAVIORAL MEDICINE

Behavioral medicine was defined at a National Academy of Sciences meeting as "the *interdisciplinary* field concerned with the development and *integration* of behavioral and biomedical science knowledge and techniques relevant to health and illness and the application of this knowledge and these techniques to prevention, diagnosis, treatment, and rehabilitation." The traditional biomedical sciences and the practice of medicine have been devoted to discovering which biomedical variables affect which other biomedical variables. Thus, identifying the pathogen that causes disease and the chemical or surgical procedure to eradicate disease has yielded considerable growth in treatment of disease in this century. The social and behavioral sciences have been devoted to discovering which social and psychological variables influence behavior and how to modify these variables in order to modify behavior, cognition, or affect of individuals. Education and advertising rely on these sciences to a considerable degree.

Behavioral medicine concerns itself with the interface of the behavioral and biomedical sciences and practices. The objectives are (1) to identify which behaviors are related directly to health and illness; (2) to develop and evaluate methods for modifying these behaviors; and (3) to determine the impact of modifications in these behaviors on the health and illness of various groups of individuals.

Health promotion, disease prevention, and effective use of alternative methods for treating disease require that individuals change their behavior and that medical organizations be reorganized to promote those changes. Effective use of the scientific principles and the strategies derived from them is critical to the success and longevity of these programs.

■ PRINCIPLES OF BEHAVIORAL CHANGE

The National Academy of Sciences was called upon recently to summarize what is known about how to change behavior to guide work in AIDS prevention. Their study yielded a generic set of principles of behavioral change that apply to virtually any situation in which the desired end is changing behavior to prevent disease. These principles, summarized in Table 1 and explained in the following paragraphs, can provide a guide for the physician in changing patient behavior.

Principle 1: Providing information is the logical starting point in any behavior change effort. Individuals must understand the risks that they incur by engaging in certain behaviors and the benefits they will realize by adopting others. However, the physician should understand that information, although necessary (and sufficient to produce behavior change in some patients), is rarely sufficient by itself to produce significant behavior change in most patients. Significant attention must be paid to how information is presented to patients. Information must be delivered in a manner that is comprehensible and relevant to the patient for whom it is intended. A major impediment to ensuring that information is given appropriately and received by the patient occurs when the physician fails to check whether or not the patient has understood and can act on the information given. This requires more than asking the patient whether or not he or she understands what is to be done. It requires that the physician take the time to ask the patient to summarize the major points that have been discussed and the plans for behavior change developed in the medical encounter.

Principle 2: Individuals are more likely to change if they believe that their behavior will lead to a disease with serious consequences. Most people have optimistic outlooks on life and are likely to deny the possibility of future disease in the absence of personal experience with that disease (e.g., in themselves or in their immediate family). In addition, patients interpret statements about their risk for disease in relation to the value they place on avoiding the health problems in question and on the incentives for engaging in alternative actions. Nonetheless, individuals may be more likely to change if they understand that the risks associated with their lifestyles are serious and likely to lead to important adverse consequences. This can be accomplished in two ways: (1) by relating an individual's family history to his or her current behaviors and risk for disease; and (2) by relating an individual's current disease symptoms to his or her behaviors (e.g., upper respiratory tract infections in a smoker).

Principle 3: Messages to patients that evoke fear about their behavior can be useful in motivating behavioral change. Behavioral change in the context of medical care has the one purpose of helping the patient to avoid the morbid and mortal consequences of his or her lifestyle. A certain level of threat and fear is necessarily involved. However, fear by itself, especially if overwhelming, can hinder rather than help the patient to change. Individuals can deny their risk, point to others who have practiced similar health-threatening behaviors and survived, or avoid medical care altogether. The National Academy of Sciences has proposed three prescriptions for using threatening messages to motivate behavioral change.

Table 1 Summary of Behavior Change Strategies

Information
- Communication is comprehensible to patient
- Information is relevant to patient
- Patient summarizes information to ensure understanding

Risk Perception and Fear
- Perception of risk is accurate
- Physician relates current symptoms to unhealthful behaviors
- A balance in the level of threat is maintained
- Patient is given specific information on steps to take to protect health

Self-Efficacy: Perceived Ability to Perform Desired Behaviors
- Self-monitoring makes patients aware of behaviors
- Incremental changes
- Substitute new behaviors rather than eliminate old ones
- Provide choices to patient

Skills Training
- Provide opportunities to plan and rehearse new behaviors

Create Environments That Encourage Change
- Help patients to identify environments associated with healthful and unhealthful behaviors
- Plan environments that encourage healthful behaviors

Expect and Plan for Slips
- Advise patients that slips are expected
- Use specific descriptions at slips to plan for future behavioral change

1. The messages to the patient should strike a balance in the level of threat that is employed. The level should be sufficiently high to motivate individuals to take action but not so high as to paralyze individuals with fear or cause them to deny their susceptibility. The fear level should be low enough so that it can be effectively managed by the adoption of the desired behavior. For example, telling smokers with upper respiratory tract infections that they may develop emphysema if they continue to smoke may evoke fear. Telling the same smokers that the risk will be lessened if they quit smoking provides an escape within reach.
2. The communication must provide specific information on steps that can be taken to protect the individual from threat to his or her health. Patients must believe that the changes being proposed will do some good. Thus, a reasonable, desirable alternative behavior that protects against the undesired health problem should be offered.
3. Attention should be paid to the short-term adverse consequences of the undesirable behavior and the short-term positive consequences of engaging in the desirable behavior. For example, smokers may know that their tobacco use is related to lung or heart disease but they may deny their risk. Drawing their

attention to the respiratory consequences of smoking when they are ill with respiratory tract infections or when they are short of breath may help them to realize the impact that smoking has and will have on their health.

4. Altruism should not be overlooked. Individuals will often do for others what they will not do for themselves. Patients will take steps to avoid adverse consequences to their spouses, children, or parents. Concern for significant others can be a powerful motivator and should not be overlooked. For example, many smokers are motivated to quit because of adverse effects on their children.

Principle 4: If an individual perceives that he or she is capable of performing desired behaviors (self-efficacy), then he or she is likely to engage in those activities. Individuals need to believe that they have a reasonable chance of achieving the changes recommended. People are not likely to engage in activities they feel they will not be able to perform successfully. Expectations of one's abilities can be changed and have been used to increase contraceptive use, help patients stop smoking, or increase sexual activity following myocardial infarctions. A patient's sense of competency and hence his or her willingness to try new behaviors can be increased in the following ways.

Helping patients to become aware of the degree to which they practice unhealthful or healthful behaviors often can motivate behavior change by itself. Self-monitoring is the most effective way to help patients become aware of the degree to which they practice healthful or unhealthful behaviors and the circumstances that are related to the practice of both. Monitoring food intake, exercise, and number of cigarettes smoked per day can help patients to gain control over those behaviors. Monitoring helps patients to set realistic goals for change, to determine the circumstances under which problem behaviors occur, and to measure accurately the degree to which change has occurred. Monitoring is best accomplished when done systematically, that is, when the patient records behaviors on a form using a standardized procedure.

Patients should choose between incremental changes and global lifestyle changes. Modifying rather than eliminating behaviors may be more effective for some patients. Incremental changes provide patients with a way to build new experiences in small steps without too much risk and allow the practitioner to reinforce patient success in accomplishing these early tasks. Incremental changes also allow patients to avoid frustrating failure experiences; they are spared the difficulties involved in aspiring to global changes and then feeling a sense of failure when they are unable to accomplish the impossible. Many patients devalue the importance of small changes such as losing 5 lb in as many weeks, making small changes in dietary intake, or taking small steps in initiating an exercise program. They need to be encouraged that such steps are realistic and important in that they will be more likely to reach long-term goals if the initial steps are successful.

It is often easier to encourage patients to substitute a behavior rather than to eliminate the unhealthful behavior altogether. Individuals engage in unhealthful behaviors because they are reinforcing (i.e., they are satisfying or pleasurable) or because they are popular. To cease engaging in such behaviors is difficult because it means giving up pleasure or behaving contrary to popular norms. Thus, if instead of giving up a behavior altogether individuals can substitute a behavior that is more healthful and at the same time likely to be satisfying or popular, they are more likely to adopt and maintain the practice of that behavior. For example, using condoms may be more acceptable to patients as protection against sexually transmitted diseases than celibacy. Intravenous drug users may be more likely to modify their injection behavior than to give up drug use altogether.

Individuals are more likely to adopt a behavioral change if they are offered choices among alternative behaviors. Patients and physicians together need to negotiate and set goals for behavioral change. Setting goals requires that the physician and patient determine exactly what is to be accomplished and that benchmarks for determining success be established. Vague or unmeasurable goals can lead to the appearance of an agreement without the patient's commitment to take specific actions to change.

Formal contracting can help both patient and physician agree on specific goals and methods for reaching them. Contracting is a process whereby the patient agrees to achieve a specific goal or behavior by a predetermined time in exchange for a reward. An example of contracting is breaking a large goal (e.g., losing 30 lb) into a series of smaller contracts (e.g., losing 5 lb by the next visit) and specifying the reward (e.g., a night out at the movies). All such contracts should be recorded in the medical chart so that follow-up is ensured at the next visit.

Principle 5: Change is more likely if individuals are taught the skills for engaging in the desired behaviors. Behavioral change requires that patients plan and rehearse in advance exactly how they will behave in a specific situation. Rehearsing an activity ahead of time builds confidence and self-efficacy by allowing the person to have the experience of the new behavior before it is actually performed. In one program designed to teach patients how to manage postoperative pain, those who learned what to expect after an operation and rehearsed how to use medication and other techniques required less analgesic medication than unrehearsed patients. Physicians can plan and rehearse difficult situations with patients, such as how to refuse the offer of an alcoholic beverage or caloric food, how to manage the offer of a cigarette, how to fit medication into a busy schedule, or how to manage an asthmatic attack or the symptoms of diabetes mellitus.

Principle 6: The physician should help the patient to create environments that encourage change. Environments influence all of us to behave in healthful and unhealthful ways. For example, it is difficult to refuse alcohol in a bar and to ignore high-calorie foods when they are stocked in the refrigerator. The objective is to avoid settings associated with unhealthful behaviors or to set up the environment so that healthful behaviors are encouraged. For example, when patients are trying to quit smoking, it is often helpful for them to avoid places such as bars or smoking areas where cigarettes are available.

Principle 7: Relapse is expected. It is unreasonable to expect that individuals will change and then maintain new behaviors perfectly. To the contrary, imperfect adherence to desired activities is more likely to be the case. Patients may be reluctant to report relapses to their physician, instead either avoiding medical encounters or seeking other providers. Two attitudes need to be conveyed to the patient by the physician. The first is that one slip does not necessarily lead to complete relapse; patients can slip and then get back on their programs of behavioral change. The second is that talking about relapses does not encourage them to occur. To the contrary, patients can be advised that relapses may occur, and if they do they should not be regarded as "failures" but rather as opportunities to learn how to change behavior more effectively in the future. In the case of smoking, for example, the more times that patients have tried to quit, the more likely they are to be successful at quitting. Advice will be more effective if the relapses are analyzed very specifically, for example, determining where the first cigarettes or drink came from and what circumstances surrounded the "slip," coupled with description and rehearsal of how such slips might be avoided in the future.

■ THE PHYSICIAN'S PERSPECTIVE

These strategies for behavioral change are based on the optimistic premise that individuals can introduce and maintain changes in their lives. The practicing physician may not always feel such optimism. Change is difficult for anyone, and modifying life-long habits for the long-term goal of better health may not seem worthwhile for many patients. Two points might help the physician to maintain enthusiasm for this part of medical practice. The first is that the tools available to the physician are limited. Persuasive communication of a limited duration in the confines of the medical office cannot be expected to have an overwhelming influence on patients in comparison with the other influences in their lives. Past histories, personal preferences, the media, the family, and long-standing habits are not overcome easily, even when better health is the motivation. However, the physician can be another voice encouraging the patient to change, and the physician can take advantage of patient vulnerabilities to motivate change. Second, behavioral change should be considered for all patients. Physicians can become discouraged when the patient with extreme chronic obstructive pulmonary disease fails to quit smoking, when the patient with severe diabetes or hypertension fails to lose weight, or when the alcoholic patient cannot stop drinking. Nevertheless, even if success rates are low, these preventive efforts are as worthwhile as any therapy for prevention of chronic disease. Perhaps these patients will never change. Concentrating on patients whose problems are less severe may be more rewarding because their problems are less likely to be out of control and they are more likely to be able to change. In addition, there is the old adage of "trying harder or trying differently." We have attempted to suggest some ways of trying differently and in that way experiencing greater success in an important aspect of medical practice.

Suggested Reading

Bandura A. Self-efficacy: Toward a unifying theory of behavioral change. Psychol Rev 1977; 34:191–215.

Becker MH. Patient adherence to prescribed therapies. Med Care 1985; 23: 539–555.

Job RFS. Effective and ineffective use of fear in health promotion campaigns. Am J Pub Health 1988; 78:163–167.

Martin AR, Coates TJ. A clinician's guide to helping patients change behavior. West J Med 1987; 146:751–753.

Turner CF, Miller HG, Moses LE. AIDS, sexual behavior and intravenous drug use. Washington, D.C.: National Academy Press, 1989.

ALCOHOLISM

Enoch Gordis, M.D.
Richard K. Fuller, M.D.

Alcoholism is recognized by its complications, but the treatment of its complications is not the treatment of alcoholism. Physicians are familiar with many of the toxic consequences of alcohol abuse. In fact, 15 to 30 percent of admissions to large urban hospitals are estimated to be related to the complications of alcohol abuse and alcoholism. The management of these complications is certainly important; however, the treatment of alcoholism means the modification of alcohol-seeking and alcohol-abusing behavior (Table 1). If this behavior is not arrested, the patient goes on to repeated problems from drinking or dies. To treat the hemorrhage or the pancreatitis and not to treat the alcoholism is bad medicine, akin to treating iron-deficiency anemia without treating the colon cancer that is causing it.

Physicians, because of their authority and knowledge, are in an advantageous position to begin the management of alcoholism. Nevertheless, many physicians are reluctant to do it, for several reasons. They may believe that alcoholism is a symptom of some underlying psychologic problem and that alcoholism itself cannot be addressed directly. They may see alcoholism as a moral, not a medical, issue. They may consider the condition hopeless. These views are almost certainly incorrect. Physicians also may fear that by discussing drinking with a patient, the patient will be offended and find another doctor. This argument has some merit, but it obviously cannot justify failing to practice good medicine. Further, if all physicians managed the problem appropriately, they might gain patients, because some patients who had walked out on other physicians might now be ready for help. Finally, a

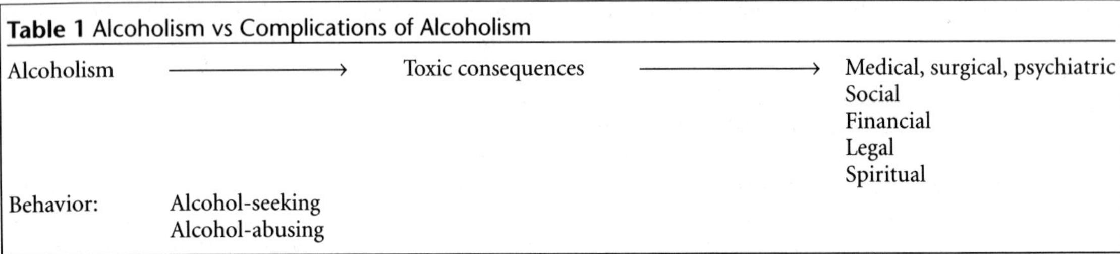

Table 1 Alcoholism vs Complications of Alcoholism

Alcoholism	⟶	Toxic consequences	⟶	Medical, surgical, psychiatric Social Financial Legal Spiritual
Behavior:	Alcohol-seeking Alcohol-abusing			

minority of physicians have problems with alcohol themselves and find it impossible to examine someone else's drinking objectively.

We have written this chapter with the following assumptions: physicians who will read it are busy, and their primary interest is in clinical medicine and its scientific basis. Yet they want to practice good medicine and are willing to take a certain amount of time to address the problem of alcoholism. Although many physicians will probably refer the patient to long-term treatment by experts, this first step is critical. The reward is the saving of many more lives than can be saved by intimate knowledge of hepatic cytoarchitecture or liberal application of sclerotherapy.

Table 2 CAGE Questionnaire

1. Have you ever felt you should **C**ut down on your drinking?
2. Have people **A**nnoyed you by criticizing your drinking?
3. Have you ever felt bad or **G**uilty about your drinking?
4. Have you ever had a drink first thing in the morning to steady your nerves or get rid of a hangover (**E**ye opener)?

From Mayfield DG, McLeod G, Hall P. The CAGE questionnaire: Validation of a new alcoholism screening instrument. Am J Psych 1974; 131:1121–1123 and Ewing JA. Detecting alcoholism, the CAGE questionnaire. JAMA 1964; 252: 1905–1907.

WHAT IS ALCOHOLISM?

Alcoholism is a chronic relapsing disease characterized by four main clinical features: (1) tolerance, a state of adaptation in which more and more alcohol is needed to produce desired effects; (2) physical dependence, which means that on interruption of drinking, a characteristic withdrawal syndrome appears that is relieved by alcohol itself (e.g., morning drinking) or by other drugs in the alcohol-sedative group; (3) impaired control, which means that the alcoholic person cannot invariably regulate total alcohol intake at any drinking occasion once drinking has begun; and (4) the dysphoria of abstinence, or "craving", which is the most elusive feature of alcoholism and which leads to relapse. Formal diagnostic criteria for alcohol use disorders can be found in two major diagnostic systems: the Diagnostic and Statistical Manual of Mental Disorders, Fourth Edition (DSM-IV), published by the American Psychiatric Association; and the International Classification of Diseases, Tenth Revision (ICD-10), published by the World Health Organization.

TREATING ALCOHOLISM

Alcoholism treatment consists of (1) recognizing alcoholism, (2) confronting the patient with the problem, (3) safe conduct through withdrawal, and (4) long-term management of the illness.

Recognizing Alcoholism

Recognizing alcoholism is no problem in the acutely ill hospitalized patient who has one of the major alcohol-related medical complications. In the office, things are more difficult. The patient is not acutely ill, will choose to hide or deny the problem, and will prefer that the medical complication be addressed and the drinking overlooked. The denial of the problem is not simply deliberate lying; much of the denial is unconscious because the thought of living without alcohol can be terrifying to one addicted to it. Here the physician must use a combination of clinical clues, laboratory clues (well-known abnormalities of bone marrow, liver, and urate metabolism), and social clues (especially job, marital, and legal problems) to make the diagnosis.

A standard alcoholism-detection questionnaire (e.g., CAGE, MAST, Short MAST) is helpful because it provides a structured and consistent means to detect individuals at risk. This information can then be used as a starting point for helping a patient confront his/her alcohol problem. For example, the CAGE questionnaire is a self-report screening instrument taking about 1 minute to complete (Table 2). ("CAGE" is a mnemonic for the four questions that comprise the instrument.) It is suitable to a busy medical setting when there is limited time for patient interviews. One "yes" response suggests an alcohol use problem; more than one is a strong indication that a problem exists.

Alcoholics are tolerant of large concentrations of alcohol. They may be ambulatory and coherent with a blood alcohol level that would be lethal to a nondrinker. The small, commercially available breath alcohol meters, which are no larger than a paperback, are very convenient and settle doubts and disagreements about recent drinking in a few seconds. When a drinking bout has ended more than 12 hours or so before the consultation, and the blood alcohol level is zero, clues to alcoholism may be provided by tremor, tachycardia, and hypertension in a usually normotensive patient. These clues are early signs of withdrawal. MCV and γ-glutamyltransferase abnormalities caused by alcohol use are familiar to internists. Newer laboratory tests, such as the carbohydrate-deficient transferrin, which could provide a clinically useful indicator of heavy alcohol consumption and does not depend on the presence of liver disease, may become available to physicians in the near future.

Discussing Alcoholism with Your Patient

Discussing alcoholism with your patient must be handled firmly but tactfully. It can be managed as a mutual exploration of the possibility that alcohol is causing many of the patient's troubles. The information gleaned from standardized questionnaires and laboratory tests is helpful because the patient sees that his/her situation is not unique and that he/she has not been singled out for harassment. If the patient consents to have the physician contact a family member or close friend, the physician can enlist the help of these relatives or friends to join in a meeting with the patient. At this meeting, the others quietly describe to the patient the impact of the patient's drinking on their lives and urge the patient to agree to treatment. The impact of such a meeting is stronger if family or friends state their intent to terminate contact with the patient unless he/she enters treatment.

If the patient agrees to be treated, and if the physician chooses not to manage the alcoholism any further, the patient should be referred immediately to another therapist or agency for help, as well as to Alcoholics Anonymous.

Safe Conduct Through Withdrawal

Many patients will be alcohol free at the time they seek treatment for their alcoholism and will be in no discomfort from withdrawal. For these patients, the approaches described in the section Long-Term Management of Alcoholism may begin promptly. Patients who still have alcohol in their system, have mild withdrawal symptoms, or are uncomfortable from withdrawal symptoms may need treatment. The aim of treatment for withdrawal is to relieve symptoms and prevent the more serious complications of withdrawal.

For clarity, we have divided the following discussion into two parts: a description of the withdrawal syndrome and then practical details about its treatment.

The Withdrawal Syndrome

Clinical Picture

On interruption of drinking, even before the blood alcohol has reached zero concentration, the patient may experience a group of adrenergic symptoms—tremor, sweating, tachycardia, systolic and diastolic hypertension, and irritability (or mild agitation). In addition, the patient may be sleepless. These symptoms vary in intensity and subside within several days or, rarely, 1 or 2 weeks. The diastolic pressure may be as high as 115. We do not recommend treating hypertension below this level, because it usually disappears within a few days as the withdrawal itself subsides. (Some patients, of course, are hypertensive as well as alcoholic, and will need treatment while sober. There is no way of knowing this beforehand, however, unless a physician had to treat the patient for hypertension during a previous period of abstinence.) The tremor is a postural tremor at about eight per second; sometimes it is hard to distinguish it from anxiety, but if the fingers continue to shake when the examiner immobilizes the wrist and elbow, it is probably alcohol withdrawal. A tongue tremor, if present, is virtually pathognomonic. The patient may be nauseated and may vomit at the beginning of withdrawal. Some patients hallucinate during the first 1 or 2 days. Hallucinations may be visual or auditory, are usually recognized by the patient as abnormal, are not associated with persistent belief (as in delusion), and are not a sign of psychosis.

Hyperglycemia

Hyperglycemia in nondiabetic patients is often seen in early withdrawal. It is probably more common in malnourished patients because normal glucose tolerance depends on adequate nourishment. In addition, alcohol is known to blunt the insulin response of the pancreas to a glucose load. With abstinence and eating, this condition rapidly clears and a diagnosis of diabetes should not be made.

Seizures

Patients may experience seizures, usually 2 or 3 days into withdrawal. They are epileptiform, are not characteristically preceded by an aura, are temporally related to the cessation of drinking, and, of course, are accompanied by a brief period of unconsciousness. Electroencephalograms and brain scans are normal. We order these tests only once in any patient. Competing causes of seizures (e.g., epilepsy, hypoglycemia, old head injury with organized seizure focus) must be considered but are rarely found.

Delirium Tremens

A minority of patients enter a severe form of withdrawal on about the third day, delirium tremens (DTs), which is characterized by disorientation, agitation, fever, fluid loss, tremulousness, and hallucinations.

Treating Withdrawal Syndrome

Assessment

A rating scale, the Clinical Institute Withdrawal Assessment for Alcohol (CIWA-Ar) has been shown to be of value in managing alcohol withdrawal in general hospitals. This scale, which takes approximately 2 to 5 minutes to administer, consists of 10 items. The first nine items are nausea/vomiting; tremor; paroxysmal sweats; anxiety; agitation; tactile, auditory, and visual disturbances; and headache or fullness in the head. These nine items are graded on a 0 to 7 Likert scale. A tenth item, disorientation and clouding of the sensorium, is scored 0 to 4. The higher the score, the greater is the severity of withdrawal. Scores of 9 or less represent minimal withdrawal, and pharmacotherapy is not necessary. Scores of 10 to 19 represent mild to moderate withdrawal, and 20 or more is severe withdrawal. Because no scaling instrument is infallible, such instruments should be used to complement, not replace, a thorough clinical evaluation of the patient.

Pharmacotherapy

For those patients who require pharmacotherapy, and who can be continually observed (usually inpatient), we recommend giving 20 mg of diazepam every 1 to 2 hours orally until the symptoms are suppressed because the benzodiazepines (BZs) have been shown to reduce the occurrence of DTs. The longer-acting BZs have an advantage over the shorter-acting BZs because the long half-lives of diazepam and chlordiazepoxide and their metabolites enable drug levels to be maintained longer, thereby reducing the necessity of additional doses. The shorter-acting BZs (e.g., oxazepam and lorazepam) are preferable for elderly patients. They also are preferable for patients with liver disease because they are glucuronidated rather than oxidized. In addition to their proven efficacy, the BZs are quite safe. However, the metabolism of the BZs may be inhibited by cimetidine, isoniazid, disulfiram (Antabuse), and oral contraceptives. The BZs should not be administered after the withdrawal syndrome is over because of the alcoholic's substantial risk for developing dependence on these medications.

Propranolol and clonidine can control many of the adrenergic manifestations of withdrawal, but we see no advantage in their use, unless the early hypertension is severe. One drug then might control both withdrawal and blood pressure, even though the alpha-2-agonists (e.g., clonidine) do not reduce the frequency of seizures. Carbamazepine was initially studied in Europe for treating alcohol withdrawal, and recent American studies have confirmed the earlier results. A recent U.S. study compared carbamazepine with oxazepam and found them to be equally safe and effective. An advantage to carbamazepine is that it does not have the problem of potential abuse. Disadvantages include no parenteral form and occasional serious hematologic (e.g., aplastic anemia) and dermatologic adverse reactions. Other medications have been studied to treat withdrawal. The addition of one such medication, the beta-blocker atenolol, to a BZ regimen resulted in smaller doses of BZ being needed to treat withdrawal.

In summary, although other agents are available, the BZs have the major advantage in that they are established as both safe and effective.

Although safe and comfortable withdrawal can be accomplished by giving tapering doses of alcohol over several days, we do not do this. True, this is the substance to which the patient is addicted, and one does not have to rely on other drugs that do not have identical pharmacology; however, the arguments against using alcohol make sense. First, nurses would be kept busy giving alcohol around the clock. Second, it is hard to maintain an ambience conducive to serious counseling about sobriety when patients reek of alcohol. Third, there is an ethical question inherent in prescribing a known liver and marrow toxin to patients already sick with these complications. Finally, disulfiram therapy cannot be started while ethanol is used for detoxification.

Sometimes it is safer to let the patient shake rather than to risk drug toxicity. Sedation should be avoided, if possible, in patients with chronic obstructive pulmonary disease. With advanced liver disease, we use very little sedative or none, because the metabolism of BZs is retarded in this state. Alcohol and BZs make depression worse, and, in a severely depressed patient, it is better to avoid sedatives. Note that a mild depression during alcohol withdrawal is expected and appropriate and is almost always self-limited.

Seizures

Whether withdrawal seizures are an indication for phenytoin (Dilantin) therapy in addition to the standard use of BZs is controversial. We do not recommend phenytoin because we believe that the seizures are controlled for the entire period of withdrawal with adequate BZ therapy. (There is no controversy about the fact that anticonvulsants have no role in long-term management in the abstinent state. The long-term treatment for withdrawal seizures is abstinence.)

Delirium Tremens

If the patient is experiencing DTs, supporting the airway and maintaining fluid and electrolyte balance are essential. For the patient's safety and that of others, it is important to control the patient's agitation. Administering diazepam intravenously is effective. The dose should be carefully titrated to the patient's level of agitation. The patient should be calm but not somnolent. In one controlled study of DTs, the initial doses required for calming varied from 15 mg to 160 mg, and repeated doses were often required.

Nutrition

The physician should be concerned with nutrition. Middle-class alcoholics are generally not particularly malnourished. Among patients who are, the commonest deficiencies are folate, thiamine, and magnesium. Many physicians routinely administer all three, and this can do no harm. Magnesium deficiency manifested by low serum magnesium levels must be corrected promptly because magnesium depletion lowers the threshold for withdrawal seizures. Claims that magnesium alone is a suitable regimen for withdrawal have not been validated. Thiamine must be administered to malnourished patients before glucose; failure to do so may precipitate Wernicke's syndrome.

Table 3 summarizes management choices based on the condition of the patient when seen in the office. (Patients hospitalized for complications of alcohol may undergo withdrawal at the same time and may need treatment for it.)

Long-Term Management of Alcoholism (Table 4)

The goal of long-term management is the maximum restoration of physical and social functioning. Complete abstinence

Table 3 Office Management of the Alcoholic Patient

Sober (no alcohol present):
Verify with breath meter.

Comfortable, can listen:
Tactful, but firm discussion; then long-term management (see text). Consider use of disulfiram or naltrexone (see text).

Uncomfortable, in withdrawal: Administer CIWA-Ar
- Withdrawal mild: Prescribe 1 day's sedative dosage (e.g., 5–20 mg diazepam) with return to physician next day. Next day proceed with confrontation and long-term management. The mistake here is to prescribe a whole bottle of diazepam. This accomplishes nothing, and the patient is likely to drink and use the pills together.
- Withdrawal troublesome (or patient has had seizures or DTs during a prior withdrawal): admit for detoxification

Alcohol present:
- Can stop drinking: Return sober next day, continue as under "Sober." It is safer not to offer sedatives to a drinking patient.
- Cannot stop drinking: Admit for detoxification. The physician may choose to manage the inpatient withdrawal on a general service, or may admit the patient to a specialized unit. Insurance coverage for alcoholism detoxification is now provided in many policies. Do not admit the patient under a false diagnosis such as "gastritis." That fuels the patient's denial and impedes recovery. The advantage of a specialized detoxification unit is that nonmedical services, such as Alcoholics Anonymous, counseling, and group therapy, are generally available.

is the only recommendation that can ethically be made at present. The commonly offered advice, "You should try to cut down on your drinking," is not worth the breath it takes to give it. Nor can the memory of past pains alone be relied on to turn the tide. Because alcoholism is a chronic, relapsing illness, it is not unusual for even patients who eventually do well to suffer one or several relapses before achieving abstinence.

The physician is the most competent person to describe the health consequences of alcoholism, and this should be done in detail. The physician also can counsel, e.g., he/she can indicate to the patient those other areas in life that are being damaged by alcohol. For the patient merely to know all this is not enough, the patient must also be persuaded that the struggle for a better life is worthwhile despite the fluctuating discomfort of abstinence. Joining with others in a self-help organization can be a potent force. The largest and perhaps best known of these organizations is the fellowship of Alcoholics Anonymous (AA). AA is neither an encounter group nor a religious denomination. Its sole aim is to help drinkers to stay sober. All patients should be encouraged to attend. Although not all patients will respond to AAs style and message, many will benefit from the sense of dignity and personal worth that AA imparts. Every physician should have available the names and telephone numbers of several AA members of diverse backgrounds who, with the patient's consent, can be called while the patient is in the office. The patient often can be taken to his/her first meeting that evening.

Table 4 Checklist: What the Concerned Physician Should Know and Have Available in the Practice to Manage Alcoholism

TO KNOW:

1. The pharmacology of alcohol: its distribution, metabolism, tolerance, physical dependence
2. The pharmacology of one sedative, e.g., diazepam, and how to use it
3. The pharmacology of disulfiram and how to use it
4. The pharmacology of naltrexone

TO HAVE AVAILABLE:

1. If the decision is made to offer disulfiram, a supply of the medication to be offered in the office so that it can be started immediately on acceptance. The remainder of the patient's supply is prescribed in the usual way.
2. A small alcohol breath analyzer. Test for heavy drinking and tolerance.
3. Photocopies of one standard questionnaire (e.g., CAGE, MAST, short MAST, and so forth) so patient can be engaged in a neutral way.
4. The following telephone numbers:
   - Several willing members of AA of both sexes and various ethnic and occupational backgrounds who will respond to a telephone call, if possible while the patient is in the office.
   - The local AA Intergroup Office (see telephone directory) for help in finding AA members as above, and also for other members if those known are unavailable. The AA Intergroup office often knows which detoxification units have available beds.
   - A list (obtained from the telephone directory) of other alcoholism support groups in your area.
   - The local National Council on Alcoholism and Drug Dependence affiliate group for further screening and referral, especially to outpatient services.
   - Three or four of the available public and private inpatient detoxification units.
   - Three or four of the available public and private outpatient multidisciplinary programs.

Pharmacotherapy

Two medications are currently used in treating alcohol dependence: disulfiram (Antabuse), which has been in use since the 1940s, and the more recently approved naltrexone (Revia).

Disulfiram

Although disulfiram has been used for more than 40 years to treat alcoholism, only recently have carefully controlled studies of its efficacy been done. This research indicates that when the patient is given disulfiram to take at his/her discretion, disulfiram, in addition to standard treatment, does not result in longer periods of abstinence than that achieved by standard treatment alone. This outcome is because compliance with the medication is often poor. However, this same research indicated that more socially stable, middle-aged men drink less frequently if prescribed disulfiram. Strategies have been devised to improve compliance with the disulfiram regimen. A recent controlled study has shown that having, for example, spouses or friends observe ingestion of the medication two to three times per week improves efficacy. Whatever its long-term value, disulfiram buys time initially by putting up a "chemical fence" so the patient knows he/she cannot drink that day, and even for 3 or 4 days after stopping it. Ambivalence about taking disulfiram is common, and the physician can point out to the patient that this indicates a less-than-total commitment to sobriety. Such a discussion may help patients to overcome their ambivalence and elect to take disulfiram.

Disulfiram can be given as soon as 12 hours after the last drink. Nowadays, the dosage is designed first for safety and then for efficacy. A common routine, which is based more on clinical experience than on pharmacokinetic evidence, is 0.5 g daily for 5 days, then 0.25 g daily. A full-blown alcohol-disulfiram reaction includes immediate flushing of the face and neck (sometimes the rest of the body as well), an initial hypertension, tachycardia, and conjunctival injection. Within minutes the flush resolves, the blood pressure falls, and the patient feels faint, and often nauseated, chilled, and generally sick. Convulsions are not part of the usual reaction. Finally, after a variable amount of time, but not more than 2 hours, the patient becomes sleepy and may sleep for several hours. On awakening, the patient is well. Compensated liver disease and diabetes are not contraindications to therapy.

Disulfiram is a safe drug; the most common side effect is sedation, which wears off usually in the first 2 weeks. Other side effects, including a rare but well-documented drug-induced hepatitis, are seen infrequently. Because disulfiram hepatitis is an idiosyncratic reaction that usually occurs early in administration, it is important to obtain liver tests on a regular basis when first prescribing the drug. A recommended schedule is that liver tests be obtained before treatment, at 2-week intervals for 2 months, and at 3- to 6-month intervals thereafter. Because liver tests may indicate a resumption of drinking as well as incipient hepatitis, a discussion with the patient is necessary. Unless it is evident that the patient has been drinking, the medication should be stopped if an increase in liver tests occurs.

Absolute contraindications to disulfiram are pregnancy, severe depression, organic brain syndrome, severe active liver disease, and cardio- or cerebrovascular disease. The last two are contraindications not because disulfiram is in itself toxic to the heart or the brain, but because the rare patient who drinks while taking disulfiram (most stop it several days before drinking) will undergo a hypotensive episode. Disulfiram interferes with the biotransformation of certain medications including phenytoin, isoniazid, diazepam, chlordiazepoxide, warfarin, imipramine, and desipramine. This contraindication has to be kept in mind when prescribing disulfiram. We must emphasize again, however, that for the vast majority of alcoholic patients, disulfiram is easy and safe to prescribe.

Naltrexone

The outlook for recovery from alcoholism may be seen to hinge on the outcome of a struggle between two functional parts of the brain—the part that determines appetite and the part that can understand the consequences of surrendering to that appetite and can decide not to. Research is continuing on pharmacologic interventions to control the appetite—or craving—for alcohol. One such medication recently approved by the Food and Drug Administration (FDA) for this purpose is naltrexone, an opiate antagonist that has been used for many years to treat heroin addiction.

Naltrexone appears to reduce craving in many abstinent patients and to block the reinforcing effects of alcohol in many patients who drink. The latter effect often enables patients who drink a small amount of alcohol to avoid full-blown relapse and lessens the likelihood of their return to heavy drinking. However, the mechanism of naltrexone's effect in alcoholism has not been conclusively demonstrated.

The initial clinical trials of naltrexone's effectiveness in treating alcohol dependence found that naltrexone cut the rate of patient relapse by about 50 percent. In addition, patients who receive naltrexone reported less alcohol craving, fewer drinking days, and less severe alcohol-related problems than patients treated with a placebo. It is important to note that in each trial, naltrexone was used *in combination with counseling*, an important part of the treatment regimen.

Naltrexone has been established as safe at the prescribed dose (50 mg per day) in a large heterogeneous population of alcoholics in diverse treatment modalities and settings. Clinical trials are currently underway to determine the patient type, dose, therapy combinations, and treatment duration with which naltrexone works best. Until results from those studies are available, it is recommended that only those physicians who are familiar with addiction treatment prescribe naltrexone, only in the context of psychosocial treatments, and only for the FDA-recommended time period. Physicians will rely on clinical judgment to determine whether and at what point in treatment a patient should be started on conventional treatments or conventional treatments accompanied by naltrexone.

Other Aspects of Patient Care

Patients frequently attribute relapse to stress. In many cases this may be true, however, it is often used as an excuse for drinking. Patients taking disulfiram who relapse have almost all stopped disulfiram several days before the alleged drink-provoking stress occurred. Counseling and social work are valuable because they help the patient undo the damage that drinking has done and help the patient adjust to a sober routine. When life has some rewards, the patient is more likely to view the struggle for sobriety as worthwhile.

In general, a psychiatric diagnosis cannot be made while the patient is either drinking or in early withdrawal. Most alcoholics do not need treatment for psychiatric illness; they are drunk, but not mentally ill. Once sober, however, a minority will need treatment by a psychiatrist for an affective disorder, manic-depressive disorder, or panic attacks. In the sober state, they can respond to competent psychiatry as do nonalcoholics.

There is no role for sedation in the long-term management of alcoholism. It does not control the drinking, and it sets up the patient for a possible second drug habit. Insomnia may persist many months after withdrawal; the sleep electroencephalogram may not become normal in a year's time. Sleeping pills should not be prescribed. The patient should be told that the condition will improve in time if he/she does not take pills. The commonest cause of insomnia, however, is caffeine, and most insomnia will respond to the cessation of all caffeine, including coffee, tea, and cola beverages.

We know physicians who genuinely enjoy the long-term management of alcoholism, including nonmedical counseling. Most, however, prefer not to do this management and will choose to refer their patients to a competently run alcoholism treatment program. There, a variety of counseling and social work services are frequently available, and many of these programs will also handle the prescription of disulfiram and have AA meetings on their premises. More recently developed techniques such as cognitive behavioral therapy, which are useful for some patients, are available through these programs. These specialized techniques are usually beyond the available time and expertise of many internists.

When voluntary approaches fail, coercion may become necessary. Sometimes it has already been applied by others. The spouse may be contemplating divorce. The job may be in danger. There may be court pressure after driving while intoxicated or an incidence of family violence. In many states, legislation has tightened the requirement for prompt reporting to medical licensing agencies of alcoholic physicians. In these situations, the added use of mandatory disulfiram can be very helpful. Finally, a trusted physician confronted with a patient's repeated alcoholic hemorrhage or pancreatitis may tell the patient that after the acute episode is over, he/she will no longer be responsible for the patient's care if the patient does not immediately begin disulfiram under supervision and enter treatment for alcoholism. Coercive measures may seem harsh but the stakes are very high—alcoholism is a malignant disease.

Suggested Reading

Ewing JA. Detecting alcoholism, the CAGE questionnaire. JAMA 1984; 252:1905–1907.

Fuller RK, Branchey L, Brightwell DR, et al. Disulfiram treatment of alcoholism: A Veterans Administration cooperative study. JAMA 1986; 256: 1449–1489.

Kadden RM, Cooney NL, Geffer H, Litt MD. Matching alcoholics to coping skills or interactional therapies: Post treatment results. J Consult Clin Psychol 1989; 57:698–704.

Mayfield DG, McLeod G, Hall P. The CAGE questionnaire: Validation of a new alcoholism screening instrument. Am J Psych 1974; 131:1121–1123.
Moore RD, Bone LR, Geller G, et al. Prevalence, detection, and treatment of alcoholism in hospitalized patients. JAMA 1989; 261(3):403–407.
O'Malley SS, Jaffe AJ, Chang G, et al. Naltrexone and coping skills therapy for alcohol dependence: A controlled study. Arch Gen Psychiatry 1992; 49:881–887.
Sellers EM, Naranjo CA, Harrison M, et al. Diazepam loading: Simplified treatment of alcohol withdrawal. Clin Pharmacol Ther 1983; 34:822–826.
Volpicelli JR, Alterman AI, Hayashida M, O'Brien CP. Naltrexone in the treatment of alcohol dependence. Arch Gen Psychiatry 1992; 49:876–880.

SMOKING CESSATION

Harry L. Greene II, M.D.

Cigarette smoking has been a major health hazard throughout the 20th century and will continue as the major health problem into the new millennium. It is the most important preventable cause of premature death, with an annual loss of 420,000 lives and the sacrifice of 5,000,000 potential years of life. It is responsible for one in every five deaths in the United States. Prior to 1900 tobacco use was largely in the form of snuff or cigars, with few cigarettes used. By 1910 the process for manufacturing cigarettes was perfected, and from that time until approximately 1965 smoking prevalence increased. It peaked in 1965, a time when 40 percent of adult Americans were smoking. Following the Surgeon General's report of the hazards of smoking in that year tobacco use rates have progressively declined, falling at the rate of approximately 0.5 percent per year until the mid-1990s. At its peak in 1965, 50 percent of men and 32 percent of adult women were smoking. The fall for men has been much faster than for women. In 1992, 24 percent of adult women and 20 percent of adult men were smoking. Tobacco use for men is still higher, with men being much more likely to smoke cigars or pipes or to use snuff. The number of young men and women initiating smoking underwent a progressive decline since the 1960s, with the drop being greater in boys than in girls. During the mid-1980s more women and girls than men and boys were initiating smoking, a trend that has persisted to the present.

Smoking behavior is universally correlated with education, with college graduates smoking less than half as frequently as high school drop-outs. Lower socioeconomic status is also highly correlated with current day smokers. Blue-collar workers are more likely than white-collar workers to smoke. Native Americans and Alaskan Natives also have high rates of use.

■ HEALTH CONSEQUENCES OF TOBACCO USE

It is well known that tobacco and its constituents are among the most potent of human carcinogens as well as being highly atherogenic. It is no surprise with these two properties that each year there are 148,000 deaths from smoking-related cancers, 100,000 deaths from coronary heart disease, and 23,000 deaths due to stroke. An additional 85,000 deaths per year are due to respiratory illnesses, specifically chronic obstructive pulmonary disease and pneumonia. Among the cancers caused by smoking are those of the lung, trachea, bronchus, larynx, pharynx, oral cavity, and esophagus. Smoking also contributes to cancer of the pancreas, kidney, bladder, and uterine cervix. It interacts with other substances such as alcohol to increase the risk of laryngeal, oral cavity, and esophageal cancer and with asbestos and radon to substantially increase the risk of lung cancer. Children and adolescents who are active smokers have an increased prevalence and severity of respiratory illness and respiratory symptoms, decreased physical fitness, and decreased rate of lung growth. Tobacco, perhaps through its effect on estrogen, is believed to contribute to the development of osteoporosis. In addition, smokers have higher rates of peptic ulcer disease, poor wound healing, and increased occurrence of cataracts and are more likely to experience impotence or premature menopause. For both sexes smoking gives premature aging of the skin with wrinkling and loss of elasticity.

The effects of passive smoking on those persons who are near the smoker include lung cancer, increased rates of coronary artery disease, increasing middle ear effusions and infection of the lower respiratory tract in children, and a small but measurable decrease in lung function and a role in the exacerbation of asthma. Passive smoking has also been associated with sudden infant death syndrome.

Cigarette smoking contributes to 25 percent of the deaths from residential fires, most of these occurring in children, and 33,300 other fire-related injuries per year. Smoking during pregnancy is believed to contribute to up to 6 percent of perinatal deaths, contribute to low birth weight, and is a factor in up to 10 percent of preterm deliveries. It increases a woman's risk of miscarriage and fetal growth retardation. Smoking also interacts with other medications, specifically oral contraceptives, and increases the risk of cerebral infarct, subarachnoid hemorrhage, and stroke, as well as causing a tenfold increase in the likelihood of myocardial infarction.

■ BENEFITS OF QUITTING

Increasing epidemiologic data show that there are health benefits for quitting smoking at virtually any age. Even those smokers who stop smoking beyond age 65 years or who quit after the development of smoking-related diseases may derive some measurable advantages from smoking cessation. The most dramatic improvement is in cardiovascular risk reduction, which occurs almost immediately for rhythm disturbances, and in the risk of sudden death. Up to half of the excess risk of cardiac mortality is slashed in the first year after quitting. For lung cancer 30 percent to 50 percent of the excess risk is still evident at 10 years, and even at 15 years there is some measurable residual risk. The risks of cancer never return completely to the level of a nonsmoker but approach it with continued years of cessation. Clearly, those persons who quit when they are young and have fewer pack-years of smoking exposure and stop before developing smoking-related disease have the greatest health benefits in terms of morbidity and mortality. In a recent nurses health study, it was shown that there was a 24 percent reduction in cardiovascular death within 2 years of quitting smoking. According to that study, the total risks from cardiovascular mortality and total cancer among former smokers approached the level of that for the general nonsmoking population between 10 and 14 years after cessation. Those persons who stop smoking before pregnancy or during the first trimester have infants who are the same size as those born to women who are nonsmokers. Women who stop at any time up to the 30th week of gestation seem to have infants with higher birth weights than those who continue to smoke for the duration of their pregnancy.

■ SMOKING CESSATION

Roughly half of living Americans who were reported to ever have smoked have quit. Most of those smokers remaining in the survey have suggested that they would like to quit, and most have made at least one or more serious attempts to quit. Without question, most former smokers cite fear of illness or concern about health as a major factor for quitting. More recent data suggest that social acceptability, social pressure, and legislative initiatives are increasing in importance for the contemplation of smoking cessation. More than 90 percent of smokers know that smoking is harmful, yet this knowledge alone may not be enough to prompt action. The chance of symptoms, chest pain, breathlessness, esophageal pain, and the fear of the development of cancer or heart disease are often potent stimuli to consider discontinuing smoking. Illness in a family member, a loved one, or a friend also may act as a trigger to motivate interest in smoking cessation.

Most former smokers have used quitting "cold turkey" as a method, others have cut their cigarette use on a daily basis, and still others have used formal programs for help. The evidence suggests that a multicomponent program, featuring behavior modification, is probably the most successful. A number of studies have been performed looking at the value of hypnosis with variable results. In those studies that were randomized, the success rate is disappointing. This result is true for acupuncture as well.

Quitting smoking is a learning process, with most former smokers having to try several times before achieving success. A helpful paradigm for smoking cessation was developed in which cessation is viewed as a series of cognitive stages. The program begins with a precontemplation stage in which one is not thinking about quitting, a contemplation stage in which one is actually thinking about the health risks or other reasons for quitting, a pre-action state in which one is preparing to quit within the next month, an action stage in which one is in the process of quitting smoking, and finally the maintenance of a nonsmoking state from which one may relapse or become a permanent nonsmoker. All of these stages may be interactive, and a person may go from one stage back to another or may skip a stage depending on what factor prompts the subject's attention. Throughout the early maintenance period and indeed for many smokers throughout life, there are a number of triggers that can lead to the resumption of smoking.

■ BARRIERS TO SMOKING CESSATION

The U.S. Surgeon General, after a review of the data, announced that tobacco use was addicting and that the specific agent most closely linked to the addiction was nicotine. Tobacco use satisfied the addictive potential by illustrating tolerance in those who used it frequently, creation of physical dependence, and occurrence of a withdrawal syndrome in those who discontinued its use.

The challenge of therapy for smoking stems from the withdrawal symptoms, which include cravings, irritability, anxiety, anger, difficulty concentrating, increasing appetite, sleep disturbances, and dysphoric dreams. Symptoms begin within hours of the last cigarette, peak within 2 to 3 days, and rapidly dissipate over the next 2 weeks, although individual symptoms may recur and be quite overpowering for a substantial period, in some individuals for up to 1 year. The severity of symptoms depends on the length of use and the number of cigarettes and amount of nicotine. Symptoms vary from individual to individual. There is some evidence that nicotine withdrawal symptoms may be worse during the luteal phase of the menstrual cycle.

It is this extreme combination of signs and symptoms constituting nicotine withdrawal that makes it so difficult for smokers to quit. In addition to nicotine addiction, a number of behavioral factors must be addressed during the smoking cessation attempt. Smoking is often viewed as an attractive attribute, stemming from billions of advertising dollars being spent to create an association between elegance and smoking. It is also a habit, frequently coupled with other things one does, e.g., following a meal, after a cup of coffee, following sex. It is easy then for the use of the cigarette to be coupled with each of these activities so that every time one has a cup of coffee a cigarette is automatically reached for.

Others who smoke in the car may reach for a cigarette as soon as they get in the car. For others, breaks at work may be associated with smoking. Smoking becomes inextricably entwined with the other activity. One of the elements of behavioral therapy is to make smokers aware of these triggers to smoking, to help them understand the cues to smoking and why and where they smoke, and to learn alternative, more helpful coping behaviors.

■ SOCIAL SUPPORT

Those therapists experienced in smoking cessation programs recognize that people attempting to smoke who live with other smokers have the greatest challenge to quitting. Social support from partners, family, friends, and co-workers is extremely important. For those persons who are living with a smoker, establishing smoke-free zones within the house and/or encouraging the smoker to smoke outside the house can be helpful. The most likely person for the nonsmoking neophyte to get a cigarette is from his or her smoking spouse.

■ WEIGHT GAIN

Smokers in general weigh from 5 to 10 lb less than their nonsmoking counterparts. After quitting, the average individual will regain from 5 to 8 lb, with up to 10 percent of individuals gaining 25 lb or more. The amount of weight gain is in direct proportion to the amount of nicotine consumed, e.g., heavy smokers generally gain more weight than light smokers. The mechanism is believed to be a decrease in metabolic rate and/or action on lipoprotein lipase and in some individuals an increase in food intake. Although weight gain occurs in both sexes, it is a much greater concern for women and often must be addressed as part of the cessation attempt in order to have sustained cessation. For those individuals who are using nicotine replacement, weight gain generally does not occur until after the nicotine replacement has been discontinued.

■ MOOD CHANGES

Discontinuation of smoking is viewed as a loss for many smokers. Some refer to cigarettes as their best friend—asking nothing but being there when they need them. This common sadness is reported by many smokers and can occur some months after cessation. Smokers also have been noted to have more depressive symptoms than nonsmokers and may well have had a history of major depression. This observation has led to a hypothesis suggesting that smokers and other addicted individuals may use their drug of choice to help regulate their mood. It is important to monitor a person undergoing smoking cessation for any mood changes and if depression becomes apparent to treat it appropriately.

■ OTHER ADDICTIONS

Smokers are more likely to use other medications and have other addictions. Specifically, alcohol is frequently part of the co-addiction and may be a principal factor in a smoker's relapse. The physician or therapist must be aware of alcohol, marijuana, cocaine, heroin, and other addicting substances as possible contributing factors in repeatedly failed smoking cessation attempts.

■ THE PHYSICIAN'S ROLE IN SMOKING CESSATION

Studies have shown that most individuals visit a physician at least one time per year, giving the physician an opportunity to broach the subject of smoking at that time. More detailed studies have shown that heavy smokers visit the physician more than once a year, allowing other opportunities for smoking behavior discussions. Although most physicians report that they ask about smoking, surveys of smokers show that only half of them admit to having been advised to quit smoking and an additional 50 percent do not recall the subject being mentioned. Whether this discrepancy is due to a lack of total recall on the part of the smoker or whether it is due to a lack of reaction on the part of the physician is unknown, but it is clear that there is room for improvement. The reasons physicians are not more aggressive in smoking cessation advice are probably manifold and include a lack of knowledge and skills or in many cases unrealistic expectations. Although it is known that increasing the number of interventions brought to bear on the problem increases the likelihood of success, less than half of physicians are familiar with or use combination strategies in smoking cessation. Less than 30 percent of physicians spend 5 minutes or more counseling their patients who smoke. This trend is likely to get worse under managed care. The most frustrating thing for many physicians is the patient who does not want to quit smoking. Often physicians who confront these patients repeatedly stop asking them about smoking behavior. This result is in spite of data that have clearly shown that smokers expect to be asked about their smoking behavior and feel abandoned or that the physician has lost interest in them if they stop asking. Finally, the expectations of physicians that simple advice will lead to a very high likelihood of cessation contradicts the actual data. Although there is a seventeenfold increase in cessation or starting the cessation attempt with simple advice, the highest 1-year cessation rates of 25 percent to 30 percent are only obtained with multimodality efforts and are unusual and not the rule. Abnormal and unrealistic expectation rates on behalf of the patient and the physician may lead to frustration for both.

One of the more successful physician education programs has focused on simply getting physicians to advise patients to stop smoking, using brief advice and supplementing that advice with brief counseling if possible; encouraging the patient to select a quit date; providing written materials to support the decision; suggesting ways to overcome the barriers and triggers to smoking; offering nicotine replacement therapy, prescribing it, and talking about its use for those who select this modality; and finally, scheduling follow-up visits. All of these methods increase the likelihood of smoking cessation. Studies looking at cost-effectiveness analysis have shown that there is clear benefit for taking the time to do this type of counseling.

A schematic approach to office-based smoking prevention is shown in Figure 1.

■ ASSESSMENT OF TOBACCO USE

It is well known that there are psychologic, behavioral, and environmental factors that help initiate and maintain smoking behavior. Using this knowledge, an assessment is done with the goals of characterizing the stage of change for the particular patient and evaluating the motivation to stop smoking. An assessment of the severity of nicotine dependence and understanding of the reasons for smoking, the triggers to its use, the environmental factors that help precipitate it, and any other co-morbid conditions such as depression or other substance use that may make it more difficult to quit.

The National Cancer Institute (NCI) has organized and developed an elegant but simple approach to the common elements for effect smoking cessation in its four-step protocol, which is designed to be delivered in 3 minutes of an office visit. The four steps are ask, advise, assist, and arrange.

Under *ask*, physicians should ask all patients at every visit whether they smoke or not. Additionally, they should ask about whether the patient is interested in quitting smoking and how he or she feels about being a smoker. This helps set the stage for understanding which counseling strategy is appropriate to use and which elements of that strategy are likely to move the patient to the next step of readiness of change. Although the overall goal is clearly to assist a smoker in stopping permanently, realistic goals are to attempt to move a smoker from one stage of readiness to another. Focused query can include timeline questions, such as "Do you intend to quit smoking within the next 6 months?" When answered no, the patient is in the precontemplation stage. Another question, "Do you intend to quit smoking within the next month?" If the answer to the first question, thinking about quitting, was yes, and to this question is no, the patient is really contemplating change. If, on the other hand, the patient states that he or she intends to quit within the next month, he or she is really in a preparation stage. It is important to note that as many as 40 percent of smokers seen in office practice are in the precontemplation stage and need to have interventions that will increase their awareness of the damage of smoking and its negative aspects, as well as to present some of the positive material that would be gained by smoking cessation. Another 40 percent are in the contemplative phase and have given serious thought to quitting or have attempted to quit in the past. These individuals need to be moved toward the preparation stage with the counseling that is delivered. Only one-fifth of smokers that come in for medical care are in the preparation stage and have taken steps toward quitting, such as delaying, brand switching, decreasing the number of cigarettes per day, or smoking later in the morning. These individuals are those who are most likely to respond to interventions that will actually help them manage a subsequent cessation attempt. It is this group for whom nicotine replacement, self-help manuals, behavioral skill training, contracting, frequent visits, and referral to a formal treatment program may be indicated.

Under the NCI program, after asking about smoking behavior, clear *advice* to quit is given. The message is described as being strong and unequivocal with examples such as, "Quitting smoking is the most important action you can take to live a long and healthy life. As your physician, I must give you strong advice to quit. I'd be willing to help you if you would like to try to do that."

The third step in the NCI program is *assisting* the smoker in quitting. From the clinical standpoint, this phase includes moving the smoker along the stages of change. If a smoker is not contemplating quitting, providing information and increasing awareness of smoking behavior and its negative aspects as well as the positive benefits of cessation may be shared in a brochure form. The physician should also offer to help the patient at any time in the future if the patient decides he or she wants to quit. For the patients actually interested in quitting smoking, a question about whether or not they are ready to set a quit date within the next month is important. Again, the person who is unwilling to set a quit date often lacks the confidence of success and time may be spent on exploring the barriers that are perceived by this individual. The physician can explore a cafeteria of options and allow the patient to select the type of smoking cessation program that he or she feels would be most helpful. These options can vary from cold turkey quitting on the patient's own to self-help booklets, video tapes, or working with office staff or with the physician himself or herself. This visit should include exploring the barriers to cessation and overcoming them with client-centered suggestions supplemented by professional ideas. Intensive treatment is needed for those smokers who have been unsuccessful in previous attempts. One option is for the patients in this category to be referred to a formal smoking cessation program. They also are candidates for nicotine replacement therapy.

Nicotine replacement therapy is appropriate for those patients who have severe nicotine withdrawal symptoms. Withdrawal symptoms include craving, anxiety, irritability, frustration, anger, difficulty concentrating, restlessness, increased appetite, weight gain, decreased heart rate, disrupted sleep, and dysphoric moods. These symptoms can be ascertained by simple questioning and by quantitating the number of cigarettes smoked: if the patient smokes more than 25 per day, smokes within 30 minutes of arising, smokes when ill, and cannot refrain from smoking for more than a few hours, he or she is a candidate. Frequently mentioned in the literature is the Fagerstrom Tolerance Questionnaire, a seven-item self-administered form that identifies behaviors that reflect nicotine dependence. In fact, in clinical practice this questionnaire is often not necessary. Most patients can give the physician a clear indication of their addiction to nicotine by describing what has happened in their prior cessation attempts. The result of all this questioning is to determine clearly that the patient is smoking to control the withdrawal symptoms resulting from abstinence. Careful questioning about previous cessation attempts can be very helpful in learning about the reasons for relapse and in helping to plan to deal with these signs and symptoms. Tests have been developed to ascertain levels of nicotine exposure. These tests vary from measuring nicotine levels or its metabolites in urine or blood to measurement of carbon monoxide in expired breath samples. Although these tests may add some physiologic

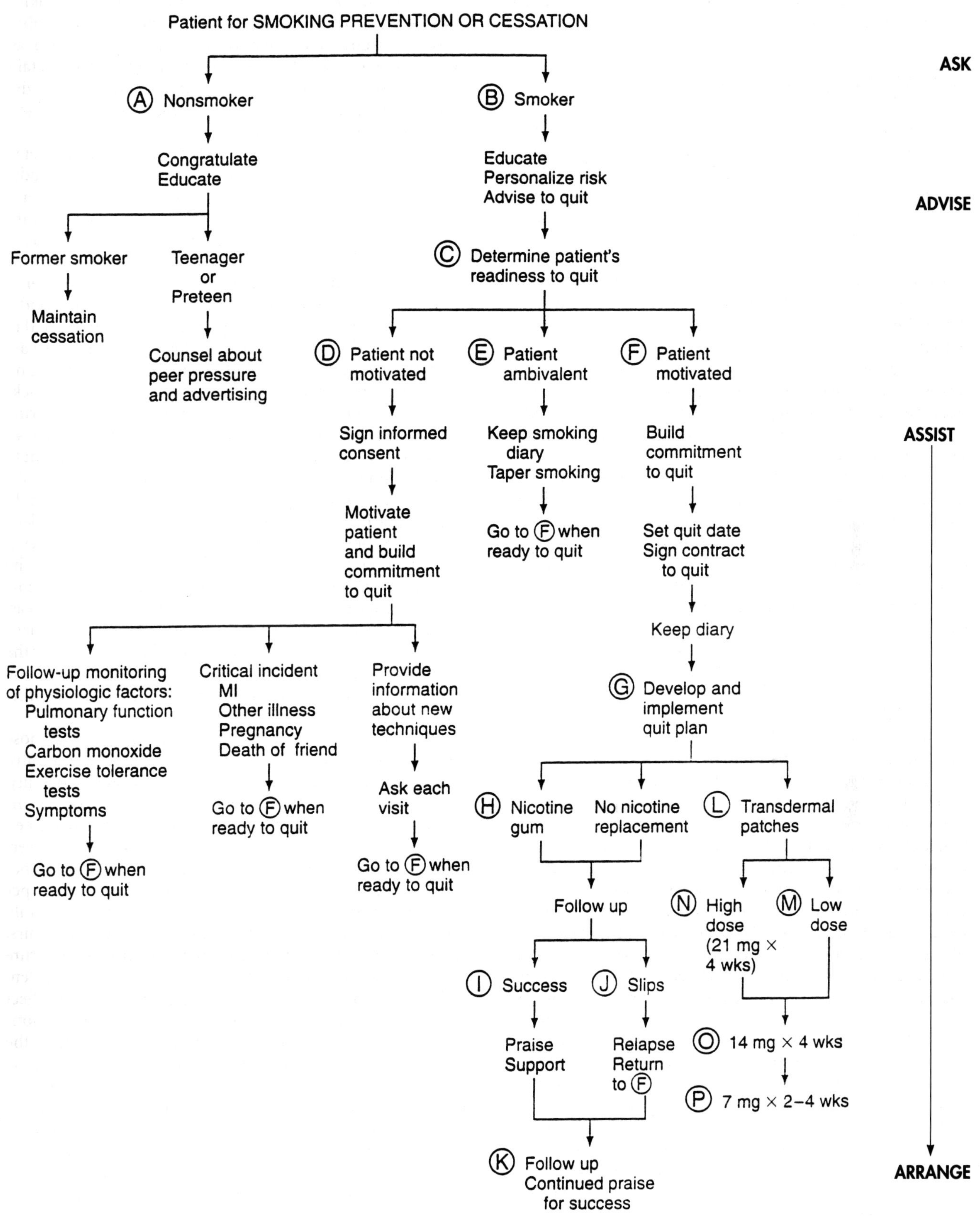

Figure 1
Algorithm for office-based programs of smoking prevention or cessation. *(From Greene HL, Johnson WP, Maricic MJ, eds. Decision making in medicine. St. Louis: Mosby–Year Book, 1993:505.)*

measurements, they increase cost and time and, in most cases, are probably not necessary.

The last step in the NCI program is *arranging* follow-up visits. Most people will relapse within the first week after their quit date, and many will find the first 48 to 72 hours the most difficult. Simple telephone availability for support may be extremely valuable during this period, although it has not been studied in detail. Most physicians would recommend that the follow-up appointment occur within 1 week after the quit date and include questions about smoking status, congratulations for those who have been successful, brainstorming any high-risk situations that are coming up, and rehearsing the coping strategies for these situations. For those smokers who have slipped during this period, it is helpful to discuss the triggers for the slip and what was learned from the experience and to review the new quit date in anticipation of success. Trials have shown that offering follow-up visits to discuss smoking increases the success of physician counseling and leads to increased 1-year and long-term cessation rates. If withdrawal symptoms are significant, they may be treated as appropriate. If the smoker has been unable to remain abstinent, reframing the issues to present some measure of success is often helpful: "Look you made it for 1 week—that's a good start!" The physician's counseling can be supplemented by the use of office personnel who have an interest in smoking. These individuals can help, for example, by asking about smoking at the time the patient checks in or while weight and blood pressure are being taken. They also can assist in labeling the chart to identify the smoker, and they can arrange reading materials in the waiting room so that smoking cessation brochures are available.

■ PHARMACOLOGIC TREATMENT

Nicotine replacement therapy is designed to replace the blood levels of nicotine in a form other than tobacco in order to block the withdrawal symptoms while the smoker is learning to break the habit of cigarette handling and inhalation of tobacco smoke. It allows the smoker to break the habit first and to taper the nicotine dependence at a later date. Currently in the United States, nicotine replacement is available in the form of gum and transdermal patches. The supply of nicotine via the gum and the patch is in most cases at a lower level and without the initial spike that seems to be associated with the pleasure of smoking. The blood levels obtained are, however, adequate to blunt the nicotine withdrawal symptoms and are the major rationale for its use. Multirandomized placebo control trials have shown the effectiveness of both patches and gum if used appropriately. The randomized control trials of the patches have shown greater levels of success than have those of the gum. Part of the problem with the gum is adequate and timed use. In either case, it is critical for the patient to understand how nicotine replacement works and how the gum or patches are to be used. Contraindications to nicotine replacement include acute or recent cardiovascular events, myocardial infarctions, unstable angina, serious arrhythmia, or pregnancy. Although there have been anecdotal reports of myocardial infarction in patients who were smoking while simultaneously using the patch, these reports do not seem to have occurred in enough numbers to be attributed to more than chance. One recent study (Joseph and co-workers, 1996) has shown the safety of transdermal nicotine in a high-risk cardiac population. The gum should not be used in those patients with temporomandibular joint disease and should be discussed with a dentist before being used in the presence of extensive dental appliances. Nicotine replacement is probably safer than smoking cigarettes, but approved labels and medicolegal concerns discourage use in other than approved settings. Some clinicians have used it in pregnant patients who are unable to stop smoking after behavioral programs but have done so only after carefully documenting a risk-benefit discussion with the patient and obtaining a signed informed consent.

Transdermal nicotine patches are designed to continuously release a fixed dose, which gradually ebbs and which is absorbed through the skin and into the bloodstream. The products that are available have all been shown to be more effective than placebo, and although there are arguments among manufacturers about the efficacy of one over the other, clear studies have not shown an advantage of one patch over another. The common side effects include erythema and skin irritation; the latter can be treated with topical steroids. Reports of vivid dreams, insomnia, and nervousness are also fairly common but are not significant enough to cause discontinuance in most cases. When these side effects occur patches can be removed at bedtime, a 16-hour patch can be used, or a lower-dose nicotine patch can be prescribed. The smoker applies the patch in the morning to a clean spot of skin and rotates the skin sites each morning afterward. Product doses are described in Table 1. Most of the patches are available in different doses to allow for tapering, and most patch manufacturers recommend continuing the use for several months. The starting dose is lower depending on the individual's weight. The patient should review the product information and prescribing information before use.

Nicotine gum is available in both 2 mg and 4 mg dosages. The gum should be used regularly at a timed interval and must be chewed in a specific way. A piece of gum is chewed until the nicotine is released, which produces a tart or pepper-like taste, and is then "parked" between the gum and the buccal mucosa to allow for nicotine absorption. Eating and drinking while the gum is in place should be discouraged, and the patient should avoid acidic beverages prior to gum use because this alters absorption. Reactions to the gum include stomach upset, hiccups, dizziness, nausea, and reflux, as well as jaw soreness and occasional local ulcerations. Clinicians who specialize in smoking cessation in general believe that the fixed-dose schedule and chewing a piece every 30 minutes each hour while awake will help achieve adequate blood levels and prevent the withdrawal symptoms. In most of the early drug trials, many of the patients did not even get the prescription filled and many others did not use the medication as suggested, thus leading to a lack of efficacy. This result highlights the importance of the physician spending time to discuss the gum use with the patient.

Because both of these products are now available over the counter, the impact of patient understanding of the use of both patches and gum is clear. It would be worthwhile for the physician to take time to explain gum and/or patch use or to provide information on this for patient reading.

Table 1 Nicotine Replacement Products

BRAND NAME (MANUFACTURER)	NICOTINE CONTENT (MG)	DOSAGE PER DAY	RECOMMENDED DURATION OF USE
Transdermal nicotine patch			
Habitrol (*Ciba-Geigy*)			
21 mg	52.5	21 mg/24 hr	4–8 wk
14 mg	35.0	14 mg/24 hr	2–4 wk
7 mg	17.5	7 mg/24 hr	2–4 wk
Nicoderm (*Marion Merrell Dow*)			
21 mg	114.0	21 mg/24 hr	4–8 wk
14 mg	78.0	14 mg/24 hr	2–4 wk
7 mg	36.0	7 mg/24 hr	2–4 wk
Nicotrol (*Parke-Davis*)			
15 mg	24.9	15 mg/16 hr	4–12 wk
10 mg	16.6	10 mg/16 hr	2–4 wk
5 mg	8.3	5 mg/16 hr	2–4 wk
Nicotine gum			
Nicorette 2 mg (*Marion Merrell Dow*)	2.0	9–12 pieces/day* (maximum 30)	2–3 mo (maximum 6)
Nicorette DS (*Marion Merrell Dow*)	4.0	9–12 pieces/day* (maximum 20)	2–3 mo (maximum 6)

*Chew as needed or one piece every 1 to 2 hours while awake.
Modified from Nicotine patches, Med Lett 1992; 34:37.

■ OTHER PHARMACOLOGIC AGENTS

A number of pharmacologic agents from tranquilizers to sleeping pills to clonidine have been used with some reports of success. Overall, however, these agents have not been found to be beneficial in long-term cessation, and the quest for a silver bullet for smoking cessation continues. One agent that is currently undergoing testing is the serotonin reuptake inhibitor fluoxetine, which has the additional benefit of treating depression. It is currently undergoing placebo control trials to determine if it adds to smoking cessation success. Early reports are that it does, and it is currently being considered for release by the Food and Drug Administration.

■ NEW DEVICES

Nicotine administration via nasal spray and inhaler is currently being evaluated. These routes of administration have the advantage of producing nicotine peaks that more closely simulate those produced by smoking. This feature theoretically may make them more likely to be subject to abuse or to habituation in place of cigarettes. The latter case may be better because of the absence of the carcinogen in smoke and would certainly eliminate the problem of passive smoke for others in the nicotine-addicted person's environment.

Suggested Reading

Albright CL, Farquhar JW. Principles of behavioral change. In: Greene HL, Glassock RJ, Kelly MA, eds. Introduction to clinical medicine. Philadelphia: BC Decker, 1991:596.

Bartecchi CE, MacKenzie TD, Schrier RW. The human costs of tobacco use. N Engl J Med 1994; 907–911, 975–980.

Bronson DC, et al. Smoking cessation counseling during periodic health exams. Arch Intern Med 1989; 149:1653.

Cummings SR, et al. Training physicians in counseling about smoking cessation: A randomized trial of the "quit for life" program. Ann Intern Med 1989; 110:640.

DeNelsky GY. Smoking cessation strategies that work. Cleve Clin J Med 1990; 57:416.

Greene HL, Garcia LA. Smoking cessation. In: Greene HL, Johnson WP, Maricic MJ, eds. Decision making in medicine. St. Louis: Mosby–Year Book, 1993:502.

Guise BJ, Goldstein MG, Clark MM, Thebarge RW. Behavior change: The example of smoking. In: Noble J, Greene HL, Levenson W, eds. Primary care medicine. St. Louis: Mosby–Year Book, 1996:1650.

Huston CG, et al. How to help your patients stop smoking. Am Fam Physician 1990; 42:1017.

Joseph AM, Norman SM, Ferry LH. The safety of transdermal nicotine as an aid to smoking cessation in patients with cardiac disease. N Engl J Med 1996; 335:1792–1798.

Ockene JK. Cigarette smoking. In: Greene HL, Glassock RJ, Kelly MA, eds. Introduction to clinical medicine. Philadelphia: BC Decker, 1991:589.

Ockene JK, Kristeller J, Goldbert R. Increasing the efficacy of physician delivered smoking interventions: A randomized clinical trial. J Gen Med 1991; 6:1.

CHRONIC FATIGUE SYNDROME

Gary P. Holmes, M.D.

The chronic fatigue syndrome (CFS) is a complex, often severely debilitating condition that continues to discourage and bewilder affected patients and their physicians. In the mid-1980s several reports described a nonspecific, chronic debilitating illness associated with elevated serum levels of Epstein-Barr virus (EBV) antibodies, but this association has since been disproved in several studies. The promulgation of competing case definitions and numerous unproven diagnostic tests and treatments has added to the confusion for the average physician evaluating chronically fatigued patients. An international working group convened by the Centers for Disease Control and Prevention (CDC) has developed a new, unified, and updated case definition, which is aimed at research applications but incorporates recent knowledge gained from the better scientific studies and clarifies the complex nature of the syndrome. It includes an algorithm for evaluation that has not been clinically validated but is reasonable and straightforward (Fig. 1). Several studies have identified no significant clinical or laboratory differences between patients who fulfill CFS criteria and chronically fatigued patients not fulfilling the CFS criteria. The new guidelines acknowledge this concept by defining a broad illness, idio-

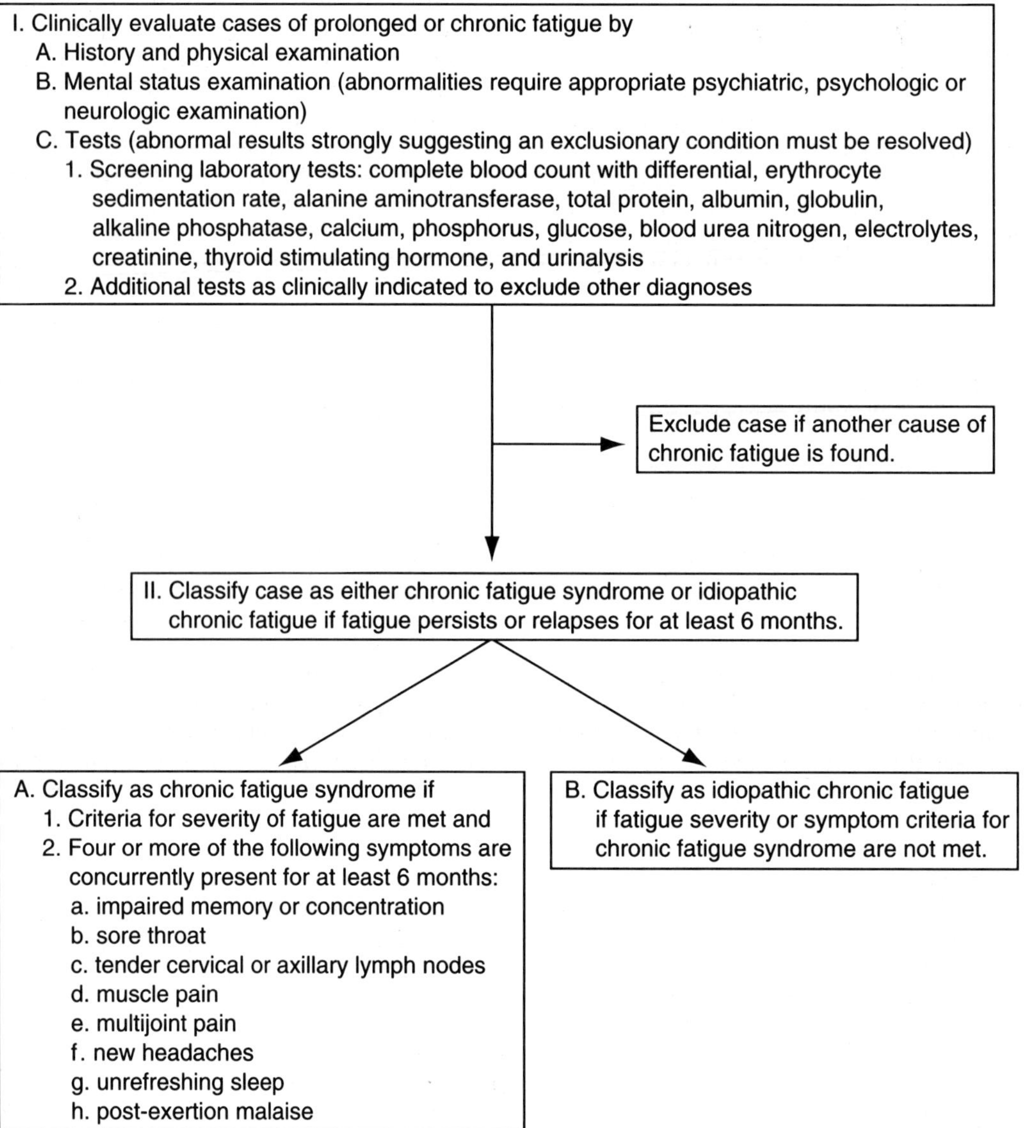

Figure 1
Algorithm for evaluating patients with chronic fatigue. *(From Fukuda K, Straus SE, Hickie I, et al. Chronic fatigue syndrome: A comprehensive approach to its definition and study, Ann Intern Med 1994; 121:953–959).*

pathic chronic fatigue, within which the more specific illness of CFS resides. Idiopathic chronic fatigue, probably more diagnostically appropriate than CFS for routine clinical use, is the basis for the following diagnostic and therapeutic approach.

■ BACKGROUND

Etiologic Studies

Numerous hypotheses, including systemic candidiasis, human herpesvirus-6, retroviruses, and enteroviruses, have failed to withstand rigorous studies. No specific immunologic defects, such as decreased numbers or function of specific subsets of lymphocytes or immunoglobulin subset deficiencies, have been reproducibly detected. The most consistent correlations have been identified with emotional disorders, including major depression, dysthymia, atypical depression, somatization, and anxiety disorders.

Therapeutic Studies

Numerous treatments for CFS, including acyclovir, intravenous immunoglobulin, a synthetic RNA oligopeptide, and a host of questionable and often bizarre alternative therapies, have been promoted. To date those that have been subjected to controlled trials have not produced consistent benefit. The most promising treatments appear to center on education, antidepressants, and psychiatric therapy as indicated, and progressive exercise regimens.

■ CLINICAL EVALUATION

General Medical History

Most patients describe a panoply of chronic or recurring symptoms that are usually vaguely defined, nonspecific, and unmeasurable. Generally they suggest no specific pathologic process. Most are common to the human condition, such as vague aches and pains, headaches, or tiredness from overexertion or lack of sleep, but have become incapacitating due to a perception of excessive severity or chronicity. Complaints of recurrent sore throat and upper respiratory infections rarely exceed the normal range of three to five infections per year, and complaints of fever or perceived feverishness are rarely documented to exceed the normal temperature range.

Several factors should be kept in mind during the evaluation (Table 1). The physician's responsibility is to identify symptoms suggesting a focal abnormality that should lead to further evaluation for any diagnosable medical condition such as hypothyroidism, autoimmune disorder, or other organ system disease. Taking a detailed clinical history often requires 30 to 60 minutes, but it is an absolute necessity. Emphasis should be placed on identifying previous episodes of similar illnesses or symptoms; medical, psychiatric, and substance abuse histories; and detailed descriptions of the most significant symptoms (e.g., frequency, severity, duration, progressive worsening or improvement, inciting events). Many patients are highly defensive and distrustful of physicians, and they may hold tightly to preconceived ideas regarding the causes of their symptoms. Breaking through this defensive barrier requires tact but is critical to a reasonable diagnostic and therapeutic outcome, and it can be accomplished in most cases with a logical discussion of pertinent research results. In my experience, most CFS patients have been evaluated by several other physicians and describe a generally negative impression of the medical profession. In some cases this results from unreasonable expectations on the part of the patient, but all too often it is because the physician did not take time to listen to the complaints and rationally address the concerns. This cycle of doctor shopping may be broken by an understanding and caring physician who takes time to listen.

Psychiatric History

Extensive evidence now indicates that any of several psychiatric disorders may be detectable in up to 50 percent of patients with chronic fatigue. These must be actively sought in the initial evaluation of all patients. A careful history will often identify previous episodes of similar symptoms and not uncommonly will identify previous episodes of depression, suicide attempts, or drug or alcohol abuse. Formal evaluation may identify major psychological stressors ranging from excessively demanding bosses to physical or sexual abuse in some patients who fail to describe such events as part of their routine medical histories. Social isolation is a common problem that probably contributes to perpetuation of symptoms. This may be self-imposed as a result of depression with anhedonia or chronic illness, or it may result from the progressive alienation of family and friends who believe the person is feigning illness or who simply give up attempting to involve the person in their activities. Spouses often perceive such persons as failing to support their responsibilities to the family, leading to marital discord and often to divorce. Such events undoubtedly contribute to the emotional aspects of the illness.

Unfortunately, physicians often have difficulty in diagnosing depression and other emotional disorders in patients with chronic fatigue, and many patients refuse to consider the possibility unless a reasonable justification is provided them. As a result it is often easier to provide an alternative, albeit useless, diagnosis such as a chronic viral infection or immunologic disorder. This disservice to the patient occurs all too commonly and perpetuates the cycle of doctor shopping. The newly revised CFS guidelines now recommend at least a formal mental status examination for all patients being evaluated for chronic fatigue (see Fig. 1). This limited recommendation reflects concerns about the availability of psychologi-

Table 1 Concepts in Evaluating Patients with Idiopathic Chronic Fatigue

1. A detailed history and physical examination are required.
2. All chronic fatigue patients should be referred for formal psychological testing.
3. A basic laboratory evaluation is sufficient in the absence of specific localizing symptoms and signs (see Fig. 1).
4. Viral serologic studies, including Epstein-Barr virus antibodies, and immunologic studies such as immunoglobulin levels and lymphocyte enumeration and function panels are not indicated in the absence of recent prolonged febrile illness or recurrent atypical infections suggesting possible immunodeficiency states.

cal testing to the average physician—the view of most experts is that formal psychological testing is a mandatory step in the initial evaluation of all chronic fatigue patients.

Not all patients with idiopathic chronic fatigue have psychiatric illness. While some patients are obviously clinically depressed, a significant number may have no evidence of significant psychiatric illness after formal evaluation. This distinction is important in determining a treatment approach. Obviously, those with overt psychiatric disease require specific treatment, regardless of whatever other conditions may be contributing to their symptoms. For most patients who have overt psychiatric diseases amenable to specific treatment, therapy will lead to marked improvement and occasionally to complete resolution of symptoms.

Physical Examination

Physical examination rarely identifies significant abnormalities suggesting a cause of the symptoms, but may detect the occasional patient with previously undiagnosed hypothyroidism, subacute endocarditis, autoimmune disease, congestive heart failure, diabetes mellitus, or other chronic systemic disease.

Laboratory Evaluation

In the absence of focal symptoms or signs, laboratory evaluation should be directed toward ruling out the more common organic causes (see Fig. 1). In this setting, cultures and serologic tests for viruses, lymphocyte function and enumeration studies, immunoglobulin electrophoresis, and computed tomography or magnetic resonance imaging studies are of no diagnostic value. Numerous patients with idiopathic chronic fatigue continue to be told they suffer from chronic EBV infection due to inappropriate use of EBV serologic tests. The physician must explain to the patient that such tests have no apparent clinical value for diagnosis, prognosis, or therapy.

■ THERAPY

Clearly, no two CFS patients are alike, and no standard treatment will be helpful to all patients (Table 2). Assuming no specific physical or psychiatric abnormalities were detected during the initial evaluation, the most important aspect of treatment is to reassure the patient that there is no evidence for a chronic, incurable viral illness or immunologic disorder. The patient may also be reassured that the illness can often be overcome with a concerted personal effort and appropriate medical and psychiatric therapy. Most patients' concerns may be alleviated by the simple assurance that there is no detectable serious chronic, progressive, or life-threatening disorder.

This accomplished, the next step is aggressive treatment of any diagnosed psychiatric condition. Some, such as major depression, dysthymia, and atypical depression, are directly treatable with antidepressants. Although no adequate controlled studies confirm this approach, the most effective agents with the best levels of tolerance appear to be the selective serotonin reuptake inhibitors. Low doses of fluoxetine or paroxetine (20 mg orally every morning) or sertraline (50 mg orally every morning) will produce significant improvement in many patients. Most patients who are going to respond will notice at least some improvement at these dosages within a month. Those who derive incomplete benefit after a month of therapy should be advised to increase the dosage to two tablets every morning for another month, and so forth until maximal benefit, maximal recommended dosage, or intolerable side effects are apparent. If the first agent tried is ineffective, another of these agents will often be therapeutic. In general, the only significant side effects of these medications are related to overstimulation (agitation, sleeplessness), and usually resolve with dose reduction. Sleeplessness often responds to addition of doxepin or amitriptyline 10 to 25 mg orally at bedtime.

Table 2 Concepts in Treating Patients with Idiopathic Chronic Fatigue

1. There is no single therapeutic approach. Treatment is multidimensional and is highly dependent upon the motivation of the patient.
2. Reassurance is therapeutically important:
   a. There is no evidence of any serious organic condition based upon the history, examination, and laboratory testing.
   b. There is no apparent infectious or immunologic cause.
   c. There is no evidence of transmissibility to others.
3. Psychiatric conditions, such as dysthymia, depression, anxiety, and personality disorders, must be treated if they are present.
4. A slowly progressive exercise program should be encouraged.
5. Isolation contributes to the illness. Reentry into society must be strongly encouraged.

Other psychiatric disorders, such as anxiety and somatization disorders, various personality disorders, and other complex conditions, usually are much more resistant to therapy and should be referred for psychiatric follow-up. Spouse abuse or any other detected social problems should be referred to appropriate resources for intervention. For those who have no identifiable psychiatric disorder, I have little specific advice. Reassurance and symptomatic therapy are probably the only interventions indicated for these patients, many of whom feel much better after being told they have no evidence of chronic viral disease.

Most of the physical complaints in CFS patients with diagnosed psychiatric disorders are so tightly interlinked with emotional factors that other therapeutic intervention should be deferred until specific psychiatric or antidepressant therapy has been maximized. While awaiting clinical responses from these interventions, head and body aches, myalgia, and arthralgia may be managed with nonsteroidal anti-inflammatory agents. There is clearly no indication for the use of experimental or alternative therapy in managing idiopathic chronic fatigue.

Exercise is an important adjunctive treatment for essentially all CFS patients. Many patients have been advised to rest by their physicians under the old belief that physical exertion may worsen any active chronic infection. Given that no such chronic infection has been detected in most CFS patients, such limitation of exertion has limited usefulness and probably exacerbates the condition. Physical deconditioning, which is to be expected in patients who are inactive secondary to depression, lack of motivation, or any prolonged illness, will lead to progressively reduced exercise tolerance that is easily misinterpreted as part of the underlying disease process.

Depressed patients cannot be expected to attempt physical exercise until their depressive symptoms have improved, and an exercise program should be deferred until antidepressant therapy has produced some benefit. Patients should be advised not to attempt levels of exercise they may have been able to accomplish before they became ill, because they will undoubtedly fail and feel more fatigued for several days afterward. Initial efforts should aim for achievable goals of 5 to 10 minutes of steady walking every 2 to 3 days for 1 or 2 weeks, depending upon the level of deconditioning. As tolerated, the duration of exertion should be extended by 10 to 15 minutes every 2 weeks and the pace increased, with a goal of 30 to 45 minutes of fairly brisk walking or similar exercise at least every other day. The effect of this slowly progressive program is to improve muscle and cardiovascular tone, but it also generates an overall sense of well-being, inspires confidence, and allows the patient to set achievable short-term and long-term goals. Patients should also be encouraged to increase social contacts with family and friends. Cognitive behavioral therapy, a formal approach to increasing physical and social activity, has yielded significant benefit in some studies, but in other studies it has been matched by a less formal physician-initiated approach similar to that described previously.

Regular follow-up is helpful and is necessary for patients who are begun on antidepressant therapy. A compassionate physician who is available to answer questions and concerns will often provide sufficient reassurance and support, especially during the critical first few months of therapy, while the patient remains unconvinced that the illness can be mitigated or conquered. Periodic follow-up evaluations are also advisable, especially in the group with no identifiable psychiatric diagnoses, to detect previously undiagnosed indolent disease processes.

Suggested Reading

Blondel-Hill E, Shafran SD. Treatment of the chronic fatigue syndrome: A review and practical guide. Drugs 1993; 46:639–651.

Fukuda K, Straus SE, Hickie I, et al. Chronic fatigue syndrome: A comprehensive approach to its definition and study. Ann Intern Med 1994; 121:953–959.

Goodnick PJ, Sandoval R. Psychotropic treatment of chronic fatigue syndrome and related disorders. J Clin Psychiatry 1993; 54:13–20.

Wilson A, Hickie I, Lloyd A, Wakefield D. The treatment of chronic fatigue syndrome: Science and speculation. Am J Med 1994; 96:544–550.

ADVICE FOR TRAVELERS

Phyllis E. Kozarsky, M.D.

Studies show that 50 to 75 percent of short-term travelers to the tropics or subtropics develop some health impairment. Fortunately, most problems are minor, with only 5 percent requiring medical attention and fewer than 1 percent requiring hospitalization. Valuable sources of information for travel health advisers are found in Table 1.

All travelers should be encouraged to carry a travel health kit, which should always remain with the traveler and never be stowed with baggage (Table 2).

IMMUNIZATIONS

Immunizations may be divided into those of worldwide importance and those of special importance to certain travelers. Those of worldwide importance should be considered by physicians not only for travelers but also for the general public who are at risk. Examples of those having worldwide importance include diphtheria, tetanus, polio, measles, mumps, and rubella (MMR), influenza, pneumococcus, and hepatitis B vaccines (see the chapter *Immunizations*) Immunizations of special importance for certain travelers include yellow fever, typhoid, cholera, rabies, meningococcal meningitis, Japanese B encephalitis, and hepatitis A. Two vaccines rarely indicated are plague and tick-borne encephalitis, the latter of which is not available in the United States. Immunizations should always be recommended according to risk of disease and not according to the country visited.

Most vaccines may be administered simultaneously. A notable exception is measles vaccine, which should be administered at least 2 weeks before or 6 weeks after the receipt of immunoglobulin for hepatitis A protection. In addition, if measles and yellow fever vaccines are not administered simultaneously, they should be separated by an interval of at least 30 days. When both cholera and yellow fever vaccines are indicated, antibody levels have been highest when their administration was separated by at least 3 weeks. Table 3 lists the immunizations of special importance and their schedules.

Immunizations of Worldwide Importance

Diphtheria and Tetanus

Diphtheria continues to be a problem worldwide, with recent outbreaks affecting areas in eastern Europe. Serosurveys have shown that tetanus titers are lacking in many Americans, particularly in women and in adults over 50. A diphtheria-tetanus booster should be administered at 10 year intervals. Physicians may encourage frequent high-risk travelers to receive a tetanus booster alone every 5 years, since a tetanus-prone wound does not necessitate a booster, or tetanus immunoglobulin if tetanus toxoid has been given within 5 years.

Table 1 Sources of Information for Travel Health Advisers

Health Information for International Travel. Published by the U.S. Department of Health and Human Services (CDC) 1997. Available from the Superintendent of Documents, Government Printing Office, Washington, D.C. 20402. Telephone 202-783-3238. A yearly updated book reviewing malaria chemoprophylaxis, immunization requirements, and recommendations for international travel.

Centers for Disease Control and Prevention Voice Information System, Atlanta. A computer-assisted telephone information hotline for worldwide travel health advice. Telephone 404-332-4559. Fax capability available.

International Association for Medical Assistance to Travelers (IAMAT), 736 Center Street, Lewiston, NY 14092. Telephone 716-754-4883. Provides information on tropical diseases, climate charts, list of English-speaking physicians.

Travel Medicine Advisor. Published by American Health Consultants, Atlanta, GA. This comprehensive looseleaf text, continually revised, provides bimonthly updates and alerts. Telephone 404-262-7436.

Health Hints for the Tropics. Published by the American Society of Tropical Medicine and Hygiene (ASTM&H) and written by several of its members. Authoritative source of information for the travel health adviser and for the traveler. Available from ASTM&H Headquarters, 60 Revere Drive, Suite 500, Northbrook, IL 60062. Telephone 708-480-9592.

International Society of Travel Medicine (ISTM). An association of travel health advisers. The ISTM sponsors biannual meetings. Members receive a quarterly journal and newsletter. For information fax 770-736-6732.

Polio

Studies in the United States have found varying levels of immunity to polio in the general population, with recent data revealing 12 percent of adult American travelers unprotected against at least one serogroup. The Centers for Disease Control and Prevention (CDC) recommends that all adults complete a primary series if they have never received one, and also receive a booster dose of polio vaccine once only prior to travel to an endemic area. If time permits, infants and children under 2 years of age should receive at least three doses of oral polio vaccine. Intervals between doses may be reduced to 4 weeks to maximize immunization status before departure.

Countries considered free of endemic wild poliovirus circulation are the United States, Canada, Japan, Australia, New Zealand, and most of eastern and western Europe. The western hemisphere may indeed be polio free, as there have been no reported cases of paralytic disease caused by wild poliovirus in the Americas in several years.

Measles, Mumps, and Rubella

Measles continues to be a major cause of morbidity and mortality in the developing world. Outbreaks of measles in the United States have been linked to cases of imported measles. In the 1980s, it was estimated that over 25 percent of cases of measles in the United States could be attributed directly or epidemiologically to importations. Because the rate of primary failure with the vaccine was somewhat greater in persons born after 1956 and vaccinated before 1980, the CDC recommends that travelers in this group be revaccinated. A recent serosurvey found that almost 10 percent of

Table 2 Travel Health Kit

- Usual prescription drugs
- Aspirin (Tylenol, NSAID)
- Bismuth subsalicylate
- Sunscreen
- Antihistamine, decongestant
- Insect repellent
- Rehydration solution packets
- Steroid cream
- Loperamide
- Codeine tablets
- Mild sedative
- High-altitude sickness prophylaxis
- Antimalarial chemoprophylaxis
- Thermometer
- Bandages, gauze, adhesive
- Antiseptic solution
- Antacid
- Anti-motion sickness medication
- Laxative
- Cough preparation
- Topical antifungal, antibacterial cream or ointment
- Antibiotic for self-treatment of traveler's diarrhea

American travelers born after 1956 were seronegative for measles. Immunization may be given at 6 months of age if necessary for travel, followed by a booster injection at 15 months.

Mumps and rubella are less of a health threat to travelers, though both diseases may have serious complications. A report of aseptic meningitis due to mumps in an American returning from Kenya, and reports of rubella outbreaks in the late 1980s in the Pacific, reawaken the need to consider protection for all travelers against these illnesses.

Pneumococcus and Influenza

The pneumococcus and influenza vaccines should be administered to those at risk for severe illness due to these infections. Bear in mind that influenza may occur year round, depending on the traveler's destination.

Hepatitis B

Hepatitis B vaccine has typically been reserved for persons such as health care workers in contact with blood or body fluid secretions in developing countries and for long-term travelers to countries with a high prevalence of infection. Ideally, however, everyone should be immunized against this most important cause of acute and chronic liver disease. In Asia and Africa up to 20 percent of children and adults are hepatitis B carriers. As of November 1991 the vaccine has been recommended in the United States for all infants.

Immunizations of Special Importance for the Traveler

Yellow Fever

Yellow fever is a viral illness transmitted by mosquitoes in tropical Africa and South America. It is rare in travelers, but because of its high mortality, individuals journeying to endemic areas require protection. Some countries require evidence of vaccination from all entering travelers and even from individuals whose destination is a noninfected area but

Table 3 Immunizations for Foreign Travel

VACCINE	ADULT DOSE	DURATION OF EFFICACY
LIVE ATTENUATED		
Yellow fever	1 (0.5 ml) SC 10 days to 10 years before travel	Booster q10yr
Typhoid	1 enteric-coated capsule taken on alternate days for 4 doses with cool liquid 1 hour before a meal	Booster series q5yr
INACTIVATED		
Typhoid	1 dose (0.5 ml) IM	Booster q2yr
Cholera	2 doses (0.5 ml) SC or IM 1 wk to 1 mo or more apart and at least 6 days before travel	Booster q6mo
Rabies pre-exposure* (HDCV or rabies vaccine adsorbed)	3 doses (1.0 ml) IM (deltoid) on days 0, 7, and 21 or 28 (HDCV may be administered ID 0.1 ml days 0, 7, and 21 or 28)	1 dose (1 ml) IM (deltoid)† (or HDCV 0.1 ml ID) q2yr
Meningococcal (quadrivalent A/C/Y/W-135)	1 dose (0.5 ml) SC	Duration of immunity unknown; booster recommended q3yr
Japanese B encephalitis	3 doses (1 ml) SC days 0, 7, 30	Duration of immunity unknown; booster recommended at 3 yr
Hepatitis A	2 doses, at 0 and 6–12 mo	Unknown
PASSIVE PROPHYLAXIS		
Immunoglobulin for protection against hepatitis A	0.02 ml/kg for travel <3 mo 0.04 ml/kg for travel 4–6 mo	Repeat dose q4–6mo

*If traveler is taking chloroquine or mefloquine for malaria chemoprophylaxis, the series must be completed prior to initiation of antimalarial treatment. If not possible, IM dosing must be used.
†If risk is high and continuous, serology should be checked every 6 mo. Acceptable antibody level is ≥1.5 titer by rapid fluorescent focus inhibition test.
SC, subcutaneous; IM, intramuscular; HDCV, human diploid cell vaccine; ID, intradermal.

who will be crossing the yellow fever zone. The vaccine can be administered only at an approved yellow fever vaccination center. State and local health departments may administer the vaccine or can advise where it can be obtained. Documentation of yellow fever vaccination should be placed on the International Certificate of Vaccination card, which may be obtained from the U.S. Government Printing Office, 412-644-2721, and which should be carried with the passport. Individuals for whom the vaccine is contraindicated must carry a waiver on a physician's letterhead to prevent the possibility of requiring an injection at a border.

Typhoid

Though *Salmonella typhi* is prevalent in many countries in Africa, Asia, and Central and South America, typhoid fever is not common in travelers. The Inactivated Vi polysaccharide (Pasteur Merieux) vaccine, or the oral Ty21a (Berna) vaccine, the products of choice, should be used by travelers to endemic areas who are going off tourist routes or who are particularly adventuresome with regard to their food and beverage intake. In addition, long-term and frequent short-term travelers to developing countries should receive vaccine.

Cholera

Cholera is caused by ingestion of food or beverage contaminated with *Vibrio cholera,* an organism found in raw sewage. The risk of cholera to travelers is extremely low, estimated to be about 1 case per 500,000 journeys to endemic regions. Most cases occur in travelers returning from visits to family, relatives, and friends in endemic countries. These groups tend to have a greater likelihood of dietary indiscretion. Drinking safe beverages and eating well-cooked food, especially seafood, is the best prevention.

The vaccine requires two injections for a maximum protection of 30 percent to 50 percent for only 3 to 6 months. Because of its poor efficacy, the vaccine is not cost effective for most travelers, even those who will be in endemic areas for long periods. Those for whom the vaccine may be appropriate are those living and working in an epidemic area, travelers with achlorhydria, and those who have had a gastrectomy. An oral cholera vaccine is now available in some countries in Europe and in Canada. Its usefulness is yet to be determined for most travelers.

Rabies

The pre-exposure rabies vaccine series should be administered to those spending more than 30 days where rabies is a constant threat. The risk is highest where dog rabies is highly endemic, such as Mexico, El Salvador, Guatemala, Peru, Colombia, Ecuador, India, Nepal, the Philippines, Sri Lanka, Thailand, and Vietnam. Of the 20 cases reported in the United States since 1980, 10 were acquired outside the country. Travelers should avoid contact with domestic animals, and if bitten, should wash the wound immediately with soap and water and seek medical care. Even if a pre-exposure rabies series has been administered, postexposure prophylaxis with rabies immunoglobulin and vaccine must be given.

Meningococcal Meningitis

The meningococcal meningitis vaccine is very protective against disease due to *Neisseria meningitidis* serogroups A, C, Y, and W-135. The vaccine is recommended for long-term travelers to the meningitis belt in sub-Saharan Africa and for short-term travelers during the dry season. It is also recommended for travelers to areas where outbreaks have occurred in the past decade, such as northern India, Nepal, Mecca, Chad, Burundi, Kenya, and Tanzania.

Japanese Encephalitis

Japanese encephalitis (JE) occurs in Asia during the summer and autumn in temperate regions and primarily during the rainy season in the tropics. It is transmitted by night-biting mosquitoes in rural rice-growing, pig-farming areas. Since 1981, 11 U.S. residents have been infected, eight of whom were military personnel or their dependents. Most travelers to Asia should not be immunized unless they are spending more than 4 weeks in an endemic area during transmission season.

Hepatitis A and Immunoglobulin

Hepatitis A is the most common immunizable infection in travelers. In contrast to other serious food-borne illnesses, many travel-related cases have occurred with standard tourist itineraries. In fact, the estimated incidence of symptomatic hepatitis A in travelers to the developing world per month of stay abroad is as high as 20 per 1,000 in some destinations. The new hepatitis A vaccine is highly immunogenic and will probably give years of protection. Immune globulin may also be used for short-term prophylaxis.

Malaria

For prevention of malaria, see the chapter *Malaria.*

Traveler's Diarrhea

Prevention of diarrhea requires careful selection of food and beverages while traveling in the developing world. Foods that are well-cooked and still hot or steaming are safe. Fruits peeled by the traveler are safe. Since vegetables such as lettuce and tomatoes grow in areas where human fertilizer may be used, and since they cannot be peeled, salads should be avoided unless washed carefully with purified water. Commercially bottled carbonated beverages, alcohol, hot tea, and coffee are also safe. The purity of plain bottled water is not regulated, so this is best avoided. Ice cubes should also be avoided, since they are often made with tap water. Milk and dairy products should be pasteurized, cooked, or avoided. Disinfection requires brief boiling or the use of halogens (e.g., chlorine, iodine), though the protozoan cysts of *Giardia lamblia* and *Entamoeba histolytica* are resistant to the latter. A variety of inexpensive portable purifiers that contain effective iodination are available from camping stores.

Prophylaxis of diarrhea with a daily dose of a quinolone antibiotic (e.g., 500 mg ciprofloxacin) or trimethoprim-sulfamethoxazole (one double-strength tablet) may be appropriate for short-term travelers who are at very high risk of illness or of serious complications of diarrhea. For more detail, see the chapter *Traveler's Diarrhea.*

Schistosomiasis

Schistosomiasis is caused by infection with a blood fluke, *Schistosoma mansoni, Schistosoma haematobium, or Schistosoma japonicum,* which in one part of its life cycle can penetrate the human skin without causing symptoms. A subacute illness similar to serum sickness may occur about 6 weeks after exposure, and chronic problems such as portal hypertension, urinary obstruction, and bladder cancer may result. In recent years reports of American travelers contracting schistosomiasis and developing unusual central nervous system findings such as transverse myelitis from aberrant egg deposition have heightened the awareness of this disease. Travelers to endemic areas put themselves at risk when they wade, swim, or bathe in freshwater lakes, streams, or rivers containing the reservoir snails.

If exposure to possibly infected water sources is unavoidable, towel-drying the skin immediately after contact may be protective.

■ MISCELLANEOUS CONSIDERATIONS

The human immunodeficiency virus (HIV)-infected traveler confronts several potential problems. The live oral polio and yellow fever vaccines are generally contraindicated because of the theoretic risk of infection from the vaccine strains of these viruses. The enhanced inactivated polio vaccine may be substituted, but there is no alternative for yellow fever protection. A physician may give a waiver if the yellow fever vaccine is required by the destination, but if the traveler will be in an area of high endemicity and if he or she is asymptomatic with a CD4 lymphocyte above 200 per cubic millimeter, it may be reasonable to give the vaccine. When it was inadvertently administered to HIV-infected military personnel, there were no adverse events. The new inactivated typhoid vaccine may be used if *Salmonella typhi* exposure is a possibility. Bacille Calmette-Guérin (BCG) is contraindicated because of the possibility of disseminated disease. Protection against measles is important, and thus immunization with measles, mumps, and rubella (MMR) is recommended; despite its being a live vaccine, there have been no severe complications from its use in these patients. Some countries have regulations preventing the entry of HIV-infected individuals, including tourists.

Even the most experienced travelers suffer jet lag. It is estimated that the body takes about one day to adjust for each time zone crossed. Adequate hydration while traveling, resting after arrival, and judicious use of short-acting benzodiazepines assist the adjustment. A variety of other maneuvers may be helpful as well. Few advocate the jet-lag diet, which alternates high- and low-protein meals and limits caffeine. Bright light can reset the internal clock. For travel eastward it is recommended that travelers seek bright light in the early morning, and for westward travel they should be in bright light in the late afternoon. Artificial light sources with the appropriate lux intensity may also be used. The use of melatonin is being investigated for this purpose, and results are promising; however, the melatonin tablets available in health food stores may not contain standardized amount of hormone and therefore cannot be recommended.

Suggested Reading

Gardner P, ed. Health issues of international travelers. Infect Dis Clin North Am 1992; 6:275–510.

Wolfe MS, ed. Travel medicine. Med Clin North Am 1992; 76:1261–1497.

Public Health Service. Health Information for international travel 1995 Atlanta: Health and Human Services Publication No. (CDC) 95:8280

Wyler DJ. Malaria chemoprophylaxis for the traveler. N Engl J Med 1993; 329:31–37.

IMMUNIZATIONS

Elaine C. Jong, M.D.

Immunizations, or vaccines, are important to the prevention of infectious diseases. Protective immunity against many serious diseases can be elicited through active immunization, the administration of specific antigens (killed or attenuated micro-organisms; purified polysaccharides, proteins, or other components; or recombinant antigens produced by genetic engineering) that stimulate the host's production of protective antibodies. Antigens may be given orally or by intradermal, subcutaneous, or intramuscular injection. In addition, through passive immunization, protective immunity may be obtained through transfer of preformed antibodies from an immune host to a nonimmune recipient, either as immunoglobulin or antibody-specific immunoglobulin.

Protective efficacy resulting from active immunization with a vaccine depends on several factors: the age of the host, with decreased efficacy of certain vaccines observed in the very young and very old; the immune status of the host, with decreased efficacy observed in persons with immunosuppression due to disease or therapy; and the characteristics of the vaccine itself.

The protection elicited by active immunization is relatively long lasting. Protective levels of specific antibodies usually develop within 2 to 4 weeks of primary immunization, and the antibody response can be recalled and boosted when the immune system is challenged by additional doses of the vaccine antigen or by the actual infection. Passive immunization can confer rapid protection, but serum levels of specific antibody in recipients are highest immediately after transfer, decreasing with the passage of time, and there is no immune recall upon challenge.

Active or passive immunization may be used for preexposure protection against certain diseases, and the two forms may be administered simultaneously at different sites for postexposure therapy. Tetanus, hepatitis A, hepatitis B, and rabies are examples of diseases for which active and passive immunization may be used together postexposure.

Several vaccines may be given at separate sites concomitantly without decreased efficacy, although the timing and sequence of vaccines have to be taken into account. For example, although immunoglobulin is usually given for passive immunization against hepatitis A, antibodies against several common infections are present in sufficient amounts to interfere with the response to certain other vaccines. Vaccines against measles, mumps, rubella (MMR), and varicella may be given on the same day, but immunoglobulin should not be given for 3 months before or for 3 weeks after MMR vaccines and not for 2 months after varicella vaccine.

However, vaccines against tetanus, diphtheria, yellow fever, typhoid fever, hepatitis B, rabies, and meningococcal meningitis can be given on the same day as immunoglobulin. If immunoglobulin is given on the same day as hepatitis A vaccine, the vaccine is still efficacious, although the resulting peak antibody titer is lower than when the vaccine is given alone.

Tolerance to minor adverse effects associated with each vaccine and the potential for more serious vaccine-associated symptoms must also be taken into account in the person who is a candidate for multiple doses on the same day.

Concurrent therapy with antibiotics can inhibit the activity of live attenuated bacterial vaccines, such as oral typhoid vaccine. Concurrent antimalarial therapy (chloroquine and possibly mefloquine) decreases the immune response to intradermal rabies vaccine.

■ CHILDHOOD IMMUNIZATIONS

The routine immunizations recommended during childhood and adolescence prevent nine communicable diseases of public health importance: diphtheria, pertussis (whooping cough), tetanus, polio, *Haemophilus influenzae* type b, hepatitis B, measles, mumps, and rubella (German measles). Table 1 shows the immunization schedules for these diseases according to recommendations from the Centers for Disease Control and Prevention Advisory Committee on Immunization Practices (CDC ACIP) and the American Academy of Pediatrics (AAP).

Varicella virus (chickenpox) vaccine and hepatitis A virus vaccine have recently been licensed in the United States, but neither vaccine was included in the group of targeted childhood immunizations at the time of this writing. Hepatitis A vaccine is recommended for high-risk children in the following categories: all foster children, children attending therapeutic child care programs, Native American children and Alaskan Native children, homeless children, street teens, migrant Hispanic children, male teenagers who have sex with men, those with clotting factor disorders, those with chronic liver disease, and illicit drug users. Table 2 provides trade names and licensed distributors, and Table 3 gives special notes and additional details on indications and dosing.

■ SCHEDULING OF PEDIATRIC IMMUNIZATIONS

The number of recommended early childhood immunizations creates issues of compliance and scheduling for parents, patients, and health care providers. Depending on the use of combination vaccines and coordination of immunization schedules, the vaccines can be delivered with only one or two injections per visit if oral polio vaccine is selected or in as many as four injections per visit if inactivated polio vaccine is used.

The approved use of vaccine combinations (different vaccines mixed and administered through the same syringe) depends on efficacy data from clinical trials, whether compatible vaccines from a single supplier are used, and the relative costs of commercially prepared combination vaccines compared with the costs of each vaccine purchased separately. Examples of this comparison are the relative costs of the diphtheria, tetanus, pertussis (DTP) plus HbOC combination vaccine (Tetramune, Lederle) compared with the DTP plus PRP-T vaccines (DTP adsorbed plus ActHIB, Connaught)

Table 1 Recommended Childhood Immunization Schedule*

VACCINE	BIRTH	2 MONTHS	4 MONTHS	6 MONTHS	12§ MONTHS	15 MONTHS	18 MONTHS	4–6 YEARS	11–12 YEARS	14–16 YEARS
	HB-1									
Hepatitis B¶		HB-2		HB-3						
Diphtheria-Tetanus-Pertussis (DTP)**		DTP	DTP	DTP	DTP or DTaP at ≥15 months			DTP or DTaP	Td	
Haemophilus influenzae TYPE b††		Hib	Hib	Hib	Hib					
Poliovirus		IPV or OPV	IPV or OPV		OPV			OPV		
Measles-Mumps-Rubella§§					MMR			MMR or	MMR	

*Recommended vaccines are listed under the routinely recommended ages. Bars indicate range of acceptable ages for vaccination.
†Although no changes have been made to this schedule since publication in *MMWR* weekly in January 1995, this table has been revised to more accurately reflect the recommendations.
§Vaccines recommended for administration at 12–15 months of age may be administered at either one or two visits.
¶Infants born to hepatitis B surface antigen (HBsAg)-negative mothers should receive the second dose of hepatitis B vaccine between 1 and 4 months of age, provided at least 1 month has elapsed since receipt of the first dose. The third dose is recommended between 6 and 18 months of age. Infants born to HBsAg-positive mothers should receive immunoprophylaxis for hepatitis B with 0.5 ml Hepatitis B Immune Globulin (HBIG) within 12 hours of birth, and 5 μg of either Merck, Sharpe, & Dohme (West Point, Pennsylvania) vaccine (Recombivax HB®) or 10 μg of SmithKline Beecham (Philadelphia) vaccine (Engerix-B®) at a separate site. For these infants, the second dose of vaccine is recommended at 1 month of age and the third dose at 6 months of age. All pregnant women should be screened for HBsAg during an early prenatal visit.
**The fourth dose of DTP may be administered as early as 12 months of age, provided at least 6 months have elapsed since the third dose of DTP. Combined DTP-Hib products may be used when these two vaccines are administered simultaneously. Diphtheria and tetanus toxoids and acellular pertussis vaccine (DTaP) is licensed for use for the fourth and/or fifth dose of DTP in children aged ≥15 months and may be preferred for these doses in children in this age group.
††Three *H. influenzae* type b conjugate vaccines are available for use in infants: a) oligosaccharide conjugate Hib vaccine (HbOC) (HibTITER®, manufactured by Praxis Biologics, Inc. [West Henrietta, New York] and distributed by Lederle-Praxis Biologicals [Wayne, New Jersey]) ; b) polyribosylribitol phosphate-tetanus toxoid conjugate (PRP-T) (ActHIB™, manufactured by Pasteur Mérieux Sérums & Vaccins. S.A. [Lyon, France] and distributed by Connaught Laboratories, Inc. [Swiftwater, Pennsylvannia], and OmniHIB™, manufactured by Pasteur Mérieux Sérums & Vaccins. S.A. and distributed by SmithKline Beecham); and c) *Haemophilus* b conjugate vaccine (Meningococcal Protein Conjugate) (PRP-OMP) (PedvaxHIB®, manufactured by Merck, Sharp, & Dohme). Children who have received PRP-OMP at 2 and 4 months of age do not require a dose at 6 months of age. After the primary infant Hib conjugate vaccine series is completed, any licensed Hib conjugate vaccine may be administered as a booster dose at age 12–15 months.
§§The second dose of MMR vaccine should be administered EITHER at 4–6 years of age OR at 11–12 years of age.
Source: Advisory Committee on Immunization Practices, American Academy of Pediatrics, and American Academy of Family Physicians.

and with DTP plus PRP-T vaccines (DTP adsorbed plus OmniHIB, SmithKline Beecham) (Table 2).

■ ADULT IMMUNIZATIONS

Adults should have their immunization history reviewed, updated, and documented at the time of initial intake into a primary care plan, interim health maintenance visits, employment in one of the health care professions, and/or prior to international travel.

Primary series or booster doses of a given vaccine may be needed to update immunity to tetanus, diphtheria, measles, mumps, rubella, polio, and chickenpox. Hepatitis A and B vaccines are recommended if anticipated lifestyle, occupation, or international travel will expose the person to risk. Table 3 lists the schedules for routine immunizations in older children and adults, according to recommendations from the CDC ACIP, the AAP, and the American College of Physicians.

■ VACCINE RECOMMENDATIONS FOR SPECIAL PATIENTS

Attenuated live viral or bacterial vaccines are generally contraindicated for pregnant women and patients with immune compromise. Exceptions are the recommendation for giving the measles, mumps, and rubella vaccine to children with human immunodeficiency virus (HIV) infection and giving the yellow fever and oral polio vaccines to pregnant women

Table 2 Vaccine Trade Names for Identification

VACCINE	TRADE NAME	MANUFACTURER
Cholera Vaccine		
Cholera	Cholera Vaccine	Wyeth-Ayerst
Diphtheria, Tetanus, Pertussis for Pediatric Use		
DTP	DTP Adsorbed	Connaught
DTP	Tri-Immunol Adsorbed	Lederle
DTP	DTP Adsorbed	SmithKline Beecham
DTaP	Acel-Immune	Lederle
DTaP	Tripedia	Connaught
DTP-HbOC	Tetramune	Lederle
Haemophilus Influenzae b		
HbOC	HibTITER	Lederle
PRP-D	Pro-HIBiT	Connaught
PRP-OMP	PedvaxHIB	Merck
PRP-T*	ActHIB	Connaught
PRP-T†	OmniHIB	SmithKline Beecham
Hepatitis A		
Hepatitis A	Havrix	SmithKline Beecham
Hepatitis A	Vaqta	Merck
Hepatitis B		
Hepatitis B	Engerix-B	SmithKline Beecham
Hepatitis B	Recombivax HB	Merck
Human Immunoglobulin (Intramuscular Route)		
Immunoglobulin	Gammar	Armour
Immunoglobulin		Michigan Department of Public Health (1-517-335-8120)
Influenza		
Influenza	Fluzone	Connaught
Influenza, trivalent, types A and B	FluShield	Wyeth-Ayerst
Measles, Mumps, Rubella		
Measles	Attenuvax	Merck
Mumps	Mumpsvax	Merck
Rubella	Meruvax	Merck
Measles, mumps	Biavax II	Merck
Measles, rubella	M-R-Vax II	Merck
Measles, mumps, rubella	M-M-R II	Merck
Meningococcus		
Meningococcus	Menomune-A/C/Y/W-135	Connaught
Pneumococcus		
Pneumococcus	Pneumovax 23	Merck
Pneumococcus	Pnu-Immune 23	Lederle
Polio		
Poliovirus, inactivated, trivalent, types 1, 2, 3	IPOL Poliovirus	Connaught
Poliovirus, live oral, trivalent, types 1, 2, 3	Orimmune	Lederle
Tetanus, Diphtheria (for Adult Use)		
Tetanus	TE Anatoxal Berna	Berna
Tetanus	Tetanus Toxoid Adsorbed	Lederle
Tetanus	Tetanus Toxoid Adsorbed	Wyeth-Ayerst
Tetanus	Tetanus Toxoid Fluid	Wyeth-Ayerst
Td	Tetanus & Diphtheria Toxoids Adsorbed	Connaught
Td	Tetanus & Diphtheria Toxoids Adsorbed	Lederle
Td	Tetanus & Diphtheria Toxoids Adsorbed	Wyeth-Ayerst
Typhoid		
Typhoid, live oral Ty21A	Vivotif	Berna
Typhoid	Typhim vi	Connaught
Typhoid	Typhoid vaccine	Wyeth-Ayerst
Varicella (Chickenpox)		
Varicella, live attenuated	Varivax	Merck

*May be reconstituted with DTP vaccine (Connaught) in the same vial.

†ActHIB and OmniHIB are the same vaccine, manufactured by Pasteur Merieux, and may be used interchangeably.

Td, adsorbed tetanus and diphtheria toxoids.

Table 3 Schedules for Routine Immunizations of Older Children & Adults

Hib	1 dose	≥15 mo of age or for splenectomized host
Influenza		
MMR*	1 dose† SC at age 12–15 mo or older	Boost measles vaccine at 10–12 yr old routinely or give dose 2 at least 1 mo after first; second measles vaccine dose should be given before international travel for people born after1956 and before 1980
eIPV (killed vaccine, safe for all ages)	Doses† 1 and 2 SC or IM 4–8 wk apart; dose 3 6–12 mo after dose 2; give dose 4 children aged 4–6 yr	Booster dose before travel in areas of risk every 5 years
OPV (attenuated live virus)*	Doses† 1 and 2 PO 6–8 wk apart; dose 3 6 wk–12 mo after dose 2; dose 4 to children 4–6 yrs of age	One booster dose to people ≤18 yr old or to previously immunized adults 19 yr or older prior to travel in areas of risk
Td (for persons over age 7)	3 doses (0.5 ml SC or IM), doses 1 and 2 4–8 wk apart, dose 3 6–12 mo later	Routine booster dose every 10 yr; booster dose after 5yr for prophylaxis of a dirty wound
Pneumococcus polysaccharide 23-valent		
Varicella (chickenpox) (live attenuated virus)†	0.5 ml SC 12 mos–12 yrs of age; 2 doses (0.5 ml SC) 4–8 wk apart for persons at least 13 years of age	May be given concurrently with measles, mumps, and rubella, using separate sites and syringes; may also be given with diphtheria, tetanus, and polio. Lower antivaricella titers when given concomitantly with DTaP or PedvaxHIB

*Caution; may be contraindicated in patients with any of the following conditions: pregnancy, leukemia, lymphoma, generalized malignancy, immunosuppression due to human immunodeficiency virus infection or treatment with corticosteroids, alkylating drugs, antimetabolites or radiation therapy.

†See package insert for recommendations on dosage.

Hib, *Haemophilus influenzae* type b; MMR, measles, mumps, and rubella; eIPV, enhanced, inactivated poliomyelitis; OPV, oral poliomyelitis; Td, adsorbed tetanus and diphtheria toxoids.

with imminent unavoidable travel to high-risk destinations in foreign countries. In both cases the theoretic risk of serious adverse vaccine complications may be outweighed by the anticipated benefit of vaccination.

Annual doses of influenza and pneumococcal vaccines are recommended for persons 65 years or older and for persons with cardiovascular or pulmonary disease. The vaccines against encapsulated bacteria (*H. influenzae* type b, pneumococcal, and meningococcal vaccines) are recommended for persons who have a history of functional asplenia or of splenectomy because of the risk of overwhelming sepsis associated with infections from these agents.

Vaccine efficacy can be affected by various conditions and therapies that lead to compromise of the immune system. In hemodialysis patients, the suboptimal immune response to hepatitis A and B vaccines necessitates higher than standard antigen doses, given as a special vaccine formulation or as additional doses after the standard series. Tests for measuring protective serum antibody levels are widely available for both vaccines.

■ TRAVEL IMMUNIZATIONS

The patient seeking vaccine advice for international travel presents an opportunity to review and update routine immunizations as well as assess the risk of exposure to exotic diseases during the trip. See the chapter *Advice for Travelers.*

Suggested Reading

American College of Physicians. Guide for adult immunization. 3rd ed. Philadelphia: American College of Physicians, 1994.

Centers for Disease Control. Diphtheria, tetanus, and pertussis: Recommendations for vaccine use and other preventive measures. Recommendations of the Immunizations Practices Advisory Committee (ACIP). MMWR 1991; 40(RR-10):1–28.

Centers for Disease Control. Hepatitis B virus: A comprehensive strategy for eliminating transmission in the United States through universal childhood vaccination: Recommendations of the Immunization Practices Advisory Committee (ACIP). MMWR 1991; 40:1–25.

Centers for Disease Control. Update on adult immunization: Recommendations of the Immunization Practices Advisory Committee (ACIP). MMWR 1991; 40(RR-12):1–94.

Centers for Disease Control. Pertussis vaccination: Acellular pertussis vaccine for reinforcing and booster use—supplementary ACIP statement. Recommendations of the Immunization Practices Advisory Committee (ACIP). MMWR 1992; 41(RR-1):1–10.

Centers for Disease Control and Prevention. Committee on Immunization Practices. Use of vaccines and immune globulins in persons with altered immunocompetence. MMWR 1993; 42(RR-4):1–18.

Centers for Disease Control and Prevention. Standards for pediatric immunization practices recommended by the National Vaccine Advisory Committee, approved by the U.S. Public Health Service. MMWR 1993; 42(RR-5):1–13.

Jong EC, McMullen R (eds): The travel and tropical medicine manual. 2nd ed. Philadelphia: WB Saunders, 1995.

FOOD POISONING

Andrew T. Pavia, M.D.

Food-borne illnesses are caused by ingestion of foods containing microbial and chemical toxins or pathogenic microorganisms. This chapter concentrates on toxin-mediated syndromes, usually called food poisoning, rather than on syndromes reflecting enteric infection, such as salmonellosis, shigellosis, vibriosis, and *Escherichia coli* O157:H7 infection. Treatment of these infections is covered in the chapter *Gastroenteritis.*

■ CLINICAL PRESENTATION AND DIAGNOSIS

Initially the diagnosis of specific food poisoning syndromes is suggested by the clinical presentation, the incubation period from exposure to onset of symptoms, and the food. The incubation periods, symptoms, and commonly associated foods for specific syndromes are shown in Table 1. Incubation periods range from a few hours or less in the case of preformed chemical and bacterial toxins such as histamine (scombroid), staphylococcal food poisoning, and *Bacillus cereus,* to several days for bacterial infections (e.g., *Campylobacter jejuni, Salmonella, Yersinia enterocolitica,* and *E. coli* O157:H7 or other enterohemorrhagic *E. coli*) and some types of mushroom poisoning. It is essential, therefore, to obtain a diet history covering 3 to 4 days before onset of symptoms. A careful history of illness in meal companions may help point to the responsible food.

It is clinically useful to consider syndromes grouped by incubation period and symptoms.

Nausea and Vomiting Within 1 Hour

Symptoms developing within 5 to 15 minutes of exposure that resolve over 1 to 2 hours are typical of contamination of food or drink with heavy metals or other nonspecific chemical irritants.

Nausea, Vomiting, or Diarrhea Within 1 to 16 Hours

When gastrointestinal symptoms develop 1 to 16 hours after exposure, the likely agents include *Staphylococcus aureus, B. cereus,* and *Clostridium perfringens.* Vomiting is the dominant feature of *S. aureus* and short-incubation, or emetic, *B. cereus* food poisoning. These syndromes are due to preformed centrally acting toxins elaborated by the organisms in food when the food is mishandled. In contrast, abdominal cramps and diarrhea are most prominent in long-incubation, or diarrheal, *B. cereus* poisoning and *C. perfringens* food poisoning. In these syndromes toxins are also elaborated in the small intestine. The duration of illness is usually less than 24 hours. Diagnosis of these syndromes is usually made on epidemiologic and clinical grounds. Laboratory confirmation of *S. aureus* food poisoning is based on isolation of *S. aureus* from food handlers and demonstration of more than 10^5 colonies per gram of the same strain in food or enterotoxin production. Laboratory confirmation of *B. cereus* and

Table 1 Incubation Period, Symptoms, and Common Vehicles for Microbial Causes of Food Poisoning

ORGANISM	INCUBATION PERIOD (IN HOURS) MEDIAN (RANGE)	VOMITING	DIARRHEA	FEVER	COMMON VEHICLES
Staphylococcus aureus	3 (1–6)	+++	++	0	Ham, poultry, cream-filled pastries, potato and egg salad
Bacillus cereus (emetic syndrome)	2 (1–6)	+++	++	0	Fried rice
B. cereus (diarrheal syndrome)	9 (6–16)	+	+++	0	Beef, pork, chicken, vanilla sauce
Clostridium perfringens	12 (6–24)	+	+++	0	Beef, poultry, gravy
Vibrio parahemolyticus	15 (4–96)	++	+++	++	Fish, shellfish
Vibrio cholerae O1 and non-O1	24 (12–120)	++	+++	+	Shellfish
Norwalk virus	24 (12–48)	+++	++	++	Shellfish, salads, ice
Shigella	24 (7–168)	+	+++	+++	Egg salads, lettuce
Clostridium botulinum	24 (12–168)	++	+	0	Canned vegetables, fruits, and fish; salted fish; bottled garlic
Salmonella	36 (12–72)	+	+++	++	Beef, poultry, pork, eggs, dairy products, fruit and vegetables
Campylobacter jejuni	48 (24–168)	+	+++	+++	Poultry, raw milk
Enterohemorrhagic *Escherichia coli* (e.g., O157:H7)	96 (48–120)	++	+++	+	Beef (esp. hamburger), raw milk, salad dressings
Yersinia enterocolitica	96 (48–240)	+	+++	+++	Pork, chitterlings, tofu, raw milk

0, rare (<10%); +, infrequent (11%–33%); ++, frequent (33%–66%); +++, classic (>67%).

Table 2 Clinical Features of Fish and Shellfish Poisoning

SYNDROME	INCUBATION PERIOD	SYMPTOMS	VEHICLES	DURATION
Histamine (scombroid)	5 min–1 hr	Facial flushing, headache, nausea, cramps, diarrhea, urticaria	Tuna, mackerel, bonito, mahi-mahi, bluefish	Hours
Ciguatera	1–6 hr	Diarrhea, nausea, vomiting, myalgia, arthralgia, shooting pains, perioral and extremity paresthesias, hot-cold reversal, fatigue	Barracuda, snapper, grouper, amberjack	Days to months
Neurotoxic shellfish poisoning	5 min–4 hr	Paresthesias, nausea, vomiting, ataxia	Shellfish	Hours to days
Paralytic shellfish poisoning	5 min–4 hr	Paresthesias, cranial nerve weakness, ataxia, muscle weakness, respiratory paralysis	Shellfish	Hours to days
Domoic acid	15 min–38 hr	Vomiting, cramps, diarrhea, confusion, ammesia, cardiac irritability	Mussels	Indefinite

C. perfringens can be performed in epidemiologic investigations; it requires collection of food and stool for quantitative cultures.

Watery Diarrhea and Cramps Within 16 to 48 Hours

Diarrhea following a slightly longer incubation period is typical of viral food-borne illness, particularly Norwalk virus, and enterotoxin-producing bacteria, including enterotoxigenic *E. coli* (ETEC), *Vibrio cholerae* O1 and non-O1, and other *Vibrio* species. Most microbiology laboratories can diagnose *Vibrio* infections from stool culture provided the lab is aware that *Vibrio* is being considered. Diagnosis of ETEC infection requires detection of enterotoxin production by *E. coli* isolates and is limited to reference labs. Antigen detection-based enzyme immunoassays have been developed for the diagnosis of Norwalk and other gastroenteritis-causing viruses; these are limited to research labs but may soon become commercially available.

Fever, Diarrhea, and Abdominal Cramps Within 16 to 96 Hours

Bacterial infections of the gastrointestinal tract and gut-associated lymphatics with *Salmonella, Shigella, C. jejuni, Y. enterocolitica,* and enterohemorrhagic *E. coli* typically follow a longer incubation period and are marked by more prominent signs of colonic inflammation or systemic illness. Diarrhea that becomes bloody after 12 to 36 hours is typical of *E. coli* O157:H7 and other enterohemorrhagic *E. coli.* These organisms are now among the most common causes of bacterial gastroenteritis in North America (see the chapter *Gastroenteritis*). Food-borne infection with *Listeria monocytogenes* and *Cyclospora catetensis* have been recently reported as causes of this syndrome.

Paresthesias Within 6 Hours

Chemical food poisoning due to niacin, Chinese restaurant syndrome (monosodium glutamate), histamine fish poisoning, ciguatera poisoning, and neurotoxic and paralytic shellfish poisoning present with paresthesias and other symptoms after a brief incubation period.

Chinese restaurant syndrome is characterized by a burning sensation in the neck, chest, and abdomen with chest tightness and occasionally facial flushing, headache, nausea, and abdominal cramps.

The features of fish and shellfish poisoning are summarized in Table 2. Histamine fish poisoning (scombroid) is due to bacterial decarboxylation of histidine in fish that are inadequately refrigerated, resulting in production of large amounts of histamine. Signs and symptoms are facial flushing, headache, nausea, and less commonly urticaria or diarrhea. The fish is often reported to have a peppery or bitter taste. Demonstration of high levels of histamine in the implicated fish confirms the diagnosis.

Ciguatera fish poisoning results from ingestion of fish containing toxins produced by the dinoflagellate *Gambierdiscus toxicus.* Predatory fish such as amberjack, snapper, and barracuda are usually implicated. The symptoms, which are quite distinctive, usually involve the combination of gastrointestinal and neurologic symptoms, most commonly perioral and distal extremity paresthesias, and reversal of hot and cold sensation. Other symptoms include sensation of loose teeth, arthralgias, headaches, muscle weakness, pruritus, lancinating pains, and hallucinations. Bradycardia, hypotension, and respiratory paralysis may occur. The symptoms may last from a few days to 6 months. The diagnosis is based on the clinical picture; detection of ciguatoxin in the fish by radio-immunoassay (RIA) or enzyme-linked immunoassay (EIA) (stick test), or by bioassay is confirmatory.

Paralytic shellfish poisoning (PSP) and neurotoxic shellfish poisoning (NSP) are closely related syndromes caused by heat-stable neurotoxins produced by dinoflagellates (*Gonyaulax catonella* and *Gonyaulax tamarensis* cause PSP; *Gymnodinium breve* causes NSP). During periodic blooms of the dinoflagellates, which may cause red tides, shellfish concentrate the heat-stable toxins. PSP is more severe and occurs in colder waters. Patients develop symptoms a median of 30 minutes after exposure. Symptoms consist of paresthesias and dysesthesias, beginning with the lips, mouth, and face and progressing to the extremities; then dysphonia, dysphagia, ataxia, muscle weakness, and in severe cases respiratory paralysis. NSP occurs primarily near warmer waters and is

Table 3 Clinical Syndromes of Mushroom Poisoning

SYNDROME (TOXINS)	INCUBATION PERIOD	SYMPTOMS	MUSHROOMS
Parasympathetic (muscarine)	30 min–2 hr	Sweating, salivation, lacrimation, blurred vision, diarrhea, bradycardia, hypotension	*Inocybe* sp., *Clitocybe* sp.
Delirium (ibotenic acid, muscimol)	30 min–2 hr	Dizziness, incoordination, ataxia, hyperactivity, visual disturbance, stupor	*Amanita muscaria, Amanita pantherinia*
Disulfiram-like (coprine)	30 min after alcohol or up to 24 hr after mushrooms	Flushing, metallic taste, nausea, vomiting, sweating, hypotension	*Coprinus atramentarius, Clitocybe clavipes*
Hallucinations (psilocybin)	30–60 min	Mood elevation, anxiety, muscle weakness, hallucination	*Psilocybe cubensis, Panaleolus* sp.
Gastroenteritis	30 min–2 yr	Nausea, vomiting, abdominal cramps, diarrhea	Various
Methemoglobin poisoning (monomethyl hydrazine gyromitrin)	6–12 hr	Nausea, vomiting, bloody diarrhea, abdominal pain, convulsion, coma, liver failure, hemolysis	*Gyromitra* sp.
Hepatorenal failure (amatoxins, phallotoxins)	6–24 hr	Nausea, vomiting, abdominal pain, diarrhea; then jaundice, liver and kidney failure, coma, death	*Amanita phalloides, A. verna, A. virosa, Galerina automnalis, G. marginata*
Tubulointerstitial nephritis (orellanine)	36 hr–14 days	Thirst, nausea, vomiting, flank pain, chills, oliguria	*Cortinarius orellanus, C. speciosissimus*

characterized by similar paresthesias, reversal of hot and cold sensation, nausea, vomiting, and ataxia. Toxin can be detected in samples of the shellfish by bioassay.

Anamnestic shellfish poisoning is a recently described syndrome associated with mussels contaminated with domoic acid elaborated by *Nitzchia pungens.* Gastrointestinal symptoms are followed, in some patients, by memory loss, coma, cardiac arrhythmias, and death.

Nausea, Vomiting, Diarrhea, and Paralysis Within 18 to 36 Hours

Food-borne botulism results from exposure to one of three distinct botulinum toxins, A, B, and E, produced when *Clostridium botulinum* spores germinate in food in an anaerobic environment. Gastrointestinal symptoms occur before the onset of neurologic symptoms in about 50 percent of patients with acute food-borne botulism. Descending paralysis begins with cranial nerve weakness manifested as dysphonia, dysphagia, diplopia, and blurred vision, followed by muscle weakness and respiratory insufficiency. Larger doses of toxin result in shorter incubation periods and more severe symptoms. Botulism can be differentiated from acute myasthenia gravis and Guillain-Barré syndrome (which may follow *C. jejuni* infection) by normal cerebrospinal fluid protein, the descending nature of the paralysis, absence of sensory symptoms, normal nerve conduction studies, and typical electromyographic findings of increase in the action potential with rapid repetitive stimulation. Confirmation is based on detection of toxin in food or in serum or stool of patients by mouse toxicity assay or of *C. botulinum* spores in the stool by selective culture.

Mushroom Poisoning Syndromes

Syndromes of food poisoning due to mushrooms fall into eight major categories, outlined in Table 3. Parasympatheticsyndromes, delirium, disulfiram (Antabuse)-like symptoms, hallucinations, or gastroenteritis may occur after a short incubation period. The more serious syndromes of monomethyl-hydrazine poisoning, hepatorenal failure due to amatoxin-containing mushrooms, and tubulointerstitial nephritis develop after longer incubation periods and may not be initially suspected. If available, specimens of the mushrooms should be examined promptly by a mycologist or poison control expert to confirm the diagnosis. Toxins can be detected in gastric contents, blood, or urine by thin-layer chromatography.

■ THERAPY

Nonspecific Therapy

Assessment

Most food poisoning syndromes are self-limited, and for the majority of episodes nonspecific supportive therapy is all that is required. Exceptions include botulism, listeriosis, some enteric infections in infants and compromised hosts, and some types of mushroom poisoning.

The mainstay of treatment is fluid and electrolyte replacement to prevent and treat dehydration. The first step is to assess the degree of volume depletion by examining the skin turgor, mucous membranes, vital signs, and mental status. Measuring postural changes in pulse and blood pressure is also helpful in quantifying the volume loss. Slightly dry mucous membranes and thirst indicate mild dehydration (5 to 6 percent deficit, or 50 to 60 ml per kilogram); loss of skin turgor, very dry mucous membranes, postural pulse increases, and sunken eyes indicate moderate dehydration (7 to 9 percent); and the additional presence of weak pulse, postural hypotension, cold extremities, or depressed consciousness indicates severe volume depletion, above 10 percent.

Treatment

Most children and adults with diarrhea can be successfully treated with oral rehydration. This therapy is possible because of the coupled transport of glucose with water and sodium even in severely damaged small bowel. Diarrheal stool contains significant concentrations of sodium, potassium, and bicarbonate, and fluid therapy should replace these losses.

One liter of the World Health Organization's recommended replacement solution contains 90 mmol of sodium, 20 g of glucose, 20 mmol of potassium, 80 mmol of chloride, and 30 mmol of citrate (as a bicarbonate source); this is close to an ideal solution. Commercial solutions such as Rehydralyte, Ricelyte, and Pedialyte have a slightly lower sodium concentration, but they are convenient and readily available, if expensive. A homemade approximation of the oral solution can be made by adding a pinch of salt, a pinch of baking soda, and a spoonful of sugar or honey to an 8-ounce glass of fruit juice. For patients with altered consciousness or uncontrolled vomiting, intravenous rehydration with Ringer's lactate should be used initially. The estimated volume deficit should be replaced over 4 hours; after that, ongoing losses should be replaced. Gatorade and commercial soft drinks are poor choices because the low sodium content can lead to hyponatremia and the high osmolarity can exacerbate diarrhea.

Water intake should be allowed ad lib, and solid food can be introduced as soon as it is tolerated. Some patients will develop lactose intolerance after severe or protracted diarrhea, and dairy products should be avoided if they appear to exacerbate symptoms.

Phenothiazine antiemetics may be useful for severe or prolonged vomiting. Promethazine (Phenergan) 12.5 to 25 mg and prochlorperazine (Compazine) 5 to 10 mg orally or IM, 25 mg rectally, can be given orally, as suppositories, or intramuscularly. Alternatively, droperidol (Inapsine) 1 to 2 ml can be used intravenously. Antidiarrheals are probably best avoided if enteric infection is suspected, especially in children. Pepto-Bismol 30 ml orally every 4 to 6 hours may be a reasonable choice if an antidiarrheal is used, since it has been shown to bind some enterotoxins. Care must be taken because of the salicylate content.

Table 4 Specific Treatment for Food Poisoning Syndromes

SYNDROME	FIRST-LINE TREATMENT	COMMENT
S. aureus, B. cereus, C. perfringens, Norwalk virus	Fluid replacement, antiemetics, e.g., promethazine (Phenergan), prochlorperazine (Compazine), droperidol (Inapsine)	Oral rehydration is usually adequate if vomiting can be controlled.
Bacterial gastroenteritis	Fluid replacement; antimicrobials helpful for some syndromes	See the chapter *Gastroenteritis* for specific antimicrobial therapy.
C. botulinum	Gastric emptying, cathartics if food still in gut; respiratory support, polyvalent antitoxin*	Antitoxin should be given as soon as possible.
Histamine (scombroid)	Antihistamine, e.g., diphenhydramine 25–50 mg IM or IV	H_2 receptor antagonists (cimetidine) have been helpful for refractory symptoms.
Ciguatera	Empty stomach if vomiting has not occurred; analgesia, antiemetics, supportive measures; atropine for symptomatic bradycardia	Amitriptyline 25–50 mg daily or tocainide may help paresthesias. Mannitol infusion, calcium gluconate infusion have been used.
Neurotoxic shellfish poisoning	Supportive therapy	
Paralytic shellfish poisoning	Supportive therapy; monitor vital capacity	
Muscarine-containing mushrooms	Gastric emptying, activated charcoal, cathartics; atropine 0.01 mg/kg IV up to 1 mg	Titrate atropine to drying of secretions.
Muscimol- and ibotenic acid-containing mushrooms	Gastric emptying, activated charcoal, cathartics; supportive measures	Physostigmine may be used if anticholinergic symptoms are severe.
Hallucinogen-containing mushrooms	Reassurance, quiet room; diazepam for severe agitation	
Monomethyl-hydrazine-containing mushrooms (*Gyromitra* spp.)	Gastric emptying, activated charcoal, cathartics; for delirium, pyridoxine 25 mg/kg IV	For methemoglobinemia, methylene blue 1% solution 0.1–0.2 ml/kg over 5 minutes
Amatoxin-containing mushrooms	Gastric emptying, activated charcoal, cathartics; correction of fluid and electrolytes; monitor glucose, liver and renal function	Thioctic acid may be useful.† High doses of steroids and IV penicillin have been advocated, but controlled data are lacking.
Orellanine-containing mushrooms	Gastric emptying, activated charcoal, cathartics; cautious correction of fluid and electrolyte problems	Hemodialysis is frequently necessary.

*Available through state health department or Foodborne and Diarrheal Diseases Branch, Centers for Disease Control and Prevention, 404-639-2206, 8:00 to 4:30 Eastern Time workdays; 404-639-2888 nights, weekends, and holidays.

†Assistance in obtaining thioctic acid can be sought through regional Poison Control Centers or by contacting Berton M. Berkson, M.D., Ph.D., Las Cruces, New Mexico, 505-678-2321 or 505-521-1609.

Specific Therapy

Specific therapies for food poisoning are outlined in Table 4. Gastric emptying and administration of active charcoal and cathartics are important for virtually all mushroom poisoning. If vomiting has not occurred spontaneously in patients with botulism or ciguatera, the remaining food should be removed from the gut. In botulism, paralytic shellfish poisoning, and ciguatera, death from respiratory failure is the major risk, and monitoring the vital capacity can be lifesaving.

Polyvalent equine antitoxin, which binds botulinum toxins A, B, and E, is available in the United States through state health departments and the Centers for Disease Control and Prevention (404-639-2206, 8:00 to 4:30 Eastern Time workdays; 404-639-2888 nights, weekends, and holidays). It may prevent further paralysis but does not reverse established symptoms. To be effective it should be administered early. Dosage and a protocol for desensitization in the case of a positive skin test are listed in the package insert.

In ciguatera poisoning, analgesia and avoidance of unpleasant stimuli such as warm baths are usually adequate. Anecdotal reports in the literature suggest that amitriptyline 25 to 50 mg orally daily and tocainide may be useful for dysesthesias. Intravenous mannitol has also been reported to be effective for severe neurologic manifestations. For histamine fish poisoning conventional antihistamines, such as diphenhydramine 25 to 50 mg IM or IV, are helpful. Epinephrine or albuterol should be given for bronchospasm. Intravenous cimetidine can be tried for refractory symptoms.

Atropine is a specific antidote for poisoning due to muscarine-containing mushrooms, but the dose (0.01 mg per kilogram up to a maximum of 1 mg) should be titrated to control excess respiratory secretions and bradycardia rather than other symptoms.

Specific treatment is usually not necessary for poisoning due to ibotenic acid-containing or muscimol-containing mushrooms. If severe anticholinergic symptoms such as hyperpyrexia, hypertension, or severe agitation are present, physostigmine 0.01 mg per kilogram IV should be used. Cardiac and blood pressure monitoring are necessary, since hypotension and bradycardia can result.

For poisoning due to monomethyl-hydrazine-containing mushrooms, pyridoxine 25 mg per kilogram IV should be given; the dose can be repeated every 5 to 10 minutes. The methemoglobin level should be measured if possible. If there is symptomatic methemoglobinemia with central cyanosis, methylene blue 0.1 to 0.2 ml per kilogram of a 1 percent solution should be given over 5 minutes.

The high fatality rate associated with poisoning by *Amanita phalloides* and related amatoxin-containing mushrooms makes it a special concern. Toxin removal should be attempted with activated charcoal and cathartics even after several days because of the extensive enterohepatic cycling. During the initial phase, gastrointestinal symptoms may cause hypotension. This first stage is often followed by a stage of apparent improvement, but hepatic transaminases usually are elevated by 24 to 48 hours. Fulminant hepatic necrosis and acute renal failure begin after 48 to 96 hours. Supportive treatment consists of careful fluid replacement and monitoring of serum glucose and liver function tests. Thioctic acid may be partially effective at 300 mg per kilogram per day IV with glucose infusion in divided doses every 6 hours; contact the regional poison control center for help in obtaining it. The roles of intravenous penicillin and high-dose steroids are unclear. Charcoal hemoperfusion is theoretically attractive if it can be begun within the first 10 to 16 hours.

Reporting

Reporting of suspected food-borne outbreaks to local or state health departments is an important part of management, since epidemiologic investigation can clearly establish the responsible food and may prevent many additional cases.

Suggested Reading

Avery ME, Snyder JD. Oral therapy for acute diarrhea: The underused simple solution. N Engl J Med 1990; 323:891–894.

Hall AH, Spoërke DG, Rumack BH. Mushroom poisoning: Identification, diagnosis and treatment. Pediatr Rev 1987; 8:291–298.

Hedberg CW, MacDonald KL, Osterholm MT. Changing epidemiology of food-borne disease: A Minnesota perspective. Clin Infect Dis 1994; 18: 671–680.

Hughes JM, Merson MH. Fish and shellfish poisoning. N Engl J Med 1976; 295:1117–1120.

Pavia AT. Approach to acute foodborne and waterborne disease. Semin Pediatr Infect Dis 1994; 5:222–230.

NONSURGICAL ANTIMICROBIAL PROPHYLAXIS

James P. Steinberg, M.D.
Mitchell A. Blass, M.D.

Chemoprophylaxis is the use of an antimicrobial agent to prevent infection. Prophylaxis is often administered after exposure to a virulent pathogen or before a procedure associated with risk of infection. Chronic prophylaxis is sometimes administered to persons with underlying conditions that predispose to recurrent or severe infection. Antibiotics can also be used to prevent clinical disease in persons infected with a microorganism such as *Mycobacterium tuberculosis.* This chapter discusses the specific areas where antimicrobial prophylaxis is generally accepted. For information on prophylaxis of bacterial endocarditis see the chapter *Endocarditis of Natural and Prosthetic Valves;* for information on prophylaxis in persons infected with the human immunodeficiency virus (HIV) see the chapter *HIV Disease: Prophylaxis of Opportunistic Infections;* for malaria prophylaxis see the chapter *Malaria;* and for surgical prophylaxis see the chapter that follows this one.

Several concepts are important in determining whether or not chemoprophylaxis is appropriate for a particular situation. In general, prophylaxis is recommended when the risk of infection is high or the consequences significant. The nature of the pathogen, type of exposure, and immunocompetence of the host are important determinants of the need for prophylaxis. The antimicrobial agent should eliminate or reduce the probability of infection or if infection occurs, reduce the associated morbidity. The ideal agent is inexpensive and orally administered in most circumstances and has few adverse effects. The ability to alter the normal microbial flora and select for antimicrobial resistance should be limited, so duration of prophylaxis as well as choice of agents is critical. The emerging crisis of antibiotic-resistant bacteria underscores the importance of rational and not indiscriminate use of antimicrobial agents. In addition, the development of antibiotic-resistant pathogens necessitates reassessment of many of the established prophylactic regimens.

The efficacy of chemoprophylaxis is well established in situations such as perioperative antibiotic administration, exposure to invasive meningococcal disease, prevention of recurrent rheumatic fever, and prevention of tuberculosis. Chemoprophylaxis is accepted in other situations without supporting data. When the risk of infection is low, such as with bacterial endocarditis following dental procedures, clinical trials of prophylaxis are not feasible. However, the consequences of infection may be catastrophic, providing a compelling argument for chemoprophylaxis despite the low risk of infection. When prophylaxis is advocated without data confirming efficacy, there should be a scientific rationale to support the use of a particular antimicrobial agent.

Table 1 lists the situations in which antimicrobial prophy-

Table 1 Prophylaxis Following Selected Exposures

EXPOSURE	PATHOGEN	PROPHYLAXIS*	COMMENTS
Meningitis, meningocccal bacteremia	*Neisseria meningitidis*	Ciprofloxacin 500 mg b.i.d. for 5 days (adults only) or ceftriaxone 250 mg IM Rifampin 600 mg (10 mg/kg for children) q12h for four doses (see the chapter *Meningococcus*)	Recommended for close contacts only (e.g., family members, roommates, day-care contacts); prophylaxis not recommended for health care workers unless very close contact such as mouth-to-mouth resuscitation occurred; secondary cases reported with meningococcal pneumonia, but role of prophylaxis is uncertain; sulfonamide resistance precludes routine use of sulfadiazine
Meningitis	*Haemophilus influenzae*	Rifampin 600 mg (20 mg/kg for children) daily for 4 days	Recommended for children <4 years old after exposure at home or day care; when such a child is present, prophylaxis should be given to all exposed individuals regardless of age; index case should receive prophylaxis to eradicate nasopharyngeal colonization

*All regimens are administered orally unless otherwise specified.

Table 1 Prophylaxis Following Selected Exposures—cont'd

EXPOSURE	PATHOGEN	PROPHYLAXIS*	COMMENTS
Human bite	Viridans and other streptococci, oral anaerobes, *Staphylococcus aureus, Eikenella corrodens*	Amoxicillin-clavulanic acid 250 mg t.i.d. for 3–5 days	Risk of infection high; no clear alternative for penicillin allergy; *Eikenella* is resistant to clindamycin and first-generation cephalosporins; clindamycin 300 mg q.i.d. is a reasonable alternative in many situations; clenched-fist injuries often require parenteral antibiotics
Cat bite	*Pasteurella multocida, S. aureus,* streptococci	Penicillin V 500 mg q.i.d. or amoxicillin-clavulanic acid 250 mg t.i.d. for 3–5 days; for penicillin allergy consider doxycycline 100 mg b.i.d.	First-generation cephalosporins not as active as penicillin against *P. multocida,* which is present in oral flora of 50–70% of cats
Dog bite	Viridans streptococci, oral anaerobes, *S. aureus, P. multocida, Capnocytophaga canimorsus* (formerly DF-2)	Penicillin V 500 mg q.i.d. or amoxicillin-clavulanic acid 250 mg t.i.d. for 3–5 days; for penicillin allergy consider doxycycline 100 mg b.i.d.	Infection less frequent than with cat or human bites; need for routine prophylaxis for all bites uncertain; persons without spleens at risk of overwhelming *Capnocytophaga* sepsis should receive prophylaxis following any dog bite
Sexual assault	*Trichomonas vaginalis, Chlamydia trachomatis, Treponema pallidum, Neisseria gonorrhoeae*	Ceftriaxone 250 mg IM single dose plus doxycycline 100 mg b.i.d. for 7 days plus metronidazole 2 g, single dose; may substitute single dose azithromycin 1 g for doxycycline	For pregnant victim erythromycin 500 mg q.i.d. for 7 days in place of doxycycline or azithromycin; metronidazole acceptable after first trimester
Syphilis exposure	*T. pallidum*	Benzathine penicillin G 2.4 million units IM	Treat if exposed within the previous 90 days
Sexual contacts (urethritis and cervicitis)	*N. gonorrhoeae, C. trachomatis*	Ceftriaxone 250 mg IM single dose plus doxycycline 100 mg b.i.d. for 7 days	Ceftriaxone probably effective against incubating syphilis
Sexual contacts	*T. vaginalis*	Metronidazole 2 g single dose	No satisfactory alternatives available in the United States
Influenza	Influenza A	Amantadine or rimantadine 100 mg b.i.d. for 5–7 weeks or for 2 weeks if given concurrently with vaccination; use 100 mg daily for those >65 years old	Recommended for high-risk individuals (elderly, immunocompromised) during outbreaks; usually given to unvaccinated individuals but provides additive protection for the vaccinated; consider for unvaccinated health care workers; two agents have equal efficacy but fewer neurologic side effects with rimantadine
Whooping cough	*Bordetella pertussis*	Erythromycin 500 mg q.i.d. (50 mg/kg q.i.d. in children) for 14 days	Secondary attack rate often over 50%; erythromycin prophylaxis not 100% effective, reduces transmission, is important in aborting outbreaks; trimethoprim-sulfamethoxazole an alternative, although efficacy data not available
Plague	*Yersinia pestis*	Tetracycline 500 mg b.i.d. for 5 days	Resistance not a problem

*All regimens are administered orally unless otherwise specified.

laxis is indicated after exposure to certain pathogens. Because the duration of exposure is usually brief, the duration of chemoprophylaxis is short, which helps limit adverse reactions, minimizes the potential for resistance, and limits cost. Some of these pathogens are virulent and can produce serious disease in normal hosts. With exposure to pathogens that cause meningitis, the decision whether to use prophylaxis can be complicated. Because of fear and anxiety provoked by these illnesses there is a tendency to provide prophylaxis to persons outside the high-risk populations.

Persons with an underlying predisposition to infection may benefit from prophylactic antimicrobial agents (Table 2). In contrast to short-term prophylaxis administered after exposures, chronic prophylaxis is often required. Because of the duration of antibiotic administration, the complications of chemoprophylaxis, including alteration of the microflora and antibiotic resistance, are major considerations. The emergence of antibiotic-resistant *Streptococcus pneumoniae* may force reassessment of the standard chemoprophylactic recommendations when pneumococcus is a prominent pathogen, as with anatomic or functional asplenia and recurrent otitis.

Chemoprophylaxis for tuberculosis is generally administered to those already infected with *Mycobacterium tuberculosis*

Table 2 Chronic Prophylaxis in Specific Clinical Settings

UNDERLYING CONDITION	PATHOGENS	PROPHYLAXIS*	COMMENTS
Acute rheumatic fever (prevention of recurrences)	*Streptococcus pyogenes*	Penicillin G 12 million units IM every 4 weeks; alternatives penicillin V 125 or 250 mg b.i.d.; erythromycin 250 mg b.i.d., sulfadiazine 1 g daily (0.5 g if weight <60 lb)	Risk diminishes with increasing age and time since initial attack; optimal duration unknown but continue prophylaxis at least until the early 20s or for 5 years after most recent attack; some authorities advocate lifelong prophylaxis, especially after rheumatic carditis
Recurrent UTI	Gram-negative bacilli	TMP-SMX ½ tablet (40 mg, 200 mg) daily single strength or trimethoprim 100 mg or nitrofurantoin 50 mg daily or postcoital TMP-SMX 1 tablet	For selected patients with more than 3 infections yearly; consider prophylaxis for 6–12 months
Chronic bronchitis, bronchiectasis	*Streptococcus pneumoniae, Haemophilus influenzae, Moraxella catarrhalis*	Amoxicillin 500 mg t.i.d. or TMP-SMX 1 DS b.i.d. or erythromycin 250 mg q.i.d. or tetracycline 500 mg q.i.d.	May be useful in selected patients with frequent exacerbations (>4 per year); some authorities prefer antibiotics at first sign of infection
Asplenia including sickle cell disease	Predominantly *Str. pneumoniae*, also *H. influenzae*, meningococci	Penicillin V 250 mg b.i.d. (125 mg b.i.d. for children <5 years old) or benzathine penicillin G 1.2 million units IM every 4 weeks; Prophylaxis generally continued 2 years after splenectomy; for children with sickle cell disease, prophylaxis continued at least until age 5 years	Efficacy of chemoprophylaxis clearly established for children with sickle cell disease; some authorities recommend amoxicillin or TMP-SMX for children <5 years old because of increased risk of *H. influenzae* infection; chemoprophylaxis generally not recommended for adults (lower risk); penicillin-resistant pneumococcus diminishes attractiveness of antibiotic prophylaxis, increases importance of vaccination
Recurrent otitis media	*Str. pneumoniae, H. influenzae, M. catarrhalis*	Sulfisoxazole 50 mg/kg or amoxicillin 20 mg/kg daily hs	Recommended for children with >3 infections in 6 mo; usually during peak infection season (winter and spring) or for 6 mo
Lymphedema with recurrent cellulitis	*Str. pyogenes*	Benzathine penicillin G 1.2 million units IM monthly	Only for frequent episodes of cellulitis

*All regimens are administered orally unless otherwise specified.
UTI, urinary tract infection; TMP-SMX, trimethoprim-sulfamethoxazole; DS, double-strength.

Table 3 Criteria for Preventive Therapy for Persons with Positive PPD Skin Tests

SITUATION	PPD SIZE (5 TU)	AGE GROUP
Recent PPD converter (negative PPD within the previous 2 years, excluding booster phenomenon)	PPD ≥10 mm except ≥5 mm after exposure to active tuberculosis	All ages
Identified risk factors including HIV infection, immunosuppressive illnesses, abnormal chest radiograph, silicosis, intravenous drug abuse	PPD ≥10 mm except ≥5 mm if HIV seropositive or if radiograph shows fibrotic disease suggestive of old tuberculosis	All ages
Normal hosts from high-incidence groups: indigent patients, residents of extended-care facilities, immigrants from endemic areas	PPD ≥10 mm	Age <35
Normal hosts from low-incidence groups	PPD ≥15 mm	Age <35
Exposure to tuberculosis	HIV seropositive and anergic Initial PPD nonreactive*	All ages Age 0–5 years

*Repeat PPD in 3 months; if negative, stop chemoprophylaxis.
PPD, purified protein derivative (tuberculin test); TU, tuberculin unit.

losis (i.e., have a positive tuberculin—purified protein derivative, or PPD—skin test), in an attempt to prevent active tuberculosis (Table 3). Preventive therapy with 6 months of isoniazid (INH) 300 mg daily (10 mg per kilogram daily in children) is nearly as effective as the 12 month standard and is associated with a lower incidence of hepatitis. Thus, 6 months of prophylactic INH may have a preferable risk-benefit ratio, especially for those at high risk for INH hepatitis (age over 35). Patients coinfected with HIV should receive at least 12 months of prophylaxis, and some authorities recommend lifelong prophylaxis. Pyridoxine 50 mg daily is usually given with INH to prevent peripheral neuropathy. The criteria in Table 3 take into account that (1) the risk of developing active tuberculosis is greatest in the first 2 years following PPD conversion, (2) the risk of INH hepatitis in those over 35 years of age is greater than the risk of developing tuberculosis except in high-risk individuals, including recent skin test converters, and (3) PPD skin testing may produce false-positive and false-negative results. Consequently, different diameters of induration are used according to the prevalence of *M. tuberculosis* infection in the population tested.

When infection with INH-resistant *M. tuberculosis* is suspected, the optimal chemoprophylactic regimen is unknown. Rifampin 600 mg daily for 1 year is usually recommended. A possible alternative is rifampin 600 mg daily plus pyrazinamide 25 mg per kilogram daily for 2 months. In the setting of suspected infection with multidrug-resistant *M. tuberculosis,* the prophylactic regimen should be based on the susceptibility pattern of the prevalent multiresistant strain.

Chemoprophylaxis has been advocated for other situations, but at this time it cannot be considered standard practice (Table 4). Although data are limited, it is likely that cost-benefit analyses would not favor routine prophylaxis in these settings or that the benefits of prophylaxis in the short

Table 4 Controversial Areas Regarding the Use of Prophylactic Antibiotics

CONDITION	COMMENTS
Prosthetic device infections	Routine chemoprophylaxis prior to dental work, other procedures that cause transient bacteremia in patients with prosthetic joints or vascular prostheses probably not warranted; prosthetic joint infections caused by oral flora including α-streptococci uncommon, with rate approaching that of endocarditis in patients with mitral valve prolapse without regurgitation, for which chemoprophylaxis is not recommended
Traveler's diarrhea	Most authorities do not recommned antibiotic prophylaxis for traveler's diarrhea because of possible adverse reactions, potential for development of resistance, and cost; preferable strategy is judicious use of antimotility agents and empiric fluoroquinolone (ciprofloxacin 500 mg b.i.d., ofloxacin 300 mg b.i.d., or norfloxacin 400 mg b.i.d. for 3–5 days) for moderate diarrhea; prophylactic bismuth subsalicylate 2 tablets q.i.d. is alternative
Lyme disease	Risk of Lyme disease following bite by an *Ixodes* tick <3% even where Lyme disease endemic; routine chemoprophylaxis is not recommended; to transmit Lyme spirochete, *Ixodes* tick must be attached >24 hours
Catheter-associated UTI	Systemic antibiotics reduce incidence of UTI during initial 4–5 days after Foley catheter insertion; with prolonged catheterization antibiotic-resistant bacteria appear in urine with increasing frequency, dissuading most authorities from routine use of prophylaxis; prophylactic antibiotics possibly useful in selected high-risk patients during short-term catheterization
Intravenous catheter-associated infections	Flushing central venous catheters with an antibiotic solution, usually vancomycin (antibiotic lock) proposed to reduce catheter-associated bacteremia; vancomycin-resistant enterococci led most authorities, including Centers for Disease Control and Prevention, to oppose this strategy.

UTI, urinary tract infection.

term would be outweighed by long-term consequences such as the development of antibiotic-resistant organisms.

Suggested Reading

Centers for Disease Control and Prevention. The use of preventative therapy for tuberculosis infection in the United States: Recommendations of the Advisory Committee for Elimination of Tuberculosis. MMWR 1990; 39(RR-8):9–12.

Centers for Disease Control and Prevention. 1993 sexually transmitted diseases treatment guidelines. MMWR 1993; 42(RR-14):1–99.

DuPont HL, Ericsson CD. Prevention and treatment of traveler's diarrhea. N Engl J Med 1993; 328:1821–1827.

Murphy TV, Clements JF, Breedlove JA, et al. Risk of subsequent disease among day-care contact of patients with systemic *Haemophilus influnzae* type B disease. N Engl J Med 1987; 316:5–10.

Shapiro GD, Gerber MA, Holabird NB, et al. A controlled trial of antimicrobial prophylaxis for Lyme disease after deer tick bites. N Engl J Med 1992; 327:1769–1773.

Stamm WE. Catheter-associated urinary tract infections: Epidemiology, pathogenesis, and prevention. Am J Med 1991; 91: 65S–71S.

SURGICAL PROPHYLAXIS

N. Joel Ehrenkranz, M.D.

Prevention of postoperative infections complicating surgical procedures involves the totality of surgical patient care, beginning with preoperative assessment and ending with postoperative management of the patient. A reliable surveillance system for each type of operation to identify all postoperative infections—primary bacteremia, pneumonia, and symptomatic urinary tract infection as well as infections of the operative site—is essential to assess the efficacy of efforts to limit infections. The patient should be watched for all types of postoperative infection during hospitalization and for an appropriate period after discharge.

■ PREOPERATIVE ASSESSMENT OF THE PATIENT

To the extent possible, the level of bacterial contamination at the operative site should be defined preoperatively or at the time of surgical incision. The usual classifications of procedures are clean (nontraumatic uninfected site; no mucosal surfaces incised), clean contaminated (nontraumatic, uninfected site; mucosal surfaces incised), contaminated (open and fresh trauma, intestinal spillage, or acute nonpurulent inflammation at site), and dirty (old traumatic wounds, perforated viscera, or active purulent bacterial infection at site). These classifications describe surgical risk across all types of operations. However, they do not stand alone. Reporting combined infection rates of different groups of operations stratified only by these classifications is meaningless.

A prime consideration in preoperative evaluation of the patient is to identify treatable infections and colonizations that may promote postoperative infection. Clinical assessment reveals which patients need preoperative treatment. For example, persons with urinary tract infection require antimicrobial treatment prior to genitourinary surgery, and nasal carriers of *Staphylococcus aureus* need treatment with mupirocin intranasally before implantation of vascular access shunts for hemodialysis. Preoperative antimicrobial treatment of skin conditions such as pustular dermatitis or cellulitis, bronchopulmonary infections, and any infection that may possibly contaminate the planned surgical site by direct extension or venolymphatic drainage, decreases the opportunity for postoperative infection. The adage that time spent in antimicrobial treatment is more valuable before surgery than after it has much truth.

In the instance of nonelective cesarean section it may be impossible to treat pre-existing infection by a single dose of an antimicrobial, and there may be no opportunity for more than one preoperative dose. Repeated postoperative therapeutic doses are then necessary; failure to provide them is likely to account for postpartum endomyometritis in certain patients, despite a dose of prophylactic antimicrobial. Gram stain of amniotic fluid taken at the time of uterine incision may indicate which patients, should receive postoperative treatment for several days. Microscopy showing bacteria in the amniotic fluid indicates a patient at increased risk for postoperative endometritis. This test is a useful predictor of postpartum infection when bacteria are seen; if they are not, however, endometritis is still possible.

Failure of beta-lactam antimicrobials to prevent incisional cesarean section wound infection may be due to presence of genital mycoplasmas (*Ureaplasma* and *Mycoplasma* spp.) not susceptible to these drugs.

■ PREPARATION FOR SURGERY

Patients do not require preoperative antiseptic bathing to reduce postoperative infection. If it is absolutely necessary to remove body hair, it should be clipped immediately before operation. Shaving at any time increases the risk of infection.

In a classic study, Burke demonstrated a golden period of decreasing antimicrobial efficacy lasting somewhat longer than 3 hours after experimental bacterial contamination of an open incision. Although a study by Classen and associates revealed considerable variation in actual practice in timing of prophylactic antimicrobials for elective surgery, the clinical findings were quite in keeping with Burke's results. When antimicrobials were given within 2 hours of incision, the surgical wound infection rate was 0.6 percent, and when given up to 3 hours after incision, 1.4 percent; there is no statistically significant difference between these rates ($p = 0.12$). Based on the foregoing studies I define surgical prophylaxis as pharmacologically active antimicrobial presence at the operative site or available to the site in serum any time within approximately 3 hours after incision and prior to closure. To be effective in prophylaxis, antimicrobial activity should be present at wound closure. This is best accomplished by giving the antimicrobial immediately before incision and repeating the dose as necessary every two serum half-lives during operation or at the time of major hemorrhage. For cefazolin, two serum half-lives equals approximately 4 hours. There is no evidence that administration of an antimicrobial after wound closure serves any prophylactic purpose. By contrast, I define early therapy as pharmacologically active antimicrobial presence at the operative site, initiated more than 3 hours following surgical incision or at any time after closure. The theoretic purpose of early therapy in clean operations is to deal with bacteria that may have already attached themselves to prosthetic material, and in contaminated operations it is to contain infection due to bacteria dispersed within the operative field.

Antimicrobial prophylaxis is indicated in cardiac and certain other clean operations, especially those that include implantation of prostheses, and in clean-contaminated and generally contaminated operations (Tables 1 to 3). Cefazolin is the recommended parenteral cephalosporin for routine surgical prophylaxis. In prevention of endometritis after cesarean section, 2 g of cefazolin has been found to be more effective than 1 g. Extrapolating this finding to other operations, I suggest that the 2 g dose be routine. The postoperative duration of early therapy as defined here should be no more than 18 to 24 hours. For cardiac surgery, 18 to 24 hours of postoperative antimicrobials is as good as any regimen, although many cardiac surgeons administer antimicrobials prophylactically for a total of 2 days. Prolonged or unnecessary use of antimicrobials is a factor in promoting resistance. This is particularly true of the broad-spectrum antimicrobials.

I do not routinely recommend cefoxitin in prophylaxis of clean or clean-contaminated procedures except for simple appendectomy, despite its broad aerobic and anaerobic bacterial range of efficacy. It has a short half-life and generally requires doses at 3 hour intervals to maintain an appropriate serum level. It is not effective in prophylaxis of percutaneous endoscopic gastrotomy, and cefazolin is. It provides no clinical advantages over cefazolin in prophylaxis of clean-contaminated gynecologic and obstetric operations. Finally, it has an increased potential for inducing *Clostridium difficile* colitis because it decreases colonization resistance through reduction in numbers of anaerobic bowel flora. The last consideration also applies to other second- and third-generation cephalosporins.

Brief early therapy is effective in early management of trauma. In one study of early surgical treatment (within 4 hours of injury) of penetrating abdominal and visceral injuries, patients were randomized to receive either 12 hours or 5 days of antimicrobial therapy after laparotomy. The two programs were quite comparable in outcome. Similar findings have been reported for early therapy of open fractures.

The major determinant of postoperative infection in abdominal operations is intestinal penetration. The need for prophylaxis of bowel content spillage is clear in planned bowel operations but may be overlooked in operations with other primary objectives, as for example when incidental appendectomy is done in gallbladder operations, when the bowel may be inadvertently entered in the course of certain pelvic operations for cancer, or when the ureter is diverted into an ileal pouch. In elective operations there generally is an opportunity for mechanical bowel preparation and oral antimicrobial prophylaxis. The purpose of the mechanical bowel cleansing is to eliminate gross fecal material with its high content of aerobic and anaerobic bacteria. Following this, administration of oral antimicrobials reduces numbers of mucosal-

Table 1 Routine Indications for Standard Parenteral Surgical Antimicrobial Prophylaxis and Early Treatment*

Clean Operation I (No postoperative doses)
Craniotomy
Laminectomy including vertebral fusion
Vascular operations in abdomen or lower extremities
Emergency vascular shunt operation for dialysis use (e.g., clotted shunt)
Clean Operation II (no more than two postoperative doses at 8 hour intervals)
Joint replacement†
Routine penile prosthesis implantation
Clean Contaminated Operations (no postoperative doses)
Abdominal hysterectomy (no likelihood of bowel entry or appendectomy)
Biliary tract surgery in high-risk patients‡
Percutaneous endoscopic gastrotomy
Primary ccsarean section§
Gastric bypass operation
Small bowel operation
Thoracic operation
Vaginal hysterectomy
Contaminated Operations (no more than two postoperative doses at 8 hour intervals)
Open compound fracture‖
Lower-extremity amputation with distal ulceration

*Cefazolin 2 g IV immediately preoperatively; dosage repeated every 4 hours of operating time. No oral drugs.
†If a repeat joint replacement is being done, antimicrobial prophylaxis may be given after the existing joint prosthesis is removed for culture.
‡High risk = age ≥60 years; findings of biliary stones, obstructive jaundice, cholecystitis.
§Antimicrobial is administered after cord is clamped. Note: for prophylaxis of group B streptococcal infection of the newborn, an intrapartum antibiotic should be administered to high-risk mothers.
‖For operations done within 6 hours of trauma.

Table 2 Optional Indications for Standard Parenteral Surgical Antimicrobial Prophylaxis*

Breast operation
Cerebrospinal fluid shunt operation
Simple laminectomy or spinal stenosis

*Cefazolin 2 g IV immediately preoperatively, dosage repeated every 4 hours of operating time, no postoperative doses. No oral drugs.

Table 3 Routine Indications for Special Surgical Antimicrobial Prophylaxis and Early Treatment

- Cardiac operations I (first operation)
  - Cefazolin 2 g IV immediately preoperatively
  - Cefazolin 2 g IV immediately after cardiopulmonary bypass is complete; two additional doses q8h postoperatively thereafter
  - Many cardiac surgeons administer five additional doses q8h preoperatively. This is the maximum.
- Cardiac operations II (reoperation of recently closed incision, as for bleeding); the incision may be colonized with bacteria, and acute non-purulent cellutic inflammation may also be present, reflecting a contaminated operation.
  - Cefotaxime 2 g IV and metronidazole 1 g IV immediately postoperatively and q12h for a total of 2–4 doses
- Colorectal operations I (elective operations planned to begin between 8 and 10 AM, operation lasting less than 3 hours)
  - Mechanical intestinal preparation day before
  - Neomycin and erythromycin 1 g PO* day before: at 1 PM, 2 PM, 11 PM
  - Acephalosporin 2 g IV immediately before incision
- For operation extending past 12 noon, starting past 11 AM or likely to last more than 3 hours: cefotaxime 2 g and metronidazole 1 g one time
- Colorectal operations II (colostomy present)
  - Mechanical intestinal preparation and neomycin–erythromycin as in colorectal operations I
  - Cleansing enemas if possible
  - Cefotaxime 2 g IV, metronidazole 1 g IV immediately before incision and 12 hours later (to deal with possible spillage of enteric content from bowel distal to colostomy)
- Colorectal operations III (urgent, no mechanical intestinal preparation or oral medications possible); includes appendectomy in presence of abscess, gangrene, or frank perforation
  - Cefotaxime 2 g IV, metronidazole 1 g immediately before incision and 12 hours later
- Head and neck operations
  - Clindamycin 600 mg every 8 hours for three doses
- Hysterectomy for cancer (Wertheim procedure)
- Possibility of bowel entry: as in colorectal operations I
- Ophthalmologic surgery
  - Tobramycin—several drops locally q2h for 6 to 12 doses.
- Penetrating abdominal trauma, surgery less than 4 hours after trauma
  - Bowel intact: cefazolin 2 g IV immediately before operation and again every 8 hours for a total of three doses
  - Bowel perforated: cefotaxime 2 g immediately before operation or as soon as perforation is identified and again q8h for a total of three doses; metronidazole 1 g q12h for two doses, starting as soon as perforation is identified
- Penile prosthesis implantation for patients who may be colonized with enteric flora on perineal skin (e.g., men with paraplegia or major vascular insufficiency)
  - Cefotaxime 2 g and metronidazole 1 g immediately before operation and q12h for a total of two doses
- Prostate surgery for benign prostatic hypertrophy
  - Gentamicin 80 mg IV immediately before operation; no postoperative treatment
  - or
  - Treat patient for specific microorganisms cultured from urine; give one dose of an effective antimicrobial immediately preoperatively
- Simple appendectomy
  - Cefoxitin 2 g IV immediately preoperatively and q3h of operating time
- Small bowel operations with incidental appendectomy
  - As in colorectal operations I
- Ureteroileoconduit urinary bladder bypass operation
  - As in colorectal operations I, plus treatment for specific pathogens cultured in urine or gentamicin as in prostate surgery for benign prostatic hypertrophy
- Vascular shunt implantation for hemodialysis
  - Mupirocin ointment applied intranasally twice daily up to 5 days before operation; and once per week after operation for *S. aureus* nasal carriers

*This is the only set of oral medication.
Note: for beta-lactam-allergic patients: clindamycin 600–900 mg IV or trimethoprim-sulfamethoxazole 5 mg trimethoprim component per kilogram IV may be given instead of beta-lactam.

associated colonizing bacteria from a high level to fewer than 10^5 per gram of mucosa, which usually does not initiate infection. Even in dirty colorectal operations it is often necessary to administer timely prophylaxis despite the fact that the patient is already receiving antimicrobial treatment. This is particularly true when parenteral beta-lactams and aminoglycosides are being used together. The short postantibiotic effect of beta-lactam antibiotics is likely to leave little or no antimicrobial activity against bowel flora at the time of wound closure unless specific timed prophylaxis is also given, and parenterally dosed aminoglycosides do not have a biliary-enteric excretion pathway to diminish numbers of bowel flora.

There is a myth that highly protein-bound beta-lactams are to be preferred in surgical management of biliary disease because of their biliary excretion pathway. This must be debunked for these reasons: (1) if the biliary tract is obstructed, concentrations of an antimicrobial in the bile are diminished to ineffective levels even if this is the usual excretion pathway; (2) antimicrobials having high biliary concentrations but lacking effective serum concentrations fail to decrease operative site infections complicating biliary operations when the biliary tract is unobstructed; and (3) antimicrobials such as gentamicin, having high serum concentrations but no biliary excretion pathway, are highly effective in reducing wound infection rates complicating biliary tract operations in unobstructed as well as obstructed conditions.

In prophylaxis of biliary tract instrumentation, the value of antimicrobial prophylaxis for endoscopic retrograde cholangiopancreaticography (ERCP), in absence of cholestasis, appears to relate primarily to its efficacy in reducing asymptomatic bacteremia originating from mucosal lesions of the oropharynx, caused by manipulation during passage of the instrument. In this setting the frequency of cholangitis following ERCP is not significantly reduced by antimicrobial prophylaxis, which is not indicated for surgical purposes unless bilary tract obstruction exists. By contrast, in the presence of cholestasis, a recent publication indicates that antimicrobial prophylaxis and early treatment with piperacillin reduces the frequency of symptomatic bacteremia.

There are conflicting reports as to the benefit of antimicrobial prophylaxis in decreasing the totality of infections after clean operations without a prosthetic implant, such as herniorrhaphy and breast operations. This may be a result of the quality of postdischarge surveillance to identify all types of postoperative infections.

In light of the problem of hospital dissemination of vancomycin-resistant enterococci, vancomycin should not be used in surgical antimicrobial prophylaxis.

■ INTRAOPERATIVE MANAGEMENT

Full adherence to maximal barrier techniques is important for operations done within or outside an operating room. Use of maximal barrier techniques in an outpatient setting for insertion of central venous catheters has reduced subsequent bloodstream infection to one-sixth of previous levels. Minimizing extraneous traffic and maintaining an adequate air exchange in the operating room are important in prevention of postoperative infection.

As long as prophylactic antimicrobials are administered correctly, there is no evidence that laminar flow or ultraclean operating room ventilation offers any benefit in preventing infections at sites of total joint replacement. Charnley's original studies demonstrating efficacy of laminar air flow ventilation were done without antimicrobials in the 1960s, before the usefulness of prophylactic antimicrobials in joint replacement operations was established. Since then, findings of two large studies revealed that whether antimicrobial prophylaxis of patients with joint replacement operations was done either in an operating room with conventional ventilation or in a laminar air flow setting, the result was similar low frequencies of postoperative infection.

Avoidance of homologous whole blood transfusion, or, if possible, use of autologous blood, is important in prevention of operative site infections, as demonstrated in a number of studies. The mechanism by which transfused homologous whole blood promotes infection is not known.

Surgical skills consistent with application of the best Halsteadian principles of technique are paramount. These include sharp dissection, gentle handling of tissues, proper hemostasis, and avoidance of dead spaces that permit fluid collections.

■ POSTOPERATIVE MANAGEMENT

Acquisition of infection after operation does occur. Patients having orthopedic and cardiac operations are especially vulnerable, but infection may be acquired postoperatively in other types of operations. For example, in one episode after cardiac operations, *Legionella* spp. sternal wound infections were initiated during care; these bacteria were present in tap water in the intensive care unit, and were carried from there by personnel to the wound site during dressings. Operative site infection such as mediastinitis may result secondarily from spread of postoperative infections at other sites, such as primary bacteremia or pneumonia acquired after operation.

Postoperative soft-tissue edema after radical breast operation or extremity amputation may be an avenue for direct bacterial invasion. In this setting some physicians use low doses of older antimicrobials, intermittently on a more or less permanent basis, to prevent recurrent soft-tissue infection and destructive lymphangitis; however, reports of success are only anecdotal. Similarly, repeated antimicrobial suppression of bacteremia may be effective when recurrent cholangitis cannot be surgically corrected. Residual hematoma or seroma in operative sites may promote postoperative infection, and these collections should be drained to limit the opportunity for infection.

Primary bloodstream infection and pneumonia may have an especially grievous effect on postoperative patients. Aggressive infection control measures are necessary among susceptible individuals. The main protection against postoperative spread of bacteria among high-risk surgical patients is the health care workers' use of hand antisepsis with alcohol or chlorhexidine (not bland soap hand washing), along with protective gloves for contact with devices, body fluids and secretions, mucous surfaces, nonintact skin, and skin likely to be colonized with unusual flora. It has not been demonstrated that segregating patients in special units with personnel limited to care of uninfected fresh postoperative patients is required or even preferred, as long as infection control services are adequate to prevent bacterial transmission by hands of health care personnel. However, in a few clinical situations, postoperative patients should be confined to a single room. These include patients who are likely to cause high levels of environmental contamination such as those with infected burns or who have diarrhea, especially when *C. difficile* or vancomycin-resistant enterococci may be present, and patients who are uniquely susceptible to infection because of therapeutically induced profound granulocytopenia in association with bone marrow or solid organ transplantation. In the last instance, special positive-pressure air handling is also necessary.

Postoperative treatment with intravenous immunoglobulins and/or glutamine-supplemented parenteral nutrition offers promise to prevent infections of the primary bloodstream and at other sites. These studies need to be explored further. Oral feedings reduce the likelihood of bloodstream infection. Anatomic changes evident in the villi of the resting or unfed bowel appear to be associated with a facilitation of microbial translocation from the bowel to abdominal lymphatics and the bloodstream. In patients receiving parenteral nutrition, this route of infection may be confused with primary bloodstream infection. If possible, enteric nutrition, including use of proximal small-bowel feeding tubes placed during surgery, is recommended in place of parenteral nutrition to minimize the risk of micro-organism translocation and infection. However, aspiration pneumonia and purulent sinusitis may occur in this setting, so watchful care is necessary. Elevating the angle of the head of bed to 30 to 45 degrees helps prevent aspiration. Prevention of primary postoperative bloodstream infections has broad implications for prevention of blood-borne abscess, osteomyelitis, septic arthritis, and endocarditis as well as infections of the operative site.

Suggested Reading

Burke JF. The effective period of preventive antibiotic action in experimental incisions and dermal lesions. Surgery 1961; 50:161–168.

Classen DC, Evans RS, Pestotnik SL, et al. The timing of prophylactic administration of antibiotics and the risk of surgical-wound infection. N Engl J Med 1992; 32:281–286.

Faro S, Martens MG, Hammill HA, et al. Antibiotic prophylaxis: Is there a difference? Am J Obstet Gynecol 1990; 162:900–909.

Lowry PW, Blankenship RJ, Gridley W, et al. A cluster of *Legionella* sternal wound infections due to postoperative topical exposure to contaminated tap water. N Engl J Med 1991; 324:111–113.

Page CP, Bohnen JMA, Fletcher JR, et al. Antimicrobial prophylaxis for surgical wounds: Guidelines for clinical care. Arch Surg 1993; 128:79–88.

Platt R, Kaiser AB. International symposium on perioperative antibiotic prophylaxis. Rev Infect Dis 1991; 13(Suppl 10): S779–S894.

DRUG REACTIONS

Richard D. DeShazo, M.D.
David L. Smith, M.D.

EPIDEMIOLOGY

Adverse reactions to drugs (ADRs) occur in 15 to 30 percent of hospitalized patients. Most of these reactions are not severe, although deaths occur in up to 0.1 percent. No more than 10 percent of ADRs are due to drug allergy. The worst of these, anaphylaxis, has been most often reported with beta-lactam antibiotics. For instance, anaphylaxis to penicillin occurs in 0.002 percent of drug courses. Adverse drug reactions are a special problem in the elderly.

CLASSIFICATION OF DRUG REACTIONS AND SOME GENERAL PRINCIPLES

ADRs are classified as predictable or unpredictable (Table 1). A *predictable drug reaction* is related to the pharmacologic actions of the drug, is seen in otherwise normal patients, and although uncommon, is known to occur. *Unpredictable reactions* are related to immunologic responses (hypersensitivity reactions) or to genetic differences in susceptible patients (idiosyncrasy or intolerance). A subtype, the *pseudoallergic* reaction, mimics an allergic reaction, but has nonimmunologic mechanisms (Table 2).

RISK FACTORS FOR DRUG REACTIONS

A variety of *abnormalities of drug metabolism* occur and predispose to idiosyncratic and immunologic reactions (Table 3). In patients with the slow acetylator phenotype, drug metabolism may proceed by alternative pathways predisposing to the production of toxic metabolites. These metabolites

Table 1 Classification of Adverse Drug Reactions with Some Representative Examples

Predictable Adverse Reactions
- I. Toxicity due to overdosage; seizures secondary to theophylline
- II. Side effects: immediate or delayed; sedation with antihistamines
- III. Secondary or indirect effects
  - A. Related to drug alone; disturbance of bacterial flora
  - B. Related to both disease and drugs; maculopapular rash to ampicillin with viral infections
- IV. Interactions between or among drugs: bleeding with warfarin and cimetidine

Unpredictable Reactions
- I. Intolerance: a known effect occurring with an unusually small dose; tinnitus due to small doses of aspirin
- II. Idiosyncratic reactions in patients with abnormal metabolism (see Table 3)
- III. Allergic (immunologic) or pseudoallergic reactions (see Table 2)

Modified from DeSwarte RD. Drug allergy. In: Patterson R, ed. Allergic diseases: Diagnosis and management. 4th ed. Philadelphia: JB Lippincott, 1993:395.

can form haptens with tissue proteins and produce neoantigens. This occurs in the metabolism of sulfonamides to reactive hydroxylamines. Drug-induced lupus is also more common in slow acetylators. Serum sickness-like reactions to cefaclor may be due to variant metabolism because patients with this response usually tolerate other beta-lactam antibiotics.

Age-related abnormalities in drug pharmacology contribute to the fact that ADRs increase with age. Psychotropic and cardiovascular agents are the more common causes of serious ADRs in the elderly, perhaps because of the narrow therapeutic-toxic window with these drugs. Although drug absorption is probably normal in most elderly patients, abnormalities of drug distribution, metabolism, excretion, and cellular response to drugs are present. For instance, age-related decreases in serum albumin increase serum levels of highly protein-bound drugs. Changes in total body weight and lean body mass affect the volume of distribution and drug half-life. First-pass drug metabolism (oxidation, reduction, and hydroxylation) decreases with age while second-pass metabolism (biotransformation, acetylation, glucuronidation) is less affected. Age-related changes in creatinine clearance also have profound changes on serum drug concentrations.

Specific HLA haplotypes are linked to an increased risk of developing immunologic reactions to certain medications (Table 3). Although atopy per se is not strongly linked to a risk for drug reactions, there may be a familial tendency to drug allergy independent of specific HLA associations. A multiple-drug allergy syndrome has been described in a group of patients who have had IgE-mediated reactions to many drugs. Drug allergy also appears to be more common in females than males.

Other risk factors include *bronchial hyper-reactivity* and *HIV infection*. Patients with bronchial hyper-reactivity may be sensitive to beta-blockers, including those in eye drops. Beta-blockers may also increase the severity of anaphylactic reactions and decrease the response to epinephrine used to treat them. Patients with HIV infections, especially those with AIDS, have frequent immunologic drug reactions, perhaps related to a deficiency of glutathione, which detoxifies hydroxylamines.

■ PATTERNS OF ADVERSE DRUG REACTIONS

Certain drugs predictably produce patterns of adverse drug reactions often involving specific organ systems. At least seven of these patterns exist (Table 4) and are briefly reviewed below:

Multisystem Patterns

Anaphylactic (IgE-mediated) or *anaphylactoid* (mast cell degranulation by mechanisms other than IgE) reactions frequently involve multiple organ systems. Common manifestations include urticaria and/or angioedema, itching, bronchospasm, laryngeal obstruction, and hypotension. Anaphylactic reactions may occur in response to any foreign protein to which the patient has been previously exposed. Most drugs have been reported to cause anaphylaxis and cross-allergenicity among chemically similar drugs appears common. For instance, patients with hypersensitivity reactions to sulfonamide antimicrobial agents may react to oral hypoglycemic drugs or thiazide diuretics. Administration of opiates may activate dermal opiate receptors, which may lead to anaphylactoid reactions, primarily urticaria and hypotension. Iodinated radiocontrast media may cause ana-

Table 3 Examples of Genetic Variants in Drug Metabolism Predisposing to Drug Reactions

G6PD deficiency
- Hemolytic anemia: sulfonamides, nitrofurans, vitamin K analogues, sulfones, 8-aminoquinolones, aminosalicylic acid, probenecid, quinidine, aminopyrine, chloramphenicol, aspirin

Slow acetylation
- Drug-induced lupus: isoniazid, hydralazine, ? procainamide
- Drug toxicity: isoniazid

Slow acetylation or oxygenated amine detoxification phenotype
- Increased toxic oxidative metabolites: sulfonamides

Fast acetylation
- Hepatotoxicity: isoniazid (increased likelihood with rifampin, decreased with para-aminosalicylic acid)

Abnormal plasma cholinesterase
- Prolonged paralysis: succinylcholine

Epoxide hydrolase deficiency
- Toxicity: phenytoin

Hemoglobin Zurich
- Methemoglobinemia, hemolysis: sulfonamides

Hemoglobin H
- Hemolytic anemia: sulfonamides, nitrites, methylene blue

Subclinical myopathy with elevated CPK
- Malignant hyperthermia: succinylcholine, halothane

Coumarin resistance
- Decreased sensitivity: coumarin

Protein C deficiency
- Skin necrosis: coumarin

Selective IgA deficiency
- Anaphylaxis: blood products containing IgA

Specific HLA types
- Toxic epidermal necrolysis: sulfonamides (HLA B12)
- Agranulocytosis: levamisole (HLA B27)
- Drug-induced lupus: hydralazine (HLA DR4)
- Nephrotoxicity: gold, penicillamine (HLA DR3)
- Thrombocytopenia: gold (HLA DR3)

Developed partly from data of Van Arsdel PP Jr. Classification and risk factors for drug allergy. Immunol Allergy Clin North Am 1991; 11:475.

Table 2 Pseudoallergic Reactions with Some Representative Examples

A. Anaphylactoid reactions (mast cell mediator release without IgE involvement): opiates, radiocontrast media, desferoxamine, vancomycin
B. Probably involving accumulation of bradykinin: cough, angioedema due to ACE inhibitors
C. Probably due to excess leukotriene production: aspirin-induced asthma or urticaria
D. Bronchospasm: inhaled or ingested sulfites, beta-blockade

Table 4 Some Organ-Specific Patterns of Adverse Drug Reactions

I. *Multisystem Patterns*
- Anaphylactic-anaphylactoid: antimicrobials, proteins, iodinated contrast media, NSAIDs, ethylene oxide, taxol
- Stevens-Johnson syndrome or toxic epidermal necrolysis: sulfonamides, beta-lactam antibiotics, hydantoins, carbamazepine
- Hypersensitivity syndrome: anticonvulsants, sulfonamides, allopurinol
- Serum sickness or vasculitis: proteins, antimicrobials, allopurinol, thiazides, pyrazolones, hydantoins, propylthiouracil
- Drug fever: bleomycin, amphotericin B, sulfonamides, beta-lactam antibiotics, methyldopa, quinidine, procainamide
- Drug-induced lupus: hydralazine, procainamide, isoniazid, methyldopa, chlorpromazine, quinidine, anticonvulsants

II. *Dermatologic Patterns*
- Urticaria-angioedema: same as for anaphylactic reactions, plus opiates. Isolated angioedema: ACE inhibitors
- Pruritus without urticaria: gold, sulfonamides
- Morbilliform rashes: penicillins, sulfonamides, barbiturates, antituberculosis drugs, anticonvulsants, quinidine
- Fixed eruption: phenolphthalein, analgesic-antipyretics, barbiturates, beta-lactam antibiotics, sulfonamides, tetracycline
- Photoallergic photosensitivity: phenothiazines, sulfonamides, griseofulvin
- Phototoxic photosensitivity: tetracycline, sulfanilamide, chlorpromazine, psoralens
- Contact dermatitis: local anesthetics, neomycin, paraben esters, ethylenediamine, antihistamines, mercurials

III. *Hepatic Patterns*
- Cholestasis: macrolides, phenothiazines, hypoglycemics, imipramine, nitrofurantoin
- Hepatocellular: valproic acid, halothane, isoniazid, methyldopa, quinidine, nitrofurantoin, phenytoin, sulfonylureas
- Granulomatous: quinidine, allopurinol, methyldopa, sulfonamides

IV. *Renal Patterns*
- Nephrosis (membranous glomerulonephritis): gold, captopril, NSAIDs, penicillamine, probenecid, anticonvulsants
- Acute interstitial nephritis: beta-lactams (especially methicillin), rifampin, NSAIDs, sulfonamides, captopril, allopurinol

V. *Respiratory Patterns*
- Rhinitis: reserpine, hydralazine, alpha-receptor blockers, anticholinesterases, iodides, levodopa, triethanolamine
- Asthma: inhaled proteins (pancreatic extract, psyllium), beta-lactam antibiotics, sulfites, NSAIDs, β-receptor blockers
- Cough: ACE inhibitors
- Pulmonary infiltrates with eosinophilia: nitrofurantoin, methotrexate, NSAIDs, sulfonamides, tetracycline, isoniazid
- Chronic fibrotic reactions: nitrofurantoin, cytotoxic chemotherapeutics

VI. *Hematologic Patterns*
- Eosinophilia: gold, allopurinol, 5-ASA, ampicillin, tricyclics, capreomycin, carbamazepine, digitalis, phenytoin
- Thrombocytopenia: quinidine, sulfonamides, gold, heparin
- Hemolytic anemia (Coombs' positive)
  - Hapten-carrier mechanism: penicillin, cisplatin
  - "Innocent bystander," sulfonamides, quinines, chlorpromazine, para-aminosalicylic acid
  - Drug-induced autoimmune antibodies: methyldopa, penicillin
- Granulocytopenia: sulfasalazine, procainamide, penicillins, phenothiazines

VII. *Reticuloendothelial Patterns*
- Phenytoin, penicillin, aminosalicylic acid, dapsone

Modified from DeSwarte RD. Drug allergy. In: Patterson R, ed. Allergic diseases: Diagnosis and management. 4th ed. Philadelphia: JB Lippincott, 1993:395.

phylactoid reactions, perhaps by activation of the complement system with subsequent mast cell degranulation via mast cell complement receptors. Other agents causing anaphylactoid reactions include vancomycin, dextran, and polymyxin B.

Adverse reactions to local anesthetics, neuromuscular blockers, and nonsteroidal anti-inflammatory compounds (NSAIDs) require specific comments. Although frequently discussed, true anaphylaxis or anaphylactoid reactions to local anesthetics is rare or nonexistent. The usual causes of ADRs to these agents include vasovagal syncope and inadvertent systemic administration. Serious reactions to neuromuscular blockers may occur via specific IgE. However, some neuromuscular blockers such as tubocurarine have intrinsic histamine-releasing activity.

The *Stevens-Johnson syndrome* (SJS), which may occur after the administration of penicillin, sulfa-based antimicrobials, and other drugs, is characterized by a macular rash (sometimes with necrotic centers), fever, stomatitis, and conjunctivitis. It overlaps with and may evolve into the syndrome of *toxic epidermal necrolysis* (TEN) associated with extensive epidermal loss and a scalded skin appearance. SJS and TEN are absolute contraindications to readministration of suspect drugs. The *hypersensitivity syndrome* is an ADR to aromatic antiepileptic agents and sulfonamides and is associated with an exanthematous to purpuric rash with one or more systemic manifestations. These include fever, lymphadenopathy, hepatitis, nephritis, carditis, eosinophilia, and atypical lymphocytes in the peripheral blood. It most frequently appears after 2 to 6 weeks of drug administration. *Serum sickness* is an immune complex reaction characterized by fever, lymphadenopathy, and cutaneous vasculitis beginning 10 to 14 days after administration of xenogenic proteins. Similar vasculitic reactions occur to beta-lactam antibiotics and may last up to several months. Cutaneous vasculitis is characterized by palpable purpura and may be accompanied by vasculitis in other organs. *Drug fever* may be associated with maculopapular or urticarial rashes and leukocytosis, or may occur alone. The latter is the case with bleomycin and amphotericin B.

Dermatologic Patterns

Cutaneous reactions to drugs occur in 2 to 3 percent of hospitalized patients. Certain patterns occur predictably to certain drugs. However, *urticaria* and/or *angioedema* has been reported with almost all drugs. Angiotensin converting enzyme (ACE) inhibitors may cause isolated angioedema, which begins as late as several months after beginning therapy, probably by increasing tissue levels of bradykinin. The pathophysiology of the *drug-related morbilliform dermatitis* associated with beta-lactam antibiotics is poorly understood. Most patients with this response remain otherwise asymptomatic, but in a small number, the rash may proceed to more serious reactions. The *fixed eruption,* a nummular eczema reoccurring in the same area on re-exposure to a drug, is thought to be lymphocyte-mediated. Eczematous *photoallergic reactions* are thought to be due to ultraviolet-induced immunogenic alterations of drugs in the skin, whereas blistering *phototoxic reactions* appear to be due to absorption and transmission of light energy by drugs. Numerous drugs, even diphenhydramine, applied topically may produce *contact dermatitis.* In a given medicinal, the culprit may be a preservative or other excipient rather than the active drug. After contact sensitivity occurs, administration of the drug by another route may lead to a generalized eczematoid reaction as is the case with contact dermatitis to ethylenediamine followed by a generalized dermatitis to aminophylline.

Hepatic Patterns

Hepatic reactions may mimic any acute or chronic hepatobiliary disease. *Cholestatic reactions* are characterized by jaundice without elevation of enzymes other than alkaline phosphatase; however, fever, rash, and eosinophilia may be present. Recovery is not always rapid after withdrawal of the drug and chronic cholestasis has been described. Erythromycin estolate has been implicated in such reactions more often than other erythromycin salts, probably because it is better absorbed. *Hepatocellular reactions* to drugs are characterized by hepatic enzyme elevations and may cause fulminant hepatic failure. Both hepatotoxic metabolites and immunologic mechanisms have been suggested, and antinuclear and smooth muscle antibodies are sometimes seen. Mixed patterns of cholestatic and hepatocellular disease occur, and variable hepatic necrosis may be seen with *granulomatous reactions.* Methotrexate may produce *cirrhosis* without prodromal enzyme elevations.

Renal Patterns

Drug-induced *nephrotic syndrome* appears related to drug-induced immune complexes. Resolution is usually rapid on drug withdrawal, but proteinuria may persist for several years. Drug-induced *interstitial nephritis* is a common cause of renal failure and hypersensitivity manifestations such as fever, rash, arthralgia, and eosinophilia, and eosinophiluria may coexist.

Respiratory Patterns

With the exception of reactions to triethanolamine, *drug-associated rhinitis* is felt to occur on a nonimmunologic basis. *Asthmatic reactions* to inhaled proteins are almost always IgE-mediated, but asthmatic reactions to inhaled or ingested sulfite generally occur by nonimmunologic mechanisms. *Cough* is the predominant symptom in the syndrome of drug-induced pulmonary infiltrates with eosinophilia (PIE). Cough also occurs as a response to ACE inhibitors. Reactions to nitrofurantoin are associated with cough and pleural effusions; pulmonary fibrosis occurs in as many as 1 of 750 long-term users. *Pulmonary edema* may occur in opiate overdoses, with toxic doses of salicylates, and with hydrochlorothiazide (but not other thiazide diuretics). Aspirin and other NSAIDs are prostaglandin synthetase inhibitors and may induce overproduction of leukotrienes, causing urticaria, anaphylaxis, or *exacerbations of rhinosinusitis and asthma* in some individuals. NSAIDs also cause a syndrome of *aseptic meningitis.*

Hematologic Patterns

Eosinophilia occurs with or without other manifestations of drug allergy. Eosinophilia without other manifestations requires observation but not necessarily drug withdrawal. Drug-induced *thrombocytopenia* and Coomb's positive *hemolytic anemia* include the "hapten-carrier" (chemical combination of a drug metabolite with cell surface) and the "innocent bystander" (antigen-antibody complexes associated with cell surface, with subsequent complement activation) types. In addition, some drugs induce anti-red cell antibodies. Modification of the RBC membrane by cephalosporins results in nonspecific uptake of immunoglobulins and a positive Coombs' test without hemolysis.

Reticuloendothelial Patterns

Phenytoin may produce *depression of serum IgA* and cell-mediated immunity, leukopenia and lymphadenopathy. Rarely patients develop lymphoma even when the drug is stopped. *Angioimmunoblastic* (hyperglobulinemic) *lymphadenopathy* has been described with penicillin and phenytoin.

■ APPROACH TO THE PATIENT WITH A HISTORY OF A DRUG REACTION WHO REQUIRES DRUG TREATMENT FOR THE SAME INDICATION

For most patients with a history of drug reaction who require drug treatment for the same indication a systematic approach resolves the problem. This approach requires a knowledge of the material previously discussed and is outlined in Figure 1.

First, *determine what type of ADR the patient had experienced.* More often than not, the patient seen for evaluation of drug allergy has had a *predictable* drug reaction such as a side effect. In such a case the problem may resolve with a modification in dose or change in agent. Taking a more detailed history may reveal only a poorly characterized rash that occurred in early childhood, which is unlikely to recur. The physician should correct erroneous chart entries and stickers and educate the patient. If, after review of the history, a serious reaction on readministration is considered highly unlikely but further security is desired, the consenting patient may be given an initial small dose in a setting where anaphylaxis can be adequately treated. *Intolerance or idiosyncratic* reactions are not amenable to immunologic manipulation and require avoidance of the responsible drug and others of the same chemical class.

Evaluation and therapy for an *immunologic* drug reaction,

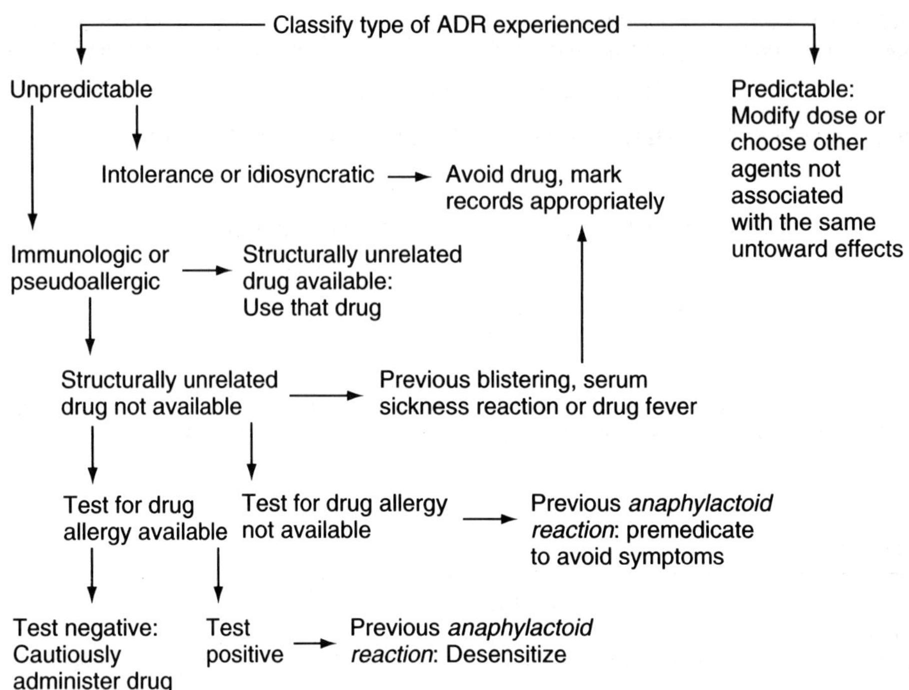

Figure 1
Approach to the patient with a previous ADR who requires treatment for the same indication.

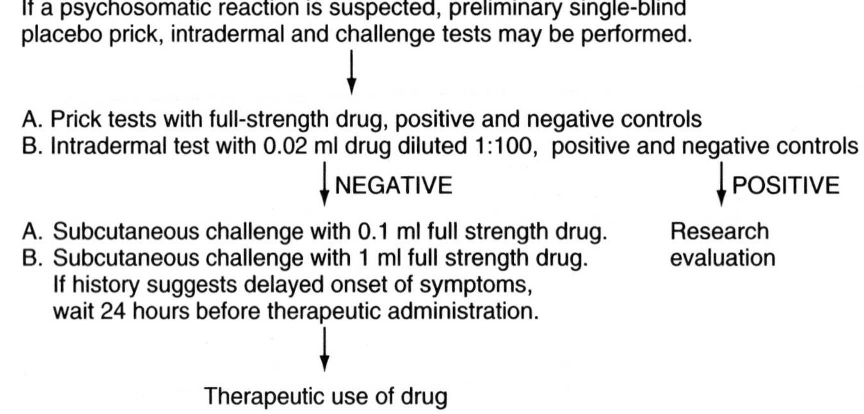

Figure 2
Method of skin testing and provocative dose challenge for local anesthetics. *(Modified from deShazo RD, Nelson HS. An approach to the patient with a history of local anesthetic hypersensitivity: Experience with 90 patients. J Allergy Clin Immunol 1979; 63:387.)*

such as with skin testing and/or desensitization, may result in anaphylaxis. Personnel familiar with and equipped to treat anaphylaxis must be available throughout the procedure, which should not be undertaken unless the drug is absolutely necessary. For instance, penicillin skin testing is not required if the patient does not require the drug. The patient should be assured that the physician is available if further consultation is required. If an alternative structurally unrelated drug is available, that drug may be used without further evaluation. If the reaction consisted of SJS, TEN, serum sickness, or a drug fever, avoid further administration of the drug. In the absence of a suitable alternate drug, evaluation usually consists of skin testing for IgE-mediated hypersensitivity where available; in vitro tests may be substituted in some cases but are generally regarded as being less reliable. For instance, skin testing has been successfully used to find a nonreacting neuromuscular blocker for patients with IgE-mediated sensitivity to one or more of these agents while in vitro testing frequently gives false-positive results (see Suggested Reading). Skin testing is often immediately followed by a challenge procedure if nega-

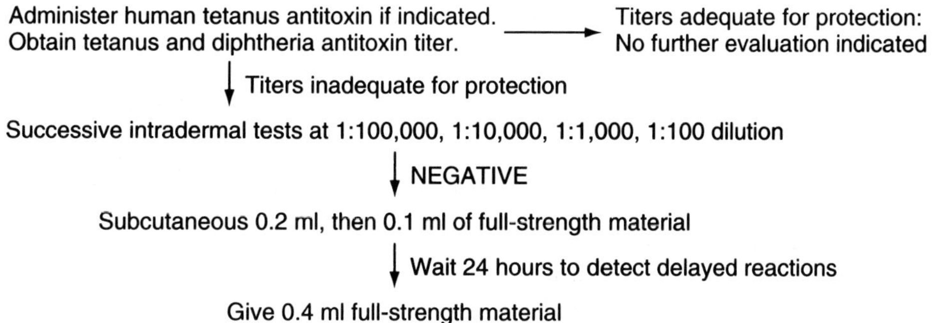

Figure 3
Suggested skin testing/challenge procedure for patients with possible hypersensitivity to tetanus/diphtheria toxoid. *(Modified from Jacobs RL, Lowe RS, Lanier BQ. Adverse reactions to tetanus toxoid. JAMA 1982; 247:40).*

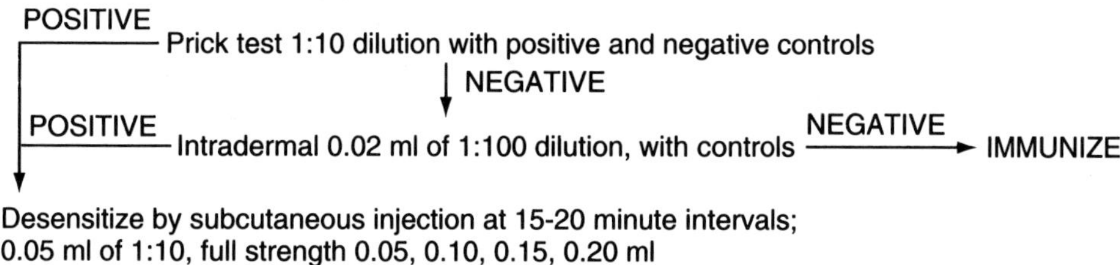

Figure 4
Suggested skin testing/desensitization procedure for patients with possible sensitivity to MMR, influenza, and yellow fever vaccines. *(Modified from Peter G, ed. Report of the Committee on Infectious Diseases. 24th ed. Elk Grove Village, Ill: American Academy of Pediatrics, 1997:33.)*

Table 5 A Protocol for Intravenous Desensitization to an Aminoglycoside Using Tobramycin

DOSE NO.*	TOBRAMYCIN DOSE (MG)	DOSE NO.	TOBRAMYCIN DOSE (MG)
1	0.001	10	0.512
2	0.002	11	1
3	0.004	12	2
4	0.008	13	4
5	0.016	14	8
6	0.032	15	16
7	0.064	16	32
8	0.128	17	16
9	0.256	(Total dose of 80 mg)	

Modified from Earl HS, Sullivan TJ. Acute desensitization of a patient with cystic fibrosis allergic to both beta-lactam and aminoglycoside antibiotics. J Allergy Clin Immunol 1987; 79:477.
*Doses are given 30 minutes apart.

Table 6 A Protocol for Desensitization to Trimethoprim-Sulfamethoxazole (T/S)

DAY	DOSE	T/S
1	1 ml of 1 : 20 pediatric suspension	0.4/2 mg
2	2 ml of 1 : 20 pediatric suspension	0.8/4 mg
3	4 ml of 1 : 20 pediatric suspension	1.6/8 mg
4	8 ml of 1 : 20 pediatric suspension	3.2/16 mg
5	1 ml of undiluted pediatric suspension	8/40 mg
6	2 ml of pediatric suspension	16/80 mg
7	4 ml of pediatric suspension	32/160 mg
8	8 ml of pediatric suspension	64/320 mg
9	1 tablet	80/400 mg
10	1 double-strength (DS) tablet	160/800 mg

Modified from Absar N, Daneshvar H, Beall G. Desensitization to trimethoprim-sulfamethoxazole in HIV-infected patients. J Allergy Clin Immunol 1994; 93:1001.

tive or desensitization if positive. Drugs for which skin testing may be followed by graduated challenge include local anesthetics (Fig. 2) and tetanus toxoid (Fig. 3). A skin test-challenge protocol for streptokinase consists of 0.1 ml of 1,000 IU per milliliter, with positive and negative controls. Testing and challenge-desensitization to MMR, yellow fever, and influenza vaccines (Fig. 4) may be undertaken in the patient with clinical sensitivity (unable to eat) to eggs but is not required merely because of a positive skin test to egg. Drugs for which a positive skin test is often followed by desensitization include beta-lactam antibiotics (see the chapter *Penicillin Allergy*) and proteins, such as insulin. Package inserts for heterologous serums give appropriate procedures for skin testing and desensitization.

Desensitization to a limited number of drugs has been successful even when skin testing is not available or is unreliable. Most regimens for prevention of anaphylactic re-

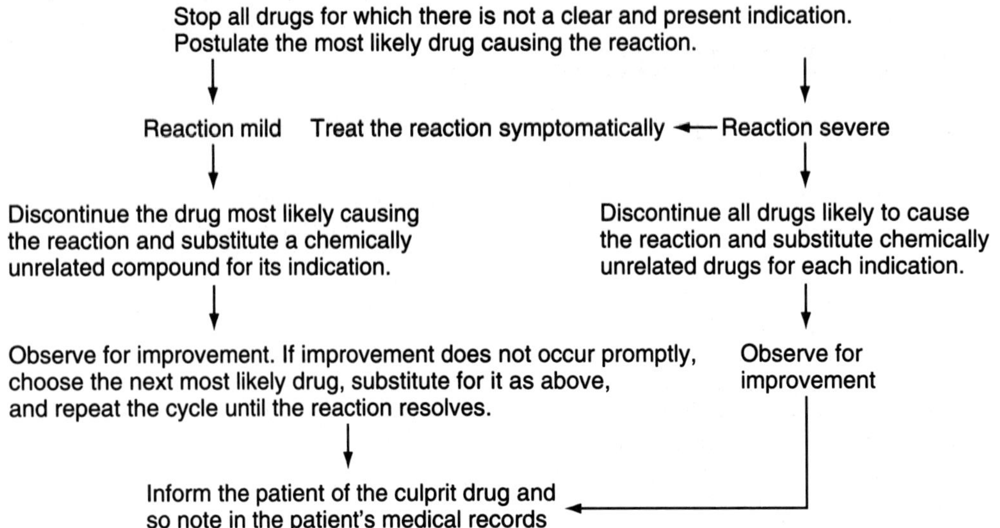

Figure 5
Approach to the patient with a drug reaction while on multiple drugs.

Table 7 A Combination Regimen to Prevent Reactions to Radiocontrast Agents in Patients with Previous Reactions

Prednisone 50 mg PO or hydrocortisone 200 mg IV 13, 7, and 1 hour before radiocontrast procedure
PLUS
Diphenhydramine 50 mg PO or IV, 1 hour before procedure
PLUS
Ephedrine 25 mg PO, 1 hour before procedure (may be withheld in patient with contraindications such as angina)
PLUS
Use lower osmolarity radiocontrast media (e.g., iopamidol or iohexol)

Modified from Greenberger PA, Patterson R. The prevention of immediate generalized reactions to radiocontrast media in high-risk patients. J Allergy Clin Immunol 1991; 87:867.

actions to such drugs, such as aminoglycosides (Table 5), give a doubling dose every 15 to 20 minutes such that a full therapeutic dose has been given after 3 to 8 hours. The patient will usually remain desensitized as long as the drug is administered at least every 12 hours, but if therapy is interrupted, desensitization may have to be repeated. Oral desensitization appears to be safer than parenteral desensitization. Desensitization for less acute immunologic reactions such as to trimethoprim-sulfamethoxazole has been most successfully performed over a period of several days to weeks (Table 6). Desensitization to NSAIDs has been successful for asthmatic but not urticarial drug reactions. If the reaction was anaphylactoid in nature, premedication may serve to minimize or prevent symptoms on readministration. Premedication with corticosteroid and antihistamines has been shown to reduce the reaction rate to radiocontrast media to less than 5 percent (Table 7), and may be similarly effective for other anaphylactoid reactions such as those to taxol. Although premedication has not been shown to be similarly effective for anaphylaxis, it may be used when there is no choice but to give the drug.

APPROACH TO THE PATIENT EXPERIENCING A DRUG REACTION WHILE ON MULTIPLE DRUGS

Management of the patient who experiences a drug reaction while receiving multiple drugs may be difficult. The most recently administered drug is more often the culprit, but delayed-onset reactions such as serum sickness may occur to a drug previously administered. The clinical approach should be organized in such a way as to facilitate a resolution of the reaction, while at the same time providing useful information as to the culprit drug responsible for the reaction, if possible. One such approach is as outlined in Figure 5. The information provided in the preceding paragraphs and tables provides the basis for postulating the most likely drug causing the reaction. For instance, the most likely drugs causing multisystem reactions are antibiotics, including antituberculosis and antifungal drugs, diuretics, anticonvulsants, allopurinol, coumarin, heparin, oral hypoglycemics, and antiarrhythmic agents. The ADR provides an opportunity to review the patient's therapy and eliminate nonessential drugs.

Suggested Reading

Absar N, Daneshvar H, Beall G. Desensitization to trimethoprim/sulfamethoxazole in HIV-infected patients. J Allergy Clin Immunol 1994; 93:1001.

Anderson JA. Allergic reactions to drugs and biological agents. JAMA 1992; 268:2845.

DeSwarte RD. Drug Allergy. In: Patterson R, ed. Allergic diseases, diagnosis and management. 4th ed. Philadelphia: JB Lippincott, 1993:395.

Smith DL, deShazo RD. Systemic reactions to local anesthetics and neuromuscular blocking agents. Immunol Allergy Clin North Am 1995; 15: 613–634.

Sullivan TJ. Drug allergy. In: Middleton E Jr, Reed CE, Ellis EF, Adkinson NF Jr, et al., eds. Allergy: principles and practice. 4th ed. St Louis: Mosby, 1993:1726.

ACUTE DRUG INTOXICATION

Eben I. Feinstein, M.D.

Drug overdosage, either suicidal or accidental, is a major health problem in the United States with an estimated incidence of 7.5 million cases per year and more than 10,000 deaths. However, the number of patients who may require extracorporeal methods (hemodialysis or hemoperfusion) for the removal of the toxic agent is considerably smaller. One estimate is that 10 to 15 percent of patients hospitalized for treatment of an overdose have intoxications severe enough to be considered for either hemodialysis or hemoperfusion. The number that receive such therapy is smaller still, based on the estimated 1,000 hemoperfusion devices used each year in this country. The efficacy of extracorporeal removal is well documented for a number of important drugs and poisons. The use of hemodialysis or hemoperfusion in cases of severe poisoning requires no special technical skill, other than that required for the treatment of acute or chronic renal failure. These techniques in most cases entail no significant morbidity. Nonetheless, there is still a difference of opinion as to the role of these techniques in the treatment of poisoning. The arguments pro and con will be considered after a discussion of the therapeutic alternatives, the usual indications for extracorporeal devices, and their side effects.

CLINICAL APPROACH TO THE PATIENT WITH ACUTE DRUG INTOXICATION

The initial evaluation of the patient with suspected or witnessed drug overdosage is outlined in Table 1. A witness to the drug ingestion or an empty drug container is helpful in estimating the type and amount of drug ingested. A history of prior ingestion of drugs may be important.

Physical examination reveals crucial information. Vital signs and the level of consciousness should be immediately assessed. If stupor or coma is present, signs of head trauma should be looked for. The size of the pupils is often an important clue: constricted pupils suggest an opiate intoxication, dilated pupils may be due to an anticholinergic agent. The integument should be inspected for needle tracks (from intravenous drug injection) or bullae (secondary to chronic barbiturate use).

Routine laboratory analyses can at times point to a specific intoxicant in addition to supplying important data regarding the general clinical condition of the patient. The clinician should strongly suspect ethylene glycol poisoning in the patient with an acute brain syndrome and acute renal failure who has calcium oxalate crystals in the urine. An elevation of the anion gap may suggest several types of intoxicating substances in the patient with metabolic acidosis. Once uremia and diabetic ketoacidosis are ruled out, salicylate, methanol, and ethylene glycol ingestion should be considered. An osmolal gap (measured plasma osmolality minus calculated osmolality) of greater than 15 mOsm per kilogram is another clue to an alcohol or ethylene glycol intoxication. Finally, analysis of urine and blood can provide qualitative and quantitative information about specific intoxicating agents. These data are usually available several hours after the initial assessment and treatment has been instituted.

Table 1 Initial Evaluation of the Patient

History
Witnessed ingestion
Empty drug bottles
Physical Examination
Vital signs
Level of consciousness
Signs of trauma, especially to the head
Other neurologic signs, e.g.:
Constricted pupils (narcotic overdose)
Dilated pupils (anticholinergic drugs)
Skin
Barbiturate-induced skin blisters
Laboratory Tests
Nonspecific analyses
Complete blood count
Urinalysis
Serum electrolytes
Serum urea nitrogen and creatinine
Serum glucose
Serum bilirubin and transaminases
Serum osmolality
Specific toxicology analyses
Qualitative toxicology screening tests of blood or urine
Qualitative assays
Barbiturates and other sedatives
Antidepressants
Lithium
Cardiac glycosides and other cardiac active drugs, e.g., quinidine, theophylline

The early treatment of acute drug intoxications depends upon the vital signs and level of consciousness of the patient. The comatose patient (Table 2) should be carefully observed for the rate of respiration and the patency of the airway. All patients with coma of unknown cause should receive intravenous glucose and naloxone. Intravenous thiamine is also recommended to treat possible Wernicke's encephalopathy. Supplemental oxygen is helpful in patients with depressed respirations. In many instances these therapies are given by paramedical personnel on the scene where the patient is discovered. Treatment of a suspected intoxication can also begin before arrival at the hospital.

Techniques of Active Drug Removal

The oral administration of activated charcoal is the most commonly used method of enhancing the removal from the body of ingested toxins. Prepared as a slurry of charcoal powder and water (1.0 g of charcoal per kilogram of body weight), the charcoal is either swallowed or given via a gastric tube lavage. If the patient is stuporous, protection of the airway with prior endotracheal intubation is required. Charcoal absorbs many drugs before they can leave the gastrointestinal tract and may later enhance elimination from the body of

Table 2 Initial Management of the Comatose Patient with a Suspected Drug Overdose

Ensure patient airway
Administer:
  Intravenous glucose
  Intravenous naloxone
  Thiamine hydrochloride
  Oxygen
Prevent gastrointestinal absorption with activated charcoal and a cathartic
Treat hypotension with infusion of normal saline

substances that diffuse back into the gastrointestinal tract from the circulation. However, charcoal may also interfere with the action of orally administered antidotes (e.g., acetylcysteine). A laxative is frequently administered with the sorbent to avoid obstipation; 70 percent sorbitol is effective and avoids possible hypermagnesemia from other laxatives in patients with renal failure.

Enhanced excretion of certain substances by the kidneys can be produced by forced diuresis and alteration in the urinary pH. To be effectively removed in this manner, the substance must be filtered by the glomerulus, must not be highly lipid-soluble or highly protein-bound, and must undergo significant elimination via glomerular filtration and/or tubular secretion. Changing the urinary pH increases drug elimination of those drugs that are weak acids or bases. Their transport across the renal tubular cell depends on the pH of the tubular luminal fluid, which in turn determines the fraction of the drug existing in a nonionized form. As luminal pH rises, the fraction of a weakly acidic substance that is ionized will increase, thus reducing its tubular reabsorption. The ionized fraction of weakly basic drugs similarly is greater at an acidic luminal pH. Forced alkaline diuresis has been advocated for the treatment of *phenobarbital* and *salicylate* overdosage. Acid diuresis is used less frequently; it has been shown to promote renal excretion of amphetamines, fenfluramine, phencyclidine, and quinine. Both methods require administration of large amounts of intravenous fluids and close monitoring of urine flow and systemic and urinary pH. Even with careful monitoring, serious side effects may occur, such as hyponatremia, pulmonary edema, alkalemia, or acidemia. In summary, although a theoretically attractive mode of therapy requiring no invasive techniques, forced diuresis has a minor role in current therapy of most severe intoxications.

Extracorporeal Methods of Drug Removal

Of the extracorporeal methods available for treating intoxication, the two most commonly used are hemodialysis and hemoperfusion. Peritoneal dialysis offers little advantage over forced diuresis. Hemodialysis has been employed for treating intoxications for 30 years. Since its first reported use, data have been gathered concerning the removal of most of the common intoxicating substances. Effective removal by hemodialysis depends upon the nature of the toxin and the properties of the dialysis system. For optimal removal by dialysis, a substance should be of low molecular weight (less than 300 daltons), not highly protein-bound or highly lipid-soluble, and found in adequate concentration in the extracellular fluid. Factors governing removal of poisons by hemodialysis are similar to those affecting removal of uremic toxins; i.e., removal varies with the surface area of the membrane, its permeability, the flow rates of dialysate and blood, and the concentration gradient between blood and dialysate. The removal of molecular weight solutes is usually greatest at blood flow rates of 200 to 300 ml per minute.

Hemoperfusion entered routine clinical use later than hemodialysis and its major use is now for treatment of poisoning. Activated charcoal is the sorbent in common use, but hemoperfusion using the XAD-4 polystyrene resin is also effective, although not in clinical use currently. Charcoal that is "activated" has a large number of pores with multiple ramifications that greatly increase the surface area available for adsorption. Compared to hemodialysis, charcoal hemoperfusion has the capacity to remove both larger molecular weight substances (up to 40,000 daltons) and highly lipid-soluble drugs.

Complications of Extracorporeal Therapy

Hemodialysis, whether used in the treatment of renal failure or exogenous intoxication, entails certain risks. Hypotension is one of the most common complications. In most patients, the fall in blood pressure responds to the administration of normal saline. However, there are other causes for dialysis-induced hypotension. The acetate buffer used in dialysate has been implicated as a vasodepressant factor. Therefore, many nephrologists prefer to use a bicarbonate-buffered dialysate in the critically ill patient. It should also be remembered that the poisoning agent may cause hypotension. In such cases it may be necessary to use vasoactive agents such as dopamine to maintain a blood pressure adequate for the patient and for sufficient blood flow through the dialyzer. Another complication of hemodialysis is hypoxemia which is usually not profound. The fall in arterial Po_2 seen with acetate dialysate is reduced when bicarbonate dialysate is used. Dialysis with cellulose-based membranes leads to an early, transient fall in the peripheral leukocyte count. This is usually not clinically significant and can be avoided by using noncellulosic membranes. Bleeding during or after the treatment is another potential problem because heparin is required for anticoagulation during hemodialysis. Finally, in addition to removing the toxic agent, hemodialysis also removes electrolytes, such as potassium, phosphate, and other small, non-protein-bound substances in the circulation. However, hypokalemia and hypophosphatemia are usually not clinically significant problems in the treatment of drug intoxications.

Hemoperfusion shares many of the complications of hemodialysis. Bleeding is a more important concern with hemoperfusion because platelets and clotting factors are absorbed to the cartridge. Although coating of the charcoal with albumin or polymer solutions has reduced the degree of thrombocytopenia, a fall of about 30 percent in the platelet count during the treatment can still be expected. Hemoperfusion is also similar to hemodialysis in removing substances other than those desired for therapeutic effect. Serum glucose, phosphate, and calcium may decline. Hypoglycemia is avoided by infusing dextrose and/or water during the treatment. Clinically important hypocalcemia and hypophosphatemia usually do not occur. Hypotension is less often a problem with hemoperfusion, but it should be kept in mind that vasopressor substances can be taken up by the sorbent. If the blood pressure is being maintained with dopamine or other vasopressor infusions, they should be given into the tubing returning blood to the patient.

There are certain problems with hemoperfusion that are not seen with hemodialysis. Because the blood tubing and sorbent cartridge are usually not heated, body temperature may drop. The alert patient may complain of feeling cold. In the comatose patient, body temperature should be monitored frequently. Another potential problem with charcoal is embolization of the sorbent. With sorbent cartridges now in use, the charcoal is either coated or fixed to a mesh. This method of preparation, along with filters in the blood circuit, have eliminated the danger of significant microembolization.

Access to the circulation is required for both hemoperfusion and hemodialysis. For rapid institution of therapy, insertion of a large catheter(s) into either the femoral or subclavian vein is the commonly used approach. In experienced hands, catheter placement is quick, safe, and relatively painless (many patients will not experience pain in their comatose state). Because of the risks of bleeding during hemoperfusion, particular attention must be paid to adequate hemostasis if the catheters are removed soon after the end of treatment. Large hematomas have developed when adequate local pressure was not applied to the insertion site after catheter removal.

Indications for Extracorporeal Drug Removal

Once the nature of the intoxicant is known and the blood level is determined (where possible), appropriate further therapy can be started. The clinical guidelines for further therapy are given in Table 3. The decision to use an extracorporeal method for drug elimination is based on the clinical condition of the patient and the nature of the drug. Most patients in otherwise good health with blood levels of barbiturates or other hypnotics exceeding those given in Table 4 will survive if treated in an intensive care unit where respiratory and blood pressure support are given. Many physicians, however, prefer to use hemodialysis or hemoperfusion in the deeply comatose patient with profound depression of respiration and blood pressure with the aim of reducing the duration of coma. Certainly, when a patient who is being managed conservatively shows further deterioration or develops other complications such as pneumonia or pneumothorax, then extracorporeal methods are indicated.

Knowledge of the intoxicating substance is also essential for appropriate management. Where specific antidotes or antagonists exist, they should be employed as soon as possible. Examples of such drugs are acetaminophen, methanol, digoxin, and cyanide.

It is generally accepted that intoxications with agents that can cause delayed and often permanent tissue damage should be treated with hemodialysis or hemoperfusion. Ethylene glycol is such a substance; it is metabolized to oxalic acid, which can cause irreversible renal failure and central nervous system damage. Methyl alcohol intoxication causes blindness as a result of the toxic effects of its metabolites formaldehyde and formic acid. Other examples of substances with delayed toxic effects include paraquat (pulmonary fibrosis), lithium carbonate, and theophylline (central nervous system damage).

Table 3 Indications for the Use of Hemodialysis or Hemoperfusion in Patients with Drug Intoxications

- Clinical condition of the patient
  - Stage III or IV coma
  - Respiratory failure
  - Hypotension
  - Progressive deterioration of vital signs during conservative therapy
  - Development of potentially life-threatening complications
  - Presence of pre-existing conditions that may predispose to complications
  - Impaired normal routes of drug excretion
- Nature of the drug
  - The substance can be eliminated by extracorporeal methods at a rate exceeding that of the hepatic or renal routes
  - The drug produces late toxic effects either directly or via a metabolic product
  - Ingestion of more than one intoxicating substance which have similar effects

Table 4 Extracorporeal Drug Removal in Common Drug Intoxications

	POTENTIALLY LETHAL SERUM LEVEL (MG/DL)	PREFERRED TREATMENT
Sedatives and tranquilizers		
Barbiturates		
Long-acting	10	HP
Short-acting	5	HP
Glutethimide	3	HP
Ethchlorvynol	10	HP
Methaqualone	3	HP
Methyprylon	5	HP
Meprobamate	10	HP
Analgesics		
Salicylates	100	HD
Acetaminophen	150 (μg/ml)	HP
Theophylline	50 (μg/ml)	HP
Paraquat	0.2 (μg/ml)	HD
Lithium	3.0 (mEq/L)	HD
Alcohols		
Ethanol	500	HD
Methanol	50	HD
Ethylene glycol		HD

HD, hemodialysis; HP, hemoperfusion.

Treatment of Specific Intoxications

Table 4 lists the common intoxications, the preferred method of removal, and the blood levels above which hemodialysis or hemoperfusion should be considered. The treatment of several commonly encountered intoxications are discussed in this section.

Barbiturates

These drugs are commonly used in attempted suicide. They are prescribed as hypnotic and anticonvulsant agents. Patients who are chronically using barbiturates may develop a tolerance to them and at high blood concentrations may not demonstrate all of the toxic effects that may be seen in a patient who does not have drug tolerance.

Barbiturate overdosage impairs central nervous system function, leading to coma and depression of respiration, blood pressure, and temperature. Treatment of the patient should include prompt gastric lavage and administration of activated charcoal for intestinal adsorption. The patient with coma, respiratory depression, or hypotension needs supportive care in an intensive care unit. Although the overall mortality in barbiturate poisoning is low, patients with profound coma have a mortality rate as high as 34 percent. Therefore these patients should be treated with forced alkaline diuresis, and preferably charcoal hemoperfusion. Forced diuresis will be effective only with phenobarbital-like drugs and not with short-acting barbiturates such as secobarbital.

Other Hypnotics and Sedatives

Glutethimide and ethchlorvynol are nonbarbiturate hypnotic drugs that have significant lipid solubility. Both drugs can cause deep coma, respiratory depression, and hypotension. The treatment of choice for patients with these findings is hemoperfusion. It is important to bear in mind that rebound of blood levels following hemoperfusion can occur. Therefore repetitive treatment with hemoperfusion may be needed as the drug is released from tissue stores.

The benzodiazepine group of drugs includes several commonly prescribed sedatives. Fortunately, severe toxicity following overdosage is rare. When respiratory failure or hypotension occurs, it is likely to be in the setting of a multiple drug overdose. The use of gastric lavage and gastrointestinal absorption usually suffices for the treatment of benzodiazepine overdose. Neither hemoperfusion nor hemodialysis has been well studied in this situation.

Lithium

Lithium carbonate is a mainstay of the treatment of bipolar affective disorders. The drug has significant toxic effects on the kidneys and central nervous system. Lithium antagonizes the action of antidiuretic hormone, leading to impaired urinary concentrating ability. Some patients may develop chronic interstitial renal disease, but significant renal toxicity is seen only in a small percentage of patients treated with lithium. Central nervous system toxicity includes muscular hyperirritability, parkinsonian movement disorders, delirium, seizures, and coma. Treatment of severe intoxication should include restoration of extracellular fluid volume by saline infusion in the volume-depleted patient. However, enhanced elimination by saline diuresis is not an effective treatment in potentially life-threatening cases. Lithium is highly dialyzable and hemodialysis is indicated in patients with potentially lethal blood levels of the drug. In patients with renal insufficiency, urinary elimination may be impaired; such patients should also be considered for treatment with hemodialysis.

Tricyclic Antidepressants

The tricyclic antidepressants are in common clinical use and are a frequent cause of drug overdosage. The major toxicity of these drugs involves the heart and includes arrhythmias and depressed myocardial contractility. Coma may develop with severe intoxication. Electrocardiographic signs of toxicity include prolongation of the QRS interval, intraventricular conduction defects, and ventricular tachycardia. Patients with serious tricyclic overdosage should have continuous cardiac monitoring. Repeated doses of activated charcoal help to eliminate the drug from the gastrointestinal tract. Alkalinization therapy with intravenous sodium bicarbonate is indicated to control cardiac arrhythmias. Physostigmine is also advocated (2 mg IV given slowly and repeated up to 4 times at 15- to 30-minute intervals), but serious side effects include bradycardia and cardiac arrest. It should not be used when conduction defects are present. Diphenylhydantoin and propranolol may also be used in treatment of ventricular arrhythmias. Extracorporeal therapy to remove these drugs is ineffective owing to their protein binding.

Acetaminophen

Acetaminophen is a widely used analgesic and is a component of numerous over-the-counter medications. The drug itself is nontoxic, however, it is converted to a metabolite which, in high concentrations, causes liver cell necrosis. Since the drug is rapidly absorbed from the gastrointestinal tract, it is imperative that treatment for acute intoxication be instituted within 24 hours (preferably within 16 hours) of ingestion. The plasma level declines sharply in the first 24 hours, so a decision as to the severity of the overdosage must take into account the time interval after the drug was taken. The antidote for acetaminophen poisoning is N-acetylcysteine. This is given orally at an initial dose of 140 mg per kilogram, and 70 mg per kilogram for repeated doses. Signs of liver damage (elevated serum transaminases and bilirubin) should be monitored frequently.

Salicylates

Salicylates can be fairly described as ubiquitous, being found in a myriad of over-the-counter oral analgesics and other preparations. The common symptoms of salicylate poisoning include tinnitus, diaphoresis, and hyperventilation. Agitation is frequently observed, and coma is uncommon. There are several associated disorders of acid-base balance. Respiratory alkalosis occurs as a result of hyperventilation. There may be a concomitant metabolic acidosis producing a mixed acid-base disorder. Salicylate intoxication should be considered (along with ethylene glycol and methanol) in the intoxicated patient with an elevated anion gap acidosis. Salicylates are rapidly absorbed, highly protein-bound, and excreted in a conjugated form in the urine. Treatment of drug overdose includes the standard methods for preventing intestinal absorption. Salicylate excretion in the urine can be effectively enhanced by forced alkaline diuresis. Many patients may require large quantities of sodium bicarbonate to achieve an alkaline urine. For this reason, careful monitoring of the patient is mandatory to prevent circulatory volume overload. In patients with renal insufficiency or pulmonary edema, treatment with hemodialysis should be considered. Hemodialysis not only removes the drug efficiently, but can correct an associated metabolic acidosis.

Theophylline

Theophylline is used mainly in the treatment of acute and chronic obstructive airway disease. Symptoms of toxicity include nausea, seizures, and tachycardia. The liver is the site of theophylline metabolism and the metabolites are excreted in the urine. The treatment of theophylline toxicity should be guided by the serum concentration and the clinical state of the patient. However, in patients who have serum concentrations greater than 50 μg per milliliter, without signs of severe toxicity, hemoperfusion is indicated because of the danger of permanent central nervous system damage. Hemoperfusion is also indicated in elderly patients, and in the presence of heart failure or hepatic insufficiency.

Digoxin

Digoxin toxicity is a common clinical problem. The drug acts as an inhibitor of Na-K-ATPase. Its major toxicity is cardiac: conduction defects, suppression of the sinus node, and stimulation of ectopic pacemaker activity. In severe overdoses, hyperkalemia develops as the Na-K ATPase-dependent cellular transport systems are blocked, preventing cellular uptake of potassium. Treatment for digoxin poisoning includes correction of any precipitating factors, especially hypokalemia. Specific therapy for cardiac arrhythmias may require antiarrhythmic drugs or cardioversion. Hemodialysis and hemoperfusion are not effective owing to the significant tissue binding of the drug. In fact, hemodialysis may be dangerous because it can produce a drop in serum potassium while raising the serum calcium concentration. A specific antidote, digoxin antibody (Fab fragments), reverses digoxin toxicity and enhances drug elimination.

The treatment of acute drug intoxications requires a systematic approach that couples a careful assessment of the individual patient with knowledge of the nature of the intoxicating agent and its metabolism. Extracorporeal methods for drug elimination should be reserved for those situations in which such methods will prevent serious organ damage. In many cases of hypnotic and sedative overdosage, intensive support of the patient during the period of coma and respiratory failure may suffice. In support of this approach, some investigators argue that most of these patients have developed side effects such as aspiration pneumonia before they come to the hospital and their stay in the intensive care unit is usually short. Therefore, extracorporeal drug elimination is largely unnecessary. However, there are no suitable guidelines for predicting which patients will require a lengthy period of intensive care (more than 3 days). With the level of technical expertise that is currently available for the use of extracorporeal methods of drug removal, it is likely that in most cases the risks of the procedure are far smaller than the benefits of accelerated drug removal.

ILLICIT DRUG INTOXICATION

Adrienne N. Knopf, M.D.

The use of illicit drugs has continued to be a major public health problem. In 1994, approximately 10 percent of all toxic deaths reported to the American Association of Poison Control Centers were related to the use of cocaine, heroin, amphetamines, and other street drugs.

The medical management of these patients is similar to the management of all poisoned patients. Immediate treatment of all life-threatening complications is followed by efforts at decontamination and enhancement of elimination of the poison, use of specific antidotes in the rare poisoning that has a specific pharmacologic antagonist, general supportive care, and appropriate use of laboratory services to corroborate clinical findings.

This chapter describes the treatment of the more common illicit drug intoxications as well as acute alcohol intoxication. The common drugs of abuse are outlined in Table 1.

■ AMPHETAMINES (CENTRAL NERVOUS SYSTEM STIMULANTS)

Amphetamines are approved for use in the treatment of narcolepsy, hyperkinetic behavior in children, and short-term weight reduction. These agents have strong, long-lasting central nervous system stimulatory effects. "Ice," a form of methamphetamine, or "speed," which comes in crystal form and is smoked, creates an 8- to 24-hour "high" and is widely abused.

Amphetamines are taken orally, inhaled, and administered intravenously, subcutaneously, and intravaginally. An acute overdose of an amphetamine or one of its analogues manifests as an enhancement of its usual sympathomimetic and hallucinogenic effects. The major systems affected are the central nervous and cardiovascular systems. The patient may demonstrate hyperactivity, mydriasis, diaphoresis, confusion, hypertension, hyperpyrexia, and rhabdomyolysis. More severe reactions include seizures, acute vascular spasm, arrhythmias, myocardial infarction, hypotension, cardiomyopathy, or coma. Intracranial hemorrhage and transient Gilles de la Tourette-type syndromes have been precipitated by amphetamine use.

As is the case with other abused drugs, the amount of the drug ingested and the route of use do not correlate well with

Table 1 Common Drugs of Abuse

TYPE	STREET NAME
Hashish	
Marijuana	Sensimilla, pot, Acapulco gold, Mary Jane, MJ, weed, grass
DEPRESSANTS	
Barbiturates	Barbs
Benzodiazepines	
Chloral hydrate	With alcohol = Mickey Finn
Glutethimide (Doriden)	With codeine = packs, loads
Methaqualone	Quaalude
HALLUCINOGENS	
Lysergic acid diethylamide (LSD)	Acid, blue dots, D
Mescaline-amphetamine hybrids	
MDA	Zen
MDEA	Eve
MDMA	Love pill, ecstasy, Adam
PMA	
Phencyclidine	PCP, angel dust, hog, star search = cocaine and PCP
NARCOTICS	
Codeine	
Fentanyl (analogues)	China white
Fentanyl (Sublimaze)	"Sub"
Heroin (diacetylmorphine)	H, scag, horse, smack, junk Speedball = heroin and cocaine or heroin and amphetamines
Hydrocodone	
Hydromorphone (Dilaudid)	Little d
Meperidine (Demerol)	Big D
Methadone	Meth, fizzies
Morphine	Dreamer, Miss Emma
MPTP (meperidine analogue)	
MPPP (meperidine analogue)	
Opium	Dover's powder, big O, black-stuff
Oxycodone (Percodan, Percocet)	Perks
Pentazocine (Talwin)	t's and blues = Talwin and tripelennamine
Propoxyphene (Darvon)	Dummies
STIMULANTS	
Amphetamines	Ice
Cocaine (benzoylecgonine)	Coke, flake, snow, speedball = heroin and cocaine Crack = free-base form of cocaine

the toxic reactions. Blood urine samples can confirm the presence of amphetamines but should not be used to guide patient management.

Treatment consists primarily of stabilization and supportive care aimed at specific manifestations. Stomach emptying and charcoal administration are recommended for those who ingested the drug orally. Amphetamines are weak bases and acidification of the urine increases the excretion of unmetabolized drug, but the major metabolism occurs in the liver. Acid diuresis can worsen seizures, arrhythmias, or rhabdomyolysis and is not recommended.

Supportive treatment is similar to that discussed for cocaine intoxication. The agitation and psychosis seen with amphetamines may be more severe than with cocaine intoxication and may require aggressive treatment. Droperidol (0.1 mg per kilogram given at 2.5 mg per minute) is an intravenous butyrophenone that has been used for amphetamine-associated psychosis. Dystonia, hypotension, and respiratory depression can occur with droperidol.

Inadvertent intra-arterial administration of an amphetamine can cause acute vascular spasm and threaten tissue viability. An axillary nerve block, intra-arterial tolazoline, and intravenous nitroprusside have been used in these instances.

■ COCAINE (BENZOYLECGONINE)

Cocaine is a local anesthetic as well as a sympathomimetic agent that blocks the presynaptic uptake of norepinephrine and dopamine. It is currently the most abused major stimulant in the United States, with an estimated 22 million users. The major clinical use for cocaine is as a topical anesthetic and vasoconstrictor in rhinolaryngologic procedures. Illicit cocaine may be sold on the streets adulterated with other white powders, such as mannitol, lidocaine, sugars, phencyclidine, or amphetamines. The purity of "street cocaine" ranges from 20 to 70 percent. It is most commonly used intranasally or intravenously. A purer, more potent form of cocaine, crack (the free-base form) is now readily available and has been implicated in many deaths. Crack is not water-soluble and is generally smoked. Complications of cocaine and crack use include angina, myocardial infarction, chest pain syndromes, ventricular arrhythmias, seizures, intracranial hemorrhage, hypertensive emergencies, acute aortic dissection, and rhabdomyolysis.

Cocaine and crack have rapid onsets of action and cause immediate central nervous stimulation with a sense of euphoria and excitement associated with pupillary dilation, tachycardia, and an elevated blood pressure and respiratory rate. There is usually a typical biphasic response, the "caine reaction," characterized by initial excitation followed by depression with coma and circulatory failure.

The major life-threatening risks of cocaine intoxication are intractable seizures, respiratory arrest, hyperthermia, and dysrhythmias. Even at pharmacologic doses used in rhinolaryngologic procedures, cocaine can cause coronary vasoconstriction and a decrease in coronary blood flow despite an increase in myocardial oxygen demand via alpha-adrenergic-mediated stimulation.

Cocaine-induced seizures can be controlled with diazepam, 2 to 10 mg intravenously. Phenobarbital and phenytoin are second-line agents. Pancuronium bromide in combination with a short-acting barbiturate such as thiopental may be required for status epilepticus. Because succinylcholine administration can cause muscle fasciculation and thus worsen hyperthermia, it should be avoided.

Cocaine-induced hypertension probably is the consequence of beta-adrenergic-mediated tachycardia and alpha-adrenergic-mediated vasoconstriction. Mild hypertension does not require treatment. Labetalol is an adrenergic receptor blocking agent that has both alpha-1 and nonselective beta-blocking activity and can be given as an intravenous bolus or infusion, beginning with 20 mg intravenously. Propranolol, 1 mg intravenously every 5 minutes, also can be used. Esmolol is a short-acting parenteral beta-blocker agent. Its effects wear off quickly after discontinuance if adverse reactions, such as bradycardia, develop. The usual dose of esmolol is 500 μg per kilogram over 1 minute as a loading dose, followed by 50 to 100 μg per kilogram per minute. The pure alpha-adrenergic blocker, phentolamine, at a dose of 5 mg intravenously or intramuscularly, may be used alone or in conjunction with a beta blocker. Sodium nitroprusside at a dose of 0.5 to 10 μg per kilogram per minute is the best treatment for hypertensive emergencies because its antihypertensive effects can be titrated immediately.

Cocaine-associated tachyarrhythmias can be treated with standard agents, remembering the usefulness of beta-adrenergic blockade to decrease the adrenergic cardiac stimulation. One should recall that lidocaine is not an uncommon adulterant of cocaine, and thus there is the potential for producing lidocaine toxicity when administering this drug. Some evidence suggests that alkalinization protects the myocardium against cocaine-induced arrhythmias.

Hypotension is treated with fluids while other coexisting conditions or toxins are considered. Naloxone should be administered to rule out a coexisting narcotic overdose. If hypotension exists despite aggressive fluid administration (i.e., rapid infusion of 2 L), a vasopressor, such as norepinephrine or dopamine, should be given.

Hyperthermia can be treated with passive cooling with a cooling blanket to keep body temperature lower than 39°C.

Unstable angina related to cocaine use can be treated with nitrates or calcium channel blockers. The use of aspirin, anticoagulant, or thrombolytic therapy must be individualized.

For mild toxic psychosis, sedative doses of diazepam at 2.5 to 5.0 mg intravenously may be used. Providing a quiet environment and reassurance also can be helpful. For schizophreniform psychosis, haloperidol, 2 to 5 mg intramuscularly, can be used. It is generally safe but can lower the seizure threshold.

Treatment of cocaine-associated rhabdomyolysis is with hydration, alkalinization, and metabolic monitoring.

There is no effective means of decreasing absorption or enhancing elimination of cocaine, and there is no specific antidote. Cocaine is rapidly absorbed from all routes and is rapidly metabolized by serum and liver cholinesterases. The serum half-life is approximately 1 hour. Laboratory detection generally depends on detecting a cocaine metabolite in the urine. Blood levels do not correlate well with the severity of the reaction or with the occurrence of death.

■ DESIGNER DRUGS

Designer drugs are the products of pharmacologic manipulations of legal drugs by black market chemists and are specifically created to mimic the effects of illicit drugs, including narcotics, stimulants, and hallucinogens. As with other illicit drugs, there are no controls over purity or potency.

Fentanyl and Its Derivatives

Fentanyl and its legal derivatives are synthetic opioids that are used as anesthetics and analgesics preoperatively. As a group, they are about 200 times more potent than morphine. Many illicit analogues are available on the streets. "China white," "synthetic heroin," and "Mexican brown" are common street names for fentanyl derivatives.

These drugs are rapidly distributed, metabolized, and excreted by the body. They can cause rapid respiratory depression, bradycardia, hypotension, hypothermia, and seizures. Many deaths have been associated with the most potent of the fentanyl derivatives, 3-methyl-fentanyl, which is 7,000 times more potent than morphine.

The treatment for a fentanyl overdose is identical to that for a heroin overdose, except that very high doses of the narcotic antagonist naloxone hydrochloride (more than 10 mg) may be needed. Laboratory tests are usually not helpful because these drugs are rapidly cleared in the serum.

Meperidine Analogues

Methylphenyltetrahydropyridine (MPTP) and methylphenylpropenylpiperidinol (MPPP) are also synthetic opiate derivatives. Symptoms associated with this group of narcotics are burning along the course of the injection site, blurred vision, a metallic taste in the mouth, myoclonus, athetoid movement, and muscle rigidity. The treatment for the overdose is identical to that for the narcotic overdose.

These drugs resulted in rapid development of a severe, irreversible parkinsonian syndrome in drug abusers in the 1980s.

Mescaline-Amphetamine Hybrids

These hybrids of hallucinogens and stimulants include MDA, 3,4-methylene dioxyamphetamine ("zen"); MDMA, 3,4-methylene dioxymethamphetamine ("ecstasy," "Adam"); MDEA, 3,4-methylene dioxyethamphetamine ("Eve"); and PMA, p-methoxyamphetamine.

Many of these drugs were introduced in the 1970s as "disinhibitors," popularized by some therapists as adjuncts to facilitate psychotherapy. MDMA is less hallucinogenic and has less sympathomimetic effects at lower "therapeutic" doses, but in high doses it can cause all the effects of a typical amphetamine overdose, with hypertension, seizures, tachycardia, and dysphoria.

Treatment consists primarily of supportive care. Acidification has been suggested to enhance clearance but can worsen the potential complications of rhabdomyolysis and seizures and should be avoided.

■ ETHANOL

The most common of all intoxications requiring treatment is the acute ethanol intoxication. Ethanol is a central nervous system depressant. Enhanced toxicity occurs with the coingestion of other central nervous system depressants, such as barbiturates or benzodiazepines. A blood alcohol level of 100 mg per deciliter correlates with the legal level of intoxication in most states, and at this level, most patients have lack of coordination. Higher levels produce stupor. Levels higher than 500 to 700 mg per deciliter can produce coma and death, although chronic alcoholics can tolerate these higher levels.

These patients must be evaluated for associated trauma, coingestions, and other causes of stupor or coma. Airway or circulatory compromise can occur and requires immediate therapy. Treatment then involves thiamine, 100 mg intravenously, to avoid the Wernicke-Korsakoff syndrome, glucose for the comatose patient or the patient with a serum glucose level less than 60 mg per deciliter, hydration, positioning of the patient to help avoid aspiration, administration of benzodiazepines for seizures, and serial neurologic examinations to detect focal abnormalities suggesting a comorbid event that requires additional studies.

A patient may be considered safe for discharge if he or she is fully oriented and ambulatory without ataxia. Ideally, patients should be offered treatment for alcoholism.

■ MARIJUANA

Marijuana is the most commonly used recreational drug. The active agent is tetrahydrocannabinol. The average marijuana cigarette has 500 mg of marijuana, 1 percent of which is tetrahydrocannabinol. Hashish is a more potent form of marijuana. Marijuana has been used to diminish the nausea and enhance the appetite of patients undergoing chemotherapy and to decrease intraocular pressure in glaucoma patients.

Marijuana produces euphoria, passivity, and an enhanced appetite. Higher doses can produce disturbed thought processes, hallucinations, headache, tachycardia, tremor, and ataxia. The effects begin minutes after inhalation and last for several hours. Urine testing for cannabinoid confirms its presence.

Marijuana users seldom seek medical attention, since their symptoms resolve spontaneously. Treatment of the patient who does seek medical attention involves ruling out other more serious mind-altering toxins, such as phencyclidine (PCP). Benzodiazepines or haloperidol can be used to control agitation. Primary psychiatric illness may need to be excluded.

The toxicity of acute and chronic marijuana use is a subject of great controversy.

■ NARCOTICS

The clinical effects of a narcotic overdose are pinpoint pupils, depressed respirations, and coma. Seizures may occur, especially with meperidine (Demerol) and propoxyphene (Darvon). Routes of overdose may be intravenous ("mainlining"), subcutaneous ("skin popping"), oral, sniffing, or smoking.

The treatment of the patient with a narcotic overdose and coma begins with establishing an airway, assuring ventilation with initiation of assisted ventilation if necessary, and administering 100 mg of thiamine and 50 ml of 50 percent glucose, followed by the specific antidote, naloxone hydrochloride. Gastrointestinal decontamination is useful if the drug was taken orally.

Naloxone (Narcan) is a synthetic congener of oxymorphone and is a specific narcotic antagonist at all three opioid receptors—mu, kappa, and sigma. Ampules containing 0.4, 0.8, and 2.0 mg of naloxone are available. Although naloxone usually is administered intravenously, it can be given subcutaneously, intramuscularly, sublingually, and by endotracheal instillation, an important fact to remember in a comatose intravenous drug user with poor venous access. An initial bolus of 0.4 to 0.8 mg is given, with expected lightening of coma and increased respiratory rate within 15 to 30 seconds. If there is no response, repeated doses should be given every 1 to 2 minutes, up to 10 mg, allowing for assessment of response between doses to avoid using too much naloxone and precipitating acute withdrawal. If acute withdrawal does occur, it can be reversed with cautious administration of 2 mg of morphine sulfate every 2 to 3 minutes until the withdrawal symptoms become tolerable.

If there is no response after 10 mg of naloxone, alternative causes of the coma, such as other toxins or head trauma, must be considered. These higher doses of naloxone (6 to 10 mg) are needed to antagonize the very potent fentanyl derivatives as well as overdoses with meperidine, codeine, propoxyphene, and methadone.

Naloxone has a duration of action of 1 to 3 hours. Repeated doses of naloxone may be required after an initial favorable response. A continuous intravenous infusion may be needed and can easily be formulated by adding 4.0 to 8.0 mg of naloxone to 1,000 ml of 5 percent dextrose in water and administering at 100 ml per hour. Longer-acting narcotics, such as methadone, may require a naloxone infusion for several days. When the infusion is discontinued, the patient should be observed for 2 hours in the intensive care unit for relapse of coma.

A common clinical question arises regarding the appropriate medical disposition of the narcotics user with an accidental overdose who awakens after naloxone and refuses further therapy. Given that the duration of action of naloxone is 2 to 3 hours, it should be safe to allow such a patient to leave the emergency room if he or she has been observed for 4 to 6 hours after the last dose of naloxone and has no other problems necessitating hospitalization.

Naloxone is a well-tolerated and safe drug. The only common adverse reaction is acute withdrawal.

■ NITRITES

Methemoglobinemia, vasodilation, and hypoxemia complicate nitrite poisoning. Many nitrites are abused as aphrodisiacs ("rush") and stimulants. Stupor, respiratory depression, seizures, and arrhythmias can occur. Venous blood may appear "chocolate brown."

Oxygen should be administered. Levels of methemoglobin higher than 30 percent, as measured by arterial blood gas sample, should be treated with methylene blue, 1 to 2 mg per kilogram of 1 percent solution intravenously. Methylene blue should not be used in glucose-6-phosphate dehydrogenase-deficient patients because it can induce a severe hemolytic anemia in these patients.

■ PHENCYCLIDINE [1-(1-PHENYLCYCLOHEXYL)PIPERIDINE]

Phencyclidine (PCP) is a synthetic hallucinogen with no medical use. It is the most commonly abused major hallucinogen. A powdered or liquefied form of the drug usually is mixed with tobacco or marijuana and smoked. It is rapidly absorbed, conjugated in the liver, and excreted in its free and conjugated form in the urine. Its half-life varies from 7 to 46 hours.

Nystagmus, hypertension, altered mental status, and psychotic behavior are common manifestations, but other effects occur, including cholinergic, anticholinergic, adrenergic, and dopaminergic reactions. Major intoxication often progresses rapidly to coma.

Treatment must be individualized because of the wide spectrum of manifestations. Gastric lavage and repeated charcoal administration are useful (even when PCP is smoked) because PCP does undergo enterohepatic clearance. Although PCP is a weak base, acidification is generally not indicated because 90 percent is cleared in the liver. Acidification can worsen preexisting metabolic acidosis and is contraindicated if rhabdomyolysis is present.

Behavior modification is an important part of the treatment. Many patients are acutely agitated and require quiet rooms and haloperidol, 5 to 10 mg intramuscularly every hour. Restraints on the extremities can increase the probability of the patient's developing rhabdomyolysis. Phenothiazines should be avoided because they can lower the seizure threshold, accentuate anticholinergic effects, and precipitate hypotension. These patients may be violent and may be potentially harmful to themselves and others.

The laboratory can usually detect urinary PCP, but the clinical severity of intoxication does not correlate well with the drug level.

■ SEDATIVE-HYPNOTICS

The most serious complications of intoxication with a sedative-hypnotic include respiratory and cardiovascular compromise and hypothermia. Treatment includes airway protection, assisted ventilation, monitoring for sudden apnea, vasopressors and fluids for hypotension, and warming measures for hypothermia. This class of drugs is associated with myocardial depression. Fluid status should be closely monitored to avoid pulmonary edema.

The illicit drugs in this class include methaqualone and glutethimide-codeine combinations.

Methaqualone (Quaalude) is regarded as the street aphrodisiac and creates a sense of indestructibility in the user. In addition to the complications of sedative-hypnotics, methaqualone may induce bleeding diathesis from platelet dysfunction and prolonged prothrombin time and partial thromboplastin time and may require blood product support. Severe muscle rigidity can also occur and can be treated with muscle relaxants.

Glutethimide (Doriden)-codeine combinations are known on the street as "packs" or "loads." Effects such as cerebral edema, seizures, and prominent anticholinergic properties of these agents may require treatment.

Suggested Reading

Goldfrank LR. Toxicologic emergencies section IV: Alcohols and drugs of abuse. Norwalk, CT: Appleton & Lange, 1994.

Leikin JB, Palovcek FP. Poisoning and toxicology handbook, 1995–1996. Hudson, Lexi-Comp, 1995.

Litouitz TL, et al. 1994 Annual Report of the American Association of Poison Control Centers Toxic Exposure Surveillance System. Am J Emerg Med 1995; 5:551–597.

PARENTERAL AND ENTERAL NUTRITION*

Margaret Malone, Ph.D., M.R.Pharm.S., F.C.C.P.
Lyn Howard, M.B., F.R.C.P., F.A.C.P.

Over the centuries, many heroic attempts have been made to feed malnourished patients through enteral tubes or by vein infusion. However, these therapies did not become widely used until certain technical developments made such artificial feeding clinically feasible, more acceptable to patients, and safer. Tube enteral nutrition (EN) expanded once soft, small-bore, nasally inserted tubes and endoscopic gastrostomies were developed. Parenteral nutrition (PN) expanded once the technique of central vein catheterization and more complete intravenous (IV) nutrient solutions became available. Both therapies expanded from the "acute" care hospital setting to the more "chronic" care ambulatory setting, after this transfer was shown to be safe. Reimbursement mechanisms were established and home infusion services were developed to support and monitor these off-site patients. Table 1 provides an estimate of the total number of United States patients on EN and PN therapy in 1992 and the approximate number of dollars spent. This amounted to 18.5 million patients at an approximate cost of $8.5 billion: a little over 1 percent of the entire health care budget.

Like respiratory support, cardiac monitoring, or dialysis treatment, PN is often part of the management of high-acuity patients in an intensive care unit (ICU). In such patients, it is very difficult to demonstrate that specialized nutrition support (SNS) is cost effective. Many of these patients die despite high-intensity care. In fact, a study showed that patients requiring SNS had four times the average hospital stay and stayed 2.7 times longer than patients in the same diagnosis-related group who were not receiving SNS. Despite these unfavorable statistics, SNS is the cornerstone in many clinical situations to bringing patients through major surgery and other severe illness. An important challenge is to demonstrate clinical and cost benefit in well-designed prospective randomized controlled trials (PRCTs). In the present climate of health cost constraint, such trials must measure hard clinical end points such as mortality rate, length of hospital stay, and frequency of complications. It has been shown that a major complication such as wound dehiscence or pulmonary embolism increases the cost of a patient's hospital care by about $50,000. For SNS to be cost effective, it must not only reduce mortality rate, hospital stay, and complications but also induce these positive results without adding serious therapy-related complications such as pneumothorax from subclavian line placement or aspiration pneumonia from tube feeding. With this in mind, the section of this chapter that discusses indications for SNS emphasizes the findings of PRCTs and points out where an evaluable trial has not been done.

Before looking at how and when to provide SNS, it is important to consider the rationale for the use of nutritional therapy. There are perhaps three reasons for using SNS. The first is to support a patient through an illness associated with a prolonged inability to eat. A simple example is a young man with a ruptured appendix, peritonitis, and ileus. It may be weeks before his gastrointestinal (GI) tract tolerates a regular diet, but if he is adequately supported, complete recovery can be expected. Second, SNS may be used to treat established malnutrition and redress the complications of malnutrition such as impaired wound healing, compromised immunity, and delayed mobilization. The third rationale is the least established; it involves nutritional manipulations that can alter metabolic functioning and may therefore provide adjunctive treatment. An example is the use of branched-chain amino acids (BCAAs) in portal encephalopathy or early enteral feeding which may prevent bacterial translocation and reduce the systemic hypercatabolic response.

To maintain realistic expectations of SNS, it is important to

*Editor's Note: This is the chapter we've been seeking for those of us who serve as "pseudo"-nutritionists. It includes information for both medical and surgical conditions.

Table 1 Estimated Cost and Number of Persons Receiving Parenteral and Tube Enteral Nutrition in 1992

	NO. OF PERSONS (THOUSANDS)		ESTIMATED COST ($ MILLIONS)	
	PARENTERAL	ENTERAL	PARENTERAL	ENTERAL
Hospital	500	1,000	6,000	1,200
Home	42	148	636	287
Nursing home	1	160	6	410
Dialysis centers	3	<1	20	<1
	Total persons = 1,854,000		Total cost = $8.56 billion	

Hospital estimate based on Infusion Industry market data and on data from Anderson AF, Steinberg EP. JPEN 1986;10: 3–8, with the dollars increased by 11.6% per year, the quoted growth rate. Nonhospital estimate based on Medicare data and North American HPEN Registry information, Oley Foundation, Albany, NY.

keep a rationale in mind. Most well-nourished patients can survive 10 days of marginal postoperative nutrition; hence, routine postoperative PN is likely to be associated with more harm than benefit and may be unwarranted. Likewise, patients with metastatic cancer are frequently cachectic, but currently available formulations apparently cannot reduce cytokine-induced wasting, so again SNS is likely to cause more harm than benefit.

After much ethical and legal processing, SNS has been deemed active treatment and not a comfort measure. This is appropriate, since SNS is invariably associated with some degree of discomfort. This means that a patient or the legal guardian must formally consent to SNS.

At least 20 percent of hospitalized patients show evidence of malnutrition. Many of these patients can benefit from SNS, but some cannot. In those who are terminally ill, wasting is often an inherent part of the disease course. Distinguishing between reversible and irreversible clinical situations requires knowledge and experience: knowledge of the remediable features of the primary pathologic process and experience with the benefits and hazards of SNS. Figure 1 is an algorithm to help clinicians determine where SNS is indicated, emphasizing the point at which it is essential to involve the patient and family in the decision. This algorithm does not address the question of withdrawing SNS. For a conscious patient, the physician makes this decision with the patient and family. For a patient who is unconscious or for other reasons unable to make medical decisions, withdrawal of SNS requires a written directive or the approval of a previously appointed health care proxy. For this reason, before initiating SNS, it is important to make sure the patient has written a living will and has appointed a health care proxy, and that the SNS stopping point is clearly addressed.

■ ASSESSMENT OF NUTRITIONAL STATUS

Evaluation of nutritional status is important in order to identify patients who are severely malnourished and also to predict those likely to be at risk for clinically significant nutritional impairment. However, difficulties arise because none of the measurements used in practice are indicators solely of nutritional status. Some of the common criteria used to monitor and assess nutritional status are described in Table 2. As a general guideline, any patient who is 25 percent below ideal body weight, shows evidence of significant muscle wasting, and has a serum albumin level of 2.8 g per deciliter or less is seriously malnourished.

Most of these measures are static, i.e., they do not reflect functional status and rarely alter significantly during short-term SNS. For this reason, alternative methods of assessment continue to be evaluated. Tests of muscle function and respiratory function reserve may be useful in predicting clinically significant nutritional impairment. New technologies using dual energy x-ray absorption (DEXA) allow independent measurement of total body fat and the mineral compartment of the body. A combination of DEXA, in vivo neutron activation analysis measurements of nitrogen and chloride, and tritium dilution (injection of tritiated water) allows a complete assessment of the body compartments.

■ GENERAL NUTRITIONAL REQUIREMENTS

Fluid Requirements

Fluid requirements can be estimated as 35 to 40 ml per kilogram per day or 1,500 ml for the first 20 kg plus 20 ml per kilogram for body weight greater than 20 kg plus any additional abnormal fluid losses.

On average, most adults drink 1,000 to 1,500 ml of liquids per day. A commonly overlooked additional source of fluid is that which comes from solid food intake, which is around 1 liter per day, giving an actual fluid intake closer to 2,500 ml per day. In addition, the metabolism of ingested fuels produces another 500 ml of water.

Calorie Requirements

Although estimations of caloric requirements are based on measures of energy expenditure, there is evidence that in the stressed state the body cannot always effectively use a similar amount of exogenously supplied calories.

In practice, for most purposes, general calorie requirements can be estimated using the values in Table 3. A second more tailored method of calculating resting energy expenditure (REE) is based on the Harris-Benedict equation, which takes into account additional patient variables:

$$\text{REE Males} = 66 + [13.7 \times \text{wt (kg)}] - [5 \times \text{ht (cm)}] - [6.8 \times \text{age (yr)}]$$
$$\text{REE Females} = 655 + [9.6 \times \text{wt (kg)}] + [1.7 \times \text{ht (cm)}] - [4.7 \times \text{age (yr)}]$$

The calculated REE is then modified on the basis of activity and stress factors that increase calorie requirements.

$$\text{Energy requirement} = \text{REE} \times \text{activity factor} \times \text{injury factor}$$

Activity factor: 1.2 (in bed), 1.3 (ambulatory)
Stress factor: 1.2 (minor operation), 1.35 (trauma), 1.6 (sepsis), 2.1 (burns)

Where available, a more sophisticated approach may be adopted using indirect calorimetry, which estimates expenditure based on oxygen utilization and carbon dioxide production during metabolism:

$$\text{Calorie expenditure} = [(3.78 \times VO_2\ \text{L/min}] + [1.16 \times VCO_2\ \text{L/min})] \times 1{,}440\ \text{min/day},$$ where VO_2 = oxygen consumption and VCO_2 = carbon dioxide production

VO_2 is invalid in patients requiring mechanical ventilation who have chest tubes and/or when FIO_2 (fractional inspired oxygen) is greater than 50 percent. Values are also inaccurate when the nutritional regimen of the patient is unstable. Interpretation of respiratory quotient, $RQ = VCO_2/VO_2$, may be of value in assessing the impact of Nutrition Support as indicated in Table 4.

Protein Requirements

The adult daily requirements for protein in hospitalized patients are:

Maintenance	1.0 g/kg/day
Mild stress	1.2 g/kg/day
Moderate stress	1.5 g/kg/day
Severe stress	2.0 g/kg/day

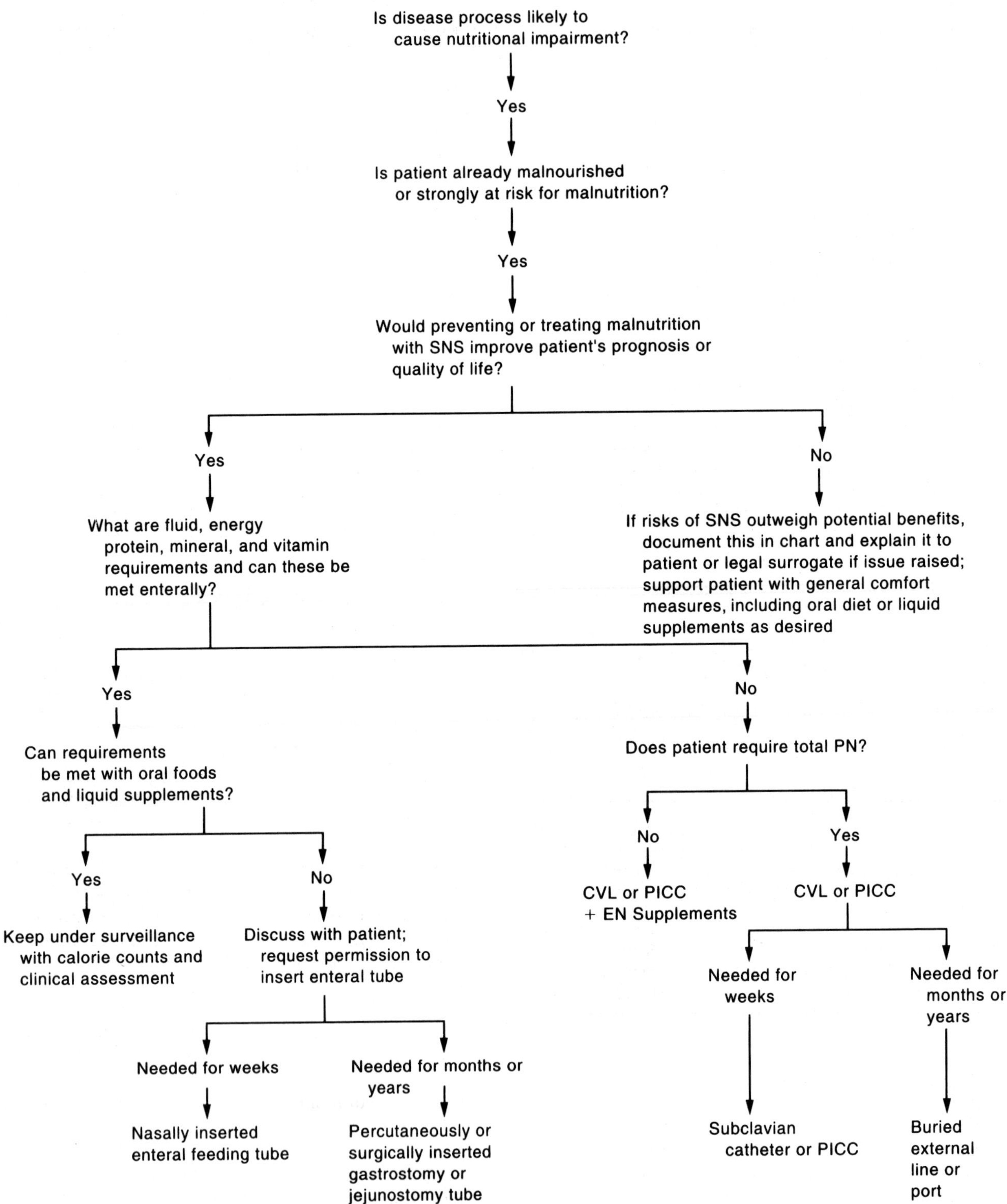

Figure 1

Algorithm for deciding whether specialized nutrition support (SNS) is indicated. CVL, central venous line; PICC, peripherally inserted central catheter. *(From Howard L. Chapter 76. In: Isselbacher KJ, Braunwald E, Wilson JD, et al, eds. Harrison's principles of internal medicine, 13th ed. New York: McGraw-Hill, Inc., 1995; with permission.)*

Table 2 Assessment of Nutritional Status

METHOD OF ASSESSMENT	DEGREE OF MALNUTRITION NORMAL	MODERATE	SEVERE
Routine Methods			
Ideal weight (IBW) (%)*	100	60–80	<60
Creatinine height index	100	60–80	<60
Triceps skinfold thickness (TSF, mm)	M 12.5	7.5–11.3	<7.5
	F 16.5	9.9–14.9	<9.9
Midarm muscle circumference (MAMC, cm)	M 29.3	17.6–26.4	<17.6
	F 28.5	17.1–25.7	<17.1
Serum albumin (g/dl)	3.5–5.0	2.1–3.0	<2.1
Serum prealbumin (mg/dl)	>20	10–15	<10
Serum transferrin (mg/dl)	200–400	100–150	<100
Retinol binding protein (mg/dl)	3–6	2–3	<2
Total lymphocyte count 10^6/l	1.8–3.0	0.8–1.2	<0.8
Delayed hypersensitivity index (DHI)†	2	1	0
Experimental Methods (Functional Tests)			
Prognostic nutritional index (PNI) %‡	<40	40–50	>50
Subjective global assessment (SGA)§	A	B	C
Grip strength/skeletal muscle function	82	65	50

*IBW (male) = 50 kg + 2.3 kg for each inch >60″; IBW (female) = 45.5 kg + 2.3 kg for each inch >60″.
†DHI quantitates the amount of induration elicited by skin tested with a common antigen such as *Candida*, PPD, or mumps. Induration grade 0 = <0.5 cm, 1 = 0.5 cm, 2 = 1.0 cm.
‡PNI % is a weighted combination = 158 − 16.6 × albumin (g/l) − 0.78 × TSF (mm) − 2 × transferrin (g/l) − 5.8 × DHI.
§SGA: clinical assessment based on weight change, dietary intake change, GI symptoms >2 weeks, functional capacity, disease and relation to nutritional status, physical findings.

Table 3 General Calorie Requirements

Normal maintenance/elective surgery	25 kcal/kg/day
Trauma, acute pancreatitis, inflammatory bowel disease	30 kcal/kg/day
Sepsis, minor burns	35 kcal/kg/day
Major burns, severe trauma	40 kcal/kg/day

Table 4 Interpretation of Respiratory Quotient (RQ) Values

RQ	INTERPRETATION	RECOMMENDED ACTION
0.7	Fat catabolism	Increase calories
0.8	Protein catabolism	Increase calories
0.9	Normal state	Maintain
1.0	Carbohydrate catabolism	Maintain
>1.0	Fat synthesis	Decrease calories

Electrolyte Requirements

For the average patient with no abnormal losses, the daily electrolyte requirements for enteral and parenteral intake are outlined in Table 5. Modifications are necessary to take account of abnormal GI fluid losses (Table 6) and altered disease state and severity.

Micronutrient Requirements

There are commercially available multivitamins, multi-trace element preparations, and also EN formulations that follow the American Medical Association guidelines for daily maintenance requirements. In the case of enteral tube feeds, a minimum of 1,500 kcal should be given to provide sufficient micronutrients. Additional quantities of specific individual micronutrients may be needed to correct a particular deficiency or correct for abnormal losses. The daily micronutrient requirements, associated signs of depletion, and appropriate monitoring tests in adults are described in Table 7.

Table 5 Adult Electrolyte Requirements per 24 Hours

ELECTROLYTE	ENTERAL (G)	PARENTERAL (MMOL)
Sodium	1–3	50
Potassium	2–5	80–120
Magnesium	0.3	5–10
Phosphorus	0.8–1.2	20–45
Calcium	0.8–1.2	5–7.5
Chloride	2-5	150–180

■ MANAGEMENT OF THE PATIENT REQUIRING NUTRITIONAL SUPPORT

The purposes of monitoring are (1) to ensure early recognition of metabolic, mechanical, and infectious problems; and (2) to follow the patient's progress in meeting the goal of therapy. As mentioned earlier, the assessment of nutritional depletion and repletion is difficult, and the clinician must often rely on broad clinical end points, e.g., a previously debilitated patient now being able to clear secretions, get out of bed, or be self-caring indicates improvement in strength and well-being.

The monitoring of patients who require SNS varies with their clinical status and the route of nutrient administration. A typical monitoring schedule is described in Table 8. While

Table 6 Enteric Fluid Volumes (L/day) and Their Sodium, Potassium, Chloride, and Bicarbonate Content (mmol/L)

	L/DAY	NA	K	CL	HCO_3
Enteric secretions					
Saliva	1–2	10	30	10	30
Gastric juice	2	60	9	90	0
Pancreatic fluid	?	130	10	75	90
Bile	2–3	150	10	90	70
Small bowel	1	100	5	100	20
Colon	Variable	40	100	15	60

Enteric secretions are also rich in magnesium, calcium, zinc, and copper. Losses are increased by steatorrhea and diarrhea. Potassium losses are small except in secretions distal to the ileocecal valve. The regulation of Na-K exchange in the bowel is partially controlled by aldosterone's influence on the colon. Bicarbonate losses must be replaced as acetate or lactate in TPN solutions to avoid large alterations in the pH of the final solution.

Table 7 Vitamin and Micronutrient Requirements in Adults

NUTRIENT	DAILY REQUIREMENT ENTERAL	DAILY REQUIREMENT PARENTERAL	SIGNS OF DEFICIENCY	METHOD OF ASSESSMENT
Iron (mg)	10	1–2	Hypochromic, microcytic anemia	Serum iron, ferritin, TIBC
Zinc (mg)	15	3–12 +15 mg/l of diarrheal or ileostomy output	Growth retardation, diarrhea, alopecia, hypogonadism, skin lesions, immune deficiencies, night blindness, taste disturbances, and wound healing	Serum zinc, metallothionine 2 activity
Copper (mg)	2–3	0.3–0.5	Anemia, neutropenia, depigmentation of hair and skin, defective elastin synthesis—bone defects, CNS changes, hypotonia, hypothermia	Serum copper
Iodine (mg)	0.15	0.15	Hypothyroidism	Thyroid function tests
Manganese (mg)	2–5	2–5	Defective growth, bony anomalies, reproductive dysfunction, CNS abnormalities	Serum manganese
Chromium (μg)	15	15 +20 μg for GI losses	Glucose intolerance, peripheral neuropathy, metabolic encephalopathy, cardiovascular disease	Serum chromium
Molybdenum (μg)	50–300	10–500	Headache, night blindness, cholestasis, lethargy, coma, abnormal purine and amino acid metabolism	Serum molybdenum
Selenium (μg)	50–200	50–100	Myalgia, muscle tenderness, red blood cell fragility, cardiomyopathy, weakness, hair loss	Serum selenium, RBC glutathione peroxidase activity
Ascorbic acid (mg)	60	100	Poor wound healing, capillary fragility, hemorrhage, aching joints, loose teeth, bleeding gums if teeth present	Serum vitamin C, WBC vitamin C
Thiamine (mg)	1.4	3.0	Beri-beri, cardiomyopathy, neuropathy, Wernicke-Korsakoff syndrome, fatigue, depression, encephalopathy	Transketolase activity
Riboflavin (mg)	1.6	3.6	Angular stomatitis, cheilosis, glossitis, nasolabial dermatitis, dry eyes, achlorhydria	Serum vitamin B_2
Niacin (mg)	18	40	Pellagra, dermatitis, diarrhea, dementia, glossitis, fissuring and swelling of tongue	NAD and NADP levels
Biotin (μg)	60	60	Dermatitis, alopecia, neuritis	Serum biotin
Pantothenic acid (mg)	5	15	Usually seen only with severe B complex deficiency	
Pyridoxine (mg)	2	4	Dermatitis, cheilosis, glossitis, megaloblastic anemia	
Folic acid (μg)	400	400	Macrocytic anemia, glossitis	Serum and RBC folate
Cobalamin (μg)	3	5	Macrocytic anemia, neuropathy, dementia	Serum B_{12}
Vitamin A (IU)	1,000	3,300	Xerophthalmia, keratomalacia, night blindness	Serum vitamin A
Vitamin D (μg)	10	5	Rickets, osteomalacia, bone pain	Serum 25(OH) vitamin D
Vitamin E (mg)	8–10	10–15	Cardiomyopathy, hemolysis, anemia, edema, neuropathy, retinopathy	Serum vitamin E
Vitamin K (μg)	70–140	200	Prolonged prothrombin time	Prothrombin time

TIBC, total iron-binding capacity; NAD, nicotinamide-adenine dinucleotide; NADP, NAD phosphate.

the adage "if the gut works, use it" holds up well, it is essential when using the enteral route to ensure that the prescribed amount of feed is being infused and that feeding is not constantly interrupted or discontinued, leading to inadequate intake.

COMPLICATIONS OF NUTRITIONAL SUPPORT

Complications are often classified as mechanical, metabolic, or infectious. Acute complications occurring in the first few days of therapy are usually metabolic because of fluid or electrolyte imbalance or associated with catheter insertion or enteral tube placement. Infectious complications can occur any time, although line sepsis rarely accounts for fever within the first 48 to 72 hours. Later complications after 3 months of therapy are micronutrient deficiencies or physical damage to the catheter or feeding tube. Multiple-lumen catheters are associated with an increased risk of infection owing to more frequent connections and disconnections for intravenous access. Safe management requires strict adherence to aseptic techniques. Some complications associated with PN catheters can be resolved without removing the catheter (Table 9).

SNS teams have shown their cost effectiveness by reducing the incidence of catheter-related sepsis, decreasing wastage of solutions, and encouraging EN rather than PN, whenever feasible.

Table 8 Monitoring Patients Receiving Nutritional Support

ASSESSMENT PARAMETER	FREQUENCY
Clinical Well-being	
Vital signs	
Body weight	Daily
Fluid and nutrient intake	
Laboratory Data	
Urine glucose	Four times daily first 24 hr
Blood glucose by capillary stick	then daily
Serum glucose, Na, K, Cl, HCO_3, BUN	Daily until stable then twice weekly
Serum albumin, liver function tests, serum Ca, P, Mg, creatinine	Baseline then weekly
Hematology Data	
Hemoglobin, hematocrit, WBC, differential, prothrombin time, partial thromboplastin time	Baseline then weekly
Folate, vitamin B_{12}, Fe, transferrin	As indicated
Micronutrient assays	
Serum lipids	
Nitrogen balance	

INDICATIONS AND CONTRAINDICATIONS IN SPECIFIC CLINICAL CONDITIONS

Since SNS is an expensive therapy, particularly when administered parenterally, it is important to know where clinical benefit is likely to occur. In the following sections, various clinical conditions are reviewed and the important issues highlighted.

Perioperative Nutrition

Clinical Issues:

1. What are the risks and benefits of pre- and/or postoperative nutrition, particularly in terms of morbidity and mortality?
2. What is the most effective route of nutrient administration?

A large cooperative Veterans Administration study and a meta-analysis of 18 smaller studies showed that preoperative nutrition is of benefit in severely malnourished patients only. Patients with mild to moderate malnutrition in the nutritionally supported treatment group showed no clear benefit and a greater incidence of complications than the control patients.

The duration of preoperative support has also been investigated in several PRCTs. Two to 3 days of IV nutrition before

Table 9 Catheter-Related Complications

COMPLICATION	MANAGEMENT
Thrombosis	*Urokinase lock:* 5,000 units urokinase dissolved in 2 ml saline, instilled into catheter, left in situ for 30–60 min, then withdrawn; if unsuccessful, may attempt urokinase infusion, 40,000 units/hr for 6 hr
	Streptokinase lock: 5,000 units/ml instilled to fill internal volume of catheter, dwell time 30 min then withdrawn
	Tissue plasminogen activator: Used on an investigational basis in urokinase failures, 2 mg/2 ml with a 4 hr dwell time
Infection	*Antibiotic lock technique:* Limited studies have reported the efficacy of treating cather-related sepsis with a high concentration of an appropriate antibiotic, e.g., amikacin, 1.5 mg/ml; minocycline, 0.2 mg/ml; vancomycin, 1–5 mg/ml, left in situ for 12 hr
Occlusion	*With lipid:* Limited experience in clearing lipid-occluded catheters with 3 ml 70% ethanol, dwell time 1 hr
	With drug/electrolytes: Where alteration of pH will improve the occluding agent's solubility, 1 ml 0.1 N hydrochloric acid or 8.4% sodium bicarbonate may be instilled, dwell time 1 hr

surgery does not influence surgical outcome, and 5 to 7 days produces equivocal results, but in several studies 7 to 10 days of preoperative PN resulted in a significant reduction in postoperative complications and mortality in severely malnourished patients.

Postoperative SNS administered parenterally or enterally in critically ill patients has been demonstrated in PRCTs to reduce mortality, infectious complications, and length of ICU stay. A number of studies have indicated that early enteral feeding via a jejunostomy within the first 24 to 48 hours, even with small amounts, improves patient outcomes with decreased length of hospital stay, and reduces proinflammatory cytokine responses. These studies showed that jejunal feeding is tolerated even though the patient frequently has gastric atony and colonic ileus.

Inflammatory Bowel Disease

Clinical Issues:

1. Does SNS have a primary role in treating inflammatory bowel disease (IBD) or is the role simply one of correcting secondary complications of malnutrition?
2. Does the route of administration make a difference?

IBD, particularly Crohn's disease, is often associated with severe hypoalbuminemia and weight loss. Anemia and vitamin and mineral deficiencies are also common.

Some new data suggest a possible role for a modified oral diet in the maintenance of disease remission. Several studies have compared steroid therapy with elemental diets and have found that steroids are somewhat more effective in inducing and maintaining a remission in Crohn's disease. However, in some clinical situations, particularly with children or in preoperative build-up, avoidance of steroids is preferred, and elemental diets may be more appropriate therapy, even though these usually involve a nasogastric tube.

Recent studies found no difference between elemental and polymeric diets. Several small studies have demonstrated no substantial benefit from the parenteral route. We interpret these data as tending to refute the hypothesis of food acting as an allergen in the pathogenesis of IBD. In fact, "bowel rest" is essentially bowel starvation, and depriving the gut of all substrates may be detrimental.

The possible value of soluble fiber in sustaining colonic short-chain fatty acid levels, the preferred fuel of the colonocyte; the role of glutamine as the preferred fuel for the enterocyte; and the anti-inflammatory role of omega-3 fatty acids, nucleotides, and arginine are all under investigation.

Pancreatitis

Clinical Issues:

1. Can the gut be used without exacerbating the pancreatitis?
2. Should SNS be a routine part of management?
3. Are there any contraindications to the use of IV fat as a calorie source?

Pancreatic secretion is stimulated by IV feeding and enteral nutrients that are delivered proximal to the ligament of Treitz. J-tube feeding appears to be well tolerated in up to 80 percent of patients with acute pancreatitis.

PN does not alter medical outcome in mild to moderate pancreatitis. In severe pancreatitis, malnutrition is associated with a poor outcome. Several studies have demonstrated benefit of SNS started early in the disease course.

In the absence of hyperlipidemia and impaired triglyceride clearance or thrombocytopenia, IV lipids can be administered without exacerbating pancreatitis, and provide a useful calorie source in a patient who may have impaired insulin secretion. Careful monitoring of acid-base balance is essential in patients with pancreatic fistulas or surgical drains, owing to loss of large amounts of bicarbonate in the pancreatic fluid.

Liver Disease

Clinical Issues:

1. Is there a role for BCAA-enriched formulas?
2. What are the constraints for SNS in a patient with acute or chronic liver dysfunction?

Malnutrition is common with advanced liver disease. Adequate protein intake may be constrained by the development of portal encephalopathy. Several studies have shown benefit from branched-chain (leucine, isoleucine, and valine) amino acid-enriched solutions in patients who cannot tolerate enough protein to achieve nitrogen balance. The rationale behind BCAA therapy is that patients with liver impairment have increased muscle breakdown for gluconeogenesis and reduced muscle and plasma BCAA levels, with a relative increase in aromatic amino acid (AAA) levels. This imbalance favors the transport of tryptophan, an aromatic amino acid, across the blood-brain barrier, leading to an increase in brain serotonin, which is a tryptophan breakdown product and a central nervous system (CNS) depressant. Since BCAA-enriched formulas are very expensive, they should be reserved for patients who cannot tolerate adequate protein intake (0.5 to 0.8 g per kilogram per day) without developing encephalopathy. These are only occasional liver failure patients.

In less severe liver disease, the protein intake should ideally be between 0.8 and 1 g per kilogram per day. The aim should be to meet the caloric requirement while keeping the serum glucose below 200 mg per deciliter. Fat emulsions must be used cautiously because of decreased lipid clearance. Sufficient fat must be provided to meet essential fatty acid requirements (5 percent of daily calories or 200 ml of 20 percent lipid emulsion twice weekly). A recent randomized study of alcoholic cirrhotic patients showed that the provision of a modest daily enteral oral supplement, on an outpatient basis, significantly reduced morbidity and hospitalization rates. This benefit appeared to relate primarily to a decrease in the incidence of infection.

Limited data suggest that aggressive post-liver transplant nutrition (1.5 g per kilogram per day of protein and 35 kcal per kilogram per day) is beneficial. Since many candidates for transplantation are malnourished, preoperative build-up is desirable. The ratio of plasma BCAA to AAA appears to be predictive of graft survival. To date, the benefit of post-transplant BCAA infusions has not been fully investigated. Infusion of BCAA increases the BCAA:AAA ratio, as would be expected, but no differences in outcome or encephalopathy have been demonstrated.

Table 10 Nutritional Requirements of Dialysis Patients

TYPE OF DIALYSIS	CALORIE REQUIREMENTS	PROTEIN REQUIREMENTS	COMMENTS
Hemodialysis	Intake and loss from hemodialysis fluid minimal	1–1.2 g/kg/day	Water-soluble vitamins lost in dialysate; iron required with erythropoietin: micronutrients (e.g., copper and zinc) lost in dialysate
Peritoneal	Patients absorb 60%–80% of dialysate glucose, average 8 kcal/kg/day	1.2–1.5 g/kg/day	Increased protein loss in peritonitis by 50–100 to 3.6 g water-soluble micronutrients lost in peritoneal dialysis fluid
Hemofiltration	Limited data available: 43% of infused glucose retained	Estimated losses around 11 g/day	

Alterations in Liver Function Tests in Patients on Parenteral Nutrition

The incidence of abnormal liver function test results (raised alkaline phosphatase and transaminase levels) is reported to be 25 to 100 percent in patients on PN. Peak levels usually occur within 1 to 4 weeks of starting PN and then remain stable or decline despite continued therapy. A raised bilirubin level is less frequent (0 to 46 percent). Histologically, steatosis is more common in adults and cholestasis in children. Periportal fibrosis advancing to cirrhosis is a rare but serious complication of long-term PN that occurs more often in infants than in adults. Many etiologic factors have been proposed, including excessive administration of dextrose; lithocholic acid toxicity after bacterial overgrowth; bacterial translocation; and inadequate provision of sulfur-containing amino acids, to sustain normal levels, and of cytoplasmic antioxidants such as selenium and vitamin E. The presence of sodium bisulfite in the PN solutions may be an oxidant stress. Methods of reducing liver abnormalities have included the avoidance of overfeeding by accurate estimation of requirements, cyclic feeding with periods off the PN each 24 hours, maintenance of some enteral intake whenever possible to stimulate bile flow, and the use of oral antibiotics to reduce bacterial overgrowth.

Renal Disease

Clinical Issues:

1. Does SNS improve the outcome in acute renal failure (ARF)?
2. What is the role of essential amino acid solutions?
3. What is the role of SNS in the support of malnourished dialysis patients?
4. What is the place in therapy of novel methods of nutrient delivery during dialysis?

Acute Renal Failure

ARF in patients with major trauma is associated with a high mortality rate. Many of these patients have multiorgan failure that makes SNS very complex in terms of fluid and electrolyte monitoring. Early studies demonstrated an improved outcome in patients who received PN that supplied both essential amino acids and dextrose, compared with dextrose-only solutions. As a consequence, expensive specialized renal support solutions, rich in essential amino acids or their keto analogues, have been advocated. More recent randomized studies have shown no greater benefit of these special amino acid formulas compared with more standard amino acid solutions. In general, patients with ARF who are not on dialysis require a reduced fluid and protein intake (0.5 to 0.6 g per kilogram per day of protein) with normal calorie requirements and generous micronutrients except for vitamin A, which accumulates.

Chronic Renal Failure Patients on Dialysis

A summary of nutritional requirements associated with different methods of dialysis is presented in Table 10.

Intradialytic Parenteral Nutrition (IDPN). IDPN is usually administered in the last 90 minutes of the hemodialysis treatment period. Limited data are available from a few studies that evaluated intradialytic infusion of calories, essential amino acids, and histidine along with a high protein–high calorie oral intake. These studies have shown improved appetite, serum protein levels, and body weight in malnourished patients. Problems may be experienced with postinfusion hypoglycemia when PN is abruptly halted at the end of dialysis. Glucose administration should not exceed the known maximal oxidation rate of 1.2 g per kilogram per dialysis treatment. Replacing some of the calories with lipid may limit glycemic problems, but hypertriglyceridemia should be avoided. Patients with end-stage renal disease have around 75 percent of normal lipid clearance. Lipid infusions should not be administered at more than 1 g per kilogram per hour and should be withheld if serum triglycerides are more than 300 mg per deciliter before dialysis. There are no studies comparing IDPN with improved enteral intake alone as might be achieved by cycled tube EN.

Peritoneal Dialysis. Amino acids are a good osmotic agent providing twice the osmotic load of glucose. The benefits of using some amino acids rather than just glucose in the peritoneal dialysis solution are the reduction in glucose load, reduced hypertriglyceridemia, and decreased protein loss with normalization of serum amino acids. Standard continuous ambulatory peritoneal dialysis (CAPD) solutions contain either a high glucose (4.25 percent, 486 mOsm) or a low glucose (1.5 percent, 347 mOsm) concentration. Amino acid CAPD solutions are glucose free and contain high amino acids (2.5 percent, 460 mOsm) or low amino acids (1.0 percent, 364 mOsm) with standard electrolyte concentrations. Acidosis may occur, possibly because of free sulfur from methionine in the amino acid solutions. Small studies have used one amino acid exchange followed by three glucose exchanges per day, or alternating amino acid and glucose solutions. The peritoneal use of solutions containing lipid has so far been evaluated only in animal studies.

Lung Disease

Clinical Issues:

1. Is an increased REE associated with lung disease?
2. What is the optimal fuel source in patients with severe lung disease?

Patients with severe lung disease have a 15 to 20 percent increase in energy expenditure owing to the increased work of breathing. If this increased expenditure is not taken into account, patients with chronic lung disease gradually lose weight. Loss of any excess weight may be desirable, but if the weight loss impairs the respiratory muscle strength, ciliary clearance function, and immunocompetence, the patient is at greater risk for acute exacerbations. In patients who are being weaned off a ventilator, glucose should be given at no more than 5 mg per kilogram per minute and lipid at no more than 1 to 1.5 g per kilogram per 24 hours. The provision of excessive carbohydrate calories increases carbon dioxide production both by increasing metabolic rate and by stimulating lipogenesis. This may lead to worsening of the respiratory status. Lipids should not provide more than 40 percent of the nonprotein calories and should be discontinued if serum triglyceride levels are higher than 250 mg per liter. Controversy exists over the use of lipids with regard to impaired lung diffusion due to coating of red blood cells, deposition in the alveolar wall, and increased blood viscosity. The effect of lipids on the inflammatory response appears to be dose- and rate-related. Slow infusions (for more than 10 hours) are predominantly vasodilatory; fast infusions (for less than 5 hours) exhibit vasopressor and proinflammatory changes. Protein intake should be between 1.2 and 1.5 g per kilogram per day. A protein meal is known to enhance the ventilatory response to carbon dioxide. Electrolytes should be monitored closely, particularly potassium, phosphorus, calcium, and magnesium, as deficiency adversely affects respiratory muscle function.

Chronic pulmonary disease patients who are less than 90 percent of their ideal body weight demonstrate a greater 5 year mortality, independent of their pulmonary status. Since these patients have been shown to be hypermetabolic, the recommended calorie intake is 1.7 times the REE. Short-term studies over 3 months have demonstrated improved respiratory muscle function with improved nutritional intake.

Patients with cystic fibrosis (CF) are often undernourished because of malabsorption, anorexia, and increased expenditure (30 percent greater than normal) caused by the work of breathing and repeated infections. Although prognosis is most related to the patient's pulmonary function, nutritional status is also important. Data from studies in children and adolescents suggest improvement in pulmonary function in the very young and stabilization of lung disease in older children, with better nutritional status achieved by using tube EN delivered through a gastrostomy. The psychological consequences of this aggressive approach have not been properly assessed. Also, most CF patients have reduced GI motility and are at risk for gastroesophageal reflux and aspiration. This should be assessed before a gastrostomy is inserted, since an antireflux procedure may also be needed.

Cancer

Clinical Issues:

1. Does SNS improve the outcome in cachectic cancer patients?
2. Does SNS in cancer patients increase lean body mass?
3. Does SNS improve patients' tolerance of cancer therapy?

One of the most striking forms of malnutrition is that seen in cancer cachexia. Most PRCTs designed to evaluate the risk-benefit ratio of SNS are too small to avoid a type II error, in which an important benefit is missed. From the limited data available, there appears to be no place for routine use of PN in patients with cancer. In fact there is a fourfold increase in the incidence of infection in cancer patients who receive PN, and a meta-analysis of available studies failed to demonstrate any clinical benefit in terms of survival, treatment tolerance, or tumor response. Despite this seeming lack of benefit, SNS may be justified for a finite period if normal intake is totally inadequate, such as during aggressive chemotherapy or in the severely malnourished cancer patient undergoing surgery.

Well-nourished bone marrow transplant recipients receiving prophylactic SNS before and during transplantation were shown to have significantly better late survival. EN appears to be as effective as PN where it is tolerated.

Human Immunodeficiency Virus-Positive Patients

Clinical Issues:

1. Does SNS early in the disease delay progression to symptomatic illness?
2. Does SNS late in the disease process alter survival or improve the quality of life?

The answers to these important clinical questions are not yet known. It is clear that from the moment of infection the virus is constantly replicating and that the immune status of the patient influences the disease-free interval. Thus, children who contracted human immunodeficiency virus (HIV) from Factor VIII have a longer disease-free interval than drug addicts, who are immunologically stressed by other diseases such as hepatitis. Nutritional status has a major influence on immune function. AIDS patients with HIV GI disease or an opportunistic GI infection often have fat and bile acid malabsorption, lactase deficiency, increased zinc and protein losses, and (in the presence of terminal ileal disease) vitamin B_{12} deficiency. General recommendations are that when nutritional intake meets more than two-thirds of the needs, only counseling is appropriate. If less than two-thirds of the required intake is being met, SNS may be indicated, preferably by the enteral route. There is no evidence that sterile supplements or elemental feeds are especially beneficial. Currently, data showing benefit from nutritional intervention are very limited, and large multicenter studies are needed to ensure best use of the available health care resources. Where malnu-

Table 11 Summary of Outcome on Home Parenteral and Enteral Nutrition

DIAGNOSIS	NO. OF PTS	AVERAGE AGE (YR)	MORTALITY* RATE ON RX	TIME ON RX (% ON >1 YR)	COMPS PER YR† RX REL.	COMPS PER YR† DX REL.	REHABILITATION‡ C	REHABILITATION‡ P	REHABILITATION‡ M	COMMENTS
HOME PARENTERAL NUTRITION										
Crohn's disease	480	35	5% p.a.	25	0.9	1.1	70	27	3	Usually justified
Ischemic bowel disease	274	60	10% p.a.	52	1.3	1.0	50	40	10	Usually justified
Motility disorder	264	45	10% p.a.	50	1.2	1.0	50	40	10	Usually justified
Radiation enteritis	123	57	15% p.a.	48	0.7	1.0	40	50	10	Usually justified
Congenital bowel defect	127	4	6% p.a.	44	2.0	1.0	65	25	10	Usually justified
Chronic adhesive obstructions	94	52	15% p.a.	40	1.5	1.3	30	65	5	Usually justified
Hyperemesis gravidarum	85	27	0% p.a.	Aver. dur. 8 wk (2–30)	1.5	3.5	69	13	1	Usually justified
Cystic fibrosis	46	16	50% p.a.	50	0.8	3.7	20	60	20	Occasionally justified
Chronic pancreatitis	102	37	10% p.a.	20	1.2	2.5	60	30	10	Occasionally justified
AIDS	200	30	50% in 6 mo 20% survival rate >1 yr	5	1.4	3.2	6	64	30	Occasionally justified
Active cancer	1,672	42	50% in 6 mo 25% survival rate >1 yr	7	1.0	4.0	30	65	15	Justified in patients with treatable disease (e.g., in bone marrow transplant patients) or if the cancer is indolent; rarely justified in nontreatable metastatic bowel obstruction
HOME ENTERAL NUTRITION										
Active cancer	1,296	60	50% in 6/12 30% SR >1 yr	5	0.4	2.8	20	60	20	Justified in patients with treatable disease or an obstructing cancer that can be bypassed by a feeding tube
Neurologic disorders of swallowing	918	65	40% first yr then levels off	30	0.3	1.0	10	20	70	Usually justified

*The cause of death in >95% of patients is the underlying illness or other causes unrelated to an HPEN complication.
†Refers only to those complications that result in rehospitalization.
‡Rehabilitation is designated as Complete (C), Partial (P), or Minimal (M), in relation to the patient's ability to sustain normal age-related activity. "Complete" means normal functioning; "partial" implies some limitation of activity; "minimal" indicates barely ambulatory or bedridden.
Data derived from North American HPEN Registry, 1985–1991.
Reproduced with permission from Oley Foundation, Albany, NY.

Table 12 Indications for Home Parenteral and Enteral Nutrition

Home Parenteral Nutrition (HPN) is an appropriate therapy if the patient meets all the following criteria:
1. The patient has severe bowel dysfunction that is expected to persist for a long time
2. The patient cannot be maintained by oral feeding or tube enteral nutrition alone
3. The therapy will restore, or sustain the patient at, a normal nutritional status
4. The therapy will restore, or sustain the patient at, a partial or complete level of rehabilitation
5. The patient has sufficient home support to manage HPN therapy comfortably and without undue hazard

Home Tube Enteral Nutrition (HEN) is an appropriate therapy if the patient meets all the following conditions:
1. The patient cannot be maintained through dietary adjustment or oral supplements alone
2. The patient has severe bowel dysfunction that is expected to persist for a long time
3. The patient can experience sufficient nutritional benefit and rehabilitation so that the undertaking makes sense to the patient and family
4. The patient is medically stable and has sufficient home support to be managed on HEN therapy comfortably and without due hazard

trition is a result of inadequate intake or malabsorption SNS is associated with restoration of protein mass. Where the cachexia is due to the cytokine response to systemic infection, SNS increases fat and water weight but not protein mass.

HOME PARENTERAL AND ENTERAL NUTRITION (HPEN)

A few patients require long-term SNS, which can be administered at home. Table 11 summarizes outcome data for 12 HPEN treated disorders, and Table 12 presents the currently accepted indications for HPEN. Since HEN is about one-tenth the cost of HPN, it is the most desirable route where feasible. HPN complications result in an average rehospitalization rate of once a year, half of these admissions being due to suspected or confirmed sepsis. With greater HPN experience over the past 20 years, metabolic complications have decreased, particularly for patients managed by nutrition specialists from large teaching centers. Important issues currently facing long-term HPN patients are thrombosis of PN catheters, metabolic bone disorders, liver disease, and micronutrient deficiencies including those of conditionally essential nutrients such as choline, taurine, s-adenosyl-L-methionine, and carnitine.

Psychosocial Issues

Patients requiring HPEN report feelings of anger and frustration, as well as altered body image. It is important to consider the impact of SNS on the quality as well as the quantity of life. Patients describe feelings of being unsupported in their home environment, particularly after the first 6 to 12 months when the assumption is often made that they are coping well. Support groups coordinated by the Oley Foundation offer a valuable contact point and reference source for HPEN patients, the parents of children requiring HPEN, and their physicians. In addition, self-help groups and support associations exist for specific disease states (e.g., CF, IBD, and pseudo-obstruction). These groups may have both local and national contact points.

Suggested Reading

Alp-Ikizler T, Wingard RL, Harkin RM. Malnutrition in peritoneal dialysis patients: Etiologic factors and treatment options. Perit Dial Int 1995; 15(5S):S63–S66.

Grant JP. Nutrition care of patients with acute and chronic respiratory failure. Nutr Clin Pract 1994; 9:11–17.

Hill GL. Body composition research: implications for the practice of clinical nutrition. JPEN 1992; 16:197–218.

Howard L, Ament R, Fleming CR, et al. Current use and clinical outcome of home parenteral and enteral nutrition therapies in the United States. Gastroenterology 1995; 109:355–365.

Jones MR, Intraperitoneal amino acids: a therapy whose time has come? Perit Dial Int 1995; 15(5S):S67–S74.

Klein S, Koretz RL. Nutrition support in patients with cancer: what do the data really show? Nutr Clin Pract 1994; 9:91–100.

Quigley EMM, Marsh MN, Shaffer JL, Martin RS. Hepatobiliary complications of TPN. Gastroenterology 1993; 104:286–301.

White BJ, Madara EJ. The self help source book. 4th ed. Denville NJ: American Self Help Clearinghouse, St. Clare's Riverside Medical Center, 1991.

FEVER OF UNKNOWN ORIGIN

Natalie C. Klein, M.D., Ph.D.
Burke A. Cunha, M.D.

The classic definition of fever of unknown origin (FUO), formulated by Petersdorf and Beeson in 1961, is an illness characterized by fever above 38.3°C (101°F), lasting more than 3 weeks without a diagnosis after 1 week of investigation in a hospital. This definition remains useful even after over 30 years.

A new classification developed by Durack and Street includes classical, nosocomial, neutropenic, and HIV-associated FUO (Table 1). Rather than being considered new categories of FUO, it seems more useful to consider these FUO categories as prolonged fevers in special populations. An alternate definition of classical FUO no longer requires a week of hospital investigation but instead 3 days of investigation of the source of fever either in the hospital or as an outpatient.

Table 1 Fever of Unknown Origin in Special Populations

Classical FUO
Fever 38.3°C (101°F) or higher on several occasions.
Fever of more than 3 weeks' duration.
Diagnosis uncertain despite appropriate investigation after at least three outpatient visits or at least 3 days in hospital.
Prolonged Fever in Hospitalized Patients
Fever 38.0°C (100.4°F) or higher on several occasions in a hospitalized patient receiving acute care.
Infection not present or incubating on admission.
Diagnosis uncertain after 3 days despite appropriate investigation, including at least 2 days' incubation of microbiologic cultures.
Prolonged Fever and Neutropenia
Fever 38.0°C (100.4°F) or higher on several occasions.
Patient has fewer than 500 neutrophils per cubic millimeter in peripheral blood or expected to fall below 500/mm^3 within 1 or 2 days.
Diagnosis uncertain after 3 days despite appropriate investigation, including at least 2 days' incubation of microbiologic cultures.
Prolonged Fever and HIV
Fever 38.0°C (100.4°F) or higher on several occasions.
Confirmed positive serology for HIV infection.
Fever of more than 4 weeks' duration for outpatients or more than 3 days' duration in hospital.
Diagnosis uncertain after 3 days despite appropriate investigation, including at least 2 days' incubation of microbiologic cultures.

Adapted from Durack DT, Street AC. Fever of unknown origin—reexamined and redefined. In: Remington JS, Swartz MN, eds. Current clinical topics in infectious diseases. Boston: Blackwell Scientific Publications, 1991:37.

■ FUO

The three major causes of FUO in adults (infections, neoplasms, and collagen vascular disease) account for about 70 percent of FUO. Infections were the most common cause of FUO in the Petersdorf and Beeson series in 1961, and neoplasms accounted for slightly more FUO in the 1982 series by Larson and associates. Causes of FUO include drug fever, granulomatous hepatitis, pulmonary embolism, inflammatory bowel disease, sarcoidosis, familial Mediterranean fever, and factitious fever (Table 2). Some cases of FUO remain undiagnosed even after thorough investigation.

Approach to the Patient

The approach to the patient with FUO begins with a careful history and physical examination to exclude common causes of fever such as urinary or respiratory tract infections, phlebitis, wound infection, viral infections, and drug fever. A patient should be questioned about travel, exposure to animals, tick bites, and occupational hazards. Physical examination should be thorough, including a search for rashes, heart murmur, lymphadenopathy, hepatosplenomegaly, nail lesions, and a complete ophthalmologic exam. Repeated physical examinations are necessary because new physical findings may appear late in the course of the disease.

Laboratory tests should include cultures of blood, urine, sputum, stool, pleural and peritoneal fluid if present, and cerebrospinal fluid if indicated. Biopsies of enlarged lymph nodes, liver, bone marrow, and any skin nodules should be considered. Direct examination of the blood smear should be performed to exclude malaria, relapsing fever, and trypanosomiasis if there is travel or transfusion history. An intermediate purified protein derivative (PPD) test along with an energy panel should be performed. Serum samples should be obtained from the patient and a portion frozen for subsequent viral titers. Serologic tests that should be considered in a patient with an FUO include cytomegalovirus (CMV) and Epstein-Barr virus (EBV) serology, and *Toxoplasma, Legionella, Brucella,* and psittacosis titers. Screening for collagen vascular disease should include sedimentation rate, antinuclear antibody, and rheumatoid factor.

A chest film; computed tomography (CT) scan of abdomen, pelvis, and perhaps chest; and radionuclide scans such as technetium-99m, sulfur colloid, indium-111, and gallium citrate may be helpful in individual cases. Magnetic resonance imaging is preferred to CT scanning for detection of sources of FUO in the central nervous system unless calcifications are present. Echocardiography including transesophageal echocardiography should be performed if endocarditis is suspected. Advances in diagnostic radiology have markedly reduced the need for exploratory laparotomy in patients with FUO. Diagnostic laparotomy should be reserved for collecting biopsy specimens to study abnormalities seen on scans not approachable by percutaneous route or as a final step in the work-up of a patient with FUO in whom an abdominal process is strongly suspected.

Therapy

The use of empiric therapy of the patient with FUO should be discouraged. The mortality of patients with FUO who are

Table 2 Diseases Causing FUO

	COMMON	UNCOMMON	RARE
Malignancy	Lymphoma Metastases to liver/CNS Hypernephromas	Hepatomas Pancreatic carcinoma Preleukemias Colon carcinoma	Atrial myxomas CNS tumors Myelodysplastic diseases
Infections	Extrapulmonary TB Renal TB TB meningitis Milliary TB Intra-abdominal abscesses Subdiaphragmatic abscesses Peri-appendiceal Peri-colonic Hepatic Pelvic abscesses	SBE CMV Toxoplasmosis Salmonella enteric fevers Intra/perinephric abscess Splenic abscess	Periapical dental abscesses Small brain abscesses Chronic sinusitis Subacute vertebral osteomyelitis Chronic meningitis/encephalitis *Listeria* *Yersinia* Brucellosis Relapsing fever Rat-Bite fever Chronic Q fever Cat-Scratch fever HIV EBV mononucleosis (elderly) Malaria *Leptospirosis* *Blastomycosis* *Histoplasmosis* *Coccidiodomycosis* *Cryptococcosis* Infected aortic aneurysm Infected vascular grafts RMSF Lyme disease *Leischmaniasis* *Trypanosomiasis* LGV Permanently placed central IV-line infections Trichinosis Prosthetic device infections Relapsing mastoiditis Septic jugular phlebitis
Rheumatologic	Still's disease (Adult JRA) Temporal arteritis (elderly)	PAN Rheumatoid arthritis (elderly)	SLE Vasculitis (e.g., Takyasu's arteritis hypersensitivity vasculitis) Felty's syndrome Pseudogout (CPPD) Acute rheumatic fever Sjögren's syndrome Behçet's disease FMF

From Cunha BA: Fever of Unknown Origin (FUO). In: Gorbach SL, Bartlett JB, Blacklow NR, eds. Infectious diseases in medicine and surgery. Philadelphia: W.B. Saunders, 1991.

otherwise well is low. The continued observation of the patient with monitoring of temperature curves and avoidance of antipyretics that may alter the temperature chart is of utmost importance. The use of empiric antibiotics that may partially treat an occult infection should be avoided. However, if after careful and thorough investigation a definitive diagnosis cannot be made, a therapeutic trial with antibiotics or anti-inflammatory agents may be indicated in a few select patients (Table 3). In patients with granulomatous hepatitis, a short course of antituberculous therapy should be initiated. If fevers are unresponsive to antituberculous medication, a trial of steroids should be considered. In a patient in whom a neoplastic disease is suspected, an empiric trial of naproxen or steroids, which supress tumor fever, may be attempted. In a patient in whom mycobacterial disease is strongly suspected, an empiric trial of antituberculosis therapy for several weeks may cause defervescence. This is best done with antituberculous drugs that are specific for mycobacteria, e.g., isoniazid, ethambutol and pyrazinamide. Finally, a patient with culture-negative endocarditis should receive a course of empiric antibiotics, usually penicillin with gentamicin.

Table 2 Diseases Causing FUO—cont'd

	COMMON	UNCOMMON	RARE
Miscellaneous Causes	Drug fever Cirrhosis Alcoholic hepatitis	Granulomatous hepatitis	Regional enteritis Whipple's disease Fabray's disease Hyperthyroidism Hyperparathyroidism Pheochromocytomas Addison's disease Subacute thyroiditis Cyclic neutropenias Polymyositis Wegener's granulomatosis Occult hematomas Subacute aortic dissecting aneurysm Weger-Christian disease Sarcoidosis (e.g., basilar meningitis, hepatic granulomas) Pulmonary emboli (multiple, recurrent) Hypothalmic dysfunction Habitual hyperthermia Factitious fever Giant hepatic hemanigomas Mesenteric fibromatosis Pseudolymphomas Idiopathic granulomatosis Kikuchi's disease Malakoplakia Hyper IgD syndrome

Table 3 Empiric Management of FUO

SUSPECTED DIAGNOSIS	THERAPY
Granulomatous hepatitis	Antituberculous therapy followed by steroids
Tuberculosis	Antituberculous therapy
Culture-negative endocarditis	Penicillin and gentamicin
Tumor fever	Naproxen or steroids

■ PROLONGED FEVERS IN HOSPITALIZED PATIENTS

Patients with prolonged hospital-acquired fevers commonly are elderly; have major underlying medical problems such as diabetes, heart disease, chronic lung disease, or cancer; or have undergone recent surgery. They are commonly hospitalized in an intensive care unit. The presence of foreign bodies such as central indwelling catheters or endotracheal tubes increases the likelihood that an infection is the cause. Management includes a thorough review of culture results, appropriate radiologic procedures such as CT scan of abdomen and pelvis, sinus films, hepatitis serology, echocardiograph of the heart, and bronchoscopy with biopsy and/or brushing for a lung infiltrate. Often empiric antibiotics are begun based on a presumptive diagnosis. Common causes of nosocomial FUO include candidiasis, chronic sinusitis, hepatitis, acalculous cholecystitis, *Clostridium difficile* colitis, septic thrombophlebitis, and drug fever.

■ PROLONGED FEVER IN NEUTROPENIC PATIENTS

Fever in the neutropenic patient is most often caused by bacteremias, pneumonia, mucositis, perianal infection, skin or soft-tissue infection, candidemia, or aspergillosis. The management of neutropenic patients with FUO differs completely from that of the patient with classical FUO. Empiric broad-spectrum antimicrobial therapy must be begun immediately in the neutropenic patient with fever. The most common regimens used are beta-lactam plus an aminoglycoside, although in institutions with frequent staphylococcal isolates or if the patient has an indwelling central catheter, vancomycin may be part of the empiric regimen.

In a neutropenic patient fever occurring 1–2 weeks after antimicrobial therapy suggests fungemia-invasive fungal disease.

■ PROLONGED FEVERS IN HIV PATIENTS

The major causes of FUO in the HIV-positive patient are HIV infection itself, disseminated *Mycobacterium avium-intracellulare* disease, disseminated CMV infection, extrapulmonary tuberculosis, non-Hodgkin's lymphoma, and drug fever. Management of FUO in an HIV-positive patient is similar to that in classical FUO. It is important to obtain a current CD4 lymphocyte count, since a patient with a CD4 count of less than 200 per cubic millimeter has advanced HIV infection, so the risk of opportunistic disease is high (Table 4).

Table 4 Infectious Causes of Prolonged Fevers in HIV-Positive Individuals

CD_4 COUNT	CAUSES OF PROLONGED FEVER
>500/mm^3	Acute HIV
200–500/mm^3	*Mycobacterium tuberculosis*
	HIV
<200/mm^3	Dissseminated *Mycobacterium avium-intracellulare*
	Disseminated CMV
	Toxoplasmosis
	Cryptococcosis
	HIV

Usually there is no need for immediate empiric antimicrobial therapy unless the patient has a neutrophil count less than 500 per microliter. The febrile neutropenic HIV-positive patient should receive immediate empiric broad-spectrum antibiotics and should be treated like the non-HIV-positive patient with neutropenia.

Suggested Reading

Chang JC, Gross HM. Utility of naproxen in the differential diagnosis of fever of undetermined origin in patients with cancer. Am J Med 1984; 76:597–603.

Cunha BA. Fever of unknown origin (FUO). In: Gorbach SL, Bartlett JB, Blacklow NR, eds. Infectious diseases in medicine and surgery. Philadelphia: WB Saunders, 1991.

Durack DT, Street AC. Fever of unknown origin—reexamined and redefined. In: Remington J, Swartz M, eds. Current clinical topics of infectious diseases. Boston: Blackwell Scientific, 1991:35.

Goetz MB. Fever of unknown origin in the elderly. Infect Dis Clin Prac 1993; 2:377–380.

Larson EB, Featherstone HJ, Petersdorf RG. Fever of undetermined origin: Diagnosis and follow-up of 105 cases 1970–1980. Medicine 1982; 61: 269–292.

Petersdorf RG, Beeson PB. Fever of unexplained origin: Report on 100 cases. Medicine 1961; 40:1–30.

PRINCIPLES OF PAIN MANAGEMENT

Gregory W. Albers, M.D.
Stephen J. Peroutka, M.D., Ph.D.

The management of pain is one of the most common and difficult problems facing neurologists. Pain is a nonspecific symptom which may be a manifestation of a diverse array of pathologic conditions. Therefore, identification of the cause of pain is always the first objective of a patient evaluation. Once a tentative diagnosis has been established, a wide variety of treatment options may be considered. In general, the most common and effective mode of treatment for pain is pharmacologic. Surgical options are sometimes available for selected pain syndromes or for conditions refractory to standard treatment approaches. In some patients, therapeutic success may be achieved with alternative modalities such as physical therapy, biofeedback, and/or psychiatric intervention. A summary of the major options available to the physician is provided in Table 1.

Table 1 Overview of Pain Management Options

- Pharmacologic
  - Prostaglandin inhibitors
  - Atypical analgesics
  - Narcotics
  - Combination analgesics
- Surgical
  - Local anesthesia
  - Epidural injections
  - Nerve decompression
  - Thalamotomy
- Alternative options
  - Psychological/psychiatric interventions
  - Electrical stimulation (TENS)
  - Biofeedback
  - Physical therapy

■ DIAGNOSIS

The classification of pain syndromes is difficult, and pain terminology is often confusing. However, some simple generalizations are useful. Pain produced by activation of peripheral pain receptors (somatic or nociceptive pain) usually responds well to standard analgesics. Central pain (pain associated with central nervous system lesions) and neuropathic pain (pain associated with peripheral nerve damage) often respond best to atypical analgesics.

A second important diagnostic consideration concerns the differentiation of chronic pain disorders from acute pain disorders. Chronic pain differs from acute pain both symptomatically and pathophysiologically. For example, patients with chronic pain usually adapt to constant pain and therefore may appear to be quite comfortable. Unfortunately, this lack of apparent distress may lead the physician to question the validity of the patient's complaints. Generally, pharmacologic therapies aimed at treating patients with chronic pain must avoid the use of addicting substances such as narcotics.

■ PHARMACOLOGIC OPTIONS

The selection of an appropriate pharmacologic agent for the management of pain can seem quite difficult. Because the number of drugs used for pain may appear overwhelming, it is useful to classify these medications into four major categories: (1) prostaglandin inhibitors; (2) atypical analgesics; (3) narcotics; and (4) combination analgesics. Selection of an appropriate medication for pain relief requires knowledge of the pharmacologic properties and side effect profiles of each of these four drug groups.

Prostaglandin Inhibitors

Prostaglandin inhibitors are the drugs of choice for the management of mild to moderate pain. This group of agents includes aspirin, acetaminophen, and the nonsteroidal anti-inflammatory drugs (NSAIDs). Their mechanism of action involves the inhibition of prostaglandin synthesis primarily through the inhibition of the enzyme cyclooxygenase. These medications have principally analgesic, antipyretic and anti-inflammatory properties. However, it is important to note that the anti-inflammatory potency of acetaminophen is quite weak compared with that of aspirin and the NSAIDs.

Aspirin remains the prototypical prostaglandin inhibitor analgesic. It also remains the drug of choice for mild to moderate pain from headache, neuralgia, or myalgia. Nonetheless, the analgesic potency of aspirin tends to be underrated by most patients and physicians. In blinded studies, for example, 650 mg of aspirin is usually as effective as or more effective than 65 mg of codeine. The extremely low cost and effectiveness of aspirin make it an ideal analgesic for patients who can tolerate its gastrointestinal effects.

Acetaminophen is an excellent alternative for patients who are unable to tolerate aspirin. In general, acetaminophen appears to be equipotent to aspirin in its analgesic effects. However, because of its lack of significant anti-inflammatory actions, it is less effective for pain related to inflammation. Although acetaminophen has minimal gastrointestinal toxicity, it does carry the risk of hepatic necrosis, which may occur with chronic doses as low as 5 to 8 g per day or with an acute overdose of only 10 to 15 g.

NSAIDs offer several potential advantages over aspirin and acetaminophen. First, they have less gastrointestinal toxicity than aspirin. Second, because NSAIDs cause reversible inhibition of cyclooxygenase, their antiplatelet activity is of shorter duration. Third, their analgesic potency is often slightly better than that of aspirin or acetaminophen. Otherwise, NSAIDs have a mechanism of action and side effect profile similar to that of aspirin. Unfortunately, NSAIDs differ from aspirin and acetaminophen also in that they are considerably more expensive.

Although insufficient data are available to differentiate the various NSAIDs in terms of analgesic potency or risk of gastrointestinal hemorrhage, there are many significant differences among agents. For example, piroxicam (Feldene) has the longest half-life (approximately 45 hours), and this allows for once daily dosing. Diflunisal (Dolobid), sulindac (Clinoril), and naproxen (Naprosyn) can be administered in twice daily doses. Indomethacin (Indocin) has superior anti-inflammatory activity but appears to cause more frequent side effects than other NSAIDs. Meclofenamate (Meclomen) is associated with incidence of diarrhea as high as 30 percent.

All NSAIDs carry a small risk of renal toxicity because of the role of prostaglandins in modulating renal blood flow. This risk is greatly accentuated in patients with pre-existing renal disease, congestive heart failure, or hepatic dysfunction. Several studies have suggested that sulindac (Clinoril) has minimal effects on renal prostaglandin synthesis and therefore appears to carry a relatively reduced risk of renal toxicity.

Since most NSAID side effects are dose-related, a low dose should be chosen initially and increased gradually as required. NSAIDs are highly bound to serum albumin (most are greater than 99 percent bound) and can potentially displace other highly protein-bound drugs such as coumarin anticoagulants, phenytoin, methotrexate, and oral hypoglycemics. Obviously, such interactions could potentially lead to toxicity.

Atypical Analgesics

Several drugs that were originally developed for other conditions such as depression or epilepsy have been found to be useful in pain management. These agents are primarily useful in treating chronic pain syndromes, particularly conditions involving central or neuropathic pain. For example, a substantial amount of data suggest that antidepressants can provide significant pain relief in both depressed and nondepressed patients. Although the exact mechanism remains unclear, effects on descending monoamine pathways involved in the modulation of pain transmission appear to be important.

Before pain therapy with antidepressant drugs is initiated, the rationale for using these agents for pain control, as opposed to depression, should be stressed to the patient. Patients with pain syndromes are often offended by the implication that they are depressed. Therefore, the physician should clearly state the reasons for using these agents for pain. Low doses should be used initially (Table 2). If pain relief is not obtained after 6 to 8 weeks of therapy, the dosage should be increased slowly to full antidepressant doses and continued for at least another 6 to 8 weeks. When a positive response is obtained, drug therapy should be continued for 3 to 6 months, after which a gradual withdrawal of the medication is attempted. If the pain recurs after medication withdrawal, treatment should be reinstituted.

As with the NSAIDs, there are insufficient data to rank the analgesic potency of the antidepressants. Many of the controlled trials have involved the use of agents associated with a high incidence of side effects, such as amitriptyline (Elavil) and imipramine (Tofranil). However, significant analgesic effects also occur with better-tolerated agents such as nortriptyline (Pamelor) and desipramine (Norpramin).

A second major class of atypical analgesics is that of the anticonvulsants. Carbamazepine (Tegretol), phenytoin (Dilantin), valproic acid (Depakene), and clonazepam (Klonopin) are the anticonvulsants most frequently used for pain. These agents may be effective in the treatment of a variety of pain syndromes, including various neuropathies, neuralgias, and pain in multiple sclerosis or Guillain-Barré syndrome. Carbamazepine (Tegretol) has proven to be the most effective agent for the treatment of trigeminal neuralgia. However, the data are limited on comparisons of the anticonvulsants in treating other painful conditions. Although the exact mechanism of action for pain control is unclear, a

Table 2 Commonly Used Analgesics

DRUG	BRAND NAME*	TYPICAL STARTING DOSE
Prostaglandin inhibitors		
Aspirin		650 mg q4–6h
Acetaminophen	Tylenol	650 mg q4–6h
Ibuprofen	Motrin	400 mg q4–6h
Naproxen	Naprosyn	375 mg q12h
Sulindac	Clinoril	150 mg q12h
Diflunisal	Dolobid	500 mg q12h
Piroxicam	Feldene	20 mg q24h
Atypical analgesics		
Amitripyline	Elavil	25 mg qhs
Nortriptyline	Pamelor	25 mg qhs
Carbamazepine	Tegretol	100 mg q12h
Narcotics		
Codeine		30 mg q4–6h
Pentazocine	Talwin Nx	1 tab q4h–6h
Meperidine	Demerol	100 mg IM q4–6h
Combination analgesics		
Aspirin/butalbital/caffeine	Fiorinal	1 tab q4h
Aspirin/butalbital	Axotal	1 tab q4h
Acetaminophen/chlorzoxazone	Parafon Forte DSC	2 tabs q6h
Acetaminophen/codeine	Tylenol #3	1 tab q4h
Acetaminophen/hydrocodone	Vicodin	1 tab q6h
Aspirin/oxycodone	Percodan	1 tab q6h

*Several brand names are available for some of these analgesics.

reduction of excitatory synaptic transmission within pain-modulating circuits has been postulated.

Several other medications such as anticholinergics, phenothiazines, and baclofen have been advocated for the management of various painful conditions. Unfortunately, very little data from controlled studies are available regarding the use of these drugs. The short-term use of anti-anxiety agents may also be helpful, particularly if pain is accompanied by significant anxiety.

Narcotic Analgesics

Although narcotics are the most effective analgesics available, we strongly believe that narcotic use should be restricted to the short-term relief of moderate to severe pain. We believe that narcotics should rarely be used for chronic pain control in neurologic patients. Quite simply, the problems encountered with long-term narcotic use (e.g., tolerance and addiction) far outweigh their benefits in patients with chronic pain disorders.

For the short-term relief of acute pain, codeine is usually the oral narcotic of choice. Its advantages include a relatively low dependence liability and good oral bioavailability. Unfortunately, like many narcotics, codeine has a short plasma half-life (only about 3.5 hours), necessitating frequent dosing. Codeine, as well as the other orally active narcotics, should generally be administered in combination with a prostaglandin inhibitor, as discussed in the following section of this chapter.

Propoxyphene (Darvon) is one of the least potent narcotics. In many studies it has proven to be less effective than aspirin or acetaminophen. We find that there is little use for this agent in treating neurologic patients. If more potent orally active narcotics are required, hydrocodone (Vicodin) or oxycodone (Percodan) may be considered. These agents are available only in combination with nonopioid analgesics. Of these, oxycodone is the more potent and appears to have higher abuse potential.

For parenteral use, meperidine (Demerol) is a recommended choice because of its relatively low incidence of gastrointestinal side effects. Meperidine hydrochloride (Demerol) can occasionally produce central nervous system side effects, including excitement and seizures, and should not be used for patients on monoamine oxidase inhibitors. Several mixed agonists-antagonists such as pentazocine (Talwin), butorphanol (Stadol), and nalbuphine (Nubain) appear to offer the advantage of less abuse potential than other potent narcotics. Their disadvantages, however, include the risk of precipitation of a withdrawal reaction in patients being treated with other opioids and occasional psychotomimetic effects.

Combination Analgesics

A variety of combination analgesics are available for use in moderate pain disorders. Aspirin or acetaminophen is frequently combined with caffeine and/or a barbiturate for the treatment of headaches (e.g., Excedrin, Fiorinal, Axotal) or with a muscle relaxant for acute musculoskeletal strain (e.g., Norgesic, Soma, Parafon Forte DSC). Certain analgesic combinations appear to offer synergistic effects greater than those obtained by doubling the dose of either individual agent. For example, the most successful combinations involve a prostaglandin inhibitor (usually aspirin or acetaminophen) coupled with an oral narcotic—for example, propoxyphene (Darvon compound), codeine (Tylenol with codeine), hydrocodone bitartrate (Vicodin), and oxycodone (Percodan, Tylox).

■ SURGICAL OPTIONS

A large variety of surgical or anesthetic procedures are available for specific pain syndromes. Focal neuropathies such as occipital neuralgia, painful neuromas, and carpal tunnel syndrome can be treated with local injections of anesthetic agents and corticosteroids. Occasionally, the pain relief that follows local infiltration is long lasting. Epidural or intrathecal injections may also provide pain relief for selected patients, and standard orthopedic and neurosurgical procedures such as laminectomy and peripheral nerve decompression are available for specific syndromes. For example, reflex sympathetic dystrophy often responds to sympathectomy and/or sympathetic blocking agents. More invasive procedures such as gangliolysis, posterior rhizotomy, cordotomy, or thalamotomy should be performed only in specialized centers.

■ ALTERNATIVE OPTIONS

A diverse variety of alternative (i.e., nonpharmacologic and nonsurgical) therapies are also available for patients with pain syndromes. In certain chronic pain patients, psychological factors may play a primary role in the pain syndrome and can severely complicate patient management. Fear and depression are also frequently associated with pain and sometimes need to be addressed specifically. For these individuals, psychological and/or psychiatric evaluations may be most appropriate.

Physical therapy and exercise are important options and may be particularly useful in treating pain syndromes related to muscle contraction or spasm. Other therapeutic options such as biofeedback, relaxation training, hypnosis, and transcutaneous nerve stimulation (i.e., TENS) are helpful for selected patients. Depending on the clinical situation, multimodality therapy may be more successful than any single therapeutic option used alone. For instance, chronic headaches often respond well to a combination of drug therapy, cervical exercises, and psychological or psychiatric intervention.

Suggested Reading

Boynton CS, Dick CF, Mayor GH. NSAIDs: an overview. J Clin Pharmacol 1988; 28:512–517.

Beaver WT. Combination analgesics. Am J Med 1984; 77:38–53.

Hackett TP, Bouckoms A. The pain patient: evaluation and treatment. In: Hackett TP, Cassem NH, eds. Massachusetts General Hospital handbook of general hospital psychiatry. 2nd ed. Littleton, MA: PSG Publishing, 1987:42.

The International Association for the Study of Pain, Subcommittee on Taxonomy. Classification of chronic pain: descriptions of chronic pain syndromes and definitions of pain terms. Pain 1986; 3(suppl):S1–S226.

Malone MD, Strube MJ. Meta-analysis of non-medical treatments for chronic pain. Pain 1988, 34:231–244.

DECISIONS TO FORGO LIFE-SUSTAINING TREATMENT

Peter A. Singer, M.D., M.P.H., F.R.C.P.C.
Mark Siegler, M.D.

There is a broad consensus in medicine, law, and ethics that mentally competent adult patients may decline all treatments, including life-sustaining treatment (LST). Patients may decide to forgo a treatment that has been proposed (i.e., to have treatment withheld) or one that has already been started (i.e., to have treatment withdrawn). The patient may decide to forgo a wide range of potentially lifesaving treatments, including cardiopulmonary resuscitation, mechanical ventilation, dialysis, antibiotic therapy, and tube feeding. The right of patients to make their own health care decisions regarding LST is founded in the legal right of self-determination and the ethical principle of individual autonomy. It should be noted that the right to forgo LST does not extend to active euthanasia, such as by lethal injection, which remains illegal in all jurisdictions of the United States.

Although in the American legal context the right to forgo LST applies to both competent and incompetent adult patients, the right is effectuated very differently in these two clinical situations. Competent patients can express their wishes regarding life-sustaining treatment directly to their physicians. Incompetent patients must exercise this right through a process of substitute decision making (see below).

Clinicians should be prepared to assist patients and families to deal with the following five clinical situations that relate to forgoing LST: (1) brain death; (2) the determination of patient competency; (3) decision making with competent patients; (4) substitute decision making for incompetent patients; and (5) the use of advance directives. This chapter aims to describe the principles of management in these five clinical situations.

■ BRAIN DEATH

If the patient is brain dead, treatment may be discontinued. The family should be informed that the patient has died and that mechanical ventilation and other forms of life support will be stopped. There is no need to ask the family's permission to do so. In three specific circumstances, the physician may choose to continue LST for a limited period even though the patient is brain dead. These circumstances include organ procurement, supporting the patient until the family arrives, and maintaining a brain-dead pregnant woman in an attempt to deliver a viable baby. In all cases of brain death, the physician must remain sensitive to the emotions of the family and should counsel and support them.

Brain death is a clinical diagnosis. The following criteria may be useful in determining brain death in adult patients: (1) absent cortical function as manifested by a patient in a coma who has no spontaneous movement, no response to verbal commands, no response to deep pain, and no seizures; (2) absent brain stem function as manifested by the absence of pupillary, corneal, oculocephalic (doll's eyes), and oculovestibular (ice-water calorics) reflexes and a "negative" apnea test (i.e., absent respiratory effort, hypercarbia, and acidosis in the oxygenated patient who has been taken off the ventilator for 5 to 10 minutes); (3) either the cause of coma is known (e.g., head trauma) and precludes improvement in brain function, or a sufficient period of observation has passed to permit solid prognostication; and (4) other conditions that may be confused with brain death, such as drug intoxications, other metabolic problems, and hypothermia, have been excluded.

The principal clinical justification for using the brain-death standard is futility: no treatment can reverse the pathophysiologic damage in brain-dead patients. Moreover, at least

45 states have laws or judicial opinions recognizing the brain-death standard, and physicians should be familiar with the law in their own state. [Note: At least one state, New Jersey, provides for a specific exemption from the brain-death standard based on a family's religious beliefs.] The specific clinical procedures for determining brain death are generally not prescribed by law. Often, institutional policies outline local guidelines such as those listed previously. These policies may also suggest a variety of confirmatory procedures including two or more separate observers, consultation with a neurologist or neurosurgeon, two separate examinations 6 to 12 hours apart, and supplementary tests including an electroencephalogram or cerebral blood flow studies. Most policies suggest that the declaration of death be made by physicians who are not involved in the potential transplantation of the organs of the deceased and who have no other economic or legal conflicts of interest.

■ ASSESSMENT OF COMPETENCY

When decisions arise about using or forgoing LST, the physician's first task is to determine whether the patient is competent to make decisions for him- or herself. The assessment of competency plays a pivotal role in patient management. Respect for the ethical and legal rights of patients means that physicians accede to the requests of competent patients to forgo treatment, even if it results in the patient's death. On the other hand, physicians may overrule requests to forgo treatment made by incompetent patients because they do not want such patients to suffer serious harm not intended by the patient if he or she were competent. Whether a physician finds a patient competent or incompetent often determines whether or not the doctor accepts the patient's stated wishes about LST or takes steps to override the decision. With so much at stake, it would be desirable to have well-developed clinical standards for the determination of competency. Unfortunately, at present, there are no reliable and valid measures for the determination of competency at the bedside.

The President's Commission for the Study of Ethical Problems in Medicine and Biomedical and Behavioral Research has identified three elements of competency: possession of a set of values and goals, the ability to communicate and understand information, and the ability to reason and deliberate about one's choices. The Commission also noted that competency was specific to "the person's actual functioning in situations in which a decision about health care was to be made." In other words, whether the physician acts on a patient's request to stop LST should not depend primarily on whether the patient is oriented to time, place, and person but rather on whether the patient understands that he or she will die without LST. More recently, Appelbaum and Grisso have suggested that the competent patient should be able to communicate choices, understand relevant information, appreciate the situation and its consequences, and manipulate information rationally. An effective clinical index of patient competency to decide about LST, however, would require a listing of specific questions for the physician to ask the patient, clearly stipulated criteria for the appraisal of patient responses, and a mechanism for combining the responses on individual questions into an overall assessment. Until such an index has been developed and evaluated, physicians must continue to rely on ad hoc assessments of competency.

At the extremes, doctors can usually establish whether a patient is competent or incompetent. Moreover, the clinician can sometimes restore patients to a state of competency by treating reversible causes of cognitive dysfunction, including a wide range of metabolic encephalopathies or psychoactive drug use. If uncertainty remains about the patient's competency, we recommend consultation with colleagues. Appropriate consultants include psychiatrists, neurologists, institutional ethics committees, ethics consultation services, or hospital attorneys. At present, it is unclear which of these groups is the preferred consultant, and this may vary in different clinical cases and institutional settings. In controversial cases, judicial review may be indicated. After physicians have determined whether the patient is competent or incompetent, patient management proceeds as described below.

■ DECISION MAKING WITH COMPETENT PATIENTS

Patients who are competent should be permitted to make their own health care decisions, including the decision to forgo life-sustaining medical treatments. This does not mean that the physician must casually accept the patient's treatment refusal without further discussion. The physician should enter into a dialogue with the patient to ensure that the patient's desire to stop treatment is an authentic reflection of his or her wishes and goals. Further, the physician should try to persuade the patient to pursue a medically reasonable course of treatment. If, after such discussion, the patient remains adamant in refusing treatment, the physician should respect the competent patient's wish and accede to the request to forgo treatment. If conflicts arise, consultation with the institutional ethics committee or even judicial referral may be advisable, but it is preferable to resolve such cases without recourse to a court. If a physician is unable to carry out a competent patient's request to forgo LST on the grounds of the physician's personal conscientious standards, the physician may withdraw from the case after ensuring that another source of care is available to the patient.

■ SUBSTITUTE DECISION MAKING FOR INCOMPETENT PATIENTS

If the patient is incompetent, the physician should search for reversible causes of cognitive dysfunction. Sometimes, the correction of electrolyte disturbances, acidemia, hypoxemia, uremia, or other metabolic, infectious, or structural causes will restore the patient's competency and allow the patient to speak for him- or herself. Frequently, drugs such as analgesics or sedatives may be the cause of the patient's incompetence.

Incompetent patients whose competency cannot be restored present a troubling ethical problem. This group includes both permanently unconscious patients and patients who are conscious but have severe and irreversible cognitive impairments (such as Alzheimer's disease, congenital mental retardation, or anoxic encephalopathy). Because incompetent patients cannot speak for themselves, courts and legislatures since the 1976 Quinlan decision have developed an approach to end-of-life decisions that allows other parties (substitute decision-maker) to make decisions for the incompetent person. The underlying philosophic and legal assumption that permits substitute decision making is that incompetent patients have the same autonomy claims and right of self-determination (for example, in the refusal of treatment) that competent patients possess. This philosophic and legal fiction views the incompetent person as an autonomous competent decision maker and requires that the substitute make choices that are in accord with the choices that the now incompetent individual would make if he or she were competent.

In practice, substitute decision making raises two key questions: who should decide on behalf of the incompetent patient, and on what basis should the decision be made? In addressing these questions, it is important to remember that the goal of substitute decision making is to project the incompetent patient's wishes onto the current clinical situation.

Who Should Decide?

The best substitute decision maker is someone identified and trusted by the patient to represent the patient's own wishes. It is the responsibility of the physician to find out whether the patient has appointed such a substitute. The patient may have done so formally using a proxy advance directive. In the absence of a formally executed legal document, the physician should still attempt to discover whether the patient had previously designated a surrogate. This may have been done through written or oral statements. Although such surrogates may not have the legal status of a durable power of attorney, they may still have an ethically acceptable standing allowing them to participate in decisions.

In many cases, the patient has not designated a substitute decision maker. Many states have enacted laws recognizing the decisional authority of family substitute decision makers even in the absence of a proxy advance directive.

The patient with no readily identifiable surrogate decision maker presents a particularly difficult clinical management problem. There is no consensus on how to manage these difficult cases. Health care facilities should address this situation prospectively through institutional policies. Moreover, it may be desirable to refer such cases to the institutional ethics committee or ethics consultation service. Some jurisdictions have legislation providing for a public official or a guardian to make decisions in these circumstances.

Another clinically challenging situation occurs when family members disagree about decisions to forgo LST. Some family members may want treatment stopped, whereas others want it continued. When such conflicts arise, ethics committees and consultants may provide an effective, extrajudicial mechanism for mediation. If the "ethical impasse" persists, judicial referral may be necessary.

Once a substitute decision maker has been identified, a second question arises. On what grounds should the substitute reach a decision? Again, the physician should remember that the goal of substitute decision making is to project the incompetent patient's wishes onto the current clinical situation.

On What Basis Should the Decision Be Made?

Whenever possible, the substitute should follow the incompetent patient's general wishes about LST. In the absence of explicit written (see Instruction Directives) or oral prior wishes, two main standards for substitute decision making have been developed: substituted judgment and best interests.

Substituted Judgment

With substituted judgment, the substitute applies the patient's values and beliefs to his or her actual clinical situation. The goal of substituted judgment is "to reach the decision that the incapacitated person would make if he or she were able to choose."

A weakness of the substituted judgment approach is highlighted by empirical data that show low rates of agreement between patients and their likely surrogates regarding resuscitation and other end-of-life decisions. Such data raise troubling questions about the adequacy of the substituted judgment approach and should provide impetus for the broader use of advance directives.

Best Interests

When there is no available information about an incompetent patient's prior wishes or values and beliefs, physicians and courts have relied on "best interests." This approach is used for patients who have never been competent (such as an adult with severe, congenital mental retardation), or perhaps for patients who were previously competent but never discussed their wishes regarding end-of-life care. The best interests approach involves a balancing of benefits and burdens: the substitute chooses as a reasonable person in the patient's circumstance would choose. It requires a set of "objective, societally shared criteria" to rank burdens and benefits.

The problem with the best interests approach is that it requires societal consensus on burdens and benefits. In a pluralistic society, such a consensus is difficult to achieve. The best interests approach requires one person to judge the quality of life of another, opening the door to discrimination against those with disabilities. There is empirical evidence that third parties undervalue the quality of life of chronically ill patients relative to the value these patients place on their own quality of life. The potential for discrimination on the basis of third-party quality-of-life judgments is a serious limitation of the best interests approach.

■ ADVANCE DIRECTIVES

Advance directives permit patients to project their wishes regarding LST onto a future situation when they have become incompetent. Therefore, advance directives reduce the vagaries of clinical decision making for incompetent patients who cannot tell the physician at the time what medical care they want. There are two types of advance directives: instruction directives and proxy directives.

Proxy Directives

In a proxy directive, a now incompetent patient has appointed, while still competent, another person to make health-care decisions on his or her behalf. The focus here is not on the specific details of the decision but rather on having the patient appoint an agent whom he or she trusts to represent his or her values. The advantage of the proxy directive is that decisions about the use of LSTs can be based on the actual clinical circumstances, since a competent decision maker (i.e., the proxy) is at hand. The disadvantage is that although the patient chose the proxy to represent his or her wishes, the proxy's decision on behalf of the patient in a specific clinical situation may not reflect what the patient would choose if he or she were competent. In many jurisdictions, proxy directives have been legally formalized as "durable powers of attorney for health care."

Instruction Directives

In an instruction directive, such as a "living will," the now incompetent patient, while still competent, has recorded his or her preferences regarding LST so that these wishes can guide medical care if and when the patient becomes incompetent. The instruction directive focuses on what treatments the patient would want if he or she were unable to participate in decision making in various health states in the future. The advantage is that the patient's preferences for withholding and withdrawing care are explicitly stated in the instruction directive. The disadvantage is that these stated preferences may not apply to the patient's actual clinical situation.

Ideally, proxy and instruction directives will be used together. More importantly, the writing of advance directives should be embedded in a process of communication involving patients, their proxies, and their physicians.

■ THE FUTURE

In the future, several powerful forces will shape policy about decisions to forgo LST.

Attempts to limit the spiraling costs of health care may influence policies regarding LST. The United States spend about $1 trillion on health care, almost 15 percent of its gross national product. An earlier study in the Medicare population showed that almost 30 percent of annual spending flowed to the 6 percent of enrollees who died during the year. Physicians can expect cost-containment policies aimed to reduce this "high cost of dying." These pressures may be especially pronounced in some managed care organizations. Faced with these policies, the clinical-ethical challenge for physicians will be to maintain their fiduciary commitment to the patient's good.

Policies about LST will also be affected by recent initiatives to legalize physician-assisted suicide (PAS) and euthanasia (U) which have been introduced in a number of states. (The state of Oregon passed a referendum in 1994 permitting PAS, but this practice is currently enjoined in federal court pending a formal judicial resolution.) During the past year, state courts in New York, Michigan, and Oregon and federal courts in Washington State and the ninth Circuit have rejected claims that there is a constitutionally protected "right to die" that includes PAS and U. A recent report from the Council on Scientific Affairs of the American Medical Association reaffirmed the AMA's opposition to PAS and U and stated: "The pertinent public policy question now is, 'What strategies should this society pursue to improve the care of persons who are dying?'"

The failure of the recently published SUPPORT study, which was designed to improve end-of-life care for dying patients highlights the complexity of dealing clinically with issues of death and dying in the United States. In the first phase of the SUPPORT study, investigators documented that many dying patients were treated aggressively even though the patients had expressed wishes to avoid aggressive life-sustaining treatment. The SUPPORT study's phase II intervention, which used trained nurses to try to effect changes in physician behavior, was also a complete failure. As the SUPPORT Principal Investigators noted: "In phase II of SUPPORT, improved information, enhanced conversation, and an explicit effort to encourage use of outcome data and preferences in decision making were completely ineffectual, despite the fact that the study had enough power to detect effects." These negative results remind us once again that patients, families, and clinicians have great difficulty reaching decisions about death and dying and that even though we have guidelines and rules in place, actual practices around the issue of death are very complex and often are in tension with formal guidelines.

We believe, however, that enduring solutions to the problems posed by decisions to forgo LST must come from within the profession. Physicians must learn to discuss the elective use of LSTs with patients and to elicit patients' wishes about LST. Physicians should be taught during medical school, post-graduate training, and continuing education how and when to discuss with patients and their appointed substitute decision-makers their wishes for end-of-life care.

Fundamental clinical research challenges remain for example the design and evaluation of an index of patient competency and more research to improve the care of dying patients. Despite the immense political, social, and economic importance of clinical policies to guide decisions to forgo LST, this research has not been a high priority for traditional biomedical granting agencies. Moreover, professional education about decisions to forgo LST has been inadequate. We hope that the medical profession will meet these basic research and educational challenges before external solutions are imposed by bureaucrats, administrators, regulators, and payors.

Suggested Reading

Appelbaum PS, Grisso T. Assessing patients' capacities to consent to treatment. N Engl J Med 1988; 319:1635–1638.

Council on Scientific Affairs, American Medical Association. Good care of the dying patient. JAMA 1996; 275:474–478.

Emanuel EJ, Weinberg DS, Gonin R, Hummel LR. How well is the Patient Self-Determination Act working? An early assessment. Am J Med 1993; 95:619–628.

Jonsen AR, Siegler M, Winslade WJ. Clinical ethics: A practical approach to ethical decisions in clinical medicine. 3rd ed. New York: McGraw-Hill, 1992.

Menikoff JA, Sachs GA, Siegler M. Beyond advance directives. Health care surrogate laws. N Engl J Med 1992; 327:1165–69.

President's Commission for the Study of Ethical Problems in Medicine and Biomedical and Behavioral Research. Deciding to forgo life-sustaining treatment: Ethical, medical, and legal issues in treatment decisions. Washington, DC: U.S. Government Printing Office, 1983.

Singer PA, Siegler M. Euthanasia: A critique. N Engl J Med 1990; 322:1881–1883.

The SUPPORT Principal Investigators. A controlled trial to improve care for seriously ill hospitalized patients. JAMA 1995; 274:1591–1598.

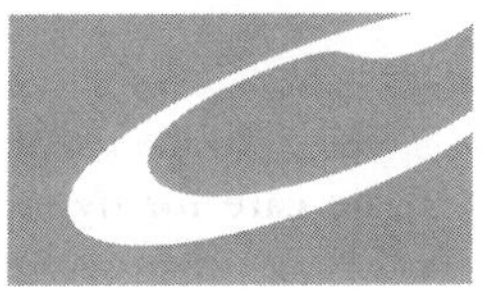

WOMEN'S HEALTH

DELAYED PUBERTY IN GIRLS AND PRIMARY AMENORRHEA

Michael A. Thomas, M.D.
Robert W. Rebar, M.D.

■ DEFINITION AND NORMAL PUBERTAL MATURATION

Delayed (or interrupted) puberty is generally defined as the absence of any secondary sex characteristics by the age of 13 years, menarche by age 16, or the passage of 5 years or more from breast budding to menarche. Because primary amenorrhea is generally defined as the failure to have any spontaneous menstrual bleeding by age 16 regardless of the development of other secondary sex characteristics, individuals with primary amenorrhea form a subset of those with delayed puberty.

To understand the pathophysiology of delayed puberty, it is important to be familiar with the normal sequence of pubertal maturation. Perhaps the most important aspect of pubertal development is that the numerous physical changes occur in an orderly sequence over a definite time frame. Breast budding in girls is usually the first obvious pubertal change, typically beginning after 8 years of age, followed shortly by the appearance of pubic hair, with menarche occurring late in pubertal development. In general, the interval from breast budding (so-called thelarche) to menarche is about 2 years, and the entire pubertal sequence of accelerated growth, breast development, and menarche covers a period of 4.5 years (with a range of 1.5 to 6 years). The peak growth rate associated with puberty is achieved 2 years after thelarche and 1 year prior to menarche. Clinically, the stages described by Marshall and Tanner are commonly utilized to describe breast and pubic hair development.

As might be expected, numerous hormonal changes occur during pubertal development, with a number of these changes beginning even before any physical changes become apparent. Early in puberty there is increased sensitivity of luteinizing hormone (LH) to gonadotropin-releasing hormone (GnRH). Sleep-entrained secretion of both LH and follicle-stimulating hormone (FSH) with increased nocturnal secretion is accompanied early in puberty by increased secretion of estradiol the following morning. Investigators have noted a 5.7 to 9.3 hour time lag between LH secretion and estradiol production during this peripubertal time period.

Estradiol secretion increases steadily through puberty. In addition, progressive increases in the major adrenal androgens dehydroepiandrosterone and its sulfate begin as early as 2 years of age, accelerate at 7 to 8 years of age, and continue until 13 to 15 years of age. Thus, increases in adrenal androgens occur at least 2 years before the increases in gonadotropins and gonadal sex steroids at a time when the hypothalamic-pituitary-gonadal axis is still functioning at a low prepubertal level. Also, recent studies suggest that both melatonin and growth hormone (GH) may play active roles in the initiation and continuation of normal pubertal development.

■ CLINICAL EVALUATION AND TREATMENT

Most important in the evaluation of the young woman with delayed or interrupted pubertal development is the history and physical examination (Fig. 1).

Perhaps most common are the young women who present with mature secondary sex characteristics on examination but who have failed to undergo menarche by age 16. The most frequent cause of such "anatomic" amenorrhea is müllerian dysgenesis, sometimes referred to as the Rokitansky-Küster-Hauser syndrome, which is typified by hypoplasia and failure of fusion of the müllerian anlagen and may be associated with total or partial vaginal agenesis. Any or all parts of the müllerian system may fail to develop or to fuse in the midline. In addition, distal genital tract obstruction, either because of an imperforate hymen or a transverse vaginal septum, may occur. Obstruction to the normal efflux of menstrual blood can result in hematocolpos and hematometra. Although a bulging perineum and a bulging mass are commonly present in such circumstances, differentiating a vaginal septum from an imperforate hymen may be very difficult. The occurrence of intermittent (cyclic) abdominal pain may suggest intraabdominal bleeding. Surgical excision of an imperforate hymen or vaginal septum is required.

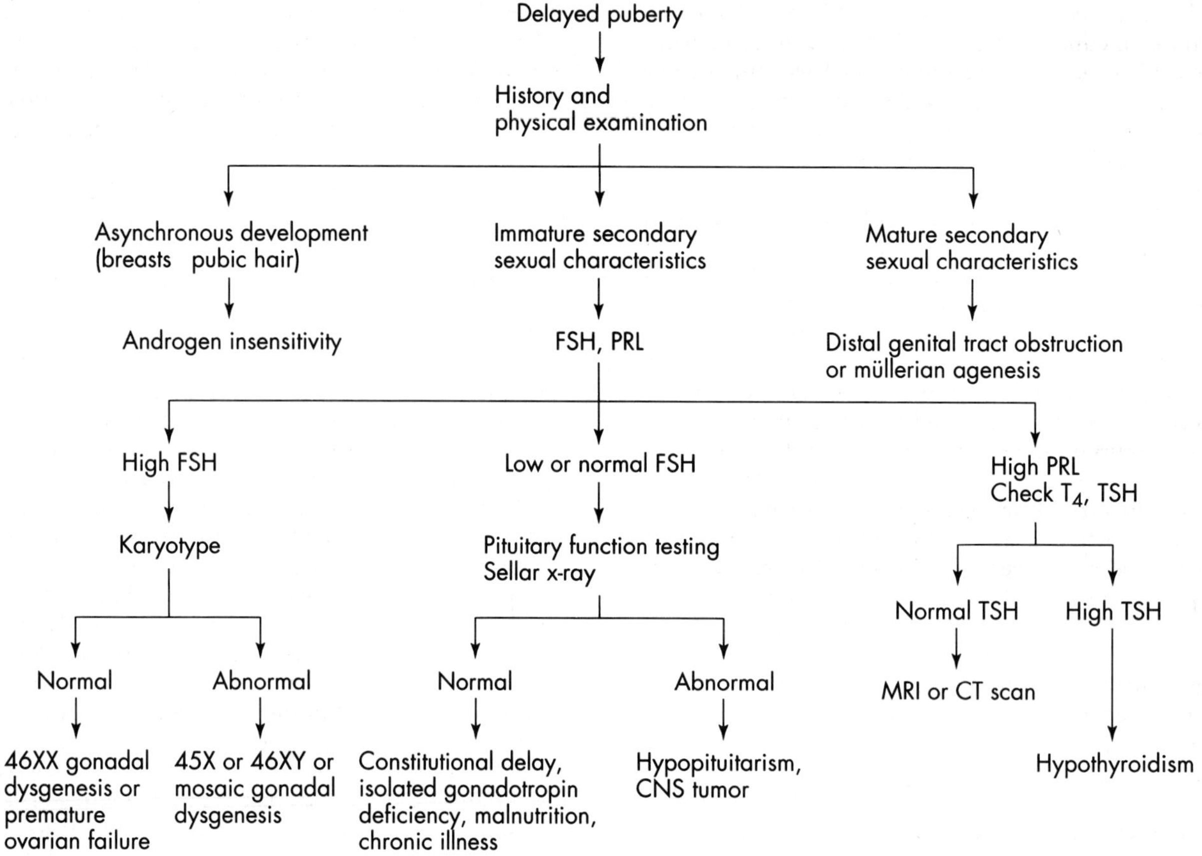

Figure 1
A possible flow diagram for the evaluation of delayed puberty. *(From Rebar RW. Normal and abnormal sexual differentiation and pubertal development. In: Moore T, et al., eds. Gynecology and obstetrics: An integrated approach. New York: Churchill Livingstone, 1993:97; with permission.)*

Similarly, intra-abdominal bleeding from any endometrial cavity in which efflux is blocked will require a surgical approach.

Differentiation of obstruction or malformation of the genital tract from androgen insensitivity (i.e., testicular feminization) is generally straightforward because the rare individuals with this latter syndrome present with "asynchronous" pubertal development with advanced breast development (Tanner stage 3) relative to pubic hair development (stage 1 or 2). An absent or foreshortened vagina may be present. The diagnosis may be confirmed by documenting a 46XY karyotype and circulating levels of testosterone in the male range. Removal of the gonads is warranted after the normal age of puberty to eliminate any potential for malignant degeneration. Estrogen replacement is then required. An explanation of the problem to the patient and her family requires much sensitivity on the part of the health care provider.

Individuals who fail to develop secondary sex characteristics should have basal levels of FSH and prolactin determined. In addition, bone age should be estimated by obtaining an x-ray of the nondominant hand to predict final adult height. Elevations in prolactin may suggest primary hypothyroidism, which may be diagnosed by documenting elevated levels of thyroid-stimulating hormone (TSH). If thyroid function is normal, a hypothalamic or a pituitary tumor is possible. TSH-secreting neoplasms are extremely rare and probably should be considered only if the patient does not respond to thyroid hormone replacement.

A karyotype should be obtained in any individual with delayed puberty and increased basal FSH concentrations. The individual with hypergonadotropic hypogonadism (with FSH concentrations greater than 30 mIU per milliliter) has some form of ovarian "failure," with failure of gonadal steroid secretion leading to the increase in gonadotropin secretion.

The most common form of hypergonadotropic hypogonadism with sexual infantilism is gonadal dysgenesis with or without the stigmata of Turner's syndrome (including among other physical features short stature, a webbed neck, low-set ears, an increased carrying angle of the arms, and a shieldlike chest). These features may be minimal or absent in patients who have sex chromosome mosaicism or structural deletions of the X chromosome, and some degree of pubertal maturation may be present. Patients with chromosomes bearing a Y cell line are at increased risk for gonadal neoplastic transformation, and in such individuals the gonads should be removed.

Treatment for patients with gonadal dysgenesis is directed toward increasing their predicted adult height and correcting their estrogen deficiency so that development of secondary sexual characteristics can take place. Multicenter studies have shown that methionyl human GH, alone or in combination with oxandrolone, stimulates linear growth with minimal side effects. However, comparative studies will be needed to ascertain whether the increase in height is greater with very low doses of estradiol alone or when estradiol is added to oxandrolone and GH.

In girls with hypergonadotropic hypogonadism, induction of secondary sexual characteristics is usually required. Deciding when to begin hormone therapy is difficult, but starting between 12 and 13 years of age (if the patient and her family are psychologically prepared) will help to approximate the secondary sexual development of her peers. We initiate treatment with low doses of estrogen (conjugated estrogens, 0.3 mg orally every other day) until breakthrough bleeding occurs or for no longer than 6 months. Use of lower doses than are readily available may have a greater beneficial effect on growth. Medroxyprogesterone acetate (2.5 to 5.0 mg orally) is then added for 12 to 14 days every 1 to 2 months so that withdrawal bleeding is induced. The dosage of estrogen then can be gradually increased at 6-month intervals to more adult levels, with progestin administered for 12 to 14 days every 1 to 2 months as well. Estrogen ultimately can be given daily (micronized estradiol-17β, 1 to 2 mg, or estrone sulfate, 1.2 to 2.5 mg orally each day or estradiol-17β, 0.1 mg transdermally changed as directed) with medroxyprogesterone acetate (5 to 10 mg) added for the first 12 to 14 days of every 1 to 2 months. The recent availability of second generation matrix transdermal estradiol-17β patches in the United States allows this form of estrogen to be used exclusively for pubertal maturation. The quantity of estradiol absorbed is directly proportional to the surface area of the patch. The smaller (0.05 mg) patches can be quartered, then halved, and finally used wholly to deliver increasing quantities of estradiol to the patient.

If adult doses of estrogen are given from the onset, most breast development occurs in the subareolar region and is cosmetically unacceptable because of the development of tubular breasts. Administration of the sex steroids, as outlined, will enhance the development of secondary sexual characteristics. It also will allow the adolescent to have regular menses like her peers and protect her from problems such as atrophic vaginitis, hot flashes, and osteoporosis. The prevention of coronary heart disease may be an even greater benefit. It is current practice to administer progestin to every woman with a uterus to prevent the endometrial hyperplasia and cancer that may result from therapy with unopposed estrogen. The final dose of estrogen utilized depends upon the patient. The first sign that too much estrogen is being given is continuous breast tenderness.

Later, when conception becomes an issue, fertility can be achieved in the group of hypergonadotropic patients who have intact uteri with the use of oocytes that have been donated by either known or anonymous donors. The recipient's uterus can be stimulated with varying doses of estrogen to mimic the proliferative phase of the normal menstrual cycle, while the donor's ovaries are hyperstimulated with human menopausal gonadotropins. After fertilization in vitro, embryos can be implanted in the recipient's uterus in the induced luteal phase.

The differential diagnosis of individuals with low or normal levels of FSH is more complex. It is now recognized that puberty can be delayed by any abnormality that will cause secondary amenorrhea in older females. Whenever pubertal development begins and is then interrupted, the etiology is almost invariably central. Pituitary function testing and sellar x-rays may be required to differentiate central lesions from isolated gonadotropin deficiency and panhypopituitarism. Girls with anorexia nervosa and hypogonadism secondary to malnutrition or chronic illness are generally identified easily. Constitutional delay, perhaps the most common cause of delayed puberty, remains of necessity a diagnosis of exclusion. Appropriate management is dependent on the etiology. Individuals requiring induction of secondary sex characteristics can be treated as previously delineated for girls with gonadal dysgenesis. Individuals with an intact pituitary also can have pubertal maturation induced with pulsatile GnRH, but such therapy is far more cumbersome for the patient. Regardless of the therapy, once mature secondary sex characteristics have been attained, cyclic menses can be induced either with sequential estrogen-progestin therapy as outlined or, alternatively, low-dose combination oral contraceptive agents can be used. Accumulating data indicate that young women with hypoestrogenic forms of amenorrhea (including many with low or normal levels of FSH) have an increased incidence of scoliosis and osteoporosis unless treated with exogenous estrogen. There is no evidence that administration of estrogen impairs "recovery" of the hypothalamic-pituitary axis. Thus, the estrogen can be discontinued when the patient desires fertility. If ovulatory cycles do not begin spontaneously, ovulation induction is warranted.

Those women desiring pregnancy who have intact pituitary function can have ovulation induced either with pulsatile GnRH or with human menopausal gonadotropins (hMG). Women with abnormal pituitary function may have ovulation induced with hMG after the primary problem has been treated appropriately.

For individuals with constitutional delay, reassurance that appropriate development will occur is the only therapy warranted. Administration of estrogen to these girls can lead to premature epiphyseal closure and impairment of ultimate adult height. Such girls will ultimately achieve their full genetic potential in height and attain full sexual maturity, but it will take them longer than their peers. Although we do not favor their use, some clinicians recommend low doses of estrogen (not more than the equivalent of 0.3 mg conjugated estrogens) for a short period of time (1 to 3 months) to "accelerate" the onset of pubertal development.

Suggested Reading

Albanese A, Stanhope R. Investigation of delayed puberty. Clin Endocrinol 1995; 43:105–110.

Bridges NA, Hindmarsh PC, Matthews DR, Brook CG. The effect of changing gonadotropin-releasing hormone pulse frequency on puberty. J Clin Endocrinol Metab 1994; 841–847.

Cavallo A, Richards GE, Smith ER. Relation between nocturnal melatonin profile and hormonal markers of puberty in humans. Horm Res 1992; 37:185–189.

Goji K. Twenty-four-hour concentration profiles of gonadotropin and estradiol (E2) in prepubertal and early pubertal girls: The diurnal rise of E2 is opposite the nocturnal rise of gonadotropin. J Clin Endocrinol Metab 1993; 77:1629–1635.

Kasa-Vubu JZ, Padmanabhan V, Kletter GB, et al. Serum bioactive luteinizing and follicle-stimulating hormone concentrations in girls increase during puberty. Pediatr Res 1993; 34:829–833.

Marshall WA, Tanner JM. Variation in patterns of pubertal changes in girls. Arch Dis Child 1969; 44:291.

Saggese G, Cesaretti G, Giannessi N, et al. Stimulated growth hormone (GH) secretion in children with delays in pubertal development before and after the onset of puberty: Relationship with peripheral plasma GH-releasing hormone and somatostatin levels. J Clin Endocrinol Metab 1992; 74:272–278.

DYSMENORRHEA

Rapin Osathanondh, M.D.

Dysmenorrhea, or painful menstruation, is characterized by cramping pain in the lower abdomen before and/or during menstrual flow. It may be accompanied by a constellation of symptoms such as sweating, weakness, lack of energy, insomnia, nausea and vomiting, diarrhea, lower backache, headache, dizziness, and syncope, which together are called dysmenorrhea syndrome. Management protocols are traditionally divided into whether the dysmenorrhea is of the primary type (i.e., without identifiable pelvic lesions) or of the secondary type (i.e., due to an organic pelvic disease). These may be two separate conditions for which different types of endocrine or surgical therapy are specifically indicated.

Dysmenorrhea represents a major public health problem because of its common incidence among women of reproductive age and because the monthly moderate to severe pain leads to poor quality of life and decreased productivity. Furthermore, some women with secondary dysmenorrhea, despite mild symptoms, may have extensive pelvic disease that can lead to infertility.

Another incapacitating condition, which is partly related to cyclic ovarian function and dysmenorrhea, is premenstrual syndrome (PMS). PMS is characterized by a combination of symptoms that occur during the 5 to 10 days before menses and, in some cases, through the week after menses. Physical complaints may include bloating, slight weight gain, edema of the hands and feet, vasomotor flushes, tender or swollen breasts, acne, and gastrointestinal disturbances. Subjective symptoms may include anxiety, fatigue, exhaustion, depression, aggression, nervous tension, headache, mood swings and irritability, food cravings, and change in libido. PMS, together with dysmenorrhea, are major contributors to the three most common complaints in medicine, namely, headache, depression, and low back pain. Over one-half of women with PMS benefit from monthly or daily pharmacotherapy. Favorable drug responses should be judged on an individual basis and over three menstrual cycles because symptoms vary from woman to woman and from one month to the next in the same woman. Many patients report cycle-to-cycle variabilities in both the number of their symptoms and the degree of severity.

■ PRIMARY DYSMENORRHEA

Primary dysmenorrhea is diagnosed in the absence of any discernible pelvic lesion: the work-up and plan of management are summarized stepwise in Table 1. These steps begin with a routine office investigation and treatment (or therapeutic diagnosis); abdominal plus transvaginal ultrasound; chlamydia and gonorrhea cultures; screening blood tests (CA-125, C-reactive protein); and invasive ambulatory investigations such as laparoscopy, hysteroscopy, dilation and curettage, or hysterosalpingography. Following this management scheme, a physician can distinguish primary from secondary dysmenorrhea and provide appropriate pharmacotherapy. Primary dysmenorrhea can be effectively treated with the use of an oral contraceptive or a nonsteroidal anti-inflammatory drug (NSAID). The latter class of drugs inhibits the endometrial production and release of prostaglandins of the E and F series. These prostaglandins are responsible for the symptoms of dysmenorrhea such as the increased myometrial activity and for the unpleasant systemic effects on other target organs such as the gastrointestinal tract.

The most appropriate choice among an abundance of NSAIDs for the treatment of primary dysmenorrhea is an over-the-counter (OTC) alkanoic (arylpropionic) acid derivative such as ibuprofen or naproxen sodium. A practical difference between these two OTC drugs is in their elimination half-lives (2 hours for ibuprofen versus 13 hours for naproxen sodium). These two NSAIDS are "type I" inhibitors of "prostaglandin synthetase" enzymes. Other effective type I inhibitors are fenamate derivatives such as flufenamic acid and mefanamic acid. The latter has also been shown to relieve some PMS symptoms. However, I do not recommend a fenamate derivative for monthly therapy because of its high incidence of bone marrow toxicity. Not all of the type I inhibitors can be recommended for the treatment of dysmenorrhea. For example, aspirin (a benzoic acid derivative) is not potent enough in the usual dose, and high doses produce unpleasant side effects; and the risks from indomethacin (an indole-acetic acid derivative) in the long-term monthly treatment outweigh the benefits. Type II prostaglandin synthetase inhibitors such as a buterophenone (oxyphenbutazone or phenylbutazone) may not be effective in the treatment of dysmenorrhea because they do not reduce the cyclic endoperoxides, which are also potent uterotonic substances. Note

Table 1 Work-Up of Dysmenorrhea

Step I	*Routine Office Investigations* 1. History and physical examination 2. Internal examination Pelvic examination including Papanicolaou test Rectovaginal examination Rectal examination if age >40 for occult blood 3. Appropriate treatment Positive finding(s): treat secondary dysmenorrhea Negative finding: therapeutic trial with an NSAID for 3 months *or* a combination oral contraceptive (COC) if birth control is also required Satisfactory response → continue therapy and yearly follow-up Unsatisfactory response → Step II
Step II	*Noninvasive Ambulatory Investigations* 1. Abdominal and transvaginal ultrasound 2. Complete blood count plus serum CA-125 and C-reactive protein 3. Repeat internal examination with genital cultures (or a rapid immunogenetic multiple screen) for chlamydia and gonorrhea Positive finding(s): treat the cause(s) of secondary dysmenorrhea Negative finding: switch to another NSAID, or NSAID plus COC for 3 months Satisfactory response → continue therapy and yearly follow-up Unsatisfactory response → Step III
Step III	*Invasive Ambulatory Investigations* 1. The following procedure(s) may be indicated: Laparoscopy Hysteroscopy Dilation and curettage Hysterosalpingography

that factors other than prostaglandins, such as serotonin, opioid neuropeptides, dopamine, and decreased blood levels of magnesium, may play some etiologic roles in these cyclic symptoms.

The effective use of NSAIDs for dysmenorrhea in the last 2 decades signified the beginning of a new era of pharmacologic manipulations at the end-organ (uterus) level. Eighty percent of patients with primary dysmenorrhea respond favorably to NSAIDs. Other agents such as nifedipine (a calcium channel blocker) have also been prescribed with success in a limited number of cases. However, nifedipine may produce headache and facial flushing, and should conception occur, this drug could be embryotoxic. Because most NSAIDs do not adequately reduce the central nervous system symptoms or other associated symptoms in a well-defined group of women with primary dysmenorrhea, investigators are constantly searching for agents that will eliminate the central effects of dysmenorrhea syndrome. A patient with dysmenorrhea may respond to one NSAID better than another drug of the same class. Thus, if an adequate dose (400 to 800 mg orally every 6 hours) of ibuprofen, a common OTC alkanoic acid derivative, does not provide relief, switching to another NSAID such as naproxen sodium (275 to 550 mg orally every 8 hours) is advised instead of increasing the dose of the same drug. This advice is based on the fact that there is a plateau analgesic effect for most NSAIDs tested and that side effects of such drugs are inherently dose related. Adverse effects of NSAIDs include a variety of gastrointestinal and central nervous system symptoms, as well as allergic reactions (from rash, edema, and bronchospasm to hepatic, renal, and marrow toxicity). Patients with impaired renal function will not tolerate a regular dose of such drugs, which inhibit essential renal prostaglandins.

NSAIDs are contraindicated in women with a history of hypersensitivity to aspirin or similar agents and in the presence of gastrointestinal ulcers. There is no proven therapeutic value in taking any NSAID before the onset of the symptoms. NSAIDs do not alter the cyclic pituitary-ovarian function or induce metabolic effects, as seen with oral contraceptives. However, like the effect of a combination oral contraceptive (COC), the amount of menstrual bleeding is decreased with prolonged use of an NSAID. Like aspirin, NSAIDs inhibit some platelet functions and chronic surreptitious use leads to prolonged bleeding time. Thus, a history should be carefully obtained regarding the recent use of any OTC analgesics. Patients should not undergo invasive procedures within 48 hours of the cessation of NSAID therapy.

Primary dysmenorrhea can be effectively and appropriately treated by inhibiting monthly ovulation. Therefore, a patient with dysmenorrhea who desires a birth control method should be treated with a COC. Most adolescents (over 90 percent of the cases) are provided adequate relief of symptoms with a COC. However, if needed, an NSAID can be added to the regimen. Patients who do not respond after 6 months of pharmacotherapeutic trials require further investigation in order to search for an occult pelvic disease. COCs have a longer history of use for reducing menstrual cramps than NSAIDs. Impressively, COCs have withstood the test of time during which their possible and probable adverse effects have been continuously studied over 4 decades. Patients receiving a COC should sign an informed consent form that explains the drug's benefits and risks.

■ SECONDARY DYSMENORRHEA

Secondary dysmenorrhea is diagnosed when a macroscopic lesion or inflammation of the upper genital tract is identified by way of a pelvic examination and confirmed by ultrasound imaging or laparoscopic, bacteriologic, radiographic contrast, or histopathologic studies. The most common cause of secondary dysmenorrhea is pelvic endometriosis. Surgical and endocrine therapies are usually required to relieve dysmenorrhea caused by endometriosis; these two methods of treatment are complementary or adjunctive. A triad of dysmenorrhea, persistent septated ovarian cyst(s) greater than 3 cm in diameter, and serum CA-125 levels greater than 40 U per milliliter may suggest organic pathology such as ovarian endometrioma (chocolate cyst). CA-125 is an embryonic antigen that can be measured by specific radioimmunoassay. Serum CA-125 levels are elevated in patients with nonmucinous epithelial ovarian cancer and other types of adenocarcinoma, as well as in healthy women during menstruation and pregnancy.

Other causes of secondary dysmenorrhea are anatomic lesions such as imperforate hymen, congenital stricture of the cervix, intrauterine adhesions or synechiae (Asherman's syndrome), uterine leiomyoma or polyp, adenomyosis, or ovarian cysts. Inflammatory lesions such as pelvic inflammatory disease (PID) or the presence of an intrauterine device may produce, or often aggravate, the dysmenorrhea syndrome. Treatment of secondary dysmenorrhea is aimed at pain relief, as well as removing or inhibiting the underlying pathologic process to maintain or restore the patient's reproductive capability. Gynecologic surgery is often indicated for such purposes.

Synthetic hormonal steroids have been used successfully in the treatment of pelvic endometriosis. This disease is diagnosed by positive identification of the ectopic endometrial tissues, which are found outside the inner lining of the uterine wall. Such tissues may be felt on pelvic examination (bimanual and rectovaginal palpations) as tender nodules in the cul-de-sac or as cysts in the ovary. The definitive diagnosis is obtained by the laparoscopic visualization of hemosiderin plaques (eschars) on the surface of the ovaries or visceral peritoneum. These lesions are chronically stimulated by cyclic ovarian steroids with resultant hemorrhagic cysts (chocolate cysts), local irritations, and adhesions. Many patients with this disease suffer dysmenorrhea, deep dyspareunia, and, in some cases, involuntary infertility. The latter results from functional disturbance or anatomic damage of the oviducts as well as oligo-ovulation, luteal phase insufficiency, or even anovulation. Treatment of this type of dysmenorrhea requires prolonged suppression of menstrual bleeding and ovarian function for 3 to 12 months. The duration of the induced amenorrhea depends on the extent of the lesions, the patient's history regarding duration of the disease, previous treatment methods, drug response, and her desire to conceive. Drugs that can be used for inducing prolonged amenorrhea are norgestrel-containing COCs administered continuously (and in increasing doses if necessary) to inhibit the menstrual bleeding and cyclic ovarian function (the so-called pseudopregnancy therapy) and danazol, which is an androgen derivative that suppresses both the pituitary and the ovarian functions. In selected cases a synthetic progestin alone or high doses of a gonadotropin-releasing hormone (GnRH) analogue (e.g., leuprolide or nafarelin acetate) may be used for short-term therapy for 6 to 9 months. A COC for pseudopregnancy therapy produces decidual changes in all endometrial tissues. Progressive necrosis, liquefaction, and absorption follow. An NSAID can be prescribed for pain relief in conjunction with hormonal therapy. If, however, the secondary dysmenorrhea is due to adenomyosis, pain would generally be worsened with the use of a COC and may be relieved by danazol or dl-norgestrel. Adenomyosis denotes the presence of endometrial glands and stroma inside the myometrium (endometriosis interna), a condition that often occurs in multiparous women. It poses a therapeutic dilemma because, in conventional practice, this diagnosis can be confirmed only by the histologic examination of hysterectomy specimens.

Surgery is usually indicated for patients with moderate or severe endometriosis (classified by the American Society for Reproductive Medicine as stage III or IV disease,* respectively) and for patients with mild (stage II) disease whose pain or infertility has proved unresponsive to medical treatment for one year. Bleeding time should be checked before the patient undergoes any surgical procedure for chronic pain if OTC analgesics containing aspirin or an NSAID have been regularly consumed. When conservative surgery is performed to relieve pain, ablation of the lesions by means of CO_2 laser or electrocautery may be combined with a presacral neurectomy or transection of the uterosacral ligaments to ensure pain relief. On the other hand, many women with severe (stage IV) disease of long duration may no longer experience dysmenorrhea or pelvic pain and conservative surgery may not restore or bring back their fertility. Most of the time, however, extirpative surgery is indicated for stage IV disease to treat sequelae such as a partial intestinal obstruction caused by endometriosis of the intestinal wall. Surgery for these patients may involve not only removal or debulking of lesions but also removal of the uterus and ovaries. Bilateral oophorectomy ensures cessation of the disease process, because the remaining microscopic lesions (aberrant or ectopic endometrial glands) regress into the state of atrophy (burnt-out spots). Following extirpative surgery, 0.5 to 1 mg micronized estradiol is administered vaginally every second or third night to control vasomotor flush and prevent osteoporosis. The dose is titrated to achieve adequate relief of symptoms with the minimum amount of estradiol. Some patients later produce sufficient levels of endogenous estrogens from peripheral conversion (aromatization) of adrenocortical precursors. Alternatively, transdermal estradiol as a skin patch may be used (Climara once a week, Estraderm twice a week, or Vivelle twice a week) to deliver 0.05 to 0.1 mg per day. Five to

---

*A scoring system based on the size of all endometriotic lesions and adhesions found on the peritoneum, ovaries, and oviducts. A score of 1, 2, or 3 is given for less than 1 cm, 1 to 3 cm, or greater than 3 cm lesions, respectively. Stage I (minimal), II (mild), III (moderate), or IV (severe) indicates a total score of 1–5, 6–15, 16–40, or greater than 40, respectively.

10 percent of patients discontinued this mode of treatment or switched the brand of estradiol patch because of skin rash. Both the vaginal and transdermal estradiol routes of administration avoid significant first-pass hepatic metabolism.

Adverse effects from estrogen replacement therapy after hysterectomy with bilateral ovariectomy are breast tenderness, abdominal bloating, and irritability. Interestingly, nausea, which may occur with oral estrogen therapy, is noted relatively infrequently with the lowest effective dose of transdermal or vaginal estradiol. Oral estrogens have been effectively utilized for replacement therapy for 5 decades in the form of conjugated equine estrogens (Premarin) made from pregnant mare urine (0.6 to 1.2 mg per day). When estrogen therapy is not well tolerated or contraindicated, transdermal clonidine, oral dl-norgestrel (minipill), or medroxyprogesterone acetate can be prescribed for the relief of vasomotor symptoms (but they are not useful to prevent osteoporosis). Although there are no published data on the efficacy of dl-norgestrel, some practitioners and I prefer this minipill to other progestins based on patients' subjective preference perhaps due to its mild androgenic effects. However, patients should be informed of the possible side effects from prolonged use of mild androgens.

Not all patients with endometriosis are infertile. Intrauterine pregnancy, which by itself represents a prolonged (9-month) cessation of menstruation, may provide a hormonal milieu that retards the progress of this disease. In fact, ameliorative effects of pregnancy have been observed in some women with endometriosis. Conversely, women with endometriosis who conceive are at increased risk of miscarriage and ectopic pregnancy. Retarded follicular growth, luteal phase insufficiency, and anovulatory cycles are not uncommon in patients with endometriosis. Daily recording of the basal body temperature is advised, and ovulation induction may be required if pregnancy is desired. If surgery is anticipated for treating female infertility, a male infertility factor must be ruled out before that woman is subjected to surgery. After conservative surgery, short-term (3-month) endocrine therapy may be indicated for selected cases. In general, minimal (stage I) disease responds to treatment with continued suppression of endometrial and ovarian function for 6 to 9 months using either danazol or a long-acting GnRH analogue for temporary medical castration. Prolonged use of the potent GnRH may lead to significant sex steroid deprivation in young women, with resultant adverse sequelae such as decreased mineral density of the vertebrae. Long-term effects of temporary estrogen deprivation have not been clearly established. However, once the treatment is discontinued, menstruation resumes within 4 to 6 weeks in most women. Alternatively, synthetic progestins (mostly androgen derivatives) can be used as well for continued suppression of menses. These agents are norgestrel with ethinyl estradiol, dl-norgestrel, medroxyprogesterone acetate, or norethindrone acetate. The risks and adverse effects of synthetic progestins are similar to those of oral contraceptives. However, patients should be warned of the sleepiness, tiredness, light-headedness, muscle cramps, and constipation. Side effects of danazol include weight gain, fluid retention, mood swings, change of libido, vasomotor flush, sweating, muscle cramps, dizziness, atrophic vaginitis, androgenic effects such as reduced breast size, and decreased level of plasma high-density lipoprotein (HDL) cholesterol, most of which are reversible. Patients with borderline hepatic or adrenocortical function should not receive the full dose of danazol (800 mg per day) because this drug is cleared through the liver and has been shown to inhibit certain adrenal enzymes. When prescribing danazol, I advise the patient against swimming alone because of the possible development of sudden muscle cramping. These occasional muscle cramps may be relieved by drinking Gatorade, tonic (quinine) water, or Pedialyte. I also monitor the patient's serum aminotransferase and HDL-cholesterol levels every other month while she is on high doses of danazol. Possible adverse effects of danazol are rash, gastrointestinal upset, hepatic dysfunction, and, in rare cases, Addisonian-like symptoms. Danazol should be started at 400 mg per day and increased to 800 mg per day within 1 to 2 weeks as tolerated. Most women do not ovulate when receiving danazol in dosages of 400 mg (or more) per day. Prolonged amenorrhea of 28 months' duration has been observed in one woman following 9 months of therapy with 800 mg per day.

Some patients with dysmenorrhea will seek help only after their symptoms have been aggravated by a concomitant PID. The latter is usually diagnosed by internal examination (acute pain on cervical motion and severe pelvic tenderness). However, when in doubt, a questionable diagnosis of PID can be confirmed by a highly elevated serum C-reactive protein level. Usual treatment is oral doxycycline 100 mg twice a day for 1 to 2 weeks. Doxycycline may induce nausea or hypersensitive skin to ultraviolet light (sunburn). Patients with known hypersensitivity to doxycycline may benefit from azithromycin or ofloxacin.

■ PREMENSTRUAL SYNDROME

PMS, like primary dysmenorrhea, is characterized by its cyclicity, which is partly related to ovarian function, and by the fact that its severity may vary greatly from one month to the next in the same woman. However, unlike primary dysmenorrhea, there is no single drug treatment that has proved to be as effective as an NSAID or COC is for primary dysmenorrhea. There are two likely reasons to explain this problem. First, an etiologic factor(s) responsible for the cyclic symptoms of PMS is believed to be different from that of primary dysmenorrhea but may be a result of an interplay between estrogen(s) and central neurotransmitter(s) such as serotonin. NSAIDs or oral contraceptives relieve primary dysmenorrhea in 80 percent of the patients, but they usually do not modify the symptoms of PMS. These cyclic symptoms persist after hysterectomy or temporary medical castration with GnRH. Second, there is no confirmatory diagnostic test available except for "therapeutic diagnosis" using a "selective serotonin reuptake inhibitor" (SSRI). Personality profiles, psychological testing, or classifying patients into various types or categories by the "symptoms cluster" has not been helpful or practical. Behavior modification programs or support groups, while helpful for certain patients, may mask an underlying endocrine disorder in other cases. Currently useful drugs for alleviating many PMS symptoms are venlafaxine hydrochloride (Effexor), 12.5 to 25 mg per day, fluoxetine hydrochloride (Prozac), 5 to 10 mg per day, or sertraline hydrochloride (Zoloft), 25 to 50 mg per day. While their conventional antidepression dosage increases serotonin at the postsynaptic membrane, their actual mechanism(s) in controlling PMS symptoms has not been clearly elucidated. I start my patients with one-half of the smallest available tablet of SSRI per day. Therapeutic response at this low dose may surprisingly occur within one to two weeks without side effects except for nausea (less than 10 percent). The patient is instructed to call me within 2 weeks if the drug works well so that she can continue at that lowest effective dose for 6 months. If there is no relief, I will double her daily dose once or twice every 2 weeks providing there are no side effects. Like NSAID or COC for dysmenorrhea, some patients will respond to one brand of SSRI better than another brand. Fluoxetine, which has been used for a relatively long period, appears to be nonteratogenic in human offsprings thus far. The other two SSRIs have shorter elimination half-lives than fluoxetine, but they have been available only recently. Dosage of all SSRIs must be reduced in patients with hepatorenal impairment. They must not be combined with a monoamine oxidase (MAO) inhibitor or a diuretic because fatal drug reactions could occur. In some circumstances, venlafaxine may provide an advantage over fluoxetine and sertraline since venlafaxine is not highly bound to plasma proteins and thus will not cause increased free concentrations of a drug such as Coumadin or digitoxin when used concomitantly.

Several other agents have been shown, in controlled studies, to be effective in the treatment of PMS. Spironolactone, alprazolam, micronized estradiol, and bromocriptine mesylate are prescription drugs that have been separately used to relieve the following symptoms of PMS: fluid retention, central nervous system disturbances, vasomotor flushes, and breast tenderness, respectively. Additionally, pyridoxine hydrochloride (vitamin B_6) and gammalinolenic acid (evening primrose oil), both of which are OTC drugs, may be effective if breast tenderness is the strongest complaint. However, not all women with PMS respond to these drugs or even to the combination of different agents. Only half of the patients respond to one or a combination of such drugs. Spironolactone may be effective at a dose of 25 mg orally three to four times per day during the last half of every menstrual cycle. Spironolactone is an antagonist of aldosterone, a hormone that is structurally related to progesterone. It can be used in combination with hydrochlorothiazide (Aldactazide). Pyridoxine hydrochloride is generally recommended at a dose of 200 to 400 mg daily throughout every cycle. This dose must be strictly adhered to because of the reported neurotoxicity if more than 1 g per day is consumed. Alprazolam, a short-acting anxiolytic, has been shown to be effective only in low doses (i.e., not exceeding 0.75 mg per day in the perimenstrual period). A high dose of alprazolam (supposedly a "downer") may produce a "high" paradoxically without pronounced sedation when taken along with certain opioid drugs, and patients with a history of alcohol or substance abuse should not be given alprazolam. Micronized estradiol and gammalinolenic acid should be tried in the lowest effective dose and only during the premenstrual week because long-term untoward effects have not been established.

Two related products that have been used for relieving PMS symptoms in selected cases are bromocriptine mesylate and ergotamine tartrate. The former is an ergot derivative used for a small number of women with PMS who have slightly elevated serum prolactin or fasting growth hormone levels. The latter is an old drug (Cafergot) used for treating migraine and may be beneficial for certain PMS patients whose strongest complaint is migraine headache. It is also an ergot derivative with no stimulatory effect on the myometrium and is sometimes used in combination with a mild sedative plus an anticholinergic (Bellergal). However, because of the chronicity of PMS (and dysmenorrhea) symptoms, the use of a narcotic or long-acting anxiolytic drug should be discouraged. Patients should be advised to read package inserts and to adhere strictly to all the precautions.

There are OTC drugs for self-administration in the treatment of PMS, but their efficacy has not been proven in well-controlled clinical trials. In the United States, several OTC drugs for this purpose contain a combination of acetaminophen, pamabrom (a mild diuretic), and pyrilamine maleate (an antihistamine with anticholinergic plus sedative effects). Indirect evidence suggests that acetaminophen may strongly potentiate the NSAID's effect in inhibiting prostaglandin synthesis. I warn my patients against combining acetaminophen with any NSAID for fear of cumulative adverse effects on renal function. This cautionary advice is based on the reported renal insufficiency following chronic ingestion of aspirin combined with acetaminophen. Another type of OTC drug for PMS combines aspirin, caffeine, and cinnamedrine hydrochloride (a smooth muscle relaxant). Other neuroactive agents that have been shown to relieve PMS symptoms are buspirone, fenfluramine, naltrexone, and clonidine. Buspirone and fenfluramine are serotoninergic drugs that should not be used in conjunction with another tranquilizer or an MAO inhibitor. I also monitor the eosinophil count whenever serotoninergic drugs are prescribed. Patients with food cravings and/or late luteal cognitive and mood disturbances may benefit from a proprietary beverage, InterNutria. This concoction of simple and complex carbohydrates reportedly increases serum tryptophan levels.

Suggested Reading

Osathanondh R. Dysmenorrhea. In: Bardin CW, ed. Current therapy in endocrinology and metabolism. 4th ed. Philadelphia: BC Decker, 1991:195.

Osathanondh R. Combination oral contraceptives. In: Bardin CW, ed. Current therapy in endocrinology and metabolism. 5th ed. St. Louis: BC Decker/Mosby–Year Book, 1994:250.

Osathanondh R. Conception control. In: Ryan KJ, Berkowitz R, Barbieri RL, eds. Kistner's gynecology. 6th ed. St. Louis: Mosby–Year Book, 1995:532.

Sayegh R, Schiff I, Wurtman J, et al. The effect of a carbohydrate-rich beverage on mood, appetite, and cognitive function in women with premenstrual syndrome. Obstet Gynecol 1995; 86:520.

PREMENSTRUAL SYNDROME

Joseph F. Mortola, M.D.

Recent advances in the understanding of premenstrual syndrome (PMS) have provided sufficient elucidation of its pathophysiology to permit the development of sound pharmacologic interventions. Prior to the initiation of therapy, careful consideration should be given to accurate diagnosis of the syndrome and its differentiation from other medical and psychiatric disorders. Although at present there are no Food and Drug Administration (FDA)–approved medications for this indication, several well-designed studies have been conducted that guide the clinician's treatment of PMS. As a result, less-proven nonpharmacologic modalities, such as dietary modification, exercise regimens, and psychotherapy, are more quickly supplanted by the use of medication. Three classes of agents have been proven efficacious and are widely used to treat the disorder. These include benzodiazepines (especially alprazolam), serotonin-reuptake inhibitors (especially fluoxetine), and gonadotropin-releasing hormone (GnRH) agonists. In addition to these medications, which are used to treat the generalized syndrome of PMS, a variety of other drugs are used in the treatment of specific aspects of this disorder. In addition, a variety of less well-proven pharmacologic remedies are commonly in use. In these cases, the side effects of the medications may well outweigh their benefits.

As understanding of the pathophysiology of PMS has improved, increasingly specific treatments are being devised based on these insights. At present the treatments with demonstrated efficacy are directed at either reduction of circulating steroid levels or neurotransmitter modulation. Each of these strategies has sound rationale, because it is increasingly apparent that the neurobehavioral symptoms of PMS are the result of the interaction of ovarian steroids with central neurotransmitters. Although attempts to discern differences in circulating estrogen, progesterone, or androgen levels in women with PMS have been unsuccessful, it is likely that women have varying central nervous system sensitivities to the alterations in neurotransmitter economy that result from the normal cyclic fluctuations in sex steroids that occur during the reproductive years. Moreover, there is evidence that these susceptibilities are different from those seen in affective disorders or anxiety disorders. It is therefore optimal to accurately diagnose PMS prior to initiation of therapy. Once this has been accomplished, focused treatment regimens can be instituted.

■ DIAGNOSIS

Symptoms

Although more than 150 symptoms have been ascribed to PMS, it is now apparent that the symptom constellation is rather specific and well defined. The repeated occurrence of either irritability or depression and fatigue during the luteal phase of the cycle accompanied by bloated sensations in the abdomen or extremities, breast tenderness, or headache is seen in almost all patients. In addition, a select group of other symptoms occur with sufficient frequency to merit their inclusion in the syndrome. The behavioral symptoms include labile mood with alternating sadness and anger (81 percent), oversensitivity (69 percent), crying spells (65 percent), social withdrawal (65 percent), forgetfulness (56 percent), and difficulty concentrating (47 percent). The common physical symptoms include acne (71 percent) and gastrointestinal upset (48 percent). Appetite changes and food cravings are seen in 70 percent of women with PMS. Vasomotor flushes (18 percent), heart palpitations (13 percent), and dizziness (13 percent) are less commonly observed.

Temporal Patterns

None of the symptoms of PMS is unique to the syndrome. What is diagnostic of the disorder is the marked fluctuation of symptoms with the menstrual cycle. During the time from the fourth day after the onset of menses, until at least cycle day 12, symptoms, if they occur at all, are sporadic and no more frequent than those seen in the general population. This criterion is applicable to the vast majority of reproductive age women, although women with cycles that are typically shorter than 26 days may have the onset of symptoms slightly earlier than day 12. Using prospective recording of symptoms, the pattern of symptom severity in women with PMS has been defined. Mean symptom severity increases gradually throughout the luteal phase, reaches a peak just prior to the onset of menses, and subsequently declines rapidly over the first 4 days following the onset of menses.

Level of Impairment

Diagnosis of PMS also requires assessment of symptom severity. Therefore, a measurement of the degree of impairment should be ascertained. With respect to the physical symptoms of breast tenderness and bloating, for instance, their occurrence is so common as to be considered no more than a normal sign of ovulation. Such symptoms should be more accurately referred to as premenstrual molimina. In contrast, headaches in some women occur so severely as to prohibit work. Because there is no "gold standard" by which to compare the severity of a self-reported symptom in one individual with that in another, more objective external manifestations of the disorder are required. This permits differentiation of PMS as a distinct syndrome at one end of the continuum between women who discern no physical and emotional differences during the course of the menstrual cycle and those who become incapacitated during the luteal phase. The assessment is most verifiable if objective criteria for impairment are based on socioeconomic performance. Identifiable disruption in performance can be ascertained by (1) marital or relationship discord confirmed by the partner, (2) difficulties in parenting children manifested by behavioral disturbance in the child, (3) poor work or school performance, (4) increased social isolation, (5) legal difficulties, (6) expressed suicidal ideation, or (7) seeking medical attention for a somatic symptom (Table 1).

In addition to the application of criteria for symptom

Table 1 UCSD Diagnostic Criteria for Premenstrual Syndrome

1. The presence of self-report of at least one of the following affective and somatic symptoms during the 5 days prior to menses in each of the three prior menstrual cycles:

Affective	*Somatic*
Depression	Breast tenderness
Angry outbursts	Abdominal bloating
Irritability	Headache
Anxiety	Swelling
Confusion	
Social withdrawal	

2. Relief of the above symptoms within 4 days of the onset of menses, without recurrence until at least cycle day 12.
3. The symptoms are present in the absence of any pharmacologic therapy, hormone ingestion, or drug or alcohol use.
4. The symptoms occur reproducibly during two cycles of prospective recording.
5. Identifiable dysfunction in social or economic performance by one of the following criteria:
   - Marital or relationship discord confirmed by partner
   - Difficulties in parenting
   - Poor work or school performance, attendance/tardiness
   - Increased social isolation
   - Legal difficulties
   - Suicidal ideation
   - Seeking medical attention for a somatic symptom(s)

From Mortola JF, Girton L, Beck L, et al. Depressive episodes in premenstrual syndrome. Am J Obstet Gynecol 1984; 161: 1682-1686.

timing and degree of impairment, the diagnosis of PMS can only be made in the presence of spontaneous menstrual cycles. Frequently, oral contraceptive pills may mimic the symptoms of PMS. In such patients, accurate diagnosis depends on discontinuation of the oral contraceptive and assessing symptoms in the absence of any pharmacologic intervention. In addition, self-prescribed substances such as alcohol or marijuana may obscure the ability to assess the progression of symptoms during the course of the menstrual cycle.

■ DIFFERENTIAL DIAGNOSIS

Several prospective rating scales are available to aid in the diagnosis of PMS. Because of the inability to diagnose PMS based on the symptoms themselves as opposed to the timing of the symptoms, the importance of prospective recording has become apparent. Although specific criteria for the diagnosis of PMS vary among the particular instrument used, in general a twofold increase in symptom severity scores is required to make the diagnosis. In addition, the severity of symptoms during the luteal phase should remain lower than those expected in psychiatric disorders such as dysphoric disorder or generalized anxiety disorder.

The use of prospective symptom inventories is particularly useful in distinguishing PMS from a variety of disorders that may mimic PMS. The pathognomonic finding in PMS using prospective symptom inventories is the presence of a relatively symptom-free interval between days 4 and 12 of the menstrual cycle. The disorders from which PMS must be separated include a rather large number of medical and psychiatric entities such as hypothyroidism, perimenopausal symptoms, and pheochromocytoma. In addition, several reports have indicated a high incidence of affective disorder in patients with premenstrual syndrome. Moreover, premenstrual exacerbations of anxiety disorders have been observed.

Table 2 Pharmacologic Agents for PMS

Treatments Based on Neurotransmitters
- Serotonin reuptake inhibitors
- Alprazolam

Treatments Based on Sex Steroid Suppression
- GnRH agonists

Treatments for Specific Symptoms
- Danazol
- Diuretics

Ineffective Treatments
- Progesterone
- Vitamin B_6
- Linoleic acid (evening primrose oil)
- Oral contraceptive pills

■ THERAPY

Within the past decade several treatments for PMS have been shown to be efficacious through well-controlled, blinded, randomized clinical trials (Table 2). This type of scientific rigor is absolutely essential in studies of treatment modalities to be applied to syndromes such as PMS, where the predominant symptoms are affective and behavioral. Such entities are notoriously subject to dramatic placebo effects. Unfortunately, the lack of well-controlled studies prior to those in the past decade has subjected and continues to subject women to a plethora of ineffective and sometimes deleterious remedies.

Treatments with proven efficacy based on alteration of hormonal status are limited to those employing GnRH agonists or, in extreme cases, oophorectomy. Oral contraceptives, while anecdotally helpful to some women, do not have proven efficacy in treating PMS. In fact, there is substantial evidence to indicate that oral contraceptives may induce a PMS-like syndrome in some women. Progesterone treatments have also been shown to be ineffective.

With respect to treatments directed at altering neurotransmitter levels, selective serotonin reuptake inhibitors and alprazolam have been shown to be effective. Although there continues to be interest in the possibility that alterations in the endogenous opioid and adrenergic systems may play a role in PMS symptomatology, these hypotheses remain unproven. To date, they have not yielded effective treatment interventions.

In addition to the treatments outlined above, several other treatments may have a role in the treatment of specific symptoms. These include spironolactone or other diuretics in the symptoms of water retention and danazol in the treatment of premenstrual migraines.

Selective Serotonin Reuptake Inhibitors

The largest body of both laboratory and clinical evidence suggests that serotonin (5-hydroxytryptamine) is the neuroactive agent with the greatest influence on PMS symptoms. This has led to extensive use of selective serotonin reuptake inhibitors (SSRIs) as the first-line treatment for PMS.

Interest in a 5-hydroxytryptamine mechanism in the appearance of PMS symptoms was generated by the evidence for interaction of progesterone with the 5-hydroxytryptamine system. There is substantial evidence that progesterone is a key mediator of PMS symptoms. In the rat, serial injection of progesterone results in increased 5-hydroxytryptamine uptake in several areas of the brain, as well as increased 5-hydroxytryptamine turnover. During the normal estrus cycle, 5-hydroxytryptamine receptors in the median forebrain undergo cyclic fluctuations, being upregulated after ovulation. Primate data support the mediation of 5-hydroxytryptamine by progesterone. In the macaque, extensive localization of progesterone receptors has been discerned in median raphe 5-hydroxytryptamine-positive neurons. In humans, decreased 5-hydroxytryptamine uptake by platelets has been reported in the premenstrual phase of the cycle following steroid withdrawal and to be correlated with the severity of some PMS symptoms. Differences in platelet 5-hydroxytryptamine uptake mechanism have also been noted in women with PMS. Similar alterations have been demonstrated in whole blood 5-hydroxytryptamine. In addition, the 5-hydroxytryptamine metabolite 5-hydroxyindoleacetic acid has been measured in urine across the menstrual cycle and found to be highest at the mid-luteal phase and lower in the late luteal phase.

In addition to data showing that progesterone modulates 5-hydroxytryptamine, it is apparent that the symptoms of PMS may be 5-hydroxytryptamine mediated. Decreased serotonergic activity, as is found in the late luteal phase of the cycle, has been implicated in increased appetite, psychomotor activity, and depression. In rats, m-chlorophenylpiperazine, a postsynaptic serotonin agonist, produces profound anorexia as does the serotonin agonist fenfluramine, when injected into the medial hypothalamus. In humans, cyproheptadine, a serotonin receptor antagonist, increases appetite in anorexia nervosa and potentiates hyperphagia in bulimia. In addition to producing anorexia, m-chlorophenylpiperazine has been shown in mice and rhesus monkeys to decrease locomotor activity. In humans, decreased CSF levels of 5-hydroxyindoleacetic acid are associated with depression.

Several SSRIs are available that are currently being actively studied in the treatment of PMS. These include fluoxetine, paroxetine, and sertraline, as well as SSRI-related compounds such as clomipramine and nafazadone.

Fluoxetine (Prozac) was initially demonstrated in small, independent double-blind, placebo-controlled studies to be effective in the treatment of PMS. More recently, these results have been confirmed by a large multicenter trial in Canada. When compared with tricyclic antidepressants, the efficacy of fluoxetine has been demonstrated to be superior. Conventional tricyclic antidepressants have been studied only to a limited degree in PMS. Investigators have been dissuaded from conducting large, appropriately controlled trials of tricyclics as a result of their relatively erratic performance in open trials.

The dose of fluoxetine that has been demonstrated to be effective is 20 mg daily. In the Canadian multicenter trial the use of higher doses resulted in greater side effects without a statistically significant improvement of symptoms as compared with the 20 mg dose. However, in clinical practice, some women do respond better to higher doses. There is also preliminary evidence that a 20 mg dose may be equally effective when administration is restricted to the luteal phase of the menstrual cycle. In contrast, in the treatment of depression, although many patients respond to the 20 mg daily dose, doses up to 60 mg and occasionally 80 mg are not uncommonly required for therapeutic response.

Widely publicized reports of an increased risk of suicidal or homicidal behavior on fluoxetine have been refuted in careful studies. Nonetheless, patient acceptance of the drug continues to be a problem for the clinician. Reassurance that the earlier reports of bizarre behaviors as a result of fluoxetine are unsubstantiated is often required.

Approximately 15 percent of patients taking fluoxetine experience side effects of sufficient severity or discomfort to warrant discontinuation of the drug. These include insomnia (5 percent), gastrointestinal disturbance (5 percent), and headache (5 percent). Although only 5 percent of patients have agitation or insomnia of sufficient severity to discontinue treatment, a much larger percentage (15 percent) experience this symptom to some degree. Some patients on fluoxetine experience drowsiness and fatigue rather than agitation. In these patients changing to a nighttime regimen is highly successful.

The incidence of a decline in libido during fluoxetine treatment is reported at approximately 2 percent in studies of depressed patients. However, this may be falsely low due to the already decreased libido that usually accompanies depression. In nondepressed patients, it appears that decreased libido is more commonly noted, and occurs in up to 30 percent of women with PMS.

Although large doses of fluoxetine given to animals have not been associated with birth defects, human studies, although highly encouraging, are not yet conclusive. Fluoxetine should be taken by pregnant or breast-feeding patients only with careful informed consent.

Alprazolam

Given that the most commonly observed symptom of PMS is fatigue, the steroid fluctuations during the menstrual cycle have been examined with respect to inhibitory neurotransmitters. Of these, gamma-amino-butyric acid (GABA) is the most studied. The GABA receptor complex constitutes the major site of action of benzodiazepines, where they serve to promote binding of GABA agonists to receptors. It is now apparent that progesterone and its metabolites bind to the GABA receptor complex at a site distinct from the GABA binding site and consequently influence GABA effect. In addition, both estrogen and progestin may serve to regulate GABA activity by attenuation of the number of GABA receptors or modulation of GABA release. This finding has led to exploration of the role of GABA-active agents in PMS.

At least two double-blind studies have demonstrated the

efficacy of a particular benzodiazepine, alprazolam, in the treatment of PMS. The usual dose range is 0.25 mg four times a day during the luteal phase of the cycle. Occasionally, higher doses of 0.5 mg up to four times a day are required. Although efficacy has been demonstrated at these doses, clinically many patients report significant improvement when the medication is taken during the luteal phase on an as-needed basis.

The side effect of greatest concern with alprazolam is its addictive potential. This has prompted a number of clinicians to substitute other benzodiazepines for alprazolam in the treatment of PMS. While there is sound theoretical rationale to posit that other benzodiazepines may have efficacy similar to alprazolam based on their biochemical similarity, this has not been demonstrated in controlled studies. Moreover, while alprazolam may be more addictive than some other benzodiazepines, all agents in this class carry a substantial risk of addiction. For this reason the use of benzodiazepines in PMS should be carefully restricted to luteal phase administration in the reliable patient. Addiction to alprazolam has not been reported when restricted to use during this prescribed time interval.

Alprazolam is associated with drowsiness in up to 40 percent of patients and with light-headedness in 5 percent of individuals. Administration of alprazolam has not been demonstrated to be safe in pregnancy and has been reported to cause lethargy in the infants of nursing mothers. Women on this agent for PMS should be instructed to use reliable methods of birth control. Because of the variable effects of oral contraceptives on PMS symptoms, barrier methods are preferred.

GnRH Agonists

In 1984 Muse et al. published the first results demonstrating a dramatic reduction of symptoms in women with PMS using daily injections of a GnRH agonist. Since that time, several other reports using different GnRH agonists have confirmed these results. The use of GnRH agonist for this indication depends on its ability to cause pituitary desensitization to GnRH, thought to be the result of internalization of the GnRH receptor. Depending on the potency of the agonist, the desensitization phase, or down-regulation, requires 7 to 21 days. Once down-regulation has been established, it persists for as long as the agonist is administered. During down-regulation, luteinizing hormone (LH) and follicle-stimulating hormone (FSH) secretion by the pituitary is substantially reduced. As a result, there is insufficient stimulation of the ovary for normal sex steroid production. Circulating estrogen levels are therefore in the postmenopausal range, and progesterone levels are similarly low.

The daily subcutaneous injection form of GnRH agonists as described by Muse et al. (1984) is cumbersome for the patient. Administration of GnRH analogues may be associated with localized pain and irritation at the injection site. More recently, depot formulations of the compounds have become available. These are administered as monthly intramuscular injections. A nasal spray has also been formulated, which is available for twice-daily or three-times-daily use. Although less uncomfortable than intramuscular administration, absorption may be somewhat more erratic and patient reliability becomes a greater concern.

In women, the side-effect profile of GnRH agonists is largely the result of hypoestrogenism. Most women on the medication experience significant hot flashes. These are generally classic postmenopausal hot flashes that last a few minutes and tend to be more pronounced on the upper torso and face. The hot flash is accompanied by an increased pulse rate and vasomotor instability. Often, the patient reports awakening in the middle of the night drenched in perspiration. These hot flashes tend to be most bothersome at the initiation of the down-regulation phase. In some women, they continue to be highly disturbing, whereas in others their perceived severity decreases over weeks to months.

In addition to hot flashes, the acute menopausal syndrome includes emotional lability and insomnia. In general these symptoms tend to be less disturbing than the symptoms of severe PMS.

The long-term use of GnRH analogues is limited by the effects of chronic hypoestrogenism. The most pronounced of these is osteoporosis. As a result, use of GnRH analogues is limited to 6 months unless accompanied by serial bone densitometry studies to demonstrate maintenance of bone integrity. In premarketing trials, bone pain has been reported in some men. The incidence of this symptom in women is not well known. In addition to osteoporosis, there is concern about the long-term consequences of negating the putative protective effect of estrogen against cardiovascular disease in women.

To reverse the potential side effects of GnRH agonist administration, low-dose estrogen and progestin replacement therapy, similar to that used in postmenopausal women, has been advocated. Because almost all short-term and long-term side effects of the therapy are the result of this hypoestrogenism, this is based on a sound rationale. Preliminary evidence suggests that this "add-back" therapy may maintain most of the beneficial effects of GnRH agonists on the symptoms of PMS. Larger scale studies are required before this can be widely advocated.

■ INEFFECTIVE TREATMENTS

Progesterone

Until recently, progesterone in the form of vaginal or rectal suppositories was widely prescribed for PMS. This was based on uncontrolled studies. More recently, progesterone has been shown to be no more effective than placebo in treating PMS symptoms. Moreover, there is evidence that both the physical and emotional symptoms of PMS may be progesterone induced. Thus administration of progesterone commonly results in increased breast tenderness, bloating of the abdomen and extremities, and emotional lability. The use of progesterone in treatment of PMS therefore cannot be advocated.

Oral Contraceptives

Oral contraceptives contain higher than physiologic doses of the hormones that are believed to produce many of the symptoms of PMS. As a result they should not be used for treatment, and other forms of contraception should be selected if possible.

■ TREATMENTS FOR SPECIFIC SYMPTOMS

Diuretics

The efficacy of diuretics in treating PMS remains to be conclusively established. There have been some reports that both spironolactone in doses of 25 to 50 mg per day and hydrochlorothiazide in doses of 25 mg per day may be beneficial. In the carefully monitored patient, there are few contraindications to these treatments when limited to the luteal phase of the cycle. Such treatments are indicated when fluid retention symptoms predominate.

Danazol

Although some investigators have reported the efficacy of the use of danazol in PMS, this treatment has more widespread support for use in premenstrual migraines. Danazol is a derivative of the synthetic androgen 17-α-ethinyl testosterone. As such, it possesses significant androgenic properties. Administration of danazol results in amenorrhea in most women. The objective of therapy is to obtain the beneficial effects that occur secondary to this amenorrhea. The usual dose required to achieve this is 600 to 800 mg per day in divided doses.

The side effect profile of danazol is considerable. This results from the androgenic activity and antiestrogen properties of danazol. Acne and weight gain are commonly reported. Decreased breast size is a particularly disturbing complaint for many women. More rarely, overtly masculinizing side effects are noted. These include deepening of the voice and clitoromegaly. Fluid retention on danazol therapy is particularly disturbing to women with PMS.

The antiestrogenic side effects, while better tolerated by most women than the androgen effects, are at times quite bothersome. These are the same side effects as those observed on GnRH analogues and include hot flashes, vaginal dryness, and emotional lability. Although the osteoporosis that accompanies GnRH agonist therapy is less of a concern with danazol, the effects on lipid profiles are more worrisome than with GnRH agonists. This is because of the combined adverse effects of hypoestrogenism and hyperandrogenism. For this reason the use of danazol should be accompanied by monitoring of lipid profiles.

Danazol is contraindicated during pregnancy because of in utero female pseudohermaphroditism. There have also been reports of hepatotoxicity, manifested by increased liver function tests while on danazol. Liver function studies should be monitored periodically in patients taking this drug.

■ NONSPECIFIC TREATMENTS

In the absence of an understanding of the pathophysiology of PMS, nonspecific attempts to alleviate symptoms achieved popularity. These included dietary restrictions, including the elimination of caffeine, chocolate, and sweet and salty foods. There is little evidence to demonstrate the efficacy of these treatments. Dietary supplements including vitamin B_6, magnesium, and calcium have also been advocated. While some studies have shown benefit of the treatments, their efficacy has not been proven. Some uncontrolled studies suggest that women engaged in aerobic exercise have a decreased severity of PMS symptoms compared with women with PMS who do not exercise. Because of the reported benefits of this treatment, an exercise program with its overall health benefits appears a reasonable prescription for women with a low degree of symptom severity.

Suggested Reading

Casson P, Hahn PM, Van Vugt DA, Reid RL. Lasting response to ovariectomy in severe intractable premenstrual syndrome. Am J Obstet Gynecol 1990; 162:99.

DeJong R, Rubinow DR, Roy-Byrne P, et al. Premenstrual mood disorder and psychiatric illness. Am J Psychiatry 1985; 142:1359–1363.

Hammarback S, Backstrom T. Induced anovulation as treatment of premenstrual tension syndrome. A double-blind cross-over study with GnRH-agonist versus placebo. Acta Obstet Gynecol Scand 1988; 67:159.

Mortola JF, Girton L, Beck L, et al. Diagnosis of premenstrual syndrome by a simple prospective, and reliable instrument: The calendar of premenstrual experiences. Obstet Gynecol 1990; 76:302.

Mortola JF, Girton L, Fischer U. Successful treatment of severe premenstrual syndrome by use of gonadotropin-releasing hormone agonist and estrogen/progestin. J Clin Endocrinol Metab 1991; 71:252A–252F.

Muse KN, Cetel NS, Futterman LA, Yen SSC. The premenstrual syndrome: Effects of medical ovariectomy. N Engl J Med 1984; 311:1345–1349.

Smith S, Rinehart JS, Ruddick VE, Schiff I. Treatment of premenstrual syndrome with alprazolam: Results of a double-blind, placebo-controlled, randomized crossover clinical trial. Obstet Gynecol 1987; 70:37–43.

Steiner M, Steinberg S, Stewart D, et al. Fluoxetine in the treatment of premenstrual dysphoria. N Engl J Med 1995; 332:1529–1534.

MENOPAUSE

Sanjay K. Agarwal, M.B., B.S.
Howard L. Judd, M.D.

After menopause, most women sustain a marked decrease of endogenous estradiol production of ovarian origin. The resultant hypoestrogenic state can lead to the production of a variety of symptoms. Estrogen replacement therapy can alleviate many of these problems, but its use is associated with a number of potentially harmful side effects. Consequently, it is essential that physicians caring for women understand the potential benefits and risks of this type of therapy. This chapter contains a brief review of indications, as well as potential complications and contraindications of estrogen replacement therapy. We recommend specific methods of administering estrogen replacement as well as alternative forms of therapy.

■ FOOD AND DRUG ADMINISTRATION (FDA)–APPROVED INDICATIONS FOR ESTROGEN REPLACEMENT

Hot Flashes

The hot flash or flush is the most common symptom compelling postmenopausal women to seek medical attention. Two-thirds to three-quarters of women experience flashes at the time of either natural or surgical menopause. Eighty percent of those having hot flashes complain of them for more than 1 year and 25 to 50 percent for longer than 5 years. The symptom is real; changes of skin temperature, skin resistance, core temperature, and pulse rate have been measured at the time of symptoms. At night, hot flashes are associated with waking episodes that contribute to the insomnia and resultant cognitive (memory) and affective (anxiety) changes seen in older women. Hot flashes likely result from a disruption of function of thermoregulatory centers within the hypothalamus as a consequence of enhanced hypothalamic activity secondary to loss of ovarian hormonal feedback. The brain chemicals that most likely have causative roles in the development of hot flashes are increased norepinephrine and reduced endorphins levels. Estrogen therapy effectively decreases the frequency and severity of the symptoms and improves sleep patterns.

Genitourinary Changes

Following menopause, the vagina undergoes atrophic changes which are accompanied by vaginal dryness, burning, itching, dyspareunia, discharge, and, occasionally, bleeding. It is well recognized that estrogens are effective in ameliorating atrophy of the vaginal epithelium and associated symptoms. Women can also experience dysuria and urinary frequency, even though urine cultures are negative for infection. The epithelia of the urethra, bladder trigone, and the vagina have a common origin in the urogenital sinus and all exhibit estrogen receptors. In addition, it has been reported that there is an increase in the number of superficial cells of the urethral epithelium with estrogen administration. A recent randomized, double-blind, placebo-controlled study found the use of intravaginal estriol to be efficacious in the treatment of postmenopausal women with recurrent urinary tract infections.

Bone Changes

Osteoporosis is one of the two most important health hazards associated with the climacteric. It is a disorder characterized by a reduction in the quantity of bone without changes in its chemical composition. This process is accelerated by the loss of ovarian function, resulting in a greater prevalence of osteoporosis in women than men. Several other risk factors have been identified including immobilization, white race, slender body habitus, excessive alcohol consumption, low calcium uptake, and cigarette smoking.

By itself, the loss of bone mass produces minimal symptoms, but it does lead to reduced skeletal strength and fractures. The vertebral body is the most common site of fracture, although fractures of the humerus, distal radius, and upper femur are also enhanced. This last fracture is of particular concern, resulting in appreciable mortality and substantial morbidity. It has recently been reported that 1.5 million new fractures attributable to osteoporosis occur annually in America, with women experiencing about two-thirds of them. These fractures are associated with appreciable morbidity and mortality, with up to 20 percent of hip fracture patients dying within a year of the fracture. The annual cost of osteoporosis-related fractures is more than $10 billion in health care dollars for acute and chronic care. In addition to this, there is the cost of lost productivity and other indirect costs.

The diagnosis of osteoporosis can be reliably made by noninvasive techniques. The modalities currently available provide an accurate measurement of bone mass or density and can be used for the assessment of fracture risk and to monitor therapy. It has been shown that for each standard deviation reduction in bone mass density the risk of fracture doubles.

The mechanisms responsible for enhanced bone loss with menopause have not been completely defined. It is clear that reduction of ovarian estrogen production plays a key role, with bone resorption exceeding formation in osteoporotic patients. Because estrogen receptors exist in osteoblasts, osteoclasts, macrophages, and T cells, it is likely that estrogens have direct effects on bone. This concept is supported by the measurement of increased bone loss with discontinuation of ovarian function and reduction in parameters of bone resorption with estrogen replacement. Several studies indicate that low-dose estrogen therapy can arrest bone loss and reduce the incidence of fractures if treatment is begun shortly after menopause. Even if treatment is begun later in life (e.g., after age 65) or after an interruption of treatment, bone loss can be substantially retarded.

Several alternative, nonhormonal therapies for the prevention of postmenopausal osteoporosis-related bone fractures have recently been developed for women who are either unable or unwilling to take hormone replacement therapy. These will be reviewed later.

■ NON-FDA–APPROVED INDICATIONS FOR ESTROGEN REPLACEMENT

Cardiovascular Disease

Cardiovascular disease is the leading cause of death of women in this and most other developed countries. Coronary heart disease is much more prevalent in men than women before the age of 55, but the difference begins to disappear after this age, and the ratio approaches unity by the ninth decade of life. The presence of ovarian activity in younger women has been suggested to be protective, and the loss of this function at the menopause is thought to be responsible, in part, for the increased deaths resulting from myocardial infarction in older women.

Many cohort and case-controlled studies have examined the connection between loss of ovarian function and the occurrence of heart disease. The preponderance of evidence supports the hypothesis that loss of ovarian function increases the occurrence of coronary heart disease.

The role that estrogen replacement plays in the prevention of heart disease also is not fully established. Case control studies using hospital controls have reported relative risks between 0.6 and 4.2. Results of these studies are difficult to interpret, because estrogen use may be associated either directly or inversely with diseases or injuries leading to hospitalization. Use of the general population as a comparison group tends to avoid this problem, and the relative risk of heart disease in estrogen users has always been less than 1 (protection) when this type of control was used. Numerous cohort studies evaluating the effect of estrogen in preventing nonfatal infarctions and deaths attributable to coronary heart disease have been published. The majority have demonstrated a substantial protective effect.

Concerns have been raised about epidemiologic studies because it is likely that women who use estrogens are different from those who do not in regard to other cardiovascular risk factors. Thus, it appears essential that randomized drug trials be performed to determine if estrogens reduce heart attacks and/or deaths due to heart attacks. Two such trials have begun. The HERS Trial is determining if estrogen and progestin replacement will prevent heart disease events in women who already have coronary artery disease, a secondary prevention trial. The Women's Health Initiative is doing the same in postmenopausal women without heart disease, a primary prevention trial.

Until these studies are completed, the major approach to determining the action of hormone replacement on heart disease is to examine their influence on cardiovascular disease risk factors. The recently published Postmenopausal Estrogen/Progestin Interventions (PEPI) Trial showed in a large 3-year randomized trial that conjugated equine estrogens at a daily dosage of 0.625 mg raised high-density lipoprotein (HDL) cholesterol and lowered low-density lipoprotein (LDL) cholesterol and plasma fibrinogen levels in comparison to placebo. The addition of medroxyprogesterone acetate given cyclically or continuously prevented much of the increase of HDL cholesterol whereas cyclic micronized progesterone did not. The other risk factors for heart disease were not influenced by the addition of progestins.

Although most of these data suggest estrogen use prevents heart disease, it should be noted that the FDA has not yet approved the prevention of heart disease as an indication for any estrogen preparation. If this association is conclusively established, it will become the primary reason for giving estrogen replacement.

There are several possible mechanisms by which estrogens could have a favorable impact on heart disease. As mentioned, estrogens increase HDL and lower LDL cholesterol levels. In animals, estrogens have also been shown to retard atherogenesis, decrease cholesterol deposition in vascular walls, increase coronary blood flow, and prevent paradoxical vasoconstriction of the coronary arteries at the sites of atheromatous plaques when exposed to acetyl choline. Each of these could explain the probable benefit estrogen exerts on heart disease.

Integument

With aging, noticeable changes in the skin occur. There is a generalized thinning accompanied by a loss of elasticity, which results in wrinkling and increased fragility. This occurs particularly in the sun-exposed areas. Following menopause, decreases in skin thickness and collagen content have been identified in the skin of the thigh and forearm of women. The presence of estrogen receptors in certain elements of the skin suggests that estrogens could affect the skin directly. Estrogen replacement has been shown to increase both the thickness and collagen content of skin, with the effects being greatest in women with low values before therapy. These observations have been interpreted to indicate that in women with reduced skin thickness and collagen content, estrogen therapy may be therapeutic as well as prophylactic; in women with high values (just after the menopause), however, it can only prevent loss. Although these studies are of great interest, they are flawed by the lack of placebo-controlled, randomized study design. These studies are also troubled by the lack of assessment of skin of the face and neck, the areas of greatest cosmetic concern for women. Until this is accomplished, these drug trials cannot be considered conclusive.

Psychological Factors

The climacteric does not appear to be associated with an increased incidence of serious mental illness. Nevertheless, this period of a woman's life is a psychological as well as a physical milestone in the aging process. Such times of transition are usually stressful. The climacteric has been associated with an increase in overall psychological symptom reporting. An array of affective symptoms are reported, including nervousness, irritability, anxiety, depression, and tearfulness. Increased consultations for psychological problems and enhanced use of psychotropic drugs have also been documented. Alterations of cognitive functions have been described, including decreases in concentration and memory. The mechanisms responsible for these changes in brain function have not been identified, but several changes in brain chemistry have been observed in animals given estrogen.

In good randomized studies, estrogen therapy has improved affective and cognitive functions in postmenopausal women. Estrogens also decrease sleep latency and the number of waking episodes while increasing sleep length and rapid-eye-movement sleep. These effects may be the result of the suppression of flashes. Certainly, overt flashes can occur nightly, impair sleep, and be a cause of chronic fatigue. Improvement in sleep patterns, therefore, can be achieved by estrogen replacement through alleviation of this common physical symptom.

There have been several reports over the last 5 years suggesting that estrogen replacement therapy can improve short-term memory, and can have positive effects on sexually dimorphic cognitive skills in which women typically excel, such as articulation and fine motor movements. The beneficial effects of estrogen on memory loss have been particularly noted in women with Alzheimer's disease, and it has been suggested by several studies that estrogen replacement therapy may even help to prevent the development of this devastating condition. While the exact mechanism for this effect remains to be clarified, it is possible that estrogen works via either one or several of the following mechanisms: a direct antidepressant effect, an improvement in cerebral blood flow, or suppression of apolipoprotein E.

Sexual Factors

Menopause is associated with changes in sexual expectations, libido, and behavior. These are brought about by the complex interaction of both physical and psychological changes. The vaginal atrophy seen in the menopause can lead to dyspareunia and decreased sensation. Reduced self-esteem, depression, and other emotional changes created by the menopause can also interfere with normal sexual functioning.

Treatment of genital atrophy with estrogen can certainly alleviate some of the problems derived from genital atrophy. The impact of estrogen on libido per se remains unclear. There are scattered reports of testosterone treatment improving libido. However, there is a paucity of well-conducted, randomized, placebo-controlled studies. Care should be taken to counsel the patient with regard to the potential side effects before embarking on this unproven therapy.

■ THERAPY

As long as ovarian function is sufficient to maintain some uterine bleeding, no treatment is usually required. As menopause approaches, the menstrual pattern alters because of increased frequency of anovulatory cycles, and symptoms from the hypoestrogenic state prompt patients to seek help. This provides an opportunity to discuss the treatment of menopause.

Each woman, whether she has climacteric symptoms or not, deserves an adequate explanation of the physiologic event she is experiencing in order to dispel her fears and minimize symptoms such as anxiety, depression, sleep disturbances, and so on. Reassurance should emphasize what the climacteric is not—that is, contrary to anything the patient may have heard, she need not expect sudden aging or personal disasters of any sort. Specific reassurance about continued sexual activity is important.

Estrogen replacement is the hallmark of treatment of the climacteric. Before administering this form of therapy, a discussion of the advantages, as well as the complications of and contraindications to estrogen replacement therapy, should be held.

■ COMPLICATIONS OF ESTROGEN THERAPY

Hyperplasia and Endometrial Cancer

The possibility of a causal relationship between unopposed estrogen therapy and endometrial cancer was first recognized in the mid-1970s. Many epidemiologic studies reported an association between the prolonged use of unopposed estrogens by postmenopausal women and increased risk of endometrial cancer. Endometrial cancer associated with estrogen intake is usually well differentiated and has a high cure rate. The risk has been correlated to dose and duration of treatment. Administration of estrogen in a cyclic fashion provides little or no protection. Protection can be achieved by periodic administration of a progestin. The minimum number of days required to reduce the risk of endometrial cancer to zero in all women is not known. Some studies suggest that longer intervals of exposure increase the likelihood of protection and that most patients would be protected by a regimen of 12 to 13 days of progestin administration each month. Dosage also plays a role, with most patients being protected with a dose of 10 mg medroxyprogesterone acetate. Lower doses also afford some protection, particularly when used daily with an estrogen. The PEPI Trial has recently shown that one-third of the women given 0.625 mg conjugated estrogens daily will develop complex and/or atypical hyperplasia within 3 years. The addition of a progestin given cyclically or continuously will prevent most of this hyperplasia.

Breast Cancer

The single greatest concern of women regarding estrogen replacement therapy is its possible association with the development of breast cancer. The much greater occurrence of breast cancer in women than men, coupled with the extensive animal data incriminating estrogens in the development of breast tumors, have heightened everyone's awareness of the possible role of exogenous estrogen therapy in the development of breast cancer in older women. However, it has been surprisingly difficult to substantiate a risk of estrogen replacement and breast cancer. More than 40 epidemiologic studies have been published since 1974 in an effort to determine the relationship, if any, between postmenopausal estrogen replacement and breast cancer. Subtle increases in risk have been observed in some studies with prolonged use of the medication. The relative risk has rarely exceeded 2, and statistically significant differences reported in one study are often not confirmed in the next. At least six meta-analyses have been published concerning this issue. None showed an increase of overall risk of breast cancer with estrogen usage. However, several reported an increased risk of 20 to 30 percent with long-term use. Because estrogen replacement is now being proposed for long-term administration, this apparent increase is of concern.

Questions have been raised about these studies, particularly the possibility that a detection bias may exist. Women who take estrogen are more likely to have had mammography than those who do not. Supporting this view are the observations that four of five studies have found similar rates of death attributable to breast cancer in women who do or do not take estrogen. It is likely that we will not know if estrogen use is a risk for this tumor until the results of the Women's Health Initiative are known.

The addition of a progestin to estrogen therapy has also been examined for risks. The results of these studies have been inconsistent. It must be mentioned that in vitro studies have shown breast ductal epithelial growth is greatest during the luteal phase of the cycle, suggesting progestins may increase growth of this cell type. In the nurses study, progestins were not found to decrease the overall risk of developing breast cancer in estrogen takers. Because of these data and because of the detrimental effects of progestins on the serum lipid profile, a majority of experts do not recommend the use of progestin in women without a uterus.

Physicians who prescribe hormone replacement should be diligent in assessing the patient's breasts with regular examinations and mammograms as recommended by the American Cancer Society. Physicians also need to be alert to any new findings regarding this issue but can be reassured that to date hormone replacement appears to elicit little if any risk of the development of breast cancer.

Hypertension

Oral contraceptive (OC) use has been associated with an increase in blood pressure by several investigators. Large population studies have reported elevated blood pressure occurring more frequently in OC users than in controls. The mean increment of blood pressure has been statistically significant but small in magnitude (5 mm Hg systolic and 1 mm Hg diastolic). There have been many attempts to link hormone replacement with hypertension. Several case-controlled studies have been published in the last 2 decades. At least seven prospective drug trials also have been conducted, of which five were randomized. The PEPI study is one of two notable prospective studies published over the last 2 years that has shown no increase in blood pressure with hormone replacement therapy. In this large study, there was slight increase in both systolic and diastolic blood pressures over the course of the 3 years of study. This rise in blood pressures paralleled a concurrent increase in body weight but was not different between the treatment and placebo groups. Thus, it appears that the increase in blood pressure observed with OC usage cannot be identified with replacement therapy.

Thromboembolic Disease

The administration of synthetic estrogens in OCs also increases the risk of overt vascular thromboembolic disease and the occurrence of subclinical thrombosis. In uncontrolled studies, thrombophlebitis has been reported with estrogen replacement therapy, whereas this association has not been present in controlled experiments.

Although no evidence exists to incriminate hormone replacement with clotting episodes, it must be remembered that estrogens exert several effects on the clotting mechanism, including increased vascular endothelial proliferation, decreased venous blood flow, and increased coagulability of blood with changes in the platelet, coagulation, and fibrinolytic systems. The Framingham study has reported a strong positive correlation between fibrinogen levels and cardiovascular disease including strokes. The PEPI study found an increase in serum fibrinogen with age in the placebo group. This was not seen in the estrogen alone or estrogen plus either medroxyprogesterone acetate or micronized progesterone groups. Interpretation of this elimination of the age-related increase in fibrinogen concentration is unclear at present, other than to say that standard dose estrogen replacement can influence the coagulation system. Thus, caution should be exercised when administering hormone replacement to women who have recently experienced a vascular thrombosis or embolism.

Hepatic Problems

Estrogens have an impact on both protein and lipid metabolism by hepatocytes. These effects are exaggerated when estrogen is given by mouth, absorbed by the gastrointestinal organs, then delivered directly to the liver through the portal circulation, where it acts on the hepatocytes before it is partially metabolized to less active compounds. Estrogen stimulates the hepatic synthesis of angiotensinogen, the renin substrate, and certain clotting factors, while suppressing synthesis of some anticlotting factors. At doses recommended for replacement therapy (0.625 mg conjugated estrogens or its equivalent), the effects seem to elicit few if any problems.

Orally administered estrogens also alter hepatic lipid metabolism. Low-density lipoprotein cholesterol metabolism is enhanced, leading to a lowering of its circulating level by increasing the entry of cholesterol into bile. This, possibly coupled with mild alterations of bile acids, may lead to supersaturation of cholesterol in bile and possibly stone formation. This last problem appears to be a consequence of OC therapy. Whether it is a consequence of hormone replacement needs to be established. The nonoral administration of estradiol reduces the hepatic actions of the hormone by bypassing the "first pass" effect. Whether this confers long-range benefit to women has yet to be established.

Contraindications and Precautions

Contraindications to estrogen replacement therapy include undiagnosed vaginal bleeding, acute liver disease, chronic impaired liver function, a recent vascular thrombosis (with or without emboli), and carcinoma of the breast or endometrium. Estrogens may also have adverse effects on some patients with fibrocystic disease of the breast, uterine leiomyoma, familial hyperlipidemias, migraine headaches, chronic thrombophlebitis, endometriosis, and gallbladder disease.

■ PRINCIPLES OF ESTROGEN REPLACEMENT

Generalized guidelines of hormone replacement for all postmenopausal patients cannot be outlined. Each patient needs to be evaluated individually, and her symptoms and risk factors must be considered. Current replacement therapy should be directed toward the relief of hot flashes and atrophic vaginitis and the prevention of osteoporosis. Different treatment strategies are required for each of these indications.

Therapy for Hot Flashes

Menopausal hot flashes characteristically occur at irregular intervals, as frequently as every 20 minutes, and each episode lasts 3 to 4 minutes. There is usually a sensation of heat or flushing in the face, neck, and upper trunk. Perspiration is also a frequent complaint. Unlike all other problems associated with the menopause, hot flashes usually become less problematic with time from menopause. For disabling hot flashes, estrogen replacement should be considered. If flashes are minimal or absent, then the need for treatment is reduced. Transdermal estradiol by skin patches at a dose of 0.05 mg has been shown to reduce objectively measured hot flashes by 40 percent. It is a clinical impression that conjugated equine estrogens at a dose of 0.625 mg elicit a similar suppression. Thus, higher doses of estrogen are required in the remainder of patients, and in isolated women very high estrogen doses are needed to provide relief. This is the one symptom that we "chase" with higher doses of estrogen to provide relief. Occasionally as much as 0.4 mg transdermal estradiol or 5 mg conjugated estrogens may be necessary. When giving large doses of estrogen, it is important to be sure that the patient is experiencing menopausal hot flashes. Careful questioning of the patient often can elicit documentation that this is indeed the problem. If higher than usual doses of estrogens are required to reduce the symptoms, efforts should be made to wean the patient off the higher doses as soon as feasible. A gradual reduction of the dosage is usually effective.

In a woman who cannot take estrogens because of contraindications, progestins have also been shown to relieve hot flashes. This therapy is also appropriate for women with a history of endometrial cancer. Medroxyprogesterone acetate at doses of 20 to 40 mg and megestrol acetate at doses of 40 to 80 mg per day have been shown to provide substantial relief of the symptom. In women with a history of breast cancer, it is inappropriate to use either estrogens or progestins. The hypertensive medications, clonidine (0.2 to 0.4 mg per day) or alpha-methyldopa (375 to 1,125 mg per day at bedtime), have also been shown to give partial relief of hot flashes. These therapies may be associated with their own side effects. Sedatives and psychopharmacologic agents have been used to reduce the symptoms, but their efficacies have not been studied critically.

Therapy for Atrophic Vaginitis

For vaginal atrophy, both orally and vaginally administered estrogens can be effective. Conjugated estrogens at dosages of 0.625 to 1.25 mg and transdermal estradiol at dosages of 0.05 to 0.1 mg have been shown to revert the vaginal epithelium to that seen in premenopausal women. Vaginal cream containing conjugated estrogens comes in a concentration of 0.625 mg per gram of cream. One gram of cream given every other day or less frequently converts the vaginal epithelium back to a premenopausal state in the average woman. At this dosage, minimal hormone is absorbed and has limited or no systemic biologic actions. In the drug insert, it is recommended that 2 to 4 g cream be administered on a daily basis. This dosage is almost never required but, if utilized, systemic actions can be expected.

When giving vaginal estrogen cream to a woman with a uterus, we usually administer 10 mg medroxyprogesterone acetate for 12 days once a year. At the dosage of cream recommended above (1 g every other day or less), we have yet to find a patient who has experienced vaginal bleeding. If one were to have this side effect, we would then administer the progestin at monthly intervals.

Prevention of Osteoporosis

For the prevention of osteoporosis, an effective dose is 0.625 mg conjugated estrogens daily. This dosage prevents bone loss from the spine and hips. One report indicates that 0.3 mg conjugated estrogens coupled with 1,500 mg calcium daily also prevents bone loss. This observation has yet to be confirmed by other investigators. Daily piperazine estrone sulfate (1.25 mg) and transdermal estradiol (0.05 mg) have also been shown to prevent bone loss from the spine and the hip. Micronized estradiol at a dose of 0.5 mg daily will prevent bone loss from the spine. However, we recommend the 1 mg dose daily in hopes of preventing bone loss from the hip.

It is recommended that estrogen therapy commence within 1 year of cessation of ovarian function. If begun later, some bone loss will have already occurred, and estrogen replacement does not replace this previous loss. Long-term studies have indicated bone loss can be retarded for at least 10 years.

If a patient cannot or will not take hormone replacement, several other options can be considered to prevent bone loss. Calcium therapy at a dose of 1,500 mg per day is recommended in women who do not take estrogens and 1,000 mg per day in women who do. There are now several studies that have shown that calcium alone prevents bone loss, particularly from the spine, more than placebo, and it appears to reduce spinal fractures. It should be noted that calcium does not prevent the bone loss associated with menopause. Thus, its effects are greatest in women who are several years postmenopausal.

Vitamin D at doses between 400 to 800 U per day has also been shown to prevent bone loss in older postmenopausal women (over age 70). This is likely because many of these subjects are vitamin D deficient. The diphosphonates etidronate and alendronate have also been shown to increase bone density. The former is given at a dosage of 400 mg per day for 14 days, followed by calcium carbonate 500 mg per day for 10 weeks. The latter is given as a 10 mg daily dosage with a 500 mg daily supplement of calcium carbonate.

Salmon calcitonin, as a subcutaneous or intramuscular injection (100 IU) every other day or as a daily nasal spray (200 IU), has been shown to prevent bone loss from the spine in conjunction with calcium carbonate (1.5 g daily) and vitamin D (400 U daily) in women at least 5 years after the menopause. On the horizon is the use of slow-release sodium fluoride which actually increases bone density.

It must be remembered that only a minority of women will experience an osteoporotic fracture sometime in their lives. Thus, therapy should be directed at those individuals who appear to have greater risk than the average woman for development of fractures. There are no definitive biochemical tests to diagnose osteoporosis or to assess risk of fracture. The most commonly used technique to screen and diagnose osteoporosis is the measurement of bone density. Several techniques are currently available, including dual-energy X-ray absorptiometry (DEXA), dual-photon absorptiometry, computed tomography, and single-photon absorptiometry.

The last assesses density of the wrist while the others assess density of the spine and hip. The DEXA technique is considered the standard because of high precision, low-radiation exposure, and better resolution.

According to the World Health Organization, osteoporosis is defined as bone mineral density (BMD) that is greater than 2.5 standard deviations below the mean of young adult women, and osteopenia is defined as BMD greater than 1 but less than 2.5 standard deviations below the mean for young adult women. Prevention of bone loss should be undertaken in women with osteoporosis and strongly considered in women with osteopenia.

Factors Influencing Complications

If estrogens are given, there are certain factors that seem to influence the incidence of complications. It does not seem to make any difference which preparation is prescribed. All have been incriminated in the genesis of side effects, particularly the development of endometrial hyperplasia. Results indicate there is little or no benefit to interrupted schedules. Also, these schedules confuse patients, and symptoms can return during the medication-free intervals. For these reasons, we usually prescribe estrogens continuously.

Estrogen and progestin therapy can be administered in either a sequential or continuous fashion. Both forms of therapy markedly reduce the occurrence of endometrial hyperplasia and endometrial cancer. When employing sequential therapy, an estrogen is usually taken daily and 10 mg medroxyprogesterone acetate is administered for 12 to 13 days each month. This form of therapy usually results in periodic vaginal bleeding, a condition that is unacceptable to some postmenopausal patients. Continuous daily estrogen plus progesterone therapy has recently gained in popularity. The same estrogen can be used as with sequential therapy but with the daily administration of a reduced amount of medroxyprogesterone acetate (2.5 mg). This schedule frequently leads to amenorrhea secondary to endometrial atrophy but can produce unpredictable bleeding. If present, the total bleeding with continuous therapy is usually less than that with sequential therapy. Estrogen-only therapy can be given, but pretreatment and yearly endometrial biopsies are recommended. If endometrial hyperplasia is identified on any of these biopsies, estrogen-only therapy should either not be started or be discontinued.

When considering estrogen and progestin administration, it must be remembered that progestins have their own set of potential problems. These include depression, anxiety, mood changes, headaches, and breast tenderness. Some women just cannot take them.

■ ENDOMETRIAL SURVEILLANCE

The traditional procedure for diagnosis of endometrial hyperplasia or cancer has been the fractional dilation and curettage. This has been shown to produce adequate material for histological evaluation in up to 94 percent of cases. Major problems with this diagnostic procedure include cost, possible medical complications, and inconvenience, and it is for these reasons that alternative screening procedures have been sought.

Less expensive and invasive office endometrial sampling procedures, such as those employing the Pipelle device, are replacing the formal dilation and curettage. In a study of 40 patients already known to have endometrial carcinoma as diagnosed by other procedures, 39 (97.5 percent) were confirmed as having endometrial carcinoma by Pipelle biopsy specimens. Although this sensitivity is similar to that reported for dilation and curettage, isolated reports of women with endometrial cancer missed by the Pipelle instrument continue to trouble gynecologists.

Use of ultrasound could help avoid some of the negative curettages that are performed because cervical stenosis prevents the performance of office endometrial biopsy. The data suggest that in postmenopausal women, an endometrial thickness of less than 4 mm is highly unlikely to be neoplastic and, thus, does not warrant endometrial sampling. The practice of histologically assessing only women with an endometrium that is thicker than 4 mm has been shown in one study to have a sensitivity approaching 100 percent at detecting endometrial hyperplasia and carcinoma. This also avoids the need for sampling the majority of women with benign histology. Further refinements such as the use of color Doppler with pulsatility and resistance indices are currently under evaluation.

■ MANAGEMENT OF ESTROGEN THERAPY

Prior to the institution of estrogen replacement therapy, a complete and thorough evaluation of the patient should be performed. This examination should include, first, a history, with specific reference to contraindications and precautions, and, second, a physical examination, including blood pressure, breast, and pelvic examinations (including cervical smears) for cancer detection.

Following this, a careful analysis of the potential benefits and risks of estrogen replacement individualized for each patient must be undertaken. If, on the basis of this information, the patient wishes to receive estrogen replacement therapy, the following recommendations should be followed.

1. Estrogen therapy should be given utilizing the lowest dosage compatible with effective treatment of the indicated symptom (e.g., hot flashes, atrophic vaginitis, or osteoporosis).
2. For women with a uterus, most use medroxyprogesterone acetate, and either sequential or continuous addition of a progestin is recommended. The 19-norprogestins are likely to be safe at low doses, but this awaits documentation. There are no data available to substantiate that progestin therapy is beneficial to women without a uterus.
3. If treatment with estrogen and progestin therapy is instituted, it is our view that endometrial biopsy is not required prior to institution of therapy (unless other indications exist, such as postmenopausal bleeding). Scheduled withdrawal bleeding is expected with sequential estrogen and progestin. The patient should be alerted to this probability. She should be counseled concerning the benign nature of this anticipated event. If break-

through bleeding occurs, an endometrial biopsy should be performed to exclude the development of abnormal histology. The timing of further biopsies, should any be needed, is a clinical decision based on the results of the histologic examination of the endometrium obtained. The presence of endometrial hyperplasia dictates more prolonged use of the progestin or discontinuation of estrogen and progestin therapy. Patients begun on continuous estrogen and progestin therapy should be counseled regarding the possibility of irregular vaginal bleeding. This is most troublesome during the first year of therapy and decreases in incidence with prolonged use. We perform an endometrial biopsy if the bleeding either lasts longer, is heavier, and/or is more frequent than a normal period.

4. Some patients may not accept the addition of progestin to their estrogen replacement regimen; others may experience adverse reactions to this combination and request removal of the progestin component. In the absence of progestin, estrogen replacement therapy carries markedly increased risk of development of endometrial hyperplasia and, with time, the possibility of endometrial carcinoma. With this in mind, the physician should observe the following guidelines carefully:
   a. An endometrial biopsy should be performed before initiating estrogen-only therapy. If hyperplasia is present, estrogen-only therapy should not be instituted.
   b. An endometrial biopsy should be performed annually.
   c. An endometrial biopsy should be performed with any unusual bleeding. The presence of endometrial hyperplasia requires discontinuation of estrogen-only therapy.
5. Treatment programs for hot flashes should be discontinued and re-evaluated every 12 to 18 months. The prophylaxis and treatment of osteoporosis, if successful, requires more prolonged therapy. The exact length of time estrogen should be administered for this purpose has not been defined beyond 10 years. Treatment of atrophic vaginitis should be continued until the patient is no longer sexually active.
6. At the present time, oral therapy is the most common route of estrogen and progestin therapy. In women who experience side effects such as nausea, vomiting, or headaches, it is sometimes effective to try another form of therapy such as a transdermal estradiol patch. Injectable therapy, while effective, is not recommended for routine use on the basis of cost, dose effectiveness, and the hazards of prolonged action.

Suggested Reading

Black DM, Palermo L, Nevitt MC, et al. Comparison of methods for defining prevalent vertebral deformities: the study of osteoporotic fractures. J Bone Miner Res 1995; 10:890–902.

The Postmenopausal Estrogen/Progestin Interventions (PEPI) Trial. Effects of estrogen or estrogen/progestin regimens on heart disease risk factors in postmenopausal women. JAMA 1995; 273:199–208.

Sherwin BB. Sex hormones and psychological functioning in postmenopausal women. Exp Gerontol 1994; 29:423–430.

Stovall TG, Photopulos GJ, Poston WM, et al. Pipelle endometrial sampling in patients with known endometrial carcinoma. Obstet Gynecol 1991; 77:954–956.

IMPLANTABLE CONTRACEPTION

C. Wayne Bardin, M.D.

Research on contraceptive implants began with the demonstration that steroids could be released from Silastic capsules. Various progestins were investigated, and by 1974 the six-capsule Silastic drug delivery system, which was to be termed the Norplant* contraceptive system, was perfected and made ready for clinical trials. By 1978 sufficient data were available from this clinical study to indicate that the failure rate of Norplant implants was unexpectedly low: 0.6 percent after 2 years. In 1983 Leiras Pharmaceuticals of Turku, Finland, was licensed to manufacture Norplant, and Finland became the first country to give regulatory approval for the distribution of this new contraceptive. In 1984 the World Health Organization (WHO) evaluated the Norplant method in response to a request by the United Nations Fund for Population Activities (UNFPA) for technical evaluation. The WHO concluded that Norplant implants are an effective, reversible, long-term method of fertility regulation that has particular advantage for women who wish to have an extended period of contraceptive protection. After approval of Norplant implants by the Food and Drug Administration (FDA), Wyeth-Ayerst Laboratories began to distribute this implantable contraceptive in the United States as the Norplant system. More than fifty countries have now approved Norplant implants for distribution for use in women.

■ WHAT IS THE NORPLANT CONTRACEPTIVE SYSTEM?

Norplant implants are a method of providing a progestin-only contraceptive for women. They consist of six soft, flexible

*Norplant is a registered trademark of The Population Council.

capsules of Silastic rubber that contain levonorgestrel. This hormone is also used in other contraceptives such as the progestin-only minipill and in several widely used progestin-estrogen combination pills. The capsules are inserted in a superficial plane beneath the skin on the inside of the upper arm. It is recommended that Norplant implants be inserted at the time of menstruation. Once in place, levonorgestrel diffuses through the wall of the Silastic capsule into blood and provides effective protection against pregnancy during the first month and through 5 years of use.

Immediately after implantation, the dose of levonorgestrel provided by Norplant implants is about 85 μg per day. This declines to about 50 μg per day by 9 months, to about 35 μg per day by 18 months, and to about 30 μg per day over the remaining 5 years of use.

The blood levels of levonorgestrel that result as this progestin diffuses out of the Silastic capsules are lower than those usually observed in women using combined oral contraceptives containing 100 to 150 μg levonorgestrel. As noted below, however, the greater effectiveness of the implants relates to the constancy of the blood levels rather than the peaks and valleys that occur after the use of each pill. The concentrations of levonorgestrel in women show considerable variation, depending on individual clearance rates, body weight, and possible other factors. Nonetheless, levels in an individual remain relatively consistent; i.e., women with high levels tend to maintain such levels and women with low levels tend to maintain low levels.

■ MECHANISM OF ACTION

The mechanism of action of Norplant implants is of interest in view of the high effectiveness that results from a low dose of levonorgestrel. Every-other-day blood samples from a randomly selected group of users show serum progesterone levels compatible with ovulation in some women. Furthermore, the percentage of women with elevated serum progesterone levels suggestive of ovulation increases with longer durations of Norplant implant use. After 3 to 5 years, approximately 50 percent of women using implants have progesterone levels consistent with ovulation. Thus, ovulation suppression cannot account entirely for this method's extremely high effectiveness.

Norplant implant users with regular menstrual periods are more likely to have elevated progesterone consistent with ovulation. In such women the progesterone levels are 50 percent lower than in ovulatory women who are not taking hormonal contraceptives. In these latter Norplant users, the mid-cycle surges of luteinizing hormone are blunted even though cyclic estradiol secretion by the ovary continues. These results suggest that not all Norplant implant users who have elevated progesterone ovulate. Such individuals may secrete progesterone from a luteinized follicle or from an "inadequate corpus luteum." Ultrasonic studies show that many women who have regular menses while using Norplant implants develop a follicle that does not rupture but regresses over several weeks.

Examination of cervical mucus from Norplant implant users shows that most women have scanty mucus that is extremely viscous, and thus sperm penetration is impaired. These observations suggest that levonorgestrel increases the viscosity of cervical mucus, thus changing its structure. As a result, sperm cannot enter the uterus and fertilization cannot occur.

Norplant implants therefore mediate their effects on fertility by a variety of mechanisms, including suppression of ovulation, alteration of cervical mucus, and possible other effects. These actions of levonorgestrel are mediated on the cervix and on the pituitary-gonadal axis and are the principal mechanisms by which Norplant implants provide extremely effective contraception.

To ensure that the woman is not pregnant at the time of capsule placement and to ensure contraceptive effectiveness during the first cycle of use, it is advisable that insertion be done during the first 7 days of the menstrual cycle or immediately following an abortion. However, Norplant implants may be inserted at any time during the cycle provided pregnancy has been excluded and a nonhormonal contraceptive method is used for at least 7 days following insertion. Insertion is not recommended before 6 weeks postpartum in breast-feeding women.

Insertion and removal are not difficult procedures, but instructions must be followed closely. It is strongly advised that all health care professionals who insert and remove Norplant implant capsules be instructed in the procedures before they attempt them. A proper insertion just under the skin (Fig. 1) will ensure that implants are not displaced from the site of insertion and will facilitate removals (Fig. 2). Proper implant insertion and removal should result in minimal scarring. If the capsules are placed too deeply, they can be harder to remove. The method of removal illustrated in Figure 2 was developed by a group of physicians with extensive experience in Norplant use. As is the case with many medical procedures, other physicians have had ideas about how removal could be performed. As a result, several modifications of the removal procedure have been described in the medical literature including the pop-out method, the U-technique, and the hook-traction technique. Physicians who have used multiple procedures report that implants are relatively easy to remove with all procedures when they have been inserted correctly and difficult with any technique when they have been inserted improperly. There have been infrequent reports of the use of general anesthesia during the removal procedure; this is generally not required.

Before initiating the removal procedure, all Norplant capsules should be located via palpation. If all six capsules cannot be palpated, they may be localized via ultrasound (7 MHz), x-ray, or compression mammography. If all capsules cannot be removed at the first attempt, removal should be attempted later when the site has healed. Bruising may occur at the implant site during insertion or removal. Other cutaneous reactions that have been reported include blistering, ulcerations, and sloughing. There have been reports of arm pain, numbness, and tingling following these procedures. In some women, hyperpigmentation occurs over the implantation site but is usually reversible following removal.

There have been reports of capsule displacement (i.e., movement), most of which involve minor changes in the positioning of the capsules. However, infrequent reports of significant displacement (a few to several inches) have been received. In some instances displacement is associated with

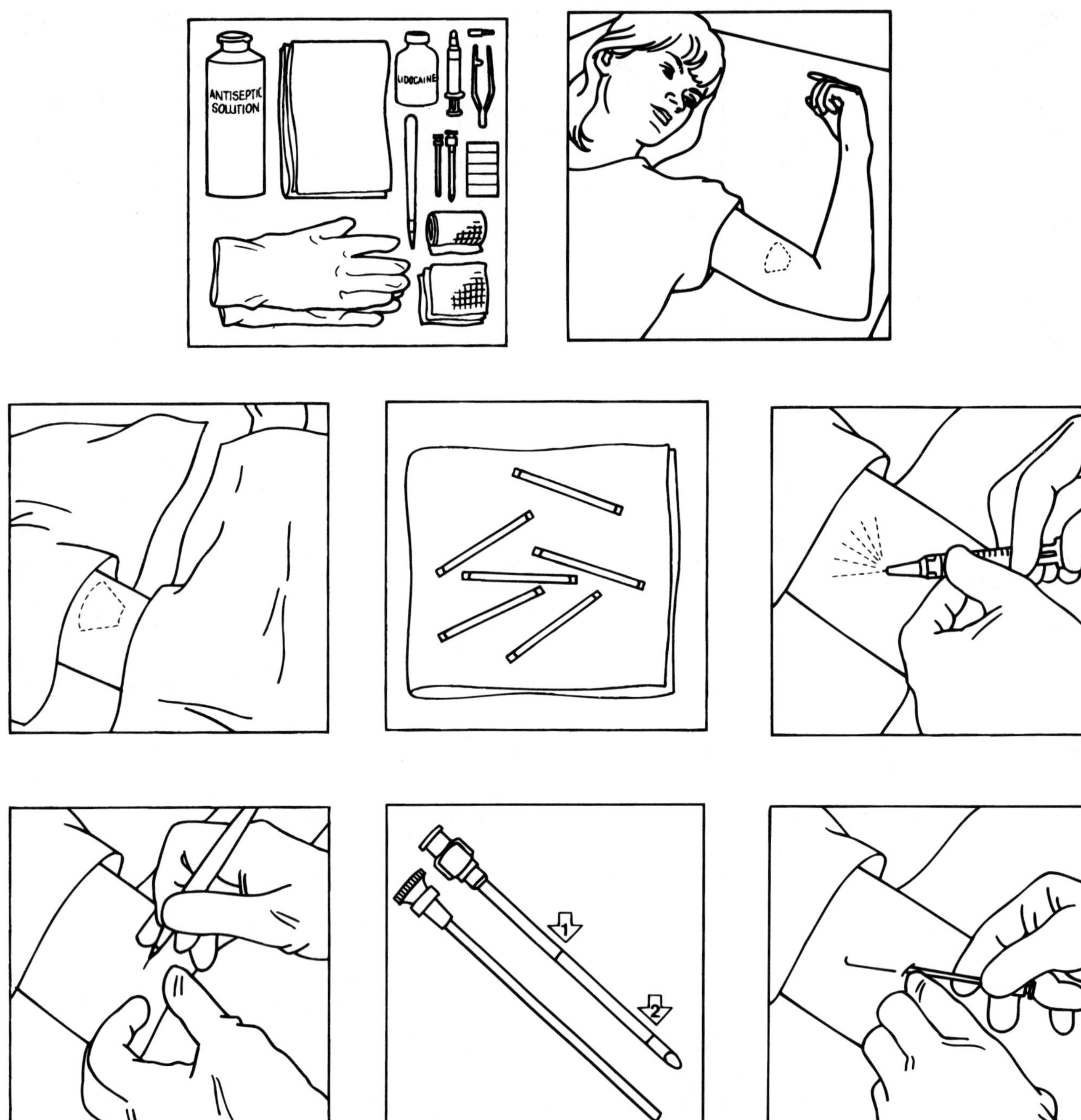

Figure 1
Insertion of Norplant implants. For a more detailed legend, see the labeling for the Norplant system that is published in the Physicians Desk Reference. *(Courtesy of Wyeth-Ayerst Laboratories.)*
Continued

improper insertion. For example, in one woman a Norplant implant that was inserted into a muscle migrated along the muscle to the end of the arm. Such displacement is sometimes associated with pain or discomfort. In the event that capsule movement occurs, the removal technique may need to be modified, such as additional incisions or visits.

Dunson et al. (1995) recently reported the complications associated with removal of Norplant implants in 3,416 users from 11 countries. More than three-fourths of all complications were due to implants that were broken by the health care provider doing the removal (1.7 percent), embedded implants below the subdermal plane (1.2 percent), and displaced implants (0.6 percent). Removal complications occurred in 4.6 percent of women in this study. Most complications resulted in longer removal times. The mean removal times were 11.5 minutes and 29.7 minutes for implants without and

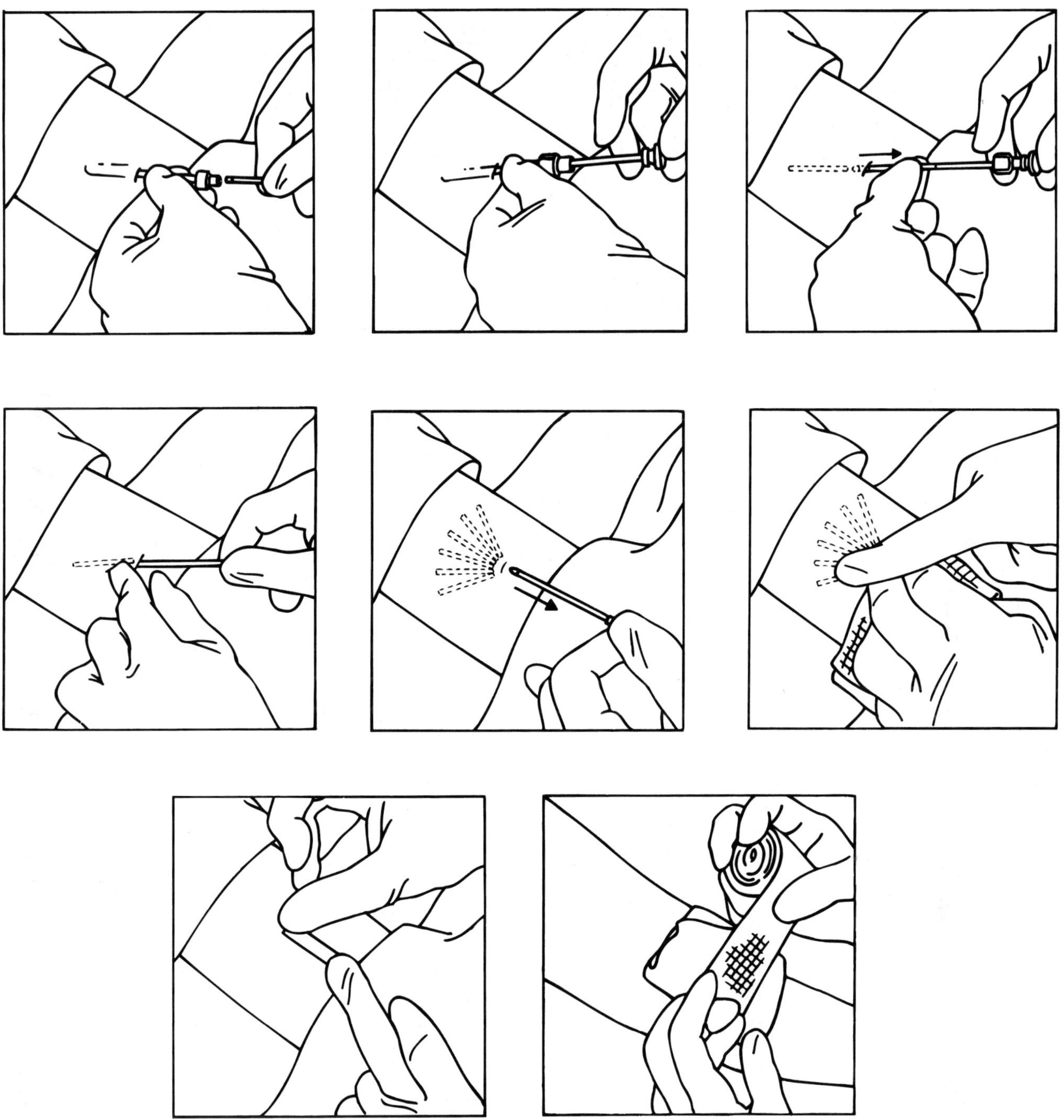

Figure 1, cont'd.
For legend see opposite page.

with complications, respectively. It was concluded that proper insertion by well-trained health care providers will reduce the number of difficult removals.

■ EFFECTIVENESS

During the first year of use, only 0.2 percent of all continuing users became pregnant. In the second year, the pregnancy rate was 0.5 percent for all users. During years 3 to 5, the pregnancy rates rose to over 1 percent. After 2 years of use, differences in pregnancy rates were noted among women of differing weights. For example, in women less than 50 kg, there were almost no pregnancies, even after 5 years of use while in women greater than 70 kg, the yearly pregnancy rate rose to 2.5 to 5.1 percent in years 3 and 4. In the clinical trials from which these data were derived, Norplant implants were manufactured from two types of silicone rubber tubing. Approximately, one-fourth of the women used Norplant implants manufactured from silicone rubber that was slightly

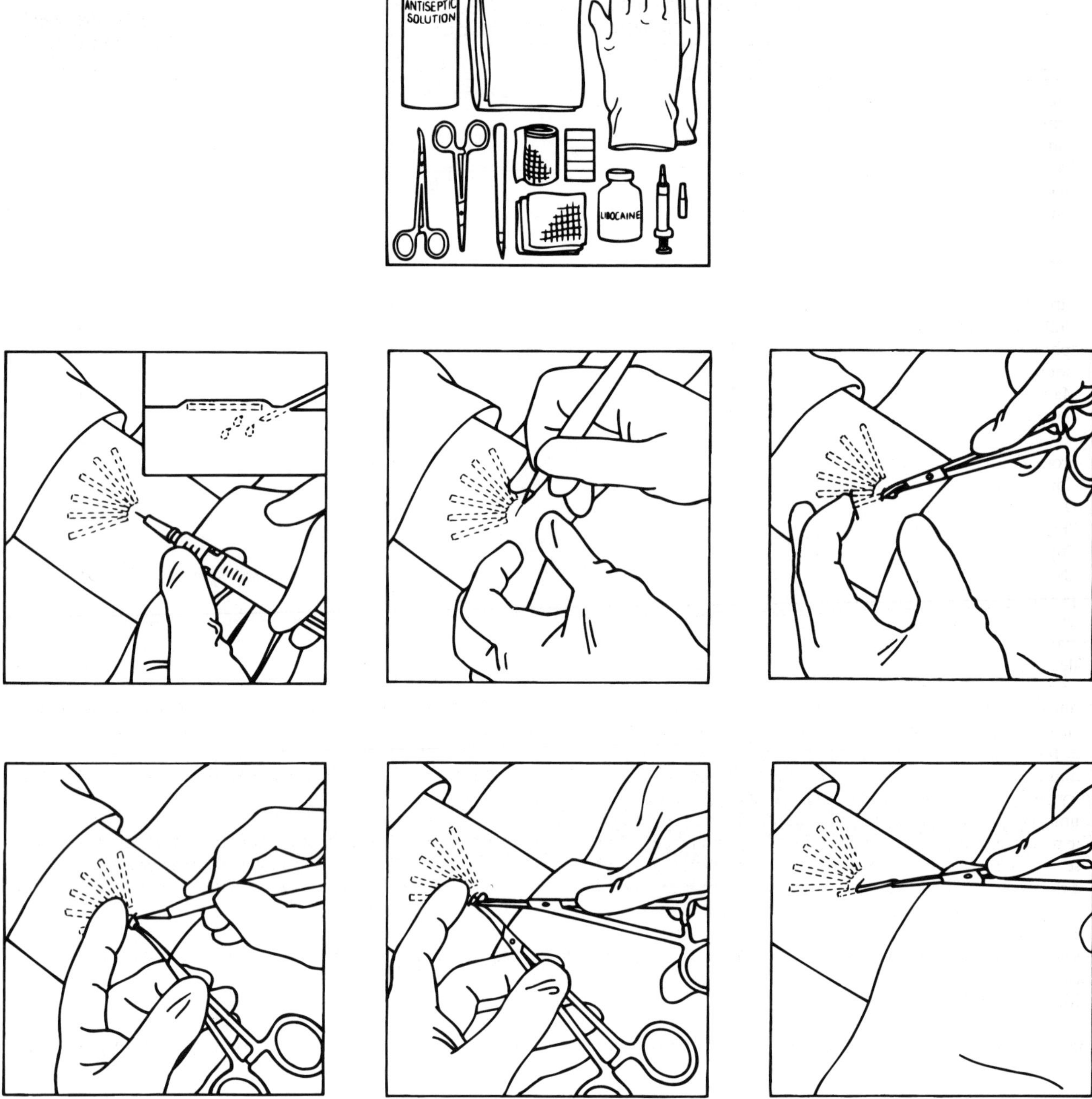

Figure 2
Removal of Norplant implants. For a more detailed legend, see the labeling for the Norplant system that is published in the Physicians Desk Reference. *(Courtesy of Wyeth-Ayerst Laboratories.)*

more flexible (soft tubing) and that released slightly more levonorgestrel than the implants made from less flexible or hard tubing that were used in the other three-fourths of the women. The study showed that women using implants manufactured from soft tubing had fewer pregnancies than those who used implants made with hard tubing. Since the majority of the results in the pivotal trials were from women using implants made from hard tubing, the efficacy data used in the labeling reflect the results of hard tubing. Subsequent clinical trials have confirmed that the effectiveness of Norplant implants made with soft tubing is much greater than that of implants made with hard tubing. The increased effectiveness of Norplant implants made with soft tubing was noted regardless of the weight of the user. Implants made with soft tubing are the contraceptive devices that are marketed throughout the world.

Table 1 Percentage of Women Experiencing a Contraceptive Failure During the First Year of Perfect Use and the First Year of Typical Use and the Percentage Continuing Use at the End of the First Year, United States

METHOD	% OF WOMEN EXPERIENCING ACCIDENTAL PREGNANCY WITHIN THE 1ST YR OF USE		% OF WOMEN CONTINUING USE AT 1 YR[3]
	TYPICAL USE[1]	PERFECT USE[2]	
Chance[4]	85	85	
Spermicides[5]	21	6	43
Periodic abstinence	20		67
Calendar		9	
Ovulation method		3	
Symptothermal[6]		2	
Postovulation		1	
Withdrawal	19	4	
Cap[7]			
Parous women	36	26	45
Nulliparous women	18	9	58
Diaphragm[7]	18	6	58
Condom[8]			
Male	12	3	63
Female (Reality)	21	5	56
Pill	3		72
Progestin only		0.5	
Combined		0.1	
IUD			
Progestasert	2.0	1.5	81
Copper T 380A	0.8	0.6	78
LNg 20	0.1	0.1	81
Depo-Provera	0.3	0.3	70
Norplant (6 capsules)	0.09	0.09	85
Female sterilization	0.4	0.4	100
Male sterilization	0.15	0.10	100

[1]Among couples who initiate use of a method (not necessarily for the first time) and who use it *perfectly* (both consistently and correctly), the authors' best guess of the percentage expected to experience an accidental pregnancy during the first year if they do not stop use for any other reason.
[2]Among *typical* couples who initiate use of a method (not necessarily for the first time), the percentage who experience an accidental pregnancy during the first year if they do not stop use for any other reason.
[3]Among couples attempting to avoid pregnancy, the percentage who continue to use a method for one year.
[4]The percentage failing in columns (2) and (3) are based on data from populations where contraception is not used and from women who cease using contraception in order to become pregnant. Among such populations, about 89% become pregnant within 1 year. We lowered this estimate slightly (to 85%) to represent our best guess of the percentage who would become pregnant within 1 year among women now relying on reversible methods of contraception if they abandoned contraception altogether.
[5]Foams and vaginal suppositories.
[6]Cervical mucus (ovulation) method supplemented by calendar in the preovulatory and basal body temperature in the postovulatory phases.
[7]With spermicidal cream or jelly.
[8]Without spermicides.
From Hatcher RA, Trussell J, Stewart F, et al. Contraceptive technology, 17th ed. New York: Irvington Publishers, in press; with permission.

When implants were used for longer than 5 years, the yearly pregnancy rate rose to 2.5 to 3.0 percent for all users. The latter rates are comparable with those for oral contraceptives (OCs) and are higher than during the previous years. Therefore, Norplant implants are replaced at the end of 5 years. This schedule provides a 1 year margin for noncompliance in which the protection afforded is equivalent to that of OCs.

To place the effectiveness of Norplant implants in perspective, typical pregnancy rates in various contraceptive methods for the first year of use are summarized in Table 1. The efficacy of most methods depends on the reliability of use. By contrast, the efficacy of Norplant implants, like that of intrauterine devices (IUDs) and sterilization, does not depend on patient compliance.

The effects of Norplant implants are completely reversible. Observations in women who terminated use because they desired to become pregnant suggested that fecundity is about the same as it was at the time of marriage. The life table pregnancy rates were 24 percent at 1 month after removal, 90 percent at 1 year, and 95 percent at 2 years.

■ CONTRAINDICATIONS

Who should not use Norplant implants? Until greater experience is available, clinical judgment and experience with other hormonal contraceptives suggest that Norplant implants should not be used in women with active thrombophle-

Table 2 Annual and 5-Year Cumulative Discontinuation Rates per 100 Users

	YEAR 1	YEAR 2	YEAR 3	YEAR 4	YEAR 5	CUMULATIVE
Pregnancy	0.2	0.5	1.2	1.6	0.4	3.9
Bleeding irregularities	9.1	7.9	4.9	3.3	2.9	25.1
Medical reasons (excluding bleeding irregularities)	6.0	5.6	4.1	4.0	5.1	22.4
Personal reasons	4.6	7.7	11.7	10.7	11.7	38.7
Continuation	81.0	77.4	79.2	76.7	77.6	29.5

bitis or thromboembolic disorders, undiagnosed abnormal genital bleeding, known or suspected pregnancy, acute liver disease, benign or malignant liver tumors, known or suspected carcinoma of the breast, history of idiopathic intracranial hypertension, or hypersensitivity to levonorgestrel or any of the components of the Norplant implants.

■ ADVERSE EFFECTS

Menstrual Problems

The major reason women with Norplant implants discontinue their use is because of menstrual problems similar to those associated with other progestin-only methods. Women must therefore be warned of the possibility of irregular bleeding and/or spotting. A typical woman is likely to have increases in the numbers of bleeding and/or spotting days per cycle. Menstrual diaries show that women who eventually terminate Norplant implant usage because of menstrual problems tend to have more bleeding days than do other users. Even though menometrorrhagia is the prime reason for terminating implant use, hemoglobin values are not usually lower in women who stop use because of menstrual problems. Furthermore, anemia is a rare side effect of the implants. These findings are consistent with the observations that menstrual flow volume decreases during implant use. Thus, women who keep menstrual diaries over a 5-year period document an overall decrease in bleeding events. The total number of bleeding days per year declines significantly from a mean of 54 days per year in year 1 to 44 in year 5. The total number of spotting days per year also decreases significantly after the first year.

Disruption of the normal cycle during implant use produces long intervals without frank bleeding, although spotting often occurs in such intervals. Because delayed menses can be interpreted as pregnancy, a long interval of amenorrhea may be stressful for women who are not counseled in advance and who are not reassured that the Norplant implants are unlikely to fail. In fact, the typical woman who becomes pregnant while using Norplant implants has regular menstrual bleeding that is then interrupted by a period of amenorrhea, which signals the onset of pregnancy. Thus, women with oligomenorrhea are not likely to become pregnant and should be counseled accordingly.

Medical Problems

A significant number of women stop using the implants for medical reasons other than menstrual problems (Table 2).

Delayed Follicular Atresia and Ovarian Cysts

Ovarian cysts develop in some women using Norplant implants. These cysts, some of which are 7 to 10 cm in diameter, are detected by palpation at the time of routine pelvic examination, and regress over several weeks. Daily ultrasonographic studies performed in Norplant implant users who had regular menses show that the following sequence occurs in some cycles: a dominant follicle is selected, ovulation does not occur, the follicle persists for up to 2 weeks past the time of expected ovulation, and involution gradually occurs. We therefore conclude that use of Norplant implants is associated with delayed follicular atresia in some women. Because the enlarged follicles may be indistinguishable from ovarian cysts of other causes to the casual examiner, women using Norplant implants and their health care providers should be advised that delayed atresia occurs and that invasive measures are not required. Rather, these women should be observed for 6 weeks or until regression occurs. If regression does not occur, the ovarian enlargement must be further evaluated. The incidence of ovarian cysts requiring surgery is no greater than that in women who do not use hormonal contraception.

Infection or Pain

Another medical reason for terminating Norplant implant use is infection at the site of insertion. This rare event (0.7 percent of users) is usually associated with inadequate asepsis and no longer occurs once health care providers gain experience. If infection occurs, suitable treatment is instituted; if infection persists, the implants should be removed. Pain or itching at the implant site occurs in 3.7 percent of users. These complaints are usually transient.

Drug Interactions

Certain drugs used to treat epilepsy increase the risk of pregnancy in implant users because they increase the rate of levonorgestrel metabolism. Evidence of drug interaction is most convincing in the case of phenytoin and carbamazepine.

Ectopic Pregnancy

Because ovulation and subsequent pregnancy do occasionally occur, there is concern that users may be subject to a heightened risk of ectopic pregnancy, a factor of marked importance in users of progestin-only contraception. Ectopic pregnancies have occurred among users of Norplant capsules at an average rate of 1.3 per 1,000 woman years. The risk of ectopic pregnancy may increase with time, with duration of use, and possibly with weight. Thus, implants must be removed after 5 years.

To put this ectopic pregnancy rate into perspective, the rate for all women in the United States in 1992 was calculated from the combined ectopic pregnancies treated in hospitals plus outpatient clinics. In that year 108,800 ectopic pregnancies were recorded in approximately 60 million women, a rate of 1.8 per 1,000. The reason that Norplant implants might reduce ectopic pregnancy rate is because this contraceptive is so effective at protecting women against all types of pregnancy. Nonetheless, a pregnancy in a Norplant implant user is more likely to be ectopic than in women not using contraception. Thus, physicians should be alert to the possibility of ectopic pregnancy in women who complain of lower abdominal pain and in those who have symptoms of pregnancy.

Foreign Body Carcinogenesis

Rarely, cancers occur at the site of foreign bodies or old scars. None has been reported in clinical trials of Norplant implants. In rodents, which are highly susceptible to such cancers, the incidence decreases with decreasing size of the foreign body. Because of the resistance of human beings to these cancers and because of the small size of the capsules, the risk to users of Norplant implants is judged to be minimal.

Idiopathic Intracranial Hypertension

Idiopathic intracranial hypertension (pseuduotumor cerebri) is a disorder of unknown etiology that is seen most commonly in obese females of reproductive age. As noted in other chapters, growth hormone treatment is associated with the appearance of this disorder. There have been reports of idiopathic intracranial hypertension in Norplant implant users. Cardinal signs include visual disturbances and headaches. The headaches are often different from those previously experienced by the women with regard to frequency patterns, severity, or duration. Of particular importance are those headaches that are unremitting in nature and obese patients with these symptoms with recent weight gain. These women should be screened for papilledema, and, if present, the patient should be referred to a neurologist for further diagnosis and care. Norplant implants should be removed from patients experiencing this disorder.

Other Adverse Reactions

Approximately 50 percent of Norplant users with medical problems (see Table 2) have complaints commonly associated with other steroid-containing contraceptives. Comparative clinical trials suggest that the following adverse reactions occurring during the first year are probably associated with use of Norplant implants: headache, nervousness, nausea, dizziness, adnexal enlargement, acne, mastalgia, weight gain, and hirsutism. In addition, the following adverse reactions have been reported with a frequency of 5 percent or more during the first year and possibly may be related to Norplant implant use: breast discharge, cervicitis, musculoskeletal pain, abdominal discomfort, leukorrhea, and vaginitis.

The pivotal studies used to define the adverse reactions to Norplant implants involved 2,470 women. This exposure, even though quite large for a newly introduced method, is not sufficient to determine whether Norplant implants are associated with many of the rare but serious risks of combined OCs.

■ BENEFITS

Contraception

Pregnancy and abortion are leading causes of death in women under age 35 in developing countries. To put this into perspective, women in the United States are 38 times more likely to die in an automobile accident than from pregnancy or abortion. Nonetheless, contraception can also reduce mortality even in the United States. Child mortality can also be significantly reduced by preventing teenage pregnancy and by spacing of births. Thus, in addition to allowing women to have children when they want, contraception has a beneficial effect on both maternal and child health. One might argue that the more effective the contraceptive, the greater is this health effect. As noted in Table 1, the Norplant implant system is one of the most effective contraceptives yet devised, ranking with sterilization and modern IUDs (such as the TCu 380A), for preventing pregnancy.

Convenience

When women are questioned on what they liked best about Norplant implants after 5 years of use, the majority respond "convenience." That is, after insertion, implants promoted long-term contraception that does not require daily intake, use with each intercourse, or frequent return to the clinic for new supplies.

Reduction of Adverse Reactions

Many women who choose to use Norplant implants do so because they previously discontinued OCs because of annoying medical problems such as nausea, light-headedness, and weight gain. Many former users of OCs continued to use Norplant because they felt there were fewer adverse reactions.

Prevention of Anemia

As noted above, the average blood loss during the first year of implant use was not increased even though bleeding and spotting did increase. After the first year, menstrual blood loss was reduced and hemoglobin levels rose.

■ WHO MAY WISH TO USE NORPLANT IMPLANTS

1. Women who desire highly effective, low-dose hormonal contraception
2. Women who want long-term contraception after completing their family but do not want sterilization
3. Women who wish to delay having children for long periods
4. Women who cannot use estrogen
5. Women who are unhappy with other forms of contraception

■ WHO MAY NOT WISH TO USE NORPLANT IMPLANTS

1. Women who are happy with their present method of contraception
2. Women who do not want to use a method that requires a visit to a health care provider to discontinue
3. Women who do not wish to or cannot pay the upfront cost of Norplant implants, even though they know that the overall cost over 5 years is lower
4. Women who do not wish to tolerate irregular menstrual bleeding, should it occur

■ NORPLANT II

During the development of the Norplant implant system, clinicians involved in the clinical trials realized that an implant system with fewer than six capsules would likely be much easier to insert and remove. After many studies, implants were structurally modified from capsules to covered rods and lengthened so that two 4 cm covered rods (Norplant II) could release the same amount of levonorgestrel as six 3 cm capsules. Three-year clinical trials showed that the safety and efficacy of Norplant II implants was the same as the Norplant implant manufactured with soft tubing. These clinical trials also confirmed that Norplant II implants were easier to insert and remove. In 1995 an application was made to the FDA to market Norplant II implants in the United States.

Suggested Reading

Alvarez-Sanchez F, Brache V, Tejada AS, Faundes A. Abnormal endocrine profile among women with confirmed or presumed ovulation during long-term Norplant use. Contraception 1986; 33:111–119.

Bardin CW. Long-acting steroidal contraception: An update. Int J Fertil 1989; 34(Suppl):88–95.

Croxatto HB, Diaz S, Salvatierra AM, et al. Treatment with Norplant subdermal implants inhibits sperm penetration through cervical mucus in vitro. Contraception 1987; 36:192–201.

Dunson TR, Amatya RN, Krueger SL. Complications and risk factors associated with the removal of Norplant implants. Obstet Gynecol 1995; 85:543–548.

Nilsson CG, Holma P. Menstrual blood loss with contraceptive subdermal levonorgestrel implants. Fertil Steril 1981; 35:304–306.

Trussell J, Hatcher RA, Cates W Jr, et al. Contraceptive failure in the United States: An update. Stud Fam Plann 1990; 21:51–54.

INTRAUTERINE DEVICES

Daniel R. Mishell Jr., M.D.

The main benefits of intrauterine devices (IUDs) are (1) a high level of effectiveness, (2) a lack of associated systemic metabolic effects, and (3) the need for only a single act of motivation for long-term use. Despite these advantages less than 1 percent of married women of reproductive age use the IUD for contraception in the United States, compared with 15 to 30 percent in most European countries and Canada. In contrast to other types of contraception, there is no need for frequent motivation to ingest a pill daily or to use a coitus-related method consistently. These characteristics, as well as the necessity for a visit to a health care facility to discontinue the method, account for the fact that IUDs have the highest continuation rate of all currently available reversible methods of contraception.

Unlike other contraceptives, such as the barrier methods, which rely on frequent use by the individual to be effective and therefore have higher use-failure rates than method-failure rates, the IUD has similar method-effectiveness and use-effectiveness rates. First-year failure rates with the Copper T 380A IUD are less than 1 percent and with the progesterone-releasing IUD are 1.8 percent. Pregnancy rates are related to the skill of the clinician inserting the device. With experience, correct high-fundal insertion occurs more frequently, and there is a lower incidence of partial or complete expulsion, with resultant lower pregnancy rates. Furthermore, the annual incidence of accidental pregnancy decreases steadily after the first year of IUD use. The cumulative pregnancy rate of the Copper T 380A IUD after 7 years of use is only 1.6 percent. The incidence of all major adverse events with IUDs, including pregnancy, expulsion, or removal for bleeding and/or pain, steadily decrease with increasing age. Thus, the IUD is especially suited for older parous women who wish to prevent further pregnancies.

■ TYPES OF IUDs

In the past 35 years many types of IUDs have been designed and used clinically. The devices developed and initially used in the 1960s were made of a plastic, polyethylene, impregnated with barium sulfate to make them radiographic. In the 1970s, in order to diminish the frequency of the side effects of increased uterine bleeding and pain, smaller plastic devices covered with copper were developed and widely utilized. In the 1980s devices bearing a larger amount of copper, including sleeves on the horizontal arm, such as the Copper T 380A and the Copper T 220C were developed as well as the Multiload Cu 250 and Cu 375. These devices have a longer duration of high effectiveness and thus need to be reinserted at less frequent intervals than the devices bearing a smaller amount of copper. Only the Copper T 380A IUD is marketed in the United States, but the Multiload Cu 375 is widely used in Europe.

Because of the constant dissolution of copper, which amounts daily to less than that ingested in the normal diet, all copper IUDs have to be replaced periodically. The Copper T 380A is currently approved for use in the United States for 10 years and may maintain its effectiveness for a longer time. At the scheduled time of removal, the device can be removed and another inserted during the same office visit.

Adding a reservoir of progesterone to the vertical arm also increases the effectiveness of the T-shaped devices. The currently marketed progesterone-releasing IUD allows 65 mg progesterone to diffuse into the endometrial cavity each day. This amount is sufficient to prevent pregnancy by local action within the endometrial cavity but is not enough to cause a measurable increase in peripheral serum progesterone levels. Because of the progestational effect on the endometrium, the amount of uterine bleeding is reduced with use of this device and it has been used therapeutically to treat menorrhagia. The currently approved progesterone-releasing IUD needs to be replaced annually, because the reservoir of progesterone becomes depleted after about 18 months of use and the surface area of plastic in this small device is insufficient to produce a sufficiently large leukocytic response to yield a high level of contraceptive effectiveness.

A T-shaped device containing a reservoir of levonorgestrel on the vertical arm has been developed and undergone extensive clinical testing. A large comparative trial of the Copper T 380A and the levonorgestrel-releasing IUD found that the effectiveness and continuation rates of both devices were similar. Because of the slower rate of release of levonorgestrel than progesterone, the levonorgestrel-releasing IUD has an estimated duration of use of at least 5 years. The levonorgestrel-releasing IUD also reduces menstrual blood loss and has been used therapeutically to treat abnormal uterine bleeding. This device is currently marketed in only a few European countries (see the chapter *Progestin-releasing Intrauterine Devices*).

Unlike the medicated IUDs, there is no need to change a nonmedicated plastic IUD unless the patient develops increased bleeding after it has been in place for more than a year. Calcium salts are deposited on the plastic over time, and their roughness can cause ulceration and bleeding of the endometrium. If increased bleeding develops after a nonmedicated IUD has been in the uterus for several years, the old IUD should be removed and a new device inserted.

■ MECHANISM OF ACTION

The IUD's main mechanism of contraceptive action in the human is spermicidal. This effect is caused by a local sterile inflammatory reaction produced by the presence of the foreign body in the uterine cavity. There is about 1,000 percent increase in the number of leukocytes in washings of the human endometrial cavity 18 weeks after the insertion of an IUD, compared with washings obtained before insertion. In addition to causing phagocytosis of spermatozoa, tissue breakdown products of these leukocytes are toxic to all cells, including spermatozoa and the blastocyst. The amount of inflammatory reaction, and thus contraceptive effectiveness, is directly related to the size of the intrauterine foreign body. Copper markedly increases the extent of the inflammatory reaction, so this metal has been added to the small sized frame of T-shaped devices. In addition, copper impedes sperm transport and viability in the cervical mucus. Sperm transport from the cervix to the oviduct in the first 24 hours after coitus is markedly impaired in women wearing IUDs. Because of the spermicidal action of IUDs, very few, if any, sperm reach the oviducts, and the ovum usually does not become fertilized.

Further evidence for this spermicidal action of IUDs was reported by a group of investigators who performed oviductal flushing in 56 women wearing IUDs and 45 using no method of contraception who were sterilized by salpingectomy soon after ovulation. These women had unprotected sexual intercourse shortly before ovulation. Normally cleaving, fertilized ova were found in the tubal flushings of about half of the women not wearing IUDs, whereas no eggs having the microscopic appearance of a normally developing embryo were found in the oviducts of the women wearing IUDs.

A long-term study of women wearing the TCu 380A IUD revealed that while the intrauterine pregnancy rate gradually increased with duration of IUD use, the ectopic pregnancy rate remained low and constant after the first year of use. If fertilization occurred frequently with IUD use and its main mechanism of action was to prevent uterine implantation of the blastocyst, the ectopic pregnancy rate would be expected to increase at a rate more rapid than the intrauterine pregnancy rate, and this outcome did not occur. Thus, the principal mechanism of action of the Copper T 380A IUD is as a spermicide, preventing fertilization of the ovum. The progesterone-releasing IUD has a much higher ectopic pregnancy rate than the copper IUD and probably acts mainly by slowing tubal transport of the embryo, as well as preventing implantation of the fertilized ova due to the presence of a high level of progesterone in the uterine cavity.

Upon removal of the IUD, the inflammatory reaction rapidly disappears. Resumption of fertility following IUD removal is prompt and occurs at the same rate as resumption of fertility following discontinuation of the barrier methods of contraception. The incidence of term deliveries, spontaneous abortion, and ectopic pregnancies in conceptions occurring after IUD removal is the same as in the general noncontraceptive-using population.

■ TIME OF INSERTION

Although it is widely believed that the optimal time for insertion of an IUD is during the menses, there are data indicating that if a woman is not pregnant, the IUD can be safely inserted on any day of the cycle. An analysis was made of 2-month event rates of about 10,000 women who had TCu 200s inserted on various days of the cycle. Differences in event rates with insertion occurring on different days of the cycle were small and of little clinical relevance. Therefore, the IUD can be inserted on any day of the cycle. Since bacteria are introduced into the endometrial cavity at the time of IUD insertion, it may be preferable to insert the IUD after the menses cease in order to avoid providing a good environment for bacterial growth.

It has also been recommended that IUDs not be inserted until more than 2 to 3 months have elapsed after completing a term pregnancy. However, in 1982 we analyzed event rates in our clinic among women who had Copper T IUDs inserted between 4 and 8 weeks postpartum and more than 8 weeks postpartum. The 1- and 2-year event rates for all causes were similar for the two groups, indicating that Copper T IUDs can be safely inserted at the time of the routine postpartum visit. No uterine perforations occurred in this series, in which the withdrawal technique of insertion was used. Although one report suggested that the uterine perforation rate was increased if the IUD is inserted when a woman is lactating, this finding has not been confirmed in several other studies.

The effect of breast-feeding on performance of the Copper T 380A IUD was evaluated from data obtained from a large multicenter clinical trial in which the device was inserted into

559 breast-feeding women and 590 non-breast-feeding women, all of whom were at least 6 weeks postpartum. There were significantly fewer problems with pain and bleeding at the time of insertion in the group that was breast-feeding. The expulsion rate, which was low, and the continuation rate, which was high, were similar in the breast-feeding and non-breast-feeding groups 6 months after insertion. Therefore, insertion of the IUD can be performed in postpartum women who are breast-feeding their infants, as well as those who are not nursing at the time of the routine postpartum visit.

ADVERSE EFFECTS

Incidence

In general, in the first year of use IUDs have about a 1 percent pregnancy rate, a 10 percent expulsion rate, and a 15 percent rate of removal for medical reasons, mainly bleeding and pain. The incidence of each of these events, especially expulsion, diminishes steadily in subsequent years.

In an ongoing World Health Organization study of the Copper T 380A, termination rates for adverse effects continued to decline annually following the first year after insertion for each of the 7 years in which sufficient data had been accumulated. In this study the cumulative percentage discontinuation rate for pregnancy, bleeding and pain, and expulsion at the end of 7 years was 1.6, 22.7, and 8.6, respectively.

Uterine Bleeding

Most women who discontinue this method of contraception do so for medical reasons. Nearly all the medical reasons accounting for removal of copper-bearing or inert IUDs involve one or more types of abnormal bleeding: heavy and/or prolonged menses or intermenstrual bleeding. The heavy bleeding may be produced by a premature and increased rate of local release of prostaglandins brought about by the presence of the intrauterine foreign body. The stimulation of uterine contractions by excessive levels of prostaglandins may prolong the duration of the menstrual flow, which is significantly longer in women wearing IUDs than normally cycling women.

The amount of blood lost in each menstrual cycle is significantly greater in women using inert as well as copper-bearing IUDs than in nonusers. In a normal menstrual cycle, the mean amount of menstrual blood loss was previously reported to be about 35 ml, but with improved techniques of extraction of blood from sanitary napkins it is now estimated to be about 60 ml.

After insertion of a loop IUD, the mean menstrual blood loss is increased by about 110 to 130 percent. The increase is less with copper-bearing devices. With the smaller Copper 7 and Copper T 200 IUD, the mean menstrual blood loss was reported to increase by about 40 to 85 percent. The Copper T 380A IUD is associated with about a 55 percent increase in menstrual blood loss. In contrast, with the progesterone-releasing IUD, the amount of blood loss is significantly reduced to about 25 ml per cycle. There is also reduced blood loss with the levonorgestrel-releasing IUD.

In a study of Swedish women inserted with the TCu 380A there was no significant change in mean measurements of several hematologic parameters including hemoglobin, hematocrit, and erythrocyte count 3, 6, and 12 months after IUD insertion when compared with mean values before insertion.

A sensitive indicator of tissue iron stores is the serum ferritin level. Earlier studies reported that use of nonmedicated plastic IUDs was associated with significant decreases in serum ferritin levels and an increase in the percentage of women with extremely low ferritin levels, indicative of iron deficiency in the bone marrow. Low serum ferritin levels are therefore a good predictor of the development of anemia, and levels less than 4 mg per liter require oral iron supplementation to prevent anemia. In the recent study of women wearing the Copper T 380A IUD there was no significant change in serum ferritin levels at 3, 6, and 12 months after IUD insertion. None of the women with low ferritin levels had a decrease in hemoglobin levels. They probably had an increase in intestinal iron absorption to compensate for the increased menstrual blood loss as none of these women developed anemia.

Excessive bleeding in the first few months following IUD insertion should be treated with reassurance and supplemental oral iron. The bleeding may diminish with time as the uterus adjusts to the presence of the foreign body. Excessive bleeding that continues or develops several months or more after IUD insertion is best treated by systemic administration of one of the prostaglandin synthetase inhibitors during menses.

Mefenamic acid ingested in a dosage of 500 mg three times a day during the days of menstruation has been shown to reduce menstrual blood loss significantly in IUD users. If excessive bleeding continues despite this treatment, the device should be removed. After a 1-month interval, another type of device may be inserted if the woman still wishes to use an IUD for contraception. Consideration should be given to using a progestin-releasing IUD, because this device is associated with less blood loss than the copper-bearing IUDs.

Perforation

Although uncommon, one of the potentially serious complications associated with use of the IUD is perforation of the uterine fundus. Perforation always occurs at the time of insertion. Sometimes only the distal portion of the IUD penetrates the uterine muscle at insertion. Then uterine contractions over the next few months force the IUD into the peritoneal cavity. IUDs correctly inserted entirely within the endometrial cavity do not wander through the uterine muscle into the peritoneal cavity. The incidence of perforation is generally related to the shape of the device and/or amount of force used during its insertion, as well as the experience of the clinician performing the insertion. IUDs inserted within the uterine cavity do not perforate the uterus. Perforation of the uterus is best prevented by straightening the uterine axis with a tenaculum and then probing the cavity with a uterine sound before IUD insertion.

In large multiclinic studies, perforation rates for the Copper 7 were about 1 in 1,000 insertions, but perforation rates for the Copper T 380A were only about 1 in 3,000 insertions. Because the perforations occurring at the time of insertion are nearly always asymptomatic, the clinician should always suspect that perforation has occurred if the user cannot feel the appendage but did not observe that the device was expelled. One should not assume that an unnoticed expulsion has occurred when the appendage is not visualized. Sometimes the IUD is still in its correct position in the uterine cavity but the appendage has been withdrawn into the cavity as the position of the IUD has changed. In this situation, after pelvic examination has been performed and the possibility of pregnancy excluded, the uterine cavity should be probed.

If the device cannot be felt with a uterine sound or biopsy instrument, a pelvic sonogram or x-ray should be obtained. If the device is not visualized with pelvic ultrasonography, an x-ray visualizing the entire abdominal cavity should be performed as IUDs that have been pushed through the uterus may be located anywhere in the peritoneal cavity, even in the subdiaphragmatic area.

Any type of IUD found to be outside the uterus even if asymptomatic should be removed from the peritoneal cavity because complications such as severe adhesions and bowel obstruction have been reported with intraperitoneal IUDs. Therefore, it is best to remove intraperitoneal IUDs shortly after the diagnosis of perforation is made. Unless severe adhesions have developed, most intraperitoneal IUDs can be removed by means of laparoscopy.

Perforation of the cervix has also been reported with devices having a straight vertical arm such as the Copper T or Copper 7. The incidence of downward perforation into the cervix has been reported to range from about 1 in 600 to 1 in 1,000 insertions. A plastic ball has been added to the distal vertical arm of the TCu 380A to reduce the rate of cervical perforation. When follow-up examinations are performed after IUD insertion, the cervix should be carefully inspected and palpated, because often perforations do not extend completely through the ectocervical epithelium. Cervical perforation is not a major problem, but devices that have perforated downward should be removed through the endocervical canal with uterine packing forceps. Their downward displacement is associated with reduced contraceptive effectiveness.

■ COMPLICATIONS RELATED TO PREGNANCY

Congenital Anomalies

When pregnancy occurs with an IUD in place, implantation takes place away from the device itself, so the device is always extra-amniotic. Although there is a paucity of published data, so far there is no evidence of an increased incidence of congenital anomalies in infants born with a plastic, copper-bearing, or progesterone-releasing IUD in utero.

Data from two studies of more than 300 babies conceived with a copper IUD in utero suggest that its presence does not exert a deleterious effect on fetal development or increase the risk of birth defects. Although relatively few infants have been born with a progesterone-releasing IUD in the uterus during their gestation, examination of these infants has revealed no evidence of cardiac or other anomalies.

Spontaneous Abortion

In all reported series of pregnancies with any type of IUD in situ, the incidence of fetal death was not significantly increased; however, a significant increase in spontaneous abortion has been consistently observed. If a woman conceives while wearing an IUD that is not subsequently removed, the incidence of spontaneous abortion is about 55 percent, approximately three times greater than would occur in pregnancies without an IUD.

After conception, if the IUD is spontaneously expelled or if the appendage is visible and the IUD is removed by traction, the incidence of spontaneous abortion is significantly reduced. In one study of women who conceived with Copper T devices in place, the incidence of spontaneous abortion was only 20 percent if the device was removed or spontaneously expelled. This figure is similar to the normal incidence of spontaneous abortion and significantly less than the 54 percent incidence of abortion reported in the same study among women retaining the devices in utero. Thus, if a woman conceives with an IUD in place and wishes to continue the pregnancy, the IUD should be removed if the appendage is visible, to significantly reduce the chance of spontaneous abortion. If the appendage is not visible, blind probing of the uterine cavity may increase the chance of abortion as well as sepsis. However, several recent reports indicate that during early gestation with sonographic guidance it is possible to remove IUDs in the lower uterine cavity without a visible appendage and not adversely affect the outcome of the pregnancy.

Septic Abortion

If the IUD cannot be removed from the uterine cavity during early gestation, there is some evidence that suggests the risk of septic abortion may be increased if the IUD remains in place. Most of the evidence was based on data from women who conceived while wearing the shield type of IUD. This device, with its multifilament tail, was extensively used in the United States during the 1970s. The structure of the shield's appendage allowed vaginal bacteria to steadily enter the spaces between the filaments of the tail beneath the surrounding sheath. This action differs from the inability of bacteria to enter the monofilament tails or migrate along their surface through the cervical mucus barrier. During pregnancy, when the shield was drawn upward into the uterine cavity as gestation advanced, the bacteria in the tail string could exit into the uterine cavity and cause a severe and sometimes fatal uterine and systemic infection. This infection usually became manifest during the second trimester of pregnancy.

Although there are data indicating that there is an increased risk of septic abortion if a patient conceived with a shield IUD in place due to the structure of the appendage of the shield, there is no firm evidence that IUDs with monofilament tail strings cause sepsis during pregnancy. In a British study, there was no significant difference in the incidence of septic abortion among women who conceived with an IUD in place and those who conceived while using other methods. In a study of 918 women who conceived with the Copper T in situ, there were only two cases of septic abortion, both occurring in the first trimester. These data indicate that there is no increase in sepsis in pregnancy due to the presence of an IUD except for the shield device. However, about 2 percent of all spontaneous abortions are septic, and the continued presence of an IUD is associated with about a 50 percent risk of having a spontaneous abortion. Therefore, the overall incidence of septic abortion may be increased with any IUD in place because the incidence of spontaneous abortion is increased, not because the presence of the IUD increases the risk of sepsis by itself.

Ectopic Pregnancy

As stated above, the IUD's main mechanism of contraceptive action is the production of a continuous sterile inflammatory reaction in the uterine cavity due to the presence of a foreign body. As the large numbers of leukocytes are catabolized, their breakdown products exert a toxic effect on sperm and the blastocyst. If the egg is fertilized, effects of this foreign body reaction act to prevent implantation of the embryo into the endometrium. Because more inflammatory reaction is present in the endometrial cavity than the oviducts if fertilization occurs, the IUD prevents intrauterine pregnancy more effectively than it prevents ectopic pregnancy.

Several epidemiologic studies have confirmed the fact that if pregnancy occurs with an IUD in place it is more likely to be ectopic than if pregnancy occurs in the absence of an IUD. If a patient conceives with an IUD in place, her chances of having an ectopic pregnancy range from 3 to 9 percent. This incidence is about ten times greater than the reported ectopic pregnancy frequency of 0.3 to 0.7 percent of total births in similar populations. Despite the increased incidence of ectopic pregnancy in women conceiving with an IUD in place, because the IUD is such an effective contraceptive, the overall incidence of ectopic pregnancy is reduced in IUD users compared with women using no contraceptives. A large U.S. study reported that women using nonmedicated IUDs have only about 40 percent as great a chance of developing ectopic pregnancy as sexually active women using no method of contraception. This degree of reduction of risk of ectopic pregnancy is similar to that provided by barrier methods but not as effective as that with use of oral contraceptives.

In two large studies, the ectopic pregnancy rate for nonmedicated IUD wearers was 1.2 per 1,000 woman years. With the Copper T 380A IUD it was only 0.34, and with the progesterone-releasing IUD the ectopic pregnancy rate was 3.6 per 1,000 woman years. The rate in sexually active reproductive age women using barrier contraceptives was reported to be 1.15 per 1,000 woman years. Therefore the rate for the Copper T 380A was one-fourth as much as the latter group due to its high level of contraceptive effectiveness.

Thus, if a patient conceives with an IUD in place, ectopic pregnancy should be suspected and pelvic sonography should be performed early in gestation. If any patient with an IUD has an elective termination of pregnancy, the evacuated tissue should be examined histologically to be certain that the gestation was intrauterine.

The increased risk of ectopic pregnancy if a woman conceives with an IUD is temporary and does not persist after removal of the IUD. In two large European studies, it was reported that women wishing to conceive after they had an ectopic pregnancy had a much greater chance of having an intrauterine pregnancy if they were using an IUD at the time of their ectopic pregnancy than those who had an ectopic pregnancy without an IUD.

Prematurity

In the previously cited study of conceptions occurring in the presence of Copper T devices, the rate of prematurity among live births was four times greater when the Copper T was left in place than when it was removed. A higher incidence of prematurity with IUDs in utero was also noted in a British study, which reported that 13.6 percent of infants conceived during IUD use weighed less than 2,800 g at birth, compared with 3 percent of infants conceived during the use of other contraceptive methods.

If a pregnant patient has an IUD in place and the device cannot be removed but the patient wishes to continue her gestation, she should be warned of the increased risk of prematurity as well as that of spontaneous abortion and ectopic pregnancy. She should also be informed of the possible increased risk of septic abortion and advised to report promptly the first signs of pelvic pain or fever. There is no evidence that pregnancies with IUDs in utero are associated with an increased incidence of other obstetric complications. There is also no evidence that prior use of an IUD results in a greater incidence of complications in pregnancies occurring after its removal.

■ INFECTION IN THE NONPREGNANT IUD USER

In the 1960s, despite great concern among clinicians that use of the IUD would markedly increase the incidence of salpingitis, or pelvic inflammatory disease (PID), there was little evidence that such an increase did occur. During that decade, the IUD was inserted mainly into parous women, and the incidence of sexually transmitted disease was not as high as occurred subsequently. In 1966 a study was performed in which aerobic and anaerobic cultures were made of homogenates of endometrial tissue obtained transfundally from uteri removed by vaginal hysterectomy at various intervals after insertion of the loop IUD. During the first 24 hours after IUD insertion, the normally sterile endometrial cavity was consistently infected with bacteria. Nevertheless, in 80 percent of uteri removed during the following 24 hours, the women's natural defenses had destroyed these bacteria and the endometrial cavities were sterile. In this study, when transfundal cultures were obtained more than 30 days after IUD insertion, the endometrial cavity, the IUD, and the portion of the thread within the cavity were always found to be sterile. These findings indicate that development of PID more than a month after insertion of the IUD is due to infection with a sexually transmitted pathogen and is unrelated to the presence of the device.

These findings agree with the incidence of clinically diagnosed PID found in a group of 23,977 mainly parous women wearing non-copper-bearing IUDs in the 1960s. When PID rates were computed according to the duration of IUD use, the rates were highest in the first 2 weeks after insertion and then steadily diminished. PID rates during the interval of 2 months until 6 years after insertion remained in the range of 1 to 2.5 per 100 woman years. Results of a large multicenter study coordinated by the WHO revealed similar findings. In this study of 22,908 women inserted with IUDs the PID rate was highest in the first 3 weeks after insertion but remained lower and constant during the 8 years thereafter at 0.5 per 1,000 woman years. The results of both of these studies indicate that an IUD should not be inserted into a patient who may have been recently infected with gonococci or *Chlamydia*. Insertion of the device will transport these pathogens from the cervix into the upper genital tract where the large number of organisms may overcome the host defense and cause salpingitis. If there is clinical suspicion of infectious endocervicitis, cultures should be obtained and the IUD insertion delayed until the results reveal no pathogenic organisms are present. It does not appear to be cost effective to administer systemic antibiotics routinely with every IUD insertion, but the insertion procedure should be as aseptic as possible.

A preliminary analysis of an ongoing prospective study comparing use of an antibiotic ingested just prior to insertion with placebo control reported that there was no significant difference in the subsequent rate of pelvic inflammation. In a recent study of the Copper T 380A IUD, the rate of removal for infection in the first year of use was only 0.3 percent.

Following the introduction and widespread use of the shield device, particularly among nulliparous women (in whom IUDs were previously inserted only occasionally), several studies published in the late 1970s suggested that IUD use itself increased the relative risk of PID from threefold to sevenfold.

There were several problems with these studies. One is that uniform guidelines were not used for the diagnosis of PID (or salpingitis). Differences in diagnostic criteria may have increased the frequency of the diagnosis among IUD users. Women with lower abdominal pain and only minimal or no elevation of temperature may have been given the diagnosis of PID more often when an IUD was in the uterus, resulting in diagnostic bias.

A second problem is the evidence that use of oral contraceptives (OCs), condoms, and diaphragms provide protection against development of PID. The data from numerous studies indicate that the incidence of both febrile and nonfebrile PID is about half as much in women using OCs and barrier methods as in women using no method of contraception. Most sexually active women use contraception, mainly OCs, barriers, or the IUD. The increased risk of infection reported with the IUD was due in large part to the protective effect of the other contraceptives.

A third problem is that in most of the studies performed in the 1970s, a high percentage of IUD wearers were using the shield. This device was more likely than other types to have a causal relationship to PID. Examination of the sheaths of the appendages of both new shields in their sterile packages and shields removed from women showed that 9 percent of the new shields and 34 percent of the used shields had breaks in the sheath around the knot attaching it to the device. These breaks could allow bacteria to have continuous access from the vagina to the endometrial cavity and thus increase the risk of upper genital tract infection.

Finally, none of these early studies differentiated between episodes of PID developing in the first month after IUD insertion and episodes developing later. In 1987 investigators from the Centers for Disease Control and Prevention reported results from a multicenter case-control study of the relationship of the IUD and PID. They found the overall risk of PID in IUD contraceptive users versus nonusers to be 1.9. The risk in shield users was 8.3; in other IUD users, it was only 1.6. When the risk of PID in IUD users (other than shield users) was correlated with duration of use, it was found that a significantly increased risk of PID with the loop and Copper 7 was present only during the first 4 months after insertion. Beyond 4 months there was no significantly increased risk in IUD users other than those with shields. Thus, this report is in agreement with our bacteriologic study and the two large prospective studies of PID in IUD users mentioned above. These data provide additional evidence that aside from the insertion process, the presence of an IUD with monofilament tail strings does not increase the incidence of PID.

Analysis of a large amount of data indicates that PID occurring more than a month following insertion of IUDs with monofilament tail strings is due to a sexually transmitted pathogen and not related to the presence of the IUD.

The increased risk of impairment of future fertility from PID developing in the first month after IUD insertion, as well as the possibility of ectopic pregnancy in the event of contraceptive failure, must be considered when deciding whether to use an IUD in a nulliparous woman, especially if she has multiple sexual partners. Contraceptive steroids reduce the risk of developing salpingitis in women infected with gonorrhea and should be offered to such women. However, for women with medical reasons for not using contraceptive steroids, the IUD is the only other effective reversible method of contraception that can be used. Condoms should be advised to reduce the risk of transmission of pathogens.

Symptomatic PID can usually be successfully treated with antibiotics without removing the IUD until the woman becomes symptom free. For women with clinical evidence of a tubo-ovarian abscess, the IUD should be removed only after a therapeutic serum level of appropriate parenteral antibiotics has been reached, preferably after a clinical response has been observed. An alternative method of contraception should be substituted in women who develop PID with an IUD in place.

There is evidence that IUD users may have an increased risk for colonizing actinomycosis organisms in the upper genital tract. The relationship of actinomycosis to PID is unclear, as many women without IUDs have actinomycosis in their vagina and are asymptomatic. If actinomycosis organisms are identified on the routine examination of cervical cytology and the woman is asymptomatic, she may be treated with appropriate antimicrobal therapy to eradicate the organisms or be followed without therapy. The IUD should not be removed from an asymptomatic woman who is colonized but not infected with actinomycosis.

■ CONTRAINDICATIONS

It is logical and consistent with good medical practice that IUDs not be inserted into women with the following seven conditions listed as contraindications to IUD insertion in the United States: (1) pregnancy or suspicion of pregnancy; (2) acute pelvic inflammatory disease; (3) postpartum endometritis or infected abortion in the past 3 months; (4) known or suspected uterine or cervical malignancy; (5) genital bleeding of unknown etiology; (6) untreated acute cervicitis; or (7) a previously inserted IUD that has not been removed. However, there are little data available to indicate that the complications of Wilson's disease, allergy to copper, and genital actinomycosis are true contraindications for insertion of copper-bearing IUDs and, because of the infrequency of these conditions, it is unlikely that data will ever become available.

The remaining contraindications for IUD use listed in the

product labeling—(1) abnormalities of the uterus resulting in distortion of the uterine cavity; (2) history of pelvic inflammatory disease; (3) vaginitis, including bacterial vaginosis, until infection is controlled; (4) patient or her partner has multiple sexual partners; and (5) conditions associated with increased susceptibility to infections with microorganisms—remain questionable because of the lack of clinical studies of copper IUD use in women with these conditions.

The reason the IUD is stated to be contraindicated in women who have multiple sexual partners or whose partner has multiple sexual partners is unclear. Such couples should be counseled to use condoms to protect against transmission of these diseases and to use the IUD to effectively prevent pregnancy if they so desire.

Prospective studies need to be undertaken to determine whether the absolute contraindications listed in the product labeling, such as a remote history of PID, and conditions that might predispose to infections, such as diabetes mellitus, are indeed contraindications to IUD use. Three studies of IUD use in women with either type 1 or type 2 diabetes mellitus indicate that the IUD does not increase the risk of salpingitis or contraceptive failure in diabetic women compared with healthy controls.

■ OVERALL SAFETY

Several long-term studies have indicated that the IUD is not associated with an increased incidence of endometrial or cervical carcinoma and may actually be associated with a reduction in risk of developing these neoplasms during and following its insertion. The IUD is a particularly useful method of contraception for women who have completed their families and do not wish permanent sterilization and have contraindications to, or do not wish to use, other effective methods of reversible contraception. A recent analysis reported that after 5 years of use, the IUD was the most cost-effective method of all methods of contraception including sterilization. Women in the United States who use an IUD have a higher level of satisfaction with their method of contraception than women using any of the other methods of reversible contraception.

Suggested Reading

Lee NC, Rubin GL. The intrauterine device and pelvic inflammatory disease revisited: New results from the women's health study. Obstet Gynecol 1988; 72:1.

Farley TM, et al. Intrauterine devices and pelvic inflammatory disease: an international perspective. Lancet 1992; 339:785.

Sivin I: Dose- and age-depenent ectopic pregnancy risks with intrauterine contraception. Obstet Gynecol 1991; 78:291–298.

White MK, Ory HW, Rooks JB, et al. Intrauterine device termination rates and the menstrual cycle day of insertion. Obstet Gynecol 1980; 55:220.

World Health Organization. The TCu220C, Multiload 250 and Nova T IUDs at 3, 5, and 7 years of use. Results from three randomized multicentre trials.

World Health Organization Special Programme of Research, Development and Research Training in Human Reproduction. Task Force on the Safety and Efficacy of Fertility Regulating Methods: The TCu380A, TCu220C, Multiload 250 and Nova T IUDs at 3, 5, and 7 years of use. Results from three randomized multicentre trials. Contraception 1990; 42:141–158.

INFERTILITY IN WOMEN

Snunit Ben-Ozer, M.D.
Arlene J. Morales, M.D., F.A.C.O.G.

Infertility is defined as the failure to conceive after 1 year of unprotected intercourse. Today couples often proceed directly from contraception to active pursuit of pregnancy, timing intercourse by basal body temperatures (BBT) or urinary luteinizing hormone (LH) detection kits. Infertility, in a milieu of "active" conception attempts, remains undefined. In the United States, 15 percent of couples experience infertility. A female factor is present in approximately 60 percent of infertile couples.

Most couples with infertility are subfertile rather than absolutely infertile. Absolute infertility, implying a treatment-independent pregnancy rate of zero, encompasses bilateral tubal occlusion, amenorrhea secondary to gonadotropic cell destruction, ovarian or endometrial failure, as well as azoospermia. Subfertility is manifest in nonstatic conditions such as chronic anovulation, functional amenorrheas, endometriosis, endocrinopathies, decreased ovarian reserve, as well as oligoasthenospermia. Controversial etiologies of subfertility include cervical mucus abnormalities, luteinized unruptured follicle (LUF) syndrome, leukospermia, and decreased sperm "function."

This chapter is limited to a discussion of the rationale and treatment of infertility attributable to the wide spectrum of ovulatory dysfunctions, the most severe of which is anovulation.

■ CHOOSING A THERAPEUTIC APPROACH: CATEGORIZING THE OVULATORY DYSFUNCTION

The appropriate timing of initiating medical intervention must account for the age-related decline in fertility, which is most pronounced in women older than 35. Thus, we investigate infertility after 1 year of unprotected intercourse or

Table 1 Categorization of Ovulatory Dysfunctions

Hyperandrogenic Anovulation
Polycystic ovarian syndrome (PCOS)
Late-onset congenital adrenal hyperplasias (LOCAH)
Ovarian hyperthecosis
Androgen-producing ovarian tumors
Androgen-producing adrenal tumors
Cushing's syndrome
Hypoestrogenic Anovulation (hypothalamic or pituitary etiology)
Hypogonadotropic hypoestrogenic states
Reversible:
Functional hypothalamic amenorrheas (FHA)
Eating disorders (anorexia nervosa, excessive weight loss)
Excessive athletic training
Neoplastic
Craniopharyngioma
Pituitary stalk compression
Infiltrative diseases
Histiocytosis-X
Sarcoidosis
Hypophysitis
Pituitary adenomas
Hyperprolactinemia
Euprolactinemic galactorrhea
Endocrinopathies
Hypothyroidism/hyperthyroidism
Cushing's disease
Irreversible:
Kallmann's syndrome
Isolated gonadotropin deficiency (IGD, hypothalamic or pituitary origin)
Panhypopituitarism/pituitary insufficiency
Sheehan's syndrome, pituitary apoplexy
Pituitary irradiation or ablation
Hypergonadotropic hypoestrogenic states
Physiologic states
Menopause
Perimenopause
Premature ovarian failure (POF)
Immune-related
Radiation/chemotherapy-induced
Ovarian dysgenesis
Turner's syndrome
46XX with mutations of X
Androgen insensitivity syndrome (AIS)
Miscellaneous
Endometriosis
Luteal phase defect (LPD)

"active" pursuit of conception in women younger than 35. In women 35 years of age or older, we initiate the evaluation after 6 months to 1 year of attempted conception.

The goal of an infertility evaluation is to define the underlying pathophysiology so that diagnosis-specific therapy may be applied. Pregnancy is commonly achieved when such an approach is applied to infertility of ovulatory origin. Ovulatory dysfunctions are characterized as described in Table 1.

Ovulatory dysfunction associated with hyperandrogenemia is ideally treated by normalizing androgen levels, as in the surgical management of ovarian or adrenal tumors. The optimal approach to polycystic ovarian syndrome (PCOS) and ovarian hyperthecosis is more controversial. Ovulation induction in these patients is usually attempted with clomiphene, although spontaneous ovulation may occur after progestin withdrawal. If necessary, ovulation is induced with exogenous gonadotropins. Successful treatment of endocrinopathies with hyperandrogenemia, such as Cushing's syndrome and late-onset congenital adrenal hyperplasia (LOCAH), often leads to resumption of ovulatory status. Moderate weight reduction in obese anovulatory women may be the only "infertility treatment" required. Weight loss is associated with the return of ovulatory status, as well as a reduction in gestational complications. We strongly encourage this approach as the first step of therapy in patients younger than 35. If no conception occurs, ovulation induction may be pharmaceutically induced with gonadotropin-releasing hormone (GnRH) pulsatile therapy, clomiphene, or menotropins.

Hypogonadotropic hypoestrogenic ovulatory dysfunctions are of central origin. Anatomic causes of hypothalamic GnRH neuronal dysfunction, such as isolated gonadotropin deficiency (IGD, which may also be of pituitary origin) and Kallmann's syndrome, are irreversible and require ovulation induction with GnRH pulsatile therapy or controlled ovarian hyperstimulation (COH) with gonadotropins. In contrast, successful treatment of the underlying cause of functional hypothalamic amenorrheas (FHA) allows for resumed menses and ovulation in 75 percent of patients. Examples of FHA are anorexia nervosa, rapid weight loss, excessive athletic activity, psychological stress, and depression. Patients who remain amenorrheic require therapy with GnRH pump or gonadotropins. Clomiphene is usually ineffective in these hypoestrogenic states. Neoplasms and infiltrative diseases must be specifically treated. GnRH neuronal function and ovulation may return, depending on the degree of injury sustained.

Pituitary etiologies of ovulatory dysfunction present as irreversible or reversible hypogonadotropic hypoestrogenic states. Irreversible etiologies include IGD and hypopituitarism, and require gonadotropin-induced COH. Reversible processes causing anovulation, such as pituitary stalk compression, hypophysitis, hypothyroidism or hyperthyroidism, Cushing's disease, and hyperprolactinemia (or euprolactinemic galactorrhea) require specific treatment of the underlying condition.

Hypergonadotropic hypoestrogenic anovulatory states may be physiologic, e.g., menopause and perimenopause, or pathophysiologic, such as the various premature ovarian failure (POF) and ovarian dysgenesis syndromes. Elevated gonadotropin levels mirror ovarian resistance. To interpret results appropriately, physicians must be familiar with the assay used by their institution. At our institution, women with day 3 FSH levels greater than 30 IU per liter are resistant to ovulation induction, thus requiring oocyte donation or adoption. The absolute prognostic value of moderately elevated baseline FSH levels (20 to 30 IU per liter) is less clear, but most clinicians agree it is indicative of significant ovarian resistance. Fertility centers must establish their own guidelines to therapy exclusion. At our center, the decision reflects the worst of 2 to 3 recent cycle day 3 FSH values, the duration and etiology of ovarian resistance, and the couple's emotional need for therapy to put "closure" on matters. If treatment is pursued, high gonadotropin doses or assisted reproductive techniques (ART) often serve patients best.

Table 2 Diagnosis of Ovulation

- Menstrual history
  - Prospective for 3–6 months preferred
  - Normal: regular cycles, 24–35 days in length
- Basal body temperature charting (before out of bed in AM)
  - Normal: biphasic
    - Lowest temperature indicative of ovulation:
    - >0.4°F elevation for 12–15 days indicative of adequate luteal phase
- Urinary LH detection kits
  - Normal: detectable LH surge (kit positive during most of LH surge)
- Late-luteal phase endometrial biopsy (2 consecutive cycles)
  - Normal: <2 days lag in endometrial dating
- Serum midluteal progesterone (not indicative of endometrial histology)
  - Normal: >6.5–10 ng/ml (21–32 nmol/L)
- Three post-ovulatory serum progesterone levels
  - Normal: sum of the three levels >30 ng/ml (96 nmol/L)
- Urinary pregnanediol glucuronide (PdG) levels daily (not readily available)
  - Normal: 14 days of luteal phase elevation
- Frequent periovulatory pelvic ultrasounds
  - Normal: follicular collapse

Of the etiologies mentioned, undulating ovarian status may exist in the perimenopause, in the recovery stages of radiation- or chemotherapy-induced ovarian resistance, and in autoimmune-related POF. Coordinating gonadotropin therapy with cycles of lower baseline FSH levels in ovarian resistance states is alluring but not supported by data. In autoimmune-related POF, corticosteroid use is discouraged, because risks (including aseptic necrosis of the hip) are significant and benefits are not established. Patients with vacillating ovarian status and chromosomal abnormalities, e.g., mosaic Turner's syndrome or other mutations of the X chromosome, often find oocyte donation or adoption necessary. Preconception counseling stressing the increased risk of abnormal fetal karyotype and miscarriage rates is important. In contrast, patients with androgen insensitivity syndrome (AIS) cannot conceive or gestate.

■ PREFERRED THERAPEUTIC APPROACHES

The diagnosis of anovulation and ovulatory dysfunction is based on history, physical exam and laboratory evaluation (Table 2). Oligomenorrhea, or irregular menstrual cycles greater than 35 to 40 days in length, is a sign of anovulation commonly established by history. Less severe ovulatory dysfunctions manifest as varying cycle lengths of 21 to 35 days and can go unnoticed by patients until prospective menstrual charting has been done. When ovulatory dysfunction is suspected, one of two laboratory schemes is chosen, according to the expected pathophysiology. In presumed hyperandrogenic anovulatory states, gonadotropins (LH, FSH), prolactin, sensitive TSH (sTSH), androgens (T, DHEAS, 17-OHP) and progesterone (P, confirming proliferative phase) are obtained. In presumed hypoestrogenic anovulatory states, gonadotropins, prolactin, and sTSH are evaluated initially.

Table 3 Therapeutic Options in Ovulatory Dysfunction

- *Progesterone*
  - Luteal phase defect (LPD)
  - Polycystic ovarian syndrome (PCOS)
- *Bromocriptine*
  - Hyperprolactinema, euprolactinemic galactorrhea
- *Ovulation Induction*
  - Clomiphene citrate—requires adequate estrogenic millieu
    - Chronic anovulation
    - PCOS
    - LPD
    - Unexplained infertility
    - Unfavorable cervical mucous
  - GnRH—requires an intact adenohypophysis
    - Anatomical hypothalamic amenorrheas
    - Functional hypothalamic amenorrheas
    - PCOS—less effective
  - Gonadotropins
    - Failed clomiphene or GnRH therapy
    - PCOS usually require lower doses
    - Hypopituitarism
- *Assisted Reproductive Techniques (ART)*
  - Failed gonadotropin controlled ovarian hyperstimulation (COH)
  - In vitro fertilization (IVF)
  - Gamete intrafallopian transfer
  - Zygote intrafallopian transfer
  - Intracytoplasmic sperm injection
- *Oocyte Donation*
  - Failed gonadotropin COH, or ART
  - FSH >30 IU/L (POF, menopause, unresponsive perimenopause, ovarian dysgenesis)

Diagnosis-specific therapy is instituted, as will be discussed in this chapter, and is summarized in Table 3.

■ DRUG MANAGEMENT OF OVULATORY DYSFUNCTIONS

Table 4 summarizes proprietary names of drugs used in infertility therapy.

Clomiphene Citrate (Clomid, Serophene)

Indications

Clomiphene is the first-line drug for treatment of chronic anovulation, luteal phase defect (LPD), and unexplained infertility in euestrogenic patients with intact anterior pituitary function. The goal of chronic anovulation or LPD therapy is induction of a single mature follicle. In contrast, with unexplained infertility (implying normal ovulation), the goal is the development of 2 to 4 mature follicles per cycle.

Pharmacology

Clomiphene is a nonsteroidal relative of diethylstilbesterol, with predominantly antiestrogenic effects. At the hypothalamus and pituitary, clomiphene blocks estrogen-to-estrogen-receptor binding, thereby preventing estrogen negative feedback. GnRH secretion is enhanced, elevating gonadotropin secretion, and thereby stimulating follicular recruitment and maturation. Clomiphene may also directly affect ovarian steroid production.

Table 4 Proprietary Names for Fertility Drugs

Clomiphene Citrate	*hCG*
Clomid	Profasi
Serophene	*GnRH Agonists*
GnRH	Lupron
Lutrepulse	Buserelin
Factrel	Nafaralin
Gonadotropins	Synarel
Metrodin	Zoladex
Humegon	*Bronocriptine*
Pergonal	Parlodel

Administration and Monitoring

Clomiphene is available in 50 mg oral tablets and is administered for 5 consecutive days beginning on cycle days 3, 4, or 5. We usually prescribe clomiphene for cycle days 3 through 7. Most of our anovulatory patients require a progestin (medroxyprogesterone acetate, 10 mg for 10 days) to induce a withdrawal bleed. In the initial cycle, clomiphene (50 mg per day) is prescribed, inclusive of obese or older patients who often, but unpredictably, have higher drug requirements. A transvaginal ultrasonographic (TVUS) evaluation 1 to 2 days prior to expected ovulation (cycle days 10 to 12) helps to determine whether follicular development goals were attained. If so, and the patient does not conceive, the same dose is used in the next cycle. If follicular development, and thus ovulation, did not occur, the dose is increased by 50 mg each cycle up to a maximum dose of 200 to 250 mg per day.

Ovulation is monitored by over-the-counter urinary LH-detection kits. Most women spontaneously ovulate on clomiphene, if follicles are successfully recruited. Infrequently, a patient with documented follicular recruitment does not have a spontaneous LH surge by cycle day 15. We evaluate follicular status by TVUS and rarely need to induce ovulation with human chorionic gonadotropin (hCG, 10,000 U IM) within 1 to 2 days of follicular maturation (18 to 24 mm). Intrauterine insemination (IUI) is usually reserved for patients who receive clomiphene for COH.

We recommend separating each 3-month treatment block with a drug-free month to minimize the antiestrogenic effects of clomiphene on the endometrium. After three nonconceptive cycles in which the ovulatory goal was achieved, we re-evaluate options with the couple. Depending on age, as well as follicular and endometrial response, we decide whether to repeat three cycles of clomiphene or to initiate gonadotropin therapy.

Results

In the absence of multiple infertility factors, successful treatment with clomiphene yields cycle fecundability of 15 to 20 percent per cycle in anovulatory patients. In patients with LPD, cycle fecundability is approximately 10 to 15 percent, compared with 10 to 12 percent in patients with unexplained infertility.

Side Effects and Complications

We minimize the antiestrogenic endometrial effects of clomiphene with drug-free intervals. If inadequate, conjugated estrogen (0.625 mg daily on cycle days 8 to 14) may be useful. Antiestrogenic effects on cervical mucus are bypassed by IUI, which we recommend after three ovulatory, nonconceptive cycles.

Generally, clomiphene is well tolerated. Most common complaints include flushing (about 10 percent) and pelvic, gastrointestinal (GI), or breast discomfort (less than 5 percent). These symptoms resolve spontaneously. The drug should be discontinued if visual disturbances develop (less than 2 percent).

Multiple pregnancy risk is increased with clomiphene: 8 percent twins, less than 0.5 percent risk of triplets or higher multiples. Preconception therapy does not increase congenital malformations or abortion rates.

Ovarian hyperstimulation is rare, most commonly seen in PCOS patients. TVUS monitoring virtually eliminates this complication, because withholding hCG and avoiding exposure to sperm in high-risk patients typically leads to an uneventful resolution of the signs and symptoms of hyperstimulation.

A possible association between clomiphene and ovarian cancer has been proposed, although not supported by the most recent data analysis. Further studies are ongoing.

Cost Issues

Clomiphene is a relatively inexpensive drug. In the above protocol, the expense is accrued mostly in cycle monitoring. In financially limited patients, the following protocol can reduce cost:

- Bimanual exam to confirm normal ovarian size
- Clomiphene given 5 consecutive days
- Ovulation monitoring with BBT or LH kits
- If ovulation was induced, do not change dose if no conception
- If ovulation did not occur, increase dose by 50 mg in next cycle

Using this protocol, multiple follicular recruitment to optimize therapy in unexplained infertility cannot be confirmed. This protocol is safest, and therefore most appropriate, in ovulatory patients in whom multiple follicular recruitment, and thus hyperstimulation, is rare. Ovarian examination prior to cycle initiation is stressed, especially in women with risk factors for PCOS.

GnRH Therapy (Lutrepulse, Factrel)

Indications

GnRH pulsatile therapy is the preferred mode of ovulation induction in patients with hypothalamic amenorrhea and an intact anterior pituitary. It can also be used in anovulatory states such as PCOS and obesity, although success rates are significantly reduced.

Pharmacology

A synthetic GnRH decapeptide, with a sequence identical to the natural GnRH, stimulates pituitary gonadotropin production and secretion. Follicular recruitment, selection, maturation, and all the feedback loops operate spontaneously.

Administration and Monitoring

GnRH is available as vials of Lutrepulse (800 μg, 3200 μg), or Factrel (100 μg, 500 μg) which are used in an automated portable IV infusion pump. Pulse frequency and dose are adjustable (5–10 μg every 90 to 120 minutes; we prefer 5 μg every 90 min). Subcutaneous injections can be used, but results are uniformly disappointing.

Ovulation is monitored with LH kits, and occurs spontaneously when follicular recruitment is successful. Luteal support is necessary in patients with hypothalamic amenorrhea. It can be achieved by continuing the GnRH treatment through the first 10 weeks of the pregnancy, or by supplementing with progesterone suppositories if GnRH infusion is to be discontinued upon ovulation.

Results

GnRH pulse therapy may be more accepted by patients, who often think of it as a "natural induction." Patients with hypothalamic amenorrhea achieve a 20 to 30 percent pregnancy rate per cycle with pulsatile GnRH administration, with a cumulative pregnancy rate of 93 percent after 12 months. In anovulatory states such as PCOS and obesity, cumulative pregnancy rates achieved (40 to 60 percent) are significantly lower.

Side Effects and Complications

Although GnRH is very well tolerated, occasional phlebitis mandates changing the site of the injection port. In contrast with hMG COI I, treatment with the GnRH pump carries only a minimally increased risk of multiple pregnancies and a negligible risk of severe OHSS. Spontaneous abortion rates are approximately 20 percent higher than those in normal cycles.

Cost Issues

Per cycle, GnRH pump therapy is comparable to the cost of menotropins. Overall cost may be lower with GnRH secondary to a reduction in monitoring and in the risk of multiple pregnancies and subsequent gestational complications.

COH with Human Menopausal Gonadotropins (Humegon, Pergonal) or Purified FSH (Metrodin)

Indications

Human gonadotropins are used for COH in hypogonadotropic hypogonadal states and in women who did not conceive with clomiphene or GnRH therapy. Neither a hypoestrogenic environment nor LPD preclude use of this modality. The ovulatory goal is 4 to 6 mature (18 to 20 mm) follicles, with ovulation occurring after cycle day 10.

Pharmacology

Gonadotropins directly act on the ovary, stimulating follicular recruitment, selection, and maturation.

Administration and Monitoring

The gonadotropins are available as lyophilized Humegon and Pergonal (75 IU LH plus 75 IU FSH per vial), and Metrodin (partially purified FSH, 75 IU per vial). The drug powder is mixed in 1 cc of diluent and injected intramuscularly. A common initial daily dose is 2 ampules. Higher doses may be used in women with an elevated day 3 FSH level and in those with an inadequate response in a prior cycle. Lower doses should be considered in women with PCOS.

TVUS is used to determine ovarian quiescence at onset of therapy, to monitor follicular development, and to define when to trigger ovulation with hCG. Large residual follicles (larger than 2.5 cm) present at baseline evaluation (cycle days 2 to 3) may secrete estrogen and interfere with COH. Delaying the cycle for a month is recommended. If multiple follicles of intermediate size (1.5 to 2.5 cm) are present at baseline, we consider postponing the cycle because, even in the absence of estrogen secretion, their size alone may hinder monitoring.

Nightly gonadotropin injections usually begin on cycle day 2 or 3. Preovulatory follicles are evaluated by TVUS on cycle day 8. Twelve or more intermediate-size follicles on each ovary indicates an increased risk of ovarian hyperstimulation syndrome (OHSS) and the need for close monitoring. In the absence of alarming findings, patients return for TVUS monitoring of periovulatory follicles. When the dominant follicles mature (16–18 mm), 10,000 IU hCG is administered intramuscularly and is followed by intrauterine insemination 36 hours later. In the event of significant follicular lag in some dominant follicles, ovulation may be delayed by withholding menotropins for 24 hours prior to hCG administration. If spontaneous LH surge is evidenced by urinary kits during this interval, we supplement with 10,000 IU hCG and perform intrauterine insemination 36 hours later.

Results

Overall, pregnancy rates are 15 to 20 percent per cycle. Pregnancy rates are generally lower in PCOS patients than in patients with hypoestrogenic amenorrheas. Cycle fecundity declines substantially after the first 3 to 4 cycles of COH/IUI, especially in nonhypoestrogenic patients; thus, we review options and plans with patients after each three treatment cycles.

Side Effects and Complications

Patients commonly note periovulatory pelvic heaviness and discomfort, as well as bruising and soreness at injection sites. Occasionally, patients experience low-grade fevers or increased emotional liability.

OHSS is the most serious gonadotropin therapy complication. Manifestations range from mild to severe. Mild OHSS is most common. Patients are given warning signs and are managed as outpatients, with daily measurement of weight, fluid intake, urine output, and abdominal girth, as well as activity restrictions.

Patients with severe OHSS may suffer from the consequences of extreme ovarian enlargement (pain, hemorrhagic cysts, torsion), vasculature hyperpermeability (ascites, hypoproteinemia, electrolyte imbalance, hemoconcentration, oliguria, and pulmonary edema). These patients are hospitalized and are given symptomatic supportive therapy. Surgical exploration is very rarely required, and is reserved for patients with ovarian torsion or active hemoperitoneum.

Severe OHSS most commonly occurs in patients who achieve pregnancy. Additionally, if ovulation does not occur, the syndrome is much milder. Thus, hCG is withheld, and exposure to sperm is prevented in high risk patients. Each center must determine its own criteria for OHSS risk management. At our center, we usually withhold hCG and IUI for serum estradiol levels greater than 2,000 pg per milliliter, although this is highly individualized.

Multiple gestations are significantly increased, with twins occurring in 20 to 30 percent of pregnancies, triplets in 1 to 2 percent, and quadruplets in less than 1 percent. Congenital malformations are not increased by gonadotropin therapy. Spontaneous abortions occur in up to 25 percent of gonadotropin-induced pregnancies, representing an increase over the abortion frequency in natural cycles.

The possibility that gonadotropin COH enhances the risk of borderline or epitheial ovarian cancer is supported by some studies, although definite causality has not been shown. Further studies are necessary and ongoing. We inform our patients of the possible enhanced risk of ovarian cancer, but stress that even if substantiated, the overall risk of ovarian cancer remains low. In patients younger than 30, the increased ovarian cancer risk may be minimized by eliminating the risk associated with nulliparity.

Cost Issues

This method of ovulation induction is expensive, as well as more invasive and time consuming than the other modalities of COH.

Progesterone or hCG Therapy for Luteal Phase Support

Indications

Luteal phase support is necessary in patients with LPD or hypothalamic amenorrhea, over the lifetime of the corpus luteum, i.e., through the eighth gestational week. We also prescribe luteal phase support in patients undergoing gonadotropin COH.

Pharmacology

Progesterone directly supports the pregnancy, while hCG stimulates corpus luteal secretion of progesterone.

Administration and Monitoring

Progesterone is adequately absorbed with intramuscular or transmucosal delivery. Oral administration is fraught by inconsistent bioavailability and is not recommended. We commonly prescribe vaginal progesterone suppositories (25 to 50 mg twice a day). Alternative regimens are progesterone oil (12.5 mg per day IM) or hCG (5,000 IU IM, injected on alternating days). Luteal support is initiated on the third postovulatory day, and is discontinued at the completion of the tenth gestational week or at the onset of menses. We obtain a serum hCG on the fifteenth postovulatory day if menses has not begun, to differentiate between a pregnancy and a progesterone-related delay. Progesterone is discontinued if pregnancy is not detected.

In patients with LPD, an endometrial biopsy (EMB) during a progesterone treatment cycle is needed to confirm that in-phase endometrium is achieved. We offer patients the option of performing this EMB in a "mock" cycle in which no exposure to sperm is planned, or a "real" cycle, accepting the very small risk of biopsy-related pregnancy injury.

Results

Most studies of luteal phase support in LPD are small, with reported pregnancy rates ranging from 10 to 50 percent per cycle. Luteal phase support is commonly used in COH although clinical trials do not clearly demonstrate an improvement in pregnancy rates.

Side Effects and Complications

Progesterone therapy may slightly delay menses. Some patients experience premenstrual syndrome–like symptoms, which resolve spontaneously. Occasionally, patients become depressed, and therapy may need to be discontinued.

Cost Issues

Progesterone is relatively inexpensive. Vaginal suppository preparations must be prepared by the local pharmacist.

GnRH Agonist (Lupron, Buserelin, Nafarelin) Therapy in COH

Indications

GnRH agonists can be used to prevent premature spontaneous ovulation in patients undergoing COH.

Pharmacology

GnRH agonists bind to gonadotrope GnRH receptors, inciting an initial phase of enhanced secretion of LH and FSH, and subsequently enhance ovarian steroid secretion, the "flare," for 2 to 3 weeks. The second phase, "down-regulation" of pituitary gonadotropin secretion, is sustained for the remainder of the therapeutic course.

Administration and Monitoring

Two types of protocols are available. In the down-regulation protocol, leuprolide (0.5 to 1 mg SQ daily) is followed by gonadotropin therapy after serum gonadotropins and estradiol levels are suppressed. This protocol increases the gonadotropin requirement by approximately 2 ampules per day. We favor this protocol when premature LH surges interfere with effective COH.

In the "flare" protocol, leuprolide (0.5 to 0.75 mg SQ daily) and daily gonadotropins are initiated simultaneously in the first three days of the cycle (usually day 2 or 3). This approach takes advantage of the endogenous gonadotropin flare, and may be useful in reducing gonadotropin requirements in highly resistant ovaries. The extent of the flare, however, is unpredictable. In both protocols, leuprolide is discontinued after ovulation is triggered, and luteal phase support is commonly provided.

Results

Evidence of benefits from GnRH agonist use in hMG COH protocols, without assisted reproductive technologies, is limited; therefore GnRH agonist therapy is reserved for patients with proven premature ovulation.

Side Effects and Complications

Patients experience menopausal symptoms, including hot flushing, emotional liability, or disturbances of sleep and memory. These symptoms remit with cessation of therapy. Leuprolide has not been shown to increase congenital malformations or spontaneous abortion rates.

Cost Issues

GnRH agonist therapy raises the cost of COH cycles, but the reduction of cycle cancellations may be overall cost effective.

Bromocriptine (Parlodel)

Indications

Bromocriptine is indicated in hyperprolactinemic patients and in euprolactinemic patients with galactorrhea and ovulatory dysfunctions.

Pharmacology

Hyperprolactinemia diminishes GnRH secretion, leading to ovulatory disturbances and infertility. Bromocriptine is an ergot derivative with dopamine (type II) receptor agonist properties. It normalizes the prolactin levels in hyperprolactinemic patients by inhibiting both prolactin gene transcription and mRNA accumulation in lactotrophs. Return of ovulation in euprolactinemic galactorrheic patients probably involves the reduction of bioavailable, nonimmunoreactive, prolactin.

Administration and Monitoring

We initiate therapy with a daily dose of 2.5 mg oral bromocriptine and adjust as needed after 2 weeks of therapy. The intravaginal route is used in patients with GI side effects. Bromocriptine therapy is further discussed in the chapter *Prolactinoma.*

Results

Ovulation is re-established in most patients. In the absence of other fertility factors, pregnancy often occurs with no further therapy.

Side Effects and Complications

Bedtime administration of bromocriptine minimizes dizziness until tolerance develops, usually within a couple of weeks. GI complaints are minimized by vaginal transmucosal absorption, which is very efficient and requires about half the oral dose.

Cost Issues

Bromocriptine is relatively inexpensive.

■ SURGICAL APPROACH TO PCOS

The surgical approach to correcting the hyperandrogenemia in PCOS is reserved for patients who fail medical therapy with clomiphene and gonadotropins. Patients who do not conceive spontaneously postoperatively are often rendered sensitive to clomiphene therapy despite their prior resistance. Ovarian wedge resection in PCOS eliminates at least one-fourth of the ovarian cortex in order to significantly decrease ovarian stromal volume and androgen secretion. The reduction in testosterone levels is maintained for months and is associated with return of menses and fertility. Pregnancy rates as high as 63 percent have been reported. Laparoscopic "ovarian drilling" with laser or electrocautery achieves similar hormonal and fertility results and is favored today if surgery must be done. Postoperative adhesive disease, with inherent risks of infertility and pelvic pain, is an undesired complication seen with both techniques. Additionally, the long-term effects of extensive ovarian cortical damage have not been elucidated.

Suggested Reading

Donesky BW, Adashi EY. Surgically induced ovulation in the polycystic ovary syndrome: Wedge resection revisited in the age of laparoscopy. Fertil Steril 1995; 63:439.

Healy DL, Trounson AO, Andersen AN. Female infertility: Causes and treatment. Lancet 1994; 343:1539.

Jacobs HS. Polycystic ovary syndrome: Aetiology and management. Curr Opin Obstet Gynecol 1995; 7:203.

Keye WR Jr, Chang RJ, Rebar RW, Soules MR. Infertility evaluation and treatment. Philadelphia: WB Saunders, 1995.

Morris RS, Sauer MV. New advances in the treatment of infertility in women with ovarian failure. Curr Opin Obstet Gynecol 1993; 5:368.

Olive DL. The role of gonadotropins in ovulation induction. Am J Obstet Gynecol 1995; 172:759.

Saenger P. Clinical review 48: The current status of diagnosis and therapeutic intervention in Turner's syndrome. J Clin Endocrinol Metab 1993; 77:297.

Santoro N, Elzahr D. Pulsatile gonadotropin-releasing hormone therapy for ovulatory disorders. Clin Obstet Gynecol 1993; 36:727.

Shushan A, Paltiel O, Isocovich J, et al. Human menopausal gonadotropin and the risk of epithelial ovarian cancer. Fertil Steril 1996; 65:13.

Speroff L. The effect of aging on fertility. Curr Opin Obstet Gynecol 1994; 6:115.

Speroff L, Glass RH, Kase NG. Clinical gynecologic endocrinology and infertility. 5th ed. Baltimore: Williams & Wilkins, 1994.

Van der Meer M, Hompes PG, Scheele F, et al. Follicle stimulating hormone (FSH) dynamics of low dose step-up ovulation induction with FSH in patients with polycystic ovary syndrome. Hum Reprod 1994; 9:1612.

ENDOMETRIOSIS

Richard J. Falk, M.D.
Preston C. Sacks, M.D.

Endometriosis is the presence of endometrial-like glands and stroma in a location other than the lining of the uterine cavity. Responsive to cyclical ovarian hormones, the small blister-like implants are colored by trapped blood pigments and have been compared, in a less politically correct era, to "tobacco-spit" or "gunpowder burns." More recently, small nonpigmented lesions have been described and are felt to be early forms of the disease. Large ovarian endometriotic cysts (endometriomas) are called "chocolate cysts" because of their brown, viscous contents.

Symptoms of endometriosis are related to the location of lesions and their associated and often dense adhesions. The most common symptoms, dysmenorrhea and dyspareunia, reflect involvement of the pelvic peritoneum, ovaries, and uterosacral ligaments. Intestinal involvement may result in tenesmus, melena, or obstruction. Cyclical hematuria or dysuria, or ureteral obstruction can result from urinary tract endometriosis. Rarely, endometriosis may be found in the pleural cavity, resulting in catamenial hemothorax or pneumothorax. Palpating a retroverted, fixed uterus with tender, nodular uterosacral ligaments or the presence of a persistent ovarian cyst suggests endometriosis. Many women with endometriosis, however, have no obvious symptoms and present only with infertility. Although traditionally associated with infertility, endometriosis is clearly the cause only when extensive lesions or adhesions impede ovum pickup or transport. The relationship of minimal disease with infertility is less clear.

Diagnosis is definitively made by direct observation or biopsy, usually via laparoscopy. It is generally felt that 10 to 15 percent of fertile women and 25 to 35 percent of infertile women are affected, making endometriosis one of the most prevalent disorders in gynecology. Some tumor markers, notably CA-125, are often elevated in women with endometriosis. The wide variety of reasons for CA-125 elevation limits its specificity as a marker for endometriosis. The greatest utility of tumor markers appears to be in the long-term management of patients known to have endometriosis. Once a baseline value is obtained, increases in disease activity may be identified by noting an increase in the serum level of CA-125. This is particularly helpful in distinguishing whether exacerbations in pelvic pain are related to increased endometriosis activity or to an unrelated condition.

Several clinical observations indicate an association between endometriosis and gonadal steroids: (1) endometriosis is rarely found before menarche, (2) the symptoms fluctuate with the menstrual cycle, and (3) symptoms and objective physical findings frequently improve during pregnancy and regress after menopause. In view of this relationship, surgical castration was an early therapy for severe endometriosis. Good symptomatic relief was usually achieved, at the expense of rendering the woman sterile.

Surgery still plays a significant role in the therapy of endometriosis. Milder forms of the disease are often diagnosed by laparoscopy, and destruction of the lesions, by excision, electrocautery, or laser vaporization is usually carried out concomitantly. More extensive endometriosis, with ovarian endometriomas, and/or extensive adhesions, neither of which responds well to hormonal therapy, are best treated by surgery as well. The approach may be laparotomy or laparoscopy, depending on the extent of the disease and the experience of the surgeon. Bowel and ureteral obstruction are also indications for surgery. Surgical castration still plays a role when more conservative methods have failed and fertility is no longer desired.

■ HORMONAL THERAPY

Nonsurgical manipulation of the hormonal environment has been used to treat endometriosis for over 50 years. The object of all available hormonal therapies is the inhibition of cyclical ovarian function, with resultant atrophy of the implants. Estrogens, androgens, progestins, and gonadotropin-releasing hormone (GnRH) analogues have all been widely used, both alone and as adjuncts to surgery (Table 1).

Estrogens

Estrogen in high doses can suppress ovulation. In the 1940s and 1950s high doses of estrogen were utilized to treat endometriosis-related symptoms. There were reported clinical successes, though the stimulatory effect of estrogens on the endometrium frequently resulted in hyperplasia and breakthrough bleeding. Today, estrogens have no place in the management of the disease, except in combination with other agents.

Androgens

Androgens have been employed in the treatment of endometriosis. Ten milligrams of oral methyltestosterone daily for 30 days, followed by 5 mg daily for 2 to 3 months, can result in symptomatic relief. Interestingly, ovulation is frequently not inhibited at these doses, suggesting a direct effect of androgen on the lesion. Side effects of androgenization (e.g., hirsutism, increased muscle mass, voice deepening) make this treatment undesirable for most patients. We have seen the occasional patient whose discomfort responded poorly to other medical therapy and for whom surgery was not feasible but who responded well to methyltestosterone.

Estrogen-Progestin Combinations (Birth Control Pills)

In the late 1950s, appreciation of the potent gonadotropin-suppressing activity of oral contraceptives spurred the use of these estrogen-progestin combinations for the treatment of endometriosis. Administered continuously for 6 to 9 months instead of cyclically (as for contraception), they produce a pharmacologic "pseudopregnancy." Birth control pills were the principal hormonal treatment for endometriosis in the 1960s and 1970s. The variety of preparations available allows individualization of treatment to minimize breakthrough

Table 1 Drugs Used for the Treatment of Endometriosis

MEDICATION	DOSAGE AND ADMINISTRATION	SIDE EFFECTS	ESTIMATED COST PER MONTH*
Androgen	Methyltestosterone 10 mg PO q day for 30 days, then 5 mg q day for 2-3 months	Acne, weight gain, hirsutism, changes in lipid profile	$25
Oral contraceptives	Active pill every day	Bloating, breakthrough bleeding	$20-25
Progestational agents	Medroxyprogesterone acetate 10 mg t.i.d.	Bloating, breakthrough bleeding	$30-50
Oral			
Depot	Depot medroxyprogesterone acetate 400 mg IM every 2 weeks for 4 doses, then 400 mg IM every 4 weeks	Bloating, breakthrough bleeding, prolonged anovulation	$40-80
Danazol	200-400 mg PO b.i.d.	Acne, weight gain, hirsutism, voice deepening, changes in lipid profile	$200-400
GnRH agonists		Hot flushes, vaginal dryness, loss of libido, sleep disturbances, loss of bone density	
Nafarelin	Synarel 200 μg intranasally b.i.d.		$325
Goserelin	Zoladex 3.6 mg SC every 28 days		$360
Lueprolide injection	Lupron 1 mg SC daily		$540
Leuprolide depot	Lupron depot 3.75 mg IM monthly		$380

*Average wholesale price. From Drug topics red book. Montvale, NJ: Medical Economics, 1995; with permission.

bleeding, which is more common with the low estrogen pills. There is no convincing evidence that any single preparation is therapeutically superior. It is therefore our policy to begin treatment with a pill of moderate strength, containing the equivalent of 35 μg ethinyl estradiol and 1 mg norethindrone. Although breakthrough bleeding occurs invariably in the first few months of treatment, continued administration usually produces the desired amenorrhea. Should amenorrhea not occur, or if the patient is upset by the inconvenience of the spotting, a preparation with 50 μg ethinyl estradiol may be substituted. Should the vaginal bleeding continue, the patient is advised to double the dosage for a few days. If this proves unsuccessful, endometrial pathology should be ruled out before continuing the therapy. Ultrasonography may demonstrate a submucous leiomyoma or endometrial polyp, and endometrial biopsy will rule out endometrial hyperplasia or carcinoma.

Efficacy of birth control pills is difficult to assess, due to the paucity of large controlled studies. It is reasonably clear that pain relief is attained in 80 to 90 percent of patients, although the rate of recurrence of symptoms is high upon cessation of treatment. The pregnancy rate following therapy in infertile patients is approximately 40 percent, not significantly different from expectant management in some studies.

Contraindications to this therapy, including hepatic disease, a history of thromboembolic phenomena, hypertension, and the presence of estrogen-sensitive neoplasms, have been exhaustively reviewed. If the patient has or is at risk for such conditions, progestins may be employed without estrogen.

Prophylaxis of recurrence by means of lower dose, cyclical oral contraceptives has been widely used, and although statistically significant proof of efficacy is lacking, it seems a reasonable approach in the young patient who does not desire pregnancy.

Progestins

Oral medroxyprogesterone acetate, 10 mg three times daily, is sufficient to inhibit ovulation and has been utilized to treat dysmenorrhea and dyspareunia related to endometriosis. Most studies show good relief from pain but no impact on subsequent fertility rates.

The principal problem with progestin therapy is irregular breakthrough bleeding. This may be minimized by using the depot form of the drug, which is administered 400 mg IM every 2 weeks for four doses, then every 4 weeks for another 5 months. Serious complications with "progestin-only" therapy, such as thromboembolic phenomena, have been reported only rarely. A monthly injection may be seen as an advantage over the large number of pills necessary by the oral route, but the long half-life of the depot form results in a prolonged amenorrhea following cessation of treatment. This may create a problem for those women whose therapeutic goal is fertility in addition to pain relief. Furthermore, studies have failed to show improved pregnancy rates following cessation of therapy. We therefore utilize progestins mainly in the older woman with severe symptomatic disease who does not desire pregnancy and in whom the use of combined estrogen-progestin preparations is ill advised, who cannot undergo surgery, and for whom the financial burdens of other medications (see below) is too great.

Danazol

An isoxazol derivative of 17-ethinyl testosterone, danazol was originally believed to reduce gonadotropin levels with concomitant reduction in estrogen and little or no demonstrable estrogenic or progestational activity; indeed, it was felt to induce a "pseudomenopause." In actuality, however, studies on the hormonal effects of the drug show it to block the mid-cycle FSH and LH surge, without lowering the baseline levels of the gonadotropins. It exhibits significant androgenic activity, as suggested by its structure, and binds not only to androgen receptors but to progesterone and glucocorticoid receptors as well. A progestin-like effect on the endometrium has also been demonstrated. Recent studies have shown danazol to inhibit in vitro stimulation of endometrial cells by monocyte-derived growth stimulating factors. The action of danazol on endometriosis is therefore probably via several mechanisms.

Side effects are primarily androgenic and include weight gain, muscle cramps, reduced breast size, flushing, mood changes, oily skin, depression, edema, acne, hirsutism, and voice deepening. It is effective in controlling pain in about 90 percent of patients, but symptoms recur in about one-third of them. Although some studies show a response superior to progestin therapy, others show similar results. Its effect on infertility ascribed to endometriosis has some theoretical validity. Peritoneal fluid of endometriosis patients is toxic to mouse embryos, but not after treatment with danazol. Despite this, clinical pregnancy rates after treatment are about 40 percent, similar to those seen with expectant management.

GnRH Agonists

A variety of GnRH agonists have been synthesized, many of which bind more readily than native GnRH to the receptor and have reduced susceptibility to the peptidases. This results in greater potency than native GnRH (about 100×) with a longer half-life (~2.5×). These agonists bind to receptors in the pituitary gland and initially stimulate release of follicle-stimulating hormone and luteinizing hormone. With continued administration, receptor down-regulation occurs, and within 2 to 4 weeks a hypogonadotropic hypoestrogenic state is achieved. This hormonal suppression is maintained as long as administration of the agonist continues. The benefits of GnRH agonist administration result from the reduction in estrogenic stimulation of the endometriotic implants. As would be expected, there is no significant effect on adhesions or endometriomas. The hypoestrogenic state leads to significant side effects, such as hot flushes, vaginal dryness, and loss of trabecular bone, limiting long-term clinical utility. In particular, administration of GnRH agonists for 6 months leads to a 3 to 14 percent decrease in bone density. While there may be some recovery following cessation of therapy, it is not usually complete, resulting in an increased risk for osteoporosis.

There are three GnRH analogues approved by the Food and Drug Administration (FDA) for the treatment of endometriosis-related symptoms—nafarelin acetate, leuprolide acetate, and goserelin acetate. These medications are indicated for the short-term (6 months) treatment of endometriosis-related symptoms. The major differences among these agents are the routes of administration and frequency of dosage.

Nafarelin acetate (Synarel), which has a D-Naphthyl-Ala(2) substitution at position 6, is available as a nasal spray that delivers a metered dose of 200 µg. Synarel is administered twice daily. While the nasal route of administration may be attractive to patients, compliance is a problem with long-term administration.

Leuprolide acetate (Lupron) has a D-Leu at position 6 and an ethylamide substitution at position 10. It is available as a daily subcutaneous injection or in depot form (Lupron Depot) as a monthly intramuscular injection. Localized reactions at the site of injection occur in less than 5 percent of patients and may be treated with anti-inflammatory agents and antihistamines.

Goserelin acetate (Zoladex) is a available as a 1 mm diameter cylinder containing goserelin dispersed in a lactic and glycolic acid matrix. Goserelin contains a D-Ser(Bu) substitution at position 6 and a modification of position 10, making it particularly long acting. The cylinder containing goserelin is inserted monthly into the subcutaneous tissue of the upper abdominal wall with a preloaded syringe with a 16-gauge needle. As with Lupron, localized reactions are rare and easily treated with anti-inflammatory agents and antihistamines.

GnRH analogues have gained widespread acceptance in the medical management of endometriosis-related symptoms. In controlled trials, these agents show benefits similar to danazol; the major difference is in the side effects. Danazol use is associated with androgenic side effects, whereas use of GnRH agonists produces hypoestrogenic side effects.

In an effort to improve compliance and counteract the hypoestrogenic side effects, physicians have utilized a regimen known as "add-back" therapy. In add-back therapy, additional medications are given in order to combat the hot flushes and vaginal dryness associated with GnRH agonist use. Generally women will respond to small doses of estrogen without exacerbation of the symptoms associated with endometriosis. There is favorable experience with both transdermal estradiol 0.05 mg and oral estrogen (equivalent of 0.625 mg conjugated estrogens). Clinical data, however, show these dosages may not be adequate to prevent bone loss with extended GnRH agonist therapy. It is our practice to follow women on add-back therapy with a bone density measurement 6 months following initiation of therapy to identify those persons who will continue to lose bone mass. In these cases, one may increase the dosage of estrogen or add another medication, such as a bisphosphonate.

There is some experience with the use of bisphosphonates as adjuvant therapy in women receiving GnRH analogues. In one study, cyclic sodium etidronate and norethindrone were administered to women along with GnRH agonist for 12 months. There was good relief of endometriosis symptoms and no change in bone density. Recently, alendronate (Fosamax) was approved by the FDA for the treatment of osteoporosis. The dose of alendronate is 10 mg PO daily. Side effects are mostly related to gastrointestinal disturbances and may be minimized by taking the medication first thing in the morning on an empty stomach. There is much hope that the combination of GnRH agonist, low-dose estrogen, and alendronate may allow for safe and effective long-term medical management of the patient with endometriosis.

Suggested Reading

Dawood MY, Ramos J, Khan-Dawood FS. Depot leuprolide acetate versus danazol for treatment of pelvic endometriosis: Changes in vertebral bone mass and serum estradiol and calcitonin. Fertil Steril 1995; 6:1177–1183.

Howell R, Edmonds DK, Dowsett M, et al. Gonadotropin-releasing hormone analogue (goserelin) plus hormone replacement therapy for the treatment of endometriosis: A randomized controlled trial. Fertil Steril 1995; 3:474–481.

Keefe DL. Endometriosis and reproductive function. Assisted Reprod Rev 1995; 5:224–230.

Lemay A, Surrey, Friedman. Extending the use of gonadotropin-releasing hormone agonists: The emerging role of steroidal and nonsteroidal agents. Fertil Steril 1994; 1:21–34.

Surrey ES, Voigt B, Fournet N, Judd HL. Prolonged gonadotropin-releasing hormone agonist treatment of symptomatic endometriosis: The role of cyclic sodium etidronate and low-dose norethindrone "add-back" therapy. Fertil Steril 1995; 4:747–755.

PELVIC INFLAMMATORY DISEASE

William J. Ledger, M.D.

Any assessment of the therapy of pelvic inflammatory disease (PID) has to acknowledge several shortfalls in our knowledge. In many instances, physicians have difficulty making the diagnosis of PID. In addition, our knowledge of treatment outcomes with antibiotics is limited to the patient's acute response. The long-term effects of these therapeutic interventions on tubal potency and fertility have not been studied in detail.

■ MICROBIOLOGY

The two organisms that are clearly pathogens for the genital tract of sexually active women are *Neisseria gonorrhoeae* and *Chlamydia trachomatis.* Any scheme for the evaluation of patients with suspected PID must include antimicrobial agents effective against both of these organisms. Unfortunately for the physician who wants a straightforward agenda, most patients with PID do not have either of these organisms. PID usually involves a wide variety of gram-positive and gram-negative aerobic and anaerobic organisms. This microbial complexity has influenced the recommendations to use more than one antibiotic in its treatment.

■ DIAGNOSIS

It is often difficult to diagnose PID. When I make this statement to residents in training at city hospitals with many poor patients, my remarks are greeted with skepticism. These trainees have extensive experience in emergency room PID in which the patient is febrile, has a purulent discharge from the cervix, and has uncontrolled tenderness when the adnexa are palpated during the initial pelvic examination. "What difficulty?" they wonder. This spectrum of obvious pelvic infection in nonpregnant women has been documented in women with PID in whom *N. gonorrhoeae* has been isolated.

In contrast to these obvious cases, most women with acute PID have few or no symptoms. The classic clinical and laboratory signs of acute PID are lower abdominal pain, fever, tender adnexal swelling or a mass, and an elevated white blood cell count or sedimentation rate. The shortcomings of these criteria, however, are obvious; too many women with PID would not be diagnosed. Therefore, there have been continued attempts to loosen diagnostic requirements. The Centers for Disease Control and Prevention (CDC) has as minimum criteria lower abdominal tenderness, adnexal tenderness, and cervical motion tenderness. Additional laboratory and imaging studies may detect a specific pathogen or determine whether a tubo-ovarian abscess (TOA) is present. All of these attempts to broaden the indications for treatment increase the number of women who will receive antibiotic therapy. They do not address the problem of the asymptomatic patient who does not seek medical care.

■ MEDICAL THERAPY

Criteria for the admission of women to the hospital for the treatment of PID have not been based upon prospective studies. In general, admission is reserved for the patient judged by the physician to be seriously ill, for example, with a TOA or failure to respond to outpatient medical treatment.

Most women with a diagnosis of PID are treated as outpatients. These are the variety of treatment alternatives recommended by the CDC:

1. Cefoxitin 2 g IM plus 1 g probenecid orally or ceftriaxone 250 mg IM or other third-generation parenteral cephalosporin plus doxycycline 100 mg orally twice a day for 14 days.

This regimen effectively covers *N. gonorrhoeae* and *C. trachomatis.* I believe this coverage is inadequate for the treatment of gram-negative anaerobes, as I have seen women with a pelvic abscess days or weeks after receiving this regimen.

2. Ofloxacin 400 mg orally twice a day for 14 days plus clindamycin 450 mg orally four times a day for 14 days or metronidazole 500 mg orally twice a day for 14 days.

This provides much better anaerobic coverage. How well this regimen will be tolerated awaits the clinical experience of a large prospective study.

These are the recommended inpatient regimens:

1. Cefoxitin 2 g IV every six hours or cefotetan 2 g IV every 12 hours; either of these drugs continued for at least 48 hours after significant clinical improvement plus doxycycline 100 mg IV or orally every 12 hours; after significant clinical improvement the oral dosage should be continued to complete a total of 14 days of therapy.

This popular inpatient treatment regimen effectively covers *N. gonorrhoeae* and *C. trachomatis.*

2. Clindamycin 900 mg IV every 8 hours plus gentamicin 2 mg per kilogram IV or IM loading dose followed by 1.5 mg per kg every 8 hours; this combination should be continued for at least 48 hours after significant clinical improvement and followed by either clindamycin 450 mg orally four times a day or doxycycline 100 mg orally twice a day for a total of 14 days of therapy.

This is also a popular inpatient regimen because obstetrician-gynecologists have been using this combination for the treatment of soft-tissue pelvic infections, particularly postpartum endomyometritis, for over a decade. However, oral clindamycin can be problematic if diarrhea develops, and some clinicians do not like to complete therapy with a third antibiotic different from the two that resulted in clinical cure.

3. Ampicillin-sulbactam plus doxycycline or ofloxacin intravenously plus clindamycin or metronidazole. All of these combinations have theoretic appeal. Clinical studies are needed to document treatment outcomes.

■ SURGICAL THERAPY

There has been a steady evolution in the operative care of patients with severe PID. Because of mortality associated with intra-abdominal rupture of TOA, the operative philosophy of the 1950s was complete pelvic organ extirpation. A whole series of discoveries has modified this approach. New knowledge about the importance of gram-negative anaerobes in pelvic abscess formation led to the use of antibiotics effective against this group of bacteria. The presentation of pelvic infection changed with the documentation of unilateral pelvic abscesses as opposed to the all-encompassing bilateral pelvic infection concept of the past. Clearly, complete tissue removal is not needed if the infection is selective, with its attack on adnexa. As a result, a number of gynecologists experimented with abscess aspiration rather than removal of the pelvic organs. To the surprise of conservative American gynecologists, this approach worked. Finally, the explosion of assisted reproductive technology meant that future pregnancy could be achieved even when both tubes were irreversibly blocked, so operative care today is very conservative, with aspiration of selected abscesses under laparoscopic guidance, broad antibiotic coverage, and conservation of all the pelvic organs possible.

Suggested Reading

Centers for Disease Control and Prevention. 1993 sexually transmitted diseases treatment guidelines. MMWR. 1993; 42 (RR-14):75–81.

Golde SH, Israel R, Ledger WJ. Unilateral tubo-ovarian abscess: A distinct entity. Am J Obstet Gynecol 1977; 127:807–810.

Henry-Suchet J, Soler A, Loffredo V. Laparoscopic treatment of tubo-ovarian abscesses. J Reprod Med 1984; 29:579–582.

Jacobson L, Westrom L. Objectivized diagnosis of pelvic inflammatory disease: Diagnostic and prognostic value of routine laparoscopy. Am J Obstet Gynecol 1969; 105:1088–1098.

Ledger WJ. Anaerobic infections. Am J Obstet Gynecol 1975; 123:111–118.

Soper DE, Brockwell NJ, Dalton HP, Johnson D. Observations concerning the microbial etiology of acute salpingitis. Am J Obstet Gynecol 1994; 170:1008–1017.

Vermeeren J, TeLinde RW. Intra-abdominal rupture of pelvic abscesses. Am J Obstet Gynecol 1954; 68:402–408.

VAGINITIS AND CERVICITIS

James L. Breeling, M.D.

Lower genitourinary symptoms are common among adult women in primary care settings, accounting for up to 10 percent of office visits. Symptoms and signs of abnormal vaginal discharge may be caused by a variety of conditions. However, despite inexpensive, simple diagnostic tests and the widespread use of topical antimicrobial preparations, clinicians continue to encounter difficulties because of atypical, recurrent, or mixed infections that respond poorly to treatment. Most important, potentially serious but asymptomatic infection (cervicitis or upper genital tract) should be excluded.

■ HISTORY AND EXAMINATION

Vaginal discharge by itself does not indicate a pathologic process. It is important to concentrate on the presence or absence of intermenstrual or postcoital spotting suggestive of cervicitis, abdominal pain and fever suggestive of pelvic inflammatory disease, and multisystemic complaints suggestive of toxic shock syndrome. A complete and detailed sexual history performed in a skilled and confidential manner is particularly important. Data should include exposure to new sexual partners, patterns of sexual behavior, previous sexually transmitted diseases, and the partner's sexual history.

Physical examination should include a search for evidence of sexually transmitted disease and peritoneal signs suggestive of pelvic inflammatory disease. The pelvic examination should pay attention to the labia and perineum. After insertion of the speculum, the most important finding is any mucopurulent cervical discharge suggestive of *Chlamydia trachomatis, Neisseria gonorrhoeae,* or herpes simplex virus. Vaginal and cervical infection frequently coexist, especially with trichomonal vaginitis. Descriptions of yellow-green discharge *(Trichomonas),* frothy discharge *(Gardnerella),* and curdy discharge *(Candida)* are given but in practice are relatively nonspecific and unreliable. Algorithms based on the clinical findings have low sensitivity and specificity.

■ ROUTINE OFFICE AND LABORATORY TESTING

Rapid tests for the office diagnosis of vaginitis are summarized in Table 1. Routine cultures of vaginal secretions should not be obtained because of wide variety of micro-organisms that can be isolated. Pathogens such as *Gardnerella* and *Candida,* even in high concentrations, in asymptomatic or symptomatic women are not specific for the diagnosis of vaginitis. However, cervical secretions should be routinely examined for *N. gonorrhoeae* by appropriate culture and can be screened for *C. trachomatis* by enzyme-linked immunosorbent assay (ELISA) or other rapid technique.

Table 1 Office Tests for Diagnosis of Vaginitis

	NORMAL	VAGINOSIS	CANDIDIASIS	TRICHOMONIASIS
Cause	None	*Gardnerella* and others	*Candida* spp.	*T. vaginalis*
Symptoms	None	Odor	Itching, discharge	Discharge, odor
Vulvitis	None	Rare	Common with erythema	Rare
Discharge				
Color	Clear, white	Gray	White	Yellow
Type	Floccular	Frothy	Clumped	Profuse
pH	<4.5	>5.0	<4.5	>5.0
Whiff test	None	Positive	None	Positive or none
Microscopic	Normal epithelial cells, gram-positive rods	Clue cells, few PMN, mixed flora	PMN, epithelial cells, yeast	PMN, motile, trichomonads

PMN, polymorphonuclear leukocytes.

BACTERIAL VAGINOSIS

Bacterial vaginosis has been suggested as the proper name for what used to be called nonspecific vaginitis, since there are few clinical signs of inflammation and the cause seems to be a diverse population of organisms including *Gardnerella vaginalis, Mobiluncus* spp., *Mycoplasma hominis,* coliforms, and anaerobic bacteria like *Bacteroides.* Few inflammatory cells are present, and the regular *Lactobacillus* population appears depressed. The four diagnostic criteria for bacterial vaginosis are (1) gray-white homogeneous discharge; (2) pH > 5; (3) fishy amine odor on mixing the discharge with 10 percent potassium hydroxide (KOH); and (4) clue cells on wet mount. Originally attributed to *Gardnerella,* since 95 percent of women with this infection were culture positive, it is now thought to be a mixed infection because 40 to 50 percent of healthy asymptomatic women are culture positive. Microscopic examination of clue cells suggests that most are covered with *Gardnerella,* but occasional clue cells are composed mainly of curved gram-negative rods compatible with *Mobiluncus.* These atypical clue cells have recently been termed comma cells.

Bacterial vaginosis is not usually considered a sexually transmitted disease even though male partners of patients with vaginosis carry urethral *Gardnerella.* Therapy of male partners with metronidazole does not influence the recurrence rate in women. (The exceptions may be men with clinical balanitis and women with refractory symptoms or multiple relapses.) It can also be found in up to 15 percent of prepubertal girls.

Metronidazole is the most effective treatment. This is consistent with the polymicrobial cause of bacterial vaginosis because metronidazole is very active against *Bacteroides fragilis* but only moderately active against *Gardnerella* and *Mobiluncus* and inactive against *Mycoplasma hominis.* Although metronidazole is not active against *Lactobacillus* and therefore is theoretically capable of allowing regrowth of this endogenous species while suppressing anaerobes, in the subpopulation of women with recurrent bacterial vaginosis the normal *Lactobacillus*-dominated flora fails to repopulate. Metronidazole 500 mg orally twice daily for 7 days results in 90 percent cure; 2 g orally as a single dose or on day 1 and 3 as a single dose is associated with similar cure rates but has a high rate of adverse effects, mainly nausea, dysgeusia, and vomiting. Although ampicillin is highly active against *Gardnerella* in vitro, the regimen of 500 mg orally four times a day for 7 days is not as effective as metronidazole; most regimens show a 20 to 30 percent relapse rate when patients are followed for longer than 6 months after cure. Ineffective drugs include erythromycin, tetracycline, and sulfonamide creams. This means that during the first trimester of pregnancy the less effective ampicillin regimen should be used to avoid theoretic concerns over metronidazole's potential for teratogenicity. However, usage of metronidazole in the second and third trimesters appears to be safe. An interesting report found clindamycin 300 mg orally twice daily for 7 days effective in 94 percent of women, but only 49 patients were studied. If further studies support this efficacy, clindamycin may become the drug of choice in pregnancy. Local application of metronidazole-impregnated sponges or a clindamycin cream appear as effective as systemic therapy with fewer side effects and offer a safe option in the pregnant patient.

TRICHOMONAS VAGINITIS

Trichomonas vaginalis is a sexually transmitted vaginal infection. The organism is a motile protozoan specific to humans (*Trichomonas tenax* is found in the mouth, *Trichomonas hominis* in the colon). *T. vaginalis* attaches itself to the vaginal mucosa via a specific receptor also found in the urethra, bladder, prostate, Skene's glands, and ectocervix, leading to multifocal infection requiring systemic therapy for cure.

The signs and symptoms of *T. vaginalis* infection vary considerably with the severity of the inflammatory response. Some 50 to 75 percent of women complain of a profuse frothy yellow discharge. The discharge has a pH above 5 and a foul odor. Vulvar itching is another common complaint. A strawberry cervix is rather specific. A saline wet mount to identify the characteristic jerky motility is very helpful. The sensitivity of microscopy is about 70 percent and the specificity is 100 percent.

T. vaginalis is highly sensitive to metronidazole. A single 2 g dose will cure 90 percent of women if the male sexual partner is simultaneously treated. Topical therapy does not eliminate the organism from the periurethral glands, bladder, and urethra, hence should not be used. Failure to eliminate the organism has also been associated with rare metronidazole-resistant organisms. These may respond to metronidazole 750 mg orally twice daily for 2 weeks, but some have required intravenous metronidazole for cure. If resistance is suspected, culture and sensitivity testing should be done, and the patient advised to use condoms to prevent the spread of the resistant organisms.

First-trimester *T. vaginalis* infections may respond to clotrimazole suppositories for 7 days, but response rates are only 40 to 50 percent. This may palliate the patient until the second or third trimester, when metronidazole may be less of a risk. Metronidazole may be given to a breast-feeding mother, since the infant will only receive about 25 mg of the drug from a single 2 g dose, or breast-feeding can be suspended for 24 hours.

■ VULVOVAGINAL CANDIDIASIS

Candida (spp., including *C. albicans, Torulopsis glabrata, C. tropicalis,* and *C. parapsilosis*) are carried by up to 50 percent of asymptomatic women in the vagina and by 80 to 90 percent of all adults in the gastrointestinal tract. Yeast therefore is an integral part of human microflora. The factors that lead to development of symptomatic vaginal irritation are unknown, although the relative pathogenicity of *Candida* correlates with its ability to adhere to vaginal epithelial cells, with filamentous forms adhering better than yeast forms. Women with symptomatic vulvovaginal candidiasis do not appear to have a higher yeast load than asymptomatic women, but active disease appears to be linked to a predominance of filamentous forms known as pseudohyphae and a paucity of yeast forms. The dissociation of inoculum and symptoms has led some to postulate an allergic or immunologic mechanism, supported by the observation that some men develop penile irritation within hours of sexual contact with infected women.

Risk factors for development of *Candida* vaginitis include antibiotic use, pregnancy, oral contraceptives, diabetes mellitus, immunosuppression, and corticosteroids. Since *Candida* can be part of the normal flora, the condition is not thought to be a sexually transmitted disease, although yeast can infect men causing inflammation of the glans and prepuce. Most forms of topical therapy in women treat male carriers if coitus continues during treatment.

Candidal vulvovaginitis is characterized by vulvar itching, burning, or other irritation, often associated with external dysuria and with scant, nonmalodorous discharge. The discharge is usually clumpy and adherent to an inflamed mucosa. Diagnosis is based on 10 percent KOH preparation; adding one or two drops of 10 percent KOH to a drop of discharge, stirring, adding a cover slip and allowing digestion of the debris for 60 seconds or heating gently over a flame for 10 seconds. The sensitivity of this test ranges from 40 to 70 percent, depending on the skill of the observer; however, almost all women are culture positive even if asymptomatic. This leads one to offer treatment to symptomatic women with no other diagnosis with prominent vulvar itching and a normal vaginal pH even if the KOH prep is negative. Reliance on culture data will result in overtreatment of patients and possibly lead to further imbalance in the vaginal ecology.

With the imidazole topical antifungal agents, superior results can be obtained with daily application for 7 days than with older regimens using nystatin or mycostatin twice daily for 2 weeks. The drugs of choice are miconazole or clotrimazole cream 100 mg at bedtime daily for 7 days. Follow-up cultures should not be performed because cultures usually remain positive even when symptoms resolve. Prevention of recurrent symptomatic infection is one of the major problems in the management of vaginitis. The idea that rectal carriage of *Candida* is associated with relapse is not correct: studies of oral nonabsorbable antifungal therapy in conjunction with vaginal therapy have failed to show fewer relapses. Some women have regular recurrences linked to the menstrual cycle and should keep a log of symptoms. If a distinct pattern can be seen, self-diagnosis and prophylactic treatment with 3 to 5 days of clotrimazole or miconazole at the same time each month may be the best strategy. Topical treatment of the skin under the prepuce of the clitoris may reduce the frequency of symptoms. Oral ketoconazole prophylaxis of 100 mg orally daily has been studied and is very effective for women with the most severe symptoms, but relapse occurs and the drug has been associated with serious hepatotoxicity. Oral fluconazole offers a significant advance, since this drug is more potent in vitro against most *Candida* strains and produces less hepatotoxicity. Vaginitis has been studied with a dose 50 mg orally for three days or a single 150 mg oral dose has been found to have a similar cure rate as topical clotrimazole.

■ CERVICITIS

Yellowish, thick secretions in the cervical canal or a large number of polymorphonuclear leukocytes on gram stain of cervical secretions is evidence of mucopurulent cervicitis. The major infectious causes are *C. trachomatis, N. gonorrhoeae,* and herpes simplex. A swab of the endocervical mucus should be obtained for gram stain to diagnose gonorrhea (sensitivity for gram-negative diplococci 50–70 percent, sensitivity of culture 90 percent). *Chlamydia* can be identified by immunofluorescence, ELISA, or DNA probe using commercial kits. However, routine testing for *Chlamydia* is not necessary to initiate therapy when *Chlamydia* is suspected.

Because 30 to 60 percent of women with cervicitis may have coinfection with *Neisseria* and *Chlamydia,* simultaneous treatment of both conditions is recommended. Gonorrhea can be treated with a single dose of one of the following: ceftriaxone 125 mg IM, cefixime 400 mg orally, ciprofloxacin 500 mg orally, or ofloxacin 400 mg. (See the chapter on *Neisseria gonorrhoeae.*) *Chlamydia* is treated with doxycycline 100 mg orally twice daily for 7 days or azithromycin 1 g orally in a single dose. Alternative regimens are ofloxacin 300 mg orally twice daily for 7 days or erythromycin base 500 mg orally 4 times a day for 7 days or erythromycin ethylsuccinate 800 mg orally 4 times daily for 7 to 14 days. Only the latter two erythromycin regimens are acceptable for treatment of *Chlamydia* in pregnant women. If erythromycin cannot be tolerated by the pregnant woman, amoxicillin 500 mg orally 3 times daily for 7 to 10 days is acceptable.

Suggested Reading

Lossick JG. Treatment of sexually transmitted vaginosis/vaginitis. Rev Infect Dis 1990; 12(Suppl 6):S665–S681.

Lugo-Miro VI, Green M, Mazur L. Comparison of different metronidazole therapeutic regimens for bacterial vaginosis. JAMA 1992; 268:92–95.
Schmitt C, Sobel JD, Meriwether C. Bacterial vaginosis: Treatment with clindamycin cream versus oral metronidazole. Obstet Gynecol 1992; 79:1020–1023.
Sobel JD. Bacterial vaginosis—an ecologic mystery. Ann Intern Med 1989; 111:551–553.
Vuylsteke B, Laga M, Alary M, et al. Are clinical algorithms useful to screen women for the presence of gonococcal and chlamydial infection? Clin Infect Dis 1993; 17:82–88.

BENIGN BREAST DISEASE

Régine Sitruk-Ware, M.D.

Although for many years breast disease of benign origin was considered unimportant, the established relationship between benign breast disease and breast cancer has justified detection and treatment. Benign breast lesions are now considered an evolutionary link between the normal and the cancerous breast. Epidemiologic data suggest an increased risk of breast cancer in women in whom a breast biopsy has confirmed a benign breast lesion, especially if there was proliferative disease with atypia. Therefore properly diagnosing benign breast disease and offering a therapy to these patients is highly justified.

Clinical examination is essential for the differential diagnosis of breast disease and, together with the breast x-ray and the breast biopsy, allows the physician to make an accurate diagnosis in 99 percent of the cases. The causes of benign breast disease are essentially hormonal. There is good evidence from in vivo and in vitro studies to support the hypothesis of luteal insufficiency as a common denominator in most types of benign breast disease and especially those with an epithelial proliferative component.

Hormonal imbalance because of spontaneous irregular cycles, oral contraceptive (OC) use, or hormonal replacement therapy (albeit rarely) can lead to breast mastalgia as a short-term consequence and to development of benign breast disease if the same hormonal imbalance persists uncorrected for several months or years.

Mastalgia appears to be a marker for those who are susceptible, and the appearance of this symptom signifies the onset of benign breast disease. It should not be left untreated, especially when its intensity impairs the woman's daily life during the 7 or more days preceding menstruation.

Controversy remains about the role of progestins in breast cell multiplication. Strong arguments favor their main role as a factor in breast cell differentiation and growth arrest. This is supported by the observation of the therapeutic efficacy of relatively high doses of progestogens given to women with benign breast disease.

Among the therapies proposed for the treatment of benign breast disease, antigonadotropic agents are effective as they decrease estrogen secretion. Progestogens, danazol (an androgenic compound), and gonadotropin-releasing hormone agonists have been proposed, progestogens being the most efficacious and well tolerated. Bromocriptine is not universally efficacious in relief of mastalgia.

The use of the antiestrogen tamoxifen and its active derivative 4-hydroxy-tamoxifen has been proposed to control breast cell proliferation and as a preventive therapy in patients at high risk for breast cancer. At present it is premature to treat premenopausal women, free from cancer, with these compounds, especially in view of an increased stimulatory effect on the endometrium. Only long-term prospective studies can determine the risks and benefits of such treatment.

Because the breasts are situated on the surface of the body, they are readily accessible to examination. A systematic examination of the breasts must be included in any general physical examination of the patient, and women should be taught how to examine their own breasts. The characteristic features of physiologic findings and any cyclical pattern should be explained in order to avoid unnecessary anxiety if a woman discovers an apparent abnormality.

The patient herself may seek medical advice either because of pain or because she has accidentally discovered a lump or a nipple discharge. Alternatively the physician may detect a lump(s) or nipple discharge in the course of a general examination. In general, bilateral nodularities are most likely to be benign, whereas an isolated lump is more suspect. A green or yellow nipple discharge is generally benign; a bloody discharge is more likely to reveal a malignant intraductal lesion.

■ CLINICAL CHARACTERISTICS OF BENIGN BREAST DISEASE

Mastalgia

Cyclic pain (mastalgia or mastodynia) must be defined and differentiated from unilateral thoracic pain or intercostal neuralgia. Painful bilateral swelling of the breasts, starting toward the end of the cycle and lasting at least 4 days and up to 3 weeks before menstruation, but which is alleviated after menstruation, is most likely hormone dependent.

In a case-control study of 210 newly diagnosed breast cancers and 210 controls matched for age, age at first full-term pregnancy (FFTP), and socioeconomic status, Plu-Bureau et al. (1992) found a strong association between a previous history of cyclic mastalgia and increased risk of breast cancer. The adjusted relative risk of breast cancer was 2.1 (95 percent confidence interval 1.3 to 3.4) for a history of mastalgia after adjustment for a familial history of breast cancer, personal history of benign breast disease, and age at menarche. Mastalgia, therefore, appears to be a marker of breast cell susceptibility and should not be left untreated, especially when women are incapacitated by severe pain.

Isolated Breast Lumps

The discovery of an isolated breast lump by the patient or her physician often generates anxiety as breast cancer is presumed to be the main differential diagnosis. If, however, the lump is regular, mobile and nonadherent to the skin, it is often found to be either a cyst or a fibroadenoma. The latter usually occurs in young women and varies in size with the cycle, decreasing during the first days, whereas cysts tend to be round or ovoid and fluctuant, their consistency varying according to fluid pressure. This labile characteristic helps to differentiate cysts from carcinoma or an adenoma. They are more frequent in women during the perimenopausal period. Cysts and fibroadenomas can be multiple. Bilaterality is always reassuring, indicating a benign origin.

The endocrine origin of fibroadenomas has been demonstrated by in vitro studies showing the presence of estrogen and progesterone receptors especially in tumors with a high content of epithelial cells. Isolated cysts are found when dilation of epithelial ducts occurs in older women. Their hormone dependence is controversial.

Bilateral Nodularities

The most common decision clinicians have to make is that of distinguishing increased physiologic nodularity from true breast disease. Most women experience increased nodularity of the breasts during the few days before menstruation. The symptoms usually abate after menstruation. The bilateral characteristic of such breast nodules is always reassuring and generally reflects nodular hyperplasia of mammary tissue. Irregular small, round, and regular nodules may be palpated in the upper outer sector of both glands. In practice, increased nodular hyperplasia is found more often in very young patients, whereas cystic disease occurs in the women aged 35 or over.

Cysts and Fibrocystic Disease

Clinically, fibrocystic disease (FCD) presents as bilateral nodularities of different sizes, with some very hard areas perceived on palpation as small, round, regular nodules, or larger "stony" areas. A precise diagnosis is made by histologic examination when both microcysts and fibrotic areas are found, often associated with edema and some proliferative tissue.

Cysts of the breast can be isolated or multiple. They are usually round and well delineated. They are less easy to appreciate when they are deep in a thick breast. Their consistency depends on the fluid pressure within them, soft or firm when tightly distended and usually mobile in the surrounding tissue.

Cysts can suddenly become apparent to the patient, as when a sudden increase in fluid content occurs, usually after a psychological stress. The sudden discovery of such a "tumor" often alarms women. They can be readily reassured, however, when a careful fluid aspiration made at the time of examination by the breast consultant induces an immediate reduction in the swelling.

Nipple Discharge

Spontaneous discharge from the nipple is not a frequent phenomenon, but in many women gentle squeezing of the nipple may produce a drop of greyish material. This is not abnormal and is produced by terminal ectatic ducts. The appearance of a nipple discharge is an important distinguishing feature. A milky discharge—galactorrhea—usually leads to diagnoses other than benign breast disease, e.g., a prolactinoma or drug-induced elevated prolactin secretion. Nipple discharge smears are recommended in all cases of serous or bloody discharge but not with bilateral thin, watery material. Microscopical study of smears enables the diagnosis of papilloma as well as of carcinoma in a considerable number of cases (see the chapter *Galactorrhea*).

■ BREAST CANCER: DIFFERENTIAL DIAGNOSIS

As mentioned above, the differential diagnosis of a benign or a malignant lesion can be made at the clinical examination. The examiner must identify the characteristics that tumors exhibit, namely, size, shape, boundary, consistency, and mobility within the breast.

The shape and boundaries of a tumor may indicate the diagnosis—a rounded and well-defined cyst or adenoma or an irregular and poorly defined cancerous lesion. The consistency may differentiate cysts (elastic and soft) from firm carcinomas, but a calcified fibroadenoma is also hard. The degree of mobility of the tumor is the best guide to its nature. Benign tumors are usually freely mobile, whereas carcinomas are relatively fixed and may induce surrounding tissue retraction.

Only diagnostic tests, however, can definitively determine the diagnosis. The recommended triad to secure diagnosis includes clinical examination, mammography, and breast biopsy. Small cancers cannot be detected by palpation, especially when they are situated deep in the breast and are only revealed by x-ray screening.

■ HORMONE DEPENDENCE OF HUMAN BREAST: CONTROVERSIES

Experimental Data

The human breast is a target organ for the main steroids secreted by the ovary, estradiol (E_2) and progesterone (P). During the menstrual cycle, the mammary gland exhibits physiologic changes that appear to be related to the variation in the secretion of these steroids.

From animal experiments, it seems likely that E_2 stimulates the epithelial cells and the duct growth, whereas P induces the development of acini and counteracts the action of E_2 on the mesenchymal part of the gland. The continuous administration of E_2 to castrated female rodents has been shown to induce proliferation of the tubular system, followed by dilation of ducts, formation of cysts, and stimulation of the connective tissue. These changes are comparable with fibrocystic disease observed in the human.

It has been suggested that long-term exposure to disturbed hormonal balance may result in proliferative lesions with edema leading to mastalgia as the first symptom of breast disease. Dilation of ducts, formation of cysts, and fibrosis then take place.

In women the effects of sex steroids on breast tissue are less well known than their effects on the endometrium, essentially because normal breast tissue is not easy to collect in humans.

In experiments conducted on human breast adenoma cells, it was shown that P regulates E_2 and P receptors in epithelial cells. It was also demonstrated that P stimulates 17-β-dehydrogenase activity, which converts E_2 into E_1, a less active metabolite. The hormone dependence of those adenomas was confirmed in tumors with a high epithelial content. It was also shown that progestins that are 19-norpregnane derivatives decreased cell multiplication in normal human breast cells in culture. These findings, however, have been criticized as being obtained under experimental conditions, and it was argued that under physiologic conditions both E_2 and P stimulate epithelial cell proliferation, contrary to the antiestrogenic effect of P observed in the endometrium.

Analysis of human breast tissue obtained from women undergoing breast surgery for a variety of reasons, but mainly for benign breast disease, showed that mitoses in surrounding "normal tissue" were more frequent in tissue collected during the luteal phase than in tissue collected in the follicular phase. On the other hand, examination of breast tissue from women undergoing plastic surgery for correction of hyperplastic breasts showed a higher number of mitoses in the follicular phase, after which there was a decline and then absence of mitoses during the luteal phase, in which there also seemed to be secretory activity.

It must be stressed that in all models used for breast tissue collection the women cannot be considered as having a normal breast, because they underwent surgery for a specific breast problem. Normal women have no reason to undergo a breast biopsy. Furthermore, breast tissue is permanent, in contrast to the endometrium, which is shed monthly. Hence, a biopsy taken at a given day of the menstrual cycle does not necessarily reflect the effect of steroid secretion on that day but more probably reflects the cumulative effect of several months of hormonal fluctuation.

Luteal Phase Insufficiency as an Endocrine Cause of Breast Disease

It has been suggested that women with benign breast disease have low levels of circulating P together with normal or elevated E_2 plasma levels. On the basis of these findings, the hypothesis was generated that luteal phase insufficiency was a common denominator in the physiopathology of benign breast disease.

Oral Contraceptives and Risk of Benign Breast Disease

Previous epidemiologic findings have indicated a protective role of OCs against fibroadenomas. This effect was observed in users of standard OCs containing 50 μg of ethinyl estradiol (EE) and relatively high doses of progestins. The large Royal College of General Practitioners Study, performed in the early 1970s in 46,000 women, showed that for a fixed dose of EE in the OCs, increasing doses of the same progestogen (a 19-nortestosterone derivative) led to a decreased risk of fibroadenomas in young women. Further studies showed that OCs containing lower doses of steroids did not influence the overall risk for fibroadenomas. A lower risk of FCD was also found in standard OC users, compared with low-dose steroids containing OC.

It must be remembered, however, that the changes in composition of OCs since the mid-1970s may have led to a different hormonal balance at target level and could modify the response of breast tissue. These variations in response may explain the occurrence of mastalgia in a considerable percentage of OC users.

Hormonal Replacement Therapy and Benign Breast Disease

Although mastalgia is a relatively common side effect of postmenopausal estrogen therapy (ET) sometimes related to overdosage, there are few data suggesting that postmenopausal women receiving estrogen replacement therapy may develop benign breast disease.

Recently, a large meta-analysis of epidemiologic studies evaluating the relationship between ET and breast cancer found no association between ET and breast cancer in women with a previous history of benign breast disease. The risk ratio of users versus nonusers was 1.16 (95 percent confidence interval; 0.89 to 1.5), which was not statistically significant.

Some discrepancies between the various epidemiologic studies may be related to the fact that a previous history of benign breast disease is defined differently according to the studies. A history of breast biopsy is usually considered as a marker of benign breast disease, but this may not be the case. Also, the term *fibrocystic disease* has been incorrectly used as a general denomination of any breast condition.

ET should nevertheless be prescribed cautiously in women with a previous history of benign breast disease especially if they had a histologically documented fibrocystic disease with atypia and a history of breast cancer in a first-degree relative (mother or sister).

Postmenopausal Estrogen Therapy and Breast Cancer

The relationship between long-term ET and risk of breast cancer remains controversial. Based on the controversy regarding the role of progesterone and progestins in breast cell proliferation, opinions are divided on whether women receiving ET should receive concomitant sequential progestogen therapy, especially if they have undergone a hysterectomy.

■ RATIONALE FOR TREATMENT OF BENIGN BREAST DISEASE

Benign Breast Disease and Breast Cancer Risk

Since the early 1960s, long-term prospective studies have indicated that women with a previous breast biopsy for benign breast disease were at increased risk of breast cancer. Recently, epidemiologic studies have indicated that the risk was increased, especially in those women who exhibited proliferative lesions associated with fibrocystic disease when atypia was identified. Cysts or fibrosis alone were not associated with an increased risk of breast cancer.

Although, as already discussed, controversy exists as to the effect of steroids on the breast tissue, it has been demonstrated that estrogens can act as promoters of cells previously transformed into intermediate cells under the action of a carcinogenic "initiator" factor. Hence agents able to maintain the mammary cells in a resting state, without increased cell multiplication, might act as "antipromoter" agents, preventing DNA transcription errors leading to increased cell replication.

The justification for the treatment of benign breast disease must be considered in terms of correction of breast cell overproliferation. The fact that only benign breast disease with proliferative lesions leads to an increase in breast cancer risk argues for the necessity for treating these lesions and maintaining breast cells in a low rate of proliferation.

Experimental Approach for Prevention of Breast Tumors

In animal experiments it was found that chemically induced breast cancer is prevented when the mammary gland is completely differentiated by an FFTP prior to exposure to a carcinogen. This observation has led workers to test the hypothesis that synthetic steroids contained in OCs might drive the mammary gland to differentiation and protect it from carcinogen-induced neoplastic transformation.

Experimentally it was found that dimethylbenz[a]anthracene (DMBA)-induced tumor incidence was significantly decreased when animals were previously treated with E_2, P, or both in an increasing efficacy. It was also shown that administration of both steroids induced tissue differentiation similar to the state observed after an FFTP, i.e., rapid and complete differentiation of all terminal end buds into alveolar buds and these to lobules. Although such experiments are not feasible in the human, it is well known that an FFTP at an early age (below the age of 25) leads to decreased risk of breast cancer while nulliparity or a late FFTP (after the age of 35) exposes the woman to a higher risk. The key factor appears to be the full differentiation of the mammary gland. Attempts to stimulate pharmacologically an early differentiation of the gland are, however, premature and further research is urgently needed in this area.

■ THERAPEUTIC OPTIONS

Progesterone and Progestins

The therapeutic approach is based on the fact that in vivo benign breast disease is characterized, at least at the beginning, by a hormonal milieu of inadequate luteal function. In addition, it has been shown that progesterone and progestogen administration in patients with fibroadenoma leads to an increase in 17-β-hydroxysteroid dehydrogenase activity and to an increased retention of progesterone receptors in the nucleus of breast epithelial cells.

Estrane derivatives are particularly effective, acting both as antigonadotropic agents at the pituitary level and as antiestrogenic agents on the breast cell. Also, progesterone dissolved in a hydroalcoholic gel has been shown to be absorbed through the skin and to be concentrated in the mammary tissue. Topical daily application of this gel throughout the cycle has been shown to stimulate 17-β-hydroxysteroid dehydrogenase activity in human breast fibroadenomas. More recently it was shown in Europe that 19-norpregnane derivatives, such as nomegestrol acetate or R5020, also acted to decrease cell proliferation. The former, acting also as an antigonadotropic agent, has been recommended for therapy.

The best treatment for benign breast disease consists of 9 months of cyclic administration of a progestin with antigonadotropic effects, from day 10 to day 25 of the menstrual cycle. Normal cycles will return in most cases after therapy is withdrawn. With irregular cycles, there is a risk of relapse of mastalgia and, later, of breast nodularities, especially if the hormonal imbalance persists for several months. A fresh course of progestin therapy is then advised, with careful follow-up of breast symptoms, lipid and high-density lipoprotein (HDL)-cholesterol levels in plasma, body weight, and blood pressure.

In a cohort study of 1,150 women (20 to 50 years old) with a diagnosis of benign breast disease, it was shown that the use of 19-norsteroid derivatives was significantly associated with a lower risk of breast cancer as compared with untreated women (relative risk 0.48 [95 percent confidence interval 0.25 to 0.90]). In addition, there was a significant linear relationship between the duration of use and the decrease in breast cancer risk (p for trend = 0.02).

Antiestrogens

Tamoxifen has been proposed for treatment of benign breast disease; theoretically it should be effective. In premenopausal women, however, it increases pituitary gonadotropin secretion, as occurs with clomiphene citrate, and hence an increase in ovarian estradiol secretion. The hypersecretion of E_2 displaces the antiestrogen binding to the receptor and can lead to a loss of effect. Moreover, hypersecretion of LH and FSH can lead to formation of ovarian cysts. It has therefore been proposed that antiestrogens be combined with an antigonadotropic agent.

Topical therapy using the active derivative of tamoxifen (4-hydroxy-tamoxifen) has also been proposed. The absorption of this compound through the skin of the breast has been demonstrated; no systemic side effects were observed. Although this treatment looks promising, until the safety of this compound has been proved in long-term trials, it cannot be recommended for young women without cancer.

Antigonadotropic Agents

Danazol

A derivative of 17α-ethyltestosterone has been suggested as an antigonadotropic alternative for the treatment of benign breast disease. High doses of 400 to 600 mg per day are necessary to achieve gonadotropin suppression, but such doses lead to many drawbacks, in particular to a dramatic decrease in HDL cholesterol of 40 to 60 percent. Moreover, the effects of the therapy on benign breast disease are very poor compared with those obtained with 19-norsteroid progestins (see Vorherr, 1986).

Luteinizing Hormone–Releasing Hormone Analogues

The use of luteinizing hormone–releasing hormone agonists or antagonists capable of inducing a reversible chemical castration might be useful in decreasing the circulating levels of E_2. It is not advisable, however, to prescribe such treatments in young women who could develop hypoestrogenic symptoms or bone loss as side effects. Moreover, these drugs do not induce the transformation of the breast tissue into a secretory state nor do they induce the progestin-receptor–mediated effects.

Bromocriptine

Because prolactin is involved in the genesis and growth of mammary cancer in rodents, extensive research has been devoted to prolactin secretion in women with benign breast disease, and bromocriptine was proposed as a therapeutic option. The main indication proposed for bromocriptine was in mastalgia. However, the results obtained have been contradictory, and the side effects of the drug, essentially dizziness, nausea, and vomiting, make its long-term use impractical in the treatment of benign breast disease. Some patients do, however, obtain symptomatic relief, especially if the drug is given vaginally.

Suggested Reading

Clarke CL, Sutherland RL. Progestin regulation of cellular proliferation. Update 1993. Endocr Rev 1993; 11:132–135.

Mauvais-Jarvis P, Sitruk-Ware R, Kuttenn F. The role of hormones in the pathogenesis of benign breast disease. In: Grunfest-Broniatowski S, Esselstyn CB, eds. Controversies in breast disease—Diagnosis and management. New York: Marcel Dekker, 1988:43.

Plu-Bureau G, Thalabard JC, Sitruk-Ware R, et al. Cyclical mastalgia as a marker of breast cancer susceptibility: Results of a case-control study among French women. Br J Cancer, 1992; 65:945–949.

Russo IH, Russo J. Hormone prevention of mammary carcinogenesis: A new approach in anticancer research. Anticancer Res 1988; 8:1247–1264.

Sitruk-Ware R. Estrogens, progestins and breast cancer risk in postmenopausal women: State of the ongoing controversy in 1992. Maturitas 1992; 15:129–139.

Vorherr H. Fibrocystic breast disease: Pathophysiology pathomorphology, clinical picture and management. Am J Obstet Gynecol 1986; 154:161–179.

HEART DISEASE AND PREGNANCY

John H. McAnulty, M.D.

A woman may first develop heart disease as a result of pregnancy, but most cardiovascular abnormalities exist before conception. Treatment should preferably begin at that time. Therapy before and during pregnancy is unique because it so directly affects the health of two individuals. When treating all pregnant women with heart disease, it is essential to address the following issues: establish health priorities, provide counseling, and balance the potential benefits and risks of diagnostic procedures.

Maternal safety is the highest priority. The well-being of the fetus should be considered when treating maternal heart disease, but procedures and medications necessary to protect the mother should be used.

The woman and her family should understand the heart disease. In selected cases the risk of pregnancy to the woman is so great that avoidance is recommended or, if pregnancy has occurred, interruption is advisable (Table 1). The parents should understand the potential for fetal loss and the potential for abnormalities in the newborn infant. Parents with congenital heart disease should be advised that their offspring have an increased chance of being born with a cardiac abnormality (Table 2).

Desirable activity levels should be reviewed in each case. In healthy women, the heart is able to meet maternal needs as well as those of the fetus. In the woman with heart disease, however, uterine blood flow may be compromised, even at rest. Although the effects of exercise have not been well studied, pregnant women with heart disease should be advised to keep their exercise level below that which causes symptoms.

The electrocardiogram and echocardiogram are safe for the mother and fetus, but interpretation should be done by an individual who recognizes the changes of a normal pregnancy. Radiographic procedures are best deferred until after pregnancy or to as late in pregnancy as possible, when fetal development is complete. Optimal shielding of the fetus is required. Radionuclide studies should be avoided unless absolutely essential for maternal safety.

Table 1 Cardiovascular Abnormalities Placing a Mother and Fetus at Extremely High Risk

Advise avoidance or interruption of pregnancy
Pulmonary hypertension
Dilated cardiomyopathy with congestive failure
Marfan's syndrome with dilated aortic root
Cyanotic congenital heart disease
Symptomatic obstructive lesions
Prepregnancy counseling and close clinical follow-up required
Prosthetic valve
Coarctation of the aorta
Marfan's syndrome
Dilated cardiomyopathy in asymptomatic women
Obstructive lesions

From McAnulty JH, Morton MJ, Ueland K. The heart and pregnancy. Curr Probl Cardiol 1988; 13:595; with permission.

Table 2 Congenital Heart Disease in the Offspring of a Parent with Congenital Heart Disease

CONGENITAL HEART DEFECT IN PARENT	RISK OF CONGENITAL HEART DISEASE IN OFFSPRING IF ONE PARENT IS AFFECTED (%)
Intracardiac shunts	
ASD	3–11
VSD	4–22
PDA	4–11
Obstruction to flow	
Left-sided obstruction*	3–26
Right-sided obstruction	3–22
Complex abnormalities	
Tetralogy of Fallot	4–15
Ebstein's anomaly	Uncertain
Transposition of the great arteries	Uncertain

Note: The higher number in each range comes from one large series. The incidence of congenital heart disease in the offspring tends to be closer to the lower numbers for most other reported series.

The risk in obstructive lesions is decreased by corrective surgery prior to pregnancy.

*Includes coarctation, aortic stenosis, discrete subaortic stenosis, supravalvular stenosis. It does not include idiopathic hypertrophic subaortic stenosis (IHSS); with this the child has a 50 percent chance of having IHSS.

ASD, Atrial septal defect; PDA, patent ductus arteriosus; VSD, ventricular septal defect.

From McAnulty JH, Metcalfe J, Ueland K. Cardiovascular disease. In: Burrow GN, Ferris TF, eds. Medical complications during pregnancy. Philadelphia: WB Saunders, 1988; with permission.

■ USE OF CARDIOVASCULAR MEDICATIONS DURING PREGNANCY

Cardiovascular drugs may be essential for maternal safety. However, in addition to causing side effects in the mother, they may adversely affect the fetus. They may depress uterine blood flow and may adversely affect labor and delivery. Most cardiovascular drugs cross the placenta. Some are potential teratogens. Many drugs are secreted in breast milk, thereby continuing to expose nursing infants to potential problems. Information about drug use during pregnancy is incomplete, but recommendations for use of selected cardiovascular drugs are presented in Table 3. Doses used should be similar to those in nonpregnant women. If a desired effect is not achieved, blood levels should be evaluated.

■ MANAGEMENT OF CARDIOVASCULAR SYNDROMES DURING PREGNANCY

Congestive Heart Failure

Pulmonary edema is as much an emergency during pregnancy as at other times. Therapy with oxygen, diuretics, morphine sulfate, or preload- and afterload-reducing agents should be initiated. Arrhythmias should be controlled with drugs if necessary. Occasionally, pulmonary edema is caused by drugs used to quiet the uterus (e.g., ritodrine, terbutaline). Although the value of these "tocolytic" drugs is unproven, if pulmonary edema occurs as they are used, treatment should consist of stopping the drug and use of diuretics.

Chronic congestive heart failure should also be treated in a standard fashion by limiting sodium intake, restricting activity, and, if necessary, medication. If chronic congestive heart failure cannot be controlled and the condition is due to a potentially correctable anatomic lesion, surgery (or potentially a balloon valvuloplasty if a valve is involved) should be performed.

Low Cardiac Output Syndromes

Traditionally, volume excess is a cautionary symptom, but in pregnancy sudden loss or depletion of intravascular volume is more dangerous. This is true in all pregnant women with heart disease, but it is of particular concern in those with pulmonary artery hypertension, right and left ventricular outflow tract obstructive lesions, or mitral stenosis. Support stockings should be used when the woman stands, and leg elevation should be encouraged when she is sitting. Dehydration should be avoided. Diuretics and vasodilator agents should be used cautiously. Bleeding should be avoided, with rapid repletion if it occurs. In middle to late pregnancy, the enlarged uterus compresses the inferior vena cava. In some women, especially when they are in the supine position, this compression is not followed by a compensatory increase in heart rate and vascular tone. Syncope may therefore occur. Resting on the side, particularly the left side, can prevent this syndrome.

If hypotension occurs, err on the side of the volume repletion. At the time of labor and delivery, administer 1,000 to 1,500 ml of saline just prior to the administration of anesthesia. The anesthesia should be selected with the aim of minimizing venous pooling. In women with a high-risk cardiovascular condition, pulmonary capillary wedge and arterial pressure monitoring lines should be inserted at the beginning of labor, and pressures should be followed during labor and for 24 to 48 hours after delivery.

Systemic Arterial Hypertension

Hypertension during pregnancy is defined as a systolic blood pressure exceeding 130 mm Hg or a diastolic pressure greater than 80 mm Hg. The condition may precede pregnancy. With it, women have a fivefold greater risk of developing toxemia (pre-eclampsia or eclampsia) during pregnancy than do normotensive women. Treatment should include limitation of sodium intake in the diet to less than 2 g daily. If the blood pressure does not normalize, atenolol (50 to 100 mg), hydrochlorothiazide (50 to 100 mg), or both should be given daily. Hydralazine 25 to 50 mg four times daily should be added if control is not achieved. The safety of angiotensin converting enzyme inhibitors has not been established.

Pre-eclampsia (hypertension associated with proteinuria and with mild central nervous system instability) makes blood pressure control even more essential. Limitation of activity is required, and diuretics should be stopped as they may worsen the syndrome. If hypertension is associated with visual disturbances, pulmonary edema, convulsions, or vascular accidents (i.e., the syndrome of eclampsia), immediate hospitalization is required. Magnesium sulfate (1 g intrave-

Table 3 Cardiovascular Drugs Used During Pregnancy

DRUG GROUP	USE DURING PREGNANCY	ADVERSE EFFECTS
Diuretics	Use as in nonpregnant women; should not be used prophylactically or to treat pedal edema unless there is associated pulmonary vascular congestion	May exacerbate pre-eclampsia by reducing uterine blood flow
Inotropic agents	Pregnancy does not alter the indications for digitalis therapy; an increased dose may be required to achieve acceptable serum levels; digitalis crosses the placenta and is excreted in breast milk but fetal or infant toxicity is unusual	Labor potentially earlier and shorter in women on digitalis
	Beta-stimulation or dopaminergic agents should be reserved for life-threatening situations	May decrease uterine blood flow
Vasodilator agents	Afterload-reducing agents; adverse fetal effects not reported with hydralazine; there is little experience during pregnancy with clonidine or diazoxide	Hypotension may jeopardize uterine blood flow The angiotensin converting enzyme inhibitors may cause fetal renal abnormalities
	Preload reducing agents: nitrates indicated as in nonpregnant state; nitroprusside justified in life-threatening situations; there is little experience with prazosin	Concern about but no documentation of cyanide toxicity with nitroprusside
Antiarrhythmic agents	Indications for use as in nonpregnant state; greatest experience with quinidine but procainamide and disopyramide not clearly inferior; lidocaine crosses placenta but no teratogenic effects reported; little information is available on tocainide, mexiletine, flecainide, encainide, propafenone, or amiodarone	Potential fetal arrhythmias Phenytoin can cause fetal abnormalities and should be avoided
Beta-blocking agents	May be used to treat hypertension, angina, and supraventricular tachyarrhythmias when there are no reasonable alternatives; close fetal and neonate monitoring required	May depress intrauterine growth Newborn bradycardia, hypotension, hypoglycemia, and respiratory depression
Calcium channel blockers	Use verapamil and nifedipine as with nonpregnant patients; there is little information on diltiazem hydrochloride or nicardipine	
Anticoagulants	Warfarin in *contraindicated* at time of conception and during pregnancy because of teratogenic effects and placental and fetal bleeding	10–20% teratogenic effect in first trimester
	When anticoagulation is required, heparin via subcutaneous administration at home is preferred; it does not cross the placenta	Maternal, placenta bleeding
	Acetylsalicylic acid may be used but there is some increased risk of bleeding	Maternal plus fetal bleeding
	There is no reported experience with dipyridamole or sulfinpyrazone	Potential premature closure of ductus arteriosus by prostaglandin inhibition

Modified from McAnulty JH, Metcalfe J, Ueland K. Pregnancy in the cardiac patient. In: Parmley WW, Chatterjee K, eds. Cardiology. Philadelphia: JB Lippincott, 1987; with permission.

nously each hour) may effectively treat both the hypertension and the symptoms. If they persist, nitroprusside should be started and titrated to the level of blood pressure control. Intravenous diazepam (5 to 20 mg) should be given for convulsions. When blood pressure control has been achieved and the patient is stable, delivery, which is the ultimate treatment, should be performed as soon as the fetus is considered mature.

Arrhythmias

Pregnancy should not significantly alter the approach to arrhythmia treatment. The urgency of therapy for symptomatic arrhythmias should increase slightly because they are likely to be causing hemodynamic embarrassment to the fetus. If an arrhythmia is recognized, it is essential to determine whether treatment is worth any hoped-for benefits. No treatment should be given until the rhythm abnormality is documented and defined.

Tachyarrhythmias

Treatment for the tachyarrhythmia should be the same as in the nonpregnant woman. If at all possible, drugs should be avoided because all cross the placenta. If the woman is in significant distress, cardioversion can be used without adverse effects to the fetus.

Sinus tachycardia is a reason to search for a cause (the heart rate at rest should not exceed 100 beats per minute, even at term, in the normal pregnancy), but treatment of the rhythm itself is not appropriate. Premature atrial and ventricular beats do not require treatment, no matter what their frequency, unless they cause intolerable symptoms.

Paroxysmal supraventricular tachycardia can be treated

with a vagal maneuver. If this is unsuccessful, intravenous verapamil (5 to 10 mg) or adenosine (6 to 12 mg) can quickly convert the rhythm without compromise to the fetus. A rare arrhythmic event does not justify daily medication. Some women can use oral verapamil (120 to 160 mg) on an as-needed basis if the rhythm recurs (with warnings about hypotension). If there are frequent recurrences, daily drug therapy with digoxin (0.25 to 0.5 mg) is appropriate. Sustained-release verapamil preparations (240 to 480 mg) or the selective beta-blocking agents (atenolol 50 to 100 mg) are reasonable alternatives. Suspicion of an accessory atrioventricular pathway would make the beta-blocker the preferred drug. Intolerable recurrent rhythms justify the use of a class 1 agent. Quinidine (900 to 1,800 mg daily in three divided doses) has been used most often without adverse effects on the fetus.

Atrial fibrillation and flutter suggest the presence of underlying heart disease. It is appropriate to consider other explanations (particularly drugs or hyperthyroidism). If ventricular rate control is required, intravenous verapamil or digoxin can be given or cardioversion performed. If fibrillation or flutter persists after rate control, one attempt at DC cardioversion is indicated. Persistence or recurrence is a reason to institute daily digoxin therapy for rate control. Thromboembolic complications are of concern, but the risk in women of this age is low. Still, the consequences are great enough to recommend one aspirin tablet (325 mg) daily.

Treatment of ventricular tachyarrhythmias should be no different than in the nonpregnant woman. Recurrent symptomatic nonsustained ventricular tachycardia or sustained ventricular tachycardias justify anti-arrhythmic drug therapy. Quinidine therapy, beta-blocker therapy, or both should be used first. If they are ineffective, use of agents less thoroughly evaluated during pregnancy is necessary.

Bradyarrhythmias

Therapy for bradyarrhythmias should not be influenced by pregnancy. If a reversible cause of arrhythmias cannot be found and if the rhythms are symptomatic, pacemaker insertion is required. If this is necessary early in pregnancy, efforts to shield the fetus from radiation during pacemaker insertion are essential.

Endocarditis

Prevention of endocarditis is preferable to treatment. Although infective endocarditis occurs in less than 0.1 percent of deliveries, bacteremia is estimated to occur in 5 percent of women with normal labor and delivery and in up to 20 percent of patients undergoing cesarean section. Because of this, and because endocarditis continues to be associated with a high morbidity and mortality, antibiotic prophylaxis with penicillin (vancomycin if patient is penicillin-allergic) and an aminoglycoside should be initiated at the onset of labor and continued for 24 hours after delivery. A false labor will make this recommendation difficult in some select cases, but in most it can be applied. If endocarditis occurs during pregnancy, evaluation and treatment should be treated as aggressively as at other times. If urgent surgery is required, it too should be performed. Depending on fetal maturity, cesarean section can be performed in concurrence with the cardiac surgery.

Pulmonary Hypertension

Primary or secondary pulmonary artery hypertension is a contraindication to pregnancy. When first documented during pregnancy, interruption should be recommended. Maternal mortality approaches 50 percent, with many of the deaths occurring at the time of interruption of the pregnancy or labor and delivery. If pregnancy occurs and interruption is not accepted by the mother, close clinical follow-up is essential. Activity should be kept at an absolute minimum. Hypovolemic states should be avoided. Capillary wedge pressure and arterial monitoring lines are appropriate during labor and for 24 to 48 hours after delivery. The anesthesiologist should take all measures to avoid venous pooling.

■ CONGENITAL HEART DISEASE

Effective surgery is making maternal congenital heart disease more common. Because these women have children with an increased chance of congenital heart disease, this trend will continue (see Table 2).

Intracardiac Shunts

Whether due to an atrial septal defect, a ventricular septal defect, or a patent ductus arteriosus, left-to-right shunts are generally well tolerated by the mother. This is probably because the fall in vascular resistance during pregnancy is similar in the pulmonary and systemic beds and there is no significant alteration in shunting. Surgical closure of the defects is generally preferable before delivery, but this does not decrease the chance that the offspring will have heart disease. In the rare case when heart failure or symptomatic arrhythmias develop, they should be treated as described earlier.

Whether they are due to right ventricular outflow obstruction with normal pulmonary vascular resistance or to elevated pulmonary vascular resistance syndromes, right-to-left shunts are associated with high maternal and fetal morbidity and mortality. They are often associated with complex heart disease and associated cyanosis. Until they are corrected, it is advised that pregnancy should be avoided and, if pregnancy occurs, interruption is recommended. Tetralogy of Fallot is the most common cause of shunting caused by obstruction to pulmonary outflow. Once surgical correction has been performed, pregnancy can be completed with almost no maternal mortality and a small (10 to 20 percent) incidence of spontaneous abortions. Ebstein's anomaly may occasionally be associated with severe right-to-left shunting. Milder forms of the syndromes, with little shunting, are associated with a well-tolerated pregnancy.

Obstructive Lesions to Ventricular Outflow Tracts

Right and left ventricular outflow tract obstructions are associated with increased maternal and fetal mortality and with an increased chance of congenital heart disease in the offspring. Surgical correction before pregnancy alleviates each of these problems. If pregnancy occurs and these lesions are recognized, activity should be limited to the level below which symptoms occur and, if symptoms accelerate despite this curtailment, surgical intervention may be necessary to protect the mother.

One syndrome of left outflow tract obstruction, coarctation of the aorta, is associated with a 3 to 9 percent maternal mortality rate. Surgical correction before pregnancy is advisable. Balloon dilation is an alternative; there is no information on the effects of the vasculature changes of pregnancy on the dilation site. If severe coarctation is noted when a patient is pregnant, interruption is recommended. If the woman does not wish to accept this recommendation, strict limitation of activity and control of systemic hypertension are indicated.

Another cause of outflow tract obstruction is idiopathic hypertrophic subaortic stenosis. Affected women may have increased symptoms during pregnancy; there has been only one reported death. Treatment of the symptoms is as difficult as at any other time, but, if they are severe, beta-blocker therapy (atenolol 50 to 100 mg daily) should be instituted.

Marfan's Syndrome

Complications of Marfan's syndrome frequently occur at the time of pregnancy with reported maternal mortality rates varying from 4 to 50 percent. Because of this and because long-term survival is uncommon and the offspring have a 50 percent chance of having the same abnormality, avoidance of pregnancy is recommended. Interruption should be considered if the syndrome is recognized after a woman is pregnant. This recommendation should be made more strongly if there is evidence of aortic root dilation (>40 mm by echocardiography). If this advice is unacceptable to the mother, activity should be strictly limited, blood pressure well controlled, and a beta-selective blocking agent instituted. Cesarean section is preferable to labor and vaginal delivery.

Valve Disease

Management of valve disease, addressing the issues of endocarditis prophylaxis, prophylaxis against rheumatic fever, the need for anticoagulation, and treatment of complications, should be the same during pregnancy as at other times.

Mitral Stenosis

Recognition and mechanical correction of mitral stenosis before pregnancy is the preferred approach. The more severe the hemodynamic abnormality, the greater the risk of pregnancy. Mitral commissurotomy is preferable to prosthesis insertion (see discussion of prosthetic heart valves later in this chapter). If a woman with mitral stenosis becomes pregnant, symptoms and complications should be treated in the standard fashion. Prophylactic digoxin should be given to minimize the fast ventricular response if she develops atrial fibrillation. If severe symptoms persist despite limitation of activity and use of medications, mitral commissurotomy or balloon valvuloplasty is required.

Mitral Regurgitation

This lesion is generally well tolerated during pregnancy. Arrhythmias or congestive heart failure should be treated in the standard fashion.

Mitral valve prolapse is common in women of childbearing age. The incidence of symptoms, arrhythmias, endocarditis, or emboli does not alter during pregnancy. Antibiotic prophylaxis at the time of labor and delivery is recommended for those women with a murmur.

Aortic Stenosis

Maternal mortality as high as 10 percent makes surgical correction (preferably a valvotomy) before pregnancy desirable. No treatment is necessary for women with aortic stenosis who become pregnant and are asymptomatic. Symptomatic women should limit activity; again, it is important to avoid hypovolemia. If congestive heart failure occurs and cannot be controlled, surgical or balloon valvuloplasty should be considered.

Aortic Regurgitation

This lesion is well tolerated during pregnancy. In those who do develop congestive heart failure or arrhythmias, standard treatment should be used. If acute aortic regurgitation occurs owing to bacterial endocarditis or to aortic dissection, emergency treatment, even surgery, is required despite the pregnancy.

Pulmonic Valve Disease

Pulmonic stenosis should be corrected before conception. If first recognized during pregnancy, hypovolemia should be avoided. Pulmonic insufficiency is uncommon except after previous heart surgery. No specific treatment is needed during pregnancy.

Tricuspid Valve Disease

Isolated tricuspid valve stenosis is rare, and treatment should be individualized. The incidence of regurgitation is increasing (because of illicit drug use), but the lesion is well tolerated during pregnancy and no specific therapy is required.

Prosthetic Heart Valves

Insertion of a prosthetic heart valve commits an individual to a 3 to 6 percent chance per year of a major complication. Pregnancy may increase this risk, and a prosthetic valve is a relative contraindication to pregnancy. Complications occurring in pregnant women with a prosthetic valve require standard urgent therapy.

Selecting a prosthesis for a woman who desires subsequent pregnancies is difficult. A tissue valve lessens the need for anticoagulation therapy, but pregnancy may accelerate the already high incidence of early valve degeneration, making early reoperation likely. A mechanical prosthesis mandates the need for anticoagulation therapy. Because warfarin is contraindicated (see previous section on drugs), the woman must administer heparin subcutaneously throughout the pregnancy. The choice of prosthesis must be individualized, but, in balance, the long-term durability makes a mechanical prosthesis the preferable choice despite the issue of anticoagulation therapy.

Myocardial Disease

A woman with dilated cardiomyopathy has a 30 percent chance of congestive heart failure and an increased mortality rate with pregnancy. These and her guarded long-term prognosis make the diagnosis a relative contraindication to pregnancy. If pregnancy occurs, interruption is advisable. If the woman chooses to proceed with pregnancy, heart failure, arrhythmias, and thromboembolic complications require treatment.

If dilated cardiomyopathy develops late in pregnancy or

in the first 6 weeks after delivery, the pregnancy itself is considered the cause. This is a peripartum cardiomyopathy. Treatment for myocarditis as a cause is reasonable if the disease is rapidly progressive and the diagnosis is proved by biopsy.

Coronary Artery Disease

Coronary artery obstruction occurs on rare occasions during pregnancy. Spasms, dissection, thromboemboli, and, rarely, atherosclerosis are the presumed causes. Complications of a myocardial infarction require standard treatment. The risk of thrombolytic therapy has not been defined, and it should be reserved for those likely to get the very highest benefit.

Implanted Electronic Devices

Women with permanent pacemakers and cardioverter-defibrillators do not require specific treatment. If a defibrillator is discharging inappropriately, a doughnut magnet can be taped over the device to shut it off (this is true for all manufacturers' models).

Cardiac Transplantation

There have been reports of successful pregnancies following transplantation. Care for the mother should be directed toward her safety with treatment of complications (e.g., congestive heart failure, infections) as would normally be done.

Pericardial Disease

Pregnancy should not alter the treatment of pericardial disease syndromes.

Suggested Reading

McAnulty JH, Metcalfe J, Ueland K. The heart and certain physiological conditions. In: Hurst JW, Rackley CE, Schlant RC, et al, eds. The heart. 7th ed. New York: McGraw-Hill, 1990:1465.

McAnulty JH, Morton MJ, Ueland K. The heart and pregnancy. Curr Probl Cardiol 1988; 13:595.

Whittemore R, Hobbins JC, Engle MA. Pregnancy and its outcome in women with and without surgical treatment of congenital heart disease. Am J Cardiol 1982; 50:641.

ANOREXIA NERVOSA AND BULIMIA NERVOSA

Bruce S. Rothschild, M.D.
Joseph M. Nesta, M.D.

Anorexia nervosa and bulimia nervosa are eating disorders of increasing prevalence, with a female-to-male ratio of 20:1. The rate of occurrence in high school and college age women is 0.5 percent for anorexia and 3 percent for bulimia.

The cause of these disorders is unknown, although a multifactorial perspective taking into account biologic perturbations, societal pressures, and psychological issues is empirically most useful. Briefly, women with these disorders often have a proclivity for weight instability, exist in a social context that overly prizes thinness, and need to cope with destructive personality patterns, family relationships, and/or traumatic life events.

Anorexia nervosa is a disorder of willful and dramatic starvation (Table 1). Patients lose body weight by starvation, compulsive exercise, and, at times, purging, with laxative and diuretic abuse. Their thoughts are marked by an overwhelming fear of fatness, and their perception is altered by a distorted body image. Thus, a 5 ft, 4 inch, 80 pound woman might not recognize the medical danger in which she is putting herself, as insight tends to atrophy along with body fat. Indeed, this difficulty in getting the patient to recognize she has a serious problem is one of the most challenging aspects of the disorder.

Bulimia nervosa is a disorder of binge eating and purging (Table 2). The diagnosis is made irrespective of body weight and is defined by ingestion of huge amounts of calories in a short period in an uncontrollable fashion. This is usually followed by self-induced vomiting and is often accompanied by laxative or diuretic abuse.

Table 1 DSM-IV: Diagnostic Criteria for Anorexia Nervosa

A. Refusal to maintain body weight at or above a minimally normal weight for age and height (e.g., weight loss leading to maintenance of body weight less than 85% of that expected; or failure to make expected weight gain during period of growth, leading to body weight less than 85% of that expected).
B. Intense fear of gaining weight or becoming fat, even though underweight.
C. Disturbance in the way in which one's body weight or shape is experienced, undue influence of body weight or shape on self-evaluation, or denial of the seriousness of the low current body weight.
D. In postmenarcheal females, amenorrhea, i.e., the absence of at least three consecutive menstrual cycles. (A woman is considered to have amenorrhea if her periods occur only following hormone, e.g., estrogen, administration.)

Specify Type

Restricting Type: during the current episode of Anorexia Nervosa, the person has not regularly engaged in binge-eating or purging behavior (i.e., self-induced vomiting or the misuse of laxatives, diuretics, or enemas)

Binge-Eating/Purging Type: during the current episode of Anorexia Nervosa, the person has regularly engaged in binge-eating or purging behavior (i.e., self-induced vomiting or the misuse of laxatives, diuretics, or enemas)

From Diagnostic and Statistical Manual of Mental Disorders, 4th ed. Washington, DC: American Psychiatric Association, 1995; with permission

Mortality rates for the two disorders range from 1 to 5 percent. Early detection and treatment by professionals

Table 2 DSM-IV-R: Diagnostic Criteria for Bulimia Nervosa

A. Recurrent episodes of binge eating (rapid consumption of a large amount of food in a discrete period)
B. A feeling of lack of control over eating behavior during the eating binges
C. The person regularly engages in self-induced vomiting, use of laxatives or diuretics, strict dieting or fasting, or vigorous exercise in order to prevent weight gain
D. A minimal average of two binge-eating episodes a week for at least 3 months
E. Persistent overconcern with body shape and weight

who are informed both psychiatrically and medically improve the prognosis.

The remainder of this chapter focuses on treatment. General aspects of psychiatric treatment are covered, followed by more specific recommendations regarding the gastrointestinal (GI) complications associated with these disorders.

■ ANOREXIA NERVOSA

The level of severity of illness dictates the treatment setting. The percentage of ideal body weight may be the most important factor in this regard. We believe optimal inpatient treatment occurs with a psychiatric admission to a specialty eating disorder unit. This unit should be in a hospital and have access to experienced medical physicians and ancillary services.

The most basic function of intensive treatment for anorexia nervosa is helping the patient to begin to eat normally again. As anyone who has tried to "kick a habit" will attest, changing basic biologic behaviors is no easy feat. These patients need the imposed structure and support of a well-trained staff knowledgeable in eating disorders. Inpatient treatment is necessary for the most severely ill patients. Day hospital treatment, where available, is a less restrictive approach for patients able to muster some self-control and motivation. Indeed, the day hospital (in which, for example, patients attend a program 7 hours a day, 5 days a week) offers the advantage of providing structure and support for part of the week while allowing the patient to work on "self-feeding" while away from the program.

Weight restoration is the first order of business for the starved patient. Many abnormal eating habits, food preoccupations, rigid thinking patterns, and tendencies to depression can be reversed solely with the approximation of body weight back to the normal range.

What is the proper goal weight range for an individual patient? A combined approach using Metropolitan Life Table data along with the patient's personal weight history, particularly in regard to loss and resumption of menses, is crucial. A goal weight range slightly below normal can be a realistic compromise in that the patient is able to accept it and yet is spared medical complications.

Once a patient is in a safer weight range, treatment can ensue on an outpatient basis. This should occur at least once weekly, and the patient should be weighed regularly by the treating physician. She should be exhorted to refrain from weighing herself, as weight gains can precipitate panic and weight loss can lead to a downward spiral (the new lower weight becomes the maximal weight "allowed").

Psychotherapy usually occurs on a one-to-one basis, although there is evidence suggesting that family therapy is more useful for younger patients. Psychological issues are explored, but never at the expense of attending to weight and medical issues.

The utility of pharmacotherapy for anorexia nervosa is limited. Early trials of neuroleptics targeted at the "delusional" distorted body image proved to be without benefit. The best "antidepressant" for these patients tends to be food and normalization of body weight. Occasional use of a short-acting benzodiazepine, e.g., alprazolam, 0.25 mg 30 minutes before meals, for patients who are extremely anxious around mealtime can be beneficial.

Recently, there has been some suggestion through case reports that the serotonin reuptake blocker fluoxetine can aid anorectic patients with weight gain. This is counterintuitive, given fluoxetine's tendency to promote mild weight loss in several depressed patients for whom it was prescribed. However, it is possible that this agent has the ability to free the patient somewhat from rigid obsessional thinking. A daily dose of 20 mg would be likely, although 10 mg might be safer in a severely emaciated patient. Ultimately, up to 60 mg daily might be needed. Again, support for this approach remains anecdotal, and controlled studies need to be performed.

Finally, what about the patient who is not taking responsibility for getting better? A patient may see her psychiatrist weekly and the internist monthly and still continue to lose weight. The treating physicians can make all the right recommendations, including hospitalization, but it is ultimately the patient's decision whether to follow through with these. It is not in the patient's best interest to continue in therapy indefinitely in the face of noncompliance with the treatment plan of weight gain. If the patient cannot be kept medically safe as an outpatient, hospitalization is warranted. Involuntary psychiatric hospitalization is justified only in very rare circumstances and usually results in little benefit, because treatment alliance between physician and patient is needed to effect behavioral change. Patients who have become significantly medically compromised, but lack the insight or desire to work on their problem, are probably best served by a short-term medical admission to correct medical complications and reverse weight loss. Similarly, in the outpatient setting, if a patient is not able or willing to work on her eating disorder in therapy, the internist may remain involved to provide medical support and surveillance of the patient, e.g., on a monthly basis. Referral back to the psychiatrist for further therapy may be made when the patient is better able to actively work on her problem.

■ BULIMIA NERVOSA

Although patients with bulimia nervosa tend not to lose weight down to dangerously low levels, their health can be seriously jeopardized by their bulimic behaviors. Significant metabolic abnormalities can result from vomiting, laxative abuse, and diuretic abuse. The most common metabolic abnormality is a hypochloremic metabolic alkalosis. Hypokalemia is also common. Severe disturbances of this kind can lead to seizures, cardiac arrhythmia, and death.

In general, bulimic patients can be treated outside the hospital setting. However, patients who are binge eating and purging numerous times daily, and experiencing frequent medical complications, need inpatient or perhaps day hospital treatment. In ambulatory treatment, laboratories should be checked on a regular basis, depending on the symptoms of the patient. This may range from following electrolytes once monthly to once every 6 months.

Psychotherapy for bulimia often includes the patient's keeping a meal record or a food journal that is reviewed weekly. Along with this focus on food intake, the therapy tries to correct cognitive distortions involving diet, weight, and esteem. Emphasis is placed on improving destructive interpersonal relationship patterns, which usually have a role in initiating and maintaining the disorder.

Comorbid diagnoses are more common with bulimia nervosa than with anorexia nervosa. The experienced clinician will be on the lookout for substance abuse, major depression, or borderline personality disorders in patients with bulimia. These conditions need to be diagnosed, and then properly treated, in order to maximize therapeutic impact.

Unlike anorexia nervosa, there is clearly a strong role for medication in the treatment of these patients. Numerous antidepressant trials have been run, and essentially have all shown effect compared with placebo. Antidepressants of all types are included: tricyclics, monoamine oxidase inhibitors, trazodone, buproprion, and the selective serotonin reuptake inhibitors (SSRIs), such as fluoxetine, sertraline, and paroxetine. These medications are useful independent of a comorbid diagnosis of major depression. Thus, it is important to stress that all the agents marketed as antidepressants are also effective antibulimic drugs.

Which agent to choose? The advent of fluoxetine and the SSRIs that have followed have changed prescription habits immensely. The SSRIs generally do not promote weight gain as most of the other antidepressants potentially do. This is an extremely important selling point in trying to convince a reluctant patient to take medication when she is already overconcerned about body weight. Also, SSRIs tend to be better tolerated in general than the older antidepressants. A special warning should be made for buproprion: it is generally contraindicated in this population, as pretrial studies resulted in a significantly higher incidence of seizures in bulimic patients.

Laboratory tests should be made upon initiating a medication (complete blood count, SMAC, and one set of thyroid function tests should suffice). Fluoxetine is a good first-line drug and is started at 20 mg daily; if, after 1 month, only marginal improvement has occurred, the dosage can be doubled. This is often the maximal dose needed, but some patients require 60 mg daily in a single morning dose. When the medication is effective, patients report a decrease in their desire to binge and general improvement in mood stability.

For patients who do not respond to fluoxetine, it is reasonable to try another SSRI such as sertraline, 50 to 100 mg daily, or a tricyclic antidepressant with a relatively favorable side effect profile such as nortriptyline or desipramine. For example, nortriptyline can be started at 25 mg at bedtime, increased to 50 mg after 4 days, and then increased to 75 mg after another 4 days. This last dose is frequently sufficient to reach the targeted therapeutic blood level (between 50 and 150 mg per milliliter). A blood level should be drawn 5 days after reaching this dose, and future dosing adjustments should be made accordingly. Potential side effects of lightheadedness, dry mouth, and constipation should be discussed with the patient. For patients who are actively bulimic, an electrocardiogram should be obtained either before or at the start of treatment.

Some patients with bulimia represent a significant suicidal risk. All such patients, of course, should be seen concurrently by a psychiatrist. Prescribing for these patients is often best done by the psychiatrist so that the prescription of the medication can be incorporated into the psychotherapeutic process. Two week supplies with one refill are usually a safe way to dispense for this higher-risk population.

■ GASTROINTESTINAL MANAGEMENT

The evaluation of a patient with a suspected eating disorder requires a comprehensive medical assessment, including history, physical examination, laboratory blood studies, and anthropometric measurements. The most useful of these measurements are the patient's height, current weight, and percentage of ideal body weight. The patient's usual weight also has clinical significance. A weight loss greater than 10 percent of usual weight occurring within 1 to 2 months, or a weight less than 70 percent of usual weight, is a concern. Calorie and protein requirements are determined per individual patient. The patient's weight is consistently monitored. A typical initial diet is 1,200 to 1,500 calories per day and 50 to 70 g protein per day. Caloric adjustments are made weekly to ensure a weight gain of 2 to 4 pounds per week. When the goal weight is achieved, a maintenance caloric diet is utilized.

Anorectic patients are fed orally. If they are unable to tolerate regular food, oral liquid nutritional supplements are used. Rare patients who refuse to eat and are medically compromised as a result of this malnutrition, or consistently fail to gain satisfactory weight, may require enteric tube feedings or intravenous (IV) fluids.

GI problems encountered in patients with an eating disorder are reviewed by organ involvement. Bulimic patients, with their characteristic history of ingesting large quantities of food with high carbohydrate content and repetitive volitional vomiting, can develop significant dental disease. Injury to the lingual surfaces of teeth precipitated by the chemical action of the regurgitated gastric contents, and aggravated by the mechanical action of the tongue against the teeth, causes loss of dentin and enamel. This is perimylolysis. Patients with perimylolysis complain of hot and cold temperature sensitivity and have an increased incidence of dental caries. The incidence of dental caries may also be affected by bulimics' high carbohydrate intake. Evaluation by a dentist is recommended when these conditions are present.

Enlargement of parotid glands is commonly noted in patients with eating disorders. It may be painless or painful, and the exact pathophysiology remains unresolved. The observation that benign parotid enlargement occurs in obese patients, and in patients with restrictive diets without anorexia nervosa or bulimia nervosa, has led to the speculation that for bulimic patients, this is secondary to their commonly noted underlying obesity, while for anorectic patients, this is secondary to underlying malnutrition.

Hyperamylasemia is also common in these patients. When the amylase has been analyzed, it is frequently the salivary-type isoamylase. In bulimic patients, this elevated serum amylase has been observed during periods of active purging, with resolution of the hyperamylasemia when this behavior has resolved. It is postulated that repeated vomiting may injure the salivary glands or induce hypersalivation, causing this hyperamylasemic state.

Hyperamylasemia with abdominal pain may also represent acute pancreatitis. Acute pancreatitis, although infrequent, has been documented in patients with anorexia nervosa. When reported, pancreatitis occurs in severely malnourished patients during the refeeding phase of treatment. It responds to conventional therapy for acute pancreatitis.

Rumination can also occur in patients with eating disorders. Recently ingested food fills the oral cavity 10 to 15 minutes after eating; this can be expectorated, rechewed, or reswallowed, only to reappear in a cyclic fashion. This is an involuntary action that lasts approximately 30 minutes and then ceases. It is not associated with nausea; it can be associated with a neuromotility disorder of the esophagus and stomach. Rumination can be extremely difficult to treat. Biofeedback techniques have been used.

It is not unexpected that symptoms suggestive of esophageal disease are seen in patients with eating disorders. Anorectics, with their delayed gastric emptying, and bulimics, with their frequent purging, may experience heartburn, regurgitation, and chest pain (classic symptoms of gastroesophageal reflux disease). Thus, esophagitis, esophageal erosions, esophageal strictures, and Barrett's esophagus can develop. Gastroesophageal reflux, with its complications, respond in this population to conventional therapy. Bulimics, with their repeated retching and vomiting, are at risk for esophageal ruption (Boerhaave's syndrome), gastric rupture, and Mallory-Weiss tears.

Acute gastric retention can occur with refeeding or binge eating and can result in gastric rupture. The usual clinical presentation for acute gastric retention is rapid onset of nausea, vomiting, and abdominal pain with abdominal distention, with gastric or gastroenteric dilation seen radiographically. This distention responds to making the patient NPO, with nasogastric suction and IV fluids. If peritoneal signs are present, or free air is seen radiographically, IV antibiotics and surgical consultation are indicated.

Gastric motility disorders are very common in anorexia nervosa. Delayed gastric emptying occurs in at least 80 percent of patients with this disease and may involve solid or solid and liquid phase emptying. It is unclear whether this is primary, secondary, or an epiphenomenon of this disorder. The observation that the severity of the malnutrition influences the magnitude of these symptoms, and that refeeding anorectic patients often improves their symptoms, suggests that dysfunctional emptying may be secondary to the anorexia nervosa. The delayed gastric emptying may not be totally reversible after restoration of body weight. Pharmacologic intervention may be required with severe symptoms. Bethanechol, 25 mg orally four times a day, or metoclopramide, 10 mg orally 30 minutes before meals and at bedtime, have been utilized. Both drugs have limitations. Bethanechol can cause abdominal cramping, urinary frequency, and blurred vision in these dosages. Depression and tardive dyskinesia can occur with metoclopramide. Cisapride or domperidone may prove more effective with this population.

Basal and stimulated gastric acid output are decreased in anorexia nervosa, as noted in the limited literature studies, in which both measurements failed to return to control levels with refeeding.

No consistent structural abnormalities of the stomach or small intestine in patients with anorexia nervosa have been seen radiographically.

The most commonly encountered symptoms of colonic dysfunction are constipation and diarrhea. Frequently, underlying laxative abuse is the cause. This can occur in an anorectic patient but is more often seen in bulimics. These patients commonly complain of constipation, or alternating diarrhea and constipation, often associated with nausea, vomiting, and weight loss. Concomitant usage of diuretics and vomiting can complicate their management.

Chronic laxative abuse leads to a "cathartic colon": a dilated, hypotonic colon with loss of haustrations, often on only one side. Histologic damage to the ganglion cells in Auerbach's plexus may be seen and can contribute to poor colonic tone and the often present constipation. Chronic ingestion of anthraquinone laxatives can cause a brownish-black discoloration of the colonic mucosa (melanosis coli).

Constipation can be difficult to manage in these patients. It has been our practice to start most eating disorder patients on docusate sodium, 100 mg orally twice a day. Any electrolyte or volume imbalances are corrected. All medications are reviewed. If an agent produces a high incidence of constipation, an alternative is suggested. Consideration is given to exclude other conditions that may present with constipation, such as hypothyroidism. Judicious intake of fluids and exercise is encouraged. Bulk laxatives are initially tried unless the patient has a known cathartic colon or has prominent symptoms of delayed gastric emptying. In these cases, a low-residue diet is employed. If these interventions fail, subsequent therapies include use of osmotic laxatives, enemas, or polyethylene glycol agents. On initial presentation, patients who consume large amounts of laxatives are tapered off these agents. We try to minimize use of stimulant laxatives.

In refractory cases, or cases with alarming presentations such as Hemoccult-positive stools or high clinical suspicion of intestinal obstruction, further evaluation is required. This entails radiographic investigation: abdominal x-rays, barium studies or serial KUBs after ingestion of radiopaque markers, endoscopy, or manometry.

There are isolated case reports of laxative abuse causing protein-losing enteropathy and steatorrhea.

Finally, significant elevations of liver function test results have not been routinely seen in patients with eating disorders. Mild elevations in transaminase may be noted while anorectic patients are refed. This probably reflects mild steatosis or hepatic glycogen deposition, and tends to normalize with time.

It is important to realize that GI complaints are extremely common in patients with eating disorders. Waldholtz and

Andersen studied GI symptoms in 16 consecutive anorexia nervosa patients. They noted that, with refeeding and psychiatric treatment, statistically significant symptom improvement occurred in the anorexia, constipation, diarrhea, vomiting, and early and late meal-associated bloating. Abdominal pain, nausea, and heartburn improved, but not to statistically significant levels. This conclusion is confirmed in our clinical experience. Aggressive initial evaluation of all GI symptoms may not be warranted and in fact may be counterproductive to therapy. The fasting required to perform many of these tests, and the additional time needed, can cause these patients to miss meals, which can lead to additional loss of nutritional support. This is not to imply that these symptoms should be neglected. Persistent and unprovoked vomiting, persistent reflux symptoms refractory to conventional therapy, inappropriate weight gain, Hemoccult-positive stools, exacerbation of symptoms associated with well-documented previous GI diseases, and hemodynamically compromised GI bleedings or refractory constipation require further evaluation.

A comprehensive initial evaluation with a conservative approach to medical therapy, combined with medical monitoring for contributory pathologic states, provide the best clinical outcome for patients with eating disorders.

Suggested Reading

Comerci GD. Medical complications of anorexia nervosa and bulimia nervosa. Med Clin North Am 1990; 74:1293–1310.

Cuellar RE, Van Thiel DH. Gastrointestinal consequences of the eating disorders: anorexia nervosa and bulimia. Am J Gastroenterol 1986; 7:1113–1121.

Herzog DB, Copeland PM. Eating disorders. N Engl J Med 1985; 313:295–303.

Lucas AR, Callaway CW. Anorexia nervosa and bulimia in Bockus' gastroenterology 1985; 7:4416–4434.

Waldholtz BD, Andersen AE. Gastrointestinal symptoms in anorexia nervosa: a prospective study. Gastroenterology 1990; 98:1415–1419.

Webb WL. A clinical review of developments in the diagnosis and treatment of anorexia nervosa and bulimia. Psychiatr Med 1988; 6:24–38.

Diagnostic and statistical manual of mental disorders. 4th ed. Revised 1994. Washington, D.C.: American Psychiatric Association, 1987.

CERVICAL AND ENDOMETRIAL CANCER

Tate Thigpen, M.D.

Cancers of the endometrium and uterine cervix, two of the three most common malignant lesions of the female genital tract, will account for 49,400 new cases and 10,800 deaths in the United States in 1997. The relatively low ratio of deaths to new cases reflects the high frequency with which both diseases are diagnosed at an early stage of development and the reasonable success of surgery and/or radiotherapy in achieving cure of limited disease. The fact that over 10,000 deaths from these two neoplasms are expected in 1997 points out, however, the need for effective systemic therapy to deal with advanced or recurrent disease. This discussion focuses on the status of management of cancers of the cervix and endometrium with an emphasis on the role of systemic therapy.

■ CANCER OF THE UTERINE CERVIX

Cancers of the uterine cervix will cause 14,500 new cases of invasive disease and 4,800 deaths in the United States in 1997. Far more cases will be detected at a preinvasive stage. Results of treatment in the combined population of preinvasive cases and invasive cases detected at a limited stage are excellent, with cure rates ranging from 80 to 100 percent. Decisions regarding the appropriate management of cervix cancer are based on the extent of disease at the time of diagnosis as expressed in the International Federation of Gynecologists and Obstetricians (FIGO) staging system (Tables 1 and 2).

General Considerations

Carcinoma of the uterine cervix exhibits the epidemiology of a venereal disease. Associated factors include relatively low socioeconomic status, onset of coitus at an early age, frequent coitus, multiple sexual partners, and coitus with a partner who is uncircumcised or practices poor genital hygiene. There is also a connection with human papilloma virus (HPV).

Squamous cell carcinoma of the uterine cervix, by far the most common histologic type, is the focus of this discussion. Other histologic types are sufficiently uncommon that management is essentially the same for all histologies. These lesions are associated with a well-described premalignant state variously described as cervical intraepithelial neoplasia (CIN 1–3) or a squamous intraepithelial lesion (SIL—low grade, or LGSIL, and high grade, or HGSIL). Cervical cytology constitutes a very effective screening test for carcinomas of the cervix. The process by which cells go from mild through severe dysplasia and carcinoma in situ to frankly invasive cancer usually takes years; hence, there is a high probability of early diagnosis and cure with the widespread use of cervical cytology.

The most important prognostic feature of invasive lesions is the FIGO stage. An appropriate staging evaluation should include careful history and physical to include a thorough pelvic and rectal examination, complete blood count, tests to evaluate hepatic and renal status, urinalysis, flexible sigmoidoscopy, barium enema, intravenous pyelogram, and com-

Table 1 FIGO Staging System for Cancer of the Uterine Cervix

STAGE	DESCRIPTION
0	Carcinoma in situ
I	Cervix carcinoma confined to uterus (disregard extension to corpus)
IA	Invasive carcinoma diagnosed by microscopy only
IA1	Minimal microscopic stromal invasion
IA2	Invasive component less than 5 mm depth from base of epithelium and 7 mm or less horizontal spread
IB	Larger than IA2
II	Invasion beyond uterus but not to pelvic wall or lower third of vagina
IIA	No parametrial invasion
IIB	Parametrial invasion
III	Extension to pelvic wall and/or involvement of lower third of vagina or hydronephrosis or nonfunctioning kidney
IIIA	Lower third of vagina only
IIIB	Pelvic wall involvement or hydronephrosis or nonfunctioning kidney
IVA	Involvement of mucosa of bladder or rectum
IVB	Extension beyond true pelvis

Table 2 Management Recommendations for Cervix Cancer

DISEASE STATUS	RECOMMENDATIONS
Preinvasive or IA	Total abdominal hysterectomy; lesser procedures in selected cases of preinvasive disease
Stage IB, IIA	Radiotherapy for bulkier lesions; radical hysterectomy for smaller stage IB lesions; role of chemotherapy unclear
Stage IIB, III, IVA	Radiotherapy; randomized trials support the use of concomitant hydroxyurea, particularly in stage IIIB and IVA
Stage IVB or recurrent	Systemic therapy; platinum compounds, ifosfamide, doxorubicin

puted tomographic (CT) scan of the abdomen and pelvis. Histologic diagnosis of malignancy, which is mandatory, may require cytologic smears, colposcopy, conization, punch biopsies of four quadrants of the cervix, and dilatation and curettage as well as cystoscopy.

Limited Disease (Stage 0 or IA)

Patients with disease confined to the cervix, detectable by microscopy only, and limited to 5 mm or less in depth taken from the base of the epithelium and 7 mm or less in horizontal spread are in stage 0 (carcinoma in situ), stage IA1 (minimal microscopic stromal invasion), or stage IA2 (more invasion). Definitive treatment is total abdominal hysterectomy; nonsurgical candidates can be treated with radiotherapy. Patients with carcinoma in situ or lesions with invasion less than 1 mm deep can be managed with more conservative measures such as conization if all margins are clear. The cure rate for this group of patients should approach 100 percent.

Locoregionally Advanced Disease (Stages IB to IVA)

Patients with stage IB or IVA disease traditionally are treated with pelvic radiotherapy. Exceptions to this rule include selected patients with stage IB disease deemed eligible for radical hysterectomy. Recent studies, however, have pointed to several important refinements of the treatment approach: determination of para-aortic node status, neoadjuvant chemotherapy in stage IB surgical candidates, and the use of concomitant chemotherapy as a radiation sensitizer in patients with stage IIB through IVA disease.

Para-Aortic Node Status

Fewer than 15 percent of patients with stage IB through IVA disease have evidence of metastases to para-aortic lymph nodes. Because standard therapy for such patients requires extension of the field of radiotherapy to include the para-aortic node region, however, knowledge of node status is important for therapeutic decision making. Accurate assessment of involvement can be accomplished only by surgical sampling of the para-aortic nodes; hence, such a procedure has become an important part of clinical trials.

The role of surgical assessment of node status in routine clinical practice is not so clear. Patients with positive nodes have a significantly poorer survival than those with negative ones; hence, surgical assessment can accurately identify a high-risk patient subset. Unfortunately, no treatment option has been shown to improve outcome in the subset with positive para-aortic nodes. Extended-field radiation may decrease recurrence in the para-aortic area, but overall survival appears to be unaffected. No systemic treatment option has been shown to improve results. It is therefore difficult to recommend surgical staging of these nodes as a part of routine clinical practice in the absence of meaningful therapeutic intervention.

Neoadjuvant Chemotherapy in Stage IB to IIA Disease

The use of chemotherapy prior to either surgery or radiation has been evaluated in phase II trials in stages IB through IVA disease. A total of 11 studies yield two important observations. First, such an approach with platinum-based chemotherapy is feasible. Second, response rates to chemotherapy in a population with no prior radiotherapy are high (range from 23 to 100 percent). From these studies it is not possible to assess the relative merits of this approach versus radiation alone.

Three randomized trials have been reported. All three studies employed a platinum-based combination regimen preceding radiotherapy versus radiation alone. Two of these show no differences in survival between radiation alone and radiation preceded by cisplatin plus methotrexate plus chlorambucil plus vincristine or by cisplatin plus bleomycin plus vinblastine. The third actually shows an inferior 5 year survival (23 versus 39 percent) for mitomycin plus vincristine plus bleomycin plus cisplatin followed by radiation versus radiation alone. These results do not recommend the use of neoadjuvant chemotherapy followed by radiation. No randomized trials of neoadjuvant chemotherapy followed by surgery have been reported.

Chemoradiation for Stage IIB to IVA Disease

The use of concomitant chemotherapy and radiation in patients with stages IIB through IVA disease has received extensive study in both phase II and phase III trials. Of particular importance to rational treatment planning are the results of the phase III trials of the Gynecologic Oncology Group (GOG). The initial such study, GOG protocol 4, was initiated in 1970 and completed in 1976. A total of 97 patients with clinical stage IIIB or IVA disease were randomized to receive radiotherapy (5,000 cGy external radiation plus 3,000 cGy intracavitary radiation) to point A plus either placebo or hydroxyurea 80 mg per kilogram twice weekly during radiation. Patients receiving hydroxyurea had a higher complete response rate (68 versus 48 percent), longer progression-free interval (median 13.6 versus 7.6 months), and longer survival (median 19.5 versus 10.7 months) with all differences statistically significant ($p < .05$).

A second trial, GOG protocol 56, compared radiation plus hydroxyurea in the same dose and schedule with radiation plus misonidazole, a promising hypoxic cell sensitizer, 1 gram per square meter twice weekly during radiation. Patients on both regimens received 4,000 cGy (stage IIB) or 5,000 to 6,000 cGy (stage III to IVA) of external radiation. Stage IIB patients were given intracavitary radiation 4,000 cGy to point A; stage IIIB to IVA patients received 2,000 to 3,500 cGy intracavitary radiation to point A. Only patients with negative para-aortic nodes as demonstrated by limited para-aortic sampling were entered, in contrast to the lack of node sampling in protocol 4. Some 60 percent of the patients had stage IIB disease. Among the 296 patients, no significant difference was observed between the two arms. Subset analysis produced perhaps the most significant observation. The progression-free survival curves for both stage IIB groups and the stage IIIB to IVA hydroxyurea subset essentially overlapped, but the stage IIIB to IVA misonidazole subset had a poorer progression-free survival. This tends to confirm the observations of GOG protocol 4 and suggests that observed benefit from concomitant hydroxyurea and radiation may be limited to those with stage IIIB or IVA disease.

A third trial, GOG protocol 85, employed the same entry criteria and radiation regimen as in protocol 56 and randomized patients either to hydroxyurea 80 mg per kilogram orally twice weekly during radiation or to cisplatin 50 mg per square meter intravenously on days 1 and 29 and 5-fluorouracil 1 g per square meter as a continuous intravenous infusion days 2 to 5 and 30 to 33 of radiation. No statistically significant differences in either progression-free or overall survival were observed.

These results support the role of chemoradiation, at least in patients with stage IIIB and IVA disease. Both hydroxyurea and the combination of cisplatin and 5-fluorouracil as given in the GOG trials are reasonable choices for combination with radiation, but toxicity findings favor hydroxyurea. No evidence supports the value of such an approach in patients with earlier stage disease.

Current Recommendations and Future Directions

Radical hysterectomy is the treatment of choice for patients with stage IB small lesions (less than 3 to 4 cm), radiotherapy for larger lesions. At least one study suggests the addition of an extrafascial hysterectomy following the completion of radiation. There is no evidence to support the use of chemotherapy as a part of routine clinical practice for these patients. For patients with stage II, III, and IVA disease, radiotherapy is the mainstay of treatment. Based on randomized trials, concomitant chemotherapy in the form of either hydroxyurea 80 mg per kilogram twice weekly during radiation or cisplatin 50 mg per square meter on days 1 and 29 and 5-fluorouracil 1 g per square meter as a continuous infusion daily on days 2 to 5 and 30 to 33 during radiation should be used in patients with stage IIIB or IVA disease.

For the immediate future, several randomized trials of GOG may affect treatment decisions. In patients with stage IIB through IVA disease, GOG protocol 120 evaluates radiation with concomitant chemotherapy consisting of either hydroxyurea, weekly cisplatin, or hydroxyurea plus cisplatin plus 5-fluorouracil. In patients with stage IB disease, GOG protocol 71, now completed, compared radiation with or without subsequent extrafascial hysterectomy. This study is under analysis. In this same population GOG protocol 123 compares radiotherapy with and without weekly cisplatin followed by extrafascial hysterectomy, whereas GOG protocol 141 randomizes patients with small lesions to radical hysterectomy alone or preceded by cisplatin plus vincristine. The results of these studies should better define treatment for locoregionally advanced disease.

Advanced or Recurrent Disease

The management of patients with advanced or recurrent disease depends entirely on the use of systemic therapy. There are three essentials to the development of effective treatment: a thorough understanding of patient characteristics that might influence choice of therapy, identification of drugs with a high order of activity against cervix cancer, and evolution of combinations of drugs that yield a high frequency of durable responses.

Patient Characteristics

The patient population considered for the use of systemic therapy as definitive treatment presents several challenges to the development of effective regimens. First, the majority of patients will have received pelvic radiotherapy as a part of initial management. This poses two problems. Patients will have an impaired bone marrow reserve as a result of radiation-induced damage to the pelvic marrow and hence will not tolerate dose-intense regimens. In addition, blood supply to foci of cancer will be altered by radiation and can limit drug access to tumor cells. Even active drugs may yield low response rates because of these two factors.

Second, most patients have extensive pelvic involvement. Ureteral obstruction, a common complication of pelvic tumor, leads to renal impairment in a significant number of patients. Since many drugs are excreted renally, drug dosing becomes problematic in patients with impaired renal function.

Finally, although a variety of histologic types make up the overall population, squamous cell carcinomas account for 85 percent of all patients. These lesions typically are moderately responsive to numerous drugs, but the duration of response is characteristically short and patient benefit limited even when combinations of agents are used.

These characteristics dictate certain approaches to the use

Table 3 Single Agents Active in Cervix Carcinoma

DRUG	RESPONSE (%)
ALKYLATING AGENTS	
Cyclophosphamide	38/251 (15)
Chlorambucil	11/44 (25)
Melphalan	4/20 (20)
Ifosfamide	25/157 (15)
Dibromodulcitol	23/102 (29)
Galactitol	7/36 (19)
PLATINUM COMPOUNDS	
Cisplatin	190/815 (23)
Carboplatin	27/175 (15)
Antibiotics	
Doxorubicin	45/266 (20)
Porfiromycin	17/78 (22)
ANTIMETABOLITES	
5-Fluorouracil	29/142 (20)
Methotrexate	17/96 (18)
Baker's Antifol	5/32 (16)
VINCA ALKALOIDS	
Vincristine	10/55 (18)
Vindesine	5/21 (24)
Other Agents	
ICRF-159	5/28 (18)
Hexamethylmelamine	12/64 (19)

of systemic therapy. Because of the increased likelihood of significant adverse effects, drugs should have clearly demonstrated activity. Initial doses must take into account the high probability of impaired marrow reserve in previously radiated patients. Drugs excreted by the kidneys or producing renal toxicity should be avoided in patients with ureteral obstruction. If these cautions are heeded, systemic therapy can be safely and effectively used.

Single-Agent Therapy

For practical purposes, reports of trials of chemotherapy in cervix cancer are actually trials in patients with squamous cell carcinoma. A number of drugs have demonstrated activity in such testing over the past 2 decades (Table 3). Four agents or groups of agents in particular have shown consistent activity at the 20 percent or greater level in well-designed trials with appropriate definitions of response: the platinum compounds, ifosfamide, dibromodulcitol, and doxorubicin.

The platinum compounds are the most extensively studied agents. Both cisplatin and carboplatin have received attention. GOG has conducted one phase II and two phase III trials of single-agent cisplatin at various doses and schedules. These studies permit several conclusions. First, the drug clearly has activity, as demonstrated by an overall response rate of 23 percent among 785 patients with no previous exposure to chemotherapy. The median duration of response is relatively short at 4 to 6 months, as is survival at 7 to 10 months. This activity has been confirmed by non-GOG trials. Even in patients with prior chemotherapy, cisplatin yields response rates of 20 percent. Second, there is no major advantage to a doubling of dose intensity, as evidenced by the absence of both a 15 percent difference in response between 50 mg per square meter every 3 weeks and 100 mg per square meter every 3 weeks and a response duration and survival difference. Third, a prolonged infusion over 24 hours yields no difference in response rate, duration of response, or survival, but the prolonged infusion is associated with a reduction in nausea and vomiting. This observation of a toxicity difference predated the availability of ondansetron and metoclopramide; hence, its relevance to current therapy probably is minimal.

Carboplatin. Because of reduced frequency of nephrotoxicity and neurotoxicity, carboplatin was subsequently tested by the GOG in comparison with another platinum compound, iproplatin, as a part of a randomized trial. The overall response rate to carboplatin was 15 percent, somewhat lower than that observed with cisplatin. Response duration and survival were similarly short. There are no data to permit a reliable judgment regarding the relative efficacy of carboplatin versus cisplatin.

Ifosfamide. Though chemically similar to its cousin, the alkylating agent cyclophosphamide, ifosfamide produces response rates that appear to be of a higher order than those observed with cyclophosphamide. Both in a fractionated 5 day schedule of 1.5 g per square meter per day every 3 to 4 weeks and in a 24 hour infusion schedule of 5 g per square meter every 3 to 4 weeks, response rates range from 33 to 50 percent in patients with no prior chemotherapy. In patients with prior platinum-based chemotherapy, response rates are considerably lower, from 0 to 11 percent.

Dibromodulcitol. A halogenated sugar, dibromodulcitol demonstrated activity in small trials. A more recent GOG phase II trial of 180 mg per square meter per day orally for 10 days every 4 weeks in patients with no prior chemotherapy yielded a 29 percent response rate. Clearly, the drug has activity, but reports of leukemia in patients with breast carcinoma treated with adjuvant dibromodulcitol may well prevent it from being released for use in the United States.

Doxorubicin. An anthracycline, doxorubicin was tested extensively by the GOG in patients with no prior exposure to chemotherapy. The overall response rate was 17 percent, with response duration and survival of a similar short duration to that seen with the platinum compounds. Other series confirm an observed activity in the range of a 20 percent response rate.

Other Drugs. Other drugs with some demonstrated activity fall into one of two categories. Some have shown significant activity in a single relatively small trial, activity not corroborated by other studies. Others have moderate activity with response rates ranging from 10 to 15 percent. Some of these drugs may prove to be useful as a part of combination chemotherapy in future trials, but their role in current therapy is questionable at best.

Combination Chemotherapy

Numerous combinations of drugs have been tested in uncontrolled series with varying results. Response rates ranging from 0 to 100 percent have been reported. Higher reported response rates have generally not held up when larger confirmatory series are undertaken or when randomized trials are conducted. Response durations and survivals, furthermore, have remained relatively short in both phase II and phase III trials. No evidence to date supports scientifically the superiority of combination chemotherapy over single agents. Despite the lack of concrete proof of superiority, certain combinations are used frequently in practice, and they deserve further discussion.

Cisplatin with 5-Fluorouracil. Cisplatin in combination with prolonged infusion of 5-fluorouracil, because of its activity in squamous cell carcinomas of other sites, has been of prime interest in squamous cell carcinoma of the cervix. Seven nonrandomized trials have been conducted. In patients with no prior radiotherapy or chemotherapy, response rates in two series were 68 and 69 percent. Four series involving patients with prior radiotherapy but no prior chemotherapy yield response rates ranging from 15 to 27 percent. An additional series in patients with prior radiotherapy reported a response rate of 61 percent, the only report of a high response rate in previously radiated patients. In all series response duration and survival are of the same magnitude as that seen with a platinum compound alone.

These results lead to two conclusions. First, the results with cisplatin plus 5-fluorouracil in previously irradiated patients are similar to those with cisplatin alone. This suggests that the combination is of little value in this setting. Second, in patients not previously exposed to radiation, the combination produces high response rates. This points to a possible role for cisplatin plus 5-fluorouracil in more limited disease, whether prior to or in combination with radiation.

Ifosfamide with Platinum. Certain combinations include ifosfamide plus a platinum compound on the basis of the significant single-agent activity noted with both drugs and reports of high response rates with combinations. Five phase II trials of ifosfamide-platinum combinations, most commonly also including bleomycin, have been reported. In patients not previously exposed to radiotherapy, response rates range from 59 to 100 percent. These rates are significantly lower in previously irradiated patients. In both groups, response and survival durations are relatively brief and similar to those achieved with single agents. Determining whether such combinations offer advantages over single-agent therapy requires a randomized trial.

Other Combinations. Other regimens viewed as having some potential include doxorubicin plus cisplatin and 13-*cis*-retinoic acid plus interferon. Neither has been extensively investigated. The GOG completed a phase II trial of doxorubicin 60 mg per square meter plus cisplatin 50 mg per square meter every 3 weeks with an overall response rate of 32 percent and response duration and survival similar to that achieved with either agent alone. Investigators at M.D. Anderson Hospital and Tumor Institute reported a 47 percent response rate with 13-*cis*-retinoic acid 1 mg per kilogram per day orally plus interferon-alpha 6 million units per day subcutaneously, but response durations were again similar to those seen with single agents. Neither combination can be recommended for routine clinical use.

Current Recommendations and Future Directions

Patients with advanced or recurrent carcinoma of the cervix should be offered systemic therapy. Since there is no clear demonstration of the superiority of combination chemotherapy over single agents, it is acceptable to use either a platinum compound or ifosfamide alone. A reasonable dose and schedule is either cisplatin 50 to 100 mg per square meter intravenously every 3 weeks or ifosfamide 1.5 g per square meter intravenously daily for 5 days every 3 weeks in combination with Mesna 300 mg per square meter prior to and 4 and 8 hours after ifosfamide. With such an approach, response rates will range between 20 and 30 percent with response durations in previously radiated patients of 4 to 9 months and survival of 9 to 12 months.

Should combination chemotherapy be used at present? Although no randomized trials demonstrate clear superiority for combination regimens, response rates in phase II trials appear higher with combinations including ifosfamide and a platinum compound. If such a combination is to be recommended, ifosfamide should be given over 3 to 5 days to decrease the likelihood of central nervous system toxicity. One such dose and schedule is as follows: ifosfamide 1.5 g per square meter per day plus cisplatin 15 mg per square meter per day over 5 days.

For the immediate future, two important randomized trials seek to evaluate promising combinations. GOG protocol 110, which was recently completed and is still under analysis, randomized patients with advanced or recurrent squamous cell carcinoma of the uterine cervix to cisplatin 50 mg per square meter on day 1 and every 3 weeks alone or with either ifosfamide 5 g per square meter over 24 hours on day 1 every 3 weeks or dibromodulcitol 180 mg per square meter orally days 2 through 6 every 3 weeks. GOG protocol 149 randomizes patients to either the same ifosfamide-cisplatin regimen used in protocol 110 or the same two-drug schedule plus bleomycin 30 mg on day 1 every 3 weeks. Long-range plans in advanced disease focus on the identification of new active agents and the exploration of the possible role of the biologic regimen 13-*cis*-retinoic acid plus interferon.

■ ENDOMETRIAL CARCINOMA

Endometrial carcinoma is the most common invasive neoplasm of the female genital tract. In 1994 over 34,900 new cases are expected in the United States. The number of deaths is much lower than might be expected (approximately 6,000 in 1997 in the United States) because of certain important characteristics of the disease. Management can be rationally based on these characteristics.

General Disease Characteristics

Endometrial carcinoma is primarily a disease of menopausal and postmenopausal women. Unopposed, continuous estrogen stimulation of the endometrium has been implicated in the origin of the lesion in the form of both endogenous estrogen imbalance and exogenous estrogen and/or tamoxifen. Associated problems include diabetes, hypertension, and obesity. Patients usually present with abnormal or postmenopausal uterine bleeding, a fact that accounts for early diagnosis in the majority of patients.

The vast majority of lesions are adenocarcinomas, but adenosquamous carcinomas, adenoacanthomas, and a variety of rarer histologic types are reported. Two facts regarding

Table 4 FIGO Staging System for Endometrial Carcinoma

STAGE	DESCRIPTION
Stage 0	Carcinoma in situ; histologic findings suspicious for malignancy
Stage I	Carcinoma confined to corpus
IAG123	Tumor limited to endometrium
IBG123	Invasion to <½ myometrium
ICG123	Invasion to >½ myometrium
Stage II	Carcinoma involving corpus and cervix but not extending outside uterus
IIAG123	Endocervical glandular involvement only
IIBG123	Cervical stromal invasion
Stage III	Carcinoma extending outside uterus but not outside true pelvis
IIIAG123	Tumor invades serosa or adnexae or positive peritoneal cytology
IIIBG123	Vaginal metastases
IIICG123	Metastases to pelvic or para-aortic lymph nodes
Stage IV	Carcinoma extending outside true pelvis or involving bladder or rectal mucosa
IVAG123	Tumor invasion of bladder and/or bowel mucosa
IVB	Distant metastases including intra-abdominal and/or inguinal lymph nodes

Table 5 Recommendations for Patients with Endometrial Carcinoma

DISEASE STATUS	RECOMMENDATIONS
Stage I and II	Total abdominal hysterectomy plus surgical staging of adnexae, pelvic and para-aortic lymph nodes, peritoneal cytology; consider radiotherapy in cases with grade 3 disease, deep myometrial invasion, or involvement of cervical stroma
Stage III and IVA	If amenable to surgical resection to no or minimal residual disease, surgery followed by radiotherapy tailored to disease extent
Stage IVB and recurrent	Include bulky residual stage III and IVA as well as IVB and recurrent disease; systemic therapy with progestins or tamoxifen if grade 1 and/or receptor-positive disease; doxorubicin plus cisplatin if grade 3 and/or receptor-negative or progressive on hormones

pathology are worthy of note. First, the degree of differentiation is an important prognostic feature, particularly of stage I lesions. Well-differentiated tumors are much less likely to recur than are poorly differentiated lesions. Second, two cell types are associated with a poor prognosis: clear cell and papillary serous carcinomas.

The most important determinant of outcome is the extent of disease at diagnosis. This is expressed in the FIGO staging system (Table 4), a surgical-pathologic staging system in its recent revision, which defines stage I disease as confined to the corpus, stage II disease as involving the cervix, stage III disease as extending beyond the uterus to involve adnexa, the vagina, or pelvic and/or para-aortic lymph nodes, and stage IV disease as extension to the bladder or rectal mucosa or to extrapelvic structures other than para-aortic nodes. Within each stage further subdivision of patients on the basis of such features as depth of myometrial invasion (stage I), nature of cervix involvement (stage II), type of extension (stage III), and local or distant dissemination (stage IV) permits separation of groups of patients according to prognosis. Stages I through III are further subdivided by grade. Patients with stage I disease account for 75 percent of all cases, stage II 13 percent, and stages III and IV only 12 percent. Not only are most cases stage I, but most stage I cases are grade 1 with minimal or no myometrial invasion.

Design of an appropriate management plan requires that all of these surgical-pathologic factors be taken into account (Table 5). Subsequent discussion will use the staging system as a basis for the development of a rational approach to management. Patients with stage III or IV disease will be referred to as having advanced disease, and the management of these patients as well as those with recurrent disease will be discussed first. Management of patients with stage I or II disease, hereinafter called limited disease, will be described last.

Advanced or Recurrent Disease

The FIGO staging system recognizes three distinct groups of patients with advanced disease: those with stage III disease, those with stage IV disease confined to the pelvis, and those with disseminated stage IV disease. To this must be added patients with disease recurrent after initial therapy. From the standpoint of therapeutic decision making, the first two groups should be considered together, although the precise details of treatment may vary. In a similar fashion, the latter two groups, those with extrapelvic stage IV disease and those who have recurred, can be taken together.

Locoregionally Advanced Disease (Stages III and IVA)

Patients in this group have disease confined to the pelvis and/or para-aortic lymph nodes. The standard of care for this group is surgery and/or radiotherapy. Overall 5-year survival rates of 25 to 50 percent have been reported. Management principles based on more recent data focus on surgical resection of gross disease, if possible, followed by radiotherapy.

Selected patients with stage III or stage IV disease are amenable to surgical resection of gross disease to the point that no or only minimal residual disease remains. The great majority of these patients will recur or progress and should be considered for further treatment after resection. Therapeutic options for postoperative treatment include radiation and/or chemotherapy. Although it is difficult to make firm specific recommendations because of the lack of data from randomized trials, general guidelines for management can be based on prognostic features of the disease.

For patients with stage III disease by virtue of adnexal involvement or positive peritoneal cytology (favorable advanced disease), complete surgical resection of gross disease followed by adjuvant radiation is a rational approach. Those whose disease was confined to the pelvis may be considered for pelvic radiation, whereas more extensive involvement (positive peritoneal cytology) logically dictates an enlarged treatment volume with abdominopelvic radiation.

For patients with stage III disease by virtue of lymph node involvement, surgical resection of known disease followed by radiotherapy should be employed. If nodal involvement is confined to pelvic nodes, pelvic radiation is acceptable, al-

Table 6 Active Single Drugs in Endometrial Carcinoma

DRUG	PATIENTS	RESPONSE RATE
Medroxyproges-terone acetate	609	20%
Tamoxifen	52	24
Doxorubicin	161	26
Cisplatin	124	24
Carboplatin	52	31
Paclitaxel (Taxol)	28	36

though abdominopelvic radiation has been recommended by some. In patients with positive para-aortic nodes, the standard approach to postoperative therapy is extension of the radiation field to include the node area.

A number of studies, including an ongoing major randomized GOG trial, are evaluating abdominopelvic radiation as an option for all patients who can be surgically resected to the point that no or minimal residual disease remains. In studies to date, radiation to 3,000 cGy to the whole abdomen followed by a boost of 1,980 cGy to the pelvis is used. For those with para-aortic node involvement, the boost to the para-aortic area is 1,500 cGy. The GOG phase III trial randomizes patients to abdominopelvic radiation as described versus chemotherapy (doxorubicin plus cisplatin).

Bulky, Disseminated, or Recurrent Disease

Patients who have bulky residual or extrapelvic dissemination or who recur after initial therapy will require systemic hormonal therapy or chemotherapy.

Hormonal Therapy. Endometrial carcinoma is clearly a hormonally influenced disease (Table 6). Older literature reports objective regression of disease in 33 percent of patients with endometrial carcinoma treated with progestational agents. Responses correlate with histologic grade and receptor status. Well-differentiated lesions are more likely to respond and to be positive for estrogen and progesterone receptors than poorly differentiated lesions. Receptor-positive lesions are more likely to respond to progestin therapy than receptor-negative ones.

With dose and schedule based on a pilot study demonstrating that serum levels of progestin were comparable for oral and parenteral medroxyprogesterone acetate (MPA), a study of oral MPA 150 mg per day in patients with advanced or recurrent endometrial carcinoma not previously treated with systemic therapy reported 32 complete (10 percent) and 26 partial (8 percent) responses among 331 patients with measurable disease. Median progression-free interval was 4 months, median survival 10.4 months. In the 102 patients with known receptor status, response to MPA occurred more frequently and progression-free interval and survival lasted longer in patients with tumors positive for both estrogen and progesterone receptors.

A follow-up study randomized patients to receive either 200 mg or 1 g per day of MPA and required that blood levels of progestin be assessed. Blood levels confirmed compliance. The lower dose of MPA offered a marginal advantage in terms of progression-free interval with a similar response rate. Frequency of response correlated with both grade and receptor status, as expected.

Table 7 GOG Protocol 107: Doxorubicin With or Without Cisplatin

RESPONSE STATUS	DOXORUBICIN 60 MG/M² Q 3 WK (%)	DOXORUBICIN-CISPLATIN 60 MG/M²-50 MG/M² Q 3 WK (%)
Complete response	10 (8)	23 (21)
Partial response	25 (20)	25 (23)
Stable disease	60 (47)	46 (42)
Increasing disease	32 (25)	16 (15)
Total	127 (100)	110 (100)

The overall response rate of 44% with the combination is significantly superior to the 28% with doxorubicin. Progression-free survival with the combination is also superior (6 versus 3.8 months).

Based on these data, hormonal therapy should be considered in advanced or recurrent disease, particularly for patients with known receptor positivity or well-differentiated neoplasms. The hormone of choice is a progestin. The only other agent to be tested in a significant number of patients is tamoxifen, which demonstrated activity in two of three trials.

Chemotherapy. With regard to chemotherapy, three clearly active drugs have been identified: the platinum compounds, doxorubicin, and paclitaxel (Taxol) (see Table 6). Each agent produces response rates ranging from 20 to 30 percent, median duration of responses of 4 to 7 months, and median survival of 9 to 12 months. Most attempts at evaluating combination regimens for endometrial carcinoma have consisted of small series with no control arm and hence no opportunity to assess the relative merits of the combination versus single-agent therapy. Randomized trials of the GOG have compared doxorubicin 60 mg per square meter with or without cyclophosphamide 500 mg per square meter every 3 weeks (GOG protocol 48) and doxorubicin 60 mg per square meter with or without cisplatin 50 mg per square meter every 3 weeks (GOG protocol 107).

In GOG protocol 48, among 202 patients with measurable disease the single agent produced a response rate of 22 percent and median survival of 6.8 months compared with 32 percent and 7.6 months for the combination. The response rate difference was marginally significant, but survival was not different.

In GOG protocol 107 (Table 7), among 261 patients with measurable disease the combination produced responses in 44 percent with a median progression-free survival of 6 months and median survival of 9 months. Doxorubicin alone yielded a response rate of 28 percent with a median progression-free survival of 3.8 months and median survival of 9 months. The differences in response and progression-free survival are both significant, while survival is obviously not different.

Current Recommendations and Future Directions

Patients with advanced or recurrent disease should be divided into those with disease amenable to surgical resection such that only minimal residual or no disease remains and those with bulky, disseminated, or recurrent disease. The first group should be managed with surgical resection followed by radiation. The extent of the radiation will be dictated by disease sites. The second group should be managed with systemic therapy. For patients with well-differentiated or receptor-positive disease, medroxyprogesterone acetate 150 to 200 mg per day orally or megestrol acetate 160 mg per day orally is appropriate. For those with poorly differentiated or receptor-negative disease or with disease progressive on hormones, doxorubicin 60 mg per square meter plus cisplatin 50 mg per square meter every 3 weeks should be used.

For the future, several questions are under study. GOG protocol 122 randomizes patients with advanced disease with minimal residual or no disease after surgery to either abdominopelvic radiation or doxorubicin plus cisplatin. GOG protocol 139 randomizes patients with disseminated or recurrent disease to standard doxorubicin plus cisplatin or timed doxorubicin at 6 AM plus cisplatin at 6 PM. Studies to follow will evaluate the role of paclitaxel in front-line combination chemotherapy as well as continue the search for new active agents.

Limited Disease

Patients with stage I or II disease constitute the vast majority of newly diagnosed endometrial carcinoma. The mainstay of treatment for these patients is hysterectomy. Estimation of risk of recurrence is based on the pathologic features of the primary lesion at the time of surgery: degree of differentiation (grade), histologic type, depth of myometrial invasion, and, in the case of patients with stage II disease, whether the involvement of the cervix includes invasion of cervical stroma or simply extension to endocervical glands. These factors have already been discussed.

The vast majority (75 percent) of patients with limited disease will be at low risk for recurrence because of the presence of well-differentiated lesions with little or no myometrial invasion and disease confined to the corpus of the uterus. For these, surgery alone is appropriate therapy. For patients with poorly differentiated lesions, deep myometrial invasion, or cervical stromal involvement, risk of recurrence rises significantly. These patients are candidates for adjuvant therapy, with options including radiotherapy, hormones, and chemotherapy.

The case for adjuvant radiotherapy is not clear. No definitive, well-designed, randomized trial explores the various options in a way that permits firm conclusions. Only two statements can be made with confidence. First, radiation to the upper vagina probably decreases the incidence of vaginal cuff recurrence. Second, external beam therapy appears to reduce the frequency of pelvic recurrence. However, there does not appear to be any change in ultimate survival. Efforts to study preoperative, postoperative, and tailored radiotherapy have been unsuccessful because of lack of accrual; a principal reason seems to be the unwillingness of investigators to randomize patients among these three approaches because of preconceived bias. For the present it is reasonable to consider limited-disease patients with poorly differentiated lesions, deep myometrial invasion, or cervical stromal involvement for adjuvant radiotherapy with the understanding that no statement can be made as to its ultimate effect on outcome.

No evidence supports the use of adjuvant systemic therapy in limited disease. Adjuvant progestins were evaluated in a large study prior to understanding of hormone receptors and prior to the availability of surgical-pathologic data defining prognostic factors. The study showed no advantage for the use of progestins, but the overall survival of all patients was very high as a result of inclusion of mostly low-risk patients in the trial. Whether adjuvant hormonal therapy would fare better in a high-risk population is not known. Adjuvant doxorubicin was evaluated in a randomized trial versus no systemic adjuvant therapy in high-risk stage I patients who had undergone hysterectomy and postoperative external beam radiotherapy; no differences were observed. No other controlled trials of adjuvant hormonal or cytotoxic therapy have been reported in limited endometrial carcinoma.

Current Recommendations and Future Directions

Patients with limited (stage I or II) endometrial carcinoma should undergo a total abdominal hysterectomy and bilateral hysterectomy. Patients with grade 2 or 3 lesions, deep myometrial invasion, or cervical stromal invasion should be considered for postoperative radiation tailored to the specific circumstances of the patient. No systemic adjuvant therapy is indicated at present.

For the future, one ongoing randomized trial addresses the important question of the role of radiation. GOG protocol 99 randomizes patients with myometrial invasion to postoperative radiotherapy or no adjuvant treatment to determine whether radiation has any role in these patients. Randomized trials are needed to evaluate the role of radiation, hormones, and combination chemotherapy in high-risk patients, although no such trials are under way at present.

Suggested Reading

Benda J. Pathology of cervical carcinoma and its prognostic implications. Semin Oncol 1994; 21:3–11.

Burke T, Wolfson A. Limited endometrial carcinoma: Adjuvant therapy. Semin Oncol 1994; 21:84–90.

Creasman W. Limited disease: Role of surgery. Semin Oncol 1994; 21:79–83.

Gordon M, Ireland K. Pathology of hyperplasia and carcinoma of the endometrium. Semin Oncol 1994; 21:64–70.

Hatch K. Preinvasive cervical neoplasia. Semin Oncol 1994; 21:12–16.

Homesley H, Zaino R. Endometrial cancer: Prognostic factors. Semin Oncol 1994; 21:71–78.

Hoskins W, Perez C, Young R, eds. Principles and practice of gynecologic oncology. Philadelphia: JB Lippincott, 1992.

Lentz S. Advanced and recurrent endometrial carcinoma: Hormonal therapy. Semin Oncol 1994; 21:100–106.

Muss H. Chemotherapy of metastatic endometrial cancer. Semin Oncol 1994; 21:107–113.

Omura G. Chemotherapy for cervix cancer. Semin Oncol 1994; 21:54–62.

Randall M, Reisinger S. Radiation therapy and combined chemo-irradiation in advanced and recurrent endometrial carcinoma. Semin Oncol 1994; 21:91–99.

Rose P. Locally advanced cervical carcinoma: The role of chemoradiation. Semin Oncol 1994; 21:47–53.

Stehman F, Thomas G. Prognostic factors in locally advanced carcinoma of the cervix treated with radiation therapy. Semin Oncol 1994; 21:25–29.

Thigpen T. Chemotherapy of gynecologic cancer. In: Perry M, ed. The chemotherapy sourcebook. Baltimore: Williams & Wilkins, 1992; 1039–1067.

Thigpen T, Vance R, Khansur T. Carcinoma of the uterine cervix: Current status and future directions. Semin Oncol 1994; 21:43–56.

Thomas G, Stehman F. Early invasive disease: Risk assessment and management. Semin Oncol 1994; 21:17–24.

HIRSUTISM

Roger S. Rittmaster, M.D.

Hirsutism is excess hair growth in women. It is not a disease. Although hirsutism may rarely be a manifestation of a serious underlying disorder, most often it results from a combination of increased androgen production (compared with nonhirsute women) and increased skin sensitivity to androgens.

Not all hirsutism is androgen dependent. Several drugs (e.g., glucocorticoids, cyclosporine, diazoxide, and minoxidil) can cause diffusely increased hair growth. Androgen-independent hirsutism can also be inherited as a familial trait, particularly in women of East Indian origin. The key to determining the hormonal dependency of hair growth is the physical examination. Androgen-dependent hirsutism occurs in areas where men typically develop hair growth. Hirsutism consisting of long, fine hairs located diffusely over the trunk and face, including the forehead, is not androgen dependent, and medical therapy will not benefit such women.

■ PRINCIPLES OF MEDICAL THERAPY

Women gradually develop more body and facial hair with age. Therefore, if hirsutism is left untreated, it tends to become gradually worse with time. Although most women will respond to medical therapy, it is easier to prevent hair growth than to treat established hirsutism. Adolescent girls who are beginning to develop hirsutism and who have a family history of excessive hair growth are excellent candidates for medical therapy. Nevertheless, most women experience some improvement with treatment.

Mechanical hair removal (shaving, plucking, waxing, dipilatory creams, electrolysis) can control hirsutism, but usually does not change the underlying natural history. Although electrolysis is advertised as permanent hair removal, in many women regrowth occurs. Nevertheless, the combination of mechanical hair removal and medical therapy offers a speedier improvement than medications alone. A common misconception is that mechanical hair removal, especially shaving, causes hair to grow more rapidly. Women begin to shave because of worsening hirsutism. When the hair growth continues to worsen, shaving is blamed.

As noted in the introduction, hirsutism is usually caused by a combination of increased androgen secretion and increased skin sensitivity to androgens. In women with severe polycystic ovarian syndrome (PCOS), ovarian androgen secretion predominates. In such women it is important to lower serum testosterone levels (with an oral contraceptive, for example) to achieve optimal improvement. In women with hirsutism and low- or mid-normal testosterone levels, adding an oral contraceptive to an antiandrogen such as spironolactone is usually no more effective than the antiandrogen alone.

In women with PCOS the onset of hirsutism may coincide with weight gain and the onset of irregular menses. Although weight loss may restore ovulation and cyclic menses, usually medical therapy is necessary for a satisfactory improvement in the hirsutism to occur.

The primary determinant of whether a woman's hirsutism is going to improve is the intrinsic sensitivity of the hair growth to androgen suppression or blockade. Typically, long-standing facial hirsutism responds slowly to medical treatment—even if androgens are suppressed to undetectable levels. More commonly, hirsutism improves over the first 6 to 12 months of medical therapy and then reaches a new plateau. The dose-response relationship for most medications is relatively shallow, and maximal doses are often only slightly more effective than mid-range doses. When starting a medication, it may take as long as 6 months for a woman to note an improvement in hirsutism, especially if she is not mechanically removing hairs at the same time. If after 6 months of medical therapy no improvement is seen, either a higher dose or a second medication should be used. Treatment needs to be continued indefinitely. If medical therapy is stopped the hirsutism is likely to recur.

For clinical purposes, the best indication that a treatment is effective is a reduction in the time a patient spends in mechanically removing the hair. If a woman shaves, how often? If she plucks or has electrolysis, for how many minutes each day or week? If such questions are asked routinely during the initial evaluation and follow-up, the physician will have a good estimate of the effectiveness of the treatment.

One of the difficulties in evaluating the literature on the treatment of hirsutism is the lack of rigor in the scientific evaluation of the response to treatment in many studies. Most frequently hirsutism scoring is used as the principal method of evaluation. This involves grading the amount of hair growth in androgen-dependent areas, usually on a scale of 0 to 4. Such scoring systems are semiquantitative at best and subject to large observer variation, even when done by the same individual. To be credible, hirsutism scoring should only be used in published studies when the scorer is blinded to treatment status. Measurement of hair shaft diameter or hair weights is more objective. However, even these methods need to be adequately validated. Two to three baseline evaluations in each patient are essential to determine the variability of the method. Theoretically, the measurement of hair weight should be more accurate than hair shaft diameter (the latter measures changes in only one dimension). However, serially shaving an area of excess hair growth requires careful measurements of the area being shaved and is labor intensive.

The medical treatment of hirsutism involves either suppressing ovarian or adrenal androgen secretion or blocking the action of androgens in the skin with androgen receptor blockers (antiandrogens) or 5α-reductase inhibitors (Table 1).

Reprinted with modifications from Rittmaster RS. 1995 Clinical Review 73:Medical treatment of androgen-dependent hirsutism. J Clin Endocrinol Metab 1995; 80:2559–2563; © The Endocrine Society.

Table 1 Medical Treatments of Hirsutism

- Ovarian suppressants
  - Oral contraceptives
  - Cyproterone acetate
  - Gonadotropin-releasing hormone analogues
- Adrenal suppressants
  - Glucocorticoids
- Antiandrogens
  - Spironolactone
  - Flutamide
  - Cyproterone acetate
- 5α-reductase inhibitors
  - Finasteride

■ OVARIAN ANDROGEN SUPPRESSION

Oral Contraceptives

Birth control pills are designed to prevent ovulation, not to maximally suppress ovarian androgen secretion. The progestin component decreases ovarian estrogen and androgen production by inhibiting gonadotropin secretion. The estrogen component increases sex hormone–binding globulin (SHBG) through a direct effect on the liver. In women with PCOS, coexisting hyperinsulinemia can suppress SHBG and limit the ability of estrogens to increase serum SHBG concentrations. Progestins also may bind weakly to the glucocorticoid receptor and cause a modest decrease in adrenal androgen secretion. Many progestins (e.g., norethindrone, levonorgestrel, ethynodiol diacetate, desogestrel) are 19-nortestosterone derivatives and have androgenic activity when given in high doses to castrated rats. The relevance of this property to women has never been demonstrated when progestins are used in low dose as part of an oral contraceptive. Cyproterone acetate is both a progestin and an antiandrogen. When used to prevent ovulation, low doses (2 mg daily) are effective; for maximal ovarian androgen suppression and antiandrogenic activity, 25 to 50 mg daily are required. Other progestins (gestodine and norgestimate) are less androgenic and have no antiandrogenic activity. On a theoretical basis, an oral contraceptive containing an antiandrogenic progestin such as cyproterone acetate would be best for hirsute women. Such a pill (Diane) is available in Europe and elsewhere but is not available in the United States or Canada. Despite these considerations, no birth control pill has ever been shown to be more effective than another for the treatment of hirsutism. Perhaps at the doses used in oral contraceptives, the relative androgenicity of the progestin is inconsequential.

How effective are oral contraceptives for the treatment of hirsutism? Although many studies describe improvement in hirsutism with oral contraceptives, these studies have usually been unblinded and uncontrolled, using either subjective criteria or hirsutism scoring as end points. In my experience, only about 10 percent of hirsute women will have significant improvement and 40 percent will continue to develop more hair growth with oral contraceptives alone. Some women do note the onset or worsening of hirsutism after stopping a birth control pill, indicating that they do have a beneficial effect. However, this effect is modest when compared with antiandrogens. The women most likely to benefit from oral contraceptives are those with anovulation and elevated testosterone levels. In such women, the ability of the progestin to maximally suppress luteinizing hormone (LH) is probably the most important feature. Outside the United States, this can be best accomplished by adding cyproterone acetate to an oral contraceptive (see the section Antiandrogens). An alternative is to use an oral contraceptive with a high progestin content, such as one of the newer pills containing 0.15 mg desogestrel. Oral contraceptives are also useful for cycle control and contraception in women receiving antiandrogens.

Gonadotropin-Releasing Hormone Analogues

Gonadotropin-releasing hormone (GnRH) analogues decrease ovarian steroid production by suppressing pituitary LH and follicle-stimulating hormone secretion. Depending on the preparation used, they are given by daily subcutaneous injection (buserelin, leuprolide), two or three times daily nasal spray (buserelin, nafarelin), monthly intramuscular depot injection (leuprolide), or monthly subcutaneous implant (goserelin). Provided that a sufficient dose is used to maximally suppress ovarian androgens, all of the commercially available preparations should be adequate for clinical use. From a practical standpoint, however, it is difficult to deliver enough of the intranasal preparations to cause complete ovarian androgen suppression. Otherwise, the choice of GnRH analogue depends on the availability, cost, and convenience of the preparation. In research studies, I have found that 3.75 mg depot leuprolide is sufficient to maximally suppress ovarian androgen secretion. Dose-response studies for other GnRH analogues have not been published using androgen suppression as an end point.

The greater the increase in ovarian androgen secretion in a hyperandrogenic woman, the greater will be the decrease in androgen production with a GnRH analogue. Therefore, GnRH analogues are most effective in women with PCOS and severe ovarian hyperandrogenism. GnRH analogues have no effect on adrenal androgen secretion. Women with normal or near normal serum testosterone levels and adrenal hyperandrogenism do not usually respond well to GnRH analogues. The likelihood of a good clinical response can be predicted by determining the percent decrease in serum testosterone and androstenedione after 4 to 6 weeks of analogue therapy.

When given alone, GnRH analogues suppress estrogens to castrate levels. Because there is no need to suppress both androgens and estrogens when treating hyperandrogensim, estrogen/progestin replacement is usually given, either as an oral contraceptive or as one of the postmenopausal treatment regimens. Such combined treatment prevents the decrease in bone density and symptoms of estrogen deprivation that occur with GnRH analogues alone. In this regard, the dose of estrogen necessary to preserve bone density and prevent symptoms of estrogen deficiency in young women is somewhat higher than that required in postmenopausal women. As long as the dose of GnRH analogue is sufficient to maximally suppress ovarian androgens, female hormone replacement does not result in a greater improvement in hirsutism (compared with the analogue alone).

Because the relative contribution of the ovaries and adrenal glands to androgen secretion varies among women, the clinical efficacy of GnRH analogues also varies greatly. Substantial improvement in hirsutism can occur in women with severe PCOS. Because adrenal androgen secretion is unaffected, it may be beneficial to add an antiandrogen, especially in women whose testosterone is not suppressed into the low-normal range by the analogue alone. The major disadvantage to using GnRH analogues is cost (in excess of $400 per month). In my experience, the combination of cyproterone acetate and an oral contraceptive is as effective as a GnRH analogue in women with ovarian hyperandrogenism, making this combination the treatment of choice for hirsute women with severe PCOS (in countries where cyproterone acetate is available).

■ ADRENAL ANDROGEN SUPPRESSION

Glucocorticoids

Most hirsute women, including those with PCOS, have some degree of adrenal hyperandrogenism compared to nonhirsute women. Glucocorticoids reduce adrenal androgen secretion, but the clinical efficacy of glucocorticoids in hirsute women has been a subject of much debate. Because adrenal androgens are somewhat more easily suppressed than cortisol and remain suppressed longer, clinicians have attempted to find a dose of exogenous glucocorticoid that would adequately suppress adrenal androgen secretion without causing excessive adrenal suppression or symptoms of glucocorticoid excess. This has led to a wide range of treatments, including 10 to 20 mg hydrocortisone or 2.5 to 5 mg prednisone nightly (or divided into morning and evening doses) or 0.25 to 0.5 mg dexamethasone nightly. Low doses generally cause little or no suppression of serum testosterone (although dehydroepiandrosterone sulfate levels decrease), and higher doses are often associated with subtle signs of glucocorticoid excess such as weight gain or nocturia. Although some women do note improvement in hirsutism, especially when glucocorticoids are combined with other medical treatments, the response rate is not nearly as great as when antiandrogens are used.

About 1 percent of hirsute women have nonclassic 21-hydroxylase deficiency, a form of congenital adrenal hyperplasia. Such women have well-defined adrenal hyperandrogenism that can lead to anovulation and the clinical features of PCOS. They have normal or near-normal cortisol secretion. In such women, glucocorticoid therapy can restore ovulation and fertility. Nevertheless, the hirsutism in women with late-onset 21-hydroxylase deficiency often responds better to antiandrogens than to glucocorticoids. Many women with this disorder have normal menses and are fertile; in such women, there is usually no need to use glucocorticoids.

■ ANTIANDROGENS

Antiandrogens competitively inhibit binding of testosterone and dihydrotestosterone to the androgen receptor. All antiandrogens have other hormonal effects and/or toxicity. Therefore, the particular choice of antiandrogen will depend on patient characteristics, availability and cost of drug, and potential side effects. Although each antiandrogen has its proponents who proclaim it to be better than any other, no antiandrogen has been shown to be unequivocally superior in a well-designed randomized clinical trial with objective end points.

Spironolactone

Spironolactone is an aldosterone antagonist originally used to treat hypertension. Subsequently it was found to bind competitively to the androgen receptor with an affinity of 67 percent compared with dihydrotestosterone. It is also a weak progestin and a weak inhibitor of testosterone biosynthesis. After oral administration it is rapidly converted to canrenone, a less potent antiandrogen.

Numerous studies have demonstrated the efficacy of spironolactone in a wide variety of hirsute patients. Usually 25 to 100 mg is given orally twice daily. Higher doses are somewhat more effective, but also have an increased frequency of side effects. In healthy adult women, I recommend starting at a dose of 50 mg twice daily. At this dose, 70 to 75 percent of women will note an improvement in hirsutism within 6 months, and it is rare for women to have worsening hirsutism while taking spironolactone. It is my impression that spironolactone works best in ovulatory women with normal testosterone levels. In women with PCOS the addition of an oral contraceptive will improve response rates. In women who do not improve within 6 months and who are having no side effects, the dose can be doubled. Up to 400 mg daily has been used, but I do not recommend this dose because of the frequency of side effects. Topical spironolactone is usually ineffective.

The only common side effect of spironolactone is more frequent menses, usually every 2 weeks, which occurs in 20 to 25 percent of women who are not using an oral contraceptive. This can be treated by adding a birth control pill or by reducing the dose to 25 mg two or three times daily. Some authors recommend giving spironolactone for only 3 of every 4 weeks. Menstrual irregularity can still occur on this regimen, and efficacy should be better when androgens are blocked continuously. Nausea, dyspepsia, or fatigue can occur with high doses of spironolactone. The drug is excreted through the kidneys, and life-threatening hyperkalemia can occur in patients with renal insufficiency. Spironolactone should be used with caution in elderly women, patients with diabetes, and women taking other drugs that can increase serum potassium. Allergic reactions (rash, hives) occur infrequently and may not recur when a different brand is used. Although there is appropriate concern about giving spironolactone to pregnant women, I know of one patient with Bartter's syndrome who delivered two male infants with normal genitalia while taking 400 mg spironolactone daily. The retail cost of generic spironolactone in Nova Scotia is about $23 (U.S. $17.02) per 100 for 25 mg tablets and $48 (U.S. $35.52) per 100 for 100 mg tablets (which can be broken in half).

Flutamide

Flutamide is an antiandrogen used to treat prostate cancer. It has about 20 percent of the affinity of spironolactone for the androgen receptor, but it is used in higher dose (125 to 250 mg twice daily for hirsutism; 250 mg three times daily for prostate cancer). It is metabolized to active and inactive metabolites by the liver and is excreted primarily in the urine. Its efficacy is similar to that of spironolactone. Although some uncontrolled studies have reported dramatic improvement in hirsutism with flutamide, I have not found it to be better than other antiandrogens.

The most common side effect of flutamide is dry skin. Increased appetite has been reported in several studies, although it is unclear whether this was associated with weight gain. Other gastrointestinal complaints are reported in men receiving 250 mg flutamide three times daily for prostate cancer, but these are uncommon in the lower doses used in women. The major concern with flutamide is a potentially fatal drug-induced hepatitis, which occurs in less than 0.5 percent of patients given this drug. Flutamide can cause ambiguous genitalia in male offspring of rats given very high doses; its safety in pregnant women has not been established. The retail cost of flutamide (in Nova Scotia) is about $300 per 100 for 250 mg tablets. Because of its high cost and potential hepatotoxicity, I do not recommend flutamide in the routine treatment of hirsutism.

Cyproterone Acetate

Cyproterone acetate is a potent progestin, a moderately potent antiandrogen and a weak glucocorticoid. It also induces hepatic metabolism and increases testosterone clearance. It has a long biologic half-life, partly because it is stored in adipose tissue. It is metabolized by the liver and its half-life is reduced in patients receiving other hepatic enzyme inducers such as anticonvulsants. It is excreted in both the feces and urine. Cyproterone acetate is not available in the United States, but is available throughout the world including Europe, Canada, and Mexico. It is used in an oral contraceptive (2 mg in combination with 35 or 50 µg ethinyl estradiol) or as a 50 mg tablet for the treatment of prostate cancer (only the latter formulation is available in Canada). Although the oral contraceptive decreases hair growth in many women, higher doses are usually used to treat hirsutism. Originally, 25 to 100 mg cyproterone acetate daily was given during the first 10 to 11 days of a cyclic 21-day course of estrogen with 7 days off both medications. More recently, the same doses have been given during the first 10 days of a low-progestin oral contraceptive pill cycle, with 50 mg being the most frequent starting dose. Because of its long biologic half-life and potent progestational activity, amenorrhea is common when 50 mg cyproterone acetate is given for more than the first 10 days of the birth control pill cycle. Its progestational activity should enhance the contraceptive efficacy of the birth control pill, although this has not been formally evaluated. Cyproterone acetate can also be given continuously (e.g., 25 mg daily or every other day) in women who do not have a uterus.

In unselected hirsute women, the efficacy of cyproterone acetate and spironolactone are similar. On theoretical grounds, cyproterone acetate is best for women with PCOS and elevated testosterone levels. My personal experience indicates that 50 mg cyproterone acetate daily for 10 days (with an oral contraceptive) suppresses serum LH and testosterone at least as much as a GnRH analogue. On the other hand, because cyproterone acetate can only be given for the first part of the menstrual cycle, its antiandrogenic activity will be less during the latter part of the cycle. Therefore, for hirsute women with normal menses and normal testosterone levels, spironolactone may be a better alternative. Because low doses of cyproterone acetate are almost as effective as higher doses, once the maximum improvement in hirsutism is reached, a low dose of the drug will likely prevent worsening hair growth.

In women who are already using an oral contraceptive, the addition of 50 mg cyproterone acetate for 10 days is usually tolerated well. There is often a 2- to 3-day delay in the onset of menses, and amenorrhea can occur. Higher doses can cause weight gain and edema, probably due to its glucocorticoid activity. Drug-induced hepatitis has been reported, and, although this complication is rare with cyclic administration of 25 to 50 mg daily for 10 days each month, it is prudent to monitor liver enzymes. A transient mild elevation of liver enzymes is more commonly seen, if one monitors liver enzymes closely. The retail cost of cyproterone acetate in Nova Scotia is about $310 (U.S. $229.40) per 100 for 50 mg tablets (only 5 to 10 tablets per month are needed).

■ 5α-REDUCTASE INHIBITORS

Finasteride is used for the treatment of benign prostatic hyperplasia and is the only 5α-reductase inhibitor currently available. It has no other known hormonal activity. The dose recommended for treatment of benign prostatic hyperplasia is 5 mg (1 tablet) daily, although 1 mg daily is almost as effective. The biologic half-life is at least 24 hours. Doses of up to 100 mg daily have been given to men without serious adverse effects but also with no greater reduction in serum dihydrotestosterone levels.

One controlled study has found 5 mg finasteride daily to be as effective as 100 mg spironolactone daily in reducing hair shaft diameter (14 percent reduction after 6 months). Other uncontrolled studies have found more marked improvement in hirsutism scores with finasteride. No side effects have been noted in women, and the drug has a good safety profile when given to men. Finasteride causes ambiguous genitalia in male offspring of female rats given finasteride, and one would expect the same to occur in humans, if finasteride were taken throughout the first trimester of pregnancy.

I consider finasteride to be a reasonable option for the treatment of hirsutism in women who cannot become pregnant. For that reason, it may be especially useful in postmenopausal women. One mg daily may be as effective as 5 mg daily, although this hypothesis has yet to be tested. The retail cost of finasteride in Nova Scotia is about $210 (U.S. $155.40) per 100 for 5 mg tablets.

■ COMMENTS

Although hirsutism is more a cosmetic and psychosocial problem than a disease, hirsute women are often some of the most grateful patients in an endocrinologist's practice. The combination of mechanical hair removal and judicious use of medications will improve hair growth in most women. Unfortunately, no drug is approved by regulatory agencies in North America for treatment of hirsutism. Well-designed comparative studies with objective end points are needed to demonstrate which drugs work best in which hirsute women. Because pharmaceutic companies are reluctant to market drugs for women of child-bearing age, there has been little industry support for such studies.

Suggested Reading

Barth JH. ACP broadsheet 131. Hirsute women: Should they be investigated? J Clin Pathol 1992; 45:188–192.

Jeffcoate W. The treatment of women with hirsutism. Clin Endocrinol 1993; 39:143–150.

Rittmaster RS. Evaluation and treatment of hirsutism. Infertil Reprod Med Clin North Am 1991; 2:511–529.

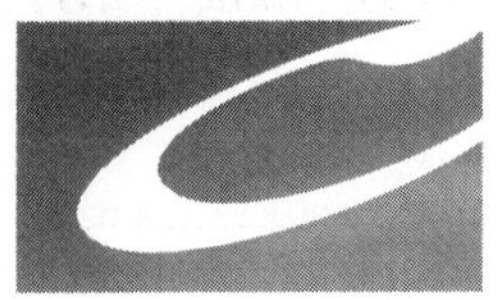

THE ACQUIRED IMMUNODEFICIENCY SYNDROME

HIV INFECTION: INITIAL EVALUATION AND MONITORING

Ahmed S. Rabbat, M.D.
Aaron E. Glatt, M.D., F.A.C.P., F.C.C.P., F.I.D.S.A.

Human immunodeficiency virus (HIV) infection is a major catastrophic event in a patient's life, bringing fear, frustration, and challenge to the physician and society. More than 1 million people in the United States are infected with HIV, with hundreds of thousands more expected to become infected during the next few years.

Primary care physicians will care for most of these patients, especially in the earliest stages of infection. Thus, they need to know which elements of the history and physical examination hold particular importance, which screening and diagnostic studies are necessary, when and how to begin antiretroviral therapy, which preventive measures should be offered, and how to provide appropriate counseling on many other important issues. Therefore, a major goal of initial evaluation is to assess what level of immunocompromise is present.

■ HIV SEROCONVERSION

Patients may develop an acute illness shortly after primary infection with HIV-1 or HIV-2. Individuals may have nonspecific symptoms characterized by lymphadenopathy, malaise, fever, anorexia, diarrhea, headache, and rash; rarely opportunistic infections have been reported. Many persons do not seek medical attention. An estimated date of initial HIV infection may be helpful to assess disease progression. This is possible to document when there has been an isolated known exposure such as an occupational injury, short period of substance abuse, or a single new sexual partner.

Establish the route and risks of acquisition of HIV with open, nonjudgmental questions, as this is important for reducing further transmission and recognizing complications.

■ HISTORY AND PHYSICAL EXAMINATION

HIV disease causes and predisposes to multiple organ disease; evaluation should be systematic and comprehensive. After obtaining a detailed chief complaint and history of present illness, a thorough review of systems of all patients is necessary. Detailed physical examination with careful documentation of baseline observations is essential for early recognition of new problems.

Available data suggest that zidovudine (AZT) may be somewhat effective in preventing and/or ameliorating occupational HIV infection; the optimal dosing and regimen (alone or in combination) remain to be determined.

Review of Systems

General

Fever, weight loss, malaise, fatigue, shaking, chills, night sweats, and loss of appetite can be initial findings of significant illness. They are less common in early HIV infection. They may signify worsening immunosuppression. Weight and nutritional assessment should be recorded at each visit.

Skin

The skin of nearly all HIV-infected persons will eventually be affected secondary to infectious and noninfectious dermatologic disorders. Skin or nail pigmentation and rashes of all varieties can occur in disseminated or sporadic fashion, and they may be clues to underlying serious illness, coinfection, or worsening immunosuppression (Table 1).

Lymph Nodes

Nonspecific small, symmetric, mobile nodes, frequently seen in patients with HIV infection, frequently reflect nonspecific reactive hyperplasia. Acute generalized lymphadenopathy can be seen during seroconversion. Non-Hodgkin's lymphoma (NHL) and infectious pathogens can present as single or multiple nodes.

Table 1 Common Cutaneous Manifestations in HIV Patients

CAUSE	CLINICAL FEATURES
Bacterial Infection	
Bacillary angiomatosis	Numerous angiomatous nodules associated with fever, chills, weight loss
Staphylococcus aureus	Folliculitis, ecthyma, impetigo, bullous impetigo, furuncles, carbuncles
Syphilis	May occur in different forms (primary, secondary, tertiary); chancre may become painful due to secondary infection
Fungal Infection	
Candidiasis	Mucous membranes (oral, valvovaginal), less commonly candida intertrigo or paronychia
Cryptococcoses	Papules or nodules that strongly resemble molluscum contagiosum; other forms include pustules, purpuric papules, and vegetating plaques
Seborrheic dermatitis	Scaling and erythema in the hair-bearing areas (eyebrows, scalp, chest, and pubic area)
Arthropod Infestations	
Scabies	Pruritus with or without rash, usually generalized but can be limited to a single digit
Viral Infection	
Herpes simplex	Vesicular lesion in clusters; perianal, genital, orofacial, or digital; can be disseminated
Herpes zoster	Painful dermatomal vesicles that may ulcerate or disseminate
HIV	Discrete erythematous macules and papules on the upper trunk, palms, and soles are the most characteristic cutaneous finding of acute HIV infection
Human papilloma virus	Genital warts (may become unusually extensive)
Kaposi's sarcoma (herpesvirus)	Erythematous macules or papules; enlarge at varying rates; violaceous nodules or plaques; occasionally painful
Molluscum contagiosum	Discrete umbilicated papules commonly on the face, neck, and intertriginous sites (axilla, groin, or buttocks)
Noninfectious	
Drug reactions	More frequent and severe in HIV patients
Nutritional deficiencies	Mainly seen in children and patients with chronic diarrhea; diffuse skin manifestations, depending upon the deficiency
Psoriasis	Scaly lesions; diffuse or localized; can be associated with arthritis
Vasculitis	Palpable purpuric eruption (can resemble septic emboli)

At each visit lymph node groups should be assessed for size, quantity, texture, and tenderness. Biopsy is not helpful unless nodes are rapidly enlarging or are associated with fever and weight loss.

Head, Eyes, Ears, Nose, and Throat

Candida and herpes simplex virus frequently cause painful cheilitis, stomatitis, or pharyngitis and can manifest at any stage of HIV infection. Cytomegalovirus (CMV), Epstein-Barr virus (EBV; oral hairy leukoplakia), varicella zoster virus, mycobacterial infection, *Cryptococcus neoformans, Histoplasma capsulatum,* Kaposi's sarcoma, squamous cell carcinoma, and non-Hodgkin's lymphoma may be visible on oral examination, and idiopathic aphthous ulcers are a significant cause of troublesome oral pain. Toothache and dental tenderness may indicate periodontal disease or abscess and may cause both fever and headache. Gingival and periodontal infection are particularly aggressive in patients with HIV infection.

Facial pain, nasal obstruction, postnasal drip, and headache can be due to sinusitis, which occurs frequently in HIV infection. Atopy may coexist.

Blurred vision, scotoma, or decreased visual acuity suggests CMV retinitis. Complete eye exams at baseline and when retinitis is a consideration are essential, especially in hosts with CD4 cell count below 50 per milliliter.

Headache of new onset or changing character may be an early manifestation of a central nervous system opportunistic process.

Cardiopulmonary

Precise baseline pulmonary and cardiovascular examinations are important because of increasing pulmonary and cardiac complications in advancing HIV disease. Shortness of breath at rest or with exertion, its duration and progression, whether a cough is dry or productive, sputum color, amount, and odor may help with the differential diagnosis. Hemoptysis can be due to tuberculosis, thrombocytopenia, bacterial pneumonia, or other lung pathology. Chest pain can be due to pneumonia, spontaneous pneumothorax (often *Pneumocystis*-related), pericarditis, herpes zoster, or HIV-related cardiomyopathy. Palpitation and postural hypotension suggest symptomatic anemia.

Gastrointestinal

Gastrointestinal diseases are increasingly frequent as HIV disease progresses.

Odynophagia, dysphagia, retrosternal chest pain, nausea, anorexia, and weight loss are commonly associated with esophagitis due to *Candida,* herpes simplex, CMV, or more rarely, lymphoma. Hepatic or splenic enlargement may be an early manifestation of HIV-related complications; the baseline size should be documented.

Right upper quadrant pain associated with fever and elevated alkaline phosphatase may indicate viral or drug-induced hepatitis, cholelithiasis, or acalculous cholecystitis related to *Mycobacterium avium* complex (MAC) or cryptosporidiosis.

Epigastric or left upper quadrant pain may indicate pancreatitis. Abdominal distention, tenderness, masses, constipation, or fecal incontinence may be due to Kaposi's sarcoma, lymphoma, carcinoma, gastrointestinal opportunistic infections (CMV, histoplasmosis, tuberculosis), or parasitic infestation. Diarrhea occurs in 30 to 66 percent of adults with HIV. *Salmonella, Cryptosporidium, Isospora,* CMV, microsporidia, and other enteric pathogens occur frequently. Constipation is commonly seen in patients on methadone, heroin, or opioids, as well as other medicines.

Painful defecation or rectal pain can be caused by trauma, perirectal abscess, herpes, or other sexually transmitted diseases. Careful sexual and social histories may help identify the pathogens. Perirectal areas should be carefully examined for lesions, abscess, fissures, proctitis, and ulcerations. Stool should be tested for occult blood.

Genitourinary, Obstetric, and Gynecologic Manifestations

Painful, frequent urination may indicate urinary tract infection, sexually transmitted disease, or vulvovaginitis. The latter are more frequent and possibly more difficult to treat in HIV infection. Recurrent or severe vaginitis, vaginal discharge, and pruritus are common and may not be related solely to sexual practices. Prompt evaluation of all genital discharges, ulcers, and lesions will allow correct identification of any sexually transmitted disease.

Women should be queried regarding menstrual history, fertility, method of birth control, and numbers and dates of pregnancies and abortions. Menstruation may become irregular in worsening HIV infection, and fertility declines as well. Prior tubal scarring from salpingitis or pelvic inflammatory disease predisposes to ectopic pregnancy and infertility. An external genital, rectal, and complete pelvic exam (speculum and bimanual), including Pap tests and appropriate cultures and stains, should be performed initially and at least annually.

Neurologic

Neuropsychiatric complications eventually occur in up to 80 percent of patients, yet symptoms may go unrecognized because of coping strategies and the large reserve available till significant deterioration is noted. Subtle neurologic deterioration, memory loss, and poor concentration may be the only early signs of HIV dementia. Central and peripheral neurologic complications may be due to HIV infection, opportunistic infections, medications, or malignancy. Illness can occur at any stage of HIV infection, albeit with different manifestations. Symptoms depend greatly on the location of the abnormality and the pathophysiology involved. Progressive encephalopathy or peripheral neuropathy can occur years or even decades post seroconversion; intracranial mass lesions are usually a late complication of HIV disease.

Distal predominantly sensory polyneuropathy, chronic inflammatory demyelinating polyneuropathy, mononeuropathy, herpesvirus and CMV radiculitis, and neuropathies of vitamin deficiency are frequently seen. Neurologic evaluation and appropriate diagnostic testing may differentiate treatable from less responsive pathology. A carefully documented baseline neurologic examination, including mental status assessment, cranial nerve testing, and evaluation of sensation, strength, coordination, and reflexes, should be part of an initial and yearly comprehensive evaluation. Mini-mental status test results should be clearly documented.

Musculoskeletal

Myalgia and proximal muscle weakness, tenderness, and wasting may be manifestations of primary HIV or drug-related myositis. Severe, persistent oligoarthritis, primarily affecting the large lower limb joints with exquisite pain, psoriatic arthritis with erosive changes and crippling deformities, and septic arthritis caused by *Staphylococcus aureus,* especially in substance abusers, are not uncommon.

Medical History

A clear history of prior HIV-related events, CD4 cell counts, complications, opportunistic infections, and malignancies will help stage HIV infection, provide prognostic information, and clarify therapeutic options. Opportunistic infections signify marked immunocompromise and are discussed at length in a subsequent chapter.

HIV infection significantly increases the risk of tuberculosis. Purified protein derivative (PPD) status, previous exposure to tuberculosis, and previous prophylaxis or treatment (date, duration, and medications) are critical. Noncompliance, prior hospitalizations, and geographic and social factors play major roles in development of drug resistance and empiric management.

Medications

Polypharmacy with prescription agents; vitamin, mineral, and herbal supplements; and alternative medications are very common. They can cause or change disease manifestations and be associated with adverse effects and toxicity, which can be confused with symptoms of HIV-related disease. For example, vitamin overdosing may cause diarrhea, abdominal cramps, peripheral neuropathy, increased intracranial pressure, headache, anorexia, nausea, and vomiting. Drug interactions are also common and must be diligently sought for both prescription and nonprescription medicines.

Allergy

The physician should differentiate between allergic reaction and intolerance, which is commonly misinterpreted as allergy. The specific reaction, duration, and resolution of toxicity for each medication should be noted. Rash and fevers are the most common type of adverse drug manifestations.

Social History

Particular attention must be given to all aspects of the psychosocial history, especially residence status, occupational history, substance abuse, and sexual history. A complete sexual history should be obtained, including orientation, practices, lifetime number of partners, prostitution, and any sexually transmitted diseases. Dietary habits and water sources are important for certain pathogens.

Travel History

Because certain opportunistic infections occur predominantly in particular geographic regions, place of birth and travel history are particularly useful in formulating a differential diagnosis (e.g., southwestern United States for coccidioidomycosis, Ohio River Valley for histoplasmosis). History of travel to developing or tropical countries may raise suspicion of traveler's diarrhea, malaria, leishmania, kalaazar, strongyloidiasis, *Penicillium* infection, HIV-2, and so on.

Pets

Certain opportunistic infections have been associated with particular animals. Patients should be queried regarding exposure to animals and advised about methods of avoiding zoonoses. *Bartonella* (formerly *Rochalimea*) spp. have been associated with cat-scratch disease and bacillary angiomatosis, and exposure to cats may be associated with toxoplasmosis.

Table 2 Purposes of Laboratory Testing in HIV Infection

- Establish baseline parameters
- Identify underlying disease
- Determine appropriate therapy
- Estimate the likelihood and rate of disease progression
- Monitor response to therapy
- Monitor adverse reactions and toxicities
- Screen for common and preventable illnesses

Laboratory Studies

Laboratory testing, while invasive, uncomfortable, and expensive, is frequently the only way to establish or confirm a diagnosis. Laboratory studies should be individualized, but several general principles apply (Tables 2 and 3).

A complete blood count may reveal mild normocytic, normochromic anemia, which often develops as HIV progresses. Macrocytosis develops on zidovudine and can help assess compliance. Pancytopenia may suggest bone marrow involvement or infiltration; isolated thrombocytopenia may be an early finding of HIV infection; and leukopenia and/or a blunted neutrophil response to infection is a common finding. Neutropenia frequently becomes more pronounced with various drug therapies (zidovudine, trimethoprim-sulfamethoxazole, pentamidine, and others).

Assessment of chemistries, liver function, and hepatitis tests are useful in diagnosing concurrent illness and as a guide to monitoring drug toxicities or development of new illness.

A nonspecific syphilis test, such as the rapid plasma reagin (RPR) or the Venereal Disease Research Laboratory (VDRL) tests, with confirmatory fluorescent treponemal antibody absorbed (FTA-abs) tests, should be performed initially, and repeated annually in patients at risk. Lumbar puncture may be indicated for patients with reactive serologies of uncertain duration and/or symptoms.

Table 3 Routine Laboratory Studies for HIV-Infected Adults

TEST	INDICATIONS	INTERVAL
Antitoxoplasma antibody (IgG)	Screen for previous exposure Guide diagnostic and empiric management	Baseline (?) Yearly in patients with negative results
Chemistry and liver functions	Evaluation of baseline renal and liver functions and nutritional status Diagnosis of concurrent hepatitis Monitor efficacy of therapy	Baseline Every 6–12 mo More frequently in patients with advanced disease, baseline abnormalities, or with drug toxicity
Cervical swabs	Screening for chlamydial and gonorrheal infection	Baseline Yearly in patients at risk
Chest radiograph	Screen for disease Diagnosis of active disease	Baseline If pulmonary disease suspected
Complete blood count	Evaluate for anemia, leukopenia, thrombocytopenia Monitor drug toxicities Monitor efficacy of therapy Assess compliance	Baseline Every 6 mo More frequently in patients with abnormalities or on marrow-suppressing agents
Hepatitis profile	Diagnose viral hepatitis Evaluate for vaccination Response to vaccination	Baseline During potential acute infection Post vaccination
Lymphocyte subset testing (CD4 cells)	Guide initiation of prophylactic, antiretrovial therapy Prognostic information Monitor efficacy of therapy	Baseline Every 6 mo if >500 Every 3 mo if <500 Discontinue when <50
Pap smear	Screening for dysplasia/cancer	Baseline Every 6–12 mo
RPR or VDRL	Screening for syphilis Monitor response to therapy Use specific test (i.e., FTA) for confirmation, false-negative specimen	Baseline Yearly (at least) in patients at risk or with prior infection Monthly for 6 mo, 9 to 12 mo post therapy During new symptoms
Tuberculosis skin test (PPD)	Screen for infection or previous exposure Identify new converters	Baseline if negative history Yearly if negative history More frequently if at greater risk

Table 4 Vaccination Guidelines for HIV-Infected Adults

VACCINE	FREQUENCY
Pneumococcal vaccine	Once; booster at 5 years?
Hepatitis B vaccine series	Series of three at 0, 1, 6 mo; booster in 5 years?
Influenza	Yearly in autumn
Inactivated polio vaccine	Per standard guidelines
Diphtheria, tetanus	Per standard guidelines
Measles (MMR)	Per standard guidelines
Haemophilus influenzae vaccine	Once?

A PPD should be placed on initial evaluation and at least annually except in patients with a history of tuberculosis or reactive PPD. Baseline chest x-ray film is recommended regardless of PPD status.

Baseline antitoxoplasma immunoglobulin (Ig)G antibodies may influence prophylaxis decisions and help with the evaluation and empiric treatment of central nervous system mass lesions. CMV and EBV serologies and baseline cryptococcal antigen testing have no value.

Pelvic examination, including cervical swabs for detection of *N. gonorrhoeae* and chlamydia, and pap smears for early identification of cervical dysplasia should be performed at baseline, and repeated every 6–12 months in at-risk patients. Other sexually transmitted illnesses also should be sought.

CD4 lymphocyte counts, useful markers of immune status, should be obtained every 3 to 6 months as a guide for treatment and prophylactic interventions. CD4 monitoring should be discontinued when clinical decisions are no longer based on the results. There is significant variability in CD4 cell counts; the aggregate picture over weeks or months is more useful than a single reading for major therapy decisions.

Accumulating data suggest that quantitative measurements of HIV-RNA in the blood may be a more accurate marker of immune status and viral load than CD4 cell counts. They may be useful as an independent marker of disease progression, and may replace CD4 cell count measurements in terms of intervention strategies. Cost remains a significant disadvantage at present.

■ VACCINATIONS

Patients should receive immunizations as early as possible in the course of HIV infection to optimize response (Table 4), although clinical efficacy is difficult to assess.

Pneumococcal vaccine should be given. The merit of a booster in 5 years is controversial. It is unknown whether *Haemophilus influenzae* vaccination is indicated for HIV-infected adults.

Patients without serologic evidence of hepatitis B exposure or immunity should be given hepatitis B vaccine. It is unknown when and whether any booster is necessary.

Influenza vaccine is recommended annually.

Inactivated polio vaccine, standard childhood vaccinations, and booster diphtheria and tetanus immunizations can be given as per published guidelines.

■ BEHAVIORAL ADVICE

As part of the routine initial comprehensive visit, as well as at future visits, the physician should discuss modification of risk activities and behaviors. This should include discussions regarding sexual, occupational and environmental risks; pets, foods, water, and travel issues; and any additional factors that may contribute to repeated HIV exposure or exposure to opportunistic pathogens.

■ GUIDELINES FOR FOLLOW-UP

Stable asymptomatic HIV patients should be examined and re-evaluated at least every 6 months, more frequently as immunocompromise worsens. Follow-up of symptomatic patients should be individualized. Most patients have numerous psychosocial needs that also must be addressed; referral to the appropriate staff is essential for complete and compassionate care.

Suggested Reading

Centers for Disease Control and Prevention. 1993 Revised classification system for HIV infection and expanded surveillance case definition for AIDS among adolescents and adults. MMWR 1992; 41:1.

Centers for Disease Control and Prevention. USPHS/IDSA guidelines for the prevention of opportunistic infections in persons infected with human immunodeficiency virus. MMWR 1995; 44:1–34

Cohen PT, Sande M, Volberding PA, eds. The AIDS knowledge base. 2nd ed. Boston: Little, Brown, 1995.

Gold J. HIV-1 infection, diagnosis, and management. Med Clin North Am 1992; 76:1–18

Ong K, Iftikhar S, Glatt AE. Medical evaluation of the adult with HIV infection. Infect Dis Clin North Am 1994; 8:289–301.

HIV INFECTION: THERAPY

John P. Phair, M.D.

The availability of effective antiretroviral agents enabled Ho and colleagues and Wei and co-workers to elucidate the dynamics of the human immunodeficiency virus (HIV) replication in the human host. The publication of these investigations, in January 1995, was paralleled by an increase in the number and type of effective agents available to physicians for treatment of this retroviral infection. The result of the increase in our understanding of the biology of this virus and access to new and more effective treatment regimens has resulted in a major change in the management of persons infected with HIV.

In addition to the nucleoside reverse transcriptase inhibitors (RTI), zidovudine (ZVD), didanosine (ddI), zalcitabine (ddC), stavudine (d4T), lamivudine (3TC), nevirapine (NVP), and three protease inhibitors (saquinavir, retonavir and indinavir) are currently available to physicians for use in treatment of HIV infection (Table 1). In addition, a number of agents are in clinical development (Table 2). In parallel with the increased number of effective antiretroviral agents, the understanding that the number of copies of HIV-RNA in plasma accurately reflects the rate of viral replication and that this rate correlates with clinical progression has enabled physicians to accurately provide a prognosis for an infected individual. Further demonstration that reducing the viral burden is associated with slowing of progression and enhanced survival has provided physicians for the first time with a means of monitoring and altering therapy effectively.

The current goal of antiretroviral therapy is to reduce levels of plasma HIV-RNA to undetectable levels. This can be achieved by combining RTIs, combining RTIs with a protease inhibitor (PI), or using two PIs. Monotherapy with any of the available agents leads—rapidly in the case of 3TC or NVP, or more slowly with ZVD, ddI, and the PIs—to selection of resistant variants.

Combination therapy that maximally reduces viral replication is thought to minimize selection of such variants. Finally, the effectiveness of combination therapy in inhibiting viral replication has increased the possibility that therapy initiated early in the course of infection could result in eradication of the virus from the host. Currently, trials evaluating this possibility are under way.

Clinical trials have shown that combinations of RTIs benefit patients naive to therapy. In the AIDS Clinical Trials Group (ACTG) trial 175, ZVD naive and experienced participants received ZVD monotherapy, ddI monotherapy, the combinations of ZVD plus ddI, or ZVD plus ddC. The ZVD naive participants receiving ddI alone or either of the combinations demonstrated less progression and improved survival as compared to persons taking ZVD alone. For ZVD experienced patients, ddI monotherapy and ZVD plus ddI were more effective than ZVD alone. The combination of ZVD plus ddC prevented a 50 percent decline in CD4+ lymphocytes, but progression to AIDS or death was similar to results achieved with ZVD monotherapy. A subgroup of participants were included in a virology study demonstrating that clinical and immunologic results paralleled reduction in viral load. The clinical results of ACTG 175 were confirmed in the Delta trial conducted in Europe and Australia and the NuCombo study in the United States. Another trial evaluating the triple combination of ZVD, ddI, and NVP for treatment of naive participants demonstrated that two-thirds of the individuals receiving the triple combination had undetectable HIV-RNA levels at one year (Table 3).

Table 1 Unavailable Antiretrovial Agents

DRUG	DOSE
Nucleoside RTIs	
ddI	300 mg q12hr
ddC	0.75 mg q8hr
d4T	40 mg q12hr
3TC	150 mg q12hr
Non-nucleoside RTI	
Nevirapine	20 mg qd induction 400 mg qd
Protease inhibitors	
Saquinavir	600 mg q8hr with food
Indinavir	800 mg q8hr on empty stomach
Retonavir	600 mg q12hr

Table 2 Antiviral Agents in Clinical Development

AGENT	CLASS
1502U89	Nucleoside RTI
Delavirdine	Non-nucleoside RTI
DMP-266	Non-nucleoside RTI
Adefovir	Nucleoside phosphonate RTI
Nelfinavir	Protease inhibitor
VX-478	Protease inhibitor

In treatment of experienced patients, the most encouraging results have been seen in trials combining two RTIs with a PI. The first trial that demonstrated a survival benefit was conducted in persons with less than 50 CD4+ lymphocytes. The participants were allowed to continue their current therapy and randomly receive retonavir or a placebo. There was a significant reduction in the deaths in the group receiving the PI. In the viral substudy, a slow rise in viral RNA was noted after six months, suggesting that the benefit was primarily due to monotherapy with the PI and that, with time, resistant variants were being selected. This experience and the initial trials of PIs as monotherapy demonstrating selection of resistant virions has led to the belief that an effective alteration in therapy requires a PI and a new RTI. Therefore, this approach is similar to management of therapy in a patient with tuberculosis.

Overall, the results of triple therapy combining two RTIs plus a PI in naive or treatment experienced patients have been extremely encouraging, demonstrating survival benefits and/or prolonged suppression of plasma HIV-RNA. Similar results have been demonstrated in small trials com-

Table 3 Combinations of Antiretroviral Agents with Proven Clinical Efficacy

TREATMENT NAIVE
ZVD + ddI
ZVD + ddC
ZVD + 3TC
TREATMENT EXPERIENCED
ZVD & ddI
Retonavir + RTI
Saquinavir + ddC

Table 4 Combination with Sustained Antiviral Effects

TREATMENT NAIVE
ZVD + ddI + nevirapine
ZVD + 3TC + indinavir
ZVD + ddI + retonavir
d4T + ddI
TREATMENT EXPERIENCED
ZVD + ddI + indinavir or retonavir
ZVD + 3TC + indinavir or retonavir
Saquinavir + retonavir

bining the two PIs, saquinavir and retonavir (Table 4). The rational for combining these two PIs lies in the fact that PIs are metabolized by the hepatic cytochrome P4503A enzyme system. Saquinavir has low bioavailability; only four percent on average is measurable in blood after administration of the recommended dose. Retonavir, because of effects upon the hepatic enzyme system, inhibits the metabolism of saquinavir. The result of combining the two agents is a marked increase in saquinavir blood levels, a significant reduction in plasma HIV-RNA and, it is expected, a prolonged clinical benefit.

This synergistic effect also illustrates a major concern with the use of PIs in the treatment of patients. Many of the drugs used to prevent or treat opportunistic complications of the immunodeficiency resulting from HIV infection are also metabolized by this hepatic enzyme system. Therefore, knowledge of the drug-drug interactions by physicians is necessary to prevent induction of toxic levels of drugs such as rifabutin or terfenadine (Seldane). Some agents that inhibit p450, such as ketoconazole, enhance blood levels of the PIs. The non-nucleoside, NVP, lowers blood levels slightly while the investigational non-nucleoside RTI, delavirdine, increases blood levels of saquinavir and indinavir. Certain drugs, such as terfenadine are contraindicated for use in patients receiving PIs since the increased blood levels of this agent, resulting from concomitant administration with a PI, have been associated with fatal cardiac arrhythmias (Table 5).

All effective antiretroviral agents have been associated with adverse effects. ZVD and 3TC suppress the bone marrow, and in some patients, when these two drugs are used in combination, anemia is profound. Neuropathy limits the use of ddC, d4T, and ddI. Use of the latter agent also has been associated with pancreatitis. Nevirapine and delavirdine are each associated with development of rash, although the incidence of serious reactions such as Stevens-Johnson syndrome is uncommon. The majority of patients receiving these non-nucleoside RTIs ultimately tolerate these drugs. Saquinavir is generally well tolerated. Indinavir is associated with a benign hyperbilirubinemia, but 4 percent of treated patients develop renal calculi. The calculi are composed of drug precipitation in renal tubules of patients who become dehydrated. Retonavir administration is initially associated with severe gastrointestinal side effects and perioral parasthesias. To reduce the incidence of these problems, which can limit adherence to therapeutic regimens, therapy is initiated with half the recommended dose (300 mg twice daily) and gradually increased to the full dose (600 mg twice daily) over a period of 2 weeks. The 300 mg dose given twice a day produces a therapeutic blood level initially. As the administration of the agent is continued, the cytochrome p450 enzyme system is induced, increasing drug metabolism and allowing a gradual increase in the total daily dose. A similar induction of the cytochrome p450 enzyme, using a half dose of NVP, reduces the incidence of the rash associated with administration of this agent.

Table 5 Classes of Drugs Metabolized by the Cytochrosome P450 Hepatic Enzyme System

CLASS	EXAMPLE
Analgesics	Meperidine
Anti-arrhythmia	Amiodarone
Rifampicins	Rifabutin
Calcium channel blockers	Bepridel
Antihistamines	Terfenadine
Ergot alkaloids	Ergotamine
Gastrointestinal	Cisapride
Antidepressants	Bupropion
Neuroleptics	Clozapine
Hypnotics	Alprazolam
Antifungals	Fluconazole
Antibiotics	Clarithromycin
Xanthines	Theophylline

The recommendations of the consensus conference of 1993 have been rendered obsolete by the rapidly expanding understanding of the biology and natural history of HIV infection. Antiretroviral therapy should be initiated in all infected individuals regardless of the level of the CD4+ lymphocyte count if plasma HIV-RNA is detectable. The goal of treatment is to determine the combination of agents capable of reducing the rate of viral replication maximally in the individual patient. Periodic monitoring of plasma HIV-RNA is necessary to ascertain whether or not the treatment continues to be effective. If the number of copies of HIV-RNA in plasma increases, it is assumed that the current administered combination is losing efficacy. At least two agents, which the patient has not previously received, should be administered in the next combination.

The most experience to date with RTIs and a PI combination has been with ZVD, 3TC, and a PI or ZVD, ddI plus a PI. Currently studies of ddI, d4T and, a PI are underway. Specific combinations of RTIs differ in their effectiveness. ZVD plus 3TC has been widely used, as the rapid selection of a 3TC-resistant variant is associated with sustained susceptibility of the predominant variant to ZVD. In contrast, 3TC plus d4T has been reported to be a less effective combination, implying antagonism with use of these two drugs.

The durability of the effect of the various combinations of antiretroviral agents remains to be determined. To date, effectiveness has been documented to persist for between 18 and 24 months. The goal of managing HIV infection as a chronic disease and prolonging AIDS-free time from the median of 8 to 11 years to 20 or 30 years is dependent upon a sustained benefit from combination therapy. While a greater understanding of adverse effects of such therapy in the short run is accumulating, long-range limitations of treatment are still unknown.

A major caveat in the use of PIs in combination with RTIs is the need for the physician to make the patient understand that adherence to the therapeutic regimen is required. Intermittent compliance will lead to selection of resistant variants, and cross resistance between the available PIs has been documented. Thus, failure to adhere to the therapy will lead to virologic and clinical failure.

Suggested Reading

Coffin JM. HIV Viral dynamics. AIDS 1996;10 (Suppl 3):S75–S84.

Hammer SM, Katzenstein DA, Hughes MD, et al. A trial comparing nucleoside monotherapy with combination therapy in HIV-infected adults with CD4 counts from 200 to 500 per cubic millimeter. N Engl J Med 1996; 335:1081–1090.

Hammer SM. Advances in antiretroviral therapy and viral load monitoring. AIDS 1996; 10 (Suppl 3): S1–S11.

Ho DD, Neumann AU, Perelson AS, et al. Rapid turnover of plasma virions and CD4 lymphocytes in HIV-1 infection. Nature 1995; 373:123–126.

Katzenstein DA, Hammer S, Hughes MD, et al. The relation of virologic and immunologic markers to clinical outcome after nucleoside therapy in HIV-infected adults with 200–500 CD4 cells per cubic millimeter. N Engl J Med 1996; 335:1091–1098.

Mellors JW, Munõz A, Giorgi JU et al. Plasma viral load and CD4+ lymphocytes as prognostic makers of HIV-1 infection. Ann Int Med, in press.

Mulder J, McKinney N, Christopherson C, et al. Rapid and simple PCR assay for quantitation of human immunodeficiency virus type-1 RNA in plasma: application to acute retroviral infection, J Clin Microbiol 1994; 32:292–300.

O'Brien TR, Blattner WA, Walker D, et al. Serum HIV-1 RNA levels and time to development of AIDS in the Multicenter Hemophilia Cohort Study. JAMA 1996; 276:105–110.

Pachl C, Todd JA, Kern DG et al. Rapid and precise quantification of HIV-1 RNA in plasma using a branched DNA (bDNA) signal amplification assay. J AIDS Hum Retro 1995; 8:446–54.

Perelson AS, Neumann AV, Markowitz M, Leonard JM, Ho DD: HIV-1 dynamics in vivo virion clearance rate, infected cell life-span, and viral generation time. *Science* 371:1582–1586, 1996.

Wei X, Ghosh S, Taylor ME, at al. Viral Dynamics in human immunodeficiency virus type-1 infection. Nature 1995; 373:117–122.

AIDS: THERAPY FOR OPPORTUNISTIC INFECTIONS

Noppamas Rojanasthien, M.D.*

Belle L. Lee, Pharm.D.

Merle A. Sande, M.D.

This chapter discusses therapy of opportunistic infection in AIDS. Recommendations for primary and secondary prophylaxis of opportunistic infection are found in the next chapter.

■ PNEUMOCYSTIS CARINII

Pneumocystis carinii is the most common cause of pulmonary infection in AIDS patients. However, its incidence has been decreasing as a result of effective prophylaxis and therapy. The clinical manifestations of *P. carinii* infection are changing; extrapulmonary involvement and atypical pneumonitis are becoming more common.

For patients with mild to moderate disease or Pao_2 above 70 mm Hg, oral trimethoprim-sulfamethoxazole (TMP-SMX) remains the drug of choice (Fig. 1). The major disadvantage of this regimen is its high incidence of adverse reactions in patients with acquired immunodeficiency disease (AIDS). These include fever, rash, nausea, azotemia, hepatitis, leukopenia, and thrombocytopenia. Rechallenge treatment with TMP-SMX may be attempted in patients who have mild adverse reactions. However, this drug should not be given to patients with a history of Stevens-Johnson syndrome, exfoliative dermatitis, or anaphylaxis caused by sulfa drugs. Concurrent use of TMP-SMX with another myelotoxic drug such as zidovudine or ganciclovir may cause severe bone marrow suppression. Complete blood counts (CBC) and absolute neutrophil counts should be closely monitored if TMP-SMX is used concurrently with other myelotoxic drugs. Dapsone-trimethoprim and clindamycin-primaquine work about as well as TMP-SMX. These two combination regimens are contraindicated in patients with glucose-6, phosphate dehydrogenase (G6PD) deficiency. Dapsone and primaquine may cause methemoglobinemia, and monitoring of methemoglobin levels is required, especially in patients with marginal oxygenation. Other adverse effects of clindamycin-primaquine include rash, *Clostridium difficile* colitis, and diarrhea. Atovaquone is a well-tolerated oral drug; however, its variable absorption keeps response rates lower than those of TMP-SMX, and relapses are more common. Aerosol pentamidine may be useful in limited cases. Inhaled pentamidine is not effective against extrapulmonary *P. carinii* infection, and parenteral administration may be required.

For patients with moderate to severe disease or Pao_2 below

Dr. Rojanasthien has received a Merck Fellowship in Clinical Pharmacology.

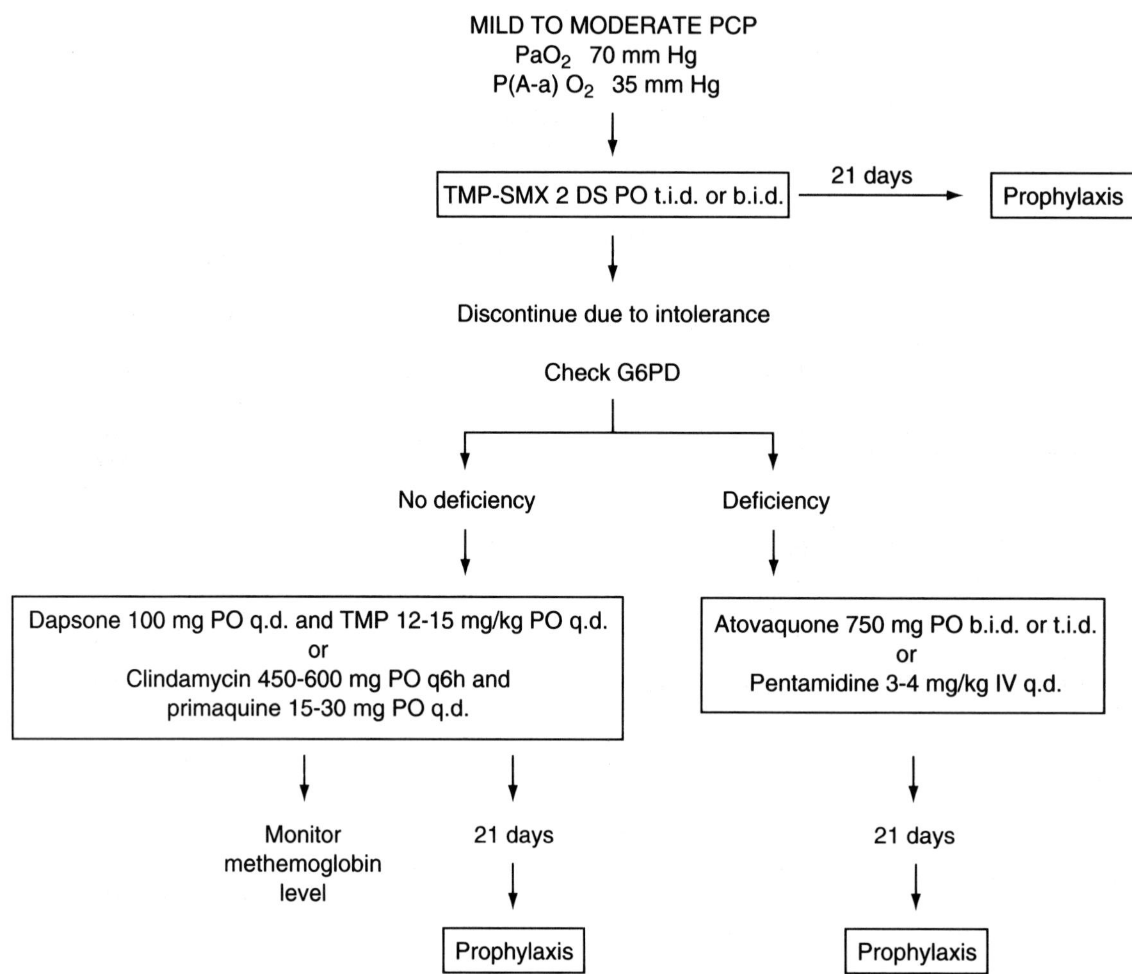

Figure 1
Algorithm for the treatment of mild to moderate PCP.

70 mm Hg, the arterial-alveolar (A-a) gradient above 35 mm Hg, intravenous TMP-SMX and pentamidine are therapeutic options (Fig. 2). The administration of TMP-SMX requires a large volume of fluid (1 L per day) that may worsen respiratory distress. However, concurrent use of diuretic may alleviate volume overload. Pentamidine is comparable in efficacy to TMP-SMX. However, it is associated with more serious side effects such as nephrotoxicity, alteration of glucose metabolism, pancreatitis, neutropenia, thrombocytopenia, and hypotension. Thus, its use is usually limited to patients who cannot tolerate TMP-SMX. Pentamidine is generally given via slow intravenous infusion, as a more rapid rate may cause hypotension and arrhythmia. Alteration in glucose metabolism may result in either hyperglycemia or hypoglycemia, frequently seen in patients who develop concomitant renal toxicity. Blood glucose monitoring is required during therapy and for 2 weeks afterward. Clindamycin-primaquine and trimetrexate-leucovorin are alternative therapies for patients with moderately severe *P. carinii* pneumonia (PCP). Trimetrexate and Eflornithine, which have some efficacy as a salvage treatment, should be reserved for patients unable to tolerate or failing other forms of treatment.

A course of treatment for PCP is generally 21 days for any regimen. Survival and response of the patients depend on the severity of pulmonary dysfunction and tolerance to treatment. Clinical response to therapy generally occurs at the end of the first week. Treatment should not be considered to have failed unless there is no improvement after days 7 to 10 or there is continued worsening after 5 days of treatment. Adverse drug reactions, which are very common in AIDS patients, tend to appear in the second week of therapy. If therapy must be changed, switching the regimen is preferred, since adding a new drug is no more effective than a single regimen. During the first 5 days of treatment patients with moderate to severe disease often deteriorate clinically or develop respiratory failure, presumably due to the inflammatory response to the damaged organisms in the lung. Adjunctive corticosteroid therapy has been shown to reduce this inflammatory response and to decrease mortality and the number of patients requiring respiratory support. Corticosteroid therapy should begin at the same time or within 1 or 2 days of initiation of treatment in patients with PCP who have Pao_2 below 70 mm Hg or the A-a gradient above 35 mm Hg. Delaying corticosteroid therapy until after 72 hours has no clinical benefit and may be associated with an increased risk of other opportunistic infections. The recommended dose is 40 mg of predisone

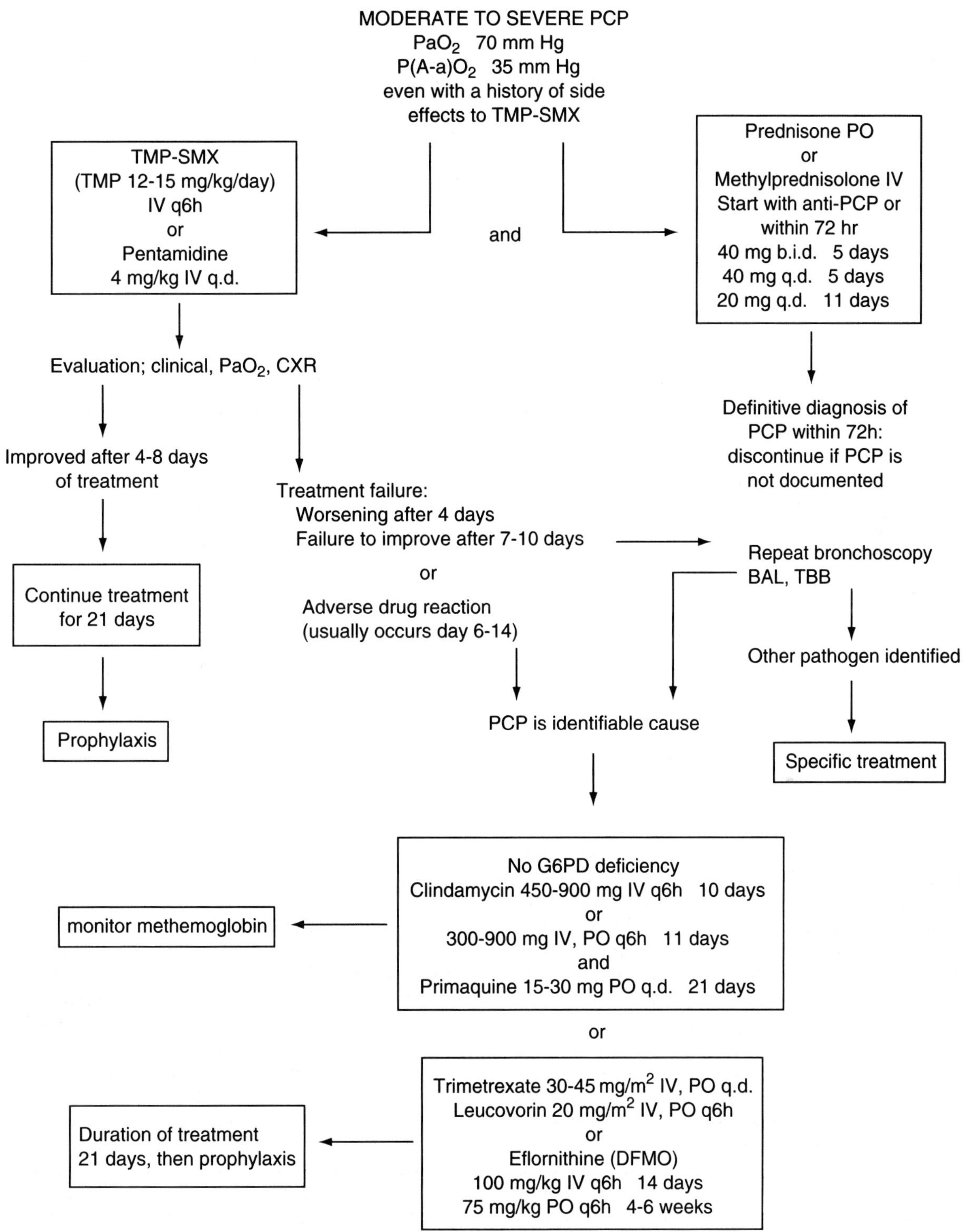

Figure 2
Algorithm for the treatment of moderate to severe PCP, *Pneumocystis carinii* pneumonia. CXR, chest x-ray; BAL, bronchoalveolar lavage; TBB, transbronchial biopsy.

twice daily for 5 days, then 40 mg daily for 5 days, then 20 mg daily until completion of therapy. Adverse effects of corticosteroid use in this clinical setting are surprisingly few, but there is an increased incidence of thrush and reactivation of localized herpetic lesions.

■ MYCOBACTERIUM AVIUM COMPLEX

Disseminated *mycobacterium avium* complex (MAC) infection usually develops late in the course of HIV disease, when the CD4 cell counts are under 100 per cubic millimeter. MAC may be acquired via gastrointestinal or respiratory route, as the organisms are ubiquitous in food, water, and soil. MAC infection usually accompanies other opportunistic infections, thus, the patient's symptoms may be nonspecific.

The initial treatment regimens for MAC infection should include clarithromycin or azithromycin with ethambutol (Table 1). Rifabutin, clofazimine, amikacin, and fluoroquinolones (ciprofloxacin, ofloxacin, sparfloxacin) may be added as a third or fourth drug. The goals of treatment are to reduce the symptoms and improve the quality of life. Effective MAC therapy may be needed for life, since disseminated infection cannot be eradicated.

■ TUBERCULOSIS

The increasing incidence of tuberculosis (TB) is probably due to both reactivation of latent infection and rapid progression of symptoms after acquiring a new infection in human immunodeficiency virus (HIV)-infected patients. Tuberculosis can spread rapidly through casual contact and respiratory droplets. The emergence of multidrug-resistant (MDR) organisms and an increased risk of nosocomial transmission have intensified the problem, and aggressive efforts are being made to control these outbreaks. Purified protein derivative (PPD) skin tests in patients with early-stage HIV disease are likely to be reactive, and reaction of more than 5 mm of induration may indicate infection with *Mycobacterium tuberculosis.* In patients with advanced immunosuppression anergy is more common, and a negative PPD skin test does not rule out tuberculosis. MDR tuberculosis is likely to be diagnosed in foreign-born patients, patients from areas where MDR TB has become a problem (New York, Florida), and patients who have a history of inadequate treatment. Patients with cavitary lesions also have a high frequency of MDR organisms, since they harbor greater numbers of mycobacteria.

An initial four-drug regimen consisting of isoniazid 300 mg per day, rifampin 450 to 600 mg per day, pyrazinamide 20 to 30 mg per kilogram per day, and ethambutol 15 mg per kilogram per day is recommended for the first 2 months. Isoniazid and rifampin should be continued for at least another 4 months if organisms are shown to be sensitive to these drugs. Patients who cannot take concurrent isoniazid and rifampin should receive either isoniazid or rifampin and ethambutol plus pyrazinamide for a minimum of 18 months. With an effective drug regimen and an adequate duration of chemotherapy, nearly all patients can be cured. Nevertheless, treatment may fail, usually because of noncompliance with the treatment regimen. Treatment may be complicated by frequent adverse drug reactions and drug interactions. Both isoniazid and rifampin may lower the serum levels of ketoconazole and fluconazole. Ketoconazole can interfere with the absorption of rifampin.

Treatment of MDR TB requires a five- or six-drug regimen based on the prevailing patterns of resistance (Table 2). These regimens usually include the fluoroquinolones (ofloxacin, ciprofloxacin) and amikacin. Therapy should begin with at least two agents to which the organisms are susceptible in small doses, with increasing doses over 3 to 10 days while observing toxicity and tolerance to these drugs. Determination of peak and trough serum concentration may improve therapy, since bioavailability and clearance of these drugs are not predictable.

Table 1 Treatment for Disseminated MAC

Clarithromycin 500 mg PO b.i.d.
or
Azithromycin 500 mg PO qd
plus
Ethambutol 15–25 mg/kg/day PO
One or more of the following agents are recommended by some authorities:
Rifabutin 300–600 mg/day PO
Clofazimine 100–200 mg/day PO
Ciprofloxacin 750 mg/day PO
Amikacin 7.5 mg/kg/day or twice a day

Table 2 Antituberculosis Agents

DRUG	DOSE PER DAY	SIDE EFFECTS
FIRST-LINE DRUGS		
Isoniazid (with B_6 25–30 mg/day	300 mg	Hepatitis, neuritis, rash, drug interactions
Rifampin	450–600 mg	Hepatitis, rash, drug interactions
Ethambutol	15–25 mg/kg	Optic neuritis
Pyrazinamide	30 mg/kg	Hepatitis, arthralgia, hyperuricemia
PARENTERAL DRUGS		
Amikacin	15 mg/kg	Ototoxicity and nephrotoxicity
Streptomycin	15 mg/kg	
Kanamycin	15 mg/kg	
Capreomycin	15 mg/kg	
SECOND-LINE DRUGS		
Ofloxacin	400 mg b.i.d.	GI distress
Ciprofloxacin	750 mg b.i.d.	GI distress
Ethionamide	250 mg b.i.d. or t.i.d.	GI distress, hepatitis
Para-aminosalicylic acid	3 g t.i.d.	GI distress
Cycloserine	250 mg b.i.d. or t.i.d.	CNS toxicity, seizure, psychosis

GI, gastrointestinal; CNS, central nervous system.

■ FUNGAL DISEASES (TABLE 3)

Cryptococcus Neoformans

Cryptococcus neoformans is a common cause of life-threatening meningitis in AIDS patients. The disease is global, since the fungus is ubiquitous in soil and bird excrement (pigeon droppings). Cryptococcal infection is generally acquired via the respiratory route but may cause infection in any organ. The most common site of infection is the meninges and brain. Mortality of patients diagnosed with cryptococcal meningitis is great in the first 2 to 6 weeks of therapy. Altered mentation (confusion, lethargy, obtudation), cranial nerve deficits, cerebrospinal fluid (CSF) cryptococcal antigen (CRAG) titers above 1:1024, and CSF white blood cell (WBC) counts below 20 per cubic millimeter are risk factors associated with poor outcome.

Initial treatment for high-risk patients is slow intravenous infusion of amphotericin B 0.6 to 0.8 mg per kilogram per day. Hydrocortisone 25 mg and heparin 500 to 1,000 U may be added with each dose to decrease fever, chills, and thrombophlebitis. The total dose and length of amphotericin B therapy depend on the clinical response of the patient. Generally, at least 1 to 2 weeks of administration is required. If there is definite clinical improvement after that, therapy may be switched to fluconazole 400 mg daily for 8 to 10 weeks or amphotericin B may be continued to a total dose of 1.5–2.5 g over 6 to 8 weeks. Flucytosine (5-FC) 150 mg per kilogram per day in four divided doses can be given in combination with amphotericin B 0.3 mg per kilogram per day for 6 to 8 weeks or for 2 weeks followed by fluconazole. This combined regimen is associated with an increase in myelosuppression, especially in patients with impaired renal function, and usu-

Table 3 Antifungal Treatment

DISEASE	DRUG AND DOSE	ADVERSE EFFECTS
Cryptococcosis	Amphotericin B 0.7 mg/kg/day IV qd for 2 weeks followed by	Nephrotoxicity, fever, chills, vomiting
High-risk group		
Altered mentation	Fluconazole 400 mg PO qd for 8–10 weeks	Hepatotoxicity, GI disturbance
CSF CRAG >1 : 1024	Amphotericin B 0.7 mg/kg/day, IV; cumulative dose, 2.5 g	Nephrotoxicity, electrolyte imbalance
CSF WBC <20/mm^3	Amphotericin B 0.3 mg/kg IV qd and	
	5-FC 150 mg/kg PO qd for 6 weeks	Bone marrow toxicity
Low-risk group	Fluconazole 400 mg PO qd for 8-10 weeks	
Normal mentation		
Maintenance therapy	Fluconazole 100–200 mg PO qd	
Candidiasis	Clotrimazole troches 10 mg dissolved in mouth 15 minutes 3–5 times/day	Hepatotoxicity, abdominal pain
Oropharyngeal and vaginal infection (duration of therapy 10–14 days)	Nystatin 200,000 U 1–2 pastilles dissolved in mouth 5 times/day	Nausea, vomiting, diarrhea
	Ketoconazole 200 mg PO qd; absorption requires gastric acid	GI disturbance, hepatotoxicity, drug interactions, inhibits steroid synthesis antacid and H_2 blocker impair absorption
	Fluconazole 100–200 gm PO qd	
Candida esophagitis	Ketoconazole 200–400 mg PO qd for 14 days, then 200 mg/day indefinitely	
	Fluconazole 200 mg PO qd for 14 days, then 100 mg/day indefinitely	
	Amphotericin B 10–20 mg IV qd for 10-14 days followed by fluconazole 100 mg/day	
Histoplasmosis	Amphotericin B 50 mg IV qd, total dose of 1–2 g	
	Itraconazole 300 mg PO b.i.d. for 3 days, then 200 mg PO b.i.d. for 12 weeks	GI disturbance, hepatitis
Maintenance therapy	Itraconazole 200 mg/d PO qd	
Coccidioidomycosis	Amphotericin B 1 mg/kg IV qd total dose of 1.5–2.5 g	Nephrotoxicity, fever, chills, vomiting
	Fluconazole 400 mg PO qd	Hepatotoxicity, GI disturbance
Maintenance therapy	Fluconazole 200–400 mg PO qd	Hepatotoxicity, GI disturbance
	Itraconazole 300–400 mg PO qd	GI disturbance, hepatitis

CSF, cerebrospinal fluid; CRAG, cryptococcal antigen; WBC, white blood cell count; GI, gastrointestinal.

ally requires discontinuation of 5-FC. Its value has yet to be clearly demonstrated. Adverse effects of amphotericin B include reversible impairment of renal function, hypokalemia, hypomagnesemia, anemia, fever with chills, nausea, and vomiting. Adequate hydration with saline and dosage modification of amphotericin B may alleviate renal toxicity. Amphotericin B should be discontinued if serum creatinine (Cr) is above 2.5 mg/dl and can be restarted after Cr drops below 1.5 mg/dl. Premedication with acetaminophen or meperidine 25 to 50 mg, antiemetics, potassium, and magnesium supplements may also be needed.

Fluconazole can be used as initial treatment of patients with moderate disease and normal mentation. The drug is well absorbed and penetrates well into the CSF. The recommended dose is 400 mg per day orally for 8 to 10 weeks. The combination of oral fluconazole and flucytosine is now under investigation for safety and efficacy. Adverse effects of fluconazole are mainly gastrointestinal intolerance, rash, and impaired hepatic function. Fluconazole increases serum levels of phenytoin, warfarin, and sulfonylureas, and its serum level may be lowered by rifampin and raised by thiazide.

Initial treatment with itraconazole 200 mg twice daily is less effective than with amphotericin B. This may be due to poor CSF penetration. Clinical trials comparing the efficacy of itraconazole and fluconazole as maintenance therapy are under way. Ketoconazole is not effective for cryptococcal disease. Increased intracranial pressure may develop as an early or late complication of cryptococcal meningitis. Shunt placement should be considered in patients with noncommunicating hydrocephalus. Daily repeated lumbar puncture with removal of 15 to 30 ml of CSF may be required in communicating hydrocephalus. Acetazolamide 250 mg orally four times a day is a possible therapy if repeated lumbar puncture fails to reduce intracranial pressure.

Serum and CSF CRAG titers frequently increase after initiation of antifungal treatment; however, the increased titers do not correlate with treatment failure. The serum CRAG titers often stabilize in the second month; thus, the CRAG titer may be useful for following the response of therapy. A stable or declined CRAG titer may indicate quiescent disease and a rise in titer with clinical evidence of disease, recrudescence of infection.

Fluconazole 200 mg per day is an effective and convenient regimen for maintenance therapy. Amphotericin B as a maintenance therapy has a high relapse rate, and it is associated with a significantly higher rate of drug toxicity and central venous catheter infections.

Figure 3 is an algorithm for the diagnosis and management of cryptococcal meningitis.

Candida Infection

Oral and vaginal candidiasis are often seen as the CD4 count drops down to the 200 to 300 per cubic millimeter range. Oral candidiasis (thrush) may indicate progression to AIDS and herald other opportunistic infections. Treatment with topical nystatin or clotrimazole troches for 10 to 14 days may be initially adequate. Recurrent infection is common, especially in patients who receive prolonged antibiotic medication. Oral ketoconazole or fluconazole is used in recurrent cases or cases that fail to respond to topical therapy. Fluconazole is more effective and less toxic than ketoconazole and provides a longer disease-free period than clotrimazole. However, prolonged use of fluconazole has been associated with resistance.

Candida esophagitis in AIDS patients may or may not accompany oral thrush. Empiric treatment with ketoconazole 200 to 400 mg per day or fluconazole 200 mg per day may be given. If the patient improves, medication should be continued for 14 to 21 days. If no clinical improvement occurs after 1 week, endoscopy should be performed to rule out other causes. If endoscopic findings confirm *Candida* infection while on oral drug therapy, amphotericin B 10 to 20 mg per day for 10 to 14 days may be useful. Maintenance therapy consists of ketoconazole 200 mg per day or fluconazole 100 mg per day for life to prevent relapse.

Invasive *Candida infection, or candidemia,* is rare. It is associated with iatrogenic causes such as indwelling catheter, prolonged use of broad-spectrum antibiotics, and drug-induced neutropenia. Amphotericin B is the drug of choice for systemic *Candida* infection. The dose and duration of amphotericin B should match the immune status of the patients and the severity of the infection. Removal of the catheter is necessary in catheter-related candidemia. Fluconazole may be effective therapy in hepatosplenic and renal candidiasis in patients without neutropenia. A recent study has shown that fluconazole and amphotericin B are not significantly different in their effectiveness in treating candidemia of patients with neither neutropenia nor major immunodeficiency.

Histoplasmosis

The endemic areas of histoplasmosis are the Mississippi and Ohio river valleys, Puerto Rico, the Dominican Republic, and South America. AIDS patients who reside in or travel to the endemic areas may acquire the infection via inhalation of organisms from soil containing droppings of birds and bats.

Amphotericin B and itraconazole are effective for both initial and maintenance therapy. The initial dose of amphotericin B is 0.5 to 0.6 mg per kilogram per day. The goal of amphotericin B treatment is to reach the 1 to 2 g cumulative dose as rapidly as the patient can tolerate and then switch to maintenance therapy. Thereafter a maintenance dose of 50 to 80 mg weekly or every other week should be given indefinitely. Clinical response to amphotericin B usually occurs by 7 days of treatment. An alternative is itraconazole 300 mg twice daily for 3 days followed by 200 mg twice daily for 12 weeks. Clinical improvement will usually be observed within 2 weeks. Maintenance therapy with itraconazole 200 mg per day indefinitely is necessary to prevent relapse.

Coccidioidomycosis

Coccidioides immitis is an endemic mycosis of the southwestern United States. A fungus, it exists in the soil and causes primary pulmonary infection via inhalation. Acquired or reactivated coccidioidal infection may develop early in the course of HIV disease. Treatment of choice is amphotericin B 1 mg per kilogram per day to a total dose of 1.5 to 2.5 g. Fluconazole 400 mg per kilogram per day also provides good response in patients with coccidioidal meningitis. Indefinite maintenance therapy is necessary with fluconazole 200 to 400 mg per day or itraconazole 300 to 400 mg per day to prevent relapse.

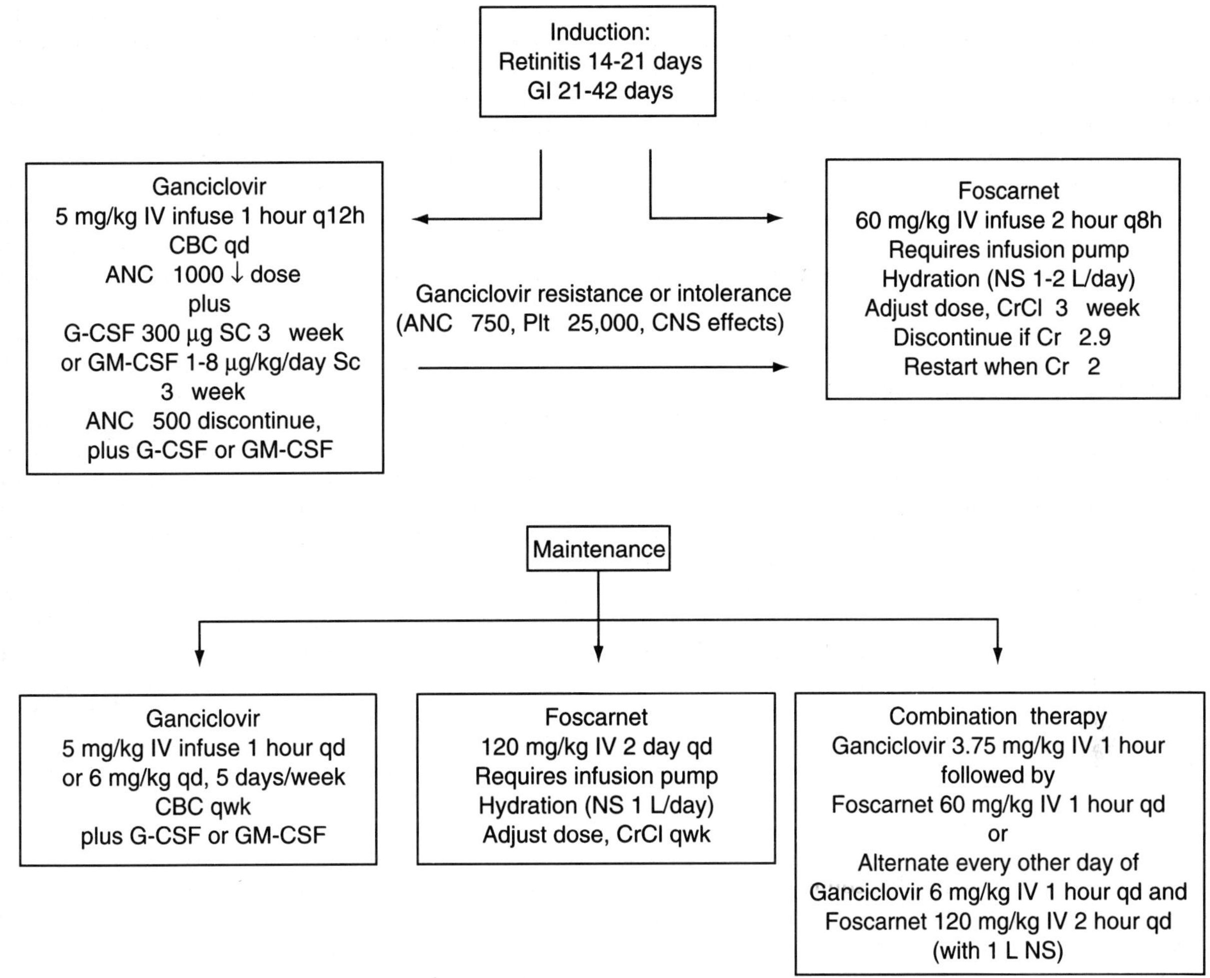

Figure 3
Algorithm for the diagnosis and treatment of cryptococcal meningitis. CT, computed tomography; CRAG, cryptococcal antigen; LP, lumbar puncture; CSF, cerebrospinal fluid; SBC, white blood cell count.

Toxoplasmosis

Toxoplasma gondii is the most common cause of central nervous system (CNS) infection in AIDS patients. The incidence is high in the Caribbean, Haiti, France, Germany, and the developing world. Toxoplasmosis is usually reactivation of infection. Positive *Toxoplasma* serology and a low CD4 count strongly predict a potential to develop *Toxoplasma* encephalitis. Infection may be acquired by exposure to a cat or by eating undercooked pork, mutton, or beef contaminated by the organisms.

A presumptive diagnosis consists of the characteristic computed tomography (CT) or magnetic resonance imaging (MRI) findings, multiple enhancing mass lesions in more than one location, and a positive immunoglobulin (Ig)G antitoxoplasma titer above 1:64. Nevertheless, a solitary mass lesion on MRI study or a negative serology for antitoxoplasma antibody should not be used as an exclusion criterion. In suspected cases a trial of empiric antitoxoplasma treatment should be considered. Most patients show clinical improvement within 7 to 10 days. A patient who fails to respond or deteriorates after 1 week of therapy is a candidate for brain biopsy to rule out lymphoma or another infectious process.

Ninety percent of patients respond to the combination of pyrimethamine and sulfadiazine. The major disadvantage of this regimen is dose-related bone marrow suppression, which requires concomitant use of folinic acid. Folic acid must not be given, since it will inhibit pyrimethamine activity. Patients who receive other myelosuppressive agents (i.e., zidovudine or ganciclovir) should have dosage modification and hematologic monitoring. Other adverse effects, including fever, rash, crystalluria, and hepatitis, usually develop within 7 to 10 days. An alternative regimen with comparable efficacy is pyrimethamine, folinic acid, and clindamycin. Although this regimen is associated with gastrointestinal disturbance, it has less hematologic toxicity than sulfadiazine plus pyrimethamine. Initial treatment should be continued for 6 weeks. Maintenance therapy with pyrimethamine plus folinic acid and either sulfadiazine or clindamycin should continue indefinitely. Recent data show that pyrimethamine plus sulfadiazine is superior to pyrimethamine plus clindamycin for maintenance therapy. Patients with seizures at presentation

Table 4 Treatment of Cytomegalovirus Infection

DRUG	ADVERSE EFFECTS	COMMENTS
Ganciclovir	Neutropenia, thrombocytopenia CNS: confusion, convulsion, psychosis, headache, dizziness GI: nausea, vomiting, diarrhea Others: abnormal LFT, rash, phlebitis	More convenient to administer drug induction Avoid other myelotoxic drugs, e.g., AZT (consider ddI or ddC) Ganciclovir-resistant CMV may develop after 3 months of ganciclovir monotherapy
Foscarnet	Nephrotoxicity Electrolyte imbalance hypocalcemia, hypokalemia hypomagnesemia hypo- or hyperphosphatemia	Rapid IV infusion may cause fatal hypocalcemia, arrhythmia, and seizure (need infusion pump); requires electrolyte supplement; Cr should be ≤2 mg/dl to start foscarnet; avoid other nephrotoxic drugs, e.g., amphoteracin B, aminoglycoside, pentamidine

AZT, zidovudine; ddI, didanosine; ddC, zalcitabine; GI, gastrointestinal; LFT, liver function test.

should also receive anticonvulsant drugs at least during the initial treatment period. Patients with intracranial hypertension and impending herniation may need a short course of dexamethasone 10 mg every 6 hours.

■ VIRAL INFECTIONS

Cytomegalovirus

The clinical manifestations of cytomegalovirus (CMV) infection generally occur late in the course of HIV disease. Retinitis and polyradiculomyelitis usually respond well to therapy; however, if left untreated, the disease may cause irreversible blindness and neurologic deficits. CMV can be isolated from blood, urine, pulmonary secretions, and lung tissue in AIDS patients with other opportunistic infections such as PCP. These patients usually respond to therapy of PCP alone. CMV pneumonitis is extremely rare. Ganciclovir and foscarnet are the drugs of choice for treatment of CMV infection (Table 4). In addition to anti-CMV activity, both ganciclovir and foscarnet are active against herpes simplex virus (HSV) and varicella zoster virus (VZV). Foscarnet is effective against ganciclovir-resistant CMV and has anti-HIV activity.

Initial treatment for CMV (Fig. 4) consists of ganciclovir 5 mg per kilogram infused over 1 hour twice a day; the dose should be reduced in patients with impaired renal function. Ganciclovir is more convenient to administer than foscarnet and is therefore the first line of treatment for CMV disease. The major adverse effect of ganciclovir is myelosuppression. The dose should be reduced when the absolute neutrophil count (ANC) falls below 1,000 per cubic millimeter or discontinued when ANC is under 500 per cubic millimeter and platelet counts are under 25,000 per cubic millimeter. The drug can be restarted when ANC rises above 750 per cubic millimeter. Granulocyte colony-stimulating factor (G-CSF) 300 mg subcutaneously three times per week may reverse ganciclovir-induced neutropenia. Concurrent use of other myelotoxic drugs (i.e., zidovudine, TMP-SMX) should be temporarily discontinued. Other adverse effects of ganciclovir include confusion, dizziness, headache, convulsion, nausea, vomiting, diarrhea, and abnormal liver function tests.

Foscarnet must be delivered by an intravenous infusion pump over 2 hours. Rapid infusion of foscarnet may reduce the serum ionized calcium level since the drug chelates calcium. The initial dose of foscarnet is 60 mg per kilogram every 8 hours; again, the dose should be reduced in patients with impaired renal function. Foscarnet, although generally free of myelotoxicity, is associated with renal and electrolyte disorders, especially in dehydrated patients. The drug may lower serum calcium, magnesium, and potassium, and it requires frequent monitoring of renal function and serum electrolytes. To minimize nephrotoxicity prehydration or concurrent administration of isotonic saline should be given daily during therapy. Other nephrotoxic drugs (i.e., amphotericin B, aminoglycosides, and pentamidine) should be avoided if possible. Foscarnet should be interrupted if serum Cr is above 2.9 mg/dl and restarted if Cr is less than 2 mg/dl.

Duration of induction therapy for CMV retinitis is 14 to 21 days. Initial response rates for retinitis is approximately 80 to 90 percent with either ganciclovir or foscarnet therapy. Decrease in visual acuity caused by edema of the macula may improve with treatment, but visual-field deficits from damaged retina are not reversible. Relapse rates are extremely high. Since the drugs are virostatic against CMV, infection may continue to progress, and patients must receive long-term maintenance therapy. CMV esophagitis and enterocolitis may or may not respond to ganciclovir or foscarnet treatment.

CMV disease that is refractory to single treatment with either ganciclovir or foscarnet may respond to a combination of these drugs. Toxicities between the two drugs do not overlap; lowering the doses of these two agents may be possible, and associated toxicities may be reduced.

Maintenance therapy (see Fig. 4) requires permanent installation of a central venous catheter to administer the drug. Maintenance therapy can be ganciclovir 5 mg per kilogram per day, 7 days a week or 6 mg per kilogram per day, 5 days a week or foscarnet 90 to 120 mg per kilogram per day (with 1 L saline). Recent data have shown that foscarnet is effective and less toxic, and it is the drug of choice for maintenance therapy. Oral ganciclovir is well tolerated, but its bioavailability is low. Ganciclovir-resistant CMV may develop, often after 3 months of continuous ganciclovir therapy; foscarnet is the drug of choice in this situation.

Herpes Simplex Virus

HSV infection in HIV-infected patients commonly presents as recurrent orolabial, genital, and anorectal lesions. The frequency and severity of the disease depend on the degree of immunosuppression. In AIDS patients reactivation of HSV is frequent and is associated with severe symptoms including disseminated infections. HSV encephalitis is rare.

HSV is treated with acyclovir (ACV) 200 to 400 mg orally 5 times a day for 7 to 14 days (Table 5). Local care of the lesion

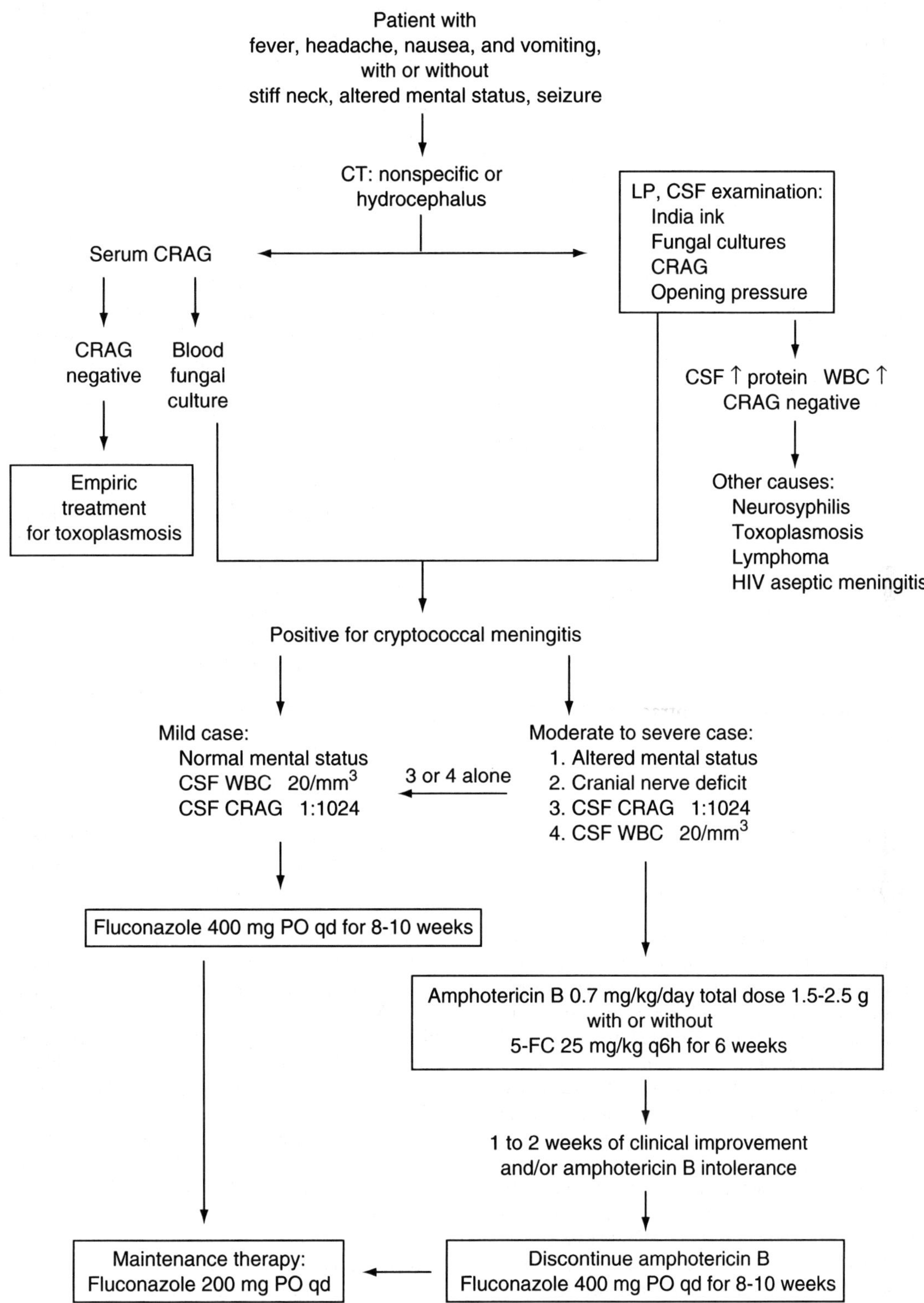

Figure 4
Algorithm for the treatment of cytomegalovirus infection. GI, gastrointestinal; CBC, complete blood count; ANC, absolute neutrophil count; G-CSF, granulocyte colony-stimulating factor; GM-CSF, granulocyte-macrophage colony-stimulating factor; Plt, platelet count; NS, normal saline; CrCl, creatinine clearance.

Table 5 Treatment of Herpes Simplex Infections

Mild mucocutaneous infection	ACV 200–400 mg PO 5 times/day for 10–14 days
Severe mucocutanoeus infection	ACV 5 mg/kg IV (1 hour) q8h for 10–14 days
Visceral organ infection	ACV 10 mg/kg IV (1 hour) q8h for at least 10 days
Suspected ACV-resistant HSV	ACV 400 mg PO 5 times/day Observe 3–5 days; if not improved, ACV 800 mg PO 5 times/day Observe 5–7 days; if not improved, topical trifluridine q8h until complete healing or Foscarnet 60 mg/kg b.i.d. or 40 mg/kg t.i.d. IV (2 hours)
Chronic prophylaxis	ACV 200–400 mg PO t.i.d. or Foscarnet 40 mg/kg/day IV

ACV, Acyclovir.

and topical antibiotic application are important for comfort and prevention of secondary infection. Clinical improvement should be observed within 1 to 2 weeks after therapy in ACV-sensitive HSV infection. However, recurrence frequently develops shortly after ACV is discontinued; thus, oral ACV 400 mg twice a day may be required for maintenance. Oral ACV occasionally causes mild toxicities such as nausea, vomiting, and headache. In severe cases ACV 5 mg per kilogram IV may be infused over 1 hour every 8 hours. A serious infection such as retinitis, esophagitis, or CNS infection may require a dose of up to 10 mg per kilogram IV every 8 hours. Most patients can tolerate intravenous ACV treatment, but phlebitis, nausea, hematuria, nephropathy, hypotension, and encephalopathy may develop. These toxicities are generally associated with renal insufficiency and high drug level in the plasma. Dosage adjustment is necessary for patients with impaired renal function. Other rare adverse effects of ACV that may be serious include CNS symptoms, confusion, tremor, delirium, psychosis, seizure, and coma.

ACV-resistant HSV can emerge during ACV treatment and cause lesions refractory to therapy. These ACV-resistant HSV are usually sensitive to foscarnet. The treatment of suspected ACV-resistant infection the response is poor or the patient is still forming new lesions after 3 to 5 days of therapy, the dosage should be increased to 800 mg five times a day. If no response is seen after 5 to 7 days, the disease probably will not respond to intravenous ACV. An alternative topical treatment is with trifluridine (TFT) applied with an occlusive dressing every 8 hours. In inaccessible lesions or lesions that fail to respond to topical TFT, therapy with intravenous foscarnet 60 mg per kilogram twice daily or 40 mg per kilogram three times a day

Table 6 Treatment of Varicella Zoster Virus

Shingles	ACV 800 mg PO 5 times/day for 10–14 days
Disseminated infection	ACV 10 mg/kg IV (1 hour) q8h for at least 10 days
Primary infection	ACV 10 mg/kg IV (1 hour) q8h for at least 10 days
Suspected ACV-resistant HSV	ACV 10 mg/kg IV (1 hour) q8h Observe 7–10 days; if not improved, foscarnet 60 mg/kg IV (2 hours) b.i.d. or 40 mg/kg t.i.d.

ACV, Acyclovir; HSV, herpes simplex virus.

is required until complete healing of the lesions, usually 10 days to 3 weeks. HSV lesions recurring at the same site as previous ACV-resistant HSV lesions are likely to be caused by ACV-resistant strains, so the patient should be given oral ACV 800 mg five times a day or intravenous foscarnet. However, if lesions recur at a different location, the strain of HSV may be susceptible to ACV and the patient may be treated initially with a standard dose of oral ACV.

Varicella Zoster Virus

HIV-infected patients are at increased risk for shingles or recurrent dermatomal varicella (VZV) infection at any time in the course of HIV disease. As with HSV, most adult AIDS patients usually have had primary VZV infection (chickenpox) and are not susceptible to primary infection. Primary infection disease may be more severe and complicated by disseminated visceral organ infection.

Treatment of VZV infections requires ACV 800 mg PO 5 times daily for 7 to 10 days (Table 6). This regimen may be poorly tolerated because of gastrointestinal side effects. Patients with disseminated infection should be treated with ACV 10 to 12 mg per kilogram IV infused over 1 hour every 8 hours for 7 to 14 days. Acyclovir treatment has been shown to reduce the duration of viral shedding, new lesion formation, and disseminated infection. ACV-resistant VZV may have characteristic findings of hyperkeratotic or nodular lesions that respond poorly to adequate doses of ACV therapy. ACV-resistant VZV calls for intravenous foscarnet 40 mg per kilogram three times daily or 60 mg per kilogram twice daily until the lesions are completely healed.

Suggested Reading

Cohen PT, Sande MA, Volberding PA. The AIDS knowledge base. 2nd ed. Boston: Little, Brown, 1994.

Sande MA, Volberding PA. The medical management of AIDS. 4th ed. Philadelphia: WB Saunders, 1995.

Sanford JP, Sande MA, Gilbert DN, Gerberding JL. The Sanford guide to HIV/AIDS therapy, 1994.

PROPHYLAXIS OF OPPORTUNISTIC INFECTIONS IN HIV DISEASE

Evelyn J. Fisher, M.D.

Table 1 Major Primary Prophylaxis Decision Points

All patients	TB px if indicated; Pneumococcal vaccine q3–5 yr; PCP px if indicated (indications 2–5, Table 2)
CD4 <200	Above plus PCP px for all patients; toxoplasmosis px if indicated (Table 2)
CD4 <100	Above; consider adding MAC px; Fungal px; (CMV px)

CD4, CD4+ T lymphocytes per microliter; TBS, tuberculosis; px, prophylaxis; PCP, *Pneumocystis carinii* pneumonia; MAC, disseminated *Mycobacterium avium* complex; CMV, cytomegalovirus.

The use of infection prophylaxis has been a major advance in HIV disease. This chapter presents the state of the art. Research is ongoing in this area, and it is to be hoped that even better prophylaxis—fewer drugs with greater efficacy—can be achieved in the future.

Primary prophylaxis is given before an infection develops. The two best known and most effective are trimethoprim-sulfamethoxazole (TMP-SMX) prophylaxis against *Pneumocystis carinii* pneumonia (PCP) (estimated to add a year to survival in late HIV disease), and isoniazid (INH) prophylaxis of tuberculosis (TB). Primary prophylaxis against other opportunistic infections is more controversial at present because of the lower efficacy of available drugs and concerns about cost and development of drug resistance. Compared with more than 90 percent efficacy of the PCP and TB prophylaxis, some other prophylaxes, such as those for disseminated *Mycobacterium avium* complex (MAC) and cytomegalovirus (CMV), have reduced disease only by about 50 percent.

Secondary prophylaxis is given after acute treatment of an opportunistic infection to prevent or reduce the incidence of relapse. For some refractory infections this is more accurately called maintenance or chronic suppressive therapy. A common error of clinicians not experienced in HIV is to omit secondary prophylaxis. Secondary prophylaxis is optional only if (1) the infection is not life threatening, such as mucocutaneous herpes simplex or *Candida* esophagitis; (2) the patient refuses it; or (3) the patient cannot tolerate any prophylaxis regimen.

An outline of major primary prophylaxis decision points is presented in Table 1. Tables 2 and 3 list major primary and secondary prophylactic drugs and their indications, efficacy status, and doses. Table 4 presents the major toxicities, drug interactions, and status of use in pregnancy.

■ *PNEUMOCYSTIS CARINII* PNEUMONIA

Primary and Secondary Prophylaxis

TMP-SMX is the drug of choice; it is also effective prophylaxis for *Toxoplasma* and bacterial infections. Dose-limiting toxicity, mainly rash or fever, occurs in 25 percent of patients on one double-strength (DS) tab daily and in 10 percent on one DS tablet thrice weekly. Patients having mild to moderate reactions to higher doses of TMP-SMX can be rechallenged after 2 weeks off drug; about half will tolerate the lower dose. Several regimens for oral desensitization to TMP-SMX have been published.

Dapsone, a sulfone used in leprosy treatment, the next choice, is tolerated by up to two-thirds of patients allergic to TMP-SMX, but is best avoided if the patient has had a severe TMP-SMX reaction (exfoliation or erythema multiforme). Ideally, one should test for glucose-6-phosphate dehydrogenase (G6PD) deficiency prior to dapsone use, although severe hemolysis is rare. Less effective than TMP-SMX, dapsone is as effective as or more effective than aerosolized pentamidine. Dapsone requires gastric acid for absorption; hence, attention to drug interactions is critical. The value of attempting to increase the efficacy of dapsone by adding a second drug, particularly in breakthrough PCP, is as yet unproven, but commonly done. Second drugs being added to dapsone include pyrimethamine, trimethoprim, aerosol pentamidine, and atovaquone.

Aerosolized pentamidine should be reserved for patients who cannot tolerate these oral drugs. Its disadvantages include lower efficacy, expense, inconvenience, lack of prevention of extrapulmonary pneumocystis, and risk of TB transmission via cough during treatment. About half of patients require pretreatment and sometimes post-treatment bronchodilator therapy (e.g., inhaled albuterol) to prevent bronchospasm and cough. Pentamidine can be used intravenously, but it is cumbersome and has a cumulative pancreatic islet cell toxicity.

There are no data for atovaquone as PCP prophylaxis, only for treatment. Nevertheless, it is being used as an alternative by a number of clinicians. Atovaquone requires fatty food for absorption, and some patients absorb it poorly. A liquid suspension being developed may improve absorption.

■ TOXOPLASMA

Primary Prophylaxis

Patients with fewer than 100 CD4 and IgG *Toxoplasma* antibodies run a one in three risk of developing cerebral toxoplasmosis. About 15 to 30 percent of HIV-infected persons in North America are *Toxoplasma* seropositive. Therefore, clinicians must consider trying to achieve some anti-*Toxoplasma* activity in PCP prophylaxis regimens for *Toxoplasma*-seropositive patients. TMP-SMX 160–800 mg once or twice a day has been shown effective; the efficacy of dosing three times a week is unproven. If *Toxoplasma*-seropositive patients are on aerosolized pentamidine because of sulfa and dapsone intolerance, consider adding an unproven alternative to aerosolized pentamidine, since the latter offers no protection against toxoplasmosis.

Table 2 Primary Prophylaxis

INFECTION	INDICATION	EFFICACY STATUS	REGIMEN
PCP	CD4 <200 CD4 <15%	Proven; standard of care	TMP-SMX DS 160–800 mg qd or 3×/wk
	Unexplained fever ≥2 wk Thrush	Proven	Dapsone 50–100 mg qd ± pyrimethamine 50 mg 1–3×/wk or trimethoprim 300 mg qd
	Chemotherapy		Aerosol pentamidine 300 mg q1mo
		Probable	IV pentamidine 4 mg/kg q2–4 wk
		Unknown	Atovaquone 750 mg b.i.d.
TB	Positive PPD or history of such Recent exposure to active TB High-risk anergic	Proven; standard of care	INH 300 mg with pyridoxine 50 mg qd × 12 mo, or for directly observed px, INH 900 mg with pyridoxine 50 mg 2 × week
	Alternative: For INH intolerance or exposure to INH-resistant but rifampin-sensitive TB	Probable (proven in non-HIV)	Rifampin 600 mg qd × 12 mo
	Alternative: For exposure to TB resistant to both INH and rifampin	Unknown	Three-drug regimen × 6 mo: PZA 1.5 g qd plus ethambutol 15–25 mg/kg qd or either ofloxacin 400 mg b.i.d. or ciprofloxacin 750 mg b.i.d. To the extent possible, regimens should be based on likely sensitivities of the exposed strain.
MAC	CD4 <75	Proven	Rifabutin 300 mg qd
			Clarithromycin 500 mg b.i.d.
		Possible	Azithromycin 500 or 600 mg qd
Toxoplasma	CD4 <100 and *Toxoplasma* IgG antibody-positive	Proven	TMP-SMX DS 160–800 mg qd
		Probable	Dapsone 50 mg qd plus pyrimethamine 50 mg 1–2×/wk with leukovorin 25 mg/wk
		Unknown	Atovaquone 750 mg b.i.d.
			Clarithromycin 500 mg b.i.d.
			Azithromycin 500 mg qd
			Consider adding pyrimethamine 50 mg 2–3×/wk with leukovorin 25 mg/wk to any of the above.
Herpes simplex	Recurrent herpes simplex	Proven; possible survival benefit	Acyclovir 400 mg b.i.d.
Candida esophagitis and cryptococcus	CD4 <100	Proven	Fluconazole 100–200 mg qd
		Probable	Ketoconazole 200 mg qd
			Itraconazole 100–200 mg qd
CMV	CD4 <100 and evidence of CMV carriage	Uncertain	Oral ganciclovir 1 g t.i.d.
Bacterial infections	Frequent bacterial pneumonia	Probable	TMP-SMX DS 160–800 mg qd or b.i.d.

Duration is rest of patient's life unless otherwise specified.
All drugs are oral unless otherwise specified.
PCP, *Pneumocystis carinii* pneumonia; TMP-SMX, trimethoprim-sulfamethoxazole; DS, double strength; CD4, CD4+ lymphocyte; TB, tuberculosis; PPD, purified protein derivative; INH, isoniazid; PZA, pyrazinamide; MAC, disseminated *Mycobacterium avium* complex; Ig, immunoglobulin.

Secondary Prophylaxis

Optimal doses have not been established. Half of the treatment dose of sulfadiazine and pyrimethamine is most commonly used. TMP-SMX is probably also effective, but data are lacking. For the sulfa-intolerant, clindamycin 450 mg four times a day with pyrimethamine is usually effective. There are isolated case reports of use of minocycline or doxycycline 100 mg twice a day for acute treatment and suppression. Although clarithromycin and azithromycin have some anti-*Toxoplasma* activity, their use has been disappointing. Whether combining these azalides with another drug, such as pyrimethamine or minocycline, would improve efficacy is unknown.

■ FUNGAL INFECTIONS

Primary Prophylaxis

The risks and benefits are unclear for primary prophylaxis of *Candida* esophagitis and cryptococcal disease, mainly meningitis, because of the cost and drug resistance issues. Fluconazole and even ketoconazole probably reduce the incidence of these fungal infections, but *Candida,* resistance to the oral azole antifungal drugs is being seen with increasing frequency, mainly in patients with fewer than 50 CD4 cells per microliter. It is unknown whether lowering or raising the prophylactic dose of fluconazole would reduce emergence of resistance. In areas highly endemic for *Histoplasma* or *Coccid-*

Table 3 Secondary Prophylaxis: Chronic Maintenance or Suppression

INFECTION	INDICATED INDEFINITELY	EFFICACY OF REGIMEN	REGIMEN
PCP	Yes	Proven	Same as primary prophylaxis
TB	Unknown	Unknown	INH 300 mg qd with pyridoxine 50 mg/day Rifampin 600 mg qd
MAC	Yes	Proven	Continue acute treatment indefinitely: Clarithromycin 500 mg b.i.d. plus ethambutol 15–25 mg/kg/day with or without additional drugs, e.g., rifabutin 300 mg qd or clofazimine 100 mg qd
Toxoplasma	Yes	Proven	Sulfadiazine 500 mg q6h plus pyrimethamine 50 mg/day with leukovorin 10 mg qd
		Probable	TMP-SMX DS 160–800 mg b.i.d.
		Somewhat less effective	Clindamycin 450 mg q.i.d. plus pyrimethamine 50 mg/qd with leukovorin 10 mg/day
		Unknown	Atovaquone 750 mg b.i.d. Clarithromycin 0.5–1 g b.i.d. or azithromycin 1 g load, then 500 mg qd With any regimen of unknown efficacy, consider adding pyrimethamine 50 mg/day with leukovorin 10 mg/day or minocycline 100 mg b.i.d.
Herpes simplex	Recurrent herpes simplex	Proven	Acyclovir 400 mg b.i.d.
Candida esophagitis	Uncertain value if recurrences not frequent	Proven	Fluconazole 100–200 mg qd
		Probable	Ketoconazole 200–400 mg qd
		Probable	Itraconazole 200–400 mg qd
Cryptococcus	Yes	Proven	Fluconazole 200 mg qd
		Less effective	Itraconazole 200 mg b.i.d.
Fungal, other			
Histoplasma, Aspergillus	Yes	Proven for histoplasmosis	Itraconazole 200 mg b.i.d.
Coccidioides	Yes	Probable	Fluconazole 400 mg qd
CMV	Always for retinitis	Proven	Ganciclovir IV 5 mg/kg/day
	Need unpredictable for other CMV disease	Proven	Foscarnet IV 90–120 mg/kg/day (120 mg more effective)
		Proven for retinitis	Oral ganciclovir 1–1.5 g t.i.d.
Bacterial			
Frequent bacterial pneumonia	Uncertain, but patients often on drug for PCP prophylaxis	Proven for b.i.d. dose	TMP-SMX DS160–800 mg b.i.d., qd or 3× wk

All drugs are oral unless otherwise stated.
PCP, *Pneumocystis carinii* pneumonia; TB, tuberculosis; INH, isoniazid; MAC, disseminated *Mycobacterium avium* complex; TMP-SMX, trimethoprim-sulfamethoxazole; DS, double strength; CMV, cytomegalovirus.

ioides disseminated disease due to these soil fungi may account for 25 percent of opportunistic infections. In such areas prophylaxis should be discussed with patients, although efficacy is unclear. Theoretically, one would choose itraconazole 200 mg per day for *Histoplasma* and fluconazole 200 mg per day for *Coccidioides.*

Secondary Prophylaxis

Fluconazole is more effective than amphotericin B for cryptococcus suppression. If breakthrough has occurred, higher doses of fluconazole can be tried, up to 800 mg per day. For fluconazole intolerance, itraconazole 400 mg per day can be used, although it is probably less effective. For *Histoplasma,* itraconazole 400 mg per day provides very effective suppression. It is possible to give higher doses of itraconazole, 600 or 800 mg per day, for *Histoplasma* and *Aspergillus,* but toxicity is more likely.

■ *MYCOBACTERIUM AVIUM* COMPLEX

Primary Prophylaxis

Disseminated MAC occurs in 30 percent or more of persons with AIDS, almost always when CD4 cells are below 50 per microliter. It causes extreme fever, rigors, drenching night sweats, anemia, and severe wasting. Because it is difficult to treat, prophylaxis is appealing.

Rifabutin prophylaxis reduces MAC by at least 50 percent and does not select for rifabutin-resistant MAC. Clarithromycin in an initial study reduced MAC by two-thirds and may have improved survival. However, clarithromycin resistance occurred in 9 of 15 (40 percent) of disseminated MAC that did occur (thus rendering our best MAC drug useless). There is a theoretic possibility that prophylactic rifabutin use selects for rifampin-resistant TB. However, data to date have not indicated it. Trials are continuing to look

Table 4 Toxicities and Interactions of Drugs Used in HIV Prophylaxis

ANTIMICROBIAL AGENT	MAJOR ADVERSE REACTIONS	MAJOR DRUG INTERACTIONS: EFFECT ON DRUG ACTIVITY	USE IN PREGNANCY*
Acyclovir	GI and renal at high dose	None to date	Yes (C)
Atovaquone	Rash, often clearing on treatment	Decreased by rifampin and metoclopramide	No data (C)
Azithromycin	GI upset, rarely hepatitis, hearing loss with very high doses	See clarithromycin; interacts less than clarithromycin	Yes (B)
Ciprofloxacin	GI upset, photosensitivity	Increases theophylline; absorption decreased by antacids, ddI, sucralfate, iron, magnesium, zinc	Probably safe (no human arthropathy reported (C)
Clarithromycin	GI upset, rarely hepatitis or hearing loss with very high doses	Increases terfenidine and astemizole (potential for cardiac arrhythmias), rifabutin (increased uveitis), and carbamazepine	No data (C)
Dapsone	Rash, fever, hepatitis, anemia (hemolysis, methemoglobinemia)	Decreased by rifampin and antacid drugs (H_2 blockers, ddI buffer)	Yes (C)
Ethambutol	GI upset, optic neuritis, elevated uric acid	Decreased by aluminum antacids; give 2 h apart	Yes (B)
Fluconazole	GI upset, rash, rarely hepatitis	Decreased by rifampin; increases terfenidine and astemizole (cardiac arrhythmias), rifabutin (uveitis), carbamazepine, phenytoin, sulfonylurea hypoglycemics, warfarin	Yes (C)
Foscarnet	Nephrotoxicity; decreased calcium, potassium, magnesium; nausea; anemia; rarely mucosal ulcers	Increased nephrotoxicity with other drugs causing same; increased hypocalcemia with pentamidine	If absolutely necessary (C)
Ganciclovir	Neutropenia, fatigue, some decrease in renal function	Increased neutropenia with other drugs causing same; increases ddI levels	No (marked embryo toxicity in animals) (C)
INH	Peripheral neuropathy, hepatitis, CNS effects	Increases carbamazepine and vice versa; disulfiram, phenytoin; absorption decreased by aluminum antacids	Yes (NA)
Itraconazole	GI upset; rash, rarely hepatitis; hypertension and hyperkalemia with high doses	Absorption decreased by antacids, ddI, and sucralfate; see fluconazole for other important interactions	No data (C)
Ketoconazole	Adrenocortical and sex hormone suppression with high doses; rarely hepatitis	Absorption decreased by antacids, ddI, and sucralfate; see fluconazole	No data (C)
Ofloxacin: See Ciprofloxacin			
Pentamidine, aerosol	Bronchospasm, cough	None reported	No data
Pentamidine IV	Hypoglycemia, nephrotoxicity, hypotension, pancreatitis, hypocalcemia	Increased nephrotoxicity with other drugs causing same; increased hypocalcemia with foscarnet	No animal data (C)
PZA	Hepatitis, elevated uric acid	Decreased markedly by AZT	No animal data (C)
Pyrimethamine	Neutropenia		Yes (C)
Rifabutin	Uveitis, neutropenia, orange urine	Increased by clarithromycin and fluconazole, leading to more uveitis	Yes (B)
Rifampin	Hepatitis, rash, orange urine	Decreases atovaquone, oral contraceptives, dapsone, ketoconazole, itraconazole, fluconazole, oral hypoglycemics, methadone, phenytoin, warfarin	Yes (C)
TMP-SMX	Nausea, rash, fever, hepatitis, neutropenia, photosensitivity	Increases warfarin	Yes (C)

*FDA Pregnancy categories: B, Animal studies indicate no fetal risk, but there are no human studies; or animal studies show fetal risk, but adequate studies in pregnant women have shown no adverse effects, including in the first trimester. C, Animal studies demonstrate fetal risk but there are no human trials; or neither human nor animal studies are available. D, Evidence exists for fetal risk in humans, but benefit may outweigh risk. NA, Not available (drug approved prior to need for such testing).
Yes, category B, or C where there has been sufficient experience to say any fetal risk must be very low. If necessary, insufficient experience, but drug is theoretically safer than alternative. No data, insufficient experience; may have to be used if disease is serious.
GI, gastrointestinal; ddI, didanosine; INH, isoniazid; CNS, central nervous system; PZA, pyrazinamide; AZT, zidovudine; TMP-SMX, trimethoprim-sulfamethoxazole.

for even more effective prophylaxis, including combinations of drugs.

Secondary Prophylaxis

Treatment is continued for life with at least two drugs, unless patient does not wish to continue treatment.

■ TUBERCULOSIS

Primary Prophylaxis

No other medical condition so predisposes to the development of active TB as HIV infection. In tuberculin-positive patients the risk of active TB is 5 to 10 percent per year for HIV-positive persons versus 5 to 10 percent per lifetime for HIV-negative ones.

Indications include the following:

1. Positive tuberculin skin test: purified protein derivative (PPD) at least 5 mm
2. History of positive tuberculin test
3. Recent contact with person who has active TB (household or nosocomial)
4. High-risk anergics: injection drug users, homeless persons, prisoners, other institutionalized persons, elderly persons, migrant workers, persons from developing countries where TB is common

It is critical to rule out active TB prior to starting prophylaxis. Chest x-ray film is sufficient for asymptomatic patients. If chest film shows parenchymal infiltrate or fibrotic scarring, obtain three sputum cultures. If there is no other explanation for infiltrate, start on full multidrug treatment for TB. After 2 months of treatment, if cultures are negative *and* chest x-ray is unchanged, cut back to INH alone.

Alternatives to INH are problematic, but their use seems justified due to the extraordinary risk of TB in HIV disease.

Secondary Prophylaxis

Treatment of TB in HIV patients results in very high cure rates if the organism is drug sensitive and the patient compliant. However, when TB treatment is suboptimal, relapse rates are significantly higher in HIV than non-HIV patients. Some clinicians are keeping HIV patients on indefinite INH after treatment for tuberculosis because of concern over lack of long-term (beyond 2 years) post-treatment data and the patient's anticipated further immune decline.

■ HERPES ZOSTER

Herpes zoster usually does not recur, so secondary prophylaxis is not routinely used. Theoretically, the new drug famciclovir is more convenient, requiring fewer pills, for those few patients with multiple recurrences, e.g., 500 mg two or three times a day, but there are no data on efficacy.

■ HERPES SIMPLEX

Primary Prophylaxis

Technically, primary prophylaxis is not used, since acyclovir suppression is used only in patients who have a history of herpes outbreaks. Interestingly, in patients with AIDS or fewer than 200 CD4 per microliter on zidovudine, concomitant acyclovir in doses as low as 600 to 800 mg per day appeared to improve survival in three studies not designed to look for this effect; there are no data for acyclovir alone or acyclovir with didanosine, zalcitabine, or stavudine. If the effect is real, the mechanism is unknown: speculation centers on possible effect on molecular interaction between HIV and either human herpesvirus 6 or herpes simplex. The use of acyclovir for this putative purpose can be discussed with patients.

Secondary Prophylaxis

The options are acyclovir suppression and re-treating each episode. In very late disease, chronic suppression is usually necessary, often at high doses. Partially treated large anogenital herpetic ulcers promote development of acyclovir-resistant herpes. Efforts should be made to avoid this by giving high enough doses of acyclovir to keep ulcers healed. Oral doses of up to 800 mg five times a day may be used. If these doses do not work, acyclovir resistance is likely.

■ CYTOMEGALOVIRUS

Primary Prophylaxis

CMV disease, mainly retinitis and GI, is diagnosed in about 10 to 25 percent of AIDS patients in life and in a much higher percent at autopsy. CMV disease almost always occurs with fewer than 50 CD4 cells per microliter. Evidence of CMV carriage is either positive CMV IgG antibody or history of positive CMV culture from any site. Homosexual men are about 99 percent CMV-seropositive, but adults with other HIV risk behaviors are only 75 to 90 percent positive. Efficacy versus toxicity of prophylaxis is uncertain at present. An initial prophylactic study showed a 50 percent reduction in CMV disease, mainly retinitis, in patients on oral ganciclovir versus placebo, but interim analysis of another similar study has not so far confirmed this beneficial result. Ganciclovir is less toxic orally than intravenously, but neutropenia occurs in 20 percent on 3 g per day. The oral form is on the market, but only for suppression of retinitis. Therefore, third-party payors may not cover its use for prophylaxis.

Secondary Prophylaxis

CMV drugs slow down but do not halt progression of CMV retinitis. Higher doses of ganciclovir or foscarnet may be needed later in the course of disease. For ganciclovir maintenance doses of up to 7.5 mg per kilogram per day or 5 to 7.5 mg every 12 hours have been used, generally with granulocyte colony-stimulating factor support. With foscarnet single daily maintenance doses above 120 mg per kilogram per day cannot be used, but the induction doses of 90 mg per kilogram to every 12 hours can be maintained if tolerated. The combination of ganciclovir and foscarnet is being explored. Doses of both these drugs must be altered if renal function is abnormal. In other forms of CMV disease, such as gastrointestinal, wasting syndrome (viremia, fever, and weight loss), hepatitis, and pneumonia, spontaneous remission may occur. Therefore, until more data are available, patients with a good response to treatment of these nonretinitis conditions can be presented with the option of continuing suppression after acute treatment.

Initial studies suggest that oral ganciclovir is effective for suppression of CMV retinitis, with no significant difference between intravenous and oral administration. Since blood levels are lower with oral use, the theoretic concern is that the oral route may prove in the long run to be less effective or lead to more resistance than the intravenous. Nevertheless, oral use is clearly more convenient and avoids the risks of indwelling intravenous access.

■ BACTERIAL INFECTIONS

Primary and Secondary Prophylaxis

One study showed a decreased rate of serious bacterial infections in patients on TMP-SMX DS twice a day for PCP prophylaxis. In some patients, especially injection drug users, bacterial pneumonia is a common cause of death. Some clinicians use IVIg (intravenous immunoglobulin) 200 to 400 mg per kilogram per month for adults with frequently recurring infections due to *Pneumococcus* or *Haemophilus influenzae,* but efficacy is uncertain and the cost is very high.

Suggested Reading

Decker CF, Masur H. Current status of prophylaxis for opportunistic infections in HIV-infected patients. AIDS 1994; 8:11–20.

Gallant JE, Moore RD, Chaisson RE. Prophylaxis for opportunistic infections in patients with HIV infection. Ann Intern Med 1994; 120:932–944.

Jewett JF, Hecht FM. Preventive health care for adults with HIV infection. JAMA 1993; 269:1144–1153.

Lane HC, Laughon BE, Falloon J. NIH Conference. Recent advances in the management of AIDS-related opportunistic infections. Ann Intern Med 1994; 120:945–955.

Sande MA, Volberding PA. The medical management of AIDS. 4th ed. Philadelphia: WB Saunders, 1994.

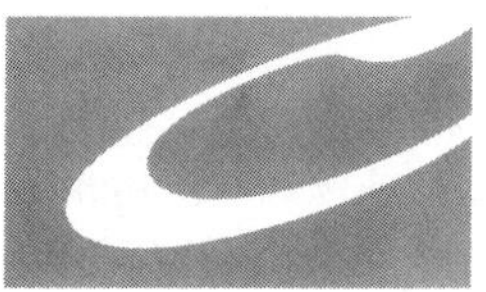

INFECTIOUS DISEASE

INFECTION IN THE NEUTROPENIC PATIENT

Judith E. Karp, M.D.
William G. Merz, Ph.D.
James D. Dick, Ph.D.

Various cellular and humoral surveillance mechanisms protect the host from overwhelming infections by microorganisms. While humoral mechanisms neutralize and prepare microbes for eventual destruction, the final arbiter of microbial eradication is the phagocytic cell with microbiocidal capabilities. It is not surprising, therefore, that the severely granulocytopenic (or neutropenic) host has highly compromised ability to contain infectious pathogens, even those of the normal flora. Further, the risk is directly proportional to the depth and duration of neutropenia.

Nowhere is the critical role of the granulocyte in host surveillance so clearly demonstrable as in the patient with acute leukemia with resultant profound bone marrow failure. The lessons learned from these patients have contributed in a major way to the ability to design and deliver curative therapies not only to leukemia patients but to patients with other types of malignancies as well. Indeed, the principles guiding the empiric antibiotic therapy for fever and infection in the neutropenic host have remained constant since they were formulated over 2 decades ago (Table 1). In such patients the absence or impairment of a localizing inflammatory response resulting from neutropenia plus lack of rapid diagnostic tests to identify any causative organisms necessitates the prompt empiric implementation of broad-spectrum antibiotics against potential pathogens.

Today there are new options due to advances in several major areas: an expanding armamentarium of both broad and targeted coverage, an increasing capacity to define the specific drug susceptibility profiles of diverse organisms, the advent of hematopoietic and immune system biomodulators, and innovative methods of drug delivery. Counterbalancing this progress is the continuing emergence of resistant microbes, which require new agents with novel mechanisms implemented in innovative approaches.

Table 1 Principles of Empiric Antibiotic Therapy During Finite Chemotherapy-Induced Neutropenia

Recognition of commonly occurring pathogens, commonly infected sites, link between specific pathogens and specific sites, drug- and/or tumor-related barrier breakdown
Broad coverage directed against the most common pathogenic organisms arising in the specific clinical setting and at the specific timing during intensive chemotherapy
Prevention of development of multiply resistant organisms
Hold the fort until the underlying lesion is corrected by the return of neutrophils

■ ANTIBACTERIAL APPROACHES

Gram-Negative Infections

Gram-negative bacterial infections arising from the gastrointestinal (GI) tract have been a major cause of morbidity and mortality in persons with neutropenia. Mucosal destruction from cytotoxic drugs permits dissemination of the indigenous bacterial flora, in particular *Escherichia coli, Klebsiella* spp., and *Pseudomonas aeruginosa.* Life-threatening infections by these bacteria early in the course of profound cytotoxic drug-induced marrow aplasia led to the concept of oral GI prophylaxis to prevent early-onset GI-based infection and inhibit late-onset GI colonization with drug-resistant pathogens. Initial studies were limited by host intolerance and emergence of resistant bacteria. More recently the oral fluoroquinolones have been shown to provide broad-spectrum activity against aerobic gram-negative pathogens, including *P. aeruginosa.* Their mechanism of action, inhibition of bacterial DNA gyrase, may prevent acquisition of plasmid-mediated resistance to other agents.

Oral norfloxacin, although not well absorbed, provides high concentrations locally within the GI tract while preserving the anaerobic GI flora and thus colonization resistance against fungal overgrowth or acquisition of new aerobic pathogens. Recent randomized, controlled trials in adults with leukemia and bone marrow transplant (BMT) patients demonstrate the efficacy of the quinolones in preventing

GI-based gram-negative infections. With regard to norfloxacin, late colonization of the GI tract and local or systemic GI-based infections from resistant gram-negative bacteria have not emerged, even in centers where prophylactic norfloxacin is used routinely. However, some quinolones, such as ciprofloxacin, are more completely absorbed and are used for systemic treatment of both local and disseminated infections. Such usage in both neutropenic and non-neutropenic individuals has led to the emergence of quinolone-resistant organisms.

Fever without obvious precipitating causes in the neutropenic host must be interpreted as a sign of infection, even in the absence of other localizing or systemic symptoms, and must prompt the empiric institution of antibacterial antibiotics. Numerous trials continue to validate this concept using agents directed against aerobic and facultative gram-negative bacteria, especially *P. aeruginosa.* To this end, the non-cross-resistant combination of aminoglycoside and an anti-pseudomonal penicillin provides noncompetitive mechanisms of action and potential antibacterial synergy. However, the renal, auditory, and vestibular toxicities that may be associated with prolonged aminoglycoside use are substantial. Nephrotoxicity is a particular concern in the setting of cyclosporin A after allogeneic BMT.

The role of single-agent antibiotics in infection management in neutropenic patients continues to be assessed. Several beta-lactam antibiotics (e.g., aztreonam, ceftazidime, and imipenem) offer broad-spectrum activity against gram-negative bacteria, including *P. aeruginosa.* These drugs are resistant to beta-lactamase hydrolysis, and with their potentially wide range of activity they offer an attractive alternative to aminoglycoside-containing regimens. Meta-analysis of recent clinical trials demonstrated equivalent efficacy in terms of both microbiologic and clinical responses for empiric ceftazidime monotherapy and combination regimens of ceftazidime or another beta-lactam plus aminoglycoside. The trials showed no clear advantage of adding aminoglycoside empirically. However, these trials consistently demonstrate the lack of efficacy of ceftazidime against gram-positive and anaerobic bacteria. In contrast, imipenem monotherapy provides comprehensive activity against gram-negative and anaerobic bacteria and some degree of coverage of gram-positive organisms, with response rates ranging from 40 percent to more than 80 percent in various series.

Continuous infusion of beta-lactam antibiotics provides maximal exposure to active drug levels, avoids periods of subtherapeutic drug concentrations, and overcomes the lack of postantibiotic effect typical of beta-lactams. These factors are especially advantageous for neutropenic patients. Preliminary clinical trials suggest that drug delivery by continuous infusion significantly improves the clinical outcome. Further trials should provide definitive data regarding the benefits of this modality in compromised hosts.

Gram-Positive Infections

Recently there has been an increasing prevalence of gram-positive infections, resulting in substantial morbidity. Factors underlying this increase are delineated in Table 2. In particular, gram-positive organisms resistant to beta-lactams but susceptible to vancomycin, specifically *Staphylococcus* and *Corynebacterium* spp., have emerged as important pathogens.

Table 2 Increased Incidence of Gram-Positive and Fungal Infection Complications During Induced Neutropenia

- Effective empiric antibacterial coverage of potentially life-threatening gram-negative infections at the time of first infectious fever
- Heightened ability to deliver dose-intensive therapies, with resultant increase in skin, oropharyneal, and gastrointestinal mucosal cytotoxicities
- Increased use of indwelling catheters, leading to increased skin barrier breakdown
- Increased use of parenteral hyperalimentation
- Development of beta-lactam antibiotic resistance and vancomycin resistance by gram-positive organisms
- Fungal overgrowth due to antibacterial antibiotic-induced imbalance in normal flora

Vancomycin is a cell wall–acting glycopeptide antibiotic with efficacy against a broad spectrum of gram-positive organisms. The frequency of local and disseminated gram-positive infections in these compromised hosts has led to a number of trials evaluating the therapeutic role of empiric vancomycin during deep aplasia. In prospective clinical trials at centers where gram-positive infections have been particularly prevalent, empiric vancomycin therapy begun at the time of first infectious fever results in prompt fever resolution, rapid clearance of local and/or disseminated gram-positive infections, and prevention of late-onset gram-positive infections in acute leukemia patients with indwelling venous catheters and chemotherapy-induced neutropenia. In centers where gram-positive infections have been less prevalent, the role for early empiric vancomycin has been less clear. In these settings, vancomycin has been effective in treating and eradicating established infection in a timely fashion, suggesting that the drug can be added selectively and nonempirically in some instances.

Prospective, randomized trials of vancomycin administered prophylactically to patients undergoing intensive antileukemic chemotherapy and BMT demonstrate that such prophylaxis prevents the vast majority of early gram-positive infections and delays the onset of first infectious fever. Continuation of vancomycin throughout profound marrow aplasia also suppresses late-onset gram-positive infections without resistance by staphylococci and streptococci to date. The use of vancomycin either prophylactically or therapeutically for gram-positive infections prolongs the length of indwelling catheter life in the deeply aplastic host and prevents the occurrence and/or propagation of infection-related thrombophlebitis.

In addition to skin invasion by indwelling catheters, chemotherapy-induced cytotoxicity to skin and oropharyngeal mucosal barriers is a significant factor in development of first fever gram-positive infection. The dissemination of gram-positive organisms from any of these possible sites of barrier breakdown can be suppressed by effective prophylactic therapy. The recent recognition of overwhelming infections caused by *Streptococcus mitis* in association with high-dose chemotherapy- and/or radiation therapy-induced oropharyngeal mucositis further supports a prophylactic approach.

Since 1986 vancomycin-resistant enterococci have

emerged as an increasingly visible clinical problem, with a twentyfold increase in resistance noted for all enterococci associated with nosocomial infections over the past 4 years. The mechanism of resistance for this glycopeptide is a genetic transposition that encodes a cell wall peptidoglycan incapable of glycopeptide binding and subsequent cell wall disruption. Importantly, these enterococci exhibit a pattern of antimicrobial resistance that spans virtually all antibiotic classes including beta-lactams, aminoglycosides, and the glycopeptides (vancomycin and teicoplanin), leaving few if any therapeutic options. The establishment and maintenance of vigorous infection control procedures is essential in dealing with this group of organisms, not only to limit their dissemination but also to prevent glycopeptide resistance in other more virulent gram-positive pathogens such as *Staphylococcus aureus.* A combination of careful and innovative antibiotic use and strict adherence to appropriate infection control procedures are the only current means for dealing with the expanding problems of antibiotic resistance in gram-positive bacteria in the compromised host.

■ ANTIFUNGAL APPROACHES

Fungal infection is an increasingly frequent cause of morbidity and mortality among patients compromised by neutropenia, especially those with acute leukemia and prolonged, therapy-induced bone marrow aplasia. Ironically, this increase is in part due to the higher rate of survival during early aplasia resulting from improved control of overwhelming bacterial infections. Additional factors include therapy-induced mucosal toxicities, invasion of skin barriers by indwelling catheters, hyperalimentation, and the prolonged use of broad-spectrum antibiotics, which in turn leads to imbalance in GI flora (see Table 2).

Antifungal Prophylaxis

Several studies have examined the role of antifungal agents given prophylactically. Trials of local polyene and local or systemic azole antifungals to control oropharyngeal or disseminated candidiasis have produced variable results. Even when decreases in systemic candidal infections have been detected, these agents have not reduced the incidence or severity of infections caused by filamentous fungi. In this regard, recent trials of low-dose (0.1 to 0.3 mg per kilogram per day) amphotericin B prophylaxis in acute leukemia and BMT patients demonstrate results that vary from major decreases in incidence and mortality of fungus infections, including invasive aspergillosis, to no effect whatsoever. The value of amphotericin B prophylaxis, the optimal dose and schedule to achieve effective suppression of fungus infections, and the specific patient populations most likely to benefit from this approach are important questions that require further clinical investigation.

The new triazole antifungal agents fluconazole and itraconazole are being examined for efficacy in preventing fungal infection during profound therapy-induced bone marrow aplasia. Fluconazole suppresses *Candida albicans* and *Candida tropicalis* colonization and superficial infections and protects BMT patients against candidemia. However, fluconazole prophylaxis may predispose to acquisition and superinfection with drug-selected pathogens, e.g., *Candida krusei* and *Torulopsis glabrata.* Fluconazole has had no demonstrable prophylactic effect against infections caused by filamentous fungi, particularly *Aspergillus* spp., and has not had a measurable effect on overall mortality from fungal infection. Itraconazole demonstrates some promising activity against invasive aspergillosis in animal models and early clinical trials, but this requires confirmation in extended trials. However, resistant yeasts may also become a problem.

Empiric Antifungal Therapy

Use of empiric antifungal therapy has gained support from the documentation of tissue and/or blood stream fungal invasion in 25 to 40 percent of persistently febrile persons with neutropenia, high mortality when treatment is not instituted until the time of specific diagnosis, the clinical response of refractory fevers when amphotericin B is instituted, and the lack of laboratory tests providing rapid and sensitive results. At present tests aimed at early detection of specific *Candida* or *Aspergillus* antigens, fungal metabolites, and nucleic acids are being evaluated for rapid, noninvasive diagnosis of these important mycoses. Invasive procedures to establish the diagnosis are often contraindicated in the clinical setting of deep marrow aplasia and may be unreliable in establishing a specific diagnosis. The significance of positive fungal cultures obtained noninvasively from respiratory, GI, or urinary tract with respect to colonization versus infection is controversial. Radiographic studies with computed tomography are useful in the early detection of deep tissue invasion, particularly pulmonary aspergillosis, but do not provide absolute or specific identification of the responsible pathogen.

Thus, the rationale for prompt amphotericin B use for refractory fever or fever that recurs 3 to 7 days after response to antibacterial therapy is based upon two factors: the inability to detect fungal infection rapidly and accurately early in a patient with multiple predisposing factors, and the finding that delayed institution of amphotericin B can be associated with a poor clinical outcome. Empiric amphotericin B at moderate doses (0.5 mg per kilogram per day) has produced responses in 50 to 70 percent of patients so treated and provides good antifungal therapy for common yeast pathogens (e.g., *C. albicans* and *T. glabrata*). High-dose empiric therapy may be initiated in patients colonized with non-*C. albicans* spp. who have refractory fever.

A critical determinant of survival following disseminated fungus infections during profound marrow aplasia is prompt and aggressive therapy with amphotericin B. Investigators at several centers have demonstrated that prompt detection and institution of aggressive fungicidal therapy with high-dose (1 to 1.25 mg per kilogram per day) amphotericin B alone or in combination with 5-flucytosine (5-FC) results in enhanced survival in infections caused by filamentous organisms such as *Aspergillus* and *Fusarium* species and non-*C. albicans* yeasts. The effect of this approach is most clearly seen in documented infection caused by filamentous fungi; the survival rate decreases from above 80 percent when amphotericin B is instituted before definitive diagnosis to 44 percent when amphotericin B institution is delayed. The timing of such empiric intervention may not differ from a late prophylaxis approach, in which antifungal treatment is started before there is clear clinical evidence of infection, on the basis of nonspecific clinical findings. Although this approach may be inadequate to prevent overt infection in the absence of granulocytes and/or the presence of damaged barriers, it may result in a reduced microbial burden even when only moderate doses of amphotericin B (0.5 mg per kilogram per day) are employed initially.

Patients with prior fungal infections are at risk for reactivation during repeated neutropenic courses. Reactivation rates as high as 50 percent have been reported for deep-seated fungal infections during cycles of therapy-induced aplasia. In the leukemia patient receiving high-dose chemotherapy with or without autologous BMT, prophylactic amphotericin B has been clinically effective without irreversible nephrotoxicity, prolonged marrow suppression, alteration of antileukemic treatment, or negative effect on clinical outcome. Realistically, however, some patients may be unable to tolerate this aggressive approach and may require attenuated doses or even discontinuation, particularly since cyclosporin A and amphotericin B may have compounding renal toxicities. The role of itraconazole in this setting warrants clinical investigation.

New vehicles for local and systemic amphotericin B administration—aerosolized amphotericin B liposomes (L-amphotericin B) and lipid emulsions (LE-amphotericin B)—are designed to deliver higher concentrations of drug to sites of active infection and to spare the host from the well-documented amphotericin B-related multiorgan toxicities. To date studies in compromised patient cohorts substantiate that lipid-based amphotericin B preparations are more tolerable and at least as efficacious as traditional amphotericin B, especially for candidiasis. Large prospective clinical trials will define the role of lipid-modified amphotericin B in prophylaxis and therapy (both empiric and definitive) in the neutropenic patient population, relative to unmodified amphotericin B and to the triazole antifungals.

■ BIOMODULATION: A NEW COMPONENT OF INFECTION MANAGEMENT

The enhancement of cellular and humoral host defense mechanisms through the use of recombinant human hematopoietic growth factors (cytokines) such as the colony-stimulating factors (CSF) and interleukins (IL) is an important direction of clinical investigation. Clinical trials have demonstrated that the administration of granulocyte (G) and granulocyte-macrophage (GM) CSF during cytotoxic chemotherapy with or without BMT for diverse malignancies is associated with acceleration of bone marrow recovery, fewer episodes of antibiotic-requiring fevers and documented infections, and in some cases shorter hospital stays.

In addition to their effects on maturating myeloid cohorts, G-CSF and GM-CSF mobilize and prime the growth and differentiation of easily obtainable peripheral blood stem cells (PBSC) in vivo. Recent studies demonstrate that cytokine-primed PBSC used alone or in combination with autologous marrow cells for autotransplantation and in conjunction with systemic CSFs lead to faster marrow engraftment, reduction in the duration of profound neutropenia (below 100 per cubic millimeter), and earlier granulocyte and platelet recoveries. As a result, numbers and duration of antibiotic usage are significantly decreased; hence, so are use of hospital resources, hospitalizations, and hospital costs.

Multi-CSF, or IL-3, stimulates the growth and differentiation of multipotential hematopoietic precursors, leading to an increase in multiple lineages including granulocytes, monocytes, eosinophils, lymphocytes, and platelets. Since IL-3 acts primarily on primordial cell cohorts, its full effects might be most evident in combination with cytokines such as G-CSF and GM-CSF, which act on more committed precursors. On the basis of its ability to recruit monocytes, eosinophils, and lymphocytes as well as granulocytes, IL-3 may have a special role in the management of fungal and perhaps viral infections. Further, IL-3 may effectively mobilize PBSC for autologous marrow reconstitution following intensive cytotoxic chemotherapy.

Monocyte/macrophage (M) CSF specifically targets monocytes and macrophages, stimulating their proliferation, survival, and functional activation, enhancing antifungal effects in particular. Some of this enhancement may relate to the ability of M-CSF-perturbed monocytes to produce a cascade of immunoreactive cytokines including GM-CSF, IL-1, and tumor necrosis factor, all of which may augment fungicidal acitivity. In a historically controlled series of allogeneic BMT patients, M-CSF 2,000 μg per square meter per day for 28 days from the time of detection of infection in conjunction with amphotericin B resulted in dramatic improvements in survival for the entire cohort of patients (from 5 percent to 27 percent with M-CSF), an increase due to long-lasting suppression of fungal infection and an associated 50 percent survival rate for M-CSF-treated patients with *Candida* infections. These findings substantiate the crucial role of monocyte/macrophage cells in suppressing fungal infections and define a promising new modality, namely M-CSF, that overcomes the monocyte defects known to characterize allogeneic BMT and synergizes with systemic antifungal agents to substantially decrease mortality. Still, *Aspergillus* infections remained relatively refractory in these compromised hosts, suggesting that other cytokines play important roles in the control of this resistant pathogen.

■ FUTURE DIRECTIONS

The strategies for prevention, diagnosis, and therapy of infections in the neutropenic host are continually being refined, with the realistic possibility of tailoring such interventions to the particular infecting pathogen and the specific host determinants (Table 3). An increasing complement of new antibiotics has some unique mechanisms of action and novel delivery systems designed to provide pathogen-directed toxicity while sparing host tissues. Emerging modalities reconstitute or augment elements of host surveillance that in turn protect against the establishment or extension of infection. For example, various hematopoietic growth factors have the potential to enhance cellular and humoral host defenses directed against bacterial and most recently fungal infections in the hematopoietically compromised patient. Additional novel antifungal approaches include new vehicles for local and systemic amphotericin B administration (aerosolized and lipid-based preparations, as examples), designed to deliver higher concentrations of drug

Table 3 Guidelines for the Prevention and Management of Infections in Neutropenic Hosts

Prophylaxis	
Started at day 0 or at day of granulocytes <500 × 10^9/l Maintain throughout granulocytopenia	Norfloxacin 400 mg orally q12h for prevention of GN sepsis. Acyclovir 250 mg/m^2 IV q8h for prevention of HSV reactivation.
Additional Options	Addition of GP coverage, e.g., vancomycin 500 mg intravenously q12h if GP infection rate is high. Addition of antifungal prophylaxis, e.g., low-dose Amp-B, azoles. Addition of cytokines, e.g., G- or GM-CSF, IL-3, M-CSF (especially for fungal infections).
First Infectious Fever	*Antipseudomonal penicillin,* e.g., ticarcillin 270 mg/kg/24h (continuous infusion) provides GN, anaerobic, and some GP coverage; and aminoglycoside, e.g., gentamicin 2 mg/kg IV q6h provides broad-spectrum coverage and synergistic effect with penicillins; *or* Single agent, new beta-lactam antibiotics, e.g., ceftazidime 2g q8h.
Progressive Disease	
No response within 48–72 hours of starting first fever coverage	With clinical suspicion of smoldering bacterial infection, substitute TMP-SMX for gentamicin. Add vancomycin if not already started. Clinical evidence of more rapidly deteriorating condition: substitute amikacin 8 mg/kg IV q6h and piperacillin 270 mg/kg/24h (continuous infusion). With clinical suspicion of fungal infections (~5 = n10% of first fever), add Amp-B 0.5 mg/kg/day IV.
Recrudescent Fever	
>72 hours after starting first fever coverage without microbial documentation	Add Amp-B (0.5 mg/kg/day) if not started already. Switch to amikacin/piperacillin if bacterial sepsis suspected.
Specific treatment of microbiologically documented infection	Bacterial-specific antibiotic or combinations of antibiotics. Fungal species-dependent: Amp-B 0.5 mg/kg/day Amp-B 1.0–1.25 mg/kg/day + 5-FC 25 mg/kg orally q6h* for more refractory yeast species and all filamentous mycoses.

*To achieve serum level of 30–60 μg/ml to avoid 5-FC related toxicity.
Amp-B, amphotericin B; 5-FC, 5-flucytosine; CSF, colony-stimulating factor (G, granulocyte; GM, granulocyte-macrophage; M, monocyte/macrophage); GN, gram-negative; GP, gram-positive; HSV, herpes simplex virus; IL, interleukin; TMP-SMX, trimethoprim-sulfamethoxazole (Bactrim).

to sites of active infection and to spare the host from the well-documented drug-related multiorgan toxicities. These innovative strategies may modify and improve the overall scheme aimed at preventing and eradicating infections in these compromised hosts. Yet the emergence of resistant pathogens, exemplified by vancomycin-resistant enterococci and amphotericin B-resistant fungi, continues to challenge the therapeutic armamentarium and the ability to eradicate and prevent infections in compromised hosts. Such challenges will be addressed through the development of structurally and functionally novel antibiotics that target molecular pathways that are critical to survival of the offending organism, coupled with innovative approaches to antibiotic use and rigorous adherence to methods that physically limit the spread of these pathogens among patients and caregivers.

Suggested Reading

Beyer J, Schwartz S, Heinemann V, Siegert W. Strategies in prevention of invasive pulmonary aspergillosis in immunosuppressed or neutropenic patients. Antimicrob Agents Chemother 1994; 38:911–917.

Craig WA, Ebert SC. Continuous infusion of beta-lactam antibiotics. Antimicrob Agents Chemother 1992; 36:2577–2583.

Francis P, Walsh TJ. Current approaches to the management of fungal infections in cancer patients. Oncology 1992; 6:81–91, 133–144.

Karp JE, Merz WG, Charache P. Response to empiric amphotericin B during antileukemic therapy-induced granulocytopenia. Rev Infect Dis 1991; 13:592–599.

Karp JE, Merz WG, Dick JD. Management of infections in neutropenic patients: Advances in therapy and prevention. Curr Opin Infect Dis 1993; 6:405–411.

Karp JE, Merz WG, Dick JD. Management of infections in neutropenic patients: new opportunities and emerging challenges. Curr Opin Infect Dis 1994; 7:430–435.

Klastersky J. Empiric treatment of infection during granulocytopenia: A comprehensive approach. Infection 1989; 17:59–64.

Roilides E, Pizzo PA. Perspectives on the use of cytokines in the management of infectious complications of cancer. Clin Infect Dis 1993, 17 (Suppl 2):S385–389.

Shlaes DM, Binczewski B, Rice LB. Emerging antimicrobial resistance and the immunocompromised host. Clin Infect Dis 1993; 17(Suppl 2): 5527–5536.

BACTERIAL MENINGITIS

Allan R. Tunkel, M.D., Ph.D.

■ CLINICAL PRESENTATION

The classic clinical presentation in patients with bacterial meningitis is fever, headache, meningismus, and signs of cerebral dysfunction (confusion, delirium, a declining level of consciousness). The meningismus may be subtle, marked, or accompanied by Kernig's and/or Brudzinski's signs; however, these signs are elicited in only about 50 percent of adult patients with bacterial meningitis, so their absence never rules out the diagnosis. Cranial nerve palsies and focal cerebral signs are seen in 10 to 20 percent of cases. Seizures occur in about 30 percent of patients. Papilledema is observed in fewer than 1 percent of patients early in infection, and it should suggest an alternative diagnosis. As meningitis progresses, patients may develop signs of increased intracranial pressure (e.g., coma, hypertension, bradycardia, and palsy of cranial nerve III).

Certain symptoms or signs may suggest causation in patients with bacterial meningitis. About half of the patients with meningococcemia, with or without meningitis, develop a prominent rash localized principally to the extremities. The rash is typically macular and erythematous early in the course of illness but quickly evolves into a petechial phase with further coalescence into a purpuric form; the rash may evolve rapidly, with new petechiae appearing during the physical examination. Patients with *Listeria monocytogenes* meningitis have an increased tendency to focal deficits and seizures early in the course of infection; some patients may have ataxia, cranial nerve palsies, or nystagmus as a result of rhomboencephalitis.

Furthermore, some patients may not show many of the classic symptoms or signs of bacterial meningitis. Disease in elderly patients, particularly those with underlying medical conditions (e.g., diabetes mellitus or cardiopulmonary disease) may develop insidiously with lethargy or obtundation, no fever, and variable signs of meningeal inflammation. Neutropenic patients may also develop disease in a subtle manner because of impaired ability to mount a subarachnoid space inflammatory response.

■ DIAGNOSIS

Bacterial meningitis is diagnosed by examination of cerebrospinal fluid (CSF) obtained via lumbar puncture. In virtually all patients with bacterial meningitis, the opening pressure is above 180 mm H_2O, with values over 600 mm H_2O suggesting cerebral edema, intracranial suppurative foci, or communicating hydrocephalus. The CSF white blood cell count (WBC) is elevated, usually 1,000 to 5,000 cells per cubic millimeter, with a range of fewer than 100 to more than 10,000 per cubic millimeter; patients with low CSF WBC up to 20 per cubic millimeter, despite high CSF bacterial concentrations, tend to have a poor prognosis. There is usually a neutrophilic predominance (at least 80 percent), although approximately 10 percent of patients with acute bacterial meningitis present with a lymphocytic predominance in CSF (more common in neonates with gram-negative bacillary meningitis and patients with *L. monocytogenes* meningitis). A CSF glucose concentration below 40 mg per deciliter is found in about 60 percent of patients. The CSF protein is elevated in virtually all cases (usually 100 to 500 mg per deciliter). Gram stain examination of CSF permits a rapid, accurate identification of the causative micro-organism in about 60 to 90 percent of patients with bacterial meningitis; the specificity is nearly 100 percent, with the likelihood of detecting the organism greater with higher CSF bacterial densities. CSF cultures are positive in 70 to 85 percent of patients with bacterial meningitis; the yield of culture is lower in patients who have received prior antimicrobial therapy.

Patients with bacterial meningitis and a negative CSF Gram stain may benefit from any of several rapid tests for specific bacterial antigens in CSF. Latex agglutination techniques have a sensitivity of 50 to 100 percent, although these tests are highly specific. They detect the antigens of *Haemophilus influenzae* type b (Hib), *Streptococcus pneumoniae, Neisseria meningitidis, Escherichia coli* K1, and *Streptococcus agalactiae.* One of these tests should be performed on CSF samples from all patients with presumed bacterial meningitis and a negative CSF Gram stain, although a negative test never rules out meningitis caused by a specific bacterial pathogen. Polymerase chain reaction (PCR) has been used to amplify DNA from patients with meningococcal meningitis; in one study the sensitivity and specificity were both 91 percent. However, there are problems with false-positive results with PCR, and further refinements are needed before this technique is useful in patients with presumed bacterial meningitis when CSF Gram stain, bacterial antigen tests, and cultures are negative.

■ THERAPY

Initial Approach

The initial management of patients with the clinical presentation of acute bacterial meningitis includes lumbar puncture. If the CSF formula is consistent with the diagnosis of bacterial meningitis, empiric antimicrobial therapy should be initiated according to results of Gram stain or rapid bacterial antigen tests. However, if no causative agent can be identified on initial CSF analysis, empiric antimicrobial therapy should be rapidly initiated according to the patient's age (Table 1). A computed tomographic (CT) scan of the head should be performed on patients with a clinical presentation of bacterial meningitis who have focal neurologic deficits or papilledema on funduscopic examination prior to lumbar puncture to avoid herniation if an intracranial mass lesion is present. However, because the time involved in obtaining a CT scan can significantly delay lumbar puncture, empiric antimicrobial therapy should be initiated before sending the patient to the CT scanner to reduce the potential for morbidity and mortality. Although the yield of positive CSF cultures may decrease with initiation of antimicrobial therapy prior to obtaining CSF for analysis, the pretreatment blood cultures,

Table 1 Common Bacterial Pathogens and Empiric Therapeutic Recommendations

AGE	COMMON BACTERIAL PATHOGENS	EMPIRIC ANTIMICROBIAL THERAPY*
0–4 weeks	*Streptococcus agalactiae, Escherichia coli, Listeria monocytogenes, Klebsiella pneumoniae*	Ampicillin plus cefotaxime or ampicillin plus an aminoglycoside
4–12 weeks	*S. agalactiae, E. coli, L. monocytogenes, Haemophilus influenzae, Streptococcus pneumoniae, Neisseria meningitis*	Ampicillin plus a third-generation cephalosporin†
3 months–18 years	*H. influenzae, N. meningitis, Str. pneumoniae*	Third-generation cephalosporin† or ampicillin plus chloramphenicol
18–50 years	*S. pneumoniae, N. meningitidis*	Third-generation cephalosporin† with or without ampicillin‡
Older than 50 years	*S. pneumoniae, N. meningitidis, L. monocytogenes,* aerobic gram-negative bacilli	Ampicillin plus a third-generation cephalosporin†

*Vancomycin should be added to empiric therapeutic regimens when highly penicillin- or cephalosporin-resistant pneumococcal meningitis is suspected.
†Cefotaxime or ceftriaxone.
‡Add ampicillin if *Listeria monocytogenes* meningitis is suspected.

Table 2 Specific Antimicrobial Therapy for Acute Bacterial Meningitis

MICRO-ORGANISM	STANDARD THERAPY	DURATION OF THERAPY
Haemophilus influenzae		7 days
β-Lactamase negative	Ampicillin	
β-Lactamase positive	Third-generation cephalosporin*	
Neisseria meningitidis	Penicillin G or ampicillin	7 days
Streptococcus pneumoniae		10–14 days
Penicillin MIC <0.1 μg/ml	Penicillin G or ampicillin	
Penicillin MIC 0.1–1 μg/ml	Third-generation cephalosporin*	
Penicillin MIC ≥2 μg/ml	Vancomycin plus a third-generation cephalosporin*†	
Enterobacteriaceae	Third-generation cephalosporin*	21 days
Pseudomonas aeruginosa	Ceftazidime‡	21 days
Listeria monocytogenes	Ampicillin or penicillin G‡	14–21 days
Streptococcus agalactiae	Ampicillin or penicillin G‡	14–21 days
Staphylococcus aureus		10–14 days
Methicillin sensitive	Nafcillin or oxacillin	
Methicillin resistant	Vancomycin	
Staphylococcus epidermidis	Vancomycin†	10–14 days

*Cefrotaxime or ceftriaxone.
†Addition of rifampin should be considered.
‡Addition of an aminoglycoside should be considered.
MIC, minimal inhibitory concentration.

CSF formula, Gram stain, and/or bacterial antigen tests will likely provide evidence for or against a diagnosis of bacterial meningitis.

Antimicrobial Therapy

Once the infecting meningeal pathogen is isolated and susceptibility testing known, antimicrobial therapy can be modified for optimal treatment (Table 2). Recommended antimicrobial dosages for meningitis in adults with normal renal and hepatic function are shown in Table 3. The following sections review recommendations for antimicrobial therapy in patients with bacterial meningitis based on the isolated meningeal pathogen.

Haemophilus Influenzae

A third-generation cephalosporin should be used as empiric therapy in all patients in whom Hib is a possible pathogen. Chloramphenicol is not recommended because resistant isolates have been reported throughout the world, and even in patients with sensitive isolates, a recent prospective study found chloramphenicol to be bacteriologically and clinically inferior to ampicillin, ceftriaxone, or cefotaxime in the therapy of childhood bacterial meningitis caused predominantly by Hib. Although cefuroxime, a second-generation cephalosporin, initially appeared to be efficacious in the therapy of Hib meningitis, a recent study comparing cefuroxime and ceftriaxone for childhood bacterial meningitis documented delayed CSF sterilization and a higher incidence of hearing impairment in the patients receiving cefuroxime; other studies have reported the development of *H. influenzae* meningitis in patients receiving cefuroxime for non-meningeal *H. influenzae* disease.

Neisseria Meningitidis

The antimicrobial agent of choice for therapy of *N. meningitidis* meningitis is penicillin G or ampicillin. These recom-

Table 3 Recommended Dosages of Antimicrobial Agents for Meningitis in Adults with Normal Renal and Hepatic Function

ANTIMICROBIAL AGENT	TOTAL DAILY DOSE	DOSING INTERVAL (HOURS)
Amikacin[a]	15 mg/kg	8
Ampicillin	12 g	4
Cefotaxime	8–12 g	4–6
Ceftrazidime	6 g	8
Ceftriaxone	4 g	12–24
Chloramphenicol[b]	4–6 g	6
Gentamicin[a,c]	3–5 mg/kg	8
Nafcillin	9–12 g	4
Oxacillin	9–12 g	4
Penicillin G	24 million units	4
Rifampin[d]	600 mg	24
Tobramycin[a]	3–5 mg/kg	8
Trimethoprim-sulfamethoxazole[e]	10 mg/kg	12
Vancomycin[a,f]	2–3 g	8–12

[a]Monitor peak and trough serum concentrations.
[b]Higher dose recommended for pneumococcal meningitis.
[c]Intrathecal dosage is 4–8 mg daily; intrathecal dosing should always be used in combination with a parenteral agent.
[d]Oral administration.
[e]Dosage based on trimethoprim component.
[f]May have to monitor CSF concentrations in severely ill patients.

mendations may change as a result of the emergence of meningococcal strains resistant to penicillin G, with a minimal inhibitory concentration (MIC) range of 0.1 to 1 µg per milliliter. However, the clinical significance of these isolates is unclear because patients with meningitis caused by these organisms have recovered with standard penicillin therapy. Based on in vitro susceptibility data, ceftriaxone is recommended as an alternative agent against relatively resistant meningococcal strains.

Streptococcus Pneumoniae

The recommended therapy for pneumococcal meningitis has recently been changed because of recent penicillin susceptibility patterns. Strains with MIC below 0.1 µg per milliliter are considered susceptible to penicillin; those with MIC ranging from 0.1 to 1 µg per milliliter are relatively resistant; and those with MIC of at least 2 µg per milliliter are highly resistant. Resistant strains have been reported throughout the world, including the United States. Because initial CSF concentrations of penicillin are only approximately 1 µg per milliliter following parenteral administration of standard high dosages, penicillin can no longer be recommended as empiric antimicrobial therapy when *S. pneumoniae* is considered a likely infecting pathogen in patients with purulent meningitis. A third-generation cephalosporin, cefotaxime or ceftriaxone, should be used where relatively penicillin-resistant strains are found, and vancomycin should be used when highly resistant strains are suspected or isolated. A recent report has suggested that vancomycin may be suboptimal for therapy of pneumococcal meningitis. Therefore, it is recommended that for empiric therapy of suspected meningitis in areas where highly penicillin- and cephalosporin-resistant pneumococcal isolates have been reported, the combination of vancomycin and a third-generation cephalosporin should be used pending susceptibility results. If highly resistant strains are documented by susceptibility testing, some investigators have also recommended the addition of rifampin, although no clinical data support this recommendation.

Listeria Monocytogenes

Despite their broad range of in vitro activity, the third-generation cephalosporins are inactive against *L. monocytogenes.* Therapy for *Listeria* meningitis should consist of ampicillin or penicillin G, with consideration of adding an aminoglycoside in proven infection because of documented in vitro synergy. In the penicillin-allergic patient trimethoprim-sulfamethoxazole (TMP-SMX), which is bactericidal against *Listeria* in vitro, should be used. Despite favorable in vitro susceptibility results, chloramphenicol and vancomycin are associated with unacceptable high failure rates, although intraventricular vancomycin was efficacious in one case of recurrent *L. monocytogenes* meningitis.

Aerobic Gram-Negative Bacilli

Outcome from meningitis caused by enteric gram-negative bacilli has been greatly improved with the availability of the third-generation cephalosporins (cure rates of 78 to 94 percent). Ceftazidime, a third-generation cephalosporin with enhanced in vitro activity against *Pseudomonas aeruginosa,* led to cure in 19 of 24 patients with *P. aeruginosa* meningitis in one study when used alone or in combination with an aminoglycoside; similar results were observed in a study of 10 children, of whom 7 were cured clinically and 9 were cured bacteriologically when receiving ceftazidime-containing regimens. In patients with enteric gram-negative bacillary meningitis not responding to conventional parenteral antimicrobial therapy, concomitant intraventricular or intrathecal aminoglycoside therapy should be considered, although this mode of therapy was associated with a higher mortality rate than systemic therapy alone in infants with gram-negative meningitis and ventriculitis.

Other antimicrobial agents have also been used in patients with aerobic gram-negative meningitis. Imipenem has been efficacious in some isolated cases and larger series, although a high rate of seizure activity (33 percent in one study) limits its usefulness. Meropenem, a drug with less seizure proclivity than imipenem, has also been evaluated with promising results. The fluoroquinolones (ciprofloxacin, pefloxacin) have also been used in some patients, although their primary usefulness is for therapy of meningitis caused by multidrug-resistant gram-negative organisms or when the response to conventional therapy is inadequate; these agents should never be used as first-line empiric therapy in patients with meningitis of unknown cause because of their poor in vitro activity against *Str. pneumoniae* and *L. monocytogenes.*

Staphylococci and Streptococci

Meningitis caused by *Staphylococcus aureus* should be treated with nafcillin or oxacillin; vancomycin is used for patients who are allergic to penicillin or when the organism is methicillin-resistant. For meningitis caused by coagulase-negative staphylococci (e.g., *Staphylococcus epidermidis*), vancomycin is recommended; rifampin should be added if the patient fails to improve. In patients with meningitis caused by *Streptococcus agalactiae,* ampicillin plus an aminoglycoside is recommended because of its documented in vitro synergy and the emergence of penicillin-tolerant strains; alternatives include the third-generation cephalosporins and vancomycin.

Adjunctive Therapy

Clinical data support the routine use of adjunctive dexamethasone 0.15 mg per kilogram every 6 hours for 2 to 4 days in infants and children with bacterial meningitis caused by Hib. In adults or in patients with meningitis caused by other bacteria, the routine use of adjunctive dexamethasone is controversial. The subgroup of patients that may benefit from adjunctive dexamethasone are those with severely impaired mental status, documented cerebral edema by radiographic studies, and/or markedly elevated intracranial pressure. The timing of administration is crucial; administration before or concomitant with the first dose of the antimicrobial agent is optimal for maximal attenuation of the subarachnoid space inflammatory response.

■ PREVENTION

It is clear that the spread of several types of bacterial meningitis can be prevented by chemoprophylaxis of contacts of patients with meningitis. The rationale is for eradication of nasopharyngeal colonization, which prevents transmission to susceptible contacts and the development of invasive disease in those already colonized. For *H. influenzae,* chemoprophylaxis is recommended for all individuals, including adults, in households with at least one child younger than 4 years of age; the index case should also receive prophylaxis if the antimicrobial agent given for the invasive infection does not eliminate nasopharyngeal colonization. Chemoprophylaxis is not recommended for day care contacts 2 years of age or older unless two or more cases occur in the center within 60 days. For children younger than 2 years of age, whether to administer prophylaxis must be individualized and should be more strongly considered in centers that resemble households, where children have prolonged contact. To prevent transmission of Hib, the recommended chemoprophylactic agent of choice is rifampin 20 mg per kilogram daily for 4 days.

Chemoprophylaxis is also recommended for contacts of a person with meningococcal meningitis. Therapy is recommended for close contacts of the index patient, defined as household contacts or day care center members who eat or sleep in the same dwelling, close contacts in a closed community (e.g., a military barracks or boarding school), and medical personnel performing mouth-to-mouth resuscitation; the index patient may also need prophylaxis. The optimal regimen to prevent invasive meningococcal disease is controversial. At present, the Centers for Disease Control and Prevention recommend rifampin 600 mg in adults, 10 mg per kilogram in children beyond the neonatal period, and 5 mg per kilogram in infants less than 1 month of age at 12-hour intervals for 2 days. However, eradication rates are only 80 percent with rifampin, and adverse events, need for multiple dosing, and emergence of resistant organisms have made it less than an ideal agent. Alternatively, ceftriaxone 250 mg IM in adults and 125 mg IM in children or a single dose of oral ciprofloxacin 500 or 750 mg has been found efficacious. Ceftriaxone is probably the safest choice in the pregnant patient. Ciprofloxacin is not recommended for use in children because of the concerns of cartilage damage.

Suggested Reading

Gray LD, Fedorko DP. Laboratory diagnosis of bacterial meningitis. Clin Microbiol Rev 1992; 5:130–145.

Roos KL, Tunkel AR, Scheld WM. Acute bacterial meningitis in children and adults. In: Scheld WM, Whitley RJ, Durack DT, eds. Infections of the central nervous system. 2nd ed. Philadelphia: Lippincott–Raven Publishers, 1997: 335–401.

Tunkel AR, Scheld WM. Acute meningitis. In: Mandell GL, Bennett JE, Dolin R, eds. Principles and practice of infectious disease. 4th ed. New York: Churchill-Livingstone, 1995: 831–865.

Tunkel AR, Wispelwey B, Scheld WM. Bacterial meningitis: Recent advances in pathophysiology and treatment. Ann Intern Med 1990; 112:610–623.

Tunkel AR, Scheld WM. Acute bacterial meningitis. Lancet 1995; 346:1675–1680.

ACUTE AND CHRONIC BRONCHITIS

Sanford Chodosh, M.D.

Bronchial infections with viral and bacterial microorganisms are responsible for a significant percentage of ambulatory care visits and are the principal cause of time lost from work. These occur in individuals with and without underlying chronic bronchial disease, each with important differences in origin, clinical presentation, laboratory findings, and requirements for therapy.

■ ACUTE BRONCHITIS WITHOUT UNDERLYING LUNG DISEASE

Acute infectious bronchitis in individuals without underlying chronic lung disease is most commonly due to viral pathogens, with a lesser contribution by *Mycoplasma, Chlamydia,* and *Legionella.* The relative frequencies of these pathogens vary with time and place, and they have epidemic-like characteristics in the population. The clinical onset is usually abrupt and is characterized by cough, which may produce scanty sputum. The variable associated symptoms include coryza, sore throat, burning sensation in tracheal area, malaise, feverishness, chilliness, and other symptoms of viremia. Wheezing and dyspnea are unusual in adults but may be present in young children.

All of these symptoms are most troublesome in the first few days of the infection and should significantly improve or resolve within 1 week. These rarely require medical intervention and are usually treated with symptomatic therapy. Laboratory studies are rarely indicated and are likely to be normal. If the patient does produce sputum, the cytologic findings are of neutrophils with swollen bronchial epithelial cells, which may demonstrate vacuolization. A Gram stain is characteristically free of bacteria. However, if symptoms worsen or persist beyond a week, a nonviral cause should be suspected. If the Gram stain now reveals significant bacterial types morphologically consistent with *Haemophilus, Streptococcus pneumoniae,* or *Moraxella,* antimicrobial therapy is appropriate. The choice of agent is similar to what will be covered under acute exacerbations of chronic bronchitis, but the duration of therapy can be halved. If *Mycoplasma* infection is suspected, a 7 day course of a macrolide, tetracycline, or newer quinolone is appropriate. Patients who seek medical care for acute bronchitis should be suspected of having underlying chronic bronchial disease, which may be revealed with careful questioning.

■ ACUTE BRONCHITIS ASSOCIATED WITH CHRONIC BRONCHIAL DISEASE

Exacerbations due to bacterial bronchitis are more frequent and more severe in patients with chronic bronchitis and chronic bronchial asthma. Since the incidence of both diseases is common, bacterial exacerbations are one of the most frequent infectious syndromes seen by clinicians. Despite this, the diagnosis and therapy of such episodes are often haphazard. The pathologic and physiologic abnormalities of the bronchial system that may predispose these patients to bacterial infection include impaired mucociliary clearance, bronchi obstructed by abnormal secretions and bronchoconstriction, and in chronic bronchitis, indolent pathogenic bacteria in the bronchial epithelium, as well as impaired host defenses. Bacterial phagocytosis and intracellular bactericidal activity by polymorphonuclear neutrophils is impaired, macrophage recruitment is decreased, and sputum immunoglobulin (Ig) A levels are subnormal.

Most acute bacterial exacerbations (ABE) have no identifiable precipitating event. However, many follow acute viral respiratory infections, excessive cigarette smoking, thickened secretions secondary to reduced humidity associated with winter heating, alcohol consumption, and anesthesia. The last factor likely accounts for the increased frequency of postoperative bronchopulmonary infections noted in patients with underlying chronic bronchitis. The presenting bronchopulmonary symptoms, although not diagnostic of bacterial infection, include increased frequency and severity of cough; greater sputum production, usually purulent; chest congestion and discomfort; increased dyspnea and wheezing; and scant hemoptysis. Systemic symptoms of malaise, anorexia, chilliness, or feverishness may also be present. However, shaking chills, fever, or pleuritic pain usually indicates pneumonia. Physical examination may reveal rhonchi, coarse rales, wheezes, decreased breath sounds, tachypnea, and tachycardia. Such exacerbations are a common cause for hospitalization of these patients, particularly those with pre-existing compromise of pulmonary function.

The signs and symptoms of ABE should be significantly improved within 5 to 7 days after starting antimicrobial therapy. Patients should be re-evaluated if this does not occur, and therapy may have to be modified.

Laboratory tests are essential to identify the likely cause of each acute exacerbation, even though bacterial infection is responsible in most instances. Other common causes are acute viral tracheobronchitis, inhalation of toxic gases or particles (e.g., cigarette smoke), thickened secretions, inhalation of allergens, and discontinuation of background therapy. The differentiation of ABE from other types of exacerbations is rarely accomplished from examination of blood, urine, chest roentgenograph, pulmonary function tests, or the gross appearance of the sputum. Purulence of the sputum is often equated with infection. However, the characteristic yellow to green color of purulence is due to myeloperoxidase released from polymorphonuclear neutrophils and eosinophils, and it reflects the stasis of secretions in the bronchial tree, a common factor in most types of exacerbations.

Microscopic assessment of the sputum by means of a Gram stain and simple wet preparation reveal the two essential characteristics of bacterial infection, increased numbers of bacteria, and increased bronchial neutrophilic inflammation. The Gram stain must have bacteria in numbers significantly above levels present when the patient is stable, which is less than two per oil immersion field. In addition, the wet preparation of the sputum should reveal that most of the inflammatory cells are neutrophils. This, with an associated increase of the volume of sputum expectorated, reflects the outpouring of neutrophils into the bronchial lumen in response to the bacterial infection. Microscopic screening of the sputum is essential to the selection for evaluation of aliquots that are free of oropharyngeal admixture. Much of the distrust of sputum findings commented on in the literature can be related to the failure to adhere to this simple procedure.

Table 1 details the unique cellular population characteristics and Gram stain findings in each type of acute exacerbation seen in chronic bronchitis or asthma. The identification of the specific cause allows for selection of appropriate therapy and avoids the adverse effects associated with unnecessary medications.

Bacteriologic cultures and sensitivity testing are rarely indicated to determine treatment for ambulatory ABE. Exceptions to this rule are when gram-negative bacilli other than *Haemophilus*-like organisms or staphylococcus-like bacteria are noted on Gram stain. Staphylococcal ABE are virtually never seen in ambulatory outpatients. False-positive culture results are not infrequent in chronic bronchitis patients and can lead to inappropriate choice of therapy.

Table 2 details the critical primary treatment modalities for the various types of acute exacerbations as well as important supportive measures. Antimicrobials are not indicated for any of the non-ABE; they can only add adverse side effects. A

Table 1 Key Sputum Characteristics in the Differential Diagnosis of Acute Exacerbations of Chronic Bronchitis or Asthma

	NEUTROPHILS*	EOSINOPHILS*	TYPE OF BRONCHIAL EPITHELIAL CELLS†	BACTERIA ON GRAM STAIN§
Acute bacterial bronchitis	Increased	No change	Pyknotic	Increased
Acute viral bronchitis	Increased	No change	Swollen	No change
Inhalation of toxic gases or particles	Increased	No change	Pyknotic	No change
Thickened secretions	No change	No change	Pyknotic	No change
Inhalation of allergens	Variable	Increased	Swollen	No change
Discontinuation of background therapy	No change	No change	Pyknotic	No change

*Percentage of all cell types and numbers excreted per day as observed in wet sputum preparations.
†As observed in wet sputum preparations.
§Numbers per oil immersion field, with 0 to 2 seen in nonacute patients.

recent trend to treat all types of exacerbations empirically with both antimicrobials and corticosteroids should be discouraged. The decrease of host defenses associated with corticosteroids can be detrimental if the bacteria responsible for the ABE are not covered by the arbitrarily chosen antimicrobial.

The two main goals in the therapy of ABE are prompt resolution of the acute infection and a long infection-free post-therapy period. The chosen antimicrobial should cover the major pathogens causative in ABE, have a dosage regimen that favors compliance, and have a low incidence of undesirable side effects. Educating patients at risk for ABE to recognize early symptoms can lead to early initiation of adequate antimicrobial therapy, which decreases morbidity, unnecessary visits to emergency rooms, and expensive hospitalizations.

Table 3 provides data concerning efficacy of various oral antimicrobials. These results correlate with the efficacy of each agent in eradicating the four major bacteria causative in ABE; namely, *Haemophilus influenzae, S. pneumoniae, Moraxella catarrhalis,* and *Haemophilus parainfluenzae.* It is helpful if the antimicrobial also covers the bacteria occurring with lesser frequency such as *Pseudomonas aeruginosa* and *Klebsiella pneumoniae.* Unfortunately, few direct data compare the efficacy of different doses or duration of therapy for any single antimicrobial. Infections in chronic bronchitis seem to be more difficult to treat, as manifested by the tendency for relapses and frequent recurrences over the course of the disease. Experience suggests that this should be managed with a longer duration of therapy (10 to 14 days) and that higher doses should be employed. An example demonstrating this difference in efficacy can be noted for ciprofloxacin (see Table 3) in the results with 750 mg twice a day compared with 500 mg twice a day.

All of the data in Table 3 are based on both clinical and bacteriologic efficacy. Except for the cephalosporins, all of the drugs provide 89 to 100 percent efficacy. However, when early relapses and the length of the infection-free period are taken into consideration, the separation of first-line and second-line antimicrobials is more rational.

The first-line antimicrobials are ciprofloxacin 750 mg twice a day and ampicillin 500 mg four times a day. Ciprofloxacin has the disadvantage of cost and a tendency to increase theophylline serum levels. The latter is easily overcome by reducing the dose of theophylline by 30 to 50 percent during therapy. Ampicillin may be a problem if there is a high incidence of beta-lactamase-active *Haemophilus* or *Moraxella* in the population to be treated. Although bacampicillin has a higher incidence of early relapses, the infection-free period is comparable to those of ciprofloxacin and ampicillin. This suggests that if treatment is adequate, the patient can remain infection free for a long period. Although ofloxacin has not been critically examined in well-controlled studies, it may be considered in this select group.

The second-line antimicrobials include doxycycline 100 mg twice a day, amoxicillin 500 mg three times a day, ciprofloxacin 500 mg twice a day, and possibly minocycline 100 mg twice a day. Amoxicillin with clavulanic acid and clarithromycin are close but have a somewhat higher incidence of early relapses. Co-trimoxazole (trimethoprim-sulfamethoxazole) has been popular for treating ABE because of cost factors. Indeed, it is an excellent agent with respect to prompt resolution. However, the infection-free period is only half that attained with ampicillin or the higher dose of ciprofloxacin. It is very useful to the patient requiring longer periods of treatment. The place of the macrolide azithromycin has not yet been established for ABE therapy. Its long half-life and consequently shorter period of therapy may be quite advantageous.

The literature on the efficacy of oral cephalosporins for treating ABE is generally not helpful. There is, however, sufficient evidence other than that noted in Table 3 to indicate that the commonly prescribed cefaclor is not a satisfactory agent for ABE therapy.

When parenteral therapy is necessary for hospitalized patients, it is more important to identify causative pathogens. Depending on the pathogen, ampicillin, ciprofloxacin (particularly for gram-negatives infections), and doxycycline are common choices. Occasionally multiple-drug therapy including cephalosporins and aminoglycosides may be necessary. Oral therapy should be considered as early as possible in these circumstances.

Antimicrobial therapy should always be accompanied by good supportive therapy. This should include avoidance of smoking and other inhalation irritants, hydration, humidification, expectorants, bronchodilators, and adequate treatment of any associated asthma. When secretion clearance is particularly difficult, chest physiotherapy and mucolytic

Table 2 Therapy for Acute Exacerbations of Chronic Bronchitis With or Without Asthma

	ANTIMICROBIAL	CORTICOSTEROIDS	HYDRATION & HUMIDIFICATION	AVOIDANCE OF INHALED IRRITANTS	EXPECTORANT	BRONCHODILATOR
Acute bacterial bronchitis	1	NA	2	2	2	2
Acute viral bronchitis	NA	NA	2	2	2	2
Inhalation of toxic gas or particles	NA	NA*	2	1	2	2
Thickened secretions	NA	NA	1	2	1	2
Inhalation of allergens	NA	1	2	2	2	1
Discontinuation of background therapy	NA	NA		Renew appropriate background therapy		

1, primary or very important therapy
2, secondary or supportive therapy
NA, not applicable
*Exception for acute inhalation of toxic materials known to cause serious acute inflammatory response.

Table 3 Oral Antimicrobials for Acute Bacterial Exacerbations in Chronic Bronchial Disease*

	DOSAGE SCHEDULES (14 DAYS' THERAPY)	TREATMENT FAILURES (%)†		INADEQUATE TREATMENT (%)‡		INFECTION-FREE PERIOD§ (RATIO)
		DBCO‖	ALL CASES¶	DBCO[E]	ALL CASES[F]	
Ciprofloxacin	750 mg b.i.d.	0.0	0.0	15.8	10.7	1.05
Ampicillin	500 mg q.i.d.	0.0	0.0	15.6	12.5	1.00
Bacampicillin	800 mg b.i.d.	0.0	0.0	29.0	20.3	1.01
Bacampicillin	1,600 mg b.i.d.	0.0	0.0	43.8	33.3	1.21
Amoxicillin	500 mg t.i.d.	11.8	5.1	11.8	10.3	0.86
Doxycycline	100 mg b.i.d.	6.1	6.5	16.3	14.5	0.85
Ciprofloxacin	500 mg b.i.d.	0.0	1.9	22.2	21.2	0.79
Amoxicillin/ clavulanic acid	500 mg, 125 mg b.i.d.	5.5	7.1	27.8	25.9	0.83
Clarithromycin	500 mg b.i.d.	11.1	8.7	33.3	26.1	0.80
Minocycline	100 mg b.i.d.	0.0	4.8	20.0	23.8	0.72
Enoxacin	400 mg b.i.d.	0.0	0.0	26.3	23.1	0.58
Co-trimoxazole	2 tablets b.i.d.	0.0	0.0	23.5	19.0	0.51
Cefixime	400 mg daily	ND	18.2	ND	36.4	ND
Cefalexin	500 mg q.i.d.	20.0	17.6	40.0	35.3	0.31
Cefaclor	500 mg t.i.d.	50.0	46.2	61.1	53.8	0.31
Cefaclor	250 mg t.i.d.	29.4	35.0	70.6	70.0	0.31

*Drugs are listed in order of choice based on percentage of unsatisfactory results and relative infection-free periods.
†Defined as failure to respond during treatment period.
‡Defined as failure to respond during treatment or rebound within 2 weeks after treatment.
§From double-blind cross-over studies. Ratios calculated relative to ampicillin, with which the infection-free periods varied from 117 to 302 days in separate studies.
‖Cases only from double-blind cross-over studies.
¶All cases from double-blind studies.
b.i.d, twice daily; q.i.d., 4 times daily; t.i.d., 3 times daily; ND, no data; DBCO, double-blind cross-over.

therapy are appropriate. Patients who have both chronic bronchitis and asthma will often note an exacerbation of asthmatic symptoms as the infection is controlled. Prompt recognition of this possibility should lead to vigorous treatment of the asthma and not be misdiagnosed as a failure of the antimicrobial. This can easily be detected by examination of the sputum, which shows a shift to a predominance of eosinophils and an absence of significant bacterial flora on Gram stain.

Suggested Reading

Chodosh S. Sputum examination. In: Fishman AP, ed. Pulmonary diseases and disorders. 2nd ed. New York: McGraw-Hill, 1988:411.

Chodosh S. Bronchitis and asthma. In: Gorbach SL, Bartlett JG, Blacklow NR, eds. Infectious diseases. Philadelphia: WB Saunders, 1992:476.

Chodosh S. Sputum production and chronic bronchitis. In: Takishima T, Shimura S, eds. Airway secretion: Physiological bases for the control of mucus hypersecretion. New York: Marcel Dekker, 1994:579.

INTRAVASCULAR CATHETER-RELATED INFECTION

David C. Dugdale, M.D.
Paul G. Ramsey, M.D.

Intravascular catheters (Table 1) are an essential part of modern medical therapy, but they cause significant morbidity and mortality, largely due to associated infections. The range of infectious complications varies from superficial exit site infections to bacteremia and septic thrombophlebitis. Therapy should be individualized to the patient while maintaining the goal of salvage of implanted catheters.

TYPES OF CATHETER-RELATED INFECTIONS

Infusion phlebitis, characterized by inflammation of the cannulated vein, is often a noninfectious condition. Many factors, including large or long catheters, certain types of intravenous fluids, and host-related factors, promote infusion phlebitis. Less than half of patients with intravenous catheter-related bacteremia have signs of infusion phlebitis, but infusion phlebitis may progress to infection and is an indication for removal of the catheter.

Exit site infections are suspected on the basis of inflammatory signs, especially expressible pus.

Tunnel infections are diagnosed when inflammatory signs extend more than 2 cm proximal to the exit site of a tunneled catheter.

Catheter-related bacteremia is suggested by local inflammatory signs associated with a positive blood culture. However, catheter-related bacteremia often occurs in the absence of local inflammation and may be suspected because of differential quantitative blood cultures (see the next section).

Septic thrombophlebitis indicates an infected clot at the site of the intravenous catheter; this may occur with a peripheral or central catheter. It should be suspected when bacteremia persists after catheter removal.

Endarteritis is suggested by signs of tissue ischemia or embolism distal to an arterial catheter.

Table 1 Vascular Access Devices

- Peripheral intravenous catheters
- Peripherally inserted central catheters
- Central intravenous catheters
  - Percutaneously inserted devices
  - Tunneled catheters
  - Implanted infusion ports
- Arterial catheters

DIAGNOSIS

Catheter-related infections are diagnosed by a combination of clinical findings and microbiologic studies. Rigors and shock may accompany peripheral or central septic thrombophlebitis, especially when the infectious agent is a gram-negative bacillus, but these clinical findings are not common in patients with catheter-related infections. Inflammation or exudate at a catheter insertion site denotes at least local infection, and in the setting of bacteremia either one implicates the catheter. However, only half of patients with peripheral catheter-related bacteremia have a local inflammatory response. Other clinical findings that support the diagnosis of a catheter-related infection include embolic events or other signs of metastatic infection (e.g., *Candida* endophthalmitis) or signs of venous obstruction distal to central venous catheters. A radiopaque dye study through the venous catheter or an ultrasonic duplex venous Doppler study may provide evidence of fibrin sheath or intraluminal obstruction that may implicate the catheter.

Bacteremia due to an organism commonly associated with catheter infections suggests a catheter-related source (Table 2). Bacteremia due to *Streptococcus* or anaerobic spp. is rarely catheter related. Infection due to a contaminated infusate can mimic a catheter-related bacteremia. The microbiologic spectrum of infusate-related bacteremia includes *Klebsiella, Enterobacter, Serratia, Pseudomonas,* and *Citrobacter* spp.

The following sources of culture should be used to aid in the diagnosis. Exudate from the site of the catheter should be Gram-stained and cultured. The catheter itself, if removed, should be cultured using the semiquantitative technique

Table 2 Microbiology of Intravascular Catheter-Related Infections

PATHOGEN	PREVALENCE
Peripheral IV catheters	
Coagulase-negative staphyloccci	92%
Staphylococcus aureus	4
Candida spp.	2
Nontunneled silastic central venous catheters	
Coagulase-negative staphyloccci	27
Candida albicans	27
S. aureus	18
Serratia marcescens	9
Streptococcus faecalis	9
Acinetobacter anitratus	9
Tunneled central venous catheters	
Coagulase-negative staphyloccci	54
S. aureus	20
Candida spp.	7
Pseudomonas aeruginosa	6
Corynebacterium spp. (especially JK-1)	5
Klebsiella species	4
S. faecalis	2
Arterial catheters	
Coagulase-negative staphyloccci	82
Pseudomonas aeruginosa	8
Enterobacter agglomerans	8

Note: In AIDS patients, *Staphylococcus aureus* is the most common pathogen.

described by Maki and associates. The catheter tip is prone to contamination at the time of removal, so a simple culture of it is less specific. Prior to removal of a catheter the skin should be cleaned to reduce flora. For short catheters the entire length should be cut off just distal to the skin insertion site and cultured by rolling it across an agar plate. For longer catheters the tip and the intracutaneous sections should be separately cultured in a similar fashion. In either case a growth of 15 or more colony-forming units on a semiquantitative plate suggests an infected catheter. If the catheter cannot be removed, Gram stain or quantitative culture of the skin insertion site combined with a culture of the catheter hub may be beneficial in diagnosis.

Blood cultures should be performed when catheter-related infection is suspected. For patients with an implanted vascular access device, cultures of blood drawn from the device and from a different venous site should be performed at the time of the first symptoms or signs of infection (e.g., febrile episode); subsequent febrile episodes can usually be evaluated with blood cultures drawn only from the vascular access device. If pour-plate quantitative blood cultures can be done, comparison of the results from blood drawn from the catheter with peripherally obtained blood may be useful. In patients with implanted vascular access devices, a tenfold increase of quantitative blood culture colony counts from the venipuncture site to the catheter strongly implicates a catheter source.

■ THERAPY

In general, antimicrobial treatment of catheter-related infections should be as specific as possible. Use of Gram stain or culture results to guide therapy is preferred, but in many cases severity of infection or other circumstances warrant empiric therapy prior to specific microbiologic results. When empiric therapy is needed, choice of drugs and routes should be based on severity of infection, type of catheter, degree of immunocompromise of the patient, and availability of exudate for Gram stain. Specific recommendations are listed next.

Peripheral Intravenous Catheters

Infusion Phlebitis. The catheter should be removed; in the absence of other signs of infection (e.g., fever or expressible pus), no antibiotic therapy is required. Local heat should be applied to accelerate resolution of the phlebitis.

Exit Site Infection. The catheter should be removed. Antibiotic therapy should be directed against pathogens seen on Gram stain and/or culture of the exit site exudate. For empiric therapy, until culture results are available, use an oral antistaphylococcal antibiotic; if signs of systemic infection, such as fever, are present, use intravenous vancomycin. Treatment should continue for 7 days.

Bacteremia. The catheter should be removed. Antibiotic therapy should be directed against pathogens found on culture. Treat for 14 days unless signs of endocarditis, metastatic infection, or prolonged bacteremia are present; in such cases, longer therapy (e.g., 4 weeks) will be needed.

Septic Thrombophlebitis. The catheter should be removed. Antibiotic therapy should be directed against pathogens seen on Gram stain and/or culture of the exit site exudate or against pathogens isolated from blood cultures. For empiric therapy, use vancomycin; add coverage for gram-negative pathogens in neutropenic patients. Treat for 14 days unless signs of endocarditis, metastatic infection, or prolonged bacteremia are present; in such cases, longer therapy (e.g., 4 weeks) will be needed. (For specific recommendations for treatment, see the chapter *Endocarditis.*) Surgical excision may be required to cure the infection. A perivenous abscess should be excluded by ultrasound examination.

Central Percutaneous Catheters with Central or Peripheral Placement

Exit Site Infection. The catheter should be removed. Antibiotic therapy should be directed against pathogens seen on Gram stain and/or culture of the exit site exudate. For empiric therapy, use intravenous vancomycin and coverage for gram-negative pathogens. Treat for 14 days; part of therapy may be oral if the infection is mild.

Bacteremia. The catheter should be removed. Antibiotic therapy should be directed against pathogens found on culture. Treat for 14 days unless signs of endocarditis, metastatic infection, or prolonged bacteremia are present; in such cases, longer therapy (e.g., 4 weeks) will be needed.

Septic Thrombophlebitis. The catheter should be removed. Antibiotic therapy should be directed against pathogens seen on Gram stain and/or culture of the exit site exudate or against pathogens isolated from blood cultures. For empiric therapy, use intravenous vancomycin and coverage for gram-negative pathogens. Treat for 14 days unless signs of endocarditis, metastatic infection, or prolonged bacteremia are present; in such cases, longer therapy (e.g., 4 weeks) will be needed. Full-dose anticoagulation with heparin should be considered as an adjunct to antibiotic therapy. For refractory infections, surgical excision may be required.

Tunneled Catheters and Infusion Ports

Exit Site Infection. Antibiotic therapy should be directed against pathogens seen on Gram stain and/or culture of the exit site exudate. For empiric therapy if there are no systemic signs of infection and the patient is not neutropenic, an oral antistaphylococcal antibiotic may be used. If fever or other signs of systemic infection *or* neutropenia is present, empiric therapy should be intravenous vancomycin. Treatment should be given for 14 days and may be exclusively oral if the infection is mild. Most (80 percent) infections can be cured without catheter removal, but some infections (e.g., *Staphylococcus aureus*) may recur with significant morbidity.

Tunnel Infection. Antibiotic therapy should be directed against pathogens seen on Gram stain and/or culture of the exit site exudate. For empiric therapy use intravenous vancomycin and coverage for gram-negative pathogens. Duration of treatment should be 14 days past the resolution of local inflammatory signs. Catheter removal is required in over 70

Table 3 Indications for Removal of Tunneled or Implantable Catheters

Tunnel infection
Bacteremic infection with selected pathogens
Staphylococcus aureus
Candida or *Aspergillus* spp.
Septic thrombophlebitis
Failure of 48 hours of appropriate antibiotic therapy to reduce signs of infection
Frequently recurrent exit site infections
Peripheral embolic events

percent of cases. Removal is especially likely to be required for cure if *S. aureus* or *Pseudomonas* spp. are cultured from the exit site or the patient is neutropenic.

Bacteremia. Antibiotic therapy should be directed against pathogens found on culture. If culture is positive only for coagulase-negative staphylococci and clinical and microbiologic response occurs in 48 hours, treat for 14 days with intravenous vancomycin but leave the catheter in place; if signs of endocarditis, metastatic infection, or prolonged bacteremia are present, longer therapy (e.g., 4 weeks) will be needed and catheter removal required. Infection with other pathogens may require catheter removal (see Table 3) to prevent serious complications. Cure without catheter removal may be attempted in hemodynamically stable patients with low-level bacteremia by pathogens other than *S. aureus* and *Candida* or *Aspergillus* spp.

Septic Thrombophlebitis. The catheter should be removed. Antibiotic therapy should be directed against pathogens seen on Gram stain and/or culture of the exit site exudate or against pathogens isolated from blood cultures. For empiric therapy, use intravenous vancomycin and coverage for gram-negative pathogens. Treat for 14 days unless signs of endocarditis, metastatic infection, or prolonged bacteremia are present; in such cases, longer therapy (e.g., 4 weeks) will be needed. Full-dose anticoagulation with heparin should be considered as an adjunct to antibiotic therapy. For refractory infections, surgical excision may be required.

Arterial Catheters

Exit Site Infection. The catheter should be removed. Antibiotic therapy should be directed against pathogens seen on Gram stain and/or culture of the exit site exudate. For empiric therapy, use IV vancomycin and coverage for gram-negative pathogens. Treat for 14 days unless signs of endocarditis, metastatic infection, or prolonged bacteremia are present; in such cases, longer therapy (e.g., 4 weeks) will be needed. For mild infections, part of the course of therapy may be oral.

Bacteremia. The catheter should be removed. Antibiotic therapy should be directed against pathogens found on culture. Treat for 14 days unless signs of endocarditis, metastatic infection, or prolonged bacteremia are present; in such cases, longer therapy (e.g., 4 weeks) will be needed.

Suggested Reading

Barnes JR, Lucus N, Broadwater JR, Hauer-Jensen M. When should the "infected" subcutaneous infusion reservoir be removed? Am Surg 1996; 62:203–206.

Dugdale DC, Ramsey PG. *Staphylococcus aureus* bacteremia in patients with Hickman catheters. Am J Med 1990; 89:137–141.

Maki DG, Alvarado CJ, Ringer MA. A prospective, randomized trial of povidone-iodine, alcohol, and chlorhexidene for prevention of infection with central venous and arterial catheters. Lancet 1991; 338:339–343.

Maki DG, Ringer M. Risk factors for infusion-related phlebitis with small peripheral venous catheters. Ann Intern Med 1991; 114:845–854.

Maki DG, Weise CF, Sarafin HW. A semiquantitative culture method for identifying intravenous-catheter infection. N Engl J Med 1977; 296: 1305–1309.

Raad I, Davis S, Becker M, et al. Low infection rate and long durability of nontunneled silastic catheters. Arch Intern Med 1993; 153:1791–1796.

CELLULITIS AND ERYSIPELAS

Daniel B. Dubin, M.D.
Richard Allen Johnson, M.D.

In the preantibiotic era the treatment of lower-extremity cellulitis often required amputation to prevent progression to disseminated infection and death. The list of agents causing cellulitis has grown in proportion to the increasing number of immunocompromised patients enduring intensive cancer chemotherapy regimens, organ transplantation, and HIV disease. Timely diagnosis and treatment cure most cases of soft-tissue infection. However, necrotizing cellulitides, focal abscesses, or opportunistic antimicrobial-resistant pathogens require surgical intervention. Factors such as moderate to severe facial or hand infections, tissue necrosis, crepitance, systemic toxicity, atypical pathogens, and complicating premorbid medical diseases are indications for inpatient treatment of soft-tissue infections (Fig. 1).

■ CLINICAL FINDINGS

Erysipelas

Erysipelas, a clinical variant of cellulitis, is characterized by well-demarcated erythema, tenderness, and swelling and is

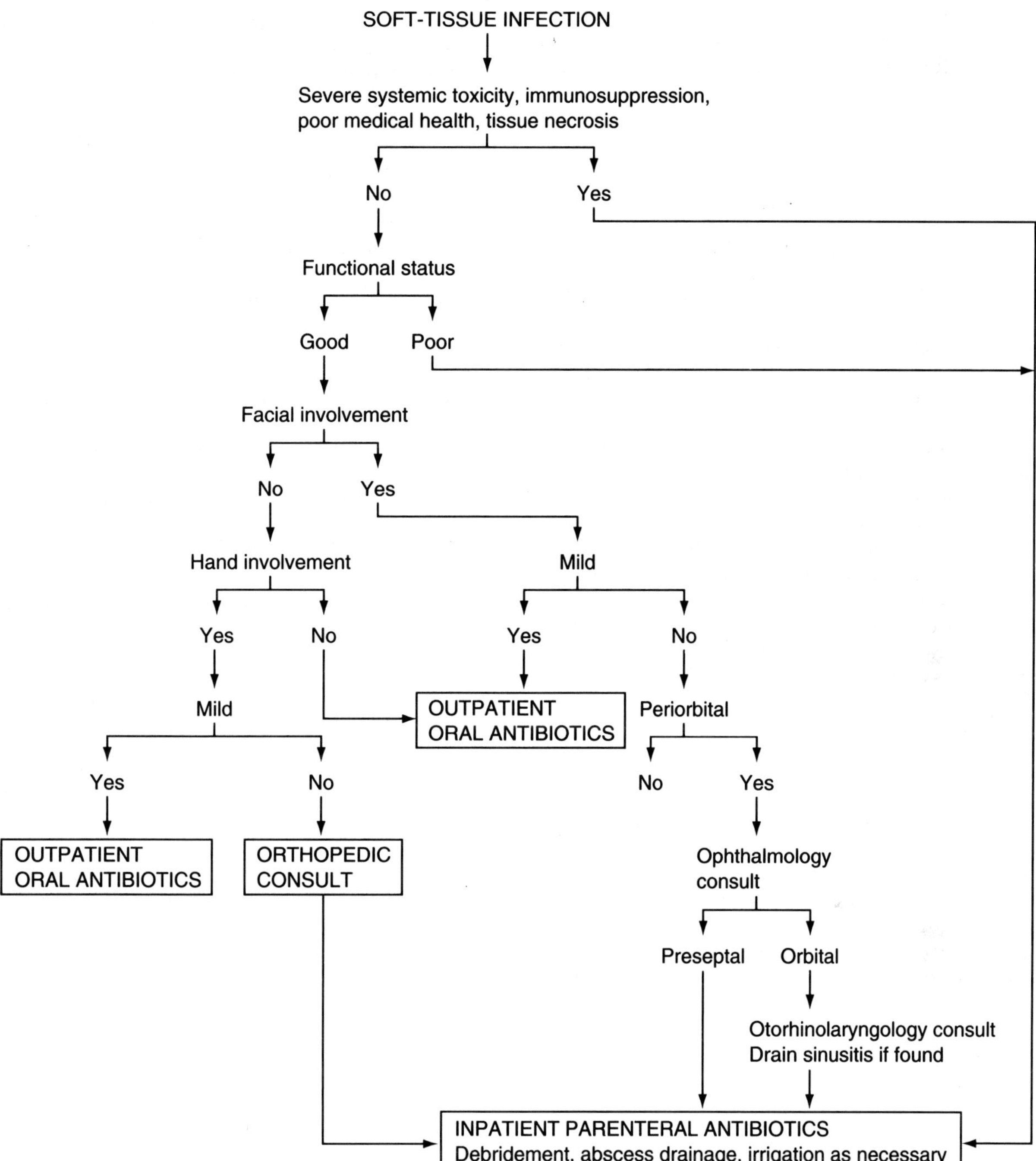

Figure 1
Algorithm for determining need for inpatient management of a patient with soft-tissue infection.

distinguished from other types of cellulitis by its discrete raised border. Dermal and lymphatic infection without significant subcutaneous involvement results in a sharp border of demarcation. Conditions that compromise skin and soft-tissue antimicrobial defenses predispose to erysipelas. They include wounds, erosive or fissuring dermatophyte infections, arterial insufficiency, venous insufficiency, chronic lymphedema, diabetes mellitus, and immunodeficiency.

Before the advent of antibiotics, erysipelas usually affected the face; however, recent series report that erysipelas most commonly arises on the extremities. Group A beta-hemolytic streptococci (GAS) cause most cases of erysipelas. Less common pathogens include group B, C, and G streptococci, *Staphylococcus aureus, Streptococcus pneumoniae, Haemophilus influenzae,* and *Yersinia enterocolitica.*

Cellulitis

Cellulitis is an infection of the skin and subcutaneous tissue without involvement of fascial planes or muscle. It is marked by redness, tenderness, swelling, and a poorly defined border. Fever, leukocytosis, lymphangitis, regional lymphadenopathy, hematogenous dissemination, and focal abscesses or bullae may accompany these infections. The factors that predispose to cellulitis are similar to those cited for erysipelas. Overall, GAS and *S. aureus* account for most cellulitic infections. *H. influenzae* may cause both facial and extremity cellulitis in young children. Other bacterial causes of cellulitis include enteric gram-negative rods, *Pseudomonas* spp. (hot tubs), anaerobes, and other streptococci.

Facial Cellulitis and Erysipelas

Most facial cellulitis in persons over 5 years of age is related to cutaneous trauma and is caused by *S. aureus* and *Streptococcus pyogenes.* A well-demarcated raised border suggests facial erysipelas and GAS infection. Preseptal and orbital cellulitis, subsets of facial cellulitis, merit special consideration.

Both preseptal and orbital cellulitis cause marked eyelid inflammation and swelling. However, decreased visual acuity, decreased extraocular eye movement, marked chemosis, pain on eye movement, or significant axial proptosis indicates orbital cellulitis, which can permanently damage the optic nerve as well as extend centrally and cause cavernous sinus thrombosis. Superficial eyelid trauma and gland infection are associated with preseptal cellulitis, and underlying sinusitis and deep orbital trauma are the most likely causes of orbital cellulitis. In immunocompromised patients and poorly controlled diabetics zygomycotic sinus infections can perforate the sinus wall and invade the orbital space.

Necrotizing Soft-Tissue Infections (Table 1)

Necrotizing cellulitis is a subset of soft-tissue infections marked by frank cutaneous and subcutaneous necrosis yet lacking involvement of fascial planes. Initially the systemic toxicity associated with necrotizing cellulitis is less than that of its more lethal cousin necrotizing fasciitis (see the chapter *Sinusitis*). However, left untreated, necrotizing cellulitis can progress to sepsis with or without invasion of underlying fascia or muscle.

In immunocompetent hosts GAS, *Clostridium, Vibrio,* and *Aeromonas* spp. may cause necrotizing cellulitis as solo pathogens. Superficial puncture injuries that introduce nonsterile material into relatively devitalized soft tissue predispose to infections with gas-forming anaerobes, such as clostridia, *Bacteroides,* and peptostreptococci; *Klebsiella* and *Escherichia coli* can also produce a crepitant cellulitis. *Aeromonas* infections are associated with outdoor freshwater injuries that introduce this aqueous pathogen into the soft tissues. While *Aeromonas* may act alone in causing necrotizing cellulitis, more frequently it is aided by coinfecting pathogens. Progressive synergistic gangrenous cellulitis occurs in association with surgical or traumatic wounds and requires mixed infection with anaerobic streptococcal species and either *S. aureus* or *Proteus.*

Marine *Vibrio* spp. can cause sepsis and soft-tissue infections, particularly in patients with alcoholism, cirrhosis, hemochromatosis, and other chronic illnesses such as diabetes mellitus. Either ingestion of raw seafood or exposure of an open wound to seawater can result in *Vibrio* soft-tissue infection. It has been recommended that cirrhotics, diabetics, and other patients with chronic disease avoid eating raw seafood. However, unlike *V. vulnificus* and *Vibrio alginolyticus,* which prey on compromised hosts, *Vibrio damselae* may cause fulminant necrotizing infections in immunocompetent patients.

In immunocompromised hosts *Pseudomonas aeruginosa* can cause a cellulitis that may have a necrotizing component, ecthyma gangrenosum (EG). Absolute neutropenia and poor neutrophil function predispose to pseudomonal cellulitis and EG. Most often arising in the axillae or anogenital region, *P. aeruginosa* gains entry into the dermis and subcutaneous tissues via adnexal epidermal structures. Bacteremia occurs soon after the onset of EG and may result in metastatic spread of *P. aeruginosa* infection. Most cases of EG are a consequence of primary soft-tissue infection; however, metastatic seeding from an internal infectious source may also cause a necrotizing cellulitis.

In the family Mucoracea are the genera *Rhizopus, Absidia,* and *Mucor,* the most common zygomycotic human pathogens. Individuals with thermal burns, recent trauma, and uncontrolled diabetes mellitus are at highest risk for mycotic necrotizing cellulitis. Mucormycoses are characterized by vascular invasion and occlusion with subsequent tissue infarction and hematogenous dissemination of the invading fungus. Early diagnosis is key, for these infections can rapidly progress to involve deeper soft tissues.

■ THERAPY

Nonfacial Cellulitis and Erysipelas

Nonfacial cellulitis or erysipelas in a patient of reasonable functional status and immunocompetence can be managed on an outpatient basis. Abscesses complicating cellulitis must be incised and drained. The purulent contents should be sent for Gram stain and culture to confirm the appropriateness of empiric treatment. Attempting to culture routine cellulitides without focal abscess formation results in low yield and does not significantly improve treatment.

Depending on the suspected pathogens, the extent of infection, and the status of the patient, the following outpatient options (Fig. 2) are reasonable: (1) oral dicloxacillin or cephalexin for 7 to 10 days; (2) a single dose of IV cefazolin followed by oral dicloxacillin or cephalexin for 7 to 10 days; or (3) a single dose of cefazolin followed by daily home parenteral ceftriaxone 50 mg per kilogram per day until significant improvement is noted, then completion of therapy with 7 to 10 days of oral dicloxacillin or cephalexin. If gram-negative rods are a concern, as in diabetic foot ulcer-related cellulitis, amoxicillin clavulanate potassium 250 to 500 mg four times a day for 7 to 10 days is recommended.

Some clinicians prefer to use inpatient parenteral antibiotics for even uncomplicated cellulitis until significant improvement is observed. If outpatient therapy is undertaken, education of the patient regarding the signs of progressing infection is essential to efficacy and safety. Services administering parenteral therapies are readily available in many localities for home intravenous antibiotic treatment.

Facial Cellulitis and Erysipelas

All patients with moderate to severe nonperiocular facial cellulitides should initially be hospitalized to monitor for progression to a necrotizing infection, which if not managed urgently by surgical debridement may result in significant

Table 1 Synopsis of Necrotizing Cellulitides

INFECTION	PREDISPOSING FACTORS	CLINICAL FINDINGS	BACTERIOLOGY	PATHOLOGIC FINDINGS	ANTIMICROBIAL TREATMENT
Streptococcal necrotizing cellulitis	Usually arising at the site of an epithelial break, traumatic or surgical GBS; patients often elderly but otherwise healthy	Fever; overlying skin becomes dusky blue with or without bullae; may progress to necrosis of tissue; initially very painful; gangenous areas become anesthetic	Usually GAS, occasionally GBS, in wound with or without blood	Vasculitis, fibrin thrombi; necrosis of epidermis and dermis; heavy infiltrate of neutrophils; gram-positive cocci	Penicillin G
Synergistic necrotizing cellulitis	Diabetes, perineal involvement, peripheral vascular disease, renal disease; may extend to involve fascia and muscle	Dishwater pus or edema, crepitus, fever, blebs, necrosis, central ulcer that slowly enlarges	Microaerophilic or anaerobic streptocci; *S. aureus*	Dense leukocytic infiltration and edema of dermis from edematous margin	Vancomycin plus gentamicin
Pseudomonas aeruginosa cellulitis and ecthyma gangrenosum	Neutropenia	Cellulitis with central necrosis in axillae or anogenital regions; fever, sepsis	*P. aeruginosa*	Cellulitis with vasculitis	Gentamicin plus antipseudomonal PCN or CEPH
Vibrio vulnificus cellulitis	Diabetes, alcoholism, cirrhosis; ingestion of raw seafood; trauma while in aquatic environment	Fever, blebs, edema, pain	*Vibrio vulnificus,* other species	Neutrophilic cellulitis	TCN with or without gentamicin
Aeromonas hydrophila cellulitis	Trauma in freshwater; most patients are immunocompetent; 90% are male	Cellulitis, necrotizing fasciitis, or myonecrosis	*A. hydrophila,* may be polymicrobial	Neutrophilic cellulitis, fasciitis	Cefotaxime or gentamicin or TMP-SMX
Clostridial cellulitis	Trauma	Fever, crepitus, blebs, red-brown fluid, edema, extreme wound pain, relatively mild toxicity	Clostridia, mixed gram-positive and gram-negative organisms	Dense leukocytic dermal infiltrate with necrosis of vessels and sweat glands	High-dose penicillin G with or without clindamycin or chloramphenicol
Mucormycosis (zogymycosis, phycomycosis)	Diabetes with ketoacidosis; trauma to soft tissue; immunocompromise	May occur as primary cutaneous at site of injury or extension from deeper focus to overlying skin	Mucoracea	Large branched nonseptate hyphae invading blood vessel walls	Amphotericin B
Cryptococcal cellulitis	Immunocompromise	Vesiculobullous, erythematous eruption	*Cryptococcus neoformans*	Encapsulated budding yeast	Amphotericin B

CEPH, Cephalexin; GAS, group A streptococci; GBS, group B streptococci; PCN, penicillin; TCN, tetracycline; TMP-SMX, trimethoprim-sulfamethoxazole.

facial disfigurement and dysfunction. Obvious facial erysipelas should be treated with parenteral penicillin G 2 million units every 4 hours, as GAS causes the vast majority of these infections. Once the patient is afebrile for 24 hours, oral penicillin VK 500 mg every 6 hours for 7 to 10 days will complete therapy. Adults with established facial cellulitis should receive a parenteral semisynthetic penicillin (e.g., nafcillin 1 to 1.5 g every 4 hours) or first-generation cephalosporin (e.g., cefazolin 1 g every 8 hours) until significant clinical improvement is noted; completion of therapy should include 7 to 10 days of oral dicloxacillin or cephalexin.

Periocular soft tissue infections require thorough ophthalmologic evaluation to distinguish preseptal from orbital cellulitis. Moderate to severe preseptal cellulitis in older children

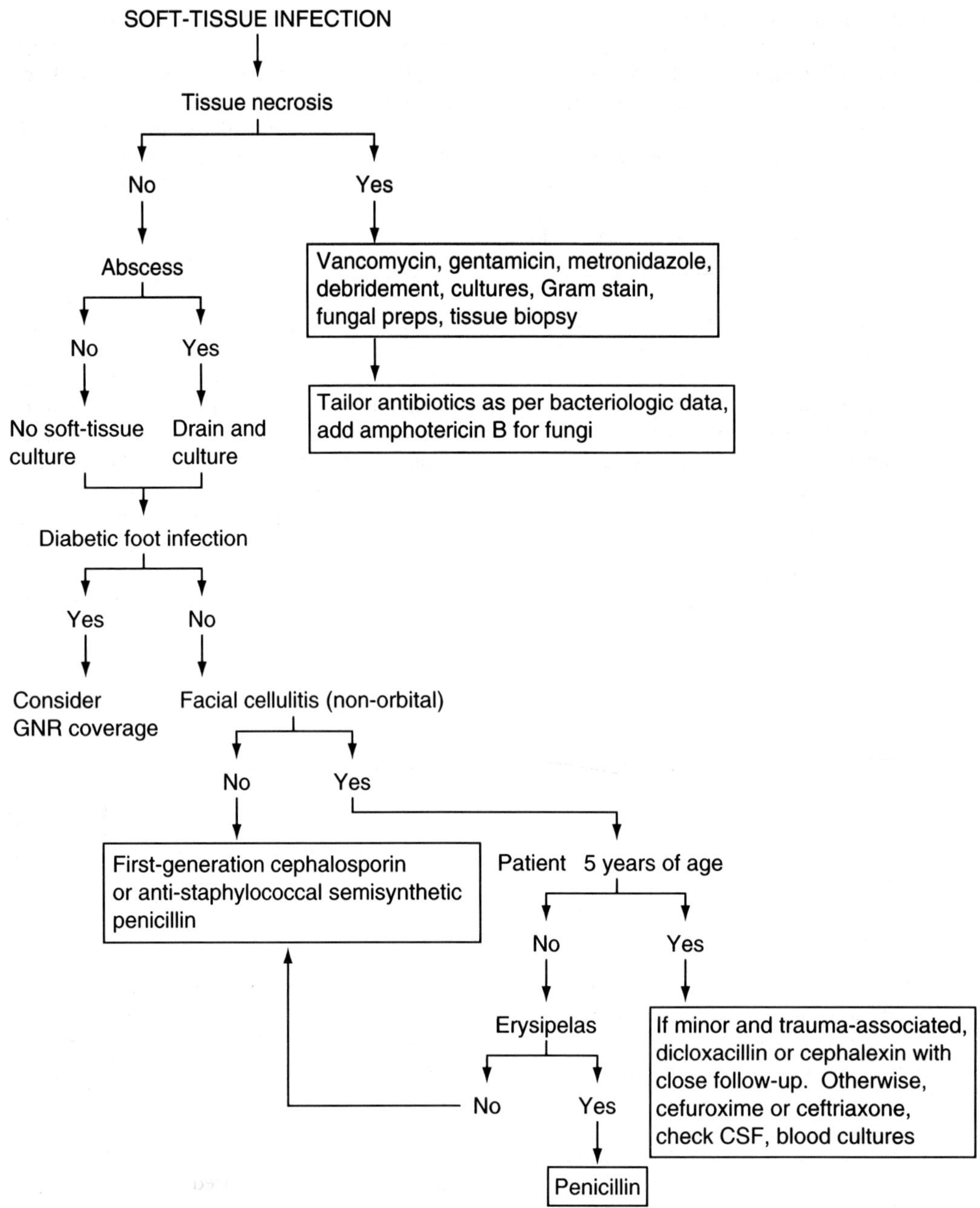

Figure 2
Algorithm for initial antibiotic selection in soft-tissue infection.

and adults can progress to a necrotizing infection that requires urgent surgical debridement; hence, these patients should be initially managed with parenteral semisynthetic penicillin or first-generation cephalosporin until significant improvement is noted.

Orbital cellulitis, a medical emergency, should be managed initially with parenteral semisynthetic penicillin and ceftriaxone. Clindamycin may be substituted for the penicillin if anaerobic infection is suspected. Orbital collections of pus must be drained immediately. Otorhinolaryngologic consultation is indicated to help search for underlying sinusitis, which must be drained. Close ophthalmologic follow-up is necessary to assess the response to treatment.

Hand Cellulitis

Group A streptococci and *S. aureus* account for most hand cellulitides. Mild early soft-tissue infections of the hand in immunocompetent patients can be managed on an outpatient basis with elevation, splinting, and oral dicloxacillin or cephalexin; penicillin, clindamycin, or metronidazole should be added if anaerobic coinfection is suspected. Established infections of the hand warrant consultation by a hand specialist to evaluate for joint, tendon sheath, deep palmar space, and muscular involvement. Delay in the treatment of hand infections of deeper structures can result in significant manual disability.

Patients admitted with hand cellulitis should initially be

treated with parenteral oxacillin, nafcillin, or cefazolin, limb elevation, and observation until significant clinical improvement is noted. All pus collections must be drained and involved tendon sheaths irrigated by a skilled hand surgeon. Immunocompromised patients with even mild superficial hand cellulitis merit initial hospitalization, observation, and parenteral antibiotics. Human and animal bite infections of the hand, which are addressed in detail in the chapter *Human and Animal Bites,* require additional coverage against organisms such as mouth anaerobes, *Haemophilus,* and *Pasteurella multocida.*

Butchers and fishermen are susceptible to erysipeloid, a manual cutaneous infection of *Erysipelothrix rhusiopathiae.* This infection is marked by a red-purple tender plaque, usually over the hand. Fever and lymphadenopathy are rare. Untreated, some cases resolve spontaneously over weeks. Erysipeloid responds to treatment with oral penicillin VK 250 mg four times a day for 10 days or erythromycin 250 mg four times a day for 7 days.

Necrotizing Soft-Tissue Infections

Tissue necrosis mandates hospitalization and immediate surgical consultation. Soft-tissue crepitance or radiographic evidence of subcutaneous air suggests infection with anaerobic gas-forming organisms. The degree of systemic toxicity and the integument examination may help differentiate a superficial necrotizing cellulitis from an established deeper necrotizing soft-tissue infection. However, given the necessity for early complete debridement of necrotic tissue, a low threshhold for proceeding with surgical investigation should be maintained.

The following factors are indications for at least an open biopsy to rule out a deep necrotizing soft-tissue infection: confusion, tachycardia, tachypnea, ketoacidosis or hyperglycemia, gangrenous skin changes, bronzing of the skin, severe pain or spreading areas of anesthesia, thin reddish discharge with undermining of wound edges, crepitus, an abscess with multiple tracks, and a cellulitis that progresses despite antibiotics, has extensive surrounding edema, or complicates a surgical wound. Since necrotizing cellulitis does not involve fascial planes, the surrounding unaffected skin will resist undermining upon exploration with a surgical probe or gloved finger.

Bacteriologic evaluation of wound exudate, bulla fluid, excised tissue, and blood is essential. Isolation of pathogens from clinical specimens usually takes days; however, Gram stains and fungal wet preps can provide useful data within minutes. A wound exudate with gram-positive rods and few polymorphonuclear leukocytes is nearly pathognomonic of clostridial infection. Fungal wet prep of crushed tissue can identify hyphal forms and prompt the early administration of antifungal therapy. Gram stains may also be useful in tailoring antibiotic therapy for polymicrobial necrotizing infections.

Treatment of necrotizing cellulitis centers on early and complete surgical debridement of necrotic tissue in combination with high-dose antibiotics. Until bacteriologic data identify the causative pathogens, broad coverage is recommended. Parenteral vancomycin, gentamicin, and either metronidazole or clindamycin constitute an effective initial regimen for treating suspected nonclostridial necrotizing cellulitis. Penicillin G at least 20 million units a day either alone or in combination with clindamycin or chloramphenicol should be instituted when crepitance or Gram stain indicates clostridial infection.

Most *Vibrio* soft-tissue infections are superficial and can be adequately treated with debridement of necrotic tissue in conjunction with parenteral tetracycline 0.5 to 1 g every 12 hours with or without gentamicin. The duration of therapy is guided by clinical response. Third-generation cephalosporins such as cefoperazone and cefotaxime, the aminoglycosides (with the exception of streptomycin), trimethoprim-sulfamethoxazole, and the quinolones have proved to be the most active agents against *Aeromonas.* Necrotizing cellulitis and bacteremia secondary to *P. aeruginosa* require debridement of necrotic tissue in conjunction with parenteral aminoglycosides and an antipseudomonal penicillin (ticarcillin, piperacillin) or ceftazidime or ciprofloxacin. Early diagnosis of mucormycosis can be made on lesional biopsy specimen identifying broad nonseptate hyphae that branch at right angles. Once mucormycosis is identified, surgical debridement and intravenous amphotericin B are indicated.

Cryptococcal Cellulitis

Immunosuppressed patients are also susceptible to cryptococcal cellulitis, which often presents as a vesiculobullous, erythematous eruption. Since cryptococcal infection typically enters the host via the respiratory tract, cutaneous involvement indicates a careful search for extracutaneous disease. Untreated, cryptococcosis is nearly uniformly fatal among these patients.

The most sensitive tests for cryptococcal cellulitis are histopathology demonstrating encapsulated budding yeasts and culture data. The serum cryptococcal antigen is helpful if positive but not sensitive enough to exclude this diagnosis if negative. A search should be made for extracutaneous sites of infection, including cultures of sputum, prostatic secretions, urine, blood, and CSF. Treatment requires parenteral amphotericin B 0.4–0.6 mg per kilogram for 6 to 10 weeks; debridement is not usually required.

Suggested Reading

Anderson DJ, et al. Cryptococcal disease presenting as cellulitis. Clin Infect Dis 1992; 14:666–672.

Dubin D, Johnson RA. Necrotizing soft tissue infections. Curr Opin Dermatol 1994; 235–42.

Lindbeek G, Powers R. Cellulitis. Hosp Pract 1993; 28 (Suppl 2):10–14.

Ochs MW, Dolwick MF. Facial erysipelas: Report of a case and review of the literature. J Oral Maxilofac Surg 1991; 49(10):1116–1120.

Phipps AR, Blanshard J. A review of in-patient hand infections. Arch Emerg Med 1992; 9:299–300.

Swartz MN. Skin and soft tissue infections. In: Mandell F, et al. Principles and practice of infectious disease. 3rd ed. New York: Churchill Livingstone, 1990: 796.

CHRONIC HEPATITIS

William N. Katkov, M.D.
Gary Gitnick, M.D.

Chronic hepatitis is a broad term encompassing a number of infectious and noninfectious diagnoses. The consequences of chronic hepatitis include cirrhosis, end-stage liver disease, and hepatocellular carcinoma. Until recently there were no effective therapies for patients with chronic liver disease. Orthotopic liver transplantation was the first major advance in treatment. Within the past decade other dramatic developments in the medical treatment of chronic liver diseases, including chronic viral hepatitis, have occurred. Indeed, the era of antiviral therapy for chronic viral hepatitis B and C (HBV, HCV) has arrived. Therapy for infection-related causes of chronic hepatitis is the subject of this chapter.

INTERFERONS

Recombinant interferon alfa-2b is the only agent licensed in the United States for the treatment of chronic viral hepatitis B and C. Interferons are endogenous, naturally occurring glycoproteins. Their antiviral and immunomodulatory effects make them ideal candidates for the treatment of chronic viral hepatitis. The initial trials used small amounts of relatively unstable interferon and reported benefits in viral hepatitis patients. Recombinant DNA techniques enabled the production of large quantities of stable pure interferon, which has been used in multicenter clinical trials. Of the three types of interferon, alpha, beta, and gamma, most clinical experience and study have employed interferon alpha, of which there are more than 20 subtypes. Interferon alpha is derived from monocytes; interferon beta is made by activated fibroblasts and interferon gamma, from stimulated T cells. Interferons alpha and beta are similar in molecular structure, suggesting that they exert comparable antiviral and immunomodulatory effects. Interferon gamma tends to have fewer antiviral effects.

Chronic Hepatitis B

A large, randomized U.S. multicenter trial of interferon alfa-2b involving 169 patients included 43 patients who were untreated controls, permitting a comparison of the natural history of chronic hepatitis B with the interferon treatment and follow-up periods. When treated with 5 million units of interferon alfa-2b daily by subcutaneous injection for 16 weeks, 37 percent of patients lost hepatitis B e antigen (HBeAg) and HBV DNA. These results have been reproduced in a number of clinical trials from a number of countries.

Loss of HBV DNA during interferon therapy is usually accompanied by normalization of aminotransferase levels. Follow-up has demonstrated that most responses to treatment are sustained. Reactivation occurs in a small number of patients, who often can be successfully re-treated. Loss of hepatitis B surface antigen (HBsAg) either during treatment or after 1 year of follow-up is uncommon, occurring in 10 to 15 percent of responders. A report from Korenman and associates of the National Institutes of Health (NIH) reported on 5 to 7 years of follow-up and found a strikingly high frequency of HBsAg loss among interferon treatment responders. In the NIH study 13 of 20 (65 percent) responders lost HBsAg during a mean follow-up period of 4 years. In many of the HBsAg-negative patients, HBV DNA became undetectable in serum by polymerase chain reaction.

Perrillo and associates have presented evidence that histologic improvement in the liver follows successful therapy with interferon. This improvement is more apparent 4 or more years after treatment than within the first year.

The U.S. multicenter trial identified variables that influence the likelihood of response to interferon. In general patients with high pretreatment alanine aminotransferase (ALT) values and low HBV DNA levels (below 200 pg per milliliter) were more likely to respond. Among patients with HBV DNA levels less than 100 pg per milliliter approximately 50 percent responded to 5 million units of interferon compared with approximately 7 percent of those with HBV DNA levels greater than 200 pg per milliliter ($p < 0.0001$). Thus, a favorable pretreatment profile consisted of an active immune response to HBV and a relatively low level of viral replication as measured by HBV DNA.

An important feature of interferon therapy for chronic HBV among most responders is a flare, or transient rise of ALT during treatment. This elevation, most commonly seen during the second or third month of therapy, is associated with a decrease in HBV DNA levels. This flare can mimic acute hepatitis clinically and can precipitate hepatic failure in a marginally compensated liver. Consequently, interferon is not recommended for patients with decompensated chronic HBV (prolonged prothrombin time, elevated serum bilirubin level, hypoalbuminemia), and all patients require close monitoring during and following interferon therapy.

Antiviral agents other than interferon have been tried in the treatment of chronic hepatitis B. Acyclovir is ineffective; adenine arabinoside (ARA-A) and its monophosphate, ARA-AMP, are limited by unacceptable neurotoxicity. Ribavirin, a synthetic nucleoside, appears to have some antiviral activity and is being studied. As a class of agents nucleoside analogues show promise and are under investigation in the treatment of chronic hepatitis B. Fialuridine (FIAU) initially showed promise but was found to lead to lactic acidosis and liver failure in a number of patients. Lamivudine, or 3TC, is administered orally, appears to have few side effects, and suppresses hepatitis B viral replication during therapy. For most if not all patients HBV replication resumes when lamivudine is discontinued. Longer-term therapy is under investigation. A pilot study of thymosin in patients with chronic HBV showed promise, and a larger-scale multicenter trial is in progress.

Hepatitis D (Delta) Virus

Hepatitis D virus (HDV) is a defective RNA virus that infects the liver in the presence of HBV infection. HDV can infect a person either concomitantly with acute HBV infection or as a superinfection after chronic HBV infection is established. The experience with antiviral therapy for HDV is limited. Interferon often leads to a decrease in aminotransferase levels; however, elimination of the infection is uncommon. Effective treatment of HDV with interferon may require higher doses and longer duration of therapy than those established for the treatment of chronic HBV infection. When HBsAg is cleared, HDV infection does not recur. Recurrence of HBV infection after liver transplantation appears to be unlikely when a patient is coinfected with HDV.

Chronic Hepatitis C

Early promising reports of the beneficial use of interferon for the treatment of chronic HBV spawned small clinical trials of interferon therapy for chronic non-A, non-B hepatitis (NANBH). These studies, including a subsequent large U.S. multicenter trial, were undertaken before the hepatitis C virus (HCV) had been identified. Retrospective analysis confirmed that most patients enrolled in these trials with a diagnosis of chronic NANBH had chronic HCV infection. Results from the earlier studies have been reproducible since the discovery of HCV.

Until recently no diagnostic tools to assess HCV viremia or replicative activity have been available. Thus, in the major trials of interferon for the treatment of chronic HCV, responsiveness has been measured by ALT levels alone. In the U.S. multicenter trial 166 patients were randomly assigned to receive 3 million units of interferon alfa-2b three times weekly by subcutaneous injection for 6 months or 1 million units for the same period or no treatment. Normalization of ALT levels occurred in 38 percent of the 3 million unit group, 16 percent of the 1 million unit group, and only 4 percent of untreated controls. The response among patients receiving 3 million units was significantly better than in either of the other two groups. Numerous additional studies have had similar results.

The encouraging response rate after 6 months of interferon therapy stands in contrast to the frequency of relapse once interferon is discontinued. During follow-up ALT elevations recur in 50 to 80 percent of responders. When HCV RNA levels are monitored during interferon therapy, they become undetectable in most patients with normal ALT levels. Unfortunately, HCV RNA levels commonly rise after cessation of therapy, a phenomenon that can precede ALT elevations.

There are few reliable predictors of response to interferon among patients with chronic HCV. In general, individuals with a mild histologic picture (precirrhotic) and low levels of HCV RNA are most likely to respond. HCV genotype, which varies geographically, has emerged as possibly a major predictor of the clinical behavior of HCV, and it may influence responsiveness to interferon.

Adjuncts and Alternatives to Interferon

The search for novel therapeutic agents to treat chronic HCV infection is challenging because of the biology of HCV and the lack of an in vitro tissue culture system. Several possible adjuncts to interferon therapy have been investigated in small uncontrolled studies. Ursodeoxycholic acid may prolong the time to relapse of ALT elevation after interferon therapy is discontinued.

Iron depletion by phlebotomy may increase the likelihood of response to interferon in some individuals with chronic HCV.

Ribavirin, a synthetic nucleoside, appears to affect ALT levels in some patients with chronic HCV while not clearly suppressing RNA levels.

The effect on aminotransferase levels is not sustained after ribavirin is discontinued. Therefore, while ribavirin alone may have a limited role in treating patients with chronic HCV, further study of its use as an adjuvant to interferon is under way.

New treatment strategies to enhance response rates and to sustain responses are being investigated. While higher-dose regimens and longer therapy have not been shown to increase the likelihood of response, if a response has occurred, lengthening treatment to a year or more may prolong ALT depression. Future strategies for the treatment of chronic HCV are likely to include prolonged therapy and/or maintenance regimens.

Selection of Patients

The natural history of chronic HCV remains unpredictable. Initially, the lack of serologic tools to monitor and characterize HCV infection virologically made treatment decisions difficult, and physicians have been reluctant to treat patients with mild clinical disease. HCV RNA testing combined with more insight into the predictive role of viral genotype will allow better-informed treatment decisions.

Side Effects of Interferons

The use of interferon as a therapeutic agent is frequently associated with side effects. While most interferon-related effects are identifiable and manageable, they necessitate regular and close monitoring during therapy. Initially, subcutaneously injected interferon can be accompanied by myalgias, fever, malaise, and nausea. These flu-like effects are most pronounced at the initiation of treatment and become milder and more tolerable after a week or two. Acetaminophen and bedtime dosing are usually sufficient management.

Bone marrow suppression with associated cytopenias is a more serious effect of interferon therapy. Leukopenia and thrombocytopenia occasionally warrant a reduction in dose or even cessation of therapy.

Interferon commonly affects a patient's mood and emotional life. These effects may become dominant issues during treatment. Patients may be subject to some degree of malaise and moodiness. Less commonly interferon exacerbates depression and rarely has been associated with psychosis. In patients with a history of psychiatric illness interferon therapy should be instituted with great care, if at all.

In its role as an immunomodulating agent, in theory interferon can enhance autoimmune activity. Some patients treated with interferon have developed hypothyroidism caused by an autoimmune process and have required hormone replacement therapy. Hypothyroidism associated with interferon therapy appears to be reversible in most cases.

■ LIVER TRANSPLANTATION

Chronic viral hepatitis is a frequent cause of advanced liver disease necessitating liver transplantation. The short-term prognosis of patients with chronic viral hepatitis after liver transplantation is no different from that of patients with other diagnoses. The short-term risk of transplantation is increased predominantly by serious multisystem failure and/or infection.

HBV infection frequently recurs after liver transplantation. Post-transplantation immunosuppression allows viral replication to thrive, and very high HBV DNA levels may be found. When liver transplantation is undertaken in patients with fulminant hepatitis B and/or coexistent hepatitis delta virus (HDV) infection, the likelihood of post-transplantation HBV recurrence is much lower. For patients with chronic HBV facing liver transplantation the most important variable predicting post-transplantation recurrence is the pretransplant viral replicative status. The likelihood of recurrence is significantly lower in patients negative for HBeAg and HBV DNA than in patients positive for these measures of viral replicative activity.

Strategies to prevent HBV recurrence after transplantation have included pretransplant antiviral therapy with interferon. Interferon in decompensated HBV must be administered with caution, if at all. The ALT flare often seen with therapy can precipitate further decompensation and hepatic failure. Administration of hepatitis B surface antibody immunoglobulin (anti-HBsIg) in the perioperative and postoperative periods has been the most effective means of preventing HBV recurrence after liver transplantation.

Like hepatitis B, hepatitis C frequently recurs in patients undergoing liver transplantation for chronic hepatitis. The clinical course following liver transplantation varies from mild aminotransferase elevations to an aggressive hepatitis rapidly leading to liver failure. The efficacy of interferon therapy in post transplantation patients remains unclear. One pilot study administered 3 million units of interferon three times weekly for 4 months to 18 post-liver transplant patients. Five (28 percent) had normalization of ALT levels. While responders and nonresponders had decreased HCV RNA levels, all patients had a recurrence of HCV viremia after interferon was stopped. Controlled trials now under way will further define the role of interferon in this setting. Interferon following organ transplantation has been used very cautiously because of the concern that an immunomodulatory agent that enhances human leukocyte antigen (HLA) class I and II molecules on cell surfaces might stimulate allograft rejection. This has not been a problem thus far in liver transplantation. In renal transplant recipients some data suggest that interferon therapy may contribute to rejection and allograft dysfunction.

■ AUTOIMMUNE CHRONIC ACTIVE HEPATITIS

Several types of autoimmune hepatitis have been identified recently, and HCV appears to play an important role in the pathogenesis of some cases of this disease. The classic case of autoimmune chronic active hepatitis (ACAH) is found in young to middle-aged women who present with elevated aminotransferases, hyperglobulinemia, and high-titer antinuclear antibodies (ANA). This disorder is designated type 1 autoimmune hepatitis.

Type 2 autoimmune hepatitis, described mainly in Europe, is characterized by circulating antibodies to liver-kidney microsome type 1 (anti-LKM1). Most patients with type 2 are children, and many have extrahepatic autoimmune phenomena. A large proportion of type 2 patients have evidence of HCV infection which leads to speculation that HCV plays a causative role in this disease.

Type 3 autoimmune hepatitis is associated with antibodies to soluble liver antigen (anti-SLA). Except for the presence of anti-SLA and absence of ANA, the clinical picture of type 3 is very similar to that of type 1.

The link between hepatitis C infection and some cases of autoimmune hepatitis has important therapeutic implications. Corticosteroids, the cornerstone of treatment for severe type 1 ACAH, may have a deleterious effect on patients with chronic HCV. Attempts must be made to distinguish patients with autoimmune hepatitis and a false-positive anti-HCV from those with a true viral infection and associated autoimmune hepatitis. The issue is complicated by the fact that autoantibodies are common in patients with chronic viral hepatitis. In patients with autoantibodies and a false-positive anti-HCV, treatment with corticosteroids is warranted. Antiviral therapy is indicated for those with chronic HCV and low-titer autoantibodies. Thus, chronic HCV with active autoimmune disease requires careful evaluation before treatment.

Suggested Reading

Clarke BE. Approaches to the development of novel inhibitors of hepatitis C replication. J Viral Hepatitis 1995; 2:1–8.

Czaja CJ, Carpenter HA, Santrach PJ, et al. Immunologic features and HLA associations in chronic viral hepatitis. Gastroenterology 1995; 108:157–164.

Davis GL, Lau JYN, Lim HL. Therapy for chronic hepatitis C. Gastroenterol Clin North Am 1994; 603–613.

Davis GL, Lindsay K, Albrecht J, et al. Clinical predictors of response to recombinant interferon-alfa treatment in patients with chronic non-A, non-B hepatitis (hepatitis C). J Viral Hepatitis 1994; 1:55–63.

Di Bisceglie AM, Conjeevaram HS, Fried MW, et al. Ribavirin as therapy for chronic hepatitis C. A randomized, double-blind, placebo-controlled trial. Ann Int Med 1995; 123:897–903.

Katkov WN, Dienstag JL. Prevention and therapy of viral hepatitis. Semin Liver Dis 1991; 11:165–174.

Korenman J, Baker B, Waggoner J, et al. Long-term remission of chronic hepatitis B after alpha-interferon therapy. Ann Int Med 1991; 114:629–634.

Perrillo RP, Brunt EM. Hepatic histologic and immunohistochemical changes in chronic hepatitis B after prolonged clearance of hepatitis B e antigen and hepatitis B surface antigen. Ann Int Med 1991; 115:113–115.

Perrillo RP, Schiff ER, Davis GL, et al. A randomized, controlled trial of interferon alpha-2b alone and after prednisone withdrawal for the treatment of chronic hepatitis B. N Engl J Med 1990; 323:291–305.

Poynard T, Bedossa P, Chevallier M, et al. A comparison of three interferon alfa-2b regimens for the long-term treatment of chronic non-A, non-B hepatitis. N Engl J Med 1995; 332:1457–1462.

Renault PF, Hoofnagle JH. Side effects of alpha interferon. Semin Liver Dis 1989; 9:273–277.

MYOCARDITIS

Darryl M. See, M.D.
Jeremiah G. Tilles, M.D.

Stedman's Medical Dictionary defines myocarditis as "inflammation of the muscular walls of the heart." Although myocarditis was first recognized as a distinct clinical entity in the early nineteenth century, the pathogenesis remains incompletely understood, diagnosis is often uncertain, and definitive therapy has not been established. Although most patients are probably asymptomatic, severe cases may result in heart failure, arrhythmias, or sudden death. Evidence suggests that some cases progress to dilated cardiomyopathy.

Myocarditis can be caused by a variety of infectious agents, drugs, chemicals, toxins, endocrine disorders, and autoimmune diseases (Table 1). Among otherwise normal individuals residing in the United States, viruses are believed to be the most common cause, with the enteroviruses predominating. The Coxsackie group B viruses account for more than 50 percent of all cases of myocarditis for which the agent has been identified. In immunocompromised patients, myocarditis is frequently a consequence of disseminated infection with opportunistic pathogens. The most frequently confirmed diagnoses have been herpes simplex virus, cytomegalovirus, *Mycobacterium tuberculosis, Cryptococcus neoformans, Histoplasma capsulatum, Aspergillus fumigatus,* and *Toxoplasma gondii.* Autopsy reports have documented a 25 to 50 percent incidence of myocarditis in patients with AIDS. Most of these were not clinically evident before death. The cause in most of these cases is thought to be the human immunodeficiency virus itself. Occasionally metastatic Kaposi's sarcoma and lymphoma have caused myocarditis in AIDS patients.

The myocardial injury occurring in acute myocarditis may be the result of any of several mechanisms including primary cellular damage from micro-organisms, drugs, chemicals, or toxins and secondary events such as autoimmune damage, ischemia, and deposition of calcium into myocytes. Murine models of viral-induced myocarditis have suggested a biphasic pathologic process. Mice infected with cardiotropic strains of Coxsackie virus B3 develop acute myocarditis, with high titers of virus in the myocardial tissue and direct cellular damage. Virus replication in surviving animals is controlled by immune mechanisms. Later, chronic myocarditis characterized by autoimmune damage from activated cytolytic T cells supervenes.

Table 1 Most Frequently Identified Causes of Myocarditis Reported in the United States

INFECTIOUS	NONINFECTIOUS
Viral	*Autoimmune disease*
Coxsackie virus group A*, B*	Systemic lupus erythematosus
Echovirus*	Sarcoidosis
Adenovirus*	Rheumatic fever
Influenza virus A, B*	
Varicella zoster virus	*Chemicals and poisons*
Herpes simplex virus	Lead
Cytomegalovirus	Arsenic
Lymphocytic choriomeningitis*	Carbon monoxide
	Venoms
	Phosphorus
Human immunodeficiency virus	
Bacterial	
Corynebacterium diphtheriae	*Drugs*
Salmonella spp.	Cocaine
Neisseria meningitidis	Norepinephrine
Mycobacterium tuberculosis	Methyldopa
Streptococcus spp.	Adriamycin
Fungal	Alcohol
Cryptococcus neoformans	*Idiopathic disorders*
Blastomycosis hominis	Kawasaki disease
Aspergillus spp.	Giant cell myocarditis
Parasitic	*Endocrine diseases*
Trichinella spiralis	Thyrotoxicosis
Toxoplasma gondii	Pheochromocytoma
Trypanosoma cruzi	

*No specific chemotherapy available

PRESENTATION

Infectious myocarditis detected in infants usually occurs in the setting of severe generalized infection. Affected patients often show mental status changes, tachypnea, fever, respiratory distress, tachycardia, and cardiac failure. Leukocytosis and elevated hepatic and cardiac enzymes are frequently present. Laboratory investigation may also reveal cerebrospinal fluid pleiocytosis and/or pancreatitis. Often there is radiographic evidence of pneumonitis. The causative organism commonly can be cultured from blood, cerebrospinal fluid, throat, or stool.

Viral myocarditis in adults is usually detected after systemic symptoms and signs of virus infection have subsided. In contrast, generalized manifestations of infection may still be present when myocarditis becomes manifest in patients with nonviral causes. Common symptoms include chest pain, palpitations, fevers, malaise, and antecedent respiratory symptoms (Table 2). Characteristic physical findings include pericardial friction rub due to accompanying pericarditis, gallop rhythm, tachycardia, arrhythmias, and signs of heart failure. On laboratory examination, elevated serum glutamic-oxaloacetic transaminase (SGOT), creatine phosphokinase (CPK), peripheral leukocyte count, and erythrocyte sedimentation rate are commonly found. Electrocardiographic abnormalities may include ST segment depression or elevation and T wave inversions. Imaging studies may be helpful in confirming a diagnosis. Echocardiograms often show abnormal wall motion. Chest roentgenograms may reveal an enlarged cardiac silhouette, and magnetic resonance imaging may suggest inflammation. Abnormal uptake may be noted on gallium, technetium-99m pyrophosphate, or indium-111 antimyosin scan.

Definitive diagnosis of myocarditis is based upon histo-

Table 2 Clinical and Laboratory Abnormalities in Myocarditis

SYMPTOMS
Chest pain
Arthralgias
Palpitations
Fever
Malaise
Antecedent respiratory symptoms

PHYSICAL FINDINGS
Pericardial friction rub
Gallop rhythm
Tachycardia
Arrhythmias
Signs of heart failure

LABORATORY TESTING
Blood: increased cardiac enzymes, leukocyte count, and/or erythrocyte sedimentation rate
Electrocardiogram: ST segment elevation or depression, T wave inversion, heart block, arrhythmias
Biopsy: inflammation and necrosis by light microscopy
Imaging: inflammation by magnetic resonance imaging; increased uptake by technetium pyrophosphate, indium-111 antimyosin, and/or gallium scan; increased heart size by chest radiograph
Identification of specific organisms: positive culture from cerebrospinal fluid, throat, blood, or stool (presumptive diagnosis); fourfold rise in antibody titer or positive immunoglobin-M titer (presumptive diagnosis); polymerase chain reaction amplification or positive culture from heart biopsy tissue (definitive diagnosis)

logic evidence of myocardial inflammation and necrosis on biopsy specimens. Unfortunately, the causative organism can only occasionally be isolated from the tissue, rendering specific diagnosis difficult. Identification of organisms from cardiac tissue with polymerase chain reaction amplification has shown promise in recent studies. In immunocompromised patients, demonstration of opportunistic microbial agents in cardiac tissue by culture or specific stains is more likely. Thus, in these patients aggressive attempts should be made to procure cardiac tissue by right heart biopsy. The causative agent should be sought in the tissue by viral, bacterial, fungal, and mycobacterial cultures; tissue stains for bacteria, fungi, Mycobacteria, and parasites; and histologic examination for giant cells or inclusion bodies.

■ THERAPY

For acute infectious myocarditis specific therapy should be directed against the implicated organism whenever possible; organism-specific regimens are detailed in their respective chapters. Unfortunately, in most patients either the organism is never identified or no specific antimicrobial therapy is available for it. Although definitive therapy has not been established for enterovirus infections in humans, there is optimism since interferon-alpha, ribavirin, and experimental antiviral drugs such as WIN 54954 were successfully used during the acute stage of infection in mice with Coxsackie virus B3, encephalomyocarditis virus, and Coxsackie virus A9, respectively. Several types of nonspecific therapy warrant consideration in all patients with acute myocarditis. Supplemental oxygen should be provided, and the importance of bed rest is supported by studies in animals. On the other hand, studies in animals have indicated that therapy with anti-inflammatory or immunosuppressive agents may be harmful during the acute stage of infection. Intravenous immunoglobulin (IVIG) at a single dose of 2 g per kilogram has been successfully used in children, but no studies of IVIG in adults have been performed.

The functional manifestations of cardiac injury must be addressed. The appearance of congestive heart failure should be managed by standard therapy such as diuretics, inotropic agents, and afterload reduction. In addition, anticoagulation may be considered. Likewise, serious arryhthmias must be treated with appropriate drugs, and even temporary transvenous pacing may be required for heart block. Finally, in cases of circulatory collapse, mechanical support in the form of intra-aortic balloon pump or ventricular assist device should be considered.

Chronic myocarditis is thought to be autoimmune. Thus, a variety of single and combination drug regimens with immunosuppressive agents have been studied. Prednisone, azathioprine, cyclosporine, cyclophosphamide, and antilymphocyte antibody have been investigated. Unfortunately, trials of these agents have been uncontrolled, and results have been variable. Empiric therapy with immunosuppressive agents does not appear to be warranted until the results of controlled studies are available. Fortunately, most patients with acute or chronic myocarditis recover without sequelae. In the few patients with severe, refractory myocardial dysfunction, transplantation should be considered.

Suggested Reading

Grody WW, Cheng L, Lewis W. Infection of the heart by the human immunodeficiency virus. Am J Cardiol 1990; 66:203–206.

Lerner AM, Wilson FM. Virus cardiomyopathy. Prog Med Virol 1973; 15: 63–91.

Maisch B, Herzum M, Schonian U. Immunomodulating factors and immunosuppressive drugs in the therapy of myocarditis. Scand J Infect Dis 1993; 88:149–162.

Martin AB, Webber S, Fricker FJ, et al. Acute myocarditis: Rapid diagnosis by PCR in children. Circulation 1994; 90:330–339.

See DM, Tilles JG. Viral myocarditis. Rev Infect Dis 1991; 13:951–956.

INFLUENZA

Neil Fishman, M.D.
Harvey M. Friedman, M.D.

Influenza is an important epidemic viral infection that has caused significant morbidity and mortality throughout history. The first worldwide pandemic was documented in 1580, and 31 pandemics have been described since that time. The most severe occurred in 1918–1919, when 21 million deaths were recorded worldwide, including 549,000 in the United States. The last pandemic was in 1977, but milder epidemics continue to occur every 1 to 3 years. The Centers for Disease Control and Prevention (CDC) documented 10,000 to 40,000 excess deaths in the United States during each of the 19 epidemics from 1957 through 1986. The major causes of death are pneumonia and exacerbation of chronic cardiopulmonary conditions; 80 to 90 percent of those who die are 65 years of age or older.

INFLUENZA VIRAL STRUCTURE AND PATHOPHYSIOLOGY

Influenza viruses are medium-sized enveloped RNA viruses belonging to the family Orthomyxoviridae. Three genera, influenza virus types A, B, and C, have been described. Influenza A and B viruses are important causes of human disease, while influenza C virus causes only sporadic upper respiratory infections.

The morphologic characteristics of all influenza virus types are similar. The envelope is composed of a lipid bilayer, with a layer of matrix protein on the inner surface and spikelike surface projections of glycoproteins on the outer surface. These glycoproteins have either hemagglutinin or neuraminidase activity and are responsible both for the attachment of the virus to human cells and for the stimulation of the host immune response. Hemagglutinins initiate the infectious process by binding to surface receptors on respiratory epithelial cells; after proteolytic cleavage, the hemagglutinins fuse with the host cell membrane. The neuraminidase cleaves sialic acid that is present on the host cell surface and appears to promote release of viral particles from infected cells. Within the envelope are eight segmented pieces of nucleocapsid composed of a nucleoprotein and segmented single-stranded RNA.

EPIDEMIOLOGY

One of the most remarkable features of influenza virus is the frequency of changes in antigenicity. Antigenic variation is annual with influenza A virus, but less frequent with influenza B virus. Therefore, immunity to the influenza viruses is partial and temporary; this phenomenon explains why influenza remains a major epidemic disease of humans. Two types of antigenic variation have been described, principally involving the two external glycoproteins of the virus, hemagglutinin and neuraminidase. The more dramatic but less common alteration, antigenic shift, results from genetic reassortment. Shifts that produce immunologically novel strains of the influenza A virus herald the larger epidemics and worldwide pandemics; they tend to occur sporadically. Between World War I and the last pandemic in 1977, antigenic shifts occurred approximately every 10 to 15 years. The second and more common change, antigenic drift, is produced by a single point mutation in the hemagglutinin or neuraminidase genes that results in a change of just one or two amino acids. Antigenic shift is seen only with influenza A virus. Although antigenic drift affects both influenza A and B viruses, changes in the latter occur less frequently. Three subtypes of hemagglutinin, H1 (variants H0, H1, Hsw1), H2, and H3, and two subtypes of neuraminidase, N1 and N2, are recognized among influenza A viruses. Only a few strains of either virus tend to dominate during each annual influenza season.

The vast majority of human infections are acquired through human-to-human transmission of small-particle aerosols. Localized epidemics begin rather abruptly, usually in children, reach a sharp peak in 2 to 3 weeks, and last 5 to 6 weeks; attack rates during such outbreaks can approach 10 to 40 percent. Although influenza is virtually always active somewhere in the world, infection is most common during the winter. The peak influenza season extends from December through April in the Northern Hemisphere. Influenza season is defined by viral isolation, and an epidemic is defined by a rise in pneumonia and influenza deaths above the epidemic threshold in the CDC's 121-city mortality surveillance system. Although influenza affects all segments of the population, severe infections and major complications are most common in patients who are young, elderly, or debilitated.

CLINICAL MANIFESTATIONS

Uncomplicated Influenza

Classic influenza is characterized by abrupt onset of symptoms after an incubation period of 1 to 2 days. Many patients can pinpoint the hour of onset. Systemic signs and symptoms predominate initially. They include fever, chills or rigors, headaches, myalgias, malaise, and anorexia. Myalgias and headache are the most troublesome symptoms, with severity related to the height of the febrile response. Severe pain of the intraocular muscles frequently can be elicited on lateral gaze. Myalgias in the calf muscles may be particularly prominent in children. The systemic symptoms and fever usually persist for 3 days. Respiratory symptoms such as dry cough and nasal discharge, also present at the onset of illness, begin to dominate the clinical presentation as systemic signs and symptoms diminish. Cough, the most frequent and troublesome of these later complaints, can take 2 or more weeks to resolve completely.

Complications of Influenza

The complications of influenza, which can be classified as pulmonary and nonpulmonary, result either from progression of the viral process itself or from secondary bacterial infections.

Two manifestations of pneumonia associated with influenza, primary influenza viral pneumonia and secondary bacterial pneumonia, are well recognized (Table 1). Extrapulmonary complications of influenza occur less frequently and are most prevalent during larger, more severe outbreaks. These include myositis (more common with influenza B infection), myocarditis, pericarditis, transverse myelitis, encephalitis, and Guillain-Barré syndrome. A toxic shock-like syndrome has occurred in previously healthy children and adults during recent outbreaks of influenza A or B; this has been attributed to the effects of the viral infection on the colonization and replication characteristics of toxin-producing staphylococcus. Reye's syndrome has also been described in children treated with aspirin during influenza outbreaks.

Table 1 Pulmonary Complications of Influenza

FEATURE	PRIMARY VIRAL PNEUMONIA	SECONDARY BACTERIAL PNEUMONIA
Setting	Cardiovascular disease Pregnancy Young adults (in large outbreaks)	Age >65 years Chronic pulmonary, cardiac, or metabolic disease
History	Rapid progression after typical onset	Biphasic illness, with worsening after clinical improvement
Physical examination	Diffuse crackles	Consolidation
Sputum culture	Normal oral flora	*Streptococcus pneumoniae* *Staphylococcus aureus* *Haemophilus influenzae*
Isolation of influenza virus	Yes	No
Chest radiograph	Diffuse bilateral interstitial disease	Consolidation
Response to antibiotics	No	Yes
Mortality	Variable, high during some pandemics	Variable, generally low

■ DIAGNOSIS

Isolation of virus and detection of viral antigen in respiratory secretions offer the greatest utility for diagnosis in the setting of acute illness. Serologic tests such as hemagglutinin inhibition antibody titers that compare acute and convalescent sera are sensitive and specific but do not yield data in time to affect clinical decisions. In clinical practice, however, the diagnosis is usually established on epidemiologic grounds. A clinical presentation with fever, headache, myalgias, and cough is usually sufficient to diagnose influenza during a winter outbreak. Several studies have documented the accuracy of clinical diagnosis during an influenza outbreak to be as high as 85 percent.

■ THERAPY (TABLE 2)

Amantadine and rimantadine are approved in the United States for the treatment of influenza A. Amantadine has been shown to reduce the duration of signs and symptoms of clinical influenza by approximately 50 percent if therapy is instituted within 48 hours of onset. It also accelerates the resolution of small-airway dysfunction. However, amantadine causes several minor reversible central nervous system

Table 2 Recommended Dosage for Amantadine and Rimantidine

ANTIVIRAL AGENT	1–9 YEARS	10–13 YEARS	14–64 YEARS	≥65 YEARS
Amantadine*				
Treatment†	5 mg/kg/day up to 150 mg in two divided doses	100 mg twice daily‡	100 mg twice daily	≤100 mg/day
Prophylaxis	5 mg/kg/day up to 150 mg in two divided doses	100 mg twice daily‡	100 mg twice daily	≤100 mg/day
Rimantadine§				
Treatment†	NA‖	NA‖	100 mg twice daily	100 or 200 mg/day¶
Prophylaxis	5 mg/kg/day up to 150 mg in two divided doses	100 mg twice daily‡	100 mg twice daily	100 or 200 mg/day¶

*The drug package insert should be consulted for dosage recommendations for administering amantadine to persons with a creatinine clearance of 50 ml/min or less.
†Treatment should be instituted within 48 hours of the onset of symptoms and continued for 7 days.
‡Children 10 years of age or older who weigh under 40 kg should be administered amantadine or rimantadine 5 mg/kg/day.
§A reduction in dose to 100 mg/day of rimantadine is recommended for persons who have severe hepatic dysfunction or those with a creatinine clearance ≤10 ml/min. Other persons with less severe hepatic or renal dysfunction taking more than 100 mg/day of rimantadine should be observed closely, and the dosage should be reduced or the drug discontinued, if necessary.
‖NA, Not applicable (not approved for this indication).
¶Elderly nursing home residents should be administered only 100 mg/day of rimantadine. A reduction in dose to 100 mg/day should be considered for all persons 65 years of age or over if they have side effects when taking 200 mg/day.
Adapted from recommendations of the Advisory Committe on Immunization Practices, Centers for Disease Control and Prevention, 1995.

(CNS) toxicities, including insomnia, dizziness, nervousness, and difficulty concentrating. Additionally, amantadine use is associated with an increased incidence of seizures in individuals with known seizure disorders. Rimantadine is structurally related to amantadine and appears to be of equal efficacy in the treatment of uncomplicated influenza. It may offer some advantages over amantadine in the management of elderly patients, because CNS side effects occur less frequently (amantadine, 14 percent; rimantadine, 6 percent; placebo, 4 percent).

There are several important pharmacokinetic differences between amantadine and rimantadine. Amantadine is excreted unchanged in the urine; therefore, renal clearance is reduced substantially both in persons with renal insufficiency and in the elderly. In contrast, rimantadine undergoes extensive hepatic metabolism; less than 15 percent of the drug is excreted unchanged in the urine. Both drugs require adjustment of dosage in the setting of renal insufficiency, but rimantadine may be a safer choice in this setting. On the other hand, the clearance of rimantadine is decreased by 50 percent in patients with hepatic dysfunction; therefore, amantadine may be a better agent for patients with underlying liver disease. Finally, rimantadine is approximately 50 percent more expensive than amantadine, with the average wholesale prices being $1.28 per 100 mg and $0.85 per 100 mg, respectively. Dosing guidelines are listed in Table 2. Amantadine and rimantadine are active only against influenza A; therefore, since influenza A and B frequently cocirculate, treatment may not be effective in any given season. Resistance to both drugs emerges rapidly and has been described in influenza A isolates from treated patients. The isolation of resistant virus is not associated with a change in severity or duration of illness, but it does temper the enthusiasm of many clinicians for treating influenza with either drug.

PREVENTION

Vaccine

Inactivated virus vaccines are the mainstay of the prevention of influenza. Efficacy has ranged between 67 and 92 percent. Because influenza viruses undergo frequent antigenic alterations, a new vaccine containing antigens expected to predominate in the winter epidemic is prepared each year. In general, vaccines have contained both an A and a B virus. Two subtypes of influenza A have circulated in recent years; both have been included in the vaccine, since the predominant strain cannot be predicted reliably. Influenza vaccination has been shown to reduce hospital admissions for influenza and pneumonia by 32 to 39 percent, and to decrease mortality from these conditions by 43 to 65 percent. Recommendations for the use of influenza vaccine are listed in Table 3. The only contraindication to vaccination is hypersensitivity to hens' eggs, in which the vaccine virus is grown. Adults with acute febrile illnesses usually should not be vaccinated until their symptoms have abated. However, minor illnesses with or without fever are not a contraindication. The optimal time for organized vaccination campaigns for persons in high-risk groups is usually mid-October through mid-November.

Table 3 Recommended Recipients of Influenza Vaccine

Groups at Increased Risk for Influenza-Related Complications
Persons ≥65 years of age
Residents of nursing homes and other chronic-care facilities that house persons of any age with chronic medical conditions
Adults and children with chronic disorders of the pulmonary or cardiovascular systems, including asthma
Adults and children who have required regular medical follow-up or hospitalization during the preceding year because of chronic metabolic diseases, including diabetes mellitus, renal dysfunction, hemoglobinopathies, or immunosuppression
Children 6 months to 18 years of age who are receiving long-term aspirin therapy and therefore might be at risk for developing Reye's syndrome after influenza
Groups That Can Transmit Influenza to Persons at High Risk
Physicians, nurses, and other personnel in both hospital and outpatient settings
Employees of nursing homes and chronic-care facilities who have contact with patients or residents
Providers of home care to persons at high risk (e.g., visiting nurses and volunteer workers)
Household members (including children) of persons in high-risk groups
Anyone who wishes to avoid influenza

Adapted from recommendations of the Advisory Committe on Immunization Practices, Centers for Disease Control and Prevention, 1995.

The vaccine should not be administered simultaneously with cytotoxic chemotherapy; the efficacy drops by 50 percent in this setting. Patients with HIV infection, particularly those with advanced disease, respond poorly to the vaccine, but there are no contraindications to vaccination. Influenza-associated excess mortality among pregnant women has not been documented except during the pandemics of 1918–1919 and 1957–1958. However, additional case reports and limited studies suggest that women in the third trimester of pregnancy and early puerperium, including women without underlying risk factors, may be at increased risk for serious complications from influenza. Therefore, since the influenza vaccine has been proved safe at any stage of pregnancy, vaccination is recommended for women who would be in the third trimester of pregnancy or early puerperium during the influenza season and for those who are otherwise at increased risk for influenza.

Chemoprophylaxis

Amantadine and rimantadine are approved for use as prophylactic agents against influenza. Their level of efficacy is about 50 to 80 percent, and protection may be additive to that of the vaccine. These drugs should be considered for prophylaxis for selected individuals for 5 to 7 weeks during an outbreak of influenza A virus but not influenza B, particularly for high-risk individuals who have not been vaccinated. In such situations either drug may be administered for just 2 weeks if vaccine is given simultaneously. Chemoprophylaxis may also be used to supplement protection offered by the vaccine in patients who may be expected to have a poor antibody response (see Table 2).

Suggested Reading

Betts RF. Influenza virus. In: Mandell GL, Bennett JE, Dolin R, eds. Mandell, Douglas and Bennett's principles and practices of infectious diseases. 4th ed. New York: Churchill Livingstone, 1995:1546.

Dolin R, Reichman RC, Madore HP, et al. A controlled trial of amantadine and rimantadine in the prophylaxis of influenza A infection. N Engl J Med 1982; 307:580–583.

Douglas RG. Drug therapy: Prophylaxis and treatment of influenza. N Engl J Med 1990, 322:443–450.

Recommendations and Reports. Prevention and control of influenza: Recommendations of the advisory committee on immunization practices. MMWR 1995;44:RR-3.

ACUTE AND CHRONIC OSTEOMYELITIS

Daniel P. Lew, M.D.
Francis A. Waldvogel, M.D.

Osteomyelitis is an infection of any of the various components of bone, namely periosteum, medullary cavity, and cortical bone. It is characterized by progressive, inflammatory destruction of bone, by necrosis, and by new bone apposition.

Acute osteomyelitis evolves over several days to weeks: the term "acute" is used in opposition to chronic osteomyelitis, a disease characterized by clinical symptoms that persist for several weeks followed by long-standing infection that evolves over months or even years, by the persistence of micro-organisms, by low-grade inflammation, by the presence of necrotic bone (sequestra) and foreign material, and by fistulous tracts.

CLINICAL MANIFESTATIONS AND CHARACTERISTICS OF THE PATHOGEN

From a practical point of view it is useful to distinguish three types of osteomyelitis, described separately. Hematogenous osteomyelitis follows bacteremic spread, is seen mostly in prepubertal children and in elderly patients, and is characterized by local multiplication of bacteria within bone during septicemia. In most cases infection is located in the metaphyseal area of long bones or in the spine.

Osteomyelitis secondary to a contiguous focus of infection without vascular insufficiency follows trauma or an orthopedic procedure. It implies a first infection, which by continuity gains access to bone. By definition it can occur at any age and can involve any bone. It is useful to distinguish in this group patients with a foreign body implant because of its high susceptibility and necessity to remove the prosthesis to achieve cure.

Osteomyelitis secondary to vascular insufficiency is the consequence of poor blood supply, usually to the lower extremities. Often associated with diabetes, this disease entity has several important contributing factors; diabetes and its metabolic consequences, bone ischemia, neuropathy, and infection probably all contribute to bone destruction.

THERAPY

Basic Principles

Except for the fluoroquinolones, which penetrate unusually well into bone, bone antibiotic levels 3 to 4 hours after administration are usually quite low compared with serum levels; antibiotic treatment given parenterally has to be given for several weeks to achieve an acceptable cure rate, and early antibiotic treatment before extensive bone destruction has occurred produces the best results. Finally, a combined antimicrobial and surgical approach should at least be discussed in all cases. At one end of the spectrum (e.g., hematogenous osteomyelitis) surgery usually is unnecessary, but at the other end (a consolidated infected fracture) cure may be achieved with minimal antibiotic treatment provided the foreign material is removed.

Microbiologic and Pathologic Criteria

Adequate sampling of deep infected tissue is extremely useful, in contrast to specimens obtained superficially from ulcers or from fistula, which are often misleading. Results of Gram stain and culture, obtained ideally before therapy, should be carefully analyzed.

Antimicrobial Therapy

Single-agent chemotherapy is usually adequate for the treatment of osteomyelitis of any type (Table 1). As a general principle these antibiotics should be given parenterally for 4 to 6 weeks, as substantiated by experimental models.

In recent years new approaches to antimicrobial therapy have been developed experimentally and validated clinically. Thus, in hematogenous osteomyelitis of childhood, parenteral administration of antibiotics for a few days may be followed by oral therapy for several weeks, provided that the organism is known, clinical signs abate rapidly, compliance is good, and serum antibiotic levels can be monitored. This approach has only been validated in small series of adult patients.

However, effective as it is for hematogenous osteomyelitis, the question remains whether this mode can be used for postsurgical osteomyelitis. Oral therapy extending over months (and more rarely, years) is aimed at palliation of acute

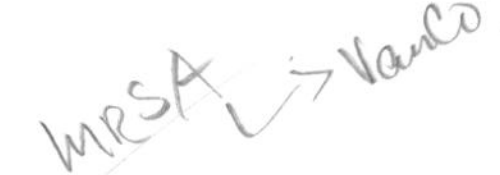

Table 1 Antibiotic Treatment of Hematogenous Osteomyelitis in Adults

MICRO-ORGANISMS	TREATMENT OF CHOICE	ALTERNATIVES
Staphylococcus aureus		
Penicillin sensitive	Penicillin G 4 million units q6h	A cephalosporin II, clindamycin 600 mg q6h, or vancomycin
Penicillin resistant	Nafcillin* 2 g q6h	A cephalosporin II, clindamycin 600 mg q6h, or vancomycin
Methicillin resistant	Vancomycin 1 g q12h⁺	Teicoplanin† 400 mg q24h; first day q12h
Various streptococci (group A or B, β-hemolytic; *S. pneumoniae*)	Penicillin G 3 million units q4–6h	Clindamycin 600 mg q6h, erythromycin 500 mg q6h, or vancomycin
Enteric gram-negative rods	Quinolone (ciprofloxacin 500–750 mg q12h, IV or oral)	A cephalosporin III
Serratia spp. *Pseudomonas aeruginosa*	Piperacillin‡ 2–4 g q4h and gentamicin 1.5 mg/kg/day	A cephalosporin III or a quinolone with aminoglycosides
Anaerobes	Clindamycin 600 mg q6h	Amoxicillin-clavulanic acid 2.2 g q8h or metronidazole 500 mg q8h for gram-negative anaerobes
Mixed infection (aerobic and anaerobic microorganisms)	Amoxicillin-clavulanic acid 2.2 g q8h	Imipenem§ 500 mg q6h

II, second generation; III, third generation.
*Flucloxacillin in Europe.
†Teiocoplanin is available only in Europe.
‡Depends on sensitivities; piperacillin-tazobactam and imipenem are useful alteratives.
§For aerobic gram-negative microorganisms resistant to amoxicillin-clavulanic acid.
⁺Dose adjustment necessary if renal failure.

flare-ups of chronic, refractory osteomyelitis. Another approach that is gaining acceptance because of its relatively low cost is parenteral administration of antibiotics, first in hospital, then on an outpatient basis. Local administration of antibiotics, either by instillation or by gentamicin-laden beads, has its advocates both in the United States and in Europe, but it has not been submitted to controlled critical studies; antibiotic diffusion is limited in time and space but may be of some additional benefit in osteomyelitis secondary to a contiguous focus of infection. The 4-fluoroquinolones have been one of the most interesting developments in this domain and have been shown to be effective in experimental infections and in several randomized and nonrandomized studies in adults. Their efficacy in the treatment of osteomyelitis due to most Enterobacteriaceae seems undisputed, but their advantage over conventional therapy in osteomyelitis due to *Pseudomonas* or *Serratia* spp. as well as gram-positive organisms, in particular *Staphylococcus aureus,* remains to be demonstrated.

Hematogenous Osteomyelitis

Historically, hematogenous osteomyelitis has been described in children. It involves mostly the metaphysis of long bones, particularly the tibia and femur, usually as a single focus. Although rare in adults, it most frequently involves the vertebral bodies.

The clinical features of hematogenous osteomyelitis in long bones are quite typical: chills, fever, and malaise reflect the bacteremic spread of micro-organisms; pain and local swelling are the hallmarks of the local infectious process.

Bacteria responsible for hematogenous osteomyelitis reflect essentially their bacteremic incidence as a function of age, so the organisms most frequently encountered in neonates include *S. aureus* and group B streptococci; in infants, the majority of infections are due to *S. aureus,* coagulase-negative staphylococci, and various streptococci. Later in life *S. aureus* predominates; in elderly persons, who are frequently subject to gram-negative bacteremias, an increased incidence of vertebral osteomyelitis due to gram-negative rods is found.

Fungal osteomyelitis is a complication of intravenous device infections, neutropenia, or profound immune deficiency; *Pseudomonas aeruginosa* hematogenous osteomyelitis is often seen in drug addicts and has a predilection for the cervical vertebrae.

When hematogenous osteomyelitis occurs in adults, debridement and/or incision and drainage of soft-tissue abscesses are usually required. Appropriate deep-tissue samples should be obtained, and in vitro susceptibility testing can be done as a guide to treatment. The standard of care is parenteral antimicrobial treatment for 4 to 6 weeks, with the start of this interval dating from the first day of treatment judged to be appropriate in light of in vitro susceptibility results.

Vertebral Osteomyelitis

The management of vertebral osteomyelitis requires effective antimicrobial therapy and may necessitate early surgery and stabilization of the spine. The choice of an antimicrobial drug is guided by the results of cultures of specimens obtained by biopsy or debridement. Needle biopsy obtained through computed tomographic (CT) guidance is the procedure of choice to obtain samples to be submitted in parallel to bacteriologic and pathologic evaluation.

Depending on its pharmacologic characteristics, the drug may be administered orally or parenterally. The antimicrobial agent should be given for 4 to 6 weeks. The duration of treatment is usually dated either from the initial use of an effective antimicrobial agent or from the last major debridement. The indications for surgery in vertebral osteomyelitis are similar to those in hematogenous infections of bone: failure of medical management, formation of soft-tissue abscesses, impending instability, or neurologic signs indicating spinal cord compression. In the latter case, surgery is an emergency procedure. Eventual fusion of adjacent infected vertebral bodies is a major goal of therapy.

Osteomyelitis Secondary to a Contiguous Infection Without Vascular Disease

The situation and the clinical picture are more complex in cases of osteomyelitis associated with a contiguous focus of infection, for example as a complication of the insertion of a total hip prosthesis. After a few days' pain following usual surgery, the situation improves and the patient is progressively mobilized. During that period pain reappears, mostly on weight bearing. The patient is mildly febrile and the wound is slightly erythematous with a slight discharge.

In the past, *S. aureaus* and coagulase-negative staphylococci were the most frequently reported micro-organisms. In recent years, various types of streptococci, *Propionibacterium acnes,* anaerobic micro-organisms, Enterobacteriaceae, and *P. aeruginosa* (the latter mostly in the setting of chronic osteomyelitis, comminuted fractures, and puncture wounds to the heel) are being encountered. Osteomyelitis of the mandible and secondary to pressure sores also frequently contains anaerobic flora, as do human and animal bites.

Adequate drainage, thorough debridement, obliteration of dead space, wound protection, and specific antimicrobial therapy are the mainstays of management. Debridement includes removal of all orthopedic appliances except those deemed absolutely necessary for stability.

Post-traumatic infected fractures are especially difficult to treat. A variety of techniques have evolved for management of the exposed bone and/or any dead space created by the trauma and debridement, i.e., use of local tissue flaps and of vascularized tissue transferred from a distant site. Other experimental modalities include cancellous bone grafting and implantation of acrylic beads impregnated with one or more antibacterial agents. Overall, considerable progress has been achieved in the development of novel surgical approaches (bone graft, revascularization procedure, muscle flaps) that allow more rapid formation of new bone. Finally, in patients with osteomyelitis, the Ilizarov fixation device allows major segmental resections, in combination with new bone growth, to fill in the defect.

Antimicrobial agents are used to treat viable infected bone and to protect revascularizing bone. Since revascularization of bone after debridement takes 3 to 4 weeks, the patient should be treated with parenteral antimicrobial agents for 4 to 6 weeks. The start of this therapy is usually dated from the last major debridement.

■ CHRONIC OSTEOMYELITIS CONTIGUOUS TO INFECTED PROSTHESES

Diagnosis

Most patients with chronic contiguous and hematogenous infections have no elevation in temperature and present with a painful joint that is found to be unstable by physical examination and/or radiography. Because of the difficulty of distinguishing loosening of the joint due to mechanical failure from that caused by infection, a positive culture of fluid aspirated from the artificial joint space and/or of bone from the bone-cement interface is required and remains the diagnostic method of choice. Since the micro-organisms responsible for these infections colonize the skin, Gram stain and quantitative cultures from deep tissues are very useful to distinguish colonization from infection.

Infections following total replacement of the hip joint are divided into three categories on the basis of time course and pathogenesis: (1) Acute contiguous infections are recognized within the first 6 months after surgery and are often evident within the first few days or weeks. These infections result directly from infected skin, subcutaneous tissue, or muscle, and/or from operative hematoma. (2) Chronic contiguous infections are diagnosed 6 to 24 months after surgery, usually because of persistent pain. In most cases infection is believed to result from contamination at the time of surgery with micro-organisms of lower pathogenicity. The infection progresses slowly to a chronic form before it is recognized. (3) The hematogenous infections discussed herein, which are diagnosed more than 2 years after surgery, arise from late transient bacteremia with selective persistence of the micro-organisms in the joint.

Coagulase-positive and coagulase-negative staphylococci, the micro-organisms most often isolated from infected prosthetic hip joints, account for three-fourths of the bacteria cultured.

Therapy

Two approaches to treatment exist. With one-stage exchange arthroplasty, the infected components are excised, surgical debridement is performed, and a new prosthesis is immediately put in place. Buchholz and associates, the chief proponents of this technique, use cement containing an antimicrobial drug, a factor that may contribute to the high success rate reported for the procedure.

A second approach, described by investigators at the Mayo Clinic, requires surgical removal of all foreign bodies, debridement of the bone and soft tissues, and a minimum of 4 weeks of parenteral antimicrobial therapy. Reconstruction is performed at least 3 months after the end of therapy for "less virulent infections" but is delayed for at least 1 year for "a more virulent infection."

Early in infection, when the prosthesis is still firmly in place, it is possible to attempt cure with antibiotics without removal of the prosthesis.

■ OSTEOMYELITIS SECONDARY TO VASCULAR INSUFFICIENCY

Osteomyelitis secondary to vascular insufficiency, a special entity observed in patients with diabetes and/or vascular impairment, occurs almost exclusively on the lower extremities. The disease starts insidiously in a patient who has complained of intermittent claudication in an area of traumatized skin. Cellulitis may be kept at a minimum, and infection progressively burrows its way to the underlying bone (e.g., toe, metatarsal head, tarsal bone). Physical examination elicits either no pain (with advanced neuropathy) or excruciating pain if bone destruction has been acute; an area of cellulitis may or may not be present; crepitus can be felt occasionally, which suggests either anaerobes or Enterobacteriaceae. *S. aureus* still predominates, but any other gram-positive or gram-negative, aerobic or anaerobic bacteria may be involved, particularly in severe infection.

The ability to reach bone by gently advancing a sterile surgical probe combined with a plain radiograph is the best initial approach to the diagnosis of osteomyelitis. If bone is detected on probing, treatment for osteomyelitis is recommended. If bone cannot be detected by probing and the plain radiography does not suggest osteomyelitis, the recommended treatment is a course of antibiotics directed at soft-tissue infection. Because occult osteomyelitis may be present, radiography should be repeated in 2 weeks. Further studies such as magnetic resonance imaging are recommended in doubtful cases.

Practical Approach and Therapy

The prognosis for cure of osteomyelitis associated with vascular insufficiency is poor because of the impaired ability of the host to assist in the eradication of the infectious agent.

It is important to determine the amount of vascular compromise. Because of impaired vascular perfusion, a case may be managed by antimicrobial therapy, debridement surgery, or ablative surgery. The type of treatment offered depends on the oxygen tensions of tissue at the infected site, the extent of osteomyelitis and time since damage, the potential for revascularization, and the preference of the patient. Revascularization often proves useful before amputation is considered. There is no convincing evidence that hyperbaric oxygen is useful for the treatment of diabetic osteomyelitis.

Debridement and 4 to 6 weeks of antimicrobial therapy may benefit the patient with localized osteomyelitis and good oxygen tension at the infected site. In the presence of a well-defined pathogen (usually *S. aureus*), 6 weeks of parenteral therapy sometimes followed by oral antibiotics can lead to a high cure rate. If these conditions do not exist, the wound often fails to heal and an amputation of infected bone is ultimately required. Digital and ray resections, transmetatarsal amputations, midfoot disarticulations, and Syme amputations allow the patient to walk without a prosthesis. The patient should be treated with antimicrobial agents for 4 weeks when infected bone is transected surgically. Two weeks of anti-infective therapy should be given when the infected bone is completely removed because there may be some residual soft-tissue infection. When the site of amputation is proximal to infected bone and soft tissue, the patient is given standard antimicrobial prophylaxis. In contrast, prolonged therapy is recommended for tarsal or calcaneal osteomyelitis, since the infected bone is debrided and not totally removed.

Suggested Reading

Caputo GM, Cavanagh PR, Ulbrecht JS, et al. Assessment and management of foot disease in patients with diabetes. N Engl J Med 1994; 331(13): 854–860.

Gentry LO. Approach to the patient with chronic osteomyelitis. In: Current clinical topics in infectious diseases 8. New York: McGraw-Hill, 1987:62.

Lew DP, Waldvogel FA. Use of quinolones for treatment of osteomyelitis and septic arthritis. In: Hooper DC, Wolfson JS, eds. Quinolone antimicrobial agents. Washington, D.C.: American Society for Microbiology, 1993: 371.

Mader JT, Norden C, Nelson JD, Calandra GB. Evaluation of new anti-infective drugs for the treatment of osteomyelitis in adults. Infectious Diseases Society of America and the Food and Drug Administration. Clin Infect Dis 1992; 15(Suppl 1):S155–S161.

Waldvogel FA, Vasey H. Osteomyelitis: The past decade. N Engl J Med 1980; 303:360–370.

NOSOCOMIAL PNEUMONIA

Burke A. Cunha, M.D.

Nosocomial organisms, acquired in the hospital, colonize the respiratory passages. Bacteria colonize the respiratory tract rapidly; thus, sputum cultures from intubated patients do not always reflect the lower respiratory tract. *Enterobacter, Serratia,* or *Pseudomonas aeruginosa* cultured via an endotracheal tube in a patient with pulmonary infiltrates or pneumonia does not necessarily mean that the patient has pneumonia due to these organisms. Most patients with nosocomial pneumonia do not have a specific microbiologic diagnosis. Usual pathogens are the aerobic gram-negative bacilli that live in water. Colonization is common because interventions put selective pressure on the patient's flora, resulting in gram-negative bacillary colonization of the respiratory tract. The usual organisms of nosocomial pneumonia are *Klebsiella pneumoniae, Serratia marcescens,* and *Pseudomonas aeruginosa* (Table 1).

■ DIAGNOSIS

The main problem with nosocomial pneumonias is diagnosis, i.e., differentiating noninfectious from infectious pulmonary infiltrates. Nosocomial pneumonia should be considered in any patient developing a pulmonary infiltrate resembling a bacterial pneumonia after a week or more of hospitalization. This definition excludes the peripheral white count and temperature of the patient, which are usually unhelpful in deciding whether an infiltrate is infectious or not. Most

Table 1 Nosocomial Colonizers and Pathogens

COMMON SPUTUM COLONIZERS	COMMON PATHOGENS IN NOSOCOMIAL PNEUMONIAS
*Enterobacter**	*Pseudomonas aeruginosa*†
Non-aeruginosa *Pseudomonas**	*Klebsiella*
*Xanthomonas**	*Serratia*
*Enterococcus**	*Escherichia coli*
*Citrobacter**	*Actinobacter*
*Acinetobacter**	
Pseudomonas aeruginosa	Uncommon
*Staphylococcus aureus**	*Legionella*
	Staphylococcus aureus‡

*Rarely if ever causes nosocomial pneumonia.
†Double-drug coverage should be directed against *Pseudomonas aeruginosa,* which covers most other nosocomial and community-acquired pathogens.
‡Occurs predominantly after viral influenza, in patients with diabetes mellitus, and in intravenous drug abusers.

Table 2 Antibiotic Selection in the Treatment of Nosocomial Pneumonia

Significant Factors
- *Double-drug antipseudomonal therapy*
  - *Proven susceptibility and clinical effectiveness in vivo*
    - Choose the agents with highest susceptibility (percent susceptible) against *P. aeruginosa* in your hospital, not the most active in vitro
    - No need to cover non-nosocomial organisms, e.g., *Enterobacter,* Non-aeruginosa *Pseudomonas, Staphylococcus aureus, Xanthomonas, Enterococcus*
  - *Favorable pharmacokinetic features*
    - Antibiotic concentrates in infected pulmonary tissues (all antibiotics concentrate well in the lungs)
    - Longest possible dosing interval
    - Minimal or no monitoring needed
  - *Safety profile*
    - Minimal side effects
  - *Resistance potential*
    - Low resistance potential; especially avoid ceftazidime plus ciprofloxacin
    - Not associated with the emergence of MRSA, or VRE.

Unimportant Factors
- *Age of patient*
  - Affects dosage of antibiotic e.g., decreased renal or hepatic function but not choice of therapy
- *Severity of illness*
  - Determines prognosis, length of hospital stay, but not initial coverage
  - Neither associated bacteremia, lobar involvement, or intubation affects the choice of empiric therapy
- *In vitro antipseudomonal activity*
  - Percent susceptible is more important than degree of antipseudomonal activity, i.e., piperacillin plus an aminoglycoside is as efficacious as ceftazidime plus ciprofloxacin
- *Other associated medical conditions*
  - May determine the most likely pathogen but does not change initial antibiotic therapy

MRSA, methicillin-resistant *S. aureus.*
VRE, Vancomycin-resistant enterococci.

Table 3 Empiric Therapy of Nosocomial Pneumonia in Normal Hosts

BACTERIAL PNEUMONIA* (NO EXTRAPULMONARY FEATURES)	ATYPICAL PNEUMONIA (EXTRAPULMONARY FEATURES)
Double-drug antipseudomonal regimens†	
APP + aminoglycoside or aztreonam	Doxycycline or macrolide
APC (cefepime or ceftazidime) + aminoglycoside or aztreonam	
APQ + APP or APC or aminoglycoside or aztreonam‡	
Single-drug regimens (suboptimal)	
APQ	
Imipenem	

*Nosocomial aspiration pneumonia should be treated the same as hospital-acquired pneumonia, and specific antianaerobic coverage is not usually necessary.
†Other antibiotics and combinations are possible, but the above choices are the most effective, proven safe, and least expensive. Given equal efficacy, selections within a group should be based on cost.
‡Avoid ceftazidime plus ciprofloxacin on the basis of greatest resistance potential and highest cost.
APP, antipseudomonal penicillin; APC, antipseudomonal cephalosporin; APQ, antipseudomonal quinolone.

patients with newly developing pulmonary infiltrates in the hospital have heart failure, adult respiratory distress syndrome, noncardiogenic pulmonary edema, or multisystem diseases mimicking bacterial pneumonia, and nosocomial pneumonias are probably overdiagnosed. If infection cannot be ruled out as the cause of the pulmonary infiltrates, empiric treatment for presumed nosocomial pneumonia is reasonable. Treatment should be based on presumed pathogens and not severity of illness or comorbid factors.

■ THERAPY

Therapy should be directed against the common nosocomial pathogens, of which *P. aeruginosa* is the most important. Although *P. aeruginosa* is a frequent colonizer, when it causes pulmonary infection, it is always severe. Double antipseudomonal coverage for the empiric treatment of nosocomial pneumonias is the preferred therapeutic approach (Table 2). No good data prove the therapeutic superiority of any combination regimen over another. Double antipseudomonal regimens need not be synergistic against *P. aeruginosa* to be effective. Therefore, the least expensive of these double-drug regimens should be selected, since none is any better than any other (Table 3).

The optimal duration of therapy has not been determined. In patients with normal host defense mechanisms usually a 2-week course is sufficient; however, longer courses may be required by patients with impaired defenses. Lung penetration of double antipseudomonal regimens is not an issue, since the lungs are well vascularized, permitting a rapid and complete distribution of all antibiotics into the lungs. Antimediator therapy has no role in the treatment of nosocomial pneumonias.

Failure to respond to this empiric approach to therapy should prompt consideration of a less common bacterial pathogen via sputum culture or of one of the agents of atypical pneumonia.

LEGIONNAIRE'S DISEASE

Atypical pneumonias occur in the hospital but are less common, excluding outbreaks, than in the community. Nosocomial Legionnaire's disease occurs if the organism is in the hospital water supply. The difficulty in diagnosing nosocomial Legionnaire's disease is complicated by the fact that many hospitalized patients have extrapulmonary findings attributable to their underlying medical conditions. A hospital-acquired pneumonia unresponsive to beta-lactam antibiotic therapy with a pulse-temperature deficit and otherwise unexplained mild elevation of serum transaminases should suggest nosocomial Legionnaire's disease. Optimal therapy includes erythromycin or azithromycin (see the chapter *Legionellosis*).

Suggested Reading

Cunha BA. Antibiotic pharmacokinetic considerations in pulmonary infections. Semin Respir Infect 1991; 6:168–182.

Cunha BA. Antibiotic therapy of pulmonary infections. In: Karetzky M, Cunha BA, Brandstetter RD, eds. The pneumonias. New York: Springer-Verlag, 1993: 255–276.

Cunha BA. The antibiotic treatment of community-acquired, atypical, and nosocomial pneumonias. Clin N Amer 1995; 79:581–97.

LaForce FM. Systemic antimicrobial therapy of nosocomial pneumonia: Monotherapy versus combination therapy. Eur J Clin Microbiol Infect Dis 1989; 8:61–68.

Lynn WA, Cohen J. Adjunctive therapy for septic shock: A review of experimental approaches. Clin Infect Dis 1995; 20:143–158.

Schrank JH Jr, Kelly, McCallister CK. Randomized comparison of cefepime and ceftazidime for treatment of hospitalized patients with gram-negative bacteremia. Clin Infect Dis 1995; 20:56–58.

COMMUNITY-ACQUIRED PNEUMONIA

Rebecca Edge Martin, M.D.
Joseph H. Bates, M.D.

Community-acquired pneumonia is a significant cause of morbidity and mortality in the United States. An estimated 4 million episodes occur annually, and at least 750,000 require hospitalization. Mortality among those admitted to a hospital ranges between 10 and 25 percent. Making the diagnosis of pneumonia is usually not difficult; selecting appropriate therapy, however, can be challenging. The purpose of this chapter is to assist the clinician in the selection of antibiotic therapy for community-acquired pneumonia in immunocompetent patients who are not residents of chronic care facilities.

DIAGNOSIS AND CAUSES

The diagnosis of pneumonia is suspected on one or more of the following clinical grounds: cough, purulent sputum, dyspnea, pleuritic pain, fever, leukocytosis, and a new pulmonary infiltrate. Once the diagnosis is made, the physician must decide whether hospitalization is necessary. A number of risk factors predict a complicated course (Table 1). The patient with pneumonia should usually be hospitalized when one of these factors is present. The risk of death increases as the number of complicating features mounts.

The exact microbial cause of an episode of community-acquired pneumonia is rarely known when treatment is started. Accurate historical information, including occupation, travel, exposure to animals, birds, and insects; recent dental work; and history of alcohol or drug abuse may suggest a cause. However, no unique clinical features of bacterial pathogens allow a specific identification. The studies listed in Table 2 may be useful in the diagnosis and management of community-acquired pneumonia. The extent of the evaluation should depend on the degree of illness and response to therapy. Many common diagnostic methods are expensive and technically difficult to perform. Simple tools, such as Gram stain and culture of expectorated sputum for usual aerobic bacteria, are helpful at times but may be misleading, in that organisms seen on Gram stain frequently do not correlate with organisms grown in sputum culture. Sputum studies can be diagnostic for *Legionella*, Mycobacteria, fungi, and *Pneumocystis carinii.* Some 10 to 15 percent of blood cultures performed on patients hospitalized with community-acquired pneumonia identify a causative organism. Bacteremia is associated with a more complicated course. Any pleural effusion should be aspirated and appropriate stains and cultures obtained. Bronchial alveolar lavage may provide useful information but should not be relied on to determine a bacterial agent. Protected brush specimens obtained by bronchoscopy are more accurate than expectorated sputum. The gold standards of transthoracic needle aspiration and open lung biopsy are definitive when an organism is found, but they place the patient at added risk. Several weeks are usually required for an appropriate serologic response. Cross-reactivity among some organisms lessens the specificity of

Table 1 Predictors of a Complicated Course in Patients with Community-Acquired Pneumonia

Suspicion of high-risk cause (Staphylococcus, gram-negative bacilli, aspiration, or postobstructive process)
Age over 60 years
Consolidation or multilobe involvement on chest radiograph
Abnormalities on physical examination
Temperature >101°F (38.3°C)
Systolic or diastolic blood pressures <100 mm Hg or 60 mm Hg, respectively
Respiratory rate >30/minute
Extrapulmonary areas of infection
Laboratory factors
Abnormal renal function (BUN >20 mg/dl or serum creatinine >1.2 mg/dl)
Hematocrit <30%
WBC <4 × 10^9l or >30 × 10^9l
Metabolic acidosis
PA_{O_2} <60 mm Hg breathing room air
Comorbid conditions
Renal insufficiency
Congestive heart failure
Chronic obstructive pulmonary disease
Liver disease
Diabetes mellitus
Altered mental status
Alcoholism
Immunosuppression
Splenectomy
No responsible person in the home to assist the patient

Table 2 Studies Useful in the Diagnosis and Management of Community-Acquired Pneumonia

Complete blood count with differential
Chest x-ray (posteroanterior and lateral)
Arterial blood gas values
Blood cultures
Pleural fluid stain and culture
Sputum studies (for pneumonia unresponsive to usual antibiotics)
Acid-fast stain and culture
Fungal stains and culture
Immunofluorescent monoclonal antibody stain for *Pneumocystis carinii*
A Gram stain examined by an expert may be of value to some patients.
Legionella DFA
Serology
Legionella species
Francisella tularensis
Chlamydia (TWAR and psittacosis) species
Mycoplasma pneumoniae
Coxiella burnetii
Urinary antigen for *Legionella*

Table 3 Guidelines for Community-Acquired Pneumonia in Patients Under 60 Years Old with No Comorbid Illnesses

COMMON PATHOGENS
Streptococcus pneumoniae
Legionella spp.
Mycoplasma pneumoniae
Respiratory viruses
Chlamydia pneumoniae
ANTIBIOTICS
Erythromycin 500 mg PO q.i.d.
Azithromycin 500 mg PO day 1, 250 mg qd × 4 days
Clarithromycin 250 mg PO b.i.d.
If macrolide-intolerant and less than 30 years old, doxycycline 100 mg PO b.i.d.
If macrolide-intolerant and over 30 years old, amoxicillin 250 mg PO t.i.d. or cephalexin 500 mg PO q.i.d.

serology. A definitive microbial cause can be identified in only 50 percent of patients, even after exhaustive investigation employing many diagnostic methods.

RECOMMENDATIONS FOR EMPIRIC SELECTION OF ANTIMICROBIAL AGENTS

Because a definitive pathogen for pneumonia usually has not been identified when therapy must begin, empiric selection of antimicrobials is usually necessary. It is often useful to categorize patients according to age and severity of illness. Some microbes cause disease in all ages and types of patients; others are common only in patients with certain comorbidities. Tables 3 to 6 list these categories of patients along with the usual pathogens and appropriate antibiotic therapy.

Among previously healthy patients with relatively mild pneumonia (see Table 3), *Streptococcus pneumoniae* is still the principal bacterial pathogen, especially during influenza season. In some areas of the United States up to 25 percent of *S. pneumoniae* isolates are resistant to penicillin, which may influence empiric antibiotic choices for hospitalized patients. The atypical pneumonias (*Mycoplasma pneumoniae* and *Chlamydia pneumoniae*) are more frequent in patients not requiring hospitalization and are generally benign, with systemic complaints often more prominent than respiratory ones. Fever, headache, and myalgia are common. Leukocytosis is rare, and chest infiltrates consist primarily of segmental, lower-lobe, or hilar infiltrates. Although *M. pneumoniae* is more common among patients less than 30 years of age, it is being recognized with increasing frequency in older persons as well. It is characterized by a prominent cough, often occurs in epidemics, and can precipitate reactive airway disease, especially in children. *C. pneumoniae* (TWAR) is a cause of mild infection consisting of a biphasic illness with initial upper respiratory symptoms and pharyngitis, recovery, then pneumonia 2 or 3 weeks later. Erythromycin is the preferred antibiotic for outpatient pneumonia. Azithromycin and clarithromycin, the newer macrolides, have fewer gastrointestinal side effects and are often better tolerated than erythromycin, although much more expensive. Tetracycline and doxycycline are effective substitutes for treatment of *Mycoplasma* or chlamydial infections. An oral beta-lactam antibiotic is adequate treatment when *Mycoplasma* and chlamydial pathogens are considered unlikely.

Patients who are older than 60 years or have comorbid illnesses (see Table 4) are more likely to require hospital-

Table 4 Guidelines for Community-Acquired Pneumonia in Patients Over 60 Years and/or with Comorbid Illness

COMMON PATHOGENS

Streptococcus pneumoniae
Legionella spp.
Haemophilus influenzae
Moraxella catarrhalis
Other gram-negative bacilli
Respiratory viruses
Chlamydia pneumoniae

ANTIBIOTICS

Azithromycin 500 mg PO day 1, then 250 mg PO qd or clarithromycin 250 mg b.i.d.
and
Trimethoprim-sulfamethoxazole 1 DS b.i.d. or ciprofloxacin 750 mg PO b.i.d. or amoxicillin/clavulanate 1 g PO t.i.d.

Table 5 Guidelines for Community-Acquired Pneumonia of Moderate Degree in Patients Requiring Hospitalization

COMMON PATHOGENS

Streptococcus pneumoniae
Legionella spp.
Haemophilus influenzae
Staphylococcus aureus
Moraxella catarrhalis
Mycoplasma pneumoniae
Chlamydia pneumoniae
Other gram-negative bacilli
Respiratory viruses

ANTIBIOTICS

Erythromycin 1 g IV q6h
and
Ampicillin/sulbactam 1.5–3 g IV q6h or cefuroxime 0.75–1.5 g IV q8h or ceftriaxone 1 g q24h or cefotaxime 2 g q6h

ization. Some can be managed as outpatients but will require frequent follow-up visits. Gram-negative organisms, such as *Moraxella (Branhamella) catarrhalis* and *Haemophilus influenzae* are more common in this group, particularly in persons who smoke or have chronic obstructive pulmonary disease. About 80 to 90 percent of *Moraxella* isolates are beta-lactamase producers, as are an increasing number of *H. influenzae* strains. Azithromycin and clarithromycin act against these more resistant bacteria; however, these bacteria may be resistant to erythromycin. The macrolide drugs should be combined with another antibiotic active against gram-negative organisms. Up to 20 percent of patients in this group may eventually need hospitalization.

Patients admitted to the hospital with pneumonia of moderate severity require empiric therapy for the organisms listed in Table 5. Again, erythromycin is necessary, especially for *Legionella.* The incidence of *Legionella* in community-acquired pneumonia is as high as 23 percent in some studies, particularly those focusing on severe pneumonia. *Str. pneumoniae, Staphylococcus aureus,* and *H. influenzae* are more common during influenza outbreaks. Anaerobic infections, although uncommon, may be of concern in elderly patients and alcoholics. Respiratory syncytial virus may cause pneumonitis in elderly patients, especially those who live in nursing homes

Table 6 Guidelines for Severe Community-Acquired Pneumonia Requiring Admission to the Intensive Care Unit

COMMON PATHOGENS

*Streptococcus pneumoniae**
Legionella spp.
Staphylococcus aureus
Haemophilus influenzae
Mycoplasma pneumoniae
Other gram-negative bacilli
Respiratory viruses

ANTIBIOTICS

Erythromycin 1 g q6h IV (Plus rifampin 600 mg qd PO or IV if *Legionella* is strongly suspected)
and
Ceftriaxone 1 g q12h IV or Cefotaxime 2 g q6h IV or imipenem 500 mg q6h IV or Piperacillin/tazobactam 3/0.375 g q6h
and
Vancomycin 1 g q12h or Nafcillin 2g q4h IV if *S. aureus* is strongly suspected

*In areas with a significant incidence of penicillin-resistant pneumococci, vancomycin 1 g q12h.

or have contact with young children. Second- or third-generation cephalosporins or beta-lactam–beta-lactamase inhibitor combinations are necessary adjuncts to erythromycin for adequate coverage.

The importance of subdividing hospital admissions for pneumonia into moderate and severe illness lies in the recognition of increased mortality in patients with severe pneumonia, especially during the first 7 days. Mortality ranges from 50 to 70 percent in some studies. Severe pneumonia manifests as hypoxia, tachypnea, multilobe involvement or consolidation, and signs of septic shock. These patients should be managed in an intensive care unit. Organisms listed in Table 6 may cause more severe disease. Antibiotic coverage should be expanded to include a third-generation cephalosporin, imipenem, or piperacillin-tazobactam in combination with erythromycin. Vancomycin should be added in areas where penicillin-resistant pneumococci are seen. Antistaphylococcal coverage should be included during influenza season or when a chest radiograph suggests *S. aureus,* i.e., pneumatoceles or necrotizing changes.

A few other organisms deserve special mention. Although rare in most of the United States, tularemic pneumonia should be considered in endemic areas among patients with exposure to wild mammals, especially rabbits, and ticks. Intravenous gentamicin should be given to a hospitalized patient when tularemic pneumonia is in the differential. *Coxiella burnetii* causes an atypical pneumonia frequently accompanied by hepatosplenomegaly. It is endemic in many hot, dry areas such as southern Texas. The most common reservoirs are sheep, goats, cattle, and ticks. Tetracycline 500 mg four times a day is the recommended therapy. *Chlamydia psittaci* is another atypical pneumonia that should be considered in patients with exposure to infected birds, especially parrots. Splenomegaly in conjunction with an atypical pneumonia suggests psittacosis. Again, the drug of choice is tetracycline 2 g per day. *Mycobacterium tuberculosis* should be considered early in the differential diagnosis of a pneumonia not responding to usual antibiotics. Endemic fungal infections, such as blastomycosis, histoplasmosis, cryptococcosis, and coccidioidomycosis may also present as a community-acquired pneumonia.

■ THERAPY

Antibiotic therapy should not be altered during the first few days unless there is marked deterioration. Usually 48 to 72 hours are required for significant clinical improvement. Fever usually lasts 2 to 4 days, and the white blood cell count generally returns to normal after 4 days. Duration of therapy should be individualized to the infecting organism and the overall health of the patient. Generally, treatment of bacterial pneumonia requires 7 to 10 days of antibiotics, whereas atypical pneumonia calls for at least 14 days. Immunocompromised patients usually require 21 days of treatment. When the patient is stable and afebrile, oral antimicrobials may be substituted, assuming the patient has normal absorption.

Resolution of abnormal radiographic findings usually lags behind clinical improvement. However, if abnormalities have not resolved or greatly improved by 6 weeks after completion of therapy, the patient should be referred for possible bronchoscopic evaluation. All patients with pneumonia should be followed until there has been radiographic resolution of the infiltrate. Resolution is slower in elderly patients, those with comorbidities or multilobe involvement, and smokers.

There are a number of reasons for therapeutic failure in community-acquired pneumonia. The serum level of the chosen antibiotics may not be high enough. Some antibiotics, such as the aminoglycosides, do not penetrate well into lung tissue. The agent may be resistant to the antibiotics or, less likely, the organisms may develop resistance during drug therapy. Lack of clinical improvement should raise the suspicion of a cause other than routine bacteria, such as viruses, Mycobacteria, fungi, or parasites. Clinicians should always keep in mind the possibility of noninfectious illness that mimics pneumonia such as pulmonary infarction, carcinoma, pulmonary edema, atelectasis, sarcoidosis, eosinophilic infiltrates, and drug reactions.

Suggested Reading

American Thoracic Society. Guideline for the initial management of adults with community-acquired pneumonia: Diagnosis, assessment of severity, and initial antimicrobial therapy. Am Rev Respir Dis 1993; 148: 1418–1426.

Bates JH, Campbell GD, Barron AL, et al. Microbial etiology of acute pneumonia in hospitalized patients. Chest 1992; 101:1005–1012.

Fine AJ, Smith DN, Singer DE. Hospitalization decision in patients with community-acquired pneumonia: A prospective cohort study. Am J Med 1990; 89:713–721.

LaForce FM. Antibacterial therapy for lower respiratory tract infections in adults: A review. Clin Infect Dis 1992; 14(Suppl 2):S233–237.

Mittl RL, Schwab RJ, Duchin JS, et al. Radiographic resolution of community-acquired pneumonia. Am J Respir Crit Care Med 1994; 149:630–635.

PROSTATITIS

Jonathan M. Zenilman, M.D.

Prostatitis, a common clinical problem, can have an infectious or noninfectious cause. Data from the U.S. National Center for Health Statistics suggest that over 25 percent of men seen for lower genitourinary complaints were diagnosed with prostatitis. In the preantibiotic era, prostatitis was a potentially fatal complication of untreated gonorrhea. Today most cases of bacterial prostatitis are complications of lower urinary tract infection (UTI).

Prostatitis is the clinical expression of inflammatory exudate within the ducts and prostate gland tissue. In acute prostatitis the inflammatory cells are polymorphonuclear leukocytes (PMN). In chronic prostatitis a lymphocytic and mononuclear inflammatory process is present. Chronic prostatitis is often focal. Furthermore, noninfectious events may contribute to the chronic prostatitis syndrome. For example, prostatic concretions may serve as a nidus for the development of chronic bacterial prostatitis. Focal prostatic necrosis as part of benign prostatic hyperplasia may cause prostatic inflammation even without infection.

Most cases of bacterial prostatitis result from reflux of infected urine into the prostatic ducts and canaliculi. Although large-scale formal epidemiologic studies have not been done, prostatitis is seen most commonly in older men. Bacterial prostatitis is most common in patients with previous prostate disease, diabetes mellitus, and a history of urethral instrumentation such as catheterization.

Infectious prostatitis is rarely caused by sexually transmitted organisms. Since urethritis is the initial symptom of gonococcal and chlamydial infection, patients seek care early, and with the widespread availability of effective treatments, the infections are eradicated. Prostatitis due to hematogenously disseminated organisms is usually seen as part of those disease syndromes. Implicated organisms include *Mycobacterium tuberculosis, Cryptococcus neoformans, Coccidioides immitis, Histoplasma capsulatum,* and *Candida* spp. With the exception of *Candida,* these infections present as granulomatous disease and are often confused with malignancy.

The long-term sequelae of bacterial prostatitis are not well described. Some authorities believe that prostatitis may contribute to male infertility.

■ CLINICAL SYNDROMES

Except for acute disease, the accurate clinical diagnosis of prostatitis is difficult. Clinical symptoms are typically nonspecific, and the differential diagnosis often includes a host of noninfectious urologic problems. Many patients seek urologic or infectious disease consultation for prostatitis evaluation after previous diagnoses of lower UTI or STD syndromes; therefore, they have often been treated with antibiotics. Because of the gland's location, definitive histopathologic diagnosis by biopsy is rarely an option unless malignancy is strongly suspected.

Acute prostatitis is characterized by an abrupt febrile illness with symptoms referable to the lower genitourinary tract. Chills, leukocytosis, urinary frequency, and occasional bladder outlet obstruction are present. A rectal examination typically shows an enlarged, boggy, exquisitely tender prostate.

Men with chronic prostatitis have a large variety of presenting symptoms, including urinary urgency, frequency, nocturia, and dysuria. Lower back pain or pain in the inguinal, suprapubic, or scrotal area may be present. Hematospermia or hematuria is seen in approximately 10 percent of patients. Systemic symptoms are unusual. Rectal examination of the prostate is typically unremarkable. In practice, most men come for evaluation after being treated initially with antibiotics for community-acquired UTI.

The differential diagnosis includes noninfectious prostatitis, UTI due to cystitis, prostatic hyperplasia due to either benign prostatic hypertrophy or tumor, and urethral stricture due to previous undertreated urethritis. Carcinoma of the bladder should be considered, especially in patients with hematuria. Urine cytology is useful in ruling out this diagnosis. Neuromuscular urologic disorders should be considered in consultation with the urologist if laboratory investigations fail to reveal cause of the symptoms.

■ LABORATORY EVALUATION

The only way chronic bacterial prostatitis can be diagnosed with certainty is by evaluating the expressed prostatic secretions for inflammatory cells and bacterial pathogens. Stamey and Meares's technique of segmental urinary tract culture is widely accepted.

Procedure

The patient should have a full bladder and should not have taken antibiotics for 48 hours. The penis is washed with sterile water; no antibacterials are used because they may reduce culture yield. Uncircumcised men retract the foreskin. The patient then voids. The first 10 ml (VB_1) and a midstream sample (VB_2) are collected. After voiding 200 ml, the patient is instructed to kneel. The physician vigorously massages the prostate, and the expressed prostatic secretions (EPS) are collected in a sterile container as they drip from the urethral meatus. The patient is then asked to empty his bladder, and the first 10 ml of this final void (VB_3) is collected. Gram stain smear is prepared from the EPS specimens; the midstream urine and prostatic secretions are sent chilled to the laboratory for culture. The laboratory should be asked to perform low colony count cultures.

Table 1 Differential Diagnosis of Prostatitis

	MIDSTREAM URINE		EPS	
	WBC	CULTURE	WBC	CULTURE
Acute bacterial prostatitis	++	+	++	+
Chronic bacterial prostatitis	+	+	+	+
Chronic nonbacterial prostatitis	–	–	+	–
Prostadynia	–	–	–	–

Adapted from Meares EM, Stamey EA. Bacteriologic localization patterns in bacterial prostatitis and urethritis. Invest Urol 1968; 5:492-518. EPS, expressed prostatic secretions.

Evaluation of Results

Differential diagnosis of prostatitis, achieved by using the data from the expressed prostatic secretions and VB_2, are summarized in Table 1. The number of white blood cells (WBC) in prostatic secretions necessary to make the diagnosis varies in the literature. However, nearly all have at least 12 WBC per high-power field. Acute bacterial prostatitis has a large number of organisms and PMN; the diagnosis is seldom subtle. Chronic prostatitis is diagnosed by presence of PMN in the expressed prostatic secretions. Culture results from the EPS differentiate bacterial and nonbacterial causes. Nonbacterial chronic prostatitis should be referred to the urologist for further evaluation. A sexually transmitted organism such as *Chlamydia* or *Trichomonas* is rarely implicated. Prostadynia is diagnosed when the prostatic secretions demonstrate no inflammation and cultures are negative. In some studies as many as 40 percent of patients have prostadynia. Delineation of this syndrome is important because antimicrobials have no effect and should not be prescribed.

■ BACTERIAL CAUSES

Determination of bacterial cause is desirable, since antimicrobial therapy for prostatitis is usually required for at least 4 weeks. If the patient has taken antibiotics, false-negative cultures will occur. Except in cases of acute prostatitis the clinician may want to consider discontinuing antibiotics, waiting for 48 to 72 hours, and then obtaining the prostatic fluid and urine cultures.

The organisms typically isolated are those associated with lower UTI (Table 2). Enteric gram-negative rods are most common, followed by *Enterococcus* spp., *Staphylococcus saprophyticus,* and *Pseudomonas* spp. Streptococci and anaerobes are rarely involved. If the patient has been recently instrumented or catheterized in a hospital, especially if he has been treated with antibiotics, *Pseudomonas* and *Enterococcus* are the major concerns. In some studies, *Mycoplasma hominis* and *Ureaplasma urealyticum* have been cultured in up to 25 percent of cases. Routine culture for these organisms is not

Table 2 Organisms Implicated in Bacterial Prostatitis

GRAM-NEGATIVE
Escherichia coli
Proteus mirabilis
Klebsiella
Pseudomonas aeruginosa
GRAM-POSITIVE
Enterococcus
Staphylococcus saprophyticus

recommended, as special media and bacteriologic techniques are required. Furthermore, both organisms are found frequently as commensals in normal hosts, and their role as pathogens is controversial.

In sexually active patients, especially those with multiple partners, *Chlamydia* and *Trichomonas* are rarely found. These organisms are difficult to culture. Fungal and mycobacterial causes can usually be diagnosed only by prostatic biopsy.

■ THERAPY

Evaluating treatment efficacy of prostatitis is complicated by the following:

1. The difficulties in making an accurate clinical diagnosis, especially in the substantial fraction of patients with prior antibiotic therapy for lower tract UTI.
2. The lack of a standard definition of cure. Most studies of treatment, even those that evaluate prostatic secretions for bacteriology, do not repeat the procedure at post-therapy evaluation.
3. The optimal duration of therapy is not defined.
4. Few longitudinal, randomized controlled trials have evaluated prostatitis treatment.

Acknowledging these difficulties, most authorities believe that treatment regimens for bacterial prostatitis should include the following elements:

1. An antimicrobial effective against the most likely organisms.
2. An antimicrobial well absorbed into prostate tissue with an acid dissociation coefficient (pK_a) favorable to trap the drug in prostate tissue compared with the acidic urinary tract environment.
3. Treatment lasting for 1 month; drugs that require relatively infrequent dosing are preferred to facilitate compliance.

Table 3 Therapy Recommended for Prostatitis

TMP-SMX DS (160 and 800 mg) b.i.d.
Ciprofloxacin 500 mg b.i.d. or norfloxacin 400 mg b.i.d.*
Oral therapy lasts 4 weeks.

*Other quinolones are probably effective, but there are limited data at this writing.
TMP-SMX, trimethoprim-sulfamethoxazole; DS, double strength.

The quinolones and trimethoprim-sulfamethoxazole (TMP-SMX) (Table 3) meet these criteria. I prefer to use the quinolones because they are associated with fewer side effects, especially in older patients, and are more active against the gram-positive organisms. However, they are 2 to 5 times as costly as TMP-SMX. Quinolones are also poorly absorbed if the gastric pH is greater than 5, a consideration in patients who are taking antacids or H_2 blockers.

Since many patients are referred for evaluation after a course of antibiotics, accurate bacteriologic evaluation may not be possible. The trap is that antibiotic treatment of nonbacterial chronic prostatitis is ineffective. One option is to discontinue antibiotics and evaluate 72 hours after discontinuation.

Recurrent disease is reported is as many as 40 percent of patients. Patients with well-documented disease should resume antimicrobials for a minimum of 3 months. If there is a second recurrence, chronic prophylaxis should be considered. Recurrence after cessation of antibiotics in patients with poorly documented disease should prompt full re-evaluation of the syndrome.

Suggested Reading

Colleen S, Mardh P-A. Prostatitis. In: Holmes KK, ed. Sexually transmitted diseases. 2nd ed. New York: McGraw-Hill, 1990:653.
del la Rosette JJMC, Hubregtse MR, Meuleman EJH, et al. Diagnosis and treatment of 409 patients with prostatitis syndromes. Urology 1993; 41:301–307.
Doble A. Chronic prostatitis. Br J Urol 1994; 74:537–541.
Krieger JN, McGonagle LA. Diagnostic considerations and interpretation of microbiological findings for evaluation of chronic prostatitis. J Clin Microbiol 1989; 27:2240–2244.
Meares EM, Stamey EA. Bacteriologic localisation patterns in bacterial prostatitis and urethritis. Invest Urol 1968; 5:492–518.

OTITIS EXTERNA

Harris R. Stutman, M.D.

Acute otitis externa (swimmer's ear) is the most common infectious disease of the external ear. It usually follows prolonged exposure of the ear canal to moisture, with maceration leading to secondary bacterial infection. The most common pathogen is *Pseudomonas aeruginosa,* although other gram-negative bacilli, such as *Escherichia coli* and *Proteus,* are occasional pathogens and gram-positive cocci, including *Staphylococcus aureus,* are not infrequent. Chronic otitis externa is usually secondary to a persistent suppurative condition of the middle ear following tympanic membrane (TM) perforation and chronic drainage. The flora is similar in the acute and chronic conditions.

In the earliest phases of otitis externa the canal is edematous and symptoms are limited to otorrhea. Later, pruritus and otalgia may be noted and the ear drainage may progress from clear to purulent. Finally, the canal may be filled with purulent debris leading to diminished hearing. Tenderness of the earlobe and severe pain noted with earlobe traction are common at this point. In addition to the common inflammatory condition, foreign bodies in the ear canal, acute otitis media with perforation, malignant otitis externa, and mastoiditis should be considered.

■ THERAPY

Therapy for acute otitis externa centers on thorough drying and debridement of the external canal, with a topical antibiotic solution used to help eliminate the secondary bacterial pathogens. In minor infections the ear canal is easily rinsed with Burow's solution and dried with cotton-tipped swabs. The patient should avoid getting water into the ear canal during treatment. Ear plugs or cotton pledgets can be used during showers and shampooing, although these should be removed as soon as possible. Swimming should be avoided, even with ear plugs. In more serious infections purulent material may obstruct an edematous ear canal and should be removed with gentle irrigation and suctioning. If the TM is not perforated, a warmed saline or 2 percent acetic acid solution may be useful in removing debris. This may be followed with a gentle rinse with a vinegar-isopropyl alcohol solution followed by drying with cotton-tipped swabs or a hair dryer. This procedure of suctioning and irrigation should probably be repeated daily or every other day until the inflammation remits. The 2 percent acetic acid solution is usually all that is necessary to provide appropriate antibacterial activity, although a variety of pharmaceutical agents (colistin, gentamicin, and others) are available. When the TM is perforated, acetic acid solutions are not well tolerated and are best replaced by commercially available solutions such as neomycin-polymyxin B-hydrocortisone. If there is cellulitis, consider adding an oral antistaphylococcal agent to the regimen.

If otic drops are to be effective, they must be appropriately instilled. Generally, this is best accomplished by having the patient lie with the affected ear up and the canal straightened with gentle tugging of the earlobe. After the drops are instilled, the patient should remain in this position for at least 1 full minute. If the drops do not easily flow down the canal because of edema or inflammation, a cotton wick can be used. Insert the wick about 1 cm into the canal and put the drops on it. The medication swells the wick, ensuring that the drops remain in the canal until they can diffuse down the inflamed lumen. Drops are typically used 3 or 4 times a day until the inflammation has resolved, generally about 7 days. If pain is severe, systemic analgesics should be used. Acetaminophen or ibuprofen is usually sufficient, although codeine occasionally is necessary.

If infection is severe or associated with a chronic draining middle ear infection, consultation with an otolaryngologist is appropriate. After cultures are obtained for specific microbiologic diagnosis, daily irrigation and debridement are needed. Patients should typically be started on systemic therapy effective against *Pseudomonas,* since this is the pathogen most commonly involved. Several investigators have suggested that *S. aureus* is frequent enough to be included in the initial regimen, but I have not found that routinely necessary unless culture results suggest it. Intravenous ceftazidime with or without gentamicin or tobramycin is an appropriate initial regimen. In malignant otitis externa the infection invades cartilage and bone and may cause neurologic complications such as seventh nerve palsy, meningitis, and brain abscess. It is typically seen in elderly diabetic patients, and diagnosis is best established by computed tomography or magnetic resonance imaging. Treatment requires surgical debridement as well as systemic antibiotics. The causative agent is almost always *Pseudomonas.*

If contiguous cellulitis is present or the results of initial cultures document *S. aureus,* nafcillin or cefazolin should be added. For reasons that are not entirely clear, some patients are prone to recurrent external otitis, usually associated with swimming. These patients should avoid prolonged stays in the water under any circumstances, although dermatologic conditions such as eczema and seborrhea may also be considered. In patients who cannot avoid the water, such as competitive swimmers, recurrent otitis externa can usually be prevented by the instillation of a 2 percent acetic acid solution into the ear canals after swimming and at bedtime.

Suggested Reading

Bojrab DI, Bruderly T, Abdulrazzak Y. Otitis externa. Otolaryngol Clin North Am 1996; 29:761–782.

Cantor RM. Otitis media and otitis externa: a new look at old problems. Emerg Med Clin North Am 1995; 13:445–455.

Evans P, Hofmann L. Malignant external otitis: a case report and review. Am Fam Physician 1994; 49:427–431.

Kimmelman CP. Office management of the draining ear. Otolaryngol Clin North Am 1992; 25:739–744.

SPONTANEOUS BACTERIAL PERITONITIS

William G. Rector Jr., M.D.

Spontaneous bacterial peritonitis (SBP) is the most serious complication of ascites formation. Earlier recognition and improved therapy have resulted in better survival. Even today, however, over a third of patients with this infection die.

Ascites infection may be divided into several categories based upon the ascites polymorphonuclear (PMN) cell count and the results of culture (Table 1). Culture-negative neutrocytic ascites usually occurs either in patients with SBP in whom antibiotics already have been administered or patients in whom optimal culture methods (bedside inoculation of blood culture bottles) have not been used. Monomicrobial bacterascites represents either early or transient ascites infection. Polymicrobial bacterascites indicates that bowel contents have been inadvertently sampled with the needle. Secondary bacterial peritonitis is ascites infection due to gut perforation.

The usual flora of SBP are facultative gram-negative aerobes and gram-positive streptococci (Table 2). Noteworthy because of their rarity are enterococci, staphylococci, and anaerobes.

Table 1 Usual Flora of Spontaneous Bacterial Peritonitis (SBP)

ORGANISMS	FREQUENCY
Enterobacteriaceae	Common
Non-group D streptococci	Common
Group D streptococci	Uncommon
Staphylococcus aureus	Rare
Anaerobes	Rare

Table 2 Categories of Spontaneous Bacterial Peritonitis (SBP)

CATEGORY	ASCITES PMN COUNT	CULTURE	ORGANISMS
SBP	>250/ml	Positive	One
Culture-negative neutrocytic ascites	>250/ml	Negative	None
Monomicrobial bacterascites	<250/ml	Positive	One
Polymicrobial bacterascites	<250/ml	Positive	Many
Secondary bacterial peritonitis	>250/ml	Positive	Many

PMN, polymorphonuclear neutrophil leukocytes.

THERAPEUTIC ALTERNATIVES

SBP is treated with antibiotics. All five categories of ascites infection may be treated. Physicians who wish simply to observe patients with monomicrobial bacterascites or polymicrobial bacterascites are obliged to repeat the paracentesis in 24 to 48 hours to assess the course of the infection.

PREFERRED APPROACH

SBP should be treated with cefotaxime 2 g intravenously three times daily for 5 days. Aminoglycosides should be avoided. Calculation of the appropriate dose is difficult owing to distortion of body mass by excess fluid. Also, muscle mass is reduced in patients with cirrhosis. Moreover, renal function may be labile. For these reasons, the serum creatinine concentration may not be an accurate reflection of glomerular filtration rate. Also, patients with cirrhosis may be abnormally sensitive to the nephrotoxic effects of aminoglycosides. Follow-up paracentesis should be done in patients who do not have a rapid clinical response to treatment. The ascites PMN count falls exponentially in adequately treated patients.

Polymicrobial bacterascites and secondary bacterial peritonitis also require coverage for anaerobes, for example with metronidazole.

Antibiotic therapy is modified appropriately when culture and sensitivity information become available.

Prevention

Prevention has recently been recognized as an important measure. SBP usually arises as a result of seeding of ascites during transient bacteremia. The commonest and most important cause of bacteremia in the hospital is catheterization of the bladder. Urinary catheters should be scrupulously avoided in patients with cirrhosis. Infections elsewhere such as cellulitis and pneumonia can also lead to SBP and should be aggressively treated. Severe upper gastrointestinal bleeding is associated with a heightened risk of ascites infection, perhaps as a result of the extensive instrumentation undergone by such patients.

A protein concentration of ascites less than 1 g per deciliter is also associated with enhanced risk of SBP, probably as a result of diminished concentration of opsonins. Diuretic therapy raises the protein concentration of ascites and may help prevent SBP.

The role of continuous oral prophylactic therapy with quinolone antibiotics in patients with recurrent SBP is not fully defined, but early reports suggest it to be safe and effective.

Suggested Reading

Runyon BA, Hoefs JC. Ascitic fluid analysis before, during, and after spontaneous bacterial peritonitis. Hepatology 1985; 5:257–259.

Runyon BA. McHutchison JG, Antillon MR, et al. Short-course vs long-course antibiotic treatment of spontaneous bacterial peritonitis. Gastroenterology 1991; 100:1737–1742.

Runyon BA, Umland ET, Merlin T. Inoculation of blood culture bottles with ascitic fluid: improved detection of spontaneous bacterial peritonitis. Arch Intern Med 1987; 147:73–75.

PHARYNGOTONSILLITIS

Itzhak Brook, M.D., M.Sc.

Pharyngotonsillitis (PT) is characterized by pharyngeal erythema and an exudate, ulceration, or a membrane covering the tonsils. Because the pharynx is surrounded by lymphoid tissues of the Waldeyer ring, an infection can spread to various parts of the ring such as the nasopharynx, uvula, soft palate, tonsils, adenoids, and the cervical lymph glands. According to its extent, the infection can be described as pharyngitis, tonsillitis, tonsillopharyngitis, or nasopharyngitis. The duration of any of these illnesses can be *acute, subacute, chronic,* or *recurrent.*

■ CAUSES

The finding of PT generally requires the consideration of a group A beta-hemolytic streptococcal (GABHS) infection. However, numerous other infectious and noninfectious causes should be considered. Recognition of the cause and choice of appropriate therapy are of utmost importance in assuring rapid recovery and preventing complications.

Table 1 lists the different causative agents and their characteristic clinical features. The occurrence of any agent depends on numerous variables that include environmental conditions (season, geographic location, exposure) and individual variables (age, host resistance, immunity). The most prevalent agents accounting for PT are GABHS, adenovirus, influenza, parainfluenza, Epstein-Barr virus (EBV), and enterovirus. However, the exact cause is generally not determined, and the role of some pathogens is not certain.

Recent studies suggest that interactions among various organisms, including GABHS, other aerobic and anaerobic bacteria, and viruses may occur during PT. Some of these interactions (e.g., between EBV and anaerobic bacteria) may be synergistic, enhancing the virulence of some pathogens, while others (e.g., between GABHS and certain interfering alpha-hemolytic streptococci) may be antagonistic. Furthermore, beta-lactamase-producing bacteria can protect themselves and other bacteria from beta-lactam antibiotics.

Table 1 Infectious Agents of Pharyngotonsillitis

BACTERIA	CLINICAL LESIONS	CLINICAL FREQUENCY
AEROBIC		
Group A, B, C, and G streptococci	F, Er, Ex, P	A
Streptococcus pneumoniae	E	C
Staphylococcus aureus	F, ER, Ex	C
Neisseria meningitidis	Er, Ex	C
Corynebacterium diphtheriae	Er, Ex	C
Corynebacterium hemolyticum	Er, Ex	C
Bordetella pertussis	Er, Er	C
Haemophilus influenzae	Er, Ex	C
Haemophilus parainfluenzae	Er, Ex	C
Salmonella typhi	Er	C
Francisella tularensis	Er, Ex	C
Yersinia pseudotuberculosis	Er	C
Treponema pallidum	F, Er	C
Mycobacterium sp.	Er	C
ANAEROBIC		
Peptostreptococcus sp.	Er, E	C
Actinomyces sp.	Er U	C
Pigmented *Prevotella* and *Porphromonas*	Er, Ex, U	B
Bacteroides sp.	Er, Ex, U	C
MYCOPLASMA		
Mycoplasma pneumoniae	F, Er, Ex	B
Mycoplasma hominis	Er, Ex	C
VIRUSES AND CHLAMYDIA		
Adenovirus	F, Er, Ex	A
Enteroviruses (polio, echo, coxsackie)	Er, Ex, U	A
Parainfluenzae	Er	A
Epstein-Barr	F, Er, Ex	B
Herpes hominis	Er, Ex, U	C
Respiratory syncytial	Er	C
Influenza A and *B*	Er	A
Cytomegalovirus	Er	C
Reovirus	Er	C
Measles	Er, P	C
Rubella	P	C
Rhinovirus	Er	C
Chlamydia trachomatis		C
Chlamydia pneumoniae		C
FUNGI		
Candida sp.	Er, Ex	B
PARASITES		
Toxoplasma gondii	Er	C
RICKETTSIA		
Coxiella burnetii	Er	C

Clinical lesions: F, follicular; Er, erythematous; Ex, exudative; U, ulcerative; P, petechial.
Frequency: A, most frequent (more than 66% of cases); B, frequent (between 66% and 33% of cases); C, uncommon (fewer than 33% of cases).

Aerobic Bacteria

Because of the potential for serious suppurative and nonsuppurative sequelae, GABHS are the best known cause of sore throat. Occasionally groups B, C, and G beta-hemolytic streptococci are responsible. Streptococcal tonsillitis can be serious because it may lead to rheumatic fever and because of the increased virulence of GABHS in recent years. Increasing numbers of cases of sepsis and toxic shock syndrome due to streptococci have been observed in the past decade. The clinical presentation of PT due to all types of streptococci is generally identical: it is characterized by exudation, petechiae, and follicles. The isolation rate of GABHS varies with patient's age, with the highest prevalence of recovery in school years. The isolation rate of non-GABHS is higher in adults than in children.

Streptococci can be involved in suppurative complications of tonsillitis such as peritonsillar, retrotonsillar, and retropharyngeal abscesses. *Streptococcus pneumoniae* can also be involved in PT, and it may either subside or spread to other sites.

Corynebacterium diphtheriae and *Corynebacterium hemolyticum* cause an early exudative PT with grayish-green thick membrane that may be difficult to dislodge. It often leaves a bleeding surface when torn off. The infection can spread to the throat, palate, and larynx. *C. hemolyticum* produces a lethal systemic exotoxin.

Neisseria gonorrhoeae is common in homosexual men and can be detected in adolescents with pharyngitis. The infection is often asymptomatic, but it may result in bacteremia and can persist after treatment. *Neisseria meningitidis* can cause symptomatic or asymptomatic PT that is a prodrome for septicemia or meningitis.

Nontypable *Haemophilus influenzae* and *Haemophilus parainfluenzae* can be recovered from inflamed tonsils. These organisms can cause invasive disease in infants, as well as acute epiglottitis, otitis media, and sinusitis.

Staphylococcus aureus is often recovered from chronically inflamed tonsils and peritonsillar abscesses. It can produce the enzyme beta-lactamase, which may interfere with the eradication of GABHS.

Rare causes of PT are *Francisella tularemia, Treponema pallidum, Mycobacterium* sp. and *Toxoplasma gondii.*

Mycoplasma

Mycoplasma pneumoniae and *Mycoplasma hominis* can cause PT, usually as a manifestation of a generalized infection. The prevalence of *Mycoplasma* infection increases with age.

Anaerobic Bacteria

The anaerobic species that have been implicated in PT are *Actinomyces* sp., *Fusobacterium* sp., and pigmented *Prevotella* and *Porphyromonas* sp. The classical infection caused by anaerobes is Vincent's angina. However, anaerobes can be involved in complications of PT such as peritonsillar retropharyngeal abscess.

Viruses and Chlamydia

The viruses known to cause PT are adenovirus, Coxsackie A virus, parainfluenza virus, enteroviruses, EBV, herpes simplex, respiratory syncytial virus, and cytomegalovirus. *Chlamydia trachomatis* has been associated with nasopharyngeal infections and pneumonia in infants as well as with PT following fellatio. *Chlamydia pneumoniae* may cause pharyngitis, often accompanying pneumonia or bronchitis.

■ CLINICAL FINDINGS

PT generally has a sudden onset, with fever and sore throat, nausea, vomiting, headache, and rarely, abdominal pain. At an early stage redness of throat and tonsils is observed, and the cervical lymph glands swell. The clinical manifestations may vary by causative agent (see Table 1) but are rarely specific. Erythema is common to most agents; however the occurrence of ulceration, petechiae, exudation, and follicles varies. The common features are exudative pharyngitis in GABHS infection, ulcerative lesions in enteroviruses, and membranous pharyngitis in *C. diphtheriae.* Petechiae can often be seen in GABHS, EBV, measles, and rubella virus infections.

Viral disease is generally self-limited and lasts 4 to 10 days. Bacterial illness lasts longer if untreated. The definitive features of anaerobic tonsillitis or PT are enlargement and ulceration of the tonsils associated with fetid or foul odor and the presence of fusiform bacilli, spirochetes, and other organisms on Gram stain.

■ DIAGNOSIS

Throat cultures generally identify GABHS by either direct growth that may take 24 to 48 hours or by one of the rapid methods of identification that takes 10 to 60 minutes. These rapid methods are associated with 5 to 15 percent false-negative results. It is therefore recommended that a bacterial culture be performed if the rapid streptococcal test is negative. Hemolysis can be best detected in sheep or horse blood agar plate, especially in an anaerobic environment. Attempts to identify beta-hemolytic streptococci other than group A may be worthwhile for older individuals. More than 10 colonies of GABHS per plate are considered to represent a true infection rather than colonization. A rise in antistreptolysin (ASO) streptococcal antibody titer after 3 to 6 weeks can provide retrospective evidence for GABHS infection and assist in differentiating the carrier state.

Other pathogens should be identified when no GABHS is found or when a search of other organisms is warranted. Since many other pathogens are part of the normal pharyngeal flora, interpretation of the data is difficult.

Attempts to identify corynebacteria should be made whenever a membrane is observed. Cultures should be obtained from beneath the membrane, using a special moisture-reducing transport medium. A Loeffler slant, a tellurite plate, and a blood agar plate should be inoculated. Identification by fluorescent antibody technique is possible.

Viral cultures and rapid tests for some viruses (e.g., respiratory syncytial virus) are available. A heterophile slide test or another rapid test for infectious mononucleosis can provide a specific diagnosis.

■ THERAPY

Many antibiotics are available for the treatment of PT caused by GABHS. However, the recommended optimal treatment for GABHS infection is penicillin administered three times a day for 10 days (Table 2). Oral penicillin VK is used more often than intramuscular benzathine penicillin G. However, intramuscular penicillin can be given as initial therapy in those who cannot tolerate oral medication or to ensure compliance. An alternative medication is amoxicillin, which is as active against GABHS. Blood levels are higher, plasma half-life is longer, and protein binding is lower, giving it theoretic advantages. Furthermore, oral amoxicillin has better compliance (better taste). Penicillin and other beta-lactam antibiotics should not be used in patients suspected of infectious mononucleosis because they can produce a skin rash.

Alternative agents for the treatment of acute GABHS tonsillitis are the macrolides (e.g., erythromycin if GABHS resistance to them is low) and a first- and second-generation oral cephalosporin. The success rate of therapy with cephalosporins was consistently found to be higher than the one with penicillin. Their increased efficacy may be due to their activity against aerobic beta-lactamase-producing bacteria (BLPB) such as *S. aureus* and *Haemophilus* sp. Another possible reason is that the nonpathogenic alpha-hemolytic streptococci that compete with GABHS and help to eliminate them are more resistant to cephalosporins than to penicillin. These streptococci are therefore more likely to survive cephalosporin therapy.

The length of therapy of acute tonsillitis with medication other than penicillin has not been determined by controlled studies. Until such studies are done, it is safe to use a 10-day regimen, as with penicillin (Tables 2 and 3).

When *C. diphtheriae* infection is suspected, erythromycin is the drug of choice and penicillin and rifampin are alternatives.

Supportive therapy of PT includes antipyretics and analgesics such as aspirin or acetaminophen and attention to proper hydration.

Prevention of recurrent tonsillitis due to GABHS by prophylactic administration of daily oral or monthly benzathine penicillin should be attempted in patients who suffered from rheumatic fever. American Heart Committee guidelines on the prevention of rheumatic fever should be followed, and if any family members are carrying GABHS, the disease should be eradicated and the carrier state monitored.

Table 2 Oral Antibiotics for the Treatment of Acute GABHS Pharyngotonsillitis

GENERIC NAME	DOSAGE (MG/KG/DAY)	ADULT DAILY DOSAGE (MG)
Penicillin V	25–50 q6-8h	250 q6–8h
Amoxicillin	40 q8h	250 q8h
Cephalexin*	25–50 q6–8h	250 q6h
Cefadroxil*	30 q12h	1,000 q24h
Cefaclor*	40 q8h	250 q8h
Cefuroxime-axetil*	30 q12h	250 q12h
Cefpodoxime-proxetil*	30 q12h	500 q12h
Cefprozil*	30 q12h	250 q6h
Erythromycin	40 q6–8h	500 q12h
Clarithromycin*	7.5 q12h	250 q8h
Amoxicillin-clavulanate†	40 q8h	150 q8h
Clindamycin†	20–30 q6–8h	

*Effective also against aerobic BLPB.
†Effective also against aerobic and anaerobic BLPB.

Recurrent and Chronic Tonsillitis

Recent studies documented bacteriologic failure rates of 25 percent or more in penicillin-treated patients with acute GABHS tonsillitis and even higher rates in re-treatment. Although about half of the patients who harbor GABHS following therapy may be carriers, the rest may still show signs of infection and represent true clinical failure. The increased treatment failure rates necessitated the consideration of alternative therapies for patients who failed penicillin therapy.

Penicillin failure in eradicating GABHS tonsillitis has several explanations (Table 4). These include noncompliance with 10-day course of therapy, carrier state, reinfection, bacterial interference, and penicillin tolerance. One explanation is that repeated penicillin administration results in a shift in the oral microflora with selection of beta-lactamase-producing strains of *S. aureus, Haemophilus* sp., *Moraxella catarrhalis, Fusobacterium* sp., pigmented *Prevotella* and *Porphyromonas* spp. and *Bacteroides* sp.

It is possible that BLPB can protect the GABHS from penicillin by inactivating the antibiotic. Such organisms in a localized soft-tissue infection may degrade penicillin in the area of the infection, protecting not only themselves but also penicillin-susceptible pathogens such as GABHS. Thus, penicillin therapy directed against a susceptible pathogen can be rendered ineffective.

An increase in in vitro resistance of GABHS to penicillin was observed when GABHS was inoculated with *S. aureus, Haemophilus* sp., and pigmented *Prevotella* and *Porphyromonas* spp. *Bacteroides* sp. protected a penicillin-sensitive GABHS from penicillin therapy in mice. Both clindamycin and the combination of penicillin and clavulanic acid (a beta-lactamase inhibitor), which are active against both GABHS and gram-negative anaerobic bacilli eradicated the infection.

Several clinical studies demonstrated the superiority of lincomycin, clindamycin, and amoxicillin-clavulanic acid over penicillin. These antimicrobial agents are effective against aerobic as well as anaerobic BLPB and GABHS in eradicating recurrent tonsillar infection. However, no studies showed them to be superior to penicillin in treatment of acute tonsillitis. Other drugs that may also be effective in the therapy of recurrent or chronic tonsillitis are penicillin plus rifampin and a macrolide (e.g., erythromycin) plus metronidazole (see Table 3). Referral of a patient for tonsillectomy should be

Table 3 Oral Antimicrobials in Treatment of GABHS Tonsillitis

	ACUTE	RECURRENT CHRONIC	CARRIER STATE
First line	Penicillin (Amoxicillin)	Clindamycin Amoxicillin-clavulanate	Clindamycin Penicillin and rifampin
Second line	Cephalosporin*, clindamycin amoxicillin-clavulanate, macrolides†	Metronidazole and macrolide Penicillin and rifampin	

*First and second generation
†GABHS may be resistant

Table 4 Possible Reasons for Antibiotic Failure or Relapse in GABHS Tonsillitis

Beta-lactamase-producing oral microflora.
Resistance (e.g., erythromycin) or tolerance (e.g., penicillin) to antibiotic.
Lack of bacterial interference or production of bacteriocins by oral flora (generally by alpha-hemolytic streptococci).
Inappropriate dose, duration of therapy, or choice of antibiotic.
Poor compliance with medication regimen.
Reacquisition from close contact or vomit.
Carrier state, no disease.

considered only after these medical therapeutic modalities have failed.

Suggested Reading

Brook I. The role of beta-lactamase-producing bacteria in the persistence of streptococcal tonsillar infection. Rev Infect Dis 1984; 6:601–607.

Brook I. Treatment of recurrent tonsillitis, penicillin vs. amoxicillin plus clavulanic-potassium. J Antimicrob Chemother 1989; 24:221–233.

Brook I, Foote PA Jr, Slote J, Johnson W. Immune response to *Prevotella intermedia* in patients with recurrent non-streptococcal tonsillitis. Ann Otol Rhinol Laryngol 102:113–116, 1993.

Brook I, Yocum P, Foote PA Jr.: Changes in the core tonsillar bacteriology of recurrent tonsillitis: 1977–1993. *Clinical Infect Dis* 21:171–176, 1995.

Committee on the Prevention of Rheumatic Fever, Bacterial Endocarditis, and Kawasaki Disease of the American Heart Association. Prevention of bacterial endocarditis. Recommendations by the American Heart Association, JAMA 1991; 264:2919–2923.

Kaplan EL. The rapid identification of group A beta-hemolytic streptococci in the upper respiratory tract. Pediatr Clin North Am 1988; 35: 535–313.

Pichichero ME, Margolis PA. A comparison of cephalosporins and penicillins in the treatment of group A beta-hemolytic streptococcal pharyngitis: A meta-analysis supporting the concept of microbial copathogenicity. Pediatr Infect Dis J 1991; 10:275–281.

Roos K, Grahm E, Holm SE. Evaluation of beta-lactamase activity and microbial interference in treatment of acute streptococcal tonsillitis. Scand J Infect Dis 1986; 18:313–319.

SEPSIS, SIRS, AND SEPTIC SHOCK

Rodger D. MacArthur, M.D.
Roger C. Bone, M.D., Ph.D.(Hon), M.A.C.C.P., M.A.C.P.

Sepsis is the systemic response to infection. Septic shock occurs with significant hypotension in the presence of sepsis. These and other related terms and diagnostic criteria (Tables 1 and 2), were developed at a consensus conference sponsored by the American College of Chest Physicians and the Society for Critical Care Medicine in August 1991. The consensus conference recommended against using the term *septicemia* because it is ambiguous and used too often to imply bacteremia.

The clinical manifestations of sepsis are due to the body's inflammatory response to toxins and other components of micro-organisms. For example, infusion of endotoxin into humans is sufficient to initiate the cascade of inflammatory mediators seen in sepsis. Endotoxin is the lipoidal acylated glucosamine disaccharide core of the cell wall of many aerobic gram-negative bacteria. Known as lipid A, this moiety exhibits all of the hemodynamic and inflammatory characteristics associated with endotoxicity. Lipid A is highly conserved among the Enterobacteriaceae and to a lesser extent among the Pseudomonodaceae. Anaerobic gram-negative bacteria, such as *Bacteroides fragilis,* lack lipid A, perhaps explaining why sepsis is not commonly seen when infection is due solely to this anaerobe.

Cytokines and other immune modulators that are released in response to Lipid A and other bacterial products mediate the clinical manifestations of sepsis. Interleukin-(IL) 1 and other interleukins, tumor necrosis factor alpha (TNF-α), interferon gamma (IFN-γ), and several colony-stimulating factors are produced rapidly (minutes to hours) after the interaction of monocytes and macrophages with lipid A. Endotoxin prompts the release of TNF-α, IL-1, IL-6, IL-8, other interleukins, IFN-γ platelet activating factor (PAF) and several colony-stimulating factors from mononuclear phagocytes and other cells, including the endothelial cells themselves. Arachidonic acid is metabolized to form leukotrienes, thromboxane A_2, and prostaglandin E_2 (PGE_2) and prostaglandin I_2 (PGI_2). Endotoxin, TNF-α, PAF, leukotrienes, and thromboxane A_2 each increase the endothelial permeability. Endothelium, in turn, releases two additional substances, endothelium-derived relaxing factor (EDRF) and endothelin-1. These two substances counterbalance each other. EDRF relaxes smooth muscle and inhibits platelet aggregation, whereas endothelin-1 is a potent vasoconstrictor. Activation of the complement cascade (fragments C3a and C5a) and IL-8 release result in neutrophil activation.

A derivative of platelets, transforming growth factor β_1 and IL-4, IL-10, and IL-13 are activated and counteract the inflammatory effects of IL-1 and TNF-2. Other agents that may be part of the sepsis cascade include adhesion molecules, kinins, thrombin, myocardial depressant substance, beta-endorphin, and heat shock protein. Adhesion molecules and thrombin may help promote endothelial damage; interleukin-4, interleukin-8, and heat shock protein may protect against it.

While TNF-α appears to be a potent mediator of gram-

Table 1 Terminology and Definitions

Infection	A microbial phenomenon characterized by an inflammatory response to micro-organisms or the invasion of normally sterile host tissue by those organisms.
Bacteremia	Viable bacteria in the blood.
SIRS	Systemic inflammatory response syndrome, which follows a variety of severe clinical insults, including infection, pancreatitis, ischemia, multiple trauma and tissue injury, hemorrhagic shock, immune-mediated organ injury, and exogenous administration of inflammatory mediators such as TNF and other cytokines.
Sepsis	The systemic response to infection. This response is identical to SIRS except that it must result from infection.
Septic Shock	Sepsis with hypotension (systolic blood pressure <90 mm Hg or a reduction of >40 mm Hg from baseline) despite adequate fluid resuscitation, in conjunction with organ dysfunction and perfusion abnormalities (e.g., lactic acidosis, oliguria, obtundation), in the absence of other known causes.
MODS	Multiple organ dysfunction syndrome. Altered organ function in an acutely ill patient such that homeostasis cannot be maintained without intervention. Primary MODS is the direct result of a well-defined insult in which organ dysfunction occurs early and can be directly attributable to the insult itself. Secondary MODS is a consequence of a host response and is identified within the context of SIRS

Table 2 Numeric Criteria for SIRS*

Temperature	>38°C (100.4°F) or < 36°C (96.8°F)
Heart Rate	>90 beats/min
Respiratory Rate	>20 breaths/min or $PaCO_2$ < 32 mm Hg
White Blood Cells	>12,000 cells/μl or < 4,000 cells/μl or >10% immature (band) forms

*Two or more are required to establish the diagnosis. These changes represent acute alterations from baseline in the absence of other known causes of the abnormalities.

negative sepsis, many other immune modulators interact with TNF-α, host defense mechanisms, and bacterial pathogens in very complex ways. IL-6 often is elevated in sepsis and may serve to down-regulate IL-1 and TNF-α. IL-8 is a chemotactic and activating factor for neutrophils. IL-10 acts on macrophages to down-regulate IL-1 and TNF-α release. Paradoxically, low doses of TNF-α and IL-1 appear to be protective against subsequent bacterial challenge. Finally, host tissue injury may not be a result of cytokine release per se but may occur through cytokine-stimulated production of nitric oxide. Recently, the term "compensatory anti-inflammatory response syndrome" (CARS) has been used to refer to the persistent release of anti-inflammatory mediators which occurs in response to SIRS. If balance between the bio-inflammatory and the anti-inflammatory cytokines cannot be restored, the result is a state of immunologic dissonance from which the patient typically does not recover.

Sepsis caused by gram-positive organisms is clinically identical to sepsis caused by gram-negative organisms. Gram-positive organisms initiate sepsis by at least two mechanisms. Components of the gram-positive cell wall, such as peptidoglycan, teichoic acids, and surface proteins, have a variety of effects on the host immune system. Both peptidoglycan and teichoic acid can activate the alternate complement pathway. Peptidoglycan precursors and staphylococcal lipoteichoic acids can stimulate IL-1 release from human monocytes. In addition, some investigators have shown that lipoteichoic acids from many gram-positive organisms elicit the release of TNF-α and IL-6. The second way in which gram-positive organisms initiate the inflammatory cascade is by the release of various toxins. For example, the *Staphylococcus aureus* toxin, toxic shock syndrome toxin 1 (TSST-1), is a more potent stimulator of IL-1 release from human monocytes than is lipid A. Various other gram-positive exotoxins and enterotoxins stimulate the release of TNF-α, IL-6, and arachidonate metabolites implicated in the pathophysiology of sepsis.

Historically, antibiotic recommendations for therapy of sepsis and septic shock were based primarily on coverage of gram-negative organisms. The incidence of gram-negative infections, especially nosocomial bacteremias, increased dramatically in the 1950s and 1960s as bacteria became resistant to the antibiotics available at that time and advances in critical care medicine resulted in severely ill and injured patients surviving after prolonged hospitalizations. In addition, early research on sepsis focused on the role of endotoxin, perhaps because lipid A was relatively easy to purify and inject.

During the 1970s and 1980s the incidence of nosocomial infections due to gram-positive organisms began to increase. In 1984 the Centers for Disease Control (CDC) reported that gram-positive infections were responsible for fewer than 30 percent of all nosocomial infections, although they caused 37 percent of all bacteremias. Coagulase-negative staphylococci (e.g., *Staphylococcus epidermidis*) were the most frequently isolated organisms from blood. In 1989 the CDC reported that gram-positive organisms were found in at least 55 percent of all cases of nosocomial bacteremia. Coagulase-negative staphylococci were found in 27 percent of bacteremias.

The incidence of gram-negative nosocomial bacteremias did not decrease in the 1980s concurrent with the increase in gram-positive nosocomial bacteremias. In fact, *Escherichia coli*, *Enterobacter* species, and *Pseudomonas aeruginosa* were the fourth, fifth, and sixth leading causes of nosocomial bacteremias in the mid to late 1980s. Consequently, the total number of cases of nosocomial bacteremias had increased dramatically by 1989, to around 500,000 cases per year in the United States alone.

It is likely that the 1990s will see further increases in the number of cases of nosocomial bacteremias. Many will be due to organisms resistant to commonly used antibiotics, such as *S. epidermidis* (often in association with long-term indwelling venous catheters), methicillin-resistant *S. aureus*, enterococci, *Enterobacter* species, *P. aeruginosa*, and *Candida* species. It should be noted that resistant nosocomial bacteria typically

Table 3 Special Circumstances of Septic Patients

CIRCUMSTANCE	POSSIBLE PATHOGENS
Splenectomy, traumatic or functional	*S. pneumoniae, Haemophilus influenzae, Neisseria meningitidis*
Neutropenia (<500 neutrophils/µl)	Gram-negatives, including *P. aeruginosa;* gram-positives, including *S. aureus;* fungi, especially *Candida* species
Hypogammaglobulinemia (e.g., chronic lymphocytic leukemia)	*S. pneumoniae, E. coli*
Burns	*S. aureus* (methicillin resistant), *P. aeruginosa,* restraint gram-negatives
AIDS	*P. aeruginosa, S. pneumoniae, P. carinii* (pneumonia)
Intravascular devices	*S. aureus, S. epidermidis*
Nosocomial infections	*S. aureus* (methicillin resistant), *Enterococcus* species, resistant gram-negatives, *Candida* species

are resistant to several antibiotics, making therapy even more difficult. Sepsis caused by community-acquired organisms such as *E. coli* and *Streptococcus pneumoniae* will continue to show clinical manifestations similar to those of nosocomially acquired sepsis. Finally, sepsis and bacteremia are not synonymous. Only a minority of patients with sepsis have bacteremia, and some bacteremic patients have no clinical manifestations of sepsis.

DIAGNOSIS

Sepsis should be considered whenever a patient meets the numeric criteria for sepsis and the systemic inflammatory response syndrome (SIRS) (see Table 2). Unfortunately, no bedside tests quickly and reliably differentiate infectious causes of SIRS from noninfectious causes. Furthermore, the mortality from septic shock or sepsis with the multiple organ dysfunction syndrome (MODS; see Table 2) is between 20 and 50 percent. Consequently, prompt empiric administration of antibiotics is appropriate in most situations. However, every effort should be made to diagnose the precise cause of sepsis. Often, various underlying risk factors predispose individuals to infection with specific organisms. Some of these conditions and associated pathogens are listed in Table 3. (See also the chapters on these conditions.) A thorough history and physical examination are crucial to the diagnosis of sepsis; their importance cannot be overemphasized. Several cultures from several sites must be obtained whenever infection is suspected. All culture material must be delivered promptly to the microbiology laboratory. Gram stains should be made and read as soon as possible on all specimens submitted for culture. Ideally, cultures should be obtained prior to the initiation of antibiotics. However, the administration of antibiotics should not be delayed by more than 10 to 20 minutes for patients who are clinically or hemodynamically unstable.

At least two sets of blood cultures, drawn from different sites, should be obtained from all patients suspected of having sepsis. Each blood culture set consists of one aerobic and one anaerobic bottle. At least 7 to 10 ml of blood must be injected into each bottle. A culture bottle containing an antibiotic binding resin or other antibiotic binding substance should be included with each culture set for patients who are receiving antibiotics at the time of evaluation. If an indwelling venous or arterial catheter is present, it may be helpful to obtain additional cultures through each port of the device.

Sputum for culture can be spontaneously expectorated, induced with 3 percent saline, or obtained by nasotracheal, endotracheal, or transtracheal techniques. Specimens should have fewer than 25 squamous epithelial cells per low-power (100×) microscopic field to decrease the chance that the specimen is contaminated with upper airway flora. However, contamination can occur even with the best techniques. Clinical judgment often is necessary to differentiate between contamination and colonization and true infection.

Urine should be obtained for culture whenever possible. Clean-catch specimens are preferred. Urine that has been in a closed collection system for more than an hour should not be sent for culture. If necessary, urine can be obtained directly from the catheter tubing or bladder (suprapubic aspiration) using a syringe and a small-gauge needle.

Many bacteriuric patients, especially those with indwelling urinary catheters, may have sepsis from another source. While the presence of more than 100,000 bacteria on culture suggests infection, this criterion has been validated only for ambulatory young adults with gram-negative bacillary organisms.

Cultures from other sites should be obtained if clinically indicated. Computed tomography scans of the abdomen and sinuses often reveal previously overlooked fluid collections that may be accessible by needle aspiration. All patients with diarrhea should have stool sent for culture and for a cytotoxic assay for *Clostridium difficile* toxin. Ultrasonography is useful for detecting ascites and biliary, hepatic, and pancreatic pathology. A portable (bedside) ultrasound can be used with critically ill patients who are too unstable to be transported to the radiology department. A lumbar puncture for cell count, protein, glucose, bacterial antigens, and culture should be performed on any septic patient with unexplained altered mentation.

THERAPY

Antibiotics form the cornerstone of therapy for sepsis. Most authorities believe that outcome is improved if the diagnosis is suspected early and appropriate antibiotics are started without delay. In addition, appropriate surgical intervention often is as important as the initial choice of antibiotics. Recommendations for specific antibiotics are listed in Table 4. Although some antibiotics administered orally achieve good serum and tissue levels, septic hospitalized patients initially should receive intravenous antibiotics to optimize serum and tissue levels and to ensure absorption.

The duration of therapy depends upon the clinical response and occasionally the infecting pathogen. A typical course of antibiotics is given for 7 to 14 days. A good rule of thumb is to administer the antibiotics for 3 days beyond the

Table 4 Recommended Initial Antibiotic Regimens for Septic Patients with Normal Renal Function

CLINICAL SITUATION	REGIMEN
Empiric coverage	Vancomycin 1g q12h + tobramycin 2–3 mg/kg q8h
Community-acquired pneumonia	Cefuroxime 1.5g q8h + erythromycin 500 mg q6h
Community-acquired urosepsis	Piperacillin 2g q8h + tobramycin 2–3 mg/kg q8h
Nosocomial infections or burns or neutropenia	Vancomycin 1g q12h + tobramycin 2–3 mg/kg q8h + 1 of the following: Piperacillin 3g q6–8h, ceftazidime 2g q8h, imipenem 750 mg q6–8h, Ciprofloxacin 400/mg q12h, ticarcillin/clavulanate 3.1g q6h, piperacillin/tazobactam 3.375 gQ6°
HIV with pneumonia	Trimethoprim-sulfamethoxazole 5 mg/kg q6h or pentamidine 4 mg/kg q24h Either one with erythromycin 500 mg q6h Add prednisone for room air Po_2 <70 mm Hg

Amikacin at 8–10 mg/kg q12h can be substituted for tobramycin at institutions with significant bacterial resistance to tobramycin. Tobramycin can be dosed at 5 mg/kg/d and amikacin dosed at 15–20 mg/kg/d without apparent increased toxicity in recent studies.

point at which the patient becomes afebrile or has normalization of laboratory values. The total course should rarely be less than 7 days. There are some important exceptions:

1. Neutropenic (absolute neutrophil count below 500 cells/µl) patients should receive 14 days of antibiotic therapy. This is a compromise between stopping antibiotics shortly after the patient becomes afebrile and continuing the antibiotics for the entire duration of neutropenia. If a previously febrile neutropenic patient becomes afebrile and is no longer neutropenic, a shorter course of antibiotic therapy can be considered.
2. Patients with *S. aureus* bacteremia should receive at least 21 to 28 days of antibiotics.
3. Patients with *P. carinii* pneumonia should receive 14 to 21 days of therapy. At least 7 days of intravenous therapy is standard.

The persistently febrile neutropenic patient represents an especially challenging problem. Intravenous amphotericin B 0.5–0.8 mg per kilogram per day should be started if fever persists despite broad-spectrum antibiotic coverage for more than 5 to 7 days. Liposome-encapsulated preparations or intralipid added to amphotericin B infusions may decrease the number and severity of side effects, but these approaches have not been compared with standard amphotericin B infusions in large clinical trials. Although the optimal duration of therapy is unknown, it is prudent to continue antifungal therapy at least as long as neutropenia exists or to a minimum total dose of 500 mg. The imidazole derivatives—ketoconazole, fluconazole, and itraconazole—show promise but cannot be recommended in place of amphotericin B at this time.

Isolation of *Candida* species from sputum, urine, stool, or drainage fluid is not necessarily synonymous with infection. On the other hand, isolation of *Candida* species from three or more nonblood sites has been shown to correlate with disseminated candidiasis in neutropenic patients. Isolation of this organism from the blood of any patient is always significant and requires immediate therapy. Isolation of *Candida* species from catheter tips usually warrants at least a short course of therapy, even though the catheter has been removed. Any macronodular skin lesions shown on biopsy to be consistent with candidal infection is tantamount to dissemination.

The combination of vancomycin and tobramycin will suffice for initial empiric coverage in most situations. It covers the majority of aerobic pathogens likely to cause sepsis, including methicillin-resistant *Staphylococcus* species and resistant gram-negative organisms. Sepsis due to anaerobic organisms is considerably less common. While both vancomycin and tobramycin are potentially nephrotoxic, several days of empiric therapy pending culture results are unlikely to cause significant or irreversible damage. Less nephrotoxic agents typically do not cover as many nosocomial organisms as does the combination of vancomycin and tobramycin.

While most antibiotics are given in doses sufficient to result in sustained serum levels well above those necessary to kill infecting pathogens, aminoglycosides are an exception. Because of concerns about nephrotoxicity, aminoglycosides typically are underdosed. This problem is compounded by the relatively poor penetration of aminoglycosides into abscesses and lung parenchyma. The doses listed in Table 4 should yield appropriate serum levels in most cases.

There is increasing concern about antibiotic resistance among bacteria, perhaps exacerbated by inappropriate empiric antibiotic use. For instance, *Enterobacter* species (e.g., *E. cloacae* and *E. aerogenes*) develop resistance to the cephalosporins very rapidly after exposure, by increasing by 100- to 1,000-fold their production of beta-lactamases. For this reason the use of cephalosporins is discouraged when these organisms are isolated. Many hospitals are reporting substantial rates of penicillin and second-generation cephalosporin tolerant strains of streprococcus pneumoniae. The third generation cephalosporin cefotaxime still works well against this organism for all infections other than meningitis. The only antibiotic with reliable activity against the pneumococcus with high-level penicillin resistance is vancomylin. It also should be noted that ampicillin- and piperacillin-resistant enteroccoci are common, and vancomycin resistant enteroccoci also are seen with increasing frequency. Unfortunately, the use of multiple antibiotics has not decreased the development of resistance by bacteria to certain classes of antibiotics. Antibiotics such as vancomycin and the aminoglycosides, on the other hand, have maintained effectiveness against many bacteria despite years of widespread use.

Septic patients have increased fluid and electrolyte needs, and close attention should be paid to this aspect of their care. It is crucial that adequate perfusion of vital organs be maintained. The insertion of pressure-monitoring devices, such as

Swan-Ganz catheters, often is very useful. Sympathomimetic amines, such as dopamine at doses of 2 to 25 μg per kilogram per minute, help to maintain adequate perfusion pressures. Intubation and mechanical ventilation may be necessary in patients with pneumonia or acute respiratory distress syndrome.

Other therapeutic approaches to sepsis and septic shock have included attempts to lessen the sequelae of SIRS by modifying the inflammatory response. None of these attempts have been successful. The largest controlled trial of methylprednisolone for severe sepsis and septic shock, published in 1987, failed to demonstrate any efficacy of that agent. Several large, well-controlled trials have failed to demonstrate any efficacy of monoclonal antibodies directed against lipid A and other components of the gram-negative bacterial cell wall. Anti-TNF-α antibodies also have not been shown to improve survival. Trials with other anti-TNF-α antibodies and modulators of TNF-α (e.g., pentoxyfylline) are ongoing. Trials of other products, such as granulocyte macrophage-colony-stimulating factor (GM-CSF), also are being planned.

Sepsis is complex, involving many mediators that we just now are starting to appreciate. Attempts to improve survival by counteracting just one mediator of the syndrome likely will continue to fail. The search for a magic bullet may be ill-advised at present. Better identification of the subset of patients likely to benefit from these products is necessary, as are rapid diagnostic assays for endotoxin, tumor necrosis factor, and various cytokines. For now, we must continue to improve patient survival by aggressively diagnosing the cause of sepsis and treating the manifestations of sepsis with antibiotics, fluids, vasoactive drugs, and surgical intervention when indicated.

Suggested Reading

American College of Chest Physicians/Society of Critical Care Medicine Consensus Conference Committee. Definitions for sepsis and organ failure and guidelines for the use of innovative therapies in sepsis. Crit Care Med 1992; 20:864–874.

Bone RC. Toward an epidemiology and natural history of SIRS (systemic inflammatory response syndrome). JAMA 1992; 268:3452–3455.

Bone RC. Sepsis syndrome: New insights into its pathogenesis and treatment. Infect Dis Clin North Am 1991; 5:793–805.

Bone RC. The pathogenesis of sepsis. Ann Intern Med 1991; 115:457–469.

Bone RC. Why sepsis trims fail. JAMA 1996; 276:565–566.

Bone RC. Immunologic dissonance: a continuing evolution in our understanding of the systematic inflammatory response syndrome (SIRS) and the multiple organ dysfunction syndrome (MODS). Ann Intern Med 1996; 125:680–687.

Natanson C, Hoffman WD, Suffredini AF, et al. Selected treatment strategies for septic shock based on proposed mechanisms of pathogenesis. Ann Intern Med 1994; 120:771–783.

Parker MM, Parillo JE. Septic shock: Hemodynamics and pathogenesis. JAMA 1983; 250:3324–3327.

Rangle-Frausto MS, Pittet D, Costigan M, et al. The natural history of the systemic inflammatory response syndrome (SIRS). A Prospective study. JAMA 1995; 273:117–123.

Young LS. Sepsis syndrome. In: Mandell GL, Bennett JE, Dolin R, eds. Principles and practice of infectious diseases. 4th ed. New York: Churchill Livingstone, 1995:690.

SINUSITIS

Andrew M. Shapiro, M.D.
Charles D. Bluestone, M.D.

Sinusitis is among the most common conditions confronting physicians, and yet diagnostic criteria remain elusive, therapy is not standardized, and misconceptions regarding prognosis remain. The approach to this disease should be individualized to account for the duration and severity of symptoms, the patient's age, the status of the immune system, and the presence of any complications.

Sinusitis usually develops because of impaired clearance of secretions resulting from obstruction of the sinus ostia by inflammation or anatomic abnormalities, increased viscosity of secretions, or disturbances in ciliary function. These conditions allow an overgrowth of pathogenic bacteria within the sinuses (Table 1). Less commonly, direct inoculation of bacteria into the sinuses may occur secondary to a dental infection or during swimming. The bacteriology of sinusitis in both children and adults has been demonstrated in a number of studies (Table 2). Patients with diabetes, uremia, or compromised immune function may be at risk for infection with unusual bacteria or invasive fungi. Patients who develop nosocomial sinusitis associated with endotracheal or gastric tubes are at risk for infection with the resident hospital flora, which is often resistant.

Table 1 Risk Factors for Sinusitis

INFLAMMATORY
Viral upper respiratory infection
Allergy
ANATOMIC
Nasal septal deformity
Concha bullosa
Hypoplastic sinus
Polyps
Foreign bodies, including endotracheal and gastric tubes
SYSTEMIC DISEASE
Immunodeficiency
Cystic fibrosis
Ciliary dyskinesia
Down syndrome

Table 2 Causative Organisms of Sinusitis

	PERCENT OF ADULT CASES BY SINUS ASPIRATE	
	ACUTE	CHRONIC
BACTERIA		
Streptococcus pneumoniae	40	7
Haemophilus influenzae	30	10
Moraxella catarrhalis	7	—
Anaerobic bacteria	8	50–100
Staphylococcus aureus	3	17
Streptococcus pyogenes	3	—
α-hemolytic streptococci	3	15
Gram-negative bacteria	—	5
VIRUSES		
Rhinovirus		
Influenza virus		
Parainfluenza virus		
Adenovirus		

Adapted from Evans FO, Syndor JB, Moore WEC, et al. Sinusitis of the maxillary antrum. N Engl J Med 1975; 293:735–739.

■ DIAGNOSIS

The diagnosis of sinusitis is based on a constellation of historical and physical findings, supported by radiologic imaging, and in selected cases, aspiration of sinus contents. It is essential but often difficult to differentiate the symptoms of a routine viral upper respiratory infection from sinusitis. Common complaints, such as purulent rhinorrhea, nasal congestion, cough, and headache, may reflect either disorder. Although pain localized to a sinus or maxillary toothache may be more specific for sinusitis, these complaints are less frequently encountered. Physical examination should include a search for purulent secretions originating from the sinus ostia, nasal polyps, deviated nasal septum, and tenderness to sinus palpation. Anterior rhinoscopy, which may be inadequate, may be supplemented by endoscopic intranasal examination. Transillumination of the sinuses may be helpful in adults when complete opacification or normal transillumination is present; however, this technique is unreliable when used in children, patients with ethmoid sinusitis, or when other sinus pathology (tumors, hypoplasia) may exist.

Plain sinus films may help to confirm the diagnosis when acute sinusitis is suspected, but they are not required. In contrast, the diagnosis of chronic sinusitis based on clinical suspicion should always be confirmed with coronal computed tomographic (CT) scans of the sinuses. It is particularly important that this study be obtained only after an appropriate course of therapy (see next section) so that the resultant images reflect the location and extent of persistent disease and may serve as a road map if surgical intervention is required. CT scans are also essential when complications are present.

■ THERAPY

The treatment of acute sinusitis should be based on improvement of sinus ventilation and appropriate antimicrobial therapy. Topical decongestants (Table 3) may reduce mucosal edema, resulting in improved drainage and symptomatic relief. However, there is evidence that these agents produce ciliary dysfunction, and usage longer than a week may lead to persistent mucosal congestion. Systemic decongestants and mucolytic agents may also provide benefit. Antihistamines should not be used for acute sinusitis because they tend to increase the viscosity of sinus secretions and impair drainage.

Antimicrobial therapy for uncomplicated acute sinusitis may be initiated on an empiric basis with an oral agent effective against the common causative organisms (Table 4). Amoxicillin is a good first choice with proven efficacy, safety, and reasonable cost. Significant improvement in symptoms within 48 to 72 hours should be expected. If symptoms persist, an antibiotic with beta-lactamase resistance, for example amoxicillin-clavulanate, cefuroxime axetil, or trimethoprim with sulfamethoxazole (TMP-SMX), should be prescribed. Two weeks of therapy should be sufficient. Severe or persistent symptoms following a trial of antimicrobial therapy warrants

Table 3 Adjunctive Therapy of Sinusitis

Decongestants
- Topical
  - Oxymetazoline
- Systemic
  - Pseudoephedrine
  - Phenylpropylamine

Mucolytic Agents
- Guaifenesin
- Organic iodides

Humidifers and Irrigants
- Saline
- Steam

Glucocorticoids
- Topical
  - Beclomethasone 2 puffs both nares b.i.d.
  - Flunisolide 2 sprays both nares b.i.d.
  - Triamcinolone 2 sprays once daily
- Systemic

Antihistamines (allergic patients)
- Sedating
- Nonsedating
  - Terfenadine 60 mg PO b.i.d.
  - Astemizole 10 mg PO daily
- Topical-Cromolyn

Immunotherapy
- Removal of endotracheal or gastric tube

Table 4 Antimicrobial Therapy for Sinusitis

FIRST LINE	
Amoxicillin	500 mg q8h
Trimethoprim with sulfamethoxazole 160/800 (Bactrim, Septra)	1 tab q12h
SECOND LINE	
Amoxicillin-clavulanate (Augmentin)	500 mg q8h
Cefuroxime axetil (Ceftin)	250 mg q12h
Loracarbef (Lorabid)	200 mg q12h
Cefpodoxime proxetil (Vantin)	200 mg q12h
Cefprozil (Cefzil)	500 mg q12h
Clarithromycin (Biaxin)	500 mg q12h
Azithromycin (Zithromax)	250 mg qd

aspiration of maxillary sinus contents for identification of the causative organism, particularly in light of the emergence of resistant organisms.

Chronic sinusitis may be arbitrarily defined as inflammation of the sinuses persisting beyond 90 days. It is a common misconception that chronic sinusitis represents irreversible mucosal disease for which no treatment is available. Decongestants and nasal irrigations often provide symptomatic relief. Antibiotic coverage for anaerobes and *Staphylococcus aureus* is often effective, so the agents used for second-line therapy of acute sinusitis can be used. Although not established in clinical trials, a course longer than the routine 10 days is probably beneficial in chronic sinusitis; frequently the treatment is continued for approximately 4 weeks. Furthermore, the management of chronic sinusitis must account for the underlying risk factors. Anatomic abnormalities such as a deviated nasal septum or concha bullosa may require correction. Allergies should be considered; therapy with antihistamines and topical nasal steroids or cromolyn is often effective. Testing for specific irritants followed by desensitization may be beneficial to selected patients. The possibility of immune dysfunction, cystic fibrosis, or ciliary dyskinesia should be considered, particularly in children.

Patients with chronic sinusitis or recurrent acute sinusitis who have failed aggressive medical management are candidates for surgery. Today paranasal sinus surgery emphasizes the restoration of normal physiology by addressing the anatomic features that contribute to impaired sinus drainage. In particular these techniques stress the importance of the ostiomeatal complex and the ethmoid sinuses, in contrast to traditional techniques focusing on the maxillary sinuses. The procedures are generally safe, well tolerated, and associated with satisfaction rates more than 80 percent.

■ FUNGAL INFECTIONS

Fungal infections of the sinuses generally present in one of three patterns. Noninvasive fungal sinusitis occurs in patients with chronic sinusitis who have failed to improve on long courses of oral antibiotic therapy. Allergic fungal sinusitis occurs in patients with symptoms of atopy, often with nasal polyps. Finally, invasive fungal infections occur in immunocompromised hosts, typically debilitated diabetic or oncologic patients. This disease is often fatal. The management of fungal sinusitis is typically surgical, followed by systemic antifungal agents in cases of invasion.

■ COMPLICATIONS

Complications of sinusitis are usually associated with acute infections of the ethmoid and frontal sinus, typically involving the orbit or intracranial space. Aspiration of the sinus for culture, intravenous antibiotic therapy, and surgical drainage form the basis of therapy.

Suggested Reading

Williams JW, Simel DL, Roberts MD, Samsa GP. Clinical evaluation for sinusitis. Ann Intern Med 1992; 117:705–710.

Winther B, Gwaltney JM. Therapeutic approach to sinusitis: Anti-infectious therapy as the baseline of management. Otolaryngol Head Neck Surg 1990; 103(Suppl):876–878.

URETHRITIS AND DYSURIA

William R. Bowie, M.D., F.R.C.P.C.

Dysuria, or burning on urination, strongly suggests urethritis or cystitis but can be associated with other infectious and noninfectious diseases. Management differs between genders, but most individuals with acute or recent onset of dysuria can be managed appropriately when they are first seen.

■ DYSURIA IN FEMALE PATIENTS

Management of dysuria in women is particularly complicated because of the overlap in symptoms of urinary tract infection (UTI) and sexually transmitted diseases (STD). The distinction is helped by differentiation of internal dysuria, in which discomfort is perceived as urine passes through the urethra, from external dysuria, in which the discomfort is felt as urine passes over the meatal or introital region. Internal dysuria strongly suggests urethritis or cystitis due to classical urinary tract pathogens or less frequently STD such as *Chlamydia trachomatis, Neisseria gonorrhoeae,* or herpes simplex virus. UTI is further suggested by acute onset of frequency, hematuria, nocturia, urgency, incontinence, suprapubic or pelvic discomfort, and possibly fever and flank pain. In a third of these no UTI is present, and about half of this subset has an STD. When a UTI is considered in a woman, initial treatment decisions depend on making the distinction between uncomplicated and complicated UTI.

External dysuria is strongly suggestive of vulvovaginitis, most often due to infection with herpes simplex virus, yeasts, or *Trichomonas vaginalis.* Vaginitis or vulvovaginitis is further suggested by a new or changed vaginal discharge, vaginal odor, itch, and genital edema, erythema, or lesions, particularly after intercourse with a new sexual partner. The differentiation can often be strongly suggested by history, but it may require examination and microbiologic testing, and some women have UTI and STD. Presentations of STD in women are discussed in the chapter *Vaginitis and Cervicitis.*

Uncomplicated Urinary Tract Infection

Uncomplicated UTI mainly occurs in otherwise healthy women with structurally normal urinary tracts and normal voiding mechanisms. There is usually only a single organism isolated, and infection responds readily to antimicrobials to which the pathogen is susceptible. Initial treatment should be a short course. Single-dose therapy has been extensively evaluated, but recommended empiric therapy for uncomplicated infection is 3 days of therapy with trimethoprim-sulfamethoxazole (TMP-SMX), 160 mg and 800 mg twice a day, trimethoprim 100 mg twice a day, or nitrofurantoin 100 mg four times a day. These regimens are as effective as longer courses and more effective than single-dose therapy. Treatment with more than 3 days of TMP-SMX results in increased adverse drug reactions. For ampicillin or amoxicillin, 5 days of therapy is more effective than single-dose or 3 day regimens.

Complicated Urinary Tract Infection

With complicated UTI there is usually a structural or functional abnormality or underlying disease. It is typically associated with more resistant organisms and several pathogens, and it responds less well to treatment. The major goal of treatment is to correct or ameliorate the underlying anatomic or physiologic problem. The duration of treatment depends on the underlying cause. In some cases no treatment is to be preferred. Choice of anti-infective agent depends on the microbiology.

Upper Tract Infection

The most useful guide to diagnosis of upper tract infection is clinical: fever, flank and/or low back pain, systemic symptoms, pyuria, and bacteriuria in conjunction with dysuria and related symptoms. Treatment of acute uncomplicated pyelonephritis may be with an oral or parenteral regimen, depending upon the severity, and on any nausea, vomiting, or ileus. TMP-SMX is highly effective and more reliable than ampicillin or amoxicillin. Other agents, such as aminoglycosides, cephalosporins, expanded spectrum penicillins, and quinolones, can be used initially with results modified according to the susceptibility pattern. The usual total duration of therapy is no more than 2 weeks.

Recurrent Urinary Tract Infection

When women have frequent episodes of proven infections (three or more per year), other approaches can be used for their management. The first option is to allow self-treatment at the onset of typical symptoms. A second option is to use long-term (6 or more months) therapy with half a tablet of trimethoprim or nitrofurantoin at bedtime on a daily basis or a full dose three times per week. When infection is temporally related to sexual intercourse, a third option is to take a dose just before or after sexual intercourse.

■ DYSURIA IN MALE PATIENTS

Acute onset of dysuria in male patients strongly suggests urethritis and is usually associated with urethral discharge, the classical sign of urethritis in men. An itch in the meatus or distal urethra is also frequently present. Urethral discharge may be apparent or hard to detect. Urethral secretions show increased numbers of polymorphonuclear leukocytes (PMN). The most important causes of urethritis in men are *C. trachomatis* and *N. gonorrhoeae.* Diagnosis of urethritis and microbiologic detection of *C. trachomatis* and *N. gonorrhoeae* are not synonymous. Infection can be present without evident urethral inflammation, and there are other causes of urethritis.

Causes and Changing Epidemiology

Gonorrhea or gonococcal urethritis is diagnosed when *N. gonorrhoeae* is detected, usually by Gram stain or culture. Approximately 20 to 30 percent of those with gonococcal urethritis have concurrent infection with *C. trachomatis.* Nongonococcal urethritis (NGU) is diagnosed in men with increased numbers of PMN in urethral secretions where *N. gonorrhoeae* is not detected. *C. trachomatis* is the most important cause of NGU, but whereas in the 1970s it was recovered from 30 to 50 percent of cases, it is now recovered in 15 to 25 percent of cases. A less important but frequent cause of NGU is *Ureaplasma urealyticum.* However, in many men neither organism is detected. In most of these cases the cause is not apparent, but infrequently *Trichomonas vaginalis* and herpes simplex virus are detected.

In developed countries NGU is many times more frequent than gonococcal urethritis. The reported number of cases of infection with *N. gonorrhoeae* has fallen in almost all areas. However, the proportion of cases of *N. gonorrhoeae* due to isolates resistant to penicillin and tetracycline has reached such levels that neither is recommended for treatment of gonorrhea because of unacceptable rates of failure.

Clinical and Laboratory Diagnosis

Detection of urethritis is usually straightforward. When examined under optimal conditions, most men with the onset of new symptoms of dysuria or urethral discharge will have objective evidence of urethritis (increased numbers of PMN in urethral secretions detected by a Gram stain or in first voided urine). Of those with symptoms, most will also have a detectable urethral discharge. The more pronounced the discharge and the more acute the symptoms, the greater the likelihood of gonorrhea. Despite these differences, distinguishing between gonorrhea and NGU in a specific patient requires laboratory evaluation.

Strictly speaking, all that is required to detect urethritis is documentation of increased numbers of PMN. However, specimens should usually be taken for detection of *N. gonorrhoeae,* preferably by culture, and for detection of *C. trachomatis.* Routine initial evaluation for *U. urealyticum* and other less usual causes is not indicated. Absence of symptoms does not exclude urethral infection. Symptomatic men who do not have urethritis documented at an initial visit should be re-evaluated, preferably when they have not voided overnight but at least when they have not voided for 4 or more hours.

Therapy at Initial Presentation

Urethritis is readily managed on a syndromic basis. This allows a rational choice of therapy, treatment at the time the man is seen, and initiation of efforts to ensure diagnosis and treatment of sexual partners. The key determinants for choice of the specific therapy are whether or not urethritis is documented and whether or not infection with *N. gonorrhoeae* has been excluded.

Regimens for Neisseria Gonorrhoeae

Treatment for proven or suspected gonorrhea has become more complex because of the recognition of the high prevalence of concurrent infection with *C. trachomatis* and of increasing resistance of *N. gonorrhoeae* to both penicillins and tetracyclines. Penicillins can no longer be relied on to treat gonorrhea. However, many newer agents provide safe and effective coverage. Recommended are a single injection of ceftriaxone 125 mg rather than the previously recommended dose of 250 mg or a single oral dose of cefixime 400 mg, ciprofloxacin 500 mg, or ofloxacin 400 mg. All are followed by an appropriate (usually doxycycline) regimen active against *C. trachomatis.* Quinolones are not recommended for patients under age 17. (See the chapter *Neisseria gonorrhoeae* for more details of therapy.)

Regimens for Chlamydia Trachomatis and Nonchlamydial, Nongonococcal Urethritis

Doxycycline 100 mg orally twice daily for 7 days is recommended. Because generic doxycycline is now sufficiently inexpensive, tetracycline hydrochloride is no longer recommended. The alternative recommended regimen is erythromycin in doses comparable to 500 mg of base orally four times daily for 7 days. For children under 9, erythromycins in appropriate doses are recommended.

Azithromycin as a single dose of 1 g orally is recommended for treatment of *C. trachomatis* but was not recommended by the CDC for treatment of NGU or for use in conjunction with a single-dose regimen active against *N. gonorrhoeae.* However, there is increasing evidence that azithromycin is effective for treatment of NGU. The single oral dose with azithromycin has considerable appeal because its administration is assumed to result in 100 percent compliance. Cost remains an impediment, although cost-effectiveness studies support its use in high-risk settings. Few data are available on the tolerability of azithromycin used in conjunction with single-dose regimens active against *N. gonorrhoeae,* so it is not recommended.

Ofloxacin 300 mg orally twice daily for 7 days is also recommended for treatment of NGU and is active against *N. gonorrhoeae,* but it is much more expensive and has no significant advantages over other regimens.

Expected Microbiologic Outcomes

When recommended regimens are used as prescribed and men are not exposed to new or untreated partners, persistence of *N. gonorrhoeae* and *C. trachomatis* is so unusual that routine diagnostic tests of cure evaluations are not recommended. Positive tests post treatment usually indicate reinfection from an inadequately treated or new sexual partner, poor compliance, or false-positive results. This situation may change with the increasing detection of isolates of *N. gonorrhoeae* demonstrating in vitro resistance to fluoroquinolones.

Therapy when Symptoms Continue

Almost all men with gonorrhea will improve and remain clinically cured. In contrast, although over 95 percent of men with NGU will initially improve, up to one-third will have symptoms that recur or fail to resolve entirely. In the small group who show no improvement, infection with *T. vaginalis,* herpes simplex virus, or tetracycline-resistant isolates of *U. urealyticum* account for approximately half of infections. In the larger group who show initial improvement, a small proportion may be due to infection with *U. urealyticum,* but in the vast majority no cause is apparent.

Management is complicated by the persistence of symptoms in some men without objective evidence of urethritis and increased numbers of PMN in others without symptoms. Clear or mucoid urethral discharge at follow-up is not necessarily abnormal. This type of discharge or symptoms of dysuria or an itch in the absence of a PMN response does not constitute failure. For men who have documented persistent or recurrent urethritis in whom no apparent cause is detected, recommended treatment is erythromycin 500 mg orally four times daily for 2 weeks if a tetracycline was used initially. Alternatively, doxycycline 100 mg orally twice daily for 2 weeks seems reasonable, particularly if azithromycin or erythromycin had been used initially. However, no studies have conclusively shown that such an approach expedites recovery.

Most men will again improve with use of the second regimen, but approximately one-third will have symptoms that recur or incompletely resolve. At this point further antimicrobial therapy does not appear warranted. There is also little benefit from conducting urologic investigations unless there are other indications to do so. Because many of these men have additional concerns, a careful explanation of the frequency of residual minimal urethritis and the apparent absence of long-term physical consequences to the patient and any partners is often beneficial in allaying concerns.

Treatment of Partners

Recommendations for detection and initial treatment of urethritis are aggressive, mainly to decrease consequences for women. Men can have infection with *N. gonorrhoeae* or *C. trachomatis* for long periods with little risk of significant sequelae. Fewer than 1 percent will develop epididymitis, and even this is unlikely to result in sterility. In contrast, a high proportion of women who are infected with *C. trachomatis* or *N. gonorrhoeae* are at significant risk for spread of infection to the endometrium or above, with the associated risk of sterility, ectopic pregnancy, or chronic pelvic pain. These sequelae can arise without any evident symptoms or signs in the woman.

Thus detection of urethritis in men should result in urgent evaluation and treatment of any sexual partners with a regimen similar to that used for the man. Although evaluation is strongly recommended, if it will impede treatment or cannot be arranged in a timely manner, medication is sometimes prescribed to contacts even without evaluation. Unprotected intercourse should be avoided until the index case and any partners have been treated.

Other Presentations with Dysuria

Symptoms other than dysuria, urethral discharge, and itch in the urethra are unusual in men with urethritis. When associated with fever, abdominal or flank pain, hematuria, irritative symptoms such as frequency or nocturia, or problems with the flow of urine, including difficulty initiating the urinary stream or with postvoid dribbling, a disease such as prostatitis or pyelonephritis is much more likely. These are discussed in the chapters *Prostatitis* and *Urinary Tract Infection.* The small proportion who develop epididymitis are more likely to present with findings of epididymitis, and the urethritis is recognized subsequently.

Suggested Reading

Bowie WR. Urethritis in males. In: Holmes KK, Mardh PA, Sparling PF, Wiesner PJ, eds. Sexually transmitted diseases. 2nd ed. New York: McGraw-Hill, 1990: 627.

Centers for Disease Control and Prevention. 1993 Sexually transmitted diseases treatment guidelines. MMWR 1993; 42(RR-14):1–102.

Kunin CM. Urinary tract infections in females. Clin Infect Dis 1994; 18:1–12.

Norrby SR. Short-term treatment of uncomplicated lower urinary tract infections in women. Rev Infect Dis 1990; 12:458–467.

URINARY TRACT INFECTION

Judith A. O'Donnell, M.D.
Elias Abrutyn, M.D.

Urinary tract infections (UTI) are exceedingly common in both the outpatient and inpatient settings. They occur in patients of all ages, affecting women throughout life and male patients at each end of the age spectrum. It is estimated that over 6 million visits annually to physicians' offices are for evaluation of symptoms such as dysuria and urinary frequency or urgency. Additionally, UTI is the leading cause of gram-negative bacillary sepsis in hospitalized patients. The phrase "urinary tract infection" encompasses a broad array of diagnoses including cystitis, pyelonephritis, asymptomatic bacteriuria, complicated infections associated with nephrolithiasis or bladder catheters, and recurrent infections. Appropriate management of a patient with UTI depends on many factors such as the age and sex of the patient, the presence of underlying disease or pregnancy, the history and timing of prior UTI, differentiation between cystitis and pyelonephritis, and the microbial pathogen.

The delineation of upper and lower tract infection is essential to understanding the approach to therapy. Lower urinary tract infection involves the bladder (cystitis) and describes the syndrome of dysuria, pyuria, and increased urinary frequency or urgency. Upper tract infection, or pyelonephritis, involves bladder and kidney. Clinically it presents with fever, flank pain or tenderness, and the signs and symptoms of lower tract infection. The pathogenesis in most cases of upper and lower UTI is related to the ability of microorganisms to establish colonization in the periurethral area and ascend into the urinary tract, thus causing infection. The hematogenous route is less common.

The majority of both upper and lower tract infections are monomicrobial. *Escherichia coli* is the single most common pathogen; however, other Enterobacteriaceae such as *Proteus* spp., *Enterobacter* spp., and *Klebsiella* spp. are also uropathogens. *Enterococcus* spp. and *Staphylococcus saprophyticus* are the most common gram-positive pathogens; however, they are isolated much less often than enteric gram-negative rods. Many other bacteria can cause UTI in the appropriate clinical setting. A polymicrobial infection in the absence of a bladder catheter may suggest an enterovesical fistula.

The distinction between uncomplicated and complicated UTI is of paramount importance. An uncomplicated UTI occurs in an individual who has no functional or structural abnormalities of kidneys, ureters, bladder, or urethra. Most women fall into this category. Complicated UTI occurs in the setting of functional or anatomic abnormalities of the upper or lower tract, are associated with nephrolithiasis, accompany an indwelling bladder catheter, or are seen in patients with underlying conditions such as pregnancy, diabetes mellitus, renal transplantation, or sickle cell anemia. Although these conditions are recognized as influencing response to therapy, a consistent definition of complicated infection has not yet been developed.

It is necessary to determine whether the patient has an uncomplicated or complicated infection. This differentiation will determine the management and duration of therapy. Uncomplicated lower UTI responds well to 3 days of therapy and is not associated with sequelae. Complicated infections may require 10 days or more of therapy and are more likely to be associated with bacteremia and recurrence of infection.

■ CYSTITIS

Women are much more likely to develop cystitis than men, in part because bacteria more easily ascend into the bladder of women. Diagnosis can be made by microscopic examination of the sediment from a mid-stream clean-voided urine sample for pyuria (defined as at least 10 white blood cells per high-power field) and significant bacteriuria (more than 10^5 organisms per milliliter of urine). Quantitative culture of the specimen can provide a specific microbiologic diagnosis, and susceptibility testing can offer the most effective means for determining adequate therapy. Bacteria can be readily seen by examining a wet-mount preparation or by Gram stain of uncentrifuged urine. The Gram-stained preparations are particularly useful in differentiating vaginal flora from gram-negative rods and for determining whether the likely uropathogen is a gram-positive organism. In most women with uncomplicated UTI the diagnosis can be established by finding pyuria and bacteriuria. A urine culture need not be performed for a young woman with an uncomplicated UTI, as presumptive therapy for the expected uropathogens (*E. coli, S. saprophyticus*) is usually successful.

Therapy of uncomplicated cystitis is directed at eradicating pathogenic bacteria from the bladder and periurethral area, and it can be accomplished with a short course of an effective antimicrobial agent. Regimens composed of either a fluoroquinolone (ciprofloxacin, ofloxacin, norfloxacin, enoxacin, lomefloxacin) or trimethoprim-sulfamethoxazole (TMP-SMX) are more effective than those containing a beta-lactam or tetracycline. TMP-SMX given as one double-strength tablet orally every 12 hours; trimethoprim 100 mg orally every 12 hours; ciprofloxacin 250 to 500 mg orally every 12 hours; norfloxacin 400 mg orally every 12 hours; and ofloxacin 300 to 400 mg orally every 12 hours are all equally effective when prescribed for a 3-day course of therapy (Table 1). In well-designed clinical studies, 3-day regimens have been shown to be significantly more effective than 1-day regimens. Short-course therapy can be recommended only for women with acute uncomplicated cystitis, as there have been no clinical studies in men with UTI.

Ampicillin and amoxicillin have been mainstays of therapy for uncomplicated lower UTI in the past, but they should no longer be considered first-line agents. Some 30 to 40 percent of community-acquired *E. coli* strains produce beta-lactamase and are resistant to these beta-lactam drugs, and recent studies have shown that these agents have poor ability to eradicate uropathogens from perineal and perianal colonization sites compared with the fluoroquinolones and TMP-SMX. Moreover, TMP-SMX and the fluoroquinolones, given for 3 days, will eliminate *E. coli* and other pathogens from the vaginal reservoir without disturbing the normal vaginal and fecal flora. The beta-lactam drugs cannot achieve this.

Those less likely to respond adequately to short-course therapy include men with UTI, women with more than 1 week of symptoms at the time of presentation, women with a history of recurrent infections, pregnant women, and patients with infection due to resistant bacteria. The management of patients with complicated lower UTI must include a urine culture and susceptibility testing, the results of which should be used to guide the choice of an antimicrobial regimen. Fluoroquinolones and TMP-SMX are often appropriate anti-infectives in this setting because of their superior tissue levels. Successful therapy of complicated lower UTI hinges upon the duration of treatment. Regimens given for a 10 to 14 day course are preferred.

■ PYELONEPHRITIS

The diagnosis of pyelonephritis, which remains clinical, includes fever, flank pain or tenderness, pyuria, and bacteriuria. The decision to hospitalize a patient with pyelonephritis should be based upon the likelihood of bacteremia associated with the infection (presence of hypotension, rigors, or septic

Table 1 Summary of Treatment Recommendations for Urinary Tract Infections

INFECTION	THERAPY	DURATION	MISCELLANEOUS
Uncomplicated lower tract infection in women	TMP-SMX one DS tab q12h	3 days	
	TMP-SMX 100 mg q12h	3 days	
	Ciprofloxacin 250–500 mg q12h	3 days	Avoid divalent, trivalent cations
	Ofloxacin 200–300 mg q12h	3 days	Avoid divalent, trivalent cations
	Norfloxacin 400 mg q12h	3 days	Avoid divalent, trivalent cations
	Levofloxacin 500 mg daily		
Complicated lower tract infections	Same as uncomplicated	14 days	Therapy guided by C&S
Pyelonephritis			
Outpatient	Therapy directed by urine Gram stain		Follow-up in 72 hours to determine response
	Same as uncomplicated	14 days	
Hospital	TMP-SMX 10 mg/kg/day in 2–4 divided doses	14 days	Therapy should be streamlined according to C&S data; switch to oral therapy once patient responds
	Ceftriaxone 1 g q24h	14 days	
	Ciprofloxacin 400 mg IV q12h	14 days	
Asymptomatic bacteriuria in pregnancy	Amoxicillin 500 mg t.i.d.	7 days	Follow-up urine culture must be obtained
	Cephalexin 500 mg q.i.d.	7 days	

C&S, culture and sensitivity; DS, double strength; TMP-SMX, trimethoprim-sulfamethoxazole shock), as well as the patient's ability to tolerate and be compliant with an oral antimicrobial regimen.

If the patient is deemed an appropriate candidate for outpatient oral therapy, any of a number of antimicrobials can be prescribed after a urine Gram stain is performed and culture is obtained (see Table 1). Again, either TMP-SMX or a fluoroquinolone in the doses discussed previously would be an appropriate empiric choice when Gram stain reveals gram-negative bacilli. When gram-positive cocci in chains and pairs are identified, amoxicillin 500 mg three times daily is a reasonable empiric therapy. If gram-positive cocci in clusters are present, antistaphylococcal therapy with dicloxacillin 500 mg four times daily or cephalexin 500 mg four times daily should be instituted. All regimens should be given for a 14-day course. Patients should have clinical follow-up within 48 to 72 hours after beginning antimicrobial therapy to ensure clinical response and confirm the diagnosis. If the patient does not improve clinically, i.e., has persistent fever, pyuria, or flank pain, further diagnostic evaluation of the kidneys and urinary tract is warranted to seek out any abscess or obstruction. Hospitalization and intravenous therapy should be considered as well.

Patients who require hospitalization for management and initial treatment of pyelonephritis can be given parenteral therapy with any of several anti-infectives. TMP-SMX 10 mg per kilogram per day in two to four divided doses; ciprofloxacin 400 mg every 12 hours; a third-generation cephalosporin such as cefotaxime 1 g every 8 hours or ceftriaxone 1 g every 24 hours; aztreonam 1 g every 8 hours; an aminoglycoside; an extended-spectrum penicillin such as piperacillin are all possible choices for the initial empiric therapy of pyelonephritis (see Table 1). Empiric therapy should be re-evaluated once the microbiologic diagnosis and susceptibilities are known. Therapy should be tailored to the specific pathogen with cost-effectiveness in mind. Patients can be switched to oral therapy once clinical response has been documented. A 14-day course of therapy is necessary to ensure cure. In the event that there is no response to therapy within the first 72 hours, renal ultrasound to evaluate for obstruction, abscess, or other infectious complication is suggested.

■ ASYMPTOMATIC BACTERIURIA

Asymptomatic bacteriuria is defined as significant bacteria in the urine in the absence of signs or symptoms of UTI. The diagnosis of asymptomatic bacteriuria is certain only after two separate urine specimens demonstrate more than 10^5 colony-forming units (CFU) per milliliter of the same organism. The appropriate management of this entity depends on the age of the patient and the presence or absence of pregnancy. Some 1 percent of neonates, 1 to 3 percent of nonpregnant women aged 15 to 24, 4 to 10 percent of pregnant women, and 10 percent of women in the sixth and seventh decades of life have significant bacteriuria. Children who are found to have asymptomatic bacteriuria should be treated as for complicated UTI. Asymptomatic bacteriuria in the elderly should be neither sought nor treated. Pyuria in the elderly is not always a predictor of infection, and incontinence or a perceived change in the pattern of incontinence is not an indication for therapy.

Pregnant women and candidates for urologic surgery are the only two subsets of the adult population who have been shown to derive benefit from treatment of asymptomatic bacteriuria. Patients undergoing urologic procedures should be screened and if culture positive, treated to lower their risk of post procedure infection. As many as 60 percent of pregnant women with asymptomatic bacteriuria develop symptomatic lower or upper UTI during pregnancy. Moreover, acute pyelonephritis in this setting has been associated with premature birth. For these reasons pregnant women with asymptomatic bacteriuria should be treated with antimicrobials that are safe for use in pregnancy. Fluoroquinolones and tetracyclines should be avoided throughout gestation and sulfonamide-containing preparations avoided in the third trimester. Empiric choices include amoxicillin 500 mg orally three times daily; cephalexin 500 mg orally four times daily. Duration of therapy should be 7 days, with follow-up urine cultures obtained at the completion of therapy to document sterilization of urine. If bacteriuria persists or recurs, 4 to 6 weeks of therapy may be necessary.

■ RECURRENT UTI

Recurrent UTI are defined as three or more infections per year. There are two distinct types: reinfection with different bacterial pathogens and relapse of infection with the same pathogen. Reinfection, which accounts for 80 percent of recurrent infections, can be seen weeks to months after initial infection. Relapse accounts for 20 percent of recurrent infections and usually occurs within 2 weeks of initial therapy. Relapsing UTI are usually due to inadequate length of therapy, structural abnormalities, or chronic bacterial prostatitis. Relapse, however, may be difficult to distinguish from reinfection in the clinical situation without specialized tests which are not generically available.

Treatment of relapse is as follows: failure of short-course therapy necessitates a 2-week regimen; failure of 2-week therapy, a 6-week regimen; failure of 6-week therapy suggests a 6-month regimen. For women with frequent reinfection antimicrobial prophylaxis for 6 to 12 months with trimethoprim 100 mg, nitrofurantoin 50 to 100 mg, or TMP-SMX one single-strength tablet, all prescribed either nightly or three times weekly, can be considered. The same regimens can also be used as postcoital prophylaxis for the subset of women who develop UTI symptoms in association with sexual intercourse.

Suggested Reading

Hooton TM, Winter C, Tiu F, Stamm WE. Randomized comparative trial and cost analysis of 3-day antimicrobial regimens for treatment of acute cystitis in women. JAMA 1995; 273:41.

Kunin CM. Urinary tract infections in females. Clin Infect Dis 1994; 18:1.

Lipsky BA. Urinary tract infections in men: Epidemiology, pathophysiology, diagnosis, and treatment. Ann Intern Med 1989; 110:138.

Mittendorf R, Williams MA, Kass EH. Prevention of preterm delivery and low birth weight associated with asymptomatic bacteriuria. Clin Infect Dis 1992; 14:927.

Rubin RH, Tolkoff-Rubin NE, Cotrans RS. Urinary tract infections, pyelonephritis, and reflux nephropathy. In: Brenner BR, Rector FC Jr, eds. The kidney. 4th ed. Philadelphia: WB Saunders, 1991: 1369.

Stamm WE, Hooton TM. Management of urinary tract infections in adults. New Engl J Med 1993; 329:1328.

INFECTIONS ASSOCIATED WITH URINARY CATHETERS

Luis M. Valdez, M.D.
Edward J. Septimus, M.D., F.A.C.P.

Each year millions of urinary catheters are used in acute and chronic care facilities, rehabilitation units, and nursing homes across the United States for indications such as urine output measurement, acute urinary retention, urinary incontinence, and neurogenic bladder. Urinary tract infections (UTI) are the most common complication of urinary catheters, and despite the fact that most catheter-associated UTI are asymptomatic, catheter-induced bacteriuria is the most common source of nosocomial gram-negative bacteremia in hospitalized and other institutionalized patients.

PATHOGENESIS

Urinary catheters lead to chemically or mechanically induced inflammation of the urethra and bladder mucosa and offer bacteria a niche on its lumen and external surface. A biofilm that coats catheters, drainage bags, and uroepithelium will protect bacteria from local host defenses. In addition, the catheter may impair the normal flow of urine, which may impede the normal washout of bacteria. Catheters may also impair normal local host defenses by blunting adequate polymorphonuclear leukocyte function. More important, the catheter assists bacteria in gaining access to the urinary tract in three ways:

1. During insertion. The bacterial flora that colonizes the urethra may be carried into the bladder during insertion.
2. Intralumenally. The closed catheter system may be opened at two points, the filling and emptying joints of the collection bag. If either of these points is contaminated with bacteria, the organisms will start multiplying and may ascend the collection tube and catheter through the urine itself or by growth along internal surfaces.
3. Extralumenally. Bacteria colonizing the periurethral area may ascend into the bladder through the space between the external catheter and the urethral mucosa. Rectal and periurethral colonization often precedes catheter-associated bacteriuria, especially in women, and such colonization precedes bacteriuria with the same strain in up to two-thirds of patients.

RISK FACTORS FOR BACTERIURIA

In a prospective study carried out by Platt and colleagues, multiple logistic regression analysis identified nine factors significantly associated with infection: duration of catheterization, lack of systemic antibiotic during short catheter courses, lack of urinemeter drainage, female sex, diabetes mellitus, microbial colonization of the drainage bag, serum creatinine greater than 2 mg/dl at the time of catheterization, indication for catheterization, and the use of catheters with sealed collection junctions when no antibiotic was administered. The duration of catheterization is the most important risk factor. The daily increase in prevalence of bacteriuria is 3 to 10 percent, and almost all patients will have bacteriuria after 30 days.

MICROBIOLOGY

Among patients with short-term catheterization many studies have required at least 100,000 colony-forming units per milliliter of urine to establish the diagnosis, but some who consider the urinary tract of catheterized patients to be highly susceptible to infection once small numbers of microorganisms gain access believe that a concentration considerably below 10^5 organisms per milliliter may be clinically and epidemiologically important in this setting. In one study low-level bacteriuria or candiduria (fewer than 10^5 organisms per milliliter) progressed to concentrations above 10^5 organisms per milliliter 96 percent of the time, usually within 3 days of the initial culture, unless the patient received intercurrent suppressive antimicrobial therapy. *Escherichia coli* is the most common species isolated in patients with short-term catheterization. Other common organisms are *Proteus mirabilis*, *Pseudomonas aeruginosa*, *Klebsiella pneumoniae*, enterococci, and *Staphylococcus epidermidis*. Most cases of bacteriuria associated with short-term catheterization are caused by a single organism, although on occasion the process is polymicrobial. Yeast also may be isolated, particularly from patients receiving broad-spectrum antibiotics.

Bacteriuria in patients with long-term catheterization is commonly polymicrobial. Studies have shown that many bacteria have relatively similar access to the lumen of the catheter or bladder, but the subsequent fate of the organism varies greatly by species. *Providentia stuartii* tends to persist once it gains access, probably establishing a niche within the urinary catheter, and other organisms, such as *E. coli* and *K. pneumoniae*, appear to reside in the urinary tract itself, bound to the uroepithelium. *P. mirabilis* and *Morganella morganii* probably behave in a similar way to *P. stuartii* within the urinary catheter, increasing their ability to cause subsequent bacteriuria. Other organisms such as coagulase-negative staphylococci, nonenterococcal streptococci, and diphtheroids are present only transiently and are apparently unable to persist in either the urinary catheter or the urinary tract.

THERAPY

Most patients with bacteriuria are asymptomatic, and these patients should not be treated while the catheter remains in place (Table 1). Therapy may be indicated if certain bacterial strains are known to cause a high incidence of bacteremia (*Serratia marcescens*) or to control outbreaks by resistant organisms in a medical unit. In patients with short-term

Table 1 Management of Infections Associated with Urinary Catheters

INFECTION	MANAGEMENT
Asymptomatic Bacteriuria	No antibiotic treatment needed. Catheter should be removed if possible in patients with STC. LTC: No need for routine surveillance cultures. STC: May culture urine after catheter removal. If culture remains positive, treat with oral antibiotics per sensitivities.
Symptomatic bacteriuria Fever Urinary symptoms Acute pyelonephritis Bacteremia	Antibiotic therapy. Intravenous therapy if signs of bacteremia or unable to take oral antibiotics. In upper UTI (pyelonephritis) treat for 10–14 days. In uncomplicated lower UTI 3–7 days. Modify therapy to match susceptibility. Other sources of infection should be ruled out. Urine and blood cultures should be obtained. Rule out catheter obstruction, stones, and periurethral infection. Some recommend removal or replacement of catheter.
Candiduria	Uncomplicated: Removal (STC) or change (LTC) of catheter. If persistent, consider treatment. 1) Amphotericin B bladder irrigation. 50 mg in 1 L of sterile water. Irrigation may be intermittent (200–300 ml instilled with clamping of the catheter for 1–2 hours), or continuous (40 ml/hr). 2) Fluconazole 200 mg the first day, then 100 mg a day for 3–5 days. If candiduria persists after treatment, rule out fungus ball or invasive renal infection.

STC, short-term catheterization; LTC, long-term catheterization; UTI, urinary tract infection.

catheterization bacteriuria will resolve after catheter removal. A small group of patients, however, will develop persistent bacteriuria and have an increased risk of developing symptomatic UTI. For this reason some recommend a urine culture after catheter removal and a short course of oral antibiotics if there is persistent bacteriuria. In asymptomatic long-term catheterized patients there is no need for routine surveillance cultures.

Patients with symptomatic catheter-related infections often present with fever, urinary symptoms, acute pyelonephritis, and bacteremia. If the patient develops only fever or signs of bacteremia, sources of infection outside the urinary tract must be ruled out, and urine and blood cultures should be obtained. Catheters should be checked for obstruction, and the periurethral area should be examined, especially among men. Initial antibiotic therapy should be based on knowledge of organisms common in the medical facility and Gram stain of the patient's urine. The dosages are the same as in noncatheterized patients with UTI. In case of fever and signs of bacteremia, intravenous therapy should be started. Therapy should be modified once susceptibility patterns of the urine and blood isolates are available. In complicated cases (pyelonephritis, bacteremia) therapy for 10 to 14 days is recommended. For patients with symptoms limited to the bladder and without fever or evidence of systemic infection, oral therapy can be used for 3 to 7 days. Catheters should be removed if possible, and in patients with long-term catheterization, because of the presence of bacteria in biofilm on the catheter, changing the catheter is recommended by some.

Candiduria may develop in catheterized patients, especially those receiving antibiotics. The fact that most cases of candiduria are benign is supported by the disappearance of yeast from the urine following catheter removal or replacement. In the opinion of some, the persistence of candiduria after removal or replacement of the catheter should prompt therapy. Certainly, if the candiduria is symptomatic, therapy is indicated.

■ PREVENTION

No catheterization is obviously the most direct way of preventing catheter-related infections. Urinary catheters should not be used unnecessarily, and it is important to recognize alternatives, such as external collection devices (condom catheters), intermittent catheterization, suprapubic catheterization, intraurethral catheters, and urinary diversions. Intermittent catheterization in particular has been widely accepted as the method of choice for urologic rehabilitation of persons with spinal cord injury who have neurogenic bladder and in the long-term management of some of these individuals, although the majority will develop recurrent or continuous bacteriuria.

Prevention of bacteriuria is another approach. If a catheter must be used, it is important to maintain the closed system and minimize the duration of catheterization. Systemic antibacterial agents may postpone bacteriuria, but most authorities think they are not indicated because of the potential for side effects, cost, and emergence of resistant bacteria. Silver oxide-coated catheters have also been studied but were beneficial in only a small subgroup of patients.

Suggested Reading

Platt R, Polk BF, Murdock B, Rosner B. Risk factors for nosocomial urinary tract infection. Am J Epidemiol 1986; 124(6):977–985.

Sanford JP. The enigma of candiduria: Evolution of bladder irrigation with amphotericin B for management from anecdote to dogma and a lesson from Machiavelli. Clin Infect Dis 1993; 16(1):145–147.

Stamm WE. Catheter-associated urinary tract infections: Epidemiology, pathogenesis, and prevention. Am J Med 1991; 91(Suppl 3B):65S–71S.

Warren JW. The catheter and urinary tract infection. Med Clin North Am 1991; 75:481–493.

ENTEROBACTERIACEAE

Thomas Butler, M.D.

The Enterobacteriaceae are a family of gram-negative bacteria that normally reside in the intestines of humans and other animals. Members of these genera are the leading causes of human infectious diseases affecting the urinary tract, intestine, lung, and nervous system, and of the production of localized inflammation in the form of abscesses and the generalized systemic illness known as sepsis, or systemic inflammatory response syndrome. These diverse infections are common causes of severe disease and death, and accordingly, they require prompt antimicrobial therapy and sometimes surgical intervention.

This chapter covers genera that are important causes of human illness (Table 1). Some genera in the Enterobacteriaceae family—*Salmonella, Shigella,* and *Yersinia*—are not included here because they are covered in other chapters.

CLINICAL PRESENTATION AND DIAGNOSIS

Most patients with infections caused by members of Enterobacteriaceae have fever, often with chills, sweating, headache, and malaise. Other symptoms are more variable, depending on the site of infection. Although all the pathogenic species of Enterobacteriaceae can cause infection at any bodily site, each species is associated preferentially with certain clinical presentations (Table 1). The most common site is the urinary tract, which gives rise to increased urinary frequency, dysuria, suprapubic or back pain, and sometimes hematuria. Physical examination may reveal tenderness localized to the suprapubic or costovertebral regions over the kidneys or a generalized abdominal tenderness. The prostate gland may be enlarged or tender. Localization of infection in the urinary tract occurs in one or both kidneys (pyelonephritis), in the bladder (cystitis), or in the prostate (prostatitis), but precise localization by symptoms or signs of localized tenderness often cannot be accomplished by the examining physician. The diagnostic proof of urinary tract infection is urine showing microscopic pyuria and bacteriuria.

Another common infection caused by Enterobacteriaceae is sepsis. The symptoms include fever, chills, anorexia, vomiting, headache, diminished mental alertness, and prostration. There is often an antecedent or concomitant urinary infection, but the symptoms are more severe than in uncomplicated urinary infections, necessitating hospitalization and sometimes intensive care for intravenous fluids and monitoring of vital signs. Patients with sepsis show fever (temperature above 38°C, or 100.4°F) or hypothermia (temperature below 36°C, or 96.8°F), tachycardia, and tachypnea. The white blood cell count is usually above 12,000 per cubic millimeter or may be below 4,000 per cubic millimeter, and the percentage of band forms of polymorphonuclear leukocytes (PML) is often greater than 10. In some cases the systolic blood pressure is below 90. When the blood pressure remains low after an intravenous fluid bolus of at least 500 ml of normal saline, this is called septic shock. The diagnostic proof of sepsis is a positive blood culture. Sepsis is most likely to occur in immunocompromised patients, such as those with cancer receiving chemotherapy, patients receiving corticosteroids, patients with renal failure, and patients with cirrhosis. Mortality in severe sepsis or septic shock is about 50 percent and is highest in patients with underlying disease such as malignancy, cardiac disease, emphysema, cirrhosis, and renal failure.

Infections of the gastrointestinal tract with *Escherichia coli* may cause gastroenteritis with fever, vomiting, and diarrhea. Only strains of *E. coli* that are enterotoxigenic by virtue of carrying certain plasmids cause acute watery diarrhea. Persons are at increased risk for acquiring these infections when traveling in countries such as Mexico and Guatemala. The serotype of *E. coli* 0157:H7 is enterohemorrhagic; it can cause bloody diarrhea after ingestion of incompletely cooked beef or foods contaminated with juices of infected beef. This infection can result in the serious complication of the hemolytic-uremic syndrome.

Table 1 Enterobacteriaceae

PATHOGEN	CLINICAL SYNDROMES
Citrobacter diversus freundnii amalonaticus	Nosocomial infections of urinary tract, lung; neonatal meningitis, brain abscess
Edwardsiella tarda	Rare cause of gastroenteritis, abscess, menigitis; septicemia
Enterobacter cloacae aerogenes agglomerans	Nosocomial infections of urinary tract, lung, surgical wounds, burns; septicemia; diabetic ulcers
Escherichia coli	Most common cause of community-acquired urinary tract infection, and urosepsis; common cause of gastroenteritis; nosocomial lung infection, septicemia; neonatal meningitis, abscess, peritonitis
Hafnia alvei	Rare cause of nosocomial infection
Klebsiella pneumoniae ozaenae rhinoscleromatis oxytoca	Occasional cause of lung infection, empyema, urinary tract infection, sepsis; nosocomial infections of lung, urinary tract, surgical wounds, intravenous catheters, biliary tract, septicemia
Morganella morganii	Rare cause of nosocomial infections of urinary tract, lung, septicemia
Proteus mirabilis vulgaris myxofaciens	Occasional cause of urinary tract infection, lung infection, sepsis; nosocomial infections of urinary tract, lungs, surgical wounds, septicemia
Providencia alcalifaciens stuartii rettgeri	Nosocomial infections of urinary tract, septicemia
Serratia marcescens liquifaciens rubidaea odorifera	Nosocomial infection of lungs, urinary tract, surgical wounds, skin, septicemia; endocarditis, osteomyelitis in drug addicts

Excluding *Salmonella, Shigella,* and *Yersinia,* which are covered elsewhere.

Less common clinical presentations of Enterobacteriaceae include pneumonia, abscesses, and meningitis. Community-acquired pneumonia caused by *Klebsiella pneumoniae* sometimes occurs in debilitated persons such as alcoholics. Patients who are placed on mechanical ventilators in intensive care units are at high risk for bacterial pneumonia; the most common causative organisms are *Pseudomonas aeruginosa* and Enterobacteriaceae including *K. pneumoniae, Enterobacter aerogenes,* and *Serratia marcescens.* The presentation of pneumonia usually includes cough productive of purulent yellow or green or blood-tinged sputum, dyspnea, and pleuritic pain. For hospitalized patients on mechanical ventilators, pneumonia is suspected when fever appears and suction of the endotracheal tube produces copious fluid with a yellow, green, or red coloration. The proof of pneumonia is radiographic infiltrates. Enterobacteriaceae as the cause of pneumonia is established by a Gram stain of sputum or tracheal aspirate showing plentiful PML with a predominance of gram-negative bacilli. The culture of sputum is used to confirm the results of the Gram stain. Abscesses caused by Enterobacteriaceae manifest as abdominal pain, fever, diarrhea, ileus, intestinal perforation, or jaundice. The abscesses are localized in places such as in the liver, spleen, intestinal wall, peritoneum, or retroperitoneum. Most abscesses in these abdominal locations originate from the intestine, either by translocation of bacteria or by direct extension or perforation, and they frequently contain anaerobic bacteria (*Bacteroides* spp., peptostreptococci, or *Clostridium* spp.) in addition to Enterobacteriaceae. Enterobacteriaceae rarely cause meningitis except for neonatal meningitis caused by *E. coli.* In adults Enterobacteriaceae may cause meningitis in the elderly and sometimes after trauma or surgical procedures affecting the brain or spinal cord.

Spontaneous bacterial peritonitis may accompany pre-existing ascites. The two most common causes of spontaneous bacterial peritonitis are *Streptococcus pneumoniae* and *E. coli.*

Enterobacteriaceae may cause localized infections in other sites. These clinical presentations include septic arthritis, pericarditis, endocarditis, empyema, myositis, osteomyelitis, and cholecystitis. When the common bile duct is occluded by a stone or tumor, Enterobacteriaceae may cause ascending cholangitis.

The diagnosis of these infections can be rapidly made by Gram stain of appropriate fluid. A Gram stain of uncentrifuged urine is advised. One or more gram-negative rod per oil immersion field suggests Enterobacteriaceae urinary tract infection. Likewise, Gram stain of sputum, spinal fluid, and other relevant fluids can provide diagnostic information on the day of the first examination.

Quantitative cultures of urine using a calibrated loop should be done in cases of suspected urinary tract infection. A clean-catch midstream collection is advised to reduce likelihood of contamination. In patients who are incontinent, uncooperative, or showing abnormal urinary retention, the bladder should be catheterized to obtain urine. Counts of a single bacterial species of at least 10^5 per milliliter of voided urine suggest a significant infection; counts between 10^4 and 10^5 may represent a significant infection but should be repeated to confirm the infection. Bacterial counts less than 10^4 per milliliter of urine obtained by catheter or suprapubic aspiration should be considered significant because bladder urine is normally sterile. In a patient with an indwelling urinary catheter in place for more than 48 hours, a specimen for culture is preferably obtained after removal of the catheter to exclude bacterial colonization of the catheter lumen.

Blood should be cultured by venipuncture in patients with sepsis or fever with suspected infection at any of several sites. Standard techniques of skin cleansing should be followed to decrease likelihood of contamination. Blood should be obtained from at least two venipuncture sites to show reproducible results and to exclude contamination in the event that a possible contaminant is obtained from only one site. About 10 milliliters of blood should be obtained from each venipuncture, with 5 milliliters placed into each of two bottles, one for aerobic and one for anaerobic growth. The bottles should contain adequate broth volume to dilute the blood 10:1 to reduce concentrations of antibiotic and other growth-inhibiting substances in plasma. As the Enterobacteriaceae are both aerobic and facultatively anaerobic, they grow under both aerobic and anaerobic conditions. A positive blood culture for Enterobacteriaceae is useful not only for the diagnosis of sepsis, but also for determining which pathogen originating from a site such as the lung or wound—which sometimes show growth of multiple organisms—is the most significant pathogen, and hence has the highest priority for specific antimicrobial therapy.

■ THERAPY

Antimicrobial therapy should be guided by susceptibility testing. Most laboratories use disk diffusion in agar to report whether an organism shows susceptibility, resistance, or intermediate susceptibility to any specified drug. These designations are based on achievable serum concentrations of drug after administration of a usual dose. Urinary concentrations usually exceed these levels, but concentrations in other fluids, such as cerebrospinal fluid, may be considerably less.

The drugs listed in Table 2 are recommended as initial choices pending the results of culture and susceptibility testing. In the absence of Gram stain results, empiric therapies sometimes have to be started before any diagnostic information is available. After results of culture and antimicrobial susceptibilities are available, the therapy can often be changed to a narrower-spectrum drug that is preferably less toxic and less expensive than the initial therapy. For example, a patient with urosepsis caused by *E. coli* susceptible to ampicillin or cefazolin should be treated with one of these agents in place of the more nephrotoxic aminoglycoside or the more expensive third-generation cephalosporin, aztreonam, or imipenem.

Once the drug of choice has been determined, the duration of therapy must be decided. Three days of therapy is optimal for uncomplicated urinary infections in women. For complicated urinary infections with suspected sepsis or for urinary tract infections in men, courses of 7 to 14 days are appropriate to ensure cure and to prevent relapse. To establish that a urinary tract infection has been effectively treated, a quantitative urine culture should be repeated after 3 or more days of therapy and should show no growth or fewer than 10^4 organisms per milliliter. For infection of soft tissue, including pneumonia, bronchitis, abscesses after drainage, meningitis, arthritis, and peritonitis, the duration of therapy should be

Table 2 Antimicrobial Drugs for Therapy of Infections Caused by Selected Species of *Enterobacteriaceae*

INFECTION	DRUG OF CHOICE	ALTERNATIVE
Escherichia coli		
Acute uncomplicated urinary tract infection in female patient	TMP-SMX orally	Amoxicillin-clavulanate, ampicillin, fluoroquinolone*, tetracycline†
Pyelonephritis, complicated urinary infection, urinary infection in male patient, sepsis	Third-generation cephalosporin‡ intravenously	Gentamicin§, ampicillin, ampicillin-sulbactam, amoxicillin, amoxicillin-clavulante
Diarrhea due to enterotoxigenic or enterohemorrhagic strains	TMP-SMX orally	Tetracycline†, fluoroquinolone*
Klebsiella pneumoniae	Third-generation cephalosporin‡ or gentamicin§	Cefazolin, cefoxitin, piperacillin‖, imipenem, aztreonam, TMP-SMX, fluoroquinolone*, tetracycline†
Enterobacter aerogenes	Gentamicin§, imipenem	Third-generation cephalosporin‡, ticarcillin¶, piperacillin‖, aztreonam, fluoroquinolone*
Proteus mirabilis	Ampicillin	Gentamicin, cefazolin
Proteus vulgaris, Morganella morganii, Providencia spp.	Gentamicin§, third-generation cephalosporin‡	Ticarcillin¶, piperacillin‖, imipenem, aztreonam, TMP-SMX, fluoroquinolone*
Serratia marcescens	Third-generation cephalosporin‡	Gentamicin§, imipenem, aztreonam, fluoroquinolone*, ticarcillin¶, piperacillin‖, TMP-SMX
Citrobacter spp.	Gentamicin§	Cefazolin, ticarcillin¶
Hafnia alvei	Same as for *Enterobacter aerogenes*	
Edwardsiella tarda	Treatment not indicated for gastroenteritis	
Gastroenteritis, bacteremia, abscess, meningitis	Gentamicin§	Tetracycline†, cefazolin, ampicillin

*Fluoroquinolone indicates choice of ciprofloxacin, norfloxacin, ofloxacin, enoxacin, or lomefloxacin.
†Doxycycline may be substituted for tetracycline and is preferred sometimes for its twice daily dosing and greater ease of use in renal failure.
‡Third-generation cephalosporins are cefotaxime, ceftriaxone, ceftazidime, ceftizoxime, and cefoperazone. Third-generation cephalosporins should be used with caution or avoided when *Enterobacter* infections are suspected or present because they induce beta-lactamase production, rendering these organisms multiresistant and causing an associated increase in mortality.
§Other aminoglycosides, including tobramycin, amikacin, and netilmicin, may be substituted for gentamicin.
‖Mezlocillin may be substituted for piperacillin.
¶Carbenicillin may be substituted for ticarcillin. Both antibiotics have the same spectrum of activity, but the lower recommended doses of ticarcillin expose patients to lesser amounts of the sodium salt.
TMP-SMX, trimethoprim-sulfamethoxazole.

about 7 to 14 days, individualized to the speed of resolution. Therapy may be continued until 2 to 4 days after fever and other signs of disease have disappeared. For patients with endocarditis or osteomyelitis, treatment is recommended to continue for about 6 weeks.

Oral administration of antimicrobials is the most convenient and least expensive for outpatients with most forms of infection that are not clinically severe. For uncomplicated urinary infection and soft-tissue infections of lung, skin, and intestine of mild to moderate degrees of severity, the oral route is preferred. For patients requiring hospitalization because of greater clinical severity, age over 60 years, or underlying disease, the intravenous or intramuscular route is preferred to ensure adequate tissue concentrations of drug. After a few days of parenteral therapy and clinical improvement, most patients may be safely switched to oral therapy, usually in the outpatient setting. For patients with endocarditis or osteomyelitis, the full course of therapy is usually given parenterally because of the requirement of high blood concentrations of drug for about 6 weeks for cure.

Surgical drainage is an essential part of the therapy of localized infections caused by Enterobacteriaceae. Abscesses in common areas such as the liver and other intra-abdominal or retroperitoneal sites, including perinephric, diverticular, and appendiceal sites, should be promptly drained in the operating room. Similarly, infected fluids such as empyema and septic arthritis require drainage by insertion of a chest tube and by arthrotomy or aspiration, respectively.

Doses of antimicrobial drugs vary with body weight and renal function. The usual dosages and other pharmacologic data are supplied in the appendix *Antimicrobial Agent Tables.* For gentamicin and other aminoglycosides, blood levels should be monitored periodically for adjustment of dosage. For gentamicin, tobramycin, and netilmicin, peak concentrations of 4 to 10 μg per milliliter and trough concentrations less than 2 μg per milliliter are advised. For amikacin, peak concentrations should be 15–30 μg per milliliter and trough less than 10 μg per milliliter.

Certain groups of patients with infections caused by Enterobacteriaceae have to be treated differently from others. Pregnant women should never receive tetracycline, doxycycline, chloramphenicol, ciprofloxacin, or any other fluoroquinolone because of their toxicity to bony development in the fetus. Trimethoprim-sulfamethoxazole (TMP-SMX) should be used with caution during pregnancy and is contraindicated at term. Tetracycline and doxycycline should be avoided in children under 10 years old to avoid staining of teeth. Ciprofloxacin and other fluoroquinolones are not approved for use in children until age 18 years because they may affect cartilage development in growing bones.

The cost of antimicrobial therapies can be very great for the patient or insurer and should be minimized in a manner that does not compromise therapeutic efficacy. The cost of a course of treatment varies with the route of administration, whether a drug is off patent and available in generic form, the duration of treatment, and the practice of local pharmacies to buy large lots of drugs at discounted prices. In general, oral drugs are significantly less expensive than parenteral ones. Generic preparations of oral drugs are the least expensive. They include (see Table 2) TMP-SMX, ampicillin, amoxicillin, tetracycline, doxycycline, and cephalexin. Oral drugs that remain on patent and are more expensive include amoxicillin-clavulanate, the fluoroquinolones, cefaclor, cefuroxime-axetil, and cefixime. For intravenous therapies the generic drugs that should be used when possible include ampicillin, cefazolin, gentamicin or tobramycin, and tetracycline. The remaining parenteral drugs, such as ampicillin-sulbactam, ticarcillin-clavulanate, piperacillin-tazobactam, imipenem, aztreonam, and third-generation cephalosporins, remain the most expensive and should be used only when less expensive alternatives are unsatisfactory.

The management of severe sepsis or septic shock due to Enterobacteriaceae requires admission to an intensive care unit. Intravenous normal saline or lactated Ringer's solution to expand plasma volume is given in volumes of at least 500 milliliters to adults to ensure adequate intravascular fluid volume. Oxygen should be administered to obtain at least 90 percent saturation of hemoglobin. In severe cases mechanical ventilation will be required to achieve adequate oxygenation. In cases of shock, vasopressors such as dopamine, epinephrine, and norepinephrine are needed to raise the blood pressure. Because of the high mortality associated with severe sepsis, new drugs are being developed to block certain bacterial products and certain cytokine mediators of severe sepsis. These new drugs include monoclonal antibodies against endotoxin of gram-negative bacteria, monoclonal antibodies against tumor necrosis factor (TNF), TNF receptors, and interleukin-1 receptor antagonists. Some of these drugs now in clinical trials offer promise when combined with antibiotics and fluid therapy for reducing mortality and organ failure caused by sepsis.

Suggested Reading

Eisenstein BI. *Enterobacteriaceae.* In: Mandell GL, Bennett JE, Dollin R, eds. Mandell, Douglas, and Bennett's principles and practice of infectious diseases. 4th ed. New York: Churchill Livingstone, 1995: 1964.

Greenman RL, Schein RMH, Martin MA, et al. A controlled clinical trial of E5 murine monoclonal IgM antibody to endotoxin in the treatment of gram-negative sepsis. JAMA 1991; 266:1097–1102.

Janda JM, Abbott SL. Infections associated with the genus *Edwardsiella:* The role of *Edwarsiella tarda* in human disease. Clin Infect Dis 1993; 17:742–748.

Medical Letter of Drugs and Therapeutics. Handbook of antimicrobial therapy 1994. New Rochelle, NY: Medical Letter.

Natanson C, Hoffman WD, Suffredini AF, et al. Selected treatment strategies for septic shock based on proposed mechanisms of pathogenesis. Ann Intern Med 1994; 120:771–783.

Sirot DL, Goldstein FW, Soussy CJ, et al. Resistance to cefotaxime and seven other β-lactams in members of the family *Enterobacteriaceae:* A 3-year survey in France. Antimicrob Agents Chemother 1992; 36:1677–1681.

ENTEROCOCCUS

Ronald N. Jones, M.D.

In the past decade the enterococci have emerged as major hospital-acquired (nosocomial) pathogens. They are now the third most common cause of nosocomial bloodstream infection and the second most common cause of nosocomial wound and urinary tract infection. The emergence of this genus may in part be related to patterns of general antimicrobial use in the hospital and in particular to widespread use of extended-spectrum cephalosporins, monobactams, carbapenems, and aminoglycosides.

Cephalosporins are not potent or bactericidal against enterococci, and they may therefore result in a selective advantage for this genus. *Enterococcus faecalis* accounts for most human infections (60 to 95 percent) and *Enterococcus faecium* accounts for most (8 to 16 percent) of the remainder. Antimicrobial resistance is a particular problem among *E. faecium* isolates. Other species of interest are *Enterococcus casseliflavus* and *Enterococcus gallinarum,* not because of the frequency with which they are isolated (usually among top five), but because of the intrinsic low-level resistance to vancomycin, e.g., the *vanC* genotype and resultant resistant or intermediate phenotype.

In addition to the problems posed by the increasing frequency of enterococcal infection, the therapy of these infections has become very difficult as resistance to ampicillin, high-level resistance to aminoglycosides, and most recently glycopeptide (vancomycin and teicoplanin) resistance have narrowed the proven therapeutic drug options. In addition, the value (because of risk of failure) of trimethoprim-sulfamethoxazole (TMP-SMX) in therapy even for urinary tract infection has become controversial. All enterococci are intrinsically resistant to achievable in vivo levels of aminoglycosides; however, synergic killing may occur when aminoglycosides are combined with a cell wall–active agent such as a penicillin or a glycopeptide. Strains resistant to high levels of aminoglycoside (more than 500 µg per milliliter of gentamicin or more than 1,000 µg per milliliter of streptomycin) are not susceptible to the synergic codrug activity of the aminoglycosides. It is clinically significant that cross-resistance to the synergic activity of the aminoglycosides is incomplete between gentamicin (and the related compounds tobramycin, netilmicin, amikacin, kanamycin, and isepamicin) and streptomycin. Streptomycin may be used successfully in combination to treat some high-level gentamicin-resistant strains. The selection of the appropriate aminoglycoside codrug should be directed by validated and standardized in vitro susceptibility tests.

Resistance to vancomycin is more common with *E. faecium* isolates than with *E. faecalis,* but it may occur with either species. Comprehensive multicenter reports in 1995 and 1996 suggest that the overall vancomycin-resistant rate for enterococci is approaching 15 percent, and higher resistance rates for some other drugs and species limit therapeutic choices (Table 1). Acquired vancomycin resistance is often associated with resistance to teicoplanin (Van A phenotype or *vanA* genotype) or may occur in the absence of cross-resistance to teicoplanin (Van B phenotype or *vanB* genotype), and this difference may be clinically significant. Intrinsic low-level resistance to both glycopeptides has been observed in *E. casseliflavus* and in *E. gallinarum,* and is called the Van C phenotype that has species-specific genotypes. Other enterococci such as *E. dorons, E. raftinosus, and E. avium* have also been observed to be resistant to glycopeptides.

For the clinician the problems posed by the emergence of resistance have been exacerbated by the technical difficulties in reliable in vitro detection of these resistances. In vitro resistance to TMP-SMX due to the ability of the most prevalent enterococci to use thymidine or thymine in the susceptibility test medium has been addressed by the use of media free of or low in concentration for these antagonists. However, there are significant amounts of antagonists, for example, in the urine, and therefore, the meaning of test results performed in these "improved" media is doubtful. Routine testing against ampicillin without testing for organism beta-lactamase production may result in false-susceptible results. However, beta-lactamase production is an exceedingly uncommon mechanism of resistance (less than 0.1 percent) among *E. faecalis* isolates. A number of problems with the detection of high-level aminoglycoside resistance using the most prevalent automated and commercial broth microdilution susceptibility test systems (Vitek, MicroScan) have been reported, although in some cases these now appear to have been resolved. Similarly, with vancomycin resistance both automated susceptibility tests and disk diffusion tests interpretive criteria have required modification to enable consistent, accurate detection of resistant strains.

Empiric therapy of enterococcal infection is not satisfactory given the complexity of resistance patterns, and therefore, availability of prompt, reliable susceptibility test results is indispensable. At present, disk diffusion susceptibility testing, Etest (AB biodisk Solna, Sweden), Vitek System (personal experience), and the reference broth microdilution or agar dilution methods are reliable methods for detection of important enterococcal drug resistances.

■ ENTEROCOCCAL BLOODSTREAM INFECTION

Isolation of enterococci from the blood may occur with or without endocarditis. In community-acquired enterococcal bloodstream infection approximately one-third of cases are associated with endocarditis, as compared with fewer than 5 percent of nosocomial enterococcal bacteremias. These nosocomial infections are usually associated with urinary tract disease or instrumentation, intra-abdominal infection, intravascular devices, neoplastic disease, and significant neutropenia.

Infective endocarditis, even when caused by more susceptible strains of enterococci, is more difficult to treat than endocarditis due to viridans group streptococci. Only two-thirds of patients will be cured if a penicillin is used alone. A combination of a cell wall–active agent (a penicillin or glycopeptide) with an aminoglycoside for 4 to 6 weeks is recommended. In general, ampicillin (two or four times as active) is used in preference to penicillin; however, the scientific basis for this pattern of use is less than compelling on potency issues alone. High-dose penicillins (ampicillin 2 grams every 4 hours or penicillin G 18–30 million U/day) are appropriate, combined with gentamicin 1 mg/kg every 8 hours. Limited clinical information at this time supports the use of once-daily aminoglycosides in this clinical setting. Monitoring of aminoglycoside serum concentrations is essential to ensure adequate therapeutic levels and to minimize toxicity during the extended therapeutic course. (See also the chapter *Endocarditis of Natural and Prosthetic Valves: Treatment and Prophylaxis.*)

Table 1 Susceptibility Rates for 1,936 Enterococci Isolated from Patients with Numerous Types of Infection at 97 Medical Centers in 1992–1993

	PERCENT SUSCEPTIBLE		
ANTIMICROBIAL AGENT	*E. FAECALIS* (NO. = 1428)	*E. FAECIUM* (NO. = 306)	*OTHER SPECIES* (NO. = 202)
Ampicillin	>99	41	81
Gentamicin	74	69	73
Streptomycin	69	44	65
Vancomycin	98	78	93
Teicoplanin	>99	84	94

Modified from Jones RN, Sader HS, Erwin ME, et al. Emerging multiple resistant enterococci among clinical isolates: I. Prevalence data from a 97 medical center surveillance study in the United States. Diag Microbiol Infect Dis 1995; 21:85–94.

The choice of an aminoglycoside for combination therapy is between gentamicin and streptomycin. Gentamicin is generally preferred, as synergic killing is more consistent, ototoxicity is less, and facilities to measure serum levels are more easily available. Enterococcal strains resistant to high levels of aminoglycoside in vitro are not susceptible to synergic killing with a penicillin or glycopeptide, and in such patients use of aminoglycosides constitutes exposure to potential toxicity for no apparent clinical benefit. Cross-resistance between gentamicin and streptomycin is not universal, and strains resistant to one should be tested against the other. Optimal therapy is not well defined for strains resistant to high levels of both aminoglycosides. Prolonged therapy with high doses of a penicillin, possibly by continuous infusion, may be successful in some cases. Combination therapy with vancomycin and a penicillin has also been reported successful.

Enterococcal resistance to penicillin and vancomycin and to high levels of aminoglycoside will be increasingly encountered in hospital practice and possibly in clinic patients. There is no established therapy for this group of organisms. Vancomycin-resistant enterococci of the Van B phenotype remain susceptible to teicoplanin, which is not available in the United States but may be obtainable for compassionate use for patients with this type of infecting organism. Teicoplanin is not bactericidal alone, and combinations with an aminoglycoside appear appropriate for strains for which the combination will be synergistic. It is important that teicoplanin be used in adequate dose, particularly if used alone. Not less than 6 mg per kilogram twice on the first day and once daily thereafter is required for effective therapy of serious infection, and doses of 10 to 15 mg per kilogram have been used without serious toxicity. Monitoring for adequacy of trough levels (at least 20 μg per milliliter) is important where feasible, although facilities for such monitoring may not be available. Serum inhibitory and bactericidal titers may be as useful. Teicoplanin resistance has emerged on chemotherapy.

Therapy with teicoplanin is not an option for Van A strains, and this is the predominant phenotype of vancomycin resistance in the United States. Various therapeutic approaches have been suggested, but none are widely accepted. Chloramphenicol and doxycycline have demonstrated a high degree of activity (over 90 percent susceptible by NCCLS criteria; Table 2) against the multidrug-resistant enterococci. Case reports indicate that these drugs used alone or with codrugs have been successful in a high percentage of cases, but each is only bacteriostatic. Combinations of both

Table 2 In Vitro Susceptibility of Alternative Antimicrobials for *E. Faecalis* Isolates (42 Strains Tested) with Resistance to Glycopeptides, Penicillins, and Both Aminoglycosides

ANTIMICROBIAL AGENT	SUSCEPTIBLE	INTERMEDIATE	RESISTANT
Fluoroquinolones			
Ciprofloxacin	0%	55%	45%
Clinafloxacin*	64	2	34
DU-6859a*	76	19	5
DV-7551a	67	2	31
Levofloxacin	57	7	36
Ofloxacin	57	5	38
Sparfloxacin	62	0	38
Trovafloxacin*	62	2	36
Everninomycins			
SCH 27899	100	0	0
Glycylcyclines			
Cl-331,928	100	0	0
Cl-344,677	100	0	0
Oxazolidinones			
Eperzolid (U-100592)	100	0	0
Linezolid (U-100766)	100	0	0
Pristinomycins			
Quinupristin-dalfopristin*	100	0	0
Other classes			
Chloramphenicol	100	0	0
Clindamycin	0	0	100
Doxycycline	93	7	0
Erythromycin	0	0	100
Imipenem	0	0	100
Novobiocin*	100	0	0
Rifampin	21	0	79
TMP-SMX	2	0	98

These strains represent approximately 2 percent of all organisms isolated among a sample of nearly 2,000 strains from 97 medical centers.

*May be available by compassionate use protocol; contact manufacturer.

TMP-SMX, trimethoprim-sulfamethoxazole.

Modified from Sader HS, Pfaller MA, Tenover FC, et al. Evaluation and characterization of multi-resistant *Enterococcus faecium* from 12 U.S. medical centers. J Clin Microbiol 1994; 32:2840–2842.

drugs are also not bactericidal. Even with eradication of enterococci from the bloodstream, mortality remains high (30 to 50 percent). Fluoroquinolones (ciprofloxacin and ofloxacin) may have value for tested susceptible strains (see Table 2), although resistance may emerge rapidly when these drugs are used alone. Their action on susceptible strains is usually bactericidal. Combinations of ampicillin and ciprofloxacin have been found bactericidal for some strains. In vitro and animal studies support the use of a combination of novobiocin and a fluoroquinolone for some isolates, although in our experience the high degree of protein binding for novobiocin (above 95 percent) significantly reduces its perceived activity. Pristinomycins (quinupristin-dalfopristin or Synercid) are generally bacteriostatic agents available for compassionate use for therapy of *E. faecium* infection. These agents are not active against most *E. faecalis* strains. A variety of other fluoroquinolones in development (see Table 2) are more active against enterococci than ciprofloxacin and may have expanded potential for future use. Everninomicin, oxazolidinones, and glycylcyclines are other highly effective investigational compounds of recent interest (see Table 2). However, most of these drugs demonstrate little or inconsistent bactericidal action against multidrug-resistant enterococci.

Therapy for enterococcal bloodstream infection in the absence of endocarditis follows the same general principles as for endocarditis except that bactericidal therapy may not be necessary. Bactericidal effect should be sought in the immunocompromised patient. Empiric therapy for such patients should be initiated with vancomycin, since patients likely to develop nosocomial enterococcal infection are also at risk for infection with methicillin-resistant, coagulase-negative staphylococci. As with all other pathogens, removal of potential foci of infection, such as an indwelling device, and drainage of an abscess, is essential for successful therapy.

■ THERAPY OF MODERATE INFECTION AND URINARY TRACT INFECTION

In the absence of immediate susceptibility test results, ampicillin or amoxicillin is still a reasonable option for therapy of moderate infections and particularly for urinary tract infection, given the high levels of ampicillin achieved in urine. Nitrofurantoin is also active against most enterococci and is useful in therapy of urinary tract infection. Clearly these approaches must be modified in the context of local epidemiology and emergence of resistant strains. In centers with very high incidence of infection with ampicillin-resistant enterococci, usually *E. faecium*, this may not be appropriate therapy. For infection with drug-resistant organisms, the options are similar to those discussed for bloodstream infection, except that synergic combinations are usually not necessary.

■ ENTEROCOCCAL CARRIAGE

There is no general acceptance that fecal carriage of multidrug-resistant enterococci is an indication for therapy; however, given the risk to the patient of subsequent disseminated infection, there is high epidemiologic interest in this issue. It seems reasonable to review the patient's therapy with a view toward discontinuation of any nonessential antimicrobials that might confer a selective advantage for the enterococci. There have been reports of the successful use of oral bacitracin to eradicate fecal carriage of vancomycin- and ampicillin-resistant enterococci.

■ COMMENTS

Therapy of enterococcal infections is one of the most challenging areas in the contemporary treatment of infectious disease. Good laboratory support is essential to management of these infections in the most appropriate manner with minimal toxicity. Given the emerging inadequacies of our therapeutic armamentarium and the clear evidence that nosocomial spread of this pathogen can occur, an aggressive stance with respect to hospital environment surveillance and infection control are of critical importance. Also, more study will be required to develop new therapeutic agents and to focus our treatments on existing antimicrobial agents that produce acceptable enterococcus infection eradication.

Suggested Reading

Arthur M, Reynolds PE, Depardieu F, Evers S, Dutka-Malen S, Quintiliani R Jr, Courvalin P. Mechanisms of glycopeptide resistance in enterococci. *J Infect* 1996; 32:11–16.

Centers for Disease Control. Nosocomial enterococci resistant to vancomycin: United States, 1989–1993. MMWR 1993; 42:597–599.

Centers for Disease Control. Addressing emerging infectious disease threats: a prevention strategy for the United States. Executive summary. MMWR 1994; 43(RR-5):1–18.

Cormican MG, Jones RN. The role of teicoplanin in contemporary therapy of enterococcal infection. *Chemother J* 1996; 5:174–179.

Emori TG, Gaynes RP. An overview of nosocomial infections, including the role of the microbiology laboratory. Clin Microbiol Rev 1993; 6:428–442.

Federal Register Preventing the spread of vancomycin resistance: quarterly report from the Hospital Infection Control Practices Advisory Committee. Fed Reg 1994 May 17;59:25758–25763.

Freeman C, Robinson A, Cooper B, et al. In vitro antimicrobial susceptibility of glycopeptide-resistant enterococci. Diag Microbio Infect Dis 1994; 21:47–50.

Frieden TR, Munsiff SS, Low DE, et al. Emergence of vancomycin-resistant enterococci in New York City. Lancet 1993; 342(8863):76–79.

Jones RN, Sader HS, Erwin ME, et al. Emerging multiple resistant enterococci among clinical isolates: l. Prevalence data from a 9 medical center surveillance study in the United States. Diag Microbiol Infect Dis 1995; 21:85–94.

Moellering RC Jr. Emergence of Enterococcus as a significant pathogen. Clin Infect Dis 1992;14:1173–1176.

Sader HS, Pfaller MA, Tenover FC, et al. Evaluation and characterization of multi-resistant *Enterococcus faecium* from 12 U.S. medical centers. J Clin Microbiol 1994; 32:2840–2842.

Woodford N, Johnson AP, Morrison D, Speller DCE. Current perspectives on glycopeptide resistance. *Clin Microbiol Rev* 1995; 8:585–615.

HAEMOPHILUS

Feng-Yee Chang, M.B., D.M.S.
Victor L. Yu, M.D.

Members of the genus *Haemophilus* are gram-negative bacteria that constitute part of the normal flora of the respiratory tract of humans and many animal species. The *Haemophilus* spp. *H. influenzae, H. parainfluenzae, H. aphrophilus, H. paraphrophilus, H. aegyptius,* and *H. ducreyi* are well documented human pathogens, and *H. haemolyticus, H. segnis,* and *H. parahaemolyticus* have been implicated infrequently.

H. influenzae is indigenous to humans only. *H. influenzae* in cultures obtained from the upper (but not from the lower) respiratory tract is a normal finding, because up to 80 percent of persons are carriers. Although most people are colonized with unencapsulated strains, 3 to 5 percent of individuals are colonized with encapsulated strains, most commonly serotype b. The type b capsule is a major virulence factor, and type b strains cause 95 percent of systemic *H. influenzae* infections in children.

Two clinical patterns of *H. influenzae* disease are seen: the most serious is invasive infection such as meningitis, septic arthritis, epiglottitis, and cellulitis; bacteremia is common. Invasive infections are usually caused by type b strains and are seen in young children during the winter. The second presentation is less serious but occurs more frequently as a result of contiguous spread of *H. influenzae* within the respiratory tract, leading to otitis media, sinusitis, conjunctivitis, or pneumonia. These infections are usually caused by unencapsulated strains.

Haemophilus spp. other than *H. influenzae* cause a variety of diseases including respiratory tract infection, endocarditis, septicemia, meningitis, brain abscess, and soft-tissue infections. *H. ducreyi* is the causative agent of chancroid. *H. influenzae aegyptius* causes Brazilian purpuric fever, which arises as conjunctivitis in young children and then progresses to sepsis with purpura.

The correct diagnosis of *Haemophilus* infections relies on isolation of the organism or detection of capsular antigen. Nasopharyngeal culture for *H. influenzae* is not helpful because of the high carriage rate among healthy persons. Cultures of blood, cerebrospinal fluid (CSF), and other normally sterile fluids (e.g., from joints or pleural, subdural, or pericardial spaces) are diagnostic. Cultures in cases of epiglottitis are generally positive but should be taken only when the airway can be protected. Needle aspiration of the middle ear (tympanocentesis), maxillary sinus, an area of cellulitis, or lung may occasionally yield the organism. Specimens should also be Gram stained. *Haemophilus* varies morphologically, appearing as coccobacilli or filamentous rods. Pleomorphic character, small size, and inconsistent uptake of dyes often render identification by stains difficult. In about 70 percent of cases of meningitis CSF smears reveal small coccobacillary organisms. Detection of capsular antigen in serum, CSF, or concentrated urine using immunoelectrophoresis, latex agglutination, or enzyme-linked immunosorbent assay (ELISA) may be diagnostic and can be found in up to 90 percent of culture-proved cases of meningitis. It may be especially useful in patients who have received empiric antibiotic therapy, because even if the culture is negative, antigen after antibiotic therapy is detectable in infected pleural, pericardial, or joint fluid, as well as in CSF.

Table 1 Treatment for *Haemophilus* Infections

ORGANISMS	DISEASES	PREFERRED ANTIBIOTICS	ALTERNATIVES
H. influenzae, H. parainfluenzae, H. aphrophilus, H. paraphrophilus	Serious infection, pneumonia, cellulitis	Ceftriaxone, ceftizoxime, cefotaxime	Ampicillin (if β-lactamase negative) or cefuroxime or chloramphenicol
	Meningitis	Ceftriaxone/cefotaxime	Ampicillin (if β-lactamase negative) or chloramphenicol
	Otitis, sinusitis	Amoxicillin (if β-lactamase negative) or amoxicillin-clavulanate or cefuroxime axetil, cefuroxime	TMP-SMX or Cefaclor, cefixime, loracarbef, cefprozil, cefpodoxime, or azithromycin
	Exacerbations of chronic bronchitis	TMP-SMX or doxycycline	Amoxicillin (if β-lactamase negative) or Amoxicillin-clavulanate or Cefaclor, cefixime, or Azithromycin, clarithromycin
H. parainfluenzae, H. aphrophilus, H. paraphrophilus	Endocarditis	Ampicillin (if β-lactamase negative) with gentamicin or ceftriaxone	
H. ducreyi	Chancroid	Ceftriaxone or erythromycin	TMP-SMX or amoxicillin-clavulanate or ciprofloxacin, ofloxacin

TMP-SMX, trimethoprim-sulfamethoxazole.

Table 2 Recommended Dosages of Antibiotic Therapy in *Haemophilus* Infections in Adults

DRUG	DOSE, INTERVAL	DAILY DOSE FOR SERIOUS INFECTION
Amoxicillin	0.25–0.5 g q8h PO	1.5 g
Ampicillin	0.5–1 g q6h PO	4 g
	1–2 g q4–6h IV/IM	8–(12)*g
Amoxicillin-clavulanate	0.25–0.5 g q8h PO	1.5 g
Cefaclor	0.25–0.5 g q8h PO	1.5 g
Cefixime	0.4 g/day q12–24 PO	0.4 g
Cefpodoxime	0.2–0.4 g q12h PO	0.4–0.8 g
Cefuroxime axetil	0.125–0.5 g q12h PO	0.5–1 g
Cefuroxime	0.75–1.5 g q8h IV/IM	4.5 g
Cefprozil	0.25–0.5 g q12h PO	0.5–1 g
Loracarbef	0.2–0.4 g q12h PO	0.4–0.8 g
Cefotaxime	1–2 g q4–12h IV/IM	6–(12)* g
Ceftizoxime	1–4 g q8–12h IV/IM	6–(12)* g
Ceftriaxone	1–2 g q12–24h IV/IM	2–(4)* g
Chloramphenicol	12.5–(25)* mg/kg q6h IV/IM	4 g*
Erythromycin	0.25–.5 g q6h PO	2 g
	0.25–1 g q6h IV	4 g
Azithromycin	0.25–0.5 g q24h	0.5 g
Clarithromycin	0.25–0.5 g q12h PO	0.5–1 g
Doxycycline†	0.1 g q12–24h PO/IV/IM	0.2 g
Ciprofloxacin	0.25–0.75 g q12h PO	1.5 g
	0.2–0.4 g q12h IV	0.8 g
Ofloxacin	0.2–0.4 g q12h PO or IV (infuse over 60 min)	0.8 g
TMP-SMX	4–5 mg/kg q6–12h (as TMP) IV	1.2 g TMP, 6 g SMX IV
Gentamicin	1–1.7 mg/kg q8h IV/IM	3–5 mg/kg

*For meningitis or life-threatening infections.
†Use in children older than 7 years.
TMP-SMX, trimethoprim-sulfamethoxazole.

■ ANTIBIOTIC THERAPY

Meningitis and epiglottitis due to *H. influenzae* type b can be rapidly fatal. For many years ampicillin and chloramphenicol have been the mainstays of therapy. However, increasing resistance to both ampicillin and chloramphenicol has necessitated major changes in antibiotic therapy. Third-generation cephalosporins (e.g., cefotaxime and ceftriaxone) are now recommended as initial therapy for meningitis in children beyond the neonatal period. The usual duration of therapy is 7 to 10 days, depending on clinical response. Repeat CSF culture to validate cure is usually unnecessary in patients who have a clinical response.

Use of corticosteroid therapy to reduce cerebral edema and other complications has been controversial. However, one study has suggested that deafness was decreased by dexamethasone.

Treatment of serious infection caused by nontypeable *H. influenzae,* such as meningitis, lower respiratory tract infections, tubal abscess, and neonatal sepsis, requires systemic antibiotics. Cephalosporins, including second-generation (cefuroxime) and third-generation agents, are most commonly used. Chloramphenicol is also effective, but blood concentrations must be monitored in premature infants. Sinusitis and otitis media caused by nontypeable *H. influenzae* can usually be treated with oral amoxicillin. If ampicillin resistance is common in the geographic area, then amoxicillin-clavulanate, trimethoprim-sulfamethoxazole (TMP-SMX), an oral second-generation cephalosporin, or azithromycin is effective (Tables 1 and 2).

H. influenzae is often implicated with other respiratory pathogens in chronic bronchitis. Antibiotic therapy for exacerbations of chronic bronchitis is commonly used in adult patients with chronic obstructive pulmonary disease, although efficacy is uncertain. Worsening cough with increasing purulence of sputum is the primary indication. We recommend the cheapest oral agents, including TMP-SMX or the tetracyclines, especially doxycycline. Amoxicillin, amoxicillin-clavulanate, oral cephalosporins, and azithromycin are alternatives. Duration is 7 to 10 days. Some authorities recommend sputum culture prior to initiation of therapy, but we do not, since results do not necessarily correlate with clinical response.

■ PREVENTION

Four vaccines are licensed for active immunization against invasive type b infections. Conjugate vaccines are administered at the same time as diphtheria-pertussis-tetanus and polio immunizations as part of the routine program of childhood immunizations. The inclusion of a conjugate type b vaccine in the routine immunization schedule has resulted in a dramatic decline in invasive type b disease in young children in the United States. Chemoprophylaxis for those with close contact to patients with *H. influenzae* meningitis, such as day care or household contact, is indicated. The drug of choice is oral rifampin 20 mg per kilogram (maximum 600 mg) in a single daily dose for 4 days.

Individuals with immunodeficiencies, especially those with primary deficiency of antibody synthesis, have increased susceptibility to infection with *H. influenzae,* particularly nontypeable strains. They may benefit from passive infusion of immunoglobulin preparations administered either intramuscularly or intravenously.

Suggested Reading

Isada CM. Antibiotics for chronic bronchitis with exacerbations. Semin Resp Infect 1993; 8:243–253.

Moxon ER. *Haemophilus influenzae.* In: Mandell G, Bennett JE, Dolin R (eds) Principles and practice of infectious diseases. 4th ed. New York: Churchill Livingstone, 1995: 2039.

LEGIONELLOSIS

Lutfiye Mulazimoglu, M.D.
Victor L. Yu, M.D.

Legionellosis defines the clinical syndromes Pontiac fever and Legionnaires' disease, which are caused by members of the Legionellaceae family. The most prominent species is *Legionella pneumophila,* but there are over 35 other species. *L. pneumophila* causes about 90 percent of human infections and contains 14 serogroups, but serogroup 1 is the predominant pathogen. *Legionella micdadei* (Pittsburgh pneumonia agent) causes 6 percent of infections. The other species cause the remaining 4 percent of cases.

L. pneumophila can be found in natural aquatic habitats, including rivers and lakes. Man-made water distribution systems are the primary reservoir for dissemination of the organism. Cooling towers have been implicated in some reports, but their actual role in disseminating the organism has been questioned. Air conditioning systems have never been implicated in cases of Legionnaires' disease. The mode of transmission is aspiration, aerosolization, or instillation of water contaminated with *Legionella* into the respiratory tract.

■ CLINICAL MANIFESTATIONS

Legionnaires' disease is pneumonia caused by *Legionella* spp. The clinical presentation is that of an acute pneumonia. Cigarette smoking, chronic lung disease, advanced age, immunosuppression, especially with corticosteroids, and transplant surgery are the major risk factors.

Fever is virtually always present, and 20 percent of patients have temperatures in excess of 40°C (104°F). Some 80 percent of patients cough, initially mildly and only slightly productively. In about 10 percent of cases sputum may be streaked with blood. Chest pain, pleuritic and nonpleuritic, is a prominent feature for 10 percent of patients. Watery diarrhea, nausea, vomiting, and abdominal pain are seen in 25 to 50 percent of cases. Headache and mental status changes are the most common neurologic symptoms.

The initial finding on chest radiograph is usually a unilateral alveolar infiltrate, which can progress to other lobes with consolidation. Diffuse interstitial infiltrates were seen in 25 percent of those affected at the original American Legionnaires' outbreak in 1976. Circumscribed peripheral opacities with cavitation tend to occur in immunosuppressed patients receiving corticosteroids. Radiologic improvement lags behind clinical improvement. Although there are a few clinical clues suggestive of Legionnaires' disease (Table 1), the presentation is actually nonspecific, and specialized laboratory tests are necessary for definitive diagnosis.

Pontiac fever is an acute, self-limiting, flulike illness with 24 to 48 hours' incubation period and high attack rate.

Table 1 Clinical SIgns Suggestive of Legionnaires' Disease

High fever, often over 40°C (104°F)
Diarrhea
Hyponatremia (serum sodium less than 131 mEq per liter)
Gram stain of respiratory specimens showing numerous neutrophils but no organisms
Failure to respond to beta-lactam agents or aminoglycosides

Pneumonia does not occur. The predominant symptoms are malaise, myalgias, fever, chills, and headache. Complete recovery is the rule even without any specific therapy.

■ LABORATORY FINDINGS

Patients often have moderate leukocytosis. Hyponatremia (serum sodium value below 131 mEq per liter) occurs more often in Legionnaires' disease than in pneumonias of other causes.

Legionellae are small gram-negative rods and usually cannot be seen in Gram stain of sputa, although they are occasionally visualized in pleural fluid. Isolation of the organism by culture from respiratory secretions is the definitive method of diagnosis. Buffered charcoal yeast extract agar supplemented with antibiotics and dyes is the most sensitive medium. Macroscopically visible colonies are seen in 3 to 5 days. Culture using multiple selective media has a sensitivity of 80 percent. Direct fluorescent antibody stain of the specimen is rapid and highly specific. Sensitivity is 50 percent to 70 percent; large numbers of organisms (10^4 to 10^5 per milliliter) within the specimen are required for microscopic visualization. Antibody titers were often used in the past prior to the advent of culture, but they require both acute and convalescent sera. A single titer of 1:128 is presumptive evidence of disease, and a fourfold rise in titer is diagnostic. The sensitivity of serology is about 40 percent.

Detection of *Legionella*-soluble antigens in urine is a rapid diagnostic test that is highly sensitive but available only for *L. pneumophila* serogroup 1. This drawback may be minor because this serogroup causes about 80 percent of *Legionella* infections. Antigen in urine is detectable 3 days after the onset of clinical disease, even if specific antibiotic therapy is given, and it persists for several weeks.

■ ANTIBIOTIC THERAPY (TABLE 2)

Erythromycin has been the historic antibiotic of choice. However, erratic responses is severely ill patients and intolerance of erythromycin has been problematic. Adverse effects of erythromycin therapy include thrombophlebitis, gastric intolerance (nausea, vomiting, abdominal discomfort), and ototoxicity at the 4 g (but not the 2 g) dose. In the hospitalized patient the requirement for large volumes of fluid with the administration of the 4 g dose is problematic. Patients with Legionnaires' disease are likely to have underlying heart and lung disease and not likely to tolerate large fluid loads. With the appearance of newer macrolides, it is likely that erythromycin will be displaced by other more efficacious and less

Table 2 Antibiotic Therapy for *Legionella* Infections

ANTIMICROBIAL AGENTS	DOSE	ROUTE	FREQUENCY
Erythromycin	1 g	IV	q6h
	500 mg	PO	q6h
Rifampin*	600 mg	PO	q12h or 24h
	600 mg	IV	q12h or 24h
TMP-SMX	160/800 mg	IV	q8h
	160/800 mg	PO	q12h
Doxycycline	100 mg	IV, PO	q12h
Tetracycline	500 mg	IV, PO	q6h
Ciprofloxacin	400 mg	IV	q8h
	750 mg	PO	q12h
Azithromycin	500 mg	PO	q24h
Clarithromycin	500 mg	PO	q12h

*Rifampin must be given in combination with another agent.
TMP-SMX, trimethoprim-sulfamethoxazole.

toxic antibiotics. The recommended dosage for erythromycin is 2 g orally or 4 g intravenously daily.

Although oral antibiotics may be adequate for nontoxic and immunocompetent patients, abrupt deterioration has been observed in some patients who appeared stable at the time of diagnosis. Furthermore, gastrointestinal dysfunction commonly seen in Legionnaires' disease may compromise absorption of any oral antibiotic; thus, initial parenteral administration is prudent. Clinical response, including defervescence and feeling of well-being, usually occurs within 3 to 5 days. Once a clinical response has been documented, oral therapy can replace parenteral therapy. Duration of therapy is 10 to 14 days, although 3 weeks has been recommended for immunosuppressed patients.

For confirmed cases of Legionnaires' disease we recommend combination therapy with a macrolide or quinolone combined with rifampin as initial treatment. We also suggest that a macrolide (erythromycin, azithromycin, clarithromycin) may be the antibiotic of choice for immunocompetent patients with community-acquired pneumonia in whom the Gram stain of sputum shows many neutrophils but a paucity or absence of organisms. Such a Gram stain also suggests *Mycoplasma pneumoniae* or *Chlamydia pneumoniae,* and these infections are also covered by a macrolide. We now use azithromycin as the drug of choice for *Legionella* infections. In vitro intracellular penetration models show that azithromycin is much more active than erythromycin, and anecdotal cases of such therapy have been successful. Furthermore, the gastrointestinal intolerance seen with the newer macrolides is much less than that of erythromycin.

Ciprofloxacin is the antibiotic of choice for transplant recipients because both macrolides and rifampin interact pharmacologically with transplant immunosuppressive medications, including cyclosporine and tacrolimus.

Pontiac fever need only be treated symptomatically; no antibiotic therapy is required.

■ PREVENTION

Disinfection of the water supply is the ultimate preventive measure. The superheat and flush method requires heating the water so that the distal outlet temperature is 70° to 80°C (158° to 176°F) and rinsing the outlets (faucets, shower heads) with hot water for at least 30 minutes. This method is easy to implement and highly effective but logistically tedious because of the necessity to run hot water through all the distal outlets. A commercial copper and silver ionization has proved highly effective in numerous hospitals. Chlorination is no longer recommended.

Suggested Reading

Edelstein PH. Legionnaires' disease. Clin Infect Dis 1993; 16:741–749.
Nguyen MH, Stout JE, Yu VL. Legionellosis. Infect Dis Clin N Am 1991; 5:561–584.
Roig J, Domingo C, Morera J. Legionnaires' disease. Chest 1994; 105:1817–1825.
Yu VL. *Legionella pneumophila* (Legionnaires' disease). In: Mandell GL, Bennett JE, Dolin R eds. Mandell, Douglas, and Bennett's principles and practice of infectious disease. 4th ed. New York: Churchill Livingstone, 1995:2087.

GONOCOCCUS

John H. Powers, M.D.
Michael F. Rein, M.D.

Neisseria gonorrhoeae, a sexually transmitted pathogen, causes disease by attachment to columnar or cuboidal epithelial cells. Attachment is mediated by pili and outer membrane proteins. The organism penetrates between and through the cells to submucosal areas, where it elicits a neutrophilic host response. Definitive diagnosis is based on isolation of the organism in culture or identification by one of the newer noncultural techniques such as enzyme-linked immunosorbent assay (ELISA) or DNA probe.

Acute urethritis, presenting as some combination of urethral discharge and dysuria, is the primary manifestation of disease in men. Gram stain of a smear of urethral discharge may be used for presumptive diagnosis of gonococcal urethritis. Gram-negative diplococci in neutrophils are found in 90 percent of men with this disease, and the finding is 98 percent specific.

In women the primary site of infection is the endocervix. Although the organism can be isolated from the urethra and the periurethral (Skene's) and Bartholin's glands, these are rarely the sole site of infection. In women, Gram stains of cervical smears have a specificity of 97 percent when intracellular organisms are present but a sensitivity of only 50 to 70 percent, which probably obviates the use of the Gram stain in women.

Anorectal gonorrhea occurs in up to 40 percent of women with endocervical disease and in homosexual men. Most patients with *N. gonorrhoeae* cultured from this site are asymptomatic, but acute proctitis may be present. Most patients with pharyngeal infection are also asymptomatic. Gonococcal conjunctivitis in the adult produces a range of degrees of inflammation.

Disseminated gonococcal infection is uncommon overall, occurring in 0.5 to 3 percent of infected patients. The predominant clinical entity of disseminated infection is the arthritis-dermatitis syndrome, which usually manifests as asymmetric migratory polyarthritis, arthralgias, or tenosynovitis accompanied in 33 to 50 percent of cases by small painful papules or pustules on an erythematous base. Complement deficiency has been noted in up to 13 percent of patients with disseminated disease.

■ THERAPY

Uncomplicated anogenital infection with *N. gonorrhoeae* can be treated with a single dose of an appropriate medication. Treatment has been complicated in recent years by the emergence of resistance to various antimicrobials. The susceptibility of the gonococcus to penicillin has been severely compromised by the organism's acquisition of a plasmid that codes for the production of beta-lactamase, yielding the so-called penicillinase-producing strains of *N. gonorrhoeae* (PPNG). Chromosomally mediated resistance, which codes for alteration of the penicillin-binding proteins, has also resulted in decreased sensitivity of the organism, to the point that penicillin is no longer recommended for the treatment of gonococcal infections. Chromosomal and plasmid-mediated resistance to tetracyclines, also noted worldwide, has precluded the use of tetracyclines in the treatment of gonorrhea. Up to half of isolates demonstrating chromosomal resistance to penicillin are also resistant to trimethoprim-sulfamethoxazole (TMP-SMX), and this drug should be avoided if alternatives are available. Given the public health implications of spread of the organism in the population and the potential for the emergence of further resistance to antimicrobials, regimens with less than 95 percent efficacy are considered unacceptable. The treatment of gonococcal disease is further complicated by frequent coinfection with *Chlamydia trachomatis* in genital infections, proctitis, and conjunctivitis.

Oral Therapy (Table 1)

The fluoroquinolone antibiotics have demonstrated efficacy in all forms of uncomplicated anogenital gonococcal disease and can all be given as a single oral dose. These agents can be used in patients with immediate hypersensitivity reactions to beta-lactam antibiotics but are contraindicated in pregnant women and children because of the possibility of toxicity at the epiphyseal growth plate. Resistance of *N. gonorrhoeae* to the quinolones has been noted but is still rare in the United States. Oral cephalosporins are also effective treatment. Cefixime and cefpodoxime have been studied, although clinical experience is greater with the former drug. Cefixime seems to have efficacy in the treatment of pharyngeal gonorrhea, but this regimen has been tested in only a few patients for this indication. There have been unacceptably high failure rates in pharyngeal gonorrhea with other oral cephalosporin regimens.

Parenteral Therapy

Third-generation cephalosporins such as ceftriaxone, cefotaxime, cefotetan, and ceftizoxime appear to have equal efficacy when given as a single intramuscular dose (Table 2). Clinical experience is greatest with ceftriaxone. This drug has the longest half-life and is injected in the smallest volume. A dose of 125 mg of ceftriaxone is effective, and this regimen is recommended by the Centers for Disease Control. However, concern has been expressed that routine use of the lower dose may lead to the emergence of resistance of the gonococcus to this agent. Only the higher dose of ceftriaxone has been studied in pregnant women. The smallest vial of ceftriaxone available for clinical use contains 250 mg, and unless more than one patient is to be treated, the use of the lower dose does not result in cost savings. Resistance to cefoxitin has developed in several areas, often in association with high-level tetracycline resistance; it should therefore no longer be used in the treatment of uncomplicated gonorrhea.

The aminocyclitol spectinomycin is an alternative for patients who are pregnant or for children who have a history

Table 1 Oral Regimens for Treatment of Localized Gonococcal Infection Including Urethritis, Cervicitis, Pharyngitis, Proctitis

DRUG	REGIMEN (SINGLE DOSES)	CDC RECOMMENDATION	SAFETY IN PREGNANCY	SAFETY IN AGE ≤16 YEARS	EFFECTIVE IN PHARYNX	COMMENTS
Ciprofloxacin	500 mg	Yes	No	No	Yes	
Ofloxacin	400 mg	Yes	No	No	Possibly effective	300 mg twice daily for 7 days covers gonorrhea and chlamydial infection
Norfloxacin	800 mg	Alternative	No	No	No	Limited data
Enoxacin	400 mg	Alternative	No	No	Limited data	Resistance rapidly developing in some areas of the Far East
Lomefloxacin	400 mg	Alternative	No	No	Limited data	Very limited experience
Cefixime	400 mg	Yes	Yes	Yes	Limited data but probably effective	
Cefpodoxime proxetil	200 mg	No	Yes	Yes	Probably not	Limited experience
Azithromycin	1–2 g	No	Yes	Yes	Very limited data	May cause GI upset at this dose; effective against chlamydial infection as well

All regimens for localized disease should be accompanied by appropriate therapy for concomitant chlamydial infection, e.g., doxycycline 100 mg PO b.i.d. for 7 days or a single dose of 1 g of azithromycin.
CDC, Centers for Disease Control; GI, gastrointestinal.

Table 2 Parenteral Regimens for Treatment of Localized Gonococcal Infection Including Urethritis, Cervicitis, Pharyngitis, Proctitis

DRUG	REGIMEN (SINGLE DOSE, IM)	CDC RECOMMENDATION	SAFETY IN PREGNANCY	SAFETY IN AGE ≤16 YEARS	EFFECTIVE IN PHARYNX	COMMENTS
Ceftriaxone	125 mg	Yes	Yes*	Yes	Yes	
Ceftriaxone	250 mg	Formerly	Yes	Yes	Yes	Partial activity against coincident incubating syphilis
Ceftizoxime	500 mg	Alternative	Yes	Yes	Probably	
Cefotaxime	500 mg	Alternative	Yes	Yes	Probably	
Cefotetan	1 g	Alternative	Yes	Yes	Probably	
Spectinomycin	2 g	Alternative	Yes	Yes	No	

All regimens for localized disease should be accompanied by appropriate therapy for concomitant chlamydial infection, e.g., doxycycline 100 mg PO b.i.d. for 7 days or a single dose of 1 g of azithromycin.
CDC, Centers for Disease Control.
*This dose has not been studied in pregnant women (see text).

of immediate hypersensitivity to the beta-lactams. Resistance has been noted in Korea, and the drug does not reach adequate concentrations in saliva, rendering it ineffective in the treatment of pharyngeal disease. Parenteral aminoglycosides, especially gentamicin, have been included in inpatient regimens for the treatment of pelvic inflammatory disease.

Nonstandard Therapy

The monobactam aztreonam and the carbapenem imipenem-cilastatin regimens are uniformly effective against *N. gonorrhoeae* but are costly and available only in intravenous form. These drugs are never primary therapy for gonorrhea. Penicillins formulated with a beta-lactamase inhibitor (i.e., amoxicillin-clavulanate, ampicillin-sulbactam, ticarcillin-clavulanate, and piperacillin-tazobactam) are costly, and although they are effective against PPNG strains, they may not be effective against isolates with chromosomally mediated resistance.

The dose of the newer macrolide azithromycin required to eradicate the gonococcus (2 g orally) is twice that used in the

Table 3 Regimens for Treatment of Disseminated Gonococcal Infection

DRUG	REGIMEN	CDC RECOMMENDATION	SAFETY IN PREGNANCY	SAFETY IN AGE ≤16 YEARS	COMMENTS
Ceftriaxone	1 g IM or IV q24h	Yes	Yes	Yes	Use until clinical improvement, then complete 7–10 days of therapy with cefixime 400 mg PO b.i.d., ciprofloxacin 500 mg PO b.i.d., or ofloxacin 400 mg PO b.i.d. Use cefixime for patients under 17 years of age.
Ceftizoxime	1 g IV q8h	Alternative	Yes	Yes	Use until clinical improvement, then complete 7–10 days of therapy with cefixime 400 mg PO b.i.d., ciprofloxacin 500 mg PO b.i.d., or ofloxacin 400 mg PO b.i.d. Use cefixime for patients under 17 years of age.
Cefotaxime	1 g IV q8h	Alternative	Yes	Yes	Use until clinical improvement, then complete 7–10 days of therapy with cefixime 400 mg PO b.i.d., ciprofloxacin 500 mg PO b.i.d., or ofloxacin 400 mg PO b.i.d. Use cefixime for patients under 17 years of age.
Spectinomycin	2 g IM b.i.d.	Alternative	Yes	Yes	Primarily for use in the setting of allergy to the beta-lactams. Use until clinical improvement, then complete 7–10 days of therapy with ciprofloxacin 500 mg PO b.i.d. or ofloxacin 400 mg PO b.i.d.

As with localized disease, therapy for disseminated gonococcal infection should be accompanied by appropriate therapy for concomitant chlamydial infection e.g., doxycycline 100 mg PO b.i.d. for 7 days or a single dose of 1 g of azithromycin. Seven days of ofloxacin as part of an above regimen will cover chlamydial infection.
CDC, Centers for Disease Control.

single-dose treatment of nongonococcal urethritis. This high dose frequently causes gastrointestinal upset and is far more expensive than alternative regimens. Limited data suggest that a 1 g dose may be effective.

Extragenital Disease

A single dose of ceftriaxone 125 mg IM in children or 1 g IM in adults cures gonococcal conjunctivitis, but long-term follow-up is lacking, and 7 to 10 days of a parenteral drug may be the safest alternative. Although saline flushing of the conjunctiva has been employed, topical antibiotics have no proven additional benefit.

No prospective studies on the treatment of disseminated gonococcal infection have been performed since 1976; hence, recommendations are empiric because the worldwide spread of resistant gonococci occurred after that time. The gonococcal arthritis-dermatitis syndrome should be treated with ceftriaxone. Regimens employing other third-generation cephalosporins should be equally effective. If frank septic arthritis is not present, the patient can be switched to oral cefixime or ciprofloxacin or an equivalent dose of another oral cephalosporin or quinolone after initial clinical improvement to complete 7 to 10 days of therapy. Spectinomycin is an alternative for pregnant women, children, and those who are allergic to beta-lactams. Gonococcal endocarditis should be treated with 4 weeks of an appropriate parenteral regimen, preferably ceftriaxone or another third-generation cephalosporin. Meningitis should be treated for 10 to 14 days. Penicillin therapy may still be used if the isolate in question is found to be susceptible to the drug, with a minimum inhibitory concentration (MIC) of 2 μg/ml or less. (Table 3)

Any regimen used to treat genital infections, conjunctivitis, or proctitis must include treatment for possible coinfection with *C. trachomatis.* It is also important to treat sexual contacts of patients with gonorrhea to prevent spread in the population as well as reinfection of the patient.

Suggested Reading

Centers for Disease Control and Prevention. 1993 sexually transmitted diseases treatment guidelines. MMWR 1993; 42(RR-14):56–60.

Centers for Disease Control and Prevention. Fluroquinolone resistance in *Neisseria gonorrhoeae*—Colorado and Washington, 1995. MMWR 1995; 44:761–764.

Moran JS, Levine WC. Drugs of choice for the treatment of uncomplicated gonococcal infections. Clin Infect Dis 1995; 20(Suppl 1):S47–S65.

Moran JS. Treating uncomplicated *Neisseria gonorrhoeae* infections: is the anatomic site of infection important? Sex Transm Dis 1995; 22:39–47.

Rein MF. Gonorrhea. Curr Opin Infect Dis 1991; 4:12–21.

MENINGOCOCCUS

Joann Pfundstein, M.D.
Edmund C. Tramont, M.D.

MENINGOCOCCAL INFECTION

Meningococcal infections are a worldwide health problem, with most cases occurring in children between 6 months and 5 years of age and in young adults 16 to 25 years of age. Epidemic cerebrospinal fever, the historical term for meningococcal meningitis, has been recognized for almost 2 centuries. Epidemics of meningococcal disease have been well described, especially in closed populations such as military recruits and in small towns. They are usually caused by serogroups A and C, while sporadic cases are more often associated with serogroups B and Y. Individuals with terminal complement component deficiencies are at an increased risk for developing meningococcal infections because their serum loses the ability to lyse the bacteria.

Clinical Features

The clinical manifestations of meningococcal disease can be quite varied. The mildest form is a transient bacteremia that usually begins insidiously, with fever, malaise, and symptoms of an upper respiratory infection. A few petechial skin lesions may appear, but neither signs nor symptoms of sepsis or meningitis develop. Symptoms usually resolve spontaneously within 24 to 48 hours. Acute meningococcemia, which often follows several days of upper respiratory infection symptoms, is heralded by fever, chills, malaise, weakness, headache, myalgias, nausea, and/or vomiting. The most remarkable manifestation is the characteristic petechial skin lesions, which usually appear in crops on the ankles and wrists and in the axilla. The palms, soles, neck, and face are usually spared. Fulminant meningococcemia, also referred to as Waterhouse-Friderichsen syndrome or purpura fulminans, complicates acute meningococcemia in 5 to 15 percent of cases and is associated with vascular collapse and high mortality. Meningitis may occur with or without any manifestations of meningococcemia. Clinically, meningococcal meningitis resembles an acute bacterial meningitis of any cause presenting with headache, fever, and a clouded sensorium, but it progresses to obtundation and death more rapidly than most other infections. On rare occasions a chronic meningococcemia develops. This is characterized by intermittent febrile episodes that last 2 to 10 days and are associated with a variety of skin lesions, macular, maculopapular, or pustular rash, as well as migratory arthralgias and myalgias. The infection may last months and can be fatal, but it usually resolves spontaneously. Occasionally meningococci may produce oropharyngitis, pneumonia, conjunctivitis, proctitis, or a genital tract infection; except in advanced acute cases, the response to appropriate antibiotic treatment is dramatic.

Culture and Laboratory Findings

Neisseria meningitidis is an aerobic oxidase-positive, gram-negative diplococcus that grows best at 35° to 37°C (95° to 98.6°F) in a moist environment of 5 to 7 percent CO_2 (candle jar). Oxidative metabolism of glucose and maltose but not of sucrose, lactose, or fructose is the major means for differentiating *N. meningitidis* from other *Neisseria* spp. The organism is surrounded by a polysaccharide capsule that provides the basis for serogrouping. With very rare exceptions invasive meningococci are encapsulated, attesting to the virulence conveyed by the polysaccharide capsule, but meningococci colonizing mucous membranes frequently are not. To date, 13 serogroups have been identified: serogroups A, B, C, W135, and Y are responsible for the overwhelming majority of cases of invasive disease.

Whenever possible, specimens should be cultured for *N. meningitidis* before instituting antibiotics. For culture of a normally sterile site, such as blood or cerebrospinal fluid (CSF), nonselective chocolate agar is preferred. A selective antibiotic-containing medium, such as a modified Thayer-Martin or New York City, is necessary when the culture specimen is obtained from a nonsterile site such as the oropharynx.

As in any patient with an acute bacterial meningitis, an abnormal CSF is accompanied by an elevated leukocyte count consisting predominantly of polymorphonuclear neutrophils associated with a low glucose level. A CSF Gram stain is positive for gram-negative diplococci in about 75 percent of cases. For a definitive diagnosis of meningococcal disease, isolation from a sterile body fluid site is required. CSF and blood are the most frequent sources of positive cultures. Nasopharyngeal cultures of *N. meningitidis* must be interpreted with caution. A positive throat culture may reveal serogroupable *N. meningitidis* in patients with invasive disease, but that alone should not be considered proof of a meningococcal infection, because patients with other causes of meningitis may be coincidental carriers of *N. meningitidis.* A Gram stain of scrapings from petechial lesions will demonstrate the pathogen in up to 70 percent of cases, since the petechial lesions are microabscesses. Rapid identification of *N. meningitidis* capsular polysaccharide in blood and CSF by latex particle agglutination (LPA) is also available, but its sensitivity is about the same as that of a Gram stain, so it offers little advantage.

Therapy

The introduction of antimicrobial agents dramatically transformed this highly fatal disease into a curable one, particularly when the diagnosis is made early. The era of chemotherapy for meningococcal infection began in 1937, when sulfonamides were successfully used to treat meningococcal meningitis and meningococcemia. However, resistance to sulfonamides rapidly developed, and today they have only a limited role in the treatment of meningococcal infections. Penicillin has remained the treatment of choice for more than 50 years.

Penicillin G therapy for meningococcal infections should be administered intravenously, at least initially. Adults should receive 300,000 U per kilogram per day divided q4h IV; the dose can be reduced after a few days, depending on the patient's clinical response. Infants and children should receive 250,000 U per kilogram per day IV in divided doses every 4 hours (Table 1).

Table 1 Treatment of Meningococcal Meningitis

ANTIBIOTIC	INTRAVENOUS DOSE	COMMENT
Penicillin G	Adults: 300,000 U/kg/day divided q4h Children: 250,000 U/kg divided q4h	Remains drug of choice; exceeds usual MIC with meningeal inflammation; relatively resistant strains reported
Ampicillin	Adults: 12 g qd divided q4h Children: 50–75 mg/kg q6h	As effective as penicillin; exceeds usual MIC with meningeal inflammation
Ceftriaxone	Adults: 1 g q12h Children: 8–150 mg/kg/qd divided q12h or qd	Good CNS penetration; exceeds usual MIC
Cefotaxime	Adults: 8–12 g/qd divided q4h Children: 200 mg/kg/day divided q6–8h	Exceeds usual MIC with meningeal inflammation
Ceftazidime	Adults: 1–2 g q8–12h Children: 125–150 mg/kg/qd divided q8h	Exceeds usual MIC with meningeal inflammation
Chloramphenicol	Adults: 25 mg/kg q6h Children: 25 mg/kg q6h	Concentrates in CSF; because of potential to cause irreversible aplastic anemia (1:10,000 to 1:40,000), it is rarely used in U.S. but is used more frequently in emerging countries
Ciprofloxacin	Adults: 400–600 mg q12h Children: 10–15 mg/kg/q12h	Appropriate spectrum and pharmacokinetics but few clinical data; no studies in children

In all instances treatment should extend 7 to 10 days.
MIC, minimum inhibitory concentration; CNS, central nervous system; CSF, cerebrospinal fluid.

For children the recommended empiric treatment with ampicillin plus an aminoglycoside is appropriate and adequate. The third-generation cephalosporins ceftriaxone, cefotaxime, and ceftazidime have been used for the empiric treatment of bacterial meningitis, primarily in children, and have cured meningococcal meningitis in a small number of patients. Nevertheless, these agents should be used only when drug hypersensitivity precludes the use of penicillin or a relatively penicillin-resistant meningococcus is isolated.

The duration of antibiotic therapy varies somewhat with the presentation of the disease and the patient's response to therapy. About 7 to 10 days of therapy is sufficient to sterilize the patient. Supportive therapy is vitally important for a successful outcome. Steroid therapy is indicated when acute adrenal insufficiency is a consequence of the Waterhouse-Friderichsen syndrome. Dexamethasone 0.15 mg per kilogram every 6 hours in infants and 8 to 12 mg every 12 hours in children and adults is recommended. Other uses of steroid therapy in meningococcal infection are unproven but probably not harmful.

Chloramphenicol has primarily historical importance; however, it remains a time-proven effective substitute in the patient allergic to penicillin; the dosage is 100 mg per kilogram per day in divided doses every 6 hours up to 4 g per day.

There have been rare reports from Spain and the United Kingdom of clinical isolates with resistance to penicillin (MIC greater than 1 mg/dl). Clinical isolates of *N. meningitidis* with relative resistance to penicillin (MIC 0.1 to 1 mg/dl) have also been found worldwide, including documented cases of invasive disease from geographically distinct areas in the United States. If *N. meningitidis* follows the trend of *Neisseria gonorrhoeae* and *Streptococcus pneumoniae*, the prevalence of penicillin resistance among meningococci will increase over the next decade, making antimicrobial therapy for meningococcal infection more complicated. While such resistant meningococcal strains have been infrequent to date, clinicians should be alerted to the possibility of them in unexplained treatment failures or in cases of slowly resolving documented meningococcal infections.

Prevention

Antimicrobial prophylaxis continues to play an important role in the management of meningococcal infection (Table 2). The need for prophylaxis is based on the demonstration that close contacts of patients with invasive meningococcal disease are at 500 to 1,000 times greater risk for developing the disease than the normal population. The primary factor determining the effectiveness of a meningococcal prophylactic agent is the ability of that agent to achieve bactericidal levels in the upper respiratory tract and thus interrupt transmission. The standard practice is to prescribe an antibiotic course that will eradicate the meningococcus from the throat of all household contacts, defined as persons residing in the same house, dorm, barracks, and so on, with the index case or spending more than 4 hours a day with the index case for 5 to 7 days before the onset of illness in the index case. Therefore, chemoprophylaxis is given to children and personnel in day care centers after a case has been identified. Medical personnel who perform cardiopulmonary resuscitation on an index patient should also receive prophylaxis.

A number of antibiotics for prophylaxis have been studied. A single injection of ceftriaxone 250 mg IM in adults and 125 mg IM in children is 97 percent effective in eradicating meningococcus from throat carriers; but the cost, availability, and route of administration limit worldwide use. Ciprofloxacin 500 mg orally twice a day for 5 days has an efficacy rate of 93 to 100 percent. A single 400 mg oral dose of ofloxacin was found to be 97.2 percent effective in eradicating carriage for 33 days in a Norwegian outbreak.

Rifampin 600 mg orally every 12 hours for 2 days for adults or 10 mg per kilogram every 12 hours for 2 days for children eradicates meningococci for 75 to 90 percent of carriers. Failure has been associated with rifampin-resistant strains, and rifampin treatment can result in the emergence of rifampin-resistant meningococci in 10 to 27 percent of patients. Minocycline can be given at 100 mg orally twice a day for 5 days as an alternative. Eradication rates approximate those of rifampin, and resistance does not readily emerge, although vestibular side effects limit its use. Spectinomycin

Table 2 Prophylaxis for Meningococcal Carrier State

ANTIBIOTIC	DOSE	COMMENT
Ciprofloxacin	Adults: 500 mg PO b.i.d. × 5 days Children: 250 mg PO b.i.d. × 5 days	Drug of choice Well tolerated
Minocycline	Adults: 100 mg PO q12h × 5 days Children: 1 mg/kg PO q12h × 5 days	Proved effective but vestibular toxicity
Rifampin	Adults: 600 mg PO q12h × 2 days Children: 10 mg/kg PO q12h × 2 days	Proved effective but rapid emergence of resistance
Ofloxacin	Adults: 400 mg PO × 1 Children: 200 mg PO × 1	Has not been tested in children
Ceftriaxone	Adults: 250 mg IM × 1 Children: 125 mg IM × 1	Ceftriaxone more effective than rifampin against group A meningococci
Spectinomycin	Adults: 500 mg PO q.i.d. × 5 days Children: 10 mg/kg PO q.i.d. × 5 days	Primary treatment in many European countries
Sulfadiazine	Adults: 1 g IV q8h × 3 days Children: 50 mg IV q12h × 2 days	Excellent CSF penetration; cannot be given to persons with G6PD deficiency; resistance limits its use

CSF, cerebrospinal fluid; G6PD, glucose-6 phosphate dehydrogenase.

(Spiramycin), the primary prophylactic agent used in Europe, can be given at 500 mg orally four times a day for 5 days to adults and 10 mg per kilogram orally four times a day for 5 days to children. Despite the efficacy of penicillin in treating invasive disease, it does not predictably eradicate the carrier state and therefore transmission.

Vaccine immunoprophylaxis is recommended for persons at high risk for meningococcal disease, primarily military recruits, populations residing in an epidemic focus, and persons traveling to an endemic area. Licensed meningococcal vaccine consists of a mixture of purified high molecular weight capsular polysaccharides from serogroups A, C, Y, and W135. This tetravalent vaccine has virtually eliminated meningococcal disease due to these serogroups in U.S. military recruits. There is no vaccine to prevent group B disease. The duration of immunity to the capsular polysaccharide vaccines is not precisely known but is estimated to be at least 2 to 3 years. Licensed meningococcal vaccine is poorly immunogenic in children under 2 years of age; therefore, only chemoprophylaxis can be relied on for the prevention of secondary cases of meningococcal disease in this age group.

■ INFECTION WITH OTHER *NEISSERIA* SPECIES

The nonpathogenic *Neisseria* spp. include *N. lactamica*, *N. sicca*, *N. subflava*, *N. mucosa*, *N. flavescens*, *N. cinerea*, and *N. polysaccharea*. Infections caused by these organisms are extremely rare, occurring primarily in immunosuppressed hosts, especially those who are hypogammaglobulinemic or have defective antibody production, i.e., chronic lymphocytic leukemia. This is because these organisms are not encapsulated and hence have no predilection for the meninges and are easily controlled by normal nonspecific host defense mechanisms. Since these organisms normally reside in the oropharynx, local extension to the human ear, sinuses, and lungs make these sites the most commonly infected. Conjunctivitis, meningitis, endophthalmitis, endocarditis, and urethritis have also been reported, attesting to the common tropism that these sites share with the oropharynx. Like their more virulent cousins, these nonpathogenic *Neisseria* are easily treated with penicillin, cephalosporin, or quinoline antibiotics.

Suggested Reading

Boslego JW, Tramont EC. *Neisseria meningitidis*. In: Gorbach SL, Bartlett J, Blacklow N, eds. Infectious diseases. Philadelphia: WB Saunders, 1992:1452.

De Voe IW. The meningococcus and mechanisms of pathogenicity. Microbiol Rev 1982; 46:162.

McCracken GH Jr, Lebel MH. Dexamethasone therapy for bacterial meningitis in infants and children. Am J Dis Child. 1989; 143:387.

Peltola H. Meningococcal disease: Still with us. Rev Infect Dis. 1983; 5:71.

PNEUMOCOCCUS

Jeffrey N. Weiser, M.D.

Treatment of pneumonia caused by *Streptococcus pneumoniae* began in the early decades of this century with the use of type-specific antisera, which required the accurate typing of organisms obtained from sputum. With the availability of antibiotics, first the sulfa drugs and later penicillin, therapy of pneumococcal infections became relatively straightforward. This success led to an underestimation of the continued importance of this pathogen, and as a result, decreased vigilance in establishing a specific diagnosis, particularly from expectorated sputum. Although the widespread use of antibiotics has significantly decreased the mortality of pneumococcal infection, pneumococci remain the cause of an estimated 40,000 deaths annually in the United States. Of this total, 6,000 to 7,000 are caused by invasive pneumococcal disease, i.e., bacteremia and meningitis. The morbidity and mortality from pneumococcal meningitis remain high despite the use of antimicrobial therapy. Pneumococci are the causative agent in 30 to 50 percent of community-acquired pneumonias requiring hospitalization and are associated with especially high mortality in the elderly. It is the leading cause of acute bacterial otitis media among children, the most common reason for physician visits by children.

We now face a third phase in the therapy of pneumococcal disease because of the development and widespread dissemination of penicillin- and multiantibiotic-resistant strains. Resistance of pneumococci to penicillin, first reported in 1967, considerably complicates treatment and raises issues in diagnosis and prevention that received little attention when susceptibility to antibiotics was taken for granted. Although pneumococcal disease has remained a serious public health problem, there is now concern that antibiotic resistance may lead to increased morbidity and cost associated with diseases caused by pneumococci.

■ CLINICAL MANIFESTATIONS

Pneumococci are common inhabitants of the human nasopharynx and may be isolated from 5 to 70 percent of a normal population. Although carriage is generally asymptomatic, it may result in upper respiratory tract disease such as sinusitis or acute otitis media. Lower respiratory tract infection, generally bronchopneumonia in children and lobar pneumonia in adults, follows the aspiration of secretions containing the organism. Patients at highest risk are those with impairment of normal defenses of the respiratory tract. Pneumococcal pneumonia frequently follows viral respiratory tract infection. The most common symptoms of pneumococcal pneumonia include fever and cough productive of rust-colored sputum. On physical examination the patient typically appears acutely ill with signs of bronchopneumonia or lobar consolidation on examination of the chest. Bacteremia is common in young children and is found in approximately 25 percent of cases of pneumonia in adults. Dissemination of the infection to the central nervous system is a result of bacteremic spread. Since humoral immunity is the essential component of host defense against the pneumococcus, patients with qualitative or quantitative defects in serum antibody are at increased risk for severe infection.

Presumptive diagnosis is suggested by gram-positive diplococci in purulent sputum and confirmed by culture. It is critical to pursue aggressively a microbiologic diagnosis because of the uncertainties in clinical management in this period of increasing antibiotic resistance. Blood cultures and purulent sputum obtained for Gram stain and culture are important in establishing an accurate diagnosis. Because of the prevalence of resistant strains, sensitivity to penicillin may no longer be presumed. Susceptibility testing of all suspected isolates from sputum and normally sterile sites is recommended. Screening for penicillin resistance is performed by disk diffusion using a 1 μg oxacillin disk. Isolates with an oxacillin disk zone of 19 mm or more should be tested to determine the minimum inhibitory concentration (MIC) of penicillin and other drugs used in treatment.

■ ANTIBIOTIC RESISTANCE

It appears that within the United States and throughout the world, the distribution of penicillin- and multidrug-resistant strains varies considerably. It is important, therefore, that resistance patterns be determined by regional surveillance and that practitioners be aware of local resistance patterns. It is of special concern that in populations frequently exposed to antibiotics, such as young children, penicillin resistance has been reported in up to 60 percent of isolates from the nasopharynx. Rates of resistance have been much lower in isolates from normally sterile sites. There have been numerous reports of poor outcomes caused by the use of agents to which isolates were later shown to be resistant. Mortality in pneumonia caused by penicillin-resistant isolates has been reported to be twice as high as in pneumonia caused by penicillin-sensitive strains. When pneumococcus is known or suspected to be the causative agent, treatment failure should raise as a possibility resistance of the organism to the antibiotic in use.

Penicillins

Penicillin G remains the drug of choice for penicillin-sensitive isolates, defined as those with MIC below 0.1 μg per milliliter. Resistance to penicillin as well as to other beta-lactam antibiotics is mediated by altered penicillin-binding proteins, and therefore, beta-lactamase-resistant forms of penicillin offer no therapeutic advantage. Intermediate resistance is defined as an MIC between 0.1 and 2.0 μg per milliliter, and highly resistant strains are those with MIC at least 2 μg per milliliter. Recent surveys of isolates from different regions of the United States have shown about 5 to 10 percent intermediate resistance and 1 to 3 percent high resistance (Table 1).

Cephalosporins

Although resistance to cephalosporins, also a result of mutations in penicillin-binding proteins, has been rising, many of these agents are active against penicillin-resistant strains. Resistance to the cephalosporins generally increases in parallel to penicillin, but for a given isolate the MIC to cephalosporins may be higher or lower than the MIC to penicillin. Among the parenterally administered cephalosporins, cefuroxime, a second-generation drug, and cefotaxime and ceftriaxone, third-generation drugs, have good activity in vitro. The activity of ceftazidime is inferior to that of the other third-generation agents. The activity of oral first-, second-, and third-generation cephalosporins is lower than that of the oral penicillins. In addition, drug levels in middle ear effusions are below the MIC of a substantial proportion of penicillin-resistant strains, making questionable the use of these agents for upper respiratory tract infections caused by penicillin-resistant strains.

Table 1 Prevalence of Resistance to Anti-pneumococcal Drugs

ANTIBIOTIC	MIC (μG/ML) FOR RESISTANT ISOLATES	ESTIMATED INCIDENCE OF RESISTANCE*
Penicillin†	0.1–2 (intermediate)	5–10%
	≥2 (high)	1–3
Cefotaxime	≥1	1–5
	≥2	0.6
Erythromycin†	>4	3–7
Azithromycin	>4	1–2
Tetracycline†	>2	2–10
TMP-SMX	>0.5/>9.5	6–12
Chloramphenicol†	>4	1–2
Rifampin‡	not established	
Imipenem	>1	<1
Vancomycin†	>4	0

*Estimates are based on various recent surveys of U.S. isolates from normally sterile sites. Rates of resistance for nasopharyngeal isolates in different regions in the U.S. and in other parts of the world may be considerably higher.
†MIC is based on the guidelines of the National Committee for Clinical Laboratory Standards for susceptibility.
‡Resistance documented but incidence unknown.
TMP-SMX, trimethoprim-sulfamethoxazole.

Macrolides

Although the activity of the macrolide antibiotics against pneumococci is usually high, resistance to this class of antibiotics is now common. Erythromycin has been the drug of choice for patients allergic to penicillin. Rates of erythromycin resistance are higher among penicillin-resistant strains, making it a poor choice in infections caused by penicillin-resistant pneumococci. The rates of resistance to the newer macrolides appear to be lower than that of erythromycin.

Vancomycin

Empiric administration of vancomycin, the only agent to which resistance has not been documented, should be minimized to avoid promoting acquisition of vancomycin resistance already established in other streptococci, by unnecessary selective pressure.

Others

Resistance to tetracycline and to trimethoprim-sulfamethoxazole (TMP-SMX) is relatively common. Rates of chloramphenicol resistance have remained low in this country. Imipenem-cilastatin is very active against the pneumococcus, although resistance has been observed in isolates with high resistance to penicillin. The activity of ciprofloxacin is low, and experience with the newer fluoroquinolones is inadequate to support their use.

■ THERAPY (TABLE 2)

Lower Respiratory Tract Infection

Empiric therapy should take into account the severity of the infection and the local frequency of intermediate and highly resistant strains. Therapeutic decisions should be based on the results of diagnostic tests, including antibiotic susceptibility tests on isolates from cultures of sputum and blood. If the causative agent of a community-acquired pneumonia is un-

Table 2 Recommended Therapy for Pneumococcal Infections

INFECTION	ROUTE	CHOICES FOR EMPIRIC THERAPY*	CHOICES FOR PENICILLIN-SENSITIVE ISOLATES†	CHOICES FOR PENICILLIN-RESISTANT ISOLATES†‡
Mild pneumonia, acute sinusitis, otitis media	Oral	Amoxicillin, erythromycin	600,000 U procaine penicillin IM, then Pen VK 250 mg PO q.i.d.	Erythromycin, clindamycin, azithromycin
Pneumonia	Intravenous	Penicillin G 8–12 million U/day in 4–6 doses§	Penicillin G 600,000–1.2 million U/day in 4–6 doses	Penicillin G high dose unless highly resistant, cefuroxime, cefotaxime or ceftriaxone
Meningitis, serous cavity infections‖	Intravenous	Cefotaxime or ceftriaxone with or without rifampin or vancomycin	Penicillin G 20 million U/day in 4–6 doses	Cefotaxime or ceftriaxone, vancomycin, imipenem

*Choice of empiric therapy should take into account organisms other than *Streptococcus pneumoniae.*
†Choice of agents should be determined by susceptibility testing.
‡Choices for penicillin-resistant isolates may also be considered for patients allergic to penicillin.
§Empiric therapy of pneumonia with penicillin should be based on sputum examination.
‖Infections of serous cavities (pleural, pericardial, peritoneal, and joint) may require surgical drainage and longer therapy.

known, therapeutic options should take into consideration other common pathogens, such as *Mycoplasma pneumoniae* and *Haemophilus influenzae,* for which penicillin is not the drug of choice. If sputum examination shows gram-positive diplococci and polymorphonuclear leukocytes, penicillin is recommended. For patients requiring parenteral therapy, penicillin G 8–12 million units a day should provide sufficient serum levels to treat all but highly penicillin-resistant isolates. For isolates with MIC below 0.1 μg per milliliter, penicillin 300,000 to 600,000 U IM or IV two to four times daily until the patient has been afebrile for 48 hours may be used. Outpatient therapy with procaine penicillin 600,000 U IM followed by phenoxymethyl penicillin (Pen VK) 250 mg orally four times a day is an alternative approach for mild cases. Other choices for parenteral therapy include cefuroxime and cefotaxime or ceftriaxone. No studies compare outcomes of different antibiotic regimens for pneumonia caused by penicillin- and multiple-resistant pneumococci.

Upper Respiratory Tract Infection

Pneumococci are a leading cause of acute otitis media and acute sinusitis. Cases of chronic sinusitis are more likely to be caused by other organisms. A bacteriologic diagnosis is seldom made for these conditions, and rates of pneumococcal resistance appear to be higher for upper respiratory tract isolates, although surveys have focused on the pediatric population. Oral therapy for otitis media or sinusitis and for milder cases of community-acquired pneumonia with ampicillin, amoxicillin, or macrolide antibiotics should be adequate for the majority of pneumococcal isolates. Duration of therapy is generally 21 days for sinusitis and 10 days for otitis media, although the duration of therapy has not been specifically determined for pneumococcal infection of these sites. The MIC of many resistant pneumococci is above the achievable drug levels with oral agents. Nasopharyngeal isolates are commonly resistant to tetracycline and to TMP-SMX. Drug levels in middle ear effusion following administration of oral clindamycin are particularly high, and this drug should be considered for the treatment of upper respiratory tract infections with resistant pneumococci when first-line agents fail.

Pneumococcal Meningitis

Treatment of meningitis is complicated by the difficulty in achieving drug levels above the mean bactericidal concentration of pneumococci in the central nervous system. In addition, it is difficult to compare outcomes with different therapeutic regimens, since such studies require large numbers of patients and treatment failures are difficult to assess because the case-fatality ratio in pneumococcal meningitis is high even when penicillin is used to treat infection with penicillin-sensitive strains. Treatment failures have been reported with most agents, including vancomycin. Judging by the prevalence of penicillin resistance, penicillin alone is no longer recommended for use without first establishing susceptibility of the infecting organism (MIC below 0.1 μg per milliliter). The third-generation cephalosporins cefotaxime and ceftriaxone are suggested for the initial empiric coverage because resistance to these agents is still uncommon. Some centers use a combination of vancomycin and cefotaxime or ceftriaxone until susceptibilities are known because of the possibility of cephalosporin resistance. It has been suggested that if the MIC to cefotaxime or ceftriaxone is at least 1 μg per milliliter, these agents should not be used alone. The inclusion of vancomycin is not suggested if the patient is receiving steroids, which decreases penetration of this drug into the cerebrospinal fluid. Recent evidence suggests that rifampin in combination with ceftriaxone may be a useful alternative in treating infection with cephalosporin-resistant strains, although there is little experience with rifampin in pneumococcal meningitis, and resistance to rifampin has followed its use. Most strains are sensitive to chloramphenicol, but the clinical efficacy of this drug for treatment of pneumococcal meningitis has been questioned. Treatment of meningitis caused by penicillin-sensitive strains should be with penicillin G 20 million units per day IV for 10 to 14 days.

The poor outcome of pneumococcal meningitis despite adequate antimicrobial therapy has led to efforts to prevent neurologic damage caused largely by the host immune response to bacterial components resulting from the rapid cell lysis following administration of antibiotics. However, the use of steroids in pneumococcal meningitis remains controversial. Although some reports suggest that dexamethasone administered prior to antibiotics may improve the neurologic outcome in pneumococcal meningitis, clear-cut benefit has been demonstrated only for meningitis caused by *H. influenzae* type b.

■ PREVENTION

In 1977, a vaccine based on purified capsular polysaccharide of 14 common pneumococcal types was introduced; it was subsequently expanded to the current 23 valent product. Although 84 serotypes have been identified, the 23 valent vaccine includes serotypes accounting for over 90 percent of invasive pneumococcal infection in this country. The recommendation of the Advisory Committee on Immunization Practices is for administration to all persons over 65 years of age and to those over 2 years of age with medical conditions associated with increased risk of serious pneumococcal disease. The duration of the protection provided by the vaccine has not been established in any population. Young children and those with immunodeficiency may not respond effectively to polysaccharide antigens. This finding has led to recent efforts to conjugate these antigens to protein carriers as in the case of vaccines for *H. influenzae* type b. Pneumococcal conjugate vaccines based on five and seven of the most prevalent serotypes are now being tested in clinical trials.

A 14 year retrospective indirect cohort analysis by the Centers for Disease Control indicated that the aggregate effectiveness of the 23 valent vaccine was 57 percent overall and 75 percent for those over age 65. Compliance in the adult population, however, has been disappointing. A recent survey showed that 27 percent of the elderly with an underlying disease or disorder and only 9 percent of the healthy elderly had received the vaccine. The low use may be in part caused by controversy about its efficacy, duration of protection, and cost effectiveness. Some experts have suggested that there are insufficient data to recommend its use, while others think immunization should be given to the population 50 years of age and older, in whom more than half of bacteremic infections occur. An additional reason for earlier immunization is that the immune response to the vaccine may be more effective if given prior to the seventh decade of life. Widespread use of the vaccine may have to be re-examined in light of the increasing complexity of anti-pneumococcal therapy.

Suggested Reading

Austrian R. Confronting drug-resistant pneumococci. Ann Intern Med 1994; 121:807–809.

Breiman RF, Butler JC, Tenover FC, et al. Emergence of drug-resistance pneumococcal infections in the United States. JAMA 1994; 271: 1831–1835.

Butler JC, Breiman RF, Campell JF, et al. Pneumococcal polysaccharide vaccine efficacy. JAMA 1993; 270:1826–1831.

Friedland IR, McCracken GH. Management of infections caused by antibiotic-resistant *Streptococcus pneumoniae.* N Engl J Med 1994; 331:377–382.

Klugman K. Pneumococcal resistance to antibiotics. Clin Microbiol Rev 1990; 3:171–196.

STAPHYLOCOCCAL AND STREPTOCOCCAL TOXIC SHOCK SYNDROME

Aris P. Assimacopoulos, M.D.
Patrick M. Schlievert, Ph.D.

Staphylococcal and streptococcal toxic shock syndromes (TSS) are acute-onset multiorgan illnesses defined by criteria listed in Tables 1 and 2. Staphylococcal TSS is caused by *Staphylococcus aureus* strains that make pyogenic toxin superantigens (PTSAgs); coagulase-negative strains do not make the causative toxins. Streptococcal TSS is caused mainly by toxin-producing group A strains but occasionally by groups B, C, F, and G strains. There are several subsets of staphylococcal TSS, two major categories being menstrual and nonmenstrual.

Menstrual TSS, which occurs within a day or two of and during menstruation, has primarily been associated with use of certain tampons, notably those of high absorbency, and is associated with production of TSS toxin-1 (TSST-1) by the causative bacterium. Three theories have been proposed to explain the role of tampons in menstrual TSS: (1) tampons introduce oxygen, which is required for production of TSST-1, into the vagina; (2) tampons bind magnesium, which alters growth kinetics of *S. aureus* and thus alters the time when TSST-1 is made; (3) pluronic L-92, a surfactant present in the Rely tampon, which was highly associated with TSS, amplifies production of TSST-1. It is possible other surfactants have similar effects.

Nonmenstrual TSS occurs in both male and female adults and children and is associated with *S. aureus* strains that make TSST-1 or staphylococcal enterotoxins, notably enterotoxin serotypes B and C. It occurs in association with nearly any kind of staphylococcal infection, but four major forms have been identified: postsurgical TSS, influenza-associated TSS, recalcitrant erythematous desquamating (RED) syndrome, and occasionally TSS with use of a contraceptive diaphragm. Postsurgical TSS is often associated with *S. aureus* infections that do not result in pyogenic responses, and thus the source of infection may be difficult to find. Influenza TSS may be a consequence of influenza or parainfluenza damage to the

Table 1 Diagnostic Criteria for Staphylococcal Toxic Shock Syndrome

1. Temperature above 38.9°C (102°F)
2. Systolic blood pressure below 90 mmHg for adults, less than the fifth percentile for children, or more than a 15 mmHg orthostatic drop in diastolic blood pressure, or orthostatic dizziness or syncope or both
3. Diffuse macular rash with subsequent desquamation
4. Three of the following organ systems involved:
   Liver: bilirubin AST, ALT more than twice the upper normal limit
   Blood: platelets below 100,000/mm^3
   Renal: BUN or creatinine more than twice the upper normal limit or pyuria without urinary tract infection
   Mucous membranes: hyperemia of the vagina, oropharynx, or conjunctivae
   Gastrointestinal: diarrhea or vomiting
   Muscular: myalgias or CPK more than twice the normal upper limit
   Central nervous system: disorientation or lowered level of consciousness in the absence of hypotension, fever, or focal neurologic deficits
5. Negative serologies for measles, leptospirosis, and Rocky Mountain spotted fever; blood or CSF cultures negative for organisms other than *Staphylococcus aureus*

AST, aspartate transaminase; ALT, alanine aminotransferase; BUN, blood urea nitrogen; CPK, creatine phosphokinase; CSF, cerebrospinal fluid.

Table 2 Diagnostic Criteria for Streptococcal Toxic Shock Syndrome

1. Isolation of group A streptococci
   From a sterile site for a *definite* case
   From a nonsterile site for a *probable* case
2. Clinical criteria
   Hypotension and two of the following:

Renal dysfunction	Coagulopathy
Liver involvement	Adult respiratory distress syndrome
Erythematous macular rash	Soft-tissue necrosis

respiratory tract epithelium and superinfection with toxin-producing *S. aureus*. This illness is highly fatal in children. RED syndrome, a disorder in AIDS patients, may last 70 or more days or until the patient dies. Finally, nonmenstrual TSS associated with use of a diaphragm may be similar to menstrual TSS, though the reason for the association is unclear.

Streptococcal TSS is primarily associated with group A streptococcal infections, particularly M types 1 and 3; it may or may not be associated with necrotizing fasciitis and myositis. Occasionally streptococcal TSS is caused by other groups of streptococci, primarily groups B, C, and G.

Group A streptococcal strains that cause TSS make streptococcal pyogenic exotoxins (SPEs). The major association has been with SPE serotype A, but other members of the family, including SPE B and C, streptococcal superantigen, and SPE F, may also contribute significantly. Non-group A streptococci associated with TSS also make PTSAgs, only one of which—that made by some group B strains—has been characterized.

Major risk factors for development of streptococcal TSS include chickenpox in children, wounds, use of nonsteroidal anti-inflammatory agents, and pregnancy.

■ THERAPY

Staphylococcal Toxic Shock Syndrome

The differential diagnosis of toxic shock syndrome comprises viral disease, including measles, rubella, parvovirus B19; spotted fever group rickettsiosis; leptospirosis; drug reactions, including Stevens-Johnson syndrome; collagen-vascular diseases, including systemic lupus erythematosus and Still's disease; scarlet and rheumatic fever; syphilis; and typhoid fever. During the initial evaluation, identify possible sources of infection. Perform a vaginal examination, removing any tampon, and culture for *S. aureus*. Remove any wound packing.

Supportive care is of primary importance. Patients often require large amounts of intravenous fluids and vasopressors as well as management of associated problems such as acute renal failure, adult respiratory distress syndrome, disseminated intravascular coagulation, and myocardial suppression.

Antistaphylococcal therapy decreases the risk of recurrence. One of the antistaphylococcal penicillins such as nafcillin (adults 2 g IV every 4 hours; children 150 mg per kilogram per day IV divided every 6 hours) is an appropriate choice. For penicillin-allergic patients, cefazolin (adults 1 to 2 g IV every 8 hours; children 50 to 100 mg per kilogram per day IV divided every 8 hours) or vancomycin (adults 1 g IV every 12 hours; children 40 mg per kilogram per day IV divided every 6 hours) can be used. Some support the use of clindamycin (adults 900 mg IV every 8 hours; children 40 mg per kilogram per day IV divided every 6 to 8 hours) because experimental data suggest that it inhibits toxin production. Dosage adjustments for renal failure may be required.

Surgical intervention includes draining any obvious source of infection and maintaining a low threshold for exploring possible sites even if they lack signs of significant inflammation.

Up to 30 percent recurrence has been suggested. A course of rifampin is sometimes given in hopes of eliminating colonization. Avoidance of further tampon use is prudent after menstrual TSS. Although there are no controlled trials, intravenous immunoglobulin (IVIG) and steroids have been used in TSS.

Streptococcal Toxic Shock Syndrome and Myositis

The differential diagnosis is as described for staphylococcal TSS. Consider myositis in any patient who has severe local pain, especially in an extremity, and few other findings.

In the initial evaluation, look for a skin or soft-tissue focus. Attend to any painful or tender areas, even in the absence of inflammatory signs. Unpack and inspect any wounds. There may be no obvious site of infection.

Patients often require large amounts of intravenous fluids and vasopressors as well as management of associated problems such as acute renal failure, adult respiratory distress syndrome, disseminated intravascular coagulation, and myocardial suppression. Treatment of group A streptococcal TSS includes a combination of a beta-lactam and a protein synthesis inhibitor: penicillin (adults 4 million units IV every 4 hours; children 250,000 U per kilogram per day IV divided every 4 hours) or ceftriaxone (adults 2 g IV every 24 hours; children 50 to 75 mg per kilogram per day IV divided every 12 to 24 hours) in combination with clindamycin (adults 900 mg IV every 8 hours; children 40 mg per kilogram per day IV divided every 6 to 8 hours) or erythromycin (adults 1 g every 6 hours IV; children 20 to 40 mg per kilogram per day IV divided every 6 hours).

Surgical intervention includes draining any obvious source of infection and maintaining a low threshold to explore other sites. Remember that expected signs of inflammation may be absent in streptococcal myositis.

Appropriate cleansing of any wounds is important in the prevention of streptococcal TSS. There is no controlled experience with antibiotic prophylaxis. As expected, anecdotal experience indicates that close contacts of an index case of streptococcal TSS may carry toxin-producing streptococci in the nasopharynx. There are no data on the beneficial or adverse effects of prophylactic treatment in these patients. Group A streptococci can also colonize the skin, vagina, and anus.

IVIG has been used as therapy in some patients. Experience indicates there may be some benefit. IVIG may act to neutralize toxins elaborated by the streptococci.

Suggested Reading

Barry W, Hudgins L, Donta ST, Pesanti EL. Intravenous immunoglobulin therapy for toxic shock syndrome. JAMA 1992; 267:3315–3316.

Stevens DL. Invasive group A streptococcus infections. Clin Infect Dis 1992; 14:2–13.

Todd JK. Therapy of toxic shock syndrome. Drugs 1990; 39:856.

The toxic shock syndrome: A conference sponsored by the Institute of Medicine, National Academy of Sciences. Ann Intern Med 1982; 96:831–996.

STAPHYLOCOCCUS

Carol A. Kauffman, M.D.
Suzanne F. Bradley, M.D.

Staphylococci are ubiquitous micro-organisms. The species causing most serious infections is *Staphylococcus aureus* (coagulase-positive), but infections due to coagulase-negative staphylococci (e.g., *Staphylococcus epidermidis*) appear to be increasing. Treatment of staphylococcal infection depends on the site and severity of infection and the antibiotic susceptibility pattern of the organism. *S. aureus* is a highly invasive pathogen, but coagulase-negative staphylococci generally require prosthetic material to gain a foothold and cause infection. Once *S. aureus* invades deeper structures, it often spreads hematogenously to other organ systems, leading to metastatic infection.

Staphylococci have a propensity to develop resistance to antibiotics relatively quickly. Penicillinase-resistant penicillins (nafcillin, oxacillin, methicillin) are the drugs of choice for most staphylococcal infections. Virtually all staphylococci should be considered resistant to all penicillins susceptible to penicillinase (e.g., amoxicillin, ampicillin, piperacillin, mezlocillin, ticarcillin). However, the addition of clavulanic acid, sulbactam, or tazobactam to several of the above penicillins renders them resistant to penicillinase, and thus useful for treating staphylococcal infections. Examples are amoxicillin-clavulanic acid (Augmentin) and ampicillin-sulbactam (Unasyn).

Cephalosporins also are useful for the treatment of staphylococcal infections. First-generation cephalosporins (e.g., cefazolin, cephalexin) are the most active, followed by second-generation (e.g., cefuroxime, cefotetan, cefoxitin), and then third-generation (e.g., ceftriaxone, ceftazidime). Only first-generation cephalosporins should be used for serious staphylococcal infection.

Since the 1970s, *S. aureus* and coagulase-negative staphylococci have become increasingly resistant to penicillinase-resistant penicillins (nafcillin, methicillin, oxacillin) and those penicillins combined with sulbactam, tazobactam, and clavulanic acid. These so-called methicillin-resistant staphylococci, *S. aureus* and *S. epidermidis* (MRSA and MRSE respectively), are common in hospitals throughout the United States, and in some centers they account for as many as 50 percent of all *S. aureus* isolates causing nosocomial infection. These organisms are usually resistant to several other classes of antibiotics also, and vancomycin is often the only effective treatment. Although it is tempting to treat all staphylococcal infections with vancomycin, there is anecdotal evidence that infection is cleared less quickly by vancomycin than a beta-lactam antibiotic. Thus, organisms that are identified as methicillin-susceptible *S. aureus* (MSSA) should be treated with a beta-lactam antibiotic, such as nafcillin, and if the infecting organism is MRSA, vancomycin should be given.

For patients allergic to beta-lactam antibiotics, other antimicrobial agents for staphylococcal infections include trimethoprim-sulfamethoxazole (TMP-SMX), quinolones such as ofloxacin and ciprofloxacin, clindamycin, erythromycin, and vancomycin. With the exception of vancomycin, the use of these antistaphylococcal agents should generally be restricted to the treatment of localized, uncomplicated infections. Organisms that are resistant to erythromycin but susceptible to clindamycin should not be treated with clindamycin because resistance to this antibiotic is almost always induced within several days.

■ INFECTIONS DUE TO *S. AUREUS*

Skin and Soft-Tissue Infections

The most common infections caused by *S. aureus* afflict the skin and soft tissue. Folliculitis, furuncles, abscesses, and wound infections are common and can often be treated with oral antibiotics. Beta-lactam antibiotics (penicillinase-resistant penicillins and cephalosporins) are the most effective drugs for treating these infections (Table 1). In addition to antibiotic therapy, incision and drainage of abscesses are crucial to early resolution of infection.

Cellulitis due to *S. aureus* may be difficult to differentiate from that due to beta-hemolytic streptococci. Initial treatment of cellulitis should always include drugs effective against both *S. aureus* and beta-hemolytic streptococci. Therefore, penicillinase-resistant penicillins or cephalosporins are used until susceptibilities are reported. Many patients will require intravenous administration of antibiotics until the acute illness has improved, and then can be switched to oral antibiotics. Initial therapy with nafcillin or cefazolin followed by dicloxicillin or cephalexin is preferred.

Osteoarticular Infections

S. aureus is the leading cause of osteoarticular infections; these are difficult to treat and frequently require long-term therapy with intravenous antibiotics. In the case of septic arthritis, drainage of infected fluid is essential to preserve joint function and eradicate infection. Therapy should continue for at least 3 weeks. For treatment of osteomyelitis, antimicrobial therapy should be given for a minimum of 4–6 weeks. Nafcillin or vancomycin should be used until antibiotic susceptibilities are available.

Pulmonary Infections

Staphylococcal pneumonia, now uncommon, is mostly seen in elderly patients with underlying illnesses. It has a high mortality rate. Empyema may be present in up to 50 percent of patients with staphylococcal pneumonia, and it must be drained. Treatment of staphylococcal pneumonia should be nafcillin or vancomycin based on available susceptibilities, and should continue for 2 to 4 weeks.

Endocarditis

The most serious infection due to *S. aureus* is endocarditis. Patients with left-sided cardiac lesions frequently have metastatic abscesses in the spleen, brain, kidney, and myocardium, and mortality is 25 to 70 percent. The patient must be monitored closely for symptoms and signs of septic complications that may require surgical intervention.

Table 1 Treatment of Noncardiac Infections Due to *Staphylococcus aureus*

INFECTION	FIRST-LINE DRUGS*	SECOND-LINE DRUGS†	COMMENTS
Folliculitis, furunculosis, minor abscesses, wound infections	Dicloxacillin 250 mg or cephalexin 250 mg q6h PO for 7–10 days	Clindamycin 300 mg or erythromycin 250 mg q6h PO for 7–10 days	Usually community acquired, rarely due to MRSA
Cellulitis	Nafcillin 1 g q4h or cefazolin 1 g q8h IV for 10–14 days	Vancomyin 1 g q12h IV for 10–14 days	Usually community acquired, rarely due to MRSA; after patient afebrile and nontoxic, switch to oral cephalexin or dicloxacillin
Major abscesses and wound infections			
MSSA	Nafcillin 2 g q4h or cefazolin 2 g q8h IV for 2 weeks	Vancomycin 1 g q12h IV for 2 weeks	Drainage of abscesses important
MRSA	Vancomycin 1 g q12h for 2 weeks		
Osteomyelitis			
MSSA	Nafcillin 2 g q4h or cefazolin 2 g q8h IV for 4–6 weeks	Vancomycin 1 g q12h IV for 4–6 weeks	
MRSA	Vancomycin 1 g q12h IV for 4–6 weeks		
Septic arthritis			
MSSA	Nafcillin 2 g q4h or cefazolin 2 g q8h IV for 3 weeks	Vancomycin 1 g q12h IV for 3 weeks	Repeated needle aspiration, arthroscopic drainage, or operative drainage of joint fluid essential
MRSA	Vancomycin 1 g q12h IV for 3 weeks		
Pneumonia			
MSSA	Nafcillin 2 g q4h IV for 2–4 weeks	Vancomycin 1 g q12h IV for 2–4 weeks	
MRSA	Vancomycin 1 g q12h IV for 2–4 weeks		
Catheter-associated bacteremia			
MSSA	Nafcillin 2 g q4h IV for 2 weeks or longer	Vancomycin 1 g q12h IV for 2 weeks or longer	Treat for 2 weeks only if blood cultures drawn after device removed are negative, patient becomes afebrile within 1–2 days, *and* no metastatic foci of infection found; otherwise treatment should be for 4–6 weeks
MRSA	Vancomycin 1 g q12h IV for 2 weeks or longer (see comment)		

*Usual adult doses. Doses of cephazolin and vancomycin depend on renal function. Vancomycin levels should be checked to ensure proper dosing.
†Second-line drugs used mostly for patients allergic or intolerant to beta-lactam antibiotics.
MSSA, methicillin-susceptible *Staphylococcus aureus;* MRSA, methicillin-resistant *Staphylococcus aureus.*

For details of specific antibiotic regimens for endocarditis, see the chapter *Endocarditis of Natural and Prosthetic Valves.*

Catheter-Associated Bacteremia

In the past, 4 to 6 weeks of therapy for staphylococcal bacteremia has been recommended. Recent debate has focused on whether sometimes the duration of treatment can be shortened. If there is a removable focus of infection and it has been promptly removed with rapid documented resolution of the bacteremia, it may be possible to treat selected patients with 2 weeks of antibiotic therapy with nafcillin, cefazolin, or vancomycin. It is necessary to be absolutely certain that there is no metastatic focus of infection and that the bacteremia resolved as soon as the device was removed. For patients with persistent fever and/or bacteremia following the removal of the intravenous device, therapy for only 2 weeks is contraindicated. Under no circumstances should patients simply have the catheter removed without antibiotic treatment, because of the propensity of *S. aureus* to seed to several organs, including the brain, spleen, kidney, joints, and bones.

Toxic Shock Syndrome

Through the elaboration of toxins, *S. aureus* may cause multiorgan system disease in the absence of bacteremia. Rash associated with renal failure, anemia, thrombocytopenia, and central nervous system and hepatic dysfunction may be present. Conditions associated with toxin production in staphylococci include the use of tampons in menstruating women, and the packing of surgical wounds. Treatment of shock and the removal of tampons or surgical packing are primary therapy. Antistaphylococcal therapy is initiated primarily for the eradication of carriage of toxin-producing strains.

INFECTIONS DUE TO COAGULASE-NEGATIVE STAPHYLOCOCCI

Infections due to coagulase-negative staphylococci are often hospital acquired and are usually associated with prosthetic devices. Coagulase-negative staphylococci are frequently resistant to many antibiotics. In general, the most consistently reliable antibiotic is vancomycin, but nafcillin can be used if the organism is susceptible. Rifampin is an important adjunctive agent in the treatment of infected prosthetic devices. The recommended treatment regimen for prosthetic valve endocarditis is vancomycin or nafcillin combined with rifampin for 6 weeks; gentamicin for 2 weeks may be added if the organism is susceptible (see the chapter *Endocarditis of Natural and Prosthetic Valves*). A trial of 6 weeks of vancomycin or nafcillin with or without rifampin is usually tried in patients with infected prosthetic joints. For both infections it is possible that therapy will fail or that the infection will relapse, necessitating the removal of the device for cure. For infected intravenous devices, such as Hickman catheters, a 2 week trial of vancomycin or nafcillin may be adequate unless tunnel infection or septic phlebitis is present. However, if relapse occurs, the catheter should be removed (see the chapter *Intravascular Catheter-Related Infection*).

Suggested Reading

Jernigan JA, Farr BM. Short-course therapy of catheter-related *Staphylococcus aureus* bacteremia: A meta-analysis. Ann Intern Med 1993; 119:304–311.

Musher DM, Lamm N, Darouiche RO, et al. The current spectrum of *Staphylococcus aureus* infection in a tertiary care hospital. Medicine 1994; 73:186–208.

Rupp ME, Archer GL. Coagulase negative staphylococci: Pathogens associated with medical progress. Clin Infect Dis 1994; 19: 231–245.

Turnidge J, Grayson ML. Optimum treatment of staphylococcal infection. Drugs 1993; 45:353–366.

Wilson WR, Karchmer AW, Dajani AS, et al. Antibiotic treatment of adults with infective endocarditis due to streptococci, interococci, staphylococci, and HACEK microorganisms. JAMA 1995; 274:1706–1713.

STREPTOCOCCUS GROUPS A, B, C, D, AND G

Dennis L. Stevens, M.D., Ph.D.

GROUP A

Pharyngitis

All group A streptococcal infections have their highest incidence in children younger than age 10. About 5 to 20 percent of the population harbor group A streptococci in their pharynx, and some are colonized on their skin. Thus, group A streptococcus is ubiquitous in the environment, but with rare exceptions is exclusively found in or on the human host. Streptococcal pharyngitis, the most common infection of this organism, causes abrupt onset of sore throat, fever, submandibular adenopathy, painful swallowing, and chilliness. These symptoms combined with submandibular adenopathy, pharyngeal erythema, and exudates correlate with positive throat cultures in 85 to 90 percent of cases. Sore throat without fever or any of the other signs and symptoms has a low predictive value for pharyngitis caused by group A streptococcus. Rapid strep tests correlate with positive cultures in 68 to 99 percent of cases, but results depend greatly on the individual performing the test as well as the bacterial colony count. Colony counts greater than 100 correlated with positive rapid strep test in 95 percent of patients, and counts less than 100 correlated with positive rapid strep tests for only 68 percent of patients.

Therapy

Penicillin remains the drug of choice for group A streptococcal pharyngitis and tonsillitis (Table 1). In the past, treatment of streptococcal pharyngitis was largely to prevent postinfectious sequelae such as rheumatic fever and post-streptococcal glomerulonephritis. However, because some patients with pharyngitis have subsequently developed streptococcal toxic shock syndrome with or without necrotizing fasciitis, it seems prudent to diagnose and treat streptococcal pharyngitis aggressively in an attempt to prevent this complication as well. Antibiotic treatment of strep pharyngitis reduces pharyngeal pain and fever by approximately 24 hours. Penicillin treatment within 10 days of the onset of pharyngitis is extremely effective in the prevention of rheumatic fever, though it is unclear whether it prevents post-streptococcal glomerulonephritis. Penicillin fails to eradicate streptococcus from the pharynx in 5 to 25 percent of patients with pharyngitis or tonsillitis. Penicillin tolerance has been documented in some cases, yet the most popular explanation for such failure, particularly in patients with tonsillitis, is the inactivation of penicillin by beta-lactamases produced by co-colonizing organisms such as *Staphylococcus aureus, Haemophilus influenzae, Moraxella catarrhalis,* and *Bacteroides fragilis.* A second course of penicillin fails in more than 50 percent of cases, and treatment with dicloxacillin, a cephalosporin, augmentin, erythromycin, or clindamycin cures 90 to 95 percent of patients. Preparations containing procaine penicillin G plus benzathine penicillin are as effective as benzathine alone and less painful on injection. Ceftriaxone is under study for this indication. Resistance to erythromycin is about 5 percent in the United States, but in 1970 reached a prevalence of 70 percent in Japan during a period of tremendous erythromycin usage in that country. Cefpodoxime proxetil, cefuroxime axetil, cephalexin, cephradine, cephadroxil, cefaclor, clarithromycin, and azithromycin

Table 1 Streptococcal Infections

ORGANISM	LANCEFIELD GROUP	TYPE OF INFECTION	THERAPY
Streptococcus pyogenes	A	Pharyngitis and impetigo	Benzathine penicillin IM 1.2 million units for adults; 600,000 U for children <60 lb Penicillin G or V PO 400,000 U q.i.d. for 10 days for adults; 200,000 U q.i.d. for children <60 lb Erythromycin ethyl succinate PO 40 mg/kg/day
		Recurrent streptococcal pharyngitis, tonsillitis	Same as above or Ampicillin + clavulanic acid PO 20–40 mg/kg/day Oral cephalosporin Clindamycin PO 10 mg/kg/day in 4 doses
		Cellulitis and erysipelas	Nafcillin IV 8–12 g/day for 7–10 days Penicillin G or V PO 200,000 U q.i.d. for 10 days Dicloxacillin PO 500 mg q.i.d. for 10 days for adults
		Necrotizing fasciitis, myositis, and streptococcal toxic shock syndrome	Clindamycin IV, 900 mg q8h in adults and Penicillin IV 4 million U q4h for adults
		Prophylaxis of rheumatic fever	Benzathine penicillin IM 1.2 million U every 28 days Penicillin G PO 200,000 U b.i.d. for children <60 lb Sulfadiazine 1 g/day for patients over 27 kg; 500 mg/day for patients under 27 kg Erythromycin PO 250 mg b.i.d.
Streptococcus agalactiae	B	Neonatal sepsis	Penicillin IV 100,000–150,000 U/kg/day in 2–3 divided doses for infants <7 days of age Penicillin IV 200,000–250,000 U/kg/day in 4 divided doses for infants >7 days of age Ampicillin IV 100 mg/kg/day in 2–3 divided doses for infants <7 days of age Ampicillin IV 150–200 mg/kg/day in 4 divided doses for infants >7 days of age
		Postpartum sepsis	Ampicillin IV 8–12 g in 4–6 divided doses or penicillin 12–24 million U/d for adults
		Septic arthritis	Penicillin or ampicillin as for neonatal sepsis or postpartum sepsis above
		Soft-tissue infection Osteomyelitis	Penicillin or ampicillin as for postpartum sepsis above
Streptococcus equi		Bacteremia Cellulitis Pharyngitis	Penicillin as for streptococcal toxic shock syndrome above
Enterococcus faecalis[1]	D	Endocarditis Bacteremia Urinary tract infection Gastrointestinal abscess	Ampicillin + gentamicin
Streptococcus bovis	D	Bacteremia Abscesses	Penicillin as for streptococcus equi above
Streptococcus canis	G	Bacteremia Cellulitis Pharyngitis	Penicillin as for streptococcus equi above

[1]See the chapter *Enterococcus* for more details.

also have indications for streptococcal pharyngitis, though expense may limit usage.

Prophylactic treatment is indicated during epidemics of streptococcal pharyngitis when rheumatic fever is prevalent, and in individuals with a history of rheumatic fever. Benzathine penicillin given intramuscularly once each month has the greatest efficacy, though oral agents such as phenoxymethyl penicillin are also effective. In recent years, the U.S. military has demonstrated that such prophylaxis, particularly benzathine penicillin, prevents epidemics of streptococcal infections among young soldiers living in crowded conditions.

Pyoderma (Impetigo Contagiosa)

Impetigo is most common in patients with poor hygiene or malnutrition. Colonization of the unbroken skin occurs first; then intradermal inoculation is initiated by minor abrasions, insect bites, and so on. Single or multiple thick, crusted, golden-yellow lesions develop within 10 to 14 days. Penicillin orally or parenterally, or bacitracin or mupirocin topically, is effective for impetigo; these treatments also reduce transmission of streptococci to susceptible individuals. None of these treatments, including penicillin, prevents poststreptococcal glomerulonephritis.

Erysipelas

Erysipelas occurs most commonly in the elderly and very young, is caused almost exclusively by group A streptococcus, and is characterized by an abrupt onset of fiery red swelling of the face or extremities. Distinctive features are well-defined margins, particularly along the nasolabial fold, scarlet or salmon red rash, rapid progression, and intense pain. Flaccid bullae may develop during the second to third day of illness, and desquamation of the involved skin occurs 5 to 10 days into the illness. Treatment with penicillin, a cephalosporin, or nafcillin is effective. Swelling may progress despite treatment, though fever, pain, and the intense redness usually diminish.

Cellulitis

Clinical clues to the category of cellulitis such as dog bite (DF-2), cat bite (*Pasteurella multocida*), freshwater injury (*Aeromonas hydrophila*), seawater (*Vibrio Vulnificus*), and furuncles (*Staphylococcus aureus*) are extremely important because definitive diagnosis in the absence of such factors rests on aspiration of the leading edge, of the cellulitic lesion, and at best, bacterial cause is established in only 15 percent of cases. Streptococcus is the most common cause of cellulitis, and though group A is the most frequent, groups B, C, and G also cause cellulitis in specific clinical settings. Patients with chronic venous stasis or lymphedema are predisposed to develop recurrent cellulitis due to streptococci. Cellulitis due to group A streptococcus responds to penicillin, nafcillin, erythromycin, clindamycin, and a variety of cephalosporins. Ceftriaxone, cefpodoxime proxetil, and cefuroxime axetil have the greatest in vitro susceptibility, and all have FDA-approved indications for streptococcal cellulitis. Though quinolones have efficacy in the treatment of the clinical entity of cellulitis, because of their poor in vitro activity against streptococci in general, other agents should be used.

Invasive Group A

In the past 10 years there has been an increase in the number of severe soft-tissue infections and bacteremia, associated with shock and death in 30 to 70 percent of cases. Shock and organ failure early in the course of infection define streptococcal toxic shock syndrome (strep TSS), and the inciting infection may be necrotizing fasciitis, myositis, pneumonia, peritonitis, septic arthritis, uterine infection, and so on. Predisposing factors include varicella virus infections, penetrating or blunt trauma, and nonsteroidal anti-inflammatory agents.

Therapy

In severe infections when large numbers of streptococci are found, the remarkable efficacy of penicillin appears somewhat diminished, likely due to the Eagle phenomenon: where large numbers of streptococci accumulate, organisms are likely in stationary phase. Decreased expression of critical penicillin-binding proteins in such slow-growing bacteria likely explains the lack of efficacy of penicillin. In vitro clindamycin—but not penicillin—prevents synthesis of toxins. Interestingly, in experimental necrotizing fasciitis and myositis, clindamycin has markedly better efficacy than penicillin.

■ GROUP B

Streptococcus agalactiae (group B streptococci) colonize the vagina, gastrointestinal tract, and occasionally the upper respiratory tract of normal humans. Group B streptococci are the most common cause of neonatal pneumonia, sepsis, and meningitis in the United States and Western Europe, with an incidence of 1.8 to 3.2 cases per 1,000 live births. Preterm infants born to mothers who are colonized with group B streptococci and have premature rupture of the membranes are at highest risk for early-onset pneumonia and sepsis. The mean time of onset is 20 hours, and symptoms are respiratory distress, apnea, and fever or hypothermia. Ascent of the streptococcus from the vagina to the amniotic cavity causes amnionitis. Infants may aspirate streptococci either from the birth canal during parturition or from amniotic fluid in utero. Radiographic evidence of pneumonia and/or hyaline membrane disease is present in 40 percent of neonates with infection, and meningitis occurs in 30 to 40 percent of cases. Type III group B streptococcus causes most meningitis.

Late-onset neonatal sepsis occurs 7 to 90 days post partum. Symptoms are fever, poor feeding, lethargy, and irritability. Bacteremia is common, and meningitis occurs in 80 percent of cases.

Adults with group B infections include postpartum women and patients with peripheral vascular disease, diabetes, or malignancy. Soft-tissue infection, septic arthritis, and osteomyelitis are the most common presentations.

Therapy

Adults should receive 12 million to 24 million units of penicillin per day for bacteremia, soft-tissue infection, or osteomyelitis; the dose should be 8–12 grams of ampicillin or 24 million units per day for meningitis (Table 1). Vancomycin or a first-generation cephalosporin is the alternative for patients allergic to penicillin. Intrapartum administration of ampicillin to women colonized with group B streptococcus who had premature labor or prolonged rupture of the membranes prevents group B neonatal sepsis. Infants should continue to receive ampicillin for 36 hours post partum. It is imperative that women during the third trimester be screened for risk factors for premature labor, and those with high risk should be cultured. Women presenting in labor without such definition can be screened with a rapid antigen detecting kit, though the false-negative rate may be 10 to 30 percent. Both passive immunization with intravenous immunoglobulin and active immunization with multivalent polysaccharide vaccine show promise and will likely become the best approach to prevent neonatal sepsis as well as postpartum infection in the mother.

■ GROUPS C AND G

These organisms, which may be isolated from the throats of both humans and dogs, produce streptolysin O and resemble group A in colony morphology and spectrum of clinical disease. Before rapid identification tests were developed, many infections caused by groups C and G, such as pharyngitis, cellulitis, skin and wound infections, endocarditis, meningitis, osteomyelitis, and arthritis, were mistakenly attributed to group A. Rheumatic fever following group C or G infection has not been described. These strains also cause recurrent cellulitis at the saphenous vein donor site in patients who have undergone coronary artery bypass surgery. Both organisms are susceptible to penicillin, erythromycin, vancomycin, and clindamycin.

■ GROUP D

These gram-positive, facultatively anaerobic bacteria are usually nonhemolytic but may demonstrate alpha- or beta-hemolysis. *Streptococcus faecalis,* renamed *Enterococcus faecalis,* was previously classified as group D because it hydrolyzes bile esculin and possesses the group D antigen. *Streptococcus bovis* is also a cause of subacute bacterial endocarditis and bacteremia in patients with underlying gastrointestinal malignancy. Enterococci are commonly isolated from stool, urine, and sites of intra-abdominal and lower-extremity infection. Enterococci cause subacute bacterial endocarditis and have become an important cause of nosocomial infection, not because of increased virulence, but because of antibiotic resistance. First, person-to-person transfer of multidrug-resistant enterococci is a major concern to hospital epidemiologists. Second, superinfections and spontaneous bacteremia from endogenous sites of enterococcal colonization are described in patients receiving quinolone or moxalactam antibiotics. Last, conjugational transfer of plasmids and transposons between enterococci in the face of intense antibiotic pressure within the hospital milieu have created multidrug-resistant strains, including some with vancomycin and teicoplanin resistance.

Therapy

Serious infections with enterococci, such as endocarditis or bacteremia, require a synergistic combination of antimicrobials such as ampicillin or vancomycin together with an aminoglycoside. Beta-lactamase-positive (Nitrocefin disk positive) strains can be treated with ampicillin and sulbactam (see also the chapter *Enterococcus*). Unlike enterococci, *S. bovis* remains highly sensitive to penicillin.

Suggested Reading

Bisno AL. Group A streptococcal infections and acute rheumatic fever. N Engl J Med 1991; 325:783–793.

Gossling R. Occurrence and pathogenicity of the *Streptococcus milleri* group. Rev Infect Dis 1988; 10:257–285.

Murray BE. The life and times of the *Enterococcus.* Clin Microbiol Rev 1990; 3:46–65.

Stevens DL. Invasive group A streptococcus infections. Clin Infect Dis 1992; 14:2–13.

Stevens DL. Invasive group A streptococcal disease. Infect Agents Dis 1996; 5:157–166.

Stevens DL, Bryant AE, Hackett SP, et al. Group A streptococcal bacteremia: the role of tumor necrosis factor in shock and organ failure. J Infect Dis 1996; 173:619–626.

Stevens DL, Tanner MH, Winship J, et al. Severe group A streptococcal infections associated with a toxic shock-like syndrome and scarlet fever toxin A. N Engl J Med 1989; 321:1–8.

PSEUDOMONAS

Barbara Menzies, M.D.
David W. Gregory, M.D.

Infections with *Pseudomonas* spp. cause substantial morbidity and mortality and are difficult to treat. Four species of *Pseudomonas* are considered important human pathogens: *P. aeruginosa, P. cepacia, P. pseudomallei,* and *P. mallei.* The first two are common pathogens in the United States. *P. aeruginosa,* an aerobic gram-negative rod and the fourth most frequently isolated nosocomial pathogen, commonly causes pneumonia, urinary tract infections, and surgical wound infections (Table 1). *Xanthomonas maltophilia,* formerly *Pseudomonas maltophilia,* another opportunistic pathogen, is briefly discussed here.

■ EPIDEMIOLOGY

The epidemiology of *P. aeruginosa* infections reflects its predilection for moist environments. In hospitals *P. aeruginosa* has been isolated from respiratory devices, disinfectants, distilled and tap water, and sinks. *P. aeruginosa* colonizes respiratory tracts of intubated patients, burn wounds, and the gastrointestinal tracts of patients receiving chemotherapy or antibiotics. Colonization usually precedes invasion.

■ ANTIMICROBIAL THERAPY

Over the past 15 years several antipseudomonal antibiotics have been introduced (Table 2). Beta-lactam antibiotics active against *P. aeruginosa* include the carboxypenicillins and ureidopenicillins, some third-generation cephalosporins, the carbapenems, and the monobactam aztreonam. Initial selection of an antipseudomonal beta-lactam should be guided by the site of infection, the patient's allergy history, and the institution's antibiogram if known. Subsequent modification may be based on the susceptibility profile of the isolate.

The aminoglycosides gentamicin, tobramycin, and amikacin have excellent in vitro activity against *P. aeruginosa.* The concentration-dependent bactericidal activity and the post-antibiotic effect of aminoglycosides provide the rationale for single daily dosing (i.e., high dosages of aminoglycosides at extended intervals).

Table 1 Infections Caused by *P. aeruginosa*

TYPE OF INFECTION	SETTING
Bacteremia	Neutropenia, pulmonary or urinary tract focus
Pneumonia	Mechanical ventilation, neutropenia, cystic fibrosis
Endocarditis	Intravenous drug abuse, prosthetic heart valve
Meningitis, brain abscess	Hematogenous or contiguous spread
Urinary tract infection	Bladder instrumentation
Osteomyelitis, septic arthritis	Contiguous spread of local infection, hematogenous spread, intravenous drug abuse (e.g., sternoclavicular joint)
Osteochondritis	Puncture wounds of the feet
Malignant external otitis	Advanced age, diabetes
Green nail syndrome	Wet skin, immersion

Table 2 Antimicrobial Agents for *P. aeruginosa**

β-lactams	*Quinolones*
Piperacillin 3–4 g IV q4–6h	Ciprofloxacin 200–400 mg IV q12h or 500–750 mg PO q12h
Azlocillin 3–4 g IV q6h	Ofloxacin 200–400 mg IV q12h or 200–400 mg PO q12h
Ticarcillin 3.0 g IV q3–6h	Norfloxacin 400 mg PO q12h
Timentin 3.1 g IV q4–6h	*Aminoglycosides†‡*
Mezlocillin 3.0 g IV q4h	Tobramycin 3–5 mg/kg/day IV in 3 divided doses
Aztreonam 1–2 g IV q8h	Gentamicin 3–5 mg/kg/day IV in 3 divided doses
Imipenem 0.5–1 g IV q6h	Amikacin 15 mg/kg/day IV in 2 divided doses
Meropenem 0.5–1 g IV q6h	
Cephalosporins	
Ceftazidime 1–2 g IV q8h	
Cefoperazone 2–4 g IV q6h	
Cefipime 1–2 g IV q8h	

*Suggested dosing in adult patients with normal renal function.
†Suggested loading doses: tobramycin and gentamicin, 2 mg/kg; amikacin, 7.5 mg/kg.
‡Once-daily administration may be just as efficacious, less nephrotoxic, and less ototoxic.

Combination therapy with a beta-lactam and an aminoglycoside agent is recommended for most serious infections. In vitro synergy between the two agents and postponement of antibiotic resistance form the basis of the practice.

The quinolone antibiotics have become popular for treatment of *Pseudomonas* infections. Ciprofloxacin, the most active quinolone against *P. aeruginosa,* has high bioavailability (approximately 70 percent) with oral dosing. Synergy between quinolones and aminoglycosides has not been observed in vitro.

■ MANAGEMENT OF SPECIFIC INFECTIONS (TABLE 3)

Respiratory Infections

P. aeruginosa pneumonia may follow colonization of patients in the setting of mechanical ventilation, antibiotic administration, neutropenia, chronic pulmonary disease, and congestive heart failure. Lower respiratory tract infection may be distinguished from airway colonization by an increase in quantity and purulence of respiratory secretions. Clinical manifestations may be fulminant, with fever, chills, dyspnea, productive cough, and systemic toxicity. Diffuse bronchopneumonia with nodular infiltrates is commonly seen on chest radiograph. Pneumonia may be accompanied by bacteremia, particularly in neutropenic patients. Empiric antimicrobial treatment for *P. aeruginosa* should be included in initial management of the neutropenic patient with fever and lung infiltrate.

Conventional antimicrobial therapy for *P. aeruginosa* pneumonia includes an antipseudomonal beta-lactam agent combined with an aminoglycoside. Ciprofloxacin appears to be comparable to ceftazidime for the therapy of *Pseudomonas* pneumonia; however, few patients have been studied. Endobronchial administration of aminoglycosides has been used as an adjunct to systemic therapy with improved bacteriologic outcome but little or no improvement in clinical outcome.

Patients with cystic fibrosis are prone to chronic lower respiratory infections with mucoid strains of *P. aeruginosa.* These infections usually persist for a lifetime, with frequent acute exacerbations manifested by decreased exercise tolerance, increased cough and sputum, and weight loss. Therapy consists of a semisynthetic penicillin such as ticarcillin or piperacillin and an aminoglycoside. These patients may require large doses because of altered pharmacokinetics. Aggressive physiotherapy, nutrition, and hydration are also essential.

Table 3 Management of *P. aeruginosa* Infections

INFECTION	ANTIBIOTICS	ADJUNCTIVE
Bacteremia	AP β-lactam + AG	Identify source
Pneumonia	AP β-lactam + AG	Pulmonary toilet
Endocarditis	Ticarcillin + tobramycin 8 mg/kg/day	Valvulectomy for persistent bacteremia
Meningitis	Ceftazidime + AG	Intrathecal AG
Urinary tract	Monotherapy (e.g., AP β-lactam, AG, quinolone)	Remove urinary catheter if possible
Malignant external otitis	AP β-lactam + AG ciprofloxacin	Surgery usually unnecessary
Osteomyelitis	AP β-lactam + AG (ciprofloxacin?)	Surgical debridement

AG, aminoglycoside; AP, antipseudomonal.

Bacteremia

Bacteremia may complicate *P. aeruginosa* infections at other sites. Predisposing factors include neutropenia, hematologic malignancy, organ transplantation, vascular and urinary tract catheterization, and antibiotic use. The respiratory tract is the most frequent source of *Pseudomonas* bacteremia, followed by skin, soft tissues, and the urinary tract.

No distinct clinical characteristics differentiate *P. aeruginosa* bacteremia from other gram-negative bacteremias. Most patients have fever, tachycardia, and tachypnea. Many have signs of systemic toxicity, with hypotension, shock, DIC, and altered mental status. Skin manifestations include papules and rarely, ecthyma gangrenosum (Fig. 1). Prompt initiation of combination therapy is crucial. Therapy should be for 2 to 3 weeks in seriously ill patients. An aggressive search for the source for the bacteremia is important.

Infective Endocarditis

Endocarditis due to *P. aeruginosa* occurs primarily in the setting of intravenous drug abuse and less frequently with prosthetic heart valves. Intravenous drug users acquire *P. aeruginosa* from nonsterile diluents such as tap water or nonsterile paraphernalia. Fever and bacteremia are invariably present. Tricuspid valve infection, which is typical, commonly presents with signs of septic pulmonary embolism. If treated early and aggressively with effective antibiotics, cure may be achieved without surgery. Tricuspid valvulectomy may be necessary in the event of bacteriologic failure or recurrence. Involvement of the aortic or mitral valves may manifest as a severe acute illness with sepsis and large arterial emboli necessitating early surgical valve replacement in addition to antimicrobial treatment. Combination therapy with a beta-lactam agent and an aminoglycoside in high doses (e.g. tobramycin 8 mg per kilogram per day) is recommended. Renal function and aminoglycoside levels should be monitored. (See the chapter *Endocarditis of Natural and Prosthetic Valves.*)

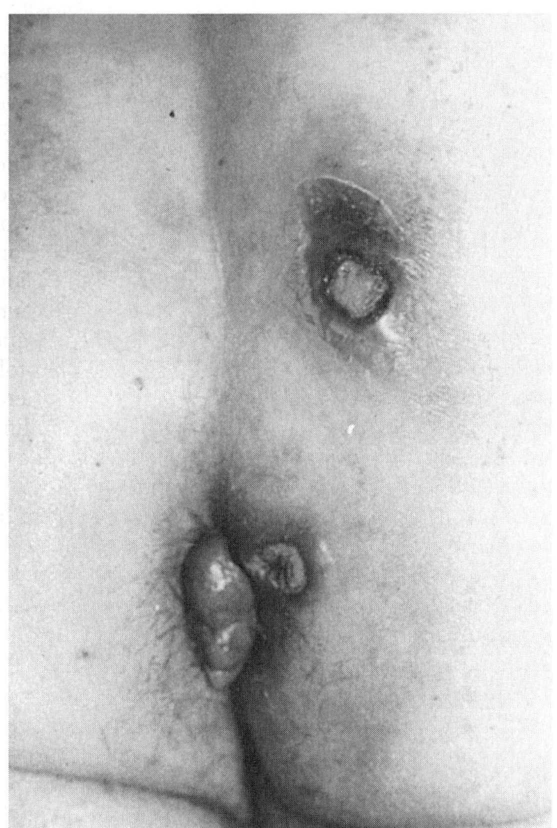

Figure 1
Ecthyma gangrenosum in patient with *Pseudomonas* bacteremia.

Urinary Tract Infections

P. aeruginosa is the third most common nosocomial urinary pathogen. These infections are associated with indwelling urinary catheters. Bacteremia, a common complication, may lead to metastatic infection (e.g., vertebral osteomyelitis). Symptomatic urinary tract infections should be treated by removing the catheter when possible and administering an antibiotic. Monotherapy with a beta-lactam antipseudomonal agent, an aminoglycoside, or a quinolone suffices unless there is complicating bacteremia or upper tract infection. Oral ciprofloxacin may be successfully used even in complicated urinary tract infections. However, emergence of strains resistant to quinolone is a concern. A 7 to 10 day course of treatment is adequate for uncomplicated cases. Longer courses, at least 2 to 3 weeks, are necessary for pyelonephritis or complicating bacteremia.

Meningitis

P. aeruginosa is a rare cause of meningitis and brain abscess. Infection may occur by (1) extension from a contiguous structure such as the ear, mastoid, or sinuses; (2) direct inoculation from trauma or neurosurgical procedures; and (3) metastatic spread from a distant site. Ceftazidime is the antimicrobial of choice because of its excellent in vitro activity and its ability to penetrate cerebrospinal fluid (CSF). Aztreonam has good in vitro activity and adequate CSF penetration, but experience with this agent is limited. Addition of an aminoglycoside may be justified on the basis of possibly conferring synergy and preventing resistance. Because of poor penetration of aminoglycosides into CSF, intrathecal or intraventricular doses may be required. There are anecdotal reports of successful therapy with parenteral ciprofloxacin, but quinolones should be used only when other drugs have failed or when organisms are resistant to beta-lactam agents. Cure of *Pseudomonas* central nervous system infections may require surgical drainage of brain abscesses, debridement of infected tissues, and removal of prosthetic materials. A minimum of 2 and as many as 6 weeks of antimicrobial therapy may be necessary.

Bone and Joint Infections

P. aeruginosa causes osteomyelitis and septic arthritis as a result of hematogenous dissemination or contiguous spread. Surgical debridement and removal of prosthetic materials are usually necessary, and combination antibiotic therapy with a beta-lactam and an aminoglycoside for a minimum of 4 to 6 weeks is the standard of care. The quinolone agents achieve sustained concentrations in bone tissue well above bactericidal levels for most strains of *P. aeruginosa.* These may play a role as single-agent oral therapy following a course of com-

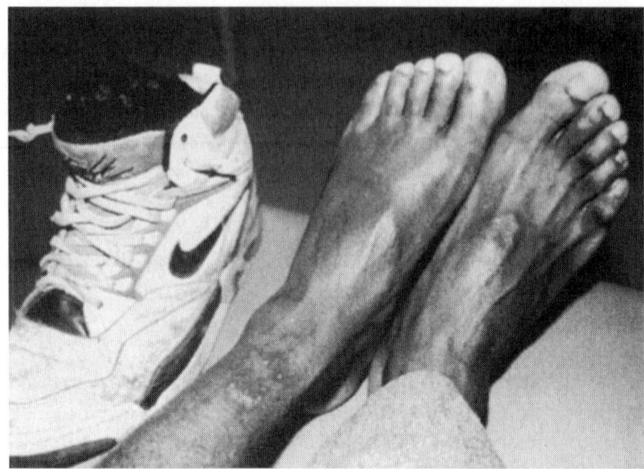

Figure 2
Acute *pseudomonas* osteochondritis with cellulitis following nail puncture wound of sole. Note swelling of left foot.

bination parenteral therapy. Osteochondritis of the foot, seen following nail puncture wounds through the soles of footwear colonized by *P. aeruginosa,* may be treated with shorter courses (Fig. 2).

Ear Infections

External otitis is most commonly caused by *P. aeruginosa* and is usually associated with immersion (swimmer's ear). Patients complain of pain and pruritus; examination reveals edema, exudate, and erythema of the pinna and external canal. This infection is treated with topical agents such as antibiotic drops (polymyxin, neomycin, and hydrocortisone) or dilute acetic acid.

In elderly diabetic patients external otitis may become invasive, with necrosis of bone and soft tissues—malignant external otitis (Fig. 3). There is purulent drainage from the external canal but usually no fever or leukocytosis.

Neurologic complications such as cranial nerve palsies may become manifest. Computed tomography or magnetic resonance imaging is useful to delineate the extent of bone and soft-tissue destruction. Although radical surgical debridement is not always necessary, ear, nose, and throat consultation is advised. Combination treatment is recommended. There are reports of success with oral ciprofloxacin with and without rifampin.

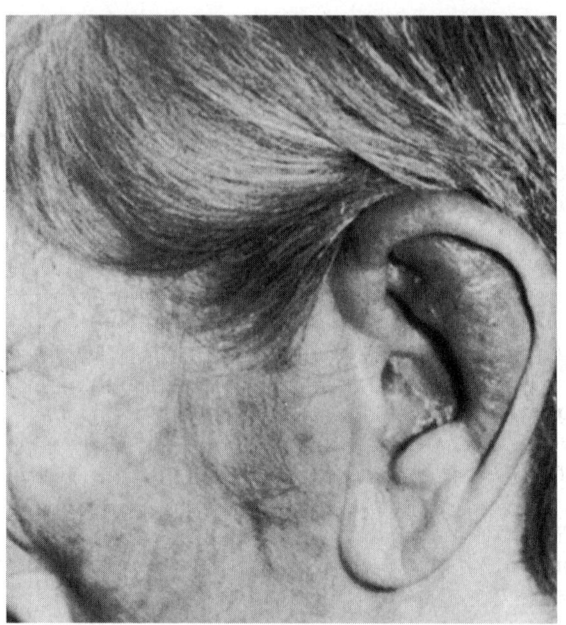

Figure 3
Invasive external otitis in elderly diabetic patient.

Skin Infections

Exposure to contaminated whirlpools, hot tubs, and swimming pools may produce *P. aeruginosa* folliculitis, a diffuse red maculopapular or vesiculopustular rash (Fig. 4). The eruption is self-limited and does not require specific antimicrobial treatment.

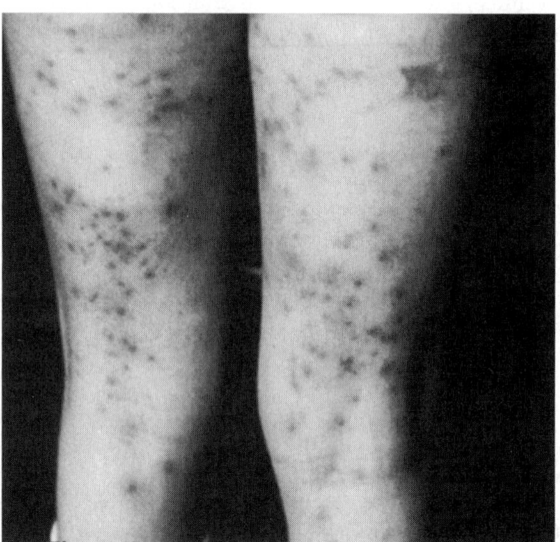

Figure 4
Red papular rash of *Pseudomonas* folliculitis.

Burn wounds may become colonized and later infected with *P. aeruginosa,* resulting in sepsis. Systemic antibiotic combinations should be administered. A topical agent such as mafenide acetate or silver sulfadiazine should be used to reduce burn wound colonization.

Persons with a history of submersion of the hands may develop greenish discoloration of the nail plates and *Pseudomonas* nail bed infection. This condition has been called green nail syndrome (Fig. 5). Treatment requires elimination of the exposure; orally administered ciprofloxin is a useful adjunct.

■ INFECTIONS CAUSED BY OTHER *PSEUDOMONAS* SPECIES

X. maltophilia is a nosocomial gram-negative pathogen that may cause bacteremia, pneumonia, and wound infection. It is resistant to most antipseudomonal beta-lactam agents. Infection may be treated with trimethoprim-sulfamethoxazole

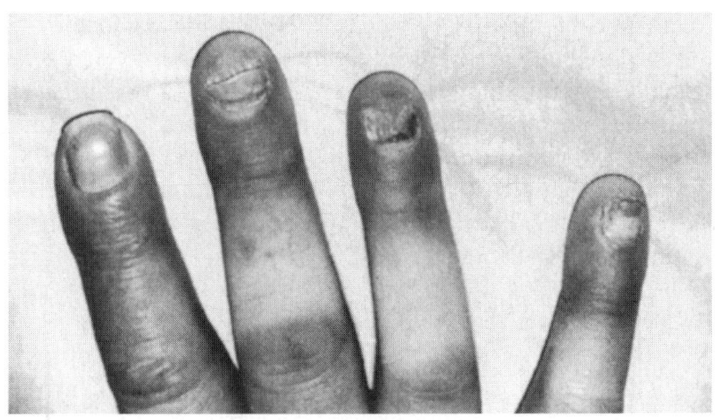

Figure 5
Nails of digits discolored by green pigment of *Pseudomonas aeruginosa.*

(TMP-SMX) alone or in combination with an antipseudomonal penicillin or rifampin. Ceftazidime may be used if susceptibility is documented.

P. cepacia is an opportunistic pathogen that may colonize the respiratory tract of a patient with cystic fibrosis and lead to persistent disease with progressive respiratory failure. Therapy is thwarted by antibiotic resistance and by variable susceptibility to antipseudomonal beta-lactam agents, quinolones, and aminoglycosides. TMP-SMX and chloramphenicol may have activity. Combination therapy should be used.

P. pseudomallei causes melioidosis, an epizootic disease endemic in Southeast Asia. Melioidosis produces septicemia, pneumonia, and local suppurative infections. The choice of antibiotics should be based on susceptibility studies, and treatment should be given for at least 30 days. Combination therapy with ceftazidime and another active agent such as TMP-SMX is recommended. Imipenem and amoxicillin clavulanate are other options.

Suggested Reading

Baltch AL, Smith RP, eds. *Pseudomonas aeruginosa:* Infections and treatment. New York: Marcel Dekker, 1994.

Hilf M, Yu VL, Sharp J, et al. Antibiotic therapy for *Pseudomonas aeruginosa* bacteremia: Outcome correlations in a prospective study of 200 patients. Am J Med 1989; 87:540–546.

Korvick JA, Victor Yu. Antimicrobial agent therapy for *Pseudomonas aeruginosa:* Minireview. Antimicrob Agents Chemother 1991; 35:2167–2172.

SYPHILIS AND OTHER TREPONEMATOSES

Adaora A. Adimora, M.D., M.P.H.

Treponemes are members of the family Spirochaetaceae, which also contains *Borrelia* and *Leptospira.* Although most treponemes do not cause disease in human beings, a few cause substantial morbidity. This chapter briefly reviews the clinical manifestations and treatment of syphilis in adults and the nonvenereal treponematoses, yaws, pinta, and bejel.

■ SYPHILIS

Clinical Manifestations

As with other treponemal diseases, the clinical manifestations of syphilis are divided into early and late stages. Early syphilis is further divided into primary, secondary, and early latent stages. The Centers for Disease Control and Prevention use 1 year as the dividing point between early and late latent disease. However, although clinical staging is useful for diagnosis and treatment, it is also imprecise; overlap between stages is relatively common.

Primary and Secondary Syphilis

Treponema pallidum, the causative agent of syphilis, usually enters the body through breaks in the epithelium during sexual contact. Some organisms persist at the site of entry, and others disseminate via the lymphatic system, proliferating and stimulating an immune response. The incubation period of primary syphilis is usually about 21 days, although extremes of 10 to 90 days have been noted.

The first clinical manifestation is usually a chancre at the site of genital trauma. The chancre begins as a red macule that becomes papular and then ulcerates. The painless lesion has a well-defined margin and thickened rubbery base. If untreated, the chancre persists for 3 to 6 weeks and then heals. Nontender regional lymphadenopathy also develops.

In untreated individuals *T. pallidum* disseminates throughout the body, and secondary syphilis develops about 3 to 6 weeks after the chancre's onset. Common symptoms include malaise, headaches, sore throat, fever, musculoskeletal pains, and weight loss. Physical examination reveals rash in 75 to 100 percent, regional or generalized lymphadenopathy in 50 to 85 percent, and mucosal ulceration in 5 to 30 percent of persons with secondary syphilis. The appearance of the rash can vary greatly, but lesions are frequently maculopapular or papulosquamous, and they often involve the entire body, including the palms and soles. Broad, flat lesions, known as condylomata lata, may develop in warm moist areas, such as the scrotum, vulva, or perianal region. Patchy alopecia and shallow painless mucosal ulcerations called mucous patches may also be seen. Like the chancre, these manifestations of secondary syphilis resolve spontaneously with or without therapy. A small proportion of patients develop complications, including hepatitis, syphilitic glomerulonephritis with nephrotic syndrome, anterior uveitis, choroiditis, arthritis, bursitis, and osteitis. The wide variety of neurologic complications includes meningitis, cranial nerve palsies, transverse myelitis, nerve deafness, and cerebral artery thrombosis.

Neurosyphilis

See the chapter *Neurosyphilis.*

Non-Neurologic Manifestations of Tertiary Syphilis

Syphilitic heart disease, now an uncommon cause of cardiovascular disease, occurs 15 to 30 years after initial infection. During the early phases of infection *T. pallidum* organisms disseminate to the heart and lodge in the aortic wall, where they may cause endarteritis of the vasa vasorum of the aorta, with resultant scarring and destruction of the vessel's wall. Major cardiac manifestations include thoracic aneurysm, aortic regurgitation without associated aortic stenosis, and coronary ostial stenosis.

Late benign syphilis is another now uncommon form of tertiary syphilis. It results from the chronic inflammatory response to *T. pallidum* and a granulomatous type of lesion, the gumma. Gummas may be ulcerative, nodular, or noduloulcerative. They most commonly occur in the skin and bones but may also invade the viscera, muscles, and other structures.

Laboratory Tests

Direct Microscopic Examination

Direct microscopic examination can provide immediate diagnosis of primary and secondary syphilis. Dark-field microscopy must be used because *T. pallidum's* narrow width (0.15 μm) puts it below the level of resolution of light microscopy. Wet preparations can be made from the skin or mucous membrane lesions of primary or secondary syphilis; examination reveals tightly coiled organisms 6 to 14 μm long and 0.25 to 0.30 μm wide, with corkscrew motility. When examination of specimens must be delayed or oral lesions evaluated, direct fluorescent antibody testing can be useful. This test specifically detects *T. pallidum* and eliminates confusion with oral treponemal saprophytes, whose morphology is similar to that of *T. pallidum.*

Serologic Tests

Serologic tests for syphilis measure either nonspecific nontreponemal antibody or specific treponemal antibody.

Nontreponemal antibody tests measure immunoglobulin (Ig) G and IgM antibodies formed by the host against lipid from *T. pallidum's* cell surfaces. These tests are used to screen for disease and disease activity; titers fall progressively over time and should decrease in response to therapy. The following nontreponemal tests are commonly used: VDRL test, rapid plasma reagin (RPR), automated reagin screen test (ART), unheated serum reagin test (USR), and the reagin screen test (RST). False-positive nontreponemal test results occur in 1 to 2 percent of the general population, but false-positive titers are usually less than 1:8.

Specific treponemal antibody tests are usually used to confirm current or past syphilis. These tests detect antibodies formed in response to treponemal antigens. Treponemal tests usually remain reactive after treatment, but a few infected persons become seronegative. Commonly used treponemal tests include the fluorescent antibody absorption (FTA-ABS), microhemagglutination assay for antibodies to *T. pallidum* (MHA-TP), and the hemagglutination treponemal test for syphilis (HATTS).

Cerebrospinal Fluid Evaluation

CSF of all syphilis patients with neurologic signs or symptoms should be examined, as should that of those with latent syphilis if any of the following are present: eye involvement, other evidence of active syphilis, human immunodeficiency virus (HIV) infection, or treatment failure. CSF of patients with latent syphilis should also be examined when duration of infection is known to be less than a year if nonpenicillin therapy is planned or the serum RPR or VDRL is greater than 1:32.

When CSF specimens are free of blood contamination, a positive CSF VDRL test almost always indicates neurosyphilis. Diagnosis is unclear, however, in patients with negative CSF serology, a positive blood serologic test, increased CSF protein levels, and slight pleocytosis. Although such patients may have asymptomatic neurosyphilis, other diagnoses should be considered.

Therapy and Follow-Up

Therapy and follow-up are outlined in Tables 1 and 2.

Syphilis in Persons with HIV Infection

Since syphilis and HIV infection share means of transmission and other risk factors, they frequently coexist. Moreover, increasing evidence suggests that syphilis, like other genital ulcer diseases, facilitates HIV transmission. The clinical effect of HIV infection on the course of syphilis remains controversial. However, the limited prospective data available suggest that HIV infection does not significantly change the presentation, serologic response, clinical course, or response to treatment of syphilis. Nevertheless, clinical observation and case reports suggest that some HIV-infected patients may have an aggressive course of syphilis, and neurosyphilis is common. The prevalence of CSF abnormalities among HIV-positive patients with asymptomatic syphilis appears to be high. Concerns have been raised about the adequacy of single-dose benzathine penicillin G for treatment of early syphilis in HIV-positive patients, as some investigators have isolated *T. pallidum* and identified CSF abnormalities in HIV-infected patients with secondary syphilis after this regimen. Recently investigators have questioned the effectiveness of intravenous penicillin G for treatment of neurosyphilis in HIV-positive patients after documenting clinical and laboratory evidence of treatment failure among prospectively followed patients. However, the true incidence of these events and risk of complications are difficult to determine, since most of these observations are case reports, case-control studies, retrospective studies, or based on small numbers of patients.

Nevertheless, several points remain virtually uncontested. Careful evaluation and follow-up of all HIV-positive patients with syphilis are essential. CSF should be evaluated to exclude central nervous system (CNS) involvement in all HIV-

Table 1 Management of Syphilis in Nonpregnant Adults Without Known HIV Infection

PRIMARY AND SECONDARY SYPHILIS

Treatment
- Benzathine penicillin G 2.4 million units IM once
- If penicillin allergy
  - Doxycycline 100 mg orally b.i.d. for 2 wk, or
  - Tetracycline 500 mg orally q.i.d. for 2 wk
  - Alternative if compliance is certain:
    - Erythromycin 500 mg orally q.i.d. for 2 wk

Management and follow-up
- HIV testing
- If evidence of neurologic disease, evaluate for neurosyphilis
- If evidence of eye disease, do slit-lamp examination
- Repeat serology and clinical examination at 3 mo and 6 mo

LATENT SYPHILIS

Treatment
- Early latent syphilis (duration <1 yr)
  - Benzathine penicillin G 2.4 million units IM once
  - If penicillin allergy,
    - Doxycycline 100 mg orally b.i.d. for 2 wk, or
    - Tetracycline 500 mg orally q.i.d. for 2 wk
- Late latent syphilis or latent syphilis of unknown duration
  - Benzathine penicillin G 2.4 million units IM qwk for 3 wk
  - If penicillin allergy,
    - Doxycycline 100 mg orally b.i.d. for 4 wk, or
    - Tetracycline 500 mg orally q.i.d. for 4 wk

Management and follow-up
- HIV testing
- Clinical evaluation for evidence of tertiary disease (e.g., aortitis, neurosyphilis, gumma, iritis)
- Examine CSF before treatment if any of the following are present:
  - Neurologic or ophthalmic signs or symptoms
  - Other evidence of active syphilis
  - Treatment failure
  - HIV infection
  - Serum RPR or VDRL >1:32 unless duration of infection <1 yr
  - Nonpenicillin therapy planned unless duration of infection <1 yr
- Repeat quantitative VDRL or RPR at 6 and 12 mo
  - Evaluate for neurosyphilis and re-treat if:
    - Serologic titers increase four-fold
    - An initially high titer (≥1:32) fails to fall by at least four-fold within 12–24 mo
    - Patient develops signs or symptoms consistent with syphilis

LATE SYPHILIS (GUMMA OR CARDIOVASCULAR SYPHILIS)

Treatment
- Benzathine penicillin G 2.4 million units IM weekly for 3 wk
- If penicillin allergy, use treatment for late latent syphilis

Management
- Examine CSF

HIV, human immunodeficiency virus; CSF, cerebrospinal fluid; RPR, rapid plasma region; VDRL, Venereal Disease Research Laboratory (test).

Table 2 Treatment of HIV-positive Patients with Syphilis

PRIMARY AND SECONDARY SYPHILIS

Treatment
- Benzathine penicillin G 2.4 million units IM once
- Alternative: benzathine penicillin G 2.4 million units IM weekly × 3
- If penicillin allergy, desensitize if possible, then treat with penicillin

Management
- Clinical and serologic evaluation 1, 2, 3, 6, 9, and 12 mo after therapy
- If nontreponemal titers fail to show fourfold decrease by 4 mo or there is other evidence of treatment failure, examine CSF
  - If CSF normal, re-treat with penicillin G, 2.4 million units IM weekly × 3
  - If CSF suggests neurosyphilis, treat for neurosyphilis as in Table 1

LATENT SYPHILIS

Examine CSF
- If CSF normal, give benzathine penicillin G 2.4 million units IM weekly × 3
- If CSF suggests neurosyphilis, treat for neurosyphilis as in Table 1

infected syphilis patients with latent syphilis or neurologic signs or symptoms. Vigilant follow-up is essential to document resolution of infection and allow prompt evaluation and retreatment if relapse, reinfection, or other complications occur. HIV-positive patients with syphilis should be treated with penicillin if at all possible; those with a history of hypersensitivity should undergo desensitization.

■ NONVENEREAL TREPONEMATOSES

Yaws, pinta, and bejel (endemic syphilis) are caused respectively by the *Treponema* spp. *T. pallidum pertenue*, *T. carateum*, and *T. pallidum endemicum*. These diseases, seen mainly in tropical and subtropical regions, are transmitted by direct contact with infected skin lesions and not primarily by sexual contact. Like venereal syphilis, these diseases have self-limited primary and secondary stages, a latent stage, and a late stage with destructive lesions. The causative agents are morphologically indistinguishable from *T. pallidum pallidum*, and the serologic responses they elicit are identical to those of venereal syphilis. Diagnosis can be made by dark-field examination of lesions or serologic testing. Long-acting penicillin G, the treatment of choice, has dramatically decreased the incidence of these diseases in endemic regions.

Yaws occurs in the tropical regions of Africa, Southeast Asia, South America, and Oceania. About 3 to 5 weeks after infection papules develop and enlarge, erode, and then spontaneously heal. A generalized secondary eruption of similar lesions occurs weeks to months later, sometimes in association with osteitis or periostitis. In the late stage infected persons may develop hyperkeratoses on the palms and soles; plaques, nodules, and ulcers of the skin; and gummatous bone lesions.

Pinta occurs in remote parts of Mexico, Central America,

and Colombia. About 7 to 21 days after infection small red pruritic papules develop and enlarge, become squamous, and merge with other primary lesions. These lesions eventually heal, but residual hypopigmentation persists. About 3 to 12 months after the appearance of the primary lesions small scaly papules known as pintids appear. These may eventually become brown, gray, or blue, and may recur as long as 10 years after initial infection. Depigmented lesions develop in the late stage.

Bejel occurs in Africa and western Asia. Unlike yaws and pinta, bejel is spread not only by direct contact but also through eating and drinking utensils. Primary lesions are seldom seen. Secondary manifestations include mucous patches, condylomata lata, split papules at the angles of the mouth, and lymphadenopathy. Gummatous lesions of the skin, nasopharynx, and bones are common in the late stage.

Suggested Reading

Centers for Disease Control and Prevention. 1993 Sexually transmitted disease treatment guidelines. MMWR 1993; 42(RR-14):27–46.

Chulay JD. Treponema species (yaws, pinta, bejel). In: Mandell GL, Bennett JE, Dolin R, eds. Mandell, Douglas, and Bennett's principles and practice of infectious diseases. 4th ed. New York: Churchill Livingstone, 1995:2133.

Gourevitch MN, Selwyn, PA, Davenny K, et al. Effects of HIV infection on the serologic manifestations and response to treatment of syphilis in intravenous drug users. Ann Intern Med 1993; 118:350–355.

Hook EW III, Marra C. Acquired syphilis in adults. N Engl J Med 1992; 326:1060–1069.

Rolf RT. Treatment of syphilis, 1993. Clin Infect Dis 1995; 20(Suppl 1):523–528.

NEUROSYPHILIS

Christina M. Marra, M.D.

Neurosyphilis is one of the most daunting diseases to understand because its diagnostic criteria, optimal therapy, and expected response to therapy have not been firmly established. These uncertainties are particularly troublesome now that neurosyphilis is most commonly described in patients also infected with the human immunodeficiency virus (HIV) type-1. Both HIV and neurosyphilis are associated with neurologic and cerebrospinal fluid (CSF) abnormalities, and distinguishing the contribution of each may be difficult. In addition, HIV-infected persons with neurosyphilis may be more likely to fail therapy. The goal of this chapter is to provide guidelines for diagnosis, treatment, and management of neurosyphilis, based on our current state of knowledge. Insights gained from additional study will allow these recommendations to be refined and improved in the future.

■ EARLY CENTRAL NERVOUS SYSTEM INVASION

Syphilis and neurosyphilis are caused by *Treponema pallidum*, a nonculturable bacterium that is not visualized by conventional microscopy. The organism invades the central nervous system (CNS) early in the course of the disease, as demonstrated by its identification in CSF from 10 to 30 percent of patients with early syphilis (primary, secondary, and early latent syphilis) by inoculation of samples into rabbits. In addition, 10 to 70 percent of patients with early syphilis have CSF pleocytosis; elevated CSF protein concentration, albumin ratio, or IgG index; or reactive CSF-Venereal Disease Research Laboratory (VDRL) test. Figure 1 shows the sequence of detection of CSF abnormalities in syphilis: (1) identification of *T. pallidum;* (2) pleocytosis; elevated albumin, protein, and globulin concentrations; and presence of anti–*T. pallidum* antibody; (3) reactivity of CSF-VDRL.

Unlike other bacterial CNS infections, *T. pallidum* is cleared from the CNS in approximately 70 percent of patients, and CSF abnormalities resolve. Normalization of CSF carries a good prognosis, predicting a low likelihood of developing symptomatic neurosyphilis, whereas persistence of CSF abnormalities carries a poor prognosis. Unfortunately, it is not possible to predict which patients with abnormal CSF (asymptomatic neurosyphilis) will spontaneously clear these abnormalities and which will not. Thus, all patients with asymptomatic neurosyphilis are treated to prevent progression to symptomatic disease.

■ CLINICAL FEATURES

Neurosyphilis traditionally has been categorized into specific syndromes, each occurring at an estimated time after primary infection. It is easier to envision them as the early forms (asymptomatic neurosyphilis, symptomatic meningitis, and meningovasculitis), characterized by meningeal involvement, and the late forms (general paresis and tabes dorsalis), characterized by parenchymal involvement. Early neurosyphilis occurs weeks to a few years after infection, and late neurosyphilis occurs decades after infection (Fig. 2). The key clinical features of early and late neurosyphilis are outlined in Table 1.

In the preantibiotic (and pre-HIV) era, most patients with syphilis did not develop neurosyphilis. In 1946, Merritt and coworkers reported the frequency of neurosyphilis patients with syphilis at Boston City Hospital. Symptomatic neurosyphilis was found in approximately 17.5 percent of these patients: symptomatic meningitis in less than 0.5 percent, meningovasculitis in 3 percent, general paresis in 5 percent, and tabes dorsalis in 9 percent; asymptomatic neurosyphilis

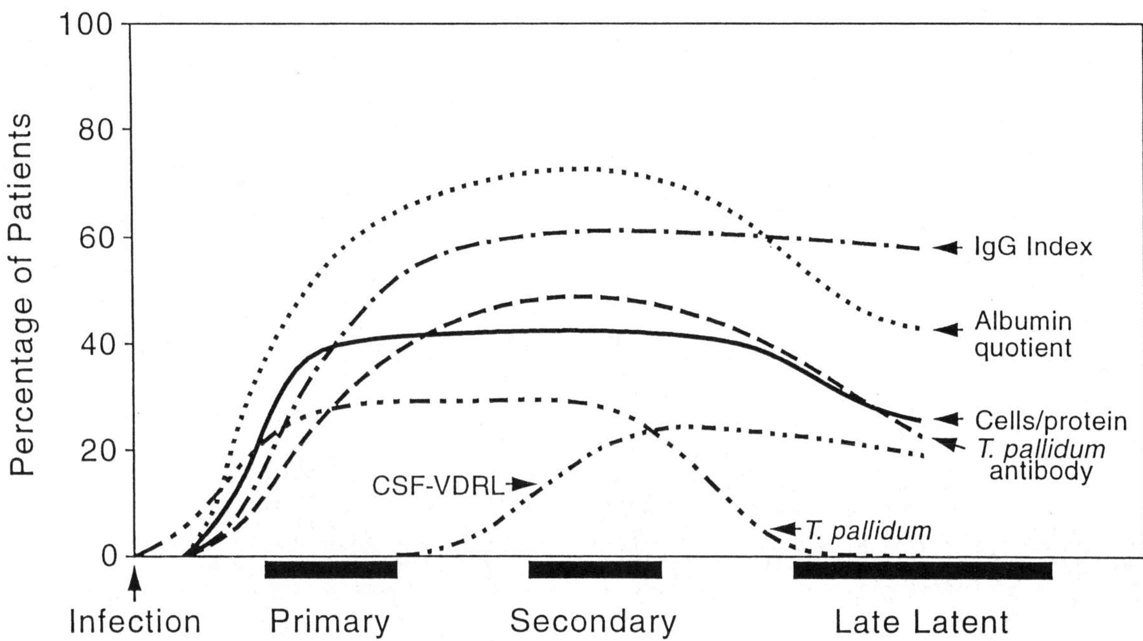

Figure 1
Time course of development of cerebrospinal fluid (CSF) abnormalities in patients with syphilis. Invasion of the CNS by *T. pallidum* occurs early, followed by pleocytosis and development of specific *T. pallidum* antibody. Reactivity of the CSF-VDRL develops after these changes. *(Modified from Lukehart SA, Marra CM. A comparison of syphilis and Lyme disease: Central nervous system involvement. In: Schutzer S, ed. Lyme disease: Molecular and immunologic approaches. New York: Cold Spring Harbor Laboratory Press, 1992:59–77; with permission.)*

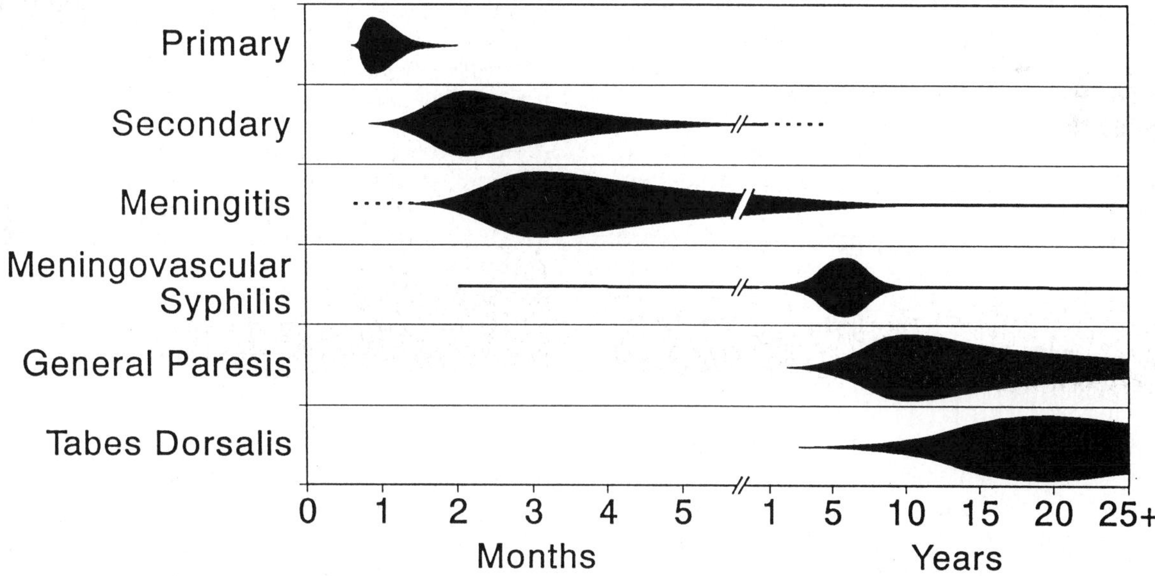

Figure 2
Approximate time course of the clinical manifestations of early syphilis and neurosyphilis. Neurosyphilis can occur at any time after primary infection. Meningeal and meningovascular disease occur early in the course of disease and may be seen in patients with primary or secondary syphilis. Paresis and tabes occur late in the course of infection. *(Modified from Hook EW III, Marra CM. Acquired syphilis in adults. N Engl J Med 1992; 326:1060–1069; with permission.)*

Table 1 Clinical Findings in the Forms of Neurosyphilis

Asymptomatic: These patients have CSF abnormalities due to CNS invasion by *T. pallidum,* but are neurologically normal. This form of neurosyphilis may occur any time after infection but is most common in the first few years. Patients with asymptomatic neurosyphilis are at risk for development of symptomatic disease and should be treated with penicillin regimens recommended for neurosyphilis to prevent this progression.

Meningeal: These patients have clinical evidence of meningitis with headache, stiff neck, nausea, and vomiting. Cranial nerve abnormalities and hydrocephalus may develop. This form of neurosyphilis is most common in the first year of infection. Treatment results in clinical improvement.

Meningovascular: These patients experience stroke, often in the middle cerebral artery territory. Other vascular distributions, including spinal cord, may be involved. Symptoms of meningitis also may be present. Peak incidence is 7 years after primary infection. Treatment results in clinical improvement, although residual deficits are common.

General Paresis: Early in the course, these patients may be forgetful and show personality changes. Psychiatric symptoms such as mania, depression, or psychosis may develop. All patients eventually become demented, often with pupillary abnormalities, hypotonia, and intention tremor. Onset is usually 10 to 20 years after primary infection. Treatment may halt progression but does not usually result in clinical improvement.

Tabes Dorsalis: These patients develop sensory loss, ataxia, and bowel and bladder dysfunction. This syndrome has the longest latent period between primary infection and onset of symptoms with an average of 20 years. Treatment may halt progression but does not usually result in clinical improvement.

From Marra CM. Neurosyphilis: A guide for clinicians. The Neurologist 1995; 1:157–166; with permission.

was identified in 25 percent of patients. In another series, only 62 (6.5 percent) of 953 patients with untreated early syphilis developed symptomatic neurosyphilis.

Today, neurosyphilis is seen most commonly in patients also infected with HIV, in large part because the two diseases share common risk factors. The reported prevalence of symptomatic neurosyphilis ranges from 5.7 to 12.5 percent of HIV-infected patients with reactive syphilis serologic tests in blood, and the prevalence of asymptomatic neurosyphilis from 2 to 54 percent. Early neurosyphilis may be more likely to develop in HIV-infected than -uninfected individuals. A retrospective study of neurosyphilis in HIV-infected and -uninfected patients performed at a single institution showed that syphilitic meningitis was significantly more common in HIV-infected patients without acquired immunodeficiency syndrome than in HIV-uninfected patients.

DIAGNOSIS

In addition to neurologic symptoms and signs, serologic tests for syphilis on serum and CSF, CSF leukocyte count, and CSF protein concentration are integral elements in the diagnosis of neurosyphilis. Although identification of *T. pallidum* DNA in CSF is possible by polymerase chain reaction, the role of this test in the diagnosis of neurosyphilis has not been established.

Nontreponemal serologic tests such as the VDRL or the rapid plasma reagin (RPR) may be nonreactive in blood, particularly in individuals with late neurosyphilis. However, specific treponemal serologic tests such as the serum microhemagglutination test for *T. pallidum* (MHA-TP) or fluorescent treponemal antibody-absorbed (FTA-ABS) test will be reactive in all patients with neurosyphilis. Thus, treponemal tests are the first step in screening patients for neurosyphilis (Fig. 3).

Mononuclear CSF pleocytosis and a modestly elevated protein concentration are characteristic of neurosyphilis. Higher cell counts and protein concentrations are more common in the early forms of neurosyphilis. Although the specificity of the CSF-VDRL is high, the sensitivity has been estimated to be 22 to 69 percent, and a nonreactive result does not exclude the diagnosis of neurosyphilis. The low sensitivity of the CSF-VDRL in the diagnosis of neurosyphilis is particularly problematic in HIV-infected patients, because mild CSF pleocytosis and elevated CSF protein concentration are common in these individuals even when they do not have syphilis. Lack of CSF FTA-ABS or CSF MHA-TP reactivity may be particularly useful in excluding the diagnosis of neurosyphilis in these cases (Fig. 3). Unlike the CSF-VDRL, lack of CSF FTA-ABS or CSF MHA-TP reactivity excludes a diagnosis of neurosyphilis with a high degree of certainty, but reactivity of these tests does not confirm the diagnosis of neurosyphilis.

TREATMENT

The Centers for Disease Control and Prevention (CDC) recommends either high-dose intravenous penicillin or a combination of intramuscular procaine penicillin and oral probenecid for the treatment of neurosyphilis (Table 2). Over the years, several alternative antibiotic regimens have been proposed based on their ability to produce treponemicidal antibiotic concentrations in CSF, not on efficacy in clinical trials. In many communities, ceftriaxone is considered to be an alternative to penicillin for the treatment of neurosyphilis. A recent retrospective study of ceftriaxone for treatment of HIV-infected patients with neurosyphilis, latent syphilis, and presumed latent syphilis (many of whom were later found to have neurosyphilis) showed an unacceptably high (23 percent) failure rate using serologic criteria for cure. Until further study proves otherwise, ceftriaxone should not be used for treatment of neurosyphilis. Patients with a history of penicillin allergy should be skin tested, desensitized if necessary, and treated with a CDC-recommended penicillin regimen.

RESPONSE TO THERAPY

The best outcomes after treatment of neurosyphilis are seen in patients with CSF pleocytosis. Treatment does not reverse parenchymal damage seen in patients with meningovascular neurosyphilis, general paresis, and tabes dorsalis, but it does prevent disease progression.

Traditionally, the criteria for assessing response to treatment of neurosyphilis have relied on improvement, or lack of progression, of neurologic findings and resolution of serum and CSF abnormalities. The CDC guidelines suggest that CSF should be examined every 6 months after neurosyphilis

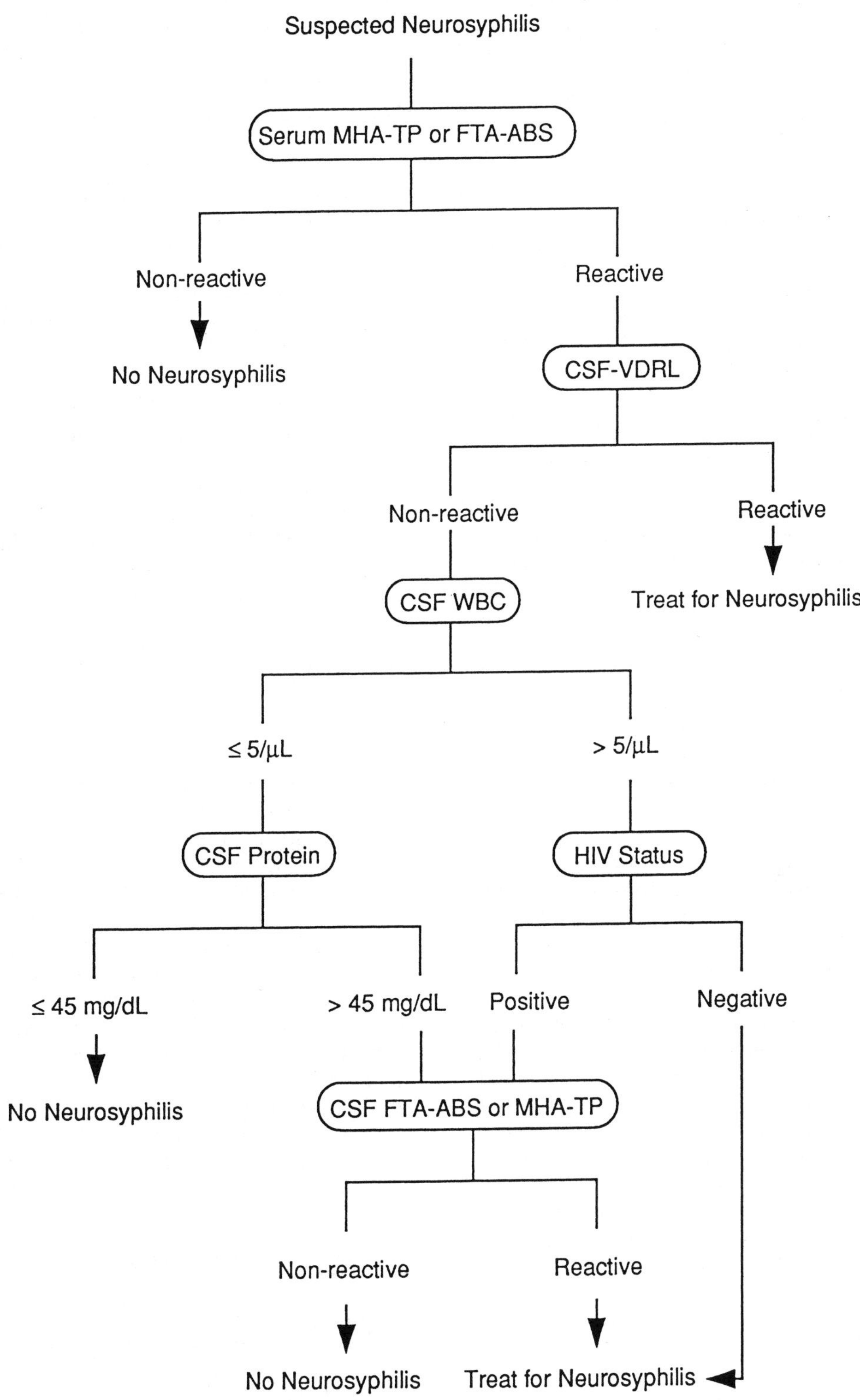

Figure 3
Algorithm for the laboratory diagnosis of neurosyphilis: MHA-TP, FTA-ABS, CSF, VDRL, leukocyte count, HIV. *(From Marra CM. Neurosyphilis: A guide for clinicians. The Neurologist 1995; 1:157–166; with permission.)*

Table 2 Recommended Therapy for Neurosyphilis

Aqueous crystalline penicillin G, 2–4 MU IV every 4 hours, for 10–14 days
or
Procaine penicillin, 2.4 MU IM once daily, plus probenecid 500 mg orally four times a day, both for 10–14 days

Many experts recommend following therapy for neurosyphilis with benzathine penicillin G, 2.4 MU IM weekly for 3 weeks. From Centers for Disease Control and Prevention. 1993 Sexually transmitted diseases treatment guidelines. MMWR 1993; 42:27–46.

treatment until the cell count is normal. Re-treatment is advised if the cell count has not declined at 6 months or if the CSF is not entirely normal by 2 years after therapy. No recommendations are provided regarding rate of decline of CSF protein concentration or of decline in CSF or serum VDRL titers.

Although I am not aware of well-documented instances of neurosyphilis treatment failure in HIV-uninfected individuals, several reports of clinical and serologic failure of high-dose intravenous penicillin therapy for neurosyphilis in HIV-infected patients have been published in the past 5 years. I recently used survival analysis to examine normalization of serum and CSF abnormalities after treatment of neurosyphilis in nine HIV-uninfected and 13 HIV-infected patients. These patients had reactive CSF-VDRLs and were treated with CDC-recommended penicillin regimens. All the HIV-uninfected patients met CDC-recommended guidelines for cure. Using the points that the survival curves intersected the x-axis, serum VDRL titer declined by two dilutions, or to nonreactive, and CSF pleocytosis and elevated protein concentration normalized by 7 months after therapy. Similarly, 87 percent of HIV-uninfected patients showed a decline in CSF-VDRL by two dilutions, or to nonreactive, at 5.6 months. In contrast, one HIV-infected patient met CDC criteria for treatment failure. Three other HIV-infected patients had persistent, mild elevation of CSF leukocyte counts 6 months or more after therapy. Compared with HIV-uninfected patients, decline in serum and CSF-VDRL titers, and in CSF leukocyte count, was significantly slower in HIV-infected patients. Taken together, these data suggest that neurosyphilis therapy may be less effective in HIV-infected individuals. In fact, some experts suggest that, because of underlying immunodeficiency, neurosyphilis is not a curable disease in HIV-infected patients.

Resolution of this issue awaits further study. In the meantime, I suggest that serum VDRL or RPR titers be determined every 3 months and CSF be examined at 3 and 6 months and then every 6 months thereafter following treatment for neurosyphilis in both HIV-uninfected and HIV-infected individuals. Serial CSF examinations should continue until all

Table 3 Suggested Criteria for Re-treatment of Neurosyphilis

Sustained increase in serum VDRL or RPR titer by two dilutions (fourfold increase)
Persistent CSF pleocytosis 6 months after therapy in an HIV-uninfected patient
Persistent CSF pleocytosis and no change in CSF-VDRL or serum VDRL titer 6 months after therapy in an HIV-infected patient
Persistence of any CSF abnormality 2 years after therapy in an HIV-uninfected patient
Persistent CSF-VDRL reactivity 2 years after therapy in an HIV-infected patient
Increase in CSF-VDRL titer by two dilutions (fourfold increase)
Worsening neurologic symptoms or signs
Development of new neurologic symptoms or signs

CSF abnormalities resolve. Serial serum examinations can be terminated when the serum VDRL or RPR becomes nonreactive or the titer drops by two dilutions (a fourfold reduction) and the CSF has normalized. CSF pleocytosis and elevated protein concentration may persist in HIV-infected individuals because of HIV infection alone, but CSF-VDRL should revert to nonreactive, or the titer drop by two dilutions. It should be remembered that, although it is easy to devise such criteria for "cure," we do not know if failure to meet these criteria is equivalent to treatment failure. Despite these limitations, suggested criteria for re-treatment are listed in Table 3.

Selected Reading

Dowell ME, Ross PG, Musher DM, et al. Response of latent syphilis or neurosyphilis to ceftriaxone therapy in persons infected with human immunodeficiency virus. Am J Med 1992; 93:481–488.

Katz DA, Berger JR, Duncan RC. Neurosyphilis: A comparative study of the effects of infection with human immunodeficiency virus. Arch Neurol 1993; 50:243–249.

Lukehart SA, Hook EW III, Baker-Zander SA, et al. Invasion of the central nervous system by *Treponema pallidum:* Implications for diagnosis and therapy. Ann Intern Med 1988; 109:855–862.

Marra CM, Critchlow CW, Hook EW III, et al. Cerebrospinal fluid treponemal antibodies in untreated early syphilis. Arch Neurol 1995; 52:68–72.

Marra CM, Longstreth WT Jr, Maxwell CL, Lukehart SA. Resolution of serum and cerebrospinal fluid abnormalities after treatment of neurosyphilis: Influence of concomitant human immunodeficiency virus infection. Sex Transm Dis 1996; 23:184–189.

Merritt HH, Adams RD, Solomon HC. Neurosyphilis. New York: Oxford, 1946.

Moore JE, Hopkins HH. Asymptomatic neurosyphilis VI: The prognosis of early and late asymptomatic neurosyphilis. JAMA 1930; 95:1637–1641.

Musher DM. Syphilis, neurosyphilis, penicillin, and AIDS. J Infect Dis 1991; 163:1201–1206.

LYME DISEASE

Janine Evans, M.D.
Stephen E. Malawista, M.D.

Lyme disease, a systemic illness caused by the spirochete *Borrelia burgdorferi,* is the most common tick-borne disease in the United States. In 1992, 45 states reported 9,677 cases of Lyme disease using the surveillance case definition of the Council of State and Territorial Epidemiologists (CSTE) and Centers for Disease Control and Prevention (CDC). Since the discovery of Lyme arthritis in the mid 1970s, the clinical spectrum has expanded to include a wide variety of organ systems, primarily the skin, joints, nervous system, and heart. Protean symptoms, uncertainty in diagnosis because of lack of definitive testing methods, and public fear of late sequelae of disease often lead to overdiagnosis and overtreatment. Although optimal therapy of many of the clinical features of Lyme disease is unclear, better understanding of the natural history, epidemiology, and pathogenesis of Lyme disease help with the decisions related to diagnosis and treatment.

B. burgdorferi has been isolated from blood, skin, cerebrospinal fluid, and rarely, other specimens from infected patients, although with the exception of skin biopsy specimens, culture of *B. burgdorferi* from sites of infection is a low-yield procedure. *B. burgdorferi* displays phenotypic and genotypic diversity and has been classified into three genospecies. Species I includes all strains studied thus far from the United States and some European and Asian strains, called *B. burgdorferi sensu stricto;* species II, *Borrelia garinii,* and species III, *Borrelia afzelii,* are found in Europe and Asia. *B. afzelii* seems primarily associated with a chronic skin lesion, acrodermatitis chronicum atrophicans; this is rare in the United States. *B. burgdorferi* is transmitted to the skin of the host via a tick bite.

Lyme disease occurs in three principal foci in the United States: the Northeast, the upper Midwest, and the Pacific Coast. These areas correspond to the distribution of the predominant tick vectors of Lyme disease in the United States, *Ixodes scapularis* in the East and Midwest and *Ixodes pacificus* in northern California. Lyme disease also occurs widely in Europe, where it is transmitted by the sheep tick, *Ixodes ricinus. I. scapularis* has a three-stage, 2 year life cycle. Transovarial passage of *B. burgdorferi* occurs at a low rate. Ticks become infected with spirochetes by feeding on a spirochetemic animal, typically a small mammal, during larval and nymphal stages. In highly endemic areas, 20 percent to more than 60 percent of *I. scapularis* carry *B. burgdorferi.* Man is only an incidental host of the tick; contact is typically made in areas of underbrush or high grasses but may occur in well-mown lawns in endemic areas. Lyme disease occurs predominantly during May through July, when *I. scapularis* nymphs feed. Animal models show that transmission is unlikely to occur before a minimum of 36 hours of tick attachment and feeding.

■ CLINICAL MANIFESTATIONS

Clinical features of Lyme disease are typically divided into three general stages: early localized, early disseminated, and late persistent infection. These stages may overlap, and most patients do not exhibit all stages. Direct invasion of the organism with a resultant vigorous inflammatory reaction is responsible for many of the clinical manifestations associated with Lyme disease, so the manifestations respond to antibiotic therapy. Some features, such as late neurologic deficits and chronic arthritis, respond poorly to treatment. It is not clear that live organisms are responsible for these later symptoms. Seroconversion can occur in asymptomatic individuals but is rare with strict surveillance.

Early Localized Disease

Erythema migrans (EM), the hallmark of Lyme disease, begins at the site of a deer tick bite after 3 to 32 days. Reported by 60 to 80 percent of patients, it appears as a centrifugally expanding erythematous macule or papule, often with central clearing. The thigh, groin, and axilla are common sites. The lesion may be warm, pruritic, and painful, but is often asymptomatic and easily missed if out of sight. Occasionally these lesions develop blistering or scabbing in the center, remain an even, intense red without clearing, or develop a bluish discoloration. Spirochetes are present in the EM lesion and can be readily cultured from the expanding edge. Mild musculoskeletal flulike symptoms such as low-grade fever, chills, malaise, headache, fatigue, arthralgias, and myalgias may accompany EM lesions. Theoretically such symptoms can occur without dissemination of the organism via local generation of cytokines. Untreated EM resolves after several weeks, and treated lesions clear within several days.

Early Disseminated Disease

In some patients the spirochete disseminates hematogenously to multiple sites, causing characteristic clinical features. Secondary annular lesions, sites of metastatic foci of *Borrelia* in the skin, develop within days of onset of EM in about half of U.S. patients. They are similar in appearance to EM but are generally smaller, migrate less, and lack indurated centers. Musculoskeletal flulike symptoms, mild hepatitis, splenomegaly, sore throat, nonproductive cough, testicular swelling, conjunctivitis, and regional and generalized lymphadenopathy may occur during early stages.

Diagnosis of early localized and early disseminated Lyme disease is based on clinical presentation, since serologic confirmation is often lacking and culture is not readily available. EM is diagnostic of Lyme disease, although atypical lesions and rashes mimicking EM may be confusing. A history of a tick bite and residence or travel in an endemic area should be sought in patients presenting with rashes compatible with EM or a flulike illness in summer. Specific immunoglobulin (Ig) M antibody responses against *B. burgdorferi* develop 2 to 6 weeks after the onset of EM. IgG antibody levels appear approximately 6 weeks after disease onset but may not peak until months or even years into the illness. The highest titers occur during arthritis. Antibodies are typically detected using indirect immunofluorescence, enzyme-linked immunosorbent assay (ELISA), and immunoblotting (Western blot).

Antibody responses may persist for months to years after infection.

■ THERAPY

Early Lyme Disease

The symptoms of early Lyme disease resolve spontaneously in most cases; therefore, the goals of therapy for early localized and mild early disseminated Lyme disease are to shorten the duration of symptoms and reduce the risk of developing serious late manifestations of infection. Treatment of these stages with oral antibiotics is adequate for most patients (Table 1). Initial studies of treatment for early Lyme disease reported that phenoxymethyl penicillin, erythromycin, and tetracycline 250 mg four times a day for 10 to 20 days shortened the duration of symptoms of early Lyme disease. Phenoxymethyl penicillin and tetracycline were superior to erythromycin in preventing serious late manifestations of disease. Subsequent clinical trials have proved amoxicillin and doxycycline to be equally efficacious. Amoxicillin has largely replaced penicillin because of greater in vitro activity against *B. burgdorferi.* Concomitant use of probenecid has not been definitively shown to improve clinical outcome and is associated with a higher incidence of side effects. Doxycycline is usually preferred to tetracycline because of its twice daily dose schedule, increased GI absorption and tolerability, and greater central nervous system penetration. Cefuroxime axetil, an oral second-generation cephalosporin, has recently been shown to be about as effective as amoxicillin and doxycycline in treating early Lyme disease; azithromycin, an azilide analogue of erythromycin, is somewhat less so. Long-term follow-up of patients treated during early stages of Lyme disease support the current dosing regimens. Patients who received a 14 to 21 day course of a recommended antibiotic rarely developed late manifestations of illness. Jarisch-Herxheimer-like reactions, increased discomfort in skin lesions, and temperature elevation within hours of the start of antibiotic treatment, have been encountered in 14 percent of patients treated for early Lyme disease. They typically occur within 2 to 4 hours of starting therapy, are most common in severe disease, and are presumably due to rapid killing of a large number of spirochetes.

Minor symptoms, including arthralgia, fatigue, headaches, and transient facial palsy, are common following treatment and generally resolve over 6 months. Patients with disseminated disease are most likely to have persistent symptoms. These symptoms may be due to retained antigen rather than ongoing infection with *B. burgdorferi,* since longer courses of antibiotics have not been shown to shorten their duration. Long courses of antibiotics should be reserved for patients with evidence of persistent infection with *B. burgdorferi.*

Table 1 Treatment of Lyme Disease

EARLY LYME DISEASE*
Amoxicillin 500 mg t.i.d. for 21 days†
Doxycycline 100 mg b.i.d. for 21 days
Cefuroxime axetil 500 mg b.i.d. for 21 days
Azithromycin 500 mg daily for 7 days‡ (less effective than other regimens)
NEUROLOGIC MANIFESTATIONS
Bell's palsy (no other neurologic abnormalities)
Oral regimens for early disease suffice
Meningitis (with or without radiculoneuropathy or encephalitis)§
Ceftriaxone 2 g daily for 14–28 days
Penicillin G 20 million units daily for 14–28 days
Doxycycline 100 mg b.i.d PO or IV for 14–28 days‖
Chloramphenicol 1 g q.i.d for 14–28 days
ARTHRITIS¶
Amoxicillin and probenecid 500 mg q.i.d. for 30 days**
Doxycycline 100 mg b.i.d. for 30 days
Ceftriaxone 2 g daily for 14–28 days
Penicillin G 20 million units daily for 14–28 days
CARDITIS
Ceftriaxone 2 g daily for 14 days
Penicillin G 20 million units daily for 14 days
Doxycycline 100 mg orally b.i.d. for 21 days††
Amoxicillin 500 mg 3 t.i.d. for 21 days††
PREGNANCY
Localized early disease
Amoxicillin 500 mg t.i.d for 21 days
Any manifestation of disseminated disease
Penicillin G 20 million units daily for 14–28 days
Asymptomatic seropositivity
No treatment necessary

*Without neurologic, cardiac, or joint involvement. For early Lyme disease limited to single erythema migrans lesion, 10 days is sufficient.
†Some experts advise addition of probenecid 500 mg 3 times daily.
‡Experience with this agent is limited; optimal duration of therapy is unclear.
§Optimal duration of therapy has not been established. There are no controlled trials of therapy longer than 4 weeks for any manifestation of Lyme disease.
‖No published experience in the United States.
¶An oral regimen should be selected only if there is no neurologic involvement.
**Amoxicillin is generally administered 3 times daily, but the only trial of this agent for Lyme arthritis used a 4-times-daily regimen.
††Oral regimens have been reserved for mild carditis limited to first-degree heart block with PR ≥0.30 seconds and normal ventricular function.
From Rahn DW, Malawista SE. Treatment of Lyme disease. In: The year book of medicine. St. Louis: Mosby–Year Book, 1994: xxi-xxxvi; with permission.

Lyme Carditis

Cardiac involvement occurs in up to 10 percent of untreated patients. Transient and varying degrees of atrioventricular block several weeks to months after a tick bite are the most common manifestations. Other features are pericarditis, myocarditis, ventricular tachycardia, and on rare occasions a dilated cardiomyopathy; valvular disease is not seen. Carditis is typically mild and self-limited, although patients may present quite dramatically with complete heart block, and some require a temporary pacemaker. In most cases carditis resolves completely, even without treatment with antibiotics. Recent studies examining endomyocardial biopsy specimens from patients with Lyme carditis have indicated that direct invasion of *B. burgdorferi* into myocardium and an associated inflammatory reaction are responsible for the clinical events.

Although optimal treatment of carditis is unknown, oral therapy for mild forms of cardiac involvement is usually sufficient. Intravenous antibiotics and cardiac monitoring are recommended for patients with varying or high-degree heart block and more serious cardiac involvement. There is no evidence of long-term cardiac abnormalities in patients treated for carditis.

Dilated cardiomyopathy is a rare complication of Lyme disease reported in Europe but not yet in the United States. Most of the patients were from areas endemic for Lyme disease, had other clinical features of disease, and were seropositive for anti-*B. burgdorferi* antibodies. Their myopathy was cured by antibiotic treatment.

Early Neurologic Disease

Early neurologic involvement occurs in 15 to 20 percent of untreated patients and appears within 2 to 8 weeks after the onset of disease. Manifestations include cranial nerve palsies, meningitis or meningoencephalitis, and peripheral neuritis or radiculoneuritis. Unilateral or bilateral seventh nerve palsies are the most common neurologic abnormalities. Presenting symptoms depend on the area of the nervous system involved: patients with meningitis have fever, headache, and stiff neck; those with Bannwarth's syndrome (primarily in Europe) develop severe and migrating radicular pain lasting weeks to several months; and those with encephalitis have concentration deficits, emotional lability, and fatigue. In patients with early central nervous system (CNS) involvement, analysis of cerebrospinal fluid (CSF) typically reveals lymphocytic pleocytosis. Specific antibodies against *B. burgdorferi* may also be concentrated in the CSF relative to the serum concentration; they are useful to confirm disease.

Intravenous antibiotics are recommended for all patients with neuroborreliosis except isolated seventh nerve palsy. Patients with Bell's palsy who have features that suggest CNS involvement, such as high fever, headache, or stiff neck, should undergo a lumbar puncture for evidence of more extensive disease. The most experience in the treatment of CNS Lyme disease has been with aqueous penicillin and third-generation cephalosporins. Although optimal duration of therapy is unknown, it is recommended that patients be treated for 2 to 4 weeks. Ceftriaxone 1 to 2 g per day is the agent of choice because of good CNS penetration and ease of administration. Patients with persistent symptoms after recommended antibiotic therapy pose a particular management problem. It is often unclear whether these symptoms are due to resolving inflammation or ongoing infection. Meningitis and sensory symptoms usually resolve within days to weeks; other features may take months to improve. In most cases it is not necessary to continue antibiotic therapy until complete recovery.

Late Manifestations

Arthritis, the dominant feature of late Lyme disease, occurs in up to 60 percent of untreated patients days to years after initial infection (mean of 6 months). The initial pattern of involvement may be migratory arthralgias early, followed in 60 percent of patients by intermittent attacks of arthritis lasting days to months. Large joints, particularly the knee, are most commonly involved. Swelling is often prominent, with large effusions and Baker's cysts. Serologic testing in patients presenting with arthritis is positive in almost all cases.

Lyme arthritis has been treated successfully with oral and intravenous antibiotics. In early studies examining response to intravenous benzathine penicillin 2.4 million units intramuscularly weekly for 3 weeks, 7 of 20 patients responded compared with none of 20 in the control group. Intravenous ceftriaxone 2 to 4 g daily for 2 to 4 weeks has been thought to be superior to benzathine penicillin. Oral regimens of doxycycline 100 mg twice a day for 4 weeks and amoxicillin plus probenecid 500 mg of each orally four times a day for 4 weeks have reported success in 18 of 20 patients and 16 of 18 patients, respectively. Response to antibiotics is typically excellent, but effusions may take months to resolve completely.

A small subgroup of Lyme arthritis patients develop a chronic, potentially erosive arthritis unresponsive to antibiotics. These patients often have major histocompatibility class II gene products, HLA DR4 accompanied by strong serum IgG responses to *Borrelia* outer surface proteins A or B (OspA or OspB). Repeated courses of antibiotics have not been shown to improve clinical outcome. Surgical synovectomy has cured a number of such patients.

Late Neurologic Lyme Disease

Chronic neurologic syndromes, which are relatively uncommon, may occur months to years after initial infection. Cognitive dysfunction, affective changes, seizures, ataxia, peripheral neuropathies, and chronic fatigue have all been reported. Because these complaints are often nonspecific and may be associated with post-Lyme syndromes, it is important to look for and document evidence of ongoing *B. burgdorferi* infection. Lymphocytic pleocytosis is uncommon in late neurologic disease, but increased intrathecal *B. burgdorferi*-specific antibodies may well be present. Careful evaluation with neuropsychological testing can help distinguish cognitive abnormalities in Lyme disease from those associated with chronic fatigue and depression. Chronic neurologic dysfunction usually improves with antibiotics but may not completely reverse. Late neurologic manifestations of Lyme disease are treated with intravenous antibiotics. Agents with demonstrated efficacy are aqueous penicillin and third-generation cephalosporins. Doxycycline, both oral and intravenous, has been reported successful in treating late CNS Lyme disease in Europe.

Ocular Disease

Ocular lesions in Lyme disease, which have involved every portion of the eye, vary with the stage of the disease. The most common ophthalmic presentations in early disease include conjunctivitis, photophobia, and neuro-ophthalmologic manifestations due to cranial nerve palsies. The most severe ocular manifestations occur in late stages; they include episcleritis, symblepharon, keratitis, iritis, choroiditis, panuveitis, and retinal vasculitis. Serologic testing in these patients is typically positive.

Experience treating late ocular lesions in Lyme disease is scanty. The most success has been with the use of ceftriaxone IV 2 to 4 g daily for 10 to 14 days.

Pregnancy

Intrauterine transmission of *B. burgdorferi* is uncommon, usually occurring in cases of obvious disseminated infection during pregnancy. No uniform pattern of congenital anomaly has been reported. Prenatal exposure to Lyme disease has not been found to be associated with an increased risk of adverse pregnancy outcome. Optimal treatment of the pregnant patient with Lyme disease is unknown, but the recommended regimens have not been associated with adverse outcomes. Oral antibiotic use for early localized disease is sufficient, and intravenous antibiotics are recommended for patients with symptoms suggesting disseminated disease.

Tick Bites

The risk of infection from a deer tick bite in a Lyme disease endemic area is low. Patients bitten by deer ticks, even those infected with *B. burgdorferi,* generally do not develop Lyme disease. In mice, infected ticks have been attached for more than 36 hours before significant risk of developing Lyme disease occurred. In a controlled double-blind study of patients with tick bites, no patient asymptomatically seroconverted, no treated patient developed EM, and the 2 of 182 untreated patients who did develop EM were successfully treated with oral antibiotics. These results support marking and watching a tick bite, and should EM develop, treating it early, when antibiotics are most effective.

Seropositive Patient with Nonspecific Symptoms

Patients with nonspecific symptoms such as myalgias, arthralgias, concentration difficulties, and fatigue are frequently tested for Lyme disease. Some patients, especially those from endemic areas, test positively and are treated for presumed Lyme disease, often without improvement in their symptoms. In several studies, over 50 percent of patients reporting to Lyme disease clinics did not have evidence of Lyme disease, and the reason for a lack of response to antibiotics was an incorrect diagnosis. Objective clinical evidence in support of the diagnosis of Lyme disease should be sought prior to initiating antibiotics; treatment should be given for the recommended duration and then discontinued; and the patient should be observed for resolution of symptoms.

■ COMMENTS

Antibiotic regimens, which are recommended according to results of clinical trials and evolving clinical judgments, depend on the stage of infection and the organ system involved. Successful eradication of the infecting organism, *B. burgdorferi,* occurs in most patients with Lyme disease using these treatment guidelines. Patients with persistent symptoms following antibiotic therapy, particularly those with previous evidence of disseminated disease, pose a difficult management problem. Most persistent symptoms are likely due to retained antigens and not the result of persistent infection or noninfectious sequelae such as fibromyalgia. In the former patients' resolution of symptoms occurs over the course of weeks to months and does not require prolonged courses of antibiotics; in the latter, treatment is for the associated syndrome. Rarely, persistent or recurrent symptoms are due to continued or recurrent infection and require additional courses of antibiotics. Such patients require careful diagnostic evaluation to determine the need for additional treatment.

Suggested Reading

Bockenstedt LK, Malawista SE. Lyme disease. In: Rich RR, Fleischer TA, Schwartz BD, et al., eds. Clinical immunology: principles and practice. St. Louis: Mosby–Year Book, 1995.

Halperin J, Volkman D, We P. Central nervous system abnormalities in Lyme neuroborreliosis. Neurology 1991; 41:1571–1582.

Logigian EL, Kaplan RF, Steere AC. Chronic neurologic manifestations of Lyme disease. N Engl J Med. 1990; 323:1438–1444.

Rahn DW, Malawista SE. Clinical judgment in Lyme disease. Hosp Prac 1990; 25:39–56.

Steere AC, Levin RE, Molloy PJ, et al. Treatment of Lyme arthritis. Arthritis Rheum 1994; 6:878–888.

TICK-BORNE DISEASE

J. Thomas Cross Jr., M.D., M.P.H.
Richard F. Jacobs, M.D., F.A.A.P.

Exposure to ticks is an important part of the history of a patient with signs and symptoms of systemic infection. Important factors include tick activity in the area, season of the year, geographic distribution of ticks known to carry specific pathogens, site of exposure, and signs and symptoms at presentation in relationship to the time of exposure. Tests for the diagnosis of tick-borne infections are frequently inadequate. Therefore, the physician must understand the epidemiology and symptoms of tick-borne infections to make a quick and accurate diagnosis. A high index of suspicion is required for the diagnosis of many tick-borne infections. Physicians must consider them during periods of high tick activity; however, cases occasionally are seen during winter. It is helpful to use epidemiologic data from local state health departments and publications such as the *Morbidity and Mortality Weekly Report* to evaluate the risk of tick-related infections.

An embedded tick found 3 days to 2 weeks before symptoms appear should alert the physician to the possibility of tick-related infections. The difficulty with determining the specific infection lies in the fact that most are initially non-

Table 1 Tick-Related Infections in the United States

DISEASE	ORGANISM	VECTOR	RESERVOIR	GEOGRAPHIC DISTRIBUTION	TYPE OF ILLNESS
Babesiosis	*Babesia microti*	*Ixodes scapularis*	*Peromyscus luecopus* (white-footed mouse)	Islands of Massachusetts, Rhode Island, New York	Malaria-like; fever, anemia, renal failure
Lyme disease	*Borrelia burgdorferi*	*Ixodes scapularis* *Ixodes pacificus*	Rodents, deer	Northeastern, midwestern, and western U.S.	Fever, erythema migrans, headache, myalgias; multiple stages
Tularemia	*Francisella tularensis*	*Ambylomma americanum, Dermacentor andersoni, D. variabilis*	Rabbits, dogs, rodents	Southern, southeastern, midwestern U.S.	Fever, lymphadenopathy, pneumonia
Rocky Mountain spotted fever (RMSF)	*Rickettsia rickettsii*	*Dermacentor variabilis, D. andersoni*	Dogs, cats, rodents	Southeastern U.S., western hemisphere	Fever, headache, rash, toxic appearance
Ehrlichiosis	*Ehrlichia chaffeensis*	*D. variabilis, A. americanum*	Dogs	South-central and south Atlantic U.S.	Fever, chills, hematologic abnormalities
	Human Granulocytic Ehrlichiosis	*D. variabilis* *A. americanum* *I. scapularis*	Unknown	Northeastern, midwestern U.S.	Fever, chills, hematologic abnormalities
Relapsing fever	*Borrelia hermsii, B. turicatae, B. parkeri*	*Ornithodoros hermsii, O. turicata, O. parkeri*	Rodents	Grand Canyon, western mountains U.S.	Fever, chills, relapsing course
Q fever	*Coxiella burnetii*	Inhalation of infected aerosols	Cattle, sheep, cats, ticks	Nova Scotia, Europe, Australia	Fever, headache, pneumonia
Colorado tick fever	Coltivirus	*Dermacentor andersoni*	Squirrels, rabbits, deer	Rocky Mountain states	Fever, headache, leukopenia
Tick paralysis	Neurotoxin	*Dermacentor andersoni, D. variabilis, A. americanum, A. maculatum, I. scapularis*		Pacific Northwest, Rocky Mountain states	Ascending flaccid paralysis, ataxia

specific in presentation (Table 1). The nonspecific signs and symptoms of most tick-borne diseases include fever, malaise, and flulike symptoms. However, it is useful to consider specific categories of symptoms. For example, Lyme disease has the characteristic rash of erythema migrans, arthritis, and neurologic abnormalities with systemic manifestations. Rocky Mountain spotted fever (RMSF) may be manifested as a classic complex of headache, photophobia, petechial rash on the wrists and ankles, thrombocytopenia, and hyponatremia. The differential diagnosis of RMSF can be quite varied: ehrlichiosis, brucellosis, salmonellosis, Epstein-Barr virus, cytomegalovirus, enterovirus, and many others. It is frequently helpful to categorize tick-borne infections according to the patient's history and presenting signs and symptoms (Table 2).

■ FEVER, HEADACHE, MYALGIAS (FLULIKE ILLNESS)

Infections associated with the triad of fever, headache, and myalgias, or more succinctly, flulike illnesses, include RMSF, other spotted fever rickettsiae, ehrlichiosis, tularemia, relapsing fever, Q fever, and Colorado tick fever. Usually travel history or residence in an endemic area will suggest the diagnosis. If the fever is persistent with a biphasic or recurring pattern, Colorado tick fever or relapsing fever should be strongly considered. If pneumonia occurs with the triad of symptoms, tularemia, RMSF, and Q fever should be considered.

■ FEVER, RASH, MULTISYSTEM INVOLVEMENT

Tick-borne infections frequently have nonspecific rashes that are not helpful in delineating the final diagnosis. However, typical rashes do occur with certain of these infections. RMSF can present 2 or 3 days after the tick bite as blanching erythematous macules on the wrists and ankles. The rash progresses rapidly to a maculopapular or petechial rash concentrated on the distal extremities, usually the palms and soles. The rash is frequently confused with meningococcemia, especially when it progresses to a confluent hemorrhagic infiltration with thrombotic disease similar to purpura fulminans. Lyme disease is classically diagnosed by its rash, erythema migrans. It occurs in about 50 percent of patients and is diagnostic for the disease; serology is not indicated, as frequently with early treatment the serology will be negative. The classic lesion is an erythematous macule that expands over several days to weeks with a warm, raised, pruritic but usually painless character. In some patients the lesion has a

Table 2 Presenting Signs and Symptoms in Tick-Borne Illnesses

Fever, Headache, Myalgias (Flulike Illness)
Rocky Mountain spotted fever (RMSF)
Ehrlichiosis
Tularemia
Relapsing fever
Q fever
Colorado tick fever
Fever, Rash, Multisystem Involvement
RMSF
Lyme disease
Ehrlichiosis
Fever, Adenopathy
Tularemia
Lyme disease
RMSF
Ehrlichiosis
Fever, Hematologic Abnormalities
Babesiosis
Colorado tick fever
RMSF
Ehrlichiosis
Fever, Neurologic Manifestations
RMSF
Colorado tick fever
Tick paralysis
Lyme disease

central clearing. Patients will frequently develop multiple secondary lesions. Ehrlichiosis can cause a rash similar to that of RMSF, but generally it is spotless.

FEVER, ADENOPATHY

Tularemia is the classic tick-borne disease associated with fever and adenopathy. The site of involvement is usually the neck in children and the groin in adults. This is thought to be related to the site of tick attachment. An ulcerative lesion at the tick-bite site with regional lymphadenopathy is characteristic of the ulceroglandular form of tularemia, the most common form of the disease. Lymphadenopathy has also been described with RMSF, Lyme disease, and ehrlichiosis.

FEVER, HEMATOLOGIC ABNORMALITIES

The hematologic manifestations of the tick-borne diseases are the most interesting and yet poorly understood presentations. Babesiosis causes hemolytic anemia similar to that of malaria. The diagnosis in endemic areas is made on the organisms using thick and thin blood smears. Leukopenia is described in Colorado tick fever and RMSF. Thrombocytopenia is associated with RMSF and its classic early rash. Ehrlichiosis due to *Ehrlichia chaffeensis* classically results in pancytopenia without a characteristic rash. It also can be diagnosed by observing the organisms (morulae) in peripheral blood smears or in bone marrow preparations.

FEVER, NEUROLOGIC MANIFESTATIONS

Neurologic manifestations in a febrile child with a history of exposure to ticks indicate RMSF, Colorado tick fever, tick-borne encephalitis, or tick paralysis. Lyme disease in its later stages has a high incidence of neurologic deficits including aseptic meningitis, cranial neuritis, motor and sensory radiculitis, peripheral neuropathies, and myelitis. However, Bell's palsy can occur early in the illness and be the only manifestation of the disease.

EMPIRIC THERAPY

The diagnosis of tick-borne infections is usually based on presumptive clinical findings at the time of diagnosis. Most specific tests are insensitive to early disease or require the physician to send tests out to a reference lab. Therefore, empiric therapy is usually undertaken before a specific serologic confirmation is obtained. In these cases acute serum should be sent for specific diagnostic testing and some saved for later studies if the initial findings are negative. Acute titers that are presumptively positive should be confirmed with convalescent titers. Empiric antibiotics are based upon the most likely diagnosis for the endemic area, the season, and the clinical manifestations of the illness. Tetracyclines are a logical choice in most tick-borne infections.

Beta-lactam antibiotics are effective for Lyme disease but are ineffective for most other tick-borne infections. For specific treatment and more detail about individual illnesses, see the specific chapters.

Suggested Reading

Cross JT, Jacobs RF. Tularemia: Treatment failures with outpatient use of ceftriaxone. Clin Infect Dis 1993; 17:976–980.

Fishbein DB, Dawson JE, Robinson LE. Human ehrlichiosis in the United States, 1985 to 1990. Ann Intern Med 1994; 120:736–743.

Goodpasture HC, Poland JD, Francy DB, et al. Colorado tick fever: Clinical, epidemiologic, and laboratory aspects of 228 cases in Colorado in 1973–1974. Ann Intern Med 1978; 88:303–310.

Horton JM, Blaser MJ. The spectrum of relapsing fever in the Rocky Mountains. Arch Intern Med 1985; 145:871–875.

Lyme disease—United States, 1991–92. MMWR 1993; 42:345–348.

Spach DH, Liles WC, Campbell GL, et al. Tick-borne diseases in the United States. N Engl J Med 1993; 329:936–947.

Weber DJ, Walker DH. Rocky Mountain spotted fever. Infect Dis Clin North Am 1991; 5:19–35.

MYCOPLASMA

Ken B. Waites, M.D.
Gail H. Cassell, Ph.D.

Mycoplasmas, the smallest free living organisms, are unique among procaryotes in that they lack a cell wall, a feature responsible for their biologic properties and lack of susceptibility to many commonly prescribed antimicrobial agents. Although there have been at least 14 species of mycoplasmas isolated from humans, 3 are responsible for most clinically significant infections. Therefore, this discussion is limited to *Mycoplasma pneumoniae, Mycoplasma hominis,* and *Ureaplasma urealyticum.*

■ *MYCOPLASMA PNEUMONIAE* RESPIRATORY DISEASE

M. pneumoniae occurs endemically and occasionally epidemically in persons of all age groups but is most common in school-aged children, adolescents, and young adults. It is perhaps best known as the primary cause of walking, or atypical, pneumonia, but in fact the most frequent clinical syndrome is tracheobronchitis, often accompanied by upper respiratory tract symptoms. Typical complaints include hoarseness, fever, cough that is initially nonproductive but later may yield small to moderate amounts of nonbloody sputum, sore throat, headache, chills, coryza, and general malaise. The throat may be erythematous, but cervical adenopathy is uncommon. Myringitis sometimes occurs. Bronchopneumonia involving one or more lobes develops in 3 to 10 percent of infected persons, accounting for a third to over half of cases of community-acquired pneumonias. Moist rales and rhonchi can be detected by chest auscultation. Abnormalities on chest radiographs often appear more severe than the clinical condition of the patient would predict. True lobar consolidation is uncommon, but pleural effusion develops in about 25 percent of cases. The incubation period is generally 2 to 3 weeks, and spread throughout households is common. Hospitalization is necessary in about 10 percent of children and adults, but recovery is almost always complete and without sequelae. Some people have extrapulmonary complications after onset of or even in the absence of respiratory illness. Such complications most commonly include skin rashes, pericarditis, hemolytic anemia, arthritis, meningoencephalitis, peripheral neuropathy, and pericarditis. Acute mycoplasmal infection may also be associated with exacerbations of chronic bronchitis and asthma.

M. pneumoniae has been isolated from extrapulmonary sites such as synovial fluid and cerebrospinal fluid (CSF), pericardial fluid, and skin lesions. The frequency of direct invasion of these sites is unknown because the organism is rarely sought. The hemogram is usually normal, and the cellular response of the sputum is mononuclear, with no bacteria visible by Gram stain. In about 50 percent of patients a cold agglutinin titer of at least 1:32 may develop by the second week of illness, but usually disappears by 6 to 8 weeks. This is not a specific test for *M. pneumoniae,* since other micro-organisms may induce similar reactions. Several viruses, *Chlamydia pneumoniae, Streptococcus pneumoniae, Haemophilus influenzae, Moraxella catarrhalis, Legionella* spp., and even some mycobacteria and fungi can produce infections that are clinically indistinguishable and may accompany mycoplasmal infection.

Because of widespread lack of readily available diagnostic services, length of time until a positive result can be obtained, impracticality of obtaining proper diagnostic specimens in some types of respiratory infections, and similarity of clinical syndromes due to several other micro-organisms that may be equally difficult to identify, clinicians often do not attempt to obtain a precise microbiologic diagnosis in mild to moderately ill outpatients. Instead they elect to treat empirically. If mycoplasmal respiratory infection is to be confirmed, culture and/or serologic tests are necessary. Clinical laboratories may offer culture service through a reference laboratory familiar with the complex cultivation requirements of mycoplasmas. Respiratory tract specimens suitable for culture include throat swabs, sputum, tracheal aspirates, bronchial lavage fluid, pleural fluid, and lung biopsy tissue, according to the patient's clinical condition. Care should be taken in collecting specimens, inoculating into a suitable transport medium such as SP4 broth—at bedside whenever possible—and not allowing desiccation. Freezing at −70°C (−94°F) is advised if specimens cannot be transported to the diagnostic laboratory immediately after collection. Growth in culture is slow, requiring at least 3 weeks in some cases.

Serology is most frequently used to confirm *M. pneumoniae* infection. Enzyme-linked immunosorbent assays are now preferred to the older complement fixation assays. Since primary infection does not guarantee protective immunity against future infections and residual antibody may remain from earlier encounters with the organism, there has been a great impetus to develop sensitive and specific tests to differentiate between acute and remote infection. Definitive diagnosis requires seroconversion documented by paired specimens obtained 2 to 4 weeks apart. Although single-titer immunoglobulin (Ig) M or IgA assays purported to detect current infection have recently become available, it is not clear how long IgM persists after acute infection, and as many as 50 percent of adults may not mount a detectable IgM response. Therefore, reliance on a single serologic test may be clinically misleading, and paired assays for both IgM and IgG are recommended. There are no commercially available rapid diagnostic methods for detecting *M. pneumoniae* in clinical specimens, but preliminary data suggest that molecular techniques such as polymerase chain reaction may eventually be the optimum method for detecting mycoplasmal infection.

Therapy

It was once believed that mycoplasmal respiratory infections were entirely self-limited and no antimicrobial treatment was indicated. More recently it has been shown that appropriate antimicrobial therapy shortens the symptomatic period and hastens radiologic resolution of pneumonia and recovery, even though organisms may be shed for several weeks. In general, the clinical efficacy of antimicrobial therapy is most apparent in severe pneumonia and with prompt initiation of treatment.

Unlike the genital mycoplasmas, *M. pneumoniae* has remained predictably susceptible to macrolides, lincosamides, and tetracyclines, so that in vitro susceptibility testing to guide therapy is not indicated. Oral erythromycin has long been the drug of choice for mycoplasmal respiratory infections. Tetracycline and its analogues are also effective in vivo and in vitro but should not be given to children because of the potential for bone and tooth toxicity. Clindamycin is effective in vitro, but limited reports suggest that it may be less active in vivo and should not be considered a first-line treatment. The beta-lactams, sulfonamides, and trimethoprim do not work in vitro or in vivo against *M. pneumoniae.* The fluoroquinolones exhibit some antimycoplasmal activity but are usually much less active in vitro than the macrolides and tetracyclines.

The new macrolide clarithromycin and the azalide azithromycin are broad-spectrum drugs used primarily for treatment of community-acquired upper and lower respiratory infections. Both are effective in vitro against *M. pneumoniae* at concentrations equivalent to or lower than those of erythromycin. They have the advantage of better tolerability, fewer gastrointestinal side effects, and longer half-life, allowing less frequent dosage. Clarithromycin has proven in vitro as well as clinical efficacy against *M. pneumoniae.* Outcomes of preliminary clinical trials with both agents are encouraging, but a drawback is their cost, which can be several times that of erythromycin treatment. As with erythromycin, administration of clarithromycin may cause an increase in serum theophylline concentrations. Neither clarithromycin nor azithromycin should be used by pregnant women if there is any other available treatment.

Mycoplasmas are slow-growing organisms, so it would be logical to expect infections to respond better to longer treatment courses than are used for other types of infections. Although most regimens are prescribed for 7 to 14 days, a 14 to 21 day course of oral therapy with most agents is also appropriate. Azithromycin given once daily for 5 days has been shown to be effective for community-acquired pneumonia because it has a long half-life. However, comparative clinical trials evaluating outcomes of patients with proven *M. pneumoniae* infections have not yet been completed, and unlike clarithromycin, azithromycin does not yet have an approved indication for treatment of *M. pneumoniae* infections.

Other measures such as cough suppressants, antipyretics, and analgesics should be given as needed to relieve the headaches and other systemic symptoms of *M. pneumoniae* infections. Corticosteroids may help some patients with severe pneumonia, erythema multiforme, or hemolytic anemia. Since most extrapulmonary manifestations are diagnosed late in the course of disease, the benefit of early treatment is unknown.

Fortunately, the treatments of choice for *M. pneumoniae* are appropriate for many of the other microbial agents responsible for upper respiratory infections and atypical pneumonia. This is especially important in view of the fact that the identity of the infectious organism of most ambulatory patients seeking medical care is never determined. The new-generation macrolide and azalide agents are superior to erythromycin against *H. influenzae* and are usually but not always active in vitro against penicillin-resistant *Str. pneumoniae.* Standard and alternative drugs and their recommended dosages for use in mycoplasmal respiratory, genitourinary, and other systemic infections are listed in Table 1.

MYCOPLASMA HOMINIS AND *UREAPLASMA UREALYTICUM* INFECTIONS

U. urealyticum and *M. hominis* can be isolated from the lower genital tract of most sexually active women; they are somewhat less frequent in men. The presence of genital mycoplasmas in asymptomatic persons has made it difficult to prove their pathogenic potential, but in recent years conditions such as urethritis have been proven unequivocally to be caused by *U. urealyticum* in some instances. Only a subgroup of otherwise healthy adult men and women who are colonized develop one or more of the genitourinary diseases described in Table 2, but the risk factors are poorly understood. Colonized women may transmit genital mycoplasmas to their offspring either in utero or at delivery. Superficial mucosal colonization in the newborn tends to be transient and without sequelae, but neonates, especially those born preterm, are susceptible to a variety of systemic conditions due to either *M. hominis* or *U. urealyticum* (see Table 2). The most significant neonatal conditions caused by these organisms are pneumonia and meningitis.

Both *M. hominis* and *U. urealyticum* grow more rapidly than *M. pneumoniae* and can therefore be detected in cultures of appropriate specimens within 2 to 5 days. Proper handling and bedside inoculation of 10B or SP4 transport broth as described for *M. pneumoniae* are recommended to enhance recovery of these organisms. Urethral or wound swabs, cervicovaginal or prostatic secretions, and urine and respiratory specimens such as those described for *M. pneumoniae,* CSF, blood, other body fluids, and tissues are appropriate for culture, depending on the clinical setting. Cultures are available mainly through reference laboratories. At present there are no commercial serologic assays or rapid detection tests for routine diagnostic studies.

Genitourinary or extragenital diseases known to be due to or associated with mycoplasmas warrant appropriate diagnostic tests when available and treatment if infection is confirmed, particularly if the organisms are recovered in the absence of other pathogens. For the same reasons as for *M. pneumoniae* infections, practitioners must often rely on familiarity with clinical syndromes typically due to genital mycoplasmas and treat empirically. Many of the conditions associated with genital mycoplasmas can be due to a variety of microbial agents, and some conditions, such as pelvic inflammatory disease, can be polymicrobial. Therefore, the selection of drugs must take into account several possible causes.

Therapy

Oral tetracyclines given for at least 7 days have historically been the drugs of choice for use against urogenital infections due to *M. hominis,* but resistance now occurs in 20 to 40 percent of *M. hominis* isolates and in 10 to 15 percent of

Table 1 Treatment of Infections Caused by *Mycoplasma pneumoniae, Mycoplasma hominis,* and *Ureaplasma urealyticum*

DRUG	ROUTE	DOSAGE: CHILDREN	DOSAGE: ADULTS	COMMENTS
STANDARD TREATMENT				
Doxycycline	PO	4 mg/kg loading dose day 1, then 2–4 mg/kg/day in 1–2 doses	200 mg loading dose day 1, then 100 mg q12h	Contraindicated in children under 8 years of age unless no other alternative; if giving IV, infuse over 60 min to prevent thrombophlebitis
	IV	Same as PO	Same as PO	
Tetracycline	PO	25–50 mg/kg/day in 4 doses	250–500 mg q6h	Same as for doxycycline
	IV	10–20 mg/kg/day in 2–4 doses	125–500 mg q6–12h	
Erythromycin	PO	20–50 mg/kg/day in 3–4 doses	250–500 mg q6h	Not for *M. hominis;* infuse over 60 min to prevent thrombophlebitis and minimize risk of cardiac toxicity; may cause elevation in serum theophylline levels
	IV	25–40 mg/kg/day in 4 doses	250–500 mg q6h	
Clindamycin	PO	10–25 mg/kg/day in 3–4 doses	150–450 mg q6h	Not for *U. urealyticum* or *M. pneumoniae*
	IV	10–40 mg/kg/day in 3–4 doses For neonates do not exceed 15–20 mg/kg/day in 3–4 doses	150-900 mg q6–8h	
ALTERNATIVE TREATMENTS				
Chloramphenicol	PO	Not recommended	Not recommended	Frequent monitoring of hematologic parameters and blood levels of the antibiotic necessary
	IV	50–100 mg/kg/day in 4 doses For neonates aged up to 2 weeks use 25 mg/kg/day in 1 dose, thereafter 50 mg/kg/day in 1 dose	25 mg/kg q6h	
Azithromycin	PO	Not recommended	1 g single dose for urogenital infection; 500 mg day 1, then 250 mg daily × 4 days for respiratory infections	Not for *M. hominis*
	IV	Not available	Not available	
Clarithromycin	PO	15 mg/kg/day in 2 doses	250–500 mg q12h	Not for *M. hominis;* may cause elevation of serum theophylline levels; not approved for use in sexually transmitted diseases
	IV	Not available	Not available	
Ofloxacin	PO	Not recommended	200–400 mg q12h	Use for *U. urealyticum* or *M. hominis;* not approved for persons under 18 years of age
	IV	Not recommended	200–400 mg q12h	
Levofloxacin	PO	Not recommended	500 mg q24h	Use for *M. pneumoniae*
	IV	Not recommended	500 mg q24h	

U. urealyticum, indicating that the susceptibility of these organisms can no longer be assumed. The degree of resistance may vary with geographic area, but alternative agents must be considered for treatment failures if tetracyclines are used as first-line drugs. Erythromycin or tetracyclines are the drugs of choice for *U. urealyticum* infections. High-level erythromycin resistance, though uncommon, has been described. Thus, it is reasonable to request in vitro susceptibility testing from reference laboratories for isolates of *M. hominis* or *U. urealyticum.* This is most important for organisms recovered from a normally sterile body site, from immunocompromised hosts, and from persons who have not responded to initial treatment. Susceptibility testing can be accomplished in 3 to 5 days once the organism is isolated.

Clindamycin is an alternative treatment for tetracycline-resistant *M. hominis.* Susceptibility of genital mycoplasmas to fluoroquinolones is not affected by tetracycline resistance mediated by the tet-M transposon. Ciprofloxacin is generally less active in vitro against both species than ofloxacin. A 7 day course of oral ofloxacin appears adequate for urethritis, but studies have focused on *Chlamydia trachomatis* rather than *U. urealyticum.* Clinical trials of women with mild uncomplicated pelvic inflammatory disease have shown that monotherapy with oral ofloxacin is effective, though the Food and Drug Administration has not yet approved it for use in this condition. A single dose of azithromycin is approved for treatment of urethritis due to *C. trachomatis* and has been shown to work as well clinically as doxycycline in persons with infection due to *U. urealyticum,* which reflects its in vitro activity against this organism. Clarithromycin, though active

Table 2 Association of *Mycoplasma hominis* and *Ureaplasma urealyticum* with Specific Pathologic Conditions

DISEASE	*M. HOMINIS*	*U. UREALYTICUM*
MEN		
Urethritis	–	+
Prostatitis	+/–	+/–
Epididymitis	–	+/–
WOMEN		
Acute urethral syndrome	–	+/–
Pelvic inflammatory disease	+	+/–
Bacterial vaginosis	+	+/–
Chorioamnionitis	+/–	+
Spontaneous abortions, stillbirth	+/–	+/–
Postpartum, postabortal fever	+	+/–
MEN AND WOMEN		
Pyelonephritis	+	+/–
Cystitis	–	+/–
Urinary calculi	–	+
Extragenital diseases*		
Septic arthritis	+	+
Osteomyelitis	+	+
Bacteremia	+	+
Soft-tissue abscesses	+	+
Wound infections	+	–
Peritonitis	+	–
Meningitis, brain abscess	+	–
Pneumonia	+	+
Pericarditis, endocarditis	+	+
NEONATES		
Prematurity	–	+
Congenital, neonatal pneumonia	+	+
Chronic lung disease of prematurity	–	+/–
Bacteremia	+	+
Soft-tissue abscesses	+	+
Meningitis	+	+

–, No association or causal role demonstrated; +, causal role; +/–, association, but causal role not proven.

*Invasive extragenital diseases due to either *M. hominis* or *U. urealyticum* are almost always associated with genitourinary manipulation or trauma, hypogammaglobulinemia, or other immunocompromised state when they occur beyond the neonatal period. The true incidence of such infections in susceptible persons is unknown, since mycoplasmas are infrequently sought.

against *U. urealyticum* in vitro at concentrations at or lower than erythromycin, has not been recommended for use in treatment of urogenital infections. *M. hominis* is resistant to erythromycin, azithromycin, and clarithromycin. For venereally transmissible infections such as urethritis, all sexual contacts of the index case should also be treated.

Experience with mycoplasmal or ureaplasmal infections in immunocompromised patients, especially those with hypogammaglobulinemia, demonstrates that even though mycoplasmas are primarily noninvasive mucosal pathogens in the normal host, they can produce destructive and progressive disease. Infections caused by resistant organisms refractory to antimicrobial therapy may require administration of a combination of intravenous antimicrobials, intravenous immunoglobulin, and/or antisera prepared specifically against the infecting species. Even with aggressive therapy, relapses are likely. Repeat cultures of affected sites may be necessary to gauge in vivo response to treatment.

Isolation of *M. hominis* or *U. urealyticum* from CSF in neonates with pleocytosis, progressive hydrocephalus, other neurologic abnormality, pericardial fluid, pleural fluid, tracheal aspirate in association with respiratory disease, abscess material, or blood is justification for specific treatment in critically ill neonates with no other verifiable pathogens. Whether to treat for a positive CSF culture when no evidence of clinical illness is observed should be decided case by case. It may be pertinent to monitor the patient, repeat lumbar puncture, and re-examine for inflammation and organisms before initiating treatment, since some cases spontaneously resolve.

Parenteral tetracyclines have been used most often to treat meningitis due to either *M. hominis* or *U. urealyticum* despite contraindications. Alternatives are erythromycin for *U. urealyticum*, clindamycin for *M. hominis*, and chloramphenicol for either species. No single drug has always eradicated these organisms from CSF of neonates. No reports have demonstrated efficacy of aminoglycosides against genital mycoplasmas. There has been no experience with quinolones or the new generation macrolides in treatment of neonatal infections, and at present none are recommended for general use in this population.

Suggested Reading

Cassell GH, Drnec J, Waites KB, et al. Efficacy of clarithromycin against *Mycoplasma pneumoniae.* J Antimicrob Chemother 1991; 27 (Suppl A):47–59.

Furr PM, Taylor-Robinson, Webster ADB. Mycoplasmas and ureaplasmas in patients with hypogammaglobulinemia and their role in arthritis: Microbiological observations over twenty years. Ann Rheum 1994; 53:183–187.

CAMPYLOBACTER

David W.K. Acheson, M.D.
Andrew G. Plaut, M.D.

Campylobacter (Greek *campylo,* curved; *bacter,* rod) are motile, non-spore-forming gram-negative rods. They are a common cause of gastrointestinal and systemic human infection in many parts of the world. *Campylobacter* was first isolated from blood in 1947 but not identified in stool until 1972, principally due to difficulty in culturing the organisms. There are many members of the genus *Campylobacter;* the major enteric pathogen for humans is *C. jejuni,* although *C. coli, C. fetus,* and *C. iaridis* are also human pathogens. *C. jejuni* is associated with gastrointestinal disease, and *C. fetus* usually causes systemic infection, often in debilitated patients.

Campylobacter is microaerophilic, and although all will grow at 37°C (98.6°F), *C. jejuni* grows best at 42°C (107.6°F). A number of selective media are in use, including Skirrows, Butzler's, and Campy-BAP. Although several serotypes of *C. jejuni* have been reported, there are few data regarding the relative virulence of these different types.

EPIDEMIOLOGY

Campylobacter is one of the main causes of bacterial diarrheal disease in the United States and Europe. It is especially common in children under a year of age and in young adults, and it occurs most frequently in the summer. *Campylobacter* spp. are found in fowl and many wild and domestic animals, and most human infections probably result from contamination of milk and other animal food sources. The organisms can also be transmitted by direct contact with infected animals and contaminated water. Small numbers of organisms may cause disease; as few as 800 have been shown to cause infection in volunteer studies, but the infecting dose is usually about 10^4. Although asymptomatic carriage of *Campylobacter* is uncommon in developed countries, in less developed nations carriage rates as high as 37 percent have been reported among children.

CLINICAL FEATURES

The incubation period for *C. jejuni* infection varies between 1 and 7 days, with most cases occurring 2 to 4 days after exposure. *C. jejuni* illness typically presents with a prodrome of fever, headache, myalgia, and malaise for up to 24 hours before intestinal symptoms develop. The fever may be as high as 40°C (104°F), and the diarrhea varies from a few loose stools to copious watery discharge. Blood is frequently present in the stool but varies in amount. The illness usually lasts less than a week, but patients untreated with antibiotics frequently continue to excrete the organisms for several weeks. Bacteremia is rare in *C. jejuni* infections, although focal infections such as endocarditis, meningitis, septic abortion, acute cholecystitis, pancreatitis, and cystitis have all been documented. Postinfectious reactive arthritis may also occur, especially in HLA B27-positive individuals.

In contrast to *C. jejuni, C. fetus* frequently produces systemic disease, often in vascular sites: endocarditis, pericarditis, and mycotic aneurysms of the abdominal aorta. Central nervous system infections such as meningoencephalitis also occur with *C. fetus,* as do other localized infections including septic arthritis, spontaneous bacterial peritonitis, salpingitis, lung abscess, empyema, cellulitis, urinary tract infection, vertebral osteomyelitis, and cholecystitis. In patients with the acquired immunodeficiency syndrome *Campylobacter* spp. other than *C. fetus* and *C. jejuni* may also cause bacteremia.

DIAGNOSIS

Campylobacter have a characteristic darting motility, and a presumptive diagnosis of *Campylobacter* infection may be made by examination of stool passed within 2 hours using direct dark-field or phase-contrast microscopy. Leukocytes and red cells are also frequently seen in stool samples, with 75 percent of patients having polymorphonuclear leukocytes in their stool. Confirmation of the diagnosis of *C. jejuni* infection is based on a positive stool or blood culture. DNA probes, polymerase chain reaction, and serologic testing have all been used to confirm diagnosis but are not routinely available. *C. fetus* may be isolated from blood held in culture up to 14 days. The fastidious nature of the organisms means that failure to culture *Campylobacter* does not rule them out as the cause of significant clinical disease.

THERAPY

As with many diarrheal diseases, fluid replacement is the most important therapy in *Campylobacter* diarrhea. Oral rehydration is usually adequate, but patients with severe dehydration should be given volume replacement with intravenous solutions of electrolytes and water.

The vast majority of *Campylobacter* infections are mild and self-limited and do not result in a visit to a physician. These mild infections require no specific treatment. Antibiotics are recommended only for patients with severe infection, including those with significant fever or volume loss, frequent bloody diarrhea, prolonged or severe symptoms, and for persons who are immunocompromised. Antibiotic therapy can have a dramatic positive effect on symptoms of *C. jejuni* infection, justifying a trial of therapy in severe or persistent illness. Another possible reason for using antibiotic therapy is to prevent infected children from spreading the infection in day care settings. *C. jejuni* is susceptible to a wide variety of antimicrobial agents in vitro, including erythromycin, tetracyclines, aminoglycosides, chloramphenicol, quinolones, nitrofurans, and clindamycin. (Table 1). Erythromycin has consistently been the drug most widely used in the treatment of *C. jejuni,* as it is inexpensive, safe, and time tested. Erythromycin treatment will terminate gastrointestinal shedding of

Table 1 Recommended Antimicrobial Agents for *C. jejuni*

	DRUG	DOSAGE AND DURATION	
Preferred	Erythromycin	Adults	250–500 mg PO q.i.d. × 7 days
		Children	30–50 mg/kg/day q.i.d. × 7 days
Alternative	Ciprofloxacin	Adults	500 mg PO b.i.d. × 7 days
Other agents	Doxycycline		
	Furazolidone		
	Ampicillin		
	Trimethoprim-sulfamethoxazole		

Campylobacter within 24 to 72 hours, which should be kept in mind when treating infections in day care or preschool settings to avoid spread of the disease.

More recently, as the quinolones became available, they have been used in the treatment of *Campylobacter.* Although ciprofloxacin and other fluoroquinolones are generally effective for *C. jejuni* infection, they are expensive and not recommended for children. There has also been a documented rise in the incidence of resistance to quinolones in Europe since 1992, with up to 57 percent of *C. jejuni* and 43 percent of *C. coli* isolates being resistant (determined by disk diffusion using nalidixic acid and ciprofloxacin). Extraintestinal infection with *C. jejuni* needs at least 10 days of treatment, and systemic infection with *C. fetus* warrants 2 to 3 weeks of therapy.

■ PROGNOSIS AND PREVENTION

The vast majority of patients recover totally following infection with *C. jejuni.* A few patients develop reactive arthritis, and an association between *Campylobacter* and Guillain-Barré syndrome has been reported. Systemic *C. fetus* infections have a significant mortality, especially in patients with underlying disease such as diabetes mellitus, cirrhosis, or immunocompromise. Transmission of *Campylobacter* infection can be reduced by careful food handling with special attention to poultry products. Proper cooking of food, pasteurization of milk, and protection of water supplies are all critical in preventing infection with *Campylobacter.*

See the chapter *Helicobacter pylori* for a discussion of that organism, once called *Campylobacter pylori.*

Suggested Reading

Blaser MJ. Campylobacter. In: Farthing MJG, Keusch GT, eds. Enteric infection. London: Chapman and Hall, 1989:298.

Blaser MJ, Berkowitz ID, LaForce FM, et al. *Campylobacter* enteritis: Clinical and epidemiological features. Ann Intern Med 1979; 91: 179–185.

Giesendorf BAJ, van Belkum A, Koeken A, et al. Development of species-specific DNA probes for *Campylobacter jejuni, Campylobacter coli,* and *Campylobacter lari* by polymerase chain reaction fingerprinting. J Clin Microbiol 1993; 31:1541–1546.

Guerrant RL, Lahita RG, Roberts RB. Campylobacteriosis in man: Pathogenic mechanisms and review of 91 bloodstream infections. Am J Med 1978; 65:584–592.

Skirrow MB. *Campylobacter* enteritis: a "new" disease. BMJ 1977; 2:9–11.

Skirrow MB, Blaser MJ. *Campylobacter jejuni.* In: Blaser MJ, Smith PD, Raudin JI, Greenberg HB, Guerrant RL, eds. Infections of the gastrointestinal tract. New York: Raven 1995:825–848.

TRAVELER'S DIARRHEA

Luis M. Valdez, M.D.
Herbert L. DuPont, M.D.

Traveler's diarrhea is a syndrome characterized by a twofold or greater increase in the frequency of unformed bowel movements in a person who normally resides in an industrialized region and who is visiting a developing, tropical or semitropical country. It is associated with one or more signs and symptoms of enteric infection: nausea, vomiting, abdominal pain or cramps, fecal urgency, and tenesmus, or the passage of bloody or mucoid stools. It may include illness during the first 7 to 10 days after returning home. Diarrhea is by far the most frequent health problem of travelers to these high-risk areas, affecting 20 to 50 percent of persons. The diarrhea can be severe enough to interfere with planned activities in up to 20 percent of the affected people. Latin America, Africa, and southern Asia are considered the high-risk areas. Attack rates are variable, but they average approximately 40 percent for travel from an industrialized region to one of the high-risk areas.

■ CAUSES

Bacterial enteropathogens cause most cases of traveler's diarrhea regardless of specific area of risk. Enterotoxigenic *Escherichia coli* (ETEC) is the single most common bacterial pathogen isolated, followed by *Shigella* spp., *Campylobacter jejuni, Aeromonas* spp., *Plesiomonas shigelloides, Salmonella* spp., and noncholera *Vibrio.* In Mexico and Morocco, where seasonal patterns of traveler's diarrhea have been studied, ETEC occurs during the warmer rainy season and largely disappears during the wintertime, when *C. jejuni* becomes more common. Parasites, such as *Giardia lamblia* and *Cryptosporidium parvum,* occur in approximately 2 to 3 percent of affected travelers to most regions. They occur more commonly during travel to mountainous areas of North America and to Russia. *Entamoeba histolytica* is an uncommon cause. *Cyclospora* has been recently described as an important agent producing chronic diarrhea in travelers to Nepal. Rotavirus and Norwalk virus cause as much as 10 percent of traveler's diarrhea occurring in Mexico. In 20 to 50 percent of episodes no agents can be identified despite complete microbiologic assessment. Most of this undefinable illness appears to be bacterial, in view of its favorable response to antimicrobial therapy.

■ THERAPY

Fluids and Electrolytes

Although this diarrhea is rarely severe enough to cause fluid and electrolyte depletion, rehydration is an important part of therapy, especially in the very young and the elderly. Consumption of fruit juices, caffeine-free soft drinks, or flavored mineral water, coupled with a source of sodium chloride (e.g., saltine crackers) is usually enough to hydrate most ill travelers. Commercial oral rehydration solutions are available in prepackaged and ready-to-use forms.

Dietary Management

Dietary management of diarrhea is also important. Staple foods such as cereals (wheat, rice, oats), potatoes, noodles, crackers, and bananas facilitate entocyte renewal. Patients should resume their usual diet once stools retain their shape. No caffeine or lactose should be taken while stools are unformed, since they may prolong diarrhea.

Symptomatic Therapy

Pharmacologic measures include the use of symptomatic agents and antimicrobials (Table 1). The commonly used symptomatic drugs include attapulgite, a nonabsorbed intraluminal drug; bismuth salicylate; and the antimotility synthetic opiate drugs such as loperamide. These agents are useful for the symptomatic treatment of mild to moderate cases. Attapulgite is nonabsorbable magnesium aluminum silicate, which binds to fluid and perhaps toxins, producing more formed stools.

Bismuth salicylate has been used as therapy for traveler's diarrhea, decreasing the number of stools passed by as much as 50 percent. Its activity is believed to be related to the antisecretory properties of the salicylate moiety. Bismuth salicylate should not be used by those who must avoid salicylates, and tinnitus has been a minor complaint in a small number of patients taking this medication. Bismuth sulfide produces harmless blackening of tongue and stools in patients taking bismuth subsalicylate.

Loperamide, an antimotility agent, reduces both the frequency of stools and the duration of illness by up to 80 percent as compared with no treatment. However, its use is not recommended for patients who have fever or blood in the stools or whenever symptoms persist for more than 48 hours.

Antimicrobial Therapy

Antimicrobial therapy (Table 2) shortens the duration of disease from an average of 59 to 93 hours to 16 to 30 hours. Therapy is indicated in moderate to severe cases. We recommend it after passage of the third unformed stool in 24 hours. The other indication for antimicrobial therapy is enteric symptoms that persist for 48 hours or longer. Fluoroquinolones are the preferred agents because of their activity against enteric pathogens in most high-risk parts of the world. Trimethoprim-sulfamethoxazole remains effective in the interior (noncoastal) areas of Mexico during the rainy season, summertime, when ETEC is the most common cause of illness. For the patient with disabling diarrhea, no fever, and no grossly bloody stools, the combination of loperamide and an antimicrobial drug is probably the best treatment. For the patient with fever or dysentery (passage of bloody stools), the antimicrobial should be given as a single agent. In most patients a single dose of the antimicrobial is sufficient. With a slow response or when the patient has particularly severe disease, fever, or dysentery, 3 days of the antimicrobial should be given.

Table 1 Treatment of Traveler's Diarrhea in Adults

SEVERITY OF ILLNESS	PREFERRED TREATMENT*	COMMENTS
Mild (no alteration of itinerary)	None	Symptomatic agents may be used.
Moderate (forced change in itinerary but able to function)	Loperamide	May use attapulgite or bismuth subsalicylate; antimicrobials should be employed with the passage of the third unformed stool in 24 hours or if symptoms persist for more than 2 days.
Severe (symptoms are incapacitating): no fever, stools are not bloody	Loperamide plus single-dose antimicrobial therapy	Continue standard dosing of antimicrobial for 3 days if symptoms are no better after 12 hours.
Severe (symptoms are incapacitating); fever >100.9° F (38.3° C) or stools are bloody	Loading dose of antimicrobial agent, standard doses for 3 days	Do not use loperamide.

*All patients should receive oral fluids and electrolytes.

Table 2 Pharmacologic Agents for Prophylaxis and Therapy of Traveler's Diarrhea in Adults

AGENT	PROPHYLACTIC DOSAGE	THERAPEUTIC DOSAGE	COMMENTS
Attapulgite	Not used	3 g initially, then 3 g after each loose stool or q2h for a total of 9 g/day	Nonabsorbed. Should be safe during pregnancy and for infants (although not approved).
Loperamide	Not used	4 mg initially, then 2 mg after each loose stool (not to exceed 16 mg/day)	Do not use with dysentery.
Bismuth subsalicylate	Two 262 mg tablets, chewed well, 4 times a day with meals and at bedtime	30 ml or two 262 mg tablets q30min for 5 doses; may be repeated on day 2	Salicylate is absorbed; avoid toxicity. Harmless darkening of tongue and stools will result. Do not use for prophylaxis when stays are for more than 3 weeks.
TMP-SMX	TMP 160 mg, SMX 800 mg qd	TMP 160 mg, SMX 800 mg b.i.d. 3 days or TMP 320 mg, SMX 1,600 mg as single dose	TMP resistance is common in most tropical areas. Effective in the non-coastal areas of Mexico during the summer.
Fluoroquinolones			
Norfloxacin	400 mg PO qd	800 mg once or 400 mg b.i.d. × 3 days	Most effective when susceptibilities are not known. Have been used as single dose.
Ciprofloxacin	500 mg PO qd	750 mg once or 500 mg b.i.d. × 3 days	
Ofloxacin	300 mg PO qd	600 mg once or 300 mg b.i.d. × 3 days	
Fleroxacin	400 mg PO qd	400 mg once or 400 mg qd × 3 days	

TMP-SMX, trimethoprim-sulfamethoxazole.

■ PREVENTION AND CHEMOPROPHYLAXIS

All travelers to high-risk areas should be educated as to the safe foods and beverages: those served steaming hot, dry foods like bread, items that have high acid content like citrus and other fruits that can be peeled, and syrups and jellies. For a limited number of persons, chemoprophylaxis may be considered. Although a National Institutes of Health Consensus Development Conference found no role for chemoprophylaxis, we consider that it has a place in preventing illness in small groups of travelers after a discussion about the risks and benefits of the approach. Antimicrobial prophylaxis will prevent 80 to 90 percent of the disease that would occur without prophylaxis. If the traveler has an important underlying health impairment or the trip would be ruined by a brief illness that might force a change in itinerary, antimicrobial prophylaxis should be considered (see Table 2). Bismuth subsalicylate has also been used as a prophylactic agent in young adults, preventing approximately 65 percent of the cases of diarrhea that would otherwise occur. Travelers should begin taking the drug on their first day in the country they are visiting and should continue to take it for 1 or 2 days after leaving the country. This approach is appropriate only for trips of 3 weeks or less.

Suggested Reading

Black RE. Epidemiology of travelers' diarrhea and relative importance of various pathogens. Rev Infect Dis 1990; 12(Suppl 1):S73–S79.

DuPont HL, Ericsson CD. Prevention and treatment of traveler's diarrhea. N Engl J Med 1993; 328:1821–1827.

Ericsson CD, DuPont HL Traveler's diarrhea: Approaches to prevention and treatment. Clin Infect Dis 1993; 16:616–626.

Gorbach SL, Edelman R, eds. Traveler's diarrhea: National Institutes of Health Consensus Development Conference. Rev Infect Dis 1986; 8(Suppl 2):S109–S233.Malaria-Treatment and Prophylaxis

MALARIA: TREATMENT AND PROPHYLAXIS

Phyllis E. Kozarsky, M.D.
Jay S. Keystone, M.D., M.Sc. (C.T.M.)

Malaria is one of the most frequent causes of fever in a returned traveler or recent immigrant from a malarious endemic area. Since death from malaria can occur within several days of the onset of symptoms, it is necessary to consider a febrile illness in a patient from a malarious endemic area to be a medical emergency. This is particularly so when symptoms begin within the first 2 months of arrival, since more than 90 percent of those with malaria due to *Plasmodium falciparum* present within this time frame. Those infected with other species, such as *Plasmodium vivax,* usually become symptomatic within a year of arrival from the tropics. An additional clue to the likely species of malaria is the area from which a traveler returns. For example, 85 percent of those with imported *P. falciparum* malaria acquire the infection in Africa, whereas *P. vivax* malaria is most frequently acquired in South Asia.

The standard approach to diagnosing malaria is the examination of thick and thin blood films, but many laboratories do not have the expertise to examine the former. Thick films are five to six times as sensitive as thin films, but thin films are better for determining the species of malaria. If the expertise to examine thick films is not available, as is usually the case in the middle of the night, thin blood films are better than none at all. Although the diagnosis may be missed on a thin blood film, a negative result will rule out a life-threatening infection, which is always associated with high parasitemia. If the initial blood films are negative, they should be repeated two or three times at 12 hour intervals.

The Becton Dickinson Company has recently developed two new diagnostic tests for malaria that do not require the degree of expertise needed to examine a thick blood film. The quantitative buffy-coat (QBC) method requires a trained technologist to examine with a fluorescent microscope the buffy-coat layer of a centrifuged specimen; malaria parasites are visible because they fluoresce with acridine dye. The parasite F test is a dip-stick test of lysed blood for falciparum antigen, which adheres to a monoclonal antibody impregnated in the stick. Both of these tests have a high degree of sensitivity and specificity for malaria.

Treating malaria appropriately requires knowledge of (1) the infecting species; (2) the likely location the infection was acquired; (3) the geographic patterns of drug resistance; and (4) the percent parasitemia in the case of *P. falciparum* malaria. Figure 1 shows the worldwide distribution of malaria. When there is any doubt about the infecting species, treat for the worst-case scenario, chloroquine-resistant *P. falciparum* (CRPF) malaria. Malaria due to *P. vivax* and *Plasmodium ovale* may leave dormant forms, hypnozoites, in the liver after the blood phase has been eradicated. Thus, treatment of these two infections requires eradication of the erythrocytic phase followed by a second drug, primaquine, to eradicate the liver phase.

Treatment of malaria has been increasingly complicated in recent years by the rapid spread of drug-resistant strains. No longer do clinicians have to be concerned only with CRPF malaria, but also with chloroquine-resistant and primaquine-resistant *P. vivax* malaria. Drug resistance has not been established in *P. ovale* or *P. malariae.* Drug regimens for treatment are provided in Table 1.

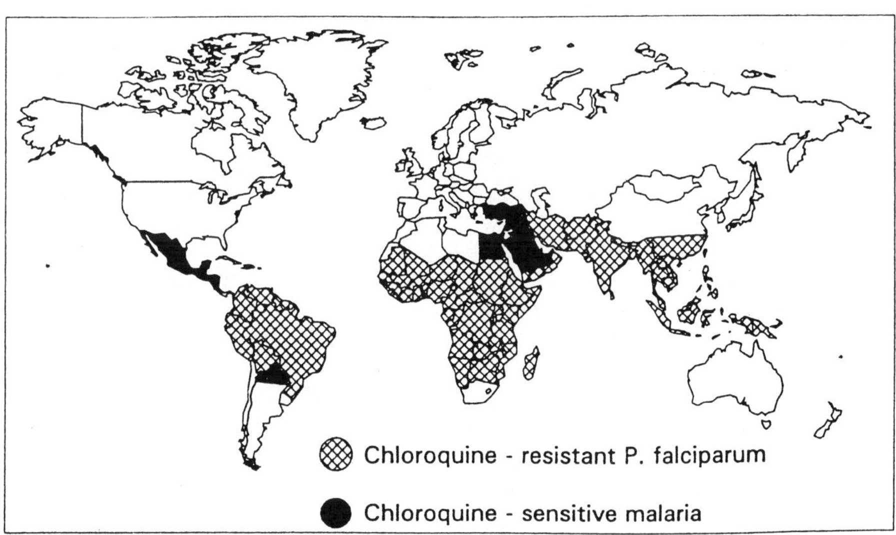

Figure 1
Distribution of malaria and chloroquine-resistant *Plasmodium falciparum,* 1994.

Table 1 Treatment of Malaria

DRUG	ADULT DOSE	PEDIATRIC DOSE
CHLOROQUINE-SENSITIVE MALARIA (ALL SPECIES)		
Chloroquine phosphate 1 tablet (150 mg base = 250 mg salt)	600 mg base (1 g) 300 mg in 6 hr, then 300 mg daily × 2 days plus in *P. vivax* and *P. ovale* only:	10 mg/kg (max. 600 mg) 5 mg/kg in 6 hr, then 5 mg/kg × 2 days
Primaquine phosphate	15 mg base/day × 14 days	0.3 mg base/kg/d × 14 days
Chloroquine-resistant P. vivax		
Chloroquine as above plus primaquine	10 mg base/kg total over 14 days or 2.5 mg base/kg total over 48 hr	Same as for adults
Halofantrine	24 mg/kg in 12 hr	Same as for adults
UNCOMPLICATED CHLOROQUINE-RESISTANT P. FALCIPARUM		
Quinine sulfate plus	650 mg t.i.d. × 3 days	24 mg/kg (base)/day in 3 doses × 3 days
Pyrimethamine/sulfadoxine (Fansidar) 25 mg/500 mg or	3 tablets in a single dose	2–11 mo, ¼ tab 1–3 yr, ½ tab 4–8 yr, 1 tab 9–14 yr, 2 tab >14 yr, adult dose
Tetracycline or	250 mg q.i.d. × 7 days	5 mg/kg q.i.d. × 7 days
Clindamycin	900 mg t.i.d. × 3 days	20–40 mg/kg/day in 3 doses × 3 days
Mefloquine	1–1.5 g (base) on individual dose over 12 hr	15 mg/kg in individual dose over 12 hr
Halofantrine	500 mg t.i.d. × 1 day; repeat in 1 week	8 mg/kg t.i.d. × 1 day; repeat in 1 week
TREATMENT OF SEVERE ILLNESS, PARENTERAL DOSE FOR ALL SPECIES		
Quinine loading	20 mg/kg (salt) [1 mg salt = 0.83 mg base] in 300 ml normal saline IV over 2–4 hr Maintenance: 10 mg/kg q8h	Same as for adults
Quinidine loading	24 mg/kg (salt) in 300 ml of normal saline IV over 2–4 h Maintenance: 12 mg/kg q8h or 10 mg/kg (salt) IV over 1–2 h, then constant infusion of 0.02 mg/kg/min by infusion pump	Same as for adults

THERAPY

P. Vivax Malaria

P. vivax malaria, which has very low mortality, is the most frequently imported malaria. The erythrocytic phase of *P. vivax* malaria is usually effectively treated with chloroquine; primaquine is then used to eradicate hepatic hypnozoites. Since primaquine is one of the most potent oxidizing agents known, a glucose-6-phosphate dehydrogenase (G6PD) level must be determined before primaquine therapy is initiated.

Chloroquine-resistant *P. vivax* malaria was first described in Indonesia in 1989. Since then it has been shown to be highly endemic in Irian Jaya and Papua New Guinea. Recently it has been described in the Amazon basin of Brazil and in Guyana. Malaria due to chloroquine-resistant *P. vivax* should be suspected when the illness recurs within 28 days after a patient has received standard therapy with chloroquine and primaquine. Recent studies from Indonesia suggest that a standard course of chloroquine combined with high-dose primaquine (2.5 mg per kilogram over 48 hours) is effective therapy for drug-resistant *P. vivax* malaria. Halofantrine alone is also effective but is not available in North America.

When a relapse of *P. vivax* occurs more than 28 days after treatment with chloroquine and primaquine, primaquine resistance should be considered. Primaquine-resistant *P. vivax* malaria is frequently reported from Papua New Guinea, Irian Jaya, other parts of Southeast Asia, and less commonly from Colombia and Somalia. Patients who fail the usual course of primaquine should receive 1½ to 2 times the standard dose over 14 days, or a total dose of 6 mg per kilogram, to prevent further relapses.

P. Ovale Malaria

Malaria due to *P. ovale,* which is found mostly in Africa, is managed as is that due to chloroquine-sensitive *P. vivax.* No drug-resistant strains of *P. ovale* have been documented.

Plasmodium Malariae and Uncomplicated Chloroquine-Sensitive *P. Falciparum* Malaria

Chloroquine-sensitive *P. falciparum* malaria is confined to Central America north of Panama, Haiti, parts of North Africa, and the Middle East. Chloroquine in standard doses should be used to treat *P. falciparum* from these areas and *P. malariae* infections from any part of the world. Chloroquine does not eradicate the gametocytes of *P. falciparum* malaria, which circulate harmlessly for several months after the other erythrocytic forms of the parasite have been eradicated.

Uncomplicated Chloroquine-Resistant *P. Falciparum* Malaria

With the exception of the regions where chloroquine-sensitive *P. falciparum* malaria remains, malaria due to *P. falciparum* should be considered chloroquine-resistant. Quinine sulfate remains the drug of choice for treatment of CRPF malaria in combination with a second agent such as pyrimethamine-sulfadoxine (Fansidar), a tetracycline derivative, or clindamycin. Pyrimethamine-sulfadoxine should not be used for treatment of strains acquired along the Thai-Cambodian or Thai-Myanmar borders or in the Amazon basin of Brazil, where multidrug-resistant strains occur. Clindamycin is usually reserved for pregnant women and for young children, in whom no tetracycline derivative is generally used. Since these second agents tend to be slower acting, it is important to institute quinine therapy as soon as the diagnosis is confirmed. Virtually everyone who takes quinine will suffer from cinchonism, and complaints of tinnitus, dizziness, headache, and possibly temporary hearing loss are common.

Mefloquine alone is a very effective therapy for uncomplicated CRPF malaria. Along the Thai borders the treatment dose must be increased from 15 to 25 mg per kilogram because of multidrug resistance. Unfortunately data confirm the development of cross-resistance among mefloquine, halofantrine, and quinine due to their chemical relatedness. Major concerns about the use of mefloquine for treatment of malaria are the severe neuropsychiatric adverse reactions (psychosis, convulsions), which occur 10 to 60 times as frequently as when the drug is used for prophylaxis; these complications are estimated to occur in 1:215 to 1:1700 users. In an attempt to decrease the gastrointestinal side effects of mefloquine, the dose may be split and administered over 12 hours.

Halofantrine, not yet available in North America, is being widely used in malarious areas throughout the world. In standard doses, however, it is not very effective along the borders of Thailand. Recent studies have documented cardiotoxicity with halofantrine, particularly in those who have taken the drug with food, as drug absorption increases sixfold with a fatty meal. Halofantrine should be taken on an empty stomach. It is contraindicated in those with a family history of prolonged QT interval or conduction disturbances or when any other QT-prolonging agent such as mefloquine or quinine has been administered. An electrocardiogram is recommended prior to halofantrine administration.

Increasingly in Southeast Asia and more recently in Africa, malaria is being treated with the oral artemisinin derivative artesunate. This drug is well tolerated, and it leads to a rapid reduction in parasitemia and fever; however, monotherapy is associated with a high rate of recrudescence. The combination of a second agent such as mefloquine or tetracycline with artesunate is necessary to ensure cure of the infection. If travelers or expatriates need to be treated with artemisinin derivatives because of treatment failures with quinine and mefloquine, therapy should be conducted under expert supervision.

Complicated *P. Falciparum* Malaria

When *P. falciparum* parasitemia reaches 5 percent or more, complications such as cerebral malaria, renal failure, adult respiratory distress syndrome (ARDS), and massive hemolysis may occur. The mortality of even appropriately treated severe *P. falciparum* malaria ranges from 10 to 20 percent. Patients with complicated malaria, and those who cannot tolerate oral quinine due to vomiting, require parenteral therapy with quinine or quinidine. Because parenteral quinine preparations are not readily available in most centers, quinidine should be used. However, because of its potential for cardiotoxicity, continuous electrocardiographic monitoring should be undertaken. Since both quinine and quinidine cause insulin to be released from the pancreas, it is very important to monitor for hypoglycemia, a frequent complication of severe malaria, especially in pregnant women and children. Fluid balance should be corrected judiciously with the aim of avoiding fluid overload because of the risk of ARDS. Lactic acidosis, a common complication of severe malaria, indicates a poor prognosis. For parasitemias above 10 percent, particularly when other complications are present, exchange transfusion with at least four units of blood may be lifesaving. When patients present with severe *P. falciparum* malaria, it is prudent to rule out other concomitant infections such as meningitis in those who are comatose and septicemia in those who are hypotensive.

■ PROPHYLAXIS

The primary goal of prophylaxis is to prevent *P. falciparum* infection in nonimmune travelers, since almost all fatal cases are associated with illness due to this species. For decades chloroquine was widely effective in the prevention and treatment of all species of malaria. However, with the spread of chloroquine resistance, recommendations for antimalarial chemoprophylaxis have become more complicated and often controversial. Figure 2 is an algorithm for determining an appropriate antimalarial chemoprophylactic regimen.

Areas within a country may differ with respect to risk. For example, travel in most areas in Kenya places travelers at risk for acquisition of chloroquine-resistant *P. falciparum*. The risk is highest near Lake Victoria, intermediate on the coast, and lowest in the game parks. However, if the traveler will be staying only in Nairobi, the capital, where there is no malaria, prophylaxis is not necessary.

Mefloquine is the agent of choice for the prevention of chloroquine-resistant *P. falciparum* infections. It is contraindicated only for those with a history of seizure disorder or depression. Mefloquine may be used in the second and third trimesters of pregnancy, and dosage regimens are available for children. Mefloquine can probably be used during the first trimester, but data are insufficient to recommend it without any reservations. Prolonged exposure to malaria in areas intensely endemic for *P. vivax* (for example, Central America, Northwest Africa, South Asia, Oceania) warrants terminal malaria prophylaxis with primaquine phosphate to eradicate the hepatic hypnozoites and prevent relapsing malaria. As noted above, G6PD levels should be checked before prescribing this drug. Primaquine is usually taken after completing chloroquine, mefloquine, or doxycycline therapy and is contraindicated during pregnancy. The adult dose is 21.5 mg salt/per day for 14 days.

Because no antimalarial regimen is 100 percent effective, all travelers to malarious regions need to be meticulous about personal protection measures. Between dusk and dawn, when the *Anopheles* mosquitoes bite, travelers should wear protective clothing (long sleeves, pants), use mosquito repellents

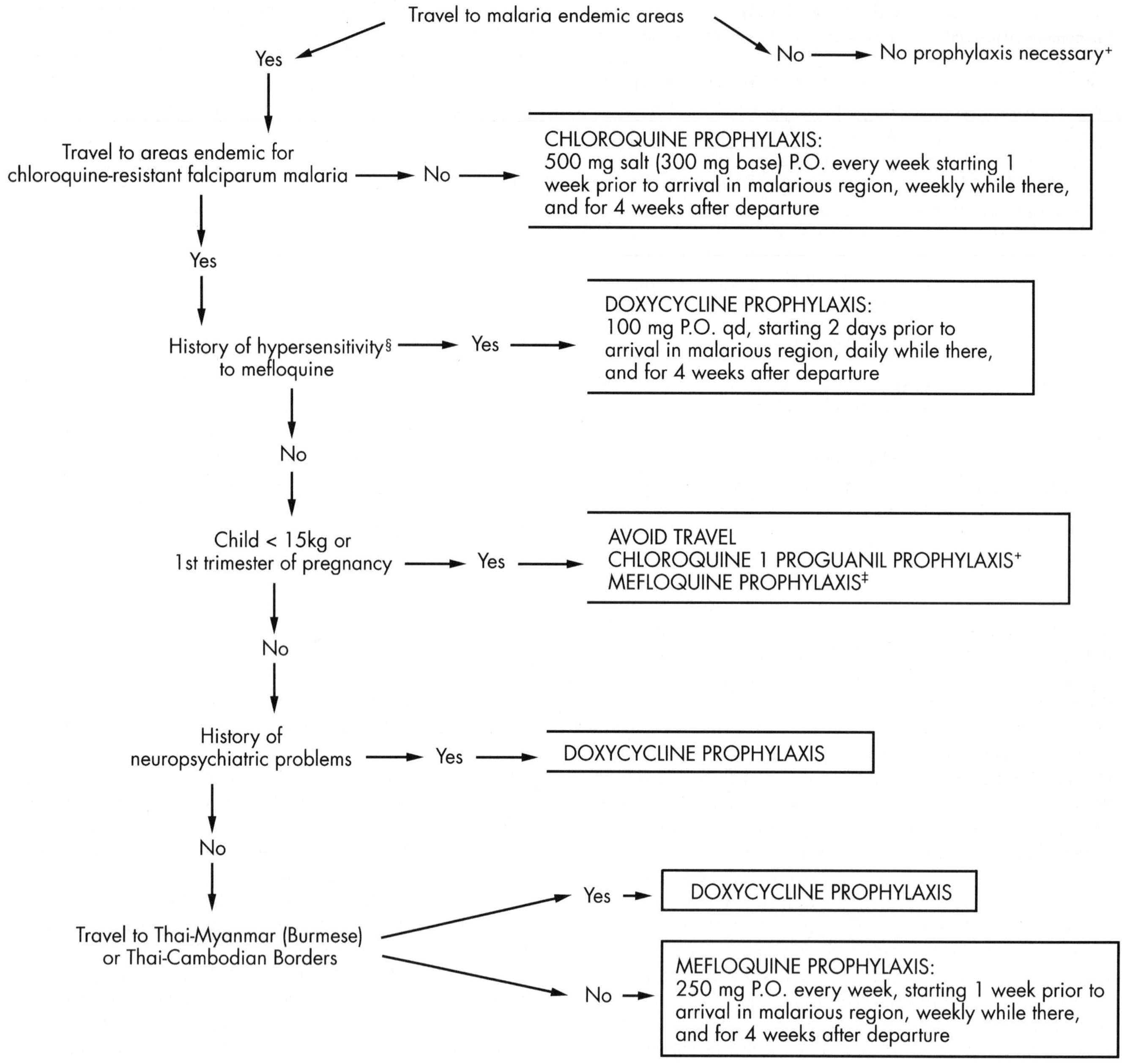

*Malaria in many countries is confined to rural areas or regions not on usual tourist itineraries.
+Probably safe, but efficacy much less than mefloquine. Proguanil not available in the United States.
‡Not enough data to support use; inadvertant use not a reason for abortion.
§Seizures, psychoses, depression, need for fine motor coordination skills (pilot, surgeons).

Figure 2
Algorithm for the chemoprophylaxis of malaria. Doses given are for adults.

and sleep under netting or in screened or air conditioned rooms. Insect repellents that contain 35 percent diethyltoluamide (deet) are very effective for 4 to 6 hours. Repellents containing 5 to 10 percent deet should be used on young children to prevent toxicity. Knock-down sprays should be used indoors and in infected areas before bedtime.

Physicians who are responsible for preventing and treating malaria will have to keep abreast of the global spread of drug resistance and the new agents being developed to combat this problem. Assistance may be sought from the malaria branch of the Centers for Disease Control and Prevention by calling 404-332-4555 (phone or fax).

Suggested Reading

Anonymous. Artemisinin. Trans R Soc Trop Med Hyg 1994: 88(Suppl 1): 1–65.

Baird JK, Basri H, Subianto B, et al. Treatment of chloroquine-resistant *P. vivax* with chloroquine and primaquine or halofantrine. J Infect Dis 1995; 171:1678–1682.

Bryson HM, Goa KL. Halofantrine: A review of its antimalarial activity, pharmacokinetic properties and therapeutic potential. Drugs 1992; 43:236–258.

Kozarsky PE, Lobel HO. Antimalarial agents: Are we running out of options? Curr Opin Infect Dis 1994; 7:701–707.

Phillips P, Nantel S, Benny WB. Exchange transfusion as an adjunct to the treatment of severe falciparum malaria: Case report and review. Rev Infect Dis 1990; 12:1100–1108.

World Health Organization. Severe and complicated malaria. Trans R Soc Top Med Hyg 1990; 84(Suppl 2):1–65.

TUBERCULOSIS

Asim K. Dutt, M.D., F.C.C.P.
William W. Stead, M.D., F.C.C.P., M.A.C.P.

In the United States, the epidemiology of tuberculosis (TB) has changed greatly. Infection by human immunodeficiency virus (HIV) and the increase in homelessness, poverty, and drug abuse are major factors in this change. TB occurs most commonly among ethnic minorities, African-Americans, and Hispanics 25 to 44 years of age. Immigrants from developing countries with a high prevalence of TB and drug resistance have contracted almost one-third of the new cases in this country in the past several years. Drug-resistant disease is a major concern.

DIAGNOSIS

Whenever there is a suspicion of pulmonary TB, three spontaneously produced sputum specimens should be examined by microscopy and culture. If necessary, sputum production may be induced by inhalation of aerosol of warm saline (Fig. 1). Methods such as early-morning gastric lavage and laryngeal swab on suction are less productive. When suspicion of TB is high and microscopy is negative on at least three specimens, a bronchial washing or transbronchial biopsy through a fiberoptic bronchoscope or postbronchoscopy sputum may be productive. In an unconscious patient, tracheal aspiration or transthoracic needle aspiration of the lung may be needed to obtain a specimen. On rare occasions diagnosis must be made by open lung biopsy.

Rapid diagnostic tests directly from sputum are now commercially available. Mycobacterium Tuberculosis Direct test (MTD) (Gene Probe, San Diego) is a transcription-mediated amplification which utilizes nucleic acid probe. Amplicor (Roche) is a Polymerase chain reaction (PCR) which is detected by a DNA probe. Both tests are performed in 5 to 6 hours and have high sensitivity and specificity.

Positive sputum microscopy suggests TB, but the only positive identification of *Mycobacterium tuberculosis* is by culture or DNA probe to distinguish it from other less virulent mycobacteria. Drug susceptibility testing should be performed.

For the diagnosis of extrapulmonary TB secretions and/or biopsy, material must be obtained from the site (Fig. 1). In the case of tuberculous meningitis it may be necessary to initiate therapy empirically because the disease may become irreversible before the diagnosis can be made.

THERAPY

Principles of Chemotherapy

Table 1 lists drugs, dosages, and major side effects. Several first-line bactericidal drugs are commonly combined initially because they reduce the bacterial population rapidly without the risk of resistance. Second-line drugs are most useful when resistance to two or more first-line drugs is found or they cannot be used because of life-threatening side effects or intolerance (Fig. 2).

The bactericidal drugs in suitable combinations actually kill actively multiplying extracellular bacilli in TB lesions. Rapid elimination of these bacilli renders the sputum bacteriologically negative, leading to cure. No bactericidal drug should be used alone to treat active TB because this inevitably leads to resistance to that drug. When initial therapy fails at this stage, the sputum bacteriology does not become negative, as shown by persistence of positive sputum smears beyond 3 months. Failure of therapy is usually due to emergence of drug-resistant organisms, most often due to poor compliance, prescription of an inadequate regimen, or inadequate dosage of individual drugs.

In the continuation phase of therapy, the drugs slowly eliminate small populations of intermittently metabolizing persisters in the closed caseous lesion or within macrophages. Incomplete therapy may lead to relapse after discontinuation of treatment, often with drug-sensitive organisms.

Drug-resistant Organisms

The inclusion of a number of drugs in a regimen should be based on the awareness of the circumstances under which drug-resistant bacilli are likely to be present (Table 2).

At the minimum, a four-drug regimen should be initiated when drug resistance is likely, until susceptibility results are available. The number of drugs in the initial regimen may have to be increased to five to seven if the organisms are resistant to three or more drugs and HIV infection is present,

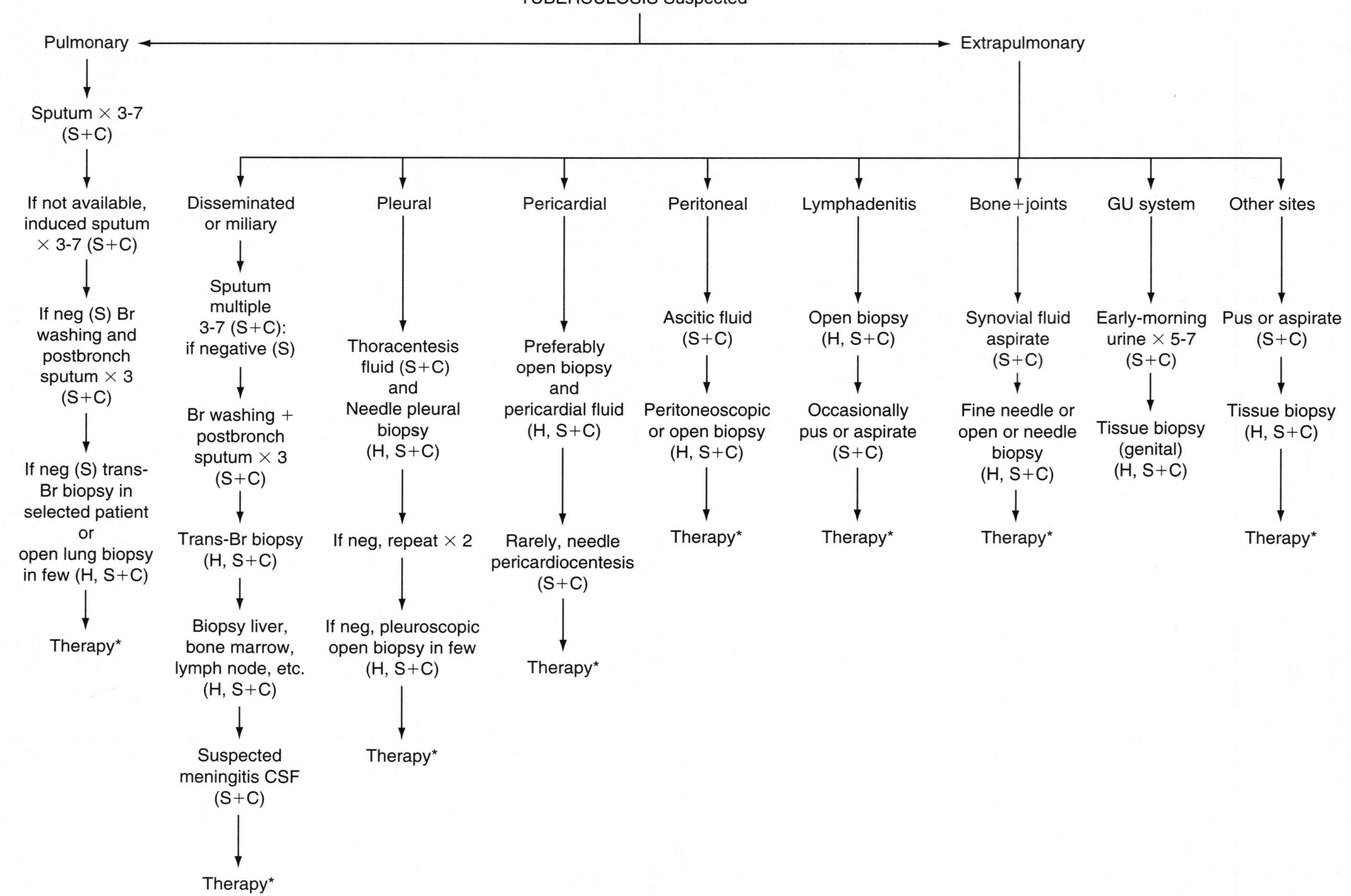

Figure 1
Diagnosis of suspected TB. S, smear; C, culture for mycobacteria; H, histology; Br, bronchial; Bronch, Bronchoscopy; CSF, cerebrospinal fluid; Bx, biopsy; neg, negative; GU, genitourinary.
*Therapy started in suspected cases, awaiting culture results and/or clinical response.

Table 1 Antituberculosis Drugs

DRUG	DAILY DOSAGE	TWICE-WEEKLY DOSAGE	SIDE EFFECTS	MODE OF ACTION
FIRST-LINE DRUGS				
Streptomycin, other aminoglycosides	10–15 mg/kg (usually 0.5–1 g) 5 days/week	20–25 mg/kg (usually 1–1.5 g) IM	Cranial nerve VIII damage (vestibular and auditory), nephrotoxicity, allergic fever, rash	Active against rapidly multiplying bacilli in neutral or slightly alkaline extracellular medium
Capreomycin	Same as aminoglycosides	Same as aminoglycosides	Same as aminoglycosides	Same as aminoglycosides
Isoniazid	5 mg/kg (usually 300 mg) PO or IM	15 mg/kg (usually 900 mg) PO	Peripheral neuritis, hepatotoxicity, allergic fever and rash, lupus erythematosus phenomenon	Acts strongly on rapidly dividing extracellular bacilli; acts weakly on slowly multiplying intracellular bacilli
Rifampin	10 mg/kg (usually 450–600 mg) PO	10 mg/kg (usually 450–600 mg) PO	Hepatotoxicity, nausea, vomiting, allergic fever and rash, flulike syndrome, petechiae with thrombocytopenia or acute renal failure during intermittent therapy	Acts on both rapidly and slowly multiplying extracellular and intracellular bacilli, particularly on slowly multiplying persisters
Rifabutin (Ansamycin)	150–300 mg PO	Not used	Same as rifampin	Same as above
Pyrazinamide	25–30 mg/kg (usually 2.5 g) PO	45–50 mg/kg (usually 3–3.5 mg) PO	Hyperuricemia, hepatotoxicity, allergic fever and rash	Active in acid pH medium on intracellular bacilli
Ethambutol	15–25 mg/kg (usually 800–1,600 mg) PO	50 mg/kg PO	Optic neuritis, skin rash, hyperuricemia	Weakly active against both extracellular and intracellular bacilli to inhibit the development of resistant bacilli
SECOND-LINE DRUGS				
Ethionamide	10–15 mg/kg (usually 500–750 mg) in divided doses PO	Not used	Nausea, vomiting, anorexia, allergic fever and rash, hepatotoxicity, neurotoxicity	Same as ethambutol
Cycloserine	15–20 mg/kg (usually 0.75–1 g) in divided doses with 200 mg pyridoxine PO	Not used	Personality changes, psychosis, convulsions, rash	Same as ethambutol
Paraminosalicylic acid	150 mg/kg (usually 12 g) in divided doses PO	Not used	Nausea, vomiting, diarrhea, hepatotoxicity, allergic rash and fever	Weak action on extracellular bacilli; inhibits development of drug-resistant organisms
Thiocetazone*	150 mg PO	Not used	Allergic rash and fever, Stevens-Johnson syndrome, blood disorders, nausea, vomiting	Same as paraminosalicylic acid
Clofazimine (antileprosy)	100 mg t.i.d. PO	Not used	Pigmentation of skin, abdominal pain	Active against *Mycobacterium intracellulare*
NEWER AGENTS				
Ofloxacin	800 mg qd	Not used	Gastrointestinal: diarrhea, nausea, abdominal pain, anorexia; central nervous system: dizziness, restlessness, nightmares, ataxia, seizures	Rapidly multiplying bacilli at neutral or alkaline pH
Ciprofloxacin	750 mg qd	Not used	Same as ofloxacin	Same as ofloxacin
Azithromycin	500 mg/day, up to 30 days	Not used	Diarrhea, nausea, abdominal pain, elevation of liver enzymes	Rapidly multiplying bacilli in macrophages against *M. intracellulare*
Clarithromycin	1 g q12h	Not used	Same as azithromycin	Same as azithromycin

*Not available in the United States.

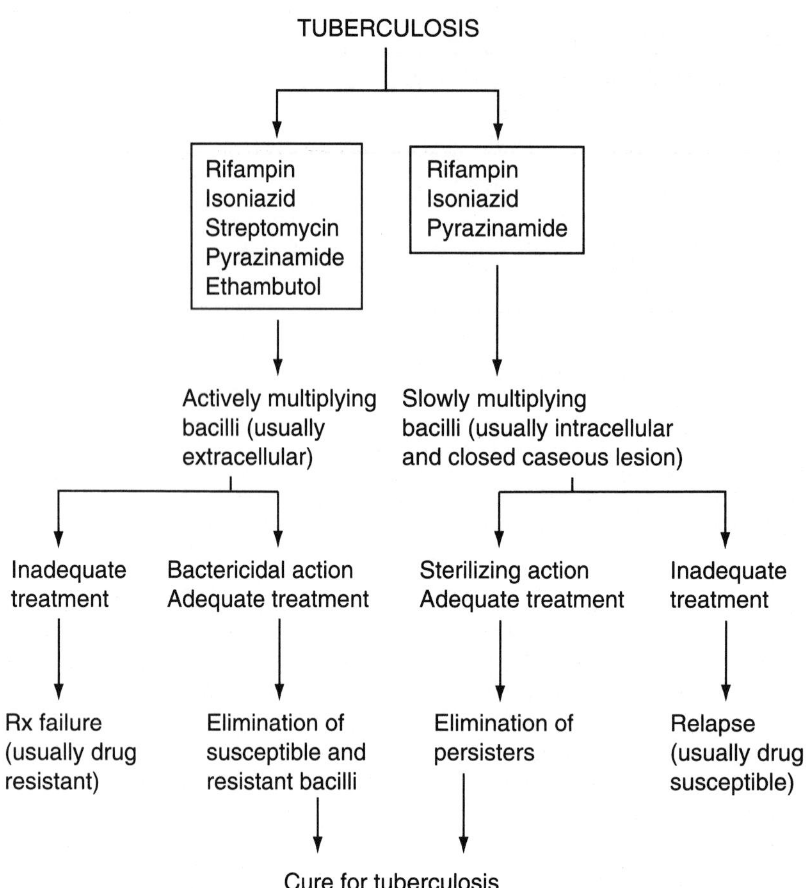

Figure 2
Principles of chemotherapy of TB.

Table 2 Conditions and Patients with Increased Risk of Drug-Resistant TB

History of treatment with anti-TB drugs, including preventive therapy
Patients from areas with high prevalence of initial or primary drug resistance (>4%), e.g., urban population in the northeastern United States, Florida, California, U.S.-Mexican border
Foreign-born persons from areas with high prevalence of drug-resistant TB, e.g., Southeast Asia, Mexico, South America, Africa
Contacts of persons with drug-resistant disease
Disease in persons who are homeless, drug abusers, and HIV infected
Persons with positive sputum smears and cultures after 3 months of chemotherapy

as often occurs in large cities in the United States and in many developing countries.

Drug Regimens

Any of several drug regimens with variable durations may be selected according to the local conditions.

Nine Month Regimen

Since the mid-1970s, Arkansas Department of Health physicians have treated patients with isoniazid (INH) and rifampin (RIF) in a combination capsule (Rifamate) for 9 months. The therapy may be administered daily or, as in most cases, twice weekly. The Arkansas regimen consists of INH-RIF two capsules daily for 1 month followed by two INH-RIF capsules and two 300 mg INH tablets twice weekly for another 8 months. Several thousand patients have been treated, and the success rate is over 95 percent. Development of drug resistance has not been a problem because the patient cannot take a single drug alone, and side effects are minimal. The cost of medication is quite reasonable.

The main objection to a two-drug regimen is possible presence of drug-resistant bacilli during initial therapy. In Arkansas the incidence of initial or primary resistance is below 3 percent. Moreover, patients with risk factors (see Table 2) are excluded from this regimen. However, the regimen should never be prescribed in large cities, in places with high prevalence of primary drug resistance, or in certain areas of the United States such as the Mexican border and areas in which Southeast Asians have settled.

We still find this regimen useful in the initial treatment of elderly persons in whom the disease is generally caused by recrudescence of an infection acquired many years ago, when drug resistance was not a problem. Moreover, the twice-weekly schedule is easily supervised when needed, either by health care personnel or by relatives or friends.

Six Month Regimen

The addition of pyrazinamide (PZA) 25 to 30 mg per kilogram to the INH 300 mg and RIF 600 mg daily for

Table 3 Regimens for the Initial Treatment of TB

TB WITHOUT HIV INFECTION			
OPTION 1	**OPTION 2**	**OPTION 3**	**TB WITH HIV INFECTION**
INH, RIF, PZA (if initial INH resistance is <4%) daily for 8 weeks, followed by INH and RIF daily or twice weekly for 16 weeks Add EMB or SM if resistance is (>4%)	INH, RIF, PZA, EMB, or SM daily for 2 weeks, then twice weekly for 6 weeks (DOT), subsequently INH and RIF twice weekly for 16 weeks (DOT)	INH, RIF, PZA, EMB, or SM 3 times a week for 6 months (DOT)	Option 1, 2, or 3 for a total of 9 months, at least 6 months beyond culture conversion
Total treatment 6 months (at least 3 months past culture conversion)	Total treatment 6 months	Total treatment 6 months	Total treatment 6–9 months

From Centers for Disease Control and Prevention: Initial therapy for tuberculosis in the era of multidrug resistance: Recommendations of the Advisory Council for the Elimination of Tuberculosis. MMWR 1993; 42(RR-7):1–8.
INH, isoniazid; RIF, rifampin; PZA, pyrazinamide; EMB, ethambutol; SM, streptomycin; DOT, directly observed therapy.

the initial 2 months, (preferably in combination capsules [Rifoter 5–6 capsules/day]) followed by INH 300 mg and RIF 600 mg daily or INH 900 mg and RIF 600 mg twice weekly (Rifamate 2 capsules and INH 2 tablets) for another 4 months (a total of 6 months), has proved highly successful. Centers for Disease Control and Prevention (CDC) American Thoracic Society guidelines recommend this regimen if the prevalence of primary drug resistance is below 4% (Table 3, option 1).

The three-drug regimen reduces the duration of therapy to 6 months. Addition of PZA accelerates reduction of the bacterial population and adds little to the toxicity of the regimen, although its cost is greater. The addition of a third drug, PZA, ensures against failure in the event of initial resistance to either INH or RIF. In clinical studies, 6 months of therapy with these drugs has been less effective in RIF-resistant cases than in INH-resistant cases.

Six Month Therapy when Resistance Is Suspected

When drug resistance is suspected or likely, at least four-drug therapy consisting of INH 300 mg, RIF 600 mg, PZA 25 to 35 mg per kilogram, and streptomycin (SM) 0.5 to 1 g IM 5 days a week or ethambutol (EMB) 25 mg per kilogram should be administered initially (option 1, Table 3). After drug susceptibility results are available, usually 2 months, the regimen is modified accordingly. If the organisms are found to be susceptible to both drugs, therapy is completed with INH-RIF daily or twice weekly for another 4 months. In cases of INH resistance therapy may consist of RIF, PZA, and EMB for another 6 to 7 months. INH should be included in the regimen because of its action on persisters, which generally remain INH sensitive. In RIF-resistant cases other bactericidal drugs should be continued for at least 10 to 12 months to prevent relapse.

Treatment of Multidrug-Resistant Disease

Where the prevalence of multidrug resistance (MDR) and HIV infection are very high, it is necessary to initiate a five- to seven-drug regimen, including second-line drugs. This is applicable to large urban populations such as New York City, Miami, parts of New Jersey, and San Francisco, as well as persons from developing countries.

In the treatment of MDR disease, i.e., resistance to INH and RIF, some basic principles must be followed: (1) a single drug must not be added to a failing regimen; (2) at least three new drugs the patient has not yet taken should replace the existing drug regimen until the susceptibility results are available; (3) the total duration of therapy must be prolonged to 24 months or more; (4) the regimen should include an injectable drug (e.g., streptomycin or capreomycin) for at least 4 months or until the culture is converted to negative to improve compliance; (5) directly observed therapy (DOT) should be used to ensure compliance, because it is the patient's last chance at a cure.

Most drugs used for MDR disease are second-line drugs (see Table 1)—ethionamide, cycloserine, para-aminosalicylic acid (PAS), capreomycin, and kanamycin. Newer drugs, fluoroquinolones (ciprofloxacin, ofloxacin, and levofloxacin), and amikacin are available but unproven. Finally, clofazimine and thiocetazone (not available in the United States) may be used but also are unproven. These second-line drugs are often rather toxic, and close monitoring is necessary. Monthly bacteriologic studies are necessary to monitor response to treatment.

Because of high failure and relapse rates in MDR TB, surgical resection of the major diseased area of the lung is again becoming necessary after reasonable medical treatment has been given to reduce the bacterial load.

Preventive therapy for recent contacts with MDR TB is controversial. However, two possible regimens are PZA plus EMB and PZA plus ciprofloxacin or ofloxacin for 12 to 24 months, during which periodic clinical, bacteriologic, and radiologic monitoring must be maintained.

Treatment Regimens for HIV-Infected Persons

Current 6 month treatment in the United States consisting of INH, RIF, PZA, and EMB or SM daily for 2 months followed by INH and RIF daily or twice weekly for another 4 months may not be adequate in HIV-infected patients. The CDC recommends that therapy for patients with HIV infection be prolonged to 9 months or for at least 6 months following conversion of sputum cultures to negative (Table 3). Treatment-limiting side effects are frequent in HIV-infected patients, and they require innovative measures. Intermittent regimens (2 or 3 doses a week) are generally well tolerated in such situations.

Smear-Negative Tuberculosis

Positive sputum smears indicate a large bacterial population and advanced disease, while negative smears generally suggest less advanced disease. We have treated a large number of patients having three initial specimens with negative smears but one or two positive cultures with INH and RIF for 6 months. Relapses are no more common than in smear-positive cases treated for 9 months. Occasionally a patient who is smear negative is also culture negative, but is treated for TB on the basis of clinical and x-ray findings. Regimens for such patients have included 4 months of INH plus RIF. Another suggested regimen for smear-negative TB is INH, RIF, PZA, and EMB for 4 months.

Extrapulmonary Tuberculosis

The bacterial load in extrapulmonary TB usually is much smaller than in cavitary pulmonary TB. Thus, 6 to 9 month regimens (see Table 3) are adequate for treatment of extrapulmonary TB. Figure 1 indicates the steps in the diagnosis of pulmonary and extrapulmonary TB. We have successfully treated many patients with extrapulmonary TB with INH and RIF, but the increasing incidence of drug resistance necessitates additional drugs. It is generally recommended that the duration of therapy be prolonged in TB spondylitis (Pott's disease).

Directly Observed Therapy in Noncompliant Patients

The fact that most of the 6 month regimens may be given intermittently two or three times per week has led to the development of some innovative regimens. The Denver regimen consists of DOT administration of daily INH, RIF, PZA, and SM or EMB for 2 weeks, followed by twice-weekly doses for 6 weeks and then twice-weekly administration of INH or RIF for another 16 weeks. Another DOT regimen is INH, RIF, PZA, and EMB or SM three times a week for 6 months (Table 3, options 2 and 3).

Therapy in Special Situations

Pregnancy

Treatment with INH, RIF, and EMB is safe in pregnancy. SM should not be used because of toxicity to eighth nerve of the fetus. Experience with PZA is limited in pregnancy, and at present it should be avoided if possible.

Renal Failure

INH and RIF dosage need not be altered in renal failure because these drugs are excreted by the liver. Renal dialysis patients should receive the drugs after dialysis. EMB dosage must be reduced to 8 to 10 mg per kilogram in advanced renal failure. SM and aminoglycosides should be avoided in these patients, and the level should be monitored if they must be used in very unusual circumstances. PZA dosage should be reduced to 15 to 20 mg per kilogram.

Liver Disease

Alcoholic liver disease does not preclude use of antituberculosis drugs. However, monitoring for side effects must be careful and regular. In overt liver failure the therapy should consist of INH and EMB until liver function returns to normal. At that time RIF and/or PZA may be added to the regimen.

Combined Preparations

In the United States, two commercial preparations of combination drugs are available. It is advantageous to use combination preparations because they preclude the taking of only one bactericidal drug, which encourages drug resistance. Rifamate is a combination capsule of INH 150 mg and RIF 300 mg, and two capsules are the recommended daily dose. Another preparation, Rifater, contains INH 50 mg, RIF 120 mg, and PZA 300 mg in each tablet; the recommended dose is 5–6 tablets daily. We strongly recommend the use of combination preparations for therapy as a safeguard against development of drug resistance, particularly for patients not on DOT.

Corticosteroid Therapy

Corticosteroids are not routinely used in the treatment of TB. Prednisone 20 to 30 mg a day may improve the general sense of well-being, reduce fever, increase appetite, and improve nutrition of markedly toxic or severely debilitated patients. The drug should be tapered off gradually after 4 to 8 weeks. In disseminated TB associated with hypoxemia and respiratory failure, prednisone 40 to 60 mg a day may improve oxygenation. Steroids have been successfully used in AIDS patients with TB, but they may promote opportunistic infections. Most authorities believe that complicated tuberculous meningitis should be treated with prednisone 60 to 80 mg a day, slowly tapered after 8 to 12 weeks. Some advise corticosteroid therapy for all cases of tuberculous pericarditis to prevent constrictive pericarditis.

■ MONITORING AND FOLLOW-UP OF PATIENTS

Intense bacteriologic monitoring is necessary during therapy of pulmonary TB. We recommend that three to five specimens of bronchial secretions (sputum) be examined initially by smear and culture, followed by drug susceptibility testing. Genetic studies with PCR methodology facilitate rapid diagnosis. During therapy, at least one specimen of sputum should be examined every 2 weeks until conversion to negative occurs. This permits early detection of noncompliance and impending failure. After completion of treatment, to detect early relapse, one specimen every 3 months three times should be examined before discharging the patient from the clinic.

Monitoring for side effects should be done monthly after explaining to the patient the symptoms of side effects for which to be alert (e.g., nausea, vomiting, anorexia, dark urine, jaundice). Blood should be collected for baseline complete blood count, renal, and hepatic function tests. We do not recommend routine monthly blood studies. Rather, the patients are advised to discontinue medication when symptomatic, and to report for repeat hepatic function studies at that time. The drugs are then adjusted to the laboratory findings. For EMB, vision and color studies are performed monthly, and for SM, monthly examination for balance and hearing loss.

■ PROPHYLAXIS

For prophylaxis, see the chapter *Nonsurgical Antimicrobial Prophylaxis.*

Suggested Reading

Centers for Disease Control. Initial therapy for tuberculosis in the era of multidrug resistance: Recommendations of the Advisory Council for the Elimination of Tuberculosis. MMWR (RR-7) 1993; 42 (RR-7): 1–8.

Dutt AK, Moers D, Stead WW. Short course chemotherapy for extrapulmonary tuberculosis. Ann Intern Med 1986; 104.

Dutt AK, Stead WW. Medical perspective: Present chemotherapy for tuberculosis. J Infect Dis 1982; 146:698–704.

Goble M, Iseman MD, Madsen LA, et al. Treatment of 171 patients with pulmonary tuberculosis resistant to isoniazid and rifampin. N Engl J Med 1993; 328:527–532.

Iseman MD. Treatment of multidrug-resistant tuberculosis. N Engl J Med 1993; 329:784–791.

Jones BE, Otaya M, Antoniskis D, et al. A prospective evaluation of antituberculosis therapy in patients with human immunodeficiency virus infection. Am J Respir Crit Care Med 1994; 150:1499–1502.

Moulding T, Dutt AK, Reichman LB. Fixed dose combination of antituberculosis medications to prevent drug resistance—a perspective. Ann Intern Med 1995; 122:951–954.

Weiss SE, Slocum PC, Blais FX, et al. The effect of directly observed therapy on the rates of drug resistance and relapse in tuberculosis. N Engl J Med 1994; 330:1179–1184.

VARICELLA-ZOSTER VIRUS

John A. Zaia, M.D.

Varicella-zoster virus (VZV) is one of the seven known herpesviruses of man, and is the cause of chickenpox (varicella) and shingles (zoster). Chickenpox, the exanthem caused by primary infection with VZV, usually occurs in children. Shingles, the clinical syndrome of segmental exanthem and pain due to reactivation of latent VZV infection, usually occurs many years after the primary infection. In the immunodeficient person both primary and reactivated VZV infection can lead to severe generalized virus dissemination, the life-threatening form of VZV infection. The availability of antiviral agents for management of VZV infection has raised the importance of recognizing this infection in high-risk groups. It is estimated that approximately 3.7 million cases of chickenpox occur each year, 83 percent in children under age 9 years. There are 300,000 cases of herpes zoster in the United States per year, and the incidence is constant for each age group through mid-adulthood. Thereafter the incidence of zoster increases with age; persons age 80 and above have a 1:100 chance per year of developing shingles.

■ CLINICAL PRESENTATION

Chickenpox

In healthy children, VZV infection manifests as a vesicular exanthem often associated with prodromal malaise, pharyngitis, rhinitis, and abdominal pain. At the median, the rash appears 15 days after VZV exposure; the range is 10 to 21 days. The vesicular eruption emerges in successive crops over the first 3 to 4 days of illness, usually with concomitant enanthem. Each skin vesicle appears on an erythematous base, resulting in the descriptive image of a dew drop on a rose petal. This stage of infection may be missed because of rupture of the vesicle, which then undergoes inflammatory changes and crusting. The exanthem usually begins on the head and quickly progresses to the trunk, arms, and finally the legs. It is common to see all stages of the exanthem, including macules, vesicles, papules, and crusts, in the same region of the skin, and this should be looked for in the examination of the patient. Fever can be expected for the first 3 to 4 days of the exanthem, and much of the morbidity is associated with the extent of the cutaneous rash. In addition, primary VZV infection invades the mucosal surfaces of respiratory, alimentary, and genitourinary systems, and the patient with chickenpox can have severe laryngitis, laryngotracheobronchitis, vaginitis, urethritis, pancreatitis, and enteritis. Severe abdominal pain or back pain is a hallmark of progressive VZV infection in the immunocompromised individual.

The rate of complications is highest in persons under 1 year old and over 15 years old. The complications that lead to hospitalization in VZV infection consist of bacterial superinfection of skin, dehydration, pneumonia, encephalitis, and hepatitis. Bacterial skin infections and bacterial pneumonias occur in the youngest groups, and before the antibiotic era severe bacterial infections, including osteomyelitis, were fairly common in association with chickenpox. Encephalitis occurs in approximately 1:11,000 cases in the age group 5 to 14 years. Reye's syndrome, once a concern in VZV infection, has become very uncommon because of the recommendation against aspirin use. With the availability of acyclovir and of varicella-zoster immunoglobulin (VZIG), VZV-associated mortality has decreased to fewer than 100 deaths per year in the United States.

Shingles

Shingles occurs when VZV infection reactivates in cranial or spinal nerve ganglia and then spreads to the cutaneous nerves. The clinical presentation and major complications of this disease derive from the neural origin of the virus infection. The most common area of involvement is the trunk, presumably because this is the area of greatest primary infection, followed by cranial dermatomes and then by cervical and lumbar dermatomes. Thus, shingles presents with pain and with a vesicular eruption in a unilateral cutaneous distribution. Pain alone, called zoster sine herpete, can be the only symptom of this disease. The pain of herpes zoster that persists after the healing of skin lesions is termed postherpetic neuralgia. This problem increases in frequency with age and is a major problem in patients over 50 years old. Virus reactivation in the spinal or cranial nerve ganglia causes intense inflammation with hemorrhagic necrosis of nerve cells, eventual destruction of portions of the ganglion, poliomyelitis of posterior spinal columns, and leptomeningitis. This intense inflammation results in nerve dysfunction manifested clinically by meningitis and myelitis, with or without paresis at sites of involved nerves. Thus, there may be weakness or paralysis of limbs, of facial muscles, and of muscles within abdominal viscera. In addition, intense inflammation of the cutaneous site of infection results in scarring of the involved epidermis. This is a particular concern when the cornea or other ophthalmic structures are involved.

■ DIAGNOSIS

The history and physical examination remain the primary methods for diagnosing chickenpox and shingles. In chickenpox, look for lesions in all stages of development, including macules, vesicles, pustules, and crusted lesions. The rash of chickenpox can be mistaken for a diverse array of entities, such as rashes due to herpes simplex virus, Coxsackie and other enteroviruses, mycoplasma, streptococcal impetigo, rickettsialpox, insect bites, and delayed-type hypersensitivity reactions such as poison ivy. In certain individuals, especially those at high risk for complications of VZV infection, specific diagnosis can be pursued by laboratory methods. The most rapid and accurate method is the direct immunofluorescent stain of a skin scraping for VZV antigen using a commercially available kit. The Tzanck prep, a method to demonstrate multinucleated giant cells in skin scrapings stained with Wright-Giemsa, has been superseded by this fluorescent antigen detection assay when the latter technique is available. Conventional methods of culture of VZV or serology for VZV antibody can also be used to confirm the diagnosis, but these are rarely necessary.

■ DETECTION OF SUSCEPTIBILITY TO VZV

The simplest method of reliably ruling out susceptibility to chickenpox is to obtain a history of chickenpox or of having cared for children with it. A positive history from adults has a 97 to 99 percent correlation with serologic confirmation. A negative history from an adult fails to conform to a negative serologic status in 72 to 93 percent. Therefore, serologic tests are necessary to determine whether a person with a negative history has been infected with VZV. Commercial assays, fluorescent or enzyme-linked immunoassays, and a very rapid latex agglutination assay are very reliable except in persons who have received blood products and have acquired passive antibody.

■ THERAPY

Chickenpox

Overall Assessment

The goal in management is to treat the symptoms of primary VZV infection and to prevent complications if possible. A flow chart describing an approach is shown in Figure 1. The three stages of management are (1) establishing the likelihood of the diagnosis; (2) determining whether antiviral therapy is indicated; and (3) ruling out secondary bacterial infection, other complications, and failure of antiviral treatment. In children chickenpox usually requires minimal medical attention, but if there is an atypical course or severe skin involvement, the patient should have a physical examination to assess the level of hydration, the need for temperature control, the baseline mental status, and other physical findings that suggest complications.

Symptomatic Therapy

Itching is the major symptom of chickenpox, and antipyretic management is important. Warm baths containing baking soda (⅓ cup per bathtub) or emulsified oatmeal (Aveeno) can temporarily relieve pruritus. This can be combined with the oral administration of either diphenhydramine (Benadryl) 1.25 mg per kilogram by mouth every 6 hours or hydroxyzine (Atarax, Vistaril) 0.5 mg per kilogram by mouth every 6 hours. In older children, cold pramoxine HCl 1 percent lotion with calamine 8 percent (Caladryl) can be used, but this should be avoided in infants because of the risk of excessive surface exposure and absorption of drug or vehicle (alcohol 2.2 percent). Fever should be controlled with acetaminophen and *salicylates should not be used* because administration of salicylates to children with chickenpox increases the risk of subsequent Reye's syndrome. A warning against the use of ibuprofen in children with chickenpox has been made in certain parts of the United States because of an association of ibuprofen with severe streptococcal infection. For severe dysuria, a cold compress on the genital area during urination will ease the pain and minimize the likelihood of a functional bladder obstruction.

Antiviral Therapy

Acyclovir (Zovirax) is the only agent licensed in the United States for the treatment of chickenpox. It is indicated for treatment of chickenpox in certain normal persons, for disseminated VZV infection in immunosuppressed persons, and for treatment of shingles (later section). Oral acyclovir should be used in otherwise healthy persons with chickenpox who are at risk for moderate to severe disease, such as those older than 12 years, those with chronic cutaneous or pulmonary disorders, those receiving chronic salicylate therapy, and persons receiving short or intermittent courses of corticosteroids or aerosolized corticosteroids (Table 1). The American Academy of Pediatrics (AAP) does not recommend that otherwise normal children under age 12 receive oral acyclovir for chickenpox. However, studies have shown that treatment of chickenpox within 24 hours of the onset of rash reduces the

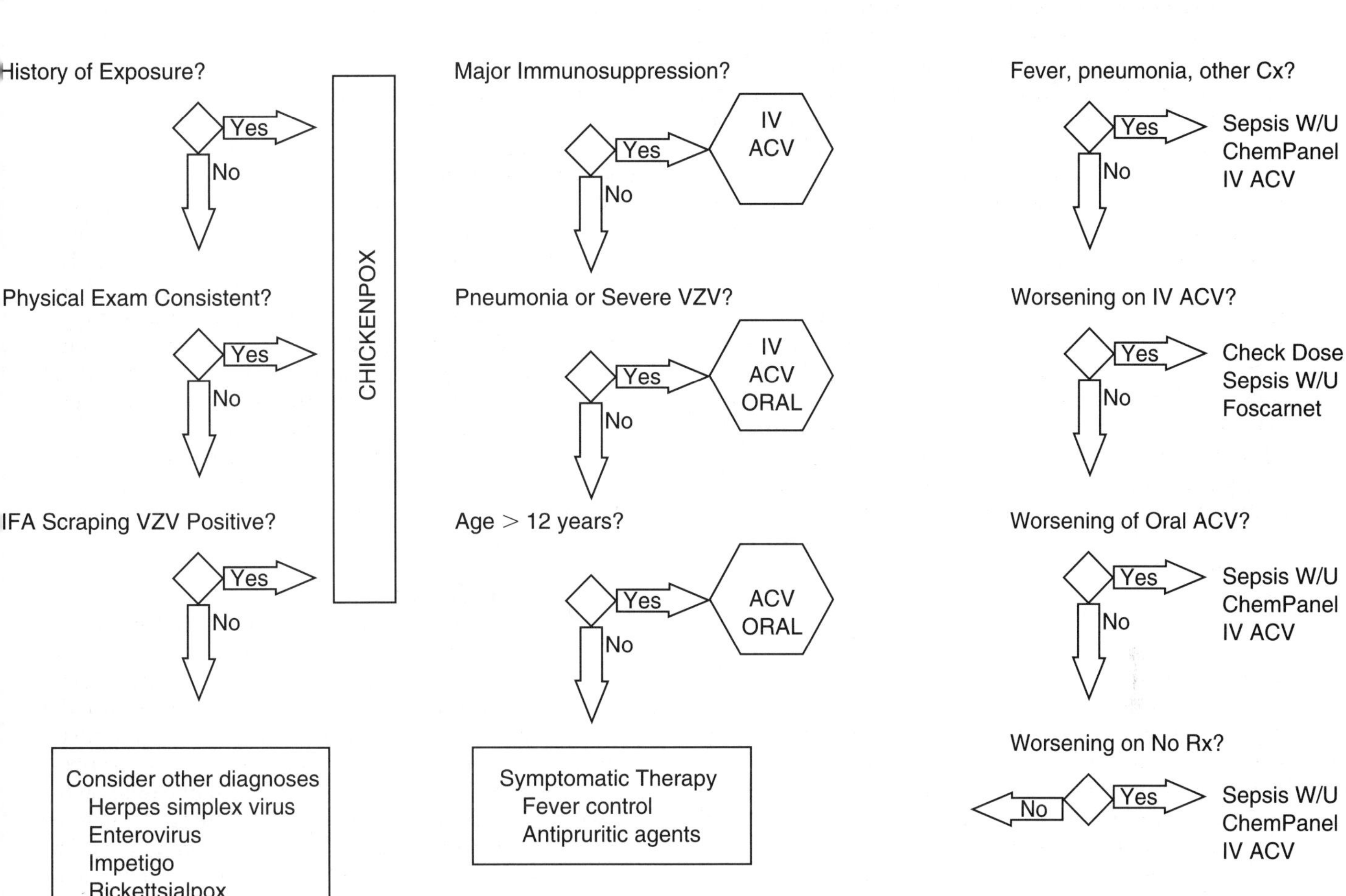

Figure 1
Algorithm for the management of chickenpox. IV, intravenous; ACV, acyclovir; Cx, complications; W/U, work-up; IFA, immunofluorescent antibody.

duration and magnitude of fever and the number and duration of skin lesions. Therefore, some experts recommend using oral acyclovir in secondary household cases because disease is usually more severe in these children. The data are insufficient regarding the safety and efficacy of acyclovir therapy for infants less than age 12 months, and it is not recommended.

All adults with chickenpox should receive oral acyclovir, and those with rapidly progressive infection should be treated with intravenous acyclovir. All immunosuppressed persons with chickenpox should be treated with intravenous acyclovir, since there is inadequate experience with the oral formulation. However, as noted by the AAP, some experts have used oral acyclovir in highly selected immunocompromised persons who are at relatively low risk for developing complications and in whom follow-up is assured. Case-by-case evaluation of risks versus benefits is necessary, but for many groups the risk of disseminating infection is sufficiently high and so unpredictable that intravenous treatment should be recommended in nearly all cases. Acyclovir should not be used by exposed persons in an attempt to prevent chickenpox. It should be considered for the pregnant patient at risk for serious complications of varicella, but oral acyclovir is not recommended for routine use by the pregnant woman with uncomplicated chickenpox, since the risk and benefits to the fetus and mother are mostly unknown. VZIg is licensed for use in high-risk individuals at the time of exposure to VZV infection but is not recommended for treatment of chickenpox.

Bacterial Infections

Pyoderma is the most frequently observed bacterial complication of varicella. It can be minimized by attention to good hygiene, including daily bathing with bacteriostatic soap, trimming of children's fingernails to minimize excoriation of itchy skin, and early recognition of superinfection. Streptococcal and staphylococcal bacterial infections can be associated with bacteremia and subsequent osteomyelitis, with scarlet fever, and with bacterial synergetic gangrene. Therefore, aggressive management of bacterial infection is warranted.

Table 1 Antiviral Treatment of VZV Infection

AGENT	INDICATION	CREATININE CLEARANCE (ML/MIN/1.73 M²)	DOSE	DOSING INTERVAL	DURATION (DAYS)
Oral acyclovir	Chickpox >age 12 yrs	>25	20 mg/kg up to 800 mg	q6h	5
	Shingles	10–25	Same	q8h	5
		0–10*	Same	q12h	5
IV acyclovir	Life-threatening VZV infection	>50	500 mg/M² or 10 mg/kg†‡	q8h	7
		25–50	Same	q12h	7
		10–25	Same	q24h	7
		0–10*	250 mg/M²	q24h	7
Famyciclovir	Shingles >age 18	>60	500 mg	q8h	7
		40–59	500 mg	q12h	7
		20–39	500 mg	q24h	7
Foscarnet	Acyclovir-resistant VZV§	>100‖	60 mg/kg	q8h	7–10

See package insert for recommended dose adjustment of all drugs.
*An additional dose is recommended after each hemodialysis treatment.
†To minimize renal toxicity an adequate urine output is required. This can be assured if the acyclovir is infused at a concentration of approximately 4 mg/ml over 1 hour and the same volume of fluid is given over the next hour.
‡Use ideal body weight for height to calculate dose in obese persons; M^2, square meter of body surface area.
§Foscarnet is recommended by experts for treatment of life-threatening acyclovir-resistant VZV infection, but this is not an FDA-approved indication for foscarnet use. Appropriate informed consent should be obtained before such use.
‖Foscarnet is nephrotoxic, and dosage should be based on creatinine clearance. Guidelines for dosage adjustment are listed in the package information.

Respiratory Tract Infection

In addition to the occasional laryngitis and laryngotracheobronchitis that can occur during chickenpox, bacterial superinfection can affect the lower respiratory tract, producing pneumonia and bronchitis. Pneumonia is most often due to the usual respiratory pathogens, including *Streptococcus pneumoniae, Haemophilus influenzae,* and *Staphylococcus aureus.* Viral pneumonia is more likely to be a problem in older persons with chickenpox.

Gastrointestinal Complications

When death occurs during VZV infection, the gastrointestinal tract is invariably involved. Specific attention must be given to bleeding, particularly in the immunosuppressed person. Vomiting is not a usual part of the clinical course of this infection, and it should alert the physician to look for abdominal or central nervous system (CNS) complications. Also, surgical emergencies such as appendicitis and intussusception can occur during varicella. Mild hepatitis is seen in a majority of children with chickenpox, usually asymptomatic elevation of hepatic enzymes for which no treatment is necessary. However, elevation of serum or urinary amylase indicates pancreatitis, which may require supportive treatment. As noted, the concomitant use of aspirin in the child with chickenpox has been associated with an increased incidence of Reye's syndrome. Although this is rare today, Reye's syndrome and other metabolic diseases must be excluded in any child with varicella in whom there is vomiting and changes in mental status.

Encephalitis

Cerebral complications may be either cerebral or cerebellar abnormalities; the latter is a more benign disease. Cerebellar ataxia, the most common syndrome associated with varicella encephalitis, is generally a benign entity thought to be due to postinfectious demyelination. There is no evidence that acyclovir treatment is necessary in postchickenpox cerebellitis, but it is prudent to include antiviral therapy in any cerebral presentation of VZV infection, especially if it may be associated with continued viral replication such as in AIDS or other immunosuppression.

Bleeding Disorders

Bleeding disorders during chickenpox are due to disseminated intravascular coagulation, vasculitis, or idiopathic thrombocytopenic purpura (ITP), which can occur during active infection or convalescence. It responds to conventional treatment for ITP.

Immunosuppressed Patients

Acyclovir is the only indicated drug for the treatment of VZV infections in the immunosuppressed patient, whether disseminated chickenpox, disseminated shingles, or localized shingles. Three other commercial antiviral drugs, vidarabine (ViraA), famciclovir (Famvir), and foscarnet (Foscavir) have activity against VZV. It has been shown in comparative studies of vidarabine and acyclovir for the treatment of zoster in immunocompromised patients that acyclovir produces a more complete clinical and antiviral response, and there is almost no indication for use of vidarabine in the treatment of VZV. Vidarabine has been used for acyclovir-resistant VZV infection, but usually only as an alternative to foscarnet. Famciclovir is not licensed for the treatment of acute zoster in immunosuppressed persons.

Shingles

Overall Assessment

The major complication of shingles is postherpetic pain. For this reason effective analgesic medication must be a principal part of treatment, and the initial assessment should be directed to a determination of general medical status and tolerance for narcotic-based therapy. In addition, there is increasing evidence that early antiviral therapy can lessen late neuralgia, and therefore, institution of specific anti-VZV agents is important in certain patients.

Symptomatic Therapy

A hallmark of shingles is intense inflammation, and the cutaneous site of disease can take weeks to heal. The patient or caretaker should be instructed to have daily soaks with salt solutions and dressing changes to minimize bacterial infection and speed healing. If the eye is involved, an ophthalmologist should be consulted for use of topical anti-inflammatory or antiviral medication and for long-term evaluation. Management of pain will vary from patient to patient, but it usually begins with acetaminophen-codeine combinations and increases to more potent analgesia if indicated. In severe postherpetic neuralgia, if there is no response to conventional pain management, tricyclic antidepressant medications such as amitriptyline (Elavil) can be tried, although this is not an indicated use. Local nerve block should be used in refractory pain. Topical pain medications are not recommended, since the source of pain stimulation is central.

Use of corticosteroids in the acute phase of disease remains controversial, but a recent controlled study indicated no effect of steroids combined with acyclovir compared with acyclovir alone on postherpetic pain. However, steroids plus acyclovir produced earlier healing and less pain in the initial 2 weeks of shingles. There were more side effects with steroid use, and therefore, the routine use of steroids for shingles cannot be recommended. It is possible that early treatment with antivirals alone can significantly reduce late postherpetic pain, and at present this must be the focus of initial therapy.

Antiviral Therapy

Both acyclovir and famciclovir are licensed in the United States for the treatment of shingles in otherwise normal persons (see Table 1). Acyclovir is the agent of choice for immunocompromised persons and is the only intravenous agent available for treatment of shingles. Famciclovir is an oral prodrug of the antiviral agent penciclovir, which has potent activity against VZV and undergoes rapid biotransformation to the active antiviral compound. Safety and efficacy in children under age 18 years has not been established. Also, because of the potential for tumorigenicity in rats, the drug should not be given to nursing mothers unless nursing is discontinued. Treatment should be given to those over age 50 years because this population is at greatest risk for postherpetic neuralgia, and the decision to treat adults less than age 50 with antiviral agents should be made on individual assessment. Except for administration of famciclovir three rather than four times per day, as for acyclovir, there is little to recommend famciclovir until there is more experience with its use.

Exposure to VZV

The spread of infectious VZV from a person with chickenpox is by air droplets from nasopharyngeal secretions, which usually requires face-to-face exposure indoors for an hour but can also be via air currents to susceptible individuals without direct contact. The period of respiratory infectivity is generally considered to begin 48 hours prior to the onset of exanthem and to continue for 4 days after onset. In addition, the vesicular fluid can spread the virus by direct contact, so infectivity by contact with skin lesions is possible until they are crusted. Shingles can also spread by direct contact or by exposure to airborne infectious material. The incubation period for chickenpox following exposure to shingles is the same as for exposure to chickenpox—15 days, range 10 to 21 days. The clinical varicella attack rate in susceptible children on household exposure to chickenpox is approximately 90 percent, and is 25 percent on exposure to household shingles.

Table 2 Groups at Risk for Complications of VZV Infection*

Susceptible persons on immunosuppressive therapy†
Persons with congenital cellular immunodeficiency
Persons with an acquired immunodeficiency, including AIDS
Persons over age 20 years
Newborn infants exposed to onset of maternal varicella less than 5 days before or 2 to 7 days after birth
Premature infants weighing less than 1 kilogram‡

*Susceptible (antibody negative) persons exposed to VZV by indoor face-to-face contact with an infected person less than 2 days before or anytime during vesiculopustular stage of chickenpox are at highest risk and should receive VZIG.
†All cytoreductive and radiotherapy is considered immunosuppressive. The immunosuppressive dose of prednisone equivalent can vary in individual cases but is in the range of 1 to 2 mg per kilogram per day.
‡The risk of complications of VZV infection in this group, which is poorly defined, is based on the likelihood of protective maternal antibody versus gestational age at birth.

Immunocompromised Host Exposed to VZV

Until the VZV vaccine became available in the United States, the only protection from VZV infection was passive immunization at the time of exposure. Even now families and school personnel must continue to be aware of exposure to VZV in high-risk persons so that VZIG can be administered within 96 hours. Any susceptible person at risk for complications of VZV (Table 2) should receive passive immunization if exposure was adequate to communicate disease and occurred within approximately 4 days after rash. Adequacy of exposure is defined as indoor face-to-face exposure for 1 hour with a person during the infectious phase. VZIG should not be used in any person with a history of chickenpox except persons who have undergone bone marrow transplantation. Immunosuppressive therapy should be stopped during the incubation period, although this precaution is waived if the underlying disease requires continued treatment, such as initial therapy for acute leukemia.

Adults Exposed to VZV

More than 90 percent of adults have had VZV, and although reinfection occurs after exposure to chickenpox, these persons do not usually develop disease, although some cutaneous lesions can occur. Susceptible adults are at risk for life-threatening chickenpox, and they are the source of unexpected epidemics. One adult population known to have a high rate of susceptibility to chickenpox is immigrants from subtropical climates. Serologic tests of susceptibility should be considered in any such immigrants working in a health care setting. The decision to use VZIG in susceptible healthy adults following close exposure to VZV should be made on an individual basis, taking into consideration the person's health, the type of exposure, and the likelihood of previous chickenpox.

Nosocomial VZV

Control of nosocomial infections requires three actions: (1) routine continuous surveillance of VZV susceptibility among hospital staff, with VZV vaccination as indicated; (2) adequate isolation of contagious VZV infections; and (3) rapid evaluation of and response to exposure. Hospitals that care for immunodeficient children should screen staff at the time of employment for susceptibility. This can be done efficiently by performing antibody tests on those who have a negative or unknown history of chickenpox. Susceptible employees should be excluded from care of patients with VZV infection. Exposed susceptible health care workers should be furloughed from the tenth day after initial exposure until 21 days after the last exposure.

If the VZV exposure is from a patient, he or she should be discharged if possible. If not, the patient should be placed in isolation designed to prevent spread of infection by both air and direct contact. Optimally this consists of a private room with negative air pressure relative to the corridor, with gown and glove precaution guidelines posted on the door and restricted entry for susceptible persons. Isolation should remain in effect until skin lesions are crusted.

After control of the source of infection, there comes quick assessment of three types of information: (1) the nature of the exposure and whether it is likely to result in secondary infections; (2) which of the exposed patients or staff are susceptible; and (3) which patients are at risk for complications. Thus, the initial step is to define the hospital areas in which a definitive VZV exposure occurred and then to focus on which patients in these areas are at risk for infection. Once susceptibility or positive history of varicella is determined and serologic evaluation of those with ambiguous or negative history is done, all susceptible patients who are exposed should be discharged if possible. Those remaining in the hospital should be placed in respiratory isolation between days 8 and 21 post exposure, or for 8 to 28 days for those receiving VZIG. Those remaining in the hospital without exposure should be placed in a cohort that protects them from exposures.

Management of the Pregnant Woman

A syndrome of congenital varicella consisting of low birth weight, cutaneous scarring, limb hypoplasia, microcephaly, and other brain and eye abnormalities can occur in the baby of a pregnant woman who has chickenpox, but not shingles. Teratogenic damage results only from first- and second-trimester infection, and clinically apparent disease occurs only in approximately 2 percent of infants born after maternal varicella in early pregnancy. For this reason experts advise that maternal chickenpox is not a medical indication for abortion. There is no reliable diagnostic method, including amniocentesis and ultrasound, for determining teratogenic intrauterine infection.

It is recommended that after exposure in pregnancy susceptibility be determined and that the susceptible person be given VZIG.

Varicella Vaccine

A live, attenuated VZV vaccine (Varivax) was approved in the United States in 1995 and is recommended for all healthy, chickenpox-negative persons older than age 12 months. In addition to normal children, it is particularly recommended for eligible health care and day care workers, college students, prisoners, military recruits, nonpregnant women of child-bearing age, and international travelers. After a single dose in children less than age 12 years and two doses one month apart in older persons, protection from chickenpox can be expected in more than 94%. The vaccine is not recommended for infants less than 1 year old, for immunosuppressed persons, for those on salicylate therapy, for pregnant women, nor for those allergic to components of the vaccine, including neomycin, gelatin, and monosodium glutamate.

Suggested Reading

Balfour HH Jr, Kelly JM, Suarez CS, et al. Acyclovir treatment of varicella in otherwise healthy children. J Pediatr 1990; 116:633–639.

Enders G, Miller E, Cradock-Watson J, et al. Consequences of varicella and herpes zoster in pregnancy: Prospective study of 1739 cases. Lancet 1994; 343:1548–1551.

Preblud SR. Age-specific risks of varicella complications. Pediatrics 1981; 68:14–17.

Prevention of varicella: Supplement to Morbid Mortal Wkly Rep. 45: pp. 11, July, 1996.

Wallace MR, Bowler WA, Murray NB, et al. Treatment of adult varicella with oral acyclovir: A randomized, placebo-controlled trial. Ann Intern Med 1993; 117:358–363.

Wood MJ, Johnson RW, McKendrick MW, et al. A randomized trial of acyclovir for 7 days or 21 days with and without prednisolone for treatment of acute herpes zoster. N Engl J Med 1994; 330:896–905.

Zaia JA, Grose C. Varicella and herpes zoster. In: Gorbach SL, Bartlett JG, Blacklow NR, eds. Infectious diseases. Philadelphia: WB Saunders, 1992:1101.

HERPES SIMPLEX VIRUSES

David W. Kimberlin, M.D.
Richard J. Whitley, M.D.

Herpesviruses are generally defined as large enveloped virions with an icosahedral nucleocapsid consisting invariably of 162 capsomeres arranged around a double-stranded DNA core. The two antigenically distinct types of herpes simplex virus (HSV) are HSV-1 and HSV-2. Considerable homology exists between the HSV-1 and HSV-2 genomes, with most of the polypeptides specified by one viral type being antigenically related to polypeptides of the other viral type. While this results in considerable cross-reactivity between the HSV-1 and HSV-2 glycoproteins (g), unique antigenic determinants exist for each virus (e.g., gG-1 and gG-2). Surrounding the viral genome and nucleocapsid is a tightly adherent membrane, the tegument. A lipid envelope containing the viral glycoproteins loosely surrounds the tegument.

PATHOLOGY AND PATHOGENESIS

Cutaneous HSV infection causes ballooning of infected epithelial cells, with nuclear degeneration and loss of intact cellular membranes. Infected epithelial cells either lyse or fuse to form multinucleated giant cells. With cell lysis, clear fluid containing large quantities of virus, cellular debris, and inflammatory cells accumulates between the epidermal and dermal layers. Multinucleated giant cells are usually present at the base of the vesicle. An intense inflammatory response extends from the base of the vesicle into the dermis. As the lesions heal, vesicular fluid becomes purulent as more inflammatory cells are recruited to the site of infection. Scab formation then follows. Scarring is uncommon.

When infection involves mucous membranes, shallow ulcers are more common than vesicles due to rapid rupture of the very thin cornified epithelium at mucosal sites. Nevertheless, the histopathologic findings of mucosal lesions are similar to those of skin lesions.

EPIDEMIOLOGY

HSV-1 is found most commonly in the oropharynx, although any organ system can be involved. Factors that influence the frequency of primary HSV-1 infection include geographic location, socioeconomic status, and age. Throughout childhood and adolescence, African-Americans maintain approximately twice the prevalence of HSV-1 antibodies as white children, with 40 percent of African-American children being seropositive for HSV-1 by 5 years of age. By age 60 years, however, both African-Americans and whites have a similarly high prevalence of HSV-1 antibody (up to 90 percent).

Recurrences of herpes labialis have been associated with physical or emotional stress, fever, exposure to ultraviolet light, tissue damage, and immunosuppression. As with primary infections, recurrent disease may occur in the absence of clinical symptoms. At any given time, 1 percent of normal children and 1 to 5 percent of normal adults asymptomatically excrete HSV-1.

HSV-2 causes 85 to 95 percent of genital HSV infections in the United States. As would be expected, antibodies to this virus are rarely found prior to the onset of sexual activity. Among adolescents and adults, factors that correlate with seroprevalence for HSV-2 include sex (higher for women than for men), race (higher for African-Americans than for whites), marital status (higher for persons previously married than for single or married persons), and income (the lower the income, the higher the prevalence).

The propensity for recurrence of genital HSV infection depends on a variety of factors, including sex (more frequent in men), viral type (more frequent with HSV-2), and the presence and titer of neutralizing antibodies (more frequent in the presence of high neutralizing antibody titers). Overall, 60 to 90 percent of patients with primary genital HSV-2 infection have clinically apparent recurrence of infection.

CLINICAL MANIFESTATIONS

Oropharyngeal HSV Infection

Primary oropharyngeal infection with HSV-1 occurs most commonly in children between 1 and 3 years of age. It is usually asymptomatic. The incubation period ranges from 2 to 12 days, with an average of 4 days. Symptomatic disease is characterized by fever to 40°C (104°F), oral lesions, sore throat, fetor oris, anorexia, cervical adenopathy, and mucosal edema. Oral lesions initially are vesicular but rapidly rupture, leaving 1 to 3 mm shallow gray-white ulcers on erythematous bases. These lesions are distributed on the hard palate, the anterior portion of the tongue, along the gingiva, and around the lips (Fig. 1). In addition, the lesions may extend down the chin and neck due to drooling. Total duration of illness is 10 to 21 days.

Primary infection in young adults has been associated with pharyngitis and, often, with a mononucleosis-like syndrome. In such patients, ulcerative lesions on erythematous bases frequently appear on the tonsils.

Primary gingivostomatitis results in viral shedding in oral secretions for an average of 7 to 10 days. Virus can be isolated from the saliva of asymptomatic children and adults. Virus is also shed in the stool.

Recurrent orolabial HSV lesions are frequently preceded by a prodrome of pain, burning, tingling, or itching. These symptoms generally last for less than 6 hours and are followed within 24 to 48 hours by painful vesicles, typically at the vermilion border of the lip (Fig. 2). Lesions usually crust within 3 to 4 days, and healing is complete within 8 to 10 days. Recurrences occur only rarely in the mouth or on the skin of the face of immunocompetent patients.

Genital HSV Infection

Genital HSV-2 disease is usually acquired by sexual contact with an infected partner. The incubation period of primary disease ranges from 2 to 12 days. Lesions persist for an

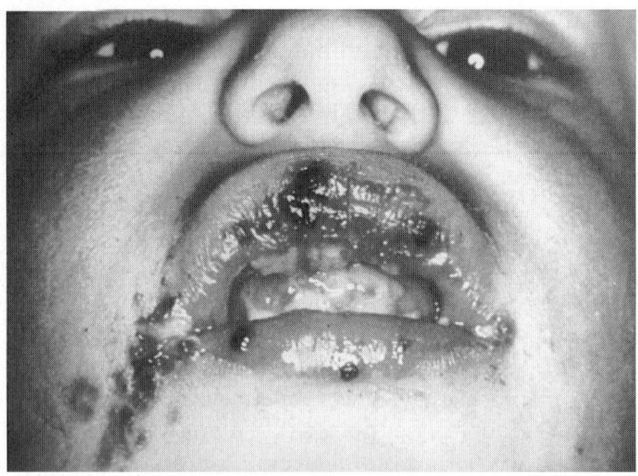

Figure 1
Herpes simplex gingivostomatitis. *(From Whitley RJ, Gnann JW. The epidemiology and clinical manifestations of herpes simplex virus infections. In: Roizman B, Whitley RJ, Lopez C, eds. The human herpesviruses. New York: Raven Press, 1993: 69; with permission.)*

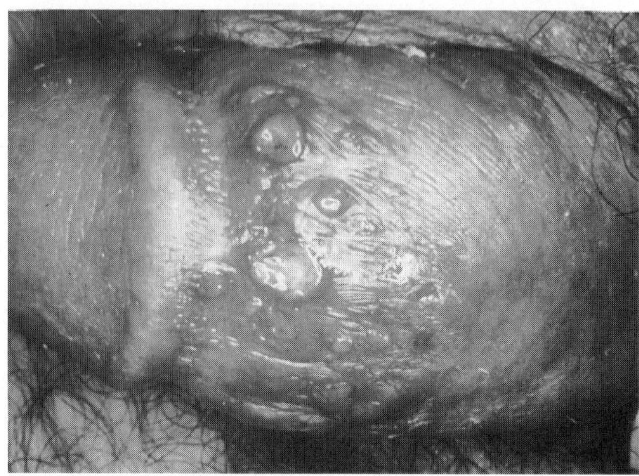

Figure 3
Primary genital HSV infection in men. *(From Whitley RJ, Gnann JW. The epidemiology and clinical manifestations of herpes simplex virus infections. In: Roizman B, Whitley RJ, Lopez C, eds. The human herpesviruses. New York: Raven Press, 1993:69; with permission.)*

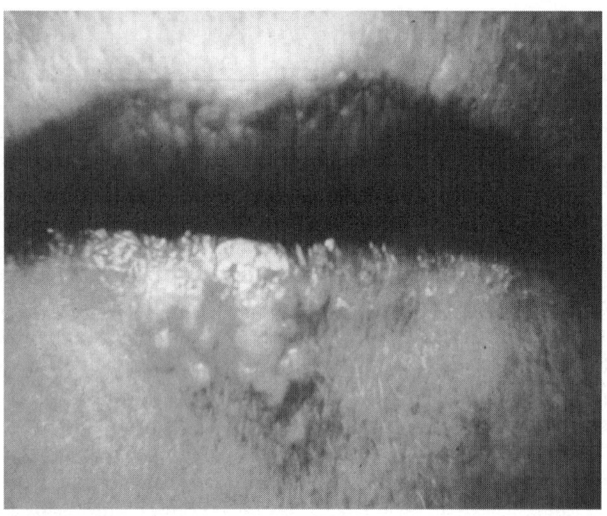

Figure 2
Recurrent herpes simplex labialis. *(From Whitley RJ, Gnann JW. The epidemiology and clinical manifestations of herpes simplex virus infections. In: Roizman B, Whitley RJ, Lopez C, eds. The human herpesviruses. New York: Raven Press, 1993:69; with permission.)*

average of 21 days. In 70 percent of patients, primary infections are associated with fever, malaise, myalgias, inguinal adenopathy, and other signs and symptoms of systemic illness. Complications include extragenital lesions, aseptic meningitis, and sacral autonomic nervous system dysfunction with associated urinary retention. Women tend to have more severe primary infections and are more likely to develop complications than men.

In men, primary genital HSV infection usually manifests as a cluster of vesicular lesions on erythematous bases on the glans or shaft of the penis (Fig. 3). In women, primary genital HSV lesions usually involve the vulva bilaterally (Fig. 4). Concomitant HSV cervicitis occurs in 90 percent of women with primary HSV-2 infection of the external genitalia. In women, the lesions rapidly ulcerate and become covered with a gray-white exudate. Such lesions may be exquisitely painful.

Recurrent genital HSV-2 infection can be either symptomatic or asymptomatic. A prodrome of itching, burning, tingling, or tenderness may be noted several hours prior to a recurrence. The duration of recurrent disease is shorter (7 to 10 days) and fewer lesions are present than with primary disease. In men, lesions usually appear on the glans or shaft of the penis. In women, lesions occur most frequently on the labia minora, labia majora, and perineum. Cervical excretion of HSV occurs in 10 percent of women with recurrent genital lesions. Systemic symptoms are uncommon in recurrent genital HSV disease.

Other Primary HSV Skin Infections

Alteration in the barrier properties of skin, as occurs in atopic dermatitis, can result in localized HSV skin infection (eczema herpeticum). Most cases resolve over 7 to 9 days without specific therapy. Localized cutaneous HSV infection following trauma is known as herpes gladiatorum (wrestler's herpes, or traumatic herpes).

HSV infection of the digits results in herpetic whitlow. Such lesions may be the result of autoinoculation, as in the case of infants, or exogenous exposure, as occurs among medical and dental personnel.

Ocular HSV Infection

Herpetic infection of the eye usually presents as either a blepharitis or a follicular conjunctivitis. As disease progresses,

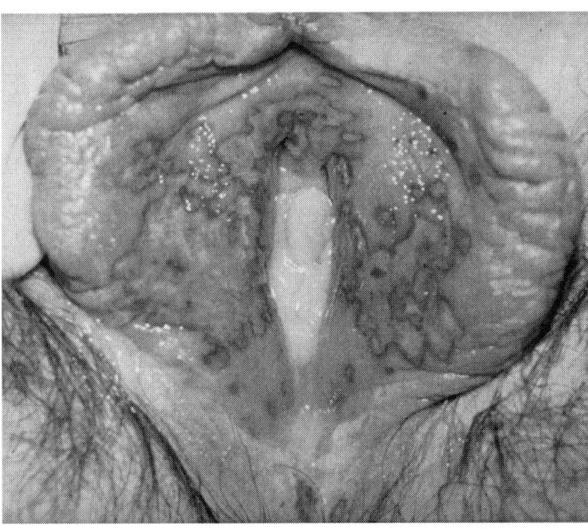
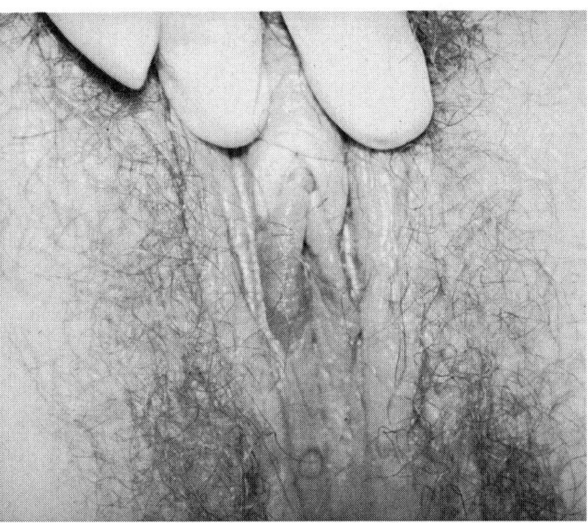

Figure 4
Genital HSV infection in women. *(From Whitley RJ, Gnann JW. The epidemiology and clinical manifestations of herpes simplex virus infections. In: Roizman B, Whitley RJ, Lopez C, eds. The human herpesviruses. New York: Raven Press, 1993: 69; with permission.)*

branching dendritic lesions develop. Symptoms include severe photophobia, tearing, chemosis, blurred vision, and preauricular lymphadenopathy. An ophthalmologist should always be involved in the care of such patients.

Central Nervous System HSV Infection

Central nervous system (CNS) signs and symptoms of HSV disease can begin suddenly or can follow a 1 to 7 day period of nonspecific influenza-like symptoms. Prominent CNS features include headache, fever, behavioral disturbances, speech disorders, altered consciousness, and focal neurologic findings such as focal seizures.

Neonatal HSV Infections

Neonatal HSV infection can be classified as: (1) disease localized to the skin, eye, and/or mouth (SEM); (2) encephalitis, with or without SEM involvement; and (3) disseminated infection that involves multiple organs including the CNS, lung, gastrointestinal tract, liver, adrenals, skin, eye, and/or mouth. Infants with HSV disease are divided roughly evenly among these three categories. Infants with disseminated and SEM disease usually require medical attention within the first 2 weeks of life, and infants with disease localized to the CNS usually present between the second and third weeks of life. Presenting signs and symptoms can include any combination of irritability, seizures (both focal and generalized), lethargy, tremors, poor feeding, temperature instability, bulging fontanelle, respiratory distress, jaundice, disseminated intravascular coagulopathy, shock, and cutaneous vesicles. More than 20 percent of infants with disseminated disease and 30 to 40 percent of infants with encephalitis never have skin vesicles during the course of illness.

HSV in the Immunocompromised Host

Patients compromised by immunosuppressive therapy, underlying disease, or malnutrition are at increased risk for severe HSV infection. Disseminated disease may occur with widespread dermal, mucosal, and visceral involvement. Alternatively, disease may remain localized but persist much longer than in immunocompetent hosts.

■ DIAGNOSIS

Serologic diagnosis of HSV infection has no great clinical value, largely because current commercial serologic assays cannot distinguish between HSV-1 and HSV-2. Isolation of HSV by culture remains the definitive diagnostic method. If skin lesions are present, a scraping of the vesicles should be transferred in an appropriate viral transport medium on ice to a diagnostic virology laboratory. Other sites from which virus may be isolated include the cerebrospinal fluid, urine, throat, nasopharynx, conjunctivae, and duodenum. Intranuclear inclusions and multinucleated giant cells on a Tzanck prep suggest but are not diagnostic for HSV infection.

In HSV encephalitis, CSF findings are variable, but they frequently include a moderate pleocytosis with a predominance of mononuclear cells, elevated protein level, and normal or slightly decreased glucose. The electroencephalogram (EEG) generally localizes spike and slow wave activity to the temporal lobe, even when obtained very early in the disease. Computed tomography (CT) of the brain may initially be normal or reveal only edema, but as the disease progresses, it can demonstrate temporal lobe involvement as well. Detection of HSV DNA by polymerase chain reaction (PCR) will likely prove very helpful in confirming this diagnosis in the future.

■ THERAPY

Herpes Labialis

Topical acyclovir is not efficacious treatment for orolabial herpes lesions. Oral acyclovir 400 mg five times daily for 5 days reduces duration of pain and time to the loss of crusts by about one-third, but only if treatment is started during the

Table 1 Antiviral Therapy in Herpes Simplex Virus Infections

TYPE OF INFECTION	DRUG	ROUTE AND DOSAGE*	COMMENTS
Genital HSV			
Initial episode	Acyclovir	200 mg PO 5 times/day × 10 days	Preferred route in normal host
		5 mg/kg IV q8h × 5 days	Reserved for severe cases
		5% ointment topically q6h × 7 days	Less effective than PO
Recurrent episode	Acyclovir	200 mg PO 5 times/day × 5 days	Limited clinical benefit
Suppression	Acyclovir	400 mg PO b.i.d.	Titrate dose as required
Mucocutaneous HSV in immunocompromised patient	Acyclovir	200–400 mg PO 5 times/day × 10 days	
		5 mg IV q8h × 7–10 days†	
		5% ointment topically q6h × 7 days	For minor lesions only
HSV encephalitis	Acyclovir	10 mg/kg IV q8h × 10–14 days‡	
Neonatal HSV	Acyclovir§	10–15 mg/kg IV q8h × 14–21 days	
Herpetic conjunctivitis	Trifluridine	1 drop q2h while awake × 7–14 days	Alternative; vidarabine ointment

*The doses are for adults with normal renal function unless otherwise noted.
†250 mg/m^2 should be given to children under 12 years of age.
‡500 mg/m^2 should be given to children over 12 years of age.
§Acyclovir is not approved by the FDA for this indication.
Adapted from Whitley RJ, Gnann J. Acyclovir: A decade later. N Engl J Med 1992; 327:782-789; with permission.

prodromal or erythematous stages of recurrent infection. Thus, oral acyclovir has a slight clinical benefit only if initiated very early after recurrence, and cannot be recommended as routine treatment for herpes labialis in immunocompetent patients. No data support the use of long-term suppressive treatment with acyclovir for the prevention of herpes labialis.

Genital Herpes

Acyclovir administered topically, orally, or intravenously treats primary genital herpes in the normal host, decreasing the duration of symptoms, viral shedding, and time to healing of lesions (Table 1). However, neither systemic nor topical treatment of primary HSV infection reduces the frequency or severity of recurrences. Episodic administration of oral or topical acyclovir for the treatment of recurrent genital HSV lesions provides only a modest benefit, with duration of lesions shortened at most by 1 to 2 days. However, daily oral acyclovir can suppress recurrences of genital herpes in 60 to 90 percent of patients. Treatment should be interrupted every 12 months to reassess the need for continued suppression.

Mucocutaneous HSV Infections in Immunocompromised Patients

In immunocompromised patients, topical, oral, and intravenous acyclovir all diminish the duration of viral shedding as well as substantially improve time to cessation of pain and to total healing of HSV lesions. In addition, prophylactic administration of oral or intravenous acyclovir to such patients significantly reduces the incidence of symptomatic HSV infection (see Table 1).

Herpes Simplex Keratoconjunctivitis

Idoxuridine (Stoxil), trifluridine (Viroptic), and vidarabine ophthalmic drops all are effective and licensed for treatment of HSV keratitis. Trifluridine is the most efficacious and the easiest to administer and so is the drug of choice for HSV ocular disease (see Table 1).

Herpes Simplex Encephalitis

In patients with HSV encephalitis, acyclovir administration greatly reduces mortality and has a modest effect on morbidity. Dose and length of therapy are shown in Table 1. Outcome is more favorable when therapy is instituted early in the disease.

Neonatal HSV Infections

Though not licensed for this indication, acyclovir is the drug of choice in the treatment of neonatal HSV infection (see Table 1). Therapy is most efficacious if instituted early in the course of illness. Due to the exceptional safety profile of acyclovir, an intravenous dose of 30 to 45 mg/kg/day divided every 8 hours should be given. Duration of therapy is 14 to 21 days.

Infants with ocular involvement caused by HSV should receive topical antiviral medication in addition to parenteral therapy. Trifluridine is the treatment of choice for ocular HSV infection in the neonate (see Table 1).

Acknowledgments

Original studies were performed by the investigators and supported under contract with the Antiviral Branch of the National Institute of Allergy and Infectious Diseases (NIAID), NO1-AI-15113 and NO1-AI-62554, and by grants from the General Clinical Research Center Program (RR-032) and the state of Alabama.

Suggested Reading

Douglas JM, Critchlow C, Benedetti J, et al. Double-blind study of oral acyclovir for suppression of recurrences of genital herpes simplex virus infection. N Engl J Med 1984; 310:1551–1556.

Whitley RJ, Corey L, Arvin A, et al. Changing presentation of neonatal herpes simplex virus infection. J Infect Dis 1988; 158:109–116.

Whitley RJ, Gnann J. Acyclovir: A decade later. N Engl J Med 1992; 327: 782–789.

Whitley RJ, Soong S-J, Hirsch MS, et al. Herpes simplex encephalitis: Vidarabine therapy and diagnostic problems. N Engl J Med 1981; 304: 313–318.

BELL'S PALSY AND HERPES ZOSTER OTICUS

Gregory Y. Chang, M.D.
James R. Keane, M.D.

■ BELL'S PALSY

To treat fallopian neuritis (Bell's palsy) a century ago, Gowers recommended that "fomentations should be applied to the region in front of and below the ear, as hot as can be borne.... In all cases, except those of very trifling degree, a blister should be applied behind the ear ... small doses of iodide of potassium may be given; with quinine and strychnine." After we smile at this regimen, we're forced to acknowledge that there is still no universally accepted treatment for Bell's palsy.

Gowers accepted cold as the usual cause of Bell's paralysis and stated that "in more than half the cases a special and considerable exposure to cold can be traced; generally a draught of cold air has blown on the side of the face and head, as in sitting in a railroad carriage opposite an open window." This "rheumatic" etiology has gradually given way to that of a viral neuritis. Herpes simplex has long been a leading contender as the causative virus and has recently shown to produce "Bell's palsy" in the mouse, with acute onset and good recovery.

Bell's palsy is a common condition, with an incidence of about 25 out of 100,000—approximately as common as parkinsonism and half as frequent as first seizures. Diabetes, pregnancy, and possibly older age increase the risk of acquiring Bell's palsy. A predisposition to cranial neuropathies, especially seventh and third nerve palsies, runs in a few families. About 5 percent of Bell's palsy cases experience recurrence; less than 1 percent of facial palsies are bilateral, and only one-fourth of these are idiopathic and self-limited.

Diagnosis

The progression of facial weakness in Bell's palsy is rapid, with maximum involvement usually reached within several days. Preceding ear pain was noted by 22 percent of patients in a retrospective study and 68 percent in a prospective study. Other symptoms of seventh nerve involvement included increased tearing in 24 percent and 68 percent, decreased tearing in 6 percent and 17 percent, taste abnormalities in 23 percent and 57 percent, abnormal facial sensation in 23 percent and 48 percent, and hyperacusis in 6 percent and 29 percent. Minor symptoms reflecting adjacent cranial nerve involvement are reportedly common when carefully sought, but frank cranial polyneuropathy indicates a need for further investigation.

Occasionally, cerebral lesions present with acute facial weakness. Absence of mastoid pain, dysarthria out of proportion to facial weakness, or subtle extremity weakness may help identify a cerebral origin.

Up to 5 percent of cases diagnosed as Bell's palsy will be due to tumors, and many of these may show a temporary response to steroid therapy. Dramatic steroid responsiveness during treatment of facial neuritis should cause the same concern about an underlying compressive lesion as it does in treating optic neuritis. Most experienced neurologists have seen resolution of facial paralysis presage a serious underlying disease. Atypical features or course may warrant an evaluation with contrast-enhanced magnetic resonance imaging (MRI) and lumbar puncture.

A less serious but diagnostically confusing situation occurs when the patient's concern about Bell's palsy being a stroke "overflows" to produce complaints of spurious weakness or sensory loss in the ipsilateral limbs. Reassurance usually returns symptoms to the face alone. A psychogenic crossed hemiparesis suggesting a pontine lesion occurred in one of our patients who confused the side of facial paralysis.

Bell's palsy is a clinical diagnosis. A focused history should include a careful review of possible contraindications to steroid therapy. A general physical examination is important to search for systemic causes of facial palsy. The neurologic examination should concentrate on evaluation of the lower cranial nerves, with special attention to hearing, vestibular function, and otoscopic examination.

Laboratory testing is not essential in straightforward cases, but certain tests may be mandated by local conditions. We test for syphilis and diabetes in our inner-city population. A chest x-ray film is useful to look for the hilar adenopathy of sarcoidosis where that disease is common. An additional use of the chest x-ray film lies in detecting tuberculosis in inner-city or appropriate immigrant populations before giving steroids. Serologic testing for Lyme disease is advisable in endemic areas.

MRI frequently shows seventh nerve enhancement in Bell's palsy, but as this finding is neither sensitive nor specific, imaging should be reserved for atypical cases. A small number of Bell's palsy cases show mild elevation of cerebrospinal fluid protein or white blood cells, but lumbar puncture is indicated only when other conditions appear likely. Electrodiagnostic studies of facial nerve function will support a bad prognosis, but as surgical decompression is ineffective, there is no rush to anticipate bad news.

Therapy

Patients should be reassured and informed that 95 percent of individuals recover satisfactorily within few months. Informing the patient that Bell's palsy is due to a virus attacking the nerve and not a stroke is helpful.

The importance of avoiding corneal drying is stressed, and patients are shown how to apply a single strip of skin tape, such as micropore paper tape, horizontally along the upper lid to keep the palpebral fissure narrowed but open. Artificial tears are of limited value due to the brief duration of action. When going outdoors, the patient may want to wear dark glasses to minimize exposure as well as for cosmetic purposes. At night, Lacrilube ophthalmic ointment should be applied and the eye kept closed by placing a strip of paper tape from upper lid to cheek.

Although the benefits of steroid therapy have not been

proven to the satisfaction of all, most studies suggest that a brief course of prednisone conveys modest benefits with minimal risk. The optimal steroid dose is not known. For simplicity, we recommend that patients with moderate or severe facial weakness, seen within the first week, take one 50 mg prednisone tablet with breakfast for 7 days. With a half-life of about 24 hours, a short course of prednisone provides its own tapered conclusion.

Benefit from acyclovir or other antiviral agents in treating Bell's palsy has not been established, and we recommend their use, at present, only in the setting of a controlled study.

In the absence of compelling evidence for the benefits of surgery, we do not recommend decompression of the facial nerve. Neither electrical stimulation nor massage of the facial muscles has been shown to have benefits beyond that of psychological support.

All patients with Bell's palsy show some recovery; 85 percent recover completely, and 95 percent are satisfied with their outcome. Persisting weakness is usually less bothersome than the effects of aberrant regeneration and is more amenable to plastic surgery. Anastomosis of the twelfth and seventh nerves may increase patients' difficulties in talking and eating and has a limited role in facial restoration.

■ HERPES ZOSTER OTICUS

Zoster facialis is less common but usually more severe than simplex facialis. Pain is nearly universal, and hyperacusis, dry eye, vertigo, tinnitus, and decreased hearing are more common than with Bell's palsy. Variants of zoster oticus consist of involvement of weakness beyond the facial nerve innervation that may result in paresis of pharynx or tongue, sometimes termed *herpes zoster cephalicus.*

Herpes zoster oticus is usually accompanied by vesicles about the ear. Occasionally, other sites such as palate, tongue, or face may be involved. Recognition of zoster oticus is difficult in the absence of characteristic skin lesions. Vesicles may be delayed until after the onset of facial weakness or may not occur at all.

The benefits of acyclovir remain unproven. Because of the worse prognosis of zoster oticus, it seems reasonable to add the small burden of the side effects and use acyclovir in combination with prednisone. Our practice is to treat patients seen within the first 2 weeks of illness with oral acyclovir (800 mg four times per day for 7 days). One 50 mg prednisone tablet is also given each morning for 7 days.

In the rare event of corneal numbness due to concomitant herpetic involvement of the ophthalmic branch of the trigeminal nerve, the cornea must be carefully protected. Lacrilube ointment should be applied frequently and the lid kept closed with paper tape. At the first sign of redness and irritation of the eye, the patient should be referred to an ophthalmologist to consider marginal tarsorrhaphy.

Suggested Reading

Adour KK. Otological complications of herpes zoster. Ann Neurol 1994; 35:S62–S64.

Adour KK, Byl FM, Hilsinger RL Jr, et al. The true nature of Bell's palsy: Analysis of 1,000 consecutive patients. Laryngoscope 1978; 88:787–799.

Katusic SK, Beard CM, Wiederholt WC, et al. Incidence, clinical features, and prognosis in Bell's palsy, Rochester, Minnesota, 1968–1982. Ann Neurol 1986; 20:622–627.

Patient Resources

American Academy of Otolaryngology—Head and Neck Surgery (AAO-HNS)
Ordering Department
One Prince Street
Alexandria, Virginia 22314
Phone: (703) 519-1528
FAX: (703) 683-5100
Brochures: A discussion of facial nerve problems
Costs: $20 member, $25 nonmember per 100 copies

Group Health Inc.
Riverside-Neurology Dept.
Attn: Bryce Droweiler
2220 Riverside Avenue, South
Minneapolis, Minnesota 55454
Phone: (612) 371-1715
Booklet: *Bell's palsy*
Cost: single copies are free

CANDIDIASIS

Thomas J. Walsh, M.D.
Philip A. Pizzo, M.D.

Candidiasis is the most common mucosal and deeply invasive mycosis. *Candida albicans* is the most common species causing such infections. Other *Candida* spp., such as *C. tropicalis, C. parapsilosis, C. krusei, Torulopsis glabrata* (considered by some authorities to be a *Candida*) also may cause infection. *Candida* is characterized morphologically by yeast forms (blastoconidia), pscudohyphac, and hyphac. *Torulopsis glabrata* has no hyphae or pseudohyphae.

C. albicans is a normal member of the flora of the alimentary tract. An opportunistic pathogen, *Candida* requires compromised immunologic or mechanical host defense to establish infection. Candidiasis as an infectious process consists of various patterns of infection including cutaneous, mucosal, and disseminated candidiasis and fungemia and single-organ infection.

■ CUTANEOUS CANDIDIASIS

The most common patterns of cutaneous candidiasis are intertriginous and diaper dermatitis. Intertriginous *Candida* dermatitis is managed by maintaining a dry skin surface and applying nystatin, miconazole, or clotrimazole cream. Diabetic patients with *Candida* dermatitis benefit from control of blood glucose levels. *Candida* diaper dermatitis is managed by maintaining a dry skin surface, frequent changing of diapers, and applying miconazole or clotrimazole cream. Nystatin powder may also help if imidazole cream is not effective.

■ MUCOSAL CANDIDIASIS

Mucosal candidiasis may develop in the oropharynx, esophagus, gastrointestinal tract, urinary tract, vaginal mucosa, or tracheobronchial tree. The risk factors for developing mucosal candidiasis include broad-spectrum antibiotic therapy, impaired cell-mediated immunity (e.g., human immunodeficiency virus [HIV] infection, chronic mucocutaneous candidiasis), corticosteroid therapy, diabetes mellitus, and oral contraceptives containing high levels of progesterone. A diagnosis of mucosal candidiasis is best established by a combination of physical examination, direct microscopic examination, and culture confirmation. The principal treatment of mucosal candidiasis consists of reversal of known risk factors and administration of antifungal therapy. Depending on the severity of disease and the underlying host defects, topical therapy of nystatin or clotrimazole is employed initially and is followed by systemic therapy if the former is not successful or appropriate. Systemic therapy may be with ketoconazole, fluconazole, or itraconazole.

Oropharyngeal Candidiasis

Initial management of oropharyngeal candidiasis consists of establishing an accurate diagnosis. Many cases of apparent thrush, particularly in granulocytopenic patients, have other causes, including herpes simplex virus and mixed oral bacterial flora. Since white mucosal plaques are not necessarily pathognomonic of oropharyngeal candidiasis, direct microscopic examination of scrapings of lesions and culture confirmation are the most reliable means of establishing this diagnosis. Such an approach becomes even more important when a patient does not respond to topical or systemic antifungal therapy.

Improvement of host defense is an integral part of managing mucosal candidiasis. Topical antifungal treatment controls most cases of oropharyngeal candidiasis and is recommended as the initial therapeutic intervention. Nystatin suspension is limited by the somewhat bitter taste, which may lead to compliance problems. Clotrimazole administered four or five times a day may help patients unresponsive to nystatin. However, the administration of clotrimazole requires compliance in retaining the troche in the oral cavity until it is completely dissolved. The longer exposure of the oral cavity to clotrimazole may contribute substantially to its antifungal activity. If a patient is not able to maintain a clotrimazole troche under the tongue or under buccal mucosa for a sustained period, the troche may be pulverized and formulated into a suspension for oral administration.

Patients with oropharyngeal candidiasis refractory to topical therapy are candidates for systemic therapy with fluconazole, ketoconazole, or 3 mg per kilogram in two divided doses for adults, or 3 mg per kilogram in two divided doses for children. Patients with particularly depressed cell-mediated immunity may have oropharyngeal and esophageal candidiasis that becomes completely refractory to topical and oral therapy, requiring a course of amphotericin B 0.5 mg per kilogram per day for approximately 3 to 7 days, depending on therapeutic response. Lower doses of amphotericin B for refractory mucosal candidiasis may not eradicate the infection. In addition to treating the oropharyngeal candidiasis, treat any concomitant infection, such as that caused by herpes simplex virus, which may accompany invasive candidiasis. Advanced stages of oropharyngeal candidiasis in HIV-infected patients and granulocytopenic hosts may be accompanied by esophageal candidiasis.

Esophageal Candidiasis

Esophageal candidiasis is associated with risk factors similar to those of oropharyngeal candidiasis, but may occur in the absence of conspicuous oropharyngeal *Candida* infection. Radiation to the mediastinum and gastroesophageal reflux are additional risk factors for esophageal candidiasis. Concomitant infections caused by herpes simplex virus, cytomegalovirus, and bacteria may coincide with or precede esophageal candidiasis.

Esophagoscopy with mucosal biopsy is the most reliable method for establishing a diagnosis of esophageal candidiasis. Although biopsy of the esophageal mucosa is the gold standard for diagnosis, it may not be feasible, practical, or safe. Accordingly, an empiric approach is often warranted. For patients with granulocytopenia it may consist of initial clotrimazole and/or a systemic azole. However, since the esophagus may be the portal of entry for candidiasis, failure of symptoms to respond promptly is an indication for empiric amphotericin B in granulocytopenic patients. Furthermore, the resolution of symptoms does not necessarily signify the eradication of esophageal candidiasis in granulocytopenic patients. Thus, a persistently febrile patient with proven esophageal candidiasis may require empiric amphotericin B therapy despite resolution of esophageal symptoms.

Genitourinary Candidiasis

Candiduria should be evaluated as involvement of either the upper or the lower urinary tract. The management of urinary candidiasis is controversial; it depends on the state of the host and the location of infection. Removal of urinary catheters and other foreign bodies (e.g., urinary stents) when possible is a basic principle of the management of urinary catheter infections. The diagnostic significance of candiduria depends on the host. Candiduria that is microbiologically proved through a reliable clean-catch specimen or a straight catheterized specimen in an immunocompromised patient should be considered on practical grounds as evidence of disseminated candidiasis until proved otherwise. By comparison, a nonimmunocompromised patient with candiduria and temporary placement of a urinary catheter most likely does not have disseminated candidiasis. Such patients are more likely to have infection restricted to the mucosa.

Several options are available for medical management of uncomplicated *Candida* cystitis: oral or intravenous fluconazole 200 to 400 mg a day, amphotericin B bladder washout (concentration of 5 μg/ml in sterile D_5W with closed continuous irrigation of 15 ml per kilogram per day for 5 days), and intravenous amphotericin B 0.3 to 0.5 mg per kilogram per day. Oral flucytosine (5-FC), which achieves high urinary concentrations, as a single agent should be discouraged because of emergence of resistance.

Fluconazole is highly effective in the treatment of urinary tract infections caused by *C. albicans* and *C. tropicalis. Torulopsis glabrata* and *C. krusei,* however, may emerge as resistant superinfecting organisms if fluconazole is used. Resistant organisms may be treated with amphotericin B. Single doses or short courses of intravenous amphotericin B achieve sufficiently high fungicidal concentrations in the urine to eradicate *Candida.* Nevertheless, candiduria may recur as long as the patient remains catheterized. Bladder irrigations with amphotericin B also may not permanently eradicate *Candida* cystitis in patients who remain catheterized.

The management of vaginal candidiasis includes establishing a direct microscopic and microbiologic diagnosis, ruling out other causes of vaginal discharge, and administering appropriate antifungal chemotherapy. Most cases of vaginal candidiasis may be treated by topical therapy such as clotrimazole or miconazole cream or clotrimazole troches. Ketoconazole or fluconazole may be used for treatment of recurrent vaginal candidiasis.

Pulmonary Candidiasis

Fever and pulmonary infiltrates in an immunocompromised patient should not be ascribed to *Candida* unless proven by biopsy. Lung biopsy often demonstrates other causes of infiltrates in such patients. True pulmonary candidiasis develops most frequently as hematogenous pulmonary candidiasis in granulocytopenic patients or *Candida* bronchopneumonia in low-birth-weight infants and elderly debilitated hosts. Hematogenous pulmonary candidiasis and *Candidiasis* bronchopneumonia are treated with amphotericin B as deeply invasive.

■ FUNGEMIA

The risk factors for hospital-acquired candidemia include the simultaneous use of more than two antibiotics, the use of Silastic chronically indwelling vascular catheters (e.g., Hickman-Broviac catheters), hemodialysis, granulocytopenia, and abdominal surgery. Diagnosis of suspected fungemia is highly dependent on the blood culture detection system. The lysis centrifugation system and nonradiometric (infrared) blood culture system with resins are two effective systems for detection of fungemia. The lysis centrifugation system is especially valuable in conveying a semiquantitative determination of the number of yeast cells per quantity of blood and is superior to many other systems for early and frequent detection of fungemia. The newer BacTAlert system, which uses an automated iterative scan for monitoring rate of CO_2 production, may further improve the detection of candidemia. Despite these important advances, deep-tissue candidiasis often evades early detection by blood culture detection systems.

Detection of *Candida* in blood cultures should be considered sufficient evidence of invasive candidiasis to warrant a course of antifungal therapy. Fungemia left untreated may be followed in nongranulocytopenic patients by an approximately 20 percent frequency of late complications, including *Candida* endophthalmitis, meningitis, osteomyelitis, arthritis, endocarditis, and renal candidiasis. Disseminated candidiasis in neonates and granulocytopenic patients, which is often reflected by fungemia, carries a high mortality. Fungemia may be followed in granulocytopenic patients by hepatosplenic candidiasis or acute disseminated candidiasis. Untreated fungemia in very low-birth-weight infants may be complicated by renal candidiasis and *Candida* meningitis. Thus the concept of transient candidemia, suggesting a benign process, is not tenable. Candidemia may reflect clinical occult deep tissue seeding. Indeed, candidemia should be considered to have the same therapeutic significance as a positive blood culture for *Staphylococcus aureus,* in which the complications following bacteremia are similar to those of candidemia.

Management of candidemia depends on the host and the organism isolated. Recent data indicate that fluconazole is as effective as amphotericin B in non-neutropenic patients with uncomplicated fungemia. Although the optimal dosage and duration of fluconazole and amphotericin B for treatment of fungemia have not been determined, several guidelines may be offered, particularly for fungemia caused by *C. albicans.* Treat uncomplicated fungemia in adult non-neutropenic patients with fluconazole 800 mg loading dose followed by 400 mg per day for 2 weeks. Treat uncomplicated candidemia with a 2 week course of amphotericin B at 0.5 mg per kilogram per day. Given the higher level of resistance of *C. tropicalis* and *C. parapsilosis,* fungemia caused by these organisms may require higher doses of amphotericin B (e.g., 0.75 to 1 mg per kilogram per day) and a course of 3 to 4 weeks. Treat persistent fungemia, particularly in granulocytopenic patients, by increasing the dosage of amphotericin B, adding 5-FC, and removing any intravascular foreign bodies.

Intravascular catheters may be the source of fungemia or the target for attachment of circulating *Candida* spp. from another portal of entry (e.g., the gastrointestinal tract). Intravascular catheters in either circumstance may continue to seed the blood stream. Thus, whenever feasible, remove intravascular catheters from patients with fungemia.

■ DISSEMINATED CANDIDIASIS

Tissue-proven disseminated candidiasis may be classified as acute or chronic. The syndromes of acute and chronic disease occupy two ends of a spectrum that is particularly well demonstrated in granulocytopenic patients. Acute disseminated candidiasis typically manifests in granulocytopenic patients as persistent fungemia, hemodynamic instability, multiple cutaneous and visceral lesions, and high mortality despite antifungal therapy. By comparison, chronic disseminated candidiasis, otherwise known as hepatosplenic candidiasis, is characterized by an indolent process of disseminated candidiasis following recovery from granulocytopenia. Patients with chronic disseminated candidiasis usually are hemodynamically stable, do not have detectable fungemia, and have a good survival rate when antifungal therapy is administered. Of course, there is a continuum of patterns of infection between these two distinctive syndromes.

Treatment of acute disease consists of amphotericin B 1 mg or more per kilogram per day plus 5-FC when possible. Prompt initiation of aggressive antifungal therapy is necessary in such patients. A characteristic syndrome of acute disseminated candidiasis, which may develop in low-birth-weight infants, manifests as apnea, hypotension, and fever or hypothermia. Aggressive antifungal therapy also is warranted in these patients. Early recognition of acute disseminated candidiasis and initiation of effective antifungal therapy are essential for optimal management and outcome.

Chronic disseminated candidiasis is a more stable condition that develops during the course of granulocytopenia but usually becomes apparent only on recovery from granulocytopenia. A computed tomographic (CT) scan or magnetic resonance imaging (MRI) performed at this time often demonstrates multiple lesions in liver, spleen, and at times other organs such as kidneys and lungs. A biopsy of hepatic lesions is important in management of these patients. Our initial approach in managing hepatosplenic candidiasis is administration of amphotericin B, usually with 5-FC. We sometimes administer fluconazole as follow-up outpatient therapy. We continue to treat patients who are receiving antineoplastic therapy or who remain chronically immunosuppressed until resolution or calcification of lesions. Such a course of therapy may require 6 months to 1 year.

■ DEEP CANDIDIASIS OF SINGLE NONMUCOSAL SITES

Candida Peritonitis

Candida peritonitis develops in two clinical settings: gastrointestinal surgery and peritoneal dialysis. Gastrointestinal surgery may be complicated by leakage of lumenal contents into the peritoneum from an anastomotic site, particularly in patients receiving broad-spectrum antibiotics and undergoing revision of the anastomosis. Management of this condition requires re-exploration of the abdominal cavity, drainage of the infection, and administration of amphotericin B. The role of fluconazole in this setting is not defined.

Chronic ambulatory peritoneal dialysis may be complicated by catheter-associated *Candida* peritonitis. This infection is best treated by removal of the catheter and administration of antifungal therapy. Failure to remove the catheter often results in relapses after discontinuation of antifungal therapy. Amphotericin B or fluconazole may be administered, depending on the organism.

Candida Meningitis

Candida meningitis is most commonly encountered in low-birth-weight infants and immunosuppressed hosts of any age. It may develop as a complication of ventricular shunts and drains. Amphotericin B plus 5-FC is the most appropriate regimen for this infection. Removal of any ventricular prosthetic device is especially important for successful eradication of *Candida* spp. from the cerebrospinal fluid (CSF). *Candida* meningitis has a high propensity for recurrence and may require several months of therapy.

Candida Osteomyelitis

Candida osteomyelitis requires surgical debridement of the bone for both diagnostic and therapeutic effects and subsequent amphotericin B. Monitoring of bone scans or MRI as well as erythrocyte sedimentation rate permits therapeutic end points to be evaluated.

Candida Endocarditis

Candida endocarditis requires an accurate diagnosis of fungemia and valvular infection. Diagnosis may be difficult to establish and may be heralded by the abrupt onset of an embolic event in a major artery. The recent introduction of transesophageal echocardiography has substantially improved detection of valvular vegetations in suspected cases with negative transthoracic echocardiograms. Definitive treatment requires resection of the valve and administration of amphotericin B plus 5-FC. Given the risk and unpredictability of lethal or neurologically catastrophic embolization, surgical resection should take place promptly.

Candida Endophthalmitis

Characteristic white vitreal opacities in a patient with candidemia signify *Candida* endophthalmitis. Management is conducted in concert with ophthalmologic consultation. Timely use of vitrectomy may be critical in saving vision. Amphotericin B plus 5-FC is recommended for this infection. Transition to fluconazole 400 to 800 mg a day in adults may be considered for subsequent outpatient therapy in carefully selected non-immunosuppressed patients who can be reliably followed. Intravitreal amphotericin B is recommended by some.

■ PREVENTION OF MUCOSAL AND DISSEMINATED CANDIDIASIS

Prevention of invasive candidiasis is most common for patients receiving intensive cytotoxic chemotherapy or ablative radiation therapy. Nystatin or clotrimazole may prevent oropharyngeal candidiasis. Our experience, however, indicates that neither agent is completely effective in preventing oropharyngeal candidiasis, so we treat oropharyngeal candidiasis when it develops.

Fluconazole has achieved an important role as an agent for prevention of invasive candidiasis in allogeneic bone marrow transplant recipients. A dose of 400 mg a day orally or intravenously initiated on day 1 of marrow-ablative chemotherapy reduces the frequency of deeply invasive candidiasis in adult bone marrow transplant recipients. While the findings are encouraging, there are several limitations to antifungal activity. For example, fluconazole at the current recommended dosages has little or no activity against *Candida krusei, Torulopsis glabrata, Aspergillus* spp., Zygomycetes, and *Fusarium* spp.

■ EMPIRIC AMPHOTERICIN B FOR PERSISTENTLY FEBRILE GRANULOCYTOPENIC PATIENTS

Granulocytopenic patients who are persistently or recurrently febrile for 7 or more days despite antibacterial therapy are at high risk for invasive candidiasis. Amphotericin B 0.5 to 0.6 mg per kilogram per day significantly reduces the likelihood of developing invasive candidiasis and may prevent invasive aspergillosis (see the chapter *Infection in the Neutropenic Patient*).

Suggested Reading

American Thoracic Society. Fungal infection in HIV-infected persons. Am J Respir Crit Care Med 1995; 152:816–822.

Fisher JF, Newman CL, Sobel JD. Yeast in the urine: solutions for a budding problem. Clin Infect Dis 1995; 20:183–189.

Lecciones JA, Lee JW, Navarro E, et al. Vascular catheter-associated fungemia in cancer patients: analysis of 155 episodes. Rev Infect Dis 1992; 14:875–883.

Reef SE, Levine WC, McNeil MM, et al. Treatment options for vulvovaginal candidiasis. Clin Infect Dis 1995; 20 Suppl 1:S80–90.

Rex JH, Bennett JE, Sugar AM, et al. A randomized trial comparing fluconazole with amphotericin B for the treatment of candidemia in patients without neutropenia. N Engl J Med 1994; 331:1325–1330.

Walsh TJ, Hiemenz J, Anaissie E. Recent progress and current problems in treatment of invasive fungal infections in neutropenic patients. Infect Dis Clin N Am 1996; 10:365–400.

Walsh TJ, Whitcomb PO, Ravankar S, et al. Successful treatment of hepatosplenic candidiasis through repeated episodes of neutropenia. Cancer 1995; 76:2357–2362.

PNEUMOCYSTIS CARINII

Walter T. Hughes, M.D.

Pneumocystis carinii is the cause of a diffuse bilateral pneumonitis in severely immunocompromised patients, including those with the acquired immunodeficiency syndrome (AIDS), congenital immunodeficiency disorders, cancer, and organ transplants. Without treatment mortality nears 100 percent. The diagnosis requires demonstration of *P. carinii* in fluid or tissue obtained by bronchoalveolar lavage, lung biopsy, or induced sputum.

■ THERAPY

All patients with *P. carinii* pneumonitis require immediate antimicrobial and supportive treatment. Trimethoprim-sulfamethoxazole (TMP-SMX) is the drug of first choice. Moderately and severely ill patients should receive 15 mg TMP and 75 mg SMX per kilogram IV per day in four doses 6 hours apart. Mild cases in patients who can take oral medication may be treated with 20 mg TMP and 100 mg SMX per kilogram per day in four divided doses by mouth. Usually 21 days of therapy is required, and most patients who qualify for prophylaxis will continue on the drug at one-fifth the therapeutic dose for life or until no longer at risk for recurrence or reinfection. Adverse reactions are infrequent in non-AIDS patients, but about 40 percent of AIDS patients have significant reactions to TMP-SMX. Rash, neutropenia, and fever are the most common treatment-limiting events. Some patients can tolerate mild reactions, and TMP-SMX is continued. Rare but life-threatening reactions to TMP-SMX include Stevens-Johnson syndrome, hepatic necrosis, aplastic anemia, agranulocytosis, and allergic reactions. Leucovorin should not be used routinely with TMP-SMX therapy.

Patients who cannot tolerate or who fail to respond to TMP-SMX may be changed to effective alternative drugs. Three drugs approved by the Food and Drug Administration (FDA) are atovaquone, pentamidine isethionate, and trimetrexate with leucovorin.

Atovaquone tablets 2,250 mg per day as three divided doses orally may be used to treat mild or moderately severe *P. carinii* pneumonitis in patients who can take medication by mouth. While this treatment is less effective than TMP-SMX, treatment-limiting events are also less frequent, resulting in similar rates of therapeutic success for the two regimens. No parenteral preparation is available at this time. A suspension formulation recently approved by the FDA provides higher plasma concentrations than the tablets. The dose is 750 mg (5 ml) twice daily.

Pentamidine isethionate 4 mg per kilogram per day as a single intravenous dose may be used for *P. carinii* pneumonitis of any severity. This drug is similar in efficacy to TMP-SMX, but more than 50 percent of patients have significant adverse effects. These include, among others, nephrotoxicity, leukopenia, hypoglycemia, hypotension, thrombocytopenia, hypocalcemia, and Stevens-Johnson syndrome. Pentamidine can be given intramuscularly, but serious injection site reactions are common. Aerosolized pentamidine has only limited therapeutic effect but is relatively safe. There is no oral preparation of pentamidine.

Trimetrexate glucuronate 45 mg per square meter is given as a single daily infusion over 60 to 90 minutes plus leucovorin 20 mg per square meter over 5 to 10 minutes every 6 hours (total daily dose, 80 mg per square meter). Leucovorin but not trimetrexate may be given orally at the same dosage. This regimen is an alternative therapy for moderate and severe cases of *P. carinii* pneumonia.

Other drugs with demonstrated efficacy are in general use but not approved by the FDA for the treatment of *P. carinii* pneumonitis. These include dapsone plus trimethoprim, and clindamycin plus primaquine. These drugs are limited to oral administration.

A recent addition to supportive therapy for moderate and severe cases of *P. carinii* pneumonia is the use of corticosteroid drugs. Studies have shown that when patients with arterial oxygen tension (Pao_2) of 70 mmHg and lower are given corticosteroids within the first 3 days of therapy, survival is significantly increased and deterioration of oxygenation is reduced. The recommendation is to administer oral prednisone 40 mg twice daily during the first 5 days of therapy, then reduce the dose to 40 mg daily for days 6 through 10 and to 20 mg daily days 11 through 21. The duration of corticosteroid therapy may be shortened for patients who respond promptly. It is important to watch for complications of corticosteroid immunosuppression. See the chapter *AIDS: Therapy for Opportunistic Infections* for more details of *Pneumocystis Carinii* pneumonitis therapy in AIDS patients.

■ PREVENTION

Chemoprophylaxis can prevent *P. carinii* pneumonitis in most high-risk patients. Prophylaxis is indicated for all patients who have been treated for an episode of *P. carinii* pneumonitis, because 30 to 50 percent of patients will have a recurrent episode without it. All adults with HIV infection and CD4+ lymphocyte counts less than 200 cells per cubic millimeter should receive prophylaxis. Infants and children with reduction in CD4+ lymphocyte counts below the range of normal for age and all HIV-infected infants less than 1 year of age should receive a prophylactic regimen as follows:

1. TMP-SMX is the preferred drug at any of the following schedules:
   - 160 mg TMP, 800 mg SMX once or twice a day to adults either daily or 3 days per week
   - Some evidence suggests 80 mg TMP, 400 mg SMX also effective in adults
   - 5 mg TMP, 25 mg SMX per kilogram per day given daily or 3 days a week to infants and children, not to exceed the adult dose
2. For patients who cannot tolerate TMP-SMX, any of the following regimens may be selected:
   - Dapsone 100 mg as a single or divided dose daily
   - Dapsone 50 mg per day plus pyrimethamine 50 mg and leucovorin 25 mg per week; also provides prophylaxis for *Toxoplasma* encephalitis
   - Dapsone 200 mg plus pyrimethamine 75 mg plus leucovorin 25 mg once a week
   - Aerosolized pentamidine 300 mg delivered by nebulizer once a month

Some physicians prefer dapsone with or without pyrimethamine to aerosolized pentamidine because of low cost and ease of administration of dapsone and because of the option to expand prophylaxis for *Toxoplasma* encephalitis with the addition of pyrimethamine. Prophylaxis must be maintained until the host is no longer immunocompromised.

Suggested Reading

Centers for Disease Control and Prevention. Recommendations for prophylaxis against *Pneumocystis carinii* pneumonia for adults and adolescents infected with human immunodeficiency virus. MMWR 1992; 41(RR-4):1–20.

Hughes WT, Keoung G, Kramer F, et al. Comparison of atovaquone (566C80) with trimethoprim-sulfamethoxazole to treat *Pneumocystis carinii* pneumonia in patients with AIDS. N Engl J Med 1993; 328:1521–1527.

Martinez A, Suffredini AF, Masur H. *Pneumocystis carinii* disease in HIV-infected persons. In: Wormser, G, ed. AIDS and other manifestation of HIV infection. 2nd ed. New York: Raven Press, 1992:225.

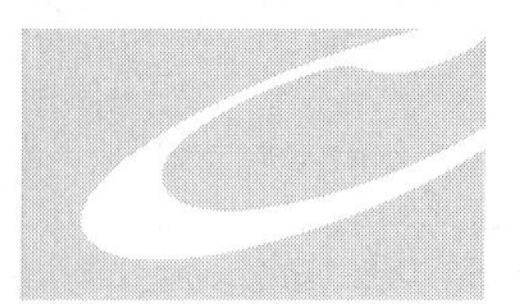

CARDIOVASCULAR DISEASES

ACUTE PULMONARY EDEMA

David T. Kawanishi, M.D.
Shahbudin H. Rahimtoola, M.B., F.R.C.P., M.A.C.P.

Acute pulmonary edema is the abrupt accumulation of fluid in the lungs resulting either from high intravascular pressure (cardiogenic pulmonary edema) or from increased permeability of the alveolar-capillary membrane, which allows rapid fluid extravasation (noncardiogenic pulmonary edema). In the clinical setting many forms of pulmonary edema have some component of both because it is difficult to affect vessel permeability without affecting pressures at the microvascular level and vice versa. However, it is important to determine the nature of the predominant underlying condition in order to guide the direction of therapy.

■ THERAPEUTIC ALTERNATIVES

Treatment of acute pulmonary edema may range from use of simple general measures to extremely invasive and costly interventional maneuvers or mechanical support (Table 1). General measures that may be employed quickly may produce a rapid improvement in comfort and in the condition of the patient and include placement of the patient in a semi-upright position, application of supplemental oxygen, careful use of intravenous morphine, and titration of intravenous aminophylline, particularly if the patient is wheezing. Simple nonpharmacologic measures for reduction of venous return to the heart, such as rotating tourniquets or phlebotomy, are used less often in the modern medical setting owing to the improved effectiveness of medications. Failure to respond to these general measures usually requires that the patient be intubated, suctioned vigorously to aid in clearing the copious secretions, and mechanically ventilated.

Subsequent specific therapy should be directed at the underlying cause of the acute pulmonary edema and any aggravating factors. Alternatives directed at improving cardiovascular hemodynamics include administration of positive inotropic medications, preload reducing agents, and afterload reducing agents. Proper selection and adjustment of dosage usually requires measurement of pulmonary vascular pressure and cardiac output using a thermodilution pulmonary artery catheter. The potential of calcium entry blockers to improve diastolic compliance may be of added benefit and may be considered as a therapeutic adjunct when they are employed for vasodilation or for heart rate control. When the underlying cardiac disorder is extreme, the pulmonary edema may not respond or may improve incompletely until definitive correction of the disorder can be achieved. In these cases, identification of the underlying disorder becomes of paramount importance. Intervention with temporary artificial pacing for bradyarrhythmias or intra-aortic balloon pumping for ischemic heart disease, for example, may help to stabilize the patient's condition temporarily. Definitive correction of such cardiac disorders, however, often requires additional maneuvers, such as implantation of a permanent pacemaker or coronary reperfusion with percutaneous coronary angioplasty or bypass surgery, respectively, unless the acute pulmonary edema was precipitated by a correctable aggravating condition. Other examples of therapy for specific disorders include surgical valve reconstruction or implantation of a prosthesis for valvular heart disease and pericardiocentesis and pericardial window or pericardiectomy for tamponade.

Table 1 General Therapeutic Measures in Acute Pulmonary Edema

Semi-upright position
Supplemental oxygen
Intravenous morphine
Intravenous aminophylline
Rotating tourniquets
Intubation, mechanical ventilation

■ PREFERRED APPROACH

Medical Treatment

Initial therapy of acute pulmonary edema is directed toward improving pulmonary gas exchange. Once the condition of acute pulmonary edema is recognized, immediate implemen-

Table 2 Measures for Improvement of Cardiac Function in Cardiogenic Pulmonary Edema

FUNCTIONAL DERANGEMENT	MEDICAL	INTERVENTIONAL/SURGICAL
Heart rate/rhythm		
Tachyarrhythmia	Digitalis, calcium entry blockers, cardioversion, antiarrhythmics	
Bradyarrhythmia	Isoproterenol	Artificial pacemaker
Loss of A-V synchrony	Cardioversion	A-V sequential pacemaker
Myocardial systolic function		
Inadequate	Digitalis, aminophylline, isoproterenol, epinephrine, norepinephrine, dopamine, dobutamine, amrinone	Intra-aortic balloon pump, coronary reperfusion via CABG
Excessive (as in hypertrophic cardiomyopathy)	Propranolol, disopyramide	A-V sequential pacing
Myocardial diastolic function	Anti-ischemic, antianginal therapy; calcium entry blockers	Intra-aortic balloon pump, coronary reperfusion via PTCA or CABG, pericardiocentesis, pericardiectomy
Volume excess or maldistribution	Diuretics, digitalis, aminophylline, nitrates, nitroprusside, angiotensin converting enzyme inhibitors, rotating tourniquets, morphine	Valve surgery, catheter balloon valvuloplasty
Hypertension or excessive resistance to ventricular outflow	Nitroprusside, phentolamine, trimethaphan, hydralazine, angiotensin converting enzyme inhibitors, morphine	Intra-aortic balloon pump, valve surgery, catheter balloon valvuloplasty
Regional wall motion abnormality due to myocardial ischemia	Improve arterial Po_2; reduce MVo_2 by slowing tachycardia, preload reduction, afterload reduction; increase cardiac output and correct hypotension	Intra-aortic balloon pump, PTCA, CABG

A-V, Atrioventricular; CABG, coronary artery bypass graft; PTCA, percutaneous transluminal coronary angioplasty.

tation of general supportive measures using semi-upright positioning of the patient and administration of supplemental oxygen is indicated. Measurement of blood pressure and assessment of peripheral perfusion should be made at the earliest opportunity because associated hypotension or hypoperfusion or both suggests the need for a more global cardiovascular approach to therapy as in the case of cardiogenic shock. In the early stages of pulmonary edema, arterial oxygen saturation is depressed with an associated hyperventilation that may decrease carbon dioxide; therefore, supplemental 50 percent oxygen administered via nasal prongs at rates of 6 to 8 liters per minute may suffice. Use of Venturi masks or reservoir bag masks may improve delivery. With progression of the condition, the patient may become cyanotic, increasingly dyspneic, and tachypneic, and pulmonary rales become more prominent. When available, measurement of blood gases should be used to guide therapy, although advanced therapy should not be delayed in the presence of clinical deterioration. Inability to maintain a Pao_2 at 60 mm Hg or better, even at high supplemental oxygen concentrations and flow rates; evidence of carbon dioxide retention; clinical evidence of hypoventilation; or inability to clear the edema fluid and secretions adequately suggests the need for endotracheal intubation, suctioning, and mechanical ventilation.

If the pulmonary edema is secondary to damage to the alveolar-capillary membranes, further medical treatment may include use of positive end-expiratory pressure (PEEP) to maintain or improve arterial blood oxygen concentrations. Use of PEEP may reduce venous return and increase the afterload of the right ventricle, with a resultant decrease of cardiac output. The depression of cardiac output may be severe when right ventricular failure is an associated condition. Monitoring pulmonary artery and wedge pressures along with cardiac output is essential in these patients. Another potential complication of PEEP is barotrauma, resulting in pneumomediastinum, pneumothorax, and subcutaneous emphysema. The patient may also benefit by maintenance of pulmonary artery wedge pressures at as low a pressure as possible, to decrease the rate of pulmonary edema fluid extravasation, as long as cardiac output is not compromised. Finally, treatment of any reversible causes of alveolar-capillary membrane injury, such as pneumonia, may hasten the healing process.

If the cause of the acute pulmonary edema is a cardiac disorder, additional measures to improve hemodynamics may be essential (Table 2). Intravenous morphine sulfate is in general very helpful as a supportive measure for cardiogenic pulmonary edema. In addition to improving patient comfort, reduction of central sympathetic activity may result in venous and arteriolar dilation. An initial dose of 3 to 5 mg repeated approximately every 15 minutes to a total of 15 mg is generally effective. Reduction of dosages is advisable in the elderly and in individuals with very small body habitus. For persons with large body habitus or for young or extremely agitated individuals, larger doses may be needed to effect improvement. Morphine sulfate may produce depression of respiratory effort and should be used cautiously or avoided entirely when ventilation may be compromised, as in patients with altered consciousness, intracranial hemorrhage, or bronchial or chronic pulmonary disease, or when there is carbon dioxide retention.

If the patient with pulmonary edema has associated bronchospasm and is wheezing, intravenous aminophylline should be considered as part of the initial treatment regimen.

Because of its bronchodilating action, it is indicated particularly if there is uncertainty whether the breathlessness is due to an attack of bronchial asthma or is a result of cardiogenic pulmonary edema. In patients with the latter, aminophylline also has the beneficial effects of stimulation of myocardial systolic function, venodilation, and production of a mild diuresis. The initial intravenous dose of aminophylline is 5 mg per kilogram given over 10 to 15 minutes, followed by an infusion of 0.9 mg per kilogram per hour in a patient not previously given aminophylline or related preparations. In patients already taking theophylline, for example, the infusion rate should be reduced to approximately 0.5 mg per kilogram per hour. The latter infusion rate, or occasionally even slower rates, may be indicated in the elderly and in those with hepatic or renal dysfunction. Agitation, marked tachycardia and arrhythmias, nausea and vomiting, hypotension, headaches, and seizures occur when aminophylline levels rise toward toxicity. With maintenance of infusion beyond 12 hours, aminophylline dosage should be adjusted according to measured blood levels of the drug.

Reduction of preload is a desirable therapeutic objective in cardiogenic pulmonary edema and can be accomplished initially by employing rotating tourniquets. Wide rubber tourniquets or, preferably, blood pressure cuffs should be used, with the objective being to inflate to just below the arterial diastolic pressure and thus to allow arterial inflow but restrict venous outflow. Placed proximally at three of the four limbs, the tourniquets should be released every 15 to 20 minutes, and one of the tourniquets should be rotated to the free extremity at that time. Although in most cases drug therapy alone may produce satisfactory improvement, rotating tourniquets may occasionally hasten or be a helpful adjunct in helping to resolve the pulmonary edema. In the field, tourniquets may be used as a bridge until medical support becomes available.

A potent loop diuretic such as furosemide may be very useful in treatment of most cases of cardiogenic pulmonary edema, and its initial beneficial effect is probably also preload reduction through venodilation. As a general rule, drugs should be administered intravenously in these patients because there may be significant constriction of many vascular beds, making absorption via oral, subcutaneous, or intramuscular routes less reliable or predictable. An initial dose of 40 to 60 mg should be given, and improvement resulting from its vasoactive property may be expected even before the onset of diuresis. Diuresis may begin as rapidly as in 5 minutes. In some patients, the diuresis may be massive, with several liters of urine being produced over 0.5 to 2 hours. In others, especially when renal function is compromised, repeated incrementally doubled doses of 80 and 160 mg of furosemide may be given until diuresis is initiated. Alternatively, intravenous ethacrynic acid at an initial dose of 50 mg or bumetanide 0.5 to 1 mg may occasionally produce diuresis when there is no response to furosemide. In some cases, as in frank renal failure, the only way to effect reduction of fluid volume may be dialysis. An early potential complication of diuretic treatment is a marked reduction of intravascular volume, resulting in a catastrophic fall of cardiac output, especially when ventricular function is depressed and is unusually preload dependent. Later, hypokalemia, hyponatremia, alkalosis, and hyperuricemia may occur. The elderly, dehydrated, or malnourished patient or those on chronic diuretic regimens may be particularly susceptible to such complications.

If diuresis is inadequate to produce a resolution or a satisfactorily rapid improvement of the pulmonary edema, or as an added initial maneuver when a rapid response is desired, additional reduction of preload may be achieved using nitrates to produce venodilation. Nitroglycerin 0.4 mg sublingually has a rapid onset of action of 2 minutes or less and may produce a reduction in pulmonary artery wedge pressure within 5 to 10 minutes. It has the advantage of not requiring vascular access for administration, but it has the disadvantage of a short (approximately 15 minutes) duration of effect. When venous access becomes available, titration of intravenous nitroglycerin as an infusion beginning at 10 μg per minute may be used to maintain venodilation. Tolerance to nitroglycerin may develop rapidly, within 24 hours, and infusion rates should be adjusted according to measured pulmonary artery wedge pressure if sustained nitrate therapy is indicated. Nitrates are very potent venodilators and may lead to excessive reduction of cardiac output when ventricular function is unusually preload dependent, as in acute myocardial infarction, especially with large infarctions of the left ventricle or when the right ventricle is involved.

When there is evidence of depressed cardiac output, and especially when systemic vascular resistance is known to be increased in the patient with pulmonary edema, intravenous nitroprusside should be used to obtain arterial dilation as well as venodilation. As a result, both systemic and pulmonary artery pressures may be lowered quickly. Preferably, arterial pressure should be directly monitored through an indwelling arterial catheter, along with pulmonary pressures and cardiac output through a thermodilution pulmonary artery catheter when using nitroprusside. However, if the patient is frankly hypertensive, nitroprusside should be initiated immediately as arrangements for monitoring are being made. In such a hypertensive patient, initial sublingual nitroglycerin immediately followed by intravenous nitroprusside may be the preferred sequence of therapy. An initial infusion of 8 to 10 μg per minute should be increased by increments of 5 to 10 μg per minute at intervals as short as 5 minutes, until the desired pulmonary artery wedge pressure, cardiac output, systemic resistance, or systemic arterial pressure is achieved. Individuals with underlying systemic hypertension may require larger doses, whereas patients with diminutive stature, the elderly, or those with severely depressed ventricular function may require very precise and careful titration of relatively small doses of nitroprusside. Although the usual maximum dose of nitroprusside is in the range of 500 μg per minute, it may be considerably less in the latter types of patients as well as in those with renal failure, in whom the thiocyanate metabolites of nitroprusside may accumulate to toxic levels.

The angiotensin converting enzyme inhibitors captopril, enalapril, and possibly lisinopril appear to have an increasingly valuable role in treatment of chronic heart failure. Some of the newer agents such as benazepril, quinipril, ramapril, and fosinopril may produce similar results. In addition to blockade of the renin-angiotensin system, they may also act by increasing the level of vasodilating prostaglandins. Although they are vasodilators, their role, if any, in the treatment of acute pulmonary edema has not been established. They may be significant, however, as a potential aggravating factor in patients with chronic underlying cardiac disease who are under chronic therapy with these agents because their use may be associated with a deterioration of renal function.

Intravenous administration of a short-acting cardiac glycoside is still a mainstay of treatment in patients with cardiogenic pulmonary edema. It should be a part of the initial regimen, particularly when the pulmonary edema is associated with atrial fibrillation or other supraventricular tachyarrhythmias in patients in whom the pulmonary vascular pressures are increased as a result of a shortened diastole and elevation of left atrial pressure. The patient with mitral stenosis is the prototypical example of this situation. Digoxin acts by increasing the effective refractory period and reducing the ventricular response rate. Occasionally, it may result in conversion to sinus rhythm. Digoxin may also be considered as initial therapy in patients with pulmonary edema and impaired systolic left ventricular function, especially when cardiomegaly is present. Such patients benefit from the positive inotropic effect and mild diuretic effect of digoxin. If the patient has not previously been receiving digoxin, an intravenous loading dose of 0.5 mg should be given over 15 minutes to avoid the possibility of systemic or coronary arterial vasoconstriction with a too-rapid infusion. Subsequently, 0.25 mg may be given every 6 hours to a total of 1 to 1.5 mg, depending on the adequacy of the clinical response. In general, even those patients previously receiving digoxin may benefit from additional drug when they develop acute pulmonary edema, as long as there is no evidence of toxicity, and especially when the deterioration is due to supraventricular tachyarrhythmias with accelerated ventricular response. However, such patients should be examined carefully prior to administration of additional digoxin for manifestations of digitalis toxicity, such as nausea and vomiting, accelerated nonparoxysmal junctional tachycardia, atrial tachycardia with intermittent atrioventricular nodal block, premature ventricular complexes, ventricular tachycardia, bradycardia, and heart block. In the presence of hypokalemia, severe renal failure, or both, extreme caution should be used when giving intravenous digitalis preparations, or it may be avoided entirely. Oral diltiazem in doses of 30 to 90 mg may provide additional blockade of the atrioventricular node and may be a useful adjunct to the digoxin regimen if additional rate-slowing is needed. Intravenous diltiazem (Cardizem) is a useful alternative, or adjunct, to digoxin. Initial dosage of diltiazem is 0.25 mg per kilogram infused over 2 minutes, followed by infusion of 5 to 15 mg per hour. If after 15 minutes the rate response is inadequate, a second bolus of 0.35 mg per kilogram may be given over 2 minutes. Diltiazem is metabolized by the liver and excreted by the kidneys and has a rare potential for negative inotropic effect. Therefore, it should be used with caution in the setting of hepatic or renal dysfunction or severe myocardial dysfunction.

If the aforementioned regimens are ineffective, use of the positive inotropic agents dopamine or dobutamine may be considered. Intravenous dopamine infused at 2 to 5 μg per kilogram per minute improves myocardial contractility, and by decreasing peripheral resistance and improving renal blood flow, it may help to initiate diuresis when previous efforts have failed. However, at higher rates of infusion, tachycardia and vasoconstriction with resultant increase of peripheral resistance may be produced. Dobutamine at intravenous infusion rates of 2 to 10 μg per kilogram per minute may have a positive inotropic effect on cardiac function, with either a small increase or a reduction of left ventricular end-diastolic pressure. Both are sympathomimetic amines and should be used with caution when the pulmonary edema is associated with ischemic coronary disease, especially acute myocardial infarction, because their use may result in an increase in myocardial oxygen demand or production of ventricular arrhythmias.

All the aforementioned therapeutic agents are generally useful, within the guidelines described in each discussion, regardless of the nature of the underlying cardiac disorder. However, the importance of an early, accurate diagnosis cannot be overemphasized. For some cardiac causes of acute pulmonary edema, specific therapy is urgently indicated. Acute pulmonary edema coincident with onset of atrial fibrillation may be quickly reversed with a minimum of pharmacotherapeutics in patients known to have disorders that are critically dependent on coordinated atrial systole, such as mitral stenosis, aortic stenosis with left ventricular hypertrophy, acute myocardial infarction, or hypertrophic cardiomyopathy, if rapid electrical cardioversion can be performed. Similarly, acute pulmonary edema associated with a bradyarrhythmia that fails to respond to isoproterenol may show minimal response to medical treatment until artificial pacing can be instituted. Pericardial tamponade may be dramatically relieved by pericardiocentesis when the response to medications is minimal. Other cardiac conditions may actually be exacerbated by some of the usual therapies. For example, in hypertrophic cardiomyopathy, the patient condition may be severely aggravated by overdiuresis or use of positive inotropic agents or arteriolar dilation. In addition to attempting to make a precise cardiac diagnosis, effort should be directed at identifying and correcting any precipitating or aggravating medical conditions while supportive measures are being applied. Appropriate and early treatment of acute infection, hyperthyroidism, renal failure, or pulmonary embolism, as examples, may greatly facilitate patient response to medical treatment of acute pulmonary edema.

Surgical Treatment

In most cases, medical treatment of acute pulmonary edema can result in satisfactory recovery of the patient. However, there are some cardiac conditions that can result in acute pulmonary edema and that are unlikely to result in more than a modest improvement, if any, with the aforementioned supportive medical approach. These usually involve a major structural alteration of some part of the cardiovascular system. Examples include acute and severe valvular insufficiency of the aortic or mitral valve and, in some cases, severe aortic or mitral stenosis or rupture of the ventricular septum or free wall. In such cases, medical treatment should be instituted as arrangements for corrective surgery are being made. In some cases of chronic heart failure, pulmonary edema may be relatively refractory to medical treatment even after identification and correction of any precipitating or aggravating factors. In such cases, the episode of pulmonary edema may be indicative of progression of the chronic disorder to a critical state. Although emergent or urgent surgery in a patient with incompletely resolved pulmonary edema may be associated with increased risk, undue delay may be associated with an equally poor prognosis. The timing and nature of the cardiac surgery and preparation of the patient should then be based on the nature and severity of the underlying disorder.

Suggested Reading

Chatterjee K, Parmley WW. The role of vasodilator therapy in heart failure. Prog Cardiovasc Dis 1976; 19:301.

DeMots H, Rahimtoola SH, McAnulty JH, Murphy ES. Acute pulmonary edema. In: Mason DT, ed. Cardiac emergencies. Baltimore: Williams & Wilkins, 1978:173.

Ellenbogen KA, Dias VC, Plumb VJ, et al. A placebo-controlled trial of continuous intravenous diltiazem infusion for 24-hour heart rate control during atrial fibrillation and atrial flutter: A multicenter study. J Am Coll Cardiol 1991; 18:891.

Nishimura H, Kubo S, Ueyama M, et al. Peripheral hemodynamic effects of captopril in patients with congestive heart failure. Am Heart J 1989; 117:100.

Spann JF, Hurst JW. Recognition and management of heart failure. In: Hurst JW, ed. The heart. 6th ed. New York: McGraw-Hill, 1990:418.

CARDIOGENIC SHOCK

David W. Ferguson, M.D., F.A.C.C., F.A.C.P., F.C.C.P., Capt. M.C. U.S.N.

Cardiogenic shock is a pathophysiologic state arising from a variety of underlying etiologies, in which the common denominator is marked inadequacy of tissue perfusion due to a primary myocardial defect. Peripheral tissue perfusion is dependent on both arterial pressure and regional vascular resistance, with systemic arterial pressure being determined by cardiac output and systemic vascular resistance. Cardiac output is the product of heart rate and stroke volume. Stroke volume is determined by three major factors: ventricular preload, ventricular afterload, and the inotropic state of the myocardium.

In common clinical usage, cardiogenic shock describes clinical conditions in which forward cardiac output is inadequate to meet peripheral metabolic demands, usually as a result of inadequate forward stroke volume rather than a primary disorder of heart rate. A strict hemodynamic definition, requiring invasive hemodynamic monitoring, is essential for defining this pathophysiologic state and for excluding nonmyocardial etiologies (e.g., hypovolemia) as the cause of the reduced stroke volume. The clinical hemodynamic definition of cardiogenic shock is summarized in Table 1.

Table 1 Hemodynamic and Clinical Essentials for Defining Cardiogenic Shock

Arterial hypotension (intra-arterial catheter)
Absolute: systolic arterial ≤90 mm Hg
Relative: systolic arterial pressure >60 mm Hg below baseline
Impaired forward cardiac output (thermodilution pulmonary arterial catheter)
Cardiac index ≤2.2 L/min/m^2
Widened arterial mixed-venous (preshunt) oxygen content difference
Adequate ventricular preload (pulmonary arterial catheter)
Left ventricular filling pressure ≥12–15 mm Hg
Clinical end-organ hypoperfusion
Depressed or altered mentation
Oliguria (urine output <30 ml/h) or anuria
Peripheral vasoconstriction and/or cyanosis
Presence of primary myocardial insult

■ ETIOLOGY AND PATHOGENESIS

Cardiogenic shock most commonly occurs as an acute deterioration of myocardial function, although this may be superimposed on chronic impairment of cardiac function. In the majority of cases, cardiogenic shock results from acute myocardial infarction, with shock complicating the clinical course in 5 to 15 percent of patients with myocardial infarction. Shock is seen more commonly following anterior wall infarctions than following inferior wall infarctions. Unfortunately, the incidence of and prognosis for cardiogenic shock complicating acute myocardial infarction have not improved during the past 15 years. Detailed postmortem studies have demonstrated that patients sustaining a myocardial infarction complicated by cardiogenic shock, in the absence of a mechanical lesion, usually have infarct involvement of at least 35 percent of their functioning left ventricular mass. However, large inferoposterior infarctions and inferior wall infarctions with significant involvement of the right ventricle may also be complicated by cardiogenic shock. Mechanical defects resulting in regurgitant lesions (e.g., ventricular septal rupture and mitral insufficiency) may produce cardiogenic shock in the setting of an acute infarction and occur with similar frequency in inferior and anterior infarctions. Other noninfarct etiologies of cardiogenic shock are summarized in Table 2.

■ DIAGNOSIS

A high index of clinical suspicion and early diagnosis are essential for effective management of the patient in cardiogenic shock. The prognosis of these patients varies both with the underlying myocardial insult and with the rapidity with which secondary consequences of the shock state develop (e.g., acidosis, multiorgan system failure). Early clinical recognition, rapid hemodynamic assessment, initiation of sup-

Table 2 Differential Diagnosis of Cardiogenic Shock

Acute Myocardial Infarction
Impairment of critical muscle mass
Large anterior left ventricular infarction
Large inferoposterior left ventricular infarction
Massive right ventricular infarction
"Global" subendocardial infarction
Acute mechanical (regurgitant) lesions
Ventricular septal rupture
Acute mitral insufficiency
Severe papillary muscle dysfunction
Rupture of mitral valvular apparatus
Left ventricular free wall rupture
Left ventricular aneurysm
Valvular Heart Disease
Critical valvular stenosis
Severe valvular insufficiency
Obstructive Nonvalvular Cardiac Lesions
Cardiac tamponade
Hypertrophic cardiomyopathy with ventricular outflow obstruction
Constrictive pericardial disorders
Atrial myxoma with ventricular inflow obstruction
Massive pulmonary embolism
Severe restrictive cardiomyopathy
Infectious Cardiac Lesions
Infective endocarditis with valvular involvement
Fulminant myocarditis
Pharmacologic or Physiologic Myocardial Depression
Pharmacologic depressants
Beta-adrenergic blocking agents
Calcium channel blocking agents
Antiarrhythmic agents
Cardiotoxic chemotherapeutic agents
Anesthetic agents
Physiologic depressants
Severe hypoxemia
Severe acidosis
Severe alkalosis
Miscellaneous
End-stage cardiomyopathy
Post-cardiopulmonary bypass myocardial depression
Myocardial depression complicating nonmyocardial disease process
Acute pancreatitis
Septicemia

portive therapy as soon as possible, and expeditious anatomic diagnosis are the keys to successful management. The major goals of therapy are to stabilize the patient hemodynamically and metabolically and to reverse the shock state prior to the development of irreversible end-stage cellular shock.

Cardiogenic shock following myocardial infarction may occur in one of three general patterns: (1) rapid onset of fulminant cardiovascular collapse within the early hours following myocardial insult, usually as a result of massive myocardial involvement or rupture of the left ventricular free wall; (2) abrupt onset of shock with pulmonary edema remote in time from the initial insult, accompanied by a new systolic murmur (papillary muscle dysfunction or rupture with mitral insufficiency or ventricular septal rupture) (Fig. 1); or (3) gradual onset of a low-flow state, culminating in low cardiac output failure and shock over many days, as a result of recurrent "piecemeal" myocardial necrosis. The presentation of other forms of cardiogenic shock varies with the underlying disease processes involved.

The physical examination of the patient with cardiogenic shock also varies with the underlying etiology. Special attention should be directed at determining the presence or absence of tachycardia, hypotension, narrowed pulse pressure, neck vein engorgement, Kussmaul's sign, pulmonary edema, ventricular gallops, murmurs of valvular stenosis or insufficiency, peripheral signs of low output, and stigmata of disease etiologies (e.g., splinter hemorrhages in the setting of endocarditis). The clinician needs to remember, however, that many auscultatory signs of cardiac pathology (e.g., murmurs) are dependent on the forward flow state and may therefore be minimal or absent in patients with severe impairment of cardiac output.

Noninvasive diagnostic studies that may be of benefit include chest roentgenogram, electrocardiogram, two-dimensional echocardiogram with Doppler flow measurement, and radionuclide angiography for assessment of both right and left ventricular function.

Certain physiologic measurements are essential in the management of patients with cardiogenic shock and are outlined in Table 3.

■ PREFERRED APPROACH

Management of the patient with cardiogenic shock needs to be directed simultaneously at correction (if possible) of the underlying myocardial insult and at reversal of the secondary consequences of the shock state. Management can be conceptualized in seven phases (Fig. 2). In reality, all seven phases of management need to overlap and to be implemented in close succession. The exact order of management varies with the condition of the patient. These phases of management include clinical suspicion, initial stabilization, invasive hemodynamic assessment, tailored pharmacologic therapy, anatomic diagnosis, mechanical circulatory support, and definitive therapy.

Initial Assessment and Stabilization

Once the clinical suspicion of cardiogenic shock is entertained, prompt initiation of invasive hemodynamic monitoring is essential. This is because the bedside physical examination is not sensitive enough to predict reliably and serially cardiac filling pressures and forward cardiac output. In addition, these patients require administration of potent pharmacologic agents, with the titration of these agents being dependent on close attention to the patient's hemodynamic response.

Initial assessment of the patient's airway patency and adequacy of ventilation is of paramount importance. The patient should be intubated if the airway cannot be protected and should be ventilated mechanically if there is failure of ventilation or severe failure of oxygenation. Intubation and mechanical ventilation should also be considered in select patients in whom the work of breathing may be too great in view of minimal or no cardiac reserve. Nonintubated patients who have either confirmed hypoxemia (increased alveolar-arterial oxygen gradient) or suspected tissue hypoxia should

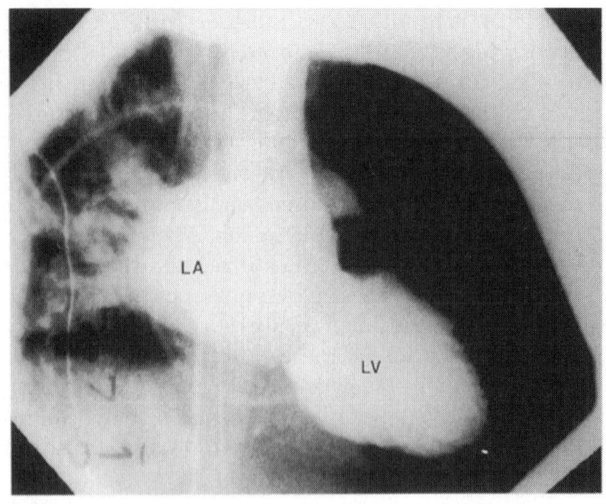

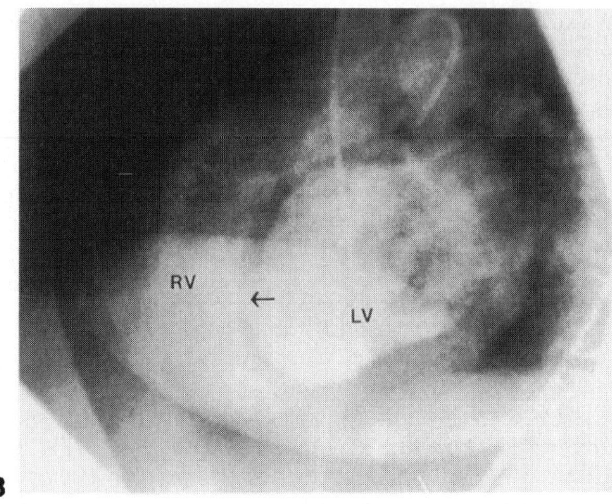

Figure 1
Angiographic definition of mechanical lesions producing cardiogenic shock following acute myocardial infarction. *A,* Left ventricular (LV) angiogram obtained in the right anterior oblique projection during end-systole in a patient with cardiogenic shock and new systolic murmur following an acute inferior wall myocardial infarction. Left ventriculography demonstrates severe mitral insufficiency, with opacification of the entire left atrium (LA) and all four pulmonary veins. *B,* Left ventricular angiogram obtained in the left anterior oblique projection with cranial angulation in a patient with cardiogenic shock and a new systolic murmur occurring 48 hours after acute anterior wall myocardial infarction. A large ventricular septal defect is visualized in the midseptal region (arrow) with left-to-right opacification of the left (LV) and right (RV) ventricles.

Table 3 Essential Physiologic Monitoring in Cardiogenic Shock

Electrocardiographic monitoring (continuous)
Intra-arterial pressure monitoring (continuous)
Pulmonary artery pressure monitoring (continuous)
Balloon flotation catheter
Thermodilution cardiac output capability
Serial (or on-line) oxygen saturation capability
Indwelling Foley catheter with hourly urimetrics
Serial physiochemical assessment
Arterial blood gases: pH, P_{CO_2}, P_{O_2}, O_2 saturation
Arterial-mixed venous oxygen content difference (preshunt)
Alveolar-arterial oxygen tension gradient
Serum electrolytes, blood urea nitrogen, creatinine
Hemoglobin and hematocrit

be maintained on a high-flow oxygen delivery system in which a continuous and known F_{IO_2} can be administered and carefully titrated (e.g., with a Venturi mask). Adequacy of systemic circulation should be assessed rapidly by the level of patient consciousness, palpation of large peripheral pulses, presence of peripheral cyanosis, and assessment of arterial pressure. Cardiopulmonary resuscitation should be implemented if adequate peripheral perfusion cannot be achieved pharmacologically.

At least two large-bore intravenous catheters (≥16 gauge) should be inserted as soon as possible, with one preferably placed centrally under optimal sterile conditions. Ideally, the central catheter should be a venous sheath with sidearm attachment (for drug administration into central circulation), which permits subsequent passage of a pulmonary artery monitoring catheter.

An indwelling arterial line, preferably in a central artery (e.g., femoral), should be inserted as rapidly as possible for accurate measurement of core blood pressure in the patient with profound shock. Accurate assessment of blood pressure in these patients requires the continuous monitoring of blood pressure from a large central artery (e.g., femoral) rather than

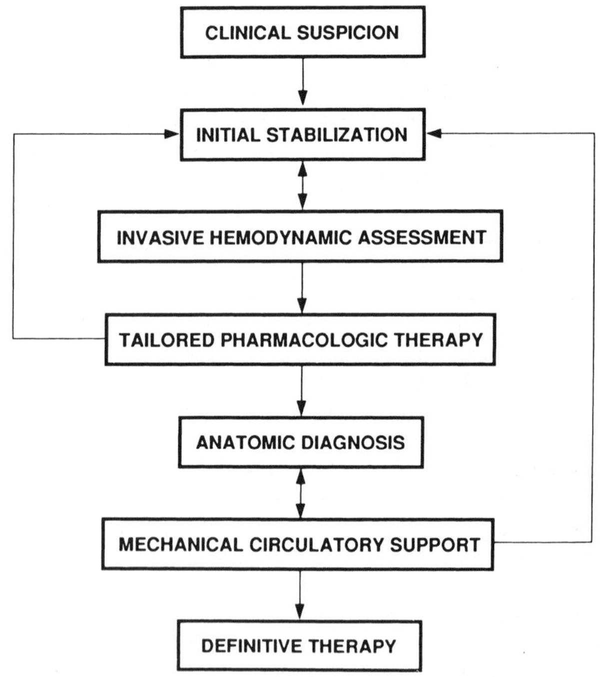

Figure 2
Therapeutic schema for the management of patients with cardiogenic shock.

from a smaller distal artery (e.g., radial). This is related to the presence of intense intrinsic or pharmacologically induced vasoconstriction in these patients, which results in inaccurate pressure waveforms for analysis. A rapid but complete right heart catheterization should be performed with assessment of right atrial, right ventricular, pulmonary arterial, and pulmonary capillary wedge pressures. Careful attention should be paid to obtaining reliable pressure tracings during end-expiration. Visual examination of the waveforms should be performed to assess for diastolic equilibration of right heart pressures (e.g., cardiac tamponade), correlation of pulmonary arterial diastolic and mean pulmonary capillary wedge pressures, ratio of mean right atrial to mean pulmonary capillary wedge pressures (e.g., elevated in right ventricular infarction), and magnitude of atrial and ventricular waveforms in the pulmonary capillary wedge tracing (large *v* waves with slow upslope in the wedge position suggest mitral insufficiency). In addition, initial oximetric assessment should be performed at the time of insertion of the pulmonary arterial catheter, with duplicate blood samples obtained from the superior vena cava, right atrium, pulmonary artery, and systemic artery.

Initial assessment of cardiac output should be performed directly by the thermodilution technique and indirectly by assessment of arterial-mixed venous oxygen content difference. In the presence of a left-to-right intracardiac shunt (e.g., ventricular septal rupture), thermodilution cardiac output will not reflect true forward left heart output, and the repeated bedside determination of an accurate preshunt mixed venous oxygen content sample is impractical. The most important information obtained from this initial hemodynamic assessment is to confirm the true systemic arterial pressure, exclude (or correct) inadequate ventricular preload (e.g., pulmonary capillary wedge pressure <12 mm Hg) as the etiology of the low stroke volume, assess for intracardiac left-to-right shunt (oxygen step-up), and provide a baseline hemodynamic profile on which to base pharmacologic therapy. If the patient is hypovolemic, rapid fluid resuscitation with isotonic saline should be administered initially to maintain the pulmonary capillary wedge pressure in the 15 to 18 mm Hg range.

This initial assessment of the patient in cardiogenic shock should be completed within the first hour of presentation. Other features of initial stabilization include correction of acidosis (or alkalosis), correction of hypoxemia (alveolar-arterial oxygen gradient ≥20 torr), and control of hemodynamically significant cardiac arrhythmias.

Pharmacologic Therapy

All pharmacologic therapy administered to patients in cardiogenic shock must be delivered through secure intravenous lines, preferably via centrally placed catheters where the risk of extravasation is minimized. Pain relief and control of anxiety can be achieved by judicious titration of a reversible narcotic agent such as morphine sulfate. Close monitoring of ventilation (arterial P_{CO_2}), blood pressure, cardiac rate and rhythm, and cardiac filling pressures is essential following administration of morphine. Antiarrhythmic agents should be administered only in the presence of hemodynamically significant cardiac arrhythmias because most of these agents have myocardial depressant actions. The use of lidocaine solely as a prophylactic agent is contraindicated in the presence of cardiogenic shock.

As noted previously, adequate ventricular preload should be maintained by volume administration with normal saline to maintain cardiac filling pressures at 12 to 15 mm Hg or greater. Sequential performance of in vivo Starling's curves with assessment of forward cardiac output at various levels of preload will be required to determine optimal preload in these patients because ventricular compliance is usually decreased and may change rapidly.

On the basis of assessment of arterial pressure, cardiac output, and cardiac filling pressure, patients can be categorized hemodynamically, and appropriate pharmacologic treatment can be tailored to the patient's hemodynamic state. In the presence of cardiogenic shock due to inotropic failure (impaired stroke volume with adequate preload) without severe hypotension, the preferred agent is the synthetic ($beta_1$ and $beta_2$) adrenergic agonist dobutamine. Dobutamine can be titrated (2 to 15 μg per kilogram per minute intravenously) to achieve the desired inotropic effect on the basis of serial measurements of cardiac output, arteriovenous oxygen content difference, and clinical effect (e.g., mentation, urine output). An alternative agent would be the phosphodiesterase inhibitor amrinone administered as an intravenous bolus of 0.75 mg per kilogram over 3 to 5 minutes, followed by an infusion of 5 to 10 μg per kilogram per minute.

In patients with cardiogenic shock manifested by marked inotropic impairment *and* arterial hypotension of more than moderate degree, the administration of dopamine would be the preferred agent. At low doses (0.5 to 2.0 μg per kilogram per minute intravenously), dopamine selectively stimulates dopaminergic receptors primarily in the kidney, with resultant renal arterial dilation and increased urine flow. At intermediate doses (2 to 10 μg per kilogram per minute intravenously), cardiac beta-adrenergic effects predominate, with increases in cardiac output and small increases in heart rate and blood pressure. At higher doses (10 to 20 μg per kilogram per minute intravenously), dopamine produces mixed beta-adrenergic effects and alpha-adrenergic–mediated vasoconstriction, with further increases in cardiac output and heart rate as well as an increase in blood pressure. At very high doses (>20 μg per kilogram per minute intravenously), dopamine acts essentially as an alpha-adrenergic agent with marked peripheral vasoconstriction. The selective dopaminergic renal vasodilating effects of dopamine achieved at low infusion rates are overcome and negated by alpha-vasoconstricting effects of the agent at the upper dose ranges.

Cardiogenic shock complicated by profound hypotension initially may require the use of more potent vasopressor agents such as norepinephrine. Because coronary artery perfusion occurs primarily during diastole, norepinephrine may be required in some patients to maintain diastolic arterial pressure within acceptable ranges to ensure adequate coronary blood flow. Norepinephrine has both beta-adrenergic inotropic and chronotropic effects, but its most profound effect is alpha-adrenergic–mediated vasoconstriction. Norepinephrine should be titrated (2 to 20 μg per minute intravenously) to achieve desired hemodynamic effects. However, as soon as possible an attempt should be made to wean the patient to either dopamine or dobutamine.

Adverse side effects can be encountered with all vasopressor and inotropic agents. Potential side effects include cardiac arrhythmias (both atrial and ventricular), nausea, aggravation of ischemia, ventilatory depression, and profound vasoconstriction. Care must be taken to monitor the patient's cardiac rhythm closely and to ensure the stability of the infusion site during the use of these agents.

Vasodilator therapy may be of significant benefit to patients with cardiogenic shock, especially when used in combination with an intravenous inotrope such as dobutamine or dopamine. However, essential hemodynamic features that must be present to permit effective utilization of vasodilators include adequate ventricular preload and absence of fixed obstruction to ventricular outflow (e.g., critical aortic stenosis). Vasodilators are of particular benefit in the management of regurgitant lesions such as ventricular septal defects and acute aortic or mitral insufficiency. The most appropriate commercially available agent for afterload reduction in the setting of cardiogenic shock is the direct-acting arteriolar vasodilator sodium nitroprusside. Nitroprusside should be administered with close monitoring of arterial pressure and can be titrated every 1 to 3 minutes from an initial intravenous infusion rate of 0.4 μg per kilogram per minute to achieve the desired hemodynamic effect. The major risks associated with nitroprusside infusion are hypotension, adverse reflex tachycardia, arterial hypoxemia due to increase in pulmonary ventilation-perfusion mismatch, and thiocyanate toxicity following prolonged administration. Intravenous nitroglycerin may be of some benefit to patients with low output state, pulmonary congestion, and ongoing myocardial ischemia as the basis for inotropic impairment. The agent is administered via intravenous infusion beginning at approximately 10 μg per minute and is titrated to achieve the desired hemodynamic and clinical effect.

Every effort should be made to stabilize the patient in cardiogenic shock rapidly within the first 2 to 3 hours of presentation. If the patient can be stabilized, further diagnostic studies should be performed to define the precise nature of the cardiac impairment as a guide to definitive therapy. If the patient cannot be stabilized, these additional studies should still be performed, although preceded by placement of mechanical circulatory support devices.

Specialized Diagnostic Studies and Support Procedures

The decision to proceed with specialized studies and mechanical support procedures is one that must be made as rapidly as possible in the course of managing the patient with cardiogenic shock, preferably within the first 4 to 6 hours following initial assessment and stabilization. The decision to proceed with these invasive procedures must be based on a number of factors, including the overall condition of the patient prior to development of cardiogenic shock, the expressed wishes of the patient and the patient's family, and the potential for reversible pathology. It must be remembered, however, that in the setting of cardiogenic shock following myocardial infarction, a survival rate of 50 to 60 percent is the best that can be achieved, even under optimal conditions and with the utilization of the most advanced support procedures. In general, in the absence of definite medical contraindications or wishes expressed by the patient or family to the contrary, it is desirable to proceed with anatomic definition as a guide to both short-term and long-term therapeutic options.

In most cases, definitive and comprehensive anatomic diagnosis requires invasive cardiac catheterization. Noninvasive studies such as echocardiography and nuclear angiography may be of benefit in directing the cardiac catheterization. For example, echocardiography is particularly useful in identifying the presence of mitral insufficiency due to papillary muscle dysfunction or rupture in the presence of ventricular septal rupture. In addition, the presence of a large pericardial effusion is rapidly identified by transthoracic echocardiography. The cardiac catheterization should include a comprehensive right heart hemodynamic study with assessment of oxygen saturations via sampling from the superior and inferior vena cava, right atrium, pulmonary artery, and left ventricle. A biplane left ventricular angiogram should be performed if at all possible, followed by selective coronary arteriography. Additional angiographic studies depend on the underlying disease processes being considered (e.g., aortic root angiography for suspected acute aortic insufficiency in a patient with endocarditis). A minimal but appropriate amount of the least toxic angiographic contrast agent should be used to ensure an adequate angiographic study.

Mechanical circulatory support may be required before, during, or after the cardiac catheterization. From a technical standpoint, the cardiac catheterization suite is probably the preferred locale for placement of such devices via the percutaneous approach. The most frequently used mode of mechanical circulatory support is the intra-aortic balloon pump (IABP). The potential clinical indications for IABP support include (1) cardiogenic shock refractory to maximal medical therapy; (2) mechanical regurgitant lesions for which the IABP may be the preferred therapeutic approach (e.g., acute severe mitral insufficiency or ventricular septal rupture); (3) perioperative support of the high-risk patient with cardiogenic shock who is to undergo surgical intervention; and (4) management of medically refractory myocardial ischemia producing ventricular dysfunction in patients with high-grade coronary lesions.

The IABP can be placed percutaneously over a guidewire from the femoral artery and can be positioned in the thoracic aorta just distal to the left subclavian artery. Under ideal operation, the IABP functions to increase coronary artery diastolic pressure (increase myocardial oxygen delivery), reduce mechanically impedance to left ventricular ejection and lower ventricular preload (reduce myocardial oxygen demand), and reduce the magnitude of regurgitant lesions, thereby improving forward ejection fraction. These effects are achieved without increasing heart rate, as would likely occur if pharmacologic means were employed to achieve the same objectives. Major complications occur in 10 to 30 percent of patients undergoing IABP support and include vascular insufficiency and trauma, infection, and bleeding. Definite contraindications to IABP include severe atherosclerotic peripheral vascular disease, aortic insufficiency, or inability of the patient to tolerate systemic anticoagulation. Other types of temporary mechanical support devices that can be considered for percutaneous placement include portable cardiopulmonary bypass apparatus. In addition to percutaneous support devices, left and right ventricular assist devices and mechanical heart devices are available but require surgical replacement via thoracotomy.

All these mechanical support devices should be considered for use only as temporizing therapy in patients who have correctable or reversible disorders of cardiac function. Every attempt should be made to proceed with definitive therapy and subsequent removal of these devices as soon as possible because complications increase with the duration of use.

Definitive Therapy

Various acute medical and surgical interventional therapies have been described for the treatment of patients with cardiogenic shock. Not unexpectedly, most of these therapeutic approaches have not undergone careful prospective, randomized, controlled trials to assess their efficacy in comparison to conventional noninvasive medical therapy in large numbers of patients with cardiogenic shock. Historical controls emphasizing a mortality rate of 80 to 90 percent in large series of patients treated with medical therapy alone for cardiogenic shock following acute myocardial infarction have been used as justification for these alternative therapies. The individual clinician should consider these alternative therapies but cannot rely on well-designed comparative studies for guidance.

Medical interventions for cardiogenic shock following myocardial infarction include thrombolytic therapy and emergent coronary angioplasty. Successful thrombolytic reperfusion has been shown clearly to improve survival following anterior myocardial infarction and has been described as effective therapy for cardiogenic shock in selected patients. Recently, emergent coronary angioplasty has been reported to offer significant benefit over medical therapy alone when compared retrospectively in a moderate-sized group of patients with acute myocardial infarction complicated by cardiogenic shock. Finally, aortic balloon valvuloplasty has been described recently as a potentially effective therapy for patients with cardiogenic shock resulting from end-stage critical aortic stenosis.

Surgical revascularization for ischemic left ventricular dysfunction and shock has been described but remains controversial. Surgical intervention for mechanical complications of acute myocardial infarction has been the best-described approach for the care of the patient with severe mitral insufficiency or large ventricular septal rupture following acute myocardial infarction. The timing of surgery remains controversial, although recent data suggest that early intervention is probably better than delayed intervention. Whether surgical repair of the defect should be accompanied by myocardial revascularization remains unclear.

Certain forms of cardiogenic shock, such as cardiac tamponade, are reversed readily by definitive intervention (e.g., pericardiocentesis). Surgical valvular replacement has been described as effective therapy in patients with severe regurgitant valvular lesions complicating endocarditis and in patients with cardiogenic shock due to severe valvular stenosis. Mechanical circulatory support may be a useful temporizing measure in the management of patients with fulminant myocarditis and cardiogenic shock.

The role of urgent cardiac transplantation for younger patients with refractory cardiogenic shock of any etiology is being evaluated. Obviously, the keys to the use of this mode of definitive therapy include adequate donor availability and timing of the transplantation. One would not wish to consider transplantation before it is clear that conventional modes of therapy are not sufficient. Yet, one would like to proceed with transplantation before secondary organ failure or complications of shock management (e.g., infection, pulmonary embolism, stress ulceration, adult respiratory distress syndrome) develop and prohibit transplantation.

Suggested Reading

Barbour DJ, Roberts WC. Rupture of a left ventricular papillary muscle during acute myocardial infarction: Analysis of 22 necropsy patients. J Am Coll Cardiol 1986; 8:558.

Ferguson DW. Shock. In: Wyngaarden JB, Smith LH Jr, Bennett JC, Plum F, eds. Cecil textbook of medicine. Philadelphia: WB Saunders, 1992:207.

Goldberg RJ, Gore JM, Alpert JS, et al. Cardiogenic shock after acute myocardial infarction: Incidence and mortality from a community-wide perspective, 1975–1988. N Engl J Med 1991; 325:1117.

Hibbard MD, Holmes DR, Bailey KR, et al. Percutaneous transluminal coronary angioplasty in patients with cardiogenic shock. J Am Coll Cardiol 1992; 19:639.

Joyce LD, Johnson KE, Toninato CJ, et al. Results of the first 100 patients who received symbion total artificial hearts as a bridge to cardiac transplantation. Circulation 1989; 80(Suppl III):192.

Moore CA, Nygaard TW, Kaiser DL, et al. Postinfarction ventricular septal rupture: The importance of location of infarction and right ventricular function in determining survival. Circulation 1986; 74:45.

Moosvi AR, Khaja F, Villanueva L, et al. Early revascularization improves survival in cardiogenic shock complicating acute myocardial infarction. J Am Coll Cardiol 1992; 19:907.

Pennington DG, Kanter KR, McBride LR, et al. Seven years' experience with the Pierce-Donachy ventricular assist device. J Thorac Cardiovasc Surg 1988; 96:901.

Schreiber TL, Miller DH, Zola B. Management of myocardial infarction shock: Current status. Am Heart J 1989; 117:435.

Stone PH, Raabe DS, Jaffe AS, et al. for the MILIS GROUP. Prognostic significance of location and type of myocardial infarction: Independent adverse outcome associated with anterior location. J Am Coll Cardiol 1988; 11:453.

Thanavaro S, Kleiger RE, Province MA, et al. Effect of infarct location on the in-hospital prognosis of patients with first transmural myocardial infarction. Circulation 1982; 66:742.

CARDIAC ARREST AND RESUSCITATION FROM SUDDEN DEATH

Corey M. Slovis, M.D., F.A.C.P., F.A.C.E.P.
Steven L. Brody, M.D.

Sudden death has been defined by various authors as death occurring instantaneously, 1, 2, or 24 hours after the onset of acute symptoms. Most sudden deaths that occur within 2 hours of the acute onset of symptoms are due to a malignant rhythm disturbance in patients with underlying coronary atherosclerotic heart disease (CASHD) or cardiomyopathy. Approximately 60 to 70 percent of these arrhythmia-induced sudden death victims have ventricular fibrillation (VF), whereas asystole or bradyasystole, electromechanical dissociation, and ventricular tachycardia (VT) each account for about 10 percent. Only one-half of patients have a known history of coronary artery disease. Pathologic evidence of an acute myocardial infarction as the terminal event is seen in only a minority of cardiac sudden death victims. The other major noncardiac causes of sudden death are ruptured aortic aneurysm, pulmonary embolism, and cerebrovascular accident.

■ RISK FACTORS

Risk factors for sudden cardiac death include a history of CASHD, especially in association with abnormal ventricular function or aneurysm; hypertension; hypercholesterolemia; diabetes mellitus; cigarette smoking; family history; male sex; black race; history of prior malignant arrhythmias, especially primary VF; hereditary prolongation of the Q-T interval; and use of any medication that has significant effects on the electrocardiogram (ECG), such as quinidine and other oral antiarrhythmic agents.

■ SURVIVAL

In general, resuscitation rates from cardiac arrest are dismal. Only 8 to 15 percent of all patients who suffer a cardiac arrest survive to hospital discharge, and up to one-half of these patients have a significant degree of functional impairment, intellectual impairment, or both. Survival of cardiac arrests in hospitalized patients is similarly poor.

Factors that favor a successful resuscitation from cardiac arrest include a witnessed arrest, well-performed bystander cardiopulmonary resuscitation (CPR), advanced life support in less than 4 to 8 minutes, VF as the underlying arrest rhythm, rapid defibrillation, and quick return of a perfusing rhythm. Additional favorable factors include a primary cardiac etiology for the arrest, no functional impairment prior to the arrest, and fewer than two major organ system diseases in hospitalized patients. Based on the results of multiple studies and the Brain Resuscitation Clinical Trials, functional survival after 10 to 15 minutes of pulselessness is highly unlikely. Due to this poor outcome, physicians and patients should establish a "code status" at the time of hospitalization. The patient's desires, as enunciated in an advanced directive or living will, should be readily available and should always be respected.

Successful resuscitation from cardiac arrest requires an organized and rapid response by any or all of the following: the victim's family, prehospital care providers, and hospital workers from all areas of the hospital, particularly the emergency department and coronary care unit. Sudden death usually occurs out of the hospital, and most cases are witnessed, often by relatives. Thus, learning basic cardiac life support (BCLS) is imperative for the entire family of patients with CASHD.

■ BASIC CARDIAC LIFE SUPPORT

Many of the recent changes in BCLS reflect a better understanding of the biomechanics involved with manual chest compression. Because of the possible coexistence of cervical spine injury, the airway should be opened with a chin lift or jaw thrust and not by hyperextending the neck. Foreign bodies in the airway should be cleared by the Heimlich maneuver and not via back slaps. After an arrest state has been established, two slow breaths, rather than the previously recommended four rapid breaths, should be provided. Chest compressions for adults should be at a depth of 1 ½ to 2 inches and given at a rate of at least 100 per minute.

■ ADVANCED CARDIAC LIFE SUPPORT

The American Heart Association's Advanced Cardiac Life Support (ACLS) recommendations serve as the basis for resuscitating patients in cardiac arrest. The ACLS guidelines are not inviolate standards of care; they are merely recommendations that should be modified, based on the most current available information. Recent data suggest that early defibrillation is the most effective therapy for improving outcome from cardiac arrest. These data have led to the development and now widespread use of automatic defibrillators in the out-of-hospital arrest setting. Several other interventions have been less effective and are no longer used.

Isoproterenol, a potent beta-agonist, had previously been recommended in the treatment of asystole and electromechanical dissociation-pulseless electrical activity (EMD-PEA). It is no longer recommended, however, because it lacks the alpha-adrenergic agonist properties necessary for coronary artery and cerebral perfusion. Calcium chloride was also commonly used in cardiac arrests. It is no longer routinely used because of a lack of proven efficacy. Calcium administration may also increase the likelihood of postarrest ischemic neuronal damage and cerebral hypoperfusion.

PREFERRED APPROACH

Asystole

The keys to treating asystole successfully are to diagnose its presence correctly, provide rapid oxygenation, and administer epinephrine quickly (Table 1). The treatment of asystole begins with confirming the diagnosis of a pulseless, electrically silent rhythm. Loss of a monitor lead, failure to increase the ECG's gain, or fine ventricular fibrillation may all simulate asystole, and all these should be ruled out rapidly. The patient's airway should then be secured, and the patient should be oxygenated and hyperventilated. Endotracheal intubation is the optimal way to secure an airway and also allows endotracheal drug administration of the patient's initial medications if a large-bore intravenous line is not yet functional (Table 2). Epinephrine, atropine, and lidocaine may all be given via the endotracheal route; calcium and bicarbonate should never be given endotracheally.

As the patient is being hyperventilated, 1 mg of epinephrine and 1 mg of atropine should be administered rapidly. Atropine may be especially useful in primary bradyasystolic arrests. A single 360 watt second defibrillation should be performed whenever presumed asystole could also potentially be interpreted as fine ventricular fibrillation, i.e., in a moving ambulance.

Table 1 Five-Step Protocol for Treating Asystole

STEP 1:	Confirm Asystole 1. Check monitor and lead connections 2. Switch to two or more leads
STEP 2:	Oxygenate Intubate, oxygenate, and hyperventilate with 100% oxygen
STEP 3:	Begin Therapy 1. Epinephrine 1 mg 2. Atropine 1 mg 3. Defibrillate at 360 ws*
STEP 4:	Continue Epinephrine Therapy Epinephrine 1 mg q 3–5 minutes
STEP 5:	Re-evaluate Resuscitation 1. Evaluate $ETCo_2$ reading 2. Consider termination of code

1 mg of epinephrine = 1 cc of 1:1,000 or 10 cc of 1:10,000
*if fine ventricular fibullation is a possibility
Modified from Slovis CM, Wrenn KD: The technique of managing asystole. J Crit Illness. 1995;10:363.

Table 2 Guidelines for Endotracheal Medications Given in Cardiac Arrests

- Stop manual cardiac compressions for 5 sec postadministration
- Use the maximum recommended drug dosage
- Either dilute to 10 to 20 ml or flush the medication with 5 to 10 ml of saline
- Inject the medication into the distal portion of the endotracheal tube using a plastic intravenous catheter (not a needle) affixed to the syringe
- Hyperventilate the patient

From Slovis CM, Brody SL. The technique of reversing ventricular fibrillation. J Crit Illness 1988; 3:93; with permission.

At least 1 mg epinephrine should be repeated every 3 to 5 minutes. Higher doses of epinephrine may still be utilized by some; however, the efficacy of high-dose alpha stimulation remains unproven.

A 1 mg dose of epinephrine was used with small mongrel dogs in the landmark studies of Redding and Pearson during the 1960s. This 1 mg dose has long been used for adult humans weighing 70 to 100 kg. More recent studies have demonstrated that a dose of 0.2 mg per kilogram of epinephrine is required to raise aortic diastolic pressure to 25 to 27 mm Hg. This is the minimum pressure required to perfuse coronary and cerebral blood vessels during manual CPR. Based on these data, many acute care clinicians and EMS agencies switched to "high-dose" epinephrine and began using doses of 5 to 15 mg every few minutes. Unfortunately, a number of recent human studies have failed to show any improvement in neurologic outcome or survival with the use of high-dose epinephrine. Patients were more likely to regain a perfusing rhythm with high-dose epinephrine, but this did not affect their chances for survival or a better neurologic outcome.

The role of pH correction by bicarbonate administration in cardiac arrest victims is not yet clearly established. Based on data from Weil and co-workers, very selective use of bicarbonate appears to be most appropriate for pulseless patients in asystole, EMD-PEA, and VF. This is because the acidosis seen early in cardiac arrest is predominantly a respiratory acidosis that should be treated by hyperventilation. Because bicarbonate and carbon dioxide ions attempt to equilibrate ($HCO_3 \leftrightarrow HCO_3 \leftrightarrow H_2O + CO_2$), bicarbonate administration has the potential of paradoxically lowering the pH as a result of a cellular increase in carbon dioxide. At present, bicarbonate administration (1 mEq per kilogram) should be reserved for those patients who are known to be acidotic prior to their cardiac arrests such as those in diabetic ketoacidosis or septic shock.

The survival rate for victims of asystole is less than 1 to 2 percent. Pacemaker insertion, calcium chloride administration, and isoproterenol infusion have all proven to be ineffective. It seems morally and ethically justified to discontinue CPR in these arrest victims after 10 to 15 minutes of advanced life support that has included optimal oxygenation, hyperventilation, attempts at pH correction if appropriate, and multiple doses of epinephrine. Patients who receive appropriate prehospital ACLS will not survive if they remain in asystole or EMD-PEA throughout transport. Consideration should be given to pronouncing these patients dead on arrival. We highly recommend the use of an end-tidal CO_2 ($ETCO_2$) detector to help provide objective evidence of the futility of continued CPR. Disposable $ETCO_2$ detectors are now readily available. Patients with low or no detectable $ETCO_2$ who persist in asystole or EMD-PEA should have their arrests terminated after 10 to 15 minutes of advanced life support whether performed in the field or hospital.

Ventricular Fibrillation

The successful treatment of VF is based on rapid defibrillation. All other therapy rendered for VF is merely an attempt to make the myocardium more responsive to electrical reversion. Patients found in VF should be immediately shocked at

Table 3 Treatment of Ventricular Fibrillation (and Pulseless V Tach)

PHASE I:	*Electrical Reversion Phase*
	1. Shock 200 ws
	2. Reshock 300 ws
	3. **Reshock 360 ws**
PHASE II:	*Correct Correctable Causes Phase*
	1. Intubate, oxygenate, and hyperventilate with 100% O_2
	2. 10 cc of epinephrine 1:10,000 via large-bore IV or ET tube
	3. **Shock at 360 ws**
PHASE III:	*Lidocaine Phase*
	1. 1.5 mg/kg lidocaine (75–150 mg) IV push
	2. **Shock at 360 ws**
PHASE IV:	*Antiarrhythmic Phase*
	1. 500 mg Bretylium (one amp) IV push, and
	2. 2 g $MgSO_4$ (4 cc of 50%) IV push
	3. **Shock 360 ws**
PHASE V:	*Refractory Phase*
	1. Readminister additional antiarrhythmics
	2. Repeat epinephrine q 5 minutes
	3. **Reshock at 360 ws q 1 minute**
	ANTIARRHYTHMICS FOR REFRACTORY V-FIB
	Double-dose—two ampules **bretylium** (1,000 mg) IV Push
	and/or
	1-2 grams of $MgSO_4$ (2–4 cc of 50%) q 1 minute
	and/or
	20 mg/min **procainamide**
	and/or
	1 mg IV **propranolol** q 1 minute
	and/or
	amiodarone 150 mgs IV over 10 minutes
	and/or
	Repeat **lidocaine** 1–1.5 mg/kg (75–150 mg) IV push

Modified from Slovis CM, Wrenn KD: The technique of reversing ventricular fibrillation. J Crit Illness. 1994;9:878.

200 watt-seconds. Time should not be wasted attempting to secure the airway or administering medications. It is easiest to remember the treatment of VF by using a five-phase protocol (Table 3).

Phase I of the VF protocol is the electrical reversion phase. Patients are successively shocked at 200, 300, and 360 watt-seconds if VF continues. A 200 watt-second initial shock maximizes the chance for a successful defibrillation without increasing the likelihood of electrically induced myocardial damage. Firm paddle pressure should be applied (25 lb per square inch) as the patient is defibrillated, and it is imperative that no one be in contact with the patient or stretcher-bed at the time the shock is delivered.

Phase II is the reversible causes phase. Potentially reversible causes of VF, including hypoxia, acidosis, vasodilation, and coronary hypoperfusion, are treated by intubation, oxygenation, hyperventilation, and administration of 1 mg of epinephrine (10 ml of 1:10,000). This phase, like all others, ends with a 360 watt-second shock.

Phase III in the management of VF is the lidocaine phase. One or more antiarrhythmic agents should be administered rapidly and briefly allowed to circulate, and the patient should be reshocked with 360 watt-seconds. A bolus dose of lidocaine (1.5 mg per kilogram) is currently the best initial antiarrhythmic choice. Lidocaine has a long history of use in malignant ventricular arrhythmias, although its use in ischemic VF is not well studied. It works by depressing excitability and normalizing conduction in ischemic myocardial cells.

Phase IV is the antiarrhythmic phase where the antiarrhythmics bretylium and/or magnesium are rapidly administered. Bretylium, which works via a poorly understood mechanism as an antifibrillant, seems to have similar efficacy to lidocaine in VF. The combined use of these two agents may have additive or synergistic effects in VF. Magnesium's role in the treatment of VF has not yet been clearly defined. It has calcium blocking effects, speeds repolarization, and stimulates the sodium-potassium adenosine triphosphatase (ATPase)-mediated pump. It shortens the duration of phase II and increases the negativity of the resting membrane potential (phase V), thus making spontaneous depolarization less likely. It has been successful in reversing VF that was refractory to other antiarrhythmic agents. We recommend its use early in the therapy of VF because of its potential efficacy and nearly complete lack of toxicity in arrest victims. Intravenous amiodarone has recently become available and may prove useful in the treatment of refractory VF. The initial loading dose for VF is 150 mg over 10 minutes.

In phase V, refractory VF is treated by attempts at defibrillation at least every 60 seconds, checking for and correcting arterial blood gas abnormalities, repeating epinephrine, and trying additional antiarrhythmic agents. Repeat doses of lidocaine (75 to 100 mg), double-dose bretylium (1,000 mg), and magnesium (1 g every minute to a total dose of 5 to 10 g) should be considered. Consideration should be given to trying propranolol (1 mg) every minute for three to five doses. Beta-blockers such as propranolol increase the relative refractory period of ischemic myocardium and have membrane stabilizing effects when given intravenously. Procainamide may also be tried as bolus doses of 100 mg every 5 minutes. Propranolol may be especially useful for patients in refactory VF due to cocaine intoxication or those arrest victims who have previously received multiple doses of epinephrine.

Survival rates in VF may approach 50 percent in patients who are rapidly defibrillated, and most survivors usually respond to the first few shocks. Patients with prolonged VF rarely survive and may convert to asystole or EMD-PEA after defibrillation. Pulseless idioventricular rhythms after defibrillation should be observed for up to 30 seconds to allow for spontaneous reversion to a perfusing rhythm.

Ventricular Tachycardia

The therapy of VT is determined by patient stability. It is most helpful to think of the treatment of VT along a continuum that ranges from the administration of antiarrhythmic medications to immediate electrical conversion (Table 4). Patients who are pulseless are treated exactly like those patients in VF (see Table 3). Patients who are unstable as evidenced by hypotension, chest pain, or alterations in mental status should be electrically converted with 100 watt-seconds. Although VT is electrically responsive and may respond with as little as 5 to

Table 4 Initial Treatment of Ventricular Tachycardia

STABLE (NO CHEST PAIN, NORMAL BLOOD PRESSURE)	BORDERLINE (CHEST PAIN, BORDERLINE BLOOD PRESSURE, ELDERLY)	UNSTABLE (HYPOTENSIVE, UNCONSCIOUS, PULMONARY EDEMA)	ARREST
Lidocaine 1.5 mg/kg over 1 min	Lidocaine 1.5 mg/kg over 1 min *and* Shock at 100 ws if no response to lidocaine (premedicate with IV diazepam)	Shock at 100 ws *and* Administer lidocaine 1.5 mg/kg rapidly	Treat as ventricular fibrillation
ONCE CONVERTED			
Maintain patient on antiarrhythmic(s) (i.e., lidocaine 3 mg/min *and/or* magnesium 1–2g/hour)			

Table 5 Treatment of Refractory Ventricular Tachycardia

STABLE			BORDERLINE OR UNSTABLE
Antiarrhythmic(s) and consider shock		*Antiarrhythmics*	Reshock at 200 ws *and* Begin antiarrhythmic(s)
	Magnesium sulfate	2 g (4 ml of 50%) over 1–5 min *and/or*	
	Procainamide	20 mg/min *and/or*	
	Propranolol	0.5–1 mg every 1–5 min *and/or*	
	Bretylium	25–50 mg/min *and/or*	
	Lidocaine	0.5 mg/kg over 1 min (if 1 mg/kg given 10 min previously)	

10 watt-seconds, a 100 watt-second shock maximizes the likelihood of a one-shock conversion.

Progressively lower electrical energy settings should be used in patients who revert back to VT after an initial 100 watt-second shock. Unless a separate and distinct T wave is apparent in a stable patient with a heart rate below 160 beats per minute, the unsynchronized mode is recommended for cardioverting VT.

Stable patients in VT should be treated initially with antiarrhythmic agents. Lidocaine in an intravenous dose of 1.5 mg per kilogram (75 to 100 mg) is the best initial choice. It has a very high safety profile in single-dose administration, works rapidly, and is very effective in VT associated with acute myocardial infarction. Lidocaine is not as effective in cases of torsades de pointes VT or in VT that is recurrent or chronic. Patients who respond to a bolus of lidocaine should be placed on a lidocaine drip at 2 to 3 mg per minute. A rebolus of lidocaine at one-half the initial loading dose has been recommended 8 to 10 minutes after the first administration. This dose must be slowly administered over 30 to 60 seconds to minimize lidocaine toxicity.

Most of the side effects of lidocaine have occurred at the time of the rebolus or when the patient is left on a drip for more than 6 to 12 hours. Patients with heart failure, liver failure, or renal failure; who are older than age 74; and who are taking medications that decrease the hepatic metabolism of lidocaine, such as erythromycin, cimetidine, and propranolol, are at highest risk for lidocaine toxicity. Clinicians must make a risk-benefit analysis before choosing to rebolus stable patients.

Patients who do not respond to a single dose of lidocaine should receive a second agent or be cardioverted (Table 5). The use of a concurrent lidocaine drip is at the physician's discretion. The efficacy of a continued lidocaine infusion is minimal in the patient who has failed to respond to a bolus dose.

Procainamide and magnesium sulfate are the two second-line agents that are most likely to be effective in patients with VT in the acute setting. Procainamide is an electrically stabilizing agent that works by decreasing rates of conduction through the conducting system and ventricular tissue. It is administered at a dose of 20 mg per minute or as a 100 mg bolus every 5 minutes until the VT abates. It must be discontinued temporarily if hypotension or QRS widening (of 50 percent or more) occurs. A slow intravenous infusion of bretylium (5 mg per kilogram, 25 to 50 mg per minute) may also be tried. The side effects of nausea, vomiting, and hypotension make this drug less attractive. Adenosine (6 to

12 mg IV push) should be considered for patients with presumed VT that is refractory to multiple antiarrhythmic agents, as it may convert aberrantly conducted SVT.

Magnesium is the drug of choice for the torsades de pointes variant of VT. It works immediately and has reversed torsades de pointes in patients who had been previously unresponsive to treatment with multiple agents. Magnesium is also very effective for patients with VT associated with hypokalemia, cyclic antidepressant overdose, or digitalis toxicity and for patients with prolonged Q-T intervals. Magnesium should be given as a 2 g rapid infusion. It may be pushed as a bolus in less stable patients or infused over 1 to 5 minutes in relatively stable patients. An infusion of 2 g per hour should be started in any patient who initially responds to magnesium. Flushing or dysphoria may be experienced temporarily by patients, but serious side effects of magnesium at these doses are nearly nonexistent in patients with normal renal function.

Beta-blocking agents, including propranolol or esmolol, may be used in the acute setting of VT. These agents work by decreasing sympathetic tone and decreasing the rate of impulse conduction. Patients with VT associated with cocaine overdose or VT after epinephrine use are most likely to benefit from propranolol (0.5 to 1 mg every 1 minute) or esmolol (0.5 mg per kilogram IV push).

A brief attempt at pharmacologic control of VT prior to a 100 watt-second shock seems most appropriate in patients who border on instability. A single bolus of lidocaine and a brief trial of procainamide or magnesium sulfate may be appropriate for this group of patients. In general, conscious, alert patients should be sedated with low doses of an intravenous benzodiazepine prior to electrical reversion. The risks of sedation prior to elective cardioversion and possible intubation must be weighed against delaying cardioversion.

Patients who have recurrent ventricular ectopy or VT must have reversible causes of ventricular instability ruled out. These include hypoxia, hypokalemia, hypomagnesemia, profound acidosis or alkalosis, and concurrent arrhythmogenic medication administration or device insertion (e.g., isoproterenol or theophylline administration and pacemaker or Swan-Ganz catheter insertion).

Pulseless Electrical Activity and Electromechanical Disassociation

Pulseless electrical activity (PEA) is defined as organized electrical activity without evidence of perfusion. Electromechanical dissociation (EMD) is defined as organized electrical activity in the absence of ventricular contractions. PEA is now the preferred term as a number of patients previously considered in EMD (though unable to generate a pulse or decrease in blood pressure), have been shown to have regular ventricular contractions. Whether the patient has EMD or PEA is trivial as compared to finding and treating potentially reversible causes of this often agonal rhythm. There are numerous irreversible causes of EMD-PEA, including aortic dissection, free wall rupture, and massive pulmonary embolus. The reversible causes fall into five categories (Table 6). Therapy is directed toward ruling out each category in an orderly fashion (Table 7). An epinephrine titration should be administered rapidly if no reversible cause can be established.

Patients in EMD-PEA should be rapidly intubated, oxygenated, and hyperventilated. This practice corrects both hypoxia and acidosis; it also allows assessment of breath sounds and ease of Ambu-bag compressions, two keys in identifying a tension pneumothorax. EMD-PEA in a patient with asthma or chronic obstructive pulmonary disease should be considered due to a tension pneumothorax until proved otherwise. Patients at increased risk for a tension pneumothorax such as those with bronchospasm, positive pressure ventilation or those who develop EMD-PEA after a central line insertion should have a 14 gauge needle inserted in their second intercostal spaces of each midclavicular line in an attempt to relieve a possible tension pneumothorax.

Table 6 Reversible Causes of EMD-PEA

Hypoxia
Tension pneumothorax
Hypotension
Cardiac tamponade
Toxic metabolic causes

Table 7 Treatment of EMD-PEA

1. Intubate, Oxygenate, and Hyperventilate
   a. Consider Tension Pneumothorax
2. Consider Reversible Causes
   a. Evaluate ECG for hyperkalemia*
   b. Evaluate neck veins; consider tamponade and hypovolemia
   c. Evaluate patient's temperature; consider hypo- and hyperthermia
3. Begin High Flow IV Normal Saline solution
4. Begin Pharmacologic Therapy
   a. Administer 1 mg epinephrine (10 cc of 1:10,000) every 3 minutes
   b. Administer 1 mg Atropine every 3 minutes if heart rate is below 60
5. Reconsider Reversible Causes
   a. Reconsider the 5 reversible causes of EMD-PEA
   b. Evaluate $ETCO_2$ readings
   c. Consider blood gas evaluation
   d. Consider termination of code

*Administer 5 ml of 10% CaCl IV push if hyperkalemia is suspected

Once the patient in EMD-PEA is intubated, the ECG should be evaluated closely for evidence of hyperkalemia and bradycardia. Hyperkalemia should be strongly suspected in patients with renal failure or in others at risk for hyperkalemia. Calcium at a starting dose of 5 ml of 10 percent calcium chloride should be administered to patients with wide complex electromechanical dissociation and suspected hyperkalemia as evidenced by tall-peaked T waves or a sine wavelike ECG. It should be followed immediately by glucose (100 ml of 50 percent) and insulin (10 units IV push). Atropine (1 mg IV push) should be given to patients in electromechanical dissociation with a heart rate of less than 60.

The patient's neck veins should also be evaluated rapidly. Hypovolemia is assumed if the neck veins are not prominent and should be treated by aggressive volume repletion (two large-bore intravenous lines of crystalloid, run wide open). Pericardial tamponade should be suspected in patients with electromechanical dissociation and elevated neck veins. Tamponade is a relatively rare cause of electromechanical dissociation but should be strongly suspected in patients with a history of renal failure, lymphoma, tuberculosis, pericarditis, or open heart surgery. Pericardiocentesis is required in these patients. A palpable pulse will return when as little as 10 to 30 ml of blood is removed from the pericardium. Patients should have their body temperatures rapidly assessed by touch and subsequently by a rectal thermaprobe.

If the patient persists in EMD-PEA, high-flow intravenous lines should be initiated and epinephrine at a dose of 1.0 mg administered every 3 minutes. Atropine should also be administered at a dose of 1.0 mg every 3 minutes if the patient's heart rate remains below 60 beats per minute. As the epinephrine and atropine are being administered, all potentially reversible causes, especially toxic-metabolic etiologies should be reconsidered.

Potentially toxic metabolic reversible causes of EMD-PEA include drug overdoses with digitalis, cyclic antidepressants, beta-blockers, and calcium blockers; hypothermia; and hyperthermia. If no return of circulation is obtained after all reversible causes have been ruled out and epinephrine in appropriate doses has been administered, the resuscitation should be terminated. The survival rate of patients with electromechanical dissociation is similar to the less than 1 to 2 percent survival rate reported in patients with asystole. A low or undetectable $ETCO_2$ reading is helpful in supporting a decision to discontinue CPR.

Special Cardiac Arrest Situations

Drowning

Drowning victims who suffer cardiac arrest should be evaluated for concomitant hypothermia, cervical spine injury, head trauma, other occult injuries, tension pneumothorax, and profound acidosis. Early bicarbonate administration is usually indicated, owing to the likelihood of a combined metabolic and respiratory acidosis.

Drug Overdose

Cardiac arrest from an overdose of digitalis, cyclic antidepressant, calcium channel blocker, or beta-blocker should be treated by attempting to reverse the pharmacologic actions of the offending agent. Digitalis-induced arrests should be treated by Fab fragment antibodies, magnesium, and evaluation for digitalis-induced hyperkalemia. Magnesium stimulates the sodium-potassium ATPase pump, which digitalis poisons. Phenytoin's efficacy in ventricular arrhythmia associated with digitalis toxicity is predominantly anecdotal, and its role in life-threatening overdoses is unclear.

Cardiac arrests due to cyclic antidepressant overdose should be treated by attempting to alkalinize the patient to an arterial pH of 7.5 to 7.55 via both sodium bicarbonate administration and hyperventilation. Sodium bicarbonate helps normalize conduction in poisoned sodium channels, and alkalinization increases the percentage of protein-bound inactive drug. Magnesium is very effective in ventricular arrhythmias due to cyclic toxicity because of its ability to shorten the prolonged Q-T interval (phase 2 prolongation) associated with the antidepressants.

Beta-blockers and calcium blocking agents may cause arrests by inducing bradycardias and hypotension. Both may be treated by an epinephrine drip (1 mg in 250 ml D_5W). Calcium blocker toxicity should also be treated by immediate calcium chloride infusion (1 to 20 ml of 10 percent calcium chloride). Beta-blocker toxicity may also respond to calcium. Glucagon (2 to 5 mg IV) has been effective in refractory cases of beta-blocker and calcium blocker overdose. Its mechanism of action appears to be via the stimulation of nonalpha, nonbeta myocardial receptors. If readily available, cardiopulmonary bypass may be lifesaving. Isoproterenol is of little value in these overdoses.

Hypothermia and Hyperthermia

Cardiac arrests due to hypothermia should be treated by aggressive core-rewarming techniques, including heated mist and heated peritoneal, orogastric, or rectal lavage. If readily available, cardiopulmonary bypass provides the highest likelihood for successful resuscitation from hypothermia. Cardiac arrests due to hyperthermia may respond to aggressive volume resuscitation in association with rapid cooling, using evaporative heat loss. Fans should be directed onto the hyperthermic patient, and the patient's skin should be kept constantly wet.

Traumatic Arrests

Patients suffering traumatic cardiac arrests should be rapidly intubated and evaluated for tension pneumothorax and pericardial tamponade. Thoracotomy and open chest compressions are indicated for penetrating chest injuries that result in cardiac arrest. Patients who suffer a cardiac arrest after penetrating chest injuries may be successfully resuscitated neurologically intact if they have early open chest CPR and thoracic exploration for aortic cross-clamping and ventricular repair. Patients rarely survive cardiac arrest due to blunt trauma; open thoracotomy in these patients is not beneficial.

Postarrest Management

Attention should be focused on optimizing oxygenation, ventilation, and hemodynamic status while minimizing metabolic demands following the successful resuscitation from cardiac arrest. A constant infusion of 2 to 3 mg per minute of lidocaine should be maintained if VT or VF was the arrest rhythm. Serum levels of magnesium and potassium along with arterial blood gases should be evaluated in surviving patients. Possible acute myocardial infarction should be ruled out, although an elevated serum creatine kinase MB fraction must be interpreted with caution in patients who have received prolonged chest compressions or multiple defibrillations. Unstable patients, especially those with a depressed level of consciousness, should remain intubated and fully supported by mechanical ventilation. Ventilator settings that provide an FIO_2 of 90 percent, a tidal volume of 12 ml per kilogram, and a rate of 12 are appropriate for most patients immediately following arrest. Mean arterial pressures should be tightly controlled within the 100 to 200 mm Hg range to maximize cerebral and coronary artery perfusion. An arterial catheter should be placed for continuous blood pressure monitoring and arterial blood gas sampling. Hypotension should be treated with crystalloid infusion or, if unsuccessful, with dopamine infusion (starting at 5 μg per kilogram per minute). Hypertension should be treated with nitroprusside or nitroglycerin infusion, rapidly titrating upward from 5 to 10 μg per minute. A pulmonary artery catheter may be useful in the unstable patient. Metabolic demands should be minimized by providing sedation, controlling temperature, maintaining normoglycemia, providing nutrition, and aggressively treating seizures with a benzodiazepine and phenytoin. Prophylaxis for deep vein thrombophlebitis should be initiated.

Careful serial examination of neurologic status is mandatory in postarrest patients. To date, no specific drug has been found to improve cerebral outcome. The deeply comatose patient with minimal brainstem function after 3 to 4 days is unlikely to have a normal outcome, and consideration of further life support should be discussed with the patient's family.

Suggested Reading

Bialecki, L, Woodward RS. Predicting Death After CPR. Chest. 1995; 108: 1009–1017.

Brown CG, Martin DR, Pepe PE, et al. A comparison of standard-dose epinephrine in cardiac arrest outside the hospital. N Engl J Med 1992; 15: 1051.

Brown CG, Wesman HA. Adrenergic agonists during cardiopulmonary resuscitation. Resuscitation 1990; 19:1.

Callaham M, Madsen CD, Barton CW, et al. A randomized clinical trial of high-dose epinephrine and norepinephrine vs standard-dose epinephrine in prehospital cardiac arrest. JAMA 1992; 19:2667.

Cummins RO (ed): Textbook of advanced cardiac life support. Dallas, American Heart Association, 1994.

Fulton RL, Voigt WJ, Hilakos AS. Confusion surrounding the treatment of traumatic cardiac arrest. J Am Coll Surg. 1995; 181:209–214.

Gallagher EJ, Lombardi G, Gennis P. Effectiveness of bystander cardiopulmonary resuscitation and survival following out-of-hospital cardiac arrest. JAMA 1995; 274:1922–1925.

Gray W, Capone RJ, Most AS. Unsuccessful emergency medical resuscitation: are continued efforts in the emergency department justified? N Engl J Med 1991; 20:1393.

Niemann JT. Cardiopulmonary resuscitation. N Engl J Med 1992; 15:1075.

Pepe PE, Levine RL, Fromm Jr., RE, et al. Cardiac arrest presenting with rhythms other than ventricular fibrillation: contribution of resuscitative efforts toward total survivorship. Crit Care Med 1993; 21:1838–1843.

Rogove HJ, Safar P, Sutton-Tyrrell K, Abramson NS. Brain Resuscitation Clinical Trial 1 and II Study Groups: old age does not negate good cerebral outcome after cardiopulmonary resuscitation: analyses from the Brain Resuscitation Clinical Trials. Crit Care Med 1995; 23:18–25.

Standards and guidelines for cardiopulmonary resuscitation and emergency cardiac care. JAMA 1992; 268:2171.

Stiell IG, Hebert PC, Weitzman BN, et al. High-dose epinephrine in adult cardiac arrest. N Engl J Med 1992; 15:1045.

Tzivoni D, Banai S, Schuger C, et al. Treatment of torsades de pointes with magnesium sulfate. Circulation 1988; 77:392.

Wayne MA, Levine RL, Miller CC. Use of end-tidal carbon dioxide to predict outcome in prehospital cardiac arrest. Ann Emerg Med 1995; 25:762–767.

SINOATRIAL BLOCK: BRADYCARDIA-TACHYCARDIA SYNDROME

Scott E. Hessen, M.D.
Leonard S. Dreifus, M.D.

Dysfunction of the sinoatrial node is a common cardiovascular disorder that is responsible for a galaxy of symptoms including light-headedness, syncope, drop attacks, fatigue, shortness of breath, and periods of rapid heart action alternating with sinus arrest or bradycardia. Lown (1966) first used the term *sick sinus syndrome* to describe certain postcardioversion arrhythmias as well as pacemaker activity in subsidiary pacemakers following cardioversion. He also recognized the association of asystolic periods with tachycardia.

Sinus node dysfunction, sometimes described as sick sinus syndrome, consists of (1) persistent, severe, and unexpected sinus bradycardia; (2) sinus arrest, brief or sustained, with escape atrial or atrioventricular (AV) junctional rhythm; (3) prolonged sinus arrest with failure of subsidiary pacemaker, resulting in total cardiac asystole; (4) chronic atrial fibrillation with slow ventricular responses not caused by drug therapy; (5) inability of the heart to resume sinus rhythm following an electroconversion for atrial fibrillation; and (6) alternating bradyarrhythmias and tachyarrhythmias. The carotid sinus syndrome includes marked slowing of the sinus rate or arrest greater than 3 seconds, fall in systemic blood pressure of more than 50 mm Hg with carotid sinus stimulation, or both.

Three types of carotid sinus syndrome are recognized: a cardioinhibitory type with bradycardia or asystole, a vasodepressive type with hypotension but minimal change in the sinus rate, and a primarily cerebral type. The disease is usually seen in elderly individuals, although rarely it may occur in childhood or adolescence. The majority of patients in the older age groups also suffer from hypertensive or coronary heart disease. Sinus dysfunction may result from abnormal autonomic tone, particularly increased vagal activity. It can be associated with acute myocardial infarction or coronary ischemia. A sclerodegenerative process has been observed to result in sinus node dysfunction. Sinus node dysfunction may also result from surgical trauma, active myocardial or pericardial disease, drug excess with agents such as digitalis, sensitivity to beta-adrenergic and calcium channel blocking agents, electrolyte imbalance, and other metabolic diseases.

Systemic embolization may occur in up to 16 percent of patients with the sick sinus syndrome, especially in those individuals with the bradycardia-tachycardia syndrome.

Sinus node dysfunction may be due to either failure of impulse formation within the sinus node or exit block from

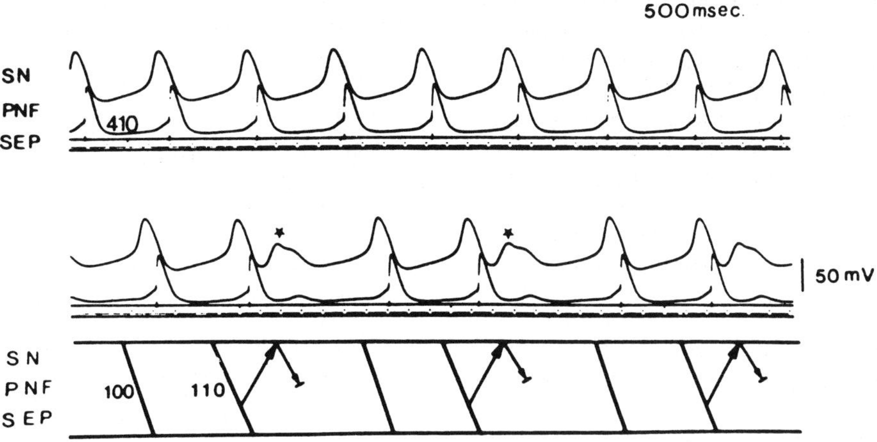

Figure 1
Concealed re-entry from the perinodal to the sinus nodal fibers causing periods of sinus node arrest. SN, Sinus node intracellular electrogram; PNF, perinodal cell intracellular electrogram; SEP, atrial septal electrogram.

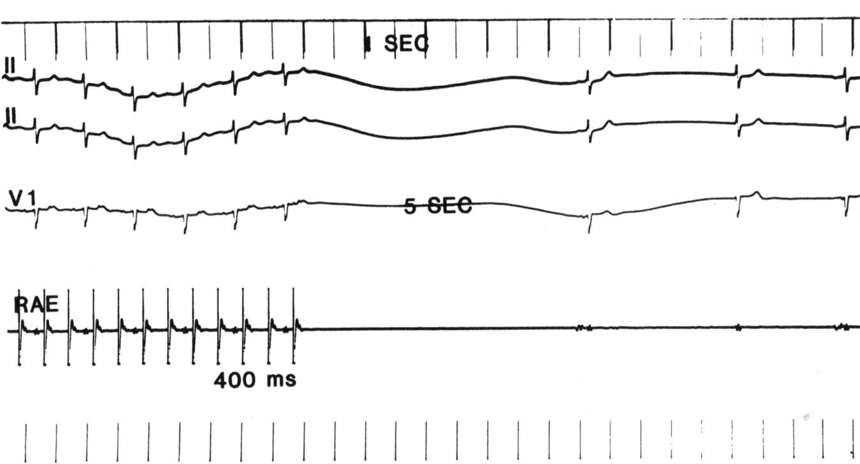

Figure 2
Atrial pacing at 400 milliseconds (150 beats per minute) with 2:1 atrioventricular conduction. There is a 5 second pause following cessation of pacing (sinus node recovery time = 5,000 msec, basic sinus cycle length = 900 msec, corrected sinus node recovery time = 4,100 msec). A secondary pause is also seen.

the sinus node to perinodal atrial tissue as a result of conduction abnormalities. The fact that conduction disturbances from the sinus node to the perinodal cells can lead to sinus node re-entry and tachycardia as seen in Figure 1 suggests that the bradycardia-tachycardia syndrome may be related to conduction abnormalities in and near the sinus node. In addition, supraventricular tachycardias that suppress sinus node function due to so-called overdrive suppression may result in long periods of sinus arrest, which also characterize the bradycardia-tachycardia syndrome (Fig. 2).

■ DIAGNOSIS

The diagnosis of sinus node dysfunction should be suspected when neurologic symptoms of light-headedness, dizziness, or frank syncope occur. In addition, the association of resting heart rates below 50 beats per minute, atrial tachyarrhythmias, and neurologic symptoms often alerts the clinician to the presence of sinus node disease. Existent and unexplained sinus bradycardia and an inability to increase the heart rate with exercise may also be clues to the presence of sinus node dysfunction. It is important to emphasize that asymptomatic individuals with sinus bradycardia at rest, especially if young, generally will not have sick sinus syndrome. The presence of long periods of cardiac asystole either following the termination of tachycardia in the bradycardia-tachycardia syndrome or due to sinus node dysfunction or exit block implies failure of a subsidiary pacemaker as well (Fig. 3).

Although it is possible to record electrograms directly from the region of the sinus node by using closely spaced bipolar catheters, diagnosis of sinus node dysfunction is often apparent from the surface electrocardiogram, Holter monitor, or rhythm strips in many cases (Fig. 4). Because most episodes of syncope or dizziness are paroxysmal, a 24 hour or longer Holter monitor may be necessary to document the arrhythmia. However, unexplained sinus bradycardia in the presence of an exaggerated response to carotid sinus pressure or the presence of various degrees of sinoatrial exit block can be diagnostic (Fig. 5). The asystolic periods associated with symptoms can obviate the need for expensive invasive electrophysiologic studies (see Figs. 3 and 4). The inability to increase the heart rate above 90 beats per minute with moderate exercise can also lead the clinician to suspect the presence of sinus node dysfunction. Because symptoms resulting from sinus node dysfunction are unpredictable and often difficult to document, specific electrophysiologic studies can be used to aid the clinician in the diagnosis of this disorder. In addition, in patients suspected of having sinus node dysfunction, electrophysiologic testing may document other etiologies for clinical symptoms, such as transient AV block or ventricular tachyarrhythmias.

The following electrophysiologic tests of sinus node function may be performed on patients suspected of having symptomatic sick sinus syndrome when the diagnosis is not apparent from long-term electrocardiographic monitoring, particularly when a decision regarding pacemaker implantation is entertained (Table 1).

Electrophysiologic Testing

The most useful test of sinus node function is the measurement of the sinus node recovery time (SNRT) (Fig. 6). Atrial pacing is performed near the sinus node at rates above the sinus rate to approximately 150 to 200 beats per minute. Pacing should be performed for 30 seconds to 1 minute at each cycle length, with at least 1 minute of recovery time between paced drives. The interval from the last paced atrial complex to the first sinus node escape beat is the SNRT. Subtracting the basic sinus cycle length from the SNRT yields an SNRT corrected for the prevailing sinus rate, the corrected SNRT (CSNRT). The CSNRT should be measured at several different paced cycle lengths. Normally, the maximal CSNRT is less than or equal to 550 milliseconds. An abnormal CSNRT has been found in 35 to 93 percent of patients suspected of having sinus node dysfunction. Abnormal responses are commonly seen in patients with symptomatic tachycardia-bradycardia syndrome. Another measure of sinus node recovery is the time required to return to basic sinus cycle length after pacing, the total recovery time. Normally, this is less than 5 seconds and occurs between the fourth to sixth recovery beat.

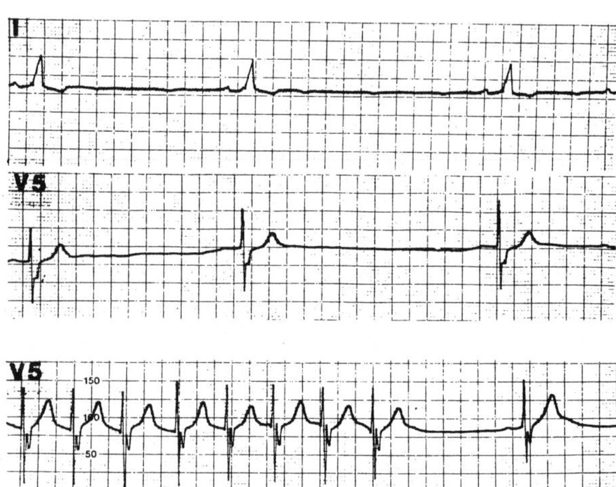

Figure 4
Sinus node dysfunction in a 70-year-old man, demonstrated by periods of sinus tachycardia alternating with sinus bradycardia.

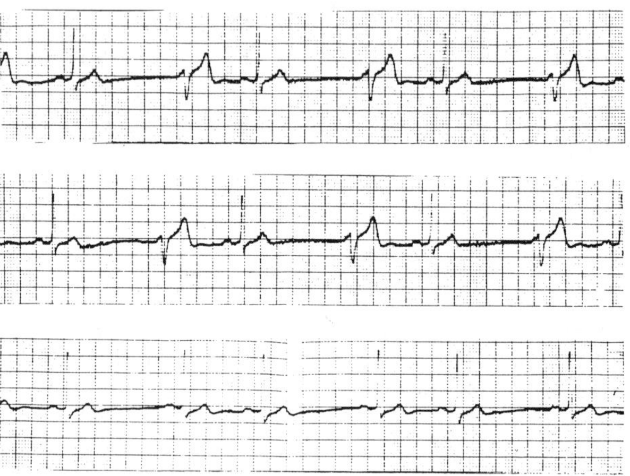

Figure 5
Escape capture bigeminy. Lower two tracings demonstrate a bigeminal rhythm due to 3:2 sinoatrial (SA) exit block. Sinus cycle length = 780 milliseconds. This accounts for 2:1 SA exit block seen in the upper two tracings. Ventricular escape complexes are also noted.

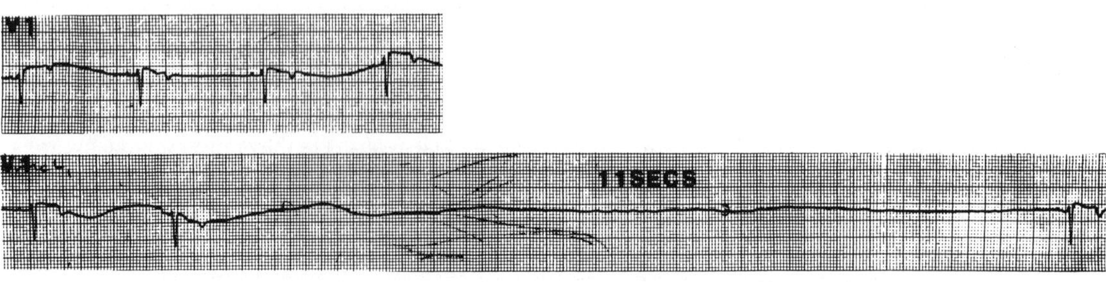

Figure 3
Sinus arrest of 11 seconds in an 18-year-old male.

The sinoatrial conduction time (SACT) may be measured either directly or indirectly by several techniques. One indirect method involves pacing the atria minimally faster than the basic sinus rate for eight beats and measuring the interval from the last paced atrial beat to the first sinus escape beat as shown in Figure 7*A* (method of Narula). When subtracted from the prevailing sinus cycle length, this measurement approximates two times the SACT. Another indirect method involves scanning the diastolic period with atrial extrastimuli as shown in Figure 7*B* (method of Strauss). The intervals from the extrastimulus to the return sinus beat are measured. Four patterns of behavior are seen: collision, reset, interpolation, and re-entry. During the reset zone, the return cycle interval minus the prevailing sinus cycle interval approximates two times the SACT. Atrial extrastimulation may also initiate sinus node re-entry tachycardia in some patients. Normal SACT intervals range from 50 to 125 milliseconds. Measurement of the SACT is not a sensitive test for sinus node dysfunction because only 40 percent of patients with clinical sinus node dysfunction have abnormal SACTs.

Table 1 Sinus Node Function Tests

AUTOMATICITY	
SNRT	A pace near SN for 1 min at incremental rates: "overdrive suppression" (normal = 1,300 to 1,500 msec or 130–150% of BCL)
CSNRT	SNRT – BCL (normal <550 msec)
TRT	5 beats <5 sec total
CSP	Normal <3 sec pause
IHR	117.2 – (0.53 × age in years) ± 16
CONDUCTION	
SACT	A pace minimally faster than BCL for 8 beats (method of Narula), or atrial extrastimulus method: $\frac{\text{A2A3} - \text{A1A1 (BCL)}}{2} < 125$ msec
CSP	SA exit block
SN re-entry	Atrial extrastimulus method

A, atrial; BCL, basic sinus cycle length; CSNRT, corrected sinus node recovery time; CSP, carotid sinus pressure; IHR, intrinsic heart rate; SA, sinoatrial; SACT, sinoatrial conduction time; SN, sinus node; SNRT, sinus node recovery time; TRT, total recovery time.

Autonomic control of sinus node function may be measured by the effect of intravenous atropine (1 to 3 mg) to assess parasympathetic tone. The heart rate should increase to greater than 90 beats per minute or at least 20 to 50 percent above the control rate following injection of atropine. To assess sympathetic responsiveness, isoproterenol may be infused at a rate of 1 to 3 μg per minute; the heart rate should accelerate by at least 25 percent. An absent or blunted response to atropine or isoproterenol suggests sinus node dysfunction.

Pharmacologic denervation using atropine 0.04 mg per kilogram and propranolol 0.2 mg per kilogram allows measurement of the sinus rate unaffected by autonomic tone. Between the ages of 15 and 70 years, this basic or intrinsic heart rate (IHR) normally decreases with age according to the regression equation IHR = 117.2 – (0.53 × age in years). A depressed IHR correlates well with other abnormalities of sinus node function and can differentiate patients with isolated sinus bradycardia due to increased vagal tone from those with true sinus node dysfunction.

The use of sinus node function testing can be important in patient management. Clearly, if the symptoms are associated with electrophysiologic abnormalities reproduced during testing, it can be of extreme importance for further management. Notably, patients presenting with syncope and an abnormality in the sinus node during electrophysiologic studies are usually rendered free of syncope following the implantation of a cardiac pacemaker. Unfortunately, electrophysiologic testing of sinus node function is not always predictive of outcome. Even considering the battery of studies discussed, an exact prognostic implication cannot always be ascertained.

Recommendations for electrophysiologic studies have been published by the Joint Task Force of the American Heart Association and the American College of Cardiology (ACC/AHA Task Force Report, 1989).

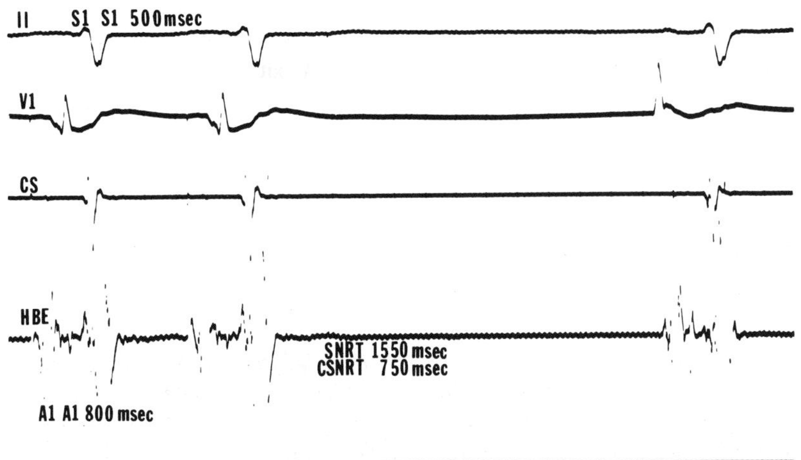

Figure 6
Sinus node recovery time (SNRT) and corrected sinus node recovery time (CSNRT).

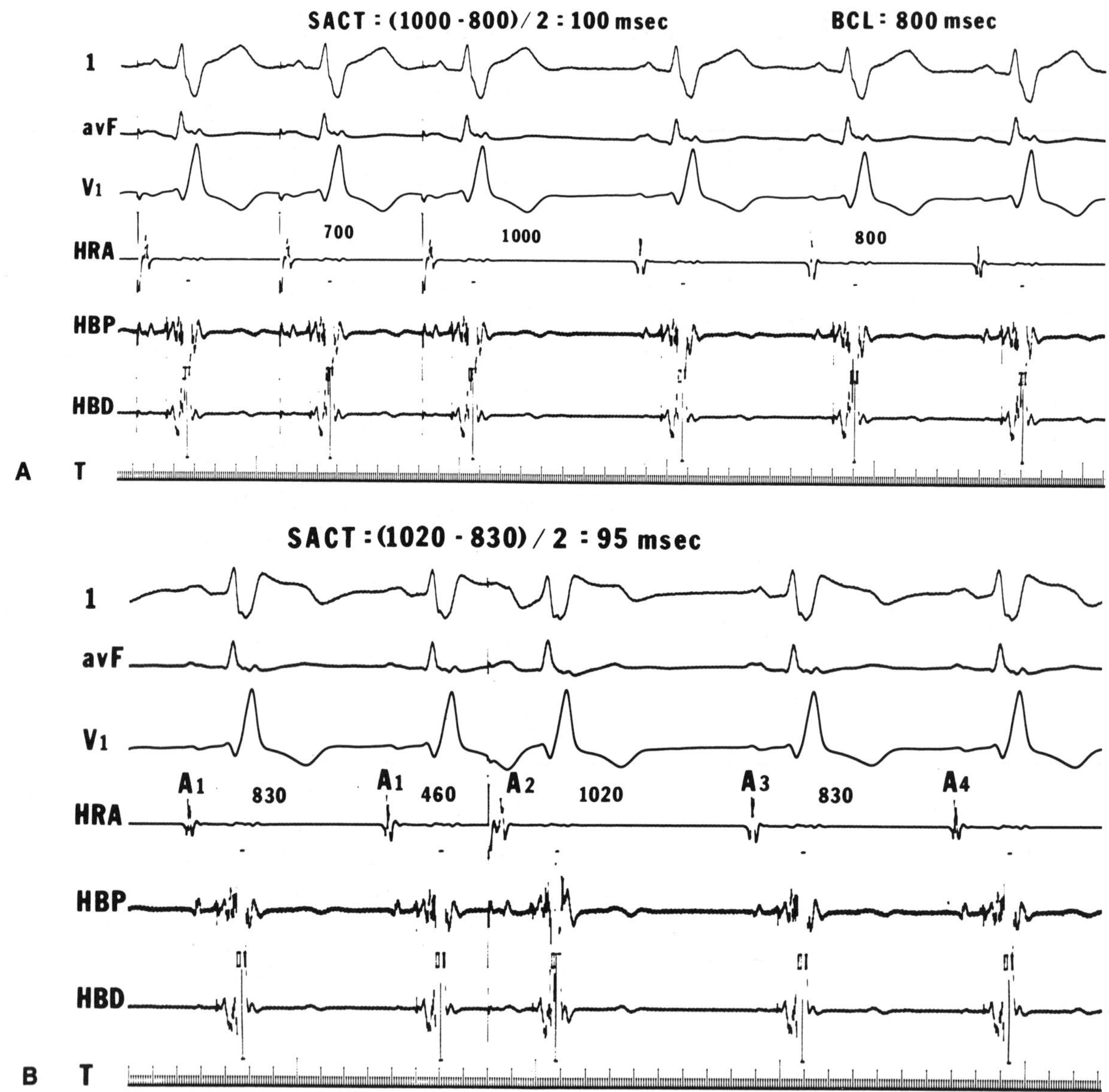

Figure 7
A, Sinus node conduction time as measured by the method of Narula. *B,* Sinus node conduction time as measured by the atrial extrastimulus method (Strauss) in the same patient. HRA, high right atrium, HBP, proximal His bundle electrogram, HBD, distal His bundle electrogram.

Neurovascular Syncope

In about 25 percent of cases of syncope, the cause remains undetermined despite an extensive diagnostic work-up. Transient global cerebral hypoperfusion results from a complex interplay between multiple biologic mechanisms involving autonomic neurocontrols, cardiac factors, and peripheral hemodynamic alterations. In the absence of obvious sinus node dysfunction or AV heart block, the neurovascular cause of syncope should be investigated. Head-up tilt testing (HUT) is now used as a hemodynamic screen, particularly in patients with unexplained syncope. It is now recognized that upright posture in conjunction with the administration of exogenous catecholamine may be used to reproduce neurally mediated syncopal spells.

The mechanism for neurovascular syncope can be explained by stimulation of afferent C-fibers in the base of the left and right ventricles (the cardiac mechanicoreceptors). Activation of these receptors through cardiac extension and vigorous systolic contraction resulting from decreased venous return to the ventricles or increased heart rate due to catecholamines or isoproterenol infusion triggers a reflex similar to the Bezold-Jarisch reflex and is closely related to the mechanism of carotid sinus stimulation that would induce bradycardia and vasodilation and ultimately due to the marked cholinergic effect, resulting in severe hypotension and syncope (Fig. 8).

The test is performed on a tilt table, and the patient is placed in the supine position initially for at least 10 minutes. The patient then is tilted to 60 or 80 degrees for a maximum of 60 minutes or until symptoms develop. Frequently, symp-

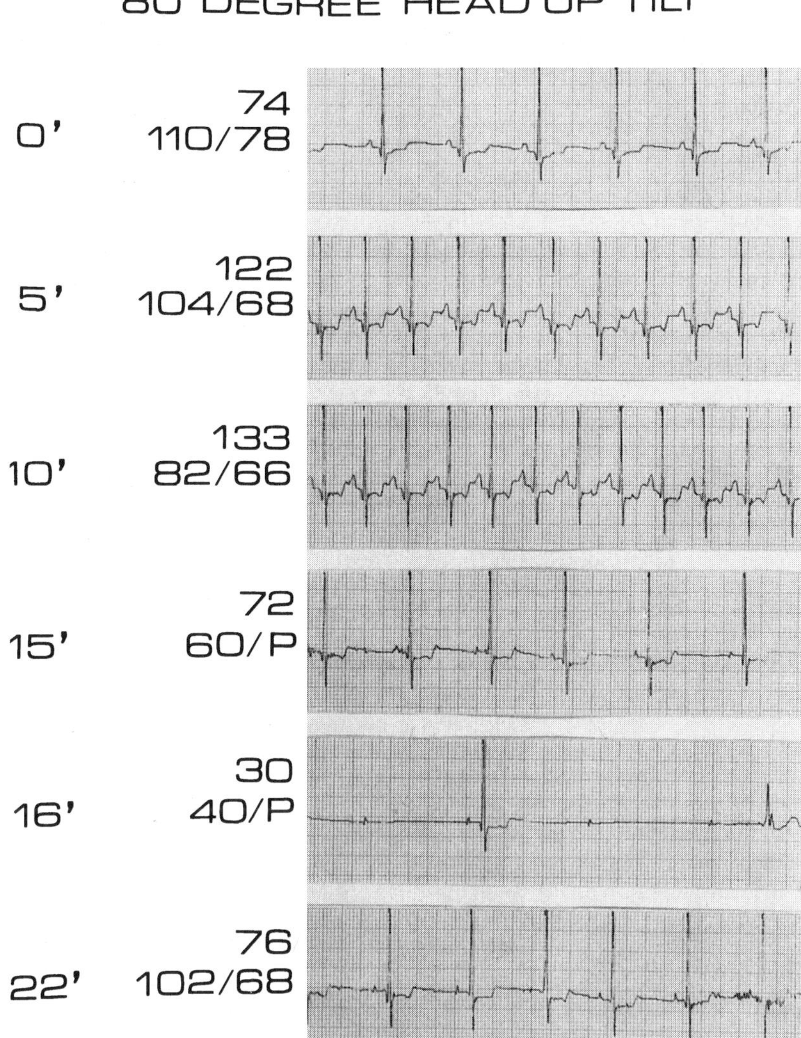

Figure 8
Positive tilt table response. Initial tachycardia at 5 to 10 minutes, followed by severe hypotension and bradycardia leading to high-grade AV block after 16 minutes. *(Reprinted from Hahnemann University with permission from Cardiac Electrophysiology for the Practicing Physician 1992; 2:1–8.)*

toms develop between 10 and 15 minutes after tilting. In the presence of a negative study, isoproterenol, 1 to 3 μg per minute, is infused for 10 minutes. A fall in the heart rate below 60 beats per minute or a drop in blood pressure of 30 mm Hg constitutes a positive response to tilt testing either alone or in conjunction with isoproterenol.

These patients usually respond to beta-blockade using propranolol or metoprolol. Alternatively, disopyramide has been utilized. The patient should be warned against certain changes in posture and prolonged standing and should have adequate fluid intake.

■ PREFERRED APPROACH

Medical Treatment

A meticulous drug history must be obtained in patients suspected of sinus node dysfunction. Drugs such as digitalis, beta-adrenergic blocking agents, calcium channel antagonists, and antiarrhythmic agents such as quinidine, procainamide, disopyramide, flecainide, propafenone, and amiodarone can be potent suppressors of sinus node automaticity in patients with sinus node dysfunction. Patients receiving beta-blocking eye drops for glaucoma may have sufficient systemic absorption to provoke sinus node dysfunction. Drugs known to depress sinus node function should be discontinued in patients with sick sinus syndrome unless a permanent pacemaker is present. Patients with the tachycardia-bradycardia syndrome may benefit from antiarrhythmic agents if tachyarrhythmias can be suppressed and if bradyarrhythmias are not significantly worsened.

In general, pharmacologic therapy usually fails to control symptoms and can never be absolutely depended on to manage patients with sinus node disease.

Commonly, patients develop atrial flutter or fibrillation in the presence of sinus node dysfunction, which may alleviate symptoms related to bradycardia or pauses, but patients require AV nodal blocking agents for control of ventricular rate and may be at increased risk of systemic embolization. At least one-half of patients experiencing symptoms from sinus node dysfunction require permanent cardiac pacing.

Although ventricular demand pacing may alleviate symptoms in many patients with sick sinus syndrome, many retrospective studies and one prospective study have shown that the rate of atrial fibrillation and systemic embolization may be decreased by using either pacemakers that both stimulate and sense in the atria (AAI) or AV sequential pacing modes. In a review of previous studies encompassing 1,171 patients followed for a mean of 38 months, 3.9 percent of patients treated with AAI pacing developed atrial fibrillation compared with 22.3 percent treated with pacemakers pacing and sensing only in the ventricles (VVI). A similar low incidence has been reported using AV sequential pacing modes. Similarly, the incidence of systemic embolization was 1.3 percent with AAI pacing compared with 13 percent with VVI pacing.

Several retrospective studies have suggested decreased mortality among patients with sinus node dysfunction when treated with AAI or AV sequential pacing. Although these patients were similar with regard to baseline characteristics to patients treated with VVI pacing, these results must be interpreted cautiously, because the studies are retrospective and an implantation bias cannot be excluded.

Atrial demand pacing offers the advantages of a simple pacing system, decreased cost, and maintenance of AV synchrony, and it allows a normal sequence of ventricular conduction and contraction. The development of atrial fibrillation and advanced grade AV block may limit the usefulness of this modality, however. Atrial demand pacemakers should not be implanted in patients with sustained or frequent paroxysms of atrial fibrillation or in those patients whose AV nodal Wenckebach point is reached at pacing rates less than 120 beats per minute.

Dual-chamber AV sequential pacing alleviates concern about the future development of AV block and maintains AV synchrony, but these devices are more complicated and more expensive than single-chamber pacemakers. In addition, universal AV sequential pacemakers, devices that pace and sense in both the atria and ventricles (DDD), may track atrial tachyarrhythmias and may produce pacemaker-mediated tachycardias, resulting in rapid ventricular pacing. Dual-chamber inhibited (DDI) mode pacemakers are perhaps ideal for patients with sinus node dysfunction because AV synchrony is maintained but atrial tachyarrhythmias are not sensed and pacemaker-mediated tachycardias cannot occur.

More recently, electrophysiologists have recognized the importance of chronotropic incompetence among patients with sinus node dysfunction. In these individuals, there is a failure to increase the sinus rate appropriately for the patient's metabolic needs. These patients, especially younger individuals, may not be capable of increasing their physical activity. Consequently, rate-adaptive single- and dual-chamber pacing are now available using a physiologic sensor such as vibration (activity), temperature, pH, bioimpedance, ventricular gradient, and Po_2.

Patients with sick sinus syndrome should be considered candidates for permanent pacing if they have symptoms related to sinus bradycardia or sinus pauses that are unrelated to medications. In view of the studies showing a decreased incidence of atrial fibrillation and systemic embolization, and possibly increased survival with atrial (AAI) or AV sequential pacing modalities, these pacemakers should be used whenever possible. Patients with documented chronotropic incompetence should have atrial or AV sequential rate-adaptive systems implanted (AAIR, DDIR, or DDDR). In carefully selected patients without evidence of significant AV nodal disease, AAI or AAIR pacing may be the modality of choice.

Complications of cardiac pacing are relatively uncommon and are related mainly to premature battery failure, infection, lead displacement or fracture, or problems associated with the physiologic sensing mechanism of rate-responsive pacemakers.

Suggested Reading

ACC/AHA Task Force Report. Guidelines for clinical electrophysiologic studies: A report of the American College of Cardiology/American Heart Association Task Force on assessment of diagnostic and therapeutic cardiovascular procedures (subcommittee to assess clinical intracardiac electrophysiologic studies). J Am Coll Cardiol 1989; 14:1827.

Anderson HR, Thuesen L, Bagger JP, et al. Prospective randomised trial of atrial versus ventricular pacing in sick sinus syndrome. Lancet 1994; 344:1523–1528.

Bigger JT, Reiffel JA. Sick sinus syndrome. Am Rev Med 1979; 30:91.

Dhingra RC. Sinus node dysfunction. PACE 1983; 6:1062.

Fitzpatrick AP, Theodorakis G, Vardos P, Sutton R. Methodology of head-up tilt testing in patients with unexplained syncope. J Am Coll Cardiol 1991; 17:125–130.

Hatano K, Kato R, Hayashi H, et al. Usefulness of rate responsive atrial pacing in patients with sick sinus syndrome. PACE 1989; 12:16.

Lown B. In: Dreifus LS, Likoft W, Mayer J, eds. Fourteenth symposium on mechanisms and therapy of cardiac arrhythmias. New York: Grune & Stratton, 1966:185.

Mazgalev T, Dreifus LS, Michelson EL. Modulation of the effects of post-ganglionic nasal stimulation in the sinus and atrioventricular nodes by cardioactive agents and electrolytes. In: Mazgacev T, Dreifus LS, Michelson EL, eds. Electrophysiology of the sinoatrial and atrioventricular nodes. New York: Alan R. Liss, 1988:207.

Reiffel JA, Bigger JT Jr. Current status of direct recordings of the sinus node electrogram in man. PACE 1983; 6:1143.

Reiffel JA, Livelli F, Gliklide J, Bigger JT Jr. Indirectly estimated sinoatrial conduction time by the atrial premature stimulus technique: Patterns of error and the degree of associated inaccuracy as assessed by direct sinus node electrography. Am Heart J 1983; 106:459.

Rosenqvist M, Brandt J, Schuller H. Long-term pacing in sinus node disease: Effects of stimulation mode on cardiovascular morbidity and mortality. Am Heart J 1988; 116:16.

Strauss HC, Saroff AL, Bigger JT Jr, Grardina EGV. Premature atrial stimulation as a key to the understanding of sinoatrial conduction in man: Presentation of data and critical review of the literature. Circulation 1973; 47:86.

Sutton R, Kenny RA. The natural history of sick sinus syndrome. PACE 1986; 9:1110.

ATRIOVENTRICULAR BLOCK

David P. Rardon, M.D.
Charles Fisch, M.D.

Atrioventricular (AV) block occurs when atrial impulse transmission to the ventricle is delayed or blocked secondary to pathologic refractoriness or interruption of AV pathways. The normal cardiac impulse originates in the sinus node and conducts through the atrium, AV node, and His-Purkinje system to the ventricle. The sinus node discharge is not recorded on the surface electrocardiogram but is inferred from the presence of upright P waves in electrocardiographic leads II, III, and AV_F. The P-R interval, therefore, represents conduction through the atrium, AV node, and His-Purkinje system. Atrioventricular block may result from conduction delay or block at one or more of these sites.

His bundle recordings allow delineation of three anatomic sites of AV block: (1) proximal (above the His bundle), representing delay or block in the AV node; (2) intra-Hisian, representing delay within the His bundle; and (3) infra-Hisian or distal to the His bundle, representing block or delay distal to the His bundle either in the distal His bundle or in the bundle branches. Although the His bundle potential is not recorded on the surface electrocardiogram, the electrocardiographic patterns of AV block correlate with the anatomic site of block. In general, the prognosis of patients with AV block is dependent on the site of block. Block within the AV node proximal to the His bundle implies a favorable prognosis, whereas block distal to the His bundle implies a more onerous prognosis. In most cases the electrocardiogram, without need for electrophysiologic testing, provides enough information to make appropriate decisions concerning the prognosis and management of patients with AV block.

■ PREFERRED APPROACH

First-Degree Atrioventricular Block

By definition, AV block is classified as first, second, or third degree. First-degree AV block is present when the P-R interval exceeds 0.2 second. When first-degree AV block occurs with a QRS of normal duration, the site of delay is most often within the AV node and only rarely within the atrium, His bundle, or bundle branches. In the presence of a bundle branch block, the site of conduction delay can be localized to the AV node with less certainty. Regardless of the site of conduction delay, the prognosis of patients with first-degree AV block is excellent, and no specific therapy is indicated. Even when first-degree AV block is associated with chronic bifascicular block, the rate of progression to complete or third-degree AV block is slow, and prophylactic ventricular pacing is not indicated in the asymptomatic patient.

Second-Degree Atrioventricular Block

Second-degree AV block is divided into two types: type I (Mobitz I or Wenckebach AV block) and type II (Mobitz II AV block). Type I Wenckebach AV block is characterized typically by a progressive prolongation of the P-R interval, with the largest increment following the second conducted P wave. The gradual prolongation of the P-R interval is at progressively decreasing increments, and thus the R-R intervals gradually shorten. The pause that follows the blocked P wave is less than the sum of two basic sinus cycles (Fig. 1). In type I second-degree AV block with a QRS of normal duration, block is usually within the AV node and only rarely within or distal to the His bundle. When the QRS duration is prolonged, block may be within the AV node or below the His bundle.

The prognosis and management of type I second-degree AV block are dependent on the clinical setting and the presence of associated organic heart disease. Ambulatory electrocardiographic monitoring has demonstrated that type I second-degree AV block occurs in a small percentage of normal persons during sleep and with some increased frequency in well-trained athletes. In asymptomatic individuals without organic heart disease, type I second-degree AV block has an excellent prognosis and no therapy is required.

Second-degree type I AV block occurs in 4 to 10 percent of all patients admitted to the coronary care unit with acute myocardial infarction (Meltzer and Kitchell, 1966). Type I block occurs more commonly in association with inferior versus anterior myocardial infarctions. In the setting of an acute inferior myocardial infarction, the QRS duration is usually normal, and the block occurs within the AV node. Type I block in this setting is usually transient and commonly resolves within the first 48 to 72 hours after the infarction. Most patients are asymptomatic, and rarely does type I AV block progress to advanced second-degree or third-degree block. Therefore, no specific therapy is warranted. Rarely, because of symptomatic bradycardia associated with hypotension, ventricular arrhythmias, or myocardial ischemia, therapy may be required. Because type I second-degree AV block is often secondary to increased vagal tone in the setting of an acute inferior infarction, patients may respond to atropine. Atropine is given in 0.5 mg aliquots intravenously every 5 minutes until the desired response is achieved (i.e., an increased heart rate of usually 60 to 80 beats per minute or abatement of signs and symptoms). Two milligrams of intravenous atropine is a fully vagolytic dose in most patients. Doses of atropine smaller than 0.5 mg can produce a paradoxical bradycardia as a result of the central or peripheral parasympathomimetic effects of low doses. Rarely, temporary transvenous ventricular pacing is required for persistent bradycardia or hypotension that fails to respond to atropine, or if the required dose of atropine produces intolerable side effects such as dry mouth, urinary retention, disorientation, or confusion.

Although type I second-degree AV block in general is associated with a good prognosis, occasional patients with organic heart disease and elderly patients have a worse prognosis. When type I AV block complicates organic heart disease, the clinical course tends to be more malignant, but the worsened clinical course is secondary to the extent and severity of the organic heart disease and not to the presence of AV nodal block. Currently routine prophylactic pacing is not

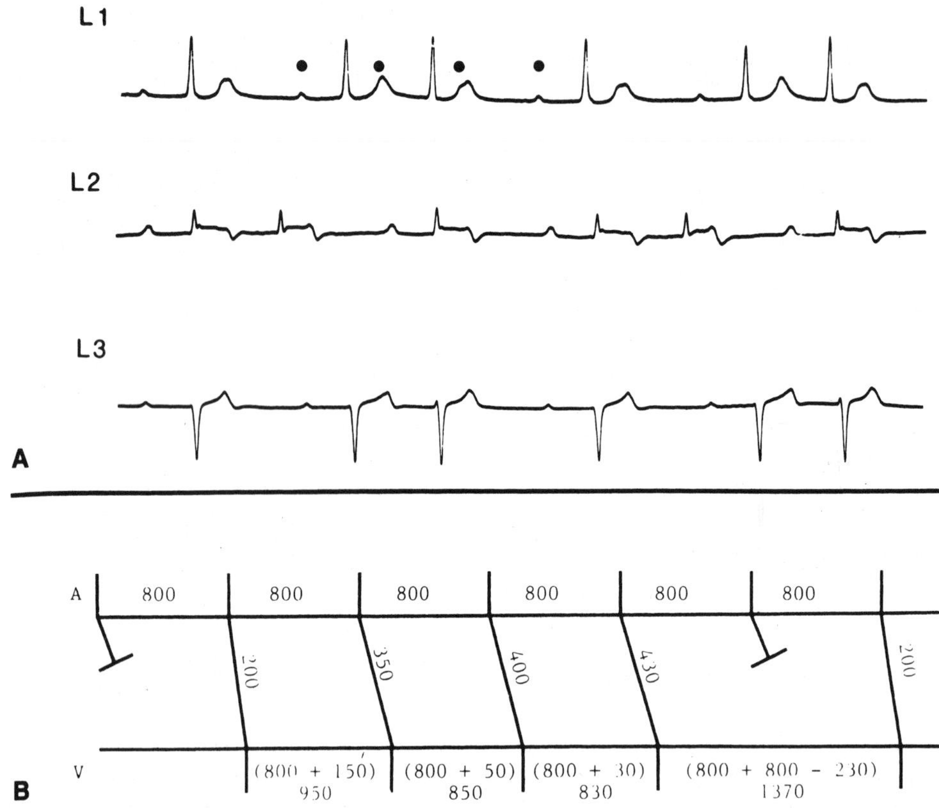

Figure 1
Type I second-degree atrioventricular (AV) block. *A,* Type I second-degree AV block in a patient with an acute inferior myocardial infarction. The P waves are denoted by bullets. Both 3:2 and 2:1 Wenckebach cycles are present in this record. *B,* the structure of a "typical" Wenckebach cycle. The P-P interval is constant at 800 msec. The P-R interval progressively lengthens, with the greatest prolongation occurring with the second conducted P wave. Therefore, the R-R intervals progressively shorten. The pause encompassing the blocked P wave is less than the sum of two basic cycles by an amount equal to the total delay at the AV node (800 + 800 – 150 – 50 – 30 = 1,370 msec).

recommended in patients with AV nodal Wenckebach block and organic heart disease, unless they are symptomatic with recurrent syncope, near syncope, or bradycardia that exacerbates congestive heart failure. Occasionally, type I second-degree AV block is present in patients with syncope. The QRS is usually widened, and either block occurs below the His bundle or delay occurs both within the AV node and distal to the His bundle. In these patients, permanent ventricular or atrioventricular sequential pacing is indicated.

Type II second-degree AV block (Mobitz II) is characterized by constant P-R intervals preceding the nonconducted P wave (Fig. 2). Type II AV block is seen most frequently in association with a bundle branch block, and the anatomic site of block is almost always within or below the His bundle. Type II AV block often progresses to complete AV block and Adams-Stokes attacks. Therefore, prophylactic ventricular or atrioventricular sequential pacing is indicated in most patients.

Type II second-degree AV block occurs in less than 1 percent of patients with acute myocardial infarction (Meltzer and Kitchell, 1966). In contrast to type I block, type II second-degree AV block occurs more commonly with anterior as opposed to inferior myocardial infarctions. There is usually an associated bundle branch block, and the anatomic site of block is distal to the His bundle. Because of the potential for progression to complete heart block, patients with type II second-degree AV block should be treated with temporary transvenous ventricular demand pacemakers set initially to pace at 50 to 60 beats per minute.

A 2:1 AV block may be either type I or type II, and the differential diagnosis may be difficult or impossible. Although the P-R interval is generally not helpful in differentiating the site of AV block except when it is very long, the QRS duration may be. A 2:1 block with a normal QRS duration supports block within the AV node, and a prolonged QRS favors, but is not diagnostic of, block below His. More prolonged electrocardiographic recording at times helps to delineate 2:1 AV block as type I or II because the 2:1 block may become 3:2 AV block, allowing determination of whether the second conducted P wave in the series maintains a constant (type II AV block) or incremental (type I AV block) P-R interval. In general, the management does not differ from that outlined for type I or type II AV block, respectively, as outlined here.

"Advanced" Second-Degree Atrioventricular Block

This form of AV block, a variant of either type I or II AV block, is manifest by block of two or more consecutive P waves, and

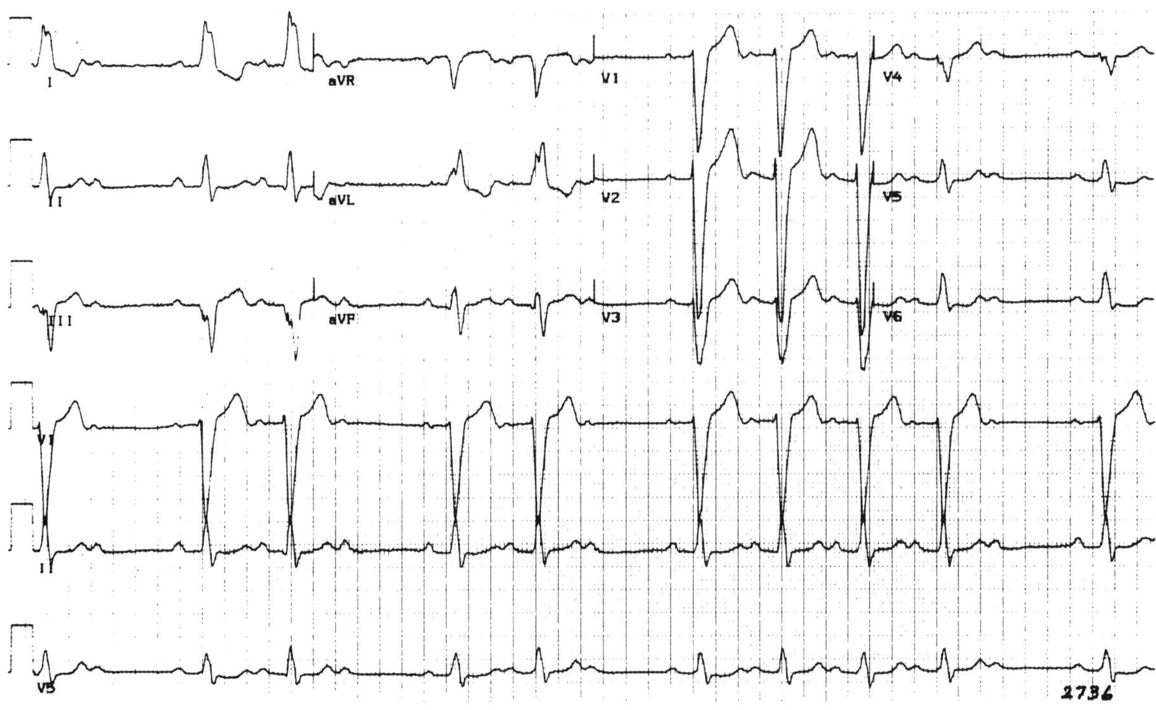

Figure 2
Type II second-degree atrioventricular block. This record demonstrates sinus rhythm with left bundle block. There is intermittent unexpected failure of P waves to conduct to the ventricle. This occurs without preceding gradual P-R interval prolongation. Type II block usually occurs in association with a bundle branch block, and the site of block is almost always distal to the His bundle.

may be interrupted by occasional isolated junctional or ventricular escape or intermittent AV dissociation with short runs of junctional or ventricular rhythm. When complicating type II AV block, permanent pacing is indicated.

Paroxysmal Atrioventricular Block (PAVB)

PAVB is manifest by an abrupt AV block of varying duration in the presence of an otherwise normal AV conduction. Dizziness and syncope are common. Occasionally the cause of PAVB is evident, as for example ischemia, but most often the etiology is unclear. As a rule, permanent pacing is indicated.

Third-Degree Atrioventricular Block

Third-degree or complete AV block is characterized by the failure of all the P waves to conduct, resulting in complete dissociation of P waves and QRS complexes. The rate of the subsidiary pacemaker is slow, approximately 40 to 60 beats per minute, in the presence of a junctional pacemaker (narrow complex QRS in the absence of a pre-existing bundle branch block) and is approximately 30 beats per minute if the impulse originates in the Purkinje fibers (wide complex QRS) (Fig. 3). Complete AV block may result from block within the AV node (usually congenital), block within the bundle of His, or block distal to the His bundle in the Purkinje system (usually acquired).

Acquired third-degree AV block is usually due to drug intoxication, coronary artery disease, or sclerotic degeneration of the AV conduction system. Sclerotic degeneration produces partial or complete anatomic or electrical disruption within the AV node, the His bundle, or both bundle branches. In patients in whom sclerosis of the conduction system produces third-degree AV block, there is general agreement that permanent pacing is indicated, with symptomatic bradycardia manifesting as transient dizziness, lightheadedness, near syncope, frank syncope, or more generalized symptoms such as marked exercise intolerance or frank congestive heart failure. Even in asymptomatic patients with complete heart block and ventricular rates greater than 40 beats per minute, the natural history appears to be one of progression to the point of symptoms, and prophylactic ventricular or atrioventricular pacing is recommended.

The choice of the appropriate permanent pacing modality for patients with either type II second-degree AV block or third-degree AV block should be considered on a case-by-case basis. Ventricular (VVI) pacing provides symptomatic improvement in the majority of patients with impaired AV conduction by establishing a basal ventricular rate that ensures an adequate cardiac output. However, ventricular pacing has several disadvantages. This pacing mode does not allow physiologic increases in heart rate and cardiac output to meet the demands of normal daily living. Inappropriately timed atrial systole may impair cardiac output, and consistent ventriculoatrial activation may produce significant hemodynamic compromise. Atrioventricular pacing has been shown to increase cardiac output and work capacity substantially compared with ventricular pacing. Table 1 summarizes current recommendations regarding preferred pacing modes for patients with AV block. We emphasize that a patient's overall

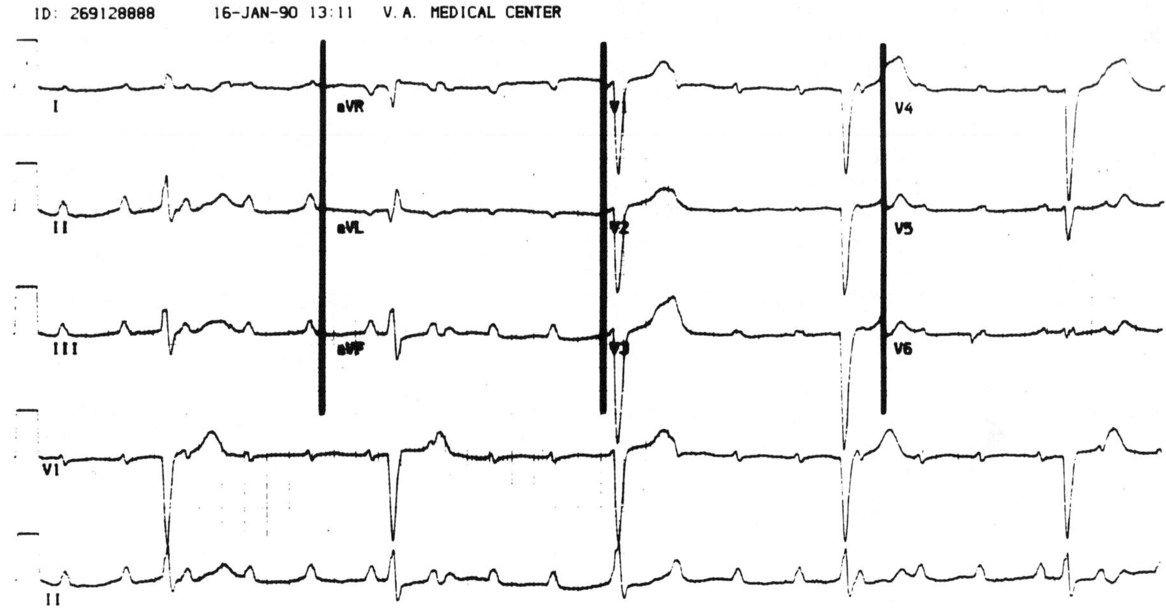

Figure 3
Third-degree atrioventricular (AV) block. There is sinus tachycardia at a rate of 107 beats per minute. There is no relationship between the P waves and the QRS complexes. The ventricular rate is 30 beats per minute, and the QRS has a left bundle branch block morphology. This suggests that the ventricular focus arises in the Purkinje system.

Table 1 Preferred Pacing Modalities for Atrioventricular Block

	ATRIAL RHYTHM		
AV CONDUCTION	NORMAL	BRADYCARDIA	BRADYCARDIA/ TACHYCARDIA
AV block without prolonged retrograde VA conduction time	DDD	DDD or VVI-RR	VVI-RR or DDI
AV block with prolonged retrograde VA conduction time	VVI-RR or DVI	VVI-RR or DVI	VVI-RR or DDD

DDD, AV universal pacemaker with dual chamber pacing and inhibited on channel sensed and triggered on alternate channel. DDI, AV sequential pacemaker with dual-chamber pacing and dual chamber inhibited sensing. DVI, AV sequential pacemaker with dual chamber pacing and ventricular inhibited sensing. VVI-RR, rate-responsive ventricular demand pacemaker.
Modified from Zipes DP, Duffin EG. Cardiac pacemakers. In: Braunwald E, ed. Heart disease: A textbook of cardiovascular medicine. 3rd ed. Philadelphia: WB Saunders, 1988:717; with permission.

physical and mental state, including the presence of associated diseases that might result in a limited prognosis for life, should influence both the decision to pace and the pacing modality selected.

Complete heart block develops in 5 to 8 percent of patients with acute myocardial infarction (Meltzer and Kitchell, 1966). Complete heart block can occur in patients with both inferior and anterior myocardial infarctions. With inferior infarctions, complete heart block usually develops secondary to AV nodal block. The escape rhythm is often junctional with a rate exceeding 40 beats per minute and a narrow QRS complex. It is generally agreed that temporary ventricular demand pacing is indicated in most patients with acute inferior myocardial infarctions and complete AV block, particularly if the ventricular rate is slow (less than 45 beats per minute) or if there is associated hypotension. Atropine may be used in this setting but is rarely of value. In patients with anterior myocardial infarction, complete AV block is often preceded by intraventricular block or type II AV block. The escape rhythm is often ventricular with rates less than 40 beats per minute. The block is usually distal to the His bundle. Temporary transvenous ventricular demand pacing is indicated in all patients with anterior infarctions and complete heart block. This patient population has a high mortality secondary to large infarctions and impaired left ventricular function.

The need for permanent pacing in the small group of patients with anterior myocardial infarction complicated by conduction defects and transient complete heart block is controversial. These patients have a high incidence of sudden death due to either ventricular fibrillation or complete heart block. A retrospective study suggests that this incidence may be reduced by a permanent ventricular demand pacemaker, suggesting a role for prophylactic permanent pacing in patients with acute myocardial infarction and bundle branch block with transient third-degree AV block.

Congenital complete heart block is secondary to discontinuity between the atrial musculature and the AV node or the His bundle, if the AV node is absent. No known etiology exists for the majority of cases, but fetal myocarditis, idiopathic hemorrhage, and necrosis of the conduction tissue and transplacental passage of immune complexes from mothers with systemic lupus erythematosus are all entities capable of causing congenital heart block. Treatment is not required for the asymptomatic infant. Patients usually remain asymptomatic during childhood and adolescence, with some patients developing symptoms later in life. Pacing is indicated for patients with congenital second-degree or third-degree AV block with symptomatic bradycardia. It is difficult to predict which children will develop symptoms; therefore, pacing has been recommended for congenital AV block with a wide QRS escape rhythm or for asymptomatic patients with a ventricular rate of less than 45 beats per minute. Additionally, pacing has been recommended for patients with documented infra-Hisian block. Pacing is not recommended for asymptomatic congenital heart block without profound bradycardia in relation to age.

Suggested Reading

Fisch C. Electrocardiography of arrhythmias. Philadelphia: Lea & Febiger, 1990.

Frye RL, Collins JJ, DeSanctis RW, et al. Guidelines for permanent cardiac pacemaker implantation, May 1984. J Am Coll Cardiol 1984; 4:434.

Hindman MC, Wagner GS, Jaro M, et al. The clinical significance of bundle branch block complicating acute myocardial infarction: 2. Indications for temporary and permanent pacemaker insertion. Circulation 1978; 58:689.

Kugler JD, Danford DA. Pacemakers in children: An update. Am Heart J 1989; 117:665.

Langendorf R, Pick A. Atrioventricular block, type II (Mobitz): Its nature and clinical significance. Circulation 1968; 38:819.

Meltzer LE, Kitchell JB. The incidence of arrhythmias associated with acute myocardial infarction. Prog Cardiovasc Dis 1966; 9:50.

Mullins CB, Atkins JM. Prognosis and management of ventricular conduction blocks in acute myocardial infarction. Mod Concepts Cardiovasc Dis 1976;45:129.

ATRIAL PREMATURE DEPOLARIZATION, ATRIAL TACHYCARDIA, ATRIAL FLUTTER, AND ATRIAL FIBRILLATION

Yoshio Watanabe, M.D., D.M.Sc.
Masao Nishimura, M.D.
Takakazu Katoh, M.D.

■ ATRIAL PREMATURE DEPOLARIZATION

Atrial premature depolarization (or atrial premature systole) is defined as an ectopic impulse formation in the atria occurring earlier than an expected sinus node discharge. An enhanced physiologic automaticity (phase 4 depolarization), the development of abnormal automaticity (including triggered activity), and re-entry have been suggested as possible electrophysiologic mechanisms underlying this arrhythmia. The premature depolarization may occur either singly or in pairs (couplets).

Therapeutic Alternatives

Atrial premature depolarizations usually do not require treatment, regardless of their number, unless the patient is markedly symptomatic. However, underlying cardiac, pulmonary, or other systemic diseases must be treated because they may predispose the patients to ectopic impulse formation. Similarly, when certain predisposing factors such as smoking, alcohol, caffeine, or emotional stress can be identified, an attempt must be made to reduce those factors. The therapeutic approach to symptomatic patients should begin with reassurance and a full explanation of the benign nature of this arrhythmia. If the patients still complain of severe palpitation and chest discomfort, administration of minor tranquilizers or beta-adrenergic blocking agents often successfully ameliorates these symptoms. An antiarrhythmic drug should be administered only when all these measures have failed. Although sporadic appearance of atrial premature depolarizations would not cause significant hemodynamic derangements, nonconducted premature depolarizations occurring in bigeminal pattern could sometimes produce lightheadedness or even syncope and must be treated.

Preferred Approach

Table 1 shows the commonly accepted classification and dosage of antiarrhythmic agents. Generally, class II agents (beta-adrenergic blockers) are effective in suppressing a majority of atrial premature depolarizations. Class I (sodium channel blocker) and class III (potassium channel blocker) drugs may exert a potent inhibitory action on atrial premature depolarizations as they directly block ionic channels of the cardiac cell membrane. Conversely, class IV drugs (calcium channel blockers) appear to be less effective in suppressing atrial premature depolarizations. These antiarrhythmic agents should be administered when atrial premature depolarizations are responsible for the initiation of supraventricular tachyarrhythmias such as atrial tachycardia, atrial flutter and fibrillation, and paroxysmal supraventricular tachycardia. In other words, the management of atrial premature depolarizations should be directed at (1) reducing the asso-

Table 1 Classification, Dosage, and Side Effects of Antiarrhythmic Agents

CLASS	AGENT	ORAL DOSAGE	INTRAVENOUS DOSAGE	SIDE EFFECTS
IA	Quinidine sulfate	200–400 mg q6h		Prolongation of Q-T interval, ventricular tachycardia (torsades de pointes), conduction block, enhanced AV nodal conduction due to anticholinergic action, hypotension, diarrhea, vomiting, thrombocytopenia
	Procainamide	250–500 mg q6–8h	25–50 mg/min up to 15 mg/kg	Ventricular tachycardia (torsades de pointes), conduction block, lupus-like syndrome (arthralgia, positive antinuclear antibodies), agranulocytosis
	Disopyramide	100–200 mg q6–8h	10–15 mg/min up to 3 mg/kg	Congestive heart failure, anticholinergic action (urinary retention, constipation)
IB	Lidocaine		20–50 mg/min up to 1–3 mg/kg, then infusion at a rate of 2–4 mg/min	Central nervous system symptoms (seizures, drowsiness, dysarthria, paresthesia)
	Mexiletine	100–200 mg q8h		Neurologic symptoms (tremor, blurred vision, dizziness), rash, thrombocytopenia, bradycardia
	Tocainide	400–600 mg q8–12h	10–20 mg/min up to 10 mg/kg	Hypotension, congestive heart failure, nausea, vomiting, paresthesia, tremor, dizziness
IC	Flecainide	100–200 mg q12h	10–15 mg/min up to 2 mg/kg	Conduction block, congestive heart failure, aggravation of arrhythmia, increased pacing threshold, hypotension, cardiac arrest, paresthesia, visual disturbance, tremor, insomnia, blurred vision
	Encainide	25–50 mg q8h	5–10 mg/min up to 1 mg/kg	Ventricular tachycardia, conduction block, worsened arrhythmia, congestive heart failure, increase in defibrillation threshold, cardiac arrest, dizziness, blurred vision, ataxia, slurred speech
	Propafenone	100–300 mg q8h	10–20 mg/min up to 2 mg/kg	Hypotension, conduction block, nausea, vomiting, headache, tremor
II	Propranolol	10–60 mg q6h	1 mg/min up to 0.1 mg/kg	Bronchial asthma, congestive heart failure, sinus bradycardia, SA and AV block, hypotension, hypoglycemia, Raynaud's phenomenon, carcinogenesis, oculomucocutaneous reaction
	Metoprolol	50–100 mg q12h	2 mg/min up to 0.2 mg/kg	Identical to those with propranolol, but lesser adverse effects on bronchial and vascular beta-adrenoreceptors
III	Amiodarone	800–1,600 mg/day for 2 wk, then 200–600 mg/day	3–5 mg/kg over 30 min	Hypotension, interstitial pneumonitis, hyperthyroidism or hypothyroidism, corneal microdeposits, photosensitivity of the skin
IV	Verapamil	80–120 mg q8h	0.075–0.15 mg/kg over 1–2 min. If unsuccessful, repeat IV 10 min later	Sinus bradycardia, SA and AV block, hypotension, congestive heart failure, constipation
	Diltiazem	30–90 mg q6–8h	0.15–0.30 mg/kg over 3 min. If unsuccessful, repeat IV 10 min later	Sinus bradycardia, SA and AV block, hypotension, congestive heart failure, headache
Others	Digoxin	0.25–0.5 mg q24h	0.75–1.0 mg over 3 min	Atrial and ventricular premature depolarizations, nonparoxysmal atrial, AV junctional and ventricular tachycardias, AV block, enhanced conduction in the accessory pathway, nausea, vomiting, diarrhea, gynecomastia
	Deslanoside	—	0.4–0.8 mg over 3 min	Similar to those with digoxin
	ATP	—	10 mg in less than 1 sec. If unsuccessful, 20 mg IV 2 min later	Transient nausea, headache, dyspnea, flushing, sinus bradycardia, AV block, atrial and ventricular premature depolarizations and tachycardias
	Adenosine	—	5 mg in less than 1 sec. If unsuccessful, 10 mg IV 2 min later	Similar to those with ATP
	Coumarin	15 mg for 3 days, then 2–10 mg daily depending on prothrombin time		Systemic hemorrhage

ATP, adenosine triphosphate; AV, atrioventricular; IV, intravenous; SA, sinoatrial.

ciated symptoms and (2) preventing the induction of more serious tachyarrhythmias.

■ ATRIAL TACHYCARDIA

Atrial tachycardia is usually defined as a consecutive appearance of three or more atrial premature depolarizations. Its electrophysiologic mechanism is either sinus node or intra-atrial re-entry, enhanced physiologic automaticity, or abnormal automaticity due to a triggered activity occurring in an ectopic focus within the atria. Infrequently occurring atrial tachycardias of a short duration (10 seconds or less) are usually asymptomatic and do not require medical treatment. Indeed, many patients in whom brief periods of atrial tachycardia were recorded on 24 hour ambulatory electrocardiograms failed to note such episodes.

Ectopic Atrial Tachycardia

Ectopic atrial tachycardias of either persistent or incessant type should be treated because, if untreated, they may eventually lead to the development of cardiomyopathy in certain instances. To make a correct diagnosis, one must distinguish this entity from so-called paroxysmal supraventricular tachycardias involving the atrioventricular node in their re-entry circuit. Because vagotonic maneuvers such as breath-holding, eyeball pressure, and carotid sinus massage depress conduction through the atrioventricular node, paroxysmal supraventricular tachycardias can be interrupted by these maneuvers, whereas atrial tachycardia usually is not terminated despite the development of atrioventricular block. However, it is possible that paroxysmal atrial tachycardia due to sinus node re-entry is terminated by vagal stimulation because its re-entry circuit is richly innervated by vagal nerve fibers.

Preferred Approach

To treat atrial tachycardia pharmacologically, intravenous administration of digoxin or deslanoside may be indicated, especially in patients with congestive heart failure. Although this therapy may not always terminate the tachycardia, its beneficial effects on coexisting heart failure can be expected. If atrial tachycardia is accompanied by atrioventricular block, cardiac glycosides should not be administered because such an arrhythmia most often results from digitalis overdose. The initial treatment for digitalis-induced atrial tachycardia is to discontinue the drug and correct serum electrolyte imbalance (especially hypopotassemia) if such a condition exists. When the aforementioned treatment does not convert the tachycardia to sinus rhythm, an antiarrhythmic drug therapy should be considered.

It is well known that atrial tachycardias are often refractory to drug treatment. Indeed, most of the class IA and IB antiarrhythmic drugs are usually ineffective against this arrhythmia. Quinidine and procainamide (class IA) may even accelerate the tachycardia, probably as a result of their anticholinergic action. For an acute termination of persistent or incessant atrial tachycardia, intravenous administration of propranolol (class II) is probably the first choice (Table 1). This drug is successful in approximately half the patients but cannot be applied to patients with lung disease. Intravenous amiodarone (class III) is also quite effective in terminating tachycardia without significant adverse effects. We have observed a permanent suppression of chronic ectopic atrial tachycardia in a young, postmyocarditic patient with oral amiodarone treatment (Fig. 1). Intravenous flecainide or encainide (class IC drugs) has been reported to be as potent as amiodarone, but further clinical evaluation may be necessary before these drugs can be considered as first-line agents. Among class IB agents, ethmozin appears to be the only drug that suppresses atrial tachycardia, but its clinical efficacy has not yet been established. Because all these class I drugs more or less cause conduction disturbances in both the atria and the ventricles and lower the blood pressure, continuous electrocardiographic monitoring and frequent blood pressure measurements are mandatory during their intravenous administration. If QRS complexes in sinus beats become widened to 0.12 second or longer, or if arrhythmogenic side effects (either the development of a new tachyarrhythmia or aggravation of the initial arrhythmia) are observed, the drug injection should be discontinued immediately. If the patient has a pre-existing intraventricular conduction disturbance, class I drugs are contraindicated for the same reason. Verapamil (class IV) also should not be used because this agent seldom terminates the tachycardia and may even accelerate it after an intravenous administration.

Following a successful termination of the episode of atrial tachycardia, long-term pharmacologic therapy is often required to prevent its recurrence. In most instances, an acute intravenous drug test is helpful in predicting the clinical response to long-term oral drug therapy. Hence, oral administration of those intravenously effective drugs can be initiated. Such a drug may well be taken in combination with oral digoxin because the latter agent is beneficial in the management of heart failure. Adverse effects that might be observed on long-term administration of these drugs are listed in Table 1.

For those ectopic atrial tachycardias entirely refractory to these pharmacologic approaches, surgical resection of the arrhythmogenic atrial foci may provide a complete cure. The operative risk of this procedure is low, with generally good results for left atrial foci but rather inconsistent success for right atrial foci. However, the recurrence of tachycardia has been observed in 30 to 50 percent of the cases. Thus, surgical ablation should be considered for patients whose ectopic atrial tachycardia proves refractory to antiarrhythmic drug therapy and in whom the rapid heart action causes hemodynamic deterioration.

Recently, new techniques such as cryoablation and catheter electroablation of the arrhythmogenic foci have been reported to abolish the tachycardia successfully. The transcatheter ablation, especially using radiofrequency currents, appears to be a safe and effective therapeutic option with a 92 percent success rate, and it may be recommended as first-line therapy for those patients with a depressed ventricular function. However, further experience is needed to establish their feasibility and clinical values. Electrical treatments such as atrial or ventricular pacing and direct current cardioversion are generally not indicated against ectopic atrial tachycardia.

Multifocal (or Chaotic) Atrial Tachycardia

Multifocal or chaotic atrial tachycardia is another form of atrial tachycardia often resistant to medical treatment. This arrhythmia is characterized by a relatively slow atrial rate of

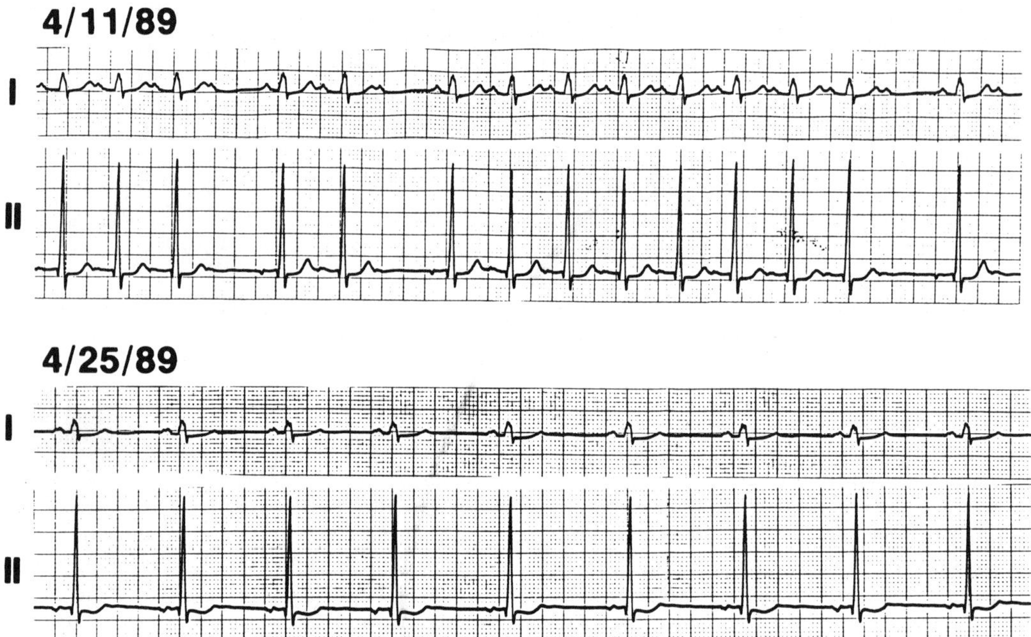

Figure 1
Treatment of persistent atrial tachycardia with oral amiodarone. This 19-year-old male student developed a rapid heart action 6 months after suffering from acute myocarditis. The tachycardia had rates ranging from 110 to 140 beats per minute and was diagnosed as an ectopic atrial tachycardia. It was resistant to various antiarrhythmic drugs, including quinidine, disopyramide, propranolol, and verapamil, and persisted for more than 2 years before these electrocardiograms were recorded. Simultaneous records of leads I and II in the upper panel (4/11/89) reveal an atrial tachycardia at the rate of 115 beats per minute associated with a Wenckebach type second-degree atrioventricular (AV) block. Such an AV block was observed only in the supine position. Oral administration of 200 mg per day of amiodarone was started on this day, and the tachycardia was completely suppressed in 2 weeks as shown in the bottom panel (4/25/89).

100 to 150 beats per minute, three or more P wave morphologies, and varying P-P and P-R intervals. Triggered activity caused by an increased intracellular calcium concentration has been suggested as a possible electrophysiologic mechanism. Endogenous or exogenous catecholamines are likely to facilitate the development of this arrhythmia by increasing the calcium current in the atria.

Preferred Approach

Multifocal atrial tachycardia is associated most often with chronic obstructive pulmonary disease, followed by congestive heart failure and coronary artery disease. Hence, the initial treatment should be focused on the correction of these precipitating factors. For instance, improved ventilation with better oxygenation of the blood, correction of serum electrolyte imbalance, and amelioration of congestive heart failure must be attempted. If multifocal atrial tachycardia persists despite such measures, pharmacologic therapy should be instituted because the prognosis of patients with this arrhythmia is quite grave, as evidenced by the average in-hospital mortality rate of 38 to 62 percent. As in the case of persistent or incessant ectopic atrial tachycardia, class IA and IB drugs and digitalis glycosides are usually ineffective, whereas intravenous injection of up to 0.2 mg per kilogram metoprolol (a cardioselective $beta_1$-adrenergic receptor blocking agent) has been shown to terminate the tachycardia without significant adverse effects, even in patients with pulmonary disease. However, utmost caution should be exercised when metoprolol is administered to such patients. Intravenous propranolol is also effective against this arrhythmia, but this drug should not be used in the presence of chronic pulmonary disease because of its adverse action on the respiratory function. Hypotension constitutes another serious side effect of class II agents. Hence, one must be careful in administering these agents to patients with congestive heart failure.

The drug of second choice against multifocal atrial tachycardia is either verapamil (class IV) or amiodarone (class III). Intravenous administration of verapamil may convert the tachycardia to sinus rhythm without major complications. Although this agent appears less potent than metoprolol in terminating the tachycardia, it has an additional benefit of slowing the ventricular response when the tachycardia persists. Hence, verapamil may be selected for patients who are resistant to class II agents. Intravenous amiodarone is also known to terminate multifocal atrial tachycardia. Because an acute administration of this drug usually does not cause any adverse side effects, amiodarone may be used for any patient regardless of underlying disease. However, amiodarone therapy against this arrhythmia has not yet been widely accepted, and we should await further clinical investigation to establish its usefulness.

Long-term management of multifocal atrial tachycardia should be directed primarily at the correction of underlying disease. It must be supplemented by the oral administration

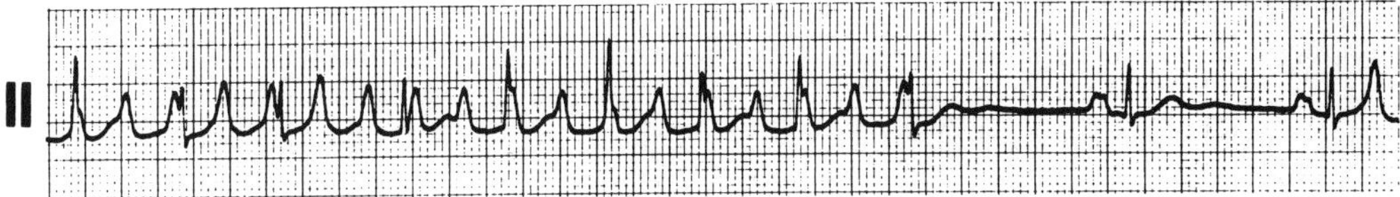

Figure 2
Treatment of paroxysmal atrial flutter with intravenous disopyramide. The patient was a 57-year-old woman who complained of severe palpitation for more than 5 hours. The patient initially showed large sawtooth undulations of the baseline, with their amplitude almost equaling the QRS complexes. After an intravenous injection of 100 mg of disopyramide over 5 minutes, the flutter rate was slowed from 282 to 228 beats per minute, with the maintenance of a 2:1 AV conduction ratio. Sinus rhythm was re-established 2 minutes after the injection was over, although a single atrial premature depolarization occurred on the T wave of the last beat.

of drugs initially proven to be effective in terminating the tachycardia with intravenous injection. As has been described previously, metoprolol, verapamil, and amiodarone are the drugs of choice. Because the former two drugs may sometimes show adverse effects, including hypotension, aggravation of pre-existing pulmonary disease, and congestive heart failure, careful patient selection is mandatory. Chronic amiodarone therapy may cause asymptomatic corneal microdeposits, thyroid dysfunction, pulmonary fibrosis, or congestive heart failure, but these changes can usually be reversed by discontinuation of the drug therapy.

There is a report that an overdrive ventricular pacing was successful in suppressing this arrhythmia in some cases, but this treatment is probably not feasible against multifocal atrial tachycardia with high rates. Electrical cardioversion has been associated with rather poor results in terminating the tachycardia. Surgical resection and radiofrequency or microwave catheter ablation of arrhythmogenic atrial foci have not yet been successful, probably because of the widespread pathologic changes in the entire atrial tissue.

■ ATRIAL FLUTTER

Atrial flutter is rapid, regular, and repetitive atrial depolarizations at rates ranging from 250 to 400 beats per minute. Electrocardiographically, it is characterized by sawtooth undulations of the baseline without being separated by a horizontal isoelectric segment in typical cases (Fig. 2). This arrhythmia is usually initiated by an atrial premature depolarization. A macro re-entry movement involving the bulk of the atrial tissue is generally considered responsible for the maintenance of atrial flutter.

Paroxysmal and Persistent Atrial Flutter

Paroxysmal and persistent atrial flutter should be treated, although it is frequently resistant to pharmacologic treatment. When atrial flutter is associated with an atrioventricular conduction ratio of 1:1, an Adams-Stokes attack may develop because the rapid ventricular rate of more than 250 beats per minute can compromise the cardiac output. Even in the presence of a more common atrioventricular conduction ratio of 2:1, the ventricular rate can be too high to maintain adequate cardiac hemodynamics. Hence, the treatment must be aimed initially at slowing the ventricular response by depressing atrioventricular conduction.

Preferred Approach

Although intravenous injection of cardiac glycosides (digoxin or deslanoside) is a classic approach for this purpose, the drug action is not sufficiently rapid. Therefore, when the ventricular rate is higher than 150 beats per minute and the patient is symptomatic, intravenous injection of verapamil or diltiazem should be given promptly to prevent the development of hypotension, congestive heart failure, and ventricular fibrillation. Although these calcium antagonists are not potent in converting atrial flutter to sinus rhythm, they can immediately decrease the ventricular rate.

Following this treatment or when the ventricular rate is relatively slow without any medication, antiarrhythmic agents can be used to restore a sinus rhythm. Class IA drugs are considered the first choice, and oral quinidine has been used most frequently to achieve this goal. More recently, however, quinidine has been replaced by newer antiarrhythmic agents because (1) it takes more than several hours or even a few days to convert flutter to sinus rhythm; (2) there is a possibility of quinidine toxicity causing more serious ventricular arrhythmias; and (3) its anticholinergic action may cause an atrioventricular conduction ratio of 1:1. Hence, class IA drugs currently recommended include intravenous disopyramide and procainamide. Because these two agents also possess an anticholinergic action, the patient should always be pretreated with digitalis glycosides or calcium antagonists to prevent the acceleration of ventricular response. Reversion of atrial flutter to sinus rhythm with these drugs is often preceded by a period of atrial fibrillation. Although atrial fibrillation may persist in some instances, the ventricular response can be controlled much more easily in atrial fibrillation than in atrial flutter. Intravenous administration of class IC drugs (flecainide, encainide, or propafenone) may be more potent than class IA drugs in terminating atrial flutter, with reported success rates of 10 to 40 percent, whereas class IB drugs are usually ineffective against this arrhythmia. However, some investigators point out a possible risk of class IA and IC drugs in treating this arrhythmia because theoretically these agents may shorten the wavelength in the re-entry circuit (determined as the product of conduction velocity and refractory period), may widen the excitable gap, and may make the re-entry movement more stable. If this assumption turns out to be valid, intravenous amiodarone (potassium channel blocker) may be considered a drug of choice in restoring sinus rhythm because this drug markedly prolongs the refractory period. However, its clinical efficacy has not yet been established, and another class III agent, sotalol, and class II and IV agents appear generally ineffective in terminating atrial flutter.

The most effective way to convert atrial flutter to sinus rhythm is electrical cardioversion. If the patient is in the state of circulatory failure because of an extremely rapid ventricular rate, synchronized direct current shock of 5 to 10 joules should be applied immediately. If unsuccessful, the energy is increased stepwise to 50 joules. In this way, almost 95 percent of patients can be converted to sinus rhythm. When the patient is fully digitalized, withhold the glycoside before cardioversion. In the absence of such an emergency, rapid atrial pacing can also be used to convert atrial flutter to either sinus rhythm or atrial fibrillation. For this purpose, transesophageal atrial pacing is recommended because it is a noninvasive procedure and still shows the same success rate as transvenous right atrial pacing. Termination of atrial flutter is best achieved by applying atrial overdrive pacing at a cycle length 20 ms shorter than the spontaneous flutter cycle, followed by two atrial extrastimuli 10 ms shorter than the drive train. As has been pointed out previously class IA and IC agents may widen the excitable gap in the re-entry circuit. It can then be suggested that, in the presence of these agents, electrical stimuli would more easily enter the excitable gap and interrupt the re-entry movement. Indeed, successful conversion of refractory atrial flutter to sinus rhythm with a combination of intravenous procainamide and rapid atrial pacing has been reported (Olshansky and co-workers, 1988).

Prophylactic treatment of paroxysmal and persistent atrial flutter is different from that aimed at their termination. If the arrhythmia develops in the presence of either valvular heart disease, cardiomyopathy, coronary artery disease, pulmonary embolism, or hyperthyroidism, such an underlying disease must be treated intensively. Because atrial flutter is initiated by atrial premature depolarizations, oral administration of class IA, IC, II, or III drugs is recommended to reduce the number of premature depolarizations. Oral digitalis or a class IV agent such as verapamil or diltiazem may be added to the aforementioned antiarrhythmic drugs in the hope that the former would effectively control the ventricular rate by depressing atrioventricular conduction even when atrial flutter does develop. Electrical or surgical treatment is not indicated for prophylaxis.

Chronic Atrial Flutter

Preferred Approach

In certain cases, atrial flutter is quite refractory to pharmacologic treatment and tends to recur shortly after an electrical cardioversion. The term *chronic atrial flutter* is applied to those cases, and no further attempts should be made to terminate this arrhythmia. The only therapy is to control the ventricular rate by depressing atrioventricular conduction with a maintenance oral dose of either digitalis glycosides, beta-adrenergic blockers, or calcium antagonists, and an optimal ventricular rate of 60 to 80 beats per minute can be obtained by producing an atrioventricular conduction ratio of 4:1. Drug selection should be based on the underlying disease. For instance, if chronic atrial flutter is associated with congestive heart failure, digitalis is the drug of choice and calcium antagonists are contraindicated. In the presence of a pulmonary disease, digitalis or calcium antagonists should be administered but not beta-blockers. For this type of atrial flutter, class IA drugs with an anticholinergic action as well as class IC drugs are not desirable because a resultant slowing of the flutter rate may permit a better atrioventricular conduction and increase the ventricular rate.

There is no indication for rapid atrial pacing. However, radiofrequency catheter ablation is now available for the treatment of type 1 atrial flutter. Radiofrequency energy applied either inferior or posterior to the coronary sinus ostium can interrupt the re-entry circuit, terminate the flutter, and prevent its recurrence. Long-term follow-up is definitely required to confirm the efficacy of this technique.

It has become increasingly apparent that anticoagulation therapy is desirable for chronic atrial flutter.

■ ATRIAL FIBRILLATION

Atrial fibrillation is a completely disorganized, rapid atrial excitation. Electrocardiographically, the isoelectric line is replaced by rapid, irregular undulations called *f waves*, usually having rates higher than 400 beats per minute. Because of the filtering action of the atrioventricular node, many atrial impulses are blocked in this node, and only some of the depolarization waves are conducted to the ventricles, causing an entirely irregular ventricular response. Atrial fibrillation is initiated usually by an atrial premature depolarization occurring in the vulnerable period of atrial excitability. Numerous micro-re-entry circuits are considered to sustain this arrhythmia. More recently, however, nonstationary vortexlike reentrant activity has been proposed as the mechanism of cardiac fibrillation.

Paroxysmal and Persistent Atrial Fibrillation

Preferred Approach

An attempt must be made to convert paroxysmal and persistent atrial fibrillation to sinus rhythm. If the patient has an underlying disorder such as valvular heart disease, coronary heart disease, cardiomyopathy, or thyrotoxicosis, its treatment is necessary. However, regardless of the type of underlying diseases (except for Wolff-Parkinson-White [WPW] syndrome), the initial treatment for atrial fibrillation is generally intravenous digitalis. This drug is expected to slow the ventricular response by depressing atrioventricular conduction and often successfully converts paroxysmal atrial fibrillation to sinus rhythm. If paroxysmal atrial fibrillation is not terminated, intravenous disopyramide or procainamide (class IA drugs) should be given. Although not mandatory, combination with digitalis is recommended to prevent the occurrence of a rapid ventricular response before the restoration of sinus rhythm. Oral quinidine is also very potent to convert atrial fibrillation to sinus rhythm, but this treatment is not encouraged for the reason described in the treatment of atrial flutter. If this mode of treatment is chosen, the patient should be pretreated with digitalis or verapamil. The combination of oral quinidine and verapamil is more effective in restoring sinus rhythm and in regularizing atrioventricular conduction even if atrial fibrillation persists despite these medications. Intravenous flecainide, encainide, propafenone (class IC), or amiodarone (class III) has also been reported as successful in restoring sinus rhythm without significant adverse effects. The success rate for chemical cardioversion with these drugs (60 to 80 percent) is equal to or slightly better than that with class IA drugs, although individual success rates largely depend on the duration of atrial fibrillation, the atrial size, and the underlying heart diseases. Recently, flecainide has been said to be the most potent oral antifibrillatory drug. Indeed, this drug administered orally in a single loading dose of 300 mg was highly effective in converting recent onset atrial fibrillation to sinus rhythm with a success rate of 91 percent.

Propranolol (class II) and verapamil (class IV) are not effective in terminating atrial fibrillation and are used mainly to control the ventricular response. When atrial fibrillation is accompanied by WPW syndrome, cardiac glycosides and, to a lesser extent, verapamil are contraindicated because they tend to enhance conduction in the accessory pathway and may induce ventricular fibrillation. In such cases, class IA, IC, or III drugs should be administered intravenously to depress conduction or prolong refractoriness in the accessory pathway and to restore a sinus rhythm.

Another excellent way of treating this arrhythmia is electrical cardioversion. This treatment is indicated for any type of atrial fibrillation. Above all, atrial fibrillation with a rapid ventricular response due to accessory atrioventricular conduction (WPW syndrome) or with congestive heart failure is best treated with this method. A synchronized, direct current shock of 50 joules should be applied initially. If the current is not sufficient to terminate fibrillation, its energy is increased stepwise to 200 joules, and a normal sinus rhythm can be established in 95 percent of cases. Conversely, electrical pacing is useless to terminate atrial fibrillation or to control the ventricular rate during fibrillation. No surgical treatment is indicated for this arrhythmia. Recently, however, catheter ablation of the atrioventricular junction has been used in cases of refractory paroxysmal atrial fibrillation. Although this procedure does not cure atrial fibrillation and permanent ventricular pacing is required, the patient's quality of life and exercise capacity appear to be improved significantly.

After a successful conversion of atrial fibrillation to sinus rhythm, treatment of underlying diseases should be maintained. Efforts must also be made to reduce the precipitating factors such as smoking, alcohol, caffeine, mental stress, and fatigue. If atrial fibrillation recurs in spite of these measures, the patients should be treated pharmacologically. Because atrial fibrillation is initiated by atrial premature depolarizations in most cases, and occasionally by ventricular premature systoles in cases of WPW syndrome, prophylactic therapy should be focused on the prevention of these premature systoles. In general, class IA drugs (especially disopyramide) are recommended for these purposes. Although class IC and class III drugs may be more potent, they should be used only when class IA drugs fail to maintain sinus rhythm because their long-term administration may cause adverse side effects as listed in Table 1.

Patients with atrial fibrillation have a 5 to 10 times higher risk of systemic embolization compared with patients with a regular sinus rhythm. Hence, even when thrombus formation is not demonstrated by echocardiography, anticoagulation therapy must be used in cases of persistent and recurrent atrial fibrillation associated with valvular heart disease, cardiomyopathy, prosthetic valves, or a history of embolism. Although it has been said classically that atrial fibrillation in the absence of underlying heart diseases (so-called lone atrial fibrillation) would not cause thromboembolism, systemic embolization does occasionally develop in those cases as well. Coumarin is usually administered for 3 weeks prior to pharmacologic or electrical cardioversion. Its dosage should be determined according to the prothrombin time. Because hemorrhagic complications may develop when the prothrombin time is prolonged to more than twice the control, it should be maintained at approximately 1.5 times the control level. After cardioversion, anticoagulation therapy should be continued for another week or two, including those patients who were not pretreated with coumarin because of an emergency cardioversion. No convincing evidence has been presented so far that aspirin or dipyridamole provides sufficient protection against thromboembolism.

Chronic Atrial Fibrillation

Preferred Approach

Chronic atrial fibrillation is defined as atrial fibrillation that cannot be converted to sinus rhythm or prevented from recurrence by any means. Hence, its treatment should be focused on controlling the ventricular rate. Drugs to be used are those that depress atrioventricular conduction, including digitalis, beta-adrenoceptor blockers (class II), and calcium antagonists (class IV). They should be administered depending on the types of underlying diseases. There is no way to treat chronic atrial fibrillation with electrical measures, except that VVI pacing has been shown to achieve slower, more stable ventricular rhythms. Recently, it has been reported that surgical isolation of a conducting pathway between the sinus and atrioventricular nodes by multiple incisions to and suturing of the atrial tissue could produce a slower and stable "sinus" rhythm in certain instances. So-called maze operation, in which multiple incisions in the atrial tissue are expected to interrupt re-entry movements and re-establish regular sinus rhythm has also become quite popular. However, more extensive studies are definitely needed before this procedure is accepted as an effective treatment against chronic atrial fibrillation.

Catheter ablation or surgical section of either the atrioventricular node or the His bundle may have to be considered for patients in whom a good atrioventricular conduction is maintained despite the aforementioned drug therapies. Because these ablative procedures cause a complete atrioventricular block, a permanent artificial pacemaker must be implanted to provide a stable ventricular rhythm. Anticoagulant therapy should be applied to those patients as discussed previously. However, care should be taken when coumarin is administered to hypertensive or elderly patients because they have a greater risk of developing cerebral hemorrhage.

Suggested Reading

Bianconi L, Boccadamo R, Pappalardo A, et al. Effectiveness of intravenous propafenone for conversion of atrial fibrillation and flutter of recent onset. Am J Cardiol 1989; 64:335.

Feld GK, Fleck RP, Chen P-S, et al. Radiofrequency catheter ablation for the treatment of human type 1 atrial flutter: Identification of a critical zone in the re-entrant circuit by endocardial mapping techniques. Circulation 1992; 86:1233.

McGuire MA, Johnson DC, Nunn GR, et al. Surgical therapy for atrial tachycardia in adults. J Am Coll Cardiol 1989; 14:1777.

Olshansky B, Okumura K, Hess PG, et al. Use of procainamide with rapid atrial pacing for successful cardioversion of atrial flutter to sinus rhythm. J Am Coll Cardiol 1988; 11:359.

Scher DL, Arsura EL. Multifocal atrial tachycardia: Mechanisms, clinical correlates, and treatment. Am Heart J 1989; 118:574.

Van Gelder IC, Crijns HJGM, Van Gilst WH, et al. Efficacy and safety of flecainide acetate in the maintenance of sinus rhythm after electrical cardioversion of chronic atrial fibrillation or atrial flutter. Am J Cardiol 1989; 64:1317.

Walsh EP, Saul JP, Hulse JE, et al. Transcatheter ablation of ectopic atrial tachycardia in young patients using radiofrequency current. Circulation 1992; 86:1138.

Watanabe Y, Dreifus LS. Cardiac arrhythmias: Electrophysiologic basis for clinical interpretation. New York: Grune & Stratton, 1977.

VENTRICULAR PREMATURE DEPOLARIZATIONS AND VENTRICULAR TACHYCARDIA

Alfred E. Buxton, M.D.

The approach to the evaluation and therapy of patients with ventricular premature depolarizations (VPD) and ventricular tachycardia (VT) varies widely. This variation undoubtedly reflects the fact that much is unknown regarding the relative risks versus benefits of available therapies for certain of these arrhythmias. Furthermore, a range of techniques has been used to evaluate therapy for these arrhythmias, including noninvasive methods (e.g., ambulatory electrocardiographic monitoring, exercise testing) and invasive methods (e.g., programmed stimulation), none of which has been proven to be superior to the others. The arrhythmias considered in this chapter include VPD, nonsustained VT (defined as three or more sequential premature depolarizations at rates of 100 or more beats per minute and terminating spontaneously within 30 seconds), and sustained VT (defined as tachycardias lasting more than 30 seconds or requiring termination in less than 30 seconds because of loss of consciousness).

There are two primary reasons why we treat patients with ventricular arrhythmias: (1) to make the patient feel better when the arrhythmia causes annoying or disabling symptoms and (2) to prolong the patient's life in the case of arrhythmias that result in severe hemodynamic compromise or cardiac arrest. Many have advocated the treatment of asymptomatic arrhythmias (VPD and nonsustained VT) on the theory that it will prevent sustained tachyarrhythmias causing cardiac arrest. To date, no evidence suggests a cause-and-effect relationship between VPD and sustained ventricular tachyarrhythmias, and data do not demonstrate that eradication of asymptomatic arrhythmias will prevent sudden death. Because all available antiarrhythmic therapies carry significant toxicity—both cardiac and noncardiac—it is imperative before initiating antiarrhythmic therapy to be certain that the risks of the arrhythmia to the patient far exceed the risks of therapy.

■ THERAPEUTIC ALTERNATIVES

Before initiating specific antiarrhythmic therapy, the physician must be certain that the arrhythmia to be treated represents a primary electrophysiologic abnormality and is not occurring secondary to other factors. A number of pharmacologic agents, including both cardiovascular drugs (e.g., all antiarrhythmic agents, digitalis preparations) and noncardiac drugs (e.g., phenothiazines, certain antibiotics), may precipitate isolated VPD and VT. Second, determine whether a metabolic disturbance such as an electrolyte abnormality or myocardial ischemia could be responsible for precipitating the ventricular arrhythmia. Arrhythmias precipitated by any of these factors are unlikely to respond favorably to specific antiarrhythmic therapy without correction of the underlying primary abnormality: withdrawing the responsible pharmacologic agent, correcting myocardial ischemia or electrolyte abnormalities, or optimizing the hemodynamic state of patients with severe congestive heart failure.

The next decision the physician must make prior to initiating specific antiarrhythmic therapy is how to assess the efficacy of therapy. Therapeutic efficacy may be assessed directly by observing the effects of treatment on the actual spontaneous arrhythmia. This empiric method of expectantly observing the patients for spontaneous recurrence is satisfactory in the case of arrhythmias that do not cause severe hemodynamic compromise, such as cardiac arrest or syncope. It is less than satisfactory when failure of therapy is revealed by a life-threatening arrhythmic event. This method is also less than optimal for patients whose arrhythmias occur infrequently, with spontaneous events separated by months to years.

Two general techniques have evolved to evaluate efficacy of therapy. *Indirect methods* of assessing antiarrhythmic efficacy include ambulatory electrocardiographic monitoring to observe the effect of drugs on spontaneous ventricular ectopy. This method has a number of disadvantages, including the fact that there is frequently enormous spontaneous variation in the frequency of spontaneous ventricular depolarizations and nonsustained ventricular tachycardias that may mimic changes in arrhythmia frequency caused by antiarrhythmic therapy. Furthermore, in many patients there is a dissociation between the effects of antiarrhythmic drugs on spontaneous ectopy and symptomatic sustained arrhythmias. Finally, there is no proof that the effect of a drug on spontaneous ectopy will mimic its effect, both beneficial and potentially harmful, on the sustained tachyarrhythmias at which treatment is primarily aimed. In fact, the Cardiac Arrhythmia Suppression Trial (CAST) has demonstrated that suppression of ventricular ectopy, as assessed by rigorous criteria during ambulatory electrocardiographic monitoring, does not prevent sudden cardiac death in patients with asymptomatic arrhythmias after recent myocardial infarction.

In an attempt to circumvent the limitations of passive electrocardiographic monitoring, *direct methods* have been developed by using various techniques to provoke the patient's sustained clinical tachycardia. They include exercise testing; infusion of sympathomimetic amines, such as isoproterenol; and programmed stimulation. Exercise testing works well for some patients whose arrhythmias are precipitated by exercise. Unfortunately, most sustained ventricular tachyarrhythmias are not precipitated by exercise, and, in those cases associated with exercise, the provocation with exercise is often not reproducible. Isoproterenol infusion also precipitates only a minority of sustained ventricular tachyarrhythmias but may be useful for certain patients. Programmed stimulation utilizes pacing techniques to induce and reproduce a patient's spontaneous arrhythmias. The sensitivity and specificity of this technique vary, depending on the type of arrhythmia, anatomic substrate, and skill of the operator. To interpret the results of programmed stimulation appropriately, one must demonstrate that the patient's clinical arrhythmia can be induced reproducibly, first in the absence of antiarrhythmic drugs. The patient is then treated with an antiarrhythmic agent, and programmed stimulation is repeated, the end point being absence of induction of the same arrhythmia. A number of studies have demonstrated that eradication of inducibility following treatment with an antiarrhythmic agent correlates well with prevention of spontaneous recurrent arrhythmias. Some have suggested that an alteration in the mode of induction by an antiarrhythmic agent may also be a favorable end point, but no systematic data exist to support this concept.

■ PREFERRED APPROACH

Medical Treatment

Having arrived at a decision to initiate treatment, the physician must decide among several available modes of antiarrhythmic therapy, including pharmacologic agents, implanted antiarrhythmic devices, and potentially curative therapy such as surgery or catheter ablation. Some general statements about each of these modes are warranted.

Pharmacologic therapy for ventricular arrhythmias is palliative, as the substrate for the arrhythmia remains. Thus, the patient is always subject to recurrences if levels of the antiarrhythmic drug drop below those that are therapeutic for the individual patient. In addition, in some cases the antiarrhythmic effect may be overridden by changes in autonomic nervous system tone or increased levels of circulating catecholamines. In spite of numerous laboratory studies demonstrating the effects of antiarrhythmic drugs on various measurable electrophysiologic parameters, the mechanisms by which these drugs act in humans are unknown. Thus, although many of these drugs slow conduction and prolong refractoriness, which, if either, of these effects accounts for antiarrhythmic efficacy has not yet been determined. Furthermore, many of these agents have direct or indirect effects on the autonomic nervous system that may account in part for antiarrhythmic actions. A further caveat is the observation that, under the proper circumstances, the actions of pharmacologic agents to slow conduction and prolong refractoriness may facilitate the development of arrhythmias. These effects may or may not be predictable.

Finally, it is important to realize that in some cases, the disease substrate may evolve with time, or be subject to transient changes that may alter the efficacy and toxicity of antiarrhythmic agents, or create substrates for arrhythmias. Examples of the evolution of disease effecting new arrhythmia mechanisms would be the development of congestive heart failure or progression of left ventricular hypertrophy. An example of the latter phenomenon is transient myocardial ischemia in patients with coronary artery disease. Myocardial ischemia may facilitate the development of "proarrhythmic" effects with certain antiarrhythmic agents. Ischemia may also precipitate arrhythmias independent of antiarrhythmic drugs.

Unfortunately, the efficacy of antiarrhythmic drugs is frequently limited in the patients who are most dependent on them. Several studies have documented that patients with increasingly severe underlying heart disease are progressively less likely to respond to drug therapy. The overall response rates of patients with recurrent sustained VT to pharmacologic therapy have been between 30 and 40 percent. Moreover, the chance of cardiac side effects, especially paradoxical facilitation of arrhythmias ("proarrhythmia"), may be increased in patients with severe cardiac disease. As a general principle, whatever method is used to judge antiarrhythmic efficacy, when serum drug levels are available, they should be checked at the time that the antiarrhythmic effect is noted, and these levels should be maintained chronically in each patient in order to ensure continued efficacy. Published "therapeutic" and "toxic" drug levels are useful only as a general guide and may be totally irrelevant in an individual patient. The physician treating a patient can judge what drug level is therapeutic only by correlating the serum level with the desired effect. Likewise, the toxic level for an individual patient is any level that results in an undesired side effect. Our lack of understanding of the mechanisms by which antiarrhythmic agents exert beneficial and harmful actions means that pharmacologic therapy of ventricular arrhythmias today remains largely empiric, with no antiarrhythmic agent clearly superior to any others, and no specific antiarrhythmic agent or group of agents can be specifically recommended for most ventricular arrhythmias.

Implantable Antitachycardia Devices

A second type of palliative therapy is the *implantable* cardioverter-defibrillator.

Patients whose tachyarrhythmias result in cardiac arrest may be candidates for implantable cardioverter-defibrillators. These devices have the capability of automatically sensing the onset of VT or fibrillation and delivering a direct current shock that may terminate the arrhythmia. Limitations to the use of these devices include the fact that they do not prevent the onset of tachyarrhythmias but merely terminate them. Therefore, they may not prevent loss of consciousness associated with tachyarrhythmia. Loss of consciousness may also occur if the delivered therapy accelerates the initial arrhythmia. Another common problem is inappropriate delivery of therapy for supraventricular tachyarrhythmias. Furthermore, patients with frequent episodes of tachycardia frequently require concomitant pharmacologic treatment to decrease the frequency of spontaneous episodes. Pharmacologic therapy is also frequently required with currently available devices in order to suppress brief runs of asymptomatic tachycardia, which can trigger the device unnecessarily.

Technical advances now permit the implantation of cardioverter-defibrillators in most patients without sternotomy or thoracotomy. Transvenous lead systems and progressive decrease in the size of devices now make implantation only slightly more complicated from a technical standpoint than implanting permanent pacemakers. The greatest hazard from the devices undoubtedly remains an infection rate of 3 percent.

Most current implantable cardioverter-defibrillators have multiple tiers of therapy, including antitachycardia pacing as well as shock therapy. These instruments are capable of recognizing ventricular tachyarrhythmias with different rates and of delivering differential therapies tailored to the specific arrhythmia. Thus, VT not causing loss of consciousness may be treated with overdrive pacing or low-energy shocks; more rapid tachycardias can be treated by higher-energy shocks. In addition, these devices include provision for backup bradycardia pacing. They allow for varying arrhythmia detection criteria, reducing the chance of delivering therapy for nonsustained tachycardias. These devices extend the range of arrhythmias suitable for therapy to ventricular tachycardias that do not precipitate cardiac arrest. Extensive electrophysiologic testing is required both before and after implantation in order to assure appropriate device selection and programming.

Ablative Treatments

Two types of therapy offer the chance for cure of VT. Several approaches to surgical cure of VT have been developed. All are based on the evidence supporting re-entry as the mechanism underlying sustained VT and depend on the ability to initiate VT by using programmed stimulation in the catheterization laboratory and/or operating room. The ability to initiate and terminate VT reproducibly permits mapping the sequence of ventricular excitation during a single cycle of VT. Based on these observations, a critical portion of the circuit may be identified. Once identified, this area may be ablated with cryosurgical techniques, resected mechanically (the subendocardial resection), or isolated from the remaining viable myocardium with a procedure called *encircling ventriculotomy.* The most successful of these procedures has been the subendocardial resection, combined in some cases with supplementary cryoablation. This approach is limited to patients who have a uniform tachycardia morphology. Polymorphic tachycardias, in general, have not been amenable to this approach. Limitations to the surgical approach are the obvious requirements for open heart surgery with an operative mortality of 5 to 15 percent. Cure rates have been as high as 75 percent in the absence of further antiarrhythmic therapy.

The advent of radiofrequency catheter ablation has now permitted the cure of certain monomorphic VT in the electrophysiology laboratory with a low risk. Cure rates with this technique approach 100 percent in patients with VT in the absence of structural heart disease in experienced laboratories. Monomorphic VT complicating chronic coronary artery disease and cardiomyopathy is being cured with increasing success by catheter ablation, but the presence of multiple tachycardia morphologies and progression of the underlying disease has resulted in lower cure rates (approximating 40 percent in our laboratory, for example).

■ APPROACH TO THERAPY OF SPECIFIC VENTRICULAR ARRHYTHMIAS

Ventricular Premature Depolarizations

The vast majority of patients with VPD are unaware of them. Therefore, I do not treat such patients, regardless of the presence or absence of structural heart disease. Patients complaining of palpitations are frequently discovered to have VPD; most often the symptoms do not correlate with the occurrence of VPD. In patients in whom VPD causes annoying symptoms, I make every effort to treat with reassurance. When reassurance does not suffice, my next line of therapy, regardless of the presence or absence of structural heart disease, is to institute therapy with beta-adrenergic blocking agents. I believe that these work as often by decreasing the patient's awareness of the VPD as by actually suppressing the VPD. Only as a last resort would I institute therapy with specific antiarrhythmic drugs. My reasoning is that, regardless of the presence, absence, or severity of underlying heart disease, the potential risks of antiarrhythmic therapy outweigh its benefits in these patients.

Nonsustained Ventricular Tachycardia

Nonsustained VT is not often found in patients without structural heart disease. Most commonly, when it does occur in patients without structural heart disease, it appears as a syndrome called *repetitive monomorphic VT,* which consists of frequent paroxysms of uniform VT, usually arising from the right ventricular outflow tract. It appears electrocardiographically as a left bundle branch block pattern with a normal (inferior) frontal plane QRS axis. In most cases, nonsustained VT is discovered fortuitously during a routine physical exam or electrocardiogram and is not associated with symptoms. In such cases, I reassure the patient and do not institute antiarrhythmic therapy. Occasional patients have disabling symptoms associated with nonsustained VT in the absence of structural heart disease. In such cases, pharmacologic therapy may suppress these arrhythmias. Frequently, patients with repetitive monomorphic VT arising from the right ventricular outflow tract have the arrhythmia provoked by exercise or isoproterenol. These patients constitute some of the rare cases in which beta-adrenergic blocking therapy may actually suppress the arrhythmia. Other specific antiarrhythmic agents such as verapamil may also suppress VT in such patients. These patients often have such frequent spontaneous arrhythmias that the efficacy of therapy may be judged from the ambulatory electrocardiogram. Repetitive monomorphic VT from the right ventricular outflow tract is usually not inducible by programmed stimulation, although bursts of atrial or ventricular pacing initiate the arrhythmia in approximately one-third of cases. In these patients, the pacing induction of VT may be used to assess antiarrhythmic efficacy. Because repetitive monomorphic VT is most often not associated with symptoms and does not place patients at risk for sudden death, I make every effort to avoid pharmacologic antiarrhythmic therapy in these patients. Radiofrequency catheter ablation is highly successful in curing patients with symptoms refractory to other therapies.

Nonsustained VT is frequently found in patients with severe ventricular dysfunction due to noncoronary heart disease. Twenty-four hour Holter monitors in patients with valvular disease and with both hypertrophic and dilated cardiomyopathies have shown nonsustained VT in at least 50 percent of cases. Most often these arrhythmias are not associated with symptoms. In such patients, they may indicate a higher risk for sudden death, but their utility as a specific marker for sudden (rather than nonsudden) cardiac death is unproven. No data suggest that prophylactic antiarrhythmic therapy in such patients is beneficial. Programmed stimulation in such patients induces sustained uniform VT in only 10 percent of patients and appears to be of no utility to predict sudden death at present (Buxton and co-workers, 1983; Poll and co-workers, 1986). I do not treat patients who are asymptomatic with nonsustained VT in the setting of noncoronary heart disease with ventricular dysfunction.

Patients with coronary artery disease are not infrequently found to have nonsustained VT, especially when left ventricular dysfunction is present (ejection fraction ≤40). Although nonsustained VT discovered late after myocardial infarction is associated with an increased risk for sudden death, these patients are at a similarly increased risk for nonsudden cardiac death. A number of studies suggest that, when nonsustained VT is found in patients with coronary artery disease and ejection fractions greater than 40 percent, the risk for sudden death is very low. Therefore, I do not evaluate such patients or treat them. Patients with nonsustained VT and ejection fractions of 40 percent or less present a difficult problem at present. Even when asymptomatic with regard to the arrhythmia, some of these patients are at increased risk for sudden death. The predictive value of frequent VPDs and nonsustained VT has recently been confirmed in patients receiving thrombolytic therapy. A number of studies have suggested that programmed stimulation in these patients may be useful in stratifying risk for sudden death. About 36 percent of such patients have sustained VT inducible by programmed stimulation. Those without inducible VT appear to be at low risk for sudden death and do not warrant therapy with antiarrhythmic agents. Patients with inducible sustained VT are clearly at increased risk for sudden death, but whether antiarrhythmic treatment will reduce this risk is unclear at present.

Patients who have nonsustained VT that is clearly documented to cause symptoms such as syncope should receive antiarrhythmic therapy. The manner in which to guide therapy depends in large part on the frequency of spontaneous episodes of nonsustained VT and on the anatomic substrate associated with the VT. Patients with syncope and nonsustained VT associated with structural heart disease should undergo electrophysiologic studies; if sustained VT is induced, the results of these studies may be used to guide antiarrhythmic therapy. Patients with severe symptoms due to nonsustained VT associated with nonischemic heart disease are less likely than those with chronic coronary artery disease to have inducible VT when they are subjected to programmed stimulation. However, about 10 percent of patients with dilated cardiomyopathies and up to 50% of those with coronary disease and nonsustained VT have inducible sustained uniform VT, and in these patients programmed stimulation may help to identify appropriate antiarrhythmic therapy. Patients with frequent (more than 20 to 30 daily) episodes of nonsustained VT associated with intolerable symptoms may undergo trials of pharmacologic therapy with assessment by continuous electrocardiographic monitoring, regardless of the presence, absence, or type of underlying heart disease.

Sustained Ventricular Tachycardia

The treatment of sustained VT must be based on the impact of the arrhythmia on the clinical state of the patient. Patients with VT who remain conscious without angina or severe congestive heart failure may be treated pharmacologically, acutely, whereas those experiencing marked hypotension, severe heart failure, or angina should be cardioverted immediately. Our initial choice is usually procainamide, administered at a rate of 50 mg per minute to a total dose of 15 mg per kilogram. When administered at this rate, procainamide may cause hypotension, and the blood pressure must be monitored every 5 minutes. If hypotension occurs, the rate of infusion is slowed to 10 to 25 mg per minute. If the arrhythmia terminates during the loading dose, a maintenance infusion is not usually necessary; most patients have discrete episodes of sustained VT, and continued drug administration in certain cases may facilitate spontaneous development of the arrhythmias by converting paroxysmal into incessant tachycardias. If continued antiarrhythmic medication is desired following the loading dose, procainamide must be administered at a rate of 0.11 mg per kilogram per minute in order to maintain levels that are likely to be therapeutic. Even when procainamide infusion fails to terminate VT, it usually slows the arrhythmia and stabilizes the hemodynamic status. If the tachycardia fails to convert to sinus rhythm following the loading dose of procainamide, cardioversion is performed.

An intravenous formulation of amiodarone has been approved recently for patients with hemodynamically unstable VT refractory to other acute therapies. An initial loading dose of 150 mg over 10 minutes is infused, followed by continuous IV infusion of 700 to 800 mg per 24 hours. The principal limitation of this mode of administration is hypotension. In addition, its prolonged half-life makes management of side effects difficult.

Following the restoration of sinus rhythm after an acute episode of sustained VT, several diagnostic and therapeutic avenues may be pursued. If the tachycardia did not result in severe symptomatology and a stable hemodynamic state was maintained, after the first episode of sustained VT, the physician may choose not to pursue further diagnostic studies or institute specific antiarrhythmic therapy. The natural history of paroxysmal sustained VT is extremely variable, with some patients experiencing gaps of many months or years between spontaneous episodes, even in the absence of treatment. In some cases, institution of empiric therapy may increase the frequency of episodes of spontaneous tachycardia. If a patient has had more than one episode or the initial episode caused severe hemodynamic embarrassment, the optimal method to guide therapy is then electrophysiologic study because I believe it permits the most objective evaluation of the effects of pharmacologic and nonpharmacologic therapy. A baseline electrophysiologic study in the absence of antiarrhythmic drugs is likely to induce sustained VT in more than 90 percent of patients with spontaneous sustained VT (Buxton and co-workers, 1984). If antiarrhythmic drugs are then administered, programmed stimulation may be repeated, with the end point being eradication of inducible sustained VT.

A recent multicenter trial demonstrated that the use of Holter monitors was equal to electrophysiologic studies in predicting efficacy of pharmacologic therapy. Holter-guided therapy resulted in shorter hospitalizations. However, less than half the patients entering the trial had spontaneous ectopy at a frequency high enough to permit use of Holter monitoring. Furthermore, the trial did not evaluate the utility of ablative therapy or implantable devices, both of which require the use of electrophysiologic testing. Finally, the methodology used in this study resulted in a greater than 60 percent rate of arrhythmia recurrence.

In some patients who have either failed multiple trials of antiarrhythmic drugs or in whom curative therapy appears preferable, catheter ablation or surgical resection of the arrhythmia may be undertaken after performing activation mapping of spontaneous or induced VT in the electrophysiology laboratory. If surgical therapy is not desired or accepted, patients are generally given pharmacologic therapy, which results in the greatest degree of hemodynamic stability during the tachycardia. Usually this means the drug or combination of drugs that results in the greatest slowing of the tachycardia when induced by programmed stimulation. In some cases, no drug regimen can be found that produces an acceptable hemodynamic state during tachycardia. These patients are then usually offered an antitachycardia device such as an implantable cardioverter-defibrillator with antitachycardia pacing capability either alone or in combination with pharmacologic therapy.

The choice of pharmacologic therapy for recurrent sustained VT is entirely empiric. For chronic therapy, my usual initial choice is either quinidine, disopyramide, procainamide, or sotalol. I avoid disopyramide in patients with left ventricular ejection fractions of less than 30 percent or a history of congestive heart failure due to systolic ventricular dysfunction. I avoid the use of sotalol in patients with a history of congestive heart failure, and those whose left ventricular ejection fraction is less than 20 percent. Because of its beta-adrenergic blocking activity its use is also limited in patients with bronchospastic pulmonary disease. Sotalol is administered in doses of 80 to 160 mg b.i.d. I usually initiate therapy with a standard, short-acting preparation of one of these agents, aiming for plasma concentrations of 3.5 to 5 mg per liter for quinidine, 8 to 10 mg per liter for procainamide, and 2 to 5 mg per liter for disopyramide. I avoid the long-acting preparations initially because attainment of adequate serum drug levels is often delayed with these preparations. I avoid the use of disopyramide in older men because of frequent side effects of bladder outlet obstruction. Quinidine administration is limited in some patients by gastrointestinal side effects and the occasional development of anemia or thrombocytopenia. The utility of quinidine is frequently limited in patients who require phenytoin because of an interaction between the two drugs that limits attainment of adequate serum quinidine levels. Chronic procainamide administration is usually limited by development of the systemic lupus syndrome. Patients may also complain of insomnia. Although serum procainamide levels of 10 to 20 mg per liter may occasionally be necessary to suppress spontaneous and inducible sustained tachycardias, levels greater than 10 are rarely tolerated chronically.

During chronic therapy amiodarone continuously accumulates in body tissues. Thus, if toxicity develops, months may be required before drug effects dissipate. For this reason, we are reluctant to use this agent in young persons who are likely to require years of therapy. When given orally, it requires several days to attain therapeutic effects, and weeks to reach full effects.

An accelerated effect may be obtained with large oral loading doses (2 to 3 g daily). When a decision is made to give amiodarone for chronic recurrent VT, I usually administer it as a single dose of 1,400 mg per day for 1 week, followed by a maintenance dose of 400 mg per day. Occasionally patients experience marked symptomatic sinus slowing on the loading dose and require a lower loading dose. The utility of electrophysiologic studies to judge the efficacy of amiodarone therapy is controversial, but the weight of evidence would suggest that suppression of induction of tachycardia by amiodarone is meaningful in most cases, whereas failure to suppress induction by programmed stimulation correlates with eventual recurrence of tachycardias. Patients in my laboratory are studied with programmed stimulation after 1 to 4 weeks of amiodarone therapy. The hemodynamic stability of induced tachycardias may be predictive of the hemodynamic stability of spontaneous recurrences, should they occur. Amiodarone therapy is limited by side effects of hypothyroidism or hyperthyroidism, symptomatic hepatitis (and frequent asymptomatic elevations in liver enzymes), a pulmonary fibrosis, myopathy, and peripheral neuropathy. It causes photosensitivity, and patients must be warned to avoid sun exposure. It is also a common cause of incessant VT.

I follow thyroid and liver studies and chest roentgenograms three to four times yearly in patients on amiodarone. Serial pulmonary function studies may also be useful in predicting amiodarone pulmonary toxicity. Chronic amiodarone therapy frequently causes corneal microdeposits visible on slit lamp exam, but they rarely cause symptoms. Occasionally patients appear to benefit from a combination of mexiletine and amiodarone when VT recurs in the presence of amiodarone alone. However, other combinations of antiarrhythmic drugs plus amiodarone have not been very useful and seem only to increase the chance of drug toxicity.

Suggested Reading

Brugada P, Talajic M, Smeets J, et al. The value of the clinical history to assess prognosis of patients with ventricular tachycardia or ventricular fibrillation after myocardial infarction. Eur Heart J 1989; 10:747.

Buxton AE, Waxman HL, Marchlinski FE, Josephson ME. Electrophysiologic studies in nonsustained ventricular tachycardia: relation to underlying heart disease, Am J Cardiol 1983; 52:985.

Buxton AE, Waxman HL, Marchlinski FE, et al. Right ventricular tachycardia: Clinical and electrophysiologic characteristics. Circulation 1983; 68:917.

Buxton AE, Waxman HL, Marchlinski FE, et al. Role of triple extrastimuli during electrophysiologic study of patients with documented sustained ventricular tachyarrhythmias. Circulation 1984; 69:532.

The Cardiac Arrhythmia Suppression Trial (CAST) Investigators. Increased mortality due to encainide or flecainide in a randomized trial of arrhythmia suppression after myocardial infarction. N Engl J Med 1989; 321:406.

The Cardiac Arrhythmia Suppression Trial II Investigators. Effect of the antiarrhythmic agent moricizine on survival after myocardial infarction. N Engl J Med 1992; 327:227.

Denes P, Gillis AM, Pawitan Y, et al. Prevalence, characteristics and significance of ventricular premature complexes and ventricular tachycardia detected by 24-hour continuous electrocardiographic recording in the Cardiac Arrhythmia Suppression Trial. Am J Cardiol 1991; 68:887.

Epstein AE, Bigger TJ, Wyse DG, et al. Events in the Cardiac Arrhythmia Suppression Trial (CAST): Mortality in the entire population enrolled. J Am Coll Cardiol 1991; 18:14.

Kadish AH, Buxton AE, Waxman HL, et al. Usefulness of electrophysiology study to determine the clinical tolerance of arrhythmia recurrences during amiodarone therapy. J Am Coll Cardiol 1987; 10:90.

Kuchar DL, Rottman J, Berger E, et al. Prediction of success of sustained ventricular tachyarrhythmias by serial drug testing from data derived at the initial electrophysiologic study. J Am Coll Cardiol 1988; 12:982.

Maggioni AP, Zuanetti G, Franzosi MG, Rovelli F, Santoro E, Staszewsky L, Tavazzi L, Tognoni G, on behalf of GISSI-2 Investigators. Prevalence and prognostic significance of ventricular arrhythmias after acute myocardial infarction in the fibrinolytic era: GISSI-2 results. Circulation. 1993; 87:312–322.

Mason JW, for the Electrophysiologic Study versus Electrocardiographic Monitoring Investigators. A comparison of electrophysiologic testing with Holter monitoring to predict antiarrhythmic-drug efficacy for ventricular tachyarrhythmias. N Engl J Med 1993; 329:445–451.

Marchlinski FE. Ventricular tachycardia associated with coronary artery disease. Prog Cardiol 1988; 1:231.

Miller JM. The many manifestations of ventricular tachycardia. J Cardiovasc Electrophysiol 1992; 3:88.

Mitchell LB, Duff HJ, Manyari DE, Wyse DG. A randomized clinical trial of the noninvasive and invasive approaches to drug therapy of ventricular tachycardia. N Engl J Med 1987; 317:1681.

Poll DS, Marchlinski FE, Buxton AE, Josephson ME. Usefulness of programmed stimulation in idiopathic dilated cardiomyopathy. Am J Cardiol 1986; 58:992.

Pratt CM, Theroux P, Slymen D, et al. Spontaneous variability of ventricular arrhythmias in patients at increased risk for sudden death after acute myocardial infarction: Consecutive ambulatory electrocardiographic recordings of 88 patients. Am J Cardiol 1987; 59:276.

Pratt CM, Thornton BC, Magro SA, Wyndham CR. Spontaneous arrhythmia detected on ambulatory electrocardiographic recordings lacks precision in predicting inducibility of ventricular tachycardia during electrophysiologic study. J Am Coll Cardiol 1987; 10:97.

Ward DE, Camm AJ. Dangerous ventricular arrhythmias—can we predict drug efficacy? N Engl J Med 1993; 329:498–499.

Wilber DJ, Garan H, Finkelstein D, et al. Out-of-hospital cardiac arrest: Use of electrophysiologic testing in the prediction of long-term outcome. N Engl J Med 1988; 318:19.

PRE-EXCITATION SYNDROMES

William M. Miles, M.D.
Douglas P. Zipes, M.D.

Pre-excitation syndrome occurs when an atrial impulse activates all or part of the ventricles (or a ventricular impulse activates all or part of the atria) earlier than would be expected if the impulse traveled via the normal conduction system only. Pre-excitation is caused by abnormal electrical connections, the most common being an accessory atrioventricular (AV) connection (pathway) between the atrial muscle and ventricular muscle, bypassing the normal AV node-His bundle. When such a pathway exists, the QRS complexes during sinus rhythm may represent fusion between activation via the normal pathway and activation via the rapidly conducting accessory pathway, usually resulting in a P-R interval of less than 120 milliseconds, a QRS duration of greater than 120 milliseconds with a slurred onset (delta wave), and secondary ST-T changes directed opposite to the major delta and QRS vectors. When these electrocardiographic findings are associated with symptoms of tachyarrhythmias, the Wolff-Parkinson-White syndrome is said to exist. Although these pathways usually conduct both anterogradely and retrogradely, some pathways may be capable of only retrograde conduction (concealed accessory pathways), and therefore the electrocardiogram during sinus rhythm may be normal. Approximately 10 percent of patients have more than one accessory pathway. Other more unusual forms of pre-excitation (e.g., atriofascicular fibers) are not discussed in this chapter.

The two most common arrhythmias associated with accessory pathways are orthodromic reciprocating tachycardia (RT) and atrial fibrillation with rapid ventricular response. Orthodromic RT is a re-entrant tachycardia during which the impulse travels anterogradely through the normal AV node and His-Purkinje system and returns to the atrium retrogradely via the accessory pathway. There is no delta wave during tachycardia, and the QRS complexes are usually of normal contour and duration, although functional left or right bundle branch block may occur. Atrial fibrillation usually results from disorganization of pre-existing RT and can be associated with extremely rapid ventricular rates owing to the lack of AV conduction delay in the accessory pathway (Fig. 1). On rare occasions, the ventricular response can be so rapid that ventricular fibrillation results. Antidromic RT, when the impulse travels anterogradely via the accessory pathway and retrogradely via the His-Purkinje system and AV node, is less common and is not discussed here.

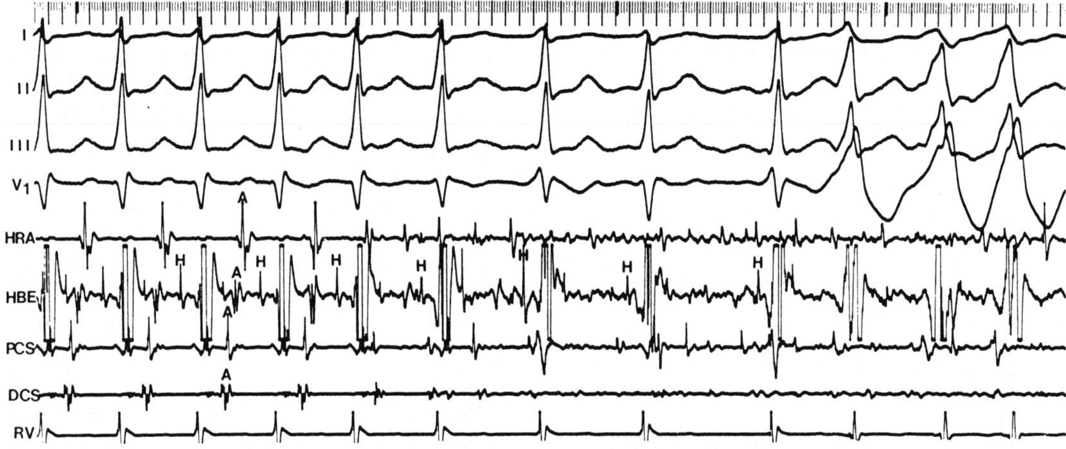

Figure 1
Disorganization of orthodromic reciprocating tachycardia (RT) into atrial fibrillation. Surface leads I, II, III, and V_1 are displayed along with intracardiac high right atrial (HRA), His bundle (HBE), proximal and distal coronary sinus (PCS, DCS), and right ventricular (RV) electrograms. On the left, orthodromic RT is present; the atrioventricular (AV) node and His-Purkinje system comprise the anterograde limb, and a left-sided accessory pathway comprises the retrograde limb of the tachycardia circuit (note the early atrial activation [A] recorded from the coronary sinus, representing left atrial activation). H, His bundle activation. After the fourth atrial depolarization, disorganized atrial activity (atrial fibrillation) occurs; AV conduction initially is via the normal pathway (each narrow QRS complex is preceded by a His bundle electrogram), but conduction subsequently occurs via the accessory pathway (the last three wide QRS complexes are not preceded by a His bundle electrogram).

■ THERAPEUTIC ALTERNATIVES

Therapeutic alternatives for patients with arrhythmias due to pre-excitation syndromes include (1) no therapy, or instruction in performing vagal maneuvers such as Valsalva or carotid sinus massage; (2) pharmacologic therapy; (3) antitachycardia pacing; and (4) surgical or catheter ablation of the accessory pathway. Therapy may be directed toward the acute termination of a tachyarrhythmia or the long-term prevention of its recurrence.

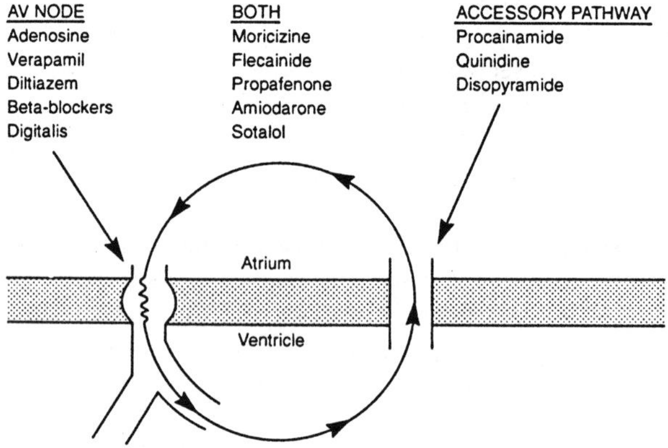

Figure 2
Schematic of the site of drug action in the pre-excitation syndromes.

■ PREFERRED APPROACH

Medical Treatment

Mechanism of Drug Action in the Pre-excitation Syndromes

Drugs for treating arrhythmias related to pre-excitation syndromes prolong conduction time or refractoriness in the AV node, the accessory pathway, or both (Fig. 2). Drugs that exert their major effect on the AV node include beta-adrenoceptor blockers (e.g., propranolol, metoprolol, or atenolol), calcium channel blockers (e.g., verapamil or diltiazem), and adenosine. Beta-blockers and calcium channel blockers are available for either intravenous or oral administration, whereas adenosine is effective only by an intravenous bolus. Drugs that predominantly affect the accessory pathway include procainamide, disopyramide, and quinidine. Lidocaine may prolong conduction and refractoriness in some pathways but may actually shorten refractoriness in certain pathways with preexisting short refractory periods. Drugs that prolong refractoriness and conduction time in both AV nodal and accessory pathway tissues include flecainide, propafenone, sotalol, and amiodarone. If single-drug therapy is not effective, combining a drug that prolongs AV nodal conduction time and refractoriness with one that does the same to the accessory pathway may be successful.

Digitalis glycosides prolong conduction and refractoriness in the AV node and may terminate or prevent RT. However, digitalis decreases accessory pathway refractoriness in approximately one-third of patients and thus may increase the ventricular response during atrial fibrillation. Therefore, digitalis can be used for RT in patients with concealed accessory pathways (no anterograde conduction) but should not be used in patients with manifest (anterogradely conducting)

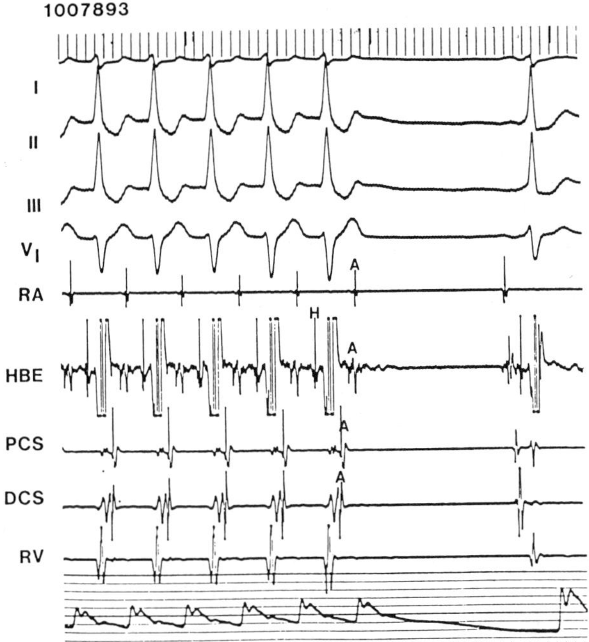

Figure 3
Termination of orthodromic reciprocating tachycardia (RT) by adenosine. This format is the same as in Figure 1; femoral arterial blood pressure is displayed at the bottom. On the left, orthodromic RT using a left-sided accessory pathway for retrograde conduction is present (H, His bundle activation, A, atrial activation). Adenosine, given approximately 10 seconds previously, causes sudden termination of tachycardia via anterograde block in the atrioventricular node, with subsequent resumption of sinus rhythm.

accessory pathways, unless it has been demonstrated that the patient is not prone to rapid ventricular rates during atrial fibrillation or that digitalis does not shorten the accessory pathway refractory period in that particular patient.

In addition to prolonging conduction time and refractoriness in the AV node or accessory pathway, antiarrhythmic drugs may prevent tachycardia in some patients by suppressing the premature atrial or ventricular complexes that initiate the RT.

Acute Therapy for Termination of Arrhythmias

Reciprocating tachycardia can usually be terminated by vagal maneuvers or drugs that transiently block AV nodal conduction. When one atrial impulse fails to conduct through the AV node to the ventricles, RT terminates suddenly. Vagal maneuvers such as Valsalva or carotid sinus massage should be the initial therapy to terminate RT if hemodynamic compromise is not present. Some patients can be taught to perform these maneuvers on occurrence of tachycardia. If vagal maneuvers are unsuccessful, more than 90 percent of episodes can be terminated with intravenous adenosine or verapamil (Fig. 3). Adenosine is the initial drug of choice to terminate RT because it does not have the negative inotropic or vasodilator effects of verapamil and a more rapid onset of action. Adenosine is given as a very rapid 6 mg intravenous bolus; if ineffective, another intravenous bolus of 12 mg can be given 2 to 5 minutes later. It should be emphasized that the bolus must be given as rapidly as possible because adenosine is metabolized very quickly (half-life of less than 10 seconds). Occasionally, atrial fibrillation can result, and subsequent rapid ventricular rates over the accessory pathway may necessitate cardioversion. Adverse effects are minor and short-lived and most commonly include transient dyspnea, facial flushing, or chest tightness. Adenosine effects are antagonized by theophylline preparations and potentiated by dipyridamole. Patients receiving dipyridamole should be given lower doses of adenosine.

Intravenous verapamil is given as a 5 to 10 mg bolus administered over 2 minutes under continuous electrocardiographic and blood pressure monitoring. Reciprocating tachycardia is usually terminated 5 to 10 minutes after the dose. If the first dose is ineffective, a second dose of 10 mg can be given 30 minutes after the initial dose. If verapamil fails to terminate the arrhythmia, a repeat attempt at vagal maneuvers may be successful. Verapamil administration can exacerbate heart failure, hypotension, or coexisting sinus nodal dysfunction. Intravenous verapamil should not be given to a patient with atrial fibrillation and an anterogradely conducting accessory pathway because it may result in vasodilation, reflex sympathetic stimulation, and acceleration of the ventricular response via the accessory pathway, leading to hemodynamic collapse, ventricular fibrillation, or both. Therefore, if a patient with RT is known to have rapid anterograde conduction over the accessory pathway and is prone to developing atrial fibrillation, intravenous adenosine would be preferred over intravenous verapamil. It is important to remember that the vagomimetic action of adenosine can also precipitate atrial fibrillation. If either adenosine or verapamil fails to terminate RT, the drug not used initially may be tried subsequently in the usual doses.

The availability of intravenous adenosine, verapamil, and diltiazem has reduced the need for other drugs to block AV nodal conduction to terminate RT. These other drugs include the cholinesterase inhibitor edrophonium, given intravenously as a test dose of 2 mg, followed after 45 seconds by the remaining 8 mg to a total dose of 10 mg. Edrophonium may cause bronchospasm in susceptible patients and commonly causes nausea. Phenylephrine is an alpha-adrenergic agonist that increases systemic blood pressure and reflexively activates the vagus. It is given as 200 to 500 μg intravenous boluses to titrate a blood pressure increase of 30 to 60 mm Hg. It may be useful in patients with mild to moderate hypotension during tachycardia and is otherwise generally not used.

In rare cases when RT cannot be terminated with adenosine or verapamil, or if tachycardia repetitively recurs after a short period of sinus rhythm, intravenous procainamide can be administered to slow or block retrograde conduction in the accessory pathway. Procainamide dosage is 10 to 15 mg per kilogram, given no faster than 50 mg per minute while blood pressure is monitored closely. Intravenous procainamide causes a mild decrease in blood pressure that can be exaggerated in some patients during tachycardia. Intravenous beta-blockers can also terminate and prevent recurrence of RT in selected patients. Propranolol (0.1 mg per kilogram no faster than 1 mg per minute), metoprolol (15 mg intravenously in three divided doses over 15 minutes), or esmolol (50 to 200 μg per kilogram per minute after a loading dose of 500 μg per kilogram over 1 minute) can be used. Potential adverse effects of the beta-blocking agents include hypotension, congestive heart failure, bronchospasm, and bradycardia. Likewise, verapamil can be given as an intravenous bolus or a continuous intravenous infusion (0.005 mg per kilogram per minute). In rare cases when tachycardia continues to recur despite drug therapy, a temporary atrial or ventricular pacemaker may be introduced to terminate the RT by pacing each time it occurs. If hypotension, angina, congestive heart failure, or other hemodynamic symptoms occur at any time, direct current shock should be employed, generally beginning with a synchronous shock of 10 joules. Rarely, incessant RT may be treated with emergent accessory pathway ablation.

Infrequently occurring, mildly symptomatic episodes of RT can also be managed by having the patient take an oral dose of calcium blocker or beta-blocker at the onset of the tachycardia (e.g., verapamil 120 mg orally at the onset of attack; if the episode does not terminate within 1 hour, a second dose can be given).

Atrial fibrillation with a rapid ventricular response is a medical emergency; however, many patients with pre-excitation syndromes are young with normal hearts and tolerate very rapid ventricular rates surprisingly well. If hemodynamic compromise is present, the therapy of choice is to obtain a 12-lead electrocardiogram quickly for documentation of QRS morphology and then terminate tachycardia with direct current cardioversion. If the patient is relatively stable, a trial of intravenous procainamide in the doses listed previously is often successful in either blocking anterograde accessory pathway conduction (decreasing the resultant ventricular response) or terminating the atrial fibrillation (Fig. 4). Intravenous verapamil should *never* be administered to patients with atrial fibrillation and ventricular pre-excitation. Intravenous adenosine is probably not harmful to patients with atrial fibrillation but is not effective and therefore should not be used. Intravenous lidocaine has been reported to increase the ventricular response during atrial fibrillation in patients who have a short anterograde effective refractory period of the accessory pathway and should not be used.

Long-Term Medical Therapy for Prevention of Tachyaarhythmias

Asymptomatic Patients with Delta Waves. Patients who have evidence of pre-excitation on their electrocardiograms but who have had no tachyarrhythmias or only very rare episodes of RT associated with insignificant symptoms require no therapy and should probably not undergo electrophysiologic study. The concern in these patients is detecting those who may be prone to developing atrial fibrillation with a rapid ventricular response leading to sudden death. The incidence of sudden death in patients with pre-excitation is extremely low, approximately 1 in 1,000 patient years of follow-up. Patients resuscitated from sudden death almost always have a rapid ventricular response during atrial fibrillation, with the minimum interval between two pre-excited QRS complexes (shortest pre-excited R-R interval) during atrial fibrillation of less than 250 milliseconds at drug-free electrophysiologic study. Most patients with sudden death have a history of RT, and many have multiple accessory pathways; however, 12 percent of these patients have been entirely asymptomatic before their arrest. Therefore, attempts have been made to identify those patients at high risk for sudden death.

Noninvasive tests that establish a low-risk group include documentation of intermittent sudden anterograde conduction block in the accessory pathway, either at rest or during exercise, and loss of pre-excitation after intravenous administration of type I antiarrhythmic drugs such as procainamide (500 to 1,000 mg). Patients with these responses usually have accessory pathways with longer refractory periods and are less likely to conduct rapidly during atrial fibrillation. Indeed, some authors advocate determining the shortest pre-excited R-R interval in all patients who show evidence of anterograde pre-excitation by inducing atrial fibrillation with either transvenous or transesophageal pacing. However, because approximately 15 to 20 percent of asymptomatic patients with delta waves have a shortest pre-excited R-R interval of less than 250 milliseconds, one cannot justify treatment in this large number of patients, considering the small incidence of sudden death. Electrophysiologic study might be indicated in selected asymptomatic patients who participate in competitive athletics, in certain high-risk occupations such as airline pilots, in patients for whom digitalis therapy is considered (e.g., for congestive heart failure), or in patients who are undergoing cardiac surgery for other indications in whom concomitant surgical ablation of the accessory pathway might be considered.

Symptomatic Patients. Patients with minimally symptomatic or very infrequent episodes of RT may require no long-term antiarrhythmic therapy. They may benefit from instruction in methods of vagal stimulation or intermittent oral drug therapy upon recurrence of tachycardia. However, patients with frequent or symptomatic episodes of RT require therapy. In most of these patients, catheter ablation of the accessory pathway is preferable to long-term antiarrhythmic drug therapy, certainly before considering treatment with class I or III antiarrhythmic agents.

If the symptoms are not life threatening, drug therapy can be administered empirically and efficacy can be judged by absence of tachycardia on follow-up. Drugs that prolong conduction time and refractoriness in the AV node or the accessory pathway may be used alone or in combination. Digitalis should be avoided if anterograde accessory pathway conduction is present, unless the effects of digitalis on that specific accessory pathway are known. Flecainide (100 to 200 mg twice a day) and propafenone (150 to 300 mg three times a day) are highly effective and very well tolerated; these were our drugs of choice until the results of the Cardiac Arrhythmia Suppression Trial (CAST) were revealed. We now reserve these drugs for patients in whom other drugs (oral beta-blockers, calcium channel blockers) have failed and who have no evidence of ischemic heart disease. Amiodarone is very effective, but its side effect profile precludes its use in most patients.

The remaining concern in patients with RT without life-threatening symptoms is the possibility that RT may disorganize into atrial fibrillation. Patients whose shortest pre-excited R-R interval during atrial fibrillation is less than 250 milliseconds are considered at risk for hemodynamic collapse

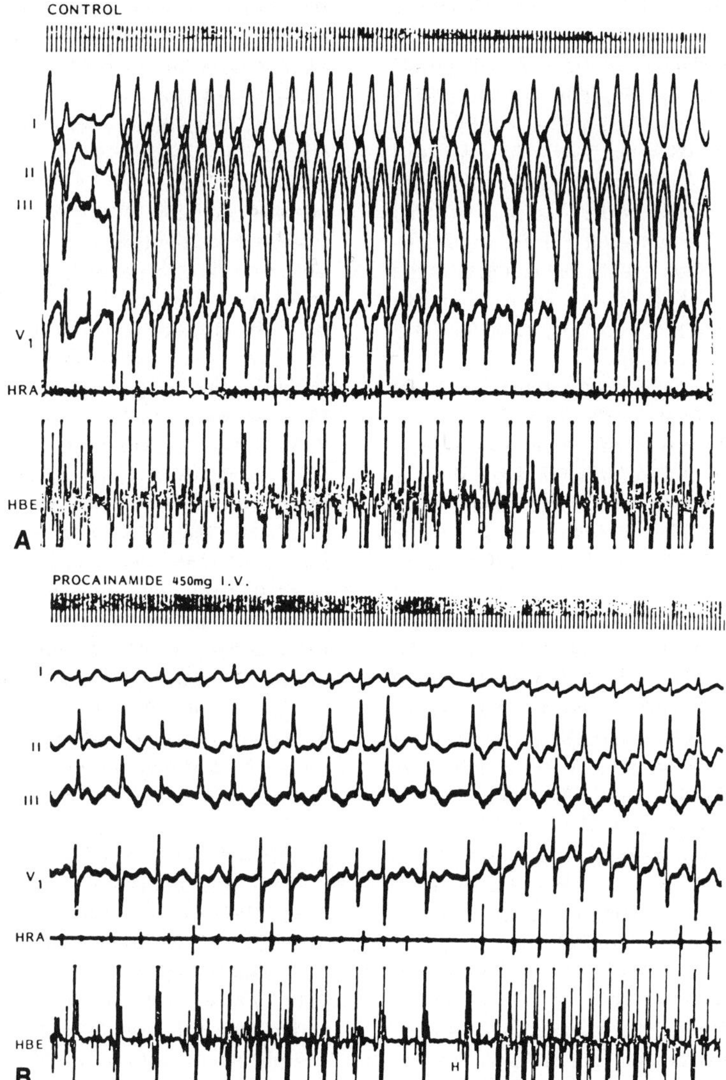

Figure 4

Response of atrial fibrillation to procainamide infusion. Surface leads I, II, III, and V_1 are displayed along with high right atrial (HRA) and His bundle (HBE) electrograms. *A,* Atrial fibrillation with a rapid ventricular response. Except for the second and third complexes, atrioventricular (AV) conduction is via an accessory pathway as demonstrated by the wide QRS complexes. The shortest pre-excited R-R interval is 180 milliseconds. *B,* After the intravenous administration of procainamide, atrial fibrillation persists but anterograde accessory pathway conduction has been blocked; the narrow QRS complexes result from conduction via the normal AV node and His-Purkinje system. On the right of the panel, atrial fibrillation stops; a junctional complex (H) following termination of atrial fibrillation initiates orthodromic reciprocating tachycardia. *(From Prystowsky EN, Miles WM, Heger JJ, Zipes DP. Preexcitation syndromes: Mechanisms and management. Med Clin North Am 1984; 68:831; with permission.)*

during atrial fibrillation. We therefore recommend that most patients with RT and manifest anterograde accessory pathway conduction undergo induction of atrial fibrillation with either transvenous or transesophageal pacing (unless the pre-excitation is intermittent). If the shortest pre-excited R-R interval is less than 250 milliseconds, atrial fibrillation should be induced after drug therapy is initiated to make sure that the ventricular response has been slowed and that the resultant arrhythmia is tolerated hemodynamically. Catheter ablation should be considered if the ventricular response is still rapid.

In some patients, drug therapy can potentially increase the frequency of RT by prolonging anterograde refractoriness of the accessory pathway with little change retrogradely. This makes anterograde block of a premature atrial impulse in the accessory pathway more likely and widens the tachycardia echo zone.

Patients who have serious hemodynamic symptoms (e.g., syncope or presyncope) during arrhythmias should undergo electrophysiologic study. In some patients, reciprocating tachycardia may be so rapid that hemodynamic compromise occurs. However, in most patients atrial fibrillation is the more hazardous arrhythmia. Patients in whom the shortest pre-excited R-R intervals are less than 250 milliseconds are not likely to respond adequately to drug therapy and should be considered for accessory pathway ablation. Electrophysiologic study is used to confirm the presence of an accessory pathway (especially in patients with concealed accessory pathways) to confirm that the accessory pathway participates in the tachycardia (i.e., is not just a bystander), to exclude other tachycardia mechanisms such as AV nodal re-entry and atrial tachycardia as a cause of symptoms, to determine the conduction characteristics of the accessory pathway (especially the shortest pre-excited R-R interval during atrial fibrillation), to confirm the location and number of accessory pathways, and to perform accessory pathway ablation.

Assessment of the therapeutic response depends on the symptoms and the frequency of the arrhythmia in the individual patient. If tachycardia is very frequent (e.g., daily), telemetry monitoring during initiation of antiarrhythmic drug therapy may be adequate to assess a therapeutic response. If arrhythmias are not life threatening but still occur relatively frequently (e.g., weeks), then clinical follow-up of arrhythmia symptoms with or without an electrocardiographic event recorder may be adequate. If the tachycardia is life threatening or potentially life threatening or if episodes are very infrequent (e.g., months to years), electrophysiologic study once the patient is receiving drug therapy is indicated to confirm the desired drug effects. It is especially important to confirm that the shortest pre-excited R-R interval has increased after drug therapy and that atrial fibrillation is tolerated hemodynamically. In patients with very infrequent tachycardia episodes, electrophysiologic study may be the only way of determining drug efficacy without waiting long periods of time for arrhythmia recurrence while the patient is receiving a drug that has potential adverse effects.

Nonpharmacologic Treatment

Antitachycardia Pacing

Implantable antitachycardia pacemakers are useful in very few patients with pre-excitation syndrome and are mentioned here primarily to complete the survey of therapeutic options. Reciprocating tachycardia can usually be terminated by atrial pacing. However, ease of terminating tachycardia varies with changes in autonomic tone, posture, and the tachycardia rate, so that antitachycardia pacing devices are not always effective for terminating every spontaneous episode of tachycardia. Even if it were always successful, antitachycardia pacing has the disadvantage that it does not prevent episodes of tachycardia. Furthermore, attempts to terminate RT using atrial pacing may inadvertently induce atrial fibrillation; atrial fibrillation cannot be terminated by antitachycardia pacing and is a dangerous rhythm in patients with anterograde accessory pathway conduction. Therefore, antitachycardia pacing should be used only in patients with RT whose pathway is concealed, or in a patient with a manifest accessory pathway who is unlikely to have atrial fibrillation (from clinical history or electrophysiologic data) and in whom the ventricular response to induced atrial fibrillation is slow. In general, we do not advocate treatment with antitachycardia pacing devices, especially since the advent of ablative therapies.

Accessory Pathway Ablation

Catheter Ablation. The success and safety of catheter ablation of accessory pathways have become so great that we recommend this nonpharmacologic approach as an initial option to any patient with pre-excitation syndrome who has recurrent symptomatic arrhythmias. The risks and benefits of catheter ablation compare favorably with long-term drug therapy, which may be associated with side effects, incomplete efficacy, and poor patient compliance, especially in young patients facing a lifetime of drug therapy or women wishing to become pregnant. Catheter ablation should be strongly considered for patients who have frequent symptomatic arrhythmias unresponsive to drug therapy, patients with rapid accessory pathway conduction during atrial fibrillation that cannot be adequately slowed with drugs, and patients presenting with life-threatening arrhythmias such as ventricular fibrillation, atrial fibrillation with a very rapid ventricular response, very rapid RT, or syncope.

With the development and refinement of radiofrequency (RF) energy for ablation, accessory pathways in any location can be successfully ablated by energy delivered from the tip of a catheter (Figs. 5 and 6). Radiofrequency energy (similar to cautery used in surgery) creates a discrete small scar, can be carefully regulated, and does not require general anesthesia. It is not associated with the barotrauma (pressure shock wave) using direct current ablation energy sources, and perforation of cardiac chambers or damage to valve tissue is rare. Because the lesion created by RF current is very small (3 to 5 mm diameter), precise localization of the catheter adjacent to the accessory pathway either along the mitral ring, along the tricuspid ring, or near the origin of the coronary sinus (including possibly the recording of an accessory pathway potential) is necessary to effect successful ablation.

Radiofrequency ablation eliminates accessory pathway conduction in approximately 95 percent of patients. Accessory pathway conduction recurs within the first 2 months after ablation in approximately 6 percent of patients with initially successful RF ablations, but the vast majority of these patients are able to undergo successful reablation. The risk of complications from RF catheter ablation of accessory pathways appears to be 2 to 4 percent, including femoral arterial occlusion or pseudoaneurysm, cardiac tamponade, atrioventricular block, myocardial infarction, cerebrovascular or pulmonary embolism, or damage to a cardiac valve, each of which occurs in less than 1 percent of patients.

In patients who had atrial fibrillation prior to ablation, recurrent atrial fibrillation after the ablation procedure is unusual unless structural heart disease is present. This emphasizes that atrial fibrillation in patients with Wolff-Parkinson-White syndrome is usually a result of RT.

Surgical Ablation. Accessory pathways can be divided surgically by using either an endocardial or an epicardial approach to the AV groove; the results and complications of these two techniques are similar. Mortality approaches 0 in most series except for patients who have serious concomitant cardiac disease. Successful accessory pathway ablation using surgical techniques exceeds 95 percent. The incidence of postoperative AV block in recent series is close to 0, although early series reported a higher incidence of AV block in patients with septal accessory pathways. It is important that any other arrhythmias that can also be treated surgically (such as AV nodal re-entry) are identified.

With the advent of effective and safe RF catheter ablation techniques, surgical indications have narrowed considerably.

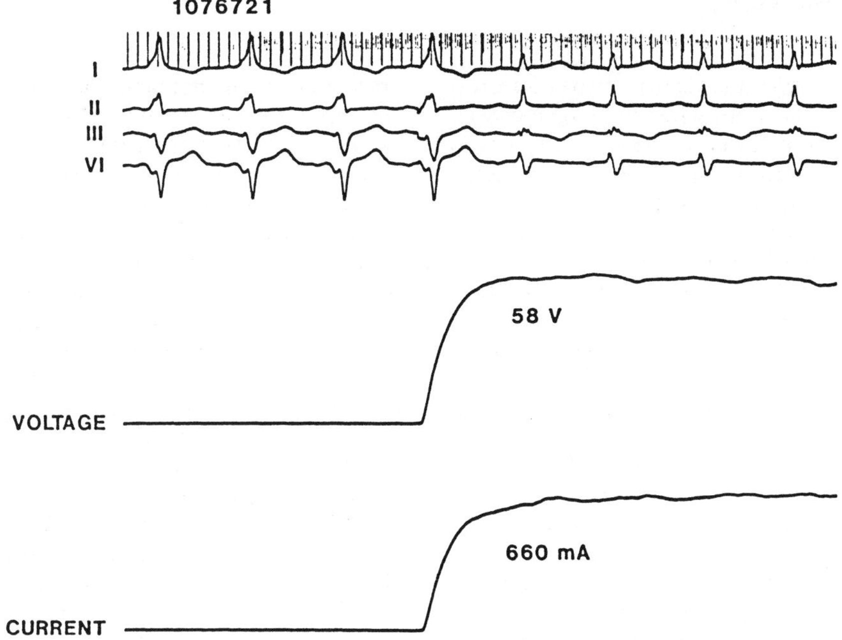

Figure 5
Radiofrequency catheter ablation of a right free wall accessory pathway. Surface leads I, II, III, and V_1 are displayed along with radiofrequency current and voltage. The delta wave is eliminated almost immediately after the onset of radiofrequency energy delivery. *(From Zipes DP, Klein LS, Miles WM. Nonpharmacologic therapy: Can it replace antiarrhythmic drug therapy? J Cardiovasc Electrophysiology 1991; 2:S255; with permission.)*

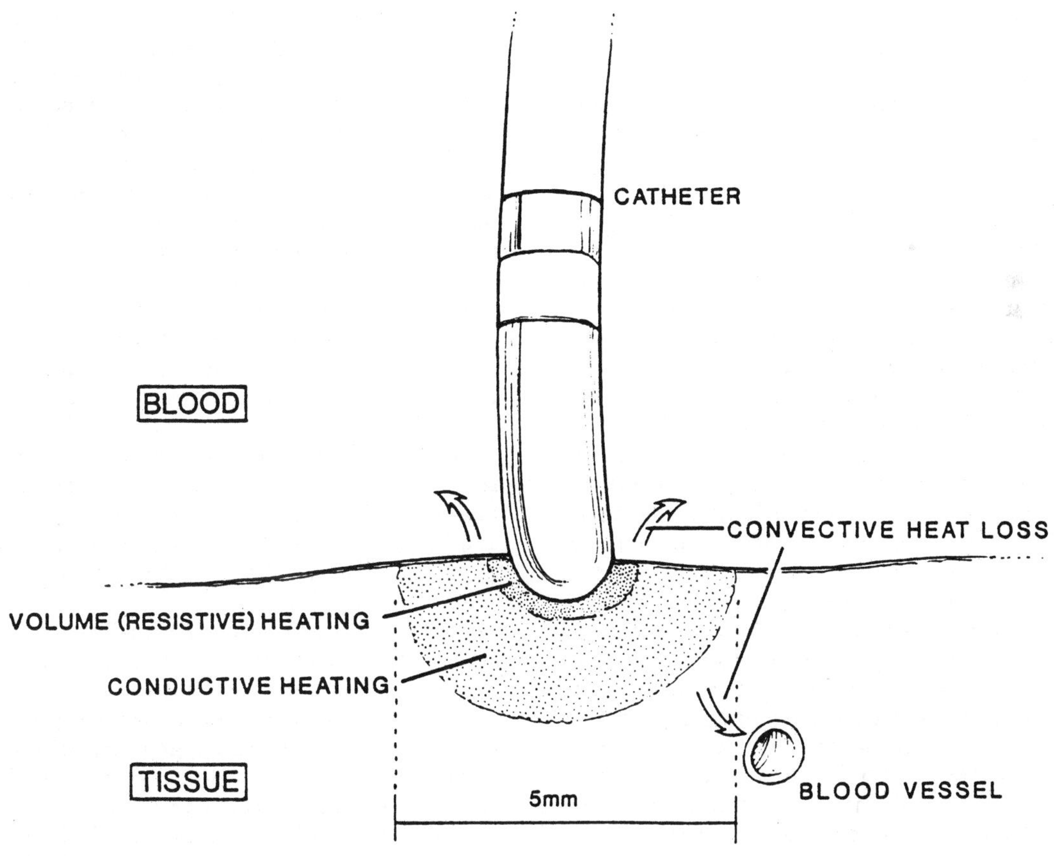

Figure 6
Lesion formation during delivery of radiofrequency (RF) current. A large-tipped catheter located in the blood pool is in contact with the endocardium. When RF energy is delivered through the distal catheter electrode, the temperature of the tissue adjacent to the electrode is increased by volume (resistive) heating as the RF energy passes through the tissue resistance; more distant tissue is heated by conduction from the rim of tissue surrounding the electrode. There is convective heat loss into the blood pool and via myocardial blood vessels. Myocardial tissue that is heated to a temperature greater than approximately 50°C is irreversibly damaged. The resultant lesion is approximately 5 mm in diameter and 3 mm deep.

Candidates are patients who have a concomitant indication for cardiac surgery that allows surgical ablation of the accessory pathway at the same session, as well as the rare patient in whom one or more catheter ablation sessions have failed to interrupt the accessory pathway.

Suggested Reading

Benditt DG, Benson DW, eds. Cardiac preexcitation syndromes: Origins, evaluation, and treatment. Boston: Martinus Nijhoff, 1986.

DiMarco JP, Miles WM, Akhtar M, et al. Adenosine for paroxysmal supraventricular tachycardia: Dose ranging and comparison with verapamil. Ann Intern Med 1990; 113:104.

Gallagher JJ, Selle JG, Svenson RH, et al. Surgical treatment of arrhythmias. Am J Cardiol 1988; 61:27A.

Jackman WM, Wang X, Friday KJ, et al. Catheter ablation of accessory atrioventricular pathways (Wolff-Parkinson-White syndrome) by radiofrequency current. N Engl J Med 1991; 324:1605.

Klein GJ, Prystowsky EN, Yee R, et al. Asymptomatic Wolff-Parkinson-White: Should we intervene? Circulation 1989; 80:1902.

Miles WM, Klein LS, Rardon DP, et al. Atrioventricular reentry and variants: Mechanisms, clinical features and management. In: Zipes DP, Jalife J, eds. Cardiac Electrophysiology: From cell to bedside. 2nd ed. Philadelphia: WB Saunders, 1995:638.

Wolff L, Parkinson J, White PD. Bundle branch block with short P-R interval in healthy young people prone to paroxysmal tachycardia. Am Heart J 1950; 5:685.

Zipes DP, ed. Catheter Ablation of Arrhythmias. Armonk, NY: Futura Publishing, 1994.

Zipes DP. Specific arrhythmias: Diagnosis and treatment. In: Braunwald E, ed. Heart disease: A textbook of cardiovascular medicine. 4th ed. Philadelphia: WB Saunders, 1992:667.

Zipes DP, DiMarco JP, Gillette PC, et al. Guidelines for clinical intracardiac electrophysiology and catheter ablation procedures: A report of the American College of Cardiology/American Heart Association Task Force on Practice Guidelines (Committee on Clinical Intracardiac Electrophysiologic and Catheter Ablation Procedures), developed in collaboration with the North American Society of Pacing and Electrophysiology. J Am Coll Cardiol 1995; 26:555.

PROLONGED REPOLARIZATION SYNDROMES

Deborah J. Statters, B.M., B.Ch, M.A.
A. John Camm, M.D.
Nicholas J. Linker, M.D.

The term *prolonged repolarization syndrome* conveniently describes the observed association between prolongation of the QT interval on the surface electrocardiogram (ECG) or an alternative measure of repolarization and a tendency, often familial, to syncope or to sudden cardiac death. Syncope frequently occurs in children with the syndrome and can be associated with fitting. This association has led to several cases being misdiagnosed as epilepsy, while attacks are allowed to continue, occasionally resulting in avoidable mortality. QT interval measurement is, however, fast becoming part of the routine assessment of patients with newly diagnosed epilepsy, particularly if other features are not entirely typical of that condition. The prolonged repolarization syndromes are often referred to as the long QT syndromes. However, a normal resting QT value does not exclude the condition, with abnormalities of repolarization sometimes only becoming obvious under particular conditions.

■ ETIOLOGY

Prolonged repolarization syndromes may be congenital or acquired. The congenital condition usually is inherited, but does appear to also occur sporadically. The pattern of inheritance may be autosomal recessive or autosomal dominant. The recessive form, known as the Jervell and Lange-Nielsen syndrome, is associated with neural deafness. Deafness is not a feature of the autosomal dominant Romano-Ward syndrome. Techniques of gene mapping have demonstrated that a number of different genetic abnormalities may result in the latter condition. In some families the condition appears to be linked to a locus on the short arm of chromosome 11 (11p15.5). In other families the condition is linked to chromosome 7 (7q11.23 or 7q35–36) and in others to chromosome 3 (3p21–24). Additional loci are also being evaluated.

Genetic heterogeneity is not really surprising when one considers the number of ionic channels involved in determining the duration of myocardial action potentials and hence the timing of repolarization. The locus on chromosome 7 may be part of the cardiac potassium channel gene, whereas the locus on chromosome 3 may be part of the gene for the cardiac sodium channel.

The identification of different genetic linkage patterns in patients with the prolonged repolarization syndromes suggests that there may be a group of different conditions resulting in similar clinical features and may explain why these patients do not all respond similarly to treatment.

When syncope occurs during ECG recording, the cause is usually a form of ventricular tachycardia known as torsades de pointes (Fig. 1). This type of arrhythmia is usually self-terminating but can deteriorate into ventricular fibrillation. Acquired repolarization syndromes have been reported in a number of contexts (Table 1) but most commonly occur after drug therapy. Several drugs (Table 2) have been reported as being responsible for the condition, which is reversible when drug treatment is stopped. Most patients who develop drug-related torsades de pointes do so within 4 days of the initiation of therapy, but the condition can manifest itself after months or years of therapy. Late-onset drug-related torsades de pointes may occur due to an increase in serum drug levels, which is often caused by the introduction of a second drug

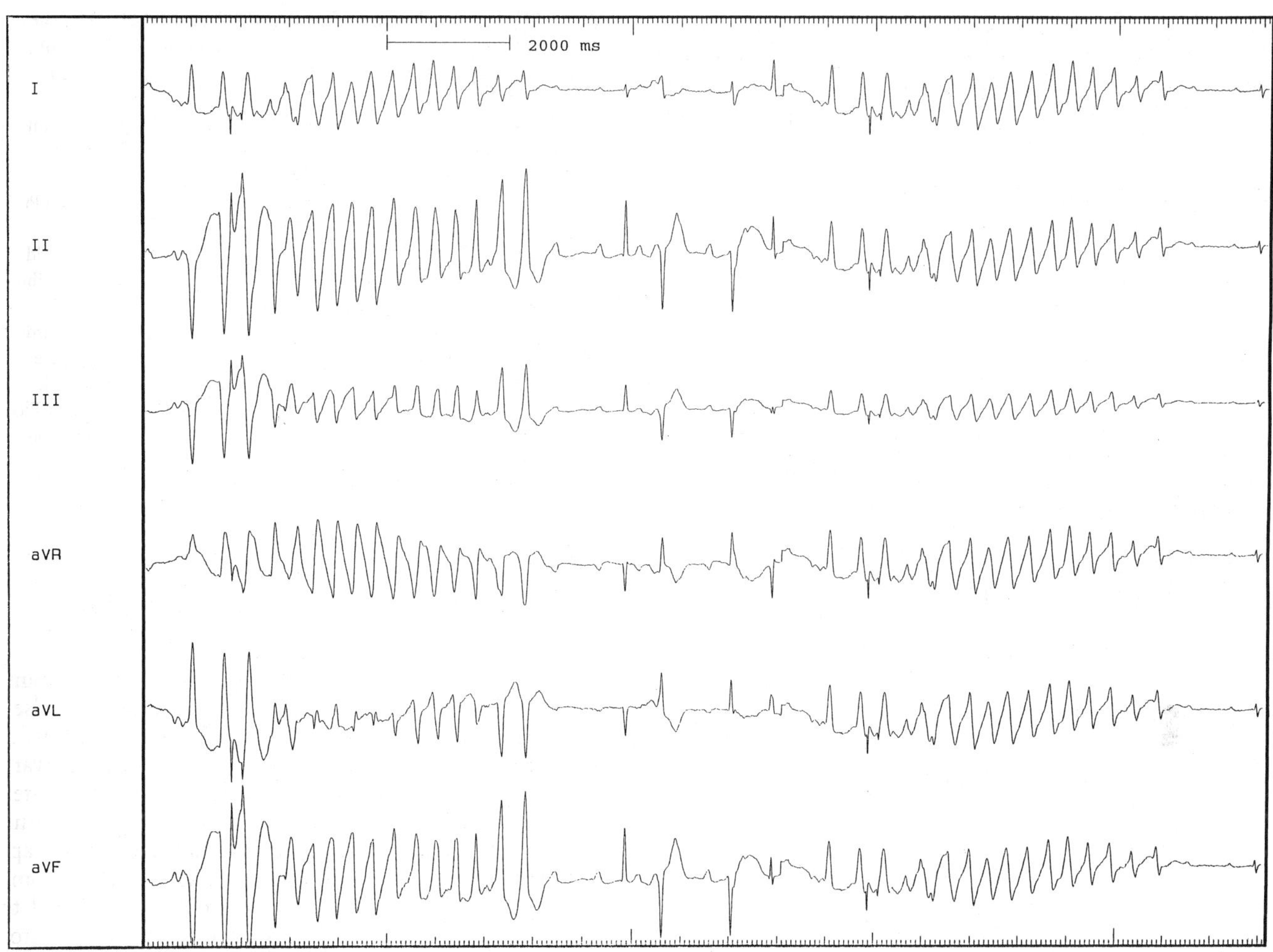

Figure 1
Torsades de pointes.

Table 1 Conditions Associated with Prolonged Repolarization Syndromes

Conditions
Drugs and toxins
Myocardial ischemia/infarction
Intracoronary contrast media
Mitral valve prolapse
Myocarditis
Left ventricular dysfunction
Rheumatic fever
Pacemaker malfunction
Bradycardias (sinoatrial disease, atrioventricular block)
Hypothyroidism
Electrolyte deficiencies (hypokalemia, hypomagnesemia, hypocalcemia)
Anorexia nervosa
Central nervous system disturbance (e.g., cerebral hemorrhage)
Postoperative complication

affecting the metabolism of the responsible agent, although the effect is idiosyncratic and levels outside the therapeutic range are not usually involved. In other instances, drug-related torsades de pointes may occur during a period of electrolyte imbalance.

■ THERAPY

In patients with the acquired repolarization syndromes, the treatment is therapy for or withdrawal of the causal factor. Suppression of torsades de pointes during treatment of the underlying cause can occasionally be achieved by intravenous magnesium, high-rate pacing, and occasionally by class III antiarrhythmic agents such as amiodarone. In patients with the congenital condition, syncope usually occurs during periods of heightened sympathetic activity such as sudden exertion, startling by loud noises, or pain. Untreated, the prognosis is relatively poor, although family screening occasionally turns up affected members who have been largely or entirely asymptomatic for many decades. Increased risk is associated with sudden death in a first-degree relative, a history of prior syncope, QTc value greater than 500 $ms^{1/2}$, and a resting heart rate of less than 60 beats per minute. The frequency of arrhythmias and survival can be improved by treatment with beta-blockers. If arrhythmias continue despite adequate beta-blockade, pacing the heart in addition to beta-blockade to prevent bradycardias is often effective. Patients refractory to this therapy also are usually considered for left stellate ganglionectomy. This latter treatment was devised

Table 2 Drugs and Toxins Associated with Prolongation of QT Intervals or Torsades de Pointes (Not Usually in Patients With the Inherited Long QT Syndromes)*

ANTIARRHYTHMIC AGENTS		
Class Ia	**Class Ib**	**Class Ic**
Procainamide	Aprindine	Encainide
Quinidine	Mexiletine	
Disopyramide		
Ajmaline		
Class III		**Other**
NAPA (N-acetyl-procainamide)		Isoprenaline
		Atropine
Amiodarone		
Sotalol		
ALLERGIC DISORDERS		**ANTIBIOTICS**
Astemizole		Erythromycin
Terfenidine		Pentamidine
Promethazine		Bactrim
Corticosteroids		Spiramycin
		Ampicillin
ANTIMALARIALS		**GASTROINTESTINAL**
Halofantrine		Cisapride
Chloroquine		
ANTIDEPRESSANTS		**ANTIPSYCHOTIC DRUGS**
Tricyclic anti-depressants		Phenothiazines
Amitriptyline		Chlorpromazine
Imipramine		Thioridazine
Protriptyline		Trifluoperizine
Nortriptyline		Mesoridazine
Doxepin		Pimozide
Maprotiline		**VASODILATORS**
Zimelidine		Prenylamine
Fluoxetine		Lidoflazine
ANTIHYPERTENSIVE/ DIURETICS		Fenoxidil
		Bepridil
Indapamide		
Ketanserin		
Nifedipine		
Furosemide		
OTHER		**TOXINS**
Glycyrrhizin	Synthroid	Arsenic
Probucol	Chloral hydrate	Organophosphates
Doxorubicin	Suxamethonium	Liquid protein diets
Vasopressin	Amantadine	
Terodiline		

*This list is not intended to be comprehensive.

because of a theory that the disorder may be caused by an imbalance in the sympathetic input to the ventricular myocardium caused by subnormal activity of the right stellate ganglion. Reducing left-sided cardiac sympathetic input may partially restore this balance. In support of this theory, some patients with repolarization syndromes have been found to have inflammation of the right stellate ganglion. Stimulation of the left stellate ganglion can result in prolongation of the QT interval, whereas stimulation of the right stellate ganglion decreases the QT interval. Abnormality of cardiac autonomic control in congenital long QT syndrome patients is also suggested by low resting heart rates and reduced heart rate increment during exercise and the administration of atropine.

■ ARRHYTHMOGENIC MECHANISMS

Delay in myocardial repolarization is not always arrhythmogenic. Occasionally, delay in repolarization, with associated QT interval prolongation, is the mechanism by which an antiarrhythmic agent achieves its protective effect. Prolongation of the QT interval will occur when repolarization in all or part of the myocardium is delayed. If repolarization is delayed only in some regions of myocardium, either due to delay in activation or due to prolonged action potential duration, this provides a potential substrate for re-entry circuits within the myocardium and thus encourages arrhythmias. A relationship has been demonstrated between inhomogeneous timing of ventricular repolarization and vulnerability to ventricular arrhythmias and a reduced ventricular fibrillation threshold. If repolarization and hence refractoriness of all areas of myocardium are equally delayed, this may prevent re-entrant circuits from forming and provide an antiarrhythmic effect. Myocardial action potential duration can be directly measured from monophasic action potential (MAP) recordings. These recordings are obtained using invasive techniques and are not widely available. Such recordings have demonstrated increased regional variation in MAP duration in patients with arrhythmogenic QT prolongation (in one study, up to 270 ms in patients with the congenital long QT syndrome compared with up to 40 ms in normal controls), but homogeneous MAP duration in those patients with QT prolongation caused by antiarrhythmic agents such as amiodarone. A noninvasive measure of regional variation in action potential duration is clearly needed to assess arrhythmia risk.

QT interval duration varies between the 12 leads of the ECG. This interlead variation, known as QT dispersion, may reflect differences in repolarization time between areas of underlying myocardium, thus providing a noninvasive measure of these differences and thus of arrhythmia substrate. Many studies have supported this hypothesis. However, methodologic inconsistencies complicate the interpretation of this research and have so far prevented QT dispersion from becoming a clinically useful tool. Although QT dispersion is significantly increased in patients with congenital long QT syndromes, there does not appear to be any correlation between QT dispersion and arrhythmia occurrence within this group of patients.

Increased dispersion of repolarization timing may provide a substrate for arrhythmia propagation. However, arrhythmias also need to be initiated. MAP recordings of some patients with repolarization syndromes show morphologic changes consisting of "humps" known as afterdepolarizations (Fig. 2). These humps are depolarizing shifts of membrane potential occurring during repolarization (early afterdepolarizations) or following completion of repolarization (delayed afterdepolarizations). Afterdepolarizations may result from enhancement of depolarizing sodium or calcium currents flowing late in the action potential or a reduction in the repolarizing potassium current. Afterdepolarizations have been recorded in patients suffering from torsade de pointes due to both congenital long QT syndromes and drug-induced prolonged repolarization syndromes. Figure 2 shows that afterdepolarizations can reach threshold for initiating ven-

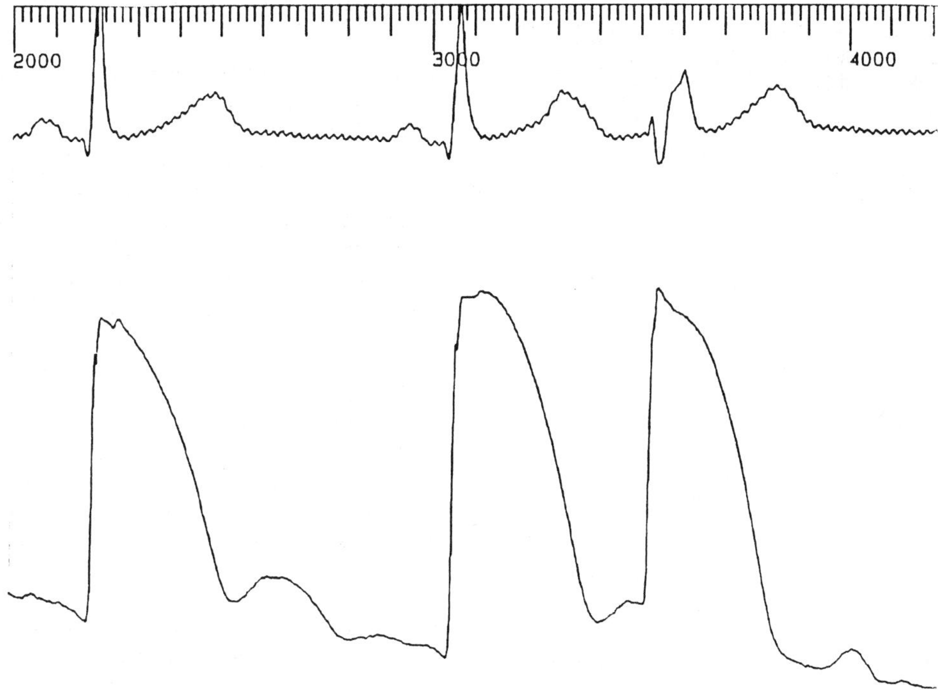

Figure 2
Monophasic action potentials demonstrating afterdepolarizations, one of which has reached threshold and resulted in a ventricular ectopic beat.

tricular ectopy and may provide the trigger for more sustained arrhythmias. Afterdepolarizations, when present, are often more pronounced during bradycardias or in the complex following a pause (such as the compensatory pause after an ectopic beat). The role of afterdepolarizations in initiating tachycardias is supported by the classic onset sequence of arrhythmias in the prolonged repolarization syndromes. There is usually a pause followed by an early ectopic beat that initiates tachycardia, the so-called "long-short" initiation sequence. When a long-short sequence does not result in a sustained tachycardia it can be seen instead to result in marked abnormalities of T-U morphology.

THE FUTURE

An understanding of the genetic background to the abnormalities in prolonged repolarization syndromes is likely to prove important in the development of therapy targeting the specific ionic channel defects in individual patients after genotyping. Eventually it is hoped that genetic therapy will be developed to reverse the underlying genetic abnormality. Although this form of treatment may be some way off, advances in this field are progressing rapidly and offer a great deal of hope for the future.

Suggested Reading

Bonatti V, Rolli A. Recording of monophasic action potentials of the right ventricle in long QT syndromes complicated by severe ventricular arrhythmias. Eur Heart J 1983; 4:168.

Jackman WM, Friday KJ, Anderson JL, et al. The long QT syndromes: A critical review, new clinical observations and a unifying hypothesis. Prog Cardiovasc Dis 1988; 31:115.

Schwartz PJ, Locati E. The idiopathic long QT syndrome: Pathogenic mechanisms and therapy. Eur Heart J 1985; 6(Suppl D):103.

Surawicz B. Electrophysiologic substrate of torsade de pointes: Dispersion of repolarization or early afterdepolarizations? J Am Coll Cardiol 1989; 14:172.

Statters DJ, Malik M, Ward DE, Camm AJ. QT dispersion: Problems of methodology and clinical significance. J Cardiovasc Electrophysiol 1994; 5:672.

SURGICAL AND CATHETER ABLATIVE THERAPY OF SUPRAVENTRICULAR ARRHYTHMIAS

Samuel J. DeMaio Jr., M.D.
Eric H. Stocker, M.D.

Most patients with supraventricular arrhythmias can be successfully treated with medical therapy. However, those patients who are poorly controlled or who are intolerant to medical therapy can now be successfully treated by surgical and catheter ablative techniques. In considering any patient for surgical or catheter ablative therapy, the patient's age and general medical condition, along with the clinical arrhythmia and its response to medical therapy, should be evaluated.

Although surgical ablation of supraventricular arrhythmias has been quite successful, this technique has been largely replaced by percutaneous transcatheter ablation. As discussed later, transcatheter ablation (particularly utilizing radiofrequency energy) has been proven highly effective for both accessory pathway ablation as well as the treatment of atrioventricular (AV) node re-entry arrhythmias. Although the mortality of surgical therapy can be as high as 5 percent with a 4 percent reoperation rate (Jackman and co-workers, 1991), the morbidity of radiofrequency ablation of supraventricular arrhythmias has been quite low, with no mortality reported to date. Furthermore, the risks of general anesthesia and open heart surgery are obviated with catheter ablation. Surgical treatments are reviewed, because they are still performed in the event that transcatheter ablation fails.

■ SURGICAL THERAPY

Accessory Pathways

Surgical therapy for patients with Wolff-Parkinson-White syndrome has been performed since 1968. Initially, the procedure was limited to those patients with intractable supraventricular tachycardia. The indications for this procedure have subsequently broadened to include patients (1) with poorly tolerated rhythms on antiarrhythmic medication; (2) who have intolerable side effects from their medication; (3) who have life-threatening arrhythmias, such as atrial fibrillation or atrial flutter with hemodynamically intolerable ventricular response with or without antiarrhythmic medications; (4) who may be asymptomatic with regard to the bypass tract but who are undergoing cardiac surgery for other indications; or (5) who are young and would prefer not taking antiarrhythmic medications for a long period of time.

Preoperative Preparation

Prior to surgery, all cardiac anomalies should be elucidated. This goal is usually accomplished by physical examination, echocardiography, or both. Male patients over the age of 35 years and female patients over the age of 40 years should undergo coronary arteriography to assess the presence or absence of coronary artery disease. Most important, all patients in whom ablative therapy is contemplated should undergo electrophysiologic study.

Electrophysiologic testing is useful in identifying the mechanism and susceptibility of the patient to the arrhythmia; defining the role, if any, for pharmacologic therapy; determining the function of the accessory pathway by measuring the effective refractory period; and determining the ventricular response over this pathway during atrial fibrillation or atrial flutter. In those patients who are candidates for ablative therapy, preoperative localization of the accessory pathway is imperative because these findings determine the cannulation techniques during surgery and are used to direct the surgical procedure if an adequate intraoperative map cannot be performed. The preoperative map is not a substitute for intraoperative mapping, which may more precisely localize the accessory pathway and may identify additional pathways not apparent preoperatively.

Intraoperative Mapping

Intraoperative mapping is performed during sinus rhythm and orthodromic tachycardia to determine the atrial and ventricular insertion sites of the accessory pathway. The intraoperative map has been conventionally performed by a hand-held bipolar probe sampling selective sites on the atrial and ventricular side of the AV groove. Recently, a computer-guided mapping system using a nylon mesh containing multiple bipolar electrodes placed around the AV groove has become available. Using this computer-generated map, only a single beat in sinus rhythm and a simple cycle of orthodromic tachycardia are needed to generate a complete intraoperative map. Some patients do not tolerate orthodromic tachycardia hemodynamically, and, if point-by-point mapping is required with a standard hand-held bipolar probe, cardiopulmonary bypass may be required. Also, some patients do not have stable tachycardia, and multiple reinductions of this rhythm may be needed if the hand-held probe is used, which may greatly limit the ability to perform a complete map. Therefore, this computerized mapping system, requiring only one beat during orthodromic tachycardia, is of obvious benefit. With this system, complete atrial and ventricular mapping with data analysis may be performed in less than 10 minutes.

Surgical Technique

Currently, two surgical approaches are used to disrupt the accessory pathway. The approach most widely used, which is the one employed at our institution, utilizes an endocardial approach to all pathways. All pathways, including the left and right free wall, anterior and posterior septal, and the atypical pathways including interseptal and Mahaim fibers, may be approached in this manner. The disadvantage of this approach is that it requires hypothermic cardiopulmonary bypass and cardioplegic arrest. A second approach, described by Guiraudon and co-workers in 1984, uses an epicardial

Table 1 Surgical Therapy of Accessory Pathways: Results

	PATIENTS/ ACCESSORY PATHWAYS	SUCCESSFUL DIVISION—ACCESSORY PATHWAYS				
		LEFT FREE WALL	POSTEROSEPTAL	RIGHT FREE WALL	ANTEROSEPTAL	TOTAL
Endocardial						
Gallagher	200/221	93/101	42/58	39/41	17/21	191/221
Cox	118/149	85/86	36/36	19/19	8/8	148/149
Epicardial						
Guiraudon	105/108	74/74	23/23	10/11	—	107/108

From Gallagher JJ, Sealy WC, Cox JL, Kasell JH. Results of surgery for preexcitation in 200 cases. Circulation 1981; (abstract) 64:146.
Cox JL, Gallagher JJ, Cain ME. Experience with 118 consecutive patients undergoing operation for the Wolff-Parkinson-White syndrome. J Thorac Cardiovasc Surg 1985;90:490.
Guiraudon GM, Klein GJ, Sharma AD, et al. Closed-heart technique for Wolff-Parkinson-White syndrome: Further experience and potential limitations. Ann Thorac Surg 1986; 42:651; with permission.

approach with dissection in the fat pad over the AV groove in conjunction with cryosurgery at the site of atrial and ventricular insertions of the accessory pathway. This procedure may be used when the pathway is localized to the left and right free wall or to the posteroseptal area. If the pathway is localized in the anteroseptal area or if there is coexistence of a Mahaim fiber, the endocardial approach should be used.

The major advantage of this procedure is that a cardiopulmonary bypass is not required for right free wall and posteroseptal pathways. Ablation of the left free wall and anteroseptal pathways does require cardiopulmonary bypass but not cardioplegic arrest (i.e., it may be performed on a warm, beating heart). This procedure is advantageous because it allows continuous monitoring of antegrade conduction of the bypass tract, the surgical effects on the accessory pathway, and potential damage to the AV node.

Results

Gallagher and co-workers (1981) reported on the first 200 patients undergoing surgery for Wolff-Parkinson-White syndrome at Duke University Medical Center. Surgical division of the accessory pathway was successful in 92 percent of patients with left free wall pathways, 98 percent with right free wall pathways, and 77 percent with posteroseptal pathways. The overall success rate in this population is 86 percent, with a reoperative rate of 19.5 percent. After 1981, the surgical technique was modified, and the results of 118 consecutive patients undergoing surgical division of the accessory pathway were reported by Cox and co-workers in 1985. They reported a 99 percent success rate in the surgical division of left free wall pathways and a 100 percent success rate in the surgical division of posteroseptal, right ventricular free wall, and anteroseptal pathways, with an overall success rate of 99 percent. Using the closed heart technique, Guiraudon and co-workers (1984) were successful in the surgical division of all but one pathway in 105 patients undergoing surgical division of 108 accessory pathways (Table 1).

Prystowsky and co-workers (1987) reported on the quality of life and the arrhythmia status after surgery for Wolff-Parkinson-White syndrome. From May 1968 to May 1986, 357 patients underwent surgery for Wolff-Parkinson-White syndrome. Follow-up data were obtained in 88 percent of patients by questionnaire and telephone. They found that the quality of life was markedly improved following surgery: 93 percent of patients had less frequent hospitalization, 92 percent were satisfied with the results of surgery, and 98 percent would recommend surgery to other patients. All patients were taking antiarrhythmic drug therapy preoperatively, whereas only 23 percent of patients were taking antiarrhythmic drug therapy postoperatively. However, 52 percent of patients, including 37 percent who were taking antiarrhythmic drugs, reported an arrhythmia after surgery. The potential problem of new onset atrial fibrillation was seen in only 2 percent of patients, half of whom required antiarrhythmic therapy.

Complications

The complication rate in patients undergoing surgical division of accessory pathways has improved significantly from the initial reports to those procedures performed after 1981. The overall success rate increased from 86 percent to 99 percent, the reoperative rate decreased from 19.5 percent to 0.5 percent, and the incidence of heart block decreased from 10.5 percent to 1 percent (Cox and co-workers, 1985) (Table 2).

Postoperative Evaluation

After postoperative recovery and prior to discharge from the hospital, all patients should undergo electrophysiologic study to evaluate the success of the procedure and to direct further therapy, if needed.

Other Supraventricular Arrhythmias

A number of surgical procedures have been performed on patients with supraventricular arrhythmias other than those due to accessory pathways. They are listed in Table 3 and are discussed in subsequent paragraphs.

Atrioventricular Nodal Re-entrant Tachycardia

Although atrioventricular nodal re-entrant tachycardia (AVNRT) usually is treated with antiarrhythmic agents, interruption or modification of AV conduction occasionally is required in patients who are refractory to medical therapy. The first operative procedure involved surgical ablation of the bundle of His, which required implantation of a permanent pacemaker. Cox and co-workers (1987), using a cryosurgical technique to modify AV nodal conduction, reported on eight patients undergoing operative therapy for AV nodal re-entrant tachycardia. Under conditions of normothermic cardiopulmonary bypass and during atrial pacing, nine separate

Table 2 Surgical Therapy of Accessory Pathways: Complications

	MORTALITY (%)					
	TOTAL	ABNORMAL	PPS (%)	AF (%)	3RD AVB (%)	REOPERATION (%)
Endocardial						
Gallagher	2.5	—	—	—	10.5	19.5
Cox	5	0.8	6.7	4.2	2.5	0
Epicardial						
Guiraudon	0	0	1	0	0	4.7

AF, Atrial fibrillation and atrial flutter; AVB, atrioventricular block; PPS, postpericardiectomy syndrome.
From Gallagher JJ, Sealy WC, Cox JL, Kasell JH. Results of surgery for preexcitation in 200 cases. Circulation 1981; (abstract) 64:146.
Cox JL, Gallagher JJ, Cain ME. Experience with 118 consecutive patients undergoing operation for the Wolff-Parkinson-White syndrome. J Thorac Cardiovasc Surg 1985;90:490.
Guiraudon GM, Klein GJ, Sharma AD, et al. Closed-heart technique for Wolff-Parkinson-White syndrome: Further experience and potential limitations. Ann Thorac Surg 1986; 42:651; with permission.

Table 3 Surgical Procedures for Supraventricular Arrhythmias

ARRHYTHMIAS	THERAPY
AV node re-entry	Cryoablation of normal AV conduction Cryosurgical attenuation of AV node conduction
Atrial fibrillation/ flutter	Cryoablation of normal AV conduction Cryosurgical attenuation of AV node conduction Atrial isolation Atrial cryoablation
Ectopic atrial tachycardia	Cryoablation—ectopic focus Atrial isolation Cryoablation/attenuation of normal AV conduction

3 mm cryolesions (–60°C for 2 minutes) were placed at predetermined sites around the triangle of Koch in the lower right atrial septum. Postoperatively, no patient had AVNRT induced or had experienced AVNRT clinically during follow-up of up to 5 years. They found that the cryosurgical procedure had no detrimental effects on the atrial-His or His-ventricular intervals or on the paced cycle length at which AV node Wenckebach occurred. More recently, Bredikis and Bredikis (1990) reported a 96 percent success rate (51 of 53 patients) using cryoablation to treat atrioventricular tachycardia. This and other surgical techniques for AVNRT have been described with favorable preliminary results, all obviating the need for permanent pacemaker implantation.

Atrial Flutter

Atrial flutter is believed to be associated with a re-entrant circuit around the fossa ovalis and is associated with a critical area of slow conduction or block in the region of the coronary sinus os. Guiraudon and co-workers (1986) performed cryoablation on the area of slow conduction in three patients with atrial flutter. This procedure resulted in successful attenuation of the atrial flutter in two patients, whereas the third patient developed symptomatic atrial fibrillation after the operation. Indirect control of the arrhythmias by AV nodal attenuation or ablation has also been used with success. However, because of the success of catheter ablation and modification of the AV node, these procedures should be reserved for those patients undergoing other operative procedures.

Atrial Fibrillation

Surgery for atrial fibrillation had been directed at alleviating hemodynamic effects of the arrhythmia rather than toward ablation of the arrhythmia itself. Elective surgical interruption or modification of AV conduction has been effective in controlling the ventricular response during atrial fibrillation. Two new surgical methods are being studied, however, which focus on curing the arrhythmia and restoring normal sinus rhythm. One of these new methods is the Maze procedure, which involves performing multiple atriotomies; the other is a corridoring procedure in which a corridor between the sinoatrial and AV nodes is created along with AV electrical isolation of the atria. The preliminary results of these procedures are encouraging. However, because of the success of catheter ablation or modification of the AV node, the operative treatment of these patients is reserved for those patients undergoing other operative procedures.

Ectopic Atrial Tachycardia

Ectopic atrial tachycardia is believed to result from derangements in automaticity, which most likely originate in cells comprising the specialized intra-atrial conduction system. These arrhythmias appear to have a focal origin and have been shown to originate from the right atrium, left atrium, or interatrial septum. These arrhythmias are often incessant and difficult to control by standard antiarrhythmic medications. Direct AV nodal ablation is useful in controlling the ventricular response in those patients with ectopic atrial tachycardias in whom the ventricular response cannot be controlled with medications; however, it does not eliminate the atrial arrhythmia. Surgical techniques aimed at removing or excluding the arrhythmogenic substrate have been proposed and reported. Preoperative mapping to locate the arrhythmogenic focus is of paramount importance because the ectopic focus becomes quiescent during general anesthesia and the arrhythmia cannot be mapped intraoperatively in up to 50 percent of the patients. Clinical experience with this operative technique has been limited. Although the numbers have been small, the results of surgical therapy have been disappointing with a high percentage of patients having recurrence of the arrhythmia or atrial fibrillation after the procedure.

■ CATHETER ABLATION TECHNIQUES

The term *catheter ablation* refers to the placement of catheters percutaneously via the femoral, subclavian, or internal jugular vessels; the ablating tip directed against the arrhythmogenic myocardium; and some form of energy being used to destroy that focus. The most frequently used form of energy is radiofrequency (RF) energy, which has rapidly replaced the use of direct current (DC) energy. Both methods are reviewed, because some institutions still utilize DC energy as the ablative energy source.

Catheter ablation may be performed at the time of the diagnostic electrophysiologic study. In addition to recording and stimulating electrodes placed in the routine course of the electrophysiologic study, a recording-ablating catheter is placed against the arrhythmogenic focus. An indifferent electrode in the form of a skin patch is placed between the patient's scapulae, and RF current is passed from the large-tipped RF catheter to the patch electrode. The destruction of the tissue is believed to be due to resistive heating, and lesions 8 to 12 mm in diameter and 5 to 10 mm deep are usually produced. Usually mild to moderate sedation is necessary, because patients experience either no discomfort or only a mild burning sensation; however, deep sedation is commonly given when a longer procedure is anticipated.

The application of high-energy direct current to potentially arrhythmogenic areas of the myocardium was the first method used to percutaneously ablate supraventricular arrhythmias. This technique is very similar to RF ablation in terms of the catheter placement and preprocedure diagnostic evaluation. A standard defibrillator acts as the current source and is delivered in the range of 100 to 300 joules, given over 4 to 8 ms. The destruction of tissue is believed to be due to primary electrical energy, and lesions 2 to 3 cm deep are usually produced. Because there is significant discomfort to the patient at this time, general anesthesia or heavy sedation must be used.

Preliminary studies suggested that the use of DC energy is associated with an increased risk of left ventricular dysfunction, arrhythmias, coronary sinus rupture, and mortality (Evans, 1988; Calkins and co-workers, 1991; Jackman and co-workers, 1991; Huang and co-workers, 1991). Given the success of radiofrequency ablation (RFA) over the past several years and its improved safety profile, DC energy is now only rarely used.

Atrioventricular Nodal Re-entrant Tachycardia

The most common form of paroxysmal supraventricular tachycardia, AVNRT, has been successfully treated with RF ablation. Recent studies show that modification of the AV node with radiofrequency energy is highly effective, with very low morbidity and no reported mortality.

The AV node re-entry pathway has two forms: "common" and "uncommon." The common form is seen in 90 percent of patients with tachycardia secondary to AV nodal re-entry and is comprised of an anterograde conducting "slow" pathway and a retrograde "fast" conducting pathway that connects the atrium to the His bundle. Both pathways are located outside the AV node. The slow pathway is usually posterior to the AV node near the coronary sinus ostium, and the fast pathway anterior. Selective ablation of the slow pathway is considered the preferred, more efficacious approach and should be considered initially because of its decreased risk of AV block and decreased need for pacemaker placement. The techniques, results, and complications are outlined in the following section.

Techniques

Prior to catheter ablation with either RF or direct current, the cardiac anatomy must be elucidated as for presurgical preparation. Echocardiography should be performed, and angiography should be considered in male patients over the age of 35 years and in female patients over the age of 40 years. The diagnostic electrophysiologic study must always be performed prior to the ablative procedure and may be done in the same session.

The patient is anesthetized with fentanyl (50 to 150 μg per hour) and midazolam (2 to 6 mg per hour). Multipolar electrode catheters are inserted percutaneously for programmed atrial and ventricular stimulation and for localization of the slow pathway. Usually, recording and stimulating electrodes are placed in the coronary sinus via the left subclavian vein and in the high right atrium, at the bundle of His, and right ventricular apex via the femoral vein. Intravenous (IV) heparin is given to all patients, usually an initial 5,000 U bolus followed by a 1,000 U per hour IV drip.

Under fluoroscopic guidance, the ablation catheter is advanced through the femoral vein across the tricuspid annulus to record the largest His potential possible, which indicates that the recording-ablating electrode is very close to the His bundle. The catheter is then withdrawn in such a way as to maximize the atrial electrogram, while minimizing the His potential. This result indicates that the catheter is along the AV conduction pathway with the ablating electrode sufficiently far from the His bundle, decreasing the risk of unintentionally destroying the His bundle and leading to complete AV block. This maneuver also positions the ablating electrode near the coronary sinus ostium above the tricuspid annulus, the area most likely to contain the slow pathway.

Radiofrequency current is delivered at 20 to 60 ws between the ablation electrode and a skin electrode positioned on the chest wall. The current is delivered for up to 60 seconds. The electrogram is continuously monitored during delivery of the destructive energy. Impedance that abruptly rises between the catheter tip and the endocardium suggests the formation of coagulum on the tip of the catheter. In this event, the current is immediately discontinued, the tip is cleaned and repositioned, and ablation is attempted again if necessary.

Programmed atrial and ventricular stimulation is employed after each application of RF current to assess slow pathway conduction. If AVNRT or slow pathway conduction is still present, either RF current is reapplied to the same area or the catheter is repositioned higher along the tricuspid annulus. If it is not possible to ablate the slow pathway, the fast pathway is ablated. This procedure, however, increases the risk of inducing complete AV block. The ablation procedure is discontinued when AVNRT or slow pathway conduction can no longer be elicited.

Postablation Management

The recommended time of in-patient postablation monitoring depends on whether slow or fast pathway ablation is performed. Slow pathway ablation requires approximately 24

Table 4 Results of RF Catheter Ablation: AV Node Re-Entry

	STUDY				
	JACKMAN ET AL (1991)	MANOLIS ET AL (1994)	LANGBERG ET AL (1992)	CHEN ET AL (1993)	KAY ET AL (1994)
No. of patients	80	55	88	100	245
No. (%) with "common" form	69 (86%)	55 (100%)	88 (100%)	95 (95%)	235 (96%)
Clinical success, No. (%)	80 (100%)	55 (100%)	81 (92%)	98 (98%)	244 (99.6%)
Selective ablation of slow pathway	78 (98%)	55 (100%)	0 (0%)	68 (68%)	234 (95.5%)
Mean follow-up, mo	15.5 ± 11.3	12 ± 7.0	12 ± 3.0	12 ± 6.0	8.4 ± 5.9
Recurrence requiring 2nd treatment, No. (%)	0 (0%)	7 (12.5%)	0 (0%)	2 (2%)	16 (6.5%)
No. of complications/mortality	5/0	1/0	—	3/0	5/0
No. requiring antiarrhythmics	0	0	0	0	2

hours, whereas fast pathway ablation requires 48 to 72 hours postablation monitoring because of the potential risk for heart block within the first 48 hours after the procedure. An electrocardiogram is obtained the following morning. Routine cardiac enzymes are checked after the procedure, but serial enzymes are not usually performed. Creatine kinase levels can underestimate the degree of myocardial injury because radiofrequency ablation may inactivate this enzyme. Follow-up electrophysiologic testing is performed only if clinically indicated.

Results

Of the 568 patients treated for AVNRT as described in this chapter, initial success was reported in 558 (98 percent) (Table 4). Recurrence of the tachycardia requiring a second treatment occurred in 0 to 12.5 percent (average, 4 percent), all with successful second treatments. There was no reported mortality associated with the treatment, and only two of the patients required antiarrhythmic medication to control residual tachycardia.

Complications

In the studies presented in this chapter, the incidence of complications ranged from 2 percent (Manolis and co-workers, 1994; Kay and co-workers, 1994) to 6 percent (Jackman and co-workers, 1991). Complications included a total of six patients who experienced complete AV block requiring placement of a pacemaker (1 percent); one patient with transient AV block—a small pulmonary embolus occurring 3 days after the ablative procedure; one patient with an asymptomatic pulmonary embolus detected by pulmonary ventilation-perfusion scanning, which showed a right lower lobe abnormal perfusion defect that resolved in a follow-up study done one month later; three patients with asymptomatic thrombi discovered by routine transesophageal echocardiography; and two patients who developed large groin hematomas requiring blood transfusion (Table 5).

Accessory Pathways

Catheter ablation offers an alternative nonpharmacologic approach to those patients with accessory pathways as well. Catheter ablative management of patients with Wolff-Parkinson-White syndrome is appropriate when the patient meets the criteria defined for surgical ablation. Additionally, patients who may be ineligible for surgical repair may be appropriate candidates for catheter ablation, particularly patients with pulmonary disease or dilated cardiomyopathy (Jackman and co-workers, 1991).

Various methods for accessory pathway ablation have been reported. In general, success rates have been high and the complication rates low, particularly when RF current is used. Initial reports used ablation of the bundle of His to prevent orthodromic reciprocating tachycardia by interrupting the antegrade limb of the tachycardia circuit. This procedure produced third-degree AV block and required permanent pacemaker implantation. However, conduction over the accessory pathways and the risk of atrial fibrillation with rapid conduction to the ventricle remained a potential hazard. Therefore, this procedure has been replaced by newer methods of direct ablation of the accessory pathway.

As mentioned previously, several studies have suggested that ablation with RF current has lower morbidity and mortality as compared with DC shocks. Therefore, the subsequent discussion is restricted to the use of RF current with references to the earlier techniques of direct current.

Technique

The initial evaluation of cardiac anatomy as noted previously for the preablation workup of AVNRT is identical. Once the diagnosis of paroxysmal supraventricular tachycardia due to an accessory pathway has been made, the patient is anesthetized in the appropriate manner. Multipolar electrode catheters are inserted percutaneously for programmed atrial and ventricular stimulation and for localization of the accessory pathway. Placement of recording and stimulating electrodes is as described for AVNRT. The ablating catheter is guided retrogradely into the left ventricle via the left femoral artery if a left-sided pathway is suspected or to the region of the tricuspid valve if a right-sided pathway is suspected. Intravenous heparin is given to all patients, usually an initial 5,000 U bolus, followed by a 1,000 U per hour intravenous drip.

The accessory pathway is localized best by inducing an orthodromic tachycardia and locating (with the recording electrodes in place) that part of the myocardium with the shortest ventricle-to-atrium conduction time. The area with the shortest ventricle-to-atrium conduction time is most likely the area that allowed for the rapid conduction of excitation to the ventricles ("pre-excitation"), which bypasses the normal delay caused by the AV node. The orthodromic tachycardia is induced by providing a programmed train of

Table 5 Complications with RF Catheter Ablation

STUDY	COMPLICATIONS
Manolis—AVNRT (1994)	(1) Transient complete AVB
Langberg AVNRT (1992)	No complications
Chen—AVNRT (1993)	(2) Complete AVB→pacemaker
Kay—AVNRT (1993)	(3) Complete AVB→pacemaker
	(2) Groin hematoma
Jackman—AVNRT (1992)	(1) Complete AVB→pacemaker
	(1) Small pulmonary embolus 3 days after ablation
	(3) Asymptomatic coronary thrombi
Kay—AP (1993)	(2) Cardiac tamponade
	(1) Transient complete AVB
	(1) Femoral artery thrombosis→surgery
Swartz—AP (1993)	(1) Occlusion of branch of circumflex coronary artery from spasm
	(1) Complete AVB→pacemaker
Lesh—AP (1992)	(1) Cardiac tamponade
	(1) Groin hematoma
	(1) 15-year-old boy with foot pain (? microembolism)
	(1) Chest pain and transient sinus tachycardia elevation from coronary spasm
Calkins—AP (1992)	(3) Complete AVB→(2) pacemaker
	(1) Chest pain and diffuse sinus tachycardia depression from coronary spasm
	(1) Thrombotic occlusion of circumflex artery→small myocardial infarction
	(1) Valvular damage
	(1) Transient ischemic attack
	(1) Pelvic hematoma
	(1) Thigh hematoma→surgery
Jackman—AP (1991)	(1) Complete AVB→pacemaker
	(1) Hemopericardium and tamponade
	(1) Pericarditis
	(1) Pseudoaneurysm at femoral site
	(1) Femoral hematoma
	(1) Thrombus high right atrium
Feld—AFib (1994)	No complications
Williamson—AFib (1994)	(4) Complete AVB→pacemaker
Poty—AFlut (1995)	No complications
Steinberg—AFlut (1995)	No complications
Fischer—AFlut (1995)	(6) Groin hematoma

AP, accessory pathways; AVB, atrioventricular block; AVNRT, atrioventricular nodal re-entrant tachycardia; AFib, atrial fibrillation; AFlut, atrial flutter.

extrastimuli to the atria or ventricles with stimulating electrodes. If this procedure is not successful, intravenous isoproterenol may be given to increase cathecholaminergenic effects on the conduction system, potentially unmasking accessory pathways.

Ablation of Accessory Pathways

After localization of the accessory pathway, the probe-ablation catheter is positioned, with the aid of fluoroscopy, as close to the pathway as possible. The site of insertion is dependent on the location of the pathway across the AV ring. For example, left-sided pathways require advancement of the ablation catheter via the right femoral artery, passed retrogradely into the left ventricle and positioned just above or beneath the mitral leaflet. They also can be ablated using the trans-septal approach from the atrial side of the mitral annulus. Right free wall accessory pathways require advancement of the ablation catheter via the right subclavian vein to a site above or beneath the tricuspid leaflet.

Anteroseptal pathways require placement of the ablation catheter via the right subclavian vein to a site beneath the septal or anterior tricuspid leaflet. Finally, posteroseptal pathways may be approached by the right subclavian vein, placing the tip against the tricuspid annulus or near the coronary sinus ostium or by placing the tip in a venous branch of the proximal coronary sinus (associated with a higher risk of tamponade and pericarditis, as noted in the paragraph on complications). A posteroseptal pathway also may be reached by passing a catheter through the right femoral artery and placing the tip against the mitral annulus.

Radiofrequency current is delivered at 45 to 60 ws between the large-tip ablation electrode and a skin electrode positioned on the chest wall. The current is delivered for up to 60 seconds. If successful, conduction across the accessory pathway should disappear in approximately 15 seconds. Impedance (which is continuously monitored) that abruptly rises between the catheter tip and the endocardium suggests the formation of coagulum on the tip of the catheter. Current is immediately discontinued, the tip is cleaned and repositioned, and ablation is attempted again, if necessary.

Postablation Management

It is imperative to be certain that the accessory pathway has been successfully ablated to exclude the possibility of the

Table 6 Results of RF Catheter Ablation: Accessory Pathways

	STUDY				
	JACKMAN ET AL (1991)	CALKINS ET AL (1992)	LESH ET AL (1992)	SWARTZ ET AL (1993)	KAY ET AL (1993)
No. of patients	166 (177 pathways)	250 (267 pathways)	100 (109 pathways)	114 (122 pathways)	363 (384 pathways)
Clinical success, No. (%)	175 (99%)	252 (94%)	98 (90%)	116 (95%)	367 (95%)
Location of failed pathway	Posteroseptal (2)	Left free wall (9) Posteroseptal (3) Right free wall (1) Anteroseptal (2)	Septal (7) Right free wall (4) Left free wall (1)	Right free wall (4) Left anterior (1) Left free wall (1)	Left free wall (1) Right free wall (5) Posteroseptal (8) Midseptal (1) Mahaim (2)
Length of procedure, hr	8.3 ± 3.5	2.2 ± 1.3	6 ± 4.0	4.9 ± 2.2	—
Recurrence requiring 2nd treatment, No. (%)	15 (9%)	23 (9%)	12 (12%)	10 (9%)	19 (5%)
Mean follow-up, mo	8 ± 5.4	10 ± 4	10.2 ± 0.5	21.2 ± 4.6	9 ± 7.0
No. requiring antiarrhythmics	0	10	0	3	7
No. of complications/mortality	6/0	9/0	4/0	2/0	4/2

presence of a second pathway or AVNRT. For this reason, 30 to 60 minutes after ablation the patient is retested, usually after the administration of isoproterenol. The patient should be monitored by continuous electrocardiography for at least 24 hours, and a 12-lead electrocardiogram should be checked immediately after the procedure and at least the next morning. Patients usually can be discharged 48 hours after the procedure. Follow-up electrophysiologic testing is performed when clinically indicated.

Results

Long-term success of RF ablation of supraventricular arrhythmias due to accessory pathway conduction ranges from 90 to 99 percent (Table 6). In one study of 166 patients (177 pathways), Jackman and co-workers (1991) had a 99 percent initial success rate, with tachycardia returning in 15 patients within 4.7 months of the initial procedure. A second session eliminated the arrhythmia in all of these patients. The procedure lasted 8.3 ± 3.5 hours and was well tolerated in all patients. Thirty-five percent of patients also were undergoing their first diagnostic electrophysiologic testing. Late electrophysiologic studies in 75 patients (46 percent) confirmed the absence of accessory pathway conduction in all of the patients.

Calkins and co-workers (1992) had a 94 percent success rate in 235 of 250 patients with Wolff-Parkinson-White syndrome. Of these patients, 217 (87 percent) had all accessory AV connections ablated during the initial attempt at catheter ablation. Twenty-three of the 33 patients who failed an initial attempt at catheter ablation underwent a second attempt that was successful in 17 patients. A total of 15 accessory AV connections were not successfully ablated. Nine accessory AV connections were located in the left free wall, three were posteroseptal, two were anteroseptal, and one was located on the right free wall. Two patients with left-sided accessory AV connections went on to require surgical ablation. Two patients with anteroseptal accessory AV connections developed AV nodal block during the procedure (they remained asymptomatic), and a second attempt at catheter ablation was not undertaken because their accessory AV connections were either concealed or not capable of rapid anterograde conduction. One patient underwent successful catheter ablation at another institution. Ten patients required treatment with antiarrhythmic agents.

Lesh and co-workers (1992) reported on 100 patients, 90 percent of whom had successful ablation. Twelve patients required two sessions, and all others required only a single session. Seven patients had previously failed direct current surgical ablation of posteroseptal accessory pathways, but RFA was successful in five. Of the failed pathways, seven were septal, four were located on the right free wall, and one was on the left free wall. None of the patients developed AV block or other cardiac arrhythmias.

A study of 114 patients (122 pathways) by Swartz and co-workers (1993) reported a 95 percent success rate, ablating 116 of 122 pathways. Recurrent conduction requiring repeat ablation occurred in 10 accessory pathways within 1 month of the ablation procedure. After up to 2 years of follow-up, 95 percent of patients were asymptomatic and without evidence of AP conduction. Three patients required antiarrhythmic medications.

A 95 percent success rate was also reported in a large study of 363 patients (384 pathways) by Kay and co-workers (1993). The probability of successful ablation was significantly related to the location of the accessory pathway. Left free wall and anteroseptal pathways were successfully ablated more than 99 percent of the time, whereas right free wall, posteroseptal, and midseptal pathways were successfully ablated just more than 91 percent of the time. Most of the 346 patients who were successfully ablated required one ablation session; only 10 patients required two sessions. Of the 17 patients in whom catheter ablation was unsuccessful, eight were referred for surgery, seven were managed with antiarrhythmic drugs, one was effectively managed with ablation of the AV node, and one underwent successful catheter ablation at another institution.

Complications

Complications occurred in 25 of the 993 patients treated in the five recent studies cited here (Table 6). Two deaths were attributed to other cardiac causes rather than a consequence of catheter ablation. These complications included (1) six patients who developed complete atrioventricular block, four of whom underwent permanent pacemaker implantation; (2) three patients with large femoral hematomas, one of whom required surgical repair of a damaged femoral artery; (3) four patients with cardiac tamponade, one of whom had fluoroscopic evidence of penetration of a right ventricular catheter and another of whom had RF current applied in a small venous branch of the coronary sinus; (4) pericarditis in one patient after receiving RF current in a venous branch of the coronary sinus; (5) two patients with acute chest pain, one of whom who had diffuse ST T-wave segment depression and the other of whom had ST segment elevation, but both were suspected of having coronary artery spasm; (6) a small pseudoaneurysm of the right femoral artery; (7) an occlusion of a posterolateral segmental branch of a left dominant circumflex coronary artery immediately after delivery of RF energy to a left posterior paraseptal accessory pathway accomplished from within the coronary sinus via a small posterior vein—further evaluation suggested coronary spasm as the initial cause of coronary closure; (8) a thrombus found in the high right atrium by transesophageal echocardiography and believed to be secondary to the ablation procedure; (9) aortic valve damage as a consequence of catheter trauma following successful ablation of a left-sided accessory AV connection; (10) a transient neurologic deficit manifested by transient right-sided weakness and aphasia, which lasted 5 minutes and occurred 5 days after a successful ablation of a concealed left lateral accessory AV connection; (11) a large pelvic hematoma with an 8-point drop in hematocrit; (12) acute thrombosis of the circumflex coronary artery as a result of inadvertent delivery of RF current within the left coronary artery in a patient with a concealed left lateral accessory AV connection—patency of the vessel was restored within 30 minutes after angioplasty, but the patient did sustain a small myocardial infarction (peak MB isoenzyme concentration was 228 IU/l with normal being 0 to 10 IU/l) and had an uneventful recovery; (13) a 15-year-old boy who developed foot pain—results of blood flow studies were normal but microembolism could not be excluded, and he recovered promptly with no treatment; and (14) femoral artery thrombosis requiring surgical repair.

Atrial Fibrillation

The most common arrhythmia encountered in clinical practice is atrial fibrillation. The recent concept of chronic tachycardia with fast or irregular rhythms contributing to a reversible form of heart failure has led investigators to pursue a more definitive form of treatment, given the often disappointing efficacy of drug therapy. RFA has been used successfully to treat recurrent atrial fibrillation in patients who have (1) a rapid ventricular response rate that cannot be controlled with drug therapy or (2) adequate rate control but are unable to tolerate the drug therapy itself. Currently, there are two methods of RFA used for ventricular rate control. One method is AV node ablation with pacemaker implantation. The other method involves AV node modification using the same technique discussed previously, only the RF energy is applied specifically in the low middle or posterior septal right atrium near the tricuspid valve annulus. AV node ablation is effective approximately 100% of the time, whereas AV node modification, as later discussed, has been effective in approximately 70 percent of cases. AV node modification has been suggested prior to attempted ablation to avoid the need for permanent pacemaker implantation.

Recent studies have shown successful reduction in ventricular rate during atrial fibrillation or flutter by ablating the "slow" AV node pathway in patients with AV nodal dual-pathway physiology and inducible or sustained AV nodal re-entrant tachycardia (Blanck and co-workers, 1995; Tebbenjohanns and co-workers, 1995). Della Bella and co-workers (1995), however, reported that dual AV node physiology also can occur without AV node re-entrant tachycardia, implying that the slow pathway is part of the "normal" AV node. By selectively ablating the slow pathway noted to be in the posteroinferior atrial septum, they also reported success in reducing the ventricular rate during atrial fibrillation or flutter without affecting AV conduction during sinus rhythm.

Attempts to "cure" atrial fibrillation and restore normal sinus rhythm have, until recently, only been done surgically using the Maze and corridor procedures discussed previously. Swartz and co-workers (1994) have shown that a curative approach to atrial fibrillation is possible using RFA to emulate the atrial Maze procedure. More studies using this approach are needed.

Table 7 Results of RF Catheter Ablation: Atrial Fibrillation

	STUDY	
	FELD (1994)	WILLIAMSON (1994)
No. of patients	10	19
Clinical success, No. (%)	7 (70%)	14 (74%)
Mean follow-up, mo	14 ± 8	8 ± 2
Recurrence of AV conduction, No. (%)	0 (0%)	1 (5%)
No. of complications/mortality	0/0	4/1
No. requiring permanent pacemaker, No. (%)	2 (2%)	4 (21%)

Results

Success in reducing rapid ventricular response to atrial fibrillation ranged from 70 to 74 percent (Table 7). Feld and co-workers (1994) ablated the AV nodal slow pathway in 10 patients with symptomatic, medically refractory atrial fibrillation. Seven patients (70 percent) have remained symptom-free from rapid ventricular response during a mean follow-up period of 14 ± 8 months. Complete AV node ablation followed by permanent pacemaker implantation was performed in two of the three patients who did not respond to AV node modification. The third patient underwent amiodarone loading followed by DC cardioversion.

Table 8 Results of RF Catheter Ablation: Atrial Flutter

	STUDY		
	FISCHER (1995)	POTY (1995)	STEINBERG (1995)
No. of patients	80	12	16
Clinical success, No. (%)	72 (90%)	11 (92%)	16 (100%)
Mean follow-up, mo	20 ± 8	9 ± 3.4	8 ± 5.0
Recurrence of AV conduction, No. (%)	14 (17%)	1 (8%)	4 (25%)
No. of complications/mortality	6/0	0/0	0/0
No. requiring AV nodal ablation and permanent pacemaker, No. (%)	—	0 (0%)	0 (0%)

Nineteen patients with uncontrolled ventricular rates underwent catheter modification with a reported success rate of 74 percent (14 patients) in a study by Williamson and co-workers (1994). One patient had a recurrence of rapid ventricular rate after 3 months and became asymptomatic after a second ablation session. Interestingly, during the first 3 months of follow-up after a successful initial modification procedure, the mean maximal ventricular rate during exercise increased by 25 percent. This increase was believed to be secondary to partial recovery of AV conduction following the immediate effects of RF energy. The mean maximal rate was still 25 percent lower than at baseline, however, and patients remained asymptomatic.

Complications

The only complication directly attributable to the procedure was complete AV block, which inadvertently occurred in four patients in Williamson's study. Two patients in Feld's study underwent AV node ablation after not responding to modification procedures. All these patients received permanent pacemakers. One patient in Williamson's study died suddenly 5 months after a successful modification procedure. Although the patient had an idiopathic dilated cardiomyopathy and a left ventricular ejection fraction of 0.20, it is unknown if the patient's death was secondary to a late complication of the modification procedure. Other complications such as severe ventricular arrhythmias and sudden cardiac death have been reported in earlier studies. Recent studies have shown that these complications usually can be prevented by postablation rapid ventricular pacing (up to 120 bpm) tapered gradually over a 24-hour period.

Atrial Flutter

Type I ("classic") atrial flutter is a common, usually benign rhythm disturbance, which usually is found in the setting of structural heart disease. The electrophysiologic mechanism has become better understood as evidenced by several recent reports documenting increased cure rates using selective RFA. The indication for RFA is the same as for atrial fibrillation. Although there is no known substrate for the re-entry circuit of atrial flutter, the circuit is confined to the right atrium and involves a functional area of slow conduction. This area includes the right atrial free wall, the isthmus between the inferior vena cava and tricuspid valve, the low posteromedial atrial wall, and the interatrial septum. After successful ablation of atrial flutter, late recurrence of atrial flutter or atrial fibrillation has been shown to be a long-term risk. Philippon and co-workers (1995) reported a 26% incidence (14 of 53 patients) of atrial fibrillation following successful ablation of typical atrial flutter in 53 of 59 patients (90 percent). This risk was especially high for patients who had inducible, sustained atrial fibrillation after ablation of atrial flutter. Also at risk for late recurrence of atrial fibrillation are patients with a history of atrial fibrillation, those with a greater number of antiarrhythmic drug failures, and those with structural heart disease.

Results

Fischer and co-workers successfully ablated 72 of 80 patients (90 percent) with common atrial flutter after a single session (Table 8). Of the 72, 14 patients (17 percent) had recurrences of atrial flutter approximately 3 months after the first ablation session. Ten of these patients underwent successful repeat ablations without recurrence. Four patients (5 percent) developed new episodes of atrial fibrillation, and 54 patients (68 percent) remained asymptomatic and without recurrence of atrial flutter during a mean follow-up period of 20 ± 8 months. This study also used three different target sites in the right atrium for ablation. The most successful site was in the isthmus between the inferior vena cava orifice and tricuspid valve.

Poty and co-workers (1995) reported a 92 percent initial success rate in a study of 12 patients with type I atrial flutter. Although long-term recurrence rates have approached 50% in earlier studies, this study suggested that achieving block at the inferior vena cava–tricuspid annulus isthmus may be beneficial in preventing recurrences after RFA of atrial flutter. The only recurrence in this study, at a mean follow-up of 9 ± 3.4 months, occurred when block at this isthmus was not achieved.

A 100 percent success rate was reported by Steinberg and co-workers (1995) in a recent study of 16 patients. Four patients (25 percent) developed a recurrence of atrial flutter 48 hours to 20 weeks after the initial procedure. Three of these patients had successful repeat ablations, and one was placed on antiarrhythmic drugs. Over a mean follow-up period of 8 ± 5 months, one patient had an episode of atrial fibrillation, one had an episode of AV nodal re-entry, and one developed asymptomatic complete heart block that did not require a pacemaker.

Complications

No complications were reported in either Poty's or Steinberg's study. The patient in Steinberg's study with complete heart block was completely asymptomatic in a junctional escape rhythm with a resting heart rate of 40 to 50 beats per minute.

The patient's performance on an exercise treadmill was appropriate for age. All six patients in Fischer's study had a groin hematoma.

Cost

In the long term, transcatheter RFA, when compared with surgery and long-term antiarrhythmic therapy, has been shown to be the most cost-effective treatment strategy for patients with refractory paroxysmal supraventricular tachycardia (deBuitleir and co-workers, 1991; Kalbfleisch and co-workers, 1992; Ikeda and co-workers, 1994; Weerasooriya and co-workers, 1994). When evaluating cost effectiveness, it is important to consider not only financial costs, but also success and complication rates, duration of hospitalization, quality of life, and time lost from work as a result of the various treatments. In a Japanese study by Ikeda and co-workers, the total ablation charge was approximately 14% of the total estimated charges of medical treatment that would be incurred throughout the patient's life. In the Australian study by Weerasooriya and co-workers, the total cost of medical treatment in 20 years has been estimated to be greater than that for catheter ablation. Although surgery was actually more effective than catheter ablation in terms of success rates, the estimated mean cost of surgery was approximately 4.5 times that of catheter ablation. Surgery also was associated with a higher complication rate and greater morbidity as reflected by the longer duration of hospitalization. deBuitlier and co-workers reported that RFA promotes cost containment because it represents a new application of an old technology. Interestingly, they noted with RFA that a curative procedure could be offered to a much broader spectrum of patients, including patients who would not otherwise have been considered suitable candidates for surgical ablation therapy because of a much higher prevalence of general medical diseases in an older population. In comparison with drug therapy, their figures indicated that RFA would pay for itself in less than 15 years.

Suggested Reading

Bardy GH, Ivey TD, Coltorti F, et al. Developments, complications, and limitations of catheter mediated electrical ablation of posterior accessory atrial ventricular pathways. Am J Cardiol 1988; 61:309.

Blanck Z, Dhala AA, Sra J, et al. Characterization of atrioventricular nodal behavior and ventricular response during atrial fibrillation before and after a selective slow pathway ablation. Circulation 1995; 91(4):1086–1094.

Bredikis JJ, Bredikis AJ. Surgery of tachyarrhythmia: Intracardiac closed heart cryoablation. PACE 1990; 13:1980.

Cain ME, Cox JL. Surgical treatment of supraventricular tachyarrhythmias. In: Platia EV, ed. Management of cardiac arrhythmias: The nonpharmacologic approach. Philadelphia: JB Lippincott, 1987.

Calkins H, Langberg J, Sousa J, et al. Radiofrequency catheter ablation of accessory atrioventricular connections in 250 patients. Abbreviated therapeutic approach to Wolff-Parkinson-White syndrome. Circulation 1992; 85:1337–1346.

Chen S-A, Chiang C-E, Tsang W-P, et al. Selective radiofrequency catheter ablation of fast and slow pathways in 100 patients with atrioventricular nodal reentrant tachycardia. Am Heart J 1993; 125:1–10.

Cox JL, Gallagher JJ, Cain ME. Experience with 118 consecutive patients undergoing operation for Wolff-Parkinson-White syndrome. J Thorac Cardiovasc Surg 1985; 90:490.

Cox JL, Holman WL, Cain ME. Cryosurgical treatment of atrioventricular node reentrant tachycardia. Circulation 1987; 76:1329.

deBuitlier M, Sousa J, Bolling SF, et al. Reduction in medical care cost associated with radiofrequency catheter ablation of accessory pathways. Am J Cardiol 1991; 68:1656–1661.

Della Bella P, Carbucicchio C, Tondo C, Riva S. Modulation of atrioventricular conduction by ablation of the "slow" atrioventricular node pathway in patients with drug-refractory atrial fibrillation or flutter. J Am Coll Cardiol 1995; 25(1):39–46.

Deshpande S, Jazayeri M, Dhala A, et al. Catheter ablation in supraventricular tachycardia. Ann Rev Med 1995; 46:413–430.

Evans GT Jr. The percutaneous cardiac mapping and ablation registry: Final summary and results. PACE 1988; 11:1621.

Feld GK, Fleck RP, Fujimura O, et al. Control of rapid ventricular response by radiofrequency catheter modification of the atrioventricular node in patients with medically refractory atrial fibrillation. Circulation 1994; 90(5):2299–2307.

Fenelon G, Andries E, Brugada P. Current trends in transcatheter treatment of cardiac arryhthmias. Indian Heart J 1994; 46(3):123–128.

Fischer B, Haissaguerre M, Garrigues S, et al. Radiofrequency catheter ablation of common atrial flutter in 80 patients. J Am Coll Cardiol 1995; 25(6):1365–1372.

Gallagher JJ, Sealy WC, Cox JL, Kasell JH. Results of surgery for preexcitation in 200 cases. Circulation 1981; 64:146 (abstract).

Geelen P, Andries E, Brugada P. New developments and treatment strategies in patients with supraventricular tachyarrhythmias. Acta Clin Belg 1995; 50(2):103–113.

Guiraudon GM, Klein GJ, Gulamhusein S, et al. Surgical repair of Wolff-Parkinson-White syndrome: A new closed heart technique. Ann Thorac Surg 1984; 37:67.

Guiraudon GM, Klein GJ, Sharma AD, et al. Closed-heart technique for Wolff-Parkinson-White syndrome: Further experience and potential limitations. Ann Thorac Surg 1986; 42:651.

Haines DE. Current and future modalities of catheter ablation for the treatment of cardiac arrhythmias. J Invas Cardiol 1992; 4:291.

Haissaguerre M, Gaita F, Fischer B, et al. Radiofrequency catheter ablation of left lateral accessory pathways via the coronary sinus. Circulation 1992; 86:1464.

Haissaguerre M, Saoudi N. Role of catheter ablation for supraventricular tachyarrhythmias, with emphasis on atrial flutter and atrial tachycardia. Am Opin Cardiol 1994; 9:40–52.

Huang SKS, Graham AR, Lee MA, et al. Comparison of catheter ablation using radiofrequency versus direct current energy: Biophysical, electrophysiologic and pathologic observations. J Am Coll Cardiol 1991; 18: 1091.

Ikeda T, Sugi K, Enjoji Y, et al. Cost effectiveness of radiofrequency catheter ablation versus medical treatment for paroxysmal supraventricular tachycardia in Japan. J Cardiol 1994; 24:461–468.

Jackman WM, Beckman KJ, McClelland JH, et al. Treatment of supraventricular tachycardia due to atrioventricular nodal reentry by radiofrequency catheter ablation of slow-pathway conduction. N Engl J Med 1992; 327:313–318.

Jackman WM, Wang X, Friday KJ, et al. Catheter ablation of accessory atrioventricular pathways (Wolff-Parkinson-White syndrome) by radiofrequency current. N Engl J Med 1991; 324:1605–1611.

Kalbfleisch SJ, Calkins H, Langberg JJ, et al. Comparison of the cost of radiofrequency catheter modification of the atrioventricular node reentrant tachycardia. J Am Coll Cardiol 1992; 19:1583–1587.

Kay GN, Epstein AE, Dailey SM, Plumb VJ. Role of radiofrequency ablation in the management of supraventricular arrhythmias: Experience in 760 consecutive patients. J Cardiovasc Electrophysiol 1993; 4:371–389.

Kou WH, Morady F. Radiofrequency catheter ablation in the treatment of cardiac arrhythmias. Adv Intern Med 195; 40:533–571.

Langberg JJ, Calkins H, El-Atassi R, et al. Temperature monitoring during radiofrequency catheter ablation of accessory pathways. Circulation 1992; 86:1469.

Langberg JJ, Kim YN, Goyal R, et al. Conversion of typical to atypical atrioventricular nodal reentrant tachycardia after radiofrequency catheter modification of the atrioventricular junction. Am J Cardiol 1992; 69:503–508.

Lesh MD, Van Hare GF, Schamp DJ, et al. Curative percutaneous catheter ablation using radiofrequency energy for accessory pathways in all locations: Results in 100 consecutive patients. J Am Coll Cardiol 1992; 19:1303–1309.

Manolis AS, Wang PJ, Estes III NAM. Radiofrequency ablation of slow pathway in patients with atrioventricular nodal reentrant tachycardia. Do arrhythmia recurrences correlate with persistent slow pathway conduction site of successful ablation? Circulation 1994; 90(6):2815–2819.

Manolis AS, Wang PJ, Estes III NAM. Radiofrequency catheter ablation for cardiac tachyarrhythmias. Ann Intern Med 1994; 121(6):452–461.

McGuire MA, Johnson DC, Nunn GR, et al. Surgical therapy for atrial tachycardia in adults. J Am Coll Cardiol 1989; 14:1777.

Philippon F, Plumb VK, Epstein AE, Kay GN. The risk of atrial fibrillation following radiofrequency catheter ablation of atrial flutter. Circulation 1995; 92(3):430–405.

Poty H, Saoudi N, Aziz AA, et al. Radiofrequency catheter ablation of type I atrial flutter. Prediction of late success by electrophysiological criteria. Circulation 1995; 92(6):1389–1392.

Prystowsky EN, Pressley JC, Gallagher JJ, et al. The quality of life and arrhythmia status after surgery for Wolff-Parkinson-White syndrome: An 18 year prospective. J Am Coll Cardiol 1987; 9:100A.

Ruder MA, Mead RH, Gaudiani V, et al. Transvenous catheter ablation of extra nodal accessory pathways. J Am Coll Cardiol 1988; 11:1245.

Scheinman M. Supraventricular tachyarrhythmias: drug therapy versus catheter ablation. Clin Cardiol 1994; 17(Suppl. II):II-11–II-15.

Steinberg JS, Prasher S, Zolonkofske S, Ehlert FA. Radiofrequency catheter ablation of atrial flutter: Procedural success and long-term outcome. Am Heart J 1995; 130(1):85–92.

Suwalski K, Pytkowski M, Zelazny P, et al. Surgery as an effective nonpharmacological mode of treatment of atrial fibrillation resistant to standard therapy PACE 1994; 17(11 Pt 2):2167–2171.

Swartz JF, Pellersels G, Silvers J, et al. A catheter-based curative approach to atrial fibrillation in humans. Circulation 1994; 90(Suppl I):I-225 (abstract).

Swartz JF, Tracy CM, Fletcher RD. Radiofrequency catheter ablation of accessory atrioventricular pathway atrial insertion sites. Circulation 1993; 87:487–499.

Tebbenjohanns J, Pfeiffer D, Schumacher B, et al. Slowing of the ventricular rate during atrial fibrillation by ablation of the slow pathway of AV nodal reentrant tachycardia. J Card Electrophys 1995; 6(9):711–715.

Touboul P, Saoudi N, Atalla H, Kirkorin G. Electrophysiological basis of catheter ablation in atrial flutter. Am J Cardiol 1989; 64:79J.

Weerasooriya HR, Murdock CJ, Harris AH, Davis MJE. The cost-effectiveness of treatment of supraventricular arrhythmias related to an accessory atrioventricular pathway: Comparison of catheter ablation, surgical division and medical treatment. Aust NZ J Med 1994; 24:161–167.

Williamson BD, Man KC, Daoud E, et al. Radiofrequency catheter modification of atrioventricular condition to control the ventricular rate during atrial fibrillation. N Engl J Med 1994; 331(14):910–917.

SURGICAL AND CATHETER ABLATIVE THERAPY OF VENTRICULAR ARRHYTHMIAS

Samuel J. DeMaio Jr., M.D.
Eric H. Stocker, M.D.

Patients with malignant ventricular arrhythmias and left ventricular dysfunction represent an especially high-risk group for sudden death. Ventricular arrhythmias may be treated by antiarrhythmic drugs, surgical ablation, percutaneous electrical ablation, the automatic implantable cardioverter defibrillator (ICD), and percoronary chemical ablation.

Conventional antiarrhythmic drug therapy for life-threatening ventricular arrhythmias successfully controls 20 to 50 percent of such patients. The remaining patients require further therapy to lessen the risk of sudden death, which approaches 20 percent at 1 year. The ICD has been shown to reduce the risk of sudden death at 1 year to 2 percent (Tchou and co-workers, 1988; Kelly and co-workers, 1988). Antitachycardia pacing also has been used to treat these arrhythmias; however, it has limited applicability in patients with ventricular tachycardia (VT) because of the possible induction of ventricular fibrillation. Newer devices are now available that combine features of the ICD and antitachycardia pacing. Neither antiarrhythmic drug therapy nor the ICD-antitachycardia pacing system offers a cure of the ventricular arrhythmia.

■ PREFERRED APPROACH

Surgical and catheter ablative therapies offer an opportunity for cure of these arrhythmias. Surgical therapy for ischemic ventricular tachyarrhythmias has been used for more than 10 years. Indirect approaches including left stellate ganglion ablation (except in patients with long QT syndrome), mitral valve replacement, isolated coronary vascularization, and aneurysmectomy have been disappointing in their ability to control ventricular arrhythmias, with a success rate of approximately 50 percent (Cox, 1989). Because we do not perform these procedures as a definitive therapy for ventricular arrhythmias, they are not discussed further.

Surgical or catheter ablative therapy is aimed at removing or destroying the arrhythmogenic substrate. In patients with ischemic heart disease, the substrate is believed to be located in the border zones between viable and necrotic myocardium.

Removal or ablation of this area has been shown to be effective in terminating the arrhythmia.

Surgical Treatment

Ideal candidates for direct surgical ablation include those patients with (1) a drug-refractory VT; (2) a discrete left ventricular aneurysm, preferably located in the anteroapical area with good function of the remaining myocardium; (3) arrhythmogenic foci origination from only one or two areas of ventricular myocardium; and (4) a stable ventricular rhythm that would allow preoperative endocardial mapping. The only absolute contraindication to surgery appears to be left ventricular dysfunction so severe that the operative risk is prohibitive. These patients may be candidates for the ICD, percutaneous catheter ablation, or cardiac transplantation. Additionally, patients with incessant VT should be treated surgically, not with an ICD.

Preoperative Evaluation

Preoperatively, patients should have cardiac angiography to determine the potential for myocardial ischemia and the need for revascularization. Evaluation of left ventricular function is important to determine the presence or absence of an aneurysm and the function of the remaining myocardium. If the arrhythmia is believed to be due to the ongoing ischemia, revascularization should be performed prior to electrophysiologic testing. This procedure may be accomplished by either percutaneous transluminal coronary angioplasty (PTCA) or coronary artery bypass grafting. If PTCA is performed, standard electrophysiologic testing should then be undertaken to evaluate the potential arrhythmogenic substrate. If the patient is not a candidate for PTCA and the coronary anatomy precludes preoperative electrophysiologic testing, such as in the case of critical left main stenosis, intraoperative electrophysiologic testing, surgical ablation, and coronary artery bypass grafting may be performed concomitantly.

In those patients who are candidates for electrophysiologic testing, left ventricular endocardial mapping is performed in an attempt to identify the number and origin of arrhythmogenic foci. Catheter mapping during tachycardia most consistently and precisely localizes the arrhythmogenic focus. However, it is possible preoperatively only if the tachyarrhythmia is hemodynamically stable. The site of the arrhythmogenic focus is determined by the site of earliest presystolic electrical activity in the latter half of diastole. This can localize the arrhythmogenic area to within 5 cm of the area determined by direct intraoperative endocardial mapping. Other techniques using activation mapping, attempts to entrain the arrhythmia, or attempts to find areas of latency also have been used with success to localize the arrhythmogenic focus.

Pace mapping, which attempts to localize the arrhythmogenic foci by reproducing the morphology of the tachycardia on a 12-lead electrogram, and catheter mapping during sinus rhythm, which looks for fractionated, high-frequency electrograms after the inscription of the QRS complex, have corroborative value but should not replace the aforementioned techniques.

Because a significant number of patients do not have their clinical arrhythmia induced intraoperatively, owing to the left ventriculotomy or the general anesthesia, it is important to obtain a preoperative endocardial map.

Direct Operative Procedures for Ischemic Ventricular Tachycardia

Surgical techniques in the treatment of ventricular arrhythmias include encircling endocardial resection, extended endocardial resection, and map-guided subendocardial resection. These procedures are performed alone or in combination and, most recently, with the adjunctive use of cryoablation. Each of these procedures is discussed here, with major attention to the technique of map-guided subendocardial resection with cryoablation because it is the procedure most commonly performed at our institution. However, with the advent of the newer antitachycardia pacing-ICD devices, much less surgical ablative therapy is currently performed.

Map-Guided Subendocardial Resection. Map-guided subendocardial resection is the surgical procedure performed at our institution when operative therapy of ventricular arrhythmias is warranted.

Technique. Normothermic cardiopulmonary bypass is initiated. Reference electrodes are sutured to the right and left ventricle for recording a reference electrogram and for ventricular stimulation. A left ventriculotomy is made through the aneurysm or area of scar. Tachycardia initiation is attempted to reproduce all clinical arrhythmias. Endocardial mapping with a hand-held probe or ring electrode in as many positions as possible (usually 48) is performed. A new computerized mapping system, now under investigation, incorporates multiple electrodes on a balloon that is inserted through the mitral valve from the left atrium, allowing simultaneous recordings and the avoidance of a ventriculotomy. This system allows for rapid intraoperative mapping and mapping of nonsustained ventricular tachyarrhythmias. If the tachycardia cannot be initiated intraoperatively, the preoperative map in conjunction with the intraoperative mapping during sinus rhythm is used to determine the area for resection. Once the arrhythmogenic foci are identified, the patient is cooled and cardioplegia is introduced. The subendocardium is undermined and resected. The area of resection usually encompasses 10 to 15 cm of tissue (Fig. 1).

Cryoablation is a valuable adjunctive tool in areas where endocardial resection is technically difficult to perform, such as through an inferior ventriculotomy, or in areas in which preservation of functional integrity is important, such as papillary muscles, near valve rings, or in the interventricular septum. Cryoablation destroys electrically active tissue while leaving major structural elements intact. It is performed by cooling a selected area of myocardium with a hand-held probe to −60°C for 2 minutes. It may be performed in multiple and overlapping locations.

Results. The operative mortality in patients undergoing map-directed subendocardial resection remains high (approximately 12 percent). It is significantly higher in patients undergoing emergent surgery, patients with left ventricular dysfunction, and patients undergoing surgery within 6 weeks of an acute myocardial infarction.

Postoperative recurrence of arrhythmias is significant (range 0 to 33 percent, average 23 percent; Cox, 1989); however, many of these patients may be controlled with antiarrhythmic medications, which were not previously ef-

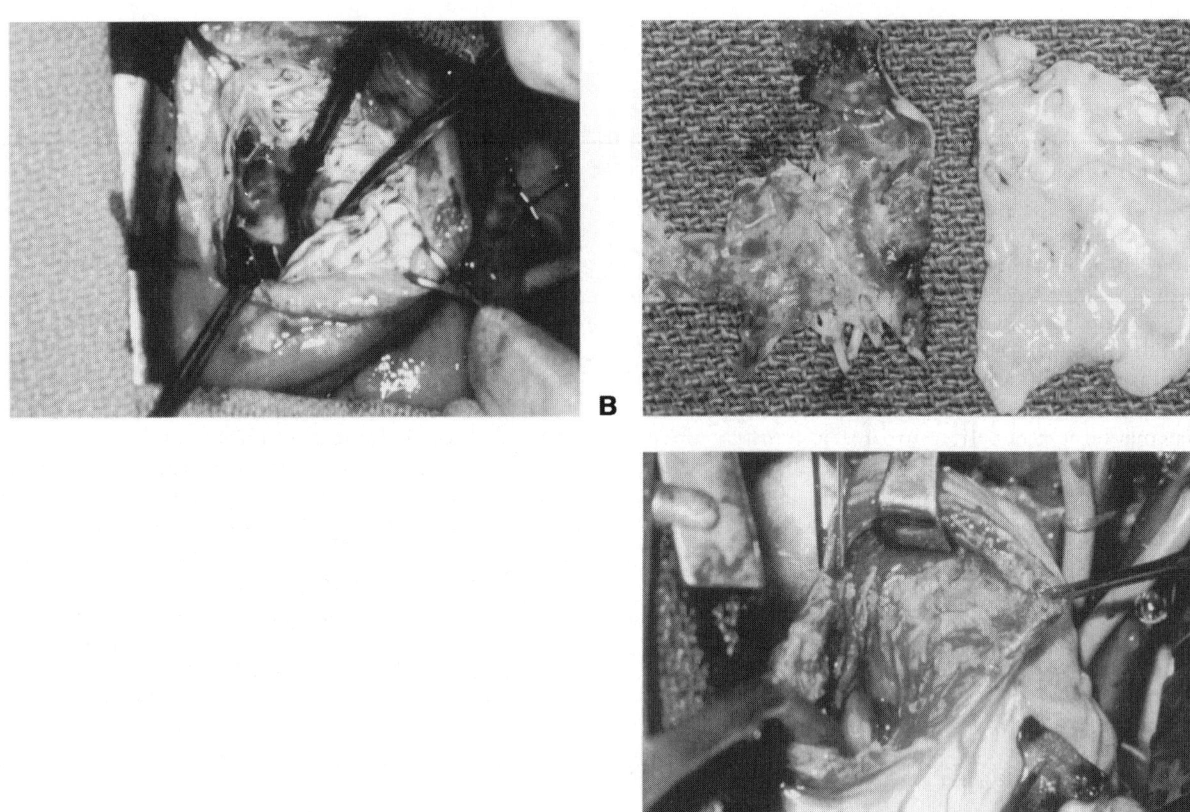

Figure 1
A, Exposure of the endocardium through the left ventricular aneurysm. *B,* The endocardial surface that has been resected. *C,* Left ventricular surface after the endocardial resection. *(Courtesy of Ellis L. Jones, M.D.)*

fective. Deterioration of left ventricular function, especially in those patients without a discrete left ventricular aneurysm, remains an important problem.

Encircling Endocardial Resection. Encircling endocardial resection has advantages over subendocardial resection in that no mapping techniques are required. The area of scar believed to contain the arrhythmogenic focus is isolated from the remaining ventricle by a ventriculotomy extending from the endocardium to the subpericardium. This condition results in a decreased blood flow to the encircled myocardium, with loss of both systolic contraction and diastolic compliance, leading to hemodynamic deterioration and a significant increase in congestive heart failure.

Extended Endocardial Resection. Extended endocardial resection suggests removal of all endocardial fibrosis. This procedure requires a more extensive operative procedure and longer cardiopulmonary bypass time than map-guided subendocardial resection. Because subendocardial fibrosis commonly involves the papillary muscles (10 to 20 percent), resection of the subendocardium in this area damages the papillary muscles to a degree requiring mitral valve replacement in approximately 13 percent of patients (Marchlinskin and Josephson, 1987). This procedure has advantages, however, in that it does not require preoperative or intraoperative mapping, therefore reducing the need for sophisticated equipment and personnel experienced in electrophysiology. The operative mortality and morbidity of this procedure are similar to those of map-guided subendocardial resection, and the incidence of arrhythmia recurrence may be just slightly greater.

Postoperative Evaluation

After postoperative recovery and prior to discharge from the hospital, all patients, regardless of the surgical procedure or the adequacy of intracardiac mapping, should undergo programmed electrical stimulation to evaluate the success of the procedure and to direct further therapy, if needed.

Operative Procedures in Patients Without Coronary Artery Disease

Surgery Following Repair of Tetralogy of Fallot. The VT in those patients undergoing repair of tetralogy of Fallot usually arises from the region of the healed right ventriculotomy site. Confirmation that this is the site of the arrhythmogenic focus is accomplished by preoperative and intraoperative mapping techniques. Once this confirmation is accomplished, the right ventricle is opened through the previous ventriculotomy site and the incision is widely excised and replaced by a pericardial patch. This technique has been shown to be useful in preventing recurrent ventricular tachyarrhythmias in these patients.

Arrhythmogenic Right Ventricular Dysplasia. Arrhythmogenic right ventricular dysplasia is a myopathy involving the right ventricle that is frequently associated with VT. The surgical procedure, as described by Guiraudon and co-workers (1983), involves the total disconnection of the right ventricular free wall from its left ventricular attachments. This procedure has been shown to control the ventricular arrhythmias in a small number of patients with this disorder.

Nonischemic Dilated Cardiomyopathy. Surgical reports have been limited in the treatment of this disorder. The substrate for the arrhythmogenesis in dilated cardiomyopathies may be very difficult to localize because it may arise in the endocardium, in the epicardium, or intramurally. Because of the diffuse nature of the disease, multiple areas of arrhythmogenisis may be present and require resection that can cause further deterioration of left ventricular function. Also, potential exists that following surgery other areas involved in the diffuse myopathic process may act as arrhythmogenic foci. Therefore, we do not recommend arrhythmia surgery in these patients, but we do recommend implantation of the ICD or, in those patients with severe left ventricular dysfunction or incessant ventricular arrhythmia, cardiac transplantation.

Catheter Ablation of Ventricular Arrhythmias

As discussed under Surgical Therapy, excision or destruction of normal myocardium is useful in the management of ventricular arrhythmias. Hartzler (1983) reported the first three cases of percutaneous electrical ablation of ventricular arrhythmias, thereby avoiding a surgical procedure.

Percutaneous catheter ablation utilizing either radiofrequency (RF) energy or direct current (DC) energy remains an experimental procedure. As such, its use should be limited to those patients with recurrent symptomatic VT who are unresponsive to antiarrhythmic drug therapy, who are not candidates for or refuse surgical therapy, and whose arrhythmia is too frequent for the ICD and are not pace-terminable with antitachycardia-ICD devices. The patients also must have an inducible, hemodynamically well-tolerated tachycardia to allow adequate endocardial mapping of the arrhythmogenic focus. Those patients with tachycardias of more than one morphology, and therefore more than one arrhythmogenic focus, are not good candidates for percutaneous endocardial ablation because of the technical difficulty in isolating more than one arrhythmogenic focus. This condition also would increase the risks of the procedure because it would necessitate multiple shocks in more than one area. In some instances, however, VT with different morphologies may use the same area of "slow" conduction, a portion of the arrhythmia circuit that is usually the vulnerable region for radiofrequency ablation (RFA).

Electrode catheter ablation has been the most frequently used technique in the treatment of malignant ventricular arrhythmias. Recently, RF ablation also has been shown to be more effective in patients with sustained monomorphic VT without structural heart disease and in bundle branch reentry VT. It also has been occasionally used in patients with VT caused by arrhythmogenic right ventricular dysplasia (discussed previously under Operative Procedures), and may be considered a useful option in patients who have one predominant tachycardia morphology that can be induced and is hemodynamically stable. Catheter ablation also has shown some success in the setting of structural heart disease, mainly in patients with coronary artery disease. Although it has been attempted in patients with dilated cardiomyopathy, long-term cure is still presumed unlikely and it is therefore not considered a viable option in these patients. Additionally, transcoronary delivery of ethanol has been shown to be very effective in the treatment of patients for whom surgery or the ICD is not appropriate.

Techniques of Endocardial Catheter Ablation

The most important determinant of a successful catheter ablation is precise localization of the arrhythmogenic focus. This procedure is performed by endocardial mapping techniques as described in the previous section. No single criterion has yet been found to be universally successful in predicting a successful site for VT ablation.

In the electrophysiology laboratory a standard quadripolar catheter (usually 5 or 6 Fr) is placed into the right ventricle for tachycardia initiation, right ventricular septal mapping, and backup bradycardiac pacing. A mapping catheter is then placed retrograde across the aortic valve for mapping the left ventricular endocardium. Heparin is given to lessen the risk of thrombus formation and embolization. Arterial pressure is monitored throughout the procedure by an indwelling arterial catheter. In the left ventricle, the distal endocardial electrode is placed at the site of the arrhythmogenic focus. If the arrhythmogenic focus is located on the left ventricular free wall, this electrode is connected to the cathodal output of a defibrillator, whereas the anodal output is connected to a patch on the anterior or posterior chest wall.

If the arrhythmogenic focus is located on the intraventricular septum, the left ventricular endocardial catheter is placed and connected to the cathodal output as described previously. The right ventricular catheter is then placed on the septum, directly across from the left ventricular catheter. The distal electrode of this catheter is then connected to the anodal output of the energy source.

Anesthesia is then induced with a short-acting barbiturate or etomidate, and a shock of 150 to 200 joules is delivered and repeated once. After the shocks are delivered, programmed electrical stimulation is performed to assess the success of the procedure. If the same tachycardia remains inducible, repeat mapping is done and catheter ablation is again attempted.

If DC energy is used, the patient should be observed in the coronary care unit for 24 hours to monitor the possible complications (see Complications). Because of the risks of malignant ventricular arrhythmias, the patient should have continuous electrocardiographic monitoring for 3 days. If the ablation procedure was successful, prior to discharge from the hospital the patient should undergo programmed electrical stimulation to assess inducibility of the arrhythmogenic substrate. This arrhythmogenic substrate may be the initial one on which ablation was attempted or a new one formed by the ablation procedure itself. If VT is not inducible, the patient is discharged without antiarrhythmic medications. If the tachycardia is inducible, pharmacologic testing is then performed.

When RF is the energy source, the current is again passed from the catheter tip to a skin patch electrode placed on the patient's chest wall with a voltage between 45 and 50 ws. Current applications should be effective by 30 seconds. A sudden rise in the impedance during ablation suggests formation of coagulum on the tip of the catheter, and the current should be immediately turned off, the catheter cleaned, and

Table 1 Catheter Ablation of VT: Results

	PCMAR NO. (%)	FONTAINE NO. (%)	KLEIN NO. (%)	STEVENSON NO. (%)	NAKAGAWA NO. (%)
No. of patients	164	43	51	15	8
Success (no VT/no antiarrhythmic drugs)	30 (18%)	22 (51%)	45 (88%)	6 (40%)	8 (100%)
Partial success (no VT/antiarrhythmic drugs)	67 (41%)	17 (39%)	5 (10%)	4 (27%)	0 (0%)
Unsuccessful (recurrent VT or death)	67 (41%)	4 (9%)	1 (2%)	5 (33%)	0 (0%)

From Evans GT, Scheinman MM, Zipes DP, et al. The percutaneous cardiac mapping and ablation registry: Final summary of results. PACE 1988; 11:1621. Fontaine G, Tonet JL, Frank R, Rougier I. Clinical experience with fulguration and antiarrhythmic therapy for the treatment of ventricular tachycardia. Chest 1989; 95:785. Klein LS, Miles WM. Ablative therapy for ventricular arrhythmias. Prog Cardiovasc Dis 1995; 37(4):225–242. Stevenson WG, Khan H, Sager P, et al. Identification of reentry circuit sites during catheter mapping and radiofrequency ablation of ventricular tachycardia late after myocardial infarction. Circulation 1993; 88(1):1647–1670. Nakagawa H, Beckman KJ, McClelland JH, et al. Radiofrequency catheter ablation of idiopathic left ventricular tachycardia guided by a Purkinje potential. Circulation 1993; 88:2607–2617; with permission.

ablation reattempted, if necessary. This problem has been reported to occur when the catheter tip's temperature reaches or exceeds 100°C. It may be prevented by monitoring the temperature of the electrode catheter tip using a thermistor or thermocouple embedded in the electrode. Good catheter tip tissue contact also may be verified using catheter tip temperature monitoring and also may aid the physician in titrating power delivery. Mild sedation is usually all that is necessary, because patients experience only a mild burning sensation at the time of energy delivery.

The use of RF energy to ablate VT has been associated with fewer complications and can be highly successful in selected patients as described. Immediately after the procedure, the patient is retested for inducible VT. If VT is no longer inducible, the patient should be monitored for 24 hours on a telemetry unit. The patient may be discharged to home on the second day after treatment without antiarrhythmic medication and is generally restudied only if clinically indicated.

Results

To evaluate the risks and benefits of percutaneous electrical ablation, the Percutaneous Cardiac Mapping and Ablation Registry (PCMAR) was formed in 1986 (Evans and co-workers, 1988). The registry has since reported on 164 patients who have undergone attempted electrical ablation of ventricular arrhythmias using DC shocks. The success rate, defined as no recurrent VT after electrical ablation, was 18 percent. Forty-one percent of patients had partial success, defined as the ablation plus antiarrhythmic drugs, which were previously unsuccessful. Another 41 percent of patients had an unsuccessful procedure, defined as recurrent VT, sudden death, or procedure-related death (Table 1). This low success rate was probably due to the small amount of myocardial damage that could be achieved with the electric shock or to generation of new arrhythmogenic foci.

Fontaine and co-workers (1989) have since reported on 43 consecutive patients undergoing catheter ablation for drug-refractory VT. After one ablative session, 13 patients (30 percent) had a successful procedure (see previous definitions). Eight patients (18 percent) had partial success, and 22 patients (52 percent) had an unsuccessful procedure. Those patients surviving the first procedure who had an unsuccessful response underwent up to three additional ablative sessions. After up to four procedures, the success rate was 49 percent and the partial success rate was 51 percent in the surviving patients.

Recent data regarding the use of RF energy to ablate VT have shown varying results depending on which type of VT the patient has and at which site the ablation is performed. Success rates of RFA for monomorphic VT in the absence of structural heart disease have been very encouraging, especially at the more common right ventricular outflow tract site. Klein and co-workers (1995) studied a total of 51 patients without evidence of coronary artery disease or right ventricular dysplasia, successfully treating 45 patients (88 percent) with RFA alone. The arrhythmia was eliminated in all of the patients whose arrhythmia was believed to arise from the right ventricular outflow tract (31 patients). Of the six patients who had a failed ablation, one received an implantable antitachycardia device and the other five were given antiarrhythmic medications. Nakagawa and co-workers (1993) reported a 100 percent success rate in a small study of eight patients without structural heart disease in whom the sites of successful ablation were all located at the posterior half of the left ventricular septum. Although similar success rates have been reported in the use of RFA for bundle branch block re-entrant tachycardias, results in patients with structural heart disease have not been as impressive. Stevenson and co-workers (1993) studied 15 patients with drug refractory VT late after myocardial infarction. Ten patients, four of whom required previously ineffective antiarrhythmic medications, did not suffer arrhythmia recurrences during a follow-up period of 10.5 ± 6.6 months.

Complications

Percutaneous electrical ablation is an alternative treatment of malignant ventricular arrhythmias that is associated with a significant number and frequency of complications. These complications include procedure-related deaths, acute pulmonary edema, cardiac tamponade, and new arrhythmias, including atrioventricular block and VT (Table 2). Because of these complications, this procedure should be considered experimental and a procedure of last resort. New techniques with the use of radiofrequency, cryoablation, and laser energy are now being studied with the hope of increasing procedural success and decreasing the procedure related complications.

The limited data published regarding the use of RF cath-

Table 2 Catheter Ablation of Ventricular Tachycardia: Follow-up

	PCMAR NO. (%)	FONTAINE NO. (%)	KLEIN NO. (%)	STEVENSON NO. (%)	NAKAGAWA NO. (%)
Follow-up, mo	12 ± 11	29 ± 12	20.2	10.5 ± 6.6	1 to 67
Early death, No.	11	5	0	2	0
Late death, No.	29	8	0	1	0
Cardiac tamponade, No.	2	0	0	0	0
Pulmonary edema, No.	3	3	0	0	0
Myocardial infarction, No.	1	1	0	0	0
Three atrioventricular blocks, No.	3	2	0	0	0
VT accelerated or ventricular fibrillation, No.	2	6	0	0	0
New morphology VT, No.	2	—	0	4	0
Pericardial effusion, No.	—	0	2	0	0
Torn chorda, No.	0	0	0	0	1

From Evans GT, Scheinman MM, Zipes DP, et al. The Percutaneous Cardiac Mapping and Ablation Registry: Final summary of results. PACE 1988; 11:1621. Fontaine G, Tonet JL, Frank R, Rougier I. Clinical experience with fulguration and antiarrhythmic therapy for the treatment of ventricular tachycardia. Chest 1989; 95:785. Klein LS, Miles WM. Ablative therapy for ventricular arrhythmias. Prog Cardiovasc Dis 1995; 37(4):225–242. Stevenson WG, Khan H, Sager P, et al. Identification of reentry circuit sites during catheter mapping and radiofrequency ablation of ventricular tachycardia late after myocardial infarction. Circulation 1993; 88(1):1647–1670. Nakagawa H, Beckman KJ, McClelland JH, et al. Radiofrequency catheter ablation of idiopathic left ventricular tachycardia guided by a Purkinje potential. Circulation 1993; 88:2607–2617.

eter ablation, however, appear favorable. In the study noted previously (Klein and co-workers, 1995), none of the patients experienced adverse side effects or complications as a result of their treatment, except for two patients who developed new pericardial effusions from right ventricle perforations, one of whom required catheter drainage. In fact, additional advantages to the use of RF energy include the lack of need for general anesthesia, better ability to control the delivered energy, and the apparent lack of hemodynamic embarrassment.

Animal studies comparing the effects of DC ablation versus RFA of coronary arrhythmias (Huang and co-workers, 1991) show that RFA resulted in smaller, more discrete lesions, decreased risk of ventricular dysfunction, fewer arrhythmias, and less damage to the ablation catheter. Randomized studies with larger populations of patients still need to be performed, however.

Bundle Branch Block Re-entrant Tachycardia

Macro re-entry within the His-Purkinje system, bundle branch block re-entry tachycardia, has been reported in up to 6 percent of patients who have had sustained monomorphic VT induced during electrophysiologic study. Patients with this type of VT usually have a dilated cardiomyopathy and a nonspecific interventricular conduction delay on the 12-lead electrocardiogram. During tachycardia, it may be recognized by a bundle branch block pattern (usually left) and from intracardiac electrograms by His activation preceding the onset of the QRS complex with the His-ventricular interval equal to or greater than that during the baseline rhythm. Conduction delay in the His-Purkinje system without complete block provides the substrate for bundle branch re-entry. Because the His-Purkinje system is integral to the maintenance of this ventricular arrhythmia, ablation of the right bundle, in a manner analogous to bundle of His ablation, has been shown to be effective and safe in terminating this arrhythmia. Identification of this rhythm is important because effective nonpharmacologic therapy is available.

Percoronary Chemical Ablation

Ventricular arrhythmias usually originate from islands of surviving myocardial cells in an area of prior infarction and scar; therefore, successful ablation of these surviving cells ought to terminate these arrhythmias. Because the arrhythmogenic focus is usually found in an area of previous myocardial infarction, that infarct-related artery provides a conduit through which ablation can be performed.

Technique

In the coronary angioplasty suite, the patient undergoes right and left ventricular endocardial mapping to identify the arrhythmogenic focus. Coronary arteriography is then performed to identify that coronary artery supplying the arrhythmogenic focus. That artery is selectively cannulated with a standard angioplasty guidewire and balloon. Temporary termination of the arrhythmia is then attempted with distal infusion of iced saline through the PTCA catheter. Iced saline infusion has been shown to change the electrophysiologic properties of the arrhythmogenic focus to allow temporary termination of the arrhythmia. If this "temporary chemical ablation" is successful, 2 ml of 99 percent ethanol may be infused distally through the PTCA catheter. Importantly, the angioplasty balloon should be inflated prior to distal instillation of ethanol to prevent backwash into more proximal coronary arteries and generalized cell death. Once the arrhythmia is terminated, the patient should be monitored in the coronary care unit for 24 hours and then undergo electrocardiography monitoring for an additional 5 days. Prior to discharge from the hospital, the patient should undergo electrophysiologic testing to evaluate the efficacy of the procedure.

Results

Brugada and co-workers (1989) reported the first three patients with incessant VT successfully treated with percoronary chemical ablation. All three patients have remained free of VT; however, one patient remains on medication that did not control the arrhythmia prior to the procedure. We have subsequently performed percoronary chemical ablation on one patient who presented in cardiogenic shock. He has remained free of arrhythmias on no antiarrhythmic medications after 5 months of follow-up.

Kay and co-workers (1992) have recently shown percoronary ethanol ablation to be moderately effective in select patients with incessant VT occurring after myocardial infarction. Of 10 patients given intracoronary injections of ethanol, 5 (50 percent) had long-term control of their tachycardia (mean follow-up period of 12 ± 17 months). Two patients redeveloped inducible VT 1 week after ablation.

Complications

The only reported complication of this procedure has been third-degree atrioventricular block in two patients. This complication was expected in both patients because the site of ablation was the His-Purkinje high on the intraventricular septum. Subsequently published events have included complete atrioventricular block in four of the 10 patients discussed previously (Kay and co-workers, 1992) and Dressler's syndrome developing in one of these patients who had to undergo three ablating sessions for permanent ablation of his tachyarrhythmia.

Suggested Reading

Brugada P, de Swart H, Smeets JL, Wellans HJ. Transcoronary chemical ablation of ventricular tachycardia. Circulation 1989; 79:475.

Cox JL. Patient selection criteria and results of surgery for refractory ischemic ventricular tachycardia. Circulation 1989; 79(Suppl I):163.

DeMaio SJ, Walter PF, Douglas JS. Treatment of tachycardia induced cardiogenic shock by percoronary chemical ablation. Cathet Cardiovasc Diag 1990; 21:170.

Evans GT, Scheinman MM, Zipes DP, et al. The percutaneous cardiac mapping and ablation registry: Final summary of results. PACE 1988; 11: 1621.

Fontaine G, Tonet JL, Frank R, Rougier I. Clinical experience with fulguration and antiarrhythmic therapy for the treatment of ventricular tachycardia. Chest 1989; 95:785.

Guiraudon G, Klein GJ, Gulamahusein SS, et al. Total disconnection of the right ventricular free wall: Surgical treatment of right ventricular tachycardia associated with right ventricular dysplasia. Circulation 1983; 67:463.

Hartzler GO. Electrode catheter ablation of refractory focal ventricular tachycardia. J Am Coll Cardiol 1983; 2:1107.

Huang SKS, Graham AR, Lee MA, et al. Comparison of catheter ablation using radiofrequency versus direct current energy: Biophysical, electrophysiologic and pathologic observations. J Am Coll Cardiol 1991; 18:1091.

Josephson ME, Harkin AH, Horowitz LN. Endocardial resection: A new surgical technique for the treatment of recurrent ventricular tachycardia. Circulation 1979; 60:1430.

Kay GN, Epstein AE, Bubein RS, et al. Intracoronary ethanol ablation for the treatment of recurrent sustained ventricular tachycardia. J Am Coll Cardiol 1992; 19:159.

Kelly PA, Canom DS, Garan H, et al. The automatic implantable cardioverter defibrillator: Efficacy, complications, and survival in patients with malignant ventricular arrhythmias. J Am Coll Cardiol 1988; 11: 1278.

Klein LS, Miles WM. Ablative therapy for ventricular arrhythmias. Prog Cardiovasc Dis 1995; 37(4):225–242.

Marchlinski FE, Josephson ME. Surgical treatment of ventricular tachyarrhythmias. In: Platia EV, ed. The management of cardiac arrhythmias: The nonpharmacologic approach. Philadelphia: JB Lippincott, 1987.

Miller JM, Kienzle MG, Harkin AH, Josephson ME. Subendocardial resection for ventricular tachycardia: Predictors of surgical success. Circulation 1984; 70:624.

Nakagawa H, Beckman KJ, McClelland JH, et al. Radiofrequency catheter ablation of idiopathic left ventricular tachycardia guided by a Purkinje potential. Circulation 1993; 88:2607–2617.

Newman D, Evans G, Scheinman MM. Catheter ablation of cardiac arrhythmias. Curr Prob Cardiol 1989; 14(3):117.

Stevenson WG, Khan H, Sager P, et al. Identification of reentry circuit sites during catheter mapping and radiofrequency ablation of ventricular tachycardia late after myocardial infarction. Circulation 1993; 88(1):1647–1670.

Tchou PJ, Kadri N, Anderson J, et al. Automatic implantable cardioverter defibrillators in survival of patients with left ventricular dysfunction. Ann Intern Med 1988; 109:529.

PACEMAKERS: INDICATION AND SELECTION

Steven P. Kutalek, M.D.

Permanent cardiac pacemakers provide chronotropic support for patients with symptomatic bradyarrhythmias or atrioventricular (AV) conduction disorders; newer devices are also useful for termination of sustained re-entrant tachyarrhythmias. Selection of an appropriate device and pacing mode is based on an understanding of the underlying rhythm disorder and available technology.

■ THERAPEUTIC ALTERNATIVES

Not all acquired bradyarrhythmias require permanent pacing. Some transient rhythm disorders result from conditions that respond to medical therapy, occasionally with the need for temporary pacing support. Reversible suppression of cardiac impulse generation or conduction may occur with drugs, electrolyte imbalance, infection, endocrine disorders, acute myocardial infarction, or the cardiac postoperative state. Such disorders are approached with attention to the precipitating cause, with appropriately directed medical therapy. Temporary pacing proves useful when vagolytic agents or adrenergic stimulants fail to reverse pathologic bradycardia. Permanent pacing is indicated if the cardiac rhythm disorder does not improve following resolution of the transient event.

■ PATIENT SELECTION

Permanent pacemakers are required in patients with irreversible symptomatic bradyarrhythmias and in those in whom asymptomatic bradyarrhythmias can reliably be predicted to worsen to produce symptoms. Such rhythm disorders may be fixed or intermittent. Symptomatic bradyarrhythmias lead to light-headedness, syncope, profound weakness, exacerbation of heart failure, exercise intolerance, or confusional states that clear with pacing.

Antitachyarrhythmia pacemakers are indicated for patients with symptomatic, recurrent supraventricular or ventricular tachyarrhythmias that cannot be controlled medically or by ablation. Ventricular antitachycardia pacemakers are incorporated in implantable defibrillators and should not be used without defibrillator support.

■ PREFERRED APPROACH

Antibradyarrhythmia Pacing (Table 1)

Symptomatic sick sinus syndrome requires permanent pacing. Symptoms are the result of profound sinus bradycardia, sinus arrest, sinus exit block, chronotropic incompetence, or the bradycardia-tachycardia syndrome, especially when drug therapy of supraventricular tachyarrhythmias exacerbates sinus node dysfunction. Association of symptoms with significant bradyarrhythmia (heart rate less than 40 beats per minute or sinus pauses more than 3 seconds) must be documented through ambulatory monitoring or transtelephonic electrocardiography. Patients with less severe sinus node dysfunction require permanent pacing if cerebrovascular insufficiency leads to symptomatic central nervous system hypoperfusion during bradyarrhythmia. Indications for pacing in patients with syncope and less severe sinus node dysfunction (i.e., heart rates more than 40 beats per minute or sinus pauses less than 3 seconds) are unclear when association of symptoms with bradyarrhythmias has not been documented. Rate-responsive dual chamber pacing may be indicated for symptomatic chronotropic incompetence (i.e., inability to adequately increase heart rate during exercise), occasionally in cardiac transplantation patients because of loss of normal sympathetic nervous control of cardiac rate. Electrophysiologic testing may unmask disordered sinus node function, but the accuracy of such testing to detect and quantify sinus node abnormalities is somewhat limited. Patients with syncope in whom other causes have been excluded who demonstrate pronounced sinus bradycardia within 30 minutes of 80 degree head upright tilting (positive tilt test), with or without intravenously administered isoproterenol, may require permanent pacing if medical therapy is ineffective. Medications may, however, obviate the need for pacing.

Pacing is indicated in patients with acquired complete heart block with symptomatic slow ventricular escape rates of less than 40 beats per minute, when unassociated with acute myocardial infarction and when postoperative, if persistent for more than 5 days after cardiac surgery. Patients with acquired complete heart block and syncope have an improved prognosis with permanent pacing. Congenital complete heart block with a narrow QRS escape rhythm that does not provide an adequate rate at rest or during exercise also requires permanent pacing, although the majority of such patients maintain adequate junctional rates during activity.

Table 1 Indications for Antibradyarrhythmia Pacing*

Symptomatic sick sinus syndrome
Acquired complete heart block
Symptomatic congenital heart block
Type II second-degree atrioventricular block (intra-His or infra-His)
Symptomatic type I second-degree atrioventricular block
Symptomatic carotid sinus hypersensitivity† (>3 second pause)
Positive tilt test†

*This list assumes that reversible etiologies have been excluded. These disorders may occur spontaneously or as the result of requisite drug therapy.
†With a history of symptoms that can be attributed to bradyarrhythmia.

Permanent pacing is indicated in patients with type II second-degree AV block owing to intra-His or infra-His conduction abnormalities, most commonly associated with a wide QRS complex. Delineation of the site of block and differentiation from supra-His conduction delay may require electrophysiologic testing. Symptomatic type 1 second-degree AV block, unassociated with drug therapy that retards AV conduction, also requires pacing. Likewise, patients who develop AV conduction disorders on requisite drug therapy require bradycardic support. There is no indication for pacing in patients with isolated first-degree AV block or in patients with asymptomatic, hemodynamically stable type I second-degree AV block, although preliminary data suggest that optimizing the AV interval in patients with decreased left ventricular compliance or congestive heart failure may significantly improve cardiac output and hemodynamics, particularly in those with prolonged intrinsic PR intervals.

Following acute myocardial infarction, patients with persistent complete heart block or type II second-degree AV block require permanent pacing. Pacing at rates above the intrinsic sinus rate in patients with congenitally prolonged Q-T intervals shortens ventricular repolarization. This reduces dispersion of refractoriness and decreases the incidence of life-threatening ventricular arrhythmias when combined with beta-adrenergic blocking medical therapy. Since transient AV block after anterior infarction may recur, such patients may be best served by pacing, since this condition indicates that a large part of the conduction system has been damaged. In those with transient AV block or new bifascicular conduction disorders, electrophysiologic testing defines the degree of residual dysfunction of intra-His and infra-His conduction structures. The approach is similar for patients who develop conduction disorders after cardiac surgery is performed in the His bundle area (e.g., mitral or aortic valve replacement). Spontaneous resolution of acquired AV conduction disorders may occur more than 5 to 7 days after myocardial infarction or cardiac surgery; in patients who have late recovery of conduction, electrophysiologic testing is recommended.

Table 2 Indications for Antitachyarrhythmia Overdrive Pacing*†

Supraventricular Arrhythmia‡
Atrial flutter
Intra-atrial re-entry
Atrioventricular nodal re-entry (typical or atypical)
Atrioventricular reciprocating bypass tract re-entry
Ventricular Arrhythmia§
Sustained monomorphic ventricular tachycardia

*Selection of overdrive modes and determination of efficacy require electrophysiologic testing.
†Atrial fibrillation, supraventricular re-entrant arrhythmias, atrial premature complexes, ventricular premature complexes, and torsades de pointes owing to a prolonged Q-T interval may be suppressed in some patients with antibradyarrhythmia pacing.
‡These arrhythmias may be amenable to catheter ablation.
§Requires combined unit with antitachycardia pacing and defibrillator capability.

Patients with syncope or recurrent near syncope owing to carotid sinus hypersensitivity benefit from permanent pacing. These individuals demonstrate symptomatic sinus pauses or AV block in response to carotid sinus pressure. Because this syndrome frequently is associated with a concomitant vasodepressor response (i.e., hypotension), AV sequential pacing is recommended to maximize cardiac output and blood pressure during symptomatic events. Hemodynamic improvement may be demonstrated with temporary AV sequential pacing in the electrophysiology laboratory.

Antitachyarrhythmia Pacing (Table 2)

Paroxysmal re-entrant tachyarrhythmias not responsive to drug therapy, or those that recur in patients intolerant to medication, may be alleviated through permanent pacing. Maintaining AV synchrony and performing atrial pacing, possible with atrial demand or dual-chamber *antibradyarrhythmia* pacemakers, may decrease the incidence of paroxysmal atrial fibrillation when compared with pacing through single-chamber ventricular devices, reducing associated morbidity. AV sequential pacing may also suppress intra-atrial or AV nodal re-entrant tachyarrhythmias in selected individuals. Other re-entrant arrhythmias can be terminated by programmed stimulation delivered through *antitachyarrhythmia* pacemakers. Supraventricular tachyarrhythmias amenable to pace termination include intra-atrial re-entry, atrial flutter, AV nodal re-entry, and AV reciprocating bypass tract tachycardia. Other re-entrant arrhythmias can be terminated, although these arrhythmias can now also be approached through catheter ablation. Sustained monomorphic ventricular tachycardia may also be terminated by overdrive pacing in most patients. Evaluation of antitachyarrhythmia pacing modes requires extensive electrophysiologic testing to determine the safety and efficacy of various termination algorithms and the effects of concomitant antiarrhythmic medications. The primary risk of overdrive pacing is acceleration of the tachyarrhythmia, which may be life threatening in patients with ventricular overdrive devices. An implanted defibrillator antitachycardia pacemaker system protects an individual from overdrive acceleration, which may result from automatic ventricular antitachyarrhythmia pacing.

■ DEVICE SELECTION

Single Chamber Pacemakers

Specific indications for single chamber ventricular demand (VVI) pacemakers (Table 3) include atrial fibrillation with slow ventricular response, intermittent AV block owing to His-Purkinje dysfunction or symptomatic AV nodal disease, or rarely, intermittent sinus node dysfunction in which infrequent ventricular pacing will not lead to the pacemaker syndrome. Rate-responsive ventricular (VVIR) units are particularly useful in patients who require frequent ventricular pacing and who are not dependent upon AV synchrony (e.g., chronic atrial fibrillation).

Frequent single chamber ventricular pacing during sinus rhythm can produce the pacemaker syndrome, the result of AV dyssynchrony or intact ventriculoatrial (VA) conduction with retrograde atrial activation. The pacemaker syndrome may lead to palpitations, neck vein pulsations, fatigue, exacerbation of congestive heart failure, light-headedness, or syncope. Significant symptoms that cannot be alleviated by decreasing the ventricular essentially converts the pacing mode to VVI(R) during atrial tachyarrhythmias, avoiding unnecessarily high ventricular tracking rates. This mode is inappropriate for patients with AV block and intact sinus node function who require tracking of atrial impulses at increased rates. Other algorithms for upper rate response have been developed that allow implantation of dual chamber pacemakers in patients with paroxysmal atrial tachyarrhythmias.

Pacing Leads

Concomitant with technologic advances that have led to a decrease in generator size and increased battery longevity, improvements in pacemaker leads safely allow programming output to lower voltages to maximize battery life. Active fixation, screw-in leads are appropriate for patients with large, dilated, nontrabeculated right-sided chambers or in cardiac postoperative patients with absent right atrial appendages. Passive fixation leads (tined or finned) may be used in individuals with trabeculated right ventricles and atria. These have the advantage of smaller diameter and lower chronic sensing and pacing thresholds when compared with active fixation leads. Steroid-eluting leads further improve long-term functional characteristics by decreasing fibrotic changes around the lead tip.

Both active and passive fixation leads are available in unipolar or bipolar forms. Bipolar leads are generally preferred, having the advantage of pacing a localized area of endocardium and sensing only local intracardiac electrograms. Thus, myoinhibition is avoided, and the leads can be used safely when pacemakers are required in conjunction with implanted defibrillators. Bipolar leads have a larger cross-sectional area and are somewhat stiffer than unipolar leads. Unipolar leads may be manipulated more safely in older patients with thin myocardial walls.

■ PACING COMPLICATIONS

Beyond surgical risks associated with implanting a device through subclavian access, pacemakers carry unique risks.

Lead dislodgement may occur with atrial or ventricular leads, especially passive fixation leads.

Endless loop tachycardias (pacemaker-mediated tachycardias) may develop in dual chamber systems in patients with intact VA conduction, initiated by spontaneous atrial or ventricular ectopy. In this situation, retrograde (VA) atrial activity is sensed, followed by anterograde pacemaker "conduction" to the ventricle; this leads to another retrograde atrial activation through the patient's native conduction system, establishing an endless loop. Terminating these tachyarrhythmias acutely involves magnet application over the pacemaker to establish fixed-rate pacing, followed by chronically reprogramming the postventricular atrial refractory period (PVARP) to a longer interval to avoid sensing retrograde atrial activity. Alternatively, shortening the AV delay may prevent recurrence. Some dual chamber devices incorporate automatic endless loop tachycardia termination algorithms with automatic AV delay and/or PVARP reprogramming.

Although abrupt generator malfunction is rare, the complexity of pacing systems demands careful follow-up to ensure appropriate pacing and sensing margins above threshold while maintaining output at a low enough level to maximize battery life. Loss of ventricular capture can lead to symptomatic bradyarrhythmia, whereas loss of atrial capture in dual chamber systems can produce the pacemaker syndrome. Intermittent sensing or pacing malfunction in either chamber can initiate tachyarrhythmias if impulses occur while the myocardium is partially refractory.

To ensure appropriate pacing and sensing functions, thresholds should be evaluated at 1 and 3 months after implantation, with programming of chronic values at 3 months. Semiannual threshold checks for dual chamber systems (annual for single chamber pacemakers) ensure appropriate programming, whereas monthly or bimonthly transtelephonic evaluations provide screening for generator end-of-life indicators and continued normal pacemaker function.

Suggested Reading

Ausubel K, Furman S. The pacemaker syndrome. Ann Intern Med 1985; 103:420.

Dreifus LS, Fisch C, Griffin JC, et al. Guidelines for implantation of cardiac pacemakers and antiarrhythmia devices: A report of the American College of Cardiology/American Heart Association Task Force on Assessment of Diagnostic and Therapeutic Cardiovascular Procedures (Committee on Pacemaker Implantation). J Am Coll Cardiol 1991; 18:1.

Frye RL, Collins JJ, DeSanctis RW, et al. Guidelines for permanent cardiac pacemaker implantation, May 1984. J Am Coll Cardiol 1984; 4:434.

Furman S, Schwedel JB. An intracardiac pacemaker for Stokes-Adams seizures. N Engl J Med 1959; 26:943.

Humen DP, Kostuk WJ, Klein GJ. Activity-sensing, rate-responsive pacing: Improvement in myocardial performance with exercise. PACE 1985; 8:52.

Levine PA. Physiological pacing 1988: A comparison of single- and dual-chamber pacing systems with rate adaptive single- and dual-chamber pacing systems. J Electrophys 1989; 3:167.

Rosenqvist M, Brandt J, Schuller H. Long-term pacing in sinus node disease: Effects of stimulation mode on cardiovascular morbidity and mortality. Am Heart J 1988; 116:16.

CHRONIC CONGESTIVE HEART FAILURE

Kanu Chatterjee, M.B., F.R.C.P., F.A.C.C., F.C.C.P., M.A.C.P.

Chronic congestive heart failure, a common clinical syndrome, results from various etiologies, including valvular heart disease, hypertension, ischemic heart disease, and primary myocardial and pericardial diseases. The presenting symptoms, such as dyspnea, fatigue, and edema, and the hemodynamic abnormalities, such as systemic and pulmonary venous hypertension and decreased cardiac output, may be similar, regardless of the etiology of chronic congestive heart failure. During the initial evaluation, it is imperative to exclude primary valvular disorders and pericardial diseases as the potential cause for chronic heart failure. Myocardial dysfunction, however, is the most frequent cause of chronic congestive heart failure, and assessment of myocardial function is necessary before a rational therapeutic approach is considered.

Both abnormal ventricular systolic and diastolic function can be the predominant mechanism of the hemodynamic abnormalities and symptoms of heart failure. Impaired systolic function, the most frequent cause of chronic heart failure, is recognized by the presence of reduced (40 percent or less) left ventricular ejection fraction, which can be assessed noninvasively by echocardiography or radionuclide ventriculography or invasively by contrast ventriculography. In ischemic or idiopathic dilated cardiomyopathy, ventricular end-systolic and end-diastolic volumes are also increased, and there is only a slight to modest increase in left ventricular wall thickness. Once dilated cardiomyopathy is diagnosed, it is desirable to investigate the presence of myocardial ischemia due to obstructive coronary artery disease (exercise testing or dipyridamole thallium scintigraphy). Pharmacologic therapy, nonpharmacologic therapy, or both for the relief of ischemia may be necessary and of benefit, in addition to antifailure treatment, for optimal management of such patients. If left ventricular ejection fraction is normal, abnormal diastolic function due to hypertrophic cardiomyopathy, hypertensive heart disease, or restrictive cardiomyopathy should be suspected as the cause of chronic heart failure, and appropriate investigations are required to establish the diagnosis. Because impaired systolic function is

Table 1 Therapeutic Options in Chronic Heart Failure

Pharmacotherapy
Diuretics
Digitalis
Vasodilators
Beta-adrenergic antagonists
New inotropic drugs
Antiarrhythmic drugs
Cytotoxic drugs
Surgical Therapy
Cardiac transplantation
Cardiomyoplasty
Coronary artery bypass surgery
Artificial heart

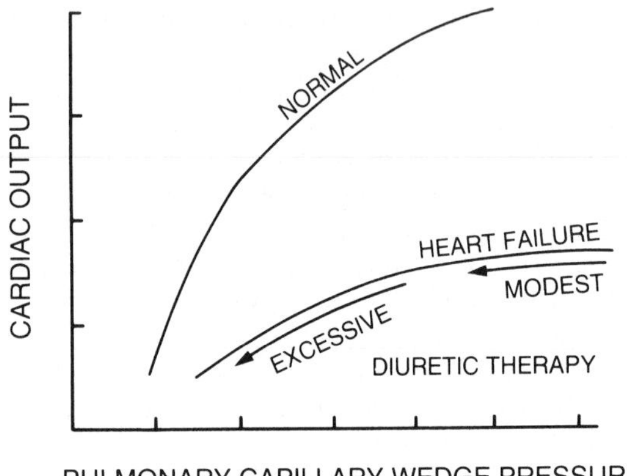

Figure 1
Diuretic therapy in chronic heart failure and expected changes in systemic hemodynamics. During diuretic therapy, with a modest reduction in pulmonary capillary wedge pressure, there is little or no decrease in cardiac output; with excessive reduction in pulmonary capillary wedge pressure, however, cardiac output will fall.

the principal cause of chronic heart failure in the majority of patients with this syndrome, therapy for chronic heart failure resulting from depressed systolic function, as in patients with dilated cardiomyopathy, is emphasized.

The objectives of pharmacotherapy in chronic heart failure are to relieve symptoms, to improve cardiac performance and exercise tolerance, and, if possible, to achieve a better prognosis. During the last two decades, several therapeutic options have been explored to achieve these goals (Table 1). Based on the results of many investigations, it is now possible to adapt a rational therapeutic approach for the management of patients with chronic congestive heart failure.

■ PREFERRED APPROACH

Medical Treatment

Diuretics

Diuretics, in general, are effective in relieving congestive symptoms and improving exercise tolerance. They decrease pulmonary and systemic venous pressures, principally by decreasing intracardiac volumes resulting from diuresis and decreased intravascular volume. Diuretics, however, do not usually increase cardiac output or improve ventricular performance. In patients with heart failure, ventricular function curve shifts downward and to the right compared with that in patients with normal ventricular function (Fig. 1). Most patients with chronic heart failure and congestive symptoms have elevated systemic and pulmonary venous pressures and lie on the flat portion of the ventricular function curve. A modest reduction of ventricular preload in these patients is associated with little or no decrease in cardiac output, although systemic venous and pulmonary capillary wedge pressures are likely to decrease. With excessive diuretic therapy, cardiac output may decrease as a result of a marked decrease in ventricular preload. Hypotension and impaired renal function may also result. Furthermore, aggressive diuretic therapy alone may activate renin-angiotensin-aldosterone and adrenergic systems, which may produce adverse effects on cardiac and renal function. *Thus, diuretic therapy alone is not recommended for treatment of chronic heart failure, and diuretics should be used in conjunction with other drugs that have the potential to increase cardiac output.*

As a guide to diuretic therapy, monitoring of renal function is helpful, and the doses of the diuretics should be reduced when there is a significant increase in blood urea nitrogen (BUN) and creatinine levels. For patients with severe resistant heart failure, with markedly elevated systemic venous pressures and peripheral edema, a combination of diuretics (e.g., furosemide and metolazone) is frequently employed. Intravenous diuretic therapy may be more effective than oral therapy in these patients. It should be emphasized, however, that concomitant vasodilator therapy, inotropic therapy, or both should always be considered to maintain adequate cardiac output.

Digitalis

The role of maintenance digitalis therapy in the management of patients with chronic heart failure in sinus rhythm remains somewhat controversial, although many recent studies have demonstrated its usefulness in improving clinical status and left ventricular function. Withdrawal of digoxin therapy is associated with an increase in pulmonary capillary wedge pressure and a decrease in left ventricular stroke work index, indicating a deterioration of left ventricular function; reinstitution of digoxin therapy increases stroke work index and decreases pulmonary capillary wedge pressure. In prospective, randomized multicenter clinical trials, when digoxin was withdrawn from the treatment regimen of digoxin, diuretics, and angiotensin converting enzyme inhibitors, symptomatic status deteriorated, with decreased exercise tolerance; the frequency of hospitalization for treatment of heart failure increased, despite continued therapy with angiotensin converting enzyme inhibitors. Left ventricular function also deteriorated after withdrawal of digoxin therapy. Compared with placebo, long-term digitalis therapy results in clinical improvement in patients with heart failure with depressed ejection fraction and S3 gallop. In patients with mild to moderate heart failure, digoxin has more potential than captopril to increase left ventricular ejection fraction, although the improvement in exercise tolerance with digoxin is less than that with captopril. In patients with more severe heart failure (New York Heart Association [NYHA] class III and IV), the magnitude of increase in exercise tolerance with digoxin is comparable to that with milrinone, a peak III phosphodiesterase inhibitor. In patients with very mild heart failure, digoxin is less effective than xamoterol, a partial $beta_1$-adrenergic agonist, in improving exercise tolerance. *Thus, except in patients with no or minimal symptoms, digoxin therapy is indicated, provided that impaired left ventricular systolic function is the principal mechanism for heart failure.*

Digoxin is also indicated to control ventricular response in the presence of atrial fibrillation complicating chronic heart failure. Digoxin should be avoided in patients with severe renal failure because of the propensity to develop toxicity. Digoxin is also contraindicated in patients with sinoatrial or atrioventricular nodal disease because it may induce unacceptable bradycardia. The prognosis of patients with chronic heart failure treated conventionally with digitalis and diuretics alone has been determined by prospective, controlled studies. In patients with mild to moderately severe heart failure, 1 year mortality is approximately 20 percent; in patients with more severe heart failure, mortality is approximately 50 percent. The addition of certain vasodilators or angiotensin converting enzyme inhibitors has been shown to improve the prognosis of such patients. *Thus, combination therapy with vasodilators or angiotensin converting enzyme inhibitors and digitalis and diuretics (triple therapy) should always be considered until specific contraindications exist, and such therapy is tolerated without adverse effects.*

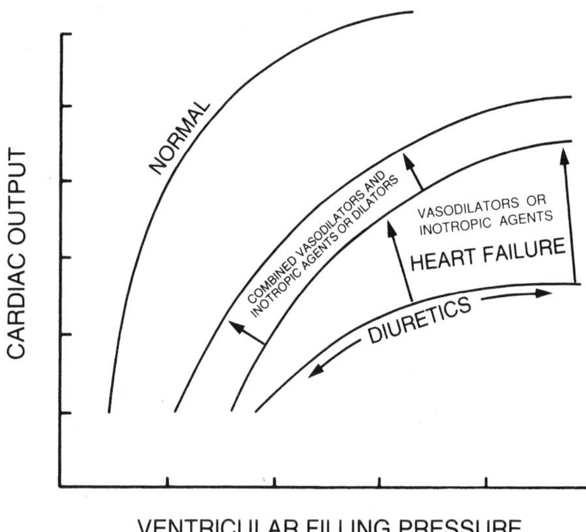

Figure 2
Effects of diuretics, vasodilators, inotropic agents, and combined vasodilators and inotropic agents on the ventricular function curve. Ventricular function curves are constructed by relating changes in cardiac output to changes in ventricular filling pressure. Compared with normal, in heart failure, the ventricular function curve is shifted downward. With diuretics, there is no shift in ventricular function curve. With vasodilator or inotropic agents, the ventricular function curve moves toward normal; cardiac output increases with a fall in ventricular filling pressures. With combined vasodilator and inotropic therapy, there is further upward and leftward shift of ventricular function curve, with a further increase in cardiac output and decrease in ventricular filling pressure.

Vasodilators and Angiotensin Converting Enzyme Inhibitors

The rationale for the use of vasodilators is to reduce afterload and preload and thereby improve cardiac performance (Fig. 2). A large number of vasodilators with different mechanisms of action have been evaluated for the management of chronic heart failure. The systemic hemodynamic effects of some of the commonly used vasodilator agents and their mechanisms of action are summarized in Table 2. The systemic hemodynamic effects of vasodilators are determined primarily by their principal site of action on the peripheral vascular bed. Drugs with predominantly arterial dilating effects, such as hydralazine and calcium entry blocking agents, increase cardiac output by decreasing systemic vascular resistance and may not cause any significant decrease in systemic and pulmonary venous pressures. Predominant venodilators, such as nitrates and nitroglycerin, decrease systemic and pulmonary venous pressures with little or no increase in cardiac output. With the combination of an arterial dilator and a venodilator, a significant increase in cardiac output and a decrease in systemic and pulmonary venous pressures are expected. Drugs with both arterial and venodilating properties, such as angiotensin converting enzyme inhibitors and alpha-adrenergic blocking drugs, produce similar hemodynamic effects. It is emphasized that there is no correlation between improvement in systemic hemodynamics and long-term clinical response and outcome.

Although systemic hemodynamic effects of various vasodilators are qualitatively similar, their effects on regional hemodynamics may differ. Angiotensin converting enzyme inhibitors and nitrates decrease myocardial oxygen consumption, whereas hydralazine and prazosin may increase oxygen consumption. Dihydropyridine, a class of calcium-entry blocking agents, may increase coronary blood flow due to primary coronary vasodilation. Renal function tends to improve with hydralazine and angiotensin converting enzyme inhibitors and remains unchanged with nitrates and prazosin. Long-term efficacy in maintaining improved clinical status and exercise tolerance has not been demonstrated with all vasodilators. In general, angiotensin converting enzyme inhibitors and nitrates have been shown to cause sustained improvement in exercise tolerance; hydralazine, prazosin, and calcium channel blocking agents usually do not cause sustained improvement in clinical status or exercise tolerance. Improved prognosis of patients with chronic heart failure has been documented only with the use of certain vasodilators. Combined hydralazine and nitrate therapy, in addition to digitalis and diuretics, decreases mortality significantly in patients with mild to moderately severe chronic heart failure. The angiotensin converting enzyme inhibitors captopril and enalapril decrease mortality not only in patients with mild to moderately severe heart failure but also in patients with severe chronic heart failure (NYHA class IV). *Thus, the addition of hydralazine, isosorbide dinitrate, or angiotensin converting en-*

Table 2 Expected Hemodynamic Effects of Vasodilators in Chronic Heart Failure

AGENTS	PRINCIPAL MECHANISM OF ACTION	PRINCIPAL SITES OF ACTION ON PERIPHERAL VASCULAR BED	CARDIAC OUTPUT	PULMONARY CAPILLARY WEDGE PRESSURE	SYSTEMIC VENOUS PRESSURE	MEAN BLOOD PRESSURE	HEART RATE
Hydralazine	Direct acting	Arterial	Increase	No change or slight decrease	No change or slight increase	No change or decrease	No change or decrease
Nitrates and nitroglycerin	Direct acting	Venous	No change or slight increase	Decrease	Decrease	No change or decrease	No change or increase
Angiotensin converting enzyme inhibitors*	Angiotensin II inhibition	Arterial and venous	Increase	Decrease	Decrease	Decrease	Decrease or no change
Alpha-adrenergic antagonists†	Alpha-receptor blockade	Arterial and venous	Increase	Decrease	Decrease	Decrease	No change or decrease
Calcium channel blocking agents‡	Calcium antagonism	Arterial	Increase or no change	No change or decrease	No change or decrease	Decrease or no change	Increase or no change

*Captopril, enalapril, lisinopril.
†Prazosin, trimazosin, terazosin.
‡Nifedipine, nicardipine, diltiazem.

zyme inhibitors should be considered in all symptomatic patients with chronic heart failure regardless of its severity—mild, moderate, or severe.

Angiotensin converting enzyme inhibitors are preferred over hydralazine-nitrates for a number of reasons. The potential benefits of angiotensin converting enzyme inhibitors are (1) consistent decrease in myocardial oxygen consumption; (2) reduction of aldosterone levels; (3) decrease in norepinephrine levels; (4) increase in prostaglandins and bradykinins; (5) improved renal function; (6) decreased ventricular arrhythmias; and (7) better tolerance. It also appears that the magnitude of reduction in mortality is greater, given treatment with angiotensin converting enzyme inhibitors, than treatments with hydralazine-isosorbide dinitrate. Thus, angiotensin converting enzyme inhibitors are preferable to hydralazine-isosorbide dinitrate, and later vasodilators should be used in patients intolerant of angiotensin converting enzyme inhibitors. Angiotensin converting enzyme inhibitors appear to prevent marked left ventricular enlargement and to delay development of congestive heart failure in asymptomatic patients with left ventricular systolic dysfunction, the important determinants of long-term prognosis. Indeed, the prognosis of asymptomatic patients with postinfarction decreased left ventricular ejection fraction improves when they are treated with angiotensin converting enzyme inhibitors. Thus, long-term angiotensin converting enzyme inhibitor therapy should be considered even in asymptomatic patients with significantly reduced ejection fraction (< 40 percent).

Approximately 30 percent of patients cannot tolerate the doses of hydralazine and nitrates that are effective in improving hemodynamics. Tachycardia, recurrence of angina, gastrointestinal intolerance, arthralgia, and lupus-like syndrome are important adverse effects. Angiotensin converting enzyme inhibitors may also not be tolerated by some patients. Hypotension, deterioration of renal function, cough, skin rash, and dysgeusia (associated with captopril) are important side effects. In patients with bilateral renal artery stenosis or even in hypotensive patients with a low cardiac output, angiotensin converting enzyme inhibitors may cause severe renal failure. In patients with hypotension, particularly in those with hyponatremia, angiotensin converting enzyme inhibitors may induce further hypotension and renal failure; in such patients, angiotensin converting enzyme inhibitor therapy should be initiated with a very small dose (captopril, 6.25 mg; enalapril or lisinopril, 2.5 mg) after hypotension and low output states are partially corrected with inotropic therapy. Frequently, a combination of angiotensin converting enzyme inhibitors or vasodilators and newer inotropic agents is required, along with digitalis and diuretics in the management of such patients.

Calcium entry blocking agents should not be used as the principal agent for vasodilator therapy for chronic heart failure. Verapamil is contraindicated in patients with overt heart failure resulting from depressed systolic function because of its pronounced negative inotropic effect. Dihydropyridines, such as nifedipine, nicardipine, and felodipine, may improve cardiac performance in some patients. Diltiazem also improves left ventricular function. Despite initial improvement in hemodynamics, mortality of patients with overt heart failure may be higher when they are treated with calcium entry blocking agents. Thus, these agents should not be considered for vasodilator therapy of heart failure. In patients with coronary artery disease and evidence of myocardial ischemia, calcium entry blocking agents such as nifedipine or diltiazem can be added to hydralazine-nitrates or angiotensin converting enzyme inhibitors in an attempt to relieve myocardial ischemia, provided that significant hypotension does not result. However, the impact of such combination therapy on prognosis remains unknown. Amlodipine, a new vasoselective, dihydropyridine calcium-entry blocking agent, has been shown to improve clinical status of patients with systemic ventricular failure and to improve prognosis of the subject with nonischemic dilated cardiomyopathy.

Alpha-adrenergic blocking agents such as prazosin, trimazosin, and terazosin produce short-term beneficial hemodynamic and clinical effects in patients with chronic heart failure; hemodynamic and clinical tolerance develops rather rapidly in response to these agents. Thus, these agents alone should not be used for the treatment of chronic heart failure. However, in some patients who cannot tolerate adequate doses of hydralazine-nitrates or angiotensin converting enzyme inhibitors, alpha-adrenergic agents may be used along with lower doses of angiotensin converting enzyme inhibitors, particularly in relatively hypertensive patients. However, the long-term benefit of such combination therapy has not been determined.

The role of newer vasodilator agents such as nicorandil, flosequinan, and atrial natriuretic peptide in the management of chronic congestive heart failure remains unclear.

Nondigitalis Inotropic Drugs

Several adrenergic and nonadrenergic agents with positive inotropic effects have been evaluated. The adrenergic agents dobutamine and dopamine and the nonadrenergic peak III phosphodiesterase inhibitor amrinone are available only for short-term intravenous use. Of many nonparenteral adrenergic agents—pirbuterol, xamoterol, ibopamine, and levodopa—currently levodopa is the only drug available that can be used for long-term management of patients with chronic heart failure. Many nonparenteral peak III phosphodiesterase inhibitors—milrinone, enoximone, piroximone, pimobendan, and others—are currently undergoing clinical trials and are not available for clinical use. Intermittent intravenous infusion of dobutamine (5 to 10 μg per kilogram per minute) can cause sustained hemodynamic and clinical improvement for a few days to a few weeks in some patients. However, the duration of sustained improvement is variable, and the more severe the heart failure and hypotension, the shorter the duration of benefit. Furthermore, improvement in prognosis has not been documented with intermittent dobutamine infusion. Similarly, although intermittent amrinone infusion improves hemodynamics and clinical status of patients with refractory failure, it does not improve prognosis in these patients.

Levodopa (1.5 to 2 g three to four times daily) is converted to dopamine by dopa-decarboxylase, and the hemodynamic effects of levodopa are similar to those of low-dose (2 to 4 μg per kilogram per minute) dopamine infusion. Usually there is a modest increase in cardiac output with little or no change in mean arterial, right atrial, and pulmonary capillary wedge pressures. Approximately 30 percent of patients do not tolerate levodopa, particularly the large doses that are required to produce beneficial effects; gastrointestinal intolerance and central nervous system side effects prohibit its use in many patients. Long-term hemodynamic or clinical benefit of other nonparenteral adrenergic agents—pirbuterol, xamoterol, and ibopamine—has not been demonstrated in patients with moderately severe or severe heart failure.

The peak III phosphodiesterase inhibitors—milrinone, enoximone, and others—exert direct positive inotropic and vasodilatory effects and thus are called *inodilators.* Following their acute administration, cardiac output increases markedly, along with a substantial decrease in systemic and pulmonary venous pressures, a slight decrease in mean arterial pressure, and a slight increase in heart rate. However, clinical deterioration occurs in a significant proportion of patients during the long-term administration of these agents, and larger doses of diuretics frequently need to be added to prevent fluid retention. Prospective, controlled studies have reported that the phosphodiesterase inhibitors enoximone and milrinone can improve clinical status and exercise tolerance in patients with moderately severe and severe heart failure during 3 months of follow-up. However, long-term treatment with phosphodiesterase inhibitors such as milrinone and enoximone is associated with increased mortality. Increased mortality has also been observed during the treatment with beta-adrenergic agonists. Thus, indications for the use of nonglycosidic inotropic agents or inodilators are limited to those patients who fail to respond to vasodilators or angiotensin converting enzyme inhibitors. These agents are also used in patients awaiting cardiac transplantation as "pharmacologic bridge" therapy. Frequently, combination therapy using vasodilators, angiotensin converting enzyme inhibitors, and newer inotropic agents is required in addition to conventional therapy in prospective cardiac transplant recipients.

Beta-Adrenergic Blocking Agents

In patients with idiopathic dilated cardiomyopathy, beta-blocker therapy has been shown to improve clinical status and left ventricular function, presumably by up-regulation of myocardial beta-adrenergic receptors. However, the precise role of beta-blocker therapy in patients with chronic heart failure remains to be established.

When beta-blocker therapy is initiated, deterioration in clinical status and hemodynamics, such as decreased cardiac output and arterial pressure and increased pulmonary capillary wedge pressure, may occur. Following maintenance therapy for 6 to 8 weeks, clinical and hemodynamic improvement may be apparent. Hemodynamic improvement is characterized by an increase in cardiac output and systolic blood pressure, decreased left ventricular end-diastolic pressure, and decreased left ventricular end-systolic volume, with little or no change in end-diastolic volume. Although the precise mechanism for the hemodynamic improvement with chronic beta-blocker therapy remains unclear, up-regulation of myocardial beta-adrenoreceptors and enhanced contractile response are likely to be contributory. A few uncontrolled studies have claimed improved prognosis with long-term beta-blocker therapy; however, controlled studies have not substantiated this claim. Uncontrolled studies have also demonstrated decreased incidence of sudden death with beta-blocker therapy. Recently, Carvestilol, a new beta-blocker vasodilator, has been shown to improve clinical states of heart failure and sudden death of stable heart failure patients. *Clinical experience suggests that certain subsets of patients with dilated cardiomyopathy with tachycardia, gallop rhythm, relatively preserved cardiac output, and elevated pulmonary capillary wedge pressure are more likely to benefit from chronic beta-blocker therapy, particularly in combination with angiotensin converting enzyme inhibitors.* To avoid initial clinical deterioration, the starting dose of beta-adrenergic blocking agent should be very low (e.g., metoprolol, 5 mg once or twice daily), and the dose should be increased slowly until the resting heart rate decreases by 10 to 15 beats per minute. The potential benefit or hazard of beta-blocker therapy has not been established.

Cytotoxic Drugs and Corticosteroids

In a few patients with active myocarditis proved by myocardial biopsy, cytotoxic drugs (azathioprine) and corticosteroids have been reported to improve left ventricular function. However, controlled studies suggest that the potential benefit of corticosteroid treatment is too little compared with the risk of developing serious side effects. Cytotoxic drug therapy also does not appear to improve survival. *Thus, corticosteroid and cytotoxic drug therapy are not recommended for the treatment of chronic heart failure.*

Amiodarone and Other Antiarrhythmic Drugs

Approximately 50 percent of patients with moderately severe or severe chronic heart failure die suddenly, and it is generally accepted that the majority of these deaths result from ventricular arrhythmias and occasionally bradyarrhythmias. As a result, antiarrhythmic drug therapy has been postulated to decrease the incidence of sudden death in these patients. However, type IA antiarrhythmic drugs have not been found to be particularly effective in patients with heart failure and asymptomatic ventricular arrhythmias. Furthermore, type IA and IB antiarrhythmic drugs may cause significant deterioration of ventricular function in patients with overt heart failure. Type IC antiarrhythmic drugs such as flecainide and encainide may enhance mortality of patients with depressed left ventricular function, presumably owing to increased incidence of drug-induced proarrhythmia in these patients. Thus, type I antiarrhythmic drugs should not be used for suppression of asymptomatic ventricular arrhythmias in patients with chronic heart failure. A few uncontrolled studies have reported that amiodarone, a type III antiarrhythmic drug, can potentially decrease the incidence of ventricular arrhythmias and mortality of patients with severe chronic congestive heart failure without causing deterioration in left ventricular function. Controlled studies have reported conflicting results in terms of changes in survival rate. Low-dose amiodarone added to angiotensin converting enzyme inhibitors may increase left ventricular ejection fraction. *Thus, it is reasonable to consider the addition of a low dose of amiodarone (200 mg per day after initial loading dose) to conventional treatment in selected patients with severe heart failure.* Amiodarone has several undesirable side effects, of which pulmonary toxicity is the most serious. *Development of pulmonary toxicity may preclude cardiac transplantation in potential can-*

Table 3 Therapeutic Approach in Chronic Heart Failure

1. To exclude valvular heart disease and pericardial disease
2. To determine whether heart failure is due primarily to abnormal ventricular diastolic function or to systolic dysfunction
3. Symptomatic chronic heart failure due to diastolic dysfunction associated with ventricular hypertrophy. Cautious use of diuretics, nitrates, and a trial of calcium entry blocking agents; cardiac transplantation in appropriate subsets who remain unresponsive to medical therapy
4. Chronic heart failure due to systolic dysfunction (reduced ejection fraction, mild to severe dilation of ventricular cavity with or without increased wall thickness)
   A. Totally asymptomatic—use angiotensin converting enzyme inhibitors
   B. Mild to moderately severe heart failure—diuretics, digitalis, and angiotensin converting enzyme inhibitors or hydralazine, nitrates, diuretics, and digitalis (when angiotensin converting enzyme inhibitors produce adverse effects or are not tolerated). Continues to be symptomatic or deterioration—consider cardiac transplant in appopriate subsets and intermittent dobutamine or amrinone therapy or newer inotropic drugs for patients awaiting cardiac transplantation or for those who are not candidates for cardiac transplantation
   C. Severe chronic heart failure—digitalis, diuretics, and angiotensin converting enzyme inhibitors. Consider cardiac transplant for patients who fail to respond quickly; intermittent dobutamine or amrinone infusion or newer inotropic agents for patients awaiting cardiac transplantation or for patients considered not suitable for cardiac transplantation; consider low-dose beta-blocker or amiodarone therapy in selected patients

didates, and thus in such patients amiodarone should be used cautiously, if at all.

Surgical Treatment

Cardiac Transplantation and Other Surgical Therapy

Cardiac transplantation is the most effective treatment to improve the prognosis in patients with severe refractory heart failure. Two year survival with medical therapy in such patients is, at best, 25 percent; in contrast, 5 year survival rate following cardiac transplantation may exceed 60 percent. *Thus, patients who remain significantly symptomatic despite aggressive medical therapy or those who fail to respond to conventional therapy including vasodilators and angiotensin converting enzyme inhibitors should be considered for cardiac transplantation, provided that there are no contraindications for transplantation.* However, the very limited availability of donor hearts does not allow such treatment for the vast majority of potential candidates. Cardiomyoplasty, a surgical technique to wrap skeletal muscle such as latissimus dorsi around the heart to improve cardiac mechanical performance, is now undergoing clinical trials, and the role of such surgery in the management of severe chronic heart failure needs to be established.

Stepwise Therapeutic Approach

Therapy of chronic congestive heart failure includes use of diuretics, digitalis, vasodilators, angiotensin converting enzyme inhibitors, newer inotropic drugs, and cardiac transplantation. However, based on available information, a stepwise therapeutic approach should be undertaken as outlined in Table 3.

Suggested Reading

Chatterjee K, Parmley WW. Vasodilator therapy for acute myocardial infarction and chronic congestive heart failure. J Am Coll Cardiol 1983; 1:133.

Chatterjee K. Digitalis, catecholamines and other positive inotropic agents. In: Parmley WW, Chatterjee K, eds. Cardiology. Philadelphia: JB Lippincott, 1988:1.

Chatterjee K. Digitalis and non-ACE inhibitors in heart failure. Cardiol Clin 1989; 7:99.

Cohn JN, Archibald DG, Ziesche S, et al. Effect of vasodilator therapy on mortality in chronic congestive heart failure: The results of a Veterans Administration cooperative study. N Engl J Med 1986; 314:1547.

Cohn JN, Johnson G, Zischi S, et al. A comparison of enalapril with hydralazine-isosorbide dinitrate in the treatment of chronic congestive heart failure. N Engl J Med 1991; 325:303.

The Consensus Trial Group. Effects of enalapril on mortality in severe congestive heart failure: Results of the cooperative north Scandinavian enalapril survival study. N Engl J Med 1987; 316:1429.

Dzau VJ, Creager MA. Progress in angiotensin converting enzyme inhibition in heart failure. Cardiol Clin 1989; 7:119.

Lee HR, O'Connell JB, Mason JW. Immunosuppression and beta blockade in heart failure. Cardiol Clin 1989; 7:171.

Pfeffer MA, Braunwald E, Moye LA, et al. Effect of captopril on mortality and morbidity in patients with left ventricular dysfunction after myocardial infarction: Results of the survival and ventricular enlargement trial. N Engl J Med 1992; 327:669.

The SOLVD Investigators. Effect of enalapril on survival in patients with reduced ejection fractions and congestive heart failure. N Engl J Med 1991; 325:293.

The SOLVD Investigators. Effect of enalapril on mortality and the development of heart failure in asymptomatic patients with reduced left ventricular ejection fractions. N Engl J Med 1992; 327:685.

DIGITALIS TOXICITY

Elliott M. Antman, M.D.
Thomas W. Smith, M.D.

Because digitalis glycosides have a relatively narrow therapeutic index, clinicians must determine which individual patients have a favorable risk-benefit ratio for digitalis use and promptly identify signs and symptoms of digitalis toxicity. Fortunately, the incidence of digitalis toxicity has dropped compared with that in the 1960s and early 1970s, probably as a result of enhanced understanding of pharmacokinetics, more widespread use of radioimmunoassays of serum digoxin levels, increased appreciation of the multitude of drug interactions that may predispose a patient to digitalis toxicity, and an appropriate tendency to use lower doses of digoxin as alternative drugs have become available for treatment of cardiovascular conditions in which digoxin was traditionally employed. Among these new drugs are verapamil (for paroxysmal supraventricular tachycardia and control of the ventricular rate in atrial fibrillation), beta-adrenergic blocking agents (for control of the ventricular rate in atrial fibrillation), adenosine (for termination of paroxysmal supraventricular tachycardia), and angiotensin converting enzyme inhibitors (for a balanced vasodilator effect in congestive heart failure).

No specific serum digoxin level can be relied on to differentiate clearly between toxic and nontoxic states; rather, such data must be interpreted in the broader clinical context, with appropriate attention to the multitude of factors that may predispose to digitalis toxicity. Electrocardiographic manifestations of digitalis toxicity are characterized by disturbances of impulse formation or conduction (at atrial, atrioventricular [AV] junctional, or ventricular levels) or a combination of both types of phenomena. Clinical symptoms of digitalis toxicity typically include anorexia, nausea and vomiting, and visual symptoms as well as a variety of nonspecific complaints such as weakness, fatigue, headache, dizziness, and psychiatric disturbances ("digitalis delirium"). Despite age-related differences in both the pharmacokinetics and pharmacodynamics of digoxin, no clinically reliable differences in presentation of toxicity or response to digoxin-specific Fab fragments have been reported.

■ THERAPEUTIC ALTERNATIVES

In addition to withholding further cardiac glycoside administration, therapeutic options in the management of digitalis toxicity range from simple observation of the patient for infrequent, asymptomatic non-life-threatening arrhythmias to administration of digoxin-specific Fab fragments for potentially life-threatening arrhythmias (ventricular tachycardia, ventricular fibrillation, high-grade AV block with a slow escape rhythm not responsive to atropine), hyperkalemia (> 5 mEq per liter), or both.

Between these extremes are found patients with mild digitalis toxicity (non-life-threatening but symptomatic cardiac arrhythmias) and those in whom the etiology of the arrhythmia is not certain but in whom the question of digitalis toxicity arises. Because clinical experience remains relatively limited and the potential hazards of repeated exposure have not been fully defined, digoxin-specific Fab fragment treatment is not indicated for mild digitalis toxicity, and conventional antiarrhythmic therapy remains appropriate in such cases. Similarly, the use of Fab fragments as both a diagnostic and potentially a therapeutic tool in cases in which the diagnosis of digitalis toxicity is uncertain remains investigational at this time. As additional experience is accumulated with digoxin-specific Fab fragments, it is possible that the indications for their use may be extended beyond overtly life-threatening cases in the future. Provided safety is borne out in further experience, broader use of Fab fragments may have useful cost-effectiveness implications by decreasing intensive care unit requirements and overall length of hospital stay.

■ PREFERRED APPROACH

Prompt identification of digitalis-toxic arrhythmias is vital to successful clinical management. We advocate the following general therapeutic measures for all patients with clinically evident digitalis toxicity.

- Cardiac glycoside administration should be discontinued, and the use of catecholamines should be avoided if possible.
- The arrhythmia and its potential impact on the patient should be evaluated. Serious rhythm disturbances (e.g., complex ventricular arrhythmias) necessitate admission to an intensive care unit, whereas less hazardous arrhythmias may be adequately treated on a general hospital floor, assuming that adequate electrocardiographic monitoring is available.
- Unless the serum potassium level is elevated when the patient is first seen (e.g., > 5 mEq per liter), renal insufficiency is present, AV block is present or conduction is prolonged (P-R interval > 0.26 second), or the patient has taken a large overdose of digitalis (in which case serum potassium may rise to dangerously high levels), potassium repletion should be considered.
- Bradyarrhythmias that cause hypotension or a significant reduction in cardiac output may be treated initially with intravenous atropine (typically 0.5 to 1 mg in adults). We insert a temporary demand ventricular pacemaker if atropine fails to resolve the problem in less than 5 minutes. Infusion of beta-adrenergic agonists such as isoproterenol is best avoided in view of the potential for provoking more serious arrhythmias.
- Cardiac arrhythmias due to enhanced automaticity that are not overtly life threatening (e.g., paroxysms of nonsustained ventricular tachycardia) may require suppression with conventional antiarrhythmic therapy (intravenous lidocaine or phenytoin) in addition to potassium supplementation.
- Cases involving large accidental or suicidal cardiac glyco-

side ingestions and those with potentially life-threatening arrhythmias, hyperkalemia, or both are treated with digoxin-specific antibody (Fab) therapy.

Potassium Repletion

Potassium repletion should be undertaken only under closely monitored conditions because of the risk of provoking more troublesome arrhythmias, marked hyperkalemia, and even death. Either the intravenous or the oral route of administration may be used. We prefer the latter when the rhythm disturbance is not immediately life threatening. The rate of intravenous infusion of potassium should be limited to less than 0.5 to 1 mEq per minute. Potassium solutions are mixed in either normal saline or D_5W but should not exceed a concentration of 120 to 160 mEq per liter. When oral potassium repletion is used, doses of 40 mEq every 1 to 4 hours are given, provided that acidosis is not present (pH > 7.3) and renal function is adequate (creatinine < 2 mg per deciliter). Regardless of the potassium administration route employed, we review the 12 lead electrocardiogram every 15 minutes to detect early evidence of impending potassium excess, and serum potassium levels are measured every 30 to 60 minutes. Because of the possibility of paradoxical worsening of hypokalemia when D_5W is used, we prefer to use normal saline in cases of severe potassium depletion (< 3.5 mEq per liter).

Conventional Antiarrhythmic Agents

Clinical reports of lidocaine use in cases of digitalis toxicity suggest that this classic antiarrhythmic drug is of value for the management of digitalis-related arrhythmias, and we continue to employ it in cases of tachyarrhythmias of less than life-threatening severity. Lidocaine is administered as serial intravenous 100 mg boluses every 3 to 5 minutes (to a total dose of 300 mg) until either a therapeutic effect or lidocaine toxicity develops. This may then be followed by continuous infusion of 15 to 50 µg per kilogram of body weight per minute if further suppression of the arrhythmia is needed. Adverse reactions to lidocaine usually involve the central nervous system and may range from feelings of dissociation to agitation or frank seizures. Several reports have indicated that the slow intravenous infusion of phenytoin 100 mg every 5 minutes (not to exceed a total dose of 1,000 mg) is also useful for digitalis-toxic arrhythmias (e.g., ectopic automatic atrial tachycardia).

Clinical experience with beta-blockers, quinidine, or procainamide has been less favorable than that with lidocaine. Because of the greater risk of cardiac toxicity (both electrophysiologic and hemodynamic) with these drugs, we do not consider them to be initial pharmacologic agents of choice to suppress non-life-threatening digitalis-induced arrhythmias. Clinical experience with newer antiarrhythmic agents (tocainide, mexiletine, amiodarone) is insufficient to evaluate their safety and efficacy in comparison with the standard agents, and we do not advocate their use for digitalis-toxic arrhythmias at the present time. However, of potential interest is verapamil, for which there are abundant experimental data indicating that it is useful for treating a specific electrophysiologic abnormality referred to as *triggered automaticity.* Triggered automaticity appears to be related to oscillations of the membrane potential during the terminal phase of repolarization known as *delayed afterdepolarizations;* the oscillatory activity is believed to be caused by release of calcium from overloaded intracellular stores. Verapamil has been shown to prevent or abort such triggered activity in experimental preparations and in scattered clinical reports. Available experience is too limited at present to permit any statement of appropriate clinical guidelines.

Cardioversion

A common clinical problem centers around direct current (DC) cardioversion in the patient receiving a digitalis preparation. It is a widely held belief that DC cardioversion can be hazardous in individuals receiving cardiac glycosides. However, this is based on earlier studies reporting that the electrical shock provoked serious ventricular arrhythmias (refractory ventricular tachycardia or fibrillation). Although near-toxic levels of digitalis can lower the threshold for postshock ventricular arrhythmias, clinical studies have shown that usual therapeutic digoxin levels do not increase the risk of serious postshock ventricular arrhythmias. Thus, an increased risk of arrhythmias does not appear to be present when transthoracic shocks are delivered in the absence of digitalis toxicity. We use the following approach when considering DC cardioversion in digitalized individuals:

- Electrolyte imbalances are corrected, fever is suppressed, and hypoxia and anxiety are treated before DC cardioversion is undertaken.
- When there is overt electrocardiographic evidence of digitalis toxicity (e.g., atrial fibrillation with very slow ventricular rate, accelerated AV junctional rhythm, multifocal ventricular premature depolarizations), elective DC cardioversion is not performed.
- Under all circumstances, the smallest amount of energy that is likely to be effective is used. Our usual schedule of energy titration starts with 25 to 50 watt-seconds, with subsequent increments of 25 to 50 watt-seconds as needed. Ventricular tachycardia can often be abolished with 10 watt-seconds or less.

Digixin-Specific Antibody (Fab Fragments) for Life-Threatening Toxicity

Hemodialysis or hemoperfusion is of limited value for prompt reversal of life-threatening toxicity because of the widespread tissue binding of digoxin. Advanced digitalis intoxication should now be treated with purified digoxin-specific polyclonal antibody fragments (Fab) obtained from sheep immunized with digoxin coupled as a hapten to a carrier protein to render it antigenic. The advantages of the smaller size of the Fab fragment (molecular weight 50,000) as compared with the whole IgG molecule (molecular weight 150,000) include a more rapid onset of action due to enhanced diffusion into the interstitial space and, in patients with normal renal function, relatively rapid renal clearance of digoxin bound to Fab fragments (with a half-life of about 16 hours). The enhanced rate of clearance by renal mechanisms minimizes the chance of late release of bound digoxin and re-emergence of toxicity. Although the average affinity constant for digoxin is thirtyfold to 100-fold higher than that for digitoxin in typical preparations, the affinity for the latter is still high enough to permit digoxin-specific Fab antibody

Table 1 Calculation of Equimolar Dose of Digoxin-Specific Fab Fragments

Calculation of Body Load of Digoxin

Ingested amount (mg) × bioavailability of digoxin tablets = mg × 0.8

$$\frac{\text{Serum digoxin concentration (ng/ml)} \times 5.6^{*} \times \text{weight in kg}}{1{,}000}$$

Calculation of Fab Fragment Dose

$$\frac{\text{MW Fab} = 50{,}000}{\text{MW Digoxin} = 781} = 64 \times \text{body load (mg)} = \text{Fab dose (in mg)}$$

$$\frac{\text{Body load of digoxin (mg)}}{\text{0.6 mg neutralized/40 mg vial}} = \text{Number of vials of Fab fragments}$$

*Volume of distribution of digoxin in average adult (liters per kilogram). For digitoxin, use 0.56 rather than 5.6.
MW, Molecular weight.
Modified from Antman EM, Wenger TL, Butler VP, et al. Treatment of 150 cases of life-threatening digitalis intoxication with digoxin-specific Fab antibody fragments: Final report of a multicenter study. Circulation 1990; 81:1744.

fragments to be used effectively for life-threatening intoxication with digitoxin as well as digoxin.

We recommend the following protocol for administration of Fab fragments.

- The dose of Fab fragments is calculated to be equal on a mole-for-mole basis to the amount of digoxin or digitoxin in the patient's body, estimated from the medical history, determinations of serum digoxin or digitoxin concentrations, or both (Table 1). Examples of the calculation of the body load of digoxin to be neutralized are shown in Table 2.
- Screening for hypersensitivity was performed during clinical trials with digoxin-specific antibody fragments, and only 1 of 150 patients developed erythema at the site of skin testing, but without a wheal reaction. In view of this statistic and because such hypersensitivity testing can delay treatment in urgent cases, we restrict skin testing to high-risk individuals, such as those with a history of allergy to sheep products and those who have previously received a course of treatment with Fab fragments. The skin test is performed by reconstituting 0.1 ml of a 10 mg per millimeter solution of Fab fragments in 10 ml of isotonic saline. Subsequently, 0.1 ml of the above 1:100 dilution (10 μg) is injected intradermally, and the patient is observed for an urticarial wheal over the next 20 minutes.
- The Fab fragments should be administered intravenously through a 0.22 μm membrane filter over 15 to 30 minutes, unless the gravity of the clinical situation demands more rapid infusion.
- It is important to note that in states of advanced digitalis toxicity, potassium excretion through renal mechanisms coupled with efforts to reduce hyperkalemia using potassium-binding resins can deplete total body potassium even though the serum potassium may be normal or even elevated. A dramatic fall in serum potassium concentration can occur after Fab administration because reversal of NaK-ATPase inhibition tends to restore the normal transmembrane potassium gradient rapidly. For this reason, serum potassium should be monitored at least every hour for the first 4 to 6 hours after Fab treatment. The decline in serum potassium (which can occur even if supplemental potassium is given) is usually complete by 4 hours.
- The sequence of events that takes place following injection of digoxin-specific Fab fragments includes prompt binding of intravascular digoxin, followed by diffusion of the Fab fragments into the interstitial space and binding of free digoxin. The decrease in free digoxin in the extracellular space to near-zero levels creates a concentration gradient promoting egress of tissue stores of digoxin into the extracellular space, where it is also rapidly bound by Fab fragments. Free digoxin molecules freshly dissociated from membrane receptors are rapidly bound and cannot reassociate with the digoxin binding (inhibitory) site on the alpha subunit of NaK-ATPase. This dissociation event and the subsequent step of binding to Fab are critically important rate-limiting events in the reversal of digitalis toxicity. Typically, the total extracellular digoxin concentration rises dramatically, but such digoxin is pharmacologically inactive because only the unbound form can associate with the inhibitory site on the alpha subunit of NaK-ATPase. For this reason as well as technical problems imposed on assay systems by the presence of high-affinity Fab fragments, measurements of serum digoxin concentration are not reliable indicators of the state of digitalization for about 1 to 2 weeks after Fab administration. We have not found this to be a noteworthy clinical problem. In those uncommon cases in which loss of the inotropic support or rate-slowing action previously provided by digitalis results in hemodynamic compromise, it is possible in principle to "back titrate" with digoxin. We have not found this necessary and do not recommend attempting it for at least 7 days after Fab administration.

We have reported the results of the initial multicenter study of 150 patients treated with purified digoxin-specific Fab fragments. These patients all had actual or potentially life-threatening cardiac rhythm disturbances or hyperkalemia (or both) caused by digitalis intoxication and were considered clinically refractory to or likely to be refractory to treatment with conventional therapeutic modalities. On the basis of the results of that trial, it can be anticipated that an initial response to Fab will be seen within 60 minutes in most patients suffering from digitalis toxicity, and complete reversal of glycoside effects will be evident within 4 hours of administration of an adequate dose of Fab fragments. Approximately 80 percent of the 150 individuals treated showed resolution of all signs and symptoms, 10 percent were definitely improved (partial resolution), and 10 percent showed no response. Only one patient was judged to have a clinical course suggesting a true lack of response; a lack of response should thus raise the suspicion that too low a dose of Fab fragments was given or, alternatively, that the clinical signs and symptoms were not the result of digitalis toxicity. In two of the 150 patients, a recrudescence of digitalis toxicity was

Table 2 Examples of Calculation of Equimolar Dose of Digoxin-Specific Fab Fragments

Case I

75-year-old man (weight 70 kg) with chronic coronary heart disease and atrial fibrillation receiving maintenance therapy with digoxin 0.25 mg daily. He becomes confused and takes two of his digoxin tablets daily for 2 weeks and presents with complaints of weakness and palpitations. ECG shows sustained ventricular tachycardia at 150 beats/min. SDC = 3 ng/ml.

$$\text{Body load of digoxin} = \frac{\text{SDC} \times 5.6 \times 70}{1{,}000} = \frac{3.0 \times 5.6 \times 70}{1{,}000} = 1{,}176\text{ mg} \approx 1.2\text{ mg}$$

$$\text{Dose of Fab fragments} = \frac{1.2\text{ mg}}{0.6\text{ mg neutralized/40 mg vial}} = 2\text{ vials}$$

Case 2

40-year-old woman (weight 70 kg) with no history of heart disease ingests 100 tablets of digoxin 0.25 mg in a suicide attempt. She presents 8 hours later with nausea, vomiting, hypotension, complete heart block, and an idioventricular escape rhythm at 35 beats/min. Serum digoxin concentration result not yet returned form laboratory (and not needed for Fab dose determination). Serum potassium = 6.1 mEq/liter.

$$\text{Body load} = [\text{ingested amount} \times 0.8] = 25\text{ mg} \times 0.8 = 20\text{ mg}$$

$$\text{Dose of Fab fragments} = \frac{20\text{ mg}}{0.6\text{ mg neutralized/40 mg vial}} = 34\text{ vials}$$

Case 3

60-year-old woman (weight 65 kg) with chronic rheumatic heart disease and mitral regurgitation maintained on digoxin 0.25 mg daily for control of the ventricular rate in atrial fibrillation. SDC = 2 ng/ml on maintenance therapy. She ingests 75 tablets of digoxin 0.25 mg during a period of depression and presents 36 hours later with fascicular tachycardia, an unusual form of ventricular tachycardia originating in or near the left anterior fascicle. Serum potassium = 5.9 mEq/liter.

Ingested amount ≈ 18 mg digoxin (tablets)

$$\text{Body load} = [\text{ingested amount} \times 0.8] + \left[\frac{\text{SDC} \times 5.6 \times 65}{1{,}000}\right] = 14.4 + 0.728 \approx 15\text{mg}$$

$$\text{Dose of Fab fragments} = \frac{15}{0.6\text{ neutralized/40 mg vial}} = 25\text{ vials}$$

SDC, serum digoxin concentration.

observed after an initial response. Neither patient had renal failure, and both appeared to have received inadequate doses of Fab to neutralize the calculated body load of digoxin.

In this multicenter trial, no acute allergic reactions or illnesses suggesting serum sickness occurred in conjunction with Fab fragment treatment. The expected adverse reactions caused by prompt reversal of digitalis effects (rapid ventricular response to atrial fibrillation, deterioration of the level of left ventricular systolic function, or hypokalemia) were seen in less than 10 percent of patients and were generally manageable using conventional approaches.

Previous reports of survival in patients with life-threatening digitalis toxicity who received conventional treatment measures are strongly indicative of the therapeutic efficacy of purified digoxin-specific Fab fragments. Thus, despite the absence of a concurrent control group, the outcome with emergency use of Fab fragments in the 150 patients enrolled in the multicenter trial (12.5 percent mortality in patients with digitalis toxicity and a serum potassium > 6.4 mEq per liter) appears to be substantially better than that reported in similarly ill patients with advanced toxicity and hyperkalemia treated conventionally. Furthermore, the mortality rate was 46 percent in those patients in whom a cardiac arrest occurred as a consequence of digitalis toxicity; this result includes several patients treated only after relatively prolonged cardiopulmonary resuscitative efforts and compares favorably with the nearly 100 percent mortality reported in other series when conventional therapy alone was used.

Subsequent to the publication of this multicenter trial, an observational postmarketing surveillance study reported the experience in 717 adults receiving digoxin-specific antibodies for suspected toxicity (Hickey and co-workers, 1991). The rapid time course of resolution of toxicity over 1 to 4 hours after treatment was confirmed, and patient care was greatly facilitated. Important differences from the prospective multicenter study included an older patient population and a slightly higher rate of nonresponse to treatment. Nonresponse to treatment was seen in 14 percent in patients with suspected toxicity while on maintenance digoxin, 20 percent in patients receiving loading doses or who were in the hospital during treatment, and 15 percent in patients with heart disease ingesting a single large overdose. In the majority of instances, nonresponse to Fab fragments was due to a combination of inadequate dosing, moribund clinical status, or incorrect diagnosis. Adverse reactions of clinical interest consisted of an allergic response in 0.8 percent of patients and recrudescence of digitalis toxicity (usually within 3 days) in 2.8 percent of patients.

Intoxication with cardiac glycosides other than digoxin and digitoxin occurs sporadically, particularly in areas of the world where tea brewed from leaves found in the wild is ingested. The diagnosis of intoxication with extracts of plants such as oleander should be suspected when patients present with a combination of gastrointestinal, neurologic, and cardiac symptoms along with unexplained hyperkalemia. Routine immunoassays may report a measurable amount of "digoxin" because of varying degrees of cross reactivity between the antibodies used in the immunoassays and the different cardiac glycosides present in plant extracts. Isolated case reports of dramatic responses to digoxin-specific Fab antibody fragments in oleander intoxication have been reported, particularly in patients refractory to the conventional measures. Calculation of the dose of digoxin-specific Fab fragments required is not easily accomplished and therefore an empiric dose of a large quantity (e.g., at least 10 vials—equivalent to approximately 400 mg) should be administered in such patients.

Clinical Implications

On the basis of the results of the multicenter trial completed in 1986, the United States Food and Drug Administration approved the marketing of purified ovine digoxin-specific Fab fragments (Digibind, Burroughs Wellcome Co.) as an orphan drug for treatment of potentially life-threatening digitalis toxicity.

Because of the specificity of the antibody preparation, the safety record in patients treated for life-threatening digitalis intoxication, and the dramatic reversal of clinical signs of toxicity, we believe that consideration should now be given to treating patients with more moderate degrees of digitalis intoxication, even though the cost-effectiveness of such an approach has not been established in a prospective trial. However, the cost and potential immunogenicity of the current preparation argue against the routine use of digoxin-specific Fab fragments for the diagnosis or treatment of suspected digoxin intoxication in patients with only minimal signs of toxicity.

Future clinical applications under consideration include production of even smaller immunoglobulin fragments with reduced immunogenicity in humans, possible diagnostic as well as therapeutic use of new antibody preparations, and extension of this immunotherapeutic approach to antibody reversal of toxicity from other drugs or endogenous substances.

Suggested Reading

Antman EM, Smith TW. "Digitalis toxicity. An overview of mechanisms, manifestations, and management." In: Mandel W (ed.). Cardiac Arrhythmias. Philadelphia: Lippincott-Raven, 1995:1051–1073.

Antman EM, Wenger TL, Butler VP, et al. Treatment of 150 cases of life-threatening digitalis intoxication with digoxin-specific Fab antibody fragments: Final report of a multicenter study. Circulation 1990: 81;1744.

Hickey AR, Wenger TL, Carpenter VP, et al. Antibody therapy in the management of digitalis intoxication: Safety and efficacy: Results of an observational surveillance study. J Am Coll Cardiol 1991; 17:590.

Safadi R, Levy I, Amitai Y, et al. Beneficial effect of digoxin-specific Fab antibody fragments in oleander intoxication. Arch Intern Med 1995; 155:2121.

Wofford JL, Hickey AR, Ettinger WH, Furberg CD. Lack of age-related differences in the clinical presentation of digoxin toxicity. Arch Intern Med 1992; 152:2261.

ANGINA PECTORIS: STABLE

Michael A. Kutcher, M.D.

Stable angina pectoris may be defined as a chest pain syndrome, usually precipitated by exertion, the pattern of which is essentially unchanged for 60 days or more.

Obstructive coronary atherosclerotic heart disease is the etiology in the great majority of patients with stable angina. The pathophysiologic mechanism is based on a directly proportionate relationship between an increase in myocardial oxygen demand and the development of myocardial ischemia. Significant fixed obstructive coronary lesions may cause a distinct mechanical impediment to coronary blood flow that prevents adequate delivery of oxygen to the myocardium at predictable levels of exertion.

■ THERAPEUTIC ALTERNATIVES

Symptoms, signs, physiologic data, and anatomic data should be used to identify coronary atherosclerotic heart disease. Once the extent of disease has been quantitated, the three major goals to which therapy for stable angina must be directed are

- Relief of angina
- Prevention of myocardial infarction
- Promotion of longevity

The three major therapeutic "weapons" available are

- Medical therapy
- Coronary angioplasty
- Coronary bypass surgery

Each therapeutic option must address the supply and demand problem of stable angina. Ideally, the best therapy for each individual patient is that which can most effectively achieve the three goals with the minimum of risk.

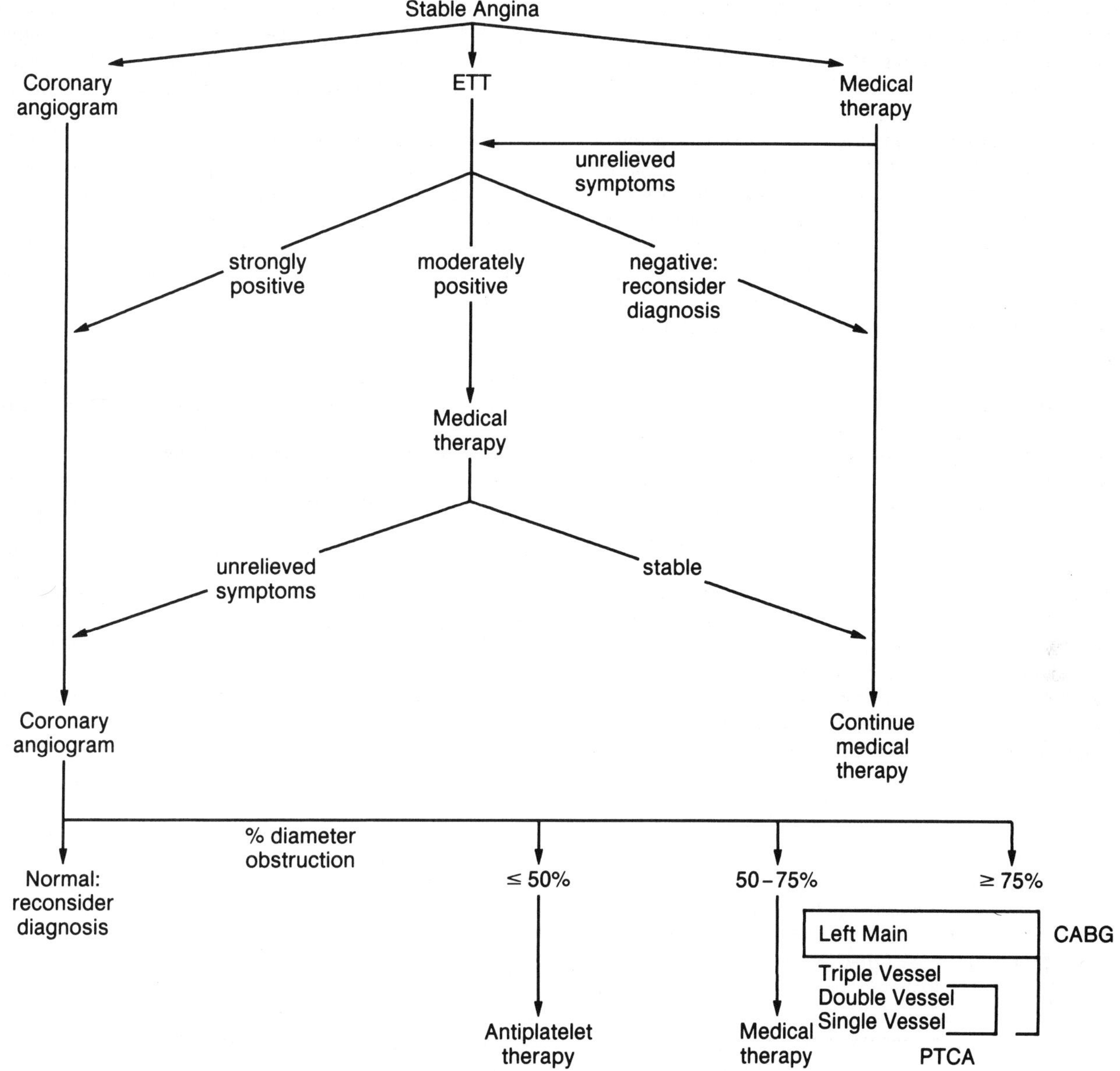

Figure 1
Schema for stable angina pectoris. CABG, coronary artery bypass graft; ETT, exercise tolerance test; PTCA, percutaneous transluminal coronary angioplasty.

■ PREFERRED APPROACH

Figure 1 is a flow diagram that represents a diagnostic strategy to select therapy for patients with stable angina pectoris.

Medical Treatment

Most patients with stable angina should be managed at least initially with medical therapy directed toward reducing myocardial oxygen demand and improving coronary blood flow. Long-term medical therapy is acceptable in patients with a low Canadian Classification angina score, good exercise tolerance test, and moderately obstructive coronaries in the range of 50 to 75 percent diameter reduction. The more elderly the patient, the more acceptable a medical regimen may be for the goal of promoting longevity with the disease stabilized. Patients who have poor vessels for revascularization or prohibitive left ventricular function may have no alternative but medication.

The three major antianginal pharmacologic groups are listed in Table 1.

Nitrates

Long-acting nitrates in oral, sublingual, or patch form represent the first line of therapy in stable angina. They primarily work by dilating coronary arteries and thus improving blood flow. A moderate preload reduction and a minor afterload reduction effect may also be beneficial by reducing demands made on the myocardium.

In view of the controversy regarding nitrate tolerance, it may be better to skip the nighttime dose of a long-acting oral

Table 1 Antianginal Pharmacologic Groups

GENERIC NAME	TOTAL DAILY DOSE RANGE (MG)	ROUTE	DOSING FREQUENCY
Long-acting nitrates			
Isosorbide dinitrate	40–240	SL or PO	q.i.d.
Isosorbide mononitrate	20–40	PO	b.i.d.
Nitroglycerin patch	5–20	Topically	q.d.
Beta-blockers			
Propranolol	40–360	PO	t.i.d./q.i.d.
Metoprolol	50–200	PO	b.i.d.
Atenolol	25–100	PO	q.d.
Nadolol	40–240	PO	q.d.
Calcium channel blockers			
Nifedipine	30–120	PO	q.d.*/t.i.d./q.i.d.
Diltiazem	90–360	PO	q.d.*/t.i.d./q.i.d.
Verapamil	120–480	PO	q.d.*/t.i.d./q.i.d.
Amlodipine	5–10	PO	q.d.
Nicardipine	60–120	PO	t.i.d.

SL, sublingually; PO, orally; q.i.d., four times per day; q.d., every day; t.i.d., three times per day; b.i.d., twice a day.
*Sustained-release preparation.
Readers are advised to check the product information sheet prior to administration of any drug to confirm accuracy of indications and dosage.

or sublingual preparation. If 24 hour patches are prescribed, removal at nighttime and reinstitution of a new patch in the morning would be an appropriate approach.

Nitrates may cause flushing, headache, dizziness, hypotension, and tinnitus. A lower dose may be better tolerated but less effective.

Short-acting sublingual or spray nitroglycerin may be used to dissipate or forestall periodic anginal attacks. The patient should be cautioned to sit or recline after administration of a dose (usually 0.4 mg sublingually) to obviate the potential hypotensive and orthostatic effects. If a protracted episode of angina lasts longer than 45 minutes and is unrelieved by three nitroglycerin tablets, the patient should be instructed to report to the nearest emergency room for evaluation.

Quantification of the amount and frequency of nitroglycerin administration by the patient may be used as a barometer to indicate effectiveness of the therapeutic plan or to alert the physician that additions to the pharmacologic regimen may be necessary.

Beta-Blockers

Beta-blockers work by blocking the beta-adrenergic pathway. This results in a reduction of heart rate, myocardial contractility, and blood pressure—all favorable maneuvers to decrease myocardial oxygen demand.

In patients with stable angina and relatively good left ventricular function, the combination of beta-blocker with nitrates is a logical step. Beta-blockers are a particularly good choice for patients who also have hypertension, tachycardia, ventricular arrhythmias, or a combination of these disorders. In individuals who have a previous history of myocardial infarction but who now have stable angina, beta-blockers are the treatment of choice in view of the impressive mortality and morbidity results in several randomized postinfarction trials.

Congestive heart failure, hypotension, bradycardia, and asthma are contraindications to beta-blocker therapy. Side effects of therapy may include worsening of heart failure, hypotension, bradycardia, advanced atrioventricular block, impotency, insomnia, nightmares, and excessive tiredness. Beta-blocker therapy may also mask the hypoglycemic response of insulin-dependent diabetes. These side effects may be less likely with the more cardioselective agents such as metoprolol or atenolol.

It is a better strategy to start with a basic beta-blocker in divided doses, titrate the effect, and then observe the long-term anginal response before trying the patient on a single or reduced-frequency beta-blocker agent.

Calcium Channel Blockers

This biochemically disparate group of agents acts by interfering with the calcium channel kinetics of smooth muscle and specialized cells. In stable angina, they work by dilating coronary arteries and preventing spasm, thus improving coronary blood flow. To different degrees, the individual calcium channel blockers may also reduce blood pressure, afterload, heart rate, and contractility to relieve myocardial oxygen demand.

Nifedipine is the best direct coronary and vasodilating agent of the group. It may also have benefit as an afterload reducing agent in patients with impaired left ventricular function. Used alone it may cause a reflex tachycardia and a paradoxical increase in angina. If possible, it could be combined with a beta-blocker to counteract these side effects.

Diltiazem has a good multidimensional capacity to vasodilate, reduce heart rate, and to some extent reduce contractility. It is an effective monotherapy agent. If necessary, it may be combined with a beta-blocker, but this should be done with caution in view of the potential cumulative effects on the heart rate and atrioventricular node.

Verapamil has the least vasodilatory action and the greatest effects on the atrioventricular node. It is an appropriate agent in stable angina patients who have atrial tachyarrhythmias as a component of their presentation. Patients with congestive heart failure and borderline left ventricular function may be worsened by the reduced contractility effects of verapamil. Verapamil should be used with extreme caution, or not at all, with beta-blockers owing to potential profound conduction disturbances.

Amlodipine and nicardipine are second-generation calcium channel blocking agents that have more selective coronary dilatory effects with minimal changes in inotropy and chronotropy. Other second-generation agents such as felodipine, isradipine, nisoldipine, and nitrendipine each have specific attractive properties but are still in the process of being evaluated for their role in the therapy of angina.

Side effects of calcium channel blockers in general include flushing, pedal edema, dizziness, hypotension, increased atrioventricular block, nausea, and vomiting. Pedal edema and flushing are particular problems with nifedipine as they reflect its strong vasodilatory action.

As with beta-blockers, it is better to use a basic calcium channel blocker agent in divided doses, titrate therapy, and observe response before committing the patient to the newer continuous delivery or sustained-release formulations of nifedipine, diltiazem, and verapamil.

Antiplatelet Therapy

In view of recent studies documenting improved mortality and morbidity in patients with unstable angina or myocardial infarction treated with aspirin, it is appropriate to consider long-term aspirin therapy as a prophylactic strategy in patients with stable angina. If no contraindications exist, a dose of 80 to 325 mg every day or every other day may be used. Therapy should be discontinued if gastrointestinal intolerance, bleeding, or other side effects occur.

Coronary Angioplasty

In patients with stable angina, coronary angioplasty should be considered if symptoms and signs of ischemia persist and restrict life-style in spite of optimal medical therapy.

Mildly symptomatic patients who have critical stenoses (> 90 percent diameter reduction) in a very proximal major artery or arteries, with a great deal of myocardium at jeopardy, should be considered for coronary angioplasty. However, the goals of preventing myocardial infarction and promoting longevity have not been substantiated as yet by large-scale randomized trials comparing this approach with either medical therapy or coronary bypass surgery.

Although coronary balloon angioplasty has a high primary success rate (90 to 95 percent) and a low morbidity (2 to 3 percent myocardial infarction or emergency bypass surgery, < 1 percent mortality), it must be weighed against the high restenosis rate (25 to 35 percent).

Newer percutaneous transluminal technology such as atherectomy, laser angioplasty, and intracoronary stents have not significantly reduced this restenosis rate, but each of these new modalities has shown promise in difficult subsets that are not easily amenable to balloon dilation. Clinical trials defining the role of these new technologies are still in progress.

Several hours prior to coronary angioplasty, patients should receive aspirin (650 mg) to prevent acute platelet activation. Long-acting nitrates and a calcium channel blocker (diltiazem if the patient has had no previous therapy, or nifedipine if the patient is already on a beta-blocker) should be started prior to and continued for at least 1 month after angioplasty to obviate the problem of reactive coronary artery spasm. Recent studies have indicated that an antiplatelet regimen after angioplasty does not reduce the long-term restenosis rate. However, if there are no contraindications, aspirin (325 mg every day) is reasonable to continue for 6 months after angioplasty, especially if the patient has had a previous myocardial infarction or an unstable anginal pattern in the past. In these cases, indefinite use may be warranted. Controversy still exists over the benefits of dipyridamole.

Successful coronary angioplasty should be followed up with an exercise tolerance test within a week after the procedure to serve as a baseline if questions of restenosis arise in the future. A negative exercise test 6 months after angioplasty may be an indirect prognostic sign that long-term patency of the dilated vessel has persisted. Thereafter, yearly evaluation and exercise testing are appropriate to rule out progression of disease elsewhere or late restenosis.

Coronary Bypass Surgery

Both randomized and observational trials have documented the effectiveness of coronary bypass surgery over medical therapy in either completely alleviating or at least significantly relieving the frequency and severity of angina. Assuming acceptable coronary anatomy and reasonable left ventricular function, coronary bypass surgery is an appropriate alternative if a stable anginal pattern does not respond to medical therapy or if it interferes with a patient's life-style and expectations. However, in patients with mild anginal symptoms and single, double, or triple vessel disease with good left ventricular function, randomized trials have not shown a benefit of improved mortality rates with surgery over medicine.

Randomized trials have shown a definite advantage of coronary bypass surgery over medical therapy in reducing mortality in mildly symptomatic patients with significant left main or with significant triple vessel disease and reduced left ventricular function.

The risks of coronary bypass surgery must be weighed against the expected benefits and the three major goals of therapy. Complications of surgery include a 2 percent mortality, 2.5 percent myocardial infarction, 2 percent reoperation for postoperative bleeding, 1 percent infection, 1 percent cerebrovascular accident, and 10 percent postoperative arrhythmia. There is a 5 to 10 percent yearly attrition rate with saphenous vein graft conduits. Internal mammary grafts have a 10 year patency rate of 95 percent compared with a 50 percent patency rate for saphenous vein grafts (ACC/AHA Task Force, 1991).

Preoperative and postoperative care of patients undergoing coronary bypass graft surgery are discussed in other chapters of this book.

Risk Factor Reduction

A strong attempt at risk factor reduction is imperative to ensure success of the overall therapeutic plan. Patients should be couraged to stop smoking, maintain reasonable body weight, control blood pressure, and achieve acceptable blood lipid levels. An individualized exercise program is an essential component of any long-range patient strategy. These preventive principles are just as important as the vast pharmacopeia and high technology in effectively treating individuals with stable angina pectoris.

Suggested Reading

ACC/AHA guidelines and indications for coronary artery bypass graft surgery: A report of the American College of Cardiology/American Heart Association Task Force on Assessment of Diagnostic and Therapeutic Cardiovascular Procedures (Subcommittee on Coronary Artery Bypass Graft Surgery). Circulation 1991; 83:1125.

DeMots H, Glasser SP. Intermittent transdermal nitroglycerin therapy in the treatment of chronic stable angina. J Am Coll Cardiol 1989; 13:786.

Packer M. Combined beta-adrenergic and calcium-entry blockade in angina pectoris. N Engl J Med 1989; 320:709.

Parisi AF, Folland ED, Hartigan P. A comparison of angioplasty with medical therapy in the treatment of single-vessel coronary artery disease. N Engl J Med 1992; 326:10.

Parker JO. Nitrate therapy in stable angina pectoris. N Engl J Med 1987; 316:1635.

Ridker PM, Manson JE, Gaziano JM, et al. Low-dose aspirin therapy for chronic stable angina: A randomized clinical trial. Ann Intern Med 1991; 114:835.

Stone PH, Gibson RS, Glasser SP, et al. Comparison of propranolol, diltiazem, and nifedipine in the treatment of ambulatory ischemia in patients with stable angina: Differential effects on ambulatory ischemia, exercise performance, and anginal symptoms. Circulation 1990; 82:1962.

Wong JB, Sonnenberg FA, Salem DN, et al. Myocardial revascularization for chronic stable angina: Analysis of the role of percutaneous transluminal coronary angioplasty based on data available in 1989. Ann Intern Med 1990; 113:852.

ANGINA PECTORIS: UNSTABLE

Craig M. Pratt, M.D.
Robert Roberts, M.D.

Unstable angina has been defined in a variety of ways and encompasses a wide spectrum of patients with coronary artery disease.* The unstable angina syndrome describes the clinical features of patients presenting with a symptom complex intermediate to that of chronic stable angina and acute myocardial infarction. However, the distinction is more than semantic because patients presenting with unstable angina have a severalfold higher incidence of myocardial infarction and death than patients with chronic stable angina. A reasonable estimate of the 1 year mortality of patients presenting with unstable angina is 5 percent, and a larger number develop an acute myocardial infarction within weeks after the clinical presentation. The syndrome of unstable angina, therefore, represents a state of increasing myocardial ischemia. The various presentations in Table 1 have common temporal and prognostic elements and represent high-risk patients who should be targets for intensive diagnostic evaluation and aggressive medical management.

In the purest sense, unstable angina occurs in the absence of recent myocardial infarction and without the presence of other noncardiac conditions that might precipitate or heighten myocardial ischemia. Postinfarction angina is presented as a separate category because of differences in pathophysiology and treatment. Unstable angina includes patients presenting with new onset of severe and prolonged episodes of angina or patients with previous stable exertional angina pectoris who developed more prolonged, intense chest pains at lower levels of activity. Patients may also present with either new onset or heightened episodes of chest pain that occur at rest or that wake the patient out of sleep (nocturnal angina). In general, the clinical situation is more urgent if the patient has documented transient ischemia as evidenced by electrocardiographic (ECG) changes (transient ST-segment shifts or T wave changes) during the anginal episode, which normalize after the cessation of pain. Likewise, the clinical situation is more severe if the patient develops unstable angina while already taking conventional doses of pharmacologic agents for ischemia.

A reasonable question to ask is, How do these clinical presentations differ from acute myocardial infarction? In fact, there is considerable overlap, such that the working diagnosis

Table 1 Clinical Presentations of Unstable Angina Syndrome

New onset of angina pectoris*
As first manifestation of coronary artery disease
Worsened prognosis with:
Rest angina/nocturnal angina
With evidence of reversible electrocardiographic changes (T wave and ST-segment changes)
Recent exacerbation of frequency, duration, or severity of angina pectoris*
Less responsive to sublingual nitroglycerin/anti-ischemic therapy
New rest or nocturnal angina
With evidence of reversible electrocardiographic changes
Angina within days/weeks of acute myocardial infarction*
With evidence of reversible electrocardiographic changes

*May be exacerbated by noncardiac disorders (see text).

*Editor's note: The term *stable angina pectoris* is used when a patient has had no increase in frequency or severity of angina within the last 60 days. Unstable angina pectoris should be viewed within this context and time frame.—J.W.H.

of unstable angina rests on the premise that the diagnosis of acute myocardial infarction has been ruled out by obtaining serial ECGs and serial CK-MB enzymatic assays. In addition, these definitions assume that the chest pain is due to structural or functional abnormalities in the coronary arteries, either from fixed atherosclerotic coronary stenosis or altered vasomotor tone or coronary thrombus. However, even with a careful clinical history, at least 10 percent of patients who present with "unstable angina" turn out to have angiographically normal coronary arteries, most of which do not have demonstrable coronary spasm during provocative ergonovine testing. Also, some of the patients presenting initially with unstable angina develop an acute non-Q wave myocardial infarction within the first 24 to 48 hours of observation. The overlap of patients with normal coronary arteries and patients developing non-Q wave infarction is inevitable because of the heterogeneity of the clinical presentations characterizing the unstable angina syndrome.

ETIOLOGY AND PATHOGENESIS OF UNSTABLE ANGINA

Unstable angina occurs in the clinical setting of significant atherosclerotic coronary artery disease. In most cases, the coronary stenosis involves 50 percent or greater stenosis of the intraluminal diameter of the involved coronary artery. At times, in patients with multivessel disease it is unclear as to which coronary artery represents the "culprit lesion." Pathophysiologic mechanisms implicated in the unstable angina syndrome include rapid progression of fixed coronary atherosclerosis, the contribution of increased vasomotor tone in the area of a fixed coronary stenosis, and subtotal or partially occlusive thrombus in the area of a fixed coronary stenosis. Intracoronary thrombus has been documented to play a role in certain patients with unstable angina, although the observed frequency of reported thrombus has been highly variable, ranging from 30 to 50 percent of patients. Coronary angioscopy has revealed that intraluminal coronary lesions frequently have a pattern described as eccentric and irregular with fissured plaques, often containing visible thrombus. The activation of platelets and of the clotting system is also likely to be of importance in the pathogenesis of unstable angina. Coronary spasm in the presence of angiographically normal coronary arteries is often accompanied by transient ST-segment elevation and is covered as part of the variant angina or Prinzmetal's angina syndrome. Given the variety of contributing factors believed involved in the pathogenesis of unstable angina, it should not be surprising that the therapeutic approaches are myriad.

THERAPEUTIC ALTERNATIVES

Patients fitting the aforementioned clinical descriptions should be hospitalized in a coronary care unit for monitoring and definitive therapy. The wide variety of therapeutic alternatives reflects the large number of potentially contributory pathophysiologic mechanisms involved in unstable angina. Therapeutic options include antiplatelet therapy, especially aspirin; intravenous heparin; elimination of myocardial ischemia with nitrates, calcium channel blockers, and beta-blockers; the use of intravenous thrombolytic agents such as tissue plasminogen activator (rt-PA) and streptokinase; and, in some instances, coronary artery angioplasty, coronary artery bypass surgery, or both. A presentation of our preferred approach is followed by a discussion of each of the medical and invasive alternatives in the treatment of unstable angina.

PREFERRED APPROACH

Unstable angina should be considered a medical emergency, and the patient should be put in a monitored bed in a coronary care unit as expeditiously as possible. A number of general issues should be addressed immediately. First, the patient should be in a calm environment and, if necessary, sedated. The therapeutic goal is to render the patient free of chest pain with pharmacologic therapy as soon as possible. A rapid screen for noncardiac contributions to myocardial ischemia should be made. It should include a search for anemia, thyrotoxicosis, hypotension or dehydration, tachyarrhythmias, hypoxemia, fever, and infection. Appropriate tests should be performed to confirm the presence or absence of these contributing factors and, if found, corrected. Even if an ECG was obtained in the emergency room, a repeat 12-lead ECG should be obtained immediately to identify expeditiously a few patients whose ECGs evolve rapidly, revealing ST-segment elevation signifying acute myocardial infarction. These patients merit immediate consideration of thrombolytic therapy if no contraindications exist. Serial CK-MB enzymes should be obtained every 4 to 6 hours for 24 hours.

Medical therapy should begin immediately. First and most important is the administration of oral aspirin, one 325 mg tablet. Aspirin should be continued daily on an indefinite basis. Although the aspirin may seem a trivial part of this regimen, it is the mainstay of therapy for unstable angina, as demonstrated in large American and Canadian trials in which aspirin reduced the incidence of myocardial infarction and mortality by 50 percent (Cairns and co-workers, 1985; Lewis and co-workers, 1983). Administration of intravenous heparin is a reasonable alternative and, in comparative trials, is nearly as effective as aspirin but not more effective, nor is the combination more effective. Therefore, we prefer aspirin alone. It is easier to administer, has fewer potential side effects, and will be one of the medications that the patient will be discharged on regardless of the initial therapy.

In addition, pharmacologic therapy should be initiated immediately and aimed to render the patient free of angina and eliminate objective evidence of myocardial ischemia. A combination of nitrates, calcium channel blockers, and beta-blockers may be necessary and administered as described subsequently. Because a majority of these patients have a critical stenosis in at least one of the major coronary arteries, the goal should be a "cooling off" phase in which the patient is rendered free of angina for 24 to 48 hours, after which coronary angiography should be performed. It is our belief that coronary angiography is mandatory; ideally, however, the timing should be on an elective basis before hospital discharge. In some cases, the patient cannot be rendered free of angina or ischemia, mandating immediate cardiac catheter-

Table 2 Intravenous Pharmacologic Therapy for Unstable Angina

DRUG	DOSE	MONITORING	CONTRAINDICATIONS
Nitroglycerin*	10–200 μg/min IV	Dose sufficient to lower arterial pressure 10–15 mm Hg, not <100 mm Hg systolic	Hypotension
Beta-blockers*			
Metoprolol†	5 mg IV every 5 min for 3 doses, re-evaluating patient after each dose	Dose not to exceed 10 mm Hg; fall in systolic BP or <100 mm Hg or heart rate <55	Hypotension, bradycardia, heart block, congestive heart failure, asthma
Propranolol	0.025–0.05 mg/kg IV over 15–30 min, re-evaluating patient after each dose	Dose not to exceed 10 mm Hg; fall in systolic BP or <100 mm Hg or heart rate <55	Hypotension, bradycardia, heart block, congestive heart failure, asthma

*Must be individually tailored with frequent and careful clinical evaluation (see text).
†Dosing interval will vary with individual patients. Transition to oral therapy recommended in first 6 to 12 hours.

ization and coronary angiography, with the alternatives of angioplasty and bypass surgery ultimately considered. We consider the role of intravenous thrombolytic therapy such as rt-PA and streptokinase to be applicable only in selected patients rather than "routine" at this time and describe their roles later.

Medical Therapy of Unstable Angina and Postinfarction Angina

The therapeutic goal of medical therapy is to alleviate all episodes of clinical angina pectoris as well as to eliminate objective evidence of myocardial ischemia as rapidly as possible. Therefore, intravenous therapy is frequently chosen initially. Intravenous nitroglycerin is a mainstay of therapy for patients with unstable angina. As an initial therapy, we recommend intravenous nitroglycerin to be administered in doses ranging from 10 to 200 μg per minute, with the end point being the elimination of all episodes of chest pain. In general, the dose should be sufficient to lower the observed intra-arterial pressure by 10 or 15 mm Hg, with care not to lower the systolic blood pressure below 100 to 110 mm Hg. Obviously, there is more flexibility in patients who are hypertensive. Also, attention must be given to the heart rate during intravenous nitroglycerin therapy because patients with low filling pressures may develop a tachycardia that would increase myocardial oxygen consumption. A summary of the dose and administration information for intravenous nitroglycerin as well as for intravenous beta-blockers is included in Table 2.

Intravenous beta-blockers may make an important contribution to the therapy of individual patients with unstable angina, especially patients presenting with hypertension and tachycardia. In such patients, the initial therapy with beta-blockers should be either intravenous metoprolol or intravenous propranolol (see Table 2), with the goal of transition to oral beta-blockers within 12 hours. However, in most patients with unstable angina, we initially use an oral beta-blocker because we do not believe that there are clear-cut demonstrated advantages to administering intravenous beta-blockers in most patients. The use of intravenous beta-blockers is more complicated than intravenous nitroglycerin and requires close attention to contraindications (see Table 2) and careful administration. The resting heart rate represents a reliable index to follow, and repeat examination for signs of congestive heart failure is mandatory.

After the patient has been stabilized and rendered free of chest pain for 12 to 24 hours, transition to oral therapy is recommended. The dose ranges of oral beta-blockers, calcium channel blockers, and long-acting nitrates are presented in Table 3. We believe that calcium channel blockers play a useful role in the oral therapy of the unstable angina syndrome as a result of the important pathophysiologic contribution of increased vasomotor tone. The disadvantage of oral nitrates is that there must be a nitrate-free interval during long-term therapy to avoid the development of nitrate tolerance. The implications of using oral nitrates with a nitrate-free dosing interval in a clinical syndrome that is unstable are unknown. Frequently, intravenous nitroglycerin is maintained for 1 to 3 days until coronary angiography is performed for decisions regarding definitive therapy.

With regard to the calcium channel blockers, nifedipine (or nicardipine) may not be preferable because the dihydropyridine calcium blockers increase heart rate as a result of their vasodilatory effects. A number of clinical trials using nifedipine in patients with unstable angina have failed to demonstrate a therapeutic benefit. If nifedipine is the selected calcium channel blocker, it should be used in combination with a beta-blocker. Nifedipine, verapamil, and diltiazem should be used with caution in patients with left ventricular dysfunction. Verapamil should not be used with beta-blockers. Diltiazem is effective alone or in combination with beta-blockers, is well tolerated, and does not result in a reflex tachycardia. Diltiazem is our preferred calcium channel blocker for use in the treatment of the unstable angina syndrome.

Oral beta-blocker therapy should be considered, especially in patients with hypertension, tachycardia, and preserved left ventricular function. The doses of selected oral beta-blockers are presented in Table 3. The heart rate at rest, during normal activity, and with peak exercise all serve as good clinical indices of adequate beta-blockade. We believe that the shorter-acting nonselective beta-blockers are preferable in this clinical situation.

Other Pharmacologic Approaches to Unstable Angina

A number of clinical trials have addressed the issue of the administration of intravenous thrombolytic therapy to patients with unstable angina. The majority of these trials have used intravenous rt-PA and have failed to demonstrate a

Table 3 Oral Pharmacologic Therapy for Unstable Angina

PHARMACOLOGIC CLASS	GENERIC/BRAND NAME(S)	TOTAL DAILY DOSE (MG)	DOSING FREQUENCY
Selected beta-blockers	Propranolol (Inderal)	120–360	t.i.d./q.i.d.
			b.i.d.
	Metoprolol (Lopressor)	100–200	b.i.d.
			q.d.
	Timolol (Blocadren)	20–60	q.d.
	Atenolol (Tenormin)	50–100	
	Nadolol (Corgard)	40–240	
Selected calcium blockers	Nifedipine (Procardia)	30–120	t.i.d./q.i.d.
			t.i.d./q.i.d.
	Diltiazem (Cardizem)	90–360	t.i.d./q.i.d.
	Verapamil (Isoptin, Calan)	240–480	
Selected long-acting nitrates*	Isosorbide dinitrate (Isordil, Sorbitrate)	40–240	q4–6h*
	Nitroglycerin (Nitro-Bid)	10–50	q4–6h*
	Pentaerythritol tetranitrate (Penitrate)	40–160	q4–6h*

*With long-term use, tolerance may develop without a nitrate-free interval (see text).

clinical benefit. As previously mentioned, it appears that the majority of patients presenting with unstable angina do not have objective evidence of a partial or totally occluding thrombus at the time of coronary angiography. Thus, although administration of thrombolytic agents appears to be a promising approach in this syndrome, we do not recommend it as routine therapy. Thrombolytic agents should be administered to any patient who has objective evidence of coronary thrombus at the time of coronary angiography. It may be that the failure to show a clinical benefit of thrombolytic agents is due to the small number of patients in clinical trials reported. A definitive trial of more than 1,500 patients with unstable angina will be completed in 1991.

Although presented separately, *postinfarction angina* occurring in the initial days or weeks following acute myocardial infarction has prognostic similarities to other types of unstable angina. Postinfarction angina is more common in patients incurring a non-Q wave infarction than in those with a Q wave infarction; likewise, the incidence of recurrent infarction is at least fourfold higher in non-Q wave infarction. In these patients, it is important to obtain a 12-lead ECG during chest pain. It has been demonstrated that the combination of postinfarction angina and transient ECG changes identifies high-risk patients in whom aggressive therapy and coronary angiography are mandatory. In the largest trial reported studying non-Q wave infarcts, prophylactic diltiazem was effective in reducing both the incidence of postinfarction angina and the incidence of recurrent acute myocardial infarction by approximately 50 percent. We believe that effectiveness of diltiazem in this clinical setting is consistent with the hypothesis that patients with non-Q wave infarction have a larger component of increased vasomotor tone than do those with Q wave infarcts, in whom thrombosis is the primary pathophysiologic mechanism.

The management of postinfarction angina is quite similar to other unstable angina syndromes. However, we routinely recommend oral diltiazem because it has documented effectiveness in this clinical situation. Also, coronary angiography is recommended in all cases when transient ECG changes are documented during the anginal episode or objective ischemia is documented during predischarge exercise testing or thallium imaging.

Table 4 Indications for Angioplasty or Bypass Surgery for Unstable Angina

Continued angina despite aggressive medical therapy (emergency)
- Angioplasty considered for a single critical coronary stenosis meeting generally accepted anatomic criteria; consideration of multivessel angioplasty instead of coronary artery bypass surgery in this clinical setting made on an individual case basis*
- Coronary artery bypass surgery for single-vessel coronary stenoses not amenable to angioplasty and multivessel disease, left main coronary artery disease, or its equivalent

Patients responding to initial pharmacologic management (elective)
- Angioplasty considered for single critical coronary stenoses, especially for proximal left anterior descending lesions and proximal dominant right lesions†
- Coronary artery bypass surgery considered for multivessel disease, especially with some left ventricular dysfunction; triple-vessel disease or left main coronary stenosis†

*See text for discussion.
†Decision usually based on demonstration of objective evidence of ischemia rather than anatomy alone.

Coronary Angioplasty

We believe that all patients who present with the unstable angina syndrome should undergo coronary angiography prior to hospital discharge because of the relatively high incidence of myocardial infarction and death within the first few weeks after this clinical presentation. Thus, coronary angiography is performed to identify those patients with left main coronary artery disease or multivessel disease prior to hospital discharge. Continued chest pain, especially with ECG changes despite aggressive medical therapy, is an indication for immediate coronary angiography.

A number of high-risk subgroups may be considered candidates for coronary artery angioplasty (Table 4). One such subgroup is patients not responding to aggressive medical therapy who have coronary angiographic evidence of a single critical coronary stenosis appropriate to an approach with angioplasty as judged by accepted anatomic criteria. In addition to unstable patients, certain patients who are rendered asymptomatic by aggressive medical therapy may also be considered as candidates for elective coronary angioplasty prior to hospital discharge. We should emphasize that there are no well-controlled clinical trials establishing the superiority of angioplasty over conventional anti-ischemic therapy in such patients, but patients should be considered who have critical lesions in the proximal left anterior descending artery that are considered anatomically appropriate for coronary angioplasty. Although we would recommend angioplasty in most cases involving the proximal left anterior descending coronary artery, single-vessel stenoses of either the right coronary artery or the circumflex coronary artery represent more difficult and nebulous decisions. In these cases, we rely heavily on an assessment of the extent of myocardial ischemia by single photon emission computed tomography (SPECT) thallium imaging, during treadmill exercise or with intravenous adenosine administration. Asymptomatic patients with large perfusion defects, despite optimal medical therapy, are reasonable candidates for coronary angioplasty. The choice of angioplasty for patients with unstable angina and multivessel critical stenoses is more controversial. Although we do not believe that angioplasty should be considered routinely, it may be considered in individual institutions that have the appropriate skill and experience.

Coronary Bypass Surgery

In general, for coronary artery bypass surgery we select patients with unstable angina who are in one of the following categories. First, there are patients who do not respond to aggressive medical management and who continue to have significant angina, especially with transient ECG changes. In such cases, we recommend bypass surgery for patients with multivessel coronary artery disease, especially if they have some degree of left ventricular dysfunction (see Table 4). In cases in which ischemia is pharmacologically controlled, coronary artery bypass surgery should be limited primarily to patients with left ventricular dysfunction and multivessel disease and patients with left main coronary artery stenosis. In selected cases, patients with single or multiple critical stenoses who have normal left ventricular function are selected for bypass surgery, especially if the lesions are in such a location or severity that angioplasty cannot be considered. As is the case with decisions regarding angioplasty, objective assessment of the extent of myocardial ischemia with quantitative SPECT thallium imaging is useful in patient selection.

Suggested Reading

Ambrose JA, Alexopoulos D. Thrombolysis in unstable angina: Will the beneficial effects of thrombolytic therapy in myocardial infarction apply to patients with unstable angina? J Am Coll Cardiol 1989; 13:1666.

Braunwald E. Unstable angina. Circulation 1989; 80:410.

Cairns JA, Gent M, Singer J, et al. Aspirin, sulfinpyrazone, or both in unstable angina: Results of a Canadian multicenter trial. N Engl J Med 1985; 313:1369.

Lewis HD, Davis JW, Archibald DG, et al. Protective effects of aspirin against acute myocardial infarction and death in men with unstable angina. N Engl J Med 1983; 309:396.

Theroux P, Quimet H, McCan J, et al. Aspirin, heparin or both to treat acute unstable angina. N Engl J Med 1988; 319:1105.

Yusuf S, Wittes J, Friedman L. Overview of results of randomized clinical trials in heart disease: II. Unstable angina, heart failure, primary prevention with aspirin and risk factor modification. JAMA 1988; 260:2259.

EARLY MYOCARDIAL INFARCTION: THROMBOLYTIC THERAPY

Alan D. Guerci, M.D.

The timely administration of thrombolytic therapy to patients with acute myocardial infarction may preserve ventricular function and definitely reduces mortality. At the same time, thrombolytic therapy increases the incidence of stroke in some patient subgroups. This tension—between favorable myocardial effects and the risk of bleeding—defines the indications for thrombolytic therapy.

■ PRINCIPLES OF THERAPY

Benefits

Proper selection of patients for thrombolytic therapy is perhaps best served by describing the benefits and risks of therapy where they are most clearly established. This step should lead to the enunciation of some principles that can be applied to situations in which the benefit-risk ratio is somewhat ambiguous.

Meta-analysis of the large placebo-controlled, randomized trials of thrombolytic therapy demonstrates dramatic benefits when thrombolytic agents are given within 6 hours of symptom onset to patients with ST-segment elevation or bundle branch block (GISSI, 1986; ISIS-2, 1987). Mortality rates are reduced by about 35 percent in these patients. A lesser but still significant reduction in mortality has been observed among patients with ST-segment elevation or bundle branch block treated at 6 to 12 hours. In these patients mortality is reduced by about 20 percent. Treatment beyond 12 hours does not reduce mortality.

Table 1 Contraindications to Thrombolytic Therapy

Absolute Contraindications
Any active internal bleeding
Any intracranial neoplasm or arteriovenous malformation
Any intracranial surgery in past 6 months
Any stroke in past year
Any head trauma with loss of consciousness in past 6 months
Surgery in noncompressible location in past 6 weeks
Any alteration of mental status
Infectious endocarditis
Relative Contraindications
Gastrointestinal or genitourinary bleeding in past 6 months (normal menstruation excluded)
Any previous stroke
Any compressible arterial puncture in past week
Any puncture of noncompressible artery in past month
Any transient ischemic attack in past 6 months
Systolic blood pressure is greater than 175 mm Hg after nitrates and analgesics
Surgery in noncompressible extracranial location occuring between 6 and 12 weeks prior to contemplated administration of thrombolytic agent

With the likely exception of patients with deep anterior precordial ST depressions indicative of total occlusion of a nondominant circumflex artery, thrombolytic therapy does not reduce mortality among patients with ischemic myocardial pain and ST-segment depressions. Thrombolytic therapy is also of no value to patients with chest pain and normal electrocardiograms, nonspecific ST-T changes, or deep T wave inversions.

Risks

In the absence of thrombolytic therapy, acute myocardial infarction is associated with an incidence of ischemic stroke that approaches 1 percent. Most of these strokes are the result of left ventricular mural thrombus formation and subsequent systemic embolization. Thrombolytic therapy carries a risk of intracranial hemorrhage of 0.5 percent (streptokinase) to 0.7 percent (tPA) (GUSTO, 1993). In large series of patients treated with streptokinase, the overall incidence of stroke has remained unchanged; i.e., the increased risk of intracranial hemorrhage has been offset by a corresponding reduction in embolic stroke, presumably because of preservation of ventricular function and a reduced incidence of mural thrombus formation. However, neither the risk of mural thrombus formation nor the risk of intracranial hemorrhage is the same for all patients. For example, mural thrombus formation is common among patients with large anterior infarctions but rare among patients with small inferior infarctions. Intracranial hemorrhage occurs as a function of age and blood pressure, particularly among patients treated with tPA, in whom the incidence increases from 0.3 percent among patients younger than 65 or those with systolic blood pressure below 125 mm Hg to above 1 percent for patients older than 75 or with systolic blood pressure above 175 mm Hg. Thus, for patients in whom the benefit of thrombolytic therapy is marginal or the risks substantial, individualization of therapy is mandatory.

A list of absolute and relative contraindications to thrombolytic therapy appears in Table 1. Most of these recommendations are based on an understanding of potential side effects rather than well-defined experience. Nevertheless, I have witnessed or am aware of the following examples of bleeding induced by thrombolytic therapy: intracranial hemorrhage in a patient with acute myocardial infarction, syncope, and blunt facial trauma; intracranial hemorrhage in a patient with endocarditis, myocardial infarction, and unrecognized mycotic aneurysm; uncontrolled retro-orbital bleeding in a diabetic 1 week following laser retinal surgery; and cardiac tamponade in a patient with pulmonary embolism 1 week after coronary bypass surgery.

Bleeding complications increase with age. Advanced age is not, however, a contraindication to thrombolytic therapy. Among patients 75 and older, thrombolytic therapy reduces mortality from all causes by around 4 percentage points (i.e., approximately 1 life is saved for every 25 patients treated). Elderly subjects considered for thrombolytic therapy should be vigorous and in good general health.

■ PATIENT SELECTION

In the absence of a specific contraindication, the following patients should be given thrombolytic therapy:

- Patients with anterior infarction presenting within 12 hours of symptom onset
- Patients with bundle branch block not known to be old, presenting within 12 hours of symptom onset
- Patients with inferior, lateral, or true posterior infarction presenting within 6 hours of symptom onset
- Patients with inferior, lateral, or true posterior infarction and hemodynamic compromise who present 6 to 12 hours after symptom onset, i.e., patients with large ischemic regions, including patients with massive right ventricular infarctions.

Because the benefit of therapy diminishes with time, treatment at 6 to 12 hours requires careful consideration of relative contraindications and discussion of the risks and benefits with the patient.

Miscellaneous Considerations

Cardiopulmonary resuscitation (CPR) is not a contraindication to therapy, provided that the patient is awake and chest wall trauma, if any, is minimal.

The TAMI investigators reported on their experience with 62 patients who received less than 10 minutes of cardiopulmonary resuscitation, who awoke immediately after the cardiopulmonary resuscitation, and who did not have obvious chest wall trauma (Califf and co-workers, 1988). These patients were enrolled in trials of thrombolytic therapy and represented 9 percent of the population of these studies. Among the 62 patients with pretreatment cardiac arrest and CPR, there were no cases of cardiac tamponade or hemothorax. Blood loss and transfusion requirements were similar for patients with or without CPR. Predischarge ejection fraction was lower in patients requiring pretreatment CPR and mortality was higher, but these adverse outcomes were a consequence of large infarctions rather than the combination of CPR and thrombolytic therapy. The outcome is likely to have been even worse had these patients been treated with thrombolytic agents.

Premenopausal women infrequently sustain acute myocardial infarction. Nevertheless, the question as to whether menstruating women can safely be given thrombolytic agents does arise from time to time. Experience with the use of thrombolytic agents for pulmonary embolism indicates that menstruation is also a minor and relative contraindication to thrombolytic therapy. This observation is consistent with the fact that menstrual bleeding is regulated more by vasospasm than by protein-mediated hemostasis.

As in the case of patients with recent surgery or major trauma, when doubt exists in these situations, primary angioplasty should be considered.

■ ADJUNCTIVE THERAPY

The decision to treat a patient with thrombolytic therapy for acute myocardial infarction should include consideration of adjunctive mechanical therapy to maximize reperfusion and adjunctive medical therapy to minimize reocclusion.

Although salvage angioplasty, i.e., angioplasty of infarct-related arteries that remain occluded despite thrombolytic therapy, has not been proved beneficial, it should be considered in patients who present early in the course of large myocardial infarctions. This recommendation is based on two lines of reasoning. First, 15 to 20 percent of patients treated with tPA have persistent total occlusion of the infarct-related artery 90 to 120 minutes after the initiation of therapy, and most of these vessels will not be recanalized over the next 24 hours. With streptokinase, 35 to 40 percent of infarct-related arteries remain totally occluded 90 to 120 minutes after the initiation of therapy. Although many of these vessels recanalize over the next 24 to 48 hours, approximately half do not. In view of the morbidity and mortality risks associated with nonreperfusion among patients who present to hospitals early in the course of large infarcts and the potential benefit of reperfusion, these nonreperfusion rates may be considered unacceptable. Second, the conclusion that salvage angioplasty is not routinely beneficial is an inference derived from a European cooperative study of emergency angioplasty for patent and occluded infarct-related arteries, rather than a direct result of a randomized trial of salvage angioplasty (Simoons and co-workers, 1988). The benefit of salvage angioplasty in this study may have been obscured by adverse effects of emergency angioplasty of patent infarct-related arteries and the relatively small penalty associated with nonreperfusion or reocclusion in patients with small to intermediate myocardial infarctions treated with thrombolytic agents at 3 to 4 hours.

On the basis of these considerations and in view of the overwhelming evidence of benefit of reperfusion in large infarcts, it seems advisable to screen all patients with large infarcts for emergency angiography and, if necessary, salvage angioplasty. *Large infarct* may be defined as any myocardial infarction with hemodynamic compromise unresponsive to atropine or any anterior infarction with widespread ST-segment elevation (Mauri and co-workers, 1989). Given the frequent difficulty of distinguishing reperfusion from nonreperfusion on the basis of clinical or electrocardiographic criteria, and in recognition of the opportunity for salvage of ischemic myocardium that may be lost by 1 or 2 hours of observation, it is probably best to begin to make arrangements for emergency angiography and, if necessary, salvage angioplasty immediately after initiation of thrombolytic therapy in such patients. These plans may be changed later if there is evidence of reperfusion.

In conjunction with streptokinase, aspirin has been shown to reduce the incidence of nonfatal and fatal recurrent infarction. Aspirin also promotes patency of the infarct-related artery among patients treated with tPA. Intravenous heparin prevents reocclusion and is believed to reduce mortality in patients treated with tPA. Neither intravenous or intermittent subcutaneous heparin reduces mortality in patients treated with streptokinase.

■ DRUG OF CHOICE

Among patients treated within 6 hours of symptom onset, tPA reduces mortality by 1 percentage point (10 lives saved per 1,000 patients treated) when compared to streptokinase (GUSTO, 1993). Because most of the intracranial hemorrhages occurring with any thrombolytic agent are fatal, tPA also reduced the incidence of death or disabling stroke when compared to streptokinase (6.9 percent vs. 7.8 percent, $p = 0.006$). The survival advantage of tPA is greatest in high-risk patients, those with larger rather than smaller infarcts and also older rather than younger patients. Given that the survival advantage of tPA is directly related to more rapid reperfusion, it does not make sense to use tPA routinely in patients treated at 6 to 12 hours. The benefit of treatment at 6 to 12 hours appears to be more closely related to acceleration of the healing process in infarcted myocardium rather than salvage of infarcted myocardium. Therefore, the 30 to 60 minute advantage of tPA with respect to time to reperfusion is believed to make little or no difference among such patients. On the other hand, streptokinase probably should not be given to patients who have received it more than 1 week and less than 2 years ago. Such patients have high titers of neutralizing antibodies, and it is not known whether streptokinase is effective in the face of these antibodies.

Suggested Reading

Califf RM, Topol EJ, Kereiakes DJ, et al. Cardiac resuscitation should not be a contraindication to thrombolytic therapy for myocardial infarction. Circulation 1988; 78(II):127.

Fibrinolytic Therapy Trialists' Collaborative Group. Indications for fibrinolytic therapy in suspected acute myocardial infarction: collaborative overview of early mortality in major morbidity results from all randomized trials of more than 1,000 patients. Lancet 1994; 343:311.

Gruppo Italiano per lo Studio della Streptochinasi nell' Infarto Miocardico (GISSI). Effectiveness of intravenous thrombolytic treatment in acute myocardial infarction. Lancet 1986; 1:397.

GUSTO Angiographic Investigators. The effects of tissue plasminogen activator, streptokinase, or both on coronary artery patency, ventricular function, and survival after acute myocardial infarction. N Engl J Med 1993; 329:1615.

The GUSTO Investigators. An international randomized trial comparing 4 thrombolytic strategies for acute myocardial infarction. N Engl J Med 1993; 329:673.

ISIS-2 (Second International Study of Infarct Survival) Collaborative

Group. Randomized trial of intravenous streptokinase, oral aspirin, both or neither among 17,187 cases of suspected acute myocardial infarction: ISIS-2. Lancet 1988; 2:349.
Mauri F, Gasparini M, Barbonaglia L, et al. Prognostic significance of the extent of myocardial injury in acute myocardial infarction treated by streptokinase (the GISSI trial). Am J Cardiol 1989; 63:1291.
Simoons ML, Arnold AER, Betriu A, et al. Thrombolysis with tissue plasminogen activator in acute myocardial infarction: No additional benefit from immediate percutaneous coronary angioplasty. Lancet 1988; 1:197.

MYOCARDIAL INFARCTION: UNCOMPLICATED

Germano DiSciascio, M.D.
George W. Vetrovec, M.D.

The management of transmural myocardial infarction has changed dramatically with the advent of thrombolytic therapy, resulting in an increase in the frequency of uncomplicated infarctions. Uncomplicated infarction refers to no severe pump failure, cardiogenic shock, or life-threatening arrhythmias. Likewise, the recognition that a nontransmural (non-Q) infarction is not a "small event" but is a warning of worse short-term risk, prompting more aggressive drug and invasive therapy, has led to a further reduction in short-term adverse outcomes. Thus, although management strategies may be more complex, the overall outcome results in a higher proportion of uncomplicated infarctions.

■ THERAPEUTIC ALTERNATIVES

The therapy of uncomplicated myocardial infarction involves the use of certain drugs and, after coronary arteriography, a consideration of angioplasty or surgery.

■ PREFERRED APPROACH

Medical Treatment

Myocardial Infarction in the Era of Thrombolytic Therapy

The efficacy of acute thrombolytic therapy during evolving myocardial infarction is well established, and in future years thrombolysis will be primary treatment for most infarct patients without major contraindications. Therefore, the subacute and late management of myocardial infarction through the 1990s will largely involve patients after thrombolytic therapy. Clinical recognition of reperfusion is somewhat limited, making the definition of patients who fail to reperfuse difficult. Although acute invasive intervention may be appropriate for patients who fail to reperfuse, those who have strong clinical suspicion of reperfusion, such as improvement of chest pain (although chest pain frequently may not disappear completely and may sometimes be difficult to differentiate from pericardial pain), abatement of ST-segment elevation, and early (less than 16 hours) peak of creatine kinase, may be treated expectantly. Risk is stratified according to the outline described subsequently. However, successful thrombolysis is also associated with recurrent in-hospital ischemic events and the possibility of in-hospital, infarction-related artery reclosure, which occurs most frequently after heparin is discontinued (usually after 3 to 4 days) or if heparinization is subtherapeutic (activated partial thromboplastin time more than twice that of control). Those patients with acute reclosure comprise 5 to 20 percent of successfully reperfused patients. However, because of recurrent infarction, such patients often are candidates for urgent angiography and/or retreatment with thrombolytic therapy potentially to salvage the benefits of initial early reperfusion.

Risk Stratifications and Prognosis

Several factors are associated with increased mortality risk after myocardial infarction, and their recognition is of paramount importance in optimal management after infarction. Patients at increased risk may account for up to 55 percent of the population under 75 years of age experiencing myocardial infarction. Ischemia during the hospital phase beyond the initial 24 hour period after infarction is associated with an 18 percent mortality between day 6 and 1 year. Patients with a previous myocardial infarction and evidence of congestive heart failure carry a 25 percent 1 year mortality after discharge; patients with left ventricular ejection fraction between 20 and 44 percent have a 12 percent 1 year mortality (Ross and co-workers, 1989). Predischarge exercise testing may further characterize higher risk groups; ability to achieve 4 METs without ischemic changes is associated with a 1 to 3 percent 1 year mortality; a positive test or inability to achieve a 4 MET workload identifies a subgroup with higher risk (11 percent 1 year mortality). In all these groups, coronary angiography is indicated vis-à-vis possible revascularization and improvement in mortality rate.

Coronary Care Unit

The original goal of coronary care units was to provide arrhythmia monitoring and treatment before catastrophic events occur. In addition, the ability to observe patients closely and to monitor hemodynamic status is a continuously evolving use of the coronary care unit, with availability of invasive hemodynamic monitoring and intra-aortic balloon pump support.

Practical considerations in the coronary care unit include appropriate patient sedation for anxiety when necessary.

Likewise, pain management for the completed, uncomplicated myocardial infarction often requires utilization of nonsteroidal analgesics for the moderate discomfort that patients may continue to experience for the first 24 to 48 hours. In some instances, this discomfort may be associated with a pericardial rub.

Decisions about transfer from the coronary care unit are made relative to the stability of the patient. In general, patients with successful reperfusion and no evidence of life-threatening arrhythmia once antiarrhythmic therapy has been discontinued are candidates for transfer by 72 hours. The risk of serious arrhythmia is decreased substantially by this time, even for patients who have failed to reperfuse but who are otherwise uncomplicated.

Cardiovascular Drug Therapy

Anticoagulants. Following infarction all patients, even those receiving heparin, should be maintained on aspirin, unless it is contraindicated, such as in the case of adult asthma and nasal polyps. Although recommended dosages are variable, we favor using one adult enteric-coated aspirin daily for dosing convenience, which is maintained indefinitely.

Patients receiving thrombolytic therapy should be started and maintained on intravenous heparin therapy, unless it is contraindicated by risk or occurrence of bleeding, with dosage titrated to a partial thromboplastin time of twice control. Our practice is to maintain heparin for at least 48 hours or longer if ischemic symptoms recur or until coronary angiography if an early angiogram is anticipated. Longer heparinization may be warranted for documented intracoronary thrombus; following angioplasty for persistent, severe congestive failure; or because of prolonged bed rest, systemic embolic events, or echo-documented left ventricular thrombus. Heparin in the last conditions is maintained until oral sodium warfarin (Coumadin) anticoagulation is therapeutic.

Dipyridamole (Persantine) is not currently thought to be superior to or additive to aspirin in ischemic and infarction syndromes, and thus it is not routinely used except for patients unable to take aspirin. A dose of 75 mg twice daily is believed to be sufficient in such circumstances.

Indications for Coumadin are limited to documented left ventricular thrombus, systemic embolization, and severe congestive failure. The risk-benefit ratio of chronic anticoagulation with Coumadin must always be considered. Recent evidence is emerging that less stringent Coumadin anticoagulation may be equally effective with a lower risk of bleeding complications. A prothrombin time of 1.5 times control is usually quite satisfactory and is safer than higher levels. Coumadin is begun at 5 mg daily without loading. Heparin needs to be maintained until therapeutic effects from Coumadin administration are seen, usually by 5 days. Early, once or twice weekly, outpatient observation is necessary to assess any significant variation in prothrombin level. Patient education regarding increased bleeding tendency, especially from trauma or changes in associated drug therapy including nonprescription agents, is imperative.

Beta-Blockers. Prior to the era of thrombolytic therapy, beta-blockers in significant dosages (e.g., propranolol 120 mg per day) were demonstrated to reduce the risk of subsequent mortality and reinfarction, with beneficial effects decreasing over time, such that the efficacy abated 18 to 24 months following transmural infarction. Such beneficial effects of beta-blockers are unknown following thrombolytic therapy. The TIMI IIB Trial (1989) demonstrated the efficacy of intravenous beta-blockers followed by oral beta-blockers in reducing the incidence of early recurrent ischemic events in the first 6 weeks without effect on mortality. Oral beta-blockers alone had no effect on short-term outcome.

Our current bias is to maintain beta-blockers in patients begun acutely on intravenous beta-blocker therapy and to institute late oral beta-blockers only in patients not receiving thrombolytic therapy, particularly patients with large or anterior infarction without contraindications. Alternatively, beta-blockers may be used as an anti-ischemic agent in patients having continued anginal symptoms, persistent hypertension, or both.

Contraindications to beta-blockers include a history of asthma and severe congestive failure. Common side effects include fatigue, lethargy, bad dreams, and impotence. Because of frequent troublesome side effects, the popularity of routine beta-blocker treatment after thrombolysis in an uncomplicated infarction seems to be waning.

Calcium Blockers. Most studies have not shown that routine administration of calcium blockers following transmural infarction is useful in preventing major ischemic events. Although in one study patients without congestive failure receiving diltiazem had fewer recurrent adverse ischemic events, patients with congestive failure had an overall worse survival. Likewise, nifedipine has not been shown to have preventive properties following transmural infarction. However, one study of verapamil has suggested late postinfarction efficacy. Thus, routine use of calcium blockers after transmural infarction is usually limited to the treatment of hypertension or ischemia.

Nifedipine is particularly effective for rapidly reducing severe hypertension, which is useful in the face of ongoing ischemia, anticoagulation, or thrombolytic therapy. Likewise, nifedipine's marked vasodilation potentially produces the least acute depression of left ventricular function. Amlodipine, a new dihydropyridine, may be better for the management of patients with ischemia and mild to moderate left ventricular dysfunction, as recent data suggest this drug may be most favorable relative to neurohumoral responses.

Diltiazem has been demonstrated to reduce the risk of subsequent ischemic events in patients after nontransmural infarction. Because many of these patients undergo coronary angiography and subsequent intervention owing to known increased short-term risk of an adverse outcome, there is no evidence that continued calcium blocker therapy after intervention has any benefit. Thus, calcium blocker treatment seems prudent for most nontransmural infarctions, at least until angiographic documentation of limited extent or revascularization of underlying coronary disease is completed. Subsequent therapy should be indicated for continuing ischemia; if revascularization is complete, however, calcium blockers are not necessary except for blood pressure control. The usual effective dose of diltiazem is 240 to 360 mg every 24 hours. Side effects include nausea, headache, and edema. Occasional patients develop marked bradycardia, sinus node block, or atrioventricular node block, which may be exacerbated by digoxin.

Angiotensin Converting Enzyme Inhibitors. Recent evidence suggests a beneficial effect for angiotensin converting enzyme (ACE) inhibitors following infarction for reducing subsequent morbidity and mortality, presumably by supporting more favorable ventricular remodeling. The impact of ACE inhibitors seems greatest in patients with the most severe ventricular impairment. Although hypotension may be an acute side effect of these agents, subsequent subacute effects on kidney function of white blood counts are of concern. Therapy probably is best instituted later during hospitalization rather than acutely. Although not life-threatening, a persistent dry cough limits therapy in more than 10 percent of patients.

Antiarrhythmic Drugs. Lidocaine is often begun on admission to the coronary care unit, although routine use is less popular. If necessary, lidocaine is given later for increasing frequency of ventricular premature beats (> 8 per minute, couplets, R-on-T phenomena, nonsustained ventricular tachycardia), maintained for 48 hours, and then discontinued while monitoring is available. Elderly patients and patients with hepatic disease are at increased risk of toxicity. Seizures, mental confusion, or both should prompt one to discontinue lidocaine and obtain a blood level. Lidocaine is instituted with a 50 to 75 mg bolus and is continued with a 2 mg per minute drip. If by blood level or clinical efficacy the dosage needs to be increased, an increase in the drip rate to 3 to 4 mg per minute should be preceded by an additional bolus of 50 to 75 mg. Further antiarrhythmic management is discussed in the chapter *Cardiac Arrhythmias Following Myocardial Infarction.*

Patient Education

The reality of coronary artery disease manifested by myocardial infarction produces significant psychological effects in most patients, whether expressed or not. Education and discussion of feelings are important to allay anxiety. Simply reassuring a patient that feelings of anxiety or depression are common is often helpful.

Patients should be given basic explanations for the anatomic causes of coronary disease and myocardial infarction. Patient concerns regarding prevention of future coronary events are probably greatest at this time. Thus, education of risk factors should be instituted early and continued throughout hospitalization.

The anxiety of future activity and life expectancy are common concerns. Early discussion of the potential rehabilitation of most patients back to a normal life-style is helpful in allaying anxiety and limiting early concerns regarding disability.

Prior to discharge, patient education should be directed to understanding prescribed medications, including actions and potential side effects.

Following hospitalization, patient education should persist, reinforcing earlier teaching, which may have been forgotten perhaps as a result of distraction because of anxiety during hospitalization. The potential for and timing of return to work should be clearly based on the patient's progress. Likewise, reinforcement of risk factor modification remains a lifetime goal.

Lipid Screening

The importance of cholesterol as a potentially reversible risk factor is now well documented and recognized by many patients. Questions regarding cholesterol are common, and we therefore always discuss cholesterol and diet with patients. It is important to point out that cholesterol levels drawn at the time of a major illness such as myocardial infarction do not represent baseline values. Thus, early therapy is directed toward diet, with plans for lipid evaluation following hospitalization. Conversely, for patients with extraordinarily high or known lipid abnormalities, drug treatment should be initiated during hospitalization.

Activity

Early mobilization decreases the disability of bed rest and reduces the risk of thrombophlebitis. Following myocardial infarction patients should be mobilized as rapidly as possible. Sitting is easier on myocardial function even early, and thus patients may sit up within the first 24 hours if they are stable. Sitting in a chair is appropriate beyond 24 hours following infarction.

For the successfully reperfused patient, ambulation in the hospital can be quite brisk. Conversely, patients with marked congestive failure or large infarction even with successful reperfusion have to be mobilized somewhat more slowly. Because the major time frame of myocardial rupture is in the first 7 days, only moderate activity should be considered reasonable until at least 2 weeks after the event.

Hospital Discharge

Timing of hospital discharge should be based on the complexity of the infarction. Preliminary studies have demonstrated safe discharge as early as 5 days following successfully reperfused infarctions without residual significant coronary artery disease. Conversely, patients with more extensive left ventricular dysfunction, residual ischemia, or both should be observed longer, with discharge at approximately 12 days.

Management After Hospitalization

In those patients who leave the hospital without evidence of residual ischemia or need for early revascularization, continued outpatient follow-up remains important to recognize subsequent ischemia, which may develop with increasing activities. Four to 6 weeks after an uncomplicated myocardial infarction, a full-level exercise test is warranted for evidence of ischemia. If there is no evidence, the patient can resume normal activities within the context of his or her cardiac and general medical history. Conversely, if there is evidence of ischemia, we recommend angiography for those patients not undergoing catheterization during hospitalization to assess the extent of myocardium in jeopardy. Patients who have angioplasty should have a baseline stress test performed early, with a follow-up study at 6 months to document any evidence of asymptomatic restenosis. Furthermore, effective rehabilitation, risk factor modification, and patient education are important aspects of management following hospitalization.

Surgical Treatment

Coronary Angiography and Revascularization

Coronary angiography is recommended for the higher risk subgroups outlined previously because coronary bypass surgery may enhance survival in patients with depressed left ventricular function, three-vessel coronary artery disease, or postinfarction angina. Furthermore, coronary angiography following nontransmural infarction is important to document extent of disease and need for intervention. Coronary angiography after successful thrombolysis is more controversial. The TIMI IIB trial (1989) indicates that for patients who sustain a myocardial infarction there is generally no significant benefit to urgent angiography and angioplasty. Thus, the recommendations from that study are that patients be considered for angiography and possible intervention only if there is evidence of recurrent ischemia in the hospital, a positive low-level exercise treadmill before discharge, or both. However, in hospitals with available catheterization laboratories, early angiography may be the most efficient and useful method to assess patients fully following thrombolytic therapy. Benefits include identifying patients with nonsevere residual occlusions, which require no further interventions, and patients with limited coronary artery disease who may, on the basis of this anatomic information, be returned safely to earlier activity and hospital discharge. Conversely, patients with multivessel disease and depressed left ventricular function may be more readily triaged to revascularization. Although angiography may be an acceptable alternative screening technique, the recognition of a lesion is not an automatic indication for angioplasty without evidence of ischemia. Patients whose arteries reocclude after reperfusion have a higher in-hospital mortality than those whose arteries remain open, but identification of patients at risk for early reocclusion is not possible at present. Finally, the potential benefits of nonacute reopening of occluded arteries to enhance recovery of "stunned" myocardium or to enhance ventricular remodeling are under investigation.

Suggested Reading

Ross J, Gilpin EA, Madsen EB, et al. A decision schema for coronary angiography after acute myocardial infarction. Circulation 1989; 79:292.

TIMI Study Group. Comparison of invasive and conservative strategies after treatment with intravenous tissue plasminogen activator in acute myocardial infarction: Results of the thrombolysis in myocardial infarction (TIMI) phase II trial. N Engl J Med 1989; 320:618.

RIGHT VENTRICULAR INFARCTION

Louis J. Dell'Italia, M.D.

Right ventricular myocardial infarction occurs after occlusion of a dominant right coronary artery in the clinical setting of acute inferoposterior myocardial infarction. When extensive infarction of the right ventricle is present, the patient may present with a unique combination of clinical findings, including hypotension, an elevated jugular venous pressure, and clear lung fields. However, not all right coronary artery occlusions result in significant right ventricular necrosis and dysfunction. Nevertheless, when predominant right ventricular infarction occurs, the clinical sequelae require a unique form of therapy clearly distinct from that of hypotension associated with predominant infarction of the left ventricle.

Prompt clinical recognition of acute right ventricular myocardial infarction in patients is extremely important because appropriate therapy of hypotension and shock oftentimes must be started before performance of invasive hemodynamic monitoring or noninvasive tests. In an evaluation of 53 consecutive patients with acute inferior myocardial infarction (MI) within 36 hours of the onset of symptoms, physical examination findings of both an elevated jugular venous pressure (≥ 8 cm H_2O) and Kussmaul's sign were sensitive (88 percent) and specific (100 percent) markers for identifying hemodynamically important right ventricular myocardial infarction (Dell'Italia and co-workers, 1983). These findings provided accurate clinical markers of significant right ventricular dysfunction when compared with subsequent hemodynamics obtained from right-heart catheterization. Therefore, the physical examination provides an important initial guide for appropriate therapy of patients who present with acute inferior wall MI.

The hemodynamic markers of right ventricular myocardial infarction include a low cardiac output and a disproportionate elevation of the right atrial pressure (RAP) compared to the pulmonary arterial wedge pressure (PAWP) (Lopez-Sendon and co-workers, (1981). Any patient with an acute inferior wall MI should be suspected of having right ventricular dysfunction; however, less than 10 percent of these patients suffer from hypotension and shock. Data from clinical studies demonstrate that patients with right ventricular myocardial infarction may present with a spectrum of hemodynamic findings that are best summarized as follows (Lopez-Sendon and co-workers, 1981):

- RAP $\geq$ 10 mm Hg and RAP:PAW ratio > 0.8 and SAP* <100 mm Hg

---

*SAP, systolic arterial pressure.

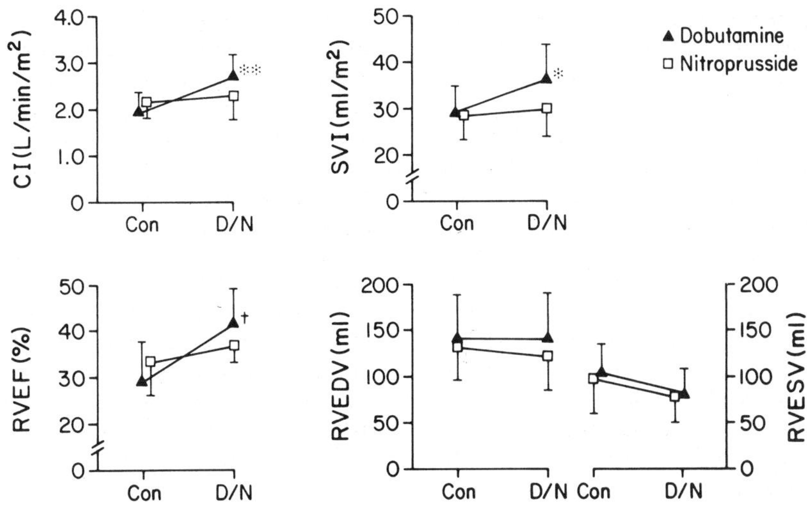

Figure 1
Results of two-way analysis of variance comparing the effects of dobutamine (D) and nitroprusside (N) therapy on cardiac index (CI), stroke volume index (SVI), right ventricular ejection fraction (RVEF), right ventricular end-diastolic volume (RVEDV), and right ventricular end-systolic volume (RVESV). Significant differences are noted as follows: $^{**}p < .001$; $^{*}p = .02$; $^{\dagger}p < .01$. *(From Dell'Italia LJ, Starling MR, Blumhardt R, et al. Comparative effects of volume loading, dobutamine and nitroprusside in patients with predominant right ventricular infarction. Circulation 1985; 72:1330; with permission of the American Heart Association and author.)*

- RAP ≥ 10 mm Hg and RAP:PAW > 0.8 and SAP > 100 mm Hg
- RAP ≥ 10 mm Hg and RAP:PAW > 0.8 only after volume loading, with or without hypotension
- RAP ≥ 10 mm Hg and RAP:PAW < 0.8 due to marked elevation of the PAW and greater amount of left ventricular damage

In a study of 53 consecutive patients with inferior MI, we demonstrated that approximately 25 percent of patients exhibited these hemodynamic patterns. Therefore, the majority of patients do not present with hemodynamic or physical examination findings of significant right ventricular dysfunction (Dell'Italia and co-workers, 1984). Other noninvasive means of diagnosing right ventricular myocardial infarction include electrocardiography (V_4R lead), echocardiography, and radionuclide angiography. Each of these tests is highly sensitive and specific for documenting right ventricular ischemia or necrosis given proper criteria (Dell'Italia and co-workers, 1984). However, careful examination of the jugular venous pressure provides the most expedient initial guide for appropriate therapy in patients who present with hypotension or shock.

■ THERAPEUTIC ALTERNATIVES

The goals of therapy are to reverse hypotension or shock and to restore circulatory stability. Volume loading has been the mainstay of therapy; however, a number of clinical studies have demonstrated that volume infusion does not uniformly produce an increase in cardiac output when given to patients who present with the hemodynamic criteria of right ventricular myocardial infarction (Dell'Italia and co-workers, 1985). Other therapeutic alternatives include inotropic agents to improve cardiac output and systemic arterial pressure or afterload reducing agents in addition to volume to improve right ventricular forward stroke volume. To determine the relative efficacy of inotropic therapy or afterload reduction as adjunctive therapy to volume infusion, the effects of dobutamine and nitroprusside were studied in 13 patients with right ventricular myocardial infarction after volume loading with normal saline (Dell'Italia and co-workers, 1985). Dobutamine produced a statistically significant increase in cardiac index, stroke volume index, and right ventricular ejection fraction when compared with nitroprusside (Fig. 1). From this study, it was concluded that nitroprusside deleteriously decreased preload so that right ventricular stroke volume was unchanged, whereas dobutamine maintained preload and augmented systolic performance, resulting in an increase in stroke output. Other studies have reported improvement in cardiac index and mean arterial pressure after atrioventricular sequential pacing in patients with right ventricular myocardial infarction. These studies demonstrate the salutary effect of atrial contraction to both ventricular filling and stroke volume in the setting of acute MI. This form of therapy may be beneficial to those patients who manifest persistent hypotension and high-grade atrioventricular block despite maximal therapy with inotropic agents and volume infusion.

The pathophysiologic mechanisms that produce hypotension include decreased right ventricular systolic performance and ventricular interdependence. The role of ventricular interdependence in the genesis of the low cardiac output state is nicely demonstrated in a closed-pericardial canine model of right ventricular myocardial infarction (Goldstein and co-workers, 1982). Right coronary artery occlusion produced typical right ventricular myocardial infarction hemodynamics: (1) elevation and equalization of right-sided and left-sided filling pressures; (2) increase in right ventricular cavity size and decrease in left ventricular end-diastolic size; and (3) decrease in cardiac output. Subsequent volume loading increased the left ventricular end-diastolic pressure from 7 to 12 mm Hg, resulting in minimal change in left ventricular cavity size, an increase in right ventricular cavity size, and a small increase in cardiac output. However, after the pericardium was removed, equalization of right and left ventricular filling pressures resolved, left ventricular end-diastolic pressure decreased as diastolic cavity size increased, and cardiac output increased significantly. Thus, despite a significant increase in left ventricular end-diastolic pressure after volume, the true distending pressure of the left ventricle was diminished due to an increased pericardial pressure. These findings in the animal laboratory corroborate the clinical studies that demonstrate that volume infusion does not uniformly produce an increase in cardiac output when given to patients who present with hemodynamic criteria of right ventricular myocardial infarction. This finding is explained by the mechanism of ventricular interaction whereby acute enlargement of the right ventricle within a fixed intrapericardial space encroaches on the left ventricle and impairs left ventricular filling.

Acute right ventricular ischemia or infarction results in decreased stroke output of the right ventricle. Stroke output from the normal right ventricle results from contraction of the right ventricular free wall, conus, and interventricular septum. Studies in animal models and in humans demonstrate that the severity of hypotension is related to the extent of decreased shortening in each of these three areas. Radionuclide angiographic studies in patients with acute right ventricular myocardial infarction demonstrate that the conus or outflow tract is relatively preserved in most patients with right ventricular MI (Dell'Italia and co-workers, 1985). Preserved function in this region results from the unique anatomy of the conus artery, which protects it from occlusion. In 40 percent of cases, it arises as a separate origin from the aorta; in the remainder of cases, it arises as an early branch off the right coronary artery. In addition to the role of systolic performance of the right ventricle, recent data in patients (Goldstein and co-workers, 1990) and in an animal model (Goldstein and co-workers, 1991) demonstrate the importance of ischemic depression of right atrial contractility in the depression of cardiac output in the setting of acute right ventricular myocardial infarction. The finding of an augmented A wave (atrial systolic contraction) on the right atrial pressure wave form, as opposed to a depressed A wave, identified those patients with significantly higher right ventricular pressures, better cardiac output, more favorable response to volume and inotropic therapy, and less frequent shock.

■ PREFERRED APPROACH

In the approach to the patient who presents with an acute inferior MI, one should assume that all patients have the potential to present with or to develop significant right ventricular dysfunction. However, only a small percentage of these patients (< 10 percent) present with hypotension or cardiogenic shock initially. Diagnosis of this condition is essential for proper management, and the initial data base should provide one with enough information to proceed with appropriate therapy. Other clinical conditions that may simulate this pattern include pulmonary embolism and cardiac tamponade. The finding of electrocardiographic evidence of acute inferior MI along with elevation of the jugular venous pressure, Kussmaul's sign, clear lung fields, and a chest film that demonstrates a normal pulmonary venous pattern and a normal or nearly normal cardiac silhouette are all consistent with acute right ventricular myocardial infarction. However, as outlined in the hemodynamic subsets, patients presenting with inferior MI may present with a normal jugular venous pressure and hypotension with right ventricular ischemia or infarction. This presentation results from increased venous capacitance due to high vagal tone and/or relative volume depletion due to nausea and vomiting. In this subset of patients a volume infusion (300 to 500 ml normal saline over 10 minutes) augments right ventricular preload (jugular venous pressure) and may quickly improve systemic arterial pressure.

In the patient who presents with acute right ventricular myocardial infarction and hypotension, immediate therapy should be aimed at increasing the mean arterial pressure to above 70 mm Hg. A rapid infusion of normal saline of 300 to 500 ml over approximately 10 to 15 minutes should be instituted through a central line or through a large-bore peripheral intravenous site. In our experience we have found that this initial therapy increases both right and left heart filling pressures and may improve cardiac output and systemic arterial pressure in some patients initially. If this initial infusion does not improve arterial pressure, further volume infusion will not improve arterial pressure because the acutely dilated right ventricle prevents adequate left ventricular filling. Therefore, therapy with an inotropic agent is necessary to improve left ventricular filling by augmenting right ventricular systolic function and decreasing right ventricular distention.

In patients who present with hypotension (SAP < 100 mm Hg), dobutamine is the drug of choice after a volume infusion has failed to improve mean arterial pressure above 70 mm Hg. In our study, dobutamine produced a significant improvement in stroke volume index and maintained SAP while decreasing systemic vascular resistance. These effects were accomplished in doses ranging between 5 and 15 μg per kilogram per minute. In the patient without a Swan-Ganz catheter in place, peak effect is achieved when systemic arterial pressure rises above baseline to achieve a mean pressure greater than 70 mm Hg. This effect should be achieved with less than a 10 percent increase in heart rate and may restore atrioventricular synchrony in patients presenting with atrioventricular block. There are a few complications of therapy. In those patients who have predominant right ventricular infarction resulting from an occlusion of the right coronary artery in addition to having significant disease of the left anterior descending artery or circumflex artery, treatment with an inotropic agent may precipitate angina in the nondilated left ventricle. Therefore, the assessment of therapeutic response must be emphasized because the primary goal should be improvement of systemic arterial pressure. Further increases in the dose of inotropes may only exacerbate an imbalance of myocardial oxygen supply and demand by increasing inotropy and heart rate and thereby precipitate angina.

In the patient who presents with cardiogenic shock or is unresponsive to more than 20 μg per kilogram per minute of dobutamine, dopamine is the drug of choice because it has significantly greater alpha-constrictive effects than dobutamine. Starting doses should range between 3 and 5 μg per kilogram per minute, and the dose should be increased until the desired systemic arterial pressure is achieved. Because dopamine has greater chronotropic effects than dobutamine, its use may result in untoward increases in heart rate, which may further exacerbate angina.

Usually these methods restore systemic arterial pressure in most patients who present with hemodynamically important right ventricular myocardial infarction. However, some patients may present with hemodynamically important right ventricular myocardial infarction and pulmonary venous congestion resulting from significant left ventricular dysfunction due to a previous anterior MI or significant ischemia in the distribution of the left anterior descending artery. In our experience, these patients have significant ST-segment depression in the anterior precordial leads that is disproportionate to the amount of ST-segment elevation in the inferior limb leads (Dell'Italia and co-workers, 1987). These patients require inotropic support to improve both right and left ventricular systolic function. In addition, intravenous nitroglycerin must be utilized to improve coronary blood flow and decrease pulmonary venous congestion. However, dosage should be adjusted carefully so that a decrease in right ventricular preload does not precipitate hypotension. Treatment of such patients should include Swan-Ganz catheterization as a therapeutic guide to maintain right- and left-heart filling pressures at levels that produce optimal cardiac index and systemic arterial pressure. These patients represent the highest risk acutely and should undergo early cardiac catheterization to define coronary anatomy and ventricular function for potential surgery or percutaneous transluminal angioplasty (Dell'Italia and co-workers, 1987).

Complications of right ventricular myocardial infarction may preclude achieving an optimal hemodynamic status with volume infusion and inotropic support. Severe hypoxemia and arterial desaturation may result from right-to-left shunting across an atrial septal defect or patent foramen ovale. Diagnosis may be confirmed by using current color-flow Doppler echocardiographic technique at the bedside. In this situation surgical correction of the shunt is indicated because prolonged therapy with high-percentage oxygen results in pulmonary toxicity. The differential diagnosis of hypoxemia in the patient who presents with hemodynamically important right ventricular myocardial infarction must include pulmonary embolism because right ventricular thrombus is a potential source for pulmonary emboli. Perfusion scanning of the lung with macroaggregated albumin may be used in the diagnosis of acute pulmonary embolism and is also a very sensitive technique for detection of intracardiac shunting across a patent foramen ovale manifested by uptake of radionuclide in the brain, thyroid, and kidneys. If pulmonary embolism is documented, therapy with intravenous heparin should be instituted.

Rupture of the intraventricular septum may be manifested by a new systolic murmur auscultated along the lower left sternal border and must be differentiated from murmurs of tricuspid regurgitation and mitral regurgitation resulting from posterior papillary muscle dysfunction. Again, a bedside Doppler echocardiographic study is very helpful in distinguishing each of these cardiac complications. The timing of surgery in this condition should be determined by the patient's hemodynamic status, as in the routine treatment of ventricular septal defect associated with acute MI. However, several surgical series have reported that acute and perioperative mortality may be determined by the severity of right ventricular dysfunction.

Suggested Reading

Dell'Italia LJ, Lembo NJ, Starling MR, et al. Hemodynamically important right ventricular infarction: Follow-up evaluation of right ventricular systolic function at rest and during exercise with radionuclide ventriculography and respiratory gas exchange. Circulation 1987; 75:996.

Dell'Italia LJ, Starling MR, Blumhardt R, et al. Comparative effects of volume loading, dobutamine and nitroprusside in patients with predominant right ventricular infarction. Circulation 1985; 72:1327.

Dell'Italia LJ, Starling MR, Crawford MH, et al. Right ventricular infarction: Identification by hemodynamic measurements before and after volume loading and correlation with noninvasive techniques. J Am Coll Cardiol 1984; 4:931.

Dell'Italia LJ, Starling MR, O'Rourke RA. Physical examination for exclusion of hemodynamically important right ventricular infarction. Ann Intern Med 1983; 99:608.

Goldstein JA, Barzilai B, Rosamond TL, et al. Determinants of hemodynamic compromise with severe right ventricular infarction. Circulation 1990; 82:359.

Goldstein JA, Tweddell JS, Barzilai B, et al. Right atrial ischemia exacerbates hemodynamic compromise associated with experimental right ventricular dysfunction. J Am Coll Cardiol 1991; 18:1564.

Goldstein JA, Vlahakes GJ, Verrier ED, et al. The role of right ventricular systolic dysfunction and elevated intrapericardial pressure in the genesis of low output in experimental right ventricular infarction. Circulation 1982; 65:513.

Lopez-Sendon J, Coma-Canella L, Gamallo C. Sensitivity and specificity of hemodynamic criteria in the diagnosis of acute right ventricular infarction. Circulation 1981; 64:515.

CARDIAC ARRHYTHMIAS FOLLOWING MYOCARDIAL INFARCTION

Kenneth M. Kessler, M.D.

Cardiac arrhythmias are common following acute myocardial infarction (Table 1). Mechanisms include increased automaticity, re-entry related to focal conduction slowing or inhomogenous refractoriness, and enhanced sympathetic and parasympathetic tone. Approaches to therapy depend on the presence or absence of symptoms and whether the arrhythmia occurs in the early phase (first 72 hours) or recovery phase of the infarction process. The acute goal of therapy is usually hemodynamic stabilization, whereas long-range therapy often relates to the more elusive end point of improving survival. For additional information on the treatment of arrhythmias, see the section on Cardiac Arrhythmias.

■ THERAPEUTIC ALTERNATIVES

Symptomatic arrhythmias deserve prompt treatment (Fig. 1). Symptoms may be overt and include syncope, hypotension, angina, and heart failure. However, symptoms of hypoperfusion may be more occult and include clouding of the sensorium, coolness of the skin, and decreased urinary output. An arrhythmia must not be considered to be well tolerated simply because the patient has normal blood pressure. The arrhythmia per se, the signs of tissue perfusion, and the general condition of the patient must be considered when determining the need for, and urgency of, treatment. Symptomatic tachyarrhythmias almost always deserve prompt electrical conversion (alternative initial strategies may be indicated in the rare cases of digitalis toxicity). Symptomatic bradyarrhythmias require rate support and are best approached in a logical sequence: atropine, external pacemaker, and temporary transvenous pacemaker. The goal of therapy of early symptomatic arrhythmias is the restoration of normal circulatory function. In treating chronic asymptomatic arrhythmias, the direction of therapy is often preventive, and solid therapeutic information is often lacking. In general, the treatment of arrhythmias can be approached using a hierarchy of therapies (Table 2). In each case the physician should be thoroughly aware of the indications, dosage, and contraindications of therapy. The following sections may serve as a guide to such treatment.

Table 1 Cardiac Arrhythmias

Persistent, early tachyarrhythmias
Sinus tachycardia
Atrial flutter and fibrillation
Ventricular tachycardia and fibrillation
Persistent, early bradycardias
Sinus bradycardia
Atrioventricular conduction disturbances and block
Transient, early arrhythmias
Atrial arrhythmias
Accelerated atrioventricular junctional rhythms
Accelerated idioventricular rhythm
Torsades de pointes
Ventricular premature complexes
Reperfusion arrhythmias
Late arrhythmias
Ventricular tachycardia and fibrillation
Nonsustained ventricular tachycardia
Premature ventricular complexes

■ PREFERRED APPROACH

Persistent, Early Tachyarrhythmias

In general, acute tachyarrhythmias are best treated by prompt cardioversion or defibrillation. Hemodynamic instability caused by such arrhythmias is not tolerated in the acute ischemic setting. Hesitation is justified only in the case of digoxin toxicity, in which correction of hypokalemia and other metabolic factors and the use of intravenous lidocaine, intravenous phenytoin, digitalis antibodies, or a combination of therapies are preferred. Cardioversion in the clinical setting of digitalis toxicity may lead to irreversible ventricular fibrillation.

Sinus tachycardia often accompanies acute myocardial infarction. Therapy must first address aggravating conditions, including hypoperfusion, heart failure, pain, fever, anxiety, pericarditis, and pulmonary embolus. When the sinus rate is increased disproportionally and is not compensatory to a low cardiac output, beta-adrenergic blocking agents can lower heart rate and improve myocardial oxygen utilization. Metoprolol in standard dosage is often adequate (Table 3). Esmolol has the advantage of being short-acting (Table 3), although if heart failure or bronchospasm is precipitated, it may persist beyond the half-life of the drug. Beta-adrenergic blocking agents should be avoided in patients with overt heart failure or bronchospasm or in those in whom sympathetic support is required to maintain perfusion. When fever is a contributory factor to sinus tachycardia, suppression of fever with an antipyretic such as acetaminophen is indicated after the possibility of infection is evaluated. Drugs with positive chronotropic effects, e.g., theophylline or vasodilators, which promote reflex tachycardia, should be avoided when possible (Table 4).

Atrial flutter and atrial fibrillation may occur as the consequences of atrial hypertension, sinus node ischemia, or pericarditis. The ventricular response is often uncontrolled, and an increase in myocardial oxygen demand resulting in further hemodynamic impairment may occur. Atrial flutter is often drug resistant and is usually best treated with cardioversion. Although 25 to 50 joules may be successful, 102 joules is almost always successful and is not harmful. Digitalis, beta-adrenergic blocking agents, verapamil, or diltiazem may be used to increase atrioventricular block and thereby slow the ventricular response in less urgent cases or if repeated cardioversion fails. Digitalis has the disadvantage of a relatively slow onset of action, and atrial flutter is often resistant to digitalis. Beta-adrenergic blocking agents should be used cautiously and avoided in overt heart failure because they worsen the failure if the arrhythmia is not controlled adequately. Esmolol has the advantage of a rapid onset and offset of action. Verapamil or diltiazem can slow the rate and at times aid in the maintenance of sinus rhythm; however, negative inotropic and peripheral vasodilatory effects may be disadvantageous. Drugs that enhance atrioventricular conduction, such as lidocaine and quinidine, are contraindicated in initial management.

Atrial fibrillation is not uncommon in the early phases of acute myocardial infarction. Heart failure that may be independent of the arrhythmia may be evident and must be addressed separately. Drugs that block the atrioventricular node such as digitalis, beta-adrenergic blocking agents, verapamil or diltiazem are more efficacious for treatment of atrial fibrillation than for atrial flutter. However, the same cautions hold (see previously), and the unstable patient should be cardioverted. Cardioversion should commence with low energy levels, e.g., 25 to 50 joules; however, higher levels are often needed. Care should be taken to avoid cardioversion in patients with digitalis excess. Atrial fibrillation with a wide QRS complex may be confused with ventricular tachycardia. If lidocaine is administered to such patients, an alarming increase in ventricular response due to enhanced atrioventricular conduction may occur. Calcium channel and beta-adrenergic blocking agents have additive negative chronotropic and negative inotropic actions; their simultaneous intravenous use is discouraged.

Ventricular tachycardia and ventricular fibrillation occur commonly in the acute phase of myocardial infarction, in which they are life threatening, may be accompanied by an increased in-hospital mortality, but paradoxically do not necessarily indicate an increased risk of mortality after hospital discharge. Ventricular tachycardia may occur intermittently, in which case control of ischemia including the use of beta-adrenergic blocking agents and antiarrhythmic therapy using lidocaine, procainamide, bretylium, or a combination of agents (see later in this article) are addressed simultaneously. In rare cases, intermittent arrhythmias are related to spasm associated with ST-segment elevation; this situation is treated with nitrates and cautious administration of calcium channel blocking agents. Symptomatic, sustained ventricular tachycardia is best treated with cardioversion beginning at low energy levels, e.g., 25 joules; increased energies are used as needed. Lidocaine can be considered as primary therapy for ventricular tachycardia in awake patients who are hemodynamically stable. Ischemia and contributory factors, especially hypokalemia, are meticulously explored and corrected. Ventricular fibrillation requires immediate electrical defibrillation: 300 to 400 joules may be needed, although repeated lower-energy shocks (e.g., 100 to 200 joules) may be effective and are preferred by some to prevent the adverse effects of high energies.

Table 2 Hierarchy of Treatment Modalities*

No treatment: Preferred whenever medically sound
Alleviate aggravating factors: Treat ischemia, hypotension, heart failure, hypoxemia, hypokalemia, anemia, drug side effects, and other conditions
Modulate sympathetic or parasympathetic tone: Beta-adrenergic blocking agents or atropine are simple and relatively safe
Electrons: Pacing, cardioversion, and defibrillation are relatively safe and potentially life-saving procedures
Antiarrhythmic drugs: Because of the side effects and proarrhythmic potential of all the group I, III, and some group IV antiarrhythmic agents, they should be used with caution
Implantable devices and antiarrhythmic surgery: Because of the necessity for invasion, these are listed last, although in given circumstances these modalities may become the approach of choice

*Least to most potential for side effects

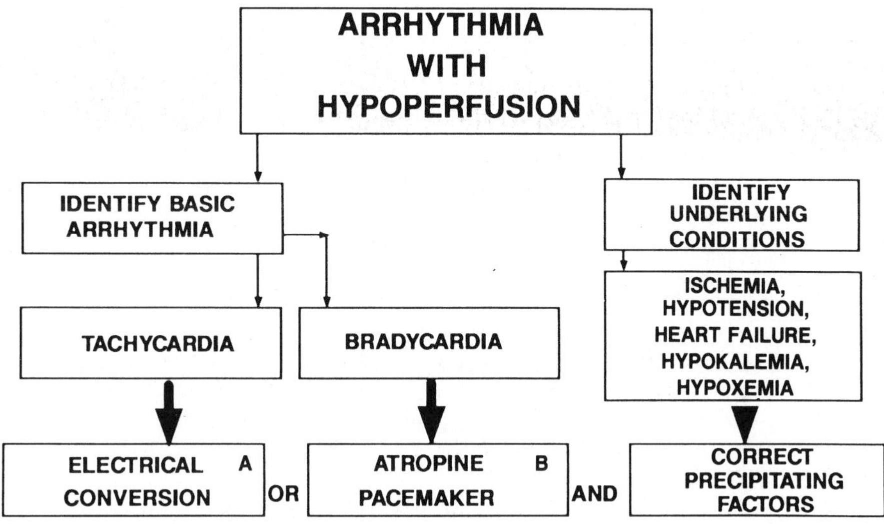

Figure 1
Simplified approach to the treatment of arrhythmias associated with signs of hypoperfusion. *A,* Electrical conversion should be avoided in arrhythmias associated with digitalis toxicity. *B,* Underdosing with atropine may induce a paradoxical bradycardia.

Table 3 Antiarrhythmic Drug Dosage and Kinetics*

	USUAL DOSING RANGE	HALF-LIFE (H)	THERAPEUTIC RANGE (μG/ML)	MAJOR ROUTE OF EXCRETION
CLASS IA				
Quinidine (Quinaglute, Quinidex)	Oral sulfate: 200–600 mg q6h	5–7	2.3–5	H
	Oral long-acting: 330–660 mg q8h or q6h			
Procainamide (Pronestyl, Procan SR)	Oral: 250–750 mg q4h or q6h	3–5	4–10	R
	Oral long-acting: 500–1500 q8h or q6h			
	IV: 10–15 mg/kg at 25 mg/min; then 1–6 mg/min			
Disopyramide (Norpace)	Oral: 100–200 mg q8h or q6h	8–9	2–5	H/R
Moricizine (Ethmozine)†	Oral: 150–300 mg q12h or q8h	6–13	—	H
CLASS IB				
Lidocaine (Xylocaine)	IV: 1–3 mg/kg at 20–50 mg/min; then 1–4 mg/min	1–2	1–5	H
Tocainide (Tonocard)	Oral: 400–600 q8–12h	15	4–10	H
Mexiletine (Mexitil)	Oral: 200–400 mg q8h	10–12	0.5–2	H
CLASS IC				
Flecainide (Tambocor)	Oral: 100–200 mg q12h	20	.02–1	H
Propafenone (Rythmol)	Oral: 150–300 mg q8h	2–10‡	0.5–1.5‡	H
CLASS II				
Propranolol (Inderal)	Oral: 10–100 mg q6h	4–6	0.04–0.1	H
	IV: 0.1 mg/kg in divided 1 mg doses			
Esmolol (Brevibloc)	IV/ 500 mg/kg/min for 1 min, followed by 50 mg/kg/min for 4 min. Repeat with 50 mg increments to maintenance dose of 200 mg/kg/min	9 min	—	H
Metoprolol (Lopressor)	Oral: 50–200 mg b.i.d.	3–4	0.5–0.1	H
	IV: (dosing for acute MI with careful monitoring) 5 mg q 2 min × 3; if tolerated 50 mg q6 × 48h then 100 mg b.i.d.			
Acebutolol (Sectral)	Oral: 200–600 mg b.i.d.	3–4	—	H/R
CLASS III				
Amiodarone (Cordarone)	Oral: 800–1,600 mg/day × 1–3 weeks; then 600–800/day × 2–4 weeks; then 200–400 mg/day	50 days	1–2.5	H
	IV: loading: 150 mg at 15 mg/min, then 360 mg at 1 mg/min			
	Maintenance: 540 mg at 0.5 mg/min			
Bretylium (Bretylol)	IV: 5–10 mg/kg at 1–2 mg/kg/min; then 0.5–2.0 mg/min	8–14	0.5–1.5	R
CLASS IV				
Verapamil (Isoptin, Calan)	Oral: 80–120 mg q6–8h	3–8	0.1–0.15	H
Diltiazem (Cardizem)	IV: 0.25 mg/kg over 2 min, at 15 min if needed 0.35 mg/kg over 2 min followed by an infusion at 10–15 mg/h	3.4	—	H
OTHER				
Digoxin (Lanoxin)	Oral: 1.25–1.5 mg in divided doses over 24 hours, followed by 0.125–0.375 mg/day	36	0.8–1.4 (ng/ml)	R
	IV: approximately 70% of oral dose			
Adenosine (Adenocard)	IV: 6 mg rapidly; if unsuccessful in 1–2 min, 12 mg rapidly	10 sec	—	—

*All dosing should follow Food and Drug Administration approved guidelines as outlined in package insert or *Physician's Desk Reference.*
†Also classified variably as IC or mixed IA and IB agent.
‡Active metabolites and genetic differences in metabolic rates limit the significance of these measurements.
H, hepatic; R, renal; MI, myocardial infarction.
Modified from Myerburg RJ, Kessler KM. Clinical assessment and management of arrhythmias and conduction disturbances. In: Hurst JW, ed. The heart. 7th ed. New York: McGraw-Hill, 1990:538; with permission.

Table 4 Antiarrhythmic Drug Interactions and Side Effects

	SELECTED DRUG INTERACTIONS	SELECTED SIDE EFFECTS	CAUTIONS		
			QTC	CHF	SN/AVN
CLASS IA					
Quinidine	Amiodarone, cimetidine, coumarin anticoagulants, digoxin, verapamil	Nausea, diarrhea, cinchonism, thrombocytopenia, hemolytic anemia	***		
Procainamide	Cimetidine, trimethoprim-sulfamethoxazole	Rash, fever, lupus syndrome, agranulocytosis	**		
Disopyramide	Cimetidine, hepatic enzyme inducers	Blurred vision, dry mouth, constipation, urinary retention	**	***	
Moricizine	Cimetidine	Tremor, dizziness, gastrointestinal upset			
CLASS IB					
Lidocaine	Cimetidine, halothane, propranolol	Drowsiness, hallucinations, seizures, hypotension, respiratory arrest			
Tocainide	—	Paresthesias, ataxia, tremor, hematologic abnormalities			
Mexiletine	Hepatic enzyme inducers	Gastrointestinal upset, liver dysfunction			
CLASS IC					
Flecainide	Amiodarone, cimetidine			***	**
Propafenone	Digoxin	Dizziness, gastrointestinal upset, bronchospasm		*	**
CLASS II					
Propranolol	Cimetidine, lidocaine, indomethacin, NSAID	Depression, fatigue, bronchospasm, heart failure, bradycardia		***	***
Esmolol	—	Depression, fatigue, bronchospasm, heart failure, bradycardia		***	***
Metoprolol	Verapamil, cimetidine	Depression, fatigue, bronchospasm, heart failure, bradycardia		***	***
Acebutolol	Procainamide, hydralazine, captopril	Depression, fatigue, bronchospasm, heart failure, bradycardia		***	***
CLASS III					
Amiodarone	Quinidine, procainamide	Multiple	**		
Bretylium	—	Transient hypertension, postural hypotension, nausea			
CLASS IV					
Verapamil	Cimetidine, digoxin, prazosin, quinidine, theophylline	Constipation, bradycardia, heart failure		***	***
Diltiazem	Cimetidine, cyclosporine, digoxin, flecainide, beta-adrenergic blocking agents	Hypotension, flushing		**	***
OTHER					
Digoxin	Antacids, erythromycin, tetracycline, cholestyramine, amiodarone, captopril, diltiazem, nifedipine, prazosin, propafenone, quinidine, verapamil	Anorexia, nausea, vomiting, neurologic symptoms, cardiac arrhythmias, gynecomastia			**
Adenosine	Dipyridamole, methylxanthines	Transient flushing, dyspnea, chest pain			**

QTc, avoid or use cautiously with other agents that prolong QTc.
CHF (congestive heart failure), negative inotrope; use with caution, if at all, in combination with other negative inotropic agents.
SN/AVN (sinus node/atrioventricular node), negative chronotrope; use with caution with other drugs that depress sinoatrial or atrioventricular nodal activity.
*, **, *** denote increasing need for caution.
NSAID, nonsteroidal anti-inflammatory drug.

Recurrences are common; close monitoring and antiarrhythmic medications are indicated to prevent further events. Antiarrhythmic medications often begin with lidocaine; a variety of regimens have been recommended. Lidocaine may be administered as a 75 mg bolus over 3 to 5 minutes, followed by a 50 mg bolus over 2 to 3 minutes at 15 minutes; if needed, 50 mg is administered again at 30 minutes. A 2 to 4 mg per minute drip is initiated after the first bolus. A decreased loading dose, given more slowly, is recommended in elderly patients or when the volume of distribution of lidocaine is known to be decreased, as in patients with heart failure or shock. Both lidocaine levels and lidocaine binding increase during acute myocardial infarction, probably rendering free drug form constant and obviating the need to taper dosing routinely for this reason alone. If lidocaine is ineffective, procainamide can be given intravenously. A commonly used regimen is a loading dose of 750 to 1,000 mg administered at 25 mg per minute, followed by a 3 to 4 mg per minute drip. Hypotension may occur but most often responds to leg-up positioning and fluids. If symptomatic ventricular arrhythmias remain troublesome, 5 to 10 mg per kilogram of bretylium may be given intravenously at a rate of 1 to 2 mg per kilogram per minute and may be followed with a drip at 0.5 to 2.0 mg per minute. These three drugs have additive vasodilatory effects; hypotension caused by these drugs may be accentuated by other antiarrhythmic and anti-ischemic therapies and by volume depletion, especially that associated with chronic diuretic therapy. The decision to discontinue bretylium after 24 hours of rhythm control may be appropriate, but the patient should be carefully monitored for the return of aggressive arrhythmias. Beta-adrenergic blocking agents are being used more routinely for the control of ischemia, antiarrhythmic effects and to improve the short- and long-term prognosis. Overdrive pacing has a role in patients with resistant ventricular arrhythmias. Verapamil is to be avoided in wide complex tachycardias: It is not generally efficacious for ventricular tachycardia, it can cause hemodynamic instability, and deaths have been reported.

Persistent, Early Bradyarrhythmias

Sinus bradycardia may be related to enhanced vagal tone, ischemia, and medications (including beta-adrenergic blocking agents and calcium channel blocking agents). Although bradycardia is relatively protective in the ischemic setting, overt and occult signs of hypoperfusion may occur, especially when rates fall into the 40s. Slower rates with hemodynamic impairment may also foster ventricular ectopy or allow the expression of accelerated idioventricular rhythms (see subsequently). Although most episodes of sinus bradycardia are asymptomatic, symptoms of hypoperfusion and the emergence of significant ventricular ectopy are indications for treatment. Atropine sulfate 0.4 to 0.6 mg may be given intravenously and repeated. Doses above 1.5 to 2 mg rarely add to the effectiveness. Small doses of atropine, 0.1 to 0.3 mg, should be avoided because these doses parodoxically may slow the heart rate. Atropine may be ineffective or, at times, too effective, with unacceptable increases in heart rate. Its effects are of uncertain duration. Most often, more reliable, longer-term rate control is needed, and a temporary transvenous pacemaker is inserted. External pacing may be used as a temporary procedure. In borderline situations a bedside external pacing unit on standby is helpful. It is important to identify the fact that the primary rhythm problem is a bradycardia and to treat it as such because treatment of bradycardia-aggravated ventricular ectopy with antiarrhythmic agents may slow the underlying rhythm and actually worsen the problem. Volume and mechanical issues as well as ongoing ischemia should be addressed simultaneously.

Atrioventricular conduction disturbances and block are noted commonly during the course of acute myocardial infarction, and the treatment varies as a function of the site of infarction. Progressive conduction disturbances may occur with inferior wall infarction, and when symptomatic, the institution of atropine, external pacing, temporary transvenous pacing, or a combination of modalities is indicated. Most often the escape pacemaker shows a relatively normal QRS complex at a rate of 40 to 60 beats per minute, and the patient remains asymptomatic. Block often improves in hours to days, and permanent pacing is rarely needed. With anterior wall infarction, heart block usually denotes extensive necrosis. Escape pacemakers are often lower and consequently slower, with resultant symptoms. Treatment with atropine is often less successful for block associated with anterior wall infarction than for block associated with inferior wall infarction, and temporary transvenous pacing and meticulous attention to mechanical factors are indicated. Because of the rapid progression to complete heart block, prophylactic pacing has been advocated for new right bundle branch block associated with hemiblock, new left bundle branch block, or Mobitz type II second-degree heart block. The indication for pacing new right bundle branch block with first-degree atrioventricular block, alternating bundle branch block or pre-existing left bundle branch block is debatable. Permanent pacing is recommended for those patients with anteroseptal myocardial infarction who manifest complete heart block or Mobitz type II block, even if these conduction disturbances are transient. The benefits of these pacing recommendations are clouded by the high mortality of such patients as a result of pump failure.

Transient, Early Arrhythmias

Atrial arrhythmias including premature atrial depolarizations, sinus node dysfunction, and atrial tachycardias are often transient and are best treated by optimizing the hemodynamic and metabolic milieu. When a dominant symptomatic rhythm is noted, therapy is indicated. Rapid supraventricular tachycardias are best treated with cardioversion (carotid sinus massage may precipitate untoward bradycardia on conversion in the acute infarction setting). Tachycardia-bradycardia symptoms are best treated by the combined use of pacing (to treat underlying and drug-induced bradycardia) and antiarrhythmic drugs (directed to the treatment of the atrial tachyarrhythmias).

Accelerated atrioventricular junctional rhythms generally are noted in inferior wall infarction when sinus node depression is coupled with increased automaticity of the junction. The patient is often asymptomatic because the rate is often at the lower side of the 60 to 100 beats per minute range. Occasionally symptoms are noted because of inadequate rate or loss of synchronized atrial contraction. In such cases, atropine or the more reliable approach of temporary transvenous pacing (including the option of dual chamber pacing) may be helpful. If symptoms are due to an increased rate (especially in anterior infarction, in which this rhythm is associated with an excess mortality), class I antiarrhythmic drugs may be tried, but their efficacy may be marginal and caution should be used. Digitalis, propranolol, and verapamil are other options. Elements of left and right ventricular dysfunction should be addressed, and digitalis toxicity, another cause for this arrhythmia, should be excluded.

Accelerated idioventricular rhythms, or so-called slow ventricular tachycardia, may appear intermittently during the early course of myocardial infarction particularly involving the inferior wall. Most often the rate is controlled, the rhythm transiently appears and disappears often as a function of the underlying sinus bradycardia and sinus arrhythmia, and the patient is asymptomatic. Such rhythms are best carefully observed but left untreated. In fact, treatment with antiarrhythmic agents may further suppress pacemaker function and lead to potentially deleterious vasodilation and left ventricular dysfunction. Most often when symptoms occur they relate to a slow rate or lack of synchronized atrial contraction. Treatment is directed to speeding the heart rate by the use of atropine or transvenous pacing (including the option of dual chamber pacing). The rhythm may become faster and symptomatic; at such times it is treated as any other ventricular tachycardia.

Torsades de pointes may occur rarely as a direct result of ischemia per se and also as a side effect of many of the agents used to treat arrhythmias. Hypokalemia, bradycardia, and other factors that prolong the Q-T interval should be eliminated. Treatment using isoproterenol, which is advised in some cases of torsades de pointes, is contraindicated in the setting of ischemia. Lidocaine, acute cardioversion, magnesium, and overdrive pacing have roles in therapy. However, correction of underlying causes, including ischemia, is the primary direction of therapy.

Premature ventricular complexes occur in the majority of patients early in the course of acute myocardial infarction. Premature ventricular complexes have been considered a warning sign for more malignant ventricular arrhythmias. However, ventricular tachycardia and ventricular fibrillation may occur without warning, and only rarely do patients with premature ventricular complexes go on to develop life-threatening forms. The R-on-T phenomenon, particularly in the early acute ischemic setting, may initiate ventricular fibrillation, but this relationship does not have as strong a predictive value as once thought. Premature ventricular complexes may reflect automatic foci and are aggravated by hemodynamic instability and hypokalemia, such that primary therapy should correct underlying abnormalities. Lidocaine can prevent ventricular tachycardia and ventricular fibrillation but does not improve hospital mortality. Because of the lack of a one-to-one relationship between warning arrhythmias and life-threatening arrhythmias and because of the failure of lidocaine regimens to change hospital mortality (when patients are in the equivalent of a coronary care unit setting), the routine use of prophylactic therapy for premature ventricular complexes has been challenged. Lidocaine therapy is potentially more helpful early in the course of the therapy of patients with acute myocardial infarction (e.g., within 6 hours), when the incidence of primary ventricular fibrillation is highest, and for those with evident, especially symptomatic, advanced forms (e.g., R-on-T phenomenon, multiform, couplets, salvos). Lidocaine therapy may not be warranted when the risk of adverse effects is high such as in the elderly and in patients with shock, hypotension, moderate to severe heart failure, or primary liver disease. Dosing should be decreased in patients with hypotension or heart failure or in those patients receiving cimetidine. Low- to moderate-grade ectopy is often preferable to drug side effects. Careful dosing and monitoring are required.

Spontaneous and therapeutically induced reperfusion is commonly recognized to be associated with arrhythmias, although the relatively high frequency of arrhythmias in early infarction often makes a cause-and-effect relationship uncertain. Arrhythmias associated with reperfusion include premature ventricular complexes, couplets, and runs of accelerated idioventricular rhythm. At times ventricular tachycardia or ventricular fibrillation is seen. Treatment guidelines are as previously mentioned; the potential transient nature of the disturbance should be recognized.

Chronic Arrhythmias

In general, the tachyarrhythmias and bradyarrhythmias of the acute infarction period resolve over the first 24 to 72 hours. Heart block associated with anterior infarction is an indication for permanent pacemaker placement (see previously). Symptomatic ventricular tachyarrhythmias and bundle branch block that appear after the first 72 hours of infarction portend a poor prognosis and are approached aggressively. The most vexing problem is how to evaluate and treat low- and moderate-grade ventricular arrhythmias that occur after the initial 72 hours of acute myocardial infarction. Such arrhythmias appear to be associated with risk, but guidelines for therapy are scarce and conflicting. Because of the beneficial effects of beta-blocking agents, their use should be considered routine except when specifically contraindicated.

Late ventricular tachycardia or ventricular fibrillation occurs rarely but is associated with a substantial excess mortality. A logical stepwise approach is useful. Noncardiac causes are identified and corrected. Cardiac anatomy, hemodynamics, and electrophysiology are defined. Therapy guided by electrophysiologic study has been preferred. The hierarchy of therapies is the alleviation of ischemic potential, including revascularization, antiarrhythmic drugs, and antiarrhythmic surgery and implantable devices. Ambulatory monitoring to guide therapy is an alternative in those patients (about one-third) who show adequate baseline ectopy both as a reflection of risk and as an adequate end point for therapy. Suppression is recommended for 90 percent or greater of repetitive forms and more than 70 percent of premature ventricular complexes. Patients with bundle branch block and anterior myocardial infarction have a high rate of ventricular fibrillation independent of warning arrhythmias. This risk window is of about 6 weeks' duration. Antiarrhythmic therapy in this unique subgroup should be individualized, and its empiric nature must be noted.

Nonsustained ventricular tachycardia is unusual but appears to be associated with an excess mortality, especially in patients with depressed left ventricular function. Symptomatic patients may undergo electrophysiologic testing when risk (inducibility into sustained ventricular tachycardia) and therapy can be addressed. The benefits of therapy are not as clear as in patients with sustained ventricular tachycardia. In patients at lower risk, those found not to be inducible, cautious therapy may still be warranted to address symptoms. Late potentials detected by signal-averaged electrocardiography appear to predict risk but are not directly affected by antiarrhythmic therapy and therefore cannot serve as an end point to guide treatment.

Premature ventricular contractions are seen in about 20 percent of patients in the recovery phase of acute myocardial infarction. This is a particularly confusing area in which risk appears defined, and proof of the benefit of therapy has eluded investigators for decades. Risk relates independently to both ventricular function, for which patients with the greatest impairment of ventricular function have the highest risk, and ventricular ectopy. Risk increases virtually with the appearance of premature ventricular complexes, becomes significant at 6 to 10 premature ventricular complexes per hour, and then plateaus. This risk occurs independently of form, although symptomatic nonsustained ventricular tachycardia is considered a more important form when it is noted.

Ambulatory monitoring of patients following acute myocardial infarction to identify ventricular ectopy followed by suppression of such ectopy by antiarrhythmic drugs has been advocated. Although there is some consensus on the degree of suppression of premature ventricular complexes required for statistical significance (70 to 85 percent comparing a 24 hour predrug to a 24 hour postdrug monitoring period), the grade of ectopy that needs treatment is unclear. Clinical trials focusing on the use of specific antiarrhythmic agents or the suppression of premature ventricular complexes have been disappointing. The results of the Cardiac Arrhythmia Suppression Trial (CAST) (Echt and co-workers, 1991; CAST II investigators, 1992) suggest that high-grade suppression of ventricular ectopy by flecainide, encainide, or moricizine may actually be deleterious. Most efforts are now being concentrated on the need to treat nonsustained forms, leaving the issue of the treatment of premature ventricular complexes more unclear than ever. Symptomatic patients may be treated with caution.

First-line therapy is beta-adrenergic blocking agents, but all eligible patients should be receiving these drugs.

Suggested Reading

Antman EM. Berlin JA. Declining incidence of ventricular fibrillation in myocardial infarction. Implications for the prophylactic use of lidocaine. Circulation 1992; 86:764.

The Cardiac Arrhythmia Suppression Trial II Investigators. Effect of the antiarrhythmic agent moricizine on survival after myocardial infarction. N Engl J Med 1992; 323:227.

Echt DS, Liebson PR, Mitchell B, et al. Mortality and morbidity in patients receiving encainide, flecainide or placebo: The cardiac arrhythmia suppression trial. N Engl J Med 1991; 324:781.

Gunnar RM, Bourdillon PDV, Dixon DW, et al. A report of the American College of Cardiology/American Heart Association Task Force on Assessment of Diagnostic and Therapeutic Cardiovascular Procedures (Subcommittee to Develop Guidelines for the Early Management of Patients with Acute Myocardial Infarction). Circulation 1990; 82:664.

Myerburg RJ, Kessler KM, Castellanos A. Recognition, clinical assessment and management of arrhythmias and conduction disturbances. In: Schlant RC, Alexander RW, eds. The heart. 8th ed. New York: McGraw-Hill, 1994:705.

Opie LH. Adverse cardiovascular drug interactions. In: Schlant RC and Alexander RW ed. The heart. 8th ed. New York: McGraw-Hill, 1994:1971.

Stewart RB, Bardy GH, Greene LH. Wide complex tachycardia: Misdiagnosis and outcome after emergent therapy. Ann Intern Med 1986; 104:766.

Woosley RL. Antiarrhythmic agents. In: Schlant RC, Alexander RW, eds. The heart, 8th ed. New York: McGraw-Hill, 1994:775.

CORONARY ANGIOPLASTY

John S. Douglas Jr., M.D., F.A.C.C., F.A.C.P., F.A.C.S.

Percutaneous transluminal coronary angioplasty (PTCA) was first performed by Gruentzig in 1977 to relieve myocardial ischemia in a patient with discrete single-vessel coronary artery disease. During the subsequent years, improvements in PTCA technology, radiographic imaging systems, and operator experience permitted a substantial broadening of indications for the technique, which today is a revascularization alternative for many patients with symptomatic coronary artery stenosis in one or more coronary arteries.

THERAPEUTIC ALTERNATIVES

The risk of angioplasty and its ability to relieve symptoms and favorably influence a patient's quality of life are important issues that help to determine the place of this technique compared with that of bypass surgery and, in some patients, compared with medical therapy. A randomized trial has recently been reported from the Veterans Administration that compared the efficacy of medical therapy and balloon angioplasty in relief of chronic stable angina pectoris in patients with single-vessel disease. This study, which analyzed patient outcome at 6 months, showed that symptomatic status and treadmill exercise time were superior in patients treated initially with PTCA. It also indicated, however, that bypass surgery was utilized more frequently in patients initially treated with PTCA. Results of randomized trials comparing PTCA with coronary artery bypass grafting (CABG) are, unfortunately, not available. However, long-term observational studies of patients undergoing PTCA in Zurich (Gruentzig and co-workers, 1987) and Atlanta (Talley and co-workers, 1988) have indicated an acceptable degree of safety and efficacy in the patients treated. Of the initial 169 Zurich patients, 133 were treated successfully with no procedural deaths and with follow-up of up to 8 years; 68 percent of the successful patients were asymptomatic and only five cardiac deaths were recorded. Restenosis occurred in 30 percent of patients, leading to CABG in 19 patients and PTCA in 27 patients. Of 427 patients who underwent PTCA at Emory University Hospital in 1981, 5 year cardiac survival was 98 percent, and 85 percent were asymptomatic at last follow-up. Repeat PTCA was required in 20 percent and CABG in 15 percent of patients. Actuarial event-free survival (freedom from cardiac death, myocardial infarction, and CABG) at 5 years was 79 percent. Single-vessel disease was present in a majority of patients in both series (58 percent and 86 percent).

In recent years, PTCA has been applied increasingly in multivessel disease. In the 1985 National Heart, Lung, and Blood Institute (NHLBI) PTCA Registry, twice as many multivessel disease patients were entered compared with those in the 1982 registry (53 percent versus 25 percent), with a higher procedural success and fewer complications (Detre and co-workers, 1989). However, long-term follow-up studies of patients with multivessel disease to analyze the impact of incomplete revascularization and restenosis are limited. In more than 1,000 patients with multivessel disease who underwent PTCA at Emory University Hospital, 77 percent of patients were asymptomatic at last follow-up, and freedom from cardiac death, myocardial infarction, and bypass surgery at 5 years was 95 percent, 90 percent, and 76 percent, respectively. In the 1985 NHLBI Registry, 75 percent of 402 multivessel patients were free of cardiac events (death, myocardial infarction, or CABG) at 1 year follow-up.

Because PTCA is applied most often as an alternative to CABG, the excellent symptomatic relief and long-term outlook following surgery must be considered. Operative mortality in most active centers is approximately 1 percent for the most favorable candidates, and symptomatic benefit is maintained for 5 years in approximately 70 percent of patients. However, up to 5 percent of patients require reoperation at 5 years, and the risk of in-hospital death and myocardial infarction is at least triple that encountered with the first operation. Symptomatic benefit and long-term survival following reoperation are also less favorable than with primary procedures. These facts have fostered a strategy of delaying surgery when adequate palliation can be achieved with less invasive methods.

Table 1 Results of the First 10,168 Consecutive Coronary Angioplasty Procedures at Emory University Hospital*

	NUMBER	PERCENTAGE
Patients	10,168	—
Arterial segments dilated	13,011	—
Initial success†	9,355	92
Complication-free success‡	9,151	90
Single-vessel disease	6,202	61
Multivessel disease§	3,965	39
Multivessel PTCA‖	956	9.4
Emergency CABG	305	3
Q wave acute myocardial infarction	142	1.4
In-hospital death	30	0.3

*Patients with evolving infarction are excluded.
†<50% residual stenosis.
‡<50% residual stenosis and freedom from complications.
§>50% stenosis of LAD + RCA, LAD + CIRC, CIRC + RCA, or LAD + CIRC + RCA.
‖Dilation of LAD + RCA, LAD + CIRC, CIRC + RCA, or LAD + CIRC + RCA.
PTCA, percutaneous transluminal coronary angioplasty; CABG, coronary artery bypass grafting; LAD, left anterior descending artery; RCA, right coronary artery; CIRC, circumflex coronary artery.

PREFERRED APPROACH

The decision to offer PTCA to an individual patient must be made with the knowledge of the potential impact of multiple clinical variables on procedural success, risk, and long-term benefit. The risk associated with PTCA should be equal to or less than that encountered with bypass surgery or medical therapy during early and long-term follow-up. Initial results of PTCA in the first 10,168 patients at Emory University Hospital are shown in Table 1. Factors favoring success of PTCA are age younger than 65 years, male gender, single-vessel disease, single-lesion PTCA, subtotal occlusion, absence of calcification, accessibility of the lesion, and normal left ventricular function.

Because acute coronary occlusion is the most common serious complication of PTCA, accounting for most of the in-hospital morbidity and mortality, the risk of the procedure is related closely to the probability of acute occlusion and the adverse consequences if this should occur. The following factors are associated with an increased risk of acute occlusion: lesion length, female gender, bend point or branch point stenosis, thrombus in situ, multiple stenoses in the vessel dilated, and multivessel disease. After completion of angioplasty, the presence of an intimal tear or dissection and a high residual translesional pressure gradient are predictors of acute closure. For patients who experience acute occlusion, the clinical variables associated with an increased mortality include age older than 65 years, female gender, hypertension, diabetes, prior myocardial infarction, previous bypass surgery, multivessel disease, left main coronary disease, a large area of myocardium at risk, poor left ventricular function, and collaterals originating from the vessel to be dilated.

Restenosis following PTCA, observed in approximately 30 percent of patients within 3 months, is a fibrocellular proliferative reaction that is more common in the presence of certain clinical variables. These variables include unstable angina, diabetes, variant angina, multivessel disease, ostial lesions, stenoses in a proximal or midsaphenous vein graft, total occlusions, intracoronary thrombus, and suboptimal angioplasty results as indicated by a residual stenosis greater than 30 percent.

As with any treatment, selection of PTCA involves an analysis of risks and benefits for the individual patient, incorporating clinical and anatomic factors known to influence outcome. Estimates must be made of the likelihood of successful dilation, acute closure with consequent morbidity and mortality, and restenosis. The skill of the angioplasty operator and of the backup surgical and anesthesia teams must also be considered.

Recognizing the critical importance of lesion morphology in predicting procedural success or failure, the American College of Cardiology/American Heart Association (ACC/AHA) Task Force subcommittee developed a risk-stratified classification of coronary artery lesions (Ryan and coworkers, 1988) (Table 2).

Type A lesions have characteristics that permit an anticipated procedural success rate of at least 85 percent and a low risk of acute closure.

Type B lesions have characteristics that predict a lower success rate (60 to 85 percent), a moderate risk of acute closure, or both. Because the presence of multiple adverse lesion features increases the probability of procedural failure and acute closure, the term *complex B lesions* is used to describe a lesion with two or more adverse features.

Type C lesions have characteristics that result in a low success rate (<60 percent), that have a high risk of acute closure, or both.

This lesion classification is imperfect in that some B characteristics seem to be more powerful predictors than others (thrombus, lesion length, bend point, and bifurca-

Table 2 Lesion-Specific Characteristics of Type A, B, and C Lesions

TYPE A LESIONS	
Discrete (<10 mm in length)	Little or no calcification
Concentric	Less than totally occlusive
Readily accessible	Nonostial in location
Nonangulated segment, <45 degrees	No major branch involvement
Smooth contour	Absence of thrombus
TYPE B LESIONS	
Tubular (10 to 20 mm in length)	Moderate to heavy calcification
Eccentric	Total occlusion <3 mo old
Moderate tortuosity of proximal segment	Ostial in location
Moderately angulated segment >45 degrees <90 degrees	Bifurcation lesions requiring double guidewires
Irregular contour	Some thrombus present
TYPE C LESIONS	
Diffuse (>2 cm in length)	Total occlusions >3 mo old
Excessive tortuosity of proximal segment	Inability to protect major side branches
Extremely angulated segments >90 degrees	Degenerated vein grafts with friable lesion

From the ACC/AHA Task Force Report: Guidelines for percutaneous transluminal coronary angioplasty. J Am Coll Cardiol 1988; 12:529; with permission.

tion). In addition, improvements in technology (balloon catheters, stents, lasers, atherectomy) have resulted in higher success rates of approximately 95% for type A lesions and 85 to 90% for most B lesions, as well as permitted success in some type C lesions. It should be recognized in certain instances that the likelihood of acute closure may be high, but the risk to the patient is low; examples include total occlusions and well-collateralized vessels.

Currently, the level of angioplasty experience and skill is not uniform. A patient with relatively complex anatomy selected for PTCA in an experienced angioplasty center may receive a more effective surgical revascularization if he or she were in a strong surgical center without extensive angioplasty experience. In centers with excellent PTCA and surgical skills, most patients with proximal single-vessel disease who require revascularization are treated initially with PTCA; patients with triple-vessel disease who are suitable for surgery undergo bypass grafting. Between these extremes, there is little standardization of therapy. Strategies recommended in the following patient subgroups reflect current practices at Emory University Hospital and guidelines of the ACC/AHA Task Force Report on angioplasty.

Single-Vessel Disease: Asymptomatic or Mildly Symptomatic

Percutaneous transluminal coronary angioplasty has become the treatment of choice for many minimally symptomatic patients with significant stenosis (≥ 50 percent diameter reduction) in a major coronary artery that serves at least a moderate-sized area of viable myocardium. These patients should (1) have objective evidence of myocardial ischemia; (2) have been resuscitated from cardiac arrest or sustained ventricular tachycardia in the absence of acute myocardial infarction; or (3) must undergo noncardiac surgery such as repair of aortic aneurysm, iliofemoral bypass, or carotid artery surgery. Patients with few or no symptoms should have a lesion that would predict a high probability of angioplasty success and a low risk for morbidity (acute closure probability < 5 percent) and mortality (< 0.5 percent), i.e., a type A or type B lesion with favorable features. An example of a favorable type B lesion is one with a single negative feature, such as eccentricity, irregular contour, or a bifurcation lesion. In some cases, occupation or life-style may influence the selection process in favor of PTCA over medical therapy, especially if the safety of others is involved (e.g., pilots, air traffic controllers, firefighters, policemen, athletes).

Patients with asymptomatic or mildly symptomatic single-vessel disease who should not undergo PTCA include those who (1) have only a small area of viable myocardium at risk; (2) do not have objective evidence of myocardial ischemia; (3) have lesions of less than 50 percent diameter reduction; (4) have type C lesions; or (5) are in a moderate-risk or high-risk group for morbidity or mortality.

Single-Vessel Disease: Symptomatic

Among the ideal patients for PTCA are those with angina pectoris (functional classes II to IV and unstable angina) and single-vessel disease who have one or more significant lesions in a major epicardial artery that subtends at least a moderate area of viable myocardium. These patients (1) have objective evidence of myocardial ischemia; (2) have angina pectoris that is inadequately controlled on medical therapy; or (3) are intolerant to the side effects of medical therapy. These patients have a high likelihood for success and low risk of procedure-related morbidity and mortality; i.e., they have type A or more favorable type B lesions.

Patients with single-vessel disease for whom there is some divergence of opinion with respect to indications for PTCA include those who have a significant stenosis in a major coronary artery that supplies at least a moderate area of viable myocardium and have objective evidence of ischemia or disabling symptoms on medical therapy. Disease in these patients has the following characteristics: (1) one or more lesions predicted to have a moderate risk of morbidity (acute closure <8 percent) and mortality (<1 percent), i.e., complex type B or a favorable type C lesion; (2) disabling symptoms and a small area of viable myocardium at risk and at least a moderate likelihood for successful PTCA with low procedural risk predicted, i.e., a type A or B lesion; or (3) despite significant angina, no objective evidence of myocardial ischemia and at least a moderate likelihood for PTCA success and low procedure risk, i.e., type A or B lesions.

Patients with symptomatic single-vessel disease in whom PTCA is not indicated include those who (1) have only a small area of viable myocardium at risk in the absence of disabling symptoms; (2) have clinical symptoms not likely indicating ischemia; (3) have unfavorable lesions for PTCA; or (4) are in a high-risk group for morbidity and mortality.

Because of the excellent prognosis of single-vessel disease treated medically, it is important that the risk-benefit ratio of a PTCA procedure be carefully analyzed and that the symptoms are indeed due to the lesion targeted for dilation.

Multivessel Coronary Artery Disease: Asymptomatic or Mildly Symptomatic (Functional Class I)

The most clear-cut indication for PTCA in this patient subgroup is in the individual with one significant lesion in a major coronary artery, the successful dilation of which would result in a nearly complete revascularization because other lesions subtend small or nonviable areas of myocardium. For PTCA to be indicated, patients must (1) have a large area of viable myocardium at risk; and (2) have objective evidence of ischemia; or (3) have been resuscitated from cardiac arrest or sustained ventricular tachycardia in the absence of myocardial infarction; or (4) need to undergo high-risk noncardiac surgery. All patients in this category should have type A or favorable type B lesions and be in a low-risk group for morbidity and mortality.

Indications for PTCA are more controversial when patient characteristics are similar to those previously described; however, these patients have (1) moderate-sized (rather than large) areas of myocardium at risk or (2) significant lesions in two or more major epicardial coronary arteries, each supplying at least a moderate-sized area of viable myocardium. These patients should have objective evidence of myocardial ischemia and one or more type A or favorable type B lesions, the dilation of which would relieve ischemia. They should be in a low-risk group for morbidity and mortality.

Patients with asymptomatic or mildly symptomatic multivessel disease in whom PTCA is not indicated include those who (1) have only a small amount of myocardium at risk; (2) have a PTCA-targeted vessel, the occlusion of which would result in cardiogenic shock; (3) have two or more major arteries with complex type B lesions; (4) have type C lesions in a major coronary artery supplying a moderate or large area of viable myocardium; or (5) are in a high-risk group owing to extreme left ventricular dysfunction or diffuse coronary atherosclerosis.

Multivessel Coronary Artery Disease: Symptomatic

Patients with symptomatic multivessel disease in whom PTCA is indicated include those with one dilatable lesion in a major coronary artery, which would result in nearly complete revascularization, and those with significant stenoses in each of two major coronary arteries, both subtending at least moderate-sized areas of the viable myocardium. These patients with symptomatic disease should have (1) objective evidence of myocardial ischemia; (2) angina pectoris that is poorly responsive to medical therapy; or (3) intolerable side effects on medical therapy; or (4) been judged by their attending cardiologist to need revascularization. These patients should have type A and B lesions, for which successful dilation would provide complete or nearly complete relief of ischemia, and should be in a low-risk to moderate-risk group for morbidity (<10 percent risk of acute occlusion) and mortality (<1 percent).

An increasing number of symptomatic patients are referred for PTCA because they are considered poor candidates for bypass surgery as a result of advanced physiologic age, coexisting medical problems, multiple prior cardiac operations, or extremely poor left ventricular function. These so-called salvage patients should have one or more type A or B lesions that could be dilated, with resultant complete or partial relief of ischemia. Lesions selected for PTCA should have a low risk of acute closure because surgical intervention may be impossible or may carry a high risk. Many patients in this category present ethical dilemmas to the PTCA operator because of the high risk if PTCA fails.

In general, patients with multivessel disease require more intensive scrutiny prior to PTCA, with the goal of achieving symptomatic and ischemia relief at an acceptable risk. Morphologic characteristics of each lesion must be considered relative to all other lesions and to the amount of myocardium subtended. An estimate must be made of the likelihood of acute closure and the consequences likely to ensue if any or all of the dilated segments closed. For example, type B lesions with multiple adverse features in major coronary arteries supplying a large proportion of the remaining viable myocardium may be inappropriate targets if surgery is feasible.

Patients with symptomatic multivessel disease who are not suitable for PTCA include those who (1) have only a small area of myocardium at risk in the absence of disabling symptoms, (2) have a type C lesion in a major coronary artery serving moderate or large areas of viable myocardium, or (3) are in an unacceptably high risk group for morbidity and mortality.

Acute Myocardial Infarction

There is overwhelming evidence of the benefit of intravenous thrombolytic therapy in acute myocardial infarction. Because improved survival has been documented for this strategy, intravenous thrombolytic therapy has become the treatment of choice for most patients with acute myocardial infarction. The place of angioplasty in the treatment of acute myocardial infarction has been studied for the past decade, and many questions remain. Although direct PTCA appears to be extremely effective (≥ 90 percent patency rate) in skilled hands, the procedure cannot often be implemented immediately, and a more common question is when to intervene with angiography and angioplasty after thrombolytic therapy has been administered. Randomized trials (European, TAMI, TIMI IIA) have shown that thrombolysis and immediate PTCA were associated with increased mortality, acute closure, emergency bypass surgery, and bleeding complications, with no improvement in left ventricular function when compared with thrombolysis and deferred PTCA. More recently, the TIMI IIB trial indicated that thrombolytic therapy and watchful waiting with utilization of angiography and PTCA only for recurrent or inducible ischemia may be a satisfactory approach.

Unfortunately, the most effective intravenous thrombolytic agents fail to re-establish flow in approximately 25 percent of patients, and reocclusion following thrombolytic therapy occurs in about 15 percent of patients with severe consequences (a twofold increase in mortality and a decrement in left ventricular function). Selection of patients for angiography and PTCA, therefore, should be carried out in a way that would include patients in whom thrombolytic therapy has failed, those who are not candidates for thrombolytic therapy (patients with hypertension, active peptic ulcer disease, or recent surgery), and patients with successful thrombolytic therapy but with ischemia producing atherosclerotic lesions. In general, PTCA in the setting of acute myocardial infarction should be confined to the infarct-related artery.

Patients referred for angiography and PTCA in our practice include those who (1) have severe, persisting angina in spite of thrombolytic therapy (reperfusion failures), recurrent ischemia following thrombolytic therapy (reocclusion), or inducible ischemia by stress testing at 5 to 7 days following thrombolytic therapy; (2) present in cardiogenic shock; (3) have symptoms compatible with acute myocardial infarction but have conditions that prevent a definitive diagnosis (permanent pacemaker or left bundle branch block); (4) present at a time when immediate angiography and direct PTCA would be possible; (5) have recurrent ventricular tachycardia, ventricular fibrillation, or both in spite of antiarrhythmic therapy; (6) experience non-Q wave infarction; or (7) are relatively young or have physically demanding jobs or life-styles.

Patients in whom angioplasty is not performed are those who (1) have residual stenosis of less than 50 percent, (2) have type C lesions, (3) have high-risk lesions for PTCA (for which bypass surgery or medical therapy would be a better option), or (4) have PTCA targets in vessels other than the infarct-related artery.

Angioplasty Procedure

Patients undergoing elective PTCA may be admitted to the hospital the day of the procedure in a fasting state. Aspirin 160 to 325 mg and diltiazem 60 mg are administered orally prior to angioplasty. In patients with very unstable angina and in those with lesion-associated thrombus or recent infarction, attempts are made to stabilize the patient on intravenous heparin, aspirin, and intensive medical treatment for 3 to 7 days before the PTCA. There is an increased risk of acute occlusion in patients who cannot be stabilized and in whom emergency PTCA is required. Patients generally receive 10,000 units of heparin intravenously after vascular access is achieved and 5,000 units of heparin per hour during the procedure. Intravascular sheaths are usually removed 3 hours after the angioplasty in elective patients, and patients with ideal angioplasty results are discharged the next morning. Many patients receive overnight heparinization when intracoronary thrombus is recognized, if a very unstable lesion necessitates emergency PTCA, or if considerable intimal disruption or dissection is induced. In multivessel PTCA, dilation of one or more lesions may be deferred to the following day, if the initial PTCA results are not optimal, if procedural time or the amount of contrast media administered is excessive, or if acute closure of all dilated sites would result in cardiogenic shock. Following PTCA, patients receive aspirin 160 to 325 mg daily, diltiazem 60 mg four times a day, and topical nitrates during their hospitalization. Prior to discharge, patients receive instructions regarding a low-fat diet, exercise, cessation of smoking, and a follow-up procedure plan. In some patients, a stress evaluation may be appropriate before discharge to assess the results of angioplasty. Following discharge, patients take aspirin 160 to 325 mg once daily. If all areas of myocardial ischemia have been relieved by angioplasty, antiangina medications may be discontinued.

Suggested Reading

Detre K, Holubkov R, Kelsey S, et al. One-year follow-up results of the 1985–1986 National Heart, Lung, and Blood Institute's percutaneous transluminal coronary angioplasty registry. Circulation 1989; 80:421.

Gruentzig AR, King SB, Schlumpf M, Siegenthaler W. Long-term follow-up after percutaneous transluminal coronary angioplasty, the early Zurich experience. N Engl J Med 1987; 316:1127.

Gunner RM, Bourdillon PD, Dixon DW, et al. Guidelines for the early management of patients with acute myocardial infarction. J Am Coll Cardiol 1990; 16:249.

Kirklin JW, Akins CW, Blackstone EH, et al. ACC/AHA guidelines and indications for coronary artery bypass graft surgery. Circulation 1991; 83:1125.

Parisi AF, Folland ED, Hartigan P. A comparison of angioplasty with medical therapy in the treatment of single-vessel coronary artery disease. N Engl J Med 1992; 326:10.

Ryan TJ, Faxon DP, Gunnar RM, et al. ACC/AHA task force report guidelines for percutaneous transluminal coronary angioplasty. J Am Coll Cardiol 1988; 12:529.

Talley JD, Hurst JW, King SB, et al. Clinical outcome 5 years after attempted percutaneous coronary angioplasty in 427 patients. Circulation 1988; 77:372.

CORONARY BYPASS SURGERY

Michael A. Kutcher, M.D.

Coronary bypass surgery is a therapeutic alternative to treat significant obstructive coronary atherosclerotic heart disease by improving coronary blood flow via surgically placed bypass conduits.

In 1967, Favaloro and co-workers (1970) reported the successful use of aortocoronary artery saphenous vein grafts in patients with severe obstructive coronary disease. Since that time, improvements in anesthesia, cardiopulmonary bypass, myocardial preservation, preparation of graft material, surgical technique, and postoperative care have made coronary bypass surgery acceptable, safe, and effective in appropriate patients.

■ THERAPEUTIC ALTERNATIVES

Once coronary atherosclerotic heart disease has been identified and the extent of disease has been documented by physiologic and anatomic parameters, the three major goals of therapy are

- Relief of angina
- Prevention of myocardial infarction
- Promotion of longevity

To determine which modality may best achieve the three goals in an individual patient—the safest, most effective way—coronary bypass surgery must be compared with medical therapy and coronary angioplasty.

PREFERRED APPROACH

Appropriate clinical settings for the application of coronary bypass surgery are outlined in Table 1.

Assessment

Key technical issues to consider in assessing patients for bypass surgery include the suitability of distal coronary vessels for grafting, the degree of anticipated revascularization (complete versus incomplete), and a reasonable left ventricular function to permit successful disengagement of cardiopulmonary bypass. Additional clinical factors include age, body habitus, functional state, and presence of other major medical problems, which may preclude the benefits of the procedure by increasing the risk of complications.

Results of Trials

As a result of several randomized and observational trials, coronary bypass surgery is accepted as superior to medical therapy in eliminating or improving the quantity and quality of angina. Furthermore, successful surgery results in improved objective indices of functional capacity and myocardial ischemia (Hultgren and co-workers, 1985). However, patients with significant single-vessel disease may be served as well by percutaneous transluminal coronary angioplasty as by revascularization, but subsets of significant double-vessel and triple-vessel disease may be served with either coronary angioplasty or coronary bypass surgery. The results of several major randomized trials comparing angioplasty with surgery for angina relief, morbidity, mortality, and long-term patency will be available by the mid-1990s. The major American trials in progress include the Emory Angioplasty and Surgery Trial (EAST) and the Bypass Angioplasty Revascularization Investigation (BARI). Until definitive recommendations come from these trials, the indications, risks, and benefits of the two revascularization alternatives must be weighed for each individual patient.

Coronary bypass surgery is definitely superior to medical therapy for mildly symptomatic or even asymptomatic patients with significant obstructive left main disease. In addition, recent reports of the long-term follow-up of randomized trials indicate a beneficial effect of surgery on mortality in mildly symptomatic patients with triple-vessel disease and with reduced left ventricular function (Detre and co-workers, 1981). However, these same trials have not detected a reduction in mortality in surgically treated patients with single-vessel or double-vessel disease. The subset of patients with stable angina, critical three-vessel obstructions, and excellent

Table 1 Indications for Coronary Bypass Surgery

Assume: –acceptable coronary anatomy for grafting
–not amenable to coronary angioplasty
–ejection fraction >20%

Angina unresponsive to optimal medical therapy
Significant single-, double-, or triple-vessel disease
–moderate to severe symptoms
–strongly positive exercise test
–major amount of myocardium at jeopardy
Significant triple-vessel disease
–mild symptoms
–compromised left ventricular function
Significant left main disease
–regardless of symptoms or signs
Acute myocardial infarction
–onset of chest pain within 6 hours
–thrombolytic therapy contraindicated or failed
Failed coronary angioplasty attempt
–acute or threatened vessel closure
Second restenosis of coronary angioplasty site
Adjunctive to valve or aortic surgery
–significant single-, double-, or triple-vessel disease
–regardless of symptoms or signs

left ventricular function is still controversial, but coronary bypass surgery may be acceptable in this setting, depending on individual factors.

Benefits and Risks

The benefits of coronary bypass surgery, compared with medical therapy and coronary angioplasty, are that surgery provides a more direct approach to improve coronary blood flow and a more effective or complete revascularization.

The percentages of risks and complications of a "standard" coronary bypass procedure are as follows: mortality 2 percent, myocardial infarction 2.5 percent, reoperation for bleeding 2 percent, infection 1 percent, cerebrovascular accident 1 percent, and arrhythmia 10 percent (ACC/AHA, 1991). The more complex and unstable the case, the higher the risk. Risk for an individual patient must be carefully assessed.

There is a 5 to 10 percent yearly attrition rate with saphenous vein graft conduits. The 10 year patency rate for internal mammary grafts is 95 percent compared with a 50 percent patency rate for saphenous vein grafts (ACC/AHA, 1991). Obviously, if at all possible, at least one internal mammary graft should be used in a coronary bypass procedure to ensure the best chances of long-term patency.

Preoperative Preparation

The patient should be continued on an antianginal regimen up to the time of surgery. Some surgeons have expressed concern about intraoperative and postoperative variations in systemic vascular resistance in patients treated with high-dose nifedipine. It might be well to reduce nifedipine or eliminate it if possible before coronary bypass surgery.

If surgery is elective and the patient stable, aspirin should be discontinued approximately 5 to 7 days before the procedure. This obviates the increased bleeding tendencies during surgery in patients on chronic aspirin therapy. It is still debatable whether pretreatment with dipyridamole offers any benefit in reducing platelet adhesiveness and improves chances of long-term graft patency. Continuation of a postoperative antiplatelet regimen of at least 325 mg of aspirin every day is an acceptable practice. Another acceptable option is to add dipyridamole 75 mg three times a day to the regimen.

Postoperative Care

Postoperative care is covered in the next chapter of this textbook.

Risk Factor Reduction

The long-term benefits of revascularization surgery are improved with attention paid to reduction of risk factors. Patients should stop smoking, maintain reasonable body weight, control blood pressure, and lower blood lipids. An exercise rehabilitation program after surgery is a key element in recovery. Regular exercise should be continued in the long term.

Suggested Reading

ACC/AHA guidelines and indications for coronary artery bypass graft surgery: A report of the American College of Cardiology/American Heart Association Task Force on Assessment of Diagnostic and Therapeutic Cardiovascular Procedures (Subcommittee on Coronary Artery Bypass Graft Surgery). Circulation 1991; 83:1125.

Bell MR, Gersh BJ, Schaff HV, et al. Effect of completeness of revascularization on long-term outcome of patients with three-vessel disease undergoing coronary artery bypass surgery: A report from the CASS Registry. Circulation 1992; 86:446.

Califf RM, Harrell FE, Lee KL, et al. The evolution of medical and surgical therapy for coronary artery disease: A 15 year perspective. JAMA 1989; 261:2077.

CASS Principal Investigators and Their Associates. Coronary artery surgery study: A randomized trial of coronary artery bypass surgery; survival data. Circulation 1983; 68:939.

Detre K, Peduzzi P, Murphy M, et al and the Veterans Administration Cooperative Study for Surgery for Coronary Arterial Occlusive Disease. Effect of bypass surgery on survival in patients in low- and high-risk subgroups delineated by the use of simple clinical variables. Circulation 1981; 63:1329.

Favaloro RG, Effer DB, Groves LK. Severe segmental obstruction of the left main artery and its divisions: Surgical treatment by the saphenous vein graft technic. J Thorac Cardiovasc Surg 1970; 60:469.

Hultgren HN, Peduzzi P, Detre K, et al. The five-year effect of bypass surgery on relief of angina and exercise performance. Circulation 1985; 72(Suppl V):79.

Varnauskas E and European Coronary Surgery Study Group. Twelve-year follow-up of survival in the randomized European coronary surgery study. N Engl J Med 1988; 319:332.

MITRAL STENOSIS

Robert C. Schlant, M.D.

Mitral stenosis is narrowing or obstruction of the mitral valve orifice. The normal mitral valve circumference is approximately 10 cm and the mitral valve area is approximately 4 to 6 cm^2.

Mitral stenosis almost always results from postinflammatory reactions to acute rheumatic fever, although a history of rheumatic fever is seldom obtained in more than 50 to 60 percent of patients. Rarely, mitral stenosis can be the result of congenital valve defects, infective endocarditis with a large vegetation, left atrial myxoma, calcified mitral annulus, malignant carcinoid, systemic lupus erythematosus, or methysergide therapy. A viral etiology has not been established.

■ THERAPEUTIC ALTERNATIVES

Medical therapy can lessen the symptoms in patients with mild to moderate mitral stenosis, but medical therapy is only slightly effective when the stenosis is very severe. Basic medical therapy consists of the following: advice regarding the avoidance of occupations associated with significant physical exertion, a decrease in physical activity, limited sodium intake (2 g sodium or 5 g sodium chloride per day), and diuretics to decrease pulmonary congestion or peripheral edema. If atrial fibrillation is present (either paroxysmally or chronically), it is important to avoid rapid heart rates and to control the ventricular response rate with the use of digoxin, at times in combination with a beta-blocker, diltiazem, or verapamil. Patients with atrial fibrillation should be anticoagulated with warfarin to maintain an INR of 2.0 to 3.0. When the stenosis becomes moderately severe (1 to 1.5 cm^2) or severe (< 1 cm^2), medical therapy is no longer sufficient, and it is necessary to increase the mitral orifice, either by surgery or by catheter balloon valvotomy (CBV). In general, medical therapy for patients with moderate or severe mitral stenosis is of limited value in the relief of symptoms in view of the fixed, mechanical obstruction. Two types of prophylaxis are important: prophylaxis to prevent recurrence of streptococcal infection and rheumatic fever and prophylaxis to prevent infective endocarditis during procedures potentially associated with bacteremia.

■ PREFERRED APPROACH

Medical Treatment

The normal mitral valve orifice in the adult is 4 to 6 cm^2. As the orifice becomes progressively narrowed, it produces no significant hemodynamic obstruction until it is rather markedly narrowed. The narrowing is probably hemody-

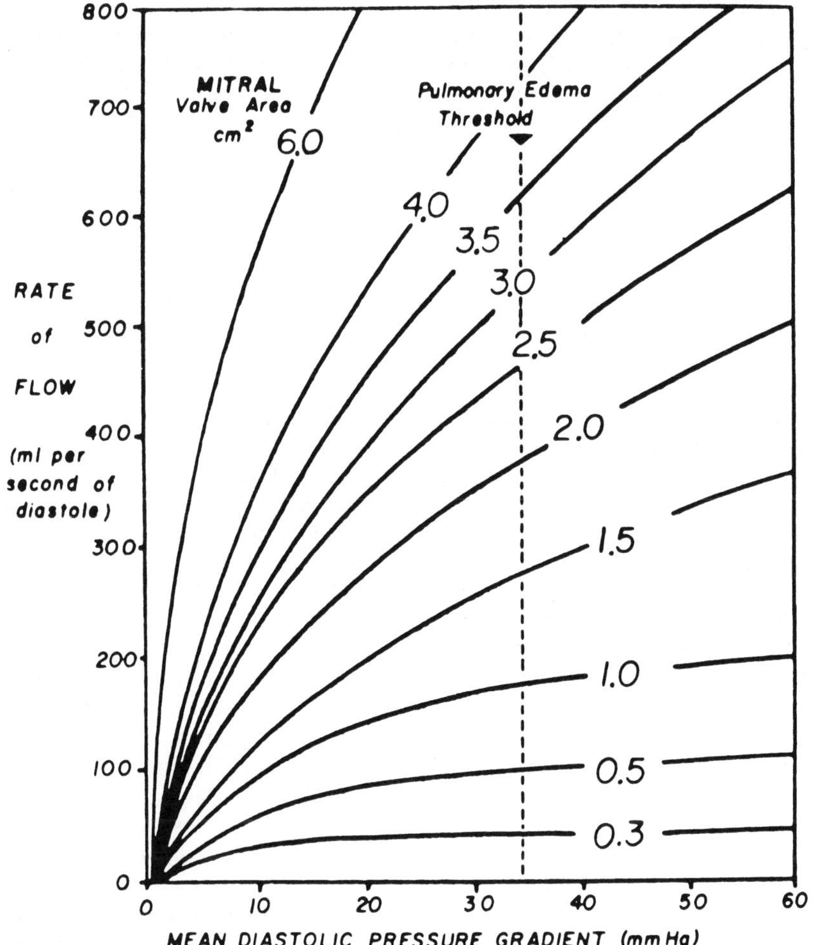

Figure 1
Diagram illustrating the relationship between mean diastolic gradient across the mitral valve and rate of flow across the mitral valve per second of diastole, as predicted by the Gorlin and Gorlin formula. Note that when the mitral valve area is 1 cm^2 or less, very little additional flow can be achieved by an increased pressure gradient. Transudation of fluid from the pulmonary capillaries and the development of pulmonary edema begins when pulmonary capillary pressure exceeds the oncotic pressure of plasma, which is about 25 to 35 mm Hg. It is also apparent that severe mitral regurgitation is incompatible with very tight mitral stenosis. *(Reproduced from Schlant RC. Altered cardiovascular function in rheumatic heart disease. In: Hurst JW, Logue RB, eds. The heart. New York: McGraw-Hill, 1966:505; with permission.)*

namically insignificant down to 2.6 cm^2; when it is between 2.1 and 2.5 cm^2 (very mild mitral stenosis), it is usually responsible for symptoms only with marked exertion, pregnancy, tachycardia, or marked anemia. Narrowing between 1.6 and 2 cm^2 (mild mitral stenosis) is associated with symptoms with moderate exertion but not with light exertion, unless this is associated with marked tachycardia, pregnancy, thyrotoxicosis, or mitral regurgitation (Fig. 1). When the valve area is narrowed to between 1 and 1.5 cm^2 (moderately severe mitral stenosis), most patients experience symptoms with light exertion. Symptoms and signs of pulmonary congestion are especially likely to occur when the area is 1.2 cm^2 or less. When the mitral valve area is reduced to the critical area of 1 cm^2 or less, symptoms occur with very mild exertion. A mitral valve area of 0.3 to 0.4 cm^2 is about the smallest area compatible with life.

At any orifice size, the patient's symptoms are influenced by the patient's total body size or body surface area, activity, heart rate and the total duration for diastolic flow per minute, and conditions (e.g., anemia, exertion, fever, emotional stress, associated mitral regurgitation) that increase flow across the mitral orifice. In some patients, mitral stenosis is very slowly progressive; in other patients, the disease is more rapid, progressive, and severe. In some areas of the world, severe mitral stenosis is not uncommonly encountered in teenage patients.

Approximately 10 to 20 percent of patients with mitral stenosis develop pulmonary vascular disease and disproportionate pulmonary hypertension. In these patients, symptoms of right heart failure (e.g., hepatomegaly, ascites, peripheral edema) may become prominent. The pulmonary hypertension, which in part is due to pulmonary arteriolar vasoconstriction, may be improved significantly with the relief of the mitral stenosis.

Although most patients with mitral stenosis have progressively severe dyspnea and fatigue with exertion, a few very rare patients unconsciously decrease their physical activity and assume that their exertional fatigue and dyspnea are normal consequences of aging. These rare, nearly asymptomatic patients must be evaluated on the basis of objective data. Exercise testing is often useful in these patients to assess the duration of exercise and to observe the patient during the exercise.

Some patients with mild or moderate mitral stenosis have episodic symptoms of pulmonary congestion only during conditions that cause an increase in cardiac output and heart rate, such as pregnancy, fever, exertion, emotional stress, anemia, or paroxysmal atrial fibrillation or flutter. Some of these patients have only mild symptoms once the precipitating event has passed and can be managed successfully medically, although the recurrence or persistence of symptoms may require surgery (or balloon valvotomy) for alleviation.

As the stenosis becomes more severe, most patients unconsciously decrease their physical activity to avoid major symptoms of dyspnea and fatigue on exertion. The progressive development of moderately severe dyspnea on exertion, decreased exercise tolerance, paroxysmal nocturnal dyspnea, peripheral edema, and acute pulmonary congestion are generally signs for the initiation of diuretic therapy, low salt diet, and the possibility of mechanical enlargement of mitral orifice.

Prophylaxis Against Rheumatic Fever and Infective Endocarditis

It is important to diagnose mitral stenosis even when the patient is asymptomatic to initiate appropriate prophylaxis against recurrent streptococcal infection. Once the diagnosis is established, I prefer to maintain the patients on prophylaxis against recurrent streptococcal infection with daily oral penicillin V 250 mg twice daily. Alternatively, one can use sulfadiazine (0.5 g twice a day) or monthly intramuscular injections of 1.2 million units of benzathine penicillin G. The latter, however, is associated with some discomfort and may also elevate the sedimentation rate. Oral erythromycin 250 mg twice daily is used for individuals allergic to penicillin and sulfadiazine. In most patients, prophylaxis is continued indefinitely; the only exceptions are the few patients older than 40 years who have very few contacts with other individuals.

Prophylaxis against infective endocarditis during dental or respiratory tract procedures is accomplished by using amoxicillin (3 g orally 1 hour before, then 1.5 g 6 hours later). Penicillin V (2 g orally 1 hour before the procedure and 1 g 6 hours later) is an acceptable alternative. For genitourinary or gastrointestinal surgery or instrumentation, one can use a combination of ampicillin (2 g intramuscularly or intravenously) and gentamicin (1.5 mg per kilogram intramuscularly or intravenously) 30 minutes to 1 hour before the procedure and repeated 8 hours later. Details of alternative regimens are discussed in the 1990 update of the American Heart Association guidelines (Committee on Rheumatic Fever, 1990).

Diet

A low-sodium diet (2 g sodium or 5 g sodium chloride) is fundamental to therapy and should be initiated early. In most instances it is also appropriate to have the patient follow a low-fat, low-cholesterol phase I American Heart Association diet. All patients should not use tobacco.

Diuretics

For most patients with any symptoms of inappropriate dyspnea on exertion, the use of a thiazide diuretic is appropriate. This can be given in doses equivalent to 25 mg of hydrochlorothiazide once a day. If patients are able to take adequate orange juice, bananas, and other fruits, potassium supplementation may not be necessary; however, serum potassium levels should be monitored to avoid hypokalemia. Some patients require the addition of a supplement of potassium chloride. In a few patients, a combination of thiazide with triamterene or amiloride to avoid hypokalemia may be useful. If the congestion does not respond to therapy with thiazide, the use of furosemide (20 to 80 mg daily) may be necessary. For severe failure, combination diuretic therapy with furosemide and either a thiazide diuretic or metolazone may be instituted. Patients on diuretics should weigh themselves each morning. This often allows patients to detect an asymptomatic weight gain and to take an extra diuretic to prevent more severe symptoms.

Heart Rate and Rhythm

An increase in heart rate results in a decreased time for diastolic flow across the mitral orifice. This, in turn, results in an increase in pressure in the left atrium and pulmonary veins and capillaries. Accordingly, an excess in heart rate both at rest and during exercise should be avoided. If the patient has normal sinus rhythm, it may be necessary to employ a beta-blocker to slow the heart rate and to prevent excessive heart rate increases during exercise. If the patient develops atrial fibrillation, digoxin should be employed to control the ventricular response rate, both at rest and during moderate exercise. An average dose of digoxin is 0.25 mg daily, with a range from 0.125 to 0.75 mg daily. In most patients, the ventricular response rate at rest and during moderate exercise (up two flights of stairs or walking a long hallway rapidly) can be used as an index of the appropriate dosage. Rare patients with atrial fibrillation treated with digoxin therapy once a day have an increase in their ventricular response rate in the early morning hours. In such patients, the institution of twice-daily therapy may provide a more uniform control of heart rate. If the ventricular response rate during exercise is not well controlled with digoxin, the addition of diltiazem, verapamil, or a beta-blocker often permits better control. The development of chronic atrial fibrillation usually signifies the presence of severe mitral stenosis.

Acute paroxysmal atrial fibrillation may precipitate acute pulmonary edema. It usually can be controlled satisfactorily with intravenous digoxin. Alternatively, intravenous diltiazem or verapamil can be used. Many patients have recurrent paroxysmal atrial fibrillation before the fibrillation becomes chronic. These patients should be maintained on therapy both with digoxin to ensure reasonable control of the ventricular response during the paroxysms and with quinidine (or procainamide) to lessen the likelihood of recurrence.

Because most patients with severe mitral stenosis who have atrial fibrillation will have recurrence of the atrial fibrillation if it is converted back to sinus rhythm (unless the severe stenosis is mechanically relieved), it is seldom appropriate to convert atrial fibrillation repeatedly either pharmacologically or electrically. The risk of systemic embolization may increase with cardioversion, even for patients who are on warfarin anticoagulation for 4 to 6 weeks. Whenever cardioversion (electrical or pharmacologic) is performed on a patient with mitral stenosis, there is a small but real risk of systemic embolization. In general, patients with mitral stenosis undergoing cardioversion of atrial fibrillation that may have been present for more than 24 hours should be on warfarin anticoagulation (INR, 2.0 to 3.0) for 3 to 4 weeks before cardioversion and for 3 to 4 weeks afterwards. Procainamide, disopyramide, or flecainide may be started 24 to 48 hours before electrical cardioversion. If the cardioversion is successful, the antiarrhythmic is continued indefinitely, as long as the patient is in normal sinus rhythm, to lessen the likelihood of recurrence of atrial fibrillation. The potential for systemic embolism each time cardioversion is performed decreases the appropriateness of conversion in patients who have recurrent episodes of atrial fibrillation despite adequate quinidine. Such patients are better left in chronic atrial fibrillation until the severe stenosis is relieved. Conversely, for patients with only mild or moderate mitral stenosis and atrial fibrillation of less than a few days' or months' duration, a trial of electrical cardioversion after anticoagulation with warfarin for 3 to 4 weeks may be successful for months or years and may improve symptoms significantly.

Arterial Vasodilators

Arterial vasodilators are of limited value to patients with isolated mitral stenosis and may occasionally increase cardiac output and worsen the symptoms of pulmonary congestion.

Anticoagulation

Patients with moderately severe or severe mitral stenosis have an increased risk of left atrial thrombus and systemic embolization even if they are in normal sinus rhythm. This risk is much greater with the onset of atrial fibrillation. The preferred medical therapy to decrease the risk of arterial embolization consists of the use of warfarin (Coumadin) in dosage to prolong the prothrombin time to an international normalized ratio (INR) of 2.0 to 3.0, which corresponds to approximately 1.3 to 1.5 times normal using North American rabbit brain thromboplastin. The relative risks of therapy with warfarin must be balanced against potential side effects, such as gastrointestinal bleeding or bruising, and consideration of patient characteristics, especially the likelihood of falling, chronic alcoholism, or noncompliance with medications. For patients in whom warfarin therapy is not appropriate, aspirin (325 mg enteric-coated daily) may be used with only a slight hazard of gastritis.

Whenever possible, thromboembolism during episodes of paroxysmal atrial fibrillation should be prevented by the prompt initiation of intravenous heparin therapy and the subsequent conversion to warfarin therapy. It is usually well to maintain the warfarin therapy for about 1 month after the reversion to normal sinus rhythm. Patients with very frequent episodes of paroxysmal atrial fibrillation or chronic atrial fibrillation should be maintained on long-term warfarin anticoagulation (INR 2 to 3) indefinitely.

Complications

Hoarseness may develop from enlargement of the left pulmonary artery and tension on the recurrent laryngeal nerve. Chest pain resembling angina pectoris can be caused by right ventricular hypertension and ischemia, coronary embolism, or associated coronary atherosclerosis. Hemoptysis should be treated with intravenous furosemide, control of the ventricular heart rate (by using a beta-blocker if there is normal sinus rhythm and by using intravenous digoxin or diltiazem and occasionally a beta-blocker if the rhythm is atrial fibrillation), sedation, and the upright position. Blood transfusion may be necessary.

Patients who have a systemic or cerebral embolus often require long-term rehabilitation. Patients who sustain a systemic embolus should be evaluated for mitral valve surgery, although some patients have systemic embolization in association with mild mitral stenosis that is no more severe than that produced by a prosthetic valve. Most patients with mitral stenosis who have had a systemic embolus should be maintained on long-term warfarin anticoagulation sufficiently to prolong the prothrombin time to an INR of 2.0 to 3.0 for at least 1 year. If an embolus recurs despite adequate anticoagulation, add daily aspirin (160 to 325 mg per day) or increase the warfarin dosage sufficiently to prolong the prothrombin time to an INR of 2.5 to 3.5.

Side Effects of Therapy

The major side effects of diuretic therapies are the development of dehydration, hypotension, hypokalemia, and hypomagnesemia and the precipitation of digitalis toxicity. The major side effects of digoxin include anorexia, nausea, and cardiac arrhythmias, particularly premature ventricular complexes, especially in a bigeminal rhythm, and atrial tachycardia, especially with atrioventricular block. In fact, virtually any cardiac rhythm disturbance can be produced by excess digitalis. One should always consider digitalis toxicity when the patient's rhythm changes either from regular to irregular or from irregular to regular.

Interventional or Surgical Treatment

The development of progressively severe symptoms and progressively decreased exertional tolerance despite medical therapy is usually an indication for mechanical relief of the mitral stenosis, by either surgery or CBV in highly selected patients. Surgical treatment consists of "open" commissurotomy, "open" valvuloplasty, or mitral valve replacement. All such therapies should be considered to be palliative.

As noted previously, most patients have minimal, if any, symptoms if the mitral orifice is greater than 2.5 cm^2. Symptoms usually develop and become progressively severe as the stenosis decreases from 2.5 cm^2 to 1.5 cm^2 which is often considered the valve orifice size below which surgery or CBV may be indicated. Mechanical relief of the stenosis is indicated in virtually all patients with an orifice of 1 cm^2 or less. The development of severe mitral stenosis may be clinically apparent by the progressive decrease in exercise tolerance with an increase in severity of dyspnea and fatigue on exertion, the occurrence of hemoptysis, the development of pulmonary congestion on chest roentgenogram, or evidence of progressive increase in the severity of the mitral stenosis on Doppler echocardiography.

Doppler echocardiography is usually the best objective test with which to follow patients who have mitral stenosis. When the stenosis is mild and slowly progressive, this can be performed at 5 year intervals; when the stenosis becomes more severe, echocardiography should be performed at 1 year or 2 year intervals or even more frequently. It is important not only to assess the estimated pressure difference across the mitral valve but also to evaluate the degree of mobility of the valve leaflets, the amount of thickening of the valve leaflets, the amount of valve calcification, the status of the subvalvular apparatus, and the presence or absence of left atrial thrombus and mitral regurgitation. These variables help determine if CBV or commissurotomy is likely to be effective.

In symptomatic younger patients who have mitral valves that are not very thickened or heavily calcified, that are still mobile, and that do not have evidence of significant subvalvular fusion of chordae tendineae or significant mitral regurgitation, CBV is an effective modality of therapy, if it can be performed by a very skilled team. Whenever possible, transesophageal echocardiography should be performed prior to CBV to detect left atrial thrombus. In most other patients, surgery is usually preferred. Surgery may be either closed or open mitral commissurotomy, open valvuloplasty, or valve replacement. In general, commissurotomy is used for patients with valvular characteristics that are similar to those desired for patients undergoing CBV. In general, mitral commissurotomy or CBV is effective in decreasing symptoms for 5 to 20 years, after which it may be necessary to implant an artificial valve, although occasionally a second commissurotomy or valvuloplasty can be performed. The long-term results of CBV are not yet available but the medium-term results are similar to the results of closed mitral commissurotomy.

In young patients with classic symptoms and signs and excellent Doppler and echocardiographic evidence of tight mitral stenosis, cardiac catheterization prior to surgery may not be necessary. In patients in whom there are any significant differences between the clinical and echocardiographic estimates of severity, cardiac catheterization is advisable. Catheterization is also advisable to evaluate the coronary arteries in older or middle-aged patients with risk factors for coronary artery disease.

Prosthetic Valve Selection

In a young female patient who wishes to become pregnant, it is advisable to implant a bioprosthesis. The patient should be informed that there is a high likelihood that the valve will have to be replaced in 7 to 25 years. It is not necessary to employ chronic warfarin anticoagulant therapy, which is teratogenic, if there is normal sinus rhythm. In such patients, however, routine warfarin anticoagulation and birth control measures are useful for 3 months after implantation to decrease thromboembolic events. If a patient with a mechanical ball or disk valve prosthesis, which requires lifelong warfarin anticoagulation (INR 2.5 to 3.5) to prevent thromboembolism, wishes to become pregnant, it is necessary to convert the warfarin therapy to subcutaneous heparin every 12 hours. This should be accomplished before the patient becomes pregnant and should be maintained at least 13 weeks during the first trimester and the last 6 to 7 weeks of pregnancy. Even this regimen is slightly teratogenic.

In other patients, the choice of a prosthetic heart valve is often determined locally based upon many variables. The major advantage of bioprostheses is the lack of need for chronic warfarin anticoagulation unless there is chronic atrial fibrillation. Bioprostheses begin to have increased fibrosis and calcification about 7 to 8 years after implantation, and they have accelerated fibrosis and calcification when inserted in young patients (up to 30 to 35 years of age) or in patients with chronic renal insufficiency. Mechanical bioprostheses have an advantage in durability, but all require lifelong anticoagulation.

Postoperative Care

Some patients with normal sinus rhythm develop atrial fibrillation at the time of mitral valve surgery. These patients should undergo cardioversion to restore the rhythm to normal either before leaving the hospital or within 4 to 8 weeks following hospitalization. If reversion is accomplished, patients should be maintained on quinidine sulfate or procainamide for 6 months following reversion to normal sinus rhythm to lessen the likelihood of reversion of atrial fibrillation. In those patients who have chronic atrial fibrillation prior to mitral valve surgery, there is less likelihood of postoperative reversion. Such patients should be maintained on long-term warfarin anticoagulation (INR of 2.0 to 3.0), and an attempt at electrical cardioversion should be made several months postoperatively. If cardioversion is successful, the patient should be maintained on both digoxin and either quinidine sulfate or procainamide. If normal sinus rhythm cannot be maintained after one or two conversions, the patient should be maintained on digoxin (and, if necessary, diltiazem or a beta-blocker) to control the ventricular rate and on chronic warfarin anticoagulation; however, quinidine or procainamide should be discontinued.

Warfarin anticoagulation should be maintained routinely for at least 3 months following open mitral commissurotomy, open valvuloplasty, insertion of a mitral bioprosthesis, or CBV. In most patients the prothrombin time should be prolonged to an INR of 2.0 to 3.0, which is approximately 1.3 to 1.5 times control using North American thromboplastin. Patients with a history of systemic embolization, evidence of thrombus at surgery, or chronic atrial fibrillation are also treated with long-term warfarin therapy (INR 2.0 to 3.0). In patients with a history of systemic embolization or evidence of thrombus at surgery, one may consider discontinuing warfarin after 3 to 12 months if the results of the procedure were thought to be satisfactory, the rhythm is normal sinus, and there is no evidence of left atrial thrombus on echocardiography. Patients with chronic atrial fibrillation are maintained indefinitely on warfarin (INR of 2.0 to 3.0).

Patients who have a mechanical prosthetic heart valve should be treated with long-term warfarin sufficiently to prolong the prothrombin time to an INR of 2.5 to 3.5, starting soon after surgery. These patients should also be considered for long-term therapy with dipyridamole (400 mg per day), particularly if there is a history of systemic embolism. Indefinite warfarin anticoagulation is indicated in all patients with mechanical bioprostheses, in patients with chronic atrial fibrillation and in many patients with a history of systemic embolization.

It is especially important to use appropriate postoperative prophylaxis against infective endocarditis whenever patients are in situations likely to be associated with bacteremia.

The postpericardiotomy syndrome is manifested by symptoms and signs of pericarditis, at times with fever, pleural effusion, and pleurisy. Most patients respond well to nonsteroidal anti-inflammatory agents, although occasional patients require corticosteroids.

Suggested Reading

Cohen DJ, Kuntz RE, Gordon PF, et al. Predictors of long-term outcome after percutaneous balloon mitral valvuloplasty. N Engl J Med 1992; 19:1329.

Dalen JE, Hirsch J, eds. Fourth ACCP Consensus Conference on Antithrombotic Therapy. Chest 1995; 108 (suppl):2255.

Dijani AS, Bisno AL, Chung KJ, et al. Prevention of bacterial endocarditis, a statement for health professionals from the Committee on Rheumatic Fever, Endocarditis, and Kawasaki Disease of the Council on Cardiovascular Disease in the Young, The American Heart Association. Circulation 1991; 83:1174–1178.

Durack DT. Prevention of infective endocarditis. N Engl J Med 1995; 332: 38–44.

Four-year follow-up of patients undergoing percutaneous balloon mitral commissurotomy: a report from the National Heart, Lung, and Blood Institute Balloon Valvuloplasty Registry. J Am Coll Cardiol 1996; 28: 1452.

Rahimtoola SH. Perspective on valvular heart disease: an update. J Am Coll Cardiol 1989; 14:1.

Reys VP, Raju BS, Wynne J, et al. Percutaneous balloon valvuloplasty compared with open surgical commissurotomy for mitral stenosis. N Engl J Med 1994; 331:961.

Schlant RC, Nutter DO. Heart failure in valvular heart disease. Medicine 1971; 50:421.

Wells FC, Shapiro LM, eds. Mitral valve disease, 2nd ed. London: Butterworth's, 1996.

Wood P. An appreciation of mitral stenosis: Part 1. Clinical features. Br Med J 1954; 1:1113.

MITRAL VALVE BILLOWING AND PROLAPSE

John B. Barlow, M.D., Hon. D.Sc. (Med.), F.R.C.P.

As a result of their cineangiographic observations of abnormal bulging of the bodies of mitral leaflets, Criley and co-workers (1966) introduced the term *prolapse of the mitral valve.* Few cardiologists or cardiac surgeons have not addressed this conundrum, and many have contributed to the scientific literature. Attempts to assess so-called mitral valve prolapse based principally on variable echocardiographic criteria and with ongoing use of Criley's terminology are misleading and compound the present confusion. Webster's dictionary defines *prolapse* as "the slipping out of place or falling of some internal organ." Prolapse, whether intermittent or permanent, implies disease and is abnormal (e.g., prolapse of hemorrhoids, the rectum, the uterus, an intervertebral disk, or the lens of the eye). It is thus regrettable that the term, which for some patients has ominous connotations, is still widely used even when the valve anomaly is mild, clinically silent, functionally normal, and should be regarded as a "normal variant."

In accord with the morphologic observations of cardiac surgeons, such as Carpentier, Duran, and Yacoub in Europe, Cosgrove, Kay, Spencer, and David in North America, and our own surgical colleagues (Antunes, 1992), who have had to evaluate functional anatomy before attempting a reconstructive procedure, we define *mitral valve prolapse* as failure of leaflet coaptation, resulting in displacement of an involved leaflet's edge toward the left atrium. Unless a leaflet is fibrosed, shortened, or retracted or has a cleft or hole in it, a mitral valve is competent throughout systole because of sustained coaptation of leaflets (Fig. 1*A* through *D*). Where leaflets are normal in size, or larger, failure of sustained apposition must result in leaflet edge prolapse and hence mitral regurgitation (Fig. 1*E* through *H*).

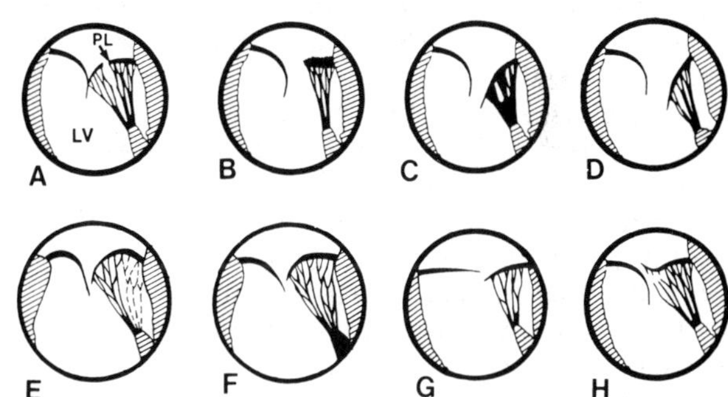

Figure 1
The mechanisms of mitral regurgitation. Some possible causes are mentioned. *A,* Perforation or cleft in a leaflet. *B,* Scarred and shortened leaflet due to chronic rheumatic heart disease or mitral annular calcification. *C,* Retracted and tethered leaflet, the result of shortened chordae tendineae in chronic rheumatic carditis. *D,* Failure of leaflet apposition because of papillary muscle retraction by a left ventricular aneurysm. *E,* Primary degeneration of mitral valve resulting in leaflet billowing, lengthened chordae tendineae, annular dilatation, and failure of leaflet edge apposition (Barlow's syndrome). *F,* Failure of leaflet apposition due to papillary muscle dysfunction secondary to occlusive coronary artery disease. *G,* Marked annular dilation causing anterior leaflet prolapse and functionally shortened PL in acute rheumatic carditis. *H,* Flail leaflet with ruptured chordae due to infective endocarditis, trauma, or unknown cause. PL, posterior leaflet; LV, left ventricle.

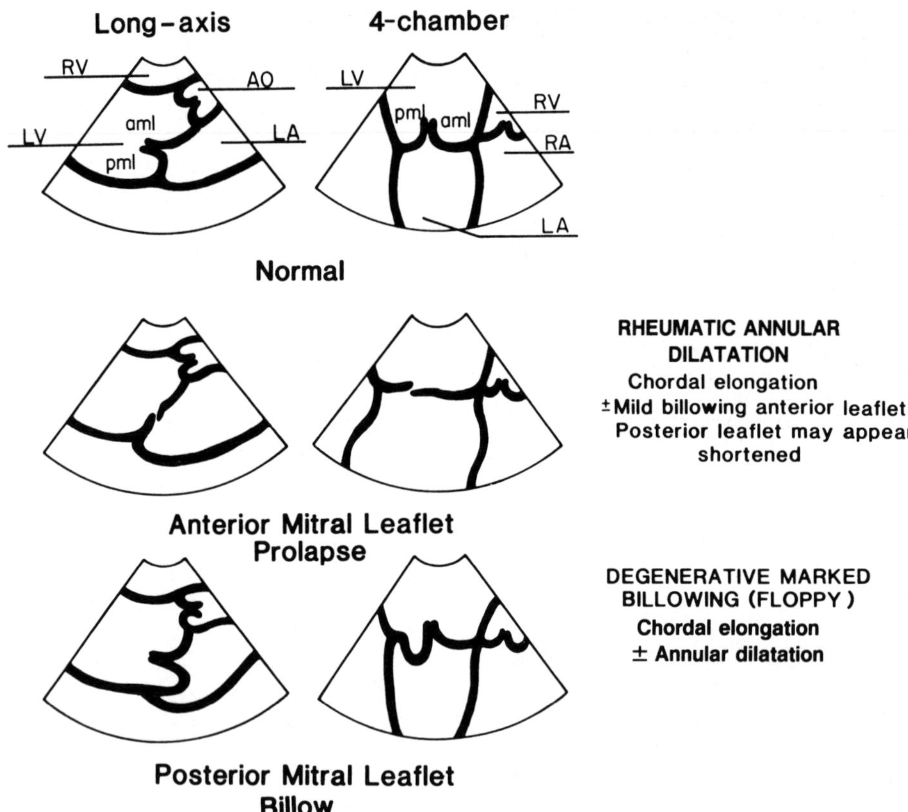

Figure 2
Two-dimensional echocardiographic appearance during systole of normal, prolapsed, and billowing mitral valves in the parasternal long axis and apical four-chamber views. In the normal valve the leaflets coapt. In rheumatic mitral prolapse, the annulus is dilated and the free edge of the prolapsing anterior leaflet is displaced beyond the line of valve closure. In degenerative mitral billow, the body of the posterior leaflet bulges into the left atrium (LA), but the leaflet margins usually appear coapted. Principal functional anatomic features are listed in the right column. Ao, aorta; LV, left ventricle; pml, posterior mitral leaflet; RA, right atrium; RV, right ventricle. *(From Barlow JB, et al. Mechanisms and management of heart failure in active rheumatic carditis. S Afr Med J 1990; 78:181; with permission.)*

The terms *billowing, floppy,* and *flail* also require definition in the context of correlating echocardiographic, cineangiocardiographic, and clinical evaluation with mitral valve functional anatomy. It is essentially the functional anatomy or pathology of the mitral valve mechanism that is evaluated by these investigations and that forms the principal basis for medical or surgical management.

Normal mitral leaflets bulge slightly, after closure, into the left atrial cavity. When this physiologic bulging is exaggerated, the term *billowing* is appropriate. *Billowing* and its more advanced form, *floppy,* are anatomic terms that describe the leaflet bodies. There is a gradation of mild billowing of near-normal leaflet bodies toward the left atrium during ventricular systole to marked displacement when the leaflets are voluminous, or floppy, and the chordae are elongated. *Prolapse* and its more advanced form, *flail,* reflect failure of leaflet edge apposition and therefore predominantly describe valve function. Two-dimensional echocardiography contributes to the evaluation of both the rheumatic and degenerative processes that may involve the complex mitral valve mechanism and result in functional prolapse, but the echocardiographic appearances are essentially different because functional anatomy is different (Fig. 2). The degenerative condition, widely and often inappropriately referred to as primary mitral valve *prolapse,* affects principally the leaflet bodies. However, in our environment, where fulminant acute rheumatic carditis remains prevalent, we have demonstrated (Marcus and co-workers, 1989, 1994) that the rheumatic process initially and predominantly causes annular dilation. The markedly dilated annulus exposes the chordae tendineae to enhanced tensile stress because of loss of the "keystone" effect during leaflet coaptation. Lengthening or rupture of chordae then supervene with consequent prolapse of the relatively normal anterior leaflet and thus mitral regurgitation. Redundancy and billowing of the leaflet bodies are not associated features.

In the degenerative nonrheumatic condition that provokes widespread interest in developed countries, billowing of the leaflet bodies, which has been the principal echocardiographic criterion for the prolapse misnomer, can range from a variant of normal to clearly pathologic floppy leaflets (Fig. 3). With markedly billowing or floppy leaflets, failure of leaflet edge apposition (prolapse) may indeed ensue, but the prolapse is obscured by the voluminous leaflet bodies and is sel-

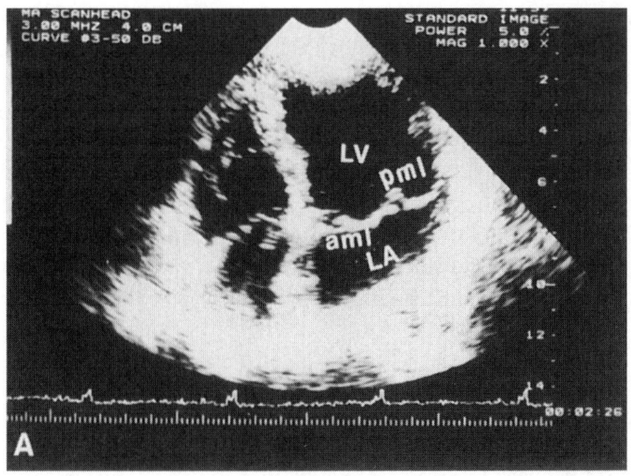

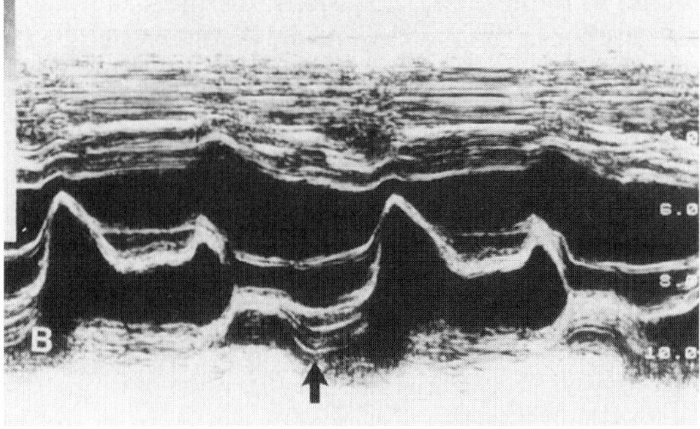

Figure 3
A, Two-dimensional echocardiogram, apical four-chamber view, demonstrates moderate billow of the anterior (aml) and posterior (pml) mitral leaflets. Both leaflets are thickened. Although the edges coapt on the ventricular side of the mitral annulus, a grade 3/6 late systolic murmur (indicative of prolapse) is present. *(From Barlow JB, Pocock WA, Mitral leaflet billowing and prolapse: Implications for management. Cardiovasc Drugs Ther 1988; 1:543; with permission.) B,* M-mode echocardiogram of the same patient illustrates marked late systolic billow of the posterior mitral leaflet. LA, left atrium; LV, left ventricle.

dom demonstrable on echocardiography until it becomes severe or a leaflet flail. Clinical examination and auscultation for the appropriate apical regurgitant murmur and third heart sound remain reliable and practical means of evaluating mitral regurgitation. Clinical cardiology as practiced in the 1990s and especially in developed countries regrettably reflects a decline in the use, accuracy, and status of auscultation. Detection and quantitative assessment of mitral regurgitation are now sought by Doppler techniques. They also have pitfalls (Bolger and co-workers, 1988), however, and the color Doppler as well as the biplane transesophageal color Doppler criteria for mild mitral regurgitation that have pathologic significance, still require clarification.

In addition to rheumatic carditis, which remains prevalent in less developed countries, many pathologic conditions affect the papillary muscles, chordae tendineae, annulus, leaflets, or the size and shape of the left ventricular cavity that may result in a billowing mitral leaflet (BML) and mitral valve prolapse (MVP). When such BML and MVP are secondary or associated entities, the prognosis is determined as much or more by the underlying or coexisting condition. This is well exemplified in Western countries by MVP secondary to hypertrophic cardiomyopathy, occlusive coronary artery disease, or Marfan's syndrome.

Discussion is confined in the remainder of this section to management of the degenerative condition that still provokes so much interest and that, in its severe form, is now recognized as the most frequent cause of pure mitral regurgitation requiring surgery in developed countries.

■ THERAPEUTIC ALTERNATIVES

Preferred Approach

Medical Treatment

The Syndrome. We use the term *BML syndrome* for what is also variously called *primary MVP, floppy valve, myxomatous leaflet, click-murmur,* or *Barlow's syndrome.* Idiopathic or primary MVP syndrome is a misnomer in the many patients who have no evidence of mitral regurgitation. A distinction between BML syndrome alone and that with MVP is crucial in formulating a management policy. The physician has to decide whether repeated auscultation, vasoactive maneuvers, echocardiography, or Doppler ultrasonography will contribute in determining whether regurgitation is present. As already intimated, echocardiographic criteria for BML are suspect, but the demonstration of advanced billowing, or floppy, bodies of leaflets would be compatible with clinically suspected mitral regurgitation and hence MVP. On the other hand, a floppy mitral valve, albeit anatomically pathologic, may still be functionally competent throughout systole.

The importance of making the diagnosis of primary BML syndrome, particularly in symptomatic patients, lies in the knowledge that in the large majority of cases reassurance can be given that there is no serious heart disease and that the prognosis for life is excellent. The BML may be focal, involving only a portion of one scallop, usually the middle scallop of the posterior leaflet, or it may be more advanced and diffuse. A constant or intermittent nonejection systolic click may be heard. Depending on the criteria used, two-dimensional echocardiography may indicate part of a leaflet body on the left atrial side of the annulus. The valve is competent and a "normal variant." Nonetheless, if the patient is symptomatic owing to chest pain or palpitations, he or she seeks assistance and the medical adviser should be wary before concluding that the symptoms are not causally related to the valve anomaly. It is now acknowledged (Boudoulas and co-workers, 1990)—and this complication is addressed later in more detail—that ventricular arrhythmias may supervene when mitral leaflets are markedly billowing or floppy. It has yet to be demonstrated that a BML does not indeed cause chest pain, albeit by an unknown mechanism or mechanisms.

Many symptomatic patients are anxious. Reasons for anxiety in patients with primary BML are not always apparent, and the role of a causally related autonomic disorder requires confirmation. Anxiety is aggravated in some patients by an incorrect diagnosis of occlusive coronary artery disease or when scant interpretation of the chest pain, sometimes allegedly severe, is involved. An explanation that there is "a very mild but also very common anomaly of a heart valve which sometimes causes ill-understood symptoms of nuisance value only" is a comprehensible explanation from which many patients derive reassurance. Excessively anxious patients who fail to respond to reassurance may improve on a small dose of a beta-adrenergic blocking drug. Chest pain and an abnormal electrocardiogram are prominent features of both the primary BML syndrome and occlusive coronary artery disease; thus the differentiation of these two conditions is a prevalent problem in clinical practice. Although this differentiation is clearly more difficult in a middle-aged man than in a young woman, careful history taking and stress electrocardiography should resolve the problem. The belief that the postexercise ST-segment and T wave changes of MVP are indistinguishable from those of myocardial ischemia, and hence are a cause of a false-positive stress test, is no longer valid. These electrocardiographic abnormalities can be reliably differentiated according to their time-course patterns after cessation of exercise (Barlow and co-workers, 1992). Radionuclide studies, other sophisticated stress test techniques, or selective coronary arteriography should infrequently be necessary.

Most patients with the BML syndrome follow a benign course, but complications may sometimes ensue. In addition to the auscultatory, electrocardiographic, and anatomic features of the syndrome originally identified in 1965 (Barlow, 1965), other components include skeletal abnormalities, arrhythmias, conduction defects, systemic emboli, hereditary factors, and, arguably, neurotic and autonomic disorders as well as myocardial dysfunction (Chesler and Gornick, 1991). A major contribution of two-dimensional echocardiography is that it can demonstrate whether the leaflet bodies are floppy and thickened (see Fig. 3). Patients with such leaflets do indeed make up a subgroup in that a majority of them have associated true MVP, with consequent mitral regurgitation, and are thus at increased risk for important complications such as infective endocarditis, spontaneous progression of the mitral regurgitation, and systemic emboli (Marks and co-workers, 1989). Moreover, voluminous leaflets and lax chordae predispose some patients to life-threatening ventricular arrhythmias.

Infective Endocarditis and Progression of Mitral Regurgitation. Whether symptomatic or not, patients with mitral regurgitation invariably have a more marked BML, and both prophylaxis against infective endocarditis and observation for progression of the mitral regurgitation are mandatory. Most nonpansystolic murmurs, whether confined to early or late systole, do not change over many years. Nonetheless, rapid progression of MVP, even in the absence of infective endocarditis may occur unpredictably. The overall incidence of such progression over a 10 year period is probably 10 percent, and this figure may be higher in middle-aged males. Then again, unequivocal billowing on echocardiography or a loud nonejection systolic click on auscultation does not imply that MVP, let alone severe MVP, will inevitably ensue.

Systemic Emboli. Bland emboli manifesting as transient ischemic attacks or partial strokes are a recognized complication of a prominent BML. Deposits of fibrin and platelet thrombi on the atrial surface of a floppy posterior leaflet may be the site of origin. We suggest that coronary embolism with coronary artery spasm is a possible mechanism for unexplained myocardial infarction in a few cases of marked BML. A purported association of MVP and migraine requires confirmation, as does a common role of increased platelet aggregability in both conditions. We recommend antithrombotic therapy only in patients who have had emboli. We have used aspirin (150 to 300 mg daily) plus dipyridamole (Persantine) (100 mg three times daily). The effectiveness of dipyridamole as an antithrombotic agent has been challenged and aspirin alone may be adequate. If systemic emboli are large or if an underlying supraventricular tachycardia is suspected, warfarin (Coumadin) therapy is suggested.

Arrhythmias and Sudden Death. Palpitations, lightheadedness, or dizziness suggests the presence of arrhythmias, but exercise electrocardiography or ambulatory monitoring is advisable for evaluation. Arrhythmias may occur without symptoms, and, conversely, dizziness and palpitations have been prominent complaints at times when electrocardiographic monitoring and clinical examination provide no objective confirmation. Orthostatic hypotension should be excluded in all patients with these symptoms. A wide variety of arrhythmias has been encountered with the primary BML syndrome, including supraventricular tachycardia, atrial fibrillation and flutter, atrial ectopic beats, ventricular tachycardia, and ventricular fibrillation. Ventricular extrasystoles are the most prevalent rhythm disturbance, may be unifocal or multifocal and may occur with or without an abnormal resting electrocardiogram. They are often precipitated or aggravated by emotion and exercise. If symptoms are troublesome, even if the arrhythmias are not potentially dangerous, patients should be given the benefit of treatment with antiarrhythmic drugs, preferably verapamil (Isoptin) (if supraventricular) or beta-blocking agents.

A reliable history of syncope, provided that it occurs outside a context of probable vasovagal syncope, is cause for major concern. Ambulatory monitoring and stress testing are then mandatory to detect multiform ventricular extrasystoles, the R-on-T phenomenon, or ventricular tachycardia. Although any beta-receptor blocking agent may contribute to therapy, in more intractable cases we have had favorable experience with the unique beta-receptor blocking agent sotalol (usual dose range 80 to 480 mg daily). Because of its important class III activity, sotalol has the potential to precipitate ventricular tachycardias of the torsades de pointes variety and should be used with caution in high dosage with concomitant diuretic therapy or in the presence of hypokalemia. Amiodarone (Cordarone), 200 to 400 mg daily after a loading dose, is highly effective in the treatment of refractory ventricular tachyarrhythmias, but serious side effects mitigate against its long-term use, especially in young patients. There are no data to justify treatment with Class IA antiarrhythmic drugs.

Over 200 patients with mitral leaflets and causally related sudden death or "sudden death syndrome" have been reported or are now known to us. Identification of patients at higher risk is crucial. A prominent BML, demonstrable on M-mode or two-dimensional echocardiography, and indisputable MVP, evaluated clinically by a constant apical late systolic murmur that becomes louder and longer on standing, are pertinent features. A family history of sudden unexpected death, abnormal T waves and ventricular ectopy detected on the resting electrocardiogram, multiform ventricular ectopy and ventricular tachyarrhythmias on exercise or ambulatory monitoring, and, most important, a history of unexpected syncope are principal risk factors. Where it is judged that the ventricular tachyarrhythmias or multifocal ventricular ectopy are causally related to the voluminous leaflets and lengthened chordae, mitral valve repair would seem the logical management. Successful short-term results have been attained with implantable defibrillators, but this approach fails to address the basic cause of the life-threatening problem.

Surgical Treatment

Severe Mitral Regurgitation. Largely because of imprecise terminology, the frequency of progressive mitral regurgitation requiring surgery in patients with BML or MVP remains unknown. Studies undertaken retrospectively or based principally on suspect echocardiographic criteria suggest that the overall frequency is approximately 5 percent, that at least two-thirds are male, and that the majority are older than 50 years. Neither we nor, to our knowledge, other investigators have followed prospectively for 10 or more years a meaningful number of unselected patients with constant late or early systolic murmurs, intermittent systolic murmurs judged mitral in origin, or isolated nonejection clicks.

The follow-up studies by Düren and co-workers in Amsterdam (1988) and You-Bing and co-workers in Japan (1990) of symptomatic patients with MVP and late or pansystolic murmurs suggest that progression to severe mitral regurgitation requiring surgery occurs in 10 to 15 percent. These higher figures relate to selected patients with established mitral regurgitation and do not provide data that dispute an anticipated excellent prognosis for patients with clinical and echocardiographic signs of a BML alone. They do confirm, however, that prognosis should be more guarded and regular observation more important in patients with MVP and constant apical late systolic murmur.

Indications for surgery in patients with severe MVP and hemodynamically important mitral regurgitation may be modified by whether or not valve repair is judged feasible. Using techniques originally described by Carpenter (1980), the degenerative floppy mitral valve is particularly amenable to a surgical repair, and the durability of such repair over at least 10 years has been confirmed. Cardiac surgeons throughout the world are now gaining meaningful and ever increasing experience with valvuloplastic procedures.

If clinical, echocardiographic, and sometimes cineangiocardiographic evaluation indicate rupture of chordae to the middle scallop of the posterior leaflet, a McGoon type valvuloplasty is reasonably certain to be successful. In such instances, and also when billowing and prolapse are confined to the posterior leaflet, we are more aggressive regarding earlier surgery and have operated on patients with class II symptoms, especially when relatively young (under about 60 years of age). When both leaflets are shown echocardiographically to be floppy and thickened, the annulus dilated, and a number of chordae elongated or ruptured, there is more difficulty in deciding on the timing of surgery. Appropriately experienced surgeons claim that mitral valve repair can be performed successfully in at least 80 percent of such cases, and this is in accord with our own observations (Barlow, 1996).

However, the prospects of a failed valvuloplasty, a long period on cardiopulmonary bypass, and obligatory valve replacement with its enhanced valve-related morbidity and mortality risks still influence a decreasing number of cardiologists and cardiac surgeons toward both postponing surgery until the patient is significantly symptomatic and insisting that the patient leave the hospital with a "normal" mitral valve, hence settling for valve replacement. We practice relatively early surgery with Carpentier ring valvuloplasty for hemodynamically important mitral regurgitation, but decisions inevitably depend much on the surgeon's ability or experience with that procedure; the overall evaluation of the patient, including age; and the presence of associated symptomatic or life-threatening arrhythmias.

Potentially Fatal Arrhythmias. A policy of surgical valvuloplasty for ventricular arrhythmias in patients with the BML syndrome without significant MVP and hemodynamically important mitral regurgitation may seem unjustified. The mechanisms proposed to explain the enhanced ventricular irritability with a floppy mitral valve include tugging on the papillary muscles, asynchronism of myocardial relaxation, endocardial friction, coronary embolism, and "diastolic dumping." Virtually all these are dependent on voluminous and excessively mobile mitral leaflets. Kligfield and co-workers (1987) observed that BML patients with mitral regurgitation had considerably more ventricular ectopy than those without mitral regurgitation. It is certain, however, that BML patients with mitral regurgitation have more advanced floppy and voluminous leaflets, and we submit that this is the relevant aspect rather than the presence or extent of the mitral regurgitation itself. Ventricular arrhythmias are not a feature of rheumatic anterior mitral leaflet prolapse, in which mitral leaflets are neither voluminous nor billowing, irrespective of the severity of the mitral regurgitation (Barlow, 1992). Successful surgical results obtained by mitral valvuloplasty have been attained in BML patients with potentially fatal ventricular arrhythmias (Pocock and co-workers, 1991), but our ongoing experience strongly suggests (Barlow, 1996) that the surgeon must reduce leaflet size significantly and shorten elongated chordae as well as eliminate the mitral regurgitation. It is the floppy leaflets and lax chordae, and not the mitral regurgitation, that predispose to the ventricular arrhythmias.

Provided that a surgeon experienced in valvuloplastic procedures is available, we therefore conclude that the combination of an advanced BML demonstrated echocardiographically, a reliable history of syncope, and potentially lethal ventricular arrhythmias are indications for mitral valve repair, even in the absence of hemodynamically important mitral regurgitation. Mitral valve replacement, with its need for anticoagulation and attendant risks of thromboembolism or hemorrhage, is probably justified only when the mitral regurgitation is severe and the surgeon unable to accomplish a successful conservative procedure.

Suggested Reading

Antunes MJ. Mitral valve repair into the 1990s. Eur J Cardiothorac Surg 1992; 6(Suppl 1):S13.

Barlow JB. Conjoint clinic on the clinical significance of late systolic murmurs and non-ejection systolic clicks. J Chron Dis 1965; 18:665.

Barlow JB. Mitral valve billowing and prolapse: An overview. Aust N Z J Med 1992; 22:541.

Barlow CW, Barlow JB, Friedman BM, Seicher ER. The importance of assessing time-course behaviour of abnormal ST/T changes after exercise. Aust N Z J Med 1992; 22:618.

Barlow JB. Mitral valve disease: A cardiologic-surgical interaction. Isr J Med 1996; 32:831.

Bolger AF, Eigler NL, Maurer G. Quantifying valvular regurgitation: Limitations and inherent assumptions of Doppler techniques. Circulation 1988; 78:1316.

Boudoulas H, Schaal SF, Stang JM, et al. Mitral valve prolapse: Cardiac arrest with long-term survival. Int J Cardiol 1990; 26:37.

Carpenter A, Chauvaud S, Fabiani JH, et al. Reconstructive surgery of mitral valve incompetence. Ten-year appraisal. J Thorac Cardiovasc Surg 1980; 79:338.

Chesler E, Gornick CC. Maladies attributed to myxomatous mitral valve. Circulation 1991; 82:328.

Criley JM, Lewis KB, Humphries JO, Ross RS. Prolapse of the mitral valve: Clinical and cine-angiocardiographic findings. Br Heart J 1966; 28:488.

Düren DR, Becker AE, Dunning AJ. Long-term follow up of idiopathic mitral valve prolapse in 300 patients: A prospective study. J Am Coll Cardiol 1988; 11:42.

Kligfield P, Levy D, Devereux RB, Savage DD. Arrhythmias and sudden death in mitral valve prolapse. Am Heart J 1987; 113:1298.

Marcus RH, Sareli P, Pocock WA, et al. Functional anatomy of severe mitral regurgitation in active rheumatic carditis. Am J Cardiol 1989; 63: 577.

Marcus RH, Sareli P, Pocock WA, Barlow JB. The spectrum of severe rheumatic mitral valve disease in a developing country. Ann Int Med 1994; 120:177.

Marks AR, Choong CY, Sanfilippo AJ, et al. Identification of high-risk and low-risk subgroups of patients with mitral-valve prolapse. N Engl J Med 1989; 320:1031.

Pocock WA, Barlow JB, Marcus RH, Barlow CW. Mitral valvuloplasty for life-threatening ventricular arrhythmias in mitral valve prolapse. Am Heart J 1991; 121:199.

You-Bing D, Takenaka K, Sakamoto T, et al. Follow-up in mitral valve prolapse by phonocardiography, M-mode and two-dimensional echocardiography and Doppler echocardiography. Am J Cardiol 1990; 65:349.

MITRAL REGURGITATION

Albert E. Raizner, M.D.
Craig O. Siegel, M.D.

Mitral regurgitation may result from acute or chronic damage to any component of the mitral valve apparatus, including the valve annulus, leaflets, chordae tendineae, and papillary muscles. Mitral regurgitation may be acute or chronic. The most common etiologies of acute mitral regurgitation are ischemic heart disease, infective endocarditis, and rupture of the chordae tendineae. The most common causes of chronic mitral regurgitation are myxomatous degeneration of the leaflets, rheumatic heart disease, ischemic heart disease, and calcification of the mitral annulus. Mitral regurgitation may also be secondary to left ventricular enlargement from any cause. The diagnosis is usually suggested by an apical systolic murmur on physical examination. Doppler echocardiography has become the mainstay of noninvasive diagnosis. Additionally, Doppler and two-dimensional echocardiography are used to estimate the severity of valvular dysfunction and left ventricular chamber size and function and thereby to follow the course of the disease and the response to treatment. In some patients with acute mitral regurgitation, a systolic murmur may not be audible and transthoracic Doppler echocardiography may fail to show severe regurgitation. If it is suspected, transesophageal Doppler echocardiography should be obtained.

Understanding the pathophysiology of mitral regurgitation is vital to the rational management of patients with the disorder. Acutely, volume overload of the left ventricle with regurgitation into a noncompliant left atrium produces pulmonary venous congestion and pulmonary hypertension. Congestive heart failure symptoms occur abruptly and are often severe. Further, the acutely volume-overloaded left ventricle cannot immediately compensate, and a low output state is often seen. In chronic mitral regurgitation, progressive dilation of the left ventricle and atrium occurs. The dilated and compliant left atrium provides a low impedance for regurgitant flow across the mitral valve. Symptoms of congestive heart failure occur late in the course of the disease and are often insidious in origin. Despite a marked increase in preload, indices of left ventricular systolic function often remain normal until late in the course of the disease. The timing of surgical intervention remains an important and challenging part of the management of patients with mitral regurgitation.

■ THERAPEUTIC ALTERNATIVES

Asymptomatic patients with mild degrees of mitral regurgitation may require little, if any, specific therapy. However, medical management is appropriate for the symptomatic patient with more severe degrees of regurgitation. Vasodilators, specifically those agents that reduce systemic arterial pressure, or afterload, are the cornerstones of treatment and may be administered intravenously in the acute setting or orally in the chronic setting. Digitalis glycosides and diuretics are used frequently as well. Arrhythmias, particularly atrial flutter and fibrillation, are encountered commonly and are treated with specific antiarrhythmic medications. In acute mitral regurgitation, intravenously administered inotropic agents and, in some cases, insertion of an intra-aortic balloon may be necessary. Patients with ischemic mitral regurgitation may be candidates for revascularization with coronary angioplasty or coronary artery bypass surgery. Surgical options include repair of the mitral valve apparatus or valve replacement using either a bioprosthetic or mechanical prosthetic valve.

■ PREFERRED APPROACH

To establish appropriate therapy, several critical questions must be addressed. (1) Is the mitral regurgitation acute or chronic? (2) Is it primary or secondary? What is the likely etiology? (3) Is the patient symptomatic? (4) What is the severity of valvular dysfunction? (5) What is the status of left ventricular function? A generalized schema of management is shown in Figure 1.

Medical Treatment

Acute Mitral Regurgitation

The patient presenting with acute mitral regurgitation should be evaluated by two-dimensional and Doppler echocardiography or by transesophageal echocardiography. By so doing, the diagnosis of mitral regurgitation can be confirmed and an estimate of its severity obtained. This is particularly important in patients with acute myocardial infarction in whom the traditional hallmark of clinical diagnosis, the systolic murmur, is often absent. Echocardiography may help to establish a specific etiology of mitral regurgitation. Transesophageal echocardiography is particularly useful in this regard in that it provides important information about valve vegetations, flail leaflets, and other factors. Additionally, the severity of valvular dysfunction, including measurement of regurgitant fraction, and qualitative and quantitative assessment of left ventricular function may be ascertained. Patients who are hemodynamically unstable require Swan-Ganz catheter insertion to monitor pulmonary artery and pulmonary capillary wedge pressure as well as to measure cardiac output. Although many of these patients require surgical intervention, initial stabilization with aggressive medical therapy is generally advisable. Central to this approach is the use of vasodilator therapy. By reducing left ventricular afterload, the regurgitant flow into the left atrium is reduced and forward cardiac output is enhanced. Additionally, left ventricular volume may decrease, thereby reducing the size of the mitral annulus and the regurgitant orifice. This latter effect may be of particular benefit to patients with secondary forms of acute mitral regurgitation.

The drug of choice for afterload reduction in the acute setting is sodium nitroprusside. A balanced vasodilator, nitroprusside relaxes both arterial and venous vascular smooth muscle. The drug is administered via a continuous intravenous infusion. It must be protected from light to prevent degradation. The initial dose is 0.5 μg per kilogram per minute. The infusion is titrated for the desired hemodynamic effect to a maximum dose of 10 μg per kilogram per minute. A fall in systemic vascular resistance, a decrease in pulmonary capillary wedge pressure, and a rise in cardiac output indicate a satisfactory hemodynamic response. Cyanide toxicity, manifested as headache, vomiting, depressed mentation, or coma, is a major concern with the use of nitroprusside; it occurs more frequently in the setting of renal insufficiency. Thiocyanate levels should be monitored during prolonged infusion and should not exceed 6 mg per deciliter.

In patients who are intolerant to nitroprusside, intravenous nitroglycerin may be used to achieve afterload reduction. The drug is particularly useful in the setting of underlying ischemic heart disease. The infusion is started at 10 μg per minute and is titrated to achieve an optimal hemodynamic effect. It is imperative to monitor cardiac output frequently when intravenous nitroglycerin is used; because nitroglycerin is a more potent venodilator, a fall in pulmonary capillary wedge pressure may occur with no change or even a decrease in cardiac output.

If the cardiac output is low or if other parameters of left ventricular systolic function are abnormal, the addition of an inotropic agent is beneficial. Dobutamine, a synthetic sympathomimetic amine that stimulates predominantly beta_1-receptors, is administered by continuous intravenous infusion. The usual starting dose is 2.5 μg per kilogram per minute and may be titrated up to 15 μg per kilogram per minute. Therapeutic doses range from 5 to 10 μg per kilogram per minute. Hemodynamically, one sees a rise in cardiac output coupled with a mild to modest fall in systemic vascular resistance; heart rate is minimally changed, and arrhythmogenic potential is negligible.

Dopamine, the catecholamine precursor of norepinephrine, is a sympathomimetic amine with multiple hemodynamic effects mediated through its binding to alpha, beta, dopaminergic, and serotonin receptors. Its hemodynamic effects depend on the dose used. In doses of 2 to 5 μg per kilogram per minute, the predominant effect is one of improved renal blood flow; cardiac contractility is only mildly enhanced. In doses ranging from 5 to 10 μg per kilogram per minute, cardiac contractility is increased with little effect on peripheral vascular resistance. Consequently, this dose range is most efficacious in patients with mitral regurgitation. Doses above 10 μg per kilogram per minute may produce a significant increase in systemic vascular resistance, an effect that may worsen mitral regurgitation. Tachyarrhythmias and increased ventricular ectopy may occur with dopamine administration and limit its usefulness.

Patients presenting with evidence of cardiogenic shock, including low cardiac output, elevated pulmonary capillary wedge pressure, and systemic hypotension, may require more aggressive management. In this setting, insertion of an intra-aortic balloon pump may be lifesaving, permitting stabilization while preparations are made for surgical interventions. Deflation of the intra-aortic balloon during systole provides effective afterload reduction while diastolic balloon expansion enhances coronary blood flow. Intra-aortic balloon counterpulsation is contraindicated in patients with concomitant aortic valve regurgitation.

Acute ischemic mitral regurgitation in the setting of myocardial infarction most commonly results from papillary muscle dysfunction. Complete or partial rupture of a papillary muscle occurs less frequently. In patients with acute ischemic mitral regurgitation, consideration should be given to reperfusion therapy with a thrombolytic agent or coronary angioplasty because this approach may restore valve competence in addition to salvaging viable myocardium. Thrombolytic therapy with tissue plasminogen activator, streptokinase, or anisoylated plasminogen streptokinase activator complex (APSAC) is indicated in the first 4 to 6 hours after the onset of infarction. Its effectiveness in establishing reperfu-

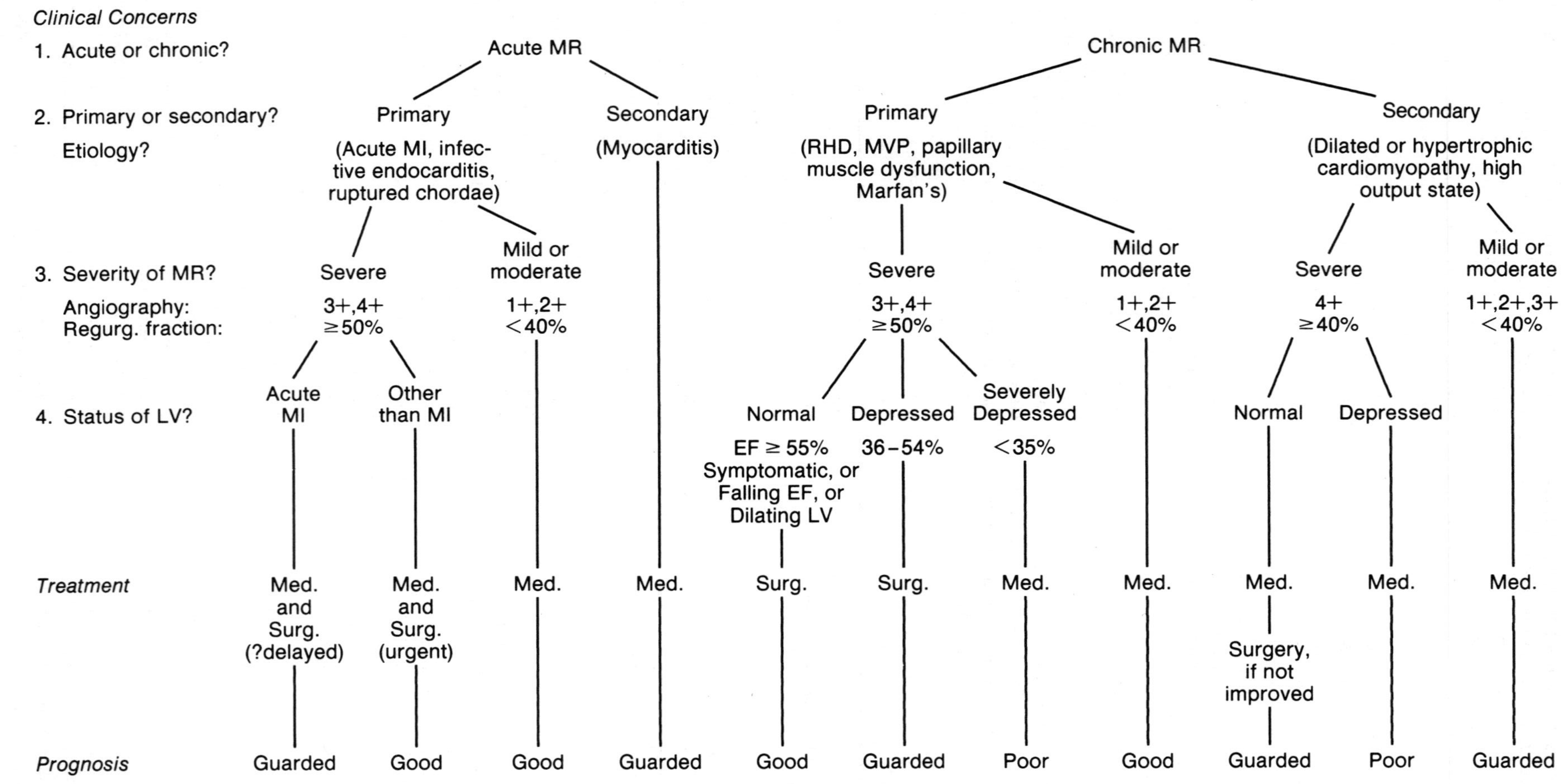

Figure 1
Management of patients with mitral regurgitation. EF, ejection fraction; LV, left ventricle; MI, myocardial infarction; MR, mitral regurgitation; MVP, mitral valve prolapse; RHD, rheumatic heart disease.

sion beyond this early time frame has not been firmly established, although some patients with persistent ischemic pain and ST segment elevation may benefit up to 24 hours after onset. Because the onset of clinically apparent ischemic mitral regurgitation may be delayed by several hours or days following infarction, the applicability of thrombolysis to such patients is limited. Coronary angioplasty, however, may be performed at any time during the course of acute myocardial infarction if the clinical need becomes manifest. It must be noted that patients with rupture of the papillary muscle are not expected to benefit from reperfusion therapy; in such patients, rapid deterioration and death often occurs within 24 hours unless mitral valve replacement is performed immediately. In contrast, patients with ischemic dysfunction of the papillary muscle may be stabilized hemodynamically with intravenous vasodilators and inotropic agents in conjunction with coronary angioplasty when anatomically appropriate. This may allow temporization of these otherwise precarious patients until definitive surgical therapy can be carried out more safely.

Patients with acute mitral regurgitation secondary to infective endocarditis are particularly troublesome. Depending on the virulence of the organism isolated and the degree of valvular dysfunction, early surgical intervention may be necessary. Although it is advantageous to eradicate the infection preoperatively with an appropriate course of antibiotics, this is not always possible. Urgent surgical intervention, regardless of the length of antibiotic treatment, should be performed if left ventricular function deteriorates or if hemodynamic measurements reveal a persistently high pulmonary capillary wedge pressure or borderline cardiac output indicating limited cardiac reserve.

Chronic Mitral Regurgitation

Medical treatment for chronic mitral regurgitation is prescribed usually for those patients with milder degrees of mitral regurgitation, for those with severely depressed left ventricular function who are believed to be poor surgical candidates, and for those with secondary forms of valvular dysfunction.

Vasodilator therapy plays a key role in managing patients with chronic mitral regurgitation. Orally administered angiotensin converting enzyme (ACE) inhibitors such as enalapril and captopril are preferred. Enalapril should be started at 2.5 mg twice a day and may be increased to 10 mg twice a day. Important side effects include orthostatic hypotension and renal dysfunction manifested as an increase in blood urea nitrogen and creatinine. This latter effect is more likely to occur when diuretics are used concomitantly. A particularly bothersome and subtle side effect is the development of a chronic, nonproductive cough. It is sometimes difficult to distinguish the cough associated with congestive heart failure from that attributed to enalapril. Discontinuation of the drug for several days should clarify the etiology; amelioration of the cough indicates a drug effect. Captopril may be started at 6.25 to 12.5 mg three times a day and should be titrated to a maximum dose of 50 mg three times a day. Its side effect profile is similar to that of enalapril.

Patients with pre-existing renal dysfunction or those who develop renal dysfunction during the course of therapy with an ACE inhibitor may be treated with hydralazine, a peripheral vasodilator that directly relaxes vascular smooth muscle. The usual initial dose is 25 mg four times a day; this may be increased to a maximum of 100 mg four times a day. Side effects include palpitations due to reflex tachycardia and hypersensitivity reactions such as arthralgias and fever. A lupus-like syndrome may occur when higher doses are used.

Digitalis glycosides and diuretics are indicated if there is evidence of left ventricular dysfunction or pulmonary venous congestion. A loading dose of digoxin, 0.75 to 1 mg, should be given over 7 to 8 hours and followed by daily maintenance therapy. Diuretics may be administered intravenously or orally, depending on the clinical circumstance. A loop diuretic such as furosemide is preferred. If an inadequate diuretic response is achieved, the addition of metolazone, which inhibits sodium reabsorption in the proximal convoluted tubule and enhances the effectiveness of loop diuretics, may be useful. It is most effective when given 1 hour before administration of furosemide. Hypokalemia, sometimes to a profound degree, may occur when this diuretic combination is used. Importantly, the hemodynamic effect of diuretics in patients with chronic mitral regurgitation must be monitored closely. Because left ventricular dilation is a compensatory mechanism to maintain cardiac output in a chronically volume-overloaded state, volume depletion resulting from diuretic usage may result in a fall in forward cardiac output manifested as fatigue, orthostatic hypotension, or progressive renal dysfunction.

Arrhythmias, particularly atrial fibrillation and atrial flutter, are encountered commonly and may herald impending hemodynamic deterioration. Attempts to control the heart rate and restore sinus rhythm should be pursued vigorously. Digoxin is the drug of choice to initiate therapy. It slows the ventricular rate and may convert the patient to sinus rhythm in some instances. Verapamil may be used concomitantly with digoxin; 5 to 10 mg intravenously over 10 to 15 minutes is usually effective in quickly slowing the ventricular rate. Oral maintenance therapy in dosages of 120 to 360 mg daily generally is required. Because verapamil is a vasodilator and has only minimal negative inotropic effects, it is particularly useful in patients with chronic mitral regurgitation. Beta-blocking drugs are also effective in slowing the ventricular rate and in converting some patients back to sinus rhythm. The negative inotropic effects of most of the drugs in this category dictate their cautious use.

Despite the effectiveness of digoxin, verapamil, and beta-blockers in slowing the ventricular rate in patients with atrial fibrillation and flutter, the ultimate goal of antiarrhythmic treatment should be conversion to sinus rhythm if the arrhythmia has been present for less than 6 months. The most effective drug in this regard is quinidine. Initial doses of 400 mg every 4 hours to a total of 2 g is generally effective in establishing sinus rhythm. Quinidine gluconate, 325 to 650 mg every 8 hours, is used for maintenance therapy. Drug levels of digoxin and quinidine should be checked periodically, particularly when changes in drugs and dosages are made, because these agents have important and potentially dangerous interactions. Gastrointestinal side effects are common with quinidine and may be severe enough to prevent its continued use. Procainamide or propafenone can be substituted as second-line drugs.

Patients with rheumatic mitral regurgitation should be

maintained on an antibiotic regimen to prevent recurrent rheumatic fever (discussed in the chapter *Prevention of Acute Rheumatic Fever*). Additionally, prophylaxis for infective endocarditis should be prescribed for patients with mitral regurgitation from any cause or for those with a prosthetic heart valve.

Surgical Treatment

The timing of surgical intervention remains one of the most difficult decisions in managing patients with mitral regurgitation. Many considerations must be taken into account, including the patient's hemodynamic and clinical status, the function of the left ventricle, the presence of other noncardiac disease, and the experience and skill of the surgical team.

In patients with severe acute mitral regurgitation, surgical intervention must be considered early in the course of the illness because deterioration of left ventricular function may occur rapidly. Initial stabilization with intravenous vasodilator and inotropic agents, along with hemodynamic monitoring, is necessary to optimize the patient's hemodynamic status in preparation for surgery. This period of stabilization may not be possible in patients with papillary muscle rupture who require immediate surgical intervention. Papillary muscle dysfunction in the setting of myocardial infarction demands surgical consideration. However, the operative mortality when performed within the first week following acute myocardial infarction is substantially higher than when performed 4 to 6 weeks later. Therefore, temporizing with aggressive medical therapy, as outlined previously, is advantageous. Some patients may even respond with a reduction in the degree of mitral regurgitation, obviating the need for surgical intervention. It must be emphasized, however, that hemodynamic parameters must be monitored attentively and surgery should be delayed only if a good hemodynamic response is achieved. Otherwise, further left ventricular deterioration and even higher operative risk result. In patients with ruptured chordae presenting with acute mitral regurgitation, surgery should be performed as soon as hemodynamic stabilization is achieved. There is little benefit to delaying surgery under these circumstances.

In patients with chronic mitral regurgitation, the timing of surgical intervention is more difficult. Hemodynamic deterioration may develop insidiously over many years. Consequently, the patient tends to adjust his or her life-style and activities, and the gradual development of symptoms may go unnoticed by the patient and physician. Symptoms that are noticeably limiting generally indicate an advanced stage of the disease. Operation is indicated in symptomatic patients, provided that left ventricular function is not severely depressed (ejection fraction < 35 percent) because left ventricular function tends to deteriorate after mitral valve surgery as the low impedence route of ventricular ejection is eliminated. Consequently, such patients often continue to deteriorate despite surgical correction.

In patients with severe regurgitation who are asymptomatic or who have only minimal symptoms, mitral valve surgery should be performed in an effort to preserve further deterioration of left ventricular function if sequential echocardiograms show (1) decreasing ejection fraction (approximately 5 units or more), or (2) enlarging left ventricular size, with end-systolic diameter approaching 50 mm or 26 mm per square meter of body surface area or end-systolic volume approaching 60 ml per square meter. Angiography is used to confirm the severity of the regurgitation, to further assess the degree of left ventricular dilation or dysfunction, and to define coronary anatomy.

Surgical options include mitral valve repair or replacement with either a bioprosthetic or mechanical prosthetic valve. Advances in surgical technique for the repair of mitral valves have enabled many or most insufficient valves with flexible leaflets to be repaired. These techniques involve annuloplasty, leaflet resection, and replacement of ruptured or elongated chordae with artificial chordae. The latter technique has been particularly valuable in preserving the native mitral valve. The major factors that prevent repair of mitral valves are heavy thickening and/or calcification of the leaflets as is seen in rheumatic mitral valve disease. Nevertheless, valve repair should be considered a serious option for any patient with mitral regurgitation. Advantages of repairing rather than replacing the valve are the avoidance of long-term anticoagulation and the preservation of left ventricular geometry, which favorably affects left ventricular function postoperatively. However, a note of caution is warranted: An inadequate or poor surgical repair is worse than no repair because a second operation to replace the inadequately repaired valve carries a higher surgical risk. Surgical expertise in repairing mitral valves varies widely depending on the skill and experience of the surgeon. Proper selection of the surgeon is as important as appropriate selection of the patient.

In choosing between a bioprosthetic or a mechanical prosthetic valve, consideration should be given to the patient's age, the presence of atrial fibrillation, and any contraindications to oral anticoagulant therapy. The older patient at increased risk for bleeding complications or the female patient of childbearing age in whom oral anticoagulants are undesirable should be considered for a bioprosthetic valve. In most other patients in whom chronic anticoagulation is feasible, we favor a mechanical prosthesis, such as the St. Jude's valve, because of long-term durability and favorable hemodynamic properties. In experienced centers, an operative mortality of less than 5 percent should be anticipated.

Postoperatively, patients should be followed for evidence of left ventricular deterioration as manifested by a reduction in ejection fraction. A reduction in ejection fraction does not necessarily imply clinical deterioration because stabilization at this level is the general rule as long as severe left ventricular dysfunction was not present preoperatively. Long-term anticoagulation with sodium warfarin should be monitored on a regular basis, with prothrombin times and INRs (International Normalized Ratio) obtained no less often than every 2 months. A prothrombin time of 1.5 to 2 times control or an INR of 2.0 to 3.0 provides satisfactory prophylaxis against thromboembolic events with a low risk of serious bleeding.

Suggested Reading

Castello R, Lenzen P, Aguirre F, Labovitz AJ. Quantification of mitral regurgitation by transesophageal echocardiography with Doppler color flow mapping: Correlation with cardiac catheterization. J Am Coll Cardiol 1992; 19:1516.

O'Rourke RA, Crawford MN. Mitral valve regurgitation. Curr Probl Cardiol 1984; 9:1.

Perloff JK, Roberts WC. The mitral apparatus: Functional anatomy of mitral regurgitation. Circulation 1972; 46:227.

Rankin JS, Hickey MStJ, Smith LR, et al. Ischemic mitral regurgitation. Circulation 1989; 79 (Suppl I):116.

Ross J. Afterload mismatch in aortic and mitral valve disease: Implications for surgical therapy. J Am Coll Cardiol 1985; 5:811.

Zile MR. Chronic aortic and mitral regurgitation: Choosing the optimal time for surgical correction. Cardiol Clin 1991; 9:239.

AORTIC STENOSIS IN ADULTS

James A. Ronan Jr., M.D.

Patients with aortic stenosis usually first become aware of it when the characteristic murmur is detected, typically on a routine examination. There is then a long asymptomatic period followed by a much shorter symptomatic period, which usually begins in middle or late life. After the onset of symptoms, most patients have surgical replacement of the aortic valve and continue active life-styles for many more years. Proper management throughout the patient's lifetime includes not only determining when and if the aortic valve needs to be replaced but also carefully attending to many other details both before and after the valve replacement.

During the many asymptomatic years, the aortic valve, although partially stenotic, has not yet reached a critical degree of narrowing. The normal aortic valve has an area of 3 to 5 cm^2. In aortic stenosis the area becomes progressively smaller over a period of many years, and it is not until it reaches about 1.5 cm^2 that a transvalvular pressure gradient is first produced. Symptoms do not usually begin until the valve narrows even further and a high pressure gradient has been present for many years. Critical aortic stenosis is often defined as a valve area of less than 0.7 cm^2, and it is usually associated with a transvalvular pressure gradient of more than 50 to 75 mm Hg.

■ THERAPEUTIC ALTERNATIVES

Medical therapy of some sort, such as the treatment of heart failure or arrhythmias, is often required. The major problem, however, is to determine if and when surgery is to be performed. Percutaneous aortic valvuloplasty is also available but has significant limitations.

■ PREFERRED APPROACH

Medical Treatment

Asymptomatic Period

Medical and surgical treatments of aortic stenosis are not merely alternative forms of therapy, but rather they are therapies used to address different goals at various stages in the natural history of the disease. During the long asymptomatic period, the patient should be educated about the aortic stenosis and its natural history; the patient should have a clear understanding that aortic valve replacement may be needed in the future. The patient should be encouraged to remain physically active, but once a critical degree of stenosis has been reached, extreme physical activities such as overly competitive sports should be avoided. To prevent endocarditis the patient should be instructed carefully in the use of prophylactic antibiotics at the time of dental work or whenever there is possible exposure to a bacteremia. For dental work 3 g amoxicillin orally 1 hour before the procedure and 1.5 g 6 hours later are advised. If the patient has had rheumatic fever, continuous prophylaxis against beta-streptococcal infections is indicated to avoid subsequent episodes of rheumatic fever. The prophylaxis should be given in the form of 200,000 units of penicillin G orally twice daily or 1.2 million units of benzathine penicillin intramuscularly each month. This should be continued until the risk of rheumatic fever is minimal, typically at about 40 years of age.

Whenever the diagnosis of aortic stenosis is established for the first time, baseline data about its severity should be obtained by a careful cardiac physical examination, a chest roentgenogram, an electrocardiogram, and an echocardiogram with Doppler studies. Cardiac catheterization is not necessary, particularly if a modern, reliable echocardiography laboratory is available. Estimate of the severity of aortic stenosis is usually as accurate by transthoracic echocardiography as by heart catheterization (Galan and co-workers, 1991). Furthermore, the echocardiogram provides additional useful information, such as the anatomy and pathology of the valve (congenital, rheumatic, or degenerative), the size and function of the left ventricle and other chambers, and the presence of additional lesions such as hypertrophic subaortic stenosis, aortic regurgitation, and mitral regurgitation. The aortic valve area can also be estimated accurately by direct planimetry of the stenotic valve during a transesophageal echocardiogram (TEE) (Stoddard and co-workers, 1991). However, in most cases the transthoracic echocardiogram is satisfactory and the TEE is not necessary. There should be a regularly scheduled longitudinal follow-up for each patient; physical examination should be repeated every 2 years and the other studies should be repeated every 3 to 5 years.

As long as the patient remains asymptomatic, aortic valve replacement is not indicated, even when the valve becomes critically stenotic, because evidence shows that mortality from aortic stenosis is extremely rare in truly asymptomatic individuals (Kelly and co-workers, 1988). However, asymptomatic patients who develop critical aortic stenosis should be seen more frequently (every 4 to 6 months) so that decisions about surgery can be made as soon as symptoms appear because ventricular function may degenerate rapidly after the onset of symptoms. Then, too, it must be remembered that occasionally patients with severe aortic stenosis remain asymptomatic simply because they are inactive.

Symptomatic Phase

The symptoms of aortic stenosis are dyspnea, syncope, and angina. By the time the symptoms appear, the aortic stenosis either is already at or approaching the critical level of narrowing, and the prognosis for survival is about 2 to 5 years. Aortic valve replacement is recommended soon after symptom onset because medical treatment provides only mild and temporary improvement in symptoms and has little effect on survival. However, during the interval before surgery, or if a patient refuses surgery, medical treatment may help temporarily. Dyspnea is the most common symptom of heart failure; it is due to left atrial pressure elevation, secondary to either systolic or diastolic dysfunction of the left ventricle. The distinction between these two types of ventricular dysfunction can be made easily by echocardiography, and it will help in the choice of the correct medical treatment. In systolic dysfunction the left ventricle is dilated and contracts poorly; in diastolic dysfunction the cavity size is normal or small and contractility is normal. In both types there is ventricular hypertrophy and left atrial enlargement. Systolic dysfunction may also be recognized by a low left ventricular ejection fraction whether measured by angiography, echocardiography, or nuclear studies. In both types of dysfunction, reduction of left atrial pressure with diuretics is usually helpful, but diuretics should be given cautiously in patients with diastolic dysfunction to avoid hypovolemia and hypotension. Inotropic agents such as digoxin may be helpful if there is left ventricular dilation and systolic dysfunction, but it will be of no value in diastolic dysfunction. Vasodilator therapy may be of limited benefit in systolic dysfunction but, if used, should be administered in low doses (such as captopril 12.5 mg one to two times daily) to avoid hypotension. It is not expected to help in diastolic dysfunction and should be avoided.

Syncope or light-headedness may be provoked by sudden physical activity or abrupt postural change. However, when syncope occurs at rest, it is often due to cardiac arrhythmia, which can be evaluated best by a 24 hour ambulatory electrocardiogram and treated accordingly. If atrial fibrillation occurs, heart failure usually follows. In such cases the rhythm should be converted back to a sinus rhythm, either by electrical cardioversion or medications, depending on the seriousness of the clinical presentation.

Angina pectoris may be due either to excessive wall tension from the high intraventricular pressure of aortic stenosis or to coexisting coronary artery disease. Coronary angiography is the optimal method for making that distinction. A thallium-201 myocardial perfusion scan and exercise electrocardiography are of some value in that assessment. Exercise treadmill testing carries a small risk in symptomatic patients with aortic stenosis, so it should always be done very carefully, avoiding hypotension and never exercising to maximum tolerance. The decision to operate can be made on clinical grounds, including echocardiography, and does not require heart catheterization. However, all patients going to surgery who are older than 40 years should have coronary angiography to ensure the absence of significant coronary artery disease.

Surgical Treatment

Critical aortic stenosis is a mechanical obstruction to left ventricular outflow, and the optimal treatment is surgical relief by aortic valve replacement; no medical therapy can relieve or overcome that obstruction. Because the prognosis is poor once symptoms begin and improves after aortic valve replacement, there is no advantage to delaying surgery. Severe congestive heart failure is not a contraindication to aortic valve replacement because in almost all cases there will be improvement in systolic ventricular function after valve replacement. The congestive heart failure in aortic stenosis is usually due to an "afterload mismatch"; i.e., the obstructed valve produces a resistance to ejection that is just too great for the contractile strength of the myocardium (a mismatch). But it is a relative, not an absolute, myocardial weakness, and the solution is to relieve the obstruction, allow the ventricle to perform to its capacity, and improve the ejection fraction. A very few patients with critical aortic stenosis have a serious primary myocardial contractile dysfunction (e.g., as a result of large myocardial infarction or after many years of heart failure); in these patients, replacing the valve is not likely to improve ventricular function. Identifying patients with that primary dysfunction is often difficult, but they characteristically have the findings of critical aortic stenosis plus left ventricular dilation, diminished contractility, and a low transvalvular aortic gradient (< 20 mm Hg). Because all aortic prosthetic valves, regardless of design, are partially obstructing and have inherent pressure gradients of 10 to 25 mm Hg, it is not likely that substituting a prosthetic valve for the native valve in this situation would effect any significant improvement. These patients should not have surgery; instead, they should continue on a medical regimen even though their prognosis is poor. Fortunately, this occurs in only a very small percentage of patients with aortic stenosis.

Age alone is not a contraindication to surgery. Because aortic stenosis is more common in older age, many patients are in their 70s and 80s, and many can have successful valve replacement (Culliford and co-workers, 1991). However, the patient's overall situation should be considered carefully before advising surgery. If there are coexisting serious diseases, which are so common in the elderly (e.g., cancer, respiratory failure, renal failure, stroke) and which by themselves severely limit life expectancy, or if the patient has so many other limitations that improving the aortic valve would not allow any improvement in overall quality of life, then the risk, stress, and discomfort that accompany aortic valve surgery may not be worthwhile. These patients should be given medical management, and it is likely that survival will be determined by other, noncardiac problems.

Choice of Prosthetic Valve

The aortic valve may be replaced with either a mechanical (nontissue) valve or a bioprosthetic (tissue) valve. However, there are no perfect prosthetic valves; all of them are more obstructive than the normal native valve, so all patients with prosthetic valves should be viewed as still having mild or moderate aortic stenosis. In general, the mechanical valve is preferred in aortic stenosis because it is more durable than the tissue valve, there is no difference in hemodynamic characteristics or risk of thromboembolism, and the risk of complications from anticoagulation is small. Tissue valves are advised over mechanical valves whenever long-term anticoagulation with warfarin is inadvisable, such as when a pregnancy is planned, if the patient has a bleeding tendency, or if there is a contraindication to anticoagulation, including the likelihood of unreliability or poor compliance.

Manangement of the Patient Following Aortic Valve Replacement

To provide careful long-term management, there should be a definite schedule of annual clinical evaluations, including a cardiovascular physical examination, a battery of laboratory tests, an electrocardiogram, a chest roentgenogram each year, and a two-dimensional echocardiogram with Doppler studies about every 2 years. The Doppler technique is not as accurate in some prosthetic valves as it is in the native aortic valve. Localized high-velocity jets can create a falsely high Doppler gradient. Therefore, if there is a suspicion that a prosthetic valve is obstructed, the decision to replace the valve should not be based on the Doppler finding alone. A cardiac catheterization should be performed (Baumgartner and co-workers, 1990).

Anticoagulation. All mechanical valves need long-term anticoagulation with warfarin, but anticoagulation is not necessary for tissue aortic valves. The prothrombin time should be checked at least monthly and maintained at 1.5 to 2 times the control value. Antiplatelet agents have not been as effective as warfarin; however, if warfarin cannot be used, dipyridamole in a dose of 100 mg four times a day offers some benefit and is clearly better than no anticoagulation at all. The major complication in patients on anticoagulation is bleeding rather than thrombosis. Minor bleeding occurs in about 2 to 4 percent of patients per year and major bleeding in about 1 to 2 percent of patients per year.

Thrombosis. When thrombosis occurs in a prosthetic valve, there is great risk of death from valvular obstruction. There is also a very high risk if surgical valve replacement is attempted. A new alternative to surgery is thrombolytic therapy with streptokinase or urokinase, and it has been effective in lysng the thrombus in the prosthetic valve. A loading dose of 250,000 to 500,000 units of streptokinase can be given over 30 to 60 minutes and then followed by an infusion of 100,000 units per hour for 24 to 72 hours. When urokinase is used, a loading dose of 150,000 units is given over 30 minutes and is followed by 75,000 to 150,000 units per hour for 24 to 48 hours. In the majority of cases this thrombolytic therapy has been successful, the patients became asymptomatic, and they did not require surgery. Complications include fever, which resolves when the drug infusion is stopped, hemorrhage, and embolization of thrombotic material. Fortunately, permanent neurologic or circulatory deficit is rare.

Prophylaxis Against Endocarditis. Whenever the patient is exposed to bacteremia, such as with dental work, genitourinary surgery, or gastrointestinal surgery, prophylactic antibiotics should be taken according to American Heart Association recommendations. The previous recommendation of the American Heart Association had been to use antibiotics by the parenteral route. However, because there are substantial logistic and financial barriers to the use of parenteral regimens and because oral regimens have been used successfully in other countries, the current recommendation is to use the standard prophylactic regimen.

Endocarditis. Prosthetic valve endocarditis is a complication with high morbidity and mortality that may lead to persistent sepsis and valvular dehiscence if treatment is unsuccessful. Medical treatment alone is usually unsuccessful but should be attempted if the organism is very sensitive to an antibiotic and if the patient does not have congestive heart failure or emboli. However, if these complications occur, the prognosis is grave and the patient should have surgical replacement of the valve immediately.

Hemolysis. All normally functioning mechanical valves cause at least a small amount of hemolysis, but the normal bioprosthetic valve causes none. However, if a perivalvular leak or prosthetic valve obstruction occurs, the rate of hemolysis may become unusually high, regardless of the type of valve. The serum lactate dehydrogenase (LDH) level is a good index of the amount of hemolysis, so the routine annual postoperative evaluation should include a complete blood count and serum LDH. In most patients with hemolysis, replacement therapy with folic acid and iron is adequate to maintain normal hemoglobin levels. Occasional refractory cases occur, and valve replacement is required.

Pregnancy. If pregnancy should occur while a mechanical valve is in place, the risk of the effect of warfarin on the fetus can be minimized by switching to subcutaneous heparin every 12 hours for the first trimester and for the last 3 weeks of pregnancy. The heparin dose is adjusted to maintain a partial thromboplastin time at 1.5 times the control value. Warfarin can be used fairly safely during the remainder of the pregnancy. Some cases of warfarin embryopathy may still appear, but the risk is reduced if it is not given in the first trimester. The prothrombin time should be kept at 1.5 times the control. Another method of anticoagulation has been to use subcutaneous heparin every 12 hours throughout the pregnancy. Neither method is without risks, but both are reasonable approaches to the problem.

Percutaneous Aortic Valvuloplasty

Since 1985 aortic valvuloplasty has been used in the treatment of selected adult patients with aortic stenosis, primarily in very elderly or debilitated patients who are considered to have prohibitive cardiac surgical risk either because of heart failure or some severe noncardiac disability. Aortic valvuloplasty clearly is not equivalent to aortic valve replacement for the treatment of severe aortic stenosis, and patients should be made aware of this so that they do not have false expectations for the procedure. Percutaneous aortic valvuloplasty is performed by passing a balloon-tipped catheter retrograde from the femoral artery into the aortic valve orifice. The balloon (which may have a diameter of 15 to 25 mm) is inflated and dilates the valve, usually by cracking the nodular calcific plaques in the leaflets or occasionally by separating commissural fusion. In most cases there has been an improvement in symptoms, a small increase in the aortic valve area (e.g., from 0.5 to 0.9 cm^2), and a reduction in the transvalvular aortic gradient (e.g., from 75 to 30 mm Hg). These results have been considered successful even though severe aortic stenosis persists. Unfortunately, the immediate improvement is often not sustained, and the stenosis may return to the previous degree of severity in weeks or months. Other complications may be aortic regurgitation, sepsis, nonfatal cardiac tamponade, transient ischemic attacks, and trauma to the artery requiring surgical repair.

Although many patients have had improvement for 1 year after valvuloplasty, symptoms have returned in more than 40 percent of patients within 9 months, and restenosis rates range from 40 to 80 percent. The risk of mortality from the valvuloplasty is less than the risk of aortic valve replacement in the perioperative period, but the mortality at 1 year generally ranges from 24 to 45 percent. A randomized, prospective trial comparing valvuloplasty with valve replacement and with nonoperative (medical) treatment for this select group of very sick patients has not yet been undertaken. The procedure's main usefulness may be to improve heart failure temporarily so that a patient might be better prepared for definitive aortic valve replacement. More experience is needed in order to make a final judgment about the long-term benefits of valvuloplasty, but the initial impression is disappointing. Still, aortic valve replacement has been proven to be an effective method of therapy and has a prolonged effect.

Suggested Reading

Baumgartner H, Khan S, DeRobertis M, et al. Discrepancies between Doppler and catheter gradients in aortic prosthetic valves in vitro: A manifestation of localized gradients and pressure recovery. Circulation 1990; 82:1467–1475.

Berland J, Cribier A, Savin T, et al. Percutaneous balloon valvuloplasty in patients with severe aortic stenosis and low ejection fraction: Immediate results and 1-year follow-up. Circulation 1989; 79:1189.

Committee on Rheumatic Fever, Endocarditis, and Kawasaki Disease of the Council on Cardiovascular Disease in the Young of the American Heart Association. Prevention of bacterial endocarditis: Recommendations by the American Heart Association. JAMA 1990; 264:2919–2922.

Culliford AT, Galloway AC, Colvin SB, et al. Aortic valve replacement for aortic stenosis in persons aged 80 years and over. Am J Cardiol 1991; 67:1256–1260.

Dalen JE. Valvular heart disease, infected valves and prosthetic heart valves. Am J Cardiol 1990; 65:29C.

Galan A, Zoghbi WA, Quinones MA. Determination of severity of valvular aortic stenosis by Doppler echocardiography and relation of findings to clinical outcome and agreement with hemodynamic measurements determined at cardiac catheterization. Am J Cardiol 1991; 67:1007–1012.

Kelly TA, Rothbart RM, Cooper CM, et al. Comparison of outcome of asymptomatic to symptomatic patients older than 20 years of age with valvular aortic stenosis. Am J Cardiol 1988; 61:123.

Rahimtoola SH. Valvular heart disease: A perspective. J Am Coll Cardiol 1983; 1:199.

Ross J, Braunwald E. Aortic stenosis. Circulation 1968; 38(Suppl 5):61.

Stein PD, Kantrowitz A. Antithrombotic therapy in mechanical and biologic prosthetic heart valves and saphenous vein bypass grafts. Chest 1989; 95(Suppl 2):107S.

Stoddard MF, Arce J, Liddell NE, et al. Two-dimensional transesophageal echocardiographic determination of aortic valve area in adults with aortic stenosis. Am Heart J 1991; 122:1415–1422.

AORTIC REGURGITATION

Charles B. Treasure, M.D.

Aortic regurgitation is manifested in acute and chronic forms. Infective endocarditis, dissection of the aortic root, and trauma are the most common causes of acute aortic regurgitation. Chronic aortic regurgitation occurs in patients with rheumatic heart disease or congenitally bicuspid aortic valves. The timing and approach to therapy depend largely on etiology and disease progression. If the valve lesion is chronic and stable, etiology becomes less important. The clinical course then depends on the left ventricle's ability to handle a progressive volume overload. Acute aortic regurgitation may demand immediate surgical intervention, whereas chronic aortic regurgitation may be managed conservatively for years before surgical intervention is considered.

The diagnosis of aortic regurgitation is made readily by history, physical examination, electrocardiography, and chest roentgenogram. Acute aortic regurgitation typically occurs with acute pulmonary edema and depressed forward cardiac output. Physical examination usually reveals tachycardia, a minimally widened aortic pulse pressure, and a medium-pitched early diastolic murmur. The first heart sound may be soft or absent. A third heart sound and a low-grade aortic systolic murmur may be present. The dramatic peripheral manifestations seen in chronic aortic regurgitation are absent. Pulmonary congestion with a normal cardiothoracic ratio is seen on chest roentgenogram. Electrocardiography may show nonspecific ST-T wave changes and P-R prolongation (in infective endocarditis).

Advances in echocardiography have allowed rapid, noninvasive diagnosis of acute aortic regurgitation. The left ventricle is hyperdynamic, and chamber dimensions are usually normal. Aortic valve vegetations or an ascending aortic dissection may be seen. Premature closure and delayed opening of the mitral valve are compatible with markedly elevated left ventricle diastolic pressures. Doppler echocardiography demonstrates a regurgitant jet below the aortic valve. Transesophageal echocardiography is particularly useful for evaluation of suspected aortic dissection.

Chronic aortic regurgitation often appears as an asymptomatic diastolic murmur. Exertional dyspnea may be present. Chest pain is a less common presentation. Pulses are

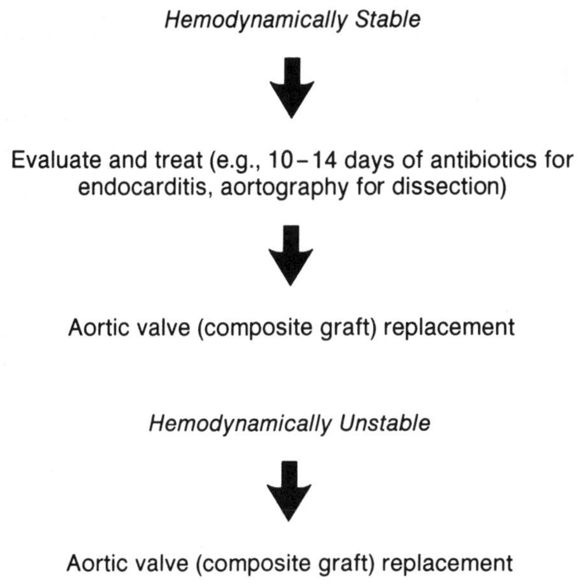

Hemodynamically Stable

Evaluate and treat (e.g., 10–14 days of antibiotics for endocarditis, aortography for dissection)

Aortic valve (composite graft) replacement

Hemodynamically Unstable

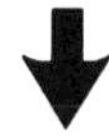

Aortic valve (composite graft) replacement

Figure 1
Management of acute aortic regurgitation.

bounding (Corrigan's pulse), and the pulse pressure is widened. The classic peripheral manifestations of chronic aortic regurgitation (Quincke's, Hill's, and Duroziez's signs among others) may be present. The chest roentgenogram may show an increased cardiothoracic ratio. Although the electrocardiogram may be normal, left ventricular hypertrophy is usually present in long-standing aortic regurgitation. Doppler and two-dimensional echocardiography confirm the diagnosis of aortic regurgitation, grades its severity, characterizes valve morphology, and allows accurate assessment of left ventricular geometry and function. The left ventricular walls may be thickened.

If aortic regurgitation is rheumatic in origin, concomitant mitral valve disease should be sought. Rheumatic mitral stenosis may mask the severity of aortic regurgitation. A combination of aortic regurgitation and mitral regurgitation may occur in endocarditis or connective tissue disease (such as Marfan's syndrome) and portends a worse prognosis than either lesion alone.

■ PREFERRED APPROACH

Management of Acute Aortic Regurgitation

Patients who present with acute aortic regurgitation and hemodynamic instability should be prepared for urgent aortic valve replacement (Fig. 1). Treatment with inotropic and afterload reduction therapy may stabilize the patient temporarily and allow time for a limited evaluation (e.g., echocardiography to define aortic valve and root anatomy, aortography in aortic root dissection). Other indications for urgent surgery include P-R prolongation or multiple emboli in patients with endocarditis. A nonstreptococcal etiology of endocarditis and large valve vegetations or early mitral valve closure seen on echocardiography are relative indications for urgent aortic valve replacement. Intra-aortic balloon counter-pulsation is contraindicated in patients with aortic regurgitation.

In acute aortic regurgitation associated with hemodynamic stability, close observation with afterload reduction therapy may be indicated to allow further evaluation and therapy. Ten to 14 days of antibiotic treatment for endocarditis will improve operative outcome and survival. Syphilitic aortitis should be treated with penicillin. Aortography may provide the surgeon a better definition of anatomy in aortic root dissection.

Better surgical results are seen in those patients with acute aortic regurgitation whose clinical condition allows appropriate medical therapy and evaluation and subsequent elective aortic valve replacement. Close preoperative observation is mandatory, including daily clinical evaluation, physical examination, and electrocardiography. Serial echocardiography may be helpful to assess for a perivalvular abscess or worsening left ventricular function. Aortic valve replacement should be performed for any evidence of hemodynamic deterioration.

Management of Chronic Aortic Regurgitation

The management of chronic aortic regurgitation presents the clinician with one of the most interesting challenges in cardiology. Substantial clinical judgment and judicious use of invasive and noninvasive tests are required to manage these patients (Fig. 2). Chronic aortic regurgitation is a relentless progression of worsening regurgitation and left ventricular dysfunction. Severe aortic regurgitation may remain asymptomatic for decades. Symptoms often are not manifest until left ventricular decompensation has occurred. Careful serial assessment of left ventricular function is critical.

The course of aortic regurgitation is marked by progressive left ventricular volume overload. With aortic regurgitation, the left ventricle must eject a large stroke volume to maintain normal forward cardiac output. The left ventricle, by dilating to increase preload, is able to maintain this large stroke volume. Cavity dilation increases left ventricular wall stress (force per unit area), and increased wall stress stimulates left ventricular hypertrophy. This myocardial adaptive response normalizes wall stress and allows systolic function to be maintained.

Eventually, the left ventricle cannot compensate (by further hypertrophy) to accommodate the large stroke volume necessary to maintain forward cardiac output. Systolic wall stress increases and left ventricular decompensation ensues as systolic function deteriorates. This turning point of left ventricular function (when elevated afterload overcomes the left ventricle's ability to compensate) has been termed *afterload mismatch.*

Because the disease progresses slowly over decades, symptoms may not appear until late in the course and may be preceded by irreversible left ventricular decompensation. Often, sedentary patients are unaware of their limitations. Standard treadmill exercise testing provides objective evidence of the patient's symptomatic status, and exercise capacity correlates significantly with survival. Undoubtedly, exercise testing is superior to the more subjective assessments of functional status (New York Heart Association and Canadian classifications). Achievement of 60 percent of functional

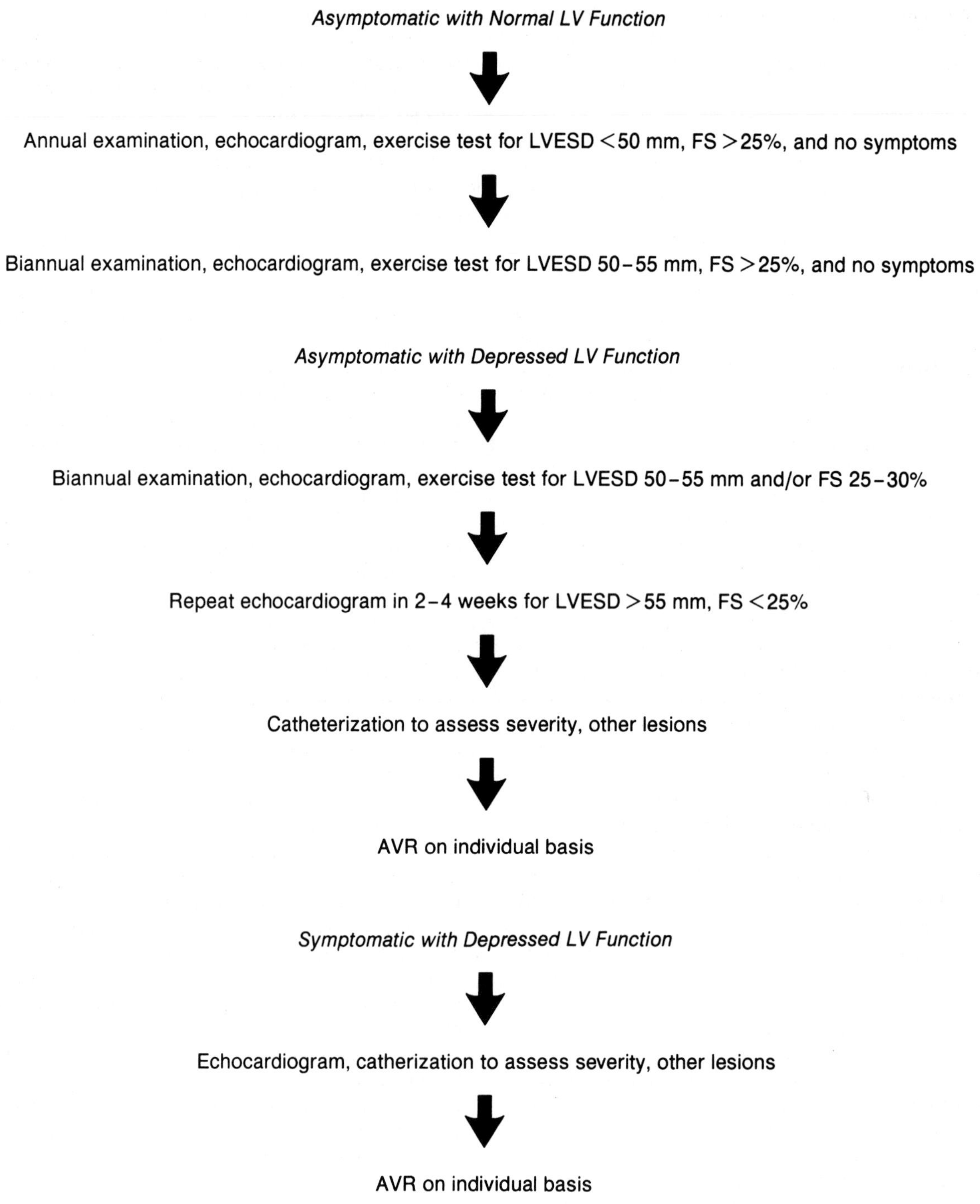

Asymptomatic with Normal LV Function

Annual examination, echocardiogram, exercise test for LVESD <50 mm, FS >25%, and no symptoms

Biannual examination, echocardiogram, exercise test for LVESD 50–55 mm, FS >25%, and no symptoms

Asymptomatic with Depressed LV Function

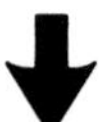

Biannual examination, echocardiogram, exercise test for LVESD 50–55 mm and/or FS 25–30%

Repeat echocardiogram in 2–4 weeks for LVESD >55 mm, FS <25%

Catheterization to assess severity, other lesions

AVR on individual basis

Symptomatic with Depressed LV Function

Echocardiogram, catherization to assess severity, other lesions

AVR on individual basis

Figure 2
Management of chronic aortic regurgitation. AVR, aortic valve replacement; FS, fractional shortening; LV, left ventricular; LVESD, left ventricular end-systolic dimension.

aerobic capacity on the exercise treadmill is good objective evidence of an asymptomatic status.

After diagnosing aortic regurgitation, and coincident with assessment of the patient's symptomatic status, one must evaluate left ventricular contractile function. Numerous parameters derived from invasive and noninvasive tests have been used to assess left ventricular contractile function and to predict postoperative left ventricular function and survival. The most useful and accepted index is derived from M-mode echocardiography. Henry and co-workers (1980) have identified left ventricular end-systolic dimension (LVESD) and fractional shortening (FS) as important determinants of postoperative left ventricular function and prognosis. A LVESD of greater than 55 mm and an FS of less than 25 percent correlate with a worse postoperative prognosis. However, Carabello and co-workers (1987) suggest that, even in the symptomatic patient with noninvasive evidence of depressed left ventricular function, postoperative outcome is not significantly worse. This improved outcome is attributed to better surgical techniques and better intraoperative techniques of myocardial preservation in the modern era. These echocardiographic parameters are probably better predictors of postoperative left ventricular function than postoperative mortality and should be used as loose guidelines for managing these patients.

Exercise radionuclide ventriculography has been touted as a predictor of postoperative outcome. A preoperative exercise ejection fraction of less than 40 percent is said to be a sensitive predictor of poor postoperative left ventricular function (Borer and co-workers, 1978). However, this has not been confirmed in subsequent studies. The limited usefulness of exercise radionuclide ventriculography is, in part, related to the complex circulatory changes associated with exercise. Exercise ejection fraction depends on many factors (e.g., systemic vascular resistance, heart rate, venous capacitance) other than the left ventricular contractile state. Clearly, patients with an abnormal response to exercise can have an excellent prognosis, provided that the resting ejection fraction is normal.

Other end-systolic indices hold promise as predictors of postoperative left ventricular function and survival. The end-systolic pressure volume relationship is an excellent indicator of the left ventricular contractile state. Unfortunately, the many assumptions necessary to make this parameter clinically useful detract from its accuracy. Because end-systolic wall stress is not completely afterload independent, its usefulness alone is limited. However, a promising contractility index is the relationship of end-systolic wall stress and the rate-corrected velocity of circumferential fiber shortening. This noninvasively determined index is preload and heart rate independent and incorporates afterload. Indices of regurgitation severity (regurgitant volume or regurgitant fraction) and preload (end-diastolic pressure, end-diastolic dimension, or end-diastolic wall stress) are unreliable predictors of surgical outcome.

Asymptomatic Patients with Good Left Ventricular Function

In addition to the initial history and physical examination, electrocardiogram, chest roentgenogram, and echocardiogram, asymptomatic patients should undergo annual examination and echocardiography to assess changes in left ventricular function and dimensions. The LVESD should increase no more than 7 mm per year in chronic aortic regurgitation. Therefore, provided that LVESD remains less than 50 mm, annual echocardiograms are adequate. When LVESD is 50 to 55 mm or FS is 25 to 30 percent, examination and echocardiography on a biannual basis are warranted. Close observation is sufficient, provided that the patient remains truly asymptomatic and left ventricular systolic function is preserved.

Medical therapy of chronic aortic regurgitation with inotropic agents and vasodilators appears to be of no proven benefit for increasing survival or deferring surgery, although adequate randomized trials have yet to be performed. Hydralazine, however, does improve systolic function and volume overload. Unfortunately, left ventricular hypertrophy, the degree of regurgitation, and left ventricular size are unaffected by this drug. Of potential benefit are other untested vasodilators (e.g., angiotensin converting enzyme inhibitors). All patients with aortic regurgitation should receive antibiotic prophylaxis.

Asymptomatic or Minimally Symptomatic Patients with Depressed Left Ventricular Function

Asymptomatic or minimally symptomatic patients pose a significant management dilemma for clinicians. The goal is to intervene with aortic valve replacement when the immediate and late risks of aortic valve replacement are less than the risk of irreversible damage to left ventricular contractility.

Currently, there are no objective data on the optimal level of left ventricular dysfunction at which to intervene with aortic valve replacement in asymptomatic patients. Because recent data indicate that asymptomatic patients with moderate left ventricular dysfunction do well after aortic valve replacement, careful observation may be appropriate. If severe left ventricular dysfunction exists, however, aortic valve replacement should be considered. Ultimately, management decisions for these patients must be made on an individual basis.

Annual exercise testing should be performed in these patients to assess symptom status and to maintain an objective yardstick on functional capacity. Biannual echocardiography (assuming LVESD is greater than 50 mm and FS is less than 30 percent) should be performed to assess LVESD, FS, and rate of change of these parameters. When LVESD and FS are confirmed at greater than 55 mm and less than 25 percent, respectively, a cardiac catheterization should be performed. If all data confirm aortic regurgitation with severe left ventricular dysfunction, aortic valve replacement should be considered. Each surgical decision must be individualized. Factors such as life-style, surgeon's experience, age, coexisting coronary artery disease, and other comorbidities must be taken into account. A decision to operate on an asymptomatic patient is difficult for both the patient and the physician, but in those patients with moderate to severe left ventricular dysfunction it is an appropriate one.

As in the asymptomatic patient with normal left ventricular function, medical therapy offers no proven survival benefit. However, vasodilators may provide symptomatic relief and some improvement of systolic function. Likewise, limitation of physical activity has not been shown to affect survival.

Symptomatic Patients with Severe Aortic Regurgitation

In general, symptomatic patients should receive aortic valve replacement. Aortic valve replacement provides symptom relief and prevents further left ventricular damage for the majority of patients. Many will experience improved left ventricular function and survival postoperatively. Although patients with severe left ventricular dysfunction are at higher risk of persistent left ventricular dysfunction and death postoperatively, it is probably never "too late" to operate on patients with aortic regurgitation. Currently, no clinical criteria identify precisely who within this subset of patients with symptoms and severe left ventricular dysfunction will suffer from persistent left ventricular failure postoperatively. Again, each patient must be evaluated individually. Age, other severe illnesses, coexisting coronary artery disease, and other factors that make operative risk higher or increased survival irrelevant must be taken into consideration. Digoxin, diuretics, and afterload reduction agents (hydralazine, nifedipine) provide symptomatic relief and hemodynamic benefit in preparation for aortic valve replacement. All patients should undergo cardiac catheterization to confirm lesion severity and to assess other valvular or coronary lesions prior to surgery. As for any patient facing prosthetic valve implantation, possible sources of infection (e.g., dental caries, urinary tract infection) should be treated prior to surgery.

Survival

One must consider the natural history of aortic regurgitation when making management decisions. Seventy-five percent of patients with moderate to severe chronic aortic regurgitation treated medically survive 5 years, and 50 percent survive 10 years after diagnosis. However, when symptoms develop, the prognosis with medical therapy worsens. Angina and heart failure portend death within 4 years and 2 years, respectively. Acute, hemodynamically significant aortic regurgitation treated medically has an in-hospital mortality rate of 50 to 90 percent.

The available survival data for patients with surgically treated chronic aortic regurgitation are from the late 1970s and early 1980s. These data may not reflect recent benefits gained from improved surgical techniques. Operative mortality for elective aortic valve replacement is 2 to 6 percent. Emergency surgery for acute aortic regurgitation secondary to endocarditis or aortic root dissection increases this operative risk to 10 percent. Increased age, preoperative heart failure, and decreased exercise capacity have been associated with increased operative and long-term mortality. Five year survival after aortic valve replacement varies from 50 to 86 percent, reflecting differences in etiology of aortic regurgitation, left ventricular function, and anticoagulation. Approximately 80 percent of patients experience symptom improvement, and in those patients with preoperative depression of left ventricular function (ejection fraction 25 to 50 percent), 50 percent experience improvement of left ventricular function.

Types of Aortic Valve Replacements

Although the 10 year failure rate for porcine valves is approximately 15 to 20 percent, these valves do not require long-term anticoagulation. In general, porcine valves are appropriate for the elderly, females of childbearing age, and patients with contraindications to anticoagulation. The cryopreserved homograft may be the most suitable valve for patients with active endocarditis. Its lack of struts and ability to be custom-fit in the left ventricular outflow tract and aortic root allow complete debridement of infection and provide resistance to reinfection. Patients with ascending aortic dissection may require a composite graft-valve consisting of an aortic valve prosthesis sewn into a Dacron graft.

The more durable mechanical prosthesis is the best choice for most other patients. Currently, the St. Jude medical prosthetic valve has the best hemodynamic performance of the mechanical valves (Gray and co-workers, 1984). The 10 year failure rate is less than 5 percent (Nair and co-workers, 1990). The risk of bleeding and thromboembolic complications related to the mechanical valve is approximately 2 to 3 percent per year. Bleeding complications are minimized with warfarin anticoagulation, maintaining the prothrombin time approximately 1.5 times control. This moderate-intensity regimen does not increase the risk of thromboembolism. Prosthetic valve endocarditis occurs in approximately 1 to 2 percent of cases. Both mechanical and biologic valves are equally susceptible to endocarditis, although bioprostheses may be more easily sterilized once infected.

Suggested Reading

Borer JS, Bacharach SL, Green MV, et al. Exercise-induced left ventricular dysfunction in symptomatic and asymptomatic patients with aortic regurgitation: Assessment with radionuclide cineangiography. Am J Cardiol 1978; 42:351.

Carabello BA, Usher BW, Hendrix GH, et al. Predictors of outcome for aortic valve replacement in patients with aortic regurgitation and left ventricular dysfunction: A change in the measuring stick. J Am Coll Cardiol 1987; 10:991.

Frankl WS, Brest AN. Valvular heart disease: Comprehensive evaluation and management. Philadelphia: FA Davis, 1986:281–312, 335–358, 361–374, 399–426.

Goldschlager N, Pfeifer J, Cohn K, et al. The natural history of aortic regurgitation: A clinical and hemodynamic study. Am J Med 1973; 54:577.

Gray RJ, Chaux A, Matloff JM, et al. Bileaflet, tilting disc and porcine aortic valve substitutes: In vivo hydrodynamic characteristics. J Am Coll Cardiol 1984; 3:321.

Henry WL, Bonow RO, Borer JS, et al. Observations on the optimum time for operative intervention for aortic regurgitation: I. Evaluation of the results of aortic valve replacement in symptomatic patients. Circulation 1980; 61:471.

Nair CK, Mohiuddin SM, Hilleman DE, et al. Ten year results with the St. Jude medical prosthesis. Am J Cardiol 1990; 65:217.

Nishimura RA, McGoon MD, Schaff HV, Giuliani ER. Chronic aortic regurgitation: Indications for operation, 1988. Mayo Clin Proc 1988; 63:270.

Saour JN, Sieck JO, Mamo LAR, Gallus AS. Trial of different intensities of anticoagulation on patients with prosthetic heart valves. N Engl J Med 1990; 332:428.

Zwischenberger JB, Sahalaby TZ, Conti VR. Viable cryopreserved aortic homograft for aortic valve endocarditis and annular abscesses. Ann Thorac Surg 1989; 48:365.

INFECTIOUS PERICARDITIS

A. Martin Lerner, M.D.

Infections and immune-mediated inflammatory lesions of the heart are common and may be life threatening. Particularly in immunosuppressed persons, the heart may be affected during bacteremias or fungemias from other sources. The pericardial sac may also be affected by contiguous spread from bacterial pneumonia with empyema involving the left lower lobe. Thoracentesis and pericardiocentesis with specific cultures is definitive evidence of the causative organism. Enteroviruses (e.g., Coxsackie viruses, echoviruses), Epstein-Barr virus, cytomegalovirus, pyogenic bacteria including *Borrelia burgdorferi* (Lyme disease), *Mycobacterium tuberculosis* and fungi are important agents.

The pericardial sac normally contains a fluid volume of 15 to 20 ml. The force of myocardial contraction is diminished by myocarditis or pericarditis. During virus and bacterial infections of the heart the pericardium and myocardium are usually simultaneously involved. Clinical signs, however, may be predominantly those of myocarditis or pericarditis. During viral myocarditis, myocardial necrosis may occur but mixed polymorphonuclear leukocytic–mononuclear cell interstitial infiltrates are usual. Acute purulent pericarditis may induce an 8 to 10 mm deep pericardium containing 500 to 2,000 ml of viscid fibrinous yellow purulent exudate containing varying quantities of granulation tissue. There may also be a fibrinous granulomatous pericarditis with no free fluid. Bacteremia or fungemia may cause myocardial abscesses. *Staphylococcus aureus* is a common cause of myocardial abscess. Fungemias, especially *Candida* or *Aspergillus*, may accompany the neutropenia of cancer chemotherapy. Abscesses may be present in the heart, kidneys, gastrointestinal tract, lungs, brain, liver, and thyroid. At histologic section stained with periodic acid-Shiff or methenamine silver, the pericardium and myocardium may contain microcolonies of fungi. Depending on the patient's underlying disease and immunologic competence, there may be marked suppuration or no inflammatory response. Myocardial fibers may show coagulative necrosis. Coronary vessels occasionally are invaded by organisms.

■ AGENTS OF DISEASE (TABLE 1)

At pericardiocentesis or pericardial biopsy, bacteria, fungi, *M. tuberculosis*, and other pathogenic organisms are regularly isolated. Enteroviruses (Coxsackie viruses and echoviruses) may also be isolated or identified by antigen capture (enzyme-linked immunoabsorbent assay, or ELISA) or DNA polymerase studies. *Streptococcus pneumoniae*, *Staphylococcus aureus*, and *Streptococcus pyogenes* are the major pathogens causing purulent pericarditis; but gram-negative bacilli are frequently encountered in immunocompromised patients.

Table 1 Infectious Causes of Pericarditis

Viruses	*Mycobacteria*
Adenoviruses	*Mycobacterium chelonei*
Cytomegalovirus	*Mycobacterium tuberculosis**
Coxsackie viruses A and B*	
Epstein-Barr	
Echoviruses*	*Fungi and Actinomycetes*
Hepatitis A	*Actinomyces israelii*
Polioviruses	*Aspergillus* species*
Herpes simplex 1 and 2	*Candida* species*
Influenza viruses A and B	*Coccidioides immitis*
Lymphocytic choriomeningitis	*Cryptococcus neoformans*
	*Histoplasma capsulatum**
Mumps	Agents of mucormycosis
Rubella	*Nocardia asteroides*
Vaccinia	
Varicella zoster	*Parasites*
	*Echinococcus granulosus**
Bacteria	*Entamoeba histolytica**
Borrelia burgdorferi	*Plasmodium* species
Corynebacterium diphtheriae	*Schistosoma* species
	*Toxoplasma gondii**
Neisseria gonorrhoeae	*Trichinella spiralis**
Neisseria meningitidis	*Trypanosoma cruzi*
Francisella tularensis	
Pseudomonas pseudomallei	*Rickettsia*
*Staphylococcus aureus**	*Coxiella burnetii*
*Streptococcus pneumoniae**	*Rickettsia typhi*
Streptococcus pyogenes	*Rickettsia rickettsii*
Treponema pallidum	
Aerobic gram-negative bacilli*	*Others*
	Chlamydia psittaci
Anaerobic bacteria, including *Bacteroides* and peptostreptococci	*Mycoplasma pneumoniae**

*These infectious agents are most frequently involved in the United States.

Cases of tuberculous pericarditis are increasing with the prevalence of isoniazid-resistant strains. Histoplasmosis may also cause a nonconstrictive or chronic constrictive pericarditis. *Candida* and *Aspergillus* pericarditis may be fulminant. Prompt pericardial drainage may be critical. Parasitic infection such as trypanosomiasis (Chagas disease), trichinosis, toxoplasmosis, amebiasis, and echinococcus during systemic disease may produce myopericarditis.

■ CLINICAL MANIFESTATIONS

Patients with pyogenic pericarditis are acutely ill, with anorexia, fever, chills, and precordial chest pain. Physical findings include increased jugular venous pulsations, an adynamic pericardium, impalpable apical pulses, and muffled decreased heart sounds. A paradoxic pulse and varying degrees of cardiac tamponade may occur. Hepatomegaly, pleural effusions, ascites, and pitting edema often follow. The cardinal physical finding of pericarditis, however, is a pericardial friction rub, which is best heard in the fourth intercostal space just to the left of the midsternal border while the patient is sitting up, leaning forward, and not breathing. Pericardial

Table 2 Treatment of Pericarditis

AGENT	MEDICAL	SURGICAL*
Viral Pericarditis		
Enteroviruses, e.g., Coxsackie virus, echoviruses; Epstein-Barr virus, cytomegalovirus, human immunodeficiency virus	Acute phase (first 14 days): Avoid corticosteroids, alcohol, β-blockers, anticoagulants, nonsteroidal anti-inflammatory agents; give digitalis, diuretics, antiarrhythmic agents; chronic phase: supportive therapy with rest (no exercise) until stable	Pericardiocentesis Pericardiocentesis or pericardiectomy
Purulent Pericarditis		
Gram-positive cocci *Staphylococcus aureus* *Staphylococcus epidermidis* *Streptococcus pneumoniae* *Streptococcus pyogenes*	For specifically sensitive organisms, penicillin G (20 million–30 million units/day IV for 4–6 weeks or nafcillin 1.5–2 g IV q4h for 4 weeks. For oxacillin-resistant *S. aureus* and all strains of *S. epidermidis*, vancomycin IV pharmacokinetic dosing guided by serum levels (C_{max} 25–35 μ/ml, C_{min} 10–15 μ/ml): All antibiotics are continued for 4–6 weeks.	Tube drainage, decortication, pericardiectomy as required
Gram-negative bacilli *Escherichia coli, Proteus, Enterobacter, Pseudomonas* spp.	Two appropriate bactericidal antibiotics according to susceptibility studies, usually a penicillin (e.g., timentin) or third-generation cephalosporin (ceftazidime) plus an aminoglycoside (e.g., timentin 3 g IV q6h; ceftazidime 2 g IV q6h; gentamicin, pharmacokinetic dosing, C_{max} 5–8 μ/ml, C_{min} 2μ/ml). All antibiotics are continued for 4–6 weeks.	Tube drainage, decortication, pericardiectomy
Fungi *Histoplasma, Aspergillus,* sporotrichosis, mucormycosis, *Blastomyces, Candida* species	The drug of choice remains amphotericin B 0.4–0.6 mg/kg IV for 10 weeks. Fluconazole and itraconazole have potential for efficacy. Dosages have not been established.	Tube drainage, decortication, pericardiectomy
Mycobacterium tuberculosis	Isoniazid-sensitive strain: A three-drug regimen daily for 12 months including INH, RIF, and PZA. Isoniazid-resistant strains: A four-drug regimen including INH, RIF, PZA, and SM or EMB; Dosages: INH, 5 mg/kg (max 300 mg); RIF 10 mg/kg (max 600 mg); PZA 15–30 mg/kg (max 2 g); EMB, 15–25 mg/kg (max 2.5 g); SM, 15 mg/kg (max 1 g)	Tube drainage, decortication, pericardiectomy

*For cardiac tamponade or constrictive pericarditis.
INH, isoniazid; RIF, rifampin; PZA, pyrazinamide; SM, streptomycin; EMB, ethambutol.

friction rubs are accentuated during inspiration or expiration and may be monophasic, diphasic, or triphasic, corresponding to atrial or ventricular systole or early ventricular diastole. At phonocardiography, a systolic murmur or click may also be detected. At times pericardial or pleuropericardial friction rubs can be palpated.

■ LABORATORY FEATURES

A sonolucent space at echocardiography (ultrasonogram) separating the ventricular wall motions from a motionless pericardial sac echo indicates a pericardial effusion. Echocardiography evaluates wall motion, estimates ejection fractions, and validates the presence of significant pericardial effusions, but a negative examination does not exclude a significant pericardial effusion. In fact, pericardiocentesis has not infrequently relieved severe cardiac tamponade when echocardiography failed to reveal a diagnostic sonolucent space. The rate of failure to determine the presence of significant pericardial effusion may be as high as 20 percent, and clinical suspicion should recognize the value of the positive tests only. Sometimes in difficult cases differential diagnosis requires coronary artery catheterization to exclude coronary artery disease.

Intravenous radioisotope (technetium-99m aggregated albumin or sodium pertechnate) outlines the intracardiac blood pool. This scan is compared with the cardiac silhouette chest x-ray film. Electrocardiograms show low voltage and ST-segment elevation or depression or both. Leukocytoses, an enlarged cardiac silhouette, increased erythrocyte sedimentation rate, and elevated C-reactive protein are frequent findings in both pyogenic and viral pericarditis. Analysis of the pericardial fluid is always helpful in reaching a specific diagnosis. Pericardiocentesis carries the risk of a resultant hemopericardium and further cardiac tamponade. The safest procedure is best done by a cardiothoracic surgeon in the operating room with concomitant electrocardiographic monitoring. Specimens must be processed promptly. Special care must be taken by the attending physician that these critical specimens are not mishandled or lost. It is best if the pericardiocentesis is done during the day, when the microbiology and immunology laboratories can freely participate without delay. At pericardiocentesis, contrast material may be injected directly into the pericardial sac. An open pericardial biopsy may be indicated for the diagnosis of chronic pericarditis.

Cultures should also be taken appropriately for the isolation and recognition of viruses. Pyogenic pericarditis is proved by the isolation of a virus, bacterium, or fungus at pericardiocentesis. Tubercle bacilli are isolated in about 40 percent of the proven cases; when a pericardial biopsy is cultured for tuberculosis, the yield is substantially higher. The pathology of tuberculosis of the pericardium with Langhans giant cells, caseation necrosis, and granulation tissue is characteristic. Special stains may recognize bacteria in these pathogenic materials. Attempts should be made to isolate both aerobic and anaerobic bacteria, fungi, and acid-fast bacilli. Gram, acid-fast, and methenamine silver stain preparations of pericardial exudates should be examined.

■ THERAPY (TABLE 2)

In patients with pyogenic or tuberculous pericarditis, pericardial drainage by pericardiostomy may be insufficient. Adequate relief of constriction may require decortication and resection. For purulent pericarditis surgical management along with intensive systemic antibacterial therapy for 4 to 6 weeks or longer is often necessary. Antibacterial treatment of tuberculous pericarditis ranges from 6 to 12 months (see Table 2). When appropriate therapy of acute tuberculous pericarditis is begun promptly, drainage procedures may not be necessary. In areas with isoniazid-resistant strains of *M. tuberculosis* initial treatment should consider a new infection to be due to a resistant strain until specific susceptibility tests are available. This may require about 6 weeks. When initiating drug treatment for tuberculous pericarditis, prednisone 80 mg per day should also be given for 6 to 8 weeks and then tapered off over several weeks. This suppresses inflammation within the pericardium, enhances reabsorption of the effusion, and retards pericardial constriction.

Serum should be collected in the acute phase and at convalescence to test for specific antibodies to viruses and fungi. Continuing fever, chest pain, and elevations in white blood cell counts, creatinine phosphokinase (CPK MB band), and serum aminotransferases (SGOT) suggest an associated myocardial necrosis.

■ PROGNOSIS

Complete recovery with no residual disease is possible. The outcome depends upon the accuracy of specific diagnosis and therapy. For treatment of noninfectious pericarditis, see the next chapter.

Suggested Reading

Cameron EWJ. Surgical management of staphylococcal pericarditis. Thorax 1975; 30:678–681.

Klacsmann PJ, Bulkley BH, Hutchins GM. The changing spectrum of purulent pericarditis, an 86 year autopsy experience in 200 patients. Am J Med 1977; 63:666–673.

Rooney JJ, Krocco JA, Lyons HA. Tuberculous pericarditis. Ann Intern Med 1970; 72:73–81.

Turner JA. Parasitic causes of pericarditis. Western J Med 1975; 122:307–309.

NONINFECTIOUS ACUTE AND RECURRENT PERICARDITIS

Noble O. Fowler, M.D.

The therapy of acute pericarditis depends on its presenting features, its etiology, its complications, and its clinical course. In some instances, symptom relief and observation for complications are enough; in others, pericarditis is a clue to a major systemic illness, such as septicemia, connective tissue disease, or cancer, which requires specific therapy. Perhaps the most common variety of pericarditis in outpatients is acute idiopathic or nonspecific pericarditis. Although most instances of this disease require only symptomatic relief and observation, cardiac tamponade requiring pericardial drainage develops in some, and approximately 15 to 32 percent have recurrences that are usually painful and often difficult to manage.

The presenting features of acute pericarditis are listed in Table 1. Chest pain, aggravated by lying, turning, or deep breathing, may be excruciating and may require urgent relief.

Table 1 Presenting Features of Acute Pericarditis

Chest pain
Precordial oppression
Dyspnea
Cardiac tamponade
Fever
Pericardial friction rub
Systemic illness (tumor, infection, connective tissue disease)
Radiologic changes
Electrocardiographic changes
An incidental echocardiographic finding

From Fowler NO. The pericardium in health and disease. Mt. Kisco, NY: Futura, 1985; with permission.

Pain is common in idiopathic pericarditis, occurring in as many as 90 percent of instances; by contrast, pain is less common in uremic pericarditis and is often absent in neoplastic pericarditis.

In hospital practice, no more than 15 percent of patients with acute pericarditis have nonspecific pericarditis. In many patients the cause is obvious, e.g., neoplasm, pneumonia, septicemia, AIDS, or end-stage renal disease. Conversely, the discovery of pericarditis may be the first clue to previously unrecognized septicemia, neoplasm, myocardial infarction, or connective tissue disease. Because pericarditis has so many causes, treatment must take into consideration the many

Table 2 Etiology of Acute Pericarditis

Neoplastic disease
Idiopathic (nonspecific)
Uremia (especially during hemodialysis)
Infections (see preceding chapter)
Drugs: anticoagulants, procainamide, hydralazine, diphenylhydantoin, and so forth
Dissecting aortic aneurysm
Connective tissue diseases, arteritis, rheumatoid arthritis, lupus, rheumatic fever
Radiation
Trauma: blunt or penetrating chest injury, pacemaker or implantable cardioverter/defibrillator placement, heart catheterization, placement of central venous lines, diagnostic cardiac puncture, injection of esophageal varices with sclerosing agents
Acute myocardial infarction
Delayed myocardial injury syndromes: Dressler's syndrome, trauma, cardiac operations, postinfectious syndromes
Chylopericardium
AIDS
Other: sarcoidosis, myxedema, amyloidosis, hypereosinophilic syndrome

possible etiologies toward which it may be directed. In some instances, no specific therapy is required; in others, specific treatment for infection, renal failure, or connective tissue disease must be carried out. In still others, treatment may consist of withdrawing a causative drug, e.g., procainamide, phenytoin, or anticoagulants. A list of the major causes of acute pericarditis is given in Table 2. In our hospital, metastatic neoplasm or lymphoma has been the most common etiology. Idiopathic pericarditis, infections (see preceding chapter), and end-stage renal disease make up the next most common group. In hospital practice, these four etiologic groups comprise approximately 50 percent of patients with acute pericarditis. However, AIDS-related pericardial disease has now become the most common cause of acute pericarditis seen in our echocardiography laboratory.

■ THERAPEUTIC ALTERNATIVES

Generally speaking, the treatment of acute pericarditis is medical. Surgical removal of the pericardium may be used occasionally for recurrent pericarditis, and surgical drainage may be necessary for cardiac tamponade or purulent pericarditis.

■ PREFERRED APPROACH

Medical Treatment of Acute Pericarditis

The patient should be hospitalized in order to relieve pain, to observe for complications (e.g., myocarditis or cardiac tamponade), and to perform a diagnostic evaluation.

Observation

Initially, if there is no evidence of cardiac tamponade (e.g., elevated systemic venous pressure, paradoxical arterial pulse, falling arterial blood pressure), the patient may be observed at bed rest in an ordinary hospital room. Observation for the development of these signs should be carried out every 6 hours for the first few days. When the patient has any of the aforementioned signs of tamponade, transfer to an intensive care unit, insertion of a Swan-Ganz catheter, and cardiac or thoracic surgical consultation should be made for the possibility of pericardiocentesis or open pericardial drainage. Persistent fever, especially with chills, and elevated white blood cell count, especially above 20,000 per cubic millimeter, suggest the need to investigate for purulent pericarditis by means of pericardial drainage. Persistent fever or increasing effusion after a week or so suggests the need for diagnostic pericardiocentesis or surgical drainage and biopsy when the cause of pericarditis is not obvious from the diagnostic evaluation. Most patients receive an initial echocardiogram to look for right atrial or right ventricular diastolic collapse as evidence for cardiac tamponade.

Pain Relief

Initial chest pain may be excruciating and resemble that of acute myocardial infarction. Aspirin 650 mg every 4 hours orally, ibuprofen 400 to 800 mg every 6 hours, or indomethacin 25 to 50 mg three times a day may provide pain relief. In the beginning, severe pain may require meperidine 50 to 100 mg intramuscularly or morphine 8 to 15 mg intramuscularly every 4 hours. Persistent pain in idiopathic and certain other varieties of pericarditis may require therapy with adrenal steroids (e.g., prednisone) as described subsequently. Ibuprofen may cause nausea, gastrointestinal ulceration, dizziness, headache, skin rash, tinnitus, pancytopenia, fluid retention, aggravation of congestive heart failure, bronchospasm, or acute renal failure. Hepatitis occurs rarely. Indomethacin may cause esophageal, gastric, or duodenal ulcer, fluid retention, gastrointestinal bleeding, headache, dizziness, somnolence, tinnitus, mental confusion, corneal deposits, retinal disturbances, and hepatitis. Drug-related dementia is a common problem in patients over 65 years.

Diagnostic Evaluation

The history should evaluate the possibility of pericarditis related to trauma, neoplasm, cardiac surgery, irradiation, renal failure, myocardial infarction, or medication. When the cause of acute pericarditis is not evident, certain tests should be carried out routinely. These include chest radiograph, electrocardiogram, blood culture, antistreptozyme titer, viral neutralizing antibody titers, especially for Coxsackie virus B, complete blood count, intermediate purified protein derivative skin test, renal profile, histoplasma complement fixation test (in endemic areas), and test for antinuclear antibodies. Serum myocardial enzyme determinations (creatine phosphokinase [CPK] and CPK-MB) performed at 6 hour intervals during the first 24 hours of pain aid in excluding the possibility of acute myocardial infarction, although minor elevations may occur with pericarditis because of associated epicarditis or myocarditis. In addition to detection of tamponade, an echocardiogram may also suggest an etiology e.g., myocardial infarction, infective endocarditis or metastatic neoplasm.

Pericardiocentesis

There are generally three indications for pericardiocentesis:

- To relieve cardiac tamponade (see the chapter *Cardiac Tamponade*)
- To evaluate suspected purulent pericarditis
- To make an etiologic diagnosis when fever, persistent or progressive effusion, or both are present after 1 to 3 weeks (perhaps sooner)

Pericardiocentesis is a major procedure, with a mortality risk of 1 to 3 percent. It should be carried out only by a skilled physician, e.g., a cardiac surgeon or a cardiologist, unless there is a life-threatening emergency due to cardiac tamponade. The procedure should be carried out after demonstration of fluid location by echocardiography and under hemodynamic and electrocardiographic monitoring. In my institution, agitated saline is injected after the aspirating needle is placed under two-dimensional echocardiographic visualization. This provides assurance that the needle tip lies within the pericardial fluid and increases the safety of aspiration. Resuscitation equipment should be at hand, and a thoracic surgeon should be available in the event of cardiac laceration by the pericardiocentesis needle. Laceration of a cardiac chamber or a coronary artery may occur. Callahan and co-workers reported no deaths among 117 consecutive patients when pericardiocentesis was guided by two-dimensional echocardiography at Mayo Clinic. As an alternative, open pericardial drainage permits pericardial biopsy as well as evaluation of the pericardial fluid and may be a safer and more definitive procedure. The pericardial fluid should be examined for infectious agents and tumor cells.

Treatment of Specific Varieties of Pericarditis

Idiopathic (Nonspecific) Pericarditis. When pain, fever, and pericardial effusion do not respond to aspirin, ibuprofen, or indomethacin as described previously, therapy with adrenal steroids may be necessary. The initial dose in adults is 60 mg of prednisone daily, given orally in a dose of 20 mg three times daily. After 5 days the dosage is reduced to 20 mg twice daily. Some patients respond to an initial dose of 20 mg twice daily; others require a total dose of 90 to 120 mg per day. After 5 days at 20 mg twice daily, the dosage is reduced to 10 mg daily for 5 days, and then to 5 mg daily for 5 days. The drug is then discontinued. Some patients have a recurrence of symptoms when the dosage is reduced below 15 to 20 mg a day. In such cases, the dose of 15 mg per day is resumed for 1 to 3 weeks, and the daily dose is reduced more slowly at a rate of 2.5 mg each week. Occasionally the prednisone may have to be continued at reduced dosages for a number of months. However, prednisone should be avoided whenever possible, since it may promote viral replication, may prolong the course of the illness, and has numerous complications.

Certain other varieties of acute pericarditis are treated in the same way as acute nonspecific pericarditis. These may include post-traumatic pericarditis and postpericardiotomy syndrome.

Pericarditis associated with an infection may persist after the infection has been controlled, e.g., in meningococcemia, histoplasmosis, and tuberculosis. In such cases prednisone may be useful. Prednisone is indicated in the pericarditis of rheumatic fever, but the patient should also receive benzathine penicillin 1.2 million units intramuscularly. Patients with Dressler's postinfarction pericarditis may respond to indomethacin or prednisone. Although these agents may delay healing in experimental myocardial infarction, this does not seem to be a practical problem in the clinical setting.

Uremic Pericarditis. Uremic pericarditis is primarily a problem in patients with end-stage renal disease who are on a hemodialysis program. The condition may respond to more frequent hemodialysis or to a change to peritoneal dialysis. Some authorities find intrapericardial instillation of triamcinolone to be useful. When there is cardiac tamponade, pericardiocentesis is needed, and persistent or recurrent effusion may require pericardial resection.

Withdrawal of Offending Agents. The patient's medication history should be reviewed for the possibility that therapeutic agents may be responsible for the pericarditis. Most common among these are procainamide, phenytoin, and anticoagulants. Antineoplastic agents, especially doxorubicin and daunorubicin, may be responsible. Hydralazine and isoniazid may cause a lupus-like syndrome that includes pericarditis. Anticoagulants, especially following myocardial infarction or in excessive dosage, can cause pericarditis and even tamponade of the heart. Minoxidil and methysergide are uncommon causes. The offending drug should be withdrawn when pericarditis complicates its use.

AIDS-Related Pericarditis. Pericarditis occurs in 5 to 15 percent of patients with AIDS. Its cause should be determined. The cause of pericarditis associated with AIDS may be viral disease, tuberculosis, neoplasm, or protozoal or fungal disease. When pericarditis is due to *Mycobacterium avium, M. tuberculosis,* or fungal infection, specific antibiotics are indicated. Lymphoma or Kaposi's sarcoma may be responsible. When the cause is a neoplasm, antineoplastic therapy is indicated. Patients with AIDS who have tuberculous pericarditis often present with cardiac tamponade and then require surgical drainage of the pericardial sac.

Fungal Pericarditis. *Histoplasma* pericarditis usually pursues a course similar to that of idiopathic pericarditis and then does not require specific therapy. However, pericarditis associated with disseminated histoplasmosis requires therapy with amphotericin B or ketoconazole. Similar therapy will be needed for pericarditis due to disseminated *Candida* or other fungal infections. Cryptococcosis may respond to amphotericin B; flucytosine may be used as additional therapy.

Neoplastic Pericarditis. When metastatic neoplastic disease is responsible for acute pericarditis, appropriate chemotherapy is indicated. In at least one-half of patients with metastatic cancer, pericardial effusion is due to another cause such as radiation, chemotherapy, or infection (Hancock, 1990). Lung cancer, breast cancer, lymphoma, and leukemia are the most common varieties of neoplastic disease leading to pericarditis. Intrapericardial instillation of tetracycline 500 to 1,000 mg in 20 ml normal saline, repeated if necessary, often prevents recurrent effusions in malignant pericardial disease. Atrial arrhythmias, pain, and fever may complicate this treatment. Cardiac tamponade is an indication for pericardiocentesis, and recurrent tamponade may be an indication for pericardial resection. Pericardial windows may be used instead of pericardial resection, but these may be ineffective owing to sealing off or widespread pericardial involvement by neoplasm. Balloon pericardiotomy is an option.

Dissecting Aneurysm. Pericarditis associated with dissecting aneurysm results from leakage or rupture from the intrapericardial portion of the ascending aorta. The treatment is immediate surgical repair of the dissection.

Radiation. Effusive or fibrinous pericarditis may follow mediastinal irradiation after a period of months or years. Ten to 50 percent of patients develop pericarditis, depending on the amount of radiation directed toward the heart. Prednisone therapy as outlined under the treatment of idiopathic pericarditis is often useful. Constrictive or effusive-constrictive pericarditis may develop eventually. Pericardial resection may be necessary, but the results may be disappointing if there is associated myocardial fibrosis resulting from radiation.

Hypothyroidism. Pericardial effusion due to myxedema usually responds to levolhydroxine therapy within a few weeks. Rarely, pericardiocentesis is required for tamponade.

Medical Treatment of Recurrent (Relapsing) Pericarditis

Recurrent pericarditis may follow idiopathic pericarditis (15 to 32 percent of instances), Dressler's post-myocardial infarction pericarditis, postpericardiotomy syndrome, intrapericardial bleeding, or traumatic pericarditis. This discussion of its treatment does not include recurrent attacks of pericarditis associated with a chronic systemic disease, such as cancer or connective tissue disease. Recurrent pericarditis may be a minor problem, with one or two relapses, which may respond to indomethacin, ibuprofen, or a brief course of prednisone. However, recurrences may be numerous and may, in our experience, take place over a period as long as 15 years. Complications after the original attack, such as cardiac tamponade, myocarditis, arrhythmias, or constrictive pericarditis, are uncommon. Treatment is therefore directed toward relief of pain, malaise, and apprehension.

Early attacks of relapsing pericarditis should be managed as described under idiopathic pericarditis, including observation in hospital for complications. Because complications are unlikely after the first few attacks, we manage most patients without hospitalization for later spells. Attacks should be managed without prednisone whenever possible. In some cases, patients are already receiving long-term adrenal steroids when first seen. Others may require long-term adrenal steroids because of almost immediate recurrences when prednisone dosage is reduced below 15 to 20 mg per day. In such cases, we reduce prednisone gradually, at a rate of 2.5 mg in daily dose per week. Flare-ups of pericarditis are treated with codeine or oxycodone rather than by increasing prednisone dosage. Because prednisone has undesirable side effects and may actually prolong the course of the illness, our ultimate goal is to withdraw the agent completely. Complete withdrawal may require as long as 1 year. The long-term dose of prednisone should be kept at a minimum, preferably 7.5 mg per day or less to minimize complications.

Adrenal steroid therapy may be complicated by infections, hypokalemia, alkalosis, fluid retention, decreased glucose tolerance, hypertension, moon facies, hirsutism, buffalo hump, peptic ulcer, poor wound healing, skeletal myopathy, osteoporosis, and aseptic necrosis of the femoral head. Emotional disorders are common. Glaucoma and cataracts may occur.

Surgical Treatment of Prolonged or Recurrent Pericarditis

Pericardiectomy may be considered for patients with prolonged and numerous attacks of pericarditis. The success rate may vary from 80 percent to under 50 percent. One study reports a 95 percent success rate (Tuna and Danielson, 1990). Because of its frequent failure and because major complications of recurrent pericarditis are uncommon, we reserve pericardiectomy for patients with prolonged disabling attacks of painful pericarditis who do not respond to nonsteroidal anti-inflammatory agents or adrenal steroids or who develop complications with prednisone therapy.

In difficult cases, other possibilities may be considered. Although azathioprine has been reported to be successful in a few instances, it was not helpful in two patients whom I treated. Colchicine 1 mg per day may be successful in some cases (Millaire et al 1994) but has been disappointing in my own experience.

Suggested Reading

Acierno LJ. Cardiac complications in acquired immunodeficiency syndrome (AIDS): A review. J Am Coll Cardiol 1989; 13:1144.

Callahan JA, Seward JB, Nishimura RA, et al. Two dimensional echocardiographically guided pericardiocentesis: Experience in 117 consecutive patients. Am J Cardiol 1985; 55:476.

Fowler NO. Tuberculous pericarditis. JAMA 1991; 266:99.

Fowler NO. Cardiac tamponade: A clinical or an electrocardiographic diagnosis? Circulation 1993; 87:1738.

Fowler NO. Pericardial disease. In: Abelmann W, ed. Cardiomyopathies, myocarditis, and pericardial disease, Vol II of Braunwald E. Atlas of heart disease. Philadelphia: Current Medicine, 1995.

Fowler NO, Harbin AD III. Recurrent acute pericarditis: Follow-up study of 31 patients. J Am Coll Cardiol 1986; 7:300.

Hancock EW. Neoplastic pericardial disease. Cardiol Clin 1990; 8:673.

Kwan T, Karve MM, Emerole D. Cardiac tamponade in patients infected with HIV. Chest 1993; 104:1059.

Millaire A, de Groote P, Decoulx E, et al. Treatment of recurrent pericarditis with colchicine. Eur Heart J 1994; 15:120.

Sagrista-Sauleda J, Barrabès JA, Permanyer-Miralda G, et al. Purulent pericarditis: Review of a 20-year experience in a general hospital. J Am Coll Cardiol 1993; 22:1661.

Tuna IC, Danielson GK. Surgical management of pericardial diseases. Cardiol Clin 1990; 8:683.

Ziskind AA, Pearce AC, Lemmon CC, et al. Percutaneous balloon pericardiotomy for the treatment of cardiac tamponade and large pericardial effusions. Description of the technique and report of the first 50 cases. J Am Coll Cardiol 1993; 21:1–5.

CARDIAC TAMPONADE

E. William Hancock, M.D.

Cardiac tamponade is a condition in which the function of the heart or circulation is compromised by the presence of fluid under increased pressure in the pericardial space. Some use the term *tamponade* only for those critical situations in which the arterial blood pressure has dropped to a definitely low level, perhaps only when cardiogenic shock is considered to be present. Others require the presence of a fall in cardiac output, to a definitely low level, as part of the definition. I prefer a broader definition, in which milder forms of compromise, such as a rise in central venous pressure, with normal arterial pressure and cardiac output, are considered to represent cardiac tamponade. Under this definition, cardiac tamponade can be mild, moderate, or severe. The severe forms can be regarded as decompensated or critical tamponade. The importance of such a definition is to indicate that the appropriate time to relieve cardiac tamponade by removing the fluid is usually when the condition is mild or moderate. Waiting until the crisis state of decompensated or critical tamponade increases the possibilities of an unsatisfactory outcome.

ETIOLOGY AND PATHOGENESIS

Cardiac tamponade can occur in any of the conditions in which pericardial effusion occurs. The etiology thus includes a wide variety of medical and surgical conditions and diverse clinical settings. The pericardial fluid may be pure blood, or it may be serosanguineous, serous, or purulent fluid. The pericardial effusion may develop rapidly or slowly. The amount of pericardial fluid is less important than the speed of its accumulation because the pericardium is resistant to sudden stretch but does stretch markedly over the course of weeks or months.

DIAGNOSIS

The diagnosis of cardiac tamponade requires two elements. It must be demonstrated that pericardial effusion is present, and it must be demonstrated that there are hemodynamic abnormalities that can be attributed to pericardial fluid under increased pressure. Ultimately, a proven diagnosis of cardiac tamponade requires the demonstration of reversal of such hemodynamic abnormalities by removal of the pericardial fluid.

Evidence from the history, physical examination, electrocardiogram, and plain chest roentgenogram can only provide suspicion, at most, of the diagnosis of pericardial effusion. An objective method of imaging is required to establish this point. Echocardiography is the most useful method of imaging because it is highly accurate and can be applied easily in almost any clinical setting. Computed tomography (CT) and magnetic resonance imaging (MRI) are also highly reliable and provide better definition of some anatomic details; they should be used as supplementary methods when echocardiography is inconclusive.

Imaging methods, however, are less reliable as a means of demonstrating that compression of the heart is necessarily present or absent. The history and physical examination are the prime methods for determining this. Patients with cardiac tamponade usually have dyspnea and other symptoms. The jugular venous pressure can virtually always be seen to be elevated if the circumstances of the examination are adequate. Paradoxical pulse is usually present, but may be difficult to assess by examination or by sphygmomanometry alone. Echocardiography does provide useful signs of compression of the heart. Imaging may show a reduced diameter of the right ventricle, inward movement of the right atrial and right ventricular walls in early systole ("systolic collapse"), and persistent full distention of the inferior vena cava throughout the respiratory cycle. Pulse-wave Doppler recordings may show exaggerated respiratory variation in the velocity of blood flow through the mitral and tricuspid valves, the analogue of paradoxical pulse. In questionable cases, direct measurements of right atrial pressure and arterial pressure should be used to confirm the presence of hemodynamic signs of tamponade.

THERAPEUTIC ALTERNATIVES

The treatment may be divided into conservative medical approach, pericardiocentesis, and surgical pericardiostomy. No one of these approaches is the most appropriate for all cases. The choice of therapy depends on many considerations. Some of the questions that should be raised in making a choice are listed in Tables 1 and 2.

PREFERRED APPROACH

Conservative Medical Approach

In moderate or severe cardiac tamponade the conservative medical approach is at best an interim and short-term approach because removal of the fluid is the only therapy that can be expected to succeed quickly and dependably. In milder forms, however, the conservative medical approach may be

Table 1 Should a Pericardial Effusion Be Drained?

- Is cardiac tamponade of more than a mild degree present?
- Is the amount of pericardial effusion increasing?
- How important is the cytologic study of the pericardial fluid?
- How important is the bacteriologic study of the pericardial fluid?
- Does the natural history of the underlying condition predict spontaneous resolution?
- Is there an effective systemic treatment for the underlying condition?
- Will draining the pericardial effusion permit a less intense level of in-hospital care?
- Will draining the pericardial effusion shorten the hospital stay?

Table 2 Should Pericardial Fluid Be Drained by Pericardiocentesis or Surgery?

How quickly are a skilled cardiologist and cardiac catheterization laboratory available?
How quickly are a skilled surgeon and operating room available?
How readily accessible is the fluid to a needle approach?
Is the fluid likely to be blood that is partially clotted?
How likely is there to be associated constrictive pericarditis?
How likely is there to be associated superior vena caval obstruction?
How likely is there to be associated congestive heart failure/fluid overload?
Does the patient have a coagulopathy?
How important is a pericardial biopsy?
How likely is there to be a site of bleeding from the heart that requires surgical control?

appropriate. Patients who are selected for this approach should have only mild elevation of jugular venous pressure, to a level equivalent to approximately 8 to 10 mm Hg (elevated to less than the angle of the jaw in the sitting upright position). They should have no symptoms attributable to the tamponade itself and should have no evidence of hypotension, pulmonary congestion, or impaired renal or cerebral perfusion. There should be confidence either that a diagnosis is known, such as neoplasm, dialysis, or a rheumatic disease, or that a diagnosis is highly unlikely to be established by studies on the pericardial fluid; e.g., the clinical picture is that of idiopathic acute pericarditis or idiopathic chronic pericardial effusion. The decision for a conservative medical approach is also supported if the natural history of the patient's illness is believed to be benign and self-limited, as in idiopathic acute pericarditis. It is also supported if the pericardial effusion is believed to be part of a systemic disorder that is responsive to systemic therapy, such as breast cancer, rheumatic disease, or uremia. Employing a conservative medical approach also implies that the patient will remain under close observation during a follow-up period, usually as a hospital inpatient initially. Thus, the conservative medical approach to mild cardiac tamponade consists of close observation of the patient for evidence of increasing tamponade, while the basic condition is treated systemically or allowed to resolve spontaneously.

Supportive Therapy in Critical Tamponade

Patients who are hypotensive because of critical cardiac tamponade may benefit from supportive therapy while the diagnosis of tamponade is being confirmed, or while the preparations for the drainage procedure are being carried out. Intravenous administration of fluid is the most important measure. Fluid should be administered even when the central venous pressure is considerably elevated, in that the right atrial pressure and the intrapericardial pressures are virtually equilibrated in tamponade. Blood, plasma, or dextran may be used for intravenous fluid administration, but simple saline solution is equally acceptable in most situations.

The systemic arterial pressure and cardiac output may be supported by the infusion of drugs such as dopamine, dobutamine, or isoproterenol. A drug that tends to reduce the size of the heart, by a combination of inotropic action and systemic vasodilation, is optimal; if the heart is made smaller, it will be compromised less by a given amount of fluid in the pericardial space. The more potent vasodilating agents such as sodium nitroprusside should generally not be used in critical cardiac tamponade because the maintenance of an adequate systemic arterial pressure is critically dependent on a reasonable level of systemic vascular tone. Support of the systemic circulation with drug infusions in cardiac tamponade does little to favor the renal, cerebral, or splanchnic circulations; its greatest importance is in supporting the coronary arterial filling pressure when the arterial pressure is markedly reduced.

Pericardiocentesis

Selection of Patients

If a skilled invasive cardiologist and a cardiac catheterization laboratory are readily available, pericardiocentesis is the preferred approach to most cases of cardiac tamponade that are seen in the medical setting. Such cases include most of those resulting from idiopathic pericarditis, tuberculous infection, neoplasm, radiotherapy, rheumatic diseases, and uremia and/or dialysis. Demonstration of the presence of pericardial effusion, usually by echocardiography, is a prerequisite. Furthermore, the fluid should be present in a significant amount over the inferior or anterolateral regions of the pericardial cavity.

Timing

Pericardiocentesis should be carried out when the jugular venous pressure has risen to approximately 10 mm Hg or higher. The procedure should be scheduled urgently, within a few hours of the time that the diagnosis has been made. It should not be carried out as an emergency, under less than optimal conditions, unless the patient is in cardiogenic shock or severe respiratory distress. Even under such emergency conditions, it is usually preferable to transfer the patient to the cardiac catheterization laboratory.

Preparation

The intravascular volume should be replenished if it is thought to be relatively or absolutely deficient. Atropine should be given as premedication, to aid in avoiding the vasodepressor response that may accompany either the insertion of the needle or the withdrawal of pericardial fluid. The apparatus for hemodynamic monitoring should be assembled, as appears appropriate for the clinical problem. At a minimum, the central venous pressure should be monitored. In many cases the direct arterial pressure should be monitored, and in some the right-heart pressures, left-heart pressures, and cardiac output should also be monitored.

Procedure

In most instances the optimal site for the insertion of the needle is in the subxiphoid area just to the left of the midline. However, it is helpful to use echocardiography in selecting the site; when this is done, an apical or parasternal site may prove to be better. The local anesthesia should be carried out to the pericardium itself; entering the pericardial space and withdrawing a few milliliters of fluid into the local anesthetic syringe identify the depth and direction for the subsequent insertion of the larger-bore pericardiocentesis needle. A long No. 16 or No. 18 needle is then passed into the pericardial space. The needle may be attached to a unipolar exploring electrocardiogram electrode to provide an indication of contact of the needle with the myocardium. However, the experienced operator will note a characteristic sensation as the needle penetrates the pericardium. An echocardiographic transducer may be attached to the needle to guide its passage into the pericardial space.

When the needle enters the pericardial space, a pressure measurement should be made within the pericardial space. In cardiac tamponade the value is nearly equivalent to the central venous pressure, and the waveform shows a monomorphic fall in systole and rise in diastole, with only minor variation with respiration. A flexible j-tipped guidewire should then be passed, the needle withdrawn, and a No. 7 pigtail catheter placed in the pericardial space over the guidewire. A sheath, passed over the needle, may also be used to place the catheter. The catheter should have multiple sideholes. In infants and children a No. 20 needle and 5 Fr catheter may be used. The pericardial fluid can then be withdrawn gradually through the catheter. At the end of the procedure, the pericardial pressure should again be measured, along with the right atrial pressure. The catheter is then secured to the skin and left indwelling with a heparin lock.

A balloon dilation catheter may be used to enlarge the needle hole to an opening that permits drainage of fluid for some period of time. This procedure usually causes an opening into the pleural space to be established as well. Balloon dilation should be considered in patients with neoplastic pericardial effusions or in other patients in whom cardiac tamponade has recurred after an initial pericardiocentesis.

Postprocedure Course

The pigtail catheter should be left in place for up to 7 days, or until there is no further pericardial fluid accumulation. The central venous pressure should be monitored especially closely during the first 24 hours after the procedure; it may not drop fully to normal immediately after the procedure but should do so by the next day as the patient has a diuresis. Persistence of an elevated central venous pressure, when the intrapericardial pressure has been restored to normal, indicates the presence of a further cardiac abnormality, often an associated visceral constrictive pericarditis.

Complications

The most important complication of pericardiocentesis is an aggravation of cardiac tamponade due to bleeding from an inadvertent puncture of the heart. The risk can be minimized by reserving the procedure for experienced operators in optimal conditions, using echocardiographic guidance and thoughtful selection of patients. Other complications include persistent pleural or pericardial pain, bleeding from the puncture site in the chest wall or pericardium, ventricular arrhythmias, vasodepressor responses that are minimized by atropine premedication, and infection associated with the indwelling catheter in the pericardial space. Acute pulmonary edema occurs occasionally after the rapid withdrawal of a large volume of pericardial fluid. Patients with this complication usually have impaired left ventricular function due to hypertension or coronary artery disease. Slow withdrawal of the fluid and frequent monitoring of the pulmonary artery pressure are indicated in such patients. Although not strictly a complication, perhaps the most frequent adverse sequelae of pericardiocentesis stem from a false sense of security about its efficacy; there must be clear documentation of how successful the procedure was and also careful observation of the patient following the procedure, so that clinical deterioration due to persistent or recurrent tamponade can be recognized and dealt with, usually by surgical pericardiostomy.

Surgical Pericardiostomy

Selection of Patients

The prime indication for surgical pericardiostomy is acute traumatic hemopericardium, as seen in the emergency room. Not only do the acuteness and severity of the condition require very quick action but also the likelihood of the presence of clotted blood and of a bleeding site in the heart that requires surgical control make pericardiocentesis a temporary delaying action at best in this situation. Postoperative cardiac tamponade after cardiac surgery and tamponade due to rupture of the heart in acute myocardial infarction or rupture of an acute dissection of the aorta into the pericardial space also call for a surgical approach. Purulent bacterial pericarditis is best managed with surgical pericardiostomy to provide adequate drainage and to prevent the development of acute constriction of the heart; however, this diagnosis is usually established first by pericardiocentesis. A surgical approach may be preferred when tuberculous pericarditis is a prominent possibility because in this condition the pericardial biopsy is superior to the fluid alone for bacteriologic diagnosis. Finally, patients with cardiac tamponade of various etiologies may require surgery if the tamponade recurs after pericardiocentesis or if the fluid is inaccessible because of location or loculation.

Timing and Preparation

Timing and preparation are similar to that of pericardiocentesis.

Procedure

The surgical approach is usually subxiphoid, which permits resection of a small area of the inferior pericardium and digital exploration of the pericardial space. A limited left thoracotomy may also be used; this permits resection of a larger area of anterolateral parietal pericardium and the establishment of a drainage pathway into the left pleural space. Pericardioscopy, with either a rigid or flexible endoscope, may be used in conjunction with subxiphoid pericardiostomy, mainly for the purpose of guiding the site of biopsies to areas that are visually suggestive of neoplasm.

Postoperative Course

The surgical drainage tubes are left in place for several days and then removed. Recurrent pericardial effusion after such procedures occurs only rarely. Complications and adverse sequelae are rare after surgical pericardiostomy. Wound infection, as in thoracotomy, is the most serious complication.

Suggested Reading

Bostman LA, Salo JA, Bostman OM. Stab wounds to the pericardium and heart: An analysis of 85 consecutive patients. Eur J Surg 1992; 158:271.

Downey RJ, Bessler M, Weissman C. Acute pulmonary edema following

pericardiocentesis for chronic cardiac tamponade secondary to trauma. Crit Care Med 1991; 19:1323.
Millaire A, Wurtz A, de Groote P, et al. Malignant pericardial effusions: Usefulness of pericardioscopy. Am Heart J 1992; 124:1030.
Shabetai R, ed. Diseases of the pericardium. Cardiol Clin 1990; 8: 579–716.
Soler-Soler J, Permanyer-Miralda G, Sagrista-Sauleda J, eds. Pericardial disease: New insights and old dilemmas. Dordrecht: Kluwer, 1990.
Taavitsainen M, Bondestam P, Manikinen P, et al. Ultrasound guidance for pericardiocentesis. Acta Radiol 1991; 32:9.
Ziskind AA, Pearce AC, Lemmon CC, et al. Percutaneous balloon pericardiotomy for the treatment of cardiac tamponade and large pericardial effusions. Description of technique and report of the first 50 cases. J Am Coll Cardiol 1993; 21:1.

CONSTRICTIVE PERICARDITIS

James J. Ferguson III, M.D.
James T. Willerson, M.D.

Constrictive pericarditis is a disorder in which there is limitation of diastolic filling of the heart as a result of the relatively fixed volume of a thickened, fibrotic pericardium. There is usually uniform restriction of filling of all heart chambers by the rigid and nondistensible pericardium, although in very unusual circumstances there can be localized pericardial thickening.

■ ETIOLOGY AND PATHOPHYSIOLOGY

Constrictive pericarditis is most frequently the result of a previous episode of acute pericarditis that subsequently progresses to a stage of chronic scarring, fibrosis, and thickening. Basically, any process that can cause acute pericarditis may ultimately result in constrictive pericarditis. The most common causes of constrictive pericarditis include neoplastic disease (especially lung cancer, breast cancer, and lymphoma), mediastinal irradiation, and chest trauma (including surgery). Other less frequent causes include chronic renal failure and dialysis, connective tissue disorders (such as rheumatoid arthritis and systemic lupus erythematosus), and bacterial pericardial infections. Tuberculosis was at one time a leading cause of constrictive pericarditis, but today it is a major cause only in underdeveloped countries. Constrictive pericarditis is also increasingly recognized as a complication of cardiac surgery.

The fundamental physiologic abnormality in constrictive pericarditis is a rigid, nondistensible pericardium that limits late diastolic filling of the ventricles. Early rapid diastolic filling is abruptly halted when it reaches the limiting volume of the rigid pericardium. The net result is impaired overall cardiac diastolic function with associated systemic and pulmonary congestion, reduced cardiac output, and hypotension. Systolic function usually remains relatively unaffected. It must be remembered that the pericardium itself has a fundamental curvilinear pressure-volume relationship, and when taken to its limits, even normal pericardium limits the filling of the ventricle (as occurs in acute right-heart failure or right ventricular infarction). The point at which limitation of filling occurs depends on the compliance (change in volume per unit change in pressure) of the pericardium, as shown in Figure 1. An understanding of this relationship serves as a basis for distinguishing "rigid" from "elastic" constriction.

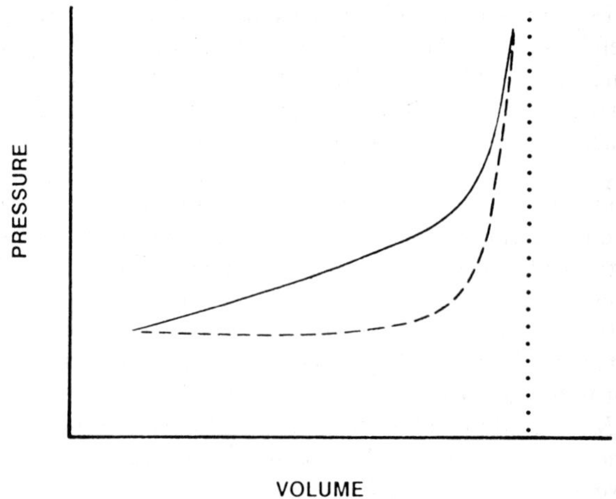

Figure 1
A schematic diagram of the curvilinear pressure-volume relationship of the pericardium. The solid line shows a curve for a rigid, calcified, nondistensible pericardium that limits further expansion as it approaches its limiting volume. The dotted line represents the absolute upper limit of pericardial volume. The dashed line shows a normal pericardium, which is more distensible but also has a limiting volume.

■ DIAGNOSIS

On physical examination, the single most striking finding in constrictive pericarditis is elevation of the jugular venous pressure, which usually has a prominent y-descent, coincident with the prominent early rapid filling of the ventricle. Patients in sinus rhythm may also have a prominent x-descent coincident with filling of the atrium as the ventricle is ejecting. Peripheral edema, hepatomegaly, and ascites are common. Kussmaul's sign (an inspiratory increase in jugular venous pressure) may be present, but pulsus paradoxus is only occasionally found with constrictive pericarditis. An early diastolic pericardial knock (high-frequency diastolic sound) coincident with the cessation of rapid ventricular filling may be noted on auscultation.

The size of the cardiac silhouette on chest film is not particularly helpful, although pericardial calcification may be seen (especially with a previous history of tuberculous pericarditis). The electrocardiogram usually demonstrates nonspecific ST-segment and T wave changes, low QRS voltages, and left atrial enlargement. The presence of ventricular hypertrophy, conduction disturbances, or Q waves suggests the presence of underlying myocardial disease and possible coronary artery involvement.

M-mode and two-dimensional echocardiography may be useful in documenting the increased pericardial thickness and abnormal ventricular diastolic function in the setting of normal systolic function. However, the sensitivity of echo images in identifying thickened pericardium is limited unless calcium is present, and with the advent of newer imaging modalities, echo images are much less useful. Doppler echocardiography may show impaired late diastolic flow across the mitral or tricuspid valves and prominent respiratory variations in left ventricular isovolumic relaxation time and peak mitral flow velocity. The sensitivity of this technique is, as yet, untested, and these findings will probably not be specific for constrictive pericarditis.

Measurements of respiratory variations in pulmonary venous flow velocity by transesophageal echocardiography have also been used to distinguish constrictive pericarditis from restrictive cardiomyopathy; constrictive pericarditis manifests relatively larger pulmonary venous systolic/diastolic flow ratios and greater respiratory variation in pulmonary venous systolic and diastolic flow velocities. Another useful echocardiographic parameter is the peak early velocity of longitudinal axis expansion (Ea), which is markedly reduced in patients with restrictive cardiomyopathy in comparison to normals and patients with constrictive pericarditis.

Both gated cardiac magnetic resonance imaging (MRI) and ultrafast cinecomputed tomography (CT) have emerged as useful techniques that allow direct measurements of pericardial thickness. Both techniques can also identify dilation of the venae cavae and hepatic veins and pericardial impingement on the right ventricle (Figs. 2 and 3).

Cardiac catheterization is the definitive technique for documenting the elevation and equalization of right and left ventricular diastolic pressures observed in constrictive pericarditis (Fig. 4). Early ventricular filling is unimpaired, but as the rapid filling phase progresses and the ventricle reaches the limits imposed by the pericardium, filling abruptly slows, resulting in the characteristic "dip-and-plateau" or "square root" sign that may be evident on right and left ventricular diastolic pressure recordings. Because the pericardium limits both left and right ventricular filling, there are equalization of the left and right ventricular pressures throughout diastole until the onset of systole. After the rapid filling phase, very little filling takes place (the diastolic plateau). In the presence of tachycardia, however, these features are difficult to identify (see Fig. 4). Recordings of right atrial pressure usually show a prominent y-descent and preservation of the x-descent (Fig. 5). Right atrial pressure may also fail to decrease (or may even

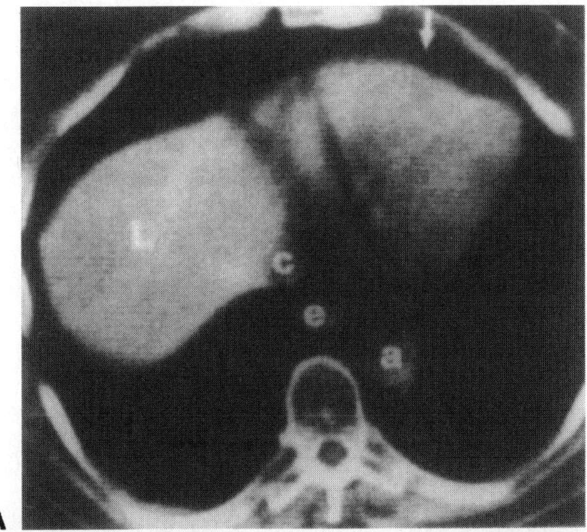

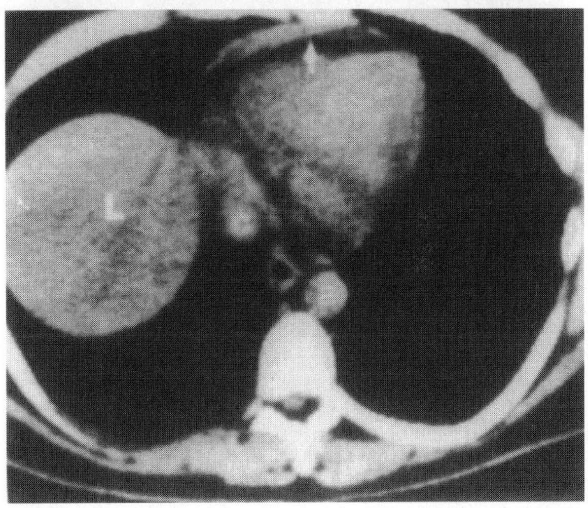

Figure 2
Ultrafast computed tomographic scans at the level of the right hemidiaphragm from a normal adult *(A)* and from a patient with constrictive pericarditis *(B)*. In contrast to the normal pericardium, which appears as a thin line *(arrow)*, the pericardium in constrictive pericarditis appears thickened. Other structures visualized include liver (L), inferior vena cava (c), esophagus (e), and descending aorta (a). *(From Sutton FJ, Whitley NO, Applefeld MM, et al. The role of echocardiography and computed tomography in the evaluation of constrictive pericarditis. Am Heart J 1985; 109: 350; with permission.)*

increase) with inspiration, the hemodynamic counterpart to Kussmaul's sign. Rapid administration of intravenous saline, exercise, or both may help bring out equalization of diastolic pressures and a dip-and-plateau contour to the ventricular pressure waveform if resting hemodynamics are nondiagnostic. The converse is also true: Volume depletion may mask the characteristic equalization of diastolic pressures. Finally, the finding of discordance between right ventricular and left ventricular pressures during inspiration (a sign of increased ventricular interdependence) may be a sensitive distinguishing feature.

The following are a number of relatively unique diagnostic

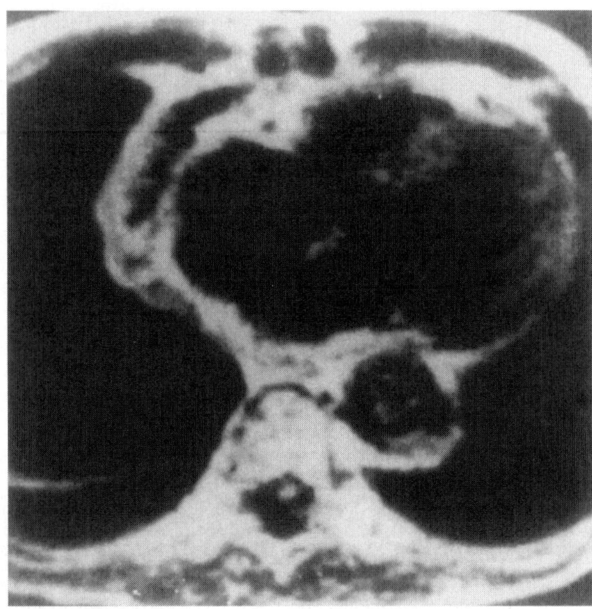

Figure 3
Magnetic resonance image from a patient with constrictive pericarditis. There is thickening of both the visceral and the parietal pericardium, with some fluid noted as well as hypertrophy of the left ventricle. *(From Soulen RL, Stark DD, Higgins CB, et al. Magnetic resonance imaging of constrictive pericardial disease. Am J Cardiol 1985; 55:480; with permission.)*

features that may help to distinguish constrictive pericarditis from other similar clinical syndromes.

Cirrhosis

Some of the clinical features of constrictive pericarditis (ascites, hepatomegaly, and abnormal liver function tests) may suggest the presence of cirrhosis. The high central venous pressures of pericardial constriction can also cause hepatic congestion and a clinical picture indistinguishable from cirrhosis. The obvious factors distinguishing cirrhosis from constrictive pericarditis are the level of central venous pressures (usually normal in cirrhosis, elevated in constriction) and the status of ventricular diastolic function (normal in cirrhosis, impaired in constriction).

Right-Sided Chronic Heart Failure

Some of the clinical features of constrictive pericarditis (i.e., elevated jugular venous pressure, edema, Kussmaul's sign, hepatomegaly, ascites) may also mimic chronic right-heart failure. In general, differentiating between the two is relatively simple by considering pulmonary artery pressures (often elevated in right-sided failure, usually normal to slightly elevated in constriction), equalization of right and left ventricular diastolic pressures (usually absent in right-sided failure, present in constriction), rapidity of the jugular venous or right atrial y-descent (normal to attenuated in right-sided failure, accentuated in constriction), "dip-and-plateau" or "square root" sign (usually absent in right-sided failure, present in constriction), and left ventricular diastolic function (usually normal in right-sided failure, abnormal in constriction). However, acute right-heart failure (as with massive

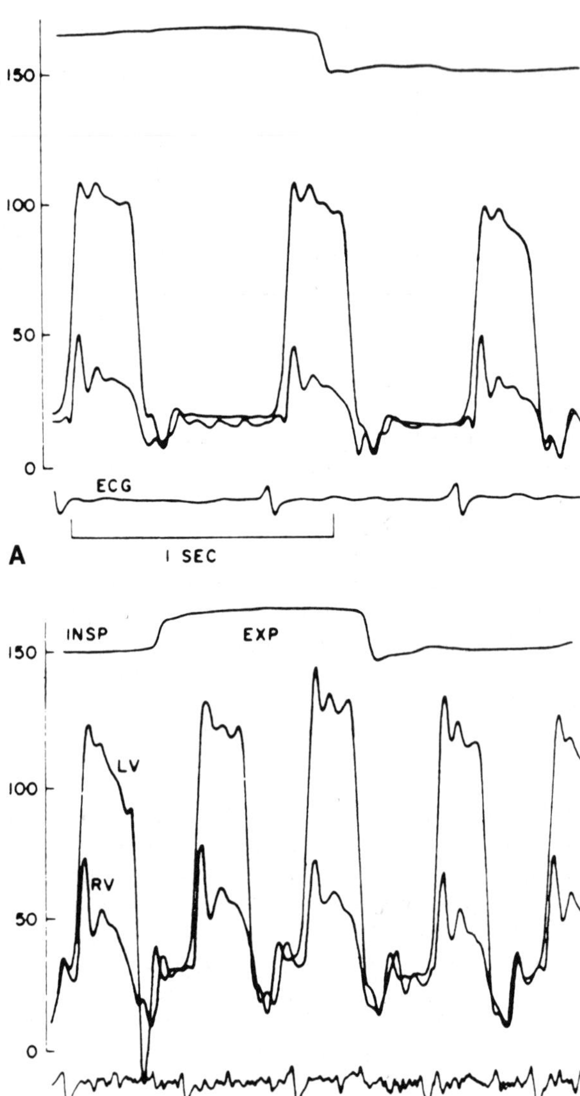

Figure 4
Simultaneous right ventricular (RV) and left ventricular (LV) pressure recordings from a patient with constrictive pericarditis. *A,* There is a characteristic "dip-and-plateau" contour in both ventricles and equalization of diastolic pressures throughout diastole at normal heart rates. *B,* With exercise, the plateau phase becomes obscured, although diastolic pressure equalization persists. *(From Shabetai R. The pericardium. New York: Grune & Stratton, 1981:181; with permission.)*

pulmonary embolus or right ventricular infarction) may cause abrupt right ventricular dilation leading to a constrictive pericarditis-like hemodynamic picture. Acute right-heart failure is also usually abrupt in onset, without any of the historical factors suggestive of pericardial constriction.

Right Ventricular Infarction

Right ventricular infarction may present a constrictive-like hemodynamic pattern. The presumptive mechanism is that sudden right ventricular dilation within the pericardium and constraint by the normal pericardium lead to the hemody-

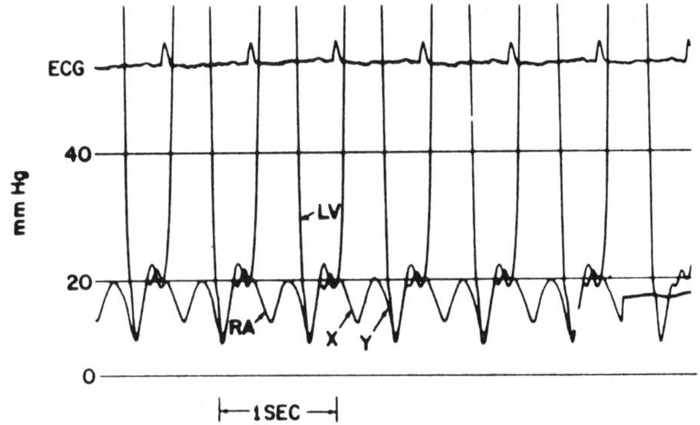

Figure 5
Simultaneous right atrial (RA) and left ventricular (LV) pressure tracings from a patient with constrictive pericarditis. There is a prominent y-descent on the RA waveform, indicating intact rapid filling and normal early diastolic ventricular function. Right atrial and left ventricular diastolic pressures are both elevated and equal throughout diastole. *(From Lorell BH, Grossman W. Profiles in constrictive pericarditis, restrictive cardiomyopathy, and cardiac tamponade. In: Grossman W, ed. Cardiac catheterization and angiography. 4th ed. Philadelphia: Lea & Febiger, 1990:636; with permission.)*

namic abnormalities that are also found with constrictive pericarditis. The hemodynamic profile may be indistinguishable from classic pericardial constriction, but the clinical setting of acute right ventricular infarction is usually obvious, with chest pain, inferior or posterior electrocardiographic changes, and hypotension as well as changes on right precordial chest leads (ST-segment elevation in V_4R–V_6R), or impairment of right ventricular function on echocardiography or gated radionuclide ventriculography.

Cardiac Tamponade

It is usually not difficult to differentiate pericardial constriction and cardiac tamponade. Among the clinical data that favor a diagnosis of constrictive pericarditis over cardiac tamponade are pulsus paradoxus (often absent in constriction, usually present in tamponade), Kussmaul's sign (usually absent in tamponade, often present in constriction), a "dip-and-plateau" or "square root" sign on ventricular pressure tracing (absent in tamponade, present in constriction), a prominent y-descent of the jugular venous or right atrial pressure (absent in tamponade, present in constriction), timing of impaired diastolic function (occurring throughout diastole in tamponade but only in the latter part of diastole in constriction) and the absolute level of pericardial pressure (high in tamponade, normal in constriction).

Restrictive Cardiomyopathy

The clinical picture of constrictive pericarditis may be extremely difficult to distinguish from restrictive cardiomyopathy. Restrictive cardiomyopathy is usually the result of some infiltrative process of the myocardium that results in diastolic dysfunction. The most important restrictive cardiomyopathies are amyloidosis, hemochromatosis, and endomyocardial fibroelastosis. Extensive radiation to the mediastinum may also lead to restrictive cardiomyopathy. Diastolic dysfunction usually occurs throughout diastole, but depending on the degree of ventricular involvement and the slope of the diastolic pressure-volume relationship, it may occur early or late in diastole. The hemodynamic picture may be indistinguishable from constrictive pericarditis. Both syndromes can exhibit equilibration of right and left ventricular diastolic pressure with a "dip-and-plateau" or "square root" sign. There may be a disparity between right ventricular and left ventricular end-diastolic pressures in restriction (that is not present in constriction), which may be brought out by exercise or fluid loading. The disparity between ventricular pressures is, to a large extent, dependent on the degree of left ventricular involvement; the more involved the left ventricle with the infiltrative process, the greater the disparity. Other data that may differentiate pericardial constriction from restrictive cardiomyopathy include right ventricular systolic hypertension (absent in constriction, present in restriction), prominent respiratory variation in left ventricular isovolumic relaxation time and peak mitral flow velocity (present in constriction, absent in restriction), timing of impaired diastolic function (occurring throughout diastole in restriction, only in the latter part of diastole in constriction), and the surface electrocardiogram (depolarization and conduction abnormalities in restriction, repolarization abnormalities in constriction). Involvement of other systems with amyloidosis (renal, gastrointestinal) and hemochromatosis (liver, skin, diabetes) may help to identify an underlying systemic cause of restrictive cardiomyopathy. Endomyocardial biopsy may also be helpful in identifying causes (amyloidosis, hemochromatosis, endomyocardial fibroelastosis) of restrictive cardiomyopathy. Ultrafast cine-CT and MRI are particularly useful in distinguishing between constrictive pericarditis and restrictive cardiomyopathy.

Effusive-Constrictive Disease

Effusive-constrictive disease is a disorder in which there is a combination of pericardial tamponade and constrictive physiology. The causes of effusive-constrictive disease are generally the same as those of constrictive pericarditis (neoplasm, previous irradiation, acute pericarditis, tuberculosis). Effusive-constrictive physiology may, in fact, be an early stage in the development of chronic constrictive pericarditis. The hemodynamic features of effusive-constrictive disease are most consistent with cardiac tamponade, and the diagnosis is confirmed with the documentation of persistently elevated right atrial pressure and equilibration of right and left ventricular diastolic pressures after pericardiocentesis and return of intrapericardial pressure to zero. Pericardiocentesis may provide temporary relief, but as with constrictive pericarditis, the definitive therapy for effusive-constrictive disease is surgical resection.

■ THERAPEUTIC ALTERNATIVES

Once the diagnosis is established, efforts should be directed toward avoiding further hemodynamic compromise prior to surgery. As with the management of acute right ventricular failure or right ventricular infarction, maintenance of an adequate preload without causing worsening constriction and further hemodynamic deterioration is crucial. Drugs that decrease preload (venodilators, nitrates, diuretics) ordinarily

Table 1 Clinical Symptoms That Mimic Pericardial Constriction

Cirrhosis
Right-sided congestive heart failure
Right ventricular infarction
Cardiac tamponade
Restrictive cardiomyopathy
Effusive-constrictive disease

Table 2 Historical and Physical Examination Features of Constrictive Pericarditis

History
Previous history of pericarditis
Tuberculosis
Renal failure
Neoplastic disease
Mediastinal irradiation
Chest trauma
Prior cardiac surgery
Physical examination
Elevated jugular venous pressure
Prominent y-descent
Peripheral edema, ascites, hepatomegaly
Kussmaul's sign
Pericardial knock
Absence of pulsus paradoxus

are not used. Drugs that decrease heart rate and increase ventricular filling (such as beta-blockers and some calcium blockers) may have theoretical disadvantages and should also be used with caution. It should be emphasized that constrictive pericarditis is not a reversible phenomenon, and the underlying problem requires surgical correction. Without surgical correction, there are no pharmacologic or hemodynamic manipulations that reverse the underlying problem, although stabilization prior to surgery is important to minimize the risks of the operative procedure. Surgical outcome is unfavorably influenced by severe clinical disability, and surgical intervention should be undertaken early in the course of symptomatic patients.

■ PREFERRED APPROACH

Surgical Treatment

Constrictive pericarditis is a progressive disorder, and the majority of patients who come to medical attention because of symptoms will, over time, become more symptomatic. The definitive therapeutic procedure for the treatment of constrictive pericarditis is surgical resection of the pericardium. This can be best accomplished with a midline thoracotomy and cardiopulmonary bypass, which allow better mobilization of the heart and total removal of the pericardium, which can be densely adherent.

Operative mortality is low, on the order of 5 percent, and the majority of patients have complete relief of symptoms. In some patients, symptomatic and hemodynamic improvement are immediately apparent, whereas in others there is more gradual improvement over days to weeks. An inadequate response to pericardiectomy is usually due to an incomplete surgical resection, especially with densely adherent pericardium and involvement of the visceral pericardium. A small number of patients have refractory and progressive cardiac failure following surgery, ending in death. In these patients, there is usually underlying myocardial disease (or atrophy) or persistent constriction of the left ventricle (due to incomplete resection). In these patients, left ventricular performance is inadequate to handle the increased pulmonary blood flow after relief of constriction of the right ventricle.

Given the fact that there is one basic treatment—surgery—for patients with constrictive pericarditis, the primary management problem lies in establishing the diagnosis and distinguishing constrictive pericarditis from the other pericardial compressive syndromes, namely, cardiac tamponade and restrictive cardiomyopathy. Other disorders involving right-sided failure may also be confused with constrictive pericarditis and must also be excluded (Table 1).

Table 3 Diagnostic Modalities Useful in the Clinical Recognition of Constrictive Pericarditis

Chest film	Pericardial calcification Left atrial enlargement
Electrocardiography	Usually nonspecific ST and T changes Low QRS voltages and left atrial abnormality may be present
Echocardiography	Increased pericardial thickness Rapid early diastolic filling Attenuated late diastolic filling Accentuated respiratory variation in isovolumic relaxation time and peak mitral flow velocity
Ultrafast cine-CT and MRI	Thickening of pericardium Dilated venae cavae or hepatic veins Impingement on right ventricle
Cardiac catheterization	Equalization of right and left ventricular diastolic pressures "Square root" sign Prominent y-descent Endomyocardial biopsy
Surgery	Pericardial histology

Factors in the history and physical examination that support a diagnosis of constrictive pericarditis are summarized in Table 2. Elevated jugular venous pressure with a prominent y-descent is strongly suggestive of either pericardial constriction or restrictive cardiomyopathy. An early diastolic pericardial knock, if present and clearly distinguishable from an S3, is virtually diagnostic. A pericardial knock is usually best heard along the left sternal border and occurs 0.09 to 0.12 second following A2. It corresponds to the abrupt cessation of ventricular filling by the limiting pericardium. It is usually higher in pitch than a typical S3, occurs somewhat earlier than S3, and may be confused with the opening snap of mitral stenosis.

The data available from other diagnostic modalities have been previously discussed and are summarized in Table 3. Electrocardiography and chest roentgenogram provide suggestive, but not definitive, diagnostic information. Echocardiography may document pericardial thickening and abnormal diastolic function, but it is relatively insensitive. Other new noninvasive diagnostic techniques for imaging the pericardium appear to be more useful, including ultrafast cine-CT and MRI. Cardiac catheterization provides the definitive hemodynamic data as well as an opportunity for endomyocardial biopsy to exclude restrictive cardiomyopathy (such as with amyloidosis, endomyocardial fibroelastosis, hemochromatosis) as a diagnostic possibility. There are still isolated cases in which a definitive diagnosis cannot be made until surgery, but fortunately with the advent of ultrafast cine-CT and MRI, they are becoming increasingly rare.

Suggested Reading

Fowler NO. Constrictive pericarditis: New aspects. Am J Cardiol 1982; 50:1014.

Fowler NO. Pericardial disease. Heart Dis Stroke 1992; 1:85.

Garcia MJ, Rodriguez L, Ares M, Griffin BP, Thomas JD, Klein AL. Differentiation of constrictive pericarditis from restrictive cardiomyopathy: Assessment of left ventricular diastolic velocities in longitudinal axis by Doppler tissue imaging. J Am Coll Cardiol 1996; 27:108–114.

Hatle LK, Appleton CP, Popp RL. Differentiation of constrictive pericarditis and restrictive cardiomyopathy by Doppler echocardiography. Circulation 1989; 79:357.

Hirschmann JV. Pericardial constriction. Am Heart J 1978; 96:110.

Hurrell DG, Nishimura RA, Higano ST, Appleton CP, Danielson GK, Holmes DR, Tajik, AJ. Value of dynamic respiratory in left and right ventricular pressures for the diagnosis of constrictive pericarditis. Circulation. 1996; 93:2007–2013.

Klein AL, Cohen GI, Pietrolungo JF, White RD, Bailey A, Pearce GL, Stewart WS, Salcedo EE. Differentiation of constrictive pericarditis from restrictive cardiomyopathy by Doppler transesophageal echocardiographic measurements of respiratory variations in pulmonary venous flow. J Am Coll Cardiol 1993; 22:1935–1943.

Oh JK, Hatle LK, Seward JB, Danielson GK, Schaff HV, Reeder GS, Tajik AJ. Diagnostic role of Doppler echocardiography in constrictive pericarditis. J Am Coll Cardiol 1994; 23:154–162.

Oren RM, Grover-McKay M, Steinford W, Weiss RM. Accurate preoperative diagnosis of pericardial constriction using one computed tomography. J Am Coll Cardiol 1993; 22:832–838.

Reddy PS, Leon DF, Shaver JA, eds. Pericardial disease. New York: Raven Press, 1982.

Shabetai R. The pericardium. New York: Grune & Stratton, 1981.

Shabetai R, Fowler NO, Guntheroth WG. The hemodynamics of cardiac tamponade and constrictive pericarditis. Am J Cardiol 1970; 26:480.

Soulen RD, Stark DD, Higgins CB, et al. Magnetic resonance imaging of constrictive pericardial disease. Am J Cardiol 1985; 55:480.

Sutton FJ, Whitley NO, Applefeld MM, et al. The role of echocardiography and computed tomography in evaluation of constrictive pericarditis. Am Heart J 1985; 109:350.

CARDIOMYOPATHY: DILATED

Celia M. Oakley, M.D., F.R.C.P., F.A.C.C., F.E.S.C.

Dilated cardiomyopathy is characterized by reduction in contractile force of the left ventricle not caused by limitation of blood flow through the extramural coronary arteries and unassociated with specific pathology. The left ventricle is dilated, and the ejection fraction is usually less than 0.40 and may be much lower. Left ventricular failure is usually the first clinical event. The right ventricle may also be dilated, and rarely the dilation affects the right ventricle alone. Disturbances of atrial and ventricular rhythm are common, and in the right ventricular form recurrent ventricular tachycardia may dominate the clinical scene, leading to the descriptive title of "arrhythmogenic right ventricular dysplasia."

■ THERAPEUTIC ALTERNATIVES

Dilated cardiomyopathy is a condition of unknown etiology, so that advances in treatment are largely a result of improvement in the management of cardiac failure. The possibility of an enterovirus etiology for some cases has followed the development of molecular cloning techniques for viruses, but until more is known neither antiviral agents nor immunosuppressive therapy is appropriate.

Therapy is therefore directed toward alleviating heart failure, improving exercise tolerance, preventing thromboembolism, treating symptomatic arrhythmias, and preventing sudden death and progressive heart failure. Despite this, cardiac transplantation offers the only hope of restoration to full activity in some patients.

■ PREFERRED APPROACH

Medical Treatment

Most patients are not seen until after their first episode of left ventricular failure. Only a few are recognized because of a third heart sound or mitral regurgitant murmur, left bundle branch block, or otherwise abnormal electrocardiogram or cardiac enlargement on chest film. Systemic embolism is occasionally the first event. In others, the onset of atrial fibrillation or the observation of frequent ventricular ectopic beats or even ventricular tachycardia may bring the underlying disease to notice.

Left Ventricular Dysfunction

Diuretics. It is rational to try to unload and to shrink the size of the left ventricle. Many patients in this category either improve or remain unchanged for years. An angiotensin converting enzyme (ACE) inhibitor alone may suffice or be combined with a thiazide diuretic, especially if the blood pressure is high.

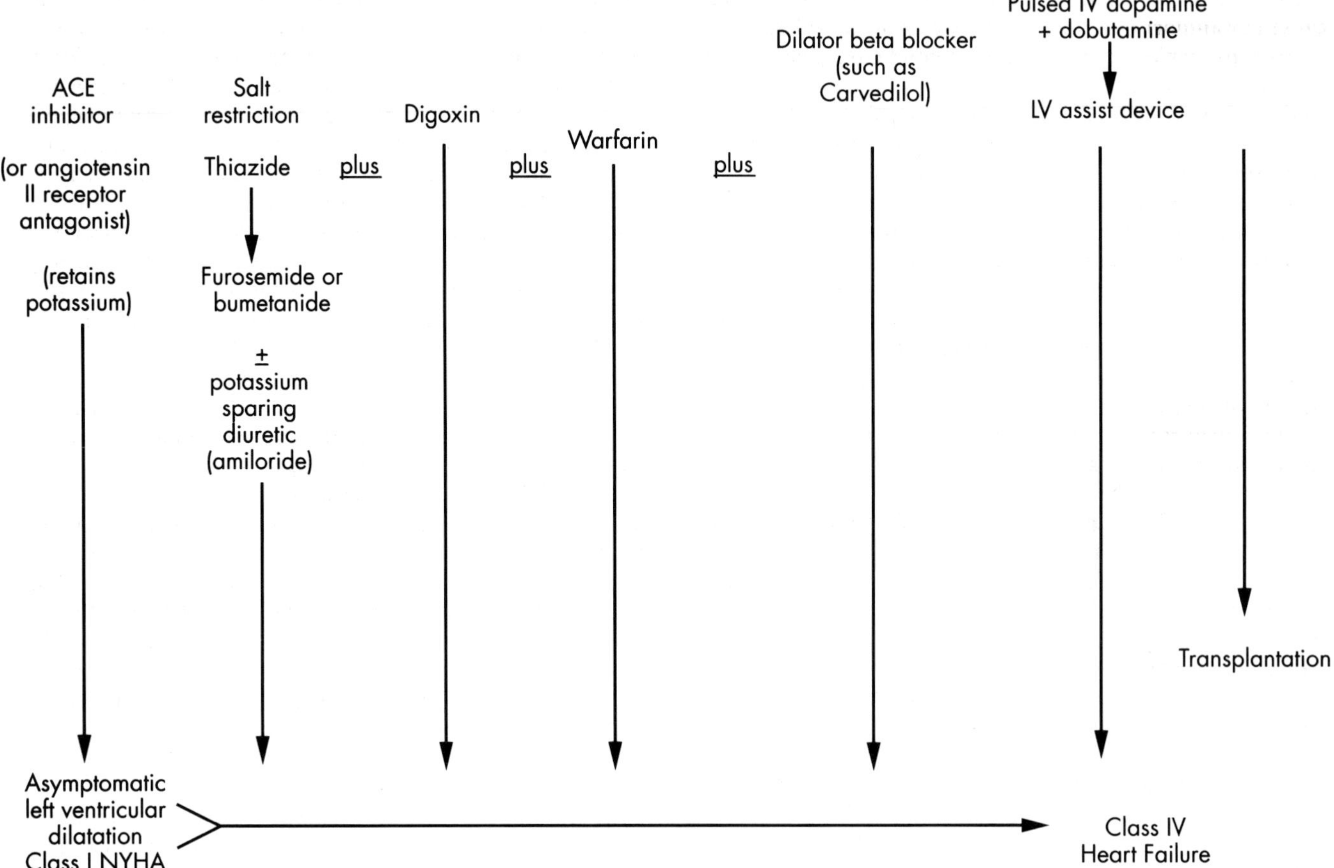

Figure 1
Management of dilated cardiomyopathy.

ACE inhibitors and a diuretic are introduced in that order according to severity (Fig. 1). If there is overt left ventricular failure, a diuretic usually removes evidence of it and improves exercise tolerance. Some patients are rendered asymptomatic, although the left ventricle remains abnormal. When fluid retention is mild, a thiazide drug is the first choice, coupled with moderate dietary sodium restriction. These drugs inhibit sodium transport proximal to the distal tubule, where sodium is reabsorbed without water. Salt excretion is affected for about 8 hours, with the exception of chlorthalidone, which has an effect lasting for over 24 hours. All thiazide drugs increase urinary potassium loss, and the diet should be high in potassium-containing fruits such as oranges and bananas. This may be sufficient, but because it is desirable to maintain potassium levels at between 4 and 5 mmol per liter, the addition of a potassium-sparing agent such as amiloride is preferable to potassium supplements that do more good to the manufacturer than to the patient. Bendrofluazide 5 mg plus amiloride 5 or 10 mg daily may be sufficient. Spironolactone is an alternative to amiloride in women but in men has a high incidence of causing painful gynecomastia. Treatment will lower blood pressure, but the aim should be to keep it low, around 100 to 110 mm Hg systolic if the patient is younger, and a little higher in older patients.

More resistant fluid retention requires a loop diuretic such as bumetanide or furosemide. They act by inhibiting sodium and chloride transport in the ascending limb of Henle's loop and promote a greater chloride than sodium diuresis. They also increase urinary potassium loss, leading to hypokalemic alkalosis. Secondary aldosteronism increases potassium depletion.

Bumetanide and furosemide have an action that peaks in about 4 hours and is complete at 6 hours, allowing the patient to choose a convenient time of day for the dose. When heart failure is more severe, the drug may need to be given twice or even three times a day, although it is usually still possible to arrange for undisturbed nights. There is a widespread tendency to use excessive doses of diuretics, which leads to hypovolemia with postural hypotension, increased fatigability, and uremia. It is often not realized that fatigue and breathlessness are symptoms of an inadequate cardiac output response to exercise and not an indication for increasing the dose of diuretic that normally should not exceed 4 mg of bumetanide or 120 mg of furosemide in patients with normal renal function and frequently may be much less.

The natriuretic effect of loop diuretics is increased by the addition of amiloride or spironolactone, and potassium loss is reduced, but the effect of ACE inhibitors introduced at an early stage is to bring up the potassium levels and usually render potassium-sparing agents unnecessary.

Both loop diuretics and thiazides can induce hyperuricemia and precipitate gout. Thiazides may cause hyperglycemia, slight hyperlipidemia, and hypercalcemia. Skin rashes may be caused by amiloride but occasionally also by thiazides.

Hyponatremia follows use of these potent drugs and is due to relative water overload and rarely, if ever, to genuine sodium depletion. Mild hyponatremia needs no treatment. More severe hyponatremia is a bad prognostic omen. Water restriction, although often advocated, can be intolerable to patients as well as not very effective. The hyponatremia reflects a shift of sodium into cells due to magnesium depletion that inhibits membrane sodium-potassium adenosine triphosphatase (ATPase). Magnesium depletion has recently come back into prominence as a problem in heart failure patients. It contributes to depression and muscular weakness and is often associated with refractory hypokalemia and rhythm disturbances.

Hypomagnesemia can be treated with a magnesium glycerophosphate in doses of 3 to 6 g daily orally.

Angiotensin Converting Enzyme Inhibitors. ACE inhibitors act as vasodilators by reducing the circulating level of angiotensin II, by inhibiting the breakdown of bradykinin, and by interacting with the sympathetic nervous system to reduce its activity. They reduce "afterload" and also lower "preload," with largely secondary effects on the heart, resulting in an increase in cardiac output and some redistribution of regional blood flow.

Numerous trials have all revealed benefit from ACE inhibitors with reduced mortality and reduced need for hospital admission. This benefit extends also to patients with subclinical left ventricular dysfunction as well as to those with overt heart failure and to patients with dilated cardiomyopathy as well as patients with coronary heart failure.

ACE inhibitors have rendered direct-acting vasodilators obsolete except in occasional patients who cannot tolerate ACE inhibitors because of hypotension, renal failure, or intractable cough. In contrast to direct-acting vasodilators, alpha-blockers, and calcium entry blocking agents, ACE inhibitors diminish aldosterone secretion, reduce sodium and water retention, increase potassium retention, antagonize angiotensin-induced vasoconstriction, reduce raised circulating spillover catecholamine levels, and reduce myocardial oxygen consumption. Coronary vasodilation may occur, subendocardial blood flow may increase, and improved ventricular function is associated with some decrease in ventricular arrhythmia.

The effect of diuresis is to stimulate aldosterone secretion, which opposes this, so diuretic dosage should be kept as low as possible and ACE inhibitors introduced early with the objective of reducing this secondary aldosteronism and improving left ventricular output. It is best to start with a short-acting drug such as captopril 6.25 mg. If starting the drug in the hospital, the first dose should be given in the morning so that the blood pressure response can be observed. If starting the drug at home, the first dose should be taken after retiring at night so that any hypotensive response is minimized. The dose can then be increased quite quickly to a maximum of 25 mg three times a day. In some patients a maximum effect is achieved with an even lower dose. Once established on a short-acting ACE inhibitor, patients can be changed onto a long-acting, once-a-day ACE inhibitor such as lisinopril in a dose of up to 20 mg per day. The blood pressure is always reduced by ACE inhibitors and in some patients hypotension, which is itself a poor prognostic omen in heart failure, may make it impossible to get the patients onto effective doses.

Hypotension is the most common and most worrisome side effect. It can be obviated to some extent by reducing the dose of diuretic or omitting it altogether for 24 hours before starting the ACE inhibitor, thus rendering it relatively ineffective so that the onset of action is gradual. Patients who are most likely to suffer a severe first-dose hypotensive response are predictable. They are on high doses of diuretics, already have low blood pressure, and are hyponatremic and may also have impaired renal function. Great caution should be exercised in such patients: The first dose should be even lower than 6.25 mg. If hypotension occurs, it should be countered by posture. Saline infusion or vasoconstrictors are undesirable and rarely necessary after captopril, but hypotension after enalapril can be severe and prolonged.

Renal function may deteriorate in the first few days following the introduction of an ACE inhibitor. This is not only in patients with renal artery stenosis or occult bilateral renal artery stenosis who are thrown into profound renal failure but also in patients with severe heart failure and reduced renal blood flow whose glomerular filtration is dependent, as in renal artery stenosis, on constriction of the efferent arterioles. In most such patients renal function gradually returns to normal after some days, but the rise in urea and creatinine can be worrying, and renal failure may be precipitated by x-ray contrast agents.

ACE inhibitors increase plasma levels of potassium, which may contribute to reduction of ventricular arrhythmias, but hyperkalemia may reach dangerous levels if potassium-sparing diuretics or potassium supplements are not stopped, particularly as the levels may continue to rise. Despite this, some patients remain hypokalemic while on ACE inhibitors and these patients still need a carefully titrated dose of amiloride. It follows that potassium levels need to be checked frequently, particularly at first and in patients with advanced failure.

"Captopril cough" is recognized early. All the ACE inhibitors can increase the sensitivity of the cough reflex and cause a dry, irritating, repetitive cough in 10 to 15 percent of patients (McEwan and Fuller, 1989). Many patients tolerate the cough because of the benefit they gain once the cause of the cough is explained. This avoids unnecessary investigations.

Skin rashes may occur. Thrombocytopenia and membranous nephritis were seen in the early days of captopril when doses of 200 mg per day and more were given. They do not seem to occur with the low doses now used.

Losartan is a specific angiotensin II receptor antagonist with similar properties to the ACE inhibitors. Possible advantages are a "cleaner" action. It does not inhibit breakdown of bradykinin or other kinins and does not cause cough. So far it has mainly been used as an antihypertensive agent.

Digitalis. Digitalis has been used in the treatment of heart failure ever since William Withering discovered that foxglove leaves were valuable in the treatment of dropsy. It is probable that most of these early patients had rheumatic heart disease and that their heart failure was precipitated by the onset of atrial fibrillation with a fast ventricular rate. The efficacy of digitalis in the treatment of heart failure with sinus rhythm has been fiercely debated in recent years, but it now seems clear that digitalis is effective as a weak inotrope in some but not all patients with heart failure. Digitalis is ineffective in mainly diastolic heart failure as occurs in the elderly, in some cases of coronary heart failure, and in hypertrophied hearts. Digitalis is most effective in thin-walled, volume-loaded, dilated left ventricles. The inotropic effect of digoxin was shown to be linear in acute studies with ouabain so that the greatest inotropic effect occurs close to the toxic dose. The problem is that in patients with sinus rhythm there is no end point as in atrial fibrillation, so the tendency is to be conservative and to use low and relatively ineffective doses. Therapy is not helped by the rather variable correlation between plasma levels and toxicity, which is enhanced in hypokalemic patients and through interaction with certain antiarrhythmic drugs including quinidine and amiodarone. Plasma levels should usually be between 1 and 3 mmol per liter.

Diet and Exercise. Obese patients should be counseled to lose weight, and the diet should be moderately low in salt and high in potassium-containing foods such as bananas and oranges. Avoidance of table salt and obviously salty foods cuts the intake to about 100 mmol per day. Patients with acute heart failure or exacerbations need bed rest, but the stable treated heart failure patient should be encouraged to take regular frequent walking exercise. This is in direct contrast to the conventional advice of only a few years ago, when heart failure patients were advised to rest as much as possible. It has been shown that exercise tolerance is slowly and steadily improved by regular exercise training with an increase in stroke volume and peak oxygen consumption and a fall in heart rate and noradrenaline. The beneficial effect can be significant. Serial exercise testing in placebo-controlled drug trials was the way in which the benefits of training were first observed. This led to studies that proved of benefit in trained compared with nonexercising patients.

Other Inotropes. No other orally active inotropes apart from digoxin have been shown to be either effective or safe. The so-called "inodilators," amrinone and milrinone, which are phosphodiesterase inhibitors, act only as vasodilators in long-term use with little evidence, if any, of continued beneficial effect on myocardial function and much concern about toxicity because of an excess of deaths in placebo-controlled trials of oral dosage. More recent drugs in this category, such as enoximone, failed to prove themselves and have been withdrawn from oral use.

Acute use of intravenous inotropes can be effective in the short term, and a combination of dopamine in renal doses with dobutamine can result in a rise in cardiac output with a fall in filling pressure, but the effects are usually only short-term because of tachyphylaxis through down-regulation of myocardial beta-receptors. Nevertheless, they may help to keep a patient going while awaiting transplantation. Pulsed doses for 48 hours every 2 weeks can be effective. Occasionally, substitution of adrenaline for dobutamine may bring about short-term further improvement, but arrhythmias may be precipitated.

Patients who require parenteral use of inotropes on account of hypotension, unresponsiveness to diuretics, or deteriorating renal function are in class IV failure with a prognosis measuring days, weeks, or months, and all should be considered for urgent transplantation unless there are contraindications.

Beta-Adrenergic Blocking Drugs. The acute use of beta-blocking drugs in patients with heart failure can cause profound loss of output with bradycardia and hypotension. There was therefore considerable incredulity and opposition when in 1975 Swedish physicians introduced the idea of using beta-blockers in heart failure (Waagstein and co-workers, 1989). They started metoprolol in very small doses of 10 mg daily, increasing only very slowly to not exceed 50 mg twice a day. Benefit was first seen in patients with coronary heart failure and tachycardia but then was found also when the treatment was extended to patients with dilated cardiomyopathy. Benefit was confined to about half of the patients and is sometimes delayed, even following early deterioration. The Swedish work has been confirmed and extended by more recent studies in Germany, in which the starting dosage was even lower, and it was suggested that benefit may not be seen for several months (Waagstein and co-workers, 1989).

The rationale for using beta-blocking drugs remains controversial. A fall in heart rate reduces metabolic demand as well as improves coronary blood flow, and up-regulation of myocardial beta-receptors may render the heart again sensitive to endogenous inotropes, particularly if calcium overload from excessive beta-stimulation has been prevented.

An interesting new beta-blocker with considerable partial agonist action, xamoterol, showed promising results in early trials but an excess of deaths in a later trial of the drug in class III and IV heart failure. Benefit in the earlier trials may have been because of inclusion of a majority of patients with coronary heart failure because xamoterol is a useful antianginal agent. In milder heart failure xamoterol caused an increase in stroke volume and cardiac index with a fall in filling pressure that was maintained without tachyphylaxis. The excess of deaths in severe heart failure is still unexplained but may have to do with the drug working as a beta-blocker during waking hours but causing tachycardia during sleep.

More recently, the vasodilating beta blocker carvedilol has been shown to reduce mortality. Clinical trials have shown impressive improvement when carvedilol was added to an ACE inhibitor and diuretic in heart failure patients. Carvedilol is a combined alpha and nonselective beta blocker which is also an antioxidant and has antiproliferative properties which may protect the myocardium.

Antiarrhythmic Drugs. Ventricular ectopic activity is common in patients with a risk of sudden death in dilated cardiomyopathy, as it is also in patients with advanced coronary disease, hypertrophic cardiomyopathy, and severe hypertensive heart disease. It is now seen as a marker of a poor myocardium rather than as an independent prognostic indicator. In the CAST study of patients with asymptomatic ventricular ectopic activity following myocardial infarction, the membrane-stabilizing antiarrhythmic effect of the class IC drugs effectively suppressed asymptomatic ventricular ectopic activity. The same effect depresses myocardial contractile activity, which may have been responsible for the increased deaths in this study. Although the results of CAST cannot necessarily be transferred to patients with dilated cardiomyopathy, there is no reason to believe that they would be different. Patients with dilated cardiomyopathy have ventricular ectopic activity whose frequency and complexity can be related to the severity of the myocardial dysfunction. Sudden death accounts for approximately half of the deaths of patients with dilated cardiomyopathy compared with about 70 percent of deaths in coronary heart failure. It has been assumed that they are caused by ventricular fibrillation precipitated by the ventricular ectopic activity, but it now seems that ventricular ectopic activity is simply a marker of a bad heart with a bad prognosis. Suppression of arrhythmia may follow improvement in left ventricular function, as was hinted at in a study of captopril (Cleland and co-workers, 1984). Certainly there is no present indication for seeking and suppressing asymptomatic ventricular arrhythmias in dilated cardiomyopathy. All the class I antiarrhythmic drugs have a myocardial depressant effect, and the results of two large trials of the class III drug amiodarone are still awaited. Only if ventricular ectopic activity is so frequent that it is having a deleterious hemodynamic effect is there an indication for amiodarone. There is some interest in the possibility that sudden death in patients being treated with class I antiarrhythmic drugs may be caused by the development of electromechanical dissociation rather than ventricular fibrillation.

In our own natural history study of dilated cardiomyopathy, sudden death was confined to patients with class III and IV heart failure (Stewart and co-workers, 1990).

There has been a revival of interest in sotalol for its combined class II and weak class III antiarrhythmic action.

Anticoagulants. There has been no controlled trial of anticoagulants in dilated cardiomyopathy. My own practice is to use anticoagulants in all patients who are in atrial fibrillation and in most patients with more than mild failure who are in sinus rhythm. This is because of a considerable incidence of systemic embolism. The source is probably the small thrombi that form in the trabecular crevices of the dilated left ventricle.

Cardiomyopathy Associated with Pregnancy and Parturition

Ventricular dilation and heart failure may follow parturition but occasionally develop in late pregnancy. Because it is rare, the literature is muddled by anecdotal cases, reviews, and heterogeneous material.

Heart failure may be sudden and catastrophic or more insidious. Treatment is for the heart failure. An immunologic interaction between mother and fetus can be postulated. This may be responsible for "myocarditis" frequently found on biopsy. Short-term immunosuppressive therapy may be given. Genuine improvement can occur from severe hypokinetic left ventricular and congestive failure with reduction in left ventricular size. Although this usually has started within weeks of delivery and is complete by 6 months, a few patients may start to improve only after more than a year. Prognosis is therefore difficult, and transplantation should be avoided if at all possible while there may still be improvement. Not all patients relapse in future pregnancies, although further childbearing is inadvisable in any patient whose left ventricular function remains significantly abnormal.

Right Ventricular Dilated Cardiomyopathy and Arrhythmogenic Right Ventricular Dysplasia

In what is probably a heterogeneous group of conditions, right ventricular dysfunction varies from subclinical to severe, but the left ventricle is apparently spared. Most common are patients with ventricular tachycardia originating from the right ventricle and showing a leftward axis and left bundle branch block pattern. These cases are sometimes familial and may show adipose replacement of myocardial tissue in the right ventricular wall. Many of these patients have excellent hemodynamic function and are asymptomatic apart from the arrhythmias, whereas others develop profound low output failure with marked systemic congestion. Apart from control of heart rate and rhythm, right ventricular failure is exceedingly difficult to treat. A very high venous pressure can often be lowered without loss of output to reduce hepatic discomfort and edema, but no attempt should be made to lower venous pressure to normal, particularly if there is evidence of tricuspid regurgitation. Normally the pulmonary artery pressure is low, and there is then no possibility of reducing right ventricular afterload, although balloon pumping of the pulmonary artery has been used in congestive heart failure with raised pulmonary vascular resistance.

Patients with arrhythmogenic right ventricular dysplasia have a high tendency to sudden death. Their symptomatic ventricular tachycardias are seen to degenerate into ventricular fibrillation and need to be treated vigorously. I have found amiodarone to be the most effective drug for this purpose and have followed some patients for up to 10 years while they remained symptom free on a low dosage of 200 mg daily. A few of these patients have shown evidence of progressive right ventricular failure.

Cardiac Toxins

Alcohol. All patients with dilated cardiomyopathy should be asked about their alcohol consumption. Macrocytosis is a useful indicator of chronically high consumption even in the absence of abnormal liver function tests. A raised gamma-glutamyltransferase may be an indicator of only recent rather than long-term intake, whereas raised levels for other liver enzymes may be due to a chronic alcohol hepatitis. There seems to be individual susceptibility to the adverse effects of alcohol on the myocardium. The heart may show dramatic improvement in function after a patient has stopped drinking. Individual susceptibility to the effects of alcohol may be shown by the finding of immunoglobulin A on the sarcolemma and in small blood vessels on biopsy of patients with alcoholic heart disease. A gratifying improvement may be an indicator of an important role for alcohol in an individual patient or of a still reversible state of myocardial depression. It seems that alcohol plays only a subsidiary role in the majority of patients with dilated cardiomyopathy who enjoy social drinking. In such patients it is still worthwhile to advise abstinence because of alcohol's adverse although mild pharmacologic effects.

Patients with alcoholic cardiomyopathy tend to be male

and beer drinkers, despite the removal of cobalt, a myocardial toxin that was included in the secret formulas of certain breweries until the 1960s, when there was an outbreak of cobalt-induced heart failure in Canadian and Belgian beer drinkers, all of whom were taking most of their calories in the form of beer.

Cocaine addiction can cause both coronary thrombosis and myocardial depression.

Other Toxins. Anthracyclines given as doxorubicin have important toxic subcellular effects that eventually lead to intracellular calcium overload and depressed cardiac function.

Surgical Treatment

Indications for Transplantation

It is obviously of great importance to be able to predict prognosis with some accuracy in patients with dilated cardiomyopathy. We have found that this is not invariably a relentlessly progressive disease with an invariably fatal outcome as has been suggested. Many patients with NYHA class I or II symptoms remain stable for many years. A few patients show unexplained and remarkable improvement. Most of them have had only moderate left ventricular dilation, but occasionally patients with greater degrees of impairment improve and become asymptomatic with good exercise tolerance, although rarely with entirely normal left ventricular function.

Patients with advanced dilated cardiomyopathy in NYHA classes III or IV usually have left ventricles measuring between 8 and 10 cm in diameter on echo with ejection fractions below 15 percent on multigated angiogram scanning (Kannel and Cupples, 1988). These patients have less than a 50 percent chance of surviving 1 year and should be considered for transplantation. Sudden death is very uncommon in patients who are stable with mild symptoms, but it accounts for about 50 percent of the deaths in patients with advanced failure. Patients with dilated cardiomyopathy do not need to be considered for transplantation until their quality of life has become considerably impaired. Because dilated cardiomyopathy behaves as though the impairment in function follows a single insult and has not shown itself to be a progressive disease, consideration for transplantation frequently is needed very soon after the patient is first referred. Such patients may have had only weeks or a few months of a downhill course. Only very rarely is the patient with dilated cardiomyopathy an "emergency" because the need for transplantation can usually be predicted. This is in contrast to coronary heart failure, in which deterioration is often abrupt owing to further myocardial necrosis, and the prognosis is unpredictable because of interruption by sudden death at almost any stage, accounting for 70 percent of the deaths in patients who reach the stage of heart failure.

Contraindications to transplantation include diseases of other organ systems that seriously limit prognosis, although multiorgan transplantation is sometimes practiced for combined cardiac and renal or cardiopulmonary and liver disease. More commonly, it is infection, usually in the lungs, or thromboembolism with pulmonary infarction that can preclude cardiac transplantation. Anticoagulant treatment, although arguable in milder heart failure, is mandatory in advanced heart failure patients.

Relative contraindications to cardiac transplantation include severe reactive pulmonary hypertension. These patients may be successfully treated in the domino procedure, whereby patients with primary pulmonary hypertension receiving heart-lung transplants donate their good hearts to patients who need a hypertrophied right ventricle in case pulmonary vascular resistance fails to fall to normal after cardiac transplantation. An alternative procedure is heterotopic transplantation, in which the patient's heart is not removed. This may be used if the donor heart is too small. Both are linked up in parallel. This procedure also allows later removal of the donor heart, which can act as an assist device in patients who may have remediable heart disease. Theoretically this might include patients with a severe postpartum cardiomyopathy or patients with a severe life-threatening acute myocarditis.

Most patients with dilated cardiomyopathy inquire about transplantation before the subject is broached by the physician, and this is always helpful. It is obvious that patients need to be highly motivated, compliant to sometimes arduous treatment regimens, and possessed of determination and confidence in success. The good results of transplantation justify their confidence, but some patients still have a difficult early postoperative course if there are complications, and, of course, hearts are in short supply so that it is improper to refer patients whose prognosis may still be relatively open-ended.

Other surgical procedures such as cardiomyoplasty, wrapping the latissimus dorsi muscle around the heart, and pacing it to augment left ventricular output are still in an experimental stage.

The wholly implanted permanent artificial heart is still some distance away, but temporary implantation has been used as a bridge to cardiac transplantation when a heart has not been available for a patient who seemed otherwise unlikely to survive. These hearts are still highly subject to thromboembolism, and survival of such patients is inversely proportional to the duration of time that the implant is used.

Left ventricular assist devices are gaining ground for the temporary support of patients who are awaiting a heart. The use of such devices is, of course, undesirable because of the risk of infection and thromboembolism.

Suggested Reading

Bouhour JB, Helias J, De Lajartre AY. Detection of myocarditis during the first year after discovery of a dilated cardiomyopathy by endomyocardial biopsy and gallium 67 myocardial scintigraphy. Prospective multi-centre French study of 91 patients. Eur Heart J 1988; 9:520–528.

Carlquist JF, Menlove RL, Murray MB, et al. HLA class I (DR and DQ) antigen associations in idiopathic dilated cardiomyopathy. Circulation 1991; 83:515–522.

Cleland JGF. The clinical course of heart failure and its modification by ACE inhibitors: insights from recent clinical trials. Eur Heart J 1994; 15:125–30.

Cleland JGF, Poole Wilson PA. ACE inhibitors for heart failure: a question of dose. Br Heart J 1995; T2(Suppl 3):S106–S110.

Dargie HJ, McMurray JJV. Diagnosis and management of heart failure. BMJ 1994; 308:321–328.

Diaz RA, Obasohan A, Oakley CM. Prediction of outcome in dilated cardiomyopathy. Br Heart J 1987; 58:393.

Jekene AD, Moreira LFP, Stolf NAG, et al. Left ventricular function changes after cardiomyopathy in patients with dilated cardiomyopathy. J Thorac Cardiovasc Surg 1991; 102:132–139.

Kannel WB, Cupples A. Epidemiology and risk profile of cardiac failure. Cardiovasc Drugs Ther 1988; 2:387.

Keogh AM, Freund J, Baron DW, Hickie JB. Timing of cardiac transplantation in idiopathic dilated cardiomyopathy. Am J Cardiol 1988; 61:418.

McEwan JR, Fuller RW. Angiotensin converting enzyme inhibitors and cough. J Cardiovasc Pharmacol 1989; 13(Suppl 3):567.

Neri R, Mestroni L, Salvi A, et al. Ventricular arrhythmias in dilated cardiomyopathy: Efficacy of amiodarone. Am Heart J 1987; 113:707.

Oakley CM. The cardiomyopathies. In: Weatherall D, Ledingham J, Warrell D, eds. Oxford textbook of medicine. 2nd ed. Oxford: Oxford University Press, 1987; 13:209.

The SOLVD Investigators. Effect of enalapril on survival in patients with reduced left ventricular ejection fractions and congestive heart failure. N Engl J Med 1991; 325:293–302.

The SOLVD Investigators. Effect of enalapril on mortality and the development of heart failure in asymptomatic patients with reduced left ventricular ejection fractions. N Engl J Med 1992; 327:685–691.

Stewart RAH, McKenna WJ, Oakley CM. A good prognosis in dilated cardiomyopathy. Q J Med 1990; 74:309.

Waagstein F, Caidahl K, Wallenten I, et al. Long-term β-blockade in dilated cardiomyopathy: Effects of short- and long-term metoprolol treatment followed by withdrawal and readministration of metoprolol. Circulation 1989; 80:551.

CARDIOMYOPATHY: HYPERTROPHIC

Thomas W. von Dohlen, M.D.
Martin J. Frank, M.D.

Hypertrophic cardiomyopathy (HC) is a primary myocardial disease characterized by asymmetric hypertrophy of the left ventricle (LV) without an identifiable cause. Symmetrical LV hypertrophy, hypertrophy of the LV apex, and involvement of the right ventricle have also been described. Autosomal dominant inheritance is most common, but some cases appear to be sporadic. The microscopic characteristics include myocyte hypertrophy and myocardial fiber disarray and varying degrees of perivascular fibrosis in all patients. Also, the majority of patients have narrowed prearteriolar intramyocardial arteries as a result of proliferation of the intimal and medial layers.

The most striking clinical manifestation of HC is sudden cardiac death, with a reported incidence as high as 2 to 3 percent per year in adults (Maron and co-workers, 1987). Also, the majority of patients seen at referral centers are symptomatic with dyspnea, chest pain, presyncope, or syncope. Multiple pathophysiologic abnormalities contribute to symptoms. These include abnormal diastolic relaxation and filling, occlusive disease of the intramyocardial coronary arteries, and excessive oxygen demand from a hypertrophied, hypercontractile LV and dynamic "obstruction" to LV outflow. As a result, myocardial ischemia and fibrosis often develop and contribute to the arrhythmogenic milieu that culminates in sudden death.

■ THERAPEUTIC ALTERNATIVES

The goals of therapy in HC are to prevent sudden death, relieve symptoms, and improve functional capacity. Medical therapy involves the use of beta-receptor blockers, calcium channel blockers, or antiarrhythmic agents, along with the judicious use of nitrates, angiotensin converting enzyme inhibitors, diuretics, and digitalis. Surgical treatment of HC—septal myotomy-myectomy or mitral valve replacement—is reserved for those with severe symptoms not controlled by medical therapy who have a significant LV outflow gradient. Unfortunately, the existing data for medical and surgical therapy of HC have not been obtained in a prospective, randomized fashion. Furthermore, it may take up to 2 years following initiation of medical therapy for maximum benefit. These limitations, the small number of patients reported in most studies, varying thresholds in the decision for medical or surgical therapy, and differing institutional referral patterns do not permit meaningful grouping or comparison of survival statistics among or within groups of HC patients.

■ PREFERRED APPROACH

Therapeutic decisions regarding patients with HC must be made on a patient-by-patient basis. In our experience, the most common reasons for "failure" of medical therapy are inadequate drug dosages and failure by the physician or patient to appreciate that treatment is a lifelong endeavor and that several years of drug therapy may be required for maximum clinical improvement.

Medical Treatment

The categories of HC patients that we believe warrant medical therapy include

- Survivors of sudden cardiac death
- Strong family history of HC associated with sudden cardiac death
- Patients symptomatic with chest pain, dyspnea, presyncope, syncope, or significant functional aerobic impairment based on exercise testing
- Multiple episodes in 24 hours of nonsustained ventricular tachycardia (VT) (at least 3 beats at a rate of at least 120 per minute) on Holter monitoring or sustained VT on electrophysiologic study
- Severe LV hypertrophy (LV wall thickness at least 20 mm on echocardiography)

- Supraventricular arrhythmias or evidence of conduction system disease (sick sinus syndrome)
- Progressive LV dilation accompanied by a declining LV ejection fraction over time
- Perfusion defect(s) on stress thallium-201 scintigraphy, regardless of symptom status

Although ventricular arrhythmias are probably the most common mechanism of sudden death in HC, findings of significant conduction system disease and supraventricular tachyarrhythmias are not uncommon. The shortening of diastole by tachycardia or loss of atrial systole may be enough to cause hemodynamic compromise, leading to syncope or sudden death in patients with severe diastolic dysfunction.

Patients at greatest risk of sudden death or syncope are young (under age 30 years), have a strong family history of sudden death, have severe LV hypertrophy, have runs of nonsustained VT on Holter monitor, or have inducible sustained VT on electrophysiologic study. However, these markers are only about 70 percent sensitive for an increased risk and lack the specificity necessary for guiding treatment decisions (McKenna, 1987).

We currently believe that increased sensitivity and specificity in predicting risk and in determining who should be treated can be achieved best by using stress or intravenous dipyridamole plus stress thallium-201 imaging. Perfusion defects seen on thallium imaging are in LV segments with near-normal wall thickness as well as those with severe hypertrophy and likely represent myocardial ischemia, fibrosis, or both. In our experience, patients who have thallium defects also are highly likely to have nonsustained ventricular tachycardia or conduction system disease, more severe LV hypertrophy, and lower LV ejection fractions. Thallium defects may occur in up to half of *asymptomatic.* HC patients, and in one study, treatment with verapamil was shown to improve or normalize such defects in most patients, strongly suggesting that they represent true myocardial ischemia.

Therefore, *before therapy is initiated,* all new HC patients require a battery of tests to provide baseline information and to assess risk. Doppler echocardiography defines the extent and distribution of LV hypertrophy, the systolic function of the LV, the presence and magnitude of an LV outflow tract gradient, and whether mitral regurgitation or other valvular disease is present. Holter monitoring for 48 to 72 hours is mandatory because 24 hour recording detects only about 50 percent of patients with runs of nonsustained VT. Electrophysiologic study is performed in all patients who have been resuscitated from sudden death and also in those with syncope who have infrequent ventricular premature contractions and no evidence of conduction system disease during 72 hours of Holter monitoring. Stress thallium scintigraphy is performed on all patients with adequate effort tolerance (heart rate × blood pressure at least 20,000) but is preceded by intravenous administration of dipyridamole (0.4 mg per kilogram over 4 minutes) in those who fail to reach this target.

The true art of treating patients with HC begins with the decision to administer medications. Given the wide array of pathophysiologic and electrical derangements that occur in this disease, it is not surprising that no single medication has been shown to provide symptomatic benefit and prevent sudden death in all patients. To rely on one drug or class of drugs for the therapy of HC is unrealistic. The often ill-defined, heterogeneous substrate of HC requires elucidation before proper management decisions are possible. Implantation of a permanent AV sequential pacemaker may be necessary in those with documented conduction system disease or significant resting bradycardia prior to medical therapy, so that adequate drug dosages can be safely administered and surgical therapy can be avoided. Dual-chamber pacing may also improve symptoms in patients with "obstructive" physiology who are refractory to adequate medical therapy by favorably altering ventricular activation and relaxation. Finally, if electrophysiologic testing or ECG monitoring documents hemodynamically significant ventricular arrhythmia, the use of an automatic implantable cardioverter-defibrillator should be considered.

The clinical management of HC also requires counseling and recommendations concerning physical activity, prophylaxis for bacterial endocarditis, and use of anticoagulants for those who have chronic or intermittent atrial fibrillation. Strenuous physical activity that exceeds the anaerobic threshold often precedes sudden cardiac death. The risk of endocarditis is greatest in patients who have systolic anterior motion of the anterior mitral leaflet (especially in association with a septal endocardial plaque that can be seen on echocardiography) and those with mitral regurgitation or other valvular abnormalities. Because antimicrobial prophylaxis has its own risks, we believe that the risk-benefit ratio must be weighed for each patient. However, for patients at risk, endocarditis prophylaxis is required for all procedures not carried out in a sterile field.

Pregnancy in HC patients is usually well tolerated. Continuation of beta-blockers has not been found to pose a major problem as far as the fetus is concerned, although small-for-date babies and fetal bradycardia are seen. There is no evidence that cesarean section is indicated or preferable to vaginal delivery.

Beta-Blockers

Beta-blockers have been the first line of therapy for HC for over 20 years. The arrhythmic nature of sudden death in HC and data confirming that beta-blockers prevent sudden death after myocardial infarction provide justification for their use. By slowing heart rate at rest, they improve diastolic LV function and allow coronary perfusion to be prolonged. Furthermore, the blunting of exercise heart rate decreases catecholamine stimulation, which may produce myocardial ischemia and lead to arrhythmias.

When using beta-blockers, the goal of therapy is to reduce the standing heart rate to 60 beats per minute and maximum exercise heart rate to less than 130 beats per minute. Initial dosing is begun with 20 to 40 mg of propranolol four times per day and titrated upward over several days. In our experience, the improvement or alleviation of symptoms is rarely achieved with daily doses of less than 320 mg of propranolol or its equivalent. The mean dose was 360 mg per day in 25 of our patients evaluated recently. Once hemodynamic endpoints are achieved, selection of other beta-blockers with a longer half-life, greater selectivity, or different lipid solubility is possible. We prefer not to use drugs that have intrinsic sympathomimetic activity because they do not reduce resting heart rate and have not been shown to be protective against sudden death in myocardial infarction patients.

We have never seen pulmonary edema due to the negative inotropic effects of beta-blockers in HC patients with normal systolic LV function. In fact, congestive symptoms correspond more with diastolic dysfunction, which these drugs tend to improve. However, excessive bradycardia or heart block may worsen congestive symptoms or lead to hypotension or syncope. Such patients may require pacemaker implantation to permit administration of adequate drug dosages. Patients with obstructive pulmonary disease should receive cardioselective drugs such as metoprolol, betaxolol, or atenolol. Betaxolol is a useful drug because it is truly a once-daily medication, which assists in patient compliance. Also, it has a good side effect profile.

Calcium Channel Blockers

Calcium channel blockers, especially verapamil, have been used extensively. All produce significant improvement in diastolic LV function, although specific mechanisms may vary. For example, verapamil decreases heart rate and the LV outflow tract gradient, whereas nifedipine may cause reflex tachycardia and provoke or exacerbate dynamic LV "obstruction." Diltiazem's pharmacologic effects appear to be between those of verapamil and nifedipine. Our use of these agents has been steadily increasing, although we still regard them as a second choice compared with beta-blockers.

We often use a combined regimen of a beta-blocker plus a calcium channel blocker, usually diltiazem because of its more benign side effect profile, in patients who are intolerant of high doses of beta-blockers. Because both drugs have beneficial hemodynamic effects, their combination is rational, allows lower doses of each drug to be given with fewer side effects, and appears to provide symptom relief in a higher percentage of patients than either drug alone.

Because verapamil or diltiazem may produce hypotension, heart block, or excessive bradycardia, combining either of these drugs with a beta-blocker must be done carefully, particularly in patients who have a resting bradycardia or decreased systolic LV function before therapy. Such patients must be followed more carefully and promptly evaluated, should their symptoms change.

Although verapamil and diltiazem tend to decrease resting and exercise heart rate, nifedipine may cause reflex tachycardia at rest, provoke or worsen an LV outflow tract gradient, or cause hypotension through its more potent peripheral dilating effects. It is much better tolerated when given with a beta-blocking drug. All calcium channel blockers cause mild increases in serum digitalis levels. Less serious side effects include edema with all drugs in this class, flushing and headache with nifedipine, and constipation with verapamil.

Antiarrhythmic Drugs

Amiodarone and disopyramide have been used as initial therapy in HC. As previously noted, the lack of randomized trials in evaluating the efficacy of these drugs does not allow any firm conclusions to be drawn. The pharmacologic effects of amiodarone include prolongation of the effective refractory period (delayed repolarization), peripheral vasodilation, decreased contractility, and decreased heart rate. Symptoms may improve in some patients independent of antiarrhythmic effects; however, worsening of symptoms by amiodarone may also occur as a result of its unpredictable hemodynamic effects. We do not consider it to be a first-line agent for treating HC because of its serious side effect profile (worsening of conduction system disease, interstitial pneumonitis, hepatotoxicity, corneal deposits, and 15 to 20 percent likelihood of discontinuation as a result of intolerance).

Although disopyramide is a class IA antiarrhythmic agent, its use in HC is primarily based on its potent negative inotropic effects. Symptomatic patients with large LV outflow gradients are given this agent as a first-line agent at some institutions. However, no long-term survival data involving a large number of patients are available. Anticholinergic side effects (urinary retention, constipation, dry mouth, blurred vision) are common and may require concomitant administration of pyridostigmine or lead to discontinuation of therapy.

Our current approach for the suppression of potentially life-threatening arrhythmias is first to combine a class IA, IB, or IC drug (most commonly mexiletine) with a beta-blocker. This approach proves to be safe and effective in the majority of patients. In others, a beta-blocker combined with a IB agent plus a IA or IC drug may be required. We have noted that the proarrhythmic effects of class IA and IC drugs are less common in patients taking a beta-blocker.

In all cases, the institution of antiarrhythmic therapy should be carried out on an inpatient basis so that proarrhythmic events may be recognized and treated promptly. Careful attention to serum electrolytes and the electrocardiographic Q-T interval are necessary when dosing any class IA drug, whereas profound prolongation of the P-R and QRS intervals may indicate toxicity with class IC drugs. If amiodarone is to be given, baseline pulmonary, hepatic, and thyroid function tests as well as ocular slit lamp examination are necessary and must be repeated during therapy.

Reassessment of arrhythmia and the efficacy of drug therapy is performed at least once per year in all patients because new, potentially lethal tachyarrhythmias and bradyarrhythmias are progressively more common with time. In fact, about 80 percent of patients followed for 10 years develop such arrhythmias. Using this approach, the annual mortality from sudden death in patients followed at our institution has been less than 0.5 percent per year.

Diuretics, Nitrates, and Angiotensin Converting Enzyme Inhibitors

Diuretics, nitrates, and angiotensin converting enzyme inhibitors, although not considered to be first-line agents, all have proven useful in the clinical management of HC. Diuretics or nitrates, if given alone, can provoke or worsen an outflow tract gradient by reducing preload. However, patients who are already receiving adequate doses of a beta-blocker or calcium channel blocker (or negative inotropic drugs such as amiodarone or disopyramide) tolerate these agents well and may have further symptomatic improvement with their addition, most likely as a result of a lowering of preload and LV end-diastolic pressure. In those patients with worsening congestive symptoms in conjunction with progressive LV dilation and systolic dysfunction, we have found that the addition of an angiotensin converting enzyme inhibitor often results in significant clinical improvement.

Digitalis

Although digitalis therapy has been associated with worsening of symptoms, a trial in certain patients is clearly justified: those with supraventricular tachyarrhythmias not controlled without digitalis and those with progressive systolic LV dysfunction.

Surgical Treatment

As noted before, patients selected for surgical procedures are those who have symptoms refractory to "adequate" medical therapy and have evidence of a significant resting or provokable (≥ 50 mm Hg) outflow tract gradient. Surgical relief of "obstruction" is performed by resecting part of the interventricular septum, inserting a prosthetic mitral valve, or both. The symptomatic benefits of the procedure are probably due to a modest decrease in LV diastolic pressure and lowering of myocardial oxygen requirements. A decrease in outflow tract gradients is seen in most patients; however, repeat procedures are required in some patients who have "recurrence."

Because the decision to perform surgery is based on symptom severity and surgery has not been shown to improve survival or prevent sudden death, it must be regarded as a *palliative* procedure only. Mortality in the perioperative period may be as high as 5 percent, although centers where the operation is performed frequently currently report mortalities of about 2 percent. In patients undergoing myotomy-myectomy, the production of iatrogenic conduction system disease, ventricular septal defect, or aortic regurgitation is not uncommon. Those who receive a mitral valve prosthesis also have the risk of thromboembolism, bleeding caused by anticoagulants, and endocarditis in addition to their pre-existing condition. Furthermore, the majority of patients who have surgical therapy still require medication to relieve symptoms or treat arrhythmias. Interestingly, one reported series emphasized that it is the patients with the most severe symptoms who are most likely not to survive the surgical procedure (Krajcer and co-workers, 1989).

Suggested Reading

Frank MJ, Watkins LO, Prisant LM. Potentially lethal arrhythmias and their management in hypertrophic cardiomyopathy. Am J Cardiol 1984; 53:1608.

Krajcer Z, Leachman RD, Cooley DA, et al. Septal myotomy-myomectomy versus mitral valve replacement in hypertrophic cardiomyopathy. Circulation 1989; 80(Suppl I):57.

Maron BJ, Bonow RO, Cannon RO, et al. Hypertrophic cardiomyopathy: Interrelations of clinical manifestations, pathophysiology, and therapy. N Engl J Med 1987; 316:780.

Maron BJ, Epstein SE, Roberts WC. Causes of sudden death in competitive athletes. Am J Cardiol 1986; 7:204.

Maron BJ, Wolfson JK, Epstein SE, et al. Intramural ("small vessel") coronary artery disease in hypertrophic cardiomyopathy. J Am Coll Cardiol 1986; 8:545.

McKenna WJ. Sudden death in hypertrophic cardiomyopathy: Identification of the "high risk" patient. In: Brugada P, Wellens HJJ, eds. Cardiac arrhythmias: Where to go from here? Mt. Kisco, NY: Futura, 1987:353.

Tanaka M, Fujiwara H, Onodera T, et al. Quantitative analysis of narrowings of intramyocardial small arteries in normal hearts, hypertensive hearts, and hearts with hypertrophic cardiomyopathy. Circulation 1987; 75:1130.

von Dohlen TW, Frank MJ. Current perspective in hypertrophic cardiomyopathy: Diagnosis, clinical management and prevention of disability and sudden cardiac death. Clin Cardiol 1990; 13:247.

von Dohlen VW, Prisant LM, Frank MJ. Significance of positive or negative thallium-201 scintigraphy in hypertrophic cardiomyopathy. Am J Cardiol 1989; 64:498.

CARDIOMYOPATHY: RESTRICTIVE

I. Sylvia Crawley, M.D.

Restrictive cardiomyopathy is characterized by structural changes in the myocardium, endocardium, or subendocardium that result in impaired ventricular filling with normal or only mildly reduced systolic function. The clinical and hemodynamic spectrum may simulate constrictive pericarditis.

Idiopathic restrictive cardiomyopathy is characterized by interstitial fibrosis. Scleroderma is also associated with interstitial fibrosis and may produce a dilated or restrictive cardiomyopathy. Interstitial infiltration and eventual replacement of the myocardium occurs in restrictive cardiomyopathy due to amyloid and sarcoid heart diseases. Restrictive cardiomyopathy is frequent in amyloid but uncommon with sarcoid. Hemochromatosis, primary or secondary, usually causes dilated cardiomyopathy, but a restrictive physiology may occur. Endocardial and subendocardial changes occur in endomyocardial fibrosis and hypereosinophilic syndrome, and restrictive cardiomyopathy is common.

Restrictive cardiomyopathy and constrictive pericarditis have similar clinical presentations. Both cause dyspnea, decreased exercise tolerance, elevated jugular venous pressure, hepatomegaly, ascites, and peripheral edema. Equal elevation of right and left ventricular filling pressures favors constrictive pericarditis but can also occur in restrictive cardiomyopathy. Impairment of left ventricular filling in both processes can be demonstrated by echo-Doppler studies, and radionuclide angiography may aid in differentiation. There is potential overlap because each has a spectrum of altered hemodynamics. Computed tomography is more helpful than echocardiography in detecting pericardial thickening. Magnetic resonance imaging offers certain advantages over echocardiography and computed tomography in the detection of pericardial thickening and myocardial changes and may prove to be especially useful in the recognition of certain forms of restrictive cardiomyopathy. Despite the plethora of comparative observations, some patients will require thoracotomy for definitive diagnosis. Transvenous endomyocardial biopsy is useful in avoiding unnecessary thoracotomy in some patients.

■ THERAPEUTIC ALTERNATIVES

Therapeutic options in restrictive cardiomyopathy are limited. Digitalis and diuretics may alleviate congestive symptoms. Specific medical or surgical therapy directed at the specific causes is currently restricted to only a few cases. Cardiac transplantation may be indicated in some patients.

Medical Treatment

Hemochromatosis

Primary hemochromatosis, a genetic disorder of iron metabolism, causes extensive iron deposits within the myocardial cells. Repeated phlebotomy can improve cardiac function, presumably as a result of removal of some of this iron accumulation. Improvement has been noted in both dilated and restrictive forms. Weekly phlebotomy of 250 to 500 ml over a 1 to 2 year period may be necessary. Studies suggest that improvement of prognosis occurs in the majority of patients. Improvement in left ventricular function has been reported in patients with mild or severe left ventricular dysfunction. The use of phlebotomy early in the course of the disease before severe symptoms develop seems appropriate and may improve survival.

The chronic anemia of secondary forms of hemochromatosis preclude the use of phlebotomy for the depletion of myocardial iron stores. Chelation therapy with deferoxamine mesylate (Desferal) has been demonstrated to decrease iron stores and improve myocardial function. Deferoxamine must be given parenterally, preferably by continuous intravenous or subcutaneous infusion, because it has a short half-life. Intramuscular injection is used but is less effective. Local chemical irritation at the injection site may interfere with patients' compliance. Ascorbic acid administration after the institution of deferoxamine may improve iron clearance but should be used with caution because of potential cardiac toxicity.

The adequacy and duration of phlebotomy or chelation therapy can be assessed by determination of serum ferritin levels, urinary clearance of iron, or liver biopsy.

Endomyocardial Fibrosis

Endomyocardial fibrosis without or with hypereosinophilia (Löffler's endocarditis) results in fibrosis of the endocardium of the inflow tract of the right and left ventricles. The papillary muscles, chordae tendineae, and atrioventricular valves are also involved, and significant tricuspid or mitral regurgitation is common. Mural thrombi in the ventricles and atria are common. Congestive symptoms may improve with digitalis, diuretics, and vasodilators. Chronic anticoagulation should be considered, although the incidence of systemic and pulmonary emboli is low. Antihypereosinophilic therapy with prednisone with or without hydroxyurea or other cytotoxic drugs has been reported to improve ventricular dysfunction significantly, slow is progression, and improve survival.

Amyloidosis

Amyloid heart disease is progressive, and there is no satisfactory therapy. Diuretics may relieve congestive symptoms but should be used cautiously to avoid detrimental reduction in ventricular filling pressures. Digitalis is not recommended because toxicity may occur with low doses. Negative inotropic agents, especially calcium blockers, are contraindicated because they may worsen myocardial dysfunction.

Sarcoidosis

Sarcoid heart disease, especially in the early phase, can produce restrictive physiology due to granulomatous interstitial infiltration of the myocardium. Corticosteroids have been used in the treatment of sarcoid heart disease with improvement in ventricular function. However, in some cases such treatment is thought to result in myocardial scar formation and ventricular aneurysm. The efficacy of corticosteroid therapy is unclear but has been recommended for biopsy-proven cases.

Surgical Treatment

Endomyocardial Fibrosis

The medical treatment of endomyocardial fibrosis without hypereosinophilia is frequently ineffective in relieving symptoms or improving prognosis. Because systolic function is preserved in many patients, surgical relief of inflow obstruction and prosthetic valve replacement of the tricuspid or mitral valves can improve symptoms and improve prognosis. Decortication of the endocardial fibrotic bands can relieve inflow obstruction. Destruction of conduction tissue related to right ventricular decortication with or without tricuspid valve replacement causes irreversible complete heart block, requiring a permanent pacemaker in a few patients. When valve replacement is indicated, a bioprosthesis is generally recommended.

Pseudoxanthoma Elasticum

A restrictive cardiomyopathy has been reported in only a few cases of pseudoxanthoma elasticum. Calcification of the endocardium, chordae tendineae, and papillary muscles results in inflow tract obstruction. Surgical correction with extensive resection of calcified tissue, requiring additional mitral valve replacement, has been reported. In this case a heterograph mitral prosthesis was placed, which became heavily calcified and stenosed within 1 year, requiring replacement with a mechanical prosthesis.

Permanent Pacemaker Therapy

Involvement of the conduction system may occur in some forms of restrictive cardiomyopathy, especially those that are infiltrative. Complete heart block may be the presenting problem in sarcoid heart disease. Amyloid heart disease may also cause complete heart block, and the pacing threshold may be quite high as a result of the extensive infiltration of amyloid in the myocardium. Idiopathic restrictive cardiomyopathy, hemochromatosis, and scleroderma may also cause complete heart block.

Suggested Reading

Ashinsky D. Hemochromatosis: It's more than skin deep. Postgrad Med 1992; 91:137.

Bousfany CW Jr, Murphy GW, Hicks GL Jr. Mitral valve replacement in idiopathic hypereosinophilic syndrome. Ann Thorac Surg 1991; 51:1007.

Challenor VF, Conway N, Monro JL. The surgical treatment of restrictive cardiomyopathy in pseudoxanthoma elasticum. Br Heart J 1988; 59:266.

Parillo JE. Heart disease and the eosinophil. N Engl J Med 1990; 323:1561.

Vaitkus PT, Kussmaul WJ. Constrictive pericarditis versus restrictive cardiomyopathy: A reappraisal and update of diagnostic criteria. Am Heart J 1991; 122:1431.

Wilmshurst PT, Katritis D. Restrictive cardiomyopathy. Br Heart J 1990; 63:323.

AORTIC DISSECTION

Joseph Lindsay Jr., M.D.

The term *aortic dissection* denotes a disease process characterized by the separation of the elastic fibers of the aortic media by a column of blood. The cleavage plane may extend for only a few centimeters or, not uncommonly, for the entire length of the aorta. Rarely, in some segments the dissection involves the entire circumference of the aorta. More often, 40 to 60 percent of the cross-section is "dissected."

This process jeopardizes the patient's life in three major ways. The aortic wall, weakened by the medial cleavage, frequently ruptures. Further, major aortic branches may be occluded if their origins and adjacent aortic segments become involved in the dissection. Finally, severe aortic regurgitation may result from involvement of the aortic root. Thus, successful therapy must prevent rupture and retard extension of the medial cleavage.

Aortic dissection should not be confused with expansion or rupture of a pre-existing atherosclerotic, luetic, or mycotic aneurysm. Although the clinical picture of such a complication may mimic aortic dissection, the pathogenetic process and the therapeutic approach differ.

Aortic dissection is encountered most commonly in the sixth decade of life or later as a complication of hypertension. Younger or normotensive victims of aortic dissection have, as a rule, underlying congenital weakness of the aortic media associated with entities such as Marfan's syndrome, coarctation of the aorta, Turner's syndrome, annuloaortic ectasia, or bicuspid aortic valve.

■ THERAPEUTIC ALTERNATIVES

Inasmuch as aortic dissection is a structural problem, surgical repair constitutes the most logical long-term remedy. Thus, the assessment in each patient of the risks and benefits of operative therapy becomes the central management decision. Teamed with a cardiovascular surgeon, the attending physician must decide whether the patient should undergo operation at once, whether it should be delayed and reconsidered at a later time, or whether operative repair can never be an option because of the patient's age, the presence of complicating illnesses, or severe neurologic injury consequent to the dissection (Table 1). Unfortunately, a substantial number of patients fall into the last of these three categories.

Table 1 Management of Patient Subsets in Aortic Dissection

Subset A: Those with syncope or hypotension
- *Assessment of prognosis:* External rupture is likely present
- *Management:* Emergency surgery

Subset B: Hypertensive patients with dissection involving the ascending aorta
- *Assessment of prognosis:* External rupture is likely within hours or days despite aggressive antihypertensive treatment
- *Management:* Urgent surgery; aggressive antihypertensive treatment preoperatively

Subset C: Hypertensive patients with dissection sparing the ascending aorta
- *Assessment of prognosis:* With aggressive antihypertensive treatment, the risk of rupture is no greater than risk of operation
- *Management:* Aggressive antihypertensive treatment; elective operative repair in younger individuals, those in good general health, and those with large aneurysms

Subset D: Complicated patients with severe aortic regurgitation or ischemia of a limb, the heart, the kidney, or the central nervous system
- *Assessment of prognosis:* Prospect for survival and recovery limited unless defect can be corrected
- *Management:* Urgent surgery in those in whom there is a reasonable expectation of correction of the problem

Subset E: Patients with advanced comorbid disease or severe ischemic complication of the dissection that precludes reasonable chance for surgical success
- *Assessment of prognosis:* Patient will not survive operation or will not benefit from it
- *Management:* Antihypertensive therapy and/or supportive care

Prior to operation and when surgery is not recommended, vigorous antihypertensive therapy is indicated to reduce stress on the aortic wall and thereby to provide protection against rupture of the wall and extension of the dissection. At least in the case of dissection involving the ascending aorta, such therapy has unfortunately failed to meet earlier expectations for long-term effectiveness.

■ PREFERRED APPROACH

Having said that operative repair is potentially the most desirable treatment for all patients with aortic dissection, it follows that the operative risk must in each case be weighed against the immediacy of the threat posed by the disease.

Before a discussion of the threat to the patient can be undertaken, the most frequently encountered anatomic variations of its aortic involvement must be described (Crawford, 1990; DeSanctis and co-workers, 1987). The most common pattern (type I of DeBakey) accounts for about two-thirds of all dissections. The proximal limit of a type I dissection lies just above the aortic valve, and an intimal ("entrance") tear is typically located near this proximal end. Type II of DeBakey is a subgroup of type I. Patients whose dissection is limited to the ascending aorta may be so categorized. Absent surgical correction and despite aggressive antihypertensive treatment, patients in these categories have an exceedingly high mortality in the acute phase. In the only other common pattern (type III of DeBakey), the medial dissection is limited to the distal arch and descending aorta. The "entrance" tear is characteristically found just distal to the left subclavian artery. These account for about one-fourth of all aortic dissections, and carry a far more favorable acute prognosis than do those involving the ascending aorta. Surgery may safely be delayed in these cases unless a life-threatening complication has occurred. The choice is less clearly defined for the small number of dissections not falling into these readily identifiable types.

In addition to the identification of the anatomic type of aortic dissection, recognition of the existence of external rupture is crucial to the choice of therapy. As is the case with any disruption of the continuity of the aortic wall, only operative management can be expected to be successful. External rupture has almost always occurred when the patient presents with syncope or is hypotensive on admission (DeSanctis and co-workers, 1987). About one-fifth of all dissections involving the ascending aorta appear in this way. External rupture most often occurs in the region of the entrance tear. Inasmuch as this tear is located in the proximal aorta in two-thirds of instances (types I and II), the rupture communicates most often with the pericardial space, hence a presentation of syncope or hypotension in the absence of appreciable blood loss. In another one-fourth of cases (type III) the intimal tear is situated just beyond the left subclavian artery. In such cases rupture occurs into the left pleural space, producing a left hemothorax.

Patients with annuloaortic ectasia, many of whom have ocular or musculoskeletal manifestations of Marfan's syndrome, constitute a discrete group. The medial dissection in such instances is usually, but not invariably, only a few centimeters in length and appears to represent a complication of the progressive dilation of the aortic root that is characteristic of this disorder. These limited dissections are usually asymptomatic until the onset of rupture.

Infrequently, aneurysmal dilation of the aorta that has developed in an aortic segment weakened by a clinically unrecognized acute dissection is the presenting evidence of this process. Most such "chronic" dissections are of the type III variety in that unrecognized and untreated dissections involving the ascending aorta are usually fatal during the acute phase. In such aneurysms the risk of rupture must be weighed against operative risk in a manner not very different from that employed in the assessment of patients with aortic aneurysm of any etiology.

Medical Treatment

General Treatment of Acute Dissection

Sudden, life-threatening complications, such as very severe hypertension, cardiac tamponade, massive hemorrhage, acute aortic regurgitation, or ischemic injury to the heart, kidneys, or central nervous system, threaten patients with acute dissection. Optimal management includes careful monitoring of vital functions in an intensive care unit. Aggressive reduction of the blood pressure, often an important part of therapy, may necessitate an intra-arterial line and careful monitoring of the urine output by means of an indwelling urinary catheter. Any uncertainty as to the status of the intravascular volume should be resolved by means of bedside right-heart catheterization.

Confirmation of the diagnosis, determination of the extent of the medial split, and identification of the site of the entrance tear must follow closely on bedside assessment and initial stabilization. Management decisions hinge on this information. Traditionally, aortography or computed tomography have been required, but transesophageal echocardiography appears to be at least as accurate and may be quicker and safer (Ballal and co-workers, 1991).

Specific Therapy in Acute Dissection

Wheat, Palmer, and associates provided an experimental and clinical foundation for the aggressive administration of antihypertensive medications to reduce the hemodynamic stress on the aortic wall and thus avert progression of the medial cleavage and external rupture of the weakened aortic wall (DeSanctis and co-workers, 1987). Their data emphasize the importance of reducing not only the aortic pressure but also its rate of rise. According to this construct, drugs that reduce arterial pressure but result in reflex augmentation of left ventricular contractility and rate of rise of aortic pressure are not useful. This approach was received with great enthusiasm at the time of its introduction in 1965, but greatly improved surgical results and disappointing clinical experience in type I patients have tempered the early enthusiasm. It is now reserved for the preoperative preparation of patients and is employed long-term only in those with uncomplicated type III dissection, and in those for whom surgical treatment cannot be recommended.

One of several drug regimens may be employed to reduce the arterial pressure and its rate of rise. Aggressive use of a beta-blocking agent may adequately reduce aortic wall stress in the majority of patients who present with relatively modest levels of hypertension. In others with more severe hypertension intravenous nitroprusside combined with a beta-blocking agent may be required. Drug therapy should aim to lower systolic arterial pressure to 100 to 120 mm Hg. Optimal blood pressure reduction may not be possible if oliguria (less than 25 ml per hour) or mental confusion appears.

In this institution, intravenous esmolol is the currently preferred beta-blocking agent for acute dissection since its effects can be readily titrated. Before infusion this agent must be diluted to a concentration of no more than 10 mg per ml because more concentrated solutions are very irritating to veins. An initial loading dose of 0.5 mg per kg is administered over one minute followed by an infusion of 0.05 mg per kg per minute. The infusion rate can be increased at four minute intervals by 0.05 mg per kg per minute. Rates beyond 0.3 mg per kg per minute have not been shown to provide added therapeutic benefit. The substantial amounts of fluid required to maintain this infusion limit the usefulness of this agent in some patients.

Alternatively, propranolol can be administered intravenously in 0.5 milligram increments at 1 to 5 minute intervals until the target blood pressure is achieved, the pulse rate slows, or a total dose of 1.5 mg per 10 kg of body weight has been given. This scheme can be repeated at 4 to 6 hour intervals. Appropriate oral doses of this agent or comparable beta-blocking agents can be given for long-term maintenance after the need for acute beta-blockade has passed.

The ability of intravenous nitroprusside to reduce arterial pressure promptly and consistently and the ease with which its hypotensive effects can be titrated recommend it as the current drug of choice for the severely hypertensive patient with acute dissection (Ashfoura and Vidt, 1991; DeSanctis and co-workers, 1987). As little as 0.5 μg per kg per minute may produce the desired result. Occasionally, as much as 10 μg per kg per minute is necessary. This dose, however, should not be exceeded and should be reduced as soon as is practical. A beta-blocking agent should nearly always be used in conjunction with nitroprusside since animal data suggest that when used alone it does not reduce and may, through reflex mechanisms, enhance the rate of rise of arterial pressure.

Reports of the use of intravenous labetalol, a drug that possesses both alpha- and beta-blocking effects, in lieu of nitroprusside, have appeared. Slow intravenous infusion of 20 mg increments and additional increments to a maximum of 80 mg has been recommended (Asfoura and Vidt, 1991). In the few reported cases, appropriate reduction in blood pressure and a favorable outcome have been cited.

Trimethaphan, the intravenous agent first employed by Wheat and Palmer, can be substituted for nitroprusside or labetalol in patients who cannot be given beta-blocking drugs because this agent reduces the rate of rise of aortic pressure. Infused at an initial rate of 1 to 2 mg per minute, this ganglionic blocker can be titrated to the same therapeutic goals as nitroprusside. When compared with nitroprusside in clinical use, this agent does not as reliably reduce the blood pressure, especially after 24 to 48 hours, when tachyphylaxis frequently appears. Because it is a ganglionic blocker, it more often than nitroprusside produces side effects such as ileus.

Other occasionally useful substitutes for nitroprusside include intravenous methyldopa and intramuscular reserpine.

As has been stated, exclusion of external rupture is the therapist's primary concern in those patients who present with a systolic blood pressure already at or below the target level for aggressive antihypertensive therapy. When rupture can be confidently excluded, intravenous beta-blocker treatment may be indicated.

Once the patient has been stabilized and a decision has been made that surgical therapy will not at once be undertaken, a plan must be developed for shifting to intramuscular and oral medications for subacute or chronic blood pressure control. Beta-blocking drugs, sympatholytic agents, and diuretics are useful, but direct vasodilators such as hydralazine, diazoxide, and minoxidil should be avoided because of the reflex sympathetic stimulation that attends their use. Experience with the angiotensin converting enzyme inhibitors and with calcium entry blockers in this context is beginning to be gained (Crawford, 1990; Asfoura and Vidt, 1991).

Treatment of Subacute and Chronic Dissection

Once several days or weeks have elapsed, the target for control of the arterial pressure may be relaxed. Blood pressure goals similar to those of any hypertensive patient are usually appropriate for long-term management.

Side Effects of Drug Therapy

Problems may arise from the therapeutic effects of the agents previously described. Oliguria, mental confusion, and postural hypotension may result from diminished perfusion pressure. The goals of treatment may have to be altered in response and the dose of the agent adjusted accordingly.

Nitroprusside possesses a specific, potentially toxic characteristic. Its metabolism produces cyanide ions that are converted to thiocyanate. Cyanide toxicity can result from overdosage. For this reason the dose of 10 μg per kilogram per minute should not be exceeded. In patients with thiosulfate depletion, lower doses may be toxic. The appearance of metabolic acidosis is a useful early sign of cyanide toxicity. Blood pH and acid-base balance should therefore be monitored. Plasma thiocyanate levels are not useful for the detection of cyanide toxicity.

Surgical Treatment

Selection for and Timing of Surgery

When a decision has been reached that the patient has no limiting comorbid conditions or complications of the dissection that preclude operative treatment, the information contained in the section Preferred Approach provides guidance for the appropriate timing of surgical intervention. Clearly the individual with evidence of external rupture must be operated on an emergency basis. Those with involvement of the ascending aorta are at high risk of rupture, and surgery should be delayed only long enough to stabilize the patient and to obtain adequate diagnostic information regarding the extent of the dissection and the location of the proximal intimal tear. Surgery may be deferred in those whose dissection is limited to the descending aorta because medical management has proved to be as efficacious as operation during the acute phase (Glower and co-workers, 1990; Neya and co-workers, 1992). Evidence of external rupture or of progression of the dissection during drug therapy may require reconsideration of this decision. A decision with regard to operation in patients who have survived for 2 weeks or more or for those who present with chronic dissection is of necessity individualized. Factors such as the age of the patient, the state of general health, and the size of the residual aneurysm must be considered.

Operative Treatment

Resection of the aorta containing the entrance tear (the intimal laceration at the proximal limit of the dissection that allows communication between the true lumen of the aorta and the false lumen created by the dissecting hematoma) is the primary objective. Reapproximation of the transected ends after closure of the false channel may be done directly or, more commonly, with a graft. In some instances revascularization of vital structures, repair of the aortic valve, or other reconstructive procedures may also be required.

Modern surgical techniques have changed such surgery from a risky, problematic enterprise to one in which success may be expected even in gravely ill individuals such as those with dissection. Better means have evolved for the preservation of vital tissue, such as the myocardium, the brain, and the spinal cord, during manipulations that might result in ischemia of these structures. Moreover, improvements in the vascular prostheses available for reapproximation of the aorta now reduce the likelihood of anastomotic leaks, formerly a major hazard of repairing the fragile aortic tissue encountered at the site of dissection.

Preoperative Preparation

For patients who present with hypotension or syncope and in whom external rupture is probable, little time is available for preoperative preparation. Restoration of blood volume and emergency treatment of other physiologic derangements should be carried out concomitantly with those diagnostic procedures essential to the surgeon for the decisions as to the operative approach.

The evaluation and correction of physiologic derangements may be a bit more deliberate for other patients with type I or type II dissection, although the presence of severe aortic regurgitation or of acute myocardial ischemia from obstruction of a coronary artery may dictate haste. Aggressive reduction of any elevation of the blood pressure (see Medical Treatment) is an important preoperative step.

For patients with type III dissections who do not have life-threatening complications, operative therapy may be delayed (Glower and co-workers, 1990; Neya and co-workers, 1992). The measures described under Medical Treatment should be implemented until the chosen time for operation.

Postoperative Course and Potential Complications

Postoperatively, the patient is at risk for all the neurologic, pulmonary, and renal complications of major cardiovascular surgery. Dysfunction of any organ system damaged as a result of preoperative shock, dissection-related arterial occlusion, or aortic valve damage may have to be reckoned with. Management of these patients challenges the skills of an experienced specialist in intensive care.

Two complications of the operation are significant. Rupture of the suture line is perhaps the most feared. The tissue that must be repaired after resection of the aortic segment is extremely friable. Creation of a firm suture line can be extraordinarily difficult even for the most experienced cardiovascular surgeon. Second, paraplegia, a consequence of interruption of the blood supply to the spinal cord, complicates repair of type III dissections in a significant percentage of patients. Fear of this outcome may play a leading part in forming a decision to avoid operation in patients with type III dissection.

Suggested Reading

Asfoura JY, Vidt DG. Acute aortic dissection. Chest 1991; 99:724.

Ballal RS, Nanda NC, Gatewood R, et al. Usefulness of transesophageal echocardiography in assessment of aortic dissection. Circulation 1991; 84:1903.

Crawford ES. The diagnosis and management of aortic dissection. JAMA 1990; 264:2537.

DeSanctis RW, Doroghazi RM, Austen WG, Buckley MJ. Aortic dissection. N Engl J Med 1987; 317:1060.

Glower DD, Fann JL, Speier RH, et al. Comparison of medical and surgical therapy for uncomplicated descending aortic dissection. Circulation 1990; 82(Suppl IV):39.

Neya K, Omoto R, Kyo S, et al. Outcome of Stanford type B acute aortic dissection. Circulation 1992; 86(Suppl II):1.

AORTIC ANEURYSM: NONDISSECTING THORACIC

E. Stanley Crawford, M.D.
Joseph S. Coselli, M.D.

Aneurysm of the thoracic aorta is a serious form of disease. Death occurs in 75 percent of untreated patients within 2 years and 90 percent within 5 years. The cause of death in more than half the patients is rupture, either by spontaneous laceration (simple bursting) or by superimposed dissection. This complication tends to be size dependent. In our series of 117 patients with acute rupture of the descending thoracic or thoracoabdominal aorta confirmed at operation, the external aortic diameter at the site of rupture was 5 to 6 cm (14 percent), 6 to 8 cm (36 percent), 8 to 10 cm (39 percent), and greater than 10 cm (12 percent). The diameter of the ruptured aneurysm in all cases was more than twice the diameter of the adjacent uninvolved aorta.

ETIOLOGY

The etiologies of aneurysms of the thoracic aorta include congenital malformations (coarctation of aorta, persistent arch abnormalities, and abnormalities of fusion of aortic root with aortic annulus), infection (mycotic), trauma, autoimmune disturbances (giant cell aortitis. Takayasu's disease, Behçet's disease), connective tissue disorders (Marfan's syndrome. Turner's syndrome, Ehlers-Danlos syndrome), atherosclerosis, aortic dissection, and medial degenerative disease. The latter two conditions are the most frequent disorders. Contrary to popular thinking, atherosclerosis is a rare etiology. To be sure, atheromatous lesions are frequently superimposed on the other diseases; however, this is a rare cause of thoracic aortic aneurysm. Aortic dissection is discussed elsewhere; this presentation concerns those aneurysms of other origins.

CLINICAL MANIFESTATIONS

The ages of our patients ranged from 15 months to 87 years. The younger patients have disease as a result of infection, trauma, congenital abnormalities, autoimmune disorders, and heritable connective tissue defects. The remaining patients (the majority), whose median age was 66 years, had aneurysms due to nonspecific medial degenerative change. Thus, aneurysmal disease of degenerative origin occurs most frequently in older patients.

Some of our patients referred for treatment were asymptomatic. Thoracic aortic aneurysm was discovered in these cases by routine chest film or computed tomographic scan that showed an abnormal mediastinal mass. Most patients were symptomatic at the time of admission. Symptoms were due to pressure of the expanding aneurysm on adjacent structures and the presence of superimposed dissection or rupture. These symptoms varied with the aortic segment involved and are discussed accordingly.

ASCENDING AND ARCH

The aortic annulus is dilated in 75 to 80 percent of patients with aneurysms of the ascending and transverse aortic arch. These patients have varying degrees of aortic valve insufficiency, and many have symptoms of heart failure. The aneurysmal mass may cause obstruction of the superior vena cava, pulmonary artery, airway, and esophagus. In rare neglected cases, the aneurysm may erode through the anterior chest wall.

Rupture occurs either by spontaneous laceration or dissection of aneurysmal wall into the pericardium, heart chamber, or mediastinum. These terminal events produce serious symptoms of hemorrhage, great vein and myocardial compression, or large left-to-right cardiac shunts.

DESCENDING AND THORACOABDOMINAL AORTA

Aneurysms of the descending thoracic and thoracoabdominal aorta produce symptoms of compression of adjacent structures, including left recurrent laryngeal nerve, esophagus, chest wall, and bronchus, such as hoarseness, dysphagia, and chest wall pain. Rupture at these levels occurs into the mediastinum, lung, bronchus, esophagus, and left chest cavity. This stage of the disease may be manifested by hypotension, increase in pain, hemoptysis, or hematemesis.

PREFERRED APPROACH

Diagnosis

Initial chest film may show a left-sided mediastinal shadow adjacent to the cardiac silhouette suggestive of an aneurysm involving the descending thoracic aorta. A right-sided anterior upper mediastinal shadow suggests an aneurysm of the ascending aorta or aortic arch. Unfortunately, even large aneurysms of the ascending aorta are frequently not visualized by this method of examination because the aneurysm is located within the normal cardiac shadow. Thus, special studies are necessary for the diagnosis in these cases and should be routinely performed to evaluate the heart in patients with high risk of aneurysms, i.e., those with connective tissue defects, valve pathology, coronary artery disease, and others who are to be treated by operation. The logic of this approach lies in the concept that the aortic root is part of the heart based on the fact that the aortic valve arises at its base and the coronary arteries that supply blood to the heart arise from it. Thus, a complete examination of the heart includes evaluation of the aortic root.

Echocardiography is an excellent method for this purpose as well as for evaluation of myocardial and valve function. The aortic root should also be routinely visualized during left-sided heart catheterization. Traditionally, echocardiography is not effective in evaluating the transverse aortic arch and descending thoracic aorta. Transesophageal echocardiography is a satisfactory method for evaluating the distal arch and descending thoracic aorta. Prototypes of equipment are now available in a few centers for evaluation of ascending, transverse, and descending thoracic aortic disease, and the method may be useful in the future in the evaluation of these cases.

The best screening methods for the diagnosis and localization of aortic aneurysms are computed tomography and magnetic resonance imaging. Computed tomographic scanning with contrast enhancement is preferable because of its general availability, ease of performance, safety, reproducibility, cost effectiveness, and reliability in determining aortic diameter. Magnetic resonance imaging is time-consuming, unpleasant to the patient, expensive, and not applicable to patients with support systems that cannot be subjected to the magnetic field.

Total aortography in three projections is the preferred method of examination in patients who are to be treated by operation. This method allows evaluation of the entire aorta, aortic valve function, the location and condition of branch vessels, the presence of fistulas, and sites of perforation or rupture. Approximately 15 percent of patients have branch vessel occlusive disease, which is best identified and evaluated by aortography. Patients with symptoms of coronary artery disease should have separate cardiac catheterization and selective coronary artery angiography with consideration for concurrent myocardial revascularization. Thus, minimal studies in our cases include computed tomographic scanning for diagnosis and estimation of aneurysmal size and total aortography for evaluation of valve function, branch vessel disease, and relationship of aneurysm position to brachiocephalic arterial origin.

Assessment of Associated Disease

Cardiac evaluation includes an estimate of myocardial and valve function with echocardiography and Doppler examination. These are usually augmented with 24 hour Holter monitor to detect cardiac arrhythmias. Patients with coronary artery disease are catheterized and selective coronary artery studies performed. Aortic valve replacement, coronary artery bypass, or both are performed at the time of ascending and arch replacement. Patients with ejection fractions of 30 percent are considered suitable for operation. Pulmonary function is assessed clinically, with room air arterial blood gases and spirometry testing. Patients whose pulmonary function is 50 percent of normal are suitable for operation. Renal function is determined by blood creatinine levels. Patients with substantial chronic reduction in renal function may be candidates for operation. In fact, more than 75 percent of patients receiving chronic hemodialysis survive operation. However, operation is reserved for such patients who have symptoms or large aneurysms.

Surgical Treatment

Graft replacement is the only treatment of thoracic aortic aneurysm that relieves the complication of the disease and prevents dissection and rupture. This operation is recommended in good risk asymptomatic patients in whom the aneurysm is twice the size of the uninvolved aorta (5 to 6 cm). Operation is performed in patients with limiting risks for symptoms or larger aneurysms.

Aortic Grafts

Tubular Dacron fabric grafts are employed to replace aneurysms of the thoracic aorta. All such grafts commercially available for use at this level are porous. To prevent bleeding through their interstices during operation, the graft walls are saturated with 25 percent human serum albumin solution and steam autoclaved at 132°C (270°F) for 3 minutes. Two pretreated grafts have been approved for use in humans on an experimental basis, and both are likely to be approved for general use in the near future. One is a knitted graft pretreated with human serum albumin solution, and the other is a woven graft pretreated with bovine collagen.

We prefer the St. Jude valve for separate valve graft replacement because of its flow characteristics and the St. Jude composite valve graft because of the matching relationship between graft diameter and valve size.

Techniques of Operation

The method of operation varies with the location and extent of aneurysm and is discussed accordingly.

Ascending Aorta and Transverse Aortic Arch. Cardiopulmonary bypass is employed to maintain circulation in patients during aortic cross-clamping for replacement of aneurysms of the ascending aorta and transverse arch. Myocardial protection is achieved with intermittent coronary artery perfusion with cold (5°C) hyperkalemic dilute blood solution, maintaining myocardial temperature less than 15°C. Using a heat exchanger in the extracorporeal circulation circuit, moderate hypothermia (25 to 28°C) is maintained during the period of aortic clamping for reconstruction of the ascending aorta. Profound hypothermia sufficient to produce electrocerebral silence (isoelectric electroencephalogram) is achieved for complete circulatory arrest during the period of graft replacement of the transverse aortic arch. After completion of the reconstruction, rewarming to 38°C (rectal) is accomplished by using cardiopulmonary bypass.

Aortic Reconstruction. The method and extent of graft replacement is dependent on the location and extent of aneurysm. Aneurysms that involve the tubular segment of ascending aorta (that segment extending from innominate artery to the insertion of the aortic valvular commissures) are replaced with a tube graft (Fig. 1). Associated aortic valvular disease in such cases is replaced by separate prosthetic aortic valve (Fig. 2), and patients with coronary artery disease are treated with bypass graft (Fig. 3). Aneurysms that extend down to involve the sinus segment of ascending aorta (the segment containing the coronary artery origins extending from the level of commissural attachment to the aortic valvular annulus) require replacement of both tubular and sinus segments to prevent progressive sinus enlargement and rupture into the right-sided heart chambers. The method of this operation is dependent on the distance between coronary artery origins and aortic annulus. The Wheat operation may be performed in cases in which the coronary arteries arise near the aortic annulus (< 2 cm) (Fig. 4). The aortic valve is usually replaced, and the ascending aorta is excised except for a

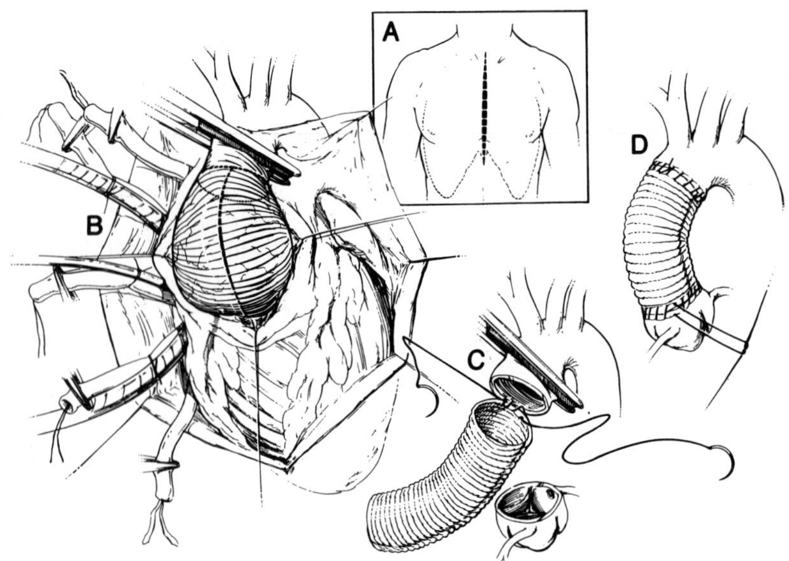

Figure 1
Graft replacement of aneurysm involving tubular segment of ascending aorta. *A,* Midsternal incision; *B,* location of aneurysm; *C,* excised aortic segment and distal anastomosis; *D,* completed reconstruction. *(Copyright 1990 by Baylor College of Medicine.)*

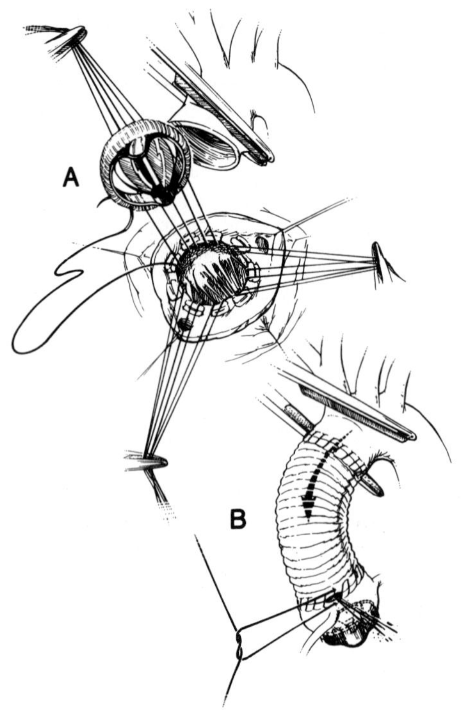

Figure 2
Separate valve-graft replacement of the ascending aorta. *A,* Tubular segment of aorta is excised and St. Jude valve being inserted. *B,* Operation is completed by graft insertion. *(Copyright 1990 by Baylor College of Medicine.)*

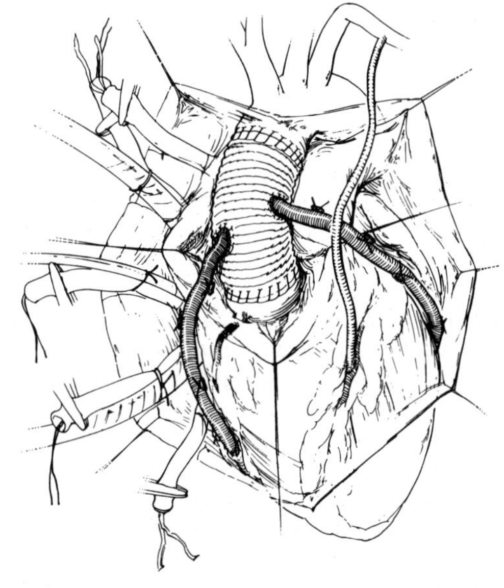

Figure 3
Position of coronary bypass grafts inserted in a patient at time of ascending aortic replacement. *(Copyright 1990 by Baylor College of Medicine.)*

tongue of aortic tissue containing the origins of the coronary arteries. The proximal end of the graft is then sutured to the aortic valve sewing ring, annulus, or residual aorta except at the tongue of aortic tissue containing the coronary arteries. The end of the graft is sutured to the aorta distal to the coronary arteries at these sites. The operation is then completed as previously described.

The other method for replacing aneurysms that involve both the sinus and tubular segments of ascending aorta is replacement of aortic valve and ascending aorta with a composite valve graft. The aortic leaflets are removed, and the valve end of the graft is attached to the aortic annulus by interrupted sutures (Figs. 5 and 6). The other end of the graft is sutured end-to-end to the distal transected uninvolved aorta. Coronary artery circulation may be restored by insertion of separate coronary artery bypass grafts (see Fig. 3), by direct

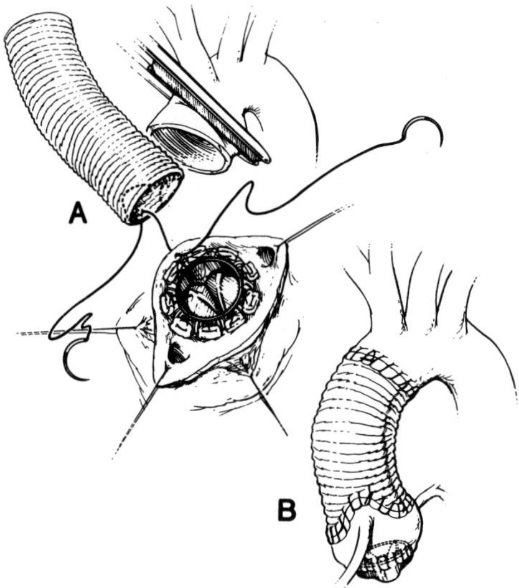

Figure 4
Separate valve-graft replacement of the aortic valve and ascending aorta after removal of most of the aorta except that from which the coronary arteries arise in a patient with sinus segment involvement and coronary artery origins located near the aortic annulus. *(Copyright 1990 by Baylor College of Medicine.)*

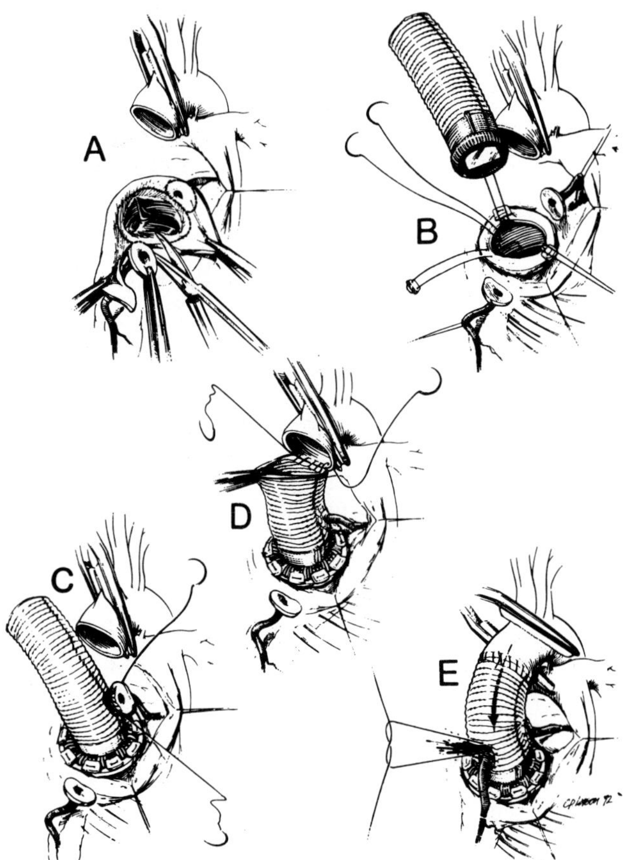

Figure 5
The steps of composite valve-graft replacement of the aortic valve and ascending aorta in which the coronary arteries are attached directly to openings made in the graft by using buttons of aortic wall. *(Copyright 1992 by Baylor College of Medicine.)*

reattachment of coronary origins to openings made in the graft (see Fig. 5), by use of a smaller Dacron tube graft (see Fig. 6), or by reattaching a button of aorta from which the coronary arteries arise directly to openings made in the graft. The ascending aorta is completely excised in the latter operation except for buttons from which the coronary arteries arise. The coronary arteries are mobilized to their first branch to obtain length and then reattached. Although we use all these methods in the replacement of diffuse aneurysms, we prefer the radical excision and separate graft replacement in patients with low-lying coronary ostia. In patients with pronounced sinus segment involvement, composite valve-graft replacement with the coronary arteries mobilized around buttons of aortic wall for reattachment without tension is utilized to avoid both operative bleeding and postoperative false aneurysm formation. Coronary artery reattachment using a smaller transversely placed Dacron tube is used in patients undergoing reoperation or composite replacement for aneurysms of extremely large diameter, where mobilization of the coronary arteries is both unsafe and time-consuming. The incidence and results of the various methods of ascending aortic reconstruction in our patients with nondissection aneurysms of the ascending aorta and transverse aortic arch are shown in Table 1.

Aortic Arch. With circulation arrested, the aneurysm is opened and the aorta transected proximally and distally and frequently excised except for an island from which the brachiocephalic vessels arise (Fig. 7). One end of the aortic graft is attached to the uninvolved distal end of the aorta. An opening is made in the side of the graft opposite the origins of the brachiocephalic vessels, and the island of aortic tissue from which the brachiocephalic vessels arise is attached to the graft. Cardiopulmonary bypass is restarted and air removed from the aorta and graft. The graft is cross-clamped proximal to the innominate artery and full bypass and rewarming begun. About two-thirds of patients with arch aneurysms have involvement of the ascending aorta (Table 1), and this segment is then reconstructed according to the principles outlined previously for ascending aortic aneurysms to complete the operation.

One-third of patients with aneurysm of the aortic arch have *diffuse aneurysms that also involve the descending thoracic aorta* or *descending thoracic aorta and abdominal aorta.* Operation is staged in these cases with the ascending aorta and arch being replaced first in most cases; the distal aneurysm is then replaced at a second operation 6 to 8 weeks later, provided the patient remains asymptomatic. The ascending aorta and arch are replaced as described previously except that a segment of free graft is left extending into the distal aneurysm to attach the proximal end of the second graft at the second operation (Fig. 8). The free end of graft is easily exposed inside the aneurysm and does not require the tedious exposure needed using conventional techniques (Fig. 8*F*).

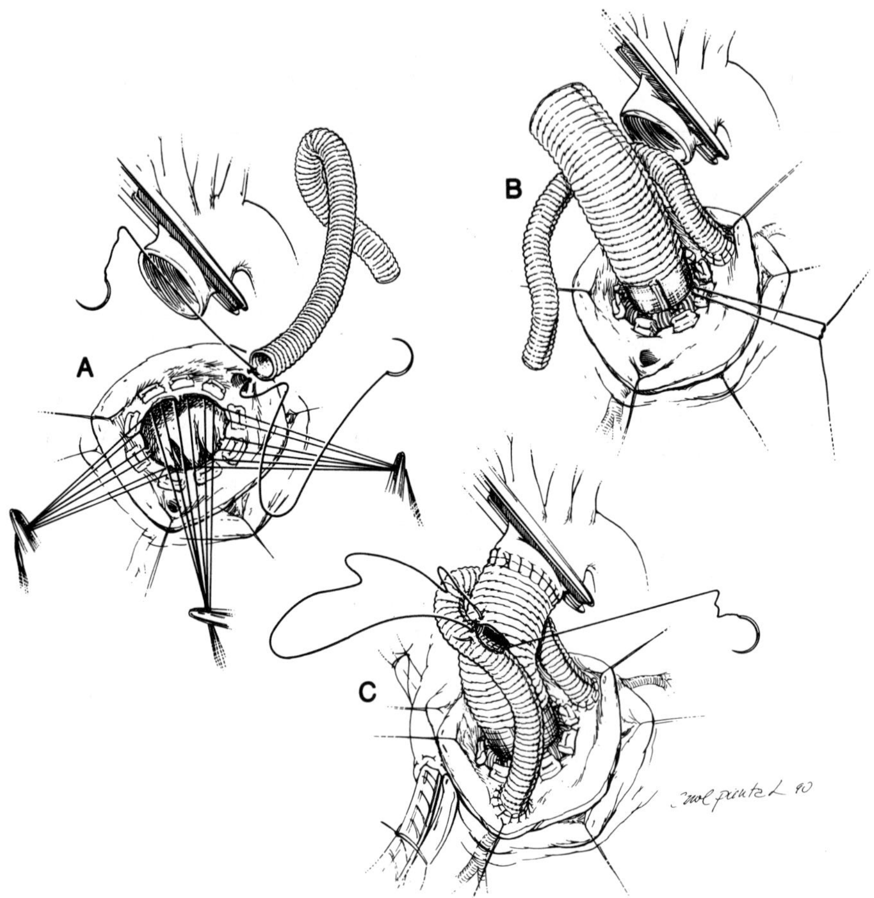

Figure 6
The steps of composite valve-graft replacement showing attachment of coronary arteries using a smaller (10 cm) Dacron tube graft. *(Copyright 1990 by Baylor College of Medicine.)*

Table 1 Survival for Nondissecting Ascending and/or Arch Aneurysms

METHOD	ASCENDING AORTA		AORTIC ARCH		ASCENDING AND ARCH	
	NO. PATIENTS	30 DAYS (%)	NO. PATIENTS	30 DAYS (%)	NO. PATIENTS	30 DAYS (%)
CVG	177	166 (93.8)	0	—	38	35 (92.1)
SVR	74	65 (87.8)	0	—	121	115 (95)
GFT	23	20 (87)	62	57 (91.9)	122	116 (95.1)
Other	21	17 (81)	66	59 (89.4)	5	5 (100)
Total	295	268 (90.8)	128	116 (90.6)	286	271 (94.8)

CVG, composite valve graft; SVR, separate aortic valve replacement; GFT, tube graft replacement.

Descending Thoracic and Thoracoabdominal Aortic Aneurysm. Although varying aortic lengths may be involved in each entity, aneurysms of the descending thoracic aorta are confined to the chest, and thoracoabdominal aortic aneurysms involve both descending thoracic aorta and abdominal aorta. Both types of aneurysms require left posterolateral thoracic chest wall incisions for exposure (Figs. 9 and 10). Exposure of thoracoabdominal aneurysms requires extension of the incision into the abdomen made by crossing the costal arch and extending downward in the midline of the abdomen. The abdominal aorta, in the latter cases, is exposed retroperitoneally first by mobilizing the peritoneum from diaphragm and abdominal wall, cutting the diaphragm, and displacing the viscera upward and to the right.

The aorta is clamped proximally and distally. To prevent heart strain with aortic clamping, proximal blood pressure is controlled with pharmacologic agents in the usual case and by temporary left atrial–left common femoral artery centrifugal pump bypass in patients with heart disease. The latter does not require the use of heparin. With the aorta clamped, the aneurysm is opened (Fig. 9*B*), the contained blood retrieved by cell saver, and the upper intercostal arteries are ligated at their origins. The aorta is transected proximally and separated from the esophagus. The proximal anastomosis is made by

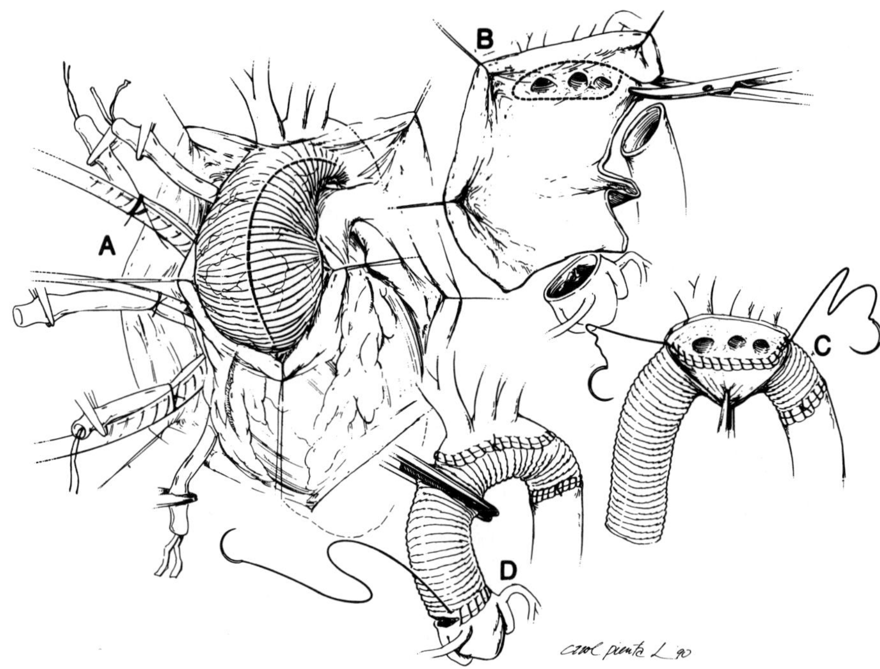

Figure 7
The common method of graft replacement of the ascending aorta and transverse aortic arch for aneurysm. *A,* The aneurysm is incised longitudinally and *(B)* excised except for a button containing the origins of the brachiocephalic arteries. *C,* The distal end of graft is inserted by end-to-end anastomosis, and the button containing the brachiocephalic vessels is attached to an opening made in the graft. *D,* The reconstruction completed by proximal anastomosis. *(Copyright 1990 by Baylor College of Medicine.)*

continuous suture, avoiding the esophagus and recurrent laryngeal nerve (Fig. 9*C*). A similar type of exposure and distal anastomosis is made in the chest in patients with aneurysm limited to the descending thoracic aorta (Fig. 9*D*). The abdominal segment of aneurysm is opened behind the left renal artery in patients with thoracoabdominal aortic aneurysms (Fig. 10*C*). An opening made in the side of the graft is sutured around the origins of the lower intercostal and upper lumbar arteries to preserve spinal cord blood supply (Fig. 10*D*). Intercostal and lumbar arteries in the region of T8 to L2, particularly those that are prominent and poorly back bleeding, are considered most important. Another opening is made in the side of the graft and sutured around the origins of the celiac axis and superior mesenteric and right renal arteries (Fig. 10*D, E*). The distal end of the graft is sutured to the uninvolved distal aorta. The origin of the left renal artery is mobilized from the aneurysm and adjacent tissues, while saving a button of aorta (Fig. 10*D*). The artery is then reattached by suturing the aortic button to a third opening made in the graft (Fig. 10*E*). In both types of cases, air is removed from the graft to prevent cerebral embolization. This is accomplished by slowly removing the clamp in the head-down position prior to completing the last anastomosis and by aspirating the uppermost segment of graft with needle and syringe.

■ RESULTS

The results of operation according to aortic segment replaced in 2,466 cases treated since January 1, 1980, are shown in Table 2. The 30 day survival varied from 90 to 95 percent, depending on segment replaced. Survival at 1 year varied from 76 to 86 percent and at 5 years, 60 to 69 percent. The causes of both early and late death were heart, lung, stroke, kidney disease, and rupture of other aneurysms, listed in order of frequency. These results are deemed very satisfactory, considering the condition of patients at time of operation, including the fact that the median age of all patients was 64 years.

The most disabling complication that occurred in patients with distal aortic reconstruction (descending thoracic aorta and thoracoabdominal aorta) was neurologic disturbances in the lower extremities. This complication varied with extent of operation and varied from 5 percent in patients with descending thoracic aortic reconstruction to 10 percent in those with thoracoabdominal aortic operation. The deficit was mild to moderate in half of these cases and permanently crippling in the other half.

An additional severe complication postoperatively is the development of renal failure, necessitating temporary or permanent hemodialysis. Important preoperative variables predictive of renal insufficiency include age, gender, rupture, renal artery occlusive disease, history of hypertension, coronary artery disease, and, importantly, preoperative renal dysfunction. Intraoperative variables affecting postoperative renal dysfunction include aortic clamp time and specifically renal artery ischemic time.

We previously evaluated cold lactated Ringer's solution as a perfusion of the renal arteries during the ischemic period required for resection and replacement of thoracoabdominal aortic aneurysms and were unable to show any significant benefit to patients with normal renal function and brief

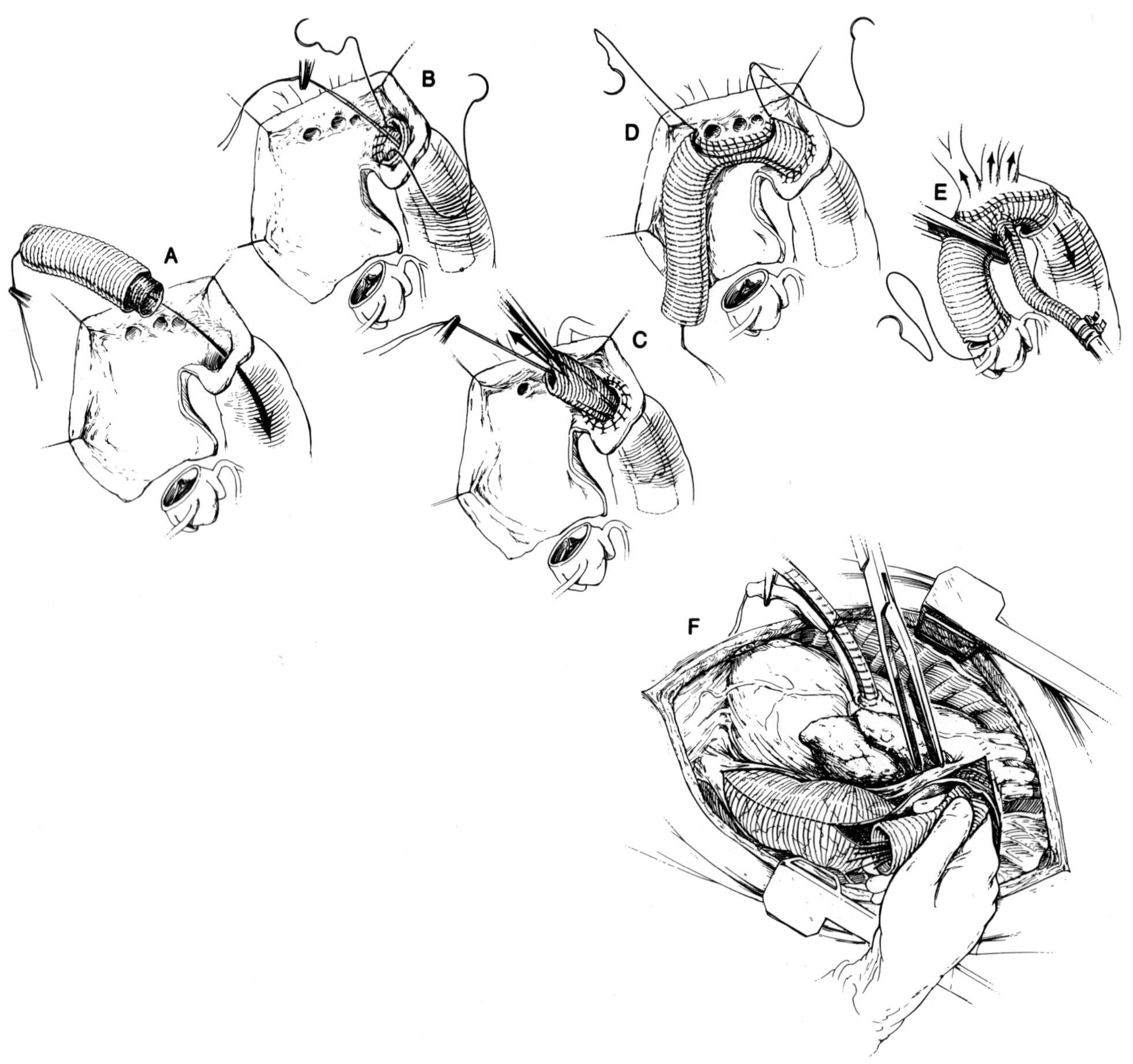

Figure 8
Elephant trunk technique, leaving a free segment of graft extending down into residual aneurysm to facilitate later graft replacement of the segment. *A,* An invaginated graft is inserted into the descending thoracic aortic aneurysm, and *B,* the proximal end of this graft is sutured circumferentially to the aorta distal to the origin of the left subclavian artery. *C,* The invaginated segment of graft is withdrawn, and *D,* an opening in the graft is sutured around the origins of the brachiocephalic arteries. *E,* Antegrade circulation to prevent cerebral emboli from the distal aorta is restored by changing femoral bypass perfusion to arch perfusion, using a separate arterial perfusion line through a small graft. *F,* The free end of the graft is exposed for operations shown in Figures 9 and 10 by making a small proximal incision in the aneurysm, inserting a finger, controlling graft flow, extending aneurysm incision, and clamping graft. *(Copyright 1990 by Baylor College of Medicine.)*

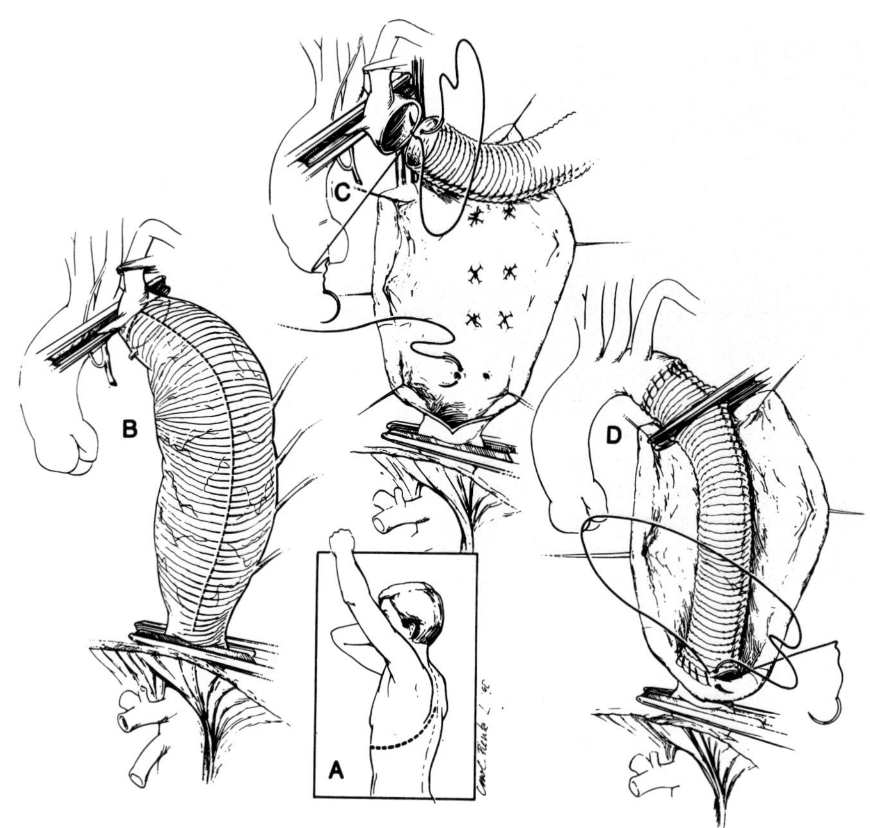

Figure 9
Graft replacement of aneurysm involving the descending thoracic aorta. For details, see text. *(Copyright 1990 by Baylor College of Medicine.)*

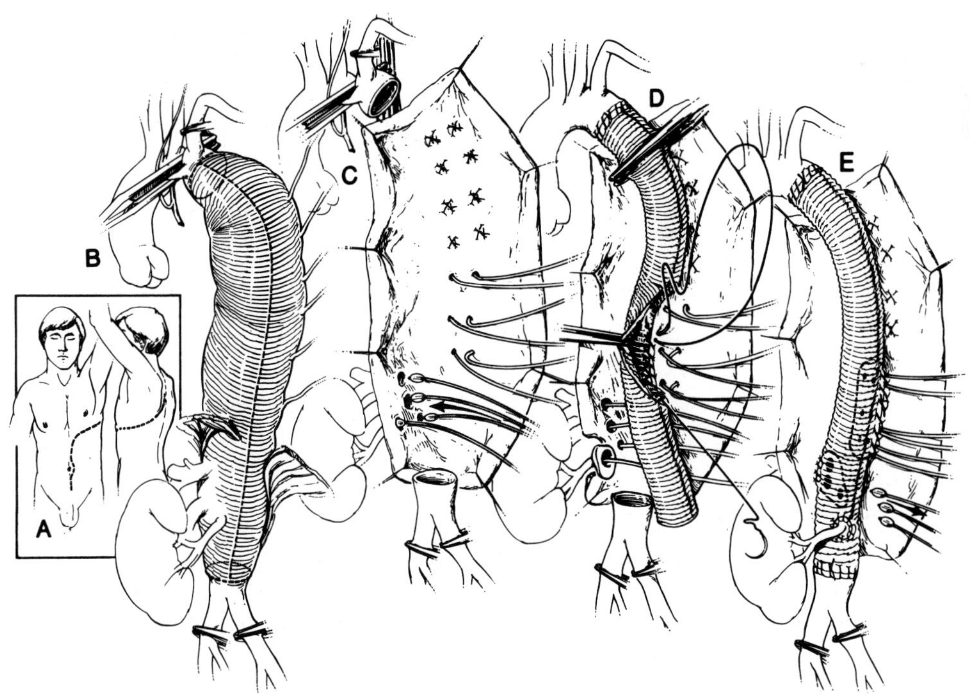

Figure 10
The author's technique for graft replacement of thoracoabdominal aortic aneurysms. For details, see text. *(Copyright 1990 by Baylor College of Medicine.)*

Table 2 Survival of Nondissectors by Aortic Segment Treated

	NO. OF PATIENTS	SURVIVAL		
		30 DAYS (%)	1 YEAR (%)	5 YEAR (%)
Ascending	295	268 (90.8)	82.1	71.6
Arch	128	116 (90.6)	80.7	68.2
Ascending and Arch	286	271 (94.8)	77.7	59.3
Descending	524	501 (95.6)	83.7	61.9
Thoracoabdominal	1,233	1,169 (94.8)	79.9	61.8
Total	2,466	2,325 (94.3)		

periods of ischemia. However, in patients with preoperative renal dysfunction and in those requiring renal ischemic periods exceeding 1 hour, there is a trend toward improved renal function with the use of either cold renal perfusion or cardiofemoral bypass. Postoperative renal failure appears to be best averted by optimization of preoperative and postoperative hemodynamic status and cardiovascular function.

This experience emphasizes that patients with aneurysmal disease of the aorta often have diffuse involvement. A total aortic evaluation allows logical planning of both the initial aortic procedure as well as postoperative surveillance with noninvasive computed tomographic scanning, magnetic resonance imaging scanning, and transesophageal echocardiography for remaining aortic segments. Long-term survival of patients with aortic aneurysmal disease is enhanced by both lifelong surveillance and an aggressive surgical approach to treatment.

Suggested Reading

Bentall H, DeBono A. A technique for complete replacement of the ascending aorta. Thorax 1968; 23:338.

Borst HG, Frank G, Schaps D. Treatment of extensive aortic aneurysms by a new multiple-stage approach. J Thorac Cardiovasc Surg 1988; 95:11.

Cabrol C, Pavie A, Mesnildrey P, et al. Long-term results with total replacement of the ascending aorta and reimplantation of the coronary arteries. J Thorac Cardiovasc Surg 1986; 91:17.

Coselli JS. Suprarenal aortic reconstruction: Endovascular repair. Semin Vasc Surg 1992; 5:180–191.

Coselli JS. Suprarenal aortic reconstruction: Perioperative management: Patient selection, patient workup, operative management, and postoperative management. Semin Vasc Surg 1992; 5:146–156.

Coselli JS, Crawford ES. Composite valve graft replacement of aortic root using separate Dacron tube for coronary artery reattachment. Ann Thorac Surg 1989; 47:558–565.

Coselli JS, Crawford ES. Thoracoabdominal aortic aneurysms. In: Yao JST, Pearce WH, eds. Vascular surgery: Long-term results, Norwalk, CT: Appleton & Lange, 1993:135.

Crawford ES, Coselli JS, Svensson LG, et al. Diffuse aneurysmal disease (chronic aortic dissection, Marfan and mega aorta syndromes) and multiple aneurysm: Treatment by subtotal and total aortic replacement emphasizing the elephant trunk technique. Ann Surg 1990; 211:521–537.

Crawford ES, Crawford JL, Safi HJ, et al. Thoracoabdominal aortic aneurysms: Preoperative and intraoperative factors determining immediate and long-term results of operation in 605 patients. J Vasc Surg 1986; 3:389.

Crawford ES, DeNatale RW. Thoracoabdominal aortic aneurysm: Observations regarding the natural course of the disease. J Vasc Surg 1986; 3:578.

Crawford ES, Hess KR, Cohen ES, et al. Ruptured aneurysm of the descending thoracic and thoracoabdominal aorta: Analysis according to size and treatment. Ann Surg 1991; 213:417–426.

Crawford ES, Saleh SA. Transverse aortic arch aneurysm: Improved results of treatment employing new modifications of aortic reconstruction and hypothermia cerebral circulatory arrest. Ann Surg 1981; 194:180.

Crawford ES, Svensson LG, Coselli JS, et al. Surgical treatment aneurysm and/or dissection of the ascending aorta, transverse aortic arch, and ascending aorta and transverse aortic arch: Factors influencing survival in 717 patients. J Thorac Cardiovasc Surg 1989; 98:659.

Maughan RE, Mohan C, Nathan IR, et al. Intrathecal perfusion of an oxygenated perfluorocarbon prevents paraplegia after aortic occlusion. Ann Thorac Surg 1992; 54:818–825.

Svensson LG, Coselli JS, Safi HJ, et al. Appraisal of adjuncts to prevent acute renal failure after surgery on the thoracic or thoracoabdominal aorta. J Vasc Surg 1989; 10:230–239.

Svensson LG, Crawford ES, Hess KR, et al. Dissection of the aorta and dissecting aortic aneurysm: Improving early and long-term surgical results. Circulation 1990; 82:IV-24–IV-38.

Wheat MN Jr, Wilson JR, Bartley TD. Successful replacement of the entire aorta and aortic valve. JAMA 1964; 188:717.

AORTIC ANEURYSM: ABDOMINAL

Thomas A. Cochran, M.D.
Robert B. Holtzman, M.D.
Arthur C. Beall Jr., M.D.

Within the last decade, research has established that the multifactorial pathogenesis of abdominal aortic aneurysms (AAAs) involves alterations in connective tissue metabolism. Histologic studies of AAA walls using immunophenotyping staining of discrete populations of inflammatory cells have identified macrophage infiltrates in the adventitia and media of the aneurysm wall. Normal aortic tissue has few inflammatory cells present. When occlusive disease of the aorta is compared to AAAs, macrophage density scores are higher in the AAA group, with inflammatory AAAs demonstrating the greatest number of macrophages infiltrating the aortic wall. Destruction of the aortic media with a corresponding loss of aortic wall elastin is a dominant histologic feature of AAAs, reflecting an abnormal balance between proteolytic and antiproteolytic activity. This homeostatic balance is influenced by genetic factors, by environmental stimuli, and by the activity of inflammatory cytokines, which are macrophage products, in the aneurysm wall. There is evidence for increased activity of interleukin-1-beta in the wall of AAAs, and this cytokine increases proteolytic activity. Patients with AAAs have an increase in cellular elastase, possibly produced by local vascular smooth muscle cells. A deficiency in the inhibition of proteolysis also is implicated. Studies have documented a deficiency in TIMP, a metalloproteinase inhibitor, in the walls of AAAs. A deficiency of alpha-1-antitrypsin activity, the major serum elastase inhibitor, also is described. Several genetic abnormalities associated with AAAs are known, including a polymorphism of the haptoglobin gene on the long arm of chromosome 16.

There is an increased prevalence of AAAs in male first-degree relatives of patients with AAAs. A familial AAA syndrome exists and accounts for approximately 15 percent of patients with AAAs. Familial AAAs are characterized by an increased percentage of women. These females are markers for an increased risk of AAAs and ruptured AAAs among male and female blood relatives of the patient. Research initiatives over the next decade will define more precisely the molecular events associated with the development of AAAs, as well as the populations at particular risk because of inherited factors.

■ PREFERRED APPROACH

Selection of Patients

Traditionally, the presence of an AAA is justification for operative repair because the natural history of more than 80 percent of AAAs is to enlarge over time, and large AAAs pose a significant risk of rupture. A report of the Joint Council of the Society for Vascular Surgery and the North American Chapter of the International Society for Cardiovascular Surgery (Hollier and co-workers, 1992) concluded that operative repair is justified for most small (4 to 5 cm) AAAs in good-risk patients because small AAAs do have a finite risk of rupture, and the general medical condition of the patient, which influences operative mortality, does not commonly remain stable with time. For patients with small AAAs and coexisting coronary artery disease, chronic obstructive pulmonary disease (COPD), or renal insufficiency, there is a gradient of influence on operative morbidity and mortality rates, depending on the severity of associated comorbid disease. The surgeon must use appropriate judgment in weighing these associated risk factors when recommending operative repair of a small AAA.

Age

The age of a patient as a solitary variable is not a contraindication to surgical treatment of an AAA. The evidence indicates that elderly patients do have a modest increase in operative risk for elective aneurysm repair. However, the contribution of associated coronary artery disease (CAD) or the presence of pulmonary and renal dysfunction, as well as the components of the surgical procedure to this increased risk, is greater than that of the patient's chronologic age. Data from the Cleveland Vascular Society Registry (Plecha and co-workers, 1987) compared mortality rates for elective AAA repair between patients younger than age 75 versus patients 75 years or older. In the younger group, the mortality was 5.6 percent; in the older group, the mortality was 11.3 percent. In a previous study involving the careful preoperative selection of octogenarians for elective AAA repair, O'Donnell and co-workers (1976) achieved a mortality rate of only 4.7 percent. Elderly patients with large AAAs should undergo elective AAA repair unless the patient has a coexisting terminal malignancy with a short anticipated survival.

High-risk Patients with Small Aneurysms

On occasion, the surgeon is confronted with a patient harboring both a small AAA and such severe associated organ system dysfunction that the operative risk of AAA repair is estimated as greater than the anticipated risk of AAA rupture. In such a circumstance, a selective rather than obligatory approach to AAA repair is indicated. Bernstein and Chan (1984) demonstrated that the prospective application of clinical selection criteria to manage a group of high-risk patients with small AAAs resulted in a low operative mortality rate and a low rate of subsequent AAA rupture. Among patients denied operation, most of the subsequent deaths were due to the progression of comorbid disease. In this approach, high-risk patients with comorbid medical conditions refractory to improvement and AAAs smaller than 6 cm in maximum transverse diameter are followed by serial computed tomographic (CT) imaging at 3 month intervals. High-risk patients include those with recent myocardial infarction, intractable congestive heart failure, dyspnea at rest, dense residual neurologic deficit from stroke, severe renal insufficiency, and terminal malignancy with an anticipated survival of less than 2 years. Rapid expansion of the AAA and/or enlargement to 6 cm in maximum transverse diameter are indications for AAA repair. CT scans are considered superior to ultrasound in characterizing aortic pathology, such as thrombus-lumen ratio, the presence of an inflammatory aneurysm, or the presence of suprarenal extension. This protocol was used to follow a series of high-risk patients with small AAAs, 41 percent of whom eventually required operative repair, with an operative mortality of 4.9 percent, whereas 34 percent of patients died of disease other than the AAA. There was a 3 percent incidence of AAA rupture. This selective operative management of high-risk patients with small AAAs results in a 5 year survival by life table analysis that approaches that of low-risk patients undergoing elective AAA repair.

Selective Operative Management of Small AAAs

For patients with small AAAs, less than 5 cm in maximum transverse diameter, the surgical approach in the United States is operative repair, because small aneurysms have a small but finite risk of rupture. In Europe and Canada, however, a more selective operative approach is popular. Recent data from Scandinavia (Johansson and co-workers, 1991) maintains that small AAAs (< 5 cm) have a risk of rupture so low that the cumulative risk imposed by AAA repair in a population of patients with small AAAs exceeds the risk of careful medical surveillance and serial CT imaging, with operation reserved for AAAs with expansion to 5 cm diameter or greater. In addition, Nevitt and co-workers (1989), in a population-based study, stated that only AAAs 5 cm or larger rupture. However, a critical review of the data indicates that approximately one-quarter of these patients with small AAAs underwent operative repair of AAAs <5 cm maximum transverse diameter. Because there exist predictors of small aneurysm rupture other than size (Cronenwett and co-workers, 1985), this policy introduces a possible selection bias in interpreting the data. In the Canadian study, Brown and co-workers (1992) reported the prospective follow-up of 268 patients with AAAs less than 5 cm in maximum diameter. As the study evolved, follow-up examination was performed using serial CT imaging. Indications for surgery included expansion to 5 cm, a rapid increase in AAA diameter of greater than 0.5 cm within 6 months, development of coexisting symptomatic aortoiliac occlusive disease, peripheral embolism, or development of a symptomatic AAA. High-risk patients with small AAAs that increased to larger than 5 cm were managed using the selective criteria of Bernstein and Chan (1984). The patients were followed for a mean of 42 months. AAAs less than 4 cm at entry demonstrated a mean expansion rate of 0.36 cm per year; AAAs greater than or equal to 4 cm at entry demonstrated a mean expansion of 0.66 cm per year. For those with an AAA 4 cm or greater at entry, 60 percent ultimately required surgery. Overall, 114 patients eventually underwent AAA repair, with two operative deaths. In the nonoperative group with a mean follow-up of 39 months, 39 of 154 patients died. However, only one patient died of a ruptured AAA (which occurred in a severely demented patient with Alzheimer's disease who had a 7.5 cm AAA).

For the patient with an AAA measuring 4 to 4.9 cm, operation is recommended for those under age 55, with low surgical risk, evidence of rapid AAA expansion, a family history of AAA, aneurysm-related complications, or CT predictors of early AAA rupture (Brown and co-workers, 1992; Hunter and co-workers, 1989). Currently there are three prospective randomized studies that will define more accurately the natural history and ideal operative management of these small AAAs.

Medical Correlates of AAA Rupture

Cronenwett and co-workers (1990) reviewed 73 patients with small AAAs managed nonoperatively over a mean of 37 months with serial ultrasound examinations. Mean initial AAA diameter was 4 cm. Operation was recommended when the aneurysm size was 5 cm. In a previous report, Cronenwett and co-workers (1985) identified three clinical variables that correlated with eventual rupture of small AAAs followed nonoperatively: COPD, hypertension, and large initial AAA size. During the 3 years of patient follow-up, only one patient suffered AAA rupture (1.3 percent); 36 percent of patients died of diseases other than the AAA, and 36 percent of patients ultimately required operative repair of the AAA due to increasing AAA size of at least 5 cm, with an operative mortality of 4 percent. There was a linear increase in the need for operation of 10 percent per year in patients with small AAAs managed nonoperatively. Advanced age at the time of presentation decreased the likelihood of eventual need for operation; large initial AAA size increased the likelihood of eventual need for operation. Higher pulse pressure was associated with rapid aneurysm expansion. Although COPD correlated with aneurysm rupture in the earlier study, it was not associated with small AAA expansion, nor did small AAA expansion correlate with initial AAA size. Statistically unconfirmed trends indicated that patients with small AAAs taking oral propranolol therapy had lower AAA expansion rates. Cronenwett and co-workers conclude that serial aortic ultrasound exams conducted at 6 month intervals in patients with small AAAs are safe, with operation considered for AAAs that become symptomatic, expand to at least 5 cm in good-risk patients, or reach 6 cm in high-risk patients. In addition, a small number of carefully selected younger patients with AAAs in the 4 to 4.9 cm range may be considered for elective AAA repair, particularly if correlates of AAA rupture are present.

In a review from the Karolinska Institute, Johansson and co-workers (1991) reported the management of 213 patients with AAAs. Those patients with AAA of 5 cm or larger underwent operative repair, unless repair was contraindicated by the presence of debilitating comorbid disease. Patients with AAAs smaller than 5 cm were followed nonoperatively with serial CT imaging. Future operation was reserved for those patients with enlarging AAAs. Of the 42 patients with small AAAs managed nonoperatively, 22 (52 percent) died during a mean follow-up period of 5 years, but only three patients died of AAA rupture. All three patients who died of AAA rupture had AAAs exceeding 5 cm in diameter at the time of rupture. Among the 134 patients who underwent AAA repair, the 30 day operative mortality rate was 7.5 percent, mostly due to associated cardiac disease. Late complications of the operation, including aortic graft infection, boosted the eventual mortality to 13.5 percent. Of the 37 patients with AAAs of 5 cm or larger who did not undergo operation, 17 died of AAA rupture, and 15 died of other comorbid disease. Based on this experience, Johansson and co-workers (1991) recommend

AAA repair for AAAs that are 5 cm in diameter or larger. Nonoperative medical management and serial CT imaging is recommended for AAAs smaller than 5 cm, in which the risk imposed by surgery exceeds the risk of rupture.

In spite of this experience, many centers in the United States report that the 30 day operative mortality rate for elective AAA repair has fallen over several decades, and in some centers averages 1 to 2 percent. In part the operative risk has fallen because of selective screening of CAD in AAA patients to identify the less than 10 percent of patients who will require preliminary coronary bypass (CAB) or transluminal coronary angioplasty (TLCA) prior to elective AAA repair. Preoperative volume loading and the routine use of Swan-Ganz catheterization to optimize intraoperative and postoperative cardiac hemodynamics also contribute to the reduction in operative mortality rate with time for patients undergoing elective AAA repair (Whittemore and co-workers, 1980). Given this more favorable outlook, more aggressive surgical intervention in otherwise healthy patients with small AAAs is justified.

Importance of Selective Screening for Coronary Artery Disease

The majority of perioperative and late deaths following AAA repair are due to myocardial infarction. Several studies have documented that prior CAB exerts a protective effect on the incidence of perioperative MI following peripheral vascular operations. Data from the Cleveland Clinic (Hertzer and co-workers, 1984), where a large number of patients with peripheral vascular disease underwent preoperative cardiac catheterization, reveal that 63 percent of patients with no antecedent history of symptomatic CAD, who had no electrocardiographic (ECG) changes suggestive of prior myocardial infarction, had normal or minimally diseased coronary arteries. Among the remaining patients, 22 percent had advanced coronary lesions with good compensatory collateral, 14 percent had severe, surgically correctable CAD, and 1 percent had severe, inoperable CAD. Among patients with either a positive history of CAD or ECG evidence of the same, 34 percent had advanced coronary lesions with good compensatory collateral, 34 percent had severe, surgically correctable CAD, and 10 percent had severe, inoperable CAD.

Therefore, one of the challenges in managing patients with AAAs is the preoperative identification and operative correction of severe CAD to lessen the perioperative risk of subsequent AAA repair. Although the Cleveland Clinic data demonstrate that a significant percentage of patients with no clinical or ECG evidence of CAD have significant clinically occult CAD, data from Brigham and Women's Hospital (Golden and co-workers, 1990) and other centers establish that this subset of patients undergoing elective AAA repair is not at high risk for perioperative myocardial infarction in spite of the certainty of some patients harboring significant subclinical CAD. Also, the routine use of CAB prior to elective AAA repair is tempered by the Coronary Artery Surgery Study (Gersh and co-workers, 1983), which demonstrated that perioperative mortality for patients undergoing CAB who were 65 years or older was 5.2 percent. The perioperative mortality for elective CAB in patients age 75 or older was 9.5 percent. Among patients younger than age 65, the perioperative mortality was 1.9 percent.

The evidence is clear that patients with AAAs need to be stratified by clinical criteria into cardiac risk groups that are selectively investigated depending on the probability of an adverse postoperative cardiac event. One screening approach is to refer all patients with AAAs and clinical or ECG evidence of CAD for coronary angiography. Those patients without clinical signs or ECG evidence consistent with CAD undergo noninvasive screening to detect clinically occult CAD. Patients with noninvasive data indicating significant CAD undergo coronary angiography. Noninvasive testing includes stress electrocardiography, radionuclide myocardial scanning, dobutamine stress echocardiography (DSE), and dipyridamole thallium imaging (DTI).

The mortality of CAB varies with the age of the patient, medical center experience, and indications for surgery. At the Mayo Clinic (Reigel and co-workers, 1987), the late survival of patients in their 70s and 80s who underwent AAA repair was studied, using a policy of selective myocardial revascularization based on disabling anginal symptoms, left main CAD, or severe three-vessel CAD with evidence of functional impairment. Patients were screened with multigated acquisition (MUGA) radionuclide scans with technetium-99m labeled red blood cells. Those elderly patients without evidence of CAD had a survival after AAA repair at 5 years that exceeded a matched control population. Those elderly patients with either surgically corrected CAD or uncorrected CAD had a survival curve as good as the control population. Given the high mortality of CAB in the elderly and the favorable 5 year survival of AAA patients undergoing elective AAA repair in spite of CAD, selective preoperative screening for severe CAD is a safe policy. Preliminary CAB prior to AAA repair in the elderly should be undertaken only in those patients with significant, symptomatic CAD identified by noninvasive screening and subsequent coronary angiography.

The management of elderly patients in the seventh and eighth decades with an AAA and moderately severe CAD requires careful surgical judgment. One must balance the known increased incidence of CAD in the elderly, the increase in mortality from CAB in the elderly, the magnitude of the aneurysm operation, the documented extent of CAD, and the knowledge that careful preoperative patient selection for AAA repair, based on clinical criteria, has achieved a satisfactory mortality rate in elderly patients (O'Donnell and co-workers, 1976). Although clinical risk factor analysis alone is not a highly sensitive means of predicting adverse perioperative cardiac events following elective AAA repair, the combination of clinical risk factors, details of aortic surgery, and noninvasive studies increases the accuracy of risk stratification.

Dipyridamole Thallium Imaging. An alternative screening approach that emphasizes clinical criteria to delimit the population of AAA patients at risk for a perioperative myocardial infarction is as follows: patients scheduled to undergo elective AAA repair are referred for perioperative DTI on a selective basis, dependent on the presence of clinical signs predictive of perioperative cardiac events. These signs have been validated by multivariate logistic regression analysis (Eagle and co-workers, 1989) and include age 70 or older, diabetes mellitus, Q waves on ECG, history of angina, or ventricular arrhythmias requiring treatment. Patients with a fixed single zone of low myocardial perfusion on DTI undergo AAA repair without preoperative coronary angiography. However, the demonstration of multiple zones of radionuclide redistribution on DTI is an indication for preoperative coronary angiography and possible CAB or TLCA. The severity and extent of thallium-201 redistribution correlates with perioperative cardiac risk. Using this selective approach to preoperative testing, Cambria and co-workers (1992) performed 202 consecutive elective aortic operations (including 151 AAA repairs) and demonstrated an overall mortality of 2 percent, with a major cardiac complication rate of 4 percent. Certain clinical criteria are independent predictors of perioperative myocardial ischemic events and select those patients requiring preoperative DTI. Such a selective policy results in only 29 percent of patients requiring DTI. Of those patients undergoing DTI, 45 percent exhibited redistribution and were considered for cardiac catheterization. All patients who underwent cardiac catheterization due to redistribution of flow identified on DTI had significant CAD. The majority of these underwent either CAB or TLCA prior to aortic reconstruction, without subsequent major morbidity. Preoperative CAB was required in only 9 percent of patients. The selective use of DTI screening increases the accuracy of risk stratification among patients with CAD and decreases the postoperative cardiac morbidity.

One argument against the nonselective use of DTI screening in all patients scheduled for elective AAA repair is the documented low perioperative mortality (≤2 percent) that occurs with the selective application of DTI in the preoperative evaluation of AAA patients. Some surgeons believe that the specificity of DTI is too low to permit its use as an obligatory screening tool and that it would lead to unnecessary invasive coronary interventions (coronary angiography, CAB, or angioplasty), with aggregate morbidity and mortality that exceed those of AAA repair alone. Using clinical predictors of perioperative cardiac ischemic events as an indication to perform preoperative DTI increases the positive predictive value of the test (Eagle and co-workers, 1989).

Surgical factors also influence the perioperative cardiac morbidity following elective AAA repair. In the data presented by Cambria and co-workers (1992), statistically significant univariate predictors of major cardiac complications include prolonged operative time (> 5 hours) ($p < .006$), and detection of intraoperative myocardial ischemia ($p < .03$). In this study, no single clinical sign of CAD was statistically significant in predicting major postoperative cardiac morbidity following aortic reconstruction.

McEnroe and co-workers (1990) studied 95 elective AAA repairs and found that DTI was a more specific test in predicting the absence of postoperative cardiac morbidity than either Goldman risk factor analysis or estimation of left ventricular ejection fraction by radionuclide angiocardiography. In contrast to other studies, patients exhibiting a fixed myocardial defect on DTI had surprisingly high postoperative cardiac morbidity (47 percent). More sensitive imaging methods, such as positron emission tomography or single photon emission computed tomography, have identified viable myocardium at risk for perioperative infarction as an area of late reversibility on thallium scintigraphy. Fixed thallium-201 defects should be evaluated by delayed imaging to assess their significance. Data suggest that the Goldman risk factor analysis underestimates perioperative cardiac risk at the time of elective aortic surgery (Jeffrey and co-workers, 1983).

Golden and co-workers (1990) reported on the selective cardiac evaluation of patients undergoing AAA repair at Brigham and Women's Hospital. Prospectively, 500 consecutive patients were stratified into one of three clinical groups based on preoperative evidence of CAD, over 16 years. Group I consisted of 260 patients with no history consistent with CAD and no ECG evidence of CAD. Group II consisted of 212 patients with either a clinical history of CAD or ECG evidence of CAD. Group III consisted of 28 patients with severe, clinically apparent, and unstable CAD. In group III 21 patients had an asymptomatic AAA (group IIIa), and 7 patients had a symptomatic AAA (group IIIb). Group IIIa patients underwent preliminary CAB, followed by staged AAA repair. Group IIIb patients underwent combined CAB and AAA repair. There were no postoperative deaths among group III patients and no postoperative myocardial infarctions. Group II patients were considered to have clinically stable CAD. At the discretion of either the vascular surgeon or the cardiologist, group II patients underwent noninvasive testing using a variety of screening techniques, including radionuclide angiography, exercise tolerance test, and DTI. The overall operative mortality was 1.6 percent (eight deaths). Acute myocardial infarction was involved in six of eight deaths and occurred in 3 percent of all patients. In group I the cardiac-related operative mortality was 0.4 percent versus 2.4 percent for group II, a statistically significant difference. Although Hertzer and co-workers (1984) at the Cleveland Clinic have demonstrated a 15 percent incidence of clinically occult, severe, surgically correctable CAD among patients with no antecedent ECG evidence or clinical history of CAD symptoms, these patients (group I) can undergo elective AAA repair with a low operative mortality and a low postoperative cardiac morbidity. Therefore, further preoperative cardiac evaluation for group I patients is not justified. Similarly, a selective policy of preoperative coronary angiography based on preliminary noninvasive evaluation using DTI to identify group II patients at risk of perioperative myocardial infarction is justified by the low operative mortality rate that characterizes such an approach. Significant perioperative cardiac morbidity and mortality are rare among patients without a clinical history or ECG evidence of CAD. Therefore, these patients need no further preoperative cardiac evaluation prior to AAA repair.

Similarly, in the Canadian Aneurysm Study reported by Johnston and Scobie (1988), among 300 patients with no clinical or ECG evidence of CAD undergoing elective AAA repair, the operative mortality rate was 0.8 percent. However, among the 366 patients with clinical history or ECG evidence of CAD who were undergoing elective AAA repair, the operative mortality was 6.8 percent. Although patients with no clinical evidence or ECG signs of CAD have a low operative mortality rate without undergoing further preoperative cardiac testing, routine intraoperative and postoperative use of a Swan-Ganz catheter is recommended, accompanied by preoperative volume loading (Whittemore and co-workers, 1980). Routine cardiac catheterization for patients with stable CAD is not indicated because the combined early mortality of CAB and AAA repair exceeds the operative mortality of AAA repair alone among the subset of patients judged to be at low risk by preoperative DTI.

Dobutamine Stress Echocardiography. DSE detects regional ventricular wall motion abnormalities. Studies indicate that dobutamine-induced regional dyssynergia has a high sensitivity and specificity for predicting significant CAD. Lalka and co-workers (1992) studied 60 patients scheduled to undergo elective aortic surgery with preoperative DSE. Of these patients, 38 had an abnormal DSE with a 29 percent postoperative cardiac event rate. Of the 22 patients with a normal preoperative DSE, only one patient had postoperative cardiac morbidity, a 4.6 percent event rate ($p < .025$). The most significant predictors of adverse postoperative cardiac events were failure to achieve target heart rate during dobutamine infusion and the development of new regional wall abnormalities that had appeared normal on echocardiography prior to dobutamine infusion. In predicting perioperative cardiac morbidity, DSE has a 92 percent sensitivity and a 44 percent specificity. Among patients with no history or ECG evidence consistent with CAD, 38 percent had abnormal DSE studies, a figure remarkably consistent with Hertzer's finding of CAD in 37 percent of vascular surgery patients with no ECG or clinical evidence of CAD undergoing preoperative coronary angiography (Hertzer and co-workers, 1984). Preoperative coronary angiography is recommended for those patients with abnormal DSE studies even in the absence of clinical cardiac symptoms. Patients with multiple dysfunctional segments also are advised to undergo coronary angiography, even if new wall motion abnormalities do not develop during dobutamine infusion.

PREOPERATIVE PREPARATION AND SURGICAL TECHNIQUE

For elective AAA repair, Bernstein and co-workers (1988) reported on the management approach used at the Scripps Clinic. In a series of 123 consecutive AAA resections there was a single death (mortality of 0.8 percent) and a single postoperative myocardial infarction. Preoperative management included careful noninvasive screening for clinically occult and significant CAD. Preliminary CAB was performed for patients with high-grade left main or triple-vessel coronary artery disease documented by coronary angiography. Preoperative duplex scans of the carotid bifurcations are performed at the discretion of the attending surgeon, particularly if the patient has an antecedent history of stroke or a carotid bruit on physical examination. Severe high-grade carotid bifurcation stenoses are considered a risk for perioperative stroke and are individually considered for prophylactic carotid endarterectomy prior to AAA repair. The patient is offered participation in an autologous blood donation program 2 weeks prior to AAA resection. Patients undergo biplane angiography with careful attention to renal, visceral, iliac, and hypogastric artery anatomy. The evening prior to operation, a Swan-Ganz catheter is placed, and the dynamics of the Starling curve titrated to optimize perioperative hemodynamics, as advocated by Whittemore and co-workers (1980). Preoperative cephalosporin antibiotics are administered intravenously on call to the operating room and continue for 24 hours postoperatively.

Operative management includes the use of epidural narcotics for postoperative pain management. Transesophageal 2-D echocardiography improves the intraoperative monitoring of cardiac performance and is a sensitive and early predictor of myocardial ischemia (Seward and co-workers, 1988). The use of a Steridrape decreases the likelihood of contact between the prosthetic graft and the skin, which is a major source of subsequent aortic graft infection. A self-retaining retractor of the Gomez or Omni type ensures uniformity of operative exposure through a transperitoneal incision, which is used routinely. After limited dissection of the anterior surface of the iliac arteries and the neck of the aneurysm just distal to the left renal vein, a knitted Dacron prosthesis is preclotted. Thereafter, the patient is administered 5,000 units of heparin intravenously. The iliac arteries are occluded with vascular clamps prior to infrarenal aortic occlusion to lessen the likelihood of atheromatous embolization. Duke's resections (aortic tube grafts) are preferred and are employed in more than 50 percent. Although some degree of coexisting common iliac artery ectasia often is encountered, it does not often eventuate in the formation of large iliac artery aneurysms. The cell saver is used routinely. The graft is sewn in place using the graft inclusion technique popularized by Creech. The aneurysm wall is closed over the graft, followed by a second layer to reconstitute the retroperitoneal tissues. Careful hemostasis is achieved, and generous irrigation with antibiotic solution containing kanamycin is done. Using this approach, the mean operative time was 2.4 hours overall and 2.2 hours for aortic tube grafts. Significantly, for the 47 patients between age 70 and 79, the 5 year life table survival probability was 67 percent, as compared with 72 percent for all patients undergoing elective AAA repair. This approaches the documented survival of 80 percent for an age- and gender-adjusted control group without aneurysm disease.

Inflammatory Aortic Aneurysms

Inflammatory aortic aneurysms account for 4.5 to 5 percent of AAAs. They are characterized by a dense, pearly white, fibrotic, "porcelain" reaction that binds the AAA wall to adjacent anatomic structures, including duodenum, vena cava, ureters, and left renal vein. Medial displacement of the ureters and ureteral obstruction may occur. Histologic examination indicates atrophy of the aortic media, with marked thickening of the adventitia, accompanied by a chronic inflammatory infiltrate composed of many plasma cells, lymphocytes, and monocytes and a perianeurysmal desmoplastic reaction. An endarteritis of the adventitial surface is common. The preoperative diagnosis is identified best by CT scan, where the anterior and lateral walls of the aneurysm are noticeably thickened, but the posterior wall is not. Patients may complain that the aneurysm is tender to palpation. The erythrocyte sedimentation rate is increased in 75 percent. A history of weight loss is given in 15 to 20 percent. In spite of the inflammatory reaction, steroid therapy does not stop the development of inflammatory aneurysms.

Modification of the usual operative techniques is required when dealing with an inflammatory aneurysm. The duodenum is not dissected off the anterior wall of the aneurysm. In 30 to 40 percent of cases, the inflammatory process is confined below the renal arteries, which permits application of the usual infrarenal aortic clamp. However, in the majority of cases, suprarenal aortic clamping is required to avoid venous injury. Supraceliac aortic occlusion as advocated by Crawford and co-workers (1985) may be required. The AAA wall is opened longitudinally, lateral to the duodenum, which remains fixed to the anterior surface of the aneurysm. The aortic graft is sewn in place using the graft inclusion technique. Ureterolysis is seldom required. In many instances, the associated ureteral obstruction slowly resolves after inflammatory AAA repair. In a review of 98 cases of inflammatory AAA, Lindblad and co-workers (1991) found no difference in the postoperative serum creatinine values among those patients who underwent ureterolysis and those who did not. Preoperative nephrostomy may be required in a few. In a series from the Mayo Clinic (Pennell and co-workers, 1985), the operative mortality was increased (7.9 percent versus 2.4 percent for standard elective AAA repair) ($p < .005$). Other centers have confirmed the increased operative risk associated with inflammatory aneurysms.

Symptomatic AAAs

The traditional management of a patient with new-onset abdominal and/or back pain, accompanied by a pulsatile abdominal mass, is an immediate AAA repair. In many series, however, the morbidity and mortality of urgent AAA repair in patients with intact AAAs exceeds that associated with elective AAA repair. To define this problem, Sullivan and co-workers (1990) reviewed 204 patients undergoing AAA operations over an 11 year period. The AAA operations were classified as elective for an asymptomatic AAA and emergent for a symptomatic but intact (expanding) AAA or for a ruptured AAA. Operative mortality was 26 percent for the expanding AAA group, and 4 of 5 patients who died in this group experienced perioperative myocardial infarctions. Operative mortality was 35 percent in the ruptured AAA group, which was quite large (69). Among patients undergoing elective AAA repair, the mortality rate was 5 percent. Significantly, 42 percent of the patients undergoing urgent repair of a symptomatic but intact AAA had a known diagnosis of AAA, but had been denied operation due to concurrent medical disease or age.

Review of operative morbidity disclosed that the patients undergoing elective AAA repair had a statistically significant lower incidence of myocardial infarction, respiratory failure, and renal insufficiency when compared to those patients operated on emergently. However, there was no significant difference in the rate of myocardial infarction, respiratory failure, or renal insufficiency between patients undergoing operation emergently for a symptomatic but intact AAA and those patients undergoing operation for AAA rupture. Sullivan and co-workers (1990) propose an algorithm for management of the patient with a symptomatic AAA that requires prospective validation. In this approach, patients with an AAA and the acute onset of abdominal and/or back pain are evaluated for hemodynamic stability. Unstable patients immediately undergo AAA repair. Patients with hemodynamic stability have an immediate contrast-enhanced CT scan. If a retroperitoneal hematoma is demonstrated, the patient undergoes immediate AAA repair. The hemodynamically stable patient with a CT scan negative for retroperitoneal hematoma who has evidence for cardiac, pulmonary, or renal disease is transferred to the intensive care unit (ICU) for an expeditious evaluation of comorbid disease and optimization of cardiac hemodynamics prior to urgent AAA repair. For this group, operation occurs within 6 hours of admission. Using this discriminating approach, Sullivan and co-workers (1990) aspire to reduce the morbidity and mortality so prevalent among patients with an intact AAA managed with an emergency operation.

Kvilekval and co-workers (1990) reviewed 95 patients evaluated over 5 years for a possible ruptured AAA. Patients were divided into four groups. Category I patients were hemodynamically unstable and underwent immediate operation. Category II patients were hemodynamically stable but had evidence of a ruptured AAA on immediate CT scanning. Category III patients were hemodynamically stable with CT evidence of an intact AAA. Category IV patients had no aneurysm detected at the time of CT scanning. The mortality for hemodynamically unstable patients with a ruptured AAA taken immediately to operation was 60 percent. For category II patients, the average duration for CT examination was 63 minutes. Of 18 patients diagnosed as having a ruptured AAA, one refused operation, and there was one false-positive CT exam (94 percent sensitivity). The operative mortality for category II patients was 25 percent, with major postoperative morbidity occurring in 31 percent. The CT scan also correctly identified four abnormalities: a left-sided inferior vena cava, an inflammatory AAA, a coexisting intact thoracic aneurysm, and a thoracoabdominal aneurysm. In category III, 59 percent of 44 patients had comorbid disease that increased their risk of emergent AAA repair. Twenty-one patients underwent a subsequent "semielective" AAA repair with no operative mortality. Thirty percent of the patients in category III were discovered to have an etiology for their pain other than the intact AAA, often involving gastrointestinal pathology. No patients with CT evidence of an intact AAA died of a ruptured AAA. Among the three patients without an AAA, the CT scan helped identify other retroperitoneal or gastrointestinal pathology. Kvilekval and co-workers (1990) conclude that the selective use of CT scanning in hemodynamically stable patients who have an AAA, accompanied by symptoms consistent with AAA expansion, does not compromise the management of those patients who are identified as having ruptured AAAs. The CT scan provides useful diagnostic information and avoids the increased morbidity and mortality associated with emergency operations for patients who have intact AAAs. The operative mortality rate for patients with CT evidence of ruptured AAA when operation was delayed briefly by the CT scan is comparable to series of patients with symptomatic aneurysms with confirmed rupture undergoing immediate operation without preliminary CT imaging. Nevertheless, the diagnosis of a ruptured AAA is made most often on the basis of clinical examination alone, with immediate transfer of the patient to the operating suite. Any delay in this effort can result in catastrophic sudden circulatory collapse.

Not all authorities agree that the selective use of rapid CT scanning in hemodynamically stable patients with symptoms consistent with expanding AAA decreases the operative mortality for patients with intact AAAs who otherwise would undergo emergency operation. Buss and co-workers (1988) reviewed 212 patients undergoing AAA repair and divided them into three groups: elective repair, emergency repair of ruptured AAA, and emergency repair of intact, symptomatic AAAs. The mean time from emergency presentation to operation was 5.2 hours for ruptured AAAs and 6.2 hours for intact, symptomatic AAAs. Between these two groups there was no significant difference in blood loss or total morbidity. The mortality for elective AAA resection was 4.5 percent versus 2.9 percent for emergency repair of an intact, symptomatic AAA. In contrast, the mortality for ruptured AAAs was 68 percent. Although the operative mortality for emergency repair of an intact symptomatic AAA was low and not statistically different from that of elective AAA repair, the incidence of perioperative myocardial infarction was five times greater in the former group and nearly identical to that of patients undergoing emergency operation for ruptured AAAs. Although the reasons for the low operative mortality among patients undergoing emergency operation for symptomatic, intact AAAs are not clear, this group was younger (mean age 66 years) than the group reported by Sullivan and co-workers (1990). In addition, 17 percent of patients undergoing emergency operation had abdominal conditions other than AAA that caused their preoperative symptoms. Buss and co-workers (1988) express concern that preoperative CT scanning will cause delay in the operative management of patients with ruptured AAAs, and thereby increase mortality. In spite of this concern, they achieved a low operative mortality in patients with symptomatic, intact AAAs, after a preoperative delay in the emergency department that represented the same time interval recommended by Sullivan and co-workers (1990) to exclude retroperitoneal hemorrhage with a CT scan and complete a preoperative hemodynamic evaluation in patients with identifiable cardiac, pulmonary, or renal disease who have negative CT scans prior to AAA repair. The increased operative mortality in the series reported by Sullivan and co-workers (1990) among patients undergoing emergency operation for intact AAAs was not due to hypotension and decompensation of the patients but rather to increased perioperative cardiac morbidity relative to patients undergoing elective AAA repair.

Ruptured AAAs

Ruptured AAAs continue to have high mortality despite the advances that have occurred in the detection of preoperative cardiac disease, preoperative volume loading, and improved anesthetic management that have contributed to a declining operative mortality among patients undergoing elective AAA repair. To characterize factors responsible for the sustained high mortality among patients with ruptured AAAs, Ouriel and co-workers (1990) at the University of Rochester reviewed 243 patients treated for ruptured AAA in Monroe County, New York, over a 10 year period. The operative mortality for the group was 55 percent. Three categories of factors were analyzed to determine variables associated with mortality: the hospital, the surgeon, and the patient. There were no differences in mortality between patients treated at a large teaching hospital versus those treated in community hospitals. There were no significant intrahospital differences in the time between the onset of symptoms and arrival at a hospital (median 8 hours). There was no mortality difference between hospitals with regard to the number of patients with ruptured AAAs treated per year. Overall, the effect of intrahospital differences on ruptured AAA mortality was limited.

When individual surgeons were considered, the surgeon's length of experience beyond residency training and the number of elective AAA resections performed per year were not significant in improving ruptured AAA mortality. However, the case mix of the individual surgeon did influence operative mortality. The most significant determinants affecting mortality from ruptured AAAs were certain pre-existing medical problems. Patients with a history of chronic obstructive pulmonary disease (COPD) or chronic renal insufficiency had a statistically significant increase in operative mortality ($p < .01$). Other factors, including pre-existing CAD, hypertension, diabetes, age greater than 70 years, hematocrit, and obesity, were not statistically significant predictors of mortality from ruptured AAA. However, the presence of hypotension did correlate with increased mortality. Although an apparent increase in mortality was observed among elderly patients, multivariate analysis indicated that a disproportionate influence of coexisting medical diseases, rather than age alone, contributes to ruptured AAA mortality.

Whereas Ouriel and co-workers (1990) demonstrated that preoperative medical status influenced survival after a ruptured AAA, both intraoperative technical factors and the development of postoperative organ system dysfunction play a significant role in patient survival. Harris and co-workers (1991) reviewed 113 patients undergoing operative treatment of ruptured AAAs at the State University of New York, Buffalo, over a 9 year period. Patient death was classified either as early, within 48 hours of operation, or late, occurring later than 48 hours postoperatively. The mean time from hospital admission to operation was 5.2 hours, and the overall operative mortality was 64 percent. Deaths occurred in a bimodal distribution, with 58 percent of 72 deaths occurring within 48 hours, and 25 percent of deaths occurring more than 2 weeks postoperatively. Using multivariate analysis, statistically significant predictors ($p <.01$) of early death included preoperative cardiac arrest and coma. The presence of preoperative hypotension (systolic BP <80) as a predictor of early postoperative death was close to statistical significance. Significant predictors of late death after operation for a ruptured AAA included postoperative renal failure and respiratory failure. Mortality varied with the degree of functional renal impairment. Among the patients developing anuria or oliguric renal failure, the mortality was 80 percent. For patients with polyuric renal insufficiency, the mortality was 66 percent. Patients with postoperative normal renal function had a 10 percent mortality. Using logistic regression analysis, the only statistically significant predictor of overall mortality was postoperative renal insufficiency. A search for preoperative variables that accurately predicted the development of postoperative renal insufficiency failed to identify any significant predictors, including preoperative renal insufficiency. A total transfusion requirement of 18 or more units of blood (reflecting intraoperative technical problems) within 24 hours and the need for reoperation due to mesenteric or lower limb ischemia correlated with overall mortality using univariate analysis. However, the significance of these factors was not confirmed on multivariate analysis.

From this study, it appears that postoperative renal failure and respiratory failure and intraoperative technical problems causing massive blood loss and/or precipitating acute visceral or acute lower extremity ischemia contribute the most to late postoperative mortality. Whereas preoperative factors, such as hypotension and cardiac arrest, are important in causing early deaths, they do not correlate well with late postoperative deaths. This may represent a statistical error because renal and respiratory failure and colon necrosis are often associated with sustained hypovolemic shock. Therefore, the preoperative prediction of those patients with ruptured AAAs who will have a complicated postoperative course, but will ultimately die late, cannot be made accurately at this time.

Screening for the presence of an AAA and timely referral for elective AAA repair are the most effective means to decrease the mortality, morbidity, and expense associated with ruptured AAAs. In spite of this, the age-adjusted incidence of AAAs in the population is rising (Bickerstaff and co-workers, 1984) and the number of elective AAA repairs is increasing, yet the incidence of ruptured AAA and its high mortality remain unchanged.

Many studies document that patients with ruptured AAAs who arrive in shock have a high mortality rate (Ouriel and co-workers, 1990; Shackelton and co-workers, 1987; Wakefield and co-workers, 1982). Those patients who suffer a preoperative cardiac arrest usually die regardless of aggressive efforts at salvage. Johansen and co-workers (1991) reviewed a 10 year experience with 186 patients treated for ruptured AAA at Harborview Medical Center, Seattle. The overall mortality was 70 percent and remained unchanged over the decade studied. Nearly all of these patients were taken to the Harborview Emergency Room by a highly trained and efficient paramedic resuscitation team that rapidly initiated prehospital care, including intravenous crystalloid infusion. The expert and rapid prehospital care ensured the delivery of critically ill patients with ruptured AAAs who might not have survived a less expeditious journey to an emergency room in a community where an organized, rapid evacuation of patients in shock to a single center did not exist. The patients arriving at Harborview were a more moribund group than reported in other series: 96 percent of the Seattle patients had a prehospital systolic blood pressure of less than 90 mm Hg.

On arrival, the patients underwent a rapid evaluation by protocol, including baseline ECG, chest x-ray, brief physical examination, and B-mode ultrasound, if the presence of an AAA was in doubt. The average delay in the emergency room prior to transfer to the operating room was 12 minutes, emphasizing the principle of obtaining rapid proximal control of the aorta as soon as possible to avoid exsanguination. Fourteen percent of the patients died in the operating room, a figure lower than the 23 percent of deaths in the operating room reported by Harris and co-workers (1991). Among the patients dying after postoperative admission to the ICU, 18 percent had colon infarction, emphasizing the concept popularized by Landreneau and Fry (1990), that the colon is a target organ for shock and is adversely affected by a sustained period of low cardiac output. In the Harborview experience, the majority of postoperative deaths were due to multiple organ failure. All patients who suffered a preoperative cardiac arrest died within the first 24 hours after operation. Ninety-two percent of patients older than age 80 died, and 92 percent of patients who remained persistently hypotensive after operative control died. Operative correlates associated with massive blood loss (hematocrit <25 on admission; total transfusion requirement of > 15 units in 24 hours) individually were associated with a 90 percent mortality.

The high mortality in the Harborview experience, which was sustained over time, cannot be attributed to delayed delivery of patients with ruptured AAAs to the operating room. Nor can the high mortality be associated with operative technical errors because inadvertent venous injuries contributed to death in only 4.4 percent of cases. The rapid resuscitative efforts of the prehospital paramedic team included the intravenous infusion of crystalloid. Such early resuscitation would help ameliorate subsequent organ system dysfunction associated with hypovolemic shock. Crawford (1991) advocates modest intravenous infusion to maintain the systolic blood pressure in a low range rather than an attempt to restore the systolic blood pressure beyond 100 mm Hg, which may cause disruption of the retroperitoneal hematoma with exsanguination. Such a policy is not widely endorsed because sustained hypotension at low levels of systolic pressure may eventuate in irreversible shock.

The concept is sound that the critical, lifesaving maneuver in managing patients with ruptured AAAs is operative control of the proximal supraceliac aorta, not preoperative restoration of systolic blood pressure via the rapid intravenous infusion of large volumes of crystalloid. In a companion editorial, Crawford reports a personal series of 87 patients with ruptured AAAs managed at Methodist Hospital in Houston. In this series, 46 percent of patients had a preoperative systolic blood pressure of less than 90 mm Hg. In this hypotensive group, the operative mortality was 42 percent. Survival of patients older than age 80 was 73 percent (8/11). The number of octogenarians presenting to the operating room with hypovolemic shock was not stated. These patients, as reported, appear different than the Harborview patients because the Texas patients were referred in many cases by other physicians to Methodist Hospital, and the majority of profoundly decompensated, moribund patients considered unstable for transfer may not have made the trip. Indeed, the efficiency of the Seattle paramedics may exceed the ability of surgeons ultimately to reverse certain undeniable correlates of eventual mortality, in spite of excellent prehospital, emergency room, and surgical care. Most prominent among these factors is irreversible shock and preoperative circulatory arrest. However, the suggestion that such patients not undergo an attempt at aneurysm repair is problematic because a few survivors are reported in other series.

Gloviczki and co-workers (1992) reviewed 231 patients admitted to the Mayo Clinic with ruptured AAAs over a 10 year period. Mean age was 74 years, and overall operative mortality was 41.6 percent. Patients were hypotensive preoperatively, less than 90 mm Hg systolic, in 67 percent of cases. Median time from arrival in the emergency room to operation was 35 minutes. The most frequent cause of death postoperatively was ongoing hemorrhage (38.6 percent), followed by multiorgan system failure (33.3 percent). Univariate analysis of clinical variables identified several parameters as statistically significant ($p < .05$) predictors of death: (1) mean APACHE II score = 19 among patients who died versus 11.3 among patients who survived; (2) preoperative hypotension; (3) low preoperative hematocrit; (4) preoperative cardiac arrest (mortality of 80 percent); (5) the extent of rupture (free intraperitoneal rupture had the highest mortality); (6) total transfusion requirement greater than 15 units of blood; (7) intraoperative cardiac arrest (mortality of 93.5 percent). Using stepwise logistic regression analysis, Gloviczki and co-workers identified four variables that most precisely predicted mortality: (1) a high APACHE II score; (2) a low preoperative hematocrit; (3) preoperative hypotension; and (4) a history of COPD. Neither age nor gender was identified by multivariate analysis as a significant predictor of death. Also, 28 percent of the patients who experienced cardiac arrest survived. Cardiac arrest was not one of the best predictors of mortality using multivariate analysis. No combination of preoperative variables permitted the accurate identification of a patient group with an exceedingly unlikely chance for survival. Therefore, no patient with a ruptured AAA should be denied an attempt at AAA repair unless the patient is in the terminal stage of a metastatic malignancy. Preoperative factors, such as advanced age, hypovolemic shock, cardiac arrest, or gender, do not contraindicate operation for a ruptured abdominal aortic aneurysm.

Suggested Reading

Bernstein EF, Chan EL. Abdominal aortic aneurysms in high risk patients: Outcome of selective management based on size and expansion rate. Ann Surg 1984; 200:255–263.

Bernstein EF, Dilley RB, Randolph HF. The improving long term outlook for patients over 70 years of age with abdominal aortic aneurysms. Ann Surg 1988; 207:318–322.

Bickerstaff LK, Hollier LH, Van Peenen HJ, et al. Abdominal aortic aneurysms: Factors affecting mortality rates. J Vasc Surg 1984; 1:6–12.

Brown PM, Pattenden R, Gutelius JR. The selective management of small abdominal aortic aneurysms: The Kingston Study. J Vasc Surg 1992; 15: 21–27.

Buss RW, Clagett GP, Fischer DF, et al. Emergency operation in patients with symptomatic abdominal aortic aneurysms. Am J Surg 1988; 156: 470–473.

Cambria RP, Brewster DC, Abbott WM, et al. The impact of selective use of dipyridamole-thallium scans and surgical factors on the current morbidity of aortic surgery. J Vasc Surg 1992; 15:43–51.

Crawford ES. Ruptured abdominal aortic aneurysm: An editorial. J Vasc Surg 1991; 13:348–350.

Crawford JL, Stowe CL, Safi HJ, et al. Inflammatory aneurysms of the aorta. J Vasc Surg 1985; 2:113–124.

Cronenwett JL, Murphy TF, Zelenock GB, et al. Actuarial analysis of variables associated with rupture of small abdominal aortic aneurysms. Surgery 1985; 98:472–483.

Cronenwell JL, Sargent SK, Wall MH, et al. Variables that affect the expansion rate and outcome of small abdominal aortic aneurysms. J Vasc Surg 1990; 11:260–269.

Eagle KA, Coley CM, Newell JB, et al. Combining clinical and thallium data optimizes preoperative assessment of cardiac risk before major vascular surgery. Ann Intern Med 1989; 110:859–866.

Gersh BJ, Kronmal RA, Frye RL, et al. Participants in the Coronary Artery Surgery Study—Coronary angiography and coronary artery bypass surgery: Morbidity and mortality in patients ages 65 years or older: A report from the coronary artery surgery study. Circulation 1983; 67: 483–492.

Gloviczki P, Pairolero PC, Mucha P, et al. Ruptured abdominal aortic aneurysms: Repair should not be denied. J Vasc Surg 1992; 15:851–859.

Golden MA, Whittemore AD, Donaldson MC, et al. Selective evaluation and management of coronary artery disease in patients undergoing repair of abdominal aortic aneurysms. Ann Surg 1990; 212:415–423.

Harris LM, Faggioli GL, Fiedler R, et al. Ruptured abdominal aortic aneurysms: Factors affecting mortality rates. J Vasc Surg 1991; 14:812–820.

Hertzer NR, Beven EG, Young JR, et al. Coronary artery disease in peripheral vascular surgery patients: A classification of 1,000 coronary angiograms and results of surgical management. Ann Surg 1984; 199:223–233.

Hollier LH, Taylor LM, Ochsner J. Recommended indications for operative treatment of abdominal aortic aneurysms. J Vasc Surg 1992; 15:1046–1056.

Hunter GC, Leong SC, Yu GS, et al. Aortic blebs: Possible site of aneurysm rupture. J Vasc Surg 1989; 10:93–99.

Jeffrey CC, Kunsman J, Cullen DJ, et al. A prospective evaluation of cardiac risk index. Anesthesiology 1983; 58:462–464.

Johansen K, Kohler TR, Nicholls SC, et al. Ruptured abdominal aortic aneurysm: The Harborview experience. J Vasc Surg 1991; 13:240–247.

Johansson G, Nydahl S, Olofsson P, et al. Selective management of abdominal aortic aneurysms. Perspect Vasc Surg 1991; 4:13–30.

Johnston KW, Scobie TK. Multicenter prospective study of nonruptured abdominal aortic aneurysms: I. Population and operative management. J Vasc Surg 1988; 7:69–81.

Kvilekval KH, Best IM, Mason RA, et al. The value of computed tomography in the management of symptomatic abdominal aortic aneurysms. J Vasc Surg 1990; 12:28–33.

Lalka SG, Sawada SG, Dalsing MC, et al. Dobutamine stress echocardiography as a predictor of cardiac events associated with aortic surgery. J Vasc Surg 1992; 15:831–842.

Landreneau RJ, Fry WJ. The right colon as a target of nonocclusive mesenteric ischemia. Arch Surg 1990; 125:591–594.

Lindblad B, Almgren B, Berqvist D, et al. Abdominal aortic aneurysm with perianeurysmal fibrosis: Experience from 11 Swedish vascular centers. J Vasc Surg 1991; 13:231–239.

McEnroe CS, O'Donnell TF, Yeager A, et al. Comparison of ejection fraction and Goldman risk factor analysis to dipyridamole thallium 201 studies in the evaluation of cardiac morbidity after aortic aneurysm surgery. J Vasc Surg 1990; 11:497–504.

Nevitt MP, Ballard DJ, Hallet JW. Prognosis of abdominal aortic aneurysm: A population based study. N Engl J Med 1989; 321:1009–1014.

O'Donnell TF, Darling RC, Linton RR. Is 80 years too old for aneurysmectomy? Arch Surg 1976; 111:1250–1254.

Ouriel K, Geary K, Green RM, et al. Factors determining survival after ruptured aortic aneurysm: The hospital, the surgeon, and the patient. J Vasc Surg 1990; 11:493–496.

Pennell RC, Hollier LR, Lie JT, et al. Inflammatory abdominal aortic aneurysms: A thirty year review. J Vasc Surg 1985; 2:859–869.

Plecha FR, Bertin VJ, Plecha EJ, et al. The early results of vascular surgery in patients 75 years of age or older: An analysis of 3529 cases. J Vasc Surg 1987; 2:769–775.

Reigel MM, Hollier LH, Kazmier FJ, et al. Late survival in abdominal aortic aneurysm patients: The role of selective myocardial revascularization on the basis of clinical symptoms. J Vasc Surg 1987; 5:222–227.

Seward JB, Khandheria BK, Oh JK, et al. Transesophageal echocardiography: Technique, anatomic correlations, implementation, and clinical applications. Mayo Clin Proc 1988; 63:649–680.

Shackleton CR, Schechter MT, Bianco R, et al. Preoperative predictors of mortality in ruptured abdominal aortic aneurysm. J Vasc Surg 1987; 6:583–589.

Sullivan CA, Roher MJ, Cutler BS. Clinical management of the symptomatic but unruptured abdominal aortic aneurysm. J Vasc Surg 1990; 11: 799–803.

Wakefield TW, Whitehouse WM, Wu SC, et al. Abdominal aortic aneurysm rupture: Statistical analysis of factors affecting outcome of surgical treatment. Surgery 1982; 91:586–596.

Whittemore AD, Clowes AW, Hechtman HB, et al. Aortic aneurysm repair: Reduced operative mortality associated with maintenance of optimal cardiac performance. Ann Surg 1980; 120:414–421.

RAYNAUD'S SYNDROME

J. Timothy Fulenwider, M.D., F.A.C.S.

Of the clinical vasospastic disorders, none incites more patient anxiety, encompasses a broader clinical disease spectrum, and invokes more etiologic and therapeutic controversy than Raynaud's syndrome (RS). Raynaud's syndrome is characterized by episodic digital arteriospasm resulting in pathognomonic biphasic or triphasic digital cutaneous color changes (Raynaud, 1988). Most patients with RS (70 to 90 percent) are women between the ages of 25 and 40 years with cold-induced or emotion-induced symmetrical finger pallor that persists in cold exposure. With rewarming, digit pallor changes to cyanosis (sluggish reperfusion) and occasionally to intense rubor (reactive hyperemia). The color changes may extend into the distal palm and may be frequently accompanied by transient, reversible digital hypothermia, mild pain, and hypesthesia. The fingers and hands are most commonly involved, although the toes, cheeks, and ears may demonstrate typical evanescent color changes. Raynaud's syndrome is often seasonal and geographic; episodes are more common and severe in northern climates during the winter months.

The clinical spectrum of RS includes "Raynaud's disease": patients with normal extremity arterial anatomy and supraphysiologic vasoconstrictor responses hypothetically due to a "local vascular fault" or exaggerated adrenergic neuroeffector activity and increased alpha$_2$-adrenergic receptors of digital arteries. "Raynaud's phenomenon" includes those patients with fixed, pressure-reducing, organic obstructive arteriopathies of the digital, palmar, or proximal extremity arteries whose superimposed normal vasoconstrictor responses effect critical arterial closure, cessation of blood flow, and the ischemic event. Although Raynaud's disease classically occurs in the absence of an identifiable clinical systemic disease, Raynaud's phenomenon is associated with a myriad of disease states (Table 1). Unfortunately, precise initial stratification of patients into such clinical subsets is arbitrary because of the well-documented long latency intervals between the onset of RS and the evolution of an associated systemic disease state. To avoid confusion, many have suggested the abandonment of the labels *Raynaud's disease* and *Raynaud's phenomenon* for the more inclusive category "Raynaud's syndrome." Raynaud's syndrome can then be pathophysiologically segregated into vasospastic and obstructive subsets.

■ THERAPEUTIC ALTERNATIVES

All therapeutic plans for RS are palliative and directed toward a reduction in the frequency and severity of digital ischemia attacks. The majority (70 to 80 percent) of patients with RS are effectively managed by explaining the involved pathophysiology of the syndrome to them and reassuring them of the favorable prognosis of RS of the purely vasospastic variety.

Table 1 Conditions Associated with Raynaud's Syndrome

Immunologic and collagen vascular diseases
Scleroderma
CREST syndrome
Systemic lupus erythematosus
Rheumatoid arthritis
Mixed connective tissue disease
Undifferentiated connective tissue disease
Dermatomyositis
Polymyositis
Hepatitis B-associated vasculitis
Drug-induced vasculitis
Sjögren's syndrome
Henoch-Schönlein purpura
Polyarteritis nodosa
Reiter's syndrome
Hypersensitivity vasculitis
Obstructive arteriopathies
Arteriosclerosis obliterans
Thromboangiitis obliterans (Buerger's disease)
Post-thromboembolic arterial obstruction
Thoracic outlet compression syndrome
Takayasu's disease
Other arteritides (giant cell, syphilitic)
Occupational or environmental trauma
Hypothenar-hammer syndrome
Vibratory tool exposure
Direct large or small arterial trauma
Cold injury, frostbite
Neurologic diseases
Central or peripheral neuropathy
Reflex sympathetic dystrophy
Carpal tunnel syndrome
Endocrinopathy
Myxedema
Graves' disease
Hypopituitarism
Addison's disease
Cushing's disease
Drug-associated conditions
Ergot alkaloids
Beta-adrenergic blockers
Oral contraceptives
Cytotoxic therapy
Nicotine
Caffeine
Sympathomimetics
Methysergide
Miscellaneous conditions
Fabry's disease
Paroxysmal hemoglobinuria
Primary pulmonary hypertension
Pheochromocytoma
Vinyl chloride exposure
Chronic renal failure
Cold agglutinins
Cryoglobulinemia
Hyperviscosity states
Malignant neoplasms
Myeloproliferative disorders (leukemia, myeloid metaplasia, polycythemia rubra vera, thrombocytosis)
Macroglobulinemia
Disseminated intravascular coagulation
Heavy metals

Digital gangrene never occurs as a consequence of vasospasm alone. Preventive measures to minimize cold exposure by wearing mittens to maintain hand warmth is an important mainstay of therapy. Additional preventive measures include proper attire for cold weather exposure to maintain central body core temperature at near-normal levels. The use of multilayered insulated garments (polypropylene, Gore-Tex, down, or Thinsulate) and battery-heated socks and gloves have proven indispensable in maintaining normal, active life-styles for patients with RS. Tobacco, in all forms, must be avoided. Ergot alkaloids, beta-blockers, oral contraceptives, and sympathomimetic medications are also relatively contraindicated. A physical measure that is alleged to be capable of aborting a prolonged episode of digital ischemia is the whirling arm maneuver. In this maneuver, the patient, while standing, rapidly whirls the affected upper extremity in a 360-degree arc for 1 to 2 minutes or for a shorter interval, should the digital ischemia subside. The avoidance of vibratory machinery (drills, sanders, chainsaws, jackhammers, grinders) is preferable; however, oscillatory trauma can be minimized by grasping the tools as lightly as possible, reducing motor speed, and wearing heavy gloves (especially those with antivibrational properties). Several investigators have reported salutary responses to stress modification instruction and biofeedback training; however, most investigators also concur that these measures should be reserved for highly motivated individuals.

A minority (20 to 30 percent) of patients with RS require pharmacologic therapy, often only during the colder months. That no single drug or combination of drugs has achieved universal acceptance as the regimen of choice is shown by the multiplicity of medications either formerly or presently endorsed as effective (Table 2). Pharmacologic investigations of patients with RS have been hampered by the paucity of objective tests that accurately quantitate the effects of medications on digital arterial flow. Accordingly, investigators have relied on subjective end responses in the majority of trials, most of which are not randomized, blinded, or placebo controlled. Nonetheless, the consensus is that pharmacotherapy does play a vital role for many patients with RS and that those with the purely vasospastic etiology respond far more favorably than those with fixed organic arterial obstructions. Medications reported to be effective in patients with RS are listed in Table 2. Favorable anecdotal responses to plasmapheresis have also been reported and are presumably related to the reduction of whole blood viscosity with improvement of red blood cell membrane deformability during microcirculatory transit.

Contemporary surgical management of RS is primarily directed toward arterial reconstruction of pressure-significant stenoses or complete occlusions because operative cervicothoracic and lumbar sympathetic denervations have been virtually abandoned. Although microsurgical palmar digital arterial sympathectomy is technically feasible, its propriety for RS is obviously dubious because of the well-documented, short-lived favorable results following conventional sympathetic denervations (Porter and co-workers, 1989). Technically incomplete sympathetic denervation, postdenervation receptor hypersensitivity, and sympathetic neural fiber regeneration have been incriminated in the late clinical failures following sympathectomy.

■ PREFERRED APPROACH

The history of episodic biphasic or triphasic digital cutaneous color changes lasting 20 to 60 minutes provoked by cold exposure or emotional stimuli is sufficient to establish the diagnosis of RS. Not infrequently, the patient's sympathoadrenal response during the initial introduction in a cool office environment is sufficient to demonstrate a typical episode of digital ischemia. Having established the historical diagnosis of RS, a detailed medical history is obtained, as at least 60 to 70 percent of individuals with symptoms and signs of the severity necessary to consult a physician will prove to have an associated illness (see Table 1) (Fitzgerald and co-workers, 1988; Porter and co-workers, 1989; Priollet and co-workers, 1987). Specific questions regarding medications are warranted and should include nonprescription remedies such as nasal aerosols and oral decongestants that if taken in sufficient quantities, have potent vasoconstrictor activities. A history of Prinzmetal's angina, migraine headaches, or abdominal migraine is important because of presumed similar "local vascular faults" creating regional episodic vasospasm. Occupational history assumes critical importance, exemplified by data suggesting that from 40 to 90 percent of loggers and 50 percent of miners using vibratory equipment experience RS (Cardelli and Kleinsmith, 1989). Additionally, the history of malignancy, neurologic disorder, blood and clotting dyscrasias, endocrinopathy, or claudication may assume etiologic significance. Approximately 30 to 40 percent of patients with RS have evidence of some associated illness and small artery obliterative disease (see Table 1). Approximately one-half of these RS-associated illnesses are autoimmune connective tissue disorders, most frequently either scleroderma or a CREST variant; therefore, the examination should include questioning for special evidence of connective tissue disease: myalgias, arthralgias, cutaneous edema or induration, dermatitis, cutaneous photosensitivity or tightening, atrophy and pigment changes, sicca complex symptoms, and dysphagia.

The complete physical examination should emphasize the integument and peripheral arterial tree. Important features include qualitative assessment of all peripheral pulses, including an attempt to palpate digital arteries of the hands. The Allen test is performed to determine patency of the palmar arches. A Doppler ultrasonographic arterial survey using a portable 10 MHz pencil transducer provides a rapid, qualitative assessment of arterial velocimetry, a method of determining patency of small arteries, and flow detection to assess segmental limb systolic pressures. The presence of digital skin ulcerations or pitted scars of healed ulcerations suggests the presence of an underlying obstructive etiology of RS because pure vasospasm of normal arterial anatomy never causes cutaneous infarction or ulceration. In the presence of chronic digital ulceration, widespread palmar and digital obliterative arteriopathy is usually present and is most likely due to vasculitis of scleroderma or CREST syndrome, hypersensitivity angiitis, or atherosclerosis obliterans, in this order of frequency.

Other physical examination clues of importance include skin eruptions, telangiectasias, and atrophy and tightening, as well as joint deformities or other manifestations of connective tissue disease.

The extent of laboratory investigation is guided by clinical

Table 2 Medications Used in Raynaud's Syndrome

CLASS	DOSE/ROUTE	RESPONSE RATE (%)	MAJOR ADVERSE EFFECTS
Calcium channel blockers			
Nifedipine	30–60 mg/d; PO	60–70	Vasomotor flushing, edema, headaches, giddiness, hypotension, late tachyphylaxis (?)
Diltiazem	90–180 mg/d; PO	60–70	Edema, hypotension, prolongation AV node conduction palpitations, syncope, vasomotor flushing
Nicardipine	60–120 mg/d; PO	60–70	Edema, headache, dizziness, asthenia, palpitations
Sympatholytics			
Reserpine	0.25–1 mg/d; PO	40–50	Depression, orthostatic hypotension, peptic ulcer disease, diarrhea, impotence, asthenia, nasal congestion
Guanethidine	10–40 mg/d; PO	40–50	Orthostatic hypotension, impotence, diarrhea, bradycardia, edema
Methyldopa	250–1,000 mg/d; PO	40–50	Impotence, orthostatic hypotension, sedation, asthenia; Coombs's positive anemia, hepatitis, systemic lupus erythematosus
Alpha-adrenergic blockers			
Prazosin	2–20 mg/d; PO	50	Dizziness, headache, asthenia, somnolence, nausea, palpitations, orthostatic hypotension
Phenoxybenzamine	20–80 mg/d; PO	40–50	Orthostatic hypotension, tachycardia, fatigue
Vasodilators			
Griseofulvin	250–1,000 mg/d; PO	30–40(?)	Photosensitivity, nausea, vomiting, diarrhea, mental confusion, paresthesias
Nicotine acid	250–2,000 mg/d; PO	40	Flushing, pruritus, diarrhea, postural hypotension, headache, hyperuricemia
Papaverine	150–450 mg/d; PO	30–40	Nausea, headache, malaise, abdominal distress, vertigo, sweating
Captopril	37.5–75 mg/d; PO	30	Hypotension, angioedema, dysgeusia, tachycardia
Nitrates	5–10 mg/d; topical 0.04 mg; sublingual	20–30	Headaches, palpitations, flushing, nausea, hypotension
Iloprost	Investigational; IV	30	Hypotension, flushing, headache, nausea, vomiting
Prostacyclin (PGI_2)	Investigational; IV	Indeterminate	Hypertension, flushing, tachycardia, nausea, vomiting
Prostaglandin E_1 (PGE_1) Alprostadil	Investigational; IV	Indeterminate	Hypertension, flushing, tachycardia, nausea, vomiting
Serotonin H_2 Receptor antagonist			
Ketanserin	10 mg IV; 60–120 mg/d PO	Indeterminate	Hypotension
Beta-receptor agonists			
Terbutaline sulfate	7.5–15 mg/d; PO	Minimal	Headache, tremor, palpitations, nausea, vomiting, sweating
Nylidrin	9–48 mg/d; PO	Minimal	Tremor, palpitations, nausea, asthenia
Isoproterenol			
Isoxsuprine*			
Fibrinolytic agents			
Stanazolol†		Indeterminate	Malaise, fluid retention, amenorrhea, acne, hirsutism, elevated liver enzymes
Miscellaneous drugs of marginal benefit			
Triiodothyronine*			
Dextran (low molecular weight)*			
Pentoxifylline*			

*No dose/route and response rate published.
†No dose/route published.

suspicions aroused by the history and physical evaluations; however, certain basic tests are routinely performed: complete blood count, erythrocyte sedimentation rate, chemistry profile, urinalysis, and antinuclear antibody. Additional investigations include the following: serum protein electrophoresis, quantitative serum immunoglobulin and complement levels, antibody to DNA, antiextractable nuclear antigens, HEP-2 ANA assay, anticentromere antibody, serum cryoglobulin and cryofibrinogen levels, hepatitis B surface antigen and antibody, chest film, nerve conduction velocities and electromyography, pulmonary function studies, and cine-esophagography.

Although the noninvasive vascular laboratory is not essential for the diagnosis of RS, its adjunctive roles include validation of the diagnosis of suspected RS patients who do not manifest typical digital color changes and the assessment of medical and surgical therapeutic efficacy. The ice water immersion test with serial fingertip thermistor probe temperature measurements is a simple and specific test for the diagnosis of RS; however, this examination suffers from low sensitivity (Jamieson and co-workers, 1971). Digital photoplethysmography with waveform analysis has been frequently used because 70 percent of patients with RS are said to exhibit a characteristic "peak waveform" (Sumner and Strandness, 1972). The digital photoplethysmography also provides excellent specificity but low sensitivity. The most accurate (97 percent) yet complex RS diagnostic test is the occlusive digital hypothermic challenge described by Nielson and Lassen (1977). This test is performed with a double inlet cuff, for local cooling, over the proximal phalanx of the test finger. Using a mercury-in-rubber strain gauge distal to the cuff, baseline pressures are determined and repeated after 5 minutes of ischemic hypothermic perfusion until pressure recovery occurs. The results are expressed as the percentage of decrease in the cool finger systolic pressure upon reperfusion compared with the reference finger. A decrease in digital pressure of 20 percent or greater is positive (Nielson and Lassen, 1977). I prefer simple digital plethysmography with waveform analysis and digital arterial pressures after ice bath immersion. These tests combined with extremity segmental air plethysmography and segmental arterial pressure determinations provide accurate, objective measurements of digital arterial flow; allow distinction between vasospastic and obstructive RS; and provide accurate, objective information regarding proximal arterial flow. Normally, the brachial-to-finger systolic pressure gradient is 10 to 15 torr. A brachial-to-finger pressure gradient of greater than 15 torr, absolute digital arterial pressure less than 70 torr, or pressure difference of more than 15 torr between any two fingers suggests the presence of significant palmar or digital arterial obstruction.

Contrast arteriography is warranted in selected patients with RS whose medical comorbidity would not contraindicate a major arterial reconstruction if remedial situations are discovered. Virtually all patients with ischemic digital ulcers should undergo complete extremity arteriography primarily to detect proximal arterial lesions (e.g., subclavian artery aneurysm) responsible for distal palmar and digital arterial occlusion (e.g., arterioarterial emboli). Magnified hand views are requested because microsurgical reconstruction techniques presently allow vein interposition grafting of small arteries, in carefully selected patients. Severely symptomatic individuals whose clinical or noninvasive laboratory investigations suggest significant proximal arterial obstruction should also undergo arteriography because revascularization in this group frequently results in the most gratifying and durable relief of RS symptoms.

The use of digital subtraction arteriographic techniques and nonionic contrast media has greatly improved small artery resolution, minimized contrast load, injection pain, hypersensitivity reactions, and nephrotoxicity. However, preangiographic crystalloid hydration and intravenous mannitol are believed to be useful in preventing risks of postangiographic small artery thrombosis and acute renal insufficiency, especially in the diabetic population.

Medical Treatment

Pharmacologic therapy is indicated in the small minority of patients for whom a 6 to 8 week trial of preventive measures provides incomplete palliation. The physician's decision to institute pharmacotherapy depends on the patient's severity of complaints, the underlying pathology of RS, and the complete understanding of potential adverse effects of medications. Numerous medications, both single and in combinations, have been used with reasonable success; however, all the sympatholytics, alpha-adrenergic blockers, beta-receptor agonists, vasodilators, and calcium channel blockers may create intolerable systemic reactions (see Table 2).

At present, most agree that the newer calcium channel blockers have yielded the greatest palliation with least toxicity when compared with previous medications (Rivers and Porter, 1987). The pharmacologic action of the slow channel blockers is smooth muscle relaxation by the selective inhibition of calcium influx into the cell. Nifedipine, having the most potent peripheral action, is presently considered the single agent of choice. The recommended starting dose of nifedipine is 10 mg orally three times a day, increasing to 20 mg orally three times a day in stepwise fashion as dictated by clinical response. The RS experience with the long-acting nifedipine preparation is presently limited; however, similarly favorable results with dosage convenience are anticipated. Diltiazem in oral doses of 90 to 180 mg per day is another leading choice of monotherapy with clinical responses that parallel those using nifedipine. Patients who remain refractory to nifedipine or diltiazem alone may benefit from the addition of prazosin, a specific alpha-adrenergic blocker; however, prazosin must be titrated in 1 mg increments every 7 to 10 days because of well-documented side effects of hypotension, palpitations, headache, dizziness, nausea, and fatigue. Another useful oral drug combination, which will rarely be required, is guanethidine (10 mg per day) with prazosin (1 to 3 mg per day). In general, palliative doses of either guanethidine or prazosin used alone are associated with intolerable side effects of impotence, fatigue, and orthostatic hypotension; therefore, these drugs are presently believed to be unsatisfactory single-agent choices for RS. Similarly, phenoxybenzamine has been followed by frequent orthostatic hypotension and has been abandoned as monotherapy for the treatment of RS.

Therapeutic responses to all medication regimens are judged clinically with the aim of reducing frequency and severity of RS attacks to tolerable levels without superimposing significant adverse effects. I have had no experience with the other proposed RS regimens listed in Table 2 but have included these medications for reader awareness of their possible effectiveness in RS patients.

Conservative management of digital ulcerations is usually successful in achieving complete secondary healing, despite the presence of underlying small-vessel occlusive disease. Limited surgical debridement of necrotic tissue with twice-daily gentle soap cleansing followed by topical antimicrobial application (1% silver sulfadiazine [Silvadene]) is a regimen that has proved successful.

Surgical Treatment

Arterial reconstruction should be reserved for those with angiographically documented large-vessel occlusive disease whose ischemic ulcers fail to heal with maximal conservative efforts or for those who suffer life-style–limiting claudication of the extremity. Rarely will reconstruction of remote radial, ulnar, or palmar arteries be necessary. Although cervicothoracic or lumbar sympathectomies are occasionally endorsed for medically refractory vasospastic RS, these procedures are virtually never indicated, particularly with the evolution and effectiveness of the slow channel calcium blockers.

Suggested Reading

Cardelli MB, Kleinsmith DM. Raynaud's phenomenon and disease. Med Clin North Am 1989; 73:1127.

Fitzgerald O, Hess EV, O'Connor GT. Prospective study of the evolution of Raynaud's phenomenon. Am J Med 1988; 84:718.

Jamieson GG, Ludbrook J, Wilson A. Cold hypersensitivity in Raynaud's phenomenon. Circulation 1971; 44:254.

Nielson SL, Lassen NA. Measurement of digital blood pressure after local cooling. J Appl Physiol 1977; 43:907.

Porter JM, Friedman EI, Mills JL. Occlusive and vasospastic diseases involving distal upper extremity arteries: Raynaud's syndrome. In: Rutherford RB, ed. Vascular surgery. Philadelphia: WB Saunders, 1989:844.

Priollet P, Vayssairat M, Housset E. How to classify Raynaud's phenomenon. Long-term follow-up study of 73 cases. Am J Med 1987; 83:494.

Raynaud M. On local asphyxia and symmetrical gangrene of the extremities (1862). New researches on the nature and treatment of local asphyxia of the extremities (1884). Translated by T. Barlow. In: Selected monographs, Vol 121. London: New Syndenham Society, 1988:1.

Rivers SP, Porter JM. Raynaud's syndrome, upper extremity vasospastic disorders, and small artery occlusive disease. In: Wilson SE, et al., eds. Vascular surgery. Principles and practice. New York: McGraw-Hill, 1987:696.

Sumner DS, Strandness DE. An abnormal finger pulse associated with cold sensitivity. Ann Surg 1972; 175:294.

ACUTE THROMBOPHLEBITIS

Joseph D. Ansley, M.D.

Acute thrombophlebitis is the clinical syndrome of venous thrombosis with or frequently without symptomatic inflammation of the superficial or deep venous systems of the extremities, neck, or occasionally the trunk. Etiologic mechanisms involve any physical or physiologic state that results in stasis of venous blood, injury to the vein wall, or hypercoagulability. The inflammatory reaction is most often noninfectious, but septic thrombophlebitis does occur secondary to intravenous lines, access procedures, or intravenous drug abuse.

The diagnosis of acute thrombophlebitis relies on the demonstration of occlusion of the venous system or inflammation of the vein and surrounding tissue. Swelling of the extremity, tenderness along the vein, or palpable venous cords may be noted on physical examination, but often symptoms are minimal, particularly in deep venous thrombosis. Clinical examination alone is not completely reliable, particularly for deep venous thrombosis; the examination should be augmented with tests for venous thrombosis including Doppler flow studies, venous plethysmography, venous duplex imaging, and radioisotope or contrast venography. Contrast venography remains the most definitive test and is recommended when placing the patient on a course of anticoagulation therapy for 3 to 6 months for deep venous thrombosis. Venous duplex imaging has become a good alternative when the study is done by experienced personnel and the findings are specific for venous thrombosis.

Therapeutic alternatives for nonseptic superficial thrombophlebitis include local warm compresses, elevation of the extremity for improved venous drainage, and nonsteroidal anti-inflammatory agents for symptomatic control in most cases. Surgical excision and ligation of the superficial venous system may be required for recurrent episodes of superficial thrombophlebitis associated with varicosities. Septic thrombophlebitis may require surgical excision and drainage when purulence is present; local warm compresses, elevation, removal of intravenous lines, and antibiotics are usually sufficient for nonpurulent cases. Deep venous thrombosis requires therapeutic anticoagulation, bed rest, and elevation of the involved extremities for 7 to 10 days, combined with oral anticoagulation therapy for 3 to 6 months in most cases. Some patients, particularly those with acute axillosubclavian vein thrombosis, may be candidates for thrombolytic therapy followed by anticoagulation therapy, and on rare occasions venous thrombectomy may be indicated.

■ THERAPEUTIC ALTERNATIVES

Medical and surgical treatments are available for the treatment of acute thrombophlebitis.

■ PREFERRED APPROACH

Medical Treatment

Management of acute thrombophlebitis is primarily medical; surgical intervention is required infrequently. Superficial thrombophlebitis not related to intravenous lines is managed by local warm compresses over the involved vein, elevation of the extremity if swelling is present, and the use of anti-inflammatory agents such as aspirin or ibuprofen if not contraindicated by a history of allergy or gastric irritation. Active exercise to increase venous flow is recommended if it does not increase discomfort. It is important to rule out concomitant deep venous thrombosis, which may be present in 10 to 15 percent of these patients, because the therapy for deep venous thrombosis requires more aggressive management with anticoagulation therapy and bed rest to decrease the risk of pulmonary embolization.

Septic thrombophlebitis requires the removal of intravenous lines when present, local warm compresses for comfort, elevation of the extremity, and antibiotics if the patient is febrile or has other evidence of sepsis. If purulence is present in the venous system, surgical consultation is necessary for consideration of excision and drainage of the involved vein.

Deep venous thrombosis is the most significant form of acute thrombophlebitis because of the associated complications of pulmonary thromboembolism, subsequent chronic venous insufficiency of the postphlebotic syndrome, and the possibility of venous gangrene with phlegmasia cerulea dolens (ileofemoral vein thrombosis) if early therapy with anticoagulation and elevation to reduce venous pressure is not effective.

Deep venous thrombosis of the lower extremities should be treated initially with full heparin anticoagulation therapy and bed rest with elevation of the lower extremities to increase venous drainage. Heparin should be given by continuous intravenous infusion after an initial bolus of 5,000 to 10,000 units. Adequate anticoagulation is obtained by prolonging the partial thromboplastin time (PTT) to 1.5 to 2 times the control value; for the average patient, approximately 1,000 to 1,200 units per hour is required but must be monitored by frequent PTT laboratory examinations and adjusted accordingly. Bed rest with elevation of the extremities by approximately 30 degrees should be continued until swelling and pain is controlled, which may take 7 to 10 days. Contraindications to anticoagulation therapy such as active gastrointestinal bleeding, recent intracranial or eye surgery, or bleeding disorders require individualized treatment with elevation of the extremity continued but consideration for prophylactic inferior vena cava interruption for thrombosis extending into the vena cava or the occurrence of pulmonary embolism.

Oral anticoagulation therapy with warfarin for 3 to 6 months is indicated for most patients with deep venous thrombosis to decrease the incidence of recurrence. The length of time varies, depending on the response to therapy and factors predisposing to recurrence such as immobility or associated disease. Warfarin therapy should be begun while the patient is on heparin therapy with a 5 to 7 day overlap to allow the protime to come into range and to preclude the potential thrombotic state that may occur because of the initial warfarin effect on protein C. Warfarin is begun at 10 mg per day and adjusted after several days when the protime is prolonged appropriately. The protime is used to control and monitor therapy, with prolongations of 1.3 to 1.5 the control value (15 to 18 seconds) effective in preventing the recurrence of thrombosis and less likely to be complicated by the bleeding that has been associated with the higher levels used in the past. If the International Normalized Ratio (INR) is used to monitor therapy, the INR should be 2.0 to 3.0.

Heparin therapy is associated with bleeding complications due to overcoagulation and to heparin-associated thrombocytopenia so that close monitoring is imperative. The PTT levels should be followed every 6 to 8 hours until stable and then daily after initial stabilization. A platelet count should be obtained every other day, and, if it falls below 100,000 cells per microliter, heparin should be discontinued and a platelet aggregation test for heparin-associated antibodies performed. With a positive test, platelet inhibition using aspirin at 300 mg twice a day or dextran solution at 20 ml per hour may be given until adequate oral anticoagulation is obtained.

Warfarin therapy is associated with bleeding if excessive prolongation of the protime occurs; therefore, proper monitoring is necessary, daily while hospitalized and then on a weekly basis as an outpatient. Skin necrosis secondary to warfarin therapy occurs in some patients and may require excision of involved areas and discontinuation of oral anticoagulation therapy. Adjusted-dose subcutaneous heparin may then be used to prevent thrombophlebitis recurrence with 10,000 to 15,000 units administered twice a day with monitoring to prolong the PTT by 15 seconds 6 hours following administration.

Surgical Treatment

Surgical treatment for acute deep vein thrombosis is necessary only when appropriate anticoagulation therapy is not effective or is contraindicated by a bleeding diathesis. Recurrent superficial thrombophlebitis may require vein ligation and stripping or excision. Septic thrombophlebitis may require excision and drainage when purulence is present or if sepsis persists despite antibiotic therapy. Ileofemoral venous thrombectomy may be indicated when impending venous gangrene occurs despite adequate anticoagulation and proper elevation of the extremity to reduce venous pressure. This procedure is associated with an increased morbidity and mortality and therefore is not widely accepted as appropriate therapy but may be indicated in selective patients.

Suggested Reading

Comerota AJ, Katz ML, Greenwald LL, et al. Venous duplex imaging: Should it replace hemodynamic test for deep venous thrombosis? J Vasc Surg 1990; 11:53.

Dalen JE, Paraskos JA, Ockene IS, et al. Venous thromboembolism: Scope of the problem. Chest 1986; 89:370S.

Lofgren EP, Lofgren KA. The surgical treatment of superficial thrombophlebitis. Surgery 1981; 90:49.

Machleder HI. The role of thrombolytic agents for acute subclavian vein thrombosis. Semin Vasc Surg 1992; 5:82.

Schafer AI. The hypercoagulable states. Ann Intern Med 1985; 102:814.

Silver D. Heparin induced thrombocytopenia and thrombosis. Semin Vasc Surg 1988; 1:228.

Wessler S, Gitel SN. Warfarin from bedside to bench. N Engl J Med 1984; 311:645.

ACUTE PULMONARY EMBOLISM

Carol M. Mason, M.D.
Warren R. Summer, M.D.

Acute pulmonary embolism (PE) affects 500,000 individuals yearly and is prominently found in 15–30% of all autopsy studies. Although the incidence of major embolism appears to be decreasing, the primary reason for its impact on mortality (30% in most series) is under diagnosis. Among patients who are diagnosed and treated, less than 5% die, and the majority of deaths have suspected recurrent PE. Clinically apparent embolism recurs in 8% of patients (Carson and co-workers, 1992) and has been attributed to delay in adequate anticoagulation.

The primary source of PE is from thrombi arising in deep veins of the lower extremities. If venous thrombosis can be diagnosed early or, better yet, prevented, PE is obviated. Thus, the initial focus should be on prevention. Unfortunately, U.S. physicians do not prescribe prophylaxis for the majority of their high-risk patients (Anderson and co-workers, 1992). The second strategy against thromboembolism is early recognition of patients at risk, accurate diagnosis, and prompt treatment. The final goal is long-term prophylaxis to prevent recurrence. Appropriate treatment is dictated by the physiologic impact of the embolus on the patient, the influence of concurrent disease, the initial risk of bleeding, and the occurrence of hemorrhagic complications. Approximately 25 percent of patients with PE die in 1 year. Most deaths are due to underlying diseases.

■ PREVENTION

It is generally believed that 90 percent of all PE originate from lower extremity deep venous thrombosis (DVT) (Moser, 1990). The most common sources are felt to be the proximal leg veins, including the iliofemoral and popliteal systems. Thrombi confined to the calf veins infrequently produce significant emboli, but 20 percent of these thrombi can propagate more proximally, posing a major threat for embolization.

The conventional view regarding prophylaxis is determined by a patient's risk for DVT. Any combination of venous stasis, vessel injury, and increased coagulation is associated with increased risk. These factors plus aging are probably additive in any combination. A patient with trauma to the lower extremity has venous injury, immobility, and increased coagulability, leading to very high risk. Similarly, hip replacement or hip fracture represents the highest risk category. High-risk patients also include those with cancer, those undergoing major surgery (general anesthesia time >30 minutes), and those with prolonged immobility, heart failure, or prior venous thrombosis. A list of moderate risk factors includes age over 70, obesity, or the use of estrogen-containing medications. A low risk would include a patient with minor (e.g., cataract or hand) surgery admitted for only 24 hours.

Several effective prophylactic options are available. We suggest the simplest and most cost-effective therapy in patients with medium risk. In patients at high risk two modalities are more effective than one, but combination prophylaxis is usually limited to special circumstances. The safest form of prophylaxis is the application of pneumatic compression devices to the lower extremities. These are best applied just before surgery or at the onset of hospitalization and continued until the patient is fully ambulatory. There are no associated complications. This modality is recommended for neurologic, urologic, ophthalmologic (retinal), and some orthopedic procedures (e.g., total knee replacement) in which any additional risk of bleeding posed by anticoagulants is problematic. Elastic stockings, although less costly and simpler, are less effective as a prophylactic modality. Additionally, to exert adequate graduated compression, they must be individually fitted, preventing early application.

Because we deal with large numbers of partially ambulatory medical patients (bathroom privileges) who are frequently transported around the hospital (numerous diagnostic tests), we rely primarily on "low-dose" heparin. This therapy is extremely effective and safe for medical patients. Our standard regimen is 5,000 units subcutaneously every 12 hours starting as soon as the patient is admitted to the hospital or intensive care unit. "Low-dose" unfractionated heparin (LDUH) is effective in most general surgical patients and is recommended for any predisposed group without substantial risk of hemorrhage. Ideally the first dose of heparin is administered as surgery commences. Low-molecular-weight heparin (LMWH) begun immediately after total hip replacement or fracture repair as enoxaparin 30 mg q12h is our preferred method of prophylaxis in this very high-risk group. Low-dose warfarin, also begun at the time of surgery (to keep the prothrombin time 1.25 to 1.5 times control), has been demonstrated to reduce the incidence of DVT in high-risk orthopedic procedures. However, this modality seems to be associated with a small risk of bleeding (≤5 percent). In patients with ischemic stroke and lower-extremity paralysis, LMWH appears superior to LDUH. We do not recommend prophylactic vena cava filters for hospitalized patients at high risk of DVT who are actively bleeding or at high risk of bleeding (pelvic and lower leg trauma, acute spinal cord injury), although this has been recommended by others. Common patient groups at moderate to high risk of thromboembolism and our recommended prophylaxes are listed in Table 1. The average estimated cost of providing prophylaxis for DVT in U.S. acute care hospitals is $50 to $100 per patient and is considered cost effective.

■ PREFERRED APPROACH

The therapy of PE can be divided into three categories: physiologic support, resolution of embolus, and prevention of recurrence (Table 2). Under most circumstances therapy is straightforward and effective. Although new emboli may

Table 1 Risk Groups for Venous Thromboembolism and Suggested Prophylaxis

PATIENT GROUP	INCIDENCE OF VENOUS THROMBOSIS (%)	INCIDENCE OF FATAL PULMONARY EMBOLISM (%)	SUGGESTED PROPHYLAXIS
Total hip replacement	40–70	1–2	Adjusted-dose heparin Low-dose warfarin; LMWH† Low-dose heparin*
Hip fracture	40–70	1–5	Any of the above
Total knee replacement	40–70	5	Pneumatic compression; LMWH
Urologic surgery	15–20	5	Pneumatic compression
General and gynecologic surgery	15–20	1	Low-dose heparin
Neurologic surgery	15–20	1	Pneumatic compression ES
Medical patients	15	1	Low-dose heparin*

LMWH, low-molecular-weight heparin; ES = elastic stocking
*Likely less effective
†Patients receiving outpatient anticancer therapy are at high risk for thrombosis and should receive low-dose warfarin to attain an INR 1.5.
†Patients with chronic central nervous catheters have less upper extremity thrombosis when warfarin 1 mg/d is used as prophylaxis.

Table 2 Treatment of Pulmonary Embolism

- Physiologic support
  - Hemodynamic
    - Fluid resuscitation
    - Vasodilators
    - Systemic vasoactive drugs
  - Respiratory
    - FiO_2
    - CPAP or PEEP
    - Bronchodilators
    - Mechanical ventilation
- Resolution of embolus
  - Thrombolytic therapy
  - Embolectomy
- Prophylaxis of recurrent embolization
  - Anticoagulation
  - Inferior vena cava interruption

CPAP, continuous positive airway pressure; PEEP, positive end-expiratory pressure.

occur during heparin administration, they are documented infrequently (< 9 percent). Although the majority of recurrences are not of major clinical significance (Girard and co-workers, 1987), they are associated with early death and are often clinically apparent in patients dying within 1 year. Of the 24 percent of patients who die within 1 year of an appropriately diagnosed and treated PE, at least half succumb due to severe underlying disease, expiring with, rather than because of, thromboemboli (Carson and co-workers, 1992).

Physiologic Support: Hemodynamic

The majority of emboli are not hemodynamically significant, although some disturbance in gas exchange (widened alveolar-arterial gradient) occurs in 90 percent of patients. Following a shower of emboli, both mechanical and humoral events result in a reduction in pulmonary vascular cross-sectional area and an increase in pulmonary vascular resistance (PVR). For pulmonary artery pressure (PAP) to rise significantly, the cross-sectional area must be extensively reduced (by 50 to 75 percent); most patients present with less extensive embolization and have normal or near-normal pressure measurements (mean PAP <25 mm Hg). With a significant increase in right ventricular afterload (mean PAP >30 to 40 mm Hg acutely), right ventricular ejection fraction decreases and right atrial pressure becomes elevated. Venous return decreases as right atrial pressure rises. This is the major reason for acute reduction in cardiac output (often resulting in syncope). To re-establish the appropriate gradient for venous return, mean systemic pressure must be increased. This is usually accomplished by peripheral and splenic venoconstriction, volume shifts, and fluid retention or administration. Recent data, however, have suggested that excess fluid infusion can reduce cardiac output, probably through the phenomenon of ventricular interdependence. An optimum goal for the management of hypotension with fluid administration is to adjust the right atrial filling pressure to approximately 8 to 10 mm Hg and no higher.

Pulmonary vasoconstriction has been demonstrated following emboli in numerous animal models and also in the clinical setting. Vasodilators can reduce elevated PVR but are rarely indicated. We have seen a few patients present with significant pulmonary hypertension, concurrent systemic hypertension, and combined left and right heart failure who responded to gentle vasodilator therapy with intravenous nitroprusside. With this therapy systemic and PVR decreased, cardiac output increased, and arterial oxygenation improved. The latter was due to improved mixed venous oxygen tension.

Physiologic Support: Treatment of Shock from Massive Pulmonary Embolism

Because increased pulmonary vascular resistance is the primary problem with massive embolism, isoproterenol has been recommended for embolic shock. Recently, it has been demonstrated that the use of noradrenaline results in a better hemodynamic profile than isoproterenol. Noradrenaline increases systemic arterial pressure, stroke volume, and cardiac output in postembolic shock without significant changes in PVR, renal blood flow, or creatinine clearance. Interestingly, right atrial pressures are lower with noradrenaline than with isoproterenol. Improved right ventricular function as a result of better coronary perfusion pressure is probably the mechanism initiating improved hemodynamics.

Physiologic Support: Respiratory

Hypoxemia is not an invariable feature of acute pulmonary embolism, although a decreased arterial oxygen tension PaO_2 and a widened alveolar-arterial oxygen gradient $P(A\text{-}a)O_2$ is common (90 percent). Abnormalities in gas exchange are due to (1) local areas of ventilation-perfusion ($\dot{V}/\dot{Q}$) mismatch caused by microatelectasis or macroatelectasis; (2) right-to-left intrapulmonary shunting; (3) reduced mixed venous oxygen tension secondary to reduced cardiac output; (4) rarely right-to-left intracardiac shunting due to opening of a patent foramen ovale. There is no straightforward relationship between the extent of vascular occlusion by the embolus and measured PaO_2. The arterial CO_2 tension ($PaCO_2$) is usually reduced because of hyperventilation in spite of the elevation in physiologic dead space. Pulmonary compliance also decreases and airway resistance is mildly increased.

Hypoxemia is usually relieved by increasing the inspired oxygen concentration (FIO_2). Fifty percent FIO_2 is usually satisfactory except following massive emboli. Tachypnea is not improved significantly by elevating the PaO_2. Improving any accompanying reduction in cardiac output with fluid infusion or vasoactive drugs reduces the peripheral tissue oxygen extraction and raises mixed venous oxygen tension. Patients who remain hypoxemic usually have large infarctions or collapse of unstable alveoli surrounding the embolized segments. Collapsed alveoli usually respond to increasing end-expiratory transpulmonary pressure, delivered as continuous positive airway pressure (CPAP) by mask or as positive end-expiratory pressure (PEEP) in those requiring mechanical ventilation.

In patients with massive embolism, extremely high minute ventilation may be necessary to overcome the large dead space produced by vascular obstruction. The combination of rapid shallow breathing, atelectasis, pleural effusion, pleurisy, increased dead space, and hypoperfusion may lead to ventilatory fatigue and hypercapnea. Patients with respiratory failure (refractory hypoxemia and/or hypercapnea) should be intubated and artificially ventilated. During the initiation of CPAP or artificial ventilation, adequate venous return and right atrial filling pressure should be ensured. Patients with audible wheezing or high peak airway pressures are given aerosolized $beta_2$-agonists to minimize airway resistance and optimize gas distribution.

Resolution of Embolus

In the presence of anticoagulation alone, emboli usually resolve slowly over days to weeks. In patients with underlying cardiopulmonary disease, resolution may take months and some patients never resolve thromboemboli. Thrombolytic therapy with streptokinase, urokinase, or recombinant tissue plasminogen activate (rt-PA) can increase the rate of resolution of emboli and lower PVR more rapidly than heparin. Major changes may be observed in hours. However, there are currently no studies demonstrating improved survival, shorter hospitalization, or better postembolus functional activity with thrombolytic treatment as compared with standard anticoagulation therapy. When properly administered, conventional anticoagulation is rarely associated with death, and PE recurs in only a small minority of patients. One week following treatment with either streptokinase or heparin, there are no differences noted in embolus resolution assessed with either angiography or lung scans.

Indications for thrombolytic therapy are massive emboli with shock or significant heart failure and hypotension. Patients with ventilation-perfusion defects involving more than 60 percent of the lung and severe hypoxemia may be candidates as well. The presence of major embolism and large or progressive iliofemoral thrombosis may benefit from thrombolytic therapy, usually with vena caval interruption. Currently streptokinase is given as a bolus of 250,000 units over 20 minutes followed by a continuous infusion of 100,000 units per hour for 24 hours. The thrombin time is measured prior to and 4 hours after initiating therapy to ensure activation of plasminogen and then repeated at 24 hours. It is not used to monitor therapeutic dosage.

Numerous variations are being examined to improve the effectiveness of thrombolytic therapy. We have given rt-PA as 50 mg over 2 hours followed by a repeat 50 mg over a second 2 hours with early reductions in PVR. Maintenance intravenous heparin is begun simultaneously at a rate of 1,000 units per hour and adjusted to maintain the activated partial thromboplastin time (APTT) at therapeutic levels after 24 hours. The repeat rt-PA dosing may not be required if significant hemodynamic improvement is observed. More recently front loading of rt-PA has been recommended with demonstrable superior resolution of emboli in experimental models. The best front-loading regimen remains to be determined but a combination of a 15 mg bolus followed by 50 mg over 30 minutes and then 35 mg over 30 to 60 minutes appears to be very effective. Alternatively, a 2 hour infusion of 100 mg rt-PA has been recommended. There is no evidence that rt-PA regimens are associated with fewer hemorrhagic complications or more clot-specific thrombolysis than streptokinase at this time.

The major problems with thrombolytic therapy are hemorrhagic complications. Bleeding is three times more common than with heparin therapy and may occur in 10 to 20 percent of cases. The high incidence of bleeding in patients with PE compared with acute myocardial infarction is due to the multiple associated underlying diseases in these patients. Also, the invasive studies recommended to confirm the presence of emboli prior to initiating thrombolytic therapy play a role. Without invasive studies, the risk of bleeding is substantially lower. However, at this time thrombolytic therapy can rarely be recommended without clot visualization. A positive Doppler study is sufficient to proceed in most cases, but pulmonary angiography is usually required. Absolute contraindications for thrombolysis are active internal bleeding, central nervous system vascular disease or surgery (within 2 months), or retinal and urologic surgery less than 48 hours previously. Numerous relative contraindications exist for possible hemorrhage and probably should obviate the use of thrombolytic therapy in all but desperate situations. Bleeding from puncture sites is to be expected, and long-term compression needs to be applied. If significant bleeding occurs, thrombolytic therapy is discontinued; if bleeding persists or is brisk, fresh frozen plasma should be administered. Rarely, cryoprecipitate or epsilon-aminocaproic acid may be necessary to stop hemorrhage. Other minor complications include

Table 3 Guidelines for Treatment of Pulmonary Embolism

THROMBOLYTIC THERAPY	
Indication:	Documented embolus on angiogram >60% vascular occlusion or hypotension requiring vasoactive drugs
Prior laboratory:	APTT, PT, platelets, and thrombin time
Dosage:	Streptokinase 250,000 U IV over 20–30 min followed by 100,000 U/h × 24 h rt-PA 50 mg over 2 h × 2; many new regimens under investigation
Monitor:	Thrombin time >1.5 × control 4 h after load and at 24 h (no adjustments in dosing based on this value) Fibrinogen levels <150 mg/dl or fibrin degradation products <400 mg/dl may be associated with increased risk of bleeding
Duration:	24 h; start heparin maintenance 2–4 h after stopping; thrombin time or APTT should be ≤1.5 × control
Complication:	Bleeding especially from puncture sites, allergic reactions (urticaria, itching, flushing), and fever Reperfusion pulmonary edema reported
Reversal:	Fresh frozen plasma or cryoprecipitate
ANTICOAGULATION	
Indication:	High probability V-Q lung scan or high clinical suspicion until studies available Occlusion >60% or shock with contraindication to thrombolytic therapy, add venous filter
Prior laboratory:	APTT, PT, and platelet count
Dosage:	100 U/kg loading dose of heparin over 10–20 min followed by maintenance of 20 U/kg/h. Use new bottle each 12 hours, may start with 5,000 U for suspected embolus and rebolus with 5,000 to 10,000 U after confirming diagnosis with test results. Large amounts of heparin are usually needed during first 24 h; then subsequently the dose is reduced
Monitor:	APTT at 4 h and every 24 h; maintain at 1.5–2 × control; hemoglobin and platelet count q.o.d.; urinalysis and stool for occult blood periodically
Duration:	Minimum of 2–3 days after achieving PT INR 2.0–3.0 (5-day course usually; 7–10 days if PE is massive)
Complication:	Bleeding, thrombocytopenia, thrombosis, hypersensitivity reaction
Reversal:	Protamine SO_4 1 mg IV for each 100 U of heparin in body Maximum at one time: 50 mg over 10 min
Warfarin	
Indication:	To follow heparin for long-term prophylaxis; a substitute for a nonhemorrhagic heparin reaction
Prior laboratory:	PT, APTT because this may interfere with PT if too high
Dosage:	Begin first 24 h after starting heparin at presumed maintenance dose: average 7 mg/day Early initiation may shorten hospitalization
Monitor:	PT and APTT until heparin stopped; keep PT INR 2.0–3.0
Duration:	First episode without ongoing risk—3 mo; use IPG to assess risk of recurrence First episode with ongoing risk—6 mo >2 episodes or continued risk (malignancy, protein C or S deficiency—indefinitely (consider venous filter)
Complication:	Bleeding, thrombosis due to early protein C deficiency hypercoagulable state (does not occur while adequately heparinized) Occult gastrointestinal or genitourinary bleeding should be investigated thoroughly
Reversal:	Fresh frozen plasma; vitamin K subcutaneously

APTT, activated partial thromboplastin time; PT, prothrombin time; U = units.

fever, pruritus, and nausea. We usually administer 40 mg of methylprednisolone with the streptokinase load to reduce possible allergic reactions.

In switching from streptokinase to heparin, the thrombolytic infusion is discontinued after 24 hours for approximately 2 to 3 hours, and then heparin is started as a maintenance infusion. A heparin load is not necessary. We always check a thrombin time immediately before beginning heparin to ensure that it is less than twice control. If the thrombin time returns higher, we slow the heparin infusion and repeat clotting studies. A summary of thrombolytic therapy appears in Table 3.

Embolectomy resolves vascular obstruction through the direct removal of central clots but is associated with very high mortality, depending on the patient's condition. Cardiopulmonary bypass is usually necessary. Embolectomy should be considered only in life-threatening situations where absolute contraindications to thrombolytic therapy exist. An inferior vena cava filter must be placed at the conclusion of embolectomy to prevent re-embolization in the early postoperative period. Anticoagulation should be instituted when the patient stabilizes, usually at 24 to 48 hours. Embolectomy for chronic unresolved pulmonary clots is recommended when persistent thrombi are associated with substantial pulmonary hypertension.

Prophylaxis

Anticoagulation has been the mainstay of therapy for thromboembolism since the introduction of heparin in the 1940s. It is now generally accepted that the majority of emboli originate in the lower extremities and that 70 percent of patients with emboli have residual venous thrombi (Moser, 1990). These residual thrombi are a potential source for recurrence in the majority of patients who experience an embolic event. Residual thrombi account for the fact that 90 percent of emboli are multiple and also for the widespread belief that death from emboli that occurs beyond the first several hours is due to recurrent embolic events. This concept dictates immediate prophylaxis, with full anticoagulation as the appropriate therapeutic choice in the vast majority of patients. Heparin does not directly prevent acute embolism or promote thrombus dissolution. Its efficacy lies in preventing thrombus growth and allowing a patient's thrombolytic system to be unopposed. Because early recurrence can still occur until remaining clot becomes organized, complete prophylaxis would include rapid anticoagulation and an inferior vena cava filter. This combination is a reasonable alternative to thrombolytic therapy in all but the most massive of emboli, and a viable alternative when thrombolytic therapy is absolutely or relatively contraindicated. Fortunately, complete prophylaxis is usually unnecessary; recurrent significant emboli are uncommon on full-dose heparin therapy.

Heparin is an acid mucopolysaccharide from porcine intestine or bovine lung. It is metabolized in the liver and excreted by the kidney. Therefore, lower maintenance dosing is reasonable in severely ill patients in shock, or those with liver and renal dysfunction. Heparin acts by promoting the binding of antithrombin III to thrombin and other clotting factors, inhibiting their function. In the absence of antithrombin III, heparin does not work, but this is a rare deficiency.

We believe that the best way to administer heparin is by a large intravenous bolus followed by a continuous infusion to maintain the APTT greater than 1.5 times the upper limit of control or a plasma heparin level of 0.2 to 0.4 U per milliliter. Failure to exceed this lower limit of therapeutic range is associated with an unacceptably high rate of recurrent venous thromboembolism. Intermittent adjusted-dose subcutaneous heparin is safe and as effective and less expensive in preventing recurrent lower extremity thrombosis (Hommes and co-workers, 1992). Fixed-dose LMWH has been reported to be as efficacious as continuous IV heparin for therapy of venous thrombosis (Leizorovicz and co-workers), and may allow early discharge home, improving the cost effectiveness of therapy (Koopman and co-workers; Levine and co-workers). Dose requirements must be individualized for each product (Lensing and co-workers, 1995), but the dose finding required with unfractionated heparin is eliminated.

Intermittent IV bolus heparin seems to result in more bleeding in some patient groups. Many patients are hypercoagulable prior to or immediately after an acute pulmonary embolus, in part due to nonspecific binding of unfractionated heparin by acute phase reactants and endothelium. This nonspecific binding of unfractionated heparin also makes dosing difficult and subject to change over time. As prevention of new clot formation as well as its detachment are the major goals of anticoagulant administration, it is imperative to reach therapeutic levels as rapidly as possible. Heparin continues to be underdosed clinically. The time to achieve adequate anticoagulation in many hospitals is 4 to 7 days, which is clearly unacceptable.

We immediately start heparin when reasonable suspicion exists that a patient has suffered an acute embolism, barring any significant contraindications to this therapy. Baseline laboratory studies include hemoglobin, platelet count, prothrombin time (PT), and APTT to ensure no underlying abnormality in the coagulation system. The initial load (bolus) should be sufficient to adequately anticoagulate the patient for at least 4 to 6 hours. For this reason we give at least 100 U per kilogram and often more, usually administering a minimum of 7,500 units and frequently giving an initial 10,000 units. Evidence that initial "overanticoagulation" is dangerous has not been documented. The bolus is followed by an infusion at 20 units per kilogram per hour or 1,400 units per hour in the average 70 kg man. Some authorities recommend administering 40,000 U per 24 hours to all subjects not at increased risk of bleeding (Hull and co-workers, 1992). Weight-based nomogram dosing of heparin may assure early adequacy of anticoagulation and simplify dose adjustments (Gunnarsson and co-workers, 1995). Administration by the subcutaneous route requires similar daily amounts of heparin in three divided doses. This is usually preceded by IV bolus of 7,500 to 10,000 units. Patients with a history of peptic ulcer disease, surgery within the previous 2 weeks, present stroke, hepatic disease, or history of urinary tract bleeding are given a 24 hour maintenance dose of 30,000 units. The APTT should be checked 4 to 6 hours after the loading dose is given and the maintenance infusion begun, and followed daily thereafter. It is used to monitor therapy and should be kept between 1.5 (the minimum effective dose) and 2 times the upper limit of control value. Although the APTT is not a direct measurement of the true antithrombotic effect of heparin, it is the best available guide at present unless plasma heparin levels are available in your institution. However, during a continuous infusion a single value may not accurately reflect the preceding 24 hours' level of anticoagulation as a result of diurnal variations in heparin binding. With this loading and maintenance regimen we almost always achieve adequate initial anticoagulation at 4 to 6 hours.

The half-life of heparin is approximately 1.5 hours, so by 4 to 6 hours after the loading dose the APTT is close to a steady-state level. Any interruption in heparin infusion for more than 2 hours will cause large APTT reductions. Knowledge of this short half-life is critical in preventing wide swings in anticoagulation and risk of renewed thrombosis. Furthermore, if APTT levels return subtherapeutic (<1.5 times control) a 3,000 to 4,000 U bolus is given, along with an increased maintenance infusion rate.

Warfarin (10 mg) is begun on the night of admission if the patient is not critically ill and given each subsequent evening; dosing adjustments are made as the PT begins to rise. The average daily warfarin dose is 7.5 mg with large individual variations. However, with daily monitoring, there is little chance of severe overdosing beginning with a 10 mg dose, and this regimen usually ensures reasonable anticoagulation for timely discharge in 7 to 10 days. Heparin is stopped after the patient's PT has been stable at an INR of 2.0 to 3.0 for at least 2 to 3 days.

The major complications of heparin anticoagulation include bleeding, thrombocytopenia, arterial thrombosis, hypersensitivity reactions, and osteoporosis. Significant hemorrhage occurs in approximately 6 percent of patients and is best predicted by concurrent illness (Landefeld and co-workers, 1987) (Table 4). In spite of a relative lack of major bleeding with heparin, approximately 20 percent of patients experience a fall in hemoglobin (Hyers and co-workers, 1989). There is no association between supratherapeutic APTT responses and bleeding. Heparin effects may be reversed by the administration of protamine sulfate. The recommended dose is 1 mg of protamine for every 100 U of heparin estimated to be in the body. No more than 50 mg

Table 4 Predictors of Major Bleeding During Heparin Therapy

Age >60 yr
Cardiac disease with acute myocardial infarction or systolic blood pressure <90 mm Hg
Liver disease with bilirubin >1 mg/dl
Renal insufficiency with creatinine >1.5 mg/dl
Cancer
Anemia (Hct <30%)
Recent surgery

should be given at one time, and it must be given slowly over 10 minutes. Excess protamine acts as an anticoagulant and can actually cause additional bleeding.

Thrombocytopenia and rarely arterial thrombi may occur during heparin therapy. These phenomena usually occur after 5 or 6 days of heparin administration but may occur earlier if heparin has been previously administered. Ensuring an early adequate PT with warfarin allows heparin to be stopped if heparin-associated thrombocytopenia should occur. This infrequent complication of heparin therapy (1 to 2 percent) cannot be effectively predicted except by monitoring platelet levels periodically. Heparin should be discontinued if the platelet count falls below 75,000 per cubic millimeter. Switching from bovine to porcine heparin or vice versa is not an established safety maneuver in the presence of worrisome thrombocytopenia, although each has its advocates. Substituting LMWH may be associated with less risk of thrombocytopenia (Warkentin, 1995). If heparin must be discontinued and warfarin anticoagulation is not yet therapeutic, a venous filter should be considered. A review of heparin therapy is outlined in Table 3.

Surgical Prophylaxis

Surgical prophylaxis is indicated for failure of anticoagulation (recurrent emboli in spite of adequate APTT), significant concurrent bleeding, or other contraindication to anticoagulation (prior severe heparin-associated thrombosis). Patients with life-threatening emboli or high risk of both thromboembolism and bleeding (pelvic fracture and lower extremity trauma) may also benefit from prophylactic venous interruption.

A Greenfield filter is the device currently recommended for venous interruption. It is usually inserted percutaneously via the right internal jugular vein into the inferior vena cava. The filter is usually positioned distal to the renal veins and proximal to the iliac veins but its ultimate positioning depends on the proximal extension of clot. Although patency does not require concurrent anticoagulation, for those patients with filters placed because of heparin or warfarin failure, anticoagulation is usually continued for a minimum of 3 to 6 months. Complications are infrequent (<6 percent) and include local venous thrombosis (usually when inserted through a femoral vein), inferior vena cava perforation, and filter migration. When migration occurs, the filter traverses the vena cava and may rarely lodge in the heart or pulmonary arteries, requiring surgical removal. Exacerbation of distal venous stasis is rare and should be managed by graduated-pressure elastic stockings.

Long-Term Anticoagulation

Heparin should be continued for a minimum of 5 to 7 days, although the optimum duration has not been determined. Heparin anticoagulation should overlap therapeutic warfarin anticoagulation for 2 to 3 days. The PT risk should be kept between 2.0 and 3.0 (see Table 3). The risk of bleeding on warfarin is only 5 percent but tends to remain at that level throughout the period of anticoagulation. Serious bleeding is treated with fresh frozen plasma after the anticoagulant is stopped. Occult bleeding from the genitourinary or gastrointestinal tract is managed by stopping therapy. However, occult bleeding is frequently associated with the presence of underlying disease and should be carefully evaluated. Therapy is usually continued for 3 to 6 months. An initial episode of thromboembolism may be treated for only 1 month if an impedance plethysmography study demonstrates no residual venous obstruction at that time. A second episode of DVT or embolism should be treated a full 6 months. Patients with more than two episodes of thromboembolism require indefinite anticoagulation.

Suggested Reading

Anderson A, Brownell W, Goldberg R, et al. The prevalence of risk factors for venous thromboembolism among hospital patients. Arch Intern Med 1992; 152:1660–1664.

Carson J, Kelley M, Duff A, et al. The clinical course of pulmonary embolism. N Engl J Med 1992; 326:1240–1245.

Clagett GP, Anderson FA Jr, Heit J, et al. Prevention of venous thromboembolism. Chest 1995; 108(Suppl 4):312S–334S.

deBoisblanc BP. Treatment of massive pulmonary embolism. Clin Pulmonary Med 1995; 2:353–358.

Girard P, Mathieu M, Simonneau G, et al. Recurrence of pulmonary embolism during anticoagulant treatment: A prospective study. Thorax 1987; 42:481.

Gunnarsson PS, Sawyer WT, Montague D, et al. Appropriate use of heparin: Empiric vs. nomogram-based dosing. Arch Int Med 1995; 155:526.

Hommes DW, Bura A, Mazzolai L, et al. Subcutaneous heparin compared with continuous heparin administration in the initial treatment of deep venous thrombosis. Ann Intern Med 1992; 116:279.

Hull R, Raskob G, Rosenbloom D, et al. Optimal therapeutic level of heparin therapy in patients with venous thrombosis. Arch Intern Med 1992; 152:1589–1595.

Hyers TM, Hull RD, Weg JG. Antithrombotic therapy for venous thromboembolic disease. Chest 1995; 108(Suppl 4):335S–351S.

Koopman MMW, et al. Treatment of venous thrombosis with intravenous unfractionated heparin administered in the hospital as compared with subcutaneous low-molecular-weight heparin administered at home. N Engl J Med 1996; 334:682.

Landefeld CS, Cook EF, Flatley M, et al. Identification and preliminary validation of predictors of major bleeding in hospitalized patients starting anticoagulant therapy. Predictors of who might bleed during anticoagulation. Am J Med 1987; 82:703.

Leizorovicz A, Simonneau G, Decousus H, Boissel JP. Comparison of efficacy and safety of low molecular weight heparins and unfractionated heparin in initial treatment of deep venous thrombosis: a meta-analysis. Brit Med J 1994; 309:299–304.

Lensing AW, Prins MH, Davidson BL, Hirsh J. Treatment of deep venous thrombosis with low-molecular-weight heparins: a meta-analysis. Arch Intern Med 1995; 155:601–607.

Levine M, et al. A comparison of low-molecular-weight heparin administered primarily at home with unfractionated heparin administered in the hospital for proximal deep-vein thrombosis. N Engl J Med 1996; 334:677–681.

Mohr DN, Ryr JH, Litin SC, Rosenow EC III. Recent advances in the management of venous thromboembolism. Mayo Clin Proc 1988; 63:281.

Moser KM. State of the art. Venous thromboembolism. Am Rev Respir Dis 1990; 141:235.

Stein PD, Alavi A. A collaborative study by the PIOPED investigators. Tissue plasminogen activator for the treatment of acute pulmonary embolism. Chest 1990; 97:528.

Warkentin TE, Levine MN, Hirsh J, et al. Heparin-induced thrombocytopenia in patients treated with low-molecular-weight heparin or unfractionated heparin. N Engl J Med 1995; 332:1330–1335.

Welch TJ, Stanson AW, Sheedy PF, et al. Percutaneous placement of the Greenfield vena caval filter. Mayo Clin Proc 1988; 63:343.

VENOUS THROMBOSIS AND USE OF ANTICOAGULANTS

Clive Kearon, M.B., M.R.C.P.I., F.R.C.P.C., Ph.D.

Jack Hirsh, M.D., F.R.C.P.C.

Pulmonary embolism (PE) is the most common preventable cause of death in hospitalized patients. Yet fewer than one-third of patients who die of this condition are diagnosed ante mortem. It is now recognized that PE and deep vein thrombosis (DVT) are not distinct entities but different manifestations and stages of the same process; venous thrombosis almost invariably starts in the lower limbs and after extending proximally to involve the larger veins, commonly detaches to cause PE. Consequently, prevention of PE is achieved by preventing or treating DVT in the legs, and anticoagulation for the two conditions does not differ. Recognizing the inseparable relationship between PE and DVT, the term *venous thromboembolism* (VTE) has been adopted for these conditions, either singly or in combination. Because PE is rarely preceded by signs and symptoms of DVT, primary prophylaxis is by far the most effective way to reduce PE mortality in hospitalized patients.

■ PREVENTION

Without prophylaxis the frequency of postoperative PE ranges from 0.1 to 0.8 percent for elective general surgery, to 0.3 to 1.7 percent for elective hip surgery, and 4 to 7 percent for emergency hip surgery. Immobilized medical patients are also at high risk for VTE, particularly if their underlying condition is associated with paralysis (e.g., stroke). A number of patient-, disease-, and surgery-specific risk factors have been identified, allowing an individual's risk of developing VTE to be established (Table 1).

Table 1 Risk Factors for VTE

Patient Factors
Previous VTE*
Age over 40
Pregnancy, puerperium
Varicose veins
Marked obesity
Underlying Condition
Malignancy*
Cancer chemotherapy
Paralysis*
Prolonged immobility
Major trauma
Lower limb injuries*
Familial hypercoagulable state
Type of Surgery
Lower limb orthopedic surgery*
General anesthesia >30 min

*Common major risk factors for VTE
Combinations of factors have at least an additive effect on the risk of VTE.

The appropriate method of prophylaxis varies according to the risk of VTE and to a lesser extent with the patient's underlying condition. Prophylaxis is directed either at suppressing coagulability or preventing venostasis. This can be achieved by using any one of the following proven prophylactic approaches: low-dose subcutaneous heparin, intermittent pneumatic compression of the legs, intravenous dextran, oral anticoagulants, adjusted doses of subcutaneous heparin, graduated compression stockings, and low molecular-weight heparins (LMWHs). Antiplatelet agents such as aspirin are relatively ineffective for preventing VTE and should not be used as the sole agent for this purpose.

Patients without any risk factors are considered to be at low risk for VTE, and early postoperative ambulation is generally considered adequate prophylaxis. An approach to VTE prophylaxis for patients at moderate or high risk is shown in Table 2. Despite improvements, the efficacy of VTE prophylaxis for the highest-risk patients remains less than ideal; close to 20 percent of patients develop DVT following major orthopedic surgery despite receiving optimum prophylaxis with LMWH, and approximately a third of these clots involve the proximal veins.

■ DIAGNOSIS

Deep Vein Thrombosis

It is well recognized that the clinical diagnosis of DVT is unreliable and that objective testing is therefore required to establish this diagnosis; nonetheless, clinical evaluation is still valuable. Clinical assessment can arouse suspicion as to the presence of DVT; it can identify an alternative explanation for symptoms in patients in whom DVT is being considered; and depending on the clinical assessment of probability of DVT

Table 2 Recommended Prophylaxes for Different Risk Categories and Surgical Groups

RISK CATEGORY	RECOMMENDED APPROACHES* (RISK REDUCTION 50–75%)
Moderate Risk (DVT rates)	
General surgery or major medical illness (~20%)	Low-dose heparin or intermittent compression
Neurologic or genitourinary surgery (~20%)	Intermittent compression
High Risk†	
Malignant disease or previous VTE (~30%)	Adjusted-dose heparin, oral anticoagulants, or LMWH
Major knee surgery (~60%)	LMWH or intermittent compression
Fractured hip or elective hip (~50%)	LMWH or oral anticoagulants

*When possible graduated compression can be added to all other forms of prophylaxis
†Low-molecular-weight heparin (LMWH) may become the prophylactic method of choice

(i.e., unlikely, possible, highly likely) it can complement the findings of noninvasive testing. Venography remains the diagnostic standard for DVT and is the only reliable method of diagnosing isolated calf vein thrombosis; however, it is not an ideal initial test because of its invasive nature, technical demands, costs, and the risk associated with contrast media.

Major advances have been made in developing noninvasive tests for the diagnosis of DVT, particularly with the use of impedance plethysmography (IPG) and venous ultrasonography (VUS). It is now recognized that the diagnostic accuracy of both IPG and VUS is influenced by the extent of the DVT and the clinical circumstances under which testing is performed. The extent of DVT is commonly categorized according to whether thrombosis is confined to the calf (calf DVT) or involves the popliteal or more proximal veins, with or without calf vein involvement (proximal DVT). The circumstances under which diagnostic testing for DVT is performed can be broadly categorized according to whether patients present for evaluation of symptoms that are suggestive of DVT (symptomatic DVT) or if testing is being performed in patients at high risk for having asymptomatic DVT (e.g., following orthopedic surgery). Over 80 percent of symptomatic outpatients with DVT are found to have proximal clots, but this proportion is generally less than 20 percent in asymptomatic inpatients. The extent of DVT, the circumstances of presentation, and the presence of symptoms are closely interrelated.

Both IPG and VUS are poor (sensitivity approximately 20 percent for IPG and 50 percent for VUS) at detecting isolated calf vein DVT, regardless of the presence or absence of symptoms. As calf vein clots rarely cause clinically important PEs, this is only a relative limitation of these noninvasive tests. However, there remains the possibility that patients with suspected DVT and no evidence of DVT on IPG or VUS may have calf vein or small proximal clot that will subsequently extend. Consequently, follow-up examinations are performed if the initial examination is normal. An approach to the diagnosis of proximal DVT in symptomatic and asymptomatic patients is outlined subsequently.

Symptomatic Patients

IPG. Studies performed in the 1970s and 1980s found that IPG was both sensitive (94 percent) and specific (95 percent) for diagnosing proximal DVT as assessed by venography. In addition, it was shown to be safe to withhold anticoagulants from patients with suspected DVT who had negative IPGs, provided serial IPGs were performed over a 2 week period to allow detection and treatment of calf vein thrombi should they extend into the proximal system. However, recent studies suggest that sensitivity of the IPG for proximal DVT is considerably lower than that found in the early studies. Some features of the earlier studies may have contributed to an overly optimistic estimate of sensitivity, but it seems most likely that, particularly in centers which have established convenient noninvasive diagnostic facilities for VTE, the spectrum of DVTs at presentation may have shifted to smaller and less occlusive clots, which are less readily detected by IPG. With heightened physician awareness of the risks of VTE, our experience is that a smaller proportion of patients who are referred for assessment for possible DVT are found to have it. The reduced sensitivity and specificity of the IPG for proximal DVT, coupled with a lower prevalence of the condition has altered the positive predictive value of this test. We estimate that the IPG now has a sensitivity of 85 percent and a specificity of 90 percent for detecting proximal DVT in symptomatic patients. If the prevalence of proximal DVT is 25 percent, the positive predictive value of the IPG will be 74 percent and the negative predictive value 95 percent. Confirmatory venography or VUS, therefore, should be performed in patients with suspected DVT and an abnormal IPG, to avoid the unnecessary anticoagulating of about one-quarter of these patients.

Clinical assessment of the probability of DVT based on clinical presentation and the presence or absence of associated risk factors for VTE can stratify patients into high and low prevalence categories prior to noninvasive testing. We have found that 85 percent of patients thought to have a high clinical suspicion of DVT have thrombosis, and 5 percent or fewer of patients who have a low clinical suspicion of DVT are found to have thrombosis at venography. Preliminary results suggest that combining clinical assessment of probability of DVT with the results of IPG improves diagnostic accuracy to a clinically important extent. In patients with a high clinical suspicion of DVT, an abnormal IPG had a positive predictive value of 95 percent, but a normal IPG had a negative predictive value of only 41 percent. Conversely, in patients with a low clinical suspicion of DVT, an abnormal IPG had a positive predictive value of only 27 percent, but a normal IPG had a negative predictive value of 98 percent. In addition to the influence of clinical assessment on prevalence, sensitivity of the IPG for proximal DVT may be higher in patients assigned a high clinical probability of disease, as large occlusive clots are expected with greater clinical manifestations. In summary, IPG can usually be relied on to direct management provided

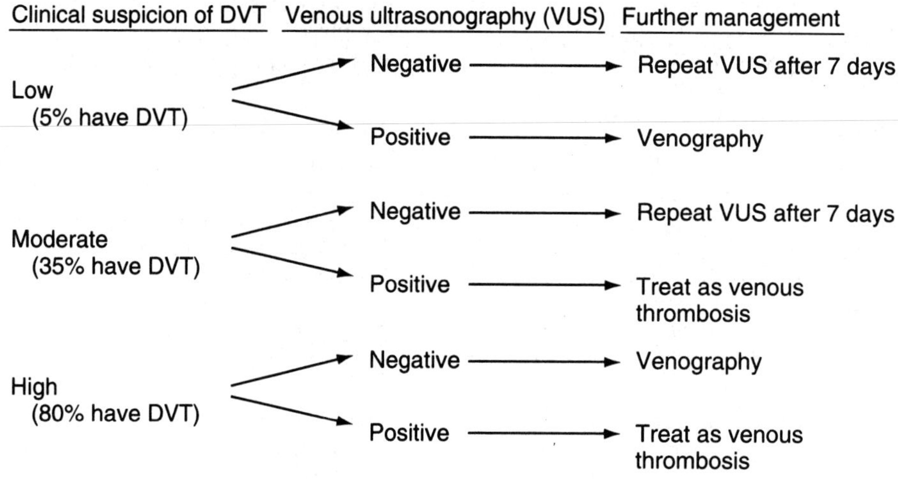

Figure 1
Approach to the diagnosis of venous thrombosis.

the clinical assessment and the IPG are in agreement, but when these two evaluations are discordant, further testing (e.g., VUS or venography) should be undertaken.

Venous Ultrasonography. VUS is becoming accepted as the noninvasive test of choice for diagnosing symptomatic proximal DVT. There are a number of techniques available vary in complexity and cost, ranging from real-time B-mode imaging alone to imaging techniques coupled with spectral and/or color imaging of flow. Current evidence suggests that for symptomatic proximal DVT, little if any diagnostic accuracy is gained by adding to real-time B-mode imaging. Furthermore, the single finding of inability to compress completely the common femoral and/or popliteal veins with the application of gentle ultrasound probe pressure appears to be the most reliable diagnostic criterion. Justification for confining ultrasonographic examination to the common femoral and popliteal veins is that the deep venous system is relatively superficial at these sites, which facilitates visualization and assessment of venous compressibility, and that isolated thrombosis of the superficial femoral vein without either popliteal or common femoral vein involvement very rarely occurs in symptomatic patients. An overview of studies that compared VUS with venography yields an overall sensitivity and specificity of 95 percent for proximal DVT. Assuming a prevalence of 25 percent, this translates to a positive predictive value of 92 percent and a negative predictive value of 99 percent, appreciably better than for IPG in this setting. However, corresponding to the analysis performed for the IPG, a positive predictive value lower than this will be obtained in patients in whom DVT is considered unlikely following clinical assessment. We perform confirmatory venography in patients with a low clinical suspicion of DVT and abnormal VUS.

Because neither IPG nor VUS is sensitive at detecting calf vein DVT, a normal initial test should be followed up with repeat examinations to detect proximal extension. This is particularly important for IPG, as the rate of conversion from normal to abnormal during a week of follow-up is more than twice as great as that seen with repeat ultrasonography during the same interval. The probable explanation for this is that repeat IPG testing, in addition to detecting proximal extension of calf DVT, also picks up smaller nonocclusive proximal DVTs that were missed at the first examination and that have extended to cause greater obstruction of venous outflow.

We consider VUS (assessment of venous compressibility) to be the noninvasive test of choice for the diagnosis of deep venous thrombosis (Fig. 1). If the patient is considered to have a moderate or high clinical suspicion of DVT and the VUS is abnormal, we accept this as evidence of deep venous thrombosis and treat accordingly. If there is a low clinical suspicion of DVT but VUS findings are abnormal, we perform confirmatory venography. If the clinical suspicion of DVT is low or moderate, we accept a negative VUS examination as excluding proximal DVT but perform a follow-up examination a week later to exclude interval proximal extension. If the clinical suspicion of DVT is high and the VUS is negative, we usually perform venography to exclude a false-negative test or isolated calf clot. While a strong argument can be made that the combination of a low clinical probability of DVT and an initial normal ultrasound examination do not require a follow-up assessment, this approach to management has yet to be tested in clinical practice.

If IPG is more readily accessible than VUS, it is reasonable to make management decisions on the basis of combined clinical and IPG assessment, provided the two are in agreement.

Asymptomatic Patients

Certain clinical situations are associated with a sufficiently high risk of DVT that screening for it may be warranted. The most important group to fall into this category are patients who have undergone major lower limb orthopedic surgery who, despite appropriate prophylaxis, have a high residual incidence of DVT. Recent studies have established that the diagnostic accuracy of noninvasive tests (e.g., IPG and VUS) for DVT is much lower in asymptomatic patients than in patients with symptomatic DVT. While most of these patients are found to have calf rather than proximal DVT, this alone does not account for the poor diagnostic yield of noninvasive testing in asymptomatic patients. Of greater clinical importance is that noninvasive tests also have a much lower sensitivity for proximal clots when they occur in asymptomatic postoperative patients. This is probably due to a higher proportion of smaller proximal thrombi, many of which do not fully occlude the vein and can be difficult to locate with VUS.

The sensitivity of the IPG for proximal DVT in asymptomatic patients is approximately 15 percent, with a specificity of about 98 percent. If the prevalence of proximal DVT in these patients is 10 percent, an abnormal IPG will have a positive predictive value of only 47 percent and a negative predictive value of 91 percent. Because these values are low, we recommend that the IPG not be used for surveillance testing in high-risk asymptomatic patients.

VUS, although better than IPG, still has marked limitations in these patients, with a sensitivity for proximal clots of approximately 60 percent and a specificity of around 97 percent. Given a 10 percent prevalence, this translates to a positive predictive value of 69 percent and negative predictive value of 96 percent. Consequently, for these patients, abnormal VUS requires confirmatory venography to avoid inappropriately anticoagulating the 3 out of 10 patients who will have false-positive tests. Given these limitations, and our recent experience that proximal DVT is very rarely detected by predischarge VUS in asymptomatic orthopedic patients who have received appropriate prophylaxis, we no longer perform routine surveillance testing.

Recurrent DVT

The diagnosis of recurrent DVT is difficult, requiring that current abnormalities on diagnostic testing be established as new, which often calls for comparison with previous tests. The change of a normal to an abnormal IPG, a new noncompressible site on ultrasonography, or a new intraluminal filling defect on venography reliably establishes recurrence. In the absence of a previous venogram for comparison, any intraluminal filling defect is accepted as evidence of recurrence provided that the last episode was not recent. When abnormalities of these tests persist from previous episodes of thrombosis, fibrinogen leg scanning may be diagnostic, but this test is not widely available. In some patients, the results of objective tests are inconclusive, and a final decision to treat or not may have to be made on clinical grounds.

A recent study suggests that measurements of residual thrombus mass, as assessed by the diameter of residual thrombus under full compression at the common femoral and popliteal sites, may be both sensitive and specific for diagnosing recurrence of DVT. To apply this method of assessing for recurrent DVT, a quantitative assessment of vein compressibility must have been performed on at least one occasion 3 months following initial diagnosis to determine baseline measurements. This approach to evaluating suspected recurrent DVT has yet to be validated by other investigators and by management studies.

Pulmonary Embolism

Clinical Evaluation

A PE is suspected initially because of clinical findings. Although the clinical manifestations of PE are often nonspecific, it is generally possible to classify patients as highly likely, possible, or unlikely to have PE on clinical grounds (prior probabilities). We believe that the essential components of such an evaluation should include an assessment of risk factors for VTE, evaluation of symptoms and signs, and interpretations of preliminary investigations (e.g., chest radiograph and electrocardiogram). We suggest the following guidelines for assigning either a highly likely or unlikely clinical probability for PE on the basis of these findings. Patients who do not fall into either of these categories are considered possible or uncertain.

Highly Likely Clinical Probability. PE is considered highly likely if the clinical features suggest PE, the patient has one or more risk factors for VTE, and there is no apparent alternative cause for the clinical manifestations.

Unlikely Clinical Probability. PE is considered unlikely if an alternative explanation for the clinical manifestation, is considered as, or more likely if clinical features are atypical, and if the patient has no risk factors for VTE.

Two large prospective studies that incorporated routine pulmonary angiography found PE in 70 to 80 percent of patients in whom the clinical suspicion of PE was highly likely; 30 to 40 percent of patients with a clinical suspicion of possible or uncertain, and 10 to 15 percent of patients with a clinical suspicion of unlikely.

Objective Testing

Because the clinical features of PE are nonspecific, objective testing to confirm or exclude acute VTE is required in patients in whom PE is considered. The diagnostic approach is influenced by the availability of investigations at the time of presentation and by the urgency of the situation. In most patients, the diagnostic process can be performed sequentially. However, heparin treatment should be commenced before the diagnosis is confirmed if there is a high clinical suspicion of PE, particularly if major embolism is suspected or when confirmatory objective tests cannot be performed quickly. The only test that can confirm a PE with certainty is the pulmonary angiogram, which is invasive, not readily available, difficult to interpret and often difficult to perform, particularly in the sickest patients. Because of these limitations, use of pulmonary angiography is usually confined to patients who after clinical assessment and noninvasive testing are still considered to have a moderate probability of having had an acute PE, particularly if underlying cardiopulmonary compromise places them at increased risk if the diagnosis of PE is missed.

Lung Scanning. Perfusion scanning is the pivotal investigation in the diagnostic workup of patients with PE, because it is relatively simple and because it can be used to rule out PE when the result is completely normal. Although the perfusion scan is highly sensitive for PE, it is nonspecific: most perfusion defects are produced by conditions other than PE. Although the specificity of perfusion scanning is improved by classifying the defects according to their size and number, the positive predictive value remains inadequate for making decisions in individual patients; only 70 percent of patients with one or more segmental or larger perfusion defects have PE at pulmonary angiography.

Table 3 Combination of Clinical Assessments and Lung Scan Patterns

STUDY	CLINICAL SUSPICION	LUNG SCAN PATTERN	NUMBER (%)‡	PE BY ANGIOGRAPHY
Hull et al. (175 patients)	Highly likely	High probability	56 (32)	96%
	Uncertain	High probability		80%
	Unlikely	Low probability*	16 (9)	5–9%
	Other combinations		103 (59)	11–71%
PIOPED (887 patients)	Highly likely	High probability	29 (3)	96%
	Possible	High probability	80 (9)	88%
	Low	Low probability	90 (10)	4%
	All three†	Normal or near normal	128 (14)	4%
	Other combinations		560 (63)	16–56%

*Segmental match, subsegmental match, indeterminate.
†All three categories of clinical suspicion.
‡Percent of total evaluable patients in each study.

Ventilation scanning was introduced in the hope that it would differentiate between perfusion defects secondary to regional hypoxia, when a matched abnormality is expected on the ventilation scan, and those due to PE, when normal ventilation is expected (mismatched defect). Studies have shown that a normal ventilation scan improves the specificity of an abnormal perfusion scan to a clinically useful degree when the perfusion defect is segmental or larger (high-probability scan), but that it has limited value when perfusion defects are smaller than this.

Two large prospective studies have shown that combining the clinical assessment of probability of having PE with ventilation-perfusion scanning improves diagnostic accuracy and allows a management decision (i.e., to treat or not to treat for VTE) to be reached in one-third to two-thirds of patients referred for evaluation of PE. The proportion of patients with different combinations of clinical assessments and lung scan patterns who had PE confirmed by angiography is shown in Table 3. In the Hull study, clinical assessment of probability was based on clinical impression, ECG, chest x-ray film, and the results of IPG in patients with abnormal (about 60 percent of total referrals) perfusion scans. In the PIOPED study, clinical assessment was based on ECG, chest x-ray film, and arterial blood gases in patients with abnormal perfusion scans (over 90% of total referrals).

Testing for occult DVT in the legs of patients with suspected PE is of great value when managing patients who have nondiagnostic combinations of clinical and lung scanning assessments.

A Practical Approach to the Diagnosis of PE

An algorithm for the diagnosis of clinically suspected PE is shown in Figure 2. If PE is still considered possible after a history, physical examination, electrocardiogram, and chest roentgenogram have been performed, the patient should undergo ventilation-perfusion lung scanning. In approximately half of these patients the combination of clinical assessment and lung scanning will either rule in or rule out PE with an acceptable degree of confidence, directing management without the need for further investigation. For practical purposes, the finding of a normal or near-normal perfusion scan rules out PE. With a lesser but still adequate degree of confidence, the diagnosis of PE can also be considered excluded by the combination of a low clinical and a low lung scan probability of PE.

The diagnosis of PE can be considered established in patients with a high probability scan with either high or uncertain (possible) clinical probabilities. With all other combinations of clinical and lung scan probabilities, PE cannot be ruled in or ruled out with an acceptable degree of confidence to justify either starting or withholding anticoagulation. Objective testing for DVT is performed in these patients.

Noninvasive testing with IPG or VUS to detect associated DVT is expected to be abnormal in close to 50 percent of patients who have symptomatic PE. The proportion of PE patients with detectable DVT increases to 70 percent if bilateral ascending venography is performed, reflecting its greater sensitivity at detecting nonocclusive proximal and calf DVTs. Therefore, if the overall prevalence of PE is 30 percent in patients whose combined clinical and lung scan assessments are nondiagnostic, 15 percent of patients will have DVT detected by noninvasive testing and can be spared further investigations.

Absence of DVT by noninvasive testing cannot exclude PE, but the prevalence of PE in patients with negative tests will be reduced to approximately half of that expected on the basis of combined clinical and lung scan probabilities alone. If bilateral venography is negative, the remaining probability of PE in these patients will be even lower.

Patients with Suspected PE who Have Nondiagnostic Clinical Assessment and Lung Scanning Without Evidence of DVT on Objective Testing

The management of this group of patients remains controversial, with a number of options available:

1. Perform pulmonary angiography to rule in or rule out PE.
2. Treat with anticoagulants despite knowing that the majority do not have PE.
3. Withhold anticoagulants despite knowing that a clinically important proportion have PE.
4. Withhold treatment and perform serial noninvasive diagnostic testing to detect and then treat recurrent proximal DVT.

Even with optimal facilities it may not be possible to perform angiography due to the patient's illness, or technical

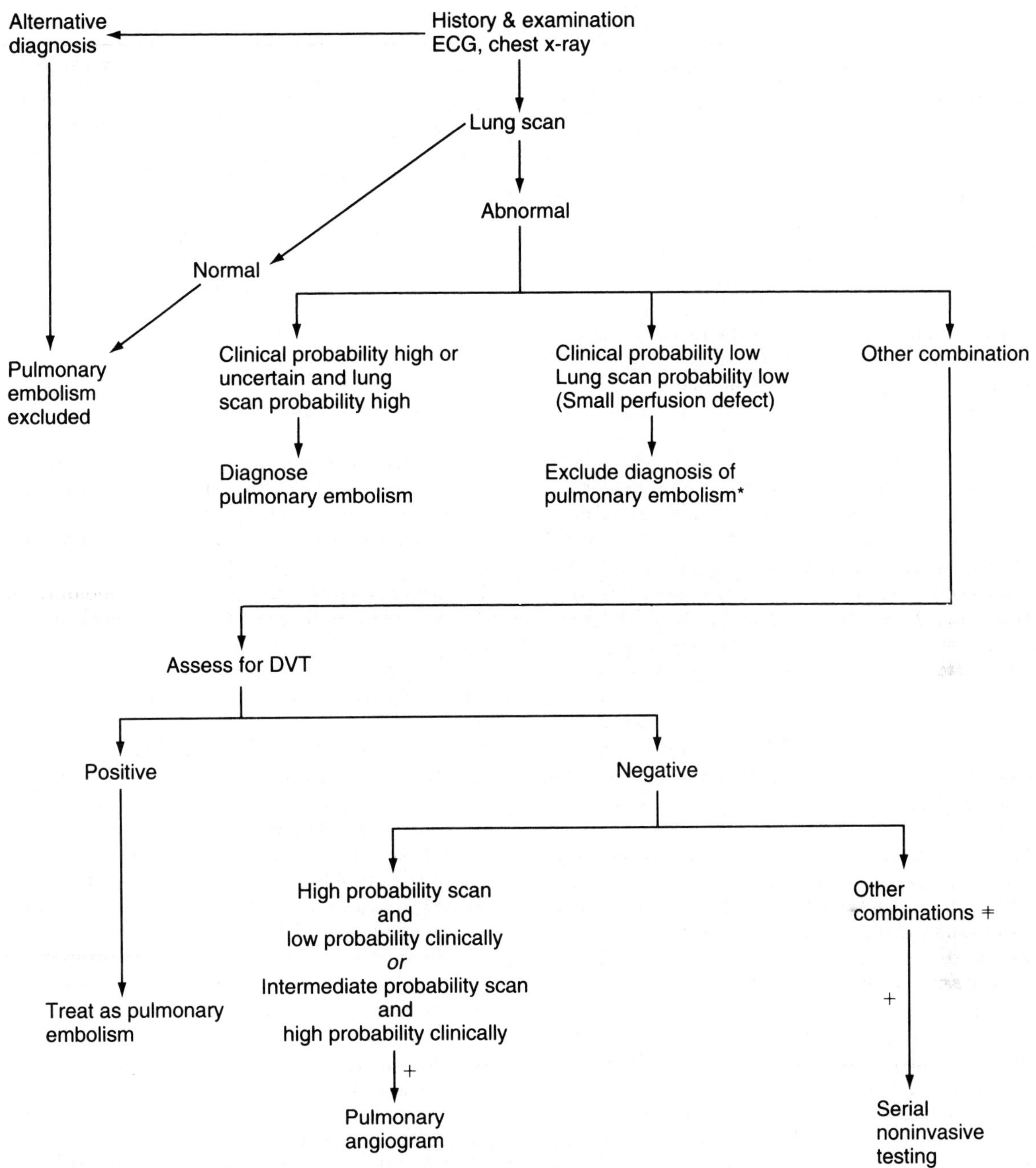

Figure 2
Diagnostic approach when PE is suspected.

difficulties encountered during the procedure. Furthermore, in patients with small perfusion defects, a negative pulmonary angiogram may not conclusively exclude PE due to the difficulty of visualizing small peripheral clots. However, the substantial risks, cost, and inconveniences associated with anticoagulant therapy do not justify treating all of these patients. Nevertheless, in occasional patients with poor cardiopulmonary reserve, a moderate or high suspicion of PE, no contraindications to anticoagulants, and in whom angiography is not feasible, empiric anticoagulant therapy may be appropriate.

The probability of having had a PE in patients with a combination of an either intermediate or indeterminate lung scan probabilities and a low clinical suspicion for PE, or a low probability lung scan and an intermediate clinical probability for PE, plus a negative noninvasive tests for DVT, is low (not more than 10 percent). Nonetheless, we prefer not to accept this risk, and we investigate these patients further. This approach is described in the next section.

Serial Noninvasive Testing for DVT in Patients with Suspected PE

Provided the initial PE does not cause severe cardiopulmonary compromise, the major risk for patients with recent PE is from further emboli. When lung scanning and tests for DVT have failed to rule in or rule out PE, an alternative to performing pulmonary angiography is to shift the focus of management from diagnosis of the presenting event to preventing recurrent PE. Some evidence suggests that this can be achieved by performing serial noninvasive testing to detect and treat evolving or recurrent proximal DVT. Our understanding of the natural history of VTE is that PEs usually originate from proximal (popliteal or larger) veins in the legs; due to their smaller size, isolated calf vein clots rarely produce clinically important emboli. Although noninvasive testing with IPG or VUS only reliably detects proximal DVT, since clinically important PE only occurs in association with proximal clots, it is safe to withhold anticoagulant therapy in patients with suspected VTE but normal noninvasive tests for DVT. However, because a proportion of these patients have isolated calf DVT that may extend into the proximal system and cause PE, it is necessary to perform serial noninvasive testing to detect proximal extension.

The safety of this approach in patients with suspected DVT has been established by large prospective studies of both inpatient and outpatient populations. These studies found that if IPG conversion is going to occur, it usually occurs early, commonly within days of presentation. Extrapolating from these studies, it has been proposed that in patients with suspected PE and nondiagnostic workups following clinical, lung scanning, and noninvasive assessments for DVT, anticoagulants can safely be withheld if serial noninvasive testing of the legs fails to detect proximal extension over a 2 week period. The object of serial noninvasive testing in this setting is not to identify patients who have already had a PE but to detect those who may have a recurrence.

One study has prospectively evaluated this approach in patients who were judged to have adequate cardiopulmonary reserve. Of 643 patients in whom this approach was used, 16 (2.5 percent) had DVT detected during 14 days of serial testing and 12 (1.9 percent) of the 627 patients whose serial IPGs remained negative had a subsequent thromboembolic event (1 fatal PE, 3 nonfatal PEs, and 8 DVTs). On the basis of this study we believe that this management option is suitable for patients with nondiagnostic assessments for PE who have reasonable cardiopulmonary reserve and in whom the probability of having sustained a PE remains below 20 percent. Because approximately 30 percent of patients with negative noninvasive testing for DVT with either (1) a low clinical probability but a high lung scan probability or (2) a high clinical probability and an intermediate lung scan probability are expected to have had a PE, we recommend performing pulmonary angiography in these patients. We perform bilateral venography prior to angiography because a positive venogram would require treatment. Alternatively, it is acceptable to perform venography followed by serial noninvasive testing, particularly if perfusion defects are small, as small emboli may be difficult to visualize at angiography. If serial noninvasive testing is being performed in patients with poor cardiopulmonary reserve and nondiagnostic assessments for PE, we recommend initial venography, as fewer patients who have had a PE will go undetected and any calf vein thrombi will be detected.

We believe that as yet there is insufficient evidence to support incorporating the results of blood tests, which assess biochemical evidence of clot formation or lysis, into the diagnostic algorithm for PE.

■ TREATMENT OF VENOUS THROMBOEMBOLISM

The long-established practice of anticoagulation with parenteral heparin followed by oral vitamin K antagonists remains the mainstay of treatment of DVT. However, prospective studies continue to refine the optimal dose, duration, and route of administration of these agents. LMWHs may represent an important advance in the treatment of established VTE, in addition to their role in primary prevention. A recent randomized trial has confirmed that an initial course of heparin therapy is required prior to oral anticoagulation in patients with DVT (recurrence rate for symptomatic VTE of 20 percent versus 6.8 percent). Two earlier studies established that the duration of heparin therapy could safely be reduced from 10 to 5 days. However, one of these studies excluded patients with large iliac vein clots or PE, and these patients made up a small proportion of the other study. The efficacy and safety of heparin therapy are similar when heparin is given by continuous intravenous infusion or by twice daily subcutaneous injections. Administration by intermittent *intravenous* bolus should be avoided because of its higher frequency of bleeding. If subcutaneous heparin is used, an initial intravenous bolus (e.g. 5,000 U) should be given followed by at least 17,500 U twice a day for rapid therapeutic anticoagulation. A recently completed randomized study has established that it is not necessary to continue escalating the dose of heparin to achieve a therapeutic activated partial thromboplastin time (APTT) in patients who are receiving large doses of heparin (more than 35,000 U per day), provided the heparin level (e.g., by anti-X_a or antithrombin activity) is therapeutic. Use of a standardized heparin nomogram, adapted to the local therapeutic range for the APTT, facilitates regulation of continuous heparin infusions. Weight adjustment, particularly of the initial continuous intravenous infusion (18u/kg/h) appears to be worthwhile.

A number of randomized trials have established that weight-adjusted, fixed-dose subcutaneous LMWH is as effective as standard heparin administered by continuous intravenous infusion for the treatment of DVT. Combining the results of these studies suggests that LMWH may also be associated with fewer bleeds. Two large randomized trials have found that DVT can be treated with LMWH on an outpatient basis.

Recent studies have led to refinements in the dose and duration of oral anticoagulant therapy for DVT. It was established in the early 1980s that less intense anticoagulation equivalent to an International Normalized Ratio—standardized expression of the prothrombin time (INR) of 2.0 to 3.0 was as effective at preventing recurrent VTE as an anticoagulant intensity equivalent to an INR of 3.0 to 4.5 but was associated with a reduced risk of bleeding (risk reduction of 81 percent). Three recent studies which evaluated the optimal duration of anticoagulation in patients with VTE found that a shorter duration of therapy (4–6 weeks) was associated with higher rates of recurrent VTE than 3–6 months of anticoagulation. These studies indicate that patients with a first episode of VTE should be anticoagulated for a minimum of 3 months. A possible exception may be in patients with a first DVT that is a complication of surgery; these patients appear to have low recurrence rates regardless of whether they were anticoagulated for longer or shorter durations.

A number of studies have established that thrombolytic therapy increases the rate of resolution of pulmonary emboli but that this is achieved at the price of increased bleeding, which occasionally is fatal. Consequently, thrombolytic therapy is usually limited to patients with confirmed massive pulmonary embolism associated with hemodynamic compromise despite adequate resuscitation with fluids, inotropes, and oxygen therapy. The use of thrombolytic therapy is further limited by the frequency with which PE occurs in the early postoperative period. We believe that there is inadequate evidence to support a net benefit of thrombolytic therapy in patients with DVT, as regimens that have been effective at achieving clot lysis are associated with high bleeding rates. The results of a randomized controlled trial recently performed at our own center showed accelerated resolution of perfusion defects and minimal bleeding t-PA for a short interval when we believe thrombolytic therapy is indicated. With this regimen, 0.6 mg of t-PA per kilogram of ideal body weight is infused over 10 minutes without interrupting therapeutic heparinization. This method of administration differs from the FDA-approved regimen of 100 mg of t-PA over 2 hours.

■ MANAGEMENT OF COMPLICATIONS OF ANTICOAGULANT THERAPY

Heparin and Bleeding

Bleeding is an important complication of heparin and oral anticoagulant therapy, occurring in approximately 5 percent of patients who receive 5 to 7 days of heparin and 5 percent of patients who then receive 3 months of oral anticoagulants. If clinically important bleeding occurs during the initial period of heparin therapy, anticoagulants are usually discontinued and an inferior vena caval filter is inserted. In the occasional patient with major bleeding and therapeutic levels of heparin and in patients who are bleeding and who have received supratherapeutic doses of heparin, protamine sulphate may be given to reverse the effect of heparin. The full neutralizing dose is 1 mg of protein sulphate for 100 U heparin. Due to the short half-life of standard heparin, the dose of protamine must be reduced to half this at one hour and to a quarter of this two hours after the heparin has been given. Protamine should be infused over 10 minutes to avoid hypotension and may have to be repeated due to its rapid clearance. Smaller repeated doses of protamine are used to reverse therapeutic doses of subcutaneous heparin.

Table 4 Antithrombotic Alternatives in Heparin-Induced Thrombocytopenia

ANCROD*

Initial infusion: 70 U (one vial) in 250 ml of normal saline administered over 6 to 8 hours.

Subsequent rates of infusion are based on fibrinogen levels (Clauss method) assayed approximately 6 hours after completion of infusions.

Fibrinogen, g/L	*Ancrod Infusion*
<0.5	0 U for 24 hrs
0.5–1.0	70 U over 24 hrs
1.0–1.5	70 U over 18 hrs
1.5–2.0	70 U over 12 hrs
>2.0	70 U over 8 hrs

ORGARAN

Bolus 2,500 U

Infusion 400 U/hr for 2 hrs, then 300 U/hr for 2 hrs, followed by 150–200 U/hr, adjusted to achieve an antiX_a activity level of 0.5–0.8 U/ml.

*This protocol acts as a guideline, to be modified according to response.

Heparin-Induced Thrombocytopenia

A fall in platelet count beginning 5 to 15 days after starting heparin (median 10 days, earlier in patients who have previously received heparin) may be due to heparin-induced thrombocytopenia, the most serious consequence of which is the risk of associated arterial and venous thrombosis. In the absence of a convincing alternative explanation for thrombocytopenia, all sources of heparin are stopped, and if indications are present for therapeutic anticoagulation, an alternative agent is used. If warfarin treatment has already been started and the INR is approaching or in the therapeutic range, warfarin can be continued without addition of an alternative treatment. Two alternative antithrombotic agents have been evaluated in descriptive studies, the defibrinogenating agent Ancrod and the heparinoid Orgaran. Dosage regimens for Ancrod and Orgaran are shown in Table 4. Heparin-induced thrombocytopenia is discussed at greater length in the chapter on drug-induced thrombocytopenia.

Warfarin and Bleeding

Clinically important bleeding while on oral anticoagulants may require slow reversal with administration of vitamin K (5 to 30 mg as single or repeated doses subcutaneously or intravenously) or rapid reversal with additional fresh frozen plasma or factor concentrates. If bleeding occurs when the patient is markedly supratherapeutic, further investigation may not be warranted and anticoagulation may be restarted subsequently. If further anticoagulation is contraindicated, the decision to insert an inferior vena caval filter is influenced by the extent of DVT, continuing risk factors for further VTE, the duration of previous anticoagulation, and the underlying cardiopulmonary reserve of the patient.

Suggested Reading

Dalen JE, Hirsh J. Fourth ACCP Consensus Conference on Antithrombotic Therapy. Chest 1995; 108:2315–2465, 2585–2905, 2135–2515.

Hull RD, Hirsh J, Carter CJ, et al. Diagnostic value of ventilation-perfusion lung scanning in patients with suspected pulmonary embolism. Chest 1985; 88:819–828.
Hull RD, Raskob GE, Coates G, et al. A new noninvasive management strategy for patients with suspected pulmonary embolism. Arch Intern Med 1989; 149:2549–2555.
Hull RD, Raskob GE, Ginsberg JS, Panju AA, Brill-Edwards P, Coates G, Pineo GF. A noninvasive strategy for the treatment of patients with suspected pulmonary embolism. Arch Intern Med 1994; 154:289–297.
Lensing AWA, Hirsh J, Buller H. Diagnosis of venous thrombosis. In: Coleman RW, Hirsch J, Marder VJ, Salzman JB, eds. Hemostasis and thrombosis: Basic principles and clinical practice. 3rd ed. Philadelphia: JB Lippincott, 1993; 1297–1321.
Levine M, Gent M, Hirsh J, et al. A comparison of low-molecular-weight heparin administered primarily at home with unfractionated heparin administered in the hospital for proximal deep-vein thrombosis. N Engl J Med 1996; 334:677–681.
The PIOPED Investigators. Value of the ventilation perfusion scan in acute pulmonary embolism. JAMA 1990; 263:2753–2759.

CHRONIC COR PULMONALE

Lewis J. Rubin, M.D.

Although many clinicians equate cor pulmonale with right-sided heart failure, it is best defined as pulmonary hypertension resulting from conditions that primarily alter the structure or function of the lung parenchyma or vasculature. Overt right-heart failure is a late manifestation of chronic cor pulmonale and need not be present either to entertain or to establish the diagnosis of cor pulmonale.

Disorders of the pulmonary circulation that result in pulmonary hypertension can be classified as either precapillary or postcapillary, based on the predominant site of the affected vasculature. The major disease processes that produce chronic cor pulmonale, which is usually precapillary in origin, are listed in Table 1. Establishing the etiology of cor pulmonale in a patient with unexplained pulmonary hypertension requires consideration of these entities; only after all known causes of pulmonary hypertension have been excluded on clinical grounds can a diagnosis of primary pulmonary hypertension (PPH) be made.

THERAPEUTIC ALTERNATIVES

Cor pulmonale is not a disease, per se, but a manifestation common to many disease states. Accordingly, a variety of medical and surgical treatments are available, but therapy must be based on the etiologic and pathophysiologic factors responsible. In addition, therapy must be individualized, taking into account the severity of symptoms and prognosis.

Table 1 Common Causes of Chronic Cor Pulmonale

Chronic obstructive pulmonary disease
Chronic pulmonary fibrosis
Alveolar hypoventilation syndromes
Chronic thromboembolic disease
Collagen vascular disease
Primary pulmonary hypertension

Treatment of the underlying disorder, if one can be identified, is the first approach to the treatment of cor pulmonale. Improving airflow, alveolar ventilation, and gas exchange through the use of bronchodilators, corticosteroids, mucolytics, and, occasionally, assisted ventilation often ameliorates the pulmonary hypertensive state in patients with parenchymal disease. Supplemental oxygen therapy reduces the degree of pulmonary hypertension in hypoxemic cor pulmonale by abolishing hypoxic vasoconstriction; indeed, low-flow continuous O_2 therapy is the only modality that has been proven to prolong life in cor pulmonale due to chronic obstructive pulmonary disease (COPD).

PREFERRED APPROACH

Medical Therapy

Timing of Therapy and Patient Selection

Because of the ominous prognosis associated with pulmonary hypertension from any cause, an aggressive approach to treatment is warranted as soon as a clinical diagnosis is made. It should be emphasized that physical findings and noninvasive studies alone are insufficient to confirm the presence and severity of pulmonary hypertension; right-heart catheterization is necessary both to establish the diagnosis and to monitor therapeutic responses.

As stated previously, therapy directed at improving gas exchange and alleviating hypoxic vasoconstriction is the initial step in the treatment for cor pulmonale secondary to parenchymal lung disease, and it should be initiated at the earliest sign of cor pulmonale. Although this approach is often successful, the maximal effects may not be clinically apparent for several months.

Patients with PPH should also be considered candidates for aggressive therapy immediately upon the establishment of a diagnosis. However, patients with severe, overt right-heart failure pose the greatest risk for adverse effects and are less likely to derive benefit from medical therapy.

Mechanisms of Action of Drugs Used

Oxygen. Low-flow supplemental O_2 therapy alleviates hypoxic pulmonary vasoconstriction and may halt the progressive vascular remodeling that is seen in patients with cor pulmonale due to severe parenchymal lung disease. Whereas it may relieve the subjective sensation of dyspnea in patients with nonhypoxemic cor pulmonale, supplemental O_2 does not usually produce hemodynamic improvement in these patients.

Methylxanthines. Theophylline, the most widely used methylxanthine derivative, has several potentially beneficial effects in cor pulmonale: Theophylline improves airflow by its bronchodilator effects and by a direct enhancement of mucociliary clearance. In addition, theophylline enhances diaphragmatic contractility, decreasing the work of breathing. It has also been suggested that theophylline improves right ventricular function in patients with COPD with cor pulmonale, possibly by a direct vasodilator effect on the pulmonary circulation. Finally, the modest diuretic effects of theophylline may limit fluid retention in patients with right ventricular dysfunction.

Vasodilators. The rationale for the use of vasodilators in pulmonary hypertension is based on the suggestion that pulmonary vasoconstriction is present, to varying degrees, and that systemic vasodilators exert comparable effects on pulmonary vascular smooth muscle. Reduction in vascular smooth muscle tone would reduce right ventricular afterload, thereby improving right ventricular function and O_2 transport to the peripheral tissues. A variety of vasodilators have been shown to reduce pulmonary vasoconstriction in experimental and clinical conditions, including the calcium channel blockers, prostaglandins I_2 and E_1 (PGI_2 and PGE_1), nitrates, and hydralazine hydrochloride. Other agents, such as the angiotensin converting enzyme inhibitors, appear far less active on the pulmonary vascular bed. It should also be emphasized that the presence or degree of reversible vasoconstriction is variable in cor pulmonale. It may be a predominant factor in some patients, especially those with hypoxemic lung disease and PPH, but it is unlikely to contribute substantially to the hypertensive state in patients with chronic thrombotic pulmonary hypertension or cor pulmonale due to connective tissue disease.

Dosage, Routes of, and Practical Considerations in Drug Administration

Oxygen. Patients with hypoxemic cor pulmonale should be treated with low-flow O_2 delivered via nasal cannula and titrated to achieve an arterial Po_2 greater than 60 to 65 torr. Oxygen therapy should be used for at least 18 hours per day, and preferably for 24 hours per day; even intermittent alveolar hypoxia is sufficient to promote ongoing pulmonary vasoconstriction. Some authors have suggested empirically increasing the flow rate by 1 liter per minute during sleep because hypoventilation with resultant hypoxemia is common in patients with cor pulmonale due to obstructive lung disease. Although oxygen concentrators are efficient and cost-effective devices for the delivery of continuous supplemental O_2, they are of limited benefit in ambulatory patients because of their size and electrical requirements. Liquid oxygen systems, which are portable albeit more expensive, allow patients to ambulate while still receiving supplemental O_2.

In some patients with pulmonary hypertension, arterial hypoxemia may be due to right-to-left shunting through a patent foramen ovale. Such patients may not substantially increase arterial Po_2 in response to supplemental O_2, but dyspnea and activity tolerance may nevertheless be improved.

Methylxanthines. I prefer to use theophylline in patients with cor pulmonale due to COPD in doses that achieve low therapeutic serum levels (10 to 12 μg per milliliter). Higher serum levels (15 to 20 μg per milliliter) may be associated with adverse effects, such as tachycardia, arrhythmias, nausea, and tremors. Oral sustained-release preparations, titrated to achieve the desired serum concentration, can be administered twice daily and provide reliable bioavailability.

Vasodilators. The use of vasodilators in pulmonary hypertension should be considered experimental, and their role in management is unclear. My approach is to withhold their use in patients with cor pulmonale due to lung disease until conventional therapy has proven inadequate. In contrast, patients with PPH are viewed as potential candidates for vasodilator therapy as soon as the diagnosis is established because no other modality of treatment has proven any more successful.

Because of the risks of sustained adverse effects when long-acting vasodilators are administered to patients with "fixed" pulmonary vascular disease, I acutely evaluate the vasoreactivity of individual patients with pulmonary hypertension during hemodynamic monitoring before embarking on long-term therapy. Prostacyclin (PGI_2) and inhaled nitric oxide (NO) are well suited for this purpose in that they are potent, titratable, short-acting agents. Individuals who manifest reductions in pulmonary artery pressure and pulmonary vascular resistance in response to the acute intravenous infusion of prostacyclin or inhaled NO are more likely to respond in a similar fashion to oral or transdermal vasodilators. [Prostacyclin is an approved drug by the Food and Drug Administration for the treatment of patients with PPH who fall into New York Heart Association Functional Classes III or IV.] Other intravenous agents, such as PGE_1 or adenosine, may be suitable alternatives for acute testing, although they may be less potent than prostacyclin or NO.

Individuals who manifest beneficial responses to intravenous prostacyclin are treated with oral or topical vasodilators. The calcium channel blockers appear to be the most potent agents, although side effects are common and may preclude their use. Nifedipine and diltiazem hydrochloride appear equally effective; verapamil is generally not used because it is less potent in the pulmonary vascular bed and it possesses negative inotropic effects. I usually begin therapy with sustained-release nifedipine in doses of 30 mg once daily, increasing the dose as tolerated; sustained-release diltiazem hydrochloride therapy is instituted in doses of 120 mg once daily, increasing as tolerated. Studies have suggested that large doses of these agents may be necessary to produce sustained responses in pulmonary hypertension, although side effects may limit the doses that can be achieved (Rich and Brundage, 1987). Survival is improved in patients who are responsive to calcium channel blocking therapy (Rich and co-workers, 1992).

If calcium channel blockers cannot be used because of adverse effects, I consider nitrates as a second line of therapy in patients with demonstrated pulmonary vasoreactivity. I prefer to use topical nitroglycerin ointment, beginning with ¼ to ½ inch every 6 hours, increasing as tolerated.

Patients who are refractory to these approaches may be considered candidates for continuous intravenous infusion of prostacyclin. This approach may be particularly useful as a bridge to transplantation in severely impaired individuals. Prostacyclin is delivered intravenously from a portable syringe pump connected to a chronic indwelling central venous catheter (Barst and co-workers, 1996).

Anticoagulation. Recent experience suggests that PPH patients who are treated with anticoagulants tend to live longer. I treat patients with PPH or chronic thrombotic pulmonary vascular disease with warfarin, adjusting the dose to achieve a prothrombin time of approximately 1.5 times control. I generally do not treat patients with other causes of cor pulmonale with anticoagulants unless a specific indication exists.

Cardiac Glycosides and Diuretics. Cardiac glycosides appear to be of limited usefulness in cor pulmonale due to parenchymal lung disease unless left ventricular dysfunction is present. Furthermore, the risk of digitalis toxicity is increased in the setting of chronic lung disease, in part because of the presence of hypoxemia, catecholamine excess, and diuretic-induced hypokalemia. Accordingly, I use cardiac glycosides in this setting only when supraventricular tachyarrhythmias requiring atrioventricular node blockade are present; verapamil may be an alternative, although its other hemodynamic effects may limit its usefulness.

Some authors have advocated combining cardiac glycosides with calcium channel blocker therapy in patients with PPH to counteract the negative inotropic effects of nifedipine or diltiazem hydrochloride (Rich and Brundage, 1987).

Diuretics should be used cautiously in patients with cor pulmonale because excessive reduction in right-heart preload may actually compromise right ventricular function. In addition, the hypokalemia and metabolic alkalosis that may result from diuretic use are poorly tolerated by patients with severe chronic lung disease. Finally, many patients with hypoxemic cor pulmonale experience a hemodynamic response to supplemental oxygen therapy, precluding the need for diuretics.

Despite these caveats, patients with persistent or severe volume overload attributable to right-heart failure should be treated with diuretics. Furosemide, in doses of 40 to 120 mg per day, are usually sufficient. In refractory situations, potent diuretics, such as metolazone in doses of 2.5 to 5 mg, may be added. Meticulous monitoring of serum electrolytes is mandatory when these agents are used, and aggressive potassium or magnesium replacement may be necessary.

Side Effects of the Drugs Used

Low-flow supplemental O_2 therapy is generally safe and is well tolerated by most patients with hypoxemic lung disease. Modest increases in P_{CO_2} can accompany its use in hypercapnic individuals with COPD, but overt suppression of respiratory drive is unlikely unless very high flow rates are used or other factors precipitating acute respiratory failure are present. The use of nasal cannulas can produce nasal mucosal drying and irritation, which can be minimized by keeping flow rates lower than 4 to 5 liters per minute and applying topical lubricants to the mucosa.

Side effects from bronchodilators are generally minor and include tachycardia, tremor, and nervousness. Selective $beta_2$-agonists and cholinergic agonists administered by inhalation are better tolerated than oral beta agonists. Oral theophylline preparations should be given in doses that achieve serum levels and that are not accompanied by side effects.

The major adverse effects of vasodilators are systemic hypotension, deterioration in gas exchange, and depression of cardiac contractility. Because there is no selective pulmonary vasodilator, most patients with cor pulmonale experience some degree of systemic vasodilation in response to the administration of a vasodilator. Patients with "fixed" pulmonary vascular disease are more likely to experience hypotension with vasodilators because cardiac output is unlikely to increase.

Some vasodilators, particularly calcium channel blockers and nitrates, can worsen gas exchange by increasing perfusion to poorly ventilated lung units. The resultant hypoxemia may be poorly tolerated by individuals with underlying parenchymal lung disease and pre-existent impaired gas exchange. Careful monitoring of arterial blood gases or saturation is important in this setting.

The calcium channel blocking agents may also precipitate a deterioration in right-heart function as a result of their negative inotropic properties. The phenomenon is more common with verapamil than with either nifedipine or diltiazem hydrochloride, but it can occur with any of these compounds and at any dose. Differentiating drug-induced heart failure from disease progression or drug-induced fluid retention (which occurs in up to 30 percent of patients taking calcium channel blockers) is often difficult and may require empirically reducing the dose or repeated right-heart catheterization (Rich and co-workers, 1987).

Assessment of Therapeutic Responses

Although improvement in symptoms, such as decreased exertional dyspnea, is suggestive of a beneficial therapeutic response, evaluation by invasive or noninvasive techniques is usually required. Echocardiography and radionuclide ventriculography are useful in providing a qualitative assessment of right ventricular function. Right ventricular catheterization, however, is the preferred approach in monitoring therapy.

The debate regarding the definition of a beneficial response to vasodilator therapy remains unsettled. I treat patients with vasodilators if they experience a sustained reduction in pulmonary vascular resistance greater than 25 to 30 percent, which is produced by a reduction in pulmonary artery pressure, an increase in cardiac output, or both. An increased pulmonary artery pressure, decreased cardiac output, symptomatic systemic hypotension, or substantial deterioration in gas exchange (usually due to either right-to-left shunting through a patent foramen ovale or increased $\dot{V}/\dot{Q}$ mismatching) constitute contraindications to vasodilator therapy.

Surgical Treatment

Patient Selection

Combined heart-lung transplantation has been successfully used in patients with PPH and patients with Eisenmenger's syndrome. Single and double lung transplants have recently been performed successfully in patients with severe emphysema and pulmonary fibrosis; preliminary experience suggests that some patients with PPH may be suitable candidates for single lung transplant as long as right ventricular function is not severely impaired. In general, patients with these disease states are considered as potential transplantation candidates as long as there is no evidence of a systemic, recurrent illness or severe, irreversible hepatic or renal disease.

Patients with pulmonary hypertension due to angiographically confirmed proximal thrombotic obstruction who have symptoms that substantially limit their life style may be considered as candidates for thromboendarterectomy.

Complications and Sequelae

The major complications of transplantation relate to the viability of the transplanted organs in the immediate postoperative period and the long-term risks of rejection and immunosuppression. Bronchiolitis obliterans, believed to be due to rejection, occurs in 20 to 30 percent of patients undergoing heart-lung transplant and can result in severe chronic respiratory disease (Reitz and co-workers, 1982). Opportunistic infections must be differentiated from acute rejection, often requiring bronchoscopy or open lung biopsy to establish a diagnosis.

Chronic immunosuppressive therapy also increases the risk for renal insufficiency and hematologic malignancies. At present, it is unknown whether diseases such as PPH will recur in transplanted lungs.

Suggested Reading

Barst RJ, Rubin LJ, Long WA, et al. A comparison of continuous intravenous epoprostenol (prostacyclin) with conventional therapy for primary pulmonary hypertension. N Engl J Med 1996; 334:269–301.

Pasque MK, Trulock EP, Kaiser LR, Cooper JD. Single lung transplantation for pulmonary hypertension: Three month hemodynamic follow up. Circulation 1991; 84:2275–2279.

Reitz BA, Wallwork JL, Hunt SA, et al. Heart-lung transplantation: Successful therapy for patients with pulmonary vascular disease. N Engl J Med 1982; 306:554.

Rich S, Brundage BH. High dose calcium-channel blocking therapy for primary pulmonary hypertension. Circulation 1987; 76:135.

Rich S, Dantzker DR, Ayres SM, et al. Primary pulmonary hypertension: A national prospective study. Ann Intern Med 1987; 107:216.

Rich R, Kaufmann E, Levy PS. The effect of high doses of calcium channel blockers on survival in primary pulmonary hypertension. N Engl J Med 1992; 327:76–81.

Rubin LJ. Current concepts: Primary pulmonary hypertension. N Engl J Med 1997; 336:111–117.

PRIMARY PULMONARY HYPERTENSION

Axel C. Matzdorff, M.D.

William R. Bell, M.D.

Primary pulmonary hypertension (PPH) is a progressive form of pulmonary arterial hypertension in which no underlying systemic or pulmonary parenchymal disorder can be identified. This disorder is also known as "unexplained plexogenic pulmonary arteriopathy," "idiopathic pulmonary hypertension" or "Ayerza's disease" after the Argentinean physician Abel Ayerza (1861–1918).

Primary pulmonary hypertension is considered a progressive and fatal illness with an average survival of 3 to 5 years after onset of clinical symptoms. The female-to-male ratio is 1.7:1 in the general population and 4.3:1 in the black population. Most patients are young, with the highest frequency between 20 and 40 years. Familial occurrence has been found in a small percentage of cases.

Clinical symptoms appear late in the course of the disease and include dyspnea, syncope, and chest pain. Raynaud's phenomenon, arthritis, and positive antinuclear antibody test have been associated with PPH.

Since 1973, there has been general agreement that the pathologic basis of PPH encompasses three different histomorphologic entities: plexogenic pulmonary arteriopathy (28 to 71 percent of patients), recurrent thromboembolic disease (20 to 57 percent), and pulmonary veno-occlusive disease (<7%). The plexogenic type is characterized by initial vasoconstriction and medial hypertrophy followed by intimal proliferation with concentric or eccentric fibrosis and plexiform lesions. Pulmonary veno-occlusive disease presents with obstructive lesions in the pulmonary venules, whereas the third type, recurrent thromboembolic disease, is defined by evidence of microscopic arterial thrombi in different stages of recanalization. These histologic findings are characteristic but not pathognomonic for PPH; similar features can be found with other diseases causing pulmonary hypertension. Lung biopsy has been recommended for subclassification and to exclude pulmonary hypertension due to other causes. Needle and transbronchial biopsy specimens are inadequate, open lung biopsy is the procedure of choice. The benefit of a biopsy would be to detect the occasional patient with an unexpected and treatable underlying disease, and it is therefore indicated when the diagnosis is still uncertain. This benefit has to be weighed against the risks of anesthesia and thoracotomy, especially because knowledge of the histologic subtype of PPH does not change the therapeutic approach. However, in the future this subclassification might provide the opportunity for more specific therapy. It has been noticed that some patients with pulmonary veno-occlusive disease do not respond satisfactorily to vasodilator therapy. Dilation of the pulmonary arterioles while the venous outflow is still obstructed increases the capillary pressure and eventually progresses to pulmonary edema in this subtype.

Recently, it has been recognized that patients with PPH have increased plasma fibrinogen concentration and diminished fibrinolytic activity compared to normal controls (Huber and co-workers, 1994), while others have demonstrated a decrease in intact von Willebrand's factor (Lopes and

Maeda, 1995). These findings may suggest new approaches to therapeutic intervention.

Patients with PPH usually present with elevated pulmonary artery pressure values of about 90 mm Hg systolic and 45 mm Hg diastolic (normal, <30/15 mm Hg). The following standard diagnostic procedures should be undertaken to exclude any underlying disease: chest radiograph, pulmonary function tests, arterial blood gas, lung perfusion scan, pulmonary angiogram, and cardiac catheterization. An echocardiogram combined with Doppler studies allows the noninvasive evaluation of pulmonary artery and right ventricular pressures. Basic data necessary for the diagnosis of PPH and to assess the effectiveness of therapy include right atrial pressure; pulmonary systolic, diastolic, and mean pressure; pulmonary capillary wedge pressure; systemic systolic and diastolic pressures; and cardiac output. It should be mentioned in this context that the pulmonary artery pressure alone does not adequately predict survival; better prognostic indicators are cardiac index and right atrial pressure as parameters for cardiac and right ventricular function (D'Alonzo and coworkers, 1991).

■ THERAPEUTIC ALTERNATIVES

As long as PPH is a primary disease, which by definition means that no causative factor has been identified, only symptomatic treatment is possible. Since the early 1950s, active vasoconstriction is considered to play a role in the pathogenesis of PPH. Systemic vasodilators that proved to be useful in treatment of systemic hypertension and left ventricular failure were expected to have similar effects on the pulmonary vasculature. About 16 drugs have been tested for therapeutic use, including captopril, diazoxide, epoprostenol, hydralazine hydrochloride, isoproterenol, minoxidil, nifedipine, nitrendipine, nitroglycerin, nitroprusside, phentolamine, phenoxybenzamine hydrochloride, prazosin hydrochloride, talazoline, terbutaline sulfate, and verapamil. This list serves as evidence for the lack of a single, totally efficacious therapeutic agent.

Although elevated pulmonary arterial pressure is the basic pathologic feature of PPH, vasodilators do not selectively affect this problem; they also alter pulmonary vascular resistance. In most cases pulmonary artery pressure stays the same or decreases just minimally, but in some patients pulmonary pressure even increases. The reason is that some vasodilators increase cardiac output. Therefore, a decrease in pulmonary vascular resistance can be offset by increased blood flow and is not necessarily accompanied by a decrease in pulmonary arterial pressure.

Heart-lung transplant is now used for the treatment of this disease.

■ PREFERRED APPROACH

Medical Treatment

The following vasodilators have been the focus of recent clinical trials and therefore are described.

Calcium Channel Blocking Drugs

Successful reduction of pulmonary vascular resistance by acute administration of nifedipine was first recognized in 1980 (Camerini and co-workers, 1980). Calcium channel blockers also inhibit proliferation of vascular smooth muscle cells and platelet aggregation. Not only short-term but also persistent effectiveness of nifedipine at rest and during exercise was found. Similar results are reported for other calcium channel blockers like verapamil and diltiazem hydrochloride. Subsequent studies could not unanimously reproduce beneficial results. Some severe adverse reactions were noted: profound hypotension, right-heart failure and even cardiogenic shock, bradycardia, and atrioventricular dissociation.

High-Dose Calcium Channel Blocking Therapy

In patients with minimal reaction to conventional doses of diltiazem hydrochloride or nifedipine, significant reduction of pulmonary arterial pressure was achieved by high-dose treatment. Not all patients tolerated this therapy (some developed hypotension, nausea, agitation), but those who did showed persistent reduction of pulmonary artery pressure and regression of right ventricular hypertrophy. At the present time, calcium channel blocking drugs seem to be one of the most promising vasodilators in PPH (Rich and coworkers, 1992). Nevertheless, the amount of data is still too small to recommend initial therapy on an empiric basis and without hemodynamic monitoring.

Hydralazine Hydrochloride and Diazoxide

Hydralazine hydrochloride and diazoxide are both direct vasodilating drugs, and initial reports noted a significant reduction of the pulmonary vascular resistance. However, these promising findings could not be repeated in larger series of patients, and serious side effects, such as hypotension, were noted. In patients with progressive stage PPH, when functional vascular stenosis has turned into structural obliteration, pulmonary vascular relaxation is minor compared with systemic vascular relaxation. This imbalance leads to increased cardiac output, increased venous return, right ventricular failure, and dyspnea. Both drugs are not commonly used in patients with PPH anymore, especially since the recent reports about the efficacy of high-dose calcium channel blocker therapy. However, it should be mentioned that diazoxide is one of the few drugs for which long-term improvement with oral treatment has been reported in a small number of patients.

Captopril

This angiotensin converting enzyme inhibitor was recommended for use in PPH. However, there are numerous studies with conflicting results that found minimal or no improvement in pulmonary hemodynamics, and systemic hypotension, near-syncope, chest pain, nausea, and vomiting are common side effects. Occasional patients experience moderate subjective relief with this treatment. This substance may be useful when pulmonary hypertension is partly caused by left ventricular insufficiency, whereas with normal left ventricle afterload it does little to increase stroke volume. In patients with PPH, when cardiac output is lowered, and with activation of the renin-angiotensin-aldosterone system, captopril might ameliorate the systemic fluid imbalance and right ventricular preload.

Nitric Oxide and Nitrovasodilators

Nitric oxide (NO) and endothelium-derived relaxing factor are the same. Inhalation of NO lowers pulmonary vascular resistance and pulmonary artery pressure. It is rapidly inactivated and has therefore no systemic vasodilating effect. NO acts as a selective pulmonary vasodilator. Recent studies in patients with PPH used inhalation of NO with a concentration of 40 ppm in air and found a decrease in pulmonary vascular resistance similar to prostacyclin (Pepke-Zaba and co-workers, 1991). Other nitrovasodilators, such as nitroprusside, nitroglycerin, or isosorbide dinitrate have been used to treat PPH. Isosorbide induced a significant reduction of right atrial pressure (McKay and co-workers, 1989). However, results of long-term treatment do not differ in comparison with other drugs such as hydralazine hydrochloride or diazoxide, and short-term response was not found to predict long-term improvement.

Nitrovasodilators and NO dilate the vessels by a mechanism different from prostacyclin. The combination of both drugs has been suggested for patients who do not respond to one drug alone.

Prostacyclin

Prostacyclin (PGI_2) is a product of arachidonic acid metabolism and a powerful vasodilator. It must be administered parenterally and has a half-life of about 1 to 2 minutes. Patients who receive a continuous infusion of PGI_2 show significant reduction of pulmonary vascular resistance. Side effects are dose related. In comparison with longer-acting drugs like diazoxide and hydralazine hydrochloride, systemic hypotension is not as severe and is quickly reversible. In PPH active vasoconstriction is believed to be the basic pathologic feature in the early stages of the disease and eventually leads to structural damage and fixed vascular stenosis in end-stage disease. Prostacyclin infusion is used to select patients with a sufficient vasodilatory potential. It is recommended that only those with markedly reduced resistance on PGI_2 should undergo prolonged catheterization for subsequent drug studies, whereas in all other patients with no responsiveness, catheterization can be stopped. Thus, the risk and potentially hazardous side effects of a prolonged diagnostic intervention would be limited to the most promising patients. Prostaglandin E_1, another arachidonic acid metabolite, is inferior to PGI_2 in predicting hemodynamic effects of vasodilators.

Besides its diagnostic potential, PGI_2 has therapeutic value. Continuous intravenous infusion of PGI_2, delivered with a portable pump, has been used in a number of patients with severe PPH to buy time until further therapy (e.g., heart-lung transplantation) could be performed (Rubin and co-workers, 1991). PGI_2 increased both cardiac output and arterial oxygen saturation, which resulted in better peripheral oxygen delivery. This might account for the patients' reduction in symptoms and improved quality of life. PGI_2 is also a potent inhibitor of platelet activation, and this may contribute to its effectiveness in PPH. Long-term infusion of iloprost, a stable PGI_2 analogue, seems to be equally effective.

Adverse Effects of Vasodilators

Severe and systemic hypotension, sometimes even shock, is a well-known adverse effect of vasodilator treatment. These agents affect both pulmonary and systemic circulation. A reduction of systemic vascular resistance that is more pronounced than a reduction of pulmonary resistance might lead to profound hypotension and syncope. Patients with progressive-stage PPH, when functional vascular stenosis has turned into structural obliteration, are particularly prone to circulatory imbalances. Some authors recommend comparing the fall in pulmonary vascular resistance with the systemic resistance to identify candidates for more beneficial treatment. However, hypotension is not as frequently observed as should be expected. This anomaly might be due to positive inotropic effects of vasodilators that to some extent compensate the decrease of systemic vascular resistance.

Another concept of vasodilator treatment is that with better intrapulmonary blood flow more oxygen is delivered to the peripheral tissues. Some investigators report relief of clinical symptoms and increased saturation after pulmonary vascular relaxation (Rubin and Petee, 1980). At the same time there are contradictory opinions regarding the possibility that pulmonary vasodilation might cause systemic hypoxemia. In pulmonary areas with reduced ventilation, active hypoxia-mediated vasoconstriction takes place. Vessels in these regions are more sensitive to vasodilators than in sufficiently ventilated areas. Vasodilation might therefore lead to an increase in perfusion of hypoxic lobuli, thereby allowing more unsaturated blood to enter the systemic circulation. However, usually vasodilators dilate not only pulmonary but also systemic vessels and increase cardiac output. Thus, the reduced saturation of left ventricular blood is offset by an augmentation of systemic blood flow. This means that a vasodilator that acts selectively on the pulmonary vasculature must be applied with great care so that the compensatory increase of cardiac output does not take place. Monitoring of systemic arterial oxygen content should be an obligatory part of any drug trial.

General Assessment of Vasodilators

It has to be mentioned in this context that the role of vasodilators in treatment of PPH is currently under reconsideration. Most publications about the effectiveness of these agents deal with changes in hemodynamic values. This does not automatically mean improved quality of life or longer survival. Even the coincidence of reduced pulmonary vascular resistance and longer survival does not prove that the latter is caused by the former. Both vasodilator response and better prognosis might be independent from each other and secondary to intrinsic factors, e.g., nonfixed, reversible vasospasm in contrast to fixed structural stenosis. The question arises why patients with PPH should undergo possibly hazardous catheterizations, drug efficacy evaluations, and subsequent treatment when the benefit is uncertain while the risks are obvious. However, one recent study seems to support the concept that long-term vasodilator treatment might be able to improve, but not completely interrupt, the course of PPH (Dantzker and co-workers, 1989).

Based on the experience that there is considerable variability regarding both clinical benefit and complications of vasodilators in patients with PPH, short-term drug testing by right ventricular catheterization is recommended. A subgroup of patients with PPH with early-stage disease and predominantly active vasoconstriction has a good response to vasodilators whereas others with progressive-stage disease and fixed obstruction are more prone to side effects. Histologic studies demonstrated that severe intimal proliferation predicts poor vasodilator response and rapid clinical deterioration.

Cardiac catheterization may be associated with hazardous, sometimes even fatal, complications. Testing the short-term response of vasodilators with right-sided cardiac catheterization should therefore be performed only in an intensive or coronary care unit. The initial catheterization may then be prolonged for subsequent drug testing. Thus, the patient is catheterized just once. It proved to be useful to wait at least 6, or even better 12 hours after catheterization before giving the first drug. During this time the patient should be kept at bed rest; an attempt should be made to relax the patient and allow the patient to become acclimated. It is essential to use this time for obtaining reliable baseline hemodynamic data by serial measurements. These values are known to have considerable variability. With one or few single-point measurements, one will never know whether the change in a value is part of natural variability or represents a drug effect.

After baseline data have been recorded, prostacyclin is administered intravenously with increasing dosage (beginning with 2 ng per kilogram per minute and increasing the dosage every 15 minutes up to a maximum of 12 ng per kilogram per minute). This infusion should be stopped if systemic blood pressure falls more than 30 percent and heart rate increases by more than 50 percent. Other side effects that might prevent further evaluation include severe headache, nausea, and vomiting. These side effects usually vanish within 1 to 5 minutes after the PGI_2 infusion is stopped. A fall in pulmonary vascular resistance of more than 30 percent should be considered as significant and due to PGI_2. The PGI_2-induced reduction of pulmonary vascular resistance is a sort of "pharmacologic biopsy," assessing reversible, nonstructural vasoconstriction and potential efficacy of vasodilators. If the patient responds, catheterization should be prolonged for subsequent short-term drug testing, whereas the decision to try vasodilators in nonresponders can be reached only on an individual basis regarding overall clinical presentation, potential side effects, facilities for close monitoring, and the fact that there is no other more effective treatment.

Most recently, iloprost, a PGI_2 analogue, and adenosine have been introduced as new alternative agents to PGI_2 for the assessment of pulmonary vasodilator responsiveness. They are short-acting and when given intravenously they affect only the pulmonary vasculature and have little to no systemic effects. Their use is still experimental.

If the decision for subsequent drug testing and prolonged catheterization has been reached, enough time should be given between each drug, at least 6 hours, even better 12 hours, to avoid overlapping drug effects or interaction between the different agents. In certain patients, vasodilators can both reduce vascular resistance and raise pulmonary artery pressure at the same time by increasing cardiac output. Those vasodilators should not be chosen for long-term treatment. Another important point of assessing vasodilator effectiveness is that an increase in cardiac output can be produced by either better ventricular function or by higher heart rate. The latter is not desirable and should be an exclusion criterion for the drug. Moreover, a comparison between the responses of pulmonary and systemic vascular resistance might help identify the most beneficial agent with the best chance for pulmonary artery pressure reduction. Besides calculating vascular resistance and cardiac output, the following "basic" values are useful in assessing the effectiveness of a vasodilator: pulmonary artery pressure, right atrial pressure, and stroke volume.

The vasodilators should be administered up to the maximally tolerated dosage. A fall of 30 percent in vascular resistance in short-term drug tests seems to correlate with longer survival. Only the agent that maximally, or at least by 30 percent, reduces both pulmonary artery pressure and vascular resistance, that produces not more than a 20 percent decrease in systemic pressure, and that maintains or increases cardiac output should be chosen for long-term treatment. Tables 1 and 2 outline the protocols for assessing short-term and long-term drug effects.

Miscellaneous Medical Treatment

General Recommendations

Patients with PPH are very sensitive to exercise and high altitudes and should avoid strenuous physical activities and traveling to the mountains. PPH has the highest incidence in women of childbearing age. The hemodynamic changes of pregnancy, such as reduced peripheral resistance and increased blood volume, are particularly detrimental, and the issue of contraception has to be addressed with the patient. It is not known whether hormonal contraceptives are free of any side effects on the thromboembolic phenomena involved in the pathogenesis of PPH; therefore, other methods of contraception should be sought.

Anticoagulants

Histopathologic studies show pulmonary thromboemboli in a large number of patients with clinical PPH. It is not clear, however, whether thrombi result from showers of minute emboli in situ or from thrombosis due to endothelial disturbances in the pulmonary microcirculation. In patients with PPH, potential sources of emboli are usually not found at autopsy.

Clinical symptoms, roentgenograms, and pulmonary function studies do not identify primary hypertension caused by pulmonary thromboemboli. Lung biopsy, which would provide sufficient tissue for histopathologic diagnosis and is so far the best method for differentiation, cannot be performed in all patients due to their sometimes fragile clinical status. At the same time cardiac catheterization and pulmonary angiogram, another approach to detect emboli and vascular thrombosis greater than 1 mm, have been reported to be hazardous and in some cases even fatal. Therefore, some authors recommend a V/Q lung scan. A normal or just slightly abnormal scan is considered to exclude pulmonary thromboembolism, whereas an abnormal lung scan does not prove

Table 1 Test Protocols to Assess Short-Term Drug Effects

DRUG	PROTOCOL
Nifedipine	(Plasma-$T_{1/2} \times$ 3–5 h): 20 mg PO with consecutive doses every hour until pulmonary artery pressure is reduced at least 33%, measurements every 30 min; depending on the amount of nifedipine that has been applied to sufficiently reduce pulmonary pressure, a cumulative dose is given every 6 to 8 h; in case of side effects, the dosage has to be reduced and given more frequently (maximum dose 240 mg/day)
Verapamil	(Plasma-$T_{1/2} \times$ 3–5 h): 5 mg; if tolerated, additional 5 mg 10 min later; measurements every 5 min for 30 min
Diltiazem	(Plasma-$T_{1/2} \times$ 2 h in first phase, 10 h in second phase): 60 mg PO with consecutive doses every hour until 33% reduction in pulmonary artery pressure; depending on the amount of diltiazem that has been applied to reduce pulmonary pressure sufficiently, a cumulative dose is given every 6 to 8 h; in case of side effects, utilize dose reduction and more frequent application; measurements every 30 min (maximum dose 720 mg/day)
Hydralazine hydrochloride	(Plasma-$T_{1/2}$ = 6 h): 0.3 mg/kg injection over 10 min with determination of hemodynamic data for 45 min
Diazoxide	(Plasma-$T_{1/2}$ = 20–70 h): first 50, then 150 and 200 mg injection (as tolerated by systemic pressure) over 15 min with subsequent measurements over 4 h
Prostacyclin	Start with 2 ng/kg/min and increase by 1 ng/kg/min every 15 minutes until 20% reduction in pulmonary vascular resistance or serious side effects (systemic hypotension, tachycardia) develop; usual average dose 5.5 ng/kg/min

Table 2 Long-Term Dose Regimens

DRUG	PROTOCOL
Nifedipine	20 mg t.i.d. up to 80 mg t.i.d. (high-dose treatment) PO
Diltiazem	60 up to 180 mg q.i.d. PO
Verapamil	Up to 120 mg q.i.d. PO
Hydralazine	25 up to 100 mg q.i.d. PO
Diazoxide	100 up to 300 mg b.i.d. PO or q.i.d. (maximum 600 mg/day)
PGI_2	Give the dose that had the greatest hemodynamic benefit during short-term testing; dose may have to be increased over time

thromboemboli but requires further investigation (Bell and Simon, 1976).

New evidence is evolving that abnormal endothelial function and platelet-endothelial interaction may be the initiating event in PPH (Christman and co-workers, 1992), which subsequently leads to the proliferative changes in the pulmonary vasculature with hemodynamic consequences. Local activation of the coagulation system in the pulmonary microcirculation and inhibition of the fibrinolytic response may also be involved. The routine administration of antiplatelet agents has been suggested. Also heparin is known to have an antiproliferative effect on vascular smooth muscle cells. Studies about the therapeutic value of these two drugs are still pending. So far only anticoagulation therapy with warfarin has been shown to be beneficial. The prothrombin time should be kept at an INR of 2.0 to 3.0. The development of right-heart failure is another indication for long-term anticoagulation because of the well-known risk to develop deep vein thrombosis from venous congestion. The consequences of a pulmonary embolus, even a small one, would be catastrophic in any patient with PPH.

Oxygen

Hypoxemia is not an etiologic cause but a common finding in PPH and a low PaO_2 has been associated with sudden death. Severe hypoxia causes myocardial ischemia, increased cardiac irritability, hypoxia-mediated pulmonary vasoconstriction, and polycythemia. In patients with low PaO_2 (<70 mm Hg) the application of O_2 should be considered as an additional treatment. Subjective relief—and in some cases even reduced pulmonary vascular resistance—has been reported. However, thus far no study has shown any statistically significant benefit from supplemental oxygen besides symptomatic improvement in some patients.

Glycosides

At a certain stage of the disease, patients with PPH develop cor pulmonale due to pressure overload. In this setting one might consider the use of an inotropic agent. Digitalis has a positive inotropic effect on the right ventricle at rest. However, there is no evidence that it is effective during exercise. Glycosides (e.g., digoxin) are usually given in combination with high-dose calcium channel blockers to compensate for the negative inotropic effects. At the same time patients with pulmonary disease are more susceptible to the toxic effects of cardiac glycosides. Besides hypoxemia, other factors not clearly identified contribute to this enhanced sensitivity. Therefore, some authors see no benefit in patients without overt right ventricular failure, whereas others recommend even prophylactic use of digoxin. In any case, digitalis should be given only under close observation.

Diuretics

Diuretics reduce volume load and elevated right atrial pressure. In patients with clinical signs of right ventricular insufficiency and dyspnea, their use has been recommended. However, close monitoring of serum electrolytes is essential.

Analgesia

PPH is sometimes associated with severe chest pain. A stellate ganglion block (10 ml bupivacaine hydrochloride 0.25 percent, on one side the first day, followed by the other side on the next day) seems to give immediate and long-standing (2 months) symptomatic relief. Although the mechanism of this treatment is not clear, the procedure might offer an additional therapeutic tool.

Surgical Treatment

Regarding the poor prognosis of patients with PPH, heart-lung transplantation, which has a perioperative mortality of about 25 percent and a 1 year survival rate of about 70 percent, seems to offer an alternative in treatment. This procedure was successfully performed in a patient with PPH in 1982 (Reitz and co-workers, 1982). Single lung transplant is an alternative to combined heart-lung transplantation when the patient's right ventricular function has not irreversibly deteriorated. Complications are fewer, and overall survival of single lung transplants seems to be better. After both single lung and combined heart-lung transplantation, the patients have long-term hemodynamic improvement and a marked increase in exercise tolerance. With increasing experience the small number of donors has become the limiting factor. In this regard it is another advantage of single lung transplants that they are more readily available than heart-lung blocks. There is currently an urgent need for an exact re-evaluation of all data regarding survival of surgically and conservatively treated patients to weigh clinical improvement and possibly longer survival against perioperative and subsequent mortality. So far only patients with class III or IV symptoms according to the New York Heart Association's criteria can be enrolled in the waiting lists for heart-lung transplantation.

It has been reported that patients with PPH and a persistent foramen ovale have longer survival. Artificial atrial septostomy has therefore been recommended as a possible palliative treatment, whereas others noticed a less favorable outcome (Rich and Lam, 1983). This treatment should be considered as an experimental short-term substitute until transplantation can be performed.

Acknowledgment

Supported in part by Research Grants no. HL36260 and HL24898 from the National Heart, Lung, and Blood Institutes of the National Institutes of Health, Bethesda, Maryland.

Suggested Reading

Bell WR, Simon TL. A comparative analysis of pulmonary perfusion scans with pulmonary angiograms. Am Heart J 1976; 92:700.

Camerini F, Alberti E, Klugman S, Salvi A. Primary pulmonary hypertension: Effects of nifedipine. Br Heart J 1980; 44:352.

Christman BW, McPherson CD, et al. An imbalance between the excretion of thromboxane and prostacyclin metabolites in pulmonary hypertension. N Engl J Med 1992; 327:70–75.

D'Alonzo GE, Barst RJ, et al. Survival in patients with primary pulmonary hypertension. Ann Intern Med 1991; 115:343–349.

Dantzker DR, D'Alonzo GE, Gianotti L, et al. Vasodilators and primary hypertension. Chest 1989; 95:1185.

Fuster V, Steele PM, Edwards WD, et al. Primary pulmonary hypertension: Natural history and the importance of thrombosis. Circulation 1984; 70:580.

Glanville AR, Burke CM, Theodore J, Robin ED. Primary pulmonary hypertension. Length of survival in patients referred for heart-lung transplantation. Chest 1987; 9:675.

Huber K, Beckman R, Frank H, et al. Fibrinogen, tPA, and PAI-1 Plasma levels in patients with pulmonary hypertension, Am J Respir Crit Care Med 1994; 150:929–933.

Lopes AAB, Maeda NY. Abnormal degradation of von Willebrand factor main subunit in pulmonary hypertension. Eur Respir J 1995; 8:530–536.

McKay CR, Brundage BH, Ports TA, et al. Long-term clinical results after vasodilator evaluation in patients with primary (unexplained) and secondary precapillary pulmonary hypertension: Acute hemodynamic comparisons and long-term survival. Int J Cardiol 1989; 22:311.

Pepke-Zaba J, Higenbottam TW, Dinh-Xuan AT, et al. Inhaled nitric oxide as a cause of selective pulmonary vasodilatation in pulmonary hypertension. Lancet 1991; 338:1173–1174.

Reitz BA, Wallwork JL, Hunt CB, et al. Heart-lung transplantation. Successful therapy for patients with pulmonary vascular disease. N Engl J Med 1982; 306:557.

Rich S. Primary pulmonary hypertension. Prog Cardiovasc Dis 1988; 31:205.

Rich S, Brundage BH, Levy PS. The effect of vasodilator therapy on the clinical outcome of patients with primary pulmonary hypertension. Circulation 1985; 71:1191.

Rich S, Dantzker DR, Ayres SM, et al. Primary pulmonary hypertension. A national prospective study. Ann Intern Med 1987; 107:216.

Rich S, Kaufmann E, Levy PS. The effect of high doses of calcium-channel blockers on survival in primary pulmonary hypertension. N Engl J Med 1992; 327:76–81.

Rich S, Lam W. Atrial septostomy as palliative therapy for refractory primary pulmonary hypertension. Am J Cardiol 1983; 51:1560.

Robin ED. The kingdom of the near-dead. The shortened unnatural life history of primary pulmonary hypertension. Chest 1987; 92:330.

Rubin LJ, Mendoza J, et al. Treatment of primary pulmonary hypertension with continuous intravenous prostacyclin (epoprostenol). Ann Intern Med 1991; 112:485–491.

Rubin LJ, Petee RH. Oral hydralazine therapy for primary pulmonary hypertension. N Engl J Med 1980; 302:69.

Wagenvoort CA, Wagenvoort N. Pathology of pulmonary hypertension. New York: Wiley, 1977:119.

TRANSIENT ISCHEMIC ATTACKS

Lewis B. Morgenstern, M.D.
James C. Grotta, M.D.

A transient ischemic attack (TIA) is defined as a cerebrovascular event that is completely reversible within 24 hours. Most TIAs, however, last a few minutes. In fact, both magnetic resonance imaging (MRI) and computed tomography confirm tissue damage in TIAs that last several hours.

A history of TIA places a patient at a tenfold increased risk of stroke. This risk is highest soon after the onset of TIA. It is sometimes difficult to recognize the critical importance of an expeditious evaluation of a patient who has had fleeting symptoms and is now neurologically normal. However, these patients have the most to gain from rapid workup and treatment. We believe that all patients with TIA should be hospitalized or at least evaluated expeditiously.

The following discussion addresses patients with atherosclerotic cerebrovascular disease. There are several other rare causes of TIA that must be excluded prior to embarking on the following diagnostic and therapeutic approach. These include brain tumor (transient tumor attacks), which is excluded by careful history and imaging; septic emboli, which are strongly suspected in patients with fever, cardiac murmur, or history of endocarditis; postseizure (Todd's) paralysis, which is excluded by history; drug use, particularly cocaine, which is excluded by a toxicology screen; or meningovascular syphilis, which is excluded by appropriate serology. Migraine is a rare cause of stroke that is suggested by clinical history.

■ APPROACH TO THE PATIENT

The three steps in evaluating TIA patients are as follows: (1) determine if the lesion is in the anterior or posterior circulation; (2) determine the mechanism of vascular insult; and (3) decide on treatment (Fig. 1). Patients with TIA may present to the emergency room (ER), call their personal physician, or, commonly, ignore their symptoms since they have resolved. Patients with vascular risk factors including hypertension, diabetes, coronary disease, atrial fibrillation, smoking, and family history should be taught the warning signs of stroke so that prompt attention by medical personnel can be ensured.

Anterior or Posterior Circulation

Localizing the lesion to the appropriate vascular territory is crucial *before* deciding on diagnostic tests and therapy. For example, patients with a lateral medullary syndrome do not need a carotid ultrasound, and patients with critical basilar stenosis should be managed quickly and carefully with anticoagulation.

Patients with anterior circulation disease have symptoms of intracranial anterior cerebral artery (ACA) or middle cerebral artery (MCA), carotid, aortic arch, or cardiac origin. Frequent symptoms include transient monocular blindness (amaurosis fugax) or altitudinal defects from branch stenoses, hemiparesis, hemisensory defects, visual field defects, dysarthria, "central" facial droop, and aphasia.

Posterior circulation TIAs originate from the intracranial basilar artery or its branches, the extracranial vertebral arteries, aortic arch, or heart. Vascular events cause long-tract, cerebellar, and cranial nerve symptoms. Patients have symptoms and signs of hemianopia or blindness, diplopia, perioral numbness, "peripheral" facial droop, tinnitus or hearing loss, dysphagia, dysarthria, hemiparesis, hemisensory loss frequently with a "crossed" pattern (i.e., loss of sensation on one side of the face and the contralateral side of the body), ataxia, gait instability, and nausea. Vertigo is a common symptom, although rarely in isolation.

Mechanism of Vascular Insult

Stroke and TIA are frequently classified as cardioembolic, large-vessel thrombotic or embolic, small-vessel or undetermined (cryptogenic). These etiologies occur in approximately equal proportions.

Patients with suspected anterior circulation TIAs should undergo carotid duplex ultrasonography. The North American Symptomatic Carotid Endarterectomy Study (NASCET) demonstrated convincingly that symptomatic patients with a greater than 70 percent ipsilateral carotid diameter stenosis benefit from carotid endarterectomy (CEA). An absolute risk reduction of 17 percent at 2 years was found for patients who had surgery compared to those randomized to best medical therapy alone. Patients with less than 30 percent stenosis should be treated medically. NASCET will soon publish data on the 30 to 70 percent stenosis group.

A cardiac history, examination, and electrocardiography (ECG) are excellent screening tests for a cardiac source of embolization. Our experience and outcomes research from Great Britain suggest that if there is no history of any cardiac disease and examination and ECG are normal, echocardiography and Holter monitoring are of low yield. We do advise that in patients without a suspected source for the vascular event (cryptogenic stroke) these tests be carried out. Cardiac history, ECG, and perhaps stress ECG are important in screening for coronary artery disease, an important cause of morbidity and mortality in cerebrovascular disease patients.

Transesophageal echocardiography (TEE) has become an important tool in detecting cardiac sources of embolization. TEE allows visualization of the left atrial appendage, a common nidus of thrombus not visualized by transthoracic echo. TEE also is better at detecting patent foramen ovale as a possible conduit for paradoxical embolization, and ventricular mural thrombus. TEE also allows visualization of a great deal of the aortic arch, a site recently recognized as an embolic source. TEE, however, is expensive, uncomfortable, and minimally risky to the patient. We reserve TEE for patients with cryptogenic stroke where we cannot completely rule out cardiac embolization on transthoracic echo. Some have found cardiac MRI a possible alternative in patients who cannot undergo TEE.

Holter monitoring is useful to detect cardiac arrhythmias,

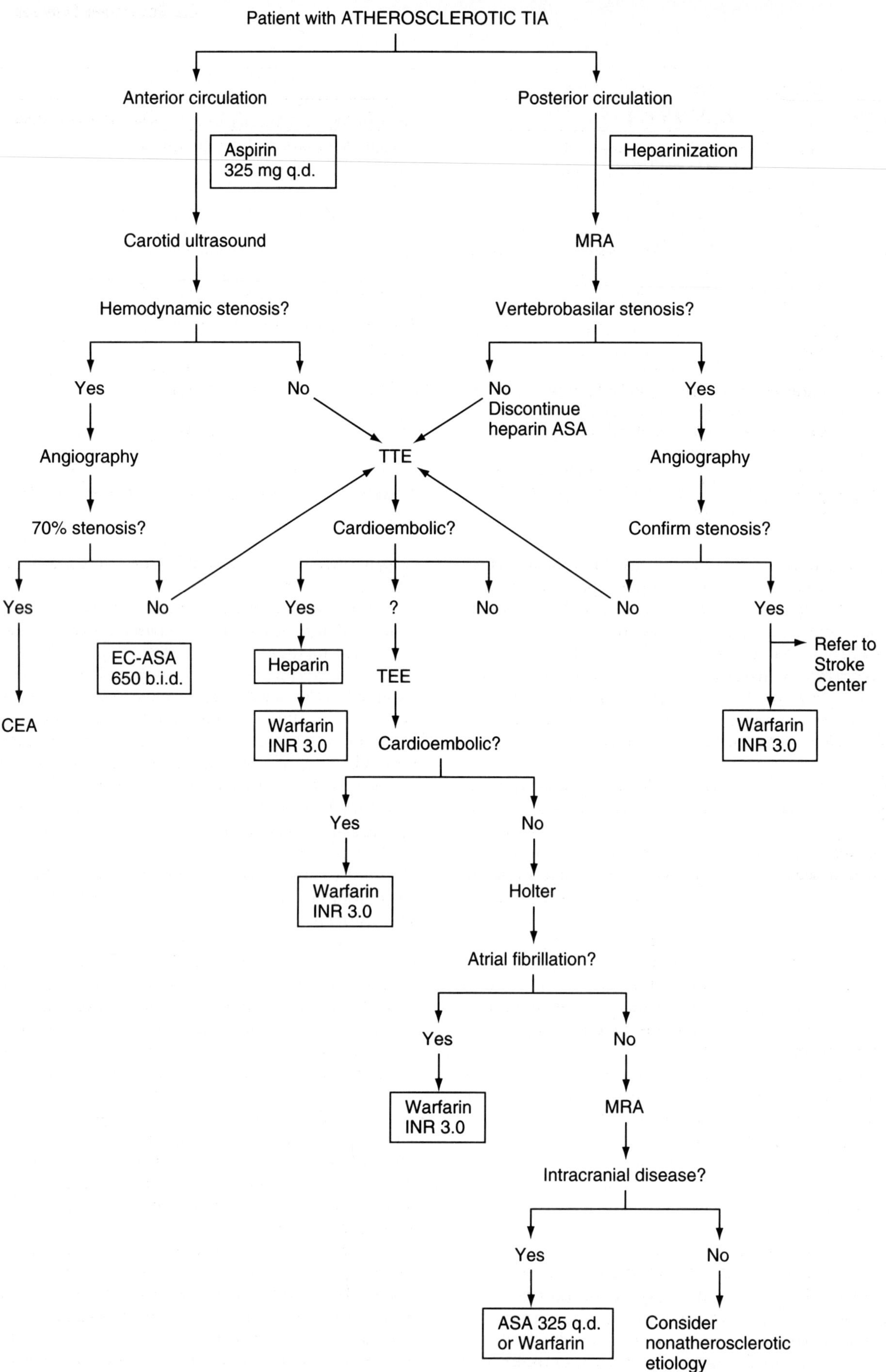

Figure 1

Algorithm for decision making in transient ischemic attacks. CEA, carotid endarterectomy; MRA, magnetic resonance angiography; TEE, transesophageal echocardiography; ASA, aspirin; EC-ASA, enteric-coated aspirin; TTE, transthoracic echocardiography; INR, international normalized ratio. For ticlopidine indications, see text.

Table 1 Therapies for Transient Ischemic Attack

THERAPY	INDICATION	REGIMEN	COMPLICATIONS
Aspirin	Noncardioembolic TIA; cardioembolic TIA in patient not amenable to warfarin treatment; chronic and acute therapy	325 mg q.d. (use enteric coated)	GI distress
	Perioperative CEA	1,300 mg b.i.d	GI distress
Warfarin	Cardioembolic TIA; vertebrobasilar stenosis or thrombus; chronic therapy	INR goal 3.0	Bleeding
	Refractory posterior circulation TIAs; chronic therapy	INR goal 3.0 plus EC-ASA 325 mg q.d.	Bleeding, GI ulcers
	Elderly patient cardioembolic TIA	2 mg warfarin and 325 mg EC-ASA	Bleeding, GI ulcers
Ticlopidine	Aspirin intolerance; event while on aspirin; chronic therapy	250 b.i.d. (at meals)	Neutropenia (rare); rash; GI distress; expensive; takes 7–10 days to work
Heparin	Cardioembolic; vertebrobasilar thrombus; acute therapy; crescendo TIA	PT goal 2.0 × control	Bleeding
CEA	Carotid stenosis >70% and ipsilateral TIA; acute therapy	—	Stroke

GI, gastrointestinal; CEA, carotid endarterectomy; TIA, transient ischemic attack; INR, international normalized ratio; EC-ASA, enteric-coated aspirin; PT, physical therapy.

notably atrial fibrillation, in patients with cerebrovascular syndromes. Magnetic resonance angiography (MRA) is a relatively new, noninvasive method of detecting vascular pathology. Although carotid ultrasound is still superior for investigation of disease at the carotid bifurcation and proximal internal carotid, MRA provides data on both the intra- and extracranial circulation and may soon obviate the need for contrast angiography. MRA, however, is still developing, specificity is low, and institutional differences in experience are high.

The gold standard of vascular radiology remains contrast angiography. In addition to enhanced sensitivity and specificity, angiography provides other useful information. Collateral circulation is delineated. The entire cerebral vascular system can be seen with one procedure including the aortic arch, carotids, intracranial circulation, and collateral flow. However, the recent data from the asymptomatic carotid endarterectomy study considering the risk of angiography are sobering. In this study the complication rate for angiography equaled the rate for CEA, just over 1 percent. We proceed to angiography in TIA patients whom we suspect, on the basis of noninvasive tests, may have a high-grade carotid stenosis amenable to urgent CEA.

Finally, transcranial Doppler ultrasonography (TCD) may have limited utility in patients with a suspected MCA stenosis. The results of TCD can be combined with MRA to yield information on intracranial disease.

■ THERAPY

Treatment for cerebrovascular disease is evolving quickly (Table 1). The underlying principal of therapy for patients who have had a TIA is recognizing that they are neurologically normal people who have just had a warning that they are at high risk for a major stroke. Time is of the essence. We begin patients on aspirin 325 mg per day while evaluation is in progress. Critical to treatment is assessment and modification of modifiable risk factors including smoking, hypertension, diabetes mellitus, coronary artery disease, atrial fibrillation, and dietary lipids.

Patients with anterior circulation TIAs should undergo carotid ultrasound as soon as possible. If a hemodynamically significant stenosis is found (>60 to 70 percent diameter or >75 to 80 percent area), cerebral angiography should be obtained to confirm the lesion and describe collateral circulation. CEA should then follow quickly. Percent stenosis on angiography is determined by calculating the ratio of the residual luminal diameter at the point of maximum stenosis over the diameter of the normal artery beyond the stenosis. There is no indication to delay surgery as you would for patients with a large ipsilateral stroke. Patients awaiting surgery should be treated with antiplatelet therapy. We use aspirin 1,300 mg per day in the perioperative period. Angioplasty is currently being investigated to treat surgically inaccessible lesions.

Patients without a carotid source of embolization should be evaluated for cardiac disease as just discussed. If a cardioembolic source is detected, heparin is often begun while the patient is started on warfarin. The goal of oral anticoagulant therapy is an international normalized ratio (INR) of 3.0. The results of the Stroke Prevention in Atrial Fibrillation II (SPAF II) study suggest that the bleeding complications of warfarin in patients older than 75 years outweigh the clinical utility of the agent. SPAF III currently is studying low-intensity warfarin plus aspirin to see if bleeding complications can be minimized without compromising efficacy. In patients over the age of 75 years with a cardioembolic source, warfarin 2 to 3 mg per day plus aspirin 325 mg per day is a plausible, but as yet unproven, therapy.

Ticlopidine is an antiplatelet agent that is a useful alternative to aspirin. Although the Ticlopidine Aspirin Stroke Study (TASS) demonstrated a slight increased benefit of ticlopidine versus aspirin in stroke prevention, the drug is best used in patients who have "failed" aspirin or are aspirin intolerant. The reason is simple: ticlopidine quite rarely causes granulocytopenia. After initiation of therapy patients must have a complete blood count every 2 weeks for 3 months to detect this potentially dangerous condition. Roche-Syntex will run these complete blood cell counts free of charge. Ticlopidine 250 mg should be given twice per day with meals to minimize gastrointestinal side effects. It takes 7 to 10 days for ticlopidine to become maximally efficacious; therefore, aspirin should be continued during this time. Despite these difficulties ticlopidine is an excellent drug, and we use it frequently in patients who are aspirin intolerant or those who have vascular events while on aspirin.

Patients with posterior circulation TIAs need urgent imaging of their vertebrobasilar circulation. In some institutions this is satisfactorily done with MRA. In others, however, cerebral angiography remains the method of choice. Imaging can identify patients with vertebrobasilar stenosis and thrombus, which necessitates emergent treatment. A vertebrobasilar thrombosis is an ominous finding on angiography. Several stroke centers have protocols for thrombolysis of these clots, and referral should be considered. Heparinization should be initiated with a goal partial thromboplastin time of 2.0 times control. Volume status should be maintained with isotonic saline and, if necessary, colloid such as albumin. Blood pressure should not be lowered; cerebral perfusion is crucial. Patients should lie flat in bed. Patients with prolonged or multiple vertebrobasilar symptoms should be managed in an intensive care unit where neurologic status, intravascular volume status, blood pressure, and anticoagulation can be carefully monitored. If the patient with proven vertebrobasilar atherothrombotic disease remains stable for several days, he or she should be switched to warfarin. An INR goal of 3.0 to 4.0 is sought. We frequently add aspirin to this regimen both acutely and in the long term.

If angiography fails to reveal a posterior circulation source, careful attention should be given to the heart, as discussed previously. If the source remains cryptogenic, these patients should be treated with antiplatelet therapy, as mentioned previously.

Patients with cerebrovascular conditions usually die from coronary artery disease. Careful attention should be paid to the patient's cardiac status during evaluation. We question patients in depth about the presence of warning signs for myocardial infarction. Patients with suspicious history or abnormal ECGs should be carefully evaluated for coronary artery disease in concert with their cerebrovascular evaluation.

Suggested Reading

Barnett HJM, Eliasziw M, Meldrum HE. Drugs and surgery in the prevention of ischemic stroke. N Engl J Med 1995; 332:238–248.

European Atrial Fibrillation Trial Study Group. Optimal oral anticoagulant therapy in patients with nonrheumatic atrial fibrillation and recent cerebral ischemia. N Engl J Med 1995; 333:5–10.

Feinberg WM, Albers GW, Barnett HJM, et al. Guidelines for the management of transient ischemic attacks. Stroke 1994; 25:1320–1335.

Matchar DB, McCrory DC, Barnett HJM, et al. Medical treatment for stroke prevention. Ann Intern Med 1994; 121:41–53.

Patient Resources

National Stroke Association, 8480 East Orchard Road, Suite 1000, Englewood, Colorado 80111, Phone: (800) STROKES

American Heart Association, National Center, 7272 Greenville Avenue, Dallas, Texas 75231-4596, Phone: (800) 242-8721

ACUTE ISCHEMIC STROKE

José Biller, M.D., F.A.C.P.
Askiel Bruno, M.D., M.S.

Stroke is the most common single neurologic cause for hospital admission. Most strokes in adults (80 to 85 percent) are cerebral infarctions, usually caused by arterial occlusion by a thrombus or embolus. Thrombotic stroke is due to either large or small artery occlusive disease, whereas embolic stroke is due to cardiogenic, aortogenic, or arteriogenic sources. Therapy of ischemic stroke is often controversial and should be individualized after careful consideration of currently available data and the risk-benefit ratio for each patient.

PATHOPHYSIOLOGY

Adequate cerebral blood flow (CBF) secures the necessary substrate for brain metabolic activity. When the CBF falls below the critical level needed to maintain tissue viability, cerebral ischemia develops. Ischemia results in impaired cellular energy metabolism, which results in toxic accumulation of glutamate and in increased permeability of ionic membrane channels. Consequently, the ionic transmembrane gradients decrease and the cells cannot function normally. Other deleterious cellular reactions include lactate accumulation, acidosis, leukocyte adhesion to the ischemic endothelium, and free radical accumulation. If the decreased CBF persists, an irreversible cerebral infarction develops.

In adults, average CBF is 50 to 55 ml per 100 g per minute. Observations in studies of focal brain ischemia have led to the concept of "ischemic flow thresholds." When the CBF falls below 18 ml per 100 g per minute, brain electrical failure occurs. When the CBF drops below 8 ml per 100 g per minute, ion pump failure occurs. The ischemic penumbra is the condition between these two thresholds, where ischemic neurons are functionally impaired but structurally intact and therefore potentially salvageable.

INITIAL MANAGEMENT AND EVALUATION

Based on animal experiments and anecdotal experience it appears that optimal outcome of acute ischemic stroke requires prompt initiation of treatment within a few hours after onset of symptoms. Best management begins with an accurate diagnosis. Stroke is a clinical diagnosis and as such includes a differential diagnosis, which must always be considered. Upon presentation, rapid differentiation between cerebral infarction and intracerebral hemorrhage is crucial if antithrombotic therapy is to be used. Other disorders in the differential diagnosis include worsening of a previous stroke due to seizures, metabolic derangements, herpes encephalitis, brain abscess, subdural hematoma, or primary or metastatic brain tumors.

All acute stroke patients should be admitted to a hospital for close observation, evaluation, and management. Initial blood tests should include complete blood count with differential, platelet count, prothrombin time with international normalized ratio (INR), partial thromboplastin time, erythrocyte sedimentation rate, Venereal Disease Research Laboratory test (VDRL), serum glucose, blood urea nitrogen, serum creatinine, serum electrolytes, cholesterol, triglycerides, and urinalysis. Chest x-ray examination and 12-lead electrocardiogram should be done primarily to evaluate the heart. Cerebral computed tomography (CT) without contrast is the test of choice to rapidly and reliably differentiate between ischemic and hemorrhagic stroke. If brainstem or cerebellar stroke is suspected, thin CT slices through the posterior fossa should be obtained. Magnetic resonance imaging and magnetic resonance angiogram (MRI and MRA) of the extracranial and intracranial circulation are performed in almost all patients.

Acute stroke patients should preferably be admitted to a specialized stroke unit, where they will receive close observation from specially trained personnel and where various monitoring devices are available should they be needed to monitor a given condition. In some patients useful information needed for optimal management may be obtained from electrocardiographic monitoring, whereas in other patients it may be obtained from monitoring the middle cerebral artery flow velocity with a transcranial Doppler or from simply monitoring the neurologic status. Vital signs and neurologic assessments are obtained every 2 hours for the first 24 hours. The need for frequent neurologic assessment and for a specific monitoring should be individualized based on the condition of the patient and the likely cause of stroke.

Evaluation should include echocardiography if cardioembolism is suspected. Transesophageal echocardiography is more likely to demonstrate left atrial, interatrial septum, and ascending aorta pathology than is transthoracic echocardiography. Carotid duplex, transcranial Doppler, and specialized hematologic studies are selectively performed to determine the underlying mechanism for acute cerebral ischemia. Cerebral angiography is indicated in possible candidates for carotid endarterectomy with moderate-to-severe carotid artery stenosis on noninvasive testing or in patients with suspected vasculitis, arterial dissection, or other intracranial vasculopathy.

ANCILLARY TREATMENT

Respiration

Supportive respiratory care is provided as needed. The airway of an obtunded patient should be protected. Some critically ill patients will need ventilatory assistance. Pulse oximetry is of value in this initial assessment. If the patient is comatose when first seen, management of the airway for maintenance of adequate ventilation and oxygenation should start immediately. Since hypoxia can also aggravate ischemic brain damage, an arterial blood gas measurement should be done and hypoxia corrected. Pulmonary hygiene measures are often needed in caring for stroke patients. Respiratory complications of acute stroke include reduced chest movements on the paretic side, inadequate or irregular respirations in brainstem stroke, atelectasis, aspiration pneumonia, and pulmonary embolism. Nosocomial pneumonia is a leading cause of death beyond the first week following cerebral infarction. Use of sucralfate in the prevention of stress ulcers may reduce the rate of nosocomial aspiration pneumonia.

Blood Pressure

During acute ischemic stroke cerebral blood flow autoregulation is impaired in the ischemic region and consequently blood flow to this region fluctuates with the blood pressure. Elevated blood pressure during the first 24 hours from stroke onset, more commonly seen in patients with pre-existing hypertension, increases blood flow to the ischemic region and a drop in the blood pressure decreases blood flow to this brain region, which may add to the ischemia and may cause neurologic worsening. This blood pressure rise during acute stroke is probably compensatory.

Normally, a minimum cerebral perfusion pressure (CPP) of 60 to 70 mm Hg is required to maintain adequate cerebral perfusion in adults. The CPP is the difference between mean arterial pressure and intracranial pressure (ICP). In patients with chronic hypertension the cerebral blood flow autoregulation is altered so that the minimum CPP needed to maintain normal CBF is higher than in normotensive subjects. Therefore, these patients are most susceptible to a fall in blood pressure during acute stroke. Severe arterial stenosis probably also increases the vulnerability of the brain region supplied by the stenosed artery to a drop in blood pressure. Therefore, during the initial 72 hours from ischemic stroke onset, an elevated blood pressure should not be lowered unless it is medically necessary to do so because of hypertensive encephalopathy, compromise of vital organs, diastolic blood pressure greater than 130 mm Hg, or in cerebral ischemia secondary to aortic dissection.

If the blood pressure needs to be lowered during acute ischemic stroke, we prefer to use the adrenergic blocker labetalol (if no contraindications) because the intravenous dose can be carefully adjusted, and it is unlikely to increase the intracranial pressure like the vasodilating antihypertensive drugs can.

Water and Electrolytes

Acute stroke predisposes to water and electrolyte disturbances. Dehydration may enhance thrombosis and predispose to hypotension. Overhydration may enhance the development of cerebral or pulmonary edema. Careful attention should be paid to vital signs, skin turgor, urine output, and other evidence of hydration problems. Free water is restricted by the use of isotonic solutions or colloids. Hyponatremia is a common electrolyte disturbance during acute stroke and may be related to inappropriate secretion of antidiuretic hormone (SIADH). Severe hyponatremia is likely to produce a confusional state and seizures. Rapid correction of hyponatremia may lead to central pontine myelinolysis.

Glucose

Both hypoglycemia and hyperglycemia appear to be detrimental to the brain. The neurologic manifestations of severe hypoglycemia and the response to the correction of hypoglycemia are well known. Most experimental studies and some anecdotal reports suggest that hyperglycemia augments cerebral ischemic injury. Hyperglycemia results in lactic acid accumulation and cellular acidosis and promotes cerebral edema in the ischemic region. This is likely to adversely affect the tissue's potential for recovery from ischemia. The deleterious effects of hyperglycemia are expected both in diabetics and in nondiabetics with "stress" hyperglycemia during the acute stroke. Despite the preponderance of experimental evidence suggesting its promise, no patient study has been done to investigate the effectiveness of controlling blood glucose in the hyperacute phase of brain infarction. We avoid hypotonic solution or fluids containing glucose. We aim to maintain the blood glucose in the range of 120 to 150 mg per deciliter.

Body Temperature

There is experimental and clinical evidence that body temperature is directly related to ischemic stroke severity. The potential for good recovery in victims of ice water drowning as compared to warm water drowning is well recognized. During acute stroke, elevations in body temperature of greater than 38°C should be treated aggressively with acetaminophen suppositories.

Gastrointestinal Function and Nutrition

Dysphagia is common in patients with brainstem and bilateral strokes, but it is often overlooked. Dysphagia increases the risk of aspiration. Standardized swallowing evaluation by a trained specialist should be done. The stress of acute stroke increases nutritional requirements and together with decreased nutrition predisposes to malnutrition. Nutritional supplementation is needed for patients who are unable to eat adequately on the third day after stroke onset. Tube feedings may be needed for some patients.

Infections

Urinary tract infection (UTI) is a common complication of acute stroke. Use of indwelling catheters increases the likelihood of UTI. Symptoms of UTI may be minimal because of decreased sensation due to the stroke. Asymptomatic bacteriuria is virtually the rule in long-standing catheterized patients. Therefore, catheterization following strict aseptic techniques should be undertaken only when other forms of catheterization are ineffective. Incontinent or comatose patients should be managed with intermittent catheterization if feasible, or a closed drainage system.

Venous Thrombosis

Because of limb paresis stroke patients have an increased risk of deep venous thrombosis (DVT). Without prophylactic measures, DVT develops in approximately 70 percent of stroke patients with hemiparesis, and lethal pulmonary embolism occurs in 2 to 3 percent. Because clinical diagnosis of DVT is unreliable, a high degree of suspicion needs to be combined with objective diagnostic tests. Early diagnosis is essential for embolism prevention. We use pneumatic compression stockings or subcutaneous heparin 5,000 units every 12 hours for DVT prophylaxis.

Seizures

Seizures can occur at any time after the onset of stroke. Seizures within hours of stroke onset are usually seen with large hemispheric infarcts. Seizures within 2 weeks of stroke are presumably caused by cytotoxic and metabolic derangements. Seizures more than 2 weeks from stroke onset are presumably caused by structural changes within the injured brain. Seizures increase blood pressure, CBF, and ICP. Late seizures following stroke place a patient at increased risk of developing epilepsy. Most poststroke seizures can be controlled with antiepileptic drug monotherapy.

Cerebral Edema

The most common cause of neurologic deterioration and death during acute ischemic stroke is cerebral edema. Cerebral edema occurs in all ischemic strokes. Ischemic brain edema is initially cytotoxic because of disturbances in cell membrane permeability to ions, and later vasogenic because of disruption of the blood-brain barrier. Both types of edema are composed of water and sodium; in addition, vasogenic brain edema consists of plasma proteins. Cytotoxic edema involves both cerebral gray and white matter, and vasogenic edema is confined usually to the cerebral white matter.

Usually the edema begins to develop soon after the onset of ischemia and it peaks 24 to 96 hours later. Usually the edema is confined to the ischemic region and does not appreciably affect the adjacent brain. However, when the edema progresses it compresses the brain regions adjacent to the ischemic zone causing neurologic worsening.

Early clinical findings after cerebral infarction that may indicate the development of cerebral edema with increased ICP include drowsiness, oculomotor or abducens paresis, periodic breathing patterns, and a Babinski sign contralateral to the hemiparesis. Several methods of treating elevated ICP during acute ischemic stroke are popular, but they remain controversial and their efficacy remains to be proven. When signs of elevated ICP are present, certain guidelines for management should be initiated (Table 1). We elevate the head of the bed 15 to 30 degrees to promote cerebral venous drainage, and the head is kept in the midline as much as possible to limit neck vein compression. However, in cases of acute carotid or basilar artery occlusion, the bed is not tilted in order to minimize the risk of hemodynamic hypoperfusion distal to the occlusion.

Table 1 Management Guidelines of Elevated ICP in Acute Ischemic Stroke

Correction of factors exacerbating increased ICP
Hypercarbia
Hypoxia
Hyperthermia
Acidosis
Hypotension
Hypovolemia
Positional
Avoid head and neck positions compressing jugular veins.
Avoid flat supine position; elevate head of bed 15–30 degrees.
Medical therapy
Endotracheal intubation and mechanical ventilation.
Hyperventilate to Pa_{CO_2} of 25 mm Hg (if herniating); gradual withdrawal.
Hyperosmolar therapy with mannitol (20% solution), 1 g/kg over 30 minutes. Maintenance dose: 0.25–0.5 g/kg over 30–60 minutes every 4–6 hours, depending on clinical course and serum osmolality.
Fluid restriction
Avoid glucose solutions. Use normal saline. Maintain euvolemia.
Replace urinary losses with normal saline in patients receiving mannitol.
Surgical therapy
Nondominant hemispheric infarction refractory to medical therapy.
Cerebellar infarction with mass effect or compression of venous or cerebrospinal fluid outflow.

ICP, intracranial pressure.

Osmotic therapy is intended to draw water out of the brain by an osmotic gradient and to decrease blood viscosity. These changes would decrease the ICP and increase the CBF. Mannitol is the most popular hyperosmotic agent for cerebral edema. Glycerol is another useful agent. When we use mannitol, we aim for a plasma osmolality 300 to 310 mOsm per liter with maintenance of adequate plasma volume.

Corticosteroids have not been proven effective in treating ischemic cerebral edema, and they have serious side effects. We do not use corticosteroids in ischemic stroke unless the stroke is caused by documented cerebral vasculitis, or to reduce peri-infarct cerebral edema in patients with stroke due to acute bacterial meningitis.

Surgical treatment is occasionally recommended in acute ischemic stroke. For large hemispheric infarcts with edema and life-threatening brain shifts, temporary ventriculostomy or craniectomy may prevent deterioration and may be lifesaving. Also, with large cerebellar infarcts with edema and life-threatening brainstem compression, surgical decompression may be life saving.

Depression

Major depression unrelated to the degree of physical disability is common during acute stroke. Depression is more common with left- than right-hemisphere stroke. Left frontal polar strokes result in more severe depression than strokes in other locations. Changes in norepinephrine-containing neurons have been implicated as the main mechanism of poststroke depression. Poststroke depression increases the morbidity, mortality, and the economic cost of stroke. It should be treated cautiously with antidepressant medications, avoiding drugs with significant anticholinergic activity to reduce the likelihood of orthostatic hypotension.

Rehabilitation

Prevention of complications is one of the main goals of rehabilitation during acute stroke. Most stroke victims benefit from consultations from one or more of the following specialists: physiatrist, physical therapist, occupational therapist, speech therapist, and neuropsychologist. Rehabilitation therapy should begin when medically and neurologically safe. Patients requiring inpatient rehabilitation are transferred to an appropriate rehabilitation facility.

■ SPECIFIC MEDICAL MANAGEMENT

Antithrombotic Therapy

Antithrombotic agents have been used extensively in patients with acute focal brain ischemia to prevent progression of thrombosis or recurrent embolization. Heparin and warfarin are the most commonly used anticoagulant agents. Beneficial antiplatelet agents include aspirin and ticlopidine.

Before beginning heparin, an activated partial thromboplastin time (aPTT), a prothrombin time, and a platelet count should be obtained for a baseline and to rule out a pre-existing bleeding diathesis. A prothrombin time and INR should be obtained before warfarin is instituted, and monitored daily until a desired INR level is achieved, thereafter once or twice on a weekly basis. Once steady levels are obtained and the patient is stable, the INR is measured every month for the duration of therapy.

In a survey of randomly selected American neurologists, 6 percent of respondents believed that heparin administration was of proven efficacy in the treatment of ischemic stroke, 16 percent felt that it was demonstrated as ineffective, and the remaining neurologists were uncertain of its therapeutic value. Despite controversy, we often use intravenous heparin in selected patients with "strokes in evolution" due to large vessel atherosclerosis; those with ischemic symptoms associated with an intraluminal thrombus; those with cervicocephalic arterial dissections; those with cerebral venous thrombosis; those with ischemic strokes associated with hypercoagulable states; and as interim measure while symptomatic patients are evaluated before surgery or initiation of maintenance medical therapy. We also use heparin in patients with recent nonseptic cardioembolic cerebral infarction in an attempt to prevent recurrences. When we use heparin, we seldom use a bolus and aim for a target aPTT of one and a half to two times control, or approximately 55 to 75 seconds.

The role of oral anticoagulation with warfarin in nonvalvular atrial fibrillation has been addressed by five major recent studies of primary prevention, all of which have demonstrated a reduced risk of stroke with warfarin therapy. In the aggregate, warfarin reduced the risk of stroke by about two-thirds compared with control patients, most of whom received placebo. This benefit was achieved at the cost of an annual risk of intracerebral bleeding of approximately 1 percent. It is generally agreed that patients with rheumatic atrial fibrillation should be given anticoagulants, in the absence of contraindications. When we use warfarin, we aim for an INR of 2.0 to 3.0, except in patients with mechanical prosthetic heart valves where we aim for an INR of 2.5 to 3.5. A large-scale randomized trial of warfarin versus aspirin for the prevention of recurrent atherothromboembolic stroke is in progress.

Meta-analyses have shown that aspirin reduces the combined risk of stroke, myocardial infarction, and vascular death by approximately 25 percent. The range of acceptable management includes daily doses of aspirin between 30 and 1,300 mg. Treatment with platelet antiaggregating drugs in acute ischemic stroke has not been thoroughly tested; however, a large-scale multicenter study of immediate aspirin administration versus subcutaneous heparin, within 48 hours from ischemic stroke onset is currently underway. Ticlopidine is superior to aspirin and placebo for prevention of stroke and recurrent stroke. Idiosyncratic neutropenia occurs in less than 1 percent of patients within 3 months of initiating ticlopidine; therefore, complete blood counts should be obtained every 2 weeks from the first 3 months of ticlopidine therapy. The recommended dose of ticlopidine is 250 mg twice per day.

Experimental Therapies

Because treatment of focal brain ischemia with heparin can be complicated by bleeding problems, thrombocytopenia, or the "white clot syndrome," the safety and possible efficacy of low-molecular-weight heparins, and low-molecular-weight heparinoids is under investigation. Low-molecular-weight heparinoids are an attractive alternative therapy because, despite a major antithrombotic effect, they have a decreased bleeding risk when compared to unfractionated heparin. These agents have a higher anti-Xa:anti-lla ratio and less effect on platelet function than unfractionated heparin. The low molecular-weight heparinoid ORG 10172, which is a mixture of sulfated glycosaminoglycans consisting mainly of heparin sulfate, and smaller amounts of dermatan sulfate and chondroitin sulfate, is being investigated in a large multicenter randomized trial in patients with acute or progressing ischemic stroke.

Prostacyclin (PG12), a derivative from arachidonic acid is a powerful vasodilator and a platelet aggregation inhibitor. Despite early encouraging studies, the administration of intravenous prostacyclin has not been therapeutically effective for victims of acute ischemic stroke.

Calcium-channel Blockers

Ischemic cell death is associated with excessive influx of extracellular calcium into the cell through defective membrane channels. Calcium may contribute to stroke by enhancing vasoconstriction, platelet aggregation, and brain susceptibility to ischemia. Calcium-channel blockers are heterogeneous compounds able to reduce the transmembrane transport of extracellular calcium ions. Irrespective of their chemical classification, they vary in their mechanism of action and in their potency to affect the cerebrovascular and cardiovascular systems. Within the dihydropyridines, nimodipine is being emphasized as a potential useful agent for cerebral ischemia. Nimodipine, a lipophilic calcium-channel blocker, crosses the blood-brain barrier and has been approved for the prevention of vasospasm following aneurysmal subarachnoid hemorrhage. In acute ischemic stroke, a combined meta-analysis suggested a positive effect when nimodipine, 120 mg daily, was given within 12 hours of ischemic stroke onset to patients with a normal CT scan. However, the usefulness of nimodipine in acute ischemic stroke has not been definitively demonstrated. Furthermore, nimodipine may decrease blood pressure, causing further cerebral ischemia. The potential beneficial effects of other L-type voltage gated calcium-entry blockers such as flunarizine, cinnarizine, nitrendipine, nicardipine, PY 108-068; isradipidine, and RS-87476 have not been established.

Opiate Antagonists

Since the discovery of opiate receptors within the central nervous system, it has been hypothesized that endogenous opiate ligands may play a role in cerebral ischemia. Naloxone, a narcotic antagonist without agonistic action, has been the most extensively studied drug. Naloxone alters transmembrane calcium flux, affects lipid peroxidation, has antioxidant actions, increases CBF, improves the cortical somatosensory evoked responses, has platelet antiaggregating effects, and may prevent cerebral edema. Despite several studies with disparate results, and very high doses given intravenously, the benefits of naloxone for patients with acute focal brain ischemia have not been conclusively demonstrated.

Excitatory Amino Acid Antagonists

Ischemia and anoxia-induced neuronal damage is mediated by high extracellular levels of excitatory amino acids such as glutamate or aspartate, which activate specific receptor-operated ion channels. These putative amino acid neurotransmitters exert their actions by interacting with distinct receptor subtypes. Numerous clinical trials evaluating the safety and potential efficacy of presynaptic agents acting on glutamate release, and postreceptor inhibitors of glutamate-induced neuronal activation in patients with occlusive cerebrovascular disease are currently in progress. Whether these agents are safe and/or effective remains to be seen.

Barbiturates

Barbiturates depress both the cerebral metabolic rate and blood flow, increase cerebrovascular resistance, limit the area of infarction following vascular occlusion, lower ICP, and have anticonvulsant properties. Barbiturates may prevent focal cerebral ischemia, particularly if therapy is administered before an ischemic insult. Notwithstanding these considerations, barbiturate therapy is of no proven benefit in the treatment of acute focal cerebral ischemia.

Thrombolytic Drugs

Cerebral angiography, when performed in the first hours after cerebral infarction, demonstrates occlusive lesions that correlate with clinical deficits in approximately 80 to 90 percent of patients. Because thrombotic and embolic arterial occlusions are the leading causes of cerebral infarction, the possibility of achieving pharmacologic cerebral arterial recanalization with thrombolytic drugs before the appearance of irreversible ischemic brain change is gaining widespread attention and enthusiasm. Pharmacologic thrombolysis can re-establish blood flow in the infarct-related vessel, improve flow to the ischemic penumbra, limit the infarct size, and thus may reduce morbidity and mortality. In addition to streptokinase and urokinase, tissue-type plasminogen activator (t-PA), acylated streptokinase-plasminogen activator complex, single-chain urokinase-type plasminogen activator complex (SCU-PA), and r-prourokinase are currently under investigation. A number of hazards exist with pharmacologic thrombolysis, mainly rethrombosis, bleeding complications, and reperfusion tissue damage with cerebral edema.

Results of current open and randomized trials have provided evidence of the tolerance of thrombolytic agents in acute ischemic stroke. Urokinase, streptokinase, and t-PA have been used intravenously and intra-arterially. A recent study showed that treatment with intravenous t-PA within 3 hours of onset of ischemic stroke improved clinical outcome at 3 months. However, treatment did not lessen death rates. Furthermore, the incidence of symptomatic intracerebral hemorrhage was tenfold greater in patients given t-PA.

At this time, we believe that a sober assessment of the available data suggest that intravenous and intra-arterial thrombolytic drugs in carefully selected patients with acute cerebral ischemia is promising. The therapeutic index of these agents has not been defined precisely, nor has optimal patient selection or the ideal thrombolytic agent. It is also unclear whether other drugs should be given with thrombolytic agents.

Hemorheologic Therapy

Therapeutic modification of hemorheologic factors is an intriguing principle in the management of cerebral ischemia. Favorable modification of hemorheologic properties may be achieved by lowering hematocrit, reducing fibrinogen concentration, and/or increasing erythrocyte deformability. Lowering hematocrit by hemodilution reduces whole blood viscosity and increases CBF. A number of studies using iso-, hypo-, or hypervolemic hemodilution paradigms failed to achieve consistent results and thus do not support the use of this type of approach in most patients with acute ischemic stroke.

Ancrod, a purified protein extract of the Malayan pit viper venom, reduces fibrinogen levels, decreases blood viscosity, and activates fibrinolysis. Small-scale randomized trials demonstrated promising results with better neurologic outcomes in the ancrod-treated groups. Large-scale randomized studies of ancrod therapy in patients with acute ischemic stroke are currently underway.

Pentoxifylline decreases whole blood viscosity, increases red blood cell deformability, decreases fibrinogen levels, inhibits platelet aggregation, and increases CBF. Pentoxifylline decreases the risk of recurrent transient ischemic attacks and stroke in patients with cerebrovascular disease but shows unsustained improvement of neurologic function in the treatment of acute ischemic stroke.

Dextran decreases platelet and erythrocyte aggregation and thus whole blood viscosity. The anticipated benefits from this agent have not been substantiated; potential life-threatening reactions due to the immunogenicity of dextran are rare. Studies carried out to investigate the effects of perfluorocarbons (Fluosol), an oxygen-carrying artificial blood substitute, failed to show consistent protection from ischemic brain injury.

Lipid Peroxidation Inhibitors

Oxygen free radical mediated lipid peroxidation is an important pathophysiologic event in ischemic or hemorrhagic stroke. Because excessive accumulation of free radicals causes lipid peroxidation, impaired function of cell membranes, and cell death, free-radical scavengers need investigation. Tirilazad mesylate, a non-glucocorticoid 21-aminosteroid, and a potent inhibitor of iron-dependent lipid peroxidation in vitro, has shown efficacy in several models of focal brain ischemia, and has been developed as a cerebroprotective agent. Results of a clinical trial of tirilazad, in acute ischemic stroke (within 6 hours from onset of symptoms), were negative.

Gangliosides

Gangliosides may promote neuronal plasticity. Monosialoganglioside (GM1) is a neuroprotective agent that has been reported to be beneficial in functional recovery following stroke; the results were only modest and unsustained. However, GM1 therapy may be associated with the Guillain-Barré syndrome and should not be used.

Other Therapies

Treatment with intravenous aminophylline and hyperbaric oxygen has been ineffective. Baclofen inhibits gamma-aminobutyric acid (GABA) and the release of glutamate but fails to protect neurons from experimental ischemia.

Although cerebral vasodilators have been widely used, several studies have produced consistently negative results. Naftidrofuryl, a promising vasodilator, spasmolytic, and enhancer of cerebral oxygen metabolism, is being investigated in a large clinical trial. Previous reports have described favorable results with the use of vasopressor agents. However, this therapeutic approach has not gained wide acceptance, except in selected complications following cerebral angiography.

Cerebrovascular disease and coronary artery disease have similar risk factors and often coexist. The observations that propranolol has protective effects in experimental myocardial ischemia, and that the long-term case fatality rate in patients with cerebrovascular disease are primarily due to coronary artery disease, has led to several investigations of the effect of beta blockers in stroke patients. Such treatment has not been found to be beneficial.

Reperfusion injury mediated by neutrophils plays an important role in the pathogenesis of ischemic stroke. Enlimomab, a murine monoclonal antibody that binds to intercellular adhesion molecule-1, is currently under investigation in patients with ischemic stroke.

■ SURGERY

The decision to perform carotid endarterectomy or pursue medical therapy should be tailored to the individual patient. Several distinctive clinical situations are encountered in daily practice that require special considerations. We outline here our current approach to three common clinical scenarios in patients with recent ischemic stroke.

The first scenario includes patients with a minor ischemic stroke who have angiographically 70 percent to 99 percent ipsilateral carotid artery stenosis. For patients who are adequate surgical candidates, we recommend endarterectomy. In the North American Symptomatic Carotid Endarterectomy Trial (NASCET) study, a 65 percent relative risk reduction in ipsilateral stroke was seen at 2 year follow-up; for the European Carotid Surgery Trial (ECST), a 39 percent risk reduction in ipsilateral stroke was observed at 3 year follow-up; and in the Veterans Affairs study, a relative reduction in all outcome events of 60 percent occurred.

The second scenario includes patients with a minor stroke who have angiographically 30 percent to 69 percent ipsilateral carotid stenosis. The optimal treatment is uncertain. We recommend enrollment in NASCET.

For the third group, patients with a minor ischemic stroke who have angiographically less than 30 percent ipsilateral carotid stenosis, we recommend platelet antiaggregants.

Suggested Reading

Adams HP Jr, Brott TG, Crowell RM, et al. Guidelines for the management of patients with acute ischemic stroke: A statement for Healthcare Professionals from a Special Writing Group of the Stroke Council, American Heart Association. Stroke 1994; 25(9):1901–1914.

Biller J. Medical management of acute cerebral ischemia. Neurol Clin 1992; 10:63–85.

European Carotid Surgery Trialists' Collaborative Group. MRC European carotid surgery trial: Interim results for symptomatic patients with severe (70–99%) or with mild (0–29%) carotid stenosis. Lancet 1991; 337:1235–1243.

Feinberg WM, Albers GW, Barnett HJM, et al. Guidelines for the management of transient ischemic attacks from the Ad Hoc Committee on Guidelines for the Management of Transient Ischemic Attacks of the Stroke Council of the American Heart Association. Stroke 1994; 25(6): 1320–1335.

Frank JI. Large hemispheric infarction, deterioration, and intracranial pressure. Neurology 1995; 45:1286–1290.

Marsh EE III, Adams HP Jr, Biller J, et al. Use of antithrombotic drugs in the treatment of acute ischemic stroke. A survey of neurologists in practice in the United States. Neurology 1989; 39:1631–1634.

Mayberg MR, Wilson SE, Yatsu F, et al. Carotid endarterectomy and prevention of cerebral ischemia in symptomatic carotid stenosis. JAMA 1991; 266:3289–3294.

Multicenter Acute Stroke Trial—Italy (MAST-I) Group. Randomized controlled trial of streptokinase, aspirin, and combination of both in treatment of acute ischemic stroke. Lancet 1995; 346:1509–1514.

The National Institute of Neurological Disorders and Stroke rt-PA Stroke Study Group. Tissue plasminogen activator for acute ischemic stroke. N Engl J Med 1995; 333:1581–1587.

North American Symptomatic Carotid Endarterectomy Trial Collaborators. Beneficial effect of carotid endarterectomy in symptomatic patients with high-grade carotid stenosis. N Engl J Med 1991; 325:445–453.

Randomized Trial of Tirilazad in Acute Stroke (RANTTAS) by the RANTTAS Investigators. The Neuroclinical Trials Center, University of Virginia, Charlottesville, VA, and the North American RANTTAS Participants. Stroke 1996; 27(1):162 (abstract #164).

CAROTID ARTERY OCCLUSIVE DISEASE

Thomas F. Dodson, M.D.
Robert B. Smith III, M.D.

The majority of transient ischemic attacks (TIAs) and cerebrovascular accidents are thought to result from the embolization of material from ulcerated plaques in the carotid bifurcation or from reduced regional blood flow related to a severely stenotic or occluded internal carotid artery. Over the past 30 years, carotid endarterectomy (CEA) has become a widely accepted, generally effective, and relatively safe operation for prophylactic intervention in the stroke-prone patient. Although it continues to be the most common vascular procedure, its apex was reached in 1985; approximately 107,000 CEAs were performed that year in the United States.

The surgical approach to atherosclerosis of the carotid artery is among the most controversial topics in medicine and surgery. Although the incidence of cardiovascular disease and cerebrovascular accidents is declining, there are still approximately 500,000 new stroke victims in the United States each year, and stroke continues to be the third leading cause of death in the United States. Although we have gained a great deal of information about carotid artery occlusive disease since the first carotid operations in the mid-1950s, the natural history of carotid disease is still not fully characterized. A number of prospective randomized trials involving patients undergoing CEA have been underway for several years. In symptomatic patients, we now have important data to support operation in patients with "high-grade" stenoses.

The results of the ACAS (Executive Committee for the Asymptomatic Carotid Atherosclerosis Study, 1995) and the VA (Hobson and co-workers, 1993) trials have helped to clarify the uncertainties of operative intervention in patients with asymptomatic carotid stenoses. CEA, carried out with less than 3% perioperative morbidity, is efficacious in patients with asymptomatic carotid lesions which cause a 60% or greater reduction in luminal diameter.

The clinical problems of the asymptomatic patient with a carotid bruit, the symptomatic patient with TIAs or amaurosis fugax, and the symptomatic patient with a completed stroke comprise the majority of carotid-related problems that physicians must evaluate. Management perspectives of each of these conditions are presented in the following sections.

■ THERAPEUTIC ALTERNATIVES

In the case of atherosclerotic occlusive disease of the carotid bifurcation, the therapeutic alternatives are limited. Essentially, the choice is between CEA and medical therapy, as there are no other practical or safe treatment modalities. Extracranial-intracranial arterial bypasses are seldom performed today, and direct disobliteration of the chronically occluded internal carotid is not a feasible approach. Remote interventional techniques such as transluminal balloon dilation, laser angioplasty, or intra-arterial atherectomy—all approaches that are used currently in other segments of the arterial system—are "investigational only" in the carotid artery at present. Medical therapy requires a choice between antiplatelet medications such as aspirin and dipyridamole versus short-term heparin and long-term sodium warfarin (Coumadin) anticoagulation. Cessation of tobacco use, control of hypertension, and reduction of elevated serum cholesterol levels are forms of "medical therapy," but they are important steps that also should be taken in surgically treated patients.

■ PREFERRED APPROACH

Asymptomatic Patient with a Carotid Bruit

It is well known that the mere presence of a carotid bruit does not signify the hemodynamically significant carotid disease in one-half of patients. The converse is also true: Patients with a hemodynamically significant lesion in their internal carotid artery have bruits only about one-half of the time. Although physician trainees are taught that auscultation of the carotids, the abdomen, and the area of the femoral arteries is an important part of the vascular exam, a bruit is an imprecise measure of the degree of stenosis of the underlying vessel. If a carotid bruit is detected, however, the next step should be an evaluation of the patient by duplex scanning of the carotid bifurcation. Whereas oculopneumoplethysmography (OPG) was formerly the noninvasive procedure of choice to evaluate carotid flow, it has now been largely supplanted by ultrasound technology. At the present time, ultrasonography results are categorized as follows: 1 to 39 percent stenosis is considered minimal; 40 to 59 percent stenosis is considered mild; 60 to 79 percent stenosis is considered moderate; and 80 to 99 percent stenosis is considered severe. These categories allow the physician to make an informed decision concerning proceeding with additional diagnostic studies. Experience from the University of Washington in Seattle suggests that the great majority of strokes, TIAs, and carotid thromboses are preceded by disease progression to an 80 percent stenosis or greater (Roederer and co-workers, 1984). Additional information pertaining to plaque morphology, also obtainable at the time of ultrasonography, may be helpful in the decision process because a greater risk of symptoms correlates with plaques of lower density or heterogeneous composition.

In those asymptomatic patients shown to have severe stenosis (80 to 99 percent) by duplex scan, the next step is to recommend arch aortography with four-vessel arteriography. Even a lesser degree of stenosis of one internal carotid warrants angiography if the opposite internal carotid is totally occluded. The carotid system is studied to its terminal intracranial branches to gain complete information concerning both extracranial and intracranial lesions. Ordinarily this portion of the workup is performed on an inpatient basis, although some centers are equipped to perform outpatient cerebral arteriography on selected patients.

It must be acknowledged at this point that some centers are altering the routine performance of contrast angiography. The data cited by Kent and colleagues (1995) concerning cost effectiveness of imaging strategies suggest that careful duplex sonography or duplex sonography plus magnetic resonance angiography could "potentially" take the place of contrast angiography alone.

In the majority of cases, angiography confirms the noninvasive duplex scan findings. If the carotid lumen is encroached by 80 percent or more, or if the lesion is severely ulcerated or irregular, operation should be considered. As a regular part of preoperative preparation, cardiologic consultation is obtained to help assess the patient's perioperative risks. Approximately 50 percent of patients with asymptomatic carotid disease have significant coronary atherosclerosis, and myocardial infarction continues to be the most common cause of death in the early postoperative period (Hertzer and coworkers, 1984). If there is any concern about the possibility of myocardial ischemia, a dipyridamole-thallium scintigraphy or dobutamine echo examination is performed to evaluate myocardial perfusion.

Once the cardiac risks of the procedure have been assessed and other factors such as underlying pulmonary disease, renal dysfunction, and uncontrolled hypertension have been addressed, a decision can be made regarding the patient's suitability for prophylactic CEA. The patient is then fully informed concerning the risks and uncertainties of operative intervention versus those associated with medical therapy. Based on the work of Roederer and co-workers (1984) in Seattle, the risk of nonoperative therapy in patients with 80 percent or greater carotid stenosis is quite high: 35 percent of such patients had a stroke, TIA, or carotid occlusion within 6 months of the discovery of the lesion, and 45 percent had similar events within 1 year. Although the ACAS data found a reduced 5 year risk of ipsilateral stroke in patients with a 60 percent reduction (or greater) in luminal diameter who underwent CEA, we have only adjusted our operative indications in the asymptomatic patient by a slight degree: we now offer endarterectomy to asymptomatic patients with a 70–75% narrowing of the carotid artery.

In the otherwise good-risk patient, that course can be contrasted with our own figures of less than 1 percent operative mortality and approximately 1 percent perioperative stroke rate in asymptomatic patients. This is obviously the most important key to the puzzle: being able to offer patients who are asymptomatic an operation that has an extremely low morbidity and mortality rate, yet one that will favorably alter their risk of serious symptoms or premature death over the ensuing years. With respect to the long-term outcome, our own statistics and those of others suggest that following operation the patient has an annual 1 percent risk of stroke in the ipsilateral cerebral hemisphere. In fact, in patients with bilateral carotid disease, the risk of stroke is five times greater in the unoperated side over time.

Increasingly, the workup of the asymptomatic patient is being done on an outpatient basis. Therefore, the patient frequently has preoperative studies completed prior to admission and may be admitted in the early morning of the day of operation. Individuals with heart disease or evidence of myocardial ischemia may have placement of a Swan-Ganz catheter or insertion of a transesophageal ultrasound probe to aid in delineating cardiac function. All patients have placement of a radial artery cannula for constant monitoring of blood pressure. The choice of anesthesia for CEA is variable in our institution. Patients who are at high risk for cardiac or pulmonary complications are usually done under monitored local anesthesia with minimal sedation. This form of anesthesia has the advantage of reducing the wide blood pressure fluctuations commonly associated with general anesthesia, and it also allows an exquisitely sensitive method of monitoring the patient neurologically during the operation. General anesthesia, on the other hand, reduces the metabolic demands of the brain while increasing cerebral perfusion, and it allows for a quiet surgical field. If general anesthesia is used, cerebral function is monitored by computed electroencephalography. Contraindications to local anesthesia are: (1) previous carotid surgery (although the senior author increasingly utilizes local anesthesia even in this situation), (2) high carotid lesions requiring extended exposure, and (3) poor patient compliance.

Although only 15 to 20 percent of patients require placement of a shunt during CEA based upon observed responses during local anesthesia, we prefer to insert a shunt in all cases. The only exception to this preference would be anatomic constraints encountered at the time of operation. Because we routinely shunt, the EEG's chief value is to assess the adequacy of flow through the shunt. An EEG that shows loss of amplitude or slowing of rhythm may indicate shunt dysfunction or occlusion.

Patients who are stable postoperatively with no neurologic changes, on no intravenous medicines to raise or lower blood pressure, and who have a stable cardiac status may safely be observed postoperatively in a non-ICU setting. Recent information from two centers in Washington state (Luna, 1995, and Kraiss, 1995) confirms our own experience in limiting utilization of the intensive care unit and in decreasing the postoperative stay to 1 or 2 days in most cases.

All who can tolerate aspirin are instructed to take 80 mg per day on a permanent basis. Follow-up plans include office visits at 6 weeks, 6 months, and 1 year, with annual assessments thereafter. A carotid duplex scan is performed annually if the patient remains asymptomatic and is not shown to have a rapidly progressive recurrent stenosis. Patients with hemodynamically significant bilateral disease have staged operations, typically undergoing the second procedure 1 to 2 months after the first. At follow-up visits, subjects are reminded to report new central nervous system symptoms or the reappearance of old deficits very promptly. They are also instructed to reduce known risk factors (smoking, hypertension, elevated cholesterol) as much as possible.

Symptomatic Patient with Transient Ischemic Attacks or Amaurosis Fugax

The presence of symptoms adds a degree of urgency to the evaluation of carotid disease patients. Prospective studies in the literature indicate that patients experiencing TIAs have a risk of stroke of about 35 percent at 5 years and that 50 percent of these strokes occur within the first year after the onset of symptoms (Wiebers and Whisnant, 1982). In light of these statistics, a TIA is a strong indicator of stroke risk. Accordingly, this clinical presentation has become the most widely accepted indication for operative intervention in patients with carotid artery occlusive disease.

The definition of a TIA is not uniform among disciplines treating patients with cartoid disease; it is generally described as a focal neurologic deficit that usually lasts only minutes, but in all cases it resolves within 24 hours without residual neurologic deficit. The 24 hour limit for resolution of symptoms must be acknowledged as arbitrary, bearing no known relationship to the underlying pathophysiology. Also important to remember is that the risk of myocardial infarction is quite high among patients who suffer from TIAs. Thus, an episode of cerebral ischemia should be interpreted as a warning signal of diffuse atherosclerosis.

With these factors in mind, when confronted with a patient who states that within the recent past he or she has experienced a brief loss of sensation or motor function of the face, arm, or leg or is reported by an observer to have suffered a brief episode of inability to speak (aphasia) or even a short period of impairment of speech (dysphasia), the physician should infer that the clinical symptoms indicate a transient loss of blood supply to an area of the cortex. Another common presentation is the patient who reports a "shade" descending over the eye for a few seconds or minutes, suggesting a diagnosis of transient monocular blindness or amaurosis fugax. In symptomatic patients, we strongly suggest prompt admission to the hospital for carotid assessment and complete neurologic evaluation.

Although the most common etiology for TIAs is atherothrombotic disease in the cervical portion of the carotid artery, a host of other disease processes can be responsible for similar symptoms. Other less common etiologies include spontaneous dissection of the carotid artery, temporal arteritis, fibromuscular dysplasia, vasculitis, coagulopathy, and cardiac pathology such as arrhythmias and valvular or ventricular emboli. A helpful clinical indicator is that embolic events from carotid atherothrombotic disease tend to be similar in repetitive episodes, whereas emboli from a cardiac source tend to be more variable in presentation. Other disease processes can masquerade as a TIA, including migraine, focal seizures, hypoglycemia, orthostatic hypotension, and simple fainting. During the patient's stay in the hospital, these other potential diagnoses are considered while the primary focus of attention is directed toward the extracranial carotid circulation. As a routine part of the vascular examination, consultation is sought from the cardiology department to assess myocardial function. Because cardiac pathology may be an important part of the differential diagnosis, the cardiologist plays a significant role in the assessment of patients with TIAs. Neurologic consultation is also requested to assist in the interpretation of neurologic symptoms and help to exclude other nonvascular neurologic disorders.

Just as in the patient who is asymptomatic, initial examinations are noninvasive and designed to provide baseline information without discomfort or risk to the patient. Thus, among the early studies are duplex ultrasound scanning of both carotids and CT of the brain, the latter preferably with contrast. If the carotid ultrasound is entirely normal and another etiology is discovered for the TIA, we may conclude our work-up after CT. If the carotid ultrasound is read as minimal or mild stenosis and no other etiology has been discovered for the patient's neurologic symptoms, however, four-vessel cerebral angiography should be performed in the search for an ulcerated atheroma that may not be identified by duplex scanning. This aggressive diagnostic approach is justified in our institution by an experienced group of neuroradiologists with a low complication rate from cerebral angiography.

The "practice guidelines" issued by Moore and co-workers (1992) suggested that CEA is indicated in symptomatic patients with at least a 70 percent diameter stenosis of the carotid artery, patients with a "low profile" but ulcerated plaque, and patients with plaques of mixed consistency. The European, North American, and Veterans Affairs trials (1991) all confirmed the efficacy of CEA in symptomatic patients with "high-grade" lesions. Patients who have experienced TIAs are at slightly greater risk of operative complications than symptomatic patients, but our experience suggests that the risk of death with operation is approximately 1 percent and the perioperative stroke risk no more than 2 percent. The surgical approach to the symptomatic patient is essentially the same as in the asymptomatic individual. Because of the greater potential for cerebral embolization during dissection of the carotid artery in such circumstances, however, it is important to "dissect the patient from the carotid, rather than the carotid from the patient." Again it should be emphasized that risk factors such as smoking, hypertension, and hypercholesterolemia should be controlled postoperatively and that the main thrust of care after operation should be educating both patient and family in risk reduction of vascular disease overall. In the case of an asymptomatic but hemodynamically significant stenosis of the carotid opposite the one requiring endarterectomy for symptoms, surgical care should be consistent with that described in the foregoing section on asymptomatic lesions. Endarterectomy on the second side, if needed, is staged a number of weeks following the initial procedure.

Symptomatic Patient with a Completed Stroke

In 1969, the Joint Study of Extracranial Arterial Occlusion was performed in an attempt to answer some of the questions surrounding early operative intervention in patients with acute neurologic deficits. Of the 50 patients who were operated upon within the first 2 weeks after their acute stroke, 42 percent died; these figures contrasted with a mortality of 20 percent among those treated medically. This study strongly suggested that operation in the acute stroke patient was dangerous and contraindicated. Since that time, additional studies have been published that question the poor results of surgical management of patients with a complete stroke, but just as in other issues related to carotid artery occlusive disease, a consensus would be hard to obtain.

The acute stroke patient is typically a referral from within the hospital or from another hospital. Usually they have already been evaluated by a neurologist and initial diagnostic studies performed. The great majority of strokes are secondary to embolic or thrombotic events, whereas intracranial hemorrhage accounts for about 20 percent of such cases. Thus, the CT of the head is an important first step in the assessment of these patients to rule out intracranial hemorrhage. The next step should be duplex scanning of the carotid bifurcation. If severe occlusive disease is identified, and if the neurologic deficit is small or fluctuating, emergency carotid arteriography is performed. This step is obviously a prelude to possible early operation and would be undertaken only if the patient was felt to be an acceptable surgical candidate. If the patient is stable and the carotid duplex scan does not indicate severe carotid stenosis, arteriography is delayed for 4 to 6 weeks, during which time the patient undergoes supportive treatment and rehabilitation. At that point, he or she is readmitted to assess completeness of recovery and suitability for operative intervention. If a good neurologic recovery has occurred, the patient should be considered for endarterectomy to prevent recurrent ipsilateral strokes. The cardiologist and neurologist are invited to re-evaluate their respective systems, and cerebral angiography is performed. If a significant lesion is confirmed by arteriography, CEA is planned during this second admission, usually about 6 weeks from the initial cerebral event.

There are obvious permutations in the presentation of patients with a completed stroke, but our overall viewpoint is to be relatively aggressive in the patient with a small or fluctuating neurologic deficit and a "dangerous lesion," namely, an ultratight stenosis or trailing intraluminal thrombus, and to be relatively conservative in patients with severe, fixed neurologic deficits. One major exception to this approach is the patient who undergoes CEA and who has the onset of a neurologic deficit during operation or in the early postoperative period. In this situation, reoperation is undertaken immediately in the effort to restore full internal carotid flow. Such occlusions are likely to be related to a technical error at the time of the initial operation, which may be identified and corrected at the second procedure. Another uncommon exception is the patient who develops an acute stroke in the hospital after having severe carotid disease identified angiographically a short time before. If carotid flow can be restored within 1 to 2 hours from the onset of symptoms, operative intervention should be considered. Some patients have dramatic neurologic clearing after an emergency thromboendarterectomy in this setting, but others fail to respond.

As emphasized at each step in this discussion, surgery for carotid artery occlusive disease continues to be a controversial topic, although it is slowly becoming less so. Many physicians, particularly those who deal with cardiovascular disorders, are confronted daily by patients with evidence of disease in the extracranial carotid circulation. It is not enough to say simply that we do not yet know the correct answers to all their problems. Physicians must manage each patient as an individual with compassion and candor by weighing the expected natural history of the disease against the risks inherent in surgical therapy. We have confidence in the system of care described but realize that all modes of therapy are subject to change as new data become available.

Suggested Reading

Blaisdell WF, Clauss RH, Galbraith JG, et al. Joint study of extracranial arterial occlusions. JAMA 1969; 209:1889.

Chambers BR, Norris JW. Outcome in patients with asymptomatic neck bruits. N Engl J Med 1986; 315:860.

European Carotid Surgery Trialists' Collaborative Group. MRC European Carotid Surgery Trial: Interim results for symptomatic patients with severe (70–99%) or with mild (0–29%) carotid stenosis. Lancet 1991; 337:1235.

Executive Committee for the Asymptomatic Carotid Atherosclerosis Study. Endarterectomy for asymptomatic carotid artery stenosis. JAMA 1995; 273:1421.

Hertzer NR, Beven EG, Young JR, et al. Coronary artery disease in peripheral vascular patients: A classification of 1000 coronary angiograms and results of surgical management. Ann Surg 1984; 199:223.

Hobson, II RW, Weiss DG, Fields WS, et al. Efficacy of carotid endarterectomy for asymptomatic carotid stenosis. N Engl J Med 1993; 328:221.

Kent KC, Kuntz KM, Patel MR, et al. Perioperative imaging strategies for carotid endarterectomy: an analysis of morbidity and cost-effectiveness in symptomatic patients. JAMA 1995; 274:888.

Kraiss LW, Kilberg L, Critch S, et al. Short-stay carotid endarterectomy is safe and cost-effective. Am J Surg 1995; 169:512.

Luna G, Adye B. Cost-effective carotid endarterectomy. Am J Surg 1995; 169:516.

Mayberg MR, Wilson SE, Yatsu F, et al. Carotid endarterectomy and prevention of cerebral ischemia in symptomatic carotid stenosis. JAMA 1991; 266:3289.

Moore WS, Mohr JP, Najafi H, et al. Carotid endarterectomy: Practice guidelines. J Vasc Surg 1992; 15:469.

North American Symptomatic Carotid Endarterectomy Trial Collaborators. Beneficial effect of carotid endarterectomy in symptomatic patients with high grade stenosis. N Engl J Med 1991; 325:445.

Roederer GO, Langlois YE, Jager KA, et al. The natural history of carotid arterial disease in asymptomatic patients with cervical bruits. Stroke 1984; 15:605.

Wiebers DO, Whisnant JP. In: Warlow C, Morris PJ, eds. Transient ischemic attacks. New York: Marcel Dekker, 1982:8.

PERIPHERAL ARTERIAL DISEASE (OTHER THAN THE AORTA AND CAROTID ARTERIES)

Thomas F. Dodson, M.D.

Cardiovascular disease continues to be the leading cause of death in the United States, and hence patients with peripheral vascular disease are endemic within our population. A new multidisciplinary field, entitled *endovascular surgery,* holds great promise for patients with vascular disease, both now and in the future. Unfortunately, with burgeoning technology, it is sometimes unclear which technique should be utilized in specific patient problems. This chapter describes my method of management in the two most common types of patient presentation: (1) the patient with claudication due to atherosclerosis and (2) the patient with rest pain or a distal lesion due to atherosclerosis.

■ APPROACH

The Patient with Claudication

Depending on the site of the obstructing lesion(s), patients with claudication may describe pain in the buttocks or thighs, as in patients with aortoiliac disease, or pain in one or both calves, as in patients with (typically) more distal disease. After listening to the initial complaints or symptoms, it is important at this point in the examination to try to gain some appreciation of the distance the patient is able to walk prior to onset of claudication. A typical clinical classification is (1) less than one block (150 meters), (2) one to two blocks (150 to 300 meters), and (3) more than two blocks.

Simple observation of the patient's extremities is also informative at this time as lack of hair, thin or shiny skin, pallor with elevation, and rubor with dependency are helpful indicators of the degree of ischemia. Careful physical examination of the patient with claudication includes not only examination of the pulses and their intensity but also palpation of the abdomen and popliteal fossa for the presence of aneurysms, and auscultation of the neck, abdomen, and groins for the presence of bruits. In the majority of patients, the physical examination reveals or suggests the site of the obstructing lesion(s).

If the patient has relatively new onset of claudication (<2 months) and the claudication does not interfere with his or her occupation or significantly with his or her lifestyle, I try to suggest alteration of any attendant risk factors that might be playing a role in this process. Therefore, I encourage cessation of smoking, treatment of hypertension (if present), loss of weight if the patient is overweight, treatment of hyperlipidemia, and increased exercise. The latter should be done to the point of pain with the patient stopping at this point, and then resumed after a few minutes of rest. Although there is still some debate about the relative benignancy of claudication, it is relatively clear that the patient has only a small risk of limb loss (about 3 percent per year) over the ensuing years (Imparato and co-workers, 1975). It should further be recognized, however, that claudication is often an indicator of diffuse atherosclerotic disease, and most studies have demonstrated an annual mortality of about 5 percent per year. Given the fact that the majority of patients die of heart disease, it is easy to appreciate the importance of risk factor reduction as a primary therapy. As a part of the initial examination of the patient with claudication, vascular laboratory arterial studies are ordered to document quantitatively the degree of the patient's ischemia. These are used both as a baseline measurement and as a predictor of future problems. As an important part of the vascular laboratory assessment, an ankle-brachial artery index (ABI) is performed on each lower extremity, and, with the exception of some diabetic patients, this is another helpful indicator of the degree of ischemia of that extremity. Although the normal ABI is greater than 1.0, most patients with claudication have a pressure index of 0.6 or less.

Even if the patient has had claudication for longer than 2 months or the claudication interferes with his or her occupation or life-style, it is rare for us to offer interventional therapy at the first visit. Most of these patients have risk factors to which some attempt at reduction should be made. Although a majority of patients will not be able to stop smoking, reduce their weight and blood pressure, and increase their exercise, a minority will be able to do so and should be given the opportunity prior to attempts at intervention. We are, however, slightly more aggressive with the patient with aortoiliac lesions and resultant buttock or thigh claudication because of the potential that a percutaneous approach to the problem may be possible.

Once we are convinced that the claudication is not responsive to attempts at risk reduction *and* (most important) it is interfering with the patient's occupation or life-style to a significant degree, we then bring the patient into the hospital for angiography. It should be re-emphasized at this point that only a minority of patients with claudication should be considered for operative intervention. The majority of such patients who do not have disabling claudication or claudication that interferes with gainful employment should rather be treated by risk reduction and exercise programs. Part of the responsibility of the attending physician at this point, particularly with so many options available to the interventional radiologist or cardiologist, is to communicate with the interventionist as to the patient's signs and symptoms and the results of the noninvasive vascular laboratory examinations. This communication lends itself to a smoother and (it is hoped) less complicated hospital course and is an important part of the "team" approach to vascular disease.

The mainstay of the interventional radiologist or cardiologist, since the mid-1960s, has been percutaneous transluminal balloon angioplasty. Although lasers are being used to recanalize arteries by either heat or vaporization, this is still an experimental technology, and the results in the literature have been equivocal at best. The burgeoning of this technology has even prompted representatives from leading vascular and radiology societies to write to a prominent medical journal to inform the readers about the "indiscriminate" use of the laser and the "experimental nature" of this approach. Other techniques that seem to hold promise and are currently undergoing investigation are the use of the atherectomy catheter, a device that allows plaque to be shaved free from the wall of the vessel, compacted into a distal chamber, and then withdrawn from the vessel; stents that can be placed across stenotic regions; and ultrasonic angioplasty that utilizes catheter-delivered ultrasound energy to permit recanalization of total arterial obstructions. All of these devices are in an early, developmental stage, although the Simpson atherectomy catheter has been approved by the Food and Drug Administration for the treatment of stenotic vessels.

In our institution, the patient with claudication due to atherosclerosis who is to undergo angiography typically comes into the hospital the night before the procedure and is placed on the vascular surgery service. Both the vascular surgeon and the radiologist visit the patient prior to the procedure to answer any questions that the patient might have. The vascular surgeon thus serves as a backup in case the radiologist encounters problems or has complications in the radiology suite.

If lesions that are amenable to balloon angioplasty are discovered during the examination, the interventional radiologist passes a guidewire through the area of stenosis or obstruction and then creates a "controlled injury" to the vessel wall by means of balloon inflation. Although the luminal diameter is increased by means of breaking or cracking the diseased intima and media, the results in selected circumstances are quite good: Iliac stenoses have a primary success rate of approximately 90 percent, with follow-up studies showing an approximate 80 percent patency; and femoral stenoses, although they do slightly less well, have initial patency rates of 70 to 85 percent with follow-up figures of 50 to 70 percent patency (Widlus and Osterman, 1989). The role of percutaneous transluminal angioplasty has recently been questioned in patients with limb-threatening ischemia because of a lack of durability of the procedure with respect to conventional bypass procedures. The Veterans Administration Cooperative Study, however, in looking primarily at patients with claudication, demonstrated that percutaneous transluminal angioplasty and bypass were similar with respect to hemodynamic results, amputations, and deaths after a mean follow-up of 2 years (Wilson and co-workers, 1989).

If lesions are discovered that are not typically amenable to angioplasty—multiple stenotic areas, short occlusions that do not allow passage of the guidewire, or lengthy occlusions—the angiogram is completed and the patient is returned to his or her room. At this point the surgeon and the patient have to discuss the options that are available from a surgical standpoint to revascularize the extremity and relieve the claudication. An important part of the decision-making process in this situation is an assessment of the cardiovascular risk of the particular procedure. If the patient will require a general or spinal anesthetic for the performance of the procedure, we then ask our cardiology colleagues to see the patient and help us assess the patient's cardiac status. The history of the patient obviously plays a significant role in this assessment, and certainly a history of a previous myocardial infarction, angina at either rest or exertion, or electrocardiographic changes suggesting either ischemia or infarction make us less enthusiastic about operating for the symptom of claudication. In this institution, dipyridamole-thallium scintigraphy (Persantine-thallium scan) is the preferred preoperative examination in patients who have evidence either by history or electrocardiogram of myocardial ischemia. It would be unusual in the patient in whom claudication was the indication for surgery to proceed to coronary artery arteriography after discovery of a "positive" dipyridamole-thallium scan. When angina is present or the cardiologist determines the dipyridamole-thallium scan indicates a serious reperfusion defect, a coronary arteriogram may be performed. When this occurs, a decision must be made as to the need for coronary bypass surgery or coronary angioplasty before the surgery on the peripheral arteries. Only after a clear evaluation of the risks and imponderables of operative intervention can a prudent decision be made for or against operation.

If the patient is a reasonable operative candidate, a procedure is planned to relieve the patient's claudication with a minimum of operative risk. The surgical approach to both aortoiliac occlusive disease and femoropopliteal occlusive disease in the patient with claudication follows.

Aortoiliac Occlusive Disease

In these patients, the claudication has to be of a very severe nature to warrant operative intervention. The reason for this restrictive approach is that these patients often require an aortobi-iliac or aortobifemoral operation, an operative procedure that carries, in the best of hands, a 1 to 2 percent perioperative mortality. Thus, one does not embark on an operation of this magnitude unless the claudication is severely limiting to the degree that the patient is unable to carry out the daily activities of living or the patient's employment is threatened. Once this degree of disability has been confirmed and the patient's cardiac risk has been assessed to be minimal, mild, or stable disease, the patient is taken to the operating room where, in the majority of patients, an arterial line and Swan-Ganz catheter are placed for careful monitoring of blood pressure and intravascular volume. We generally place a bifurcated graft, even in situations where there appears to be only minimal or moderate disease in one iliac, because the natural history of aortoiliac disease is ultimately to involve both runoff vessels. If there is evidence of disease in the external iliac, then we tend to make the distal connection to the common femoral artery in the groin and extend a portion of the prosthesis over the profunda femoris vessel, addressing at that time the potential for stenosis at the orifice of this important vessel to the musculature of the thigh. Because these patients may have or may develop occlusion of the superficial femoral artery, the runoff of the profunda femoris often becomes the main blood supply to the lower leg. After the graft has been placed and hemostasis has been obtained, the retroperitoneum is closed over the graft to decrease the risk of graft erosion into the duodenum, and the abdomen is closed. Perfusion to the lower extremities is checked postoperatively by either palpation of pulses or by use of the Doppler to assess flow. The patient is then transferred to the intensive care unit to be monitored overnight, and typically the patient is able to be transferred out of the intensive care unit the next day. The postoperative recovery period for an operation of this magnitude is usually 7 to 10 days, and we usually recommend another 2 to 4 weeks of limited activity after returning home before going back to work. The short- and long-term results of this operative procedure are quite good: the 5 year patency rate is usually greater than 80 percent, and the 10 year patency rate is about 75 percent. Patients can usually tell a difference in their perfusion while ambulating in the hospital, and an even more marked improvement is noted upon return to work or to the activities of daily living.

Femoropopliteal Occlusive Disease

In this group of patients, although we still insist upon some significant limitation of activity due to the patient's claudication, the operative procedures do not carry the same degree of risk as in patients with aortoiliac disease, and thus we are somewhat more inclined to intervene in patients with less severe claudication. It should be emphasized, however, that patients with claudication should be approached carefully and conservatively because of the potential risk of taking a relatively stable situation and converting it into one where the patient may lose either limb or life. Patients with calf claudication usually have either significant stenoses or occlusion in the superficial femoral artery of the thigh. As discussed, in selected circumstances, percutaneous transluminal angioplasty may be selected as the method of treatment. When this form of intervention is either not appropriate or not available, placement of a bypass graft from the femoral artery to the above-knee or below-knee popliteal artery is the usual technique of surgical therapy. There is currently debate within the vascular community about whether the ipsilateral saphenous vein should be saved at the initial operation for an above-knee bypass, and a prosthetic graft (usually polytetrafluoroethylene [PTFE]) used for the first bypass. A recent report by Quinones-Baldrich and colleagues (1992) at UCLA suggested that PTFE had an "important role" in bypasses performed above the knee and a "limited role" for those to the below-knee vessels. They documented a primary patency rate of 68 percent for patients with claudication who had PTFE above-the-knee bypasses at both 5 and 8 years after operation. In patients who had PTFE above-the-knee bypasses for limb salvage, the results were considerably less optimistic: primary patency rates of 50 percent and 40 percent at 5 and 8 years, respectively. Because of the superior patency of the autogenous saphenous vein grafts (77 percent patency at 5 years by Taylor and colleagues [1990]), we have preferentially used this as our conduit of choice. In situations where saphenous vein is not available (usually because of previous usage for coronary artery bypass grafts), we use prosthetic material, but generally *only* for above-knee anastomoses. The majority of patients who undergo lower-extremity procedures for claudication are transferred to the intensive care unit for monitoring overnight, primarily for potential cardiac problems. They are then transferred out the next morning and are taking a few steps in the room by the second or third postoperative day. The postoperative course requires about a week in the hospital after the operation, and another week or two with limited exertion prior to returning to work or daily activities. With careful selection of patients, the operative mortality should be less than or near 1 percent.

The Patient with Rest Pain or a Distal Lesion

Patients with these problems constitute the majority of patients that we are called upon to evaluate. This also seems appropriate in that vascular surgery carries certain inherent risks, and the patient who has limb-threatening ischemia is usually willing to accept these factors in order to preserve the limb. Rest pain is correctly described as an "intolerable symptom," and although it is a clinical finding, it is seen in patients who have ABIs of from 0.30 to 0.50. It should be noted that, as pointed out by the vascular laboratory at Southern Illinois University, patients who have an ABI of 0.30 or less have a "malignant prognosis" with respect to death and vascular-related disorders (Howell and co-workers, 1989). Thus, although we noted that claudication was an indicator of diffuse atherosclerotic disease, severe lower-limb ischemia is an even more ominous finding. Patients with rest pain or distal lesions (including nonhealing ulcers, infected sites that are not resolving, and gangrene) should undergo vascular laboratory arterial studies to quantitate the degree of ischemia, and plans should be made for admission to the hospital (sometimes urgently or even emergently if infection is a significant part of the underlying problem). Interestingly, although patients with rest pain realize the importance of timely admission to the hospital because of their unremitting discomfort, patients with diabetes and severe peripheral neuropathy may not realize the severity of their ischemia, and lesions may go undetected or unnoticed for some period of time, suggesting that education of the diabetic and daily foot examinations are an important part of the care of these patients.

Once the patient with severe lower-extremity ischemia has been admitted to the hospital, plans are made both for angiography and cardiology consultation to aid in the assessment of cardiac risk factors. Other disease processes (e.g., diabetes, hypertension, pulmonary disease) are identified and treated as necessary. As mentioned previously, the patient with a history of or electrocardiographic evidence of previous ischemia or infarction typically undergoes a dipyridamole-thallium scan in order to detect more accurately the risks of myocardial dysfunction with a pending operation. In patients who have "positive" dipyridamole-thallium scans and yet who may need or require operative intervention, it may be necessary to proceed to coronary arteriography in order to define more clearly the lesions responsible for the myocardial ischemia. These lesions may then be dealt with by either a percutaneous technique (i.e., balloon angioplasty) or directly (by cardiac surgery). In the majority of situations, cardiac catheterization is not necessary, and an assessment of myocardial risk factors can be made on the basis of history, electrocardiogram, and the dipyridamole-thallium scan. Given the sophistication of today's anesthesiology and the fact that a number of "extra-anatomic" bypasses can be constructed with reduced risk in even patients with severe heart disease, our preference is to offer operative intervention to most patients with limb-threatening ischemia. This is based on the subjective feeling that patients who have been successfully revascularized seem, in general, to recover somewhat better than patients who require amputation as the primary modality. Moreover, data from the University of Rochester group confirmed a 10 percent in-hospital mortality and a return of ambulatory abilities in less than 50 percent of survivors in patients with severe ischemia subjected to primary amputation (Ouriel and co-workers, 1988). This group also noted that patients who underwent amputation had longer hospital stays than those who had revascularization, and their long-term survival was diminished as well.

As was noted in the discussion of patients with claudication, transluminal angioplasty procedures in patients with limb-threatening ischemia are notable for their lack of durability. The group from the University of Chicago reported that their 2 year patency rate of angioplasty procedures in patients with severe ischemia was approximately 18 percent—significantly lower than their results for either femoropopliteal bypass (68 percent) or femorodistal bypass (47 percent) (Blair and co-workers, 1989). We are in agreement with their data and generally prefer bypass whenever the patient's own risk factors allow that approach. An exception to this standard is the patient with an iliac stenosis who also needs distal surgical reconstruction. We and others have successfully used iliac balloon angioplasty in combination with distal bypass to salvage limbs in jeopardy.

If a bypass procedure is required and the patient's risk factors allow either a general or a spinal anesthetic, the prime responsibility of the vascular surgeon is to ascertain that adequate inflow will be available for revascularization. In patients who have simultaneous aortoiliac disease and femoropopliteal disease (a common combination in patients with limb-threatening ischemia), it may first be necessary to perform a procedure to enhance inflow (i.e., an aortobifemoral operation) before doing the distal bypass procedure. A small percentage of patients with severe ischemia or distal gangrene may require both operations at the same procedure. If the patient is a poor operative risk and cannot undergo a general or spinal anesthetic, other options, including extra-anatomic bypasses such as an axillofemoral bypass or a femorofemoral bypass, can be done, if necessary, under local anesthesia. With the establishment of adequate or good inflow, attention is turned to enhancing the distal perfusion. Unfortunately, the distal procedures (those done at the knee or below) cannot be done with local anesthesia and require at least a spinal anesthetic. A small percentage of patients with limb-threatening ischemia have evidence on angiography of a significant stenosis of the profunda femoris orifice. This anatomic problem can be addressed under a local anesthetic if necessary and may provide enough collateral flow to relieve the rest pain or heal the nonhealing lesion.

Patients whose clinical condition allows a spinal or general anesthetic are candidates for bypass grafts to any arteriographically visualized artery of the lower extremity. Using loop magnification, the vascular surgeon now has the ability to suture to vessels of 1 to 2 mm in diameter. From a practical standpoint, this means that we are able to create a saphenous vein bypass from the groin to either of the three runoff vessels of the lower leg (anterior tibial, posterior tibial, peroneal) or, if necessary, to the vessels of the foot (posterior tibial or dorsalis pedis). In certain selected cases, even in situations with tissue loss in the lower leg or foot, we are able (in conjunction with our plastic surgery colleagues) to revascularize the extremity and then place a free flap over the defect or area of tissue loss. Our preference for distal bypass is to use the saphenous vein. When this is not available, we look for other sites of unused vein and have utilized arm vein or short saphenous vein as acceptable conduits. Although it is not clear from the literature that the "in situ" technique is superior to the previous "reversed" saphenous vein technique, it is clear to us that utilization of the vein in situ allows for less size discrepancy in the proximal and distal anastomoses and probably allows for more frequent use of veins that would otherwise be felt to be too small or inadequate. In our hands, an in situ bypass is a rather lengthy procedure and typically takes from 5 to 6 hours. If a nonhealing lesion is present, we usually debride or amputate as necessary during the same procedure to limit the number of anesthetics that the patient has to undergo. As we have done in the other instances, the patient is transferred to the intensive care unit for monitoring overnight and for careful observation of the distal perfusion because patients with distal bypasses encounter most of their problems within the first 24 hours. The patient who is doing well by the next morning is transferred to the floor, and a gradual course of increasing ambulation is started if the initial distal lesion can tolerate this plan of action. The usual hospital course for the successfully revascularized patient is approximately 7 to 10 days, and debrided open wounds are often placed on dressings and the patient is allowed some time at home prior to readmission and closure of the wound.

Suggested Reading

Ahn SS, Eton D, Moore WS. Endovascular surgery for peripheral arterial occlusive disease. Ann Surg 1992; 216:3.

Blair JM, Gewertz BL, Moosa H, et al. Percutaneous angioplasty versus surgery for limb-threatening ischemia. J Vasc Surg 1989; 9:698.

Gloviczki P, Morris SM, Bower TC, et al. Microvascular pedal bypass for salvage of the severely ischemic limb. Mayo Clin Proc 1991; 66:243.

Howell MA, Colgan MP, Seeger RW, et al. Relationship of severity of lower limb peripheral vascular disease to mortality and morbidity: A six-year follow-up study. J Vasc Surg 1989; 9:691.

Imparato AM, Kim GE, Davidson T, et al. Intermittent claudication: Its natural course. Surgery 1975; 78:795.

Ouriel K, Fiore WM, Geary JE. Limb-threatening ischemia in the medically compromised patient: Amputation or revascularization? Surgery 1988; 104:667.

Quinones-Baldrich WJ, Prego AA, Ucelay-Gomez R, et al. Long-term results of infrainguinal revascularization with polytetrafluoroethylene: A ten-year experience. J Vasc Surg 1992; 16:209.

Taylor LM, Edwards JM, Porter JM. Present status of reversed vein bypass grafting: Five-year results of a modern series. J Vasc Surg 1990; 11:193.

Widlus DM, Osterman FA. Evaluation and percutaneous management of atherosclerotic peripheral vascular disease. JAMA 1989; 261:3148.

Wilson SE, Wolf GL, Cross AP. Percutaneous transluminal angioplasty versus operation for peripheral arteriosclerosis. J Vasc Surg 1989; 9:1.

ENDOCARDITIS OF NATURAL AND PROSTHETIC VALVES: TREATMENT AND PROPHYLAXIS

Linda A. Slavoski, M.D.
Donald Kaye, M.D.

Infective endocarditis (IE) is a microbial infection of the endothelial lining of the heart. The characteristic lesion is a vegetation found on the valvular leaflets that may extend to the chordae tendineae and involve the endocardium of the ventricles, atria, or septal defects. Extracardiac endothelium may harbor the microbial infection as well.

■ NATIVE VALVE ENDOCARDITIS

Some 60 to 80 percent of persons with native valve endocarditis (NVE) who do not use parenteral drugs have an identifiable predisposing cardiac lesion. Congenital heart disease can be a predisposing factor in the development of IE in adulthood. These lesions include ventricular septal defect (VSD), bicuspid aortic valve, coarctation of the aorta, and tetralogy of Fallot. Other lesions predisposing to IE include those associated with rheumatic valvular disease, the mitral valve being the most commonly involved, followed by the aortic valve. Mitral valve prolapse (MVP) is another common predisposing entity, especially in the younger population. Degenerative heart disease, particularly calcific aortic stenosis, is important in the elderly.

Most cases of endocarditis in native valves in nondrug abusers are caused by streptococci, enterococci, and staphylococci. Viridans streptococci (*S. sanguis, S. milleri, S. mutans*) account for most streptococcal infections, and most are highly susceptible to penicillin. These are frequently reported in patients having recently undergone dental procedures.

Enterococci commonly associated with endocarditis are *Enterococcus faecalis* and *Enterococcus faecium,* which cause about 10 percent of cases of NVE. They are normal inhabitants of the lower gastrointestinal tract and anterior urethra. It is important to review the sensitivity patterns, since most are not killed by penicillin alone.

Staphylococci cause 25 percent of cases of NVE, most being *Staphylococcus aureus* (coagulase positive) and are usually resistant to penicillin due to the production of betalactamase. Endocarditis due to *S. aureus* is often fulminant, with rapid valve destruction. Many other bacteria occasionally cause IE.

Fungi rarely cause NVE in the absence of intravenous drug abuse. Other predisposing factors are a long course of antibiotics, corticosteroids, or cytotoxic agents and indwelling central venous catheters.

■ PROSTHETIC VALVE ENDOCARDITIS (PVE)

PVE is divided into early, within 60 days of valve replacement, and late, more than 60 days after valve replacement. Early PVE generally reflects contamination arising either intraoperatively or postoperatively from intravascular lines, ureteral catheters, and so on. Organisms most commonly isolated are *Staphylococcus epidermidis* followed by *S. aureus.* The remaining cases are due to gram-negative aerobic organisms, diphtheroids, enterococci, fungi, and streptococci.

Late PVE is most often the result of transient bacteremia occurring months after the valve has been implanted. However, many cases of apparent late PVE are acquired in the early period but with a very long incubation period. Thus, the bacteriology resembles a mixture of that of native valve endocarditis and early PVE. Viridans streptococci are the most common, followed by staphylococci, gram-negative bacilli, fungi, and diphtheroids.

■ ENDOCARDITIS IN INTRAVENOUS DRUG ABUSERS

Infective endocarditis in intravenous drug abusers (IVDA) occurs in normal valves, congenitally or otherwise abnormal valves, or prosthetic valves. *S. aureus* is by far most frequently isolated, followed by enterococci, streptococci, gram-negative bacilli (predominantly *Pseudomonas* and *Serratia* species), and fungi (usually a nonalbicans *Candida* species). The great majority of patients with *S. aureus* infection have right-sided endocarditis, most frequently involving the tricuspid valve. When endocarditis in the drug addict affects the left side of the heart, previous valvular abnormalities usually exist.

■ PATHOGENESIS AND PATHOPHYSIOLOGY

The hemodynamic factors that lead to endothelial damage include a high-velocity abnormal jet stream as in aortic and mitral insufficiency, flow from a high-pressure to a low-pressure chamber as in VSD, and a narrow orifice between two chambers capable of creating a pressure gradient. The damaged endothelium promotes deposition of clumps of fibrin and platelets, forming sterile vegetations or nonbacterial thrombotic endocarditis. Organisms adhere to these abnormal areas, and fibrin and platelets continue to be deposited. Underlying valve destruction occurs. Virulent organisms such as *S. aureus* can infect normal valves.

For IE to occur, micro-organisms must invade the circulation, most often from the oropharynx, the gastrointestinal tract, and the genitourinary tract. The bacteremias are transient (15 to 30 minutes). Viridans streptococcal bacteremias are associated with dental manipulations or trauma to the tissues in the mouth. Enterococcal and gram-negative bacillus bacteremias occur with trauma to the genitourinary or gastrointestinal tracts.

Pathology in the heart includes obstruction of the valve orifices from large vegetations, valve deformity, rupture of chordae, and burrowing abscesses. Extension of an abscess can lead to pericarditis. Embolization from fragmentation of vegetations can cause occlusive disease or abscesses in peripheral organs, most commonly in renal, splenic, or cerebral circulation. Mycotic aneurysms may form.

Persistent bacteremia stimulates the humoral and cellular immune systems, which accounts for much of the extracardiac manifestations. The immunologic host response includes circulating immune complexes, hypocomplementemia, and formation of rheumatoid factor. Circulating immune complexes are responsible for the glomerulonephritis as well as mucocutaneous vasculitic lesions.

■ CLINICAL MANIFESTATIONS

IE should be considered in any patient with unexplained fever. Symptoms of endocarditis generally begin within 2 weeks of the initial bacteremia. Fever is the most common finding. Chills, night sweats, and nonspecific symptoms such as fatigue, malaise, anorexia, and weight loss often accompany fever.

Cardiac murmurs are present in most patients with endocarditis; right-sided infection is an exception. Other cardiac manifestations include congestive heart failure, myocarditis, conduction disturbances, and pericarditis.

About 30 percent of IE cases have splenomegaly and about half have cutaneous or peripheral manifestations. Petechiae are the most common cutaneous findings and are generally found on the conjunctiva, palate, buccal mucosa, and the upper extremities. Splinter hemorrhages are subungual linear dark red streaks. Osler's nodes (small, tender, purple nodules) develop in the pulp of digits. Janeway lesions are small nontender hemorrhagic lesions on the palms or soles. Roth's spots appear as pale centered oval hemorrhages on the retina. Musculoskeletal complaints are frequent.

Systemic embolization occurs in about a third of IE patients. The most common site is the spleen, followed by the kidneys. Cerebral embolism is often devastating. Pulmonary emboli are common in right-sided disease.

Most patients with IE have renal disease with glomerulonephritis from immune complex deposition or infarction or abscess as a result of embolization.

■ LABORATORY FEATURES AND DIAGNOSIS

A normochromic normocytic anemia is relatively common. The white blood cell count is usually normal. The erythrocyte sedimentation rate is almost always elevated, and rheumatoid factor is present in about 50 percent of the patients. The urinalysis is usually abnormal, with hematuria and/or proteinuria. Echocardiography can provide information about valvular destruction, perivalvular involvement, and hemodynamic changes. Transesophageal echocardiography is more sensitive than transthoracic echocardiography in detecting vegetations (especially on prosthetic valves) and myocardial abscesses.

The blood culture is the single most important laboratory test. Once IE is suspected, at least three sets of blood cultures should be obtained over 24 hours at least 1 hour apart, regardless of temperature. In the case of acute endocarditis, they should be collected over 2 hours. Blood culture results may be negative in those who have received prior antibiotics or with fastidious organisms such as the HACEK group (*Haemophilus, Actinobacillus, Cardiobacterium, Eikenella, Kingella*), nutritionally deficient streptococci, *Brucella* species, *Neisseria* species, *Chlamydia, Nocardia,* and fungi. If the patient has received prior antibiotic therapy and if the clinical status allows, it may be worthwhile to obtain serial blood cultures off antibiotics. Since some organisms (e.g., HACEK) may take 3 weeks or longer to grow, cultures should be held for at least 3 to 4 weeks. Appropriate subcultures and Gram stains

Table 1 Treatment of Streptococcal and Enterococcal Endocarditis

Viridans streptococci/*S. bovis*	
Penicillin G-susceptible (MIC ≤0.1 μg/ml)	
Regimen A	Penicillin G 12 million to 18 million U/day IV (divided doses) for 4 weeks
Regimen B	Penicillin G as in A + gentamicin 1 mg/kg IV q8h, both for 2 weeks
*Regimen C	Ceftriaxone 2 g IV/IM qd for 4 weeks
†Regimen D	Vancomycin 15 mg/kg IV q12h for 4 weeks
Prosthetic valve:	Penicillin or vancomycin as above for 6 weeks with gentamicin for at least 2 weeks
Streptococci with relative penicillin resistance (MCI >0.1 μg/ml but <0.5 μg/ml)	
Regimen E	Penicillin G 18 million U/day IV for 4 weeks + gentamicin 1 mg/kg IV q8h for the first 2 weeks
Regimen D	
Enterococci or other streptococci (MIC ≥0.5 μg/ml)	
Regimen F	Penicillin G 18 million to 30 million U/day IV (divided doses) or ampicillin 2 g IV q4h plus gentamicin 1 mg/kg (max 80 mg) q8h IV/IM combination for 4–6 weeks
Regimen G:	Vancomycin 15 mg/kg IV q12h + gentamicin as in F, both for 4–6 weeks
Prosthetic valve:	As in F or G, treatment for 6–8 weeks

*Can be used for patients with history of penicillin rash.
†Anaphylaxis with penicillin.
Streptomycin 7.5 mg/kg (not to exceed 500 mg) IM q12h may be substituted for gentamicin.

Table 2 Treatment of Staphylococcal Endocarditis

NATIVE VALVE	
Methicillin susceptible (*S. epidermidis, S. aureus*)	
Regimen A	Nafcillin 2 g IV q4h for 4–6 weeks with or without gentamicin 1 mg/kg IV q8h for the first 3–5 days
*Regimen B	Cefazolin 2 g IV q8h for 4–6 weeks with or without gentamicin as in regimen A
†Regimen C	Vancomycin 15 mg/kg q12h for 4–6 weeks
Methicillin resistant	
Regimen C	
PROSTHETIC VALVE	
Methicillin susceptible	
Regimen A, B, or C for 6–8 weeks plus gentamicin 1 mg/kg IV q8h for the initial 2 weeks plus rifampin 300 mg PO q8h for 6–8 weeks	
Methicillin resistance	
Regimen C for 6–8 weeks plus gentamicin 1 mg/kg IV q8h for the initial 2 weeks plus rifampin 300 mg PO q8h for 6–8 weeks	

*History of penicillin rash.
†Anaphylaxis with penicillin.

Table 3 Treatment of Endocarditis Involving Uncommon Organisms

HACEK organisms	Ceftriaxone 2 g IV q.d. for 4 weeks
Enterobacteriaceae	Third-generation cephalosporin or imipenem 0.5–1 g IV q6h or aztreonam 2 g IV q6h plus gentamicin 1.7 mg/kg IV q8h for 4–6 weeks
Pseudomonas aeruginosa	Piperacillin 3 g IV q4h or ceftazidime 2 g IV q8h or imipenem 0.5–1 g IV q6h or aztreonam 2 g IV q6h plus tobramycin 1.7 mg/kg IV q8h for 6 weeks
*Fungi	Amphotericin B 1 mg/kg IV/day plus flucytosine 150 mg/kg/day in 4 divided doses (levels must be monitored)

*Cardiac surgery is required.
HACEK, *Haemophilus, Actinobacillus, Cardiobacterium, Eikenella, Kingella.*

of the blood cultures that would otherwise be considered negative may identify positive cultures for some of these organisms.

■ THERAPY

Antimicrobial therapy should be initiated as soon as feasible, often started empirically until the organism is isolated, then adjusted. Therapy should consist of bactericidal antimicrobial therapy in sufficient doses and for a long enough period to sterilize the vegetation. Parenteral therapy is preferable, since it achieves higher and more predictable serum levels than oral therapy.

Once isolated and identified, the infecting organism should be evaluated by susceptibility testing. Both minimum inhibitory concentration (MIC) and minimum bactericidal concentration (MBC) should be determined.

Streptococci and Enterococci

The regimens for streptococcal and enterococcal endocarditis are based on MIC to penicillin G. For streptococci inhibited by 0.1 μg/ml and for nonallergic adults, penicillin may be used in conjunction with an aminoglycoside for 2 weeks (Table 1, regimen B). If aminoglycoside therapy is problematic, a 4 week regimen of penicillin or ceftriaxone alone is adequate (regimens A and C). For penicillin-allergic patients, a cephalosporin (regimen C) or vancomycin (regimen D) is substituted or desensitization is used if suitable. Regimen C is useful for home therapy of stable patients. PVE should be treated with at least 6 weeks of penicillin with at least 2 weeks of aminoglycoside combination.

With strains that are relatively penicillin resistant (MIC between 0.1 μg per milliliter and 0.5 μg per milliliter), an aminoglycoside should be added to penicillin for the first

Table 4 Recommendations for Prophylaxis Against Endocarditis

PROCEDURE	LIMITING FACTORS	RECOMMENDED REGIMEN
Dental/upper respiratory	Not allergic to penicillin; able to take oral meds	Amoxicillin 3 g PO 1 hour before, then 1.5 g 6 hours later
	Allergic to penicillin	Erythromycin 1 g PO 2 hours before, then 0.5 g PO 6 hours later or clindamycin 300 mg PO 1 hour before, then 150 mg 6 hours later
	Unable to take oral meds	Ampicillin 2 g IV or IM 30 min before, then 1 g 6 hours later
	Unable to take oral meds, allergic to penicillin	Clindamycin 300 mg IV 30 min before, then 150 mg IV 6 hours later
	High risk optional (prosthetic valve)	Ampicillin 2 g IV or IM plus gentamicin 1.5 mg/kg 30 min prior to procedure, repeated 8 hours later*
	High risk, allergic to penicillin	Vancomycin 1 g over 1 hour starting 1 hour before; no repeat dose needed
Genitourinary/lower gastrointestinal	No allergy	Ampicillin 2 g IV or IM plus gentamicin 1.5 mg/kg 30 min before, then repeat 8 hours later*
	Allergy to penicillin	Vancomycin 1 g IV over 1 hour plus gentamicin 1.5 mg/kg 1 hour before, then repeat 8 hours later
	Low-risk patient	Amoxicillin 3 g PO 1 hour before, then 1.5 g 6 hours later

*Or amoxicillin 1.5 g orally 6 hours later.

2 weeks of therapy (regimen E). Regimen D should be used in the patient who is allergic to penicillin.

Viridans streptococci with MIC of at least 0.5 μg per milliliter, nutritionally variant streptococci, and enterococci require higher doses of penicillin or ampicillin with an aminoglycoside for the duration of therapy, provided that the organism in vitro is inhibited by 500 μg of gentamicin or 2,000 μg per milliliter of streptomycin (regimen F). Vancomycin is substituted in cases of penicillin allergy (regimen G). Therapy should be expanded to 6 to 8 weeks with a complicated course or prosthetic valve.

Enterococci should be tested for antimicrobial resistance. Strains with high resistance to one or more of the agents used for therapy have been isolated from patients with endocarditis, rendering the agent ineffective (i.e., MIC above 32 μg per milliliter for penicillin G, ampicillin or vancomycin, above 500 μg per milliliter for gentamycin, and above 2,000 μg per milliliter for streptomycin). When no aminoglycoside is active, therapy with a cell-wall active agent alone should be given for 8 to 12 weeks.

Staphylococci

Most staphylococci are resistant to penicillin due to beta-lactamase production. Drugs of choice are the semisynthetic penicillinase-resistant penicillins (nafcillin, oxacillin) or first-generation cephalosporins (Table 2, regimens A and B). Those who are allergic to penicillin or are infected with methicillin-resistant staphylococci should be treated with vancomycin (regimen C). The addition of gentamicin hastens clearing of bacteremia but should be administered only for 3 to 5 days. Therapy is usually for 4 weeks, but 6 weeks or longer may be indicated with complicated courses.

Staphylococcal prosthetic valve endocarditis with *S. epidermidis* is treated for 6 to 8 weeks with the addition of rifampin and gentamicin. If intracardiac abscess or valve dysfunction is noted, surgery is indicated. The use of rifampin and gentamicin for *S. aureus* in PVE is controversial but reasonable.

Other Organisms

Endocarditis caused by gram-negative bacilli, anaerobes, and other uncommon pathogens should be treated with the regimen that demonstrates the best activity in vitro (Table 3). Fungal endocarditis is best managed with medical and surgical therapy.

■ PREVENTION

Conditions for which prophylaxis is recommended include prosthetic valves, previous bacterial endocarditis, rheumatic and other valvular abnormalities, MVP with regurgitation, hypertrophic cardiomyopathy, and most congenital cardiac malformations. Prophylaxis is not recommended for isolated secundum atrial septal defect, prior coronary bypass graft surgery, physiologic murmurs, cardiac pacemakers, or implanted defibrillators.

Prophylaxis is recommended for invasive procedures associated with a high incidence of bacteremia with organisms likely to cause endocarditis and is advised for dental and other traumatic procedures in the mouth, nose, or esophagus. It is also recommended for genitourinary, lower gastrointestinal tract, and gallbladder procedures that are likely to cause significant trauma such as urethral dilation, prostatic surgery, vaginal hysterectomy, and colonic or gallbladder surgery. Recommended regimens are listed in Table 4.

Suggested Reading

Dajani A, Bisno A, Chung K, et al. Prevention of bacterial endocarditis: Recommendations by the American Heart Association. JAMA 1990; 264:2919–2922.

Kaye D. Infective Endocarditis. 2nd ed. New York: Raven Press, 1992.

Weinstein L. Infective Endocarditis. In: Braunwald E, ed. Heart diseases: A textbook of cardiovascular medicine. 3rd ed. Philadelphia: WB Saunders, 1988:1093.

Wilson WR, Katchmet AW, Datani AS, et al. Antibiotic treatment of adults with infective endocarditis due to streptococci, enterococci, staphylococci, and HACEK microorganisms. JAMA 1995; 224:1706–1713.

HYPERTENSION: ESSENTIAL

Edward D. Frohlich, M.D., M.A.C.P., F.A.C.C.

Arterial pressure is controlled by a fine interrelationship of physiologic mechanisms that maintain normal vessel caliber and blood flow to the organs. Essential hypertension is a common (upward of 20 percent of the general population) cardiovascular disease that results from a disregulation of those mechanisms, and it is manifested by an elevated (≥90 mm Hg) diastolic pressure. A classification of hypertension with respect to severity of essential hypertension is presented in Table 1. If essential hypertension remains untreated, it will result in functional impairment of the target organs (i.e., heart, brain, kidneys) and death. When systolic arterial pressure is elevated (≥140 mm Hg) in the absence of diastolic pressure elevation (<90 mm Hg), isolated systolic hypertension results. This is encountered more frequently in elderly individuals and is discussed elsewhere in this text.

The abnormally elevated arterial pressure in essential hypertension is produced primarily by an increased total peripheral resistance that reflects arteriolar constriction. This increased vascular resistance is more or less uniformly distributed throughout the organ circulations and particularly the target organs of the disease.

Venular constriction also occurs in hypertension and is responsible for the redistribution in the periphery circulating blood to the central cardiopulmonary area to augment or maintain cardiac output, and it is also responsible for increasing capillary hydrostatic pressure that serves to contract intravascular volume. There is a large variety of physiologic factors that may participate in increasing vascular smooth muscle tone by active constriction or reduced dilation (Table 2). A clear understanding of these mechanisms is important because, with the wide spectrum of antihypertensive agents that is presently available and under study for clinical use and because of the multifactorial nature of the disease, it is now possible to select therapy that is more appropriate for the specific patients based on their clinical, demographic, and pathophysiologic characteristics (Table 3).

Table 1 Classification of Blood Pressure for Adults 18 Years and Older

CATEGORY	SYSTOLIC (MM HG)	DIASTOLIC (MM HG)
Normal	<130	<85
High normal	130–139	85–89
Hypertension		
Stage 1 (mild)	140–159	90–99
Stage 2 (moderate)	160–179	100–109
Stage 3 (severe)	180–209	110–119
Stage 4 (very severe)	≥210	≥120

From the Joint National Committee's Fifth Report on the Detection, Evaluation and Treatment of High Blood Pressure. Arch Intern Med 1993; 153:154–183; with permission.

THERAPEUTIC ALTERNATIVES

At the present time, therapy of essential hypertension is exclusively medical in nature unless a secondary form of hypertension (e.g., aortic coarctation, renal arterial disease, hormonal producing tumor) complicates underlying essential hypertension. Medical therapy should consider nonpharmacologic as well as pharmacologic modalities. The former may be adequate in itself for controlling arterial pressure in patients with lower levels of mild essential hypertension (i.e., diastolic pressures 90 to 95 or 100 mm Hg); however, it may also be of value in patients requiring pharmacotherapy because these modalities may permit reduced doses or the number of pharmacologic agents prescribed.

Pharmacotherapy of hypertension has undergone a dramatic evolution over the past 3 decades. Initially, this involved a rational stepped-care approach in which a diuretic was prescribed followed by an antiadrenergic agent and then a direct-acting vasodilator; if necessary, a still more potent agent was used. However, at present, because of the introduction of other classes of agents (i.e., beta-adrenergic receptor blockers, alpha-adrenergic receptor and alpha-beta adrenergic receptor blockers, angiotensin converting enzyme [ACE] inhibitors, and calcium antagonists), a program of "individualized stepped care" is now possible. This approach provides a greater option for selection of initial therapeutic agents that may be more specific for that particular patient. Some have suggested that the former approach to therapy was "empiric," but actually there was an important physiologic rationale for the diuretic as the initial choice. Thus, were either the adrenergic inhibitor or the vasodilator to be used initially, intravascular volume would expand because of the reduced hydrostatic and renal perfusion pressures, thereby attenuating the immediate pressure reduction. This phenomenon of pseudotolerance does not seem to occur with the beta-blockers, ACE inhibitors, calcium antagonists, or the alpha- or $alpha_1$-beta–adrenergic receptor inhibitors when they are used as monotherapeutic agents. Moreover, these newer classes of antihypertensive agents do not provoke reflexive cardiac stimulation with arterial pressure reduction as did the direct-acting smooth muscle vasodilators.

The following discussion details the variety of nonpharmacologic and pharmacologic options available and their mechanisms of action, side effects, and potential indications in patients with essential hypertension.

MEDICAL TREATMENT

Nonpharmacologic Therapy

The basis of any pharmacologic program is a sound patient education keyed to the applicability of any (or all) of the nonpharmacologic alternatives: weight control, sodium restriction, alcohol moderation, a regular exercise program, and cessation of cigarette smoking.

Table 2 Normal Physiologic Mechanisms that Serve to Control Arterial Pressure by Altering Vascular Smooth Muscle Tone

VASCULAR CONSTRICTORS

Active

- Adrenergic stimulation
- Catecholamines (released from nerve endings, adrenal medulla, or pheochromocytoma): norepinephrine, epinephrine, dopamine
- Renopressor system: renin-angiotensin-aldosterone
- Hormonal agents: aldosterone, cortisol, and other adrenal steroids (the latter administered exogenously, produced by tumors, or induced by enzyme deficiencies); parathormone; growth hormone; other hormone excess
- Cations: calcium, potassium (high levels)
- Humoral substances: vasopressin, serotonin, certain prostaglandins

Passive

- Edema: extravascular compression
- Vessel wall "water-logging"
- Increased blood (or plasma) viscosity
- Intravascular obstruction: thrombosis, embolus
- Cold

VASCULAR DILATORS

Active

- Catecholamines: epinephrine (low-grade increases), dopamine
- Neural: acetylcholine, histaminergic, and others
- Prostaglandins (e.g., prostacyclin)
- Kinins: bradykinin, kallidin, kallikrein
- Histamine
- Peptides (more frequently as modulators of vessel tone): atrial natriuretic factor, insulin, secretin, glucagon, vasoactive intestinal polypeptide, parathormone, calcitonin gene-related peptide, endorphins, encephalins
- Renal medullary phospholipid substance
- Vasoactive metabolites: adenosine, Kreb's intermediate metabolites

Passive

- Reduced blood (or plasma) viscosity
- Increased plasma toxicity (osmolality)
- Heat

Exogenous obesity may reflect itself at times in erroneous blood pressure measurements; however, obesity and hypertension are frequently correlated. Weight control not only may result in a reduced arterial pressure in overweight (i.e., >15 percent over ideal body weight) patients with hypertension but also it may reduce antihypertensive drug doses.

Excessive alcohol consumption is directly related to pressure elevation; the greater the daily consumption of ethanol, the higher the pressure. Excessive sodium intake (i.e., ≥100 mEq per day) may play a critical role in elevating arterial pressure, at least in some patients with hypertension (35 to 50 percent), and in limiting the effectiveness of pharmacologic therapy of others. Therefore, moderation of alcohol consumption and restriction of sodium intake (<70 to 100 mEq per day) are reasonable recommendations. Nicotine raises arterial pressure transiently but is not associated with persistently increased pressure. In the heavy smoker this elevation may be long-lasting.

Smoking may also interfere with the antihypertensive benefits of certain drugs (e.g., propranolol) even though arterial pressure may be well controlled. A regular exercise program is also accepted as a useful adjunct in reducing arterial pressure, and recent studies suggest this is independent of associated weight control.

Although other nonpharmacologic modalities may be of value for good cardiovascular health (e.g., stress reduction, exercise), only perhaps regular isotonic exercise, weight reduction, alcohol moderation, sodium restriction, and tobacco cessation have positive antihypertensive effects.

Diuretics

This group of antihypertensive drugs has been available for well over 30 years; the agents indicated for patients with uncomplicated essential hypertension are the thiazides and their congeners. These agents, including chlorothiazide, hydrochlorothiazide, and chlorthalidone, and their congeners are similar in action, side effects, and dosages. One tablet of any one agent is generally equivalent to another in its antihypertensive and natriuretic potency, hypokalemic potential, and frequency of side effects. They may be initiated in doses of 12.5 mg hydrochlorothiazide, which may be increased to 25 and 50 mg daily alone or in combination with other antihypertensive drugs. Larger doses of these thiazide compounds produce little more in sodium and water excretion in patients with normal renal excretory function. In contrast, the dosage of loop diuretics may be increased progressively in patients with renal functional impairment until, eventually, diuresis may be achieved.

Arterial pressure is reduced initially by the thiazides primarily as a result of contracted extracellular (plasma and interstitial) fluid volume. Thus, after administration, there is a fall in plasma volume and cardiac output associated with a reduced total body sodium and water. Shortly thereafter,

Table 3 Basic Clinical and Laboratory Information Necessary Prior to Initiating an Antihypertensive Treatment Program

Confirmation of hypertension
- At least three confirmatory pressures in the supine and standing positions obtained on three separate occasions; in a hypertensive emergency more rapid institution of antihypertensive therapy (and even hospitalization) may be indicated

History
- In addition to symptoms of cardiac, renal, and neurologic involvement, family history of hypertension and other vascular and metabolic diseases or of premature or sudden death is important

Physical examination
- Should include retinal funduscopy, careful cardiac auscultation (extra sounds, murmurs, irregularity), and vascular (palpation and auscultation)

Laboratory
- Hemogram: including hematocrit or hemoglobin, white blood cell count
- Blood chemistries:
  - For hypertension: serum potassium, calcium, creatinine, and uric acid concentration
  - For other risk factors: plasma glucose (fasting, if possible, or 2 h postprandial lipid and lipoprotein concentrations)
- Complete urinalysis (including microscopic examination of sediment)
- Noninvasive cardiac evaluation: chest film and electrocardiographic evidence of left atrial abnormality (enlargement) presages chest film or electrocardiogram evidence of left ventricular hypertrophy; evidence of left ventricular hypertrophy, cardiac dysrhythmia, myocardial ischemia, and T wave changes; previous myocardial infarction; in special circumstances echocardiography may be necessary
- Other studies useful for excluding secondary forms of hypertension or for selecting antihypertensive therapy:
  - Urine culture (and sensitivity): urinary tract infections may be the basis of renal parenchymal hypertension
  - Serum electrolytes—sodium, potassium, chloride, carbon dioxide, calcium, phosphate—are important for consideration of hyperaldosteronisms and other steroidal forms of hypertension, hypercalcemic diseases (70% of which are associated with hypertension)
  - Urinary electrolytes may assist in the foregoing diagnoses
  - Plasma renin activity: for secondary hypertensions and for selection of antihypertensive therapy, differential renal venous renin activities are useful for diagnosis of renal arterial disease
  - Plasma (or urinary) hormones: aldosterone and other adrenal steroids; thyroid hormone; parathormone; growth hormone
  - Renal arteriography
  - Computed tomography scan of adrenal glands
  - Serum catecholamines: for pheochromocytoma, adrenergic participation in hypertension and associated diseases (e.g., mitral valve prolapse syndrome)
  - Blood volume and hemodynamic studies
  - 24 h ambulatory blood pressure assessment: in selected patients

arterial pressure falls; in time, plasma volume and cardiac output return toward pretreatment levels when the reduced-arterial pressure is related to reduced total peripheral resistance. In addition, the thiazides potentiate the depressor effects of hypotensive agents and attenuate the effects of pressor agents. Thiazides promote natriuresis at various nephron levels: inhibition of carbonic anhydrase and of sodium reabsorption in the proximal and distal tubules.

Associated with natriuresis is a loss of potassium and chloride ions; the net result is hypokalemic alkalosis and an alkaline urine (i.e., secondary hyperaldosteronism). In the presence of excessive sodium intake, this induced state of hyperaldosteronism results in exacerbation of hypokalemia. These agents also increase tubular urate reabsorption so that plasma uric acid level increases; this may be associated with gouty symptoms. If hyperuricemia is 10 to 11 mg per 100 ml or more, it may be necessary to prescribe hypouricemia therapy. This may be achieved with a uricosuric agent (e.g., probenecid) or with a xanthine oxidase inhibitor (e.g., allopurinol). Alternatively, other antihypertensive agents that are effective as initial therapy may be substituted for the diuretic.

The thiazides also produce hyperglycemia of varying degrees because of inhibition of insulin release from the beta-cell pancreatic islets. Another factor may be the "diabetogenic" propensity of hypokalemia. Should overt diabetes mellitus develop, this does not mean that the thiazide diuretic need be discontinued; it may be possible to control the problem with diet therapy, weight reduction, an oral hypoglycemic agent, or, if necessary, increasing insulin dosage if already used. Alternatively, another agent may be substituted as initial therapy.

Hypokalemia can be minimized with lower thiazide doses with equal control of pressure. Another important means is by reducing dietary sodium intake since the excessive sodium that is presented to the distal tubule is exchanged for potassium in the face of the secondary hyperaldosteronism induced by the diuretic. Spironolactone and amiloride may further reduce arterial pressure but triamterene has little, if any, additional antihypertensive effect. All three agents, however, protect potassium; they should be used with extreme caution (if at all) in patients with renal functional impairment or who are already receiving ACE inhibitors. Symptoms of hypokalemia (polyuria and nocturia, muscle weakness, and ectopic cardiac activity) should be corrected with supplemental potassium or a potassium-retaining agent. If the patient is receiving digitalis or there are other explanations for aggravating hypokalemia (e.g., chronic diarrhea), potassium levels should be corrected; alternatively, another antihypertensive agent should be considered. Hypomagnesemia (and reduced intracellular magnesium) may also complicate diuretic therapy and coincide with hypokalemia. Sometimes, correction with remission of cardiac dysrhythmias until magnesium is also corrected.

Other more frequently encountered side effects include

impotence, hyperlipidemia, hypercalcemia, and some reduction in renal function as a consequence of reduced renal blood flow. The issue of hyperlipidemia has engendered great controversy. Should it be induced significantly by diuretics, other therapeutic options may be selected.

Diuretics may be of particular value in patients who are volume-dependent and who have lower plasma renin activity; some may have a history of renal parenchymal infections (even if renal excretory function is normal). They are also of value in essential hypertension with lower plasma renin activity (e.g., blacks, obese individuals, or elderly individuals) or in steroid-dependent forms of hypertension (e.g., primary aldosteronism, Cushing's disease or syndrome, and perhaps oral-contraceptive associated). Recently, several multicenter, placebo-controlled studies have been reported from the United States and Europe that demonstrated significant reduction of total and cardiovascular morbidity and mortality (strokes as well as myocardial infarction) in elderly patients with isolated systolic hypertension.

The loop diuretics are potent agents, exerting their natriuretic action by inhibition of sodium transport at the ascending limb of the loop of Henle. Unlike the thiazides, their onset of action is more immediate (within 15 to 20 minutes). Perception and persistence of diuresis is more evident than with thiazides, rebound retention may be more noticeable, and there may be a greater potassium loss. Hence, these compounds should be reserved for patients who cannot take thiazides, in whom a more prompt onset of diuretic action is desired, with renal functional impairment, and when an intravenous diuretic is necessary.

Beta-Adrenergic Blocking Agents

These drugs inhibit stimulation of beta-adrenergic receptor sites by adrenergic neurohumoral agents (norepinephrine, epinephrine). By inhibiting beta-receptor stimulation, their effects on peripheral arterioles (i.e., dilation) and on myocardium (increased heart rate, myocardial contractility, and myocardial metabolism) are reduced; renal renin release is also inhibited. The result is a reduced arterial pressure associated with decreased cardiac output and an increased total peripheral resistance. However, even though cardiac output may be reduced by 20 to 25 percent, renal blood flow and excretory function may not be reduced. In addition, as already indicated, expansion of intravascular volume does not occur when pressure is reduced.

At present, 11 beta-blocking agents are available for antihypertensive therapy; a twelfth agent (labetalol) possesses in a single moiety both alpha-adrenergic and beta-adrenergic receptor inhibiting properties. Four agents (acebutolol, carteolol, penbutolol, and pindolol) possess cardiostimulatory (intrinsic sympathomimetic) properties; they do not reduce heart rate and cardiac output as much as the other agents and may have some value in patients with pre-existent bradycardia or low cardiac output syndromes. The cardioselective beta$_1$-blockers (acebutolol, atenolol, metoprolol) probably exceed this property when used in the doses necessary for treatment of hypertension and angina pectoris (Table 4).

These agents may be more effective as initial beta-blocking treatment in patients with hyperdynamic circulatory states having faster heart rates, symptoms of cardiac awareness, palpitations related with enhanced myocardial contractility, and extrasystoles. Young patients may be more responsive than older individuals, and patients who are lean, male, or white may be more responsive than those who are obese, female, or black, respectively. Because beta-blocking therapy is effective for other clinical conditions, it may be wise to use this therapy for initial treatment of hypertension in patients with angina pectoris, previous history of myocardial infarction, and cardiac dysrhythmias responsive to beta-blockers. Further, patients with migraine headaches, muscle tremors, and glaucoma (who already receive beta-blocking eyedrops without systemic side effects) may also respond well to beta-blockers.

Table 4 Beta-Adrenergic Receptor Blockers

AGENT	DOSE RANGE (MG PER DAY)
Adrenergic inhibition	
Beta-blockers	
Atenolol	25–100 qd
Betaxolol	5–40 qd
Bisoprolol	50–20 qd
Metoprolol	50–200 qd
Metoprolol (extended release)	50–200 qd
Nadolol	20–240 qd
Propranolol	40–240 qd
Propranolol (long-acting)	60–240 qd
Timolol	20–40 b.i.d.
Beta-blockers with intrinsic sympathomimetic activity (ISA)	
Acebutolol	200–1,200 b.i.d.
Carteolol	10–25 qd
Penbutolol	20–80 qd
Pindolol	10–60 qd
Alpha-beta blocker	
Labetalol	200–1,200 b.i.d.

Because of systemic inhibition of beta-receptors, the beta-blockers should not be used in patients with a history of asthma, chronic obstructive lung disease, cardiac failure, heart block of second degree or more, and Raynaud's phenomenon or severe peripheral arterial insufficiency.

If full doses of the chosen beta-blocking agent do not control pressure, addition of a diuretic or even a calcium antagonist may be effective. Caution must be exercised when using beta-blockers in association with calcium antagonists, lest exacerbation of negative inotrophy be produced. If side effects such as fatigue, depression, hallucination, or nightmares preclude further use of the chosen beta-blocker, the use of another beta-blocker may be wise before switching to another class of antihypertensive agents.

Adrenergic Inhibiting Compounds

With the present array of sympathetic-depressant drugs, it is now possible for the clinician to dissect the autonomic nervous system pharmacologically. The ganglion blocking agents are not used today for the treatment of essential hypertension unless in an emergency situation to lower pressure under highly controlled circumstances.

The rauwolfia alkaloids include a number of agents having varying potencies and abilities to deplete neuronal tissue (brain, adrenal, and postganglionic sympathetic nerve endings) of the biogenic amines. These compounds were used with greater frequency in earlier years of antihypertensive drug therapy. By injection (e.g., reserpine, 1 to 5 mg), they were effective in hypertensive emergencies and for thyrotoxicosis. More recently, other agents with less bothersome side effects (e.g., obtunded sensorium, nasal stuffiness, depression) have been used. When administered orally, their effect is minimal and must be used with a diuretic, a vasodilating drug, or both. They reduce arterial pressure through a fall in total peripheral resistance, with decreased heart rate and relatively unchanged cardiac output. Side effects include nasal stuffiness, postural hypotension, bradycardia, overriding parasympathetic gastrointestinal tract stimulation (increased acid production, peptic ulcerations, increased frequency of bowel movements), mental depression (often very subtle), and sexual dysfunction.

Included among the postganglionic neuronal blockers are guanethidine and guanadrel. The former agent has been used in patients with more severe hypertension for over 35 years; the latter has been made available more recently for patients with milder hypertension. Both act similarly, although with the lower doses of guanadrel, its side effects are less. Guanethidine's onset of action is frequently over 24 to 48 hours; but once achieved, its action may persist for up to 1 month after discontinuance. Both agents demonstrate similar hemodynamic effects to the ganglion blocking drugs but without parasympathetic inhibition: a fall in vascular resistance, venodilation with reduced cardiac venous return and reduced cardiac output, attenuated cardiovascular reflexive adjustments, and reduced renal blood flow that may impair excretory function. The latter, however, will adjust itself in the patient with adequate pretreatment renal functional reserve, and less completely with already impaired function. Additional side effects include bradycardia, orthostatic hypotension, increased frequency of bowel movements and diarrhea (from unopposed parasympathetic function), and retrograde ejaculation. These agents are taken up by postganglionic nerve endings to inhibit reuptake of norepinephrine and leading to its action of norepinephrine depletion. This concept is important in understanding their interaction with the tricyclic antidepressants (imipramine or desipramine derivatives) that, in turn, inhibits the neuronal uptake of guanethidine or guanadrel; the result is further elevation of arterial pressure.

The centrally acting postsynaptic alpha-adrenergic agonists include methyldopa, clonidine, guanabenz, and guanfacine. Although originally thought to reduce pressure through inhibition of the enzyme dopa decarboxylase, methyldopa was later postulated to act as a false neural transmitter through metabolism of the drug, alpha-methyldopa, to the less biologically active amine, alpha-methylnorepinephrine, that binds to alpha-adrenergic vascular smooth muscle receptor sites in competition with norepinephrine. Its antihypertensive action has now been shown to be through this "false" neurohumoral substance (alpha-methylnorepinephrine) stimulation of postsynaptic alpha-receptor sites in the brain's nuclei tractus solitarii. This reduces adrenergic outflow from the brain to the cardiovascular system and kidney to reduce pressure through a fall in arteriolar tone. Cardiac output and renal blood flow are maintained and postural hypotension is infrequently observed. Side effects include dry mouth, lethargy, easy fatigability and somnolence, and sexual dysfunction attributable to their central action. Less common side effects include Coombs' test positive reactions (and still less frequent hemolytic anemia), high fever, and hepatotoxicity, all remitting with discontinuance of the drug. The other agents in this group (although different from methyldopa) share similar pharmacologic actions but directly stimulate the same central alpha-receptors and share the same physiologic effects and many of the same side effects as methyldopa. One effect of clonidine that merits attention is a precipitous rebound of arterial pressure after its abrupt withdrawal; it may be associated with palpitations and tachycardia that can be treated with beta-blockers and reinstitution of the clonidine or another adrenergic inhibitor. Its transdermal patch formulation makes clonidine therapy less frequent and the rebound phenomenon perhaps less likely.

The presynaptic and postsynaptic (alpha$_1$ and alpha$_2$) receptor antagonists were introduced many years ago and have limited use in the treatment of most hypertensive patients. They may be used for unexplained pressor episodes that suggest excessive catecholamine release, by continuous intravenous (phentolamine) infusion in a patient with pheochromocytoma crisis, or with pressor crises-associated clonidine withdrawal. Pargyline hydrochloride and other monoamine oxidase inhibitors continue to be available as antihypertensive and antidepressant agents, and may be associated with hypertensive crisis after ingestion of certain foodstuffs (e.g., Chianti wine, marinated foods, certain processed cheeses) containing tyramine. Alpha-blockers are valuable in treating these pressor crisis episodes.

There are two types of alpha-adrenergic receptors. Postsynaptic alpha$_1$-receptors, when stimulated by catecholamines that are released from postganglionic nerve endings, respond by arteriolar and venular constriction. When presynaptic alpha$_2$-receptors are stimulated, further release of norepinephrine from the nerve ending is inhibited. In contrast to the alpha$_1$- and alpha$_2$-receptor inhibiting compounds (i.e., phentolamine and phenoxybenzamine), agents that selectively block the postsynaptic alpha$_1$-receptors (doxazosin, prazosin, and terazosin) do not prevent alpha$_2$-receptor stimulation. Other agents belonging to this class of drugs include indoramin, trimazosin, and tiodazosin (none of these drugs has been approved for this use by the Food and Drug Administration). Hemodynamically, the alpha$_1$-receptor antagonists reduce pressure by decreasing total peripheral resistance without reflex increase in heart rate, cardiac output, or myocardial contractility. These agents may produce postural hypotension, often after the first dose. Therefore, treatment may be initiated with a 1 mg dose at bedtime, with instructions to the patient not to arise for 4 to 6 hours since symptomatic hypotension may be expected 1 to 3 hours after the initial dose. With prolonged treatment, higher doses (up to 10 to 20 mg per day) may be required. Two problems may occur with pressure control: Dose titration may be associated with symptomatic orthostatic hypotension, and pseudotolerance may develop. The latter problem is offset with addition of a diuretic, but this may exacerbate the former. Recently, the alpha$_1$-adrenergic inhibitors were introduced for the treatment of patients with benign prostatic hyperplasia since they may diminish the symptoms of frequency and nocturia associated with that disease. It is important to remember that men who have these agents prescribed for that condition while receiving other antihypertensive agents may develop postural hypotension associated with nocturia. This may predispose these older men to fractures and other trauma unless precautions are taken.

Vasodilators

With the introduction of the beta-blockers interest in direct-acting smooth muscle vasodilating drugs for hypertension increased. These agents (e.g., hydralazine, diazoxide, minoxidil) decrease vascular smooth muscle tone and arteriolar resistance and arterial pressure, associated with reflex cardiac stimulation so that tachycardia and palpitations (from increased myocardial contractility) frequently result. Therefore, these agents should not be administered to hypertensive patients with myocardial infarction, angina pectoris, cardiac failure, or dissecting aortic aneurysm; the reflexive cardiac stimulation will aggravate these underlying cardiac conditions. Other side effects are headaches, nasal stuffiness, fluid retention, and in the case of hydralazine edema, a syndrome manifested by a positive lupus erythematosus (LE) test (skin rash leukopenia, thrombocytopenia, and arthralgias) that is more apt to occur in patients receiving in excess of 400 mg per day. A not infrequent side effect of minoxidil, particularly in women, is facial hair growth.

Hydralazine may be administered by injection (10 to 15 mg intravenously). Another parenteral vasodilator, diazoxide, is a thiazide congener that is not natriuretic; in fact, diazoxide may cause sodium retention. To rapidly reduce pressure diazoxide must be injected in a single bolus (300 mg, or in successive pulsed boluses of divided doses). Diazoxide also should not be administered to patients with cardiac failure, angina pectoris, myocardial infarction, or an actively dissecting aortic aneurysm for the reasons cited above, but it is of value in the patient with hypertensive encephalopathy, intracranial hemorrhage, and severe malignant or accelerated hypertension (without cardiac failure) in whom rapid and immediate reduction in arterial pressure is mandatory. Sodium nitroprusside, also an injectable vasodilator, is also useful in hypertensive emergencies. It is infused by microdrip (60 µg per milliliter) to produce an immediate pressure reduction associated with venular as well as arteriolar dilation. Thus this compound, like trimethaphan (a ganglion-blocking drug), decreases ventricular preload as well as arterial pressure and total peripheral resistance (ventricular afterload), and this has particular value in the severely hypertensive patient with myocardial infarction, cardiac failure, or dissecting aneurysm. Because the nitroprusside is metabolized to thiocyanate, and thiocyanate toxicity may become manifest with prolonged infusion, it is advisable to monitor blood thiocyanate levels in these severely sick and hypertensive patients.

Angiotensin Converting Enzyme Inhibitors

This class of antihypertensive agents is also effective as monotherapy for controlling arterial pressure in patients with mild to moderately severe hypertension as well as in those with severe, very severe, or even refractory hypertension. They reduce pressure by interfering with the generation of the hemodynamically active octapeptide angiotensin II from the inactive decapeptide angiotensin I. Therefore, these compounds inhibit the formation of angiotensin II as well as the degradation of the active, naturally occurring vasodilator bradykinin. The angiotensin converting enzyme is the same substance that inactivates the very potent and naturally occurring visodilator bradykinin. Because angiotensin II interacts with norepinephrine in the brain as well as at peripheral neurons, less angiotensin II is available for that action. Recent studies have demonstrated that the entire renin-angiotensin system (in all of its components) exists in the vascular and cardiac myocytes, thereby providing an explanation for the effectiveness of these compounds in patients with normal (or even low) plasma renin activity and in anephric patients. They reduce pressure as a result of arteriolar dilation and a reduced total peripheral resistance without reflex increase in heart rate and cardiac output, and renal blood flow may even increase. Glomerular filtration rate usually remains stable and the renal filtration fraction may even diminish, suggesting that the reduced glomerular hydrostatic pressure results primarily from efferent glomerular arteriolar dilation. Because of their effects on intrarenal homeostatic mechanisms (e.g., prostaglandins and kinins), ACE inhibitors can exacerbate renal functional impairment and elevate arterial pressure in patients with bilateral renal arterial disease and in patients with a solitary kidney who have unilateral renal arterial disease. Further, for similar reasons, they should not be used with supplemental potassium or potassium-sparing agents. In addition, these agents are contraindicated for pregnant women.

Angiotensin converting enzyme inhibitors are effective in patients with low and normal plasma renin activity as well as in patients with renin-dependent forms of hypertension (e.g., unilateral renal arterial disease and one normally functioning kidney, congestive heart failure, high-renin essential hypertension). Recent multicenter, placebo-controlled trials (SOLVD [Study on Left Ventricular Dysfunction] and SAVE [Study Against Ventricular Enlargement]) in patients with cardiac failure or myocardial infarction have shown protection against development or need for hospitalization for cardiac failure reduction in cardiovascular morbidity and mortality (including reinfarction). They are useful as monotherapeutic agents and their effectiveness is enhanced with the addition of a diuretic or a calcium antagonist. They have a low incidence of side effects. Initial studies with captopril suggested that neutropenia and proteinuria should be sought during the first few months of therapy, but long-term studies suggest that these effects are more likely in patients with impaired renal function prior to therapy or in those who were receiving immunosuppressive agents. Other side effects include rash and cough (ascribed to the inhibited degradation of the kinins); they disappear following cessation of therapy.

Because metabolic side effects (e.g., in electrolytes, carbohydrate, uric acid, and lipids) have not been reported with these agents, patients with these problems receiving other antihypertensive agents are likely beneficiaries of this class of drugs. Table 5 lists the currently available ACE inhibitors (with dose ranges).

Recently, a new class of agents that inhibits the renin-angiotensin system has been introduced for the treatment of hypertension. This agent, losartan, is an angiotensin II (type I) receptor antagonist that prevents angiotensin II from exerting its effects on vascular smooth muscle, adrenal cortex

Table 5 Angiotensin Converting Enzyme Inhibitors

AGENT	DOSE RANGE (MG PER DAY)
$Alpha_1$-receptor blockers	
Doxazosin	1–16 qd
Prazosin	1–20 b.i.d.
Terazosin	1–20 qd
ACE inhibitors	
Benazepril	10–40 qd
Captopril	12.5–150 b.i.d.
Cilazapril	2.5–5.0 qd
Enalapril	2.5–40 qd
Fosinopril	10–40 qd
Lisinopril	5–40 qd
Perindopril	1–16 qd
Quinapril	5–80 qd
Ramipril	1.25–20 qd
Spirapril	12.5–50 qd

and medulla, brain, and elsewhere. It is effective alone and with added diuretic to reduce pressure; and, since it operates without inhibiting the ACE and, hence, elevating kinins, does not produce cough.

Calcium Antagonists

These agents constitute the newest class of antihypertensive agents, although they have been available for study and clinical use for at least 25 years. These compounds are quite heterogeneous in chemical structure, action, and indications; nevertheless, they have a final commonality of action: inhibition of availability of calcium ions in cardiac and vascular smooth muscle cells, thereby diminishing contractility of the myocyte. As a result, arteriolar resistance decreases, thereby reducing total peripheral resistance and, hence, arterial pressure.

An increasing number of calcium antagonists are available in the United States (Table 6). The functional heterogeneity of these agents may be exemplified by three of the oldest agents in use. Thus verapamil, in addition to its vasodilating property, has a cardiac inhibitory action to diminish impulse conduction transmission. As a result, it is used for the treatment of certain supraventricular cardiac tachyarrhythmias. In contrast, nifedipine has an exclusive peripheral action to dilate arterioles; its cardiac effects are secondary to reflex stimulation as a result of arterial pressure reduction. Diltiazem's action is intermediate. All calcium antagonists approved for the treatment of hypertension reduce pressure without expanding intravascular volume; consequently, they also may be used alone (one calcium antagonist—nimodipine—does not reduce pressure significantly and is employed for the treatment of brain hemorrhage). Although some calcium antagonists have been associated with pedal edema, this alteration in fluid distribution is probably related to postcapillary reflex venoconstriction and increased capillary hydrostatic pressure that favors transcapillary fluid migration into extravascular tissue. Fluid retention is a highly unlikely explanation for the edema, since a natriuretic effect of calcium antagonists is well known. Reduced vascular resistance seems to be distributed throughout the vasculature, with the target organs of hypertension (heart, brain, and kidney) all sharing

Table 6 Calcium Antagonists

AGENT	DOSE RANGE (MG PER DAY)
Diltiazem	90–360 b.i.d.
Diltiazem (sustained release)	120–360 b.i.d.
Diltiazem (extended release)	180–360 qd
Verapamil	80–480 b.i.d.
Verapamil (long-acting)	120–480 qd
Dihydropyridines	
Amlodipine	2.5–10 qd
Felodipine	5–20 qd
Isradipine	2.5–10 b.i.d.
Nicardipine	60–120 t.i.d.
Nifedipine	30–120 t.i.d.
Nifedipine (GITS)	30–90 qd

in this effect. This reduced resistance may also be associated with increased organ flow; all appear to increase coronary blood flow, but diltiazem and nitrendipine (and perhaps verapamil) may increase renal blood flow without increasing glomerular filtration rate. Most calcium antagonists reduce cardiac mass; however, as indicated earlier, the clinical significance of this effect remains to be shown. Therefore, it must still be demonstrated that the increased risk due to left ventricular hypertrophy is diminished by pharmacologic reversal of that hypertrophy.

The calcium antagonists are effective in volume-dependent hypertensive patients with lower plasma renin activity. They have been recommended for older patients and black patients with hypertension, but they are also useful in young and white patients. Because they are not associated with metabolic side effects (e.g., hypokalemia, carbohydrate intolerance, hyperlipidemia, hyperuricemia), they may be also used in patients who have experienced these side effects with other agents (e.g., diuretics). More frequent side effects include constipation (primarily verapamil), flushing, headaches, and gingival hyperplasia.

It is of interest that a calcium antagonist and ACE inhibitor have been formulated in single tablets recently. The concept is intriguing and probably of value since the combination permits lower doses of each agent while possessing their dual advantages.

■ INDIVIDUALIZED THERAPY

Inherent with the newer concept of *individualized* or *tailored care* is the wise selection of an initial pharmacologic agent. This depends on the following clinical criteria: (1) the patient's medical history and physical findings (which may exclude certain agents and include others); (2) demographic criteria (e.g., age, race, gender, body habitus); (3) laboratory findings, including the presence (or absence) of biochemical risk factors; (4) presence of coexisting diseases, such as coronary arterial disease, prior myocardial infarction, hyperlipidemia, diabetes mellitus, gout, or migraine headaches; (5) previous personal experience (of the patients) with other antihypertensive drugs; and (6) the mechanism of action of the various classes of antihypertensive agents.

Once an initial antihypertensive agent is selected, it should

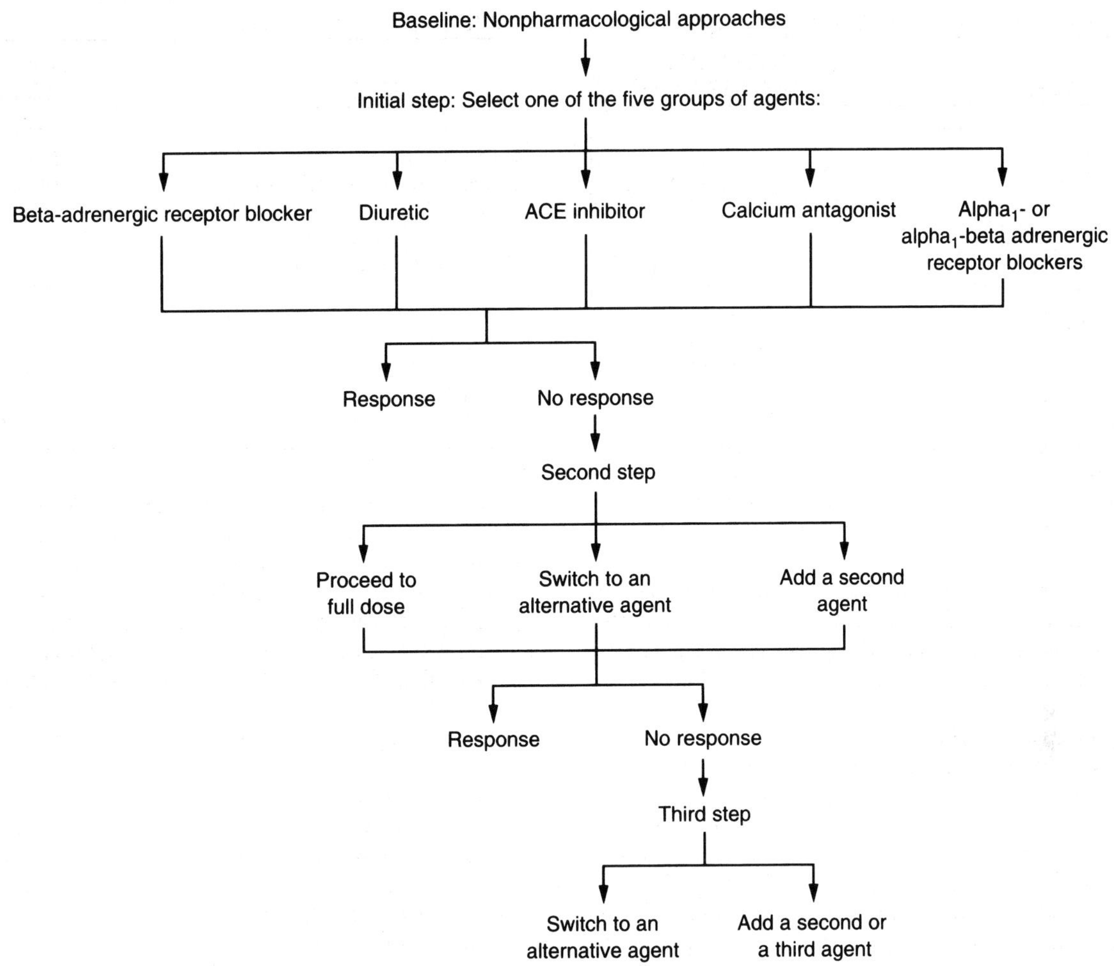

Figure 1
Individualized stepped care for hypertension.

be prescribed in less than full doses. Only one of two effects can occur: the drug may be completely effective and without unwanted effects or the drug may not be effective. Clearly, if the first alternative occurs, then therapy is maintained. If the initial option is found to be ineffective, there are then three alternatives: (1) the drug may then be prescribed at full doses; (2) a second agent may be added to the initially selected drug; or (3) the initial drug can be discontinued and an alternative first-step option prescribed (Fig. 1). The clinical steps that ensue follow the same line of thinking.

In the preceding discussion of the different classes of antihypertensive agents, I have suggested some of the likely hypertensive patient populations and clinical indications that may prompt selection of an initial therapeutic option for each class of drugs. Any of the five classes of antihypertensive agents may be selected for initial monotherapy. However, the most recent Joint National Committee's fifth report suggests that the diuretics and beta-adrenergic receptor blocking agents may be preferred since these agents have been shown, in multicenter placebo-controlled trials, to reduce total and cardiovascular morbidity and mortality. The other groups (including ACE inhibitors, calcium antagonists, and the alpha$_1$- or alpha-beta–adrenergic receptor antagonists) are equally efficacious in controlling arterial pressure, but reduced morbidity and mortality have not been reported in similar trials.

If a diuretic agent is not selected first, it may be added to any of the alternative agents. Beta-blockers have been used with the vasodilators, but consideration should be given to the patient's cardiac and renal status. The calcium antagonists and ACE inhibitors can be used alone or with one another, and clearly any of the adrenergic inhibitors (alpha-blockers or centrally active) have a long track record of efficacy with diuretics or with the vasodilators. In any event, at least 1 to 3 months should be allowed before proceeding to other therapeutic options. In addition, as indicated previously, undesired responses to one agent of a class of drugs may not always indicate that the class should be totally excluded from consideration in that patient.

If necessary, a vasodilator (direct-acting smooth muscle relaxant, ACE inhibitor, calcium antagonist, or even guanethidine) may be added as a third agent, although few patients with hypertension require more than two antihypertensive drugs. Once the therapeutic goal is achieved and maintained for some time (I usually aim for diastolic pressure less than 90 mm Hg), it may be wise to consider "stepping down" in therapy. This can be achieved by reducing the dose of the least desired agent first and eventually discontinuing its use with the goal of maintaining therapy at the lowest possible dosage of the fewest agent(s) employed.

Suggested Reading

Frohlich ED. Evaluation and management of the patient with essential hypertension. In: Parmley WW, Chatterjee K, eds. Cardiology. Philadelphia, JB Lippincott, 1994:1–17.

Frohlich ED. Pathophysiology of systemic arterial hypertension. In: Schlant RC, Alexander RW, eds. Hurst's the heart. 8th ed. New York: McGraw-Hill 1993:280.

Frohlich ED, Hypertension. In: Rakel RE, ed. Conn's current therapy. Philadelphia, WB Saunders, 1993:280–296.

Frohlich ED. Hypertension. In: Abrams WB, Beers MH, Berkow R, eds. The Merck Manual of Geriatrics. 2nd ed. New Jersey, Merck Research Laboratories 1995:454–474.

Frohlich ED, Apstein C, Chobanian AV, et al. The heart in hypertension. N Engl J Med 1992; 327:998–1008.

Frohlich ED, Gifford R Jr, Horan M, et al. Nonpharmacologic approaches to the control of high blood pressure. Report of the Subcommittee on Nonpharmacologic Therapy of the Joint National Committee on Detection, Evaluation, and Treatment of High Pressure, 1984. Hypertension 1986; 8:444.

The Joint National Committee on the Detection, Evaluation, and Treatment of High Blood Pressure (member): The 1992 Report of the Joint National Committee on Detection, Evaluation and Treatment of High Blood Pressure. Arch Intern Med 1993; 153:154.

HYPERTENSION: SECONDARY

Ray W. Gifford Jr., M.D.

It is estimated that 50 million people in the United States have hypertension (systolic blood pressure ≥140 mm Hg and/or diastolic blood pressure ≥90 mm Hg). Of these, approximately 90 percent have primary (essential) hypertension, and 10 percent have secondary hypertension. The subject of this chapter is the treatment of the causes for secondary hypertension that may lead to cure or amelioration of the hypertension (Table 1).

Table 1 Classification of Hypertension

Primary (essential) (90% of cases)
Secondary (10% of cases)
Potentially curable
Coarctation of aorta
Renal artery stenosis
Fibrous dysplasia
Atherosclerotic
Pheochromocytoma
Primary aldosteronism
Cushing's syndrome
Pre-eclampsia/eclampsia
Drug-related hypertension
Not curable
Bilateral renal parenchymal disease

■ PREFERRED APPROACH TO POTENTIALLY CURABLE CAUSES OF SECONDARY HYPERTENSION

Coarctation of the Aorta

Surgical repair is the only therapeutic approach to coarctation of the aorta, which is associated with hypertension in the upper part of the body and normotension, or even hypotension, below the level of the coarctation. The coarctation is usually located at or just distal to the origin of the left subclavian artery. Except when it leads to congestive heart failure in neonates and infants, it is preferable to defer surgical correction until age 3 or 4 years.

Occasionally the diagnosis of coarctation of the aorta is not made until patients have reached their full growth potential. In such cases the procedure of choice is end-to-end anastomosis after resection of the coarctation. The chances of curing the hypertension are much less than when the diagnosis is made and surgery performed in childhood.

Preoperatively, hypertension associated with coarctation of the aorta can be managed with the usual antihypertensive agents used for treating essential hypertension (Table 2).

Postoperative complications include hemorrhage, damage to adjacent structures (such as the vagus and recurrent laryngeal nerves, thoracic duct), infection, myocardial infarction, renal insufficiency, and stroke. The most feared complication is paraplegia related to spinal cord ischemia. This complication is more frequently encountered during reoperation for coarctation than following initial surgery.

Paradoxical hypertension sometimes occurs during the first 10 days after surgical relief of coarctation. Sodium nitroprusside, beta-adrenergic blockers, angiotensin converting enzyme (ACE) inhibitors and calcium antagonists are usually effective in managing this temporary type of hypertension.

"Postcoarctation syndrome", characterized by abdominal pain and distention, and progressing to more serious complications including necrosis of the bowel, is thought to be due to uncontrolled hypertension and seems to be less frequent with good blood pressure control postoperatively.

Long-term surveillance for hypertension and/or recurrent stenosis is indicated. Persistent or recurrent hypertension is particularly prevalent in patients whose coarctation has not been corrected until adulthood, whereas restenosis is more frequent in children, especially when resection and re-

Table 2 Some Antihypertensive Drugs Used to Treat Secondary Hypertension

AGENT	TRADE NAME	USUAL DAILY DOSE* (MG)	SIDE EFFECTS	PRECAUTIONS AND SPECIAL CONSIDERATIONS
THIAZIDES AND RELATED SULFONAMIDE DIURETICS			Hypokalemia, hypomagnesemia, hyponatremia, hypercalcemia, hyperuricemia, glucose intolerance, hypercholesterolemia, hypertriglyceridemia, sexual dysfunction, weakness, rash	Except for metolazone and indapamide, may be ineffective in renal failure; hypokalemia increases digitalis toxicity; may cause an increase in blood levels of lithium
Chlorthalidone	Hygroton	12.5–50		
Hydrochlorothiazide	HydroDIURIL	12.5–50		
	Esidrix			
Indapamide	Lozol	1.25–5		
Metolazone	Zaroxolyn	1.25–5		
	Mykrox	0.5–1		
LOOP DIURETICS†				
Bumetanide‡	Bumex	0.5–5	Same as for thiazide diuretics, but do not cause hypercalcemia	Effective in chronic renal failure
Furosemide‡	Lasix	20–320		
Torsemide	Demadex	5–20		
POTASSIUM-SPARING AGENTS			Hyperkalemia, sexual dysfunction; gynecomastia and menstrual irregularities (spironolactone), danger of renal calculi (triamterene)	Danger of hyperkalemia or renal failure in patients treated with an ACE inhibitor or a nonsteroidal anti-inflammatory drug; may increase blood levels of lithium
Amiloride	Midamor	5–10		
Spironolactone‡	Aldactone	25–100		
Triamterene‡	Dyrenium	50–150		
BETA-BLOCKERS§			Bronchospasm, may aggravate peripheral arterial insufficiency, fatigue, insomnia, sexual dysfunction, exacerbation of congestive heart failure, masking of symptoms of hypoglycemia, hypertriglyceridemia, decreased HDL cholesterol (except for those with ISA), reduced exercise tolerance	Should not be used in patients with asthma, chronic obstructive pulmonary disease (COPD), congestive heart failure with systolic dysfunction, heart block (greater than first degree), or sick sinus syndrome; use with caution in insulin-treated diabetics and patients with peripheral vascular disease; should not be discontinued abruptly in patients with ischemic heart disease
Acebutolol‡,¶	Sectral	200–1,200		
Atenolol¶	Tenormin	25–100		
Betaxolol	Kerlone	5–40		
Bisoprolol		5–20		
Carteolol¶	Cartrol	2.5–10		
Esmolol	Brevibloc	50–200 μg/kg/min IV		
Metoprolol	Lopressor Toprol XL	50–200 P.O.		
Nadolol	Corgard	40–320		
Penbutolol	Levatol	20–80		
Pindolol‡,¶	Visken	10–60		
Propranolol‡	Inderal	40–240		
Propranolol, long-acting (LA)	Inderal LA	60–240		
Timolol‡	Blocadren	20–40		
ACE INHIBITORS			Rash, cough, angioneurotic edema, hyperkalemia, dysgeusia	Can cause reversible, acute renal failure in patients with bilateral renal arterial stenosis or unilateral stenosis in a solitary kidney and in patients with cardiac failure and with volume depletion; proteinuria may occur (rare at recommended doses); hyperkalemia can develop, particularly in patients with renal insufficiency; rarely can induce neutropenia; hypotension has been observed with initiation of ACE inhibitors, especially in patients with high plasma renin activity or in those receiving diuretic therapy; absolutely contraindicated in second and third trimesters of pregnancy
Benazepril¶	Lotensin	10–40		
Captopril‡,¶	Capoten	12.5–150		
Enalapril¶	Vasotec	2.5–40		
Fosinopril	Monopril	10–40		
Lisinopril¶	Zestril	5–40		
	Prinivil	5–40		
Quinapril¶	Accupril	5–80		
Ramipril¶	Altace	1.25–20		
Moexipil	Univasc	2.5–10		
Trandolapril	Mavik	1–4		
ANGIOTENSIN II RECEPTOR ANTAGONIST				
Losartan	Cozaar	50–100	Muscle cramps, back and leg pain, dizziness, insomnia, nasal congestion, hyperkalemia	Reversible, acute renal failure in patients with bilateral renal arterial stenosis or unilateral stenosis in a solitary kidney, and in patients with cardiac failure and with volume depletion; hyperkalemia can develop, particularly in patients with renal insufficiency; hypotension especially in patients with high plasma renin activity or those receiving diuretic therapy; absolutely contraindicated in second and third trimesters of pregnancy.

Continued.

Table 2 Some Antihypertensive Drugs Used to Treat Secondary Hypertension—cont'd

AGENT	TRADE NAME	USUAL DAILY DOSE* (MG)	SIDE EFFECTS	PRECAUTIONS AND SPECIAL CONSIDERATIONS
CALCIUM ANTAGONISTS				
Benzothiazepine derivative			Headache, dizziness, asthenia, flushing, edema, atrioventricular block, bradycardia, gingival hyperplasia	Relatively contraindicated for congestive heart failure, sick sinus syndrome, or greater than first-degree heart block; may cause liver dysfunction
Diltiazem SR‡	Cardizem SR	120–360		
Diltiazem XR	Dilacor XR	180–480		
Diltiazem CD	Cardizem CD Tiazac	180–360		
Diphenylalkylamine derivative				
Verapamil‖	Calan Isoptin	120–480	As diltiazem, plus constipation	As diltiazem
Verapamil	Verelan	120–480		
Verapamil SR	Calan SR Isoptin SR Coverans	120–480		
Dihydropyridines				
Amlodipine	Norvasc	2.5–10	Dizziness, flushing, headache, weakness, nausea, heartburn, pedal edema, tachycardia	Contraindicated in CHF except Amlodipine; may aggravate angina and myocardial ischemia
Felodipine	Plendil	5–20		
Isradipine‡	DynaCirc	2.5–10		
Nifedipine (XLCC)	Procardia XL Adalat CC	30–90		
Nicardipine‖	Cardene	60–120		
Nisoldipine	Sular	20–60		
ADRENERGIC INHIBITORS				
Centrally acting $alpha_2$-agonists				
Clonidine‡	Catapres	0.1–1.2	Drowsiness, sedation, dry mouth, fatigue, sexual dysfunction; localized skin reaction to clonidine TTS patch	Rebound hypertension may occur with abrupt discontinuation, particularly with prior administration of high doses or with continuation of concomitant beta-blocker therapy
Clonidine-TTS (patch)#	Catapres-TTS	0.1–0.3		
Guanabenz	Wytensin	4–64	Same as clonidine	Same as clonidine
Guanfacine	Tenex	1–3	Same as clonidine	Same as clonidine
Methyldopa‡	Aldomet	250–2,000	Same as clonidine	May cause liver damage and Coombs'-positive hemolytic anemia; use cautiously in elderly patients because of orthostatic hypotension; interferes with measurements of urinary catecholamine levels by fluorimetric methods
Nonselective $alpha_1$-adrenergic blockers				
Phentolamine	Regitine	5–10 IV push	Acute and prolonged hypotensive episodes, tachycardia, and cardiac arrhythmias have been reported; weakness, dizziness, flushing, orthostatic hypotension, nasal stuffiness, nausea, vomiting, and diarrhea may occur	Myocardial infarction and cerebrovascular occlusion have been reported, usually in association with marked hypotensive episodes
Phenoxybenzamine‡	Dibenzyline	20–80	Nasal congestion, miosis, postural hypotension, inhibition of ejaculation	
Selective $alpha_1$-adrenergic blockers				
Doxazosin	Cardura	1–16	First-dose syncope, orthostatic hypotension, weakness, palpitations, headache	Use cautiously in elderly patients because of orthostatic hypotension
Prazosin‡	Minipress	1–20		
Terazosin	Hytrin	1–20		

Table 2 Some Antihypertensive Drugs Used to Treat Secondary Hypertension—cont'd

AGENT	TRADE NAME	USUAL DAILY DOSE* (MG)	SIDE EFFECTS	PRECAUTIONS AND SPECIAL CONSIDERATIONS
Labetalol‡,**	Normodyne Trandate	200–1,200 PO, 20–40 IV bolus	Orthostatic hypotension, dizziness, fatigue, nausea	Can occasionally cause a paradoxical increase in blood pressure in patients with pheochromocytoma or receiving other antihypertensive medications; should not be withdrawn abruptly; use with caution in patients with congestive heart failure
VASODILATORS			Headache, tachycardia, fluid retention	May precipitate angina pectoris in patients with coronary artery disease; generally, use with diuretic and beta-blocker
Hydralazine‡	Apresoline	50–200	Positive antinuclear antibody test	Lupus syndrome may occur (rare at recommended doses)
Minoxidil‡	Loniten	2.5–80	Hypertrichosis	May cause or aggravate pleural and pericardial effusions
Sodium nitroprusside	Nipride Nitropress	0.5–10 μg/kg/ min IV	Nausea, vomiting, agitation, muscle twitching, cutis anserina, thiocyanate toxicity	Close observation necessary due to rapid onset of action; rapidly degraded by exposure to light; monitor thiocyanate levels, especially with renal or liver disease

Immediate release diltiazem and nifedipine have never been approved for hypertension by FDA.
*The dosage range may differ slightly from recommended dosage in *Physicians' Desk Reference* or package insert. Given once daily unless otherwise indicated.
†Larger doses of loop diuretics may be required in patients with renal failure.
‡Usually given in divided doses twice daily.
§Atenolol, acebutolol, betaxolol, bisoprolol, and metoprolol are cardioselective; acebutolol, carteolol, penbutolol, and pindolol have intrinsic sympathomimetic activity.
¶These drugs are excreted by the kidney and require dosage reduction in the presence of renal impairment (serum creatinine ≥221 μmol/L [2.5 mg/dl]).
||Usually given in divided doses three or four times daily.
#Administered as a skin patch once weekly.
**Combined alpha- and beta-blocker.
Adapted from the 1993 report of the Joint National Committee on Detection, Evaluation, and Treatment of High Blood Pressure. Arch Intern Med 1993; 153:154.

anastomosis have been performed at an early age. Balloon angioplasty has sometimes been successful in managing recurrent stenosis. Aortic dissection may sometimes occur proximal or distal to the repair site. Prophylaxis with suitable antibiotics should be prescribed before procedures that put patients at risk for bacteremia.

Renovascular Disease

Various forms of fibrous dysplasia of one or both renal arteries and/or their branches cause hypertension in children, adolescents, or young adults, usually girls or women; atherosclerotic disease of one or both renal arteries or their branches causes hypertension in middle-aged or elderly patients, usually after age 50, who are mostly male. Because the natural history and response to treatment are different in these two forms of renal artery disease, they are discussed separately.

Fibrous Renovascular Disease

Therapeutic Alternatives. Because most of these patients are young and in good health, the treatment of choice is revascularization of the kidney when possible by either percutaneous transluminal balloon angioplasty (PTLA) or surgical revascularization, usually using a saphenous vein bypass graft. Successful revascularization spares these patients a lifetime of medical therapy with antihypertensive agents.

Medical Treatment. Antihypertensive agents are indicated to control blood pressure before PTLA or operation and afterwards if the procedure fails to normalize blood pressure. Pharmacologic treatment is indicated in lieu of PTLA or surgical treatment when the lesion is so extensive that revascularization is not possible, when the significance of the lesion in the pathogenesis of the hypertension is doubtful, or when the patient refuses invasive treatment.

Usually hypertension secondary to fibrous renal disease can be controlled with the same regimens used for primary hypertension, although it may require multiple drugs. Although ACE inhibitors or angiotensin II receptor antagonists would seem to be the drugs of choice because the renin-angiotensin system is activated in renovascular hypertension, other agents including beta-blockers, diuretics, calcium antagonists, and selective alpha$_1$-adrenergic blocking drugs are also effective (Table 2). Acute renal failure can be caused by ACE inhibitors or angiotensin II receptor antagonists in patients who have tight stenosis in both renal arteries or in the renal artery to a solitary kidney, which is much less likely to occur in fibrous renovascular disease than in atherosclerotic renovascular disease. Even with unilateral renovascular disease, it is possible for ACE inhibitors or angiotensin II receptor antagonists to reduce function dramatically in a kidney distal to a tight renal artery stenosis. This might escape detection if the opposite kidney is functioning normally, unless a technetium-99m-diethylenetriamine penta-acetic acid (technetium-99m-DTPA) renal flow scan was made after the administration of an ACE inhibitor.

Renal Revascularization. Cure of hypertension by renal revascularization can be expected in up to 85 percent of patients if hypertension is less than 5 years in duration, renal vein renin activity is higher on the side of the lesion, the lesion is unilateral and does not extend into the branches, and the technetium-99m-DTPA renogram shows slower perfusion and decreased function on the side of the lesion.

Long-term results with PTLA are encouraging, provided the lesion(s) is accessible to the balloon catheter and the pressure gradient can be greatly diminished or eliminated. Long segments of stenosis and extension of lesions into the branches make it less likely that PTLA will be successful.

Complications of PTLA include rupture, dissection, or thrombosis of the renal artery, and for this reason an experienced surgeon should be immediately available to handle these emergencies that occur in less than 2 percent of cases. Bleeding at the site of femoral artery puncture, with or without hematoma formation, occurs in 2 to 6 percent of cases when small catheter systems are used and can usually be handled by application of pressure. A late complication is false aneurysm formation at the site of arterial puncture that may have to be repaired at a later date (<1 percent).

In the absence of complications, the patient can be discharged from the hospital within 48 hours. If the patient is normotensive, only blood pressure monitoring is recommended for follow-up. If hypertension persists or recurs, medical treatment should be instituted (as previously discussed) and if correction of the stenosis was incomplete or restenosis has occurred, another attempt at PTLA may be made or surgical revascularization should be considered.

Surgical revascularization, using a saphenous vein bypass graft, should be considered if the lesion is not amenable to PTLA or if hypertension recurs after PTLA. Using microsurgical techniques and ex vivo surgery in which the kidney is removed and perfused while the surgeon reconstructs the arterial supply, followed by autotransplantation, usually into the pelvis, it is possible to repair fibrous lesions that extend into the branches. Complications include acute ischemic renal failure, renal artery thrombosis or dissection that may threaten survival of the kidney, and hemorrhage, as well as complications of general anesthesia. Mortality rate for surgical revascularization is less than 1 percent. Hospitalization is required for about 7 days following the operation.

Atherosclerotic Renovascular Disease

Therapeutic Alternatives. There is less enthusiasm for renal revascularization in atherosclerotic renovascular disease than for fibrous disease because patients with atherosclerosis are older, often have atherosclerotic complications in the coronary or cerebral circulations, the disease is more frequently bilateral, the mortality rate for operation is higher, and the cure rate for hypertension is lower (1995 Update of the Working Group Reports on Chronic Renal Failure and Renovascular Hypertension).

Transluminal angioplasty is preferable to surgical revascularization, but it carries a higher risk of complications and a lower success rate for patients with atherosclerotic renovascular disease than for patients with fibrous dysplasia of the renal arteries. Moreover, many patients are not candidates for PTLA because the atherosclerotic plaques originate in the aorta and protrude or "grow" into the renal artery, making dilation more difficult, if not impossible. Recurrence rate of stenoses and hypertension is much greater with atherosclerotic lesions than with fibrous lesions. In some series, the restenosis rate has been as high as 30 percent within 1 year. Placement of stents after transluminal angioplasty procedures offers some hope for better long-term patency rates, especially for patients with orificial lesions.

If renal function is not in jeopardy, medical treatment of hypertension is preferred for most patients with atherosclerotic renovascular disease.

Medical Treatment. For reasons discussed previously, ACE inhibitors and angiotensin II receptor blockers, although frequently effective, should be administered cautiously, if at all, to patients who have severe stenosis in both renal arteries or in the renal artery to a solitary kidney. Diuretics, beta-blockers, calcium antagonists, and selective $alpha_1$-adrenergic blocking agents are also effective in controlling atherosclerotic renovascular hypertension (see Table 2). Renal function must be monitored carefully because the renal artery lesions can progress in spite of good control of hypertension. Technetium-99m-DTPA flow scans should be obtained at least once a year to detect decreasing function in one kidney, which might not be apparent if the opposite kidney is functioning normally.

Renal Revascularization. Revascularization by PTLA or operation is indicated if hypertension is resistant to a well-designed, rational, multidrug regimen or if renal function is seriously threatened. When the lesion is short and 1 or 2 cm distal to the orifice of the renal artery, PTLA is preferred to operation. Aspirin 0.3 g every day or every other day, dipyridamole 50 mg four times a day, or both have been prescribed following PTLA by some physicians, although there is no clear-cut evidence that this prevents or delays restenosis.

Complications described for PTLA and surgical treatment of fibrous stenosis of the renal arteries are also encountered, but more frequently when atherosclerotic lesions are treated with these modalities. Moreover, the risk of precipitating atheroembolization to the kidneys and other viscera by PTLA or aortorenal bypass is not even a consideration in patients with fibrous lesions of the renal artery.

Bilateral atherosclerotic lesions of the renal artery can threaten total renal function, whereas this is seldom a concern in patients with fibrous disease. More and more, the indication for revascularizing kidneys threatened by atherosclerotic lesions is to preserve renal function and not to cure or ameliorate hypertension.

Pheochromocytoma

These chromaffin tissue tumors that occur most frequently in the adrenal medulla, but can also be found along the sympathetic chain in the thorax or abdomen, cause hypertension by secreting large amounts of the catecholamines norepinephrine and epinephrine.

Therapeutic Alternatives

The treatment of choice is surgical extirpation because 10 percent of these tumors are or can become malignant. Moreover, hypertension secondary to pheochromocytoma is notoriously resistant to pharmacologic treatment.

Medical Treatment. While pharmacotherapy is used to prepare the patient for operation and during the operation, it is not a substitute for surgical treatment unless the patient is a poor surgical risk or the tumor is malignant and cannot be removed in its entirety. Under these circumstances, the drugs of choice are calcium antagonists or alpha-adrenergic blocking agents by mouth (prazosin, terazosin, doxazosin, phenoxybenzamine, labetalol) or phentolamine intravenously (see Table 2). Sodium nitroprusside is also effective by intravenous infusion (see Table 2). Metyrosine (Demser) is a specific inhibitor of tyrosine hydroxylase and thus interferes with the synthesis of catecholamines. It is given orally in doses of 250 to 1,000 mg four times a day to control hypertension and symptoms in patients with metastatic pheochromocytoma. Sedation is a common side effect, and extrapyramidal signs occur in about 10 percent of patients. Frequent urinalyses are recommended to detect metyrosine crystalluria; if this occurs in spite of large fluid intake, the drug should be discontinued.

Some malignant pheochromocytomas are radiosensitive, but most are not. The only effective chemotherapeutic regimen has been a combination of vincristine, cyclophosphamide, and dacarbazine, which in some cases has induced short remissions.

Surgical Treatment. Using computed tomography or magnetic resonance imaging techniques, it is usually possible to localize the tumor or tumors (in 10 percent of cases they are multiple) preoperatively (Manger and Gifford, 1989). To minimize intraoperative paroxysms of hypertension and postoperative hypotension, an alpha-adrenergic blocking agent (prazosin, terazosin, doxazosin, phenoxybenzamine, or labetalol; see Table 2) can be administered for 5 to 10 days preoperatively. In addition to, or instead of, this preoperative pharmacologic regimen, some authorities recommend generous volume replacement with intravenous fluids within 6 hours of the operation to correct the hypovolemia that frequently accompanies these tumors, thus making the postoperative course smoother.

Hypertensive paroxysms are frequently precipitated by induction of anesthesia and intubation and by manipulation of the tumor during operation. These can be managed by intravenous boluses of sodium nitroprusside or phentolamine administered by the anesthesiologist (see Table 2). Catecholamine-induced arrhythmias can be treated with IV bolus injections of a beta-blocker such as propranolol or esmolol. Beta-blockade without previous alpha-blockade can result in paradoxical hypertension.

Postoperative hypotension is best managed by fluid administration rather than pressor agents, from which it is often difficult to wean the patient.

Table 3 Combination Tablets Containing Hydrochlorothiazide and a Potassium-Sparing Diuretic

PREPARATIONS CONTAINING AMILORIDE		
Preparation	*Hydrochlorothiazide*	*Amiloride*
Moduretic	50 mg	5 mg
PREPARATIONS CONTAINING SPIRONOLACTONE		
Preparation	*Hydrochlorothiazide*	*Spironolactone*
Aldactazide	25 mg	25 mg
	50 mg	50 mg
PREPARATIONS CONTAINING TRIAMTERENE		
Preparation	*Hydrochlorothiazide*	*Triamterene*
Dyazide	25 mg	37.5 mg
Maxzide	25 mg	37.5 mg
	50 mg	75 mg

If all tumor tissue is removed, the cure rate for hypertension is over 80 percent. Operative mortality should be less than 2 percent (Sheps and co-workers, 1990).

Primary Aldosteronism

Excessive secretion of aldosterone from an adrenal cortical tumor or by bilateral hyperplasia causes a syndrome characterized by hypokalemia and hypertension.

Therapeutic Alternatives

Surgical removal of an adrenocortical tumor or of a *unilateral* hypertrophied gland is usually curative and is the treatment of choice in patients who are good operative risks. Medical treatment is reserved for patients with bilateral adrenal hyperplasia and for those who have tumors but present unacceptable operative risks or who are unwilling to submit to surgical treatment.

Medical Treatment. For patients who have bilateral adrenal hyperplasia or for those who do not become normotensive after adrenalectomy, a low-sodium diet and pharmacotherapy are indicated. Because aldosterone-producing tumors of the adrenal cortex are rarely malignant, medical treatment is not unreasonable for patients who elect not to have surgical treatment. The goal of therapy is to normalize blood pressure (<140/90 mm Hg) and correct hypokalemia. Basic therapy usually consists of a thiazide–potassium-sparing combination diuretic such as hydrochlorothiazide with spironolactone or amiloride (Table 3). Triamterene can be prescribed if spironolactone and amiloride are poorly tolerated. Adjunctive therapy should include a beta-blocker or calcium antagonist if necessary (see Table 2). ACE inhibitors are not usually effective in this type of hypertension.

Surgical Treatment. Because of the vascularity of the adrenal gland, adrenalectomy is usually necessary to remove an adenoma. One must therefore be certain that the opposite adrenal gland is intact. Hypokalemia should be corrected by administration of potassium chloride orally or intravenously (up to 100 mEq daily) or by the oral administration of a potassium-sparing diuretic in larger than recommended doses (amiloride 10 to 20 mg daily, spironolactone 100 to 400 mg daily, or triamterene 100 to 400 mg daily). The operative mortality is less than 1 percent and the duration of hospitalization is 7 to 10 days.

Mild hyperkalemia is frequently observed postoperatively for several days because of suppression of aldosterone production in the remaining adrenal cortex. Potassium chloride should be omitted from the fluids given postoperatively if this occurs. Complete remission of hypertension can be expected in 60 to 80 percent of patients, although hypertension may not abate for several days or even weeks after the operation.

Cushing's Syndrome

Hypertension is an important component of Cushing's syndrome, which can be caused by tiny pituitary tumors that produce ACTH (70 percent); ectopic ACTH production by tumors, usually small cell carcinomas of the lung or carcinoid tumors (13 percent); or by carcinoma, adenoma, or ACTH-independent bilateral hyperplasia of the adrenal cortex (17 percent).

Therapeutic Alternatives

Appropriate surgical treatment, when possible, is preferred for any of these types of Cushing's syndrome.

Medical Treatment. Drugs that block secretion of ACTH (cyproheptadine and bromocriptine) or glucocorticoid synthesis (aminoglutethimide, metyrapone, mitotane, and ketoconazole) are difficult to use as long-term treatment of Cushing's syndrome. These are best used for short-term intervention. Ketoconazole 600 to 1,200 mg daily is preferred. Metyrapone blocks 11-beta-hydroxylase but does not inhibit synthesis of 11-deoxycorticosterone and can therefore lead to hypertension and hypokalemia. Consequently, it should be administered with aminoglutethimide. Mitotane is a cytotoxic agent that can lead to adrenocortical necrosis, and for this reason its primary use is in managing adrenocortical carcinoma, for which it is only palliative.

Surgical Treatment. Trans-sphenoidal pituitary microsurgery is indicated for pituitary-dependent Cushing's syndrome. The cure rate is approximately 80 to 95 percent, and recurrences are uncommon. Removal of an ectopic source of ACTH, usually a small cell carcinoma of the lung or carcinoid tumor, is the treatment of choice if the tumor can be located. Unilateral adrenalectomy is indicated for patients with cortical adenoma or carcinoma. Bilateral adrenalectomy is the treatment of choice for patients in whom Cushing's syndrome is due to ACTH-independent bilateral hyperplasia or when the site of ACTH-producing tumors cannot be identified.

Pre-Eclampsia and Eclampsia

Pre-eclampsia is characterized by onset of hypertension (≥140 mm Hg systolic and/or 90 mm Hg diastolic) in the third trimester of pregnancy, accompanied by edema and proteinuria. Most patients with this syndrome are primiparous, and the hypertension almost always subsides after delivery. Onset of convulsions (eclampsia) makes the prognosis for mother and fetus worse.

Therapeutic Alternatives

Medical treatment is indicated until the uterus can be emptied.

Medical Treatment. Bed rest is the basic treatment for pre-eclampsia. Obstetricians prefer using hydralazine 10 to 20 mg by intravenous injection whenever the blood pressure exceeds 150/105 mm Hg, or methyldopa 250 mg twice to four times a day given orally to keep blood pressure between140/90 and 150/105. ACE inhibitors are contraindicated, and diuretics and sodium nitroprusside are relatively contraindicated. Drastic reduction of blood pressure is not desirable because it can jeopardize blood flow to the placenta, which usually shows evidence of patchy infarction in women with pre-eclampsia. If gestation is less than 30 weeks, the patient can be maintained on this temporizing regimen until fetal viability is assured, although this involves hazards to mother and fetus. If the condition of either deteriorates or eclampsia supervenes, the uterus should be emptied regardless of the duration of pregnancy. Magnesium sulfate can be administered intravenously to prevent or control convulsions. The loading dose is 2 to 4 g (4 to 8 ml of a 50 percent solution) over 5 minutes, followed by a constant infusion, 1 to 2 g per hour (8 ml of 50 percent solution in 230 ml of dextrose injection 5 percent to equal 1 g $MgSO_4$ per 60 ml). Diazepam can also be administered intravenously in doses of 5 to 10 mg for this purpose.

Surgical Treatment. The treatment of choice is to empty the uterus by aggressive induction of labor or, in selected cases, cesarean section. Medical treatment as described previously is necessary in preparing the mother for delivery and in some cases to procrastinate until fetal viability is assured.

Drug-Related Causes of Hypertension

Hypertension can result from ingestion of drugs or drug-drug interactions that may be iatrogenic or self-induced.

Perhaps the most frequent cause of reversible hypertension in women of childbearing age is use of oral contraceptive drugs. Excessive ingestion of ethyl alcohol (>1 oz daily) can exacerbate pre-existing hypertension or induce hypertension de novo in susceptible persons.

Use of cyclosporine to combat rejection following solid organ transplantation is associated with hypertension in up to 100 percent of cases. Cyclosporine-associated hypertension seems to be dose related and occurs more often after cardiac transplantation than after renal transplantation.

Although therapy with nonsteroidal anti-inflammatory agents can make hypertension resistant to a previously effective regimen, it is doubtful that it can induce hypertension de novo.

Cocaine can induce acute hypertension, tachycardia, tremor, and seizures, and it causes coronary artery constriction. It can be associated with ischemic and hemorrhagic cerebrovascular accidents in young adults.

Erythropoietin increases blood pressure in one-third of patients with end-stage renal disease. It is not related to the dose or to the final hematocrit level achieved, or to the rate of increase of hematocrit.

Interaction between monoamine oxidase (MAO) inhibitors and certain drugs that release norepinephrine from sympathetic nerve endings such as ephedrine and tyramine or foods that contain tyramine can lead to a severe hypertensive crisis resembling pheochromocytoma. Sudden cessation of treatment with clonidine, especially if the dose is greater than 0.4 mg daily, can cause similar hypertensive crises.

Overdoses of sympathomimetic drugs such as phenylpropanolamine, ephedrine, or amphetamine, whether by mouth or inhalation from sprays, can cause temporary hypertension.

Therapeutic Alternatives

Usually, stopping the offending agent is all that is necessary. Occasionally, it is wise to prescribe antihypertensive agents for short periods.

Medical Treatment. Intravenous bolus injections of phentolamine (5 to 10 mg) or oral administration of prazosin, terazosin, or doxazosin (1 to 2 mg), labetalol (200 mg), or phenoxybenzamine (10 to 20 mg) is indicated to shorten the hypertensive crisis induced by interactions between MAO inhibitors and sympathomimetic agents. These antihypertensive drugs are also effective in combating clonidine withdrawal hypertension, although administration of clonidine orally is usually just as effective.

Oral contraceptive hypertension can be severe and may not abate for several weeks or months after withdrawing the offending agent. During this period it may be necessary to treat the patient with antihypertensive agents such as oral diuretics, beta-blockers, or ACE inhibitors in various combinations.

Frequently, it is inadvisable to stop therapy with cyclosporine for patients who have received allografts. If reduction in dosage of cyclosporine is contraindicated or if hypertension persists in spite of reduction in dosage, the drugs of choice are diuretics and calcium antagonists. Verapamil and diltiazem can interfere with metabolism of cyclosporine, often requiring a reduction in dosage of the cyclosporine.

The treatment of choice for acute hypertension induced by cocaine is alpha-adrenergic blockade (e.g., phentolamine intravenously). A beta-blocker should be used for complicating cardiac arrhythmias induced by the catecholamine excess.

If conventional antihypertensive therapy does not control hypertension associated with erythropoietin, the drug may have to be temporarily discontinued.

Surgical Treatment. There is no surgical treatment for drug-related causes of hypertension.

■ PREFERRED APPROACH TO INCURABLE CAUSES OF SECONDARY HYPERTENSION

Bilateral Renal Parenchymal Disease

Almost any renal parenchymal disease can and usually does cause hypertension. These include acute and chronic glomerulonephritis, chronic pyelonephritis, polycystic renal disease, collagen vascular diseases, diabetic glomerulosclerosis, and interstitial nephritis. An exception is renal amyloidosis, which may be associated with hypotension.

Therapeutic Alternatives

Medical treatment is the only choice except in unusual cases of unilateral hydronephrosis or pyelonephritis, in which nephrectomy is sometimes curative.

Medical Treatment. Hypertension associated with chronic renal disease is usually due to fluid retention and volume expansion, making a diuretic the drug of choice. When the glomerular filtration rate (GFR) is less than 30 ml per minute per 1.73 m^2 (serum creatinine >2 mg per deciliter), a loop diuretic (furosemide, torsemide, or bumetanide) or indapamide or metolazone should be prescribed because conventional thiazide diuretics are not effective when the GFR gets below this level. Additional drugs, if needed, include centrally acting $alpha_2$-agonists, direct vasodilators, beta-blockers, calcium antagonists, selective $alpha_1$-adrenergic blockers, and ACE inhibitors. In animals made azotemic by subtotal renal ablation or streptozocin-induced diabetes, ACE inhibitors reduce blood pressure and proteinuria and prolong survival. ACE inhibitors reduce proteinuria in patients with Type I diabetic glomerulosclerosis, and postpone the need for dialysis. If ACE inhibitors or angiotensin II receptor blockers are to be administered to azotemic patients, serum creatinine and potassium should be measured within a few days and at least every 2 weeks thereafter for 6 weeks because hyperkalemia with or without worsening azotemia can result.

Minoxidil is particularly effective in controlling severe and resistant hypertension associated with chronic renal failure, but large doses of a loop diuretic or metolazone must be prescribed to prevent fluid retention, and a beta-blocker should be administered to prevent reflexive tachycardia. There is reason to believe that the optimal blood pressure for preserving renal function is 130/70 mm Hg or lower.

A diet limited in sodium to 2 g and in protein to 40 or 50 g daily is indicated for most patients with hypertension and chronic renal failure.

Surgical Treatment. Except for the rare case of unilateral chronic pyelonephritis or hydronephrosis when nephrectomy may be curative, surgery has no place in the management of hypertension secondary to chronic renal disease. Bilateral nephrectomy was once advised to control severe and resistant hypertension prior to renal transplantation, but this is seldom required anymore.

Suggested Reading

1995 Update of the Working Group Reports on Chronic Renal Failure and Renovascular Hypertension. U.S. Department of Health and Human Services: National Institutes of Health and National Heart, Lung, and Blood Institute. Arch Int Med 1996; 156:1938–1947. (NIH Publication # 95-3791 October 1995.)

Boutros AR, Bravo EL, Zanettin G, Staffon RA. Perioperative management of 63 patients with pheochromocytoma. Cleve Clin J Med 1990; 57:613.

Bravo EL. Pheochromocytoma: New concepts and future trends. Kidney Int 1991; 40:544.

Bravo EL. Primary aldosteronism: Issues in diagnosis and management. Endocrinol Metab Clin North Am 1994; 23:271–283.

Gifford RW Jr, Manger WM, Bravo EL. Pheochromocytoma. Endocrinol Metab Clin North Am 1994; 23:387–404.

Klahr S, Levey AS, Beck GJ, et al. The effects of dietary protein restriction and blood-pressure control on the progression of chronic renal disease. N Engl J Med 1994; 330;877–884.

Lewis EJ, Hunsicker LG, Bain RP, Rohde RD, for the Collaborative Study Group. The effect of angiotensin-converting-enzyme inhibition on diabetic nephropathy. N Engl J Med 1993; 329:1456–1462.

Manger WM, Gifford RW. Clinical and experimental pheochromocytoma, 2nd ed. Cambridge: Blackwell Scientific, 1996.

National High Blood Pressure Education Program Working Group report on high blood pressure in pregnancy. Am J Obstet Gynecol 1990; 163:1689.

Orth DN. Cushing's syndrome [review]. N Engl J Med 1995; 332:791–803.

Peterson JC, Adler S, Burkart JM, et al. Blood pressure control, proteinuria, and the progression of renal disease: The Modification of Diet in Renal Disease Study (MDRD). Arch Int Med 1995; 123:754–762.

Rocchini AP. Cardiovascular causes of systemic hypertension. Pediatr Clin North Am 1993; 40:141–147.

The 1993 report of the Joint National Committee on Detection. Evaluation, and Treatment of High Blood Pressure. Arch Intern Med 1993; 153:154.

HYPERTENSION IN THE ELDERLY

Edward D. Frohlich, M.D., M.A.C.P., F.A.C.C

Two types of hypertension exist in the elderly population. They are isolated systolic hypertension, defined by the Joint National Committee's Fifth Report (1992) as a systolic pressure of less than 90 mm Hg; and diastolic hypertension, defined as a pressure of 90 mm Hg or greater.

Patients older than 60 years of age with systolic hypertension usually have a lower cardiac output and left ventricular ejection fraction with a significant increase in total peripheral resistance as compared to age-matched controls. Ventricular filling rate and diastolic relaxation are reduced. In addition, this population, as with most patients with essential hypertension, have a contracted plasma volume in proportion to the height of arterial pressure and total peripheral resistance when compared to controls. Systolic hypertension is a disease that involves reduced large-vessel compliance in conjunction with these preceding factors. Diastolic hypertension in elderly patients has a pathophysiology similar to those younger than age 60. Studies have shown, however, that older populations have an increased total peripheral and renal vascular resistance as well as left ventricular mass. Moreover, there is a greater likelihood of myocardial fibrosis and associated left ventricular diastolic dysfunction in elderly patients with hypertension. Furthermore, since this population has a greater likelihood of occlusive atherosclerotic disease, unilateral or bilateral renal artery stenosis may precipitate hypertension de novo or exacerbate already existing essential hypertension.

THERAPEUTIC ALTERNATIVES

Numerous studies have continued to demonstrate that lowering arterial pressure below 140 mm Hg systolic and 90 mm Hg diastolic is associated with a significant decrease in total, cardiovascular as well as cerebral morbidity and mortality. When life-style modification (i.e., weight reduction to ideal body weight, sodium restriction to less than 100 mEq per day, alcohol modification to 1 oz ethanol or its equivalent, regular exercise program, and smoking cessation) do not reduce arterial pressure to the foregoing acceptable levels, addition of various antihypertensive agents will further potentiate these pressure reduction measures. These agents include diuretics, beta-adrenergic receptor blockers, calcium antagonists, angiotensin converting enzyme (ACE) inhibitors, and alpha$_1$- or alpha-beta–adrenergic blockers. Any one of these agents is effective for reducing both isolated systolic and diastolic hypertension in the elderly. In selecting an initial agent, however, one should consider the coexistence of other pathophysiologic conditions such as peripheral vascular, lung, heart, or kidney disease, as well as a history of previous strokes, before prescribing antihypertensive medications for this population.

It is most important to recognize that since publication of the last edition, there have been several important reports concerning the feasibility, efficacy, and safety of antihypertensive therapy in elderly patients with hypertension, particularly those with isolated systolic hypertension (the SHEPS, STOP-Hypertension, and MRC trials). Each of these studies involved the use of diuretics and beta-adrenergic receptor blocking drugs, and all demonstrated reduction in morbidity as well as mortality from stroke and myocardial infarction. Thus, these studies in the elderly in addition to the Hypertension Detection and Follow-Up Program (HDFP) and the European Working Party Study reported similar beneficial responses in elderly patients having systolic or diastolic hypertension (also using diuretics, beta-adrenergic receptor blockers, or centrally acting adrenergic inhibitors). Thus, a massive body of placebo-controlled and other multicenter national and international trials demonstrated in younger adults as well as the elderly that diuretics and beta-blocking drugs were particularly effective in controlling arterial pressure and in reducing morbidity and mortality. These findings were so striking and compelling that the most recent Joint National Committee's fifth report (in the Detection, Evaluation, and Treatment of Hypertension) recommended that, for the initial selection of pharmacologic therapy in hypertension, the diuretics and beta-adrenergic receptor blockers were preferred and that, in those patients for whom that therapy was not deemed appropriate by the prescribing physician, the ACE inhibitors, calcium antagonists, alpha$_1$-adrenergic receptor and alpha-beta–adrenergic receptor blockers were also indicated for initial therapy. Notwithstanding these preliminary qualifications, it is entirely appropriate to individualize antihypertensive therapy. This tailoring of initial antihypertensive therapy would take into account the particular coexisting medical and other problems that may be specific for any particular patients.

■ PREFERRED APPROACH

Medical Treatment

Isolated Systolic and Combined Diastolic Hypertension Without End-Organ Dysfunction

As indicated, multicenter studies have shown that reduction of arterial pressure in the elderly may be achieved with any antihypertensive agent regardless of whether it is isolated systolic or diastolic hypertension. Data from the Systolic Hypertension in the Elderly Program Study (SHEPS) demonstrated that low-dose thiazide diuretics, alone or in combination with a beta-adrenergic receptor blocker, reduces elevated systolic pressures to a normal level. This was associated with a significant reduction in fatal and nonfatal strokes and nonfatal myocardial infarction. These findings are in concert with those from the Swedish Trial in Old Patients with Hypertension (STOP-Hypertension) and the British Medical Research Council trials in similar patients using similar antihypertensive drugs. When lower doses of diuretics were used than in the earlier multicenter trials with diastolic hypertension, metabolic side effects were minimal.

Diuretics may also be used in elderly patients who are either volume-expanded or who are already receiving other antihypertensive agents in order to enhance their effectiveness. They should also be employed in patients with cardiac or renal insufficiency as well as elderly subjects with hypoalbuminemia associated with massive proteinuria or cirrhosis. The thiazides are prescribed for patients without impaired renal function (i.e., serum creatinine of ≤1.6 mg per deciliter) and may be started in doses of 12.5 mg per day and can be increased to 25 to 50 mg daily. In contrast, loop diuretics (i.e., furosemide or bumetanide) are more effective in patients with renal insufficiency (i.e., serum creatinine of ≥1.7 mg per deciliter) in doses of 40 to 80 mg or 2 to 4 mg, respectively, once or twice daily. If an adequate response is not attained with these doses, they may be increased progressively until the therapeutic response is achieved. It is important to recognize that when used alone, some patients taking diuretics may be predisposed to hypokalemia and sudden cardiac death. These patients may be taking increased doses of the thiazide, have pre-existing cardiac disease, and are not protected by concomitantly prescribed agents that spare potassium.

The calcium antagonists are also effective in reducing both isolated systolic as well as diastolic pressures. Furthermore, they are available in sustained-release formulations and can therefore be given conveniently in once or twice daily doses. In general, one may begin therapy with sustained-released verapamil (120 to 240 mg daily), sustained-release diltiazem (90 mg twice daily or 180 mg once daily), or sustained-release nifedipine (30 to 60 mg daily) as single agents. These long-acting preparations are not as frequently associated with those side effects reported with multiple-dose formulations. Furthermore, some calcium antagonists decrease myocardial oxygen deficit and are more beneficial in states of coronary arterial insufficiency or renal functional impairment. The dosage of these medications, as with all medications in the elderly, should be governed by the rule "start low and go slow." The reasons for this adage are summarized in Table 1. The more prominent side effects of these agents include constipation with verapamil, headache and peripheral edema with nifedipine, and nausea or heart rate and conduction disturbances with diltiazem. A recent "case-controlled study" comparing patients receiving short-acting calcium antagonists with patients taking other antihypertensive drugs suggested increased risk of cardiac death. However, in general, calcium antagonists with short duration of action are not prescribed for patients with hypertension and prospective, controlled studies have not yet been reported. Thus, the professional societies have recommended reassurance of patients so treated, switching to other forms of therapy if requested by the patient.

Table 1 Factors Affecting Drug Disposition in Elderly Patients

AGE-RELATED DECREASES IN PHYSIOLOGIC PARAMETERS	PATHOLOGIC CONDITION
GI absorption	
Absorptive surface	Diarrhea
Gastrointestinal motility	Malabsorption syndromes
Volume of distribution	
Cardiac output	Congestive heart failure
Total body water	Dehydration
Lean body mass	Edema or ascites
Serum albumin	Hepatic failure
Metabolism	
Hepatic blood flow	Congestive heart failure
Renal function	
Renal blood flow	Hypovolemia
Glomerular filtration rate	Renal insufficiency
Tubular secretion	Renal insufficiency
Neural function	
Postprandial splanchnic blood pooling	Postural hypotension
Reduced *net* adrenergic function	Bradycardia Postural hypotension

ACE inhibitors, like the calcium antagonists, are relatively devoid of metabolic side effects and are effective in reducing arterial pressure in the elderly. Their side effects are indicated in Table 2. These agents may be of particular value in elderly patients either following a myocardial infarction or with impaired left ventricular function and cardiac failure. The SAVE (Survival and Ventricular Enlargement) and SOLVD (Studies of Left Ventricular Dysfunction) studies demonstrated myocardial remodeling and protection from development of congestive heart failure and myocardial infarction (SAVE study) and improvement of left ventricular function and reduction in hospital readmissions for cardiac failure (SOLVD) without increasing the chances for death or myocardial infarction. Furthermore, one may add a diuretic to potentiate the antihypertensive effects of ACE inhibitors, especially in patients with isolated systolic hypertension. They may also be employed as second drugs when a calcium antagonist or another agent fails to control pressure adequately or if adverse effects are experienced.

The beta-adrenoreceptor blockers reduce arterial pressure in the elderly, and they are of particular value in those patients with angina pectoris, a previous myocardial infarction, isolated systolic hypertension, and catecholamine-related ectopic beats. Those agents with intrinsic sympathomimetic activity (ISA), e.g., celiprolol, pindolol, or acebutolol, however, may not protect against a second myocardial infarction,

Table 2 General Side Effects of ACE Inhibitors

Angioedema
Hyperkalemia
Dysgeusia
Rash
Cough
Renal insufficiency
Contraindicated in bilateral renal arterial disease or unilateral disease in solitary kidney
Contraindicated in pregnant women

but may be useful in patients in whom bradycardia limits the use of non-ISA compounds.

The central alpha-adrenoreceptor agonists (methyldopa, clonidine) are effective in controlling pressure in both isolated systolic and diastolic hypertension. However, they may be associated with adverse reactions, the most frequent of which are sedation, dry mouth, and sexual dysfunction. Postganglionic neuronal inhibitors (e.g., guanethidine, guanabenz) or the alpha-adrenoreceptor antagonists (e.g., prazosin or terazosin) may be limited in the elderly patient because of their most frequent side effect of postural hypotension. However, these latter agents have been found to be helpful in men with benign prostatic hyperplasia. Hence, when they are prescribed, particular care must be exercised if the patient is already receiving other antihypertensive agents—especially diuretics—since postural hypotension may be provoked that may predispose these men to falls and fractures.

Arterial Hypertension with Myocardial Dysfunction

Patients with either left ventricular hypertrophy or moderately impaired cardiac function, defined as an ejection fraction of less than 35 percent, are at significant risk for a cardiac event (e.g., left ventricular failure, angina pectoris, potentially lethal cardiac arrhythmias, sudden death). Much has been written about the independent risk of cardiovascular morbid and mortal events in patients with left ventricular hypertrophy (over and above that from the elevated systolic or diastolic pressure). All antihypertensive therapy, no matter which class of pharmacologic agent is used, will reverse that hypertrophy if that therapy is used for a sufficiently long time. However, certain classes of agents (i.e., centrally acting adrenergic inhibitors, beta-adrenergic receptor blockers, calcium antagonists, and ACE inhibitors) reverse ventricular hypertrophy in a very short time (within a few weeks). Notwithstanding, there are no data available at this time that have demonstrated that with reduction of cardiac mass the associated risk is diminished. It seems reasonable to expect that this may occur, but when risk is shown to diminish, this must be shown to be independent of the effects of reducing arterial pressure, improving coronary blood flow and flow reserve, the potential antiarrhythmic effects of the agent, and so forth.

Even in the absence of significantly impaired left ventricular contractility patients with left ventricular hypertrophy are at considerably increased risk of premature cardiovascular morbidity and mortality. In these patients, calcium antagonists (e.g., diltiazem or a dihydropyridine congener such as nifedipine) are of value since they tend to have less negative inotropic effect upon the myocardium. Furthermore, since coronary blood flow and flow reserve are diminished and coronary vascular resistance is increased in patients with left ventricular hypertrophy, these compounds may improve these hemodynamic alterations. Alternatively, therapy might also be initiated with an ACE inhibitor. In elderly individuals, however, it might be worthwhile to begin such therapy with a relatively short-acting agent such as captopril, making sure not to administer the agent with a potassium-sparing diuretic or with potassium-sparing agents or supplemental potassium. This shorter-acting ACE agent usually does not exacerbate pre-existing renal functional impairment in patients with borderline or overt congestive heart failure as compared with the longer-acting agents benazepril (e.g., enalapril, lisinopril, quinapril, ramipril). Once pressure is controlled with the shorter-acting ACE inhibitor, one can then shift to the longer-acting agent (which can be taken once or twice daily). Both classes of agents (i.e., calcium antagonists and ACE inhibitors) may have their antihypertensive actions enhanced with the addition of a diuretic. Clearly, if cardiac failure is not corrected with the ACE inhibitors, there is no contraindication to the use of a cardiac glycoside (e.g., digoxin), prescribed either prior to or concomitant with the ACE inhibitor. Moreover, a diuretic may also be necessary in these patients—not only to control arterial pressure but also the cardiac failure. In these patients, if renal function is improved, a loop-acting agent (e.g., furosemide) should be added. Once again, however, cardiac failure is manifested by secondary hyperaldosteronism that is associated by hypokalemic alkalosis. Care must be taken to avoid cardiac dysrhythmias or inducing life-threatening hyperkalemia with potassium-sparing agents or potassium supplements. In these patients hypokalemia frequently is associated with hypomagnesemia, and evaluation and correction of this abnormality are also indicated.

It is important to reiterate that two recent studies in older patients with ischemic heart disease (but without hypertension) have demonstrated improved morbidity and mortality with angiotensin converting enzyme inhibition. The SAVE study, using captopril in patients who had a recent myocardial infarction, prevented congestive heart failure and a second infarction and also reduced deaths. SOLVD reduced the number of deaths and readmission for cardiac failure and tended to reduce deaths from myocardial infarction. These findings are particularly important to note since neither study demonstrated a J-shaped curve of increased deaths in these patients with low diastolic pressures as pressure was reduced further with the ACE inhibitor. This concept is important since such a finding has been purported to occur when hypertensive patients with or without ischemic heart disease but with lower diastolic pressure elevations had pressure reduced with antihypertensive therapy.

In these patients, with prior myocardial infarction, it is reasonable to use beta-adrenergic receptor blocking therapy to prevent a second infarction as well as to control arterial pressure elevation. If there is a contraindication to the beta-blocker or if arterial pressure is not controlled optimally with that agent, there is reason to add an ACE inhibitor to control arterial pressure and prevent further impairment of cardiac dysfunction. Alternately, if angina pectoris is not controlled well with the beta-blocker, addition of a calcium antagonist (that does not further impair contractile or chronotropic function) is also reasonable.

Arterial Hypertension with Renal Functional Impairment

Frequently in elderly patients, renal functional impairment is secondary to long-standing hypertension, diabetes mellitus, or congestive heart failure. It is wise to assess the volume status of these patients. Patients with severe renal functional impairment (creatinine ≥30 mg per deciliter) generally have intravascular volume expansion. These patients require a loop diuretic to improve volume status. Moreover, when an ACE inhibitor is also used, reduction of arterial pressure and urinary protein excretion may be expected. In recent and early studies proteinuria secondary to diabetic nephropathy suggests that certain calcium antagonists (e.g., diltiazem, verapamil, nitrendipine) may also be of value. It is important to evaluate every patient with renal functional impairment for the real possibility of bilateral renal artery stenosis (or renal artery stenosis in a solitary kidney) to prevent the adverse effect of further loss of renal function produced by ACE inhibitors. Even after initiation of therapy with this important precaution, it is important to check blood chemistries within 1 week for renal functional deterioration and then periodically thereafter to ensure that serum potassium and creatinine have not risen significantly; this is further evidence to suggest bilateral renal artery stenosis. In these patients with bilateral occlusive renal arterial disease, there is no contraindication to the use of a calcium antagonist even before transluminal angioplasty reconstructive or bypass surgery is pursued.

Suggested Reading

Amery A, Birkenhäger W, Brixko P, et al. Mortality and morbidity results from the European Working Party on High Blood Pressure in the Elderly trial. Lancet 1985; 1:1349.

Coope J, Warrender TS. Randomised trial of treatment of hypertension in elderly patients in primary care. Br Med J 1986; 293:1145.

Dahlöf B, Lindholm LH, Hanssson L, et al. Morbidity and mortality in the Swedish trial in old patients with hypertension (STOP-Hypertension). Lancet 1991; 338:1281.

Frohlich ED. Hypertension in the elderly. In: Cassel C, Walsh E, Reisenberg D, Sorenson L, eds. Geriatric medicine. New York: Springer Verlag, 1990:141.

Frohlich ED. Hypertension. In: Abrams WB, Beers MH, Berkow R, eds. The Merck manual of geriatrics. 2nd ed. New Jersey, Merck Research Laboratories 1995:454–474.

Frohlich ED. Hypertension. In: Rakel RE, ed. Conn's current therapy. Philadelphia: WB Saunders, 1993; 280–296.

Hypertension Detection and Follow-up Program Cooperative Group. The effect of treatment on mortality in "mild" hypertension: Results of the hypertension detection and follow-up program. N Engl J Med 1982; 307:976.

Joint National Committee on Detection, Evaluation, and Treatment of High Blood Pressure. The 1992 report of the Joint National Committee on Detection, Evaluation, and Treatment of High Blood Pressure. Arch Intern Med 1993; 153:154.

Management Committee. Treatment of mild hypertension in the elderly. Med J Aust 1981; 2:398.

MRC Working Party. Medical Research Council trial of treatment of hypertension in older adults: Principal results. Br Med J 1992; 304:405.

SAVE (Results of the Survival and Ventricular Enlargement Trial). Effect of captopril on mortality and morbidity in patients with left ventricular dysfunction after myocardial infarction. N Engl J Med 1992; 327:669.

SHEP Cooperative Research Group. Prevention of stroke by antihypertensive drug treatment in older persons with isolated systolic hypertension. JAMA 1991; 265:3255.

The SOLVD (Studies of Left Ventricular Dysfunction) Investigators: Effect of enalapril on mortality and the development of heart failure in asymptomatic patients with reduced left ventricular ejection fractions. N Engl J Med 1992; 327:685.

HYPERTENSIVE CRISIS

W. Dallas Hall, M.D.

There are two types of hypertensive crisis: hypertensive emergency and hypertensive urgency. A *hypertensive emergency* is defined as a clinical setting where blood pressure (BP) must be reduced effectively within minutes to 1 hour or less. Examples include accelerated and malignant hypertension, hypertensive encephalopathy, and severe diastolic hypertension (usually in the range of 120 to 160 mm Hg) that is associated with acute pulmonary edema, ischemic chest pain, dissecting aortic aneurysm, or intracerebral hemorrhage.

A *hypertensive urgency* is defined as a situation where severe elevations of BP are not causing immediate end-organ damage but should be effectively lowered within 24 hours to reduce potential risk to the patient. A typical example would be a patient with a BP of 220/134 mm Hg with minimal or no symptoms.

■ THERAPEUTIC ALTERNATIVES

Hypertensive emergencies are generally treated by hospitalization and institution of parenteral antihypertensive therapy. The drugs used most commonly are listed in Table 1, along with their recommended starting doses and infusion rates. The brand names for these drugs are included in Table 2.

Hypertensive urgencies are generally treated by short-term hospital admission and institution of oral antihypertensive therapy. The regimens used most commonly are listed in Table 3.

Table 1 Hypertensive Emergency: Options for Intravenous Therapy

DRUG (ROUTE)	MIXTURE	INITIAL ADULT DOSE	ONSET	DURATION	MAJOR ADVERSE EFFECTS	COMMENTS
Nitroprusside (continuous infusion)	50 mg dissolved in 250 ml D5W provides a solution of 200 µg/ml. Protect from light and change q12h	20–50 µg/min (0.3–0.5 µg/kg/min)	Immediate	2–5 min	Thiocyanate toxicity, acidosis, vomiting, seizures	Infusion rates greater than 8 µg/kg/min should be avoided; monitor SCN levels in presence of renal failure or with prolonged infusions
Nitroglycerine (continuous infusion)	32 µg/ml often constituted by adding 50–250 mg into 250 ml D5W in a special delivery system	32 µg/min (0.5 µg/kg/min)	Immediate	2–5 min	Headache, tachycardia, methemoglobinemia, alcohol intoxication (prolonged high-dose infusion)	Infusion rates above 50 µg/min are often necessary to achieve reduction in blood pressure
Labetalol (IV minibolus)	5 mg/ml in 20 ml ampule	20 mg (4 ml) in 2 min, then 40–80 mg (8–16 ml) at 15 min intervals	10 min	4–6 h (variable)	Dizziness, scalp tingling, orthostasis, bradycardia	Contraindicated in patients with bronchospasm, congestive heart failure, bradycardia, or heart block greater than first degree
Labetalol (continuous infusion)	100–200 mg in 1,000 ml D5W	0.5 mg/min; increase as necessary to a maximum of 2 mg/min	As above	As above	As above	As above
Enalaprilat (IV minibolus)	1.25 mg/ml in a 2 ml Vasotec IV vial; can be mixed with either dextrose or saline	1.25 mg (1 ml) in 5 min, followed by 1.25 mg q6h if effective; total daily dosage should not exceed 20 mg	5–15 min	6 h or more	Excessive hypotension; rarely, angioedema, hyperkalemia, or acute renal failure	Initial dose should be reduced to 0.625 mg (0.5 ml) if the patient is receiving diuretic therapy or has a serum creatinine level >3 mg/dl
Diltiazem hydrochloride (bolus, then infusion)		Inject 0.25 mg/kg over 2 min, followed by infusion of 0.35 mg/kg at an initial rate of 10 mg/h	3–30 min	—	Excessive hypotension; flushing; rarely, amblyopia	Approved primarily for supraventricular tachyarrhythmias but can also be useful for control of BP
Nicardipine (continuous infusion)		5–7.5 mg/h depending on body weight	5–60 min	20–40 min	Headache, flushing, phlebitis at infusion site	

SCN, serum cyanide

■ PREFERRED APPROACH

Hypertensive Emergencies
Sodium Nitroprusside

Intravenous therapy with sodium nitroprusside (SNP) allows minute-to-minute titration of BP to a desired level. The usual starting dose is 0.3 to 0.5 μg per kilogram per minute, followed by increments of 0.5 to 1.0 μg per kilogram per minute as needed. The maximum infusion rate should not exceed 8 μg per kilogram per minute. Sodium nitroprusside must be protected from photodegradation by wrapping the infusion bottle with tinfoil; the solution must be renewed every 12 hours. Administration of SNP requires careful monitoring by experienced staff in an intensive care setting.

The goal of initial therapy is often a 20 to 25 percent reduction of diastolic BP toward 110 to 120 mm Hg, or to a mean arterial BP (i.e., diastolic BP plus one-third of the pulse pressure) of 120 mm Hg, depending on the clinical setting and the course of individual patients. In general, the reduction should be slower in patients with acute cerebral infection, for whom the goal should be to maintain a BP of at least 170 to 180/100 mm Hg.

Table 2 Generic (Brand) Names of Drugs Mentioned

Captopril (Capoten)
Clonidine (Catapres)
Diltiazem (Cardizem)
Enalaprilat (Vasotec IV)
Furosemide (Lasix)
Hydroxocobalamin (alphaREDISOL)
Isosorbide dinitrate (Isordil)
Labetalol (Trandate)
Nicardipine (Cardene) (Normodyne)
Nifedipine (Procardia)
Nimodipine (Nimotop)
Nitroglycerin (Nitrol IV)
Sodium nitroprusside (Nipride, Nitropress)

Oral antihypertensive therapy can often be started once the severely elevated BP has improved, typically within 12 to 24 hours after beginning SNP. Excellent choices for the transition from parenteral to oral therapy include labetalol (200 mg every 12 hours), clonidine (0.1 to 0.2 mg every 12 hours), or captopril (12.5 mg every 12 hours).

Sodium nitroprusside reacts with cysteine to form nitrosocysteine, which activates guanylate cyclase and leads to accumulation of cyclic guanosine monophosphate (cGMP) resulting in direct vasodilation of vascular smooth muscle.

Cyanide is a metabolic by-product of the reaction, and serum thiocyanate or cyanide levels should be monitored in patients with renal insufficiency or whenever therapy with SNP is continued for 3 days or more. Thiocyanate levels above 12 mg per deciliter suggest toxicity and require discontinuation or down-titration of the SNP. Acute toxicity is flagged most readily by metabolic acidosis and can be treated with infusion of 25 mg per hour of hydroxocobalamin (a vitamin B_{12} derivative that binds cyanide) or infusion of 3 percent sodium nitrite followed by slow (15 to 20 minutes) injection of 12.5 g sodium thiosulfate.

Sodium nitroprusside therapy is associated with sodium retention and activation of the sympathetic nervous system. The latter is reflected by tachycardia (less if plasma catecholamines have already been stimulated by the underlying condition) and hyperreninemia. Both of these reflex responses

Table 3 Hypertensive Urgency: Options for Oral Therapy

DRUG/REGIMEN	INITIAL ADULT DOSE	ONSET	DURATION	MAJOR ADVERSE EFFECTS	COMMENTS
Clonidine loading	0.2 mg PO then 0.1 mg qh to a maximum total dose of 0.8 mg or until diastolic BP is reduced 20 mm or more or below 110 mm Hg	30–120 min	8–12 h	Sedation, dry mouth, dizziness, orthostasis	Contraindicated in patients with sinus bradycardia, sick sinus syndrome, or heart block. Excess hypotension can be counteracted with IV saline plus 5 mg IV tolazoline
Labetalol	200–300 mg single oral dose followed by 100–200 mg q8h	60–120 min	12–24 h	Bradycardia	See Table 1
Hospitalize and resume previous therapy for 24 h	Previous medications and dosage	—	—	Excessive hypotension	This plan will control BP in 25–50% of patients seemingly resistant to outpatient therapy; occasional quasicompliant patients can experience hypotension
Nimodipine (oral)	0.7 mg/kg initial oral dose, followed by 0.35 mg/kg q4h for 21 days	1–3 h	4 h	Hypotension, edema, headache	Indicated to improve the outcome of intracranial bleeding due to aneurysmal subarachnoid hemorrhage

can blunt the initial hypotensive effect of SNP, which can be restored by effective diuresis with furosemide and, when not contraindicated, concomitant therapy with a beta-blocker or angiotensin converting enzyme inhibitor.

Therapy with SNP can be associated with intrapulmonary shunting of blood flow, resulting in a decrease in arterial oxygenation. This effect is less prominent with infusion of nitroglycerin, which may have other advantages over SNP in some patients with chest pain and/or myocardial ischemia. When the elevation of BP is severe, however, SNP and labetalol are more potent for effective reduction of BP. Administration of isosorbide dinitrate (10 mg sublingually) is also often useful and can lead to further improvements in BP within 30 to 60 minutes.

Labetalol Minibolus

Minibolus therapy with labetalol is sometimes preferable to continuous infusion of SNP, particularly in emergency room or some perioperative settings where it is not always possible to monitor BP on a minute-to-minute basis. In addition, in patients with increased intracranial pressure (e.g., intracerebral or subarachnoid hemorrhage), reduction of systemic blood pressure and cerebral vasodilation with SNP can be associated with an increase in intracranial pressure and a decrease in cerebral perfusion pressure. Hence, some prefer minibolus labetalol to SNP therapy in this clinical setting.

Intravenous labetalol is contraindicated in the presence of sinus bradycardia, sick sinus syndrome, second- or third-degree heart block, bronchospasm, and left ventricular dysfunction. In the absence of these conditions, the appropriate initial dose of intravenous labetalol is 20 mg (4 ml), given over 2 minutes. After 15 minutes, a second bolus of 40 mg is given, increasing to 80 mg 15 to 20 minutes later as needed. Once a reasonable improvement in BP is obtained (usually within 2 to 3 hours following a total labetalol dose of 180 to 300 mg), therapy can be maintained by continuous infusion of 0.5 to 2 mg per minute of labetalol. Transition to oral therapy is best accomplished after 12 to 48 hours, beginning with an oral labetalol dose of 200 mg every 12 hours with subsequent titration to 400 mg twice a day as needed. Addition of low doses of a diuretic often facilitates control of BP.

■ PREFERRED APPROACH

Hypertensive Urgencies

Short-Acting Calcium Antagonists

Although effective in rapidly reducing marked elevations of blood pressure, short-acting calcium antagonists, such as nifedipine, are not indicated for hypertensive urgencies because of concern about precipitous decreases in blood pressure and reflex sympathetic stimulation. Alternate therapies include the clonidine loading regimen or oral doses of labetalol, each of which has an onset within 1 to 3 hours (see Table 3).

Clonidine Loading

When it is desirable to reduce BP gradually over a 6 to 24 hour period, the clonidine loading regimen is often effective, especially if intensive care unit monitoring is neither desirable nor judged necessary. An initial oral dose of 0.2 mg is followed by a dose of 0.1 mg every hour until diastolic BP is below 110 mm Hg or a total dose of 0.8 mg clonidine is reached. Therapy is effective in 80 to 90 percent of patients, and maintenance therapy can then be initiated at approximately 75 percent of the total loading dose, given in divided doses twice daily.

Suggested Reading

Battey LL Jr, Felner JM, Hall WD. Clinical manifestations of 104 patients with diastolic blood pressure ≥140 mm Hg. Emory Univ J Med 1988; 2:102.

Fagan TC. Acute reduction of blood pressure in asymptomatic patients with severe hypertension. An idea whose time has come—and gone. Arch Intern Med 1989; 149:2169.

Gifford RW Jr. Management of hypertensive crises. JAMA 1991; 266:829.

Houston MC. Treatment of hypertensive emergencies and urgencies with oral clonidine loading and titration: A review. Arch Intern Med 1986; 146:586.

Joint National Committee. The fifth report of the Joint National Committee on Detection, Evaluation, and Treatment of High Blood Pressure. Arch Intern Med 1993:154.

Wallin JD, Cook ME, Blanski L, et al. Intravenous nicardipine for the treatment of severe hypertension. Am J Med 1988; 85:331.

Weber MA. Immediate treatment of severe hypertension: Widening the options. Arch Intern Med 1989; 149:2635.

SYNCOPE

Richard P. Lewis, M.D.

Syncope is a transient loss of consciousness due to a sudden decrease in cerebral perfusion pressure. If it occurs abruptly, serious bodily injury may occur. *Presyncope* is a less precise term, and in most cases it defines those instances in which consciousness is not lost. Presyncope commonly occurs in patients with syncope, and in these cases it usually has a similar mechanism. Frequently, the mechanism of syncope is complex, requiring several factors to be present simultaneously. Table 1 lists several common predisposing factors that often determine whether syncope actually occurs. Failure to consider these factors is a major reason that the mechanism of syncope is not determined.

Syncope is a common problem that accounts for 1 to 2 percent of hospital admissions (Lewis and co-workers, 1994). Because it is a symptom, rather than a disease, it has diverse and multisystem etiologies. A useful recent approach to the categorization of the causes of syncope is shown in Table 2. Each

Table 1 Predisposing Factors for Syncope

Metabolic abnormalities (drug, electrolyte, acid base, hypoxia, anemia, alcohol)
Deconditioning (bed rest, debilitating disease)
Old age
Fatigue
Fever or high ambient temperature
Upright posture
Postprandial state
Fasting
Advanced cerebrovascular disease
Variations in autonomic tone

Table 2 Common Causes of Syncope

Noncardiac
Vasodepressor
Orthostatic
Situational
Reflex
Carotid sinus hypersensitivity
Cerebrovascular disease
Cardiac
Obstructive
Aortic and pulmonary stenosis
Hypertrophic cardiomyopathy
Pulmonary hypertension
Left atrial myxoma
Prosthetic valve dysfunction
Acute myocardial infarction
Arrhythmic
Bradyarrhythmias
Supraventricular tachycardia
Ventricular tachycardia
Unknown cause
Occult arrhythmia and vasodepressor
Combined cause
Pseudosyncope
Neurologic disorders
Psychiatric
Metabolic

of the three broad categories accounts for approximately one-third of the total cases. The 1 year mortality for each category from the study of Kapoor and co-workers (1983) is shown in Table 3. The mortality for cardiac syncope is alarmingly high. Although the mortality for the other forms of syncope is lower, it probably exceeds the expected mortality for a healthy population. It should be noted that both diagnosis and therapy have improved since 1983 such that 1 year mortality is probably lower. Nonetheless, syncope is a serious symptom. It requires an etiologic mechanism to be found, or therapy will be ineffectual.

All patients with syncope (except young individuals with obvious neurocardiogenic syncope) should undergo a complete history and physical examination, routine laboratory studies, a chest roentgenogram, and an electrocardiogram. If heart disease is suspected, a cardiac echo-Doppler study is usually also recommended. Unfortunately, the routine clinical evaluation yields a correct diagnosis in only one-half of all patients with syncope. Further laboratory evaluation is often

Table 3 1 Year Mortality for the Various Causes of Syncope

CAUSE	MORTALITY (%)
Noncardiac	12
Cardiac	30
Undetermined	6

Data from Kapoor WN, Karpf M, Weiland S, et al. A prospective evaluation and follow-up of patients with syncope. N Engl J Med 1983; 309:197.

required, and it can be costly (e.g., neurologic studies in patients with no evidence of neurologic disease or prolonged arrhythmia monitoring in the hospital). Therefore, in the following sections on therapy of various types of syncope, the appropriate laboratory evaluation is also briefly discussed.

■ PREFERRED APPROACH

Noncardiac Syncope

Vasodepressor Syncope

The most frequent cause of syncope is vasodepressor syncope, or the common faint. It occurs mainly in young individuals in response to emotional or physical stress and is often an isolated event, but the initial episode can occur at any age. Vasodepressor syncope is the result of an inappropriate autonomic nervous system reaction that involves both sympathetic withdrawal and parasympathetic discharge. Generally the sympathetic withdrawal occurs first, and the parasympathetic component is variably present. Sympathetic withdrawal causes the blood pressure to fall as a result of arterial and venous dilation, whereas parasympathetic stimulation lowers the cardiac output largely by slowing the heart rate. When parasympathetic discharge is predominant, the term *vasovagal reaction* has been used. The precipitating mechanisms of the vasodepressor reaction are still unclear. It is often preceded by an acute diminution in venous return, hypotension, or both. This, in turn, may produce excessive stimulation of intracardiac baroreceptors leading to the autonomic response. This has led some recent investigators to call vasodepressor syncope *neurocardiogenic syncope.*

Vasodepressor syncope is usually of gradual onset and is frequently preceded by autonomic symptoms such as sweating, gastrointestinal distress, pupillary dilation, and pallor. The patient usually responds promptly to the head-down position or supine position with leg elevation. Premature return to the upright posture may precipitate a recurrence.

Vasodepressor syncope can now be reproduced in the laboratory by the technique of head-up tilt, usually at 60 degrees for 30 minutes. This technique does not seem to precipitate the vasodepressor reaction in normal individuals but the precise sensitivity and specificity is still unclear. Head-up tilt can also be used to assess pharmacotherapy of vasodepressor syncope.

In general, vasodepressor syncope does not require pharmacotherapy. Simple avoidance of precipitating factors is usually sufficient. When the symptom is recurrent, various autonomic blocking agents have been used with variable success. Beta-adrenergic blockers are the most useful. Of them, the nonselective agents such as metoprolol (25 to 100 mg daily) or atenolol (25 to 100 mg daily) have been most widely used.

Orthostatic Syncope

Presyncope due to orthostatic hypotension is far more common than actual syncope. When syncope does occur, it may be the result of a superimposed vasodepressor, vasovagal reaction, or both. Orthostatic syncope can result from blood volume depletion (blood loss, dehydration, overdiuresis) or impaired vascular tone. The latter may result from neuropathic disorders (most commonly diabetes and alcoholism) or may be drug-induced. Pharmacologic agents most commonly associated with postural hypotension and syncope include antiadrenergic agents, vasodilators, and psychotropic drugs. The recent popularity of vasodilator therapy for heart failure has resulted in an increase in orthostatic syncope in this population. Patients with mitral valve prolapse syndrome often have both hypovolemia and dysautonomia and are especially prone to this type of syncope.

Therapy for orthostatic syncope consists of restoration of plasma volume and discontinuation or reduction in the dose of the causative pharmacologic agents. This treatment is usually successful unless neuropathy or other neurologic diseases are the cause. In such patients, antigravity stockings, avoidance of sudden and prolonged standing, and volume expansion with a high-salt diet or fludrocortisone acetate should be tried.

Situational Syncope

Situational syncope is usually identified by a typical history. As with postural syncope, a superimposed vasodepressor reaction may be necessary for syncope to occur. The most common events that lead to situational syncope are cough, defecation, and micturition. Therapy is directed toward the prevention of the precipitating event by treating the underlying disease. Thus, therapy of pulmonary disease when present, the addition of stool softeners and laxatives, or prostatic surgery all should be considered in individual patients.

A recently described and probably common form of syncope occurs in elderly patients after meals (postprandial syncope). This seems to involve sympathetic withdrawal. Treatment for this form of syncope has not been clearly defined, but frequent small feedings should be tried, as well as modification of any vasodilator therapy.

Reflex Syncope

Reflex syncope usually involves a vasovagal reaction producing marked sinus bradycardia, atrioventricular (AV) block, or asystole. Because parasympathetic discharge also inhibits sympathetic outflow, there may be an associated sympathetic withdrawal as well. Reflex syncope can result from painful stimulation of the oropharynx, esophagus, or tracheal-bronchial tree. It can also occur with swallowing in patients with esophageal disorders (diverticulum, stricture, achalasia, or spasm) and glossopharyngeal neuralgia.

Recently, a syndrome of paroxysmal hypervagotonia has been described, which may produce sudden death as well as syncope. It often occurs in apparently healthy young individuals. In our experience, many of these individuals have mitral valve prolapse syndrome. This form of syncope may be elicited by head-up tilt.

Reflex syncope related to manipulation of the oral cavity, esophagus, or tracheal-bronchial tree is treated by the prophylactic use of atropine sulfate (1 mg intravenously) before the procedure. In cases associated with esophageal or other disease, treatment of the underlying disease is required. However, in refractory cases or those with paroxysmal vagotonia, a pacemaker may be indicated.

Carotid Sinus Syncope

Recent studies indicate that hypersensitivity to carotid sinus stimulation is more common than has been considered in the past. In such cases, carotid sinus stimulation may elicit a vasodepressor reaction, a predominant vasovagal reaction, or both. Hypersensitivity can occur as a primary abnormality in the carotid sinus mechanism or because of excessive sensitivity of the heart due to underlying conduction system disease. Digitalis, beta-blocking agents, and calcium channel blocking agents can aggravate this syndrome.

Carotid sinus massage with blood pressure as well as arrhythmia monitoring in the head-up tilt position is indicated in all patients with syncope of unknown cause. A hypotensive response suggests carotid sinus hypersensitivity is the cause of the patient's syncope. Therapy should first be directed toward patient education and the withdrawal of the aggravating pharmacotherapy if possible. Carotid sinus denervation may be attempted when neck pathology is the cause. For patients with refractory symptoms, pacemaker therapy is required. The pacemaker syndrome commonly occurs in these patients with single-chamber (VVI) pacing so that dual-chamber (DDD or DVI) pacing is necessary. Pacemaker therapy significantly reduces the incidence of syncope despite the fact that the vasodepressor response is not directly affected.

Cerebrovascular Disease

Cerebrovascular disease produces transient ischemic attacks that usually do not produce a loss of consciousness. Thus, cerebrovascular disease generally does not produce syncope, although its presence may predispose an individual to syncope from other causes. When syncope does occur with cerebrovascular disease, there is usually vertebrobasilar system or aortic arch disease. Therapy is aimed at avoiding hypotension, but occasionally carotid artery surgery is feasible to improve cerebral blood flow. Cervical spine disease or neck deformities may mechanically compress the vertebral arteries and produce syncope with neck extension—a maneuver that should be avoided. Subclavian artery stenosis may produce syncope associated with arm effort (the "subclavian steal"), and this condition is amenable to surgical therapy. Patients with migraine headache may occasionally develop syncope (syncopal migraine). Beta-adrenergic blocking agents should be considered for these patients.

Cardiac Syncope

Obstructive Cardiac Syncope

Disorders that produce mechanical obstruction to the cardiac output may produce syncope. The syncope usually appears to be a vasodepressor reaction probably related to stimulation of intracardiac baroreceptors. This type of syncope may occur during exertion.

The most common cause of obstructive cardiac syncope is valvular aortic stenosis, and in such patients the symptom is associated with a poor prognosis. Therefore, it is generally an indication for aortic valve replacement, which usually abolishes the symptom, unless syncope was related to an arrhythmia or conduction system disease, which may also be present in more advanced cases.

Pulmonary stenosis or tetralogy of Fallot may cause syncope. Syncope in postoperative cases of tetralogy of Fallot may be due to ventricular tachycardia and suggests an unsuccessful surgical repair. Other causes of obstructive cardiac syncope include left atrial myxoma and prosthetic valve dysfunction. For all these disorders, the therapy is surgical correction.

Patients with pulmonary hypertension (primary pulmonary hypertension, Eisenmenger's syndrome, chronic pulmonary emboli) may also develop syncope. Although no good therapy other than activity limitation exists when pulmonary vascular disease is fixed, patients with acute pulmonary emboli may benefit from heparin, urokinase, or a vena caval filter if the diagnosis is established in time. In patients at high risk for pulmonary emboli (e.g., hip fracture), syncope may be an early warning sign of pulmonary embolism.

Syncope is common in hypertrophic cardiomyopathy; it may be related to outflow tract obstruction (typically postexertional) or cardiac arrhythmia. Hemodynamic syncope may require an intervention such as dual-chamber pacing or surgical myomectomy if discontinuation of aggravating drugs (digitalis and vasodilators) does not relieve the symptom. Arrhythmic syncope must be evaluated and treated aggressively (see later).

Acute Myocardial Infarction

Five to 10 percent of patients with acute myocardial infarction have syncope as their initial presentation (Lewis and coworkers, 1994). This condition largely occurs with Q wave inferior wall infarction and may be fatal. In this setting, activation of the Bezold-Jarisch reflex appears to be the mechanism. This reflex may not completely respond to atropine (0.5 mg intravenously as an initial dose) if there is associated ischemic injury to the conduction system or right ventricular infarction. Some patients with severe hypotension and bradycardia may require transient use of intravenous isoproterenol (1 to 2 μg per minute) or a temporary pacemaker. Atropine is safe and may be lifesaving in this setting, provided that the initial dose does not exceed 0.5 mg and the patient is carefully monitored. Frequently, repeat administration of atropine is required when hypotension and bradycardia recurs during the subsequent 12 to 24 hours.

Arrhythmic Syncope

An abnormal heart rate at either extreme may produce syncope, but syncope is more likely to occur in patients with limited cardiac reserve due to valvular or myocardial disease. Such patients are also more likely to have conduction system disease, which predisposes to arrhythmia. Arrhythmic syncope should be suspected if the patient has underlying heart disease, notes palpitations, or has abrupt syncope with bodily injury, or the syncope is unrelated to posture. The mechanism of arrhythmic syncope is often undocumented by routine examination, and a further diagnostic evaluation is required that may include cardiac catheterization to define coronary anatomy. It should be noted that ambulatory monitoring in excess of 24 hours has a low yield. Table 4 summarizes the use of specific laboratory tests to evaluate arrhythmic syncope.

Table 4 Laboratory Evaluation of Arrhythmic Syncope

TEST	PURPOSE
Electrocardiogram	Defines conduction system disease, Wolff-Parkinson-White syndrome, myocardial infarction, left ventricular hypertrophy, atrial and ventricular ectopy, and occasionally arrhythmia
Signal-averaged electrocardiogram	Screens for ventricular tachycardia after myocardial infarction
Ambulatory monitoring	Documents arrhythmia and relates to symptoms; aids in defining therapeutic response
Patient-activated monitoring devices	Documents paroxysmal arrhythmias in low-risk subsets
Exercise test	Reproduces exertional arrhythmias; evaluates role of ischemia
Invasive electrophysiologic study	Defines conduction system disease, elicits supraventricular and ventricular tachycardia, and measures hemodynamic effect of arrhythmias and response to pharmacologic and pacing interventions
Head-up tilt	Elicits vasodepressor response, aids in assessment of hemodynamic response to arrhythmia

Modified from Weissler AM, Boudoulas HB, Lewis RP, et al. Syncope: Pathophysiology, recognition, and treatment. In: Hurst JW, ed. The heart. 7th ed. New York: McGraw-Hill, 1990.

Unfortunately, noninvasive testing can establish a clear-cut etiology for syncope in only the minority of cases. More patients with suspected arrhythmic syncope are undergoing invasive electrophysiologic study (EPS). With appropriate patient selection (i.e., strong suspicion of arrhythmia by noninvasive testing and/or underlying heart disease), EPS defines the mechanism of syncope (and therefore proper therapy) in two-thirds of patients with suspected arrhythmic syncope who undergo the procedure.

The most common "occult" arrhythmias revealed by EPS are bradyarrhythmias and ventricular tachycardia. Supraventricular tachycardias (mostly atrial flutter and fibrillation with rapid ventricular rate or the Wolff-Parkinson-White syndrome) account for the remainder. Of note, patients with a negative study have a low short-term mortality but often have recurrent nonarrhythmic syncope.

In patients with bradyarrhythmias, the conduction system disease is usually diffuse. In our experience, the greater the number of electrophysiologic abnormalities of the conduction system found, the more likely it is that syncope is due to a bradyarrhythmia. Variations in intrinsic vagal tone probably account for the episodes of severe bradycardia that lead to syncope in such patients. Pacemaker therapy nearly always abolishes symptoms (both syncope and presyncope), provided that the proper type of pacemaker is selected to avoid the pacemaker syndrome. Furthermore, follow-up studies after pacemaker insertion indicate that progression of the conduction disease occurs in many individuals. Thus, pacemaker therapy (DDD or DVI when sinus rhythm is present) is generally indicated in patients with syncope and evidence of primary conduction system disease. However, withdrawal of drugs such as digitalis, beta-adrenergic blocking agents, verapamil, or antiarrhythmic drugs should be attempted, if appropriate, before the final decision to insert a pacemaker is made. Not infrequently, patients with conduction system disease have the "tachycardia-bradycardia syndrome" and may require a pacemaker in order to tolerate pharmacotherapy for the tachycardia. Finally, there are patients with syncope due to the pacemaker syndrome in whom the VVI pacemaker must be replaced with a dual-chamber system.

Pharmacologic therapy of supraventricular and ventricular tachycardia is considered in detail in subsequent chapters. However, a few general considerations for therapy of tachyarrhythmias in patients with syncope can be stated. When a tachyarrhythmia causes syncope, the arrhythmia is generally more rapid, more sustained, or associated with significant underlying heart disease. Thus, these patients are at high risk for both morbidity and mortality, and therapy is clearly indicated. Experience from several laboratories indicates that successful therapy, often guided by serial EPS studies, can reduce both morbidity and mortality.

Newer, nonpharmacologic techniques should be considered for individuals who are refractory to antiarrhythmic therapy. For supraventricular tachycardias, they include antitachycardia, pacemakers, radiofrequency ablation of anomalous pathways in the Wolff-Parkinson-White syndrome or for AV nodal re-entry, and occasionally AV node ablation with pacemaker insertion for atrial fibrillation. For ventricular tachycardia, implantable defibrillating devices should be considered.

When ischemia is present and may be playing a role in the arrhythmia, revascularization should be attempted first (coronary bypass or angioplasty). Beta-adrenergic blocking agents should be used as adjunctive therapy in patients with ischemic heart disease (and possibly cardiomyopathies as well) because these agents raise the ventricular fibrillation threshold and suppress arrhythmias that are aggravated by adrenergic stimulation.

Because of its antiarrhythmic efficacy, low incidence of proarrhythmia, and ease of administration, amiodarone is the antiarrhythmic agent of choice for ventricular tachycardia, especially when there is left ventricular dysfunction. Severe toxicity can be minimized by using the lowest possible dose (200 mg per day once steady state has been reached). Nonetheless, careful monitoring of thyroid and pulmonary function is required. In some patients with mitral valve prolapse, a beta-blocking agent (nadolol is useful because of its once-a-day administration) may eliminate the ventricular tachycardia.

Syncope of Unknown Cause

This category has become progressively smaller with the more widespread use of EPS and head-up tilt. Occult arrhythmias and vasodepressor syncope constituted a significant proportion of these patients in the past. Nonetheless, there is a small subset (10 to 20 percent) of patients in whom no clear-cut etiology can be established in spite of an extensive workup. In many cases, these patients probably have "syncope due to multiple causes," which is particularly common in the elderly. Counseling should be given regarding the avoidance of potentially dangerous activities and the elimination of predisposing factors. The patient should be followed carefully because up to one-third of patients have a recurrence.

Pseudosyncope

Several noncardiac disorders may produce states of altered consciousness, which in most cases are not true syncope. Seizure disorders should not usually be confused with syncope, but occasionally the distinction is difficult on clinical grounds alone. The most common error is to misdiagnose syncope as a seizure disorder. Syncope lacks a postictal state, incontinence is rare, and generalized or focal seizure activity is also rare. If seizure-like activity does occur with syncope, it occurs at the onset and is not sustained. Cerebral emboli virtually always produce focal neurologic deficits rather than syncope. These are usually platelet emboli originating from either the heart or the carotid arteries. Sleep disorders may be associated with narcolepsy or impaired wakefulness, but they are usually clearly distinguishable by history. Hysterical syncope does not involve true loss of consciousness and is often bizarre and occurs in the setting of obvious psychiatric illness. Therapy of all these disorders requires treatment of the underlying neuropsychiatric disorder.

Various metabolic abnormalities that cause syncope are rare; the syncope is probably induced by precipitating a vasodepressor reaction. More commonly, metabolic abnormalities predispose to some other form of syncope. These disorders include hypoxia, hypoglycemia, severe anemia, electrolyte disorders, hyperventilation, and carbon dioxide retention. Metabolic disorders should be appropriately treated when present in patients with syncope.

Suggested Reading

Boudoulas H, Schaal SF, Lewis RP. Electrophysiologic risk factors in syncope. J Electrocardiol 1978; 11:339.

Gibson TC, Heitzman MR. Diagnostic efficacy of 24 hour electrocardiographic monitoring for syncope. Am J Cardiol 1984; 53:1013.

Grubb BP, Temesy Arnas P, Mann M, et al. The utility of upright tilt-table testing in the evaluation and management of syncope of unknown origin. Am J Med 1991; 90:6–10.

Huang SK, Ezri MO, Hauser RG, et al. Carotid sinus hypersensitivity in patients with unexplained syncope: Chemical, electrophysiologic, and long term follow-up observations. Am Heart J 1988; 116:989.

Kapoor WN, Karpf M, Weiland S, et al. A prospective evaluation and follow-up of patients with syncope. N Engl J Med 1983; 309:197.

Klein GJ, Gersu BI, Yee R. Electrophysiological testing: The Final Court of Appeal for diagnosis of syncope? Circulation 1995; 92:1332–1335.

Kushner JA, Kou WH, Kadish AH, et al. Natural history of patients with unexplained syncope and a nondiagnostic electrophysiologic study. J Am Coll Cardiol 1989; 14:391.

Lewis RP, Boudoulas H, Schall ST, et al. Diagnosis and management of syncope. In: Schlant RS, Alexander RW, O'Rourke RA, et al, eds. The Heart. 8th ed. New York, McGraw-Hill 1994:927–945.

Sra JS, Murthy VS, Jazayeri MR, et al. Use of intravenous esmolol to pre-

dict efficacy of oral beta-adrenergic blocker therapy in patients with neurocardiogenic syncope. J Am Coll Cardiol 1991; 19:402.
Warren JV, Lewis RP. Beneficial effects of atropine in the prehospital phase of coronary care. Am J Cardiol 1976; 37:68.
Winters SL, Stewart D, Gomes A. Signal averaging the surface QRS complex predicts inducibility of ventricular tachycardia in patients with syncope of unknown origin: A perspective study. J Am Coll Cardiol 1987; 10:775.

THE ADULT WITH CYANOTIC CONGENITAL HEART DISEASE

Robert H. Franch, M.D.

Examiners should be aware that a patient may have a congenital heart anomaly that is associated with right-to-left shunting; however, clinical cyanosis may not be evident or may be overlooked. Medical treatment is primarily supportive and palliative; surgical treatment may be palliative or anatomically or physiologically corrective. The adult with cyanotic congenital heart disease has certain problems regardless of the underlying anatomy.

The cyanotic adult with symptomatic erythrocytosis or hyperviscosity syndrome has symptoms of headache, dizziness, visual disturbances, fatigue, muscle pains, paresthesias, or slow thinking. These symptoms usually appear with a hematocrit of 70 or greater. The hematocrit should be lowered only to the level that relieves symptoms, which is usually at 65 percent (Perloff and co-workers, 1988). Ordinarily, 500 ml of blood is withdrawn at a sitting and is replaced by an equal volume of normal saline or 5 percent albumin. If correction to a specific hematocrit is desired, the estimated whole blood volume to be removed equals the body weight (kilograms) times 0.11 times the initial venous hematocrit minus the desired venous hematocrit divided by the initial venous hematocrit. If venous access is difficult in the arms, a small sheath may have to be placed in the femoral vein. Iron deficiency anemia should be avoided to prevent increased rigidity and decreased deformability characteristic of hypochromic microcytic red blood cells, thus increasing resistance to capillary flow. Iron should not be given unless there are symptoms. Treatment should be limited to 200 mg of iron daily for 1 week. Symptoms and the hematocrit are then assessed. The cycle of alternate bleeding and iron replacement should be avoided. In severe polycythemia, thrombotic events, bleeding events, or both may occur. Poor clot retraction has been noted as well as a depression of thromboplastin generation, thrombocytopenia, and other abnormalities. The cyanotic polycythemic patient may have troublesome bleeding intraoperatively or postoperatively.

In our practice, a 25-year-old man with tetralogy of Fallot had prolonged bleeding following dental extraction. A liter of blood was removed and the volume replaced; the hematocrit fell from 77 percent to 65 percent. The plasma prothrombin time fell from 19.1 to 11.3 seconds and the partial thromboplastin time from 81.3 to 28.9 seconds. The platelet count rose to normal levels. Corrective surgery was performed without significant bleeding.

A 36-year-old cyanotic woman with Eisenmenger's physiology had increasing left foot and ankle rest pain over 6 weeks. The left femoral pulse was absent. The hematocrit was 56. The abdominal aortogram showed occlusion of the left common iliac and left external iliac as well as the common femoral artery (Fig. 1A). The distal left popliteal artery was also closed (Fig. 1B).

To accelerate thrombolysis, urokinase was given at a dose of 240,000 units per hour into the thrombus in the common and external iliac artery via a multilumen multiside hole catheter and via an infusion wire. Flow was re-established in the proximal arteries in 3½ hours, but the left popliteal remained closed. An infusion of 60,000 units of urokinase per hour for the next 24 hours was given via an inlying superficial femoral artery catheter and infusion wire. Heparinization was maintained at a therapeutic level. After 24 hours the popliteal artery remained closed. The infusion wire was then passed into the popliteal artery and 390,000 units of urokinase was given over an hour. The vessel opened intermittently and was responsive to nitroglycerin infusion.

Three days later an arteriogram showed the popliteal artery to be closed, and urokinase was given through the superficial femoral artery catheter and through the popliteal artery infusion wire at a total rate of 60,000 units per hour for 24 hours. No change was noted, and 80,000 units of urokinase was given the following 24 hours. The popliteal was now open to the bifurcation but a balloon catheter could not be passed into the posterior tibial and peroneal arteries. Continued ischemia required an above-the-knee amputation.

Hyperuricemia related to low fractional excretion of uric acid and less related to increased urate production tends to be present in cyanotic polycythemic patients. I have used indomethacin to treat the occasional acute case of gout. Finding uric acid crystals in joint fluid aspirate allows prompt initial treatment and helps exclude infection. Uricosuric agents have not been routinely used for asymptomatic hyperuricemia.

Cyanosis may occur if the pulmonary arteriolar resistance and pulmonary arterial pressure rise near or beyond systemic levels, allowing right-to-left shunting to occur across a preexisting septal or aortopulmonary defect. Pregnancy is contraindicated in this group of patients. Pulmonary hypertension poses a great threat to the mother, and hypoxia is a threat to the infant. In the course of the illness, which goes to the third or fourth decade, hemoptysis may occur. This does not

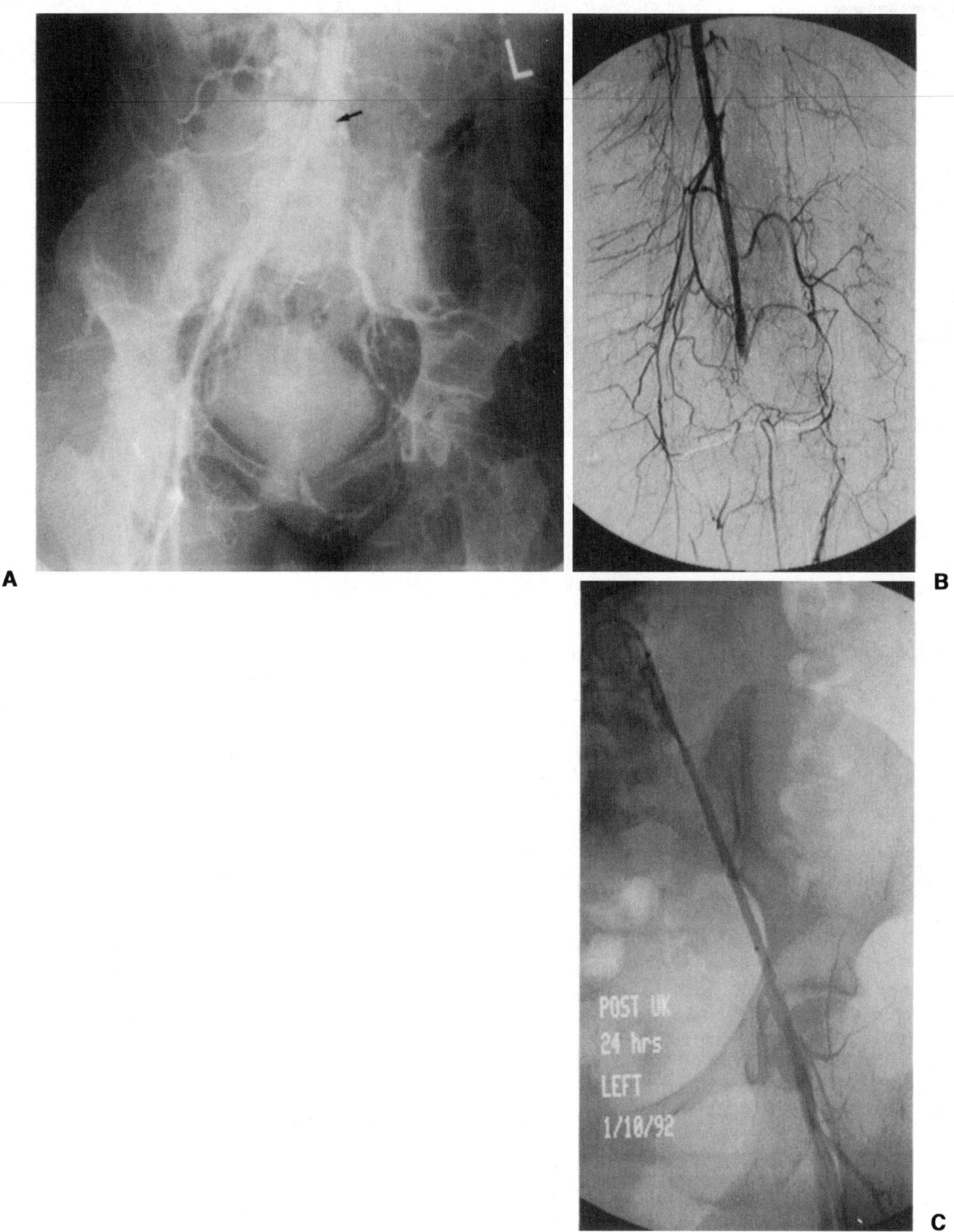

Figure 1

A, The abdominal aortogram of a 36-year-old cyanotic woman with Eisenmenger's physiology shows thrombotic occlusion of the left common (arrow) and the left external iliac arteries. The inferior mesenteric artery collateralizes the left internal iliac, which in turn collateralizes the left common femoral artery, its superior and deep branches, and the proximal popliteal artery. *B,* The distal left popliteal artery is totally closed, 3 cm above the knee joint. *C,* Selective arteriography via the infusion catheter in the left common and external iliac artery is obtained 24 hours after urokinase. Re-establishment of flow in these arteries as well as the common femoral artery was first noted at 3½ hours after infusion, and patency was maintained on all subsequent studies. The left popliteal remained occluded.

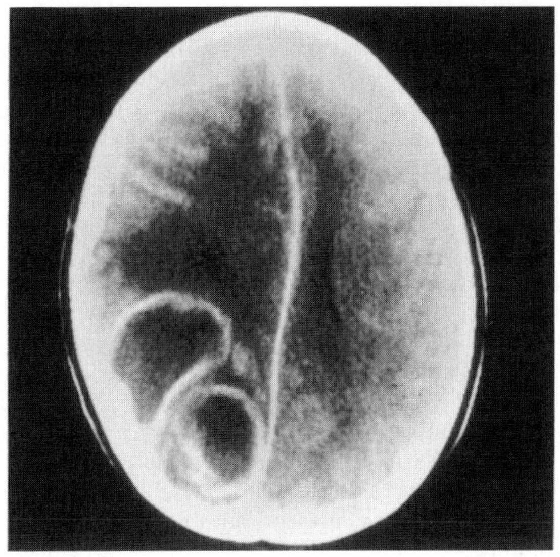
A

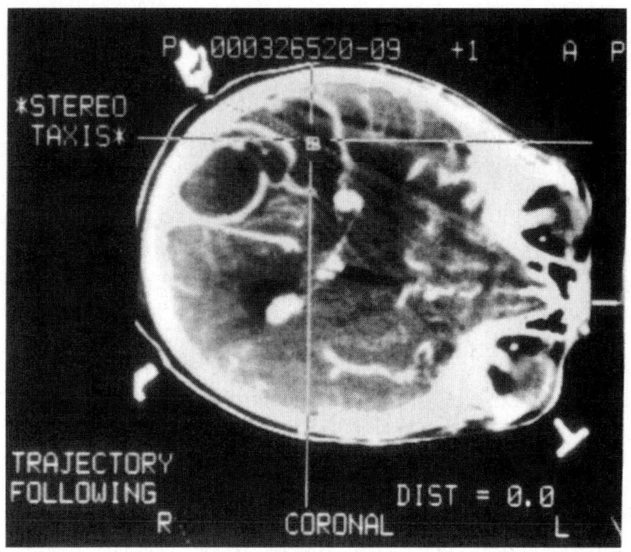

B

Figure 2
A, A 21-year-old woman with transposition of the great arteries, large ventricular septal defect, and pulmonary artery hypertension had a 1 cm midline shift and ring-enhancing hypodense lesions in the right parietal and occipital lobes. *B,* CT-directed needle aspiration drainage of the cerebral abscesses was done using a stereotactic biopsy frame. The organism was *Haemophilus paraphrophilus.* Ceftriaxone 2 g intravenously every 24 hours and metronidazole 500 mg every 6 hours were given for 6 weeks. Recovery was complete. *(Courtesy of the Department of Radiology, Emory University Hospital, Atlanta, Georgia).*

require bronchoscopy or special studies and is nearly always self-limited and thus requires reassurance. A fall in systemic blood pressure, which may occur in common faint or with standing suddenly or prolonged standing or sitting, permits increased right-to-left shunting and cyanosis. It is controlled by the squatting or supine position with elevation or flexion of the legs on the abdomen. Some patients sit in a Buddha position. If there is exertional faintness or severe hypoxia, a handicapped vehicle or wheelchair is prescribed. Sojourns to high altitudes should be avoided. One should recall that flying at an altitude of 40,000 feet produces a cabin Po_2 of 118 mm Hg, giving an arterial Po_2 of 58 mm in the normal patient. Home oxygen therapy may be offered continuously for a PaO_2 less than 55 mm Hg (O_2 Sat <88%) or intermittently for a PaO_2 of 56 to 59 mm Hg, especially with exertion, straining at stool, or nocturnally. There is no satisfactory drug therapy for pulmonary artery hypertension associated with Eisenmenger's physiology. Right ventricular failure is treated with digitalis and diuretics.

A computed tomographic (CT) scan is ordered for the cyanotic patient with headache, lethargy, and visual field deficit or other focal neurologic signs to exclude a circumscribed purulent lesion in the brain's substance. Because of the threat of increasing intracranial pressure and cerebral herniation, surgical treatment, either excision or aspiration, is usually required, followed by 6 weeks of antibiotic treatment based on culture of recovered abscess material. The CT-guided and ultrasound-guided stereotactic needle drainage of the encapsulated abscess was used successfully in our last adult case, followed by 6 weeks of antibiotic treatment (Fig. 2). Until an organism is identified, antibiotic treatment should cover a spectrum of bacteria. Nafcillin or vancomycin plus cefotaxime covers streptococci, staphylococci, and most anaerobes and gram-negative rods.

The adult patient with congenital asplenia and complex cyanotic heart disease has the potential for sepsis due to the encapsulated bacteria. Polyvalent pneumococcal vaccination may be given. The asplenic patient requires appropriate cultures and prompt antibiotic treatment for febrile illness. Initial drugs include penicillin, ampicillin, and amoxicillin; trimethoprim-sulfamethoxazole is useful against *Haemophilus influenzae.* Lifelong penicillin prophylaxis for the adult is controversial.

The cyanotic adult is susceptible to endocarditis. A 30-year-old asymptomatic housewife who had bilateral Blalock shunts done in childhood for pulmonary stenosis (PS) associated with single ventricle had four episodes of endocarditis unrelated to dental procedures, each 4 years or so apart and each caused by alpha-hemolytic streptococcus, not group D, responding to 24 million units of IV penicillin daily for 4 weeks.

■ PREFERRED APPROACH

Treatment

As the pediatric cardiologist releases adults into the mainstream, we are often confronted with patients with complex cyanotic heart disease who have had equally complex surgical procedures. To follow the adult intelligently, we must know the operations, their complications, and sequelae, especially the functional abnormalities and whether there are residual defects. Some therapeutic attention may be directed to whether reoperation is necessary. Occasionally we have the experience of seeing a cyanotic adult who, through judicious neglect, fearful parents, or other inexplicable factors, including nature's palliation with just the right amount of PS and an adequate ventricular septal defect (VSD), has had no surgery.

Glossary of Operations for Cyanotic Congenital Heart Disease

Palliative Procedures to Increase Pulmonary Blood Flow

Waterston's Procedure. Anastomosis of the ascending aorta to the right pulmonary artery (RPA) is done infrequently.

Blalock-Taussig Procedure. This involves anastomosis of the subclavian artery to the pulmonary artery. A modification uses a Goretex tube to fashion a central shunt from the ascending aorta to the pulmonary artery.

Potts's Procedure. Anastomosis of the descending aorta to the proximal left pulmonary artery has been done in the past.

Glenn's Procedure. Anastomosis of the end of the superior vena cava (SVC) to the end of the RPA is now modified by joining the end of the SVC into the side of the RPA.

Brock's Procedure. This is a closed procedure via the right ventricle to relieve pulmonary stenosis.

Palliative Procedure to Reduce Pulmonary Blood Flow

Muller-Damman Procedure. This procedure involves performing annular constriction (banding) of the main pulmonary artery.

Palliative Procedures to Increase Intracardiac Mixing or Cross-Flow

Blalock-Hanlon Procedure. This procedure involves surgical creation of an atrial septal defect by a closed technique (modified by using inflow occlusion and open atrial septectomy).

Rashkind's Procedure. This procedure involves creation of an atrial septal defect by rupture of the fossa ovale membrane with a balloon or blade catheter (medical septostomy).

Anatomic or Physiologic "Correction" Procedure for Transposition of the Great Arteries

Venous Redirection or Atrial Baffle Procedure

Mustard's Procedure. This procedure involves insertion of an interatrial baffle of pericardium or prosthetic material to direct systemic venous blood to the pulmonary ventricle and pulmonary venous blood to the systemic ventricle.

Senning's Procedure. The interatrial baffle is fashioned nearly entirely from the right atrial wall and the atrial septum. Occasionally a small piece of pericardium is used to complete the baffle.

Arterial Switch Operation (Jatene's Procedure) for Transposition of the Great Arteries. The ascending aorta and the main pulmonary artery are switched to serve the proper ventricle, and the coronary arteries are reimplanted above the pulmonic valve, which acts as the systemic semilunar valve.

Rastelli's Operation. This operation was originally devised to create a new outflow channel from the left ventricle to the pulmonary artery (in transposition of great arteries with severe pulmonic stenosis and ventricular septal defect), using a homograft of the ascending aorta that includes the aortic valve. Rastelli-type operations are now used to establish right ventricular to pulmonary artery continuity in truncus, double outlet right ventricle with ventricular septal defect committed to the aorta, and pulmonary atresia with ventricular septal defect. A synthetic conduit with a heterograft valve is commonly used. Stiffening of the valve occurs within a decade, and the Dacron conduit may develop an obstructive peel-like intima.

Fontan's Procedure. The modified procedure involves directing the entire systemic venous return from the cavae or the right atrium to the pulmonary artery in patients with tricuspid atresia or single ventricle by using a nonvalved conduit or direct anastomosis of the right atrium to the pulmonary artery or a superior vena cava to RPA end-to-side anastomosis combined with an inferior vena cava to RPA intra-atrial tunnel anastomosis.

Anatomic Types of Cyanotic Congenital Heart Disease and Their Surgical Treatment

Tetralogy of Fallot. Tetralogy of Fallot occurs as a clinical and hemodynamic spectrum based primarily on the degree of pulmonic stenosis and the size of the VSD. If PS is severe and the pulmonary artery small, a palliative shunt serves to relieve hypoxia and enlarge the pulmonary arteries. The Blalock-Taussig shunt is preferred because it rarely causes pulmonary vascular obstructive disease, aneurysm, or injury to the major pulmonary artery. Total correction is usually preferable in all ages. Patients over 40 years have shown good results. The VSD is closed with a prosthetic patch. The right ventricular outflow tract obstruction is relieved by wide resection of the infundibular muscle, and pulmonary valvotomy is needed. If obstruction persists as a result of a small annulus or hypoplastic main pulmonary artery, an elliptical Dacron or pericardial patch may be extended from the right ventricular outflow tract across the valve annulus as far as the bifurcation of the right and left pulmonary arteries. The adult who has had surgery in childhood and extensive right ventricular outflow tract reconstruction will have significant pulmonary valve regurgitation. This is usually well tolerated, but in some patients fatigue and decreased exercise tolerance result. My preference is still to manage these people medically unless progressive right ventricular enlargement or failure occurs. A porcine valve can be put in the pulmonary valve position with resultant decrease in right ventricular size in some cases.

After correction of tetralogy, a residual VSD of 1.7 : 1 or greater shunt size is repaired in the symptomatic patient with cardiomegaly. Postoperative complete right bundle branch block is the rule. Associated left anterior hemiblock and trifascicular block occurs in a small number. If in follow-up, MOBITZ II AV block occurs, a pacemaker is immediately required. A marker for potentially serious ventricular arrhythmias is the presence of frequent ventricular premature contractions. We have ablated an area adjacent to the outflow tract patch repair in order to control recurrent ventricular tachycardia. Periodic 24 hour electrocardiographic monitoring of these patients is advisable.

Pulmonary Atresia, VSD, and Systemic Artery to Pulmonary Artery Collateral. The adult with pulmonary atresia, VSD, and systemic artery to pulmonary artery collateral arising from the upper descending thoracic aorta may have been passed over as being inoperable. Every effort should be made by careful angiography to determine whether true pulmonary arteries that are confluent are present. If these can be identified and if they are small, they may be shunted for further growth. Balloon dilation of a narrow Blalock shunt results in the palliation of hypoxemia in the adult whose pulmonary artery anatomy precludes total repair. In children, the arterial oxygen saturation has increased from 71 ± 7 percent to 81 ± 4 percent following dilation of the stenotic anastomosis of the systemic artery to pulmonary artery shunt. The systemic arterial collateral can be ligated. Anatomic correction using a valved conduit and closure of the VSD may be considered in the future. Some of these patients will have hemoptysis because of vascular malformation at the junction of the systemic arterial collateral to a pulmonary artery branch or because of pulmonary artery hypertension in a lung segment. Selective embolization via a catheter can be used to occlude the culprit systemic collateral artery.

Valvular Pulmonic Stenosis with an Intact Ventricular Septum and Interatrial Right-to-Left Shunting. Balloon pulmonary valvuloplasty is successful in infants and children with valvular pulmonic stenosis with an intact ventricular septum and interatrial right-to-left shunting. In 12 patients the arterial saturation increased from 83 ± 8 percent to 94 ± 5 percent, and the peak systolic gradient fell from 105 ± 48 mm Hg to 28 ± 18 mm Hg. The intervention is also applicable to adults.

Transposition of the Great Arteries. Currently the adult patient with transposition of the great arteries (TGA) presents to the cardiologist having had physiologic correction by venous redirection using the Mustard or Senning procedure. Patients who have had this interatrial baffle procedure may have atrial arrhythmias associated with sinus node dysfunction and may require atrial pacing. Transvenous atrial automatic antitachycardia pacemakers have been used. Obstruction to pulmonary or systemic veins by the interatrial baffle has usually been resolved by reoperation in childhood. In the postatrial baffle patient, the right ventricle continues to act as the systemic ventricle. Most studies have shown that the right ventricular ejection fraction is reduced, and the long-term ability of the right ventricle to serve as the systemic ventricle is under scrutiny.

A newer operation, currently the procedure of choice for the infant with TGA in many centers, is the Jatene or arterial switch procedure. In this repair, the left ventricle now functions as the systemic ventricle; the pulmonary valve, with the coronary arteries transplanted above it, still functions as the systemic semilunar valve. There is interest in whether the main trunk of the transplanted coronary arteries will angulate or stenose with time. Left main coronary artery stenosis has been successfully dilated after this procedure.

Rarely, an adult with TGA has not had corrective surgery. We performed a Mustard procedure on a symptomatic young woman who had enough pulmonic stenosis to protect her pulmonary vascular bed and good cross-shunting via a large atrial septal defect. In an adult with TGA, VSD, and pulmonary vascular obstructive disease, we improve arterial saturation by doing a palliative atrial baffle procedure without closing the ventricular septal defect.

Tricuspid Atresia. An innovative surgical procedure for patients with tricuspid atresia was developed by Fontan of Bordeaux, France, in which the atrial septal defect is closed and a conduit is placed from the right atrium to the pulmonary artery. A direct anastomosis between the right atrium or the superior and inferior cavae and pulmonary artery has been an excellent modification. Because the right atrium acts only as a passive conduit, the left ventricle must have excellent function. The pulmonary vascular resistance and pulmonary artery pressure must also be normal and the pulmonary arteries of normal size. We have followed a number of these patients in their late teens, and they increase their cardiac output with exercise primarily by increasing the heart rate. They do well unless pulmonary artery hypertension, left atrioventricular valve regurgitation, or left ventricular dysfunction develops. Chronic afterload reduction therapy to improve or maintain LV function has not been studied prospectively. Atrial arrhythmias may occur late in 45 percent of cases. Increased caval pressure has been associated with a low serum albumin secondary to varying degrees of protein-losing enteropathy in 5 percent of cases.

The cardiologist working with adults will see some patients with tricuspid atresia who have had one or more shunt procedures or the Glenn procedure and now, because of poor left ventricular function or pulmonary artery hypertension, are not candidates for the Fontan procedure.

Truncus Arteriosus. The adult with truncus arteriosus will most likely have had an external homograft or synthetic conduit containing a homograft or heterograft valve sutured into the right ventricle and connected to the right and left pulmonary arteries. The conduit valve is subject to degenerative stenosis, and the woven Dacron develops an intimal peel that may be exuberant or become detached, obstructing the valve. There also may be stenosis at the origin of the conduit from the right ventricle, but most stenosis is at the native pulmonary artery–distal conduit anastomosis, particularly if the pulmonary artery branch is small or if one or both branches were subject to palliative banding in infancy. Residual pulmonary hypertension secondary to pulmonary obstructive vascular disease may occur. The truncal valve over the years may become regurgitant also.

Single Ventricle. The majority of patients with single ventricle have two separate atrioventricular valves that enter the large left ventricle. The right ventricle is a rudimentary outlet chamber. The surgical procedure of choice is to perform the modified Fontan procedure.

Ebstein's Anomaly. In Ebstein's anomaly, survival into adult life is common, particularly if there are no associated defects. Surgery is performed for heart failure, arrhythmia, or severe hypoxia. The surgical approach is to reconstruct the tricuspid valve if possible from the large anterior leaflet or to replace it if necessary. If there is a symptomatic anomalous atrial ventricular pathway with troublesome arrhythmias, surgical ablation of the pathway is indicated. The atrial septal defect is closed, and suture reduction of the atrialized portion of the right ventricle is done. The heart remains large after surgery, but if tricuspid valve competence is restored, function is improved.

Suggested Reading

Hu DCK, Seward J, Puga FJ, et al. Total correction of tetralogy of Fallot at age 40 years and older: Long term follow up. J Am Coll Cardiol 1985; 5:40.

Humes RA, Mair DD, Porter CJ, et al. Results of the modified Fontan operation in adults. Am J Cardiol 1988; 61:602.

Kaufman SL, Martin LG, Gilarsky BP, et al. Urokinase thrombolysis using a multiple side hole multilumen infusion catheter. Cardiovasc Intervent Radiol 1991; 14:334.

Lois JF, Gomes AS, Smith DC, Laks H. Systemic-to-pulmonary collateral vessels and shunts: Treatment with embolization. Radiology 1988; 169:671.

Mair DD, Puga FJ, Danielson GK. Late functional status of survivors of the Fontan procedure performed during the 1970's. Circulation 1992; 80(II):306.

Perloff JK, Child JS. Congenital heart disease in adults. Philadelphia: WB Saunders, 1991.

Perloff JK, Rosove MH, Child JS, Wright GB. Adults with cyanotic congenital heart disease: Hematologic management (clinical review). Ann Intern Med 1988; 109:406.

Rao PS. Transcatheter management of cyanotic congenital heart defects: A review. Clin Cardiol 1992; 15:483.

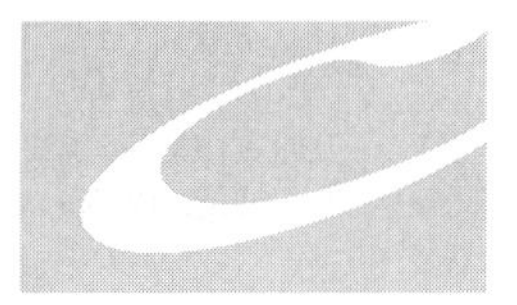

GASTROINTESTINAL DISEASES

GASTROESOPHAGEAL REFLUX: MEDICAL THERAPY

Joel E. Richter, M.D.

Gastroesophageal reflux, with its major symptom, heartburn, is the most common disorder of the esophagus, the major indication for antacid consumption in the United States, and probably the most prevalent clinical condition originating from the gastrointestinal tract. In fact, most healthy persons intermittently reflux gastric contents into the esophagus. Such episodes occur in the postprandial period, are short-lived, rarely cause symptoms, and almost never take place at night. This has been designated *physiologic reflux* in contradistinction to *pathologic reflux,* which is commonly associated with esophageal symptoms (heartburn, regurgitation, dysphagia, or water brash) and/or esophageal mucosal damage. The extent of mucosal damage is variable, ranging from histologic esophagitis to erosions, ulcerations, strictures, or Barrett's esophagus. Although symptoms are common, some patients have no complaints, especially those with Barrett's esophagus and extraesophageal manifestations of reflux disease. The latter presentations include oropharyngeal complaints such as hoarseness, sore throat, and cough as well as respiratory problems including asthma, aspiration pneumonia, bronchiectasis, and chronic bronchitis. The term *gastroesophageal reflux disease* (GERD) has been coined to encompass the constellation of problems and presentations associated with pathologic acid reflux.

In the past two decades, a consensus has developed that GERD is a multifactorial process whose pathogenesis may vary in a given patient. The major predictor of esophageal symptoms and damage is prolonged contact of refluxed gastric acid with the esophageal epithelium. In healthy individuals, the esophagus is protected from prolonged acid contact by a three-tiered defensive system: the antireflux barrier provided by the lower esophageal sphincter (LES) and crural diaphragm, acid clearance mechanisms (peristalsis, saliva, and gravity), and the intrinsic resistance of the esophageal mucosa to damage. Conceptually, GERD occurs when the noxious gastric contents, especially acid and pepsin, overwhelm the esophageal defense mechanisms. This usually takes a long time, and consequently GERD is characteristically a slowly progressive mucosal disorder in which acute life-threatening events are rare. Medical therapy alleviates symptoms and heals esophagitis, but the disease usually recurs when drug therapy is stopped. GERD is therefore a chronic disease, especially in patients with esophagitis.

■ MEDICAL TREATMENT

Medical management of GERD can be divided into two types: lifestyle modifications and drug therapy. Both of these work to improve GERD either by reducing acid secretion or by enhancing the protective mechanisms of the esophagus.

Lifestyle Modifications

Lifestyle modifications remain the cornerstone of effective antireflux treatment for all GERD patients. The cost is low and the short- and long-term benefits are great. Time spent by the physician explaining the nature of GERD and the reasons for the various therapeutic maneuvers helps enhance treatment compliance. The following maneuvers will produce a response in most patients with mild to moderate symptoms (Table 1).

Table 1 Lifestyle Modifications

Elevate head of bed (>6 inch)
Dietary modifications
Avoid:
Foods that decrease LES pressure: fats, chocolate, alcohol, carminatives
Irritants: citrus, tomato, coffee
Smaller, more frequent meals
Meals 2 hours before retiring
Reduce weight (if overweight)
Decrease or stop smoking
Avoid excessive alcohol
Avoid:
Medications that decrease LES pressure (see text)
Direct esophageal mucosa irritants

LES, lower esophageal sphincter.

Elevation of the head of the bed is simple, time-honored, and effective therapy for GERD. Findings from several studies confirm that the use of bed blocks improves acid clearance time and reduces esophageal exposure to acid. Moreover, a recent study found an additive effect in reducing symptoms and healing esophagitis when elevation of the head of the bed was combined with an H_2 blocker (ranitidine, 150 mg twice daily). The preferred way to elevate the head of the bed is on 6 to 8 inch blocks or bricks. An alternative procedure employs a firm, 10-inch wedge, particularly if the patient has a water bed. Using several pillows to elevate the head is not recommended, since the patient usually rolls off them while asleep.

Particular foods may precipitate reflux symptoms and should be avoided. Liquids with low pH or increased osmolarity (e.g., citrus juices, tomato-based products, and coffee) can evoke heartburn in patients with an acid-sensitive esophagus. Carminatives and certain food ingredients (garlic, onions, peppermint, and some after-dinner liqueurs) lower LES pressure and facilitate belching, often accompanied by reflux. Foods high in fat content and chocolates decrease LES pressure and delay gastric emptying. Patients should refrain from overeating, because increased gastric volume increases the frequency of spontaneous transient LES relaxations and associated reflux. For similar reasons, patients should not eat for several hours before retiring so as to avoid supine reflux. Patients often identify a period of weight gain that coincides with the appearance or exacerbation of reflux symptoms. Although the mechanism remains unclear, weight loss of only 10 to 15 pounds may have a dramatic effect on symptoms. Smoking and excessive alcohol use promote gastroesophageal reflux. Smoking reduces LES pressure, delays esophageal acid clearance, and increases distal esophageal acid exposure. Excessive alcohol reduces LES pressure and prolongs nocturnal acid exposure; the latter may be due to a diminished arousal response after reflux episodes.

Review of concomitant medications is crucial. Many drugs, including theophylline preparations, calcium channel blockers, nitrates, anticholinergics, antidepressants, and progesterone, reduce LES pressure. Calcium channel blockers, nitrates, and anticholinergics may also reduce esophageal contraction pressures, and the latter agents reduce salivary flow. One must also consider drugs that possibly cause esophageal mucosal irritation independent of GERD, such as doxycycline, tetracycline, quinidine, slow-release potassium chloride, iron salts, and nonsteroidal anti-inflammatory drugs (NSAIDs). One recent surgical series found that 20 percent of patients initially referred for antireflux surgery had drug-induced lesions.

Drug Therapy

Drug therapy is usually reserved for patients with symptomatic disease not responding to lifestyle modification, or for individuals with esophagitis. Drugs may act by decreasing or neutralizing acid secretion, promoting motility, or improving esophageal mucosal resistance. A list of drugs and their suggested dosages is provided in Table 2.

Table 2 Drug Therapy for GERD

DRUGS	DOSE
Antacids	
Mylanta II, Maalox TC Tums, Rolaids	15 ml, 1–2 tablets 30 min after meals and q.h.s.
Gaviscon	2–4 tablets q.i.d., p.c. and q.h.s.
Prokinetic drugs	
Bethanechol (Urecholine)	25 mg q.i.d., 30 min a.c. and q.h.s.
Metoclopramide (Reglan)	10 mg q.i.d., 30 min a.c. and q.h.s.
Cisapride (Propulsid)	10 mg q.i.d., 30 min a.c. and q.h.s.
Sucralfate (Carafate)	1 g q.i.d., 1 hr p.c. and q.h.s.
H_2-receptor antagonists	
Cimetidine (Tagamet)	800 mg b.i.d., AM and 30 min after dinner
Ranitidine (Zantac)	150 mg b.i.d., AM and 30 min after dinner
Famotidine (Pepcid)	20 mg b.i.d., AM and 30 min after dinner
Nizatidine (Axid)	150 mg b.i.d., AM and 30 min after dinner
Omeprazole (Prilosec)	20–40 mg qAM

Antacids

Used on an as-needed basis, antacids are the mainstay for rapid, safe, effective relief of heartburn symptoms. Antacids primarily work by neutralizing acid, albeit for relatively short periods. Therefore, patients need to take these agents frequently, usually 20 to 30 minutes after meals and at bedtime, depending on the severity of the symptoms. Liquid forms are preferable to tablets, although the latter are the most popular preparation of this medication. Antacids are effective in relieving mild to moderate heartburn symptoms. They are particularly useful in patients with situational episodes of heartburn brought on by lifestyle indiscretions or pregnancy. Antacids, even in high doses, are not predictably effective in healing reflux esophagitis.

Excessive use of antacids may be associated with side effects. Magnesium-containing antacids produce diarrhea, and aluminum-containing agents cause constipation. The potential for magnesium or aluminum toxicity further limits their use in patients with significant renal disease, and low sodium antacids (e.g., magaldrate [Riopan]) are preferable for individuals on salt-restricted diets. In pregnant patients, adverse effects of antacids include interference with iron absorption, and metabolic alkalosis and fluid overload, in both fetus and mother, with ingestion of sodium bicarbonate.

Gaviscon

Containing alginic acid and antacids, Gaviscon is a popular drug for treating heartburn. The active component of this medication, alginic acid, interacts with saliva to form a highly viscous solution that floats on the surface of the gastric pool, acting as a mechanical barrier. The barrier reduces the number of reflux episodes and diminishes esophageal acid exposure. Recent studies using radionuclide scintigraphy and 24 hour pH monitoring confirm that Gaviscon effectively prevents episodes of upright acid reflux but is not effective at night. Evidence concerning the clinical efficacy of Gaviscon is similar to that for antacids. Although Gaviscon is safe, it contains aluminum, magnesium, and sodium; therefore, the same precautions listed for antacids apply.

Prokinetic Drugs

Drug of this class available in the United States for treating GERD include bethanechol, metoclopramide, and (most recently) cisapride. Bethanechol is a cholinergic agonist that works by increasing LES pressure, improving esophageal peristalsis, and increasing salivary flow, which in turn improves esophageal acid clearance. In contrast, metoclopramide, a dopamine antagonist, works primarily by improving gastric emptying. Cisapride is a prokinetic agent that increases gastric emptying and LES pressure by enhancing the release of acetylcholine from the myenteric plexus.

Multiple studies show that both bethanechol and metoclopramide effectively relieve heartburn symptoms, but their efficacy in treating esophagitis is equivocal. Some physicians prefer to use these prokinetic drugs in treating patients with mild to moderate persistent reflux symptoms. However, I consider their side effect profile, especially that of metoclopramide, to be very bothersome. I therefore currently use bethanechol and metoclopramide only if there is a history of symptoms related to delayed gastric emptying (i.e., after a large meal) or possibly as adjunctive therapy with H_2-receptor antagonists when patients are not responding to acid inhibition alone. European studies have found cisapride, 10 mg four times a day, to be more effective than placebo and equal to H_2-receptor antagonists in controlling reflux symptoms and esophagitis. Studies in the United States suggest that its efficacy lies primarily in the treatment of reflux symptoms, especially those occurring at night.

Common side effects associated with bethanechol include flushing, blurred vision, headaches, abdominal cramps, and urinary frequency. It is contraindicated in a number of common disorders such as asthma, peptic ulcer disease, ischemic heart disease, and obstructive disease of the intestine or urinary tract. Cisapride is associated with minimal side effects, the most common being abdominal cramps, borborygmus, and diarrhea. The most worrisome feature of metoclopramide is its profile of possible side effects. Fatigue, lethargy, and mood and extrapyramidal problems occur with the full recommended dose (10 mg before meals and at bedtime) in 10 to 30 percent of patients. These effects are reversible on cessation of drug therapy, although tardive dyskinesia may persist. The dopamine antagonist property of metoclopramide may lead to hyperprolactinemia and galactorrhea. It is possible to decrease the frequency of side effects by lowering the dose, giving a larger dose only before troubling meals (such as the largest meal of the day) or at bedtime, or using a sustained-release tablet. Of the prokinetic drugs, only metoclopramide is safe to use during pregnancy.

Sucralfate

This drug is the basic aluminum salt of sucrose octasulfate. Sucralfate acts topically, binding to acid, pepsin, and bile. European studies have found sucralfate to be superior to placebo and equivalent to H_2 antagonists and antacid-alginate in the treatment of GERD. U.S. trials have shown only marginal benefits from sucralfate, although, interestingly, patients with the more severe erosive disease appear to benefit most from its use. This inconsistency may reflect the greater retention of sucralfate within the esophagitis of patients with erosive or ulcerative disease. Sucralfate can be used as adjunctive therapy with H_2 antagonists because, at standard doses, H_2 antagonists do not raise gastric pH high enough to prevent the acidic refluxate from activating sucralfate.

Sucralfate is a safe drug because it has limited systemic absorption, and it may therefore be used during pregnancy. The most common side effect is constipation, a reflection of its aluminum content. Since some of the aluminum may be absorbed, sucralfate should be used cautiously and at reduced dosage in patients with renal disease.

H_2-Receptor Antagonists

This family of drugs achieved the first real breakthrough in the treatment of GERD and have largely supplanted antacids for long-term relief of symptoms and healing of esophagitis. Despite advertising to the contrary, all the H_2 antagonists are equally effective when used in proper doses. H_2 antagonist therapy for GERD differs from that for peptic ulcer disease in two ways. A greater amount of acid suppression is required to control GERD than to control peptic ulcer disease, and acid suppression is needed around the clock or at least during the periods of increased reflux.

To control acid reflux, H_2 antagonists are usually given once or preferably twice a day. Recent data on patterns of acid exposure show that the bulk of acid reflux occurs during the early evening hours after dinner and decreases markedly during the sleeping hours. It may be preferable, therefore, to advise the patient to take a dose of an H_2 antagonist *30 minutes after the evening meal* rather than at bedtime. Clinical trials in patients with GERD show that heartburn (during both day and night) can be significantly decreased by H_2 antagonists in comparison with placebo, although symptoms are rarely abolished. Recent reviews found that overall esophagitis healing rates with H_2 antagonists rarely exceed 60 percent after up to 12 weeks of treatment, even when higher than standard doses are used. Healing rates differ in individual trials, depending primarily on the degree of esophagitis before therapy. Grades I and II esophagitis heal in 75 to 95 percent of patients, whereas grades III and IV esophagitis heal in only 40 to 50 percent of patients. In view of these data, I prefer to use H_2 antagonists in treating patients with moderate to severe reflux symptoms and those with grades I and II esophagitis. On the other hand, the more severe grades of ulcerative esophagitis are best treated with omeprazole.

All the H_2 antagonists are now available over-the-counter, usually at 50 percent of the prescription dose. They can be used similar to antacids for symptomatic heartburn, although the rapidity of relief is not as good as antacids. I find these drugs more helpful to prevent heartburn episodes after large meals, exercise, etc. In these prophylactic situations, the H_2 antagonist should be taken 30 minutes before the refluxogenic activity. Over-the-counter H_2 RAs should not be used continuously for more than 2 weeks. Prolonged symptoms suggest a more severe disease and the need for prescription medication.

H_2 antagonists have been used safely for nearly 20 years. Side effects, although infrequent, differ among agents. Cimetidine may cause gynecomastia, impotence, hypospermia, mental confusion, and drug interactions. Ranitidine, generally free of the antiandrogenic and central nervous system effects and drug interactions associated with cimetidine, may produce a higher incidence of hepatic injury than cimetidine. Famotidine and nizatidine are the newest members of the H_2

Table 3 General Approach to Short- and Long-Term Management of GERD

	SYMPTOMS WITHOUT ESOPHAGITIS	MILD ESOPHAGITIS (GRADES I–II)	SEVERE ESOPHAGITIS (GRADES III–IV) OR INTRACTABLE SYMPTOMS
ACUTE	1. Lifestyle changes 2. PRN medications Antacids Gaviscon Prokinetic drugs Sucralfate H_2 antagonists	1. Lifestyle changes 2. Daily medications H_2 antagonists b.i.d. Regular dose High dose H_2 antagonist + prokinetic ↓	1. Lifestyle changes 2. Strong acid suppression with PPIs Omeprazole, 20–60 mg ↓
CHRONIC	1. Medications usually not needed 2. Follow-up endoscopy not necessary	1. H_2 antagonists b.i.d., sometimes only in evening 2. Cisapride, 20 mg b.i.d. 3. Flu endoscopy usually not necessary	1. Full-dose PPI 2. Lower-dose omeprazole, 10; lansoprazole, 15 mg 3. High-dose H_2 antagonist ± prokinetic 4. Antireflux surgery 5. Endoscopy to ensure healing

antagonist category; both appear to have side effect profiles similar to that of ranitidine. Although these agents are not recommended in pregnancy, there is a large human experience with safe use of both cimetidine and ranitidine during gestation. Less common side effects are described in the *Physicians' Desk Reference.*

Proton-Pump Inhibitors (PPI)

The substituted benzimidazole, omeprazole and lansoprazole are potent and long-acting inhibitor of both basal and stimulated gastric acid secretion. They act by selective, noncompetitive inhibition of the H^+/K^+-ATPase pump located in the secretory membrane of the parietal cell. A single morning dose maintains gastric pH at 5 or more for almost 24 hours and decreases gastric volume by over 60 percent. PPIs have no effect on LES pressure. Controlled studies show that omeprazole, 20 mg or lansoprazole, 30 mg in the morning, completely abolishes reflux symptoms in most patients with severe GERD, usually within 1 to 2 weeks. Complete healing of esophagitis occurs after 8 weeks in more than 80 percent of patients. In those who do not heal after this time, prolonging therapy with the same dose or increasing the dose usually result in nearly 100 percent healing. Comparison studies consistently show that the PPIs are superior to ranitidine (150 mg) or cimetidine (800 mg) twice a day in relieving symptoms and healing esophagitis. Peptic strictures associated with esophagitis heal faster and require fewer dilatations when treated with PPIs than with H_2 antagonists.

Side effects of PPIs are minimal with short-term use, but the safety of its long-term use has not recently been established. The profound hypoacidity produced by these drugs stimulates gastrin release, promoting the proliferation of enterochromaffin-like (ECL) cells in the gastric fundus. Prolonged therapy with high-dose omeprazole or lansoprazole causes a disturbingly high frequency of carcinoid tumors in rats with gastrin concentrations exceeding 1,000 pg per milliliter but not in similarly treated mice or dogs. In humans, extreme hypergastrinemia (over 1,000 pg per milliliter) secondary to the achlorhydria of pernicious anemia is associated with ECL proliferation, but fewer than 5 percent of patients develop gastric carcinoid tumors. However, gastrin concentrations rarely exceed 500 pg per milliliter during routine proton pump therapy. Human experience with the PPIs is approaching a point where a number of patients with reflux esophagitis are taking the drug continuously for 4 to 7 years. There has not been any reported cases of gastric carcinoid-type tumor in patients receiving either omeprazole or lansoprazole, with the rare exception of cases who had MEN syndrome that was not felt to be related to the PPI. For these reasons, the FDA has recently sanctioned the long-term use of the PPI for maintenance therapy of severe esophagistis. Obviously, omeprazole is not safe for use during pregnancy.

■ GENERAL APPROACH

In many patients, the history of heartburn and regurgitation is sufficiently typical to permit a 6 to 8 week trial of therapy without the need for diagnostic tests. Patients failing initial empiric therapy should undergo endoscopy. This procedure is indicated to rule out other diseases (e.g., peptic ulcer disease), assess for the presence and severity of esophagitis, identify potentially complicating Barrett's esophagus or peptic strictures, and guide further treatment. Patients with dysphagia and normal endoscopy may require barium esophagography with a solid-bolus challenge (tablet, marshmallow, food) to help define mildly obstructive rings or strictures.

Endoscopy permits patients with symptomatic reflux disease to be subdivided into three groups (Table 3). Those with symptoms but no gross evidence of esophagitis can be considered at low risk of developing complications such as strictures, ulcers, bleeding, or Barrett's esophagus. The primary goal of therapy in these patients is the control of symptoms, and endoscopic follow-up is generally unnecessary. On the other hand, patients with esophagitis, with or without symptoms, are at high risk of developing complications accounting for the major morbidity and, in some cases, mortality from GERD. As already discussed, these patients represent two groups, with those having the more severe grades of esophagitis (III and IV) requiring more aggressive acid suppression to heal the mucosal lesions. Regardless of the degree of esophagitis, the ultimate goal is to heal or minimize the mucosal damage while attempting to prevent further complications. Since symptom relief does not always parallel the improvement in esophagitis, endoscopic follow-up is required to ensure healing.

Initial therapy for all groups is based on lifestyle modifications as outlined in Table 1 and selective use of the drugs listed in Table 2.

Symptoms Without Esophagitis

Patients with mild to moderate symptoms without esophagitis often experience marked symptom improvement with lifestyle changes only. Others may intermittently require antacids, prokinetic drugs, sucralfate, or H_2 antagonists, either over-the-counter or higher prescription doses. Only patients with more resistant symptoms require long-term therapy, usually with H_2 antagonists but occasionally with omeprazole.

Mild to Moderate Esophagitis

Patients with mild to moderate esophagitis (grades I and II) are best treated with H_2 antagonists, at least twice daily, until the esophagitis is healed. Some may require higher doses of H_2 antagonists to heal the esophagitis. This may be accomplished by doubling the dose of H_2 antagonists (e.g., ranitidine, 300 mg twice daily; famotidine, 40 mg twice daily), although recent studies suggest that more frequent dosing (e.g., ranitidine, 150 mg four times a day) may be a better approach. Other alternatives are to add a prokinetic drug or possibly sucralfate to the H_2 antagonist. Subsequently, an attempt can be made to decrease the drug to an after-evening-meal dose, but only if symptoms and esophagitis are kept under control. Chronic therapy is often required to keep these patients' esophagitis in remission. In these situations, twice daily H_2 antagonists are usually needed; most patients relapse if only an evening dose is given. Recent studies from Europe suggest that cisapride, 20 mg twice daily, may be an alternative effective therapy. Continued endoscopies are not required unless there are important changes in symptoms (dysphagia, weight loss) or evidence of bleeding.

Severe Erosive-Ulcerative Esophagitis

Patients with severe erosive-ulcerative esophagitis (grades III and IV) or intractable symptoms require strong acid suppression to control the disease in both the short and long term. Although higher doses of H_2 antagonists improve the healing rates of severe esophagitis, I believe the expense and inconvenience may not be worth the minimal gain. For this reason, PPIs has replaced H_2 antagonists for treating the more severe forms of GERD. Omeprazole, 20 mg every morning, heals over 80 percent of patients with erosive esophagitis, but higher double doses may be needed for more recalcitrant patients. With this approach, almost all cases of acute esophagitis can be healed, but maintaining these patients in remission is a major problem because nearly 80 percent relapse within 1 year of discontinuing therapy. Not surprisingly, the major predictors of relapse are low LES pressure and the initial severity of esophagitis. After the esophagitis has healed, an attempt should be made to switch the patient to a maintenance regimen consisting of a high-dose H_2 antagonist, possibly in addition to cisapride. Unfortunately, many patients experience a recurrence of symptoms and esophagitis requiring reinstitution of omeprazole. Some of these may be controlled at a lower maintenance dose such as omeprazole, 10 mg or lansoprazole, 15 mg every morning. Serial gastric levels or endoscopy to look for carcinoid tumors are not indicated based on long-term safety date with the PPIs.

Atypical Presentations

Patients with atypical reflux presentations or difficult management problems may require further esophageal testing. The acid perfusion test can be helpful in these cases. If acid but not saline infusion brings on the symptoms, acid reflux is the likely cause. A negative test, however, does not preclude GERD, and these patients should have prolonged pH monitoring. Ambulatory, 24 hour esophageal pH monitoring allows for accurate quantification of acid reflux throughout the circadian cycle as well as correlating symptoms with acid reflux episodes. After the pH electrode has been placed 5 cm above the manometrically determined LES, this study can be performed in the patient's home or work environment, thereby increasing the opportunity of replicating the symptoms. I most commonly perform 24 hour pH monitoring in patients presenting with noncardiac chest pain, suspected pulmonary or ENT complications of GERD, and intractable reflux symptoms associated with a negative work-up who are not responding to H_2 antagonists or PPIs. In the last group, about two-thirds of the patients do not have acid reflux on pH testing, suggesting that their symptoms are functional in origin. The other third have an excessive amount of acid reflux often requiring higher doses of acid-suppressing medications.

Antireflux Surgery

Although most patients with GERD can be managed medically, approximately 5 to 10 percent require antireflux surgery. In the past, the primary indication for surgery was failure of medical therapy, but this is now extremely rare with the availability of PPIs. Surgery should still be considered in younger patients with severe GERD who otherwise would require lifetime medical therapy. Other indications for antireflux surgery include recurrent difficult-to-dilate strictures, nonhealing ulcers, severe bleeding from esophagitis, and reflux-related complications of the respiratory tract or ear, nose, and throat not responding to medical therapy. The presence of Barrett's esophagus alone is not an indication for antireflux surgery. This is discussed in another chapter.

Antireflux surgical procedures are currently performed laparoscopically through the abdomen or chest. All use crural-tightening after reducing the hiatus hernia and returning the esophagogastric junction to the abdomen, as well as varying degrees of fundoplication. Two factors are paramount to successful antireflux surgery. First is the preservation of esophageal function confirmed by esophageal testing before surgery. This evaluation should include endoscopy, esophageal manometry, and ambulatory esophageal pH monitoring. Older patients with recent onset of ulcerative esophagitis and strictures should be evaluated especially carefully because some may have drug-induced disease in which the esophageal pH studies will be normal. Esophageal manometry is performed primarily to assess the functional motor capacity of the body of the esophagus; measuring the LES pressure is of secondary importance. Nonspecific disturbances of motility, such as low-amplitude peristaltic contractions and intermittent simultaneous contractions, are not contraindications to antireflux surgery because these disorders are probably secondary to the reflux disease itself. On the other hand, it is important to identify aperistalsis, whether this be a manifestation of achalasia, scleroderma, or severe end-stage reflux disease.

The second factor is the skill and experience of the surgeon, which generally is reflected by the frequency with which this operation is performed. In the hands of experienced surgeons who perform careful esophageal preoperative testing, the results of antireflux operations are generally good but not perfect: up to 80 to 90 percent of patients have good long-term outcomes.

Suggested Reading

Hogan WJ. Gastroesophageal reflux disease: an update on management. J Clin Gastroenterol 1990: 12(Suppl 2):21–28.

Kitchin LI, Castell DO. Rationale and efficacy of conservative therapy for gastroesophageal reflux disease. Arch Intern Med 1991; 151:448–454.

Koelz HR. Treatment of reflux esophagitis with H_2 blockers, antacids, and prokinetic drugs. An analysis of randomized clinical trials. Scand J Gastroenterol 1989; 24(Suppl 156):25–36.

Maton PN. Omeprazole. N Engl J Med 1991; 324:965–975.

Mattox HE, Richter JE. Prolonged ambulatory esophageal pH monitoring in the evaluation of gastroesophageal reflux disease. Am J Med 1990; 89:345–356.

Ramirez B, Richter JE. Promotility drugs in the treatment of gastroesophageal reflux disease. Aliment Pharmacol Ther 1992 (in press).

Spechler SJ. Department of Veterans Affairs Gastroesophageal Reflux Disease Study Group. Comparison of medical and surgical therapy for complicated gastroesophageal reflux disease in veterans. N Engl J Med 1992; 326:786–792.

BARRETT'S ESOPHAGUS: MANAGEMENT DECISIONS

John G. Stagias, M.D.
Morris Traube, M.D.

Barrett's esophagus is an acquired complication of gastroesophageal reflux disease (GERD) in which columnar mucosa replaces the normal stratified squamous mucosa of the esophagus through the process of metaplasia. It is found in up to 10 percent of patients with symptoms of GERD who undergo endoscopy, and autopsy series have estimated that for every case of Barrett's esophagus that is clinically diagnosed, 20 remained unrecognized. Although there have been several reports of "familial" clustering and of its development as a sequela of chemotherapy, most cases of Barrett's esophagus result from GERD.

Barrett's mucosa alone does not produce symptoms; most patients present with symptoms or complications of GERD, including heartburn, dysphagia from stricture, bleeding, or adenocarcinoma. However, in 10 to 20 percent of patients who present with dysphagia, there is no history of heartburn.

The recognition of Barrett's esophagus is clinically important because of its malignant potential. The diagnosis is usually made at endoscopy by finding characteristic velvety, salmon-pink mucosa that extends at least 2 to 3 cm proximal to the lower esophageal sphincter (LES). When fundic or junctional gastric mucosa is seen histologically, it is often difficult to ascertain whether this represents metaplasia or a gastric lip, but in the setting of chronic symptoms, it is appropriate to consider this to be Barrett's mucosa. With specialized columnar mucosa, even smaller segments are diagnostic of Barrett's esophagus.

The proper management of patients with Barrett's esophagus should be individualized according to the severity of symptoms and the endoscopic findings. It involves the control of symptoms of underlying GERD and regular endoscopic surveillance for detection of early, curable neoplasms. However, there are currently no conclusive data to suggest that optimal medical or surgical control of GERD will reduce the risk of progression to dysplasia and adenocarcinoma or lead to regression of the Barrett's epithelium.

■ MEDICAL THERAPY

Asymptomatic

In asymptomatic individuals, it is wise to recommend lifestyle changes to reduce reflux. These include elevation of the head of the bed, cessation of smoking or drinking of alcohol, and avoidance of foods that predispose to reflux. It is difficult to categorically recommend antireflux medications. If they are given to asymptomatic patients, it seems appropriate to give only standard doses of H_2-receptor antagonists (e.g., cimetidine, 400 mg twice daily; ranitidine, 150 mg twice daily; famotidine, 20 mg twice daily; or nizatidine, 150 mg twice daily), but not higher doses or omeprazole, the powerful proton pump inhibitor.

Mild to Moderate Esophagitis

In mild to moderate esophagitis (endoscopic-histologic), therapy should be focused mainly on relief of symptoms, even though this may not be a reliable indicator of healing. While lifestyle changes and H_2-receptor antagonists are an important starting point, up to 85 percent do not have symptomatic relief and require higher doses of H_2-receptor antagonists or omeprazole, 20 mg or more per day. Although one study showed a good correlation between basal acid output and the dose of ranitidine required to heal esophagitis (and alleviate pyrosis), we generally use symptoms rather than gastric analysis to guide therapy. When symptoms, or endoscopic findings, indicate lack of response, it is more practical to increase the dose or begin therapy with omeprazole than to first perform gastric analysis. Prokinetic agents (metoclopramide and the newer cisapride, 10 to 20 mg four times per day) have also been added to facilitate esophageal clearance, raise sphincter pressure, or improve gastric emptying, but may find particular use as an adjunct to H_2-receptor antagonists or omeprazole; the combination may be more effective than the antisecretory drugs alone. Although many patients experience neuropsychiatric side effects with metoclopramide, cisapride is generally well tolerated.

Severe Esophagitis and Barrett's Ulcers

In severe esophagitis or Barrett's ulcers, therapy should begin with omeprazole, 20 mg per day. However, in some patients with Barrett's ulcer, even 40 to 60 mg per day of omeprazole does not produce complete healing after 4 to 6 months of treatment. Therefore, endoscopy should be repeated at 2 to 3 month intervals until complete healing is documented. A discrete ulcer or otherwise severe esophagitis that persists despite 4 to 6 months of intensive therapy is unlikely to heal with medical therapy alone, and antireflux surgery should be considered, as described below.

Strictures

Barrett's strictures, which most commonly occur at the squamocolumnar junction, should be extensively biopsied to exclude malignancy. Once this has been excluded, the stricture can be dilated in the same fashion as other esophageal strictures, and omeprazole given to help prevent restricturing. Occasionally, strictures do not respond to multiple dilations, necessitating surgery.

Regression with Medical Therapy

Complete regression of Barrett's epithelium with medical therapy has rarely been demonstrated. In several trials using standard dose H_2-receptor antagonists, there has been no significant (>3 cm) regression. While case reports have documented regression with high-dose omeprazole therapy (40 to 60 mg per day), no data are available from large controlled trials; we therefore do not advocate routine use of omeprazole in all patients with Barrett's esophagus. Although a recent report has documented squamous cell repopulation after the columnar epithelium was ablated with a laser, there is insufficient evidence to recommend such treatment routinely.

■ SURGICAL THERAPY

Indications for Surgery

The indications for surgery in Barrett's esophagus are similar to those for GERD without Barrett's mucosa and include persistent symptoms despite maximal medical therapy, strictures unresponsive to dilation, nonhealing ulcers or esophagitis after 4 to 6 months of intensive therapy, uncontrollable bleeding, perforation, and pulmonary aspiration from reflux. Multiple factors must be considered in any decision regarding surgery; these may include the patient's operative risk because of comorbid diseases and the results of esophageal manometry. The surgical options are standard antireflux procedures (e.g., Nissen fundoplication, Belsey cardioplasty, and Hill posterior gastropexy) and involve reduction of the hiatus hernial sac in association with a gastric wrap.

Regression with Surgical Therapy

Although some earlier surgical series reported partial regression of Barrett's esophagus after antireflux procedures, those studies had methodologic flaws, and subsequent surgical series have failed to document significant (>3 cm) regression in most patients, or the prevention of complications, including dysplasia and adenocarcinoma, after surgery. Therefore, surgery should not be performed solely because of a finding of Barrett's esophagus, nor as prophylaxis against the development of carcinoma. Furthermore, patients who have undergone an antireflux procedure should be enrolled in a surveillance program at the same intervals as for other patients with Barrett's esophagus (see below).

■ DYSPLASIA, ADENOCARCINOMA, AND SURVEILLANCE

The most serious complication of Barrett's esophagus is the development of adenocarcinoma. Multiple studies have shown an incidence of adenocarcinoma at least 30 times that of the general population. Unfortunately, adenocarcinoma is often discovered at presentation, and most of these cases are unresectable for cure. Much interest has therefore focused on identifying at an early stage those patients who may ultimately progress to adenocarcinoma.

It is generally accepted that the development of adenocarcinoma follows the sequence of dysplasia, carcinoma in situ, and finally carcinoma. (The concepts of aneuploidy and p53 protein expression are discussed below.) It has therefore been considered logical to screen patients by endoscopy at set intervals so as to identify those with dysplasia before the development of adenocarcinoma. This approach is further supported by the results of large screening programs in areas of China where squamous cell carcinoma of the esophagus is endemic; these programs have been successful in detecting and curing early squamous cell carcinoma. Nevertheless, several difficulties remain with the assumption that screening is worthwhile and will reduce the frequency of lethal carcinoma: (1) it is unclear whether all patients with dysplasia will ultimately progress to carcinoma, so that dysplasia may not be the ideal marker for progression; (2) the time frame required for dysplasia to progress to adenocarcinoma is currently unknown; (3) areas of dysplasia are often endoscopically indistinguishable from nondysplastic tissue, so that small foci of dysplasia may be missed, and a consequent considerable sampling error arises; and (4) any mass screening program is costly to implement. For example, an evaluation of this cost in 1988 estimated that yearly surveillance would cost \$62,000 and 78 lost workdays per diagnosed cancer.

Despite these concerns, screening has become the acceptable approach, and several suggestions have been proposed to overcome some of these problems.

No Dysplasia

Once a patient is found to have Barrett's mucosa, multiple biopsies at different levels are recommended in order to detect dysplasia or adenocarcinoma and to assess the degree of inflammation, if any. At the time of the initial and subsequent endoscopic examinations, the locations of the distal tubular esophagus and of the squamocolumnar junction should be accurately documented to facilitate any further diagnostic studies or repeat biopsy. In the absence of dysplasia or adenocarcinoma, patients should undergo surveillance endoscopy with biopsy at 1 to 2 year intervals, unless comorbid conditions deteriorate and surgery would not be considered, making surveillance pointless. The exact timings of surveillance, whether 1 or 2 years, should be determined after considering various factors, including the length of Barrett's mucosa, the type of columnar tissue (increased malignancy mainly in those with specialized columnar tissue), and the anxiety level of the patient. The availability of flow cytometry results (see below) as well as future genetic marker alteration results may also influence the decision regarding timing of endoscopic surveillance.

Low-Grade Dysplasia

Dysplasia may be subdivided into low- and high-grade dysplasia. Since it is often difficult for the pathologist (interobserver concordance of about 70 percent) to accurately distinguish low-grade dysplasia from regenerating epithelium with inflammation, these patients should be treated intensively with lifestyle changes, omeprazole, and, if symptoms continue, prokinetic agents. The pathologic biopsy interpretation should also be confirmed by an expert pathologist. Follow-up endoscopy should be performed at an initial interval of 3 to 6 months. Any persistent finding of low-grade dysplasia should be closely followed endoscopically at subsequent 6 month intervals until there is either progression to high-grade dysplasia (see below) or two consecutive examinations negative for dysplasia. The finding of no dysplasia on two consecutive, very thorough examinations may allow for a less intensive surveillance program, as described previously.

High-Grade Dysplasia

High-grade dysplasia is a more reproducible pathologic finding, with an interobserver concordance rate of up to 87 percent. However, any finding of high-grade dysplasia should be confirmed by an expert pathologist, and endoscopy and biopsy repeated if sufficient doubt remains. If high-grade dysplasia is confirmed, surgical resection is generally advised, since esophagectomy specimens often show invasive cancer in association with high-grade dysplasia. All columnar epithelium should be removed, in view of reports of adenocarcinoma developing in the remaining columnar mucosa after incomplete surgical resection. Despite this general recommendation, the final decision regarding surgery must also take into account comorbid conditions and the age of the patient.

Flow Cytometry

Since dysplasia is not an ideal marker for the progression to adenocarcinoma, much recent interest has centered on analysis of the cellular DNA content by means of flow cytometry. The principle behind this technique is that aneuploidy (an abnormal amount of DNA per cell) and also an increased number of dividing cells (cells that are tetraploid or in the cell cycle G2/M) are found in many carcinomas. In several reports the finding of aneuploidy or an increased G2/tetraploidy on flow cytometry correlated with the subsequent development of carcinoma. However, some carcinomas may be diploid (normal DNA content), and some patients with aneuploidy did not develop dysplasia within the study period. A second approach using flow cytometry involved the identification of p53 protein expression, which is normally found on chromosome 17p and negatively regulates cell division. A mutation of this protein may lead to unregulated cell growth and carcinoma and is the most commonly seen genetic alteration in human carcinomas. One recent study has shown that p53 protein overexpression may occur in Barrett's esophagus even in the absence of dysplasia or carcinoma, but prospective studies of patients with p53 protein overexpression have not been reported. Thus, it is unclear what role such studies will ultimately play in surveillance for the development of adenocarcinoma. At the current time, and until additional information is available, flow cytometry and genetic expression studies should not replace dysplasia in the surveillance for carcinoma.

Brush Cytology

Cytologic brushings that permit a more extensive mucosal survey of the esophagus may be complementary to multiple biopsies in detecting dysplasia and adenocarcinoma. In one retrospective series of 65 concurrent biopsies and cytology specimens, the combination of brush cytology and biopsy was superior for the detection of dysplasia and adenocarcinoma to each technique alone. However, as with dysplasia, accurate interpretation of the cytology specimen is paramount, experience with cytopathologic studies in dysplasia is limited, and prospective data are lacking.

Summary Recommendations for Surveillance

Given the current available data, we recommend surveillance for patients with Barrett's esophagus at 1 to 2 year intervals, with several caveats:

1. Patients with new symptoms (e.g., dysphagia, odynophagia, or weight loss) are obviously evaluated sooner.
2. Patients with comorbid conditions who would not be suitable candidates for operative therapy if a carcinoma or dysplasia were found are excluded (at least until more efficacious nonoperative therapy is available).
3. Although a recent study has revealed the development of Barrett's esophagus in women who received chemotherapy for breast cancer, the limited data are insufficient to warrant screening such patients.
4. The finding of low-grade dysplasia should be confirmed by an expert pathologist, and the patient treated intensively. Follow-up endoscopy should be performed at an initial 3 to 6 month interval, and then at 6 month intervals until there is progression to high-grade dysplasia (see below) or two consecutive examinations negative for dysplasia, at which time the patient should be screened at 1 to 2 year intervals.
5. The finding of high-grade dysplasia should be confirmed by an expert pathologist. If it is confirmed, complete surgical resection of all the columnar-lined esophagus is generally advised.
6. As new data emerge and newer techniques become available, these recommendations will be modified so that surveillance will concentrate on patients at greatest risk for adenocarcinoma. Such surveillance recommenda-

tions may depend on techniques other than examination of tissue for dysplasia.

Suggested Reading

Cameron AJ. Barrett's esophagus and adenocarcinoma: from the family to the gene. Gastroenterology 1992; 102:1421–1424.

Levine DS, Reid BJ. Endoscopic diagnosis of esophageal neoplasms. Gastrointest Endosc Clin North Am 1992; 2:395–413.

Spechler SJ, Goyal RK. Barrett's esophagus. N Engl J Med 1986; 315:362–371.

Streitz JM, Williamson WA, Ellis H Jr. Current concepts concerning the nature and treatment of Barrett's esophagus and its complications. Ann Thorac Surg 1992; 54:586–591.

FUNCTIONAL DISORDERS OF THE UPPER GASTROINTESTINAL TRACT

William V. Harford, M.D.

Functional gastrointestinal (GI) disorders can be defined as disturbances of GI function in the absence of pathology demonstrable on customary diagnostic studies, such as radiography, endoscopy, or biopsy. The organic basis for some functional disorders may be apparent on more sophisticated studies done principally for research. For example, postprandial antral hypomotility is found on manometric studies in some patients with nonulcer dyspepsia (NUD). However, the pathophysiology of many functional disorders is unclear or unknown.

The physician's approach plays an important role in the success or failure of treatment of functional GI disorders. The absence of objective pathology on standard studies makes it difficult to arrive at a confident diagnosis. Exhaustive and repeated testing may be done in attempts to find organic pathology. The physician may tell the patient that nothing can be found or imply that the symptoms are due to psychopathology or hypochondriasis. Most functional symptoms are chronic and respond poorly to medication. Some patients may have contributing psychopathologic conditions or abnormal illness behavior and may be confused, frustrated, and demanding. These factors undermine the patient-physician relationship. A thorough history and physical examination, sensitivity to both physical and psychologic symptoms, a rational and limited workup to screen for organic illness, careful explanation, reassurance, empathy, and patience are the elements of satisfactory treatment of functional GI disorders. (See the chapter *Peptic Ulcer Disease* for ulcer-related dysphagia.)

■ NONULCER DYSPEPSIA

Clinical Features

A substantial proportion of the population suffers from symptoms related to the upper abdomen, such as epigastric discomfort or burning, fullness, bloating, distention, early satiety, belching, or nausea. These symptoms are often related to food. When no objective cause can be found, as occurs in up to 40 percent of cases, these patients are said to have nonulcer dyspepsia. There are several general patterns of NUD. Some patients have prominent associated heartburn, and may have a component of gastroesophageal reflux (GER). Others have symptoms identical to those of peptic ulcer disease, but no ulcer can be demonstrated. Other NUD patients have symptoms suggestive primarily of motility abnormalities. There is substantial overlap among these patterns. The lower GI symptoms of irritable bowel syndrome occur commonly in patients with NUD, as they do in the general population.

Pathophysiology

There is no evidence of acid hypersecretion or abnormal acid sensitivity in NUD. In one study, patients with documented acid hypersecretion and NUD were treated with vagotomy. Acid secretion was reduced but symptoms were not. Acid suppression with H_2-receptor antagonists has been of only marginal benefit compared with placebo, with the possible exception of those patients with prominent heartburn or ulcer-like symptoms.

Chronic infection with *Helicobacter pylori* is associated with chronic histologic superficial gastritis and an increased risk of peptic ulcer disease. Some studies have shown an increased prevalence of *H. pylori* infection in patients with nonulcer dyspepsia, but others have not. Most individuals infected with *H. pylori* have no symptoms. There is no evidence that chronic *H. pylori* infection is associated with any particular symptom cluster. Treatment with bismuth compounds suppresses *H. pylori* infection and improves symptoms temporarily in *H. pylori*–positive NUD patients, but bismuth has other beneficial effects on gastric mucosa. There is no strong evidence to date that *H. pylori* infection causes NUD, or that eradication of *H. pylori* infection improves symptoms of NUD (See the chapter *Helicobacter pylori infection.*)

As many as 50 percent of NUD patients have symptoms primarily suggestive of a gastric emptying disorder, such as epigastric discomfort, bloating, fullness, nausea, and belching after meals. Postprandial antral hypomotility and delayed gastric emptying (particularly of solids) have been reported in this group. However, correction of these abnormalities does not correlate strongly with relief of symptoms. It is important to exclude other causes of delayed gastric emptying such as diabetes mellitus and gastric outlet obstruction. Recently, several studies have shown that some NUD patients have a reduced threshold for discomfort with balloon distention of the stomach. This result suggests that some cases of NUD are due to a visceral sensory disorder. Agents that increase the threshold of discomfort with distention, such as the kappa opiate agonist fedotozine, are under investigation in NUD.

Of the analgesics, only acetaminophen has been associated with NUD. Nevertheless, patients with NUD who are taking aspirin or other nonsteroidal anti-inflammatory drugs (NSAIDs) should discontinue these drugs if possible.

Smoking and alcohol, coffee, and tea consumption have not been shown to be associated with NUD. There is, however, an increased frequency of anxiety, depression, and somatization in patients seeking medical care for NUD. However, these conditions are not unique to NUD, and are associated with a variety of other conditions, such as irritable bowel syndrome and noncardiac chest pain.

Diagnostic and Therapeutic Approach

The initial history and physical examination are important to screen for potential organic causes of dyspepsia. For example, certain symptoms, such as fever, persistent anorexia, and weight loss, would be worrisome and would suggest a cause other than NUD. The differential diagnosis should include gastroesophageal reflux, peptic ulcer disease, biliary disease, pancreatitis, gastric or pancreatic cancer, malabsorption, giardiasis, diabetes, thyroid disorders, hyperparathyroidism, coronary artery disease, and adverse reactions to medications, among others. Simple screening laboratory studies may be advisable, including a complete blood cell count, chemistry survey, and stool for occult blood.

Patients under the age of 45 years who do not take NSAIDs and have no worrisome symptoms have a very small risk of malignancy. Those patients who do not take NSAIDs and have a negative *H. pylori* antibody have only a small risk of duodenal ulcer. Such patients may not require any further evaluation, and a therapeutic trial could be initiated. Patients who have NUD and take NSAIDs should be advised to stop the NSAIDs if possible. Sometimes a change from one type of NSAID to another may improve dyspepsia. Patients over the age of 45 years, those with troublesome symptoms, those who cannot discontinue NSAIDs, and those who are *H. pylori* antibody–positive should all be evaluated further. Upper GI endoscopy is the preferred test, but upper GI radiographic examination may be substituted if endoscopy is not available.

When the diagnostic evaluation is negative, reassurance and a careful explanation of potential causes of NUD are important. The physician should be attentive to evidence of psychologic distress or an unvoiced concern, such as fear of cancer. If severe psychologic distress is suspected, it should be explored. If a psychiatric problem is discovered, psychiatric referral and treatment may improve the patient's ability to cope with dyspepsia. For most patients, specific treatment is not required. Few studies demonstrate that medication relieves symptoms of NUD better than placebo.

In patients with prominent complaints of heartburn or peptic-type pain, a trial of an antacid or standard-dose H_2-receptor antagonist for 4 to 6 weeks is harmless. Despite lack of evidence of efficacy in most studies, individual patients may respond. If a clear response is reported, treatment may be continued on an as-needed basis. This approach has the additional benefit of being appropriate for those patients who actually have gastroesophageal reflux or peptic ulcer disease missed on the initial evaluation.

Patients with symptoms suggestive of gastric emptying disorder may benefit from eating smaller meals more frequently and avoiding fatty foods, which delay emptying. A trial of a prokinetic agent is reasonable. Metoclopramide is a dopamine-receptor antagonist and cholinergic agent with both central antiemetic and peripheral prokinetic effects. In a dose of 5 to 20 mg 30 minutes before meals, it has been found to be better than placebo in relieving dyspeptic symptoms. However, up to 20 percent of patients have side effects, including extrapyramidal symptoms, making it unsuitable for chronic use in many patients. Cisapride is a newer prokinetic that acts by facilitating acetylcholine release from the myenteric plexus. Unlike metoclopramide, it has no significant central nervous system effects. A meta-analysis of clinical trials concluded that cisapride is significantly better than placebo for NUD. The usual dose is 5 to 10 mg 30 minutes before meals.

Some NUD patients have persistent, troublesome symptoms that are not improved by H_2-receptor antagonists or prokinetic agents. In those difficult patients who are infected with *H. pylori*, it is difficult to resist attempting to eradicate the infection. Although most studies have shown no benefit, individual patients may improve. If a decision to treat is made, a proven regimen should be used, such as bismuth subsalicylate tablets, 2 tablets four times a day, combined with tetracycline, 500 mg four times a day and metronidazole, 250 mg three times a day, all taken for 2 weeks. Potential adverse reactions should be reviewed. Patient compliance is important for success.

■ NAUSEA AND VOMITING

Vomiting is coordinated by a center in the lateral reticular formation of the medulla. This center receives afferent input from the pharynx, the vagal nerves, GI sympathetic nerves, the chemoreceptor trigger zone in the fourth ventricle, and corticobulbar tracts. Dopaminergic (D2), histaminic (H1), muscarinic cholinergic, and serotoninergic (5-HT3) receptors are all involved in the mediation of vomiting.

Some of the causes of nausea and vomiting are outlined in Table 1. It is important to exclude correctable causes. A careful history should include a review of all medications. Physical examination should include a neurologic evaluation. Laboratory studies should include tests for metabolic and endo-

Table 1 Causes of Nausea and Vomiting

ACUTE
- Gastroenteritis, enterotoxins
- Drugs, including alcohol
- Acute intestinal obstruction
- Visceral pain
- Pancreatitis
- Cholecystitis
- Anesthesia and surgery
- Metabolic disturbances
  - Diabetes
  - Adrenal insufficiency
  - Uremia
- Hepatitis
- Vestibular disorders
- Motion sickness
- Radiation

CHRONIC
- Gastric outlet obstruction
  - Peptic ulcer
  - Gastric cancer
  - Pancreatic disease
- Partial small bowel obstruction
- Motility disorders
  - Diabetic gastroparesis
  - Drug-induced delayed emptying
  - Postgastrectomy
  - Chronic intestinal pseudo-obstruction
  - Idiopathic gastroparesis
- Metabolic disorders
- Pregnancy
- Increased intracranial pressure
- Eating disorders
- Idiopathic cyclic nausea and vomiting
- Psychogenic causes

crine disorders. In all women of childbearing age, a pregnancy test should be done early. If a GI cause is suspected, endoscopy and radiographic studies are helpful. In a few patients, the cause of nausea and vomiting is not apparent even after extensive evaluation. Some of these patients have idiopathic disturbances of gastric motility and emptying that may be documented by radionuclide gastric emptying studies or electrophysiologic testing; others may have psychophysiologic disturbances.

Idiopathic Cyclic Nausea and Vomiting

There is a syndrome of functional cyclic nausea and vomiting, which is most common in children but may also occur in adults. The onset is usually abrupt. Intractable vomiting may last from several hours to several days. The episodes are separated by symptom-free intervals of days to months. The frequency and duration of episodes tend to be stereotypic for each individual patient. Complications may include volume depletion, hypokalemia, erosive esophagitis, and Mallory-Weiss syndrome. Vomiting is unrelated to food intake. It may be triggered by emotional excitement in some patients, but this is not a consistent feature. There is an increased prevalence of motion sickness, recurrent headaches, and irritable bowel syndrome in patients with cyclic nausea and vomiting. The pathogenesis of this syndrome is not known. Gastric or intestinal dysmotility can be documented even during asymptomatic intervals, but whether this is primary or secondary has not been determined. Treatment of cyclic vomiting is difficult. Once an episode has begun, treatment must be symptomatic and consists of intravenous fluids, antiemetics, sedatives, and rest or sleep. Some episodes may be aborted by the use of antiemetics at the first sign of an attack. Lorazepam 1 to 2 mg by mouth or sublingually has been used in this manner.

Postgastrectomy Nausea and Vomiting

After vagotomy or partial gastrectomy, patients may develop nausea and vomiting from a variety of mechanical causes, including recurrent ulcer, stenosis of the gastroenterostomy, and afferent loop obstruction. Dumping, bile-alkaline reflux gastritis, and gastric stasis also may cause nausea and vomiting after vagotomy-gastric surgery. Diet changes are the most effective treatment for dumping syndrome. A number of agents have been tried for bile-alkaline reflux gastritis, including aluminum hydroxide-containing antacids, sucralfate, and cholestyramine, without uniform success. Revision of the gastroenterostomy to form a Roux-en-Y jejunal limb to prevent bile reflux helps some patients, but not others, and no method for predicting success has been developed. A number of patients with stasis after vagotomy-gastric surgery improve with metoclopramide or cisapride. A Roux-en-Y limb does not help these patients, who may require a total gastrectomy if symptoms are severe and unremitting.

Table 2 lists examples of some of the medications used for treating nausea and vomiting. Different agents are useful for different situations. The histamine$_1$ blockers act on the vomiting center and the vestibular pathways. They are especially useful for motion sickness. Drowsiness is common, but serious side effects are rare. Transdermal scopolamine is effective in controlling motion sickness. It may sometimes cause dysphoria, restlessness, and confusion.

When it is not possible to correct the underlying condition, the medications most commonly used to treat nausea and vomiting are phenothiazine derivatives, which act as dopamine antagonists in the central nervous system. Phenothiazine also has antihistaminic properties. The neuroleptic droperidol is a butyrophenone that has been used as an antiemetic. Sedation, extrapyramidal reactions, and orthostatic hypotension are the most common adverse effects. These reactions are most likely to occur in the elderly.

Metoclopramide is a dopamine antagonist that acts on both central and peripheral receptors. In high doses it may have antiserotonin activity. It has antiemetic effects independent of its prokinetic action. Metoclopramide is useful in treatment of nausea and vomiting in patients with a disturbance of gastric motility. Because absorption may be delayed in patients with gastric retention, it may be advisable to start treatment with intravenous or intramuscular medication. High-dose metoclopramide has been used for prevention of nausea and vomiting associated with chemotherapy. Side effects include sedation and extrapyramidal reactions. Reports of the rare development of tardive dyskinesia have discouraged long-term use.

Ondansetron and the more recently approved granisetron are serotonin type 3-receptor antagonists. Their specific site

Table 2 Medications for Nausea and Vomiting

MEDICATIONS	INDICATIONS
Histamine$_1$ blockers	Motion sickness
Meclizine (Antivert)	Vestibular disease
25–50 mg PO once daily	
Diphenhydramine (Benadryl)	
25–50 mg PO q6–8h	
Anticholinergics	Motion sickness
Scopolamine (Transderm Scop)	
One patch q 3 days	
Phenothiazine derivatives	
Prochlorperazine (Compazine)	Various causes
5–10 mg PO q6–8h	Postoperative
25 mg rectal q12h	
5–10 mg IM q4h (daily maximum 40 mg)	
Promethazine (Phenergan)	
25 mg PO q4–6h	
12.5–25 mg rectal q4–6h	
12.5–25 mg IM q4h	
Benzamides	Chemotherapy
Metoclopramide (Reglan)	Motility disorders
Motility disorders	
10 mg PO 30 min before meals	
10 mg IM or IV q6h	
Chemotherapy	
1–2 mg/kg IV q2h × two doses, then q3h × three doses	
5HT$_3$-Receptor antagonists	Chemotherapy
Ondansetron (Zofran)	Radiation therapy
0.15 mg/kg IV 30 min before, 4 and 8h after chemotherapy, or 8 mg PO 30 min before chemotherapy, then three times a day	Postoperative

h, hour; IM, intramuscularly; IV, intravenously; PO, orally; q, every.

of action is not clear. They act both on peripheral vagal terminals and in the chemoreceptor trigger zone but have little effect on GI motility. These agents have been useful and cost effective in the treatment of chemotherapy-related nausea and vomiting, especially in cisplatin-based regimens. They also have been used in postoperative patients and in those undergoing radiation therapy. Ondansetron is available in both intravenous and oral formulations. Adverse reactions are uncommon.

■ RUMINATION

Rumination is the repeated and involuntary regurgitation of recently ingested food, usually one mouthful at a time. Part of the material may be spit out or it may be reswallowed. Regurgitation usually begins within 15 minutes of eating and may last several hours, but characteristically stops when the food becomes acidic to taste. It is effortless and not associated with abdominal discomfort, heartburn, or nausea. It must be distinguished from gastroesophageal reflux, vomiting, and bulimia. Rumination is particularly common in institutionalized retarded children. In infants and children, it may be associated with failure to thrive. It may also occur in otherwise normal adolescents and adults, for whom it does not pose a threat to health but may be a source of concern and embarrassment.

The physiology of rumination is not well understood. It may be a learned adaptation of the belch reflex, in which there is simultaneous relaxation of the lower and upper esophageal sphincters, associated with a transient increase in intra-abdominal pressure.

Reassurance and explanation of the pathophysiology are the most important aspects of therapy. Behavioral therapy also has been used. One such method consists of having the patient eat in the presence of the therapist while being encouraged to refrain from regurgitation. Neither drug therapy nor surgery is indicated.

■ GLOBUS PHARYNGEUS

Globus pharyngeus is a continuous sensation of a lump or tightness in the throat. It is not dysphagia or odynophagia. In fact, it may be transiently relieved by swallowing. Up to 45 percent of normal individuals may experience the globus sensation at some time. Typically, a careful examination does not disclose an organic cause for this symptom. The term *globus hystericus* has been used in the past, implying a psychoneurotic cause, but these patients have no higher incidence of psychopathology than normal controls.

Globus pharyngeus probably has multiple causes. A minority of patients have conditions such as sinusitis, pharyngitis, dental infection, a vallecular polyp or cyst, pharyngeal pouch, goiter, cervical bone spur, or, most importantly, squamous cell cancer. There is no evidence of upper esophageal sphincter dysfunction. Some uncontrolled studies have found a high incidence of associated esophageal motor disorders, but a cause-and-effect relationship has not been established. Several studies have noted that increased gastroesophageal reflux is found in approximately 50 percent of globus patients, a significant number of whom do not report heartburn. In one study, 15 percent of globus patients had edema of the arytenoids compatible with reflux laryngitis. Antireflux treatment for globus has been disappointing; however, there have been no studies reported in which omeprazole was used.

In young patients with a short history of globus, reassurance and a brief trial of antacids are indicated. In patients with persistent symptoms, in older patients, and in those with a history of smoking, a careful oropharyngeal examination, laryngoscopy, and fiberoptic esophagoscopy are indicated. Lateral cervical spine radiographs may show bone spurs. If available, a 24 hour esophageal pH monitoring study should be done if esophageal reflux is suspected. When evidence of abnormal reflux is found, a trial of omeprazole, 20 to 40 mg daily for 12 weeks, may clarify whether the globus symptom is reflux related.

■ HICCUPS

A hiccup is a sudden contraction of the inspiratory muscles, terminated by abrupt closure of the glottis. Coordination of hiccups occurs in the cervical spinal cord between C3 and C5. Areas of the brainstem and midbrain also are involved

Table 3 Causes of Hiccups

TRANSIENT HICCUPS

Sudden excitement, emotion
Gastric distention
Esophageal obstruction
Alcohol ingestion
Sudden change in temperature

PERSISTENT OR CHRONIC HICCUPS

Toxic/metabolic: uremia, diabetes, hyperventilation, hypokalemia, hypocalcemia, hyponatremia, gout, fever
Drugs: benzodiazepines, steroids, α-methyldopa, barbiturates
Surgery/general anesthesia
Thoracic/diaphragmatic disorders: pneumonia, lung cancer, asthma, pleuritis, pericarditis, myocardial infarction, aortic aneurysm, esophagitis (peptic or infectious), esophageal obstruction, diaphragmatic hernia or irritation
Abdominal disorders: gastric ulcer or cancer, hepatobiliary or pancreatic disease, inflammatory bowel disease, bowel obstruction, intra-abdominal or subphrenic abscess, prostatic infection or cancer
Central nervous system disorders: traumatic, infectious, vascular, structural
Ear, nose, and throat disorders: pharyngitis, laryngitis, tumor, irritation of auditory canal
Psychogenic disorders
Idiopathic disorders

in the reflex arc. Afferent input occurs through the phrenic and vagal nerves, as well as from sympathetic afferents of segments T6 to T12. Phrenic efferents innervate the glottis, accessory muscles of respiration, and the diaphragm. Vagal efferents may be responsible for the decreased esophageal contractile tone and lower esophageal sphincter pressure associated with hiccups. Hiccups usually involve one side of the diaphragm, most often the left.

Hiccups may be caused by a wide variety of disorders involving some part of the reflex arc, either central or peripheral (Table 3). Most transient hiccups have a benign cause and require no treatment. Chronic hiccups often have a discoverable cause. Every effort should be made to find this cause and correct it. In addition to the history, physical examination, and screening laboratory tests, other studies that may be appropriate depending on the clinical circumstances include chest radiograph, upper GI endoscopy, abdominal ultrasonography, and computed tomography of the head.

When the cause cannot be found or if it cannot be corrected, a variety of simple physical maneuvers should be tried (Table 4). These maneuvers have in common an attempt to disrupt the hiccup reflex arc. If these maneuvers fail, pharmacologic agents may be needed, and Table 4 lists some of the most commonly used agents. There are scores of anecdotal reports of different drugs, reflecting the inconsistent success of pharmacotherapy. One class of drugs that should not be used is the benzodiazepines, which may cause or worsen hiccups. Baclofen, a drug used to treat spasticity, has been used to improve hiccups. Several authors have described the use of hypnosis or acupuncture. Phrenic nerve block should be a measure of last resort. Fluoroscopy should be used to determine which side of the diaphragm is contracting, and a temporary block should be done before considering phrenic nerve ablation.

Table 4 Treatment of Hiccups

Nonpharmacologic methods	*Examples*
Irritation of uvula or nasopharynx	Tongue traction, lifting uvula, swabbing pharynx
Counterirritation of vagal nerve	Carotid sinus massage
Interruption of respiratory rhythm	Breath holding
Counterirritation of diaphragm	Pulling knees up to chest
Relief of gastric distention	Nasogastric suction
Pharmacologic agents	*Dosages*
Baclofen	5 mg PO t.i.d., increasing every 3 days to 80 mg/day maximum dose if needed
Chlorpromazine	25–50 mg IV q6h 25–50 mg PO q6h
Metoclopramide	10 mg IV q4h 10 mg PO q6h
Phenytoin	200 mg IV 100 mg PO q.i.d.
Quinidine sulfate	200 mg PO q.i.d.

h, hour; IV, intravenously; PO, orally; q, every; q.i.d., four times a day; t.i.d., three times a day.

■ AEROPHAGIA AND BELCHING

Normally, 2 or 3 ml of air reaches the stomach with every swallow. Anxiety, chewing gum, and smoking increase the amount of air swallowed. Carbonated beverages add to the gastric air bubble. Belching occurs when simultaneous relaxation of the lower esophageal sphincter and upper esophageal sphincter allows this air to escape.

Belching may become a dramatic and distressing symptom. It is possible to learn how to take large amounts of air into the esophagus and stomach—up to 250 ml in a fraction of a second. Patients who have learned how to belch at will can be observed to elevate the chin and extend the neck, which holds open the upper esophageal sphincter, while making an inspiratory effort with the glottis closed, thus reducing intrathoracic pressure. The swallowed air does not always go into the stomach but may stay in the esophagus, to be subsequently expelled by contraction of the chest wall and diaphragm. In some patients a substantial fraction of air enters the stomach, and from there the small bowel. Belching is sometimes a learned semivoluntary compulsive tic. Initially, the patient may have learned to associate relief of certain symptoms with belching. These symptoms may include dyspepsia from gastroesophageal reflux, peptic ulcer, biliary tract disease, irritable bowel syndrome, or even angina pectoris. Nausea or psychologic distress may increase the swallowing rate, leading to gas accumulation in the stomach. Belching relieves the distress of gastric distention, and a vicious cycle is initiated. Treatment of the underlying condition may decrease the stimulus to the learned reflex, and belching may stop. However, it may also persist even if the initial condition resolves.

Some patients with aerophagia may retain a significant amount of gastric air without belching, causing the "gas-bloat syndrome," or may pass a significant amount of gas into the small intestine, causing additional distention and discomfort. Symptoms in these patients are usually aggravated by meals, especially large meals. The gas-bloat syndrome may also be a consequence of fundoplication surgery, which may leave some patients unable to belch.

It is irrational, given the pathophysiology of belching, to use antacids, simethicone, charcoal, or pancreatic enzymes, unless they are aimed at some underlying condition. If belching persists once an underlying condition has been treated, careful explanation and reassurance may be helpful. Patients with a strong psychoneurotic component may be difficult to reassure and may not accept the physician's explanation.

FUNCTIONAL ABDOMINAL BLOATING

Abdominal bloating is a common functional GI complaint. Gastric outlet obstruction, small bowel or colonic obstruction, intestinal motility disorder, abdominal mass, or ascites must be excluded. Lactose intolerance, giardiasis, or mild malabsorption may present as dyspepsia and bloating without diarrhea. A careful history and physical examination may be sufficient evaluation in a young and otherwise healthy patient, particularly when bloating is associated with symptoms of NUD, irritable bowel syndrome, or premenstrual distress. A lactose tolerance test, stools for parasites, or fecal fat determination should be done if clinical suspicion warrants. In other cases, plain abdominal radiographs, barium studies, and sonography may be necessary.

Functional bloating is intermittent. It often follows meals, even small meals. It may be absent on arising and worsen progressively during the day. The increase in abdominal girth is visible and measurable. One group of investigators confirmed changes in abdominal cross section by computed tomographic scan in these patients. The physiology of functional abdominal bloating is unclear. Contrary to intuition, patients complaining of bloating do not have excessive intestinal gas. Subtle changes in GI motility or muscle tone may be involved.

If an organic cause can be excluded, reassurance may be sufficient. Other patients are very distressed and demand treatment. Unfortunately, no treatment is of proven efficacy. A trial of milk or fiber restriction can be considered. Patients with associated constipation obtain temporary relief from mild laxatives. Cisapride has been helpful in one small study. Antigas medications have not been shown to be better than placebo, although they are harmless.

Suggested Reading

Allan SG. Antiemetics. Gastroenterol Clin North Am 1992; 21:597–611.

Fleisher DR, Matar M. The cyclic vomiting syndrome: A report of 71 cases and literature review. J Pediatr Gastroenterol Nutr 1993; 17:361–369.

Physiology of belch (editorial). Lancet 1991; 337:23–24.

O'Brien MD, Bruce BK, Camilleri M. The rumination syndrome: Clinical features rather than manometric diagnosis. Gastroenterology 1995; 108:1024–1029.

Rousseau P. Hiccups. South Med J 1995; 88:175–181.

Sullivan SN. Functional abdominal bloating. J Clin Gastroenterol 1994; 19:23–27.

Talley NJ. Functional dyspepsia—should treatment be targeted on disturbed physiology? Aliment Pharmacol Ther 1995; 9:107–115.

GASTROPARESIS

Marvin M. Schuster, M.D., F.A.C.P., F.A.P.A., F.A.C.G.

Gastric emptying disorders may be acute or chronic and the cause may be functional or mechanical. The disorder in emptying may be either excessively rapid or delayed. Rapid emptying results most frequently from gastric surgery (vagotomy, partial gastric resection, pyloroplasty) associated with the dumping syndrome. Delayed gastric emptying can be seen with any of these disorders.

The most common cause of acute alterations in gastric motility and emptying are drugs, gastroenteritis, and metabolic disorders. Metabolic causes include ketoacidosis, hypokalemia, uremia, hepatic failure, hypothyroidism, and hypo- or hypercalcemia. Among the drugs that most commonly produce altered emptying of the stomach are anticholinergics, opiates, psychotropics, ganglionic blocking agents, and dopamine agonists. Infection of volunteers with the Norwalk agent has been demonstrated to produce acute delay in gastric emptying that may extend to a subacute period of 2 to 3 weeks, after which resolution usually occurs. However, there are reports indicating that chronic gastroparesis may also have its onset after an acute infectious (usually flulike) process.

The most common causes of chronic changes in gastric emptying are diabetes mellitus, vagotomy, and partial gastric resection. Gastric dysmotility is seen in 20 to 30 percent of diabetics. Liquids and digestible solid emptying is often normal, whereas indigestible solids empty slowly. Delayed gastric emptying can be an isolated phenomenon or part of a more generalized dysautonomia. Neuromuscular and collagen vascular disorders also may lead to gastric emptying disturbances. Patients with chronic intestinal pseudo-obstruction often have delayed gastric emptying, as do those with anorexia nervosa. Altered gastric emptying may also be seen in pregnancy.

Mechanical obstruction is usually due to peptic disease or cancer, but may also be seen in adult hypertrophic pyloric stenosis.

■ CLINICAL PRESENTATION

Symptoms of rapid emptying are sweating, weakness, giddiness, tachycardia, and occasionally orthostasis. The earliest symptom of delayed gastric emptying is early satiety, which may be associated with or followed by nausea, bloating, distention, and occasionally dyspeptic symptoms. Later, patients experience vomiting, anorexia, and weight loss.

■ DIAGNOSTIC TESTS

Upper endoscopy and upper gastrointestinal (GI) x-ray examination with contrast material, while generally inadequate to establish the presence of disordered emptying, may point to underlying etiologic or pathogenetic factors such as ulcer, inflammation, scarring, pyloric hypertrophy, or mechanical obstruction. Tests of gastric emptying rely generally on radionuclide scintigraphy. Gastric manometry with perfused tubes and electrogastrography with surface abdominal electrodes are becoming more useful as experience and technology improve, but are not available to most physicians.

■ TREATMENT

As previously noted, the optimal treatment involves correction of the underlying disorder. This may not be possible, either because the underlying disorder is unknown or because it is uncorrectable. When this is true, measures are taken to alter the pathophysiology as much as possible and to treat symptomatically.

Treatment is discussed under two broad headings: that of delayed gastric emptying and that of rapid gastric emptying. If the underlying disorder is not amenable to treatment or not immediately responsive, symptomatic therapy is instituted. When the disorder is primary, symptomatic therapy is the only treatment available.

Some disorders are more responsive to treatment than others. For example, gastric stasis associated with hypothyroidism and myxedema responds more rapidly to treatment than stasis associated with diabetic neuropathy. Nevertheless, strict diabetic control may produce some improvement, particularly when this is accompanied by correction of ketoacidosis and electrolytes. Diabetic gastroparesis, for unknown reasons, may appear episodically or even cyclically. Gastric symptoms may be independent of the blood sugar or electrolyte disturbance.

Rapid Emptying

Accelerated gastric emptying is most commonly seen in the dumping syndrome after gastric surgery (either subtotal gastrectomy or truncal vagotomy with pyloroplasty). Subtotal gastrectomy accelerates the emptying of both liquids and solids, whereas vagotomy and pyloroplasty accelerates liquid emptying but has a less predictable effect on emptying of solids. Treatment of rapid gastric emptying involves both dietary therapy and drug therapy.

Dietary Therapy

Dietary therapy involves the restriction of fluids during meals, since fluids tend to empty rapidly. Instead, dry meals, low in simple sugars (which increase osmolarity) and high in complex carbohydrates, are prescribed. In particular, hyperosmolar fluids are interdicted; so is added salt. Soluble fiber, such as psyllium seed compounds and oatmeal, may be beneficial because these can slow down gastric emptying. Pectin is a dietary fiber that has been shown to delay liquid emptying in patients with the dumping syndrome and may provide symptomatic improvement. Small, frequent feedings are recommended.

Drug Therapy

Specific drugs may slow down gastric emptying to a degree but usually are not dramatically effective. When anticholinergic agents are used, they should be given in increasing doses to the point at which side effects appear. They should be administered prophylactically one-half hour before meals to allow time for absorption before intake of food. Opiates may provide some benefit, but their addiction potential generally precludes their use except in severe instances of dumping syndrome.

Octreotide may be effective, particularly in late dumping syndrome, by delaying gastric emptying and inhibiting insulin release in response to a carbohydrate meal. Because serum serotonin has been shown to be elevated in the dumping syndrome, serotonin antagonists such as cyprohepatidine have been prescribed in doses of 4 mg administered 30 to 60 minutes before meals.

Delayed Emptying

Symptomatic Management

Acute or episodic gastroparesis, which can be seen in otherwise uncomplicated diabetes or associated with electrolyte disturbance, ketoacidosis, sepsis, or surgery, should be managed with nasogastric decompression, fluid and electrolyte replacement, and correction of any coexisting sepsis or ketoacidosis. Prolonged aspiration can also be helpful in alleviating chronic distention from accumulation of swallowed air that remains in the stomach owing to the inability to empty it. Decompression of a distended stomach may not provide relief if there is a significant central component to the nausea and vomiting. Gentle intermittent suction is preferred to continuous suction, since the latter often results in occlusion of the aspirating ports. When chronic aspiration is required, a percutaneous endoscopic gastrostomy (PEG) may be performed, or it may be combined with a percutaneous jejunostomy (PEJ) for feeding. This is discussed under diet and nutrition.

Diet and Nutrition

Since the stomach tends to empty liquids more rapidly and easily than solids, the consistency of the diet is often more important than the type of food, with the exception of fats, which may aggravate gastric stasis from any cause because they delay gastric emptying. Fats should therefore be avoided. Hypertonic solutions are not well tolerated, nor are poorly digestible fibers. In fact, the fibrous material can form bezoars that may further obstruct the gastric outlet. Meat impactions of the stomach often can be dissolved with papain (Adolph's meat tenderizer without spice). One teaspoon is mixed in a half-glass of water and sipped slowly for 10 minutes. Phytobezoars do not respond to papain digestion as meat protein does, and therefore fibrous bezoars may have to be removed endoscopically or sometimes even surgically.

The diet should be as liberal as tolerated. The best nutritional substance is food, and the ideal food is the most normal diet that can be tolerated. When only soft foods can be managed, blenderized or baby foods may have to constitute a large part of the diet. When only liquids are tolerated, adequate nutrition can be maintained by liquid formulas such as Sustacal and Ensure. However, when used in full strength, these solutions are hypertonic and therefore delay gastric emptying. Dilution may be necessary.

When gastric stasis is so severe that even liquids fail to empty, a medical trial of enteral feeding directly into the jejunum should be attempted, bypassing the stomach. Often the nasojejunal tube must be passed endoscopically because gastric motility is inadequate to propel it out of the stomach. If jejunal feeding (or direct measurement of intestinal motility) demonstrates good motility and satisfactory tolerance of jejunal tube feedings, a percutaneous jejunal feeding tube can be placed. This can be done in one of two ways. The simplest and generally most effective manner is via a PEG with a double-lumen tube placed so that one remains in the stomach while the other traverses the stomach and passes into the jejunum. The advantage of this approach is that the gastric tube can be used for decompression whenever nausea and vomiting are severe, while the jejunal tube is used for providing nutrition. The jejunal tube, by permitting fluid and electrolyte replacement at home, can diminish the need for hospitalization due to dehydration induced by vomiting. Vitamin supplements are often advisable.

Patients with PEGs and PEJs may wish to try oral liquids, soft foods, or even solids that are well chewed in small quantities to satisfy appetite needs. If these too are not tolerated, patients may derive some benefit from sham feeding (chewing soft foods or drinking liquids and aspirating the swallowed material via the gastrostomy as soon as gastric distention produces nausea and vomiting).

Enteral feeding may not be possible if dysmotility involves the small bowel as well as the stomach. In this case, total parenteral nutrition via a central line may be required. Patients who do not tolerate enteral feeding but have benefited from intermittent gastric aspiration may wish to discontinue the PEJ and keep the PEG for gastric decompression, and to provide the satisfaction that can be obtained from sham feeding.

Drug Therapy

H_2-Receptor Antagonists. Inhibition of acid production by H_2 blockers or proton-pump inhibitors (omeprazole) may be helpful for dyspeptic symptoms and gastroesophageal reflux of acid that is associated with gastric stasis.

Antiemetics. Symptomatic treatment of nausea and vomiting with phenothiazine drugs and antihistamines may be required intermittently or continuously. Prochlorperazine maleate (Compazine), although one of the more effective antiemetics, carries the risk of producing extrapyramidal symptoms when doses significantly higher than 40 mg per day are required. In rare instances, these side effects are not reversible. The scopolamine patch has the advantage of long-term gradual dosing and is preferred by some patients. Scopolamine, as well as antiemetics (most of which have anticholinergic action), may not only produce uncomfortable dryness, blurred vision, or urinary retention but may also further slow gastric emptying. When nausea and vomiting do not respond to these more common antiemetics, cannabinoids may provide relief.

Promotility Agents. In recent times, a new class of drugs has been developed. The prokinetic (promotility) agents are actually "designer" drugs whose molecular structure is based on that of haloperidol, which was noted to have, in addition to its psychotropic action, a promotility effect. Attempts were then made to design new drugs that would improve motility without producing the central nervous system (CNS) effects of haloperidol. Bethanechol, a cholinomimetic agent, should not be considered a promotility agent, since its effect is massive and uncoordinated. This may be one of the reasons it is also generally ineffective for the treatment of motility disorders, including those involving the stomach.

The first prokinetic agent approved in this country was metoclopramide (Reglan), which unfortunately crosses the blood-brain barrier and can produce hyperkinesia or somnolence in about 30 percent of patients, often to the extent that the drug has to be discontinued. The second-generation prokinetic drug domperidone was designed so that it would not cross the blood-brain barrier, and it therefore does not produce these CNS side effects. For this reason, it can also be tolerated in higher doses. Both metoclopramide and domperidone achieve their promotility effect by inhibiting the dopaminergic nervous system, which inhibits esophageal and gastric motility. Inhibition of the inhibitor results in improved motility and improved antroduodenal coordination, which is important for appropriate gastric emptying. Metoclopramide also releases acetylcholine, which may assist in stimulating GI motility. Unfortunately, however, neither of these drugs is effective distal to the ligament of Treitz, since dopamine nerves begin to disappear at that site.

Domperidone has an antiemetic effect despite the fact that it does not cross the blood-brain barrier and therefore does not enter the vomiting center. The reason is that the chemoreceptor trigger zone (which, like the vomiting center, also controls vomiting) is located in the brainstem outside the blood-brain barrier and is therefore accessible to domperidone. Both domperidone and metoclopramide are best administered one-half hour before meals to allow time for absorption by the duodenum and small bowel, which is necessary for their effectiveness. To facilitate gastric emptying and duodenal absorption, it may be necessary to initiate gastric emptying intravenously (IV) and subsequently follow up with oral administration of these agents. Only metoclopramide is available for parenteral use. A nighttime dose maintains the blood level during the hours of sleep so that the morning dose can then be more effective. Metoclopramide is generally given in doses of 10 mg, although some people tolerate only 5 mg. Domperidone can be administered in 20 mg doses or higher; its main side effect is constipation. Permanent dyskinesia has been reported with metoclopramide in rare instances.

A third-generation drug, cisapride, has become available by prescription. This is a 5-HT3 antagonist and therefore can alter motility throughout most of the GI tract. Experience has shown its effect on colonic motility to be unpredictable and usually disappointing.

Recently, Japanese investigators have demonstrated that erythromycin mimics exogenous motilin in inducing the migrating motor complex in the small intestine in dogs and in humans by competing for motilin receptors in the gut. Belgian workers have demonstrated the stimulation of antral phase III-like contractions in both normal volunteers and patients with diabetic gastroparesis, some of whom had autonomic neuropathy. A dose of 40 mg, which is effective in inducing phase III migrating motor complexes in the small bowel, was also effective in stimulating antral activity in three-fifths of patients, whereas a high dose of 200 to 350 mg was effective in all the diabetic patients. Because this high dosage has less efficacy in the small bowel than a 40 to 70 mg dose, diabetic patients with gastric and small bowel dysmotility would probably respond better to the lower dose of 50 mg (40 to 70 mg). Erythromycin is more effective when given IV but also has efficacy when administered orally 30 to 60 minutes before meals and at bedtime. Because the lowest-dose tablet contains 200 mg, a 50 mg dosage can best be achieved by using the liquid suspension (¼ tsp of the 200 mg per 5 ml strength administered one-half hour before meals and at bedtime). Two preparations of erythromycin that are readily available are ethylsuccinate EES and EryPed.

More recently, octreotide (Sandostatin), a somatostatin analogue, has been shown to induce the migrating motor complex in small bowel in patients with scleroderma. However, octreotide has its effect directly on small bowel and does not seem to stimulate gastric acidity; it may actually delay gastric emptying. Octreotide use in scleroderma is discussed in another chapter.

ENDOSCOPIC TUBE PLACEMENT

A percutaneous endoscopic gastrostomy (PEG) tube placed by upper endoscopy can serve to vent the stomach and alleviate nausea. A percutaneous endoscopic jejunostomy (PEJ) tube can be placed inside the larger diameter PEG and guided into the duodenum in order to instill fluids and electrolytes during periods of severe nausea or vomiting. Enteral feeding can also be provided through this tube. These measures may help avoid the need for hospitalization for dehydration.

SURGICAL TREATMENT

Experience with operative approaches for both gastric stasis and accelerated gastric emptying has been variable. In my experience, subtotal gastrectomy is of little help in the treatment of delayed gastric emptying, and vagotomy and pyloroplasty often worsens the situation. In drastic situations a total gastrectomy, while carrying its own problems, may improve nutrition and absorption.

The response of the dumping syndrome and other forms of rapid gastric emptying to operative intervention is also unpredictable. Both the Roux-en-Y procedure and interposition of a 10 cm segment of reversed jejunum are used with varying degrees of success.

Suggested Reading

Brown CK, Dkanderia U. Use of metoclopramide, domperidone and cisapride in the management of diabetic gastroparesis. Clin Pharm 1990; 9:357–365.

Drenth JPH, Engels LGJB. Diabetic gastroparesis: a critical reappraisal of new treatment strategies. Drugs 1992; 44:537–553.

Geldorf H, Van der Schee EJ, Van Blankenstein M, Grashuis JL. Electrogastrographic study of gastric myoelectric activity in patients with unexplained nausea and vomiting. Gut 1986; 27:799–808.

Janssens J, Peters TL, Van Trappen G, et al. Improvement of gastric emptying in diabetic gastroparesis by erythromycin. N Engl J Med 1990; 322: 1028–1032.

Koch KL. Gastric dysrhythmias and the current status of electrogastrography. Pract Gastroenterol 1989; 13:37–44.

Koch KL. Stomach. In: Schuster MM, ed. Atlas of intestinal motility. Baltimore: Williams & Wilkins. 1993:158.

PEPTIC ULCER DISEASE

Andrew H. Soll, M.D.

The normal gastric and duodenal mucosae have a remarkable ability to defend against injury from the acid of peptic activity in gastric juice. In fact, peptic ulcers would be rare if mucosal defense mechanisms were not disrupted by exogenous factors. It is now clear that the two most important factors associated with peptic ulcer are infection with *Helicobacter pylori* (HP) and use of nonsteroidal anti-inflammatory drugs (NSAIDs). Ulcers occurring in patients under protracted physiologic stress represent a distinct form of peptic ulcer. Uncommon causes of peptic ulcer include extreme acid hypersecretion (e.g., gastrinoma), rare abnormalities of the duodenum (e.g., annular pancreas), and possibly other infections (herpes simplex virus type I). Uncommonly, ulcers may reflect underlying disease processes, such as Crohn's disease or neoplasia. With clarification of the role of HP and NSAIDs, idiopathic ulcers have become the exception.

Despite the fact that most gastroduodenal ulcers are due to NSAIDs or HP, they remain peptic ulcers. With HP and NSAID ulcers, antisecretory agents accelerate healing and refractory ulcers respond to higher doses of potent antisecretory agents. The observation that continued NSAID therapy impairs healing in response to moderate acid inhibition (H_2-receptor antagonists [RA]), but not to marked acid inhibition with 40 mg of omeprazole, suggests that NSAID ulcers are superpeptic ulcers. The terms "peptic/HP ulcer" and "peptic/NSAID ulcer" are preferable.

Although understanding of pathophysiology and therapy is still incomplete, therapy must be adapted to the underlying cause of peptic ulcer. A generic approach to treating peptic ulcer disease (PUD) is no longer appropriate. Therapy will certainly be refined as understanding of pathophysiology and of the impact of therapy on natural history is advanced.

■ CLINICAL APPROACH

Especially with the present focus on cost effectiveness, the clinical history provides critical information for developing appropriate differential diagnosis and plans for assessment and management. In addition to the common functional disorders discussed below, it is important to exclude drug-induced dyspepsia (e.g., NSAIDs, digoxin, and theophylline) and disorders such as gastric cancer, pancreatic, or biliary tract disease. Especially with the initial presentation of gastric ulcer (GU), gastric carcinoma must be excluded.

Differentiating Gastric Ulcer and Gastric Cancer

Gastric cancer can masquerade as benign GU; however, visual inspection and adequate biopsy detects greater than 98 percent of gastric cancer on the first endoscopy. A thorough initial evaluation obviates the necessity of a second endoscopy to monitor ulcer healing in patients who are responding well to therapy. However, if the ulcer is giant (>2 to 3 cm) or if there were suspicious features on the initial endoscopy or inadequate biopsy, a second endoscopy is warranted. To insure adequate biopsy, the policy at UCLA is to use large biopsy forceps and train technicians to discriminate an adequate tissue sample from the debris; four such adequate biopsies have proved to be sufficient to exclude carcinoma (personal communication, W. Weinstein).

Differentiating Peptic Ulcer from Other Common Functional Disorders

Common disorders that frequently overlap with PUD must be identified (Table 1). Acid dyspepsia is an upper abdominal burning discomfort that generally occurs on an empty stomach and is relieved with food, antacids, or antisecretory agents. Although these symptoms are the classical presentation for PUD, two-thirds of such patients do not have ulcers identified. In addition to the typical nonulcer acid dyspepsia, it is useful to distinguish a second form of nonulcer dyspepsia, which I call "dysgastria," referring to symptoms of belch-bloat symptoms of indigestion (Table 1).

Although not documented by formal study, clinical experience indicates that these several functional disorders occur together in an overlapping pattern that will confound the uninitiated observer. It is my belief that this overlap reflects common underlying mechanisms, such as hypersensitivity of the afferent sensory nerve pathways. This phenomenon was first recognized in the colon in patients with the irritable bowel syndrome in whom the threshold for distention was markedly reduced compared to control subjects. A similar pattern also holds for two other of the functional bowel disorders (FBD)—the irritable esophagus and irritable stomach.

Overlap of PUD and FBD

Patients with PUD frequently (40 to 60 percent) complain of symptoms atypical for "classic" peptic ulcer, such as nausea, exacerbation by eating, belching, bloating, and fatty food intolerance. These symptoms are indicative of FBD and suggest a possible association between PUD and functional disorders outlined in Table 1. The first patient who taught me about this overlap presented initially with the classic symptoms of duodenal ulcer (DU), which responded well to H_2-RA therapy. However, after a few weeks he returned with a recurrence of epigastric pain, loss of antacid relief, and pain radiation to his back. At endoscopy his ulcer had healed, and subsequent physical examination revealed a paraspinous trigger point that reproduced his pain. Trigger point injection brought sustained relief. It appeared that the musculoskeletal symptoms developed as a spinal reflex in response to the initial visceral insult. I now try to detect such clues during my initial clinical evaluation.

Patients with intractable peptic ulcer also underline the potential overlap between PUD and FBD. Before the advent of endoscopy and effective medical therapy for PUD, such patients were frequently operated on, often with a poor outcome. This point was highlighted in a study of patients undergoing proximal gastric vagotomy; when the indication was refractory ulcer, recurrent symptoms occurred in 40 percent, but recurrent ulceration was found in only 4 percent. In contrast, in patients operated for relapsing PUD that remained responsive to medical therapy, recurrences of both symptoms and ulcers occurred in less than 5 percent. Symptoms associated with PUD may reflect mechanisms in addition to acid bathing an ulcer crater and I suspect that many of these atypical cases reflect an overlap of PUD with FBD. Peptic ulcer may serve as one of several triggers for induction of the afferent neuronal hypersensitivity that appears to bridge these overlapping functional disorders. Alternatively, peptic ulcer may result from mechanisms triggered by neuronal dysfunction associated with these other FBD syndromes.

It is essential that the clinician learn to discriminate these overlapping symptom patterns; a detailed history generally reveals clues that allow the overlap to be appreciated. Dissecting out these elements greatly simplifies diagnosis and management. Although endoscopy is the most effective approach for diagnosing PUD, for grading esophagitis, and confirming the presence of gastritis and HP, it cannot replace an expert clinical evaluation. Obviously, before concluding that symptoms are due to functional disorders, it is essential to look for "alarm" markers of serious underlying disease, such as anemia, GI blood loss, anorexia, weight loss, or liver function abnormalities.

Finding a DU in a patient who is not consuming NSAIDs is among the most sensitive "diagnostic" tests for HP. However, in patients in whom a DU is identified, HP testing may still be useful; a negative HP test shifts attention to other potential causes for ulcers such as unrecognized aspirin use or gastrinoma, and precludes therapy directed at HP eradication. It is important to recall that several medications (H^+/K^+-ATPase inhibitors, bismuth, sucralfate, antacids, and antibiotics) can suppress HP and lead to negative cultures, biopsies without organisms, and negative breath tests. The

Table 1 Differential Diagnosis of Peptic Ulcer

CLINICAL ENTITY	SYMPTOM COMPLEX	PRECIPITATING FACTORS	TIMING AND RELATION TO MEALS	RESPONSE TO INTERVENTION
Acid dyspepsia	Epigastric burning pain		Usually >2 h postprandially or in the evening or early nighttime hours.	By definition, relief with food, antacids, or antisecretory agents
"Dysgastria"	Indigestion: belching, bloating, early satiety, nausea, and epigastric pain	Often specific food triggers, especially fatty foods. Dysgastria may occur with or without gastroparesis. Must be distinguished from gastric outlet obstruction produced by ulcer or neoplasia.	Usually occurs with or shortly after eating	Decreasing gastric distention with belching or vomiting often decreases symptoms
Esophageal reflux	Epigastric burning pain with substernal radiation	Occurs in two patterns: (1) primarily postprandial, upright reflux due to transient LES relaxation (tLESR = a vagal reflux) or (2) stress or free reflux, precipitated by abdominal pressure (e.g. bending over, with late stage pregnancy) or when the protective effects of gravity are reversed (supine posture, especially soon after eating). Symptoms can be most readily explained by sensitization to esophageal distention or exposure to acid (an "irritable" esophagus).	Symptoms frequently occur 30–90 min after meals due to gastric distention with food and acid plus transient LES relaxation in upright reflux or a low resting LES in stress or free reflux.	Relief should be achieved with adequate doses of antacids or antisecretory agents. Lifestyle measures are very useful. Aggressive Rx is needed for erosive esophagitis or a very irritable esophagus.
Irritable bowel syndrome	Periumbilical or lower abdominal crampy pain associated with alteration in bowel pattern (diarrhea and/or constipation). Frequently associated with a complaint of abdominal distention and a sensation of incomplete evacuation.	Symptoms usually peak with the urge to move (colonic contraction ± distention). Usually a chronic, undulating syndrome precipitated by stress. Balloon studies reveal a low threshold to distention, i.e., the irritable bowel.	Often worse in the postprandial period, the misnamed "gastrocolic reflex"	Colonic decompression usually reduces symptoms (i.e., passing gas or stool).
"Back-gut" syndrome	Pain and tenderness of paraspinous, intercostal, or abdominal muscles	Symptoms may be exacerbated by twisting or tensing abdominal or rectus muscles and the pain (or a component thereof) may be reproduced by pressure on trigger points.	No direct relation to meals, but overlaps with other functional syndromes	Relief often produced by well-targeted local anesthesia or other physical measures

finding of chronic active gastritis without HP suggests a false-negative for HP, whereas the absence of antral gastritis confirms the absence of HP infection.

A careful history is required to assure that NSAID consumption is detected; NSAID abuse, particularly with aspirin, has been frequently associated with refractory peptic ulcer. Some patients are reluctant to admit NSAID use and this factor deserves consideration especially when peptic ulcers fail to heal. When faced with a slowly healing HP-negative ulcer, measurement of salicylate levels should be considered.

■ HP AND PEPTIC ULCER THERAPY

Although a tight epidemiologic link was quickly established between HP and peptic ulcer, the relevance of this association was unclear because HP is a very common infection, but only a small proportion of subjects infected with HP develop PUD. In contrast, Koch's postulates have been fulfilled for HP infection as the cause of the very common antral predominant chronic, active gastritis (type B). Proof that HP is a causal factor for peptic ulcer has rested upon the numerous studies indicating that eradication of HP in patients with PUD markedly reduces the otherwise high rate of recurrences. The causal factors that distinguish the small proportion of individuals with HP at risk for PUD remain to be elucidated.

Diagnosis of HP

Noninvasive testing includes serology and urea breath testing (UBT). IgG antibody testing has a specificity and sensitivity of about 90 percent in HP infected subjects. IgA antibodies are also useful, but somewhat less reliable indicators of infection. UBT testing has just been approved in the United States; ingested urea is split by bacterial urease and labeled CO_2 detected in breath. False negatives occur, especially when antibiotics, bismuth, or a proton pump inhibitor (PPI) suppress bacteria number. It takes at least 4 weeks and sometimes longer for the number of HP to recover for detection.

"Invasive" testing at endoscopy include urease testing on biopsies. Tests such as the CLO (Campylobacter-like organism) test are most widely used. It is a reliable test; positives are accurate for correctly predicting true HP infection (nearly 100 percent specificity), but negatives can be false for two reasons: (1) Low bacteria counts can result from recent treatment with antibiotics, PPI, or bismuth; and (2) In addition, the high pretest prevalence of HP in ulcer patients results in a poor predictive value of negative tests for the true absence of HP, as noted below. A practical approach to endoscopy is to take at least three biopsies: one or two for CLO testing and two for antral histology. If the CLO is positive discard the histology; if the CLO is negative confirm the absence of HP using histology. This care is particularly important for complicated or troublesome ulcer disease. Histology is also very useful, but pathologists must be focused on detecting HP; we and they ignored the organism for decades. Although standard H&E (hematoxylin and eosin) is fine for detecting high numbers of HP, special stains (Giemsa or silver stain) are helpful in reliably detecting lower numbers by making the bacteria easier to detect. False negatives are frequent in practice, especially when antibiotics, PPI or bismuth have been used within one month. HP produces chronic, active antral gastritis: inflammation with polys are present in most subjects with HP; chronic inflammation in the antrum is present in virtually all subjects with HP. The absence of this type of antral gastritis provides critical support for confidently excluding HP. Finding chronic or chronic, active gastritis with a "negative" CLO suggests a false-negative result: do histology with special stains to gain more definitive information about the presence or absence of HP.

The eradication of HP modestly accelerates initial DU healing rates, compared to standard H_2 blocker therapy. Enhanced healing per se would be a weak justification for eradicating HP at the time of initial treatment. However, it is now very clear that HP eradication decreases subsequent recurrences and the associated costs and risks, and therefore becomes a cure for what otherwise would be a chronic, relapsing disease. In the available randomized, controlled trials, the yearly ulcer recurrence rate of DU decreased from 84 percent in patients remaining HP positive to only 5 percent in patients with successful HP eradication. Numerous other trials support this conclusion, and, to my knowledge, no data to the contrary have been presented! Fewer data are available to assess the impact of HP eradication on the natural history of GU, but the response appears similar to DU; HP should be treated in patients with GU who are HP positive.

Bayes theorem impacts interpretation of HP testing in patients with known ulcers, since prevalence of HP is high in subjects undergoing testing. Therefore, a negative result has a high likelihood of being a false-negative determination. Assuming a specificity and sensitivity of 90 percent and a prevalence of HP infection of 90 percent in DU, the predictive value of a positive test for true infection is >99 percent. In contrast, at this high prevalence of HP in DU, the predictive value of a negative test for the true absence of infection is only about 50 percent. Therefore, in patients with a known ulcer, a positive HP test reliably predicts HP infection. Although alternative etiologies deserve consideration in HP test-negative ulcer patients, false-negative tests are common, and further testing to definitely exclude HP or antibiotic therapy despite the negative test result is justified. For practical management of patients with known, uncomplicated DU (without NSAID use), empiric antibiotic therapy is a reasonable alternative to HP testing because of this high prevalence of HP infection and poor predictive value of a negative test.

Although uncommon, ulcers may recur after HP eradication and can reflect NSAID use or uncommon disorders, such as gastrinoma.

Specific Regimens

HP infection is easily suppressed, but to achieve reasonable cure rates (90 percent in 7 to 10 days of therapy) requires good patient compliance with one of a few very good regimens. No regimens are simple; when a simple, highly effective, well-tolerated regimen is introduced, buy stock—it is a guaranteed winner. Although these regimens are confusing, there are only a few good combinations that really work that combine two antibiotics with either colloidal bismuth or antisecretory agents. Bismuth (B) (bismuth subsalicylate in the United States, but bismuth subcitrate in most other countries) is combined with two of four antibiotics [metronidazole (M), tetracycline (T), clarithromycin (C), or amoxicillin (A)]. BMT produces about 85 to 90 percent cure of HP, but is limited by M-resistance and is hard to take. BCT appears equally effective, but efficacy with BMA drops to about 80 percent. Efficacy with BMT and BMA will be severely compromised by metronidazole resistance, which probably occurs in about 10 to 20 percent of HP-infected patients in the United States. Studies with bismuth subcitrate suggest that 1 rather than 2 week treatment with BMT is adequate, except if there is M-resistance. However, addition of a PPI (omeprazole, 20 mg b.i.d., and probably lansoprazole, 30 mg b.i.d.) improves BMT efficacy, especially with M-resistant HP and one week therapy is adequate. A new agent RBC (ranitidine bismuth citrate = Tritec) has been approved in the United States which combines bismuth citrate with an ranitidine; adequate healing is not an issue. RBC (400 mg, b.i.d. 4 weeks) plus clarithromycin (500 mg b.i.d. or t.i.d., 2 weeks) produced cure rates >80 percent. Efficacy will probably be improved and treatment shortened by adding another antibiotic (metronidazole or amoxicillin), but no data are available to establish optimal regimens with RBC.

Regimens without bismuth combine two of three antibiotics (C, M, or A) with omeprazole (O) or lansoprazole (L). The combination of M (500 b.i.d.) O (20 b.i.d.) and C (500 bid) achieves about 90 percent cure with good compliance; this MOC regimen is probably effective with a 7 day treatment. AOC (M is replaced by A, 1 g b.i.d.) appears equally effective, whereas MOA is less effective, especially with M-resistance. Data are too limited to justify substitution of H_2RA for PPI; effectiveness may drop by 10 to 20 percent and longer therapy is probably required. M-resistance of HP compromises efficacy, especially with MOA. Although PPI pretreatment was reported to impair efficacy of an amoxicillin/PPI combination, a PPI loading dose (20 mg omeprazole × 3) 1 day prior to starting antibiotics is recommended for short-term (1 week) dual antibiotic/PPI regimens. Data are too limited, especially in the United States, to discriminate between the best regimens; current data suggest to me that three regimens (BMT + O, MOC, and AOC) are the best candidates to achieve 90 percent cure rates with a 7 to 10 day treatment. Antibiotic resistance is of concern, especially since treatment with M or C that fails to cure HP infection reliably produces M or C resistance, respectively. Therefore, it is of considerable importance to use effective regimens. In addition, patients must be informed of the importance of compliance and of the likelihood of minor side effects, such as nausea and an altered bowel pattern, which would otherwise prompt termination of therapy. I usually use a 1 day PPI loading dose; data available in the near future will clarify whether 7 day therapy is as effective as 10 or 14 day treatment courses. Monotherapy with M or C is ill-advised in HP-positive subjects, since antibiotic resistance will result.

HP and Recurrent, Refractory, or Complicated Peptic Ulcer

Eradication of HP, if present, is the first step in preventing ulcer recurrence. HP eradication reduces the recurrence of ulcer complications and will facilitate healing of refractory ulcers. HP must be coded in patients with recurrent, refractory, or complicated ulcer disease!

In individuals with a history of ulcer complications, frequent or troublesome recurrences, or refractory ulcer, maintenance therapy with H_2 blockers is indicated until HP eradication is confirmed via a negative urea breath test (which is now available) or a marked decrease of the titers of HP antibodies after 6 to 12 months. An analysis comparing pre- and post-treatment serum titers in a single assay is most likely to provide useful information. Qualitative assays are not useful, since detectable antibody titers will persist in many subjects for several years. Repeat endoscopy cannot be justified simply to confirm HP eradication in only the high-risk group. In this high-risk subgroup of ulcer patients, one cannot be faulted for continuing maintenance therapy for another 6 to 12 months, but sustained maintenance therapy is not necessary in most patients.

■ CONVENTIONAL ULCER THERAPY

Conventional ulcer therapy is indicated for HP-negative ulcers, for healing of HP-positive ulcers, and for maintenance of HP-positive ulcers pending or with failed HP eradication.

Regimens for Initial Therapy

Uncomplicated ulcers can be treated by a variety of safe and effective therapies (Table 2), including antacids, sucralfate. H_2-RA, and proton-pump inhibitors (PPI, omeprazole or lavnsoprazole). The rate of healing of DU correlates with the potency, duration of action during the day, and length of therapy with antisecretory agents. For example, healing is more rapid with omeprazole at 40 mg per day and to a lesser extent with the 20 mg per day dose than with conventional doses of H_2-RA. However, with the exception of somewhat more rapid symptom relief, the benefits of this more rapid healing on clinical outcome are of little clinical importance in uncomplicated ulcer and cost is a more relevant factor.

For healing GU, full doses of H_2 blockers provide effective initial therapy. PPI are also clearly effective alternatives approved for GU therapy in the United States. Although GU respond to antisecretory agents, the variable of most importance is the length of therapy; therefore, with the exception of continued cotherapy with NSAIDs, the most cost-effective approach is to treat with the least expensive agent for a longer time. In one study, an advantage of omeprazole over H_2 blockers was evident in subjects continuing NSAID use; in the absence of NSAIDs, ranitidine and the 20 mg dose of omeprazole produced apparently comparable healing.

Therapy on Demand

The advent of over the counter availability of H_2 blockers highlights the need for a risk to benefit analysis of "on demand" antisecretory therapy. In reality, many patients treat themselves on an "as needed" basis. However, in the HP era, this approach is not appropriate for PUD. If symptoms are recurrent due to PUD and HP is present, the organism should be treated rather than continuing intermittent therapy.

Conventional Maintenance Therapy

Maintenance therapy is currently indicated for patients pending HP eradication, in whom HP eradication has failed, or who have HP-negative ulcer disease. After initial ulcer healing, continued treatment with several medications (Table 2) reduces the high spontaneous recurrence rate found in placebo-treated patients. The goals of maintenance therapy are prevention of symptomatic recurrences and complications. Even in patients compliant with maintenance therapy, asymptomatic recurrences are frequent, but usually remain clinically silent. Therefore, with the possible exception of patients with a prior history of complications, there is no justification to pursue asymptomatic recurrences in patients with a good clinical response to maintenance therapy.

Patient Selection

Since peptic ulcer is a recurrent disease, the challenge for the physician is to base therapy on a prediction of the natural history of ulcer disease in the individual patient. Accurate predictions are difficult in individual patients, but several factors are associated with future recurrences, the most important of which is a prior history of ulcer complications. Recurrent DU hemorrhage has been observed at a rate of 1 percent per month in patients with prior GI bleeding from a DU and this rate was markedly suppressed by maintenance

Table 2 Therapies for Peptic Ulcer

DRUG	MECHANISM OF ACTION	DOSAGE REGIMEN: ULCER HEALING	DOSAGE REGIMEN: MAINTENANCE	SIDE EFFECTS
H_2-receptor antagonists	Inhibit acid secretion by blocking parietal cell H_2 receptors			Cardiac conduction abnormalities, idiosyncratic hepatic injury, immune hypersensitivity reactions, and thrombocytopenia
Cimetidine (Tagamet)		400–600 mg b.i.d. or 800 mg hs	400 mg hs	Gynecomastia, P450-mediated drug interactions with warfarin, diazepam, and phenytoin, theophylline, nifedepine, and flosequinan†
Ranitidine (Zantac)		150 mg b.i.d. or 300 mg hs	150 mg hs	Weak drug interactions, headaches, rare hypersensitivity
Famotidine (Pepcid)		20 mg b.i.d. or 40 mg hs	20 mg hs	
Nizatidine (Axid)		150 mg b.i.d. or 300 mg hs	150 mg hs	
Omeprazole (Prilosec)	Inhibits the parietal cell H^+/K^+-ATPase. Requires pH partition into the stimulated parietal cell; effectiveness markedly compromised in resting or inhibited parietal cells*	20 mg q.AM, 30 min before first meal	10–40 mg, depending on specific circumstances	P450-mediated drug interactions with warfarin, diazepam and phenytoin; rare hepatitis
Lansoprazole (Prevacid)		30 mg q.AM,. 30 min before first meal	15–60 mg depending on circumstances	Unknown, probably few
Sucralfate (Carafate)	Topical action that enhances healing; many theories such as binding growth factors and inhibiting pepsin diffusion	1 g q.i.d. or 2 g b.i.d.	1 g b.i.d.	Aluminum loading in renal failure
Antacids	Acid neutralization and possible topical action of Al-OH complexes	280–1,000 mEq daily		Aluminum loading in renal failure, diarrhea with Mg, constipation with Al

*Effectiveness of omeprazole is markedly inhibited in fasting patients, or in patients on other secretory inhibitors, such as H_2RA or somatostatin.

†Central nervous system side effects in the intensive care unit have been reported more frequently with cimetidine than with the other H_2 blockers; however, this apparent difference has not been tested in controlled trials and may reflect usage patterns and reporting biases with the first drug in a series.

H_2 blocker therapy. Other factors favoring recurrence include frequent prior ulcer recurrences, a history of refractory ulceration, continued cotherapy with NSAIDs, smoking, a deformed duodenum, and age greater than 65 years. Patients with recurrent or refractory ulcers warrant consideration for an acid hypersecretory syndrome, which can be idiopathic or secondary to gastrinoma. It is clear that persisting HP-positive status is a major determinant of recurrent ulceration.

Specific Regimens

Surprisingly, there are no data available to guide decisions regarding the optimal regimen for maintenance therapy in the subgroup who will now be treated (patients with HP-negative ulcers, or HP-positive ulcers failing eradication). The greatest experience is with H_2-RA, so that these agents are my first choice. If the patients fails maintenance doses or has a history of troublesome disease, I favor sustained full dose H_2-RA therapy. Omeprazole is another effective alternative, which is appropriate for the very small group of high-risk patients who have not responded to H_2 RA therapy and are either HP-negative or have failed HP eradication.

Duration and Sustained Efficacy

In the patients who have been studied (mostly HP-positive), maintenance therapy continues to be safe and effective for 3 to 5 years. In fact, ulcer recurrences often decrease in frequency over the course of follow-up. I favor continuing therapy for at least 3 years in high-risk patients before attempting to discontinue. There are conflicting views on the natural history of peptic ulcer—some cases seem to burn out over time, while others continue to be symptomatic for decades. We now need to reassess this situation based upon the behavior of this new subset of patients being treated.

Refractory Ulcers

It is essential to distinguish patients with intractable symptoms associated with refractory ulceration from those with intractable symptoms without active ulceration. A great advantage of current medical management is that refractory ulcers (or their absence) can be identified and virtually all such ulcers can be healed, thereby revealing symptoms due to mechanisms other than refractory ulceration and avoiding unnecessary antiulcer therapy or surgery. Two elements that are critical to the evaluation of refractory ulceration are expert clinical evaluation and endoscopy. Refractory GU require adequate biopsies to identify neoplasia and the several infectious and inflammatory conditions that can mimic peptic ulcer. With refractory DU, particularly in the absence of HP or NSAID use, endoscopic biopsy should be considered to exclude unexpected pathology.

Once it is clear that a refractory peptic ulcer is the problem at hand, look for HP and treat with antibiotics. Other factors that can potentially delay healing deserve consideration (these factors are generally similar to those precipitating ulcer recurrences). Obviously patient understanding of and compliance with therapy should be assessed. Aspirin abuse is surprisingly frequent in the setting of refractory and recurrent ulceration, including ulcers recurring after surgery. Clinical evaluation should include salicylate levels, a history from family members, or even a room search since patients frequently decline to admit this habit.

Of the available treatment options, only maximal acid inhibition with a regimen such as omeprazole 40 mg daily or therapy with colloidal bismuth subcitrate (not available in the United States) offers advantages over continued therapy with standard regimens. No difference was found when patients with DU refractory to 6 weeks of H_2 blocker therapy were randomized to subsequent therapy with omeprazole at a daily dose of 20 mg or to therapy with ranitidine (150 mg twice daily). However, 96 percent of the ulcers refractory to 3 months of H_2-RA therapy healed with 8 weeks of omeprazole (40 mg per day), while only 57 percent healing was found with continued ranitidine therapy (300 mg daily). Thus, omeprazole will heal ulcers refractory to standard doses of H_2 blockers but a 40 mg dose appears necessary for a predictable advantage over continued H_2 RA therapy.

The use of drugs with different modes of action does not enhance healing of uncomplicated or refractory ulcers and the added cost is not justified. In fact, addition of H_2 RA to omeprazole compromises the effectiveness of the PPI (Table 2).

■ NSAID ULCERS

NSAID use is widespread and endoscopic ulcers are frequent, but clinically significant ulceration occurs infrequently. The pathogenic mechanism(s) distinguishing those few individuals at risk for ulcer complications have not been defined. Differentiating endoscopic from clinical ulcers is critical when interpreting studies. Depending upon the definition, endoscopic ulcers are found at surveillance endoscopy in 10 to 25 percent of patients taking NSAIDs, whereas clinical ulcers present in clinical settings with complications or symptoms at a rate of 1 to 4 percent per patient per year of NSAID use. A selection bias distinguishes the natural history of endoscopic ulcers from clinical ulcers; most endoscopic lesions remain clinically silent. The extrapolation from investigation of endoscopic ulcers to the prevention and treatment of clinical ulcers may be justified but requires caution.

Consumption of NSAIDs appears to be both an independent cause of peptic ulcer and an exacerbating factor for individuals with an underlying ulcer diathesis. The conclusion that NSAIDs are a de novo cause of ulcer is based on the observations that about half of NSAID-associated GU presenting in a clinical setting occur in the absence of HP or its associated antral gastritis.

Prevention and treatment are discussed briefly here and in greater detail in the next chapter.

Treatment

Discontinuation of NSAIDs or a reduction in dose should be the first step when possible. If NSAIDs must be continued, uncomplicated ulcers can be treated with twice daily (b.i.d.) dosing of H_2 RA, whereas complicated, large, or slowly healing ulcers warrant high dose (40 mg) omeprazole therapy. More data are needed to allow confident selection and dosing of therapy. Although misoprostol is reasonably effective healing non-NSAID ulcers, there are no data establishing efficacy healing (in contrast to preventing) clinical NSAID ulcers.

Prevention

Preventive cotherapy with antiulcer agents is not indicated for every patient taking NSAIDs, but is appropriate in patients using both NSAIDs and steroids and in patients with a definite history of prior ulcer disease or with serious comorbid conditions that would compromise tolerance to ulcer complications. Age alone appears to be a risk factor for NSAID-induced ulcer disease but the cost of antiulcer cotherapy for all patients over 65 years of age taking NSAIDs is hard to justify with present data. However, patients over 75 to 80 years old probably warrant antiulcer cotherapy while taking NSAIDs. NSAIDs now carry a warning label regarding ulcer complications and any time NSAIDs are used, with or without these risk factors, the patient should be informed about the potential risk of ulcer complications with these drugs.

Misoprostol

Misoprostol is the only drug currently approved for the prevention of NSAID-induced endoscopic ulcers. Preliminary analysis of a recently completed randomized trial with over 9,000 patients indicates that the rate of ulcer complications was reduced by 40 to 50 percent in patients taking misoprostol (200 μg four times a day) plus NSAIDs versus those taking NSAIDs alone. Side effects of abdominal pain and diarrhea limit the use of misoprostol but these are reduced if the dose is gradually increased from 100 μg daily to 200 μg four times a day. Prevention of NSAID-induced endoscopic ulcers is dose dependent; maximal effect is observed with 200 μg four times a day. The dose relation for prevention of ulcer complications has not been determined. In light of the available data, misoprostol must be considered the first choice for ulcer prevention due to NSAID use in a high-risk patient.

Omeprazole and H_2 RA

Full-dose H_2 blockers prevent endoscopic DU and double-dose H_2-RA decrease endoscopic GU; they are a reasonable choice in patients with a history of DU responsive to these agents or in patients who cannot tolerate misoprostol. Omeprazole has not been formally tested for efficacy in preventing NSAID-induced ulceration or its complications, although this agent is the only alternative if ulcers developed during full-dose H_2 blocker therapy and misoprostol cannot be tolerated. There are no guidelines for selecting omeprazole doses in this setting. Although a 40 mg daily dose probably produces a more reliable effect, maintenance should be attempted with the 20 mg dose.

Less Toxic NSAIDs

Switching from NSAIDs to acetaminophen or salsalate provides a good alternative with a lower ulcer risk. NSAID prodrugs such as nabumetone or etodolac, which have a reduced risk of endoscopic ulceration, may also deserve consideration; however, no data from controlled trials address the risk of ulcer complications on these regimens, especially in patients who have a prior ulcer history.

■ HP AND NSAID ULCERS

About 50 percent of patients presenting in a clinical setting with NSAID-associated peptic ulcers are infected with HP. Even though causality between HP and NSAID-associated ulcer complications has not been firmly established, the NIH Consensus Development Conference concluded that antibiotics were indicated for NSAID-associated ulcer when HP-positive. However, HP cure at most will only reduce the ulcer risk during subsequent NSAID therapy. The only way to discriminate the ulcer type is to determine whether successful HP cure eliminates the ulcer risk despite continued NSAID use (an HP-induced ulcer) or whether after HP eradication the ulcer recurs upon resuming NSAID therapy (an NSAID-induced ulcer). Because HP cure will not eliminate the ulcer risk from NSAIDs, antiulcer cotherapy is probably warranted regardless of HP status if NSAIDs are continued or restarted in subjects with a history of clinically relevant peptic ulcer. In subjects without an ulcer history, long-term trials are needed to determine the extent to which NSAIDs might exacerbate an underlying, HP-associated ulcer diathesis. I suspect that preventive cure of HP infection will substantially (≈30 to 50 percent) decrease subsequent ulcer risk from NSAID use, thus justifying HP screening before initiating NSAID therapy. This is a controversial view, but I believe that patients should be offered this option.

■ SIDE EFFECTS OF THERAPY

The untoward consequences of induced hypochlorhydria remain largely theoretical. However, prolonged acid secretory inhibition should be avoided unless the clinical benefit for managing refractory ulceration or esophagitis justifies the costs and exposure to these theoretical risks. Increased risk of enteric infection with organisms such as cholera and salmonella has been reported in subjects with achlorhydria, but these events have been very infrequently reported with antisecretory therapy.

Another potential untoward effect of prolonged antisecretory therapy is the trophic consequences of the elevation of serum gastrin on the gastric mucosa and possibly on other gastrin-sensitive tissues. In rats, extensive studies have established that high-dose antisecretory therapy with omeprazole or other antisecretory agents induces hyperplasia of the histamine-containing enterochromaffin-like (ECL) cells in the oxyntic mucosa and, at the end of their 2 year life span, formation of gastric carcinoids. This sequence of events has been demonstrated to reflect the hypergastrinemia produced by the secretory inhibition. However, carcinoid formation has not been found in other species, with the exception of mastomys. Hyperplasia of ECL cells also occurs in states of extreme and sustained hypergastrinemia in man (gastrinoma and atrophic gastritis). However, carcinoids only occur with gastrinoma plus MEN-I or with chronic atrophic gastritis. Hypergastrinemia alone does not produce gastric carcinoids in sporadic gastrinoma. For most, hypergastrinemia in response to antisecretory therapy may produce modest ECL cell hyperplasia, but dysplasia and tumor formation have not been found during thousands of patient-years of monitoring and use. The risk of carcinoid formation is very remote.

Omeprazole usually produces only modest hypergastrinemia. However, in a small percentage of patients, the fasting serum gastrin concentration can exceed 500 pg per milliliter. I am not reluctant to continue omeprazole longer than 8 weeks if the benefit justifies the expense and theoretical risk. However, I favor measuring fasting serum gastrin levels after 6 months and yearly thereafter in an attempt to detect extreme hypergastrinemia. If hypergastrinemia is found, it is safe to assume that secretory suppression is excessive and need for the drug deserves reassessment or the dose reduced.

Suggested Reading

Anonymous. NIH Consensus Conference. *Helicobacter pylori* in peptic ulcer disease. NIH Consensus Development Panel on *Helicobacter* pylori in Peptic Ulcer Disease [see comments]. [Review]. *JAMA* 1994; 272:65–69.

Cantu TG, Korek JS. Central nervous system reactions to histamine-2 receptor blockers. Ann Intern Med 1991; 114:1027–1034.

Cutler AF, Havstad S, Ma CK, Blaser MJ, Perez-Perez GI, Schubert TT. Accuracy of invasive and noninvasive tests to diagnose *Helicobacter pylori* infection [see comments]. Gastroenterology 1995; 109:136–141.

Goodman AJ, Kerrigan DD, Johnson AG. Effect of the pre-operative response to H_2 receptor antagonists on the outcome of highly selective vagotomy for duodenal ulcer. Br J Surg 1987; 74:897–899.

Graham DY, Lew GM, Klein PD, et al. Effect of treatment of *Helicobacter pylori* infection on the long-term recurrence of gastric or duodenal ulcer. Ann Intern Med 1992; 116:705–708.

Griffin MR, Piper JM, Daugherty JR, et al. Nonsteroidal anti-inflammatory drug use and increased risk for peptic ulcer disease in elderly persons. Ann Intern Med 1991; 114:257–263.

Kochman ML, Elta GH. Gastric ulcers—when is enough, enough. Gastroenterology 1993; 105:1582–1584.

Mayer EA, Gebhart GF. Basic and clinical aspects of visceral hyperalgesia. Gastroenterology 1994; 107:271–293.

Ofman JJ, Etchason J, Fullerton S, Kahn KL, Soll AH. Management strategies for *Helicobacter pylori* seropositive patients with dyspepsia: clinical and economic consequences. Ann Intern Med 1997; (In Press)

Piper JM, Ray WA, Daugherty JR, Griffin MR. Corticosteroid use and peptic ulcer disease: Role of nonsteroidal anti-inflammatory drugs. Ann Intern Med 1991; 114:735–740.

Schuster MM. Irritable bowel syndrome. In: Sleisenger MH, Fordtran JS, eds. Gastrointestinal disease. 5th ed. Philadelphia: WB Saunders, 1993:917.

Soll AH. Gastric, duodenal, and stress ulcer. In: Sleisenger MH, Fordtran JS, eds. Gastrointestinal disease, 5th ed. Philadelphia: WB Saunders, 1993, p. 580.

Soll AH. Medical treatment of peptic ulcer: practice guidelines. JAMA 1996; 275:622–629.

van der Hulst RWM, Keller JJ, Rauws EAJ, Tytgat GNJ. Treatment of *H. pylori* infection in man: review of the world literature. Helicobacter 1996; 1:6–19.

Walan A, Bader J-P, Classen M, et al. Effect of omeprazole and ranitidine on ulcer healing and relapse rates in patients with benign gastric ulcer. N Engl J Med 1989; 320:69–75.

HELICOBACTER PYLORI

Kirsten J. Kinsman, M.D.
M. Brian Fennerty, M.D., F.A.C.P., F.A.C.G.

Helicobacter pylori was first identified and isolated from gastric biopsies in 1983 and has since emerged as an important gastroduodenal pathogen. It is commonly found in an asymptomatic population, with prevalence varying with socioeconomic class and age. *H. pylori* is endemic in developing countries, but prevalence is decreasing in developed countries (cohort phenomenon). *H. pylori* is the cause of type B gastritis, as eradication of the bacteria results in histologic improvement. *H. pylori* also plays an important role in the pathogenesis of duodenal ulcer and most cases of gastric ulcer. Treatment aimed at eradication of the organism favorably affects both the rate of ulcer healing and recurrence rate. Hence, the discovery of *H. pylori* has led to new therapies that alter the natural history of peptic ulcer disease and have changed our approach to peptic ulcer disease irrevocably.

■ DIAGNOSIS

Diagnosis of *H. pylori* infection can be made by a variety of invasive and noninvasive tests (Fig. 1). The organism, a 3 × 0.5 mm spiral gram-negative rod, may be detected directly by histologic examination of gastric biopsies using Giemsa or routine hematoxylin-eosin staining. Several other diagnostic tests for *H. pylori* rely on the organism's urease enzyme. Urease catalyzes the degradation of urea to bicarbonate and ammonium, which produces an alkaline microenvironment and protects the organism from gastric acid. Gastric biopsy specimens can be placed on a urea gel or substrate pad that contains a pH indicator, commonly phenol red or bromophenol blue. If the specimen contains *H. pylori,* ammonia is generated, which results in a change in pH and characteristic color change (Clotest; Pyloritek).

Urease activity can also be detected by the carbon-13 and carbon-14 urea breath tests. In these noninvasive tests the subject ingests radiolabeled urea, which in the presence of *H. pylori* results in the production of ammonium and radiolabeled bicarbonate. The bicarbonate is absorbed into the blood stream and excreted in the breath as radiolabeled carbon dioxide, which is detected by either scintillation counter (^{13}C breath test) or mass spectrography (^{14}C breath test).

Serologic studies using enzyme-linked immunoabsorbent assays detect antibodies produced against high molecular weight cell proteins of the outer membrane of *H. pylori.* A positive test does not distinguish between current and old infection. However, a fall in antibody titer resulting from eradication of the organism may be useful in assessing the efficacy of therapy for *H. pylori.* Recently introduced office-based antibody precipitin tests are inexpensive, sensitive, and specific, making them ideal for screening for *H. pylori* infection.

■ INDICATIONS FOR THERAPY

The association between peptic ulcers and *H. pylori* is well established. In patients with duodenal ulcer not due to nonsteroidal anti-inflammatory drugs or gastrinoma, more than 95 percent demonstrate *H. pylori* in gastric antral mucosa. Further evidence supporting the association of *H. pylori* and duodenal ulcer is that eradication of the organism results in a markedly reduced rate of ulcer relapse (0 to 5 percent) compared with patients treated with conventional antisecretory therapy (70 to 90 percent). Similarly, more than 70 percent of patients with gastric ulcer have evidence of *H. pylori* infection, and it appears that eradication of the organism decreases the rate of relapse of gastric ulcers as well.

The association between *H. pylori* and nonulcer dyspepsia is less clear. There is a variable association, 30 to 70 percent, of nonulcer dyspepsia and chronic active gastritis with *H. pylori.* Neither treatment of gastritis nor the eradication of *H. pylori* leads to consistent improvement in symptoms.

H. pylori has also been associated with gastric carcinoma and lymphoma. A rare lymphoma, MALT-oma, has even been shown to regress with *H. pylori* eradication. However, there is no evidence that eradication of *H. pylori* affects the development or natural history of the more common gastric tumors.

At present it is therefore appropriate to treat only *H. pylori*-associated duodenal or gastric ulcers. Patients presenting acutely with an *H. pylori*-positive duodenal or gastric ulcer should be treated with antimicrobial therapy. Patients with an ulcer previously diagnosed by endoscopy or barium radiography with recurrent symptoms or requiring maintenance therapy who have *H. pylori*-positive serology or breath testing also are candidates for *H. pylori* therapy. Data do not support the treatment of *H. pylori* in the setting of other gastroduode-

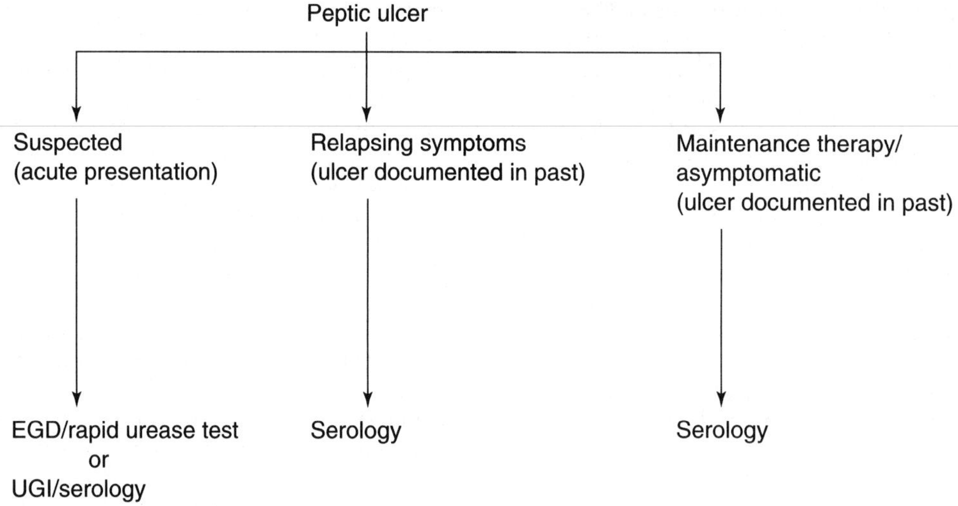

Figure 1
Diagnosis of *H. pylori.* EGD, esophogogastroduodenopathy; UGI, upper GI series.

Table 1 Therapeutic Options for Eradication of *Helicobacter pylori*

REGIMEN	DRUGS	DOSAGE	DURATION
Dual therapy with acid pump inhibitor	Omeprazole with clarithromycin	40 mg qd 500 mg t.i.d.	2 weeks
Triple therapy	Omeprazole with metronidazole* and clarithromycin	20 mg b.i.d. 500 mg b.i.d. 500 mg b.i.d.	1 week
Standard triple therapy	Pepto-Bismol with metronidazole, tetracycline, or amoxicillin	2 tablets q.i.d. 250 mg q.i.d. 500 mg q.i.d.	2 weeks
Quadruple therapy	Standard triple therapy plus Omeprazole	20 mg daily	1 week

*Amoxicillin b.i.d. can be substituted for metronidazole

nal maladies, and *H. pylori* therapy is not recommended in patients with nonulcer dyspepsia or gastric cancer.

■ THERAPY

Efficacy of therapy for *H. pylori* depends on both the sensitivity of the organism to antibiotics and the patient's compliance with the therapeutic regimen. *H. pylori* is sensitive to most antibiotics in vitro; however, results in vivo with single antimicrobial agents have been disappointing. In addition to the low rates of efficacy encountered with single-agent therapy, resistance to some antibiotics develops rapidly. In fact, resistance of *H. pylori* to metronidazole is now as high as 30 to 70 percent in some population. Due to the lack of efficacy and development of resistance, monotherapy is not considered a treatment choice for the eradication of *H. pylori.*

Combination therapy, developed in part to address the issue of antimicrobial resistance, has proven successful, with eradication rates of 50 to 90 percent. However, this approach to therapy has disadvantages. The complexity of the regimens (5 to 16 pills per day for 7 to 14 days) and the high incidence of side effects (e.g., abdominal pain, diarrhea, nausea, taste disturbance, rash) have been associated with poor compliance. Poor compliance significantly compromises therapeutic efficacy of combination therapy, and variation in specific dosing, amount, and relationship to meals all affect success.

Two-drug therapeutic regimens offer both a favorable efficacy (above 80 percent) and more tolerable side effect profiles. Improved compliance with these simpler regimens may offset the reported higher rates of efficacy of three-drug therapy, as a larger percentage of patients may complete the treatment. The cost of therapy remains an issue. The most expensive therapy is the one that does not work; therefore, seemingly more expensive but better tolerated regimens resulting in higher eradication rates may be the most cost-effective choice.

■ REGIMENS

Several specific therapeutic regimens for *H. pylori* eradication in the setting of acute and remote ulcer disease have been described (Table 1). Standard triple therapy with bismuth and two antibiotics has the highest overall efficacy and has become the gold standard with which other regimens are compared. The combination of bismuth, metronidazole, and tetracycline is most effective, with an eradication rate of 90 percent. When amoxicillin is substituted for tetracycline, eradication decreases to 80 percent. In addition to its efficacy, the cost of triple therapy is low. Disadvantages of this regimen include side effects (dyspepsia, diarrhea, nausea) in up to 60 percent and a complicated dosing schedule, both of which may affect compliance and success of therapy.

Dual therapy with the proton-pump inhibitor omeprazole and clarithromycin has an eradication rate of approximately 80 percent. (Omeprazole and amoxicillin has not proven as effective, with eradication rates in U.S. trials of 50 percent or less. Thus, a regimen of omeprazole and amoxicillin should not be used.)

While the cost of dual therapy is higher than standard triple therapy, advantages include a simpler dosing regimen, fewer side effects, and higher compliance rates. Increased compliance with dual therapy may result in overall greater eradication than triple therapy if patients are not expected to comply with triple therapy (more than 60 percent of their tablets taken).

Recently, shorter course triple therapy with omeprazole, metronidazole or amoxicillin, and clarithromycin has shown promising results. Shorter treatment duration (7 days), simpler regimen (b.i.d. dosing) and superb efficacy (>90 percent eradication of *H. pylori*) make these regimens very useful and the treatment of choice by many investigators in this field.

■ FOLLOW-UP

Eradication can be presumed to be successful in 60 to 90 percent of patients treated with an appropriate antimicrobial regimen for *H. pylori*. Documentation should rarely be necessary except in patients with a history of complicated ulcer disease, e.g., bleeding or perforation. In these patients eradication documentation is mandatory prior to discontinuing maintenance antisecretory therapy. In other patients the return of ulcer symptoms should lead one to determine *H. pylori* status. As *H. pylori* may be suppressed with antimicrobial treatment, testing for eradication should be delayed for at least 4 weeks following completion of therapy.

Biopsy of the gastric mucosa for histology is the most sensitive means of detecting *H. pylori* and determining eradication of the organism. However, unless repeat endoscopy is indicated for another reason, this approach is rarely necessary. The urea breath test offers a noninvasive test for cure but is not yet widely available and is relatively expensive. Serology is easily obtained, and a serial decline in antibody titers after therapy is evidence of eradication, though paired serologies are necessary but rarely available. Therefore, it appears that breath testing will be the primary means by which eradication is documented when such information is necessary.

Suggested Reading

Fennerty MB. *Helicobacter pylori.* Arch Intern Med 1994; 154:721–727.

Graham DY, Lew GM, Evans DG, et al. Effect of triple therapy (antibiotics plus bismuth) on duodenal ulcer healing. Ann Intern Med 1991; 115(4):266–269.

Hentschel E, Brandstatter G, Dragosics B, et al. Effect of ranitidine and amoxicillin plus metronidazole on the eradication of *Helicobacter pylori* and the recurrence on duodenal ulcer. N Engl J Med 1993; 328(5):308–312.

Labenz J, Gyenes E, Ruhl GH, Borsch G. Omeprazole plus amoxicillin: Efficacy of various regimens to eradicate *Helicobacter pylori.* Am J Gastroenterol 1993; 88(4):491–495.

Labenz J, Ruhl GH, Borsch G. Amoxicillin plus omeprazole versus triple therapy for eradication of *Helicobacter pylori* in duodenal ulcer disease: A prospective, randomized and controlled study. Gut 1993; 34:1167–1170.

Logan RPH, Gummet PA, Schaufelberger HD, et al. Eradication of *Helicobacter pylori* with clarithromycin and omeprazole. Gut 1994; 35:323–326.

UPPER GASTROINTESTINAL BLEEDING

John Baillie, M.B., Ch.B., F.R.C.P. (Glasg.)

Acute upper gastrointestinal (GI) hemorrhage is a life-threatening emergency. Early recognition and prompt and appropriate management of this condition will avoid unnecessary deaths. Mortality from GI bleeding can be divided into *avoidable* and *unavoidable* deaths. Avoidable causes of death include delayed or otherwise inadequate resuscitation, aspiration, transfusion reaction, and complications of attempted therapy (e.g., tamponade tube placement). It is particularly tragic when errors of commission or omission result in a needless death from GI bleeding, especially in a young person.

Most deaths from GI hemorrhage are unavoidable. Patients with liver disease may have GI bleeding as the agonal event. Arterial or variceal hemorrhage may be the lethal event in patients with progressive, multisystem failure. It has long been said that the mortality rate from acute GI bleeding remains static at around 10 percent. Clearly, this figure is lower and falling owing to advances in resuscitation and the benefits of diagnostic and therapeutic GI endoscopy. In many countries, gastroenterologists and surgeons jointly manage GI hemorrhage. In large, specialist referral centers, this may occur in designated GI bleeding units. The advantages of a multidisciplinary approach to GI bleeding are obvious. To ensure the best outcome for every patient, collaborative management is essential. A clear understanding of end points, defining failure of medical management, should result in the patient proceeding without delay to radiologic or surgical intervention. Although this discussion focuses principally on

Table 1 Causes of Upper Gastrointestinal (GI) Bleeding

Common Causes of Profuse Upper GI Bleeding
Duodenal ulcer
Gastric ulcer
Esophageal varices
Dieulafoy's lesion*
Common Causes of Acute Upper GI Bleeding, But Rarely Profuse
Esophagitis
Gastritis
Gastric erosions
Duodenitis
Mallory-Weiss tear
Uncommon Causes of Profuse Upper GI Bleeding
Aortoduodenal fistula
Esophageal ulcer
Hemobilia
Vascular malformation
Malignancy (carcinoma, lymphoma)
Pseudoaneurysm in pancreatitis†
Generalized hemorrhagic states (e.g., ITP, DIC)
Duodenal-small bowel varices
Ulcerated diverticulum
Common Causes of Chronic GI Bleeding (May Present as Anemia)
Gastric ulcer
Duodenal ulcer
Esophagitis, gastritis, duodenitis
Vascular malformation‡
Malignancy (carcinoma, lymphoma)
Uncommon Causes of Chronic GI Bleeding
Diffuse vascular ectasia ("watermelon stomach")
Polyps
Ampullary carcinoma
Crohn's disease

*Arterial "point" bleeder.
†Splenic artery or pancreaticoduodenal artery.
‡Telangiectasia.
ITP, idiopathic thrombocytopenic, purpura; DIC, disseminated intravascular coagulation.

upper GI hemorrhage, the general principles apply to all causes of GI bleeding.

■ CAUSES

With few exceptions, massive bleeding from the upper GI tract is arterial or variceal in origin (Table 1). Severe erosive disorders such as esophagitis, gastritis, and duodenitis may occasionally cause significant fresh hemorrhage, but the "industrial strength" bleeding that is truly life threatening suggests that an "arterial pumper" or varix is hemorrhaging. There is an important lesson to be learned from this. One should be skeptical about accepting the diagnosis of, say, "gastritis" in a patient with obviously massive hemorrhage. Small arterial bleeding points (e.g., Dieulafoy's lesion) are easily missed by the inexperienced endoscopist. One must always be prepared to reassess the patient who suffers bleeding out of proportion to the apparent endoscopic diagnosis. If necessary, several endoscopies may be necessary to establish the true cause of bleeding. Although duodenal and gastric ulcers are the prime causes of upper GI arterial bleeding, acute esophageal ulcers and Mallory-Weiss tears can also produce this dramatic effect. Indeed, the original description of the Mallory-Weiss lesion was published as an autopsy series. Immunodeficient and immunosuppressed patients, such as those with AIDS, may develop deep, penetrating esophageal ulcers secondary to infection with cytomegalovirus or herpesvirus. A special case is the patient who has undergone previous surgery for aortic aneurysm. Infection of prosthetic aortic grafts can cause aortoenteric fistulas, which mimic acute ulcer hemorrhage. Failure to make the diagnosis of aortoenteric fistula after the initial hemorrhage often results in death (the second or subsequent hemorrhage is usually fatal). Hemorrhage from esophageal, gastric, or duodenal varices is rarely less than spectacular and often life-threatening. The reluctance of varices to stop bleeding (until portal venous pressure has dropped sufficiently low) is due in part to the lack of a muscular arterial wall that can contract and contain bleeding. With the widespread use of endoscopic sclerotherapy, gastric (and more distal) varices have become more common; obliterating esophageal varices by sclerotherapy (or other endoscopic techniques) simply shifts the venous pressure problem "downstream."

As previously stated, "-itis" rarely causes life-threatening hemorrhage. However, esophagitis, gastritis, or duodenitis coupled with a clotting disorder may render a relatively benign condition more serious. Patients on anticoagulant therapy may bleed profusely from relatively unimpressive lesions. Similarly, hemorrhage in the setting of disseminated intravascular coagulation (DIC) or other coagulopathy may be brisk and difficult to contain. Chronic (often occult) upper GI blood loss may result from esophagitis, gastritis, or duodenitis as well as from ulcers, polyps, and telangiectasia. "Watermelon stomach," named after its endoscopic appearance, is a peculiar and sometimes dramatic form of vascular ectasia. A broad spectrum of disorders ranging from burns, trauma, and sepsis to the stress of the perioperative period contribute to acute gastric erosions and ulceration. These may present with acute hemorrhage. It is common in intensive care unit (ICU) practice to suppress acid with continuous infusion of antacids through a nasogastric (NG) tube or intravenous (IV) administration of H_2 blocking agents such as ranitidine or cimetidine. For reasons that are poorly understood, these prophylactic measures are often unsuccessful. Presumably, some defect in mucosal resistance must be involved in stress ulceration. The role of *Helicobacter pylori* in the causation and persistence of duodenal ulcers is now being appreciated.

Benign and malignant tumors of the upper GI tract can cause bleeding that is usually slow, resulting in progressive anemia or iron deficiency. Massive bleeding from an upper GI tumor is most unusual. However, eroding tumors (e.g., carcinoma in the pancreas) or large friable tumors (e.g., ampullary carcinoma) present a major management problem, as they may be resistant to the usual hemostatic measures. Hemorrhage from eroding tumors is often a terminal event. Foreign bodies rarely cause GI bleeding. However, sharp objects (e.g., chicken bones, toothpicks) have been reported to cause life-threatening hemorrhage by perforating the esophagus, creating a fistula into the thoracic aorta. Finally, it should not be forgotten that a story of hematemesis or hematochezia (passing blood per rectum) may be *factitious;* i.e., this may be an invention to gain sympathy or hospital admission in patients with psychiatric illness or those who are seeking shelter and food (which are usually available in hospitals). Prison inmates may claim to have vomited or passed blood and not infrequently swallow foreign bodies (e.g., a razor blade with tape covering the sharpened edge) in an attempt to gain prison hospital privileges or a brief sojourn in a pleasant hospital environment.

■ CLINICAL PRESENTATION AND MANAGEMENT

When acute upper GI bleeding presents as hematemesis (vomiting of blood), there is little doubt about the diagnosis. Hematemesis must be distinguished from hemoptysis. This is usually evident from a careful history. Unexplained syncope should always raise suspicion of occult GI bleeding, especially in the elderly. A large volume of blood may be lost into the GI tract without immediate hematemesis or passage of fresh (or altered) blood per rectum. Blood in the GI tract constitutes a protein load that is partially digested and absorbed. Elevated blood urea nitrogen (BUN) is a manifestation of this phenomenon. The protein load may be sufficient to "push" a patient with hepatic insufficiency into encephalopathy. Any stable cirrhotic patient who develops encephalopathy without obvious reason should be suspected of having had occult GI bleeding and appropriately investigated.

A careful history often suggests the underlying diagnosis. For example, repeated retching followed by hematemesis, particularly in the setting of excessive alcohol intake, is a common presentation of a Mallory-Weiss tear. An elderly patient who has been using nonsteroidal anti-inflammatory drugs (NSAIDs) may well have a lesser-curve gastric ulcer. Known liver disease or portal hypertension should raise suspicion of esophageal, gastric, or other varices as the source of a major bleed. Patients with tumors involving or impinging on the GI tract may bleed as a complication of their disease. Chronic renal failure and aortic valve disease predispose to angiodysplasia, which can cause troublesome acute or chronic GI bleeding. An appropriate history and physical examination will reveal the patient with hereditary hemorrhagic telangiectasia (Osler-Weber-Rendu disease). A detailed physical examination may be impractical or undesirable when resuscitative efforts demand immediate attention. A brief but focused initial examination suffices in these circumstances.

The management of massive, acute upper GI hemorrhage is quite different from that of chronic GI blood loss, with or without anemia. Patients with massive upper GI bleeding present sooner or later to an emergency room. Initial evaluation is very important. The number one priority in managing patients with massive GI bleeding is *resuscitation.* There is little point in having the intern (or medical student) take a wonderfully detailed history as the patient becomes dangerously hypovolemic. This is not to say that the history is unimportant, but immediate and vigorous resuscitation is the key to a favorable outcome. When the acutely bleeding patient arrives in the emergency room, at least two large-bore IV cannulas should be placed for venous access. If the patient is markedly hypotensive, it is advisable to place him or her in a head-down position to maintain cerebral perfusion. However, the patient should not be left supine, as this favors reflux of gastric contents and aspiration. If not significantly orthostatic, the patient should preferably be nursed with the head of the bed elevated, to reduce the risk of free reflux of gastric contents into the esophagus and hypopharynx.

While blood is being cross-matched and prepared for transfusion, the circulating volume should be replaced, preferably by colloid (e.g., plasma protein solution, dextran) rather than crystalloid (e.g., saline solution). However, if only standard IV solutions are available, these are certainly better than nothing. The patient who has lost a significant amount of circulating volume is often confused and agitated owing to the effects of reduced cerebral perfusion. Providing supplemental oxygen by nasal cannula or face mask is a simple measure that may improve the patient's mental state. It is a sensible precaution to pass an NG tube for aspiration of stomach contents in patients with acute bleeding. However, care should be taken to ensure that the tip of the tube is well down in the stomach before it is attached to suction. Injury to the distal esophagus when mucosa is sucked into the holes of the NG tube is common and may compound the bleeding problem.

Hemodynamic Status

It is not enough to monitor peripheral blood pressure in patients with acute GI hemorrhage. Baroreceptor reflexes will maintain blood pressure until the circulating volume drops to a dangerously low level. At this point, the reflexes channeling blood away from the periphery to maintain perfusion of vital organs can no longer cope, and circulatory collapse rapidly ensues. This phenomenon can be particularly dramatic in young patients, who are often assumed to be more resistant to the effects of hypovolemia than they actually are. The status of circulating volume can easily be assessed by simple bedside maneuvers such as measuring orthostatic changes in blood pressure (e.g., with the patient lying and sitting, or before and after raising the legs). Where available, a central venous pressure (CVP) line should be placed. CVP is an accurate reflection of circulatory return to the heart; a progressively falling value should alert the physician to volume depletion. ICUs frequently use an indwelling arterial blood pressure monitor, which is a very sensitive method for following the patient's progress.

A risk that is not often considered in resuscitating patients with acute GI hemorrhage is the possibility of overtransfusion. This is particularly problematic in patients with variceal bleeding, who should not be transfused up to their normal hematocrit volume. Restoring the normal circulating volume will elevate portal venous pressure, which may precipitate further bleeding. It is advisable to limit blood transfusion in patients with varices to that required to bring the hematocrit up to around 30 percent. Excessive infusion of colloid or crystalloid solution may push even fit young patients into pulmonary edema. I have seen a fit sailor in his twenties develop gross pulmonary edema after rapid transfusion of 4 L of physiologic saline. This was "treatment" for a syncopal episode, which was wrongly attributed to occult GI bleeding. Not all patients with active bleeding can be stabilized by initial resuscitation. Investigation should not be unduly delayed in the face of persistent hemodynamic instability.

From time to time, a patient with massive bleeding from an upper GI source presents with syncope but no overt bleeding. When bleeding is suspected, an NG tube should be passed and the stomach lavaged to assess the return. If blood is recovered, this is a useful diagnostic test. However, a negative gastric aspirate and lavage means nothing; blood gushing from a duodenal ulcer may not reflux through the pylorus if spasm is present. It is even possible for a pool of blood lying in the dependent area of the stomach to be missed if the NG tube coils in the fundus. If upper GI hemorrhage is sufficiently rapid, the patient may pass fresh bloody stool. This raises the difficulty of distinguishing upper from lower GI hemorrhage.

Again, NG aspiration and lavage, if possible, is helpful. Although most fresh rectal bleeding arises within a short distance of the anus, the possibility of an upper GI source should always be considered.

Initial Management

Patients with acute GI bleeding should be kept fasting so that endoscopy can be undertaken when appropriate. Antacids and other liquid preparations (e.g., sucralfate) should not be given, as they obscure the endoscopic view. There is absolutely no place for barium studies in the assessment of acute upper GI bleeding. A baseline electrocardiogram and chest x-ray are useful. Particularly in patients over the age of 50, the hypovolemic insult of hemorrhage may precipitate ischemic events, including myocardial infarction. Amidst the turmoil that accompanies acute GI bleeding, these events may be "silent." The patient who remains persistently hypotensive and tachycardiac despite apparently adequate volume replacement should be assessed for possible myocardial infarction. Baseline chest radiography is helpful should the patient later require evaluation for possible aspiration.

Serial estimations of hemoglobin or hematocrit provide data regarding the efficacy of transfusion. However, in the early stages of significant GI bleeding, the patient can be hypovolemic with a *normal* hematocrit volume. It is a wise precaution in all patients with massive GI bleeding to check basic blood clotting parameters such as prothrombin time, partial thromboplastin time, and platelet count. When appropriate, a screen for DIC is worthwhile. Vitamin K acts too slowly to be of use in the acute situation for correction of a prolonged prothrombin time (e.g., in patients with liver disease). Fresh frozen plasma infusion is preferable, although significantly more expensive. Platelet infusions are rarely indicated unless the peripheral platelet count is exceedingly low (e.g., less than 10,000 per cubic millimeter). Patients who have been therapeutically anticoagulated with sodium warfarin require prompt reversal of this in the face of major hemorrhage.

Empiric use of vasopressin, metoclopramide, or other agents thought to be useful in the management of variceal bleeding is not recommended without confirmation of the diagnosis. Although vasopressin infusion has been used for over 30 years in acute variceal hemorrhage, there is still no well-designed study available to confirm its efficacy. Metoclopramide and somatostatin analogue have been used with reported benefit in acute variceal bleeding. Gastric lavage with ice-cold water should be avoided altogether. Thirty years ago there was a vogue for this procedure, as it was felt that cold water would cause a bleeding artery to go into spasm and stop bleeding, but this simply does not work. Gastric lavage with ice-cold water is an excellent way to render a patient hypothermic. In addition, the enzymes of the blood clotting cascade are rendered inactive at 4°C. In short, gastric lavage with ice-cold water is potentially dangerous and has no role in modern management of GI bleeding.

■ INVESTIGATION OF UPPER GASTROINTESTINAL BLEEDING

Endoscopy is now firmly established as the "gold standard" for the investigation of upper GI bleeding. Contrast studies have little to offer in the acute setting, and barium effectively obscures the endoscopic view. Radioisotope scans and angiography have an important role in carefully selected cases. Endoscopy in the setting of massive upper GI bleeding is one of the most demanding procedures (perhaps *the* most demanding) performed by gastroenterologists. The patient is often restless despite sedation. The endoscopic view may be suboptimal; the presence of blood and clot obscures common landmarks in the upper GI tract and may quickly disorient the inexperienced endoscopist. Accordingly, endoscopy in this setting should be performed by the most experienced endoscopist available.

If the patient has been difficult to resuscitate and remains hemodynamically unstable, it is likely that there is continuing arterial or variceal hemorrhage. Despite attempts at gastric lavage, preferably using a large-bore (e.g., Ewald) tube, the stomach and esophagus may contain a significant amount of blood. A patient with this amount of active hemorrhage is at significant risk from reflux of gastric and esophageal contents and subsequent aspiration. This risk is increased by sedating the patient for endoscopy and suppressing the gag reflex with pharyngeal anesthesia. It is strongly recommended that a cuffed endotracheal tube be placed before endoscopy in this setting. Even an apparently well-sedated patient may become agitated during attempts to pass an endotracheal tube. For this reason, it is wise to enlist the help of an anesthesiologist. Endotracheal intubation is particularly useful for endoscopy in patients with acute variceal hemorrhage, when attempts may be made to perform variceal sclerotherapy. It is most important for the anesthesiologist to understand that the endotracheal tube should not be removed before withdrawal of the endoscope. Indeed, it should remain in place with the cuff inflated for at least 5 minutes after the endoscopy has finished. Unfortunately, anesthesiologists without experience of managing patients in these circumstances may follow their usual operating room practice, which is to attempt extubation just as the surgeon is finishing wound closure. If the endotracheal tube cuff is deflated and the tube withdrawn as the endoscope is being removed, the patient may still regurgitate (or vomit) and aspirate, thereby negating any benefit prior to airway protection. If endotracheal intubation is not available, it is worth considering the use of an endoscopic overtube, through which an endoscope can be repeatedly advanced and withdrawn while maintaining access to the esophagus. This affords a degree of protection against aspiration.

Endoscopy should be performed with a large-channel therapeutic gastroscope whenever possible. If food debris or blood clots are present, the suction channel of a standard endoscope quickly becomes blocked. When a large amount of particulate matter is encountered, the endoscope should be withdrawn and a large-bore aspiration tube passed for further gastric lavage. It can take a long time to render the esophagus, stomach, and duodenum sufficiently clean to obtain a satisfactory endoscopic view. Repeated aspiration of blood and washing with sterile water or saline will eventually yield results unless there is continuing massive hemorrhage. It may be necessary to turn the patient to move a pool of blood and visualize a previously obscured part of the stomach. These manipulations are rendered considerably safer when endotracheal intubation has been performed and the patient is adequately sedated or anesthetized. Sometimes it is impossible to identify the source of acute upper GI bleeding at endoscopy because of a persistently obscured view. This is

Table 2 Endoscopic Therapy for Upper GI Hemorrhage

Chemical
Epinephrine solution (usually 1:10,000)
Hypertonic (1.8%) saline
Sclerosants
Ethanolamine oleate
Sodium morrhuate
Absolute alcohol
Thermal
Monopolar, bipolar, and multipolar electrocautery
Microwave coagulation
Laser (carbon monoxide, Nd-YAG)
Mechanical
"Endoscopic sewing machine"
Clips
Banding (varices)
Topical
Ferromagnetic
Clotting factors
Cyanoacrylate (SuperGlue)

particularly problematic in the patient with a bleeding lesion close to the gastroesophageal junction in the fundus of the stomach, where blood tends to pool.

When the diagnosis cannot be made at endoscopy, the alternatives are to await further stabilization and (hopefully) cessation of bleeding. Alternatively, the patient may proceed to a selective angiographic study by an interventional radiologist. It is always impressive how much better the endoscopic view is once bleeding has stopped and some hours have passed, allowing blood and clot to move "downstream." Great care must be taken to avoid attributing massive hemorrhage to a relatively insignificant finding. For example, one must be skeptical of a diagnosis of esophagitis or gastric erosions when bleeding clearly appears arterial or variceal in origin. If necessary, the patient should undergo further endoscopy, preferably by a more experienced endoscopist, whenever doubt remains.

Although an attractive technology, radioisotope nuclear medicine scanning has proved disappointing as a means of localizing gastrointestinal hemorrhage. The Tc^{99}-red cell "tagged" scan is very sensitive but lacks specificity for the bleeding site. Interventional radiologists often require a positive radionuclide scan before they will undertake arteriography. However, angiography should not be unduly delayed in an emergency. It goes without saying that the isotope (Tc^{99}) red cell scan will be positive when blood is pouring out of the patient's mouth or anus! A falsely localizing isotope scan (e.g., implicating jejunum when left colon is the culprit) may seriously delay appropriate mangement, and therefore isotope scans should be interpreted with caution and in context.

■ ENDOSCOPIC THERAPY

Endoscopy affords the opportunity to apply therapy in suitable circumstances. There are chemical, thermal, mechanical, and topical means of hemostasis at our disposal (Table 2). Since the decision to attempt endoscopic therapy has to be made at the time of the procedure, the necessary equipment should be available. For this reason, endoscopy carts that are used to transport equipment to ICUs and other sites of emergency procedures should be suitably equipped for therapeutic intervention.

Injection

Injection of chemicals that cause vasoconstriction (e.g., epinephrine) or an intense inflammatory reaction (e.g., sclerosants) is achieved using a thin needle housed within a plastic catheter. This so-called sclerotherapy needle can be used to inject agents other than sclerosants. As with all modes of endoscopic therapy, successful application requires access to the bleeding site. If the bleeding varix or artery can be identified and targeted, injection is usually straightforward. The current trend is to use larger volumes of epinephrine solution and smaller volumes of sclerosant agents. Although epinephrine (usually given as a 1:10,000 solution) has vasoconstrictive properties, increased tissue pressure due to the volume of injection may be equally important in hemostasis. There is considerable variation in injection technique for bleeding ulcers. However, it is common practice to make a number of injections around the bleeding point before making a final injection directly into it. The risk of systemic upset from epinephrine injection is more theoretical than real.

A number of sclerosant agents are available for endoscopic use; the most commonly used in the United States are ethanolamine oleate, sodium morrhuate, and absolute alcohol. These chemicals share the property of producing an intense inflammatory reaction at the site of injection. A common by-product of this phenomenon is local ulceration, which may be responsible for delayed complications, such as bleeding and perforation. Particular risk factors for complications of endoscopic sclerotherapy include repeated treatments at intervals of only a few days, and a sclerotherapy needle length greater than 5 mm. Certain sclerosant agents, such as absolute alcohol, may be particularly prone to cause ulceration.

Sclerotherapy

The technique for endoscopic sclerotherapy varies considerably and is usually a matter of personal preference. However, most endoscopists now prefer to inject directly into the varix (intravariceal) rather than between the varices (paravariceal), as the latter is associated with significant risk of ulceration. It is often difficult to be certain that the tip of the needle is inside the varix. For this reason, some endoscopists perform sclerotherapy under fluoroscopy using radiopaque contrast media mixed with the sclerosant to help visualize the local venous anatomy. If the injection is truly intravariceal, the sclerosant will opacify and outline the venous system of the varix. Another way to monitor this therapy is to connect a manometric (pressure measuring) system to the sclerotherapy needle. There is a separate chapter on management of bleeding esophageal varices.

Ulcer Injection

There is also no "correct" technique for injection therapy of bleeding ulcers. One commonly used technique is to make injections in a ring around the offending vessel before attacking the center. As stated previously, volume may be as important as chemical content when using injection therapy for hemostasis. Accordingly, a total of 5 to 10 ml of epinephrine solution (or sclerosant) may at times be appropriate. Care should be taken when using a sclerotherapy needle in the stomach, particularly proximal to the antrum, as the wall is thin compared with the esophagus. I have seen one elderly patient develop acute abdominal pain immediately after epinephrine injection into a high, lesser-curve ulcer. As there was no evidence of perforation, the pain was probably due to serosal or peritoneal irritation from a transmural injection.

Thermal Energy

A variety of methods of applying thermal energy to coagulate or vaporize tissue have been developed for use through an endoscope. These include monopolar, bipolar, and multipolar (heater) probes, microwave probes, and, of course, laser. Electrocautery probes (e.g., the heater probe) are metal-tipped catheters through which current can be applied to heat tissue. The depth of penetration of this thermal energy varies with the design of the probe. Clearly, it is wise to avoid uncontrolled, deep tissue coagulation because of the risk of perforation. For this reason, monopolar probes have fallen out of favor, as their depth of penetration is significant and difficult to control. To facilitate washing the target lesion and prevent adherence of coagulum, most modern electrocautery probes incorporate a water jet. A high-powered jet of water can be extremely useful when attempting to dislodge blood and clot from an ulcer. The ability to coagulate an ulcer base for hemostasis depends on suitable access. It is sometimes impossible to achieve direct or even tangential contact with the target using a heater probe.

A potential means of applying thermal energy from a distance is by use of a laser. Although so-called "contact" lasers have been developed, these have not proved particularly useful or effective for GI bleeding. The most commonly used laser for endoscopic work, including hemostasis, is the neodymium-yttrium argon garnet laser (Nd-YAG) system. This has the desired tissue penetration, although the surface tends to vaporize at higher energy levels. A modification of the standard Nd-YAG laser is the "water-guided" laser, which uses a jet of water as a conduit for the light beam. The water cools the surface sufficiently to prevent vaporization and its attendant problems. The laser is theoretically more flexible than the electrocautery probe, because it can be used from a distance, but in practice there is little difference. The bleeding site must be clearly targeted before the laser can be used effectively. One disadvantage of the laser compared with the electrocautery probe is that it cannot be applied tangentially. The laser also has the disadvantages of being very expensive and not easily portable. In particular, it is difficult to transport a laser system to the ICU for emergency treatment. In view of this, most endoscopy emergency carts are equipped with an electrocautery device (e.g., a heater probe) and some form of injection system for epinephrine or sclerosants.

Mechanical Devices

A variety of ingenious mechanical devices have been developed for hemostasis at endoscopy. These include the so-called endoscopic sewing machine, in which an ingenious device attached to the tip of a standard gastroscope provides the means to insert a running suture across the base of an ulcer or other bleeding site. Despite the obvious attractions of such a system, the endoscopic sewing machine remains experimental. A modified endoscopic catheter allows the placement of small metal clips at the bleeding site. The tissue to which these clips are attached eventually sloughs, releasing the clips, which are passed through the gut in the normal way. Again, despite the simplicity and effectiveness of such clips when accurately targeted, this technique has yet to catch on. Rubber-band ligation of hemorrhoids has been around for a long time. Recently, this inexpensive and apparently low-risk therapy has been applied to esophageal and gastric varices. A small banding device is attached to the tip of a standard gastroscope. The offending varix is identified and sucked into the lumen of the banding device. With the varix snugly seated, the device is triggered by the endoscopist. A small rubber band is released over the "neck" of the varix, constricting it; the varix subsequently thromboses and sloughs off. This seems to be a simple and so far relatively uncomplicated technique, particularly when compared with its "rival," variceal sclerotherapy. (The chapter on bleeding esophageal varices provides details on banding varices as well as sclerotherapy.) For bleeding varices that do not respond to sclerotherapy and banding, a variety of surgical devascularization and ligation procedures are available. However, as expected, when these procedures are used in high-risk patients (e.g., those with Child's class C), the morbidity and mortality rates are significant.

Topical Treatment

Topical treatments for acute upper GI bleeding have been introduced and evaluated, but none have stood the test of time. In general, they are cumbersome to apply and have uncertain results. The application of SuperGlue (cyanoacrylate) to an ulcer base or other bleeding diathesis is an attractive concept but a nightmare in practice. Despite every effort to avoid contaminating the endoscope channel, this is all but impossible. At best, getting SuperGlue in the endoscope channel necessitates an expensive repair. Apart from the technical difficulty, the tendency for cyanoacrylate to fall off the treated surface is a problem. There has also been at least one report of SuperGlue embolism associated with intravascular injection of the compound. A variety of blood clotting factors have been applied to bleeding sites in the hope of stimulating clot formation; again, the results are unpredictable. Finally, the ferromagnetic treatment is, if nothing else, interesting! Iron filings are liberally applied to the bleeding site, usually an ulcer. These are then drawn tightly into the base of the ulcer with a powerful external magnet, and the patient appropriately positioned. Needless to say, this particular technique has failed to gain widespread acceptance.

■ MANAGEMENT OF CONTINUED HEMORRHAGE

Mortality from upper GI bleeding has fallen in the last 20 years, thanks to early and effective resuscitation followed by endoscopic diagnosis and therapy. In particular, surgical morbidity and mortality has decreased because few patients now undergo exploratory surgery for bleeding without a probable site having been identified by endoscopy or vascular radiology. One cannot overemphasize the need for prompt and adequate resuscitation of patients with acute GI hemorrhage. Endoscopy is a useful diagnostic and therapeutic tool, but it is a mistake to rush into an endoscopic procedure before the patient has been stabilized. Sometimes it is impossible to stabilize a patient who has profuse arterial or variceal bleeding. In these circumstances, the risks of uncontrolled volume depletion outweigh those of endoscopy in the hypotensive patient. Endoscopy is not necessarily the appropriate first-line management for acute GI bleeding. For example, if the bleeding source is known (e.g., from a previous endoscopy) or strongly suspected (e.g., hemobilia in a patient with hepatoma), endoscopy may be superfluous and may delay appropriate management, such as angiography with embolism or surgery. As is true in medicine in general, each case needs to be managed on the basis of the best information available. A recent advance in the management of rebleeding from duodenal ulcers has been the discovery that eradicating *Helicobacter pylori* greatly reduces the risk.

Interventional Radiology

If an artery is actively bleeding, it may be possible to define the site of the diathesis by angiography. Vascular radiologists are specialists in this technique, which requires placement of an arterial imaging catheter, usually by the femoral route. Extravasation of contrast material injected through the catheter into the lumen of the bowel is good evidence of an active bleeding site. Selective catheterization of the celiac axis and mesenteric arteries often identifies the source of a persistent arterial hemorrhage. Once the site has been defined, an infusion of vasopressin may be effective in stopping the hemorrhage. This treatment is not without risks, as vasopressin acts by causing local vasospasm and therefore ischemia. The risk of intestinal (and cardiac) ischemia must always be considered, especially in arteriopathic patients. Infusion of vasoactive substances is a purely temporizing maneuver. If a more permanent "fix" is desired, a variety of materials can be injected into the artery to embolize the bleeding site. Homologous blood clot can be used if the effect is not intended to be permanent. The thrombolytic system of the body will reverse the effect of clot embolus within hours to days. A foreign material that resists digestion, such as Gelfoam or metal springs, will permanently block the vessel. Again, the risks of ischemia and infarction must be considered. In addition, embolization beyond the intended site is a potential risk.

What should be done when acute GI bleeding is intermittent? This is always a difficult problem. If a bleeding site cannot be identified by endoscopy, the vascular radiologist is often invited to perform a study. However, the yield of such a study will be low if the artery is not actively bleeding. For this reason, the vascular radiologist may defer angiography until a radionuclide (e.g., technetium-labeled red cell) scan has been performed. Radionuclide scans are relatively insensitive but are often positive if bleeding exceeds 1 to 2 ml per minute. A positive radionuclide scan gives the vascular radiologist some confidence that the study will have a chance of detecting the offending vessel. If angiography is performed and a bleeding vessel cannot be defined, one alternative is to leave the catheter in place for 24 to 48 hours. This catheter can subsequently be used to perform angiography should the bleeding site "open up." In this event, it is also useful for therapy (vasopressin infusion or embolization).

Surgery for Bleeding

No surgeon likes to open a patient's abdomen to search for a source for bleeding without some idea of the task involved. Even if the exact bleeding site has not been identified, the endoscopist (or radiologist) may be able to give the surgeon a good idea of the rough vicinity of the lesion. For example, repeated pooling of blood in the gastric fundus is highly suggestive of a lesion within a few centimeters of the gastroesophageal junction. However, blood and clot may often defeat the most aggressive therapeutic endoscopist. Surgery for acute bleeding should not only address the immediate problem but prevent a recurrence. For example, if the likely cause of the bleeding is a peptic ulcer, the surgeon may wish to perform a definitive ulcer operation (e.g., including vagotomy or antrectomy). It is very rare now for a patient to undergo total gastrectomy because a bleeding site cannot be identified. This is a major operation with considerable physiologic sequelae.

For everyone involved in managing patients with acute GI bleeding, a small bowel bleeding source may be the most challenging. It is fortunate that few patients with acute upper GI hemorrhage have a source in the small bowel, as this is undoubtedly a blind area for imaging of all kinds. It is rare for small bowel bleeding to be acute, although occasionally a tumor (usually benign) may ulcerate. The legendary bleeding Meckel's diverticulum is a rare beast indeed. In my experience, a Meckel's isotope scan usually gives a false-positive result.

Intraoperative endoscopy may be of considerable help in identifying the source of small bowel bleeding. The operating room is a rather hostile environment for the gastroenterologist, so some understanding and cooperation between gastroenterologist and surgeon are essential. Using gas-sterilized equipment, a long endoscope (usually a colonoscope) can be advanced all the way down the small bowel through a high enterostomy incision. This is often made distal to the ligament of Treitz. The endoscope is advanced by the surgeon, who threads it through the loops of bowel by hand, from the outside; it usually is possible to reach all the way to the ileocecal valve. It is a wise precaution to have the surgeon cross-clamp the ileocecal valve or cecum itself to prevent massive inflation of the colon during endoscopy. This makes returning the bowel to the abdomen difficult and will win no friends in the operating room. When the endoscope is withdrawn, gas can be aspirated and the small bowel returned to the abdomen.

Intraoperative enteroscopy provides two benefits. First, abnormalities may be seen directly using the endoscope; a pathologic condition usually is more easily seen when the endoscope is withdrawn. Second, light from the endoscope transluminates the bowel wall, making it relatively simple to identify vascular abnormalities such as a large telangiectasia. Whenever an abnormality is seen by either the endoscopist or surgeon, a suture should be placed in the bowel wall at that site. After the procedure, the enterostomy incision is repaired. If an abnormality has been discovered, this may be dealt with in a variety of ways. Vascular lesions may be simply oversewn or, if they are multiple, a segment of bowel may be resected with an end-to-end anastomosis. Similarly, a small bowel tumor or Meckel's diverticulum may be dealt with by segmental resection.

Peroral enteroscopy is an evolving technique that requires a particularly long endoscope. (There is a separate chapter on enteroscopy.) The so-called sonde-type enteroscope is weighted, and once positioned in the proximal small bowel is left, often for many hours, to progress by peristalsis. When fluoroscopy reveals that the enteroscope has reached the distal ileum, it is withdrawn by slow traction and the bowel inspected. Sonde enteroscopy is time-consuming and rather unpleasant for the patient, and so-called "push" enteroscopy has come into favor. It is said that in cases of occult GI bleeding, "push" enteroscopy will yield a diagnosis in 30 percent. At present, enteroscopy is limited to specialist centers only, in view of the expense of the equipment involved and the expertise required. However, as endoscope technology continues to advance, it is likely that whole bowel endoscopy will become a reality in the not too distant future.

Bleeding as the Terminal Event in Very Ill Patients

Some deaths from GI bleeding are unavoidable. For example, acute GI hemorrhage may be the agonal event in a patient with liver failure or multisystem disease. In these circumstances, the patient may have a "living will" or similar document indicating that they do not wish to have their lives unduly prolonged. These wishes must be respected. Short of this, it is sometimes appropriate to limit the volume of transfusion. Great care has to be taken when this is done to ensure that everyone involved in the patient's care, including the family, is comfortable with the decision.

Suggested Reading

Baillie J, Yudelman P. Complications of endoscopic sclerotherapy of esophageal varices. Endoscopy 1992; 24:284–291.

Choudari CP, Elton RA, Palmer KR. Age-related mortality in patients treated endoscopically for bleeding peptic ulcer. Gastrointest Endosc 1995; 41:557–560.

Fullarton GM, Birnie GG, MacDonald A, Murray WR. The effect of introducing endoscopic therapy on surgery and mortality rates for peptic ulcer hemorrhage: a single center analysis of 1125 cases. Endoscopy 1990; 22:110–113.

Fusamoto H, Hagiwara H, Meren H, et al. A clinical study of acute gastrointestinal hemorrhage associated with various shock states. Am J Gastroenterol 1991; 86:429–433.

Koyama T, Fujimoto K, Iwakiri R, et al. Prevention of recurrent bleeding from gastric ulcer with a nonbleeding visible vessel by endoscopic injection of absolute ethanol: a prospective, controlled study. Gastrointest Endosc 1995; 42:128–131.

Laine L, El-Newihi HM, Migikovsky B, et al. Endoscopic ligation compared with sclerotherapy for the treatment of bleeding esophageal varices. Ann Intern Med 1993; 119:1–8.

Laine L. The long-term management of patients with bleeding ulcers: *Helicobacter pylori* eradication instead of maintenance antisecretory therapy (editorial). Gastrointest Endosc 1995; 41:77–79.

Lin HJ, Perng CL, Lee FY, et al. Endoscopic injection for the arrest of peptic ulcer hemorrhage: final results of a prospective, randomized comparative trial. Gastrointest Endosc 1993; 39:15–19.

Loizou LA, Bown SG. Endoscopic treatment for bleeding peptic ulcers: randomized comparison of adrenaline injection and adrenaline injection + Nd:YAG laser photocoagulation. Gut 1991; 32:1100–1103.

Oxner RB, Simmonds NJ, Gertner DJ, et al. Controlled trial of endoscopic injection treatment for bleeding from peptic ulcers with visible vessels. Lancet 1992; 339:966–968.

Panes J, Viver J, Forne M. Randomized comparison of endoscopic microwave coagulation and endoscopic sclerosis in the treatment of bleeding peptic ulcers. Gastrointest Endosc 1991; 37:611–616.

Sung JY, Chung SCS, Low JM, et al. Systemic absorption of epinephrine after submucosal injection in patients with bleeding peptic ulcers. Gastrointest Endosc 1993; 39:20–22.

Swain CP. Operative endoscopy in acute upper GI bleeding—indications, techniques, prognosis. Hepatogastroenterology 1991; 38:201–206.

GASTROENTERITIS

Douglas R. Morgan, M.D., M.P.H.
Robert L. Owen, M.D.

Strictly speaking, gastroenteritis is any inflammation of the mucous membrane of the stomach or the intestines. However, it usually refers to infectious diarrhea, an acute syndrome that may be accompanied by fever, nausea, vomiting, abdominal pain, dehydration, and weight loss. This chapter provides an overview of the infectious enteritides. Other chapters consider food poisoning, traveler's diarrhea, antibiotic-associated diarrhea, and sexually transmitted enteric infections.

In developed countries, gastroenteritis, like the common cold, is frequent and annoying but usually does not require a physician visit, laboratory evaluation, or antibiotic treatment. On a global scale it is second only to cardiovascular disease as a cause of death. It remains the leading worldwide cause of childhood death and of years of productive life lost, with approximately 12,600 deaths per day. Annual per person attack rates range from 1.5 to 5 in the United States to 7 to 20 in the Third World.

■ PATHOPHYSIOLOGY

The normal gastrointestinal (GI) tract is remarkably efficient at fluid reabsorption. Normally, of the 1 to 2 L of fluid ingested orally and the 7 L that enter the upper tract from saliva, gastric, pancreatic, and biliary sources, less than 200 ml is excreted daily in the feces. In addition, there is a net fluid flux of approximately 40 to 50 L per day secreted and absorbed across the surface of the small intestine. Thus, small increases in secretory rate or decreases in the absorptive rate can easily overwhelm the colonic absorptive capacity of 2 to 3 L per day. This leads to diarrhea, defined as more than three bowel movements or more than 300 g per day.

Infection with bacteria, viruses, and parasites that produce gastroenteritis usually follows fecal-oral transmission. Host

Table 1 Host Defenses

FACTOR	DISEASE STATE
Barrier	
Gastric acid	Achlorhydria (antisecretory agents [H_2-RA, PPI], HIV, gastric surgery, atrophic gastritis)
Mucosal integrity	Mucositis (high-dose chemotherapy)
Intestinal motility	
Peristalsis	Blind loop, antimotility drugs, hypomotility states (diabetes, scleroderma)
Enteric microflora	Recent antibiotics, infancy
Sanitation (personal, community)	Contaminated water
Intestinal immunity	
Phagocytic	Neutropenia
Cellular	HIV
Humoral	IgA deficiency

defenses that protect the human intestine are reviewed in Table 1. The principal defenses are the physical barrier of the mucosa itself and gastric acidity. A gastric pH below 4 will rapidly kill over 99 percent of ingested organisms, although rotavirus and protozoal cysts can survive. Patients with achlorhydria due to chronic atrophic gastritis, gastric surgery, human immunodeficiency virus (HIV) infection, or use of acid antisecretory agents are at increased risk for infectious diarrhea. Destruction of the mucosal barrier, as with mucositis associated with high-dose chemotherapy, predisposes to gram-negative sepsis. In gastroenteritis there is an increase in peristalsis, which propels organisms along the GI tract, analogous to the cough clearing the lungs. The intestinal flora form a critical element of the host defense, in terms of both quantity and composition. The small intestine and colon contain approximately 10^4 and 10^{11} organisms per gram, respectively. Over 99 percent of the colonic bacteria are anaerobes. Their production of fatty acids with an acidic pH, as well as their competition for mucosal attachment sites, prevent colonization by invading organisms. At the extremes of age, in children and the elderly, and after recent antibiotic use, the flora are altered, and the risk of gastroenteritis increased. Inadequate community sanitation and impairment of intestinal immunity also contribute to gastroenteritis.

Virulence plays a role in acute infectious diarrhea. Whether an individual ingests an inoculum sufficient to establish clinical gastroenteritis is directly related to community sanitation and personal hygiene. Most organisms require an inoculum of 10^5 to 10^8 to establish infection. Exceptions include *Shigella* and protozoa such as *Giardia, Cryptosporidium,* and *Entamoeba,* which may cause diarrhea when only 10 to 100 organisms are ingested. Bacteria produce several types of toxins that lead to different clinical syndromes, including enterotoxin (watery diarrhea), cytotoxin (dysentery), and neurotoxin. Botulinum toxin is the classic example of a preformed neurotoxin, but interestingly, both *Staphylococcus aureus* and *Bacillus cereus* also produce neurotoxins that act on the central nervous system to produce emesis. Adherence and invasion factors facilitate colonization and contribute to virulence. Various forms of *Escherichia coli* express the gamut of virulence factors (Table 2).

Table 2 Virulence Factors

FACTORS	EXAMPLES
Inoculum size	*Shigella, Entamoeba, Giardia*
Adherence	Cholera, EAEC
Invasion	*Shigella,* EIEC, *Salmonella typhi, Yersinia*
Toxins	
Enterotoxin	Cholera, ETEC (LT, ST), *Salmonella*
Cytotoxin	*Shigella, Clostridium difficile,* EHEC
Neurotoxin	*Clostridium botulinum, Staphylococcus aureus, Bacillus cereus*

EAEC, enteroadherent *Escherichia coli;* EIEC, enteroinvasive *E. coli;* ETEC, enterotoxigenic *E. coli;* LT, heat-labile enterotoxin; ST, heat-stable enterotoxin; EHEC, enterohemorrhagic *E. coli.*

■ CLINICAL SYNDROMES

The acute infectious diarrheas can be divided into noninflammatory, inflammatory, and invasive (Table 3). Most attacks are caused by organisms from the noninflammatory, or secretory, category. The bacteria in this group, such as *Vibrio cholerae* and enterotoxigenic *E. coli* (ETEC), typically secrete an enterotoxin that affects the small intestine, producing a large volume of watery diarrhea without fecal leukocytes. Most forms of viral gastroenteritis, e.g., rotavirus and Norwalk virus, also fall into this group. The inflammatory diarrheas affect the colon, causing frequent small-volume stools, often with fecal white cells and either gross or occult blood. Fever, tenesmus, and bloody diarrhea are characteristic of dysentery. Some bacteria causing inflammatory diarrhea produce cytotoxins. The invasive or penetrating diarrheas cause enteric fever; *Salmonella typhi* is the prototype. Typhoid bacteria invade the Peyer's patches of the distal ileum, then disseminate and multiply in the reticuloendothelial system to produce systemic disease.

Certain subpopulations of patients with gastroenteritis should be under close surveillance because of the organisms involved, the potential for severe disease, and the possibility of need for intervention (Table 4). Food-borne disease should be considered in outbreaks of acute GI symptoms affecting two or more persons. The most common causes include *Salmonella* spp., *S. aureus, Shigella* spp., and *Clostridium perfringens.* Patients with acquired immunodeficiency syndrome (AIDS) are predisposed to a number of unique infections (*Cryptosporidium,* cytomegalovirus) and severe manifestations of otherwise common infections *(Salmonella, Campylobacter).* The microbial pathogens responsible for traveler's diarrhea depend on the region visited. ETEC is the most commonly isolated organism in all locations, ranging between 20 and 60 percent of isolates in areas of Asia and Latin America, respectively. Acute infectious proctitis, which is often sexually transmitted, leads to tenesmus, hematochezia, and rectal pain. Syphilis, gonorrhea, and chlamydia must be considered in addition to the more common organisms of gastroenteritis. The incidence of sexually transmitted proctitis is decreasing in the AIDS era with safer sex practices. Other important subpopulations include patients with antibiotic-associated diarrhea and those from hospitals and chronic care facilities.

Helicobacter pylori infection is a form of gastroenteritis

Table 3 Clinical Syndromes

	NONINFLAMMATORY	INFLAMMATORY	INVASIVE
Syndrome	Watery diarrhea	Bloody dysentery	Enteric fever
Site	Small intestine	Colon	Ileum
Stool			
Volume	Large	Small	—
Fecal WBC	Absent	Present	Present
Common organisms			
Bacteria	*V. cholerae* ETEC	*Shigella* spp. *Salmonella* spp. *C. jejuni* EIEC	*Salmonella typhi* *Yersinia* spp. *Brucella*
Viruses	Rotavirus Norwalk	—	—
Parasites	*Giardia* *Cryptosporidium*	*Entamoeba*	*Entamoeba*

WBC, white blood cells; ETEC, enterotoxigenic *E. coli;* EIEC, enteroinvasive *E. coli.*

Table 4 Causative Agents by Clinical Presentation

POPULATION	BACTERIA	VIRUSES	PARASITES	OTHER
Food poisoning	*Salmonella* *Staphylococcus aureus* *Shigella* *Clostridium perfringens* *Bacillus cereus*	Norwalk Hepatitis A	*Trichinella* *Giardia* *Cryptosporidium*	Ciguatera Histamine fish
AIDS	*Salmonella* *Campylobacter* *Shigella* MAC	CMV	*Cryptosporidium* *Isospora belli* *Microsporidia*	AIDS enteropathy
Traveler's diarrhea	*Escherichia coli,* ETEC *Shigella* *Aeromonas* *E. coli,* other	Rotavirus	*Giardia*	No pathogen (40%)
Acute proctitis	*Neisseria gonorrhoeae* *Chlamydia* *Treponema pallidum* *Shigella* *Salmonella*	HSV Condyloma, HPV CMV HIV	*Entamoeba* *Cryptosporidium*	
Institutional settings	*Shigella* *Campylobacter jejuni*	Rotavirus	*Giardia* *Cryptosporidium*	
Antibiotic associated	*Clostridium difficile*			*Candida albicans*
Seafood ingestion	*Vibrio* spp.		Anisakidae	

CMV, cytomegalovirus; AIDS, acquired immunodeficiency syndrome; MAC, *Mycobacterium avium* complex; ETEC, enterotoxigenic *E. coli;* HSV, herpes simplex virus; HPV, human papilloma virus; HIV, human immunodeficiency virus.

localized to the stomach. This gram-negative spiral bacterium is a cause of acute gastritis, chronic superficial gastritis, peptic ulcer disease, and possibly gastric adenocarcinoma and mucosa-associated lymphoid tissue (MALT) lymphoma. At least 25 percent of people in the United States are infected and 50 percent worldwide. Approximately 90 percent and 65 percent of duodenal ulcers and gastric ulcers respectively are caused by *H. pylori.* There is substantial prospective evidence that eradication of the organism prevents recurrence of peptic ulcers. No convincing data demonstrate either an association between *H. pylori* and nonulcer dyspepsia or that its eradication in this setting relieves symptoms. Documentation of infection is done with serology, the urea breath test, and gastric biopsy (urease test, culture, histology).

Table 5 Focal Leukocytes

PRESENT	VARIABLE	ABSENT
Campylobacter *Shigella* EIEC, EHEC	*Salmonella* *Yersinia* *C. difficile* *Vibrio parahemolyticus* Noninfectious causes Ischemic colitis Inflammatory bowel disease	Toxigenic bacteria ETEC, EPEC, EAEC Viruses Parasites

ETEC, enterotoxigenic *Escherichia coli;* EPEC, enteropathogenic *E. coli;* EAEC, enteradhesive *E. coli;* EIEC, enteroinvasive *E. coli;* EHEC, enterohemorrhagic *E. coli.*

■ EVALUATION OF THE PATIENT

The vast majority of cases of acute gastroenteritis are self-limited and do not require laboratory evaluation or antibiotic therapy. The history, physical exam, and bedside stool examination suffice in 90 percent of attacks, as does symptomatic therapy. Only 10 percent of infectious diarrhea cases require either laboratory studies or antibiotic treatment.

The history should focus on the severity of disease and the risk factors for specific types of infectious diarrhea. The patient should be questioned about duration of symptoms, fever, abdominal pain, tenesmus, and dehydration. The description of the diarrhea is important: frequency, volume, and any blood, pus, or mucus. Diarrhea lasting longer than 2 to 3 weeks qualifies as chronic, has an alternative differential diagnosis, and should be fully investigated. Inquiry should also be made as to factors that may place the patient in a specific subpopulation at increased risk for significant infection. Examples include recent international travel, camping, antibiotic use within the past 2 months, human immunodeficiency virus (HIV) disease or risk factors, other immunosuppression including prednisone therapy, anal eroticism, raw seafood consumption, household contacts of day care workers or children, and the potential for a common source outbreak (e.g., friends or relatives with similar symptoms, such as significant vomiting).

The physical exam is important in gauging the severity of the disease. Orthostasis, tachycardia, decreased skin turgor, and dry mucous membranes are signs of significant dehydration. Any fever, abdominal tenderness, and skin rashes should be documented.

All patients should undergo a rectal examination and have a fresh stool specimen evaluated. Cup specimens are preferred, as there is evidence that swab and diaper specimens have decreased sensitivity. The stool should be described as watery or with gross blood, pus, or mucus. Microscopic examination of the stool is facilitated by the methylene blue stain. A wet mount is prepared with two drops of methylene blue mixed with fecal mucus; 2 minutes should be allowed for adequate staining of the leukocyte nuclei prior to high-power microscopy of the coverslipped slide. Table 5 lists the degree of association of the usual enteric pathogens with fecal leukocytes. With fecal leukocytes there is overlap between inflammatory and noninflammatory diarrheas.

The history, physical examination, and bedside stool evaluation are screening steps prior to further laboratory evaluation and possible need for treatment. Most patients with self-limited noninflammatory infectious diarrhea require only symptomatic therapy. Laboratory evaluation is indicated for three groups: patients with severe disease (fever higher than 38.5°C [101.3°F], dehydration, stool with gross blood or pus), patients from the aforementioned subpopulations, and patients with documented fecal leukocytes or stool occult blood. The initial laboratory evaluation should include complete blood counts, serum electrolytes, and stool processed for bacterial culture *(Salmonella, Shigella, Campylobacter)* and for ova and parasite detection (three sets). The probability of a positive stool culture is less than 5 percent for patients without occult blood or fecal leukocytes, 20 percent with either one positive, and 50 percent with both positive. Fever and fecal leukocytes also have a positive predictive value of about 50 percent for bacterial pathogens.

Additional studies depend on the clinical situation. Stool testing for *C. difficile* cytotoxin is appropriate in patients with antibiotic use within the past 2 months. Differentiation of pathogenic and nonpathogenic strains of *E. coli* requires serotyping in specialized laboratories and is not generally indicated. *Yersinia* spp. require special culture techniques. Sigmoidoscopy with biopsy should be considered for cases of acute proctitis, dysentery, and persistent infectious diarrhea. Rarely, colonoscopy, barium enema, or upper GI series with small bowel follow-through may be helpful.

The initial evaluation of AIDS-associated diarrhea should include stool acid-fast bacilli smear for *Cryptosporidium* and *Isospora belli,* and up to six sets of specimens for ova and parasites; sigmoidoscopy and endoscopy with colon and small bowel biopsies are indicated in the setting of negative studies and persistent diarrhea with or without weight loss.

■ THERAPY

Rehydration is the initial goal of management. This can usually be accomplished with oral fluids. Oral rehydration solutions (ORS) have decreased worldwide cholera mortality from 50 percent to 1 percent. The World Health Organization ORS is made up of 3.5 g sodium chloride, 2.5 g sodium bicarbonate, 1.5 g potassium chloride, and 20 g glucose per liter of water. Prepared forms are available in solution (e.g.,

Table 6 Symptomatic Therapy for Diarrhea

GENERAL	INTRALUMINAL	ANTIMOTILITY	ANTISECRETORY
Fluid therapy	Bulking agents	Opiates	Bismuth subsalicylate
ORS	Psyllium	Loperamide	Octreotide
IV	Adsorbents	Diphenoxylate	
Diet therapy	Kaolin-pectin	Codeine	
	Attapulgite	Tincture of opium	
	Cholestyramine	Anticholinergics	
	Bacterial agents	Atropine	
	Lactobacilli	Scopolamine	
	Saccharomyces		

ORS, Oral rehydration solution; IV, intravenous.

Pedialyte) and packets (e.g., Orlyte). One example of the various homemade recipes is alternating 8 oz fruit juice containing ½ tsp honey and ¼ tsp salt with 8 oz water containing ¼ tsp baking soda. Another one recommends mixing 1 quart of water with 8 oz orange juice, ¾ tsp salt, 4 tbs sugar, and 1 tsp baking soda. Recommendations vary regarding the use of commercial drinks such as Gatorade. Rice-based ORS may also be used. The goal is the passage of relatively dilute urine every 2 to 4 hours. Patients are advised to eat judiciously and to avoid dairy products (transient lactose intolerance with mucosal inflammation), alcohol (cathartic effect), caffeine (increases intestinal motility), and carbonated drinks (gastric distention with reflex colonic contraction). Diet sodas should be avoided because of insufficient sugars to facilitate transport. Patients with severe dehydration require intravenous therapy.

In addition to rehydration, symptomatic therapy includes agents to control the diarrhea. These include bulking agents, antimotility drugs, and antisecretory medications (Tables 6 and 7). Antimotility agents should not be used if there is a possibility of a severe inflammatory diarrhea. The most effective drugs are the opiates, bismuth subsalicylate (BSS), and octreotide. Loperamide (Imodium) is probably the drug of choice, as it does not cross the blood-brain barrier. Diphenoxylate atropine (Lomotil) has both antimotility and antisecretory activity. BSS also has antibacterial properties. *Saccharomyces boulardii* may have a role in recurrent *Clostridium difficile* colitis, although its mechanism of action is unknown. Psyllium may improve mild diarrhea. Despite their popularity, kaopectate, cholestyramine, lactobacilli, and the anticholinergics have not been shown to be effective.

Severe nonspecific AIDS diarrhea should be treated in stepwise fashion with loperamide (Imodium) 2 to 4 mg orally four times a day, diphenoxylate-atropine 1 or 2 tabs orally four times a day, tincture of opium (DTO 0.5 to 1 ml) orally four times a day, and octreotide 100 to 500 µg SC three times a day, increasing the dose 200 µg every 3 days until response.

Antibiotic therapy is indicated in a limited subset of cases of acute infectious diarrhea (Table 8). Standard indications include symptomatic infections with certain bacteria (*Shigella*, enteroinvasive *E. coli, C. difficile, V. cholerae,*) the sexually transmitted pathogens, and the parasites. Specific therapy is generally not recommended for *Campylobacter, Yersinia, Aeromonas,* noncholera *Vibrio*, and other strains of *E. coli* (EPEC: enteropathogenic *E. coli;* EAEC: enteroadherent *E. coli;* and EHEC: enterohemorrhagic *E. coli*). Treatment

Table 7 Nonantibiotic Therapy

AGENT	DOSING	COMMENTS
Opiates		
Diphenoxylate-atropine	2 tabs or 10 ml PO q.i.d.	
Loperamide	2 mg PO q3h prn	Maximum 16 mg/day Initial dose 4 mg
Tincture of opium	0.5–1 ml PO q4–6 h	
Antisecretory		
Bismuth subsalicylate (Pepto-Bismol)	2 tabs or 30 ml PO qh	Maximum 8 doses/day
Octreotide	100–500 µg SC t.i.d.	

Table 8 Antibiotic Therapy by Pathogen (see specific chapters for more details of therapy)

PATHOGEN	THERAPY	DURATION	COMMENTS
Bacteria			
Campylobacter	Ciprofloxacin 500 mg PO b.i.d.	5–7 days	
	Erythromycin 250–500 mg PO q.i.d.		
Clostridium difficile	Metronidazole 250 mg PO q.i.d.	7–10 days	Vancomycin use should be restricted to metronidazole registered cases to minimize vancomycin-resistant enterococcus
	Vancomycin 125 mg PO q.i.d.		
ETEC*	Ciprofloxacin 500 mg PO b.i.d.	5 days	
	TMP-SMX 160–800 mg (DS) PO b.i.d.		
Salmonella	Ciprofloxacin 500 mg PO b.i.d.	5 days	See text for treatment indications
	Amoxicillin 1 g PO q.i.d.		
	TMP-SMX 160–800 mg (DS) PO b.i.d.		
	Chloramphenicol 500 mg PO q.i.d.	(14 days)	
*Shigella**	Ciprofloxacin 500 mg PO b.i.d.	5 days	
	TMP-SMX 160–800 mg (DS) PO b.i.d.		
*Vibrio cholerae**	Tetracycline 500 mg q.i.d.	3 days	
Yersinia	Ceftriaxone 1 g IV q.d.	5 days	For severe infection
	Ciprofloxacin 500 mg PO b.i.d.		
Parasites			
*Entamoeba**	Metronidazole 750 mg PO t.i.d.	10 days	
*Giardia**	Metronidazole 250 mg PO t.i.d.	5 days	

*Treatment clearly indicated. The use of antimicrobial agents for the other listed pathogens depends on the clinical situation. See specific chapters for more details.
ETEC, enterotoxigenic *Escherichia coli;* TMP-SMX, trimethoprim-sulfamethoxazole; DS, double strength.

of *Salmonella* may prolong fecal shedding and thus is usually indicated only for typhoid fever or significant concurrent disease (e.g., immunosuppression, malignancy, sickle cell anemia, prosthetic devices, sepsis), and very young or old patients. Empiric therapy is indicated in severe diarrhea with dehydration or sepsis and symptomatic traveler's diarrhea. Suggested empiric antibiotics while awaiting stool culture results include ciprofloxacin 500 mg orally twice a day or trimethoprim-sulfamethoxazole 160–800 mg (DS) orally four times a day for 5 days. *H. pylori* eradication regimens in the setting of peptic ulcer disease are outlined in the chapter *Helicobacter pylori.*

In summary, acute gastroenteritis, while common, is usually a self-limited disease, aided in some cases by symptomatic therapy. Laboratory evaluation and possible antibiotic treatment are indicated for severe diarrhea with dehydration, inflammatory or invasive disease, and certain patient populations.

Suggested Reading

Blacklow NR, Greenberg HB. Viral gastroenteritis. N Engl J Med 1991; 325: 252–264.

Friedman SL. Gastrointestinal manifestations of the acquired immunodeficiency syndrome. In: Sleisenger MH, Fordtran JS, eds. Gastrointestinal disease. 5th ed. Philadelphia: WB Saunders, 1993: 239–267.

Gorbach SL. Infectious diarrhea and bacterial food poisoning. In: Sleisinger MH, Fordtran JS, eds. Gastrointestinal disease. 5th ed. Philadelphia: WB Saunders, 1993: 1128–1173.

Guerrant RL, Bobak DA. Bacterial and protozoal gastroenteritis. N Engl J Med 1991; 325:327–340.

Levine MM, Savarino S. The treatment of acute diarrhea. In: Surawicz C, Owen RL, eds. Gastrointestinal and hepatic infections. Philadelphia: WB Saunders, 1995: 519–536.

National Institutes of Health Consensus Development Panel. *Helicobacter pylori* in peptic ulcer disease. JAMA 1994; 272:65–69.

Powell DW, Szauter KE. Nonantibiotic therapy and pharmacotherapy of acute infectious diarrhea. Gastroenterol Clin North Am 1993; 22:683–707.

SECRETORY DIARRHEA

Judy H. Cho, M.D.
Eugene B. Chang, M.D.

Active secretion of water and electrolytes is a major component of most diarrheal diseases, including those caused by infection, inflammation, and circulating secretagogues. These conditions can be acute self-limited processes or chronic lifelong disorders. When active secretion is the major component of the disease, the diarrhea is typically profuse and watery (often more than 1,000 g per day). Although typically referred to as "secretory diarrheas," these disorders arise from impaired absorption of water and electrolytes as well as increased secretion. The diagnosis of secretory diarrhea is suggested when the concentration of stool ($Na^+ + K^+$) $\times$ 2 approximately equals total stool or blood osmolality. In addition, in most cases of secretory diarrheas, the diarrhea continues despite fasting for 24 to 48 hours.

The focus of this chapter is on general considerations in the treatment of secretory diarrheas as well as the use of more specific agents for chronic diarrheas. Infectious diarrheas make up a large percentage of diagnosed secretory diarrheas, and specific antibiotic treatments for individual disorders are discussed in other chapters. Specific therapies associated with bile acid- and fatty acid-induced diarrheas are also discussed in other chapters. In inflammatory bowel disease (IBD), the local production of inflammatory mediators that both increase secretion and decrease absorption of intestinal water and electrolytes contributes significantly to the diarrhea observed with acute flare-ups. The main treatment of secretory diarrhea associated with IBD is therefore directed toward decreasing the underlying inflammatory process. This chapter focuses on the general medical management of secretory diarrheas, including hormone-related secretory diarrheas resulting from VIPomas and the carcinoid syndrome.

■ FLUID AND ELECTROLYTE REPLACEMENT

Initial considerations in the treatment of patients with secretory diarrheas should include replacement of lost fluid and electrolytes. Typically, patients presenting with secretory diarrheas exhibit dehydration, hypokalemia, and metabolic acidosis, although metabolic alkalosis is seen in some cases of secretory diarrhea. Since hypokalemia results from intestinal losses, it should be corrected promptly with potassium replacement as total body volume is being replaced, taking advantage of the avid urinary potassium retention. However, the presence of high urinary [K^+] in the setting of diarrhea resulting from laxative abuse should suggest the possibility of concomitant diuretic abuse. The severity of initial presentation determines whether oral or intravenous replacement should be attempted. The concentration of sodium and potassium in replacement solutions is not critical in the absence of renal insufficiency. When renal insufficiency does exist, the concentrations of sodium and potassium replacement need to be lowered. In short bowel syndrome, the

Table 1 Pharmacologic Agents Used in the Treatment of Secretory Diarrheas

MEDICATION	INDICATION	SIDE EFFECTS	COMMENTS
AGENTS COMMONLY IN USE			
Opiates	First-line therapy for mild to moderate diarrheas	Abdominal discomfort, constipation, toxic megacolon, nausea, vomiting, CNS (drowsiness, respiratory depression); Lomotil has anticholinergic side effects	Minimal or no risk of physical dependence; loperamide (Imodium) does not cross BBB and does not have CNS side effects
Octreotide	Severe diarrhea not responsive to other therapy; major indications: VIPomas, carcinoid syndrome, diabetic diarrhea, AIDS enteropathy	Increased incidence of gallstones, mild abdominal pain/nausea that resolves with continued therapy, malabsorption from pancreatic insufficiency, mild hypo/hyperglycemia	Use limited by cost and subcutaneous administration
Alpha$_2$-agonists	Major use is in treatment of diabetic diarrhea; also used in short bowel syndrome	Orthostatic hypotension, drowsiness	Taper dose when discontinuing therapy
Corticosteroids	Inflammatory diarrheas, VIPomas unresponsive to octreotide alone	Standard glucocorticoid side effects	Use in secretory diarrheas limited by side effects
Prostaglandin synthetase inhibitors	Inflammatory diarrheas	Generally mild and reversible	Decrease AA metabolites, which are potent secretagogues
EXPERIMENTAL OR UNPROVED AGENTS			
Calcium channel blockers	Reported use in chronic infectious diarrheas	Cardiovascular	Often not useful as a single agent
Trifluorperazine and chlorpromazine	Reported use in cholera, VIPomas	Retinopathy, movement disorders, blood dyscrasias, abnormal liver function tests	Monitor side effects carefully

AA, arachidonic acid; AIDS, acquired immunodeficiency syndrome; BBB, blood-brain barrier; CNS, central nervous system.

concentration of sodium in replacement solutions often needs to be higher.

The principle behind oral rehydration therapy is that while absorption of sodium by some carriers is impaired in secretory diarrheas, absorption via Na-glucose and Na-amino acid cotransporters is intact. Therefore, glucose-based oral rehydration solutions improve fluid and electrolyte balance by increasing intestinal absorption. As intestinal secretion and absorption are separate processes, oral rehydration therapy may temporarily worsen diarrhea. The present World Health Organization (WHO) formulation contains 3.5 g of sodium chloride, 1.5 g of potassium chloride, 2.9 g of trisodium citrate dihydrate, and 20 g of glucose per liter of water. More recently, rice-based oral rehydration solutions containing glucose polymers have been shown to not only increase absorption, but also decrease stool volume output and provide greater caloric intake without increasing osmolality.

■ PHARMACOLOGIC AGENTS

Pharmacologic agents used to treat secretory diarrheas can be divided into those accepted agents commonly in use and experimental or unproved agents (Table 1). Currently used pharmacologic agents act by (1) increasing contact time between luminal contents and the intestine, thereby increasing absorption; (2) increasing the absorption efficiency of enterocytes directly; and (3) interrupting cellular signal transduction events (secondary messengers) that lead to intestinal secretion.

Accepted Agents Commonly in Use

Opiates

Opiates are a mainstay of treatment of mild to moderate secretory diarrheas. They increase smooth muscle tone throughout the gastrointestinal (GI) tract and decrease peristaltic contractions. Consequently, there is a decrease in gastric emptying time as well as an increase in transit time. The resultant increased contact time between intestinal contents and mucosa produces increased absorption. In addition, naturally occurring opiates and some synthetic opiates (e.g., loperamide) increase the absorptive efficiency of enterocytes and possess antisecretory properties.

Synthetic opioids such as diphenoxylate (Lomotil), 2.5 mg diphenoxylate plus 25 μg atropine per tablet, and loperamide (Imodium), 2 mg loperamide per tablet, have much more potent GI effects than morphine, and also have much fewer central nervous system (CNS) effects than morphine and thus a smaller abuse potential. The recommended maximal dose of both Imodium and Lomotil is eight tablets a day or 16 mg loperamide and 20 mg diphenoxylate a day, although 32 mg Imodium has been used without untoward effects. For acute symptoms, two tablets of Imodium are given, followed by an additional tablet with each loose stool. Two tablets of Lomotil four times a day can be given acutely for initial control and the dose tapered subsequently.

At large doses, diphenoxylate does possess some CNS effects, while loperamide does not cross the blood-brain barrier; thus, even in large doses, the latter appears to have few CNS side effects. The potential for abuse with diphenoxylate has been reduced by combining it with atropine in commercial preparations (Lomotil), so that unpleasant anticholinergic side effects will result if high doses are used. Other side effects of synthetic opiates include abdominal discomfort, nausea, intractable constipation, and, in some cases, toxic megacolon.

Octreotide

Octreotide (Sandostatin) is a synthetic octapeptide that is a long-acting somatostatin analogue. Like somatostatin, octreotide suppresses secretion of gastroenteropancreatic peptide hormones such as VIP and serotonin. Thus, a major use of octreotide has been in the treatment of severe diarrhea associated with metastatic carcinoid syndrome and VIPomas. Octreotide also inhibits VIP, serotonin, and prostaglandin E_1-induced anion secretion in both small and large intestine and has been shown to stimulate sodium chloride (NaCl) absorption in animal studies. Therefore, octreotide has also been used to treat a broad array of non–hormone-related secretory diarrheas. Acquired immunodeficiency syndrome (AIDS)-related secretory diarrhea unassociated with identifiable pathogens occurs commonly, and in nonrandomized trials octreotide has been reported to decrease stool output effectively. The effectiveness of octreotide in AIDS-associated secretory diarrheas where a specific pathogen has been identified has also been reported. Carcinomas of the medullary thyroid elaborate calcitonin, an intestinal secretagogue. Although the treatment of choice is surgical removal, cases of metastatic medullary thyroid carcinoma with severe secretory diarrhea may respond to octreotide therapy. However, in our experience, diarrhea resulting from medullary thyroid carcinoma represents one of the few predominantly secretory diarrheas not responsive to octreotide therapy. Secretory diarrheas associated with intestinal graft-versus-host disease that do not initially respond to prednisone therapy have been reported to improve with octreotide therapy. Other reported uses of octreotide in the treatment of diarrheas include therapy for intestinal amyloidosis, short bowel syndrome, chemotherapy-induced diarrheas, villous adenoma-associated secretory diarrheas, and Zollinger-Ellison syndrome.

The use of octreotide is limited to cases of severe diarrhea refractory to other treatments because of its high cost and also because it is presently available only in injectable form. The initial dosage is 50 μg subcutaneously two to four times a day up to a recommended maximal daily dose of 1500 μg per day in divided doses two to four times a day, although there is little experience with daily doses above 750 μg. The half-life of octreotide ranges from 90 to 120 minutes, and peak concentrations are attained approximately 1 hour after administration.

Side effects of octreotide include the development of nausea and mild abdominal cramping, which usually resolve on continued therapy; and pain at the injection site, which can be minimized by injecting slowly and warming the solution before injection. Mild hypo- or hyperglycemia can result from alterations in secretion of the counter-regulatory hormones insulin, glucagon, and growth hormone. Some patients report lighter stools than usual, and a few (less than 2 percent) develop fat malabsorption from decreased pancreatic enzyme secretion, which often abates with time, presumably owing to subsequent adaptation. Because octreotide inhibits gallbladder emptying, it has been associated with the development of gallbladder sludge and gallstones. No recommendations are available currently on the advisability of preventive therapy for patients requiring long-term octreotide.

Alpha$_2$-Agonists

Nonadrenergic innervation of the intestinal mucosa is known to promote absorption. Since patients with refractory diabetic diarrhea invariably have autonomic neuropathy, concomitant noradrenergic denervation in the intestine may contribute significantly to the secretory diarrhea seen in these patients. In addition, alpha$_2$-agonists increase intestinal transit time, thereby increasing contact time for absorption. Clonidine, an alpha$_2$-agonist, has been used successfully to treat diabetic diarrhea, as discussed in the chapter on diabetic diarrhea. Dosage is started at 0.1 mg per day and increased slowly. The maximal effective dose is 1.0 to 1.2 mg per day in divided doses, although lesser amounts of 0.4 to 0.6 mg per day in divided doses are usually needed. Transdermal preparations of clonidine applied weekly can also be used and provide more stable therapeutic levels. Clonidine has also been used to treat diarrhea associated with short bowel syndrome in combination with opiates, and for alcohol withdrawal.

A major limitation to the use of clonidine has been cardiovascular toxicity, especially the development of orthostatic hypotension. Newer formulations of alpha$_2$-agonists should decrease these problems in the future. When discontinuing clonidine, the dose should be tapered slowly over 4 to 5 days to avoid withdrawal symptoms of rebound hypertension, headache, nausea, and vomiting.

Corticosteroids

In addition to their anti-inflammatory actions, corticosteroids alleviate diarrhea by increasing electrolyte absorption. This effect is mediated by corticosteroid-induced increased expression of absorptive carrier proteins. Improved absorption may contribute to the early improvement in diarrhea seen in acute flare-ups of IBD treated with corticosteroids. Although side effects limit their use in most cases of secretory diarrhea, corticosteroids have been used to treat VIPoma-associated diarrhea refractory to octreotide alone.

Prostaglandin Synthetase Inhibitors

Mucosal production of arachidonic acid (AA) metabolites in inflammatory disorders such as IBD or infectious diarrheas contributes to acute exacerbations of diarrhea, as a number of inflammatory mediators are potent secretagogues. Therefore, prostaglandin synthetase inhibitors such as 5-acetylsalicylic acid (5-ASA) derivatives should be useful in the treatment of inflammatory diarrheas. While the beneficial effect of 5-ASA derivatives in the treatment of IBD is primarily through preventing and decreasing inflammation, antisecretory effects may play a significant role in the early improvement in diarrhea seen in the treatment of acute flares.

Bismuth subsalicylate (Pepto-Bismol) is used primarily for prophylaxis and treatment of acute infectious diarrheas. Its beneficial effects are mediated through both antimicrobial effects and anti-inflammatory actions of the salicylate moiety. Long-term use of bismuth compounds has been associated with the development of encephalopathy. This is a rare complication with currently available preparations, but long-term bismuth usage should be avoided and drug-free intervals introduced.

Adsorbent Agents
Adsorbent agents such as psillium husk, methylcellulose, and calcium polycarbophil avidly absorb intraluminal water, resulting in firmer stool consistency and a decreased number of stools. However, they do not affect the total amount of fluid or electrolytes excreted and may actually increase stool volume. Therefore, they are not used to treat diarrheas resulting primarily from increased secretion. An exception to this is the use of the adsorbents cholestyramine or colestipol, anion exchange resins that bind bile salts, to treat bile salt-induced secretory diarrheas.

Experimental or Unproved Agents
Calcium Channel Blockers
Since one of the intracellular mediators of intestinal secretion is calcium, calcium channel blockers, which decrease intracellular calcium, could be useful in the treatment of secretory diarrheas. In fact, one of the well-known side effects of verapamil is constipation. Although not established therapy, verapamil has been used to treat chronic infectious diarrheas. However, it is often not useful as a single agent.

Neuroleptics
Neuroleptic agents such as trifluoroperazine and chlorpromazine act to decrease intestinal secretion by binding to the calcium-calmodulin complex and inactivating it. Their use has been reported for the treatment of VIPomas and cholera. Significant side effects are common and include development of retinopathy, movement disorders, blood dyscrasias, and abnormal liver function test results, which must be monitored carefully.

Berberine
Berberine is a plant alkaloid that has been used as an antidiarrheal agent in Asia for years. Animal studies suggest that it inhibits secretion and increases absorption. In addition, it may have an antimicrobial action in infectious diarrheas. Extensive experimental trials are lacking at this point, and it remains an experimental agent.

Leukotriene Synthesis Inhibitors
An alternative mechanism for decreasing mucosal production of AA metabolites is via inhibition of the leukotriene pathway. Specific inhibitors of this pathway such as MK-886, an inhibitor of 5-lipoxygenase activating protein (FLAP), are under development and study.

■ SPECIAL CONSIDERATIONS

VIPomas
The major mediator of the pancreatic cholera syndrome of watery diarrhea and hypokalemia is VIP. Since the profuse diarrhea is inadequately controlled with traditional agents such as opioids, the mainstay of initial management is currently octreotide. Octreotide suppresses secretion of VIP and decreases intestinal secretion. Whether it affects tumor size has been somewhat controversial. Enough cases have been documented to suggest that octreotide does exert a beneficial effect on tumor growth rate, but this beneficial effect is temporary and unpredictable in individual patients.

The dosage of octreotide required to attain control of the diarrhea varies greatly, ranging from 150 to 750 μg per day in divided doses; however, doses over 450 μg per day are usually not required. After initial control of the diarrhea is attained, precise localization of the VIPoma and surgical excision should be attempted, as 50 percent of all VIPomas are benign. The tumor most often originates in the pancreas, but other sites include the stomach and upper duodenum. Bronchogenic carcinoma, ganglioneuroma, or ganglioneuroblastoma can also secrete VIP and cause this syndrome.

When surgical excision is not possible, debulking of large tumors may be helpful if symptoms are poorly controlled by medical management. The number of these cases is decreasing with the advent of octreotide. Some patients initially controlled with octreotide subsequently relapse and require higher doses or the addition of corticosteroid therapy. Prednisone, 40 mg per day, can be used for initial management, with the dose tapered as control of symptoms is maintained. 5-Fluorouracil and streptozotocin have resulted in objective improvement in metastatic disease.

Carcinoid Syndrome
The carcinoid syndrome consists of watery diarrhea, flushing, right-sided endocardial fibrosis, and bronchospasm resulting from excessive production of serotonin and/or other bioactive amines. Almost all cases of carcinoid syndrome involve metastatic disease; however, since the tumor is very slow-growing, long-term medical management of symptomatic secretory diarrhea is often required. Octreotide is the mainstay of medical management; as with VIPomas, it acts by decreasing hormonal secretion as well as through more general effects on intestinal secretion and absorption. Improvement of symptoms is observed in 92 percent of patients started on octreotide, and 66 percent exhibit biochemical evidence of diminished serotonin release, such as a decrease in urinary 5-hydroxyindoleacetic acid levels. As with VIPomas, octreotide exerts a beneficial, if temporary, effect on tumor growth.

Initial control of symptoms is usually achieved with doses between 100 and 600 μg per day. As with VIPomas, patients may relapse after achieving initial control and require higher doses. The median daily maintenance dose is 450 μg per day. In addition to producing symptomatic relief of diarrhea, octreotide improves the flushing associated with the carcinoid syndrome. Cyproheptadine, 4 to 12 mg three times a day, has also been used to treat diarrhea associated with the carcinoid syndrome, but this agent rarely improves the symptoms of flushing.

Suggested Reading

Cello JP, Grendell JH, Basuk P, et al. Effect of octreotide on refractory AIDS-associated diarrhea. Ann Intern Med 1991; 115:705–710.

Ely P, Dunitz J, Rogosheske J, Weisdorf D. Use of a somatostatin analogue, octreotide acetate, in the management of acute gastrointestinal graft-versus-host disease. Am J Med 1991; 90:707–710.

Gaginella TS, O'Dorisio TM, Fassler JE, Mekhijian HS. Treatment of endocrine and nonendocrine secretory diarrheal states with sandostatin. Metabolism 1990; 39:172–175.

Gorbach SL. Bismuth therapy in gastrointestinal diseases. Gastroenterology 1990; 99:863–875.
Kvols LK. Therapy of the malignant carcinoid syndrome. Endocrinol Metab Clin North Am 1989; 18:557–568.
O'Dorisio TM, Mekhjian HS, Gaginella TS. Medical therapy of VIPomas. Endocrinol Metab Clin North Am 1989; 18:545–555.
Proceedings, Sandostatin, State of the Art. Metabolism 1992; 41(9 Suppl 2).
Smith MB, Chang EB. Antidiarrheals and cathartics. In: Wolfe MM, ed. Gastrointestinal pharmacotherapy. Philadelphia: WB Saunders. 1993: 139–156.
Zheng BY, U KM, Lu RB, et al. Absorption of glucose polymers from rice in oral rehydration solutions by rat small intestine. Gastroenterology 1993; 104:81–85.

ANTIBIOTIC-ASSOCIATED DIARRHEA

John G. Bartlett, M.D.

Diarrhea is a relatively common complication of antibiotic use. Nearly all agents with an antibacterial spectrum of activity have been implicated. The great majority of cases are either enigmatic or due to *Clostridium difficile.*

DIAGNOSTIC STUDIES

The usual method for identifying cases of diarrhea due to *C. difficile* is the toxin assay. The standard technique is with a tissue culture assay for detection of cytotoxin for toxin B; more recently many laboratories have used alternative detection methods, most commonly the enzyme immunoassay (EIA) for detection of toxin A or toxin A plus B. Other tests include the latex test for a nontoxic protein product of *C. difficile,* polymerase chain reaction, dot-blot assay, and culture for *C. difficile.* Some authorities consider the culture to be the most sensitive, and some use it in combination with the toxin assay. Studies of the EIA compared with the tissue culture assay indicate that it is moderately sensitive and quite specific and has the advantage of providing results within 2 to 3 hours.

Other diagnostic tests include fecal leukocyte exam, preferably using lactoferrin. Anatomic studies, usually sigmoidoscopy or colonoscopy, were far more common before the general availability of *C. difficile* toxin assays in the late 1970s. This also was when pseudomembranous colitis (PMC) was a relatively common complication due to the lack of treatment to interrupt the natural history of the disease. Endoscopy is still indicated in some patients who are severely ill, have negative toxin assays, or pose other problems in diagnosis. Computed tomography (CT) and x-ray studies with contrast are sometimes done for other conditions and will occasionally show changes that are highly suggestive of antibiotic-associated colitis due to *C. difficile;* nevertheless, these are substantially less sensitive than endoscopy.

CLOSTRIDIUM DIFFICILE

The first principle of treatment is discontinuation of the implicated agent. Supportive measures include fluid and electrolyte restoration and avoidance of antiperistaltic agents such as loperamide. Many patients respond to simple withdrawal of the implicated antimicrobial agent and appropriate supportive care.

Antibiotic treatment directed against *C. difficile* is readily available and highly effective. The usual agent is vancomycin or metronidazole (Table 1). Many consider vancomycin to be the gold standard, the preferred agent for patients who are seriously ill. Response is impressive; generally fever resolves within 24 hours and diarrhea over an average of 4 to 5 days. Overall response rates are usually reported at 95 to 100 percent. This drug has ideal pharmacokinetic properties and is active against all strains of *C. difficile* in vitro. Vancomycin is poorly absorbed with oral administration, so that mean levels in the colon lumen are several hundredfold higher than the minimum inhibitory concentration. This is a disease whose putative agent is entirely restricted to the colon lumen, so that tissue levels are irrelevant to therapy. The disadvan-

Table 1 Treatment of *C. difficile* Diarrhea and Colitis

NONSPECIFIC MEASURES

Discontine antibacterial agents; if continued treatment is required, change to another agent infrequently associated with this complication or continue implicated agent while giving oral vancomycin.
Provide supportive measures.
Avoid antiperistaltic agents.
Use enteric isolation precautions for hospitalized patients.

SPECIFIC TREATMENT

Antimicrobial agents if symptoms are severe or persist
- Oral agent (preferred)
  - Vancomycin 125 mg PO q.i.d., 7–14 days*
  - Metronidazole 250 mg PO t.i.d., 7–14 days*
- Parenteral agents (only until oral agents are tolerated):
  - Metronidazole 500 mg IV q12h

Alternative treatments
- Anion exchange resins
  - Cholestyramine 4 g packet PO t.i.d., 7–14 days*
  - Cholestipol 5 g packet PO t.i.d., 7–14 days
- Alter fecal flora
  - Lactinex or alternative lactobacillus preparation 1 g packet PO q.i.d., 7–14 days

*Established efficacy.

Table 2 Methods to Manage Multiple Relapses of *C. difficile* Diarrhea or Colitis

Metrondiazole or vancomycin PO × 10–14 days followed by cholestyramine (4 g t.i.d.) with lactobacilli (as Lactinex 1 g PO q.i.d.) × 4 weeks.
Vancomycin 125 mg PO q.i.d. × 10–14 days followed by vancomycin 125 mg PO qd (once daily) × 4 weeks.
Vancomycin 125 mg PO q.i.d. × 4–6 weeks, then taper over 4–8 weeks.
Vancomycin 125 mg PO q.i.d. plus rifampin 600 mg PO qd × 10–14 days.
Vancomycin 125 mg PO q.i.d. plus *Saccharomyces boulardii* 500 mg b.i.d. (investigational drug) × 10–14 days, then *Saccharomyces boulardii* 500 mg b.i.d. for 4 weeks.
Intravenous gamma globulin 400 mg/kg q 3 weeks (reported primarily in pediatric patients).
Rectal instillation of feces: 50 g fresh stool from healthy donor in 500 ml saline delivered by enema (rare use due to concern for transmissible agents).
Broth cultures of bacteria from healthy donors: stool culture using stool from healthy donor, 10 strains selected based on in vitro inhibition of *C. difficile* grown in broth culture. 10^9/ml, 2 ml of each mixed in anaerobic glovebox with 180 ml saline and given by enema.
Lactobacillus G-G 10^{10}/day (investigational drug) or Lactinex 1 g PO q.i.d. (available over the counter) × 4 weeks.

tages of vancomycin treatment are relatively high rates of relapse, relatively high costs, occasional poor tolerance to the drug, and implication of its use in promotion of vancomycin-resistant *Enterococcus faecium.* This last problem has resulted in the strong suggestion to avoid oral administration of vancomycin to hospitalized patients.

Metronidazole is active against nearly all strains of *C. difficile* and has a track record of efficacy comparable with that of vancomycin in comparative trials. Theoretic disadvantages are that the therapeutic trials have not generally included patients with advanced disease or PMC, and the low levels of the drug in the colon lumen due to almost complete absorption. This drug is substantially less expensive than vancomycin. Most authorities recommend it as initial therapy for patients who have moderate illness and for nosocomial infections of *C. difficile.* Vancomycin is reserved for seriously ill patients and those who fail to respond to metronidazole. The rate of relapse for metronidazole is comparable with that for vancomycin.

Relapses of *C. difficile* diarrhea are seen only with antibiotic therapy. The typical clinical presentation is recurrence of the initial symptoms 3 to 10 days after discontinuation of metronidazole or vancomycin. Patients generally respond to readministration of either agent, but occasional patients have multiple relapses that can be a major therapeutic problem; several therapeutic options are summarized in Table 2. The problem of relapses has prompted many to scrutinize the necessity of treating all patients, since many resolve after simple discontinuation of the implicated agent. For this reason a common recommendation is to restrict antibiotic therapy to patients with any of the following indications: (1) persistent disease despite discontinuation of the implicated agent; (2) the necessity to continue antibiotic therapy for the infection being treated; (3) severe disease as indicated by devastating diarrhea or diarrhea associated with systemic complaints such as fever and systemic toxicity; or (4) the endoscopic demonstration of PMC or advanced colitis.

■ OTHER CAUSES

Most patients with antibiotic-associated diarrhea or colitis have negative diagnostic studies for *C. difficile* toxin and have no established agent or mechanism. Some feel the best explanation is dysbiosis of the colonic flora, which simply means a disruption in the concentrations and types of bacteria that are presumably critical for maintaining homeostasis in the colonic lumen. The antimicrobial agents implicated are the same that cause *C. difficile* disease. However, some of the clinical differences include the facts that this form of diarrhea is usually dose related, symptoms usually resolve when the implicated agent is discontinued or reduced in dose, systemic symptoms are unusual, it is rarely serious or life threatening, and colitis (fecal leukocytes, fever, or evidence of colitis by endoscopy or CT scan) is unusual. This form of diarrhea also tends to be sporadic, whereas *C. difficile* may be endemic or epidemic within hospitals or nursing homes.

The usual treatment for antibiotic-associated diarrhea with a negative toxin assay is to discontinue the implicated agent; most patients respond. Patients with serious disease, evidence of colitis, or persistent symptoms after discontinuation of antibiotics should have repeat toxin assays for *C. difficile.* The tissue culture assay rarely shows false negative results, but this degree of confidence does not apply to any of the alternative tests now used by the great majority of laboratories. Patients with persistent or serious symptoms in the face of negative assays should undergo anatomic studies using endoscopy and exploration of alternative causes, for example idiopathic inflammatory bowel disease, diarrhea due to enteric pathogens, diarrhea due to other medications, lactase deficiency, and irritable bowel syndrome.

Suggested Reading

Bartlet JG. Antibiotic-associated diarrhea. Clin Infect Dis 1992; 15:573–578.

Gerding DN, Johnson S, Peterson LR, et al. *Clostridium difficile*-associated diarrhea and colitis. Infect Control Hosp Epid 1994; 16:459–464.

Fekety R, Shah AB. Diagnosis and treatment of *Clostridium difficile* colitis. JAMA 1993; 269:71–75.

McFarland LV, Mulligan ME, Kwok RY, et al. Nosocomial acquisition of *Clostridium difficile* infection. N Engl J Med 1989; 320:204–210.

Merz CS, et al. Comparison of four commercially available rapid enzyme immunoassays with cytotoxin assay for detection of *Clostridium difficile* toxin(s) from stool specimens. J Clin Microbiol 1994; 32:1142–1147.

CROHN'S COLITIS

Mark A. Peppercorn, M.D.

Although Crohn's disease may involve any portion of the gastrointestinal (GI) tract, approximately one-third of patients have disease limited to the small intestine, about one-half have ileal and colonic involvement, and the remaining one-sixth have colitis only. Of those with colonic disease, the rectum or rectosigmoid is spared in approximately 50 percent. One-third of patients have perianal lesions and up to one-fifth may have associated manifestations of skin, joint, and liver disease.

The clinical course of this idiopathic disorder, which involves the bowel in a transmural fashion, is one of unpredictable spontaneous exacerbations characterized by episodes of crampy abdominal pain and diarrhea, with or without bleeding. Microperforations often present with an acute picture of localized peritonitis resembling appendicitis or diverticulitis. Fistula to surrounding organs such as the bladder lead to complications that may dominate the clinical picture, while progressive segmental fibrosis may lead to episodes of partial colonic obstruction. Recently, it has been appreciated that colon cancer may be as much of a long-term risk for patients with Crohn's colitis as for those with ulcerative colitis.

The diagnosis of Crohn's colitis today is usually established endoscopically with findings of focal ulcerations surrounded by edematous mucosa. Colonic biopsies show focal acute and chronic inflammation and may reveal granulomas in up to one-third of patients. Barium x-ray examinations characteristically show segmental disease with skip areas and asymmetric involvement of the bowel wall. Crohn's colitis needs to be distinguished from acute forms of colitis (bacterial, amebic, viral, ischemic) by appropriate investigations; from the other major cause of chronic colitis, ulcerative colitis, which involves only the mucosa of the colon in a continuous fashion beginning in the rectum; and from both diverticulitis and obstructing or perforating colon cancer.

■ THERAPEUTIC ALTERNATIVES

Drugs are the principal form of therapy for acute exacerbations of Crohn's colitis and may also be useful in sustaining remissions. For many years, sulfasalazine has been the mainstay for such patients, and now a variety of oral and topical aminosalicylates based on the structure of sulfasalazine can be used for those intolerant of, allergic to, or unresponsive to sulfasalazine.

Standard oral corticosteroids such as prednisone and methylprednisolone and topical hydrocortisone, used alone or in combination with sulfasalazine, have proved effective for outpatients with exacerbations of Crohn's colitis, while parenteral forms including hydrocortisone, methylprednisolone, and prednisolone as well as adrenocorticotropic hormone have been used for severe and fulminant disease. There are now emerging topical and oral preparations of rapidly metabolized steroids that may be as effective with regard to anti-inflammatory activity but with less toxicity.

There has been increasing interest in the use of antibiotics for active Crohn's disease. Metronidazole has become an established agent to treat both Crohn's colitis and perianal Crohn's disease. Ciprofloxacin appears to be useful for perianal disease and may, along with other broad-spectrum antibiotics, have a primary role in the treatment of active ileal and colonic disease. Moreover, antituberculous agents look promising for both active and remitted disease in selected patients.

The therapy for Crohn's colitis has been greatly influenced in the past decade by increasing acceptance of the immunomodulators 6-mercaptopurine (6-MP) and azathioprine, which appear effective both in active disease and in sustaining remissions of Crohn's colitis. For patients intolerant of or refractory to these agents, there have been promising results from trials with cyclosporine and methotrexate, and in very preliminary studies of anti-CD4 monoclonal antibodies as well as alpha-interferon and antibody to tumor necrosis factor alpha (TNF-α). For patients intolerant or refractory to these agents, methotrexate has become an effective alternative. Although cyclosporine has proven effective in inducing remission in active Crohn's disease, its use in low dose as a long-term maintenance agent has been disappointing. Finally early studies with an antibody to Tumor Necrosis Factor look very promising in refractory patients.

Other innovative modalities that may be of benefit in a given refractory patient include T-cell apheresis, immunoglobulin infusions, oxygen-derived free radical scavengers, and, for those with severe perineal disease, hyperbaric oxygen.

Finally, in patients with well-established symptoms, one should not forget the role of antidiarrheal drugs such as loperamide, diphenoxylate with atropine, and codeine as well as cholestyramine for those with nonstenosing ileal disease and ileal resection, and anticholinergic agents such as hyoscyamine, propantheline, and dicyclomine.

In addition to drug therapy, nutritional treatment with modification of the diet and use of enteral and parenteral feedings as primary therapy should be considered in selected patients. Behavior modification and psychotherapy, with and without the use of psychotropic agents, may be important for certain individuals. Finally, surgery may be necessary for patients with Crohn's colitis who are refractory to medical therapy or who suffer an irreversible complication of the disease.

■ PREFERRED APPROACHES TO THE USE OF SPECIFIC DRUGS

Sulfasalazine

Since its introduction into clinical medicine over 50 years ago, sulfasalazine has been a mainstay of treatment for both ulcerative colitis and Crohn's disease. Controlled trials have shown the effectiveness of the drug in active Crohn's ileocolitis and colitis. Although many physicians who use the drug are convinced that it also works in a subset of patients with ileitis alone, most controlled trials have not shown efficacy in this patient group. Similarly, although controlled trials have not shown sulfasalazine to be effective in maintaining remission in Crohn's colitis, in contrast to its accepted role as prophylaxis in remitted ulcerative colitis, many clinicians keep patients with Crohn's colitis on the drug indefinitely once they have achieved remission.

Sulfasalazine has been my therapy of choice for any patient with mild to moderate symptoms of Crohn's colitis. I begin at an initial dose of 500 mg orally twice daily, with advancement over several days to 1 g orally three to four times daily. Since sulfasalazine may interfere with dietary folate absorption, I add folic acid, 1 mg per day. Clinical improvement usually occurs within 3 to 4 weeks, at which time the dose can be tapered to 2 or 3 g per day and maintained for an additional 3 to 6 months. The response to therapy is judged almost exclusively on clinical grounds, including the signs and symptoms of abdominal pain, diarrhea, and bleeding as well as improvement in laboratory parameters, including hematocrit, white blood cell (WBC) count, sedimentation rate, and albumin. There is not a good correlation between endoscopic appearance and clinical response, so follow-up with endoscopy is generally not indicated.

If the patient achieves remission and prefers not to be on long-term treatment, the drug can be stopped. For those who wish to continue therapy despite the lack of clear evidence of long-term benefit, maintenance therapy with 2 g sulfasalazine is continued. Some, however, believe that higher doses (3 to 4 g per day) are needed to improve the long-term prophylactic effect. In patients who relapse quickly but respond to reinstitution of therapy, indefinite long-term use of sulfasalazine should be considered.

Sulfasalazine's usefulness is limited by a high incidence of intolerance and allergic reactions. Nausea, anorexia, and headache can be overcome by lowering the dosage, and dyspepsia may be decreased by using an enteric-coated form. Mild neutropenia and mild degrees of hemolysis may also be reversed by lowering the dosage. The complete blood count (CBC) should be monitored frequently at first and then periodically on chronic therapy. Minor allergic reactions such as rash and fever may be overcome in up to 75 percent of patients by a process of gradual desensitization. More serious side effects such as agranulocytosis, severe hemolysis, hepatitis, pancreatitis, pneumonitis, neuropathy, alteration of sperm count and sperm morphology, and exacerbation of colitis necessitate discontinuing the drug. Sulfasalazine can be used safely during pregnancy and nursing.

Sulfasalazine consists of sulfapyridine linked to 5-aminosalicylic acid (5-ASA) via an azo bond. The drug is partially absorbed from the proximal GI tract, and a portion of the absorbed drug is excreted unchanged in the urine. The remaining absorbed portion returns unchanged to the small intestine via the bile, where, together with the unabsorbed portion, it traverses the intestine until it encounters the bacterial flora primarily in the distal ileum and colon. The azo bond is broken by the action of the intestinal bacteria with release of sulfapyridine and 5-ASA. The sulfa portion is largely absorbed, metabolized by the liver, and excreted in the urine. The 5-ASA metabolite, in contrast, stays largely in contact with the colon and is excreted in the feces. These observations suggested that sulfasalazine might be serving as a prodrug delivering an active component (5-ASA) to distal disease sites. This hypothesis, coupled with observations that most of the drug's toxicity related to the sulfa portion, led to the development of a new group of agents, the aminosalicylates.

Aminosalicylates

Controlled trials of topical 5-ASA in both suppository and enema form (known as mesalamine in the United States and mesalazine in Europe) have clearly established its effectiveness in ulcerative proctitis and distal ulcerative colitis. Only a few patients with distal Crohn's colitis or Crohn's proctitis have been treated with topical 5-ASA in an organized fashion, although there has been the impression that the agent does not work as well in distal Crohn's disease as it does in distal ulcerative colitis. Nonetheless, I have used 5-ASA enemas in patients with Crohn's disease isolated to the rectum or the left colon with success, beginning with one enema every night and then tapering to every other night or every third night, similar to its usage in distal ulcerative colitis. The topical preparations available in the United States include Rowasa enemas and suppositories. Neither has been approved by the Food and Drug Administration (FDA) for use in Crohn's disease.

Several formulations of oral 5-ASA agents have been developed and studied. These include olsalazine (Dipentum), which links 5-ASA to itself via an azo bond; balsalazide (Colazide), which links 5-ASA to an inert polymer, also via an azo bond; and slow or delayed release forms of mesalamine, which encapsulate 5-ASA in ethylcellulous microspheres (Pentasa) or coat it with an acrylic resin (Eudragit) that dissolves at pH greater than 6 or 7 (Asacol, Claversal, Rowasa).

The oral agents have proved effective in active and remitted ulcerative colitis. Studies of the use of these oral 5-ASA drugs in Crohn's disease have been limited. In the largest and most promising study, 310 patients with mildly or moderately active Crohn's disease involving the small and large bowel were randomized to Pentasa at doses of 1, 2, or 4 g per day or to placebo over a 16 week period. In the trial, 64 percent of the patients on the 4 g dose improved, with 43 percent achieving full remission. These contrasted with a 36 percent overall improvement rate in those on placebo, with only a 11 percent remission rate. The 1 and 2 g per day dose results were comparable with those seen on placebo. Neither the disease site nor previous medication usage affected the outcome. However, two similar but as yet unpublished studies failed to show efficacy for Pentasa in Crohn's disease at any dosage.

Although the slow-release and delayed-release oral 5-ASA agents may have an advantage over sulfasalazine in small bowel Crohn's disease, it is unlikely that they will be any more effective than sulfasalazine in Crohn's colitis. The oral 5-ASA agents should be considered for patients with Crohn's colitis who are intolerant of or allergic to sulfasalazine. As suggested by the Pentasa study, the dosage may have to be pushed to the higher range (e.g., Asacol, 4.8 g; Dipentum, 3.0 g) to realize an effect in active disease. Currently, Dipentum, Asacol, and Pentasa are available in the United States but have received FDA approval only for use in ulcerative colitis.

As noted previously, it has been difficult to show efficacy for sulfasalazine in preventing relapses of Crohn's disease. Several trials have shown the potential for oral 5-ASA agents to maintain remission in Crohn's disease, but the results have been variable. In one promising trial, 34 percent of patients with Crohn's disease relapsed on Asacol (2.4 g per day) in 1 year compared with 55 percent on placebo. However, these effects were especially pronounced in patients with ileitis, not those with colitis. In another study, 161 patients with inactive Crohn's disease (90 percent of whom had colon involvement) were randomized to receive either Pentasa, 2 g per day, or placebo in a 2 year trial. Only in those patients who began therapy within 3 months of remission was there a significant difference on drug therapy, with ongoing remission rates of 45 percent and 29 percent in the Pentasa and placebo groups, respectively. This efficacy was apparently unrelated to disease location, although not specifically commented on by the authors.

I believe that further clinical experience is needed before we know the true role for the oral 5-ASA agents in Crohn's disease. For now, it seems reasonable to consider long-term maintenance therapy for patients with Crohn's colitis with one of these agents in the same manner as one might use sulfasalazine.

Although 80 to 90 percent of patients intolerant of or allergic to sulfasalazine tolerate either the topical or oral 5-ASA preparations, 10 to 20 percent of patients experience the identical reaction with 5-ASA as noted with sulfasalazine. Side effects reported with the aminosalicylates include anal irritation with the topical preparations, pancreatitis, pericarditis, pneumonitis, nephritis, exacerbation of colitis, and watery diarrhea, seen particularly with olsalazine. Although experience is limited, these agents appear to be safe during pregnancy and nursing.

The mechanism of action of the aminosalicylates and the parent drug sulfasalazine remains uncertain. Most speculation has focused on the role of these agents in inhibiting the lipoxygenase pathway of arachidonic acid metabolism, and thus decreasing the production of chemotactically active leukotrienes and hydroxy fatty acids. Other investigations have pointed to a possible role as oxygen-derived free radical scavengers and as a blocker of certain antibodies toxic to colonic epithelial cells.

Metronidazole and Other Antibiotics

Although not all investigations agree, controlled trials suggest that metronidazole is as effective as sulfasalazine and more effective than placebo in patients with mild to moderate Crohn's colitis and ileocolitis. The drug has not proved effective when only the ileum is involved. Its use as a prophylactic agent for Crohn's disease patients in remission has not been investigated. I turn to metronidazole for the patient with Crohn's colitis who is not responding to or cannot tolerate sulfasalazine or one of the oral aminosalicylates. I give the drug at a dosage of 10 mg per kilogram per day and hope to see a response within 4 weeks. I then usually continue the drug for 4 to 6 months before gradually tapering and stopping it.

As with sulfasalazine, the use of metronidazole is limited by a high incidence of side effects, including nausea, anorexia, metallic taste, furry tongue, and depression. Peripheral neuropathy is a serious problem at higher doses (greater than 1 g per day), but it can occur at lower doses and may persist when the patient is off therapy. Although the potential for carcinogenicity has been raised by in vitro and animal studies, there is no evidence that metronidazole causes malignancy in humans. It should not, however, be used. It should not be used, however, during the first trimester of pregnancy.

The way in which metronidazole works in Crohn's colitis is not clear. By decreasing the anaerobic floral burden, it may be diminishing an antigen stimulus to inflammation or decreasing the production of bacterial toxins injurious to the bowel. However, it is speculated that metronidazole may have anti-inflammatory or immunosuppressive properties independent of its antimicrobial action.

In addition to metronidazole, there has long been advocacy for the use of a wide array of broad-spectrum antibiotics in the management of mild to moderate Crohn's disease regardless of distribution. Ampicillin, tetracycline, and various cephalosporins have been reported anecdotally to be of utility. I have recently had success in treating several patients with Crohn's colitis with oral vancomycin despite negative *Clostridium difficile* toxin titers, and both ciprofloxacin and clarithromycin have produced dramatic results in a group of my patients with Crohn's ileitis and ileocolitis.

Finally, there is interest in the use of combinations of antituberculous agents. Uncontrolled trials have suggested efficacy for regimens of two and four drugs in refractory active Crohn's disease of small and large bowel, and a placebo-controlled trial showed that a four-drug regimen maintained remission in Crohn's patients. I would await the results of further trials, however, before I begin to use antituberculous therapy in any but the most refractory of patients.

Corticosteroids

Both topical and systemic steroids can play an important role in the management of patients with colonic Crohn's disease. As with the topical aminosalicylate preparations, hydrocortisone enemas (Cortenema) should be considered in patients with active Crohn's proctosigmoiditis. I begin them with one enema every night for 2 to 3 weeks and then taper to every other night for 2 to 3 weeks. Some patients continue to have smoldering symptoms and seem to benefit from continued use of the enemas every 2 to 3 nights with few systemic effects. Currently, rapidly metabolized forms of topical steroids, including budesonide and beclomethasone dipropionate, appear promising in studies of patients with distal ulcerative colitis, but their use has not been reported in patients with distal Crohn's colitis.

For patients with more extensive mild to moderate Crohn's colitis who have not fully responded to sulfasalazine, oral aminosalicylates, or metronidazole or cannot tolerate these agents, I add corticosteroids. Although controlled trials give conflicting results with regard to efficacy, most of my patients are treated with a combination of steroids and one of the other agents. I begin treatment with prednisone, 40 to 60 mg per day, and hope to see a response to the initial dose within 2 weeks. Once the desired response is obtained, the prednisone dosage is tapered by 5 mg every 7 to 10 days. Since there is no benefit in continuing prednisone as a prophylactic agent once remission is achieved, I try to withdraw patients completely from the prednisone. However, some patients begin to have mild smoldering active disease as the dosage is tapered, and benefit from continued low dosages of the drug, 5 to 10 mg per day or 10 to 20 mg on alternate days. The latter schedule may decrease the frequency of the well-known long-term side effects of steroids, including cataracts, osteoporosis, hypertension, and diabetes.

As with topical preparations, there are now studies of slow-release forms of oral budesonide. Results of two control trials in patients with Crohn's ileitis and ileocolitis support the efficacy of budesonide, with little or no impact on the pituitary-adrenal access.

Immunomodulators

6-Mercaptopurine (6-MP) and Azathioprine

Resistance to the use of the immunosuppressive drugs azathioprine (Imuran) and its metabolite 6-MP (Purinethol), resulted from the inability of several short-term controlled trials to show efficacy in patients with inflammatory bowel disease (IBD), and from concern over their potential adverse effects. Much of that concern has been allayed by subsequent long-term studies and by an enlarging experience attesting to their relative safety. In a 2 year, double-blind, placebo-controlled cross-over study of patients with Crohn's disease, 6-MP used in conjunction with sulfasalazine and/or prednisone was successful in achieving specific therapeutic goals in two-thirds of patients. Many authors have now published their experiences supporting the use of these agents in patients with Crohn's disease refractory to or dependent on steroids, and the ability to taper steroid dosage and heal fistulas. There is also evidence from controlled observations that these drugs can maintain remission in Crohn's disease.

I turn to 6-MP (the drug is the active metabolite of Imuran and the two can be used interchangeably) in patients with Crohn's colitis refractory to other drugs, those dependent on steroids, those with nonhealing fistulas, and those with early postoperative recurrence. I initiate treatment at 50 mg per day, explaining to patients that the average time for clinical response is about 3 months and that some individuals may not show benefit for 6 to 9 months. I monitor the CBC weekly for the first week of therapy, every other week for the second week, and monthly thereafter. If after 4 weeks there is no therapeutic response (e.g., decrease in symptoms, ability to slowly taper steroids), I raise the dosage but not to exceed 2 mg per kilogram per day. Some authors feel that mild leukopenia must be achieved to get a maximal response, but I lower the dose of drug if the WBC count drops below 4,000 k per microliter.

Once the desired therapeutic response is achieved, the question arises as to how long to continue therapy. Previous concerns about a malignancy risk have been allayed by large studies suggesting that patients with IBD on 6-MP or azathioprine are at no increased risk for the development of cancer. A recent study suggested that the maximal benefit from these agents is obtained at 4 years, although in patients with the most refractory disease who have had multiple surgeries these drugs are usually continued indefinitely.

The overall toxicity of 6-MP and azathioprine has been limited, and more than 90 percent of patients treated have not experienced an adverse effect. Mild allergic reactions such as fever and rash are infrequent, as are more serious reactions such as hepatitis and pancreatitis. Bone marrow depression can usually be avoided by careful monitoring, and teratogenicity has not been established, although I discourage women from becoming pregnant while on 6-MP or azathioprine. If conception occurs, the drug is stopped and the pregnancy continued.

Methotrexate

Long given to patients with rheumatologic disorders, methotrexate has recently been used with apparent success in patients with IBD. In an open trial of patients with active small bowel and colonic Crohn's disease, 30 of 37 (70 percent) improved or went into remission during a 12 week treatment period, receiving 25 mg per week intramuscularly. Eighty percent of patients previously unresponsive to 6-MP or azathioprine improved on methotrexate.

In a chronic-phase open trial in which 39 patients with Crohn's disease receive 15 mg per week of methotrexate orally with gradual tapering of the dose, 20 (51 percent) remain on methotrexate at a mean follow-up of 69 weeks. Most patients in this group remain dependent on low-dose prednisone. Adverse effects have been limited to a few patients with abnormal liver enzymes, mild leukopenia, and pneumonitis.

In a separate 52 week trial, patients with ileal and colonic Crohn's disease who were steroid dependent were randomized to either methotrexate, 15 mg per week, or placebo. At the end of the trial, there were no differences in the activity index between the two groups. In the course of the study, however, 46 percent of patients in the treatment group had flares compared with 80 percent in the placebo group.

In a more recent trial, steroid-dependent Crohn's patients were randomized to either methotrexate, 25 mg IM per week, or placebo. Remission was achieved in 40 percent of the methotrexate group compared with 20 percent in the placebo group. This effect was seen primarily in the patients dependent on greater than 20 mg of prednisone daily.

I believe there is a role for methotrexate in the patient with Crohn's colitis who has failed standard treatment, including 6-MP. If there is no evidence of small bowel disease that might compromise absorption, I begin patients on 15 mg per week and hope to see a response within 4 months. I then taper the dosage and maintain it at 5 to 7.5 mg per week for 2 years before attempting to stop it.

Cyclosporine

In a 3 month placebo-controlled trial involving patients with refractory ileal and colonic Crohn's disease, oral cyclosporine was associated with improvement in 59 percent of patients compared with a 32 percent improvement rate on placebo. However, during a 3 month period in which cyclosporine was then gradually withdrawn, only 38 percent of the original responders to cyclosporine remained well. Long-term use of low-dose cyclosporine in patients with Crohn's disease in remission has not been efficacious. Long-term side effects of hirsutism and paresthesias are common. Hypertension and renal failure are also potential problems for those on chronic cyclosporine therapy. I believe that cyclosporine has a limited role in patients with Crohn's colitis and should be reserved for those with active disease who are refractory to standard therapies and not good candidates for surgery.

■ OTHER MODALITIES

T-cell apheresis has been reported to achieve remission in 64 of 72 patients with refractory, chronic active Crohn's disease in open trials. The remission lasted 1 year in 24 patients and 5 years in one patient. The investigators report no mortality or immunoincompetence, but sepsis related to central lines was seen. In the one reported controlled trial, T-cell apheresis improved steroid weaning in Crohn's disease but had no effect on the relapse rate.

In an open trial of a small number of patients with active Crohn's disease, infusions of a chimeric monoclonal anti-CD4 antibody appeared to produce remission. Finally, intravenous immunoglobulin, alpha interferon and antibody to TNF-α given to a few patients with active Crohn's disease have been associated with improvement in disease parameters. Although these modalities can be considered for patients with Crohn's colitis in whom other therapeutic options have been unsuccessful, they should be viewed as experimental and requiring further controlled observations.

■ ANTIDIARRHEAL, ANTICHOLINERGIC, AND PSYCHOTROPIC AGENTS

Loperamide, diphenoxylate with atropine, and codeine may be of benefit in the setting of mild, chronic diarrhea due to active Crohn's colitis. These agents should not be used in unstable patients with severe degrees of activity because of the risk of precipitating ileus and even toxic megacolon. Occasional patients with Crohn's colitis have symptoms resembling the irritable bowel syndrome, with frequent small stools alternating with constipation associated with a sense of incomplete evacuation. For such patients, hydrophilic mucilloids such as psyllium may be of benefit. Similarly, the crampy pain experienced by such patients may be relieved by anticholinergic drugs such as propantheline, bromide, dicyclomine hydrochloride, and hyoscyamine sulfate given before meals and at bedtime. Although not a substitute for a concerned caregiver, minor tranquilizers such as oxazepam and diazepam, or antidepressants such as amytriptiline and doxepin, may be useful in patients in whom stress appears to be playing a pivotal role in symptom exacerbation. Behavior modification should also be considered in such patients.

■ NUTRITIONAL THERAPY

It has been difficult to prove that specific diets are effective for patients with Crohn's colitis. I always consider lactose intolerance in such patients and usually perform a lactose breath test to determine whether lactose withdrawal might benefit them. I also ask patients with gas, cramps, and diarrhea to avoid fresh fruit and fresh vegetables, carbonated beverages, and diet gum.

Controlled trials have shown that both total enteral nutrition (TEN) and total parenteral nutrition (TPN) may induce remission in Crohn's disease. Most studies suggest that patients with ileal disease derive greater benefit from this approach than do those with Crohn's colitis. In my experience, most patients have limited tolerance for prolonged TEN, but I use elemental diets to supplement caloric intake in patients with Crohn's colitis. I rarely use TPN in patients with Crohn's colitis, since in my experience the improvements are short-lived and not usually worth the risks of infection with a prolonged central venous line. Such tools are extremely useful, however, in young children with growth failure.

■ OTHER CONSIDERATIONS

Perineal Disease

For patients with perineal fistulas and abscesses who do not require surgical intervention, or for those who have persistent problems despite surgery, I administer metronidazole, 1 to 2 g per day. For patients who respond, I attempt to slowly lower the dosage, although many require indefinite maintenance therapy at doses of 500 mg to 1 g per day. Ciprofloxacin, 500 mg twice a day, can be used in a similar fashion. Finally, there is evidence from preliminary studies that continuous infusions of cyclosporine (4 mg per kilogram per day) may promptly improve refractory perineal Crohn's disease.

Fulminant Colitis

A few patients with Crohn's colitis present with severe symptoms and toxicity, with or without megacolon. Such patients are treated in a manner similar to those with severe ulcerative colitis, with intravenous (IV) fluids and electrolyte replacement and bowel rest. I use IV prednisolone as a continuous drip at 60 mg per 24 hours and add broad-spectrum antibiotics (e.g., ampicillin, gentamicin, or metronidazole). For those with dilated colons, I place a nasogastric tube and use the technique of rolling them to a prone position for 15 minutes every 2 hours. For those not improving within 72 hours, surgical intervention is advised. Whether IV cyclosporine, now shown to be of benefit in a controlled trial of patients with severe ulcerative colitis, will be of similar benefit for those with Crohn's colitis is not clear.

A more common acute presentation of the patient with Crohn's colitis is that of an acute appendicitis- or diverticulitis-like picture, with localized peritoneal signs due to a contained microperforation. I avoid corticosteroids in such patients not already on them for fear of masking sepsis, and instead use broad-spectrum antibiotics as primary therapy in such instances.

Colon Cancer

It is becoming increasingly apparent that patients with Crohn's colitis have a risk of colon cancer similar to that in their counterparts with ulcerative colitis, given the same extent and duration of disease. Although good prospective trials with large numbers of patients are lacking to support a surveillance program, I have begun to perform colonoscopies with biopsies for dysplasia in patients with Crohn's colitis who have had their disease for over 7 years, and I recommend colectomy for those with high-grade dysplasia. Unlike the situation in patients with ulcerative colitis, colon cancer in Crohn's disease may occur in grossly uninvolved areas in up to one-quarter of patients.

Surgical Options

The indications for surgery in patients with Crohn's colitis include refractoriness to medical therapy, obstruction, perforation, abscess formation, fistulas, and perineal disease. Since many patients have rectal sparing, a segmental resection with anastomosis is often possible, although the recurrence rate is extremely high. For those with disease involving most of the colon, including the rectum, panproctocolectomy is necessary. The ileoanal anastomosis and pouch is not an option for patients with Crohn's colitis because of the very high recurrence rate in the pouch. Almost 75 percent of patients who have a colectomy with ileostomy for Crohn's colitis with no obvious evidence of small bowel Crohn's disease will remain disease free.

Suggested Reading

Brynskov J, Freund L, Rasmussen JN, et al. A placebo-controlled double-blind randomized trial of cyclosporine therapy in active chronic Crohn's disease. N Engl J Med 1989; 321:845–850.

Ekbom A, Helmich C, Adams HO. Increased risk of large bowel cancer in Crohn's disease with colonic involvement. Lancet 1990; 336:357–359.

Feagan BG, Rochon J, Fedorak RN, et al. Methotrexate for the treatment of Crohn's disease. The North American Crohn's Study Group Investigators. N Engl J Med 1995; 332:292–297.

Hanauer SB. Inflammatory bowel disease. N Engl J Med 1996; 334:841–848.

Nyman M, Hansson J, Eriksson S. Long-term immunosuppressive treatment in Crohn's disease. Scand J Gastroenterol 1985; 20:1197–1203.

Peppercorn MA. Advances in the drug therapy for inflammatory bowel disease. Ann Intern Med 1990; 112:50–60.

Prantera C, Zannoni F, Scriboni ML, et al. An antibiotic regimen for the treatment of active Crohn's disease. Am J Gastroenterol 1996; 91:328–332.

Present DH, Korelitz BI, Wisch N, et al. Treatment of Crohn's disease with 6-mercaptopurine. A long-term randomized double blind study. N Engl J Med 1980; 302:981–987.

Rutgeerts P, Lofberg F, Malchow H, et al. A comparison of budesonide with prednisolone for active Crohn's disease. N Engl J Med 1994; 331:842–845.

Singleton J, Gitnick G, Hanauer SB, et al. Response of Crohn's disease to oral Pentasa as a function of disease location and prior therapy. Gastroenterology 1991; 100:A251.

Singleton JW, Hanauer SB, Gitnick GL, et al. Mesalamine capsules for the treatment of active Crohn's disease. Gastroenterology 1993; 104:1293–1301.

Summers RW, Switz DM, Sessions JT Jr, et al. National Cooperative Crohn's Disease Study: results of drug treatment. Gastroenterology 1983; 77:847–869.

Ursing B, Alm J, Barany F, et al. A comparative study of metronidazole and sulfasalazine for active Crohn's disease: the cooperative Crohn's disease study in Sweden. Gastroenterology 1982; 83:550–562.

ULCERATIVE COLITIS

Daniel H. Present, M.D.

Ulcerative colitis is a complex illness. Current knowledge indicates that there are underlying genetic factors that predispose to its development. This is suggested by the increased incidence noted in first-degree relatives and in the Jewish population, concordance in monozygotic twins, and the association with a distinctive serum antineutrophilic cytoplasmic antibody in ulcerative colitis patients as well as their first-degree relatives. Finally, there is a selective reduction in colonic glycoproteins in patients and families as well as monozygotically unaffected twins. It has been suggested that the disease may be triggered by multiple factors, including superimposed infections (*Salmonella*, viral) and the taking of nonsteroidal anti-inflammatory agents. Attacks may even occur in a seasonal pattern. Discontinuation of cigarette smoking appears to be a major factor in either initiation or worsening of the inflammatory process. Once the condition is under way, multiple alterations in patients' immune response have been noted with subsequent enhancement of cytokine release and alterations of the lipoxygenase and cyclooxygenase pathways.

Although many drugs are available to treat active ulcerative colitis, there is no standard management for this complex clinical condition, and artful individualization is required for most patients. Current therapeutic approaches are directed toward manipulation of the nonspecific inflammatory pathways as well as the more specific initial immune response.

■ VARIABLES AFFECTING MANAGEMENT

Management with available agents varies according to several factors, the most important being the extent of involvement and severity of disease. Other potential differences include whether this is an initial attack, a recurrent flare-up, or chronic refractory activity.

Extent of Disease

Almost by definition, ulcerative colitis involves the rectum, which is the most active segment in most patients, even in those in whom involvement is extensive. The clinician should carefully note the extent of the inflammatory process, i.e., proctitis (involvement up to 10 to 15 cm), proctosigmoiditis (activity up to 30 to 40 cm), left-sided colitis (up to the splenic flexure), extensive (to the hepatic flexure), or universal (to the cecum).

When disease is only distal (proctitis and proctosigmoiditis), the involved segment often must be treated more intensively, and a major error in management of extensive ulcerative colitis is failure to use topical in addition to oral or parenteral medications. The institution of concurrent rectal therapy will help more quickly alleviate symptoms such as diarrhea, bleeding, and tenesmus. For example, high-dose oral steroids may effectively treat refractory distal proctosigmoiditis, but when steroid doses are decreased exacerbation is common if concomitant rectal therapy has not been instituted and maintained. An accurate measurement of extent is important in terms of potential development of fulminant disease (rarely seen in limited proctitis and proctosigmoiditis) and increased cancer risk (also not seen in proctitis and proctosigmoiditis), but of highest risk in universal disease that has been present for 8 or more years.

There have been infrequent reports of "skip" areas in ulcerative colitis, especially in the right colon. The significance of these skip areas is uncertain, but they may serve to predict those patients in whom the disease process will extend in the future.

Proctitis and proctosigmoiditis have been reported to extend in 10 to 30 percent of patients, and endoscopic re-evaluation may be required with the passage of time. Barium enemas are not accurate in describing the extent and should mainly be used to evaluate strictures and scarring of the colon and the presence of small bowel inflammation that may suggest Crohn's disease. Colonoscopic biopsies demonstrating microscopic activity when the colon appears grossly normal are of little to no value in guiding the choice of therapy. For example, if the gross extent of the disease is 30 cm and biopsies show universal disease, distal topical therapy is often all that is required for symptomatic clinical relief. It is uncertain whether the proximal positive biopsy findings are forerunners of extension and therefore an indication for oral preventive therapy.

Activity of Disease

Ulcerative colitis disease is usually defined in terms of symptoms that are correlated with endoscopic findings. Mild disease is associated with four or fewer loose bowel movements daily with occasional blood and associated with abdominal cramps, blood, and infrequently tenesmus. Systemic symptoms are not present. Endoscopy shows erythema, edema, and mild friability of the mucosa. In moderate disease, there are movements ranging from four to eight daily with urgency, a nocturnal pattern, blood in the stool, abdominal discomfort, and some systemic symptoms such as weight loss, mild anemia, and low-grade fever of less than 100°F. Blood chemistries are usually unremarkable, and endoscopy shows spontaneous bleeding and friability, increased mucoid material in the lumen, and scattered ulcerations. Severe attacks are classically described by the passage of six or more bloody stools daily accompanied by systemic symptoms such as fevers of 100°F or greater, weight loss, tachycardia, anemia with a hemoglobin count of 10 g per deciliter or less, elevated sedimentation rate, and hypoalbuminemia. Endoscopy demonstrates all of the above-noted findings seen in moderate disease plus large amounts of blood in the lumen and large areas of ulcerated denuded mucosa. Plain abdominal x-ray films often demonstrate a column of air in the descending and/or transverse colon, or even a full-blown toxic megacolon.

I believe that treatment should be primarily directed at symptoms and not at endoscopic findings. The latter should be used as guidance for the duration of specific therapy (Table 1).

■ DIET AND NONSPECIFIC THERAPEUTIC MEDICATIONS

Although patients and families initially focus on dietary alterations in an attempt to manage ulcerative colitis, there is unfortunately little to be gained from dietary therapy. Thus far, no one specific diet or elimination of potential irritants has been successful, other than producing a mild improvement in bowel symptoms.

If diarrhea is a major symptom, bulk such as raw fruits and vegetables should be eliminated. However, in distal proctitis and proctosigmoiditis in which proximal constipation is common, extra bulk in the diet may be required or the addition of psyllium compounds that may be useful in relieving the constipation. Gas-producing foods such as beans or cabbage and stimulants, or laxatives such as caffeine or dietary (sorbitol-containing) gum are best avoided when cramps and/or diarrhea are prominent. Milk is often inappropriately withheld from patients with ulcerative colitis. Since lactase deficiency is not observed in most patients, lactose intolerance should be documented before complete exclusion is advised, especially in young children. Elemental diets and predigested supplements have never been shown to play any role in suppressing inflammation in ulcerative colitis, as contrasted with Crohn's disease, and are indicated only if there is significant nutritional depletion and a normal diet cannot be tolerated. In fact, total parenteral nutrition (TPN) has shown no efficacy in several controlled trials in the management of severe ulcerative colitis. TPN should not be used as primary therapy but only to improve the nutritional status in depleted patients before surgery or while waiting for acute therapy (such as cyclosporine) to become effective.

Emotional factors have not been shown to be etiologic and rarely worsen already active disease. Psychotherapy rarely if ever alters the clinical course and is best used as supportive therapy unless the patient has an underlying separate psychiatric disorder. Family therapy and mutual support groups (as sponsored by the Crohn's and Colitis Foundation of America) are valuable in the long-term adjustments to this chronic illness. A major benefit is a concerned and caring physician who will be available to answer questions and personal concerns, especially in the early phases of the illness and at the time of hospitalization or complications.

■ SYMPTOMATIC DRUG THERAPY

It is not unique to observe patients with ulcerative colitis who are taking a variety of medications (5-aminosalicylic [5-ASA] agents, steroids, immunosuppressives), whose main symptom is diarrhea, and who are not receiving an antidiarrheal agent. Choices include diphenoxylate, 2.5 to 5 mg; loperamide, 2 to 4 mg; deodorized tincture of opium, 5 to 15 drops;

Table 1 Drug Therapy for Active Ulcerative Colitis

MILD ACUTE RELAPSING		MODERATE ACUTE RELAPSING		SEVERE ACUTE RELAPSING	
PROCTITIS-PROCTOSIGMOIDITIS	LEFT-SIDED, UNIVERSAL	PROCTITIS-PROCTOSIGMOIDITIS	LEFT-SIDED, UNIVERSAL	PROCTITIS-PROCTOSIGMOIDITIS	LEFT-SIDED, UNIVERSAL
Symptomatic (bulk, antidiarrheals)	Symptomatic (antidiarrheals)	Symptomatic (antidiarrheals, bulk)	Symptomatic (antidiarrheals)	Symptomatic (antidiarrheals)	No antidiarrheals
Rectal steroids (or rectal 5-ASA)	Rectal steroids (or rectal 5-ASA)	Rectal steroids (? double-dose) (? combination)	Rectal steroids, Oral steroids	Double-dose rectal steroids (or rectal 5-ASA) (or combination)	Rectal steroids × 2
? Oral 5-ASA	Oral 5-ASA	Oral 5-ASA in increasing doses	Maintenance oral 5-ASA	Increased oral 5-ASA Oral steroids (? systemic ACTH or hydrocortisone)	Maintenance oral 5-ASA, IV steroids IV antibiotics IV cyclosporine (if no response to steroids)

ACTH, adrenocorticotropic hormone.

and codeine, 15 to 30 mg, all given up to four times daily. Individuals vary as to which of these agents is most effective. All are best given 15 to 30 minutes before meals and before sleep. Addiction is rare and the only major concern regarding these symptomatic agents is that during a severe, systemic attack there is the potential of triggering a toxic megacolon. This complication occurs infrequently, but antidiarrheals are best avoided with severe disease. However, when the activity is controlled, they can be reinstituted.

Irritable bowel syndrome (IBS) is a common gastrointestinal (GI) disorder and the astute clinician will observe symptoms of IBS superimposed on the symptoms of the active colitis in about 15 percent of patients. The use of anticholinergics such as dicyclomine, 10 to 20 mg, or hyoscyamine, 0.25 mg, before meals and sleep, bulking agents, and occasional antidepressants such as amytriptyline, 10 to 20 mg at sleep, may be valuable for symptomatic relief when IBS symptoms are present. Excessive bowel movements after an otherwise successful ileoanal anastomosis may occasionally be the result of a superimposed IBS and will require symptomatic medications.

■ SPECIFIC DRUG THERAPY

Salicylates (5-ASA Compounds)

Sulfasalazine

Sulfasalazine (Azulfidine) was the original and is still the foundation and should be the most commonly used drug in the treatment of ulcerative colitis. The drug consists of 5-aminosalicylic acid bound by an azo bond to sulfapyridine. About 20 percent of the parent compound is absorbed in the small intestine and excreted predominantly unmodified in bile. Colonic bacteria are responsible for azo bond reduction, thereby releasing 5-ASA and sulfapyridine. The latter is absorbed from the colon and acetylated by the liver (slow acetylation results in an increased incidence of sulfapyridine side effects). If given orally alone or uncoated, 5-ASA is rapidly absorbed in the jejunum, whereas when azo-bonded 5-ASA is released by bacteria, colonic absorption is limited, and the active moiety is thus distributed throughout the colon. 5-ASA is acetylated by colonic epithelium and excreted primarily in the stool.

The mechanism of action is uncertain and various proposals have been put forward, including inhibition of: the lipoxygenase and cyclo-oxygenase pathways, free radical scavengers, platelet activating factor, macrophage, neutrophil and mast cell function, and of production of cytokines as well as alterations in humoral immunity.

Approximately 75 to 80 percent of patients with mild to moderate ulcerative colitis are reported to be responsive to sulfasalazine, usually within 2 to 3 weeks. Some patients may require several months to show complete response. The drug should be started at 500 mg twice daily, with gradual increase over 1 to 2 weeks. Most patients respond to 3 g, but if activity persists the dose can be increased to 4 g daily or rarely higher, since most patients do not tolerate doses over 4 g. The drug is best given with meals to minimize side effects. Enteric-coated sulfasalazine is valuable and should be substituted if GI side effects are seen soon after initiation.

Of equal importance is the fact that sulfasalazine, in addition to quieting active ulcerative colitis, is effective in maintaining remission, with a three to four times lower relapse rate compared with placebo for 1 year's duration. Preventive dose-ranging studies have shown that 4 g is more effective than 2 g, which in turn is more effective than 1 g; however, the higher doses result in increased side effects. The ideal preventive dose is approximately 2 to 3 g daily for most patients. The need for frequent administration during the day often results in poor patient compliance. There are few more difficult tasks in clinical medicine than convincing teenagers or young adults who have been in clinical remission that they must remain on this drug for prevention. However, the effort is worth the rewards in terms of preventing exacerbations and possible extension of disease.

Adverse effects occur in about 20 percent of patients taking sulfasalazine, and approximately half of these will have to stop the drug. The most common side effects are related to sulfapyridine blood concentration and depend on the administered dose and the acetylator status. These include nausea and vomiting, anorexia, abdominal pain, heartburn, and occasionally diarrhea. As noted, slow increase in dosage and taking the coated preparation with meals result in increased tolerance. Other important side effects include impaired male fertility secondary to oligospermia, morphologic sperm abnormalities, and abnormal motility. All are reversible within 6 to 8 weeks of stopping the drug. Severe side effects include idiosyncratic rash (ranging from mild to Stevens-Johnson syndrome), fever, agranulocytosis, liver dysfunction (cholestasis, hepatitis, massive liver necrosis), and lupus-like phenomenon with Raynaud's syndrome and pericarditis. Pulmonary eosinophilic pneumonias, fatal fibrosing alveolitis, and severe depression have also been noted. Neutropenia may occur, making concurrent use of 6-mercaptopurine or azathioprine more difficult. Megaloblastic anemia and hemolysis have been reported. Although folate deficiency can occur, routine supplementation is not required since the deficiency is usually not clinically significant. Initial reports recommending the use of folic acid to prevent the development of dysplasia or carcinoma have not been confirmed by subsequent studies. Uniquely, there have been reports of sulfasalazine producing exacerbation of colitis. This adverse effect appears to be related to the 5-ASA moiety as it has been observed with the newer 5-ASA analogues that do not contain sulfapyridine.

New Salicylates

Since many of the adverse effects of sulfasalazine are due to the sulfapyridine moiety, and since 5-ASA has been shown to be the active agent, there has been recent rapid development of newer 5-ASA formulations. Slow desensitization to sulfasalazine, which is effective in 80 to 90 percent of allergic patients, has been abandoned in favor of these newer formulations. Alternative delivery systems either substitute a new carrier molecule for the sulfapyridine or coat the 5-ASA, protecting it from absorption in the jejunum and allowing subsequent release in the distal small intestine or colon where it can exert its effect.

Olsalazine (azodisalicylate, Dipentum) consists of two molecules of 5-ASA linked by the same azo bond as in sulfasalazine. It also requires reduction by colonic bacteria and is well tolerated in many patients who are sensitive or intolerant to the sulfapyridine component of sulfasalazine. It shows efficacy equal to that of sulfasalazine in mild attacks as well as in maintenance of remission. Therapeutic doses for active disease range from 1 to 3 g daily; the greatest effectiveness is seen with 3 g, whereas the preventive dose (which is FDA approved) is usually 1 g given as 500 mg twice daily. The major toxicity of this agent is diarrhea resulting from small bowel secretion of fluid; this is dose related and more common in patients with extensive colitis. Diarrhea can be diminished if the dose is increased gradually and given with meals. Diarrhea tends to improve with time, but in about 10 to 20 percent of patients the drug must be stopped because of this side effect.

Balsalazide (Colazide) links 5-ASA by an azo bond to 4-aminobenzoyl-β-alanine and is cleaved similarly to olsalazine and sulfasalazine, releasing the 5-ASA into the colon. Recent prevention studies suggest that higher oral doses are well tolerated and are more effective in maintenance of remission than lower doses of balsalazide. The major side effects of this agent are GI (abdominal discomfort, heartburn, and diarrhea). The maximal tolerable doses giving the greatest efficacy are yet to be determined.

Coated 5-ASA (mesalamine) contains no other compounds but is released at different sites in the small intestine, depending on the coating. Asacol is coated with Eudragit S, which dissolves at lumenal pH 7 (approximately at the terminal ileum and/or right colon). Claversal (Salofalk) is coated with Eudragit L and dissolves at a pH greater than 6. Studies have demonstrated that Asacol is effective in active mild to moderate ulcerative colitis and also in maintaining remission in ulcerative colitis patients. Of interest is the demonstrated efficacy of higher-dose Asacol (4.8 g daily, which is equal to about 10 g sulfasalazine) in over 60 percent of patients with mild to moderate ulcerative colitis, whereas 2.4 g is effective in 50 percent of patients and 1.6 g daily is no better than placebo. The drug is well tolerated and toxicity is similar to that seen with placebo. The standard dose of Asacol used by most clinicians to treat ulcerative colitis is 800 mg three times daily. This dose was approved by the FDA. Thus far, no one has determined the ideal time to give this medication in relation to meals. It has been shown that if Asacol is taken with food, the coated capsule may remain in the stomach for many hours and be released much later in the intestine. By contrast, capsules often appear intact in the stool if intestinal motility is increased in association with more active bowel inflammation.

With all the 5-ASA compounds, idiosyncratic allergy to 5-ASA can be seen in the form of pericarditis, pleuritis, pancreatitis, and nephrotic syndrome. Nephrotoxicity is a potential long-term problem, as it has been noted in animals ingesting high doses of 5-ASA. There have been some scattered reports of interstitial nephritis in patients with inflammatory bowel disease (IBD) taking mesalamine. My long-term experience indicates that sulfasalazine is safe during pregnancy and nursing, and preliminary data suggest that there are no complications with mesalamine in pregnancy, but further evidence is awaited.

Pentasa is a sustained-release preparation that contains granules of 5-ASA coated with ethylcellulose. Release occurs with time and increased pH. Efficacy has been observed (and FDA approved) in active ulcerative colitis as well as in maintenance of remission. The response rate is once again similar to the previous-mentioned preparations. Doses of 2 to 4 g daily are effective.

Despite the numerous new agents developed, none has so far proved more effective than the standard sulfasalazine. The advantage of the newer agents appears to be that of less toxicity in avoiding the sulfapyridine molecule; a major disadvantage is increased cost. Long-term data are required for accurate comparison of each of the new formulations in active disease and to establish the best dosage. It remains to be determined whether higher doses will give increased efficacy without increased toxicity. At this stage of our knowledge, perhaps more important than which formulation is given is the need to convince the patient to stay on medication for maintenance of remission.

Topical 5-ASA

Since the demonstration that 5-ASA was the active ingredient in sulfasalazine, topical 5-ASA has been used for distal disease. Initially, 5-ASA enemas (Rowasa) of 4 g daily were shown to be more effective than cortisone enemas containing 100 mg daily. In addition, 5-ASA enemas of 1 to 4 g daily have clearly proved more effective than placebo for mild to moderate disease. Clinical response is noted in about 70 to 75 percent of patients and does not appear to be dose related. Of greater importance may be the amount of fluid administered with the active ingredient. It is stated that 100 ml enemas will reach the splenic flexure in most patients, but U.S. preparations are produced as 60 ml, which may have less extensive distribution. Refractory patients may require 5-ASA enema therapy for several months to induce clinical remission, and relapse is high when the enema is discontinued in this group of patients. Prevention should be attempted, and enemas taken every other day are successful in most patients. 5-ASA suppositories (Rowasa) in doses of 200 mg, 1 g daily, are also effective for distal rectal activity, and if continued are more effective than placebo in maintaining remission. The optimal dose is yet to be determined. The toxicity of topical 5-ASA is similar to that seen with placebo and is usually idiosyncratic, in addition to occasional local irritation and pruritus.

There are no prospective studies determining the best initial topical therapy of choice for active distal ulcerative colitis. Both 5-ASA and steroid enemas have been used initially with success but it is important to remember that only the 5-ASA compounds are preventive. The short- and long-term role of oral 5-ASA in the treatment of proctitis and proctosigmoiditis is uncertain.

Corticosteroids

Steroids have become the treatment of choice for moderate to severe ulcerative colitis. The mechanism of action is uncertain, with multiple anti-inflammatory and immune effects. Inhibition of bound arachidonic acid and decreased activity of by-products of the lipoxygenase and cyclo-oxygenase pathways are noted, as well as impaired neutrophil chemotaxis and phagocytosis, inhibition of cytokine production, and decreased capillary permeability.

In the 1960s, prednisone (the most frequently used corticosteroid) proved more effective at doses of 40 to 60 mg daily than at 20 mg daily. The 60 mg doses were associated with increased toxicity, and it was concluded that most patients with active disease should be given 40 to 45 mg daily, with tapering after a good response. Although the literature suggests that a once-daily dose is as effective as multiple doses, the studies are limited to few patients and short periods. My experience is that multiple doses are more effective if the patient is very active but also result in increased side effects. For moderate to severe attacks, it is suggested that steroids be initiated in dosages three to four times daily, with a decrease to 1 to 2 times daily after a response has occurred. Overall, the response rate to oral steroids is greater than 75 percent. Tapering after response is usually in 5 mg decrements every 5 to 7 days, but this can be varied depending on the degree of clinical response and the severity of side effects. Relapse, when it occurs, is usually seen at dosages between 10 and 20 mg daily. There is no evidence that steroids are effective in maintaining remission, and therefore 5-ASA products are added (or maintained) once remission has been obtained. Steroids should then be discontinued.

For patients with severe disease, admission to the hospital is indicated with administration of intravenous (IV) steroids: hydrocortisone (Solu-Cortef), 300 mg daily, or methylprednisolone, 48 to 60 mg daily. There are no controlled trials to confirm my impression that continuous infusion is more effective than pulse administration. However, personal experience suggests that about 25 to 30 percent of all refractory patients on pulse IV steroids improve when switched to continuous infusion. In one controlled trial, adrenocorticotropic hormone (ACTH), 120 units by continuous daily infusion, was shown to be more effective than 300 mg hydrocortisone only in patients who had not been receiving previous steroids. It is suggested that ACTH be used in this situation.* It is incorrect to switch a patient who is refractory to IV hydrocortisone to ACTH in the hope of further response. The response rate to IV steroids in active colitis is better than 60 percent.

Toxicity with steroids is extensive and can result in long-term irreversible effects. Toxic effects include emotional disturbances (occasionally psychosis), a cushingoid habitus, hyperglycemia, hypertension, electrolyte disturbances with hypokalemia and metabolic alkalosis, myopathy, and increased intraocular pressure. Other long-term complications include osteoporosis, aseptic necrosis of the hip, cataracts, growth retardation in children, and impaired immunity resulting in increased infections. Steroids must be used promptly when indicated but rapidly decreased and discontinued when not needed. If exacerbation occurs when lowering the dosage or if long-term steroid use is required, consideration must be given to other therapeutic tools such as immunosuppressive agents or surgery. Steroids can be safely given in pregnancy, in which the risk to mother and child of increased bowel inflammation far outweighs any potential side effects to the fetus.

Topical Steroids

Studies starting in the late 1950s were convincing that topical steroids were about four to five times more effective than placebo in the treatment of distal colitis. A response rate of over 70 percent is usually noted within 2 weeks. Some unresponsive patients with extensive disease seem to benefit from being given two enemas at the same time at night. Many patients cannot tolerate enema preparations when the disease is active, and for these Cortifoam, which is also more effective than placebo, should be used initially. Administration of the more tolerable foam preparation twice daily for 1 week usually quiets the rectal segment sufficiently for higher-reaching enema preparations to be administered and retained. The combination of topical and oral steroids is highly effective initial therapy for moderate to severe ulcerative colitis.

Because systemic absorption with potential toxicity is noted with prolonged use of rectal steroids, several newer steroid preparations with decreased absorption or less systemic availability have been developed. These include prednisolone-metasulphobenzoate, which is poorly absorbed and comparable in efficacy with prednisolone enemas or low-dose oral steroids. This preparation is not available in the United States. Tixocortol pivalate, with replacement at the 21-hydroxylate area with a thiol group esterified to pivalic acid, is inactivated by red blood cells and first-pass metabolism through the liver. This agent therefore does not suppress the hypothalamic-pituitary-adrenal axis. Large multicenter trials have shown equal effectiveness with hydrocortisone enemas in short-term studies of 3 weeks, but approval and release of tixocortol pivalate has not occurred in the United States. Beclomethasone dipropionate, a rapidly metabolized steroid, has shown conflicting results compared with conventional topical steroids in distal disease. Fluticasone, a fluorinated steroid that is subject to first-pass metabolism, has also shown conflicting results, and further trials are ongoing.

Budesonide, a nonhalogenated glucocorticoid with potent anti-inflammatory activity, has proved more effective than placebo and prednisolone enemas in several studies. Dose-response studies suggest that a 2 mg dose is an attractive alternative to prednisolone enemas, in that minimal suppression is seen on the hypothalamic-pituitary-adrenal axis. The results of controlled trials will soon be available in the United States.

Immunosuppressive Agents

Recognition of the importance of immune system abnormalities in pathogenesis has resulted in increasing and better-defined indications for the use of immunosuppressives for ulcerative colitis.

Azathioprine/6-Mercaptopurine

Azathioprine is well absorbed and converted to 6-mercaptopurine (6-MP) in vivo, with subsequent impairment of purine synthesis. The exact mechanism of action is uncertain, especially in the low dosages used in IBD. The first successful therapeutic report occurred in the early 1960s with subsequent uncontrolled literature showing a response rate of 80 percent (84 of 105 patients). In addition to the clinical response, healing of pyoderma gangrenosum was also noted. There are several controlled trials of the use of these agents in ulcerative colitis, with a demonstrated efficacy equal to that of sulfasalazine as well as significant steroid-sparing action. Since the drug takes a mean time of over 3 months for response, its use is limited in acute ulcerative colitis, in which steroids and 5-ASA agents are the drugs of choice.

The major indication is for patients with chronic refractory colitis or steroid-dependent disease and for those with significant early steroid toxicity (e.g., psychosis, aseptic ne-

*Editor's Note: The use of ACTH should be limited to 10 to 14 days because of instances of bilateral and adrenal hemorrhage after several weeks of therapy.

crosis of the hip, uncontrollable diabetes). Uncontrolled trials have been carried out with 6-MP in which the clinical response and toxicity have been similar to those seen with azathioprine. Both drugs are for all intents and purposes similar and equally effective. 6-MP should be initiated in a dose of 50 to 75 mg daily; azathioprine at 75 to 100 mg daily. The dosage can be increased until leukopenia is observed, but most patients respond to 75 mg 6-MP (or 100 mg azathioprine). Leukopenia is not essential to obtain a clinical response. However, if they do not respond clinically with decreased requirements of steroids in 3 to 4 months, the dosage should be maximized to leukopenia and should not be considered ineffective until after at least 6 to 8 months of therapy. Recent data indicate that if there is only slight response at 6 months, continuation of 6-MP for longer periods (≥1 year) may result in complete clinical remission. There is not always a correlation of clinical response and endoscopic findings after therapy with 6-MP and azathioprine, in that it is not unique to have a clinical remission with mild scattered inflammatory changes persisting on colonoscopy. In uncontrolled trials and in a recent double-blind withdrawal trial, 6-MP and azathioprine have shown prevention of relapse in ulcerative colitis. Approximately three-quarters of patients remain in remission once this has been obtained with these agents. Relapse on these agents, when it occurs, is often mild and responds to increasing doses of immunosuppressives or 5-ASA agents or a short course of topical or oral steroids. Surgery can be prevented with 6-MP or azathioprine in more than two-thirds of refractory cases.

Acute toxicity consists of allergic reactions such as rash, fever, and joint pains in about 2 percent; pancreatitis in 3 to 4 percent; and (rarely) hepatitis. Bone marrow depression is dose related and can be avoided with close monitoring of the white blood cell count during the first 1 to 2 months. Almost all acute toxicity and allergic reactions occur in the first 3 to 4 weeks of taking these agents and disappear if the drug is stopped. Although there has been great fear of long-term immunosuppression leading to superinfections and neoplasia or lymphoma, no association or increased risk has so far been noted in the more than 25 years of using these agents for IBD. Long-term studies in transplant patients and recent studies in IBD patients have shown no increase in fetal abnormalities in women or men taking 6-MP or azathioprine at the time of conception. Some clinicians have maintained these agents throughout pregnancy with no untoward side effects noted so far.

These agents should be initiated if ulcerative colitis patients do not go into remission or cannot discontinue systemic steroids after two attempts. I believe steroid use of 3 to 6 months' duration is an indication for the institution of 6-MP or azathioprine.*

*Editor's Note: As a personal approach, I use azathioprine as described except for patients with over 8 to 10 years' duration of colitis because of an unproved (and perhaps unfounded) concern about colon neoplasia. I favor colectomy for these latter patients. Connell et al. (Abstract, Gastroenterology April 1994) cite 20 years' experience that shows no increase in colon cancer with azathioprine therapy.

Cyclosporine

Cyclosporine, a fungally derived immunosuppressive that inhibits the production of interleukin-2 as well as subsequent production of cytokines, has proved effective in ulcerative colitis as well as Crohn's disease. In uncontrolled studies and as recently confirmed in a controlled trial, continuous IV cyclosporine is effective when administered in a dose of 4 mg per kilogram daily to patients with severely active ulcerative colitis who have failed 10 or more days of IV steroids. In this group in whom colectomy was indicated, response was seen in 82 percent in 6 to 7 days, so that patients could leave the hospital well controlled on oral steroids (45 to 60 mg prednisone daily) and cyclosporine (6 to 8 mg per kilogram per day). The long-term response has been satisfactory, and approximately 60 percent of the original study group of 46 patients have gone into complete clinical and endoscopic remission and been able to discontinue both steroids and cyclosporine. They are currently being maintained predominantly on 5-ASA compounds, with an increasing number of patients taking 6-MP. A recent controlled trial of cyclosporine enemas has failed to confirm the efficacy in distal disease that was seen in several smaller uncontrolled series.

Cyclosporine has a high potential for toxicity, including hypertension, renal injury (which is dose related), hepatotoxicity, neurologic toxicity (tremors, paresthesias, and seizures), and long-term neoplasia. Pneumocystis pneumonia has been seen in some series, which is likely related to the combination of steroids and cyclosporine (with or without 6-MP). Prophylaxis with Septra DS may be indicated with long-term use of combinations of immunosuppressives. However, in series in which the drug was monitored carefully and used in the short term (less than 1 year), toxicity was not excessive. The clinician should obtain experience with this drug before using it extensively for ulcerative colitis.

Other Immunosuppressive Agents

Other immunosuppressives have yet to undergo extensive studies in patients with ulcerative colitis. In an uncontrolled study, intramuscular methotrexate, 25 mg once weekly, showed a response rate of greater than 70 percent. However, maintenance of response and significant steroid sparing have not been seen with lowering of the dose or switching to oral administration. A new potent immunosuppressive, FK506, has so far not been used extensively in ulcerative colitis. Dihydroxychloroquine (Plaquenil), a drug that inhibits lysosomal processing of antigens, was effective in a small uncontrolled series. A larger controlled trial using a dosage of 400 mg daily for 6 weeks was no more effective than placebo, but higher doses used for longer periods may be effective.

Other Agents

Space limits the discussion of a variety of agents that have been tried or are currently being studied in the management of ulcerative colitis, including topical lidocaine, acetarsol, sucralfate, short-chain fatty acids, and clonidine. A lipoxygenase inhibitor (Zileuton) has proved effective in those ulcerative colitis patients not taking sulfasalazine but is no more potent than sulfasalazine alone. Studies using higher doses of this potentially promising drug show no increased efficacy. Studies of omega$_3$ fatty acids, as found in fish oils, have produced modest clinical improvements in ulcerative colitis patients.

Although there are anecdotal reports showing efficacy, so far there is no evidence that broad-spectrum antibiotics or metronidazole are effective therapy for ulcerative colitis, whether for moderate to severe disease or distal disease, or whether administered topically, orally, or intravenously.

FULMINANT COLITIS AND TOXIC MEGACOLON

Fulminant colitis is one of the severe complications of ulcerative colitis. Colectomy occurs in about 25 percent of patients and is required in almost 50 percent of patients if the entire colon is involved at the time of the acute attack. The typical clinical picture of severe colitis, described earlier, requires careful monitoring by both gastroenterologist and surgeon and must be treated intensively with all available modalities if recovery and remission are to be obtained. Certain therapies should always be initiated, including rapid admission to the hospital, the patient being given no food or fluid by mouth, and IV fluid, electrolyte, and blood replacement. Continuous IV steroids should be administered in the form of hydrocortisone, 300 mg daily; methylprednisolone (Solu-Medrol), 48 to 60 mg daily; or ACTH, 120 units daily (if no previous steroids have been given) over a 24 hour period. Rectal hydrocortisone enemas, 100 mg, should be administered twice daily; if these cannot be retained, Cortifoam should be given twice daily. Although the use of antibiotics is controversial, in view of the potential of minute sealed-off perforations, broad-spectrum IV coverage using an aminoglycoside, ampicillin, and metronidazole should be undertaken. There is no indication to start short-term 5-ASA orally or rectally if the patient has not been receiving these agents, but they should be maintained (when feedings are restarted) in those already taking them. There is no indication for 6-MP or azathioprine, because they take too long to be effective. There is no controlled evidence nor any indication for the use of TPN in these patients, and after they have stabilized (24 to 48 hours), oral feedings are allowed as tolerated. If the patient fails to respond to this regimen in 1 week, cyclosporine should be initiated, 4 mg per kilogram per day by continuous IV infusion. Failure to show any response to cyclosporine in 7 days or deterioration is an indication for surgery.

If toxic megacolon complicates fulminant colitis, all the above therapies should be continued plus cessation of oral feedings; passage of a long, small intestinal tube with suction drainage; and use of a rolling technique in which patients lie on the abdomen for 10 to 15 minutes every 2 hours while awake. This allows for passage of gas and easier decompression of the dilated colon.

SURGERY

Indications for surgery in ulcerative colitis can be specific or occasionally less well defined. Free perforation and unstoppable hemorrhage are fortunately rare but are clear indications for urgent colectomy. The finding of either cancer or confirmed high-grade dysplasia is an indication for surgery no matter what current therapy is being employed. Surgery for low-grade dysplasia is more controversial. However, mounting evidence suggests low-grade dysplasia is also an indication for surgery. More definite is that multifocal low-grade dysplasia found at a single endoscopy, or repeat low-grade dysplasia on sequential endoscopies, is an indication for colectomy.

In fulminant colitis and toxic megacolon the indications for surgery are not clear-cut, but patients should be treated as outlined, and if there is no response after adequate medication has been initiated or if there is a rapid decline after therapy (fever, hypotension), acute colectomy is indicated. In patients with chronically active disease, surgery is not indicated until there has been a trial of 6-MP or azathioprine. This requires that the treating physician not take too long to institute immunosuppressives, because steroid toxicity may destroy patients' health and so deplete them that there is no time for the immunosuppressives to be effective. Drug therapy for refractory patients should be maximized before colectomy (Table 2).

Table 2 Drug Therapy for Chronic Refractory Ulcerative Colitis

PROCTITIS-PROCTOSIGMOIDITIS	LEFT-SIDED, UNIVERSAL
Symptomatic (bulk and/or antidiarrheals)	Antidiarrheals
Double enemas (steroid × 2 or steroid + 5-ASA)	Steroids + 5-ASA enema
Maximize oral 5-ASA	Maximize oral 5-ASA
6-MP/azathioprine	6-MP/azathioprine
Course of IV steroids	Course of IV steroids
	Possible course of IV cyclosporine
Surgery vs experimental agents	Surgery (especially if disease >8 yr)

6-MP, 6-mercaptopurine.

Suggested Reading

Biddle WL, et al. 5-Aminosalicylic acid enemas: effective agent in maintaining remission in left-sided ulcerative colitis. Gastroenterology 1988; 94:1075.

Habal FM, Hui G, Greenberg GR. Oral 5-aminosalicylic acid for inflammatory bowel disease in pregnancy. Gastroenterology 1993; 105 (in press).

Janowitz HD. Systemic corticosteroid therapy of ulcerative colitis. Gastroenterology 1985; 89:1189.

Lichtiger S, Present DH, Kornbluth A, et al. Cyclosporine in severe ulcerative colitis refractory to steroid therapy. N Engl J Med 1994; 330:1841.

Peppercorn MA. Sulfasalazine: pharmacology, clinical use, toxicity and related new drug development. Ann Intern Med 1984; 3:337.

Present DH. 6-Mercaptopurine and other immunosuppressive agents in the treatment of Crohn's disease and ulcerative colitis. Gastroenterol Clin North Am 1989; 18:57.

Sheppach W, Sommer H, Kirchner T, et al. Effect of butyrate enemas on the colonic mucosa in distal ulcerative colitis. Gastroenterology 1992; 103:51–56.

Truelove SC, Witts LJ. Cortisone in ulcerative colitis. Final report on a therapeutic trial. Br Med J 1955; 2:1041.

CROHN'S DISEASE OF THE SMALL BOWEL

Daniel H. Present, M.D.

Current treatment of Crohn's disease is as variable as the disease itself. To treat this chronic gastrointestinal (GI) disorder adequately, the clinician must be familiar with its natural history, the exact extent of the inflammatory process, the presence or absence of complications (fistulization and obstruction), the recurrence rate, and the patterns of recurrence after surgical resection.

Illustrative Cases

A presentation of a recently encountered case will set the background for my recommendations as to therapy for Crohn's disease of the small bowel. A 16-year-old white female with "no" GI symptoms developed secondary amenorrhea. A gynecologic examination was normal, and an endocrinologic consultant found normal growth, secondary sexual development, and no abnormal physical findings other than clubbing of the fingernails. Hormonal levels were normal, but the sedimentation rate was elevated to 32 mm per hour and the hemoglobin and albumin levels were lowered to 11.8 and 3.1 g, respectively. The astute clinician ordered GI radiographs, which showed Crohn's disease involving 5 inches of jejunum as well as 8 inches of the terminal ileum and the cecal tip. The question then arose, is it possible to treat clinically asymptomatic Crohn's disease and to alter the future course by any dietary change or medicinal administration? I polled ten experts in inflammatory bowel disease (IBD) and was given six different therapeutic approaches.

There are no controlled trials in the literature to answer this question, and unfortunately very few controlled clinical trials showing efficacy of the currently available medications in the treatment of Crohn's disease. With this limited data in mind, I would like to present my personal experience of treating about 1,000 patients with small bowel Crohn's disease. Many of the lessons I have learned are contrary to what is espoused in the literature as standard treatment, and some of my recommendations are controversial or unorthodox.

The most important advice I can give the clinician is to listen to the patient. We often "hear" what the patient tells us but fail to "listen" to the specifics and their meaning. Another clinical story will demonstrate this point. A 38-year-old female with Crohn's disease was seen who had 8 inches of ileitis for approximately 10 years. The symptoms were predominantly those of recurrent obstruction with limitation of food intake and subsequent weight loss. The patient had taken steroids on several occasions with good results, but she experienced significant emotional lability and relapsed on stopping oral prednisone. Treatment with sulfasalazine had failed and her gastroenterologist recommended a resection. I agreed that surgery was a reasonable alternative, but the patient asked if there was "any" medication that she had not taken that might be effective. I suggested that broad-spectrum antibiotics were effective in some patients with Crohn's disease but usually not when there was obstruction. She requested a trial and was treated with ampicillin, 500 mg four times daily. The patient's symptoms abated and she called 3 months later to ask for a renewal of ampicillin. I advised that she visit her primary gastroenterologist but she informed me he would not renew the prescription since "antibiotics did not work in Crohn's disease." I contacted her physician and tried to convince him to continue the medication, but he refused since there was no literature to support this treatment. I renewed the ampicillin and the patient has at this time been well for approximately 3 years while taking intermittent ampicillin. Clearly, the physician was not "listening" to this patient. I learned of the efficacy of antibiotics from many patients who told me of clinical improvement of their Crohn's disease while receiving antibiotics for other indications.

Information Required Before Institution of Therapy

In order to treat the patient with Crohn's disease a basic set of information is required. Most important is the history of patterns of exacerbations and remissions as well as the type of symptoms (inflammatory, fistulizing, or obstructive). The finding of a tender mass on physical examination is crucial to therapeutic decisions. Diagnostic studies must be performed for stool culture, ova and parasites, and *Clostridium difficile* to exclude other concurrent problems. Also indicated are blood studies to gauge the degree of inflammation (sedimentation rate, C-reactive protein, orosomucoid) and basic blood studies (complete blood count, SMA 6 and 12, and magnesium) to indicate malabsorption or chronicity.

A complete set of bowel x-rays is mandatory to define the extent of the disease (colon and/or small bowel) and any complications. A single contrast barium enema is the first procedure of choice; a double contrast enema is often very uncomfortable for the patient and is not absolutely required. I feel strongly that a barium enema is of greater value than a colonoscopy; the latter gives no extra information, and minimal findings such as scattered aphthous ulcers are of little value in the management of the patient. Crohn's disease affects the entire wall of the colon, and a look at the mucosa through the colonoscope does not add valuable data except in early initial diagnosis or in surveillance in the patient with Crohn's colitis over 8 to 10 years. GI series and small bowel follow-through with "spotting" of the terminal ileum or other disease sites is essential. Fistulization, shortening, and strictures as well as dilatation of the bowel proximal to the stricture are best seen with barium studies.

Severity of disease does not necessarily correlate with severity of the inflammatory process as seen on radiography or colonoscopy; for example, inability to enter the terminal ileum on colonoscopic examination does not mean obstruction, which is best diagnosed on the basis of clinical symptoms. Most important is the presence of a fistula on radiographs, which suggests a different therapeutic approach.

MEDICAL TREATMENT

General

The goal is to control the disease process while maintaining the patient's normal lifestyle as closely as possible. I therefore do not place major restrictions on the patient unless it is essential. I do not routinely advise dropping out of school to "rest" or taking off from work for long periods. Patients with small bowel Crohn's disease should try to exercise routinely, maintain a normal social life, and not be confined to home or hospital unless absolutely essential.

Nutrition

A dietary history should be obtained, but I believe the role of diet has been overemphasized to most patients. If physicians "listen" carefully, they will hear that most patients when feeling well can eat almost all foods, and that when they are going through an active phase, many foods increase symptoms. In my experience there is no increase in bowel symptoms with the ingestion of spicy or seasoned food in comparing patients with and without Crohn's disease. Patients, without their physician's advice, usually discover which foods increase their symptoms. Rather than ordering an expensive lactose tolerance test, I advise 7 to 10 days with no milk or milk products, and then a return to these foods; the patient should note any change in symptoms while on or off lactose.

A nutritional profile of blood studies may be a good academic approach, but for most patients is often expensive and unrewarding. A simple measurement of weight and height (especially in children) plus a complete blood count and check of sedimentation rate and serum albumin, will reveal as much about the nutritional status as tests of vitamin B_{12}, serum iron, serum folate, serum magnesium, and blood levels of trace minerals. If the patient is underweight, a complete history of the amounts and types of food being consumed is important. It is also important to determine whether there are audible bowel sounds suggesting obstruction. If the patient has obstructive symptoms, the diet must be modified to avoid roughage (e.g., raw fruits, raw vegetables, nuts, Chinese vegetables, popcorn) while maintaining adequate caloric intake. If there is malabsorption a diet adequate in calories while low in fat, supplemented with medium-chain triglycerides, is indicated. Vitamin supplements are indicated for patients with inadequate nutritional intake.

Elemental Diets

Elemental diets have been shown to be as effective as steroids in inducing remission in acute Crohn's disease. They are more effective in small bowel disease than in Crohn's colitis. However, there are major drawbacks to their use. Frequently, potential patients are systemically ill and too anorectic to drink these preparations. Some success has been obtained in adults with nasogastric feedings of elemental diets; however, most patients relapse after returning to normal diets, and the currently available oral preparations are not palatable for long periods. In my experience, adult patients do not follow this form of therapy for any prolonged period, and since this disorder is a chronic one, elemental diets play only a small therapeutic role in Crohn's disease of the small bowel. However, in active patients I often supplement oral intake with formulas such as Ensure or Ensure Plus, to maintain adequate caloric intake while I am treating with other medications.

Parenteral Nutrition

Parenteral nutrition, on the other hand, can play a major role in small bowel Crohn's disease if used for the appropriate indications. It must be strongly emphasized that parenteral nutrition is not a primary therapy of the bowel disease, but rather an adjunctive modality. It can be used in patients with:

1. Active Crohn's disease plus poor nutrition.
2. Major internal fistulae such as ileocolic or ileocutaneous fistulae, before treatment with immunosuppressive agents.
3. Preoperatively and postoperatively in patients with major nutritional depletion.
4. Growth retardation.
5. Short bowel syndrome.

In my experience, parenteral nutrition seems to restore the patient's responsiveness to other medications that may have failed, such as steroids and immunosuppressives, and if an extensive small bowel resection is the only alternative, a trial with parenteral nutrition plus the previously failed medications is warranted before surgery. Parenteral nutrition is not indicated (1) for chronic stenotic obstruction of the small bowel, or (2) postoperatively as a routine if the patient's nutritional status is adequate.

Recently it has been shown that total parenteral nutrition (TPN) with nothing by mouth and bowel rest is no more effective than parenteral nutrition plus added oral feedings. In fact, many patients with Crohn's disease develop worse diarrhea when they are NPO than when they are allowed one or two small feedings daily. I therefore do not stop oral intake when prescribing parenteral nutrition except when there are major enterocutaneous fistulae.

SYMPTOMATIC MEDICATIONS

It is not unusual for me to evaluate patients who are taking steroids for protracted periods, sulfasalazine, immunosuppressives and even parenteral nutrition who are having diarrhea and have not been given adequate doses of antidiarrheal agents. The currently available medications for diarrhea include diphenoxylate in dosages of 2.5 to 5 mg; loperamide, 2 to 4 mg; codeine, 15 to 30 mg; and deodorized tincture of opium, 8 to 15 drops. All of these medications are given up to four times daily depending on the severity of the process, preferentially one-half hour before meals and before sleep if the diarrhea is nocturnal. Patients should be allowed to take these medications as needed depending on their symptoms. Some patients with Crohn's disease of the small bowel may also respond to anticholinergics such as propantheline bromide (Pro-Banthine), 7.5 to 15 mg; dicyclomine (Bentyl), 10 to 20 mg; and hyoscyamine sulfate (Levsin), 0.125 to 0.25 mg. All these medications again are given one-half hour before meals and sleep as needed. None of the above agents should be given if there are signs of clinical obstruction, and patients should be advised as to the early symptoms of intestinal obstruction when they are taking these medications.

Approximately 6 percent of the population have addictive personalities, and since patients with Crohn's disease invariably have pain, the use of narcotic agents such as meperidine (Demerol), Percodan, and Percocet should be restricted and used only for short periods (1 to 2 weeks). Injectable narcotics should almost never be given to patients at home. Likewise, sedatives and tranquilizers, which are often required during high-dose steroid usage, should be carefully monitored by the physician, especially in patients who have demonstrated addictive tendencies.

Cholestyramine, often used in patients who have undergone previous ileal resection and have significant diarrhea, is presumed to counter the diarrheal effect of bile salts on the colon. The medication is available in 4 g packets and should be administered in as low a dose as will control the diarrhea: often half a packet one to three times daily, or one packet once or twice daily. Many patients have difficulty taking this medication since it does not dissolve easily in citrus juices.

Psychosocial Support

The early literature described an IBD personality. These judgments were made by physicians who saw patients mostly during hospitalizations and after they had been ill for a long time. Recent studies have not suggested an IBD personality, although it has been reported that depression is more common in Crohn's patients even after taking into account the chronicity and severity of the illness. My experience does not support this finding; I find Crohn's patients to be no different from others with chronic illness. I rarely refer patients to psychiatrists but rather rely on mutual self-help groups. The Crohn's and Colitis Foundation of America, 386 Park Avenue South, New York, NY 10016-8804 (phone 212-685-3440) can provide supportive literature and refer patients to support groups in their local areas. If a patient does need psychotherapy, I usually rely on a family therapist, since this illness is chronic and requires support of all family members.

■ SPECIFIC DRUG THERAPY

Sulfasalazine

There is disagreement among physicians as to the value of sulfasalazine in the management of Crohn's disease confined to the small bowel. Three controlled trials are available for review and none have shown statistically significant efficacy when only the ileum is involved. In contrast, two of the three studies have demonstrated efficacy in comparison with placebo when there is involvement of both small and large bowel. Other experienced clinicians have reported not only the clinical effectiveness of sulfasalazine in the treatment of small bowel Crohn's disease but also radiologic improvement and healing.

These discrepancies arise, first, from the fact that in few of the patients who were entered into these controlled trials was the disease limited to the small bowel and second, due to the metabolism of sulfasalazine. Although sulfapyridine and 5-aminosalicylic acid (5-ASA) are azo linked to produce sulfasalazine, it is only the 5-ASA that is the active therapeutic moiety. Sulfasalazine is split in the terminal ileum and right colon by bacteria, which then release the 5-ASA. Transit times through the intestine are uncertain, and narrowing of the small bowel may build up bacteria and delay transit. It is therefore possible that in different patients 5-ASA may be released in greater amounts in the small bowel, whereas in others sulfasalazine may have left the small bowel before significant cleavage occurs.

My experience agrees with that of many clinicians rather than with the controlled trials and indicates that sulfasalazine is an effective agent for mild to moderate Crohn's disease predominantly when the colon is involved. The dosage is increased slowly to 2 to 4 g daily in divided doses to be administered with food. If a patient experiences upper GI symptoms with sulfasalazine, this is a strong clue to duodenal involvement with Crohn's disease or peptic disease of the antrum or duodenum. A change to coated sulfasalazine may overcome this problem. I also maintain sulfasalazine, once again with colonic disease, in preventive doses of 2 g daily after a clinical remission has been obtained. My patients usually stay on this drug for long periods of time. If the disease exacerbates, I increase the dose to 4 g daily. Although controlled trials indicate that the combination of sulfasalazine and steroids is not of value, my experience suggests that sulfasalazine may function in a steroid-sparing role in some patients. I therefore introduce sulfasalazine to patients who have been brought under control with steroids, and at the same time attempt to decrease and discontinue the oral steroid agent.

The toxicity of sulfasalazine includes symptoms such as nausea, indigestion, and heartburn. Also noted are headache (especially in patients who are slow acetylators), allergic skin rashes, arthritis, low-grade hemolysis, and a decreased sperm count. It is rare to observe severe allergic reactions such as agranulocytosis, sulfasalazine lung, and hepatitis. Clinicians tend to treat all patients who receive sulfasalazine with folic acid since there is competitive inhibition for this vitamin. I do not prescribe folic acid supplements to all patients but instead monitor blood counts every few months; if macrocytic anemia develops, I treat with 1 mg of folic acid two to three times daily until the anemia comes under control and then maintain a preventive dose of 1 mg daily.

New Oral 5-ASA Drugs

Since 5-ASA is the active agent and 10 to 20 percent of patients are intolerant of the sulfapyridine moiety of sulfasalazine, newer formulations of 5-ASA have been developed with the thought of increased delivery to the small intestine.

Olsalazine (Dipentum) consists of two molecules of 5-ASA linked by the same azo bond as in sulfasalazine. However, delivery is primarily to the colon and there is therefore no advantage over sulfasalazine; the drug is not indicated for small bowel Crohn's disease.

Coated 5-ASA (mesalamine) contains no other carrier compounds but rather is released at different sites in the intestine depending on the coating. Asacol has a coating of Eudragit S, which dissolves at lumenal pH 7 (approximately the terminal ileum and right colon). Although this drug has not been approved by the U.S. Food and Drug Administration (FDA) for Crohn's disease, clinical experience has indicated a response rate of approximately 60 percent with doses of 2.4 to 3.6 g daily. As in ulcerative colitis, use of higher doses (4.8 g daily) may show increased response, but long-term use runs the risk of increased small intestinal absorption and potential toxicity. The drug is generaly well tolerated; however, no one has determined the ideal time to give this medication, and if taken with food the coated capsule may remain in the stomach for many hours. Capsules often appear intact in the stool if intestinal motility is increased and/or if there was prior extensive resection of small intestine.

Pentasa is a sustained-release preparation of 5-ASA granules coated with ethylcellulose. Release occurs after the drug leaves the stomach, with delivery of 5-ASA to jejunum, ileum, and colon. The drug has not been FDA approved for Crohn's disease because there have been conflicting controlled trials. The initial study demonstrated that low doses were not effective and that only 4 g daily was effective. However, a follow-up study failed to confirm efficacy greater than placebo at any dose. Nevertheless, many clinicians are treating with 3 or 4 g daily. Compliance is difficult to maintain since 16 capsules are required when giving 4 g daily.

Recently multiple studies as well as several meta-analyses have confirmed that the new 5-ASA drugs are preventative agents for both exacerbations of disease and following surgical resection. Controlled trials have shown relapse rates were decreased by just over 40 percent provided that adequate doses (>2.5 g daily) were used. The subset of patients with pure ileal involvement seems to respond better to mesalamine prevention.

Likewise, several studies using 2.4 or 3 g daily of mesalamine showed prevention of endoscopic and clinical recurrence after resection of all grossly visible Crohn's disease. Recurrence is again decreased about 40 percent.

There has been recent debate regarding routine prophylaxis with mesalamine, looking at the high long-term cost compared with moderate response as well as potential toxicity. Most clinicians await further data. However, all facts should be thoroughly discussed with patients, who should have the final decision.

Toxicity with the new 5-ASA drugs includes idiosyncratic reactions such as pericarditis, pleuritis, pancreatitis, and nephrotic syndrome. Nephrotoxicity has been observed in animals taking long-term high doses of 5-ASA, and there are scattered clinical reports of interstitial nephritis in IBD patients. True allergy to the 5-ASA compound may be observed in some patients. These drugs appear to be safe in pregnancy but data in nursing women is lacking.

Corticosteroids

If physicians were polled as to the drug of choice for active Crohn's disease of the small intestine, they would certainly select corticosteroids. Two multicenter-controlled trials confirmed the short-term efficacy of these agents. The National Cooperative Crohn's Disease Study (NCCDS) achieved control of active disease in approximately 60 percent of patients, usually within 6 weeks. A somewhat disconcerting factor regarding the accuracy of the study was the lack of response in patients with colonic Crohn's disease, since most clinicians have seen a short-term dramatic response in patients with Crohn's colitis. The European Cooperative Crohn's Disease Study (ECCDS) demonstrated the efficacy of steroids in both colonic and small bowel Crohn's disease, although only 24 patients with small bowel disease were entered into the study. It was rather disturbing that 80 percent of the deaths in the ECCDS were in patients treated with steroids, especially those with abdominal masses. Also of concern was the inability of patients to stop steroids once having started them. In the NCCDS, over 50 percent of patients could not withdraw without clinical relapse.

These factors might have been expected to cause many objections to the use of steroids in a chronic lifetime illness such as small bowel Crohn's disease. However, this has not occurred, and as noted previously, corticosteroids are used by most physicians as first-line treatment. I will suggest an alternative approach later.

If steroids are initiated, they should be administered in adequate dosage, 30 to 60 mg of prednisone daily. Physicians disagree as to whether this should be given in a single dosage in the morning or spread through the day. In my clinical experience, three or four times daily dosing works more quickly and effectively than a single administration; however, spreading the dose also produces more side effects. I prefer rapid control of the inflammatory process with a high initial dose and then quick lowering of the steroids, which is preferable to "creeping" up to higher doses. In my experience, the latter technique often results in the patient's inability to stop steroids. I have tried alternate-day dosing in moderate to severe disease and have found it ineffective. Although many physicians use alternate-day dosing to reduce side effects, I believe that it is not effective in active disease. For inactive disease my goal is to stop steroids, not "maintain" low alternate-day dosing. I therefore reject alternate-day administration of the drug until there is controlled evidence to support its use. I do not consider that prednisolone, methylprednisolone, or triamcinolone is preferable to prednisone.

When the patient has improved, steroids can be decreased rapidly from the initial 40 mg to 60 mg daily dosage. I usually decrease the dosage by 5 to 10 mg weekly until a dose of 20 mg is reached. Flare-ups invariably occur between 20 and 10 mg of daily prednisone. Therefore, at 20 mg I slow the reduction to a rate of 2.5 mg per week or 2.5 mg every other week, until the patient is able to stop steroids. Close clinical observation for an exacerbation is required at this crucial stage of management.

Should sulfasalazine be added while steroids are being reduced? The NCCDS suggests that this carries no advantage, but many experienced clinicians believe that some patients will benefit with this combination. Should other agents be added to steroids during withdrawal? The role of antibiotics and immunosuppressives will be discussed later. In my experience, there is a role for combined therapy (steroids plus antibiotics, steroids plus sulfasalazine, steroids plus antibiotics and sulfasalazine), in selected subsets. In addition, numerous trials have shown that immunosuppressive agents are specifically steroid sparing in Crohn's disease.

Patients who are severely ill with active small bowel Crohn's disease should be admitted to the hospital for parenteral medications. Although there are no controlled data regarding the use of intravenous steroids in the management of Crohn's disease, most clinicians consider them more effective than oral steroids. Patients to be considered for intravenous steroids include those with obstruction, severe weight loss, malnutrition, or systemic manifestations such as fever. I prefer hydrocortisone sodium succinate (Solu-Cortef), 300 mg daily, given by continuous intravenous infusion. In my clinical experience, the drug works more quickly and with better response when given continuously as compared to pulse administration. Intravenous adrenocorticotropic hormone (ACTH) has been shown to be more effective than intravenous Solu-Cortef in acutely ill ulcerative colitis patients who have not been taking steroids before admission to the hospital. A recent controlled trial suggests the same is not true in Crohn's colitis and that there is no advantage of one drug over the other.

I often use ACTH gel injections in outpatients for control of active small bowel Crohn's disease. I find it as effective as oral prednisone (possibly more effective in patients with malabsorption) and when administered in the following regimen it produces fewer steroid side effects. I administer 40 units of ACTH gel daily for 4 days and then on alternate days for another 2 weeks. Further tapering depends on the clinical response, but usually the drug is lowered to three times weekly and stopped in most patients in about 6 to 8 weeks. Despite the annoyance of injections, most patients report equal effectiveness and fewer steroid side effects with intermittent ACTH injections than with continuous oral prednisone. The long-term use of steroids (>4 to 6 months) is to be avoided if at all possible. There are no controlled data to support a long-term benefit of steroids for maintenance, prevention of relapse, or prevention of recurrence after surgical resection. The ECCDS suggests low-dose steroids for up to 2 to 3 years if remission has been obtained with steroids in some patients. This vague suggestion has not been confirmed in trials and my clinical experience suggests that this is a foolhardy approach. Steroid toxicity such as cosmetic side effects (especially in adolescents and young adults), thinning of the skin with easy bruisability, hypertension, diabetes, failure to grow, cataracts, aseptic necrosis of the hips, and bone collapse outweigh the unsubstantiated efficacy of long-term corticosteroids for small bowel Crohn's disease.

As regards intestinal obstruction, steroids are of limited value. Small bowel obstruction may be related to dietary indiscretion in a patient with a narrowed lumen secondary to Crohn's disease. This may be triggered by the ingestion of high-residue foods, especially raw fruits and raw vegetables. If these obstructed patients are treated with intravenous fluids and nothing by mouth (occasionally a nasogastric or Cantor tube is required for vomiting), most improve within 24 hours without the addition of intravenous steroids. I therefore do not administer steroids if I can obtain a history of dietary indiscretion and *no* history or signs of an inflammatory process (e.g., fever, aphthous ulcers, elevated erythrocyte sedimentation rate).

Conversely, in patients in whom inflammation has preceded obstruction, steroids are usually beneficial in decreasing mucosal edema and ulceration, and can be given in the form of ACTH or Solu-Cortef, depending on previous medications.

The third factor in obstruction is a fibrous stricture of the lumen. In my experience, steroids offer no "long-term" benefit (although sometimes a temporary benefit) with this type of obstruction. I believe that in this clinical situation surgical resection is inevitable. Fixed fibrotic stricture is diagnosed when there is no superimposed evidence of active inflammation and when the proximal small bowel is becoming increasingly dilated.

Active small bowel Crohn's disease with a tender abdominal mass is a special situation that requires important clinical decisions. Steroids given alone to patients with an inflammatory mass is not only contraindicated but may be deleterious. In these patients who have usually fistulized (into the mesentery, to other bowel loops, to internal organs such as bladder and vagina), many may already have an abscess or go on to develop one. As noted above, three deaths were seen in the ECCDS study in clinically active patients who received steroids in the face of an abdominal mass. I believe that steroids should be avoided until a computed tomographic (CT) scan is performed, and even if an abscess is not detected on CT scan, I rarely administer steroids to these patients. I prefer to treat with triple antibiotics (aminoglycosides, ampicillin, and metronidazole) through the entire course of the hospitalization. Most patients improve, and I add ACTH to the antibiotic regimen only in an occasional patient. After improvement, I discharge these patients on oral antibiotics alone, or antibiotics plus rapidly tapering intramuscular ACTH gel. If steroids are thought to be essential when a mass is present, antibiotics should be initiated at the same time.

Since (1) there is no evidence for long-term efficacy of steroids in Crohn's disease, (2) over 50 percent of patients cannot stop steroids after they are initiated, and (3) corticosteroids involve major toxicity, I try never to use steroids for small bowel Crohn's disease.

A new oral, rapidly metabolized steroid (budesonide) has shown efficacy when the disease is active around the ileocecal area. Further studies of efficacy and toxicity are indicated.

Antibiotics

Despite inadequate controlled data to justify the use of antibiotics in Crohn's disease, a vast underground group of clinicians are using these agents as first- or second-line therapy. A variety of antibiotic agents have been tried, with anecdotal reports on symptomatic efficacy and radiographic improvement. In one uncontrolled study, antibiotics were administered singly or in combination for over 6 months with success. In one controlled trial, a nonabsorbable antibiotic plus elemental diet was compared with steroids plus a normal diet, with equal results; this trial is too confusing to draw conclusions from it. Likewise, a trial of three antibiotic regimens—trimethoprim-sulfamethoxazole, metronidazole, and a combination of both—compared with placebo showed no long-term benefit of any group. Sites of disease (large or small bowel) were not mentioned in this study and early response was seen in both groups taking metronidazole.

By contrast, metronidazole alone has shown efficacy in both uncontrolled and several controlled trials. A European trial showed metronidazole to be more effective than sulfasalazine in small bowel disease. Another controlled trial showed both low-dose (10 mg per kilogram per day) and high-dose (20 mg per kilogram per day) metronidazole to be more effective than placebo predominantly in colonic disease. Metronidazole has also been demonstrated to be clearly effective in patients with perianal fistulae complicating both small and large bowel Crohn's disease. Metronidazole alone has never proved effective in closing internal fistulae in Crohn's disease, although as noted above it may help prevent abscess formation in patients with tender inflammatory masses that have fistulized into the mesentery. Another small controlled trial has shown the combination of metronidazole and ciprofloxacin to be effective in Crohn's disease.

With this conflicting data, should the clinician use antibiotics for small bowel Crohn's disease? I prefer antibiotics to steroids for short- and long-term use and prescribe ampicillin or cephalexin (Keflex), 500 mg four times daily, for signs of mild activity. My patients take the antibiotic for a minimum of 6 weeks, and some have continued for up to 2 years. I have not seen major superinfections in these long-term users. If the patient becomes quiescent, I gradually withdraw the antibiotics over 2 to 4 weeks; if there is a flare-up, I reintroduce or raise the dosage. If a patient becomes active while taking ampicillin, I often rotate to cephexalin or ciprofloxacin and vice versa. Broad-spectrum antibiotics are my drugs of choice if there is radiographic evidence of internal fistulae, a secondary suppurative process, or evidence of an inflammatory mass.

If the patient presents with moderately active disease, I often use metronidazole as the initial drug of choice; it appears to be more effective when there is colonic involvement. However, I have had success in patients who have ileocolitis and/or small bowel disease alone. The standard dosage in adults is 750 to 1,500 mg of metronidazole daily. The higher dose often is not well tolerated (causing nausea and loss of appetite, and having a metallic taste) and must be reduced as soon as the disease is under control. Peripheral neuropathy is a frequent complication with high doses, and patients must be forewarned to be alert to symptoms of numbness and tingling, which necessitate stopping or lowering the dose. The drug usually has to be completely discontinued when neuropathy appears. It may take over 6 to 12 months for the symptoms to reverse and I have seen tingling, albeit mild, persist for over 2 years.

Patients are usually cautioned by pharmacists and physicians not to drink alcohol while taking metronidazole because of an Antabuse-type effect. In fact, this reaction occurs in about 1 to 2 in 100 people, and I advise patients who are taking the drug for a long period, and would like to have an occasional drink, to try alcohol. This should be done at home to prevent embarrassment if vomiting should occur, but most patients experience no reaction.

Animal studies have shown an increase in tumor production with metronidazole (particularly liver and lung), although short-term administration of metronidazole has demonstrated no predisposition to neoplasm in large numbers of women who received the drug for vaginitis. There are no data showing that long-term administration of metronidazole is safe in humans. Isolated case reports of neoplasm with long-term usage suggest maintenance of low doses of 500 to 750 mg daily. Although a 6 to 8 week course of metronidazole is preferred for treatment of active small bowel disease, the condition of many patients is exacerbated with early discontinuation of the drug. The clinician must carefully weigh the need for long-term usage and try to substitute other antibiotics (broad spectrum) in patients who have continued low-grade activity or who worsen when metronidazole is lowered or stopped.

Broad-spectrum antibiotics are of value in patients with jejunoileitis with stricture, low-grade obstruction, and bacterial overgrowth. Tetracycline in doses of 250 mg twice daily helps malabsorption and often decreases symptoms of bloating, diarrhea, and abdominal discomfort.

Combination antibiotics can be used in more seriously ill hospitalized patients with inflammatory masses. For patients taking steroids long term whose condition worsens with lowered dosages, I add single or double antibiotics to the regimen before another attempt to withdraw prednisone. I have had some success in substituting antibiotics for steroids, especially in patients with internal fistulization. In a trial, metronidazole has been successful in preventing postoperative recurrence when used for 3 months. This effect did not last beyond 1 year and further studies are required.

Immunosuppressive Agents

Both 6-mercaptopurine (6-MP) and azathioprine have been studied in uncontrolled and controlled trials of patients with Crohn's disease. The uncontrolled data are convincing, showing efficacy in approximately 70 to 75 percent of cases. These studies do not specifically emphasize small or large bowel involvement, and with a wide clinical spectrum of Crohn's disease it is difficult to determine the indications for use of these agents in isolated small bowel disease. Controlled studies have shown effectiveness in four of eight trials, including those with involvement of large bowel or small bowel and/or ileocolitis. Immunosuppressives have shown healing of fistulae and prevention of exacerbation. However, in the NCCDS they were used in 49 patients with only small bowel involvement; statistical significance was "not seen but there was a trend in favor of azathioprine." The failure to show efficacy in this study was due to the design of the trial, which was prejudiced against a slow-acting drug such as azathioprine. The duration of the trial was only 4 months, and patients were taken off all other agents and randomized to azathioprine alone, which did not have enough time to show efficacy before exacerbation occurred.

In our 6-MP study, we demonstrated that the mean time to respond was 3.1 months, with 68 percent response at 3 months and 80 percent at 4 months; some patients took as long as 6 to 7 months to respond. Efficacy was seen in both small bowel and colonic disease, although the quality of the response was better in patients with Crohn's colitis and ileocolitis than in those with ileitis or ileojejunitis. We have demonstrated success in closing and improving fistulae both from the large and small bowel, including ileovesical, ileosigmoid, ileocutaneous, and perineal fistulae. Steroid sparing is seen in 70 percent of patients, and it was possible to stop prednisone completely in 50 to 60 percent of patients while maintaining clinical improvement.

In our controlled trial, we used 1.5 mg per kilogram daily as the initial dosage. When administering 6-MP I now start with a lower dosage; I give 50 mg daily and monitor the white blood cell (WBC) count (weekly for 1 month, every other week for 1 month, and then monthly). If the WBC count is maintained above 5,000, the dose can be slowly raised to 75 to 100 mg daily. A lower dose is associated with a longer time to respond, but rarely produces leukopenia. Since the drug takes a long time to act, I maintain all other medications (steroids, antibiotics, and 5-ASA agents) until the 6-MP has had an opportunity to be effective. When improvement is seen, steroids are gradually reduced. If a patient has not responded after 6 to 8 months, the 6-MP dose should be increased to produce leukopenia, which may be required in a small percentage of patients.

When should immunosuppressives be used in patients with small bowel Crohn's disease? They should be considered in patients who have already undergone resection and in whom further resection might compromise nutritional status. This also applies to patients in whom the initial resection is so extensive that it might produce a short bowel syndrome. 6-MP is indicated in patients with major internal fistulization or fistulization to the skin or bladder. 6-MP should not be introduced in these patients in the face of an active secondary infection or abscess until antibiotics have quieted the process or drainage has occurred. Immunosuppressives are indicated in patients with active small bowel disease and active perianal fistulae. They should be considered in patients on chronic steroids (≥4 months) in whom at least two attempts have been made to stop the corticosteroids. They should also be used in patients suffering from steroid toxicity and in whom surgical resection would be extensive.

I have seen marked healing of pyoderma gangrenosum in almost all patients treated with 6-MP. I have had less success with other extraintestinal manifestations such as arthritis and erythema nodosum, but my colleagues who also use 6-MP think differently and have reported success in treating these latter complications.

I do not use 6-MP in the face of obstruction due to a fibrous stricture, but it may be effective when the obstruction is due to inflammatory swelling. There has been an excellent response to recurrent ileitis in ileostomies after colectomy. Response has also been observed in internal and/or stomal fistulae with an ileostomy.

I do not administer 6-MP to patients who have limited disease in the terminal ileum and in whom a simple resection would lead to rapid recovery without the long-term close observation required with 6-MP. We are now administering 6-MP to patients who have required two to three resections within a short time (≤5 years). We hope to prevent recurrence by giving 6-MP, but at this time no data are available to assist therapeutic conclusions. I have not seen dramatic effects on growth in children, even when the 6-MP has quieted the inflammatory process. In such cases, we use 6-MP plus nutritional supplementation (elemental or parenteral feedings).

A recent study suggests that intravenous azathioprine shows efficacy in 2 weeks. Controlled trials are awaited. Antibody to TNF has recently shown efficacy in active Crohn's disease and A recent controlled trial has confirmed response in approximately two-thirds of patients.

Side Effects

There has been great fear of the long-term toxicity in IBD patients treated with 6-MP. Our studies of 396 patients (with ulcerative colitis and Crohn's disease) with a mean follow-up of over 5 years have shown few serious side effects. Unpublished data on over 800 patients have shown similar results with a 10 year follow-up. Allergic reactions (pancreatitis, rash or fever, hepatitis) occur in 6 percent of patients and rapidly disappear when the drug is stopped. Leukopenia is seen rarely when the drug is administered as advised. Care must be taken when giving 6-MP or azathioprine to patients taking allopurinol; in this situation, one-quarter to one-third the usual dosage is given.

We have seen few severe infections that might be related to 6-MP (1.8 percent) and no deaths attributable to an infectious complication. We have not seen pneumocystis pneumonia.

We have observed a number of tumors in patients taking 6-MP, but apart from one histiocytic lymphoma of the brain, these neoplasms are not associated with immunosuppressive drugs. Considering the increased risk of lymphoma in IBD (especially Crohn's disease), this single case may be a chance occurrence. Several large studies have shown no increased risk of either cancer or lymphoma with 6-MP or azathioprine.

Since 6-MP and azathioprine have shown efficacy in prevention, and since discontinuing the drug within 1 year often results in exacerbation, I advise administration for at least 4 to 5 years before the drug is stopped. Many patients have taken the drug for more than 20 years without any major secondary complication. There have been no abnormalities in children born to patients who are taking 6-MP or had taken it prior to conception. I do not advise stopping 6-MP when pregnancy is being considered. A recent United Kingdom study has confirmed the lack of abnormalities in children conceived on 6-MP; physicians did not stop the drug during pregnancy.

Cyclosporine

Cyclosporine has shown some efficacy, usually within 1 to 2 weeks, in about two-thirds of patients in uncontrolled trials in Crohn's disease. Although the initial controlled trial showed efficacy, this was not confirmed in two other controlled trials, perhaps because a lower dose was given. These uncontrolled and controlled studies as well as a controlled prevention study have shown failure of cyclosporine to maintain remission.

However, when initially administered intravenously in doses of 4 mg per kilogram, cyclosporine has shown efficacy in perianal and abdominal wall fistulae, active Crohn's colitis, and pyoderma gangrenosum. After initial intravenous use, oral doses of 6 to 8 mg per kilogram daily are given, with tapering depending on renal function. The response rate in fistulae is 88 percent (44 percent closure) with subsequent relapse of about one-third of patients. The addition of 6-MP may prevent relapse. The use of steroids is to be avoided when treating Crohn's fistula, as healing is delayed.

Toxicity of cyclosporine may be marked (occurring in about 10 percent), including nephrotoxicity, liver function abnormalities, pneumocystis pneumonia (if used with steroids), electrolyte disturbances (low magnesium, high potassium), and seizures. Experience with this drug is required, and cyclosporine administration should be limited to 6 to 12 months.

Several uncontrolled trials have shown efficacy of methotrexate given intramuscularly 25 mg weekly. In about three-quarters of Crohn's patients response at 1 year is just under 50 percent, showing relapse as the drug is switched to oral administration and the dose lowered. A controlled trial has shown statistically significant efficacy compared with placebo when patients require high-dose steroids. Methotrexate will probably serve as an interim short-term therapy for some patients, especially those allergic or unresponsive to 6-MP and azathioprine. The major potential toxicity of methotrexate is liver fibrosis and cirrhosis, with rare cases of idiosyncratic marrow depression and pneumocystis pneumonia.

The role of both cyclosporine and methotrexate in small bowel Crohn's disease is thus uncertain and will require further trials and greater experience.

T-lymphocyte apheresis is also being studied in Crohn's disease in combination with TPN. A report of 54 patients treated with this modality showed a high rate of remission (15 of 54). This study also needs controlled trials.

■ INDICATIONS FOR SURGERY

The main indications for surgery are (1) obstruction with fibrous stricture of the small bowel, (2) intra-abdominal abscess, (3) massive bleeding, (4) intractability, and (5) perianal abscess.

As noted, surgery is indicated for obstruction due to fibrous stricture but not for inflammatory spastic obstruction. Although an abscess has been considered an indication for surgery, some medical centers are performing percutaneous needle drainage of abscesses. This modality should be pursued but only in patients who can then be managed medically without surgical resection. Percutaneous drainage appears to have no value if surgery is still required after drainage. The surgeon in these situations can drain and resect at the same time.

Massive bleeding is rare (5 percent) and usually stops with intravenous steroids and transfusions.

The definition of intractability should be determined by the patient. The physician must be a partner in helping patients define their disability, and the physician must explain the risks of surgery and of recurrence. Also to be clarified are the chronic need for medications and their side effects versus patients' ability to function normally with and without resection. Patients who select surgery will usually be gratified with their postoperative status.

Postoperative diarrhea usually responds to cholestyramine or antidiarrheals agents. Vitamin B_{12} is rarely required after surgery, and there should be few dietary restrictions unless there has been substantial resection (>50 cm). In these cases, if the patient has excessive diarrhea, malabsorption should be documented with fecal fat collection and a Schilling test. Patients often undergo elective surgery to rid themselves of medications and permit a liberal diet; therefore, the fewer restrictions and the fewer medications the better for patients' emotional well being.

■ THERAPY FOR COMPLICATIONS: SPECIAL SITUATIONS

Aphthous Ulcerations. These are usually treated symptomatically with topical diphenhydramine (Benadryl) or triamcinolone (Kenalog in Orabase); some physicians have had success with topical sucralfate (Carafate). I have had little success with any therapy for these painful lesions.

Gastroduodenal Crohn's Disease. Crohn's disease involving the distal antrum or first portions of the duodenum is common (over 25 percent of patients), behaves like peptic disease, and usually responds to H_2 blockers in adequate doses. Occasionally a higher than normal dosage of H_2 blockers is required for a few weeks to control these upper GI symptoms. I have rarely had to use steroids to control symptoms. A recent study described the successful use of Ômeprazole. Obstruction is best treated with surgery. Bypass can be performed at laparotomy or by laparoscopic technique.

Erythema Nodosum. This complication usually is not associated with small bowel disease alone but with colonic or ileocolonic involvement. If the bowel disease or minimal. I treat erythema nodosum with oral aspirin, two tablets 3 to 4 times daily. If the Crohn's disease is mild, I add aspirin to current therapy such as 5-ASA agent and/or an antibiotic. I try never to use oral steroids for this self-limiting complication. Some of my colleagues report success with colchicine in patients with erythema nodosum. If the condition is refractory, injections of ACTH gel, 40 units given intramuscularly two to three times a week for 1 to 4 weeks will help to quiet this process.

Pyoderma Gangrenosum. Pyoderma is not treated like erythema nodosum and requires more intensive medical management, even though the bowel disease is quiescent or mild in over 50 percent of cases. Pyoderma gangrenosum often occurs soon after withdrawal of sulfasalazine and especially after local trauma. The patient should be restarted on sulfasalazine or the dosage should be raised, and intralesional steroids should also be given. I have also had success with hyperbaric oxygenation and with 6-MP. Most recently there have been excellent results with intravenous cyclosporine, with closures seen in 1 to 2 weeks. Resection of the bowel is not indicated for pyoderma gangrenosum.

Peripheral Arthritis. Arthritis should be treated in a similar manner to erythema nodosum, with aspirin, and if the bowel disease is active, with an oral 5-ASA agent or antibiotics. Oral steroids should be avoided, although ACTH may be helpful in refractory cases. Effusion into the knee may require drainage with injection of steroids. Nonsteroidal anti-inflammatory drugs (NSAIDs) such as sulindac, 200 mg twice daily, may be helpful, but may also upset the upper GI tract and may trigger activity of the Crohn's disease.

Ankylosing Spondylitis. This should be treated with NSAIDs; in my experience, the best is indomethocin, 25 to 50 mg three to four times daily. The activity of the spondylitis does not correlate with the activity of the IBD and therefore does not require a change in therapy for the latter.

Ocular Manifestations. Eye complications such as episcleritis and uveitis are best treated by an ophthalmologist with topical steroids. Systemic steroids are rarely required for these complications.

Cholelithiasis and Urolithiasis. These are treated in the same manner as in patients without Crohn's disease. If an ileal resection is required and the gallbladder is known to be diseased, it can be resected at the same time, if there is no complicating intra-abdominal abscess.

Sclerosing Cholangitis. There is no indication for bowel resection for this complication. The patient should be continuously monitored and a liver transplant performed for major hepatic deterioration. No drug therapy is currently available.

Table 1 Therapy for Crohn's Disease of the Small Bowel

INDICATION	PREFERRED TREATMENT OF CHOICE
Mild activity	Symptomatic drugs Sulfasalazine oral 5-ASA agent Broad-spectrum antibiotics Metronidazole Combinations of above
Moderate activity	Symptomatic drugs Sulfasalazine, oral 5-ASA agents—increased dose Metronidazole Broad-spectrum antibiotics ACTH gel intramuscular Combinations of above Hospitalization with IV antibiotics with or without ACTH Oral steroids
Severe activity	Metronidazole + broad-spectrum antibiotics Hospitalization with intravenous triple antibiotics with or without ACTH Metronidazole + broad-spectrum antibiotics + oral prednisone
Obstruction:	
inflammatory	Hospitalization with IV antibiotics with or without ACTH
stricture	Surgery
Internal fistula with tender mass and/or fever	IV triple antibiotics IV triple antibiotics + IV ACTH Addition of TPN
Chronic steroids after failure of antibiotics and 5-ASA agents:	
Short segment	Surgery
Extensive segment	6-MP Methotrexate
Perianal disease:	
Mild	Metronidazole: stop steroids
Moderate to severe	6-MP: stop steroids Cyclosporine

Hydronephrosis. This complication per se does not require surgery since it simply indicates extension of the inflammatory process by fistulization to the retroperitoneum. Secondary pyelonephritis does not occur unless the patient undergoes cystoscopy. The ileal disease should be treated as described in previous sections, especially with antibiotics.

Pregnancy. Patients do well if they become pregnant while quiescent; however, there is often an early flare-up if pregnancy occurs when the disease is clinically active. I treat these patients with sulfasalazine and broad-spectrum antibiotics, trying to avoid metronidazole. Usually the process will be subdued during the second and third trimester; there is an increased risk of exacerbation post partum. Steroids may be used safely if the process is severe. The fetus is at little risk when the mother has IBD, and fortunately in most women IBD remains under control during pregnancy.

Perianal Disease. This is generally treated in a conservative manner with topical skin therapy, sitz baths, and soaking in order to obtain adequate drainage. Metronidazole or 6-MP is administered for active perianal fistulae. If an abscess occurs and does not drain spontaneously, the surgeon may have to perform incision and drainage. Internal sphincterotomy and drainage (Park's procedure) may be required if there is severe perianal pain associated with an internal collection. Although this procedure is quite successful in alleviating symptoms, some sphincter muscle is lost and disability may result. In my experience, it should be used primarily for younger patients and should not be performed repeatedly. Intravenous cyclosporine is effective with severe forms.

There are many forms of therapy for Crohn's disease of the small bowel. A summary of the drugs of choice for mild, moderate, and severe disease is given in Table 1. Each patient must be individualized; the problem is challenging, but the rewards for the clinician are great. There are few circumstances more satisfying in medicine than to have a long-term partnership with an appreciative patient with Crohn's disease.

Suggested Reading

Bicks RO, Groshart KD, Luther RW. Total parenteral nutrition (TPN) plus T-lymphocyte apheresis (TLA) in the treatment of severe chronic active Crohn's disease. Gastroenterology 1988; 94:A34.

European Cooperative Crohn's Disease Study: Results of drug treatment. Gastroenterology 1984; 86:249–266.

Goldstein F, Farquhar S, Thornton JJ, et al. Favorable effects of sulfasalazine on small bowel Crohn's disease: a long-term study. Am J Gastroenterol 1987; 82:848–853.

Greenberg GR, Fleming CR, Jeejeebhoy KN, et al. Controlled trial of bowel rest and nutritional support in the management of Crohn's disease. Gut 1988; 29:1309–1315.

Korelitz BI, Present DH. Favorable effect of 6-mercaptopurine in fistulas of Crohn's disease. Dig Dis Sci 1985; 30:58–64.

Kozarek RA, Patterson DJ, Gelfand MD, et al. Methotrexate induces clinical and histologic remissions in refractory inflammatory bowel disease. Ann Intern Med 1989; 110:353–356.

Messori A, Brignola C, Trallori G, et al. Effectiveness of 5-ASA for maintaining remission in patients with Crohn's disease: a meta-analysis. Am J Gastro 1994; 89:692–698.

National Cooperative Crohn's Disease Study: results of drug treatment. Gastroenterology 1979; 77:847–869.

O'Donaghue DP, Dawson AW, Powell-Tuck J, et al. Double-blind withdrawal trial of azathioprine as maintenance treatment of Crohn's disease. Lancet 1978; 2:955–957.

Present DH, Korelitz BI, Wisch N, et al. Treatment of Crohn's disease with 6-MP. N Engl J Med 1980; 302:981–987.

Present DH. 6-Mercaptopurine and other immunosuppressive agents in the treatment of Crohn's disease and ulcerative colitis. Gastro Clin North Am 1989; 18:57–71.

Rasmussen SN, Lauritsen K, Tage-Jensen U, et al. 5-aminosalicylic acid in the treatment of Crohn's disease. Scand J Gastroenterol 1987.

Sandborn WJ, Tremaine WS. Cyclosporine treatment of IBD. Mayo Clin Proc 1992; 67:981–990.

Saverymuttu SH, Gupta S, Keshavarzian A, et al. Effect of a slow-release 5-aminosalicylic acid preparation on disease activity in Crohn's disease. Digestion 1986; 33:89–96.

Ursing B, Alm T, Buriny F, et al. A comparative study of metronidazole and sulfasalazine for active Crohn's disease. Gastroenterology 1982; 83:550–562.

LEFT-SIDED ULCERATIVE COLITIS AND ULCERATIVE PROCTITIS

Philip B. Miner, Jr., M.D.

Patients with left-sided ulcerative colitis or ulcerative proctitis represent a significant proportion of those seen with inflammatory bowel disease (IBD). Seventy percent of patients with ulcerative colitis have disease limited to the left side. The advent of flexible sigmoidoscopy has (1) allowed us to identify this group more efficiently, (2) improved our understanding of the natural history, and (3) permitted us to evaluate the efficacy of new modes of therapy, including topical medications. Complementing these basic diagnostic understandings, recent analysis of the anorectal physiology of IBD has improved our ability to manage and treat this often frustrating disease. One of the most important symptoms in patients who have left-sided ulcerative colitis is tenesmus (spasm of the rectum related to inflammation in the distal colon). The traditional approach to tenesmus is to decrease rectal inflammation. Improved understanding of anorectal physiology allows intervention in other important ways. The unique metabolic regulation of the left colon dependent on short-chain fatty acids, a chief energy source for colonocytes of the left colon, may explain the value of short-chain fatty acids in treating distal colitis. As we become more familiar with the physiology of inflammation, the nutrient requirements of the left colon compared with the right colon, and the characteristics of the distal colon that cause symptoms of diarrhea, we will have new tools with which to treat these diseases.

BASIC CONCEPTS

Easy access to office-based flexible sigmoidoscopy by the family practitioner or internist has made the diagnosis of left-sided ulcerative colitis far easier. In a patient presenting with bloody diarrhea of more than 2 weeks' duration associated with symptoms of tenesmus and bloody, mucoid stools, the clinician should perform flexible sigmoidoscopy. If possible, the flexible sigmoidoscope should be passed beyond the line of demarcation of the disease in order to evaluate the extent of mucosal inflammation and the inflammatory characteristics of the mucosa such as edema, erythema, granularity, and ulceration. The pattern of inflammation with areas spared of disease may suggest either a disease of infectious origin or perhaps Crohn's disease. Biopsies are useful at the line of demarcation, in the area of active disease, and above the line of demarcation of disease, but for practical purposes the extent of disease should be determined by visual recognition and not microscopic changes.

In patients with left-sided ulcerative colitis or ulcerative proctitis, the apparent paradox of diarrhea as well as constipation often occurs. This is due to the disturbed anorectal physiology that occurs with inflammation of the distal colon. In left-sided ulcerative colitis or ulcerative proctitis, the rectal tone is increased and the rectum is far more sensitive to volume distention. These changes are present even in the absence of active inflammation. Rectal reactivity and spasm induce diarrhea while impairing proximal colonic motility. This arrested stool movement permits desiccation of stool with the failure of delivery of stool into the inflamed rectum. An understanding of this concept is important for management of patients, as avoiding constipation is a critical issue in left-sided ulcerative colitis. The frequent observation that symptoms of irritable bowel syndrome (IBS) occur in conjunction with inflammatory disease may be linked to the high number of mast cells at the line of demarcation and in the proximal mucosa in left-sided disease. It has been shown that 70 percent of patients with IBS have increased numbers of mucosal mast cells, and 60 percent of those with IBD have increased mast cells at the line of demarcation of the disease. Increased mucosal mast cells may explain the symptoms of abdominal pain, urgency, and occasional incontinence associated with anorectal dysfunction.

In a separate study of patients with increased gastrointestinal mast cells, we demonstrated similar rectal reactivity to low-volume balloon distention with increased rectal tone to the changes in ulcerative colitis patients. This observation is practical with regard to management, as antihistamines often modulate the spasm and reactivity in the rectum and can be used as adjunctive therapy for managing symptoms in patients with left-sided ulcerative colitis. The strategy of using antihistamines for retention of enemas or decreasing the feeling of tenesmus has been useful in patients with active distal inflammation. It is also important to avoid using antimotility agents, which may increase the level of constipation in patients with limited ulcerative colitis. Occasionally, stool softeners are required to make sure that hard stool located above the area of inflammation does not complicate the illness. Dietary intake of sugars can have important ramifications in these patients, since disaccharide malabsorption can lead to an increase in abdominal pain and gas. Avoidance of simple sugars, including lactose, is a useful dietary adjunct for improving symptoms.

SPECIFIC TREATMENT FOR COLONIC INFLAMMATION

Sulfasalazine

Traditional treatment of IBD with sulfasalazine remains an important part of the management of left-sided ulcerative colitis and ulcerative proctitis. This inexpensive and effective drug continues to be useful in long-term management despite the emergence of new mesalamine derivatives. Sulfasalazine has a long history of safety and efficacy, although there is a significant complication rate, with headaches and nausea in approximately 20 percent of patients. In the mid-1970s, studies were conducted to distinguish between the effects of sulfapyridine and those of 5-aminosalicylic acid (5-ASA) (mesalamine); it was determined that mesalamine was effective when given in the form of enemas for left-sided disease.

Table 1 Rectal Preparations

PRODUCT	PREPARATION
Rowasa*/Salofalk/Claversal (Reid-Rowell, US) (Interfalk, Canada) (SmithKline, International)	Enemas (4 g/60 ml buffered suspension pH 4.5)* Suppository (0.5 g/1 g)*
Pentasa (Marion, U.S.) (Ferring, Denmark)	Enema (1, 2, 4, g/dl) Buffered suspension pH 4.8
4-ASA	Enema (2 g Na-5-ASA—requires reconstitution)

*Available in the United States.
From Hanauer SB. Ulcerative proctitis and left-sided colitis. In: Bayless TM, ed. Current therapy in gastoenterology and liver disease. 3rd ed. Philadelphia: BC Decker, 1990:336.

This has led to the emergence of numerous new mesalamine formulations; it is emphasized that although many new such formulations are available, sulfasalazine was the first mesalamine-based compound. It can be used in many patients as the only drug, or can modify the cost of the new mesalamine drugs by being used in conjunction with the newer agents to decrease the total cost of management. A bacterial azoreductase breaks the bond in sulfasalazine between sulfapyridine and 5-aminosalicylate.

New Salicylates

Local Therapy (Table 1)

The efficacy of mesalamine was first demonstrated via direct application of mesalamine by enemas in patients with left-sided ulcerative colitis. Mesalamine enemas (Rowasa) proved more effective than glucocorticoid enemas in managing not only symptoms but also endoscopic and histologic appearance. The formulation of effective mesalamine enemas has been a major step in the improvement of symptoms, since the response is extremely rapid and highly effective. The low toxicity and rapid onset of action will keep these enemas at the forefront of management of left-sided disease; they have been effective in as proximal a location as the splenic flexure. In addition to the enemas, local therapy may be given in the form of mesalamine suppositories, which are effective in left-sided disease and have the advantage of greater mucosal adherence and less extensive distribution. Using frequent flexible sigmoidoscopy, I have noticed that the last area of improvement after oral drugs and enemas is the rectosigmoid junction. The suppositories can apply medication to this area more effectively than the enemas. A patient with a reactive rectum must evacuate the enema either proximally into the sigmoid or descending colon or out of the rectum. Suppositories can be used to decrease the inflammation in the rectum and rectosigmoid junction to allow the enemas to be retained in a more efficient fashion. This is an important management caveat. Rectal evacuation of the enema explains why it can be effective to the splenic flexure and why there may be a delay in the therapeutic response, which can be adjudicated by suppository therapy. Although topical medication can be used for long-term management, the value of enema therapy needs to be reconciled with costs and patient preferences as new oral drugs emerge.

Oral Preparations

The observation that sulfasalazine improved patients with ulcerative colitis led to the inevitable studies to determine whether the sulfapyridine or 5-ASA component was effective in treating the inflamed colonic mucosa. Once it was understood that 5-ASA was as effective as sulfasalazine in treating ulcerative colitis, efforts were made to develop methods for delivering mesalamine to the colon (Table 2). Sulfasalazine is split by a bacterial azoreductase present in the colonic microbiologic flora; this breaks the bond between sulfapyridine and 5-ASA. The strategy of using bacterial azoreductase enzymes was used in the development of olsalazine (Dipentum), which combined two 5-ASA molecules that could be separated by bacterial diazoreductase. Although this drug is very effective for ulcerative colitis, it has the disadvantage of inducing diarrhea in 15 to 20 percent of patients through activation of small bowel fluid secretion. In patients with constipation and distal disease, this observation can be used to treat both colonic inflammation and the constipation due to impaired colonic function with dehydration of stool in the proximal colon.

Other medications are being developed that combine mesalamine with an inert carrier, which should obviate the complications of sulfapyridine and the small intestinal secretion by olsalazine. These are not currently available in the United States, although there is extensive experience with Balsalazide outside this country. Another delivery strategy encapsulates a large amount of drug with an Eudragit coating that dissolves with change in pH in the terminal ileum or cecum. Asacol uses this strategy to release the contents of the 400 mg capsule into the cecum. This is an effective way of delivering medication to the colon; however, the renal excretion of mesalamine indicates that there is probably some release proximal to the ileocecal valve, and a few patients report seeing undissolved capsules in their stools. Microencapsulation with ethylcellulose was a strategy used to develop Pentasa. With this method, there is gradual release of 5-ASA throughout the small bowel and colon from a semipermeable ethylcellulose membrane. This form of release also delivers mesalamine to the colon, but the urinary secretion of mesalamine indicates small bowel release as well. Although this is uncertain at present, release in the small bowel may be beneficial in Crohn's disease.

One of the principal advantages of the mesalamine derivatives is their relative safety compared with sulfasalazine. In contrast to the 20 percent incidence of side effects seen in patients on sulfasalazine, the side effects associated with mesalamine derivatives are a fraction of that number. The wide array of drug release profiles allows flexibility in dosing and tailoring medication release profiles to disease distribution for long-term therapy. Even in male patients without obvious disease or toxicity, sulfasalazine induces sperm changes. Male infertility can be corrected by removal of the sulfapyridine moiety. Males should discontinue sulfasalazine and initiate mesalamine or olsalazine if they wish to father children. The oral drugs provide a convenient dosage form for patients and are effective in over 70 percent of those with left-sided ulcerative colitis.

Glucocorticoids

Glucocorticoids, whether topical or systemic, have played an important role in long-term management of IBD. As with

Table 2 New Salicylates (Oral)

PRODUCT	PREPARATION	DOSE	DELIVERY
Pentasa* (Marion, U.S.) (Ferring, Denmark)	Mesalamine encapsulated in ethylcellulose microgranules	250 mg	Time/pH release 30%–55% urinary recovery
Asacol* (Norwich-Eaton, U.S.) (Tillots, U.K.)	Mesalamine coated with Eudragit-S	400 mg	Release at pH >7 20%–35% urinary recovery
Claversal/Salofalk (SmithKline/Falk)	Mesalamine in sodium/glycine buffer coated with Eudragit-L	250–500 mg	Release at pH >6 25%–45% urinary recovery
Rowasa (Reid-Rowell)	Mesalamine in enteric-coated compress, coated with coteric opadry	250–500 mg	Release at pH >4.5 ~ 60% urinary recovery
	Mesalamine in enteric-coated tablet coated with Eudragit-L100	250–500 mg	Release at pH >5 ~ 30% urinary recovery
4-ASA (Reed and Carnrick)	Enteric coated with Eudragit compound	500 mg	Time/pH release
Dipentum* (Pharmacia)	Olsalazine (azodisalicylate)	250 mg	Two molecules of 5-ASA released into colon ~25% 5-ASA urinary recovery
Balsalazide (Brorek)	4-aminobenzyl-β-alanine-5-ASA	500 mg	Inert carrier delivers 5-ASA into colon

*Available in the United States.
From Hanauer SB. Ulcerative proctitis and left-sided colitis. In: Bayless TM, ed. Current therapy in gastoenterology and liver disease. 3rd ed. Philadelphia: BC Decker, 1990:336.

mesalamine, local application of glucocorticoids rapidly improves the disease through direct contact with the mucosa with active drug, and limits the side effects. Although it was thought for many years that glucocorticoids would be rapidly absorbed by the inflamed colon, it is the mucosa in remission that rapidly absorbs glucocorticoid enemas, in contrast to limited absorption by actively inflamed mucosa. Glucocorticoids improve tenesmus and can be used as adjunct therapy with 5-ASA drugs either rectally or orally. Glucocorticoids as foam or topical cream preparations may be utilized for distal disease. As with mesalamine, enema administration extends further into the colon for use in more proximal disease. Newer glucocorticoids such as budesonide are rapidly metabolized by the liver and thus have high first-pass clearance, which limits their systemic toxicity. Although none of the new-generation glucocorticoids have been approved for use in the United States, this major advance in glucocorticoid formulation should allow local high-dose glucocorticoid therapy with limited side effects.

Immunomodulators

Immunosuppressants such as 6-mercaptopurine and azathioprine should be cautiously administered to patients with left-sided disease, in view of their potential toxicity. Approximately 50 percent of patients with left-sided disease respond, but there is a lag period of 60 to 90 days between administration and the onset of action. There is a relative prednisone-sparing effect with sufficient immunosuppressant to improve long-term symptoms.

Emerging New Therapies

A variety of new medications are being used for the treatment of distal proctitis, proctosigmoiditis, and left-sided disease. These include methotrexate (which acts as an interleukin-1 antagonist), interleukin-1 antagonists, 5-lipoxygenase inhibitors (Zileuton), hydroxychloriquine, and short-chain fatty acid enemas. Of these, only short-chain fatty acids are unique for left-sided disease. There is emerging recognition that the left and right sides of the colon use different metabolic substrates to support mucosal integrity. If these agents are confirmed as important, they may be useful adjunctive therapy for improving resistant left-sided disease in limited colitis or pancolitis.

■ MANAGEMENT DECISIONS

Management focuses on evaluation of the extent of colonic mucosal involvement and the state of the mucosa proximal to the line of demarcation. If there is considerable uninvolved colon with the possible exception of a cecal patch, the disease should be considered to be left-sided colitis. If a line of demarcation can be established and an infectious etiology excluded, the first line of treatment depends on the extent of mucosal involvement. If more than 25 cm of the colon is involved, mesalamine enemas or local glucocorticoid enemas are most useful. The superior efficacy of mesalamine enemas compared with glucocorticoid enemas suggests that mesalamine should be a first course of treatment unless there is known sensitivity to mesalamine drugs. Disease extending less than 25 cm is effectively covered by mesalamine suppositories. Even though suppositories contain only 500 mg of drug, mucosal adherence and limited migration improve their efficacy in the rectum and distal sigmoid. If disease extends to the splenic flexure, oral adjunct therapy with mesalamine-based drugs, including azulfidine, olsalazine, or the newer-release mesalamine preparations (Asacol, Pentasa) in doses of 1 to 4 g, should often help suppress the disease. As specific symptoms are elucidated, the most disconcerting symptom should be identified and treated. Tenesmus should be treated with topical therapy. The low-volume suppository or glucocorticoid cream treatment is desirable, since medication-induced tenesmus and rectal spasm are volume related. When rigid sigmoidoscopy was the only way to visualize the mucosa, the important caveat for rectal management was that the physician not be deceived by an improvement in the rectum due to local therapy. With the use of flexible sigmoidoscopy, this does not appear to be a problem, since this procedure goes well beyond the direct contact area of local treatment and can move up to the line of demarcation. I have found local therapy to be the most effective management for these patients.

■ RECURRENT DISEASE

Therapy for recurrent episodes of colitis is an interesting topic requiring special assessment. I recently reported my approach to the problem of recurrence, which I believe is often associated with a systemic or enteric infection. The hypothesis that best explains the activation of the colitis by infection is as follows: before the infectious episode, colonic inflammation was controlled by medication that suppressed the immune system sufficiently to allow mucosal recovery. The tenuous balance between controlled homeostatic inflammation (normal) and the pathobiologic inflammation that induces mucosal disease is disrupted by the stimulation of the immune system, which has been activated to protect the body against a nonintestinal infection. Generally, activation of colonic symptoms occurs within 1 week of resolution of the systemic infection, such as an upper respiratory illness. Colonic infection with *Clostridium difficile* or other enteric infectious agents also appears to be important. I approach management of a recurrent episode by careful evaluation for treatable infection while aggressively re-establishing topical treatment and stressing the importance of compliance with drugs.

■ REFRACTORY DISEASE

If the patient is refractory to treatment, re-evaluation is essential to eliminate extension of colitis or undiagnosed disease. Possible unrecognized problems include concurrent infection, solitary rectal ulcer syndrome due to the prolapse of mucosa down into the anal canal, ischemic changes, coexistent IBS, drug-induced colitis, and mesalamine sensitivity. Each of these problems may mimic active IBD. We have recently begun to recognize an emerging group of patients with typical left-sided colitis that undergoes a gradual transition from active mucosal inflammation to a refractory disease with deep ulcerations and small areas of spared mucosa while under conventional management. Although this disease looks like Crohn's disease after the transition, transmural changes or changes consistent with Crohn's disease cannot be verified on biopsy. I believe this emerging group of patients with indeterminate colitis may be a subset of IBD with mucosal changes related to the unique metabolism of the left side of the colon. The partial repression of the disease occurs as a response to medications, and the escape from control that occurs is related to differences in the mucosal metabolism of short-chain fatty acids.

A common problem with long-term local treatment is failure to retain the enema or rapid proximal migration of the enema, leaving the distal colon inadequately treated. Although suppositories are helpful, it is also important to consider the possibility of decreasing reactivity of the rectum with antihistamines or anticholinergic agents. When this strategy is attempted, it is important to avoid constipation above the area of active inflammation.

■ LONG-TERM MANAGEMENT

Two principal issues are part of long-term management. The first is colonic surveillance for dysplasia and cancer. Cancer in the left side of the colon, although delayed, is an important risk. Intermittent flexible sigmoidoscopy to the line of demarcation of the disease should be performed with biopsies for dysplasia.

The second principal issue is maintenance therapy. It has been shown that maintenance therapy with 1 g mesalamine enemas is successful in left-sided colitis. It was possible to maintain patients in remission over the entire period, and yet when the medication was decreased, they had the same flare pattern as the controls admitted to the study 1 year previously. Anecdotal experience suggests that enemas can be used every other day or every third day for long-term management. A large study, currently being evaluated, should determine whether intermittent therapy with 4 g enemas would be successful in maintaining remission. Oral therapy is an alternative, with a mesalamine dose equivalent to 2 g sulfasalazine. In patients with limited disease, I often discontinue all therapy 6 to 10 months after successful induction of remission after the first attack, to assess the possibility that the patient might be free of symptoms without medication.

Suggested Reading

Biddle WL, Greenberger NJ, Swan JT, et al. 5-Aminosalicylic acid enemas: effective agent in maintaining remission in left-sided ulcerative colitis. Gastroenterology 1988; 94:1075–1079.

Danielsson A, Lofberg R, Persson T, et al. A steroid enema, budesonide, lacking systemic effects for the treatment of distal ulcerative colitis or proctitis. Scand J Gastroenterol 1992; 27:9–12.

Hermens DJ, Miner PB Jr. Exacerbation of ulcerative colitis. Gastroenterology 1991; 101:254–262.

Miner PB Jr, Biddle WL. Maintaining remission in distal ulcerative colitis and ulcerative proctitis. Can J Gastroenterol 1990; 4:476–480.

Petitjean O, Wendling JL, Tod M, et al. Pharmacokinetics and absolute rectal bioavailability of hydrocortisone acetate in distal colitis. Aliment Pharmacol Ther 1992; 6:351–357.

Rao SSC, Read NW, Brown C, et al. Studies on the mechanism of bowel disturbance in ulcerative colitis. Gastroenterology 1987; 93:934–940.

Rao SSC, Read NW, Davison PA, et al. Anorectal sensitivity and responses to rectal distention in patients with ulcerative colitis. Gastroenterology 1987; 93:1270–1275.

Scheppach W, Sommer H, Kirchner T, et al. Effect of butyrate enemas on the colonic mucosa in distal ulcerative colitis. Gastroenterology 1992; 103:51–56.

Sutherland LR, May GR, Shaffer EA. Sulfasalazine revisited: a meta-analysis of 5-aminosalicylic acid in the treatment of ulcerative colitis. Ann Intern Med 1993; 118:540–549.

INFLAMMATORY BOWEL DISEASE AND CANCER: DECISION MAKING

John E. Lennard-Jones, M.D., F.R.C.P., F.R.C.S.

There is no doubt that ulcerative colitis and Crohn's colitis are associated with a risk of colorectal cancer greater than in the general population. Patients with inflammatory bowel disease (IBD) constitute one of the high-risk groups within the wider problem of a universal liability to this form of cancer. The problem is to measure the element of increased liability in IBD and seek to reduce it toward the background level of risk we all face.

For clarity of discussion, ulcerative colitis and Crohn's disease are dealt with separately.

■ ULCERATIVE COLITIS

Therapeutic Possibilities

For the patient with ulcerative colitis, the big decision is whether at some stage to undergo surgical treatment for removal of the diseased colon. Very often, the correct decision is clear because the inflammation is causing so much trouble that the potential benefits of operation outweigh the possible disadvantages. For cancer prevention, the decision is often difficult because the patient is well.

Colectomy not only cures ulcerative colitis but also removes the carcinoma risk. In past years, patients wished to avoid a permanent abdominal stoma. Nowadays, the proportion of patients with ulcerative colitis who need a permanent stoma is less as reservoir procedures with ileoanal anastomosis are more commonly performed. If the operation were complication free and the patient symptomless afterwards, it would be advised and accepted more commonly than it is. In fact, there is a small postoperative mortality rate, and postoperative complications such as sepsis or obstruction can occur. Furthermore, after a pouch procedure, patients tend to pass several loose stools daily, and there is a liability to recurrent "pouchitis." Every sensible person wishes to avoid the discomfort and the time of restricted activity that major surgery entails. Add to this an element of uncertainty about the postoperative result, and a patient who has few symptoms and little disability understandably requires good evidence to justify advice that surgical treatment is needed. When, if ever, should a clinician advise a patient who is well to accept surgery?

If surgery is neither advised nor accepted, is the risk of carcinoma great enough to warrant regular precautionary measures? Are there grounds for suggesting that the patient should consult a doctor regularly? Should regular investigations be undertaken?

What is the Risk of Developing Carcinoma?

The answer to this question is not easy because it depends on the proportion of the colon inflamed, possibly on the severity of inflammation, on the duration of illness, and on the patient's age.

Extent of Disease

The literature shows that the carcinoma risk is greatest among patients in whom most or all of the colon is, or has been, inflamed. The term *extensive colitis* is widely used but with different definitions. Some series restrict the term to inflammation of the whole colon, up to and including the hepatic flexure; many series take the splenic flexure as the dividing point between "extensive" and "left-sided" colitis; and a few refer to disease proximal to the rectosigmoid as "extensive." This confusion is regrettable, and I propose that in the interests of standardization, the term *extensive colitis* should mean inflammation up to and including the splenic flexure of the colon.

Population studies show that the incidence of colorectal carcinoma among all patients with ulcerative colitis is about eight times that expected. For patients with proctitis, defined as inflammation limited to the rectum, the risk is not greater than average. For those with "left-sided" disease it is about fourfold, and for those with "extensive" disease about 20 times that expected.

Patients with proctitis can therefore be reassured that unless the extent of disease changes, they need not worry about an increased risk of cancer. For those in whom inflammation has never spread above the splenic flexure, the risk is increased but low (e.g., similar to that in healthy people with a relative who developed colorectal cancer at a relatively young age). For those in whom the inflammation has at any time involved the transverse or ascending colon, the increased risk is appreciable.

Severity of Inflammation

The definition of the extent of disease depends on the mode of diagnosis. All series before the early 1970s assessed the extent by barium enema. Originally, a single contrast technique was used that is less sensitive for showing minor mucosal disease than the double air-contrast method introduced during the 1960s. Nowadays, the extent of colitis is generally judged by endoscopy with biopsy. Endoscopic assessment of the extent tends to exceed the corresponding radiologic abnormality. Biopsy evidence of inflammation tends to exceed in extent the visual changes of inflammation. Biopsies may be abnormal throughout much of the colon when the mucosa appears normal.

There is thus a gradient of severity from mucosal ulceration or other structural changes demonstrated by single contrast barium enema to abnormal biopsies but with normal radiologic and endoscopic appearances. Series from which the risks of carcinoma have been calculated mainly relied on radiologic assessment of disease extent. We do not know if the lesser degrees of inflammation shown only by endoscopy or biopsy are associated with an increased risk of carcinoma.

As a practicality, I suggest that the extent of disease be defined from abnormalities of the mucosal line on double contrast barium enema or macroscopic evidence of inflammation seen on endoscopy during or soon after an acute episode.

Duration of Disease

All published series show a very low incidence of carcinoma during the first 10 years of disease. Carcinoma can occur during this period, but the risk is so low that it need not influence clinical decisions.

After the tenth year, patients with extensive colitis have an annual risk of carcinoma of about one in 120 per year. The largest, longest, and most complete follow-up study based on defined populations showed a cumulative increase (CI [confidence interval]) up to 25 years from onset of symptoms of 3.4 percent (CI = 1 to 5.8) at 15 years; 7.2 percent (CI = 3.6 to 10.8) at 20 years; and 11.6 percent (CI = 6.4 to 16.8) at 25 years. Other series have given similar figures at 25 years.

There is controversy over whether the annual risk increases with the passage of time after 10 years. In part, there is confusion because the gradient of life table curves tends to increase with time as the number of patients observed decreases. For the same reason, the confidence intervals widen unacceptably if the number of patients followed is low after 25 years. At present, I regard all estimates over 25 years as approximate and do not base clinical decisions upon them.

Age of Onset

The literature is divided over whether early age of onset leads to a greater cancer risk than onset later in life. Confounding variables include (1) a tendency for colitis to be more often extensive in younger than in older people, (2) the potentially long period of follow-up, and (3) the fact that the relative risk is very high among young people because colorectal cancer is so uncommon in the general population at that age. For practical purposes, the risk of young people with extensive colitis should be regarded as high because they have so many years of life ahead of them. Avoidance of cancer is also particularly important because the development of carcinoma is such a tragedy in a young person.

How Great is the Risk of Dying of Carcinoma?

If cancer can often be cured when it occurs, the pressures for prevention or early diagnosis are reduced. In fact, the likelihood of surgical cure is about the same as that for colorectal carcinoma in the general population. Overall, the crude 5 year survival rate in recent series, including disseminated tumors that are inoperable or treated palliatively, is in the range of 30 to 60 percent. For Dukes A and B tumors the 5 year survival rate is about 9 percent, and for Dukes C 20 to 60 percent, depending on the extent of lymph node involvement.

Thus, although the cumulative incidence of carcinoma for a patient with extensive colitis treated medically is about one in eight (12 percent) during the period of 10 to 25 years after onset, the risk of dying is less: 8 percent if 5 year survival is 30 percent and 6 percent if it is 50 percent. Since life tables refer only to patients who survive with an intact colon, mortality from cancer is in practice less because some patients die from an unrelated illness, particularly if colitis begins later in life, e.g., after the age of 50. As discussed earlier, many patients are removed from risk by colectomy.

How Can the Risk of Carcinoma be Minimized?

Prevention by Colectomy Before Development of Precancerous Change or Carcinoma

In my opinion, prophylactic colectomy for symptomless patients without dysplasia is not warranted. However, if patients are endangered by acute disease, socially disabled by chronic disease, or persistently unwell, colectomy is advisable. This is especially the case in young people for whom conservative operations are most appropriate and surgical cure offers many years of good health. The cancer risk is a factor in encouraging operation among such young people. A recent Danish series in which surgical treatment was undertaken for 35 percent of patients with total colitis within 5 years of onset, and an overall colectomy rate of almost 25 percent at 10 years, showed no increased risk of carcinoma in the total series followed for a median of 11.7 (range 0 to 26) years.

Prevention by Colectomy After Detection of Precancerous Changes

At present the only widely used marker of precancerous change is epithelial dysplasia diagnosed on biopsy, or occasionally on cytologic brushings. It is hard to prove that dysplasia if left untreated advances to carcinoma, and if so over what time scale. Recent studies have shown that the finding of low-grade dysplasia by current criteria is followed by the development of high-grade dysplasia or carcinoma in about 50 percent of patients within 5 years. Difficulties in the grading of dysplasia, which involve interobserver variation, suggest that more than one experienced pathologist should independently agree about the presence or absence of low-grade dysplastic changes. Current evidence suggests that a finding of unequivocal low-grade dysplasia is an indication for colectomy.

High-grade dysplasia or low-grade dysplasia associated with an elevated lesion is subject to less interobserver variation. In general, both have proved to be such a good marker of malignancy that follow-up studies have not been possible for ethical reasons. There is little doubt that either of these findings is an indication of likely present or future malignancy and is an indication for colectomy.

Cure by Colectomy Before Carcinoma has Spread Beyond the Bowel Wall

In general, a carcinoma that presents with symptoms tends to be an advanced tumor. A symptomless carcinoma may be found at a curable stage on endoscopy, as an unexpected finding in the colectomy specimen after an operation performed for inflammation, or when an operation is performed for dysplasia. All grades of dysplasia can be a marker of cancer near the site of biopsy or elsewhere in the colon. In most series, high-grade dysplasia or a dysplasia-associated mass lesion are associated with undetected carcinoma in at least 40 percent of cases.

Do Regular Investigations Reduce Cancer Risk?

Screening Endoscopy

After 8–10 Years of Disease. During the early years of disease, inflammation thought initially to be distal may spread insidiously to involve much of the colon. Such patients tend not to be recognized as in the highest-risk group and thus do not receive the same attention as other patients with extensive colitis. An upper limit in distal disease can be found by flexible sigmoidoscopy. If no upper limit is reached, colonoscopy is indicated. If patients have extensive colitis, a colonoscopy at this stage excludes the presence of adenomas or dysplasia. For these reasons, I recommend a screening endoscopy for every patient with colitis 8 to 10 years after onset.

After More Than 10 Years of Disease when No Investigation has Been Undertaken for Several Years. Several series have shown that colonoscopy performed in these circumstances not only assesses the current extent and severity of inflammation but also may detect dysplasia or a carcinoma. In our own series, three patients were found to have high-grade dysplasia or a dysplastic mass at the first colonoscopy; two of these three patients had an undetected Dukes A carcinoma at operation. Among those who continued in the surveillance program, 7 of 38 others with dysplasia at the initial colonoscopy later developed carcinoma, compared with 8 of 243 patients without dysplasia initially ($p < .01$). These findings are similar to those at the Lahey Clinic and show how a screening colonoscopy in patients with a long history of disease can detect a high-risk group.

Regular Clinical Supervision

Supervision means regular clinical consultation at yearly or more frequent intervals with a facility for early consultation at other times if new symptoms develop. The object of regular supervision is to ensure optimal use of drug therapy, to encourage patients to accept surgery if their symptoms make this advisable, and to investigate whenever there is a clinical suspicion that inflammation has extended or that a carcinoma may be present. Such supervision probably prevents deaths from acute colitis and may prevent carcinoma by encouraging surgical treatment for severe or chronic inflammation. It has not been shown to benefit the patient by early diagnosis of carcinoma.

Surveillance

Surveillance is based on two premises: (1) that a precancerous phase of colitis is recognizable so that prophylactic colectomy can be undertaken; and (2) that regular investigations may detect symptomless carcinoma at a curable stage.

A surveillance program is successful only if it reduces cancer deaths; no program has been shown to achieve this aim, and the efficacy of such programs is controversial. In fact, as already shown, cancer mortality with current methods of management is likely to be low among patients with extensive colitis.

Published series fall into two groups. Series from the United States have shown a high pick-up rate at the first (screening) colonoscopy and thereafter a relatively low detection rate of dysplasia or carcinoma among those who were free of dysplasia at the first examination. Deaths from colorectal carcinoma occurred in all these series, and their value can be questioned for this reason. Studies from Scandinavia have shown a low detection rate of dysplasia and carcinoma, with no deaths, possibly in part because surveillance began at an earlier stage in the disease than in America so that patients showed no evidence of precancer initially. These results from Scandinavia and a series from England raise the issue of cost effectiveness of surveillance, because the few positive findings may not justify the effort and expense involved. Our own study from England among 332 patients, all with a disease duration greater than 10 years and all with inflammation proximal to the hepatic flexure seen and followed over 21 years, has given mixed results. Eleven patients were operated on for symptomless carcinoma found at endoscopy, or in the operation specimen after colectomy for dysplasia (Dukes A8, B1, C2); all these patients survived. Twelve patients were also operated on for dysplasia without carcinoma. However, six patients developed a symptomatic carcinoma that led to death in four.

At present, surveillance is not mandatory because its value is not proved. If a patient with extensive colitis wishes to be investigated regularly, and diagnostic facilities and costs allow, such a program probably offers the best way of reducing the cancer risk, although both patient and doctor need to recognize that it is not infallible.

How Should Regular Investigation be Organized?

Selection of Patients

Those at highest risk are likely to derive the greatest benefit, i.e., patients with extensive inflammation and a total duration of symptoms greater than 10 years.

Mode of Endoscopy

About half the carcinomas in ulcerative colitis, and almost half the biopsies showing dysplasia separate from a tumor, occur in the rectosigmoid. Flexible sigmoidoscopy therefore has a role even as the only mode of examination. Colonoscopy is needed for complete examination of the colon.

Frequency of Endoscopy

In my experience, interval cancers occurred when colonoscopy was arranged every 2 years. Ideally, annual colonoscopy appears advisable, with the interval to the next examination reduced to 6 months if indefinite (probably positive) or low-grade dysplasia in flat mucosa is detected, and surgery is not undertaken. As an alternative policy, colonoscopy alternating with flexible sigmoidoscopy at yearly intervals would probably be effective.

Number of Biopsies

A recent study suggested that 33 biopsies are needed at colonoscopy to give a 90 percent chance of detecting dysplasia if it is present. This is time consuming. Our practice has been to take an average of nine biopsies at each colonoscopy, and the detection rate of dysplasia has been satisfactory provided that results of successive endoscopies are taken into account. In view of the patchy nature of dysplasia, as many biopsies as practicable should be taken at each examination, at least between 10 and 20.

Action to be Taken on Finding Dysplasia or Adenoma

Patients need to understand the reason for regular investigation and that, if presumed precancerous changes are found, surgery will be advised. High-grade dysplasia or dysplasia on the surface of a widespread elevated or villous lesion is an indication for operation. An adenoma is, by definition, a polyp with dysplastic epithelium. The problem in colitis is to know whether it is an isolated abnormality, common in middle-aged or elderly healthy people, or a manifestation of dysplasia. A pedunculated polyp or a single sessile polyp around which there is no evidence of dysplasia on biopsy, especially if it is found beyond the limit of inflammation and/or in a patient after the fourth decade, can be removed endoscopically and the site observed at follow-up endoscopy at 6 months and annually thereafter. An isolated broad-based polyp situated in the area of colitis in a young person should be regarded with great suspicion, and multiple biopsies should be taken to exclude dysplasia around its base or elsewhere in the colon. The probability is that this lesion is a manifestation of dysplasia in colitis. The finding of more than one such polyp, or the development of further polyps, confirms this impression, and colectomy should be advised.

Low-grade or indefinite (probably positive) dysplasia is an indication for particularly careful repeat colonoscopy within 6 months, at which more biopsies than usual are taken. If low-grade dysplasia is again found, colectomy should be advised, especially if there are any supporting indications. If this advice is not accepted or indefinite dysplasia is found, a policy of annual examination can be resumed.

CROHN'S DISEASE

A population study has shown no excessive cancer mortality in Crohn's disease of the small intestine and an excessive risk in Crohn's colitis or ileocolitis similar to that found in left-sided ulcerative colitis: about four times that expected. However, a recent hospital-based study has found a cancer risk in Crohn's colitis equivalent to that in extensive ulcerative colitis. Clinical experience suggests that carcinoma in Crohn's colitis is less common than in ulcerative colitis, perhaps partly because Crohn's colitis tends to be treated by colectomy more often than ulcerative colitis.

Should Cancer Risk Influence Clinical Policy in Small Bowel Disease?

The risk is so low that the only preventive measure needed is to avoid leaving defunctioned inflamed loops of intestine at operation. Small bowel carcinomas complicating Crohn's disease usually involve areas of long-standing disease and tend to be difficult to detect at surgery, or even in an operative specimen; they are generally highly malignant.

Should Prophylactic Colectomy be Advised?

The same arguments apply as for ulcerative colitis. Dysplasia does occur in Crohn's disease but is a most unusual indication for colectomy.

Do Screening Examinations Have a Role in Crohn's Colitis?

When endoscopies are performed, biopsies should be taken and examined for dysplasia. A stricture should be examined with particular care.

Is Regular Supervision Likely to Influence Cancer Mortality?

Cancer can occur in chronic anorectal disease, either as a squamous carcinoma or as an adenocarcinoma of the distal rectum. Digital examination should be performed to search for induration in an anal fistula or an atypical anal ulcer. Sigmoidoscopy with biopsy is useful to seek strictures or dysplasia. When colonoscopic or radiographic investigation of new symptoms is arranged, the possibility of carcinoma should be kept in mind.

Is Regular Surveillance Indicated in Extensive Crohn's Colitis?

Although the incidence of carcinoma and of dysplasia may be similar to that in extensive ulcerative colitis, examination can be difficult because of strictures. No controlled evaluation of surveillance is available. At a time when the role of surveillance in ulcerative colitis is uncertain, it seems unwise to adopt a similar program in Crohn's colitis, in which the likelihood of success is less.

PROS AND CONS OF OPTIONS IN ULCERATIVE COLITIS (TABLE 1)

Active Surgical Policy for Appropriate Patients During the First Few Years of Disease

Pro: If surgical result is good, this leads to cure and eliminates cancer risk.

Con: If surgical result is poor, this leads to persistent or recurrent symptoms. A permanent stoma may be needed.

Endoscopy for All Patients with Ulcerative Colitis 8–10 Years After Onset

Pro: This may improve medical management of colitis and encourage appropriate patients with severe symptomatic and extensive disease to accept surgery. It provides a good baseline for surveillance if this is decided on.

Con: This increases the workload and may lead to unnecessary alarm among patients, especially those with proctosigmoiditis.

Screening Endoscopy for Patients with a Long History of Unsupervised Colitis

Pro: This provides good assessment both of inflammation and of possible dysplasia or carcinoma.

Con: Nil.

Regular Clinical Supervision for All Patients with Ulcerative Colitis

Pro: This allows regular assessment of symptoms and disability, checks on growth in young people, detects anemia and treatable complications, permits review of drug therapy, provides encouragement of surgical treatment for patients with severe disability, and maintains contact with patients so that relapses or new symptoms can be reported and treated or investigated early.

Con: This increases clinical workload and cost. It makes patients dependent on clinicians and may increase anxiety about illness.

Table 1 Pros and Cons of Treatment Options in Ulcerative Colitis

OPTIONS	PROS	CONS	OPINION
Colectomy for disability	Prevents cancer	Postoperative results uncertain	Outcome better than disease
Colectomy for statistical cancer risk (symptomless patient)	Prevents cancer	Postoperative results uncertain	Possible postoperative sequelae unacceptable
Colectomy for dysplasia	Prevents cancer May cure undetected cancer	Postoperative results uncertain	Postoperative sequelae acceptable
Screening colonoscopy and biopsies (occasional investigation)	Detects dysplasia and cancer	Nil	Worthwhile
Clinical supervision (investigation only for symptoms)	Optimizes medical care May encourage surgery Maintains patient contact	Symptomatic cancer tends to be advanced	Worthwhile
Surveillance (regular endoscopy and biopsy)	Colectomy for precancer and/or curable cancer in some patients	Incurable cancers occur Costly	Unproved Optional

Regular Annual Investigation by Endoscopy after 10 Years of Disease in Patients with Extensive Colitis

Pro: This may detect dysplasia and curable carcinoma.

Con: This has uncertain clinical benefit or cost effectiveness. It may reduce but does not eliminate cancer risk; it is labor intensive, and demanding on patients; and it may increase anxiety.

■ THE FUTURE

The chronic inflammation and rapid epithelial cell turnover associated with ulcerative colitis lead to genetic changes that predispose to carcinoma, and are in many patients manifested as dysplasia. Dysplasia has limitations but is clinically useful; the possible role of chromosomal change measured as aneuploidy is being investigated. Selected centers should be encouraged to test gene mutations, deletions, and expression as possible future markers of neoplastic potential. New techniques of obtaining DNA for analysis from wide areas of epithelium, e.g., by brushing, washing, or search in the stool, also need investigation.

Suggested Reading

Burmer GC, Rabinovitch PS, Haggitt RC, et al. Neoplastic progression in ulcerative colitis: histology, DNA content, and loss of a p53 allele. Gastroenterology 1992; 103:1602–1610.

Connell WR, Lennard-Jones JE, Williams CB, et al. Factors affecting the outcome of endoscopic surveillance for cancer in ulcerative colitis. Gastroenterology 1996; 107:934–1944.

Ekbom A, Helmick C, Zack M, Hans-Olov A. Increased risk of large-bowel cancer in Crohn's disease with colonic involvement. Lancet 1990; 336: 357–359.

Gyde SN, Prior P, Allan RN, et al. Colorectal cancer in ulcerative colitis: a cohort study of primary referrals from three centres. Gut 1988; 29:206–217.

Langholz E, Munkholm P, Davidsen M, Binder V. Colorectal cancer risk and mortality in patients with ulcerative colitis. Gastroenterology 1992; 103:1444–1451.

Lennard-Jones JE. Is colonoscopic cancer surveillance in ulcerative colitis essential for every patient? Eur J Cancer 1995; 31A:1178–1182.

Löfberg R, Brostrom O, Karlen P, et al. Colonoscopic surveillance in long-standing total ulcerative colitis: a 15-year follow-up study. Gastroenterology 1990; 99:1021–1031.

Lynch DAF, Lobo AJ, Sobala GM, et al. Failure of colonoscopic surveillance in ulcerative colitis. Gut 1993; 34:1075–1080.

Nugent FW, Haggitt RC, Gilpin PA. Cancer surveillance in ulcerative colitis. Gastroenterology 1991; 100:1241–1248.

Riddell RH, ed. Dysplasia and cancer in ulcerative colitis. New York: Elsevier, 1991.

Rubin CE, Haggitt RC, Burmer GC, et al. DNA aneuploidy in colonic biopsies predicts future development of dysplasia in ulcerative colitis. Gastroenterology 1992; 103:1611–1620.

Sachar DB. Cancer in Crohn's disease: Dispelling the myths. Gut 1994; 35: 1507–1508.

Taylor BA, Pemberton JH, Carpenter HA, et al. Dysplasia in chronic ulcerative colitis: implications for colonoscopic surveillance. Dis Colon Rectum 1992; 35:950–956.

IRRITABLE BOWEL SYNDROME

W. Grant Thompson, M.D. F.R.C.P.C.

As defined by the Rome criteria (Table 1), the irritable bowel syndrome (IBS) occurs in 10 to 15 percent of adults in Western countries. If other functional bowel syndromes such as functional diarrhea or functional bloating are included, the figure is much higher (Table 2). Fortunately, most individuals with IBS do not seek attention for this chronic, benign disorder, and most of those who do are satisfactorily managed by their primary care physician. The few referred to specialists constitute a large portion of their practice and often present difficult management problems. This chapter provides a management strategy for the gastroenterologist and internist.

■ PATHOGENESIS

The cause and mechanisms of IBS symptoms are unknown. IBS does not appear to be purely a motility disorder, since we are unable to measure physiologic events in the gut that are coincident with symptoms. However, the small and large intestines of IBS patients are hypersensitive or hyper-reactive to stimuli such as eating, drugs, hormones, intraluminal distention, and emotional and physical stress. The cause of IBS symptoms may someday be found in the enteric nervous system (ENS) and its signals to and from the brain. The ENS or "gut brain" is very complex. It manages gut function through the interaction of gut hormones, neurotransmitters, and nerve plexes, all modified by events in the environment, the brain, and the gut itself. Thus, IBS pain may be as much due to an abnormal perception of normal gut physiologic events as to a normal perception of abnormal gut events. The gut symptoms must therefore be seen in the context of the patient's physical and psychosocial environment.

■ CLINICAL SETTING

Any management plan must take into account the special circumstances of those who consult specialists. IBS is a chronic, recurring disorder without cure and without dire consequences. By all physical measures, it is a benign disease. IBS subjects in the community who do not see doctors have a psychological and personality profile similar to that of the unaffected population. Most of those who see a primary care physician are satisfactorily managed there. Why, then, do a small group see specialists? Patients often volunteer that their symptoms are more severe than those suffered by others, and it may be so. However, it is also well known that IBS patients seen in tertiary care centers have more psychological problems than other patients and normal controls. They are also more likely to have suffered a threatening life event in the months before consultation, such as a death in the family or loss of a job or spouse. Still others resort to illness behavior to achieve some secondary gain with family, employer, or disability insurer.

Some patients may blame psychological difficulties on the physical symptoms. In others, the often unstated psychosocial difficulties constitute a "hidden agenda" (Table 3). The somatic symptoms can be troublesome and severe in their own right, but it is their interaction with the patient's psychosocial environment that complicates management, inhibits acceptance, and prompts referral. A treatment approach that does not include measures to address the hidden agenda is likely to be unsuccessful.

Table 1 Rome Criteria

At least 3 months of continuous or recurrent symptoms of
1. abdominal pain or discomfort that is
   (a) relieved with defecation
   (b) and/or associated with a change in frequency of stool
   (c) and/or associated with a change in consistency of stool

   and
2. two or more of the following at least one-quarter of occasions or days:
   (a) altered stool frequency*
   (b) altered stool form (lumpy/hard or loose/watery stool)
   (c) altered stool passage (straining, urgency), or feeling of incomplete evacuation
   (d) passage of mucus,
   (e) bloating or feeling of abdominal distention

*For research purposes, "altered" may be defined as >3 bowel movements/day or <3 bowel movements/wk.
From Thompson WG, Creed F, Drossman DA, et al. Functional bowel disorders and chronic functional abdominal pain. Gastroent Int 1992; 5:75–91.

Table 2 Functional Disorders of the Intestines

C. Functional bowel disorders
- C1 Irritable bowel syndrome
- C2 Functional abdominal bloating
- C3 Functional constipation
- C4 Functional diarrhea
- C5 Unspecified functional bowel disorder

D. Functional abdominal pain
- D1 Functional abdominal pain syndrome
- D2 Unspecified functional abdominal pain

From Thompson WG, Creed F, Drossman DA, et al. Functional bowel disorders and chronic functional abdominal pain. Gastroent Int 1992; 5:75–91; with permission.

■ MANAGEMENT STRATEGY

The patient who is referred to a gastroenterologist is one of a minority of sufferers who have sought help from physicians, and a still smaller group who have been unsatisfied by their encounter with primary care. The following approach to such patients includes discussion at the first clinical encounter, the

Table 3 The Hidden Agenda

Insecurity with diagnosis
  Fear of serious disease
  Cancerphobia
Dissatisifaction with treatment
Threatening life event
  Loss of spouse
  Loss of job
  Death in family
  Physical or sexual abuse
Depression, anxiety, hypochondria, pain, panic
Secondary gain (illness behavior)
  Dependent relationship
  Manipulation of employer or family
  Disability pension

Table 4 Management Strategy

First clinical encounter
  Confirm diagnosis and convince patient
  Determine previous tests and treatments
  Rational use of tests—ensure clean colon
  Bran
  Determine hidden agenda and advise
Follow-up visit (6–8 wk later)
  Ensure acceptance of diagnosis
  Confirm explanation and compliance with advice
  In unimproved patient:
    Resist temptation to reinvestigate
    Stress management, relaxation (see next chapter)
    Treat depression, anxiety
    Limited use of drugs for specific symptoms (Table 5)
The difficult patient
  Regular, brief visits
  Specific referrals:
    Psychiatrist
    Esteemed colleague
    Behavior and psychology treatments if available
  Ensure continuing care with primary care physician and gastroenterologist

follow-up visit and establishment of continuing care, and the management of the especially difficult patient (Table 4).

First Clinical Encounter

Positive Diagnosis

The first task is to confirm the diagnosis as firmly and credibly as possible. The symptoms should be reviewed in detail. The Rome criteria in Table 1 serve as a guide to identify IBS features. Some patients do not quite fulfill the IBS criteria and might fit better in one of the other diagnostic groupings suggested in Table 2. History taking should include a search for symptoms that cannot be explained by IBS, such as bleeding, anemia, weight loss, or fever. One should also be suspicious of organic disease if the symptoms occur frequently at night or if they begin late in life.

Many drugs affect the gut. In particular, the physician should inquire about the use of opiates, calcium channel blockers, antibiotics, and laxatives. If diarrhea is a dominant symptom, one should consider the possibility of lactose intolerance or excessive use of caffeine or sorbitol (an artificial sugar used in diet gums). A dietary history is important to exclude fad diets and to establish whether the fiber intake is satisfactory. Beyond these factors, it is unlikely that any dietary factor is the "trigger" of IBS. Physical examination should be thorough and will be negative. These referred patients very often have abdominal scars from the removal of a normal gallbladder, appendix, or uterus.

The patient should be carefully questioned about previous consultations. Often the referred patient has visited many physicians, and tests have been done unnecessarily and repeatedly. It is usually best that they not be done again.

Ordinarily the gastroenterologist or internist will wish to perform a sigmoidoscopy. This test enables inflammatory bowel disease (IBD) or perianal disorders to be excluded, but most importantly it is of therapeutic benefit. Confidence in the diagnosis of IBS is the foundation of its management, and the patient needs to know that the physician has taken the symptoms seriously enough to look at the bowel.

Special circumstances may indicate further tests, e.g., a family history of IBD, endemic giardiasis, or suspected lactose intolerance (especially in non-Caucasians). In a typical IBS patient without symptoms or signs of organic disease, the tests should not be exhaustive. If not previously given to a patient over 40 years old, a barium enema is prudent. The Rome criteria are not symptoms of colorectal carcinoma, but it is best that the management relationship start with a clean colon.

Reassurance

Once the diagnosis is firm, the physician should set about convincing the patient. The possible reasons for the patient's concerns should be explored: for example, cancer in the family, anxiety, hypochondriasis, or pressure of friends and relatives. Diagnostic tests should be kept to the necessary minimum, since they increase anxiety and insecurity ("If the doctor is uncertain of the diagnosis, how can I be otherwise?"). Explaining IBS to a patient is difficult but important. One may start by describing its frequency in the population, its unknown cause, and its benign nature. It may be compared with a headache: just as severe pain can occur in an apparently normal head, severe abdominal pain can occur in an apparently normal gut. The complex gut contractions required to move contents through the long intestinal tract can be explained, along with the functions of the ENS and its obvious connections with the brain. The relation of symptoms to stress and anxiety can be illustrated by having the patient recall the varied gut reactions of classmates before college examinations. Once convinced of the diagnosis, the patient may be reassured of its benign nature. Reassurance may prove to be the gastroenterlolgist most effective therapeutic weapon.

Dietary Fiber

Even if the patient claims to be on a high-fiber diet or is taking a psyllium preparation, it is seldom that enough fiber is ingested to have an impact on gut function. There are no clinical trials that establish the benefit of bran for IBS. Nonetheless, bran is effective in the constipated phase of the syndrome and is a safe and inexpensive way to recruit the 40 to 60 percent placebo response. I usually start the patient on

1 tablespoon of bran three times a day with meals. I explain that the object is to use bran's water-holding capacity to expand the stool, which ensures more adequate stimulation of gut reflexes such as the urge to defecate. The result should be less hard or difficult-to-pass stools and a regularization of bowel action. There may be an increase in flatulence or bloating during the first week of bran ingestion. Commercial psyllium and fiber preparations are satisfactory alternatives, provided that they are taken regularly and in sufficient quantity. While this approach helps many people, specialists tend to see those who have failed to respond to fiber.

The Hidden Agenda

On this first visit, careful attention should be paid to the hidden agenda. Why has the patient chosen this occasion to visit a specialist? Why is he or she unsatisfied with the care of the primary care physician? Possible answers are dissatisfaction with the diagnosis, fear that some sinister disease is being missed, or the desire for a more effective treatment for the somatic symptoms. Others have mistakenly been put on a low-roughage or unnecessarily restrictive diet, have lost weight, or are sure they have cancer. More subtle, of course, are psychosocial problems. The high likelihood that the patient has suffered abuse or a threatening life event in the months leading up to the consultation indicates that these might be more important than the somatic symptoms themselves. At least, such an event may impair the patient's ability to cope with the symptoms. Many patients suffer depression or anxiety that is amenable to specific management. Although the patient seems convinced that the symptoms cause the psychological distress, it seems more likely that psychological distress complicates or exaggerates the symptoms. The patient's relationships with other family members should be explored. It is also wise to establish whether a disability pension is at issue.

Sometimes the hidden agenda is easily dealt with. A man long suffering from IBS symptoms who has a close relative die of cancer of the colon may need only to be convinced that he has no such disease. Overt depression or extreme anxiety might be managed by pharmacotherapy. Explanation of the interactions of stress with the somatic symptoms may encourage a patient to take appropriate action to relieve the stress. Some patients may benefit from relaxation therapy. Others may require more complex interventions as described later.

■ THE FOLLOW-UP VISIT

Compliance and Comprehension

It is my practice to see patients 6 to 8 weeks after the initial visit, to establish whether they have understood the explanation and are satisfied with the diagnosis. Those patients who are improved or satisfied can be returned to the care of their family physicians. They should, of course, be warned that IBS is a chronic, remitting condition and that the symptoms will recur from time to time. To deal with recurrences, the measures described previously should be reinstituted.

In unimproved patients, the symptoms should be reviewed with other diagnostic possibilities in view. The physician should, however, resist the temptation to do further tests without good reason. One should also ensure that sufficient fiber is being employed and that "gassy" foods are being avoided.

Table 5 Drugs for Certain Circumstances

INDICATION	DRUG	DOSE
Dominant diarrhea plus incontinence	Loperamide	1–2 tabs before meals, social engagements or stressful situations
	Cholestyramine	1 scoop hs
Dominant pain		
Postprandial	Anticholinergic Dicyclomine (Bentyl)	10–20 mg 10–15 min before meals
Chronic pain	Tricyclic (amitriptyline)	25 mg hs and increase
Dominant constipation	Bran, psyllium	1 tbsp t.i.d. with meals and increase p.r.n.
	Osmotic laxatives	
	Lactulose	1–2 tsp hs
	Polyethylene glycol solution	8 oz hs
	MgSO4 (Milk of Magnesia)	1–2 tbsp hs
Gas (flatus)	Simethicone	
	Beano (beta-galactosidase)	

Drug Therapy

In a chronic, benign condition, often beginning in youth and affecting nearly 15 percent of the population, drugs should be avoided when possible. Klein reviewed the controlled clinical trials of drugs used in IBS and found no convincing evidence that any are globally useful. The complex and variable symptoms seem unlikely to be cured by a single agent. In the United States, no drugs are approved for use in this syndrome by the Food and Drug Administration.

Nonetheless, certain drugs may be useful in certain circumstances. If the patient has a single dominant symptom that is causing some disability, it makes sense to use an agent to minimize that symptom (Table 5). For example, some patients have precipitous diarrhea and urgency. While they may not mention it spontaneously, the threat of incontinence can be very troubling, and such patients are reluctant to engage in social activities for fear of embarrassing themselves. Loperamide is an ideal drug for this situation, since it not only inhibits small bowel fluid secretion and gut motility, but also increases tone in the anal sphincter. One or two tablets should be given before a meal, a social engagement, or a stressful event to prevent urgency and diarrhea. Occasionally, a patient with predominant diarrhea responds to cholestyramine. Care should be taken not to use too much of an antidiarrheal drug, because it may exaggerate the constipated phase of IBS. In the United States, a 1 mg over-the-counter loperamide (Imodium) tablet is available and may be adequate.

Occasionally, when abdominal pain regularly follows meals, an anticholinergic drug may be given before the meal to interrupt the gastrocolonic response. This targets the drug for maximal effect at the time of symptoms and minimizes the side effects that a 24 hour anticholinergic blockade might incur. Some patients with dominant abdominal pain may respond to a tricyclic antidepressant even though depression is not obvious. These drugs affect the afferent nervous system and serotonin activity in the brain.

Symptoms dominated by constipation may be overcome by a bulking agent, either bran or psyllium in doses beyond those hitherto given. Some patients may take up to 10 tablespoons of bran a day before the desired effect is achieved. It is important that the bran be taken every day with ample fluids to prevent, rather than treat, constipation. Should this be ineffective, an osmotic laxative such as lactulose, Milk of Magnesia, or polyethylene glycol-electrolyte solution (Colyte, GoLYTELY) may be given in small doses at bedtime.

For the gas-prone patient, simethicone might be considered a logical placebo. As a surfactant it breaks up gas bubbles, but its efficacy in ridding the gut of gas is questionable. Activated charcoal may be given in capsule form but is awkward, messy, and of doubtful benefit. In patients producing excessive flatus who do not respond to withdrawal of gas-producing vegetables, Beano (beta-galactosidase) has achieved anecdotal but not controlled trial success.

Many drugs proposed as IBS treatments have failed to establish their efficacy over time. These include mebeverine, trimebutane, peppermint oil, domperidone, and cisapride. Newer drugs such as the calcium channel blockers, 5-hydroxytryptamine antagonists, and somatostatin should be regarded as experimental. In my opinion, they should not be used for IBS outside clinical trials. They are costly, their efficacy is doubtful, and their use may distract from the more important issues.

Continuing Care

Some patients present more difficult psychosocial problems and need some of the special interventions cited below. In any case, the gastroenterologist and primary care physician should ensure continuing care and make every effort to prevent the doctor-shopping that is so common in IBS patients. Such patients often seek alternative medicine treatments.

■ THE DIFFICULT PATIENT

Improve Functioning

Every gastroenterologist's practice has difficult IBS patients who consume much time and challenge his or her skill. Many can be successfully managed by periodic and regular visits to the primary physician and the specialist to deal with psychosocial difficulties. Such patients demand constant reassurance and are often satisfied when they get it. In such patients, cure is not likely, and improved functioning in society should be the treatment objective. They should be encouraged to engage in social events, become financially independent, and avoid abusive relationships. Those seeking disability insurance payments for IBS symptoms may place the physician in conflict. A disability pension may not encourage the independent living and improved social functioning that such patients need.

Consultative Options

Consultations with other physicians should have a specific objective. If a serious mental illness is suspected, psychiatric consultation will be necessary. If the physician feels that he or she is losing the confidence of the patient, both may benefit from a consultation with a respected colleague. This doctor should confirm the diagnosis and reaffirm the method of treatment, thus making future management easier. There are a number of behavioral and psychological options. Although these have undergone intensive study, controlled clinical trials are obviously difficult. Nonetheless, such treatments as relaxation therapy, biofeedback, hypnotism, stress management, and psychological interventions may be helpful to certain patients if there are suitable experts in the community. Some patients with chronic pain may benefit from the multidisciplinary approach of a pain clinic.

Chronic Care

In all cases the gastroenterologist and the primary care physician should maintain control of the patient's medical care. The psychiatrist, psychologist, and pain clinic personnel are ill equipped to provide such care over the long term.

Suggested Reading

Drossman DA, Thompson WG. Irritable bowel syndrome: a graduated, multicomponent treatment approach. Ann Intern Med 1992; 116:1009–1016.

Drossman DA, Sandler RS, McKee DC, Lovitz AJ. Bowel patterns among subjects not seeking health care. Use of a questionnaire to identify a population with bowel dysfunction. Gastroenterology 1982; 83:529–534.

Klein KB. Controlled treatment trials in the irritable bowel syndrome: a critique. Gastroenterology 1988; 95:232–241.

Thompson WG. The irritable bowel. Gut 1984; 25:305–320.

Thompson WG. Irritable bowel syndrome: Pathogenesis and management. Lancet 1993; 341:1568–1572.

Thompson WG. Gut Reactions. New York Plenum 1989.

Thompson WG, Creed F, Drossman DA, et al. Functional bowel disorders and chronic functional abdominal pain. Gastroenterol Int 1992; 5:75–91.

Thompson WG, Dotevall G, Drossman DA, et al. Irritable bowel syndrome: guidelines for the diagnosis. Gastroenterol Int 1989; 2:92–95.

Walker EA, Roy Byrne PP, Katon WJ. Irritable bowel syndrome and psychiatric illness. Am J Psychiatry 1990; 147:565–572.

Whitehead WE, Winget C, Fedoravicius AS, et al. Learned illness behavior in patients with irritable bowel syndrome and peptic ulcer. Dig Dis Sci 1982; 27:202–208.

ILEOSTOMY AND OSTOMY MANAGEMENT

Robin S. McLeod, M.D., F.R.C.S.C., F.A.C.S.
Zane Cohen, M.D., F.R.C.S.C., F.A.C.S.

From estimates of United Ostomy Association membership, there are over 15,000 ostomates in the United States. The most common indicators for an ileostomy are ulcerative colitis and Crohn's disease; the most common indication for a colostomy is carcinoma of the rectum. Although the quality of life of most ostomates is normal or only minimally affected by the stoma, most patients are anxious preoperatively about both the surgery and the stoma. There may be concerns about management of the appliance, diet, work, and activity restrictions as well as psychological concerns about sexuality and body image. Thus, the management of patients with a stoma must begin before the operation. At our institution, the surgical procedure is discussed, printed materials and names of individuals who have a stoma are given to the patient, and, if possible, all patients are seen by an enterostomal therapist before hospitalization.

The other aspect of ostomy management that must be considered preoperatively is stomal siting. Our studies have shown that the most common reason for ostomates having a poor quality of life is poor stoma function. In most instances, this problem can be avoided by proper marking of the stoma preoperatively, even in patients requiring emergency surgery. This is best done by the enterostomal therapist, who views the patient both sitting and lying to observe the abdominal contour and landmarks. Consideration should also be given to the patient's activities and clothing preferences when selecting the site.

■ ILEOSTOMY

Postoperative Management

The stoma is typically edematous immediately postoperatively, but this resolves within a few days to a few weeks. The normal color of the mucosa ranges from pink to deep red. If there is concern about the viability of the stoma, it is important to determine whether the ischemia is limited to the extrafascial bowel or whether the intra-abdominal bowel is affected. If it is the former, intervention is unnecessary, whereas if it is the latter, surgery is required. The viability of the stoma may be assessed by pricking the mucosa lightly with a small-gauge needle to check whether there is arterial bleeding. To determine the line of demarcation, a light may be shone into the stoma while a test tube is gently inserted into the proximal limb of the stoma. Alternatively, the ileostomy may be gently endoscoped. If only the stoma is affected, there may be sloughing of the mucosa only, and this will lead to no permanent complication. If there is full-thickness necrosis, the stoma may stricture and a stoma revision may be required at a later date.

Intestinal peristalsis usually recommences 2 to 5 days after the surgery. Not infrequently, there is an early output of intestinal content from the ileostomy while there is still an ileus in the upper intestinal tract. However, oral ingestion should not be started until there are signs, e.g., the passage of air and resumption of bowel sounds, that the ileus has resolved. Occasionally, there may be edema at the fascial level leading to a partial obstruction. Insertion of a large Foley catheter may help relieve the obstruction while the edema resolves. The normal output from an ileostomy should range between 500 and 1,000 ml. Patients need to be aware of their ileostomy output. Low outputs may indicate an obstruction; higher outputs may result in dehydration.

While in the hospital, the patient should be taught how to care for the ileostomy in order to be proficient and confident in managing the appliance before discharge. It may also be beneficial to have a visiting nurse provide assistance following discharge.

Approximately 50 percent of patients experience some dietary restrictions postoperatively, but these are severe in only about 10 percent. Initially, patients should be advised to take a low-residue diet, but within a few weeks they can begin to introduce other foods into their diet. Foods that commonly affect patients are nuts, popcorn, corn, Oriental vegetables, cabbage, and mushrooms.

Skin care is an important component of management of ileostomates. Dermatitis caused by the leakage of stool onto the peristomal skin is the most common skin problem associated with an intestinal stoma. Ileostomy effluent is very irritating to the skin because it contains pancreatic proteolytic enzymes, bile acids, and a high concentration of alkali. Leakage may cause erythema, ulceration, and, with prolonged exposure, pseudoepitheliomatous hyperplasia of the skin. This is characterized by reddish-brown nodules that may become confluent at the mucocutaneous border and may prevent adequate maintenance of the appliance because of pain and mucous sequestration. A properly fitting appliance usually allows this condition to resolve. Occasionally, a convex face plate and belt may be needed to maintain a seal around the stoma, and rarely the stoma must be resited.

Folliculitis under the face plate may occur after the hair around the stoma has been shaved with a razor blade, or if the hair follicles are injured when the face plate of the appliance is repeatedly pulled off. The condition usually resolves with local treatment and clipping of the hair with an electric razor or scissors. Contact dermatitis may occur from an allergic reaction to the appliance or tape; this should be suspected if the irritation follows the pattern of the appliance or tape. A different skin barrier may afford equal protection and eliminate the allergic reaction. Skin testing for sensitivity to appliance materials may reduce this problem in patients who have had an allergic reaction. The other common skin lesion is *Monilia* infection, which can be recognized by its characteristic appearance of well-circumscribed erythema with satellite papules and pustules. It usually responds to dusting the skin with nystatin powder before fitting the appliance.

Postoperatively, most ileostomates achieve a satisfactory quality of life and the overwhelming majority feel that they lead normal lives or experience only minor restrictions because of the stoma. Their improved physical well-being is probably the major reason for their high degree of satisfaction. In fact, it is not uncommon for patients to comment that they wished they had had surgery much earlier in their disease course. Despite these feelings, a few patients complain of problems with noise and odor. It may be difficult to eliminate these difficulties completely, but avoidance of gas-producing foods and the use of charcoal and chlorophyll tablets may be beneficial. High-volume ileostomy output is uncommon unless the patient has had a concomitant small bowel resection. However, ileostomates are prone to dehydration in hot weather or during a flulike illness and should be cautioned to increase their intake of fluid and salt at those times. Other causes of high output are recurrent Crohn's disease and partial small bowel obstruction.

From a psychological standpoint, most patients adapt well to the ileostomy. However, a few have a poor body image and may experience negative feelings from family, friends, and employers. These patients may benefit from counseling or referral to a local ostomy chapter.

Late Complications

Many patients may experience problems related to the ileostomy, but complications tend to be temporary or minor and are often eliminated by a change in appliance. However, 15 to 25 percent of patients require revisional surgery to the ileostomy. Such surgery is required more frequently in patients with Crohn's disease owing to recurrence of disease. Otherwise, the most common indications for surgery are retraction or prolapse of the stoma, stenosis, and fistula formation. Some patients may require resiting of the stoma because of problems related to leakage, a complication that should be avoided by proper placement initially. Unlike the situation with colostomies, parastomal hernia formation is infrequent.

Cases of retraction and prolapse of the stoma can be divided into those that are fixed and those that are intermittent. If the stoma is constantly retracted, it is usually because there was tension and insufficient length of bowel to evert the stoma when it was constructed. A convex appliance may be sufficient to obviate the commonly associated problem of leakage; if not, surgical revision may be necessary. A local skin level revision is often successful, but sometimes a laparotomy is required to mobilize the small bowel adequately. Retraction of the bowel at a later date often signifies recurrent Crohn's disease. Removal of the appliance and close inspection of the stoma may reveal aphthous ulcers and other features typical of Crohn's disease; if so, treatment should be directed toward the Crohn's disease. The other situation is that of the stoma intermittently retracting and prolapsing. Again, difficulty in maintaining an appliance and leakage are the most common complaints. This is usually associated with a large stomal aperture and failure of the two serosal surfaces of the bowel to fuse, allowing the bowel to intermittently retract and prolapse. A local skin level procedure, with tightening of the fascial defect and amputation of the excess bowel, may be performed. Often, however, this is unsuccessful and resiting of the ileostomy is required. Retraction and prolapse may also be associated with a parastomal hernia, which is likewise best treated by resiting the stoma.

Peristomal fistulas are uncommon and almost always a manifestation of recurrent Crohn's disease. Occasionally a fistula may occur in the absence of Crohn's disease as a result of a suture pulling out at the time of maturing the stoma. A fistula may pose a difficult problem because it typically lies at the skin level, so there is constant leakage of stool with undermining of the appliance. Medical therapy is rarely of benefit, and a laparotomy with resection of the involved bowel and resiting of the stoma is usually necessary. If there is an associated abscess, it should be drained and treated with antibiotics, if possible, before surgery.

Peristomal ulceration most commonly occurs in patients with Crohn's disease and often suggests activation of disease. Occasionally, it may be due to continued skin irritation. Treatment may be difficult, especially if there is active disease. The enterostomal therapist plays an important role in the management of these patients. The ulcer should be treated with a debriding agent and packed with gauze, and an appliance applied. The dressing and appliance should be changed daily. Often, different agents and dressings may need to be tried, as these can be quite resistant to treatment. If there is a septic component, antibiotics may be beneficial. In resistant cases, stomal resiting is necessary, with or without concomitant resection of the bowel.

Stomal blockage, which occurs not infrequently, is usually caused by ingestion of high-fiber foods such as nuts, popcorn, string vegetables, raw vegetables, corned beef, cabbage, oranges, or fruit peels. The patient experiences cramping abdominal pain, nausea and vomiting, and cessation of ileostomy output. Treatment involves rehydration with intravenous fluids and nasogastric decompression. The obstruction can occasionally be relieved by irrigating the stoma with a large-bore Foley catheter placed into the stoma. Food bolus obstructions almost always resolve spontaneously within 24 hours; if not, one should suspect a blockage from another cause (e.g., adhesions) and treat the patient accordingly.

■ KOCK POUCH

The Kock pouch or continent ileostomy consists of a reservoir and nipple valve constructed from the distal small bowel and brought out to the surface as a flush stoma. The advantage of this procedure is that the ileostomy is continent, so the need for an appliance is eliminated. Although this was a significant advance, the procedure is now performed relatively infrequently because the surgical complication rate is high and patients are still left with a stoma. Thus, for patients wishing to avoid an ileostomy, the ileoanal pouch procedure is usually preferred.

The immediate postoperative care of these patients is similar to that of anyone undergoing a major abdominal procedure. In addition, the catheter that is left in situ at surgery must be irrigated frequently, and the stoma must be checked for signs of ischemia. Most surgeons leave the catheter in place for several weeks to decompress the pouch and in hopes of allowing better fixation of the pouch and nipple valve. After this, the patient must be taught how to intubate the pouch; thereafter, the pouch may be intubated as necessary, usually three or four times a day. Between times, a gauze patch or Band-Aid may be used to cover the stoma. Rarely, patients have trouble with excessive mucous discharge from the efferent limb. Little can be done for this except to ensure that the bowel is flush with the skin and to change the bandage more frequently. If patients have trouble emptying the pouch because the stool is thick, they should be told to increase their fluid intake and drink prune juice. The pouch may also be irrigated. Dietary restrictions, if any, are usually similar to those experienced by patients with conventional ileostomies.

Complications tend to be related to the nipple valve, which is formed by intussuscepting a 10 to 12 cm segment of nipple valve. Dessusception of the valve, known as valve slippage, has been the Achilles heel of the operation, and despite modifications still occurs in 10 to 15 percent of patients. Usually, patients complain of difficulty in intubating the pouch and incontinence. The history is usually adequate to suggest the diagnosis, but it can be confirmed with a pouchogram. If the valve has slipped, surgical revision to reconstruct it is necessary. "Valve prolapse" is the term used for the situation in which the valve is intact but prolapses through the stomal aperture. This is the result of an excessively large fascial opening, and it can be corrected by a skin level revision in which the fascial defect is tightened.

One of the unique complications of both the Kock pouch and the ileoanal pouch procedures is pouchitis, which is a nonspecific inflammation of the pouch mucosa. The risk is variable, depending on the series, and ranges from 10 to 35 percent. Typically, there is an acute onset of symptoms, which include increased ileostomy effluent, fever, abdominal tenderness, nausea and vomiting, and malaise. Endoscopically, the mucosa is fiery red and edematous with areas of ulceration and punctate hemorrhages. Although the cause of pouchitis is unknown, there is evidence that the condition is due to bacterial overgrowth; patients respond well to a short course of a broad-spectrum antibiotic. Pouchitis rarely has a more chronic course; if so, Crohn's disease should be suspected. Other inflammatory agents have been used in these situations, but often with little benefit. In recalcitrant cases, excision of the pouch may be necessary.

■ ILEOANAL POUCH PROCEDURE

The ileoanal pouch or pelvic pouch procedure has been a major advance for patients with ulcerative colitis requiring surgery. The major advantage of this operation is that patients do not have a permanent stoma and they evacuate by the normal route; neither catheters nor appliances are necessary.

After surgery (or closure of the ileostomy), stool frequency tends to be erratic for about 3 months, during which time patients may evacuate 10 to 15 times per 24 hours. Bulk agents with psyllium and antidiarrheal agents such as loperamide may help decrease the number of bowel movements. Problems with perianal skin irritation because of excessive diarrhea are common. Careful hygiene and use of creams and barrier agents such as petroleum jelly and zinc oxide are usually adequate. After 3 months, the pattern of bowel evacuation stabilizes and usually does not interfere with the patient's daily activities. By 12 months, bowel function has usually stabilized at, on average, five or six bowel movements a day. Approximately one-third of patients require long-term antidiarrheal and bulk agents.

As with the other procedures, most patients do not have dietary restrictions. Initially, they should avoid high-residue foods, but these can be gradually introduced after a few weeks. If patients have had no problems with any foods while having an ileostomy, it is unlikely that they will experience difficulties with the pelvic reservoir. However, food ingestion may increase stool frequency, and some patients modify their intake accordingly. In addition, some (usually gas-producing) foods may increase stool frequency. On the other hand, bananas, mashed potatoes, boiled rice, tapioca, peanut butter, applesauce, and cheese tend to decrease stool frequency.

Complications after this procedure occur frequently. The list includes those seen with other major abdominal procedures: small bowel obstruction, intra-abdominal sepsis, and cardiac, respiratory, urinary, and thrombotic difficulties. There are also complications specific to this operation, the most significant being a leak from the ileoanal anastomosis. This may manifest as a pelvic, intra-abdominal, or perianal abscess or as a fistula to the perianal skin, abdomen, or vagina. Although it usually manifests soon after surgery, a small leak may not be detected initially, either clinically or radiologically. One should suspect a leak in patients who have poor functional results. Treatment varies, depending on the size of the anastomotic dehiscence and the symptoms.

One late complication is ileoanal anastomotic stricture. Treatment, consisting of anal dilatation, is usually necessary only in patients who have difficulty evacuating. Perianal complications such as abscesses and fistulas may occur, but if they do, one Crohn's disease must always be suspected. Generally, abscesses can be drained and superficial fistulas laid open. However, one should always be cautious about dividing even part of the anal sphincter in these patients. The other late complication of significance is pouchitis, which is manifest in a way similar to that seen in patients with Kock pouches. Again, broad-spectrum antibiotics are usually effective treatment.

■ COLOSTOMY

The early management of a colostomy is similar to that for an ileostomy. Preoperative stoma siting and counseling are as important for this group of patients as for those undergoing ileostomy surgery. However, the concerns of these patients often differ from those of ileostomates, since they are often elderly and the diagnosis is usually cancer.

As with most abdominal surgery, there tends to be an ileus that resolves several days after surgery. However, whereas one should wait until the ileostomy has passed gas and effluent before oral intake is initiated, the colostomy must often be stimulated by the ingestion of food before it begins to function. Vascular insufficiency tends to occur with greater frequency in colostomies because of abdominal wall thickness, tension placed on the mesentery, and poorer vascular supply of the colon. Steps to assess the vascular supply are similar to those described for ileostomies. Superficial necrosis of a portion of the stoma may be managed with observation in the realization that a stricture may occur and need to be revised later. Separation of the stoma at the mucocutaneous junction may arise, especially if there is tension or vascular compromise. In virtually all situations, these should be treated nonoperatively, and healing will occur with time. A stricture may result, but the stoma can be revised at a later date if it is symptomatic.

The colostomy effluent is usually solid and nonirritating, so the colostomy can be made flush with the skin unless there has been a significant bowel resection previously or there is underlying disease in the colon or small bowel. Function through a descending colostomy is similar to normal bowel function. Some patients may suffer from constipation or even fecal impaction, particularly if there is a preoperative history of constipation or irritable bowel syndrome. Bulk agents may help regulate the stoma. Fecal impaction may require treatment with a retention enema of cottonseed oil and water.

For patients wishing to eliminate the use of an appliance, there are two possible alternatives: a continent colostomy ring (such as the Erlangen magnetic colostomy device) or colostomy irrigation. Although the concept of a continence device has appeal, it has in fact had limited success. Some patients may wish to try colostomy irrigations, but these are possible only in patients with end-sigmoid colostomies. They must also be well motivated. The advantage of irrigation is that there is no soiling of stool throughout the day, so a cap can be worn. However, the irrigation procedure often takes 1 or 2 hours to complete and must be done regularly at the same time each day.

An enterostomal therapist should be consulted to instruct the patient. Usually, 1,000 ml of lukewarm water is inserted through a soft-tipped cone gently inserted into the colostomy. Caution is required to ensure that the colostomy is not injured during insertion.

Late Complications

The late complications associated with a colostomy are similar to those with an ileostomy, but they differ in frequency. Food blockages and skin irritation are uncommon in patients with colostomies, whereas parastomal hernia formation often occurs, particularly if the colostomy is of long standing. Stricture also occurs more frequently, probably because of the more tenuous blood supply. Prolapse of the stoma is commonly seen with loop colostomies, especially transverse loop colostomies, but otherwise occurs infrequently.

Stomas placed outside the rectus sheath, or those in which the fascial aperture is large, are predisposed to the formation of paracolostomy hernias. Often the colon proximal to the stoma bulges into the subcutaneous tissue and may become obstructed. The indications for surgical repair are symptoms related to entrapment of the intestine, difficulty in irrigating the stoma, parastomal pain, and problems in maintaining the appliance. The treatment of choice is to move the stoma to another site on the abdomen. This may be difficult when there are multiple previous incisions or repairs. In these situations, the stoma can be safely brought out through a synthetic mesh.

Suggested Reading

MacKeigan JM, Cataldo PA, eds. Intestinal stomas. Principles, techniques and management. St Louis: Quality Medical Publishing, 1993.

McLeod RS, Lavery IC, Leatherman JR, et al. Factors affecting quality of life with a conventional ileostomy. World J Surg 1986; 10:474–480.

Morowitz DA, Kirsner JB. Ileostomy in ulcerative colitis. A questionnaire study of 1,803 patients. Am J Surg 1981; 141:370–375.

Nicholls RJ, Bartolo DCC, Mortensen NJ, eds. Restorative proctocolectomy. London: Blackwell Scientific, 1993.

Pemberton JH. Management of conventional ileostomies. World J Surg 1988; 12:203–214.

MESENTERIC ISCHEMIA

Peter Hugh MacDonald, B.Sc., M.D., F.R.C.S.C.
Ivan T. Beck, M.D., Ph.D., F.R.C.P.C., F.A.C.P., F.A.C.G.

Ischemic bowel disease occurs when blood flow to any part of the intestine is suddenly or chronically diminished or fully interrupted. This may be caused by inadequate systemic blood flow or local vascular abnormalities. Because of the frequency of inadequate vascular supply in the elderly, ischemic bowel disease occurs most often in older patients. It may also be seen in younger patients with vascular abnormalities such as vasculitis, collagen diseases, or diabetes or in those who are taking vasoconstrictor drugs. The approach to therapy depends on the type of vessel involved. Thus, to provide appropriate treatment, it is necessary to acquire a thorough understanding of the pathophysiology of the different ischemic syndromes. Accordingly, in this chapter we provide a short review on the classification and pathophysiology of intestinal ischemia.

■ GENERAL CONCEPTS

Classification of Intestinal Ischemia

The extent of intestinal ischemia and the pathologic consequence depends on the size and location of the occluded or hypoperfused vessels. The clinical presentation is also different, depending on the acuteness or chronicity of the vascular occlusion. Because certain acute events may change to a chronic condition, a clear-cut classification of ischemic bowel disease is very difficult. From a clinical and pathologic point of view, we find it useful to classify ischemic bowel disease according to the size of the vessels that are hypoperfused or occluded. This is because the clinical picture, investigation,

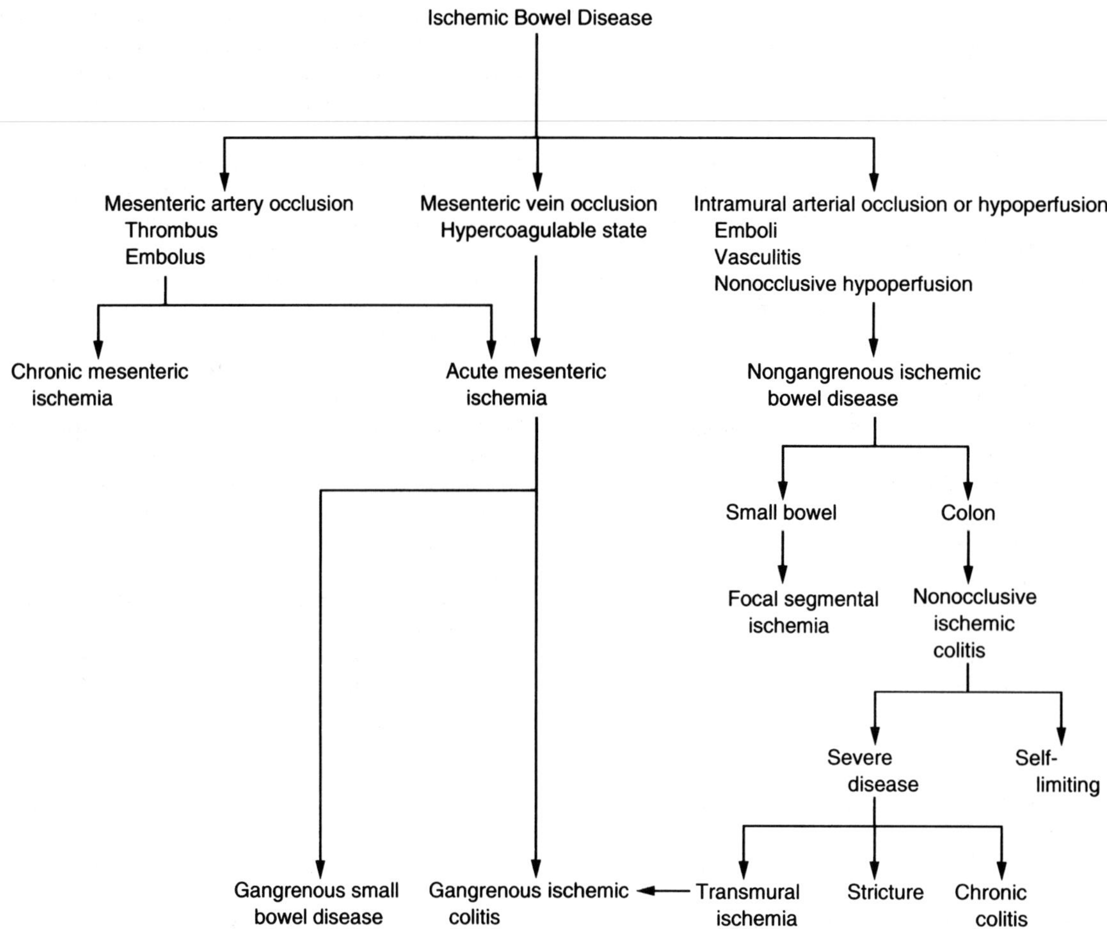

Figure 1
Classification of intestinal ischemia.

and therapy in patients with mesenteric artery or vein occlusion are often different from those in patients in whom the cause of the disease is occlusion or hypoperfusion of the intramural vessels (Fig. 1). As the classification of syndromes is based on the pathophysiologic mechanisms, we will discuss therapy based on this classification.

In our experience, ischemic colitis is more common than acute mesenteric ischemia. Overall, acute ischemia is much more common than chronic forms of the disease. Also, ischemia of arterial origin is far more frequent than that of venous disease. It is now recognized that many reported cases of mesenteric vein thrombosis were in fact incorrectly diagnosed cases of nonocclusive ischemia, and it is now believed that the true incidence of mesenteric vein thrombosis is quite low.

Pathophysiology of Intestinal Ischemia

Vascular Anatomy

The anatomy of the splanchnic circulation is complex and extremely variable. The finer details are really important only to the invasive radiologist, whereas the clinician need only be concerned with some of the more constant and important features. The blood flow to the splanchnic organs is derived from three main arterial trunks: the celiac, superior mesenteric, and inferior mesenteric arteries. The celiac artery supplies blood to the foregut (stomach and duodenum), the superior mesenteric artery to the midgut (duodenum to transverse colon), and the inferior mesenteric artery to the hindgut (transverse colon to rectum). Each arterial trunk supplies blood flow to a section of the gastrointestinal (GI) tract through a vast arcade network, a system that is generally protective against ischemia. In the event of an arterial obstruction distal to the main arterial trunk, GI blood flow can usually be maintained through collateral vessels. As shown in Figure 2, additional vascular protection is obtained from anastomotic connections between the three arterial systems.

Communication between the celiac system and the superior mesenteric system generally occurs via the superior pancreaticoduodenal and inferior pancreaticoduodenal arteries. The superior mesenteric and inferior mesenteric systems are joined by the arc of Riolan and the marginal artery of Drummond, vessels that connect the middle colic artery (a branch of the superior mesenteric artery) and the left colic artery (a branch of the inferior mesenteric artery). In addition, communication exists between the inferior mesenteric artery and branches of the internal iliac arteries via the rectum. The caliber of these anastomotic connections varies considerably, depending on the existence of vascular disease,

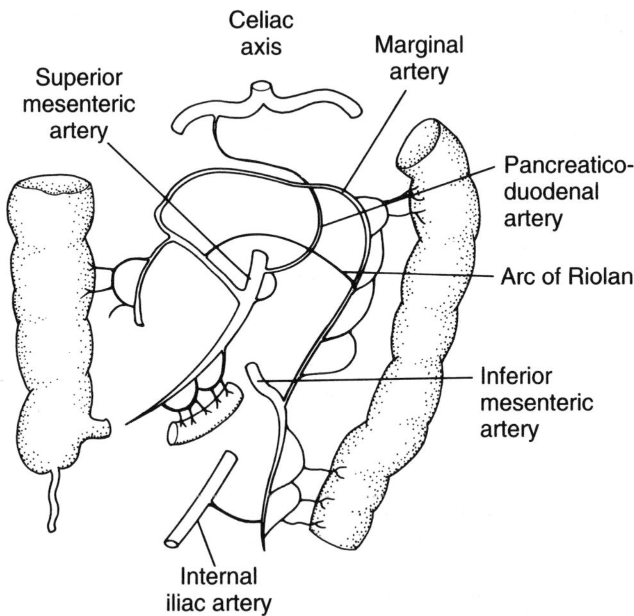

Figure 2
Splanchnic circulation.

but it is important to realize that in chronic states of vascular insufficiency, blood flow to an individual system can be maintained through these anastomotic connections even when an arterial trunk is completely obstructed. It is not uncommon to find one or even two arterial trunks completely occluded in the asymptomatic patient. In fact, there are reports of occlusion of all three trunks in patients who are still maintaining their splanchnic circulation. However, in up to 30 percent of people, the anastomotic connections between the superior and inferior mesenteric arteries, via the arc of Riolan and the marginal artery of Drummond, can be weak or nonexistent, making the area of the splenic flexure particularly vulnerable to acute ischemia or failure of a surgical anastomosis. Another area of relatively poor collateral circulation is at the rectosigmoid junction, where the anastomotic connection between the most inferior sigmoid artery and the superior rectal artery (critical point of Sudeck) is often weak. These areas of poor collateral circulation are often referred to as the *watershed areas.*

Physiology of Splanchnic Blood Flow

Splanchnic blood flow varies in the fasting and nonfasting state, but on average it receives approximately 30 percent of the cardiac output. Blood flow through the celiac and superior mesenteric trunks is about equal (approximately 700 ml per minute in adults) and is twice that which flows through the inferior mesenteric trunk. In comparison with other tissue layers of the gut, the mucosa has the highest metabolic rate and thus receives about 70 percent of the splanchnic blood flow. Per unit tissue, the small bowel receives the most blood, followed by the colon and then the stomach.

Much has been written on the control of GI blood flow and many factors are involved. It is not the intent of this chapter to review the intricacies of physiologic control, but rather to highlight some important points. Vascular resistance is proportional to $1/r^4$ (where r = the radius of the vessel). Thus, the smaller the artery, the greater is its ability to effect vascular resistance. Most blood flow control occurs at the arteriolar level, the so-called resistance vessels. Very little control of blood flow occurs at the level of the large arterial trunks. In fact, the diameter of these large arterial trunks can be compromised by 75 percent before blood flow is reduced. Additional control of blood flow occurs at the level of the precapillary sphincter. In the fasting state, only one-fifth of capillary beds are open, leaving a tremendous reserve to meet increased metabolic demands.

Among the most important control mechanisms of splanchnic blood flow are the sympathetic nervous system, humoral factors, and local factors. The sympathetic nervous system through alpha-adrenergic receptors plays an important role in maintaining basal vascular tone and in mediating vasoconstriction. Beta-adrenergic activity appears to mediate vasodilation, and it appears that the antrum of the stomach may be particularly rich in these beta receptors. Humoral factors involved in the regulation of GI blood flow include catecholamines, the renin-angiotensin system, and vasopressin. These humoral systems may play a particularly important role in shock states, and in some patients may play a role in the pathogenesis of nonocclusive ischemia. Local factors appear to be mainly involved in the matching of tissue blood flow to the metabolic demand. An increased metabolic rate may produce decreased Po_2, increased Pco_2, and an increased level of adenosine, each of which can mediate a hyperemic response. Finally, many investigators have now identified an important contribution by endothelin and endothelium-derived relaxing factor (nitric oxide) in the local control of intestinal blood flow.

The integration of these control systems, and their alteration by factors such as vascular disease, motor activity, intraluminal pressure, and pharmaceutical agents, remain poorly understood. The key to our understanding and successful treatment of intestinal ischemia lies in a better knowledge of this physiology.

Pathophysiology of Intestinal Ischemia

Intestinal ischemia occurs when the metabolic demand of the tissue supersedes the oxygen delivery. Obviously, many factors may be involved in this oxygen need/demand mismatch. These include the general hemodynamic state, the degree of atherosclerosis, the extent of collateral circulation, neurogenic/humoral/local control mechanisms of vascular resistance, and abnormal products of cellular metabolism before and after reperfusion of an ischemic segment.

Of all the intestinal wall tissue layers, the mucosa is the most metabolically active. Mechanisms that bring about redistribution of intramural blood flow have been identified. In general, they function to protect the mucosa against ischemia, but despite these mechanisms, the mucosal layer is the first tissue layer to demonstrate signs of ischemia. Changes at the cellular level begin at the tip of the villi. With ongoing ischemia, ultrastructural changes begin within 10 minutes and cellular damage is extensive by 30 minutes. Sloughing of the villus tips is followed by edema, submucosal hemorrhage, and eventual transmural necrosis.

The intestinal response to ischemia is first characterized by a hypermotility state. It is this intense motor activity that results in the patient experiencing severe pain, even though the ischemic damage may be limited to the mucosa at this stage. As the ischemia progresses, motor activity ceases and the gut mucosal permeability increases, leading to an increase in bacterial translocation. With transmural extension of the ischemia, visceral and parietal inflammation develop, resulting in peritonitis.

An important factor often responsible for or aggravating intestinal ischemia is the phenomenon of vasospasm. It has been well demonstrated that both occlusive and nonocclusive forms of arterial ischemia can result in prolonged vasospasm even after the occlusion has been removed or the perfusion pressure restored. This vasospasm may persist for several hours, resulting in prolonged ischemia. The mechanism responsible for this vasospasm is not clearly defined. To date, many of the interventional techniques used to treat mesenteric ischemia have been directed at counteracting this vasospasm.

A second factor that may be responsible for accentuating ischemic damage is reperfusion injury. In the laboratory, reperfusion has been shown to cause more cellular damage than is brought about during the actual ischemic period. Parks and Granger showed in an animal model that the injury after 1 hour of ischemia and 3 hours of reperfusion is more severe than that observed after 4 hours of continuous ischemia. The mechanism responsible for this reperfusion injury appears to be related to the release of harmful reactive oxygen metabolites, which are thought to be released from adhering polymorphonuclear leukocytes. It is not known what role ischemia reperfusion injury plays in humans with occlusive and nonocclusive disease.

■ ACUTE SUPERIOR MESENTERIC ISCHEMIA

Presentation and Diagnosis

The key to diagnosis lies in a high index of suspicion. Patients with advanced ischemia are usually not a challenge to diagnose, presenting with diffuse peritonitis, shock, and severe metabolic derangements. Often, these patients cannot be salvaged, and the mortality rate is reported to be between 70 and 90 percent. The patient with early ischemia is far more challenging to diagnose and stands to benefit most from a correct diagnosis.

The typical patient with mesenteric ischemia is usually over 50 years of age and often has a history of cardiac and peripheral vascular disease. In the early stage of ischemia the patient complains of severe abdominal pain in the absence of peritoneal findings; hence, the standard expression, "pain out of proportion to the physical findings." Other nonspecific symptoms such as nausea, vomiting, and altered bowel habit may be present but are not particularly helpful in the diagnosis.

Laboratory Findings

Many studies have attempted to identify a biochemical marker of early ischemia. Creatine kinase, alkaline phosphatase, lactate dehydrogenase, diamine oxidase, and inorganic phosphate are among the biochemical markers that have been examined. Although all of these eventually become altered with intestinal ischemia, no single marker reliably identifies early ischemia, and thus in the clinical setting they are not particularly useful.

Management

General Concepts

If a diagnosis of mesenteric ischemia is being considered, the subsequent investigation and management must proceed in an efficient and aggressive fashion if morbidity and mortality are to be reduced. Initial management of all patients consists of resuscitation, the degree of which varies widely with the degree and extent of ischemia. Patients with early ischemia require very little resuscitation, whereas those with infarcted intestine may require admission to a critical care unit for invasive monitoring. Insertion of a Swan-Ganz catheter with central pressure monitoring can be very useful in resuscitating the shocked patient with underlying cardiac disease. It must be kept in mind that in patients with extensive and advanced infarction, complete "stability" may never be obtained, and thus investigation and treatment should proceed without extensive delay. However, ongoing patient "instability" is no doubt an ominous sign. As a general rule, vasopressors to support blood pressure should be avoided as they may further increase the degree of intestinal ischemia. The role of antibiotics is not clear-cut. Our policy is to administer broad-spectrum antibiotic coverage as soon as possible to patients presenting with peritonitis. In those without peritonitis, antibiotics are used in the perioperative period should surgery be required.

Clearly, several intra-abdominal disease processes can present in a fashion identical to that of mesenteric ischemia. Thus, initial investigation is aimed at ruling out other causes of abdominal pain and peritonitis. An upright and supine plain film of the abdomen should be obtained in all patients. Although these films may support a diagnosis of ischemia, as indicated by bowel wall thickening and "thumbprinting," their main purpose is to rule out visceral perforation or bowel obstruction. In many centers, computed tomography (CT) is being used as a first-line investigation in patients with abdominal pain. Several markers of intestinal ischemia have now been described by radiologists with expertise in CT scans, including bowel wall thickening, mucosal edema, pneumatosis, and mesenteric and portal vein gas. By means of large injections of peripheral venous contrast material, mesenteric arterial and venous occlusion can now also be identified in some patients. Of course, many of these findings are not specific, and thus we do not currently advocate the CT scan as a diagnostic test for intestinal ischemia. However, in certain situations, a high index of suspicion that a disease process other than ischemia is involved will necessitate its use. For example, it is sometimes difficult to differentiate acute pancreatitis from abdominal ischemia. Both can present with hyperamylasemia and/or peritonitis. This is one situation in which an abdominal CT scan may be useful to rule out retroperitoneal inflammation.

Ultrasonography combined with Doppler assessment of blood flow in the splanchnic arterial and venous system is now being used in some centers to screen for mesenteric ischemia. Our personal experience with this technique is limited, and

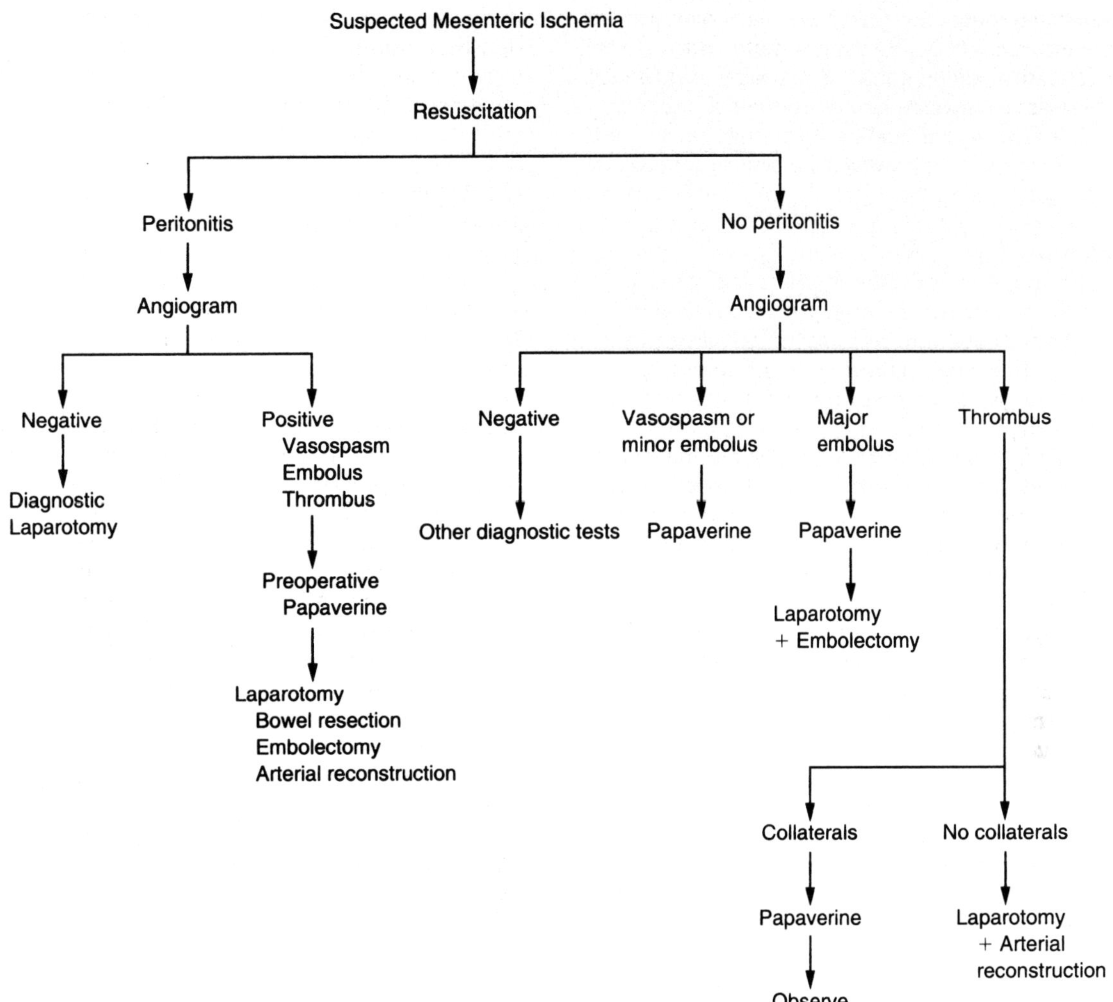

Figure 3
Treatment of mesenteric ischemia.

the exact role this technique will play is not clearly defined. There is experimental evidence from a rabbit model of ischemia that magnetic resonance imaging (MRI) may also be of significant use in the diagnosis of mesenteric ischemia. Certainly, both arterial and venous abnormalities as well as the extent of the collateral circulation can be identified in some patients through MRI technology, but further clinical experience is required before this technique can be completely evaluated.

Angiography remains the "gold standard" in the diagnosis of mesenteric ischemia and, as will be discussed, may play a significant role in the treatment of such patients. We believe that all patients with suspected mesenteric intestinal ischemia should undergo angiography to confirm the diagnosis and assist treatment planning. This approach should include those patients presenting with peritonitis. Often, there is a tendency to take patients with peritonitis straight to the operating room without performing angiography. These patients need to be treated in an expedient fashion, but the short delay involved in obtaining an angiogram may prove beneficial. Not only will it identify patients who may require embolectomy or vascular reconstruction, but it will also provide a means to treat vasospasm in the perioperative period. Such a treatment policy has two implications. First, for management to be effective, an invasive radiologist must be available at all times and a system must be in place that allows the angiography suite to function with a short lead time. Second, the physician must realize that an appreciable number of negative angiographic results should be expected with this low angiography threshold.

The treatment algorithm we recommend is outlined in Figure 3. Essentially, patients are divided into two groups: those with peritonitis and those without. Although all patients with peritonitis require laparotomy, the exact treatment plan for both groups of patients is dictated by the angiographic findings, which fall into four major categories, as outlined below.

Thrombotic Occlusion. This finding is usually identified with an aortic flush of contrast dye, but it is sometimes difficult to differentiate from a proximal arterial embolus. The other pitfall is that this finding sometimes represents a chronic obstruction not necessarily related to the patient's current symptoms and findings. Most of these patients require arterial reconstruction, although the final treatment plan will be based on the exact vascular anatomy and degree of collateral circulation. Patients with peritonitis may also require a bowel resection. Perioperative papaverine infusion in these patients may be useful; however, depending on the site of vascular obstruction, it may not be possible to secure a catheter for infusion.

Major Embolus. Major emboli are usually in the proximal portion of the superior mesenteric artery. Most of these patients should be referred to surgery for consideration of embolectomy regardless of the presence or lack of peritoneal findings. Papaverine infusion in the perioperative period should be used to reduce vasospasm-induced ischemia.

Minor Embolus. These emboli are limited to the branches of the superior mesenteric artery or to that portion of the vessel distal to the origin of the ileocolic artery. Unless peritoneal signs are present, these patients should be managed with papaverine infusion and observation.

Vasospasm (Nonocclusive Ischemia). Vasospasm may occur in response to a mechanical arterial obstruction, but when it is the sole finding it is diagnostic of nonocclusive ischemia. The recommended management is papaverine infusion.

Papaverine Infusion

Papaverine has been recommended as a mainstay of medical therapy for mesenteric ischemia. Although we support its use, it must be stressed that its efficacy has not been absolutely proved by the proper clinical trials.

Papaverine is a smooth muscle relaxant. Administered systemically, it nonspecifically dilates the vascular tree. However, since it is almost completely metabolized by a single pass through the liver, selective administration into the mesenteric circulation produces very few systemic effects. This allows vasodilatation in the mesenteric circulation to occur without a drop in systemic blood pressure. Typically, papaverine is infused into the mesenteric circulation (usually the superior mesenteric artery) after angiography-guided selective catheterization of an arterial trunk. Papaverine is dissolved in normal saline to a concentration of 1 mg per milliliter, although a higher concentration can be used. Heparin should not be added to the solution, as it will crystallize. The infusion is started at 30 mg per hour and may be increased to 60 mg per hour. In most cases the papaverine infusion is maintained for 24 hours. The catheter is then flushed with normal saline for 30 minutes and angiography is then repeated. If vasospasm persists, the cycle should be repeated every 24 hours for a maximum of 5 days. During the papaverine infusion, the patient's systemic vital signs must be monitored. A sudden drop in blood pressure usually suggests that the catheter has slipped out of the mesenteric circulation into the aorta. Repeat angiography at the bedside can be performed to confirm this. Generally, papaverine infusion is quite safe, and major complications are usually related to the initial passage of the arterial catheter. Complications include injury to the femoral artery, dislodgment of atherosclerotic plaques with embolic accidents in the lower extremities, and the formation of a false aneurysm after the catheter is removed.

Surgical Management

The role of surgery is to evaluate the viability of ischemic bowel, resect if necessary, and if possible alleviate or bypass a vascular obstruction. If possible, the vascular surgery should be performed first so that its effect on intestinal viability can be assessed.

One of the most difficult decisions the surgeon has to make is to determine whether the bowel injury is reversible or not. Subjective criteria such as bowel wall color, the presence of peristalsis, and the presence of palpable mesenteric pulses are often used. Unfortunately, these criteria can lead to an inaccurate assessment in over 50 percent of cases. This has led surgeons to adopt a second-look approach, with which only the most obviously infarcted gut is resected and any questionable bowel is left in situ. A second look within 24 hours is then used to decide on the need for further resection. More recently, several objective measurements have been employed to assess bowel viability, including fluorescence staining, laser Doppler flowmetry, surface oximetry, and intramural pH measurements. At present, no single technology has been widely adopted, but as these techniques are further refined they may eventually play a valuable role in the assessment of intestinal viability.

A second difficult situation for the surgeon is the management of patients with near-total intestinal infarction. Even with resection, the mortality rate in this group of patients is very high, and survivors are often dependent on total parenteral nutrition (TPN) indefinitely. In elderly patients with other underlying medical problems, many surgeons choose to close without resection. The approach in a younger patient with a catastrophic vascular accident tends to be more aggressive, particularly with increasing advances in bowel transplantation.

■ CHRONIC MESENTERIC ISCHEMIA

Owing to the vast collateral arterial network of the gut, chronic mesenteric ischemia is relatively uncommon. In almost all patients, the cause is related to atherosclerosis. Classically, it is written that these patients present with a similar symptom complex, namely, postprandial abdominal pain, "fear of eating," and weight loss. Unfortunately, most patients do not present with these classic symptoms, and as with other ischemic syndromes the physician must maintain a high index of suspicion. The diagnosis is made with angiography and the treatment is surgical. Because the symptoms of chronic mesenteric ischemia in the elderly often closely resemble those of functional dyspepsia, it can be difficult to decide whether arteriography with its inherent dangers is indicated. Thus, the disease may run a prolonged course before diagnosis and effective treatment is employed.

Many surgical procedures have been described for the treatment of chronic mesenteric ischemia, of which aortovisceral bypass and endarterectomy are employed most commonly. More recently, balloon angioplasty has been used, but early results suggest that the recurrence rate may be high.

■ NONGANGRENOUS ISCHEMIC BOWEL DISEASE

Etiology

Contrary to mesenteric ischemia, in which occlusion of major vessels is the cause of the disease, the ischemia in nongangrenous ischemic bowel disease is caused by hypoperfusion and occasionally secondary occlusion of intramural vessels and the gut wall microcirculation. Many factors may precipitate this disorder. Most often, hypoperfusion is caused by vascular disorders, such as collagen disease, vasculitis, and atherosclerosis or by increased viscosity of the blood in polycythemia vera. Sudden acute hypotension due to hemorrhage, acute myocardial infarct, congestive heart failure, and vasoconstricting drugs may also precipitate local ischemia in patients with already impaired local circulation. Because the disease involves the vessels of the bowel wall, localization is always segmental, and thus there is usually an adequate collateral circulation. As a result, the ischemia-induced necrosis is rarely transmural and peritonitis is a rare complication. Nongangrenous ischemic bowel disease may involve the small bowel as "focal segmental ischemia" or the colon as "nongangrenous ischemic colitis."

Focal Segmental Ischemia

The clinical course of this condition is variable and depends on the severity of the infarct. Limited necrosis may heal completely. Ongoing repeated injury may cause chronic enteritis almost indistinguishable from Crohn's disease. In other patients the necrotic ulcer may lead to late stricture formation, or may become transmural and cause peritonitis. The diagnosis is always difficult, as the symptoms may be those of chronic recurrent abdominal pain, bowel obstruction, or frank peritonitis. Unless there is complete spontaneous resolution, the treatment is surgical and the diagnosis is often made only on the resected specimen.

Nongangrenous Ischemic Colitis

Pathogenesis

Ischemic colitis was first described by Boley and co-workers in 1963. The disease was classified by Marston and colleagues in 1966 into three major forms: gangrenous, stricturing, and transient colitis. Since that time, it has become clear that there are only two major forms: gangrenous and nongangrenous ischemic colitis (see Fig. 1). These two forms are in fact two different diseases, with different etiologies and clinical courses, and require entirely different approaches to their management. Gangrenous ischemic colitis is caused by obstruction of the mesenteric vessels and was discussed in the section on acute mesenteric ischemia. Occasionally, transmural gangrene may develop when nongangrenous ischemic colitis slowly progresses to transmural necrosis. The recognition and management of this complication of nongangrenous ischemic colitis are discussed in this section.

Nonocclusive ischemia of the small bowel is rare, but there appears to be a predilection of the colon for local vascular hypoperfusion. The relative frequency of colonic involvement may be explained by the following factors: in comparison with the small intestine, the colon receives less blood, has a less well developed collateral circulation, has a different neuroendocrine control, and an ongoing motor activity that may predispose it to a temporary decrease in blood flow. Not only is the colonic blood flow quantitively smaller than that of the small intestine, but it also has fewer vascular collaterals and has susceptible "watershed areas." Recent evidence in our laboratory demonstrated that in the colon of the dog, unlike the small intestine, the major local vasoconstrictory substance is angiotensin, and the vessels of the colon respond more vigorously to hypotension than do those of the small intestine. Also, elevated intramural pressure during increased motility in patients with constipation, diverticular disease, and cancer of the colon may lead to diminished gut wall blood flow. Similarly, distention with air during colonoscopy or barium enema may temporarily reduce blood flow to the colon.

Table 1 Causes of Nonocclusive Ischemic Colitis

Acute diminution of colonic intramural blood flow
Small vessel obstruction
Collagen vascular disease
Vasculitis, diabetes
Oral contraceptives
Nonocclusive hypoperfusion
Hemorrhage
Congestive heart failure, myocardial infarction, arrhythmias
Sepsis
Vasoconstricting agents: digitalis, vasopressin, ergot, NSAIDs
Increased viscosity: polycythemia, sickle cell disease, thrombocytosis
Increased demand on marginal blood flow
Increased motility
Mass lesion, stricture
Constipation
Increased intraluminal pressure
Bowel obstruction
Colonoscopy
Barium enema

Under specific conditions, nonocclusive ischemic colitis can also occur in the young (Table 1). This sometimes has iatrogenic causes such as contraceptive medication or nonsteroid anti-inflammatory agents.

Clinical Presentation

The clinical presentation is characterized by a sudden onset of severe crampy abdominal pain, diarrhea, hematochezia, and occasionally melena. On physical examination, the abdomen may be distended. There are bowel sounds and no signs of peritoneal involvement. The patient may have one of the associated diseases such as hypotension, ischemic heart disease, or polycythemia or one of the iatrogenic causes such as oral contraceptives or digitalis (see Table 1). Occasionally, the specific event that precipitated the attack cannot be determined, especially in the elderly. The early clinical presentation is so similar to that of acute infectious colitis, ulcerative colitis, Crohn's colitis, and pseudomembranous colitis that the differentiation can be established only by excluding infection (including *Clostridium difficile*) and by demonstrating the classic radiographic or colonoscopic findings of ischemic colitis. Investigation must be carried out within 24 to 48 hours of the onset of the disease, as the typical findings tend to disappear rapidly. Because large vessels are never involved, angiography has no place in the diagnosis of nongangrenous ischemic colitis. The first radiologic examination should be an abdominal survey film, which may demonstrate "thumbprinting" in air-filled segments of the colon. Thumbprinting is caused by intramural hemorrhage but can be mimicked by severe mucosal and submucosal edema. Typically, colonic involvement is segmental. Although any part of the colon may be affected, the "watershed" areas of the splenic flexure and the rectosigmoid junction are most commonly involved. Thumbprinting can be better demonstrated by barium enema, and the submucosal hemorrhage by colonoscopy. Because distention of the colon with air may compress intramural blood vessels and decrease blood flow, barium enema and colonoscopy must be carried out carefully with minimal air insufflation. Colonoscopy is preferable to barium enema because early inspection and biopsy can differentiate between the thumbprinting caused by submucosal hemorrhage and that caused by severe edema due to inflammatory bowel disease (IBD) or colitis of other etiology. After 24 to 48 hours, the hemorrhage resolves and the mucosa becomes necrotic. If colonoscopy is performed at this stage, the endoscopist may have great difficulty in differentiating the necrosis and ulceration caused by ischemic colitis from that caused by Crohn's disease or pseudomembraneous enterocolitis. The pathologist reviewing biopsies taken a few days after the onset of the disease may have similar difficulties. Not infrequently, only time will tell whether the patient has IBD or ischemia. One cannot help but wonder what proportion of late-onset IBD or Crohn's disease in young women on contraceptive medication is actually due to ischemia.

As shown in Figure 1, the disease can progress in four ways. Mild disease may resolve spontaneously. The symptoms and physical findings subside within 24 to 48 hours and complete resolution should occur within 2 to 3 weeks. In some patients the disease does not resolve and they may suffer from ongoing or recurrent chronic colitis, indistinguishable from IBD. Since the pathologic response of colonic tissue to chronic injury is restricted to a very few factors, such as infiltration with leukocytes, crypt abscess, hemorrhage, necrosis, ulceration, and regeneration of crypts, the pathologist may have difficulty in differentiating ongoing ischemic colitis from Crohn's colitis. Hemosiderin, a sign of previous bleeding, is often considered a typical manifestation of ischemic colitis. Unfortunately, this finding is not restricted to ischemic disease; it can be seen in any type of colitis, including IBD, in which hemorrhage has occurred in the past. Furthermore, ischemia may be one of the etiologic factors involved in Crohn's disease.

Chronic disease may resolve, relapse, or progress to deeper intramural necrosis. If the necrosis stops in the submucosa or muscularis, the patient may exhibit toxic symptoms such as chills, fever, severe bloody diarrhea, abdominal distention, diminished bowel sounds, leukocytosis, anemia, elevated platelet count, and electrolyte disturbances. If it does not progress further, intramural necrosis will heal with stricture. In some instances, the necrosis results in toxic megacolon, and if the intramural necrosis becomes transmural, acute peritonitis may ensue. This usually occurs slowly and may take several days to develop. This progression must be detected early by careful follow-up.

Treatment

Appropriate treatment depends on an accurate diagnosis. Infectious causes, bacterial and amebic dysentery, and all other infectious enteropathies must be excluded. Exclusion of IBD at the early stage is less important, but other local precipitating causes of ischemia such as diverticulitis or cancer must be detected and appropriately treated. As to the immediate management of patients, we prefer to consider treatment under the following three categories: (1) nonspecific medical supportive therapy, (2) specific medical treatment, and (3) surgical therapy.

Nonspecific Medical Supportive Therapy. While investigation of the cause is progressing, fluid and electrolyte balance must be carefully maintained. Intake by mouth is restricted according to the severity of the disease. The need for nutritional support depends on the patient's overall nutritional status. Well-nourished patients can be maintained for a few days without specific support, except for what they receive in intravenous solutions. Very rarely, severely undernourished patients may have to be started on TPN at an early stage. Bleeding is rarely sufficient to require blood transfusion, but if severe anemia is present, it may be necessary to transfuse an elderly patient who has atherosclerosis, angina, or a myocardial infarct. This requires careful balancing of the cardiac and hematologic state to ensure that one does not overload an already precariously maintained circulation. Usually, patients with acute colitis request medication to relieve symptoms, but the use of analgesics and antispasmodic or antidiarrheal agents is contraindicated because these drugs may lead to an inert bowel and possibly a toxic megacolon.

Depending on the progression of the disease and the patient's response to feeding, a low-residue diet may be slowly started. In chronic ischemic colitis, enteric feeding may be required. It is our experience that diarrhea and abdominal pain may become worse on enteric nutrition in some patients. Dilution of the solution, constant slow administration over 24 hours, or the use of an iso-osmotic product may overcome this problem.

Patients must be carefully followed to detect deterioration. There is no good experimental evidence to support the value of antibiotics, but in a patient who shows signs of deterioration one should start antibiotics, using triple therapy (metronidazole, amoxicillin, and an aminoglycoside) or a beta lactam. If there is further progression and patients develop increasing peritoneal signs, surgery may become necessary, even if they appear to be a poor surgical risk. One of the major errors is to delay surgery to the point where a patient who was previously a poor risk has become so sick that successful surgery becomes impossible.

Specific Medical Treatment

Colitis. Specific therapy for colitis is not needed in mild self-limiting disease. The value of therapy for chronic ongoing disease is questionable. No experimental data are available to assess the effectiveness of drugs used in IBD for the treatment of chronic ischemic colitis. If one considers how difficult it is to ascertain by prospective double-blind studies the success of medical therapy (sulfasalazine [Azulfadine], 5-aminosalicylic acid [5-ASA], steroids, metronidazole, or immunosuppressive agents) in IBD, because of the lower incidence of ischemic colitis, there is little likelihood that controlled studies will ever be available for this disease. Taking this limitation into consideration, we believe that in long-standing progressive disease a trial with sulfasalazine or 5-ASA by oral and/or (depending on the location of the disease) rectal administration may be justified. If patients do not respond, a trial with steroids may be attempted, although it is difficult to predict the outcome. No experience exists with metronidazole and immunosuppressive agents.

One may question whether vasodilators, (e.g., papaverine, angiotensin converting enzyme [ACE] inhibitors) may be useful in the management of this disease. Once the symptoms have developed and the patient is seen by the physician, the intramural ischemic injury has already occurred. There is no evidence to indicate either that vasodilators may be useful in reverting the pathologic findings and thus facilitating recovery, or that these agents may prevent recurrence or progression to chronic disease.

Precipitating Disease. Another type of specific therapy is directed toward the condition that precipitated the ischemic attack. Treatment of heart disease, change of digitalis to other medication (e.g., ACE inhibitors), discontinuation of estrogens, management of diabetes, recognition and treatment of vasculitis and polycythemia, for example, may prevent recurrences in the future but may not necessarily alter the outcome of already established chronic disease.

Surgical Therapy

Acute Colitis. Uncontrollable hemorrhage is rare, but if it occurs, resection may be necessary. As already discussed, transmural necrosis and toxic megacolon leading to peritoneal signs require immediate surgical intervention.

Late Complications. About one-third of patients with severe ischemic colitis develop strictures, usually within 6 months after the onset of the disease. Patients present with obstructive symptoms, and barium enema and colonoscopy demonstrate an area of narrowing. If colonoscopic dilatation fails and symptoms persist, surgical resection or stricturoplasty may be necessary.

■ COMMENTS

Within the last decade, the morbidity and mortality rates of ischemic bowel disease decreased considerably. Recent advances, better radiologic and surgical techniques, new methods in measuring tissue blood flow, advances in intensive care medicine, and appropriate nutritional support have already improved the outcome of these diseases. Further research to obtain a better understanding of the physiology of the regulation of blood flow should lead to an even better approach to these patients.

Suggested Reading

Boley SJ, Brandt LJ, guest eds. Intestinal ischemia. Surg Clin North Am 1992; 72:1.

Carratu R, Parisi P, Agozzino A. Segmental ischemic colitis associated with nonsteroidal antiinflammatory drugs. J Clin Gastroenterol 1993; 16:31–34.

Kvietys PR, Barrowman JA, Granger DN. Pathophysiology of the splanchnic circulation. Vols 1 & 2. Boca Raton, FL: CRC Press, 1987.

MacDonald PH, Dinda PK, Beck IT. The role of angiotensin in the intestinal vascular response to hypotension in a canine model. Gastroenterology 1992; 103:57–64.

CONSTIPATION

Arnd Schulte-Bockholt, M.D.
Timothy R. Koch, M.D.

■ DEFINITION AND EPIDEMIOLOGY

Constipation remains difficult to define within the general population. Patients who complain of constipation may describe infrequent defecation, pain or straining with defecation, passage of firm or small-volume material, increased difficulty initiating evacuation, or a feeling of incomplete evacuation. Bowel frequency has been used as an objective criterion, and a range between three and 21 bowel movements weekly is thought to be normal defecation frequency. We define chronic constipation as a disorder lasting 6 months or longer in which individuals have two or fewer bowel movements per week. We consider a diagnosis of acute constipation in those individuals who have recently (less than 6 months previously) had either decreased frequency of bowel movements or increased difficulty initiating evacuation.

Constipation is one of the most common digestive disorders. It affects nearly 5 million people in the United States, corresponding to a prevalence rate of 2 percent, and 2.5 million people consult a physician yearly because of constipation. The occurrence of constipation increases with advancing age, rising exponentially in prevalence after the age of 65. This disorder is three times more common in women than in men. Constipation affects nonwhites more frequently than whites and is noted in people with low income or lack of formal education, indicating that environmental factors play a role in the development of constipation.

In the United States, laxatives are prescribed for more than 3 million people yearly, and 15 percent of women and 2 percent of men use laxatives on a regular basis. An estimated $250 million is spent yearly on laxatives purchased

Table 1 Causes of Constipation

Nerve disorders	Smooth muscle disorders
Hirschsprung's disease	Scleroderma
Central nervous system diseases	Amyloidosis
Heavy metal poisoning (e.g. lead/mercury)	Metabolic/endocrine disorders
	Hypothyroidism
	Diabetes mellitus with autonomic neuropathy
Mechanical obstruction	
Neoplasia and strictures	Uremia
Rectocele	Hypercalcemia/hypokalemia
Rectal prolapse	Idiopathic constipation
Endometriosis	Outlet obstruction
Medication induced	Slow transit/colonic inertia
Opiate analgesics	Normal transit/irritable bowel syndrome
Anticholinergic agents	
Calcium channel antagonists	
Calcium-containing supplements	
Aluminum-containing antacids	
Vinca alkaloids	
Polystyrene binding resins	

without a prescription, and the total amount spent on laxatives, including prescriptions, is at least $450 million yearly. These numbers are similar to those reported in European studies, and it has been noted that laxative use, as expected, increases with patient age.

■ COMMON CAUSES

Constipation is a symptom that may be present in many underlying disorders. Therefore, before beginning medical treatment, it is important to consider known treatable causes of constipation (Table 1). In general, we are more aggressive in excluding known causes of constipation in patients presenting with acute constipation (lasting less than 6 months) or with a progressive increase. In more than 50 percent of individuals seen for a complaint of constipation, it is not possible to find a specific cause. These patients are classified as having idiopathic constipation.

■ AGENTS USED FOR TREATMENT OF CONSTIPATION

Five major groups of agents have been used in the medical treatment of constipation (Table 2).

Bulk Agents

Bulk agents include soluble and insoluble fiber supplements. Fiber and fiber supplements are a diverse group of nonstarch carbohydrates that are not digestible by humans. Cellulose and lignin are fibrous and insoluble and have their greatest effect on fecal bulk. Noncellulose polysaccharides include hemicellulose, pectin, gums, algal polysaccharides such as guar, and the synthetic resin polycarbophil. These substances are viscous and soluble, have a high water-binding capacity, and appear to influence colonic motility. Most soluble fibers are digested by bacteria and may contribute to a laxative action by increasing osmotic pressure of stool and increasing fecal mass. Colonic bacterial fermentation of soluble fibers may also produce metabolites that directly influence fluid transport and motility. However, water-soluble fiber supplements may slow nutrient absorption and decrease transit through the upper gastrointestinal (GI) tract.

Colonic gas formation is a common side effect, but often subsides after a week owing to adaptation of intestinal flora. Patients with GI stenosis or intestinal pseudo-obstruction should avoid fiber. Cellulose may bind cardiac glycosides and other drugs; therefore, ingestion of drugs and laxatives should be separated in time as much as possible. Intestinal obstruction and bezoar formation are unusual complications from the use of fiber supplements. Allergic reactions have also been described, especially with plant gums, but fiber supplements generally have the fewest side effects among laxatives.

Osmotic Agents

Osmotic agents increase the water content of fecal material, an effect that may be beneficial in patients with constipation, since studies of colonic motility have suggested that transit of liquid fecal material in the human colon is more rapid than transit of solid material. Magnesium salts such as sulfate or citrate of magnesia have been extensively used and are relatively safe if used as directed. They are contraindicated for long-term use in patients with congestive heart failure or renal insufficiency. Patients receiving these agents for long-term use should periodically undergo screening of their serum magnesium level. Sodium phosphate is another salt often used as an osmotic laxative; it is more pleasant tasting than magnesium salts, but phosphate and sodium accumulation can occur in patients with diminished renal function.

In patients with renal insufficiency, poorly absorbed mono- or disaccharides or alcohol derivatives (e.g., lactulose, sorbitol, or glycerol) may be beneficial in treatment of constipation. These substances increase osmotic pressure in the colon and are metabolized by colonic bacteria to increase intraluminal bacterial mass. Sorbitol 70 percent syrup and glycerol are less expensive alternatives to lactulose. Most patients receive benefit from 30 ml of these substances once or twice daily, although the therapeutic dose has to be determined empirically; 1 to 3 days may be required before a laxative effect begins. Common side effects include gas formation due to fermentation by colonic bacteria.

Polyethyleneglycol (PEG: MW3350 daltons) electrolyte solutions are nonabsorbable polyalcohols in a saline isotonic solution containing 60 g PEG per liter. These solutions are commonly used in preparation for colonoscopy, since there is no net ion absorption or loss and dehydration does not occur because of their isotonicity. In patients with constipation, PEG solutions have been given at a dose of 3 to 4 L to obtain colonic cleansing once or twice weekly. Alternatively, these patients have been treated with 250 to 500 ml of PEG solution daily. A relative disadvantage of PEG solutions is their high price.

Stimulant Laxatives

Irritant or stimulant laxatives include anthraquinone compounds such as the extracts of senna, aloe, cascara, or rhubarb and diphenylmethane derivatives, including phenolphthalein

Table 2 Agents Used in Treatment of Constipation

GROUP	COMMENTS
1. Bulk/fiber	Least side effects but may cause obstruction
a. Soluble:	Fermentation increases flatus
psyllium, guar, pectin	
b. Insoluble/inorganic:	Not fermented
cellulose, polycarbophil salts	
2. Osmotic	May impair fluid and electrolyte balance
a. Salts:	Inexpensive
magnesium salts,	Magnesium accumulation if renal insufficiency
sodium phosphate	Phosphate accumulation if renal insufficiency
b. Sugars or sugar alcohols:	Increases flatus
Lactulose, lactose, mannitol, sorbitol, glycerol, polyethylene glycol solutions	Expensive
3. Stimulants/irritants	Tachyphylaxis occurs, electrolyte disturbances
Bisacodyl and phenolphthalein (diphenols),	Active only if bile salts and bacteria present
cascara/senna/aloe/casanthranol	Require bacterial cleavage
(anthraquinones),	
Castor oil (ricinoleic acid),	Not routinely used, poor taste
Docusate salts	Poorly effective
Chenocholic acid	Expensive
4. Prokinetic agents	Abdominal cramping; avoid in outlet obstruction
Cisapride	
Bethanecol chloride	
Neostigmine bromide	May induce cholinergic crisis
Naloxone hydrochloride	Requires parenteral delivery
Misoprostol	Expensive
Erythromycin	
5. Enema and suppository	
Sodium phosphates, glycerol, sorbitol, lactulose, mineral oil, bisacodyl, CO_2-producing suppository	Self-administered enema may produce perforation
	Mineral oil may lead to lipoid pneumonia

and bisacodyl. These substances have a prokinetic action, increase intestinal secretion, and diminish intestinal absorption. The active ingredients in the anthraquinone group are glycoside derivatives of danthron. Danthron itself has been withdrawn from the market because of its association with hepatic and intestinal tumors. Anthraquinones are nonabsorbable, and the active component, rheinanthrone, is formed by bacterial cleavage. By contrast, bisacodyl and phenolphthalein are absorbed by the small intestine, undergo glucuronidation in the liver, and are then excreted into the bile. Glucuronidated derivatives are not absorbable and will pass into the colon, where deconjugation by bacteria forms the active diphenol compound. These substances have a laxative effect only if bile flow is not obstructed and bacteria are present in the colon. Owing to the enterohepatic circulation, their laxative effect is delayed until 6 to 10 hours after ingestion.

The dosage of anthraquinones for constipation is variable, because most commercial preparations are not standardized. The adult dose for the proprietary preparation cascara sagrada (casanthranol) is 30 mg per day; the usual dose of bisacodyl is 10 to 15 mg per day, and of phenolphthalein 30 to 200 mg per day.

Stimulant laxatives, especially if used for acute constipation, cause abdominal cramping and tenesmus in 10 percent of patients. Melanosis coli is a reversible black-brown discoloration of the colonic mucosa that begins abruptly at the ileocecal valve and may progress distally to the dentate line. It is found frequently in patients who chronically use stimulant laxatives, especially anthraquinones. However, there is no present evidence that melanosis coli has a pathophysiologic importance. Stimulant agents generally should not be prescribed for longer than 2 weeks. It is presently unclear whether long-term use of these substances can damage the enteric nervous system. It is well known that patients using these substances on a long-term basis may require increasing doses. Unfortunately, older patients may develop fecal incontinence while using stimulant laxatives. Allergic reactions, including Stevens-Johnson syndrome, have been described in patients receiving stimulant laxatives.

There is a group of stimulant and irritant laxatives that we do not use in our clinical practice. Castor oil, obtained from the bean of the castor plant *Ricinus communis*, has been used since the time of the ancient Egyptians. It contains ricinoleic acid, has a terrible taste, and affects both secretion and motility. Castor oil causes cramping abdominal pain by a prokinetic effect on the small bowel. Bile acids, such as cholic acid (0.25 g three times daily) or chenodeoxycholic acid (0.25 to 0.5 g three times daily), reduce net absorption of water and electrolytes. These substances are quite expensive for use as a first-line drug in treatment of constipation. We do not use mineral oil because reflux of this material can cause lipid pneumonia. Available studies have shown minimal benefit from wetting agents or surfactants, such as docusate salts, in treatment of constipation. These docusate salts may cause increased absorption of other drugs being given concurrently.

Prokinetic Agents

Prokinetic agents or drugs that function as neurotransmitter agonists have potential use in patients with slow transit constipation, but may increase abdominal symptoms in those with constipation related to an outlet obstruction. Bethanechol chloride is a muscarinic-cholinergic agonist that increases phasic contractions in human colon at a dose of 10 to 50 mg three times daily. Neostigmine bromide is an anticholinesterase agent that is rarely used because of the possible initiation of a cholinergic crisis. A newly available prokinetic agent, cisapride, releases acetylcholine at the level of the nerve plexus and induces phasic colonic contractions. It may function as a serotonin^4-receptor agonist to stimulate GI motility. It is a promising drug for treatment of patients with mild to moderate slow transit constipation. A frequently used dosage is 10 to 20 mg up to three times daily. Cramping abdominal pain and chest pain due to its prokinetic effects on the stomach and esophagus have been noted.

The opiate antagonist naloxone hydrochloride has been used for idiopathic slow transit constipation. Its use has been limited by the necessity of parenteral administration and high cost.

Prostaglandins can induce diarrhea by altering intestinal water and electrolyte absorption and by modulating colonic motor activity. In a recent trial, a synthetic prostaglandin E_1 analogue (misoprostol) was of clinical benefit in a short term trial of patients with chronic constipation. Given at 400 µg three times a day before meals, this compound presently represents an expensive alternative for the management of chronic constipation.

Recent studies have shown no effect of oral or intravenous erythromycin on human colonic motility. Erythromycin given in a dose of 500 mg twice daily functions as a prokinetic agent in the small intestine through activation of motilin receptors. Its usefulness in selected patients with chronic constipation could be related to an increased delivery to the cecum of intestinal fluid or bile salts.

Suppositories and Enemas

The final group of agents frequently used to treat constipation are suppositories and enemas. Bisacodyl, a known stimulant laxative, is commonly used in suppository form (10 mg) or in enema form (10 mg per 30 ml). After rectal administration, it initiates defecation within 15 to 60 minutes. Some patients note cramping abdominal pain, and a burning sensation in the rectum associated with mild proctitis has been observed.

Sorbitol, glycerol, and lactulose are commercially available in both suppository and enema form. These compounds function as rectal irritants (by dehydration of exposed mucosa), and rectal discomfort or a burning sensation has been reported. Carbon dioxide-producing suppositories (a mixture of sodium bicarbonate and potassium bitartrate) distend the rectum with CO_2 and stimulate colorectal contractions. This mechanism may be beneficial in patients with chronic constipation and secondarily diminished rectal sensation of distention. We do not routinely advise patients to use enemas at home owing to the possibility of perforation of the anal canal or rectum by the enema tip.

UNPROVED THERAPY

There is little scientific evidence to support the widespread belief that increased water consumption, physical exercise, or abdominal massage is beneficial as primary therapy in patients with chronic constipation. It has been shown that water consumption has to be increased to more than 4 L daily before stool consistency is affected. This is due to the large resorptive capacity of the small and large intestine.

Psychotherapy may be helpful in coping with the irritable bowel syndrome (IBS) but has not been shown to have an effect on intestinal transit.

COMBINATION THERAPY AND HERBAL PREPARATIONS

We recommend that physicians use only one or two preparations from each main group of agents in treating constipation. This permits improved awareness of specific effects and potential side effects of different agents. There is no evidence that combinations of laxatives have an advantage over preparations containing a single ingredient. We discourage our patients from using herbal tea preparations and other "natural" laxative preparations because the substances in these preparations are poorly defined pharmacologically, are not consistent in the amount of drug that is present, and may contain hepatotoxic alkaloids.

MANAGEMENT

Standard Evaluation and Treatment

Figure 1 presents our algorithm for the laboratory investigation and treatment at the initial presentation of a patient with constipation. In the first visit, we complete a history and physical examination, including a rectal examination. Our goal is to try to differentiate among complaints of acute constipation (less than 6 months), progressive symptoms, and chronic constipation (more than 6 months).

In patients with acute constipation or progressive symptoms (especially those who are over 40 years old), metabolic or endocrine disorders associated with constipation should be excluded by examining serum potassium, calcium, glucose, creatinine, and thyroid-stimulating hormone levels. We also perform proctosigmoidoscopy and barium colon x-ray examination to exclude mechanical obstruction due to neoplasms, diverticular strictures, or endometriosis. If this laboratory evaluation provides a specific diagnosis, we treat the underlying disease. If no specific diagnosis is made, we recommend a high-fiber intake as described below.

In patients with chronic constipation, we initially recommend a high-fiber intake. The average American diet is estimated to include 15 to 20 g of fiber daily. To utilize fiber in the therapy for constipation, we recommend 30 to 50 g of total fiber intake daily. Specifically, patients can take bran (8 g fiber per 30 g serving); shredded wheat (3 g fiber per 30 g serving); corn meal (5 g fiber per 120 g serving); brown rice (5.5 g fiber per 120 g serving); whole wheat or rye bread (2 g fiber per 30 g serving); brown, Navy, or red beans (8 g fiber per 120 g serving); corn, broccoli, or peas (4 g fiber per 120 g serving); prunes (5.5 g fiber per 120 g serving); and an apple or pear (5 g fiber per medium fruit).

Since most individuals seem unable on a daily basis to reach 30 to 50 g of total fiber intake, they will require fiber

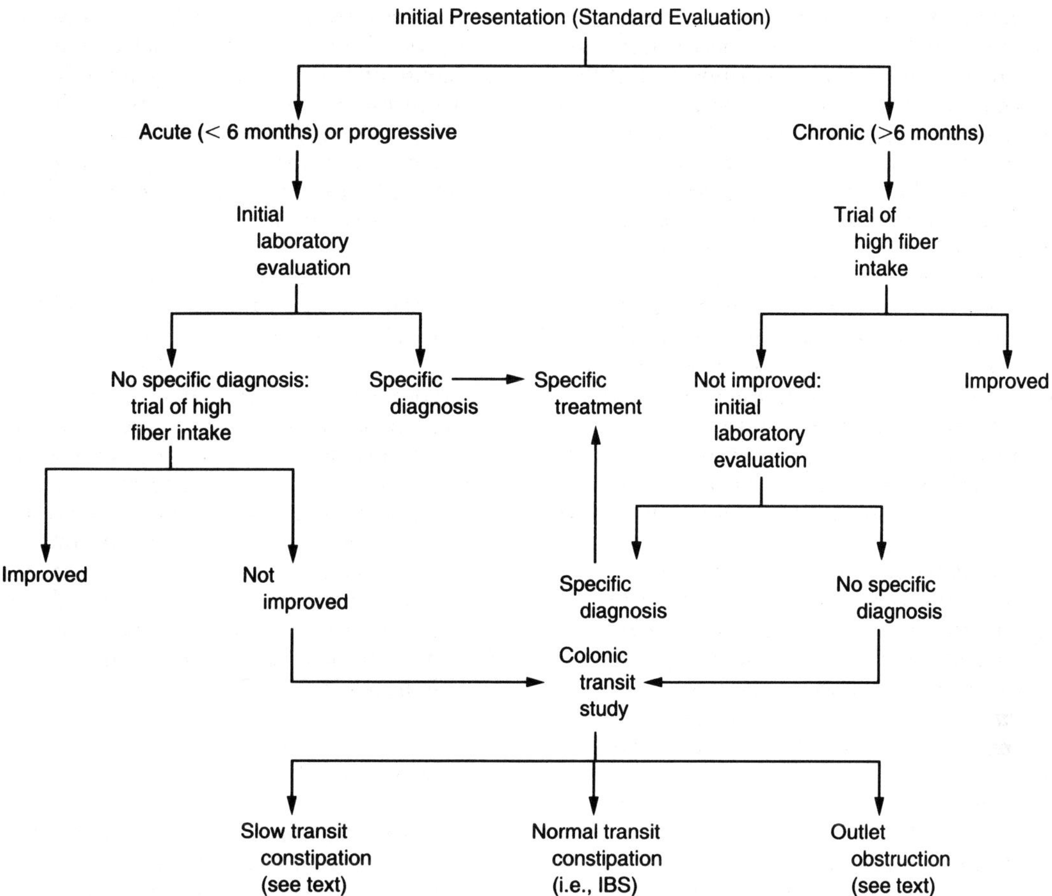

Figure 1
Algorithm for evaluation and management of constipation.

supplements, which are best taken with a meal and adequate fluid intake. Among commonly used supplements, psyllium obtained from *Plantago* seed should be taken in a dose of 3 to 4 g of fiber in at least 250 ml of fluid such as fruit juice (as a taste corrector) up to three times daily. Patients who continue to have excessive flatulence may benefit by substituting a polycarbophil salt, 1 g up to four times daily.

When we instruct patients on a high-fiber intake, we also discuss the initiation of the gastrocolonic response. In most individuals, gastric distention can increase phasic contractions of the rectosigmoid region. Because of the normal circadian rhythm of colonic motility, this response may be more pronounced in the morning. We recommend that patients eat a warm meal or drink a warm fluid after arising in the morning.

In patients with chronic constipation who have not improved with a high-fiber intake, we perform the described laboratory evaluation; if this provides a specific diagnosis, we treat the underlying disease.

Failure of Standard Treatment

In patients with constipation whose laboratory results are normal and who have not improved with a high-fiber intake, we proceed to a colonic transit study. These patients by definition have idiopathic constipation, and this test is performed to determine the subtype of constipation. Because of improved patient compliance and ease of interpretation, we use the Hinton method for examination of colonic transit. After fecal disimpaction (if appropriate), the patient ingests a single gelatin capsule containing 24 nonabsorbable markers (Sitzmarks). During the study, the patient refrains from all laxatives, suppositories, enemas, and constipation-associated medications. An abdominal flat plate x-ray film is taken at 5 days. In multiple published studies, normal individuals pass at least 80 percent of the markers at 5 days. If the study is abnormal, markers may be retained in the rectosigmoid region (consistent with a diagnosis of outlet obstruction) or more diffusely throughout the colon (consistent with slow transit constipation).

In patients with outlet obstruction, we routinely advise a low-residue diet. As supplemental therapy, the regular use of glycerol or CO_2-producing suppositories (two to three mornings a week) may be beneficial in maintaining rectal evacuation. Also, in patients with continued abdominal symptoms, we recommend addition of an osmotic agent such as citrate of magnesia, 30 to 120 ml at bedtime, or sorbitol 70 percent syrup, 30 to 60 ml at bedtime. Some patients prefer to use citrate of magnesia intermittently (120 to 240 ml twice weekly).

Some patients with rectal outlet obstruction remain symptomatic. This subset of patients may benefit from referral for a more complete evaluation. Major considerations include exclusion of Hirschsprung's disease (especially in young patients), generally by utilizing anorectal manometry which tests for a normal rectal-anal inhibitory response, and exclusion of paradoxical contraction of the external anal sphincter (termed *anismus*). Surgical therapy is indicated after a diagnosis of Hirschsprung's disease. Anismus is generally defined by specialized techniques that use cine-radiography (defecography) to examine relaxation of the levator ani muscle group during attempted defecation or electromyography (EMG) of the external anal sphincter muscle to examine myoelectric activity at rest and during attempted defecation. Selected motivated patients with anismus are candidates for anorectal neuromuscular retraining. In this type of biofeedback therapy, patients follow either pressure or EMG recordings of the external anal sphincter while learning techniques for relaxing the external anal sphincter during attempted defecation. Patients who have failed anorectal neuromuscular retraining must be referred for further evaluation before surgical therapy is considered.

In patients with normal transit constipation (probable IBS), the main goal is usually relief of chronic abdominal pain. We first try to determine whether pain is relieved after colonic cleansing with either citrate of magnesia, 120 to 240 ml, or PEG solution, 2 to 4 L. If pain relief is satisfactory, we begin the stepwise management approach for patients with outlet obstruction. Unfortunately, most individuals have continued abdominal pain after colonic cleansing.

Treatment of constipation-predominant IBS can be a challenge. Initial therapy includes a trial of a high fiber dietary intake. A clinical trial has shown that selected patients may improve after adding a polycarbophil salt, 1 g up to four times daily. In several European studies, use of a prokinetic agent such as cisapride, 20 mg two to three times daily, was of benefit. Behavioral treatments such as biofeedback, self-hypnosis, or relaxation response training may be considered in motivated patients, especially in patients with a recent onset of symptoms or a clear understanding of stress and the onset of symptoms. A subgroup of patients with chronic abdominal pain can be difficult to manage. It has been reported that for treatment of a chronic abdominal pain syndrome, a trial for at least 3 to 4 weeks of amitriptyline, 25 to 100 mg at bedtime, or trazodone, 50 to 200 mg at bedtime, may be helpful.

In patients with slow transit constipation, we routinely advise a low-residue diet. A few patients with slow transit constipation obtain relief from abdominal pain by colonic cleansing but cannot maintain colonic evacuation. These patients may obtain long-term improvement of symptoms by chronic use of a polymeric liquid diet, or an alternative treatment, a trial of a prokinetic agent such as cisapride, 10 to 20 mg up to three times daily, may be warranted. Patients with slow transit constipation are often difficult to manage in the long-term. Small studies have examined the use of PEG electrolyte solutions, 3 to 4 L once or twice weekly or 250 to 500 ml daily, or misoprostol, 400 μg times a day before meals, in order to increase fecal output. Refractory patients and patients who have radiographic evidence for the development of megacolon must be referred for examination of upper gut motility before any consideration of surgical therapy.

Laxative and Enema Dependency

After evacuation of the colon by means of a stimulant laxative or enema, it may be several days before a spontaneous bowel movement occurs. Patients may assume that they are constipated, and a vicious cycle develops in which they become dependent on the daily use of a laxative or enema to produce defecation. Secondary hyperaldosteronism, steatorrhea, hypoalbuminemia, and osteomalacia have been described as additional problems that can develop in laxative dependency.

In patients with dependency, our initial goals are to determine whether there is a treatable cause of constipation and whether there is objective evidence of colorectal dysmotility. We complete the laboratory investigation described previously and initiate proper treatment if a specific diagnosis is made. Next, if the patient has an impaction, we obtain colonic cleansing with either osmotic laxatives or prolonged use of a polymeric liquid diet. After disimpaction and in patients with no evidence of a fecal impaction, a colonic transit study is performed while the patient maintains a regular diet and avoids laxatives and enemas.

Patients with slow transit constipation or outlet obstruction are treated as described. In most patients who have normal transit constipation, we initially convert them from use of stimulant laxatives or enemas to osmotic agents or suppositories, and we discuss initiation of the gastrocolonic response as described. It is very important at this stage to reassure patients that there is no evidence for abnormal movement of solid material through the colon or rectum, and to discuss the possible side effects of continued use of stimulant laxatives or enemas. As a next step, we try to slowly increase fiber intake up to 30 to 50 g fiber daily while tapering the intake of osmotic agents or suppositories. Laxative dependency has not been well studied, but in 50 percent of cases it appears possible to discontinue stimulant laxatives after introducing a high-fiber diet. In many cases, it is possible to convert patients' stimulant laxative use to suppository use. In some patients, the believed need for routine use of stimulant laxatives and enemas cannot be overcome, and we then consider a psychiatric evaluation. In general, these patients have a great obsession about their bowel movements.

Pregnancy

Patients presenting with constipation during pregnancy should initially receive a trial of 30 to 50 g of daily fiber intake. If this is not effective, lactulose or sorbitol may be used safely. Studies examining the possible side effects of stimulant laxatives during pregnancy have been contradictory. Both the sennosides and bisacodyl have been examined for their embryonic and fetotoxic influences, and it is presently not clear whether they can be safely used in pregnancy. It has been suggested that castor oil can initiate uterine contractions and should not be used. Both bisacodyl and sennosides appear in breast milk in the postpartum period, but the concentrations are so low that no side effects should be expected in breast-feeding babies. We do not recommend the regular use of enemas. Either bisacodyl or CO_2-producing suppositories should be safe in inducing rectal evacuation.

Spinal Cord Injury

Spinal cord injuries interrupt both afferent and efferent innervation of the anal sphincter. Constipation, like urinary bladder retention, commonly occurs shortly after the injury (so-called spinal shock). In a bowel rehabilitation program, it is recommended that patients have 30 to 50 g daily of fiber intake and take daily advantage of the normal gastrocolonic response that occurs 20 minutes after breakfast. When beginning this bowel program, the spinal injury patient also has to initiate defecation by learning to apply digital rectal stimulation in combination with either a bisacodyl or glycerol suppository or a CO_2-producing suppository, to induce rectal distention. Before beginning digital stimulation, feces present in the lower rectum should be removed digitally. A well-lubricated gloved finger should be inserted 2 to 3 cm into the rectum. A gentle circular motion toward the sacrum will relax the external anal sphincter, and stimulation of the autonomic nerves in the S2-S3 segment will initiate a rectal peristaltic reflex. After 1 to 2 minutes of digital stimulation, the suppository should be inserted as high above the sphincter as possible and held in place for 15 seconds. After waiting 20 minutes, digital stimulation is repeated for periods of 3 minutes every 5 to 10 minutes until defecation occurs. During this time, the patient should attempt to use Valsalva's maneuver, if possible. Alternatively, the patient can lean forward to increase intra-abdominal pressure. If defecation is not achieved within 30 minutes, a second suppository may be inserted and the above sequence repeated.

In many patients with a spinal cord injury, an excessive amount of time is required to complete a bowel program. As an alternative, Theravac Plus mini enemas can be utilized. In this program, feces present in the lower rectum may be removed digitally. The tip of the mini enema is removed before the liquid (containing 283 mg docusate sodium and 20 mg benzocaine) is inserted into the rectum. After 10 minutes, digital stimulation is performed for 1 to 2 minutes. Digital stimulation is repeated at 10 minute intervals until rectal evacuation is completed. The use of these enemas should be discontinued in the rare patient who develops severe abdominal pain, nausea, emesis, or hematochezia.

It is important to obtain regular evacuation of the rectum at least once every 3 days, because a stool-filled colon in these patients can induce bladder spasms with urinary incontinence and autonomic hyperreflexia in patients with T4–T6 or higher lesions. The symptoms of autonomic hyperreflexia are a rise in blood pressure, headache, and profuse sweating above the lesion. If routine evacuation is not obtained in these patients, fecal impaction can cause diarrhea by leakage of fecal fluid around a rectal impaction.

Cancer Chemotherapy

Chemotherapy, especially with vinblastine or vincristine, is associated with the development of constipation. The vinca alkaloids can damage afferent and efferent rectal innervation and potentially damage the enteric nervous system. Stimulant laxatives therefore may not be effective, and osmotic laxatives such as lactulose, sorbitol, or PEG solution are alternatives. Magnesium laxatives and sodium phosphate should be avoided owing to possible magnesium retention or water and electrolyte depletion. Enemas or suppositories should not be used in view of the possible development of anal or rectal injury with resultant bleeding or infection. Fiber supplements may be helpful in patients complaining of difficulty initiating defecation or passage of hard feces.

The use of opioid agonists for pain control is also a major cause of constipation in cancer patients. Bowel obstruction must be excluded prior to a trial of therapy. It was previously suggested that as a rough estimate, ½ tablet of senna extract (an anthraquinone) would help to counteract the constipating effect of 60 mg codeine sulfate or 5 mg morphine. Alternatively, as an osmotic agent, lactulose and sorbitol syrup, 30 ml up to four times daily, has been examined in the European literature for their reversal of the constipating effect of opioid agonists. Sorbitol syrup is cheaper and is associated with less frequent complaint of nausea, but like lactulose it can induce bloating and increased flatulence. The combination of an anthraquinone laxative and an osmotic agent may be useful in patients with refractory constipation.

Suggested Reading

Andorsky R, Goldner F. Colonic lavage solution (PEG) as a treatment for chronic constipation: a double-blind, placebo controlled study. Am J Gastroenterol 1991; 85:261–265.

Camilleri M, Prather CM. The irritable bowel syndrome: mechanisms and a practical approach to management. Ann Intern Med 1992; 116:1001–1008.

Drossman DA, Thompson WG. The irritable bowel syndrome: review and a graduated multicomponent treatment approach. Ann Intern Med 1992; 116:1009–1016.

Hepner G, Hofman AF. Cholic acid therapy for constipation. Mayo Clin Proc 1973; 48:356–358.

Krevsky B, Maurer AH, Malmud LS, Fisher RS. Cisapride accelerates colonic transit in constipated patients with colonic inertia. Am J Gastroenterol 1989; 84:882–887.

Lederle FA, Busch DL, Mattox KM, et al. Cost-effective treatment of constipation in the elderly: a randomized double-blind comparison of sorbitol and lactulose. Am J Med 1990; 89:597–601.

Müller-Lissner S. Effect of wheat bran on weight of stool and gastrointestinal transit time: a meta-analysis. Br Med J 1988; 296: 615–617.

Soffer EE, Metcalf A, Launspach J. Misoprostol is effective treatment for patients with severe chronic constipation. Dig Dis Sci 1994; 39:929–933.

Snape WJ Jr, Carlson GM, Cohen S. Human colonic myoelectric activity in response to Prostigmin and the gastrointestinal hormones. Dig Dis Sci 1977; 22:881–887.

Staumont G, Frexinos J, Fioramonti J, Bueno L. Sennosides and human colonic motility. Pharmacology 1988; 36 (Suppl 1):49–56.

HEMORRHOIDS

Rama P. Venu, M.D., F.A.C.P., F.A.C.G.
John A. LoGiudice, M.D.
Stephen F. Deutsch, M.D., F.A.C.G.
Gayle M. Rosenthal, M.D.

Hemorrhoids are dilated veins located at the lower rectum and anal canal. Although not a serious illness, hemorrhoids constitute the most common abnormality affecting the anorectal region. Approximately 10 million people in the United States are affected by hemorrhoids at any time with a prevalence rate of 4.4 percent. It is estimated that about 50 percent of the population above 50 years of age suffer from hemorrhoids, costing more than $100 million annually for over-the-counter hemorrhoidal medications.

ANATOMICAL CONSIDERATIONS

The anorectal area is a highly vascular region enriched by hemorrhoidal vessels. Internal hemorrhoids arise from the superior hemorrhoidal plexus situated above the dentate line. The dentate line is an important landmark in the anorectal region for a variety of reasons. (1) It separates the mucosal surface from the cutaneous surface. (2) Autonomic nerves innervate the mucosa while the cutaneous surface below the dentate line is chiefly innervated by somatic nerves and, therefore, is very sensitive to painful stimuli. This is an important practical point to be kept in mind when nonoperative therapies are undertaken. Application of coagulation current, laser, or infrared beam in this region can cause severe pain and discomfort to the patient. (3) External hemorrhoids arise from the inferior hemorrhoidal plexus located below the dentate line.

Internal hemorrhoids are usually located at three primary sites: (1) left lateral; (2) right anterior; and (3) right posterior; at the 2 o'clock, 5 o'clock, and 9 o'clock positions of the anal ring.

PATHOGENESIS

The mechanism leading to hemorrhoid formation is not well understood. Since hemorrhoidal bleeding is characteristically bright red, hemorrhoids are considered to be a form of arteriovenous malformation. A defective anchoring mechanism resulting from submucosal connective tissue abnormalities is another postulated mechanism for hemorrhoids. Yet another view focuses on abnormality in the internal anal sphincter mechanism. Spasm involving the internal sphincter can raise rectal pressure, which in turn pushes the hemorrhoidal plexus downwards. As a proof of this theory the association between hemorrhoids and situations of high rectal pressure are often quoted. Thus, hemorrhoids are frequently seen in subjects with pregnancy, pelvic tumors, and constipation.

CLASSIFICATION

Hemorrhoids are classified as external or internal based on their anatomical location. Thus, internal hemorrhoids are located above the dentate line while external hemorrhoids are located below this line. Most hemorrhoids remain asymptomatic. A clinical classification is adopted for internal hemorrhoids on the basis of their protrusion into the lumen, prolapse through the anal canal, and reducibility.

First-degree internal hemorrhoids merely protrude into the lumen. Second-degree internal hemorrhoids prolapse through the anus during straining of defecation, but reduce spontaneously. A third-degree hemorrhoid prolapses through the anal canal and requires manual reduction. Fourth-degree hemorrhoids prolapse through the anal canal and are irreducible. This classification is useful in the proper selection of patients for appropriate therapy and to assess the efficacy of various therapeutic modalities in clinical trials.

CLINICAL MANIFESTATIONS

Internal Hemorrhoids

Bleeding per rectum is the most common and alarming symptom associated with internal hemorrhoids. Bleeding often manifests as red spots on the toilet tissue. Dripping of blood after bowel movement may also occur. Massive rectal bleeding requiring blood transfusion or chronic low-grade bleeding with iron-deficiency anemia are seldom encountered among patients with internal hemorrhoids. Pruritus ani, fecal soiling, mucous drainage, and protrusion of hemorrhoids are not uncommon symptoms associated with internal hemorrhoids. Although mild anorectal discomfort may be present with all degrees of internal hemorrhoids, strangulated hemorrhoids cause significant pain in the anorectal area. If untreated, this can lead to gangrene formation, ulceration, and infection.

External Hemorrhoids

Similar to internal hemorrhoids, external hemorrhoids often produce swelling and mild discomfort in the anal area. However, thrombosis of the external hemorrhoid can cause severe pain. The skin overlying the hemorrhoidal cushion often becomes reddened and swollen. If untreated, ulceration, infection, and abscess formation can occur. Organization of the thrombus can result in external skin tags. Such cutaneous tags are also seen in association with inflammatory bowel disease or in patients following hemorrhoidectomy.

DIAGNOSIS

Inspection

The first step in the diagnosis of anorectal abnormality is proper inspection of the perineal area. The patient should be examined in a comfortable knee-chest position. The anus and the perianal area should be examined visually after spreading the buttocks area. Inspection can be extremely helpful in differentiating hemorrhoids from other not so rare conditions such as condyloma acuminata, perianal fistulae, thrombosed external hemorrhoids, and perirectal abscesses.

Digital Examination

A proper digital examination should follow the inspection. During digital examination, hemorrhoids, polyps, and malignancy can be identified. Distinguishing a thrombosed hemorrhoid from a perianal fistula or abscess can be difficult.

Anoscopy

Anoscopic examination is the most useful procedure for the diagnosis and classification of hemorrhoids. The anoscope with the obturator in place is gently introduced into the anal canal. The obturator is then removed. The anal canal is then inspected under adequate illumination. The hemorrhoidal cushion can be seen bulging through the anoscope. All quadrants of the anal canal should be examined by reintroducing the scope.

Flexible Sigmoidoscopy

Any patient presenting with rectal bleeding or other anorectal symptoms should be carefully evaluated to rule out adenoma, adenocarcinoma, or other neoplastic disorders involving the anorectal area. Therefore, every patient with suspected hemorrhoids should eventually have flexible sigmoidoscopic examination, perhaps followed by colonoscopy or barium enema. It should always be kept in mind that all that bleed are not hemorrhoids.

■ MANAGEMENT

General Guidelines

Irrespective of the stage of internal hemorrhoids, all patients presenting with hemorrhoidal symptoms should follow certain general guidelines consisting of (1) diet, (2) anorectal hygiene, and (3) local therapy.

Diet

A diet rich in fiber seems to be beneficial for most patients with hemorrhoids. High-fiber diets can be useful in regulating bowel movements, thus avoiding straining during defecation. Quite often hydrophilic bulk agents such as psyllium or mucilloids may be necessary in addition to a standard high-fiber diet. Elimination of certain foods such as spices, citrus fruits, alcohol, caffeine, chocolate, and tomatoes may be beneficial.

Perianal Hygiene

Adequate anal hygiene can be extremely helpful for symptomatic relief. Perianal irritation and pruritus ani are often associated with residual stool soiling. After each bowel movement, moistened white toilet paper should be used for proper swabbing of the anal region. Vigorous wiping should be avoided. Cleansing pads or Tucks and perianal cleansing lotions, such as Baleonol, will provide a soothing effect. Sitz baths once or twice a day, preferably after a bowel movement, are especially useful to cleanse the perianal area and to facilitate relaxation of the internal sphincter.

Pharmacotherapy

Topical Agents

Several pharmacologic agents are available for topical use in patients with hemorrhoids. Two major components of these agents are hydrocortisone acetate and local anesthetic agents from one of the "caine" families. These agents are dispensed as ointment, cream, or foam. Such topical agents may be applied digitally using a fingercot "glove" or applicator. Although well-controlled studies are lacking, many patients claim some symptomatic improvement with these pharmacologic agents. In an occasional patient, severe allergic reaction may occur from the "caine" topical anesthetics.

Suppositories

Besides the topical agents, a variety of suppositories are also available. The chief ingredients in these suppositories are similar to the topical agents. The suppositories melt in the rectum and gravitate to the anal canal. A suppository is best utilized at bedtime. Efficacy of anal suppositories is not well studied.

Local Injection

Submucosal injection of a variety of sclerosants such as 5 percent phenol, sodium morrhuate, or hypertonic saline adjacent to the hemorrhoidal vein is one of the earliest therapies utilized for internal hemorrhoids. Some reports indicate significant success with injection therapy, especially in patients with first- and second-degree internal hemorrhoids. However, pain at the site of injection, infection, and abscess formation may complicate injection therapy.

Topical Nitroglycerine

Nitric oxide has been shown to be a mediator for anorectal inhibitory reflex. Since anal pain in hemorrhoidal disease and fissure in ano may be related to sphincteric spasm, topical application of nitroglycerine, a rich source of nitric oxide, can relieve such pain by alleviating sphincteric spasm. In a recent report, topically applied nitroglycerine ointment was noted to be effective in the treatment of thrombosed hemorrhoids by offering symptomatic relief.

Nonsurgical Treatment

Cryotherapy

Cryotherapy of hemorrhoids is accomplished by specially designed cryoprobes activated by liquid nitrogen, carbon dioxide, or nitrous oxide. Rapid freezing followed by rapid thawing leads to tissue destruction from necrosis. However, the extent of tissue necrosis is often uncontrolled, causing delayed healing and prolonged drainage or pain.

Rubberband Ligation

Rubberband ligation is the most common outpatient therapy employed in patients with symptomatic internal hemorrhoids. In this technique, the hemorrhoidal tissue is grasped, gently pulled, and a rubberband is slid over the tissue which eventually leads to necrosis and destruction of the hemorrhoidal cushion. No anesthetic agent is required, and the procedure can be performed through an anoscope. Complications such as bleeding, fever, pain, infection, and drainage are rare. Deployment of multiple rubberbands similar to endoscopic variceal banding is also a possibility.

Photocoagulation

Thermal injury through photocoagulation is utilized in some of the newer, nonoperative therapies such as infrared coagulation (IRC) and lasers.

Infrared Coagulation. A rigid light guide with a curved tip is used for IRC. A special polymer that is transparent to infrared placed at the tip of the probe allows tissue contact. A low voltage, tungsten halogen lamp (15 volt) is the source of the infrared beam. The optimal amount of energy to be delivered to the tissue can be preset using a timer. The probe is fitted onto a handle with a switch which is easy to operate. The tip can be rotated and the contact tip is replaceable.

Coagulation of the hemorrhoidal cushion causes fixation of the tissue to the submucosa with scarring and retraction. Most patients experience a sensation of heat, but severe pain is unusual. Bleeding, pain, thrombosis, and anal fissure are some of the rare complications of IRC.

Bipolar Coagulation. The equipment for bipolar coagulation (bicap) consists of a rigid rod with the active electrode at its tip. No grounding of the patient is required in this technique. The electrical energy delivered is controlled by a foot pedal. Coagulation is generated at the base of the hemorrhoidal tissue in 1 or 2 second pulses. Similar to IRC, bipolar coagulation may be occasionally associated with pain, infection, bleeding, or thrombosis.

Direct Current Coagulation. Coagulation with direct current (DC) coagulation, on the other hand, requires a grounding plate. After the electrode is applied at the base of the hemorrhoid, low-voltage current is gradually increased to 16 mA. Although DC is as effective as bicap, it takes more time and may be occasionally painful.

Laser Therapy

Both Nd:YAG laser and CO_2 laser have been used for hemorrhoidectomy. The success rate of this modality of treatment is comparable to that of surgical hemorrhoidectomy. Besides increased cost, greater degree of wound inflammation and dehiscence have been reported in patients treated with laser.

Surgical Therapy

Hemorrhoidectomy is the most definitive form of surgical therapy for internal hemorrhoids. It is especially indicated in most patients with third-degree hemorrhoids, all patients with fourth-degree hemorrhoids, strangulated hemorrhoids, and when other nonsurgical therapies are unsuccessful. However, fecal incontinence may be a rare complication from surgical therapy. This may be a problem, especially with loose or watery stools.

Ablation of the internal anal sphincter is another surgical technique sometimes employed in the treatment of internal hemorrhoids. It is especially useful in patients who have a high resting anal sphincter pressure associated with internal hemorrhoids.

Incontinence of stool can be a problem, especially after sphincter ablation. In a prospective randomized study comparing hemorrhoidectomy alone with hemorrhoidectomy and lateral sphincterotomy among patients with prolapsed hemorrhoids, no significant difference was noted in the outcome between the two groups. Routine sphincterotomy therefore seems to be unnecessary.

Thrombosis of an external hemorrhoid often requires surgical intervention. If severe pain persists more than 24 to 48 hours in patients with thrombosed external hemorrhoids, surgical evacuation is also advocated by some experts to prevent recurrent thrombus formation. The chapter on perianal surgery provides more details.

■ MANAGEMENT SUMMARY

Patients presenting with symptoms suggestive of hemorrhoids should undergo appropriate evaluation to exclude malignancy, fissure-in-ano and/or perianal abscess. Those who are constipated should be advised to use high-fiber diet supplemented with bulk agents with or without stool softener or laxative. On the other hand, patients with diarrhea, which also can make hemorrhoidal symptoms worse, should be given antidiarrheal therapy after proper evaluation to determine the etiology of diarrhea. Next the hemorrhoid should be staged, and one of many nonsurgical or surgical therapies may be undertaken. In a recently reported meta-analysis of all randomized therapeutic trials, patients treated with hemorrhoidectomy had a better response to therapy than rubber band ligation, although pain and other complications were greater in the surgical group. However, rubberband ligation was better than sclerotherapy. Patients undergoing sclerotherapy and infrared coagulation required further therapy.

Suggested Reading

Ambrose NS, Morris D, Alexander Williams J, et al. A randomized trial of photocoagulation or injection sclerotherapy for the treatment of first- and second-degree hemorrhoids. Dis Colon Rectum 1985; 28:238.

Buls JG, Goldberg SM. Modern management of hemorrhoids. Surg Clin North Am 1978; 58:469.

Dennison AR, Whiston RJ, Rooney S, Morris DL. The management of hemorrhoids. Am J Gastroenterol 1989; 84:475–481.

Gorfine SR. Treatment of benign anal disease with topical nitroglycerine. Dis Colon Rectum 1995; 38(5):453.

Leicester RJ, Nichols RJ, Mann CV. Infrared coagulation: A new treatment for hemorrhoids. Dis Colon Rectum 1981; 24:602–605.

Lieberman DA. Common anorectal disorders. Ann Intern Med 1984; 101: 837–846.

Mac Rae HM, McLeod RS. Comparison of hemorrhoidal treatment modalities. A meta-analysis. Dis Colon Rectum 1995; 38:687.

Mathai V, Ong BC, Ho YH. Randomized controlled trial of lateral internal sphincterotomy with hemorrhoidectomy. Br J Surg 1996; 83:380.

Russell Y, Migi KB, Pacher J, Loren L. Randomized, prospective trial of direct current versus bipolar electrocoagulation for bleeding internal hemorrhoids. Gastrointest Endosc 1993; 39:766–769.

Smith LE. Hemorrhoidectomy with lasers and other contemporary modalities. Surg Clinics of North America 1992; 72(3):665.

FECAL INCONTINENCE

Arnold Wald, M.D.

Fecal incontinence is an embarrassing and often socially incapacitating problem that occurs in all age groups. Incontinence may occur in otherwise healthy individuals with acute severe diarrhea, but most patients with chronic fecal soiling exhibit abnormalities of one or more of the following: mental status, stool consistency, defecation, rectal sensation, rectal storage capacity, function of the anal sphincters or anorectal reflexes, and pelvic floor muscles.

A careful medical history and physical examination should suggest the cause of fecal incontinence as well as the possible pathophysiology in most patients. In many cases, additional information of value may be obtained from diagnostic evaluation using anorectal manometry, dynamic radiographic studies of the anorectum, neurophysiologic testing of the pelvic floor, and anal ultrasonography. Manometry accurately measures anorectal sensory and motor function, including rectal sensation and compliance, resting anal sphincter tone, and squeeze pressures. Proctography employs cinefluoroscopic techniques to evaluate anorectal structure and function during rectal retention and defecation, whereas electromyographic (EMG) studies can identify innervation of the external anal sphincter and puborectal muscles in patients with suspected pelvic neuropathy. In addition, measurements of pudendal nerve conduction help to identify the presence of peripheral neuropathy.

Finally, anal ultrasonography is the optimal test to diagnose anal sphincter defects and is especially useful when considering surgical repairs. Such information helps in planning treatment for many patients with fecal incontinence and in clarifying the pathogenesis of fecal soiling associated with a variety of disorders (Table 1). Interpretation of these techniques is best when experienced individuals are available to perform and analyze the studies.

Table 1 Rectosphincteric Abnormalities Associated with Fecal Incontinence

GROUPS	RESERVOIR	SENSORY	SPHINCTER
ADULTS			
Sphincter trauma	N	N	A
Pelvic neuropathy	N	N	A
Diabetes mellitus	N	A	A
Neurogenic	N	A	A
Inflammatory bowel disease	A	N	N
Ileoanal anastomosis	A	N	N
CHILDREN			
Encopresis	A	A	N
Spina bifida	N	A	A
Imperforate anus	A	N	A

N, often or always normal; A, often or always abnormal.

■ TREATMENT STRATEGIES

The management of fecal incontinence involves strategies designed to correct abnormal continence mechanisms and to ameliorate diarrhea, if present. These approaches include measures to alter colonic function, enhance puborectal and anal sphincter function, improve rectal sensation, and correct anorectal anatomic derangements. Optimal management requires careful assessment of possible causes of fecal incontinence in each patient.

Anal Sphincter Dysfunction

Patients with rectosphincteric abnormalities include those who have sustained sphincteric trauma through injury or surgery and many patients with pelvic floor neuropathy; the latter often exhibit weakness of the puborectal muscle as well. Generally, these patients have normal rectal sensation and storage capacity and may present with or without diarrhea.

Biofeedback

Biofeedback based on the classic techniques of Engel and associates is a simple and effective treatment for patients in this category. The method utilizes the manometer used for diagnostic studies; the recording apparatus provides information (biofeedback) about anorectal responses so that the patient can tell whether anal sphincter responses are being performed appropriately. Thus, biofeedback is a trial-and-error learning process using a visual display to monitor anal sphincter responses.

Before biofeedback is performed, the importance of the external sphincter to fecal continence is explained and patients are shown how their sphincteric responses differ from normal. Biofeedback conditioning is then carried out in three phases (Fig. 1).

Phase 1. Patients are asked to contract the external anal sphincter while they watch the recording of the sphincteric responses. A normal response is illustrated and patients are praised when they produce an appropriate contraction. The ability to make an appropriate contraction is achieved through trial and error; the first phase ends when the subject produces that response repeatedly on request.

Phase 2. The appropriate contraction response is then synchronized with rectal distention (which also elicits internal sphincter relaxation). Responses are monitored by having patients watch the recording to ensure appropriate synchronization with internal sphincter relaxation.

Phase 3. Patients are weaned from the instrument by blocking their view of the recordings. During this phase, patients are informed by the instructor when sphincteric responses are appropriate. When this occurs repeatedly, the training session ends; sessions last approximately 30 to 60 minutes.

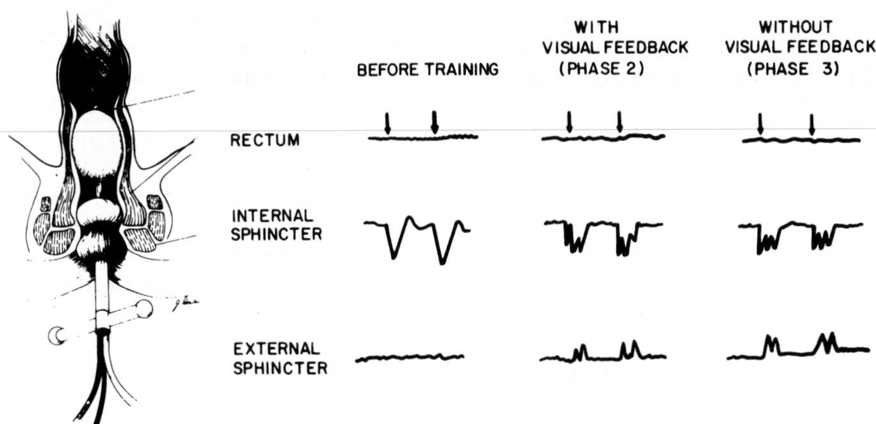

Figure 1
Three phases of biofeedback training for patients with anal sphincter dysfunction.

Subsequently, patients are instructed to practice sphincter contraction exercises three to four times daily and to contract the sphincter whenever they sense rectal distention or urgency. Routine reinforcement sessions are infrequently needed for adults and are reserved for those whose initial response is suboptimal or in whom relapses occur.

Prerequisites for successful biofeedback include appropriate motivation, ability to comprehend and follow directions, a threshold of sensing rectal distention in the normal range, and ability to contract the external anal sphincter or gluteal muscles. Success has been achieved in more than 70 percent of patients who meet these requirements.

Surgery

In general, surgery for incontinence should be considered only after conservative measures have failed. Exceptions are gross rectal prolapse, since surgical resuspension restores continence in approximately half of these patients, and acute damage to the external anal sphincter, which is best managed by direct primary repair. There is a separate chapter on surgical aspects of incontinence.

The large number of surgical procedures advocated for fecal incontinence suggests that no single technique is best for all cases. Most sphincter repairs are performed at a time remote from an identifiable injury or in the absence of an identifiable cause. After surgery, approximately 80 percent of patients regain continence of solid stool, but note somewhat poorer results with liquid stool. Because poor surgical results are associated with neuropathy of the pelvic floor, preoperative EMG and nerve conduction studies may help identify those patients who might do poorly with sphincter repair only. A recent study suggests that total pelvic floor repair is superior to either of these procedures in patients with peripheral neuropathic incontinence.

Postanal repair had been advocated in the United Kingdom to treat patients with a poorly functioning but anatomically intact sphincter. The levator ani, puborectal, and external sphincter muscles are plicated posteriorly to restore the anorectal angle and tighten the anal canal. Early studies reported that continence was satisfactory in 80 percent of patients, but subsequent studies with a longer follow-up indicated less satisfactory results. Anterior repair has been the preferred approach in the United States; satisfactory outcomes have been reported in 62 percent of patients with idiopathic fecal incontinence and 71 percent of those with a traumatic etiology. The chapter on surgical aspects provides more information.

Incontinence with Diarrhea

In some patients, fecal incontinence develops only with the occurrence of diarrhea. Liquid stool may be more difficult to perceive and, particularly when associated with urgency, more difficult to retain. Thus, diarrhea may uncover underlying abnormalities of anorectal continence mechanisms that result in fecal soiling. Rarely, massive diarrhea may overwhelm normal continence mechanisms.

Despite the presence of anorectal dysfunction, fecal incontinence can often be controlled by successfully treating the diarrhea. If a specific cause of diarrhea cannot be identified, nonspecific approaches to alter stool consistency or colonic motility often prove helpful. Therapeutic approaches include bulk laxatives, anticholinergics, antidiarrheal agents, and bile acid-binding resins.

In disorders such as diarrhea-predominant irritable bowel syndrome (IBS) and idiopathic low-volume diarrhea, bulk laxatives may help regulate bowel habits and decrease stool water content. Drinking smaller amounts of water than is usually recommended when consuming bulk laxatives may be helpful in this regard. Although anticholinergic drugs may decrease colonic motility and abdominal cramping, side effects are not uncommon. I prefer agents such as loperamide, which is prescribed in doses of 2 to 4 mg and adjusted according to the clinical response rather than administered after each episode of diarrhea. The maximum dose of 4 mg four times a day is rarely necessary, and a single morning or nighttime dose is often sufficient. I prefer diphenoxylate as a second-line agent and avoid codeine for long-term control because of its potentially addictive properties. There is some evidence that loperamide, but not diphenoxylate, improves anorectal continence mechanisms as well.

It has been suggested that bile acid-binding agents such as cholestyramine and colestipol hydrochloride may be helpful in ameliorating diarrhea and fecal incontinence in patients with radiation enteritis, IBS, choleretic enteropathy, and idiopathic diarrhea with previous cholecystectomy. Appropriate doses are 4 g cholestyramine resin or 5 g colestipol hydrochloride in the morning, or at night if the patient has undergone cholecystectomy.

Diabetes-Associated Fecal Incontinence

Fecal incontinence occurs in up to 20 percent of diabetic patients, most of whom have diarrhea as well as peripheral and autonomic neuropathy. Most of these patients have rectosphincteric abnormalities, and more than 50 percent have impairment of conscious rectal sensation.

I begin biofeedback in diabetic patients by employing rectal sensory conditioning in those who have abnormal conscious rectal sensation. I attempt to decrease the threshold of conscious rectal sensation in the following manner. Once the smallest volume of rectal distention sensed by the patient is determined, progressively smaller distention volumes are administered in decrements of 1 to 5 ml of air. When a given distention volume is sensed repeatedly, the volume is decreased and the process repeated until no further improvement can be achieved.

After sensory discrimination training, the biofeedback program proceeds in a manner identical to that for patients with normal rectal sensation. Loperamide may be helpful in those who do not respond to biofeedback. Good to excellent results have been obtained in more than 70 percent of a relatively small number of diabetic patients.

Neurogenic Injury

Fecal incontinence may occur with injury to the sacral or suprasacral spinal cord. Rectal sensation is frequently lost and external sphincter denervation is common. Sensory and motor function should be assessed by manometry in patients who appear to retain some muscle and sensory function.

Treatment of suprasacral lesions consists of attempting bowel retraining using planned regular defecation. If patients have recognizable warning symptoms of impending defecation such as dizziness or piloerection, they may be able to anticipate defecation and transfer to a toilet. In others, digital rectal stimulation or a glycerin suppository may stimulate evacuation. If such measures are ineffective, a stimulant laxative suppository such as bisacodyl may be required. If all these measures prove unsatisfactory, a low-bulk diet combined with a stool softener and small amounts of loperamide to produce constipation may decrease unwanted soiling. A weekly enema, followed if necessary by a bisacodyl suppository (Dulcolax, 10 mg) to promote colonic evacuation, should be administered to prevent fecal impaction.

Patients with sacral lesions often have fecal retention because of poor contractility of the distal colon and rectum. I prefer a low-bulk diet with stool softeners (see above) to minimize stool build-up. Bisacodyl suppositories are administered every 2 to 3 days to promote rectal emptying. This can be supplemented by digital evacuation daily to minimize fecal build-up. If continence cannot be established, a diverting colostomy can be created.

Impaired Reservoir Capacity

Patients with impaired reservoir capacity include those with idiopathic inflammatory bowel disease involving the rectum, radiation proctitis, chronic rectal ischemia, colectomy with ileoanal anastomosis, and sphincter-saving procedures for rectal lesions. Therapeutic approaches depend on the underlying disease processes. Rectal urgency and incontinence due to idiopathic proctitis often respond to steroid or 5-aminosalicylate retention enemas.

Patients with proctitis may be unable to retain an entire 5-aminosalicylate 100 ml enema when first instituted. Use of 500 mg suppositories or half of an enema for a few days may lessen inflammation and increase retentive capacity. Enemas may be supplemented with loperamide or diphenoxylate to control diarrhea and cramping. Patients with soiling associated with ileoanal anastomosis often lack localizing rectal sensation. Therapeutic approaches include reducing fecal volume through fiber restriction, use of loperamide or diphenoxylate to prolong transit and promote fluid and electrolyte intestinal absorption, and attempted defecation after meals. With time, rectal or ileal capacity may improve to restore continence in some patients.

"Overflow" Incontinence

"Overflow" soiling associated with fecal impaction is not infrequent in elderly patients who are physically immobilized. Liquid stools that seep around the obstructing fecal bolus may be misdiagnosed as diarrhea. A rectal examination to rule out impaction is mandatory before treating diarrhea or incontinence in an elderly or debilitated patient.

Treatment consists of phosphate enemas (Fleet), given once or twice daily until there is no fecal return. If the impaction is hard, a mineral oil enema (Fleet) to soften the stool should be administered. Digital removal, an unpleasant task, is rarely necessary. Failure to evacuate the colon adequately is the most frequent reason for treatment failure.

Once evacuation is complete, preventive measures should be taken. Once a week, a phosphate enema or a bisacodyl suppository will ensure periodic colonic evacuation and prevent recurrence of soiling.

Suggested Reading

Caruana BJ, Wald A, Hinds JP, et al. Anorectal sensory and motor function in neurogenic fecal incontinence. Gastroenterology 1991; 100:456–470.

Dean KI, Oya M, Ortiz J, et al. Randomized trial comparing three forms of pelvic floor repair for neuropathic faecal incontinence. Br J Surg 1993; 80:794–798.

Dean KI, Kumar D, Williams JG, et al. The prevalence of anal sphincter defects in fecal incontinence: a prospective endosonic study. Gut 1993; 34: 685–688.

Engel BT, Nikoomanesh P, Schuster MM. Operant conditioning of rectosphincteric responses in the treatment of fecal incontinence. N Engl J Med 1974; 190:645–649.

Madoff RD, Williams JG, Caushaj PF. Fecal incontinence. N Engl J Med 1992; 326:1002–1007.

Miller R, Orrom WJ, Corness H, et al. Anterior sphincter plication and levatorplasty in the treatment of faecal incontinence. Br J Surg 1989; 76:1058–1060.

Read M, Read NW, Barber DC, et al. Effects of loperamide on anal sphincter function in patients complaining of chronic diarrhea and fecal incontinence and urgency. Dig Dis Sci 1982; 27:807–814.

Wald A, Tunuguntla AK. Anorectal sensorimotor dysfunction in fecal incontinence and diabetes mellitus: modification with biofeedback therapy. N Engl J Med 1984; 310:1282–1287.

SEVERE LOWER GASTROINTESTINAL BLEEDING

Thomas J. Savides, M.D.
Dennis M. Jensen, M.D.

Lower gastrointestinal (GI) bleeding in adults is usually mild and self-limited and can be evaluated on an outpatient basis. Such bleeding is usually due to internal hemorrhoids, colonic polyps, colon cancer, or inflammatory bowel disease. At times, however, hematochezia can be severe and ongoing, requiring hospitalization, resuscitation, and therapeutic intervention. This chapter focuses on our approach to the colonoscopic diagnosis and treatment of these patients with severe lower GI bleeding.

DEFINITIONS

Hematochezia is passage per rectum of bright red blood, clots, or burgundy stools. It can originate from bleeding lesions in the upper gastrointestinal (UGI) tract, small intestine, or colon. We previously evaluated 80 consecutive patients with hematochezia who were admitted to our intensive care unit. Severe GI bleeding was associated with shock or hypotension, required intensive care unit (ICU) management for resuscitation, and needed red blood cell (RBC) transfusions. Our definition of severe ongoing hematochezia was continued blood per rectum for at least 4 hours while under ICU observation. These patients were elderly, with a mean age of 77 years, and two-thirds were male; 90 percent had other medical or surgical problems. They were evaluated with panendoscopy and urgent colonoscopy after purge. The diagnosis of a bleeding site was based on: (1) active bleeding from the lesion; (2) stigmata of recent hemorrhage, such as a visible vessel or adherent clot resistant to washing with an endoscopic catheter; or (3) blood in the area and a clean lesion without other lesions in the bowel segment to explain the bleeding. The causes of bleeding are shown in Table 1. The most common bleeding lesions were colonic angiomas and diverticula.

Table 1 Etiology of Severe Hematochezia in 80 Patients

LESION SITE	PERCENTAGE OF PATIENTS
Colonic	74
Angiomas	30
Diverticulosis	16
Polyps or cancer	11
Colitis	9
Rectal lesions	4
Bleeding polyp stalk	3
Endometriosis	1
Upper gastrointestinal	11
Small bowel*	9
No site found	6

*Diagnosis of small bowel source made when upper endoscopy and colonoscopy results were negative, but fresh blood or clots were seen coming through the ileocecal valve.

INITIAL MANAGEMENT AND DIAGNOSTIC APPROACH

Patients with severe hematochezia are admitted to an ICU and resuscitated as necessary with fluids and correction of coagulopathy or thrombocytopenia. Anoscopy with a slotted anoscope is performed to evaluate obvious rectal lesions. A nasogastric (NG) tube is placed to determine whether there is fresh blood, clots, or "coffee grounds" to implicate an UGI source. A NG lavage negative for blood does not exclude an UGI source; 11 percent of our patients in whom NG lavage revealed no blood still had an UGI source for the bleeding. However, no hematochezia patient with bile in the NG aspirate (and no blood, clots, or coffee grounds) had an UGI source. Therefore, bile and absence of blood are required to rule out an UGI source for ongoing hematochezia.

Patients with massive bleeding and shock who cannot be stabilized with ICU resuscitation should undergo urgent surgical exploration. However, nearly all patients become hemodynamically stable with fluid or transfusion resuscitation in the ICU and undergo urgent endoscopic evaluation. Figure 1 shows our algorithm for management of patients who are medically stable.

Colonoscopy and Upper Endoscopy

We perform urgent colonoscopy after a sulfate purge in hemodynamically stable patients with severe hematochezia who have a negative NG lavage and anoscopy. While in the ICU, the patient either drinks or receives 4 to 6 L of polyethelene-sulfate purge via a NG tube over 3 to 5 hours until the rectal effluent is clear of stool, blood, and clots. Metoclopramide, 10 mg intravenously given before the purge and repeated every 3 to 4 hours, may facilitate gastric emptying and reduce nausea. During the purge, the patient receives cardiac monitoring and is transfused packed RBCs, fresh-frozen plasma, and platelets as needed.

Colonoscopy is usually performed at the bedside in the ICU. Diagnosis of a colonic bleeding site is made only if active bleeding, a nonbleeding visible vessel, or a clot on a lesion resistant to washing is found. If colonoscopy does not reveal a bleeding source, an upper endoscopy is immediately performed. When fresh blood or clots are seen coming from the ileocecal valve and no lesion is found on colonoscopy or upper endoscopy, the small bowel is presumed to be the bleeding site.

Push Enteroscopy

Less than 10 percent of the time the bleeding site remains obscure after urgent upper endoscopy and colonoscopy in patients with ongoing hematochezia. If the patient has stopped bleeding and is hemodynamically stable, we reexamine the UGI tract using a 180 cm long video colonoscope

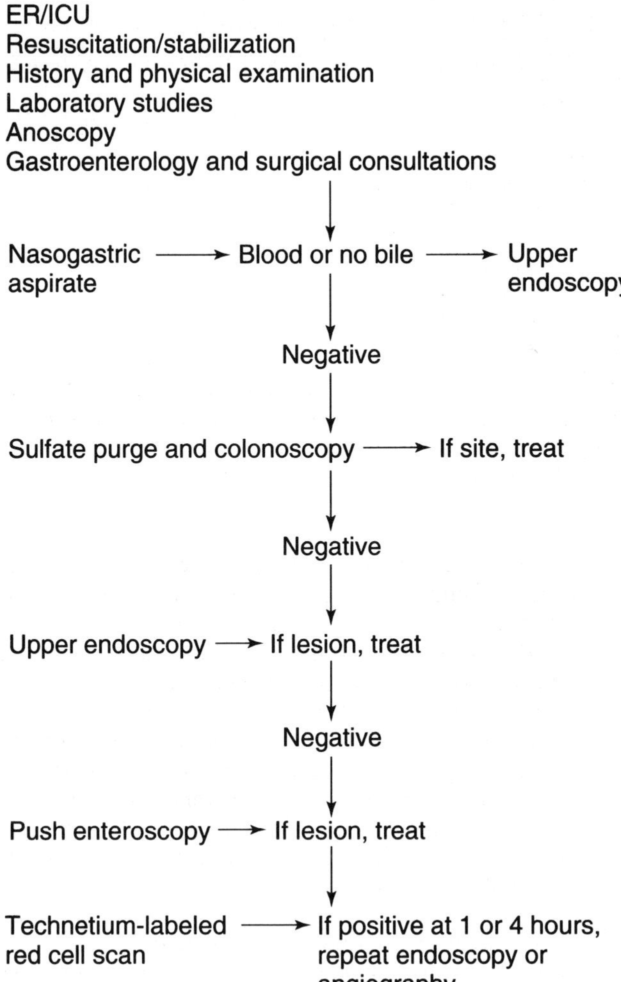

Figure 1
Diagnostic and therapeutic approach to severe lower gastrointestinal bleeding.

or enteroscope of 180–240 cm to evaluate the distal duodenum and proximal jejunum 80 to 150 cm beyond the ligament of Treitz. This "push enteroscopy" technique allows determination of lesions in 19 to 52 percent of patients with obscure bleeding sites. For emergencies, do not use the currently available 280 cm push video enteroscope or longer sonde enteroscopes in patients with acute bleeding because of the prolonged time needed for these examinations, the requirements for overtubes, and the need for fluoroscopy. Although hemostasis or biopsies cannot be performed through the sonde instrument, it is possible through longer push instruments. These techniques can be useful in determining the cause of chronic GI bleeding of obscure origin, particularly in ambulatory patients. There is a separate chapter on enteroscopy.

Technetium-99m Red Blood Cell Scanning

In patients who have intermittent lower GI bleeding in the hospital and negative endoscopic evaluations, we obtain a technetium-labeled RBC scan during the next acute bleeding episode. This test can be useful for determination of the bleeding site if the bleeding rate is more than 0.1 ml per minute. It also has a good chance of detecting an intermittently bleeding lesion, because the long intravascular half-life of the labeled RBCs allows repeated scanning to be performed over at least 24 hours without further injection of isotope. Technetium-99m RBC scanning has demonstrated active bleeding sites in 44 to 72 percent of patients with ongoing lower GI bleeding, with a sensitivity of 93 to 100 percent and a specificity of 85 to 95 percent. Early scans (<4 hours) which are positive are particularly useful for localization of GI bleeding sites. However, labeled RBC scans are less accurate for evaluating patients with occult or less severe lower GI bleeding, for whom a definite source of bleeding is often difficult to determine. In one study of the outcome in 19 patients with lower GI bleeding, it was concluded that there was incorrect localization of bleeding sites in 25 percent of patients, and that performance of a surgical procedure that relied exclusively on localization by red cell scintigraphy resulted in the wrong operation in at least 42 percent of cases.

Angiography

We rarely use selective visceral angiography as the initial test for diagnosing the site of severe lower GI bleeding. This is able to determine a source of bleeding only if there is an active arterial bleeding rate greater than 0.5 ml per minute. The diagnostic yield depends on patient selection, the timing of the procedure, and the skill of the angiographers, with positive tests ranging from 12 to 69 percent. The sensitivity for detecting a bleeding site was 36 percent with angiography compared with 100 percent for technetium-labeled scanning in one comparative study. When we compared emergency angiography with urgent colonoscopy for severe colonic or small bowel bleeding, angiography identified the lesion only 12 percent of the time compared with 82 percent with colonoscopy (Table 2). Complications of angiography can include hematomas, arterial embolization, bowel ischemia or infarction, and renal failure.

■ TREATMENT OF SEVERE HEMATOCHEZIA

Bleeding stops spontaneously in 70 to 90 percent of ambulatory patients with acute lower GI bleeding. This allows elective diagnosis and treatment in most cases. For the 10 to 30 percent with ongoing or recurrent hematochezia, urgent diagnosis and treatment are required to control the bleeding. In our large series of patients with ongoing hematochezia, 64 percent required some intervention including endoscopy (39 percent), angiography (1 percent), or surgery (24 percent) for control of continued bleeding or rebleeding.

Colonic Angiomas

Colonic angiomas can be coagulated endoscopically with bipolar electrocoagulation, monopolar electrocoagulation, heater probe, yttrium-aluminum-garnet (YAG) laser, or argon laser. In previous studies we have shown that endoscopic

Table 2 Diagnostic Yield of Emergency Colonoscopy versus Angiography in Patients With Ongoing Hematochezia

	COLONOSCOPY (%)	ANGIOGRAPHY (%)
Angioma	80	20
Diverticula	75	25
Bleeding tumor or polyp	100	0
Small bowel lesions	100	0
Blind rectal lesions	100	12
Total	82	12

Table 3 Palliative Results in 66 Patients with Colonoscopic Hemostasis of Colonic Angiomas

	BEFORE TREATMENT	AFTER TREATMENT
Mean period of comparison (yr)	2	2
Mean hematocrit (%)	26.8	37.3
Mean lower GI bleeding episodes per yr	1.3	0.6
Units of red blood cells transfused per yr	4.3	1.3

Table 4 Comparison of Treatment Techniques for Colonic Angiomas and Peptic Ulcers Using a Bipolar Probe and a 50 Watt Generator

	COLONIC ANGIOMAS	PEPTIC ULCERS
Pressure	Light	Firm
Power	2–3	3–4
Pulse	2–3 1 sec pulses	Continuous for 10 sec

coagulation can definitively control colonic angioma bleeding in 80 percent of patients. These patients often have rebleeding, and 20 percent require more than one colonoscopic treatment. However, with follow-up of over 1 year, these patients showed a significant decrease in frequency of bleeding episodes and the number of units of packed RBCs transfused per year, and an increase in mean hematocrit values (Table 3).

There have been no comparative studies in humans of the different colonoscopic modes of coagulation, nor of colonoscopic hemostasis compared with surgery. We evaluated colonic injury in a canine right colon model to simulate treatment of angiomas with various thermal modalities. These studies revealed that more frequent transmural injury and a higher rate of perforation occurred with monopolar hot biopsy forceps (HBF), monopolar probe electrocoagulation, and YAG laser than with bipolar electrocoagulation, heater probe, or argon laser. There have been reports of high complication rates from use of YAG laser and monopolar HBF in the right colon, although some experienced endoscopists have reported safer results. In view of the laboratory data and clinical reports, we advise against using YAG laser or monopolar electrocautery to treat colonic angiomas, especially in the right colon.

There have been reports of successful use of monopolar HBF to treat colon angiomas, but there have been no long-term follow-up studies of their efficacy or safety. Experimental studies in the canine right colon have shown that monopolar HBF caused greater rates of transmural injury than heater probe or bipolar electrocoagulation. A large survey of endoscopists who used monopolar HBF reported that 16 percent of patients had major complications, including significant bleeding, perforation, postcoagulation syndrome, and death.

Our current technique for treating actively bleeding colonic angiomas is to irrigate the area and then tamponade and coagulate the bleeding point. We use gentle pressure rather than the firm pressure used in treating peptic ulcers. When there is no active bleeding, we coagulate the central feeding vessels first, then coagulate the remainder of the angioma. These techniques are different from those used for treating peptic ulcers, as shown in Table 4.

The main risks of colonoscopic coagulation of angiomas are perforation, postcoagulation syndrome, and delayed bleeding. In a review of 98 patients treated for colonic angioma with an average of two treatment sessions per patient, none had perforations. Postcoagulation syndrome, as defined by abdominal pain, focal rebound tenderness, fever, and leukocytosis without evidence of perforation, occurred in 2 percent of patients. Delayed bleeding was noted in 4 percent of patients, mostly those with coagulopathies.

Diverticula

Colonic diverticular bleeding is usually self-limited but may be severe. When barium enema alone was used alone for diagnosis of diverticular hemorrhage in 50 patients with hematochezia requiring transfusions, 58 percent stopped bleeding during hospitalization and had no further short-term bleeding, 20 percent had recurrent bleeding in the hospital, and 22 percent had ongoing bleeding requiring surgery. Overall, 70 percent of patients stopped bleeding with conservative management, and of those 22 percent experienced subsequent bleeding events. The authors concluded that elective surgery should be considered only in patients who had had a second massive hemorrhage.

Mesenteric angiography has been used for diagnosis and treatment of diverticular hemorrhage. Selective arterial infusion of vasopressin can provide immediate hemostasis in massive colonic hemorrhage. However, in one study, more than 50 percent of these patients then underwent surgery for either elective resection or rebleeding. Transcatheter embolization has also been reported to stop diverticular bleeding in a few cases.

Colonoscopic treatment of bleeding diverticula was first reported in 1986, with heater probe in four patients to achieve definitive hemostasis. We recently described three patients with recurrent in-hospital lower GI bleeding from visible vessels at the necks of colonic diverticula. Because of the rebleeding, the concern over further rebleeding, and the risks involved in surgery in these elderly patients, we coagulated the visible vessels with bipolar electrocoagulation. There were no complications with treatment and none of the patients have had rebleeding with follow-up from 4 to 16 months. There have also been reports of treatment of bleeding diverticula with epinephrine injection directly into the base of the diverticulum. These colonoscopic techniques are still experimental and need to be compared with surgical resection with long-term follow-up. However, they offer a promising new nonsurgical approach to management of elderly patients with diverticular bleeding in whom surgery presents a high risk.

Polyps or Cancer

Focal ulcerations on large polyps or colonic cancers were the third most common diagnosis in our series of patients with severe hematochezia. Diagnosis and hemostasis via urgent colonoscopy are feasible with various accessories such as snares, electrocoagulation, or epinephrine injection. Patients with bleeding polyps can be definitively treated, and those with ulcerated colonic cancer can be stabilized and staged before elective surgical resection.

Ischemic Bowel Disease

Rarely, we encounter elderly patients with a history of atherosclerotic disease who present with hematochezia and on urgent colonoscopy are found to have sparing of the rectum, with sharp demarcation of abnormal mucosa, swelling, and friability. This is consistent with ischemic bowel disease. These patients are managed with supportive medical therapy only, since less than 2 percent of them will proceed to colonic gangrene.

■ COMMENTS

With currently available video colonoscopes and accessories, and the routine use of colonic purging during medical stabilization, a well-trained colonoscopist can perform a successful diagnostic colonoscopy in most patients with severe hematochezia. If no colonic bleeding site is found, upper endoscopy, push enteroscopy, RBC scanning, and angiography are important additional diagnostic tests to consider for selected patients. Therapeutic colonoscopy can achieve hemostasis of bleeding angiomas, polyps, and cancers and holds promise for treatment of some cases of diverticular bleeding.

Suggested Reading

Farrands PA, Taylor I. Management of acute lower gastrointestinal haemorrhage in a surgical unit over a 4-year period. J R Soc Med 1987; 80:79.

Jensen DM, Machicado GA. Diagnosis and treatment of severe hematochezia. Gastroenterology 1988; 95:1569–1574.

Jensen DM, Machicado GA. Techniques of hemostasis for lower GI bleeding. In: Jensen DM, Brunetaud JM, eds. Medical laser endoscopy. Dordrecht: Kluwer Academic Publishers, 1990:99–107.

Markisz JA, Front D, Royal HD, et al. An evaluation of 99m Tc-labelled red blood cell scintigraphy for the detection and localization of gastrointestinal bleeding sites. Gastroenterology 1982; 83:394–398.

McGuire HH, Haynes BW. Massive hemorrhage from diverticulosis of the colon: guidelines for therapy based on bleeding patterns observed in fifty cases. Ann Surg 1972; 175:847–853.

Nicholson ML, Neoptolemos JP, Sharp JF, et al. Localization of lower gastrointestinal bleeding using in vivo technetium-99m-labelled red blood cell scintigraphy. Br J Surg 1989; 78:358–361.

Schrock TR. Colonoscopic diagnosis and treatment of lower gastrointestinal bleeding. Surg Clin North Am 1989; 69:1309–1325.

Wadas DD, Sanowski RA. Complications of the hot biopsy forceps technique. Gastrointest Endosc 1988; 34:32–37.

ACUTE HEPATITIS: MANAGEMENT AND PREVENTION

Dominique Q. Pham, M.D.,
Leonard B. Seeff, M.D.

Advances in the treatment of acute viral hepatitis have not kept pace with the serologic and epidemiologic progress achieved over the past 2 decades. The only new efforts regarding treatment are several recent but limited studies involving interferon administration to patients with acute hepatitis B and C. The results of these studies at present are too preliminary to form an opinion with regard to efficacy. The mainstay of hepatitis management, therefore, continues to be supportive care, avoidance of liver-damaging events, and observation for progression to fulminant or subfulminant hepatitis. Indeed, the primary gains in treatment have been the omission of certain approaches that were common previously—mandatory hospitalizations, mandatory bed-rest, special diets, and treatment with corticosteroids in certain circumstances. Prevention of the disease, however, has made significant progress, and if fully implemented, could potentially eliminate or at least dramatically reduce the prevalence of some hepatitis types.

■ EVALUATION

There is no feature that is pathognomonic of acute viral hepatitis. In most instances, a presumptive diagnosis can be made from the accumulation of historical facts, physical findings, biochemical alterations, and serologic markers. In gathering the patient's history, it is important to focus on circumstances that favor exposure to viral hepatitis and on the use of all medications (prescription and over-the-counter). It must be remembered that the illness can be mimicked by drug hepatotoxicity, congestive heart failure, sudden hypotension, and acute choledocholithiasis. A similar though generally distinguishable presentation can result from infections by other agents such as cytomegalovirus, Epstein-Barr virus, autoimmune hepatitis, and metabolic disorders (Wilson's disease, $alpha_1$-antitrypsin deficiency). Physical examination should include evaluation of mental status and a search for features that might suggest the presence of chronic liver disease (spider angiomata, collateral venous pattern, gynecomastia, ascites, peripheral edema), since acute reactivation or superinfection of chronic liver disease may simulate a bout of acute hepatitis.

Minimal biochemical and serologic testing should include the serum aminotransferases, bilirubin, alkaline phosphatase, serum proteins, prothrombin time (PT), IgM anti-HAV, HBsAg, IgM anti-HBc, and anti-HCV. Additional serologic markers can be sought as necessary. Among the biochemical tests, the PT and the serum bilirubin are the most important prognostic indicators. Prolongation of the PT by more than 3 seconds and a serum bilirubin level that is greater than 20 mg per deciliter suggest the potential for the development of severe, progressive disease. Serum bilirubin values at this level should also trigger consideration of hemolysis, such as may occur in patients with underlying G6-PD deficiency or sickle cell anemia. Biochemical screening is warranted twice a week when enzyme values are rising, weekly after they have plateaued, and at 1 to 2 week intervals during the subsiding phase. Ideally, completion of evaluation requires identification of loss of HBsAg, to exclude advance to the carrier state, and return of enzymes to normal, to exclude progression to chronic hepatitis.

A routine liver biopsy is unnecessary. It can be considered when there is reason to suspect that the diagnosis might be an exacerbation of pre-existing chronic liver disease or when the disease runs an atypical, protracted course (persisting symptoms or severe biochemical abnormalities for more than 6 weeks). The finding of bridging or submassive necrosis might lead to the consideration to contact a liver transplant center.

THERAPY

Treatment Environment

Provided there is adequate family and medical support, most patients with uncomplicated acute viral hepatitis can be treated at home. Hospitalization for isolation purposes is not warranted because the most infectious period for hepatitis A and B precedes the development of clinically apparent disease. Adequate care implies that there is a household member willing to observe the patient daily for any signs of unusual physical or mental change, to supply the necessary nursing and subsistence support, and to ensure patient compliance with medical follow-up. Hospitalization will, however, need to be considered if the patient has protracted vomiting with the threat of dehydration, disturbing mental status changes, or worsening biochemical tests. The latter include rising serum bilirubin values, particularly if accompanied by rapidly declining serum enzyme activity, an increasing PT, and falling albumin levels. Elderly patients and those with significant medical problems may need to be hospitalized.

Bedrest

There is now general agreement that complete bedrest is not essential. This decision derives from studies which showed no differences in clinical outcomes when convalescing patients were subjected to strenuous activity or assigned to bedrest. However, these studies involved young and otherwise healthy men, mostly military personnel, and it is uncertain whether these results apply to older and more frail populations. The following program seems to be a reasonable approach. Bedrest with bathroom privileges should be advised when the bilirubin level is rising, if the PT is prolonged by more than 3 seconds, if the patient is severely symptomatic, or if the patient is more than 40 years of age. Gradual return to normal activity is permitted when symptoms and biochemical tests begin to improve. Patients can return to work when their biochemical tests show consistent improvement (consistent reduction of the serum enzymes preferably to less than 100 IU per liter) and they have no symptoms or jaundice.

Diet

Under normal circumstances, no specific diet restriction seems necessary. A nutritious diet should be encouraged which need not include vitamin supplementation unless there is evidence of a specific deficiency. The challenge is to induce patient to eat when anorexia and nausea are present. Because anorexia and nausea typically are least severe in the morning, it is useful to offer the major proportion of calories at this time and to provide the remainder in frequent small meals during the rest of the day. This might be accomplished with the aid of high calorie liquid formulas. Some believe a high-protein diet is beneficial but there is no obvious long-term benefit. Fatty foods need not be restricted unless they produce nausea. Severe, continued vomiting will obviously necessitate fluid and electrolyte replacement.

Drugs

As a general rule, all drugs, particularly narcotics, analgesics, and tranquilizers, should be avoided during the course of acute hepatitis. Protracted nausea and vomiting may require judicious use of small doses of metoclopramide. If sedation is necessary, oxazepam is preferred because its metabolism is not impaired by acute liver damage. Rarely, pruritis may be sufficiently severe to warrant the use of medication, such as hydroxyzine or cholestyramine. The use of vitamin K is of no benefit in acute hepatitis although it may improve abnormal PTs in patients with cholestatic liver disease. Data regarding the effects of alcohol in patients with acute hepatitis are conflicting, but the prudent approach is to proscribe its use during the acute and convalescent phase so as to reduce confusion about the meaning of subsequent enzyme abnormalities. Oral contraceptives can be continued without deleterious effect. Early studies suggested that the use of corticosteroids could hasten recovery from acute viral hepatitis accompanied by rapid reduction in serum bilirubin. Later studies comparing corticosteroids with placebos failed to substantiate a beneficial effect. Furthermore, it has been suggested that corticosteroid treatment may predispose to a higher rate of relapse and interfere with the normal immune response, particularly in persons with acute hepatitis B, and hence may promote the development of chronic hepatitis.

Accordingly, the use of corticosteroids for uncomplicated viral hepatitis is neither justified nor helpful.

Elective Surgery

Unequivocal objective evidence of the dangers of surgery is scanty. In one commonly cited study, of the 42 patients with acute viral hepatitis who were subjected to surgery, five died within 3 weeks of surgery and nonfatal major complications developed in five other patients. Elective surgery should be avoided during acute viral hepatitis.

New Forms of Treatment

A variety of specific treatment modalities have been tested in the treatment of acute viral hepatitis. Their effects are aimed directly at inhibition of viral synthesis or at alteration of the immune response. Efforts have been made to treat patients with acute viral hepatitis with ribavirin, isoprinosine, (+)-cyanidanol-3, levamisole, and anti-HBs hyperimmune globulin, with little success. Recently, based on the evidence of the partial benefit of interferon treatment in patients with chronic hepatitis B and C, efforts have begun to evaluate its efficacy for treatment of the acute illness. In one randomized, placebo-controlled trial of interferon alpha in acute hepatitis B, interferon was well tolerated. Treatment in this study appeared to shorten the period of clinical disease and induce higher titers of anti-HBs antibodies. However, there were no differences in the overall clinical and biochemical outcomes among the control and treated groups. Some preliminary studies have supported the use of interferon during acute hepatitis C infection to prevent progression to the chronic stage. These studies involved a limited number of patients, used different types and doses of interferon, and had varying durations of follow-up. Thus, it is difficult to draw any firm conclusion regarding the efficacy of interferon in preventing the progression of HCV infection to chronicity. At the present time, interferon is not recommended for treatment of acute hepatitis B or C until more data become available.

■ GENERAL PREVENTION OF VIRAL HEPATITIS

The institution of appropriate preventive public health measures depends on a thorough knowledge of the modes of transmission of hepatitis. Hepatitis A is primarily transmitted by person-to-person contact, generally through fecal contamination and oral ingestion; hence those at risk are susceptible to household or institutional contacts. The virus reaches its highest concentration in the feces from the latter half of the incubation period to approximately the time of peak illness, generally within 1 week of onset of disease. Because of this pattern of viral excretion, many of the contacts are likely to have been exposed by the time the index case is brought to medical attention. Nevertheless, to curtail further spread, the modes of disease transmission should be discussed with the patient, and strict standards of personal hygiene should be imposed. This includes regular hand washing, particularly after using the toilet (separate facilities are not required); a warning against intimate contact; and a prohibition of the sharing of food and drink. Food can be eaten using paper plates or disposable utensils although household implements are perfectly safe if washed in a dishwasher. When hospitalization is required, there is no need to impose reverse isolation procedures or enforce the use of separate bathroom facilities. Universal precautions as recommended by the Occupational Safety and Health Administration (OSHA) should be applied. Transmission of hepatitis A virus by the percutaneous route has been reported but is uncommon.

The hepatitis B virus is present in blood and in all body fluids, with the exception of the stool; presumably the same holds true for the viruses of hepatitis C and the delta agent. Thus, blood and body secretions are the source of transmission and high-risk individuals are those who are likely to come into contact with blood and its products or who have intimate contact with the index case. However, sexual transmission of hepatitis C, unlike hepatitis B, seems to be minimal. Nonpercutaneous transmission other than sexual contact also occurs but the precise mechanism often cannot be established. Consequently, preventive measures that can be adopted include the application of universal precautions, i.e., the consistent use of gloves, gown, and face mask when contamination is anticipated; the requirement that needles be properly disposed of; and that instruments in contact with blood and secretions be adequately cleaned (with soap and water), disinfected (sodium hypochlorite, formalin, glutaraldehyde), and sterilized (autoclaving, ethylene oxide). Other efforts include reduction of the number of blood transfusions; development and maintenance of hospital surveillance to identify HBsAg carriers; and the recommendation that sexual abstinence be followed during the acute disease and that sexual contact be limited by the carrier. As will be discussed, many of these problems could be avoided if immune prophylaxis is provided for all susceptible high-risk individuals.

■ IMMUNOPROPHYLAXIS

Hepatitis A

Pre-Exposure Prophylaxis

Immune globulin (IG) is recommended for all susceptible travelers to developing countries, especially those who live in or visit rural areas, or frequently eat or drink in settings of poor sanitation. A single dose of IG of 0.02 ml per kilogram of body weight is recommended if travel is for less than 3 months. For prolonged travel or residence in developing countries, 0.06 ml per kilogram should be given every 5 months (Table 1).

Table 1 Recommendations for Hepatitis A Prophylaxis*

	IG DOSES	GROUPS EXPOSED
Pre-exposure	0.02 mg/kg bw† × 1	Travelers <3 months
	0.06 ml/kg bw q5 months	Travelers >3 months
Postexposure	0.02 ml/kg bw within 2 weeks	Household, sexual, day care center contacts; outbreaks in institutions

*ACIP, CDC, 1990.
†Body weight.

Table 2 Recommended Doses of Currently Licensed Hepatitis B Vaccines*

GROUPS	DOSE MG/ML† HEPTAVAX-B‡	RECOMBIVAX HB	ENGERIX-B§
Infants of HBV-carrier mothers	10 (0.5)	5 (0.5)	10 (0.5)
Other infants and children <11 yr	10 (0.5)	2.5 (0.25)	10 (0.5)
Children and adolescents 11–19 yr	20 (1.0)	5 (0.5)	20 (1.0)
Adults >19 yr	20 (1.0)	10 (1.0)	20 (1.0)
Dialysis and immunocompromised patients	40 (2.0)	40 (1.0)	40 (2.0)

*ACIP, CDC, 1990.
†Usual schedule: three doses at 0, 1, 6 months
‡Heptavax-B: Available only for hemodialysis, immunocompromised patients, and persons with known allergy to yeast.
§Alternative schedule for Engerix-B: 0, 1, 12 months or 0, 1, 6 months for dialysis and immunocompromised patients.

Table 3 Recommendations for Hepatitis B Postexposure Prophylaxis*

EXPOSURE	HBIG	VACCINE	TIMING
Perinatal	0.5 ml IM × 1	0.5 ml IM followed by usual schedule	Within 12 hr of birth
Sexual	0.06 ml/kg bw IM × 1	1.0 ml IM followed by usual schedule	Within 14 days of last sexual contact
Infants <12 months (household contact)	0.5 ml IM × 1	0.5 ml IM followed by usual schedule	

*ACIP, CDC, 1990.
†body weight

Table 4 Recommendations for Prophylaxis Following Percutaneous/Permucosal Exposure to Hepatitis B*

EXPOSED PERSON	HBSAG STATUS OF SOURCE POSITIVE	NEGATIVE	UNKNOWN
Unvaccinated	HBIG × 1 and initiate HB vaccine	Initiate HB vaccine	Initiate HB vaccine
Previously vaccinated			
Known responder	Test for anti-HBs Adequate—no treatment Inadequate—HB vaccine booster dose	No treatment	No treatment
Known nonresponder	HBIG × 2 or HBIG × 1 plus 1 dose HB vaccine	No treatment	If high-risk source, treat as if source HBsAg positive
Unknown response	Test for anti-HBs Adequate—no treatment Inadequate—HBIG × 1 and HB vaccine booster dose	No treatment	Test for anti-HBs Adequate—no treatment Inadequate—HB vaccine booster dose

*ACIP, CDC, 1990.

Recently, two inactivated hepatitis A vaccines, Havrix and Vaqta, have been licensed by the Food and Drug Administration for persons older than 2 years of age, and have proven to be highly effective. Havrix is given to those 2 to 18 years of age in a dose of 360 enzyme-linked immunosorbent assay units (ELU) IM at 0, 1, and 6 to 12 months, and to those older than 18 years, in a dose of 1,440 ELU at 0 and 6 to 12 months. The dose for Vaqta is 25 U IM at 0 and then at 6 to 18 months for those 2 to 17 years of age, and 50 U IM at 0 and 6 months in those older than 17 years. The hepatitis A vaccine can be given together with other vaccines and toxoids without compromising immunity and can be given without adverse effect to already immune persons. Administration of the vaccine at the same time as that of IG induces lower anti-HAV titers but nevertheless appears to be at levels that are protective. Persons currently recommended for receipt of the vaccine are international travelers, men who have sex with men, parenteral drug abusers, and persons working with non-human primates. Other groups considered are those with already established chronic liver disease and those at risk of developing liver disease such as persons with clotting factor disorders.

Postexposure Prophylaxis

For postexposure IG prophylaxis, a single intramuscular dose of 0.02 ml per kilogram is recommended within 2 weeks of exposure for all household and sexual contacts, for contacts in day care centers, and for residents in institutions for custodial care (see Table 1). Serologic confirmation of the index case is recommended before contacts are treated. Serologic screening of contacts for anti-HAV is not recomended because of the cost of screening and the delay in prophylaxis administration.

Hepatitis B

Pre-Exposure Prophylaxis

Two types of hepatitis B vaccines currently licensed in the United States are (1) plasma-derived vaccine (Heptavax-B), which is no longer being produced and the use of which is now limited to hemodialysis patients, other immunocompromised hosts, and persons with known allergy to yeast; and (2) recombinant vaccine (Recombivax HB and Engerix-B). Primary vaccination consists of three intramuscular doses of vaccine at 0, 1, and 6 months. Adults and older children should be given a full 1.0 ml dose, while children less than 11 years of age should be given half (0.5 ml) this dose. Hepatitis B vaccine should be given only in the deltoid muscle for adults and children or in the anterolateral thigh muscle for infants and neonates. For hemodialysis patients and those who are immunocompromised, higher vaccine doses or an increased number of doses are required (see Table 2 for recommended doses and schedules of currently available vaccines).

Previously, groups recommended for pre-exposure vaccination included persons with occupational risk, clients and staffs of institutions for the mentally handicapped, hemodialysis patients, sexually active homosexual men, recipients of high-risk blood products, household and sexual contacts of HBV carriers, adoptees from countries with high HBV endemicity, populations with high HBV endemicity (Alaskan natives, Pacific Islanders), prison inmates, sexually active heterosexual persons, and international travelers for 6 months to endemic areas. More recently, the American Academy of Pediatrics and the Advisory Committee on Immunization Practices of the United States Public Health Service have recommended universal immunization of infants. All children should receive three doses of vaccines by the time they are 18 months of age. In our view, even nonimmune adolescents should be considered for HBV vaccination. Hepatitis B vaccine produces protective antibody (anti-HBs) in 90 percent of healthy persons. An adequate antibody response is greater than 10 milliInternational Units (mIU per milliliter) measured after completion of the vaccine series. Available data show that vaccine-induced antibody levels decline steadily over time and that up to 50 percent of vaccinees who respond adequately to vaccine may have low or undetectable levels by 7 years after vaccination. For people with normal immune status, declining antibody levels are still protective against hepatitis B infection, and hence booster doses are not routinely recommended, nor is routine serologic testing necessary within 7 years after vaccination. For immunocompromised and hemodialysis patients for whom vaccine-induced protection is less complete, antibody testing should be done annually, and booster doses be given when antibody levels decline to less than 10 mIU per milliliter.

Postexposure Prophylaxis

Prophylactic treatment to prevent hepatitis B infection after exposure to HBV should be given to newborns of HBsAg-carrier mothers (perinatal exposures), persons exposed to HBsAg-positive blood through accidental percutaneous or permucosal routes, sexual partners of persons with acute HBV infection, and infants less than 12 months of age who have been exposed to primary care givers with acute hepatitis B (Table 3). For accidental percutaneous and permucosal exposure to blood, the decision to provide prophylaxis depends on the HBsAg status of the source of exposure and the vaccination status and vaccine response of the exposed person (Table 4). Although hepatitis B immune globulin (HBIG) has been used with moderate benefit for postexposure prophylaxis, a regimen combining HBIG with hepatitis B vaccine will provide both short- and long-term protection and is the treatment of choice. For greatest effectiveness, passive prophylaxis with HBIG, when indicated, should be given within 7 days of exposure.

Delta Hepatitis

Since delta hepatitis virus (HDV) is dependent on HBV for replication, prevention of hepatitis B infection, either pre- or postexposure, will suffice to prevent HDV infection for a person susceptible to hepatitis B. At present no products are available that might prevent HDV infection in HBsAg carriers either before or after exposure.

Non-A, Non-B (Predominantly C) Hepatitis

Studies of the efficacy of immunoglobulins in prophylaxis against non-A, non-B hepatitis have provided equivocal data. For persons with percutaneous exposure to blood from a patient with non-A, non-B hepatitis, it may be reasonable to administer a single dose of immune globulin (IG) 0.06 ml per kilogram as soon as possible after exposure. No vaccine for HCV exists at the present.

Hepatitis E

There is no evidence that IG manufactured in the United States will prevent this infection. As with other enteric infections, avoidance of potentially contaminated food or water is the best means of preventing hepatitis E.

Suggested Reading

Centers for Disease Control. Protection against viral hepatitis. Recommendations of the Immunization Practices Advisory Committee (ACIP). MMWR 1990; 39(Suppl):1–26.

Seeff LB. Diagnosis, therapy and prognosis of viral hepatitis. In: Zakim D, Boyer TB, eds., Hepatology: A textbook of liver disease. Philadelphia: WB Saunders, 1990; 958.

Viral hepatitis management, standards for the future. Proceedings of a Symposium in Cannes, France, May 22–23, 1992. Gut 1993; supplement: S1–S149.

FULMINANT HEPATIC FAILURE

David H. Van Thiel, M.D.
Stefano Fagiuoli, M.D.
Paolo Caraceni, M.D.
Harlan I. Wright, M.D.

Fulminant hepatic failure (FHF) is a clinical syndrome resulting from massive necrosis of liver cells leading to a sudden and severe impairment of hepatic function. FHF was defined initially in 1970 by Trey and Davidson as the development of hepatic failure with encephalopathy occurring within 8 weeks of the onset of the acute hepatic injury in an individual without a history or evidence of pre-existing liver disease. More recently, Bernuau and colleagues in 1986 proposed an alternative definition of FHF as a condition wherein encephalopathy develops within 2 weeks of the onset of symptoms in an individual with acute hepatic injury who has no history or evidence of previous liver disease. Regardless of the specific definition used, it is generally agreed that individuals having a shorter time interval from the onset of symptoms to the point of encephalopathy (Bernuau's definition) have a better prognosis than do those who develop encephalopathy more slowly (Trey and Davidson definition). In contrast, the group defined by Bernuau is more likely to experience cerebral edema than are those with a longer time until the onset of encephalopathy (Trey and Davidson definition). Cerebral edema and brain herniation is the major cause of death in individuals who die with FHF having an early onset of encephalopathy. Conversely, in those with a later onset of encephalopathy, sepsis or renal failure is more likely to be the immediate cause of death. These confounding problems in patients with encephalopathy occurring later than 2 weeks but before 8 weeks from the onset of acute liver disease are typically the precipitating factors for the spiral of multiorgan failure that inevitably leads to the death of most of those who die of FHF.

■ ETIOLOGY

Viral

Viral liver diseases are the most common causes of FHF. Fulminant type B viral hepatitis (HBV) is the most common type of viral hepatitis that leads to FHF. Most cases of FHF due to HBV occur in young adults 20 to 40 years of age. Hepatitis C is rarely a cause of FHF. In contrast, non-A, non-B, non-C (NANBNC) hepatitis (a putative viral illness) is a common form of FHF that may account for more cases in Western and developed societies than even HBV. Hepatitis A (HAV) leads to FHF when it occurs in individuals older than 40 years of age. Because of the increasing incidence of HAV disease in adults in Western or developed societies, it may account for more cases of FHF in the near future. Hepatitis E virus (HEV) accounts for many FHF cases in central Asia and the Indian subcontinent, as well as in areas in the Western hemisphere such as Mexico and Central America. In these areas and during epidemics of HEV infection, pregnant women appear to be particularly susceptible to FHF.

The more unusual forms of viral hepatitis produce FHF primarily, if not exclusively, in individuals who are either endogenously or exogenously immunosuppressed. Examples of endogenous immunosuppression associated with FHF due to unusual causes of viral hepatitis are pregnancy, intrinsic T- and B-cell immunodeficiency states, and lymphoid neoplasms. Examples of exogenous immunosuppression associated with unusual viral forms of FHF include the use of corticosteroids or cytotoxic agents for the treatment of asthma, other autoimmune or inflammatory diseases, and neoplasms.

Drugs

Drug-induced FHF is a less common form of hepatic disease that has been increasing in incidence steadily over the past 30 to 40 years with the growth and development of the pharmaceutical industry. Halothane, antituberculous drugs, nonsteroidal anti-inflammatory drugs (NSAIDs), and antiepileptic drugs remain the major causes of drug-induced FHF. Adult women over 40 years of age, and particularly black women, appear to be particularly susceptible to this type of FHF. Acetaminophen is a common cause of self-induced FHF occurring as part of a suicide attempt. Aspirin and valproic acid are common causes of FHF in children. Acetaminophen can occasionally cause FHF in infants and toddlers who are given excessive amounts of the drug in an attempt to control fever. Similarly, alcohol abusers and occasional alcohol-intoxicated revelers experience FHF as a consequence of the use of acetaminophen to treat a hangover that under normal circumstances would not be toxic.

Other Causes

All the other causes of FHF identified in Table 1 occur much less often than do those already described in this text and are not discussed further. The particular circumstances in which these situations occur should suggest the cause of FHF in these unusual cases.

■ CLINICAL FEATURES (TABLE 2)

Acute hepatic encephalopathy is a universal feature of FHF, being an intrinsic component of the definition of the condition. Early clinical signs include a change in personality, dizziness, headaches, and nightmares. These can progress to delirium, mania, and other forms of "uncooperative" behavior. Violent acting-out behavior is common in the middle stages of acute hepatic encephalopathy. Fetor hepaticus occurs in the later stages of acute hepatic encephalopathy, whereas asterixis is transient. The clinical grades of hepatic encephalopathy merge almost indistinguishably into each other as the underlying disease progresses, but these should be distinguished whenever possible into four specific grades as shown in Table 3.

Cerebral edema occurs in late stage 3 and stage 4 acute hepatic encephalopathy. It can be recognized by the develop-

Table 1 Causes of Fulminant Hepatic Failure

Infections
Usual hepatotropic viruses
Hepatitis A
Hepatitis B
Hepatitis C
Hepatitis B + D
Hepatitis E
Hepatitis NANBNC
Unusual forms of viral hepatitis
Cytomegalovirus
Epstein-Barr virus
Herpes simplex
Varicella
Adenovirus
Drug-induced hepatic failure
Halothane
INH ± pyrazinamide
Rifampin
NSAIDs, especially diclofenac and acetaminophen
Antiepileptics
Disulfiram
Carbon tetrachloride
Amiodarone
Toxin-induced hepatic failure
Amanita phalloides
Herbal remedies
Metabolic liver disease
Fulminant Wilson's disease
Acute fatty liver pregnancy
Reye's syndrome
Vascular disease
Hepatic ischemia
Surgical shock
Acute Budd-Chiari syndrome
Miscellaneous courses
Malignant infiltration
Bacterial sepsis
Heat stroke
Autoimmune hepatitis

Table 2 Clinical Features of Fulminant Hepatic Failure

Acute hepatic encephalopathy
Cerebral edema
Coagulopathy
Hypoglycemia
Sepsis
Renal dysfunction
Acid-base disturbances
Hypotension
Hypoxia

ment of decerebrate rigidity characterized by extension and pronation of the arms and legs, dysconjugate eye movements, and a loss of pupillary reflexes. As noted earlier, it occurs in more than 80 percent of patients who die with FHF and meet the criteria of Bernuau and colleagues.

The coagulopathy associated with FHF is the most important prognostic index of the clinical syndrome. A prothrombin time greater than 20 seconds in patients with viral or drug-induced (except acetaminophen-induced) FHF or a

Table 3 Grades of Acute Hepatic Encephalopathy

Grade 1	Confused or altered mood
Grade 2	Inappropriate behavior or drowsiness
Grade 3	Stuporous but arousable, markedly confused behavior
Grade 4	Coma unresponsive to painful stimuli

prothrombin time greater than 100 seconds in individuals with acetaminophen-induced FHF, and a factor V level less than 20 percent of normal in individuals under 30 years of age and less than 30 percent of normal in those 30 years of age or older with FHF suggest a high likelihood of death. In such cases, bleeding is the usual cause of death and can occur into the lungs, gastrointestinal (GI) tract, or brain.

Hypoglycemia occurs only in patients with an extreme hepatic injury (more than 85 percent of the liver being necrotic) and is more common in children and women than in men.

Sepsis due to gram-negative organisms of enteric bacteria as well as candidiasis and/or an aspergillosis were common causes of infection in cases of FHF before the development of selective enteric decontamination protocols. Since the use of oral antibiotics has become common in patients with FHF, gram-positive organisms, particularly staphylococcus, and multidrug-resistant gram-negative organisms have become more common causes of preterminal sepsis in FHF.

The renal dysfunction seen in FHF is often functional and occurs in response to a progressive shift of renal blood flow from the cortex to the medulla. Endotoxemia occurring as a consequence of the sepsis in FHF also contributes to the high incidence of renal dysfunction. The acid-base and vasomotor consequences of FHF reflect the severity of the underlying hepatic and renal dysfunction in patients with FHF.

■ PROGNOSIS

The prognosis of FHF with medical therapy alone in cases that progress to stage 3 or 4 encephalopathy is extremely poor and varies between 20 and 40 percent, depending on the specific cause. In general, patients over 40 years of age and those under 10 years are at particular risk of dying. Other clinical signs of a poor prognosis include a rapidly shrinking liver and/or a liver volume of less than 900 ml, necrosis of more than 50 percent of the hepatic lobules assessed by liver biopsy, ascites, decerebrate rigidity, respiratory failure, and a dysconjugate gaze.

With the widespread availability of liver transplantation, it has become possible to salvage many patients with FHF who previously would have died. As a result, considerable effort has been made to identify patients with FHF who are unlikely to survive so that they can be listed for transplant before they reach a point of irreversible brain injury or experience an episode of infection that prohibits any attempt at liver transplantation. In addition to the clinical signs mentioned earlier, two groups, who have considerable experience with FHF, have developed criteria for identifying patients unlikely to survive without a liver transplant (Table 4). Although the distribution of specific etiologies of FHF differed markedly at these two centers, the criteria identified at each that characterize pa-

Table 4 Criteria Used to Identify Individuals Unlikely to Survive Without Liver Transplantation

GROUP ONE	GROUP TWO
Prothrombin time >100 sec	Factor V <20%
or	(age <30 yr)
Any three of the following:	or
Age <10 or >40 yr	Factor V <30%
Non-A, non-B hepatitis; halothane;	(age <30 yr)
or other drug reaction etiology	Coma or confusion
Duration of jaundice before onset	
of encephalopathy >2 days	
Prothrombin time >50 sec	
Serum bilirubin >20 mg/dl	
If acetaminophen induced:	
pH <7.3	
or	
Prothrombin time >100 sec	
and	
Creatinine >2 mg/dl in patients with	
grade 3 or 4 encephalopathy	

Data from O'Grady JG, Hamblay H, Williams R. Prothrombin time in fulminant hepatic failure. Gastroenterology 1991; 100:1480; and Bernuau J, Samuel D, Durand F, et al. Criteria for emergency liver transplantation in patients with acute viral hepatitis and factor V below 50% of normal: a prospective study. Hepatology 1991; 14:49A.

tients unlikely to survive are similar if one excludes patients with acetaminophen toxicity from the analysis. These criteria notwithstanding, with the development of intensive care and meticulous attention to details of good supportive care, the survival of individuals with FHF has improved considerably over the last decade and a half.

■ MANAGEMENT

General Principles

Individuals with FHF require hospitalization in specialized units prepared to manage such patients. Trained nursing personnel are essential. The immediate availability of an established liver transplant program is recommended. Because it takes time to obtain the results of diagnostic serologic testing, all patients except those with a clear-cut history of some other factor that produces FHF should be managed as if they are infectious. All nursing and hospital personnel working in such units should be vaccinated against HBV and more recently with HAV vaccines. Gloves, gowns, and eyewear are essential when patient contact is required. An arterial line can be placed if experienced personnel are available to insert it; if not, it is not essential. A central venous line should be inserted, preferably one with several ports to enable easy infusion of dextrose and other drugs and blood coagulation factors, blood to be drawn as needed, and frequent monitoring of cardiovascular status. In addition, a nasogastric tube and Foley catheter should be inserted to prevent aspiration and to monitor urinary output at regular intervals. If the patient is in grade 3 or 4 coma, endotracheal intubation is recommended to guarantee the airway and prevent aspiration. Patients are best managed in reverse Trendelenburg position to further prevent aspiration and reduce the effects of cerebral edema when advanced stages (III and IV) of acute hepatic encephalopathy are present.

The use of an H_2 blocker or omeprazole combined with a broad-spectrum antibiotic such as norfloxacin is recommended to prevent GI bleeding and translocation of enteric organisms.

Encephalopathy

Acute hepatic encephalopathy is managed by judicious use of protein, 30 to 40 g in a 70 kg individual as an oral or enteral diet, depending upon the patient's level of consciousness, and lactulose administration to produce two to four bowel movements per day. All forms of sedation are to be avoided except when used for intubation or to prevent extubation by the patient.

The use of a short-acting benzodiazepine such as midazolam and an anesthetic such as fentanyl is recommended for this purpose. Both are given intravenously (IV). Their judicious use can prevent central nervous system hemorrhage or oropharyngeal trauma and pulmonary hemorrhage in an uncooperative patient who has both severe coagulopathy and thrombocytopenia. Neomycin should not be used because of the risk of renal injury, particularly in a patient with an edematous leaky bowel due to portal hypertension and low oncotic pressure. Moreover, it is unnecessary if norfloxacin is being used to prevent bacterial translocation.

Cerebral Edema

Cerebral edema, when it occurs, can be treated with mannitol, 1 g per kilogram body weight up to a maximum of 100 g as a 20 percent solution administered as an IV bolus every 4 hours. The use of glucocorticoids to prevent cerebral edema has been shown to be unsuccessful and is associated with an increased risk of GI bleeding and infection in patients with FHF. Mannitol cannot be given in patients with renal failure, but ultrafiltration can and should be used. Thiopental infusions can be used in severe cases no longer responsive to mannitol or ultrafiltration. Extradural intracranial pressure monitoring devices have become popular recently, especially for comatose or anesthetized patients undergoing liver transplantation. Increases in intracranial pressure above 25 to 30 mm Hg that are continuous for 5 or more minutes require treatment. A cerebral perfusion pressure (systolic pressure–intracranial pressure) of 40 mm Hg is considered essential.

Nutrition

Nutrition can be maintained in the initial 3 to 4 days of hospitalization with an IV infusion of 10 percent dextrose up to 3 liters per day. Hypoglycemia often occurs and will not be detected unless frequent blood sugar determinations are made, usually every 2 to 3 hours. Hypoglycemia, when it occurs, should be treated with an emergent 50 percent glucose infusion and an increase in the rate of glucose being infused as 10 percent or, if necessary, 20 percent dextrose. IV infusions should contain sufficient potassium to maintain adequate potassium stores in a patient undergoing diuresis.

Hypotension

Hypotension can be treated early with dopamine, which also guarantees renal blood flow. In patients with a severe reduction in perpheral vascular resistance, norepinephrine (Levophed) in combination with dopamine may be necessary to maintain an adequate blood pressure.

Prostaglandins

Data from uncontrolled studies suggest that prostaglandin infusions (PGE_1) or oral prostaglandin E_2 (100 to 200 μg orally twice a day), either alone or coupled with the oral administration of acetylcysteine or *S*-adenosylmethionine, can reduce the hepatic injury that occurs regardless of the cause and hastens recovery. The use of these drugs for this purpose, however, is still investigational.

Support Systems

Very recently, the use of an extracorporeal artificial liver consisting of either porcine liver or hepatoblastoma cells contained in a hollow fiber dialysis system wherein plasma is perfused over the cells has been reported to be successful. In all of the cases to date, this therapy has been applied as a bridge to transplantation, maintaining the patient in a state that will enable liver transplantation to occur as soon as an acceptable donor organ can be identified. This usually takes 24 to 72 hours. Even more recently, human hepatocytes have been injected successfully into the spleen of patients with FHF for the same purpose.

Transplantation

The decision to transplant a specific patient is best made at the time a donor organ is identified. Such decisions, however, are usually based on the criteria identified in Table 4. Patients with NANB, drug-induced (excluding acetaminophen), and halothane-induced FHF are best served with early liver transplants, which improve the survival of these groups from 12 to 20 percent to 50 to 60 percent. Individuals with other types of FHF are chosen for liver transplantation if they meet the criteria identified in Table 4 when the donor organ is available and if they are still free of sepsis and multiorgan failure.

Suggested Reading

Bernuau J, Goudeau A, Poynard T, et al. Multivariate analysis of prognostic factors in fulminant hepatitis B. Hepatology 1986; 6:648–651.

Bernuau J, Rueff B, Benhamou JP. Fulminant and subfulminant liver failure: definition and causes. Semin Liver Dis 1986; 6:97–106.

Bernuau J, Samuel D, Durand F, et al. Criteria for emergency liver transplantation in patients with acute viral hepatitis and factor V below 50% of normal: a prospective study. Hepatology 1991; 14:49A.

Blei AT. Cerebral edema and intracranial hypertension in acute liver failure: distinct aspects of the same problem. Hepatology 1991; 13:376–379.

Emond JC, Aran PP, Whitington PF, et al. Liver transplantation in the management of fulminant hepatic failure. Gastroenterology 1989; 96:1583–1586.

Forbes A, Alexander GJM, O'Grady JE, et al. Thiopental infusion in the treatment of intracranial hypertension complicating fulminant hepatic failure. Hepatology 1989; 10:306–310.

Harrison PM, Keays R, Bray GP, et al. Improved outcome of paracetamol-induced fulminant hepatic failure by the administration of acetylcysteine. Lancet 335:1572–1573.

Klein NA, Mabie WC, Shaver DC, et al. Herpes simplex virus hepatitis in pregnancy. Gastroenterology 1991; 100:239–244.

LeRoux PD, Elliott JP, Perkins JD, Winn HR. Intracranial pressure monitoring in fulminant hepatic failure and liver transplantation. Lancet 1990; 335:1291.

Munoz SJ. Prothrombin time in fulminant hepatic failure. Gastroenterology 1991; 100:1480–1481.

O'Grady JG, Alexander GJM, Hayllar KM, et al. Early indicators of prognosis in fulminant hepatic failure. Gastroenterology 1989; 97:439–445.

Rolando N, Harvey F, Brahm J, et al. Prospective study of bacterial infection in acute liver failure: an analysis of fifty patients. Hepatology 1990; 11:49–53.

Schafer DF, Shaw BW Jr. Fulminant hepatic failure and orthotopic liver transplantation. Semin Liver Dis 1989; 9:189–194.

Van Thiel DH. When should a decision to proceed with transplantation actually be made in cases of fulminant or subfulminant hepatic failure: at admission to hospital or when a donor organ is made available? J Hepatol 1993; 17:1–2.

ASCITES AND ITS COMPLICATIONS

Anil K. Rustgi, M.D.

Lawrence S. Friedman, M.D.

The most common cause of ascites is cirrhosis of the liver. Other etiologies include neoplasms, congestive heart failure, noncirrhotic liver diseases, nephrotic syndrome, and tuberculosis. This chapter deals with the management of ascites in patients with cirrhosis of the liver as well as complications of ascites.

■ ASCITES IN CIRRHOSIS

Etiology

Several theories have been advanced to explain the development of ascites in patients with cirrhosis. The underfill hypothesis maintains that increased hepatic sinusoidal pressure leads to increased formation of hepatic lymph, which enters the abdominal cavity. Increased portal venous pressure also contributes to the formation of ascites and results in increased splanchnic blood volume. With the expansion of splanchnic extracellular fluid volume, systemic vascular resistance and effective plasma volume decrease, leading in turn to avid renal retention of sodium and water, initially with preservation of the glomerular filtration rate, creatinine clearance, and renal plasma flow. In response to the decrease in effective plasma volume, plasma renin aldosterone, norepinephrine, and vasopressin activities all increase.

In contrast, according to the overflow hypothesis renal retention of sodium and water is the primary abnormality leading to the formation of ascites in the absence of central hypovolemia. The triggering event for primary renal sodium and water retention is unclear and is postulated to involve a hepatorenal reflex, perhaps via an intrahepatic baroreceptor mechanism.

The most recent hypothesis, which attempts to reconcile the underfill and overflow hypotheses, is the peripheral arterial vasodilatation hypothesis, in which peripheral vasodilatation is thought to be the initiating event, possibly triggered by endotoxin and cytokines, which reach the portal vein as a result of increased intestinal permeability, and mediated by nitric oxide. (The same factors may account for the formation of arteriovenous shunts seen in the splanchnic, dermal, and pulmonary circulations of patients with cirrhosis.) Peripheral vasodilatation leads to sodium retention as well as a decrease in systemic blood pressure and increase in cardiac output. These physiologic changes may result in an increase in the absolute plasma volume, but not enough to refill the enlarged arterial compartment or to suppress the release of norepinephrine, renin, aldosterone, and vasopressin, all of which contribute to renal sodium and water retention. Paradoxically, plasma levels of atrial natriuretic factor are markedly elevated in patients with severe ascites refractory to diuretics, but not to levels sufficient to overcome the antinatriuretic effects of the renin-angiotensin-aldosterone system.

Ascites indicates decompensated liver disease. The 5 year survival of patients with decompensated cirrhosis is 30 percent, compared with an 80 percent survival for those with compensated cirrhosis. Parameters that correlate with a poor prognosis include small liver size, malnutrition, low urine sodium concentration, high plasma norepinephrine level, low mean arterial pressure, and low glomerular filtration rate. Ascites contributes to the morbidity and mortality associated with cirrhosis by restricting ventilation and leading to umbilical hernias, peripheral venous stasis, and spontaneous bacterial peritonitis.

Management

In any patient with new or worsening ascites, it is important first to perform an abdominal paracentesis with fluid analysis to exclude spontaneous bacterial peritonitis, malignant ascites, chylous ascites, and ascites due to hepatic congestion. Table 1 outlines routine ascitic fluid tests that are helpful. The serum-ascites albumin gradient (SAAG) is a particularly useful marker of the presence or absence of portal hypertension. A SAAG greater than or equal to 1.1 g per deciliter is suggestive of portal hypertension, whereas a SAAG of less than 1.1 g per deciliter suggests that the ascites is not caused by portal hypertension.

Table 1 Ascitic Fluid Tests

ROUTINE	OPTIONAL	SELECTED CASES
Cell count	Total protein	Smear and culture for tuberculosis
Albumin (1st tap)	Glucose	Cytology
Culture (inoculation in blood culture bottles)	Lactic dehydrogenase	Triglycerides
Gram's stain	Amylase	Bilirubin

Bed Rest and Low-Sodium Diet

Bed rest is advocated as an initial measure. Upright posture in patients with cirrhosis and ascites activates the renin-angiotensin and alpha-adrenergic systems, thereby increasing renal tubular sodium reabsorption. Theoretically, bed rest reduces the plasma renin concentration. Restriction of sodium is prescribed but alone is generally not sufficient therapy, except in outpatients with minimal ascites. Salt restriction to 1 g per day is recommended but is difficult, and many patients are unable to comply. Restriction of water to about 1,000–1,500 ml daily is necessary only if the serum sodium is less than 125 mEq per liter. Impaired water excretion in cirrhosis is due to nonosmotic hypersecretion of vasopressin, decreased delivery of filtrate to the distal tubule in the kidney, and changes in local prostaglandin metabolism in the kidney. Demeclocycline, which antagonizes the renal effects of antidiuretic hormone, may correct the impaired water excretion in these patients but frequently induces renal failure.

Diuretics

Spironolactone is generally the first diuretic agent that is used in the management of ascites. Spironolactone is a mild diuretic that is a specific aldosterone antagonist and spares renal potassium secretion. It induces diuresis in up to 75 to 80 percent of patients, but because of its long half-life and that of its active metabolites, the onset of action of spironolactone is slow. The usual starting dose is 100 to 200 mg per day, initially in divided doses and then in a single daily dose. The dose can be increased by 100 mg every 3 to 5 days as needed up to a maximum of 400 to 600 mg per day, or until the urine sodium to potassium ratio is greater than 1. Potential deleterious side effects of spironolactone include hyperkalemia and painful gynecomastia.

Loop diuretics such as furosemide and bumetanide may be added in patients who respond partially to spironolactone. (Loop diuretics given alone are generally ineffective in the treatment of ascites.) Loop diuretics cause a 20 to 25 percent excretion of filtered sodium and increase the delivery of sodium to the distal tubule, where the ability to reabsorb sodium is exceeded. The usual starting dose of furosemide is 40 mg per day, and can be increased every 1 to 2 days to a maximum of 240 mg per day. Resistance to furosemide may result from impaired furosemide transport into renal tubules. Additionally, furosemide may result in a short-term, rapid decrease in renal perfusion, intravascular volume depletion, electrolyte abnormalities, and encephalopathy.

Thiazides act at the cortical diluting site and proximal tubule to promote natriuresis. In patients with ascites resistant to the aforementioned diuretics, the addition of thiazides may promote a synergistic effect. The usual starting dose of hydrochlorothiazide is 50 to 100 mg per day. Metolazone has the same effect and can be used at a dose of 5 to 10 mg per day.

Diuresis is safer in patients with peripheral edema associated with ascites than in those with ascites alone because of the preferential mobilization of edema. Conventionally, one should aim towards a weight loss of 1 to 2 kg per day in patients with ascites and peripheral edema, whereas a diuresis of 0.5 to 0.75 kg per day should be the goal in those with ascites alone. The urine sodium concentration is a helpful parameter to follow. When the baseline urine sodium is greater than 20 to 25 mEq per liter, treatment with low-dose spironolactone usually suffices. If the urine sodium concentration is in the range of 10 to 20 mEq per liter, high-dose spironolactone with or without low-dose furosemide will likely be required. Finally, when the urine sodium is less than 10 mEq per liter, high-dose spironolactone supplemented with furosemide and possibly thiazides will likely be needed. The dosing schedule requires individualization. A typical starting regimen is spironolactone 100 mg per day with or without furosemide 40 mg per day. The spironolactone can be increased by 100 mg per day and the furosemide by 40 mg per day every 3 to 5 days if no side effects are evident and natriuresis or weight loss have not been achieved. The combination of sodium restriction and diuretic therapy is effective in nearly 90 percent of patients with cirrhotic ascites. If weight loss does not ensue after a trial of maximal doses of diuretics, ascites is considered refractory to diuretic therapy.

Therapeutic Large-Volume Paracentesis

In the 1950s, large-volume paracentesis was the standard therapeutic modality for ascites. It fell out of favor in the 1960s because it was implicated as the cause of orthostatic hypotension, renal insufficiency, symptomatic hyponatremia, and hepatic encephalopathy, especially in cirrhotic patients without peripheral edema. These complications were ascribed to a reduction in intravascular volume due to rapid re-formation of ascites. However, reports of complications were based on limited numbers of patients, and in recent years large-volume paracentesis has re-emerged as a standard therapy for ascites.

In 1985, Kao and co-workers treated 18 patients with tense ascites and peripheral edema with a 5 L paracentesis, which resulted in relief of symptoms with no changes in plasma volume, electrolytes, or hemodynamics after 24 to 48 hours. Subsequent studies from the Barcelona group concluded that patients with tense ascites treated with large-volume paracentesis had shorter durations of hospitalization without an increase in the complication rate compared to those treated with diuretics. Their observations suggested that supplementation with intravenous albumin was necessary to decrease the frequency of electrolyte and renal disturbances associated with large-volume paracentesis. They and others also demonstrated that large-volume paracentesis could be done safely in patients with ascites but without peripheral edema. In 1987, Ginés et al. randomized 117 cirrhotic patients with tense ascites to large-volume paracentesis supplemented with intravenous albumin versus diuretic therapy alone; those who failed diuretics underwent placement of a peritoneovenous (LeVeen) shunt. There was no difference in survival between the two groups, but the complication rate was lower in the large-volume paracentesis group. Salerno and co-workers., 1987 found that diuretics and large-volume paracentesis plus intravenous albumin were equally effective in mobilizing ascites in 41 patients but that the results were achieved more rapidly with large-volume paracentesis than with diuretics alone. More recently, there have been studies to indicate that tense ascites in cirrhosis can be treated with a single total paracentesis within 1 to 2 hours without adverse renal, hepatic, or hormonal effects, provided intravascular volume is expanded with intravenous albumin. Because of the expense of supplementation with intravenous albumin, alternative synthetic plasma expanders have also been investigated, including dextran-70 and Hemaccel, a polymerized synthetic gelatin, but further study is required before they can be recommended.

One mitigating effect of large-volume paracentesis is the potential to increase the risk of peritonitis. Diuresis has been shown to increase ascitic fluid opsonic activity as well as serum and ascitic fluid complement levels, thereby leading to protection from spontaneous bacterial peritonitis. By contrast, after large-volume paracentesis, ascitic fluid opsonic activity and complement levels remain stable, but serum complement levels decrease, thereby potentially increasing the risk of spontaneous bacterial peritonitis.

In general, repeated large-volume paracentesis of 4 to 6 L per tap supplemented with intravenous albumin (10 gm per liter of ascites removed) is considered the treatment of choice for tense cirrhotic ascites. Compared to diuretic therapy, large-volume paracentesis is hemodynamically safe, shortens the duration of hospitalization, and does not increase the readmission rate to the hospital. Large-volume paracentesis should be considered specifically in patients with respiratory compromise, impending rupture of an umbilical hernia, and severe peripheral venous stasis. It is also appropriate therapy in patients with ascites and peripheral edema and in those with ascites refractory to diuretics. Whether or not large-volume paracentesis is performed, those patients who excrete high amounts of sodium in the urine benefit from salt-restriction and diuretics in the conventional fashion.

The effectiveness of beta-blocker therapy in the management of ascites has not been clearly demonstrated, despite the value of beta blockers in decreasing portal venous pressure and preventing variceal bleeding. Certain other medications must be specifically avoided in patients with cirrhotic ascites. These include prostaglandin inhibitors and angiotensin converting enzyme inhibitors. Prostaglandin inhibitors diminish the renal synthesis of vasodilatory prostaglandins (PGE_2 and PGI_2), may adversely affect renal function and natriuresis, and may decrease the natriuretic response to furosemide. Angiotensin converting enzyme inhibitors reduce urinary sodium excretion and lower blood pressure. Other drugs to avoid in patients with cirrhotic ascites include aminoglycosides, which are especially nephrotoxic, and metoclopramide, which may stimulate aldosterone production.

Peritoneovenous Shunt

A variety of therapeutic modalities may be considered in patients with ascites refractory to diuretics (Table 2). Head-out water immersion (HWI) is an effective treatment in some patients with refractory ascites and acts by expanding central blood volume and suppressing renin, aldosterone, vasopressin, and norepinephrine because of reflex vasodilatation.

Table 2 Therapeutic Modalities for Refractory Ascites

Large-volume paracentesis
Head-out water immersion
Peritoneovenous shunt: LeVeen, Denver
Transjugular intrahepatic portosystemic stent shunt (TIPS)
Portosystemic surgical shunt
Liver transplantation

Table 3 Common Complications of Peritoneovenous Shunts

Consumption coagulopathy
Infection
Volume overload
Shunt occlusion

However, use of HWI is cumbersome and is advocated primarily in developing countries where other measures may be too costly.

Peritoneovenous shunts may be considered when large-volume paracentesis and diuretics have failed. The two types of peritoneovenous shunts are the LeVeen and Denver shunts. The LeVeen shunt consists of a perforated intra-abdominal tube connected through a one-way pressure-sensitive valve to a silicone tube that traverses the subcutaneous tissue up to the neck and enters one of the jugular veins. The tip of the intravenous tube is positioned in the superior vena cava near the right atrium or in the right atrium itself. When intraperitoneal pressure exceeds venous pressure by 3 to 5 cm H_2O, the valve opens and ascitic fluid flows into the circulation. Mobilization of ascitic fluid by the LeVeen shunt is associated with continuous expansion of the intravascular compartment. The Denver shunt has a valve which opens at a pressure gradient lower than that of the LeVeen shunt or when the pumping chamber is externally compressed. The Denver shunt was designed to create turbulence within the valve so as to reduce the likelihood of valve obstruction, which is frequently observed with the LeVeen shunt, but the frequency of obstruction of the two shunts is similar. Patients with high-protein ascites seem to be particularly prone to shunt obstruction.

Peritoneovenous shunts relieve ascites while simultaneously correcting most of the hemodynamic and renal alterations occurring in these patients. They increase plasma volume and cardiac index; reduce plasma renin activity and plasma levels of aldosterone, norepinephrine, and vasopressin; and lead to a reduction in portal venous pressure, as estimated by the hepatic venous pressure gradient. Immediately after insertion of a peritoneovenous shunt, central volume fluid overload is commonly observed and supplemental furosemide is routinely administered.

The complication rate of the peritoneovenous shunts is high (Table 3). Foremost among the complications are a consumptive coagulopathy caused by delivery of plasmin, plasminogen activator, thromboplastin, and fibrin degradation products to the systemic circulation, and infection, which usually requires removal of the shunt. Recurrent or persistent ascites may result from cardiac and renal failure, decreased shunt flow, or shunt occlusion. Doppler ultrasonography or scintigraphy after the intraperitoneal injection of radioactive technetium will demonstrate the absence of flow through an occluded shunt. Insertion of a 3 cm long titanium tip into the venous limb of the LeVeen shunt is of value in preventing superior vena cava thrombosis. A new heparin-coated Denver shunt has also been advocated for similar purposes.

While peritoneovenous shunts are effective for the initial relief of ascites, long-term efficacy has not been established and ultimate patient survival is not improved. In one large study by Stanley and co-workers, 1989, 299 alcoholic cirrhotic patients with ascites were randomized to medical treatment or LeVeen shunting. LeVeen shunting was associated with more rapid resolution of disabling ascites and a longer time to recurrence of ascites. However, survival was not improved by shunting and correlated instead with the severity of the underlying liver disease. Peritoneovenous shunting has not been compared in a similar fashion with large-volume paracentesis.

Transjugular Intrahepatic Portosystemic Stent Shunts

Recently, a transjugular intrahepatic portosystemic shunt using an expandable metal stent (TIPSS) has been introduced as a simple, safe, fast, and inexpensive method of creating a portosystemic shunt without the need for surgery. TIPSS is already being used widely in the management of gastroesophageal variceal hemorrhage. Because TIPSS functions as a side-to-side portacaval anastomosis, it is of potential value in the management of ascites and the hepatorenal syndrome. Preliminary reports indicate that after placement of a TIPSS, ascites disappears or is ameliorated. Clinical improvement is accompanied by an increase in creatinine clearance and improvement in nutritional status. By reducing portal venous pressure and blood flow through esophageal varices, the risk of bleeding from varices is also substantially reduced. TIPSS is a particularly attractive procedure for seriously ill patients awaiting liver transplantation.

Reports of complications of TIPSS have begun to appear. The most frequent complication is hepatic encephalopathy, which affects 20 percent of patients but tends to be mild and easily managed. Another common complication is stent stenosis, which occurs in up to 15 percent of patients and progresses to occlusion in 30 percent. Other complications include embolization of the stent to the pulmonary artery, puncture of the gallbladder, liver capsule rupture, hemobilia, intraperitoneal hemorrhage, contrast-induced transient oliguric kidney failure, bacteremia, septic shock, and fever. TIPSS may be considered in selected patients with ascites, but determining its final place in the treatment of refractory ascites will require studies comparing TIPSS with other treatment options.

Other Modalities

Portosystemic surgical shunts are used as a last resort in the management of refractory ascites. A side-to-side portacaval shunt decompresses both the splanchnic and hepatic sinusoidal bed and is therefore advantageous when compared to the end-to-side portacaval shunt, which decompresses the splanchnic bed but not the hepatic sinusoids. In selected patients with refractory ascites, liver transplantation may also be considered.

■ COMPLICATIONS OF ASCITES AND THEIR MANAGEMENT

Spontaneous Bacterial Peritonitis

Spontaneous bacterial peritonitis (SBP) may be defined as the occurrence of bacterial peritonitis in patients with ascites in the absence of a demonstrable cause of peritonitis, such as bowel perforation or intra-abdominal abscess. Among patients with cirrhotic ascites, the frequency of SBP is 10 to 27 percent. In liver units dedicated to the treatment of ascites, SBP may be diagnosed as many as three times a day and at least once a week. SBP classically occurs in patients with alcoholic cirrhosis, and, initially, it was thought that there was a special relationship between alcoholic cirrhosis and SBP. However, SBP has been reported in patients with a variety of liver disorders, including acute viral hepatitis, chronic active hepatitis, postnecrotic cirrhosis, submassive hepatic necrosis, Wilson's disease, and alpha$_1$-antitrypsin deficiency. The unifying feature of conditions that predispose to SBP is a low protein concentration in the ascitic fluid. Patients who have ascites with a high protein concentration (e.g., ascites due to heart failure or peritoneal carcinomatosis) are unlikely to develop SBP.

Other host factors predisposing to SBP include the severity of the underlying acute or chronic liver disease, which is reflected in reticuloendothelial dysfunction, neutrophil dysfunction, complement deficiency, and impairment in opsonization. Procedures that may predispose to SBP include paracentesis, bladder catheterization, nasogastric intubation, tooth extraction, endoscopic procedures including variceal sclerotherapy, and insertion of LeVeen shunts. Seeding of ascitic fluid generally occurs as a result of hematogenous transmission of organisms from the intestinal lumen or from an extraintestinal focus of infection. Common causative organisms include *Streptococcus pneumoniae,* group D streptococci, alpha-hemolytic streptococci, and gram-negative enteric organisms, whereas anaerobes rarely cause SBP.

Patients with SBP are usually men with a mean age of 50 years and severe advanced hepatic disease (varices, splenomegaly, and jaundice in greater than 85 to 90 percent of patients). The clinical features of SBP include ascites, fever, new-onset or worsening encephalopathy, abdominal pain, rebound abdominal tenderness, decreased or absent bowel sounds, and hypotension. In 10 percent of cases, fever and abdominal pain are absent, and in 30 percent of patients only subtle findings are observed, including mild hepatic encephalopathy, back pain, hypothermia, refractoriness to diuretics, and deteriorating renal function.

The diagnosis of SBP is supported by the characteristics of the ascitic fluid on paracentesis. The fluid may be cloudy and the protein content is typically low. The most reliable indicator of SBP is an ascitic fluid polymorphonuclear leukocyte (PMN) count of greater than 250 per cubic millimeter in association with characteristic clinical features. Even in the absence of signs and symptoms of SBP, an ascitic fluid PMN count of more than 500 per cubic millimeter strongly suggests SBP. Gram's stain is positive in 30 to 70 percent of centrifuged ascitic fluid specimens. It is important to submit the ascitic fluid for bacterial culture and, if indicated, cultures for tuberculosis. When ascitic fluid from patients with suspected SBP is inoculated into blood culture bottles at the bedside, up to 90 percent of specimens yield a positive diagnosis. Occasionally, blood cultures are positive while ascitic fluid cultures are negative.

Spontaneous bacterial peritonitis must be distinguished from secondary bacterial peritonitis. Features that suggest secondary bacterial peritonitis include an initial ascitic fluid white blood cell count of greater than 10,000 per cubic millimeter, an ascitic fluid protein concentration of greater than 2 per deciliter and multiple bacterial pathogens, including anaerobes.

The treatment of choice for SBP is now cefotaxime 2 g intravenously every 8 hours, pending culture results. Alternatively, amoxicillin-clavulanic acid may be used. Cefotaxime is preferable to regimens that include aminoglycosides, which are potentially nephrotoxic. Treatment is generally continued for up to 10 to 14 days, and paracentesis should be repeated after 48 hours of therapy to confirm a decline in the ascitic fluid PMN count by at least 50 percent.

The mortality of SBP in earlier reports was 80 to 90 percent. In more recent times, mortality rates of 30 to 40 percent have been reported. Adverse prognostic factors include a serum bilirubin level greater than 8 mg per deciliter, serum albumin less than 2.5 g per deciliter, serum creatinine greater than 2.1 mg per deciliter, hepatic encephalopathy, and the development of hepatorenal syndrome. Recurrence of SBP is common in patients surviving one episode, with an approximately 70 percent recurrence rate at 1 year and a high mortality rate. Recent studies suggest that the risk of recurrent SBP can be decreased greatly by the long-term prophylactic use of norfloxacin 400 mg orally once a day. In selected high-risk patients (e.g., those undergoing variceal sclerotherapy), first episodes of SBP may be prevented by initiating therapy with norfloxacin 400 mg once daily.

Hepatorenal Syndrome

The hepatorenal syndrome, the most severe alteration of renal function that occurs in patients with cirrhosis and ascites, is defined as the development of azotemia and oliguria in the absence of any known cause of renal failure. The kidneys are histologically normal or show minimal findings to account for impairment in renal function. Retrospective studies indicate that the hepatorenal syndrome is present in more than 15 percent of patients admitted to the hospital with cirrhosis and ascites. The condition is believed to be a consequence of active renal vasoconstriction leading to impaired renal perfusion and a decrease in the glomerular filtration rate. Contributory pathogenic factors include elevated thromboxane and endothelin levels, impaired renal kallikrein production, and diminished renal synthesis of vasodilating prostaglandins.

The prognosis of hepatorenal syndrome is poor. Attempts to improve renal function in patients with hepatorenal syndrome have included the infusion of renal vasodilators or prostaglandin excretion modifiers and insertion of a peritoneovenous shunt, but in most cases these measures are unsuccessful. In selected cases, patients with the hepatorenal syndrome may be considered for liver transplantation.

Suggested Reading

Arroyo V, Ginés P, Gerbes AL, et al. Definition and diagnostic criteria of refractory ascites and hepatorenal syndrome in cirrhosis. Hepatology 1996; 23:164–176.

Badalamenti S, Graziani G, Salerno F, Ponticelli C. Hepatorenal syndrome: new perspectives in pathogenesis and treatment. Arch Intern Med 1993; 153:1957–1967.

Ginés P, Arroyo V, Rodés J. Pharmacotherapy of ascites associated with cirrhosis. Drugs 1992; 43:316–332.

Kellerman PS, Linas SL. Large-volume paracentesis in treatment of ascites. Ann Intern Med 1990; 112:889–891.

Moskovitz M. The peritoneovenous shunt: expectations and reality. Am J Gastroenterol 1990; 85:917–929.

Ochs A, Rössle M, Haag K, et al. The transjugular intrahepatic portosystemic stent-shunt procedure for refractory ascites. N Engl J Med 1995; 332:1192–1197.

Runyon BA. Care of patients with ascites. N Engl J Med 1994; 330:337–342.

Runyon BA. Spontaneous bacterial peritonitis: an explosion of information. Hepatology 1988; 8:171–175.

Schrier RW, Arroyo V, Bernardi M, et al. Peripheral arterial vasodilatation hypothesis: a proposal for the initiation of renal sodium and water retention in cirrhosis. Hepatology 1988; 8:1151–1157.

Warner L, Sorecki K, Blendis L, Epstein M. Atrial natriuretic factor and liver disease. Hepatology 1993; 17:500–513.

PORTAL HYPERTENSION

Paul J. Thuluvath, M.D., M.R.C.P.

The portal vein, about 5 to 8 cm long, is formed by the union of superior mesenteric vein and the splenic vein. In a normal man, the portal blood flow is about 1,200 ml per minute and the portal pressure is less than 8 mm Hg. Although the portal pressure can be measured directly by percutaneous (transhepatic or intrasplenic) or operative catheterization, it is usually measured indirectly as the difference between the wedged and the free pressure of a hepatic venous radicle (hepatic venous pressure gradient) using a balloon catheter. The indirect pressure reading usually reflects the true portal pressure except in presinusoidal portal hypertension where it may underestimate the true pressure. Obstruction to the portal venous blood flow along its course, or rarely from increased portal blood flow as in tropical splenomegaly, results in portal hypertension. Depending on the site of lesion, the portal hypertension may be classified as prehepatic (e.g., portal vein thrombosis, tropical splenomegaly), hepatic presinusoidal (e.g., schistosomiasis, sarcoidosis, idiopathic), hepatic postsinusoidal (e.g., cirrhosis, acute alcoholic hepatitis), or posthepatic (veno-occlusive disease). A combination of clinical history, physical findings, duplex-Doppler scans, liver biopsy, wedged hepatic venous pressure readings and angiography will allow the clinician to localize the site of the lesion. A detailed discussion of the various causes of portal hypertension is beyond the scope of this chapter, but it is important to recognize that the major cause in developed countries is cirrhosis whereas schistosomiasis and noncirrhotic portal hypertension (idiopathic portal hypertension or neonatal portal vein thrombosis) account for a significant proportion of portal hypertension in the developing countries.

The pathogenesis of portal hypertension in cirrhosis is a combination of increased portal vascular resistance and a hyperdynamic circulation. The portal vascular resistance is increased in cirrhosis due to the morphological changes and the hemodynamic changes within hepatic vasculature. The hyperdynamic systemic and splanchnic circulation is caused by an increase in vasoactive mediators and a reduced sensitivity to vasoconstrictors. When portal pressure exceeds a certain level (usually 12 mm Hg), due to the unique anatomy of portal venous system, a remarkable collateral circulation develops to decompress the portal system. Despite this collateral circulation, the portal pressure is often sustained due to increased hyperdynamic splanchnic and systemic circulation, and perhaps due to enhanced portocollateral resistance.

Clinical consequences of portal hypertension include ascites, gastroesophageal varices, hypersplenism, and hepatic encephalopathy. Of all the complications of portal hypertension, variceal bleeding is perhaps the most dangerous. Approximately 30 percent of all patients with documented varices bleed during their lifetime, usually (80 percent) within 24 months after diagnosis. Of those who bleed, 30 to 50 percent die from the first bleed. Fifty to 100 percent of those who survive the first bleed will rebleed within 2 years; most bleed within 6 weeks after the first bleed. Thirty percent of all deaths in cirrhotics could be directly attributed to gastroesophageal variceal bleeding.

The prophylaxis against the initial variceal bleeding, the management of acute bleeding and the prevention of recurrent variceal bleeding are all important aspects of the management of portal hypertension and are discussed in this chapter. The management of ascites and hepatic encephalopathy are discussed elsewhere.

MANAGEMENT OF ACUTE VARICEAL BLEEDING

Management may be divided into (1) general resuscitative measures and (2) specific treatment aimed at arresting the variceal bleeding. Aspiration of blood and gastric contents is a major cause of morbidity and mortality in patients with variceal bleeding. Patients may be drowsy and may have reduced pharyngeal reflexes.

Resuscitation

Endotracheal intubation may be necessary in an encephalopathic patient particularly to safeguard the patient during the placement of balloon tamponade or for endoscopic procedures. Pulse oximetry to assess oxygen saturation and thereby to titrate supplemental oxygen through nasal canulae should be mandatory in a patient with active hemorrhage.

Venous access should be safeguarded by using two or three large-bore peripheral venous cannulae. Central venous pressure (CVP) and pulmonary capillary wedged pressure (PCWP) measures provide important hemodynamic information which facilitates optimum resuscitation but require expertise for placement and pressure recording. Assessment of blood loss by patients or family members is often inaccurate. Hematemesis is almost always overestimated; conversely, significant blood loss may occur without hematemesis. Tachycardia and postural hypotension are useful indicators, but the presence of autonomic neuropathy may influence these measurements. Repeated (over a few hours) hemoglobin and hematocrit provide important serial assessments of blood volume loss and the response to replacement. Measurement of CVP is a sensitive guide to the blood volume status but caution should be exercised in the presence of tense ascites since diaphragmatic compression of the right atrium by the ascites may lead to an overestimation of the readings. PCWP, measured using a pulmonary flotation catheter, is the most accurate guide to control blood volume and may be invaluable in the presence of major ongoing bleeding.

Blood volume restitution should be prompt and as accurate as possible to protect vital organs, particularly renal function. For practical purposes, one tries to maintain the CVP around 5 to 10 mm Hg. The ideal replacement fluid is blood to maintain the oxygen-carrying capacity of the circulation. Colloid is reserved for immediate infusion until blood becomes available. I prefer gelatin-based colloid solutions since they have less effect on platelet function, partial thromboplastin, and bleeding time, compared with dextran or hydroxy ethyl starch.

Isovolemic replacement should be the aim with care taken to avoid major overexpansion of the circulation which may precipitate further bleeding due to the associated increase in portal pressure. Furthermore, excessive transfusion may worsen thrombocytopenia and cause deficiency of clotting factors either due to disseminated intravascular coagulation or hemodilution. These abnormalities are seen usually after 9 to 15 units of blood are transfused. The role of platelets and fresh frozen plasma is not well established in the management of variceal hemorrhage, but as a general rule it is given when platelet counts are below 50,000 and prothrombin time is prolonged more than 50 percent. The use of fresh frozen plasma every 5 units of blood transfused and platelet transfusion every 8 units is a common practice. Other possible complications of massive transfusion include pulmonary microembolism, citrate toxicity, and consequent hypocalcemia and hyperkalemia.

Infection is common after hemorrhage. There is little evidence to support prophylactic antibiotics, however, care should be taken to detect such complications as aspiration pneumonia and spontaneous bacterial peritonitis at the earliest opportunity and to treat aggressively.

Specific Treatment

Since bleeding from a nonvariceal source is not uncommon in chronic liver disease, early endoscopy (after initial resuscitation) is essential to guide specific therapy. There are very few circumstances in which it is justified to initiate specific therapy for variceal bleeding without endoscopic confirmation of the bleeding point.

Endoscopic Therapy

Evidence to support injection sclerotherapy as an important technique for the treatment of active variceal bleeding came from two uncontrolled reports which claimed success rate of over 90 percent. Since then, a number of randomized controlled studies have confirmed its efficacy with control of bleeding in 75 to 90 percent of cases. It is now generally accepted that immediate sclerotherapy is the optimum treatment for active variceal bleeding, but is critically dependent upon available expertise to attain these high success rates and to minimize complications.

An important question that remained unanswered was the optimum timing of injection sclerotherapy with respect to the bleeding episode. The options are immediate treatment with the associated technical difficulties, or delayed treatment after temporary hemostasis is achieved using vasoconstrictive drugs or balloon tamponade. A recent randomized controlled study showed that at 12 hours after presentation, sclerotherapy was superior to vasoconstrictor therapy (88 percent versus 65 percent) for immediate control. The admission mortality was less in the immediate sclerotherapy group than in those managed by vasoconstrictor therapy, but it was not statistically significant (27 percent versus 39 percent).

It is disappointing to note that none of the well-designed trials have shown a consistent reduction in rebleeding (about 30 percent) or in-hospital mortality with sclerotherapy when compared to other modes of treatment. It is possible that the mortality in this group of patients (mainly Child-Pugh Grade C) is determined at an early stage of the bleeding episode, before the institution of treatment and thus masking the benefits of the therapeutic modality applied.

The last 5 years has seen the development and evaluation of two new endoscopic techniques. The tissue adhesive n-butyl-2-cyanoacrylate (Histacryl) solidifies almost instantaneously when brought into contact with blood and by intravariceal injection may produce rapid obliteration of the vessel lumen. The disadvantage is that it has to be handled very carefully, otherwise endoscopic channels may be occluded. Two studies have claimed control of bleeding in approximately 90 percent of cases and of particular note is its use to obliterate fundal varices which respond unreliably to intravarix injection of sclerosant. Reports of cerebral toxicity are a major concern and at present are a restraint on widespread use.

The ability to apply prestressed bands (endoscopic band ligation) to the varices has recently been developed with proven efficacy for both the control of active bleeder and subsequent prevention of rebleeding. A recent meta-analysis has shown that endoscopic banding achieved hemostasis comparable to sclerotherapy in patients with active variceal bleeding. However, no specific benefits have been shown for

Table 1 Control of Variceal Bleeding: Summary of Controlled Studies Using Vasopressin (VP), Glypressin (GP), VP + Nitroglycerine (NG), and Somatostatin (ST)

AUTHOR*	PLACEBO	VP	GP	VP + NG	ST
Conn 1975 (33)	25%	71%			
Fogel 1982 (33)	37%	29%			
Freeman 1989 (31)	37%		60%		
Soderland 1990 (60)	55%		84%		
Tsai 1986 (39)		47%		55% (SL)	
Gimson 1986 (72)		41%		73% (IV)	
Bosch 1990 (65)		48%		65% (TD)	
Valanzuela 1989 (84)	83%				65%
Burroughs 1990 (12)	41%				64%

*Number of bleeding episodes within parentheses.
SL, sublingual NG; IV, intravenous NG; TD, transdermal NG.

this technique over injection sclerotherapy during active bleeding.

Drug Therapy

The major benefit of pharmacologic therapy is that it can be given immediately without any specialized training. An effective agent offers immediate therapy to hospitals in which the expertise to carry out endoscopic or surgical intervention is lacking and may facilitate transfer of patients to more specialized centers. To date, the low efficacy and complications associated with drugs available have proved a major limitation. The safety margin of the newer preparations appear to be better as discussed in the following section.

Vasopressin and Glypressin. Vasopressin is a peptide hormone which has important splanchnic arterial vasoconstrictor properties, thereby reducing portal blood flow and portal pressure. Glypressin (triglycyl lysine vasopressin) is a prodrug which is converted to lysine vasopressin in vivo. The slow release from the prodrug may explain its prolonged effect (up to 6 hours). This drug has properties similar to those of vasopressin, but can be given as bolus doses (2 mg IV every 4 to 6 hours) through a peripheral line (since it is inactive before conversion) unlike vasopressin which must be given as a continuous infusion (0.4 unit per minute, increased if necessary to 0.8 unit per minute) through a central line. This may be beneficial if patients are being transferred to a specialized center.

The main side effects of vasopressin and glypressin are secondary to nonselective arterial vasoconstriction. These include ischemia of the myocardium, abdominal viscera and lower limbs, left heart failure, hypertension, and arrhythmias. In randomized, controlled studies, up to 25 percent of patients have been withdrawn because of major side effects. Selective infusion of vasopressin into the superior mesenteric artery has not been shown to overcome these adverse effects or improve efficacy.

In a number of studies, a combination of vasopressin and nitroglycerine has been shown to reduce the hemodynamic side effects of vasopressin without attenuating the effect on portal inflow (Table 1). The transdermal route may be preferred because of ease of administration.

There is a wide range (29 to 84 percent) of reported efficacy of vasopressin and glypressin which is difficult to explain (Table 1). There is now little to justify the use of vasopressin as a single agent. Despite vasopressin being the active moiety of glypressin this agent does appear to offer enhanced control of bleeding and fewer side effects. The addition of nitroglycerine to vasopressin is of proven benefit and should be an integral part of such therapy.

Somatostatin and Octreotide. Somatostatin is a 14 amino acid peptide hormone. It has a short half-life (1 to 2 minutes) and has to be given as a continuous intravenous infusion (250 μg bolus dose followed by 250 μg hourly). Octreotide (Sandostatin) is a cyclic octopeptide analogue which shares 4 amino acids with somatostatin. It has a longer half-life (1 to 2 hours) and can be used subcutaneously, but a recent study has shown that it may not be very effective given that way. For active bleeding it is administered as continuous infusion (50 μg per hour). Both drugs cause splanchnic vasoconstriction by a direct effect on vascular smooth muscle and possibly by inhibiting the release of vasodilatory peptides such as glucagon. Although both drugs reduce portosystemic collateral blood flow (measured by azygos blood flow), in cirrhotic patients the effect on portal pressure has been variable.

The results of two placebo-based, randomized, controlled studies of somatostatin have provided conflicting results. Whereas Burroughs and co-workers showed significant benefit for the somatostatin group (64 versus 41), Valanzuela et al. in a multicenter trial involving 84 patients claimed a completely opposite effect (65 percent versus 83 percent). The very high success rate in the placebo group in this latter study has not previously been observed in any study and may be artifactual reflecting recruitment into the trial of small number of patients from multiple centers. Trials comparing somatostatin with vasopressin have shown the former to be marginally superior for the control of variceal bleeding and to be associated with very few side effects (Table 1).

Two studies have compared somatostatin with tamponade and one study compared octreotide with tamponade. All three studies confirmed similar efficacy for somatostatin or its analogue as compared to balloon tamponade (58 to 71 percent versus 50 to 80 percent respectively). Two recent studies have shown that intravenous somatostatin and octreotide have similar efficacy to injection sclerotherapy. The excellent safety margin of these drugs allows their use in the emergency department while the patient is resuscitated and also over the first few days to prevent early rebleeding. A recent study confirmed that a combination of sclerotherapy and continuous infusion of octreotide for 5 days was superior to sclerotherapy alone in reducing early rebleeding and mortality. However, use of long-term subcutaneous octreotide in combination with sclerotherapy has not been shown to improve the rebleeding rate or mortality compared to sclerotherapy alone. Continuous infusion of octreotide also has been shown to be very effective in reducing bleeding from post-sclerotherapy esophageal ulceration.

Metoclopramide, Domperidone, and Pentagastrin

These drugs are known to constrict the lower esophageal sphincter and have been shown to reduce varix pressure. A single trial has suggested short-term benefit of these drugs for the control of bleeding, an observation that requires further confirmation.

Balloon Tamponade

Balloon tamponade is a highly effective method of controlling active variceal bleeding. Controlled studies have shown that, in experienced hands, it is superior to pharmacologic agents and is equivalent to sclerotherapy for the immediate control of bleeding. However, efficacy extends only to the period of application and in inexperienced hands the morbidity and mortality may be unacceptably high. Balloon tamponade is best reserved for the management of life-threatening bleeding when a risk of exsanguination exists and endoscopic intervention is unlikely to be feasible.

Surgery

While endoscopic therapy at the time of diagnostic endoscopy probably is the optimum approach to an episode of variceal bleeding, surgical intervention has an important and increasing role, particularly in patients who continue to bleed despite early injection sclerotherapy or banding. Most workers would repeat endoscopic therapy on a second occasion before considering it to have failed. However, the decision to progress to surgery should not be further delayed in order to prevent the inevitable escalation of operative risks in a deteriorating patient. Bleeding from fundal varices, frequently difficult to diagnose and even more difficult to treat, is a second major indication for surgical therapy. The types of surgery may be divided into shunt and nonshunt procedures. The choice of surgery depends on the local expertise, severity of the liver disease and suitability of the patient for future liver transplantation. There is a subsequent chapter on portal hypertension surgery.

All established shunt procedures have been used to manage active variceal bleeding although the technical difficulties and operating time associated with the selective distal splenorenal shunt makes this generally unsuitable as an emergency procedure. Shunt surgery, especially mesocaval and distal splenorenal shunts, does not preclude subsequent transplantation. The operative mortality of shunting procedures in severe liver disease has been high but in two controlled studies portocaval shunting was shown to be of equivalent benefit to injection sclerotherapy for the management of active bleeding.

Various types of nonshunting procedures are available to control variceal bleeding, but the most common is esophageal transection with varying degrees of devascularization. Three controlled trials have compared sclerotherapy with esophageal transection plus or minus devascularization for control of active variceal hemorrhage. Although there was a trend towards improved control of bleeding with esophageal transection, the survival rates were not different between the groups. However, these studies have confirmed the importance of esophageal transection as a "rescue" procedure for patients who fail endoscopic therapy. The only major concern that arises from the use of devascularization procedures is the adverse effect on liver transplantation. Extensive scar tissue or adhesions, particularly at the hilum, may markedly increase the technical difficulties of transplantation and exacerbate blood loss.

Gastric Varices

The incidence of gastric varices in published reports varies from 6 to 16 percent. Gastric varices are usually seen in association with esophageal varices or rarely in isolation as in splenic vein thrombosis (segmental portal hypertension). The overall mortality from bleeding gastric varices is over 50 percent. Although the management of gastric varices is similar to that of esophageal varices, endoscopic sclerotherapy using sclerosants should be reserved only for lesser curve varices or varices within a hiatus hernia. Tissue adhesives or thrombin may be used to inject fundal varices after the initial bleeding has stopped. It is technically difficult to inject fundal varices when they are actively bleeding. If balloon tamponade is unsuccessful in patients with bleeding fundal varices, one should proceed immediately to transjugular intrahepatic portosystemic shunting (TIPSS) or surgery. Splenectomy is curative when varices are seen in association with splenic vein thrombosis.

Ectopic Varices

Bleeding from nongastroesophageal sites varies from 1.6 to 5 percent in the large reported series. The common ectopic sites, usually seen in association with esophageal varices, are duodenum, colon, anorectum, and enterostomy. Rarely these varices may be localized, especially in the colon, and result from superior or inferior vein thrombosis, tumor infiltration, adhesions, or congenital malformation.

The management of the bleeding depends on the site of bleeding, the severity of liver disease and the local expertise. Since there are no controlled studies, it is difficult to recommend any special strategy. Shunt surgery may be the best line of management for bleeding varices in the duodenum, jejunum, ileum, and enterostomy. If the expertise for TIPSS is available, that should be considered as the first line of management before other forms of shunt surgery. Anecdotal reports suggest that duodenal varices and ileostomy varices can be managed successfully by sclerotherapy or feeding vessel embolization, but one has to consider carefully the postsclerotherapy complications like duodenal perforation and stoma dysfunction and the high recurrence rate after embolization. Colonic varices are usually localized and can be managed by local resection. Again when it is seen in association with esophageal varices, TIPSS may be a safer alternative. Anorectal varices can be safely treated with sclerotherapy or by underrunning with an absorbable suture.

Portal Hypertensive Gastropathy

The prevalence of gastrointestinal hemorrhage from gastric mucosal lesions in patients with portal hypertension has been estimated to be between 10 and 60 percent; it is the second most common cause of bleeding in portal hypertension. The risk from mucosal bleeding seems to increase after variceal obliteration by banding or sclerotherapy. The diagnosis of portal hypertensive gastropathy is based on the endoscopic appearance and the histologic features. In mild form the mucosa is hyperemic with multiple, small erythematous areas outlined by a white network (mosaic pattern) and in severe form, cherry red spots or diffuse mucosal hemorrhages are seen. These lesions are seen throughout the stomach, but rarely can be localized in the antrum when it may be difficult to distinguish it from watermelon stomach. In doubtful cases characteristic histology (mucosal dilatation of capillaries with edema but without significant inflammation, and submucosal dilatation of veins) may prove useful.

The pathogenesis of these lesions is not completely understood, but portal hypertension and increased gastric blood flow with alteration in microvascular mucosal blood flow are thought to be involved. Although the risk of death from mucosal bleeding is low compared to variceal bleeding, often bleeding is sufficient to require multiple transfusions or hepatic decompensation. Shunt surgery is very effective to arrest the bleeding from portal hypertensive gastropathy, but carries significant mortality.

Two open studies and one randomized, controlled study have shown that propranolol may significantly reduce the rebleeding rate. In the 1991 randomized study in 54 cirrhotic patients, 65 percent of those who received propranolol remained free of bleeding at 12 months and 52 percent at 30 months compared to 38 percent and 7 percent in the control group; multivariant analysis showed that the absence of propranolol treatment was the only predictive variable for rebleeding. The mode of action of propranolol in portal hypertensive gastropathy is unclear but may be a combination of reducing portal pressure and altering the blood flow pattern in gastric microcirculation. Although TIPSS has not been evaluated in any controlled studies, anecdotal evidence suggests that it is very effective and may become the standard treatment in patients who fail propranolol treatment.

■ PREVENTION OF RECURRENT VARICEAL BLEEDING (SECONDARY PROPHYLAXIS)

A number of options are available to prevent recurrent bleeding, including endoscopic sclerotherapy, endoscopic banding, propranolol, shunt surgery, esophageal transection, liver transplantation, and more recently TIPSS.

Long-Term Injection Sclerotherapy

A number of controlled trials have assessed the efficacy of this form of treatment in reducing the rebleeding rate and mortality. These trials showed an improvement in rebleeding rate, but only three studies showed improved survival. Two meta-analyses have been performed on these controlled trials to clarify the data further. Both showed a significant improvement in survival and reduction in rebleeding rate; however one must interpret these studies with caution since the meta-analysis included heterogeneous studies in which the control arm often received less effective treatment. In spite of these reservations, until recently sclerotherapy was considered the "gold standard" for prevention of recurrent variceal bleeding.

The optimal time interval between the endoscopic sessions is not known. Two studies have compared sclerotherapy at 1 and 3 week intervals and showed that 1 week was probably better than 3 weeks to reduce rebleeding rate as well as for rapid obliteration of varices. On the basis of current evidence I recommend one weekly injection during the first 3 to 4 weeks and thereafter two to three weekly depending on the size of varices and the ulceration. The duration of follow-up after the variceal obliteration is an area of controversy. There are no data to suggest that long-term endoscopic follow-up after variceal obliteration is superior to short-term treatment aimed at obliteration of varices. It may not be necessary to have endoscopic follow-up in patients who are maintained on beta blockers.

Endoscopic Banding

A number of studies have compared sclerotherapy with banding. These studies have shown that banding is similar to sclerotherapy, but banding may have a slight advantage in terms of the number of sessions required and the treatment-related complication rate. A meta-analysis performed on seven randomized, controlled studies suggested that banding was superior to sclerotherapy in reducing the rebleeding rate (odds ratio 0.52, 95 percent confidence interval [CI] 0.37 to 0.74) and the mortality rate (odds ratio 0.67, CI 0.46 to 0.98). Esophageal stricture occurred less frequently with banding, but other complications like bleeding from esophageal ulceration, pulmonary infection and peritonitis were similar. On the basis of this study, endoscopic banding is preferable to sclerotherapy for secondary prophylaxis.

Beta Blockers

Nonselective beta blockers reduce portal pressure by reducing cardiac output, and by reducing portal inflow via antagonism of the $beta_2$ receptors on the splanchnic vessels. Beta blockers also may increase porto-collateral resistance and hence reduce collateral blood flow.

Results of a meta-analysis by Hayes and co-workers of secondary prevention studies comparing propranolol with placebo showed that propranolol can reduce the bleeding rate by 39 percent (CI 30,46) and bleeding-related mortality by 40 percent (CI 17,57). The bleeding rate on propranolol in these trials was similar to that of injection sclerotherapy (about 40 percent). More recent trials comparing propranolol with sclerotherapy confirm that both forms of treatment are similar in efficacy. The limited experience with other beta blockers suggests that all noncardioselective beta blockers (e.g., nadolol) may be similar to propranolol in efficacy.

Propranolol with Endoscopic Treatment

Based on the limited data, it appears that addition of propranolol to sclerotherapy may reduce bleeding rate compared to either propranolol or sclerotherapy alone. This may be very useful in patients who are less likely to comply with medical treatment. Unless there are definite contraindications, it is my routine practice to treat patients with propranolol in addition to endoscopic band ligation.

Surgery

Long-term endoscopic sclerotherapy and beta-blocker trials suggest that a considerable proportion of patients bleed despite intensive treatment and follow-up. It is therefore important to examine the surgical trials with an open mind.

The only prospective, randomized trial of esophageal transection and gastric devascularization was reported by Triger and his colleagues in Sheffield in 1992. They found that this form of surgery conferred no benefit over endoscopic sclerotherapy in terms of long-term survival or cost effectiveness. Decompressive shunt surgery is the most effective way of preventing recurrent variceal bleeding, but it has the significant disadvantage of causing chronic hepatic encephalopathy. Since 1970, 14 randomized trials of various forms of shunt surgery have been performed. None of these trials have shown definite improvement in survival after shunt surgery. Currently, shunt surgery (preferably mesocaval shunt or distal splenorenal shunt) is reserved for patients with recurrent bleeding (without advanced liver disease) who fail all other forms of treatment.

■ TIPSS

This is the most exciting recent development in the management of portal hypertension. The role of TIPSS in the management of acute variceal bleeding is not well defined. TIPSS is an effective form of treatment for patients with variceal bleeding, but the morbidity and mortality are very high in patients with ongoing variceal bleeding. Currently TIPSS is reserved for acute gastric variceal bleeding and in patients with ongoing bleeding who are not good surgical candidates.

The preliminary data from the randomized, controlled studies suggest that TIPSS is as effective as sclerotherapy for prevention of recurrent variceal bleeding. Unlike shunt surgery, the mortality, even in most advanced cases, appears to be low; the 30 day mortality is between 2 and 16 percent and overall mortality is 6 to 26 percent. This provides the clinician an additional tool in the management of variceal bleeding.

The development of encephalopathy, contrary to expectations, appears to be low although this has not been subjected to intense study. Two large series reported new onset of hepatic encephalopathy as 18 to 20 percent, of which the majority were easily controlled with lactulose. The initial optimism for TIPSS as an effective therapy for long-term prevention of variceal bleeding is dampened by reports of very high stent stenosis (7 to 45 percent) and occlusion rate (9 to 14 percent). More randomized trials looking at the long-term outcome of TIPSS are necessary before it can be recommended for the routine management of variceal bleeding.

Liver Transplantation

The mortality after variceal bleeding and the long-term survival following the index bleed are directly related to the severity of liver disease. It is difficult to imagine that the various treatment options discussed here are likely to improve liver function and hence survival. Liver transplantation, with survival rate reaching 80 percent, is the treatment of choice for patients with advanced liver disease (Child B & C).

■ PROPHYLAXIS FOR VARICEAL BLEEDING (PRIMARY PROPHYLAXIS)

About a third of all patients with cirrhosis bleed within 2 years of the endoscopic diagnosis of esophageal varices. The chance of bleeding depends on the severity of liver disease (Childs-Pugh grade), the portal pressure (>12 mm Hg), and the severity of varices (e.g., Beppu score). Mortality depends on the severity of liver disease and varies from 30 to 50 percent. The rationale behind the prophylaxis is based on the high bleeding rate and the very high mortality associated with it. Prophylaxis may be surgical, endoscopic, or pharmacologic.

Surgery

The randomized, controlled, prophylactic shunt trials done before the endoscopic era showed significant reduction in variceal and gastric mucosal bleeding. However, the mortality and the incidence of chronic hepatic encephalopathy were significantly higher in the shunted patients compared to the control group. These poor results and the advent of endoscopy led to the abandonment of shunt surgery for prophylaxis.

A more recent, multi-center study from Japan compared devascularization versus no treatment in a group of patients with high risk of bleeding and claimed lower bleeding rate (7 percent versus 49 percent) and low mortality (22 percent versus 49 percent) in the surgical group compared to the control group. Again the deaths related to bleeding was similar in both groups. It is difficult to draw any conclusions from this study since there was a disproportionate amount of non–bleeding-related mortality in the control group. Unequal randomization due to multicenter trial design (22 centers and 112 patients) may be one explanation for this. Further trials may be necessary to validate these trial results. Moreover, this form of surgery may make future liver transplant technically more difficult.

On the basis of the current evidence, there is no role for either shunt or nonshunting surgery in the prophylaxis of variceal bleeding.

Sclerotherapy

Prophylactic sclerotherapy has been the subject of many small and large randomized, controlled studies. Earlier reports from Germany showed reduced bleeding rate and improved survival in patients who had sclerotherapy compared to controls, but more recent studies have not confirmed these results. In fact, the multicenter, Veterans Administration trial of prophylactic sclerotherapy involving 282 patients was discontinued prematurely because of the significantly high mortality in the sclerotherapy arm compared to the control group (29 percent versus 17 percent). It has been suggested that these conflicting results may have been due to the differences in patient selection. To examine this, two studies, one from Japan and the other one from Italy, carefully selected patients with high risk of bleeding. While the Japanese study showed reduced bleeding and improved survival, the North Italian study showed identical bleeding rate. However, a meta-analysis done recently on eight controlled studies showed that prophylactic sclerotherapy reduced mortality by 11 percent (95 percent CI 4 to 19 percent); the mortality rate reductions were positively correlated with the bleeding rate reduction and negatively with complication rates. The current evidence suggests that, even in high-risk patients, the benefits from prophylactic sclerotherapy may be marginal and the procedure is not cost effective.

Beta Blockers

Many trials have assessed the efficacy of propranolol for primary prophylaxis and all studies, except one, showed reduction of bleeding. A meta-analysis done on eight of these trials has shown a definite benefit in the treated group with regard to bleeding (47 percent reduction, CI 28 to 61) and mortality (45 percent reduction, CI 10 to 67). There was no evidence for heterogeneity for bleeding events in this analysis, although there was heterogeneity for the total mortality. I recommend propranolol (preferably for a long-acting preparation to improve compliance) for primary prophylaxis for all patients with advanced liver disease and large varices.

■ RECOMMENDATIONS

Active esophageal-gastric variceal bleeding is a medical emergency in which immediate and well-directed resuscitation may improve the early and possibly late outcome. Diagnostic endoscopy, as an essential part of the management, provides the optimum time for intervention by endoscopic methods.

Although sophisticated endoscopic therapy is now widely available, if the expertise for endoscopic intervention is not available, other modes of therapy, primarily pharmacologic and rarely balloon tamponade, should be tried while the patient is transferred to a center where more definitive therapy is available. Pharmacologic treatment is effective in 50 to 70 percent of cases. The choice of therapy lies between vasopressin (or glypressin) with a vasodilator (nitroglycerin) or somatostatin and its analogue octreotide. A balloon tamponade is effective in 80 to 90 percent of cases in experienced hands but has major limitations without this expertise. When pharmacologic therapy or balloon tamponade succeeds in controlling the initial bleed, it should be followed immediately by more definitive therapy, usually endoscopic treatment or surgery.

Although banding or sclerotherapy is now frequently the first choice, shunt surgery and esophageal transection are comparable in efficacy to injection sclerotherapy for the management of active bleeding. Surgery should not be delayed when injection sclerotherapy fails on two occasions. Bleeding fundal varices should be managed by early surgery if balloon tamponade fails.

For secondary prophylaxis, endoscopic treatment (banding or sclerotherapy) and propranolol are similar in terms of efficacy. Endoscopic band ligation may be marginally superior to sclerotherapy. A combination of propranolol and endoscopic treatment may be a logical approach for long-term secondary prophylaxis. TIPSS may be useful in patients with recurrent bleeding, but further long-term trials are necessary before its routine use. Shunt surgery should be reserved for patients who fail all other forms of treatment. Propranolol should be used for primary prophylaxis in patients with advanced liver disease and large varices. Liver transplantation is the treatment of choice for patients with advanced liver disease.

Suggested Reading

Bosch J. Effect of pharmacological agents on portal hypertension: a hemodynamic appraisal. Clin Gastroenterol 1985; 14:169–183.

Burroughs AK. Somatostatin and octreotide for variceal bleeding. J Hepatol 1991; 13:1–4.

Conn HO. Transjugular intrahepatic portal-systemic shunts: the state of the art. Hepatology 1993; 17:148–158.

Hayes PC, Davis JM, Lewis JA, Bouchier IAD. Meta-analysis of value of propranolol in prevention of variceal hemorrhage. Lancet 1990; 336: 153–156.

Laine L, Cook D. Endoscopic ligation compared with sclerotherapy for treatment of esophageal variceal bleeding. A meta-analysis. Ann Intern Med 1995; 123:280–287.

Lebrec D, Paynard T, Bernuau J, et al. A randomized controlled study of propranolol for prevention of recurrent gastrointestinal bleeding in patients with cirrhosis: a final report. Hepatology 1984; 6:318–331.

North Italian Endoscopic Club for the Study and Treatment of Esophageal Varices: Prediction of the first variceal hemorrhage in patients with cirrhosis of the liver and esophageal varices: a prospective multi-center study. NEJM 1988; 319:983–989.

Smart HL, Triger DR. Clinical features, pathophysiology and relevance of portal hypertensive gastropathy. Endoscopy 1991; 23:224–228.

Steigman GV, Goff JS, Michaletz-Onody PA, et al. Endoscopic sclerotherapy as compared with endoscopic ligation for bleeding esophageal varices. New Engl J Med 1992; 326:1527–1532.

Westaby D, Williams R. Status of sclerotherapy for variceal bleeding in 1990. Am J Surg 1990; 160:32–36.

HEPATIC ENCEPHALOPATHY

Andres T. Blei, M.D.

A classification of hepatic encephalopathy (Table 1) is not a mere semantic exercise. The management of changes in mental state varies according to the acute or chronic nature of the hepatic disorder. This distinction may require a vigorous diagnostic effort for patients in whom hepatic encephalopathy is the presenting symptom. In fulminant hepatic failure, where a massive necrosis of liver cells is present, severe encephalopathy carries a grave prognosis and the presence of brain edema and intracranial hypertension requires measures seldom used in patients with chronic liver disease. In cirrhosis, liver failure and portal-systemic shunting contribute in a variable degree to the development of encephalopathy, but the appearance of a precipitating factor should always be sought. Chronic hepatic encephalopathy, a fearsome complication of portacaval shunt surgery, is an uncommon clinical problem in patients receiving transjugular intrahepatic portal-systemic stents (TIPSS). While the need to treat subclinical encephalopathy is still controversial, consideration may be warranted if subtle coordination abnormalities are detected that may interfere with the ability to carry out daily activities.

Optimal treatment of hepatic encephalopathy should be based on a thorough knowledge of the pathophysiology of this syndrome. Clinical experience has taught that hepatic encephalopathy arises from gut-derived toxins which gain access to the systemic circulation in the presence of portal-systemic shunts (hence the term *portal-systemic encephalopathy, PSE*). Precipitating factors that induce coma in fact represent a large load of these putative toxins. However, many views exist as to the nature of these compounds and the mechanisms by which neurotoxicity occurs (Table 2). This has led to the testing of therapeutic agents that specifically antagonize these candidate toxins. Thus, clinical results become the arbiter of the validity of these hypotheses. With all the difficulties in studying brain metabolism in humans, the clinician's experience becomes an invaluable tool to advance research in this area.

Table 1 Classification of Hepatic Encephalopathy

- I. Associated with cirrhosis
  - A. Acute (portal-systemic) encephalopathy
    - 1. Precipitant induced
      - Gastrointestinal bleeding
      - Uremia
      - Sedatives
      - Dietary indiscretion
      - Infection
      - Constipation
      - Hypokalemia
    - 2. Spontaneous encephalopathy
  - B. Chronic hepatic encephalopathy
    - 1. Chronic recurrent
    - 2. Hepatocerebral degeneration
  - C. Subclinical encephalopathy
- II. Associated with fulminant hepatic failure
  - A. Stages similar to encephalopathy of chronic disease: lethargy (mania), confusion, stupor, coma
  - B. Brain edema evolving to intracranial hypertension at later stages

ACUTE ENCEPHALOPATHY IN CIRRHOSIS

Search for Precipitating Cause

When cirrhotic patients develop alterations in consciousness, a precipitating factor must be sought (Table 3). Gastrointestinal (GI) hemorrhage, uremia, and ingestion of sedatives are the most common factors. In addition, infection and electrolyte disturbances (especially hypokalemia) may be present. In some individuals, excess protein in the diet is enough to cause encephalopathy. Diuretics may result in volume contraction, a rise in blood urea nitrogen and hypokalemia, factors known to usher in changes in mental state.

When the precipitating factor is not clinically obvious, active testing should be pursued. This may include passage of a nasogastric tube to exclude hemorrhage, abdominal paracentesis to rule out an infected ascitic fluid as well as analysis of urinary sediment and renal ultrasonography in cases with abnormal kidney function. Treatment of the precipitating factor should be immediately started. Volume replacement, antibiotic treatment, or specific sedative antagonism (in the case of

Table 2 Pathogenesis of Hepatic Encephalopathy: Neurotoxins and Postulated Mechanisms

- I. Ammonia may act via multiple mechanisms
  - A. Direct neurotoxicity
  - B. Generation of glutamine (osmotic effect)
  - C. Alterations in neurotransmission
    - 1. Glutamatergic (excitatory)
    - 2. Serotoninergic (inhibitory)
    - 3. Gabaergic (inhibitory)
- II. Synergistic neurotoxins potentiate the effects of ammonia
  Mercaptans, short-chain fatty acids, phenols
- III. Generation of false neurotransmitters
  - A. Entry of aromatic amino acids into the brain is favored by:
    - 1. Lower levels of plasma branched-chain amino acids
    - 2. Exchange for brain glutamine, generated from ammonia metabolism
  - B. Phenylalanine, tyrosine are precursors of dopamine, catecholamines
    - 1. Generation of "false" neurotransmitters, e.g., octopamine
    - 2. Alterations in dopaminergic neurotransmission
- IV. GABA-endogenous benzodiazepines
  - A. Binding of endogenous benzodiazepines to $GABA_A$ receptor
  - B. The nature of the endogenous benzodiazepine is controversial
    - 1. Diazepam, desmethyldiazepam (small amount)
    - 2. Other compounds (endozepines)

Table 3 Management of Episode of Acute Encephalopathy

1. Removal of precipitating agent (see Table 1)
2. Lactulose
   a) By enema, 300 ml in 700 ml of water
   b) Orally, 30 ml q hour until bowel movement; then 15 to 45 ml q.i.d.
3. If unable to use lactulose, neomycin 2 to 4 g/day or metronidazole (250 mg b.i.d.–t.i.d.)
4. When able to be fed, protein is started at 40 g/day

opiates or benzodiazepines) may reverse the encephalopathic state. Although most patients hyperventilate with a primary respiratory alkalosis and have evidence of functional intrapulmonary shunts, oxygen via a nasal cannula is recommended as hypoxemia is common in cirrhosis and may aggravate the effects of the other precipitants. Intravenous fluid should be replaced with attention to electrolyte imbalance and volume status. Hypokalemia and/or hypomagnesemia (in the case of diuretic-induced encephalopathy) and intravascular volume depletion with sodium retention (as manifested by ascites and peripheral edema) may be present.

Episodes of encephalopathy, in the absence of a clear precipitating event, have been reported in patients with large spontaneous splenorenal shunts. Patients with acute alcoholic hepatitis and spontaneous encephalopathy are a subgroup whose liver disease, in the appropriate setting, may respond to corticosteroid therapy.

General Measures

Catharsis

An increase in stool frequency is a general measure to decrease the neurotoxin load arising from the gut. It acquires special importance in cases with GI bleeding, where blood in the colonic lumen may persist for days. It can be achieved via oral agents (such as lactulose) when the patient is able to swallow; oral mannitol (100 g per liter gastric lavage) has also been administered to patients with GI hemorrhage. In cases with coma, drug administration via a nasogastric tube may be necessary, with appropriate care of the airway. Cleansing enemas with tap water, in the absence of stool acidification, are of limited value.

Dietary Management

When patients are acutely encephalopathic, provision of adequate calories with intravenous dextrose is sufficient. As soon as the patient is able to tolerate oral intake, patients should be fed and protein should not be restricted to values below 0.5 g per kilogram in order to maintain body stores. It is preferable to add another medication rather than curtail protein intake. The provision of branched-chain amino acids in an intravenous formulation (30 to 40 percent of total amino acids) has been tested in cirrhotic patients with acute encephalopathy. The results are equivocal and do not warrant its use in view of its cost.

Nonabsorbable Disaccharides

These compounds benefit patients with hepatic encephalopathy via multiple mechanisms. Fermentation of the sugar by colonic bacteria results in acidification of the colonic lumen, favoring the passage of ammonia from the bloodstream, which is used by bacteria as a nitrogen source. As a consequence of this fermentation, hepatic ureagenesis is decreased. The formation of octanoic acid in the colonic lumen, implicated in the pathogenesis of encephalopathy, is reduced. Colonic acidification promotes catharsis, providing an additional mechanism of action. For patients in coma, lactulose (a synthetic disaccharide composed of fructose-galactose) does not result in immediate beneficial effects. Using a protocol where 30 ml of lactulose is administered hourly until a loose bowel movement is obtained, followed by dosing every 6 hours, 48 to 60 hours elapses before arousal occurs. For patients in whom a more rapid effect is desired, lactulose enemas (300 ml in 700 ml of water) can be administered to be retained over 1 to 2 hours, with the patient in Trendelenburg position to favor passage into the right colon.

Once the patient is awake, oral lactulose is supplied at doses of 15 to 45 ml two to four times daily, aiming for two to three loose bowel movements per day. Abdominal cramping and flatulence is common. Excessive diarrhea may result in hypertonic dehydration due to the hypotonic nature of colonic fluid. Hypernatremia with associated hyperosmolarity can induce changes in mental state and lead to the erroneous conclusion that further therapy with lactulose is necessary.

Patients who are lactase-deficient (which is common in certain parts of the world) can receive lactose as oral therapy. Lactose enemas will be effective regardless of the small bowel enzyme content. Lactitol (a new synthetic disaccharide) appears as effective as lactulose and is associated with better patient tolerance, as the taste is more palatable and appears to result in less abdominal cramping. Lactitol is currently unavailable in the United States.

Antibiotics

Antibiotic therapy is designed to reduce the population of urease-containing bacteria in the colonic lumen. Recent animal studies raise the possibility that the small bowel may be an additional target. In the case of neomycin, the activity of mucosal glutaminase may be reduced by the drug, thus decreasing the generation of ammonia from the small intestine. Neomycin is useful in acute episodes, with doses of 2 to 4 g per day, in divided doses. Although poorly absorbed, 1 to 3 percent of the dose reaches the systemic circulation, and as an aminoglycoside, its use in renal failure is not recommended. Diarrhea, fungal infections, and a malabsorption picture are potential complications. Once the precipitating factor is removed, therapy should not be prolonged beyond 1 month.

Metronidazole also appears effective as a measure to reverse PSE. The drug undergoes extensive hepatic metabolism and should be started at a lower dose, 250 mg twice daily, in patients with cirrhosis. Side effects include an Antabuse-like reaction to alcohol ingestion, peripheral neuropathy, and nausea. Oral vancomycin is an expensive choice and has no role in management. The combination of lactulose and neomycin appears theoretically contradictory in face of the need for colonic bacteria to ferment the nonabsorbed sugar. However, anaerobic species appear to mediate the latter effect and these are not affected by neomycin. Clinical studies have shown effects of combination therapy on nitrogen metabolism that are expected when ammonia moves to the colonic lumen: an increase in fecal nitrogen and a reduction of hepatic ureagenesis. Uncontrolled clinical testing has also shown efficacy and the combination can be used in face of the failure of either drug alone.

A comment is due on clinical trials in acute hepatic encephalopathy. These are extremely difficult to control, as removal of the precipitating factor is occurring at the same time that therapy is being administered. Different precipitating factors imply a different set of circumstances that require different therapeutic maneuvers. In fact, using rigid criteria, no therapy in acute encephalopathy has been compared to a true placebo.

■ CHRONIC ENCEPHALOPATHY IN CIRRHOSIS

Patients with chronic encephalopathy seldom exhibit the usual precipitating factors previously discussed and when present, dietary indiscretion or constipation are more frequent. Spontaneous episodes of encephalopathy are common. In some patients, established neurologic deficits appear, with prominent extrapyramidal symptoms (acquired hepatolenticular degeneration) or spastic paraparesis. Enthusiasm for portacaval shunt surgery has waned as the ravages of chronic hepatic encephalopathy can be devastating to the individual and family. TIPSS, the new noninvasive decompressive procedure, results in episodes of encephalopathy in up to 30 percent of individuals, but chronic changes in mental state are rare.

Measures used to treat acute encephalopathy, including protein restriction, nonabsorbable disaccharides, and/or poorly absorbable antibiotics, are also used in management of the chronic state. Vegetable protein has the benefit of providing additional fiber and promoting catharsis. Some patients do not tolerate the abdominal cramping associated with this source of protein. Supplements of fiber, such as psyllium, may be effective. The rationale for the use of oral branched-chain amino acid supplements (0.25 g per kilogram per day) has been questioned. It is based on the theory that normalization of the aromatic/branched-chain amino acid ratio will decrease the entry of the former into the brain, thus decreasing the formation of false transmitters. These supplements do not provide a major advantage, are expensive, and should be reserved for patients intolerant of oral protein.

Long-term therapy with lactulose (15 to 45 ml two to three times daily) is difficult to maintain due to subjective complaints with taste and abdominal cramping; lactitol may be more useful in this setting. Long-term use of neomycin (2 to 4 g per day) requires careful attention to potential ototoxicity, and yearly audiograms are necessary. When the first line of therapy is ineffective, metronidazole (500 to 750 mg per day) is considered. Bromocriptine (15 to 30 mg per day) has undergone testing based on its capacity to increase dopamine stores; it may be tried in patients with chronic encephalopathy. Initial enthusiasm for L-dopa has waned as clinical studies have not confirmed its efficacy.

Surgical options should be considered for the chronic patient. Occlusion of the portacaval shunt has been used for cases with intractable chronic encephalopathy. This requires additional measures to ensure that gastroesophageal varices do not recur; this may include angiographic occlusion of the coronary vein or variceal embolization via angiography prior to shunt occlusion. Another drastic surgical approach in nonshunted patients has been colonic exclusion which is seldom used nowadays, but the procedure has been effective in selected individuals. Liver transplantation is a real option for suitable candidates and chronic encephalopathy has become a clear indication for this procedure. Even reversal of chronic hepatocerebral degeneration has been recently reported after liver transplantation.

■ SUBCLINICAL ENCEPHALOPATHY

Subclinical encephalopathy is defined as the presence of abnormal neuropsychological testing in the absence of clinical signs of neurologic deficits. It is common with 30 to 70 percent of cirrhotics exhibiting such features. The need to treat these patients is controversial. Lactulose and oral zinc acetate or sulfate (200 mg three times daily) have been shown in controlled studies to improve the performance in neuropsychological testing. Whether this will represent an advantage for patients with cirrhosis is unclear. Cirrhotic patients with subclinical encephalopathy who engage in complex motor activities may be potential beneficiaries.

■ ENCEPHALOPATHY IN ACUTE LIVER FAILURE

The development of encephalopathy is a serious complication of acute liver failure. Management of encephalopathy is difficult due to the confounding presence of brain edema and intracranial hypertension. During the early stages of encephalopathy, lactulose is administered with special care to avoid electrolyte disturbances associated with catharsis in an already precarious situation. Its efficacy in preventing the progression to deeper stages of encephalopathy has not been formally tested, but does not appear important. Neomycin is not recommended in order to avoid potential deterioration of renal function.

Many patients in stages III to IV encephalopathy (stupor, coma) exhibit a distinct complication of acute liver failure—brain edema and intracranial hypertension. Management of brain edema is symptomatic; the etiology of excessive water accumulation in the brain is still controversial and therapy is thus directed at reducing intracranial pressure. Mannitol, 0.5 to 1 g per kilogram, is administered as a bolus; monitoring of intracranial pressure with epidural transducers allows optimization of therapy. Patients are kept at 30°, with avoidance of excessive mobilization. Thiopental coma and hypothermia are used in intractable cases. Liver transplantation is recommended for patients with advanced encephalopathy and poor synthetic function.

■ NEWER THERAPIES

Zinc is a cofactor for several enzymes in the urea cycle and repletion of depleted stores may improve the efficiency of ammonia conversion to urea. Administered as zinc sulfate or acetate (600 mg per day), it may be useful in patients with associated malnutrition. It has been shown to improve the results of neuropsychological testing in patients with subclinical encephalopathy and is an attractive option if treatment is considered for these individuals.

Sodium benzoate has been used in children with hyperammonemia due to urea cycle enzyme deficiencies. The drug is activated in the liver and combines with glycine (formed from ammonia, bicarbonate, and tetrahydrofolate) to form hippurate, which is now excreted in the urine. In two recent controlled evaluations, the drug was as useful as lactulose in reversing acute encephalopathy in cirrhotics. Benzoate is a ubiquitous food preservative but at this time is not commercially available as a medication. When administered, doses of 5 g twice daily are needed; this represents a sodium load and care should be exercised in patients with ascites.

Flumazenil is a benzodiazepine antagonist available for reversal of excessive sedation due to this group of drugs. Its use to reverse hepatic encephalopathy is based on experimental and clinical evidence that suggests a role for endogenous benzodiazepines in the pathogenesis of hepatic encephalopathy. It is available in an intravenous formulation, and is administered as a 1 mg bolus.

Uncontrolled studies indicate an arousal effect of flumazenil in approximately 70 percent of patients. On most occasions, this effect is transient and does not represent complete normalization of the mental state. Placebo-controlled trials indicate that 30 to 40 percent of patients ameliorate the depth of encephalopathy. These observations are important for the pathogenesis of hepatic encephalopathy. In the meantime, flumazenil is clearly indicated for patients with benzodiazepine-induced precipitation of hepatic encephalopathy. It may be tested in patients in whom other measures have failed but its exact role in the management of encephalopathy of either acute or chronic liver disease has not yet been determined.

Suggested Reading

Blei AT, Butterworth RF. Hepatic encephalopathy. Semin Liv Dis 1996.

Camma C, Fiorello F, Tine F, et al. Lactitol in the treatment of hepatic encephalopathy. A meta-analysis. Dig Dis Sci 1993; 38:916–922.

Conn HO, Bircher J. Hepatic encephalopathy. Syndromes and Therapies. Bloomington, IL: Medi-Ed Press, 1994.

Eriksson LS, Conn HO. Branched-chain aminoacids in hepatic encephalopathy. Gastroenterology 1990; 99:604–607.

Mullen KD, Weber FL Jr. Role of nutrition in hepatic encephalopathy. Semin Liver Dis 1991; 11:292–304.

ACUTE CHOLECYSTITIS

Roger G. Keith, M.D., F.R.C.S.C., F.R.C.S., F.A.C.S.

Biliary calculus disease is a very common problem facing practitioners worldwide. Gallbladder pathology is the most frequent sequela of cholelithiasis, although many patients remain asymptomatic through life. Since the advent of laparoscopic cholecystectomy, the incidence of complicated gallbladder disease has been reduced due to the increasing operative rates related to accelerated patient acceptance of surgical treatment for minimally symptomatic cholelithiasis. Nonetheless, the significant morbidity and mortality associated with acute cholecystitis remain unchanged. Understanding the spectrum of gallbladder disease and utilizing the most effective investigations and treatment while avoiding life-risking complications become a significant responsibility for the health care provider of the current decade.

SPECTRUM OF DISEASE

Calculus Related

Biliary colic is a pain syndrome related to cholelithiasis. This is the most benign form of obstructive gallbladder disease, wherein a calculus temporarily obstructs the outflow lumen of the gallbladder. This results in a short-lived episode of pain of variable severity which by spontaneous dislodgement of the gallstone terminates the clinical problem. Recurrence is the rule at unpredictable frequency related to stimulation of gallbladder contraction by food ingestion, primarily. Most patients present for cholecystectomy because of unacceptable recurrences of biliary colic.

Acute cholecystitis occurs with progressive obstruction of the gallbladder neck or duct by a gallstone, which through failure to dislodge initiates a cascade of circulatory compromise affecting the end arterial flow of the cystic artery. The complexity of inflammation and ischemia of the gallbladder wall results in local and systemic clinical findings which distinguish this process from biliary colic. Untreated ischemia leads to focal gangrenous necrosis, usually involving the fundus and Hartmann's pouch.

Perforation of the gallbladder wall by increasing secretory pressure exerted at necrotic sites may cause local or generalized spillage of contents. A pericholecystic abscess will result from localization of the leak by the regional viscera and omentum. Failure to contain the leak will lead to biliary peritonitis with risk of septic shock and 40 to 45 percent mortality if not recognized early.

Severity of inflammation of acute cholecystitis is characterized by a palpably tender, enlarged gallbladder associated with fever and leukocytosis greater than 14,000 per milliliter. Hemodynamic instability heralds bacteremia and risk of septic shock. Jaundice of mild degree is not uncommon and is usually due to extending periportal inflammation and not common duct stone. The impacted stone precipitating acute cholecystitis precludes subsequent passage of gallstones to the bile duct, unless this was a pre-existing condition.

Risk factors which lead to acceleration of the gallbladder inflammation and ischemia are related to local impairment to arterial flow such as atherosclerosis with or without diabetes mellitus and systemic factors which compromise host immune responsiveness. Advanced liver disease and portal hypertension not only blunt the response to inflammation but increase the morbidity of surgery by the derangement of local anatomy and abnormal bleeding risk.

Noncalculus Related

Acalculous cholecystitis is an acute complication of critical systemic illness. It most frequently occurs in hospitalized patients undergoing intensive care management or having immune compromising systemic therapy for unrelated diseases. Prolonged fasting and deranged gastrointestinal function are common factors in most patients who predispose to gallbladder stasis. Imaging studies delineate the pathogenetic "biliary sludge" implicated in acute acalculous cholecystitis. The other factor required to initiate the progressive necrotizing inflammation is hypoperfusion of the gallbladder relevant to critical illness caused by trauma, sepsis, or cardiopulmonary failure.

This form of cholecystitis has a more formidable course because of the blunted systemic response and the more rapid progression of gallbladder ischemia to gangrenous necrosis and perforation. Lack of awareness and compromise of signs by the pre-existing illness contribute to the delay in treatment which leads to the increased morbidity and mortality associated with the acalculous form of acute cholecystitis.

DIFFERENTIAL DIAGNOSIS

Distinction between acute cholecystitis and other causes of right upper quadrant inflammation must be based on clinical evaluation and cost effective laboratory examinations. Prior existence of gallstones lends credibility to the diagnosis of cholecystitis but does not eliminate the possibility of common bile duct stones and acute cholangitis, which may be anicteric in up to one-third of cases. Rigors and sepsis are more likely to indicate cholangitis and with high probability the gallbladder will not be palpable or tender. Immediately evident jaundice, indicating at least a threefold increase in serum bilirubin, is predictive of common duct stone not cholecystitis. Painless cholestasis with or without fever may indicate periampullary neoplasm.

Generalized peritonitis with associated cholelithiasis should be considered acute biliary pancreatitis until proved otherwise. Elevations of serum amylase greater than 1,000 IU per liter are diagnostic. Whereas normal or intermediate elevations can be found with pancreatitis, other causes of peritonitis should be ruled out. Perforation of a duodenal ulcer may mimic pancreatitis or cholecystitis. In such patients, a history of ulcer may be absent; however, most cases are confirmed by radiographic evidence of free intraperitoneal air.

Acute hepatitis of viral or toxic etiology may be difficult to differentiate from acute cholecystitis as the enlarged liver with distended Glisson's capsule may be mistaken for the gallbladder. However, the entire liver is tender to percussion over the lower chest cage on both right and left sides with acute hepatitis. Acute alcoholic hepatitis is more readily confused with extrahepatic cholestasis from stone disease as the liver tenderness is severe and the biochemical liver function tests are similar with significantly disproportionate elevation of alkaline phosphatase compared to transaminase.

Diagnostic Imaging Studies

The laboratory examination which will yield the maximal diagnostic information at least cost with greatest accessibility, is ultrasound scanning of the abdomen with reference to the gallbladder, liver, biliary tract, and pancreas. Although operator-dependent, current technology will confirm pathology of the biliary tract including gallbladder in 95 percent of cases. Cholelithiasis will be substantiated in more than 95 percent and false-negative studies should be under 5 percent.

Criteria to support the clinical diagnosis of acute cholecystitis include gallbladder distention with a thickened, edematous wall. The impacted calculus may be observed in the cystic duct or neck of the gallbladder. Pericholecystic fluid indicates transmural inflammation and gas in the gallbladder wall is an ominous finding. Empyema of the gallbladder is confirmed by finding gas in the lumen. Portal edema and lymphadenopathy indicate severity and duration of the inflammatory process. Transducer tenderness over the imaged gallbladder fundus corresponds to the findings on initial abdominal examination, but is not organ specific.

Dilatation of the intrahepatic bile ducts is most easily recognized by the ultrasonographer and suggests extrahepatic biliary obstruction. However, this is not diagnostic of common duct stones unless visualized. Distal common duct dilatation is highly suspicious for the presence of stones in the duct or the less frequent periampullary tumor, confirmed by the additional finding of a mass in the pancreas or region of the ampulla.

Acute liver disease is suggested by liver enlargement and heterogeneity of texture. Splenomegaly and a contracted liver are pathognomonic of cirrhosis.

Radionucleotide biliary scanning using technetium 99-labeled HIDA derivatives is especially valuable in acute acalculous cholecystitis or clinically apparent cholecystitis in which stones cannot be visualized on ultrasound scan. Although less readily accessible, time consuming, and more expensive, this study may confirm cystic duct obstruction and delayed bile duct emptying in selected cases. I would not recommend biliary scintigraphy as the first study for acute cholecystitis and would reserve this examination for patients in whom ultrasound proved equivocal in the face of high probability clinical findings.

Table 1 Indications for Systemic Antibiotic Therapy (One or More Criteria)

Clinical parameters on admission or within 8 hours:
Temperature >38°C
Clinical jaundice
Generalized peritonitis
Laboratory parameters:
Leukocytosis >14,000/ml
Elevated bilirubin
Amylase >500 IU/L
Elevated blood glucose
Ultrasound scan parameters:
Pericholecystic fluid
Gas in gallbladder wall or lumen
Dilated intra- or extrahepatic bile ducts

Patients with minimal leukocytosis, low-grade fever, and ultrasound evidence of extrahepatic bile duct dilatation without severe cholecystitis on scanning should have preoperative endoscopic retrograde cholangiopancreatography (ERCP) for confirmation of common duct stones, followed by endoscopic sphincterotomy and stone extraction. Subsequent cholecystectomy without operative bile duct exploration will have reduced morbidity compared to cholecystectomy with operative exploration of the duct. This is particularly important in the current era of laparoscopic biliary surgery.

Percutaneous transhepatic cholecystography is only indicated when interventional radiographic techniques will be considered for emergency therapy. Transhepatic cholangiography and biliary drainage should be considered in management of cholangitis.

The ultimate imaging study is diagnostic laparoscopy. This study should only be considered as part of definitive therapy for cholecystitis and should be conducted by a qualified abdominal surgical specialist with experience in open and laparoscopic biliary surgery.

INITIAL MANAGEMENT

Self-limited biliary colic rarely requires hospitalization and subsequent management is efficiently conducted on an ambulatory care basis. However, the clinical diagnosis of acute cholecystitis should initiate hospital admission. Baseline hemoglobin, white blood cell count, amylase, blood sugar, and liver profile biochemistry are obtained at presentation. Blood cultures should be obtained in the febrile patient after initiation of intravenous crystalloid infusions. The abdominal ultrasound scan should be obtained. Triple antibiotic therapy (aminoglycoside, metronidazole, and ampicillin) should be added when indicated (Table 1). Repeated clinical assessment including temperature and vital signs, combined with ultrasound findings, will determine the subsequent decision for or against urgent operative intervention. The criteria to guide the physician to consider urgent operation are presented in Table 2.

Clinical improvement or absence of surgical indications during the first 48 hours support the continuation of nonoperative treatment, with or without antibiotic therapy. Deterioration or presentation of surgical indications should deter the physician from further conservative management.

Table 2 Criteria Indicating Urgent Operative Intervention

Clinical and laboratory (any two at least):
Temperature 39°C or greater
BP <90 mm systolic
Jaundice and rigors
Local or generalized peritonitis
Leukocytosis 20,000/ml or greater
Ultrasound findings (at least one):
Pericholecystic fluid
Gas in gallbladder wall
Gas in gallbladder lumen
Edematous gallbladder wall and free abdominal fluid

Nonoperative treatment during initial management is proposed in order to promote resolution of acute inflammation and present an increased opportunity for minimal access surgery. This proves successful in less than one-third of cases initially diagnosed as acute cholecystitis. In this group of patients, the theoretic interval to complete resolution by 6 weeks is rarely achieved because of residual subacute inflammation or recurrent acute attacks. Therefore, I advise same admission surgery for any patient with residual pain or tenderness after the first week of otherwise effective conservative treatment. Only those with complete freedom of symptoms at 1 week will be planned for an interval cholecystectomy at 6 weeks.

NONOPERATIVE INTERVENTIONAL MANAGEMENT

Interventional Radiologic Treatment

A small percentage of patients with acute cholecystitis and surgical indications have compromising medical conditions which contraindicate general anesthesia. Although minilaparotomy for open cholecystostomy could be performed under local anesthesia, a preferable approach is ultrasound-guided percutaneous transhepatic gallbladder drainage. An 18 Fr catheter is placed for emergency decompression and left in place for continued drainage. Unaltered disease progression indicates established gallbladder necrosis and probable bacteremia. Intensive care may be successful in reversing sepsis in these critically ill patients. Failure to respond will mitigate open cholecystectomy under general anesthesia despite high risk in this selected population. Most patients respond favorably to gallbladder drainage. Subsequent management of residual cholelithiasis may utilize the established tract for graduated dilation and percutaneous extraction of stones or consideration may be given to contact lithotripsy or instillation of dissolution agents.

Interventional Endoscopic Management

Patients with acute cholecystitis associated with cholestasis and ultrasound documented dilatation of the extrahepatic biliary tract should have urgent preoperative ERCP and possible sphincterotomy with stone extraction if identified. This is particularly so if the patient is septic and the focus is not defined as gallbladder or bile duct. If stones cannot be

Table 3 Indications for Conversion to Open Cholecystectomy

At laparoscopy:
Fixed fundic adhesions
Free fundus; fixed Calot's triangle
Perforated necrotic cholecystitis
On attempted cholecystectomy:
Perforation of necrotic gallbladder on adhesiolysis
Disruption of artery or duct on dissection of obliterated porta
Nonvisualization of cystic duct—common duct junction
Inadvertent injury to common bile duct

extracted at ERCP, a nasobiliary catheter should be placed for proximal biliary decompression. Subsequent to control of sepsis, an urgent cholecystectomy and required biliary exploration should be undertaken by the appropriate open or laparoscopic route. Successful endoscopic sphincterotomy and stone extraction will quickly reverse sepsis if the cause was cholangitis. This leaves an interval opportunity before cholecystectomy, recognizing a small number of cases wherein the gallbladder stones have entirely cleared from the gallbladder without clinical incident. If the sepsis was due to cholecystitis and ERCP failed to identify common duct stones or incidental common duct stones were cleared without alteration of the septic process, urgent cholecystectomy must follow.

OPERATIVE MANAGEMENT

The developments in laparoscopic surgery have changed the approach to calculous disease of the biliary tract significantly. The recognized advantages of reduced hospital stay and earlier return to work attributed to laparoscopic cholecystectomy have driven surgeons toward minimal access surgery whenever feasible.

The documented increase in frequency of bile duct injury since the advent of laparoscopic cholecystectomy must be considered with any proposal for operative treatment of acute cholecystitis. The maximal derangement of biliary anatomy occurs with severe inflammation of the gallbladder. Technical aspects of open cholecystectomy are most significantly challenged during operation for acute cholecystitis. This has not changed with the improved visual technology of laparoscopic surgery. Thus, the initial guidelines for laparoscopic cholecystectomy contraindicated this technique for acute cholecystitis. This is no longer an absolute contraindication; however, the abdominal surgeon must be prepared to convert to open surgery at the least difficulty (Table 3).

Early Operation

Patients with indications for urgent intervention and those with unremitting pain in the hospital should proceed to cholecystectomy as soon as stabilized. Parenteral antibiotic therapy should continue after the operation for at least 20 hours. Perioperative fluid and electrolyte therapy is delivered based on maintenance requirements per body mass and measured losses. Colloid and blood products are not required unless unusual bleeding occurs during surgery.

The initial approach in most urgent cases is laparoscopic cholecystectomy. The first procedure should be to decompress the gallbladder by laparoscopic-directed percutaneous needle aspiration. Thereafter, exposure and dissection will be easier. A prograde cholecystectomy should begin at the neck of the gallbladder. The impacted stone will be readily identified and the cystic duct will be exposed by blunt dissection of the edematous tissues in Calot's triangle. Identification of the cystic artery should precede division of either structure. Then the decision for laparoscopic cholangiography must be made. I prefer selective cholangiography and perform the study through the cystic duct. Indications for selective cholangiography are outlined in Table 4. The surgeon must recognize that the impaction of a gallstone in the gallbladder neck or cystic duct causes this disease and commonly prevents migration of gallstones to the common duct.

Table 4 Indications for Selective Cholangiography in Acute Cholecystitis

Preoperative:
Ultrasound demonstration of extrahepatic duct dilatation
Ultrasound demonstration of common duct stones
Ultrasound evidence of pancreatitis or pancreatic mass
Acalculous cholecystitis
Intraoperative:
Dilated common bile duct
Palpable common duct stones
Nonimpacted gallbladder stone at neck
Empty gallbladder
Pancreatic mass or inflammation

If completion cholangiography precludes exploration of the duct, the gallbladder should be removed prograde after stepwise clipping and division of the cystic duct and artery. I prefer coagulation, not laser, for dissection and hemostasis. Removal of the severely diseased gallbladder may require extension of the umbilical incision. If the gallbladder fossa is dry and bleeding is controlled, no drainage is required.

If cholangiography reveals small common duct stones, I prefer to perform a postoperative ERCP with endoscopic sphincterotomy and stone removal. Laparoscopic duct exploration is only considered for larger stones with a wide diameter cystic duct which will allow transcystic duct introduction of a flexible choledochoscope for stone extraction or lithotripsy. If there are multiple large stones or the surgeon is not experienced with laparoscopic duct exploration, then open cholecystectomy and choledochotomy should be the procedure of choice.

Conversion to open operation should be followed by prograde or retrograde dissection according to the surgeon's preference and experience. Cholangiography should be selected by the same criteria. As open surgery will be performed in more severe cases, meticulous care should be taken during dissection around the porta. If pathology is extenuating, the decision should be taken early to perform a cholecystostomy and remove gallstones, leaving a tube exteriorized at the fundus.

Elective Operation

A small percentage of patients with acute cholecystitis settle and can return electively for definitive treatment. The same operative approach is recommended. The fibrosis of healed cholecystitis may make the adhesiolysis so difficult that the surgeon will be forced to convert to open cholecystectomy.

The advantage of preoperative ERCP must be recognized. I favor this method of study for any patient with preoperative indications for cholangiography based on ultrasound examination.

The presence of edematous inflammation should not be the reason to select early treatment if a patient is clinically improved. Most elective operations are technically satisfactory and the risks of duct injury in face of acute inflammation are reduced by the delay for resolution.

■ POSTOPERATIVE MANAGEMENT

Following laparoscopic cholecystectomy, the recovery phase is shorter than open, even with severe acute cholecystitis.

After early resolution of ileus, oral feedings are initiated without restriction of fats. Normal activity is encouraged soon after surgery, and with small laparoscopic wounds, no restriction in exertion is necessary. Return to full employment is expected after 1 week.

Laparoscopic surgery for necrotizing or perforated cholecystitis may be complicated by umbilical wound infection by the extracted gallbladder. Acute inflammation is evident about the fifth day and local drainage is effective treatment.

Intra-abdominal abscess may occur in the subhepatic or subphrenic spaces or even in the pelvis. More significant sepsis occurs without wound signs. Ultrasound scanning is the preferred first imaging technique. It is diagnostic in over 80 percent of cases. Failed localization requires CT and nuclear medical scanning.

Residual stones may be quiescent and present years after operation, or early evidence of fluctuating cholestasis may be seen within weeks. Ultrasound scans should be followed by diagnostic and therapeutic ERCP and stone extraction. Cholangitis is uncommon in the early postoperative phase, but urgent biliary decompression must be initiated under triple antibiotic coverage.

Bile duct injury presents with rapid onset of progressive cholestasis if complete occlusion of the common duct resulted from inadvertent clipping or ligation. Bile duct leaks may present as biliary fistula if open surgery was performed; or bile peritonitis or ascites may present after a delay of several weeks. Cholangiography will be required by the endoscopic or transhepatic route; in some cases both techniques may be utilized to define the exact nature and extent of the complication. Biliary intestinal continuity should be restored by reconstruction techniques using a roux-en-Y limb of jejunum. Primary end-to-end repair should only be considered when recognition of injury is apparent at the primary operation.

Open cholecystectomy prolongs hospital stay and return to full activity. Wound infection may be more frequent and cause greater morbidity. Otherwise, postoperative complications are not significantly different than for the laparoscopic procedure, except for the recognized increase of bile duct injury attributed to laparoscopic cholecystectomy.

Suggested Reading

Flowers JA, Bailey RW, Zucker KA. Laparoscopic management of acute cholecystitis. Am J Surg 1991; 161:388–392.

Hermann RE. The spectrum of biliary stone disease. Am J Surg 1989; 158: 171–173.

Jacobs M, Verdeja JC, Goldstein HS. Laparoscopic cholecystectomy in acute cholecystitis. Surg Endosc 1991; 1:174–175.

McSherry CK. Cholecystectomy: the gold standard. Am J Surg 1989; 158: 174–178.

Unger SW, Edelamn DS, Scott JS, et al. Laparoscopic treatment of acute cholecystitis. Surg Endosc 1991; 1:14–16.

CHOLELITHIASIS

Eldon A. Shaffer, M.D., F.R.C.P.C., F.A.C.P.

Gallstone disease is a major health care problem, afflicting 20 to 30 million people and resulting in over 500,000 cholecystectomies each year in the United States. It is now the most common operation after cesarean section. The resultant burden costs the U.S. economy $4 to 5 billion each year, representing 2.5 percent of all health care dollars. The variance in the performance of cholecystectomy is significant: it is sixfold to sevenfold higher in the U.S. and Canada than in Europe. The frequency of gallstone disease, though high, is not different. Such variance suggests overuse of the health care system, particularly as few patients ever become symptomatic.

The management of cholelithiasis has changed significantly with better understanding of its natural history, the introduction of new medical therapies, and advances in surgical technologies. A balanced perspective is in order.

■ NATURAL HISTORY

Cholesterol gallstones (composed of >50 percent cholesterol) are the most common type, representing over 85 percent of all stones in the Western world. They are more frequent in women especially with early menarche and parity; the obese and those undergoing rapid weight loss; older age groups and certain ethnic groups, such as American Indians. The remainder are pigment stones containing bilirubin polymers plus several insoluble calcium salts.

Cholesterol gallstones form in three stages: (1) chemical stage in which the liver secretes bile supersaturated with cholesterol; (2) physical stage in which the excess cholesterol precipitates from solution as microcrystals; and (3) gallstone growth in which these crystals aggregate and grow into macroscopic stones.

Gallstones grow at about 1 to 2 mm per year over 5 to 20 years before symptoms develop. They frequently are clinically "silent," some being incidentally detected on a routine ultrasound examination performed for another purpose. Indeed, over 80 percent of people with gallstones never develop symptoms. Problems, if they do arise, usually do so in the form of biliary pain during the first 5 to 10 years. Most will experience some symptoms for a period of time before developing a complication. No gallstone-related deaths have been reported from patients followed for asymptomatic gallstone disease. Because of this, prophylactic treatment of asymptomatic patients is no longer justified. The same applies to diabetic patients; they are not at greater risk of complications but have a high mortality if acute cholecystitis supervenes. In general, the risk of gallbladder cancer in patients with gallstones is so very low as to not justify prophylactic cholecystectomy. Prophylactic cholecystectomy is only warranted when the risk of coexistent carcinoma of the gallbladder is high, such as in the presence of a calcified gallbladder ("porcelain gallbladder"), gallstones >3 cm in diameter and possibly solitary gallbladder polyps >1 cm in diameter.

Symptomatic gallstones are best defined by the development of true biliary pain. Although termed *biliary colic*, the upper abdominal pain typically is steady, not spasmodic. It begins suddenly, becomes severe and persists for 1 to 5 hours, and then gradually disappears over 30 to 60 minutes, leaving a dull ache. Its duration may be somewhat less than 1 hour but is not as brief as 30 minutes. "Fatty food intolerance," a vague discomfort which follows a heavy or spicy meal, is not specific for biliary tract disease. Rather, biliary pain is significant enough to awaken the individual from sleep or require narcotics for relief. Episodes of pain occur irregularly, separated by pain-free intervals lasting from days to years. Symptomatic patients are likely to have recurrent episodes of biliary pain; obviously some go on to complications, such as cholecystitis or biliary obstruction. Those with symptoms warrant therapeutic intervention.

■ AVAILABLE THERAPIES

Expectant Management

No therapy other than watching is necessary for most individuals with gallstones who are not experiencing symptoms.

Medical Therapy

Oral Dissolution with Bile Acids

Chenodeoxycholic acid and ursodeoxycholic acid when taken orally can effectively dissolve cholesterol gallstones; neither works for pigment stones. The only structural difference between these two molecules is the orientation of the hydroxyl group in the seven position. This epimeric difference confers unique physical-chemical properties to each bile acid, accounting for their differences in mechanisms of action, dosage, and side effects. The 7α-hydroxyl group of chenodeoxycholic acid provides it with an axial orientation. It is therefore more soluble in water and has a greater detergent action. For ursodeoxycholic acid, the equatorial position of its 7β-hydroxyl lessens its water solubility and detergent action. Ursodeoxycholic acid is thus less injurious to biological membranes, does not cause secretory diarrhea, and is not hepatotoxic.

Both bile acids reduce the hepatic secretion of cholesterol into bile, lowering cholesterol saturation of bile. Chenodeoxycholic acid decreases hepatic cholesterol synthesis. Ursodeoxycholic acid facilitates conversion of hepatic cholesterol to bile acids and reduces cholesterol absorption in the intestine. Ursodeoxycholic acid, being less of a detergent, does not carry as much cholesterol into bile. Further, ursodeoxycholic acid may have a different mechanism by which it solubilizes cholesterol molecules from gallstones—incorporating the cholesterol into phospholipid vesicles rather than just micelles.

Pharmacologic properties also differ. Ursodeoxycholic acid is less well absorbed because of reduced water solubility, but its 7-β-OH group is removed more slowly by intestinal bacteria. This resistance to bacterial hydrolysis permits a lower therapeutic dose. Chenodeoxycholic acid should be administered at 13 to 15 mg per day, ursodeoxycholic acid at 8 to 10 mg per kilogram per day. Obese individuals may require dosages up to 50 percent higher.

Trials of clinical efficacy are controversial. Complete dissolution in patients with cholesterol gallstones varies from 0 to 64 percent for chenodeoxycholic acid and 9 to 83 percent for ursodeoxycholic acid. Methodologic differences in patient selection, sample size, and reporting bias likely account for most of these discrepancies.

The initial enthusiasm for chenodeoxycholic acid became tempered by a major National Institutes of Health study which revealed that only 14 percent of patients could expect complete dissolution of radiolucent gallstones after 2 years of therapy. Many experienced diarrhea and a few developed reversible hepatic toxicity. Although many have written off chenodeoxycholic acid based on this work, most patients in the study actually were on a subtherapeutic dose. As a result, ursodeoxycholic acid, which does not induce diarrhea or elevate serum transaminase or cholesterol levels, is now the drug of choice. Consolidating all ursodeoxycholic acid trials in a meta-analysis indicates that complete dissolution occurred in 37.3 percent of patients. Combination therapy with 7.5 mg chenodeoxycholic acid plus 6.5 mg of ursodeoxycholic acid per kilogram per day might even be faster and better, succeeding in 63 percent, although only limited studies are available.

Factors for success are patient dependent, related to gallbladder function and stone size and composition. Gallbladder visualization on an oral cholecystogram or ultrasound evidence of a decrease in gallbladder size after a fatty meal or cholescintigraphy demonstrates adequate gallbladder function and patency of the cystic duct. Gallstones should be radiolucent, indicating that they are likely composed of cholesterol. Unfortunately pigment stones are not necessarily radiopaque. Small stones with a high surface-to-volume ratio are more likely to dissolve. Ideal candidates are tiny (<5 mm), radiolucent stones which float on oral cholecystography, indicating a higher likelihood of cholesterol rather than calcium. Ninety percent of such cases will undergo total dissolution when treated for 6 to 12 months. Unfortunately only about 3 percent of all patients fall into this category. Radiolucent gallstones with diameters of 10 mm or less, representing 15 percent of all gallstones, yield a near 60 percent success rate. Dissolution rates are lower with broader selection criteria and for obese individuals.

Side effects with ursodeoxycholic acid are minimal; any symptoms likely relate to the gallstone disease per se. Biliary pain may even be less frequent while on bile acid therapy. The leading management problem is the need for prolonged therapy (up to 2 years), plus the risk of recurrence once therapy is discontinued. Fifty percent will redevelop stones over a 5 year period; most are not symptomatic and a second dissolution is quite feasible.

Oral dissolution therapy is most appropriate in those with symptomatic gallstones which are small, the informed patient who wishes to avoid surgery, or when a comorbid condition precludes a safe operation. Use of a low-cholesterol diet and ingestion of the bile acid dose at bedtime improve the success rate with chenodeoxycholic acid but are unproven for ursodeoxycholic acid where no guidelines exist. While on bile acid therapy, ultrasonographic follow-up at 6 to 9 months can determine if dissolution is proceeding. Once dissolution is complete, bile acid therapy should be continued for another 3 months to eliminate any stone remnants that might be too small for ultrasonographic detection. Then annual ultrasonography may be useful for a few years. Detection of stone recurrence indicates consideration for another course of bile acid therapy. There is no established therapy to prevent recurrent stone formation, but common sense suggests eliminating obvious risk factors such as obesity.

Bile acid therapy compared to cholecystectomy is not cost effective in younger patients. In those over 65 years, bile acids become more cost effective.

Extracorporeal Shock Wave Lithotripsy

Shock waves are an ultrashort, high pressure form of sound wave. Their multiple frequencies provide higher energy and greater tissue penetration. Generated outside the body and transmitted via water, shock-wave energy travels through human tissue with little attenuation or damage. Acoustic impedance abruptly changes at the interface between body tissues and the surface of the stone, causing wave deflection. Shock-wave energy is released, yielding tear-and-shear forces. The formation and violent collapse of macroscopic gas bubbles in the liquid bile adjacent to the stone's surface produces a cavitation effect. Fissures develop, and fragmentation leads to progressive stone disintegration.

The three techniques to generate shock waves use a spark gap, piezoelectric, or electromagnetic source. They differ in terms of the energy delivered to the stone. Higher energy produces better stone fragmentation but causes more discomfort for the patient. Current systems use a small focal volume, lessening the requirement for anesthesia or analgesia and making biliary lithotripsy an outpatient procedure.

Disintegration of gallstones into fragments permits the spontaneous passage of small particles (<2 to 3 mm) from the biliary tract into the intestine. If gallbladder contraction is impaired, mechanical ejection is less effective. Shock-wave lithotripsy therefore requires adjuvant bile acid therapy to dissolve residual fragments. The standard is a combination of 7 to 8 mg of chenodeoxycholic acid plus 6 to 7 mg ursodeoxycholic acid per kilogram per day. Several months may be necessary before clearance of stone fragments is complete.

Inclusion criteria embrace symptomatic patients with biliary pain, a functioning gallbladder, and radiolucent stones. The patient may have up to three stones, but none should be larger than 20 mm and their total diameter should be less than the equivalent of a 30 mm stone. Excluded are gallstones associated with complications (acute cholecystitis or pancreatitis), concomitant bile duct stones, coagulopathy, pregnancy, or local pathology which would either obscure targeting of the stones or present a structural risk (e.g., vascular aneurysm). Treatment times average about 1 hour; usually one to two sessions are required. The aim is to produce fragments less than 3 to 5 mm which will clear spontaneously. The ideal is a solitary, non-calcified gallstone less than 20 mm in diameter; success can be 95 percent in experienced hands. Broadening the standards to patients with 20 to 30 mm gallstones and those with up to three stones in a functioning gallbladder yields a lesser clearance rate of 60 percent. About 7 to 16 percent of all patients with symptomatic stones fall into these two categories.

Complications of shock-wave lithotripsy are minor: biliary pain (25 percent), presumably from passage of stone fragments; pancreatitis (1 to 2 percent), which usually is uncomplicated; and hematuria (3 to 5 percent). The recurrence rate is less than after bile acid dissolution, perhaps reflecting the natural history of solitary stones. Twenty percent develop stones at 4 years; most remain asymptomatic.

The procedure is not widely approved in North America. For older patients, shock-wave lithotripsy is cost effective compared to cholecystectomy but not in younger persons. It is especially useful in patients with a high surgical risk. Shock-wave lithotripsy of bile duct stones is also reasonable in selected cases in which large ductal stones cannot be crushed or extricated by ERCP or the percutaneous transhepatic route. This is discussed in the chapter *Choledocholithiasis.*

Direct Contact Dissolution

Instillation of solvents into the common bile duct to dissolve retained stones has evolved from using ether (which becomes volatile at body temperature producing pain) to a medium-chain triglyceride derivative, monooctanoin (glyceryl-1-monooctanoate), approved and marketed as Capmul 8210. Monooctanoin perfusion of the biliary tract via T-tube, nasobiliary tube, percutaneous transhepatic catheter, or cholecystectomy drain clears the common duct in 26 to 50 percent. Significant side effects including pulmonary edema, peptic ulceration, and systemic acidosis, plus the advent of sophisticated endoscopic and percutaneous methods to extract ductal stones, has obviated the need for monooctanoin infusion.

Methyl tert-butyl ether (MTBE), a liquid at body temperature, is a powerful solvent but also is potentially explosive and toxic. Its use in dissolving gallstones is invasive, requiring direct instillation via a percutaneous transhepatic catheter placed in the gallbladder. Small volumes (about 4 ml to prevent outflow from the gallbladder) are continuously infused and aspirated, facilitated by an automated pump. Dissolution occurs in 95 percent after repeated cycles lasting 6 to 7 hours. Adverse effects such as hemolysis and somnolence have been surprisingly mild. Use is limited to very highly specialized centers and then only for those who are high surgical risks.

Other percutaneous techniques are mechanical, technically demanding, and experimental. Cholecystolithotomy removes the stone from the gallbladder. Rotary contact lithotripsy crushes the stone in a metal basket containing rotary blades.

■ SURGERY

Open Cholecystectomy

Cholecystectomy via an "open" abdominal incision has been standard treatment for symptomatic gallstone disease. It is curative, removing gallstone and the gallbladder. The mortality is <0.5 percent when electively performed for biliary colic, but reaches 3 percent for emergency surgery in acute cholecystitis or for common duct procedures. It is even higher in the elderly. Hospitalization averages about 1 week. There are few contraindications to classical cholecystectomy. Variations including a mini-incision somewhat reduce the postoperative pain and shorten the convalescent time slightly. This procedure is discussed in the chapter on cholecystitis.

Laparoscopic Cholecystectomy

This new operation employs laparoscopic visualization of the gallbladder and surrounding vital tissues while the peritoneal cavity is insufflated with carbon dioxide gas. This procedure is discussed in detail in a separate chapter. The procedure is a variant of the standard cholecystectomy. Operative cholangiogram can be performed through a small incision in the cystic duct; in common practice this is only done in about 5 percent of cases. Postoperative recovery is phenomenal. Many are discharged within 24 hours and return to normal physical activity within 1 week. Patient comfort and the cosmetic effects highlight this procedure.

Contraindications are sepsis, peritonitis, and distended bowel. Conversion to an open cholecystectomy is necessary in about 5 to 10 percent of cases. The most ominous complication is bile duct injury, usually the result of mistaking the common bile duct for the cystic duct or an inaccurately placed clip. Retained common duct stones are a further problem necessitating an increased use of ERCP for their removal.

The popularity of laparoscopic cholecystectomy has spread throughout North America. About 80 percent of cholecystectomies are now performed in this manner. Critical assessment of safety, training standards, cost effectiveness, and outcome are necessary as the potential for overuse is great.

Suggested Reading

Bachrach WH, Hofmann AF. Ursodeoxycholic acid in the treatment of cholesterol cholelithiasis: Part I, II. Dig Dis Sci 1982; 27:737–761, 833–856.

May GR, Sutherland LR, Shaffer EA. Efficacy of bile acid therapy for gallstone dissolution: A meta-analysis of randomized trials. Aliment Pharmacol Ther 1993; 7:139–148.

Ransohoff DF, Gracie WA, Wolfenson LD, Neuhauser B. Prophylactic cholecystectomy or expectant management of silent gallstones: A decision analysis to assess survival. Ann Intern Med 1983; 99:199–204.

Sachmann M, Pauletzki J, Sauerbruch T, et al. The Munich gallbladder lithotripsy study: Results of the first 711 patients. Ann Intern Med 1991; 114:290–296.

Schoenfield LJ, Lachmin JM, and the National Cooperative Gallstone Study Group. Chenodiol (chenodeoxycholic acid) for dissolution of gallstones: A controlled study of efficacy and safety. Ann Intern Med 1981; 95:257–282.

Strasberg SM, Clavien P-A. Cholecystolithiasis: Lithotherapy for the 1990s. Hepatology 1992; 16:820–839.

Thistle JL, May GR, Bender CE, et al. Dissolution of cholesterol gallbladder stones by methyl-tert-butyl ether administered by percutaneous transhepatic catheter. N Engl J Med 1989; 320:633–639.

ACUTE PANCREATITIS

John H.C. Ranson, B.M., B.Ch., M.A.
Peter Shamamian, M.D.

The term *acute pancreatitis* is used to describe a broad spectrum of etiologic, pathologic, and clinical entities. Etiologic associations include factors as varied as gallstones and the bite of the black scorpion of Trinidad. Pathologic findings range from edema through hemorrhagic necrosis, and the clinical course ranges from mild, self-limiting symptoms through a fulminant, rapidly lethal illness. It is clear, therefore, that management of patients with acute pancreatitis must be individualized.

■ ETIOLOGY

Our knowledge of the actual pathogenesis of acute pancreatitis is fragmentary and incomplete. In most instances, etiologic factors have been identified primarily on the basis of epidemiologic associations. Sixty to 80 percent of patients have either *biliary lithiasis* or a history of long-standing *alcohol abuse*. Clinical pancreatitis is recognized in 0.9 percent to 9.5 percent of alcoholic patients and pathologic evidence of pancreatitis is found in 17 percent to 45 percent of this group. Cholelithiasis is present in 60 percent of nonalcoholic patients with pancreatitis and pancreatitis has occurred in 4 percent to 5 percent of patients treated surgically for biliary stones. Some of the other etiologic associations of pancreatitis are listed in Table 1.

Over 80 drugs have been implicated as causative agents of pancreatitis. Some of the more common agents implicated are asparaginase, azathioprine, didanosine, and pentamidine. Idiopathic pancreatitis is a commonly encountered entity describing patients with confirmed pancreatitis, not associated with a specific etiology as defined in Table 1.

Table 1 Etiologic Factors in Acute Pancreatitis

Metabolic:	*Vascular:*
Alcohol	Postoperative
Hyperlipoproteinemia	Atherosclerosis
Hypercalcemia	Vasculitis
Drugs	Periarteritis nodosa
Genetic	*Infection:*
Scorpion venom	Mumps
Mechanical:	Coxsackie B
Cholelithiasis	Cytomegalovirus
Postoperative	Cryptococcus
Pancreas divisum	
Post-traumatic	
Retrograde pancreatography	
Pancreatic duct obstruction	
Pancreatic ductal bleeding	
Duodenal obstruction	

CLINICAL MANIFESTATIONS AND DIAGNOSIS

An accurate diagnosis of acute pancreatitis depends primarily on a careful evaluation of the patient's history and physical examination. The clinical presentation may be variable with symptoms closely mimicking those of acute biliary disease, peptic ulcer, and intestinal obstruction or infarction. The predominant symptom is usually pain that is characteristically located in the epigastrum and may radiate to the back and to both flanks. The pain is constant in character and may be extremely severe.

Nausea and vomiting are almost invariably present and often a prominent early feature. The findings on physical examination also vary widely. Patients may be restless with a rapid pulse and respiratory rate. The blood pressure may be mildly elevated, normal, or decreased. The temperature is usually 99°F to 100°F. The abdomen is usually mildly distended and may exhibit a characteristic epigastric fullness. Tenderness is usually most marked over the epigastrum and upper abdomen. It may be diffuse, especially in more severe cases. Grey-Turner or Cullen signs are often described, yet rarely encountered in acute pancreatitis.

Laboratory Findings

Determination of serum and urine amylase levels are the most widely used tests for the diagnosis of pancreatic disease. Elevated serum levels are observed at hospital admission in 95 percent of patients with acute pancreatitis compared to only 5 percent of patients with other acute intra-abdominal conditions. Among patients with pancreatitis who have normal serum amylase levels, approximately 40 percent have hyperlipidemia with lactescent serum. In large groups of patients with acute abdominal conditions, approximately 20 percent have elevated serum amylase levels. Of these, approximately 75 percent have pancreatitis, and among the 25 percent with extrapancreatic disease, only about 50 percent have conditions that might be confused with acute pancreatitis.

Serum lipase levels are elevated in acute pancreatitis, and may represent a more accurate laboratory diagnostic test for acute pancreatitis. As with serum amylase levels, serum lipase levels are known to increase with extra pancreatic acute abdominal conditions, such as cholecystitis, intestinal obstruction, or infarction.

Radiographic Findings

Plain radiographs of the abdomen and chest demonstrate findings that may support a diagnosis of acute pancreatitis in approximately 80 percent of patients. The most common is segmental dilation or ileus of a loop of small bowel in the left upper quadrant, the so-called "sentinel loop." Dilation of the transverse colon and loss of the psoas margins are other relatively common findings.

Computed tomography (CT) provides the most accurate available noninvasive imaging of the retroperitoneum. The most frequent findings in patients with acute pancreatitis are diffuse pancreatic enlargement, obliteration of the peripancreatic fat planes, and inflammation of the left anterior pararenal space. Peripancreatic fluid collections may also be visualized. It must be recognized that early CT findings may be interpreted as normal in a significant portion of patients judged to have acute pancreatitis. In most such instances, the pancreatitis is mild.

Diagnostic Celiotomy

In most patients, the diagnosis of acute pancreatitis can be made with reasonable certainty on the basis of clinical, radiographic, and laboratory findings. In some cases, however, other diseases may closely mimic acute pancreatitis, and diagnostic celiotomy may be required to exclude or treat acute life-threatening extrapancreatic disease in up to 5 percent of patients. In this regard, it should be stressed that strong positive evidence of acute pancreatitis does not exclude the possibility of concomitant extrapancreatic disease in an occasional patient.

PROGNOSTIC ASSESSMENT

Because the spectrum of severity of acute pancreatitis ranges so widely, the early identification of the risk of life-threatening complications is helpful in permitting the appropriate application of monitoring and therapeutic interventions. For the evaluation of proposed treatments, objective means to stratify the diverse population of patients with pancreatitis are essential.

In 1974, we reported the 11 early objective prognostic criteria listed in Table 2. These signs were developed from a statistical analysis of the relationship between early measurements and overall morbidity and mortality of acute pancreatitis. The relationship between the number of signs present and morbidity in a group of 450 patients is shown in Figure 1. The acute physiology and chronic health evaluation (APACHE II) illness grading system has been applied to prognostic assessment of pancreatitis. The accuracy of this system appears to be comparable to that of the specific multiple prognostic criteria. APACHE II is more complex but has the advantage that it may be applied at times other than at diagnosis. A relationship between prognosis and the volume and color of fluid obtained by paracentesis, early hemodynamic measurements, coagulation factors, complement levels, antiproteases, and C-reactive protein have also been described.

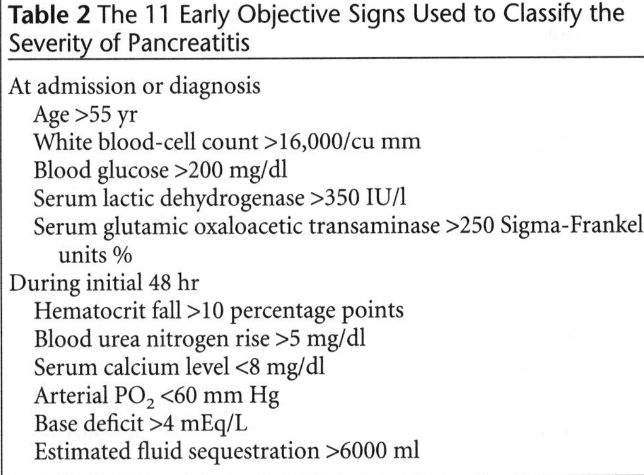

Table 2 The 11 Early Objective Signs Used to Classify the Severity of Pancreatitis

At admission or diagnosis
Age >55 yr
White blood-cell count >16,000/cu mm
Blood glucose >200 mg/dl
Serum lactic dehydrogenase >350 IU/l
Serum glutamic oxaloacetic transaminase >250 Sigma-Frankel units %
During initial 48 hr
Hematocrit fall >10 percentage points
Blood urea nitrogen rise >5 mg/dl
Serum calcium level <8 mg/dl
Arterial PO_2 <60 mm Hg
Base deficit >4 mEq/L
Estimated fluid sequestration >6000 ml

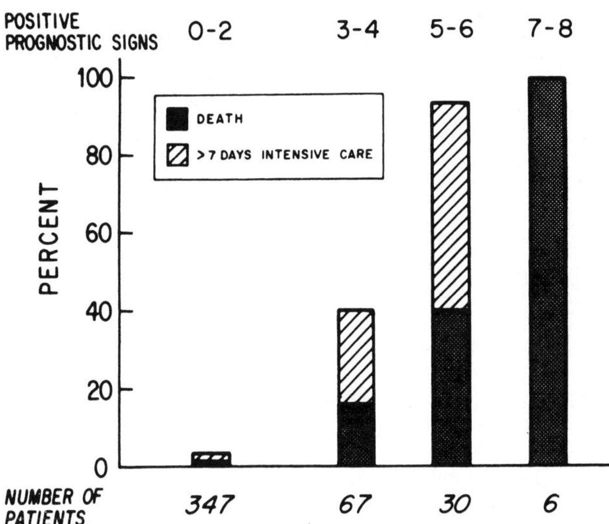

Figure 1
Correlation of positive prognostic signs and morbidity in acute pancreatitis.

In recent years, there has been renewed interest in the relationship between pancreatic necrosis and the pathogenesis of the complications of pancreatitis. Correlations have been reported to be between alpha-$_1$ protease inhibitor, alpha-$_2$ macro proteins, complement factors C3 and C4, and C-reactive protein and trypsinogen activation peptides and necrotizing pancreatitis. Most intriguing has been the use of contrast-enhanced CT.

CT appearance of the pancreas is classified as grade A, normal appearing gland; grade B, focal or diffuse enlargement of the pancreas; grade C, peripancreatic inflammation; grade D, a single peripancreatic fluid collection; and grade E, two or more fluid collections and/or the presence of gas in or adjacent to the pancreas. In our experience, patients with grade A and B pancreatitis have a mild uncomplicated course. Fluid collections can be managed expectantly, as 54 percent of these cases resolve without specific therapy. Infectious complications develop in 7 to 12 percent of patients with grade C, 17 to 25 percent of those with grade D, and 56 to 61 percent of those with grade E. The mortality rates of patients with grade D and grade E pancreatitis can approach 20 percent.

Further staging can be made by an estimation of pancreatic necrosis. Radiographic enhancement of the pancreas following contrast injection has been interpreted as evidence of tissue viability. Failure of enhancement has been interpreted as evidence of tissue necrosis. Patients without necrosis had no mortality and a 6 percent rate of morbidity, while patients with necrosis have a 23 percent mortality rate and an 82 percent rate of morbidity.

The finding of nonenhancement of pancreatic tissue is, in our experience, associated with an approximately 70 percent risk of late pancreatic sepsis.

■ TREATMENT

Multiple measures have been proposed for the treatment of patients with acute pancreatitis. It is convenient to categorize these various proposals by their therapeutic objectives. These are (1) to limit the severity of pancreatic inflammation itself; (2) to ameliorate complications by interrupting their pathogenesis; and (3) to support the patient and treat complications as they arise. Measures that have been proposed for the treatment of acute pancreatitis are listed in Table 3 under these three headings.

To Limit Severity of Inflammation

Nasogastric Suctioning and the Timing of Oral Feeding

Nasogastric suction has traditionally been instituted in patients with acute pancreatitis to reduce vomiting and abdominal distention. It has also been suggested that the aspiration of gastric acid may decrease pancreatic exocrine secretion by reducing secretin release. The therapeutic efficacy of nasogastric suction has been evaluated recently in controlled clinical trials. Although none of these trials demonstrated any significant benefit from nasogastric suction, it should be noted that the great majority of patients studied had mild, alcoholic pancreatitis. In addition, the number of patients in individual studies was small. Hence, the present data indicate that nasogastric suction is not essential for recovery from mild pancreatitis, especially that associated with alcohol abuse. I believe that further studies are needed to evaluate the role of this measure in more severe pancreatitis and in other etiologic subgroups. I continue to recommend nasogastric suction for most patients with acute pancreatitis of moderate or severe degree because of the symptomatic relief that is often reported. Inhibition of gastric acid production by the administration of H_2 blockers, and attempts to inhibit pancreatic exocrine secretion by administration of anticholinergics, calcitonin, somatostatin, and glucagon, have not been of benefit in controlled clinical trials.

In patients with mild pancreatitis, oral feedings consisting of a low-fat diet can be resumed within a few days. Patients with severe pancreatitis usually do not tolerate oral alimentation until the symptoms of acute pancreatitis have resolved and intestinal peristalsis returns.

Table 3 Measures Proposed for the Treatment of Acute Pancreatitis

A. To limit severity of pancreatic inflammation
  1. Inhibition of pancreatic secretion
    a) Nasogastric suction
    b) Pharmacologic: anticholinergics, glucagon, 5-fluorouracil, acetazolamide, cimetidine, propylthiouracil, calcitonin, somatostatin
    c) Hypothermia
    d) Pancreatic irradiation
  2. Inhibition of pancreatic enzymes
    a) Aprotinin, epsilon-aminocaproic acid, soybean typsin inhibitor, insulin, snake antivenom gabexate mesilate, camostate, fresh frozen plasma, chlorophyll, xylocaine
  3. Corticosteroids
  4. Prostaglandins
  5. Operative biliary procedures
  6. Endoscopic biliary intervention

B. To interrupt the pathogenesis of complications
  1. Antibiotics
  2. Antacids, cimetidine
  3. Heparin, fibrinolysin
  4. Low molecular-weight dextran
  5. Vasopressin
  6. Peritoneal lavage
  7. Thoracic duct drainage
  8. Operative pancreatic drainage
  9. Pancreatic resection
  10. Debridement of necrotic tissue

C. To support the patient and treat complications
  1. Restoration and maintenance of intravascular volume
  2. Electrolyte replacement
  3. Respiratory support
  4. Nutritional support
  5. Analgesia
  6. Heparin
  7. Debridement and drainage of pancreatic infection
  8. Drainage of pseudocysts

The concept that the severity of acute pancreatitis and of its complications may be reduced by inhibitors of pancreatic enzymes has received much attention over the past 30 years. The most extensively studied agent has been aprotinin. Controlled studies of this and other enzyme inhibitors have provided no convincing evidence that any of these agents would have significant clinical benefit.

Adrenocorticosteroids have been administered to patients with acute pancreatitis because of their anti-inflammatory effects. No adequate clinical studies have been reported.

Studies have recently been reported evaluating the influence of prostaglandins and drugs that influence their metabolism on the course of acute pancreatitis. A randomized double-blind clinical trial evaluated indomethacin administered by suppository (50 mg twice daily). Only 30 patients were studied, but a significant reduction in pain was reported.

Biliary Procedures

Evaluation of the treatment of patients with gallstone-associated pancreatitis has been clouded by difficulty in determining the presence or absence of actual pancreatic inflammation. Of patients who have abdominal pain, elevated serum, or urinary amylase levels and gallstones, 39 to 75 percent (60 percent average) have no significant pancreatitis demonstrable at early operation or autopsy. Such patients respond well to management of their biliary disease and behave clinically as if they had no pancreatitis. Furthermore, approximately 80 percent of patients with true pancreatitis have mild disease and will recover uneventfully. A controlled clinical trial has shown that early operative intervention to correct associated gallstones is associated with increased morbidity, especially in those who have severe pancreatitis.

Recently, endoscopic sphincterotomy and removal of stones impacted in the ampulla of Vater have been advocated for patients with gallstone-associated pancreatitis. A recent controlled clinical trial indicated that emergency endoscopic retrograde cholangiopancreatography and endoscopic papillotomy, if common bile duct stones were present, were associated with a reduction in biliary sepsis, compared to noninterventional treatment. Unfortunately, however, there was no significant difference in the incidence of either systemic or local complications of pancreatitis following early endoscopic intervention.

To Interrupt the Pathogenesis of Complications

Pharmacologic Therapy

Antibiotics have traditionally been recommended in the treatment of acute pancreatitis. Prospective controlled clinical trials of ampicillin in patients with mild acute pancreatitis have failed to effect any reduction in septic complications with this particular antibiotic. We continue to recommend broad-spectrum antibiotics in patients who have gallstone-associated pancreatitis, because of the frequency of biliary infection in this group. In addition, antibiotics may be beneficial in those patients judged to have severe pancreatitis. One trial compared patients with pancreatic necrosis randomized to receive either no antibiotic or prophylactic imipenem. There was a significant reduction of pancreatic sepsis in the imipenem group (30.3 percent vs. 12.2 percent, $p < 0.01$), although there was no effect on mortality.

Antacids or H_2 Blockers. Should be administered to patients with pancreatitis in order to reduce the frequency of acute gastroduodenal ulceration or bleeding.

Anticoagulants have been recommended on the basis of experimental studies. It has, however, been my experience that administration of heparin in the first few days of acute pancreatitis is associated with a very high risk of significant retroperitoneal hemorrhage and should be avoided, if possible. Attempts to improve pancreatic blood flow by the administration of low molecular-weight dextran and vasopressin have been recommended on the basis of experimental studies, but not evaluated clinically.

Peritoneal Lavage

Controlled clinical studies of the efficacy of peritoneal lavage in the treatment of acute pancreatitis have produced conflicting results. Our initial experience suggested that peritoneal lavage was a significant adjunct to the management of early cardiovascular and respiratory complications.

We have considered any patients who were experiencing their first or second episode of acute pancreatitis and who had "severe" pancreatitis on the basis of prognostic signs (Table 1) to be candidates for peritoneal lavage. We have attempted to minimize the risk of visceral injury by introducing lavage catheters through an open incision about 4 to 5 cm in length with direct visualization of the peritoneum. Local infiltration anesthesia is used. The lavage fluid is an approximately isotonic electrolyte solution containing 15 g per liter of dextrose (Dianeal). Potassium, 4 mEq per liter; heparin, 500 USP; and ampicillin, 125 mg are usually added to each liter of lavage fluid. In general, 2 L of the fluid are allowed to run into the peritoneal cavity over about 15 minutes to remain intraperitoneally for about 30 minutes and then drained out by gravity over 15 minutes. The cycle is usually repeated hourly using 48 liters of lavage fluid during each 24 hour period. Lavage has been instituted within 48 hours of diagnosis in all patients. It has been discontinued after 48 hours to seven days, depending upon the patient's course.

Initially we had limited the period of lavage to 4 days because of fear of introducing infection into the peritoneal cavity, if the catheters were allowed to remain longer. However, a chance observation in 1979 led to a study of the duration of peritoneal lavage that was reported in 1990. This study suggests that a longer period of lavage is associated with a reduced risk of late pancreatic infection and of death from this complication. Although this observation requires confirmation by others, the morbidity of long-term peritoneal lavage is small compared to its benefits. I would recommend peritoneal lavage for patients who have severe pancreatitis, on the basis of prognostic criteria and CT findings.

Because pancreatic enzymes can enter the blood stream by way of lymphatic channels, it has been proposed that drainage of the thoracic duct may ameliorate the course of acute pancreatitis. Reports of the efficacy of this approach have been too limited to allow evaluation.

Early Operative Drainage

Early operative drainage of the pancreas may be associated with a dramatic reduction in early cardiovascular instability. It is, however, followed by dramatically increased respiratory and pancreatic septic complications.

The concept that formal pancreatic resection may ameliorate the course of very severe pancreatitis has received extensive evaluation, especially in Europe. Recent critical evaluation of this measure has shown no convincing benefit, and this measure has, at present, few, if any, advocates.

Surgical debridement of necrotic tissue without formal pancreatic resection and with postoperative lavage of the peritoneal bed has recently been advocated. A low overall mortality has been reported. Many patients subjected to this intervention have, however, had uninfected necrosis, and it is difficult to be certain how many of these patients might have recovered without any form of surgical therapy.

To Support the Patient and Treat Complications

Until better measures are available that will limit the severity of acute pancreatitis and prevent its complications, the most important aspects of treatment are supportive and symptomatic.

Intravascular Volume Management

Evaluation and monitoring of intravascular volume and cardiovascular function require regular measurements of pulse rate and blood pressure. In most patients, a central venous catheter should be placed and an indwelling urethral catheter introduced for regular measurement of central venous pressure, venous blood gases, and hourly urine output. In those with associated cardiovascular disease, large fluid requirements, or severe respiratory complications, monitoring of pulmonary arterial pressures and cardiac output using a Swan-Ganz catheter may be essential for appropriate management. In most patients, intravascular volume can be satisfactorily restored and maintained using crystalloid solutions. Serial measurements of hematocrit may indicate the need for blood transfusion. If colloid administration is required, fresh frozen plasma may theoretically be superior to albumin because of the presence of trypsin inhibitors. Hypokalemia is frequent and potassium replacement usually is required. Intravenous replacement of calcium and magnesium has also been recommended. Symptoms and complications referable to hypocalcemia, however, are uncommon and because hypercalcemia has been implicated in the genesis of pancreatitis, calcium administration should be done cautiously.

Respiratory Monitoring and Support

Clinically occult respiratory failure is a frequent feature of acute pancreatitis and may occur in patients who do not have severe disease, by the usual clinical criteria. Changes in oxyhemoglobin affinity during acute pancreatitis may increase the physiologic consequences of respiratory failure, and hypoxemia certainly may be lethal if undiagnosed or untreated. It is essential, therefore, that arterial blood gas values be determined at the time of diagnosis and at intervals of not less than 12 hours for the initial 48 to 72 hours of treatment. Subsequent measurements depend on the patient's course.

In most patients, early hypoxemia resolves as the underlying pancreatitis subsides, and the only management necessary is close observation and administration of oxygen. Progressive pulmonary insufficiency, pulmonary infiltrates, and effusions tend to occur in those patients who have severe acute pancreatitis and following early operative intervention. They should be anticipated in these groups. The most appropriate management is early endotracheal intubation and institution of mechanical respiratory support with positive end expiratory pressure.

Nutritional Support

The occurrence of marked nutritional depletion in patients with acute pancreatitis is well known. In those with mild pancreatitis, oral feedings can usually be resumed within a few days. In patients with severe pancreatitis, oral feedings usually are not tolerated for prolonged periods of time and alternative nutritional support must be instituted as early as possible. Initially, the only possible route is intravenous alimentation. After intestinal peristalsis returns, enteral feedings are a possible alternative route.

For most patients, standard total parenteral nutrition, initiated as soon as early cardiovascular instability has subsided, is the most practical form of nutritional support. Glucose levels should be carefully monitored and insulin given as needed. The safety of intravenous lipid as a caloric source has been controversial. Although it is probably safe, we limit administration of lipids to that required to provide essential fatty acids. It should be emphasized that total parenteral nutrition is only appropriate for patients in whom oral feedings are not possible for a substantial period of time.

Table 4 Incidence of Clinical and Laboratory Features in Patients with Infected Pancreatic Necrosis

Fever >101° F	100%
Abdominal distention	94%
Palpable mass	71%
Hypotension (BP <90 mm Hg)	39%
Respirator support	39%
Renal failure	39%
Coma	28%
Elevated serum amylase	28%
White cell count >10,000/mm^3	78%
Platelet count <175,000/cm	55%
Bilirubin >1.5 mg/dl	67%
Serum albumin <3.5 g/l	75%

Analgesia

The pain associated with acute pancreatitis may be very severe and it is traditional to administer meperidine or pentazocine rather than morphine because of the spasm of the ampulla of Vater that is associated with the latter drug.

Heparin

Although early administration of heparin may be hazardous, patients with severe pancreatitis may develop a hypercoagulable state late in their course. If this occurs, heparin may be indicated during the second or third weeks of severe pancreatitis, to reduce thrombotic complications.

Diagnosis and Treatment of Infected Pancreatic Necrosis

Pancreatic infection is usually recognized after the first 14 days of treatment in patients with acute pancreatitis who have not undergone early laparotomy. The diagnosis should be suspected in all patients who have persisting fever or leukocytosis after the early phase of disease. As discussed earlier, CT scan is also helpful in identifying patients at high risk for infection. Specifically, patients who have fluid identified on their initial CT scan (grades D and E) have an approximately 50 percent risk of late infection. Furthermore, those who have more than 50 percent of their gland failing to enhance on early contrast CT scan have an approximately 70 percent risk of developing infection. The clinical and laboratory findings at the time sepsis was diagnosed in patients who developed sepsis after early nonoperative treatment of acute pancreatitis are shown in Table 4. The most prominent findings are fever, abdominal distension, and leukocytosis, with a palpable abdominal mass. Laboratory findings are nonspecific. Clearly, the occurrence of positive blood cultures that cannot be attributed to nonpancreatic sources indicates probable pancreatic sepsis. The presence of gas outside the gastrointestinal tract, either on plain abdominal film or on CT scan, usually indicates sepsis and is present in approximately 14 percent of patients with sepsis. If the presence of infection is uncertain on the basis of clinical and laboratory findings, needle aspiration of the pancreas under CT guidance with bacteriologic examination of the aspirate may be helpful in determining the presence or absence of infection.

Pancreatic infection secondary to acute pancreatitis is almost always associated with extensive necrosis of pancreatic or peripancreatic tissues. The infected material is semisolid, and attempts at percutaneous catheter drainage are usually futile. Operative treatment is, therefore, required in virtually all patients. The approach that we have favored is illustrated in Figure 2. It consists of wide exploration of the whole peripancreatic retroperitoneum and institution of sump drainage. A feeding jejunostomy is constructed, and if gallstones are identified, appropriate surgical treatment is carried out.

An alternative surgical approach has been to debride and pack infected pancreatic necrosis. Essential features of this approach are to debride necrotic tissue and cover the viscera with nonadherent porous gauze followed by packing of the wound with moist laparotomy pads. The dressings are changed under general anesthesia every 2 or 3 days, until sufficient granulation has formed to permit changes on the ward. Although adequate debridement and drainage is essential for these patients, they are usually critically ill as a result of their underlying pancreatitis and superimposed sepsis. Vigorous supportive care is, therefore, essential and includes meticulous care to respiratory management, fluid and electrolyte balance, prevention of gastroduodenal bleeding, and nutritional support. Current morbidity remains high from this complication and mortality with either closed drainage or with packing followed by an overall mortality of approximately 15 percent.

Pancreatic Pseudocysts

Pseudocysts are defined as persistent localized collections of enzyme-rich fluid with a clearly defined wall made up of fibrous tissue and adjacent viscera. They occur most commonly in patients with chronic pancreatitis. Only 1 to 2 percent of patients with acute pancreatitis develop pseudocysts. The overwhelming majority of fluid collections in acute pancreatitis resolve, if they do not become infected. Such acute collections may take weeks or months to resolve but do not require intervention.

When a symptomatic pseudocyst or enlarging pseudocyst is present following acute pancreatitis, drainage is required. External drainage, either by surgery or by percutaneous catheter placement under radiographic guidance, is the simplest approach. They are, however, associated with a significant risk of pancreatic fistula. Internal drainage of a pseudocyst into the stomach, duodenum, or jejunum is applicable to the majority of mature pseudocysts. Resection may be required for anatomical reasons or in those cysts that are accompanied by major vascular communication.

■ PREVENTION OF RECURRENCE

Biliary Lithiasis

In patients with associated cholelithiasis, the risk of recurrent pancreatitis may be reduced from 36 to 63 percent down to 2 to 8 percent by correction of the underlying biliary disease. This can usually be accomplished safely during the same hospital admission.

Pancreas Divisum

Pancreas divisum is a congenital anomaly in which there is no communication between the dorsal and pancreatic ducts. It has been suggested that in patients with this anomaly, there may be relative obstruction to drainage to the major portion

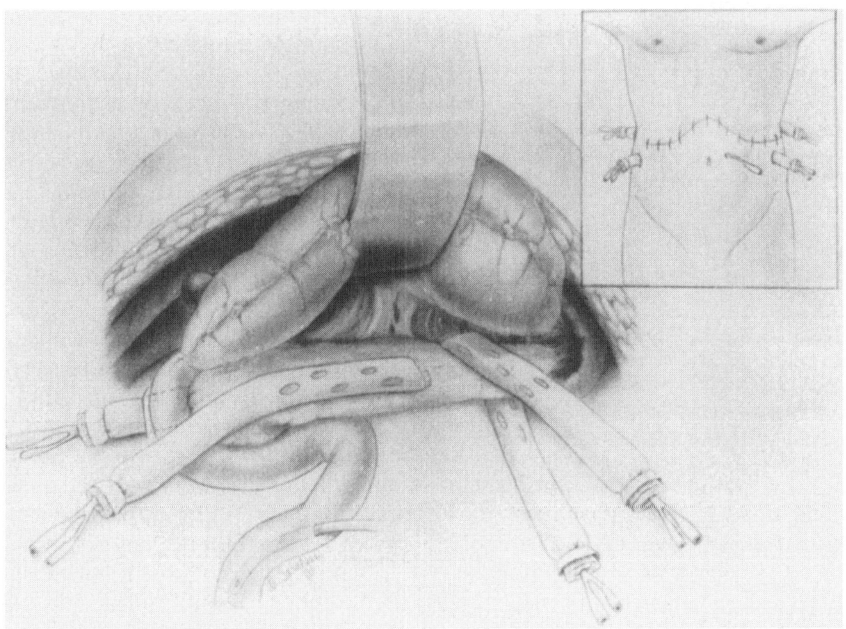

Figure 2
Operative approach in infected pancreatic necrosis.

of the pancreas served by Santorini's duct with resultant pancreatitis. There are a few well-documented cases in which the anomaly of pancreas divisum has been associated with histologically demonstrated pancreatitis with the dorsal pancreas drained by the duct of Santorini while the ventral pancreas drained by Wirsung's duct is normal. However, the frequency with which this anomaly is the primary etiology of pancreatitis and, indeed, the mechanism by which it may initiate pancreatitis, are unknown. It has been reported that transduodenal sphincteroplasty may yield good results in 50 to 68 percent of patients with pancreas divisum and recurrent acute pancreatitis. However, this therapeutic intervention can be hazardous, and further studies are required to develop criteria to identify those patients who may benefit from treatment.

■ RECOMMENDATIONS

Our current approach to the management of patients with acute pancreatitis includes close observation and reevaluation of the diagnosis. Laparotomy is reserved for those in whom there is significant concern about life-threatening extrapancreatic disease. Patients require monitoring, restoration, and maintenance of intravascular volume. Respiratory status should be closely monitored by serial measurements of arterial blood gases for at least 48 to 72 hours with the institution of respiratory support when needed. Broad-spectrum antibiotics are administered to patients who have gallstone-associated or severe acute pancreatitis. Nasogastric suction is recommended for most patients who have pancreatitis of moderate or severe degree. Oral feedings should be withheld until evidence of pancreatitis has subsided. In patients with marked cardiovascular instability or renal failure, early institution of peritoneal lavage may result in dramatic clinical improvement.

We continue to use the prognostic criteria listed in Table 2 to identify patients at a high risk of developing life-threatening complications. In patients with suspected severe disease, CT scans with contrast enhancement are helpful in delineating the anatomy of the retroperitoneum. In patients who have high risk of late complications, peritoneal lavage for 7 days may reduce this risk.

In patients who develop evidence of pancreatic infection, wide debridement, and either sump drainage or packing is required. With this approach, overall mortality from acute pancreatitis is approximately 5 percent.

Suggested Reading

Beger HG, Buchler M, Bittner R. Necrosectomy and postoperative local lavage in patients with necrotizing pancreatitis: results of a prospective clinical trial. World J Surg 1988; 12:255–262.

Bradley EL, ed. Acute Pancreatitis: Principles and Practice. New York: Raven Press, 1994.

Fan S-T, Lai ECS, Mok FPT, et al. Early treatment of acute biliary pancreatitis by endoscopic papillotomy. N Engl J Med 1993; 328:228–232.

Kelly TR. Gallstone pancreatitis: a prospective randomized trial of the timing of surgery. Surgery 1988; 104:600–604.

Pederzoli P, Bassi C, Vesentini S, Campedelli A. A randomized multicentre clinical trial of antibiotic prophylaxis of septic complications in acute pancreatitis with imipenim. Surg Gynecol Obstet 1993; 176:480–483.

Ranson JHC. Necrosis and abscess. In: Bradley EL, ed. Complications of pancreatitis. Philadelphia: WB Saunders, 1982: 72.

Ranson JHC, Berman RS. Long peritoneal lavage decreases pancreatic sepsis in acute pancreatitis. Ann Surg 1990; 211:708–716.

Ranson JHC, Spencer FC. The role of peritoneal lavage in severe acute pancreatitis. Ann Surg 1978; 187:565–575.

CHRONIC PANCREATITIS: EXOCRINE AND ENDOCRINE INSUFFICIENCY

Sudhir K. Dutta, M.D., F.A.C.P., F.A.C.G., F.A.C.N.

DIAGNOSIS

The diagnosis of chronic pancreatitis is generally considered in patients who present with upper abdominal pain, chronic diarrhea, or significant weight loss. In a given case, any combination of these symptoms may be present. Furthermore, in many cases, recurrent attacks of acute pancreatitis may precede the onset of chronic pancreatitis. However, 10 to 15 percent of patients with chronic pancreatitis present initially with only diarrhea or weight loss or both. The development of malabsorption in a patient with chronic pancreatitis indicates more than 90 percent loss of exocrine pancreatic function.

The abdominal pain associated with chronic pancreatitis is characterized by a midepigastric location, a dull and continuous nature, and radiation to the back that is relieved by forward bending. Diarrhea in these patients is chronic, with a frequency ranging from only one bowel movement per day to as many as six or more per day. Weight loss is often significant (10 lb or more) and frequently associated with clinical manifestations of uncontrolled diabetes mellitus. As a result of weight loss, protein energy malnutrition of the marasmus type is initially present in 30 to 50 percent of cases of chronic pancreatitis. It is important to assess the extent of malnutrition carefully in order to determine the response to pancreatic enzyme or nutritional therapy. It is equally important to record the symptoms in detail, because the response to medical therapy is generally evaluated in relation to the presenting symptoms.

Irreversible Structural Damage

The diagnosis of chronic pancreatitis is often difficult to establish in clinical situations, particularly in patients with early disease associated with only mild to moderate pancreatic dysfunction. Evidence of irreversible structural damage or permanent functional impairment of the pancreatic gland should be obtained by various clinical tests available. Clinical evidence of irreversible structural damage generally includes (1) pancreatic calcification, (2) pancreatic duct strictures, and (3) chronic inflammation on histologic views of the pancreatic gland. Pancreatic calcification is noted on plain radiographs of the abdomen or on computed tomographic (CT) scans. Pancreatic duct abnormality is delineated by pancreatography, which can be obtained endoscopically and occasionally at the time of surgery. Pancreatic histologic findings are available in a few patients who undergo pancreatic biopsy or resection. In clinical practice, chronic pancreatitis is frequently diagnosed on the basis of pancreatic calcification and/or abnormal pancreatographic appearance.

Permanent Functional Impairment

The presence of permanent functional impairment of the pancreatic gland can be determined by traditional tests such as the secretin stimulation test or one of the newer tests of pancreatic function, such as the bentiromide nitroblue tetrazolium-para-aminobenzoic acid (NBT-PABA) test. It should be emphasized that although the secretin stimulation test is tedious and inconvenient because of the need for duodenal intubation, it is still the most sensitive test for diagnosing early pancreatic disease in patients who have not yet developed malabsorption. Among a large number of "tubeless" pancreatic function tests, the bentiromide test appears to be the most convenient, inexpensive, and easily available for diagnosing advanced chronic pancreatitis. Because of these features, sequential bentiromide tests are being used to evaluate the response to pancreatic enzyme therapy in patients with exocrine pancreatic insufficiency. However, the bentiromide test and similar "tubeless" pancreatic function tests have low sensitivity for diagnosing early or mild pancreatic gland dysfunction. Furthermore, it is essentially a urine test, which requires normal renal function, sufficient diuresis, and proper intestinal absorption. Bentiromide is a synthetic tripeptide that is specifically cleaved by pancreatic chymotrypsin. The cleavage of this molecule by chymotrypsin in the duodenum releases para-aminobenzoic acid (PABA), which is rapidly absorbed, conjugated in the liver, and excreted in the urine. Patients with chronic pancreatitis consistently excrete less PABA in the urine than healthy controls, because of impaired chymotrypsin secretion.

TREATMENT

Treatment of patients with chronic pancreatitis is generally directed toward (1) relief of upper abdominal pain and (2) correction of diarrhea, weight loss, and malnutrition.

Treatment of Abdominal Pain

Abdominal pain is the most difficult problem to treat for several reasons. First, pain is a subjective sensation, with no objective parameter to document or monitor its occurrence. Second, alcoholism is an underlying problem in many of these patients, and alcoholics have a drug-dependent personality. Not infrequently, alcoholic patients feign abdominal pain in order to obtain analgesics, sedatives, and narcotics. Consequently, it is often difficult to determine whether the abdominal pain is truly due to an underlying organic disease. Abstinence from alcohol is obviously desirable and should be strongly recommended. In the management of abdominal pain from chronic pancreatitis, I have found a five-step strategy exceedingly helpful (Table 1). The first step is documentation of pancreatic inflammation. Biochemical or radiologic evidence of pancreatic inflammation tends to suggest a pancreatic origin for such pain. Elevated serum amylase or lipase activity or evidence of an abnormal pancreatic gland on imaging suggests active pancreatic inflammation. However, patients with chronic pancreatitis sometimes have normal serum amylase and lipase levels and a fibrotic calcified pan-

Table 1 Evaluation of Patients With Abdominal Pain Associated with Chronic Pancreatitis

Step 1	Seek evidence of active pancreatic inflammation during painful periods (elevation of serum amylase, lipase, or urinary activity).
Step 2	Seek evidence of complications of pancreatitis (pancreatic pseudocyst or phlegmon).
Step 3	Rule out other upper gastrointestinal diseases (peptic ulcer disease, gastritis, and gallstone disease).
Step 4	Re-evaluate evidence of irreversible structural abnormality or permanent functional impairment of exocrine pancreatic gland.
Step 5	Closely follow-up patient's abdominal pain for 4 to 6 months.

Table 2 Management of Abdominal Pain from Chronic Pancreatitis

Patient education (about natural history of chronic pancreatitis, risk of prolonged analgesic abuse, and need for alcohol abstinence)
Administration of non-narcotic analgesics (acetaminophen, ibuprofen, and nonsteroidal analgesics)
Exogenous pancreatic enzyme therapy
Periodic administration of narcotic analgesics
Somatostatin therapy
Endoscopic intervention
Celiac ganglionectomy
Surgical intervention
  Pancreaticojejunostomy
  Pancreatectomy

creatic gland without any evidence of edema. The second step in management of pancreatic pain involves careful evaluation of complications such as pseudocyst or phlegmon. Again, pancreatic gland imaging by ultrasonography or CT helps to confirm or rule out these complications. The third step is to rule out other gastrointestinal (GI) lesions that can present clinically with upper abdominal pain, including peptic ulcer disease, penetrating ulcer, gastritis, and cholelithiasis. Upper endoscopy, ultrasonography, and a profile of liver function tests can help the differential diagnosis. The fourth step includes careful re-evaluation of the diagnosis of chronic pancreatitis in terms of irreversible structural damage or permanent impairment of pancreatic gland function; this often involves repeat pancreatography or CT scan. The fifth and final step is a close follow-up, monitoring the severity of pain, and the analgesic needs of the patient for 4 to 6 months. Again, abstinence from alcohol is essential. Alcoholism is the subject of a separate chapter.

After a thorough evaluation of pancreatic pain, a number of treatment measures can be instituted (Table 2).

Patient Education

The first step is educating patients about the natural history of this chronic ailment, its associated complications, and its likely long-term outcome. Each patient with chronic pancreatitis should understand that after 5 to 10 years the episodes of pancreatic pain generally diminish in frequency and often disappear altogether. However, at about the time that abdominal pain diminishes, most patients with chronic pancreatitis also develop hyperglycemia and malabsorption.

Analgesics

The second step involves generous use of non-narcotic analgesics (e.g., acetaminophen, ibuprofen, and nonsteroidal analgesics) to control abdominal pain. In my experience, a large percentage of patients with chronic pancreatic pain can be managed for a long time with these two measures. Limited prescription of narcotic analgesics such as acetaminophen with codeine is also reasonable during episodes of severe abdominal pain. Patients should always be reminded that long-term use of narcotic analgesics can result in drug dependence. If a patient's requirements for narcotic analgesic appear to be gradually increasing, strong consideration should be given to possible enrollment in a pain relief program and the use of pain control by other means. Pain due to chronic pancreatitis is frequently intermittent and postprandial, but when abdominal pain becomes more frequent, persistent, and affects the lifestyle of the patient, relief of pain becomes the most crucial part of the overall management. In these situations, celiac ganglionectomy and surgical intervention should be considered.

Pancreatic Enzyme Therapy

There has been significant interest in the use of oral pancreatic enzymes to ameliorate pancreatic pain because these preparations are relatively innocuous and inexpensive. The rationale for their use is based on presence of protease-sensitive feedback regulation of exocrine pancreatic secretion in normal human subjects. It has been postulated that reduced pancreatic enzyme secretion in chronic pancreatitis causes increased and sustained stimulation of pancreatic gland, resulting in development of pancreatic pain.

The goal of pancreatic enzyme therapy in the treatment of chronic pancreatic pain is suppression of pancreatic stimulation, reduction in exocrine pancreatic secretion, decrease in pancreatic ductal and tissue pressure, and amelioration of pancreatic pain. Four clinical trials testing this hypothesis, involving a total of 69 patients with chronic pancreatitis, have been reported in the literature. Three studies (two controlled and one uncontrolled) have shown some benefit with pancreatic enzyme replacement therapy in pancreatic pain relief. Most of the benefit has been observed in patients with idiopathic chronic pancreatitis. In my experience, the use of oral pancreatic enzyme has not been effective in reducing chronic abdominal pain in patients with alcoholic pancreatitis. To examine this issue more definitively, a controlled, double blind clinical trial is needed in carefully selected patients with well-documented alcoholic and nonalcoholic chronic pancreatitis. Based on available information, a 4 week trial of oral pancreatic enzymes seems reasonable in patients with chronic abdominal pain from idiopathic pancreatitis. If abdominal pain is ameliorated or relieved, pancreatic enzyme therapy should be continued on a long-term basis. The precise dose of pancreatic enzymes necessary to restore normal feedback regulation of exocrine pancreatic secretion in patients with chronic pancreatitis has not been defined. I have used the same dose of pancreatic enzymes which is employed in the treatment of pancreatic steatorrhea (i.e., approximately 32,000 lipase units per meal).

Somatostatin Therapy

Somatostatin is a potent inhibitor of exocrine pancreatic enzyme secretion directly and indirectly via inhibition of cholecystokinin secretion. It has been proposed that a long-acting analogue of somatostatin octreotide (Sandostatin) may ameliorate pancreatic pain by reducing exocrine pancreatic secretion, diminishing pancreatic ductal pressure, and minimizing exposure of pancreatic nerves to pancreatic enzyme. However, to date there is no published controlled clinical trial evaluating the effectiveness of octreotide therapy in this group of patients. Anecdotal case reports and data from octreotide compassionate need program have provided encouraging results about amelioration of abdominal pain in patients with chronic pancreatitis. A multicenter-controlled clinical trial designed to assess the short-term efficacy of octreotide therapy in the treatment of abdominal pain associated with chronic pancreatitis, has recently been completed in the United States. In this trial, octreotide therapy was administered subcutaneously at a dose of 50 μg three times per day to a maximum of 200 μg three times per day to obtain adequate pain relief. Results of this and other similar clinical trials are eagerly awaited. Based on limited available information, it seems reasonable to consider octreotide therapy in a given case with persistent pseudocyst, pancreatic fistulae, pancreatic ascites, and chronic pancreatic pain. Limitation of octreotide therapy include lack of availability of oral preparation and development of side effects such as nausea, pain at the injection site, hyperglycemia, steatorrhea, and cholelithiasis.

Endoscopic Intervention

In the last 5 years, several published reports have documented the technical feasibility of pancreatic stent placement and pancreatic stone removal to overcome intraductal obstruction. These interventional modalities are designed to ameliorate pancreatic pain by establishing better drainage of main pancreatic duct and by reducing intrapancreatic pressure. These reports are preliminary and require further confirmation by larger controlled clinical studies. Significant concerns about the application of endoscopic techniques in this group of patients include (1) frequent occlusion of pancreatic stents, (2) distal migrations of the stent, (3) development of progressive histological changes of chronic pancreatitis, (4) development of acute pancreatitis, and (5) onset of pancreatic infection. The precise role of these endoscopic therapeutic modalities in the treatment of chronic pancreatic pain will be better defined in the next few years. The chapter on therapeutic endoscopy of the pancreas provides additional information.

Celiac Ganglionectomy

If medical treatment fails to control abdominal pain and the patient continues to consume narcotic analgesics frequently, more invasive measures should be considered. Local anesthetic agents such as lidocaine have been injected in the celiac ganglion under fluoroscopic guidance to reduce abdominal pain in patients with chronic pancreatitis. If pain relief is significant, the celiac ganglion can be destroyed by injecting alcohol at the same site (celiac ganglionectomy). Alternatively, complete destruction of celiac ganglion can be achieved surgically. The duration of pain relief after celiac ganglion destruction is approximately 6 months in the 50 percent of patients who respond to this treatment. In view of the limited long-term benefit and controlled clinical experience with this procedure, it should be used with caution in the management of chronic pancreatitis-related abdominal pain. The use of this technique for pancreatic cancer is discussed in the chapter on pancreatic and peripancreatic cancer.

Surgery

The final measure used to control pancreatic pain is surgical intervention. However, a decision for surgery is often difficult because the clinical course of this disease is unpredictable and pain frequently disappears spontaneously after a few years in a subgroup of patients. Patients should be advised of this possible outcome and encouraged to avoid surgery whenever possible.

Patients with chronic pancreatitis who have a dilated main pancreatic duct due to fibrotic strictures are generally treated by surgical drainage of the duct. Although a dilated, abnormal pancreatic duct and pancreatic pain are not well correlated, pain relief for a significant time has been well documented in some patients after a pancreatic drainage procedure. The choice of operation for abdominal pain from chronic pancreatitis includes (1) caudal pancreaticojejunostomy (DuVal procedure), (2) longitudinal pancreaticojejunostomy (Puestow procedure), and (3) subtotal pancreatectomy. The Puestow is the most popularly used drainage procedure in patients with chronic pancreatitis associated with a dilated main pancreatic duct. The entire main duct is opened in a longitudinal manner and all the pancreatic stones are extracted. A loop of jejunum is then opened longitudinally and sewn over the open duct so that the pancreatic juice can empty into the lumen of the jejunum. The results of surgery are generally better in patients who are neither alcoholic nor drug dependent. The surgical mortality rate from longitudinal pancreaticojejunostomy is less than 4 percent. As many as 50 percent of patients with chronic pancreatitis have been reported to derive relief from pain for 5 years. In those who do not respond favorably, an endoscopic pancreatogram should be obtained to verify the patency of pancreaticojejunal anastomosis. Anastomotic revision or pancreatic resection may provide pain relief in a subgroup of these patients. Marked pancreatic pain relief is achieved with distal pancreatectomy in patients with chronic pancreatic inflammation confined to the tail of the pancreas. Total and subtotal resections of the pancreatic gland have been largely abandoned by most tertiary care centers due to major metabolic and nutritional sequelae and unpredictable pain relief.

Treatment of Diarrhea and Weight Loss

Pancreatic enzyme therapy is the cornerstone of management of pancreatic malabsorption. Symptomatic diarrhea is significantly improved with oral pancreatic enzyme therapy, but complete correction of steatorrhea is exceedingly difficult even with large amounts of pancreatic enzyme supplementation. Before pancreatic enzyme therapy is prescribed a number of points should be considered (Table 3).

Type of Enzyme Preparation

Many pancreatic enzyme preparations are commercially available; only those with a significant amount of lipase should be used. Well-known preparations include Ilozyme, Cotazym, Viokase, and Ku-Zyme HP. The pH-sensitive,

Table 3 Selection of Exogenous Pancreatic Enzyme Therapy

Type of preparation: Any potent preparation that contains 8,000 units of lipase activity per capsule or more (e.g., Cotazym, Viokase, Ilozyme) can be used
Amount of preparation: Approximately 30,000 units of lipase per meal (2 to 8 capsules or tablets per meal)
Form of administration: Capsules are preferable to tablets; powder form is of dubious value
Time of administration: With meal: total dose distributed evenly during ingestion of meal (two capsules in beginning, two in middle, and two at end)
Adjuvant therapy: H_2-receptor antagonists: antacids
pH-sensitive, enteric-coated pancreatic enzyme preparations (Pancrease, Cotazym-S)
New more potent enzyme preparations: Creon, Pancrease MT25

enteric-coated preparations include Pancrease and Cotazym-S. There should be at least 8,000 units of lipase per capsule or tablet. More recently available pancreatic enzyme preparations contain as much as 10,000 to 25,000 units of lipase per capsule (Pancrease MT10, MT16, MT25; Creon 10 or 25). In general, capsules are preferable to tablets because there is no unpalatable flavor and smell in the encapsulated preparation. Smaller capsules are preferred because of the ease with which they can be swallowed. The powder form of pancreatic enzyme preparation should not be used because of extensive inactivation by the acidity in the food particles and the stomach. Low-potency enzyme preparations do not provide adequate concentrations of pancreatic enzymes in the upper small intestine. In my experience, prescription of a few potent capsules of pancreatic enzyme preparation results in better patient compliance.

Amount of Pancreatic Enzyme

The dosage of the pancreatic enzyme preparation should be adequate to reduce steatorrhea significantly and improve symptoms satisfactorily. Large amounts of these enzyme preparations are inactivated in the stomach and only 5 to 10 percent of the orally ingested enzymes reach the upper small intestine. It has been estimated that about 30,000 units of lipase are necessary with a standard meal to provide a significant reduction in steatorrhea. Once ingested, lipase activity is inactivated below a pH of 4.0 and trypsin is inactivated below a pH of 3.0. These pH values are frequently reached in the stomach and in the upper small intestine during the postprandial period in this group of patients. Clinical studies have shown that as many as six to eight tablets or capsules (24,000 to 32,000 units of lipase) of potent pancreatic enzyme preparations per meal can provide a significant concentration of pancreatic enzymes in the upper gastrointestinal tract. Adequate amount of pancreatic enzymes can be provided by 2 to 3 capsules of high-potency preparations such as Creon and Pancrease MT25. These amounts of pancreatic enzymes are generally able to reduce steatorrhea by 60 percent and fecal nitrogen loss by 75 percent.

In order to improve the efficacy of pancreatic enzyme preparations, antacids and sodium bicarbonate have also been used. It has been reported that antacids such as aluminum hydroxide and sodium bicarbonate are effective as adjuvant therapy. However, magnesium and calcium-containing antacids should not be used, because they precipitate fatty acids and bile acids. Histamine$_2$ (H_2)-receptor antagonists (H_2 blockers) as adjuncts to pancreatic enzyme supplementation have been shown by clinical studies to reduce steatorrhea significantly. H_2 blockers are likely to be more helpful in patients with hyperchlorhydria than in patients with low gastric acid secretion. H_2-blocker therapy should be added only in patients with an inadequate response to conventional pancreatic enzyme therapy alone.

Enteric-Coated Products

In order to protect pancreatic enzymes from the hostile acidic environment of the gastric acid, pH-sensitive, enteric-coated pancreatic enzyme preparations have become available. These preparations have pancreatic enzymes rolled into microspheres 1.5 to 2.5 mm in diameter, packed in a capsular form. The pH-sensitive enzyme coatings dissolve only at pH of 5.5 to 6.0 and release pancreatic enzymes into the environment. The enteric-coated preparations have been shown to be effective in reducing steatorrhea, but have not proved more effective than potent conventional enzyme preparations in alcoholic patients with pancreatic insufficiency. However, patients with cystic fibrosis seem to do better with enteric-coated preparations than with conventional preparations. The different responses of cystic fibrosis and alcoholic pancreatitis patients to enteric-coated preparations may be related to higher gastric acid secretion and gastric emptying in young patients with cystic fibrosis. The enteric-coated preparations are generally more expensive than conventional ones.

Hyperuricemia

There are no significant side effects from pancreatic enzyme therapy. Pancreatic extracts contain large amounts of nucleic acid and large doses have been reported to lead to hyperuricemia in some patients.

Poor Compliance

Compliance with pancreatic supplements is generally poor because of the large number of tablets or capsules that a patient with exocrine pancreatic insufficiency has to take with each meal. The preparations also have an unpleasant taste, so that capsules are much better tolerated by patients than the tablets. Cost can also be a factor.

Therapeutic Goals

The goal of pancreatic enzyme therapy is generally to help patients control diarrhea and gain body weight. A number of objective parameters can be used to evaluate the efficacy of pancreatic enzyme therapy in patients with exocrine pancreatic insufficiency (Table 4). With adequate pancreatic enzyme therapy, patients should gain 1 or 2 lb each week and stabilize at about 10 percent below ideal body weight. In addition, anthropometric and biochemical parameters of nutritional assessment should also show improvement. Patients who do not respond well to pancreatic enzyme therapy should be carefully evaluated for noncompliance or for the presence of other associated disorders such as celiac sprue, altered gastric emptying, or bacterial overgrowth (Table 5). Specific steps to diagnose and treat each of these disorders are necessary in such individuals.

Table 4 Parameters for Evaluation in Clinical Response to Pancreatic Enzyme Therapy in Exocrine Pancreatic Insufficiency

Weight gain and growth (in children)
Reduction in frequency and volume of bowel movements
Improvement in intestinal absorption
Decrease in fecal fat excretion
Increase in bentiromide excretion
Nutritional improvement
Height-weight relationship
Midarm muscle circumference
Serum albumin
Creatinine height index

Table 5 Management of Patients with Poor Response to Pancreatic Enzyme Therapy

Increase pancreatic enzyme therapy
Add adjuvant therapy
H_2-blocker therapy
Antacid therapy
Sodium bicarbonate
Switch to pH-sensitive, enteric-coated pancreatic enzyme therapy
Check for noncompliance
Search for other associated disorders
Celiac sprue
Altered gastric emptying (status gastric surgery)
Uncontrolled diabetes mellitus
Bacterial overgrowth
Ileal disease or resection
Pancreatic cancer

Treatment of Protein Energy Malnutrition

Nutritional support is also of paramount importance in patients with exocrine pancreatic insufficiency. As many as 40 percent of patients with chronic pancreatitis have clinically significant protein energy malnutrition.

These patients generally have diminished muscle mass as demonstrated by anthropometric and biochemical parameters of nutrition evaluation. Factors responsible for the development of protein energy malnutrition include diminished caloric intake and malabsorption due to impaired pancreatic enzyme secretion by the pancreatic gland. Not infrequently, uncontrolled diabetes mellitus and protein loss from a fistula also contribute significantly to protein energy malnutrition.

Besides generalized protein energy malnutrition due to maldigestion and malabsorption of fat, proteins, and carbohydrates, specific nutrient depletion can occur in these patients. Depletion of fat-soluble vitamins (particularly vitamins A and E) has been described in children with exocrine pancreatic insufficiency due to cystic fibrosis, and in adult patients with chronic alcoholic pancreatitis. Zinc deficiency manifesting as perioral and perianal eczematous rash has also been reported in patients with alcoholic pancreatitis. Vitamin B_{12} malabsorption can be documented in 40 to 50 percent of patients with untreated exocrine pancreatic insufficiency, but severe vitamin B_{12} deficiency and related anemia are rare in this group of patients. The physician should be aware of potential nutritional problems and should treat them appropriately when indicated. I do not routinely screen or treat patients with chronic pancreatitis for these specific nutrient deficiencies. However, patients with poor response to pancreatic enzyme therapy or with recurrent attacks of pancreatitis are carefully evaluated for deficiencies of fat-soluble vitamins and minerals.

Management of protein energy malnutrition due to exocrine pancreatic insufficiency requires not only correction of malabsorption but also administration of a high-protein–high-calorie diet. Poor caloric intake is a significant problem in some of these patients and is generally related to postprandial pain, dietary restrictions due to a recurrent flare-up of pancreatitis, and anorexia. Nutritional supplementation entails (1) assessment of the most appropriate nutritional support (e.g., total parenteral nutrition [TPN] or an elemental diet), (2) assessment of the duration of anticipated nutritional support, and (3) identification of the underlying problem contributing to the severe malnutrition.

If a patient with chronic pancreatitis is severely malnourished, early TPN may be the treatment of choice. The pancreatic gland is very nutrition sensitive, and severe malnutrition has been reported to lead to atrophy and fibrosis. Nutritional repletion in these patients is associated with an improvement in pancreatic gland function.

In patients with mild to moderate severe malnutrition, elemental diets, protein hydrolysate preparations, or other supplemental diet therapies should be carefully considered. Medium-chain triglyceride (MCT) preparations are attractive sources of lipid calories in this group of patients. Most MCT preparations contain primary fatty acids with 8 to 10 carbon chains as an energy source, and do not require lipase activity for absorption; they are derived mainly from coconut oil. However, poor taste and the development of nausea frequently limit the use of MCT in the treatment of severe malnutrition due to pancreatic insufficiency. MCT is available in a formula diet (Portagen) and also as a pure oil preparation for food. A specific nutrition supplemental therapy plan should be developed for each patient in consultation with the dietitian and nutrition support team.

Management of Diabetes Mellitus

The principal steps in the management of diabetes mellitus associated with chronic pancreatitis consist of correction of irregular food intake, malabsorption, and malnutrition and elimination of alcohol intake. Most patients require low doses of insulin, 5 to 15 units per day, to correct the hyperglycemia. The insulin requirement fluctuates between 10 and 40 units daily. Because of erratic and partial absorption of carbohydrates, these patients have a propensity to develop hypoglycemia; this may also be related to impaired glucagon secretion in chronic pancreatitis. Episodes of hypoglycemia have been reported in as many as one-third of patients being treated with insulin. The most prudent course to avoid hypoglycemia in this group of patients is to achieve higher than normal blood glucose levels, using the minimal doses of insulin necessary to avoid significant glucosuria. This approach appears to be reasonable, since the development of ketoacidosis and microvascular complications is relatively uncommon in these patients, and hypoglycemic episodes are frequent. Once the malabsorption is corrected with an appropriate diet plus pancreatic enzyme supplements, and after the body weight is stabilized, finer adjustment of blood glucose should be made. The importance of patient education about insulin administration and the management of its potential complications cannot be overemphasized.

Suggested Reading

Adsor MA, McIlrath DC. Surgical treatment of chronic pancreatitis. In: Go VLW, et al, eds. The exocrine pancrease: biology, pathobiology and diseases. New York: Raven Press, 1986:587–599.

Cremer M, Deviere J, DeMaye M, et al. Non-surgical management of severe chronic pancreatitis. Scand J Gastroenterol 1990; 25:77–84.

DiMagno EP, Go VLW, Summerskill WHJ. Relations between pancreatic enzyme outputs and malabsorption in severe pancreatic insufficiency. N Engl J Med 1973; 288:813–815.

DiMagno EP, Malajelada JR, Go VLW, Moertel CG. Fate of orally infested enzymes in pancreatic insufficiency. N Engl J Med 1977; 296:1318–1322.

Dutta SK, Hubbard VS, Appler M. Critical examination of therapeutic efficacy of a pH-sensitive enteric-coated pancreatic enzyme preparation in the treatment of exocrine pancreatic insufficiency secondary to cystic fibrosis. Dig Dis Sci 1988; 33:1237–1244.

Dutta SK, Rubin J, Harvey J. Comparative evaluation of the therapeutic efficacy of a pH-sensitive coated pancreatic enzyme preparation with conventional pancreatic enzyme therapy in the treatment of exocrine pancreatic insufficiency. Gastroenterology 1983; 84:476–482.

Graham DY. Enzyme replacement therapy of exocrine pancreatic insufficiency in man. N Eng J Med 1977; 297:1314–1317.

Owyang C, Louie D, Tatum D. Feedback regulation of pancreatic enzyme secretion. J Clin Invest 1986; 77:2042–2047.

Regan PT, Malajelada JR, DiMagno EP, et al. Comparative effects of antacids, cimetidine, and enteric coating on the therapeutic response to oral enzymes in severe pancreatic insufficiency. N Engl J Med 1977; 297: 854–858.

ACUTE APPENDICITIS

S. Frank Redo, M.D.

Acute appendicitis may occur in any age group but is most common in older children and young adults. It is rare in infants, probably because of the conical shape of the appendix, which permits easier entry and exit of stool. In children up to 4 to 6 years of age and in the elderly, diagnosis is difficult and often not made before perforation. The incidence is equal in male and female patients but increases in male patients during early adulthood, after which the sex ratio again becomes equal.

PATHOGENESIS

Acute appendicitis is initiated by obstruction of the lumen by stool (fecalith), fibrous band, lymphoid hyperplasia, or a foreign body. The normal mucosal secretion of the appendix collects distal to the site of the obstruction, which leads to an increase in intraluminal pressure. This causes interference first with venous outflow and subsequently, as pressure increases, with arterial blood inflow. Ulceration of the mucosa occurs, with infiltration of the wall of the appendix by bacteria. The resultant infection may lead to gangrene, necrosis, and perforation.

DIAGNOSIS

Symptoms and Signs

In a classic case of acute appendicitis the patient gives a history of nausea, vomiting, and periumbilical pain that migrates and localizes in the right lower quadrant. This may occur within 1 to 2 or 8 to 12 hours. Vomiting consists usually of only one or two episodes and begins after the onset of pain. If vomiting precedes the pain, the patient probably does not have appendicitis. Anorexia is common.

Unfortunately, this classic history does not exist in all cases. If the appendix is retrocecal, the pain may be described as being in the right flank or right back. When the appendix lies in the pelvis, the pain may be in the testicle or suprapubic (bladder) region. In such instances diarrhea may be a presenting associated problem.

On physical examination the abdomen is usually tense with spasm and guarding in the right lower quadrant. If the pain has had moderately long duration, the entire abdomen may be rigid, suggesting peritonitis and probable perforated appendix. Discrete tenderness at McBurney's point is diagnostic for acute appendicitis. Rebound, shake, and toe-heel tenderness indicate peritoneal irritation. When the appendix is retrocecal, rebound tenderness may not be evident. In such instances, however, there is usually a positive psoas sign.

The abdomen should be palpated for a mass in the right lower quadrant and auscultated for bowel sounds. Bowel sounds may be normal in the early phase of infection but become less active or quiet as the process progresses.

Percussion over the flank and back may cause pain when the appendix is retrocecal. Temperature rarely exceeds 38.5°C (101.3°F) unless there has been perforation and peritonitis has developed.

On rectal examination a mass may be palpable in the right lower quadrant. Pain may be elicited in this region by pressure of the examining finger on the anterior aspect of the right rectal wall.

Laboratory Findings

Laboratory work-up should begin with a complete blood count, urinalysis, serum electrolyte determinations, and supine and upright radiographs of the abdomen. The hemoglobin and hematocrit levels are helpful in assessing dehydration and hemoconcentration. The white blood cell (WBC) count is usually elevated to 15,000 or more with a differential high in polymorphonuclear cells and bands.

The urinalysis provides another clue in respect to degree of hydration. In addition, results of microscopic examination reveal WBCs, red blood cells (RBC), and bacteria content. It is not unusual to have a small number of WBC or RBC in the urine, especially when the appendix lies on or near the ureter. Large numbers of bacteria or pus in urine, not found in appendicitis, indicate probable urinary tract infection.

Abdominal radiographs rule in or out small bowel obstruction, right lower quadrant mass, and fecalith. If the presentation and clinical and laboratory findings are not diagnostic, sonography, computed tomography (CT), or barium enema may be required for the diagnosis.

Differential Diagnosis

Many conditions mimic acute appendicitis. These include gastroenteritis (particularly due to *Yersinia enterocolitica, Salmonella enteritidis,* and *Campylobacter jejuni*), mesenteric adenitis in younger patients (usually associated with *Y. enterocolitica, Yersinia pseudotuberculosis,* and occasionally with streptococcal infection), urinary tract infections, constipation, intussusception, primary peritonitis, duodenal ulcer, measles, Crohn's disease, sickle cell disease, hemophilia, leukemia, Meckel's diverticulum, pneumonia, pelvic inflammatory disease, ovarian pathology, and mittelschmerz in women. In most instances history, physical examination, and laboratory findings differentiate these problems from acute appendicitis, although the gastroenteritis and mesenteric adenitis syndromes referred to above may be particularly misleading, and their mimicry is often termed *pseudoappendicitis.* In patients with AIDS, pseudoappendicitis also may be due to bacterial typhlitis, cecal CMV infection, or tuberculosis.

■ TYPES OF APPENDICITIS

Appendicitis is seen in five forms: simple acute, suppurative, gangrenous, perforated, and abscess (Table 1).

Table 1 Types of Appendicitis

TYPE	CHARACTERISTICS
Simple acute	Mild hyperemia, edema, no serosal exudate
Suppurative	Edematous, congested vessels, fibrinopurulent exudate; peritoneal fluid increased, clear or turbid; may be early walling off by omentum and adjacent bowel or mesentery
Gangrenous	As above plus areas of gangrene, microperforations, increased and purulent peritoneal fluid
Perforated	Obvious defect in wall of appendix; peritoneal fluid thick and purulent; ileal obstruction possible
Abscess	Appendix may be sloughed; abscess at site of perforation; right iliac fossa, retrocecal, subcecal, or pelvic; may present rectally; thick, malodorous pus

■ THERAPY

The treatment of appendicitis is surgical removal of the affected organ. Surgery should be performed as soon as possible after diagnosis. Patients with signs of peritonitis with dehydration and electrolyte abnormalities should have fluid and electrolyte resuscitation for a few hours prior to surgery. This should be started promptly, but complete restoration of normality before the operation is not necessary. Ringer's lactate solution and normal saline may be infused to correct fluid and electrolyte abnormalities. If there is evidence to suggest a ruptured appendix with peritonitis, a nasogastric tube should be inserted and placed on suction.

The operation is performed using a McBurney or Rocky-Davis incision except when the diagnosis is in doubt, especially in female patients. In those cases a lower midline or right paramedian approach is preferred.

If there is an associated abscess, unless extensive dissection is required to locate the appendix, the appendix should be removed. The peritoneal cavity is irrigated copiously with saline. There is some question as to the efficacy of antibiotics in the irrigant. The value of the irrigation is to lower the inoculum of bacteria. The abscess cavity should be drained and the drains brought out through a separate stab wound, not the incision. Usually three soft rubber (Penrose) drains are placed, one up to the subhepatic region on the right, a second into the pelvis, and the third down to the right gutter near the base of the cecum. The drains are left in place for 7 days, after which they are removed over the next 2 to 3 days, by which time a definite tract should have developed. The tract should be allowed to close from the deeper to the superficial portion. The skin edges must not be allowed to seal over until the tract has closed.

If the patient is not seen early in the course of the disease, and when seen is improving, and there is a palpable (nonobstructing) right lower quadrant mass, nonoperative treatment is used by some. In such cases an interval appendectomy is usually done 2 to 3 months after the patient has recovered and is free of abdominal complaints. Similarly, in patients in whom surgery reveals a well walled-off periappendiceal abscess, some surgeons simply drain the abscess to avoid general peritoneal contamination and perform an elective appendectomy 2 to 3 months later.

In the near future laparoscopy may replace conventional appendectomy. Laparoscopic appendectomy has been reported as a safe alternative to open appendectomy in uncomplicated cases of acute appendicitis, but because of an increased rate of postlaparoscopic complications, it may be contraindicated in patients with gangrenous appendicitis, peritonitis, or abscess.

Table 2 Antibiotic Regimens in Appendicitis

TYPE OF APPENDICITIS	ANTIBIOTIC REGIMEN*
Simple acute	Triple drug, cefoxitin, or ampicillin-sulbactam alone preoperatively and for 12–24 hours postoperatively
Acute with perforation	Triple drug preoperatively and for 10 days postoperatively
Acute with abscess	Triple drug preoperatively and for as long as 21 days postoperatively

*See Table 3 for dosages.

■ ANTIBIOTIC REGIMENS

The use of antibiotic prophylaxis for appendicitis is controversial. Many surgeons think antibiotics are not needed for a patient suspected of having acute appendicitis without evidence of peritonitis to suggest perforation or abscess. However, the efficacy of preoperative antibiotics in decreasing the infectious complications of appendicitis has been reported. The possibility of perforation at the time of initial evaluation of a patient has led to almost routine use of preoperative antibiotics.

Triple drug coverage consisting of ampicillin, gentamicin, and clindamycin in appropriate dosages for age and weight should be given within 4 hours of surgery, usually 1 hour before. Some surgeons employ only a single antibiotic, cefoxitin or ampicillin-sulbactam. Further treatment depends on findings at surgery. For acute, nonperforated appendicitis antibiotics may not be necessary for more than 24 hours. In most instances the single preoperative dose is all that is given. If an acute perforated appendix is found, antibiotics are given for 10 days. If a definite abscess is encountered, in addition to adequate drainage, antibiotics should be continued for as long as 21 days. This is a conservative regimen. The patient may be discharged when there are no longer signs of active disease and continue the course of antibiotics on a home intravenous program (Tables 2 and 3).

Table 3 Recommended Dosages for Antibiotics in Appendicitis

DRUG	CHILD	ADULT
TRIPLE DRUG		
Ampicillin	100–200 mg/kg/day q6h	1–2 g q4–6h
Gentamicin	3–5 mg/kg/day q8h	1–1.7 mg/kg q8h
Clindamycin	2.5–10 mg/kg q6h	15–900 mg q6h
SINGLE DRUG*		
Cefoxitin	20–25 mg/kg q4–6h	1–2 g q6h
Ampicillin-sulbactam	25–50 mg/kg q6h	1.5–3 g q6h

*Single-drug therapy is less frequently recommended in cases of perforation or abscess.

There is no universal regimen for antibiotic use. In many institutions a single drug, cefoxitin or ampicillin-sulbactam, is employed rather than triple drug management. Ampicillin and cefoxitin have been used in combination. Metronidazole (Flagyl) has been used as an oral medication for 7 to 10 days after completion of 14 days of intravenous antibiotics in patients who have had abscess and drainage.

Basically, the choice of antibiotics depends on the results of culture and sensitivity determinations of specimens obtained at the time of surgery. Since the disease is polymicrobial, with aerobic and anaerobic organisms, the antibiotics must be effective against aerobic and anaerobic bacteria.

Suggested Reading

Bauer T, Vennits B, et al. Antibiotic prophylaxis in acute nonoperative appendicitis: The Danish multicenter study group III. Ann Surg 1989; 209:307.

Bonanni F, Reed J III, Hartzell G, et al. Laparoscopic versus conventional appendectomy. J Am Coll Surg 1994; 179:273.

Brown JJ. Acute appendicitis: The radiologist's role. Radiology 1991; 180:13.

Horattas MC. Guyton DP, Wu D. A reappraisal of appendicitis in the elderly. Am J Surg 1990; 160:291.

DIVERTICULITIS

Ronald Lee Nichols, M.D., M.S., F.A.C.S.
James Wm. C. Holmes, M.D., M.S., F.A.C.S.

Diverticulosis coli is an anatomic abnormality of the large bowel wall that manifests itself in various ways. Its occurrence varies greatly with such factors as geographic location, dietary habits, race, and age. In the United States a third of the population over age 50 is affected.

The diagnosis of diverticulosis coli is often made incidentally in otherwise asymptomatic patients at the time of routine surveillance endoscopy or barium enema x-ray examination. However, unless a stricture is present, most of these patients require only counseling about possible infectious or hemorrhagic complications of the disease and the need for prophylactic measures such as a fiber-rich diet, adequate fluid consumption, and the prevention of constipation.

When clinical manifestations of diverticulosis occur, surgical intervention is necessary in only a minority of patients. These patients may have massive, or recurrent, gastrointestinal bleeding, but more commonly have localized intra-

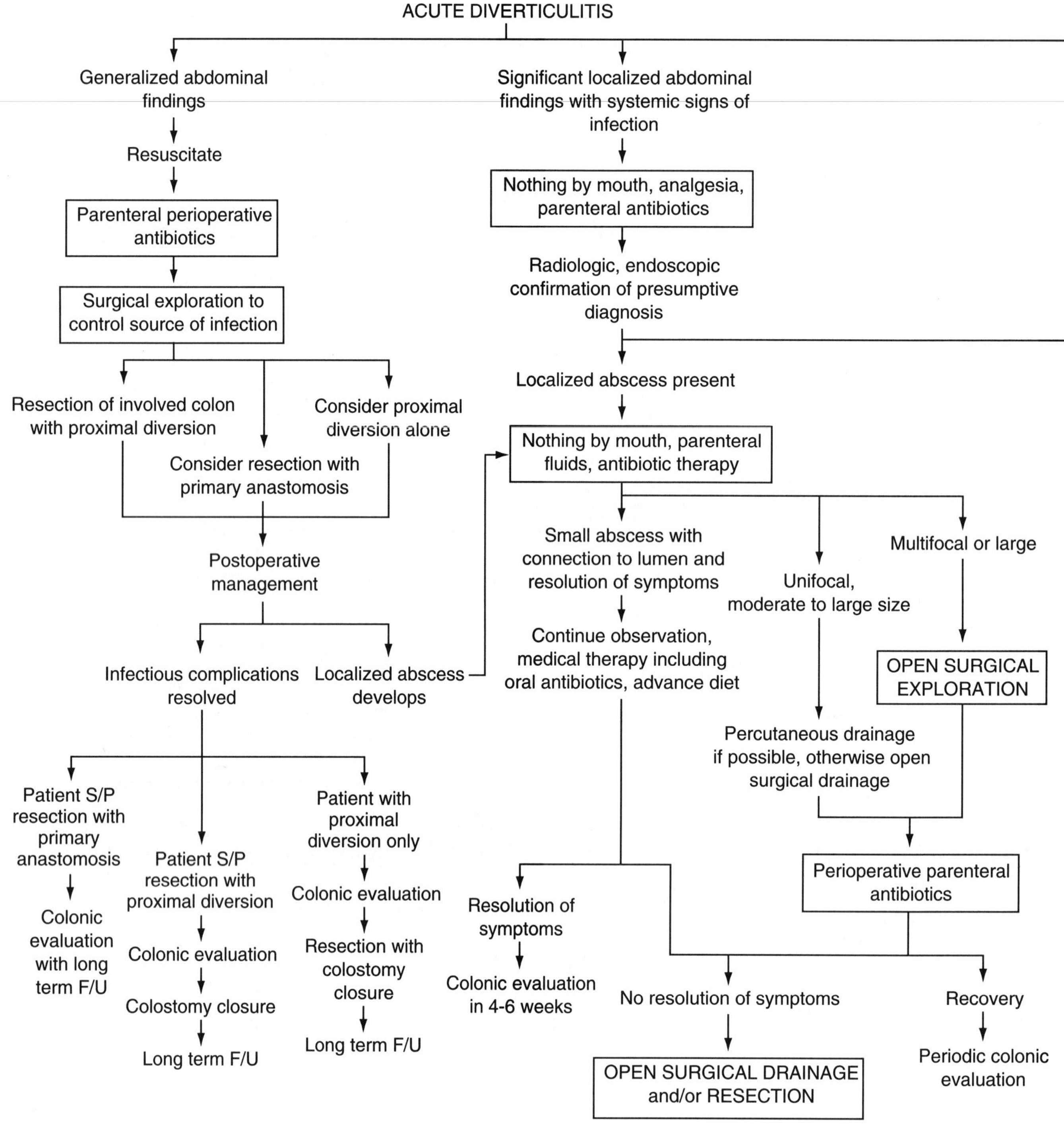

Figure 1
Algorithm for the workup and treatment of acute diverticulitis. S/P, status post; F/U, follow-up.

abdominal abscess or generalized peritonitis that has developed after diverticular perforation.

Clinically significant diverticular disease and its complications continue to tax the diagnostic and therapeutic skills of physicians. Physical findings range from diffuse slight abdominal tenderness to shock secondary to either massive hemorrhage or overwhelming sepsis. During such life-threatening emergencies the physician must be prepared to resuscitate the patient quickly and proceed to surgical intervention without benefit of a definite diagnosis.

■ DIAGNOSIS OF INFECTION

The most common clinically significant manifestations of diverticulosis are hemorrhage and infection (diverticulitis).

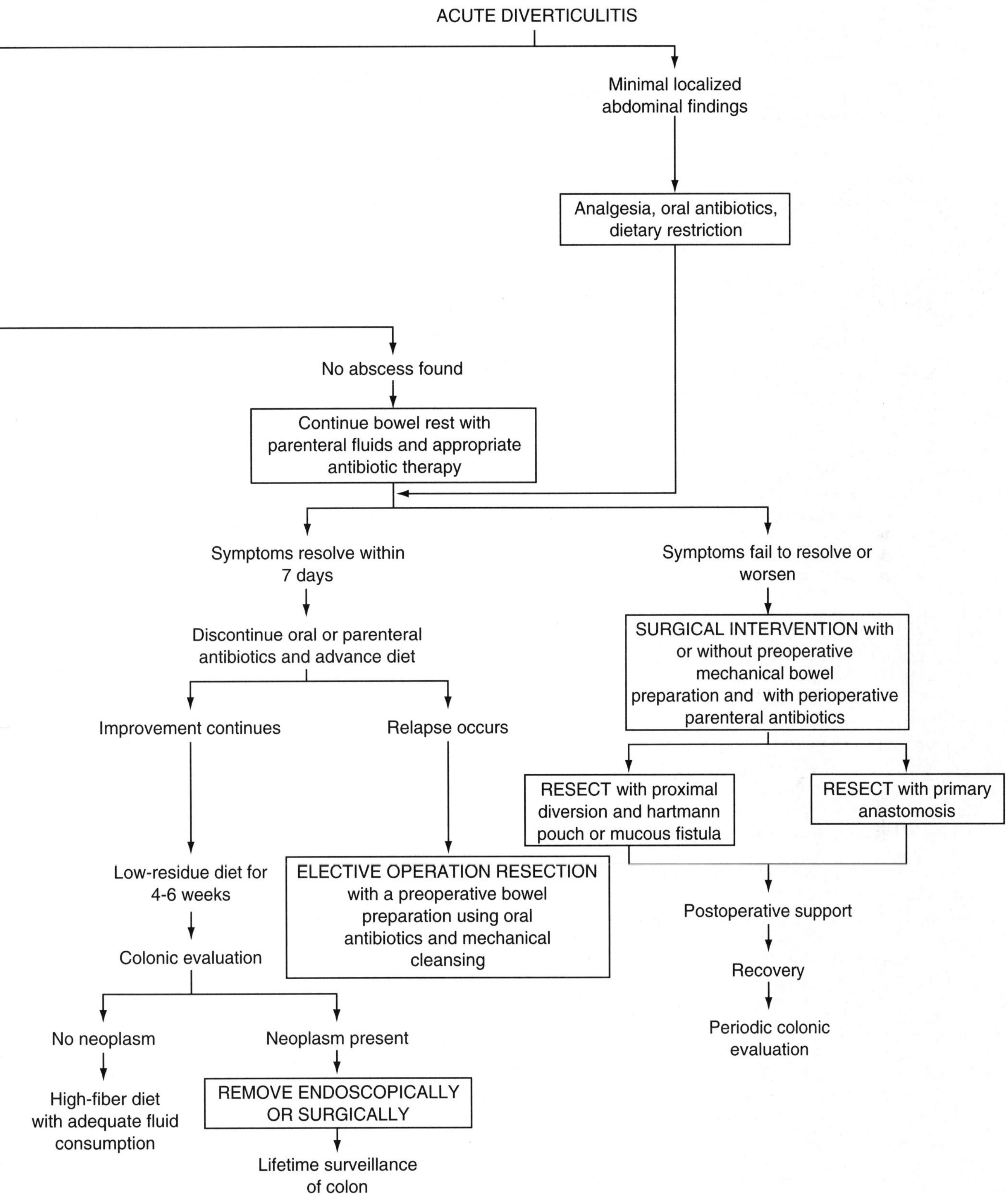
ACUTE DIVERTICULITIS
Minimal localized abdominal findings
Analgesia, oral antibiotics, dietary restriction
No abscess found
Continue bowel rest with parenteral fluids and appropriate antibiotic therapy
Symptoms resolve within 7 days
Symptoms fail to resolve or worsen
Discontinue oral or parenteral antibiotics and advance diet
SURGICAL INTERVENTION with or without preoperative mechanical bowel preparation and with perioperative parenteral antibiotics
Improvement continues
Relapse occurs
RESECT with proximal diversion and hartmann pouch or mucous fistula
RESECT with primary anastomosis
Low-residue diet for 4-6 weeks
ELECTIVE OPERATION RESECTION with a preoperative bowel preparation using oral antibiotics and mechanical cleansing
Postoperative support
Colonic evaluation
Recovery
No neoplasm
Neoplasm present
Periodic colonic evaluation
High-fiber diet with adequate fluid consumption
REMOVE ENDOSCOPICALLY OR SURGICALLY
Lifetime surveillance of colon

In patients with signs of abdominal infection, including fever and abdominal pain and tenderness, usually in the left lower quadrant, it is often possible to make a presumptive diagnosis of acute diverticulitis on the basis of history, physical examination, and initial laboratory tests. This allows for the initiation of resuscitative measures, including empiric antibiotic therapy. Although further diagnostic endoscopic and radiographic procedures can be delayed for up to 2 days, if the patient continues to show signs of improvement, it is best to perform them as soon as possible to confirm the presumptive diagnosis.

Few if any patients with acute diverticulitis will tolerate

Table 1 Intravenous Antibiotics for Aerobic and Anaerobic Human Colonic Microflora

DRUG	DOSAGE	FREQUENCY	LIFE-THREATENING
	COMBINATION THERAPY		
AEROBIC COVERAGE*			
Amikacin	15 mg/kg/day	b.i.d.–t.i.d.	
Aztreonam	1–2 g	q8–12h	2 g q6–8h
Ceftriaxone	1–2 g	qd	2 g q12h
Cefotaxime	1–2 g	q8–12h	2 g q4–6h
Ciprofloxacin	200–400 mg	q12h	
Gentamicin	3 mg/kg/day	q8h	5 mg/kg/day
Tobramycin	3 mg/kg/day	q8h	5 mg/kg/day
ANAEROBIC COVERAGE†			
Chloramphenicol	50 mg/kg/day	q6h	
Clindamycin	600–900 mg	q8h	
Metronidazole	7.5 mg/kg	q6h	
	SINGLE-DRUG THERAPY		
AEROBIC-ANAEROBIC COVERAGE			
Ampicillin-sulbactam	1.5–3 g	q6h	
Cefoxitin	1–2 g	q4–8h	
Ceftizoxime	1–2 g	q8–12h	3–4g q8h
Imipenem-cilistatin	500 mg	q6h	500–1,000 mg q6–8h
Piperacillin-tazobactam	3.375–4.5 g	q6–8h	
Ticarcillin-clavulanic acid	3.1 g	q6–8h	

*To be combined with a drug exhibiting anaerobic activity.
†To be combined with a drug exhibiting aerobic activity.

proctoscopy above 15 to 20 cm. Sigmoidoscopy is better tolerated, but force must be avoided. In addition, the examiner must be careful to avoid insufflating large amounts of air during the examination and be ready to discontinue the procedure immediately if the patient complains of abdominal pain.

Although ultrasonography is an effective and relatively inexpensive method of evaluating the abdomen and pelvis, particularly for imaging abscesses and their relationship to adnexal structures, many consider computed tomography (CT) to be superior, notably in the evaluation of right colon lesions, and safer than contrast enema studies. Nevertheless, the contrast enema is the most effective method of colonic imaging. We prefer water-soluble contrast materials to barium to avoid barium peritonitis in case of perforation or leakage.

Once diverticulitis has been documented radiographically, further clinical decisions depend on the resolution of signs and symptoms of infection. If they resolve completely and the patient is stable, examine the entire large bowel endoscopically for neoplastic disease. Colonoscopy is best performed 4 to 6 weeks after symptoms of diverticulitis have subsided, to allow time for resolution of any partial obstruction secondary to inflammatory changes in the bowel wall. We routinely perform flexible sigmoidoscopy at 4 to 6 weeks to determine whether sigmoid compliance and patency have returned to normal before preparing the patient for total colonoscopy.

■ MANAGEMENT OF COMPLICATIONS

The greatest number of complications in colonic diverticular disease result from infection. They range from localized short segments of diverticulitis to abscesses and/or fistulas, to free perforation with generalized peritonitis and overwhelming intra-abdominal sepsis (Fig. 1). The cause of the diverticular perforation is not clear. Some authorities postulate that a surge in intraluminal pressure is often the cause, while others suggest ulceration, ischemia, and foreign-body perforation.

Peridiverticulitis

When ulceration or ischemia is not accompanied by free communication with the peritoneal cavity, penetration of mixed bacterial flora into the wall initiates peridiverticular infection.

Patients with localized peridiverticular disease usually present with complaints of abdominal pain localized to the left lower quadrant. In some cases, however, a redundant sigmoid colon may have sufficient mobility to produce local symptoms in the right lower or right upper abdominal quadrant as well as in the midepigastrium. These patients are often febrile and have mild leukocytosis. However, they respond well to bowel rest, parenteral fluids, and antibiotic therapy. Nasogastric tube insertion is usually unnecessary unless obstructive signs and symptoms are present.

It is important that patients take nothing by mouth to abolish the gastrocolic reflex. Morphine sulfate should not be administered because it can increase intracolonic pressure. Most patients require a 3 to 5 day course of appropriate parenteral antimicrobials (Table 1). If they continue to improve, with normalization of the white blood cell (WBC) count, temperature, and abdominal examination, we discontinue their parenteral antibiotics and advance them to a regular diet that is devoid of poorly digestible foods (e.g., whole corn).

Patients must be followed carefully after resolution of abdominal symptoms. If no disease other than diverticulosis is found on follow-up endoscopy, each patient should follow

Table 2 Oral Antibiotic Regimens for Treatment of a Mild Episode of Acute Diverticulitis

ANTIBIOTIC	DOSAGE	FREQUENCY/ DURATION
Ciprofloxacin and	500 mg	b.i.d.
metronidazole	500 mg	t.i.d.
TMP-SMX DS and	800 mg	b.i.d.
metronidazole	500 mg	t.i.d.
Amoxicillin-clavulanate	250–500 mg	q8h
Tetracycline	250–500 mg	b.i.d.–q.i.d.

TMP-SMX DS, trimethoprim-sulfamethoxazole (Bactrim) double strength.

a fiber-supplemented diet with a generous consumption of fluids.

We do not recommend surgery after a single, uncomplicated episode of diverticulitis in otherwise healthy patients. Rather, we do recommend medical therapy when the first episode is mild and uncomplicated and advise patients under 40 years of age that a more aggressive form of the disease may develop.

Although the medical approach rarely fails to control the signs and symptoms of peridiverticulitis, surgical resection may become necessary if the infection does not resolve with prolonged parenteral antibiotic therapy. Occasionally a major complication such as liver abscess or bacteremia develops and requires colonic resection. However, patients with very limited symptoms and no signs of systemic sepsis may respond to oral regimens of antibiotics aimed at covering these colonic aerobes and anaerobes (Table 2).

Pericolic Disease

If the peridiverticular process fails to respond to antibiotic therapy or the patient presents in a late stage of the infectious process, an abscess may be present. Such a pericolic abscess can often be demonstrated by ultrasound, CT, or contrast-enhanced radiography. If any of these studies reveals a small cavity communicating freely with the colon and the patient is improving dramatically, continuation of medical therapy and antibiotics may be warranted. In selected patients percutaneous drainage of the abscess may be a useful adjunct to surgery. Decompressing the purulent contents of an abscess via CT-guided percutaneous catheter placement gains time to improve the patient's status with volume replacement, parenteral hyperalimentation, and appropriate antibiotic therapy. Once the abscess cavity has been resolved by catheter drainage, it is possible to prepare the bowel for elective resection of the diseased colon, often with primary anastomosis.

Smaller symptomatic pericolic abscesses confined to the mesocolon and larger collections associated with peritonitis are best treated surgically. There are two essential operative goals. The first is to resect the inflamed colon and control the associated septic complications; we believe surgical resection of the infectious source is superior to simple diversion of colonic contents (colostomy) and drainage. The second goal is to restore intestinal continuity. Although this may require a second procedure in some cases, we believe it can be accomplished safely during the same operation (single-stage procedure) in most patients. This is particularly true in individuals who are not hemodynamically compromised, who have localized diverticulitis, or who have diverticulitis with an associated mesocolonic abscess amenable to en bloc resection and with no intra-abdominal spillage of purulent material. Some surgeons perform an abdominal colectomy with ileorectostomy in patients who have not had preoperative mechanical bowel preparation.

A more progressive technique is resection of the involved colon, usually the sigmoid, intraoperative lavage, and primary anastomosis. This procedure requires a team effort to keep control of either the proximal or distal colon during lavage, preventing gross peritoneal fecal contamination with its accompanying disastrous effects.

In summary, if emergency surgery is necessary for localized diverticulitis, we try to remove the inflamed colon, most often performing a primary anastomosis. If this is inadvisable due to hemodynamic instability or gross evidence of peritoneal contamination, we do an end colostomy with a distal pouch, usually using the Hartmann procedure or distal mucous fistula. In modern surgery diversion alone is rarely employed.

Generalized Intra-Abdominal Sepsis

The cause of generalized abdominal findings suggesting intra-abdominal sepsis is often unknown prior to exploratory laparotomy. These patients require prompt fluid resuscitation and empiric antibiotic coverage with an agent or combination of agents that will control both aerobic and anaerobic enteric organisms (Table 1). If there is evidence of perforation or if the patient is in shock, laparotomy as soon as the patient is stable is often necessary. Laparotomy frequently reveals fibrinous exudate, free pus, or abscesses throughout the abdominal cavity. If we find diverticulitis, we resect the involved segment and perform a proximal colostomy. Under these conditions we do not consider performing a primary anastomosis. We prefer to leave a closed distal pouch, but only if a preoperative endoscopic examination has ensured that there is no other obstructing or significant neoplastic lesion present. Such a lesion could produce a blind-loop syndrome and leakage of the distal pouch, or could require another operation for its removal.

Following resection we copiously irrigate the abdominal cavity with normal saline. If a localized abscess is identified, a closed drainage system is used; however, drains are not placed if diffuse peritonitis is present. We strongly believe that if gross peritonitis is present, the skin wound should not be closed tightly, if at all. Patients who have undergone such surgery usually require careful monitoring in an intensive care unit and appropriate antibiotic coverage.

Many of these patients develop secondary intra-abdominal or pelvic abscesses, which are detectable with CT or ultrasound. If surgical drainage is required, we use an extraperitoneal approach (ribs, transvaginal, transanal) whenever possible because we believe it lowers postoperative morbidity when percutaneous drainage is not feasible. Many of these patients will also have prolonged ileus and therefore require parenteral hyperalimentation to meet the extraordinary metabolic demands of controlling intra-abdominal sepsis. Of course, enteral nutrition should be resumed as soon as possible.

Suggested Reading

Lambert ME, Knox RA, Schofield PP, et al. Management of the septic complications of diverticular disease. Br J Surg 1986; 73:576–579.

Mueller PR, Saini S, Wittenberg J, et al. Sigmoid diverticular abscesses: Percutaneous drainage as an adjunct to surgical resection in 24 cases. Radiology 1987; 164:321–325.

Nichols RL. Bowel preparation. In: Wilmore DW, Brennan MF, Harken AH, et al., eds. Care of the surgical patient. New York: Scientific American, 1995.

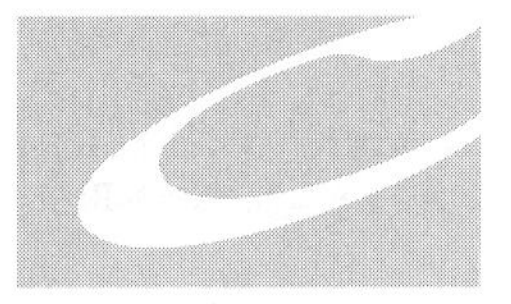

RESPIRATORY DISEASES

ASTHMA IN ADULTS

Peter S. Creticos, M.D.

Asthma is a heterogeneous disease process in which both hereditary and environmental factors contribute to the development and expression of the clinical symptoms experienced by the patient. A variety of triggering factors can incite exacerbations of symptoms. Our perception of the disease is one with a spectrum of intermittent but mild symptoms to that of persistent symptoms with chronicity.

The National Heart, Lung, and Blood Institute (NHLBI) and World Health Organization (WHO) Global Initiatives for Asthma Workshop report defines asthma as "a chronic inflammatory disorder of the airways in which many cells play a role, in particular mast cells, eosinophils, and T lymphocytes. In susceptible individuals this inflammation causes recurrent episodes of wheezing, breathlessness, chest tightness, and cough particularly at night and/or in the early morning. These symptoms are usually associated with widespread but variable airflow limitation that is at least partly reversible either spontaneously or with treatment. The inflammation also causes an associated increase in airway responsiveness to a variety of stimuli."

The key to successful management of the asthmatic disease process is to treat the acute symptomatology and, most importantly, to suppress the underlying inflammatory component, resulting in a reduction in bronchial hyperresponsiveness, attenuation of diurnal variability with improvement in lung functions, and a reduction in the chronic symptoms of asthma.

■ DIAGNOSTIC APPROACH

The workup of the asthmatic patient should include a thorough history, physical exam, and appropriate laboratory tests to corroborate the physician's clinical impression. Particular emphasis should center on the home setting, work site, occupational exposures, avocational interests, and other possible environmental influences. Asthma is one disease in which identification of the specific (allergic) triggering factor(s) and subsequent appropriate environmental manipulation to reduce exposure to the allergen burden can have a dramatic impact on the patient's disease process.

The strong association of allergy with asthma mandates an allergic evaluation of all patients with other than mild and intermittent symptoms. Skin testing to a panel of inhalant allergens relevant to the patient's geographic region provides immediate confirmation of (IgE-mediated) allergic sensitization, which correlates both with the frequency and the severity of the asthmatic's disease. An alternative to skin tests is blood testing (radioallergosorbent [RAST] testing) for specific IgE against appropriate allergens. As with any laboratory test, the findings need to be correlated with the clinical history to determine their clinical relevance.

■ THERAPEUTIC APPROACH

Successful management of the patient with allergic asthma requires an integrated approach that incorporates environmental control, the judicious use of an appropriate anti-inflammatory therapeutic agent to suppress the underlying inflammatory component, and supplemental use of a bronchodilator to treat "breakthrough" symptoms. Immunotherapy should be considered in those patients who have not responded to environmental and pharmacotherapeutic measures, who have had side effects with the medications, or who have persistent disease because of continuous exposure to allergens throughout the year (Table 1).

■ PATIENT EDUCATION

Indeed, a successful strategy for management of asthma necessitates a partnership between the patient and the health care team. Integral to this therapeutic approach is the "empowerment" of the patient in the development and implementation of any treatment strategy, which requires an appreciation of patient education as more than simple role memorization. Rather, it is a learning process in which the patient is an active participant in the management of his or her disease (Table 2). This involves helping the patient understand asthma, having the patient learn and practice the skills nec-

Table 1 Concepts in Preventive Therapy

Environmental control
"Primary" anti-inflammatory agent
Cromolyn/nedocromil
Inhaled corticosteroids
"Maintenance" bronchodilator
Long-acting β_2-agonists
Methylxanthines/theophyllines
"Rescue" bronchodilator
Short-acting β_2-agonists
Anticholinergics
Immunotherapy

From Creticos PS: Johns Hopkins Asthma and Allergy Center Press; with permission.

Table 2 Objectives of Patient Education

Helping patients understand their asthma
Learning and practicing the skills necessary to manage asthma
Positive feedback-imaging-behavior modification
Adherence to treatment plan

essary to manage asthma, establishing an open communication channel for the patient with members of the health care team, and developing a joint treatment plan. This latter point cannot be overemphasized, since a disinterested or uninformed patient is apt to spell failure for any long-term management plan.

ENVIRONMENTAL CONTROL

Cigarette smoke, aerosol sprays, and cooking odors are important irritants capable of triggering an asthmatic's symptoms in the indoor environment. Even more critical to the asthmatic patient is the role of persistent exposure to perennial indoor allergens in inducing a smoldering asthmatic process (Table 3).

House dust mites, molds, cockroaches and other insects, and animals are the primary sources contributing to the indoor allergen burden. Proteinaceous particles from decaying body parts (dust mites, roaches), fecal emanations (dust mites, roaches), dander (animals), saliva (cats, roaches), and urinary protein (rodents, cats) represent the major allergen "load."

Those particles smaller than 10 μm in diameter can easily reach the lower respiratory tract and induce asthma symptoms. Our airtight homes with wall-to-wall carpeting, indoor pets, and central heating and ventilation systems are conducive to creating an indoor environment that ensures a patient is exposed to a constant allergen burden.

Measures to reduce the allergen burden in the indoor environment have been addressed in the chapter *Allergic Rhinitis.* To reiterate, the importance of dust mite control, animal avoidance, and insect eradication cannot be overstressed because the asthmatic's disease process can be significantly attenuated or even ablated through these measures.

Not to be overlooked is the importance of pollen allergens in inducing asthmatic symptoms. Intact pollen grains (e.g.,

Table 3 Primary Allergens in Asthma

Perennial Allergens
Dust mites
Animals (e.g., cat)
Insects (e.g, cockroach)
Mold spores
Seasonal Allergens
Pollens
Trees
Grasses
Weeds
Molds

ragweed pollen, 23 μm diameter) are too large to reach the lower airways. However, a significant amount of their "total allergenic activity" is not only attributable to intact pollen but also to pollen fragments (<10 μm diameter) and microaerosol suspensions (3 to 7 μm diameter). The relevance of this is observed during the pollen season as millions of pollen grains settle to the ground; whereupon dew, rainfall, and humidity extract the relevant protein from the pollen grains, which then becomes airborne as microaerosol particles. A similar phenomenon occurs with mold in which soluble protein from the mold spores and mycelial elements is dispersed into the atmosphere.

PREVENTIVE ANTI-INFLAMMATORY THERAPY

Our recognition and understanding of the importance of inflammation in the asthmatic's disease process underscores the importance of employing a compound with anti-inflammatory properties as a primary therapeutic agent in the management of asthma. In this context, early therapeutic intervention should be aimed at suppressing mild but persistent symptoms with this primary anti-inflammatory agent in an attempt to prevent their escalation into a more moderate to severe disease process. Presently, nonsteroidal anti-inflammatory compounds (e.g., cromolyn, nedocromil) and synthetic glucocorticosteroids are choices to be considered by the physician.

Cromolyn

The compound cromolyn is a derivative of a naturally occurring antispasmodic extracted from a mediterranean weed. Cromolyn sodium has been demonstrated to be clinically efficacious in the management of seasonal allergic asthma, perennial allergic asthma, exercise-induced asthma, occupational asthma, and certain types of irritant-induced asthma. Its mechanisms are not completely understood, but it appears that one of its actions may be to stabilize mast cell membranes, inhibiting the subsequent release of inflammatory mediators. It also has been shown to interfere with the migration of eosinophils into the inflammatory site and to decrease the number of eosinophils and the concentration of eosinophilic inflammatory mediators (e.g., eosinophil cationic protein) in bronchial lavage fluids of treated asthmatics.

The most successful therapeutic approach with cromolyn is to employ the drug prophylactically, beginning 7 to 10 days

Table 4 Cromolyn: Recommended Dosages for Asthma Treatment

ROUTE	DOSE/ ACTUATION	TYPICAL DOSE	TOTAL DOSE
MDI	800 μg	2–4 puffs q.i.d.	6.4–12.8 mg
Spinhaler	20 mg/cap	1 cap q.i.d.	80 mg
Nebulized	10 mg/ml	20 mg q.i.d.	80 mg

prior to the allergen season. Because of cromolyn's safety profile, an aggressive approach to treatment can be ascribed to with an initial inhaled dose of two puffs (6,400 μg) four times daily being recommended (Table 4). Obviously, this necessitates patient compliance, but with a motivated patient instructed in the necessity of using the drug diligently in this early treatment phase, it may be possible to reduce this dosage to a regimen of two to three times a day for sustaining control of the patient's symptoms.

In symptomatic patients it is even more important to emphasize aggressive dosing of the drug, since it may be necessary to double the dose to two to four puffs four times daily during the first week or two of therapy to effect control. Furthermore, it may be necessary to extend treatment to 2 to 4 weeks before optimal efficacy occurs. Once control is achieved, it may be possible to taper the dosage to a more "user friendly" regimen that ensures patient compliance.

Clinical studies demonstrate that cromolyn-treated patients receiving 6,400 μg per day (two puffs four times daily) show improvement in daytime-nocturnal asthma, cough, peak expiratory flow, overall asthma symptoms, pulmonary function, and the need for supplemental bronchodilators. Comparative studies show cromolyn to be as efficacious as a bronchodilator in the management of asthma. However, the combination of cromolyn with a beta$_2$-agonist has been shown to result in better symptom control than cromolyn alone. Although theophylline provides similar clinical benefit, the low frequency of adverse effects associated with cromolyn represents a significant advantage in therapy.

The use of a spacer can further improve both drug delivery and clinical response in patients and a strong case can be made to employ a spacer in all cases in which inhaled cromolyn is prescribed. Likewise, the nebulized formulation of cromolyn can be employed to maintain therapeutic levels when and if a metered dose inhaler (MDI) cannot be continued. This is particularly useful in cases involving young children who cannot learn correct MDI technique, instances of severe lower airway inflammation (bronchitis, respiratory infection) that make an aerosol intolerable, or when intolerance to the aerosol propellent is a factor.

Nedocromil

Nedocromil is a nonsteroidal anti-inflammatory compound termed a pyronoquinoline (Table 5). It is a synthetically derived dicarbocylic acid with a tricyclic ring backbone. These synthetic alterations have resulted in a compound with a broader spectrum of anti-inflammatory activity as compared to cromolyn. Studies have demonstrated that nedocromil has activity on a variety of cell types involved in the asthmatic cascade (eosinophils, neutrophils, epithelial cells, mast cells), inhibits inflammatory mediator release, and has a modulatory effect on neural pathways with implications on both the immediate and late phases of the asthmatic's clinical response. Clinical studies have demonstrated efficacy in seasonal and perennial asthma, cold air-induced, SO_2-induced, exercise-induced, and cough-variant asthma.

Table 5 Nedocromil

Chemical class:
- Pyranoquinoline

Mechanism of action:
- Effects on activation of and mediator release from a variety of cells activity on neurogenic pathways

Clinical indication:
- Mild to moderate asthma

Dosage:
- 2 puffs q.i.d. until symptoms under control; then, reduce to a maintenance dosage of 2 puffs b.i.d.

From Creticos PS: Johns Hopkins Asthma and Allergy Center Press; with permission.

In studies employing bronchoprovocation, nedocromil appears comparable to beclomethasone dipropionate (BDP) in reducing the underlying bronchial hyper-responsiveness of patients with mild to moderate asthma (Fig. 1). In this context, one of the more clinically relevant features of airway inflammation is a heightened diurnal variability in peak expiratory flow (PEF). Nedocromil has been shown to both attenuate this diurnal flux and improve overall lung function (FEV_1, PEF) when used on a regular daily basis.

In contrast, maintenance therapy with a short-acting beta$_2$-agonist (e.g., albuterol) neither results in a sustained improvement in PEF nor a reduction in the diurnal variability in peak flow. The relevance of this may be correlated with bronchoalveolar lavage studies showing that nedocromil inhibits the influx of inflammatory cells (e.g., eosinophils) into the lungs, whereas a bronchodilator (albuterol) does not.

In contrast to cromolyn, nedocromil given in a dose of two puffs (4 mg) four times daily results in improvement in asthma symptoms within days of initiating therapy (Fig. 2). For optimal control, the drug should be initiated at a dose of two puffs four times daily for the first 1 to 2 weeks of therapy to ensure suppression of the bronchial hyper-responsiveness, improve lung function, and reduce symptoms. Once control is established, then the drug should be reduced to a twice-a-day maintenance regimen of two to four puffs for sustaining control.

For chronic maintenance therapy, studies show nedocromil, 4 mg four times daily, to be comparable to low-dose inhaled corticosteroids (BDP $\leq$ 400 μg per day) and superior to maintenance bronchodilator therapy (albuterol, two puffs four times daily) in reducing daytime-nocturnal asthma, wheezing, shortness of breath, and/or cough. When added to maintenance theophylline (400 to 800 μg per day) nedocromil has been shown to result in further improvement in clinical symptoms and an ability to reduce and/or replace theophylline, with no loss of therapeutic effectiveness. Various studies have shown an added benefit when nedocromil has been added to a maintenance regimen of theophylline, beta$_2$-agonists, and inhaled corticosteroids. This may be particularly beneficial in allowing patients with moderate to severe asthma

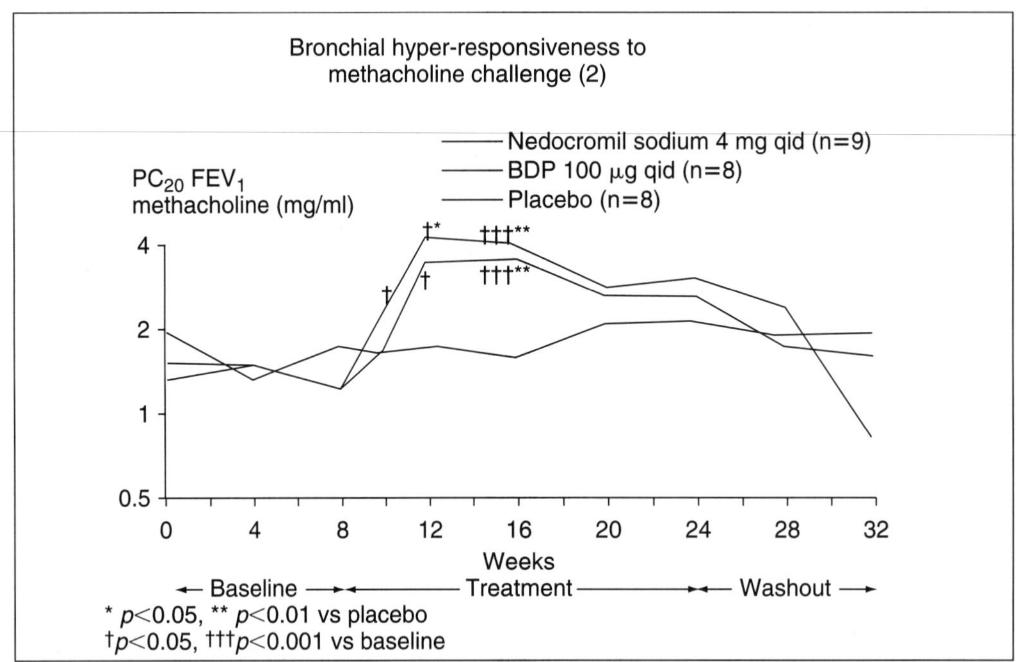

Figure 1
A second study carried out by Bel and Sterk in Holland showed a comparable reduction in bronchial hyper-responsiveness (BHR) (methacholine $PC_{20}FEV_1$) with nedocromil sodium (4 mg q.i.d.) and BDP (100 μg q.i.d.) during 16 weeks' treatment in 25 patients with intrinsic asthma previously controlled on inhaled bronchodilators. BHR decreased significantly after 4 ($p < 0.05$) and 8 ($p < 0.01$) weeks' treatment. *(From Bel EH, et al. The long term effects of nedocromil sodium and beclomethasone diproprionate on bronchial responsiveness to methacholine in nonatopic asthmatic subjects. Am Rev Respir Dis 1990; 141:21–28; with permission.)*

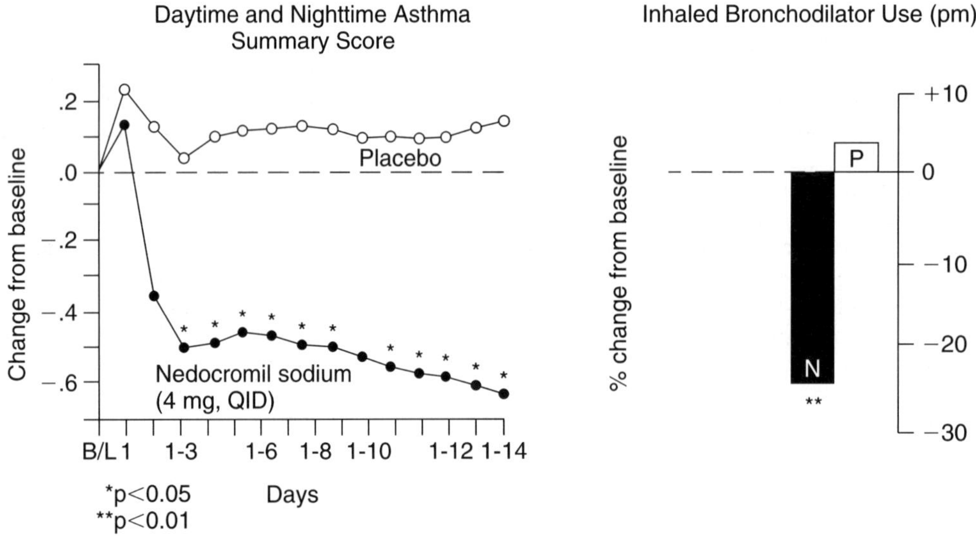

Figure 2
Change from baseline of cumulative mean asthma symptom summary scores and, as required, inhaled bronchodilator use for treatment weeks 1 and 2 (when nedocromil sodium was added to maintenance bronchodilator therapy). After a 2 week baseline period, patients maintained on sustained-release theophylline or oral β_2-agonist bronchodilators were randomized to receive 4 mg nedocromil sodium (n = 60) or placebo (n = 61) four times a day, for 16 weeks. *Closed circles* indicate nedocromil sodium *(N)*; *open circles* indicate placebo *(P)*. Statistically significant differences (*$p < 0.05$, **$p < 0.01$) favoring nedocromil sodium were determined from days 1 to 3 onward. The use of as-required inhaled bronchodilator decreased in the nedocromil sodium group and increased slightly in the placebo group during the 2 week analysis period. *(Modified from Cherniack RM, et al. A double blind multicenter group comparative study of the efficacy and safety of nedocromil sodium in the management of asthma. Chest 1990; 97:1299–1306.)*

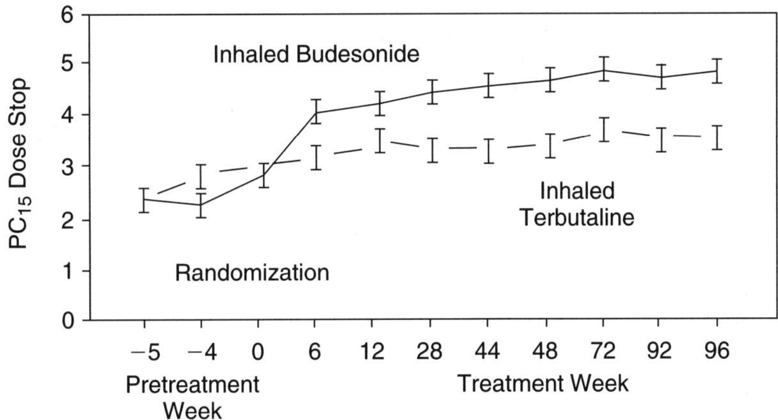

Figure 3
β_2-agonists and bronchial hyper-responsiveness. *(From Haahtela T, et al. Comparison of a beta$_2$-agonist terbutaline, with an inhaled corticosteroid, budesonide, in newly detected asthma. N Engl J Med 1991; 325:388–392; with permission.)*

Table 6 Inhaled Corticosteroid Preparations

COMPOUND	DOSE/ACTUATION	TYPICAL DOSAGE	TOTAL DOSE
Beclomethasone (Vanceril/ Beclovent)	50 µg	2–4 p q.i.d.	400 µg–800 µg
Flunsiolide (AeroBid)	250 µg	2–4 p b.i.d.	1,000 µg–2,000 µg
Triamcinolone (Azmacort)	[200] 100 µg	2–4 p q.i.d.	800 µg–1,600 µg
Budesonide* (Pulmicort)	200 µg	2–4 p b.i.d	200 µg–1,600 µg
Fluticasone* (Flovent)	100/200 µg	1–2 p b.i.d.	200 µg–1,000 µg

*Not yet approved in the U.S.; p, puff.

to reduce their total inhaled steroid requirements and yet maintain sustained control.

In direct comparison studies, nedocromil appears comparable to cromolyn in improving the asthmatic symptoms of patients with predominantly allergic asthma, but superior to cromolyn in treating predominantly nonallergic asthmatics.

In summary, nedocromil appears to represent a therapeutic agent with a broader spectrum of activity than cromolyn and, most importantly, a compound that can be reduced to a twice-a-day maintenance dosage for effective control. Its ease of administration and safety make it a reasonable choice for use in patients with mild to moderate asthma.

Inhaled Corticosteroids

Synthetic corticosteroids adapted for inhalation into the lungs have dramatically altered our approach to the treatment of asthma. Their ease of administration and their favorable risk-benefit ratio compared to oral steroids has made them the drug of choice for suppressing asthmatic inflammation.

Corticosteroids may act through several different mechanisms, including inhibition of cellular recruitment, arachidonic acid metabolism, mediator synthesis, restoration of beta$_2$-receptor responsivity, and down regulation of the effects of various inflammatory mediators on their target sites. The clinical relevance of these findings is demonstrated in properly performed provocation studies, which show that inhaled corticosteroids given for an adequate length of time block both the immediate and late phases of a (specific) allergen-induced challenge, reduce airway inflammation, and inhibit development of nonspecific airway reactivity (Fig. 3). Chronic administration results in a decrease in hyperresponsiveness to both specific (allergen) and nonspecific (irritant) stimuli.

As with the nonsteroidal anti-inflammatory preparations, prophylactic use of an inhaled steroid provides the best opportunity to prevent or disrupt the inflammatory cascade of asthma. In this context, therapy should be started 5 to 7 days prior to allergen exposure and maintained through the ensuing season. Adjustments in dosage can be made based on assessment of clinical symptoms and peak expiratory flow rates.

In symptomatic patients, judicious adherence to the treatment regimen is necessary starting with an initial dose adequate to bring symptoms under control and then tapered as tolerated to the lowest effective dose that sustains symptom control during the maintenance phase of therapy. This dose must be adequate to suppress the underlying inflammatory component, improve pulmonary function, and reduce the frequency and severity of symptoms.

Table 6 lists the topical inhaled corticosteroid preparations available in the U.S. market along with their dosing schedule. The NHLBI guidelines have given us the therapeutic approach to patients based on the severity of their disease. With this in mind, a reasonable approach for control of mild (200 to 400 µg per day), moderate (400 to 800 µg per day), and severe asthma (>800 µg per day) can be constructed.

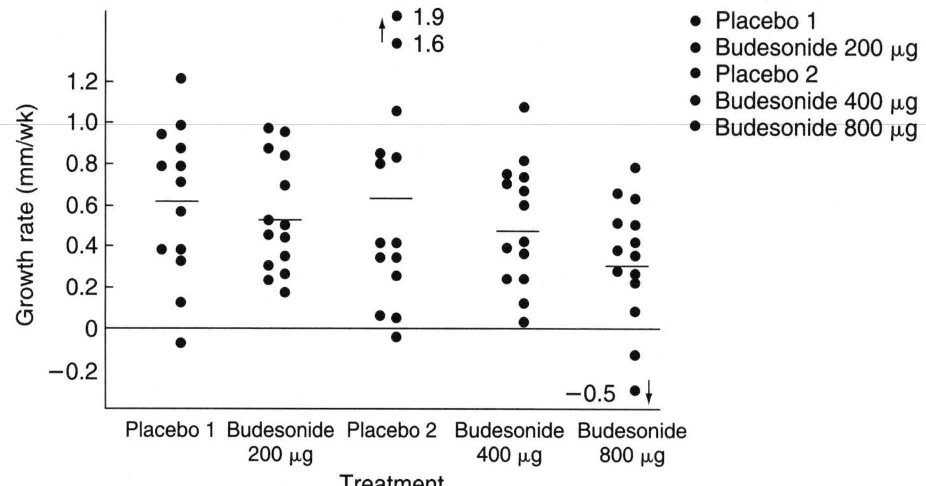

Figure 4
Effects of inhaled steroids on linear growth. *(Modified from Wolthers DH, et al. Growth of asthmatic children during treatment with budesonide: A double blind trial. BMJ 1991; 303:163–165.)*

Implicit in these suggestions is the importance of beginning therapy with a maximally recommended dose over the first 1 to 2 weeks in order to bring the inflammatory process under control quickly (800 to 1,500 μg per day), and then to reduce this to the lowest dose that still provides adequate therapeutic control (≈200 to 800 μg per day).

As with cromolyn, the key to success with inhaled corticosteroid therapy is patient compliance. Thus, dosing frequency and the number of doses (puffs) required to achieve effective control become important factors. Toogood's early studies of BDP suggested that dosing four times daily was the most efficient approach. Once control is achieved, twice-daily dosing may provide equal therapeutic benefit, especially with enhanced patient compliance. However, therapy needs to be individualized based on the patient's appreciation of symptom control, PEF readings, and periodic spirometric measurements.

A difficult issue in the United States has been the relationship of dosage among the various inhaled corticosteroid preparations. No direct clinical comparisons have been done between the three preparations presently available in the United States. However, two inhaled steroid preparations, budesonide and fluticasone, neither yet commercially available in the United States, have been extensively studied. Comparative studies of budesonide with beclomethasone have shown comparable efficacy of the two compounds at lower (400 μg per day) and higher (1,500 μg per day) dosage comparisons. The improved risk-benefit ratio of budesonide suggests that it may allow up to a 30 percent higher dosing before comparable effects on adrenal suppression are observed. Likewise, fluticasone should also improve our therapeutic armamentarium, since it appears that 30 to 40 percent less of a dose may confer a similar degree of clinical response.

The importance of this finding is in the treatment of more moderate to severe asthma where dosages of greater than or equal to 800 μg per day may be frequently necessitated. The difficulty with BDP (50 μg per puff) is that patients are unlikely to administer 20 to 30 puffs per day (1,000 to 1,500 μg per day) for any reasonable period of time. Therefore, formulations that can deliver 200 to 250 μg per puff and provide reasonable assurance of comparability on a microgram-to-microgram basis will dramatically improve our ability to manage the more difficult asthmatic.

The question of the safety of topical steroids becomes a relevant issue, especially if higher dosage therapy is required. Systemic toxicity with adrenal axis suppression, growth retardation, osteoporosis, and cataracts have all been reported with daily oral prednisone and alternate-day oral prednisone. At issue is whether these effects are likely to be seen with higher dosages of inhaled corticosteroids. Studies now provide a reasonable level of comfort in both children and adults with respect to these adverse events. The data suggest that adrenal suppression is not likely to be encountered in children until a dosage of greater than 800 μg per day is administered, and in adults at a dose greater than 1,200 μg per day. Likewise, short-term studies of growth in asthmatic children suggest that a dosage of greater than or equal to 800 μg per day of budesonide would be required before any evidence of clinically relevant growth retardation may appear (Fig. 4). Further studies are required to address the issue of whether clinically relevant findings are observed at doses of 400 to 800 μg per day of beclomethasone.

A few reported cases of posterior, subcapsular cataracts have been reported in patients taking inhaled steroids, but this risk appears to be directly related to the previous use of oral corticosteroids in these patients and not to the specific use of the inhaled steroid preparation. Local side effects attributable to topical steroid therapy include oral candidiasis, hoarseness, and dysphonia. Simply instructing the patient to rinse out the mouth after use of the inhaled steroid can minimize fungal overgrowth. Use of a spacer device with the inhaler can also obviate this concern.

As previously mentioned, the use of a spacer can further improve both drug delivery and clinical response in patients. Thus, the use of a spacer should be the first manipulation attempted in patients not demonstrating satisfactory results before considering the addition of an additional therapeutic agent. In fact, a strong case can be made for the use of a spacer device in any patient placed on a primary anti-

Table 7 Salmeterol

Entity
Long-acting β-agonist
Dosage
2 puffs (42 μg) b.i.d.
CX Uses
Maintenance treatment of asthma and prevention of bronchospasm
Prevention of nocturnal asthma
Prophylaxis against exercise-induced asthma
Contraindications
Not for relief of acute asthma symptoms
Do not exceed 2 puffs b.i.d. dosage

inflammatory therapeutic agent. In this regard, further studies that address spacer design, optimal particle size, and respirable fraction delivered to the lungs would further our progress in this area.

Bronchodilator Therapy

Preventive therapy is the desirable approach to the management of asthma. However, sympathomimetic bronchodilators are important adjunctive medicines for relief of acute symptoms or for the treatment of breakthrough symptoms in a patient already on a maintenance primary anti-inflammatory drug.

In essence, the need for bronchodilator use should be considered as an "early warning signal" for the asthmatic. That is, if a patient's asthma symptoms begin to increase in frequency or if the patient begins to note the need for a bronchodilator on a more frequent basis (>3 days in a week), then that should be an indication of worsening asthma. Steps should then be taken to identify the basis for the worsening of the asthmatic condition. In a patient who is not already on a primary anti-inflammatory agent, this would be an indication that such a drug should be started. If a patient is already on a primary anti-inflammatory agent, then the dosage of that compound should be doubled. Subsequent adjustment to the medication regimen should be based on the therapeutic response to these initial manipulations.

Maintenance Bronchodilators

Salmeterol

The recent introduction of salmeterol has provided the option of employing this long-acting, inhaled beta$_2$-sympathomimetic drug for maintenance control of asthma and prevention of bronchospasm, control of nocturnal asthma, and prevention of exercise-induced asthma (Table 7). The primary place for this therapeutic agent is in patients already maintained on a primary anti-inflammatory drug for whom addition of a "maintenance bronchodilator" would optimize control. In this context, the addition of salmeterol could obviate the need for increasing the corticosteroid dose in a less than optimally controlled patient, thus improving the risk: benefit ratio of the total drug therapy regimen.

This drug is also an appropriate therapeutic choice for control of nocturnal asthma, where the longer duration of action would provide reasonable control for a majority of patients. In contrast, short-acting bronchodilators (3- to 4 hour duration) would not be expected to provide an adequate duration of coverage through the evening hours. This would also be a superior choice in patients with gastroesophageal reflux where use of theophylline would further aggravate lower esophageal sphincter pressure and result in worsening reflux.

The final indication for this agent is in exercise-induced asthma. Indeed, because of its longer duration of action, it may provide protection against several different exercise events during a 10 to 12 hour period.

The normal dosage range is one to two puffs (42 μg per puff) twice a day. Patients should be cautioned not to exceed a twice-daily dosing frequency because the prolonged half-life of the drug may result in an exaggerated pharmacologic response with tremor, muscle cramps, headache, or adverse cardiovascular events. Furthermore, the drug should never be used to relieve acute symptoms of bronchospasm. In that regard, a short-acting selective beta$_2$ agent should be used for relief of breakthrough symptoms in a patient already on maintenance therapy with salbutamol.

Long-Acting Theophylline Preparations

Theophylline therapy has been a cornerstone of asthma therapy through the years. As with beta-adrenergic sympathomimetic agents, theophylline appears to exert its primary influence through relaxation of smooth muscle of the bronchial tree by inhibiting the breakdown of the enzyme phosphodiesterase with a resultant increase in cAMP concentrations, which results in smooth muscle cell relaxation.

As emphasized, our current approach to the treatment of asthma involves the aggressive use of an inhaled preventive therapeutic agent. As a result, theophylline is now viewed as an adjunctive, albeit important, therapeutic agent in those asthmatic patients whose condition is not easily controlled by the use of inhaled nedocromil or inhaled corticosteroids supplemented by an inhaled beta$_2$-selective sympathomimetic agent. This current strategy reflects not only the appreciated superior anti-inflammatory properties of these preventive inhaled agents but also the toxic effects associated with theophylline therapy.

In view of the small margin between therapeutic effects and toxicity, individualization of dose is mandatory with theophylline therapy (Table 8). The use of sustained-release long-acting (once or twice daily) preparations has improved this aspect of care because of the more consistent theophylline-release characteristics, which provide more consistent plasma concentration with less marked peak-trough variation. In this regard, it is important not to switch among various preparations because significant differences in serum blood levels may result because of the differences in absorption characteristics among preparations from different manufacturers.

The new once-a-day sustained-release products may be most useful in the subset of asthmatics with nocturnal symptoms who otherwise find it difficult to sleep through the night because of the short duration of activity of classic sympathomimetic agents.

Rescue Bronchodilators

Short-Acting Selective Beta$_2$ Agonists

Sympathomimetic bronchodilators have become a mainstay in the therapeutic approach to the treatment of asthma. These agents are the drug of choice for relief of acute bronchospasm. They are used effectively alone for the treatment of mild or intermittent asthma symptoms, and they are also effective in preventing or reversing exercise-induced asthma. Table 9 lists the various catecholamine and noncatecholamine compounds that are available. Improved beta$_2$ selectivity and increased duration of action are seen with the majority of the noncatecholamine derivatives.

The therapeutic effects of beta-adrenergic agents include bronchodilatation as a result of activation of a cell membrane's adenylate cyclase enzyme, which converts ATP to cAMP, resulting in sequestration of intracellular calcium. This leads to relaxation of smooth muscle; increased ciliary movement, which should improve clearance of secretions; and stabilizing effects on the mast cell to decrease mediator release. However, in regard to this last action, provocation studies demonstrate that beta-adrenergic agents can effectively ablate the immediate asthmatic response but have no demonstrable clinical effect on the late phase of airway reactivity.

Table 8 Factors Affecting Theophylline Blood Levels

CONDITIONS INCREASING THEOPHYLLINE BLOOD LEVELS
Older age (>50 years)
Obesity
Liver disease
Congestive heart failure
Chronic obstructive pulmonary disease
Acute viral infections
High-carbohydrate, low-protein diet
Influenza A vaccine
Drug use
Troleandomycin
Erythromycin preparations
Allopurinol
Cimetidine
Propranolol hydrochloride
CONDITIONS DECREASING THEOPHYLLINE BLOOD LEVELS
Young age (1–16 years)
Cigarette smoking
Eating charcoal-broiled meat
Low-carbohydrate, high-protein diet
Drug use
Phenobarbital
Phenytoins
Isoproterenol hydrochloride

From Kaliner M, Eggleston PA, Mathews KP. Primer on allergic and immunologic diseases, Ch 3: Rhinitis and asthma. JAMA 1987; 258:2851–2873. Copyright 1987, American Medical Association; with permission.

Selective beta$_2$ agonists provide better bronchodilation than do the theophylline products in both the acute and chronic state. Furthermore, the addition of aminophylline to maximum-dose inhaled beta-agonist therapy provides no further improvement in the bronchodilator response. However, in chronic therapy, receptor subsensitivity may develop. This has led to considerable discussion as to whether these agents should be administered on a regular (four times daily) maintenance dosage schedule, which again reinforces the approach that a short-acting beta$_2$ agent should be used on an as-needed basis for relief of acute symptoms. Typical dosing is one to two puffs every 4 to 6 hours because it is needed for relief of breakthrough asthma symptoms. However, it should again be reiterated that these drugs should not be overused. Their increased need should signal the need to address the underlying trigger of the asthmatic exacerbation and to make appropriate adjustments in the patient's primary anti-inflammatory regimen.

Another important point to emphasize is the proper administration of the aerosol. Careful demonstration of inhaler technique by the physician, nurse, or patient educator is mandatory and often requires repeated reinforcement. Several techniques for delivery are satisfactory, but most investigators would suggest discharging the inhaler when it is 1 to 1½ inches (two fingers) away from the open mouth (open-mouth technique). The patient should then take a slow, deep inspiration (from functional residual capacity to total lung capacity) and then hold the breath for 8 to 10 seconds. This technique improves deposition and can result in nearly doubling the amount of medication reaching the lower respiratory tract. In patients with poor technique, delivery can be improved by employing a spacer. Typically, 2 to 3 minutes

Table 9 β-Adrenergic Agonists for Inhalation

DRUG*	SELECTIVITY†	ONSET OF ACTION (MINUTES)	PEAK ACTION (MINUTES)	DURATION (HOURS)
CATECHOLAMINES				
Epinephrine (Primatene, 0.2 mg/p)	$\alpha_1, \beta_1, \beta_2$	2–7	15–20	0.5
Isoproterenol (Isuprel, 0.125 mg/p)	β_1, β_2	2–5	5	1.5–2
Isoetharine (Bronkometer, 0.34 mg/p)	β_2	2–5	15	1.5–2
NONCATECHOLAMINES				
Bitolterol (Tornalate, 0.37 mg/p)	β_2+	3–5	30–60	4–8
Metaproterenol (Alupent, 0.65 mg/p)	β_2++	5–10	120–180	3–4
Terbutaline (Brethaire, 0.25 mg/p)	β_2+++	5–10	90–120	3–4
Albuterol (Proventil, Ventolin, 0.09 mg/p)	β_2+++	5–15	60–90	4–6
Pirbuterol (Maxair, 0.2 mg/p)	β_2+++	3–5	30–60	4–6

*p, puff; Usual doses are 1–2 p every 4–6 hours; bitolterol, 2–3 p every 6–8 hours; metaproterenol, 2–3 p every 4 hours.
†+, low selectivity; ++, moderate selectivity; +++, high selectivity.
Adapted from Creticos PS. Drug therapy of asthma. In: Smith CM, Reynard AM (eds). Textbook of pharmacology. Philadelphia: WB Saunders, 1992.

should lapse between the first and second puffs from an aerosol bronchodilator, so that the maximal bronchodilating effect of the first puff can allow better penetration of the second puff.

Certainly, with the environmental concerns related to ozone depletion as a result of extensive industrial use of CFCs, the development of non-CFC and powder formulations of selected beta$_2$ agonist preparations has resulted in several new formulations that should be available soon. These may also be advantageous for patients prone to irritant effects of a freon-metered device.

Oral beta agonist preparations are available, but inhalation delivers more of the active drug directly to the mucosal surface and, at the same time, minimizes side effects. Oral therapy may be useful in certain situations (e.g., acute viral infection) in which airway irritation prevents the comfortable use of an inhaled therapeutic agent. Side effects associated with beta-agonist therapy include tremor; nervousness; and, with higher doses of even the selective beta$_2$ agents, palpitations or tachycardia.

Anticholinergic Agents

The parasympathetic nervous system appears to play a prominent role in cold air-induced asthma, SO_2-induced asthma, and cough-variant asthma. This may be a reflection of direct neural (parasympathetic) activity, reflex cholinergic bronchoconstriction, or the interplay between neural mechanisms and inflammatory mediators.

Ipratropium has been shown to be effective in reducing the cholinergic hyper-reactivity present in many patients with chronic bronchitis, emphysema, and asthma. It is administered as a metered dose inhalation of two puffs every 6 hours as needed. Although the therapeutic response obtained with ipratropium is comparable to albuterol in terms of its bronchodilating effect (increase in FEV_1), its onset of action is considerably slower (15 to 30 minutes).

Immunotherapy

Numerous studies with pollens (weeds, grasses, trees), animal allergens, and dust mites support the efficacy of immunotherapy in treating allergic rhinitis. However, only a few well-controlled studies evaluating the role of immunotherapy in treating patients with allergic asthma have been carried out.

Studies employing bronchial provocation with specific allergens (e.g., cat and/or dust mites) have demonstrated the ability to significantly shift the $PD_{20}FEV_1$ (ten fold to 100-fold) in patients immunized with an optimal dose of standardized extract. Most recently, a major study of the role of immunotherapy in adults with seasonal ragweed-induced asthma demonstrated improvement in the ragweed-immunized patients both in clinical endpoints (fewer symptoms, decreased medication usage, increased PEF readings) and in objective parameters (a reduction in skin test sensitivity, decreased bronchial responsivity to ragweed upon bronchial provocation, a rise in specific IgG ragweed antibodies, and a blunting of the usual seasonal rise in IgE ragweed antibodies). As in ragweed-induced allergic rhinitis, this study of ragweed allergic asthmatics again demonstrates that clinical success hinges upon the use of an appropriate therapeutic dose.

Suggested Reading

Barnes PJ. A new approach to the treatment of asthma. N Engl J Med 1989; 321:1517–1526.

Barnes PJ. Inhaled glucocorticoids for asthma. In: Wood AJJ, ed. Drug therapy. N Engl J Med 1995; 332(13):868–875.

Bel EH, et al. The long term effects of nedocromil sodium and beclomethasone dipropionate on bronchial responsiveness to methacholine in nonatopic asthmatic subjects. Am Rev Respir Dis 1990; 141:21–28.

Cherniack RM. A double blind multicenter group comparative study of the efficacy and safety of nedocromil sodium in the management of asthma. Chest 1990; 97:1299–1306.

Djukanovic, et al. Effect of an inhaled corticosteroid on airway symptoms in asthma. Am Rev Respir Dis 1992; 145:669–674.

Haahtela T, et al. Comparison of a β_2-agonist, terbutaline, with an inhaled corticosteroid, budesonide, in newly detected asthma. N Engl J Med 1991; 325(6):388–392.

National Institutes of Health. Global Initiative for Asthma. Global strategy for asthma management and prevention NHLBI/WHO workshop report (NIH publication # 95-3659). Bethesda, MD: US Department of Health and Human Services, Jan 1995.

National Institutes of Health. National Asthma Education Program Expert Panel Report. Executive summary: Guidelines for the diagnosis and management of asthma (NIH publication # 91-3042A). Bethesda, Md: US Department of Health and Human Services, June 1991.

Pearlman DS, et al. A comparison of salmeterol with albuterol in the treatment of mild-to-moderate asthma. N Engl J Med 1992; 327(20):1420–1425.

Petty TL. Cromolyn sodium is effective in adult chronic asthmatics. Am Rev Respir Dis 1989; 694–701.

Sears, et al. Regular inhaled beta-agonist treatment in bronchial asthma. Lancet 1990; 336:1391–1396.

Wolthers OH, et al. Growth of asthmatic children during treatment with budesonide: A double blind trial. BMJ 1991; 303:163–165.

STATUS ASTHMATICUS

J. Mark Fitzgerald, M.D., F.R.C.P.I., F.R.C.P.C.
Anton Grunfeld, M.D., F.R.C.P.C.

Status asthmaticus or acute life-threatening asthma is usually defined as a severe asthma attack necessitating care in the emergency department (ED) or hospitalization. It is a common medical emergency that in the past has been shown to be poorly managed. Its immediate optimal management is of importance, but it is also important to recognize that subjects who visit the ED are at risk for further life-threatening attacks. Therefore the opportunity should be taken not only to manage the current attack optimally, but also to initiate appropriate specialist referral and follow-up to reduce the subsequent risk for life-threatening events.

■ PATIENT EVALUATION

Certain historical features should alert the physician to be more cautious in evaluating a patient with acute asthma, and these are discussed further in the context of discharge planning. Monosyllabic speech and difficulty in completing a full sentence represent clear evidence of a severe attack. The patient's and caregivers' responses are important to document, particularly with a view to the subsequent prevention of future life-threatening events. For example, was the patient on appropriate anti-inflammatory treatment, did he or she increase medication with the first sign of deteriorating asthma, especially the use of greater than usual doses of beta-agonist?

A previous history of a life-threatening episode or current use of prednisone should also alert the examining physician to be more cautious, particularly with regard to the decision on discharge or admission.

Clinical Examination

Signs of severe life-threatening attacks of asthma include tachycardia, tachypnea, hyperinflation, wheeze, accessory muscle use, and pulsus paradoxicus, all of which should alert the physician to greater caution. Various attempts have been made to formulate a scoring index based on clinical parameters and level of airflow obstruction, but all have generally been unsuccessful in subsequent prospective validation studies. The poor correlation between these indices and subsequent need for admission highlight the fact that the assessment of the patient in the ED should be multifactorial.

Investigations

After the history, the most important investigation is the objective measurement of airflow obstruction. It not only gives the clinician information with regard to the severity of the attack at presentation, but also allows response to therapy to be monitored. Failure to use objective measurements will lead to patients with suboptimal management being discharged from the ED. Many patients poorly perceive the level of airflow obstruction and therapeutic discussions based on clinical examination, or a patient's perception of symptoms may lead patients to unacceptable risk of relapse.

Arterial Blood Gases

Routine use of arterial blood gases is not warranted, particularly with the ready availability of pulse oximetry. In patients who have very severe airflow obstruction, and in particular if the FEV_1 is less than 40 percent of predicted values, arterial blood gases are indicated. In addition, arterial blood gases should be measured if there is concern with regard to whether a patient's clinical status is deteriorating. A normal or rising P_{CO_2} should alert the physician to the possible need for intubation and mechanical ventilation.

Chest Radiograph

Similar to arterial blood gases, routine chest radiographs are not required, particularly if the patient has only a moderately severe attack and is responding appropriately to bronchodilator therapy. A chest radiograph should be ordered if there is a failure to respond, so that an unrecognized pneumothorax or pneumomediastinum is not present. Patients with airflow obstruction severe enough to require hospitalization should also receive a chest radiograph.

Electrocardiogram

In general, routine use of an electrocardiogram (ECG) is not required unless the patient is in an age group where ischemic heart disease is a possible differential diagnosis, particularly if there is some question of chest tightness that may have some features suggestive of ischemia. Previous studies have shown that during an acute attack of asthma, signs of right ventricular strain may be present on ECG, including T-wave inversion, but these promptly revert in a matter of hours, once the acute attack is under control.

Sputum Examination

The routine use of sputum examination for Gram stain and culture and sensitivity is not warranted. If the exacerbation is associated with a respiratory tract infection, it will usually be viral in origin.

■ THERAPY

Treatment of patients with severe asthma must be initiated early and aggressively and should continue while the assessment of the patient is in progress.

First-Line Drugs

The first line of treatment of patients with severe asthma consists of routine supplemental oxygen, aggressive use of bronchodilators, and, importantly, corticosteroids.

Oxygen

Oxygen should be given to all patients in status asthmaticus. In severely ill patients, extreme hypoxemia and hypercapnia are frequently seen and must be addressed urgently. Oxygen can be delivered by nasal prongs, mask, or an endotracheal

Table 1 First-Line Drugs for Treatment of Acute Asthma

AGENT	RECOMMENDED DOSAGE
Oxygen	High flow, to maintain an SaO_2 >92%–95%. Can be delivered by nasal prongs, mask, or an endotracheal tube
Beta$_2$-agonists	**MDI:** Initial dose is 4–8 puffs (albuterol 100 μg/puff). Can be repeated every 15–20 min up to 3 times. In severe disease the dose can be increased by one puff every 30–60 sec up to 20 puffs, as needed
	Wet nebulizers: Initial dose is 5–10 mg of albuterol (1–2 ml plus 3 ml of saline) every 15–20 min. For patients with severe attacks, wet nebulization can run continuously
Corticosteroids	Prednisone: 40–60 mg orally stat, then daily for 1 to 2 wk
	or
	Methylprednisolone: 125 mg IV. Repeat every 8 hr for 24 hr
	or
	Hydrocortisone: 500 mg IV. Repeat every 8 hr for 24 hr
	Parenteral therapy to be followed by 1 to 2 wk of oral prednisone

tube to maintain an SaO_2 > 92 to 95 percent (Table 1). Oxygen will not suppress the respiratory drive in acute asthma.

Bronchodilators

Sympathomimetic drugs have been used in the management of life-threatening asthma since the 1950s. Adrenaline, the original agent, has gradually been replaced by selective beta$_2$-agonists. There is little disagreement that aerosol forms of beta$_2$ agonists are the agents of first choice to relieve bronchoconstriction in acute asthma. They provide more significant bronchodilation, the most prompt relief, and they are cheaper and have fewer side effects than other agents. Aerosolized beta$_2$ agonists have also been shown to be at least equal to and often superior to parenteral therapy with the same agent, with fewer side effects. Beta$_2$ agonists have also been shown convincingly to be effective even for those patients who have pretreated themselves unsuccessfully with the same medications prior to their arrival at the ED. The reason for self-administered beta$_2$ agonists not being effective prior to arrival in the ED may be due to underdosing or improper use of metered dose inhalers. Equally effective delivery of aerosolized beta$_2$-agonists can be achieved by using nebulized medication or metered dose inhalers, preferably with a spacer device. Most physicians are accustomed to using wet nebulizers for treatment of severe asthma. These devices are also well accepted by patients. Metered dose inhalers, on the other hand, have several advantages: the medication given this way can be administered and repeated very quickly (2 minutes versus 10 to 20 minutes for the wet nebulizers). Using metered dose inhalers is cheaper, offers an opportunity to demonstrate their effectiveness, and helps physicians to educate the patient in their proper use. The dosage of beta$_2$ agonists is empiric and is titrated to patient response (see Table 1). If aerosolized therapy is used aggressively, intravenous forms of beta$_2$-agonists are usually not needed.

Corticosteroids

Corticosteroids have become a first-line drug in the treatment of acute exacerbations of asthma because of the recognition of the pivotal role of inflammation in the pathogenesis of this disease. There continues to be controversy regarding the optimum dose, route, and frequency of administration and the type of preparation used. Corticosteroids are now recommended for all but the mildest attacks of asthma. Unquestionably, the administration of steroids favorably influences the outcome of both admitted and discharged patients. What remains in doubt, in spite of a recent meta-analysis by Rowe and colleagues supporting this view, is whether or not corticosteroids, if administered early and in high doses, can prevent hospital admissions. The onset of action of corticosteroids is slow and not expected to be substantial in the first 2 hours of treatment. In addition, the decision to admit or discharge a patient is complex, involving medical and nonmedical considerations. Oral administration is cheaper and has been found to be equally effective even in severe asthmatic exacerbations. The parenteral preparations should probably be reserved for patients unable to take oral medications (see Table 1).

Second-Line Drugs

Most patients will respond to first-line drugs with significant relief of bronchoconstriction; however, for those who do not improve, there are other agents. These include anticholinergics, adrenaline, intravenous salbutamol, and methylxanthines.

Anticholinergic Agents

Ipratropium bromide, the anticholinergic agent most commonly used, has been shown to have a slower onset of action and to produce less bronchodilation when used alone than beta$_2$-agonists. There is good evidence of an additive effect of ipratropium when used in combination with aerosol beta$_2$-agonist, but this effect although statistically significant, has generally been small, and its clinical relevance is uncertain. Because of concerns regarding the cost of ipratropium solution, all patients presenting with acute asthma should not routinely receive this agent, and it should be reserved for patients failing to respond to beta agonists. The recommended dosages are empiric (Table 2).

Adrenaline

Adrenaline has been used in the treatment of acute asthma since 1951. With the current, more specific beta$_2$ agonists, adrenaline is seldom needed. In certain circumstances such as anaphylaxis with a prominent bronchospastic component, adrenaline is the drug of choice. Equally, in circumstances where inhaled bronchodilators are not available, subcutaneous adrenaline can be lifesaving (see Table 2).

Intravenous Albuterol

Aggressive treatment with inhaled albuterol eliminates the need to use intravenous albuterol. However, in severely ill

Table 2 Second-Line Drugs for Treatment of Acute Asthma

AGENT	RECOMMENDED DOSAGE
Anticholinergics	Ipratropium bromide should be given to patients with severe and near-death asthma **MDI:** Initial dose is 4–8 puffs (20 μg/puff) every 15–20 min, to be repeated 3 times. The dose can be increased by one puff every 30–60 sec to a maximun of 20 puffs, as needed **Wet nebulization:** Initial dose is 0.25 to 0.5 mg (1–2 ml in 2 to 3 ml of saline) every 15–20 min or continuous if necessary. It may be mixed with the $beta_2$-agonists
Adrenaline	Adrenaline: 0.3–0.5 ml (1 : 1,000) subcutaneously every 15–20 min, as required Adrenaline infusion: 4–8 μg/min (1 ml of 1:1,000 adrenaline in 250 ml of D5W gives 4 μg/ml solution. The infusion is started at 1–2 ml/min)
Intravenous $beta_2$ agonists	Albuterol: 4 μg/kg, over 2 to 5 minutes. Albuterol can subsequently be given as an infusion at 0.1–0.2 μg/kg/min
Aminophylline	Aminophylline loading dose: 3–6 mg/kg intravenously over ½ hr. The dose should be halved if the patient is already on theophylline. Followed by an infusion at 0.2–1 mg/kg/hr. Blood level monitoring is recommended

patients, prior to endotracheal intubation and ventilation, or in patients responding poorly to inhaled albuterol, the intravenous preparation can be tried.

Methylxanthines

Aminophylline has been used for many years in the treatment of acute asthma. It has been shown, however, that aminophylline confers no additional benefit to the use of $beta_2$ agonists alone. A recent analysis by Littenberg of 13 adequately designed studies in patients with acute, severe asthma showed that the evidence for supporting its use was inconclusive. Aminophylline has a narrow therapeutic margin and can cause significant toxicity, especially in hypoxic patients. The metabolism of theophylline is affected by multiple factors, making close monitoring of its levels during therapy imperative. The combination of the above factors has led to recent recommendations that methylxanthines should not be used during the first 4 hours of treatment of the patient in the ED. If one chooses to use aminophylline, recommended dosages are shown in Table 2.

Intubation and Mechanical Ventilation

Most patients will respond promptly to bronchodilator and corticosteroid treatment. Attention should be paid to patients who do not respond and timely preparations for intubation and mechanical ventilation should be made for the few patients who require it. The decision to intubate an asthmatic patient is ultimately made on clinical grounds. For patients in respiratory arrest, or for patients with decreased sensorium or coma who cannot protect their airways, endotracheal intubation is mandatory. Otherwise, the decision usually evolves over minutes or hours, based on the ongoing clinical observations of the patient's response to treatment. Patients who deteriorate in spite of aggressive bronchodilator therapy and become exhausted and/or confused, whose respiratory effort is decreasing, who are diaphoretic, cyanotic, or whose vital signs are unstable are not likely to improve without a period of respiratory support. These patients need endotracheal intubation and mechanical ventilation. Correctable conditions such as deterioration attributable to a pneumothorax should be sought and rapidly corrected. Arterial blood gases can be obtained to strengthen the clinical decision; their values may show hypoxia, increasing hypercapnia, and acidosis. However, the decision to intubate the patient should not be delayed while waiting to obtain arterial blood gases.

A physician experienced with airway management should proceed with the intubation, while an anesthetist should be contacted early if the attending physician is not comfortable intubating the patient. It is important to decide which patients are likely to deteriorate and to proceed expeditiously with a rapid-sequence intubation for them, thereby avoiding "crash intubations." Patients should be preoxygenated with 100 percent oxygen.

Ketamine, the induction agent of choice in asthma, is a phencyclidine analogue that induces a state of dissociative anesthesia, putting the patient in a trance like, cataleptic state. The patient maintains muscle tone, pharyngeal and laryngeal reflexes, and respiratory drive. In addition, ketamine is a bronchodilator, acting both directly and indirectly through catecholamine release. It is as effective as halothane or enflurane in preventing bronchconstriction. One-quarter to one-third of adult patients receiving ketamine experience a post-anesthesia emergence reaction, during which the patient experiences vividly dysphoric dreams and unpleasant experiences. The emergence reaction can be controlled with the use of benzodiazepines, particularly midazolam. The recommended dosage of ketamine is 1.5 mg per kilogram administered intravenously over 1 minute. The ketamine bolus can be repeated as the bronchodilating effect wears off in 20 to 30 minutes. An infusion can also be started.

Succinylcholine, a depolarizing paralytic agent, is the agent of choice for paralyzing to facilitate endotracheal intubation. It is the fastest acting agent, and it is effective and safe used in conjunction with ketamine for intubation of asthmatic patients. The recommended dosage of succinylcholine is 1.5 mg per kilogram administered intravenously as a bolus.

Vecuronium, a nondepolarizing paralytic agent, should only be used for maintenance of paralysis. Although the rate of complications for intubated asthmatic patients is high, the mortality rate is usually low. Strict attention should be paid to maintaining adequate paralysis and low flow rates or tidal volumes to reduce peak airway pressures and associated barotrauma in intubated patients. Admission and treatment in the intensive care unit is mandatory.

Table 3 Spirometric Admission and Discharge Criteria in Acute Asthma

PREBRONCHODILATOR TREATMENT

FEV_1 <1.0 L or PEFR <100 L/min or <25% predicted or best will usually require admission

POSTBRONCHODILATOR TREATMENT

FEV_1 <1.6 L or PEFR <200 L/min or <40% predicted or best, admission is recommended

FEV_1 1.6–2.1 L or PEFR 200–300 L/min, or between 40%–60% predicted or best, discharge may be possible after consideration of risk factors and follow-up care

FEV_1 >2.1 L or PEFR >300 L/min, or >60% predicted or best, discharge is likely after consideration of risk factors and follow-up care

CRITERIA FOR ADMISSION OR DISCHARGE

Most patients presenting with exacerbations of asthma respond well to treatment and are discharged safely home. Hospital admission rates vary between 10 to 25 percent and, depending on a variety of factors, between 5 and 25 percent of patients discharged suffer a relapse. Attempts have been made to predict the need for hospital admission from the initial patient evaluation. Although not entirely successful, some broad guidelines are emerging. However, in no situation is the discharge of patients with treated asthma entirely free of risk.

Spirometry

Spirometric measurements have limitations and should not be relied upon in isolation for decision making regarding the admission or discharge of asthmatic patients. However, data from several studies indicate that patients fall within discernible groups (Table 3).

Historical Risk Factors

The majority of patients who die in status asthmaticus do so prior to reaching the hospital. The best way to identify asthma patients at risk of death is to identify those who have had a recent hospital admission and in particular those who have had one or more life-threatening attacks requiring mechanical ventilation. There are at least two distinctive high-risk groups:

1. **Patients with a history of near fatal episode** regardless of the underlying severity of the disease and other risk factors, and
2. **Patients with underlying severe disease** judged by chronic severe symptoms, systemic steroid requirement, frequent regular use of bronchodilators, frequent ED visits, or hospitalization. Patients in this group also may have one or more of the following problems: recent discharge from the hospital for severe asthma, poor self-care or noncompliance with medications, depression or severe emotional disturbance, other significant psychological factors, or shortcomings in education or supervision. Patients with these characteristics (Table 4) will clearly require careful consideration and close follow-up if discharged.

Table 4 Patient Characteristics for Potentially Fatal Asthma

- Near fatal episode of asthma
- Sudden precipitous attack
- Recent ED visit
- Frequent hospitalization
- Recent use or dependence on systemic steroids
- Recent attack of prolonged duration
- Poor compliance or knowledge of asthma
- Return to the same environmental triggers

DISCHARGE PLANNING AND FOLLOW-UP

The goal of asthma therapy is the return of the patient to full function. With rare exceptions, disability is not acceptable. Patients should function with minimal or no symptoms and their asthma should not affect their school, work, or exercise. With a physician's help, each patient should have a plan on discharge from the ED and instructions on how to deal with exacerbations.

Regular use of $beta_2$ agonists is often required for at least 48 hours after discharge and patients should be advised on how to modify treatment according to symptoms. If the patient is unable to control symptoms, he should return to the ED. Patients should know the results of their pulmonary function tests, thus facilitating treatment decisions at the time of their next presentation to the ED. Prior to discharging a patient, the physician should verify that the patient knows how to use the metered dose inhaler.

Corticosteroids are indicated, upon discharge from the ED, for most patients. The treatment should be individualized, based on responses to past treatment and recent symptoms. The recommended dosage of prednisone is 30–60 mg per day for 7 to 14 days.

Steroids can usually be stopped rather than tapered as long as patients are taking maintenance inhaled corticosteroids. Patients discharged from the ED should be re-evaluated within a week by their family physician and decisions regarding maintenance anti-inflammatory therapy should be made at this time. There is also evidence that patients discharged from the ED benefit from facilitated referrals to specialists.

In summary, many acute exacerbations of asthma can be prevented with appropriate maintenance anti-inflammatory therapy and its prompt increase with the first signs of deteriorating asthma. When these acute attacks do occur, frequent bronchodilator therapy, primarily with beta agonists, systemic corticosteroids, and supplemental oxygen, should form the mainstay of treatment.

Suggested Reading

Littenberg B. Aminophylline treatment in severe acute asthma. JAMA 1988; 259:1670–1684.

Rowe BH, Keller JL, Oxman AD. Effectiveness of steroid therapy in acute exacerbation of asthma: A meta-analysis. Am J Emerg Med 1992; 10: 301–310.

Zimmerman JL, Dellinger RP, Shah AN, Taylor RW. Endotracheal intubation and mechanical ventilation in severe asthma. Crit Care Med 1993; 21:1727–1730.

ATYPICAL PNEUMONIA

James R. Tillotson, M.D.

The term *atypical pneumonias* has been attached to a group of infectious pneumonias whose manifestations differ from those of classical bacterial pneumonias, including minimal or nonproductive cough, lack of consolidation on x-ray, confusing extrapulmonary signs, pulse-temperature discrepancy, failure to isolate the pathogen on routine cultures, and lack of response to beta-lactam and aminoglycoside antibiotics. While such similarities provide a basis for the classification, distinction from common bacterial pneumonias is often difficult. The four genera most commonly considered atypical are *Mycoplasma pneumoniae; Chlamydia* spp., especially *C. pneumoniae; Legionella* spp., especially *L. pneumophila;* and *Coxiella burnetii,* the cause of Q fever, which together account for 10 to 50 percent of all community-acquired pneumonias.

MYCOPLASMA PNEUMONIAE PNEUMONIA

Mycoplasma pneumonia, once called primary atypical pneumonia, occurs predominantly in school-aged children and young adults and often is endemic in closed environments such as college dormitories and military facilities. These outbreaks and those that occur in families develop slowly because of the long incubation period, 1 to 3 weeks. Younger children are generally asymptomatic or have upper respiratory symptoms only, and older adults are generally immune, although pneumonia may rarely occur even into the 70s.

The onset is generally insidious, with constitutional symptoms preceding a pharyngitis characteristically described as a scratchy rather than a sore throat. Transient tinnitus, otalgia, or decreased hearing is common, but the more or less pathognomonic hemorrhagic bullous myringitis is rare. Rhinorrhea is much less common than with respiratory viral infections. Malaise, myalgia, arthralgia, and anorexia are common but less severe than with many viral illnesses. Various rashes have been described but are uncommon and are rarely of any diagnostic help. The initially minimal fever gradually increases but rarely exceeds 101.3°F (38.5°C). The cough later becomes productive of light yellow sputum that on stained smear has predominantly polymorphonuclear leukocytes but no bacterial pathogens. Chilliness is commonly reported with the fever, but chills are rare. Coughing may precipitate frontal headaches and retrosternal chest pains. The cough is frequently paroxysmal and often nocturnal, and the difficulty getting a night's sleep often results in the visit to the physician.

The patient generally appears quite well except during the coughing paroxysms. Findings on examination may be limited to a low-grade fever, a mildly injected pharynx, and wheezes, rhonchi, and occasional rales, although absence of findings on examination of the lung despite an infiltrate on x-ray is common. The leukocyte counts and erythrocyte sedimentation rate (ESR) are normal or minimally elevated and other laboratory values are usually normal. X-ray manifestations are variable but most commonly reveal patchy interstitial infiltrates, which may change rapidly, or homogeneous segmental pneumonias. The latter lack the density of the consolidation seen with bacterial pneumonias, an appearance that has been described as a veil effect because structures such as the ribs can be easily visualized through the infiltrate. A quarter of patients will have pleural effusions, most of which are too small to be detected on routine radiographs.

Many of the extrapulmonary manifestations, including meningitis, meningoencephalitis, cerebellar ataxia, transverse myelitis, psychosis, mononeuritis, polyneuritis, myocarditis, pericarditis, pancreatitis, ulcerative stomatitis with conjunctivitis (Stevens-Johnson syndrome), and other rashes are probably due to immunologic mechanisms, as is the pneumonia.

Erythromycin or tetracycline clears the systemic symptoms over 36 to 48 hours and may hasten resolution of respiratory manifestations. Doxycycline and the newer macrolides clarithromycin and azithromycin may be equally effective. Without antibiotics the systemic illness resolves over 7 to 10 days. The cough, however, may persist for weeks or months with or without treatment, and clearance of infiltrates on chest x-ray may require 6 weeks.

CHLAMYDIA PNEUMONIA

Three species of *Chlamydia* are implicated in acute pneumonia. *Chlamydia psittaci* was identified as the cause of psittacosis, or parrot fever, in 1930. This acute pneumonia with abrupt onset, high fever with chills, relative bradycardia, and severe headache occurs 1 to 2 weeks after exposure to infected birds. Few cases are seen in the United States, but the incidence may be rising. Response to tetracycline 500 to 750 mg four times a day and, to a lesser extent, erythromycin, occurs within 48 to 72 hours.

More recently, *Chlamydia trachomatis* has been found to be a frequent cause of afebrile pneumonia in infants who develop cough, congestion, tachypnea, and a diffuse pulmonary infiltrate shortly after birth. This species has also been implicated in infections in immunosuppressed hosts ranging from acute bronchitis to a severe diffuse interstitial pneumonia. Erythromycin, tetracyclines, and sulfonamides are active. The reported antibodies to *C. trachomatis* in other children and adults with pneumonia are apparently due to cross-reacting antibodies with *C. pneumoniae.*

The TWAR strain of *Chlamydia* has now been classified as a separate species, *C. pneumoniae.* It is estimated to be the cause of 5 to 20 percent of pneumonias. The illness is usually benign, like *Mycoplasma* infections, but more severe illnesses are reported. Person-to-person spread causes human infection, and outbreaks have been documented in families and military recruits. The average incubation period of 30 days is even longer than that of *Mycoplasma.*

The clinical picture of *C. pneumoniae* pneumonia is similar to that of *Mycoplasma* pneumonia except that the sore throat is more prominent, up to 80 percent of patients are hoarse, and fever and leukocytosis are less frequent. Some patients develop a biphasic illness with fever and a moderate to severe sore throat followed 2 to 3 weeks later by bronchitis and pneumonia, often without fever.

Sinus tenderness and abnormal breath sounds are the most common findings on examination. The white blood cell count is usually normal, although the sedimentation rate is elevated. A single subsegmental infiltrate is the most common radiologic finding, although extensive bilateral disease occurs. Pleural effusions are uncommon. Extrapulmonary manifestations include sinusitis, less commonly otitis, possibly myocarditis and pericarditis, and rashes, especially erythema nodosum. The disease is generally mild and self-limited, although recovery may be slow, with persistent cough and malaise for weeks or months after other symptoms have resolved. Reinfection may be common. Occasionally severe pneumonias, especially in the elderly or with concurrent bacterial infection or chronic disease, may be fatal.

Tetracycline and erythromycin in *Mycoplasma* dosages appear to be the drugs of choice.

■ LEGIONNAIRE'S DISEASE

Legionella infections occur in persons of all ages but are more common in older persons, up to two-thirds of whom may have an underlying illness, especially chronic lung disease, diabetes mellitus, end-stage renal disease, hematologic malignancies, immunosuppressive therapy and possibly HIV infection. *Legionella* causes 3 to 5 percent of all community-acquired pneumonias, but because of its greater severity, it may account for up to 20 percent of hospitalized pneumonias. Person-to-person spread is rare if it occurs at all. The incubation period is probably 2 to 10 days.

The onset is frequently abrupt, especially in immunocompromised patients, with malaise, myalgias, headache, and rapidly rising fever often with chills or rigors or both. Upper respiratory symptoms are rare and suggest another diagnosis. Gastrointestinal symptoms, including diarrhea in up to 50 percent of cases, and abdominal pain occur early. The cough is initially nonproductive, and later small amounts of sputum are produced. On stained smear the sputum contains few inflammatory cells, predominantly mononuclear, and no bacteria. Chest pain, often pleuritic, and dyspnea occur in about half of the cases. While headache is the most common central nervous system finding, confusion is common, and hallucination and frank psychosis occur.

The patient usually appears quite ill, often with fever of 104°F (40°C) or more. Other abnormal findings are often limited to mental status changes, a few rales, and abdominal tenderness, especially in the right upper quadrant. The leukocyte count tends to be elevated, with an increase in immature cells. Particularly helpful in diagnosis is the frequently increased ESR, often above 100 mm per hour by the Westergren method; mildly elevated creatinine, transaminases, and bilirubin; hyponatremia; and hypophosphatemia. X-ray findings are often similar to those of *Mycoplasma,* but less likely to have early patchy interstitial infiltrates. Most are alveolar from the onset and may be segmental, lobar, or more diffuse. The veil effect is also commonly seen. Later, denser nodular infiltrates may develop. Large cavitary lesions may occur in severely immunosuppressed patients.

Milder cases often present much more like *Mycoplasma* infections, with a slower onset, less fever, fewer or less severe extrapulmonary manifestations, and often faster response to therapy. Extrapulmonary disease most commonly includes encephalitis, pericarditis with or without myocarditis, pleuritis with occasional empyemas, rhabdomyolysis, and acute renal failure that may require dialysis, but virtually any organ may be involved. The mechanism is unclear, but bacteremia does occur in the more severe cases, and seeding of peripheral sites is described.

Diagnosis can be suspected clinically in the typical case by the abrupt onset, mental changes, diarrhea, and abdominal pain along with the abnormal laboratory values in a patient with atypical pneumonia.

Treatment of choice is erythromycin. Rifampin 600 mg every 12 hours can be added for patients who have severe disease.

Response to treatment may be rapid, with defervescence and significant clinical improvement within 18 to 24 hours (faster than with *Mycoplasma*), but some patients respond slowly over 7 to 10 days. In contrast to those infected with *Mycoplasma* or *Chlamydia,* most, if not all, infected patients require treatment.

■ *COXIELLA BURNETII* PNEUMONIA

Q fever is an acute zoonosis caused by the rickettsia *Coxiella burnetii.* The organism is widely distributed in nature. Human infection occurs with inhalation of aerosols of infected animal substances, especially parturient fluids. Person-to-person transmission is rare. Both sporadic and endemic infections occur. The incubation period ranges from 2 to 6 weeks and averages about 3 weeks. While infection in livestock in the United States is very common, clinical disease in humans is not. The true incidence is unknown; it is undoubtedly underdiagnosed due to lack of suspicion and appropriate diagnostic studies. Pneumonia is the predominant manifestation of *Chlamydia* and *Legionella* infections and the more severe *Mycoplasma* infections, but only 10 to 20 percent of patients with Q fever have pulmonary infiltrates.

The onset is usually abrupt with a high, spiking fever, chills or rigors or both, myalgias, and a severe headache, often retrobulbar. The cough tends to be minimal and nonproductive and may be absent. Arthralgias and diarrhea occur. Hepatosplenomegaly is common. The blood leukocyte count is usually normal. Sputum smears are predominantly mononuclear. Chest x-rays usually show patchy interstitial infiltrates similar to those of *Mycoplasma,* but occasionally segmental and lobar consolidation occur. Extrapulmonary manifestations include hepatitis, often anicteric, and rarely pleuritis, pericarditis, cerebritis, meningitis, and arthritis.

The diagnosis should be suspected if the patient develops an atypical pneumonia with an abrupt onset and splenomegaly 2 to 6 weeks after an appropriate animal exposure.

Most infections will resolve spontaneously in 2 to 4 weeks, but therapy may shorten the duration of fever and possibly prevent the development of chronic Q fever, and therefore it is generally advised. Untreated, fever persists for 2 days to

2 weeks, but antibiotics reduce temperature within 48 hours. Treatment of choice is generally considered to be tetracycline.

These four causes of so-called atypical pneumonia typically present with two different syndromes. The insidious onset with upper respiratory manifestations and less severe systemic manifestations of *Mycoplasma* and *Chlamydia* infections differs significantly from the abrupt onset with high fevers and chills seen with many *Legionella* and *Coxiella* pneumonias. With careful analysis of the presenting features it is often possible to identify a particular case as a typical *Legionella, Mycoplasma,* or other pneumonia, but a great deal of overlap occurs not only within this group but with other causes of infectious (including typical bacterial) and noninfectious pneumonias.

Most *M. pneumoniae, C. pneumoniae,* and *C. burnetii* infections resolve spontaneously without treatment, although antibiotics may shorten the duration of fever and prevent more chronic symptoms. Only *Legionella* infections typically fail to resolve untreated and even with treatment may have significant mortality.

In the absence of a strong suspicion as to a diagnosis based on clinical presentation and sputum smears, empiric therapy of community-acquired pneumonia should include a drug known to be effective against atypical pneumonias as well as other common treatable lower respiratory infections. Thus, unless epidemiologic or possibly clinical evidence suggests Q fever, erythromycin should be considered preferable to tetracyclines.

It is not reasonable to attempt to diagnose every infection using the costly cultures and/or serologic tests required for these atypical pneumonias. Properly interpreted stained smears of sputum will often demonstrate a specific bacterial pathogen as the cause of a pneumonia or if not seen, suggest an atypical, viral, or noninfectious cause. Patients with atypical pneumonia who are well enough to be treated as outpatients will generally respond with or without treatment and should require no further diagnostic testing. At the time of hospital admission, specimens of blood and sputum should be cultured on routine bacteriologic media, but it is important to consider the smear's characteristics in interpreting the culture results, since many pulmonary pathogens are normal flora of the upper respiratory tract and will contaminate poorly collected sputum. Thus, the absence of pneumococci, *Haemophilus,* or other potential pathogens on culture may be more helpful in diagnosis than their presence. Patients who have severe pneumonias or are immunosuppressed should also be evaluated for *Legionella* with sputum and possibly blood cultures as well as antigen detection in urine and sputum. Serum should be submitted for diagnosis only several days later if no diagnosis is made and only if there is some compelling epidemiologic or other reason requiring a specific diagnosis. To spend hundreds of dollars to diagnose a benign pneumonia that responded quickly to erythromycin or tetracycline is not in keeping with cost-effective practices.

Suggested Reading

Edelstein PH. Legionnaires' disease. Clin Infect Dis 1993; 16:741–749.
Grayson JT. Infections caused by *Chlamydia pneumoniae,* strain TWAR. Clin Infect Dis 1992; 15:757.
Mufson MA, Manko MA, Kingston JR, et al. Eaton agent pneumonia: Clinical features. JAMA 1961; 178:369.
Sawyer LA, Fishbein DB, McDade JE, et al. Q fever: Current concepts. Rev Infect Dis 1987; 9:935.

ASPIRATION PNEUMONIA

Elizabeth A. Williams, M.D., Ph.D.
Steven L. Berk, M.D.

Our understanding of aspiration of material into the lungs has been expanding and deepening, improving our ability to identify both the acute and long-term consequences of such aspiration, to identify the individuals at risk for aspiration, and to develop strategies to prevent and treat pathologic aspiration. However, with the increasingly common introduction of fiscal, medicolegal, and patient choice considerations into medical practice, the identification and susceptibilities of the organisms involved in aspiration episodes becomes increasingly historical. The previous "gold standard", transtracheal aspiration, is rarely used now as it carries too high a risk-benefit ratio because of the disappearance of trained practitioners. Furthermore, other reliable methods—bronchoscopy with transbronchial aspiration, protected brush, bronchoalveolar lavage, or open-lung biopsy—are expensive and invasive, and they require too long a lead time during which antibiotic therapy must be withheld. Only if a pleural effusion is present can a diagnostic thoracentesis be done rapidly and inexpensively with a reasonable chance of obtaining identifiable organisms.

This conundrum—to withhold or to treat empirically—is exacerbated by the development of new antibiotics, primarily cephalosporins, in the past 2 decades, after the seminal work on the role of anaerobes in aspiration pneumonia was done, and by their questionable efficacy in treating aspiration pneumonia because of their ability to induce resistance. Thus it is impossible to tell whether the same organisms are causing aspiration pneumonia in the same proportions as 20 years ago. However, we can tell that today's organisms are more resistant, since formerly reliable treatment regimens, e.g., penicillin G and tetracycline, now result in treatment failures. It is unlikely that this picture will change, so the average clinician will have to rely on empiric therapy in most cases of aspiration pneumonia and depend on the few centers that specialize in anaerobic research to keep the medical community abreast of the appearance of new organisms and the change in resistance and virulence patterns of pathogens.

Besides those whose lifestyle predisposes to altered levels of consciousness, poor dentition, and vomiting, most of aspiration pneumonia's victims are at the extremes of age; this is due to advances in neonatology and aggressive prolongation of life in the elderly. The very young are susceptible beginning in utero, and their airways continue to fall victim to invasion by a wide spectrum of pathogens. Similarly, the elderly develop a variety of problems because the airway protective barriers are abrogated with increasing age. The young and the elderly are subject to a number of the same risk factors for aspiration (Table 1).

Four important concepts must be considered in addressing aspiration and the pneumonia that may result: (1) the volume and concentration of the aspirate; (2) whether the aspirate is intrinsically damaging to the lung tissues, e.g., gasoline, commercial tube feedings; (3) the status of the patient (Figs. 1 and 2); and (4) the frequency, site, and timing of the aspiration. As an example of the last factor, inpatients after 72 hours may be colonized by highly resistant hospital-acquired gram-negative rods and *Staphylococcus aureus,* although their initial oropharyngeal flora may remain to complicate the picture. Intubation virtually guarantees aspiration of oropharyngeal contents, and gastric pH pharmacologically elevated above 2.5 prevents acid burn to the lung if gastric contents are aspirated but allows the colonization of that aspirate by gut flora. As outlined in Table 2, gastric contents do not have to be highly acidic to be intrinsically damaging to the lung.

Table 1 Common Conditions Predisposing to Aspiration

GENERAL
Decreased consciousness or altered mental status
Dementia
Delirium
Infection
Medications
Cerebrovascular accident
Arrhythmias
Seizures
General anesthesia
Drug or alcohol overdose
Metabolic encephalopathy
Head trauma
Esophageal disorders
Diverticulum
Motility disorders
Spasm
Connective tissue disease
Malignancy
Achalasia
Stricture
Abdominal and pelvic disorders
Gastroesophageal reflux
Vomiting
Delayed gastric emptying
Gastric outlet obstruction
Diabetic gastroparesis
Intestinal obstruction
Truncal obesity
Abdominal and pelvic masses
Tumor
Pregnancy
Disruption of the airway mechanical barrier
Tracheostomy
Endotracheal intubation
Nasogastric and feeding tubes
Neurologic disease
Decreased cough reflex
Decreased gag reflex
Incompetence of glottal structures
Malignancy
Surgery for sleep apnea
Paralyzed vocal cords
PEDIATRIC
Meconium aspiration
Overfeeding
Genetic and congenital abnormalities
Chiari syndrome
Tracheobiliary fistula
Pyloric stenosis
ELDERLY
Tube feeding
Tetanus
Brain stem infarcts
Confined supine positioning

■ PRESENTATION

Aspiration, especially of large volumes of damaging fluid, an acute event that damages the lung within minutes, is accompanied by severe cyanosis, dyspnea, tachypnea, and tachycardia with bronchospasm. Hypotension and even hypercapnia can occur if sufficient fluid shifts into the lung and/or the vagal response is overwhelming enough. Within 2 hours infiltrates may be detected on chest film, after which the syndrome may resolve over the next 72 hours or progress to full-blown adult respiratory distress syndrome with or without bacterial pneumonia. If pneumonia develops, it may be anaerobic, originating from the oropharynx; nosocomial, with resistant organisms likely, since most of these patients are intubated; or both.

An aspiration that is not witnessed or recognized, whether outpatient or inpatient, often results in an infection with a more indolent course than the usual bacterial or viral disease. The patient presents with a general failure to thrive over 10 to 14 days and may have weight loss and night sweats in addition to a low-grade fever and moderately elevated white blood cell count. Lapses in consciousness, poor dentition, and a history or production of a foul-smelling sputum or foul-tasting sputum is highly suggestive and should be followed up aggressively by examination of such material both grossly and microscopically. A Gram stain revealing many inflammatory cells, multiple bacterial forms, and rare squamous cells in such a setting is virtually pathognomonic for an anaerobic lower respiratory tract infection. Culture of the sputum should still be done to rule out aerobic pathogens that might not be covered by empiric anaerobic therapy, e.g., methicillin-resistant *S. aureus, Pseudomonas aeruginosa,* highly resistant *Streptococcus pneumoniae.*

More recently recognized is the patient with gastroesophageal reflux disease (GERD) and chronic or progressive lung disease who has developed a positive feedback loop wherein

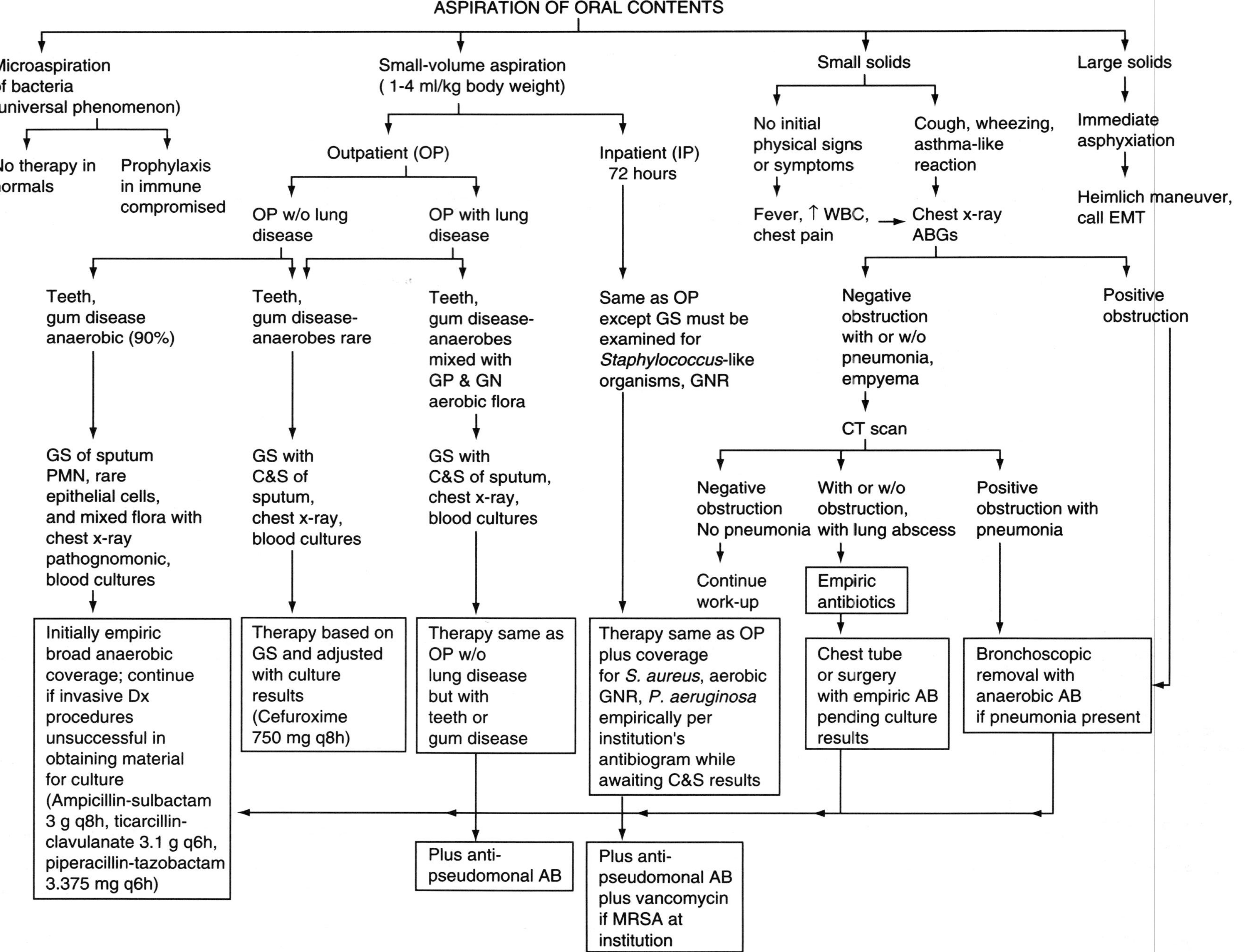

Figure 1
Algorithm for the management of aspiration of oral contents. AB, Antibiotics; ABG, arterial blood gases; C&S, culture and sensitivity; CT, computed tomography; Dx, diagnostic; EMT, emergency medical technician; GN, gram-negative; GNR, gram-negative rods; GP, gram-positive; GS, Gram stain; MRSA, methicillin-

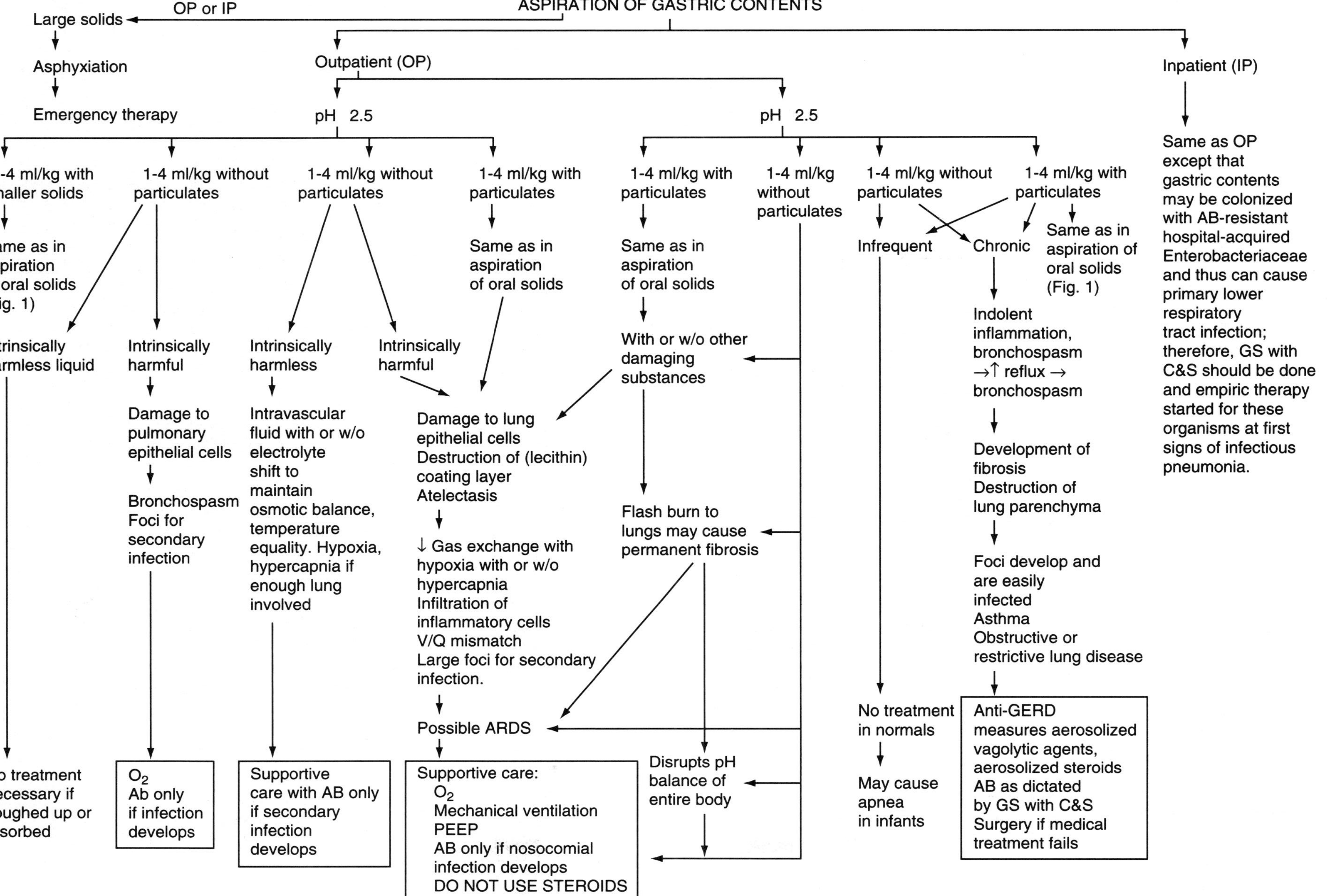

Figure 2
Algorithm for the management of aspiration of gastric contents. AB, Antibiotics; ARDS, adult respiratory distress syndrome; C&S, culture and sensitivity; GERD, gastroesophageal reflux disease; GS, Gram stain; PEEP, positive end-expiratory pressure; V/Q, ventilation-perfusion.

Table 2 Aspirates that Cause Pneumonitis and Predispose to Secondary Infection

Petroleum products, e.g., gasoline, kerosene
Edible fats, including milk, enteral feeding preparations, infant formula
Acids and alkalies, e.g., gastric secretions with pH below 2.5, lye, bleach, ammonia
Medications, e.g., sucralfate, activated charcoal

the aspiration of small amounts of acid into the lungs results in an asthmatic-like response. This in turn increases GERD until acid in the esophagus itself is enough to trigger bronchospasm. If the cycle is not interrupted, the lung can be permanently damaged, with sites that are prone to frequent infection with increased bronchospasm, and the esophagus is progressively inflamed, fibrosed, and epithelialized.

■ THERAPY

Algorithms for management of the consequences of aspiration of oral and gastric contents are given in Figures 1 and 2, respectively. Only four antimicrobial agents have been found to be entirely effective in vitro against anaerobic pleuropulmonary pathogens: amoxicillin-sulbactam, chloramphenicol, imipenem-cilastin, and ticarcillin-clavulanate. *Bacteroides fragilis* was not completely susceptible to ceftizoxime (67 percent), clindamycin (85 percent), penicillin G (8 percent), or piperacillin (77 percent). Penicillin G was also not effective against *Bacteroides* or *Prevotella* spp. (48 to 65 percent). *Clostridium* was susceptible to cefoxitin (83 percent). *Bacteroides ureolyticus* was susceptible to clindamycin (79 percent) and metronidazole (93 percent). Metronidazole was effective against only 80 and 95 percent of anaerobic gram-positive cocci and non-spore-forming gram-negative rods, respectively. Piperacillin was effective against only 89 percent of pigmented *Prevotella* spp. Piperacillin-tazobactam was not assessed, and it is possible that given its anti-beta-lactamase activity, this compound would have 100 percent activity against *B. fragilis* and *Prevotella*. However, the recommended dosing schedule of this latter drug, though adequate for *S. aureus*, is not effective against *P. aeruginosa*.

These patterns of resistance pose a dilemma for the empiric treatment of the truly beta-lactamase-allergic patient, limiting the regimen to clindamycin plus metronidazole and/or chloramphenicol. Desensitization should strongly be considered if *B. ureolyticus* is identified.

Treatment of the patient with chronic aspiration due to GERD requires a team approach, with an allergist, a gastroenterologist, an infectious diseases specialist, and a surgeon as necessary.

Near-Drowning Episodes

The paramount problem in near-drowning episodes is hypoxia secondary to either glottic lock or aspiration of large fluid volumes. If due to the latter, it is accompanied by profound intravascular and extravascular shifts in fluids and electrolytes that require intensive critical care management, which is not the subject of this discussion. Infection of the lower respiratory tract by water-borne organisms is extremely rare, and prophylactic antibiotic therapy is not recommended. The patient may develop a nosocomial aspiration pneumonia as a result of intubation and mechanical ventilation, but the organisms are those common to the intensive care unit where the patient is being treated (see the chapter *Nosocomial Pneumonia*).

Suggested Reading

Bartlett JG. Anaerobic bacterial infections of the lung and pleural space. Clin Infect Dis 1993; 16(Suppl 4):S248–S255.

Mansfield LE. Gastroesophageal reflux and respiratory disorders: A review. Ann Allergy 1989; 62:158–163.

Modell JH. Drowning and near-drowning. In: Isselbacher KJ, Braunwald E, Wilson JD, et al., eds. Harrison's principles of internal medicine. 13th ed. New York: McGraw-Hill, 1994.

HYPERSENSITIVITY PNEUMONITIS

Raymond G. Slavin, M.D.

Hypersensitivity pneumonitis is also referred to as pulmonary hypersensitivity syndrome or extrinsic allergic alveolitis. The latter term is perhaps the most appropriate because it is so descriptive. "Extrinsic" refers to an exogenous allergen as the cause of the problem. "Allergic" refers to the hypersensitivity basis for the disease. "Alveolitis" refers to the part of the lung that is most affected. Despite the different terms, they all refer to the same underlying pathogenetic entity, namely, a disease process that is caused by sensitivity to an organic dust that is inhaled. The clinical presentation of the disease depends on the circumstances and degree of exposure. In the more common acute form associated with intermittent intense exposure to the organic dust, the individual responds 4 to 6 hours after exposure with low-grade fever, chills, chest pain, cough, and dyspnea. In the chronic form associated with prolonged low-grade exposure, the clinical presentation is much more insidious, with progressively increasing cough, dyspnea, weakness, malaise, and weight loss.

The causative antigens responsible for hypersensitivity

pneumonitis can be divided into several categories. This list, with examples, includes thermophilic *Actinomycetes (Micropolyspora faeni),* fungi *(Aspergillus clavatus),* amoeba *(Naegleria gruberi),* animal products (bird droppings), and small molecular-weight chemicals (toluene diisocyanate). The majority of cases are associated with occupational exposure, such as farming, mushroom packing, or grain loading. However, offending antigens may contaminate home heating or humidification units or be associated with hobbies such as pigeon breeding.

The diagnosis of hypersensitivity pneumonitis should be suspected in any patient presenting with interstitial pneumonitis or pulmonary fibrosis. Pulmonary function testing reveals a largely restrictive dysfunction, including decreases in pulmonary compliance and in carbon monoxide diffusion capacity. A careful history eliciting the onset of symptoms following exposure with remission on avoidance, together with positive serum precipitins to the appropriate antigen, is presumptive evidence of hypersensitivity pneumonitis. In rare instances further confirmation may have to be made by inhalation challenge with the suspected antigen.

THERAPEUTIC APPROACH

Avoidance

Clearly the most important aspect in the management of hypersensitivity pneumonitis is recognition and avoidance of the causative antigen. The physician's diagnostic index of suspicion must be high, and in every case of interstitial pneumonitis or pulmonary fibrosis a careful environmental survey of the patient's occupational, home, and avocational life must be carried out, searching for the presence of offending antigens. Once the disease is diagnosed and the antigen recognized, early avoidance is the definitive therapy. Hypersensitivity pneumonitis ultimately may be a fatal disease because of progressive respiratory insufficiency. While it is not known how long or what level of exposure is required to produce irreversible pulmonary changes, it is estimated that five acute episodes will be followed by pulmonary damage and progressive disease. Therefore, it is vital to make the diagnosis early and institute proper environmental precautions to prevent the inexorable consequences of pulmonary fibrosis and irreparable tissue damage. Factors that favor a worse prognosis are repeated acute episodes, abnormalities on chest radiographs or pulmonary function tests that last more than 6 weeks, and clubbing.

Table 1 shows a general approach to the prevention of hypersensitivity pneumonitis. A number of interventions will decrease the formation of antigens in conducive environments. For example, the growth of thermophilic *Actinomycetes* spores in compost can be suppressed by treatment with a 1 percent solution of propionic acid. Water that remains for long periods of time in older air conditioning or humidification units may become a fertile source for the growth of thermophilic organisms. Therefore, the water needs to be changed and the unit cleaned on a regular basis. Contaminated ventilation systems have to be thoroughly cleaned or replaced. Blowing cool air through stored hay helps to prevent the growth of mold. Harvesting crops when the moisture content is low also results in less exposure to organic dusts.

Table 1 Prevention of Hypersensitivity Pneumonitis

Decrease formulation of antigens
Add chemicals such as 1% propionic acid to prevent growth
Change water frequently in humidification or air conditioning units and clean units regularly
Use storage dryers on hay and straw
Harvest crops when moisture content is low
Decrease exposure to organic dust
Mechanically handle dusty materials within closed spaces
Remove dusts from ambient air
Use personal respirators or masks
Remove worker from disease producing environment

Modified from Terho EO. Extrinsic allergic alveolitis—management of established cases. Eur J Respir Dis 1982; 123:101.

In occupational situations in which organic dust generation is inevitable, every effort should be made to reduce the workers' exposure. In enclosed spaces extremely dusty material should be handled mechanically. The use of particular types of silos may allow for automated feeding of cattle. Materials such as sugar cane should be stored outside and cattle fed outside as much as possible so that the associated organic dusts can be diluted by the ambient air.

In terms of removal of dusts from the air, improved ventilation may aid considerably. Electrostatic air purifiers may be of help when the concentration of dust is not too great. They would be overwhelmed in an area where moldy hay is being handled in which it is estimated that there are 1,600 million spores per cubic meter of air. A person doing light work with moldy hay inhales 10 liters of air per minute, which would deposit 750,000 spores per minute in the lung.

The use of personal dust respirators or masks is limited because of inconvenience. A type 2B filter is effective in filtering small particles but causes so much resistance to the flow of air that people hard at work are unable to wear them. An air stream helmet in which an electrical pump blows air through a filter and into the breathing zone is heavy and uncomfortable to wear. Even the best device has a maximal filtering capacity of 99 percent for fine particles. The remaining 1 percent can produce new attacks in a highly sensitive individual. If the disease is not yet manifest, even a filter with 95 percent filtering capacity is adequate. Good results have been reported with a 3M disposable mask model 8710 or reusable model 7200.

When the foregoing environmental control measures cannot be carried out or are inadequate, the patient should be removed from that work area. This may entail a change in the work place or type of work or, in extreme cases, a change in occupation. If the diffusing capacity has not returned to normal in 3 months, the individual should be advised to leave that particular workplace permanently. It should be stated that many bird breeders and farmers are unwilling or unable to avoid exposure. One should do as much as possible to educate the patient as to disease pathogenesis and the importance of avoidance.

Drug Therapy (Table 2)

In many cases no treatment is necessary other than avoidance of the causative antigen. Corticosteroid therapy, however, can greatly accelerate clinical improvement and should be considered in very ill patients with gross radiographic or physi-

Table 2 Treatment of Hypersensitivity Pneumonitis

Acute form
Remove patient from exposure; may entail hospitalization
Administer oxygen
Prednisone 40–60 mg/day with slow tapering over 10–12 days
Supportive measures—rest, antitussives, antipyretics
Repeated acute or subacute form
Decrease exposure as much as possible
Long-term corticosteroid therapy emphasizing alternate-day therapy
Chronic form
Trial with corticosteroids but continue only if radiographic findings and physiologic testing indicate a response

ologic abnormalities, such as hypoxemia. Oral therapy with prednisone in an initial daily dosage of 40 to 60 mg is usually adequate and should be continued until there is significant clinical, radiographic, and pulmonary function test evidence of improvement. The prednisone dosage then may be tapered slowly until resolution of clinical and radiologic signs is complete, generally in 10 to 12 days. The total duration of therapy should be no more than 4 to 6 weeks provided exposure to the antigen is prevented. Inhaled corticosteroids are of no value in the treatment of hypersensitivity pneumonitis, nor are bronchodilators or cromolyn unless bronchospasm is also present.

The dramatic response of hypersensitivity pneumonitis to corticosteroids may be a two-edged sword. The rapid relief afforded by steroids may result in a false sense of security, so much so that the patient may return to the same work environment. Re-exposure will result in progression of the lung disease. It therefore must be emphasized and re-emphasized to the patient that corticosteroids are not a substitute for antigen identification and avoidance.

In cases of severe hypoxemia in the acute stage, oxygen should be administered in amounts sufficient to keep the Po_2 level between 60 and 100 mm Hg. Other supportive measures include rest, antitussives, and antipyretics.

On occasion, despite the physician's best efforts, the patient may elect to return to the same work place or occupation. This seems to be especially true of farmers, who find it particularly difficult to leave farming because of age, a large financial investment, and a lack of training and skills in other occupations. In these instances long-term continuous corticosteroid therapy may have to be administered. One should strive for an alternate-day program utilizing the lowest dosage that still controls the patient's symptoms.

The chronic form of hypersensitivity pneumonitis develops insidiously and occurs either following repeated acute episodes or as a result of long-term, low-grade exposure. A therapeutic trial of steroids can be given but there are no controlled studies showing benefit. If there is clear evidence that the disease is progressive, corticosteroids can be administered but should be continued only if radiographic findings and physiologic testing indicate a beneficial response.

Appropriate treatment of the acute episode of hypersensitivity pneumonitis with avoidance of further antigen exposure results in an uneventful recovery with no progression to chronic untreatable disease.

Suggested Reading

Fink JN. Hypersensitivity pneumonitis. In: Middleton EJ Jr, Reed CE, Ellis EF, et al, eds. Allergy: Principles and practice. St Louis: Mosby, 1993.

Stankus RP, DeShazo RD. Hypersensitivity pneumonitis. In: Schwarz M, King TE Jr, eds. Interstitial lung disease. Toronto: BC Decker, 1988.

Terho EO. Extrinsic allergic alveolitis—management of stable cases. Eur J Respir Dis 1982; 123(Suppl):101.

LUNG ABSCESS

Lisa L. Dever, M.D.
Waldemar G. Johanson Jr., M.D., M.P.H.

Lung abscess is a chronic or subacute infection initiated by the aspiration of contaminated oropharyngeal secretions. The result is an indolent necrotizing infection in a segmental distribution limited by the pleura. Except for infections with unusual organisms such as *Actinomyces,* the process does not cross interlobar fissures, and pleural effusion is uncommon. The resultant cavity is usually solitary with a thick, fibrous reaction at its periphery. So defined, lung abscess is always associated with anaerobic bacteria, although aerobic bacteria may be present as well.

Diagnosis can usually be made from the clinical presentation and chest radiograph findings. Many patients have conditions that predispose them to aspiration of oropharyngeal secretions, such as seizure disorders, neuromuscular diseases, and alcoholism. Gingival disease and poor dental hygiene, which promote high concentrations of anaerobic organisms in the mouth, are common. Patients usually give a several-week history of fever and cough; putrid sputum occurs in fewer than 50 percent of patients. Many patients with chronic infection lose weight and have anemia, mimicking malignancy. Chest radiographs show consolidation in a segmental or lobar distribution with central cavitation. Air-fluid levels may be present. The lung segments most commonly involved are those that are dependent when the person is supine, i.e., posterior segment of the upper lobes and superior segment of the lower lobes. Aspiration and resulting lung abscess are uncommonly found in anterior

Table 1 Initial Antibiotic Therapy of Anaerobic Lung Abscess*

ANTIBIOTIC	DOSAGE	FREQUENCY
RECOMMENDED REGIMENS		
Penicillin G	2 million units IV	q4h
Clindamycin	600 mg IV	q6h
Penicillin G	2 million units IV	q4h
Metronidazole	500 mg IV or PO	q6h
ALTERNATIVE REGIMENS†		
Chloramphenicol	500 mg IV	q6h
Cefoxitin	2 g IV	q6h
Cefotetan	2 g IV	q12h
Piperacillin	3 g IV	q6h
Ticarcillin	3 g IV	q6h
Imipenem	500 mg IV	q6h
Ampicillin-sulbactam	3 g IV	q6h
Ticarcillin-clavulanate	3.1 g IV	q6h
Piperacillin-tazobactam	3.375 g IV	q6h

*All dosages are for adults with normal renal function.
†These regimens have not been validated by clinical trials.

lung segments due to the uphill angulation of the trachea when the subject lies prone.

Determining the cause of lung abscess is hampered by contamination of specimens by the normal anaerobic flora of the mouth. Although the Gram stain of sputum may suggest an agent, routine sputum cultures are of no value, since all contain anaerobic organisms. Techniques used to obtain uncontaminated lower-airway specimens for anaerobic cultures include transtracheal needle aspiration, transthoracic needle aspiration, and open lung biopsy. With these techniques early investigators demonstrated anaerobic bacteria in virtually all untreated patients. These invasive techniques are seldom warranted in the clinical management of patients today. More recently, investigators have used quantitative cultures of bronchoalveolar lavage or other bronchoscopically obtained lower-airway specimens, such as those obtained with a protected specimen brush, to recover anaerobic organisms. Although these methods may prove useful in the occasional patient suspected of having lung abscess, they are not needed in most.

Anaerobic organisms most commonly recovered from lung abscesses include *Bacteroides* spp., pigmented *Prevotella* spp. (formerly *Bacteroides melaninogenicus*), nonpigmented *Prevotella* spp., *Fusobacterium nucleatum*, and *Peptostreptococcus* spp. Several anaerobic organisms are frequently present along with aerobic or microaerophilic organisms. When anaerobic organisms are recovered, in vitro susceptibility testing is seldom warranted.

■ THERAPY

Most lung abscesses are treated empirically (Table 1). Traditionally penicillin is the antibiotic of choice. Penicillin has good in vitro activity against most anaerobic and microaerophilic bacteria in the oral cavity. Early studies showed excellent responses when either parenteral or oral penicillin was used as a single agent in the treatment of anaerobic lung infections. Two recent studies suggested that clindamycin is superior to penicillin. In both of these studies the time to resolution of symptoms and the failure rate were significantly lower in clindamycin-treated patients. Failure of penicillin therapy was associated with the isolation of penicillin-resistant *Bacteroides melaninogenicus* (now reclassified as *Prevotella* spp. and other species) in one of these studies. Other evidence suggests increasing penicillin resistance among oral gram-negative anaerobes, primarily due to production of beta-lactamases. For these reasons some experts now recommend that seriously ill patients take clindamycin, at least initially, for the treatment of lung abscess.

Table 2 Oral Antibiotic Therapy of Anaerobic Lung Abscess

ANTIBIOTIC	DOSAGE	FREQUENCY
Penicillin V	750 mg	q6h
Clindamycin	300 mg	q6h
Amoxicillin-clavulanate	500 mg	q8h
Penicillin V+	750 mg	q6h
Metronidazole	500 mg	q6h

The combination of metronidazole and penicillin has been used with success for the treatment of anaerobic pulmonary infections. Metronidazole has excellent bactericidal activity against gram-negative anaerobes but lacks activity against microaerophilic and aerobic streptococci, as well as *Actinomyces* spp., and therefore cannot be used as a single agent in the treatment of lung abscess.

A number of other agents have good in vitro activity against anaerobic organisms, including beta-lactamase produres, and may be useful in the treatment of lung abscess. These agents include cefoxitin, cefoletan, imipenem, anti-pseudomonal penicillins, and the beta-lactam and beta-lactamase inhibitor combination drugs ampicillin-sulbactam, amoxicillin-clavulanate, ticarcillin-clavulanate, and piperacillin-tazobactam. In addition, these drugs are attractive because of their activity against many of the aerobes that may be present in mixed infections. Chloramphenicol has excellent in vitro activity against almost all clinically significant anaerobes; however, hematologic toxicity limits its usefulness. While they are effective in vitro, it is unlikely that any of these agents will ever be studied in clinical trials due to difficulties inherent in conducting trials requiring isolation of anaerobic organisms from uncontaminated respiratory specimens. Drugs that have essentially no anaerobic activity and should not be used in the treatment of lung abscess include aminoglycosides, quinolones, and aztreonam.

Duration of Therapy

The duration of therapy for lung abscesses must be individualized, but extended therapy is usually required. Parenteral therapy is recommended initially and should be continued until the patient is afebrile and clinically improving. A prolonged course of oral antibiotics follows initial parenteral therapy (Table 2). Therapy should be continued until there is complete resolution or at least stabilization of chest radiograph lesions; this may require 8 or more weeks of therapy. Relapses have been reported when therapy was discontinued prior to resolution or stabilization of chest radiograph findings even when patients were clinically asymptomatic.

Other Therapy

As with all abscesses, the patient with lung abscess will not improve without drainage. Ideally, drainage is effected via the tracheobronchial tree. Postural drainage may be a useful adjunct. Bronchoscopy should be performed on patients who have unchanged or increasing air-fluid levels and who remain septic after 3 to 4 days of antibiotic therapy. Bronchoscopy rarely results in direct drainage of the abscess cavity; rather, drainage occurs over hours to days after suctioning of secretions and manipulation of the involved bronchopulmonary segments. A large abscess cavity (more than 6 to 8 cm diameter) requires special consideration. Some authorities prefer to drain such abscesses surgically because of the fear of an unplanned and uncontrolled sudden evacuation of the abscess contents into the bronchial tree with resultant asphyxiation. Another approach is to use a rigid bronchoscope to examine and open the involved airways because of the greater capacity for suctioning. A third approach, and the one we favor for most cases, is to perform fiberoptic bronchoscopy through an endotracheal tube with large-bore suction catheters at the ready. It must be remembered that the gross appearance of the bronchial orifice and the results of cytologic examinations may falsely suggest an underlying malignancy because of intense and long-lived inflammation. On the other hand, nearly 50 percent of lung abscesses in adults over 50 years of age are associated with carcinoma of the lung, either because of cavitation of the neoplasm or cavitation behind a proximal bronchial obstruction. Follow-up of these patients must be done with great care.

As a general rule, the pleura should not be violated unless absolutely necessary. A recent flurry of papers extolling the safety and efficacy of percutaneous catheter drainage in anecdotal series of lung abscesses has appeared in the radiology literature. The safety of this approach depends critically on the degree of synthesis of the two pleural surfaces; in the chronic stages of lung abscess this has usually been accomplished, so that passing a needle through the pleura into the lung does not result in pneumothorax. If the visceral pleura does not firmly adhere to the chest wall, a pyopneumothorax results, often with bronchopleural fistula—a true disaster. Using computed tomography to guide needle placement can minimize this complication, but it is far better avoided than treated, so our approach is to avoid the temptation to perform percutaneous drainage until attempts to achieve endobronchial drainage have clearly failed.

Suggested Reading

Bartlett JG. Anaerobic bacterial infections of the lung and pleural space. Clin Infect Dis 1993; 16(Suppl 4):S248–S255.

Bartlett JG. Antibiotics in lung abscess. Semin Respir Infect 1991; 6:103–111.

Brock RC. Lung abscess. Oxford: Blackwell Scientific, 1952.

Gudiol F, Manaresa F, Pallares R, et al. Clindamycin vs. penicillin for anaerobic lung infections: High rate of penicillin failures associated with penicillin-resistant *Bacteroides melaninogenicus.* Arch Intern Med 1990; 150:2525–2529.

PLEURAL EFFUSION AND EMPYEMA

Maurice A. Mufson, M.D.

Invasion of the pleural space by fluid (pleural effusion) and pus (empyema) as a complication of infection occurs in 40 to 50 percent of bacterial pneumonias, but much less often in mycoplasmal or viral pneumonias. It occurs with varying frequency in other infections such as pulmonary tuberculosis and fungal infections, in noninfectious conditions including carcinoma of the lung, cirrhosis, congestive heart failure, pancreatitis, and in collagen vascular diseases (Fig. 1). The initial step in the diagnosis and treatment of pleural effusion is to decide whether fluid invasion is a transudate associated with a noninfectious disease, an exudate complicating pneumonia (a parapneumonic effusion) or other infection, or an empyema (frankly purulent pleural fluid). Early recognition and therapeutic intervention are essential to achieve complete resolution of parapneumonic effusions and empyemas.

ETIOLOGY

Pleural effusions accompanying pneumonia develop most commonly in the course of bacterial pneumonias—mainly those due to *Staphylococcus aureus,* pneumococcus *(Streptococcus pneumoniae), Haemophilus influenzae,* hemolytic streptococci, anaerobic bacteria, and gram-negative bacteria—as well as in pulmonary tuberculosis. Pleural effusion, but not empyema, occurs occasionally in *Mycoplasma pneumoniae,* but rarely in viral pneumonias. The predominant bacterial pathogens of empyema are *S. aureus* and various gram-negative bacteria, such as *Klebsiella,* Enterobacteriaceae, *Pseudomonas,* and the anaerobic bacteria.

DIAGNOSIS

Physical examination and the upright chest radiograph can detect accumulations of fluid in the pleural space of at least 300 to 500 ml. The characteristic physical findings of pleural

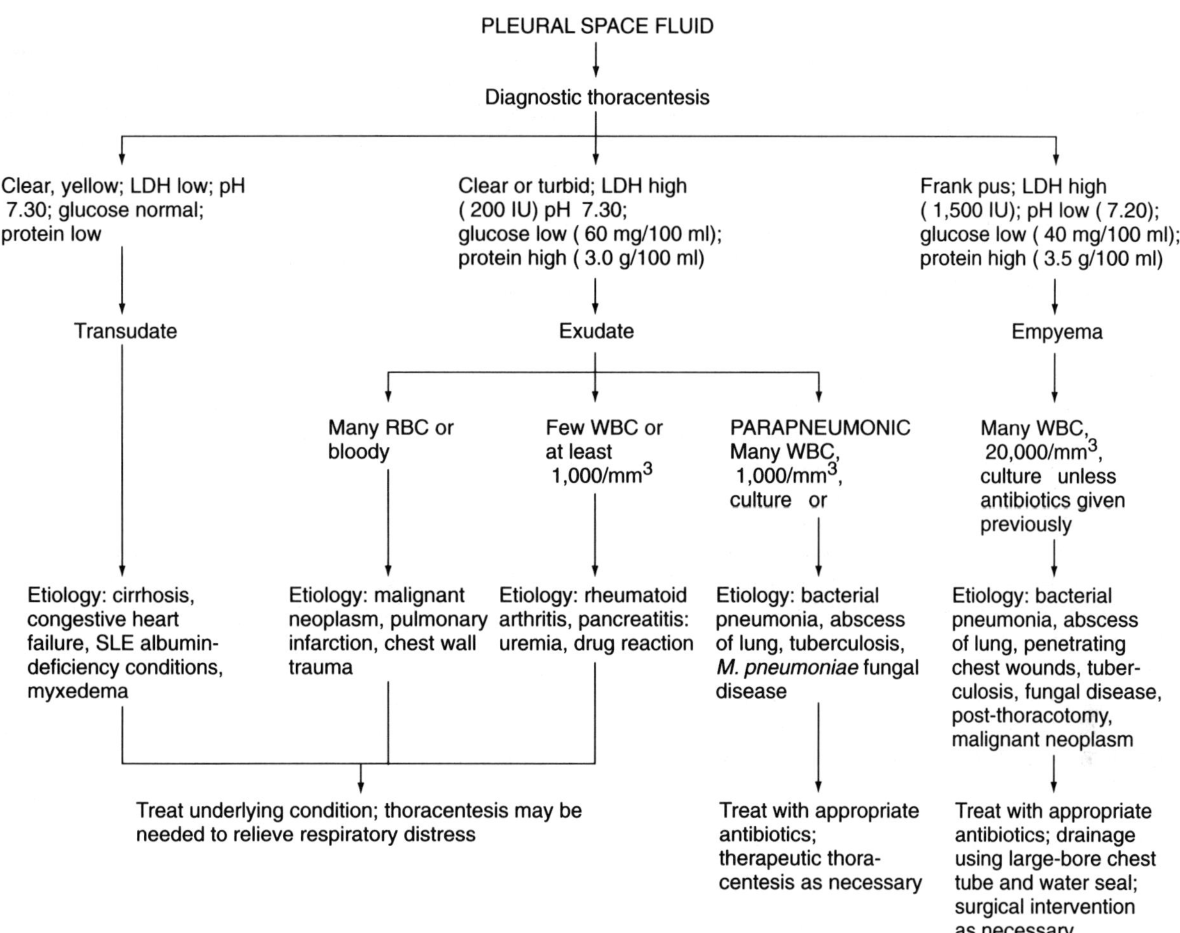

Figure 1
Evaluation, common etiologies,and management of pleural effusion and empyema. (LDH, Lactate dehydrogenase; RBC, red blood cells; WBC, white blood cells; SLE, systemic lupus erythematosus.)

effusion and empyema are decreased chest wall expansion; diminished, markedly decreased, or absent breath sounds and a flat percussion note; and, in the presence of large amounts of pleural fluid, a contralateral mediastinal shift. Fever, rapid respirations, shallow breathing, and involuntary or voluntary splinting of the affected side of the chest accompany parapneumonic effusions and empyema. Large effusions can be detected by physical examination alone. Small pleural effusions may be overlooked, however, without the aid of radiographic examination. If the patient is asymptomatic and an effusion is suspected to be small, further diagnostic tests would not be warranted to confirm its presence. However, if the patient has symptoms, e.g., fever, malaise, for which no other cause is apparent, a thorough diagnostic work up should follow. Small effusions may be recognized by comparing radiographs (lateral and anteroposterior films) of the chest that are taken upright with the lateral decubitus radiograph with the affected lung inferiorly. Small effusions should be suspected when the costophrenic angle is blunted or one hemidiaphragm is obscured. However, when an effusion or empyema is loculated, little, if any, change occurs in its configuration in the lateral decubitus position. Small or loculated effusions may need to be confirmed by diagnostic thoracentesis, by ultrasound, or by computed tomography.

A diagnostic thoracentesis should be done in all cases and 50 to 100 ml withdrawn. The tests usually done on pleural fluid include determination of lactate dehydrogenase (LDH), total protein, glucose, and pH; culture for bacteria and other micro-organisms as appropriate; Gram stain of smear, total white blood cell and differential counts; a total red blood cell count; and, when available, determination of adenosine deaminase (ADA). The selection of tests should appropriately reflect the list of diagnostic possibilities. Exudative pleural effusions contain high levels of LDH, usually greater than 200 IU (or a level more than 60 percent of the serum LDH level), total protein values of at least 50 percent of the serum protein (usually 3.0 g per 100 ml or greater in the effusion), glucose levels of less than 60 mg per 100 ml, pH less than 7.30, and a total white blood cell count of more than 1,000 to 2,000 per cubic centimeter. Polymorphonuclear leukocytes predominate in parapneumonic effusions of bacterial origin, and lymphocytes, in tuberculous effusions. The combination of an ADA value of more than 40 IU per liter and a polymorphonuclear leukocyte exudate strongly suggests a parapneumonic effusion. When pulmonary tuberculosis is suspected, a pleural biopsy should be done for identification of the organism by histologic examination and culture. Grossly bloody effusions, however, are unusual as part of infections and usually indicate malignant neoplasms, pulmonary infarction, or trauma to the chest.

■ TREATMENT

The basic approach to the treatment of parapneumonic pleural effusions and empyema involves therapy directed at both eradication of the infection and removal of accumulated fluid. The appropriate choice of antibiotic demands that the infecting organism be identified. In the treatment of parapneumonic effusions (except those caused by *M. pneumoniae*), antibiotics should be used intravenously and in adequate doses. The selection of antibiotics for the treatment of parapneumonic effusions and empyema follows these guidelines: for *S. pneumoniae* and hemolytic streptococci, use aqueous penicillin (2.4 to 6.0 million units daily in divided doses IV), or ampicillin (200 to 400 mg per kilogram per day IV), except for the penicillin-allergic patient infected with a strain of *S. pneumoniae* of intermediate resistance to penicillin, use a third-generation cephalosporin (cefotaxime 1 g every 8 hours IV or ceftriaxone 1 g daily IV) or for the penicillin-allergic patient infected with a strain of *S. pneumoniae* of high resistance to penicillin, use vancomycin (0.5 g every 6 hours IV); for *S. aureus,* use penicillin for appropriately sensitive strains, otherwise use nafcillin (2 g every 4 to 6 hours IV); for *H. influenzae,* use cefotaxime (1 g every 8 hours IV) or ceftriaxone (1 g daily IV); for anaerobic bacteria (except *Bacteroides fragilis*), use penicillin G or clindamycin (300 to 900 mg every 6 hours IV) and for *B. fragilis,* use metronidazole (500 mg every 6 to 8 hours IV); for gram-negative bacteria, tobramycin (3 to 5 mg per kilogram per day in divided doses IV) alone or in combination with piperacillin, especially for *Pseudomonas* species (4 g every 6 hours IV); and for *M. pneumoniae,* use erythromycin (1 g every 6 hours PO) or clarithromycin (500 mg every 12 hours PO).

Parapneumonic effusions usually clear without drainage procedures. However, a few of these patients may require one or more therapeutic thoracenteses. When the fluid has a pH of less than 7.00 and/or a glucose level below 40 mg per 100 ml, consideration should be given to immediate closed-tube thoracostomy. Complicated parapneumonic effusions and empyema require complete drainage using a large-bore thoracostomy tube. The tube is positioned in the most dependent portion and connected to underwater-seal drainage with continuous suction. As the volume of drainage diminishes to less than 50 ml daily or ceases, the chest tube is gradually withdrawn. Adhesions or a "lung peel" require surgical intervention. When the lung does not re-expand or when a "pleural peel" forms, thoracotomy and a decortication procedure must be performed. Such procedures are necessary in relatively few cases of empyema.

PNEUMOTHORAX

David N. Ostrow, M.D., B.Sc.(Med), M.A., F.R.C.P.C., F.C.C.P., F.A.C.P.
Bill Nelems, M.D., F.R.C.S.C.

Pneumothorax can be classified as spontaneous or traumatic. The vast majority of spontaneous pneumothoraces occur in healthy hosts, but a number of lung conditions can predispose to spontaneous pneumothorax. These include (1) eosinophilic granuloma; (2) emphysema; (3) necrotizing pneumonia, including tuberculosis; (4) usual interstitial pneumonia (in the honeycomb or end-stage phase); (5) asthma; (6) *Pneumocystis carinii* pneumonia; (7) catamenial pneumothorax; (8) cystic fibrosis; and (9) pneumothorax occurring in patients ventilated with positive airway pressure. Traumatic pneumothorax may be iatrogenic or related to chest wall trauma. Iatrogenic pneumothoraces are most commonly related to diagnostic aspiration needle biopsies and cardiopulmonary resuscitation. Thoracentesis and subclavian vein catheterization also cause this problem. Chest wall trauma may be due either to nonpenetrating blunt damage to the ribs, which in turn penetrate the lung, or to penetration of the chest wall by foreign objects.

■ SPONTANEOUS PNEUMOTHORAX

Pathogenesis

Spontaneous pneumothorax occurs most commonly in tall, thin, healthy males. Males are said to be four to eight times more susceptible to the condition than females. A number of cases of familial pneumothorax have been described. The pathogenic mechanism is likely related to rupture of subpleural blebs, which are thought to be congenital. Usually these subpleural blebs are on the surface of the lung, and their rupture causes air to dissect along the lobular septa and enter the pleural cavity. Although the onset of pneumothorax in most patients is unrelated to respiratory or physical activity, a significant number of patients describe a cough or sneeze as the initiating event. Persons with asthma, cystic fibrosis, or chronic bronchitis may have excessive mucus within the medium and small airways. This and excessive inflammation around these airways may lead to the development of check valves, which in turn may cause communicating blebs within the lungs to enlarge and subsequently to rupture. Catamenial pneumothorax occurs coincident with menses and may be related to ectopic endometrial tissue or to fenestrations in the diaphragm.

Mediastinal emphysema is presumably caused by the alveolar air tracking along the vascular bundle into the mediastinum. It may lead to pneumopericardium, pneumoperitoneum and subcutaneous emphysema without any clear-cut clinical evidence of pneumothorax.

Clinical Presentation

Nearly 90 percent of patients with spontaneous pneumothorax complain initially of sharp, pleuritic chest pain, the precise cause of which has never been adequately explained. Since the parietal pleura has the most exquisite pain sensation, it is tempting to attribute the pain to tension on adhesions between the parietal and visceral pleura. Since these adhesions are not usually present in well persons, one is tempted to draw the conclusion that many symptomatic pneumothoraces are preceded by small asymptomatic leaks that lead to the development of pleural adhesions. It is interesting that even patients who are treated conservatively, without a chest tube, notice that the pain tends to disappear or become dull within 48 to 72 hours. The reason for this is not clear. Dyspnea is present in approximately 80 percent of patients and is particularly noticeable during exercise. Cough is present in 50 percent of patients.

The physical findings are fairly classical and include tachypnea, tachycardia, shift of the trachea to the side without the pneumothorax, and decrease in tactile fremitus over the affected side. There is hyper-resonance and decreased air entry on auscultation. The cardiac apex may be shifted to the unaffected side. Occasionally, with the presence of mediastinal air, one can hear a crunch, which is synchronous with the cardiac cycle.

A tension pneumothorax is due to a check-valve phenomenon within the ruptured bleb, such that each inspiration allows more air into the pleura, and with each expiration the check-valve closes. The mediastinum is markedly shifted over to the unaffected side, and the lung is increasingly collapsed. In such patients the heart rate may exceed 150 beats per minute, and the characteristic feature on examination is a rapid fall in blood pressure. It is incorrect to believe that only a tension pneumothorax has positive intrapleural pressure within the pleural cavity. All pneumothoraces have positive pressure relative to the unaffected lung. With tension pneumothorax, the pressure is sufficient to impede venous return to the heart.

Study of arterial blood gases reveals an initial hypoxemia, because some time must elapse before there is hypoxic vasoconstriction in the collapsed lung and a leveling out of ventilation-perfusion ratios. The electrocardiogram may demonstrate a shift of the QRS axis, especially with left-sided pneumothoraces.

The diagnosis is usually fairly easily confirmed on a chest radiograph by the presence of a visceral pleural line. Occasionally, when there is some doubt, it is useful to obtain inspiratory and expiratory films. Since the air within the pneumothorax cavity does not easily communicate with the bronchi, the volume of the cavity does not decrease during expiration. This causes a relative increase in the size of the intrapleural air in an expiratory film. The diagnosis of pneumothorax can be particularly difficult in supine patients, especially those on ventilators. In supine patients approximately 500 cc of air is needed before the condition can be diagnosed and then usually when the air outlines the anterior pleural reflection or the costophrenic sulcus ("deep sulcus sign").

Estimating the size of the pneumothorax is an important step in clinical decision making. The geometry of the collapsing lung is complex, somewhat like a cylinder tethered on one side to the mediastinum. One useful way of estimating the volume of the pneumothorax is to determine the ratio of the distance from the medial aspect of the lung at the hilum to the edge of the collapsed lung (D_2) and from the hilum to the edge of the thoracic cavity (D_1). The expression

$$\frac{D_1^3 - D_2^3}{D_1^3} \times 100$$

is a fairly accurate assessment of pneumothorax size (expressed as a percentage). A more reproducible way of describing the size, although certainly not universally used, would be to describe the furthest distance from the visceral pleura to the chest wall. One centimeter of distance between pleurae corresponds to less than 20 percent pneumothorax.

Management

The approach to treatment of spontaneous pneumothorax depends on the size of the pneumothorax and on the presence of symptoms. Generally, it is estimated that a pneumothorax absorbs at the rate of approximately 1.25 percent per day (50 to 75 ml). This means that a 20 percent pneumothorax is likely to take about 2 weeks to resolve completely. The use of 100 percent inspired oxygen denitrogenates the blood and increases the gradient for nitrogen from the air within the pneumothorax to the gas within pleural tissues, which speeds recovery. However, this exposes the patient to high concentrations of oxygen and is not a practical means of therapy. It is generally accepted that pneumothoraces of less than 20 percent, especially in an asymptomatic patient, can be treated by observation. There is some evidence from Britain that larger pneumothoraces also may be treated in that fashion without any serious complications. The concern about observation as a mode of therapy is that it still leaves the patient at risk for the development of a tension pneumothorax as well as for the development of pneumonia in the atelectatic lung. Thus, many do not believe that observation is indicated if the pneumothorax is greater than 20 percent. Whatever the size of the pneumothorax, if it is secondary to an underlying pulmonary condition or associated with severe pain, an attempt should be made to drain the air.

Catheter Aspiration

Aspiration of the thoracic cavity with a small plastic catheter can be used to drain the pleural cavity. Air can be removed manually through a stopcock and syringe, or the catheter can be attached to a vacuum bottle. Polyethylene catheters attached to suction bottles tend to collapse from the negative pressure. Teflon catheters have been introduced, which have the advantage of rigid walls as well as the convenience of a narrow diameter. Aspiration of the pleural cavity is successful in 45 to 80 percent of cases. We have used it only in instances where the pneumothorax is related to trauma from the needle aspiration biopsy of a lung lesion.

Tube Thoracostomy

Tube thoracostomy is the most common technique employed to drain a large pneumothorax or a pneumothorax associated with persisting symptoms or underlying lung disease. Generally, the tube is placed in the sixth intercostal space in the midaxillary line rather than in the anterior chest wall. This placement allows the patient some mobility of the limbs without leaving a scar in a cosmetically obvious place. The technique of blunt dissection down to the pleura with the dissecting clamp, rather than inserting the plastic chest tube with a trocar, minimizes the chance of trauma to the lung, especially if there is evidence that part of the lung is tethered to the chest wall by adhesions. The chest tube is directed toward the apex of the lung. In a simple pneumothorax, a No. 20 French catheter can be used. If there is evidence of fluid or blood in the chest cavity, a No. 28 to No. 32 French catheter should be used to prevent obstruction.

The chest tube must be attached to a one-way valve to allow the egress of air from the pleura. The most commonly used valve is a tube connected to an underwater seal. Most units have the capability of providing negative suction to the pleural cavity, although for uncomplicated spontaneous pneumothoraces this may not be necessary. The patency of the tube can be monitored by watching fluctuations of the fluid level in the tube leading into the bottle. Although this system has been used for many years, it has the disadvantage of keeping the patient relatively immobile and requires hospitalization.

A one-way rubber valve within a plastic cylinder (Heimlich valve) has the advantage of being extremely light and easily portable. There are, however, two disadvantages of the Heimlich valve: (1) the collapsible rubber, which acts as a one-way valve, can become stuck if there is a significant amount of fluid or blood within the pleural cavity, and (2) it is difficult to monitor whether or not there is a continuing leak from the pneumothorax. This latter problem is overcome by attaching to the distal end of the valve a highly compliant "balloon" such as a urine drainage system. During a fixed period of time (perhaps over 4 hours), the balloon is observed by the nursing staff. If it inflates, a slow continuous leak from the lung is indicated. The method must be used only when the patient is being observed. If the balloon fills completely with air, it inactivates the one-way valve. This system is useful, especially because of the mobility it offers patients. The chest tube is usually left in place for 24 hours after the air leak has ceased. If there is evidence for air leak persisting more than 5 to 7 days, we consider that the tube thoracostomy has failed, and surgery is recommended.

The rate of recurrence of pneumothorax varies but is approximately 30 percent. A second pneumothorax has approximately an 80 percent chance of recurrence. Thus, it is recommended that a second recurrence of pneumothorax should be treated surgically. With the advent of videothoracoscopic surgery, some have argued that this should be the procedure of first choice even for first pneumothorax. We believe surgical intervention after first pneumothorax is only recommended for persons in critical occupations such as pilots and deep-sea divers.

Surgery

The surgical treatment is to oversew, staple, or laser the leaking bleb or adhesion. This can be performed through a videothoracoscopic procedure or, alternatively, via a limited third interspace transaxillary incision. To prevent further leaks from blebs that are not clearly apparent at the time of surgery, a pleuritis may be induced by vigorous abrasion of the parietal pleura with gauze to stimulate the formation of adhesions between the lung and the chest wall. Alternatively, an apical pleurectomy is performed, which separates the parietal pleura from the endothoracic fascia over the apex of the thorax. This procedure induces an even better fusion of lung to apical chest wall and further minimizes the possibility of recurrence.

Pleurodesis

Pleurodesis is associated with a decrease in recurrence of pneumothorax. Traditionally this has been performed with chemicals, but with the videothoracoscope it is possible to physically abrade just the apical pleura.

Pleurodesis with doxycycline is recommended by some, although this technique tends to be avoided until after the second pneumothorax. Generally 500 mg of doxycycline is instilled into the pleural cavity through the chest tube or thoracoscope. Talc is used as a sclerosing agent with pneumothorax associated with malignancy or malignant effusions. This is because of the concerns that even "asbestos-free" talc may not be entirely safe. We do not recommend the use of talc in spontaneous pneumothorax. If talc is used, 3 g of sterile, asbestos-free talc in a 60 cc saline slurry is instilled. This procedure initiates an extremely severe pleuritis and causes very severe pain. The pain is controlled with opiates and sedatives but is actually best controlled with aspirin or nonsteroidal anti-inflammatory agents. However, these agents are not recommended because they lessen the inflammatory process. The concomitant use of fentanyl, a short-acting anesthetic, has been recommended to avoid the severe pain. When performing a pleurodesis, pretreatment with atropine may prevent a vasovagal episode due to the pain.

■ TRAUMATIC PNEUMOTHORAX

Traumatic pneumothorax may be iatrogenic or related to chest wall trauma. Needle aspiration biopsy, which is now a popular method of obtaining tissue from peripheral pulmonary lesions, is the most common cause of this condition. Bronchoscopy and biopsies, both transbronchial and brush biopsies, can also be associated with pneumothorax. This is especially true in patients with diffuse inflammatory lung disease, such as *Pneumocystis carinii* pneumonia or other diffuse alveolar processes. Intermittent positive pressure ventilation, especially for patients with emphysema or end-stage honeycomb lung, is associated with a relatively high incidence of pneumothorax. If performed carefully, thoracentesis and pleural biopsy should not allow air to enter the pleural cavity. The insertion of subclavian vein catheters may be associated with both air and fluid within the chest. After cardiopulmonary resuscitation a significant number of rib fractures may occur, with subsequent pneumothorax.

Management

Videothoracoscopy

A tube thoracostomy or videothoracoscopic exploration is the treatment of choice for traumatic pneumothorax rather than observation, because of the greater danger that tension pneumothorax will occur. For pneumothorax caused by needle aspiration biopsy, a small noncollapsible catheter inserted in the second anterior intercostal space and attached to a vacuum bottle can be used initially.

Chest wall trauma may be associated with penetrating injuries to the chest or with blunt trauma to the ribs. Blunt trauma may cause fractured ribs to penetrate the pleural surface. In such traumatic pneumothoraces, the presence of coexistent fluid and blood requires the placement of a large-bore catheter (No. 28 to No. 32 French). An important complication of blunt trauma to the chest may be the rupture of a bronchus. This usually occurs within a few centimeters of the carina and is clinically manifested by a persisting air leak despite adequate placement of chest tubes. All trauma patients who have pneumothoraces that fail to expand should be explored with a fiberoptic bronchoscope to ascertain whether the mainstem bronchus has been damaged.

Suggested Reading

Boutin C, Astoul P, Rey F, Mathur PN. Thoracoscopy in the diagnosis and treatment of spontaneous pneumothorax. Clin Chest Med 1995; 16: 497–503.

Greene R, McLoud RC, Stark P. Pneumothorax. Semin Roentgenol 1977; 12:313–325.

Jenkinson SG. Pneumothorax. Clin Chest Med 1985; 6:153–161.

Pierson DJ. Complications associated with mechanical ventilation. Crit Care Clin 1990; 6:711–724.

Seremetis MG. The management of spontaneous pneumothorax. Chest 1970; 57:65–68.

Stradling P, Pool G. Conservative management of spontaneous pneumothorax. Thorax 1966; 21:145–149.

Verschoof AC, Ten Velde GP, Greve LV, Wouters EF. Thoracoscopic pleurodesis in the management of spontaneous pneumothorax. Respiration 1988; 53:197–200.

SARCOIDOSIS

Richard H. Winterbauer, M.D.

■ CLINICAL DECISIONS IN THE MANAGEMENT OF SARCOIDOSIS

Selection of the Patient Who Benefits from Therapy

The clinician's initial therapeutic decision regarding the patient with sarcoid is whether to treat or not. The decision process begins by recognizing subgroups with different patterns of disease progression. Approximately 75 percent of patients with sarcoidosis will have spontaneous remission or mild, stable disease not requiring steroid therapy. Indications for treatment in 10 percent will be involvement of a critical extrapulmonary organ such as the eye, brain, or heart, while only 15 percent will require treatment for progressive pulmonary disease. Recognition of the latter subgroup is important, for clinicians can then avoid giving corticosteroids to a patient who ultimately would have spontaneous resolution, and they can provide early therapy for those patients destined to have progressive pulmonary disease.

Radiographic patterns, sequential pulmonary function testing, and clinical patterns of disease have all been used to predict the outcome of sarcoidosis. Although loose correlations exist, none of these techniques has been reliable enough to become clinical dogma. For example, patients with stage 1 radiographic disease (bilateral hilar lymphadenopathy, normal lung fields) have an 80 percent frequency of spontaneous remission within 2 years of onset; patients with stage 2 (bilateral hilar lymphadenopathy with lung parenchymal disease) disease have a 65 percent chance of spontaneous remission; and those with stage 3 (lung parenchymal disease and no hilar lymphadenopathy) have a 30 percent chance. Erythema nodosum and acute arthritis indicate an excellent prognosis with an approximate 85 percent frequency of spontaneous remission. At the opposite extreme, patients with hepatomegaly, central nervous system involvement, upper airway disease, lupus pernio, bone lesions, nephrocalcinosis, or cor pulmonale all have less than a 25 percent chance of remission within 2 years, either with or without therapy. Severely symptomatic patients are more likely to have persistent disease. Persistence of symptoms for more than 2 years markedly reduces the chance of spontaneous remission. Racial factors are important since black patients are more likely to develop chronic, progressive disease. While admittedly imperfect, these clinical criteria are still the best data base on which to base treatment decisions. Laboratory tests such as serum angiotensin converting enzyme (SACE), bronchoalveolar lavage (BAL) cell populations, and gallium-67 (Ga^{67}) scans do not add significantly to treatment decisions.

Since clinical patterns, radiographic appearance, and serologic measures are imperfect in predicting the natural course of sarcoidosis, decisions regarding whom to treat remain murky. Suggested guidelines for initiation of treatment in pulmonary sarcoidosis are listed in Table 1. The suggestions are based on personal experience and patient symptoms and are offered as a general guide in patient management. Until therapy becomes available that results in cure, symptom control is a reasonable goal. Treating chest radiograph or pulmonary function abnormalities alone in the absence of symptoms is discouraged.

A caveat: a small group of patients with sarcoidosis have severe chest pain. The mechanism of the discomfort is unclear and it does not correlate with either the radiographic stage or the degree of abnormality. In my experience, the patient's pain responds better to analgesics than steroids, and chest pain is not an indication for initiation of or an increase in steroids.

Table 1 Guidelines for Initiation of Treatment in Patients with Pulmonary Sarcoidosis

1. Asymptomatic patients with pulmonary sarcoidosis should not receive corticosteroids
2. Patients with significant respiratory symptoms, abnormal pulmonary function tests, and a diffuse abnormality on chest radiograph should receive treatment
3. Patients with minimal symptoms might best be managed by serial evaluations at 2 to 3 month intervals and treatment reserved until there is evidence of disease progression
4. Patients with disease of more than 2 years' duration with deterioration in pulmonary function (FVC decrease ≥10%, DL_{CO} decrease ≥20%, increase in D[A-a] O_2 ≥5 mm Hg) over time are candidates for steroid therapy

TREATMENT

Effect of Corticosteroids

Corticosteroids are the first-line treatment in sarcoidosis. The majority of patients with sarcoidosis receiving corticosteroids show a beneficial response, usually within the first 2 weeks of treatment. Clinical experience, however, has proven that the response represents suppression, not cure. There is no indication that corticosteroid therapy increases the frequency of permanent remission of disease.

The optimal dose of corticosteroids for sarcoidosis has never been accurately defined. Generally, 30 to 40 mg of prednisone daily is adequate to start. Higher doses are rarely required. Symptomatic improvement is usually rapid, with maximum improvement frequently present at 2 weeks. Patients with acute disease (<6 months' duration) show the greatest evidence of therapeutic benefit. Improvement in vital capacity is noted more frequently than changes in the diffusing capacity. Alternate-day therapy can be very effective in maintaining improvement and may decrease side effects.

Complications of corticosteroid therapy include excessive weight gain, diabetes mellitus, aseptic necrosis, peptic ulcer, and cataracts. Tuberculosis has not been observed in more recent series as the disease has become less prevalent. Nevertheless, patients with sarcoidosis and a positive PPD who are treated with corticosteroids should receive 300 mg of isoniazid for 6 months for prophylaxis. Anergic controls are an unnecessary adjunct to tuberculin skin testing in patients with sarcoidosis.

Dose Adjustment and Duration of Therapy

In sarcoidosis, recognition of the time when the treated patient goes into remission that does not require maintenance therapy would allow therapy to be stopped. Unfortunately, there are neither clinical nor laboratory signs that identify this moment. The clinician must pick an arbitrary duration of treatment, stop the medication, and then monitor the patient's symptoms, chest radiograph, and pulmonary function tests for signs of relapse. Over 90 percent of patients treated for symptomatic pulmonary sarcoidosis show improvement in all three parameters during corticosteroid therapy, but only one-third remain improved after a year of treatment. The duration of therapy is tailored to the disease presentation and natural history of the illness. Some patients presenting with arthritis and/or erythema nodosum require steroids to control their joint or skin disease. Typically, both arthritis and erythema nodosum resolve spontaneously within 3 months, and thus steroids to control these syndromes should be stopped at 3 months. Patients with symptomatic pulmonary sarcoidosis of 2 years or longer duration have only a 20 to 25 percent chance of spontaneous remission within a year, and steroids are continued through 1 year and then stopped to see if remission has occurred.

Some clinicians worry that patients with sarcoidosis who have demonstrated a beneficial response to steroids with symptomatic, radiographic, and/or physiologic improvement may have dampened but not extinguished pulmonary inflammation. In this scenario, an unrecognized smoldering inflammatory reaction is viewed as a threat that may either spread to neighboring alveolar units and/or stimulate irreversible pulmonary fibrosis. This leads to the supposition that a measure of persistent inflammation would allow selection of a steroid dose capable of optimal disease suppression and prevent disease extension and fibrosis. It is here that BAL, Ga^{67} scanning, and SACE studies have created much heat but little light. In patients with sarcoidosis, for example, clinical improvement may occur with steroids, with SACE levels and gallium index reduced but not normal, and with BAL evidence of persistent lymphocytosis. The clinical relevance of persistent abnormalities of SACE level, gallium scan, and BAL findings in treated patients is unknown, and there is no basis for regarding persistent abnormalities of these tests as dictates of therapy at this time. SACE levels, gallium scan, and BAL have not been shown to be superior to symptoms, chest radiograph, and pulmonary function tests in following the patient with sarcoidosis.

When the Patient Fails

Lack of improvement with corticosteroid therapy should first raise the possibility of incorrect diagnosis. Multiple diseases mimic sarcoidosis, many of which are accompanied by granuloma and yet are refractory to corticosteroid treatment. Examples include histiocytosis X, Wegener's granulomatosis, fungal infection, mycobacterial infection, and neoplasm with paraneoplastic granuloma. When the patient does not improve, the diagnostic evaluation must be reviewed and the possibility of an incorrect diagnosis strongly entertained. Therapeutic failure with 30 to 40 mg of prednisone for 2 weeks is by no means incompatible with sarcoid. Patients with long-standing disease, cystic degeneration or honeycombing on chest radiograph, or striking endobronchial involvement all have a blunted response to steroids.

A second explanation for a patient's failure to show symptomatic improvement is steroid side effects negating the improvement from granuloma suppression. This patient typically shows improvement in symptoms, chest radiograph, and pulmonary function tests early but has a later recurrence of dyspnea with decreased exercise tolerance despite the improved chest radiograph. In such patients, some combination of steroid-induced weight gain, myopathy, sleep deprivation, and/or depression offset the symptomatic improvement obtained from granuloma suppression. If reduction in steroid dose does not improve the patient's symptoms, alternative therapy for steroid-sparing effect should be considered. The use of alternative therapy will almost always be dictated by the necessity to control steroid side effects. In only rare

Table 2 Alternative Therapies to Corticosteroids in the Treatment of Sarcoidosis

Nonsteroidal anti-inflammatory drugs	Cyclosporine
Chloroquine	Azathioprine
Methotrexate	Cyclophosphamide
Inhaled budesonide	Ketoconazole
Chlorambucil	

circumstances will alternative therapy offer an enhanced therapeutic effect over that of corticosteroids.

Alternative Therapies

There are only four alternative treatments for sarcoidosis that are considered adequately substantiated to incorporate into current clinical practice. These are nonsteroidal anti-inflammatory drugs for the treatment of acute arthritis and/or erythema nodosum; chloroquine, which has been especially effective in the treatment of skin disease; oral methotrexate for multisystem sarcoidosis; and inhaled budesonide for pulmonary sarcoidosis. Budesonide is not yet available in the United States, but its use in Europe and Canada has been substantial. Table 2 lists a number of other alternative therapies that are supported by anecdotal information. Kirtland and Winterbauer offer a recent in-depth discussion of alternative therapy for sarcoidosis (see Suggested Reading).

Nonsteroidal Anti-Inflammatory Drugs

Nonsteroidal anti-inflammatory drugs (NSAIDs) (indomethacin, ibuprofen, salicylates) may ameliorate the acute inflammatory symptoms of sarcoidosis presenting with arthritis and/or erythema nodosum. Anti-inflammatory agents are effective in approximately one-third of cases of acute sarcoid arthritis. Therapy should begin with a brief trial of a single agent such as indomethacin, 25 to 50 mg three times a day. If prompt symptomatic relief does not occur within 7 days, a course of systemic corticosteroids should be given. Trying a variety of NSAIDs for patients with arthritis and/or erythema nodosum who do not get adequate symptomatic improvement from a single agent is discouraged.

Chloroquine

There are 26 investigations in the medical literature in English on the efficacy of chloroquine, hydroxychloroquine, and quinacrine in the treatment of sarcoidosis. Most studies have involved patients with cutaneous sarcoidosis or combined cutaneous and pulmonary lesions and many of these studies involve patients who have previously failed a trial of corticosteroids. All but one of the studies has shown at least temporary improvement in cutaneous lesions. Pulmonary lesions have tended to show less consistent improvement. Relapse after cessation of drug treatment is typical in chloroquine treatment as with corticosteroids, confirming that chloroquine also suppresses but does not cure. Chloroquine's effectiveness in the treatment of hypercalcemia has also been demonstrated.

Chloroquine therapy has not enjoyed wide popularity, partly because of the concern over retinal toxicity. However, in comparison with corticosteroids, the side effect profile of chloroquine may be preferable. Complications of chloroquine therapy occur relatively infrequently, and most are transient and reversible with discontinuation of therapy. In patients with rheumatoid arthritis, chloroquine side effects occur in 3 percent to 7 percent of patients, with the most common complaints being nausea and diarrhea.

The most common ocular changes associated with chloroquine therapy are corneal deposition and retinopathy. Corneal deposits occur in about 95 percent of patients receiving long-term therapy of 250 mg per day of chloroquine, but over 90 percent of these patients are asymptomatic. Corneal deposition has no direct relationship to the development of retinopathy and is entirely reversible, disappearing within 6 to 8 weeks after discontinuation of therapy. The incidence of retinopathy in patients receiving chloroquine therapy is estimated to be 0.5 to 2 percent. The size of the daily dose rather than total drug exposure correlates with the development of eye disease. Daily dose must be calculated based on ideal body weight, not the actual weight of the patient. In reports in which chloroquine-induced retinopathy has occurred in patients receiving 250 mg per day or less of chloroquine, dosages usually have exceeded 4 mg per kilogram per day. Late onset chloroquine-induced retinopathy is believed by many to be less of a threat than previously suspected. However, it remains very important to have regular ocular examinations and frequent screenings to detect and prevent retinal toxicity. Ophthalmologic examination should be performed before therapy is initiated in all patients and repeated approximately every 6 months during therapy.

Chloroquine is especially effective in treating lupus pernio and cutaneous plaques, or nodules. An initial 14 day course of 500 mg per day of chloroquine phosphate followed by the smaller of either 250 mg per day or 4 mg per kilogram per day of ideal body weight as maintenance therapy is recommended. Before initiating chloroquine therapy, baseline liver function tests are recommended to assure adequate liver function necessary for normal metabolism and excretion of chloroquine. Acute toxic hepatitis can occur in patients with porphyria cutanea tarda who receive high doses of chloroquine.

Methotrexate

The most promising alternative to corticosteroids in the treatment of pulmonary sarcoidosis is low-dose methotrexate. Although its exact mechanism of action is unclear, it is unlikely that the beneficial effects of low-dose methotrexate are related to its immunosuppressive effects, which are relatively mild. Objective improvement defined as improvement on chest roentgenogram, greater than 15 percent improvement in vital capacity, greater than 50 percent reduction in skin lesions, or improvement in liver function tests has been demonstrated in several studies using methotrexate for multisystem sarcoidosis.

It appears that the risk-benefit ratio of methotrexate is quite low in comparison to prednisone. Liver disease, including cirrhosis, can be seen with methotrexate but the incidence is low and dose related. Concern has been voiced over the potential for malignancy associated with long-term use of methotrexate; however, several studies have shown no increased risk in patients followed for more than 7 years after completion of methotrexate treatment. Unfortunately, the drug has the potential to induce an allergic pneumonitis, which may complicate its use in sarcoidosis. This reaction is characterized by dyspnea, nonproductive cough, fever, and hypoxemia in association with diffuse pulmonary infiltrates. Hilar adenopathy and pleural effusions may be seen. Most patients recover with discontinuation of the drug.

Inhaled Corticosteroids

Inhaled corticosteroids became available in 1978 for the treatment of patients with bronchial asthma. Early attempts to use inhaled beclomethasone dipropionate for the treatment of pulmonary sarcoidosis were unsuccessful. However, budesonide, available since 1982 for asthma, is part of a newer generation of more potent inhaled corticosteroids. This agent has revived the enthusiasm for aerosol corticosteroid treatment in sarcoidosis. Animal studies have shown that local installation of inhaled steroids into the bronchial tree have resulted in higher tissue concentrations than systemic administration. Concentrations of budesonide are great enough to cause receptor binding and exert local anti-inflammatory effect. Budesonide is rapidly inactivated in the liver after systemic absorption, systemic bioavailability is low, and high doses can be used by inhalation with a low risk of systemic side effects.

A number of clinical trials have demonstrated improvement in the chest roentgenograms of patients with pulmonary sarcoidosis given budesonide 800 to 1,600 μg daily for 3 to 6 months. Improvement in pulmonary function, however, has been difficult to establish. Additional studies have indicated that patients initially treated with oral glucocorticosteroids who have relapsed after stopping treatment could be successfully treated with inhaled budesonide alone at a dose of 1,200 to 1,600 μg daily. Inhaled corticosteroids have also been shown to have a systemic steroid-sparing effect in patients with symptomatic pulmonary sarcoidosis treated with prednisone. The rate of improvement with aerosol therapy is slow compared to that seen with systemic steroids; frequently it takes 2 months or longer for improvement with the inhaled product. An initial combination of systemic and inhaled corticosteroids for rapid initial improvement and continuation on maintenance therapy with inhaled corticosteroids alone may prove to be best.

Patient Education

Optimal management of the sarcoid patient includes an earnest effort by the physician to educate the patient of the details of his or her illness and its management. Although written material and support groups are helpful, nothing replaces the efforts of a concerned physician speaking directly to the patient and his family. Patients should be told of their prognosis, the reasoning behind the decision to treat or not to treat, anticipated benefit of therapy, complications of therapy, and danger signals to watch for. The untreated patient must watch for cough and/or increasing dyspnea. All patients should be alerted to symptoms of ocular involvement and urged to contact their physicians immediately if they occur. Similarly, patients should be counseled about the potential ill effects from use of vitamin D and calcium supplements. The educational goals for patients receiving corticosteroids are listed in Table 3.

Table 3 Educational Goals for the Patient with Sarcoidosis Who Is to Start Corticosteroids

1. Patients must be warned of an increase in appetite and possible weight gain. Attention to caloric restriction should begin on the first day of therapy
2. Patients should be warned of the potential for water retention and instructed in dietary salt reduction
3. Patients should be urged to exercise as much as they feel comfortable with to help reduce the potential for myopathy and osteoporosis
4. Other side effects such as mood changes, including euphoria, sleep deprivation, epigastric distress, and elevation of blood sugar with polyuria and polydypsia, should be explained

Suggested Reading

Johns CJ, Zachary JB, Ball WC Jr. A 10-year study of corticosteroid treatment of pulmonary sarcoidosis. Johns Hopkins Med J 1974; 134:271–283.

Kirtland SH, Winterbauer RH. Selected aspects of sarcoidosis. In: Tierney D, ed. Current Pulmonology. Vol. 15. Chicago: Mosby, 1994:399.

Lower EE, Baughman RP. The use of low-dose methotrexate in refractory sarcoidosis. Am J Med Sci 1990; 299:153–157.

Neville E, Walker AN, James DG. Prognostic factors predicting the outcome of sarcoidosis. An analysis of 818 patient. Q J Med 1983; 52:525–533.

Winterbauer RH, Hammar SP. Sarcoidosis and idiopathic pulmonary fibrosis: A review of recent events. In: Simmons DH, ed. Current Pulmonology. Vol. 7. Chicago: Yearbook Medical Publishers, 1986:117.

Zic JA, Horowitz DH, Arzubiaga C, et al. Treatment of cutaneous sarcoidosis with chloroquine: Review of the literature. Arch Dermatol 1991; 127:1034–1041.

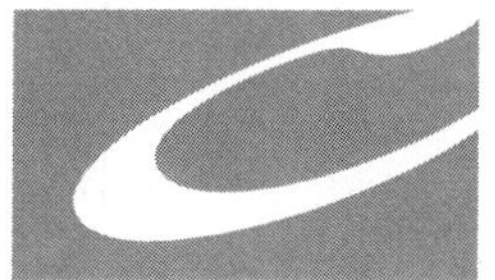

HEMATOLOGIC DISORDERS

APPROACH TO THE DIAGNOSIS AND MANAGEMENT OF ANEMIA

Bernard A. Cooper, M.D.

Anemia is a condition of inadequate hemoglobin, all of which is carried within erythrocytes. The pallor of anemia and that associated with chronic disease have been noted for centuries. Anemia may be the primary illness, as in pernicious anemia or congenital spherocytosis, or it may be a symptom of a generalized illness, such as infection, cancer, or hemorrhage. The most common cause of anemia worldwide is probably deficiency of iron.

The cause of anemia is sometimes evident, as during hemorrhage. It often is obscure.

Anemia can be diagnosed only if normal limits are defined. There are two general definitions of *normal:* (1) values within 2 standard deviations of a normalized general populations, or 95 percent of all subjects in that population, and (2) values not increased by provision of additional nutrients and factors that maintain hemoglobin concentration.

Using both definitions, Table 1 provides general guidelines for normal values for hemoglobin concentration in grams per liter of blood for several populations.

When hemoglobin concentration is less than normal, anemia is diagnosed. Anemia occurring in free-living, otherwise healthy subjects is more readily and successfully investigated and treated than is anemia in ill or hospitalized patients. Rarely, apparent anemia is caused by hemodilution due to an expanded plasma volume, as in women with hydramnios or twin pregnancies. Dilutional pseudoanemia is not physiologically true anemia because the increased blood volume induces increased cardiac output, which corrects tissue oxygenation.

Table 1 Approximate Lower Limit of Desired Hemoglobin

GROUP	HGB (GM/L)
Normal men	130
Normal women	120
>age 70	120
Children	
1 mo–2 y	110
2–11 y	115
Pregnant women	
1st trimester	120
2nd trimester	110
3rd trimester	100

RECOGNITION OF ANEMIA

Anemia may be suspected because of pallor and confirmed by blood examination. Anemia may induce cardiac failure because of reflex increased cardiac output, and so it should be suspected in elderly patients who develop dyspnea, edema, or angina pectoris.

DETERMINATION OF THE CAUSE OF ANEMIA

Otherwise Normal Subjects

The common causes of anemia in otherwise normal subjects include those listed in Table 2. When the cause of anemia is not obvious, a series of branch points can guide the investigation. All of these will, of course, be modified by the general history and associated clinical and laboratory findings. The branch points are mean corpuscular volume (MCV) very low or very high, reticulocyte count high or low, and bone marrow morphology.

If MCV is neither very high nor very low, reticulocyte count should be examined. If this is neither high nor low, bone marrow morphology is required.

Mean Corpuscular Volume

If MCV is less than 70 fl, iron deficiency or thalassemia is usually the cause. Less common causes include certain hemoglobinopathies (hemoglobin E disease, hemoglobin Lepore) and deficiency of copper.

If MCV is greater than 106 fl, the cause is almost always megaloblastic anemia, myelodysplasia, treatment with antimetabolic medications (e.g., hydroxyurea, mercaptopurine), or sometimes cold agglutinins, which give a falsely high MCV.

The investigation of patients in whom anemia is the only

obvious abnormality and in whom MCV is less than 70 or more than 106 fl is summarized in Tables 3 and 4. As indicated previously, other less common diagnoses may be present.

Reticulocytes

If MCV is neither below 70 nor above 106 fl, the reticulocytes should be counted. The total reticulocyte count per microliter is a better indication of erythropoiesis than is percentage, and counts using flow cytometry are more reproducible than those determined manually. The total reticulocyte count is obtained by multiplying the percentage of reticulocytes by the erythrocyte count.

If the reticulocyte count is greater than normal (120,000 cells per microliter of blood), the rate of erythropoiesis is increased. If associated with a rising hemoglobin concentration, it represents recovery from previous anemia. If not, it indicates compensation for shortened erythrocyte survival due to either hemolysis or continued hemorrhage (Table 5).

The causes of anemia with shortened survival of erythrocytes may be hemorrhage, when it will cause depletion of iron, or premature erythrocyte destruction because of antibodies, intrinsic defects of the erythrocyte membrane or metabolism, hemoglobinopathy, or failure of the erythrocyte to withstand the destructive effects of oxygen or drugs. Among whites the most common inherited cause of hemolytic anemia is congenital spherocytosis. Obvious spherocytes are not always present in the peripheral blood smear.

If the reticulocyte count is less than normal (50,000 per microliter), erythropoiesis is less than normal except in iron deficiency, in which reticulocytes may mature more than normal before being released into the circulation (see Table 5).

Hypoplasia of erythrocytes may be caused by erythropoietin lack, as in chronic renal failure; unresponsiveness to erythropoietin, as in chronic illness, inflammation, and in some aged persons; inadequate erythroid precursors, as in myelophthisic anemia, leukemia, and aplastic anemia; or destruction of maturing erythroid precursors, as in pure red cell aplasia, megaloblastic anemia, and some autoimmune hemolytic states.

Table 2 Common Causes of Anemia

DIMINISHED PRODUCTION OF MATURE ERYTHROCYTES

Deficiencies
- Iron
- Erythropoietin
- Cobalamin
- Folate
- Others

Replacement of Bone Marrow with Other Cells
- Myelodysplasia
- Multiple myeloma
- Cancer
- Lymphoma
- Other

Humoral or Cellular Inhibition of Normal Cells
- Antibodies
- Cytokines
- Toxic chemicals
- Undefined toxic effects

ACCELERATED LOSS OF MATURE ERYTHROCYTES FROM THE CIRCULATION
- Inherited erythrocyte defects
- Acquired erythrocyte defects
- Chemical destruction of erythrocytes
- Antibody-mediated destruction of erythrocytes
- Hemorrhage

Table 3 Investigation of Anemia with MCV Less Than 70 Fl

TEST	RESULT	INTERPRETATION
Serum ferritin	<10	Iron deficiency
Smear	Pencil RBCs	β-thalassemia or iron deficiency
FEP	Elevated	Iron deficiency
FEP	Normal	β-thalassemia
TF saturation	Low	Iron deficiency
	Normal	β-thalassemia
Bone marrow iron	0–tr	Iron deficiency
	Normal	β-thalassemia minor

FEP, free erythrocyte protoporphyrin; TF saturation, transferrin saturation (serum iron/total iron binding capacity; RBCs, red blood cells.

Bone Marrow Examination

If the reticulocyte count is between 50,000 and 120,000 per microliter and MCV is between 69 and 106 fl, aspiration, biopsy, and examination of the morphology of the bone marrow is required. The finding of megaloblastic erythropoiesis, infiltration with leukemia, multiple myeloma, cancer, or the morphology of myelodysplasia will lead to appropriate investigation. If classical morphology is not helpful, consider the tests listed in Table 6.

When all tests have been run, it is sometimes necessary to try a therapeutic trial. This is often done for iron deficiency, since in patients with mild deficiency of iron, anemia will not be microcytic. In such patients hemoglobin should increase about 2 grams per liter per week, so that a 4 to 6 week trial should be sufficient to evaluate response.

Table 4 Investigation of Anemia with MCV Greater Than 106 Fl

TEST	RESULT	PROBABLE INTERPRETATION
Serum cobalamin	<100 pg/ml	Cobalamin deficiency
RBC folate	<200 ng/ml	Folate deficiency
Blood smear	Bilobed and Hypogranular neutrophils	Myelodysplasia
Bone marrow	Megaloblastoid late, erythroid cells	Myelodysplasia*
	Megaloblastic with giant bands	Deficiency of cobalamin or folate

*If neutrophils and platelets are normal, it is defined as refractory anemia.

Patients with Other Illnesses or in Hospital

Secondary Anemia

It has been known for centuries that patients who are ill are pale, and more recently they have been shown to be anemic. The mechanism of this secondary anemia is not completely clear, but there is considerable evidence that cytokines such as the tumor necrosis factor (TNF) family, interleukin-1, and the interferons inhibit hematopoiesis. These may also cause depletion of transferrin, relative unavailability of iron stores, and reduced sensitivity to erythropoietin. Activated macrophages release ferritin into the plasma, increasing the concentration of ferritin in plasma and making this test a less reliable evaluation of iron stores than in the normal subject.

Secondary anemia usually is mild (hemoglobin greater than 80 grams per liter, often greater than 90), slightly microcytic (MCV greater than 70 fl), and unresponsive to treatment except possibly with large doses of erythropoietin. Reticulocyte count is within normal limits despite the anemia. Serum iron is normal or low, but transferrin is less than normal, and transferrin saturation with iron is usually normal but rarely is low. The concentration of transferrin receptor in plasma is normal or low. Serum ferritin is normal or high.

In hospitalized patients this mild anemia often is aggravated by acute and chronic posthemorrhagic anemia caused by the multiple venepunctures characteristic of hospital care. This is recognized by the features described, together with mild reticulocytosis (80,000 to 100,000 per microliter), which remains less than expected for the degree of anemia. This may lead to superimposition of iron deficiency on the secondary anemia. This iron deficiency is associated with decreased transferrin saturation, and serum ferritin is usually, but not always, less than 50 ng per milliliter. Bone marrow iron stores are depleted.

In patients whose illness may induce secondary anemia, bone marrow examination is usually required to define the cause of the anemia. This will reveal infiltration by neoplastic cells, aplasia, megaloblastic anemia, erythroid hyperplasia, or depletion of iron stores. In the absence of these the anemia must be presumed to be secondary to the general illness.

■ MANAGEMENT OF ANEMIA

General

When anemia causes life-threatening compromise of the circulation with consequent pulmonary edema, angina pectoris, or cerebrovascular insufficiency, correction by transfusion is required. Oxygen-carrying blood substitutes (cross-linked hemoglobin, perfluorocarbons) have not been proven effective, so transfusion of banked human blood is the only practical therapy. Such a patient should receive transfusion of 1 to 2 units of packed erythrocytes with intravenous injection of 10 to 20 mg of furosemide before and between units to prevent volume overload of the circulation. The administra-

Table 6 Investigation of Anemia with MCV 70 to 106 Fl and Reticulocyte Count Normal

TEST	RESULT	PROBABLE DIAGNOSIS
Aspirate (Bone marrow)	Erythroid hyperplasia*	Iron deficiency AIHA†
	Normal	PK deficiency‡ Uremia Secondary anemia
	Fluorescent	Protoporphyrinemia§
Iron stain (Bone marrow)	Iron absent	Iron deficiency
	Ring sideroblasts	MDS‖
Transferrin receptor	Normal/low	Secondary anemia¶

*Normal reticulocyte count and myeloid-erythroid ratio of 1:1 or less.
†With antibodies reacting against recticulocytes.
‡Pyruvate kinase deficiency. In the severe form reticulocytes accumulate in the spleen; in the milder form, elevated 2,3 DPG in erythocytes shifts the oxygen dissociation curve so that the anemia is not hemolytic.
§In congenital protoporphyrinemia young erythroid cells fluoresce due to accumulated protoporphyrinogen IX.
‖Also seen in some patients with megaloblastic anemia.
¶Usually with mild microcytosis.

Table 5 Causes of Shortened RBC Survival in the Circulation

TEST	RESULT	PROBABLE DIAGNOSIS
Splenomegaly	Present	Hemolytic anemia
Morphology	Spherocytes	Congenital spherocytosis or AIHA‡
	Ovalocytes	Ovalocytosis
	Fixed sickles	Sickle cell anemia
	Spur cells	Hepatic disease with hemolysis
	Normal	Consider congenital nonspherocytic hemolysis
DCT*	Positive	AIHA
DCT	Complement only	Cold agglutinin disease
Osmotic fragility	Abnormal	Spherocytosis§
Sugar water test†	Positive	Paroxysmal nocturnal hemoglobinuria or AIHA

*Direct antiglobulin (Coombs') test. Usually when both direct and indirect tests are positive, immune-mediated destruction of erythrocytes is occurring. In the majority of cases with positive direct and negative indirect DCT, immune-mediated destruction is absent.
†Dilution of washed erythrocytes in 5% sucrose, intubation and centrifugation.The hemoglobin content in the supernatant is compared with that of washed erythrocytes added to the same volume of water.
‡Autoimmune hemolytic anemia. This is a misnomer, since in most cases erythrocyte destruction is macrophage mediated.
§Hereditary spherocytosis, AIHA, and other uncommon causes such as *Cl. perfringens* bacteremia.

tion of oxygen may be useful to correct angina pectoris and does not retard recovery from the anemia.

In patients with chronic anemia that cannot be corrected by specific treatment, periodic transfusions may be required. These should be used to prevent cardiac failure and angina pectoris and to provide enough exercise tolerance to permit a reasonable lifestyle.

Some patients with anemia secondary to general illnesses respond to erythropoietin: patients with myeloma in whom the serum erythropoietin level is low may respond to renal doses of erythropoietin (viz 5000 units 2 times per week), whereas patients with myelodysplasia and serum erythropoietin levels less than 200 mU per milliliter, may require as much as 20,000 U daily (much more than the usual dose of 150 U per kilogram 3 times per week). In some of these, a small dose of G-CSF, sufficient to double the neutrophil count, may increase the proportion of responders.

Deficiency-Induced Anemia

Correction of the deficiency (iron, folate, cobalamin) will correct the anemia.

Iron

The cause of the iron deficiency must be determined to prevent masking of bleeding tumors in the large bowel, stomach, and urinary tract. Indiscriminate treatment with iron without assurance that blood loss can be explained is to be condemned. In adolescent children, iron deficiency may be due to a diet of insufficient iron for the increased erythron forming during rapid growth. Diet alone is never the cause of iron deficiency in adults, since only about 0.6 mg need be absorbed per day to cover nonmenstrual and nonhemorrhagic losses.

Treatment requires administration of iron in excess of daily losses. An average of 30 percent of heme iron, as in meat, is absorbed into the body, whereas only 10 percent of inorganic iron supplements or vegetable iron is absorbed. Normal women may lose 10 to 20 mg of iron per month to menstruation, so to cover normal losses, normal women must absorb 1.2 to 1.5 mg of iron a day, for which they must ingest 12 to 15 mg of inorganic iron.

In iron deficiency anemia 1 mg of iron absorbed (10 mg fed) will form about 1 ml of new normochromic erythrocytes, or 0.28 g of hemoglobin. Feeding 300 mg a day of ferrous sulfate (60 mg of iron) will generate 6 ml of the 1,400 ml of erythrocytes that normally circulate in a 50 kilo woman. It will generate 1.6 g of the about 500 g of hemoglobin normally circulating in such a patient. Correction of anemia from 70 g per liter to normal is expected to require about 150 days (10 g per liter every 3 weeks). Two tablets of iron would correct the anemia in half this period, three in a third, four in a quarter of the time, and so on. The dose of iron taken is therefore determined by the patient's tolerance to the supplement. Iron absorption is enhanced by ascorbic acid and by taking tablets remote from food, but gastric and small-bowel intolerances are increased by the latter.

I recommend treatment with 1 tablet of ferrous sulfate after dinner daily and if tolerated, increasing this to one after lunch and one after breakfast. Patients who are intolerant of iron tablets sometimes can tolerate liquid iron (e.g., Fer-in-Sol) in a glass of orange juice. A few patients who cannot tolerate oral iron supplements can gradually correct deficiency by taking a high-meat diet, including liver two or three times per week.

Iron injections are a problem. There have been deaths following intravenous infusion of iron dextran (total dose), although some physicians use this, with adrenaline and hydrocortisone available during the infusion. Some of the toxicity may be from free iron although this is unclear. *Imferon* was the iron-dextran complex available for many years and was used for intramuscular and intravenous therapy. Intramuscular injections of 100–250 mg of iron bound to dextran were given into the buttock with a long needle using a 'Z' track to reduce leakage to the skin. Tattooing from the melanocyte-stimulating properties of iron was common, and allergic reactions including arthralgias, some arthritis, adenopathy and fever were frequently seen. The occurrence of these usually precluded future use of this treatment.

There are only two injectable iron preparations available in the United States. The first is an iron dextran called *INFed* (Schein Pharmaceuticals), which contains 50 mg of iron per milliliter and is available in 2 ml (100 mg) vials. The company recommends intravenous doses of not more than 2 ml per day at no more than 50 mg per minute after a test dose. They also recommend no more than 2 ml (100 mg) per day by intramuscular injection following a successful test dose with 0.5 ml. The other is *Dexferrum* (American Regent Laboratories), an iron-dextran complex, packaged in vials of the same size as INFed and recommended for intravenous use by the manufacturer at 100 mg per dose.

In summary, injections of iron, once a common therapy, have become unusual because some form of tolerable oral supplementation can usually be found for patients who are not actively bleeding.

Cobalamin

In patients with intact absorption, 1 to 2 μg of cobalamin eaten daily will suffice to prevent anemia or macrocytosis and probably will prevent methylmalonic acidemia or homocysteinemia although this has not been tested. In patients who develop cobalamin deficiency due to achlorhydria, or other defects of absorption, oral cobalamin at a dose of 400 μg per day or more seems to maintain the serum cobalamin level well within the normal range. Cobalamin is inexpensive and so the oral tablet can be 400 to 1,000 μg per day. A sublingual cobalamin (1,000 μg) is available and although absorption from sublingual sites has been demonstrated in experiments, no data are available to evaluate its efficacy. It is recommended that when patients deficient in cobalamin are treated with oral preparations, serum cobalamin should be measured every 3 to 6 months to verify that the effect is as desired and that the medication is being reliably taken.

Folate

Oral supplements of 1 mg every second day or a diet containing 200 μg daily will prevent or correct megaloblastic anemia caused by deficiency of folate in subjects with normal guts. Those with sprue probably require 5 mg daily, and for these, cobalamin injections to maintain serum cobalamin greater than 300 pg per milliliter (230 pM) are recommended. (See the chapter *Megaloblastic Anemia* for more detailed discussion of this topic.)

Short RBC Survival

Autoimmune Hemolytic Anemia

Adrenal corticosteroids, 1 mg per kilo and then less, are standard therapy for autoimmune hemolytic anemia. Delayed responses also occur in patients receiving danazol and immunosuppressive therapy. Acute, usually transient control of erythrocyte destruction generally follows intravenous infusion of large doses of gamma globulin. Splenectomy cures some of these patients.

Congenital Spherocytosis

Splenectomy, the treatment of choice, may be delayed if anemia is absent and anemic crises associated with infection are not frequent.

Congenital Nonspherocytic Hemolytic Anemia

These usually do not respond dramatically to splenectomy, but hemoglobin level may be maintained at a higher but anemic level after this procedure.

Others

Treatment is that of the underlying illness, with care taken to apply the general principles listed previously.

Suggested Reading

Aul C, Gatterman N, Heyll A, et al. Primary myelodysplastic syndromes: Analysis of prognostic factors in 235 patients and proposals for an improved scoring system. Leukemia 1992; 6:52–59.

Brittenham GM. Disorders of iron metabolism: Iron deficiency and overload. In: Hoffmman R, Benz EJ Jr, Shattil SJ, et al., eds. Hematology: basic principles and practice. New York: Churchill Livingstone, 1991:327.

Chanarin I, England JM, Hoffbrand AW. Significance of large red blood cells. Br J Haematol 1978; 25:351–358.

Engelfriet CP, Overbeeke MAM, von dem Borne AEG. Autoimmune hemolytic anemia. Semin Hematol 1992; 29(1):3–12.

Kario K, Matsuo T, Nakao K. Serum erythropoietin levels in the elderly. Gerontology 1991; 37(6):345–348.

Miller CB, Jones RJ, Piantadosi S, et al. Decreased erythropoietin response in patients with anemia of cancer. N Engl J Med 1990; 322:1689–1692.

APLASTIC ANEMIA

Neal S. Young, M.D.

The infrequency of aplastic anemia (incidence = 2 to 6 per 10^6 in a large European epidemiologic study) does not allow most physicians to have comfortable familiarity with its treatment. Aplastic anemia is often fatal, but most patients with severe bone marrow failure can be cured. All forms of definitive therapy require adequate supportive care; these too are the subject of this chapter.

Before deciding on a therapeutic strategy, the diagnosis must be exactly established, and an estimate made of the patient's prognosis.

■ DIFFERENTIAL DIAGNOSIS

Despite the clarity of the clinical presentation in aplastic anemia—pancytopenia with an "empty" bone marrow—many patients with low blood counts are misdiagnosed because of inadequate tissue sampling, mistaken pathologic interpretation, or ignorance of pathophysiologic mechanisms. Careful examination of the aspirate smear and judgment of cellularity from a 1 cm core biopsy are minimal diagnostic requirements. Idiopathic aplastic anemia should be especially distinguished from (1) Fanconi's anemia or congenital aplastic anemia (by cytogenetic analysis of peripheral blood mononuclear cells cultured in the presence of mitomycin C or diepoxybutane); (2) paroxysmal nocturnal hemoglobinuria, which may develop from or into aplastic anemia (by Ham test or flow cytometric analysis); (3) aleukemic acute leukemia and lymphoma restricted to the bone marrow (by attention to blast cells that can be nestled close to spicules in an otherwise hypocellular specimen); (4) myelofibrosis (by remembering that failure to aspirate marrow, or a dry tap, is unusual in aplasia); and (5) dysmyelopoietic syndromes, which may be hypocellular and are often associated with chromosomal abnormalities restricted to marrow cells.

■ PROGNOSIS

Blood counts at presentation are the major determinants of survival, whereas age, sex, toxic exposures, and other historical features have had no important prognostic role in patient populations analyzed retrospectively. Patients with aplastic anemia are generally categorized as having severe disease if at clinical presentation they fulfill two of three blood count criteria: polymorphonuclear cell number less than 500 per millimeter cubed; platelets less than 20,000 per millimeter cubed; reticulocytes less than 1 percent (corrected) or less than 60,000 per millimeter cubed (absolute). Very low neutrophil counts (less than 200 per millimeter cubed) have a particularly dire significance. Severity implies a poor prognosis, with mortality untreated at 1 year of 80 to 90 percent; patients with moderate disease have a better outlook, although many ultimately die of the complications of pancytopenia or transfusional hemosiderosis. Blood count criteria

Table 1 Initial Evaluation

Complete blood counts, with differential, reticulocytes × 2
Bone marrow aspiration and 1 cm biopsy
If <30 y/o, cytogenetics of peripheral blood leukocytes
Ham test
Liver enzymes
Serology for hepatitis viruses, Epstein-Barr virus, human immunodeficiency virus-1
HLA typing

are not infallible. Some patients with low numbers of granulocytes or platelets survive for years. Conversely, a patient's blood count may fall precipitously after presentation, refractoriness to platelet transfusions may permit fatal hemorrhage, or a trivial untreated infection may become established. Patients with severe aplastic anemia require immediate definitive therapy, usually either bone marrow transplantation or horse antithymocyte globulin therapy.

INITIAL EVALUATION

A rapid initial clinical and laboratory evaluation is part of the appropriate care of the aplastic anemia patient. Severely pancytopenic patients can deteriorate quickly due to sepsis or bleeding, and curative therapy is then postponed in order to treat cascading complications. These complications and their treatments further diminish the probability of success of the definitive treatment. For example, avoidance of transfusions enhances the survival of the patient undergoing bone marrow transplantation (BMT). For either replacement therapy in the form of transplantation or immunologic therapy with horse antiserum to human lymphocytes, the patient in good general medical condition has the best opportunity of immediate survival and ultimate recovery. Table 1 summarizes the crucial laboratory studies that should be completed within the first several days of presentation.

THERAPY (FIG. 1)

Bone Marrow Transplantation

Transplantation in the form of bone marrow infusion restores normal blood counts and decreases the acute mortality. The procedure itself carries a significant expense and risk of death and acute and delayed morbidity. Patients with histocompatible (matched for class I and II human leukocyte antigens [HLA]) family members, almost always siblings, should always be considered for BMT. While patients have been successfully transplanted across HLA barriers from relatives or from HLA-identical unrelated donors, the overall success rate using alternative donors is low. Unfortunately, fewer than half of patients have identical sibling donors.

The major factors that contribute to outcome in BMT in bone marrow failure are (1) patient age, (2) transfusion history, and (3) infection at time of transplant. The incidence of graft versus host disease (GVHD), one of the major complications of BMT, increases with age and is over 90 percent in patients over 30 years. Untransfused patients have a low rate of graft rejection because their lymphocytes have not been sensitized by prior antigen exposure. Survival rates in patients receiving moderate numbers of transfusions have improved, probably due to the more common use of leukocyte-depleted blood products.

Good candidates—young, untransfused, and uninfected—have an excellent prospect of hematopoietic recovery when transplanted in experienced centers, as high as 90 percent long-term survival with hematopoietic engraftment, but survival rates of about 65 percent are more common. Death following transplantation usually results from acute GVHD, interstitial pneumonitis, other infections, or veno-occlusive disease. Chronic GVHD, even if not fatal, can be a serious multisystem disease, and it is not always responsive to immunosuppressive therapy.

Delayed complications of BMT for any indication result from irradiation and chemotherapy: diminished pulmonary function, endocrine dysfunction and infertility, cognitive disorders and leukoencephalopathy, and secondary malignancies. Patients with Fanconi's anemia have been successfully transplanted using a modified conditioning regimen; already at risk for malignancy, they may have exaggerated long-term effects.

Patients with aplastic anemia may experience graft rejection because of the underlying pathophysiology of bone marrow failure. Simple infusions of marrow from syngeneic twins without immunosuppressive therapy of the host fail about half the time. Recurrence of aplasia in identical twins who were immunosuppressed prior to transplantation is further evidence of an inhospitable environment for stem cells in some patients with bone marrow failure.

Immunosuppression

Mathé, who first noted recovery of autologous bone marrow function in some patients who had rejected their marrow grafts, suggested that aplastic anemia might be immunologically mediated. This clinical demonstration of functionally quiescent stem cells in aplastic patients indicated that the empty bone marrow contains cells capable of rescue with nonreplacement therapy. Laboratory experiments in general have supported the hypothesis of suppression of hematopoiesis by T cells and their products, but when applied to individual patients, these tests have been inadequate to predict clinical response to immunologic therapy. The decision to employ antilymphocyte sera is therefore clinical.

Two types of horse sera preparations are in wide use. Antithoracic duct lymphocyte globulin (ALG) is European and is manufactured by the Swiss Serum Institute or Institut Merieux of Lyons; they have not been approved for use in the United States. Antithymocyte globulin (ATG, ATGAM), manufactured by Upjohn, is commercially available. Although a controversial subject, there is little convincing laboratory or clinical evidence of important differences between ATG and ALG preparations or among lots. Regimens have also varied. The foreign proteins are rapidly cleared once the patient produces antihorse IgG antibodies at about 1 week; a short treatment regimen is more rational. I favor ATG at 40 mg per kilogram for 4 days.

The complications of ATG therapy are best managed by a hematologist experienced in its use; however, patients do not require routine transfer to intensive care units for ATG therapy. While rare, anaphylaxis due to horse protein allergy

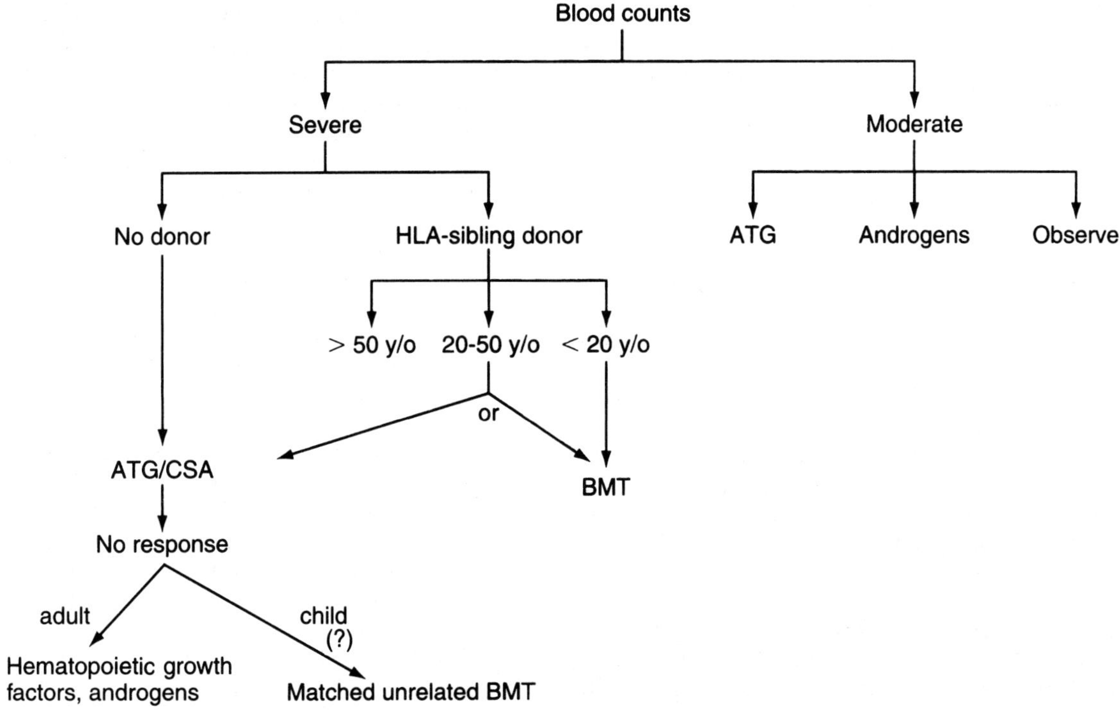

Figure 1
Treatment alternatives in aplastic anemia. ANC, absolute neutrophil count; ATG, antithymocyte globulin; CSA, cyclosporin; HLA, human leukocyte antigen; BMT, bone marrow transplant.

is the most serious consequence and has been fatal. Skin testing may predict susceptible patients. We test by epicutaneous prick testing with undiluted ATG. A wheal and flare reaction indicates the need for desensitization before ATG administration. More common allergic symptoms are fever, chills, and urticaria with the first few infusions. Serum sickness at about day 10 of therapy is also frequent and manifests usually as a flulike illness with a characteristic maculopapular eruption, fever, arthralgia and myalgia, and gastrointestinal symptoms. Serum transaminases and gastrointestinal symptoms. Generally well tolerated when corticosteroids are administered at high doses (60 to 80 mg methylprednisolone in divided daily doses), serum sickness can be temporarily incapacitating; myositis and myocarditis have been observed. Finally, as ATG binds to circulating blood elements as well as lymphocytes, lower platelet and granulocyte counts during ATG therapy should be expected and may necessitate increased numbers of transfusions or antibiotic administration; the Coombs' test may become positive during ATG therapy.

Cyclosporine, used alone or combined with ATG, is also effective in aplastic anemia. Cyclosporine can salvage about half of patients who have failed ATG treatment. ALG or ATG combined with cyclosporine as first therapy has produced hematologic remission rates of about 70 percent. Good results have been obtained with this combination in children and severely neutropenic patients. Cyclosporine is administered at 12 mg per kilogram per day in adults and 15 mg per kilogram per day in children, with dose adjustments to blood levels or creatinine, for 6 months. Nephrotoxicity can be dose limiting. Aplastic patients who are treated with cyclosporine should also receive prophylaxis for *Pneumocystis carinii.*

Patients who recover after immunosuppressive therapy often do not have normal blood counts, but improvement is sufficient so they are free of infection and the need for red cell or platelet transfusion. The likelihood of response to immunosuppression is not predicted by age, sex, presumed cause, or as noted, measurements of immune system function. Signs of hematologic improvement usually appear within a few months of starting ATG therapy. Patients who relapse can be re-treated with a second course of ATG or restarted on cyclosporine. Long-term survival after immunosuppression is comparable to results after bone marrow transplantation. Nevertheless, late clonal hematologic disease is a troubling sequela of immunosuppressive therapy in some patients. Most frequently observed is a positive Ham test, evidence of paroxysmal nocturnal hemoglobinuria without frank clinical hemolysis or thromboses; myelodysplasia and acute leukemia can also occur years after apparent recovery from aplasia.

Androgens

Often disparaged but often used, androgens have a mixed reputation, mainly because only trials from Europe have supported their use. Nonetheless, most hematologists have had at least one aplastic patient clearly respond to hormone therapy. Androgens may work best in patients with some residual hematopoiesis. Dosage is also probably important. The choice of androgen is largely individual: oxymetholone, fluoxymesterone, and nandrolone decanoate are among the more popular formulations. I employ nandrolone decanoate at 5 mg per kilogram per week, given intramuscularly (injection is well tolerated even in thrombocytopenic patients if followed by 15 minutes of local pressure); parenteral androgens avoid the hepatotoxicity associated with oral preparations. With any androgen, a fair clinical trial is at least 3 months of therapy.

Supportive Therapy

Infections

Febrile episodes and serious infections are common in severely affected patients and represent the major cause of death in aplastic anemia. Fever, local infections, and even vague symptoms such as generalized malaise that are suggestive of early sepsis must be regarded with extreme seriousness in the setting of neutropenia. The suspicion of sepsis should initiate broad-spectrum, full-dose parenteral antibiotic therapy (ceftazidime or a combination of cephalosporin, semisynthetic penicillin, and aminoglycoside). Unless a nonbacterial cause of fever becomes obvious (serum sickness, viral infection), therapy should be continued for 10 to 14 days, even with negative blood cultures. More important is the prompt institution of antibiotics than the precise choice of agents prescribed.

With the first episodes of infection, neutropenic patients defervesce and symptomatically improve within a few days of treatment. Persistent or recurrent fever despite antibiotics may respond to addition of a more specific drug that broadens bacterial coverage, such as vancomycin (resistant *Staphylococcus*) or clindamycin (anaerobes). Persistent fever in the repeatedly treated patient often signifies fungal infection and demands amphotericin B therapy. Infections due to resistant organisms, rare bacterial species, and *Pneumocystis* are uncommon in aplastic anemia patients, except in those treated with intensive immunosuppressive therapy.

Delaying antibiotics may lead to seeding of organisms, a virtually intractable problem in aplastic patients. Surgical approaches tend to spread infection across fascial planes, and concentrated collections of bacteria, even sensitive *Escherichia coli* and *Pseudomonas,* may not be eradicated even with prolonged antibiotic treatment. The role of granulocyte transfusions is uncertain.

Bleeding and Platelet Transfusions

Bleeding is common in bone marrow failure but is rarely fatal. Thrombocytopenia alone usually results in mucocutaneous hemorrhage manifesting as petechiae, ecchymoses, and gingival oozing. Spontaneous intracranial hemorrhage is the most feared complication: it is often but not invariably fatal. Major gastrointestinal, genitourinary, or pulmonary bleeding is not usually due to diminished platelet numbers alone but occurs in the setting of infection, stress, and corticosteroid therapy.

Serious bleeding is treated by transfusion of platelets as often as required for clinical effect. Four units of platelets or the donation from a single cytophoresed donor may raise the platelet count above 30,000 to 40,000 and may stem hemorrhage; transfusions as often as thrice daily may be required in other circumstances. Life-threatening hemorrhage is customarily treated with platelet transfusions even in the absence of satisfactory increments in peripheral blood platelet numbers in the hope of homing to bleeding sites.

Platelets administered prophylactically can prevent hemorrhage. A convenient goal is to maintain platelet counts at over 10,000 per millimeter cubed. There is no rationale to prophylactic transfusion to patients who have become refractory because of alloantibody formation. Bleeding in these patients may respond to Amicar (aminocaproic acid), an oral antifibrinolytic agent. Patients should, of course, be advised not to take aspirin or aspirin-like drugs, and abnormalities of coagulation factors, induced by inanition and antibiotic therapy, must be corrected.

Erythrocytes and Hemochromatosis

Blood should be transfused regularly to permit comfortable physical activity, usually achieved with a normal cardiovascular state at a hemoglobin concentration over 7 to 8 g per deciliter and in the presence of cardiac or pulmonary disease at a hemoglobin concentration over 9 g per deciliter. Complete replacement of erythropoiesis in an adult requires transfusion of about 1 unit per week of packed red blood cells. Hemochromatotic damage to the heart, liver, and endocrine glands can be expected once the transfusion burden exceeds 100 units, and deferoxamine chelation should be instituted before this point in patients with chronic disease.

Hematopoietic Growth Factors

Granulocyte colony stimulating factor (G-CSF) and granulocyte-macrophage colony stimulating factor (GM-CSF) can increase neutrophil numbers in some patients. Addition of G-CSF or GM-CSF to antibiotics is reasonable in an infected neutropenic patient; growth factors may also be useful as a regular part of an immunosuppressive regimen to promote hematopoietic regeneration. The utility of growth factor therapy is limited: severely neutropenic patients are less likely to respond than patients with only moderately depressed granulocyte numbers; continued therapy is required to sustain neutrophil numbers; and neither platelets nor reticulocytes are affected. Interleukin-1 and interleukin-3 have not shown clinical activity in aplastic anemia.

Alternative, Experimental, and Future Therapies

High-Dose Corticosteroids

Very high dose corticosteroid therapy has had comparable success rates to ALG in Europe, although it probably is most effective in patients treated within a few weeks of diagnosis. Methylprednisolone therapy has aimed at infusion of 100 mg per kilogram during the first week, 50 mg per kilogram during the second week, and gradual tapering of the dose over 30 to 40 days. Toxic effects are common, including salt and water retention, hypertension, diabetes, electrolyte imbalance, occult infection, and aseptic joint necrosis. High-dose corticosteroids should be reserved for treatment of patients when and where ATG is unavailable.

Future Therapies

Future treatment of aplastic anemia will probably take two directions. More specific attacks on immune mechanisms will utilize monoclonal antibodies or drugs to inhibit lymphokine production, lymphocyte and/or monocyte function, or the effects of specific cytokines. In addition, new hematopoietic growth factors and combinations of factors will be tested. Of the novel ones, stem cell factor is particularly interesting because its levels are low in aplastic anemia patients and it has direct action at the level of the least mature cells of the marrow compartment. In vitro and animal experiments have suggested that factors like thrombopoietin act to increase platelet counts. Combinations of hematopoietins, especially of factors that act at early and late stages of hematopoiesis, may also be useful.

References

Bacigalupo A, Broccia G, Corda G, et al. Antilymphocyte globulin, cyclosporin and granulocyte colony stimulating factor in patients with acquired severe aplastic anemia (SAA): A pilot study of the EBMT SAA Working Party. Blood 1995; 85:1348–1353.

Pizzo PA. Management of fever in patients with cancer and treatment-induced neutropenia. N Engl J Med 1993; 328:1323–1332.

Storb R, Etzioni R, Anasetti C, et al. Cyclophosphamide combined with antithymocyte globulin in preparation for allogeneic marrow transplants in patients with aplastic anemia. Blood 1994; 84:941–949.

Young NS, Alter BP. Aplastic anemia, acquired and inherited. Philadelphia: WB Saunders, 1994.

Young NS, Barrett AJ. The treatment of severe acquired aplastic anemia. Blood 1995; 85:3367–3377.

MEGALOBLASTIC ANEMIA

Dilip L. Solanki, M.D., F.A.C.P.

Megaloblastic anemias are a group of disorders having in common a selective reduction in the rate of DNA synthesis. Over 90 percent of the cases are caused by deficiency of cobalamin or folate, occasionally both, which in turn is caused by a variety of specific disorders. When megaloblastic anemia is correctly diagnosed, the treatment is safe and inexpensive and response usually prompt and complete. However, therapeutic failures due to delayed diagnosis or erroneous treatment continue to occur. Most such failures involve cobalamin deficiency, with consequent risk of irreversible neurologic damage, and they occur because of lack of appreciation of the wide clinical spectrum of cobalamin deficiency and of the pitfalls in use of the traditional laboratory tests. There is also a tendency to forgo critical diagnostic evaluation because acute care of megaloblastic anemia can be effectively handled by shotgun treatment with vitamin B_{12} and folic acid.

Pernicious anemia, the most common form of cobalamin deficiency and long regarded as a disease of whites, is as common in blacks and other racial groups. In blacks it occurs at an earlier age, with one in five cases affecting persons under age 40 and often with macrocytoses masked by high prevalence of thalassemia trait. Dietary deficiency of Cobalamin, generally considered rare in Western countries, is common in strict vegetarians and should be considered in immigrants from countries such as India.

An elevated mean cell volume (MCV), now routinely and accurately provided by automated cell counters, occurs frequently and is a useful marker of megaloblastosis. It frequently rises long before anemia occurs. However, the majority of the patients with macrocytosis do not have megaloblastic anemia but rather ill-defined macrocytosis of alcoholism or other nonmegaloblastic disorder. Conversely, a substantial number of patients with megaloblastic anemia do not have macrocytosis. In a recent study of 86 cobalamin-deficient patients, 35 percent had MCV below 100 fl. Examination of blood and bone marrow is therefore necessary in the evaluation of macrocytosis. Since the peripheral blood changes of megaloblastic anemia can be subtle and seen in other disorders, *bone marrow examination is mandatory for a definitive diagnosis of megaloblastosis.* Bone marrow examination also provides reliable morphologic diagnosis, primarily by the finding of giant metamyelocytes, when the red cell morphologic changes are masked by coexisting infection, inflammation, or iron deficiency. To be diagnostically useful, the bone marrow examination must be done early and before any therapy. This is critical when folic acid deficiency due to poor diet or alcoholism is suspected, because hospital diet and cessation of alcohol intake will quickly cause a reversal to normoblastic erythropoiesis, masking the diagnosis. Bone marrow examination is often neglected or delayed in the name of cost to the patients. However, the rewards of a well-established diagnosis are well worth the cost and minor discomfort to the patient.

Recent reports suggest that the clinical picture of cobalamin deficiency can be more varied and subtle than generally thought. This stems from the widespread use of serum cobalamin level in clinical practice and subsequent detection of many individuals with subnormal values and mild or subtle hematologic and/or neurologic features. Indeed, the textbook description of severe megaloblastic anemia and combined system disease of the nervous system seems to be the rarest presentation of the deficiency.

The idea that in cobalamin deficiency the serum cobalamin characteristically is markedly decreased (below 100 pg per milliliter) is not valid. In a recent study as many as 38 percent of cobalamin-responsive patients had levels between 100 and 199 pg per milliliter. This included patients with neuropsychiatric manifestations. Corollary to this observation is that a modest depression of serum cobalamin level should not be ignored or used to rule out cobalamin deficiency as a cause of anemia or neurologic abnormalities.

The best known neurologic disease of cobalamin deficiency is subacute combined degeneration of the dorsal and lateral spinal columns. However, symptoms of peripheral neuropathy and central nervous system abnormalities such as memory loss, dementia, somnolence, irritability, and even frank psychosis are often more prominent. Contrary to common belief, they are not manifestations of late or severe deficiency, and indeed they frequently occur with minimal or no anemia or macrocytosis. In one recent study 30 percent of 141 consecutive patients with neuropsychiatric abnormalities from cobalamin deficiency had neither clear-cut anemia nor macrocytosis, and many had only modest depression (100 to 200 pg per milliliter) of serum cobalamin. Many of these patients had high normal MCV or a low normal hemoglobin, and most had hypersegmented neutrophils and/or macro-ovalocytes in the blood smear. Folic acid deficiency is not associated with neurologic abnormalities.

Cobalamin deficiency with normal Schilling test is found in about 14 percent of patients. Food cobalamin malabsorption appears to be the cause of the deficiency in these cases. In these patients the evolving gastric atrophy causes loss of gastric acid and enzymes before a total loss of intrinsic factor. When this happens, the patient can no longer split off and absorb the vitamin B_{12} in food but can readily absorb the free, unbound vitamin B_{12} used in the classic Schilling test. Thus, a normal Schilling test should not be used to dismiss low cobalamin level as insignificant. In one in four patients with untreated pernicious anemia, Schilling test may show a pattern of intestinal malabsorption due to mucosal changes caused by the deficiency. Only when these changes revert to normal after 1 to 3 weeks of therapy can the classic malabsorption pattern of pernicious anemia be demonstrated.

The diagnosis of megaloblastic anemia has three components: (1) suspicion based on clinical and/or laboratory manifestations, (2) determination of the deficient vitamin, and (3) identification of the disorder leading to the deficiency. The serum assays of cobalamin and folate have been the laboratory tests of choice for establishing the cause of megaloblastosis. When to use assays of methylmalonic acid and homocysteine, metobolic markers of deficiency, is uncertain. Recent research using simplified serum assays does show them to be more sensitive than serum cobalamin level. However, these tests are not yet widely available and should probably be reserved for atypical or difficult cases.

Much has been written about unexplained low serum cobalamin levels in the elderly. These used to be treated as falsely low values related to advancing age. Recent research using serum methylmalonic acid and homocysteine levels shows that low cobalamin levels in the elderly reflect true deficiency and are clinically important. In light of this information it would be a mistake to attribute low serum cobalamin levels in the elderly to a mere lower normal range. This is particularly important, since recovery of cognitive defect due to cobalamin deficiency in the elderly depends on early diagnosis and treatment.

Atypical and subtle presentation of cobalamin deficiency is much more common than previously appreciated. Metabolic markers may prove helpful in such cases. However, when clinical and/or hematologic features even remotely suggest cobalamin deficiency, the most prudent course of action is a trial of cobalamin therapy.

■ TREATMENT OF THE DEFICIENCY

Megaloblastic anemia responds readily to appropriate vitamin replacement therapy. The goals of therapy are to reverse the hematologic and nonhematologic manifestations of the deficiency, to replenish body stores, and to maintain a normal vitamin balance. The last may require lifelong therapy if the causal disorder cannot be reversed. In most institutions results of tests for serum levels of the vitamins are not available for several days. In the meantime specific therapy should be withheld unless probability of one or the other vitamin deficiency seems high on clinical grounds and can be verified later by serum levels. Therapeutic trials with nonphysiologic doses are not advised because such will produce a hematologic response when either vitamin is used. If folic acid is given to a cobalamin-deficient patient, not only is there no diagnostic value, but the hematologic response (often incomplete and temporary) is usually sufficient to mislead the physician into continuing the incorrect therapy. *The real danger is that the neurologic damage of cobalamin deficiency may become manifest or progress if already present by such erroneous treatment.* If the anemia is severe or the clinical circumstance calls for immediate treatment, it is best to begin therapy with 1,000 μg of cyanocobalamin intramuscularly or subcutaneously and 1 mg of folic acid by mouth daily while awaiting results of serum assays. Once the levels are known, therapy with the deficient vitamin should be continued to replenish the stores and the other one stopped.

A high incidence (14 percent) of early mortality during the first few days of treatment of severe megaloblastic anemia (hematocrit below 25 percent) was reported in a Scottish study. The predominant cause of death was congestive heart failure. In some cases hypokalemia during the early response to vitamin therapy may have contributed to death. A sharp fall in serum potassium attributed to the uptake of potassium by rapidly proliferating marrow cells was observed in many of these patients. This has not been the experience in the United States. It is prudent to pay close attention to the metabolic and cardiopulmonary status of these patients. However, treatment of severe megaloblastic anemia per se should not be viewed as life threatening.

Transfusions

Whether or not to transfuse a severely anemic patient (hematocrit not more than 20) can be a vexing decision. Because of the slow development of anemia, most patients are well compensated even for severe anemia, and the benefit of rapidly increasing the hemoglobin level is outweighed by the danger of precipitating congestive heart failure and perhaps death. Even patients with mild cardiac decompensation may remain stable at bed rest and diuretic therapy until hematologic response occurs. In general, transfusions should be used only for immediate alleviation of symptoms truly caused or aggravated by the anemia (e.g., heart failure, angina) and not merely to treat a given hematocrit level. Mental obtundation may be another indication but is often a manifestation of cobalamin deficiency rather that cerebral hypoxia. Only packed red blood cells should be used; their transfusion should be slow, over about 4 hours, and preceded by the administration of a potent diuretic. It is best to have the patient propped up in bed throughout the transfusion as a precaution against pulmonary edema. The practice of transfusing a preset number of units is unwise and may be dangerous. The need for any subsequent transfusion should be carefully reassessed, since a single transfusion is often sufficient for relief of symptoms. Transfusion is a two-edged sword in such patients and calls for careful consideration of risks and benefits and close monitoring of those who are transfused. Platelet transfusions are rarely needed.

Cobalamin Deficiency

Initial Therapy

Definitive therapy of cobalamin deficiency is replacement with the vitamin. Because the overwhelming majority of the patients with cobalamin deficiency malabsorb the vitamin, the therapy must always be intramuscular or subcutaneous. Cyanocobalamin, a nonphysiologic form of the vitamin, is the preparation most commonly used in the United States. It is stable, inexpensive, and readily converted to physiologic forms in the body. Hydroxocobalamin is the more physiologic form of the vitamin, and its tighter binding to the transport proteins and tissue sites generally results in greater retention and more sustained serum levels after an injection. However, these advantages are of questionable practical value because of the wide variation of response in different patients and the considerably higher cost of this preparation. In specific circumstances such as optic neuritis (tobacco amblyopia), however, the hydroxocobalamin may be preferable despite its cost. Cobalamin preparations are remarkably free of toxicity. The rare allergic reactions are probably related to the preservatives.

Body stores (normal 3 to 5 mg) are easily replenished by several injections of large amounts of cyanocobalamin. The actual schedule of injections is not critical as long as 15 to 20 injections are given over a few weeks. Since many patients are hospitalized, it is convenient to administer daily injections of 1,000 μg for as long as the patient is in the hospital and then 1 to 2 injections every week for several weeks. Although a larger fraction (80 to 85 percent) of a 1,000 μg dose is lost in the urine than when a smaller dose is used, the absolute amount retained is greater, which justifies its use. Twenty injections will provide about 3 mg of vitamin stores. When severe neurologic damage is present, it is common to continue weekly injections of large doses of the vitamin for several months. Although it is not proved that such frequency and doses are necessary to produce a neurologic response, the general approach is an aggressive attempt to reverse the neurologic deficits.

Maintenance Therapy

This is begun once body stores have been repleted. A dose of 1,000 μg of cyanocobalamin monthly is recommended for this purpose. This probably exceeds the needs of most patients; 100 μg may be adequate. Higher doses are favored because optimal dose may vary considerably among patients, and the cost difference is small.

The vast majority of patients with cobalamin deficiency will require lifelong maintenance therapy to remain in normal vitamin balance because the commonest underlying causes are irreversible. Even patients with potentially reversible disorders such as sprue syndromes and intestinal bacterial overgrowth are best given indefinite maintenance therapy because relapses are frequent. Patients with total gastrectomy are obvious candidates for lifelong maintenance; those with subtotal gastrectomy and gastric bypass should be monitored, since only about 20 percent will develop cobalamin deficiency after many years. All patients with ablation, bypass, or disease of the terminal ileum also require monthly maintenance. Intrinsic factor (IF) cobalamin receptors appear to be so densely concentrated in the lower ileum that loss of only 1 to 2 feet suffices to cause cobalamin malabsorption. Rare patients with cobalamin deficiency due to malabsorption caused by drugs should receive maintenance therapy as long as the drug therapy must be continued.

Patient education is the key to the prevention of relapse, which invariably occurs if maintenance therapy is discontinued or erratic. As with other medical disorders requiring lifelong therapy, patients frequently drop out because they no longer feel ill, but they stop therapy also because the dangers of untreated cobalamin deficiency and the importance of continued maintenance have not been adequately impressed upon them and their families. In a recent analysis of relapses of cobalamin deficiency, about 30 percent could be attributed to the failure of the treating physicians to plan adequate long-term follow-up. Reinforcement during clinic visits combined with a simple explanation about the disease process can be very helpful. Another neglected aspect of the management is to train suitable patients or family members to give injections and thus save time and money spent for office and clinic visits, possibly enhancing the likelihood of compliance.

Folate Deficiency

The body stores (normal 5 to 10 mg) can be replenished by 1 mg given daily for about 4 weeks. The commonly used medicinal folate is folic acid, which because of its monoglutamate form is readily absorbed even in malabsorptive states. The oral route is satisfactory in all cases. Indeed, it is extremely rare for a patient to respond to parenteral folic acid if there has been no response to oral treatment. Thus, the only need for parenteral therapy is in patients too ill to take oral medication.

In the body folic acid is converted to various enzyme forms. An important step in the metabolic cycle of folic acid is its reduction to the tetrahydro form by the enzyme dihydrofolate reductase. Drugs such as methotrexate and trimethoprim block this conversion. The resultant folate deficiency can be treated only by folinic acid (leucovorin), the tetrahydro form. This type of deficiency is one of the few indications for this expensive preparation; other uses are the treatment and prevention of trimethoprim and nitrous oxide-induced megaloblastosis.

Lifelong therapy with folic acid is rarely needed, but if it is contemplated, cobalamin absorption must be known to be normal. Maintenance with folic acid, 1 mg daily, is needed only by patients who are unable or unwilling to change their dietary habits or have relapsing disorders such as sprue syndromes. The latter should also receive cobalamin maintenance, since many malabsorb both vitamins. In practice, drug-induced folate deficiency is seen in rare patients receiving long-term phenytoin therapy. Such patients should receive folic acid while continuing the drug. There is no evidence that such therapy increases seizure activity.

Prophylactic treatment is clearly indicated during pregnancy and in patients undergoing chronic hemodialysis. Routine prophylaxis for patients with chronic hemolytic anemias is often practiced but is probably wasteful, since megaloblastic crises are uncommon despite the increased folate requirement of these patients. Maintenance therapy is recommended for those who have had at least one documented megaloblastic crisis or are at risk because of poor dietary habits or associated medical disorders. Folic acid, like cobalamin preparations, is remarkably lacking in toxicity except for rare allergic reactions. The major adverse effect of folic acid is the progression of neurologic deficits when it is inappropriately administered to a patient with cobalamin deficiency.

As most cases of folate deficiency result from poor dietary habits, patients should be educated and encouraged to include leafy vegetables and fruits in their diet. The mode of food preparation is also important. Folates are labile and therefore largely destroyed by excessive boiling or steaming and during canning.

■ RESPONSE TO THERAPY

Objective response to therapy is the ultimate proof of deficiency and therefore must be a routine component of management.

Most patients experience a surge of well-being and alertness, and there is usually a striking improvement in appetite and painful tongue within 48 hours, long before any hematologic improvement. Other gastrointestinal symptoms such as diarrhea may take several days to 2 weeks to resolve. These changes also occur in pernicious anemia patients given folate.

Hematologic response should be monitored meticulously in all patients. In a correctly diagnosed patient, therapy with cobalamin or folic acid results in a predictable series of changes. These include a rapid reversal of the megaloblastic erythropoiesis to a normoblastic one and dramatic fall in the serum iron level within 24 to 48 hours as erythropoiesis becomes more effective. The low serum iron level persists for 1 to 2 weeks. These are followed by a rise in the reticulocyte count, which begins by about the fourth day of treatment and reaches a peak in 7 to 10 days. A gradual increase in the hematocrit begins in the second week. For an optimal response, the absolute reticulocyte count must increase to 3 to 8 times normal (or an uncorrected reticulocyte count of more than 20 percent for moderate to severe anemia) and should continue to be at least twice normal as long as the hematocrit is below 35 percent. It is, therefore, important to monitor the reticulocyte response during the first 7 to 10 days and when possible for several weeks thereafter. In most cases the hematocrit reaches normal within 8 weeks. The MCV decreases rapidly during the first 2 weeks and then more gradually to normal in 4 to 10 weeks. Neutrophil hypersegmentation and its counterpart, giant band forms in the bone marrow, persist for up to 2 weeks after therapy is begun. They thus can serve as useful morphologic clues to megaloblastic anemia in patients treated before appropriate diagnostic studies are done. Deficiency-related thrombocytopenia and leukopenia resolve within 1 to 2 weeks.

A suboptimal or delayed response is an important clue to concomitant factors that inhibit marrow response such as iron or folate deficiency, infection, inflammation, renal insufficiency, and endocrine diseases such as thyroid disorders. Concomitant use of trimethoprim-sulfamethoxazole and excessive oxygen administration may also blunt response. In all of these situations, bone marrow aspiration repeated after therapy shows a return to normoblastic erythropoiesis. If it does not and no cause for suboptimal response is found, the basic diagnostic evidence must be re-examined.

Response of neurologic abnormalities of cobalamin deficiency is variable. In general, mild and recent abnormalities respond best. A consistent response is the arrest of progression of neuropathy. Paresthesias and mild defects in vibratory and position sense usually clear rapidly. Cerebral symptoms, including psychosis, of short duration also resolve promptly and completely. Recently acquired signs and symptoms of dorsal column damage improve, but recovery from severe loss of position sense is slow and incomplete. Recovery from the full syndrome of combined system disease likewise occurs slowly for as long as 6 to 12 months after initiation of treatment, but residual dysfunction is usually permanent. Patients with lateral column damage of more than 8 to 10 weeks' duration show the least improvement, and extensor plantar responses and exaggerated tendon reflexes tend to persist. Sphincter control is usually soon regained. When visual impairment is present, improvement or return to normal can be expected in about 60 percent; the remaining 40 percent are unchanged.

■ LONG-TERM FOLLOW-UP

Megaloblastic anemias have a tendency to recur. Regular follow-up beyond the first several weeks should therefore be an essential part of management. It is one way to confirm that maintenance therapy is being administered and to impress upon the patient the importance of such therapy. More important, it allows detection of a previously unrecognized underlying disorder or recurrence of a previously treated one and of any future complications. When permanent treatment is necessary, three to four visits during the first year and then one every 6 months are adequate for most patients. A complete blood count should be obtained during each visit. Any increase in MCV or decrease in hematocrit value abnormalities may be caused by factors other than relapse of cobalamin or folate deficiency, especially in elderly patients with pernicious anemia.

That the patients with pernicious anemia are at a greater than average risk (approximately threefold) of developing gastric cancer has been confirmed in several studies. There is also an increased incidence of gastric carcinoid tumors. However, the annual risk of gastric cancer is about 0.3 percent, and no consistent premalignant gastric lesion has been identified. Therefore, the role of routine gastroscopic monitoring remains uncertain, and it is generally viewed as unwarranted. However, recent findings of benign gastric polyps in 7 to 17 percent of patients with pernicious anemia has led to the recommendation that endoscopy should be done at diagnosis with removal of any gastric polyps and the need for future examinations determined by the extent of the gastric abnormality. Regardless of the initial course followed, patients with pernicious anemia should be instructed to report promptly any anorexia, dyspepsia, or weight loss, be queried about them on each visit, and have periodic screening of stool for occult blood.

Thyroid disorders also commonly accompany pernicious anemia and should be anticipated. Patients with partial gastrectomy and gastric restriction procedures frequently have or develop concomitant iron deficiency.

■ ACUTE MEGALOBLASTOSIS

Megaloblastic anemias generally develop over months in the case of folic acid deficiency and years in the case of cobalamin deficiency. However, in certain clinical settings an acute megaloblastic state manifesting primarily as life-threatening leukopenia and/or thrombocytopenia may develop in a few days. In most cases deficiency of folate within the bone marrow cells is implicated by use of the dU suppression test. Those at risk have one or more of the following conditions: seriously ill, many in intensive care units; septic; receiving total parenteral nutrition; postoperative state after major surgery; suffering from renal failure; on dialysis and receiving weak folate antagonists such as trimethroprim. Morphologic clues such as hypersegmented neutrophils are often absent, and serum levels of folate and cobalamin may be normal. However, the bone marrow is always megaloblastic. A rapid response to folic acid is the rule. It is perhaps prudent to administer folic acid to all ill patients held in intensive care for more than 3 to 4 days along with an injection of cobalamin unless serum level of the latter is known to be normal. The increased demand for folate by the marrow cells in response to sepsis and bleeding coupled with impaired usage and slow release from stores probably explains the development of severe folate deficiency in a matter of days in patients presumed to have normal folate stores at the start of the illness.

Acute megaloblastosis has also been documented following exposure to the commonly used anesthetic nitrous oxide, which rapidly destroys methyl cobalamin, a coenzyme essential in the conversion of methyl tetrahydrofolate to tetrahydrofolate by methyl transferase. The hematologic effects of nitrous oxide can be abolished by folinic acid or cobalamin. According to some but not all workers these effects can be prevented by pretreatment with folinic acid 30 mg at the time of surgery and 12 hours later.

Suggested Reading

Carmel R. Subtle and atypical cobalamin deficiency states. Am J Hematol 1990; 34:108–114.

Hsing AW, Hansson L, McLaughlin JK, et al. Pernicious anemia and subsequent cancer: A population-based cohort study. Cancer 1993; 71:745–750.

Lindenbaum J, Healton EB, Savage DG, et al. Neuropsychiatric disorders caused by cobalamin deficiency in the absence of anemia or macrocytosis. N Engl J Med 1988; 318:1720–1728.

Lindenbaum J, Savage DG, Stabler SP, Allen RH. Diagnosis of cobalamin deficiency: II. Relative sensitivities of serum cobalamin, methylmalonic acid, and total homocysteine concentrations. Am J Hematol 1990; 34: 99–107.

Pennypacker LC, Allen RH, Kelly JP, et al. High prevalence of Cobalamin deficiency in elderly outpatients. J Am Geriatr Soc 1992; 40:1197–1204.

Stabler SP, Allen RH, Savage DG, Lindenbaum J. Clinical spectrum and diagnosis of cobalamin deficiency. Blood 1990; 76:871–881.

IRON DEFICIENCY ANEMIA

Roy D. Baynes, M.D., Ph.D., F.C.P.S.A., F.A.C.P.
James D. Cook, M.D.

Iron deficiency anemia is the end point in a spectrum of iron deficiency ranging from storage iron depletion to a significant deficit in functional iron. The latter comprises hemoglobin in circulating red cells, myoglobin in muscle, and small amounts of iron-containing enzymes in body tissues. Clinically significant liabilities of iron deficiency occur only after a reduction of iron in the functional compartment. Treatment of milder degrees of iron deficiency is therefore less important. However, in adult men and postmenopausal women, who normally have adequate iron stores, the detection of storage iron depletion should raise a concern about possible pathologic blood loss.

The three treatment modalities for the management of patients with iron deficiency anemia are oral iron, parenteral iron, and blood transfusion. In the vast majority of patients, repair of iron deficiency anemia is achieved readily with oral iron therapy. In a small subset of patients who are either intolerant of oral iron or unable to absorb iron from the gastrointestinal tract, parenteral therapy may be required. When managing patients with severe recurrent iron deficiency anemia, the primary objective is to eliminate the need for blood transfusions. This can usually be accomplished by developing an effective therapeutic iron regimen tailored to the individual patient.

■ ASSESSMENT OF IRON STATUS

Assessment of iron status in individual patients has undergone progressive refinement in recent years. The most practical and efficient means of assessing the amount of iron in the storage compartment is to measure the serum ferritin concentration, which ranges in normal subjects from 12 to 300 μg per liter. Within this range the serum ferritin concentration is quantitatively related to iron stores, 1 μg per liter being equivalent to 8 to 10 mg of storage iron. The advantage of the serum ferritin concentration is that a value less than 12 μg per liter provides unequivocal evidence of storage iron depletion. However, there is a disproportionate increase in the serum ferritin level in the presence of inflammation or liver disease, so a serum ferritin within the normal range does not completely exclude iron deficiency anemia. These patients' storage compartment is better assessed by a semiquantitative evaluation of macrophage iron observed on a bone marrow aspirate smear stained for iron.

A deficiency in iron supply to the functional compartment produces several abnormal laboratory measurements, including the serum iron, total iron-binding capacity, free erythrocyte protoproporphrin, mean cell volume, and red cell distribution width. Unfortunately, most of these measurements are also affected by the iron-deficient erythropoiesis that accompanies inflammation or infection. A new measurement, the *serum transferrin receptor concentration,* will be valuable in distinguishing iron-deficient erythropoiesis from true iron deficiency anemia. Unlike other measurements of functional iron deficiency, the serum transferrin receptor remains normal in most patients with chronic infection but is significantly increased in patients with uncomplicated iron deficiency anemia. A raised serum transferrin receptor concentration identifies functional compartment deficiency in pregnancy; serum ferritin and hematocrit have poor specificity for iron deficiency in this situation. Serum transferrin receptor is unaffected by hepatic disease.

The combination of the serum ferritin concentration as a reflection of iron stores and the serum transferrin receptor concentration as a measure of functional iron deficiency is a convenient and effective means of identifying patients with iron deficiency anemia. The hemoglobin concentration measures the severity of the deficit in the functional iron compartment. Anemia is defined as a hemoglobin concentration less than 13 g per deciliter in males and less than 12 g per deciliter in females.

The use of the serum ferritin, serum transferrin receptor, and hemoglobin concentration should identify iron deficiency in the majority of patients. However, the cost of these measurements is significant, and in certain settings there is still a place for using a therapeutic trial of iron as a diagnostic approach in patients with a high probability of iron deficiency. If you proceed directly to a therapeutic trial, it is imperative to see the patient in 4 to 6 weeks to assess the therapeutic response. If the deficit in hemoglobin concentration has not decreased by at least 50 percent within 4 to 6 weeks, a more complete laboratory evaluation is required.

■ ORAL IRON THERAPY

In a patient with significant iron deficiency anemia, oral therapy should be initiated at a level that provides 150 to 200 mg elemental iron daily in divided doses. The form of iron is relatively unimportant providing that it is in the reduced state; most ferric iron preparations have been withdrawn from the market because absorption is markedly less than that of ferrous iron. In selecting one of the numerous forms of medicinal iron, the most important consideration is the amount of elemental iron in each tablet. Ferrous sulfate tablets generally contain 60 to 65 mg elemental iron, and ferrous gluconate tablets contain about half this amount. Ferrous sulfate is the most widely prescribed oral iron at present because it is the most soluble and least expensive, especially when calculated on the basis of administered iron. Percentage of absorption is maximal with ferrous sulfate, although many forms of ferrous iron are absorbed equally well.

A number of proprietary iron preparations are promoted on the basis of either superior absorption or reduced gastrointestinal side effects, but there is little convincing evidence that these offer any therapeutic advantages. For example, many pharmaceutical preparations contain ascorbic acid, which facilitates iron absorption at the expense of more frequent gastrointestinal side effects. The higher amount of absorption from preparations containing ascorbic acid can be obtained less expensively by increasing the amount of iron in each dose.

Maximal absorption occurs when iron is taken separately from meals. The most rapid hematologic response occurs when iron tablets are taken 1 to 2 hours before each meal. Absorption is further increased by taking an additional dose at bedtime. Iron absorption from this regimen will approach 50 mg daily, or an amount that can offset blood loss in excess of 100 ml daily in chronically anemic patients. This absorption ceiling falls sharply as iron deficiency is corrected.

The major difficulty with oral iron therapy is that a significant proportion of patients develop gastrointestinal side effects at these maximal doses. It is important to distinguish between upper and lower gastrointestinal symptoms. Many patients complain of an alteration in bowel habit, either diarrhea or constipation, but these symptoms are unrelated to the dosage of administered iron. Side effects of this type can usually be treated symptomatically and seldom require alteration or discontinuation of the regimen. Symptoms of the upper intestinal tract are more significant and troublesome. When mild, these include nausea, epigastric discomfort, and heartburn. When severe, they may include vomiting and severe abdominal cramping. These symptoms usually occur within an hour of iron administration and appear to be related to the concentration of ionized iron in the lumen of the stomach or small intestine. The frequency and severity of side effects increase with the dosage of iron.

In many patients, mild nausea or epigastric discomfort can be eliminated if the iron is taken with or immediately following meals, because food binds and renders insoluble a significant proportion of the elemental iron. Taking iron with food also delays gastric emptying and reduces the concentration of unbound iron in the duodenum. When the iron is taken with meals, there is a 50 to 75 percent reduction in absorption. The magnitude of reduction varies with the diet and is much less marked when the meal contains ample quantities of meat or ascorbic acid. Since there is seldom an urgency to correct marked iron deficiency anemia, it is sometimes preferable to prescribe iron with meals initially and thereby avoid gastrointestinal symptoms.

If nausea or epigastric discomfort persists when iron is taken with meals, the amount in each dose should be reduced by switching to a preparation such as ferrous gluconate, which contains much less elemental iron. Further reductions can be accomplished by prescribing a liquid preparation of ferrous sulfate. Reducing the number of doses each day is usually less effective than decreasing the amount of iron in each dose. Another approach for patients with troublesome gastrointestinal side effects is sustained-release iron, which is aggressively promoted by many pharmaceutical firms. These preparations reduce side effects by delaying the release of iron within the gastrointestinal lumen until it is beyond the area of maximal iron assimilation in the upper small intestine. Not surprisingly, a decrease in symptoms is paralleled by a reduction in absorption. With some preparations, such as enteric-coated tablets, the resulting impairment of absorption may be profound. However, with other proprietary preparations, absorption in the presence of food may be comparable with that obtained with ferrous sulfate. Sustained-release iron is worth trying in patients with intractable gastrointestinal symptoms. A major disadvantage of these preparations is their cost, which may be 20 to 30 times that of ferrous sulfate containing the equivalent amount of iron. Sustained-release preparations should be reserved for patients who encounter side effects of conventional forms of iron and should be given with the understanding that absorption may be substantially less than with standard tablets of ferrous sulfate.

A novel approach to delaying the release of iron within the gastrointestinal tract has recently been described. With this new preparation, ferrous sulfate is combined in a gelatin capsule with materials that become buoyant on exposure to gastric secretions and are therefore retained in the stomach for long periods. While the preparation floats on the gastric secretions, the iron is slowly released from the hydrated boundary layer, providing a slow continuous infusion of iron. This gastric delivery system (GDS) has two major advantages. Food normally inhibits iron absorption, but with the GDS the bulk of the meal leaves the stomach before significant release of iron from the GDS. As a result, iron absorption is two or three times as high as with a standard preparation of ferrous sulfate. In addition, preventing the immediate release of ionized iron that occurs with conventional preparations virtually eliminates the upper gastrointestinal side effects. The advantages of less frequent administration and avoidance of nausea and vomiting should improve compliance with and efficacy of oral iron therapy.

■ RESPONSE TO IRON THERAPY

Because iron deficiency impairs proliferation of the erythroid marrow, it takes 7 to 10 days of therapy to achieve a maximal reticulocyte response. Although the degree of reticulocytosis is never dramatic, the reticulocyte count should double or triple over basal level. In patients with an initial hemoglobin below 10 g per 100 ml, full therapeutic doses of oral iron should raise the circulating hemoglobin level about 0.2 g per 100 ml whole blood daily after the first week of treatment. An increase of less than 0.1 g hemoglobin per 100 ml in blood daily is a suboptimal response, although from a clinical perspective this slower increase is usually acceptable.

By far the most common cause of failure to obtain a complete response to oral iron is poor compliance. Because of the wide distribution of iron in vitamin supplements and fortified foods, many patients regard iron as a nutritional supplement rather than a medication. The number of treatment failures can be significantly reduced if the physician takes time to explain to the patient the importance of taking iron tablets regularly. Compliance can be measured by prescribing only enough iron to last the patient until the next visit. Most patients will not ask for a refill of their prescription if they have an unused supply.

An inadequate response is commonly attributed to intestinal malabsorption, but this is an exceedingly uncommon cause of therapeutic failure. Patients who have had a partial gastrectomy absorb medicinal iron poorly when they take it with food but well when they take it between meals. Patients who have undergone a total gastrectomy or extensive resection of upper small intestine have a more profound defect in iron assimilation and do not usually respond to oral therapy. Diseases of the upper small intestine such as celiac disease may occasionally present as iron deficiency because of impaired assimilation of dietary iron. If there is any reason to suspect iron malabsorption, a convenient and simple test is to administer 100 mg elemental iron while the patient is fasting and measure the rise in serum iron level 1 and 2 hours after administration. In iron-deficient patients with a basal serum iron level below 50 μg per deciliter, an increase of 200 to 300 μg per deciliter is commonly seen. A rise of less than 100 μg per deciliter warrants a presumptive diagnosis of intestinal malabsorption and justifies a small bowel evaluation.

A more common cause of so-called refractory iron deficiency anemia is an error in the original diagnosis. The anemia of chronic disease is often mistaken for iron deficiency. This can be avoided by using the optimal measurements for assessing iron status. In some patients an inadequate response to oral iron is due to continuing blood loss. These disorders can usually be detected by a sustained reticulocytosis or by positive tests for occult blood in the feces.

Iron therapy should be continued until iron stores are replenished. A reasonable target is to increase iron reserves to 500 mg, or the amount of iron in 2 units of whole blood. In the past this has usually been obtained empirically by continuing oral iron for 4 to 6 months after the hemoglobin deficit is fully corrected. However, the replenishment of iron stores can now be determined accurately by monitoring the rise in serum ferritin levels. On this basis, oral iron should be continued until serum ferritin reaches 50 μg per liter. Ferritin measurements can subsequently be used to detect early relapse of iron deficiency.

■ PARENTERAL IRON THERAPY

A number of studies have established that repairing iron deficiency anemia with parenteral iron is no faster than with an optimal regimen of oral iron. Parenteral iron may be associated with serious and occasional fatal anaphylactic reactions. In addition to being more hazardous than oral iron, parenteral iron is more expensive because it must be administered under careful medical supervision. Therefore, parenteral iron therapy should never be undertaken to achieve a more dramatic hematologic response or as a matter of convenience to the patient or physician.

The three main indications for parenteral iron therapy are intractable gastrointestinal side effects, malabsorption, and severe recurrent iron deficiency due to uncontrollable blood loss. The most common indication is that the patient is unable or unwilling to continue with oral therapy because of persistent side effects. Some of these individuals can be treated with an oral regimen that minimizes gastrointestinal symptoms and by encouraging patients to continue with oral iron therapy despite minor symptoms. If iron requirements are not excessive, patients with some degree of impaired absorption can absorb sufficient iron to correct iron deficiency or forestall it. On the other hand, repeated courses of parenteral iron are often justified when there is large, uncontrollable blood loss, as in patients with hereditary telangiectasia. However, a word of caution is in order if patients are given parenteral iron repeatedly. Parenteral iron should never be given without careful monitoring of the serum ferritin level. At one time parenteral iron was used extensively in patients on chronic hemodialysis to offset their high requirements due to gastrointestinal bleeding, laboratory sampling, and dialyzer use. Some of these patients developed the clinical syndrome of hemochromatosis due to parenchymal iron loading.

Iron dextran is the only form used for parenteral iron therapy in the United States. Iron dextran is a complex of ferric hydroxide and dextrans of molecular weights ranging between 5,000 and 8,000. It is supplied as a dark colloidal solution containing 50 mg iron per milliliter. Iron dextran may be given either intramuscularly or intravenously. When the intramuscular route is used, it is given in the upper outer buttock at 50 to 250 mg per injection site. There are several drawbacks to intramuscular administration. Permanent skin staining may result, although this problem may be lessened by using Z-track injection. Another disadvantage is that a significant proportion of the dose may remain at the site of injection for weeks or even months. Some patients complain of persistent pain at the injection site, which may be due to an immunologic reaction to the dextran moiety. On this basis, extensive local muscle necrosis has been described in certain patients. Another concern with intramuscular administration is that sarcomas have developed in rats given massive injections of iron dextran. This prompted temporary withdrawal of iron dextran at one time, but extensive follow-up studies in humans have not provided convincing evidence of a risk of cancer.

Many of the problems of intramuscular use of iron dextran can be eliminated by giving the drug intravenously. In several early trials the undiluted preparation was administered by direct intravenous infusion over 5 to 10 minutes. Injections of 500 to 1,000 mg are repeated at weekly intervals to achieve a total dose. A more convenient and less hazardous approach is to administer the total calculated dose in a single intravenous infusion. The amount of iron required is calculated from the deficit in circulating hemoglobin, assuming that 1 g hemoglobin per deciliter whole blood corresponds to 150 mg iron in an average-sized adult. An additional 500 to 1,000 mg is given to replenish iron stores. This amount of iron dextran is diluted in normal saline to a concentration not exceeding 5 percent, and administered slowly over 2 to 3 hours.

The most serious concern with total dose infusion is anaphylaxis. Iron dextran should be given intravenously only when resuscitative measures are immediately available. To safeguard against severe anaphylaxis, the rate of intravenous infusion should be kept to less than 10 drops per minute during the first 10 to 15 minutes of administration. If no reaction occurs, the rate can be increased to several hundred milliliters per hour. For patients who have not been given iron dextran previously, it is prudent to limit the total dose to 1,000 mg on the first occasion. A variety of less serious side effects such as skin rash, fever, arthralgias, and lymphadenopathy have been reported. Although relatively uncommon, these side effects are important because they may herald more serious reactions with subsequent therapy. Iron dextran administration is contraindicated in patients with rheumatoid arthritis because it is known to exacerbate synovitis.

Iron dextran requires macrophage processing before the iron can be released to bind to transferrin. The large amount of iron passing through the macrophage after iron dextran infusion leads to some iron being diverted into insoluble sequestered forms. These may be only slowly mobilized during the subsequent recurrence of iron deficiency, thereby leading to the seemingly anomalous situation of iron deficiency anemia despite stainable iron in the macrophages in the bone marrow.

Suggested Reading

Auerback M, Witt D, Toler W, et al. Clinical use of the total dose intravenous infusion of iron dextran. J Lab Clin Med 1988; 111:566–570.

Boggs DR. Fate of a ferrous sulfate prescription. Am J Med 1987; 82:124–128.

Bothwell TH, Charlton RW, Cook JD, Finch CA. Iron metabolism in man. Oxford, UK: Blackwell Scientific, 1979.

Cook JD, Skikne BS, Baynes RD. Serum transferrin receptor. Ann Rev Med 1993; 44:63–74.

Simmons WK, Cook JD, Bingham KC, et al. Evaluation of a gastric delivery system for iron supplementation in pregnancy. Am J Clin Nutr 1993; 58:622–626.

ANEMIA OF CHRONIC DISEASE

Ronan Foley, M.D., F.R.C.P.C.
Michael C. Brain, D.M., F.R.C.P., F.R.C.P.C.

Anemia that accompanies chronic infective, inflammatory, or neoplastic disease is generally categorized as anemia of chronic disease (ACD). This type of anemia is characterized by an inability of red blood precursors to use iron, despite its presence in bone marrow stores in normal or even increased amounts. Although impaired iron use has been the most widely accepted hypothesis for ACD, a reduction in red blood cell survival and/or failure in the normal erythropoietic response to anemia have also been considered to play a role in pathogenesis. Impairment of erythropoiesis may be due to inhibition by specific cytokines, which are often elevated in chronic inflammation, or to an inadequate response to erythropoietin (EPO), because of either reduced production or reduced responsiveness. Since the cause is uncertain and may not be simple, other descriptive terms, including anemia of cellular immune response and the anemia of defective iron reutilization, have been proposed. Anemia due to chronic renal failure, hepatic or endocrine disorders requires consideration in the differential diagnosis. Other causes of anemia, including marrow replacement, hemolysis, and blood loss, must be excluded before ACD can be diagnosed.

■ DIAGNOSIS

The anemia in ACD is generally normochromic and normocytic, although hypochromic microcytes may be present. The low reticulocyte count relative to the degree of anemia reflects impaired erythropoiesis. Platelet and white cell counts are normal or increased. Marrow cellularity is normal. There is defective hemoglobinization, with iron granules absent in late erythroblasts. Iron is generally plentiful in bone marrow macrophages and fragments. A low serum iron, decreased saturation of transferrin, and normal or increased ferritin levels are evidence of impaired iron use. The low serum iron may make it difficult to differentiate iron deficiency from ACD. Serum ferritin is usually normal or increased in ACD, whereas in uncomplicated iron deficiency, a low ferritin is diagnostic. The total iron-binding capacity may be instructive. It is low in ACD and increased in iron deficiency. A transferrin saturation less than 5 percent is seen only in iron deficiency.

Patients with ACD may also be iron deficient. This has to be considered if the patient is a woman of childbearing age or at risk for gastrointestinal blood loss from erosions or ulcers when treated with steroidal and nonsteroidal anti-inflammatory drugs. In elderly patients colonic angiodysplasia, polyps, and carcinoma have to be considered. A bone marrow aspirate is the most reliable method of recognizing iron deficiency. The presence or absence of iron can be readily assessed in marrow smears stained with Prussian blue.

The severity of iron disturbance in ACD correlates with the activity of the underlying disease. The normalization of iron use may therefore depend on successful treatment of the underlying pathology. Although changes in iron use can help assess the response to treatment, it is simpler to monitor anemia.

■ CAUSES

Activation of the Reticuloendothelial System

This may be responsible for shortened red cell survival found in patients with rheumatoid arthritis (RA), a disease commonly associated with ACD, as the same cells have a normal survival when transfused into a healthy subject.

Impaired Response of Erythropoietin

EPO, a hormone produced chiefly by the kidneys, regulates erythropoiesis. In patients with RA there may be an impaired EPO response, as the increase in serum EPO levels is less than in comparably anemic patients who do not have RA. Nevertheless, about two-thirds of patients with ACD respond favorably to recombinant EPO (rEPO) treatment. Why some patients do not respond is uncertain. Other disorders, including chronic renal failure, AIDS, and cancer, respond to rEPO with an increase in hematocrit and a reduction in transfusion requirements. Recombinant EPO is generally well tolerated. However, it is expensive, and the benefits of use require further study before its routine administration can be recommended.

Role of Cytokines

States of chronic inflammation or disordered immunity are associated with elevated expression of cytokines. Cytokines mediate interactions between B and T lymphocytes and macrophages. Cytokines may contribute to the hematologic abnormalities in ACD by direct suppression of erythroid. Communication and coordination of activity is mediated through cytokines. Their contribution to the hematologic abnormalities in ACD may be mediated by direct suppression of erythroid growth and differentiation or by enhancing the ability of macrophages to store ferritin and sequester iron from developing erythroblasts. Three cytokines, tumor necrosis factor, interleukin-1, and gamma interferon, have been implicated in ACD.

Tumor necrosis factor (TNF) is increased in cancer, RA, and infection. Chronic administration of TNF to experimental animals will cause anemia characterized by a low serum iron with normal iron stores. Erythroid colony–forming units are reduced, which suggests a direct inhibition of erythropoiesis. Anemia with features of ACD has been demonstrated in human clinical trials using recombinant TNF.

Interleukin-1 (IL-1) is elevated in states of chronic inflammation and has been implicated in the suppression of erythropoiesis. Patients with RA and anemia have higher levels of IL-1-beta in their circulation than RA patients without anemia.

Interferon gamma (IFN-γ) is produced by T lymphocytes and is also increased in states of chronic immune stimulation. Macrophages are activated by IFN-γ. Activated macrophages release large amounts of a substance known as neopterin.

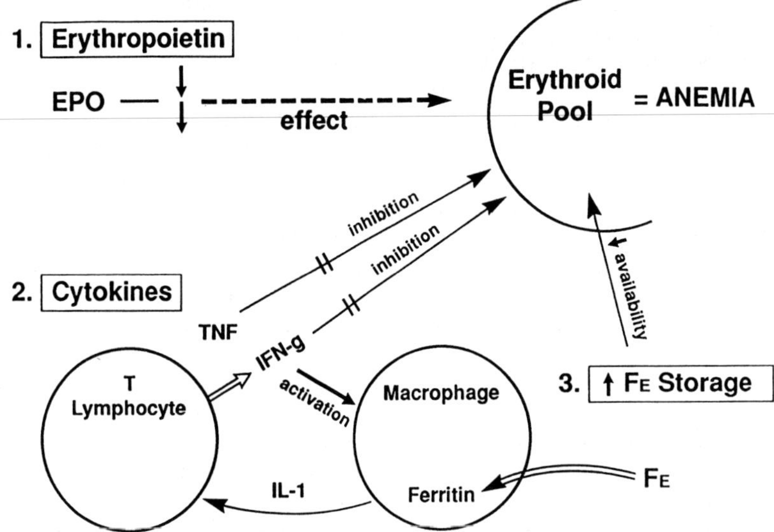

Figure 1
Summary of proposed mechanisms in ACD, with emphasis on a developing erythroid pool. The causes include (1) Erythropoietin (EPO), which may be reduced in relative amount and function; (2) cytokines elevated in states of chronic inflammation, which may have adverse effects on erythropoiesis; (3) iron, which may be stored and sequestered in macrophages, unavailable to developing erythroblasts. IFN-γ, Interferon gamma; IL-1, interleukin-1; TNF, tumor necrosis factor.

Neopterin levels in vivo are found to correlate with the degree of anemia and with decreased iron in the circulation. Compounds similar to neopterin facilitate the storage of iron in the macrophage. This process may reduce the amount of iron available to the developing erythroblasts.

Role of Activated Macrophages

An effect on increased iron storage has been explored in ACD. Lactoferrin, a protein with a strong affinity for iron, contributes to abnormalities of iron processing. Lactoferrin, released from neutrophils stimulated by IL-1, will bind iron and be taken up by macrophages; the iron is stored as ferritin. Furthermore, apoferritin may increase in chronic inflammation, similar to acute phase reactants, and sequester or trap iron in the form of ferritin. The observation that rEPO can correct anemia in some patients suggests that the lack of availability of iron is not the sole explanation for the anemia of ACD.

Figure 1 summarizes the possible causes of ACD and includes the following possibilities: (1) an impairment of erythropoietin, both in amount and function; (2) production of cytokines, which have a negative effect on erythroid growth; (3) increased storage of iron in the macrophage, effectively reducing the amount of iron available for developing erythroblasts.

■ INVESTIGATION AND TREATMENT

Recognizing the Cause

The definitive treatment of ACD requires recognition and treatment of the underlying cause. An infective, malignant, or immunologic process will commonly be discovered (Table 1). A detailed history and clinical examination may suggest the underlying process of ACD.

Table 1 Causes of Anemia of Chronic Disease

Renal failure	Erythropoietin deficiency
Endocrine	Hypothyroidism
	Panhypopituitarism
Infective	Pulmonary
	Tuberculosis, fungal infections
	Cardiac
	Endocarditis
	Pelvic inflammatory disease
	Osteomyelitis
	Chronic urinary tract infection
Inflammatory disease	Rheumatoid arthritis
	Systemic lupus erythematosus
	Sjögren's disease
	Inflammatory bowel disease
	Sarcoidosis
Neoplasia	Occult carcinoma: renal, ovarian, pancreatic, uterine
	Hodgkin's disease and non-Hodgkin's lymphoma

Seeking Alternative Explanations for Anemia

Deficiencies of folate or vitamin B_{12} should be excluded and hemolysis assessed by a reticulocyte count, analysis of the peripheral blood smear, and Coombs' test. An abnormality in the peripheral smear, such as teardrop cells, leukoerythroblastic changes, or reduction of platelets, may be indicative of a process within the marrow such as metastatic disease or a primary hematologic malignancy. This can be investigated by a bone marrow aspirate and biopsy. Renal failure will cause anemia and should be evaluated with routine screening tests early in the workup. Without direct assessment of the stores of iron in the marrow, routine indices of iron can be inconclusive. A low serum iron and low total iron-binding capacity are generally present in ACD. Assessment of thyroid and pituitary function should be completed. Disorders of immunity are assessed by history, physical examination, and laboratory evaluation (ESR, C3, C4, rheumatoid factor, antinuclear antibodies, protein electrophoresis). On occasion an occult immunologic process such as localized Crohn's disease may be responsible. Malignancy may be obvious or subtle and often requires a combination of laboratory and radiologic procedures. Finally, a chronic infection may be detected by routine blood cultures or require, as in endocarditis, an echocardiograph. Osteomyelitis can be demonstrated by radionuclide analysis.

Assessing the Clinical Significance of Anemia

In some patients with ACD, as in active rheumatoid arthritis, the anemia may not respond to treatment. It is necessary to determine whether the anemia is making a significant contribution to the patient's symptoms. In the absence of overt cardiac failure, there may be no objective clinical criteria by which this can be judged. There is evidence that muscle mass declines with anemia. However, in the absence of severe arthritis, endeavors to improve muscle function by graded exercise may be as beneficial to patients with ACD as to patients with chronic obstructive pulmonary disease.

Blood Transfusion

Correction of anemia by the transfusion of packed red cells can provide temporary benefit and may be best reserved for preparation for an elective surgical procedure or to meet some other short-term need. The survival of transfused red cells may be reduced and usually becomes progressively shorter with subsequent transfusions due to more rapid RES clearance and antigenic sensitization. Transfusion reactions, iron overload, and the risks of transfusion-transmitted diseases such as hepatitis and human immunodeficiency virus are of continuing concern, as are the possible effects of transfusion on immune regulation. The frequent transfusion of red cells is rarely an acceptable therapeutic option unless the anemia of ACD is compounded by continuing gastrointestinal blood loss due to anti-inflammatory drugs, colonic angiodysplasia, and so on.

Erythropoietin

In the absence of an effective treatment for the majority of causes of ACD and considering the risks and limited benefits of red cell transfusions, rEPO may be the treatment of choice. It has been used in clinical trials for RA, metastatic cancer, acquired immunodeficiency syndrome, and multiple myeloma as well as in patients with renal failure on dialysis. In addition to alleviating anemia, it has been shown to improve the quality of life. Of concern is the cost of long-term rEPO treatment. Recombinant EPO is available for subcutaneous or intravenous administration and is usually initiated at a dose of 50 to 100 units per kilogram three times weekly. The dose can be reduced once the desired target hematocrit is reached. An increase in biologic effect is not seen in doses beyond 300 units per kilogram three times weekly. Before therapy is initiated, iron stores should be assessed. Although rEPO is generally well tolerated, blood pressure should be controlled prior to starting rEPO therapy and monitored closely during therapy. Potential problems, generally relating to the dialysis population, include arteriovenous shunt thromboses, seizures, hypertension, and the cardiovascular changes relating to an increase in blood viscosity.

The Future

New therapeutic modalities targeting specific aspects of the inflammatory response may offer more satisfactory ways to improve hematopoiesis in symptomatic patients.

Suggested Reading

Fuch D. Immune activation and the anemia associated with chronic inflammatory disorders. Eur J Hematol 1991; 46:65–70.

Krantz SB. Pathogenesis and treatment of the anemia of chronic disease. Am J Med Sci 1994; 307:353–358.

Means RT. Progress in understanding the pathogenesis of the anemia of chronic disease. Blood 1992; 80:1639-1647.

AUTOIMMUNE HEMOLYTIC ANEMIA

John G. Kelton, M.D.
Mark A. Crowther, M.D., F.R.C.P.C.

Autoimmune hemolytic anemia (AIHA) is the second most common autoimmune cytopenia (after immune thrombocytopenic purpura [ITP]) that hematologists must manage. Its management and general principles of therapy are much the same as the management of patients with immune thrombocytopenia and readers are referred to this chapter for additional information. The way in which AIHA patients present has changed dramatically over the past decade. Some 20 years ago, a discussion on AIHA would have focused on those patients who had severe anemia as a result of their red cell destruction. Now, increasing numbers of patients with AIHA are first identified when their blood is tested in a transfusion medicine laboratory before a surgical procedure. In addition, with increased sensitivity of the reagents, particularly the anti-immunoglobulins used in indirect antiglobulin testing (IAT), more patients are discovered to have *serological* AIHA as opposed to *clinical* AIHA. It is our contention that many of these patients, like ITP patients, can be followed and do not require specific treatment. In this chapter we summarize the presentation of patients with AIHA, their investigation and management.

CLASSIFICATION

Autoimmune hemolytic anemia is anemia caused by destruction of the red cells by the patient's autoantibodies. Technically, increasing evidence suggests that some patients suspected to have AIHA are in fact reacting to antigens absorbed to the red cell surface. This is particularly true for drug-induced immune hemolytic anemia. But for the sake of thoroughness, we will also summarize this disorder in this chapter. Additionally, many patients do not become anemic despite having autoimmune hemolysis. These patients have an increased rate of red cell destruction, but the bone marrow is able to compensate for the increased red cell destruction by increased red cell production (compensated AIHA). The patients will not have anemia unless the rate of red cell destruction dramatically increases, as can happen following an infective process or a vaccination which presumably enhances autoantibody production and increases reticuloendothelial cell activity. Also, patients' hemoglobin level can drop if they have reduced red cell production because of depletion of required vitamins or minerals (typically folate or iron). Finally, some of these patients can have infection-associated marrow suppression that would prevent them from maintaining the enhanced red cell production necessary to keep up with the increased rate of red cell destruction. Recent studies have implicated the parvovirus in some episodes of viral-induced marrow suppression. Consequently, it is important for physicians to recognize that a number of factors can contribute to anemia in these patients, and that therapy is not always directed towards reducing the increased red cell destruction.

Classification of diseases typically relates to determination of the pathophysiology or mechanism responsible for the disorder, or whether the disorder is primary or secondary to an associated disorder. These classifications are useful in AIHA; however, most patients with AIHA are first diagnosed in the transfusion medicine laboratory. It is the transfusion laboratory that can be most helpful in not only classifying the type, but also in helping the physician determine the optimal treatment for the patient. Ironically, the transfusion laboratory has also contributed to confusion and sometimes delay in the management of these patients. One of the key principles in transfusion medicine is not to transfuse incompatible blood. Yet, for most patients with warm AIHA (IgG mediated), *serologically compatible* blood (as opposed to *clinically compatible* blood) cannot be obtained. Occasionally this concern can lead to an unacceptable delay in transfusion for these patients.

Frequency and Presentation

AIHA is a relatively common hematologic disorder occurring in 10 to 20 per 100,000 individuals. This relatively high frequency contrasts with the frequency of most severe hematologic malignancies, which typically occur at a rate 10 times lower. Except for cold AIHA that occurs in young children (paroxysmal cold hemoglobinuria), AIHA is a disorder of middle and old age, with the risk beginning to rise progressively and dramatically starting at age 40 to 50. Like most autoimmune disorders, women are more frequently affected than men.

Patients can present in one of three ways: first, because of symptoms of anemia resulting from red cell destruction; second, because of secondary effects of the hemolytic anemia (hepatosplenomegaly) or because of a disorder which has initiated the AIHA (such as a lymphoproliferative disorder); third, an increasing number of patients who are asymptomatic are identified during routine medical laboratory testing.

Classification According to Serologic Testing

We find the most useful classification for patients with AIHA is one that is based upon results of testing from the transfusion medicine laboratory (Table 1). The first step in transfusion testing is ABO typing. It is important for physicians managing these patients to understand the basic principles of these tests to avoid potential problems in their patients. Indeed, the two major groups of AIHA (warm and cold AIHA) have unique serologic results that are helpful in the diagnosis, but can cause problems in the treatment of these patients. The first test performed in transfusion laboratories is determination of the major blood group (A, B, AB, and O). This test, performed at room temperature, uses the patient's red cells and antisera against blood groups A and B. Patients with IgM-mediated AIHA typically have autoantibodies that will react with any red blood cells (see subsequent discussion of target antigens) at room temperature. Hence, the transfusion laboratory should suspect that the patient has AIHA mediated by IgM when all tests read positive. Sometimes, it can be difficult to

Table 1 Laboratory Characterization of Patients with AIHA*

Autoantibody	
Warm reactive (IgG)	62%
Cold reactive (IgM)	30%
(IgG-PCH)	1%
Combined (warm and cold)	7%

*The relative frequency is estimated from the reference and will vary depending upon the referral population.

determine the ABO type, particularly if the patient has a high thermal range autoantibody. These patients require blood grouping and serological testing at 37°C. The patient's red cells should be washed with warm saline before testing. Most of these IgM autoantibodies react best at temperatures cooler than the body temperature and hence are termed *cold reactive autoantibodies.* Because they almost always are of the IgM immunoglobulin class (with the notable exception of IgG, which causes PCH), they are potent agglutinators of red cells and consequently are termed *cold agglutinins.*

Most episodes of AIHA are caused by IgG, which tends to react best at body temperature. Hence, these disorders are designated *warm AIHA.* Serologic testing of these patients in the transfusion laboratory typically does not present problems during ABO typing because these procedures are performed at room temperature and the IgG autoantibody is a weak agglutinating agent. However, during the antibody screening phase of a pretransfusion testing, warm AIHA gives a characteristic panreactivity because the IgG autoantibody in the patient's serum reacts with all of the screen cells, raising the possibility of multiple alloantibodies. Also, Rh-negative patients can be mistyped as Rh positive because of the autoantibody. Techniques for overcoming this problem are summarized later in this chapter. All pretransfusion testing includes the direct antiglobulin test, in which washed red cells from the patient are tested for the presence of IgG or complement on their surface. Patients with IgM (cold) AIHA do not react with the anti-IgG but do react with anti-complement (typically anti-C3). In contrast, most but not all patients with AIHA caused by IgG autoantibodies (warm AIHA) have IgG on their own red cells. In addition, about half will have complement as well as IgG on their red cells because the IgG autoantibody (usually IgG subclass I) is an efficient activator of complement.

■ WARM AUTOIMMUNE HEMOLYTIC ANEMIA

The physician must determine whether the patient has primary AIHA (idiopathic) or secondary AIHA. The transfusion laboratory is of modest help in differentiating these two disorders. Many patients with AIHA have both IgG and complement on their red cells. The majority also have an indirect (serum) AIHA that is positive. However, there are certain high affinity autoantibodies that are only detectable on the patient's red cells. Sometimes, the transfusion laboratory can provide *inferential* information that the patient has a secondary AIHA. For example, many patients with drug-induced immune hemolytic anemia (particularly those with drug-dependent immune hemolytic anemia) will have a positive direct antiglobulin test (DAT) but a negative indirect antiglobulin test (IAT), unless the causative drug is added to the test serum. This is typically seen in patients with immune hemolytic anemia caused by penicillin and the semi-synthetic penicillins. The antihypertensive agent methyldopa can cause a true AIHA that is characterized by both a positive direct and indirect antiglobulin test that is not drug dependent. Fortunately, the majority of these patients (at least 80 percent) do not have evidence of hemolysis. Rather, they have a strongly positive DAT and IAT that is not correlated with increased red cell destruction.

Table 2 Approximate Distribution of Disease of Patients with Warm (IgG) AIHA*

Primary AIHA	
Idiopathic AIHA	60%
Secondary AIHA	
Drug induced	10%
Neoplastic Disorders	
Lymphoproliferative Disorder	10%
Chronic Lymphocytic Leukemia	
Non-Hodgkin's Lymphoma	
Hodgkin's Lymphoma	
Carcinoma (including ovarian)	5%
Myelodysplasia	2%
Immunologic Disorders	
Connective Tissue Diseases (RA and SLE)	5%
Ulcerative Colitis, Hepatitis	2%
Miscellaneous Other	6%

*This distribution varies depending upon the patient referral base.

The physical examination and history are focused on differentiating primary (idiopathic) from secondary warm AIHA. As shown in Table 2, depending upon the population studied, about 20 percent of patients with warm AIHA have a secondary cause with lymphoproliferative disorders, often chronic lymphocytic leukemia and non-Hodgkin's lymphoma. However, connective tissue disorders and certain autoimmune conditions, such as ulcerative colitis, are associated with AIHA. In most series, rheumatoid arthritis (RA) is a more common cause of immune hemolysis than is systemic lupus erythematosus (SLE), even though the relative risk per case is higher for SLE than RA. This reflects the relative differences in the frequencies of the two disorders.

Patients should be carefully examined for evidence of both primary and secondary AIHA. About 70 percent to 80 percent of patients with primary AIHA have splenomegaly, presumably because of compensatory hypertrophy due to increased red cell destruction in the spleen. This is in marked contrast with ITP, where the spleen invariably is normal sized. It has been our experience that patients with AIHA who require frequent transfusions progressively increase the size of their spleen, which may reflect increasing red cell destruction by that organ. Lymphadenopathy is not typically seen in primary AIHA and suggests the possibility of a secondary disorder such as a lymphoproliferative disorder. In patients in whom there is any question about the primary or secondary nature of the disorder, a bone marrow examination should be performed with immunofluorescent typing. Sometimes, immunophenotyping of peripheral blood will help establish the diagnosis, particularly when a monoclonal lymphocyte proliferation is identified, which would be seen in patients with chronic lymphocytic leukemia (CLL). Although a bone marrow examination is not absolutely required in every patient, we find it helpful in the investigation of these patients, particularly to distinguish secondary lymphoproliferative AIHA.

The laboratory investigation of these patients requires a measurement of the complete blood count and reticulocyte count since (as noted previously) suppression of the marrow can exacerbate the anemia in an otherwise stable patient with AIHA. The blood film shows characteristic changes including polychromasia, reflecting the increased number of reticulocytes and spherocytic red cells. Spherocytic red cells are almost always seen in patients with warm AIHA and should be carefully sought. Measurement of red cell folate and determination of iron status (ferritin), as well as serologic investigation, are important for autoimmune disorders, connective tissue disorders and infections (e.g., HIV) if the patient is considered to be at risk.

Pathophysiology and Laboratory Findings

Warm AIHA is caused by IgG autoantibodies (or IgG drug dependent antibodies). The IgG is almost always subclass I (over 98 percent of patient samples). Other subclasses are present, often in various mixtures of the four subclasses. However, some of the earlier reports of subclass restriction must be interpreted with caution because of the difficulty in obtaining subclass specific antiserum. Although IgG subclass I is invariably detected in patients with AIHA, it is polyclonal rather than monoclonal and is directed at the Rhesus blood group system with varying specificities within Rh and against band 3. Rarely, the autoantibodies mimic alloantibodies. The IgG autoantibodies have high affinity at 37°C binding to Rh determinants on the patient's red cells. Although complement is frequently found on these red cells (presumably because of the density of autoantibodies), complement-mediated hemolysis is distinctly uncommon. Rather, cell clearance is primarily mediated through the cells of the reticuloendothelial system, particularly the FcRII receptors on monocytes and macrophages in the spleen. Most of the sensitized cells will ultimately undergo partial phagocytosis by the phagocytic cells. But, phagocytosis is typically not complete, and red cells escape complete engulfment leaving a portion of their membrane behind. These cells that have lost a small portion of membrane are no longer biconcave discs but are the spherocytes that typify the disorder.

The extravascular destruction of red cells results in splenomegaly (80 percent of patients) with hepatomegaly in a smaller proportion of patients (40 percent to 50 percent). Often the bilirubin is mildly elevated (rarely to levels of visible jaundice), with the indirect being more elevated than the direct.

Rarely, there are patients who have auto-AIHA in which the red cell destruction is mediated with a particular subclass of IgG (e.g., IgG-3 or a low titer high affinity that is not detected in the direct antiglobulin test). In these patients a quantitative direct antiglobulin test (such as a radioimmunoassay) or testing for the presence of antibody from a concentrated eluate can help in the diagnosis.

Therapy

As is the case for ITP, the physician must determine if any treatment is required for a patient with AIHA. Some patients, particularly those in whom the illness is identified by an abnormal laboratory test but have normal or near-normal hemoglobin limits, may not require any specific therapy (with the exception of folic acid because of the increased red cell turnover). Patients also require an assessment of their iron stores with possible supplementation. Other patients have such severe anemia that they require red cell transfusions. The ABO typing in these patients is not difficult, but occasionally it can be difficult to be certain about their Rh typing because of the serologic target of the autoantibody. If there is doubt about the Rh-type, the patient should receive ABO group compatible, Rh-negative red cells.

Because of the panreactivity of the autoantibody, it is essentially impossible to rule out the presence of an alloantibody. Several approaches have been taken by transfusion laboratories, but the key issue is not to delay transfusing the patient while attempting to identify compatible blood. If the patient has never had a transfusion, it is important to put aside a subsample of the patient's blood for determination of the patient's phenotype in a specialized laboratory (typically a Red Cross referral laboratory). In previously nontransfused patients, the likelihood of a clinically significant alloantibody is low and the most compatible (least incompatible) red cells should be transfused. In patients who have had frequent transfusion, it is important to provide them with minor blood group compatible red cells and to try to identify alloantibodies. Typically, this is performed by looking for the presence of alloantibodies in the patient's serum after repetitive autoabsorption of the serum using the patient's own red cells. Alternatively, the IAT sample can be titred out looking for alloantibodies. The medical/surgical management of a patient with warm AIHA is essentially identical to the treatment of a patient with ITP. Corticosteroids (1 mg per kg per day) is the first line of therapy. In most patients this will result in reduced hemolysis, and a stabilization and rise in the hemoglobin concentration. The onset of action, like ITP, is about 1 to 2 weeks and we begin to taper the prednisone over a 1 to 2 month interval after the hemoglobin has begun to stabilize. As with ITP, it is best to switch to alternate-day corticosteroids to reduce side effects. The corticosteroids suppress autoantibody formation and reduce reticuloendothelial cell destruction (possibly through down regulation of the FcRII receptors in the spleen and other reticuloendothelial cell organs).

Many patients with AIHA have chronic disease that will not remit spontaneously. If the patient is steroid dependent, (as many patients are), we move to splenectomy earlier rather than later in therapy. The reason is that most of these patients (unlike typical ITP patients) are elderly, and corticosteroids can produce serious adverse reactions in this population. Splenectomy should be preceded (1 to 2 weeks) by vaccination against *Pneumococcus*. Some physicians also recommend vaccination against other encapsulated organisms that carry a higher risk of serious infection in the splenectomized patients (*Haemophilus influenzae* and *Meningococcus*). Surgery is performed with corticosteroid coverage, with care taken to identify and remove accessory spleens. To date there is no way to identify who will respond to splenectomy; overall, about one-half of patients have a significant remission or cure after splenectomy. Those patients in whom the splenectomy does not cure are more easily managed than nonsplenectomized patients.

Patients who fail splenectomy can be managed with a variety of medications. Typically, we try danazol, an attenuated androgen. The dose is 200 mg to 800 mg per day and in some patients higher doses (1,200 mg) are required. This treatment can produce some virilizing effects, but fortunately this occurs in a minority of patients. It can also cause hepatitis so all patients receiving this drug should periodically have their liver function assessed. Other agents that can be used in patients who require therapy but do not respond to splenectomy include high dose intravenous IgG to block the RE system (an expensive treatment that does not cure and may not induce a remission). More definitive treatments include other immunosuppressive agents, such as azathioprine and cyclophosphamide.

■ COLD REACTIVE (IgM) AUTOIMMUNE HEMOLYTIC ANEMIA

About 30 percent of patients have a cold reactive (IgM) autoimmune hemolytic anemia.

Serological Testing in the Transfusion Laboratory

Patients with cold (IgM) AIHA can present problems for the transfusion laboratory. Typically, the technologist will have difficulty during the major blood grouping (ABO) typing because the IgM cold agglutinin reacts at room temperature, and its potent agglutinating ability means that there will be agglutination in all tubes tested. This can be overcome by testing warm (37°C) and also by using warm saline washed red cells. The direct antiglobulin test demonstrates complement on the patient's red cells (C3d) and the indirect antiglobulin tests demonstrate the exceptionally high titer of agglutinins (IgM) that is most reactive in the cold and progressively less reactive in the warm. This is in contrast with the laboratory results in patients with warm AIHA. These patients have low titer autoantibody because most is bound to their red cells. Patients with cold AIHA have exceptionally high titer (many thousands of dilutions) of autoantibody present in their serum because the cold reactivity of the autoantibody means that most of it is not bound to their own red cells but is free in the plasma. It is helpful for the transfusion laboratory to titer out the reactivity at different temperatures. Those autoantibodies that react at progressively warmer temperatures (e.g., 22°C or higher) cause the most severe hemolysis in AIHA.

Presentation

The IgM autoantibodies react best in the cold because at low temperatures the red cell antigenic sites undergo conformational changes which make them reactive with the autoantibody. The cold-dependent nature of the autoantibody reactivity means that the coldest areas of the body (fingers, toes, tip of nose, ears, etc.) are affected. Symptoms are caused by two factors. First, the agglutination of the red cells in the extremities can cause physical sludging of the blood with reduced blood flow and decreased oxygen delivery, giving the characteristic cyanotic appearance of the fingers, ears, and nose in these patients. Rarely, the tissue ischemia can be so severe that it can lead to local gangrene. Sometimes these patients are misdiagnosed as having Raynaud's phenomenon. Second, enhanced red cell destruction can cause anemia. The red cell destruction, which is primarily extravascular, can produce severe anemia and secondary problems of generalized tissue on hypo-oxygenation (pallor, extreme fatigue, occasionally heart failure).

Pathophysiology of Red Cell Destruction

The autoantibodies bind to the red cells in the cooler regions of the body. Complement becomes deposited on the red cells and as the cells warm upon returning to the core of the body, the autoantibody elutes from the red cell and leaves complement components. Complement continues to be deposited, but seldom is the complement pathway completed, which results in intravascular red cell destruction. Rather, the red cells are removed by the phagocytic cells of the liver and other reticuloendothelial organs. Splenic clearance of the complement-sensitized red cell is minimal. In fact, intravascular red cell destruction is only likely to occur in these patients when their phagocytic system is overwhelmed, by a sudden influx of red cells sensitized by complement as occurs in patients receiving a red cell transfusion. The majority of autoantibodies are directed against the I-antigen on red cells. Certain infections (e.g., infectious mononucleosis) produce autoantibodies against I-antigen, which is seen on fetal cells and red cells recently released from the bone marrow (reticulocytes).

Evaluation of Patients with Suspected Cold AIHA

Many patients with cold AIHA seek medical attention because of complaints related to the red cell agglutination in their extremities (e.g., cyanotic fingers and toes). Splenomegaly is much less common than in patients with warm AIHA, but it is reported. Patients with cold AIHA should be investigated for evidence of a recent infection (frequently *Mycoplasma* pneumonia, infectious mononucleosis, or hepatitis). Patients should be carefully investigated for a lymphoproliferative disorder and not uncommonly a monoclonal paraprotein with cold autoantibody activity is observed. The laboratory investigation demonstrates anemia with occasional red cell agglutination (giving a falsely elevated MCV) observed on the blood film. Spherocytosis is far less common than warm AIHA but it can be observed. Polychromasia and reticulocytosis, as with warm AIHA, is also seen in most patients. As with warm AIHA, the patient's folate and ferritin should be measured.

Therapy

Frequently these patients require blood transfusion. Crossmatching these patients is seldom difficult, but occasionally the panreactivity of the cold agglutinin can lead to errors in ABO typing. Most physicians would transfuse these patients using a blood warmer and ensure that the patient is kept warm. Some physicians recommend raising the temperature in the patient's room and covering the patient with blankets. It is uncertain whether these maneuvers have a major clinical impact, but the minimal cost and noninvasive nature makes them a prudent consideration.

The nature of the autoantibody (IgM which is confined to the intravascular space) makes it an ideal candidate for treatment by plasma exchange and many patients with cold AIHA can be treated this way. However, the red cells can agglutinate during the procedure resulting in premature termination of the apheresis. Apheresis in the warm (37°C) has been used. Some patients are treated with corticosteroids, but unlike warm AIHA, corticosteroids have minimal impact on the disease. Some reports have described success with alkylating agents and occasionally splenectomy has been reported to be successful; however, splenectomy has minimal impact in most patients and seldom is used except under exceptional circumstances.

Types of Cold AIHA

The different types of cold agglutinins reflect different stimuli. For example, typical cold agglutinin disease is a *clonal* abnormality of B-lymphocytes with the agglutinin being monoclonal in nature. Certain infections such as infectious mononucleosis or *Mycoplasma* pneumonia produce polyclonal autoagglutinins.

Cold Agglutinin Disease

This rare disease is seen most frequently in elderly (over 60 to 70 years) men. The acrocyanosis is often so severe that the patient seeks medical attention because of it. Sometimes the cold agglutinin is so potent that the anticoagulated blood can be seen to sludge in the collection tube. The physical examination is normal and lymphadenopathy and hepatosplenomegaly suggest that there is an underlying lymphoproliferative disorder. These patients typically have an IgM monoclonal gammopathy that is red cell reactive (usually against the "I" antigen). Cold agglutinins against "I" usually are comprised of kappa light chains. The IgM monoclonal protein can be very high, sometimes resembling Waldenström's macroglobulinemia. Treatment includes avoidance of the cold. Immunosuppressive agents seldom are effective, but alkylating agents are often effective. Agents that have been used include cyclophosphamide and chlorambucil. The recently introduced agent, 2-chlorodeoxyadenosine, has proved very effective in some patients and could become the treatment of choice. In some patients, the cold agglutinin disease is secondary to a lymphoproliferative disorder such as a non-Hodgkin's lymphoma. These patients have lymphadenopathy, hepatosplenomegaly, or a monoclonal lymphocytic infiltration of their bone marrow. Treatment focuses on the treatment of the underlying lymphoma.

Post-Infection Cold AIHA

Cold AIHA can occur in children and adults after an infection. There are typical infections that trigger these hemolytic episodes and can include infectious mononucleosis (IgM, anti-i) and *Mycoplasma pneumoniae* (IgM anti-I). These infectious cold AIHA show major differences from the idiopathic cold AIHA including (1) their occurrence in children, young or middle aged adults (reflecting the age susceptibility of the various infectious agents); (2) the polyclonal nature of the IgM autoantibody; and (3) the usually transient nature of the cold AIHA. Treatment is supportive. If hemolysis is severe and persisting, plasma exchange therapy can be considered because it is highly effective in removing IgM, which is restricted to the intravascular compartment. The exchange fluid should be a 5 percent albumin to avoid the risk of viral infection associated with the use of plasma.

Acute Paroxysmal Cold Hemoglobinuria

This is a rare, but important, IgG-mediated cold AIHA that most frequently affects children. Like acute ITP of childhood, it follows an upper respiratory tract infection or a flulike illness. Although it is rare, it is the usual cause of acute AIHA in children (especially under the age of 5). The signs and symptoms reflect the acute intravascular hemolysis. Unlike almost all other forms of warm and cold AIHA, paroxysmal cold hemoglobinuria (PCH) is characterized by explosive *intravascular* hemolysis that results in hemoglobinuria (dark, brown urine). Jaundice is often seen and the severe anemia results in pallor. Often the children have abdominal pain, fever, and symptoms of the flu. The peripheral blood film can be normal, but polychromasia, spherocytosis, and rarely red cell fragmentation can be seen. Notably, *erythrophagocytosis* visible in the peripheral smear is often observed and while not specific for PCH, it strongly suggests the diagnosis. The low titer polyclonal IgG autoantibody of PCH is specific for the P antigen. PCH is diagnosed by the Donath-Landsteiner (DL) test. The direct (patient whole blood) or indirect (patient serum) tests have the same principle: blood is cooled (to allow the cold autoantibody to bind) and then warmed (to look for hemolysis). The test sensitivity can be enhanced by the addition of exogenous complement.

Treatment of PCH is supportive. Usually only P positive blood is available and we recommend using a blood warmer and keeping the patient warm. Seldom are other treatments, such as corticosteroids, required.

References

Engelfriet CP, Overbeeke MAM, von dem Borne AEG Jr. Autoimmune hemolytic anemia. Semin Hematol 1992; 29(1):3–12.

Heddle NM. Acute paroxysmal cold hemoglobinuria. Transfus Med Rev 1989; III(3):219–229.

Nydegger UE, Kazatchkine MD, Miescher PA. Immunopathologic and clinical features of hemolytic anemia due to cold agglutinins. Semin Hematol 1991; 28(1):66–77.

Sokol RJ, Booker DJ, Stamps R. The pathology of autoimmune haemolytic anaemia. J Clin Pathol 1992; 45:1047–1052.

SICKLE CELL DISEASE IN ADULTS

Paul F. Milner, M.D., F.R.C.Path.
Nancy F. Olivieri, M.D., F.R.C.P.C.

The sickle cell diseases are inherited anemias in which hemoglobin S (Hb S) replaces all or most of the normal hemoglobin A (Hb A). In North America the Hb S mutation is present in about 1 in 12 people of African descent. Such subjects are said to have sickle cell trait (A/S), which under normal conditions does not cause anemia or symptoms. However, at altitudes above 8,000 feet (2,500 meters), symptoms may occur. About 3 percent of persons with sickle cell traits may have one or more episodes of painless hematuria during their normal life.

Sickle cell anemia (S/S) can occur among the offspring of parents who both have sickle cell trait; the chance is 1 in 4. Similarly, if one parent is A/S and the other has a trait for Hb C (A/C), or a beta-thalassemia gene (A/β°thal or A/β^{+}thal), there is a 1 in 4 chance of an offspring with S/C, S/β°thal, or S/β^{+}thal. All these conditions can cause symptoms and anemia to various degrees (Table 1). The concomitant inheritance of an alpha-thalassemia (α-thal) gene, present in about 30 percent of patients of African descent, can modify the clinical expression of sickle cell disease, particularly of the S/S genotype. These patients are less anemic and often have a better physique but may get more frequent acute pain crises and bone infarcts. Finally, persistence of fetal hemoglobin (Hb F) in a high proportion of the red cells, which occurs in some patients, can also modify the clinical expression. The combination of alpha-thalassemia and a high level of Hb F in an S/S patient seems to be particularly beneficial.

Because of the broad spectrum of clinical expression of these inherited defects some patients will need a lot of care, while others need only to be seen for routine check-ups.

The transition from teenage dependence to adult self-reliance is difficult for the sickle cell anemia patient, and the frequency of symptoms often increases in early adult life, especially among men. Problems with getting or holding a job and poor attendance at college due to episodes of illness need medical and social service support. Hospital bills become a growing anxiety. However, many patients go for long periods without acute or severe exacerbation of their disease and with good quality of life, and some reach the sixth or seventh decade.

■ TREATMENT

Routine Care

The frequency of doctor visits and physical examinations depends very much on the type of sickle cell disease. Patients with Hb S/C or Beta^{+}thal or mild sickle cell anemia may not need to see a doctor more than once a year. However, some S/S patients require pain medication fairly frequently and need to see a doctor every 2 to 3 months. At routine visits it is important to question the patient for symptoms that can be caused by complications such as gallstones, osteonecrosis of the hips or shoulder joints, gout, or renal disease. On each occasion a thorough physical examination should be performed with these complications in mind, and blood should be drawn for a hematologic profile, including a reticulocyte count, and chemistries for liver and kidney function. Some clinical investigations should be ordered on a routine basis (see section on complications).

Contraception and Pregnancy

The use of oral contraceptives is not contraindicated in sickle cell disease. Low-estrogen preparations should be used and adjusted as necessary to prevent breakthrough bleeding and amenorrhea, which may occur frequently in those with sickle cell anemia. Alternatives are medroxyprogesterone acetate (Depo-Provera), given every 3 months, or levonorgesterel implant (Norplant), both of which suppress the menses that women frequently associate with the onset of pain crises.

Maternal mortality is low and pregnancy is not contraindicated. Most young women want to have 1 or 2 children, and with modern methods of fetal monitoring and careful prenatal care, they should be able to carry a fetus to maturity, although there is an increased incidence of spontaneous abortion in the first trimester. Symptoms may increase during pregnancy, and care of the patient should be shared between the physician and the obstetrician. Blood transfusions should be given only as clinically indicated. Early induction or cesarean section will often be needed to prevent fetal distress. Despite anecdotal reports, most Hb S/C women have an uneventful pregnancy and delivery.

Priapism

Attacks of priapism in young men can be distressing but should be managed conservatively as far as possible. They are usually self-limiting but may occur frequently. Attacks sometimes respond to nifedipine 10 mg or hydralazine 10 mg which can be repeated in about 4 hours but are usually effective in 15 to 30 minutes. The beta-adrenergic receptor agonist terbutaline (Brethine) 5 mg by mouth or by inhaler is also effective. If an acute attack persists for more than 24 hours, surgical procedures should be considered. The most successful is a corpora spongiosum shunt (Winter procedure), which should be carried out by a urologist. This involves inserting a needle or fine scalpel, under local anesthesia, through the glans into one of the corpora cavernosa and aspirating the viscous blood. After removal of the instrument a remaining communication permits continued drainage of cavernous blood from the penis to the systemic circulation. Subsequent erectile function should not be affected. Blood transfusion has little place in treatment but is often tried.

Pain Control at Home

Only about 40 percent of S/S patients and fewer S/C or S/beta-thal patients experience pain crises severe enough to require emergency treatment or hospital admission, but epi-

Table 1 Some Clinical Effects and Laboratory Values in Sickle Cell Disease

GENOTYPE	MAJOR CLINICAL EFFECTS	AVERAGE HEMATOLOGIC PROFILE	HEMOGLOBIN ELECTROPHORESIS RESULTS (%)	
S/S	Severe hemolytic anemia	Hb 6–9 g/dl*	A	0
	Stroke in childhood	PCV 18–30 g/dl*	S	80–95
	Splenic sequestration crises	MCV 85–110 fl	A_2	2–3.5*
	Aplastic crises		F	1–20
	Vaso-oclusive crises			
	Avascular necrosis of the femoral and humeral heads			
	Gallstones			
	Ankle ulcers			
S/β°thal	Moderate to severe anemia	Hb 7–10 g/dl	A	0
	Vaso-oclusive crises	PCV 20–35%	S	80–90
	Highest incidence of femoral head necrosis	MCV 65–80 fl	A_2	3–6
			F	10–20
S/C	Proliferative retinopathy	Hb 10–14 gl/dl	A	0
	Occasional vaso-oclusive crises	PCV 30–35%	S	50
	Aseptic necrosis of femoral head in about 5% of cases	MCV 75–90 fl	C	50
	Mild splenomegaly			
S/β⁺thal	Mild anemia	Hb 10–14 g/dl	A	10–25
	Rare vaso-oclusive crises	PCV 35–45%	S	70–85
	Avascular necrosis in about 5% of cases	MCV 65–80 fl	A_2	3.5–6
	Risk of proliferative retinopathy		F	1–15
S/dβ-thal	Mild anemia	Hb 10–12 g/dl	A	0
	Rare vaso-oclusive crises	PCV 36–40	S	70–80
	Rare complications	MCV 75–85 fl	A_2	1–3
			F	15–30

*S/S patients with concomitant alpha-thalassemia have Hb A_2 levels of 4 to 5 percent, a decreased mean corpuscular volume (MCV) of 75–65 fl, and a slightly higher hemoglobin and packed cell volume (PCV).

sodes of moderate pain lasting several days are not uncommon. These episodes may involve the joints, mainly the wrists, knees, and ankles, and are best treated with nonsteroidal analgesics. Joint effusions and painful bone infarcts respond well to indomethacin 25 mg three times a day. Joints need not be tapped unless septic arthritis is strongly suspected. Generalized pains may also respond to nonsteroidals but frequently require a narcotic preparation. Acetaminophen with 30 to 60 mg codeine or 7.5 mg of hydrocodone is often sufficient, but oxycodone 5 mg may sometimes be necessary. Oral meperidine and more addictive narcotics, such as oral morphine, diamorphine, and methadone, are best avoided except in special circumstances.

Narcotic Abuse

Prescriptions for narcotics should always be written for small amounts, 25 to 30 tablets at most. If more are required, the patient should return to be further evaluated. While habituation to narcotics may occur in a few patients, it is wrong to consider all patients who need narcotic pain medicine as addicts. With supporting care and continuity, narcotics can be used constructively. Emotional state and chronic anxiety are also important factors. An antidepressant, such as amitriptyline or nortriptyline 25 mg three times daily, can be useful in reducing narcotic usage. Interestingly, biofeedback-assisted relaxation methods can reduce the frequency of self-pain dosing at home while not changing the frequency of emergency room visits or hospitalizations.

The Pain Crisis

Contrary to popular belief, pain crises in adults are seldom associated with infection. Even severe infections, such as pneumococcal sepsis with high fever, may not precipitate the typical painful crisis. Severe pain is most frequently felt in the spine, the sternum, the ribs, and the long bones of the extremities. It is usually abrupt in onset, intense, and frightening. It is unpredictable and may go away within a few hours or a few days but frequently persists and gets worse until it cannot be tolerated. The patient who is used to these attacks will take oral narcotics before seeking medical assistance and will require further treatment for pain relief.

The essentials of treatment are intravenous fluid and adequate pain medication (Table 2). When managing these patients, allowance should be made for tolerance to narcotics, which reduces the duration of the analgesic effect. Although meperidine is the most popular narcotic, it is not the best. It tends to produce heavy sedation, but the patient still complains of pain. It has a short half-life and is metabolized to an inactive but toxic product, normeperidine, which can cause dysphoria, central nervous system excitation, and seizures. Morphine is a better narcotic. More hospitals are now using patient-controlled analgesic (PCA) pumps. These are ideal for sickle cell patients because their pain often comes in spasms, and with PCA they have more control over relief. The pump should be primed. It is important, whatever schedule is used, to gain the patient's confidence and provide efficient pain relief from the outset. As the patient's condition improves, the

Table 2 Treatment of the Adult Patient in Vaso-Occlusive Crisis

IN THE EMERGENCY ROOM

Hydration: Intravenous D5W at 200–250 ml/hr for the first 2 L, then D5¼NS at 100–150 ml/hr. If patient's condition has not improved after 8–12 hr, arrange admission to the hospital. If discharged, give 2 days' supply of oxycodone, 5–10 mg q 4 hr.

Pain medication: Buprenorphine* 0.3 mg by slow IV push (over 1 minute) into IV fluid line. If pain is not relieved in 30 minutes, repeat 0.3 mg deep IM injection. Pain will usually be relieved for 4–6 hr. If necessary repeat 0.3 mg IM after 4 hr. Phenergan 25 mg IM or IV prevents nausea and vomiting.

Morphine, 4 mg by slow IV push into fluid line. If there is no relief in 30 min, add 2–4 mg. Repeat the total dose after 3 and 6 hr if necessary.

Meperidine, 50–100 mg by slow IV push. If there is no relief in 60 min, repeat with 25 mg and add 75 mg to the IV bag to deliver over 4 hr. Maximum dose 200 mg.

Drugs of the nalorphine type (pentazocine, nalbuphine, butorphanol) are best avoided unless the patient's previous drug history is well known, because they can produce withdrawal symptoms in patients who have been chronically taking opiates.

IN THE HOSPITAL

Hydration: Continue D5W, alternating with D5½NS, at 100–150 ml/hr. Decrease when the patient is able to drink and eat a normal diet.

Pain medication: Morphine, 0.1–0.15 mg/kg (4–10 mg) into IV line every 2–3 hr†. If using an IV pump set to deliver at a fixed rate, the drug can be added to the infusion fluid and the dose titrated, e.g., 2.5–5 mg/hr. Meperidine 50–100 mg IV q 2–3 hr.

PCA‡: 1 mg/ml solution of morphine: After a loading dose of 2–4 mg, continuous infusion of 0.5–1.5 mg/hr to which the patient can add a bolus of 0.5–1 mg within a preset interval of 5–15 min. Maximum dose, 20 mg over 4 hr. Adjust the bolus dose and interval every 12 hr. Meperidine, 10 mg/ml solution: used in a similar manner, up to a maximum of 200 mg over 4 hr. Long-term use of meperidine may cause toxic side effects, e.g., seizures. Aspirin, 650 mg, ibuprofen, 600 mg, or indomethacin 25 mg PO or suppository, q 8 hr enhances analgesic effect.

Hydroxyizine, 50 mg deep IM or PO also effective with little extra sedation. Subcutaneous hydroxizine causes fat necrosis and is not suitable for IV use.

*For patients who use narcotics regularly, buprenorphine may not be effective.
†Using the IV route with small doses at frequent intervals, less drug is needed and unpredictable absorption and peak levels are avoided.
‡Patient-controlled analgesia.

dosage should be gradually reduced and changed to an oral preparation. In anxious patients, hydroxyzine 50 mg as necessary or amitriptyline 25 mg three times daily may be added. If there are joint effusions or swelling over bones, indomethacin 25 mg three times daily is very effective. Although informative, bone scans do not alter treatment and are usually unnecessary.

If peripheral venous access has been compromised, the external jugular vein is preferable to a central line, which carries the risk of pneumothorax. Some patients who have frequent hospitalizations and "no veins" will benefit from insertion of a Port-a-Cath. This can be placed in the external jugular under local anesthesia. The subcutaneous access port is placed just below the clavicle. It will require flushing with heparin-saline every 4 to 6 weeks.

On admission, hemoglobin and hematocrit levels may be slightly higher than steady-state levels, only to fall below these after a few days. In a patient confined to bed, blood transfusion is probably unnecessary if the hemoglobin level is above 5 g per deciliter and the reticulocyte count is elevated. When the crisis is over the hemoglobin will return to the steady-state level. There is no evidence to show that transfusion aborts or shortens an uncomplicated vaso-occlusive crisis. Fever is unusual in the first 24 hours or so, but as the crisis worsens, a mild fever frequently develops without obvious cause and is accompanied by leukocytosis.

Acute Chest Syndrome

Normal appearing lungs on the initial chest radiograph may subsequently show typical basal infiltrates as the crisis worsens. Occasionally pleurisy is a presenting symptom and a lung infiltrate with effusion is present on admission. Sputum production is often minimal, and this may help distinguish the sickle cell lung, which is due to sequestration of sickle cells or small lung infarcts, from true bacterial or viral pneumonia. A broad-spectrum antibiotic may be required to prevent secondary infection. Oxygen should be administered if blood gases show a fall in arterial PO_2 or O_2 saturation. In the rare case of a deteriorating patient, exchange transfusion is indicated and may be lifesaving.

■ COMPLICATIONS

Proliferative Sickle Retinopathy

Patients with Hb S/C or S/β^+ thal and to a lesser extent sickle cell anemia are at risk for proliferative retinopathy even in their early 20s. They should be referred to a retinal specialist and be followed at least every 2 years. Ablative laser treatment or cryotherapy is indicated for grade III disease to prevent vitreous hemorrhage and subsequent retinal detachment. S/S patients are at a much lower risk for serious eye complications but should get an initial retinal examination and a follow-up every few years, particularly if they have a relatively high hematocrit.

Gallstones

Almost 80 percent of S/S patients and 50 percent of S/C patients will develop gallstones. They consist of desiccated bilirubin or calcium bilirubinate, and only about 50 percent will be visible on a plain radiograph. It is, therefore, good practice to get a routine ultrasound examination of the upper abdomen. If gallstones are present, their significance should be discussed with the patient.

Some patients may remain symptom free for many years. Vague right upper quadrant pain and discomfort after meals can be relieved by antispasmodics such as dicyclomine 10 mg or hyoscyamine sulfate 0.125 mg per 5 ml, and symptoms may be avoided by restricting fried and fatty foods. When symptoms become chronic, elective cholecystectomy is advisable, but surgery is not indicated in the asymptomatic patient.

Osteonecrosis of the Femoral and Humeral Heads

Patients should be questioned about hip pain and shoulder pain, and the joints should be put through the full range of movement. Pain on internal rotation of the hip is an early sign indicating the need for a radiograph. If the radiograph is normal and pain persists, a bone scan or magnetic resonance imaging (MRI) examination is indicated. New orthopedic techniques are available for the treatment of osteonecrosis at an early stage, which avoids or delays for many years the necessity for total hip arthroplasty. Many patients become less symptomatic over time and may have a minimal disability despite the radiographic appearance of the femoral head.

As with the head of the femur, osteonecrosis of the humeral head can occur as early as the late teens and cause shoulder pain and decreased range of movement. The radiograph may show destruction of the humeral head. Most cases will settle down with nonsteroidal therapy, but if pain is persistent and chronic narcotics are required, arthroplasty may be advised.

Leg Ulcers

These rarely occur before the late teens but continue in patients over 40 years of age and seem to be commoner in the more anemic patients. They are essentially infarcts in the subcutaneous fat with death of overlying dermis and are most frequently seen on the lateral or medial side of the ankle. They occasionally occur higher up on the shin. The necrotic tissue becomes easily infected, and like a bed sore, they are difficult to heal.

The first goal of treatment is to eradicate the infection. The foot or leg should be immersed for 30 minutes in a tub of warm water, to each gallon of which has been added a tablespoon of salt and one or two tablespoons of hypochlorite solution (household chlorine bleach). Bathing should be done at least twice a day and the ulcer covered with a wad of gauze soaked in the same solution and kept in place with a bandage. If there is a very deep slough, the use of a proteolytic enzyme preparation such as Colaginase or Elase may be applied every night.

Once the ulcer is clean, healing can begin. A zinc oxide-impregnated bandage (Unna's boot) should then be applied to cover the ulcer and a generous area above and below. The boot can be cut up one side and removed and replaced every week until healing has occurred. The preparation Duoderm is very effective in speeding up healing when applied to a clean ulcer. It is left in place for several days and a new piece applied after bathing as described above.

Elevation of the leg and the avoidance of prolonged standing are essential for a successful outcome. Blood transfusion is unnecessary if the above regimen is followed. Topical antibiotics, except chloramphenicol, often cause allergic dermatitis and are best avoided.

Renal Insufficiency

Most patients with sickle cell disease have a low urinary specific gravity and an inability to concentrate urine while on fluid deprivation. The resulting polyuria and nocturia may be a precipitating cause of vaso-occlusive crises if fluid intake is reduced. Proteinuria is a common finding; about 30 percent of S/S patients have more than a trace. Some of this is probably attributable to papillary necrosis and is frequently associated with microscopic hematuria. Random blood urea nitrogen (BUN) and creatinine levels are usually below the normal ranges for age. A BUN of 15 mg/dl and a creatinine of 1.5 mg/dl are three times the average for sickle cell anemia and may indicate early renal insufficiency. Mild hyperuricemia is also not uncommon and may be controlled with probenecid 0.5 g twice daily. A few patients will require allopurinol 100 to 300 mg per day.

Increasing renal insufficiency, ultimately leading to renal failure, is an important cause of poor health in S/S patients over 40 years and occasionally in younger subjects. An early feature is worsening anemia with hemoglobin levels below 5 g per deciliter. Some patients can tolerate this for long periods, but others will need intermittent blood transfusion. This prolonged predialysis phase is a difficult time for these patients. The administration of erythropoietin may make a difference to their quality of life; the effective dose has to be arrived at by individual trial. Vaso-occlusive crises can be precipitated by raising the hematocrit too high, and they have been reported after renal transplants in these patients. Further developments in the therapy of sickle cell disease may help to deal with this problem.

■ SURGERY AND ANESTHESIA

No single measure can replace good clinical judgment as to whether it is necessary to transfuse a patient prior to surgery. The risk of hypoxia during induction is the same as for a normal patient because sickling does not occur instantaneously. There is no clinical basis for the much advocated formulas that call for reduction of Hb S to a predetermined level before anesthesia. Published reports of large series of patients have shown that anesthesia does not precipitate a crisis if it is properly handled. Also, anesthetic gases such as halothane, foran, and ethrane have been shown to have antisickling properties, and under anesthesia the patient is getting oxygen and intravenous hydration.

Preoperative transfusion should be considered if the hemoglobin is below 8 g per deciliter and considerable blood loss is expected. Otherwise, for most surgery lost blood should simply be replaced. In cardiothoracic or brain surgery, in which hypothermia or extracorporeal procedures will be used, exchange transfusion to remove most of the patient's red cells (to achieve about 10 to 15 percent Hb S in the post-transfusion sample) is advisable. This may require two exchanges with a few days in between. The procedure is best carried out using a cell-separating machine so as to maintain an adequate platelet count. Excessive transfusion in the absence of an exchange should be avoided because there is clear evidence that the higher the whole blood viscosity, the more likely are postoperative complications. Blood viscosity is largely a function of the hematocrit level, and this may be a concern in patients with S/C disease. Preoperative transfusion is not indicated in Hb S/β^+ thal patients who have 10 to 35 percent Hb A in every red cell. Hb S/C patients with a high hematocrit, who are at risk for cerebral complications, can be phlebotomized down to a hematocrit of about 35 percent preoperatively and any major blood loss replaced at surgery. This should be satisfactory for prolonged and bloody procedures such as total hip surgery.

When planning exchange transfusions requiring many units of blood, the risks of unexpected incompatibility must be considered. All major blood group antigens should be matched between the patient and the donors. A delayed transfusion reaction in an extensively exchanged patient may be fatal and is a tragedy if the exchange transfusion was not necessary.

■ PROGNOSIS

With good clinical care the outlook for patients with sickle cell disease is better now than at any other time, but frequent, prolonged vaso-occlusive crises, severe hemolysis, or renal insufficiency is an indication of a poor prognosis. A recently published 10 year study of more than 2,000 patients over 5 years of age found a mean age at death in sickle cell anemia of 40 years for men and 48 years for women. Several experimental approaches being explored may reduce hemolysis and decrease the frequency of vaso-occlusive crises that cause organ damage. The most promising of these is hydroxyurea, which greatly increases the proportion of fetal hemoglobin in many of the red cells. This inhibits the formation of Hb S polymers and sickling of those cells so that hemolysis is decreased, red cell life span is increased, anemia is improved, and the frequency of vaso-occlusive crises is diminished.

■ NEW THERAPEUTIC REGIMENS

Hydroxyurea

In 1993, a randomized, double-blind, placebo-controlled clinical trial was started to test the hypothesis that hydroxyurea, taken in a daily dosage of 15 to 30 mg per kilogram, could reduce the frequency of painful crises in adults with sickle cell anemia by at least 50 percent. The trial was stopped a few months short of the 24 planned for its completion, because of the compelling results which indicated that the goal of the trial had been achieved. Side effects were insignificant and easily managed. Hydroxyurea, often in a dose as low as 10–12 mg per kilogram per day, taken with 1 mg of folic acid, can raise Hb F levels to more than 20 percent. The response may be linked to genetic factors that control the synthesis of Hb F in adults. Patients vary, but most will respond to two capsules, or 1,000 mg per day in a single dose. The response is gradual over several months; the dose should not be increased until the Hb F level has reached a plateau and compliance with the daily dose schedule is assured. Body weight increases and clinical well-being improves. The mean corpuscular volume increases to 120 fl or more and the mean corpuscular hemoglobin to 40 pg or more, but the red blood cell count may decrease slightly. The reticulocyte count and serum bilirubin level also decrease, indicating decreased hemolysis. The white blood cell and neutrophil counts decrease from the usual high numbers in these patients, but care must be taken not to let the latter go too low. This is the main toxic effect for which the dose should be decreased or temporarily discontinued. The platelet count decreases but only to more normal numbers. This therapy is the greatest single advance in the treatment of patients with severe sickle cell anemia and, in some patients, can produce a dramatic improvement in overall clinical condition. The possibility of long-term malignancies is a concern, but experience with hydroxyurea in other conditions suggests the risk is very small.

Bone Marrow Transplantation

Successful allogeneic bone marrow transplantation (BMT) offers a cure to children with sickle cell disease. At the time of writing, details have been published of 55 sickle cell anemia patients aged 11 months to 26 years, who have undergone bone marrow transplantation in several centers worldwide including the United States. The results are summarized in Table 3. In all but one procedure an HLA-identical sibling or parent donated marrow. In one patient, who received a transplant from a three-antigen mismatched relative, BMT was followed by death. Sixteen (29 percent) of the patients received regular transfusions prior to BMT, and transfusion dependence for various complications of sickle cell disease, including stroke, was the most frequent indication. In three patients an unrelated condition (AML [acute myeloid leukemia], ALL [acute lymphatic leukemia], and Morquio's disease, respectively) was present. Conditioning regimens were similar to those used in patients undergoing allogeneic bone marrow transplantation for homozygous beta-thalassemia (see Table 3).

There have been five BMT-associated deaths (9 percent), and a second BMT was required in four patients for failure of engraftment. The largest series (from Belgium) reported a 14 percent incidence of graft versus host disease. Interestingly, return of splenic function, as demonstrated by absence of Howell-Jolly bodies in the blood smear and by splenic technetium 99m imaging, has been reported in 11 patients and may have occurred in others.

For the severely affected child, bone marrow transplantation from a compatible sibling may now be a feasible proposition, as advances in post-transplantation management have significantly reduced mortality. It is difficult from this early experience to establish guidelines for the use of BMT in children with sickle cell disease. Careful selection of patients is important because early data indicate that patients with sickle cell disease, especially those with prior stroke, may be at increased risk for neurologic complications in the peritransplant period. It has been suggested that symptomatic patients who lack extensive neurovascular or other end organ damage from sickle vasculopathy are likely to have the best outcomes following BMT. Unfortunately, only about 18 percent of children with sickle cell disease have an HLA-compatible sibling. Finding financial resources for adequate care for these children, many of whom come from poor families, is perhaps as important as new therapeutic approaches, which will almost certainly be expensive.

Table 3 Reported Results of Bone Marrow Transplantation in Sickle Cell Anemia

CENTER	NO. OF PATIENTS	GENOTYPE	AGE (YEARS)	PRETRANSPLANT COMPLICATIONS	DONOR	CONDITIONING REGIMEN	OUTCOME	GVHD
Pesaro, Italy	4	S/β° thal	4–11	CVA (1) Regular Tx (2)	HLA identical sib (3) 3 Ag # (1)	Bu 14, Cy 200 ALG (1)	Death (3) A&W (1)	No
Pesaro	4	SS	7–26	Regular Tx (4)	HLA identical sib	Bu 14, Cy 120–200 ALG (2)	A&W (4)	No
France	14	SS	2.2–14.8	CVA (3) Regular Tx (4)	HLA identical sib	Bu 14–16, Cy 200–60 TLI (1); ATG (1) CSA ± MTX	No engraftment →2nd BMT (1) Chimerism (3)	5 acute 3 chronic
Charleston, SC	2	SS	3.8–9.5	CVA; moyamoya (1)	HLA identical sib	BU 14, Cy 200 CSA ± Pred G-CSF	A&W (1) Seizure; extension of old CVA (1)	No
Memphis, TN	1	SS/AML	8	Frequent VOC	HLA identical sib	Cy 120 TBI; Pred + MTX	A&W	Chronic GVHD, resolved
France	1	SS/ALL	22	Tx and Chelation Rx	HLA identical sib	Cy 120; TBI; CSA	No engraftment →2nd BMT; Death	
San Francisco	1	SS/Morquio's disease	4	Frequent VOC	HLA identical sib	Bu 15; Cy 200 ATG; TBI	Successful	No
Belgium	28	SS	0.9–23	ACS (3) CVA (2) Regular Tx (5)	HLA identical sib (27) HLA identical father (1)	Bu 14–16, Cy 200 ATG (2) TAI (8) CSA + MTX	Survival 96% Disease free survival 89% No engraftment →2nd BMT (2) Death (1)	14%

A&W, alive and well; CVA, cerebrovascular accident; Tx, transfusions; ACS, acute chest syndrome; VOC, vaso-occlusive crises; Pred, prednisone; ATG, anti-thymocyte globulin; MTX, methotrexate; Bu, busulfan; Cy, cyclophosphamide; ALG, anti-lymphocyte globulin; TLI, total lymphoid irradiation; CSA, cyclosporin A; TBI, total body irradiation; GCSF, granulocyte colony stimulating factor

Suggested Reading

Embury SH, Hebbel RP, Narla M, Steinberg MH, eds. Sickle cell disease: Scientific principles and clinical practice. New York: Raven Press, 1994.

Principles of analgesic use in the treatment of acute pain and cancer pain. 3rd ed., Skokie, IL: American Pain Society.

Shapiro BS. The management of pain in sickle cell disease. Pediatr Clin North Am 1989; 36:1029–1045.

Sullivan KM, guest ed. Role of bone marrow transplantation in sickle cell anemia. Semin Hematol 1991; 28:172–267.

White PF. Use of patient-controlled analgesia for management of acute pain. JAMA 1988; 259:243–247.

POLYCYTHEMIA RUBRA VERA

Arthur I. Radin, M.D., F.A.C.P.

Polycythemia rubra vera (PRV) is a low-grade malignancy of the hematopoietic stem cell. The primary manifestation of this disease is an expansion of the red cell mass. However, its identity as a stem cell disorder is expressed in the clinical manifestations and natural history of the disease.

Polycythemia rubra vera progresses through a number of well-recognized clinical phases. It most commonly presents in the proliferative stage, characterized by the excessive production of red cells, granulocytes, and platelets. Typically the onset is insidious, and the elevated hematocrit is an incidental finding on blood tests drawn for unrelated reasons. Patients with more advanced peripheral blood abnormalities may have symptoms suggesting impaired circulation to the heart, central nervous system, or extremities. Approximately 30 percent of patients report a hemostatic complication at some time during the course. Pruritus, often made worse by bathing, and splenomegaly are characteristic of this disorder.

An appreciable minority of patients will enter the stable phase, during which essentially normal blood counts are maintained for months or years without specific therapy. Approximately 10 percent of patients will progress to post-polycythemic myeloid metaplasia with myelofibrosis, more commonly called the *spent phase* of the disease. This stage is characterized by extensive marrow fibrosis, hepatosplenomegaly, and peripheral cytopenias resembling agnogenic myeloid metaplasia clinically and pathologically. Generally the spent phase develops 2 to 13 years after the polycythemia has been manifest; but rarely, myelofibrosis may precede or appear coincident with the erythrocytosis.

■ DIAGNOSIS

The first obligation of the physician who has assumed responsibility for a patient with polycythemia is to determine its cause. PRV must be distinguished from relative (or stress) polycythemia, in which the red cell mass is in the normal or high-normal range, and from secondary polycythemia, a heterogeneous group of disorders in which the red cell mass has increased in response to factors originating beyond the bone marrow. In most cases PRV can be differentiated from these other conditions without difficulty, using the diagnostic criteria set forth by the Polycythemia Vera Study Group (Table 1). These standards are quite stringent and may exclude patients with early disease or mild manifestations of the illness. However, at a minimum the diagnosis of PRV requires confirmation of an elevated red cell mass and evidence of stem cell involvement.

Table 1 Diagnostic Criteria of the Polycythemia Vera Study Group for Polycythemia Rubra Vera

CATEGORY A

- Increased red cell volume by ^{31}chromium-labeled red cell determination
  - Men ≥36 ml/kg
  - Women ≥32 ml/kg
- Arterial oxygen saturation ≥92%
- Splenomegaly

CATEGORY B

- Thrombocytosis: platelets ≥400,000/mm^3
- Leukocytosis: WBC ≥12,000/mm^3 in the absence of fever or infection
- Elevated leukocyte alkaline phosphatase score: >100 in the absence of fever or infection
- Serum B_{12} >900 pg/ml or unbound B_{12}-binding capacity >2,200 pg/ml

CRITERIA FOR DIAGNOSIS

- All three conditions in category A are present; or
- The combination of an elevated red cell mass and normal oxygen saturation is present, along with any two conditions in category B

In equivocal cases a number of laboratory tests may help to establish the diagnosis (Table 2). Cytogenetic analysis may reveal clonal chromosomal abnormalities in approximately one-fifth of cases at presentation; most frequently complete or partial trisomy of chromosomes 1, 8, or 9; or deletions of the long arm of chromosome 20. Serum erythropoietin levels in PRV should be normal or depressed, and generally remain suppressed below the lower limits of normal, even when the patient's hemoglobin is maintained within the normal range by phlebotomy. Elevated serum erythropoietin levels suggest secondary erythrocytosis. As PRV is a stem cell disorder affecting platelets as well as the erythron, abnormalities in the platelet size distribution width (PDW) and the platelet nucleotide (ATP:ADP) ratio may also be detected. In selected

Table 2 Tests for the Evaluation of an Elevated Hematocrit

Complete blood count with WBC differential and quantitative platelet count
Leukocyte alkaline phosphatase
Serum B_{12} and B_{12} binders
Radionuclide determination of red cell mass and plasma volume
Arterial oxygen saturation
Smokers: carboxyhemoglobin level
Hemoglobin P_{50} to exclude a high oxygen-affinity hemoglobinopathy
Erythropoietin assay
Imaging of the kidneys—IVP, CT scan, or ultrasonogram
Imaging of the liver, spleen, and brain as clinically indicated
Bone marrow examination with cytogenetics
Bone marrow or peripheral blood erythroid colony formation

patients, in vitro culture of erythroid progenitors (BFU-E) may be useful. The hematopoietic stem cell in PRV is extremely sensitive to erythropoietin and will grow in culture without the addition of this growth factor, whereas normal erythroid precursors will not. As the blood of patients with PRV may contain significant numbers of circulating red blood cell precursors, these stem cell assays may be performed on samples of peripheral blood. Recently a scoring system for the diagnosis of PRV was developed based on these nonconventional criteria and was proved to be highly accurate in distinguishing PRV from secondary causes of polycythemia. At present, the in vitro assays employed in this diagnostic system are not ordinarily accessible to the clinician. However, these tests are likely to grow in importance as their availability increases.

■ CONTROL OF THE RED CELL MASS

The principal symptoms of polycythemia vera and many of its more serious complications can be related directly to the overproduction of red blood cells. This has three major effects: the total blood volume expands; the red cell mass and therefore the hematocrit increases beyond safe limits; and the metabolic demands on the patient rise. Since whole blood viscosity increases approximately as the third power of the hematocrit, even a small change in the red cell mass can have a significant effect on hemodynamics. Moreover, the greater blood volume in these patients distends their veins and increases the cross-sectional area of their blood vessels. This can reduce the mean linear rate of blood flow, so that in some vessels blood may be virtually stagnant. Together these effects more than offset the potential benefit of the increased hemoglobin in transporting oxygen to the tissues. Circulation is impaired, and the relative oxygen transport capacity of the blood is decreased.

The most direct way to reduce the red cell mass is simply to remove blood by phlebotomy. In fact, phlebotomy has proved to be the safest and most reliable means of treating patients with this disease. Prompt reduction of the hematocrit speedily relieves symptoms and substantially reduces the patient's risk of catastrophic complications. Depending on the urgency of treatment and the ability of the patient to tolerate rapid changes in blood volume, phlebotomies of one unit of blood should be performed daily or two to three times per week until the hematocrit is within normal range. Traditionally it has been said that the hematocrit should be maintained below 46 percent. However, vascular complications appear to be more frequent as the hematocrit approaches this limit, and cerebral blood flow may be impaired even at this level. It appears prudent to maintain the hematocrit closer to 40 percent.

Advanced age is not a contraindication to phlebotomy, although in elderly patients and those with cardiovascular disease, smaller volumes of blood (e.g., 200 to 300 ml) may be removed at each treatment. Some physicians prefer to treat their most fragile patients by infusing fluids in one arm while withdrawing blood from the other to avoid dehydration and rapid hemodynamic changes. In crises, such as in preparation for emergency surgery, intensive phlebotomy with plasma replacement can be lifesaving.

Patients managed by phlebotomy will rapidly deplete their iron stores, and red cell production will become impaired. Since iron absorbed from dietary sources will be used almost exclusively to produce red blood cells, patients should be advised to avoid iron supplements and medicines that contain iron. The induced iron deficiency rarely causes clinical symptoms; however, severe iron deficiency can make the red blood cell more rigid and may exacerbate the thrombotic tendency in some patients. Thus, although mild iron deficiency can facilitate the management of the red cell mass and may be desirable, severe iron deficiency should be avoided. Iron supplementation at reduced doses may be considered for patients who develop symptoms or hematologic signs of severe iron deficiency (e.g., a mean corpuscular hemoglobin less than 22 pg). Vigilant monitoring of the patient is necessary during iron treatment to avoid potentially dangerous elevations in the hematocrit.

■ MYELOSUPPRESSION

Although phlebotomy satisfactorily controls the foremost symptoms of PRV, it does not address the underlying disease process. Myelosuppressive agents, directed against the malignant clone itself, are often required to manage the other distressing and life-threatening complications of the illness. First, these agents further suppress erythropoiesis, facilitating the management of the red cell mass. Between 50 and 80 percent of patients treated with myelosuppressive agents are relieved of the need for phlebotomy. In addition, myelosuppression has proved effective in checking the hypermetabolic state in most patients, controlling the leukocytosis and thrombocytosis characteristic of this stem cell disorder, shrinking the spleen, and reducing the risk of thromboembolic complications. However, because of the risks of these drugs, most notably that of secondary malignancies, myelosuppressive therapy cannot be recommended for all patients. Therapy must be tailored to the individual, balancing the patient's risk of morbidity from the disease against the potential for immediate and long-term complications of this treatment.

Present recommendations for use of myelosuppressive agents are based principally on the experience of the Polycythemia Vera Study Group (PVSG). In a landmark multi-institutional study, 431 patients meeting the strict criteria for PRV were randomized to treatment by phlebotomy alone or by phlebotomy plus myelosuppression using either radioactive phosphorus (^{32}P) or chlorambucil. During the first 5 years of treatment the mortality rates among the three groups were similar; however, the incidence of nonfatal thrombotic episodes was significantly higher in the group managed by phlebotomy alone. Risk factors for thrombosis included advanced age, a history of thrombotic events, and a greater than average requirement for phlebotomy. During the following 10 years, however, the mortality rate of patients treated with myelosuppressive agents exceeded that of the phlebotomy group. The increase in mortality was due primarily to an increased incidence of secondary malignancies, including acute leukemia, lymphoblastic lymphoma, and various carcinomas, particularly those of the skin and gastrointestinal tract. Acute leukemia developed earlier in patients treated with chlorambucil than with ^{32}P: the median time to the development of leukemia in these two groups was approximately 5 years and 6 to 10 years, respectively.

These observations have prompted general recommendations for the treatment of PRV. In patients under age 50 with no history of thrombosis and relatively low phlebotomy requirements, myelosuppressive therapy appears ill advised. The risk of thromboembolic complications is low in these patients, and their overall survival may be diminished by the development of secondary malignancies. Phlebotomy alone appears to be the most appropriate management. In patients over age 70 the incidence of thrombotic events is considerably greater. Considering the advanced age of these patients and the long interval required for secondary malignancies to evolve, myelosuppression appears justified. In patients between ages 50 and 70 years the decision to embark on myelosuppressive therapy should be based on an assessment of that individual's symptoms and risk of thrombotic complications.

Chlorambucil is no longer considered an appropriate myelosuppressive medicine in PRV because of its inordinate carcinogenic properties. Rather, the myelosuppressive agents most commonly employed in this illness include ^{32}P, busulfan, hydroxyurea, and interferon-alpha. Recently, hydroxyurea and interferon have emerged as the agents of choice in PRV due to their low carcinogenic potential. However, ^{32}P and busulfan remain appropriate alternatives for patients who fail to achieve adequate disease control with first-line therapy, in whom compliance is doubtful, or who experience untoward effects from these drugs.

Radioactive ^{32}P is given intravenously as a bolus at 2.3 to 3 mCi per square meter, with no single dose to exceed 5 mCi. Occasionally additional doses of ^{32}P may be required to achieve optimal disease control. To avoid excessive myelosuppression, these treatments should be repeated no more frequently than every 3 to 6 months. Hematologic improvement is obtained in 75 to 85 percent of cases, with maximum effects evident approximately 10 weeks after therapy. The chief advantage of ^{32}P is its long duration of action: a single treatment may control the disease for 6 to 24 months. Thus, compliance is not an issue. Untoward effects of ^{32}P include unpredictable degrees of myelosuppression, subtle alterations in immune function, and secondary leukemias.

Busulfan is an alkanesulfonate ester with pharmacologic properties distinct from those of the classic alkylating agents such as chlorambucil and the other nitrogen mustards. Usually it is administered at 4 to 6 mg daily for 4 to 6 weeks, or until the platelet count is below 300,000/per cubic millimeter. Remissions may be obtained with this regimen in approximately 50 percent of cases. In a European cooperative group study comparing busulfan with ^{32}P as a supplement to phlebotomy, busulfan induced longer remissions and resulted in a longer median survival than ^{32}P. The leukemogenic potentials of the two agents were similar. However, the potential for cumulative, irreversible myelosuppression and a variety of nonhematologic toxicities including pulmonary fibrosis, an Addisonian-like syndrome of asthenia, and cutaneous hyperpigmentation undermine the attractiveness of this agent.

Hydroxyurea is an inhibitor of ribonucleotide reductase, an enzyme required for the synthesis of deoxyribonucleotides and ultimately of DNA. Since it does not interact with DNA directly, its mutagenic potential is considerably less than that of the alkylating agents. The incidence of leukemia in patients treated with hydroxyurea has been estimated at 1.0 to 5.9 percent, which may not be significantly greater than that of patients treated by phlebotomy alone. At doses of 15 to 30 mg per kilogram daily, approximately 70 to 80 percent of patients will achieve long-term control of their disease. The chief shortcoming of this drug is its relatively brief duration of action, which may cause peripheral blood counts to be erratic. Also, it appears to affect the production of white blood cells to a greater degree than red blood cells. Therefore, mild leukopenia may be unavoidable, and supplemental phlebotomies may be required. Other untoward effects include gastrointestinal discomfort, fevers, rash, stomatitis, hepatitis, and possibly renál dysfunction. Experience with this drug in PRV is relatively limited, and additional long-term studies will be necessary to determine its appropriate role in therapy.

The advent of the biologic response modifiers and in particular of interferon-alpha is the newest and most exciting advance in the treatment of the myeloproliferative disorders. The basis for interferon's activity in PRV is uncertain, although a general antiproliferative effect, the induction of differentiation, and potentiation of the host's immune surveillance system have been implicated. Side effects of interferon therapy include a flulike syndrome, fatigue, fevers, weight loss, myalgias, alopecia, gastrointestinal upset, and liver function test abnormalities. Rarely, neutralizing antibodies to interferon-alpha may form resulting in a loss of biologic activity. In certain cases, therapy may be continued successfully by employing a different interferon preparation (e.g., substituting interferon-alpha$_{2a}$ for interferon-alpha$_{2b}$).

As is true of the other myelosuppressive drugs that have been used to treat PRV, interferon-alpha is effective in controlling the hyperproliferative manifestations of the disease. In one series, 13 patients with PRV were treated with recombinant interferon-alpha$_{2b}$ administered at 3 million units intramuscularly three times a week for 1 year. Ten of the 13 (77 percent) needed less phlebotomy, and in 4 patients the need for phlebotomy was completely abrogated. Moreover, in all the responders, the degree of thrombocytosis and splenomegaly improved. In a second report, interferon was used in an attempt to control thrombocytosis in 31 patients with a variety of myeloproliferative disorders refractory to standard therapy. Thrombocytosis was controlled in 71 percent of patients, and the number of disease-associated symptoms, including venous and arterial thromboses, was diminished in almost all cases. Most encouraging, these responses also included improved erythropoiesis, control of leukocytosis, and improvement in bone marrow histology.

In contrast to the other myelosuppressive agents, interferon therapy may improve bone marrow histology in patients with PRV and related myeloproliferative disorders. In one study of 19 patients with PRV treated with interferon-alpha for one year, the mean cellularity of the bone marrow was reduced from a mean of 80.5 percent to 69.1 percent. Also, a decrease in the number, density, and morphometric parameters of the megakaryocytes was observed. Regression of reticulin fibrosis was appreciated in only 2 of 13 patients, so that the ability of interferon to prevent or reverse myelofibrosis was not yet established.

These benefits of interferon therapy were confirmed in a prospective, randomized, cross-over trial. Twenty-two patients with PRV were treated alternatively for 5 months each with 3 million units of interferon-alpha subcutaneously daily, or by phlebotomy alone. While the hematocrit was equally well controlled with either therapy, patients on interferon reported a significant improvement in their symptoms, primarily pruritus and paresthesias; and in 6 of 14 patients with splenomegaly, the spleen decreased in size. Bone marrow cellularity improved in 14 of 21 patients; and in one patient with a clonal chromosomal abnormality, a complete cytogenetic remission was achieved.

These effects of interferon suggest a biologic effect that distinguishes it from the other myelosuppressive agents. Potentially, these effects may modify the natural history of the disease, and delay progression to the myelofibrotic, or spent phase. Moreover, interferon has no known carcinogenic properties. For these reasons, some investigators believe that interferon therapy is appropriate for all patients with PRV, even those who traditionally have been managed by phlebotomy alone. Although the number of patients with PRV who have been treated with interferon remains small, and the duration of follow-up remains relatively short, interferon may become the drug of choice in PRV. Larger, prospective studies are in progress to confirm these results, and to determine the proper role of interferon-alpha$_2$ in the treatment of this disorder.

■ HEMOSTATIC COMPLICATIONS

Hemorrhagic and thrombotic events, the leading causes of morbidity in this disease, are reported as the cause of death in 20 to 40 percent of patients.

The prevention of hemostatic complications is the most appropriate therapeutic strategy. Fortunately, this goal can usually be achieved with proper management. Control of the red cell mass is of primary importance, using phlebotomy and/or myelosuppression as suitable. In one study the rate of thrombotic episodes was more than 10 times as great for patients with hematocrits above 60 percent than for patients with hematocrits between 40 and 44 percent. Unfortunately, the published studies were not designed to examine the contribution of thrombocytosis and/or platelet dysfunction to the hemostatic diathesis, and the effect of these factors on the incidence of thrombotic events remains controversial. Neither in vitro tests of platelet function nor the bleeding time has correlated with the risk of hemostatic complications, and neither has been of value in directing therapy. For these reasons a comprehensive evaluation of the patient's platelet function cannot be recommended in asymptomatic patients, nor should modest elevations in the platelet count cause undue concern. It is reasonable, however, to consider severe thrombocytosis (greater than 1 million per cubic millimeter) as another possible risk factor for thrombotic events when considering myelosuppressive therapy.

Antiplatelet therapy should not be recommended for antithrombotic prophylaxis regardless of the patient's platelet count. In a PVSG study, aspirin at 300 mg three times daily and dipyridamole at 75 mg three times daily as a supplement to phlebotomy failed to reduce the incidence of thrombosis. However, the incidence of significant gastrointestinal hemorrhages increased significantly. Antiplatelet therapy may be appropriate as short-term treatment for patients who have suffered recent microvascular occlusive episodes. However, myelosuppressive therapy as described remains the best therapeutic option for the prevention of thrombohemorrhagic complications.

Hemostatic complications that do arise should be treated in the usual manner, with particular attention to the correction of any pre-existing coagulation disorders. Acquired abnormalities in von Willebrand factor (VWF) and deficiencies of clotting factors V and XII are common in PRV and should be considered in the patient's evaluation. Low-grade disseminated intravascular coagulation (DIC) should also be excluded. Infusions of 1-deamino-8-D-arginine vasopressin (DDAVP) or plasma fractions may have benefit. Platelet transfusions also may be justified even in the face of a normal or elevated platelet count, since the patient's own platelets are frequently dysfunctional. Acute thrombotic episodes can be treated with heparin followed by warfarin anticoagulation. Patients with severe thrombocytosis may appear relatively resistant to heparin anticoagulation, however, due to the antiheparin effect of platelets.

Recent advances in the understanding of PRV may improve the ability to prevent and manage these hemostatic complications. It has been reported that patients with the greatest reduction in platelet serotonin content exhibit the greatest prolongation in their bleeding times following a test dose of aspirin. These patients may be at the greatest risk for complications should antiplatelet therapy be initiated. Similarly, it has been reported that individuals with PRV who additionally have abnormalities of VWF, particularly deficiencies of the high molecular-weight multimers, are at an increased risk for hemorrhage. In one study fully 75 percent of patients with VWF abnormalities reported a bleeding tendency. As our ability to determine which patients are at the greatest risk for hemorrhage or thrombosis improves, therapy can be fashioned more appropriately to the individual.

■ PRURITUS

Pruritus is one of the more common and troublesome symptoms of PRV, affecting 14 to 52 percent of patients in different reports. This symptom too commonly is dismissed by the physician as unimportant, for it has little effect on the prognosis or clinical course of the disease. However, to the afflicted patient it is one of the more distressing and even disabling aspects of the illness.

Pruritus in these patients appears to be multifactorial in origin, and no single therapeutic approach has proved uniformly successful. Two-thirds of patients with uncontrolled PRV have elevated plasma or urine histamine levels, suggesting a causative role for this factor. Serotonin and prostaglandins released by the neoplastic platelets may also mediate the itch. Customarily, the first agents employed are antihistamines, since these are relatively free of side effects. In most cases treatment is started with a histamine (H_1) blocker such as diphenhydramine hydrochloride or hydroxyzine. However, H_1 blockade alone is ineffective for most patients, and the addition of an H_2 blocker such as cimetidine may improve the response. Combined histamine and serotonin blockade using doxepin hydrochloride, trifluoroperazine hydrochloride, and cyproheptadine also has been used with success.

If these measures fail, iron supplementation may be considered. The pathogenesis of pruritus in iron deficiency is unknown, but the association is well documented, even in otherwise normal individuals with iron deficiency anemia. Iron supplements invariably accelerate erythropoiesis, however, and the patient must be monitored closely to prevent a rapid and unacceptable rise in hematocrit. Once the pruritus is controlled, the dose of iron should be reduced as much as possible to limit erythropoiesis. Anecdotal reports in the literature suggest that ultraviolet light, photochemotherapy using psoralens combined with ultraviolet A light (PUVA therapy), and cholestyramine may benefit some patients. These therapies have not been studied sufficiently to predict their response rates. Aspirin, although frequently effective, cannot be recommended because of the associated risk of life-threatening hemorrhagic complications.

When all else fails, myelosuppression or interferon therapy may be considered. Interferon-alpha has been reported to be effective, with 8 of 13 patients so treated reporting at least partial relief from their symptoms within 2 to 8 weeks of treatment. However, interferon's numerous side effects, including fatigue, myalgias, headaches, anorexia, and fevers, may be equally distressing. Three of the 13 patients in this series discontinued treatment with interferon within 1 month because of these side effects. Myelosuppression is not reliably effective, and most physicians do not consider pruritus alone sufficient reason to embark on this treatment.

■ MANAGEMENT OF THE SPENT PHASE

Treatment during the spent phase is largely supportive. As is standard in the management of bone marrow failure of any origin, the attempt should be made to correct any reversible causes of pancytopenia. Deficiencies of iron, folic acid, and vitamin B_{12} should be considered and corrected if present. If these measures are ineffective, it is reasonable to try to stimulate hematopoiesis with androgens. Oxymetholone, fluoxymesterone, and nandrolone decanoate are the most commonly used preparations. Overall, androgens are modestly effective in 50 percent of cases. In some patients red cell survival may be improved and the anemia ameliorated by glucocorticoids. Unfortunately, red cell survival studies have not proved useful in predicting which patients will respond to steroids, and a therapeutic trial of prednisone may be necessary. As hematopoiesis fails, blood transfusions may be required. The median survival of patients in the spent phase is approximately 2 years, and the long-term consequences of transfusions, such as hemochromatosis, are rarely of concern.

Massive splenomegaly may cause discomfort for the patient and exacerbate the peripheral cytopenias. Moreover, massive splenomegaly has been associated with a significant increase in portal blood flow, resulting in portal hypertension and esophageal varices. During the proliferative phase of the illness, splenomegaly usually can be controlled with myelosuppressive agents or with interferon-alpha. However, these medicines are relatively contraindicated during the spent phase, as hematopoiesis already is compromised and further myelosuppression may produce dangerous cytopenias. Radiotherapy will provide relief of splenic pain in the majority of patients. However, the benefits of radiation generally last for only 3 to 4 months.

Splenectomy may improve the quality of life in patients who do not respond to more conservative management. It is virtually 100 percent effective in alleviating the mechanical discomfort associated with a large abdominal mass and in relieving the pain associated with recurrent splenic infarctions. Its success in treating hypersplenism, refractory thrombocytopenia, and portal hypertension ranges from 30 to 80 percent in different series. Hematologic improvements following splenectomy may persist for 2 to 70 months, with a median improvement of 10 months. Although splenectomy may palliate symptoms, it is a formidable undertaking in this debilitated group of patients. In several single-institution reviews published since 1977, the immediate postoperative mortality has ranged from 0 to 18 percent and postoperative morbidity, primarily hemorrhage and infection, was reported in 35 to 75 percent of patients. Since splenectomy has not been shown to affect survival, it should be considered with extreme caution for symptomatic patients who do not respond to more conservative treatment.

Foci of extramedullary hematopoiesis may arise in organs other than the spleen. Most commonly the liver and lymph nodes are affected, but myeloid metaplasia also may develop in the lungs, kidneys, gastrointestinal tract, peritoneum, or central nervous system. Masses of hematopoietic tissue may compromise the function of these organs, simulating abscesses, disseminated carcinoma, or thrombotic events. Extramedullary hematopoiesis within the meninges has presented as increased intracranial pressure, hemiparesis, and spinal cord compression, and peritoneal involvement has caused ascites. It is important to recognize the nature of these lesions, since radiotherapy or surgical decompression is highly effective in alleviating symptoms.

In rare cases, allogeneic bone marrow transplantation has been used successfully to treat postpolycythemic myeloid metaplasia with myelofibrosis. However, this procedure is limited to younger patients with an excellent performance status and an HLA-compatible donor. As such, it is not available to the majority of patients with late stage PRV.

■ TREATMENT OF ASSOCIATED CONDITIONS

Hypermetabolism

Hypermetabolic manifestations, common during the proliferative phase of the illness, include fevers, heat intolerance, and hyperuricemia. Some patients have renal colic or hematuria caused by uric acid concretions within the urinary tract or may present with acute gouty arthritis. Once infection has been excluded, fevers and heat intolerance may be treated effectively with myelosuppression. Acute gouty arthritis is managed, as in primary gout, with colchicine, nonsteroidal anti-inflammatory drugs, or glucocorticoids. To prevent recurrences the patient should be started on allopurinol. Although myelosuppression will also reduce the incidence of gout, allopurinol is safer and generally is sufficient. Since acute gout occurs in only 10 percent of patients, the use of allopurinol for asymptomatic patients with hyperuricemia is debatable.

Erythromelalgia

Erythromelalgia, a rare complication of PRV, is characterized by intense burning pain, erythema, and elevated skin temperature in a localized acral distribution. These attacks may last for minutes to days, although between attacks the extremity seems entirely normal. This syndrome appears to be caused by platelet-mediated vascular injury, but alteration in the innervation of the skin has been implicated as well. As may be expected for a disease of the vasculature, complications of erythromelalgia include osteoporosis of the affected extremity, nonhealing skin ulcers, gangrene, and multiple cerebral infarctions. Erythromelalgia is generally treated with antiplatelet agents, particularly those that inhibit cyclooxygenase, (aspirin, indomethacin), and with cytotoxic drugs to lower the platelet count. Phlebotomy alone has been effective in some cases of erythromelalgia secondary to PRV. Other therapeutic modalities that have been used with varying success include vasodilators (nitroprusside, propranolol), surgical sympathectomy, and biofeedback.

Leukemic Transformation

Acute leukemia evolves in 2 to 15 percent of patients with PRV, generally arising 8 years or more after the onset of the primary disease. It has been suggested that transformation into acute leukemia occurs most commonly in patients who present with a higher initial hemoglobin level and in patients who are treated subsequently with one or more of the classic myelosuppressive agents. These leukemias are almost always nonlymphocytic, but occasional cases of acute lymphocytic or biphenotypic leukemia have been reported. The treatments used for these leukemias, similar to those used in de novo cases, generally include cytosine arabinoside, daunomycin, and a third agent such as 6–thioguanine, etoposidem, or amsacrine. Treatment usually is ineffective, however, and survival is short, In elderly patients it may be appropriate to provide palliative and supportive care only, rather than embarking on aggressive chemotherapy. However, this decision must be made on an individual basis.

■ INVASIVE PROCEDURES

Invasive procedures, including surgery and angiography, are dangerous in uncontrolled polycythemia, primarily because of the greatly increased risk of hemorrhagic and thrombotic complications. In an analysis of 81 major operations in patients with PRV, the perioperative mortality was seven times higher in patients with uncontrolled polycythemia (hematocrits greater than 52 percent) than in those with controlled disease. Interestingly, the duration of disease control prior to surgery affected the incidence of both fatal and nonfatal complications. There were no deaths and a morbidity rate of only 5 percent in patients with a normal hemoglobin value for 4 months or longer before their operation. However, the mortality and morbidity rates were 15 percent and 42 percent respectively for patients whose hemoglobin was normal for less than 1 week prior to surgery. Therefore, elective procedures should be postponed until the blood count has been controlled for several months. When immediate intervention is necessary, intensive isovolemic phlebotomy prior to the procedure may reduce the risk.

■ FUTURE DIRECTIONS: ANTIPLATELET AGENTS

Anagrelide is a new imidazoquinazolin compound under investigation as an antiplatelet agent. At low doses it has been shown to produce thrombocytopenia in humans. At higher concentrations it also demonstrates potent antiaggregating activity. Anagrelide has been tested in 20 patients with chronic myeloproliferative disorders and thrombocytosis to more than 800,000 per cubic millimeter; 18 of these 20 patients responded with a decrease in their platelet counts to normal levels within 12 days. Side effects included nausea, headache, and mild hypotension. Importantly, anagrelide is not a general myelosuppressive agent. No significant effect was noted on the leukocyte count or hemoglobin level, nor on the in vitro growth characteristics of the neoplastic clone. The carcinogenic potential of the drug remains unknown, but it lacked mutagenicity in preclinical tests.

Ticlopidine is another antiplatelet agent being evaluated in clinical trials. This drug is believed to act during megakaryopoiesis to alter the platelet membrane, reducing platelet reactivity. Side effects of ticlopidine include reversible neutropenia and gastrointestinal distress. In initial studies ticlopidine has proved to be superior to aspirin in preventing recurrent strokes and myocardial infarctions due to arteriosclerosis. Its efficacy in the chronic myeloproliferative disorders is still unproven, although a pilot study in PRV has recently been reported. Thirty-seven patients with PRV were treated with ticlopidine at 250 mg twice a day for 60 days, during which time venisection was continued as needed to maintain a hematocrit below 46 percent. Ticlopidine treatment resulted in a 13 percent reduction in mean plasma fibrinogen levels with no significant effect on other hematologic parameters. No bleeding events were noted. However, this study was too small and too brief to demonstrate any improvement in the morbidity of PRV. Therefore, its use in this setting remains investigational.

These drugs may prove to be important additions to the therapeutic armamentarium, reducing the incidence of hemostatic complications without the leukemogenic risk associated with ionizing radiation or alkylating agents.

Suggested Reading

Berk PD, Goldberg JD, Donovan PB, et al. Therapeutic recommendations in polycythemia vera based on polycythemia vera study group protocols. Semin Hematol 1986; 23:132–143.

Brenner B, Nagler A, Tatarsky I, Hashmonai M. Splenectomy in agnogenic myeloid metaplasia and postpolycythemic myeloid metaplasia: A study of 34 cases. Arch Intern Med 1988; 148:2501–2505.

Cimino R, Rametta V, Matera C, et al. Recombinant interferon alpha-2b in the treatment of polycythemia vera. Am J Hematol 1993; 44:155–157.

Gisslinger H, Ludwig H, Linkesch W, et al. Long-term interferon therapy for thrombocytosis in myeloproliferative diseases. Lancet 1989; 1(8639):634–637.

Hocking WG, Golde DW. Polycythemia: Evaluation and management. Blood Rev 1989; 3:59–65.

Lofvenberg W, Wahlin A. Management of polycythemia vera, essential thrombocythaemia and myelofibrosis with hydroxyurea. Eur J Haematol 1988; 41:375–381.

Sacchi S, Leoni P, Liberati M, et al. A prospective comparison between treatment with phlebotomy alone and with interferon-alpha in patients with polycythemia vera. Ann Hematol 1994; 68:247–250.

Silver RT. Interferon-alpha 2b: A new treatment for polycythemia vera. Ann Intern Med 1993; 119:1091–1092.

Silverstein MN, Petitt RM, Solberg LA, et al. Anagrelide: A new drug for treating thrombocytosis. New Engl J Med 1988; 318:1292–1294.

Westwood N, Dudley JM, Sawyer B, et al. Primary polycythemia: Diagnosis by non-conventional positive criteria. Eur J Haematology 1993; 51: 228–232.

ACUTE LYMPHOBLASTIC LEUKEMIA IN ADULTS

Dieter F. Hoelzer, M.D., Ph.D.

The outcome for acute lymphoblastic leukemia (ALL) in adults has improved substantially in recent years. After induction therapy, complete remission rates of 70 to 85 percent with disease-free survival of 30 to 40 percent at 5 years are realistic achievements. Prospective therapeutic trials in adult ALL with uniform diagnosis, intensified therapy, and an adequate number of patients have led to the definition of prognostic factors. This has resulted in risk-adapted therapy and more precise indications for bone marrow transplantation. For further improvement of cure rates some approaches remain to be evaluated, such as further intensification of therapy (carefully weighed against the increased risk of toxicity), the best modality for prophylactic central nervous system (CNS) treatment, the optimal duration of maintenance therapy, the use of biologic response modifiers, and the tailoring of treatment according to the detection of minimal residual disease (MRD). To answer such questions, it is important to include adult patients with ALL in studies whenever possible. Improved remission rates and survival have been achieved only by intensifying treatment regimens with increased toxicity. Patients should therefore be treated in hospitals by trained staff who react quickly to any complications.

DIAGNOSIS AND CLASSIFICATION

Examination of bone aspirates and blood smears confirms the diagnosis of ALL. The first bone marrow aspirates should be used for morphology, cytochemistry, immunologic phenotyping, and cytogenetic and molecular analysis. Blast cells in ALL are stained with Wright's or Wright's-Giemsa stain and are classified as L1, L2, or L3 according to the FAB (French-American-British) classification. The definitive cytochemical reactions are periodic-acid-Schiff (PAS) and acid phosphatase. The presence of the enzyme terminal deoxynucleotidyltransferase (TdT) should also be assessed for confirmation of the diagnosis of ALL.

Immunologic Phenotyping. Immunologic phenotyping is the most important classification for ALL. According to surface marker molecules, B-lineage ALL can be separated from T-lineage ALL, and within these lineages there are distinct subtypes of ALL according to their stage of differentiation. Table 1 shows the definition of ALL subtypes and their incidence in children and adults with ALL. When the ALL cells express also myeloid markers, the leukemia is termed My^+-ALL, or mixed or hybrid ALL, biphenotypic if myeloid and lymphoid markers are on the same cells and bilineal if the markers are on two blast cell populations. Less than 1 percent of ALL remains unclassifiable (null-ALL).

Cytogenetic Analysis. Cytogenetic analysis of bone marrow is essential. The most frequent cytogenetic abnormality in ALL is the Ph′ chromosome t(9;22) found in 20 to 30 percent of adults with ALL. These patients have had a very poor outcome and need specific treatment. Also the demonstration of the t(4;11) translocation is relevant for treatment decisions.

Molecular Analysis. Molecular analysis has emerged as an integral part in the diagnosis of ALL. Of particular interest in adults is the demonstration of the BCR-ABL rearrangement, the molecular correlate to the Ph′ chromosome. It can also be detected when cytogenetic analysis is difficult or unsuccessful for technical reasons. Furthermore, it may detect MRD for the follow-up to confirm remission or detect early relapse.

Lumbar puncture before therapy is necessary to determine whether or not the CNS is involved. It should be postponed as long as leukemic cells are found in the peripheral blood or when there is a risk of bleeding due to a very low platelet count (below 20×10^9 per liter). When the cell number in the spinal fluid is at a borderline level or the morphology is inconclusive, demonstration of an immunologically defined monoclonality can confirm a leukemic CNS involvement.

Table 1 Most Relevant Markers and Incidence of Immunophenotypes in ALL

SUBTYPE	MARKER	INCIDENCE (%) CHILDREN		ADULTS	
	B-LINEAGE ALL				
pre-pre-B-ALL*	HLA-DR$^+$, TdT$^+$, CD19$^+$	5		11	
common-ALL	HLA-DR$^+$, TdT$^+$, CD10$^+$, CD19$^+$	65	85	51	72
pre-B-ALL	HLA-DR$^+$, CD10$^\pm$, CD19$^+$, cyIgM$^+$	15		10	
B-ALL	HLA-DR$^+$, CD10$^\pm$, CD19$^+$, CD20$^+$, SIg$^+$		3		4
	T-LINEAGE				
pre-T-ALL	TdT$^+$, CD7$^+$, cyCD3$^+$	1		7	
T-ALL	TdT$^+$, CD7$^+$, cyCD3$^+$, CD1a/2/3$^\pm$	11	12	17	24

*Also called early pre-B-ALL.
HLA, human leukocyte antigen.

■ INITIAL COMPLICATIONS AND SUPPORTIVE THERAPY

Most patients present with indirect signs of leukemia such as infection, bleeding, anemia, and metabolic disorders rather than with symptoms due to leukemic cell infiltration. Treatment of initial complications and prophylaxis for complications expected during cytostatic therapy must be started immediately. In only a few cases is the leukemic process so far advanced that immediate treatment of the leukemia is necessary. Such an event can be dyspnea through large mediastinal masses, pleural or pericardial effusions in T-ALL, large abdominal masses with renal impairment in B-ALL and Burkitt's non-Hodgkin's lymphoma or a very high white blood cell count.

The most frequent metabolic abnormality is hyperuricemia, which further increases during therapy and exacerbates with cell destruction. To reduce the formation of uric acid and avoid urate nephropathy patients should receive allopurinol 300 mg or 600 mg per day if high leukocyte counts or organomegaly persist. Allopurinol can cause skin rashes but rarely causes severe allergic reactions.

Fluid intake should be sufficient to guarantee urine production of at least 100 ml per hour throughout induction therapy, to reduce possible uric acid formation. This may require parenteral fluid administration when the patient's oral intake is inadequate because of nausea or difficulty in swallowing. If the venous system does not offer easy access, a catheter for long-term vascular access (e.g., a Hickman catheter) is advantageous when anticipating a long period of induction therapy and is useful for therapy on an outpatient basis.

Approximately one-third of adult ALL patients present with infection and bleeding, which are major problems in the management of the disease. Bleeding is usually due to thrombocytopenia, but hyperleukocytosis and plasma clotting deficiencies may exacerbate it. Disseminated intravascular coagulation is rarely observed at diagnosis. Leukostatic hemorrhages caused by leukocyte aggregation and infiltration of small vessel walls are most severe in the brain, especially in elderly patients with high leukocyte counts. Cautious reduction of the leukocytes may but cannot always prevent fatal complications. For thrombocytopenia, platelets should be transfused when the platelet count falls below 20×10^9 per liter and/or for bleeding. Four to six packs should be given until bleeding stops, and if a longer period of platelet substitution is anticipated, platelets from human leukocyte antigen (HLA) matched single donors by apheresis is preferential.

Fever or infection present at the time of admission is mainly caused by severe granulocytopenia (granulocyte count below 0.5×10^9 per liter) but may also be due to immunologic deficiencies or mucosal lesions. Careful physical examination, chest roentgenogram, and cultures of blood, urine, sputum, and other sites of suspected infection are necessary. In patients with severe infection, broad-spectrum antibiotics should be given immediately, even before the results of cultures are available. For patients with no fever or infection, prophylactic treatment with co-trimoxazole should be initiated prior to cytostatic treatment. Co-trimoxazole in combination with prophylactic polymixin B and amphotericin B treatment apparently prevented severe infection in half of the patients in a large ALL multicenter trial.

Prophylactic measures, including the regular use of mouthwash, careful disinfection of the anogenital region, general body hygiene, sufficient fluid intake, and regular intake of oral drugs for infection prophylaxis, actively contribute to the treatment of disease.

With more intensive chemotherapy and more prolonged periods of granulocytopenia, fungal infections have markedly increased. Morbidity due to *Candida* and *Aspergillus* infections in 5 to 20 percent of patients, of which up to half may be fatal, is now a major complication in the treatment of acute leukemias. The difficulty in managing these fungal infections is not only the limited availability of effective drugs but also that of achieving a speedy confirmation of the diagnosis and prompt antimycotic treatment. Since pulmonary mycoses, particularly with *Aspergillus,* have a very unfavorable outcome, immediate diagnostic procedures with computed tomography (CT) chest scans and bronchial lavage are necessary. Early antifungal therapy, such as amphotericin B and 5-fluocytosine or new formulations of amphotericin B permitting application of higher dosages, is expected to improve the cure rates of systemic mycoses. For prophylaxis of fungal infections oral polyenes and the new triazoles, particularly fluconazole for prevention of *Candida* infections, seem effective. Aerosol application of amphotericin B is also under investigation.

Table 2 Most Used Cytostatic Drugs for Therapy of Adult ALL

Induction	Vincristine, prednisone, daunorubicin/idarubicin, L-asparaginase
	Cytosine arabinoside, cyclophosphamide, methotrexate
Postinduction	High-dose cytosine arabinoside
	High-dose methotrexate
	Teniposide, m-amsacrine, mitoxantrone
	High-dose 6-mercaptopurine ?

REMISSION INDUCTION THERAPY

When diagnosis of ALL is confirmed and the initial complications are managed, cytostatic therapy should be initiated immediately. The induction treatment in most adult ALL regimens consists of a combination of vincristine, prednisone, an anthracycline, and L-asparaginase. In some trials also cytosine arabinoside and/or cyclophosphamide are added at the beginning (Table 2).

An induction regimen for adults with ALL applied to date in 1,850 patients is given in Table 3. In patients with a large leukemic cell mass and a particularly high leukocyte count (above 25×10^9 per liter), cell reduction with a cautious pretherapy consisting of vincristine and prednisone (see Table 3) should be started. For B-ALL, a different pretherapy that includes prednisone and cyclophosphamide is recommended (see Table 7). After the pretherapy the induction treatment for T-lineage and B-lineage ALL (except mature B-ALL) consists of the combination of vincristine, prednisone, an anthracycline, and L-asparaginase (Table 3) for 4 weeks (GMALL studies 1/81 through 4/89).

To reduce the leukemic cell burden further and to avoid the early development of resistant clones, a second part of induction follows. It includes cyclophosphamide, cytarabine (ARA-C), 6-mercaptopurine, and a CNS prophylaxis consisting of cranial irradiation and intrathecal methotrexate (see Table 3). For patients in complete remission after the first 4 weeks it is a consolidation; for patients with only partial remission or failure this second part of induction treatment provides a chance to enter complete remission. This second phase of induction should be started after sufficient recovery of peripheral blood values (granulocytes above 1.5×10^9 per liter, platelets above 100×10^9 per liter, hemoglobin above 10 g per deciliter).

With this induction regimen an overall complete remission in approximately 80 percent of adult ALL patients can now be achieved, and of them only 6 to 8 percent need the second phase to enter complete remission. Also with other intensive induction regimens, the complete remission rate of 80 percent as well as the proportion requiring a second course to achieve remission are similar. In contrast to earlier studies, initial parameters such as high leukocyte count and CNS or other organ involvement have no adverse influence on the complete remission rate, except age where the remission rate has a strictly inverse correlation to increasing age (complete remission rate in children 95 percent, in adults above 60 years 40 to 60 percent).

Central Nervous System Prophylaxis

CNS prophylaxis consists of cranial irradiation (24 Gy) and intrathecal methotrexate 15 mg absolute once weekly for 4 weeks. CNS prophylaxis is given only when complete remission has been achieved; since most patients have already achieved CR during the first 4 weeks, prophylaxis is usually given during phase 2 (weeks 5 to 8). Patients with CNS involvement at diagnosis receive intrathecal treatment with a triple combination (Table 4), consisting of methotrexate 15 mg, ARA-C 40 mg, and dexamethasone 4 mg, two to three times weekly until the cerebrospinal fluid (CSF) is cleared and then three to five further consolidation doses (one to two per week). In addition the patients receive 24 Gy irradiation to the cranium and spinal column.

POSTINDUCTION THERAPY

The aim of the postinduction therapy is to eliminate clinically undetectable leukemic cells. This can be done by further chemotherapy (consolidation cycles), by bone marrow transplantation, and probably by the use of biologic response modifiers such as interleukin-2 (IL-2) or alpha-interferon, although this is not yet established in ALL.

Consolidation chemotherapy can comprise either repeated cycles of alternating drug combinations, as used in most ongoing adult ALL trials, or a reinduction therapy with drugs similar to those given in induction therapy (Table 5). Drug combinations used in consolidation cycles often include high-dose cytosine arabinoside (HD-ARA-C), high-dose methotrexate (HD-MTX), epipodophyllotoxins, or new anthracyclines such as mitoxantrone or idarubicin.

High-dose systemic chemotherapy is of particular interest in ALL, since thereby sufficient cytotoxic drug levels can be reached in the CSF which may prevent CNS relapse. Consolidation regimens including HD-ARA-C and HD-MTX used in the GMALL studies are given in Table 6. The treatment strategy is thereby stratified according to the biologic subtypes into (1) B-lineage ALL (low risk), (2) T-lineage ALL, and (3) high-risk ALL, particularly Ph′-chromosome positive ALL and mature B-ALL. The HD-ARA-C and mitoxantrone combination is included in the treatment for high-risk patients (HD-ARA-C 3 g per square meter) and for T-ALL patients (HD-ARA-C 1 g per square meter) but apparently has no advantage for standard-risk patients. The consolidation regimens HD-MTX with L-asparaginase and VM26 with ARA-C found to be effective in earlier studies are now applied in all risk groups.

TOXIC SIDE EFFECTS

In induction therapy moderate and severe neurotoxicity due to vincristine, mostly paresthesia, occurs in about one-tenth of the patients, but also occasionally a subileus can be observed in elderly patients. L-Asparaginase treatment may be discontinued if the fibrinogen level falls below 100 mg per 100 ml despite replacement or because of another infrequent complication such as pancreatitis, hypoglycemia, allergic reaction, hepatotoxicity, or bleeding complications. Toxicity caused by steroids is rare. Daunorubicin in the dosage used

Table 3 Induction Therapy

DRUG	DOSAGE	DAY
PRETHERAPY (FOR PATIENTS WITH A LARGE LEUKEMIC MASS AND/OR A HIGH LEUCOCYTE COUNT)		
Vincristine	2 mg (absolute) IV	1
Prednisone	3 × 20 mg/m² PO	1–7
PHASE I		
Vincristine	2 mg (absolute) IV	1, 8, 15, 22
Prednisone	3 × 20 mg/m² PO	1–28
Daunorubicin	45 mg/m² IV (½ hr)	1, 8, 15, 22
L-Asparaginase	5,000 U/m² IV (½ hr)	15–28
Methotrexate	15 mg (absolute) IT	1
PHASE II		
Cyclophosphamide	1,000 mg/m² IV	29, 43, 57
Cytosine arabinoside	75 mg/m² IV or SC (1 hr)	31–34, 38–41, 45–48, 52–55
6-Mercaptopurine	60 mg/m² PO	29–57
Methotrexate	15 mg (absolute) IT	31, 38, 45, 52

IT, intrathecal.

Table 4 Triple Intrathecal CNS Prophylaxis

DRUG	DOSAGE	DAY
Methotrexate	15 mg (absolute) IT	1
ARA-C	40	1
Dexamethasone	4	1

Table 5 Reinduction Therapy

DRUG	DOSAGE	DAY
PHASE 1		
Vincristine	2 mg (absolute) IV	1, 8, 15, 22
Prednisone	3 × 20 mg/m² PO	1–28
Adriamycin	25 mg/m² IV	1, 8, 15, 22
MTX, AraC, Dexa	IT	1
PHASE 2		
Cyclophosphamide	1000 mg/m² IV	29
Cytosine arabinoside	75 mg/m² IV	31–34, 38–41
Thioguanine	25 mg/m² IV	29–42
MTX, AraC, Dexa	IT	1

here for induction usually does not cause cardiotoxicity, but in elderly patients assessment of the cardiac ejection fraction may be used as a control parameter.

The most frequent and severe complications during the induction therapy are bleeding and infection, which are also the major cause of death during this treatment period. Initially bacterial or viral infections are predominant, but later fungal infections, usually candidiasis and occasionally aspergillosis, become a major problem. In phase 2 of induction, cyclophosphamide and ARA-C are myelotoxic and cause granulocytopenia and thrombocytopenia. In two-thirds of the patients these cytopenias necessitate a pause in chemotherapy, usually after the first 10 days of treatment. Hematopoietic growth factors such as G-CSF given concomitantly with the cytostatic drugs of phase 2 of induction therapy can shorten neutropenia, reduce febrile episodes, and diminish treatment delay.

Table 6 Consolidation Therapy

CYTOSTATIC DRUG	DOSAGE	DAY
HD-ARA-C*/MITOXANTRONE		
HD-ARA-C	3 g/m² IV (3h) q12h	1–4
Mitoxantrone	10 mg/m² IV (½ hr)	3–5
HD-MTX/L-ASPARAGINASE		
HD-MTX	1,500 mg/m² IV (24 hr)†	1, 15
L-Asparaginase	10,000 U/m² IV (1 hr)	2, 16
VM-26/ARA-C		
ARA-C	150 mg/m² IV (1 hr)	1–5
Teniposide	100 mg/m² IV (1 hr)	1–5

*3 g/m² in high-risk patients, 1 g/m² in T-ALL patients.
†1/10 in ½ hr, 9/10 in 23½ hr followed by leucovorin rescue (see Table 8).

■ MAINTENANCE THERAPY

After induction, reinduction, and consolidation treatment, adult ALL patients usually receive maintenance therapy, an approach transferred from childhood ALL regimens. The backbone of such maintenance treatment is 6-mercaptopurine and methotrexate, with or without reinforcement cycles. Optimal duration of maintenance therapy is not known, but in most studies it lasts 2 years. As with induction and consolidation, maintenance therapy may in future trials be related to the ALL subtype.

Dosages of 6-mercaptopurine and methotrexate should be adjusted so that granulocyte levels remain above 1.5×10^9 per liter and platelet counts above 100×10^9 per liter. Occasionally hepatotoxicity or reduced creatinine clearance also make a lowering of dose or discontinuation of therapy necessary.

■ TREATMENT REGIMENS FOR B-ALL

The results for B-ALL could be substantially improved by the use of fractionated cyclophosphamide, HD-MTX, and HD-ARA-C in combination with the conventionally used cytostatic drugs in ALL. These treatment regimens consist of four

Table 7 Therapy for Patients with B-ALL

DRUG	DOSAGE	DAY
	PRETHERAPY	
Cyclophosphamide	200 mg/m^2 IV (1 hr)	1–5
Prednisone	60 mg/m^2 PO	1–5
	BLOCK A	
Vincristine	2 mg (absolute) IV	1
HD-MTX	3 g/m^2 IV (24 hr)*	1
Ifosphamide	800 mg/m^2 IV	1–5
Teniposide	100 mg/m^2 IV (1 hr)	4, 5
ARA-C	2 × 150 mg/m^2 IV (1 hr)	4, 5
Dexamethasone	10 mg/m^2 PO	1–5
MTX, ARA-C, Dexamethasone	IT	1, 5
	BLOCK B	
Vincristine	2 mg (absolute) IV	1
HD-MTX	3 g/m^2 IV (24 hr)*	1
Cyclophosphamide	200 mg/m^2 IV	1–5
Doxorubicin	25 mg/m^2 IV (¼ hr)	4, 5
Dexamethasone	10 mg/m^2 PO	1–5
MTX, ARA-C, Dexamethasone	IT	1

*As infusion, ⅒ in ½ hr, 9/10 in 23½ hr followed by leucovorin rescue (see Table 8).

to six short intensive cycles given over 2 to 4 months without further maintenance therapy.

Such a treatment regimen for adult B-ALL consisting of six cycles and achieving leukemia-free survival (LFS) in 50 to 60 percent of patients is given in Table 7. Patients with B-ALL having a large tumor burden should initially have a safe but effective pretherapy consisting of cyclophosphamide and prednisone (Table 7). This pretherapy is then followed by six alternating 5 day cycles A and B (A, B, A, B, A, B), each with a 16 day interval. The exact timing of leucovorin rescue after HD-MTX is important (Table 8). Granulocytopenia and probably mucositis can be ameliorated by G-CSF or GM-CSF. In this treatment schedule CNS irradiation and maintenance therapy are omitted.

Table 8 Leucovorin Rescue

The dose of leucovorin depends on the methotrexate level in serum at 24, 36, 42, and 48 hours after commencement of methotrexate infusion. Desired serum methotrexate levels:

	at 24 hours	≤150 μmol/L
	36	<3.0
	42	≤1.0
	48	≤0.4
Leucovorin:	42	30 mg/m^2 IV
	48	15
	54	15

If the serum methotrexate level at 42 hours is >1 μmol/L, the dose of leucovorin is increased to 75 mg/m^2 and subsequent 6-hourly doses tapered to 15 mg/m^2 in five stages.

If the serum methotrexate level at 42 hours is >5 μmol/L, the 6-hourly leucovorin dose in mg = serum methotrexate level (μmol/L) × body weight (kg) until serum methotrexate <5 μmol/L.

Table 9 Major Adverse Prognostic Factors in Adult ALL

Delayed time to reach CR	>4 weeks
Immunologic subtype	My$^+$-ALL ?
Karyotype	t(9;22)/BCR-ABL pos. ALL t(4;11) ?
Higher age	>50 years
High initial leukocyte count	>30 × 10^9/L
Elevated LDH level	in B-ALL

■ PROGNOSTIC FACTORS

In recent larger adult ALL studies with intensive induction and consolidation therapy, similar prognostic factors for remission duration emerge (Table 9).

Favorable prognostic factors that correlate with longer remission are achievement of complete remission within 4 weeks, lower initial leukocyte count, lower age, and the immunologic subtype T-ALL or B-ALL. With increasing age, the length of remission decreases continuously. Thus it is difficult to define a particular age for stratification of patients into risk groups; formerly 25 or 35 years was used, but now stratification is often according to whether patients are candidates for bone marrow transplantation (BMT) or not (e.g., under or over 50 years). A uniform adverse risk factor in all studies is a longer time to achieve complete remission, as are higher initial leukocyte count, age above 50 years, and probably the immunologic subtype My$^+$-ALL. The poorest outcome is seen for patients with Ph′-chromosome positive ALL.

In addition, in mature B-ALL high LDH at diagnosis is an adverse prognostic factor.

These risk factors can be used to stratify adult ALL patients into standard-risk and high-risk groups. Standard-risk patients without any of the adverse factors, who form about 30 to 40 percent of patients, have a 10 year survival of approximately 50 percent; for high-risk patients survival is clearly inferior, with 10 year survival according to their risk factors between 10 and 30 percent.

Immunologic Subtypes

T-lineage ALL, which constitutes about 25 percent of adult ALL, is associated with male predominance, high leukocyte count, mediastinal tumor, extramedullary involvement, and rapid progression. The CR rate has increased from 40 to 50 percent a decade ago to 80 percent or more. Also the survival is substantially improved from less than 10 percent to cure rates of 40 to 50 percent. There is strong evidence, not proven in prospective randomized trials, that the early use of cyclophosphamide and ARA-C, which probably act synergistically, in addition to the conventional cytostatic drugs used in induction, are responsible for this improvement in outcome.

B-lineage ALL constitutes about 70 percent of adult ALL. The outcome for adult patients with pre-pre-B-ALL, mostly having the cytogenetic chromosomal aberration t(4;11) has improved, but the prognosis for common ALL and pre-B-ALL remains unchanged in most studies. This is partly due to the fact that the Ph′-chromosome/BCR-ABL positive ALL with poor prognosis is found within these two subtypes.

B-ALL, the least frequent subtype, is characterized by rapid proliferation, male predominance, frequent abdominal masses, and renal, bone, and CNS involvement. The outcome for adults as well as children with B-ALL a decade ago was very poor, with CR rates of 40 percent and survival rates of less than 10 percent. With the short, repeated cycles of very intensive chemotherapy now applied, complete remission rates have risen to 70 to 80 percent and the survival rates to 80 percent for children and 50 to 60 percent for adults.

My⁺-ALL, ALL cells expressing myeloid markers, were found in different studies with a wide variation of incidence, from 5 to 30 percent, depending on how My^+-ALL is defined. In recent studies, My^+-ALL is accepted only if more than 20 percent of the leukemic ALL blast cells express also myeloid markers. The former poor prognosis with regard to CR rate and survival in childhood as well as adult ALL has now improved in recent study protocols, and My^+-ALL may be no longer an adverse prognostic sign.

Cytogenetic Aberrations

Philadelphia chromosome-BCR-ABL rearrangement positive ALL afflicts 20 to 30 percent of adult ALL patients, in contrast to only 3 percent in childhood ALL. The CR rate has improved from 60 to 80 percent; however, it is still difficult to prevent relapse, and thus the median remission duration is only 7 months and the survival rates at 3 to 5 years are only 0 to 15 percent. Intensified chemotherapy, allogeneic or autologous bone marrow transplantation, the use of biologic modifiers such as IL-2 and alpha-interferon as maintenance are treatment options under investigation.

■ BONE MARROW TRANSPLANTATION

BMT now forms an integral part of treatment strategies in adult ALL. After allogeneic BMT the survival rate is 45 percent (weighted mean, range 21 percent to 61 percent). After autologous transplantation there is a wide range from 25 to 65 percent. It is still not solved where best to place BMT in adult ALL. When a low-risk group can be defined with a cure rate of 50 percent, BMT in first CR is recommended only to high-risk patients and to the low-risk patients in second remission. Other study groups consider all adult ALL patients as high risk and propose allogeneic or autologous transplant to all patients in first remission. Ongoing randomized studies may solve this problem.

■ RELAPSE TIMES AND SITES

Unfortunately, more than half of adult ALL patients have a recurrence of leukemia. The times when relapses in adult ALL occur are closely correlated with the immunologic subtype; in B-ALL exclusively all relapses occur within 1 year, in T-ALL within 3 to 4 years, in B-lineage ALL up to 5 years or even longer. The site of relapse is most frequently the bone marrow. Isolated CNS relapse and combined CNS and bone marrow relapses are still an obstacle, occurring together in about 8 to 10 percent of patients, whether the CNS prophylaxis consists of intrathecal therapy alone, cranial irradiation with intrathecal therapy, or systemic HD-MTX or HD-ARA-C.

Other relapse sites, such as lymph nodes, mediastinum, skin, and testes, are not frequent but are preferentially seen in T-ALL. The very low incidence of testicular relapse in adult ALL after intensified therapeutic regimens is a strong argument against prophylactic treatment of the testes.

■ RELAPSE THERAPY

The outcome after treatment for relapse in adult ALL patients is still very poor. With new induction regimens, complete remissions in up to 50 to 60 percent of ALL in first relapse can be achieved, depending on how long after remission the relapse occurs. However, the remission duration is only 3 to 6 months, and long-term prospects are poor, so patients in complete remission or good partial remission should be rescued with BMT. Treatment of first and later relapse is the place for experimental studies in ALL.

Suggested Reading

Hoelzer D, Thiel E, Ludwig WD, et al. The German multicentre trials for treatment of acute lymphoblastic leukemia in adults. Leukemia 1992; 6(Suppl 2):175–177.

Hoelzer D. Acute lymphoblastic leukemia in adults. Semin Hematol 1994; 31:1–15.

ACUTE MYELOID LEUKEMIA

Maria R. Baer, M.D.
Geoffrey P. Herzig, M.D.
Clara D. Bloomfield, M.D.

Acute myeloid leukemia (AML) is a malignancy arising in hematopoietic stem cells. It is characterized by accumulation of immature myeloid cells of clonal origin in the bone marrow, with impairment of normal hematopoiesis. Patients with AML commonly present with an acute illness due to life-threatening cytopenias and attendant complications. Patients suspected of having acute leukemia must be evaluated promptly to ensure early recognition of complications and to obtain the information needed to initiate therapy as quickly as possible. Effective treatment of AML requires intensive chemotherapy, which is best delivered in a specialized setting with meticulous supportive care. With this approach AML treatment results have improved significantly in recent years, and with appropriate management an increasing number of patients with AML now achieve long-term disease-free survival.

■ PRESENTATION AND DETECTION

Patients with AML typically come to medical attention because of the clinical consequences of abnormal hematopoiesis, including anemia, neutropenia, and thrombocytopenia. Clinical manifestations may include fatigue, pallor, dyspnea, fever, signs of localized infection, petechiae, and mucosal bleeding. Hyperleukocytosis and disseminated intravascular coagulation, if present, may result in rapidly progressive hypoxemia and neurologic changes and in diffuse bleeding and bruising, respectively. These complications are discussed later in this chapter. Lymphadenopathy and splenomegaly are present in approximately 20 percent of AML patients, and gingival hypertrophy, skin nodules, or soft tissue tumors (granulocytic sarcomas) are sometimes seen.

As noted, patients with AML present with abnormal blood counts. The total white blood cell count may be high, low, or normal, and myeloblasts may or may not be present in the blood. A bone marrow aspirate and biopsy will establish the cause of the abnormal blood counts. If AML is suspected, bone marrow samples should be obtained for cytochemical staining, immunophenotyping studies, and cytogenetic analysis in addition to morphologic study. Material should also be cryopreserved as viable cells for molecular analyses or other studies which may provide required additional information important to diagnosis and prognosis.

The diagnosis of AML is established by the presence of at least 30 percent myeloblasts in bone marrow. Blasts may be demonstrated to be of myeloid lineage by virtue of the presence of Auer rods in the cytoplasm, staining with Sudan black B or myeloperoxidase, or presence of myeloid-associated cell surface antigens, most commonly CD13 or CD33. AML is subclassified using the criteria of the French-American-British (FAB) Group. FAB types M1 through M5 include myeloblastic, promyelocytic, myelomonocytic, and monocytic leukemias, distinguished on the basis of morphology and cytochemical (peroxidase and esterase) staining. Erythroleukemia (FAB M6) is diagnosed if there are at least 50 percent nucleated red cells in the bone marrow and at least 30 percent of the nonerythroid cells are myeloblasts. A diagnosis of acute megakaryocytic leukemia (FAB M7) requires demonstration of platelet peroxidase by electron microscopy or presence of megakaryocytic cell surface antigens such as glycoprotein IIb-IIIa (CD41a). Finally, cases of acute leukemia are classified as FAB M0 AML when blasts are morphologically and cytochemically undifferentiated but have myeloid cell surface antigens.

In addition to studies performed to diagnose and classify the leukemia, patients must be rapidly assessed with respect to comorbid conditions and infectious, hemostatic, and metabolic complications. Initial evaluation should include a thorough history and physical examination. The perirectal and perineal areas should be carefully examined for signs of abscess formation and cellulitis, but digital examination of the rectum and pelvic examination should be avoided because mucosal trauma may result in infection in these areas. Baseline laboratory studies should include complete blood counts (hemoglobin, white blood cell count, platelet count, and differential white blood cell count), coagulation studies (prothrombin and partial thromboplastin times, fibrinogen and fibrin degradation products), serum electrolytes, blood urea nitrogen (BUN), creatinine, glucose, calcium, phosphate, uric acid, magnesium, liver function tests, arterial blood gases, cytomegalovirus (CMV) and herpes simplex virus (HSV) antibodies, posteroanterior and lateral chest roentgenograms, and electrocardiogram. Additional roentgenographic studies (e.g., dental, sinuses, abdomen) should be dictated by clinical findings. Blood should be sent for human leukocyte antigen (HLA) typing studies (A, B, and DR loci) so as to identify HLA-compatible platelet donors for patients who become alloimmunized as well as potential allogeneic bone marrow donors. Evaluation of ventricular function by multiple-gated acquisition blood-pool imaging is needed to decide on the feasibility of anthracycline therapy. Pretherapy lumbar puncture to obtain cerebrospinal fluid for cytologic analysis should be performed only in patients with symptoms suggestive of meningeal leukemia. Because of the possibility of introducing peripheral blood leukemia cells into the meningeal space when lumbar punctures are performed before therapy, consideration should be given to administering a dose of intrathecal chemotherapy prior to withdrawing the needle used to sample the spinal fluid.

■ PROGNOSIS

Lower complete remission rates and briefer remission durations are seen in AML patients who have antecedent hematologic disorders or who were previously treated with chemotherapy or radiation therapy (secondary AML). Advanced age is also a strong adverse factor in terms of remission rate and duration. The pretreatment bone marrow karyotype has strong independent prognostic significance in AML. Unfavorable cytogenetic findings include deletions of the long arm of chromosome 5, monosomy 7, abnormalities of 12p and 11q23, trisomy 8 and trisomy 13 as sole abnormalities, and complex karyotypes. Conversely, t(8;21)(q22;q22.3) and abnormalities of 16q22, especially inv(16)(p13q22), predict a high likelihood of achieving a complete remission and longer survival. Patients with t(8;21)(q22;q22.3) who receive high-dose cytarabine-based intensification therapy appear to have an especially high likelihood of long-term disease-free survival. Patients with t(15;17)(q22;q11-q12) have a good prognosis with therapy which includes all-*trans*-retinoic acid. Patients with a normal karyotype have an intermediate prognosis. Finally, immunophenotype and the multidrug resistance (MDR) phenotype may have prognostic significance in AML treated with current regimens. In some studies expression of CD34, an antigen expressed on early hematopoietic progenitors, is unfavorable, as is MDR expression. The prognostic significance of immunophenotype is explained in part by associations with karyotype.

■ MANAGEMENT OF EARLY COMPLICATIONS

Prompt recognition and appropriate treatment of the life-threatening problems that may be present at diagnosis or may appear with initiation of chemotherapy will reduce early deaths and may allow patients to survive long enough to receive an adequate trial of definitive chemotherapy.

Hyperleukocytosis

Vascular occlusion by aggregates of blasts may occur in patients with blood blast counts greater than 100×10^9 per liter, and AML with hyperleukocytosis is a medical emergency. Clinical manifestations of leukostasis, which are primarily pulmonary and neurologic, include dyspnea, hypoxemia, pulmonary infiltrates, lethargy, focal neurologic signs, coma, and intracerebral hemorrhage. In patients with blood blast counts approaching 100×10^9 per liter, it is imperative to rapidly lower the number of circulating blasts. Leukapheresis is an effective, albeit temporary, means of accomplishing this. To avoid rapid return of the hyperleukocytosis, chemotherapy should be started immediately after leukapheresis is completed. If it is not possible to begin definitive chemotherapy, hydroxyurea 6 to 12 g orally daily for up to 3 days can be used as a temporizing measure. If leukapheresis is not available, high-dose hydroxyurea can be used in its place. However, it is a less desirable alternative because of the lag period of 12 to 24 hours before the white blood cell count begins to decline and because of the possible metabolic consequences of tumor lysis (discussed later in this chapter). In some centers a single dose of cranial irradiation, 600 cGy, is administered with the hope of destroying intracerebral myeloblasts and lessening the risk of central nervous system (CNS) infarction and hemorrhage. Adjunctive measures include management of respiratory failure and of intracranial hypertension if present. It should be noted that Po_2, pH, and serum glucose values may be artifactually low in blood samples with high blast counts.

Disseminated Intravascular Coagulation

Laboratory evidence of disseminated intravascular coagulation (DIC)—prolonged prothrombin and partial thromboplastin times, hypofibrinogenemia, increased fibrin degradation products, thrombocytopenia—is present at diagnosis or following initiation of chemotherapy in essentially all patients with acute promyeloctyic leukemia (APL, or FAB M3 AML) as well in some patients with other subtypes of AML. Laboratory parameters generally worsen with rapid breakdown of leukemia cells following initiation of chemotherapy, and hemorrhagic complications frequently develop during this period. Coagulation parameters must be monitored prior to and for at least 3 days following initiation of chemotherapy. Remission induction therapy for APL using all-*trans*-retinoic acid instead of cytotoxic agents does not cause exacerbation of DIC. Retinoic acid induces differentiation of leukemic promyelocytes.

Patients with laboratory evidence of DIC are at high risk for life-threatening hemorrhage and must be managed aggressively. Platelet transfusions and cryoprecipitate should be administered to keep the platelet count above 50×10^9 per liter and the plasma fibrinogen level above 100 mg per milliliter at all times. Fresh frozen plasma may be given to correct prolongation of the prothrombin and partial thromboplastin times due to depletion of factors other than fibrinogen. Volume status must be carefully monitored in this setting. Low-dose heparin (10 U per kilogram per hour) is used in some centers. It is imperative that platelet counts and coagulation parameters be closely monitored. The goals of therapy are to maintain the platelet count above 50×10^9 per liter and to normalize the fibrinogen and prothrombin and partial thromboplastin times.

Tumor Lysis Syndrome

Metabolic complications of tumor lysis are uncommon in AML but may be seen with the initiation of chemotherapy in patients with hyperleukocytosis. Other risk factors include pretherapy renal insufficiency and hyperuricemia. Allopurinol and vigorous hydration with intravenous fluids should be used for rapid lowering of elevated serum uric acid levels before initiation of therapy. Alkalinization of the urine may be needed for the first 24 to 48 hours in patients with evidence of uric acid nephropathy while waiting for the allopurinol to take effect. Uric acid, potassium, calcium, phosphate, BUN, and creatinine should be closely monitored during chemotherapy. Other measures to correct metabolic abnormalities associated with tumor lysis include potassium and phosphate binding agents, and although rarely necessary in acute leukemia, dialysis. Intravenous calcium replacement is contraindicated in patients with tumor lysis syndrome because of concomitant hyperphosphatemia unless severe symptoms of hypocalcemia (e.g., tetany) are present.

■ REMISSION INDUCTION THERAPY

The first goal of therapy is rapid induction of complete remission (CR). Criteria for CR include recovery of normal blood counts; a normal bone marrow with less than 5 percent myeloblasts and no clearly leukemic blasts (e.g., with Auer rods); and absence of extramedullary leukemia. The most commonly used remission induction regimens for AML consist of combination chemotherapy with cytarabine (cytosine arabinoside) and an anthracycline. Cytarabine, an antimetabolite phosphorylated to an active triphosphate form, interferes with DNA synthesis. Anthracyclines are DNA intercalaters. Their primary mode of action is considered to be interaction with topoisomerase II leading to breakage of DNA. Cytarabine is usually administered as a continuous intravenous infusion at 100 to 200 mg per square meter per day for 7 days. Anthracycline therapy generally consists of daunorubicin 45 mg per square meter intravenously on days 1, 2, and 3 of cytarabine (7 and 3 regimen). Treatment with idarubicin, a new anthracycline, at 12 or 13 mg per square meter in conjunction with cytarabine by 7 day continuous infusion is at least as effective and may be superior to daunorubicin and cytarabine therapy, according to several recent randomized trials.

Bone marrow aspiration and biopsy may be repeated 14 days following initiation of chemotherapy to document efficacy of the chemotherapy regimen in producing bone marrow aplasia. The bone marrow is re-examined when blood counts reach normal or a plateau in order to document CR versus residual leukemia. CR is usually achieved within 4 weeks of initiation of chemotherapy. If there is unequivocal persistent or recurrent leukemia in the bone marrow on day 14 or subsequently, the patient has traditionally been treated again with cytarabine and anthracycline in doses similar to those given initially but for 5 and 2 days respectively. Our recommendation, however, is to change therapy in this setting. We prefer to give high-dose cytarabine (3 g per square meter over 1 hour every 12 hours for 12 doses, with a reduction to 1.5 g per square meter for patients over 50 years of age) and an anthracycline (e.g., idarubicin 12 mg per square meter daily for 3 days) as a second course of induction therapy for patients with clear-cut persistent or recurrent leukemia in a cellular marrow after standard dose cytarabine and anthracycline therapy. We also recommend consideration of bone marrow transplantation early in these patients' management. In APL a second course of chemotherapy should be withheld despite persistence of leukemic promyelocytes in the bone marrow on day 14, as CR frequently follows one course of therapy in this subtype of AML despite persistence of leukemia cells in the bone marrow during the initial weeks of therapy.

With the 7 and 3 cytarabine and daunorubicin regimen outlined above, CR is achieved in 65 to 75 percent of adults with de novo AML. Two-thirds achieve remission after a single course of therapy, and one-third require two courses. Approximately half of the patients who do not achieve a CR have leukemia that is resistant to the therapy administered, and half do not achieve remission because of fatal complications of bone marrow aplasia or impaired recovery of normal stem cells.

High-dose (2 to 3 g per square meter every 12 hours for 12 doses) cytarabine-based regimens have been used as initial remission induction therapy in several recent clinical trials. High-dose cytarabine and an anthracycline produce remission rates similar to those seen with standard 7 and 3 regimens, but more patients achieve remission with a single course of therapy, and remission appears to last longer. The hematologic toxicity of high-dose cytarabine-based induction regimens has typically been greater than that associated with 7 and 3 regimens. Data from Roswell Park Cancer Institute suggest that administration of recombinant human granulocyte colony-stimulating factor (G-CSF) beginning 12 hours following completion of chemotherapy accelerates count recovery following high-dose cytarabine and anthracycline induction chemotherapy, such that hematologic toxicity does not exceed and is often less than that associated with 7 and 3 regimens without growth factors. For secondary AML, treatment with high-dose cytarabine and an anthracycline has yielded better results than 7 and 3 in some but not all studies. When high-dose cytarabine regimens are used for patients over 50 years old, the cytarabine dose must be reduced (maximum dose 1.5 to 2 g per square meter) because of the higher risk of cerebellar toxicity in older patients. All patients treated with high-dose cytarabine must be closely monitored for cerebellar toxicity. Full cerebellar testing should be performed before each dose, and further high-dose cytarabine should be withheld if evidence of cerebellar toxicity develops.

Recombinant hematopoietic growth factors have recently been incorporated into clinical trials in AML. Both G-CSF and GM-CSF have been administered after completion of chemotherapy to accelerate recovery of normal stem cells. Based on results of early studies, growth factor therapy does appear to accelerate granulocyte recovery, and despite concern about potential adverse effects of stimulating growth of leukemia cells in vivo, it does not appear to have an adverse effect on remission rate. Effects on disease-free survival are not yet known. We favor the use of growth factors following chemotherapy for AML in the setting of clinical trials so that long-term follow-up data can be obtained to monitor for late adverse effects. Recombinant hematopoietic growth factors have also been administered prior to and during remission induction chemotherapy, with the goal of enhancing sensitivity to cell cycle-specific chemotherapeutic agents by increasing the numbers of cells in S phase. The impact of growth factor therapy used in this fashion (growth factor priming) on outcome of remission induction therapy in AML has not been significant in most clinical trials reported to date. We believe that at present growth factor priming should be undertaken only in a clinical trial.

Daily oral all-*trans*-retinoic acid is effective remission induction therapy in APL with rearrangements of the PML and retinoic acid receptor genes, but not in other subtypes of AML. APL cells are induced to differentiate, and complications of cytotoxic therapy (e.g., disseminated intravascular coagulation, or DIC) are averted. However all-*trans*-retinoic acid therapy is not without problems, and knowledge of its unique toxicities is required. The retinoic acid syndrome may develop within the first 3 weeks of therapy. The syndrome includes fever, chest pain, dyspnea, pulmonary infiltrates, and progressive hypoxemia. Unless reversed, it can be rapidly fatal. It must be aggressively managed, with early initiation of corticosteroid therapy and supportive care measures. Patients with elevated white blood cell counts are at particular risk for developing the syndrome but it may also develop in the setting of low white blood cell counts. Addition of chemotherapy if the white blood cell count rises above 10×10^9 per liter has been advocated by some groups. It is important that patients induced into remission with all-*trans*-retinoic acid receive consolidation chemotherapy, as essentially all patients treated with all-*trans*-retinoic acid alone relapse. We believe that consolidation chemotherapy should include an anthracycline. All-*trans*-retinoic acid is also being evaluated as maintenance therapy following consolidation chemotherapy. Early results of a recent Intergroup clinical trial appear to indicate a favorable impact of all-*trans*-retinoic acid administered in induction and/or maintenance phase of therapy on relapse rate.

■ SUPPORTIVE CARE

Adjunctive measures geared to supporting patients through several weeks of granulocytopenia and thrombocytopenia are critical to the success of AML therapy. Patients with AML should be treated in centers with availability of and expertise in supportive measures for their management.

Multilumen right atrial catheters should be inserted through a subcutaneous tunnel as soon as patients have been stabilized and should be used thereafter for administration of intravenous medications and transfusions as well as for blood drawing. The separation between the vascular access site and the exit site and the presence of a Dacron cuff in the subcutaneous channel reduce the risk of infectious complications. With meticulous attention to sterile technique in catheter placement and maintenance, catheters may often be left in place for months.

Adequate and prompt blood bank support is critical to therapy of AML. Platelet transfusions should be given as needed to maintain a platelet count above 20×10^9 per liter. We believe that the platelet count should be kept at higher levels in febrile patients and during periods of active bleeding or DIC. Measures that may be used in patients with poor post-transfusion platelet count increments include administration of platelets from HLA-matched donors and intravenous immunoglobin therapy. Red blood cell transfusions should be administered to keep the hemoglobin above 8.5 g per deciliter. Blood products leukodepleted by filtration should be used to avert or delay alloimmunization as well as febrile reactions. Blood products should also be irradiated to prevent transfusion-induced graft versus host disease. CMV-negative blood products should be used for CMV-seronegative patients who are potential candidates for allogeneic bone marrow transplantation. Leukodepleted products should be used for these patients if CMV-negative products are not available.

Infectious complications remain the major cause of morbidity and of death during induction and postinduction chemotherapy for AML. Prophylactic administration of antibacterial antibiotics is controversial. In contrast, antifungal prophylaxis (e.g. nystatin, fluconazole, or itraconazole) is generally thought to be indicated. For patients who are HSV-seropositive, acyclovir prophylaxis is effective in preventing reactivation of latent HSV infections.

Fever develops in the vast majority of patients, but infections are documented in only half of febrile patients. Early initiation of empiric broad-spectrum antibacterial and antifungal antibiotics has significantly reduced the number of patients dying of infectious complications. A combination of antibiotics adequate to treat both gram-negative and gram-positive organisms should be instituted at the onset of fever in a granulocytopenic host, following clinical evaluation and procurement of cultures and roentgenograms aimed at documenting the source of the fever. Specific antibiotic regimens should be based on antibiotic sensitivity data obtained from the institution at which the patient is being treated. We prefer to use imipenem-cilastatin with or without vancomycin as first-line therapy. Other acceptable regimens include an antipseudomonal semisynthetic penicillin (e.g., piperacillin) combined with an aminoglycoside, a third-generation cephalosporin with antipseudomonal activity (i.e., ceftazidime) or double beta-lactam combinations (ceftazidime and piperacillin), with or without vancomycin. Aminoglycosides should be avoided if possible for patients with renal insufficiency. For patients with known immediate hypersensitivity-type reactions to penicillin, aztreonam may be substituted for the beta-lactams. Aztreonam should be combined with an aminoglycoside rather than used alone. Empiric amphotericin therapy should be initiated in neutropenic patients who remain febrile without a known source or who develop new fever while on broad-spectrum antibacterial antibiotics. Antibacterial and antifungal antibiotics should be continued until patients are no longer neutropenic, regardless of whether a specific source has been found for the fever.

■ POSTINDUCTION THERAPY

Induction of a durable first remission is critical to long-term disease-free survival in AML. Once relapse has occurred, AML is generally curable only by bone marrow transplantation. A major focus of current research is detection of residual leukemia cells in the bone marrow of patients who appear to be in remission using techniques such as the polymerase chain reaction, multiparameter flow cytometry, and fluorescence in situ hybridization (FISH). The availability of sensitive and specific methods for detection of occult residual leukemia cells during CR would allow optimization of postinduction management for individual patients.

Approaches to postinduction therapy in AML have included maintenance, consolidation, and intensification regimens. The use of intensification regimens, including bone marrow transplantation, has resulted in substantial improvement, with relapse-free survival rates of up to 50 percent. Maintenance therapy, defined as treatment less myelosuppressive and intensive than induction therapy, prolongs remission but does not result in long-term disease-free survival for most patients. Median remission duration of patients receiving maintenance therapy following standard-dose cytarabine and anthracycline induction has been in the range of 8 to 18 months in various studies, compared with 4 months for patients receiving no postinduction therapy. Four year relapse-free survival is less than 20 percent. Maintenance therapy is generally no longer used in AML.

Consolidation therapy, defined as treatment of similar intensity to that used in remission induction regimens, further prolongs duration of first remission and yields 4 year disease-free survivals on the order of 20 to 30 percent. Administration of maintenance therapy following consolidation does not improve results further.

Intensification therapy is postinduction therapy more intensive than that used for induction, comprising higher doses of drugs used in the induction regimen or myelosuppressive doses of drugs other than those used in the induction regimen or both. High-dose regimens followed by allogeneic or autologous bone marrow transplantation in first remission also are a form of intensification therapy. Use of intensification regimens has consistently resulted in higher disease-free survival, on the order of 40 to 60 percent, depending on the regimen and the patient population. It is our policy to use intensification therapy in all patients with AML who achieve remission.

Several approaches to intensification appear to yield approximately equivalent relapse-free survival rates. Some 40 to 60 percent of patients undergoing allogeneic bone marrow transplantation in first remission of AML appear to be cured. Allogeneic bone marrow transplantation is generally restricted to patients under age 65 years who have an HLA-compatible family bone marrow donor or those under age 55 years with an HLA-compatible unrelated donor. Because of the age restrictions and the lack of availability of a suitable donor for many patients, allogeneic bone marrow transplantation is a therapeutic option for only approximately one-third of AML patients. Patients who undergo allogeneic bone marrow transplantation but are not cured include those who succumb to treatment-related complications including infections and graft versus host disease as well as patients who relapse. Autologous bone marrow transplantation using unmodified remission bone marrow or marrow purged of residual leukemia cells by chemical or immunologic methods has also yielded long-term disease-free survival. In addition, disease-free survival comparable with that achieved with bone marrow transplantation regimens has been achieved in clinical trials using intensive postinduction chemotherapy without transplantation. Wolff and colleagues reported a 49 percent relapse-free survival rate in 87 patients (median age, 38 years) treated with a high-dose cytarabine and daunorubicin intensification regimen, with a median follow-up of more than 3.5 years. The relapse-free survival rate was 80 percent for adult patients up to age 25 years. The principal cause of failure of the regimen was relapse; only 5 percent of patients died of therapy-related complications. A recent randomized trial by Cancer and Leukemia Group B (CALGB) demonstrated significantly better relapse-free survival in patients receiving postinduction therapy with high-dose rather than standard-dose cytarabine. Of note, relapse-free survival rates in the range of 60 to 80 percent were achieved in patients in favorable cytogenetic subgroups using high-dose cytarabine-based intensification therapy.

The approach we favor for patients in first complete remission is high-dose intensification without bone marrow transplantation, using bone marrow transplantation to salvage patients who relapse. It is important that potential bone marrow donors be identified in first remission so that transplantation will be available as soon as relapse is detected. Patients with unfavorable prognostic findings (e.g. therapy-related leukemia, antecedent hematologic disorder, cytogenetic findings with adverse prognostic significance) or with matched unrelated donors should be considered for bone marrow transplantation in first remission, although only limited data are available to support this approach. Autologous bone marrow transplantation is an option for patients for whom a suitable donor cannot be found or who are above the age limit for allogeneic transplantation. Consideration should be given to bone marrow harvesting and cryopreservation early in remission in these patients. The utility of bone marrow purging and the optimal method of purging are not yet defined. We favor allogeneic in preference to autologous bone marrow transplantation for patients of appropriate age with a suitable donor. Patients with AML should be referred to a bone marrow transplantation center for consultation in first remission or at the time of documentation of primary refractory disease, so they can discuss the optimal approach to transplantation and timing of transplantation on an individual basis.

■ MANAGEMENT OF RELAPSE

A second remission may be induced in up to 50 percent of patients with AML who relapse, especially if intensive post-remission therapy was not employed. The choice of reinduction regimen depends on the difficulty of the initial remission induction, the length of the prior CR, and the type of postinduction therapy administered. Patients with long first remissions generally relapse with drug-sensitive disease and may achieve a second remission with repetition of the original induction regimen. However long-term disease-free survival generally requires treatment with additional agents not previously received or bone marrow transplantation. Salvage regimens used for relapsed disease as well as for refractory disease include high-dose cytarabine with an anthracycline or mitoxantrone (for patients who have not received high-dose cytarabine in induction or consolidation) and high-dose etoposide in conjunction with high-dose cyclophosphamide. Patients eligible for allogeneic or autologous transplantation should be expeditiously transplanted early in first relapse or in second remission. Because long-term disease-free survival is approximately the same (30 percent) after allogeneic bone marrow transplantation in first relapse as in second remission, but fewer than 50 percent of patients achieve a second CR, bone marrow transplantation at the first sign of relapse is preferred.

■ COMMENTS

Significant progress has been achieved in the management of adult AML. Nevertheless, long-term disease-free survival is currently achieved in fewer than 50 percent of patients. Optimal therapy has not yet been defined, and therapy is only now beginning to be tailored to the individual patient according to prognostic factors. Given the intensity of therapy required for AML and the potential for excellent treatment outcome, it is essential that patients with AML be referred to specialized treatment centers. Moreover, given the substantial progress still to be made in defining optimal management of patients with AML, it is critical that patients be enrolled in therapeutic trials with the goal of optimizing therapy for AML in general as well as for particular patient subgroups.

Acknowledgment

The authors thank Dr. Brian Lipman for his helpful critique of portions of the manuscript.

Suggested Reading

Ball ED, Rybka WB. Autologous bone marrow transplantation for adult acute leukemia. Hematol Oncol Clin North Am 1993; 7:201–231.

Bishop JF, Matthews JP, Young GA, et al. A randomized study of high dose cytarabine in induction in acute myeloid leukemia. Blood 1996; 87: 1710–1717.

Christiansen NP. Allogeneic bone marrow transplantation for the treatment of adult acute leukemias. Hematol Oncol Clin North Am 1993; 7:177–200.

Mayer RJ, Davis RB, Schiffer CA, et al. Intensive post-remission chemotherapy in adults with acute myeloid leukemia. N Engl J Med 1994; 331:896–903.

Rowe JM, Andersen JM, Mazza JJ, et al. A randomized placebo-controlled phase III study of granulocyte-macrophage colony-stimulating factor in adult patients (>55 to 70 years of age) with acute myelogenous leukemia; a study of the Eastern Cooperative Oncology Group (E1490). Blood 1995; 86:457–462.

Wolff SN, Herzig RH, Fay JW, et al. High-dose cytarabine and daunorubicin as consolidation therapy for acute myeloid leukemia in first remission: Long-term follow-up and results. J Clin Oncol 1989; 7:1260–1267.

CHRONIC LYMPHOCYTIC LEUKEMIA

Kanti R. Rai, M.D., F.A.C.P.
Jagmohan Kalra, M.D., F.A.C.P.

The most common type of leukemia found in a population aged 50 years and over is chronic lymphocytic leukemia (CLL). The classic form of CLL is the B-cell type (B-CLL); only about 5 percent of cases manifest as the T-cell type or as prolymphocytic leukemia. These last two variants exhibit certain phenotypic and morphologic characteristics, and they are generally not responsive to therapy. However, no therapeutic approaches for these variants are distinct from those applied in B-CLL. This discussion focuses on management of patients with B-CLL. As is the case with many other malignancies, approach to treatment differs considerably among centers. The treatment plan practiced in our clinic is detailed here.

■ CLINICAL STAGING OF CHRONIC LYMPHOCYTIC LEUKEMIA

It is first necessary to establish the clinical stage of a patient newly diagnosed as having CLL. The criteria of staging are as follows:

Supported by grants from Helena Rubinstein Foundation, Dennis Klar Leukemia Fund, National Leukemia Association, United Leukemia Fund, Wayne Goldsmith Leukemia Fund, and Lowenstein Foundation.

Stage 0. Stage 0 manifests only with lymphocytosis in the peripheral blood and bone marrow. Although an absolute lymphocyte count of 5,000 per cubic millimeter is an acceptable definition of lymphocytosis in peripheral blood, in most instances this count is over 15,000. Bone marrow aspirate must show 30 percent or more mature-appearing lymphocytes upon differential count of all nucleated cells, or a biopsy specimen must show lymphocytic infiltration. Bone marrow is normocellular or hypercellular (i.e., not hypocellular) at the time of diagnosis.

Stage I. Stage I exhibits lymphocytosis with evidence of enlarged lymph nodes.

Stage II. Stage II exhibits lymphocytosis with evidence of enlargement of the spleen and/or the liver. Lymph nodes may or may not be enlarged.

Stage III. Stage III is characterized by lymphocytosis with anemia (hemoglobin less than 11 g per deciliter). The nodes, spleen, and liver may or may not be enlarged.

Stage IV. Stage IV exhibits lymphocytosis with thrombocytopenia (platelets below 100,000 per cubic millimeter). Anemia and enlargement of nodes, spleen, and liver may or may not be present.

The actuarial survival curves of patients with CLL show three distinct patterns rather than five. Therefore, in accordance with the survival curves, the following three risk groups have been identified: patients in stage 0 constitute the low-risk group, stages I and II constitute intermediate-risk group, and stages III and IV combined constitute high-risk group. This modified Rai staging system is being used in all clinical trials in the United States.

After the clinical stage is determined, we look for symptoms (e.g., weakness, weight loss, night sweats, fever, and increased susceptibility to infections). In addition, we monitor blood counts serially at about monthly intervals to determine the rate of increase of blood lymphocyte count, whether lymphocyte doubling time (actual or projected) is long (more than 12 months) or short (up to and including 12 months). The latter is associated with an aggressive clinical course in the low- and intermediate-risk groups.

■ OBSERVATION PHASE

We do not institute any cytotoxic therapy immediately upon making a diagnosis of CLL. A period of observation after diagnosis is advisable to determine whether any treatment is indicated.

■ INDICATIONS FOR THERAPEUTIC INTERVENTION

After an observation period of about 4 to 6 months, during which time the patient is seen regularly in the clinic, a decision is made whether therapeutic intervention is necessary. We use the following indications as guidelines and institute therapy if any one of these is present.

1. Progressive disease-related symptoms.
2. Evidence of progressive marrow failure (i.e., worsening anemia, thrombocytopenia, recurrent sepsis associated with hypogammaglobulinemia).
3. Autoimmune hemolytic anemia or immune thrombocytopenia.
4. Massive splenomegaly with or without evidence of hypersplenism.
5. Bulky disease as evidenced by large lymphoid masses.
6. Progressive hyperlymphocytosis. The rate of increase of blood lymphocyte count is usually a more reliable indicator than the absolute number. We generally do not withhold therapy when the count is higher than 150,000 per cubic millimeter. Leukostasis, which is associated with a high leukocyte count in other leukemias, is seldom encountered in CLL, but complications from hyperviscosity syndrome of hyperleukocytosis have been reported in CLL.

On rare occasions, however, the patient is markedly symptomatic at initial diagnosis. It may not be advisable to withhold therapy under such a circumstance; we institute therapy immediately in these patients.

■ THERAPEUTIC PLAN FOR SPECIFIC INDICATIONS

Progressive Disease-Related Symptoms

Usually such symptoms are controlled with chlorambucil and prednisone. We prefer to give intermittent bursts of treatment at intervals of 3 to 4 weeks rather than to treat by continuous daily regimens throughout the month. Chlorambucil is given at 0.7 mg per kilogram of body weight by mouth in a single dose on day 1, day 28, and so forth. Prednisone is given at 0.5 mg per kilogram body weight by mouth in one dose or divided in two doses daily for 7 days (days 1 through 7) in each monthly cycle. Concomitantly, allopurinol 300 mg daily by mouth is prescribed for 7 days of each cycle. Usually, symptoms (e.g., weakness, night sweats, fever) are controlled within 6 to 8 months after institution of therapy, at which time such therapy may be discontinued and the observation phase resumed.

Autoimmune Hemolytic Anemia or Immune Thrombocytopenia

Prednisone alone is given for these complications. Prednisone is started at 0.8 mg per kilogram of body weight per day by mouth for 2 weeks, and if the anemia or thrombocytopenia has started to improve, the prednisone dose is reduced by 50 percent at each 2 week interval for an overall continuous therapy time of 6 weeks. Thereafter, prednisone may be given for 1 week every month at 0.5 mg per kilogram body weight per day for an additional 4 to 6 months.

Patients with CLL are generally elderly people with a somewhat high incidence of diabetes mellitus and osteoporosis. Therefore, special attention must be given to the control of hyperglycemia and skeletal problems, which may be exaggerated with prednisone therapy.

Massive Splenomegaly with or without Evidence of Hypersplenism

Radiotherapy of the spleen is our first choice of treatment. Usually a total dose of 250 to 1,000 cGy delivered in 5 to 10 fractions is adequate to reduce spleen size and control hypersplenism. However, if there is inadequate control with radiotherapy, if the spleen again enlarges to significant proportions, or if hypersplenism remains a major problem, splenectomy is advisable. Even elderly patients (with good cardiopulmonary status) withstand this surgery without undue morbidity. However, if massive splenomegaly is not a solitary feature of a patient's disease (i.e., if adenopathy of a significant degree is also present), chemotherapy should be the initial therapeutic choice. If hypersplenism and splenomegaly persist after an adequate trial, splenic irradiation or splenectomy should be considered.

Bulky Disease of Large Lymphoid Masses

Most often chlorambucil therapy without prednisone at the dosage already detailed is adequate to shrink large lymphoid masses. Such therapy is usually necessary for 1 to 2 years on an intermittent monthly schedule. However, if the lymphoid masses are not generalized but are present at only one or two sites or if such masses are causing or likely to cause symptoms by pressing on adjacent vital organs (e.g., on a bronchus or the superior vena cava), local irradiation therapy is recommended. The total dose necessary under these circumstances ranges between 500 and 1,500 cGy delivered in 5 to 15 fractions.

Progressive Hyperlymphocytosis

Usually chlorambucil at the dosage already detailed is adequate to reduce the blood lymphocyte count. If resources are available, leukapheresis should be the first step in therapy when the starting blood count is in excess of 350,000 per cubic millimeter; chlorambucil therapy is initiated immediately after three to four treatments on a cell separator machine. Side effects of chlorambucil are usually mild nausea and minimal suppression of bone marrow function. Allopurinol should always be added while treating hyperlymphocytosis.

THERAPEUTIC GUIDELINES BASED ON CLINICAL STAGING

Low-Risk Group

Patients in this stage are generally without any symptoms, and no cytotoxic agent is prescribed. However, patients should be seen in the clinic at intervals of 1 to 3 months. Median life expectancy is in excess of 12 years.

Intermediate-Risk Group

Asymptomatic

There is no evidence that cytotoxic therapy is necessary or beneficial in these patients. We continue to observe them at monthly intervals. The median life expectancy of these patients ranges between 6 and 8 years and is probably not changed with therapy.

Symptomatic

We recommend chlorambucil on an intermittent monthly schedule at the dosage already detailed. The median life expectancy of these patients is about 5 years. It is not yet known whether therapy increases life expectancy.

High-Risk Group

Patients in these stages have a median life expectancy of 1.5 years. We give chlorambucil and prednisone to these patients at the dosage already detailed. The therapeutic objective is to achieve a partial (PR) or a complete remission (CR). Usually it takes 8 to 10 months of therapy to achieve a partial remission. Patients achieving any remission have prolongation of median survival time to about 5 years, and patients achieving less than a partial remission have a 1.5 year median survival.

ALTERNATIVE TO CHLORAMBUCIL

We use cyclophosphamide in lieu of chlorambucil if the patient cannot tolerate the latter drug or is no longer showing a satisfactory response to it. Cyclophosphamide is administered by mouth or by intravenous injection. The dose of cyclophosphamide, on intermittent schedule, is 200 mg per square meter per day by mouth for 5 days in cycles that repeat at 3 week intervals, or 750 mg per square meter on day 1 by intravenous injection every 3 weeks. Toxicity of this drug consists of controllable nausea and vomiting, hair loss, bone marrow suppression, and chemical cystitis.

An intergroup protocol is available in the United States and Canada to test whether the new drug fludarabine is better than chlorambucil in B-CLL patients who have not been previously treated with chlorambucil (front-line therapy). We offer this protocol to all eligible patients.

SECOND-LINE THERAPY

When single-agent therapy (chlorambucil or cyclophosphamide) with or without prednisone fails to control CLL-related problems, we use fludarabine phosphate. Fludarabine phosphate is administered intravenously daily for 5 days every month at 25 mg per square meter per day. Any beneficial response occurs within 6 to 8 cycles (6 to 8 months) of therapy; usual responses are PR and occasionally CR. Toxicities are dose related and generally avoidable. The second promising new drug, 2-chlorodeoxyadenosine (2-Cda), is in experimental trials. Combination chemotherapy protocols are the options to be considered for patients not responding to fludarabine or 2-CdA. These are the combinations usually administered in treatment of non-Hodgkin's lymphoma or multiple myeloma, e.g., cyclophosphamide, vincristine, and prednisone (COP); COP with doxorubicin (CHOP); and M2 protocol which consists of COP with carmustine (BCNU) and melphalan. The dosages in each combination are decided on after considering each patient's bone marrow reserve, previous exposure to and level of tolerance of cytotoxic therapy, and the overall medical status.

ASSESSMENT OF THERAPEUTIC RESPONSE

We define a CR as no symptoms and no abnormal findings on physical examination and normal values for hemogram and bone marrow studies. If all these criteria are fulfilled but serum immunoglobulin levels are still lower than normal or there is persistence of increased monoclonal B lymphocytes, we rate such a response as a CR. Achievement of even such a CR is unusual in CLL, and it is our belief that our target must be to increase the incidence of CR according to this clinical definition before we can aim to achieve a CR that includes normalization of immune function and lymphocyte subpopulation ratios as well. A partial remission is defined as a 50 percent decrease in absolute lymphocyte count in peripheral blood, hemoglobin more than 11 g per deciliter, and platelets more than 100,000 per cubic millimeter, or improvement in these values by 50 percent of their deviation from normal and decrease in palpable lymph nodes and spleen by at least 50 percent.

SUPPORTIVE THERAPY

To control signs and symptoms of anemia, transfusion of packed red cells is given as supportive therapy. Transfusions of platelets are used only in the presence of bleeding and severe thrombocytopenia. High-dose gamma globulin therapy by intravenous route, 200 to 400 mg per kilogram body weight every 21 days, benefits patients who have marked hypogammaglobulinemia or recurrent bacterial infections. There are no contraindications to giving pneumococcal or flu vaccine, but the usefulness of such immunizations is in doubt in patients with CLL. Analogues of androgens have been effective on a few occasions by stimulating erythropoiesis in patients with significant anemia. However, such therapy may be associated with adverse side effects of hepatotoxicity, fluid retention, exacerbation of symptoms of prostatic hypertrophy in men, and masculinizing effects in women. We have observed beneficial responses to cyclosporine therapy in patients with CLL whose severe anemia is found to be from pure red cell aplasia. Some patients with anemia (nonhemolytic) of CLL respond to recombinant human erythropoietin therapy.

■ TERMINAL PHASE

In CLL, death occurs most often from infectious complications secondary to disease-induced or therapy-induced neutropenia and immunodeficiency. Complications are especially difficult to control in advanced stages of CLL. The next most common causes of morbidity and mortality are bleeding complications, hepatic failure, and inanition and wasting. CLL is sometimes transformed into a large cell lymphoma (Richter's syndrome) or a prolymphocytoid cell leukemia. Such cases receive aggressive chemotherapy generally used in high-grade lymphoma, but there is little evidence that any regimen is effective in prolonging life. Even less frequently, CLL transforms into acute myelocytic leukemia, which is also refractory to intensive therapy that is used successfully in de novo acute leukemia.

Suggested Reading

Dighiero G, Travade Ph, Chevret S, et al (French Cooperative Group on CLL). B-cell chronic lymphocytic leukemia: Present status and future directions. Blood 1991; 78:1901–1914.

Foon KA, Rai KR, Gale RP. Chronic lymphocytic leukemia: New insights into biology and therapy. Ann Intern Med 1990; 113:525–539.

Gale RP, Montserrat E. Intensive therapy of chronic lymphocytic leukaemia. Baillieres Clin Haematol 1993; 6:879–885.

Rai KR. An outline of clinical management of chronic lymphocytic leukemia. In: Cheson BD, ed. Chronic lymphocytic leukemia: Scientific advances and clinical developments. New York: Marcel Dekker, 1993:241.

CHRONIC MYELOGENOUS LEUKEMIA

John M. Goldman, D.M., F.R.C.P., F.R.C.Path.

Chronic myelogenous leukemia (CML), also known as chronic myeloid leukemia or chronic granulocytic leukemia, is a relatively well defined disorder that accounts for 10 to 15 percent of all cases of leukemia. It has an incidence of about 1 per 100,000 of the population and is slightly more common in men than in women. It is thought to be a result of an acquired genetic change in a pluripotential hematopoietic stem cell and may thus be regarded as a clonal myeloproliferative disorder. Almost all patients with CML have in their leukemia cells the Philadelphia (Ph) chromosome, which is an abnormal 22q-chromosome resulting from a (9;22)(q34;q11) translocation. The Ph chromosome carries a chimeric gene, BCR-ABL, which is expressed as a protein of 210 kd, $p210^{BCR-ABL}$. The p210 is thought to play a central role in the pathogenesis of the chronic phase of CML.

Patients with CML usually present in the chronic or stable phase. In Western countries about 30 percent of patients have no symptoms at presentation; the diagnosis is based on blood tests performed for unrelated purposes, such as blood donation or routine medical tests. The remaining 70 percent have symptoms attributable to anemia, hemorrhage, or splenomegaly. The leukocyte count is typically in the range 100 to 300×10^9 per liter; platelet numbers are usually somewhat raised. The bone marrow is hypercellular and shows complete loss of normal fat spaces.

After some years in chronic phase the disease transforms spontaneously into a more advanced phase. This may take the form of an acute blast cell transformation, sometimes called *blast crisis.* In most cases the blast cells resemble to a degree those of acute myeloid leukemia; however, in about 20 percent of cases they have surface membrane and molecular features similar to those of acute lymphoblastic leukemia. In other cases the chronic phase may change more insidiously; this phase intermediate between chronic phase and blastic phase is called *accelerated.* Acceleration in due course evolves to an acute blastic phase. In 5 to 10 percent of cases the disease evolves very slowly toward myelofibrosis with increasing splenomegaly and eventual marrow failure.

■ STAGING AND PROGNOSIS

The median duration of chronic phase from the time of diagnosis is about 5 years, and the median duration of survival is about 4 to 7 years. These values, slightly longer than those quoted in the 1980s, appear to reflect the tendency to diagnose CML earlier in its natural history. It is possible that current treatment, especially the use of interferon-alpha (IFN-alpha), has resulted in prolonged survival but the notion that the disease has altered *sui generis* is extremely unlikely.

A number of efforts were made in the 1980s to identify clinical features present at diagnosis that would measure the extent and tempo of disease and therefore by implication predict duration of survival in individual patients. The most widely used system is that devised by Sokal, which takes account of patient age, spleen size, blast cell count, and platelet numbers at diagnosis; even this system discriminates relatively poorly between groups of patients and has limited value in making treatment decisions for individual patients. In practice the best determinant of survival is an assessment of the response to treatment: patients with a low leukocyte doubling time after initial treatment, patients with a low requirement for chemotherapy, and especially patients who respond to IFN-alpha all seem to survive longer than other patients.

THERAPY

Disease Presenting in Chronic Phase

As soon as the diagnosis of CML is confirmed, a treatment strategy appropriate to the patient must be devised. The first priority is a frank discussion of the prognostic implications of the diagnosis with some emphasis on the uncertainty of prognosis in individual patients. The relative roles of standard chemotherapy, treatment with IFN-alpha, allografting, and autografting should all be explained within the first few weeks of diagnosis. For example, for younger patients with HLA-identical siblings allogeneic bone marrow transplantation may be optimal treatment and should probably be performed within 6 months of diagnosis. For much older patients busulfan may be the simplest approach to treatment, and its known toxicity may be relatively unimportant. For the majority of patients the best initial treatment is probably IFN-alpha, but the details of administration and duration of treatment are complex.

The issue of fertility for younger patients who have not yet started or completed their families is of great importance. Men should be offered the opportunity to store cryopreserved semen before any treatment is initiated; women should be offered treatment that does not impair ovarian function, or if bone marrow transplantation is planned, embryo cryopreservation should be considered. Women who present with CML in pregnancy may opt for termination; more often they are keen that the pregnancy should continue. The leukocyte count can almost always be controlled by repeated leukapheresis without cytotoxic drugs.

Since there is no convincing evidence that busulfan or hydroxyurea prolongs survival, it was until very recently reasonable to defer for a while initiation of treatment for patients with relatively low leukocyte counts, e.g., less than 100×10^9 per liter. The recent recognition that IFN-alpha may prolong survival, especially in patients who achieve a major degree of cytogenetic conversion in the marrow (from Ph-positive to Ph-negative), implies that the drug should be used as soon as convenient after diagnosis.

Interferon-Alpha

IFN-alpha is one of a large family of glycoproteins that have immunosuppressive and other inhibitory functions in biologic systems. It restores the leukocyte count to normal in most patients and substantially reduces the proportion of Ph-positive marrow cells in 10 to 20 percent of cases. On the basis of two recently reported randomized studies in which treatment with IFN-alpha was compared with treatment with cytotoxic drugs, IFN-alpha seems to prolong life by perhaps 2 years. This conclusion, an important contribution to the management of CML, justifies use of the drug as primary treatment in all patients who are not already scheduled for bone marrow transplantation. However, a number of issues relating to its use are not yet resolved.

Two forms of IFN-alpha derived from recombinant DNA and one form purified from lymphoblastoid cells lines are available. All are probably broadly equivalent. It is usual to start treatment with 3 million units daily by subcutaneous injection and to increase the dose if necessary every 3 or 4 weeks until control of the leukocyte count is achieved; few patients tolerate a dose in excess of 9 million units daily. Another approach is to start with a higher dose, e.g., 5 million units per square meter body surface area daily and to reduce if toxicity is excessive. With either of these schedules 60 to 80 percent of patients will achieve normal leukocyte counts, and the counts may remain normal for months or years. In some patients IFN-alpha eventually fails to control the count and use of other drugs is required; in other cases blast transformation supervenes even though the leukocyte count is in the normal range. About 5 to 10 percent of patients achieve 100 percent Ph negativity, and this may last for a number of years. The risk of transformation is small in such patients as long as Ph negativity persists, but the ability to demonstrate in the blood persistence of BCR-ABL transcripts, albeit at low number, by the polymerase chain reaction means that such patients cannot be regarded as cured.

IFN-alpha causes influenza-like symptoms, fevers, muscle aches, sweats, and malaise, in almost all patients for the first 2 to 3 weeks after starting treatment, but these problems usually resolve spontaneously; they may recur when the dosage is increased. They may be lessened by prophylactic use of paracetamol. More severe symptoms, including anorexia, weight loss, depression, hair loss, and various cutaneous manifestations, may develop in patients who have been taking the drug for some months or longer. About 20 percent of patients cannot tolerate the drug, and it seems injudicious to insist that it be continued if the patient's quality of life is seriously impaired.

Hydroxyurea

Hydroxyurea is a ribonucleotide reductase inhibitor and thus a cell cycle-specific antagonist of DNA synthesis. It has gained popularity in the past decade because it is safe to administer and its cumulative toxicity much less than that of busulfan. It is conventional to start treatment with 2 g daily by mouth and to continue this dose until the patient's leukocyte count is normal. The dose can then be reduced to a maintenance level, typically 1 or 1.5 g daily. Some patients are well controlled on an intermediate dose, namely 1 g alternating with 1.5 g daily. Doses of 3 g or more can be given for short periods if necessary. The drug must be given continuously, since the leukocyte count rises rapidly if dosage is reduced or interrupted.

Hydroxyurea may be given to newly diagnosed patients in whom very rapid reduction of the leukocyte or platelet count is desirable. It can be given in combination with IFN-alpha. It is probably the drug of choice for patients who cannot tolerate IFN-alpha.

The major toxicities induced by hydroxyurea are nausea and diarrhea, usually dose related. Occasional patients get rashes or buccal mucosal ulcers. The red cells are macrocytic and the marrow somewhat megaloblastic. Unlike busulfan, hydroxyurea does not induce irreversible marrow failure. It is not generally regarded as mitogenic.

Busulfan

Busulfan (1,4-dimethanesulphonoxybutane) is generally classified as an alkylating agent. It was introduced into clinical practice in the 1950s and rapidly became the treatment of choice for CML. Treatment was usually started at 6 or 8 mg daily. The leukocyte count was monitored weekly and busulfan was stopped when the leukocyte count reached 20×10^9

per liter. The count would continue to fall thereafter for some weeks. The leukocyte count could then be maintained in the normal range by administration of 0.5 to 2 mg daily. The greatest danger with busulfan usage was accidental overdosage or administration of standard doses to the rare patients who were unduly sensitive to the drug; thus, the drug occasionally produced marrow aplasia culminating in death. It also induces irreversible infertility in both sexes after only a few months of treatment. Other side effects, mostly related to cumulative dosage, include cutaneous pigmentation, cataract formation, and a progressive pneumonitis, *busulfan lung*. Like other alkylating agents, it may be mitogenic and thus expedite the onset of blast transformation.

For these various reasons, busulfan is now rarely used in the primary management of CML. It may be useful in treating a patient still in chronic phase whose disease is resistant to hydroxyurea, and it can be given under supervision in single doses of 50 or 100 mg repeated at intervals of not less than 4 weeks to older patients whose compliance is thought to be poor.

Other Supportive Measures

It is conventional to give newly diagnosed patients allopurinol in additional to IFN-alpha or cytotoxic drugs. This may not be strictly necessary if the level of uric acid is not raised, and certainly the drug need not be continued after the leukocyte count has been restored to normal. Aspirin and other antiplatelet drugs are often given to patients whose platelet counts exceed 1 to 1.5×10^{12} per liter. Their value is not established.

Allogeneic Bone Marrow Transplantation

A diagnosis of CML is one of the major indications for allogeneic bone marrow transplantation. Most patients who receive transplants with marrow from HLA-identical siblings achieve durable Ph-negative hematopoiesis; the probability of leukemia-free survival at 5 years is 50 to 70 percent, and the incidence of relapse thereafter is extremely low, though relapses as late as 8 years have been seen. Most such patients reveal no BCR-ABL transcripts when blood and marrow are studied by use of the polymerase chain reaction. Thus operationally such patients may be regarded as cured.

The major cause of treatment failure is death due to graft versus host disease (GVHD). It is most common in older patients and most centers do not offer transplant to patients older than 50 or 55 years. It occurs more often and with greater severity in the presence of any degree of HLA disparity, and most centers will transplant patients only with marrow from genetically HLA-identical siblings. GVHD can be largely or completely abrogated by depletion of T lymphocytes from donor marrow before transfusion to the patient, but this technique greatly increases the risks of graft failure and of relapse: this last observation is cogent evidence for the role of a graft versus leukemia effect in the control or eradication of leukemia in the patient after transplant.

The fact that the median age of presentation for CML in the West is about 55 years and the fact that typical families in the West have two or three children mean that only about 50 percent of patients are young enough to be eligible for transplants, and only about 30 percent of these have HLA-identical siblings. Thus, only 10 percent of the total CML population can expect to be cured by bone marrow transplantation. This relative shortage of HLA-matched siblings has led some transplant centers to explore the use of partially matched family members and phenotypically HLA-matched unrelated donors for transplantation. In general transplant-related mortality is higher than when the donor is genetically HLA-identical with the patient, and the leukemia-free survival at 2 years is 40 to 60 percent.

The results of transplanting patients within 1 year of diagnosis seem to be better than results of transplanting patients who have been in chronic phase for longer periods. Moreover, the results of transplanting patients in advanced phases of CML are clearly inferior to results of transplant in chronic phase. These two points have led to the general view that any patient under the age of 50 or 55 who has an HLA-identical sibling should be offered treatment by bone marrow transplantation. Younger patients, say under 40 years, should be transplanted within 6 months of diagnosis; patients 40 to 55 years should perhaps receive an initial trial of treatment with IFN-alpha. They should receive a transplant if they do not achieve a major degree of Ph negativity.

Autologous Transplants

It has been known since 1970s that hematopoietic stem cells in the blood or marrow of patients with CML could be used for reconstitution of hematopoiesis after myeloablative treatment. Such stem cells are a mixture of Ph-positive cells and Ph-negative cells, the latter presumably nonleukemic. Thus, it may in principle be possible to treat a patient with CML in chronic phase in a way that favors reconstitution of Ph-negative hematopoiesis. It is possible also that autografting in chronic phase could be clinically beneficial merely as a result of reduction in the size of the leukemia stem cell compartment.

Anecdotal evidence together with some uncontrolled studies suggests that patients who receive autografts in chronic phase may survive longer than those who do not. Some of the patients are rendered transiently Ph-negative, and rare patients have remained Ph-negative for a year or more. It may be hoped that an autograft schedule can be developed that will induce remission in the average CML patient, as is achievable with acute leukemia.

Advanced CML

Accelerated Phase

Treatment for patients whose disease has entered an accelerated phase must be decided on an individual basis. Thus a change from hydroxyurea to busulfan may temporarily control a refractory leukocyte count. The addition of an oral antimetabolite, such as 6-mercaptopurine or 6-thioguanine, may be useful. A major degree of splenomegaly may be treated by irradiation of the spleen or perhaps by splenectomy. Bone marrow transplantation can be considered, but the risk of relapse is much higher than after transplant performed in chronic phase.

Acute Transformation

The first step in the management of CML in blastic transformation is to characterize the predominating blast cells. It should be possible to obtain preliminary information within 24 hours. If the transformation is myeloid, it can best be treated with drugs appropriate to the management of acute myeloid leukemia, i.e., some combination of an anthracycline with cytosine arabinoside with or without 6-thioguanine. The numbers of blast cells in the blood and marrow usually fall, and the patient may become hypoplastic. Unfortunately, the blast cells regenerate thereafter in more than 50 percent of cases. In 20 to 30 percent of cases it may be possible to achieve a status resembling chronic phase disease, though this is generally short-lived. In 5 to 10 percent of cases Ph-negative hematopoiesis can be re-established. Most patients die within 6 months of the diagnosis of myeloid blastic transformation.

For patients in lymphoid transformation of CML the outlook is a little less dismal. The majority will respond to treatment appropriate to acute lymphoblastic leukemia, namely vincristine, prednisone, and anthracyclines. The last drug must be given with caution to avoid prolonged hypoplasia. About 60 percent of patients will be restored to second chronic phase, and this can be maintained for months or years in some cases. All patients who respond to treatment should receive some form of neuroprophylaxis, such as a course of intrathecal methotrexate, but cranial irradiation may not be required.

Allogeneic bone marrow transplantation in advanced phases of CML is usually unsuccessful. The incidence of transplant-related complications is higher than when the transplant is performed in chronic phase, and the actuarial probability of relapse ranges from 50 to 80 percent. It can be considered, however, for the patient whose disease shows initial response to cytotoxic drugs. Autografting can restore patients to chronic phase status for a few months, but the major effort may not be justified.

Other Supportive Measures

Patients in advanced phases of CML can be helped very greatly by judicious use of various supportive measures. Transfusion of red cells may be required regularly to maintain a hemoglobin level above 10 g per deciliter. Radiotherapy may help to shrink an enlarged spleen or painful lymph nodes; it is essential as an adjunct to chemotherapy in the management of bone involvement. Special precautions must be taken to avoid the tumor lysis syndrome when initiating treatment for blastic transformation; these include use of allopurinol at full dosage, induction of an alkaline diuresis, and careful monitoring of K^+ levels and renal function. Hypercalcemia occurs very rarely and can be treated with corticosteroids or specific agents.

Suggested Reading

Allan NC, Richards SM, Shepherd PCA. UK Medical Research Council randomised multicentre trial of interferon-αn1 for chronic myeloid leukemia: improved survival irrespective of cytogenetic response. Lancet 1995; 345:1392–1397.

Derderian PM, Kantarjian HM, Talpaz M, O'Brien S, Cork A, Estey E, Pierce S, Keating M. Chronic myelogenous leukemia in the lymphoid blastic phase: characteristics, treatment response and prognosis. Amer J Med 1993; 94:69–74.

The Italian Cooperative Study Group on Chronic Myeloid Leukemia. Interferon alfa-2a as compared with conventional chemotherapy for the treatment of chronic myeloid leukemia. New Engl J Med 1994; 330: 820–825.

Goldman JM, Szydlo R, Horowitz M et al. Choice of pretransplant treatment and timing of transplants for chronic myelogenous leukemia in chronic phase. Blood 1993; 82:2235–2238.

Kantarjian HM, O'Brien S, Anderlini P, Talpaz M. Treatment of chronic myelogenous leukemia: current status and investigational options. Blood 1996; 87:3069–3081.

Sokal JE, Cox EB, Baccerani M, et al. and the Italian Cooperative CML Study Group. Prognostic discrimination in "good risk" chronic granulocytic leukemia. Blood 1984; 63:789–799.

MULTIPLE MYELOMA AND WALDENSTRÖM'S MACROGLOBULINEMIA

Francis J. Giles, M.D.

The disorders resulting from pathologic clonal expansion of plasma cells include malignancies such as multiple myeloma, plasma cell leukemia (PCL), solitary plasmacytoma of bone (SPB), extramedullary plasmacytoma, Waldenström's macroglobulinemia, immunoproliferative small intestinal disease, and heavy chain disease. More benign plasma cell proliferations may result in monoclonal gammopathy of undetermined significance (MGUS), primary systemic amyloidosis or the polyneuropathy, organomegaly, endocrinopathy, monoclonal gammopathy, skin lesions (POEMS) syndrome.

Some 99 percent of plasma cell disorders are associated with production of a monoclonal protein (M protein) and on this basis are considered distinct from other B lymphoproliferative disorders. This distinction is not absolute, as up to 10 percent of patients with chronic lymphocytic leukemia or lymphoma may have detectable M protein. Multiple myeloma accounts for 2 percent of malignancies in blacks and 1 percent in whites, with average annual age-adjusted incidence rates per 100,000 of 10.2 for black men and 6.7 for black women, 4.7 for white men and 3.2 for white women. Median age of diagnosis of multiple myeloma is 69 for men, 71 for women, with average annual age-specific incidence rates increasing sharply with age, independent of gender or race. The percentage of multiple myeloma patients less than 60 years at time of diagnosis is increasing rapidly. Patients with SPB or extramedullary plasmacytoma tend to present some 5 to 7 years younger than multiple myeloma patients.

■ PRESENTATION AND DETECTION

The clinical picture of multiple myeloma is largely dictated by a combination of effects of malignant plasma cell proliferation, M protein production, renal failure, and immunodeficiency. Plasma cell proliferation is largely confined to red bone marrow, with progressive replacement of hematopoietic tissue and tumor extension into the fatty marrow of the long bones. Both diffuse and nodular patterns of plasma cell infiltration are seen. They result in impairment or failure of bone marrow function leading to anemia, neutropenia, and thrombocytopenia.

At presentation, 60 percent of multiple myeloma patients have skeletal lytic lesions, with or without osteoporosis, wedging or collapse of vertebral bodies, or pathologic fractures; 20 percent of patients have osteoporosis alone, and the remainder have no multiple myeloma-related radiologic abnormality. Localized tumor proliferation and resultant osteoclast and osteoblast abnormalities completely destroy the fine trabeculae in cancellous bone. With further tumor expansion, the nodules encroach on cortical bone, causing sharply circumscribed punched-out lesions. Bone pain, either diffuse or localized, is the predominant presenting symptom in 60 percent of multiple myeloma patients. Because of the concentration of multiple myeloma in the axial skeleton, osteoporosis and lytic lesions are most evident in the vertebrae, pelvis, ribs, and sternum. With advanced disease pathologic fractures increasingly occur. There is no direct relationship between pain severity and the radiologic degree of skeletal involvement, apart from that associated with vertebral wedging and collapse or gross localized bone destruction. Skull lesions, although often numerous, very rarely are painful, in contrast to metastatic cancer lesions.

Mixed lytic and sclerotic bone lesions are frequently seen in patients with SPB or POEMS syndrome. Increased osteoclastic bone resorption is demonstrable in most multiple myeloma patients and is usually related to increased numbers of trabecular osteoclasts. Excessive osteoclastic activity may precede overt multiple myeloma by months or years. In early multiple myeloma abnormal bone remodeling induced by malignant plasma cells involves stimulation of both bone formation and destruction. As multiple myeloma progresses, this process is uncoupled, and along with increased osteoclast activity, decreased osteoblastic activity is found in patients with lytic lesions and advanced disease. Progressive osteoblast suppression parallels multiple myeloma progression.

Many cytokines produced by malignant B lymphocytes, stromal cells, and activated T lymphocytes, including interleukin 1-beta (IL-1-beta), multi-colony stimulating factor (M-CSF), tumor necrosis factor-beta (TNF-beta), IL-3, and IL-6, have osteoclast-activating properties. IL-6 is constitutively produced by osteoblasts, its production being stimulated by IL-1-beta and TNF-beta. IL-6 stimulates the in vitro generation and bone-resorptive activities of osteoclasts and mediates the bone-resorptive activities of IL-1 and TNF. IL-6 increases NK cell activity and in multiple myeloma, unlike the other B lymphoproliferative disorders, the marrow's NK activity is increased. While a pivotal role in the pathophysiology of multiple myeloma has been established for IL-6, it is still not clear whether it functions mainly as an autocrine or paracrine factor for plasma cell growth. Current data support the latter. Malignant plasma cells produce IL-1-beta, TNF-beta, and a functionally active truncated form of M-CSF. It is unclear whether fresh multiple myeloma cells can produce IL-6.

Net osteolysis in multiple myeloma patients causes continuing loss of skeletal calcium. At presentation, 25 percent of patients have an elevated serum calcium level. The serum alkaline phosphatase level remains normal except in the presence of healing fractures. Episodes of acute hypercalcemia leading to severe dehydration and uremia may occur abruptly at any stage in multiple myeloma patients. While acute hypercalcemia is most frequent in patients with generalized osteoporosis and extensive lytic lesions, it may occur before multiple myeloma is otherwise clinically apparent.

Anemia, usually normochromic and normocytic, is very common in multiple myeloma patients, and its symptoms may be dominant at diagnosis in some 20 percent of patients. Marrow replacement and suppression by the malignant clone, renal failure, M protein-induced plasma volume expansion, and cytotoxic therapy are key factors. Current data on serum erythropoietin (EPO) levels in multiple myeloma are inconsistent with some reporting that EPO levels are appropriately raised for the degree of anemia in patients with normal renal function and inappropriately low only in patients with uremia. Other groups have reported inappropriately low levels in both uremic and nonuremic patients.

M protein production, particularly Bence Jones protein (BJP), may result in the development of potentially irreversible functional and structural renal damage. Some 25 percent of multiple myeloma patients are uremic (blood urea concentration [BUC] at least 10 mmol per liter) at presentation, with a further 25 percent showing overt renal failure at later stages. In a minority of patients, the BUC will be normal after rehydration, but uremia persists in the great majority. Without aggressive therapy the prognosis is very poor, and 70 percent of patients with a BUC above 15 mmol per liter or a serum creatinine concentration above 200 μmol per liter die within 100 days of presentation. In over 95 percent of patients renal failure is attributable to BJP and/or hypercalcemia, with varying contributions from dehydration, sepsis, and nephrotoxic drugs. Hyperuricemia, sepsis, disseminated intravascular coagulation, and rarely, renal vein thrombosis or direct renal infiltration by plasma cells or amyloid may also be aggravating factors.

Multiple myeloma patients have a very high rate of bacterial infection, and some 10 percent present in this way, often with pneumonia. The traditional dominance of gram-positive organism infections, e.g., *Staphylococcus aureus, Streptococcus pneumoniae,* has lessened; of late gram-negative sepsis becomes increasingly prevalent. Opportunistic infections by organisms such as *Mycobacterium tuberculosis, Pneumocystis pneumoniae,* and herpesviruses, although uncommon at disease presentation, are increasing in patients with advanced disease. Fever directly attributable to multiple myeloma is said to occur in fewer than 1 percent of patients. M protein production is strongly associated with low serum concentrations of normal immunoglobulins (Ig). In about 70 percent of patients with IgG multiple myeloma at presentation, the serum concentrations of the normal immunoglobulins are less than 20 percent of normal; this is the case in 40 percent of patients with IgA multiple myeloma and in 20 percent of patients with BJP multiple myeloma. Severe immune paresis occurs in the 1 percent of patients in whom no M protein is detectable in the serum or urine. Recovery to normal immunoglobulin levels, rarely seen following conventional chemotherapy even when the concentrations of M protein fall to low levels, is increasingly documented in patients receiving alpha-interferon therapy. Immune paresis worsens with multiple myeloma progression. Cell-mediated immunity is generally intact in multiple myeloma but may be impaired, as may granulocyte function and/or complement activation. Primary immune abnormalities, uremia, neutropenia, antitumor therapy, multiple blood component transfusions, indwelling urinary and intravenous catheters, and multiple organ failure combine to cause severe immunodeficiency in many multiple myeloma patients.

In a small number of patients with multiple myeloma, soft-tissue plasma cell infiltration is seen at diagnosis, with a higher frequency of overt soft-tissue involvement in patients with IgD multiple myeloma. The most serious complications of multiple myeloma soft-tissue involvement occur when tumor extends beyond the periosteum following complete erosion of bone cortex. When this occurs from a vertebral body into the spinal theca, tumor may spread extradurally or may cause spinal cord compression by eroding the piaarachnoid. Rarely, multiple myeloma deposits occur in other tissues such as the skin, but most skin and subcutaneous involvement seems to be metastatic from extramedullary plasmacytoma. Extension of multiple myeloma tumors intraorbitally occurs frequently if the skull and facial bones are omitted from systemic irradiation fields, and soft-tissue involvement may be prominent in patients who relapse post autologous bone marrow transplantation (ABMT).

Macroglobulinemia is associated with the presence of an IgM M protein that is especially prone to cause hyperviscosity and to act as a cold agglutinin. The intrinsic viscosity of a protein is related to its concentration, size, shape, and chemical configuration. The intrinsic viscosity of IgM, which usually exists as a 900,000 dalton pentamer, is high relative to IgA and IgG, and the hyperviscosity syndrome (HVS) therefore occurs at relatively lower IgM concentrations, around 40 to 50 g per liter. In HVS associated with IgA, the M protein usually circulates in polymeric form. Polymerization is enhanced by increasing concentration and by the presence of J chains. HVS associated with IgG multiple myeloma usually occurs at very high M protein concentrations, although it may occur at lower levels if polymers or unusual molecular configurations are present.

Plasma viscosity is expressed as relative to water (normal range 1.67 to 1.94) or in absolute units (normal range 1.16 and 1.35 mPas). The symptomatic threshold varies between patients but is consistent for each. HVS rarely occurs with a relative viscosity less than 4, commonly occurring at values of 6 or greater. Common components of HVS are ocular, hemostatic, and neurologic disturbances accompanied by fatigue, malaise, or weight loss. Progression from retinal vein distention to increasing vessel tortuosity with local constrictions at arteriovenous crossings, areas of beading, and dilation of small venules may lead to a severe retinopathy with prominent hemorrhages and exudates. Visual disturbances may range from mild impairment to abrupt loss of vision.

Coagulopathy in multiple myeloma is common, while in HVS the bleeding tendency is assumed to be the result of platelet coating by the M protein. This may result in chronic, recurrent bleeding of the gums and upper respiratory and gastrointestinal tracts. The bleeding time is usually prolonged, with evident abnormalities of platelet function. Neurologic symptoms and signs, which are often prominent in HVS, include headache, fluctuating consciousness, altered mentation, dizziness, ataxia, vertigo, neuropathies, convulsions, and coma. Plasma volume increases with viscosity and may compromise cardiac function. A thrombotic tendency in patients with HVS may lead to deep venous thrombosis or pulmonary infarction.

Amyloidosis is clinically evident in less than 5 percent of multiple myeloma patients at time of diagnosis and sometimes precedes multiple myeloma diagnosis. Amyloid deposits may vary from trace amounts to quantities sufficient to cause a systemic disorder indistinguishable from primary amyloidosis. Amyloid deposits are insoluble, resist proteolysis, and have a characteristic fibrillary ultrastructure in which polypeptide chains are arrayed perpendicularly to the axis of the fibril in a beta-pleated sheet. The major component is a sequence of amino acids belonging to the variable portion of the monoclonal immunoglobulin light chain, usually lambda. Clinical manifestations may occur when the total plasma cell mass is small, because of the special properties of the amyloid material. Occasionally amyloid deposits gradually replace plasma cell infiltrates, leaving few or no traces of the original cellular lesion. Extensive amyloidosis may be found in tissues not infiltrated by multiple myeloma cells, such as ligaments, tendon sheaths, fasciae, synovial membranes, muscles, and nerves.

Common presentations of multiple myeloma–associated amyloidosis include carpal tunnel syndrome, congestive cardiac failure, macroglossia, gut disturbances, neuropathies (peripheral and autonomic), and lesions of the skin, subcutaneous tissues, tendon sheaths, and fasciae. Carpal tunnel syndromes may involve both medial nerve compression and arterial insufficiency and be part of a rheumatoid arthritis-like presentation in which ligamentous and articular involvement is prominent. Cardiac muscle deposits occur in 80 to 90 percent of patients with amyloidosis leading to enlargement without an increase in intracardiac volume. Progressive pump failure is exacerbated by conduction disturbances and coronary arterial insufficiency. Infiltration may occur in any area of the gut, causing obstruction, diarrhea, hemorrhage, malabsorption, or protein-losing enteropathy. Macroglossia may interfere with deglutition and respiration. Although liver infiltration may be massive, hepatic function is usually only mildly impaired.

The progression of renal amyloidosis may be arrested by the treatments used to control multiple myeloma, whereas the other manifestations of amyloidosis, whether primary or in association with multiple myeloma, are usually not affected by treatment. The median survival from time of diagnosis of multiple myeloma–associated amyloidosis is less than 6 months.

Table 1 comprises criteria for the diagnosis of multiple

Table 1 Diagnostic Criteria for Multiple Myeloma and MGUS

MULTIPLE MYELOMA

Major criteria
- I. Plasmacytoma on tissue biopsy
- II. Bone marrow plasmacytosis with >30% plasma cells
- III. Monoclonal globulin spike on serum electrophoresis exceeding 35 g/L for IgG peaks or 20 g/L for IgA peaks, ≥1 g/24 hr of *k* or *l* light chain excretion on urine electrophoresis in the absence of amyloidosis

Minor criteria
- I. Bone marrow plasmacytosis with 10% to 30% plasma cells
- II. Monoclonal globulin spike present but less than levels in III above
- III. Lytic bone lesions
- IV. Residual normal IgM <500 mg/L, IgA <1 g/L or IgG <6 g/L

Diagnosis is established when any of the following are documented in symptomatic patient with clearly progressive disease. The diagnosis of myeloma requires a minimum of one major plus one minor criterion or three minor criteria that must include a + b.
1. I + b, I + c, I + d (I + a is **not** diagnostic)
2. II + b, II + c, II + d
3. III + a, III + c, III + d
4. a + b + c, a + b + d

INDOLENT MYELOMA

As per multiple myeloma except
- I. No bone lesions or ≤3 lytic lesions, no compression fractures
- II. M-component levels IgA <50 g/L or IgG <70 g/L
- III. No symptoms or signs of disease
  - A. Karnofsky performance status >70%
  - B. Hemoglobin >10 g/dl
  - C. Normal serum calcium
  - D. Serum creatinine <175 μmol/L (<20 mg/L)
  - E. No persistent or recurrent infection

SMOLDERING MYELOMA

As per indolent myeloma except
- No bone lesions
- Bone marrow plasma cells 10% to 30%

Monoclonal Gammopathy of Undetermined Significance
- I. Monoclonal gammopathy
- II. M-component levels IgA <20 g/L, IgG <35 g/L, <1 g/24 hr of *k* or *l* light chain excretion on urine electrophoresis
- III. Bone marrow plasma cells <10%
- IV. No bony lesions
- V. No symptoms

myeloma. The critical distinctions are between multiple myeloma, MGUS, and smoldering multiple myeloma. Multiple myeloma should be treated only if symptomatic or rapidly progressive; neither MGUS nor smoldering multiple myeloma should be treated. Electrophoresis on cellulose acetate membrane is satisfactory for serum screening for M protein, but high-resolution agarose gel electrophoresis is necessary to detect smaller quantities of protein. Immunoelectrophoresis and/or immunofixation are vital diagnostic studies that also define the M protein heavy and light chain class. These latter tests should be performed whenever multiple myeloma, MGUS, macroglobulinemia, or amyloidosis is being considered, regardless of a normal or nonspecific electrophoretic result. Monospecific antisera to the Fc fragment of IgG, IgA, IgM, IgD, and IgE as well as antisera to *k* and *l* light chains should be employed. Rate nephelometry is the optimal method for quantitation of immunoglobulins. Sulfosalicylic acid should be used to screen urine for protein. The recognition and quantitation of BJP in the urine depend on the demonstration of a monoclonal light chain by immunoelectrophoresis or immunofixation of an adequately concentrated aliquot from a 24 hour urine collection. One of these latter tests must be performed on urine from every patient suspected of having multiple myeloma even if the sulfosalicylic acid test is negative.

A radiologic survey of the entire skeleton is mandatory in the diagnosis of multiple myeloma. Computed tomography (CT) scanning and magnetic resonance imaging (MRI) have greatly increased the sensitivity of detection of bone disease in multiple myeloma. MRI is superior to CT scanning for screening large portions of the vertebral column and spinal canal and in the visualization of soft-tissue abnormalities. MRI is particularly valuable in apparent SPB; it may detect additional sites of involvement often missed by other imaging techniques. Myelography has been the standard investigation when patients have features of cord compression, but if there is a complete block to the flow of dye, areas distal to the block will not be visualized. MRI scan should be carried out in this situation to screen for additional lesions. MRI may also demonstrate imminent cord compression in patients without localizing symptoms.

STAGING, PROGNOSIS, AND RESPONSE CRITERIA

The standard clinical staging system for multiple myeloma is that of Durie and Salmon, with stage I, II, and III differentiation as per Table 2. Some 75 percent of patients diagnosed with multiple myeloma are reported to die directly because of the disorder, this group including patients whose primary cause of death is sepsis, hypercalcemia, hemorrhage, or renal failure. Causes of death considered not directly due to multiple myeloma include 8 percent of patients who die of cardiac causes, 3 percent of central nervous system events, 2 percent of other malignancies including acute leukemia, 1 percent of pulmonary emboli, and 0.5 to 1 percent who commit suicide.

In unselected series 10 to 15 percent of patients die within the first two cycles of induction therapy. Induction regimens give an objective response rate of 50 to 60 percent. The majority of these patients will enter a clinically stable or plateau phase of an average 12 to 24 months' duration; 20 percent of patients will have stable disease, that is, will not show any dramatic response to therapy. This heterogenous group includes both patients who present in plateau phase and who have a relatively good prognosis and those destined to show early resistance to therapy, and have progressive disease and thus a poor prognosis. About 10 to 15 percent of patients will exhibit true primary resistance to induction therapy and will clinically progress while on therapy. The prognosis in this group is particularly poor. Currently, multiple myeloma patients show median survivals following induction therapy of 36 to 48 months and have a 5 year relative survival rate of approximately 25 percent, with fewer than 5 percent of patients alive 10 years post diagnosis. Relative survival rates for women are higher among both blacks and whites.

The prognosis for multiple myeloma is highly dependent on the Durie-Salmon stage and various other prognostic factors including serum beta$_2$ microglobulin and albumin levels at time of diagnosis. Other well-established independent prognostic discriminants are degree of renal failure and the plasma cell labeling index. Other prognostic factors include serum LDH, serum neopterin, serum osteocalcin, serum IL-6 or CRP, abnormal cytogenetics, H-ras expression, K-ras or N-ras mutations and aberrant myeloid, erythroid, or megakaryocytic antigens on malignant plasma cells.

Table 3 outlines the Chronic Leukemia Task Force and the Southwestern Oncology Group criteria for evaluation of response to therapy in multiple myeloma. Neither set of criteria has consistent value in predicting survival following induction therapy. The magnitude of multiple myeloma regression as assessed by M protein reduction does not correlate in a quantitative way with response or survival duration. A 75 percent regression is not necessarily better than a 25 percent regression because all responses achieved with current therapy are partial. Cytotoxic therapy has improved survival by reducing early deaths from complications and by slowing down tumor progression in some patients. Tumor bulk at presentation, intrinsic disease kinetics, and drug sensitivity in individual patients are the major determinants of survival.

Table 2 Multiple Myeloma: Clinical Staging System of Durie and Salmon

Stage I Low myeloma cell mass (<0.6 × 10^{12} cells/m^2)
All of the following:
Hb >10 g/dl
s Calcium (corrected) ≤12 mg/dl*
X-rays are normal or show single lesion
M protein production value
  IgG <5 g/dl
  IgA <3 g/dl
Urinary light chain excretion <4 g/24 hr
Stage II Intermediate myeloma cell mass
  (0.6–1.2 × 10^{12} cells/m^2)
Results fit neither stage I nor stage II
Stage III High myeloma cell mass
  (>1.2 × 10^{12} cells/m^2)
Any of the following:
Hb ≤8.5 g/dl
s Calcium (corrected) >12 mg/dl*
X-rays show multiple lesions
M protein production value
  IgG >7 g/dl
  IgA >5 g/dl
Urinary light chain excretion >12 g/24 hr
Subclassification:
A = Relatively normal renal function (serum creatinine value <2 mg/dl)
B = Abnormal renal function (serum creatinine value ≥2 mg/dl)

*Corrected calcium = calcium (mg/dl) – albumin (g/dl) + 4
From Alexanian R, Balcerak S, Bonnet JD, et al. Prognostic factors in multiple myeloma. Cancer 1975; 36(4):1192–1201.

■ THERAPY

Multiple myeloma therapy involves both cytoreduction and ancillary therapies necessary to manage disease complications. The need for therapy must be absolute, as no curative therapy for multiple myeloma has been established. Before chemotherapy, early forms of the disease and any precursor states such as MGUS, which do not require treatment, must be excluded. Two major therapeutic advances have been recently documented. Low-dose alpha-interferon regimens have been shown to prolong the plateau phase in patients who have achieved an objective response to standard induction therapy, thus markedly improving some patients' quality of life. Early high-dose consolidation therapy, e.g., high-dose melphalan therapy (200 mg per square meter) with peripheral blood stem cell (PBSC) support, has been shown to prolong remission and survival in patients who have responded to prior induction therapy and whose high-dose therapy is followed by alpha-interferon maintenance therapy.

Cytoreductive Therapy

In patients with asymptomatic stage I multiple myeloma, which may be smoldering or indolent, no specific antineoplastic or immunomodulatory therapy is indicated. Entry of such patients on prospective randomized studies involving

Table 3 Definition of Response to Therapy of Multiple Myeloma

SWOG CRITERIA

Objective response: A sustained decrease in the synthesis index of serum M protein to 25%, or less of the pretreatment value on at least two measurements separated by 4 weeks. For IgA and IgG3 M proteins the synthetic index is the same as the serum concentration. For IgG M proteins of subclasses 1, 2, and 4, the synthetic index must be estimated using a nomogram. A sustained decrease in 24 hr urine globulin to 10% or less of the pretreatment value and to less than 0.2 g/24 hr on at least two occasions separated by 4 weeks.

CHRONIC LEUKEMIA TASK FORCE CRITERIA

Complete Remission: All of the following: Disappearance of serum and/or urine M protein on cellulose acetate electrophoresis on two determinations at least 4 weeks apart. Normal marrow with <5% plasma cells, normal peripheral blood values, and no signs or symptoms. Normal serum calcium, serum proteins, normal levels of polyclonal immunoglobulins, normal serum viscosity. Resolution of all soft-tissue plasmacytomas.

Objective Response: All of the following: Reduction of serum M protein levels to ≤50% of baseline levels on two determinations at least 4 weeks apart. Significant reduction of urine M protein levels. If baseline value was >1 g/24 hr, level must be reducted by ≥50%. If baseline value was 0.5–1 g/24 hr, level must be reduced to <0.1 g/24 hr. All baseline soft-tissue plasmacytomas must reduce by ≥50% the sum of the products of the cross-diameters of each measureable lesion. Decrease in bone pain from severe or moderate to mild or none.

alpha-interferon is now indicated. Patients with asymptomatic or slowly progressive stage II or III disease should have therapy deferred for as long as possible unless entering on a clinical protocol. Patients with symptomatic or progressive multiple myeloma warrant systemic cytotoxic therapy. Commonly occurring indications for institution of therapy are bone pain, hypercalcemia, renal failure, marrow failure, and spinal cord compression. All patients should be encouraged to drink 2 to 3 L of fluid daily from time of diagnosis of multiple myeloma.

Melphalan-prednisone (MP) (Table 4) is the most widely used induction regimen. No alternate regimen has been demonstrated to offer superior long-term survival. Suggestions that poorer-prognosis patients may benefit from more complex regimens await verification in prospective studies. Whether the addition of alpha-interferon to MP adds to its therapeutic effect or not is unclear. Sequential melphalan dose escalation must be employed if necessary until moderate myelosuppression is evident. Continuous (daily) melphalan is not recommended because of the cumulative myelosuppression and increased leukemogenic potential. Nadir absolute granulocyte counts should be monitored in patients on intermittent oral alkylating agent therapy. Patients should be monitored following initial doses of therapy for effects of rapid tumor lysis, and prophylactic allopurinol therapy is indicated for at least the first cycle of chemotherapy.

Induction regimens other than MP, e.g., vincristine, doxorubicin, dexamethasone (VAD), vincristine, melphalan, cyclophosphamide, prednisone (VMCP), or VMCP-VBAP (vincristine, carmustine, doxorubicin, prednisone) are indicated in specific clinical circumstances. These regimens benefit patients with aggressive, rapidly progressive multiple myeloma. The VAD regimen should be used in patients who present with renal failure. Steroid pulses alone as induction therapy are indicated where marrow hypofunction is extreme. Alpha-interferon has been shown to increase the overall response rates to induction therapy if combined with regimens more complex than MP, particularly the VMCP regimen. The critical indication for the more complex regimens is their ability, especially if combined with alpha-interferon, to attain a 20 to 25 percent complete remission (CR) rate following induction therapy and thus serve as an optimal base for high-dose consolidation therapy (HDCT).

If the patient is suitable for HDCT, this should be performed as soon as possible following attainment of an objective response to induction therapy. HDCT should be followed by a thrice weekly 3 to 5 million unit alpha-interferon maintenance regimen continued until time of overt disease relapse. When patients are not suitable for HDCT, a documented objective response to induction therapy should be followed by a thrice weekly 3 to 5 million unit alpha-interferon maintenance regimen continued until time of overt disease relapse. Although interferon therapy defers relapse by extending plateau phase duration, it has not been shown to improve overall survival in multiple myeloma when maintenance is given post conventional therapy. Maintenance interferon given post HDCT has been shown to prolong both remission and survival.

Most HDCT involves myeloablative therapy using bone marrow and/or peripheral stem cells as rescue therapy. Total body irradiation (TBI) should not be included in initial HDCT. The use of recombinant growth factors has greatly facilitated the harvesting of a PBSC yield sufficient to support marrow recovery post myeloablative therapy. In vivo evidence of acceleration of disease by recombinant granulocyte colony stimulating factor (rhG-CSF) in multiple myeloma patients has been reported, and rhGM-CSF should be used for PBSC harvesting. Allogeneic bone marrow transplantation (Al-

Table 4 Cytoreductive Therapy

DRUG	DOSE	DAYS
MP REGIMEN (28 DAY CYCLE)		
Melphalan	6 mg/m^2/day PO × 7 days	1–7
Prednisone	100 mg/m^2/day PO × 7 days	1–7
VAD REGIMEN (28 DAY CYCLE)		
Vincristine	0.4 mg/day cIV × 4 days	1–4
Doxorubicin	9 mg/m^2/day cIV × 4 days	1–4
Dexamethasone	40 mg/day PO × 4 days	1–4, 9–12, 17–20 of the first 28 day cycle and on alternate cycles thereafter. On other cycles give days 1–4 only.
Patients should receive H_2-blocker plus trimethoprim-sulfamethoxazole.		
VMCP-VBAP REGIMEN (ALTERNATING 21 DAY CYCLES)		
Vincristine	1 mg IV	1
Melphalan	6 mg/m^2/day PO × 4 days	1–4
Cyclophosphamide	125 mg/m^2 day PO × 4 days	1–4
Prednisone	60 mg/m^2/day PO × 4 days	1–4
Vincristine	1 mg IV	1
Carmustine	30 mg/m^2 IV	1
Doxorubicin	30 mg/m^2 IV	1
Prednisone	60 mg/m^2/day PO × 4 days	1–4
Allopurinol should be prescribed for at least first cycle of chemotherapy.		
All patients should be vigorously hydrated during therapy.		

MP, Melphalan-prednisone; VAD, vincristine, doxorubicin, dexamethasone; VMCP, vincristine, melphalan, cyclophosphamide, prednisone; VBAP, vincristine, carmustine, doxorubicin, prednisone.

lo BMT) has been carried out as a consolidation procedure in a small number of patients responding to induction therapy. Age requirements (up to 55 years), need for a human leukocyte antigen (HLA)-compatible sibling donor, and other very demanding eligibility criteria mean that the procedure can be offered to very few patients. CR is achieved in 50 percent of patients with responding disease before BMT, and 30 percent of those nonresponsive before BMT. Some 30 percent of patients die within 100 days of Allo BMT, 40 percent by 6 months post transplant. Current data show a plateau of actuarial survival of 40 percent extending from 36 to 76 months. Many of these surviving patients have evidence of ongoing M protein production. The role of Allo BMT in multiple myeloma therapy awaits prospective randomized studies.

There is no role for high-dose single drug, e.g., melphalan, therapy as HDCT unless the agent is given to a level at which stem cell support is necessary. Neither autologous bone marrow transplant (ABMT) nor Allo BMT has a role for multiple myeloma patients with resistant relapse or with a combination of adverse prognostic factors. The present emphasis on PBSC, rather than the bone marrow, as the source of stem cells should be approached with some caution. The peripheral blood contains large numbers of clonogenic multiple myeloma cells, particularly after growth factor stimulation, and the optimum source of stem cells remains to be identified from prospective studies. Similarly, attempts to obtain hematopoietic stem cells and thereby to exclude multiple myeloma progenitors on the basis of CD34 positivity should be subjected to rigorous prospective study, as some data suggest that subpopulations of the multiple myeloma malignant clone may be CD34 positive.

The great majority of plateau-phase patients will ultimately develop overt disease progression. All patients stopping therapy must be closely monitored for the possibility of relapse. A complete battery of tests is necessary at 6 month intervals with an annual skeletal survey. Serum M protein levels may be insensitive for the detection of early relapse in some patients. Some 10 to 15 percent of patients relapse with Bence Jones escape, in which the serum M protein levels may drop rather than increase at the time of relapse.

It is critically important to distinguish between the categories of patient covered by the general term *relapse-refractory,* as the therapeutic approaches are different. In the first group, which includes up to 15 percent of patients with multiple myeloma, are those who are truly refractory to first-line chemotherapy (primarily resistant disease) and whose disease progresses during induction chemotherapy. In a second group are patients who relapse after an initial response. Relapse may occur while the patient is on or off therapy. If relapse occurs more than 6 months after treatment stops, the patient is said to have an unmaintained remission. All patients who are initially responsive to chemotherapy will eventually relapse if they do not first die of other causes.

There are many options for the treatment of truly refractory multiple myeloma. However, all are sufficiently ineffective to render urgent the need for progress. No relapse-refractory regimen, either cytotoxic drug or radiation based, consistently achieves a median survival greater than 1 year, and most studies record median survivals less than 9 months. A relatively effective approach is the use of simple high-dose glucocorticoids with VAD or similar regimens. The VAD regimen is recommended as second-line treatment for patients who relapse on or within 6 months of stopping first-line treatment; response rates are on the order of 75 percent. In contrast to the situation in resistant disease, this regimen is more effective than high-dose steroids alone (40 percent response rate). In addition, VAD may be effective even when other doxorubicin-containing regimens have failed. Systemic radiotherapy in multiple myeloma is used either as part of a conditioning regimen before alloBMT or ABMT or as a double hemibody irradiation (DHBI) procedure. Hemibody irradiation (HBI) is an effective, well tolerated-modality of therapy in patients with advanced disease. DHBI gives more durable responses than single HBI. DHBI prolongs the median survival in relapsed patients at least as effectively as chemotherapeutic regimens with equivalent morbidity. The entire skeleton must be included within radiation fields for optimum efficacy of DHBI. For those failing second-line therapy there are a number of experimental options, including studies of new cytotoxic agents; biologic response modifiers, e.g., anti–IL-6; different schedules of previously used drugs; and BMT. Research to overcome chemotherapeutic drug resistance includes increasing dose intensity to increase intracellular drug concentration, using non–cross-resistant regimens as proposed by the Goldie-Coldman hypothesis, targeting p-glycoprotein positive tumor cells with monoclonal antibodies, and using chemosensitizing agents or agents that inhibit p-glycoprotein function.

Supportive Therapy

Both peritoneal dialysis and hemodialysis have been used successfully in the setting of acute renal failure in multiple myeloma patients, and dialysis should be offered to all suitable patients to allow time for an adequate trial of cytotoxic therapy. Plasmapheresis is particularly effective as an emergency measure in patients with acute renal failure secondary to inability to excrete light chains and is superior to peritoneal dialysis in this circumstance. Plasmapheresis is effective at removing light chains from the blood; this cannot be achieved by dialysis. The use of plasmapheresis with dialysis may result in better overall recovery of renal function. Control of the underlying multiple myeloma is the key therapeutic goal; reversal of renal failure does not of itself confer survival benefit. However, the use of dialysis or plasmapheresis allows time for chemotherapy to take effect. In patients who are responsive to chemotherapy, renal transplantation should be considered. The use of long-term dialysis in patients with unresponsive or progressive disease is more controversial.

Vigorous hydration and diuresis are critical whenever severe or symptomatic hypercalcemia is diagnosed in multiple myeloma patients. Initial therapy of patients with severe hypercalcemia consists of rehydration with intravenous saline, with the addition of a loop diuretic such as furosemide following intravascular volume expansion. If the patient remains significantly hypercalcemic post rehydration and diuresis, a specific antiosteoclast agent, e.g., a diphosphonate, should be used. Even extremely high calcium levels frequently respond to cytotoxic therapy in newly presenting or relapsing patients. Where basic therapy is inadequate, parenteral mithramycin, diphosphonates, or calcitonin may be indicated.

Occasional patients have a paraprotein that firmly binds calcium and will thus have asymptomatic hypercalcemia with normal ionized calcium levels. No clear long-term role for agents such as the biphosphonates in multiple myeloma has been established.

Transfusion dependence in multiple myeloma is an indication for specific therapy. Anemia usually improves with response to chemotherapy but is a significant problem in patients with unresponsive or progressive disease, and rhEPO provides an alternative to blood transfusion in the management of multiple myeloma-related anemia. It offers some patients the potential for considerable improvement in quality of life. Response to rhEPO is independent of reduction in tumor mass by cytotoxic therapy, may be blunted by sepsis, and is minimal in patients with rapidly progressive disease.

■ WALDENSTRÖM'S MACROGLOBULINEMIA

Waldenström's macroglobulinemia generally behaves as a relatively indolent lymphoproliferative disorder with an IgM M protein and without bone lesions. In rare patients with disease resembling Waldenström's macroglobulinemia clinically, cytologically, and histologically, the M protein is IgG or IgA. Patients usually have fatigue, anemia, hepatosplenomegaly, lymphadenopathy, or mucosal bleeding. Serum viscosity is increased in most patients, and the HVS, evident in 70 percent of patients at some stage of the disease, is severe in 10 percent to 30 percent. Bleeding and visual disturbances are particularly common manifestations. The M protein in Waldenström's macroglobulinemia often behaves as a cryoglobulin, causing peripheral vascular abnormalities (Raynaud's phenomenon, acrocyanosis, ulceration, and gangrene of the extremities), hemolytic anemia, vascular purpura, or arthralgia. Waldenström's macroglobulinemia may involve sites outside the marrow and reticuloendothelial system in 10 percent of patients, predominantly with infiltration of skin or pulmonary tissue. Renal failure is relatively rare.

Anemia due to plasma expansion, bleeding, and marrow suppression is present at diagnosis in over 70 percent of patients and is accompanied by neutropenia and thrombocytopenia in 30 percent. Peripheral lymphocytosis is usually seen in advanced disease. The marrow is always involved, usually with a pleomorphic, diffuse infiltrate of lymphocytes, plasmacytoid lymphocytes, and plasma cells. Large, PAS-positive intranuclear inclusions (Dutcher bodies) may be seen in the lymphoid cells. Platelet function is usually abnormal, with prolonged bleeding times.

The IgM level required for the diagnosis of Waldenström's macroglobulinemia has not been standardized. It currently ranges from 10 g per liter to 30 g per liter. The M protein light chain is 1 in 75 percent of patients, and 70 percent have BJP. In patients with an IgM M protein 50 percent are associated with MGUS, 25 percent with Waldenström's macroglobulinemia and the remainder with non-Hodgkin's lymphoma (NHL), Chronic lymphocytic leukemia (CLL), primary amyloidosis, and other lymphoproliferative disorders.

Waldenström's macroglobulinemia usually behaves as an indolent lymphoproliferative disorder with a median survival of approximately 6 years. Therapy is not curative and should be deferred until necessary. Responses to chemotherapy are always transient. Chlorambucil, melphalan, or cyclophosphamide may control Waldenström's macroglobulinemia but rarely produce major durable remissions. In HVS plasmapheresis is the treatment of choice and may be extremely effective, as 90 percent of IgM is intravascular. It is usually necessary to remove 50 percent of total plasma volume, and therapy should continue until the relative serum viscosity is less than 4. Resistant Waldenström's macroglobulinemia may be treated with combination cytotoxic drugs, alpha interferon, and systemic irradiation. Fludarabine and 2-chlorodeoxyadenosine are effective agents that seem likely to become first-line agents in Waldenström's macroglobulinemia therapy.

■ SOLITARY PLASMACYTOMA OF BONE

SPB, also known as solitary myeloma of bone, may represent a very early stage in the development of multiple myeloma. The median age of diagnosis is 7 to 10 years earlier than that for multiple myeloma, with a predominance of male patients. Although any bone can be involved, SPB usually presents in the axial skeleton, with vertebral presentation in one-third of patients. It is crucial to distinguish SPB from multiple myeloma. Compared with multiple myeloma, a serum or urinary M component is found in a lower proportion of cases (approximately 50 percent). The higher proportion of nonsecretory cases may reflect a lower tumor burden. Immune paresis is generally not seen in SPB.

The most commonly used diagnostic criteria are the presence of a single bone lesion consisting of plasma cells, a normal random marrow aspirate or biopsy, and the absence of systemic disease attributable to multiple myeloma. With the use of flow cytometric marrow analysis, CT and MRI, cases that would until recently have been diagnosed as SPB are being diagnosed as multiple myeloma.

Local radiotherapy relieves bone pain and eradicates the lesion in the vast majority of patients and leads to M protein disappearance in approximately 50 percent of patients. An acute neurologic deficit requires urgent surgical decompression. At least 50 percent of SPB patients progress to multiple myeloma. The median time to multiple myeloma development is 2 to 6 years, but relapses can occur up to 20 years following initial apparently curative therapy.

Variability in diagnostic criteria may account for the apparent variability in progression rates and times. Early progression suggests that the extent of disease may simply have been underestimated at diagnosis. The disappearance of M protein after radiotherapy is a good indicator of long-term survival, with patients at greatest risk for progression being those in whom the M protein levels remain high after radiotherapy. When progression does occur, the multiple myeloma tends to be slowly progressive and is usually sensitive to chemotherapy. Adjuvant or maintenance chemotherapy after initial radiotherapy may slow progression to multiple myeloma but does not alter the overall rate of progression, and it poses the risks of drug resistance and secondary leukemia.

■ EXTRAMEDULLARY PLASMACYTOMA

Extramedullary plasmacytoma has a different natural history from multiple myeloma and SPB. The median age at diagnosis is 59, with a predominance of men. Common sites of extramedullary plasmacytoma diagnosis are the mucous membranes of the oronasopharynx and paranasal sinuses. Other sites include lung, bronchus, thyroid, skin, subcutaneous tissue, and gut, with variable local lymph node involvement. In a small minority of patients extramedullary plasmacytoma is multiple or present in nodes without evidence of a primary site. A serum M protein may be present. Treatment consists of local excision and radiotherapy, which should include regional nodes. Local recurrences occur in up to 30 percent of cases, but multiple myeloma does not necessarily follow, and most extramedullary plasmacytoma patients die of unrelated causes. Extramedullary plasmacytoma has a lower rate of conversion to multiple myeloma than SPB. Prognostic factors for progression include the size of the lesion and the presence and size of serum M protein levels. As with SPB, adjuvant chemotherapy has not been shown to be of benefit.

Suggested Reading

Alexanian R, Dimopoulous M, Smith T, et al. Limited value of myeloblative therapy for late multiple myeloma. Blood 1994; 83:512–516.

Attal M, Huguet F, Schlaifer D, et al. Intensive combined therapy for previously untreated aggressive myeloma. Blood 1992; 79:1130–1136.

Bladé J, San Miguel JF, Alcalá A, et al. Alternating combination VMCP/VBAP chemotherapy versus melphalan and prednisone in the treatment of multiple myeloma. J Clin Oncol 1993; 11:1165–1171.

Gregory WM, Richards MA, Malpas JS. Combination chemotherapy versus melphalan and prednisolone in the treatment of multiple myeloma: An overview of published trials. J Clin Oncol 1992; 10:334–340.

Jagannath S, Vesole DH, Gleen L, et al. Low-risk intensive therapy for multiple myeloma with combined autologous bone marrow transplantation and blood stem cell support. Blood 1992; 80:1666–1672.

PLASMA CELL DYSCRASIAS: BENIGN MONOCLONAL GAMMOPATHY

Robert A. Kyle, M.D.

Monoclonal gammopathies are disorders characterized by the proliferation of a single clone of plasma cells producing a homogeneous monoclonal protein (M-protein, M-component, paraprotein). Each M-protein consists of two heavy polypeptide chains of the same class designated in immunoglobulins as gamma in IgG, alpha in IgA, mu in IgM, delta in IgD, and epsilon in IgE, and two associated light chains of the same type (kappa or lambda). Although multiple myeloma (MM) constitutes the prototype of monoclonal gammopathies, the most common plasma cell disorder is benign monoclonal gammopathy (BMG), or monoclonal gammopathy of undetermined significance (MGUS). In the Mayo Clinic over 50 percent of patients with a monoclonal gammopathy have this disorder (Fig. 1). Classification of monoclonal gammopathies is provided in Table 1.

■ DETECTION OF MONOCLONAL GAMMOPATHIES

Detection of an M-protein in the Serum

Serum protein electrophoresis should be performed whenever multiple myeloma or a related disorder is suspected. However, asymptomatic patients with benign monoclonal gammopathy are found when electrophoresis is done as a screening procedure.

Agarose gel electrophoresis is a good screening technique for detection of M-proteins. Immunofixation (IF) or immunoelectrophoresis (IEP) or both should be used to confirm the presence of an M-protein and to identify the heavy-chain type and the light-chain class.

An M-protein is usually seen as a narrow peak (like a church spire) in the gamma, beta, or beta-gamma region in the densitometer tracing or as a discrete band on agarose gel. In contrast, an excess of polyclonal immunoglobulins produces a broad-based peak or a broad band and usually migrates in the gamma region. It is important to differentiate between an M-protein and a polyclonal increase in immunoglobulins, because the former is associated with a malignant or potentially malignant disorder, whereas the latter is associated with a reactive or inflammatory process such as chronic liver disease.

An M-protein may exist even when the total protein level, the globulin components, and quantitative immunoglobulin values are all within normal limits. A small M-protein may be hidden in the normal gamma or beta areas and be overlooked. A monoclonal light chain in the serum (Bence Jones proteinemia) is rarely seen on agarose gel unless the patient has severe renal insufficiency.

IF or IEP should be performed when a peak or band is observed in the electrophoretic pattern. IF, which is more sensitive, is useful when the results of the IEP are equivocal or when searching for a small M-protein in primary amyloidosis, solitary plasmacytoma, extramedullary plasmacytoma, or after successful treatment of MM or Waldenström's macroglobulinemia (WM). The kappa-lambda ratio obtained from nephelometry usually detects the light-chain type of a large monoclonal gammopathy, but small M-proteins will have a normal ratio and will not be recog-

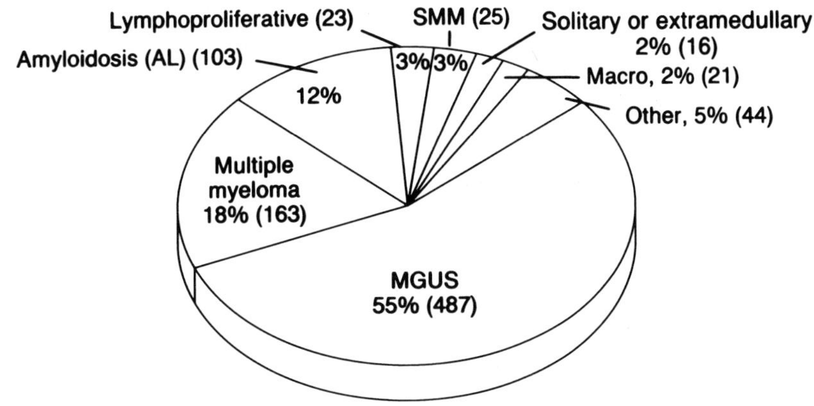

Figure 1
Monoclonal gammopathies at Mayo Clinic, 1995. AL, primary amyloidosis; SMM, smoldering Multiple myeloma; MGUS, monoclonal gammopathy of undetermined significance; CLL, chronic lymphocytic leukemia. *(From Kyle RA. Monoclonal gammopathies of undetermined significance. Baillieres Clin Haematol 1995; 8:761–781.)*; © Mayo Foundation.

Table 1 Classification of Monoclonal Gammopathies

- I. Monoclonal gammopathy of undetermined significance
  - A. Benign monoclonal gammopathy (IgG, IgA, IgD, IgM, rarely free light chains)
  - B. Biclonal gammopathies
  - C. Idiopathic Bence Jones proteinuria
- II. Malignant monoclonal gammopathies
  - A. Multiple myeloma (IgG, IgA, IgD, IgE, and free light chain)
    1. Smoldering multiple myeloma
    2. Plasma cell leukemia
    3. Nonsecretory myeloma
    4. Osteosclerotic myeloma (POEMS syndrome)
    5. Plasmacytoma
       - a. Solitary plasmacytoma of bone
       - b. Extramedullary plasmacytoma
- III. Waldenström's macroglobulinemia
- IV. Heavy-chain diseases (HCD)
  - A. Gamma-HCD
  - B. Alpha-HCD
  - C. Mu-HCD
- V. Primary amyloidosis

nized. This is particularly true for patients with a small monoclonal IgG-kappa protein. In addition, patients with biclonal gammopathy will not be recognized with nephelometry. Thus, IEP or IF is necessary.

Rate nephelometry is the preferred method for quantitation of immunoglobulins because it is not affected by the molecular size of the antigen. This is in contrast to radial immunodiffusion, which may produce spurious results because of polymers, aggregates, or pentamers of the monoclonal protein. Frequently, the nephelometry value for IgM and occasionally IgG or IgA is much higher than the value obtained with the densitometer tracing on serum protein electrophoresis. Consequently, either electrophoresis or nephelometry is necessary for follow-up of the patient rather than alternating the techniques.

Detection of an M-Protein in Urine

Dipsticks are used in many laboratories to screen for urinary proteins, but they often do not recognize Bence Jones protein (monoclonal light chains). Sulfosalicylic acid or Exton's reagent is better for light-chain detection. The heat test for Bence Jones proteinuria often produces false-positive or false-negative results. IEP or IF of an aliquot from an adequately concentrated 24 hour urine specimen reliably detects Bence Jones protein.

An M-protein appears as a tall, narrow, homogeneous peak in the densitometer tracing or as a dense, localized band on agarose gel. Its amount can be calculated on the basis of the size of the spike and the amount of total protein in the 24 hour urine specimen. It is not uncommon to find a monoclonal light chain on IF or IEP of a concentrated urine specimen even when there is a negative reaction for protein and no spike in the electrophoretic pattern.

■ DEFINITION OF BENIGN MONOCLONAL GAMMOPATHY

Benign monoclonal gammopathy indicates the presence of an M-protein in patients without evidence of MM, WM, primary amyloidosis (AL), or related disorder. Although this disorder is considered benign, it is now known that symptomatic MM, WM, AL, or a related disorder may develop in patients with an apparently benign monoclonal gammopathy. For that reason I prefer the term *monoclonal gammopathy of undetermined significance* (MGUS).

Patients with MGUS have a serum M-component below 3 g per deciliter, little or no M-protein in the urine, fewer than 10 percent plasma cells in the bone marrow, and absence of anemia, hypercalcemia, renal insufficiency, and lytic bone lesions. Discovery of an M-protein is an unexpected finding in either the laboratory evaluation of an unrelated disorder, in the investigation of an elevated erythrocyte sedimentation rate, or in a general health examination.

MGUS occurs in 3 percent of patients older than 70 years

Table 2 Findings on Follow-Up of Patients with Benign Monoclonal Gammopathy

GROUP	DESCRIPTION	NO. OF PATIENTS AT FOLLOW-UP (24–38 YR)	
1	No substantial increase of serum or urine monoclonal protein (benign)	30	12
2	Monoclonal protein ≥3 g/dl but no symptomatic myeloma or related disease	23	10
3	Died of unrelated causes	126	52
4	Development of myeloma, macroglobulinemia, amyloidosis, or related disease	62	26
Total		241	100%

and 1 percent of persons older than 50 years. The incidence increases with age, and a serum M-component is found in 4 percent to 5 percent of persons over 80 years of age. The incidence of M-components in the African-American population is higher than in whites.

■ PROGNOSIS OF BENIGN MONOCLONAL GAMMOPATHY

The prevalence of BMG is considerable, and since these patients are seen by family practitioners, internists, neurologists, dermatologists, and surgeons in various fields of clinical practice, it is of great importance to know whether the M-protein will remain stable (benign) or will progress to symptomatic MM, WM, or another malignant lymphoproliferative process or primary systemic amyloidosis.

For 20 to 35 years we at the Mayo Clinic have followed 241 patients with an apparently benign monoclonal gammopathy. The median age was 64 years at diagnosis. Any abnormal feature on physical examination such as hepatomegaly or splenomegaly as well as laboratory abnormality including anemia, thrombocytopenia, renal insufficiency, hypercalcemia, or hypoalbuminemia was due to unrelated disorders. The initial M-protein level ranged from 0.3 to 3.2 g per deciliter (median, 1.7 g per deciliter). The heavy-chain type consisted of IgG (74 percent), IgA (10 percent), and IgM (16 percent). The type of light chain was kappa in 63 percent and lambda in 37 percent. Five patients had a biclonal gammopathy. One-fourth of patients had a reduction in the uninvolved immunoglobulin level. Fifteen patients had Bence Jones proteinuria, but the amount of urinary light chain was more than 1 g per 24 hours in only three patients. The bone marrow contained 1 to 10 percent plasma cells (median, 3 percent). One-fourth of the patients had no abnormal findings at diagnosis other than the monoclonal gammopathy. The remainder had any of a wide variety of unrelated conditions such as cardiovascular or cerebrovascular disease, connective tissue disorder, inflammatory process, nonhematologic malignancy, or neurologic disorder.

After 25 to 38 years of follow-up (median, 22 years), the 241 patients were classified into four groups (Table 2).

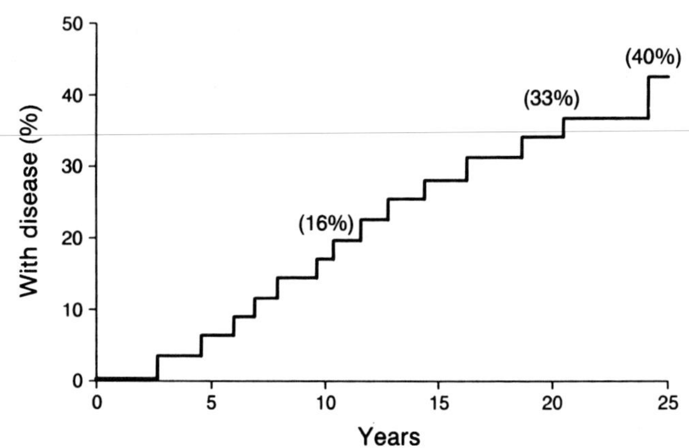

Figure 2
Rate of development of lymphoplasmacytoma during long-term follow-up of 241 patients with a serum monoclonal protein. *(From Kyle RA. Monoclonal gammopathy of undetermined significance. Baillieres Clin Haematol 1995; 8:761–781.)*

The number of patients in whom the M-component remained stable and who were classified as benign has decreased to 30 (12 percent). The patient with the longest follow-up was found to have an IgM monoclonal protein 37 years ago and at last follow-up was still alive and well with a stable M-protein at age 93 years. The M-component disappeared in two patients. The 30 patients are still at risk for developing a malignant transformation and must be followed. During follow-up, 23 patients had a serum M-protein value of 3 g per deciliter or more but did not require chemotherapy for MM, macroglobulinemia, or amyloidosis. Five of these patients are still living. The median interval from the detection of the M-protein to an increase to 3 g per deciliter was 9 years, and the median duration of follow-up after reaching this increase was 6 years. More than one-half (126) of the 241 patients (group 3) died of unrelated diseases without developing a malignant plasma cell or lymphoproliferative disorder. Cardiovascular or cerebrovascular disease accounted for half of the deaths.

One-fourth of the patients (62 of the 241, 26 percent) developed MM (42 cases), AL (8 cases), WM (7 cases), and other malignant lymphoproliferative disorders (5 cases) during the follow-up of 24 to 38 years (group 4). The actuarial rate of malignant transformation in the overall series was 16 percent at 10 years and 33 percent at 20 years (Fig. 2). The risk of malignant transformation was not significantly different whether the patient had an IgG, IgA, or IgM monoclonal gammopathy. The interval from the recognition of the M-protein to the diagnosis of a serious disease ranged from 2 to 29 years (median, 10 years). The mode of development of MM was variable. Some patients remained stable for many years and then MM gradually or suddenly developed. Others had a steady increase in the M-protein until they became symptomatic 5 to 29 years later. In seven of the patients, the diagnosis of MM was made more than 20 years after detection of the serum M-protein. The median duration of survival after the diagnosis of MM was 33 months. No features at diagnosis were useful in distinguishing patients who did not progress from those in whom a malignant change developed.

WM developed in seven patients 4 to 16 years (median, 8 years) after detection of the M-protein. All of these patients had serum values of IgM-kappa protein that ranged from 3.1 to 8.5 g per deciliter during the course of their disease. A malignant lymphoproliferative process developed in five patients 9 to 22 years (median, 10.5 years) after detection of the M-protein. These consisted of lymphoma (three cases), chronic lymphocytic leukemia (one case), and an undifferentiated lymphoproliferative process (one case). Primary systemic amyloidosis (AL) was found in eight patients 6 to 19 years (median, 9 years) after the M-protein was detected. AL was not discovered until autopsy in three cases.

Similar findings have been reported in other series. For example, the actuarial risk of development of a malignant monoclonal gammopathy was 4.5 percent at 5 years and 15 percent at 10 years in a group of 191 patients. In another series the actuarial risk was 8.5 percent and 19.2 percent at 5 and 10 years respectively in a group of 128 patients with an apparently benign monoclonal gammopathy.

DIFFERENTIATION OF MGUS FROM MULTIPLE MYELOMA OR MACROGLOBULINEMIA

A serum monoclonal protein concentration of more than 3 g per deciliter suggests MM or macroglobulinemia rather than MGUS, but some exceptions exist, such as smoldering multiple myeloma (SMM). SMM is characterized by a serum M-protein above 3 g per deciliter and more than 10 percent atypical plasma cells in the bone marrow. Frequently a small amount of monoclonal light chain is present in the urine and uninvolved immunoglobulins in the serum are reduced. These findings are consistent with those of MM or WM. However, anemia, renal insufficiency, and skeletal lesions do not develop, and the M-protein level in the serum and urine and number of bone marrow plasma cells remain stable. Furthermore, the plasma cell labeling index (PCLI) is low. Biologically, these patients have BMG, but it is not possible to make this diagnosis when the patient is initially seen because most patients with this level of M-protein in the serum and bone marrow plasma cells will have symptomatic disease. Patients with SMM should not be treated unless the abnormalities progress or symptoms of myeloma or macroglobulinemia develop.

The initial hemoglobin value, amount of serum M-protein, percentage of bone marrow plasma cells, presence of small amounts of urinary light chains, serum albumin levels, and values of uninvolved immunoglobulins are not useful in differentiating patients with a small M-protein who will remain stable with a benign condition from those in whom a malignant transformation will develop.

Although Bence Jones proteinuria is most frequently associated with MM, primary AL, WM, or another malignant lymphoproliferative disorder, it may be benign. Small amounts of monoclonal light chains (Bence Jones proteinuria) are not uncommon in BMG.

The PCLI is useful in differentiating MM from MGUS or SMM. An elevated PCLI is good evidence that a patient either has MM or will soon develop symptomatic myeloma. Circulating plasma cells in the peripheral blood are found in 80 percent of patients with symptomatic MM and in 90 percent of patients with relapsed MM, but circulating plasma cells are rarely seen in patients with MGUS or SMM.

Table 3 Tests for the Evaluation of MGUS in an Asymptomatic Patient

CBC (hemoglobin, leukocytes, and platelets)
Chemisty group (including calcium and creatinine)
Serum protein electrophoresis with IF or IEP
Quantitation of immunoglobulins
Routine urinalysis (if positive for protein, a 24 hour urine collection for electrophoresis and IF or IEP is indicated)

Elevated levels of beta$_2$-microglobulin, the presence of J chains, and elevation of plasma cell acid phosphatase levels are not reliable for differentiation between benign and malignant disease. Reduced numbers of CD4 T lymphocytes, increased numbers of monoclonal idiotype-bearing peripheral blood lymphocytes, and increased numbers of immunoglobulin-secreting cells in peripheral blood are characteristic of myeloma, but there is overlap with MGUS. No single technique differentiates benign from malignant plasma cell proliferation.

MANAGEMENT OF BENIGN MONOCLONAL GAMMOPATHY

Since it is not possible to differentiate a benign monoclonal gammopathy from one in which MM, macroglobulinemia, or a related disorder develops, the clinician must continue to observe the patient. It is essential to obtain a careful history, inquiring about skeletal pain, increased fatigue, history of recurrent infections, and bleeding diathesis. One must be alert for the symptoms of AL such as lightheadedness, change in the voice or enlargement of the tongue, weight loss, increased bruising, steatorrhea, dyspnea, edema, and paresthesias. Fever, night sweats, weight loss, blurred vision, or oronasal bleeding suggests macroglobulinemia.

The presence of a monoclonal protein and congestive heart failure, nephrotic syndrome, renal insufficiency of unknown cause, sensorimotor peripheral neuropathy, steatorrhea, carpal tunnel syndrome, or orthostatic hypotension requires appropriate biopsies to exclude the possibility of primary systemic amyloidosis.

Pallor, localized bone pain or tenderness, or subcutaneous masses suggest the possibility of MM. Hepatosplenomegaly and lymphadenopathy are characteristic of macroglobulinemia and related lymphoproliferative disorders. Periorbital purpura, macroglossia, submandibular swelling, orthostatic hypotension, hepatomegaly, and edema are all features of AL.

The patient with MGUS is asymptomatic, and the discovery of an M-protein is by chance and unexpected in a routine medical examination.

The minimal studies necessary for evaluation of MGUS in an asymptomatic patient with a normal physical examination are listed in Table 3.

If the serum M-protein is below 2 g per deciliter, the history and physical examination are noncontributory, and if the tests in Table 3 are normal, no additional studies are necessary. Serum protein electrophoresis should be rechecked in 6 months, and if stable, serum protein electrophoresis should be repeated at annual intervals.

If the initial M-protein is 2 to 2.5 g per deciliter, a 24 hour urine specimen should be obtained for determination of total protein, electrophoresis, and IF or IEP in addition to the tests in Table 3.

If the initial M-protein value is 2.5 to 3 g per deciliter, a metastatic bone survey including single views of the humeri and femurs should be obtained in addition to the tests in Table 3 and IF or IEP of urine. If the initial M-protein is above 3 g per deciliter, the patient should have a bone marrow aspirate, biopsy, and PCLI. A peripheral blood labeling index should also be done.

If MM is suspected, beta$_2$-microglobulin, C-reactive protein, and lactate dehydrogenase should be measured. If any historical or physical features suggestive of AL are found, biopsy of the subcutaneous fat and bone marrow should be performed. If these are negative and there is clinical suspicion of AL, a rectal biopsy including submucosa should be done. If this is negative and AL is still a consideration, biopsy of an involved organ should be performed.

In summary, no single parameter can differentiate a patient with BMG from those in whom a malignant plasma cell disorder will eventually develop. The most dependable means is serial measurement of the monoclonal protein in the serum and periodic reevaluation of pertinent clinical and laboratory features to determine whether MM, systemic AL, macroglobulinemia, or other lymphoplasma cell proliferative disease has developed.

■ BICLONAL GAMMOPATHIES

Biclonal gammopathies, which are characterized by the production of two different monoclonal proteins, occur in 4 percent of patients with monoclonal gammopathies. The presence of two monoclonal proteins may be due to the proliferation of two different clones of plasma cells, each giving rise to an unrelated monoclonal immunoglobulin, or it may result from the production of two monoclonal proteins by a single clone of plasma cells.

The clinical features of biclonal gammopathy are the same as those of monoclonal gammopathy. Approximately two-thirds have a biclonal gammopathy of undetermined significance. The remainder have MM, macroglobulinemia, or a malignant lymphoproliferative process. Serum protein electrophoresis shows only a single band on the acetate strip in approximately one-third of cases. The second M-protein is not recognized until IF or IEP is done. IgG and IgA are the most frequent combinations, followed by IgG and IgM monoclonal immunoglobulins. More than a dozen cases of triclonal gammopathy have been reported.

■ BENIGN (IDIOPATHIC) BENCE JONES PROTEINURIA

In most patients, a significant amount of Bence Jones proteinuria indicates MM, AL, macroglobulinemia, or another lymphoproliferative disorder. However, some patients may excrete large amounts of Bence Jones proteinuria and follow a benign course for many years. We have followed a group of patients excreting more than 1 g of Bence Jones protein daily. Most eventually develop MM or AL. In one patient MM did not require treatment until after 21 years of observation. Another patient continued to excrete the same amount of Bence Jones protein for 25 years and has developed no evidence of a serious underlying disease. Although idiopathic Bence Jones protein may follow a benign course for many years, the patient must be observed indefinitely because MM or AL eventually develops in most patients.

Suggested Reading

Bladé J, López-Guillermo A, Rozman C, et al. Malignant transformation and life expectancy in monoclonal gammopathy of undetermined significance. Br J Haematol 1992; 81:391–394.

Kyle RA. "Benign" monoclonal gammopathy—after 20 to 35 years of follow-up. Mayo Clin Proc 1993; 68:26–36.

Kyle RA, Greipp PR. "Idiopathic" Bence Jones proteinuria. Long-term follow-up in seven patients. N Engl J Med 1982; 306:564–567.

Kyle RA, Robinson RA, Katzmann JA. The clinical aspects of biclonal gammopathies: Review of 57 cases. Am J Med 1981; 71:999–1009.

CHEMOTHERAPY-INDUCED AND CHRONIC NEUTROPENIAS

Parviz Lalezari, M.D.

Leukopenia, a reduction in the total number of white blood cells, may reflect neutropenia, lymphopenia, or a decrease in all leukocyte subpopulations. This chapter focuses on the severe forms of neutropenia, in which the absolute number of neutrophils (ANC) is below 0.5×10^9 per liter. The management of these disorders requires separate strategies for correction of the underlying causes and the treatment of the acute and chronic infectious complications. The majority of the patients under treatment for severe neutropenia are the recipients of myeloreductive chemotherapy. However, a significant number of patients with selective neutropenia from other causes also require treatment. The guidelines for management of treatment-induced leukopenias are different from the rules that apply to other forms: in chemotherapy the goal of the treatment is to reduce the expected duration and severity of leukopenia and thereby allow administration of dose-intensive chemotherapy with a reduced risk of fatal infections. This goal has become attainable through various cytokines, with or without infusion of myeloid progenitor cells. The guidelines for treatment of other forms of neutropenias may be summarized as follows:

1. Treatment requirements for various pathogenetic forms of neutropenia vary. Therefore, every effort should be made to determine the pathogenesis of the disorder.
2. In some patients, especially newborn infants, chronic neutropenia is well tolerated and requires no treatment other than observation, and management of complications as they occur.
3. In most chronic neutropenias, except the transient forms, the elevation of neutrophil counts lasts only as long as the treatment is maintained.
4. Because of these considerations, treatment of neutropenia must be individualized.

In view of the importance of pathogenesis in therapeutic planning, a classification of neutropenias based on presumed or established pathogeneses is presented (Tables 1 to 4). Treatment of leukopenia caused by chemotherapy is discussed separately from other forms of bone marrow failure, diseases of the stem cells, immunologically induced neutropenias, and those caused by excessive peripheral neutrophil destruction. The important new technologies that involve mobilization, harvesting, expansion, and use of progenitor cells; gene therapy and potentials of insertion of drug-resistant genes into hematopoietic cells are not discussed because these procedures are in the developmental phase. The management of complications of neutropenias, namely infection and sepsis, is not different from treatment of other infections. This subject has been reviewed elsewhere. Therefore, only some of the complications that arise from chronic forms of neutropenia are discussed.

Table 1 Classification of Neutropenias

Failure of production or maturation
Failure of release
Margination and pooling abnormalities
Immunologic destruction
Excessive consumption
Idiopathic forms (pathogeneses not known)

CLASSIFICATION OF NEUTROPENIAS BASED ON PATHOGENESIS

The blood level of neutrophils is primarily determined by a balance between production in the bone marrow and use in peripheral blood. The neutrophil level is also influenced by changes in their release from the marrow and the distribution

Table 2 Neutropenias Caused by Failure of Production or Maturation

APLASTIC AND HYPOPLASTIC BONE MARROW
Dose-dependent chemotherapy, other myelotoxic drugs, radiation
Drug-induced idiosyncratic bone marrow failure
Idiopathic bone marrow failure: aplasia or hypoplasia

BONE MARROW REPLACEMENT
Leukemias and lymphomas
Metastatic tumors
Myelofibrosis
Gaucher's disease

METABOLIC DISORDERS
Vitamin B_{12} and folic acid deficiency
Starvation
Hyperglycinuria and other aminoacidurias

CONGENITAL NEUTROPENIAS DUE TO DISEASE OF THE STEM CELLS OR MYELOID CELL PROGENITORS
Cyclic neutropenia
Severe congenital neutropenia
Kostmann's syndrome (congenital genetic, recessive)
Schwachman-Diamond (neutropenia, dwarfism, and steatorrhea)
Congenital benign forms with dominant, recessive, or random inheritance
Dyskeratosis congenita with pancytopenia
Chediak-Higashi syndrome, myelokathexis, reticular dysgenesis

Table 3 Immunologic Causes of Neutropenias

ANTIBODY-MEDIATED ISOLATED NEUTROPENIA
Alloimmune neonatal neutropenia due to fetal-maternal incompatibility
Transitory neonatal neutropenia due to maternal autoimmune neutropenia
Autoimmune neutropenia of infancy
Primary autoimmune neutropenia in adolescents and adults
Autoimmune neutropenia due to cold-reactive antibodies
Pure white cell aplasia
Drug-associated immune neutropenias (procaine amide, aminopyrine, quinine, cephalosporin)
IMMUNE NEUTROPENIAS ASSOCIATED WITH OTHER IMMUNOLOGIC DISEASES
Neutropenia with autoimmune anemia and thrombocytopenia
Alternating autoimmune hemocytopenia
Systemic lupus, rheumatoid arthritis, Felty's syndrome
Lymphoma (T-γ, hairy cell leukemia, Hodgkin's disease)
Crohn's disease
Graves' disease
Sarcoidosis
Dysgammaglobulinemia, severe combined and IgA deficiency syndromes
Immune complexes causing neutropenia

Table 4 Neutropenias Caused by Excessive Destruction or Utilization

Bacterial infections
Sepsis
Typhoid fever, tuberculosis, brucellosis
Viral infections
Influenza; measles; rubella; varicella; AIDS; hepatitis A, B, C; infectious mononucleosis; cytomegalovirus infection; transient erythroblastopenia of childhood
Parasitic infestation

within the marginal and circulating pools. Although often a combination of factors contribute to neutropenia, an attempt should be made to identify the cause according to the general pathogenetic groups described in Table 1.

Neutropenias caused by the failure of production or maturation, which are listed in Table 2, are divided into four major pathogenetic subgroups: aplastic or hypoplastic bone marrow, bone marrow replacement, metabolic disorders, and the neutropenias that result from stem cell or myeloid progenitor cell defects.

About 30 to 40 percent of African-Americans and some Yemenite Jews have neutropenia. These and the more severe forms seen in African and West Indian blacks exemplify abnormalities in the neutrophil release mechanism. A more severe release abnormality is lazy leukocyte syndrome, in which defective neutrophil mobility leads to clinical symptoms. Examples of abnormalities related to neutrophil margination include neutropenias that develop during hypersensitivity reactions, endotoxemia, and other complement-activating immunologic reactions. Neutropenia associated with hemodialysis belongs to this group; generation of C5a activates the neutrophils, leading to their aggregation and adherence to vascular endothelium. Neutropenia found in paroxysmal nocturnal hemoglobinuria may be due to complement activation, although reduced production is also a contributory factor. Immune neutropenias in Table 3 are divided into isolated neutropenias and those associated with other immunologic diseases. Neutropenias associated with infection are described under excessive utilization (Table 4). In these cases, however, additional pathogenetic factors such as relative bone marrow failure or margination, may be contributory. Infants have relatively limited capacity to compensate for excessive utilization and therefore are predisposed to transient neutropenia with various infections. Felty's syndrome is another form of multipathogenetic neutropenia in which failure of production, excessive destruction, margination, and especially pooling are combined.

■ AN APPROACH TO INVESTIGATION OF NEUTROPENIA

Despite the complexity of neutropenia, an accurate etiologic diagnosis can be made in many patients, based on detailed clinical information that should include history of exposure to myelotoxic drugs, hepatosplenomegaly, and microscopic examination of the peripheral blood and bone marrow. One approach is to evaluate each case against a checklist (see Tables 1 to 4). The list is constantly expanding as new disorders and drugs that can cause neutropenia are identified. Bone marrow failure induced by drug therapy usually does not present a diagnostic problem. In some cases, however, despite normalization of the bone marrow after treatment, the neutrophil count does not rise for several months. The mechanism of this postchemotherapy-persistent neutropenia is obscure. In several examples investigated in this laboratory, we were unable to document any immunologic causes. In patients with chronic idiopathic neutropenia, transformation to acute leukemia is a concern. The correct diagnosis in these cases may elude clinicians for several years despite repeated bone marrow examinations and cytogenetic studies. In disorders caused by stem cell abnormalities, the key to diagnosis is the combination of diagnostic features such as age of onset, sequential blood counts, bone marrow examination, the clinical course, and the exclusion of more frequent immunologic causes. Determination of neutrophil response to injection of hydrocortisone, epinephrine, or endotoxin can be helpful in the diagnoses of release defects and margination abnormalities. The Rebuck window skin test is useful for evaluation of neutrophil mobilization. However, this technique is available only in a few centers.

In immunologically induced neutropenias (see Table 3), the diagnosis can be established by the demonstration of neutrophil antibodies. The procedures include leukoagglutination and immunofluorescence (IF) tests. Because of their subtleties, these tests should be performed only in experienced laboratories. Leukocyte agglutination test not only allows positive diagnosis of alloimmune neonatal neutropenia but can identify the specificities involved. Most of these antibodies also can be detected by IF assay, either microscopically or by flow cytometry. In certain specificities such as NB2 and 5^b (the latter is not involved in neutropenia but can cause febrile transfusion reaction), the reaction can be detected only by agglutination and not by IF. Alloimmune neonatal neutropenia usually lasts a few weeks but in exceptional cases may continue for several months. These protracted cases should be differentiated from autoimmune neutropenia of infancy. In the latter, infants are born with normal neutrophil counts but become neutropenic after 3 to 4 months and commonly before the age of 1 year. During the overlap period diagnosis is based on demonstration of maternal antibodies in alloimmune forms and autoantibodies in autoimmune forms. One of the diagnostic criteria in autoimmune neutropenia is demonstration of neutrophil-bound antibodies by direct IF assay. More recent studies in this and other laboratories have shown that neutrophil activation by infection or after administration of growth factors may induce expression of Fc-gamma-RI (FcγRI), the high affinity receptor. This receptor is absent or present in only low copy numbers on normal, not activated, neutrophils. Expression of this receptor leads to Fc-mediated binding of plasma IgG to neutrophils and development of a positive direct IF reaction. For these reasons, a positive direct IF test on neutrophils, unlike the red cells, is not an evidence for autoimmunity unless abnormal expression of FcγRI is ruled out. Expression of this marker can be tested by flow cytometry and the use of an anti-FcγRI (CD64) monoclonal antibody.

Autoimmune neutropenia of infancy is a self-limited disease, and recovery occurs within a few years. By contrast, autoimmune neutropenia in older children and in adolescence is more severe and is frequently associated with involvement of red blood cells and platelets. Anemia and thrombocytopenia, however, may be initially subclinical, and the correct diagnosis requires demonstration of platelet and red cell autoantibodies. The direct Polybrene test, performed in this laboratory on an AutoAnalyzer, is a valuable tool for detection of red cell autoantibodies in subclinical forms of the disease, especially when the antiglobulin test is negative.

■ THERAPY

Neutropenia in Myeloreductive Chemotherapy

The severity of infection in neutropenic patients is generally proportional to the neutrophil count, but it is also influenced by neutrophil availability, a phenomenon that is deficient in recipients of chemotherapy. For this reason bacterial, viral, and fungal infections are quite serious in these patients, and their management should include prophylactic and therapeutic antibacterial and antifungal treatment. Moreover, in cases of invasive fungal infections, aggressive treatment is continued even after the resolution of the neutropenia. Despite these measures, patient survival largely depends on the ultimate recovery of hematologic deficiencies, which can now be accelerated by the use of cytokines and the progenitor cells.

The clinical applications of cytokines are based on their in vitro behavior in colony assays, where their ability to support hematopoiesis can be assessed, either individually or in combination. Based on these evaluations, stem cell factor (SCF), interleukin-1 (IL-1), and interleukin-6 (IL-6) have been demonstrated to act primarily as synergistic factors. In other words, these cytokines alone do not induce colony proliferation but magnify the effects of other cytokines such as IL-2, IL-3, and the colony stimulating factors GM-CSF, G-CSF, M-CSF, erythropoietin, etc. Lineage specificity, a much desired property, is not a real feature of cytokines, although some like erythropoietin, G-CSF, and M-CSF, show predominance for the red cells, neutrophils, or monocytes, respectively. Some cytokines such as tumor necrosis factor, transforming growth factor-beta, and macrophage inflammatory protein-alpha block differentiation but not proliferation. These properties offer opportunities for developing specific mixtures for selective in vitro expansion of progenitor cells needed for clinical use without causing terminal differentiation.

In practice, the growth factors commonly in use are recombinant G-CSF produced in *Escherichia coli,* and GM-CSF produced in yeast. Both of these growth factors stimulate myeloid cells to proliferate and enhance phagocytic and microbicidal activities. Protocols for using a combination of these cytokines with synergistic factors to increase their effectiveness are being developed. One promising combination is the use of G-CSF with interferon gamma (IFN-γ), which appears to enhance fungicidal activity of neutrophils. Although in many studies significant differences in patient survival have not been established, it is clear that cytokine therapy reduces the length and severity of the expected leukopenia and thereby reduces the incidence of febrile episodes, shortens hospitalization, and decreases intravenous antibiotic usage, which in turn reduces the risks for serious fungal infections. G-CSF and other cytokines with myelostimulating effects should not be used within 24 hours before or after administration of short-acting cytotoxic chemotherapeutic agents. This is to protect the rapidly dividing normal myeloid cells. For the same reason, the simultaneous use of cytokines with long-acting myelosuppressive agents or antimetabolites is unwise. The exception may be IL-1, which may be used before chemotherapy. IL-1 is an early acting cytokine, and in this application is used for myeloprotection rather than myelorestoration.

G-CSF has an elimination half-life of 3.4 hours after subcutaneous injection and is usually given at a dose of 4 to 8 μg per kilogram per day. After chemotherapy, administration of G-CSF should continue up to 2 weeks, until a sustained normal neutrophil count is achieved. Subcutaneous or intravenous injection of G-CSF to normal individuals causes neutrophilia within 1 to 2 days without the accompanying eosinophilia that is seen with other growth factors. The neutrophils are left-shifted and may show toxic granulations, Dohle bodies, hypersegmentation, increased alkaline phosphatase staining, and a high expression of FcγRI, the high affinity IgG receptor. One of the side effects of G-CSF administration is medullary bone pain shortly after injection that lasts up to a few hours and then subsides with or without administration of common analgesics. The pain is probably due to the expansion and increased pressure within the bone marrow spaces and is milder in children whose bones are soft. In most adults the pain can be reduced by lowering the dose and gradually diminishes with continuation of treatment. Other symptoms are probably related to hypersensitivity. They include wheezing, dyspnea, hypotension, skin rashes, urticaria, and rarely more severe eruptions such as cutaneous vasculitis, erythema multiforme, and Stevens-Johnson syndrome. Capillary leak syndrome, pleuropericardial effusion, and the flu-like symptoms that limit the use of several other cytokines do not occur after G-CSF treatment. Preparations with reduced contamination with *E. coli* products may cause less severe hypersensitivity reactions. Caution should be exercised in administration of G-CSF to patients with inflammatory lung disease because neutrophilia, an occasional side effect, may increase the severity of pulmonary infiltration and aggravate hypoxia. Side effects of long-term administration of G-CSF are discussed under management of chronic neutropenias.

Recombinant GM-CSF promotes proliferation of partially committed myeloid progenitor cells, with predominant effects on differentiation and functional development of myelomonocytic cells. Because of multilineage activity, GM-CSF provides a broader hematopoietic support than G-CSF and is indicated especially for accelerating reconstruction of autologous and allogeneic bone marrow transplant. This agent is particularly effective in the treatment of lymphoid malignancies after myeloreductive therapy. Adverse effects of GM-CSF include fluid retention, pleuropericardial effusion, and capillary leak syndrome. They occur in about 1 percent of patients who receive standard treatment, which is 250 μg per square meter given by two hours intravenous infusion, 2 to 4 hours after infusion of bone marrow. The treatment is continued for 2 to 3 weeks. GM-CSF may also cause testicular atrophy, aggravate pre-existing renal and hepatic dysfunctions, and provoke hypersensitivity reactions similar to those described for G-CSF. Because of multilineage activity, potentials of cytokines to enhance the growth of myeloid-related malignant tumors remains a concern.

Congenital and Chronic Idiopathic Neutropenias

Before initiation of treatment, all of these patients must have a baseline bone marrow examination with cytogenetic evaluation and, if possible, colony assays to determine the in vitro response pattern to various hematopoietic growth factors. Patients with pre-existing cytogenetic abnormalities should be treated only symptomatically, and the growth factors such as G-CSF or GM-CSF should not be used unless the patient has a life-threatening infection. In view of risks associated with abnormal cytogenetics, it is prudent to use the growth factors in these cases only intermittently and to prepare the patients for ultimate bone marrow transplantation when the risk of leukemic transformation is known to be high.

Based on in vitro colony assays and clinical response to G-CSF, chronic neutropenic patients with normal cytogenetics can be divided into four therapeutic types: high responders who require less than 5 μg per kilogram per day of G-CSF; medium responders requiring between 5 and 10 μg per kilogram per day; low responders requiring doses above 10 μg per kilogram per day; and nonresponders, in whom the neutrophil count cannot be elevated by G-CSF, even at doses as high as 100 μg per kilogram per day. In colony assays the bone marrow of these refractory patients fails to generate normal myeloid colonies by G-CSF or by a combination of G-CSF with other growth factors. We have observed two such patients. One died of graft versus host disease and sepsis after bone marrow transplantation. Another developed monosomy-7 5 years after treatment with high doses of G-CSF. These observations suggest that severe congenital neutropenia is not a single disorder but rather it represents a heterogeneous group of diseases with different pathogeneses.

In the responder groups which constitute the majority of congenital neutropenias, G-CSF is the treatment of choice, even though it is not curative. Our general rule is that G-CSF should be given at the lowest dose that keeps the patient asymptomatic and neutrophil counts above 1×10^9 per liter.

In cyclic neutropenia daily administration of G-CSF does not eliminate the cyclic pattern, but it abrogates the clinical manifestations, shortens the duration of neutropenia, and elevates the neutrophil counts at nadir. It is not established, but it is likely that intermittent G-CSF administration, given in phase with neutropenic cycles, would be sufficient to achieve the same results. For this purpose G-CSF would be given only for 3 days before and 1 week during the neutropenic phase. Such a strategy would reduce the cost and possibly the side effects. Interestingly, many severe congenital neutropenic patients treated with G-CSF exhibit a cyclic pattern. The reason for these cycles is not clear. Possibly these patients originally have a cyclic form of neutropenia in which the neutrophil peaks are too low to be registered, but the pattern becomes apparent when production is increased, allowing cycling at a higher, and therefore detectable level. Chronic idiopathic neutropenias in adults are less symptomatic, and usually respond to G-CSF. The rules that apply to the treatment of these patients are the same: to use the lowest dose of G-CSF that keep the patient asymptomatic and the ANC above 1×10^9 per liter.

Adverse Effects of Long-Term Administration of G-CSF

In addition to the adverse effects described for short-term use of G-CSF, long-term treatment for congenital and other chronic neutropenias has been associated with a number of adverse events. In most patients the bone marrow is hypercellular, with marked increase in myeloid activity. Some develop increased fibrosis, and areas of necrosis have been observed in others. Several patients on long-term G-CSF therapy have developed a cytogenetic abnormality such as monosomy-7 or acute leukemia. The role of G-CSF in these abnormalities remains unclear, especially because the natural course of the underlying neutropenias is unknown, and several cases of leukemic transformation have been reported in congenital neutropenias before the growth factors were introduced. Until these questions are resolved, it is prudent to administer G-CSF at the lowest dose which maintains the patient in remission. Moreover, since the effects on fetuses are not known, pregnant women should not receive G-CSF. We did observe, however, a woman who gave birth to a normal infant after having received G-CSF for 6 months during her pregnancy.

Another concern is related to the possible side effects of leukocytosis, especially in patients with pulmonary infection and hypoxia. We administered G-CSF for over 6.5 months to an adult patient with Job syndrome who had no coexisting hypoxia or inflammatory lung disease. The patient maintained a persistent leukocytosis, near 40×10^9 per liter for duration of the treatment without showing any clinical or laboratory abnormality except for mild elevation of serum LDH, alkaline phosphatase, and uric acid. These abnormalities, including neutrophilia, rapidly returned to baseline when G-CSF was discontinued. Others have reported a rise in serum lysozyme level, an indication of high neutrophil turnover.

Splenomegaly, which reflects extramedullary myelopoiesis, is a common complication of chronic administration of G-CSF, especially in children with severe congenital neutropenia. The magnitude of splenomegaly is dose related. We observed massive splenomegaly in all of the rabbits injected with recombinant human G-CSF at 100 μg per kilogram per day for 6 to 9 months. Also, in a patient with refractory severe congenital neutropenia, administration of large doses of G-CSF, from 20 to 120 μg per kilogram per day, was associated with a marked enlargement of the spleen, which receded when the treatment was discontinued.

Thrombocytopenia has been observed in patients with chronic severe neutropenia who received G-CSF. Thrombocytopenia also occurred in all the rabbits which we treated with 100 μg per kilogram per day of G-CSF over several months. In one adult patient with autoimmune neutropenia, we observed a fall in platelet counts from 271×10^9 per liter to 139×10^9 per liter within 10 days after subcutaneous administration of 5 μg per kilogram per day of G-CSF. This treatment had resulted in a rise of ANC from 0.76×10^9 per liter to 16×10^9 per liter. At this point G-CSF was reduced to 2.5 μg per kilogram per day. Three days later ANC was 4.4×10^9 per liter but platelets had further dropped to 118×10^9 per liter. Continuation of treatment at this dose resulted in a gradual rise of both platelet and ANC. Subsequently, G-CSF was reduced to 2 μg per kilogram per day and 10 weeks later to 2 μg per kilogram per day every other day. The patient has been maintained at this dose for nearly 5 years with normal neutrophil and platelet counts.

Other adverse events of long term G-CSF treatment have included alopecia and mild proteinuria. Alopecia areata was a common complication in our experimental rabbits. There has been no evidence for the development of antibodies against G-CSF, but an increase in dose requirements has been observed in some children with severe congenital neutropenia.

Chloramphenicol in Congenital Neutropenias

In 1983 Adams and Pearson reported their observation on a 14-year-old child with typical clinical and hematologic features of congenital neutropenia. The child was treated with chloramphenicol on several occasions, and a marked elevation of blood neutrophils was observed within 10 to 12 days after each treatment. The patient was placed on an oral maintenance dose of 1.75 to 2 g per day, and a dose-dependent remission was achieved. Several attempts to withdraw the drug was unsuccessful, and the patient was kept on chloramphenicol for over a decade. Since that time, five more cases have been observed with similar results. Chloramphenicol has been shown to stimulate CFU-GM production in bone marrow culture at a 1 μg per milliliter concentration. Although chloramphenicol cannot be used routinely because of high toxicity, it may find an application under life-threatening circumstances when other treatments fail.

Other therapies in neutropenia include folic acid for treatment of folic acid deficiency. In addition, folic acid may be useful in treatment of leukopenia after long-term use of trimethoprim-sulfamethoxazole. Lithium carbonate at 20 to 100 mg per kilogram per day and at serum levels of 0.5 to 1 μg per milliliter is known to stimulate committed myeloid progenitor cells in the bone marrow. However, this treatment is not effective in patients who have defective or reduced bone marrow myeloid cells. Granulocyte transfusion is no longer in use, mainly because of logistic problems in preparation and frequent adverse reactions.

Immune Neutropenias

Immunologically-induced neonatal neutropenias are self-limited and do not require specific treatment other than good hygiene and protection from exposure to other children with infection. Treatment with antibiotics, when indicated, should be given for long durations, but hospitalization and reverse isolation are usually unnecessary. For severe cases with life-threatening infections, treatment with intravenous IgG (IVIgG) 1 g per kilogram per day for 3 days or G-CSF, 2 to 5 μg per kilogram per day for a few days is beneficial. Although similar rules apply to autoimmune neutropenia of infancy, which has a longer course, the affected children may require additional treatments for otitis, abscesses, mouth sores, diarrhea, and skin infections. These complications usually respond to conventional antibiotic therapy, but when they are severe, administration of IVIgG at 1 g per kilogram per day for 3 days is indicated. Neutrophil counts usually rise 2 to 5 days after initiation of IVIgG treatment, but occasionally additional courses are required for a response. The effects usually lasts for 1 to 2 weeks, but permanent recovery may occur, especially when treatment begins late in the course of the disease. Prophylactic administration of IVIgG is especially helpful for patients who may require surgery. In a retrospective study carried out in this laboratory on children treated with G-CSF for severe neutropenia, we found over 20 percent to have neutrophil antibodies. These children probably had autoimmune neutropenia, and all responded to G-CSF treatment. The mechanism by which G-CSF induces remission in immune neutropenia is unclear. A likely explanation is enhancement of myelopoiesis, which converts the neutropenia to a compensated form, as it occurs in compensated hemolytic anemia. Primary autoimmune neutropenia in older children and adolescents presents a more difficult challenge. In many of these patients other blood cells are also affected, and leukopenia may alternate with hemolytic anemia or thrombocytopenia. These conditions are usually progressive, and the patients require numerous courses of IVIgG, steroids, antibiotics, and even immunosuppression. Some of these patients respond, although temporarily, to treatment with vincristine. In one example of a protracted autoimmune disease involving neutrophils, platelets and the red cells, after long-term steroids and IVIgG administration, our patient was subjected to splenectomy at the age of 14. Splenectomy induced a remission that has thus far lasted for 4 years. Other investigators also have had similar difficulties in the management of this type of complex autoimmune disease.

Autoimmune neutropenia in adults can be severe and debilitating because of recurrent mouth sores and other forms of infection. In most of these patients, steroids have only transient effects and should be used only intermittently. Similarly, danazol and other androgens have not been beneficial, even though in some of cases of autoimmune hemolytic anemia, thrombocytopenic purpura, and paroxysmal nocturnal hemoglobinuria, danazol has been shown to reduce cell destruction and enhance the bone marrow response. IVIgG in autoimmune neutropenia of adults can induce a temporary remission but it is not cost effective. As indicated earlier, we have treated one patient with 2 μg per kilogram G-CSF given every other day for 5 years, and the patient has maintained a G-CSF–dependent normal blood count without any symptoms. A remarkable feature of the clinical response in this patient was the rapid recovery from the severe gingivitis. In view of these results, cautious use of G-CSF in neutropenias associated with other immunologic diseases may also be helpful, but long-term effects of this growth factor on autoimmunity and on the immune system are unknown. Finally, in cases of neutropenia associated with immune complex diseases, plasmapheresis may be effective. This requires several days of exchange with human serum albumin.

Complications of Chronic Neutropenia

Patients with chronic neutropenia, especially children, require treatment for recurrent otitis, sinusitis, stomatitis, and occasionally more severe acute and chronic infections such as pneumonia, lung and liver abscesses, the complications that especially occur in patients who are refractory to G-CSF.

The availability and use of effective antibiotics, cytokines, and IVIgG have changed presentation and the clinical course of acute and chronic neutropenias. In undiagnosed and improperly treated patients, however, the dramatic acute manifestations are seen occasionally. For example, appendicitis can remain undiagnosed because of reduced local inflammatory response. The failure to diagnose and treat appendicitis has catastrophic consequences, including massive bowel necrosis and perforation. The respiratory system may develop pneumonia and lung abscess, and metastatic abscesses in the brain and liver may be observed. Perirectal abscesses can lead to fistulas and recurrent diarrhea leading to wasting. In a patient with autoimmune neutropenia of infancy we observed a rapid recovery from wasting and refractory diarrhea after treatment with IVIgG. In the oral cavity periodontitis that leads to the loss of teeth and chronic hypertrophic gingivitis are the hallmarks of severe chronic neutropenia. Occasionally these patients are first seen by dentists, who should be aware of the underlying cause and should perform diagnostic blood tests. In the severe congenital forms, correction of the advanced gingivitis is difficult. In addition to treatment of neutropenia, it requires aggressive local therapy and oral hygiene. Chronic, repetitive otitis, if neglected, can cause hearing loss in these patients and in children with autoimmune neutropenia of infancy. Treatment of chronic urinary infection, especially in patients with urinary tract congenital abnormalities and obstruction, can be a challenge. In these and other chronically infected individuals, long-term prophylactic antibiotics such as trimethoprim-sulfamethoxazole may be indicated until the infection is eradicated.

Acknowledgement

Supported in part by Jimmy Pollock Research Foundation and National Foundation for Research in Blood Diseases.

Suggested Reading

Adams GR, Pearson HA. Chloramphenicol-responsive chronic neutropenia. N Engl J Med 1983; 309:1039–1041.

Bostron B, Smith K, Ramsey NKC. Stimulation of human committed bone marrow stem cells (CFU-GM) Clin Exp Hematol 1986; 14:156–161.

Calderwood S, et al. Idiopathic thrombocytopenia and neutropenia in childhood. J Pediatr Hematol Oncol 1994; 16:95–101.

Lalezari P. Autoimmune hemoloytic disease. In: Thompson RA, Rose NR. Recent advances in clinical immunology. New York: Churchill Livinstone, 1983:69.

Lalezari P, Khorshidi M. Neutrophil and platelet antibodies in immune neutropenia and thrombocytopenia. In: Rose NR, Conway DeMacario E, Fahey JL, et al. eds. Manual of clinical laboratory immunology. 4th ed. American Society for Microbiology, 1992, 344–350.

Pearson HA. Unforgettable patients. J Pediatr 1992; 121:154–155.

Wood AJJ. Management of fever in patients with cancer and treatment-induced neutropenia. N Engl J Med 1993; 328:1323.

HEMOPHILIA A AND B

Jerome Teitel, M.D., F.R.C.P.C.
Victor S. Blanchette, M.B., M.A., B.Chir., M.R.C.P., F.R.C.P. (Lon), F.R.C.P.C.

Hemophilia A and B are the X-linked congenital deficiencies of coagulation factors VIII and IX respectively. They occur with a combined frequency of approximately 1:5,000 males, hemophilia A accounting for approximately 80 percent of the total.

More hemophilia A than hemophilia B patients are severely affected, but the hemorrhagic manifestations of the two diseases are otherwise indistinguishable. The most common sites of bleeding are the joints (especially elbows, knees, and ankles), skeletal muscle, the gastrointestinal tract, the genitourinary tract, and the central nervous system. Mucocutaneous bleeding is frequent in the first 2 years of life but is not generally a major feature thereafter. Hemophilia is genetically heterogeneous, but the clinical severity correlates with the plasma factor VIII or IX activity irrespective of the genotype. Severely affected individuals, in whom factor VIII or IX activity is generally less than 1 percent of normal (less than 0.01 IU per milliter), tend to bleed frequently and spontaneously, which often causes chronic musculoskeletal problems. In moderately severe disease, factor VIII or IX activity is generally between 0.01 and 0.04 IU per milliliter, and bleeding usually follows some degree of trauma. Higher levels are generally associated with clinically mild disease. Values greater than 0.15 IU per milliliter but below the normal range are not usually associated with a clinically evident bleeding disorder.

In some patients with hemophilia A, especially mild disease, the differential diagnosis must include an inhibitory autoantibody to factor VIII (acquired hemophilia) and von Willebrand's disease (VWD), in particular those variants of VWD characterized by defective factor VIII binding sites. Hemophilia B must also be differentiated from acquired nonselective factor IX deficiency, as occurs with vitamin K deficiency.

■ GOALS AND GENERAL PRINCIPLES OF HEMOPHILIA THERAPY

The goals of hemophilia treatment are to arrest or prevent bleeding and to prevent the long-term morbidity, principally musculoskeletal, that follows repeated hemorrhages. Replacement of the deficient coagulation factor is central to treatment, but there are other useful interventions. These include lifestyle modification such as physical training to enhance joint-protective muscle bulk, avoidance of contact sports, and careful attention to dental hygiene. The latter is particularly relevant to hemophiliacs, as bleeding associated with tooth and gum disease and dental extractions can be persistent and troublesome and can require the use of large doses of factor replacement products.

The pharmaceutical and biologic agents useful in some patients are described subsequently. Nonpharmacologic modalities such as rest and the local application of cold can be of great value. Anti-inflammatory agents are valuable in the treatment of chronic hemophilic arthropathy, in which inflammation and hemorrhage occur cyclically. The antiplatelet activity of nonsteroidal agents renders their use problematic. Ibuprofen has been used safely for systemic therapy, and short courses of corticosteroids may be used in selected situations. Aspirin should not be used by hemophiliacs. Intra-articular injections of corticosteroids or of radioisotopes are emerging as useful local therapies. Surgical management for the complications of hemophilia may be undertaken to preserve life or limb (e.g., intramuscular hemorrhage with compartment syndrome), to effect long-term hemostasis (e.g., synovectomy), or to control pain (e.g., arthroplasty or arthrodesis).

Traditionally, factor replacement therapy has been given therapeutically as on-demand treatment of established bleeding or prophylactically, typically as short-term management following surgery, trauma, or repeated bleeding from a target joint. Long-term continuous prophylactic therapy by patient self-infusion has been used sparingly because of the difficulty of venous access in young children, lack (until recently) of proven efficacy in reducing chronic morbidity, inconvenience, real and perceived risks, and expense. Recently reported long-term studies have confirmed that prophylactic treatment can prevent joint debility. In light of these data and the increasing availability of safer concentrates and improved venous access devices, these prophylactic regimens will likely gain greater acceptance. Therefore, the prospect of eliminating chronic hemophilic arthropathy may now be realistic.

■ SELF-INFUSION AND HEMOPHILIA COMPREHENSIVE CARE

Despite the inconvenience and discomfort of intravenous therapy, it is both desirable and practical for people with severe hemophilia to self-infuse factor VIII or factor IX concentrate. The rationale behind home care is outlined in Table 1.

Table 1 Rationale for Hemophilia Home Care
Severe hemophiliacs bleed frequently and at unpredictable intervals.
The convenience of home care enhances compliance with treatment, thus minimizing long-term complications.
The convenience of home care facilitates prompt treatment, which optimizes hemostatic and symptomatic results.
Home care reduces disruption of day-to-day routines, improving individual achievement and productivity.
Home care liberates the hemophiliac from the hospital, promoting independence and self-reliance.
Laboratory monitoring of therapy for typical hemarthroses and intramuscular hematomas is generally unnecessary.

Hemophilia home care and clinic-based comprehensive care complement one another. Comprehensive programs are generally directed by a hematologist and supervised by a nurse coordinator. The programs also typically include a physiotherapist, a social worker, a dentist, an orthopedic surgeon, and/or a rheumatologist. A comprehensive care program must have access to a highly expert coagulation laboratory. The program should be able to provide genetic counseling and access to modern genetic testing techniques. Primary care for human immunodeficiency virus (HIV) and hepatitis may be provided at the comprehensive care hemophilia clinic or by referral, according to local practice.

■ FACTOR VIII AND IX REPLACEMENT THERAPY

Plasma-Derived Concentrates

Plasma-derived factor VIII concentrates are purified by multiple precipitation, gel filtration, ion exchange, or immunoaffinity chromatography steps. They can be categorized on the basis of purity. This is expressed quantitatively as specific activity, which ranges from less than 1 to as much as 5,000 IU per milligram protein, but the qualitative designations (low, intermediate, high, ultrahigh, purity) are not yet standardized. In this review, the term *high purity* refers to concentrates purified using immunoaffinity chromatography. Their specific activity exceeds 2,500 IU factor VIII per milligram, discounting human albumin, which is added as a stabilizer.

Factor IX complex concentrates (also known as prothrombin complex concentrates, or PCC) contain variable concentrations of the other vitamin K–dependent plasma proteins, which copurify with factor IX in adsorption and ion exchange steps. The specific activity of factor IX in PCC is generally less than 5 IU per milligram. *Factor IX concentrate* is purified using additional chromatographic or immunoaffinity steps and is largely free of other clotting factors. The specific activity of factor IX in these concentrates is approximately 50 to 200 IU per milligram. Recombinant factor IX is now being evaluated in clinical trials. Unlike high-purity factor VIII concentrates, factor IX concentrates do not require the addition of albumin as a stabilizing agent.

Table 2 Attenuation of Viral Contamination in Factor Concentrates

REDUCTION OF VIRAL LOAD IN PLASMA POOL
Exclusion of high-risk donors
Serologic screening of donor plasma for blood-borne viral pathogens
PHYSICAL PARTITIONING OF VIRUSES DURING FRACTIONATION
Purification steps designed to increase specific activity of clotting factor and concomitantly remove viruses
"Nanofiltration" applied to factor IX
APPLICATION OF A VALIDATED METHOD OF VIRAL INACTIVATION
Heat in lyophilized state, typically 80°C (176°F) for 72 hr
Heat in aqueous solution: pasteurization at 60° C (140° F) for 10 hr
Heat in wet vapor at 60°C for 10 hr at 1,160 mbar
Solvent-detergent treatment (TNBP + Tween 80 or Triton X 100 + sodium cholate)
Sodium thiocyanate + ultrafiltration (applicable to factor IX)
Combined solvent-detergent + heat treatment

Recombinant Factor VIII

Two recombinant factor VIII products are licensed in North America. Both are derived from hamster cell cultures and are immunoaffinity purified. The recombinant origin of the factor VIII provides a greater margin of safety with respect to viral transmission than do plasma-derived concentrates. Recombinant factor VIII may be contaminated with substances derived from the hamster cell cultures, the bovine proteins added to the culture media, and murine IgG, which may leach from the affinity matrix. However, in the final product the concentrations of these animal proteins are reduced to trace levels. The currently available recombinant factor VIII preparations are formulated with high concentrations of purified human albumin.

Viral Transmission by Factor VIII and IX Concentrates

All hemophiliacs should be vaccinated against blood-borne viral pathogens to which they are susceptible, i.e., not immune or actively infected. However, this approach is a reality only for hepatitis A and B among the major pathogens. Therefore, great reliance is still placed on the viral reduction strategies shown in Table 2. The efficacy of serologic testing is limited in that it is specific for known pathogens for which a screening test is available and applied. Furthermore, screening fails to identify infected donors who have not yet seroconverted. Each of the viral partitioning and virucidal procedures listed in Table 2 has been validated to inactivate HIV and hepatitis B and C viruses in vitro by viral add-back experiments and in vivo by studies involving susceptible patients. However, these procedures inactivate fixed proportions of virus regardless of the initial inoculum, so their efficacy at reducing virus contamination to numbers below the level of infectivity depends on the initial serologic screening. Process errors in any step may expose susceptible patients to the risk of disease. There have been no proven cases of transmission of HIV to susceptible patients who have exclusively used products to which these procedures have been applied and only very rare case reports of suspected transmission of hepatitis.

Table 3 Adverse Effects of Factor VIII and IX Concentrates

ADVERSE EFFECT	COMMENT
Allergic reactions	Very uncommon, even in patients allergic to plasma or cryoprecipitate; usually mild
Hemolysis	Caused by isoagglutinins in group A, B, or AB patients; usually mild, but may be clinically significant if large doses of lower purity plasma-derived concentrate are given
Inhibitor formation	Risk appears equal for plasma-derived and recombinant products
Suppressed cellular immunity	May be universal with products of less than high purity; significance uncertain, but possibly important in the presence of HIV infection
Viral transmission	Now very rare with measures shown in Table 2; less risk with recombinant products; but theoretically still possible from human or animal sources
Thrombosis	A complication unique to PCC-APCC, at least partly dose and schedule dependent; does not appear to occur with purified factor IX concentrates

Other blood-borne viruses are relatively resistant to some of the virucidal procedures shown in Table 2. Solvent-detergent treatment does not inactivate non–lipid coated viruses, such as parvovirus B19 and hepatitis A (HAV); B19 is also relatively resistant to dry heating. Infection with these agents is clinically less significant than infection with HIV or hepatitis B and C but may not be totally innocuous. HAV vaccination is recommended for seronegative hemophiliacs. Combined sequential solvent-detergent plus heat treatment is now being used in some products to broaden the range of viral inactivation. At least one manufacturer is now using filtration with hollow fiber filters (nanofiltration) to physically remove viruses from factor IX concentrate.

Human albumin is added to some factor VIII concentrates and to recombinant factor VIII preparations. Albumin has not been associated with viral transmission or other adverse effects, although there is no precedent for the frequent repetitive infusion of this protein for many months or years.

The advances in viral safety of the last decade should not give rise to complacency. Factor concentrates which are manufactured or formulated with human or animal plasma proteins retain the potential to transmit viruses or other pathogenic agents which are not yet identifed, or which are not currently prevalent in the donor population.

Other Adverse Effects of Factor VIII and IX Concentrates

The adverse affects associated with factor VIII and IX concentrates are shown in Table 3. Allergic reactions are very uncommon, and hemolysis is clinically important only rarely, in heavily treated patients.

The incidence of inhibitor antibodies in hemophiliacs treated with plasma-derived factor VIII concentrates is conventionally cited as 10 to 15 percent, but this may be an underestimate. Transient and/or low titer inhibitors may not be clinically suspected nor detected if testing is done infre-

Table 4 Use of Factor VIII and IX Concentrates

CLINICAL SITUATION	DESIRED FACTOR LEVEL (IU/ML)	INITIAL DOSE* (IU/KG) OF:	
		FACTOR VIII	FACTOR IX
Minor bleed into joint, muscle, mucosal surface, and so on	0.2–0.3	10–15	20–30
More severe bleed, especially if treatment is delayed; minor surgery	0.3–0.5	15–25	30–50
Life-threatening bleed; major surgery	0.8–1.0	40–50	80–100†

*Initial doses are based on predicted recovery in adults. Lesser recovery may be seen in children, in whom plasma volume is proportionally greater, or in the face of vigorous bleeding. For principles governing follow-up and supplemental treatment, see text.
†PCC are not recommended in these doses or for these indications.

quently. These purported incidence rates may therefore actually represent the prevalence of clinically important inhibitors. More recent prospective and retrospective observations suggest that inhibitors occur with an incidence of 22 to 33 percent (up to 52 percent in severe hemophiliacs). The incidence of inhibitors to factor IX in treated hemophilia B patients appears to be much less, in the order of 5 percent.

Recombinant factor VIII may theoretically have a greater tendency than plasma-derived factor VIII to provoke inhibitor formation, possibly due to slightly altered glycosylation. This fear has not been borne out by the clinical experience to date. The incidence of inhibitors among closely monitored previously untreated patients has been 25 to 35 percent, similar to the figures cited above for plasma-derived factor VIII. Many of the inhibitors observed in the patients treated with recombinant factor VIII have been transient and of low titer and have not precluded successful treatment with factor VIII.

Thrombosis is a risk associated with factor IX complex concentrates, but not with other concentrates used to treat hemophilia A or B. The nature of the thrombogenic stimulus is not clear. Life-threatening venous thromboembolism, disseminated intravascular coagulation (DIC), and acute myocardial infarction have occurred, although the pathophysiology of the last is not clear. Thrombotic events are unpredictable but are typically seen with PCC and activated PCC (APCC) when used in intensive treatment schedules (e.g., more than two doses of at least 75 IU per kilogram given at intervals of 12 to 18 hours), in infants, in immobilized orthopedic patients, and in the presence of crush injury or liver disease. It appears that the risk is greatly reduced or eliminated in patients treated with factor IX concentrate. Heparin is added to some PCC and factor IX concentrates by the manufacturers, and the International Committee on Thrombosis and Haemostatis recommends the addition of heparin to PCC after reconstitution. The effectiveness of heparin in reducing the thrombotic risk is not proven. Furthermore, this practice may put some patients at risk for additional adverse effects, the most important of which is heparin-induced thrombocytopenia.

Abundant data indicate a suppressive effect of factor concentrates on various aspects of cellular immune function. The clinical significance of these effects is not clear. Several studies suggest that among patients with HIV infection, those who use immunoaffinity purified plasma-derived factor VIII concentrates experience a slower rate of decline in CD4 cell numbers than those using concentrates of lower purity.

Choice of Factor VIII and IX Concentrates

Fresh frozen plasma and cryoprecipitate are no longer desirable for treating hemophilia A and B, for which viral attenuated concentrates are available. As efficacy has been established for the available factor VIII and IX concentrates, the major factors to be considered in product choice relate to cost and safety. In this regard it must not be assumed that products of higher purity are safer. All factor concentrates must be carefully scrutinized in terms of their risk-benefit ratio.

Recombinant factor VIII concentrates may be indicated for previously untreated patients and for those without evidence of infection with pathogenic retroviruses or hepatitis viruses. With respect to plasma-derived concentrates, high purity per se confers some degree of safety. The purification steps used to prepare these products complement virucidal treatments by substantially reducing the viral load. They also exclude viruses resistant to heating or to solvent-detergent treatment.

The accumulating weight of evidence concerning the immunosuppressive effects of lower-purity factor VIII concentrates favors a high-purity plasma-derived concentrate for the treatment of patients with HIV infection. This immune stabilizing effect may be related to purity, but the data demonstrating similar properties for recombinant factor VIII (which is also immunoaffinity purified) are not controlled, and there are no data for high-purity factor IX concentrates. Whether or not stabilization of CD4 cell numbers is a valid marker for long-term clinical benefit is yet to be determined.

Because of the risk of thrombosis, PCC are not recommended for hemophilia B patients who require high-dose repetitive treatment with factor IX, as is required, for example, after major surgical procedures. Their use should also be avoided in patients with severe liver disease or extensive tissue trauma.

Clinical Use of Factor VIII and IX Concentrates

The recoveries of factor VIII and factor IX concentrate are approximately 0.02 and 0.01 IU per milliliter per IU per kilogram infused respectively. The plasma half-life of factor VIII is approximately 8 to 12 hours, and that of factor IX is 24 to 36 hours. These figures are most accurately applicable to adults who are not bleeding vigorously.

Target levels and initial doses for factor VIII and IX concentrates are shown in Table 4. For treatment with factor IX, some authorities recommend somewhat lower target levels, not more than 0.5 to 0.6 IU per milliliter for major

Table 5 Use of Other Hemostatic Agents in Hemophilia

AGENT	INDICATIONS IN HEMOPHILIA	SUGGESTED ADMINISTRATION	THERAPEUTIC GOAL
DDAVP	Mild to moderate bleeding in a hemophilia A patient with a documented response to DDAVP (usually a mild hemophiliac)	0.3 μg/kg (to a maximum 20 μg) IV or SC in divided sites if necessary	Approximately 2 × to 4 × increase in factor VIII
EACA	To supplement factor replacement or DDAVP in dental extraction*	75 mg/kg (to a maximum of 4 g) PO q6h for 5 to 10 days	Prevention of secondary rebleeding after achieving hemostasis
Tranexamic acid (AMCA)	As for EACA*	25 mg/kg PO q8h; or as a mouthwash, use 10 ml of a 4.8% solution q.i.d.	As for EACA
Fibrin sealants	Incompletely defined; useful alternative to clotting factors in patients with inhibitors needing dental extraction	Local application as per directions of manufacturer	Local hemostasis

EACA, Epsilon-aminocaproic acid.
*First dose given at least 1 hour prior to extraction; efficacy in bleeding from other mucocutaneous sites has not been validated.

surgery. These cautious recommendations are appropriate when the inherently thrombogenic PCC are used.

Many uncomplicated hemarthroses and intramuscular hematomas require only a single treatment, or possibly two to three infusions given every one to two half-lives. For some indications other hemostatic agents may be used as supplements or substitutions for factor concentrate. These are described in the following section. For managing life-threatening hemorrhage or major surgery, it is essential to maintain factor levels in excess of 0.5 IU per milliliter for 1 to 2 weeks, longer in the presence of complications. This can be assured only by frequently monitoring factor VIII or IX activity levels, as the achieved responses may differ substantially from projections, especially in the face of active bleeding. Initial treatment may be given by intermittent injection at intervals of 6 to 12 hours for factor VIII and 12 to 24 hours for factor IX. After the first several days, the interval may be progressively lengthened to once daily for factor VIII and once every day or two for factor IX.

For major surgery or life-threatening hemorrhage, factor VIII may be given by continuous infusion after an initial injection to raise factor VIII to the desired peak level. The concentrates are stable for at least 12 hours after reconstitution. The initial infusion rate is 2–4 IU per kilogram per hour, adjusted to maintain the desired factor level. It is often desirable to resume an intermittent schedule several days postoperatively to enhance the patient's morbility and to avoid superficial phlebitis at the infusion site. PCC should not be given by continuous infusion. The use of factor IX concentrates by this route appears to be safe, but more confirmatory data are needed.

When used for long-term prophylaxis, the aim of factor replacement therapy is to maintain minimum factor levels above approximately 0.01 IU per milliliter. This can generally be accomplished by injecting factor VIII three times weekly or on alternate days in doses that achieve peak levels of 0.5 to 0.6 IU per milliliter. For factor IX, injections may be given twice weekly.

OTHER HEMOSTATIC AGENTS USED TO TREAT HEMOPHILIA

The use of some of these agents is summarized in Table 5. DDAVP (desmopressin) is a vasopressin analogue with greatly attenuated vasoactive and antidiuretic activity. It transiently increases plasma factor VIII as well as von Willebrand factor, tissue plasminogen activator, and urokinase, presumably by mobilizing performed stores of these proteins. Mildly or moderately affected hemophiliacs often respond to DDAVP with increases in factor VIII activity of twofold to fourfold or more. This is often sufficient to promote hemostasis in the face of hemarthroses, intramuscular hematomas, and even minor surgical procedures. DDAVP is generally given by intravenous infusion over 15 to 20 minutes or by subcutaneous injection, at 0.3–0.4 μg per kilogram. Rapid infusion may cause flushing and hypotension. More concentrated solutions for subcutaneous and for intranasal administration have recently become available. Hemophilic patients generally become tachyphylactic to repeated doses given at intervals of less than 48 hours. The residual vasopressin-like activity of DDAVP may cause serious adverse effects. Acute myocardial infarction following DDAVP infusion has been reported, usually in patients with pre-existing coronary artery disease. Sufficient water retention to cause hyponatremia and seizures has been reported in infants and in adult patients receiving intravenous crystalloids. DDAVP should be used with caution in these clinical settings.

Topical hemostatic preparations may be useful for mucocutaneous bleeding. Bovine thrombin may be used at a concentration of 100 to 1,000 IU per milliliter. It is often used in conjunction with absorbable gelatin sponges. Commercial fibrin sealant preparations are especially useful for hemophilic patients with inhibitors, for indications such as dental extractions.

Epsilon-aminocaproic acid (EACA) and tranexamic acid (AMCA) are synthetic lysine analogue with antifibrinolytic activity. Intravenous and oral forms are available. In patients with hemophilia, they are used primarily for mucosal bleeding, especially following dental extraction. In this setting tranexamic acid is also effective as a mouthwash. These agents may reduce the requirement for factor VIII or factor IX concentrate to a single preoperative dose. They are administered just before extraction and then for 5 to 10 days thereafter. Tranexamic acid tends to be better tolerated orally than EACA, which often causes nausea, and is more potent on a weight basis. Antifibrinolytic agents should probably not be given concurrently with PCC or APCC.

■ MANAGEMENT OF INHIBITORS

The optimal replacement product for an actively bleeding inhibitor patient in human factor VIII. Factor VIII can be used successfully in the presence of an inhibitor of low titer, preferably less than 5 Bethesda units but sometimes up to 10. Doses of 100 to 200 IU per kilogram may be needed to achieve clinically useful factor VIII levels. Subsequent treatment with factor VIII may be given by injection or by infusion at 3 to 15 IU per kilogram per hour.

Porcine factor VIII has only limited cross-reactivity with anti-human factor VIII antibodies. However, as the degree of interspecies cross-reactivity is variable, it is preferable to determine the anti-porcine factor VIII antibody titer before its use. Porcine factor VIII produced by polyelectrolyte fractionation (specific activity 120 to 140 IU per milligram) is substantially free of the risks of transfusion reactions, progressive resistance, and thrombocytopenia, which curtailed the use of earlier generations of these concentrates. Allergic reactions are also infrequent. Many patients develop inhibitor antibodies to porcine factor VIII at variable times after initiating therapy. These antibodies may preclude further use of this product and may cross-react with human factor VIII.

Formulas have been devised to calculate the initial dose of porcine factor VIII required to neutralize antibodies and provide therapeutic circulating factor VIII levels, but they require prospective validation. In practice, empiric doses of 50 to 150 IU per kilogram are often given, depending on the urgency of the clinical situation and the anti-porcine factor VIII inhibitor titer if known. Further doses may then be given as needed, by injection or by continuous infusion at 10 IU per kilogram per hour. The laboratory response may improve after successive infusions, and clinical hemostatic responses are sometimes seen even with small increments in plasma factor VIII activity.

Where inhibitor titers exceed approximately 10 Bethesda units, the use of human or porcine factor VIII may be facilitated by initial reduction of the inhibitor level. This may be accomplished by plasma exchange, although the resultant depletion of other clotting factors may make it necessary to replace volume with plasma rather than albumin. Extracorporeal immunoadsorption with a staphylococcal protein A column has been used as an alternative, but this approach is still experimental in North America.

Factor VIII therapy provokes an anamnestic rise in inhibitor titer over days to weeks in all but low responder patients, who constitute a minority of those with inhibitors. This must be borne in mind before embarking on any therapeutic regimen that includes factor VIII.

The factor VIII or IX deficiency in inhibitor patients may be bypassed with PCC, APCC, or recombinant human factor VIIa. PCC and APCC are given in doses of 75 to 100 IU per kilogram. This may be repeated once or twice at 8 to 12 hour intervals as needed. There is no laboratory method to monitor the efficacy of treatment with these agents. Controlled clinical studies have shown that PCC are moderately successful in bypassing factor VIII deficiency, and APCC are probably more effective. The identity of the factor VIII bypassing activity is unknown, but factor IX concentrates (as distinct from PCC) appear not to contain it. Factor VIIa bypasses factor VIII or IX deficiency by activating factor X independently of the factor IXa-VIIIa activation complex. Recombinant factor VIIa appears to be effective and generally well tolerated.

Various regimens have been reported to be successful in inducing long-term immune tolerance in at least half of inhibitor patients. The regimens are all based on frequent (usually daily) injections of factor concentrate, and in some this is combined with extracorporeal immunoadsorption and/or immunosuppressive therapy. Abolishing factor VIII or IX inhibitors may be of enormous clinical benefit. However, the tolerizing regimens are arduous and costly. They may also have substantial toxicity, particularly if alkylating agents are used in children.

■ FUTURE TRENDS IN HEMOPHILIA THERAPY

The trend toward greater reliance on high-purity plasma-derived and recombinant factor concentrates will likely continue over the coming decade, constrained by availability, cost, and caution pending long-term surveillance for adverse effects, especially inhibitor development associated with recombinant factor VIII. Further refinements in recombinant factor products will likely occur. These will include recombinant factor IX, albumin-free factor VIII, and designer molecules such as B domain-deleted factor VIII.

Radical cure of hemophilia is possible with liver transplantation, but this approach is currently appropriate only for rare individuals with end-stage liver disease. Cure in a limited sense is on the horizon with recent experimental successes with gene therapy. Hemophilia is an ideal model for this approach, as any somatic cell is a suitable target for the clotting factor gene, provided the protein has access to the circulation. Furthermore, the gene product is effective even at levels as low as 1 to 2 percent of normal.

Suggested Reading

Mannucci PM. Clinical evaluation of viral safety of coagulation factor VIII and IX concentrates. Vox Sang 1993; 64:197–203.

Kasper CK, Lusher JM, Transfusion Practice Committee A. Recent evolution of clotting factor concentrates for hemophilia A and B. Transfusion 1993; 33:422–434.

Hoyer LW. Medical progress: Hemophilia A. N Engl J Med 1994; 330:38–47.

Aledort L. Inhibitors in hemophilia patients: Current status and management. Am J Hematol 1994; 47:208–217.

Brownlee GG. Prospects for gene therapy of haemophilia A and B. Br Med Bull 1995; 51:91–105.

VON WILLEBRAND DISEASE

Zaverio M. Ruggeri, M.D.
Pier Mannuccio Mannucci, M.D.

PATHOGENESIS AND CLASSIFICATION

Von Willebrand disease (vWD) is a congenital bleeding disorder characterized by a complex hemostatic defect. Abnormal platelet function, expressed by prolonged bleeding time, is a consistent finding and may be accompanied by decreased factor VIII procoagulant activity. The pathogenesis of vWD is based on quantitative and/or qualitative abnormalities of von Willebrand factor (vWF), a large multimeric glycoprotein that circulates in plasma in complex with the factor VIII procoagulant protein. These two proteins form the factor VIII-von Willebrand factor complex. When present, the decreased factor VIII procoagulant activity is secondary to the reduced concentration of vWF. The vWF, but not the factor VIII procoagulant protein, is present in endothelial cells, the subendothelium, platelets, and megakaryocytes, as well as plasma. Factor VIII is synthesized predominantly, but not exclusively, by hepatocytes in the liver.

Different forms of vWD can be recognized by distinctive patterns of genetic transmission and by typical vWF abnormalities in plasma and platelets. Genetic mutations responsible for the molecular alterations have been identified in many cases. The classification of the different types of the disease, as outlined below, is based essentially on phenotypic characteristics, taking into account the existence of quantitative and/or functional alterations of the vWF molecule. This classification, endorsed by the von Willebrand factor Subcommittee of the International Society of Thrombosis and Hemostasis, is important for correct therapy.

Autosomal Dominant Inheritance

Type 1

Patients with type 1 vWD may represent over 70 percent of all cases. Plasma concentrations of factor VIII procoagulant and vWF are decreased to the same relative degree in most cases; the latter is usually normal in the cellular compartment, but the platelet content may be low in some patients. All sizes of vWF multimers are present, with normal structure of individual multimers. Thus, type 1 vWD is characterized by quantitative defects with no functional abnormalities of vWF. The characteristic hemostatic and laboratory abnormalities result from reduced plasma concentrations of the factor VIII-vWF complex.

The distinction between patients and normal individuals may be difficult in some cases. In particular, the levels of plasma vWF antigen are significantly different in the population depending on the ABO blood group. In individuals of group O, the lower range of normal concentration is in the order of 35 to 40 U/dL (100 U/dL or 100 percent being the "average" normal concentration), a value that is frankly abnormal in patients of different blood group. In such a situation, a careful evaluation of the patient's history is mandatory to highlight the occurrence of abnormal bleeding.

Type 2

This is a very heterogeneous group that includes all forms with abnormal structure and function of vWF, exemplified in most instances by altered relative distribution of multimers in plasma. Concentrations of factor VIII procoagulant activity and vWF may be decreased or normal in plasma. The concentration of vWF is usually normal in the cellular compartment, but it may also be decreased. In the majority of cases there are reduced plasma levels of the large multimeric forms of vWF; the extent of this defect is variable, ranging from a relative deficiency of only the largest multimers to a complete absence of large and intermediate ones. In a specific group of patients, unusually large multimers (i.e., multimers of larger size than normally seen in the circulation) are present in plasma. Several type 2 variants have been described based on distinctive alterations of vWF structure and function. Four main categories have been recognized in the classification endorsed by the International Society of Thrombosis and Hemostasis, each comprising subtypes differentiated on the basis of more specific structural and functional abnormalities. The four groups are: type 2A, characterized by decreased platelet response to ristocetin and absence of large vWF multimers; type 2B, characterized by paradoxically enhanced platelet response to ristocetin and absence of large vWF multimers; type 2M, characterized by decreased vWF-dependent platelet function not caused by lack of the larger multimers; and type 2N, characterized by an abnormally low affinity of vWF for factor VIII. In the latter case, the patients resemble mild or moderate hemophilia A patients or carriers, with disproportionally low plasma factor VIII levels as compared to vWF antigen. The differential diagnosis is, obviously, very important, and a good indication may come from the distinct modalities of genetic transmission (autosomal as opposed to X-linked).

Patients in the type 2B group, which in the new classification includes type I New York and type Malmö (actually, the same genetic abnormality), exhibit paradoxically enhanced ristocetin-induced platelet–vWF interaction resulting from an increased affinity of the abnormal vWF for the platelet glycoprotein Ib-IX-V receptor. In some families with type 2B, this heightened interaction results in chronic thrombocytopenia and the presence of platelet aggregates in the circulation. The occurrence of thrombocytopenia may be a cause for incorrect diagnosis.

Platelet-type or so-called pseudo von Willebrand disease is similar in many respects to type 2B vWD. However, the defect lies in the platelet receptor for vWF, which has an increased affinity for the protein. This disease, therefore, is a platelet abnormality distinct from vWD, although phenotypically similar to it.

Autosomal Recessive Inheritance

Type 3

Patients with type 3 disease are homozygous or double heterozygous for abnormal gene(s) inherited from both parents, who are usually clinically normal. Factor VIII procoagulant activity is markedly decreased. vWF is undetectable or present in trace amounts both in plasma and in the cellular compartment. These patients are clinically the most severely affected. A subset of patients with complete homozygous deletion of the vWF gene is prone to develop antibodies to vWF after repeated infusions of concentrates containing the protein.

GENERAL PRINCIPLES OF THERAPY

The aim of therapy in vWD is to correct the prolonged bleeding time and, if present, the abnormality of blood coagulation. To achieve this, both vWF and factor VIII procoagulant activity must be raised to normal levels in plasma. A normal concentration of a functionally normal vWF must be achieved in patients with qualitative abnormalities of the protein.

Most patients with the more common autosomal dominant form of vWD have a relatively mild bleeding tendency. In children, mucosal bleeding, particularly epistaxis and gingival bleeding, are common symptoms. Excessive blood loss following dental extraction, tonsillectomy, or other common surgical procedures is also frequent, as are cutaneous bleeding and easy bruising. Gastrointestinal bleeding is not infrequent and can be without identifiable cause. In females, menorrhagia is not uncommon, particularly after the first menses and in adolescent girls in general. Excess postpartum bleeding can also occur. However, spontaneous joint and muscular bleeding are exceptional.

Bleeding symptoms may be present in patients with normal plasma levels of factor VIII procoagulant activity. Therefore, it is not surprising that effective therapy requires correction of the quantitative and/or qualitative vWF defect. If this is not achieved, poor control of bleeding, particularly mucosal bleeding, may be observed even if concentrations of factor VIII procoagulant activity are raised to normal or above.

The clinical picture of the recessive form of vWD is more severe. Mucosal and cutaneous bleeding, as well as hemorrhages from the female genital tract, occur more frequently and are of greater severity. Excessive bleeding after dental extractions or surgery can be controlled only by replacement therapy. Hemarthroses and muscular hematomata are not uncommon, and permanent disability may ensue in some cases. In these patients, correction of both the vWF and factor VIII procoagulant defect is mandatory. In nonmucosal bleeding, particularly in cases of joint or muscle hemorrhage, raising the factor VIII procoagulant levels may be sufficient for effective hemostasis even when the bleeding time is not normalized. This is fortunate, because individuals with homozygous vWF gene deletion may develop antibodies to vWF, which may render vWF replacement therapy ineffective.

There are two main approaches to the therapy of vWD. One is replacement therapy, i.e., the infusion of exogenous factor VIII-vWF derived from normal plasma. The second is to induce release of endogenous factor VIII-vWF from tissue stores using 1-deamino-[8-D-arginine]vasopressin (DDAVP). Replacement therapy is the only possibility in patients with severe (type 3) vWD who have markedly reduced levels of the factor VIII-vWF–related activities in both plasma and tissue stores. Infusion of DDAVP may release cellular (endothelial) factor VIII-vWF into the circulation and increase its concentration to adequate levels in patients with the dominant form of vWD who have normal tissue stores of vWF. Occasional patients with type 1 and a larger percentage of those with type 2 variants do not respond to this drug.

DDAVP is considered to be contraindicated in both type 2B and platelet-type pseudo von Willebrand disease, because raising the endogenous vWF in either of these disorders results in thrombocytopenia.

REPLACEMENT THERAPY AND BLOOD DERIVATIVES

Replacement therapy is performed by infusing plasma fractions enriched in the factor VIII-vWF complex. Infusion of blood derivatives in patients with vWD promotes a delayed increase in factor VIII procoagulant activity that is disproportionate to the amount administered. After the peak reached at the end of the infusion, factor VIII procoagulant activity continues to rise for 12 to 24 hours. On the contrary, vWF starts to decrease immediately after the end of the infusion. Therefore, a discrepancy between factor VIII procoagulant activity and vWF is found between 12 to 48 hours after treatment. Correction of the bleeding time defect is even shorter than that of the vWF plasma levels. The delayed rise of factor VIII procoagulant activity is characteristically observed in all forms of vWD, with the exception of patients affected by the recessive form who have developed an inhibitor antibody to factor VIII-vWF.

Of the available sources of factor VIII-vWF, cryoprecipitate used to be considered the mainstay of treatment because it can normalize factor VIII coagulant activity, shorten or normalize the bleeding time, and stop or prevent clinical bleeding in most instances. However, virucidal methods cannot be currently applied to single-donor cryoprecipitate as produced by blood banks and this plasma fraction carries a definite risk of transmitting blood-borne viruses, such as the hepatitis viruses and the human immunodeficiency virus. This risk becomes higher when repeated infusions over time expose the recipients to a large number of different donors. The development of a variety of virucidal methods have rendered plasma concentrates containing factor VIII and vWF safer. Hence, these concentrates are currently considered by most experts in the United States the first choice in the treatment of vWD unresponsive to desmopressin. The use of cryoprecipitate has been banned in some countries, particularly in Europe, but it is still an option in others. Infusion of cryoprecipitate should be considered only if concentrates treated with virucidal methods are not available or have failed to control bleeding, and only if the product can be obtained from donors undergoing a rigorous screening program for viral infections.

Commercial concentrates of factor VIII-vWF prepared from large pools of plasma are at least as effective as cryoprecipitate in raising the levels of factor VIII procoagulant activity; however, they often fail to correct the bleeding time, even when they bring ristocetin cofactor activity up to normal levels, mainly because of the lack of larger vWF multimers that become degraded during production. Correction of the bleeding time is particularly important in cases of mucosal bleeding. In most surgical procedures, when primary hemostasis can be bypassed by surgical hemostasis, correcting the factor VIII procoagulant abnormality becomes most important. In severe bleeding episodes and to cover major surgery, a dose of virus-inactivated concentrate (or cryoprecipitate) supplying between 30 and 50 U/kg of factor VIII coagulant activity is recommended, to be repeated according to the factor VIII levels and clinical needs. This dosage should raise factor VIII procoagulant activity at hemostatic levels, but correction or significant shortening of the bleeding time may be, and usually is, inconsistent and transient. Some concentrates have been shown to contain a better representation of the whole array of vWF multimers, including the larger ones, and should be used when possible in patients with mucosal bleeding difficult to stop.

Infusion of platelet concentrates (8–10 bags) can achieve both shortening of the bleeding time and control of hemorrhages when poor correction of the bleeding time by plasma products is associated with continuing hemorrhages. Of course, platelet concentrates carry a risk of transmitting those blood-borne infections that virus-inactivated concentrates are meant to avoid. On the other hand, the pathologic conditions that truly require full normalization of the bleeding time are not frequent in clinical practice (for instance, continuing gastrointestinal or uterine bleeding, intracranial bleeding); thus, the use of platelet concentrates should be limited to few, life-threatening situations.

■ USE OF DDAVP

DDAVP (0.3 µg/kg) is the treatment of choice because of the virtual absence of serious side effects. However, it is not equally efficacious in all forms of the disorder. It is usually not effective in the severe recessive form (type 3), in which tissue stores of vWF are markedly reduced or absent. On the other hand, most patients with type 1 vWD will have a complete correction of their hemostatic abnormality lasting for 4 to 6 hours, provided that vWF concentration in plasma reaches normal levels. In type 2 disease, the bleeding time may not be corrected even though vWF levels are increased to well within normal ranges. This ineffectiveness is due to the fact that the multimeric structure of plasma vWF will not be normalized in these patients. However, factor VIII procoagulant levels will be restored to normal, and this may be sufficient for some surgical procedures in which primary hemostasis can be achieved by suturing or cautery. Where this is not possible (as in tooth extraction, gastrointestinal bleeding, or childbirth), normalization of factor VIII procoagulant activity without correction of the bleeding time will usually not secure hemostasis. Cryoprecipitate or concentrates should be used in type 2 vWD whenever primary hemostasis must be assured. It also should be used in type 1 patients who do not obtain an adequate response to DDAVP.

Because DDAVP causes thrombocytopenia in type 2B and platelet-type pseudo von Willebrand disease, its use should not be attempted in these disorders. Although few side effects have been observed in the type 2B patients in whom DDAVP has been utilized, potentially serious complications may occur in elderly patients with risk factors for thrombotic vascular occlusion. Cryoprecipitate or concentrates are usually effective in type 2B. Both should be used sparingly in platelet-type pseudo von Willebrand disease because large amounts can cause thrombocytopenia. In the latter patients, a combination of cryoprecipitate or factor VIII-vWF concentrates with normal platelet concentrates may provide the best form of therapy for severe bleeding episodes.

■ PREGNANCY AND CHILDBIRTH

During pregnancy, factor VIII-vWF levels tend to rise. In many individuals, particularly those with type 1 vWD, this is sufficient to restore hemostasis to normal. However, complete correction will not occur in patients with severe vWD (type 3) or those producing abnormal vWF (type 2). It is, therefore, recommended that the bleeding time be followed during pregnancy and, if it has not been corrected, that replacement therapy be given at the time of delivery.

■ DEVELOPMENT OF INHIBITOR ANTIBODIES AFTER REPLACEMENT THERAPY

In a subset of patients with severe (type 3) vWD, replacement therapy will induce the appearance of antibodies directed toward the factor VIII-vWF complex. The individuals so affected have a homozygous deletion of the vWF gene. These inhibitors may complicate the treatment of bleeding episodes, and correcting the abnormal hemostasis may be impossible when the inhibitor titer is too high. Since antibodies in these cases are specifically directed against vWF, inactivation of factor VIII procoagulant activity probably occurs as a result of steric hindrance. Correcting the bleeding time abnormality is therefore more difficult than correcting the coagulation abnormality. This contrasts with the inhibitors seen in hemophilia A, which are directed at the factor VIII procoagulant protein and do not characteristically affect the bleeding time.

From the clinical point of view, management of soft tissue or joint hemorrhages in the presence of vWF inhibitors may be satisfactory if plasma factor VIII procoagulant activity is raised. On the other hand, the inability of replacement therapy to shorten the bleeding time is associated with poor control of mucosal bleeding. Reactions have been described in patients with these inhibitors who are infused with factor VIII-vWF concentrates. Most of these reactions are probably due to the precipitating nature of the antibodies, with formation of circulating antigen-antibody complexes and complement activation. Infusion of factor VIII-vWF concentrates into these patients will inevitably cause anamnestic rise of the inhibitor titer. Avoiding replacement therapy, on the contrary, may lead to disappearance of the antibody. To choose the correct dosage, antibody titer should be measured before replacement therapy is administered. Plasma factor VIII procoagulant activity and ristocetin cofactor activity should be tested in vitro to evaluate in vivo recovery of infused factor VIII-vWF and to determine the successive dosage of replacement therapy often required. Post-transfusional antibody titer should also be monitored at periodic intervals.

■ ACQUIRED VWD

A bleeding diathesis similar to inherited vWD is occasionally seen on an acquired basis. This syndrome has been reported most frequently in association with lupus erythematosus, monoclonal gammopathy, hypernephroma, lymphoproliferative disorders, angiodysplastic lesions, as well as after administration of certain drugs. Antibodies to vWF have been detected in a minority of these cases. However, vWF is usually decreased in plasma, often to an impressive degree. The principles of replacement therapy usually apply to these patients as well. When antibodies have been detected, they should be monitored before and after replacement therapy. Intravenous immunoglobulins are useful in patients with acquired vWD associated with monoclonal gammopathies. Their mechanism of action probably involves blockade of Fc receptors, thus delaying the clearance of complexes formed by the monoclonal protein and vWF.

Suggested Reading

Ruggeri ZM, Zimmerman TS. von Willebrand factor and von Willebrand disease. Blood 1987; 70:895-904.
Ruggeri ZM, Ware J. von Willebrand factor. FASEB J. 1993; 7:308-316.
Ruggeri ZM, Ware J., Ginsburg D. von Willebrand factor. In Loscalzo J, Schafer AI, eds. Thrombosis and Hemorrhage. Oxford: Blackwell Scientific Publications, 1993: 305-329.
Cooney KA, Ginsburg D, Ruggeri ZM. von Willebrand disease. In Loscalzo J, Schafer AI, eds. Thrombosis and Hemorrhage. Oxford: Blackwell Scientific Publications, 1993: 657-682.

DEFICIENCIES OF THE VITAMIN K–DEPENDENT CLOTTING FACTORS

Harold R. Roberts, M.D.
Darla Liles, M.D.

Prothrombin, factors VII, IX, and X, and proteins C and S are synthesized in the liver, and vitamin K is required for their complete synthesis. Within the hepatocyte, precursor proteins of these factors undergo postribosomal modification by vitamin K–dependent hepatic carboxylase, resulting in the addition of a carboxyl group to 10 to 12 glutamyl residues on the amino terminal ends of these molecules. This results in the formation of gamma-carboxyglutamyl (GLA) residues, which are necessary for calcium-dependent phospholipid interactions. The number of GLA residues on the vitamin K–dependent clotting factors is variably reduced in the presence of warfarin drugs, vitamin K deficiency, liver disease, and some rare congenital bleeding disorders.

Proteins C and S are discussed in the chapter *Antithrombin III, Protein C, and Protein S Deficiency,* and hereditary deficiency of factor IX (hemophilia B) is discussed in the chapter *Hemophilia A and B.*

■ DIAGNOSIS

The diagnosis of these coagulation factor deficiencies is made in patients with a history of bleeding and laboratory tests that document low levels of one or more of the aforementioned clotting factors. Usually screening tests of coagulation function, i.e., the prothrombin time (PT) and activated partial thromboplastin time (APTT), are prolonged in the presence of low levels of clotting factors. Accurate diagnosis rests upon specific assays for individual clotting factors.

Clotting factor deficiencies may be congenital or acquired, as shown in Table 1. Usually only a single clotting factor is deficient in hereditary disorders, whereas in acquired disorders multiple clotting factors are usually affected.

■ CONGENITAL FACTOR DEFICIENCIES

Prothrombin

Prothrombin (factor II) deficiency is inherited as an autosomal recessive disorder. Approximately 30 cases have been described. Homozygotes for true hypoprothrombinemia have prothrombin levels of 2 percent or less. These patients may experience significant hemorrhage. Patients heterozygous for hypoprothrombinemia are asymptomatic. Dysprothrombinemias are characterized by structural abnormalities in the prothrombin molecule. Patients with dysprothrombinemia may be symptomatic in the heterozygous state. Affected patients exhibit easy bruising, epistaxis, menorrhagia, postpartum hemorrhage, and postsurgical hemorrhage. Both PT and APTT are prolonged, and functional prothrombin levels are low when measured by specific assay.

The biologic half-life of prothrombin is approximately 72 hours. To achieve normal hemostasis, the level of functional prothrombin should be raised to about 25 percent or higher. Prothrombin levels are followed to judge the frequency of infusions, but cessation of hemorrhage is the best guide to the efficacy of therapy. One method of treatment for bleeding episodes in patients with either hypoprothrombinemia or dysprothrombinemia consists of fresh frozen plasma in a loading dose of 10 to 15 ml per kilogram of body weight, followed by maintenance infusions of 3 to 6 ml per kilogram of body weight every 24 hours if necessary. Usually single doses suffice for isolated bleeding events, but in the case of surgery or sustained bleeding, replacement therapy may need to be continued for 5 to 10 days.

Commercially available prothrombin complex concentrates (PCCs) have been used for treatment of bleeding episodes (Table 2). Only PCCs that have been pasteurized or otherwise treated to inactivate viruses should be used, and those with the highest prothrombin concentrations are preferred. Some PCCs are associated with thromboembolic events. For treatment of severe hemorrhagic episodes, however, PCCs may be indicated and can be infused at a dose of 40 U per kilogram of body weight, followed by 15 U per kilogram of body weight every 24 to 36 hours.

Factor VII

Factor VII deficiency is a rare disorder; it is inherited as an autosomal recessive characteristic that occurs in about 1 in 500,000 persons. It is the only hereditary clotting factor deficiency characterized by a prolonged PT and a normal APTT. Severely affected individuals (factor VII levels below 1 percent) have hemorrhagic episodes beginning in childhood, including umbilical cord hemorrhage, epistaxis, intracranial bleeding, menorrhagia, and hemarthroses. In severely affected factor VII-deficient patients, hemorrhage is as severe as that seen in classic hemophilia. Mild and moderate forms of factor VII deficiency also occur, but the severity of bleeding with trauma or surgery varies to a surprising degree. At times no bleeding occurs in mildly affected patients, even after major surgery.

Plasma replacement therapy is the treatment of choice for bleeding episodes. Major surgery can be carried out under coverage of normal plasma. In severely affected patients, factor levels of 10 to 20 percent are considered effective for hemostasis. Plasma in a loading dose of 10 to 15 ml per kilogram of body weight is usually effective in single doses for hemarthroses, dental procedures, and other limited bleeding events. Prophylactic plasma replacement is given for dental procedures to prevent bleeding. For surgery, loading doses of plasma, as noted previously, should be followed by maintenance doses given every 6 to 12 hours for 5 to 10 days depending on the type of surgery. Like all blood products, plasma has drawbacks, as shown in Table 3. It has been suggested that major bleeding episodes in some severely affected patients may require treatment with PCCs every 6 to 12 hours. One must be certain that the PCCs contain factor VII (see Table 2). The dosage is calculated as 0.5 U (factor VII) × body weight in kilograms × desired increase (percent of normal). Some clinicians now prefer PCCs for treatment.

Highly purified recombinant factor VIIa, free of infectious agents, has been prepared by Novo Nordisk Laboratories and can be used to treat factor VII–deficient patients. Recombinant factor VIIa has been used successfully in patients with classic hemophilia and Christmas disease complicated by circulating antibodies to factors VIII and IX, respectively. It has also been used successfully in patients deficient in factor VII. Although not yet available commercially, factor VIIa has been tested in clinical trials and can be obtained on a compassionate use basis.

Factor X

Factor X deficiency is a rare disorder (approximately 1 per million of the population) and is inherited as an autosomal

Table 1 Causes of Deficiencies of the Vitamin K–Dependent Factors

CONGENITAL DEFICIENCIES
- Prothrombin: hypoprothrombinemia, dysprothrombinemia
- Factor VII deficiency
- Factor IX deficiency (Hemophilia B)
- Factor X deficiency
- Combined deficiencies: factors II, VII, IX, X

ACQUIRED DEFICIENCIES
- Hemorrhagic disease of the newborn
- Warfarin ingestion: therapeutic, toxic, surreptitious
- Superwarfarin ingestion
- Antibiotic administration
- Other drugs: cholestryamine, vitamins A and E, mineral oil, hydantoins, and salicylates
- Dietary deficiency
- Liver disease: hepatitis, cirrhosis, malignancy
- Malabsorption: pancreatic disease, small-bowel disease, biliary tract obstruction
- Other causes: amyloidosis, nephrotic syndrome, acquired inhibitors to clotting factors

Table 2 Characteristics of Prothrombin Complex Concentrates

	RISK OF VIRAL TRANSMISSION			UNITS OF PROTEIN PER 100 UNITS OF FACTOR IX			
PRODUCT (MANUFACTURER)	HEPATITIS	HIV	ASSOCIATION WITH THROMBOSIS	II	VII	IX	X
PROTHROMBIN COMPLEX CONCENTRATES							
Bebulin VH (Immuno)	No	No	No	120	13	100	139
Proplex T (Baxter-Hyland)	?	No	Yes	50	400	100	50
Profilnine HT (Alpha)	Yes	No	Yes	148	11	100	64
Konyne 80 (Cutter)	No	No	Yes	100	20	100	140
ACTIVATED PROTHROMBIN COMPLEX CONCENTRATES							
Autoplex (Baxter Hyland)	No	No	Yes	Variable amount of factors, II, VII, and X and activated factors VIIa, IXa, and Xa			
Feiba (Immuno)	No	No	Yes				

HIV, human immunodeficiency virus.

recessive characteristic. It is often heralded by umbilical cord bleeding. As with other clotting factor deficiencies, genetic heterogeneity is characteristic of the disorder, and several point mutations in the factor X gene have been reported. Depending upon the genetic abnormality, bleeding in factor X deficiency may be mild, moderate, or severe. The hemorrhagic tendency in factor X deficiency ranges from easily bruisability, epistaxis, and menorrhagia in mildly or moderately affected patients to spontaneous hemorrhages in severely affected patients.

Treatment of factor X deficiency is determined by the severity of the hemorrhage. In mild bleeding episodes, fresh frozen plasma can be given in doses sufficient to raise the factor X level to 20 to 30 percent of normal. The half-life of transfused factor X is 24 to 48 hours (mean, 40 hours), so plasma infusions every 12 to 24 hours usually result in a gradual rise in levels of factor X. A loading dose of plasma (10 to 15 ml per kilogram of body weight) is followed by 3 to 6 ml per kilogram of body weight every 12 hours when one dose will not suffice to control bleeding. In severe hemorrhagic episodes or with major surgical procedures, PCCs that are known to contain factor X (see Table 2) may be given in a dose of 50 U per kilogram every 12 to 24 hours.

Combined Deficiencies of Vitamin K–Dependent Factors

Rare combined congenital deficiencies of factors II, VII, IX, and X have been reported. These patients exhibit defective gamma-carboxylation of glutamyl residues in all the vitamin K–dependent factors. Antigenic levels of the vitamin K–dependent factors are near normal, but functional activities may be markedly decreased. Large doses of oral vitamin K should be tried in these patients, since that treatment has raised functional levels of vitamin K–dependent factors in some of them.

General Comments

Patients with hereditary deficiencies of vitamin K–dependent clotting factors should receive comprehensive care. From the time of diagnosis every attempt should be made to prevent long-term complications. While fresh frozen plasma can be used for treatment, PCCs are now safe in terms of transmission of hepatitis viruses and human immunodeficiency virus (HIV), and these products are considered by some to be the treatment of choice. Thromboembolism, including disseminated intravascular coagulation (DIC), may occur with some preparations of PCCs, so care should be exercised in using them. Prothrombin complex concentrates are usually labeled in units of factor IX per bottle. An approximation of the content of factors II, VII, and X per 100 U of factor IX in PCCs is provided in Table 2. The main advantage of PCCs is that factor levels of 50 percent or greater can be achieved without volume overload. In addition, PCCs can be stored in the lyophilized form at 4°C for prolonged periods and are easy to reconstitute. Therefore, they can be used for home therapy in patients with frequent bleeding episodes.

All patients not previously exposed to hepatitis B should be appropriately immunized.

Most severely affected patients with hereditary hemorrhagic disorders who received blood products before 1985 are seropositive for the HIV antibody. Patients infected with HIV are best managed in conjunction with an infectious disease specialist. It is particularly important to counsel these patients about safe sexual practices so that sexual partners are protected.

Home therapy, using either plasma or PCCs, is important in the management of patients with severe deficiencies of any of the blood clotting factors. Patients are taught self-infusion techniques for treatment at the earliest sign of bleeding. With hemarthroses, prompt administration of deficient factor may limit joint destruction.

Dental care is a critical part of the overall management of patients with congenital clotting factor deficiencies. Patients should receive dental cleaning every 6 months and other appropriate prophylaxis for dental problems.

Progesterone or one of the oral contraceptives should be given to affected women with menorrhagia.

Table 3 Adverse Effects of Plasma Replacement Therapy

TYPE OF ADVERSE EFFECT	RISK*
Viral Infections	
Hepatitis B	1:200,000
Hepatitis C	1:6,000
Human Immunodeficiency	1:225,000
Hepatitis Delta	1:3,000
Epstein-Barr	1:200
Allergic reactions (e.g., hives)	1:100
Anaphylaxis	1:150,000
Hypervolemia	Variable

*The risk of an adverse reaction is listed per unit of transfused plasma. Risks cited are approximate and will vary according to the donor population in a particular region. Allergic or anaphylactic reaction usually does not occur without previous exposure to blood products.

■ ACQUIRED DEFICIENCIES OF VITAMIN K–DEPENDENT FACTORS

Hemorrhagic Disease of the Newborn

Hemorrhagic disease of the newborn is an acquired deficiency of vitamin K due to poor transport of the vitamin to the fetus from the placenta, the lack of intestinal bacterial flora in the fetus, and immaturity of the fetal liver. Premature infants are at greater risk for developing vitamin K deficiency and bleeding than are term infants. Even in term infants, levels of vitamin K–dependent factors may decrease significantly on the second and third days after delivery. Human milk is a poor source of vitamin K, resulting in a greater tendency for breastfed infants to develop bleeding. The preferred prophylaxis for hemorrhagic disease of the newborn is intramuscular administration of vitamin K_1 in a dose of 0.5 to 1 mg as soon after delivery as possible.

Warfarin Therapy

One of the most common causes of decreased availability of functional levels of vitamin K in the hepatocyte is warfarin therapy. Warfarin decreases carboxylation of glutamyl residues of prothrombin and factors VII, IX, and X by inhibition of vitamin K reductase. This results in unavailability of reduced vitamin K for carboxylase activity. The most sensitive indicator of warfarin effect is a decrease in factor VII, which results in a prolonged PT. Other vitamin K–dependent factors are eventually decreased as well, resulting in a prolongation of the APTT.

The most common complication of warfarin therapy is hemorrhage. The effects of warfarin can be reversed within 4 to 12 hours by vitamin K_1 administration. In patients who are taking warfarin for therapeutic purposes, however, vitamin K should not be given unless clearly indicated, because the patient will be rendered resistant to warfarin for several days thereafter. In nonbleeding patients, overdosage of warfarin can be managed by discontinuing the drug and allowing clotting factors to increase gradually to more desirable levels. If emergent correction is necessary, fresh frozen plasma, 10 to 15 ml per kilogram of body weight, should be administered rapidly and repeated at 5 ml per kilogram of body weight every 6 to 12 hours if necessary. When temporary reversal of warfarin effect is desired, fresh frozen plasma is the treatment of choice because resumption of warfarin therapy can be initiated in the usual dose. Plasma therapy has the risks listed in Table 3.

Surreptitious Warfarin Ingestion

Surreptitious ingestion of warfarin, often by medical or paramedical personnel, must be considered in an acquired deficiency of the vitamin K–dependent factors in bleeding patients without a previous history of disease. Overdoses of warfarin have been taken in attempted suicides but are more commonly ingested for secondary gain. The treatment of choice is vitamin K_1 at a dose of 1 to 2 mg intravenously or 5 to 10 mg subcutaneously. Repeated doses of vitamin K may be required for overdoses of warfarin. If patients are bleeding in vital areas, fresh frozen plasma should be used.

Superwarfarin

Superwarfarins, such as brodifacoum and difenacoum,which were developed as rodenticides, have a very long duration of action. An ingestion of one of the superwarfarins taken for secondary gain, attempted suicide, or accidentally by a child may effectively inhibit vitamin K reductase for 50 days or more. Superwarfarins cause a marked and prolonged reduction of the vitamin K–dependent factors. Repeated large doses of vitamin K are required to control the effects of a superwarfarin. Therapy with high doses of vitamin K, e.g., 50 to 100 mg per day orally or parenterally, may be required for weeks to months. In addition, fresh frozen plasma is often necessary to control bleeding.

Antibiotic Administration

Vitamin K–dependent clotting factor deficiencies may occur as a complication of the use of certain broad-spectrum antibiotics. It is widely held that the vitamin K deficiency resulting therefrom is due to eradication of vitamin K–producing gut bacteria. Although this has not been disproved, recent evidence suggests that antibiotics containing a methyltetrazolethiol (MTT) group, such as cefamandole and cefoperazone, interfere with intrahepatic metabolism of vitamin K to cause these clotting factor deficiencies. Iatrogenic deficiency of vitamin K secondary to antibiotic administration is best reversed with parenteral vitamin K at a dose of 5 to 10 mg per day for 3 to 5 days. A slow response to therapy may occur if the offending antibiotic is continued, in which case longer supplementation with the vitamin is necessary.

Other Drugs

Other drugs interfere with vitamin K and result in clotting factor deficiencies. Cholestyramine, which binds bile acids, prevents absorption of fat-soluble vitamins, including vitamin K. Ingestion of excessive quantities of mineral oil has a similar effect. Excessive doses of vitamin A or vitamin E interfere with vitamin K absorption and possibly the metabolism of vitamin K. Salicylates and hydantoins antagonize vitamin K metabolism. In these instances withdrawal of the offending drug or supplementation with vitamin K at a dose of 5 to 10 mg daily for 3 to 5 days is the treatment of choice.

Dietary Deficiency

Dietary deficiency of vitamin K generally occurs in debilitated patients who are not eating well or who avoid eating green vegetables. Chronically ill patients on parenteral nutrition without vitamin K supplementation are especially prone to vitamin K deficiency. Dietary deficiency of vitamin K is often overlooked until bleeding occurs or the PT is noted to be prolonged. Vitamin K in doses of 5 to 10 mg corrects the defect. Green leafy vegetables, cheeses, and vegetable oils are excellent sources of vitamin K and should be added to the diet when possible.

Protein-calorie malnutrition (marasmus, kwashiorkor) may cause hypoprothrombinemia by amino acid deprivation, a condition not responsive to vitamin K administration. If bleeding occurs in these conditions, fresh frozen plasma is the treatment of choice.

Hepatocellular Disease

In hepatocellular disease, reduction in vitamin K–dependent factors results from abnormal metabolism of vitamin K or from an overall decrease in protein synthesis. Deficiencies of vitamin K–dependent factors are frequently seen in patients with hepatitis, cirrhosis, hepatic malignancy, or other type of liver disease. Vitamin K may be given to patients with liver disease, but it is usually not effective. As a general rule, the coagulopathy of liver disease requires no treatment unless the patient experiences significant hemorrhage. In this event the treatment of choice is fresh frozen plasma, which contains all of the coagulation factors. PCCs are generally not given to correct the coagulopathy of liver disease because of the danger of thromboembolic events, especially in the presence of liver dysfunction. Fresh frozen plasma in a loading dose of 10 ml per kilogram of body weight may be given, followed by maintenance doses of 3 ml per kilogram of body weight every 8 to 12 hours if necessary. With plasma therapy, there is always the danger of hypervolemia, which may contribute to increased bleeding in some patients. Deamino-arginine vasopressin (DDAVP) may be of value in the treatment of bleeding resulting from liver disease. DDAVP is given intravenously or subcutaneously in doses of 0.3 μg per kilogram of body weight. Side effects are few, but they do occur. They include nausea, vomiting, severe headache, and hyponatremia.

Malabsorption

Malabsorption may occur in a variety of conditions affecting the gastrointestinal tract. Biliary obstruction interferes with absorption of fats and fat-soluble vitamins A, D, E, and K by blocking bile acid secretion. If the obstruction has been present for several days, vitamin K 10 mg should be given by intramuscular or subcutaneous injection prior to any surgical attempt to relieve the blockage. Small-bowel disease such as regional ileitis, short-bowel syndrome, or overgrowth by intestinal bacterial flora may cause a decrease in vitamin K–dependent factors. Pancreatic insufficiency with malabsorption and steatorrhea is another cause of fat-soluble vitamin deficiency. In these cases parenteral administration of vitamin K 10 mg should correct the defect. In patients with chronic disorders, intermittent repeated doses of vitamin K may be necessary.

Acquired Deficiencies of Single Factors

Single-factor deficiencies may be acquired in a variety of conditions. Isolated acquired deficiency of prothrombin is rare but has been reported in lupus erythematosus due to an antiprothrombin antibody. Occasionally prothrombin levels are extremely low, probably because the prothrombin-antibody complex is rapidly cleared from the circulation. Treatment with steroids may be of benefit in this condition.

Acquired factor VII deficiency has been described in homocystinuria. It reportedly responds to a low-methionine diet. Factor IX levels may drop due to urinary loss in nephrotic syndrome. Acquired inhibitors to vitamin K–dependent factors are extremely rare. When they do occur, immunosuppressive therapy may be of benefit.

Amyloidosis, usually of the primary type, is occasionally associated with an isolated factor X deficiency. This deficiency is characterized by a short biologic half-life of factor X, presumably because of absorption of factor X from the plasma onto amyloid fibrils. Because production of factor X is not impaired in amyloidosis, vitamin K administration is not effective. In addition, fresh frozen plasma is ineffective because of the short in vivo half-life of factor X in the presence of amyloid. Prothrombin complex concentrates containing factor X may be necessary for profound bleeding. Splenectomy, by removing a source of the amyloid deposits, has been associated with improvement in some patients.

Suggested Reading

Alperin JB. Coagulopathy caused by vitamin K deficiency in critically ill, hospitalized patients. JAMA 1987;258:1916–1919.

Lipsky JJ. Antibiotic-associated hypoprothrombinaemia: Review. J Antimicrob Chem 1988; 21:281–300.

Menache D. New concentrates of factors VII, IX and X. In: Kasper C, ed. Recent advances in hemophilia care. New York: Alan R. Liss, 1990:177.

Olson RE. Vitamin K. In: Colman RW, Hirsh J, Marder VJ, eds. Hemostasis and thrombosis. Philadelphia: JB Lippincott, 1987:846.

Roberts HR, Lefkowitz JB. Inherited disorders of prothrombin conversion. In: Colman RW, Hirsh J, Marder VJ, eds. Hemostasis and thrombosis. Philadelphia: JB Lippincott, 1994:200.

DISSEMINATED INTRAVASCULAR COAGULATION

Craig S. Kitchens, M.D.

Disseminated intravascular coagulation (DIC) is a perversion of physiology. Theories suggesting that it might be initiated by pathophysiologic or novel mechanisms are superannuated. Rather, the day-to-day physiologic initiators of coagulation are operative in DIC. DIC is distinguished from physiologic coagulation by the sheer force of the duration and volume of generated coagulant forces which overwhelm physiologic inhibitors of coagulation, resulting in circulating, unopposed free thrombin causing platelets to be stimulated, fibrinogen to clot, and factors V, VIII, and XIII to be activated. The complexing of thrombin to endothelial-bound thrombomodulin results in brisk activation of the fibrinolytic system which then generates plasmin in quantities sufficient to overwhelm its inhibitors. Circulating, unopposed free plasmin results in lysis of fibrinogen and fibrin into characteristic high levels of serum fibrin and fibrinogen split products (FSPs). This model explains the paradox of concomitant systemic thrombosis and hemorrhage. If thrombin is dominant, the clinical picture is mainly of thrombosis; if plasmin prevails, hemorrhage is the predominant clinical manifestation. Hemorrhage is abetted by the consumption of platelets, fibrinogen, and factors V, VIII, and XIII. Indeed, a previous term for DIC, consumption coagulopathy, is descriptively correct.

■ PATHOPHYSIOLOGY

Keeping in mind that platelets and fibrinogen are consumed physiologically in repair of even the smallest cut, consider the pathophysiologic situations that result in DIC (Table 1). Factors that are produced and the manner in which they are produced are physiologic, but the stimulus is so inappropriate that pathologic events result. The release of massive amounts of procoagulant factors from tissue is one of the most common mechanisms for initiation of DIC. All tissues have within them procoagulant factors, mainly tissue factor (TF). When it gains entry into the circulation, TF serves as a powerful cofactor to coagulation, particularly the extrinsic branch of the coagulation cascade model. Massive injury of normal tissue, such as occurs in crush or burn injuries, notoriously results in a brisk yet often self-limited DIC. This is best characterized in injuries of the central nervous system. Prolonged shock with ischemia of organs and limbs can result in DIC. Release of TF is most likely the mechanism involved in DIC associated with heat stroke and the retained dead fetus syndrome. The hypercoagulability associated with neoplastic growths is due to secreted tumor procoagulants as well as necrosis of neoplastic tissue, which becomes nonviable either by outgrowing its metabolic and blood supply or through the use of cytotoxic chemotherapy.

Nearly any type of infection may initiate DIC. Notorious are the gram-negative bacteria, as DIC is actually a common part of the syndrome of gram-negative sepsis. Gram-positive organisms, particularly *Pneumococcus, Streptococcus,* and *Staphylococcus,* also can cause DIC. DIC is frequently reported in rickettsial and viral diseases and can occasionally be seen in parasitic diseases, chiefly malaria.

Occasionally the infusion of procoagulant substances into the vascular system results in DIC. This is being increasingly described following infusion of shed blood by cell savers at the time of operation. This is more common if the shed blood is contaminated, such as with bowel injury, or if the amount infused is greater than 10 to 15 units of blood. The use of shunts to infuse ascitic fluid into the intravascular system can result in DIC, particularly when severe hepatic disease is present, as a normal liver is imperative for successful weathering of a DIC challenge. Amniotic fluid occasionally gains entry into the maternal circulation during prolonged labor and other obstetric problems and can result in DIC. The venom of some exotic snakes can directly activate either factor X (boomslang, or *Dispholidus typus*) or factor II (saw-scale viper, or *Echis carinatus*), which can result in circulating thrombin and thrombosis of vital organs.

When blood clots, it may release either massive or continued amounts of thrombin, initiating DIC. This is the likely explanation for chronic DIC from large abdominal aortic aneurysms as well as the clotting of blood that takes place intravascularly in giant hemangiomas, as seen in the Kasabach-Merritt syndrome. Clotted blood beneath an abruptio placentae generates thrombin that can gain entry into the maternal circulation.

A variety of mechanisms can correct DIC. The liver is an important neutralizer of circulating activated coagulation proteins as well as the site of production of almost all coagulation factors and inhibitors of coagulation. Adequacy of circulation ensures that the products of DIC are transported to the liver to be neutralized. Inadequacy of the circulation is at least one mechanism by which shock serves to potentiate any cause of DIC.

The modern hypothesis regarding DIC requires at-large circulation of thrombin and plasmin as consequences of overpowering the physiologic inhibitors of hemostasis. Table 2 lists key hemostatic factors, the pathologic production of which can overwhelm their respective inhibitors. Massive and continued destruction of tissue results in the continued production of TF. The primary inhibitor of TF is the recently described tissue factor pathway inhibitor (TFPI), also called extrinsic pathway inhibitor (EPI) or lipoprotein-associated coagulation inhibitor (LACI). Continued production of TF after it has overwhelmed TFPI results in continued and enhanced thrombin generation. As thrombin is generated, factors V and VIII are recruited to amplify cofactors in the coagulation system. Attempting to neutralize factors V_a and VIII_a are protein C and protein S, which as they become exhausted, allow for the unabated amplification activities of activated factors V and VIII, further enhancing thrombin generation. Antithrombin III (ATIII) is the physiologic inhibitor of the activated serine proteases, chiefly activated factor X and activated factor II (thrombin). As ATIII is overwhelmed by the continued production of thrombin, thrombin accumulates and circulates freely, enhancing fibrin formation and platelet activation.

Table 1 Mechanisms for the Induction of DIC

Release of Procoagulant Factors
- CNS injury
- Crush injury
- Prolonged shock and ischemia
- Heat stroke
- Retained dead fetus syndrome
- Burns
- Neoplastic growth

Infections
- Gram-negative bacteria
- Gram-positive bacteria
- Rickettsial infections
- Viral infections
- Protozoan infections

Infusion of Procoagulant Substances
- Amniotic fluid
- Certain snake venoms
- LeVeen shunt fluid
- Transfusion by cell saver

Products of Blood Coagulation
- Abruptio placentae
- Abdominal aortic aneurysm
- Kasabach-Merritt syndrome

Table 2 Hemostatic Consequences of Subjugation of Inhibitors

KEY HEMOSTATIC FORCES	INHIBITORS	RESULTS
Tissue factor	TFPI	Enhanced thrombin generation
Activated factors V and VIII	Proteins C and S	Enhanced thrombin generation
Activated serine proteases, especially thrombin	Antithrombin III	Enhanced fibrin formation and platelet clearance
Tissue plasminogen activator	Plasminogen activator inhibitor, type 1	Enhanced fibrinolytic activation
Plasmin	Alpha-2-antiplasmin	Unopposed fibrinolysis

TFPI, tissue factor pathway inhibitor, also known as extrinsic pathway inhibitor (EPI) or lipoprotein-associated coagulation inhibitor (LACI).

The fibrinolytic system attempts to clear the vascular system of fibrin from ongoing pathologic clotting. The binding of thrombin to thrombomodulin, especially in the presence of fibrin deposition, enhances the endothelial release of tissue plasminogen activator (tPA). Its primary rapid inhibitor, plasminogen activator inhibitor type I (PAI-I), attempts to neutralize circulating tPA. As it is overwhelmed, fibrinolytic activation becomes unimpeded. Finally this results in massive amounts of circulating plasmin and eventual exhaustion of its inhibitor, alpha-2 antiplasmin (alpha$_2$-AP). At this stage fibrinolytic activity is virtually uninhibited, resulting in a massive accumulation of FSPs and a failed hemostatic system.

■ VARIATIONS

Given that the initiation of DIC may be acute or chronic and massive or slow and that there will be variable abilities of the host to neutralize circulating thrombin and plasmin, it comes as no surprise that clinical manifestations of DIC, though produced by the same basic mechanisms, may present in various patterns. Table 3 shows one example of each of three axes of DIC. DIC may be either be acute or chronic. Indeed, acute fulminant DIC is the clinical picture recalled by most clinicians when DIC is discussed. This is well represented by meningococcemia, in which a previously healthy person may within a matter of hours develop massive cutaneous thrombosis (purpura fulminans), thrombosis of various organs, adrenal insufficiency (Waterhouse-Frederickson syndrome), and massive tissue bleeding. Chronic DIC results when the stimulus for DIC is slower but sustained. A model for this end of the tempo spectrum is the syndrome of retained dead fetus in which a thrombohemorrhagic picture ensues over a protracted time, usually weeks after fetal death.

Another axis to consider is localized versus systemic initiation of DIC. An example of localized DIC activation of the coagulation system occurs in a large abdominal aortic aneurysm. In this situation a patient can appear quite well but have mild oozing and rather abnormal coagulation tests. Exhaustive workup often finds only the aneurysm. A similar situation occurs in the Kasabach-Merritt syndrome. Systemic DIC is well represented by the DIC that occurs with acute promyelocytic leukemia (APL). In this situation necrotic promyelocytes release TF directly and/or release cytokines such as interleukin-1, which then cause endothelial cells to release TF. The result is the hemorrhagic syndrome characteristic of most patients presenting with APL.

The third axis is whether patients have thrombotic or hemorrhagic episodes. Many patients have both concomitantly. Perhaps Trousseau's syndrome best presents the thrombotic model. This syndrome occurs in patients harboring cancer, particularly adenocarcinoma and even more particularly mucin-producing adenocarcinomas such as are frequently found in the gastrointestinal tract but also with hepatic and renal neoplasms. In this situation the patient usually has repeated thrombosis, whether arterial, venous, or both, which resists warfarin therapy but is at least partially manageable with heparin therapy. Abruptio placentae is a model of acute massive hemorrhagic syndrome with proportionately few thrombotic manifestations.

Table 3 Examples of Variations of DIC Syndrome

Acute	Meningococcemia
Chronic	Retained dead fetus syndrome
Localized	Abdominal aortic aneurysm
Systemic	Acute promyelocytic leukemia
Thrombotic	Trousseau's syndrome
Hemorrhagic	Abruptio placentae

■ DIFFERENTIAL DIAGNOSIS

Several situations should be considered in the differential diagnosis of DIC because their thrombotic manifestations may mimic DIC or because laboratory abnormalities may suggest DIC. Most common of these is severe hepatic cirrhosis, the laboratory coagulation abnormalities of which mimic DIC. Because severe hepatic cirrhosis results in decreased production of various hemostatic factors, including fibrinogen, ATIII, protein C, protein S, and plasminogen, these factors may well be detected in decreased quantities. However, the decrease is due to impaired production and not enhanced activation as seen in DIC. Because the liver clears the small amount of FSPs due to physiologic production, decreased clearance with hepatic disease results in an accumulation of FSPs in the serum. Portal hypertension with hypersplenism is also characteristic of advanced cirrhosis, so that thrombocytopenia frequently occurs. Bleeding varices and gastritis in these patients are due not to DIC but to hepatic failure.

Measurable decreases in plasma fibrinogen and increases in serum FSP are found in the immediate postpartum period in even uncomplicated deliveries. These measurable changes should be viewed not as pathologic but as physiologic secondary to delivery itself. In the appropriate clinical setting such as massive hemorrhage, these changes may substantiate a diagnosis of DIC.

While thrombotic thrombocytopenic purpura (TTP) is clearly a thrombotic process with major organ damage resulting from pathologic intravascular deposition of large aggregates of platelets, it is not regarded as being representative of DIC.

The venom of the Eastern diamondback rattlesnake *(Crotalus adamantus)* only partially clots fibrinogen. Also, it does not activate platelets or bind to ATIII, which distinguishes its actions from those of thrombin. Although the laboratory findings after envenomation by the Eastern diamondback rattlesnake are highly reminiscent of those of DIC, neither thrombotic nor hemorrhagic complications usually occur.

Occasionally the fibrinolytic system can be activated without prior activation of the coagulation system. Activation of the fibrinolytic system in the overwhelming majority of cases is the secondary physiologic result of thrombosis. In some circumstances the fibrinolytic system may be activated in a primary fashion. The existence of primary hyperfibrinolysis has been debated for some time and probably does exist in rare instances. Of interest, the venom of the Western diamondback rattlesnake *(Crotalus atrox)* directly activates plasminogen and may cause primary hyperfibrinolysis. In this situation bleeding may be significant, but thrombosis is not usually evident. Primary hyperfibrinolysis may also result in some cases of prostate carcinoma, as such cells may elaborate plasminogen activators. The late phases of cardiopulmonary bypass also cause the pathologic release of endogenous tPA, resulting in probably the most common cause of bleeding following cardiopulmonary bypass. Obviously infusion of pharmacologic plasminogen activators, such as streptokinase or tPA, causes a hyperfibrinolytic state.

Table 4 Difficulties in Laboratory Diagnosis of DIC

DIC remains a clinical diagnosis.
No single laboratory test is specific and sensitive enough to establish diagnosis.
DIC is a dynamic state; therefore, patterns of test results will change.
Sophisticated tests require too much time to be of routine diagnostic use.

DIAGNOSIS

As we have discussed, DIC is the result of an underlying pathophysiologic situation ranging as broad as viral infection to abdominal aortic aneurysm. It should not be viewed as an illness of itself but as a symptom of another illness. In general, the underlying illness is either blatantly obvious or not difficult to find. DIC does not spontaneously occur.

DIC remains a clinical diagnosis. Although the following paragraphs discuss laboratory manifestations of DIC, I do not view DIC as a laboratory diagnosis; rather the laboratory serves as an adjunct to bedside observations.

Patients develop DIC when some underlying mechanism provokes coagulation, acutely or chronically, locally or systemically, to such an extent that coagulation overwhelms the check-and-balance system of hemostasis. The diagnosis of DIC is predicated by the observation of a patient who is hemorrhaging, thrombosing, or both. In acute, severe DIC bleeding is usually obvious. Bleeding occurs from incisions, access sites to the vascular system, gums, nose, and at the site of any manipulation of the body, such as by urinary catheters and endotracheal tubes. Skin manifestations include the rapid production of petechiae progressing to ecchymotic areas which may become large, confluent, and even necrotic. Thrombotic complications of smaller vessels may result in purpura fulminans. Occlusion of larger vessels may result in blindness, myocardial infarction, loss of pulses in limbs, or even occlusion of major vessels such as the inferior vena cava or aorta. Major organs may suffer. As blood is an organ, DIC can be viewed as either a failed organ or an important modulator of the syndrome of multiorgan failure (MOF). Thrombosis can occur in any vessel. The astute clinician will observe for and detect manifestations of thrombosis. When thrombohemorrhagic events occur in a patient with an underlying disorder that may be characterized by the release of TF, such as shock, infection, burn, crush injury, neoplastic disease, or obstetric emergency, the diagnosis of DIC should be strongly entertained. It is at this time that the physician turns to the laboratory for confirmation of the clinical diagnosis. Indeed, this confirmation implies that laboratory tests will be employed chiefly in patients for whom there is a high index of suspicion, rather than simply as screening tests. In appropriately selected patients with DIC, positive predictive values will accordingly be high. Keep this in mind when reading more exhaustive literature on laboratory manifestations of DIC.

Laboratory Diagnosis

The difficulties in laboratory diagnosis are outlined in Table 4. DIC occurs in extremely dynamic situations during which the infusion of procoagulant substances may be episodic with more time consumed by efforts of the body to correct the effects of DIC. Accordingly, collection of blood for laboratory tests may take place during either the initiation or clearance phase of DIC. In chronic DIC there is slow activation of the coagulation system, so that changes may be much more subtle, in fact so subtle that the ability of the laboratory to discriminate these changes from normal will be lost. No single test is sensitive or specific enough to establish a diagnosis.

One may think that a battery of tests might prove the existence of DIC. After all, DIC mechanistically is thought of as enhanced clearance of platelets, fibrinogen, plasminogen, ATIII, protein S, protein C, and factors V, VIII, and XIII, and therefore decreased plasma levels should be observed. For any laboratory result to be below the broad range of normal, activation and clearance of each parameter must be faster than the ability of the host to compensate for that loss. Similarly, increases in some products, such as FSPs, may be obscured by rapid clearance by a normal hepatic system. The ability of the bone marrow to compensate for thrombocytopenia varies enormously from patient to patient. Fibrinogen is consumed in DIC, yet many of the very patients at risk for DIC (those with underlying inflammatory or neoplastic disease or who are pregnant) usually have increased plasma levels of fibrinogen such that a decrease of fibrinogen may be represented only by a decrease from elevated levels into the range of normal. The predictive value of the platelet count less than 150,000 per cubic millimeter or plasma fibrinogen less than 150 mg/dl is only slightly better than 50 percent for each test. That notwithstanding, in acute severe DIC, fibrinogen and platelets will be decreased in the vast majority of patients.

D-dimer is a specific type of FSP. This small fragment is released during fibrin degradation by plasmin and in so doing produces a neoantigen that can be detected with sensitive assays. That two D-fragments have been dimerized is the result of prior covalent bonding of fibrin, proving the previous presence of activated factor XIII. Accordingly, D-dimer is well thought of as being a footprint proving the previous activities of both thrombin and plasmin, the agents responsible for and necessary for DIC. The D-dimer assay is quite specific for DIC but is not as sensitive as the assay for FSP, which is sensitive but not specific. The combination of the two has remarkable predictive value. In patients who are at risk for DIC and have a positive screen for FSP and positive assay for D-dimer, the positive predictive value approaches 100 percent.

Other problems involving the laboratory diagnosis of DIC are that frequently the assays are too sophisticated and too time-consuming for routine bedside use. Nonetheless, such laboratory assays for DIC are important, particularly for investigational work.

Table 5 Treatment of DIC

TREATMENT	EXAMPLE	RATIONALE
Treat underlying cause	Abruptio placentae	Interrupt cause of DIC
Resuscitation	Maintain blood pressure, correct acid-base balance	Maximize blood flow from areas of activation to clearance by liver
Replacement	Fresh frozen plasma and platelet transfusions	Provide enough procoagulant materials to control hemostasis
Heparin therapy	Trousseau's syndrome, purpura fulminans, acute promyelocytic leukemia, abdominal aortic aneurysm	May decrease ongoing thrombosis
Antifibrinolytic therapy	Kasabach-Merritt syndrome, prostate cancer	Occasionally used to control fibrinolysis, but only after administration of heparin
Antithrombin III	Severe liver disease with concomitant DIC	Replace severely decreased levels of ATIII

For clinical work I use a battery of routinely available tests. These include the thrombin time (TT), prothrombin time (PT), partial thromboplastin time (PTT), platelet count, and estimation of FSP. If the FSP assay is positive, an assay for D-dimer is added. In severe acute DIC these assays are usually positive. A prolonged TT is strong evidence for hypofibrinogenemia, FSP, or both, provided the presence of heparin has been excluded. Examination of the blood smear is extremely important because of the strong predictive value of schistocytes and other findings of microangiopathic hemolysis, which can be appreciated only by looking at the blood smear. Schistocytes may be the only sign of chronic DIC such as is seen in abdominal aortic aneurysm. Although microangiopathic hemolytic anemia may be seen in other situations, such as TTP, heat stroke, or malignant hypertension, it should be sought if DIC is a possibility.

Other coagulation tests are often helpful. These include measurements of plasminogen, ATIII, protein C, protein S, and alpha$_2$-AP. These tests are rarely available for rapid turnaround but may have some confirmatory value. It has been claimed that marked decreases of plasma ATIII serve as the best single predictor for a fatal outcome in DIC, particularly DIC associated with sepsis.

I know of no data regarding any specific pattern of laboratory abnormalities or change of pattern over time in DIC that are accurate enough to depend upon for reliable prognostic use.

Histologically, DIC is strongly suggested by microvascular deposition of fibrin clots. When these are seen in biopsy specimens or at autopsy, the presence of DIC is strongly inferred. However, the reciprocal is not true; absence of vascular occlusion by fibrin clots does not disprove DIC, as the fibrinolytic system is so active that clots can be cleared in the microcirculation, leading to a false-negative biopsy. As fibrinolysis continues even post mortem, this is true even at autopsy.

■ THERAPY

The enormous variety of clinical situations that can befall a human and result in DIC makes definitive statements regarding treatment of DIC difficult (Table 5). The most effective treatment of all, of course, is treatment of the underlying disorder, inasmuch as DIC is a symptom of that disorder and not a primary diagnosis. Treatment of the underlying disorder interrupts the production of the procoagulants and the secondary generation of fibrinolytic activity. Accordingly, the levels of circulating thrombin and plasmin will decrease, and to the extent that this can be accomplished, the outlook is more favorable than if production of pathologic amounts of thrombin and plasmin continues. In experimental animals, if DIC can be reversed, multiorgan failure does not result and survival is enhanced.

Treatment of the causative process is clearly the choice in gram-negative sepsis, in which prompt therapy can not only limit DIC but can also be lifesaving. Aggressive therapy with antibiotics in the patient at risk for gram-negative sepsis is in order. Although a variety of obstetric emergencies can present as fulminant acute DIC, treatment is usually straightforward, namely, evacuation of the uterus. Interruption of the pathophysiology aided by the reparative processes of young women healthy enough to sustain pregnancy is often rewarded by rapid improvement. A patient with extremely abnormal laboratory studies and profuse hemorrhage will suddenly revert to a normal patient with normal coagulation studies following uterine evacuation. Some diseases, such as disseminated carcinoma, crush injuries, and massive burns, are clearly more difficult to treat.

The second mainstay of treatment is resuscitation of the patient. Because the liver is key in the clearance of activated coagulation products, the maintenance of hepatic circulation by maintaining blood volume and blood pressure is of prime importance. Aggressive treatment should be made to correct hypotension, arrhythmias, altered vascular resistance, decreased urine output, acid-base, fluid, and electrolyte abnormalities. Even the best therapy for DIC is enhanced by prompt resuscitation of the patient.

Replacement therapy in DIC is extremely controversial. Some advocate that treatment of thrombocytopenia with platelet transfusions, treatment of factor deficiencies with FFP, and replacement of fibrinogen by cryoprecipitate infusion merely fuels the fire by providing more substrate to the circulating enzymes plasmin and thrombin. Although this may be true in brisk DIC, it is important to maintain hemostatic parameters at levels sufficient to allow physiologic coagulation to take place. Accordingly, maintaining the platelet count in the vicinity of 50,000 per cubic millimeter, a fibrinogen level on the order of 100 mg/dl, and factor levels in the vicinity of 25 percent of normal plasma concentrations are reasonable targets. Any levels over these minimally sufficient hemostatic levels may offer more fuel than prophylaxis.

Maintenance of these reasonable levels of procoagulant activity is especially desirable if the patient requires surgery or invasive procedures. It is important to exclude TTP and heparin-induced thrombocytopenia (HIT) as diseases masquerading as DIC before the institution of platelet infusions, as it is generally regarded that TTP and HIT are contraindications for platelet transfusions.

Treatment of DIC with heparin infusions has even been more controversial. In favor of heparin treatment is that according to current understanding of the pathophysiology, if circulating thrombin is causal in DIC, it seems logical to enhance thrombin neutralization by administration of heparin. Against the use of heparin is that hemorrhage is among the leading causes of death in patients with DIC, and heparin therapy may enhance bleeding. This dilemma has never been thoroughly resolved, nor is it likely to be, considering the diverse causes and manifestations of DIC. Mant and King found in the subset of acute, severe DIC that heparin administration appeared to correlate with a poorer outcome, especially hemorrhagic death. On the other hand, the administration of heparin prophylactically before chemotherapy is regarded by many authorities as an important advancement in the treatment of acute promyelocytic leukemia. Similarly, heparin administration clearly increases levels of fibrinogen, decreases levels of FSP, and raises the platelet count in most patients with retained dead fetus syndrome, Kasabach-Merritt syndrome, and aortic aneurysms. This is particularly important because patients with these problems may be candidates for surgical procedures. Administration of heparin is clearly lifesaving in patients with Trousseau's syndrome; otherwise, most patients quickly succumb, not to their underlying malignancy, but to the intense thrombogenecity of the tumor. Heparin is also advocated for persons who have visible advancing skin necrosis such as seen in purpura fulminans.

The use of heparin has not been associated with efficacy in the treatment of DIC secondary to exotic snakebite, heat stroke, trauma, transfusion mismatches, and the acute obstetric catastrophes of amniotic fluid embolism and abruptio placentae.

Because routine coagulation studies may be perturbed in DIC, calculation of the dose of heparin to be administered is fraught with difficulties. Most authorities recommend arbitrarily giving approximately 15 U per kilogram per hour by continuous intravenous infusion. As heparin works through activation of ATIII and DIC is characteristically associated with decreased plasma levels of ATIII, it is theoretically possible for plasma concentrations of ATIII to be limiting (see below).

Antifibrinolytic therapy, chiefly epsilon-aminocaproic acid (EACA), has been advocated by some with the rationale that EACA's powerful antifibrinolytic activity would negate the effect of circulating plasmin. This works so completely that if EACA is administered, the thrombogenic activity of thrombin is unopposed and massive thrombosis may result. For that reason most experts think that EACA should not be used in the vast majority of cases of DIC. If EACA is to be used, most authorities recommend that the thrombotic action of thrombin should first be neutralized by heparin. After heparin is administered, EACA, infused at 1 g per hour following a loading dose of approximately 4 g, may be used for uncontrolled life-threatening bleeding. If efficacy is not realized within approximately 48 hours, therapy with EACA should probably not be continued.

ATIII is now commercially available as a concentrate. Theoretically, the infusion of ATIII should replenish exhausted supplies of ATIII, providing the natural inhibitor for circulating thrombin. As attractive as this sounds, at this time its use in DIC should be regarded as more theoretic than founded. Because levels of ATIII may be decreased in liver disease prior to DIC, its use is theoretically even more attractive in pre-existing liver disease complicated by DIC.

Suggested Reading

Bell WR, Starksen NF, et al. Trousseau's syndrome: Devastating coagulopathy in the absence of heparin. Am J Med 1985;79:423.

Carr JM, McKinney M, McDonagh J. Diagnosis of disseminated intravascular coagulation: Role of D-dimer. Am J Clin Pathol 1989;91:280.

Fourrier F, Chopin C, Goudemand J, et al. Septic shock, multiple organ failure, and disseminated intravascular coagulation: Compared patterns of antithrombin III, protein C and protein S deficiencies. Chest 1992; 101:816.

Horst HM, Dlugos S, Fath JJ, et al. Coagulopathy and intraoperative blood salvage (IBS). J Trauma 1992; 32:646.

Levi M, ten Cate H, van der Poll T, et al. Pathogenesis of disseminated intravascular coagulation in sepsis. JAMA 1993;280:957.

Mant MJ, King EG. Severe, acute disseminated intravascular coagulation: A reappraisal of its pathophysiology, clinical significance and therapy based on 47 patients. Am J Med 1979; 67:557.

Mombelli G, Fiori G, Monotto R, et al. Fibrinopeptide A in liver cirrhosis: Evidence against a major contribution of disseminated intravascular coagulation to coagulopathy of chronic liver disease. J Lab Clin Med 1993; 121:83.

ACQUIRED ANTICOAGULANTS

Sandor S. Shapiro, M.D.

Acquired anticoagulants are generally antibodies directed against specific coagulation factors or against negatively charged phospholipid-protein complexes (so-called lupus anticoagulants). Antibodies in the former category usually are associated with an increased risk of hemorrhage; the most common of these antibodies are directed against factor VIII (FVIII) or factor IX (FIX). Antibodies in the latter category, to the contrary, appear to be associated with a high risk of thrombosis. Therapeutic considerations in these two classes are therefore quite different, and the two classes will be discussed separately.

CIRCULATING INHIBITORS (ANTICOAGULANTS) TO SPECIFIC COAGULATION FACTORS

Although antibodies have been described against nearly all coagulation factors, the vast majority are directed against FVIII or to a lesser extent FIX. This discussion will be limited to FVIII and FIX antibodies. For a more general discussion, consult one of the references at the end of this chapter.

Antibodies to FVIII occur in 10 to 20 percent of treated patients with severe hemophilia A as a consequence of exposure to exogenous FVIII. Most inhibitors occur in patients with no immunologically detectable circulating FVIII molecules. The prevalence of FIX antibodies in severe hemophilia B is lower, perhaps 3 to 8 percent. When they occur, antibodies usually do not worsen the hemorrhagic diathesis, but they may severely complicate treatment of bleeding episodes. About 20 percent of patients with antibodies are weak responders, whose antibody levels do not exceed 2 to 5 Bethesda units (BU) per milliliter despite repeated exposure to FVIII or FIX. The remaining 80 percent behave in the manner expected for most antibodies: anamnestic responses occur 4 to 10 days after antigenic challenge, while withholding antigen results in a gradual fall in titer. Occasionally, patients with mild hemophilia A develop FVIII antibodies after treatment with FVIII. Generally such antibodies are transient but, while present, they often increase the severity of the patient's hemophilia. Individuals not suffering from genetic coagulation factor deficiencies may also develop inhibitors, most frequently against FVIII, which induce a hemorrhagic disorder; usually there is no history of exposure to blood products.

The locus of action of FVIII antibodies is the subject of current research. FVIII is a 280 Kd protein consisting of a series of domains, several closely homologous. Thus, from amino to carboxy terminus, the molecule can be pictured as a sequence of domains: A1•A2•B•A3•C1•C2. During activation by thrombin the B domain is lost. The C2 domain seems to be involved in FVIII binding to phospholipid; function of the other domains is unknown. Examination of a number of inhibitor patient plasmas shows that antibodies to the A1 and C2 domains, as well as several others to less clearly identified regions, can inhibit FVIII activity. About 75 percent of inhibitor patients have heterogeneous populations of antibodies of multiple specificities.

Acute Treatment

Proper treatment requires adequate laboratory facilities including, as a minimum, accurate quantitative assays for the coagulation factor in question and for the coagulation inhibitor. For the latter purpose, the Bethesda assay is highly recommended. Because inhibitors occur with some frequency in treated hemophiliacs, it is important to measure coagulation factor and inhibitor levels on a regular basis, including an assessment of in vivo yield after infusion of coagulation factor concentrates. Any patient whose clinical response to infusion seems suboptimal should be checked for an inhibitor.

Hemophilic patients with inhibitors who are weak responders can generally continue treatment with FVIII or FIX, although at higher doses than usual. Dose can be calculated by estimating the FVIII or FIX needed to neutralize the inhibitor and adding to that the amount needed to achieve hemostasis in the specific clinical situation. For example, a 50 kg youngster with hemophilia A and an elbow hemorrhage whose FVIII antibody is 2 BU per milliliter, would require approximately 2,000 U of FVIII to neutralize the antibody—2 BU per milliliter × 40 ml per kilogram plasma volume × 0.5 (the Bethesda unit is that concentration of antibody neutralizing 50 percent of the FVIII in an equal volume of normal plasma)—plus 700 U to treat the hemarthrosis (14 U per kilogram dose sufficient to treat a hemarthrosis in an uncomplicated hemophiliac), or a total of 2,700 U FVIII. Weak responder antibody patients can do well on home therapy.

The situation with strong responders is much more complex. Once antibody levels exceed 10 BU per milliliter, it is impractical to give replacement therapy with human FVIII or FIX. In addition, treatment can be expected to result in a substantial increase in antibody titer. Thus replacement therapy with concentrate is generally reserved for life-threatening situations. An alternative form of treatment is the use of prothrombin complex concentrates (PCCs), either the nonactivated varieties such as Konyne or Proplex or the activated types such as Autoplex or FEIBA. Although the active principle bypassing the inhibitor has not been identified, control studies have demonstrated that single infusions of nonactivated PCCs at a dose of 75 FIX U per kilogram are effective in treating hemarthroses in 50 percent of cases versus a success rate of 25 percent for placebo, while activated PCCs at a dose of 75 bypassing units per kilogram are slightly more effective (60 to 65 percent). Uncontrolled studies suggest that effectiveness may be increased with two to three doses 6 to 8 hours apart. PCCs can be used in hemophilia A patients with FVIII inhibitors and in hemophilia B patients with FIX inhibitors. Since PCCs induce a mild prothrombotic state, care must be taken to avoid their use in patients with serious liver dysfunction and to refrain from using epsilon-aminocaproic acid (EACA) concomitantly. Since variable amounts of FVIII antigen are present in PCCs, some patients show rises in FVIII antibody levels after treatment, although rarely to more than two to three times pretreatment levels. Treatment should almost always be initiated with nonactivated PCCs in view of the small difference in efficacy and the very large difference in cost. Activated PCCs should be used only after failure of the nonactivated variety. The only exception is serious cranial hemorrhage, in which the slight advantage of activated PCCs and the need for immediate treatment outweigh the cost factor.

Since FVIII therapy is by definition the treatment of choice in hemophilia A, several approaches have been taken to circumvent high antibody titers and produce circulating levels of FVIII. Plasmapheresis has been used but has not been uniformly successful. Although theoretically 60 to 85 percent of the plasma antibody can be removed with a 3 to 4 L plasmapheresis, this goal is rarely achieved and is in any event insufficient in the face of a high-titer antibody. Almost all FVIII and FIX antibodies are the immunoglobulin IgG, whose distribution is only 45 percent intravascular. Furthermore, antibody production appears to be stimulated by the procedure, since preplasmapheresis antibody levels are frequently reattained within 48 hours. Thus it may be necessary to perform daily plasmapheresis for 2 to 3 days before antibody levels are reduced by 75 percent. At that point massive doses of concentrate may neutralize the inhibitor and achieve hemostatic levels of FVIII. Until the last plasmapheresis replacement should probably be with 5 percent albumin in normal saline, since hemodynamic, metabolic, and immunologic complications have occasionally occurred when plasma was used for volume replacement.

Because of the species specificity of many FVIII antibodies, another approach to replacement therapy is the use of FVIII concentrates of animal origin. Early experience with porcine and bovine concentrates was complicated by frequent allergic reactions and thrombocytopenia. A recent polyelectrolyte-fractionated porcine FVIII (Hyate C) is largely free of these side effects. Allergic reactions, when they occur, are generally mild and easily controlled with antihistamines and/or steroids. If the use of porcine FVIII is contemplated, inhibitor titers must be measured against the porcine product and calculations of replacement quantities made on this basis. Usually a patient's antibody will react much less or not at all against the porcine material, so that hemostatic levels of FVIII can be achieved after infusion. As a rule of thumb, however, patients with Bethesda titers greater than 50 U per milliliter generally are found to have porcine antibody titers that preclude use of porcine FVIII. Because it is a foreign protein and can induce antibody formation, efficacy of porcine FVIII may decrease with repeated use, and the risk of allergic reactions may increase. Thus, this product should be reserved for life-threatening situations. In anticipation of its use and to prevent problems in emergencies, all inhibitor patients should have anti-porcine FVIII levels determined, and a small stock of porcine FVIII should be available wherever inhibitor patients are treated.

Several maneuvers have been proposed to blunt the anamnestic response when FVIII or FIX is used in patients with hemophilia A or B and inhibitors. Immunosuppressives, such as cyclophosphamide, have been administered intravenously in single doses of 10 to 20 mg per kilogram at the initiation of infusion therapy, but results have not been convincing. Immunosuppressive therapy has also been used in attempts to eradicate inhibitors, as discussed later. Recently intravenous IgG (IVIgG) has been used as an adjunct to treatment. IVIgG, made from large pools of normal plasma, has been shown to contain anti-idiotypic antibodies capable of neutralizing many patients' inhibitors in vitro and in vivo; responses may vary from patient to patient and in a given patient from lot to lot of IVIgG. The usual dose is 0.5 mg per kilogram, and infusions have been given daily for as long as 8 days. When a response is seen, a substantial fall in inhibitor occurs and may last 4 to 12 weeks. Current data suggest that in vitro testing is a good predictor of in vivo results. Thus inability of IVIgG to neutralize the inhibitor when admixed with patient plasma argues against its in vivo use.

In inhibitor patients who are capable of synthesizing FVIII to some extent (mild hemophiliacs) or normally (nonhemophiliacs), treatment with DDAVP (1-deamino-8-D-arginine vasopressin) may play a role. This drug stimulates the release of von Willebrand factor from endothelial cell stores and indirectly raises the level of FVIII. It has been used in place of FVIII or PCCs as preparation for dental extraction, for example. However, it is unlikely to be effective unless the inhibitor level is low. The drug is administered as an intravenous dose of 0.3 mg per kilogram in 50 ml normal saline over about 15 minutes. Rarely, recipients have mild vasopressin-like side effects, but usually the drug is well tolerated, with only occasional flushing or tachycardia. Antifibrinolytic therapy should be given at the same time (oral EACA, 20 g daily in four divided doses), since DDAVP also releases tissue plasminogen activator from endothelial cells, leading to an increase in blood fibrinolytic activity. DDAVP is ineffective in hemophilia B patients with FIX antibodies.

EACA alone has been used with moderate success as an adjunct to therapy in dental extractions in inhibitor and noninhibitor patients. Its use is based on the concept that the small degree of hemostasis achieved by the patient is aided by temporarily shutting off the normal fibrinolytic response at the site of extraction. EACA is given orally, 20 g per day in four divided doses, for 4 to 5 days, starting a few hours before the dental surgery. EACA should be avoided in patients with hematuria. Finally, dental extraction is much more successful in well-relaxed patients, and training patients in relaxation techniques, including hypnosis, has proven very useful.

Eradication of Antibodies

Several approaches have been taken in an attempt to eradicate antibodies. Cyclophosphamide and azathioprine, with or without steroids, have been used at the time of antigenic challenge with blood products, but success has been rare except perhaps when treatment has been given at the time of appearance of the inhibitor. Greater success has been achieved with nonhemophilic inhibitors, using long-term oral treatment. A typical regimen is 150 mg cyclophosphamide and 30 to 50 mg prednisone daily. Antibody titers fall slowly, and treatment frequently must be continued for many months. Newer regimens using combinations of drugs have also been proposed and have met with variable success.

Induction of specific tolerance has been attempted as well. Patients with hemophilia A and inhibitors have been treated with massive daily doses of FVIII—the so-called Bonn regimen—for months to years, with disappearance of antibodies, without recurrence when the regimen was stopped and FVIII therapy on a need basis was reinstituted. This regimen is enormously expensive and psychologically trying, especially for young patients, and has not found much favor. However, less stringent administration schedules may achieve similar ends. It is the general impression that patients on home treatment infusing once or twice weekly do not form antibodies at the expected rate, perhaps because of this phenomenon.

The most recent attempts at inducing tolerance have involved the use of IVIgG together with immunosuppressives and concentrates. However, a larger experience and longer follow-up will be necessary before this approach can be evaluated.

In summary, hemophiliacs with strong responder inhibitors pose a serious therapeutic challenge. The usual type of hemorrhagic events can be treated fairly successfully with PCCs. Life-threatening hemorrhage and operative procedures requiring coverage for 7 to 10 days require other approaches. Plasmaphersis may play a useful role in lowering high antibody levels so as to make replacement therapy more effective. Porcine FVIII may be very useful in these circumstances. IVIgG may be useful in some patients for similar reasons. Inhibitors in mild hemophiliacs and in nonhemophiliacs may fall after DDAVP infusion (always given with EACA), and this approach may be useful for dental extractions. Eradication of inhibitors probably involves induction of tolerance. Although not yet perfected, several promising approaches are under investigation.

■ LUPUS ANTICOAGULANTS

Lupus anticoagulants are a frequent cause of a prolonged PTT. Less frequently, they may be associated with a prolongation of the PT as well. A variety of coagulation tests have been used for their detection, none of which is absolutely specific. Of these, the dilute Russell viper venom time (dRVVT) is one of the simplest and most specific. Other tests, such as the dilute PTT, can also be used. Lupus anticoagulants interfere to a greater or lesser extent with all phospholipid-dependent coagulation tests. These anticoagulants in and of themselves are rarely if ever a cause of bleeding. To the contrary, patients with lupus anticoagulants have a high (25 to 50 percent) prevalence of thromboembolic disorders. In addition, a lupus anticoagulant is a risk factor for spontaneous abortion in women of childbearing age and is associated with thrombocytopenia, particularly in individuals with systemic lupus erythematosus. Women with histories of repeated abortion frequently have lupus anticoagulants. In roughly half the cases, patients with lupus anticoagulants have elevated levels of anticardiolipin antibodies as well. The presence of a lupus anticoagulant may be a better indicator of thrombotic risk.

The mechanism of the lupus anticoagulant effect is not known precisely, but it seems to depend on the interaction of this antibody with a complex of phospholipid with protein. Two proteins have been implicated in this regard—prothrombin and beta-2 glycoprotein I. In each case it is likely that the lupus anticoagulant binds to a neoantigen exposed when the protein binds to phospholipid. The mechanism of the thrombotic risk is unknown.

Nonpregnant patients with lupus anticoagulants and a documented history of thrombosis should receive oral anticoagulant therapy. Control of therapy can usually be achieved by following the prothrombin time, which is rarely prolonged; mild prolongations do not interfere with treatment. Patients who have had previous venous thrombosis should be anticoagulated to an International Normalized Ratio (INR) of 2.0 to 3.0. Patients who have had arterial thrombosis probably require more intense anticoagulation, to an INR of at least 3.0.

Elimination of the lupus anticoagulant can often be achieved with steroids, but the antibody tends to recur after cessation of steroids. Reduction of the lupus anticoagulant levels may not be accompanied by diminution in the titer of anticardiolipin antibodies when both phenomena are initially present. Steroids have been used to carry spontaneous aborters to term, and the rate of fetal salvage is high. However, side effects are also significant, and alternative treatments with heparin and/or aspirin appear to give equally good results with fewer complications.

Suggested Reading

Love PE, Santoro SA. Antiphospholipid antibodies: Anticardiolipin and the lupus anticoagulant in systemic lupus erythematosus (SLE) and in non-SLE disorders. Ann Int Med 1990; 112:682–698.

Aledort LM, Hoyer LW, Lusher JM, et al. Inhibitors to coagulation factors. In: Proceedings of the Second International Symposium. New York: Plenum, 1994.

Shapiro SS, Rajagopalan V. Acquired anticoagulants. In: Ratnoff OD, Forbes CD, eds. Disorders of hemostasis. 3rd ed. Philadelphia: WB Saunders, 1996.

ANTITHROMBIN III, PROTEIN C, AND PROTEIN S DEFICIENCY

Jeffrey I. Weitz, M.D., F.R.C.P.C., F.A.C.P.
Mark A. Crowther, M.D., F.R.C.P.C.

The heparin–antithrombin III system and the protein C pathway are naturally occurring anticoagulant mechanisms that regulate the hemostatic process. Protein S is a cofactor in the protein C pathway. The importance of these regulatory mechanisms is underscored by the observation that patients lacking key components of these pathways have an increased frequency of venous thrombosis. To clarify why thrombosis occurs, the mechanisms by which these pathways regulate coagulation will first be briefly reviewed. The remainder of the chapter will focus on the patterns of inheritance, clinical features, laboratory diagnosis, and the treatment of patients with deficiencies of antithrombin III, protein C, and protein S.

■ REGULATORY MECHANISMS

Heparin–Antithrombin III System

Antithrombin III is a glycoprotein inhibitor that complexes and inactivates thrombin and activated factor X (factor Xa). Heparin acts as an anticoagulant by binding to antithrombin III and accelerating these reactions about 1,000-fold. Although there is no naturally occurring heparin in the blood, the endothelium contains the anticoagulantly active glycosaminoglycan heparan sulfate, which may locally accelerate the inhibition of coagulation enzymes by antithrombin III.

Protein C Pathway

Whereas antithrombin III limits coagulation by inhibiting key clotting enzymes, activated protein C regulates the clotting process by proteolytically degrading and inactivating factors VIIIa and Va, important cofactors in the generation of factor Xa and thrombin, respectively. The activation of protein C is triggered by thrombin formed at sites of vascular injury (Fig. 1). This thrombin binds to thrombomodulin, a transmembrane protein on endothelial cells, and undergoes a conformational change that alters its substrate specificity and converts it from a procoagulant enzyme into a stimulator of a potent anticoagulant mechanism. Thus, thrombin bound to thrombomodulin loses its ability to activate platelets, convert fibrinogen to fibrin, and activate factors V and VIII. In contrast, the ability of thrombin to activate protein C is markedly enhanced when the enzyme binds to thrombomodulin. Activated protein C acts as an anticoagulant and prolongs the activated partial thromboplastin time (APTT) by degrading and inactivating factors Va and VIIIa. These reactions occur on the phospholipid surface of endothelial cells, platelets, and possibly other cells and are facilitated by protein S, which also binds to the cell membrane. The interaction of protein C and protein S with phospholipid surfaces requires gamma-carboxyglutamic acid (Gla) residues and calcium. Both protein C and protein S are vitamin K–dependent factors, and when the vitamin K cycle is blocked by warfarin, gamma-carboxylation of the glutamic acid residues does not occur and nonfunctional proteins are synthesized.

Protein S is found in plasma in two forms. About 60 percent of circulating protein S is noncovalently bound to C4b binding protein (C4bBP), a regulatory protein of the complement system, and the remaining 40 percent of protein S is free. Only the free form of protein S is functionally active. C4bBP is an acute-phase reactant the levels of which may increase postoperatively and in inflammatory states. With elevated levels of C4bBP, more protein S becomes bound, making less of it available to serve as a cofactor for protein C. This phenomenon may explain at least in part the link between thrombosis and chronic inflammatory diseases.

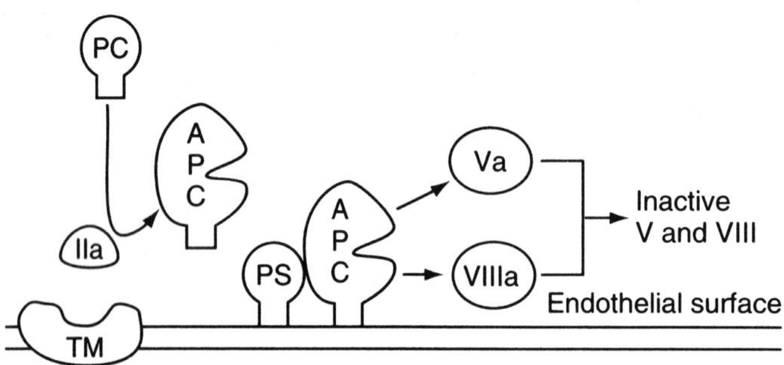

Figure 1
The protein C anticoagulant pathway. Thrombin (IIa) binds to thrombomodulin (TM) on the surface of the endothelial cells. The thrombin-thrombomodulin complex converts protein C (PC) to activated protein C (APC) which functions as an anticoagulant by proteolytically degrading and inactivating factors Va and VIIIa on a membrane surface. Protein S (PS) acts as a cofactor in these reactions. Recent evidence suggests that there is a relatively common mutation in the factor V gene that results in the synthesis of a factor V molecule that is activated normally but is resistant to proteolytic degradation by activated protein C.

Recent studies have identified a new abnormality in the protein C anticoagulant pathway. Known as activated protein C resistance (APCR), patients with this defect have a subnormal prolongation of their APTT when activated protein C is added to their plasma. In 90 percent of cases, APCR is due to a point mutation in the factor V gene (G1691A) which results in the replacement of arginine at position 506 on the factor V molecule with a glutamine reside. This mutant factor V, known as factor V Leiden, is activated normally and has normal procoagulant activity. However, activated factor V Leiden is resistant to inactivation by activated protein C, resulting in a prothrombotic state and explaining why the anticoagulant response is blunted when activated protein C is added to plasma.

■ CLINICAL FEATURES OF THE DEFICIENCY STATES

The possibility of APCR or an inherited deficiency of antithrombin III, protein C, or protein S should be considered in patients with idiopathic venous thrombosis before age 45, particularly in those with a family history of thrombosis. APCR is found in 16 to 30 percent of patients with venographically confirmed venous thrombosis, whereas only 8 percent of these patients have deficiencies of antithrombin III, protein C, or protein S. Up to 70 percent of patients with a family history of thrombosis and documented venous thromboembolism before age 45 will either have APCR or a deficiency state. In addition to those with a history of idiopathic venous thrombosis at an early age or a family history of thrombosis, patients with recurrent thromboembolic events and those with a history of thrombosis in unusual sites (such as visceral, cerebral, or cutaneous vessels) should also be investigated for APCR or a possible deficiency state.

In patients with APCR or deficiencies of antithrombin III, protein C, or protein S, thromboembolic events are unusual before puberty. From then on the annual incidence increases. Whereas patients with deficiencies of antithrombin III, protein C, or protein S usually present with venous thrombosis prior to the age of 50, those with APCR often develop thrombosis later in life. In over half of these cases an additional risk factor such as pregnancy, surgery, or immobilization can be identified as a trigger for the thrombotic event. These observations suggest that the appropriate use of prophylaxis is crucial whenever deficient individuals are exposed to a risk factor for thrombosis.

Venous thrombosis and pulmonary embolism are the most frequent clinical manifestations of APCR, antithrombin III, protein C, or protein S deficiency. Superficial phlebitis also occurs, but it appears to be less common in patients with antithrombin III deficiency than in those with APCR or a deficiency of protein C or protein S. Venous thrombosis during pregnancy is particularly frequent in patients with antithrombin III and protein C deficiency, but in all three deficiency states, the risk of venous thrombosis is higher in the postpartum period than it is during pregnancy. Although arterial thrombosis has been reported in occasional patients with APCR or antithrombin III, protein C, and protein S deficiency, it is uncertain whether the risk of arterial thrombosis is actually increased in these individuals.

Several clinical features are unique to the different deficiency states (Table 1). Patients with antithrombin III deficiency may be resistant to heparin, and those with protein C or protein S deficiency are prone to develop warfarin-induced skin necrosis. Finally, patients with homozygous protein C deficiency may develop diffuse skin necrosis or purpura fulminans.

Table 1 Clinical Features Unique to the Deficiency of Antithrombin III, Protein C, or Protein S

DEFICIENCY	CLINICAL FEATURES
Antithrombin III	Heparin resistance
Protein C	
Heterozygotes	Warfarin-induced skin necrosis
Homozygotes	Neonatal purpura fulminans
Protein S	Warfarin-induced skin necrosis

■ CONGENITAL AND ACQUIRED DEFICIENCIES

Antithrombin III

Antithrombin III deficiency may be congenital or acquired. Congenital antithrombin III deficiency is transmitted in an autosomal dominant fashion. The precise prevalence of congenital antithrombin III deficiency is unclear because few properly designed studies have been done. Based on rather limited information, it is estimated that antithrombin III deficiency occurs with a frequency of about 1 in 2,000 to 1 in 5,000 in the general population.

There are three types of congenital antithrombin III deficiency (Table 2). In type I, or classical deficiency, there is decreased production of a biologically normal antithrombin III protein so that the immunologic and biologic activities of antithrombin III are reduced to an equivalent extent. The molecular basis of this disorder is either (1) a complete deletion of one of the two autosomal genes or (2) alterations, such as nonsense mutations or base substitutions, at splice sites. The less common type II deficiency state is characterized by the synthesis of a dysfunctional protein with impaired inhibitory activity against thrombin and factor Xa. Under these circumstances, the biologic activity of the antithrombin III is reduced by about 50 percent, although its immunologic activity is virtually normal. At a molecular level these deficiencies are caused by point mutations in the gene, causing substitutions of key amino acids involved in the interaction of the inhibitor with the coagulation enzymes. Finally, in the very uncommon type III deficiency state, heparin binding to antithrombin III is defective so that heparin fails to catalyze the inhibitory activity of antithrombin III. At a molecular level the type III deficiencies are caused by point mutations in the portion of the gene that encodes the heparin-binding domain of antithrombin III. Patients with a type I or type II deficiency state can have thromboembolic events when they are heterozygous. In contrast, individuals with type III deficiency suffer from thrombosis only if they are homozygous.

Acquired antithrombin III deficiency can be caused by decreased production, increased consumption, or increased loss of the protein. At present it is unclear whether patients

Table 2 Classification of Congenital Antithrombin III Deficiency

Type I	Quantitative defect	Immunologic and functional activity reduced
Type II	Qualitative defect	Functional activity reduced; immunologic activity normal
Type III	Abnormal heparin binding	Functional activity reduced in the presence of heparin; immunologic activity normal

with an acquired deficiency are predisposed to thrombosis. Since antithrombin III is synthesized in the liver, decreased production occurs in patients with severe liver disease. Increased thrombin generation in patients with intravascular coagulation or extensive thrombosis can lead to antithrombin III consumption. Heparin accelerates antithrombin III clearance, causing a modest loss of the protein; large amounts of antithrombin III may be lost in the urine of patients with the nephrotic syndrome. Treatment with L-asparaginase also lowers plasma levels of antithrombin III. Finally, the levels of antithrombin III are decreased to about 50 percent of the adult values in the newborn and gradually reach adult levels by 6 months.

Although reductions in antithrombin III levels were reported in women taking birth control pills containing high doses of estrogen, this may be less of a problem with the newer oral contraceptive agents that contain considerably smaller amounts of estrogen. Low-dose estrogen used for postmenopausal replacement therapy does not appear to reduce antithrombin III levels.

Protein C

Congenital protein C deficiency occurs in 1 in 200 to 300 individuals within the general population. In some kindreds with protein C deficiency there is a high incidence of venous thrombosis in affected individuals, and inheritance is thought to follow an autosomal dominant pattern. However, in other families heterozygous protein C–deficient individuals do not appear to have an increased risk of thrombosis. This finding has led to the suggestion that there are two patterns of inheritance that differ in phenotypic expression. Thus, in families where thrombosis is rare in affected individuals there may be a recessive pattern of inheritance, with thrombosis developing only in subjects who are double heterozygotes or homozygotes.

Acquired protein C deficiency can be caused by decreased production or increased consumption. Protein C is synthesized in the liver, where it undergoes post-translational gamma-carboxylation through a vitamin K–dependent process. Decreased production occurs in patients with severe liver disease and in those who are vitamin K deficient or are taking vitamin K antagonists such as warfarin. Consumption of protein C occurs in disorders associated with increased thrombin generation such as intravascular coagulation and massive thrombosis. Protein C levels are lower in neonates (about 20 to 40 percent of adult values) and rise slowly after birth, reaching adult levels in adolescence.

Protein S

Congenital protein S deficiency is transmitted in an autosomal dominant fashion. Two forms of the deficiency are often encountered. Some kindreds have an approximately 50 percent reduction in total protein S associated with an appropriate decrease in the amount of free protein S. Other families have little or no reduction in the levels of total protein S but have markedly reduced free protein S because most of the protein is complexed to C4bBP. The shift in protein S to the bound form is not the result of elevated levels of C4bBP, and it may reflect an increased affinity of the protein S for its binding protein. The molecular basis for this type of an alteration remains to be determined.

Acquired deficiency of protein S may be more common than congenital deficiencies because increased levels of C4bBP will decrease the proportion of free protein S. The levels of C4bBP are increased in patients with systemic lupus erythematosus and other diseases of the connective tissues. Although total protein S levels are increased in patients with nephrotic syndrome, the amount of free protein S is actually reduced because of the marked elevation in the levels of C4bBP. There is a slight decrease in free protein S during pregnancy. Oral contraceptives cause a decrease in total protein S levels, but because of a concomitant decrease in the levels of C4bBP, the free protein S levels remain unchanged. Finally, as with protein C, protein S levels are decreased with liver disease, vitamin K deficiency, warfarin administration, massive thrombosis, or intravascular coagulation. Neonates have little or no C4bBP, so most of the protein S is in the free form.

■ DIAGNOSIS

General Principles of Laboratory Testing

Whenever possible, laboratory testing for antithrombin III, protein C, or protein S deficiency should be performed when the patient is not receiving anticoagulants. If anticoagulant therapy is indicated because of an acute thrombotic event, the optimal time for testing is prior to starting treatment. In patients already receiving anticoagulant therapy, assays are best done during heparin therapy because oral anticoagulants decrease the levels of protein C and protein S. Since heparin can reduce the levels of antithrombin III, a low value should be confirmed when the patient is taking oral anticoagulants. However, there are reports that warfarin therapy can increase antithrombin III levels to normal in occasional patients with congenital antithrombin III deficiency. Family studies may be necessary to exclude this possibility.

Before making the diagnosis of a deficiency state, the tests should be repeated on at least three occasions, and comorbid conditions that can cause a falsely low result should be excluded. Once the diagnosis is established, family studies are needed to identify carriers. This is important because asymptomatic carriers will require counseling about the need for prophylaxis in high-risk situations.

Both functional and immunologic assays for antithrombin III and protein C are available and should be used to identify the type I and type II deficiency states. Since type I deficiency states are the result of decreased synthesis of the protein, there is a parallel reduction in functional and immunologic activity. In contrast, the dysfunctional protein synthesized in type II deficiency states has decreased functional activity despite normal immunologic activity.

Testing for Antithrombin III Deficiency

Assays for antithrombin III activity should be performed in the presence of heparin so that type III deficiencies can be identified. Chromogenic assays are superior to clotting assays, and tests of factor Xa inhibition may be better than assays of thrombin neutralization in this setting because tests of thrombin inhibition may overestimate the levels of antithrombin III. This occurs because heparin cofactor II can inhibit the added thrombin when the antithrombin III levels are decreased. One of two methods can be used to circumvent this potential problem. First, the neutralization of factor Xa rather than thrombin can be measured, since unlike antithrombin III, heparin cofactor II does not inhibit factor Xa. Alternatively, if a test of thrombin inhibition is used to measure antithrombin III activity, bovine thrombin should be used in place of human thrombin because the bovine enzyme is not readily neutralized by human heparin cofactor II.

Testing for Protein C Deficiency

Like antithrombin III, protein C activity in plasma can be measured with either a chromogenic substrate or with a clotting assay. In both cases, protein C is first activated by the venom from the Southern copperhead snake *(Agkistrodon contortrix)*. The levels of resultant activated protein C are then measured chromogenically or by monitoring the extent to which the APTT is prolonged.

Assays for activated protein C resistance depend on measurements of the anticoagulant response to activated protein C. Thus, the extent to which the addition of activated protein C prolongs the APTT in patient plasma is compared with its effect in pooled plasma from healthy volunteers. Since the ratio of the APTT before and after activated protein C addition is calculated, even patients receiving anticoagulants can be evaluated for this defect.

Testing for Protein S Deficiency

Protein S levels are most often measured immunologically. Although antigenic determinations will measure both free and bound protein S, the free protein S fraction can be quantified after the protein S bound to C4bBP has been precipitated with polyethylene glycol. Functional assays for protein S also are available and are based on its capacity to serve as a cofactor for activated protein C. Thus, patient plasma is added to protein S–depleted plasma, and tests of protein C activity are performed.

■ MANAGEMENT

Treatment decisions in patients with antithrombin III, protein C, or protein S deficiency center on the management of acute events, the need for long-term anticoagulant therapy, the role of anticoagulants in asymptomatic patients, and the management of any high-risk situation such as pregnancy or surgery.

Acute Events

In addition to treatment of acute thrombosis in patients with deficiencies of antithrombin III, protein C, or protein S, the management of patients with warfarin-induced skin necrosis and purpura fulminans will be considered.

Acute Thrombosis

As with any patient with documented thromboembolic disease, heparin is used for the treatment of acute events, and warfarin is used for secondary prophylaxis. In patients with antithrombin III deficiency, heparin is given for 5 to 10 days, and warfarin is started after 24 to 48 hours using a regimen that produces an INR of 2.0 to 3.0. Since patients with known protein C or protein S deficiency are at risk for the development of warfarin-induced skin necrosis, warfarin should be delayed in these individuals until the heparin has produced a therapeutic anticoagulant response. It is also reasonable to use lower doses of warfarin at the outset in patients with protein C or protein S deficiency. Thus, warfarin can be started at maintenance doses of 5 mg daily rather than the usual 10 mg per day. Heparin treatment should be continued until the INR has been therapeutic for 3 to 4 days. Using this approach, the two anticoagulants should be overlapped for at least 7 days.

Since heparin acts as an anticoagulant by catalyzing antithrombin III, patients with antithrombin III deficiency may be expected to be resistant to heparin. Although this can occur in rare individuals with marked antithrombin III deficiency, most patients will have a satisfactory anticoagulant response to heparin, although they may require higher doses. The possibility of heparin resistance can be excluded by measuring the APTT 15 to 30 minutes after 5,000 U of heparin is given intravenously as a bolus. If there is no prolongation of the APTT, antithrombin III concentrate or plasma should be given concomitantly with the heparin. Infusion of antithrombin III concentrate at a dose of 50 U per kilogram will usually raise the plasma antithrombin III level to about 120 percent in a congenitally deficient individual with a baseline level that is 50 percent of normal. Since the biologic half-life of antithrombin III is about 48 hours, daily infusions of antithrombin III concentrates are usually adequate. Thus, to maintain the plasma antithrombin III level above 80 percent, infusions of 60 percent of the initial dose are recommended at 24 hour intervals.

Warfarin-Induced Skin Necrosis

Patients with protein C deficiency and to a lesser extent those with deficiencies of protein S are at increased risk for warfarin-induced skin necrosis during the first week of therapy. The disorder frequently affects the skin of the flanks, breasts, or thighs and is characterized by well-demarcated erythematous lesions with necrotic centers. Histologically there is thrombosis of the venules and capillaries of the skin, which may reflect a transient hypercoagulable state that occurs shortly after the initiation of warfarin. This can occur because like factor VII, protein C has a relatively short half-life, so its level decreases rapidly after warfarin is started. In contrast, the other vitamin K–dependent clotting factors have longer half-lives and disappear more slowly. In patients with pre-existing protein C deficiency, therefore, the further decrease in the protein C level produced by warfarin leads to a transient loss of the regulatory pathway before the anticoagulant effects of warfarin are fully established. The loss of the protein C anticoagulant pathway causes a hypercoagulable state that can lead to thrombosis.

Even in patients with protein C or protein S deficiency, warfarin-induced skin necrosis is relatively uncommon. These observations suggest that in addition to a transient hypercoagulable state, other factors may be involved. In particular, concurrent inflammation may play a role, because the skin necrosis frequently occurs in areas involved in an inflammatory process. This may reflect the internalization of thrombomodulin in the capillaries of the skin that can occur in response to inflammatory cytokines. In conjunction with warfarin-induced protein C or protein S deficiency, the loss of local thrombomodulin further promotes thrombosis at these sites.

Warfarin should be discontinued and vitamin K should be given to patients with established skin necrosis. Heparin should be started if there is a need for continued anticoagulant therapy. However, heparin therapy will not reverse the skin necrosis, and surgical debridement and grafting may be necessary if the necrosis involves the full thickness of the skin.

If available, protein C concentrates should be given to patients with protein C deficiency who develop warfarin-induced skin necrosis. A test dose of 10 U per kilogram is given intravenously over 10 minutes, and if there is no allergic reaction, the product is given intravenously at a dose of 40 U per kilogram, aiming for a plasma protein C level of 80 to 100 percent of the normal adult value. This dose is based on the estimate that 1 U per kilogram of protein C concentrate increases the plasma protein C level by 2 percent. The frequency of protein C administration will depend on the half-life of the protein, which should be measured in each patient. Since protein C usually has a half-life of about 6 hours, the concentrate will have to be given two to three times daily. At present there are no commercially available protein S concentrates. Although fresh frozen plasma can be used as a source of protein S in protein S–deficient patients with warfarin-induced skin necrosis, the value of this approach is uncertain.

Patients with documented warfarin-induced skin necrosis who require long-term anticoagulant therapy can be maintained on therapeutic doses of subcutaneous heparin, but this approach is not only inconvenient, it also is associated with a risk of osteoporosis. As an alternative, it may be safe to reintroduce warfarin once the skin necrosis has completely resolved provided that it is started in low doses (e.g., 2 mg per day) and concomitant heparin is given in therapeutic amounts until the INR has been therapeutic for 4 to 5 days.

Purpura Fulminans Neonatalis

Infants with homozygous protein C deficiency or double heterozygotes with virtually undetectable levels of protein C may develop extensive cutaneous thrombosis on the first or second day after birth. Disseminated intravascular coagulation may accompany the skin lesions, and thrombosis in the cerebral and ophthalmic vessels can cause seizures, hydrocephalus, or blindness.

Protein C concentrates are the treatment of choice for purpura fulminans neonatalis. Concentrates are given two to three times daily, in amounts sufficient to raise the plasma protein C level to 100 percent. If protein C concentrates are not immediately available, fresh frozen plasma should be given at 15 ml per kilogram twice daily as a temporary source of protein C. Treatment with protein C concentrates is continued until the skin lesions resolve and definitive therapy with warfarin is given. Warfarin can be started at 3 to 6 months of age in doses sufficient to prolong the INR to 3.0 to 4.5. A higher intensity of anticoagulation is recommended to prevent recurrent thrombotic events and skin necrosis. Protein C concentrates can be discontinued once the INR has been therapeutic for several days.

Patients with homozygous protein C deficiency require indefinite anticoagulant therapy. If oral anticoagulants must be discontinued because of hemorrhagic complications or in preparation for surgery, replacement therapy with protein C concentrates should be given and prophylactic measures should be used to prevent thrombotic complications. For example, if the patient is bleeding, intermittent pneumatic compression can be used in conjunction with protein C replacement to prevent deep vein thrombosis, and adjusted-dose standard heparin or low molecular-weight heparin can be used as prophylaxis in surgical patients.

Duration of Anticoagulant Therapy

Patients with antithrombin III, protein C, or protein S deficiency who have had a documented episode of thrombosis should be considered as candidates for lifelong anticoagulant therapy. This is particularly important for patients whose thrombosis occurred spontaneously or for those with recurrent thrombotic events. A possible exception may be patients with a single episode of thrombosis that occurred after major surgery or trauma. Rather than subjecting these individuals to the possible side effects of long-term anticoagulant therapy, consideration should be given to vigorous prophylaxis at times of risk.

In general, patients with antithrombin III, protein C, or protein S deficiency respond well to anticoagulant therapy with warfarin, and recurrences are unusual. A moderate-intensity regimen is recommended, with the warfarin dose adjusted to achieve an INR of 2.0 to 3.0. If the patient remains free of recurrence for several years, it may be reasonable to lower the intensity of warfarin therapy to achieve an INR of 1.5 to 2.0. Although the lower-intensity regimen will reduce the risk of bleeding, it has not yet been proven to be effective in this patient population.

Heparin should be given to patients who develop documented recurrent thrombosis despite an INR of 2.0 to 3.0. Initially, full doses of heparin should be given intravenously. The patient can then be switched to subcutaneous heparin given twice daily in doses that produce a therapeutic APTT 6 hours after heparin injection. The heparin dose should be sufficient to achieve a heparin level of 0.2 to 0.4 U per milliliter as measured by protamine titration. The usual mean daily dose needed to reach this heparin level is 30,000 to 35,000 U. Long-term subcutaneous heparin in therapeutic doses can cause bruising and discomfort at the injection sites, which can be reduced by giving the heparin through an indwelling subcutaneous catheter that contains an injection port. These catheters, which are often used by diabetics for insulin administration, are inserted into the subcutaneous fat of the abdomen and are changed every 5 to 7 days.

Since long-term subcutaneous heparin is inconvenient and can produce osteoporosis, it may be reasonable to restart warfarin after 6 to 8 weeks, aiming for an INR of 3.0 to 4.5. If there is documented recurrent thrombosis on this warfarin regimen, long-term treatment with subcutaneous heparin may be necessary. Low molecular-weight heparin may be better than standard heparin in this setting because less frequent laboratory monitoring is needed. In addition, the low molecular-weight heparin can be given once daily, and the risk of osteoporosis may be lower.

Management of Asymptomatic Patients

There is considerable uncertainty as to the optimal management of asymptomatic individuals with deficiencies of antithrombin III, protein C, or protein S. To a large extent this uncertainty reflects a lack of reliable information on the true risk of unprovoked thromboembolic events in asymptomatic carriers. To make a rational decision as to whether or not lifelong anticoagulant therapy is indicated, three critical pieces of information are needed. These are (1) the total incidence of thrombosis in patients with a deficiency of antithrombin III, protein C, or protein S, (2) the proportion of thrombotic events that are idiopathic and the proportion that are secondary to well-recognized risk factors, and (3) the probability that the presenting thrombotic event will be fatal. This information is vital to rational decision making. If, for example, the overall event rate is low, the risks and inconvenience of long-term anticoagulant therapy will outweigh any benefits. Continuous anticoagulant therapy also could be avoided if a large proportion of thrombotic events were secondary to well-defined risk factors, since in this case effective primary prophylaxis would be sufficient to prevent clinically important thrombotic events in most patients. Finally, if only a very small proportion of presenting events are unprovoked and fatal, it can be argued that it would be preferable to begin treatment after the first nonfatal event rather than expose asymptomatic carriers to the risks of primary prophylaxis over the course of many years.

Using the best estimates available from a critical review of the literature, answers to these questions are beginning to emerge. The reported incidence of thrombosis appears to be similar in all three of the deficiency states. The risk of thrombosis is low in the first 15 years of life (about 0.1 to 0.2 percent per year) and then increases to a reported average of 3 percent per year. After age 15 the risk appears to be continuous throughout life , with no evidence of a decrease in later years.

It is quite likely that the event rates reported in the literature are falsely high for at least two reasons. First, families with large numbers of affected individuals are more likely to be reported than those with only a few affected family members. Second, the diagnosis of thrombosis has often been based on clinical findings that are not specific. Support for the concept that thrombotic events are over-reported in the literature comes from the observation that the incidence of thrombosis in nonaffected family members of patients with antithrombin III, protein C, or protein S deficiency is considerably higher than what would be expected in the general population. After correction for this apparent over-reporting, the incidence of thromboembolic events in patients with antithrombin III, protein C, or protein S deficiency decreases from 3 percent per year to somewhere between 0.4 and 1.2 percent per year.

Recognizable risk factors are identified in 30 to 70 percent of patients presenting with their first thrombotic event. Most of these events are likely to respond to therapy, and therefore, the frequency of fatal events is exceedingly low. Based on these considerations, it is reasonable to withhold anticoagulants until a thrombotic event occurs, sparing the patient the inconvenience and the potential complications of long-term anticoagulant therapy. Exceptions include patients with a family history of fatal thrombotic events or other serious thromboembolic problems. If a watch-and-wait approach is used, however, prophylaxis should be given whenever the patient is at risk for thrombosis.

Management of High-Risk Situations

Patients with deficiencies of antithrombin III, protein C, or protein S require vigorous prophylaxis perioperatively and during periods of immobilization or bed rest. Pregnancy may also be a risk factor for thrombotic events, particularly in those with antithrombin III or protein C deficiency. Each of these situations will be discussed in turn.

Prophylaxis

Asymptomatic individuals with antithrombin III, protein C, or protein S deficiency who are not on anticoagulants require vigorous prophylaxis perioperatively or when immobilized because of medical illness. Effective methods of prophylaxis include oral anticoagulants, adjusted-dose standard heparin, and low molecular-weight heparin, but warfarin should be avoided in patients with protein C or protein S deficiency because of the risk of skin necrosis. In patients undergoing major surgical procedures, prophylaxis with warfarin or low molecular-weight heparin is usually started postoperatively to avoid excessive bleeding. Warfarin is started on the first postoperative day and is given in amounts sufficient to prolong the INR to 2.0 to 3.0. Low molecular-weight heparin is started 12 to 24 hours after surgery in doses that depend on the preparation. For enoxaparin the recommended prophylactic dose is 30 mg subcutaneously twice daily. When standard heparin is given in adjusted doses, it is started 2 days prior to surgery at 3,500 U subcutaneously three times daily. The dose is then adjusted to maintain the APTT at the upper limit of the normal range. Antiembolic stockings can be used in conjunction with any of these methods of prophylaxis, and early mobilization should be encouraged. Prophylaxis should be continued until the patient is fully ambulatory.

Patients on long-term anticoagulant therapy are more complicated to manage. For minor surgical procedures, such as dental extractions, the warfarin dose can be decreased preoperatively and the procedure done when the INR is between 1.5 and 1.8. The warfarin dose can then be increased postoperatively to achieve a therapeutic INR.

For major surgical procedures the warfarin will have to be discontinued, and reversal with vitamin K_1 may be needed for those who require urgent surgery. Once warfarin is stopped, therapeutic doses of heparin can be given intravenously for anticoagulant coverage prior to surgery. The heparin should be discontinued 3 to 4 hours preoperatively and can be restarted 12 to 24 hours after surgery once hemostasis is obtained. It is reasonable to restart heparin at maintenance doses, without giving a bolus, to reduce the bleeding risk. Warfarin can be restarted postoperatively, and the heparin can be discontinued when the INR has been therapeutic for several days. Patients with protein C or protein S deficiency should be started on lower doses of warfarin (e.g., 5 mg per day) to prevent skin necrosis, and heparin should be continued until the INR has been therapeutic for 3 to 4 days.

Pregnancy

Antithrombin III, protein C, or protein S deficiency in women has special implications with regards to pregnancy. Descriptive studies suggest that there is a risk of thrombosis during pregnancy in patients with antithrombin III and protein C deficiency and that patients with all three deficiency states are at high risk for thrombosis in the postpartum period. However, the correct approach to management is uncertain because properly designed clinical trials have yet to be done.

Patients on lifelong oral anticoagulants who wish to become pregnant should be advised of the risks. If pregnancy is still desired, a reasonable and practical approach is to recommend frequent home pregnancy tests after the first missed period. Once the test is positive, oral anticoagulants should be discontinued, because warfarin has fetopathic effects, particularly when taken between 6 and 12 weeks of gestation. Heparin is then given in therapeutic doses by subcutaneous injection. Starting with 15,000 U twice daily, the dose of heparin should be adjusted to maintain the midinterval APTT in the therapeutic range.

Although practical, this approach assumes that warfarin is safe during the first 4 to 6 weeks of gestation. Evidence in the literature suggests that the risk of warfarin embryopathy is highest between 6 and 12 weeks gestation, but the possibility that it can produce defects when given earlier in pregnancy cannot be fully excluded. Warfarin can be totally avoided during pregnancy by giving heparin, or by the infusion of antithrombin III or protein C concentrates as soon as the patient wishes to become pregnant. However, these approaches are impractical and may have adverse side effects. The use of subcutaneous heparin while awaiting conception and throughout the pregnancy will expose the patient to many months of heparin treatment,increasing the risk of osteoporosis. Replacement therapy with antithrombin III or protein C concentrates until conception occurs is not an attractive alternative because these products require such frequent administration.

Heparin should be given throughout pregnancy and discontinued when labor starts. Since the anticoagulant effects of subcutaneous heparin can persist for more than 24 hours in this patient population, my approach is to stop the heparin 24 hours before elective induction of labor. If an anticoagulant effect is encountered during delivery, protamine sulfate can be given to neutralize the heparin. To prevent thrombosis during delivery, consideration can be given to the use of antithrombin III or protein C concentrates, although these may not be necessary if anticoagulants are discontinued for only a short time.

Heparin should be restarted after delivery and continued for at least an additional 6 weeks, because these patients are at high risk for thrombosis in the postpartum period. In antithrombin III-deficient subjects, warfarin can be given in place of heparin in the postpartum period, since it does not produce an anticoagulant effect in the breastfed infant. Warfarin should not be used in patients with protein C or protein S deficiency because of the risk of skin necrosis.

The best approach for the management of asymptomatic individuals with antithrombin III, protein C, or protein S deficiency who were not on anticoagulants prior to pregnancy is uncertain. A reasonable approach is to give low-dose subcutaneous heparin (5,000 U twice daily) throughout the pregnancy. If subcutaneous heparin is not well tolerated, an alternative is to monitor these patients for the development of deep vein thrombosis using impedance plethysmography or duplex ultrasound imaging. This should be done at regular intervals throughout the pregnancy. After delivery, prophylaxis with subcutaneous heparin should be given for 6 weeks. Warfarin can be used in place of heparin in patients with antithrombin III deficiency.

Other Considerations

In general, oral contraceptives should not be used in asymptomatic patients with antithrombin III, protein C, or protein S deficiency, although the thrombotic risks associated with oral contraceptives that contain low doses of estrogen are unknown. If the patient is receiving warfarin, it is probably safe to give oral contraceptives, even though this approach has never been evaluated in clinical trials. In any case, because of the potential teratogenic effects of warfarin, effective birth control is mandatory in women of childbearing potential who are receiving oral anticoagulants.

The doses of estrogen used for replacement therapy in postmenopausal women are in the physiologic range and are considerably lower than those found in oral contraceptives. Thus, it is our belief that estrogen replacement therapy is not contraindicated in this patient population. Further studies are needed to test this concept.

Suggested Reading

Blajechman MA, Austin RC, Fernandes-Rachubinski F, Sheffield WP. Molecular basis of inherited human antithrombin III deficiency. Blood 1992; 80:2159–2171.

Conrad J, Horellou MH, Van Dreden P, et al. Thrombosis and pregnancy in congenital deficiencies in AT III, protein C or protein S: Study of 78 women. Thromb Haemos 1990; 63:319–320.

Dahlback B. Physiological anticoagulation: Resistance to activated protein C and venous thromboembolism. J Clin Invest 1994; 94:923–927.

Dahlback B, Carlsson M, Svensson PJ. Familial thrombophilia due to a previously unrecognized mechanism characterized by poor anticoagulant response to activated protein C: Prediction of a cofactor to activated protein C. Proc Natl Acad Sci (USA) 1993; 90:1004–1008.

Esmon CT. The roles of protein C and thrombomodulin in the regulation of blood coagulation. J Biol Chem 1989; 264:743–746.

Griffin JH, Evatt B, Wideman C, Fernandez JA. Anticoagulant protein C pathway defective in majority of thrombophilia patients. Blood 1993; 82:1989–1993.

Heijboer H, Brandjes DPM, Buller HR, et al. Deficiencies of coagulation-inhibiting and fibrinolytic proteins in outpatients with deep vein thrombosis. N Engl J Med 1990; 323:1512–1516.

DRUG-INDUCED THROMBOCYTOPENIA (INCLUDING HEPARIN-INDUCED THROMBOCYTOPENIA)

John G. Kelton, M.D.
Theodore E. Warkentin, M.D., F.A.C.P.C., F.A.C.P.

Drug-induced thrombocytopenia should be considered in any patient who develops unexpected thrombocytopenia. Virtually any drug can produce an idiosyncratic (immune-mediated) destructive thrombocytopenia, but only a few drugs appear to be responsible for most episodes. There are two prototypic drug-induced syndromes. Heparin-induced thrombocytopenia usually presents in hospitalized patients. The other, drug-induced immune thrombocytopenic purpura, often occurs in outpatients and is best exemplified by quinine and quinidine.

In addition to dramatically different clinical presentations (Table 1), it is now clear that these two drug-induced syndromes have very different pathophysiologic bases. In quinine-induced thrombocytopenia the antigen-recognizing arms of the pathogenic IgG interact with a quinine-platelet antigen complex, leaving the IgG Fc tail to be recognized by the Fc receptors of reticuloendothelial cells. This leads to rapid IgG-mediated platelet clearance and results in severe thrombocytopenia and bleeding. This contrasts markedly with heparin-induced thrombocytopenia. Here the pathogenic IgG also recognizes a drug-platelet complex. In contrast, however, the IgG Fc component interacts with the platelet Fc receptors, which is a potent trigger of platelet activation. Thus, although the severity of thrombocytopenia is usually much less in heparin-induced thrombocytopenia, paradoxic thrombotic complications rather than bleeding can result.

■ DRUG-INDUCED IMMUNE THROMBOCYTOPENIC PURPURA

Many drugs can cause an abrupt-onset thrombocytopenic syndrome that closely resembles acute idiopathic (immune) thrombocytopenic purpura. Although many dozens of drugs have been implicated, relatively few drugs have been well characterized both clinically and in the laboratory as causing this syndrome. These include quinine, quinidine, sulfa drugs, rifampin, vancomycin, ampicillin, gold, digoxin, and ibuprofen. A recent case-control study examined the use of drugs in patients presenting with acute drug-induced thrombocytopenia. This study found the following drugs to be the most likely explanations for the thrombocytopenia: trimethoprim or sulfamethoxazole, quinine, quinidine, dipyridamole, sulfonylureas, and aspirin. Many patients are not aware of their exposure to quinine, a substance found in a variety of foods such as tonic water *(cocktail purpura).*

Typically, patients present with mucocutaneous bleeding symptoms. Physical signs are usually limited to purpura and mucosal hemorrhages. The platelet count is usually less than 20×10^9 per liter, with normal hemoglobin and white count. Deaths from intracranial or pulmonary hemorrhage have been reported.

As drug-induced thrombocytopenia is a life-threatening disorder, the clinician must discontinue all suspect drugs, substituting them with molecularly distinct replacement agents as needed. The diagnosis is usually made on clinical grounds alone, as in vitro laboratory confirmation is not always available or reliable. This is because drug-dependent platelet antibody testing is usually performed only in very specialized laboratories. Moreover, the responsible antigen may be a drug metabolite that is not readily available for in vitro testing.

For actively bleeding patients, the combination of platelet transfusions and high-dose intravenous IgG (IVIgG) can be effective in raising the platelet count. We give platelet transfusions followed by IVIgG 1 g per kilogram over 6 hours. After the IVIgG infusion further platelet transfusions may be required. In most instances this approach will raise the platelet count to safe levels. Sometimes further IVIgG will be needed 1 or 2 days later. We try IVIgG alone in patients without active bleeding who are judged to be at high risk for life-threatening bleeding (e.g., numerous petechiae and oral mucosal hemorrhages). Prednisone is often given, but its benefit in this disorder remains unproven.

■ HEPARIN-INDUCED THROMBOCYTOPENIA

Heparin-induced thrombocytopenia (HIT) for several reasons is the most important allergic drug reaction that most physicians encounter. First, it has a relatively high frequency, particularly compared with other immune drug-induced thrombocytopenic disorders. For example, about 1 in 20 patients receiving therapeutic doses of heparin for more than

Table 1 A Comparison Between Quinine or Quinidine-Induced Thrombocytopenia and Heparin-Induced Thrombocytopenia

	FREQUENCY	PLATELET NADIR	THROMBOTIC COMPLICATIONS
Quinine, quinidine	0.1–0.2%	$<20 \times 10^9$/L	No*
Heparin	1–10%	$20–100 \times 10^9$/L	Yes (10–20% of thrombocytopenic patients†)

*Rarely, patients develop a disorder resembling hemolytic-uremic syndrome secondary to quinine.
†The risk of thrombosis varies with the patient population.

Table 2 Risk of Heparin-Induced Thrombocytopenia for Different Heparin Preparations Given at Different Doses*

HEPARIN PREPARATION	DOSE (UNITS PER 24 HOURS)	RISK OF HIT
Bovine	Full dose (20,000–40,000)	10%
Porcine	Full dose (20,000–40,000)	5
Porcine	Intermediate dose (15,000)	3
Porcine	Low dose (5,000–10,000)	<1
Low molecular-weight heparin	Intermediate	<1

*Note that the risk for HIT does not generally begin until the patient has received heparin for at least five days.

5 days will develop HIT. In contrast, about 1 in 1,000 patients treated with quinine develop thrombocytopenia. Second, the indications for heparin use are broadening, since heparin is the major readily available antithrombotic agent with rapid onset of action. Third, HIT is unique among immune thrombocytopenic disorders in that it is often complicated by paradoxic thrombosis.

Frequency

The risk of HIT varies among heparin preparations and doses (Table 2). For example, heparin of bovine origin carries a higher risk of thrombocytopenia than porcine heparin. The frequency of HIT also depends upon the platelet count definition used. Consequently, if 100×10^9 per liter is used to define thrombocytopenia, the risk of HIT is approximately 5 percent for bovine heparin and 2 to 3 percent for porcine heparin (therapeutic doses). However, the frequency increases if a higher platelet count threshold is used (e.g., 150×10^9 per liter). Indeed, it is our experience that some patients with laboratory-proven heparin-dependent IgG can develop a platelet count fall plus an unexpected thrombotic event, although the platelet count nadir never falls below 150×10^9 per liter.

The risk of HIT is higher for patients receiving therapeutic doses of heparin (typically 20,000 to 40,000 U in 24 hours). The frequency declines with lower doses of heparin, but the syndrome can occur even in patients receiving small doses of heparin to maintain intravascular catheters. Recognizing this risk, we believe it is not acceptable to use heparin flushes to maintain venous catheters.

Diagnosis

The diagnosis of HIT is usually made on clinical grounds. In our experience a patient whose platelet count begins to fall 5 to 8 days after starting heparin is likely to have HIT. The platelet count can decrease earlier if the patient has been previously exposed to heparin, particularly during the previous few weeks or months. Sometimes the platelet count fall is dramatic. At other times it falls gradually, taking several days to reach thrombocytopenic levels if it ever does. In contrast to the drug-induced immune thrombocytopenic purpura syndrome, the platelet count usually does not fall below 20×10^9 per liter. Most often it varies from 20 to 150×10^9 per liter (median nadir reported in the literature approximately 50×10^9 per liter). The occasional HIT patient with a platelet count below 20×10^9 per liter in our experience usually has laboratory evidence of disseminated intravascular coagulation (DIC).

Because of the danger of thrombotic sequelae in HIT, the physician should err on the side of overdiagnosing the condition and stop the heparin as soon as possible. But, unfortunately many patients will still develop thrombotic complications even after the heparin is stopped. A number of laboratory tests have been investigated for their usefulness in diagnosing HIT. The measurement of platelet aggregation using platelet-rich plasma or heparin-dependent binding of IgG to normal platelets has relatively poor sensitivity and specificity for HIT. However, the laboratory diagnosis of HIT is improved dramatically by using washed platelets in the test system. A characteristic pattern of platelet activation is produced by positive HIT sera-platelet activation at therapeutic heparin concentrations (0.1 to 0.3 U per milliliter) but absent platelet activation at very high heparin concentrations (100 U per milliliter). The "gold standard" assay for diagnosing HIT uses platelet release of radioactive serotonin as the marker of activation. It is important to use carefully selected platelet donors because platelets from different donors vary with respect to their ability to be activated by heparin-dependent IgG. Because of the complexity of this test and the requirement for radioactive markers, most laboratories do not use it. Consequently, HIT is frequently diagnosed on clinical grounds. It is important to recognize that the pathogenic antibody (an IgG) rapidly disappears from the circulation, and if there is an interval of several weeks to months following an episode of HIT, the test is invariably negative. A negative test for HIT using such a late serum sample cannot be relied on to rule out the previous diagnosis of HIT.

Thrombotic Complications

HIT is unique among drug-induced thrombocytopenic syndromes because it can be complicated by venous or arterial thrombotic events. In our experience venous thrombotic complications (proximal deep vein thrombosis, pulmonary embolism) are the most frequent complications observed in HIT patients. Arterial thrombosis most characteristically involves the distal aorta or major lower limb arteries, but thrombotic stroke, myocardial infarction, and mesenteric artery thrombosis are all well-described sequelae of HIT. HIT also causes other bizarre events such as adrenal hemorrhagic infarction (usually bilateral and therefore an important cause of acute or chronic adrenal failure), cerebral dural sinus thrombosis, and painful red lesions or even skin necrosis at sites of heparin injection. We have also observed abrupt falls in the platelet count accompanied by dramatic systemic reactions (including fever, chills, tachycardia, flushing, and dyspnea) and even transient global amnesia (a self-limited syndrome of severe anterograde amnesia) following intravenous bolus heparin administration to HIT patients. Indeed, the more unusual the thrombotic event in a patient receiving heparin, the higher should be the index of suspicion for HIT.

The risk of thrombosis appears to vary with the patient population. Thrombotic events may occur in as many as 50 percent of patients already at high risk for venous thrombosis (e.g., postoperative orthopedic patients). Although thrombotic events can occur during the early phases of a platelet count fall, in many patients the thrombocytopenia precedes the thrombosis by several days. Consequently, it is important to monitor the platelet count frequently (we recommend daily platelet counts) in patients receiving heparin and to be prepared to stop the heparin if thrombocytopenia occurs.

Therapy

It is important for clinicians to have a high level of awareness of HIT. Often patients with HIT are not diagnosed until they have developed a thrombotic complication. Our clinical approach to treatment depends on whether patients have a thrombosis that requires further anticoagulation or whether isolated thrombocytopenia has occurred in a patient who was receiving heparin for prophylaxis. We recommend that oral anticoagulants (e.g., warfarin) not be started in patients with acute HIT. This is because our experience suggests that a warfarin-induced drop in protein C (a natural anticoagulant) level can trigger or worsen thrombotic complications in these patients.

Patients who require further anticoagulation because of a confirmed venous thrombotic event should receive an alternative anticoagulant, discussed subsequently. For patients without proven or suspected thrombosis, we discontinue the heparin and closely monitor the HIT patients with isolated thrombocytopenia. However, some of these patients can subsequently develop a new thrombotic event, which has included sudden pulmonary embolism, particularly during the first week following recognition of the HIT. It is possible that alternative prophylactic anticoagulation is indicated even for these patients with isolated HIT. However, the lack of readily available alternative anticoagulant agents with a rapid onset of action and the risk that accompanies warfarin in this setting means that most of these patients are managed by discontinuation of the heparin alone.

There are several approaches for patients with a proven thrombosis who definitely require further anticoagulation. We have experience with the snake venom ancrod (Arvin). This agent produces a controlled defibrinogenation of the patient. A dose of 1 U per kilogram given slowly over 8 to 12 hours reduces the fibrinogen to below 0.5 g per liter, anticoagulating the patient. Smaller doses often must be administered every 1 to 2 days to maintain anticoagulation. It is important not to administer ancrod quickly, as microvascular thrombosis can result from overwhelming the natural clearance mechanisms for the fibrin polymers generated. Monitoring requires using an assay for clottable fibrinogen (Clauss assay) rather than determination of a derived fibrinogen; these latter optically based techniques can dramatically overestimate the true fibrinogen level following use of ancrod. We have some experience with this treatment and have found it an acceptable way to anticoagulate many patients with HIT. We would not use ancrod in those patients with severe HIT who already are hypofibrinogenemic secondary to DIC.

Some physicians have treated HIT patients with a heparinoid, Org 10172 (Orgaran). This is a mixture of glycosaminoglycans (particularly low-sulfated heparan and dermatan sulfate) with anticoagulant activity. We generally administer a loading dose (400 U per hour for 4 hours, then 300 U per hour for 4 hours), followed by maintenance doses starting at 200 U per hour, with subsequent dose adjustments made using anti-Xa levels; target range is 0.5 to 0.8 anti-Xa units. A potential advantage of this agent is its anti-Xa anticoagulant activity, which can inhibit the marked thrombin generation seen in some patients with severe HIT. A disadvantage of Org 10172 is that it sometimes cross-reacts with the pathogenic heparin-dependent IgG, which can result in persisting thrombocytopenia or even initiation of new thrombotic events (estimated at 10 percent). Another disadvantage is that monitoring of the anticoagulant effect involves measurement of anti-Xa levels.

Neither ancrod nor Org 10172 is as yet available in the United States, although either can be obtained in appropriate circumstances (compassionate release) from the manufacturer. No comparative trials have been performed to indicate which treatment is more effective for HIT.

In appropriate clinical circumstances, the clinician should also consider certain adjunct therapies such as thrombolytic therapy or thrombectomy-embolectomy. High-dose IVIgG has successfully raised the platelet count in some HIT patients. Plasmapheresis has been used successfully in some patients. This treatment may work both by removing pathogenic antibody and by improving coagulation factor and inhibitor imbalances. The synthetic antithrombin hirulog has also been used to treat HIT.

We never administer platelets for prophylactic reasons to HIT patients. This is because bleeding is very rare for patients with HIT and because platelet transfusions may increase the risk of platelet-mediated thrombosis. Also, even though low molecular-weight heparin may be less likely to cause HIT, these preparations are virtually 100 percent cross-reactive with the pathogenic IgG in vitro, and we do not recommend their use in the treatment of patients with acute HIT.

Prevention

Because heparin-induced thrombocytopenia typically develops on day 5 or later of heparin therapy, at least some episodes can be prevented by the early institution of oral anticoagulation and discontinuation of heparin whenever possible. However, warfarin should be withheld from patients with acute HIT for several days, until the platelet count has normalized, to avoid triggering thrombotic complications.

■ OTHER DRUG-INDUCED THROMBOCYTOPENIC SYNDROMES

Nonidiosyncratic Drug-Induced Pancytopenia

Most antineoplastic drugs produce a dose-dependent pancytopenia caused by dose-dependent nonidiosyncratic injury to hematopoietic progenitor cells. Typically, pancytopenia occurs and recovers at relatively predictable times following use of these drugs. Rarely, certain antineoplastic drugs (e.g., actinomycin D) can cause idiosyncratic thrombocytopenia.

Drug-Induced Thrombotic Microangiopathy

Several drugs appear to trigger a syndrome of thrombocytopenia, fragmentation hemolysis, and renal failure (drug-induced hemolytic uremic syndrome, or HUS). This syndrome has been most convincingly established for quinine, although it may also be caused by mitomycin C, an antineoplastic agent, or cyclosporine, an immunosuppressive drug. However, many patients receiving mitomycin C or cyclosporine have other possible explanations for microangiopathy (adenocarcinoma and transplant rejection, respectively). Thrombotic thrombocytopenic purpura (TTP) has recently been reported in patients receiving the antiplatelet agent ticlopidine.

Drug-Induced Immune Bicytopenia and Pancytopenia

Rarely, drug-dependent IgG causes peripheral destruction of more than one blood cell line. For example, quinidine has been reported to cause severe thrombocytopenia and leukopenia by distinct populations of drug-dependent IgG. Sometimes drugs produce severe pancytopenia, together with marrow hypoplasia or aplasia, via immune-mediated destruction of a pluripotent hematopoietic stem cell (e.g., idiosyncratic pancytopenia caused by gold, quinidine, or chloramphenicol). A bone marrow assay must always be performed in patients with suspected drug-induced pancytopenia, as a hypoplastic marrow strongly suggests the serious complication of drug-induced aplastic anemia.

Immediate Drug-Induced Thrombocytopenia

Some drugs result in immediate but generally mild and transient drops in the platelet count. These include large doses of protamine, bleomycin, hematin, ristocetin (no longer clinically used because of this effect), desmopressin (particularly in patients with type IIB von Willebrand disease) and porcine factor VIII. Although some of these drugs may produce mild in vivo platelet agglutination, no adverse clinical sequelae have been established.

Drug Hypersensitivity Reactions

Mild to moderate thrombocytopenia can occur in patients with systemic drug hypersensitivity reactions. Affected patients may also have generalized rashes, fever, cholestasis, and leukopenia. Allopurinol, isoniazid, sulfasalazine, and phenothiazines have been implicated in these types of reactions.

Thrombocytopenia Secondary to Biologic Response Modifiers

Thrombocytopenia has been observed in clinical trials of purified or recombinant biologic response modifiers, including interferon, interleukin-2, and certain colony-stimulating factors. Antilymphocyte globulins can also produce severe thrombocytopenia in some patients. The pathogenesis of the thrombocytopenia is not known in these patients.

Suggested Reading

Kaufman DW, Kelly JP, Johannes CB, et al. Acute thrombocytopenic purpura in relation to the use of drugs. Blood 1993; 82:2714–2718.

Boshkov LK, Warkentin TE, Hayward CPM, et al. Heparin-induced thrombocytopenia and thrombosis: Clinical and laboratory studies. Br J Haematol 1993; 84:322 328.

Warkentin TE, Hayward CPM, Boshkov KL, et al. Sera from patients with heparin-induced thrombocytopenia generate platelet-derived microparticles with procoagulant activity: An explanation for the thrombotic complications of heparin-induced thrombocytopenia. Blood 1994; 84:3691–3699.

Warkentin TE, Kelton JG. Heparin-induced thrombocytopenia. Prog Hemostas Thromb 1991; 10:1–34.

Warkentin TE, Kelton JG. Interaction of heparin with platelets, including heparin-induced thrombocytopenia. In: Henri Bounameaux, ed. Low molecular-weight heparins in prophylaxis and therapy of thromboembolic diseases. New York: Marcel Dekker, 1994:75.

IMMUNE THROMBOCYTOPENIA: IDIOPATHIC THROMBOCYTOPENIC PURPURA

José O. Bordin, M.D.
John G. Kelton, M.D.

Thrombocytopenia can be caused by underproduction, sequestration, or increased destruction of platelets. *Immune thrombocytopenia* is the broad description of any platelet destructive disorder caused by immune mechanisms. The destruction is almost always caused by antibodies to gamma globulin (IgG) directed at the mature cellular elements of the megakaryocytic cell line—the platelets. Thus, the diagnosis of destructive thrombocytopenia is usually made by demonstrating destructive thrombocytopenia associated with normal or increased numbers of megakaryocytes in the bone marrow.

The disease-related classification system for immune thrombocytopenia includes primary immune thrombocytopenia caused by antiplatelet autoantibodies. In this group is idiopathic thrombocytopenic purpura (ITP). Immune thrombocytopenia can be secondary to a lymphoproliferative disorder, systemic lupus erythematosus (SLE), or another autoimmune disorder. Immune thrombocytopenia as exemplified by alloantibodies can also cause alloimmune neonatal thrombocytopenia and refractoriness to platelet transfusions. Finally, immune thrombocytopenia can be associated with a variety of disorders including bacterial or viral infection, notably the human immunodeficiency virus (HIV) (Table 1).

The clinical and laboratory investigation of the patient

Table 1 Immune Thrombocytopenias

TYPE OF ANTIBODY (USUALLY IgG)	CLASSIFICATION
Autoantibody	*Primary Autoantibody*
	ITP
	Acute
	Chronic
	Secondary Autoantibody
	SLE
	Rheumatoid arthritis
	Sarcoidosis
	Lymphoproliferative disorders
Alloantibody	*Passive Alloantibody*
	Alloimmune neonatal thrombocytopenia
	Active Alloantibody
	PTP
	Refractoriness to platelet transfusions
Drug-Dependent Antibody	Quinine, quinidine
	HIT

ITP, idiopathic thrombocytopenia purpura; SLE, systemic lupus erythematosus; PTP, post-transfusion purpura; HIT, heparin-induced thrombocytopenia.

with thrombocytopenia must enable the physician to confirm the diagnosis, estimate the hemostatic risk, determine the cause, and initiate the treatment. Thus, the accurate categorization of the mechanism of thrombocytopenia allows the physician to select the most appropriate therapy. This chapter focuses on therapeutic approaches to immune thrombocytopenia, with a particular focus on ITP.

■ ITP

ITP, a common disorder in adults, is characterized by autoimmune platelet destruction. ITP is a diagnosis of exclusion and must be distinguished from secondary immune thrombocytopenia complicating a variety of diseases, including SLE, lymphoproliferative disorders, and so on (Table 1).

Pathogenesis

Most cases of ITP are mediated by the binding of IgG autoantibodies to the platelet membrane, resulting in phagocytosis of the platelets by macrophages carrying the Fc II receptors in the spleen. Thus, the spleen is critical in the pathophysiology in ITP, since it is an important site of antibody production and is the predominant organ of platelet destruction. Although the plasma antiplatelet autoantibody is usually IgG, in some patients IgM and IgA have been identified. Since the amounts of PAIgG and albumin usually parallel the plasma concentration of IgG and albumin, it is possible that some of the PAIgG does not represent true antiplatelet antibody. This suggests that a membrane alteration caused by the autoantibody may be followed by secondary binding of plasma proteins, including nonspecific IgG and albumin. The IgG antibody is bound to the platelets via its Fab terminus, and in about half of ITP patients the plasma antiplatelet autoantibodies bind to platelet membrane glycoproteins, including the III, IIIa, and Ib/IX complexes.

The basic immunobiologic dysregulation leading to autoantibody formation in ITP remains unclear. Findings of increased populations of $CD5^+$ β-lymphocytes, functional defects in natural killer cells, and alteration in the T-cell subpopulation distribution suggests an intrinsic lymphocyte defect.

Clinical Presentation

In adults ITP can present in one of three ways: (1) the patient can have bleeding that is symptomatic and occurs spontaneously or that follows ingestion of an antiplatelet drug such as aspirin or alcohol; (2) the patient can have a long history of easy bruising; or (3) the ITP is identified in an asymptomatic patient by the laboratory finding of isolated thrombocytopenia during routine blood screening.

Among adult ITP patients, women aged 20 to 50 years are most commonly affected. Typically the onset of the disease is insidious, with petechiae and ecchymosis developing for weeks spontaneously or after minor trauma. Mucosal bleeding, also called *wet purpura,* may occur, but intracranial hemorrhage is rare. In women, menorrhagia is often observed. Except for the signs of hemostatic dysfunction, the physical examination is normal. Thus, splenomegaly in a patient with immune thrombocytopenia indicates that the thrombocytopenia is secondary to another disorder.

Laboratory Investigation

Patients with ITP usually have isolated thrombocytopenia (platelet count commonly between 5 and 100 × 10^9 per liter). Abnormalities of the other blood cells suggest other diseases, unless the chronic bleeding has caused iron deficiency anemia. The finding of an increased proportion of large (mean platelet volume above 10 fl) young platelets is consistent with the diagnosis of ITP. The bone marrow examination shows either normal or increased numbers of megakaryocytes. Increased plasma glycocalicin also reflects the increased platelet destruction. The bleeding time test is elevated if there is marked thrombocytopenia or abnormal platelet function.

PAIgG tests are elevated in about 90 percent of ITP patients, and they usually correlate with the severity of the thrombocytopenia. However, a positive result is not necessarily diagnostic, since the levels of PAIgG as measured by these assays are also elevated in patients with other thrombocytopenic conditions. Conceivably the recently introduced phase III assays (immunoblotting, radioimmunoprecipitation, and protein capture assays), which can detect the binding of antiplatelet autoantibodies to individual platelet glycoproteins, may be a more specific diagnostic test for ITP.

The normal lifespan of a platelet is approximately 7 to 10 days, but in ITP the platelet survival is usually markedly reduced, often less than 12 hours. Thus, platelet life span measurements performed with indium-111 are a definitive test for diagnosing increased platelet destruction. However, a small proportion of patients with ITP have a nearly normal platelet survival.

ITP remains a diagnosis of exclusion. Since several disorders resemble ITP and can complicate it, we measure the following: antinuclear antibody; HIV antibody; thyroid function assays; direct antiglobulin test; quantitative immunoglobulins; serum proteins electrophoresis; and liver enzymes.

Principles of Therapy

In contrast with children, about 90 percent of affected adults develop chronic ITP; therefore, the long-term risks of treatment must be balanced against the long-term risk of life-threatening bleeding. One of the most important issues in the management of ITP is to determine whether any treatment is required. The goal of treatment is to achieve a hemostatically safe but not necessarily normal platelet count.

Corticosteroids

Corticosteroids are the first-line therapy for adult patients with ITP. Most patients with ITP requiring treatment have an initial clinical response to corticosteroids. Prednisone (1 mg per kilogram of body weight daily) increases the platelet count in about 80 percent of patients, but the platelet count usually falls when the medication is gradually tapered. Only about 10 to 15 percent of adult ITP patients have a complete remission or maintain adequate hemostasis with acceptably low dose of corticosteroids. It is likely that corticosteroids cause a rise in the platelet count through several mechanisms, including (1) reduction of autoantibody synthesis; (2) impairment of megakaryocyte-antibody binding, allowing increased bone marrow platelet production; and (3) modulation of the reticuloendothelial-macrophage removal of platelets from the bone marrow. Short cycles of high-dose methylprednisolone (30 mg per kilogram of body weight daily over 3 to 5 days), or dexamethasone (40 mg per day for 4 sequential days every 28 days) may induce remissions in patients with chronic resistant ITP, but large controlled prospective trials have not been reported. The side effects associated with the chronic use of corticosteroids include weight gain (Cushingoid face), risk of infection, osteoporosis, gastric complications, hypertension, diabetes, and psychosis.

IVIgG

The administration of IVIgG leads to a temporary rise in the platelet count in most adults with ITP and may be particularly useful before surgical procedures. In addition, it has been suggested that the presplenectomy infusion of IVIgG may increase the postsplenectomy remission rate in patients with corticosteroid-resistant ITP. Acute reactions, including vasomotor symptoms, headache, and muscle pain, may occur in approximately 5 percent of infusions. They can be minimized by premedication with acetaminophen or nonsteroidal anti-inflammatory drugs. More severe complications such as anaphylactic reactions, hemolysis, and thrombotic episodes are uncommon.

Anti-D

Alternatively to IVIgG, the reticuloendothelial system in Rh-positive patients can be blocked by the administration of intravenous anti-D (20 μg per kilogram of body weight IV every 7 days for 4 to 6 weeks). This well-tolerated treatment raises platelet count associated with subclinical extravascular hemolysis.

Splenectomy

Splenectomy is the definitive treatment for adult patients with ITP. Most patients have a partial or complete response to splenectomy. Even though splenectomy is removal of the predominant site for both platelet destruction and autoantibody production, it is not possible to predict which patients will respond to splenectomy. Most patients will not have excess bleeding at the time of splenectomy; however, the platelet count should be raised preoperatively with corticosteroids or IVIgG. The platelet count usually rises quickly after the splenectomy, and a remission or cure is induced within 4 to 6 weeks in approximately 75 percent of the patients with chronic ITP. In a further 5 to 10 percent of patients a partial remission is achieved. About 10 percent of patients may relapse months or years after surgery, and accessory spleens may be found in about 20 percent of the splenectomized patients who respond but subsequently relapse. Splenectomy is a relatively safe surgical procedure for young and middle-aged adults. For older patients, especially those with pulmonary or cardiac disease, the morbidity rate of about 10 percent is usually caused by pneumonia, thromboembolism, or another infectious complication. The risk of postsplenectomy septicemia in the adult is lower than in children, but polyvalent pneumococcal vaccine should be administered at least 2 weeks before surgery.

Chemotherapy

Symptomatic patients with refractory disease that fails to respond to corticosteroids and splenectomy are candidates for more aggressive therapy. The use of vincristine 1 to 2 mg IV every 7 days for 4 weeks has been associated with transient response in some patients, particularly when the drug is infused over a 6 hour period. However, repeated infusion of vincristine increases the risk of neurotoxicity. Elevation in platelet count may also be achieved with cyclophosphamide 2 to 3 mg per kilogram of body weight per day orally. However, the long-term risk of this agent makes most physicians reluctant to use it.

The overall response rate of about 25 percent achieved with azathioprine 100 to 150 mg daily may take several months and last for several months. The more common side effects include myelosuppression and liver dysfunction that respond to dose reduction or discontinuation of the drug.

Persistent (11 to 126 months) complete remission has been reported in a subset of refractory ITP patients with the use of cyclophosphamide 400 to 650 mg per square meter of body surface area IV, plus prednisone 40 mg per square meter orally, combined with either vincristine 2 mg IV, vincristine plus procarbazine 100 mg per square meter orally, or etoposide 100 mg per square meter IV. However, the risks of the combined chemotherapy, including infection associated with neutropenia and development of secondary cancers, must be taken into account when considering such a regimen.

Other Treatments

Danazol, a weak modified androgen, can cause a drug-dependent remission in a small proportion of ITP patients. The response is gradual and is usually more evident when the drug (600 to 800 mg per day orally) is administered for several months. Danazol appears to reduce platelet destruction by decreasing the number of IgG Fc receptors on macrophages. Side effects include fluid retention, myalgia, nausea, amenorrhea, headache, and virilizing effects. Danazol is contraindicated during pregnancy.

Although still considered an unproven therapy, colchicine 0.6 to 1.2 mg four times daily has been reported to inhibit macrophage function and may be used to raise platelet level in refractory patients. The response is better evaluated after 4 to 6 weeks, but the gastrointestinal toxicity may limit its use in some individuals.

Splenic radiation (600 cGy of radiation, delivered in 6 doses over 3 weeks) can be used to raise the platelet count in older patients with corticosteroid-resistant ITP in whom the risks associated with splenectomy and/or corticosteroid therapy are clinically significant. Other novel treatments, including ascorbic acid, cyclosporine, recombinant interferon, dapsone, and anti-Fc receptor monoclonal antibody have only recently been used for treatment of refractory ITP, and the available data are mainly limited to case reports.

Emergency Treatment of a Bleeding Patient

Patients with extremely low platelet counts are at risk for life-threatening bleeding such as intracranial hemorrhage or severe gastrointestinal bleeding. Such patients must be hospitalized and treated aggressively. Platelet transfusions (6 to 12 units) should be administered every 6 hours until the platelet count is raised to safe levels. IVIgG 1 to 2 g per kilogram of body weight daily will rapidly raise the platelet count and helps maximize the efficacy of the platelet transfusions. Other treatments, such as corticosteroids and/or immunosuppressive agents, should be instituted simultaneously.

■ ITP IN PREGNANCY

A common cause of thrombocytopenia in pregnancy is ITP following incidental thrombocytopenia of pregnancy and pre-eclampsia. Most pregnant ITP patients do not require specific treatment; however, if the platelet count falls to less than 20–50 × 10^9 per liter or if there is clinical evidence of a hemostatic defect, the platelet count should be raised. We prefer to use intermittent IVIgG 1 to 2 g per kilogram of body weight. Seldom is splenectomy during pregnancy required or indicated.

Since the maternal IgG antiplatelet autoantibody can cross the placenta, it may cause thrombocytopenia in the neonate. The likelihood of thrombocytopenia in the neonate depends on the capacity of the fetal megakaryocytes to compensate the accelerated platelet destruction and the phagocytic activity of the fetal reticuloendothelial system. Unfortunately, to date, it is not possible to predict which neonate born to a mother with ITP will be severely thrombocytopenic. The determination of the fetal platelet count by cord sampling is not justified, since it probably carries higher risks of fetal morbidity and mortality than the risk of life-threatening hemorrhage of the infant. Moreover, the determination of the platelet count by fetal scalp sampling frequently fails for technical reasons. The overall risk of neonatal thrombocytopenia is about 8 percent. However, the risk of severe thrombocytopenia, defined as a platelet count of less than 20 × 10^9 per liter, is only 4 percent. Therefore, if the mother has had previous uncomplicated deliveries, a spontaneous vaginal delivery can be safely performed. On the other hand, if a difficult delivery is anticipated, a cesarean section may be indicated. The infant's platelet count should be performed immediately after delivery and monitored over the next several days. IVIgG or prednisone may be indicated for severely affected infants.

Suggested Reading

Berchtold P, McMillan R. Therapy of chronic idiopathic thrombocytopenic purpura in adults. Blood 1989; 74:2309–2317.

Burrows RF, Kelton JG. Fetal thrombocytopenia and its relation to maternal thrombocytopenia. N Engl J Med 1993; 329:1463–1466.

Collins PW, Newland AC. Treatment modalities of autoimmune blood disorders. Semin Hematol 1992; 29:64–74.

Juliá A, Araguás C, Rosselló J, et al. Lack of useful clinical predictors of response to splenectomy in patients with chronic idiopathic thrombocytopenic purpura. Br J Haematol 1990; 76:250–255.

Pizzuto J, Ambriz R. Therapeutic experience on 934 adults with idiopathic thrombocytopenic purpura: Multicentric trial of the Cooperative Latin American Group on Hemostasis and Thrombosis. Blood 1984; 64:1179–1183.

Warkentin TE, Kelton JG. Current concepts in the treatment of immune thrombocytopenia. Drugs 1990; 40:531–542.

THROMBOTIC THROMBOCYTOPENIC PURPURA

John G. Kelton, M.D.

Thrombotic thrombocytopenic purpura (TTP) is an important disorder for two reasons. First, it represents the prototypic platelet-mediated thrombotic illness. Most of the arterial thrombotic disorders are caused by platelets, but for the most part these involve chronic thrombotic processes that develop over many years. Examples include myocardial infarctions and ischemic strokes caused by atherosclerosis. These atherosclerotic disorders are the consequence of many years of platelets interacting with the vessel wall. The causes of these are multifactorial and can include heredity, hypertension, hyperlipidemia, tobacco abuse, and others. In contrast, TTP is an acute and often explosive platelet disorder in which the patients develop life-threatening platelet-mediated thrombi throughout the microcirculation. TTP is important for yet another reason. The rapid diagnosis of TTP and the institution of appropriate therapy can dramatically reduce the morbidity and mortality of what untreated is a frequently fatal disease.

■ CLINICAL PRESENTATION

Most patients who develop TTP are young to middle-aged adults with a slight female to male preponderance. The presentation of the illness can be insidious or acute. Typically the patient describes several days of feeling unwell and may seek medical attention because of generalized malaise, fatigue, or focal ischemic problems. The focal ischemic problems can include sudden weakness or other neurologic symptoms such as paresthesias and confusion. Occasionally there is abdominal pain. While ischemic damage to the myocardium is not rare, it is uncommon for these patients to present with an acute myocardial infarction. TTP has been associated with a pentad of findings including destructive thrombocytopenia, schistocytic hemolytic anemia, fever, renal impairment, and ischemic neurologic events. All patients have destructive thrombocytopenia and schistocytic hemolytic anemia. About half of patients have a neurologic event. Fever and evidence of renal impairment are less commonly observed. In patients followed longitudinally, sometimes the thrombocytopenia precedes the schistocytic hemolytic anemia. Indeed, the thrombocytopenia is the best evidence of both disease activity and remission (see subsequent section). The diagnosis of TTP is usually apparent but occasionally obscure. This is most likely to occur when the thrombocytopenia is mild and the amount of hemolysis is minimal, with relatively few fragmented red cells.

TTP must be differentiated from other destructive thrombocytopenic syndromes such as idiopathic thrombocytopenic purpura (ITP), drug-induced thrombocytopenia, and the thrombocytopenia of infection. Unless these disorders are accompanied by disseminated intravascular coagulation (DIC), red cell fragmentation is not observed. Similarly, TTP must be distinguished from other disorders characterized by fragmentation hemolysis (Table 1). These disorders can include large vessel fragmentation hemolysis such as malignant hypertension and malfunctioning prosthetic valves as well as microvascular fragmentation hemolytic disorders, which are typified by vasculitis (e.g., systemic lupus erythematosus, or SLE, Goodpasture's syndrome) and DIC. Schistocytic hemolytic anemia that accompanies malignant hypertension is characterized by very severe hypertension. Patients with TTP, especially if they have renal impairment, can have a moderate rise in their blood pressure, but seldom does it reach the levels seen in malignant hypertension. Patients with vasculitic, schistocytic hemolytic anemia usually have a history of a vasculitic disorder such as SLE. The thrombocytopenia in these disorders usually is not as severe as the thrombocytopenia of TTP. DIC can closely resemble TTP and must be differentiated by appropriate laboratory tests (PTT, PT, FDP, and paracoagulation assays). DIC is always initiated by an underlying disorder such as cancer, amniotic fluid embolism, septicemia, and so on. Hence the diagnosis of DIC usually is not difficult to make. Rarely TTP can be complicated by DIC, particularly if the ischemic events are widespread. In these patients the DIC resolves during the treatment of the TTP. This does not occur in patients with DIC caused by other disorders.

Table 1 Types of Schistocytic Hemolytic Anemias

GENERAL GROUP	SPECIFIC EXAMPLES	SEVERITY OF HEMOLYSIS	SEVERITY OF THE THROMBOCYTOPENIA	ABNORMAL COAGULATION TESTS
Large vessel schistocytic hemolytic anemia	Malignant hypertension	Moderate to severe	Mild to moderate	No
	Prosthetic heart valves	Mild to moderate	Mild	No
Small vessel schistocytic hemolytic anemia	March hemoglobinuria	Mild	Mild	No
	Vasculitis (SLE)	Mild to moderate	Mild to moderate	Rarely
	DIC	Moderate	Moderate to severe	Yes
	TTP-hemolytic uremic syndrome	Moderate to severe	Moderate to severe	Rarely

DISEASES ASSOCIATED WITH TTP

Most adult patients with TTP have no associated underlying disease (Table 2). Nonetheless, the initial investigation of a TTP patient should exclude diseases associated with TTP such as autoimmune conditions, malignancies, drugs, and bone marrow transplantation. The TTP associated with bone marrow transplantation is particularly aggressive and poorly responsive to therapy. Unfortunately, most of these patients will have a fatal outcome. TTP also has been associated with the treatment of adenocarcinoma by mithramycin. There is debate whether mithramycin-associated TTP is triggered by the drug or whether the underlying malignancy is the precipitating cause. This type of TTP is notoriously difficult to manage and often is fatal. A strong association has been made with quinidine and TTP. Fortunately this is an exceptionally rare syndrome, but patients with TTP should be questioned about having taken quinine quinidine.

A large number of conditions not associated with TTP may trigger an episode of it. These disorders, similar to conditions that can trigger an episode of ITP, include infections, pregnancy, vaccinations, and other immunologic challenges (see Table 2).

Some investigators have suggested that patients who have relapsing episodes of TTP may have a different disease. I suggest a different explanation: because of improved management most patients survive their episode of TTP. Consequently, in an increasing number of patients (perhaps 20 to 40 percent) the TTP recurs. It is possible that these patients have a different type of TTP. Alternatively, they may relapse simply because they now survive their initial episode of TTP and have the opportunity.

An uncommon but important variant of TTP is familial TTP–hemolytic uremic syndrome (HUS). These patients typically present in infancy or childhood with intermittent episodes of thrombocytopenia and schistocytic hemolytic anemia with episodes of abdominal pain and oliguric renal failure resembling HUS or episodes of neurologic ischemia resembling TTP. Sometimes the same patient will have different target organs at different times during the illness, which suggests that TTP and HUS are clinically and possibly pathologically related. These patients can be managed with plasma infusion (see subsequent section).

Table 2 Classification of Thrombotic Thrombocytopenic Purpura

Primary (no disease associations)
Primary but triggered by a disorder or condition
Vaccination
Viral infection (Coxsackie B, Echo, Epstein-Barr)
Bacterial infection
Verotoxin-producing infections
Non–verotoxin-producing infections
Secondary
ITP
Human immunodeficiency virus
Collagen vascular disease
Carcinoma (typically adenocarcinoma)
Chemotherapy of carcinoma (mitomycin)
Drug associated (quinidine)
Bone marrow transplantation

LABORATORY INVESTIGATION

An accurate platelet count is important. A rise or fall in the platelet count is the first sign of response or relapse to therapy. Because most laboratories measure platelet counts with automated article counters, there is a chance of obtaining a spuriously high platelet count because of the red cell fragmentation: the fragment red cells are erroneously counted as platelets. When in doubt about the accuracy of the platelet count, it is important to confirm it using a direct count (phase contrast). Along with the platelet count, a complete blood count with hemoglobin determination and white cell count is also performed. Often the hemolytic anemia is sufficiently severe to cause a drop in the hemoglobin level. Leukocytosis is not unusual. The blood film should be reviewed for fragmented red blood cells. Although fragmented red cells (schistocytic hemolytic anemia) is required for the diagnosis, the relative number of fragments and their persistence in the circulation is not a marker of the severity or the activity of disease. I have observed patients who achieved a remission with a rise in the platelet count and resolution of the symptoms but who continue to have fragmented red cells in their circulation. I wonder if the persisting fragmented red cells are not cleared by the cells of the reticuloendothelial (RE) system because the RE cells are saturated. The lactate dehydrogenase (LDH) is almost always elevated in patients with active TTP because of the release of red cell LDH into the circulation due to the hemolysis. The LDH is a good marker of disease activity, and persistently elevated LDH levels mean the disease is still active and ongoing treatment is required. It is my experience that the LDH is a parallel but possibly less sensitive marker of disease activity compared with the platelet count. All patients should also have liver enzyme, electrolyte, and renal function tests. About 60 percent of patients with TTP will have evidence of renal impairment (Table 3). However, oliguric renal failure is far less common in TTP than in HUS.

Other laboratory tests should look for associated diseases, including human immunodeficiency virus (HIV), and antinuclear antibodies (ANA) among others (depending on possible associated illnesses). I also perform coagulation tests to exclude the possibility of DIC masquerading as TTP.

THERAPY

Plasma Exchange

The mainstay of treatment is plasma exchange using plasma. Plasma exchange has been demonstrated in a randomized prospective trial to improve significantly the survival of TTP patients over plasma infusion alone. It remains unknown whether the plasma exchange is advantageous because it removes a toxic factor, which a plasma infusion could not do, or whether the infused plasma contains a deficient factor that neutralizes the platelet aggregation factor of TTP (see subsequent section). It is my opinion that it does both. For example, there is no doubt that some patients with TTP will respond to

Table 3 Clinical Characteristics of Patients with Primary TTP

	CHARACTERISTIC	PERCENT	AVERAGE
Clinical	Female	67	40 years
	Neurologic impairment	64	
	Fever	25	
	Impaired renal function	50–60	
Laboratory	Thrombocytopenia	100	23,000/μl
	Anemia	Most	9 g/dl
	Elevated LDH	Most	1,200–1,400 (<225)
	ANA	24	

plasma infusion only. Indeed, familial TTP is perhaps best managed by plasma infusion only.

An acute episode of TTP is one of the few emergency indications for plasma exchange. As the exchange is being organized, the patient should receive plasma intravenously at 100 to 150 ml per hour for an average-size adult. Plasma infusion cannot be given to patients with azotemia because it will cause fluid overload; however, plasma exchange can readily be used in such patients. A typical plasma exchange treatment replaces one to two plasma volumes (2 to 3 liters) in the average adult. There is anecdotal evidence that patients with more severe disease (multiple thrombotic episodes) or who are failing therapy can benefit from larger exchanges administered more frequently. The therapy is administered daily until the patient enters into remission, which is evidenced by a rise in the platelet count and a fall in the LDH level. Typically this occurs after 3 to 10 plasma exchanges. I have observed that many patients have a relapse following an initial rise in the platelet count, and sometimes this relapse is more difficult to manage than the initial episode of TTP. Once the patient has responded to plasma exchange therapy, I extend the plasma exchange to every other day for 1 to 2 weeks and then once to twice per week for approximately a month. I believe that this tapered approach may result in fewer relapses.

Choice of the Plasma Product

The choice of fluid for replacement is plasma rather than albumin. Anecdotal studies have showed that albumin was not an acceptable replacement fluid but that plasma was. There is also increasing evidence that cyrosupernatant plasma is the optimum replacement fluid, and it is now my treatment of choice. Cryosupernatant is the plasma that remains following the extraction of cryoprecipitate (fibrinogen and von Willebrand factor) from a frozen-thawed unit of fresh frozen plasma. It is likely that the cryosupernatant plasma is more effective than standard plasma; experimental evidence from a number of laboratories suggests that the von Willebrand factor is a participant in the disease process. Heat-treated (virus-inactivated) plasma is not widely available. I vaccinate patients against hepatitis B after the exchange. The absolute requirement for this is uncertain given that the actual risk of hepatitis B transmission by blood is exceptionally low (about 1:200,000 per unit).

Adjunctive Therapy

Once the platelet count is above 50×10^9 per liter, I begin antiplatelet therapy (325 mg aspirin per day). Some physicians administer antiplatelet agents (aspirin with or without dipyridamole) at lower platelet counts. However, it is likely that the actual benefit from aspirin is modest, and the use of aspirin at low platelet counts may put the person at risk for hemorrhage. I have no experience with other antiplatelet agents.

A number of anecdotal reports and one large retrospective study suggest that corticosteroids may help patients with TTP. This seems a reasonable approach given that many aspects of TTP resemble ITP, which responds to corticosteroids. However, I do not use corticosteroids in a patient with uncomplicated TTP unless there is a strong autoimmune association (history of ITP, SLE, and so on). I do add corticosteroids to the regimen if the patient has a poor response to treatment or an initial relapse.

Other treatments that have been shown not to be effective are anticoagulants (heparin or warfarin) and intravenous gamma-immunoglobulin. Some reports have suggested that vincristine may be helpful.

Patients with TTP should not receive platelet transfusions, which have been associated with acute neurologic events and sudden exacerbation of the illness. Unless the patient has a life-threatening bleed (e.g., an intracranial hemorrhage), the risks of platelet transfusions outweigh any benefit.

■ MANAGEMENT OF THE REFRACTORY PATIENT

A small proportion of patients with TTP are extremely refractory to therapy, and it is almost impossible to raise their platelet count through plasma exchange. These patients should receive combined therapy (antiplatelet agents if the platelet count is sufficiently high plus corticosteroids). But it is critical that these patients continue to receive plasma exchange therapy. Patients with ongoing TTP who have their plasma exchange discontinued for any reason (most frequently loss of vascular access) are at very high risk for dying of their illness. Just as a physician managing a patient with renal failure continues dialysis treatment, physicians managing patients with refractory TTP should not be impatient about failure to respond. Plasma exchange treatment must be continued until remission is achieved.

■ MANAGEMENT OF THE PATIENT WITH RELAPSING TTP

I sometimes observe patients who have episodes of TTP weeks to months apart. These patients respond to plasma exchange, but several months later they have a relapse. Often the relapse follows an immunologic stimulus such as a viral infection. I have tried different maneuvers in these patients and had variable success with each. First, intermittent exchange on a regular basis (e.g., every 2 weeks) may help prevent relapses. Second, corticosteroids may be useful. Finally, I have achieved long-term remissions in several patients using splenectomy. This should be performed only when the patient is in remission.

■ TTP AND PREGNANCY

TTP can occur in pregnant women, and some large series of TTP patients have indicated that pregnancy is associated with about 25 percent of TTP cases. TTP also has occurred in women taking the birth control pill, which suggests that hormonal factors may trigger the syndrome. Sometimes the TTP in pregnancy is very difficult to distinguish from pre-eclampsia-toxemia (PET). The reason is that both can occur late in the pregnancy and both can be associated with thrombocytopenia and schistocytic hemolytic anemia. Often the pre-eclampsia is apparent because of severe hypertension; however, some patients with TTP have impaired renal function and hypertension because of the TTP. In patients in whom it is impossible to distinguish the two disorders, I assume that the patient has both disorders and act accordingly. Urgent delivery is the treatment of choice for pre-eclampsia except rarely, when PET develops early in pregnancy. Simultaneously, I consider using plasma exchange therapy, particularly in patients whose diagnosis of pre-eclampsia is uncertain and who clinically appear to have TTP. Sometimes the TTP relapses in subsequent pregnancies, so the woman must be warned about the risks of TTP in future pregnancies.

■ PATHOGENESIS

The observation of disseminated platelet thrombi in the vasculature of patients with TTP has long suggested that the illness is caused by a platelet-aggregating factor. However, its identity remains uncertain. One group of investigators identified a small (37 kDa) platelet aggregating factor in plasma of patients with TTP. The observations of our group have been somewhat different: We have observed an unregulated calcium-dependent protease (calpain) in the plasma and serum of TTP patients. This enzyme is present on microparticles in the circulation of these patients. We have also observed that the calpain can cleave von Willebrand factor (vWF), rendering it intensely platelet reactive. However, the mechanism of the generation of the calpain in the TTP remains unresolved.

Numerous laboratories have demonstrated abnormalities of vWF in many but not all patients with TTP. Typically the patient has absent large multimers of vWF during the acute episode. It is assumed that these multimers are bound to the patient's platelets, causing them to aggregate. During convalescence there can be an overabundance of very large multimers of vWF in these patients' plasma. This association of large multimers during recovery and predominance of small multimers during the acute episode is particularly strong in patients with familial TTP-HUS.

■ LONG-TERM FOLLOW-UP

Because a large percentage of patients (estimated at 20 to 40 percent) will relapse following initial remission of TTP, it is important to monitor recovered TTP patients for several months after the initial episode. Relapses tend to occur close to the acute episode but can occur some time later. I recommend a weekly platelet count for several months following remission and then intermittently thereafter. If the patient has some of the symptoms of the initial episode of TTP, a repeat complete blood count and platelet count should be performed immediately.

Suggested Reading

Bell WR, Braine HG, Ness PM, Kickler TS. Improved survival in thrombotic thrombocytopenic purpura-hemolytic uremic syndromes. N Engl J Med 1991; 325:398–403.

Rock G, Shumak K, Kelton J, et al. Thrombotic thrombocytopenic purpura: Outcome in 24 patients with renal impairment treated with plasma exchange. Transfusion 1992; 32:710–714.

Rock GA, Shumak KH, Buskard NA, et al. Comparison of plasma exchange with plasma infusion in the treatment of thrombotic thrombocytopenic purpura. N Engl J Med 1991; 325:393–397.

Rose M, Rowe JM, Eldor A. The changing course of thrombotic thrombocytopenic purpura and modern therapy. Blood Rev 1993; 7(2):94–103.

LONG-TERM ANTICOAGULATION

Peder M. Shea, M.D.

Long-term anticoagulation is indicated in a widening range of illnesses. With the advent of thrombolytic therapy in ischemic syndromes and the recognition of the incidence of thromboemboli in atrial fibrillation, an increasing number of patients are prescribed "chronic anticoagulation," implying at least 3 months of therapy. Even the intensity of anticoagulation has been modified in recent years. This chapter considers these changes in the indications for therapy and the level of anticoagulation in specific clinical settings.

■ PREFERRED APPROACH

Drugs Used for Anticoagulation

Several classes of medications are used for chronic anticoagulation. The drugs and their use are discussed in subsequent paragraphs.

Warfarin

The principal oral anticoagulants are antagonists of vitamin–K, the most common of which is warfarin. Warfarin prevents vitamin K–dependent carboxylation of factors II, VII, IX, and X, thus depleting the bulk of procoagulants. The onset of activity depends on the half-life of the remaining, circulating levels of these same factors, of which factor II is the shortest.

Other vitamin K–dependent and warfarin-sensitive proteins are natural anticoagulants known as protein C and S. As the half-life of protein C is shorter even than factor II, for the "first day" the effect of warfarin may be paradoxical and shift the balance of hemostasis toward coagulation. Clinically, such a hypercoagulable state is manifested as skin and fat necrosis. For this reason a loading dose of warfarin is not advisable.

The hepatic effects of warfarin and vitamin K are in strict competition; thus, warfarin can be "reversed" by loading with vitamin K, usually given intravenously. There appears to be little or no evidence of a hypercoagulable state with such vitamin K administration. Likewise, patients with low levels of vitamin K, as seen in severe fasting states or with antibiotic suppression of vitamin K absorption, require lower doses of warfarin.

Warfarin therapy is best monitored with the prothrombin time (PT), usually expressed as a ratio of the patient's PT to the normal PT for that laboratory. The PT is obtained daily while initiating warfarin therapy. Once stabilized and therapeutic, the PT is monitored every 2 to 4 weeks. Home PT monitoring, akin to home glucose monitoring, is currently in clinical trials and promises to increase the safety and reduce the cost of warfarin therapy.

The intensity of anticoagulation with warfarin as reflected by the PT has recently been clarified. The PT utilizes a reagent, thromboplastin, to stimulate in vitro coagulation. Thromboplastin is extracted from tissues, usually lung, brain, or placenta, each having a different "responsiveness." A "more responsive" thromboplastin results in a greater prolongation of the PT than a "less responsive" thromboplastin on the same sample. The thromboplastins used in North America today are less responsive than those used between 1940 and 1960 and those used in Europe. Using the same recommended target range for the PT established in the 1950s would result today in a significantly increased level of anticoagulation because of today's "less responsive" thromboplastin.

The World Health Organization has provided a standard thromboplastin, and current manufacturers provide a comparison with this standard, the International Sensitivity Index for each batch of thromboplastin. Using the International Sensitivity Index, a standardized PT ratio, the International Normalized Ratio (INR), can be obtained. Reviewing recommended levels of anticoagulation expressed in comparable terms of the INR has resulted in a less intense level of anticoagulation and fewer bleeding complications, and it more accurately reflects the intentions of the original investigators.

Heparin

Heparin is a true anticoagulant in that it inhibits coagulation by its action on antithrombin III, a natural inhibitor of factors XIIa, XIa, Xa, IXa, thrombin (IIa), and plasmin. At least some of its effect is due to the strong negative charge of heparin and can be reversed by the strong positive charge of protamine. Heparin has an immediate onset of action and its half-life is less than 1 hour. Aside from bleeding, the most significant side effect is thrombocytopenia. The most common variety occurs in approximately 10 percent of patients, is mild and not progressive, and is not associated with thrombosis (King and Kelton, 1984). A severe, progressive variety occurs with thrombosis. Fortunately, both resolve if recognized and if the heparin is stopped completely, including that in flush solutions of indwelling catheters.

The activated partial thromboplastin time (APTT) is used to monitor heparin therapy. A therapeutic range for full anticoagulation with heparin is achieved when the APTT is between 1.5 and 2 times the control. As an initial estimate of the dose required for full anticoagulation with heparin, 10 units per kilogram per hour is given intravenously. A clinical observation has been that when there is a large "clot burden," a larger dose of heparin is required to reach a therapeutic APTT than is required toward the end of a therapeutic intervention. It is not uncommon for the APTT to be significantly prolonged with the addition of warfarin to a stable dose of heparin while switching to oral therapy. Monitoring the APTT in unstable situations treated with intermittent injections may not reduce the risk of bleeding, thus the emphasis on a continuous infusion in the hospitalized patient. In the outpatient setting, heparin is administered by subcutaneous injection, usually in a dose of 12,000 to 15,000 units every 12 hours. The APTT is sampled 6 hours after injection and, if therapeutic, will remain above the target range during the entire 12 hours.

Table 1 Intensity of Anticoagulation and Risk of Hemorrhage in Major Disease Categories

INDICATION	LEVEL OF WARFARIN		BLEEDS (%)	MAJOR BLEED/100 PATIENT-YEARS
	PT RATIO	INR		
Thromboembolism	1.3–1.5	2.0–3.0	4–22	—
Bioprosthetic valves	1.3–1.5	2.0–3.0	5–7	—
Ischemic heart	1.3–1.5	2.0–3.0	17–36	0–4.8
Cerebrovascular	1.3–1.5	2.0–3.0	11–28	2–22
Atrial fibrillation	1.3–1.5	2.0–3.0	15	—
Mechanical valve	1.5–2.0	3.0–4.5	8–13	0.7–0.8
Recurrent emboli	1.5–2.0	3.0–4.5	—	—

PT, Prothrombin time; INR, International Normalized Ratio.
Modified from Hirsh I, et al. Optimal therapeutic range for oral anticoagulants. Chest 1989; 95:5S; and Levine MN, et al. Hemorrhagic complications of long-term anticoagulant therapy. Chest 1989; 95:26S.

Platelet-Inhibitory Drugs

Aspirin irreversibly inhibits the enzyme cyclo-oxygenase, thereby inhibiting platelet aggregation, platelet synthesis of vasoactive substances such as thromboxane A_2, and endothelial prostacyclin synthesis. This enzymatic inactivation lasts for the entire platelet lifespan. Aspirin dosages remain unclear because experimental results show a variety of effects at differing doses and clinical results use a wide range of doses. Ibuprofen and other nonsteroidal anti-inflammatory agents also inhibit cyclo-oxygenase.

Dipyridamole inhibits phosphodiesterase, which reduces the availability of calcium and decreases platelet aggregation. Its effects are additive to those of aspirin in theory and in some clinical experience. There is evidence that some of these effects are mediated by endothelial prostacyclin.

Anticoagulation Problems During Pregnancy

Because warfarin crosses the placental barrier and is teratogenic, a change in anticoagulant therapy is required with the onset of pregnancy. Warfarin is particularly dangerous in the first trimester as it causes central nervous system abnormalities. Later in pregnancy, hemorrhage threatens the fetus as well as the mother. Thus, women of childbearing age must take precautions to prevent pregnancy while taking warfarin. Once pregnancy is planned or confirmed, a switch to heparin is required.

Heparin does not cross the placental barrier, nor is it teratogenic. The safest time for changing to heparin is before conception but certainly in the first trimester. Intermittent, subcutaneous injection is continued throughout pregnancy, keeping the APTT in the therapeutic range. Elective induction is ideal in allowing the heparin to be stopped early in labor to allow full coagulant potential during this vulnerable time. Heparin is restarted after hemostasis is achieved and continued until a therapeutic warfarin dose is achieved. Fortunately, heparin does not cross into breast milk, and warfarin does so at such a low level that the child's coagulation potential is not affected. An alternative approach is to prescribe heparin in the first trimester and during the last 2 weeks of the pregnancy but to allow oral warfarin during the rest of the pregnancy. If labor should begin before warfarin is stopped, fresh frozen plasma should be given to normalize the PT.

■ INDICATIONS FOR ANTICOAGULATION THERAPY

Venous Thromboembolic Disease

Long-term anticoagulation is essential in the management of venous thromboembolic disease (see also the chapter *Acute Thrombophlebitis*) as short-term heparin therapy, even up to 14 days, does not prevent recurrent thrombophlebitis. Warfarin is started, without a loading dose, at day 5 of heparin therapy. The two are continued simultaneously until the PT is in the therapeutic range; the heparin is then stopped. It is not uncommon for the subsequent PT values to be slightly shorter as a result of the combined effect of warfarin and heparin on some of the clotting factors reflected by the PT. Hospitalized patients are usually kept 1 to 2 days further to establish a stable dose of warfarin. In those patients with massive pulmonary emboli in which thrombolytic therapy (streptokinase, urokinase, or tissue plasminogen activator [tPA]) has been used, the duration of heparin therapy and the timing of warfarin initiation is still not clear.

The intensity of long-term warfarin therapy has recently been adjusted downward (Table 1). If transient or reversible etiologies of the venous disease such as immobilization or estrogen use are present, 3 months of therapy should be sufficient. When venous thrombosis is documented at the time of initial presentation, a repeat study is indicated just before discontinuation of warfarin. Venous patency shown by Doppler echo with both visible flow and venous compression is a reassuring result, although its predictive value is not known. For long-term immobilization, severe heart failure, tumors, antithrombin III or protein C deficiencies, life-threatening pulmonary emboli, or recurrent venous thromboembolism, treatment should be lifelong.

Long-term subcutaneous heparin is an alternate therapeutic approach, although it suffers from problems of repeated injections and patient compliance, as well as severe osteopenia. The dose should prolong the APTT to at least 1.5 to 2 times the control time. If the APTT is prolonged to 2.9 times the control time, the risk of bleeding is increased threefold. For APTTs greater than three times the control time, the risk of bleeding increases eightfold.

Valvular Heart Disease

Rheumatic Mitral Valve Disease

Both rheumatic mitral stenosis and mitral regurgitation can be complicated by arterial emboli at a rate of 1.5 to 4.7 percent per patient year (Levine and co-workers, 1989). Atrial fibrillation dramatically increases the risk of emboli sevenfold. After the first embolus, a recurrent event is likely (30 to 60 percent) with the majority occurring in the first 6 months. Although never subjected to a randomized trial, the value of anticoagulation has been shown by a recurrent emboli rate of 9.4 percent per patient year without anticoagulation, which is reduced to 3.4 percent per patient-year with warfarin therapy (Levine and co-workers, 1989).

Warfarin therapy (INR = 2.0 to 3.0) is indicated prophylactically for patients with mitral valve disease in both paroxysmal and chronic atrial fibrillation as well as those in sinus rhythm with a left atrium of 5.5 cm or larger. More intense therapy (INR = 3.0 to 4.5) is required if documented emboli have occurred. Dipyridamole (225 mg to 400 mg daily) may reduce further emboli if they should occur in spite of the more intense regimen.

Aortic Valve Disease

Thromboemboli from isolated aortic valve disease is uncommon although calcific emboli may occur in as many as 19 percent of patients. Likewise, in the absence of mitral valve disease, atrial fibrillation is uncommon in aortic valve disease. Thus, prophylactic anticoagulant therapy is not recommended.

Mitral Valve Prolapse

In recent years clinicians have recognized transient ischemic attacks (TIA) in patients with mitral valve prolapse and no other identifiable etiology. One estimate of the risk of stroke in young adults with prolapse is 1 per 6,000 adults per year. In the absence of atrial fibrillation or documented stroke, prophylactic anticoagulant therapy is not indicated at such a low incidence. Patients with documented TIAs but with no other diagnosis than prolapse are given aspirin (325 mg to 1 g daily). Patients with recurrent emboli events despite aspirin therapy require warfarin (INR = 2.0 to 3.0) for life. Patients with mitral valve prolapse and atrial fibrillation have not been studied but experience with other mitral valve disease would suggest that chronic warfarin therapy is likely to prevent thromboemboli.

Mitral Annular Calcification

Mitral annular calcification is an increasingly recognized source of embolic events due to both calcific spicules and thromboemboli. There are no studies on the use of anticoagulant therapy in uncomplicated mitral annular calcification; however, in the setting of mitral annular calcification associated with mitral stenosis or regurgitation, with or without atrial fibrillation, thromboembolic events are likely and anticoagulation is rational. There is no information on the usefulness of antiplatelet drugs in this disease.

Cardiomyopathy

Atrial fibrillation complicates both the hypertrophic and dilated forms of cardiomyopathy when there is left atrial enlargement and mitral regurgitation. Prompt cardioversion is usually necessary to improve cardiac symptoms. This is best performed after full anticoagulation with heparin for as long as the patient's clinical status will allow. Lifelong warfarin therapy (INR = 2.0 to 3.0) is initiated before discontinuing heparin, whether or not the cardioversion is successful. In patients with the end-stage dilated cardiomyopathy, venous thromboembolism is very frequently a cause of clinical deterioration and is preventable with chronic warfarin therapy.

Mechanical Prosthetic Valves

With warfarin anticoagulation, the rate of thromboembolic events in mechanical valve prostheses such as the Starr-Edwards, Lillehei-Kaster, and Bjork-Shiley valves is reduced from approximately 23 episodes per 100 patients per year to 2.5 episodes per 100 patients per year with a wide range of results in multiple studies (Levine and co-workers, 1989). With the addition of aspirin (1 g per day) or dipyridamole (400 mg per day) a further reduction of embolic events to 1.8 percent per year can be achieved. Unfortunately, aspirin also increases the risk of bleeding. The intensity of warfarin therapy is increased with these prostheses (see Table 1). For patients with bleeding on the full dose of warfarin therapy, lower doses (INR = 2.0 to 3.0), often with dipyridamole (400 mg per day), have been used with success.

The St. Jude valve, especially in the aortic position, has been studied with antiplatelet therapy alone. Yet the short-term incidence of emboli may be as high as 12.5 percent in 4 years. Until this is further clarified, full anticoagulant therapy is still prescribed for St. Jude valves even in the aortic position.

Bioprosthetic Valves

After implantation, the risk of thromboembolism ranges from 10 percent for patients in sinus rhythm to 16 percent for those in atrial fibrillation followed over 36 months. Although patients with a prosthetic mitral valve are more likely to embolize than those with valves in the aortic position, warfarin for 6 to 12 weeks (INR = 2.0 to 3.0) is prescribed for both. Longer courses of warfarin are under study for prevention of calcific degeneration by blocking the vitamin K–dependent binding of calcium to prosthesis.

Ischemic Cerebrovascular Disease

Cerebral Emboli

In several studies on ischemic cerebral events, approximately 15 percent had a cardiac source of cerebral emboli (Sherman and co-workers, 1989). Symptoms of a TIA and amaurosis fugax can occur with cardiac emboli as well as the more common hemispheric and hemorrhagic infarction. Prophylactic anticoagulant recommendations with warfarin have been outlined in Table 1; however, once a cerebral embolus has occurred, the timing of anticoagulant therapy is difficult. The risk of extending the area of damage by hemorrhage must be balanced with the risk of recurrent embolic events occurring at a rate of roughly 1 percent per day. At this time no clear parameters other than the presence of hemorrhage and the size of the infarct on computed tomographic scan will predict the risk of hemorrhage. In the presence of large infarctions, anticoagulation is delayed 5 to 7 days to reduce the risk of delayed hemorrhage. If hemorrhage is already present, the anticoagulation is delayed at least 10 days in hopes of reducing the risk of extension.

In the setting of infective endocarditis and septic emboli, anticoagulant therapy is not indicated.

For patients presenting with TIAs or minor strokes, there is very good evidence that antiplatelet agents, particularly aspirin (1 g per day), will reduce the rate of recurrent, nonfatal stroke by 25 percent (Sherman and co-workers, 1989). However, in a completed stroke, antiplatelet therapy is not conclusively shown to alter recurrence rates. Finally in primary prevention studies in patients free of cerebrovascular disease, strokes were uncommon yet the risk of disabling and fatal strokes was increased fivefold with aspirin therapy. Thus, antiplatelet therapy is limited to TIAs and incomplete strokes. Dipyridamole has not been shown to add additional safety or benefit to aspirin therapy.

Ischemic Coronary Heart Disease

Angina Pectoris

Recent research has focused attention on the thrombotic process in the progression from stable to unstable angina and to myocardial infarction (see also the chapters *Angina Pectoris: Stable* and *Angina Pectoris: Unstable*).

As a means of preventing the initial development of ischemic syndromes, aspirin (325 mg per day) is shown to reduce the risk of myocardial infarction in previously healthy individuals by 47 percent. There was, however, a concomitant 15 percent increase in strokes (Steering Committee, 1988). Thus, enthusiasm is tempered for broad recommendations for aspirin therapy to the general population. It remains useful to recommend aspirin to high-risk individuals, particularly smokers and patients with significant hyperlipidemia. In patients with hypertension, even this recommendation includes a discussion with the patient of the increased risk of hemorrhagic stroke.

When results of five major, randomized trials of antiplatelet agents after a myocardial infarction are pooled, the risk of cardiovascular death is reduced 16 percent and the risk of subsequent myocardial infarction is reduced by 21 percent. Dipyridamole does not increase the benefits seen with aspirin and is not routinely prescribed. No benefit has been shown with sulfinpyrazone in this population. Likewise long-term anticoagulation with warfarin or heparin is not supported in the current literature.

Myocardial Infarction

Significant reductions, ranging from 39 to 55 percent, in the rate of recurrent myocardial infarction with warfarin therapy have reopened the discussion of long-term anticoagulation following a myocardial infarction (Resnekov and co-workers, 1989; Sixty Plus, 1980) (see also the chapter *Early Myocardial Infarction: Thrombolytic Therapy*). Although not yet "standard therapy" for all survivors, in certain subgroups of patients warfarin is recommended. Patients with large anterior myocardial infarctions have a risk of embolic stroke of 2 to 6 percent, usually in the presence of a mural thrombus (Resnekov and co-workers, 1989). Thus, early heparinization followed by warfarin therapy (INR = 2.0 to 3.0) for at least 3 months is justified. Longer-term anticoagulation is not necessary because once the thrombus is well incorporated into the chamber wall the risk of embolic episodes is so low as not to justify the risk of significant hemorrhage due to warfarin.

Atrial Fibrillation

The Framingham study has focused attention on the risks of cerebral thromboembolic events in the setting of atrial fibrillation, even in the absence of valvular heart disease. The incidence of stroke in patients 60 to 69 years of age without atrial fibrillation is 9 per 1,000 and 43 per 1,000 when atrial fibrillation is present, increasing further with age. Unfortunately, 17 percent die and many have severe permanent neurologic deficits with the first embolus (Wolf and co-workers, 1987). Current data support an aggressive, prophylactic approach to anticoagulation to reduce these risks. The Boston Area Anticoagulation Trial for Atrial Fibrillation showed that warfarin reduced the incidence of embolic stroke from 3 percent per year to 0.4 percent per year—an 86 percent reduction. The Copenhagen AFASAK Study found a comparable 64 percent reduction in strokes. The intensity of anticoagulant therapy is kept in the low range (INR = 2.0 to 3.0), particularly in light of the largely elderly patient population. Once undertaken, the risk of anticoagulant-induced intracranial hemorrhage is one-half the risk of stroke in untreated patients with atrial fibrillation. Only one of three randomized studies found aspirin to be of any benefit in prevention of strokes in the patient in atrial fibrillation. Comparison studies of aspirin and warfarin are underway.

Thyrotoxicosis is associated with atrial fibrillation in as many as 30 percent of patients, and one-third of these will have a cerebral embolus. This can occur early in the course of this disease as well as weeks after conversion to sinus rhythm, even in the euthyroid state. Consequently, early warfarin therapy is recommended and therapy continued at least 4 weeks after achieving both a euthyroid state and sinus rhythm.

"Lone" atrial fibrillation occurs in young patients with no identifiable heart disease. Thromboemboli are thought to be rare in this setting, and anticoagulant therapy is not required in the absence of documented emboli.

Cardioversion

Because the risk of an embolic complication with direct current cardioversion for atrial fibrillation is 5 percent, anticoagulant therapy has been recommended to reduce this risk. Although there are no controlled trials, an incidence of emboli as low as 0.8 percent has been reported for cardioversion while anticoagulated and supports this recommendation (Bjerkelund and Orning, 1969). On theoretical grounds alone, patients with atrial fibrillation of less than 3 days' duration, in the absence of valvular heart disease or documented emboli, have not been anticoagulated. For elective direct current cardioversion of more sustained atrial fibrillation, 2 to 3 weeks of adequate warfarin therapy (INR = 2.0 to 3.0) is recommended prior to cardioversion, followed by 4 weeks of therapy after successful cardioversion. This is prophylactic for those patients who will quickly return to atrial fibrillation as well as the rare patients with "late" emboli.

Risk of Bleeding

In a retrospective review of the risk of bleeding while taking warfarin, Fihn and colleagues observed a cumulative incidence of fatal bleeding of 1 percent at 1 year and 2 percent at 3 years. Expressed as a rate, the frequency of fatal bleeding complications was 0.2 events per 100 patient-years. Serious bleeding occurred in 12 percent at 1 year, 20 percent at 2 years, 40 percent at 8 years, and at a rate of 11.6 events per 100 patient-years. Four risk factors for bleeding were identified: a mean PT ratio of 2.0 or greater, a shorter duration of anticoagulation, a greater variability in the PT ratio, and the presence of three or more comorbid conditions. In this study age was not an independent risk factor.

Suggested Reading

Bjerkelund C, Orning OM. The efficacy of anti-coagulant therapy in preventing embolism related to DC electrical cardioversion of atrial fibrillation. Am J Cardiol 1969; 23:208.

Fihn SD, McDonell M, Martin M, et al. Risk factors for complications of chronic anticoagulation: A multicenter study. Ann Intern Med 1993; 118:511.

Hirsh J, Poller L, Deykin D, et al. Optimal therapeutic range for oral anticoagulants. Chest 1989; 95:5S.

King DJ, Kelton JG. Heparin associated thrombocytopenia. Ann Intern Med 1984; 100:535.

Kitchens CS, Mehta JL. Pharmacology of platelet-inhibitory drugs, anticoagulants, and thrombolytic agents. Cardiovasc Clin 1987; 18:195.

Levine HJ, Pauker SG, Salzman EW. Antithrombotic therapy in valvular heart disease. Chest 1989; 95:98S.

Levine MN, Raskob G, Hirsh J. Hemorrhagic complications of long-term anticoagulant therapy. Chest 1989; 95:26S.

O'Reilly A. Vitamin K antagonists. In: Coleman, ed. Hemostasis and thrombosis: Basic principles and clinical practice. Philadelphia: JB Lippincott, 1987:1367.

Petersen P, Godtfredsen J, Boysen G, et al. Placebo-controlled, randomized trial of warfarin and aspirin for prevention of thromboembolic complications in chronic atrial fibrillation: The Copenhagen AFASAK Study. Lancet 1989; 1:175–179.

Resnekov L, Chediak J, Hirsh J, Lewis DH. Antithrombotic agents in coronary artery disease. Chest 1989; 95:52S.

Sherman DG, Dyken ML, Fisher M, et al. Antithrombotic therapy for cerebrovascular disorders. Chest 1989; 95:140S.

Sixty Plus Reinfarction Study Group. A double blind trial to assess long-term oral anticoagulant therapy in elderly patients after a myocardial infarction. Lancet 1980; 2:989.

The Boston Area Anticoagulation Trial for Atrial Fibrillation Investigators. The effect of low-dose warfarin on the risk of stroke in patients with nonrheumatic atrial fibrillation. N Engl J Med 1990; 323:1505–1511.

The Steering Committee of the Physicians Health Study Research Group. Preliminary report: Findings from the aspirin component of the ongoing Physician's Health Study. N Engl J Med 1988; 318:262.

Stein PD, Kantrowitz A. Antithrombotic therapy in mechanical and biological prosthetic heart valves and saphenous vein bypass grafts. Chest 1989; 95:107S.

Wolf PA, Abbott RD, Kannel WB. Atrial fibrillation: A major contributor to stroke in the elderly. The Framingham Study. Arch Intern Med 1987; 147:1561.

NONINFECTIOUS ADVERSE REACTIONS TO BLOOD TRANSFUSION

Nancy M. Heddle, M.Sc., A.R.T.

Noninfectious adverse effects to blood transfusions occur in approximately 10 percent of transfusion recipients. These reactions may occur during or within a few hours of the transfusion or several days, sometimes months, after the transfusion (Table 1). Most reactions are relatively minor; however, a few result in severe morbidity or mortality. Thus, early recognition followed by an appropriate intervention is important.

■ IMMEDIATE ADVERSE EFFECTS

Bacteria-Contaminated Blood

The frequency of bacterial contamination of blood products decreased to less than 0.1 percent during the 1970s with the introduction of the plastic bag for blood collection. However, during the past decade there has been an increasing number of reports of bacterial contamination in red cell and platelet products. The contaminants isolated from red cell concentrates are frequently gram-negative bacteria, some of which grow at cold temperatures (Table 2). Bacteria in platelets can be an even greater problem, as platelets are stored for up to 5 days at room temperature before transfusion; thus, bacteria in platelet concentrates can proliferate and cause gross contamination.

When contaminated blood products are transfused, the patient often develops a high fever, chills, vomiting, hypotension, shock, hemoglobinuria, renal failure, and disseminated intravascular coagulation (DIC). Symptoms of shock include flushing, dry skin, gastrointestinal distress, and generalized muscle aches. The rapid onset of shock suggests that the symptoms may be related to bacterial endotoxins in the blood product. The signs and symptoms typical of this reaction appear within the first few minutes of the transfusion, after only a few milliliters of blood being transfused. Morbidity is often severe, and the overall mortality rate is estimated at 26 percent. If this reaction is suspected, the blood product should be stopped immediately and returned to the laboratory for microbiologic investigation. The patient's symptoms should be treated and appropriate antibiotics administered (see Table 2).

Immune-Mediated Hemolytic Transfusion Reactions

An immune-mediated hemolytic transfusion reaction occurs when the recipient has a red cell antibody that reacts with the transfused red cells, causing intravascular and/or extravascular red cell lysis. Intravascular hemolysis activates complement, the kinin system, and the coagulation system. Activation of complement proteins produces anaphylatoxins, which stimulate mast cells to release histamine and serotonin. Together these bioreactive substances can cause a precipitous fall in the patient's blood pressure (shock). The kinin system is often activated, causing hormone production by the adrenal glands and the sympathetic nervous system. These hormones act on alpha receptors in blood vessels, causing vasoconstriction primarily in the blood vessels within the kidney, viscera, lungs, and skin, hence decreased blood flow to these vital organs. Finally, the coagulation system can be activated by the antigen-antibody complexes, resulting in DIC.

Table 1 Immediate and Delayed Noninfectious Adverse Effects to Blood Transfusion

IMMEDIATE
- Immune-mediated hemolysis
- Nonimmune hemolysis
- Bacterial contamination
- Febrile nonhemolytic transfusion reactions
- Acute respiratory distress
  - IgA deficiency
  - Leukoagglutinin reaction
- Allergic reactions
- Metabolic reactions
  - Hyperkalemia
  - Citrate toxicity
  - Hypothermia
  - Hyperglycemia
- Circulatory overload

DELAYED
- Alloimmunization
- Delayed hemolytic transfusion reaction
- Post-transfusion purpura
- Transfusion-associated graft versus host disease

Fortunately, only a few blood group antibodies can cause intravascular lysis. This reaction is associated most frequently with the transfusion of ABO-incompatible blood, usually resulting from a clerical error such as specimen mislabeling, serologic testing with the wrong specimen, or inaccurate identification of the recipient before transfusion. Thus, policies and procedures to ensure correct identification of the patient and the donor unit before transfusion are critical.

Hemolytic transfusion reactions tend to occur toward the start of the transfusion; however, a minimum of 50 to 100 ml of transfused blood is usually required before the patient becomes symptomatic. This characteristic time frame can be useful to differentiate hemolytic transfusion reactions from reactions to bacterial contamination or IgA (immunoglobulin) deficiency, which usually occur with smaller transfusion volumes.

No one set of symptoms is typical of acute intravascular hemolytic transfusion reactions. During the first stage of the reaction the patient may have nausea, flushing, back pain, an uneasy feeling, fever, and chills. Fever, one of the most common symptoms, is reported to occur in approximately 75 percent of patients; about half of the patients with fever also have chills. During the second phase of the reaction the patient has dyspnea, flank pain, hypotension, renal failure, and uncontrollable bleeding due to DIC. Mortality is estimated at 3 percent for patients who receive ABO-incompatible blood.

The transfusion must be stopped at the first sign of a hemolytic reaction, because the degree of morbidity is directly proportional to the amount of blood transfused. A clerical check should be performed immediately at the bedside to determine whether an error has occurred. If a labeling discrepancy is noted, the laboratory must be informed, as there may be another patient in the hospital who is also receiving the wrong blood. The treatment of a hemolytic transfusion reaction includes intravenous support to maintain adequate urine output, treatment for shock, monitoring

Table 2 Organisms Most Frequently Isolated from Red Cell and Platelet Concentrates and Antibiotics Suggested for Treatment

PRODUCT	ORGANISMS	ANTIBIOTICS
Platelet concentrates	*Staphylococcus epidermidis*	Vancomycin
	Diphtheroids*	
	S. aureus	Cloxacillin, vancomycin
	Escherichia cloacal	Aminoglycoside
	Coliforms	Aminoglycoside
	Pseudomonas species	Aminoglycoside
Red cell concentrates	*Yersinia enterocolitica*	Quinolone
	P. fluorescens	Aminoglycoside or 3rd generation cephalosporin

*Not reported to cause post-transfusion sepsis.

of the hemostatic system, and consideration of coagulation cofactor replacement if DIC occurs.

Laboratory investigation of a suspected hemolytic transfusion reaction should include the following tests on a posttransfusion specimen: a direct antiglobulin test, visual examination of the plasma for free plasma hemoglobin, and a clerical check to ensure that there has not been a mix-up of specimens during compatibility testing. If these tests are negative, a hemolytic reaction is unlikely.

Nonimmune Hemolytic Reactions

Hemoglobinuria, or free plasma hemoglobin, is not always associated with immune-mediated red cell hemolysis. Numerous causes of intravascular hemolysis have been attributed to mechanical or environmental red cell destruction or lysis due to membrane abnormalities of the transfused red cells. Mechanical or environmental hemolysis may follow excess exposure to heat or cold, infusion (often under high pressure) through a small-gauge needle, or the use of an extracorporeal infusion device. Red cell abnormalities associated with hemolysis include glucose 6 phosphate dehydrogenase (G6PD) deficiency, sickle cell disease, polyagglutinable red cells (T activation), and paroxysmal nocturnal hemoglobinuria. Hemolysis via these mechanisms is not usually associated with morbidity or mortality; however, a careful clinical and laboratory assessment must be performed to exclude an immune-mediated event.

Febrile Nonhemolytic Transfusion Reactions

Febrile nonhemolytic transfusion reactions are traditionally defined as a rise in temperature (greater than 1°C), usually accompanied by chills, cold, rigors, or discomfort. The frequent use of antipyretics has resulted in many patients having signs and symptoms without the fever. These reactions tend to occur toward the end of or within a few hours of receiving red cells or platelets. These very common reactions are associated with 1 to 6 percent of red cell transfusions, depending on the patient population and the degree of surveillance, and 20 to 30 percent of platelet transfusions. The cause of these reactions is probably multifactorial; however, increasing evidence suggests that many of the reactions associated with platelet transfusions may be caused by biologic mediators, possibly cytokines, that accumulate in the plasma supernatant during storage of the platelets. Several studies have demonstrated a correlation between reactions and the level of interleukin-1-beta, interleukin-6, and tumor necrosis factor. A small percentage of reactions may be caused by an immune-mediated interaction between leukocyte antibodies in the patient's plasma and leukocytes present in the blood product.

The traditional way of preventing these reactions is administration of antipyretics to prevent symptoms and poststorage leukodepletion of the blood product using centrifugation or filtration. Poststorage leukodepletion of red cell concentrates (less than 5×10^8 cells per product) is effective for preventing most reactions to red cell concentrates but appears to be less effective for preventing reactions to platelets. If cytokines are the primary inducers of reactions to platelets, prestorage leukodepletion or concentration (plasma depletion) of the platelet concentrate before transfusion may be more effective. Because there is a direct correlation between duration of storage and cytokine concentration in platelet concentrates, reactions are less common with fresher blood products.

Although fever is the characteristic sign of a febrile reaction, it is not specific to this type of reaction. As discussed previously, fever also accompanies many types of immediate transfusion reactions; hence, it is important to exclude hemolysis, bacteria-contaminated blood, and noncardiogenic pulmonary edema when fever develops, as the degree of morbidity and the frequency of mortality are much higher with these reactions. The patient should be treated with antipyretic drugs such as acetaminophen when a febrile nonhemolytic transfusion reaction occurs. Patients who have a history of repeated febrile transfusion reactions should be premedicated with an antipyretic drug. Slowing the rate of infusion has also been shown to decrease the symptoms associated with this type of reaction.

Acute Respiratory Distress

Reactions characterized by acute respiratory distress have two primary causes: IgA deficiency and leukoagglutinins.

IgA Deficiency

An IgA-deficient patient can have an anaphylactic reaction after the infusion of a small volume of blood or plasma. Typical patients develop abrupt hypertension followed by hypotension, asthma, and gastrointestinal symptoms (nausea, vomiting, abdominal cramps, and diarrhea). In contrast to reactions due to bacterial contamination, fever does not occur. Thus, the presence or absence of fever can be useful to distinguish between these two events. Patients who develop anaphylaxis following a blood transfusion are usually IgA deficient and have developed an IgG antibody against IgA. When they are transfused with donor blood containing IgA, an antigen-antibody complex is formed, complement is activated, and severe anaphylaxis can occur. Although IgA deficiency occurs in approximately 1 in 700 individuals, it is estimated that only 1 in 25,000 transfused patients will have this type of reaction, as some IgA-deficient patients are not alloimmunized or have low concentrations of anti-IgA antibodies.

A patient who has a history of an anaphylactic reaction or who is known to be IgA deficient should be given IgA-deficient blood products. Alternatively, red cell concentrates or platelet concentrates can be washed to remove the plasma containing IgA. When an anaphylactic reaction occurs, the blood product must be stopped immediately, and the remainder of the product must not be given. Mortality can occur unless the situation is recognized and the patient treated immediately with intravenous epinephrine.

Leukoagglutinin Reaction

The second mechanism of transfusion-associated acute respiratory distress involves acute pulmonary edema without cardiac involvement. This reaction is associated with white cell antibodies (leukoagglutinins), which are most frequently directed against granulocytes. The leukoagglutinins are usually in the donor's plasma reacting with the patient's leukocytes in the pulmonary circulation. These pulmonary infiltrates become trapped in the microcirculation, causing vascular obstruction and symptoms of acute respiratory distress. The patient usually has dyspnea, cyanosis, chills, fever, and hypotension, and unless treated immediately, this type of reaction can be fatal. Symptoms can present during the transfusion or within 1 to 8 hours post transfusion. Treatment includes diuretics, oxygen administration, and intravenous administration of corticosteroids and epinephrine. With appropriate treatment, symptoms usually resolve within 12 to 24 hours. A potent antigranulocyte antibody can usually be demonstrated in the donor plasma; however, the technology for detecting these antibodies is not routinely available in most centers, so the diagnosis is usually made on clinical grounds. Although this type of reaction is extremely rare, it is important that it be reported to the transfusion laboratory, as it is critical that no other blood from this donor be used for transfusion.

Allergic (Urticarial) Reactions

Allergic reactions occur in approximately 1 to 3 percent of transfused patients. These reactions are caused by plasma; hence, the use of concentrated red cells has dramatically decreased the frequency of this event. Most of these reactions are thought to be caused by IgE antibodies, which react with soluble antigens present in the transfused plasma. As IgE antibodies are bound to mast cells, the antigen-antibody interaction results in release of histamine and symptoms related to the skin (hives, itching, and erythema). Other signs and symptoms, including fever, are not present.

An allergic (urticarial) transfusion reaction does not always require that the administration of the blood product be stopped, nor should the product be discarded. In most patients the rate of transfusion can be slowed and an antihistamine administered. For patients who have more severe reactions, the infusion can be temporarily interrupted while medication is administered. After 15 to 20 minutes the infusion can be restarted. Patients who have a history of allergic reactions should be premedicated with an antihistamine prior to the transfusion.

Metabolic Complications

Hyperkalemia

During storage of red cell concentrates potassium concentrations increase due to the leakage of intracellular potassium associated with inhibition of the membrane adenosine triphosphatase pump. This membrane defect is reversible once the red cells are infused. Complications related to transfusion-associated hyperkalemia are unusual with current transfusion practices. The potential for problems arises primarily during large-volume transfusions and exchange transfusions; thus, careful monitoring of cardiac function is essential in these situations.

Citrate Toxicity

The anticoagulant used for blood collection contains citrate, which chelates calcium, preventing clot formation. The rapid infusion of large volumes of citrate can decrease ionized calcium, causing convulsions, arrhythmia, and heart block. Although citrate toxicity is rare, the risk increases with concomitant factors such as hepatic dysfunction, hypothermia, and rapid infusion. Citrate toxicity can be avoided with careful cardiac monitoring during large-volume transfusion and appropriate administration of intravenous calcium.

Hypothermia

Transfusion of large volumes of cold blood can produce hypothermia with subsequent microvascular changes that can affect platelet function and blood clotting. Hypothermia can be avoided by warming the blood product before transfusion with a temperature-controlled warming coil or blood warmer.

Hyperglycemia

Blood collected and processed with preservative additive systems such as Adsol and Nutricel contain higher concentrations of dextrose than blood collected and stored in CPDA-1. This is a theoretic concern for neonatal exchange transfusions, but few clinical studies have addressed the clinical effects.

Circulatory Overload

Circulatory overload following blood transfusion is most frequently encountered in patients with cardiac failure and in premature neonates. To prevent this complication in susceptible patients, the rate of infusion should be slow. If platelet concentrates are required, the volume of the product can be reduced by removing some of the supernatant plasma before transfusion. In neonates, exchange transfusion has also been used to replace the required blood component without an overall increase in blood volume.

Investigation of Immediate Transfusion Reactions

Because the signs and symptoms associated with the different types of immediate transfusion reactions are not specific and because laboratory tests for diagnostic confirmation may not be readily available, the physician is often confronted with the decision to discard the remainder of the blood product, which may result in additional donor exposures, or to continue the transfusion. A practical approach for investigating these reactions is important to ensure optimal patient care.

Allergic reactions are easily characterized, as the only symptom is urticaria. In this situation the rate of infusion should be slowed or temporarily stopped and an antihistamine administered; the remainder of the blood product can usually be transfused. Differentiation of other immediate reactions is more difficult; however, the following approach can be useful:

1. While the reaction is being investigated, the transfusion should be stopped and the intravenous line kept open with saline. An identity check of the patient and the blood product should be performed at the bedside to rule out the possibility of immune-mediated hemolysis due to a clerical error.
2. Ask when during the transfusion the reaction occurred. Anaphylactic reactions and reactions caused by bacterial contamination usually occur after the infusion of 10 to 15 ml of the product. Hemolytic reactions to red cells also occur early during the course of the transfusion; however, 50 to 100 ml of blood is usually required before the patient becomes symptomatic. In contrast, symptoms of febrile transfusion reactions traditionally present at the end of the transfusion.
3. Hemolysis can be confirmed or ruled out by performing

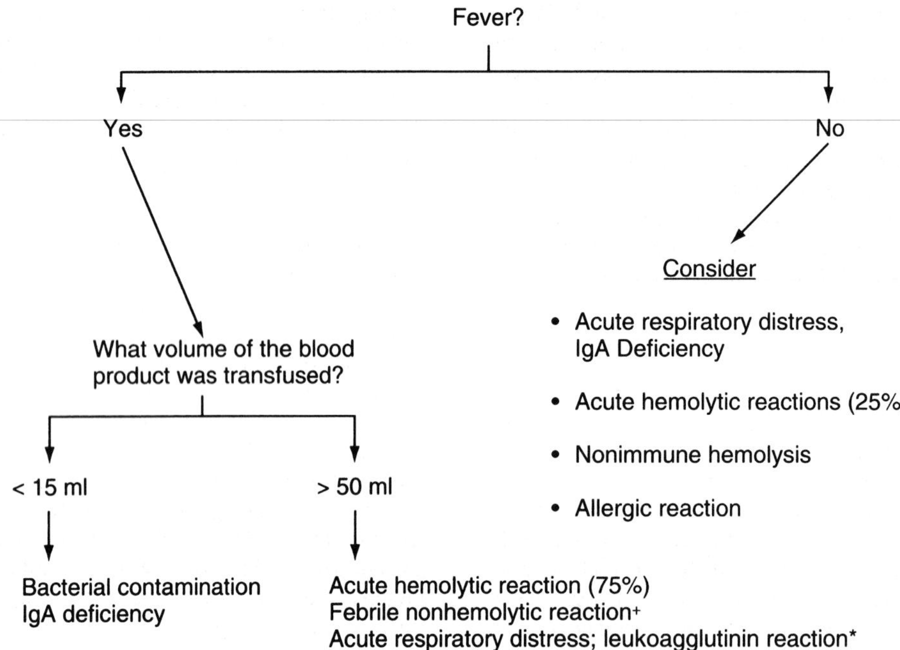

Figure 1
Algorithm for the differential diagnosis of immediate transfusion reactions.

the following tests on a post-transfusion blood sample: a direct antiglobulin test, a visual check for free plasma hemoglobin, and a clerical check of laboratory records and blood samples. If these three tests are negative, a hemolytic reaction is extremely unlikely.

There is no quick confirmation to differentiate bacterial sepsis from a hemolytic reaction; however, the symptoms associated with bacterial sepsis usually occur earlier and are more dramatic than those seen with a hemolytic or a febrile transfusion reaction. The presence or absence of fever can also be useful in differentiating the cause of immediate reactions. For example, anaphylaxis associated with IgA deficiency can be differentiated from the other types of reactions, as fever does not occur. Figure 1 provides a flow diagram to assist in the investigation of immediate transfusion reactions based on the presence or absence of fever and the volume of blood transfused.

■ DELAYED ADVERSE EFFECTS

Alloimmunization

Exposure to foreign antigens in plasma and on blood cells results in alloantibody formation in approximately 5 percent of transfused individuals. In specific patient populations who receive chronic transfusion therapy, the frequency of red cell or HLA alloimmunization may be even higher (patients with thalassemia or acute leukemia). The primary response to a foreign antigen results in predominantly IgM antibody, which is usually not detectable for 10 to 14 days following exposure. IgG antibody may be produced in low (usually undetectable) concentrations during a primary response but can rise within 48 to 72 hours following a secondary exposure.

Alloimmunization to red cell antigens can make it difficult to find compatible blood for future transfusions and can result in hemolytic disease of the newborn. Alloimmunization to leukocyte antigens may be associated with a poor response to platelet transfusions (refractoriness), transfusion-associated acute lung injury, and febrile nonhemolytic transfusion reactions. Leukodepletion of blood products below a threshold of 5×10^6 per product appears to prevent human leukocyte antigen (HLA) alloimmunization; however, the clinical relevance of this is still under investigation. Alloimmunization to platelet-specific antigens can result in post-transfusion purpura and neonatal alloimmune thrombocytopenia. It may also decrease the survival of transfused platelets.

Delayed Hemolytic Transfusion Reactions

Delayed hemolytic transfusion reactions typically occur 4 to 14 days post transfusion. The patient becomes alloimmunized to foreign antigens on the transfused donor red cells (most frequently specific for the E, C, K, Jk^a and Fy^a antigens). This alloantibody binds to the transfused red cells in the patient's circulation and in some situations can destroy these cells.

If the patient has been previously exposed to the antigen, antibody production can occur within a few days of the transfusion. If this is the primary exposure, antibody is not usually detected for 10 to 14 days or longer. Typical laboratory findings include a positive antibody screen with a specific red cell antibody and a positive direct antiglobulin test, often showing a mixed field reaction. This serologic evidence of alloimmunization occurs frequently (1 in every 100 transfused patients), but is infrequently associated with clinical evidence of hemolysis. Clinical signs of hemolysis (fever, an unexpected fall in hemoglobin, and hyperbilirubinemia) are rare, occurring in approximately 1 in 3,000 patients transfused.

Post-Transfusion Purpura

Post-transfusion purpura is characterized by severe thrombocytopenia (less than 10×10^9 per liter) approximately 7 days after transfusion. A platelet-specific alloantibody, most frequently anti-PLA_1, is usually detected in the patient's plasma and is thought to be involved in platelet destruction; however, the mechanism by which this occurs is not well understood. It has been postulated that the platelet-specific alloantibody initially interacts with the transfused platelets, destroying them, then attacks the patient's platelets. The patient must be previously sensitized to platelet-specific antigens, and consequently almost all patients with post-transfusion purpura are women who have had children. The diagnosis is confirmed by typing the patient's platelets after recovery. Treatment includes the physical removal of the alloantibody by plasma exchange and blockade of the reticuloendothelial system via high-dose intravenous gamma globulin (2 g per kilogram).

Transfusion-Associated Graft Versus Host Disease

Transfusion-associated graft versus host disease (TA-GVHD) occurs when transfused allogeneic lymphocytes (T cells) become engrafted, causing an immunologic reaction in the recipient that is directed against the host's HLA antigens. Engraftment of transfused T cells is most likely to occur in individuals who are immunosuppressed by a congenital cause such as severe combined immunodeficiency disease, DiGeorge syndrome, Wiskott-Aldrich syndrome, thymic hypoplasia, or purine nucleoside phosphorylase deficiency; patients with therapeutic immunosuppression (bone marrow transplantation and patients receiving treatment for neuroblastoma); low birth weight premature neonates who require exchange transfusion; and the fetus who requires intrauterine transfusion. However, TA-GVHD has also been reported in patients with no known predisposing factors and in infants with neonatal alloimmune thrombocytopenia. The risk of TA-GVHD is also increased when transfused donor lymphocytes share a HLA haplotype with the recipient even when an immune disturbance is absent.

TA-GVHD often results in dysfunction of skin, liver, bone marrow, and the gastrointestinal tract. Clinical signs and symptoms include a maculopapular erythematous skin rash, fever, cough, diarrhea, and vomiting. Hepatocellular damage is characterized by abnormal liver function tests, and the patient becomes aplastic with severe pancytopenia. Severe bacterial and viral infections, impaired ventilation and perfusion, and electrolyte imbalances are also frequently seen in patients with TA-GVHD. Clinical symptoms usually develop 10 to 12 days post transfusion. The outcome is invariably fatal, with death occurring within 1 month of onset. Diagnostic confirmation has been performed by skin biopsy, bone marrow chimerism, karyotype analysis, differences in the HLA phenotype of peripheral blood lymphocytes compared with other tissues, DNA probes, and autopsy. Prevention of TA-GVHD includes irradiation (2,500 cGy) of all cellular blood products being transfused to high-risk patients and irradiation of blood products that are directed donations from first-degree relatives.

Suggested Reading

Anderson KC. Clinical indications for blood component irradiation. In: Baldwin ML, Jefferies LC, eds. Irradiation of blood components. Bethesda, MD: American Association of Blood Banks, 1992:31.

Bordin JO, Heddle NM, Blajchman MA. Biologic effects of leukocytes present in transfused cellular blood products. Blood, 1994; 84:1703–1721.

Capon SM, Goldfinger D. New insights into the pathophysiology and treatment of acute hemolytic transfusion reactions. In: Nance SJ, ed. Alloimmunity: 1993 and beyond. Bethesda, MD: American Association of Blood Banks, 1993:141.

Goldman M, Blajchman MA. Blood product-associated bacterial sepsis. Transfus Med Rev 1991; 5(1):73–83.

Heddle NM, Klama L, Singer J, et al. The role of the plasma from platelet concentrates in transfusion reactions. N Engl J Med 1994; 331:625–628.

Shirey RS, Ness PM. New concepts of delayed hemolytic transfusion reactions. In: Nance SJ, ed. Clinical and basic science aspects of immunohematology. Arlington, VA: American Association of Blood Banks, 1991:179.

INFECTIOUS MONONUCLEOSIS AND RELATED SYNDROMES

Fiona Smaill, M.B., Ch.B.

Infectious mononucleosis is an acute febrile illness associated with sore throat and lymphadenopathy caused by Epstein-Barr virus (EBV). Usually there is lymphocytosis with so-called atypical changes in the peripheral blood and a heterophile antibody response. Mononucleosis-like syndromes include a heterogenous group of acute illnesses with overlapping clinical and hematologic findings that are not associated with heterophile antibody. Cytomegalovirus infection is the most frequent cause of heterophile-negative mononucleosis, but other infections, including toxoplasmosis, acute viral hepatitis, rubella, primary human herpesvirus 6, and acute human immunodeficiency virus (HIV), can produce a mononucleosis-like syndrome.

■ INFECTIOUS MONONUCLEOSIS

EBV is a double-stranded DNA virus of the herpesvirus group. By adulthood, 90 to 95 percent of most populations have evidence of previous infection with EBV. Lower socioeconomic groups have a higher prevalence of EBV antibody. In the United States and Great Britain, about half of EBV infections occur before age 5, with a second peak of seroconversion occurring in young adults. After the person recovers from acute infection, the virus persists in the oropharynx for as long as 18 months. It can be cultured from the throat washings of up to 20 percent of seropositive healthy adults. The virus is generally transmitted through close contact. Among young adults spread of the virus may be facilitated by the transfer of saliva with kissing. EBV has also been transmitted by blood transfusion. The virus remains latent in circulating B lymphocytes. Immunocompromised patients have a higher frequency of viral shedding, and the virus can be cultured from 50 percent of renal transplant recipients and up to 90 percent of leukemia and lymphoma patients.

Classical infectious mononucleosis typically is a self-limited infection in adolescents characterized by sore throat, fever, fatigue, and anorexia. Clinical findings supporting the diagnosis include (1) an exudative pharyngitis, which is indistinguishable from the acute pharyngitis caused by group A streptococcus; (2) lymphadenopathy, which most commonly involves the posterior cervical area; (3) hepatosplenomegaly; and (4) periorbital edema (Table 1). A maculopapular rash usually develops if ampicillin is given during the acute phase of the infection. In infants and young children, primary EBV infection is frequently asymptomatic, but when there are clinical findings, symptoms of respiratory tract infection can be prominent. EBV infection in older adults can be severe, with debilitating fever, malaise, and fatigue. Pharyngitis, adenopathy, and splenomegaly are less commonly observed in the elderly.

A typical infection is self-limited and lasts 2 to 3 weeks, although resolution of fatigue may take longer. Severe but rare complications include splenic rupture (estimated to occur in 0.1 to 0.2 percent of cases), fulminant hepatitis, and airway obstruction secondary to severe pharyngitis. Although clinical jaundice is unusual, laboratory evidence of hepatitis and elevated bilirubin are very common (see Table 1). Mild thrombocytopenia and granulocytopenia are frequent, but profound thrombocytopenia associated with bleeding can occur. Some patients (0.5 to 3 percent) will develop an autoimmune hemolytic anemia mediated by IgM cold-agglutinin antibodies. Neurologic manifestations in the absence of the typical findings associated with infectious mononucleosis sometimes dominate the clinical picture.

The chronic fatigue syndrome sometimes called chronic

Table 1 Clinical and Laboratory Findings in Mononucleosis-Like Syndromes

FINDING	EBV INFECTION	CMV INFECTION	TOXOPLASMOSIS
SYMPTOMS			
Fever	87%	100%	43%
Sore throat	82	21	22
SIGNS			
Lymphadenopathy	83	19	81
Exudative pharyngitis	~33–50	—	—
Palatal petechiae	~33	—	—
Rash (not related to ampicillin)	8	7	5
Rash (with ampicillin)	~90	increased	—
Splenomegaly	43	17	25
Hepatomegaly	11	31	25
Periorbital edema	~33	—	—
LABORATORY ABNORMALITIES			
Elevated serum transaminases	95	92	<1
Thrombocytopenia	50	<1	<1
Chorioretinitis	0	0	5
Neurologic complications	<1	<1	2
Myocarditis	<1	4	4

mononucleosis is an illness of unknown cause defined by extreme fatigue. Recurrent fevers, lymphadenopathy, sore throat, myalgias, headache, difficulty concentrating, and psychological disorders are associated with this condition. There is no convincing evidence that EBV infection affects most patients given this diagnosis. Serologic studies are not useful for these patients.

Rare patients have chronic or persistent EBV infection characterized by objective clinical findings (e.g., chronic lymphadenopathy, hepatosplenomegaly, interstitial pneumonia) and extraordinarily high titers of EBV antibodies. Very high antibody levels to EBV are also found in patients with African Burkitt's lymphoma and nasopharyngeal carcinoma, suggesting a role for EBV infection in these malignancies. EBV lymphoproliferative syndromes have been observed in association with the immunosuppression of renal and bone marrow transplantation and in HIV infection.

Diagnosis

The hematologic criteria that support a diagnosis of infectious mononucleosis include (1) a relative (more than half of the total leukocyte count) and absolute (more than 4,500 per cubic millimeter) mononuclear lymphocytosis and (2) atypical lymphocytes, also called Downey cells, constituting at least 10 percent of the total leukocyte count or more than 1,000 per cubic millimeter. In about 70 percent of patients with infectious mononucleosis, these findings are present at the onset of symptoms. The lymphocytosis peaks during the second or third week of illness. There is, however, a wide range in the atypical lymphocytosis. While some patients show none or only a few atypical lymphocytes, 90 percent or more of the circulating lymphocytes may be atypical in other cases. The atypical lymphocyte is a lymphoblast. These cells vary in size but tend to be large, with vacuolated cytoplasm, loose nuclear chromatin, and indentation of the cell membrane by adjacent erythrocytes. Atypical lymphocytosis in infectious mononucleosis results from the stimulation of T cells, principally those of the cytotoxic or suppressor (CD8+) phenotype, by EBV-infected and transformed B cells.

EBV cannot be cultured with routine viral culture methods. Acute EBV infection is confirmed by heterophile antibody or virus-specific antibodies. The heterophile antibody that develops as a nonspecific response to EBV infection is an IgM antibody that reacts with the surface antigen of sheep and horse red blood cells but not guinea pig kidney cells. A number of commercial tests to detect heterophile antibodies, most commonly using a slide agglutination assay (e.g., Monospot), are available for the rapid diagnosis of infectious mononucleosis. The sensitivities and specificities of these rapid tests vary from 63 to 84 percent and 84 to 100 percent, respectively. Titers of heterophile antibody can remain detectable for as long as a year after acute infection. Rare false-positive results have been reported in patients with lymphoma or hepatitis. A negative result early in infection is common. A week after the onset of infection, antibodies are detected in 40 percent of cases, but by the third week 80 to 90 percent will be positive. Many infants and young children with primary EBV infection do not have heterophile antibodies. In only 25 percent of infants 10 to 24 months of age are heterophile antibodies detected, increasing to 75 percent among children aged 24 to 28 months.

It is rarely necessary to measure EBV-specific antibodies to diagnose classic infectious mononucleosis (Table 2). Determining the antibody response to specific EBV antigens can help to confirm acute infection if repeat heterophile antibody testing is negative, particularly in children or if the clinical presentation is atypical, and to differentiate recent from remote infection. Although the tests to detect antibody to viral capsid antigen (VCA) and early antigen (EA) using an indirect immunofluorescent assay are widely available, they are cumbersome to perform and their reproducibility has been reported to be poor; the end point is subjective and results can vary with laboratory experience. An enzyme-linked immunoabsorbent assay ELISA now available for the detection of antibodies to Epstein-Barr nuclear antigen (EBNA) improves the sensitivity of this test. Table 3 shows examples of the interpretation of the results of EBV serology.

Management

There is no specific therapy for most cases of infectious mononucleosis. Supportive treatment includes salicylates or acetaminophen to control fever, headache, and sore throat. Antibiotics are not indicated in uncomplicated cases. A peritonsillar abscess with infectious mononucleosis is an indication for drainage and antibiotic therapy; penicillin is appropriate.

Table 2 Antibodies to EBV

ANTIBODY	PERSISTENCE	POSITIVE, %	COMMENTS
Viral capsid antigens			
IgM VCA	4–8 weeks	100%	Present in high titer in primary infection; may not be routinely available.
IgG VCA	Lifelong	100	Present in primary, recent, and remote infections; high titer at presentation, but level of antibody generally not helpful in differentiating recent from remote infection.
Early antigen			
Anti-D	Low titer up to 1:40 can persist for years	70	Present in 70% of acute IM; persistence correlated with severe disease.
Anti-R	Up to 3 years	low	Not routinely available; present in high titers in African Burkitt's lymphoma.
EBNA	Lifelong	100	Appears within 3–4 weeks of onset of acute IM.

VCA, viral capsid antigen;
IM, Infectious mononucleosis; EBNA, Epstein-Barr nuclear antigen.

Table 3 Interpretation of EBV Serology

EBV-SPECIFIC SEROLOGY		INTERPRETATIONS
VCA-IgG	<1:40	No prior exposure to EBV
EA	<1:40	
EBNA	Absent	
VCA-IgG	≥1:40	Probable recent primary infection
EA	<1:40	
EBNA	Absent	
VCA-IgG	≥1:40	Either recent primary infection or remote infection
EA	≥1:40	
EBNA	Present or equivocal	
VCA-IgG	≥1:40	Likely remote infection
EA	<1:40	
EBNA	Present or equivocal	
VCA-IgG	≥1:40	Likely recent primary infection
EA	≥1:40	
EBNA	Absent	
VCA-IgM	Present	Acute primary infection
VCA-IgG	≥1:40	
EA	<1:40 or ≥1:40	
EBNA	Absent	

VCA, viral capsid antigen; EA, early antigen; EBNA, Epstein-Barr nuclear antigen.

Although there is evidence from randomized studies that the course of fever is shortened by corticosteroid treatment, corticosteroids are not indicated for patients with uncomplicated disease. Corticosteroids are appropriate for patients with severe complications associated with infectious mononucleosis, including pharyngeal edema with impending airway obstruction, severe thrombocytopenia, and hemolytic anemia; however, controlled studies have not evaluated their efficacy. A dose equivalent to 60 to 80 mg of prednisone, tapered quickly over 1 to 2 weeks, is used. Corticosteroids have also been advocated when neurologic involvement, myocarditis, or pericarditis complicates EBV infection. Although there is no evidence to support the use of corticosteroids in patients whose infection is only associated with severe and prolonged fatigue, a short tapering course of lower-dose prednisone (initial dose of 40 mg) may shorten the clinical illness. There are case reports of the successful use of intravenous immunoglobulin for the treatment of thrombocytopenia. Plasmapheresis has been used in steroid-resistant hemolysis associated with EBV infection.

The antiviral agent acyclovir has been shown to inhibit EBV replication and may suppress oropharyngeal viral shedding, but randomized, placebo-controlled trials of acyclovir for the treatment of acute infectious mononucleosis have not demonstrated a benefit.

■ CYTOMEGALOVIRUS INFECTION

About half of all cases of heterophile-negative mononucleosis in adults are caused by cytomegalovirus (CMV), although most episodes of CMV infection in normal individuals are asymptomatic. Depending on the socioeconomic status of the population, the prevalence of antibodies to CMV in adults ranges from 40 to 100 percent. Transmission of CMV occurs through close personal contact, most commonly by oral and sexual routes. Ordinarily the virus is not detectable in normal adults, but asymptomatic viral shedding from the cervix is common in women, and CMV can be detected in semen in men. Infected children tend to carry the virus in the oropharynx and urine for long periods.

Infection can occur in utero or during the perinatal period, either when the infant comes in contact with infected cervical secretions at birth or through breast milk. Spread of CMV among young children in day care or in the family is common. Infection peaks again during early adulthood and is associated with sexual transmission. Exposure to CMV through blood transfusion or organ transplantation can result in clinical illness. In renal, cardiac, liver, lung, and bone marrow transplantation, clinical disease can result either from the primary acquisition of CMV from the transplanted tissue in an individual not previously exposed to CMV or from reactivation or reinfection in an individual known to be CMV antibody positive.

Acute CMV infection is difficult to recognize clinically and to differentiate from EBV-associated mononucleosis. In the normal host the most frequent finding is fever accompanied by profound fatigue. Sore throat, lymphadenopathy, and splenomegaly are less frequent than in EBV-associated mononucleosis, and pharyngitis is unusual (see Table 1). A rash can occur, either with or without the administration of ampicillin. A relative and absolute lymphocytosis with abundant atypical lymphocytes (more than 10 percent) develops in more than 90 percent of cases, often 1 to 2 weeks after the onset of fever. The atypical lymphocyte in CMV mononucleosis is a CD8+ suppressor or cytotoxic cell, similar to that of EBV infection.

In most patients liver transaminases are mildly elevated. A hepatitis-like presentation with significant abnormality of liver function tests occurs in approximately 15 to 20 percent of patients. The Guillain-Barré syndrome is recognized as a complication of CMV-induced mononucleosis. Rarely, meningoencephalitis, myocarditis, thrombocytopenia, and hemolytic anemia have been observed in the normal host.

In the immunosuppressed host, CMV infection is most often asymptomatic, but when disease occurs, extensive organ involvement can dominate the clinical picture. Laboratory abnormalities observed include leukopenia, lymphocytosis with atypical lymphocytes, and abnormal liver function tests. Pneumonitis has been described in the immunocompetent host, and next to fever it is the most common manifestation of CMV infection in the immunosuppressed patient. Hepatitis, disease of the gastrointestinal tract, retinitis, meningoencephalitis, and involvement of various endocrine organs are complications. Primary CMV infection in pregnancy, usually unrecognized, can lead to the devastating consequences of congenital infection in the infant, although most congenitally infected children have no obvious signs at birth.

Diagnosis

It can be difficult to establish the diagnosis of CMV-associated mononucleosis. The virus can be easily cultured from urine, throat, cervical swabs, and peripheral white blood cells. The traditional method of isolating CMV, detecting a cytopathic effect in human fibroblast cultures, has been replaced by a more rapid technique that involves a centrifugation step and immunofluorescent staining to detect early antigen. Results are usually available within 24 hours. New methods being developed such as the polymerase chain reaction (PCR), as well as tests to detect CMV antigen directly from clinical specimens, promise improved sensitivity and faster turnaround. During acute infection CMV shedding can be detected in saliva or urine, but the mere detection of the virus is not sufficient evidence of causation. CMV shares with other herpesviruses the capacity to remain latent in tissues after recovery from acute infection. The site of latency of CMV is not known but is probably the circulating peripheral mononuclear leukocyte. Although CMV is usually not detectable in normal hosts, the factors leading to reactivation of infection and viral shedding are unknown; after any acute infection shedding of CMV in the normal host can be prolonged. Immunosuppressed patients with transplants or HIV infection are likely to be chronically shedding virus, and the isolation of the virus from such patients requires careful interpretation.

A number of commercial tests using various methods measure antibody to CMV and have largely replaced the complement-fixing antibody test. While a fourfold or greater change in titer between acute and convalescent sera suggests primary infection, most patients by the time they are investigated for CMV mononucleosis will already have detectable or peak antibody. A negative test may be useful in excluding the diagnosis. The presence of CMV immunoglobulin M (IgM) antibody may be used to support a diagnosis of acute infection, but the test lacks specificity and may be positive with asymptomatic reactivation of infection. In pregnant women the sensitivity of the IgM antibody test for detecting primary CMV infection has been reported as 73 percent with a false-positive rate of 11 percent.

Management

Therapy is not indicated in most cases of CMV mononucleosis. The antiviral drugs ganciclovir and foscarnet, with activity against CMV, effectively treat serious CMV infections in immunocompromised patients. An aggressive approach to identify and treat bone marrow transplant patients at risk for developing CMV infection is advocated. Standard management includes prophylactic immunoglobulin, routine bronchoalveolar lavage after engraftment to detect viral shedding, and early treatment with ganciclovir. Transmission of CMV by blood can be prevented by the use of CMV antibody-negative products. In addition to bone marrow transplant patients, CMV-negative blood products should be available for HIV-positive persons who are CMV antibody negative.

Patients with CMV infection can transmit infection. Because asymptomatic shedding of CMV is so widespread, no specific infection control precautions apart from the usual close attention to hand washing are required in the hospital setting.

TOXOPLASMOSIS

Infection with the protozoan parasite *Toxoplasma gondii* is usually asymptomatic, but acute toxoplasmosis can be associated with a mononucleosis-like syndrome. The most common clinical finding in acute toxoplasmosis is asymptomatic cervical lymphadenopathy. Consequently, diagnostic confusion with Hodgkin's disease and the lymphomas can occur. Fever, malaise, night sweats, myalgia, sore throat, maculopapular rash, or hepatosplenomegaly may be present (see Table 1). In contrast with EBV-associated infectious mononucleosis, pharyngitis is not prominent. Patients should be examined for chorioretinitis, which although more often recognized following congenital toxoplasmosis infection, can occur in up to 5 percent of acute acquired infection and warrants treatment. Small numbers of atypical lymphocytes (up to 10 percent) are found in the peripheral blood; the heterophile antibody test is negative. The clinical course of acute toxoplasmosis is usually benign and self-limited, although lymphadenopathy may persist for months. Complications of acute infection, more commonly seen in immunocompromised individuals, include myocarditis, encephalitis, and pneumonia.

There are considerable geographic differences in the prevalence of infection. While in France 87 percent of adults are positive for antibody to *Toxoplasma,* in North America the prevalence ranges from 5 to 45 percent. Most of the variation in prevalence and incidence has not been explained, but dietary habits and exposure to cat feces are important in transmission. Cats are the definitive host of *T. gondii;* the intermediate hosts include humans, cattle, and sheep. Humans acquire *Toxoplasma* infection either through the ingestion of raw or inadequately cooked meat containing infectious oocysts or the ingestion of oocysts from cat feces. Maternal-fetal transmission can occur during acute infection in the pregnant woman, with congenital toxoplasmosis as a consequence. *Toxoplasma* organisms have been recovered from leukocytes, and the potential exists for transmission by blood transfusion or transplantation. The tissue cysts of *T. gondii* persist in a latent form in the host for life. Reactivation can occur in the immunocompromised host. CNS toxoplasmosis is a common opportunistic infection in patients with advanced HIV infection.

Diagnosis

It is rare to diagnose acute toxoplasmosis by isolating the organism from blood, body fluids, or tissue. Although the diagnosis is usually made serologically, the high prevalence of antibodies to *Toxoplasma* in the normal population can make interpretation of serology difficult. In most laboratories an indirect immunofluorescent antibody test has replaced the classic Sabin-Feldman dye test for the detection of IgG antibody to *Toxoplasma.* When acute acquired toxoplasmosis is suspected, a negative IFA-IgG virtually excludes the diagnosis. Recently acquired infection is confirmed if there is seroconversion or a fourfold rise in antibody titer in sera drawn 3 weeks apart. Because elevated titers may persist indefinitely, one high titer is suggestive but not diagnostic of acute infection. Several assays measure IgM

Table 4 Conditions Associated with Mononucleosis-like Syndrome

EBV infection
CMV infection
Toxoplasmosis
Rubella
Acute viral hepatitis
Acute HIV infection
Acute HHV-6 infection
Mumps
Pertussis
Infectious lymphocytosis of childhood
Cat-scratch disease
Drug reactions
Hantavirus pulmonary syndrome

antibody, but the IFA-IgM test that is routinely available lacks sensitivity and specificity. Nonetheless, a positive IgM antibody with a single high IgG antibody titer can help support the diagnosis where the clinical presentation suggests acute *Toxoplasma* infection.

Management

Therapy for most immunocompetent individuals with acute toxoplasmosis is not necessary unless symptoms are severe. Treatment is indicated for active chorioretinitis and for patients whose resistance to infection is compromised by underlying disease or by therapy. A combination of pyrimethamine 25 to 50 mg daily and sulfadiazine 2 to 4 g daily with folinic acid supplementation remains the standard regimen, although spiramycin, clindamycin, and the new macrolide azithromycin are alternatives. Bone marrow toxicity and skin rashes frequently complicate the treatment regimens, particularly in HIV patients, for whom long-term maintenance therapy is required to prevent recurrent disease. Studies are still needed to determine the best way to screen for and treat acute *Toxoplasma* infection in pregnancy. If a diagnosis of acute *Toxoplasma* infection in pregnancy is made, treatment of the mother with spiramycin or a sulfonamide and pyrimethamine (avoiding this drug during the first trimester) will probably decrease the likelihood of fetal infection.

■ OTHER SYNDROMES

Conditions associated with a heterophile-negative mononucleosis syndrome, in which the clinical and hematologic findings may overlap with those of EBV-related infectious mononucleosis, are listed in Table 4.

Because of the widespread implementation of an effective immunization program, rubella infection is now uncommon. Acute rubella infection can be associated with fever, sore throat, posterior cervical adenopathy, and a mild atypical lymphocytosis. Splenomegaly is uncommon, and unlike EBV-associated infectious mononucleosis, the clinical illness is brief. A laboratory diagnosis of acute rubella infection can readily be made by demonstrating seroconversion in paired sera or by detection of rubella-specific IgM antibody.

Infection with the recently identified herpesvirus human herpesvirus 6 (HHV-6) is usually asymptomatic, although primary infection with HHV-6 is the cause of roseola, a mild self-limited febrile exanthem in infants. Recently acute infection with HHV-6 has been reported to be associated with a severe infectious mononucleosis-like syndrome. Because diagnostic tests for infection with HHV-6 are not routinely available, the role of HHV-6 infection in heterophile-negative mononucleosis syndromes is unknown.

Viral hepatitis may result in fever, lymphadenopathy, malaise, and an atypical lymphocytosis. Usually hepatocellular enzymes are markedly elevated. Specific serologic tests to detect infection with hepatitis A, B, and C are available. Acute HIV infection, although often not clinically recognized, can be associated with a mononucleosis-like syndrome with fever, rash, generalized lymphadenopathy, and peripheral blood lymphocytosis. Although the results of an ELISA test to detect HIV antibody may be negative in the first few weeks, almost all patients will be positive within 2 to 4 months of HIV acquisition.

The cause of infectious lymphocytosis of childhood is unknown; it probably is an infection with an unidentified virus. This benign self-limited illness is characterized by fever, lymphadenopathy, and a leukocytosis with a predominance of small lymphocytes.

Hematologic neoplasms may be confused with mononucleosis-like syndromes, and a lymph node biopsy may be needed to establish the diagnosis. Cat-scratch disease, a bacterial infection putatively caused by *Bartonella henselae,* is characterized by regional lymphadenopathy after recent contact with cats. Low-grade fever and malaise may cause confusion in distinguishing this disease from infectious mononucleosis. In the immunocompetent host infection is benign and self-limited. The diagnosis is easily confirmed if lymph node biopsy demonstrates pleomorphic bacilli in silver-stained sections. Serologic testing for antibodies to *B. henselae* is available.

Atypical lymphocytosis is a characteristic finding in the peripheral blood smear of patients with pertussis infection. The clinical findings are usually characteristic, and culture of the organism *Bordetella pertussis* will confirm the diagnosis.

Atypical lymphocytosis is described in patients with the hantavirus pulmonary syndrome; leukocytosis with a left shift is common. Symptoms related to the adult respiratory distress syndrome and shock usually dominate the clinical picture.

Suggested Reading

Akashi K, Eizuru Y, Sumiyoshi Y, et al. Brief report: Severe infectious mononucleosis-like syndrome and primary human herpesvirus 6 infection in an adult. N Engl J Med 1993; 329:168–171.

Evans AS. Infectious mononucleosis and related syndromes. Am J Med Sci 1978; 276:325–339.

Fiala M, Heiner DC, Turner JA, et al. Infectious mononucleosis and mononucleosis syndrome. West J Med 1977; 126:445–459.

Remington JS, McLeod R. Toxoplasmosis. In: Gorbach SL, Bartlett JG, Blacklow NR, eds. Infectious diseases. Philadelphia: WB Saunders, 1992:1328.

Schooley RT. Epstein-Barr virus (Infectious mononucleosis). In: Mandell GL, Bennett JE, Dolin R, eds. Principles and practice of infectious diseases. 4th ed. New York: Churchill Livingstone, 1995:1364.

Straus SE, Cohen JI, Tosato G, et al. Epstein-Barr virus infections: biology, pathogenesis and management. Ann Intern Med 1993; 118:45–58.

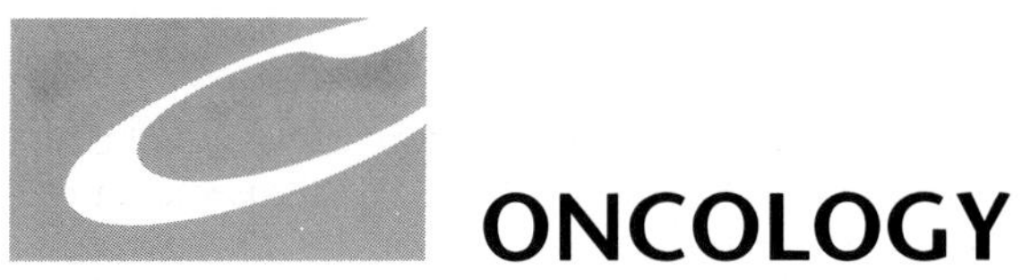

ONCOLOGY

CANCER PREVENTION

Peter Greenwald, M.D., Dr.P.H.

Health promotion and disease prevention, two fundamental objectives of health care professionals, received renewed emphasis with the publication of the U.S. Public Health Service's (PHS) report *Healthy People 2000: National Health Promotion and Disease Prevention Objectives.* This report presented a national strategy for significantly improving the nation's health during the 1990s and addressed the prevention of injuries, infectious diseases, and major chronic diseases including cancer. The last was identified as a priority area for prevention. Physicians and other health care professionals are considered by the public to be authoritative sources of health- and disease-related information. In fact, studies show that intervention by physicians can influence patients' cancer prevention practices. For example, direct advice to patients from a physician about the risks of smoking can result in cessation of smoking by 7 to 10 percent of patients who smoke. The average American makes 3.3 physician office visits each year, giving the physician several opportunities to counsel patients about lifestyle and behavior changes that have the potential to reduce cancer risk.

Both tobacco use and diet, major contributors to cancer incidence and mortality, are lifestyle factors that can be controlled and thus are a focus of cancer prevention strategies. Cigarette smoking, which leads to more than 30 percent of all cancer deaths in the United States, is a primary cause of cancers of the lung, larynx, oral cavity, and esophagus and contributes to the development of cancers of the pancreas, bladder, kidney, and uterine cervix. In addition, because an estimated 35 percent of cancers may be related to dietary factors, appropriate dietary modification has significant potential to reduce cancer incidence and mortality rates.

Chemoprevention, a recent approach to cancer prevention that uses chemical agents—including micronutrients, natural products, and synthetic compounds—to inhibit or reverse the carcinogenic process, has captured the interest of many investigators and is a rapidly growing research area. Numerous chemical agents show considerable potential as chemopreventive agents in defined high-risk groups and in the general population. The chemopreventive approach promises to bring exciting developments to cancer prevention.

This chapter highlights the recommendations of the National Cancer Institute (NCI) for physicians with respect to smoking prevention and cessation; the relationship between diet and cancer, with a focus on breast cancer; and a brief overview and update of chemoprevention research at the NCI.

■ SMOKING PREVENTION AND CESSATION

Prevalence of Smoking and Tobacco Use

Cigarette smoking is the most common form of tobacco use in the United States. The National Health Interview Survey (NHIS) data show that cigarette smoking among adults aged 18 and over declined 40 percent—from 42 to 2 percent—between 1965 and 1990. Between 1990 and 1994, however, the overall smoking prevalence among adults was essentially unchanged—although smoking among adolescents has increased. In 1994, 48 million adults (25 million men and 22.7 million women) were current smokers in the United States. In general, smoking is most prevalent among persons aged 25 to 44 years, is higher among men than women, decreases with increasing education, and is higher among persons below the poverty level. A recent analysis of regional trends in cigarette smoking and tobacco use from 1965 to 1987, based on data from national health interview surveys conducted by the National Center for Health Statistics (NCHS), indicated that trends in prevalence and initiation of cigarette smoking varied significantly among regions of the United States. The South had the smallest increase in quitting (8 percent) and the smallest decrease in initiation (11 percent), and the Northeast had the greatest increase in quitting (15 percent) and the greatest decline in initiation (21 percent). The finding of a high prevalence of cigarette smoking in the South is supported by data from the 1985 Current Population Survey (CPS), which showed that the South had the highest prevalence of both men cigarette smokers (36 percent) and tobacco users (44.6 percent). It is clear that although significant progress has been made in reducing tobacco use in the United States, much remains to be done to foster changes leading to a smoke-free society.

Table 1 Synopsis for Physicians: How to Help Your Patients Stop Smoking

Ask about smoking at every opportunity.
  a. "Do you smoke?"
  b. "How much?"
  c. "How soon after waking do you have your first cigarette?"
  d. "Are you interested in stopping smoking?"
  e. "Have you ever tried to stop before?" If so, "What happened?"

Advise all smokers to stop.
  a. State your advice clearly, for example, "As your physician, I must advise you to stop smoking now."
  b. Personalize the message to quit. Refer to the patient's clinical condition, smoking history, personal interests, or social roles.

Assist the patient in stopping.
  a. Set a quit date. Help the patient pick a date within the next 4 weeks, acknowledging that no time is ideal.
  b. Provide self-help materials. The smoking cessation coordinator or support staff member can review the materials with the patient if desired (call 1-800-4-CANCER for NCI's *Quit for Good* materials).
  c. Consider prescribing nicotine gum, especially for highly addicted patients (those who smoke one pack a day or more or who smoke their first cigarette within 30 minutes of waking).
  d. Consider signing a stop-smoking contract with the patient.
  e. If the patient is not willing to stop now:
     Provide motivating literature (call 1-800-4-CANCER for NCI's *Why Do You Smoke?* pamphlet). Ask again at the next visit.

Arrange follow-up visits.
  a. Set a follow-up visit within 1 to 2 weeks after the quit date.
  b. Have a member of the office staff call or write the patient within 7 days after the initial visit, reinforcing the decision to stop and reminding the patient of the quit date.
  c. At the first follow-up visit, ask about the patient's smoking status to provide support and help prevent relapse. Relapse is common; if it happens, encourage the patient to try again immediately.
  d. Set a second follow-up visit in 1 to 2 months. For patients who have relapsed, discuss the circumstances of the relapse and other special concerns.

From Glynn T, Manley M. How to help your patients stop smoking: A National Cancer Institute manual for physicians. Bethesda, MD: National Institutes of Health, 1989.

A goal of the PHS, as specified in *Healthy People 2000,* is that 75 percent of all U.S. physicians routinely provide antismoking counseling to all of their patients.

NCI Trials of Training and Intervention Protocols for Physicians

Recognizing the importance of strong physician involvement in efforts to reduce national smoking prevalence rates, the NCI in 1984 initiated five randomized, controlled intervention trials of physician training protocols and intervention protocols for physicians to use with patients who smoke. These trials, conducted in the United States and Canada in a variety of outpatient medical care settings, involved more than 1,000 physicians and 30,000 patients. The results demonstrated that (1) training physicians to treat nicotine dependence leads to more consistent and effective patient care; (2) when trained physicians are reminded to intervene with patients who smoke, significant reductions in smoking prevalence can be achieved; and (3) patients of trained physicians (who are reminded) were up to six times as likely to stop smoking as patients of control physicians. The necessity for combining physician training with reminders for physicians was an important finding. Although training increased the use of smoking cessation interventions by physicians, training alone did not result in increased smoking cessation rates among patients. Smoking cessation rates increased significantly only when trained physicians were routinely reminded to intervene with all smoking patients. Over all trials, cessation rates of up to 15 percent were achieved for all smokers seen in the offices of trained physicians.

NCI Recommendations for Physicians

In 1989, based on trial results and consensus development, NCI formulated recommendations for practicing physicians treating patients who smoke. These recommendations were included in a manual of practical smoking cessation techniques for physicians, *How to Help Your Patients Stop Smoking: A National Cancer Institute Manual for Physicians* (Office of Cancer Communications, NCI, Bethesda, MD 20892). The NCI-recommended intervention plan, which can be carried out in about 3 minutes, is often called "the four As": (1) *ask* about smoking; (2) *advise* smokers to stop; (3) *assist* patients willing to stop; and (4) *arrange* follow-up. Table 1 outlines each element of the intervention. (See also the chapter *Smoking Cessation.*)

Physicians who care for children can influence them not to start tobacco use. The NCI recommends that such physicians include a fifth "A," *anticipatory guidance,* and has prepared a supplement to the *Manual for Physicians* that outlines clinical interventions to prevent tobacco use for three different age periods: infancy and early childhood, late childhood, and adolescence and early adulthood. In brief, for physicians who treat children, the recommended intervention activities are: *anticipate* the risk for tobacco use at each developmental stage; *ask* about exposure to tobacco smoke and tobacco use at each visit; *advise* all smoking parents to stop and all children not to use tobacco products; *assist* children in resisting tobacco use and assist tobacco users in quitting; and *arrange* follow-up visits as required.

The physician's office staff, working as a team with specific roles and responsibilities, can contribute significantly to

Table 2 Synopsis for Office Staff: How to Develop Office Procedures to Help Patients Stop Smoking

Select an office smoking cessation coordinator to be responsible for seeing that the office smoking cessation program is carried out.
Create a smoke-free office.
  a. Select a date for the office to become smoke free.
  b. Advise all staff and patients of this plan.
  c. Post no-smoking signs in all office areas.
  d. Remove ashtrays.
  e. Display nonsmoking materials and cessation information prominently.
  f. Eliminate all tobacco advertising from the waiting room.
Identify all patients who smoke.
  a. Ask all patients, "Do you smoke?" or "Are you still smoking?" at each visit.
  b. Prominently place a "Smoker" identifier on the charts of all smoking patients.
  c. Attach a permanent progress card to each patient's chart.
Review self-help materials (provided by either the physician or the coordinator) and nicotine gum use (if a prescription has been given) with each smoking patient.
Assist the physician in making follow-up visits.
  a. With each patient who has agreed to a quit date, schedule a follow-up visit 1 to 2 weeks after the quit date.
  b. Call or write the patient within 7 days after the initial visit to reinforce the decision to quit.
  c. Schedule a second follow-up visit approximately 1 to 2 months after the first follow-up visit.

From Glynn T. Manley M. *How to help your patients stop smoking: A National Cancer Institute manual for physicians.* Bethesda, MD: National Institutes of Health, 1989.

the success of the smoking intervention. Office procedures that can increase the physician's effectiveness in treating patients who smoke include selecting a smoking-cessation coordinator (usually a nurse), making the office tobacco free, systematically identifying and monitoring patients who smoke, providing self-help information for patients, and actively involving office staff members with the intervention and follow-up. These procedures are outlined in Table 2.

In 1992, the nicotine transdermal delivery system, or nicotine patch, was introduced to help treat dependence on nicotine. The patch has been approved by the U.S. Food and Drug Administration (FDA) and has been vigorously marketed by the pharmaceutical industry. As with nicotine gum, data suggest that success rates for smoking cessation are higher when the nicotine patch is used as *part* of a comprehensive smoking cessation program that includes physician counseling.

In addition to advising and educating their patients about prevention and cessation of smoking, physicians can promote school- and community-based tobacco-control strategies. For example, they can work with school programs to counteract tobacco use and promotion and can actively support antitobacco legislation. A national organization founded in 1977, Doctors Ought to Care (DOC), has effectively countered tobacco advertising, especially that associated with sports events, and has promoted antismoking events. Wide-ranging physician efforts in smoking prevention and cessation have the potential to contribute significantly to the realization of the nation's goal to curtail tobacco use.

■ DIETARY MODIFICATION

Although causal relationships between specific dietary factors and cancer have not been definitively established, comprehensive evaluations of available evidence supporting associations between diet and cancer have led to the conclusion that considerable potential exists for reducing the risk of cancer by modifying the dietary patterns of Americans. While research on the link between diet and cancer continues, dietary guidelines directed at reducing the risk of cancer as well as other chronic diseases have been proposed by the NCI and a number of other scientific organizations. These guidelines emphasize eating foods rich in potential cancer-inhibiting components and recommend reducing foods that may be cancer promoting. They are highly likely to benefit overall health, with no discernible risk, while being consistent with good nutritional practices. Therefore, it is prudent for physicians to advise their patients to adhere to the guidelines; nurses, dietitians, and nutritionists also should provide advice, counseling, and educational materials to assist patients in modifying their diets.

NCI Dietary Guidelines

The scientific evidence supporting a direct association between dietary fat and cancer incidence, particularly for colon, postmenopausal breast, and prostate cancers, is compelling. Further, epidemiologic studies indicate that a high intake of dietary fiber from vegetables, fruits, legumes, and whole-grain products may protect against cancers at many sites. The evidence also suggests that constituents of vegetables and fruits other than fiber, such as antioxidant vitamins, including vitamins A, C, and E, and nonnutrient phytochemicals, such as indoles, isothiocyanates, flavonoids, and terpenes, may protect against cancer. The six dietary guidelines issued by the NCI include recommendations for reducing fat intake; increasing the consumption of vegetables, fruits, and other fiber-rich foods; avoiding obesity; and limiting consumption of alcoholic beverages and salt-cured, salt-pickled, and smoked foods (Table 3). These guidelines, derived in part from the National Academy of Science's 1982 committee report *Diet, Nutrition, and Cancer,* were augmented by NCI workshops and a comprehensive review of fiber data. These

Table 3 National Cancer Institute Dietary Guidelines

Reduce fat intake to no more than 30 percent of calories.
Increase fiber intake to 20 to 30 g per day, with an upper limit of 35 g.
Include a variety of vegetables and fruits in the daily diet.
Avoid obesity.
Consume alcoholic beverages in moderation, if at all.
Minimize consumption of salt-cured, salt-pickled, and smoked foods.

sources still are timely; subsequent data further support their conclusions.

The average American adult consumes about 34 percent of daily calories from fat, as compared with the NCI's recommended upper level of 30 percent. Further, at approximately 17.01 grams for men and 12.75 grams for women, the average dietary fiber intake of Americans falls short of the recommended level of 20 to 30 grams per day. The average American consumes only 3.4 servings of vegetables and fruits combined, according to the 1991 *5 A Day for Better Health* Baseline Study. To encourage Americans to increase their vegetable and fruit consumption to five or more servings a day, NCI and the Produce for Better Health Foundation launched the *5 A Day for Better Health* campaign, which provides consumers with information about how to translate the recommendation into dietary practices.

The following section briefly reviews the scientific evidence on the association between diet and breast cancer, followed by a summary of selected trials assessing dietary intervention as an approach to the primary prevention of cancer.

Diet and Breast Cancer

International correlation studies suggest a strong positive relationship between breast cancer risk and percent of dietary calories as fat, total fat intake, and/or high consumption of animal fat. For example, breast cancer incidence and mortality rates among Japanese women are about four times lower than rates for American women—a difference attributed in part to the significantly lower fat and calorie intake of the Japanese. Evidence from migrant and time-trend studies also support the effect of dietary fat on breast cancer risk. Breast cancer mortality rates in Japan have increased as the Japanese diet becomes more westernized and higher in fat. Further, Japanese migrants to the United States, and especially their children, are at greater risk for breast cancer than Japanese who remain in Japan, suggesting that environmental factors, including diet, may affect breast cancer risk.

Not every type of high-fat diet necessarily translates into high risk for breast cancer. The type of fat consumed also may be important. Although breast cancer has a strong positive association with diets high in saturated fats and in polyunsaturated omega-6 fatty acids, polyunsaturated omega-3 fatty acids, derived primarily from fish oils, may protect against breast cancer. Further, reduced risk of breast cancer is seen in countries where large quantities of monounsaturated olive oil, high in oleic acid, and low in omega-6 fatty acids, are consumed.

Despite strong evidence from descriptive epidemiologic and experimental studies supporting a role for dietary fat in breast cancer risk, results from case-control and cohort studies are mixed. A combined analysis of 12 case-control studies conducted in populations with very different breast cancer risks and dietary habits found a strong positive association between breast cancer risk and both total fat and saturated fat consumption in postmenopausal, but not premenopausal, women. In contrast, the Nurses' Health Study, a cohort study that included about 90,000 women, found no association between breast cancer incidence or mortality and total fat, saturated fat, linoleic acid, or cholesterol in either premenopausal or postmenopausal women. Divergent results may be due to the limitations and inadequacies inherent in the conduct of nutritionally-related epidemiologic research, including inexact dietary assessment techniques, small variation in the fat intake levels of comparison groups, and confounding by other dietary factors, such as fiber intake.

A high intake of dietary fiber also has been hypothesized to protect against the development of breast cancer. It is notable that Finland has a lower breast cancer mortality rate than the United States, although, like Americans, Finns consume high-fat diets (more than 30 percent of total calories). Unlike Americans, however, Finns consume large amounts of dietary fiber—more than 30 grams per day.

Dietary fat has been shown to affect chemically induced mammary carcinogenesis, both independently of and interactively with fiber. For example, a study in rats demonstrated that fat promotes and fiber protects against mammary tumors. The promotional phase of N-methyl-N′-nitrosourea (MNU)-induced mammary carcinogenesis was inhibited by supplemental wheat bran fiber in rats fed a high-fat diet. Rats fed a high-fat, low-fiber diet had the highest incidence of mammary tumors, and those fed either a high-fat, high-fiber or low-fat, low-fiber diet had an intermediate number of tumors. The fewest mammary tumors were seen among rats fed a low-fat, high-fiber diet.

Although the specific mechanisms by which dietary fat enhances the development of mammary tumors have not yet been clarified, possibilities include increased prostaglandin synthesis, which may affect cell proliferation; increased levels of certain lipid peroxy radicals and/or oxygen radicals, possible activators of cell proliferation; enhanced cell membrane fluidity associated with increased cell division; inhibition of the passage of low molecular weight, possibly growth-regulatory molecules through membrane structures; increased levels of sex steroid hormones, believed to play a role in breast cancer development; enhanced hormone-induced mammary gland growth responsiveness; and inhibition of immune system activity. Experimental and clinical evidence indicates that a low-fat diet may, via induction of a 2-hydroxylase cytochrome P450 mono-oxygenase, shift estradiol metabolism away from the production of estriol, which is biologically active and potentially carcinogenic, to the formation of inactive 2-hydroxycatechol estrogens, possibly reducing breast cancer risk.

Fruit and vegetable intake, alcohol consumption, and obesity also have been associated with breast cancer. In a combined analysis of 12 case-control studies, statistically significant inverse associations were found between fiber, vitamin A, beta-carotene, and vitamin C, all markers of vegetable and fruit intake, and breast cancer risk in postmenopausal women. Results of studies on alcohol consumption and breast cancer risk are mixed. A review of epidemiologic studies published between 1977 and 1989 that examined the association between breast cancer risk and alcohol intake reported that results from 10 to 16 case-control studies and 5 of 6 cohort studies support a weak positive association. A 1994 update of a meta-analysis of 38 case-control and cohort studies of the alcohol–breast cancer hypothesis indicated a positive association between alcohol consumption and breast cancer risk (approximately 25 percent increase in risk with daily intake of the equivalent of two drinks) and a clear dose-response relationship. Finally, a review of more than 35 correlational, case-control, and cohort studies investigating body weight and breast cancer risk found that fatness, as measured by body weight and body mass indices, generally was directly related to breast cancer incidence, particularly among postmenopausal women, and adversely affected breast cancer survival.

Selected Dietary Intervention Trials

Large-scale dietary intervention trials are the best means available to test objectively the hypotheses related to dietary modification and cancer risk that have been developed from epidemiologic and laboratory leads; examples of selected trials, described below, include the Women's Health Initiative, the Women's Intervention Nutrition Study, and the Polyp Prevention Trial.

The Women's Health Initiative (WHI), a large, 10 year trial supported by the National Institutes of Health, is examining the effects of (1) a low-fat eating pattern (20 percent of calories from fat) that is high in fruits, vegetables, and dietary fiber, (2) hormone replacement therapy, and (3) calcium supplementation on the prevention of cancer, cardiovascular disease, and osteoporosis in more than 63,000 postmenopausal women of all races and socioeconomic strata. In addition to the randomized clinical trial, the WHI includes a large prospective surveillance study and a community prevention and intervention study that will seek effective ways to promote behaviors aimed at preventing cancer, cardiovascular disease, and osteoporosis within local communities. Sixteen vanguard centers launched the WHI in the fall of 1993.

The Women's Intervention Nutrition Study (WINS) is a clinical trial to test whether dietary fat reduction, in conjunction with chemotherapy or hormonal therapy, will reduce breast cancer recurrence and increase survival in postmenopausal stage II breast cancer patients. The study will examine adherence to a dietary modification program, in which fat intake will be reduced to 15 percent of total calories, and will attempt to identify a set of behavioral and psychosocial variables that can be used as predictors of dietary change. This, randomized, multicenter 5 year clinical trial will randomize 2,000 women to either the dietary intervention group (60 percent of women) or the control group (40 percent of women). To be eligible for the trial, women must be over age 50 and postmenopausal and must have consumed, prior to the study, a diet that is 25 percent or more of calories from fat. Recurrence of breast cancer is the end point of this study.

Based on a large body of scientific evidence, it is generally accepted that several dietary factors, including fat, fiber, and fruits and vegetables, are associated with colon cancer risk. The NCI is conducting the multi-institution randomized, controlled Polyp Prevention Trial to test whether a low-fat, high-fiber, and vegetable- and fruit-enriched eating plan will prevent the recurrence of large-bowel adenomatous polyps in approximately 2,000 otherwise healthy women and men over age 35 who have had a polypectomy. Because there is a strong association between colon polyps and the development of colon cancer, an intervention that reduces the recurrence of large-bowel polyps has a strong likelihood of reducing the incidence of large-bowel cancer. Half of the participants are being randomized to a control group with no intervention except for information on basic nutrition; the other half are being assigned to the dietary intervention group. The daily intervention target goals are 20 percent of calories from fat, 18 grams of fiber per 1,000 calories, and 5 to 8 servings of vegetables and fruits. Participants in the intervention group will be counseled individually on how to meet their target goals, with a strong emphasis on behavior modification. The recurrence of polyps will be assessed in both groups at years 1 and 4 to determine the effect of this dietary intervention.

Physicians and other health care professionals should be aware of ongoing clinical trials to ensure that patients who may benefit from participation in these trials are informed about appropriate and available opportunities. The NCI's Physician's Data Query (PDQ) directory of patient and physician treatment information, which contains information on state-of-the-art treatment and current NCI-sponsored trials, may be particularly useful; it is directly accessible through office-based personal computers. In addition, the Cancer Information Service (CIS) maintains regional cancer information centers accessible through a toll-free telephone number (1-800-4-CANCER).

■ CHEMOPREVENTION

Over the past decade, chemoprevention has developed from an interesting theoretic model into a realistic approach to cancer prevention that has broad implications for public health benefits. The rationale for chemoprevention research is based on the convergence of strong laboratory and epidemiologic evidence indicating that various natural and synthetic agents can halt or reverse cancer progression in animals and reduce risk in humans. This approach to cancer prevention is becoming more clearly defined as researchers gain new insights into the molecular biology of the multistage process of carcinogenesis.

NCI's Approach to Chemoprevention

At the NCI, agents that appear to be promising are evaluated preclinically for compound efficacy and toxicity using in vitro and in vivo screening systems. In vitro screening facilitates the selection and prioritization of agents for in vivo testing. A battery of in vivo screening models, representing various target organs, is used to develop a profile of a potential agent's target specificity, efficacy, safety, tolerability, and bioavailability. Agents that show chemopreventive activity in screening tests undergo further safety evaluation in acute, subchronic, and chronic toxicity studies in animals; those that demonstrate high efficacy and low toxicity are selected for assessment in clinical trials. In contrast to

Table 4 Selected National Cancer Institute–Sponsored Clinical Trials

ORGAN	AGENT	PHASE	POPULATION	DURATION
Breast	Tamoxifen & 4-HPR*	II	Women with atypical ductal hyperplasia, DCIS†, or a familial risk pattern	2 years
	Tamoxifen	III	Women ≥35 years of age at increased risk	10 years
	4-HPR*		Previously resected unilateral stage I/II breast cancer patients	5 years
Prostate	4-HPR*	II	Biopsy negative & PSA‡ ≥4 ng/ml	1 year
	Finasteride	III	Men age ≥55, normal digital rectal exam, PSA‡ ≥3 ng/ml no prostatic carcinoma	10 years
Colon	Piroxicam	II	Patients with previous adenoma—40–80 years of age	3 years
	Sulindac		Familial adenomatous	9 mos§
	Sulindac	III	History of multiple polyposis	3 years
	Aspirin		Patients with previously resected adenomatous colon polyps	3 years
	Avarbose (α-glucosidase inhibitor)		Subjects at risk for colon cancer	1 year
	Calcium carbonate		Patients with previous adenoma	4 years
Bladder	DFMO¶	II	Resected superficial bladder cancer patients	1 year
Cervix	DFMO¶	II	Patients with cervical intraepithelial neoplasia (CIN) Grade III	1 year
	4-HPR*			
Lung	4-HPR*	II	Chronic smokers with prior resected head/neck, lung, or bladder cancers with bronchial dysplasia	6 mos
	Beta-carotene & Retinol	III	Heavy smokers & asbestos-exposed (men) & asbestosis patients	5–10 years#
	Beta-carotene & Vitamin E		Heavy smokers 50–60 years of age (Finland)	5–8 years§
	Vitamin E & Aspirin		Female nurses ≥45 years of age	4 years
Oral cavity	13-cis Retinoic acid, Beta-carotene & Retinol	III	Oral leukoplakia	4 years
Skin	Beta-carotene	III	Previous BCC** or SCC†† of the skin	5 years
	Retinol	III	Previous BCC** of skin; acitinic keratosis	5 years
	4-HPR*	II	Actinic keratosis	6 mos
Multiple sites	Beta-carotene & Aspirin	III	Healthy physicians	12 years§

*4-HPR, all-*trans*-*N*-4-hydroxyphenyl) retinamide
†DCIS, ductal carcinoma in situ
‡PSA, prostate-specific antigen
§Trial completed
¶DFMO, 2-Difluoromethylornithine
#Trial ended after 4 years
**BCC, basal cell carcinoma
††SCC, squamous cell carcinoma

cancer treatment trials, where use of toxic agents is acceptable for malignant disease not otherwise treatable, chemoprevention trials must select agents with negligible toxicity because the study populations are either high- or average-risk healthy people. For example, the synthetic retinoid N-(4-hydroxyphenyl) retinamide (4-HPR) has proved to be safer than many other retinoids. Both 4-HPR and the antiestrogen tamoxifen, when used alone, result in approximately a 25 percent reduction in rat mammary tumor incidence. It is noteworthy, however, that when these two agents are used in combination, mammary tumor incidence in rats is reduced by almost 80 percent, suggesting that coadministration of 4-HPR and tamoxifen may be beneficial, particularly for women at high risk for developing breast cancer.

Following preclinical studies, clinical evaluation of potential chemopreventive agents is conducted in phase I, phase II, and phase III trials. The phase I trial, usually conducted in a limited number of subjects, establishes a safe dose for humans on the basis of preclinical data; establishes toxicity patterns and whether the toxicity is predictive, tolerable, and reversible; determines pharmacokinetic information, including distribution, metabolism, and elimination of the agent; and estimates the dose range in which biologic activity may be expected. Phase II trials, normally conducted in a high-risk cohort, provide further data on efficacy and safety in the selected population and determine whether an agent has biologic activity affecting some stage of carcinogenesis. Objectives of a phase II chemoprevention trial include (1) identifying biochemical, genetic, and cellular or tissue markers of cancer that can be used to estimate reliably the potential for neoplastic progression and (2) determining whether the chemopreventive agent being tested can affect the incidence of that marker. Once an agent is found to have high efficacy and low toxicity in a phase II trial, prospective placebo-controlled phase III intervention trials are conducted over an extended period in a large number of subjects who initially show no obvious signs of malignancy. End points in phase III trials may include intermediate end points of cancer as well as incidence of specific cancers and overall cancer incidence.

The NCI's Division of Cancer Prevention and Control

(DCPC) has developed a Prevention Trials Decision Network to streamline the management of the growing research efforts in chemoprevention. Three network subcommittees—agent selection, end points and biomarkers, and large trials—are staffed with scientists working in related areas. Selection and prioritization of agents are facilitated by effective coordination among the NCI, pharmaceutical agencies, and FDA. In addition, the NCI is establishing a biomarkers database that can be used to evaluate the efficacy of biomarkers in ongoing or completed prevention studies and to prioritize the biomarkers for future applications. Finally, the NCI is formulating an overall strategy to assist in planning, reviewing, implementing, and monitoring large-scale phase III clinical trials.

Selected Chemoprevention Trials

Chemoprevention trials supported by the NCI, mostly in high-risk groups and in medical settings, are investigating cancer prevention at various sites, including the breast, colon, cervix, lung, prostate, head and neck, oral cavity, and skin. Potential chemopreventive agents that have advanced significantly in clinical evaluation include beta-carotene, the retinoids (13-*cis* retinoic acid, 4-HPR), and certain calcium compounds. Promising new agents entered into phase I or phase II trials include piroxicam, ibuprofen, and sulindac, which are nonsteroidal anti-inflammatory drugs (NSAIDs); oltipraz; difluoromethylornithine (DFMO); glycyrrhetinic acid; and N-acetylcysteine. Selected chemoprevention trials are presented in Table 4.

Breast cancer studies include the Breast Cancer Prevention Trial (BCPT), a 10 year study designed to test the ability of tamoxifen, an antiestrogen used in postsurgical treatment of early-stage breast cancer, to prevent breast cancer in healthy high-risk women. Approximately 16,000 women over age 35 are being randomized across the United States and Canada to receive either tamoxifen (20 mg per day) or placebo for an initial period of 5 years. The BCPT was initiated in 1992 and by April 1994 had enrolled almost 11,000 women. The efficacy of tamoxifen as a chemopreventive agent for breast cancer also is being investigated in the United Kingdom and in Italy. Further, in a study supported by the NCI, 4-HPR is being evaluated in Italy in a 5 year clinical trial plus a 2 year follow-up period, for the prevention of contralateral primary lesions in 3,000 women who have had breast cancer. If 4-HPR succeeds in preventing contralateral breast cancer in breast cancer patients, it may be useful for disease-free women at high risk for breast cancer.

Colon cancer is the focus of more chemoprevention trials than any other cancer site. The targeted study populations are primarily high-risk individuals who have had previous adenomatous colon polyps. Potential chemopreventive agents for colon cancer under study include piroxicam, sulindac, and aspirin (antiproliferative NSAIDs); DFMO, an inhibitor of ornithine decarboxylase (ODC); calcium, which suppresses the hyperproliferation of colonic epithelium; fiber (wheat bran); beta-carotene; and vitamins C and E.

Many chemoprevention trials, particularly phase II trials, are of special interest because they investigate the use of intermediate end points as cancer surrogates. Examples of possible prevention intermediate end point markers include reversal of abnormal cytology, prevention or reversal of nuclear aberrations such as micronuclei, inhibition of ODC and/or prostaglandin synthetase activity, decreases in fecal mutagens, DNA ploidy alterations, changes in mucosal or epithelial proliferation, altered status of precancerous lesions or other histologic changes, and evidence of changes in oncogene or suppressor gene activities. A specific example is the [^{3}H] thymidine labeling index, a measure of the rate at which tritium-labeled thymidine is taken up by epithelial cells lining colonic crypts and thus a measure of colonic mucosal cell proliferation. This index is being used extensively in clinical studies to establish its reliability as a possible biomarker to monitor the progress and/or success of intervention regimens, including calcium supplementation. Despite the identification of potential biomarkers, none have been validated as intermediate end points for predicting incidence of cancer. The validation of specific and sensitive biomarkers for cancer would make it possible to conduct trials on fewer subjects and for shorter durations than are required for cancer end point studies and thus to use available resources more effectively.

Suggested Reading

Blum A. Curtailing the tobacco pandemic. In: DeVita VT Jr, Hellman S, Rosenberg SA, eds. Cancer: Principles and practice of oncology. 4th ed. Philadelphia: JB Lippincott, 1993:480.

Buring JE, Hennekens CH. Retinoids and carotenoids. In: DeVita VT Jr, Hellman S, Rosenberg SA, eds. Cancer: Principles and practice of oncology. 4th ed. Philadelphia: JB Lippincott, 1993:464.

Cancer Facts & Figures—1997. Atlanta: American Cancer Society, 1997.

Flay BR, Ockene JK, Tager IB. Smoking: Epidemiology, cessation and prevention. Chest 1992; 102(3):277S–301S.

Greenwald P, Dietary fiber. In: DeVita VT Jr, Hellman S, Rosenberg SA, eds. Cancer: Principles and practice of oncology. 5th ed. Philadelphia: JB Lippincott, 1997:566.

Greenwald P, Clifford C. Dietary fat and cancer. In: DeVita VT Jr, Hellman S, Rosenberg SA, eds. Cancer: Principles and practice of oncology. 4th ed. Philadelphia: Lippincott, 1993:443.

Greenwald P, Kelloff G. The chemoprevention of cancer. In: Fortner JG, Rhoads JE, eds. Accomplishments in cancer research 1992. General Motors Cancer Research Foundation. Philadelphia: JB Lippincott, 1993:242.

Henderson BE, Bernstein L, Ross R. Hormones. In: DeVita VT Jr, Hellman S, Rosenberg SA, eds. Cancer: Principles and practice of oncology. 4th ed. Philadelphia: JB Lippincott, 1993:474.

Micozzi MS, Moon TE, eds. Macronutrients: Investigating their role in cancer. New York: Marcel Dekker, 1992.

National Academy of Sciences, National Research Council, Committee on Diet, Nutrition, and Cancer. Assembly of Life Sciences. Diet, nutrition, and cancer. Washington, DC: National Academy Press, 1982.

National Academy of Sciences, National Research Council, Food and Nutrition Board, Council on Life Sciences. Diet and health: Implications for reducing chronic disease risk. Washington, DC: National Academy Press, 1989.

Wattenberg L, Lipkin M, Boone CW, Kelloff GJ, eds. Cancer chemoprevention. Boca Raton: CRC Press, 1992.

SYMPTOM MANAGEMENT IN PATIENTS WITH CANCER

Roland T. Skeel, M.D.
Janelle Tipton, M.S.N., R.N., A.O.C.N.

Control of symptoms caused by cancer and its treatment is a major concern of both patients and physicians. It is particularly important when cure is not possible and the primary focus of treatment shifts to maintaining the best quality of life as long as possible. While physical complaints such as pain, nausea, vomiting, bowel dysfunction, poor appetite, fatigue, weakness, shortness of breath, and hair loss are most commonly expressed by patients, other aspects of function such as social interactions, sexual activity, and mood changes may distress the patient. The latter are less commonly addressed by the physician but nonetheless are also important components of quality of life for the patient with cancer.

Although there is some overlap between the physical symptoms caused by the cancer and those caused by the treatment, several problems commonly associated with chemotherapy or biologic response modifiers may be distressing enough to cause the patient to withdraw from therapy or wish never to have started. The most common of these acute treatment-related symptoms are listed in Table 1.

Because treatment-associated symptoms can be very severe and may lead to a reluctance of patients to initiate or continue treatment, both patients and physicians have an interest in devising means to minimize their impact. Techniques most commonly used have been pharmacologic or physical, though for problems such as nausea, vomiting, and mood disorders, biofeedback and other psychological means have been used as well.

■ NAUSEA AND VOMITING

Among the questions most commonly asked by patients who are about to begin chemotherapy are. "How sick will I get?" and, "Can you do anything about it?" Fortunately, the advent of more effective antiemetic agents in the past 10 years, coupled with carefully designed and controlled clinical trials of antiemetic regimens, has helped the oncologist to control and often completely prevent significant nausea and vomiting in most patients receiving chemotherapy.

Table 1 Most Common Acute Treatment-Related Symptoms of Chemotherapy and Biologic Therapy

Appetite change
Bowel dysfunction
Fatigue
Flulike symptoms
Hair loss
Nausea and vomiting
Stomatitis

Nausea and vomiting in patients with cancer most commonly arise as a result of chemotherapy, biologic therapy, or radiotherapy, but the oncologist is well advised to consider other possible causes (Table 2). For many of the causes other than the treatment of the cancer, the basis for the nausea and vomiting can be established and corrected, ameliorating the symptom. For other origins such as intra-abdominal metastatic disease or autonomic dysfunction, the underlying problem is less easily delineated and often cannot be corrected.

The pathophysiologic basis for nausea and vomiting subsequent to chemotherapy and the disparate effect of similar chemotherapeutic agents is poorly understood. Several anatomic areas appear to be involved, including the vomiting center, which is found in the lateral reticular formation of the medulla; the chemoreceptor trigger zone (CTZ) in the floor of the fourth ventricle (area postrema); receptors in the gastrointestinal tract; and the cerebral cortex. Study of neuroreceptors in the gastrointestinal tract and the central nervous system has improved our understanding of chemotherapy-induced nausea and vomiting and has led to agents with considerably more effectiveness than were available just 10 years ago.

Chemotherapy-Induced Nausea and Vomiting

Chemotherapy agents vary widely in their propensity to cause nausea and vomiting. Factors related to the chemotherapy that can affect the likelihood and severity of the symptoms, in addition to the specific agent, are the dose of drug used, the schedule and route of administration, additional agents used, and previous history with this and other chemotherapy. To plan a rational approach to control of nausea and vomiting, an understanding of these factors is essential. It is also helpful to group chemotherapeutic agents according to their emeto-

Table 2 Causes of Nausea and Vomiting Not Related to Chemotherapy but of Concern in Patients with Cancer

Intestinal obstruction
Intra-abdominal inflammation
Peptic ulceration
Disordered gastrointestinal motility
Intra-abdominal metastases
Autonomic dysfunction
Metabolic disturbances
Ketoacidosis
Hypercalcemia
Uremia
Adrenal insufficiency
Gastrointestinal infections
Intracranial tumor or infection
Sepsis with hypotension
Congestive heart failure
Pain
Medications
Antibiotics
Bronchodilators
Biologic response modifiers
Analgesics, particularly narcotics
Radiotherapy to the abdomen or head

genic potential (Table 3). Such a listing is helpful in making decisions about how aggressive an antiemetic regimen to use to prevent nausea and vomiting in a patient who is first being treated with a given regimen. Subsequent antiemetic treatment decisions will be based both on the chemotherapy regimen and the vomiting history from previous chemotherapy.

It is also helpful to remember that other factors not related specifically to the drug may affect nausea and vomiting occurring with chemotherapy and its control. These include age, gender, disease status, alcohol intake history, and psychological propensity.

Nausea and vomiting from chemotherapy may occur before the treatment is administered (anticipatory), within the first 24 hours of chemotherapy (acute), and after 24 hours (delayed). The treatment of each of these is different in emphasis, based largely on empirical evidence of effectiveness.

Table 3 Emetogenic Potential for Commonly Used Chemotherapeutic Agents

Highly Emetogenic: 75% or Greater Potential for Nausea, Vomiting, or Both
Carmustine
Cisplatin ≥40 mg/m^2
Cyclophosphamide ≥1 g/m^2
Cytarabine ≥1 g/m^2
Dacarbazine (days 1, 2 only)
Dactinomycin
Ifosfamide ≥1.2 g/m^2
Mechlorethamine
Methotrexate ≥1.2 g/m^2
Mitomycin ≥15 mg/m^2
Moderately Emetogenic: 50% to 75% Potential for Nausea, Vomiting, or Both
Carboplatin
Cisplatin <40 mg/m^2
Cyclophosphamide 200 mg/m^2 to 1 g/m^2
Cytarabine 200 mg/m^2 to 1 g/m^2
Daunorubicin
Doxorubicin (Adriamycin)
Gemcitabine
Ifosfamide <1.2 g/m^2
Irinotecan
Methotrexate 100 mg/m^2 to 1.2 g/m^2
Mitomycin <15 mg/m^2
Topotecan
Weakly Emetogenic: 20% to 50% Potential for Nausea, Vomiting, or Both
Asparaginase
Bleomycin
Cyclophosphamide <200 mg/m^2
Cytarabine <200 mg/m^2 daily
Docetaxel (Taxotere)
Etoposide
Fluorouracil
Fludarabine
Melphalan
Methotrexate <100 mg/m^2
Paclitaxel (Taxol)
Thioguanine or mercaptopurine
Thiotepa
Vinblastine
Vinorelbine
Minimally Emetogenic: Less Than 20% Potential for Nausea, Vomiting, or Both
Busulfan
Chlorambucil
Hydroxyurea
Vincristine

*Agents used in very high "transplant" doses may become highly emetogenic.

Prevention and Treatment

Agents effective in the treatment of nausea and vomiting (Table 4) come from several pharmacologic classes. For many years agents that bind to dopamine receptors, including, prochlorperazine, haloperidol, and metoclopramide were the mainstays of antiemetic regimens. These agents are moderately effective, but side effects can be a problem when dose escalations are used with highly emetogenic regimens, particularly those containing cisplatin. Prominent among these side effects are postural hypotension seen with prochlorperazine and a high frequency of extrapyramidal side effects associated with haloperidol and metoclopramide. The latter can be largely alleviated with simultaneous diphenhydramine, but this may result in excessive somnolence.

High-dose corticosteroids have been used effectively in the past 10 years, usually in combination with other antiemetics. The reasons that they are effective is not clear. Toxicity with short courses is usually mild, but gastrointestinal bleeding, agitation, delirium, and cataracts (rare) may occur.

Benzodiazepines such as lorazepam are also commonly used adjuncts to effective antiemetic regimens. They seem to have subjective benefits of reducing anxiety about the chemotherapy, and they reduce akathisia that may be induced by the dopamine antagonists. Dronabinol and smoked marijuana had short popularity several years ago, but dysphoric reactions, particularly in older patients, and variable efficacy have limited their use.

A major advance in the prevention of chemotherapy-induced nausea and vomiting has come with the discovery that blockade of the type 3 serotonin (5-hydroxytryptamine 5-HT) receptors (5-HT$_3$) rather than the blockade of dopamine receptors by metoclopramide appeared to account for its greater efficacy than that of other dopamine receptor antagonists. Subsequently other more specific serotonin antagonists have been found to be superior to any previously used antiemetics in the prevention of the acute phase of nausea and vomiting after chemotherapy. Ondansetron, the first of the serotonin antagonists to be approved for use in the United States, and subsequently granisetron, have rapidly become the mainstays of antiemetic regimens for chemotherapy with high potential for emesis. They have also rapidly become one of the highest-cost items in many hospital pharmacies around the United States.

Nausea and vomiting resulting from radiotherapy to the abdominal area or to the head can usually be alleviated by prochlorperazine 10 mg every 4 to 6 hours. If this is not successful, reducing the dose rate of the radiation may be helpful. Emesis resulting from biologic therapy such as high-dose interferon may also be helped by prochlorperazine but often is refractory and requires a reduction in the dose of the biologic agent.

The goal of therapy for nausea and vomiting associated

Table 4 Antiemetics Commonly Used for Prevention and Treatment of Chemotherapy-Induced Nausea and Vomiting

AGENT	ROUTE OF ADMINISTRATION	DOSAGE (ADULT)	COMMENTS
Prochlorperazine (Compazine)	PO	10–20 mg q4–6h	Some extrapyramidal reactions. Increased potential for severe postural hypotension when the agent is given IV. The patient must therefore be closely observed and assisted when attempting to sit up or get out of bed.
	IV (slow)	2–10 mg q4h	
	PR	25 mg q4–6h	
Thiethylperazine (Torecan)	PO, PR	10 mg q6–8h	Some extrapyramidal reactions.
	IM	2 mg q6–8h	
Trimethobenzamide (Tigan)	PO	250 mg q4–6h	Some extrapyramidal reactions.
	IM or PR	200 mg q4–6h	
Haloperidol (Haldol)	IV	1–3 mg q2–4h for 2–3 doses	Extrapyramidal reactions common.
Metoclopramide (Reglan)	PO	10–40 mg q6h	Extrapyramidal reactions common, particularly at high doses. Worse in younger patients. Diarrhea may occur.
	IV over 20 minutes	1–2 mg/kg at 2 hr intervals	
Lorazepam (Ativan)	IM, IV, or PO	1–2 mg q4–6h	Sedation is frequent.
Dexamethasone (Decadron, Hexadrol)	IV or PO	10–20 mg to start, then 4 mg PO q4–6h in tapering doses	Potential for agitation, delirium, gastrointestinal bleeding, cataracts (rare).
Ondansetron (Zofran)	IV over 15 minutes	0.15 mg/kg prior to and at 4 and 8 hours after chemotherapy *or* 30–32 mg once	For highly emetogenic therapy. Mild headache, mild transient transaminase elevation most common side effects.
	PO	8 mg 2 or 3 times in 24 hr	For moderately emetogenic therapy.
Granisetron	IV	0.4 mg/m^2 (10 μg/kg) prior to chemotherapy	For highly emetogenic therapy.
		2 mg PO prior to chemotherapy	

with chemotherapy is to prevent all three components—anticipatory, acute, and delayed. Not surprisingly, if acute and delayed emesis can be prevented in the first several cycles, anticipatory emesis is less likely to occur. The greatest challenge, therefore, is to select an appropriate antiemetic regimen at the outset that will prevent both early and delayed nausea and vomiting. This is particularly important for a patient receiving a highly emetogenic regimen such as one containing cisplatin.

There is no universally agreed formula for the most rational use of antiemetics, but several principles should be applied. Combinations of antiemetics have been shown to be more effective than single agents. It is common to use two or more agents together in the prevention or treatment of chemotherapy-induced emesis. It is easier to prevent emesis than to control it once it has begun; thus antiemetics are started prior to the chemotherapy. Some components, such as lorazepam, may best be given the evening before chemotherapy, particularly to patients who are prone to anticipatory nausea and vomiting. High cost of both the drugs and intravenous administration are important factors when using ondansetron, granisetron, and metoclopramide. Our recommendations for the prevention of nausea and vomiting with chemotherapy, according to the likelihood of emesis, are shown in Table 5. Because the greater efficacy of ondansetron compared with metoclopramide for the acute phase of emesis (first 24 hours) does not persist for the delayed phase (2 to 5 days), it is generally not used longer than 24 hours after the last day of chemotherapy. However, when a multiple-day cisplatin-based regimen is being used, ondansetron is still superior to metoclopramide so long as the chemotherapy is being administered.

Complications of Antiemetic Therapy

The most frequent complications of antiemetic therapy are shown in Table 4. Prochlorperazine, thiethylperazine, trimethobenzamide, haloperidol, and metoclopramide may cause extrapyramidal reactions, hypotension, and anticholinergic effects. The likelihood of complications depends on dose, route of administration, and the age of the patient. For example, high doses of metoclopramide are much more likely to cause akathisia than low doses, intravenous prochlorperazine is more likely to cause hypotension than oral treatment, and younger patients are more likely to have dystonic reactions than older ones. Extrapyramidal reactions can be reduced by the concomitant use of oral diphenhydramine, 25 to 50 mg every 6 hours. Ativan (lorazepam) 1 to 2 mg PO will help to alleviate akathisia. Diarrhea may result from metoclopramide because it increases bowel motility. This can be reduced by dexamethasone or with drugs that specifically reduce bowel motility such as oral diphenoxylate (Lomotil) 5 mg four times a day. Headache that is seen with ondansetron is usually well controlled with oral acetaminophen 650 mg every 4 hours. Sedation with lorazepam is frequently a desirable effect, as is the partial amnesia that may occur. The agitation that occurs with dexamethasone is usually tolerable and self-limited but may be alleviated with benzodiazepines. If delirium occurs with dexamethasone, it usually requires

Table 5 Recommendations for Antiemetic Prevention of Chemotherapy-Induced Nausea and Vomiting

DOSES FOR PATIENTS 1.5 TO 2.5 M²

Highly Emetogenic Chemotherapy

Ondansetron 30 mg IV ½ hour prior to chemotherapy. (Alternative = granisetron 0.4 μg/kg IV or 2 mg PO) For a regimen in which each day's therapy is expected to be highly emetogenic, may be repeated daily. *And*

Dexamethasone 10–20 mg IV ½ hour prior to first dose of chemotherapy. (Alternatively may give 10 mg PO evening prior and morning of therapy.) Repeat dexamethasone at 10–20 mg/day on each day highly emetogenic therapy is to be continued. Taper over 2–3 days after chemotherapy, e.g., 4 mg PO q6h × 4 doses, 4 mg q12h × 2 doses. *And*

Lorazepam 1 mg IV ½ hour prior to each dose of chemotherapy, then 1 mg IV or PO q4–6h prn nausea or vomiting. May wish to give 1–2 mg PO the evening prior and the morning of therapy. *And*

Metoclopramide 40 mg PO q6h × 3 starting 6 hr after each dose of ondansetron. May continue for 72 hours after last dose of ondansetron.

Moderately Emetogenic Chemotherapy

Ondansetron 10 mg IV ½ hour prior to chemotherapy. (Alternative = granisetron 1 mg PO) For a regimen in which each day's therapy is expected to be moderately emetogenic, may be repeated daily. *And*

Dexamethasone 10 mg IV ½ hour prior to first dose of chemotherapy. (Alternatively may give 10 mg PO evening prior to therapy.) Repeat dexamethasone at 10–20 mg/day on each day moderately emetogenic therapy is to be continued. Taper over 2–3 days after chemotherapy, e.g., 4 mg PO q6h × 4 doses, 4 mg q12h × 2 doses. *And*

Prochlorperazine 10–20 mg PO or 25 mg PR q6h for 48–72 hr. May be effective to use prochlorperazine spansules 15–30 mg the evening prior to chemotherapy and q12h for 48–72 hr. *And*

Lorazepam 1 mg PO or IV ½ hour prior to each dose of chemotherapy, then 1 mg IV or PO q4–6h prn nausea or vomiting. May wish to give 1–2 mg PO the evening prior to and the morning of therapy.

Weakly Emetogenic Chemotherapy

Prochlorperazine 10 mg PO 4 hr prior to chemotherapy, then 10 mg PO or 25 mg PR q4–6h × 48 hrs. *With or without*

Decadron 8 mg PO 1 hr prior to start of chemotherapy. *And*

Lorazepam 1 mg PO q6h prn

If the patient fails to have adequate control of nausea and vomiting on regimen 2 or 3, move to the next higher intensity of antiemetic therapy on the next cycle.

If the patient is on a multiple-day regimen, use highest level of antiemetics recommended on basis of current day's chemotherapy. However, if the previous day's regimen called for a more potent regimen, that should be followed.

Alternatives to Prochlorperazine include metoclopramide 10–40 mg PO or IV q4–6h, thiethylperazine (Torecan) 10 mg PO q6–8h, trimethobenzamide (Tigan) 250 mg PO, 200 mg PR, or 200 mg IM q4–6h, dimenhydrinate (Dramamine) 50 mg PO q4h.

dose reduction and occasionally the use of an antipsychotic medication such as oral haloperidol 1 to 2 mg as a single dose or up to four times daily.

The goal of complete control of nausea and vomiting from chemotherapy is achievable in most patients receiving chemotherapy. If an initial regimen is less successful than the patient and physician wish, modifications can be made, within limits imposed by the severity of side effects, to attain the greatest degree of freedom from nausea and vomiting with minimal adverse effects from the antiemetic regimen.

■ CONSTIPATION

Constipation is common in patients with advanced cancer. It is a particular problem in patients whose cancer has resulted in debility or immobility and in those who require narcotic analgesics or anticholinergic medications. It may also be seen in patients who have received neurotoxic chemotherapy agents, including the vinca alkaloids, etoposide, and cisplatin, each of which may cause autonomic dysfunction. Decreased bowel motility with constipation may also be seen in patients who have intra-abdominal metastatic disease without actual obstruction, dehydration, and hypercalcemia. It is promoted by lack of dietary bulk or fresh fruits and vegetables and inadequate fluid intake.

Sepsis may also result in constipation. In its extreme form, bowel motility is so impaired that the patient presents with colicky lower abdominal pain, nausea and vomiting, and an acutely distended abdomen that mimics mechanical obstruction. If the diameter of the colon exceeds 8 cm, this acute pseudo-obstruction of the intestines, known as Ogilvie's syndrome, requires urgent decompression either with colonoscopy or surgical intervention to avoid ischemic necrosis and perforation.

Of course it is critically important to consider mechanical bowel obstruction if one sees (1) changes in the stools to suggest narrowing of the lumen, (2) the development of constipation unexplained by other causes, or (3) an acutely distended abdomen with colicky pain (usually with nausea and vomiting). The treatment includes decompression from above, management of fluid and electrolyte imbalance, and surgical intervention if the obstruction is complete.

Chronic constipation in patients with cancer is more easily prevented than treated. It is worthwhile for the physician to anticipate circumstances when defecation may become a problem so that appropriate preventive measures can be taken. For example, it is important that prevention of constipation be initiated as soon as a patient is started on narcotic analgesics. One should begin with a mild regimen, such as stool softeners or bulk laxatives, but be willing to proceed to stimulant or osmotic laxatives if the simpler regimens are not effective. An appropriate goal is for the patient to have at least one soft stool daily (or less often if that has been the bowel habit pattern and the stool remains soft). Bowel management involves an assessment of the patient's previous and current

Table 6 Intervention to Prevent and Treat Constipation

INTERVENTIONS	COMMENTS, PRECAUTIONS
NONMEDICAL	
Increase fluid intake to 2 quarts daily if possible	Desirability must be balanced against problems with fluid retention or congestive heart failure.
Encourage regular exercise	May be difficult or impossible in bedridden patients.
Increase dietary fiber (5–10 g/d) using fruits, vegetables, and grains	Often difficult in patients whose appetite is already poor.
MEDICAL (BRAND NAME EXAMPLES)	
Docusate sodium (Colace), 100–300 mg daily	Stool softener.
Psyllium (Metamucil), 1 teaspoon to 2 tablespoons daily with 8–16 oz fluid	Bulk producer; must be taken with adequate fluid.
Senna (Senokot), 2–8 tablets daily	Stimulant laxative; may be habit forming.
Bisacodyl (Dulcolax), 1–3 tablets (5 mg) or one suppository (10 mg) at bedtime	Stimulant laxative; may be habit forming.
Metoclopramide (Reglan), 10–40 mg q.i.d.	Promotes gastric emptying and appears to enhance bowel peristalsis.
Milk of Magnesia, 15–60 ml	Osmotic laxative; can alter fluid and electrolyte balance. Magnesium-containing laxatives contraindicated in renal disease.
Lactulose (Chronulac), 1–4 tablespoons daily	Osmotic laxative; excessive amounts can lead to diarrhea and electrolyte losses.
Golytely (Colyte), 5 packets in 1 gallon of water	Clears bowel with minimal sodium or water imbalance (rarely used).

dietary and bowel habits and evaluation of anticipated changes in disease status or treatment that may affect bowel function. With this assessment the physician and patient together can develop a plan that will fit with the patient's ability to exercise, eat, consume fluids, and adjust medications. Suggested interventions for the prevention and management are shown in Table 6.

DIARRHEA

Among the common causes of diarrhea in patients who have cancer are chemotherapy, immunotherapy, radiotherapy, the cancer itself, and overgrowth of bacteria such as *Clostridium difficile* with resultant pseudomembranous colitis. Other causes may include medications, lactose intolerance, malnutrition, supplemental feedings, anxiety, and stress. Diarrhea may be characterized by an alteration in stool frequency, an alteration in stool fluidity, and abnormal stool constituents. This problem not only is uncomfortable for patients; it may also affect social activity and overall quality of life. If left untreated, prolonged diarrhea can cause serious electrolyte abnormalities. Taking the patient's history is the best way to distinguish among these possibilities.

Assessment

When a patient complains of diarrhea, it is important to establish usual elimination patterns. Presenting signs and symptoms include cramping, flatus, and distention. Frequency, onset, duration, and amount of diarrhea should be determined. It is also relevant to obtain a history of concurrent medical conditions and prior surgeries. Current treatments such as chemotherapy and radiotherapy, especially in combination, are important causes of diarrhea. Other medications, diet, and nutritional status also may affect gastrointestinal motility. Physical examination should include a good abdominal assessment and evaluation for signs of dehydration.

Baseline tests to be conducted in addition to history and physical examination include a complete blood count (CBC) and electrolytes. Stool should be obtained to check for *C. difficile*, ova, parasites, and enteropathic bacteria. If bowel obstruction is suspected, abdominal films may be ordered.

Management

Diarrhea Not Caused by Cancer Treatment

Diarrhea that results from the cancer itself is managed according to the particular cancer. Patients who have diarrhea associated with inoperable or metastatic secretory islet cell carcinomas of the pancreas or carcinoid tumors are treated with subcutaneous octreotide 0.05 mg twice a day to 0.1 mg three times a day. Successful chemotherapy (streptozocin) is also beneficial. Rectal villous adenomas may require fluid and electrolyte support prior to removal of the neoplasm.

Diarrhea from *C. difficile*–induced pseudomembranous colitis usually occurs only in patients who have previously been treated with systemic antibiotics. Mild to moderate leukocytosis and fever to 38.5°C are typically part of the syndrome. Any patient who is at risk should have stool sent for cytotoxic assay for *C. difficile* toxin. After obtaining the test, patients in whom this diagnosis is highly suspect should be started on oral metronidazole 500 mg PO three times a day, or oral vancomycin 125 mg four times a day; either one for 2 weeks. Metronidazole is much less expensive and the difference in efficacy is minimal, so it is the drug of first choice in most patients with this diagnosis. If the diagnosis is not confirmed, the antibiotic should be stopped and other causes investigated. It is recommended that the patient not be given loperamide or diphenoxylate (Lomotil) unless the diagnosis is effectively ruled out, as they may slow the clearance of the *C. difficile* toxin from the gut and exacerbate the problem with toxic megacolon.

Treatment-Related Diarrhea

When diarrhea is directly related to cancer treatment, the patient often requires symptomatic treatment and may need alteration in the cancer therapy. Nonpharmacologic strate-

Table 7 Interventions to Prevent and Treat Diarrhea

INTERVENTIONS	COMMENTS
NONPHARMACOLOGIC	
Low-residue diet	Avoid foods with whole grains, nuts, seeds, raw fruits and vegetables
Increase fluid intake to 3 L/day	
Ingest food at room temperature	
PHARMACOLOGIC	
Kaopectate	30–60 ml PO after each loose stool
Loperamide hydrochloride (Imodium)	2 capsules (4 mg) PO q4h initially, then add 1 capsule (2 mg) after each loose stool. Should not exceed 16 capsules daily.
Diphenoxylate hydrochloride with atropine sulfate (Lomotil)	1–2 tablets PO every 4 hours prn not to exceed 8 tablets daily. There may be anticholinergic side effects due to atropine.
Paregoric	1 tsp PO q.i.d. May alternate with Lomotil.
Belladona alkaloids (Donnatal)	Anticholinergic, antispasmodic; may help relieve bowel cramping. Dose: 1–2 tabs PO q4h
Octreotide (Sandostatin)	May be useful for chemotherapy-induced diarrhea Dose: 0.05–0.1 mg SC tid

gies to help reduce the diarrhea are included in Table 7. It is important to note that certain foods may worsen the diarrhea and should be avoided. Increasing fluid intake is significant consideration while the diarrhea is continuing. Some medications may help minimize the frequency of diarrhea (see Table 7). Lomotil (diphenoxylate HCl with atropine) and Imodium (loperamide) have been the mainstay for treatment of diarrhea. More recently it is noted that octreotide may have value in controlling the chemotherapy-related diarrhea associated with fluorouracil regimens.

Diarrhea that results from radiotherapy may first be treated with a low-residue diet or a gluten-free diet. If this is ineffective, the diarrhea can be treated with loperamide (Imodium), 4 mg to start, then 2 mg every 6 hours or diphenoxylate 2.5 mg with atropine 0.025 mg (Lomotil), 2 tabs four times a day. Radiotherapy is usually held if the diarrhea does not respond to these measures.

Chemotherapy agents that are associated with diarrhea are listed in Table 8. For most of the agents the diarrhea is not severe and is self-limited to a few days. For some agents such as fluorouracil, particularly when it is given by continuous infusion or together with leucovorin, the diarrhea may be more severe and can lead to dehydration, electrolyte imbalance, and death.

To assess the potential problems from the diarrhea, the patient must be questioned about the consistency of the diarrhea (watery or not), the number of episodes a day, and whether or not blood is present. If the patient has 2 or 3 stools per day over baseline (grade 1), it is sufficient to hold therapy. If there are four to six stools per day over baseline (grade 2), intravenous fluids should be administered and therapy held until complete resolution of the diarrhea. Dose reductions are then made, depending on the drug. If there are more than seven to nine stools daily over baseline or incontinence or severe cramping (grade 3), the patient should be hospitalized for hydration and monitored for electrolyte imbalance. If the patient has 10 or more stools in 24 hours or grossly bloody diarrhea, is clinically dehydrated, or has electrolyte imbalance (grade 4), aggressive hydration is critical to prevent a fatal outcome. Patients with less severe diarrhea (grade 1 or 2) can be treated with loperamide (Imodium) 4 mg to start, then 2 mg every 6 hours or diphenoxylate 2.5 mg with atropine 0.025 mg (Lomotil), 2 tabs four times a day. If the diarrhea persists for more than a few days or is more severe, serious consideration should be given to octreotide acetate therapy, 0.05 to 0.1 mg SC three times a day.

Table 8 Chemotherapy Drugs That Cause Diarrhea

Drugs with Which Diarrhea Is Relatively Common; More Than 10%
Aldesleukin (interleukin-2) (75%)
Cytarabine
Floxuridine*
Fludarabine (15%)
Fluorouracil*
Idarubicin
Irinotecan (50–80%)
Interferon-alpha
Mithramycin
Mitoxantrone
Paclitaxel (Taxol) (43%)
Pentostatin
Drugs with Which Diarrhea Occurs Occasionally: 10% or Less
Azacytidine
Cladribine (2-chlorodeoxyadenosine) (10%)
Dactinomycin
Daunorubicin
Doxorubicin
Etoposide
Flutamide
Methotrexate
Tamoxifen

*Diarrhea is a sign of toxicity that requires temporary discontinuation of drug therapy. With other drugs, discontinuation or dose reduction on subsequent cycles will be indicated, depending on the severity of the diarrhea and the schedule of chemotherapy.

ORAL COMPLICATIONS

Oral complications of cancer treatment are common and contribute to overall morbidity. The oral mucosa is very vulnerable to treatment-related effects due to its high mitotic rate and rapid epithelial cell turnover. Oral complications, if not effectively managed, can jeopardize therapy due to treatment delay or dose reduction. The patient may also have mild to severe discomfort, which can affect quality of life and prompt the decision to withdraw from treatment. In addition, the disruption in the oral mucosa can place the myelosuppressed and immunocompromised patient at serious risk for secondary and systemic infections.

High-Risk Populations

The identification of patients at high risk for oral complications allows for initiation of prophylactic measures and early management of complications. The type and location of the malignancy, the type and intensity of therapy, pre-existing medical and oral conditions, the patient's age, tobacco and alcohol use, and lack of self-care ability predispose the patient to oral complications. Patients with head and neck cancers or hematologic malignancies are particularly prone to develop oral complications. The degree of oral complications associated with radiotherapy is related to the dose received, the duration of therapy, and the site irradiated. Several chemotherapy agents have a direct stomatoxic effect, and higher dosages may cause more severe oral complications (Table 9).

Table 9 Chemotherapy Agents That May Cause Oral Ulcerations

Antimetabolites
Methotrexate
Fluorouracil
Cytarabine
Antitumor antibiotics
Adriamycin (doxorubicin)
Dactinomycin
Mitoxantrone
Mitomycin
Bleomycin
Plant alkaloids
Vinblastine
Vincristine
Etoposide
Others
Hydroxyurea
High doses of alkylating agents
Biologic agents
Interleukins
LAK cell therapy

Prevention

Primary preventive measures, such as nutrition and good oral hygiene, are important during the pretreatment period. Dental consultation prior to radiotherapy or chemotherapy in which oral complications are anticipated is also recommended to determine the condition of the oral mucosa and to initiate an oral care program. Antiviral and antifungal agents have been incorporated into oral care protocols of patients expected to become severely immunocompromised, but the effectiveness of the prophylactic use of these agents is not established. Because mucositis is a common dose-limiting side effect of fluorouracil when combined with leucovorin, oral cryotherapy has been used with some success in reducing the extent of mucositis. This is done by having the patient chew ice 15 minutes prior to and during the chemotherapy administration.

Early Detection

The initial assessment of each patient with cancer should include a thorough oral assessment. After treatment is initi-

Table 10 Agents for Oral Care

ORAL AGENT	COMMENTS
CLEANSING AGENTS	
Normal saline	½ tsp salt in 8 oz water Economical, nondamaging
Hydrogen peroxide	Dilute with normal saline or tap water Germicidal, debriding
Sodium bicarbonate	Nonirritating, neutralizes acid in mouth
Chlorhexidine (Peridex)	Antimicrobial, can stain teeth
LUBRICATING AGENTS	
Saliva substitutes	Decreases dryness, similar to human saliva
Water- or oil-based lubricants	Useful emollient. Oil-based lubricants should not be used in mouth due to danger of aspiration
ANALGESIC AGENTS	
Healing and coating agents	
Sucralfate	Binds to mucosa, forms protective coating
Vitamin E	Protection to mucosa, healing properties
Zilactin	Reduces discomfort by coating, safe
Antacids	Enhance comfort, coat mucosa Examples: Maalox, Milk of Magnesia, Kaopectate
Topical anesthetics	
Lidocaine viscous	Transient pain relief, absorbed systemically
Diclonine hydrochloride	Transient pain relief, minimal systemic absorption
Benzocaine	Transient pain relief, minimal systemic absorption
Systemic analgesics	
Nonsteroidal-anti-inflammatory drugs	
Narcotics	Taken before meals and prn

ated, a systematic oral assessment should be a regular part of the physical examination. During the oral examination, a good source of light and a tongue blade are important tools to help visualize the oral cavity. Special attention should be given to the anterior and lateral surfaces of the tongue, the gingiva, the soft palate, the buccal mucosa, and the lips. It is important to assess the patient for soreness, erythema, and ulcerations, which may be infected. The recognition of oral complications in the myelosuppressed or immunocompromised patient may be difficult due to atypical clinical appearance. Nonetheless, early detection is crucial for proper diagnosis and treatment of oral complications.

Management

Once oral complications have developed, the focus of care should be on meticulous oral hygiene and treatment of symptoms. Oral assessments should be done twice daily on hospitalized patients, and oral care should be done at least every 4 hours while awake and at bedtime. Agents used for oral care can be categorized according to function: cleansing agents, lubricating agents, and analgesic agents. Several commonly used oral agents are listed in Table 10. Commercial mouthwashes are not recommended because of their high alcohol content and irritation to the oral tissues. Lemon glycerin swabs are to be avoided as well because of the irritating and drying effects on the oral mucosa.

An oral care protocol should be individualized but should include a cleansing agent, a lubricating agent, and analgesics. An example oral protocol consisting of Peridex 15 ml swish and expectorate after meals and at bedtime and petrolatum jelly applied to the lips as needed has been helpful. If painful oral ulcerations do develop swishing and swallowing a stomatitis mixture combining diphenhydramine (Benadryl) elixir 5 ml, Maalox 30 ml, and lidocaine (Xylocaine) viscous 5 ml, prior to meals is often helpful. Systemic pain control measures are indicated if the topical anesthetics are ineffective. Acetaminophen 325 mg with codeine 30 mg (Tylenol #3) 1 or 2 tablets orally every 4 hours as needed, or other pain medications can be administered. Severe ulcerations may require parenteral narcotics, such as morphine, intermittently or as a continuous infusion.

Oral infections must be treated promptly and as accurately as possible. Fungal infections caused by the various species of *Candida* are common in patients with cancer. Initial treatment for oral fungal infections may include nystatin suspension or clotrimazole (Mycelex) troches. If the medications are poorly tolerated or the potential for systemic dissemination is likely, ketoconazole or fluconazole can be administered orally. Viral infections in the immunocompromised patient may resurface due to reactivation of herpes simplex virus (HSV). Systemic treatment with acyclovir (Zovirax) or an alternative antiviral agent is recommended in intravenous or oral form. Table 11 provides dosing guidelines for the medications used in the treatment of fungal and viral infections. Bacterial infections arising in the oral cavity may develop as primary or secondary infections. Oral cultures are helpful in identifying the predominant bacterial growth. Topical or systemic antibiotics are usually effective when based on the culture and sensitivity results.

The prevention and management of oral complications is truly a collaborative effort. The patient, the family, the nurse, the oncologist, and the dentist are all key in the promotion of oral hygiene and the prompt identification and management of oral complications.

Table 11 Topical and Systemic Medications in the Treatment of Infection for Oral Complications

FUNGAL INFECTIONS	
Nystatin (Mycostatin)	400,000–600,000 U swish and swallow q.i.d. Must be held against the affected mucosa for 5 min
Clotrimazole (Mycelex)	10 mg troches 5 times a day. Must be held in the mouth until dissolved
Ketoconazole (Nizoral)	200 mg PO qd
Fluconazole (Diflucan)	100–200 mg PO qd
VIRAL INFECTIONS	
Acyclovir (Zovirax)	1–2 g/day PO or 5 mg/kg q8h IV
Famcyclovir (Faxivir)	250 mg PO q8h × 5 d (minimum)
BACTERIAL INFECTIONS	
Systemic antibiotics	Antibiotics based on oral culture and sensitivity

Table 12 Medications Used for Pruritus

Antihistamines	
Diphenhydramine hydrochloride (Benadryl)	25–50 mg PO q6 hr
Hydroxyzine hydrochloride (Vistaril)	25–50 mg PO q6–8 hr
Cyproheptadine hydrochloride (Periactin)	4 mg PO q6–8 hr

■ PRURITUS

Pruritus, or itching, is an unpleasant sensation of some patients with cancer. Not only is it uncomfortable, but scratching may cause a disruption in the protective barrier, the skin. Pruritis may be caused by things such as dry skin, cancer treatments, or a cancer itself. It is pertinent for the health care professional to discern which of various factors is most likely responsible for the pruritis and then to treat it appropriately.

Assessment

When obtaining a history from a patient with itching, consider the possibility of underlying or known liver disease, renal disease, hematologic disorder, iron deficiency, or diabetes. Pruritis can be a clinical manifestation of various malignancies, including AIDS-related Kaposi's sarcoma, Hodgkin's lymphoma, and less commonly, adenocarcinomas and squamous cell carcinomas. Certain medications, such as interleukin-2, narcotics, phenothiazines, hormones, antibiotics, and vitamin B complex, may also be associated with pruritus. Hypersensitivity reactions in response to some cytotoxic agents may also result in pruritus. These agents include doxorubicin, cytarabine, daunorubicin, L-asparaginase, and cisplatin.

Physical examination should provide data regarding signs of infection, evidence of skin changes, and presence of lesions.

All skin surfaces should be examined as well as sites of scratching.

Treatment

Treatment of pruritus may involve a variety of interventions. Initially the patient may need to be educated on factors that may enhance the itching. Physical interventions such as cool compresses may also help minimize the itching. Topical application of medications and systemic medications may also be useful (Table 12). Elimination of provoking factors may assist in some reduction of pruritus. Good cleansing practices, protection from the environment, and optimal nutrition and hydration may promote healthy skin. Extensive bathing and hot baths may aggravate the itching, whereas tepid baths may cause vasoconstriction and decreased itching. Mild soaps should be used, for example Dove or Neutrogena.

Topical agents such as Aveeno ointment are typically used to keep the skin hydrated and moist. Product selection should be made after a consideration of the patient's needs. Topical agents that include talc, perfumes, or cornstarch may irritate the skin further. If the above interventions are unsuccessful, medications may provide some relief. Oral antihistamines are most commonly used for treatment of pruritus. Other medications may be useful if anxiety seems to be a complicating factor.

Suggested Reading

Beck TM, Hesketh PH, Madajewicz S, et al. Stratified, randomized, double-blind comparison of intravenous ondansetron administered as a multiple-dose regimen versus two single-dose regimens in the prevention of cisplatin-induced nausea and vomiting. J Clin Oncol 1992; 10:1969–1975.

Cascinu S, Fedeli A, Fedeli SL, et al. Octreotide versus loperamide in the treatment of fluorouracil induced diarrhea: A randomized trial. J Clin Oncol 1993; 11:148–151.

De Mulder PHM, Seynaeve C, Vermorken JB, et al. Ondansetron compared with high-dose metoclopramide in prophylaxis of acute and delayed cisplatin-induced nausea and vomiting. Ann Intern Med 1990; 113:834–840.

Fraschini G, Ciociola A, Asparza L, et al. Evaluation of three oral dosages of ondansetron in the prevention of nausea and emesis associated with cyclophosphamide-doxorubicin chemotherapy. J Clin Oncol 1991; 9:1268–1274.

Hesketh PJ, Beck T, Uhlenhopp M. Adjusting the dose of intravenous ondansetron plus dexamethasone to th emetogenic potential of the chemotherapy regimen. J Clin Oncol 1995 13: 2117–2122.

Kris MG, Gralla RJ, Tyson LB, et al. Controlling delayed vomiting: Double-blind, randomized trial comparing placebo, dexamethasone alone, and metoclopramide plus dexamethasone in patients receiving cisplatin. J Clin Oncol 1989; 7:108–114.

Morrow GR, Hickok JT, Rosenthal SN. Progress in reducing nausea and emesis: Comparisons of Ondansetron (Zofran), granisetron (Kytril) and tropisetron (Navoban). Cancer 1995 76: 343–357.

Navari RM, Madajewicz S, Anderson N, et al. Oral ondansetron for the control of cisplatin-induced delayed emesis: a large multicenter, double-blind, randomized comparative trial of ondansetron versus placebo. J Clin Oncol 1995 13: 2408–2416.

Poland J. Prevention and treatment of oral complications in the cancer patient. Oncology 1991; 5(8):45–50.

Razavi D, Delvaux N, Farvacques C, et al. Prevention of adjustment disorders and anticipatory nausea secondary to adjuvant chemotherapy: A double blind, placebo-controlled study assessing the usefulness of alprazolam. J Clin Oncol 1993; 11:1384–1390.

Sledge GW, Einhorn L, Nagy C, House K. Phase III double-blind comparison of intravenous ondansetron and metoclopramide as antiemetic therapy for patients receiving multiple-day cisplatin based chemotherapy. Cancer 1992; 70:2524–2528.

Sonis S, Clark J. Prevention and management of oral mucositis induced by antineoplastic therapy. Oncology 1991; 5:11–18.

MANAGING CANCER PAIN

Charles S. Cleeland, Ph.D.
Eduardo Bruera, M.D.

Pain from cancer can be adequately controlled with analgesics given by mouth for most patients most of the time. When this is not possible, a variety of more sophisticated pain management techniques can provide control, and it is estimated that approximately 95 percent of patients could be free of significant pain, at least until the last week or two of life. Unfortunately, many patients do not benefit from adequate pain control. Estimates based on surveys in the United States indicate that only 40 percent of all cancer patients obtain optimal pain control. Poorly controlled pain has such catastrophic effects on the patient and his or her family that proper management of pain must have the highest priority for those who routinely care for cancer patients. Mood and quality of life deteriorate in the presence of pain, and pain has adverse effects on such measures of disease status as appetite and activity. Severe pain may be a primary reason why patients and their families stop treatment. Improving the practice of anticipating, evaluating, and treating pain will benefit many patients.

■ PREVALENCE

The majority of cancer patients with terminal disease will need careful pain management; between 60 and 80 percent of such patients will have significant pain. Less attention, however, has been paid to pain, as a problem for patients before the terminal phase of the disease, when patients with months or years to live may have function compromised by poorly controlled pain. Persistent pain is rarely a problem before metastatic cancer is present. Most immediate postoperative pain can be managed without difficulty. When the cancer has metastasized, however, the percentage of patients with pain increases dramatically. In the United States, even with the availability of a full range of analgesics and other pain treatments, one-third of patients with metastatic cancer report pain so severe that it significantly impairs their quality of life.

Mild pain is often well tolerated with minimal impact on a patient's activities. However, there is a threshold beyond which pain is disproportionately disruptive. This threshold has been reached when patients rate the severity of their pain at the midpoint or higher on any of the commonly used pain severity scales. When pain is too great, it becomes the primary focus of attention and prohibits most activity not directly related to pain.

■ PHYSICAL BASIS OF CANCER PAIN

Direct tumor involvement is the most common cause of pain in approximately two-thirds of patients with pain from metastatic cancer. Tumor invasion of bone is the physical basis of pain in about 50 percent of these patients. The remaining 50 percent experience tumor-related pain that is due to nerve compression or infiltration or involvement of the gastrointestinal tract or soft tissue. Persistent post-therapy pain from long-term effects of surgery, radiotherapy, and chemotherapy accounts for an additional 20 percent of all who report pain with metastatic cancer, with a small residual group experiencing pain from non–cancer-related conditions. Most patients with advanced cancer have pain that develops through multiple mechanisms. A new complaint of pain in a patient with metastatic cancer should first be thought of as disease related, but indirectly related manageable causes should always be considered and ruled out.

The sensation of pain is generated either by stimulation of peripheral pain receptors or by damage to afferent nerve fibers. Peripheral pain receptors can be stimulated by pressure, compression, and traction as well as by disease-related chemical changes. Pain due to stimulation of pain receptors is *nociceptive pain.* Damage to visceral, somatic, or autonomic nerve trunks produces *neurogenic* or *neuropathic pain.* Spontaneous activity in these damaged nerves is the probable cause of the painful sensation. Damage to nerves can be caused by treatment or by the disease itself. Cancer patients often have nociceptive and neuropathic pain simultaneously. The physical basis of the pain is especially important because neuropathic pain is less responsive to opiod analgesics and will require the additional use of other drugs.

■ ASSESSMENT OF PAIN

It is essential to have a clear understanding of the characteristics of the pain and its physical basis for proper management. The changing expression of cancer pain demands repeated assessment, as new causes for pain can emerge rapidly. In advanced cancer cases, pain of multiple origins may be the rule and not the exception. A careful history includes questions concerning the location, severity, and quality of the pain, as well as its effects on the patient's life.

Inadequate assessment and poor physician-patient communication about pain are major barriers to good care. A small minority of cancer patients may complain of pain in a dramatic fashion, but many more patients under-report the severity of their pain and the lack of adequate pain relief. There are several reasons for this reluctance to report pain, including not wanting to acknowledge that the disease is progressing, not wanting to divert the physician's attention from treating the disease, and not wanting to tell the physician that pain treatments are not working. Patients may not want to take opioid analgesics because they do not want to become addicted, because they fear psychoactive components of opioids, because they are concerned that using opioids too early will endanger pain relief when they have more pain, or because they fear that being placed on opioids signals that death is near. Presenting information that addresses these concerns in a straightforward manner will allay most of these fears and should be considered an essential step in providing pain control. It is important for patients to understand that they will function better if their pain is controlled.

Communication about pain is greatly aided by having the patient use a scale to report it. A simple rating scale ranges from 0 to 10, with 0 being no pain and 10 being pain as bad as you can imagine. Used properly, pain severity scales can be invaluable in titrating analgesics and in monitoring for increases in pain with progressive disease.

Those who treat cancer patients should be familiar with the common pain syndromes associated with the disease. Having the patient show the area of pain on a drawing of a human figure may aid diagnosis. This can be particularly helpful in indicating areas of referred pain, common with nerve compression. Careful questioning concerning the characteristics of the pain is essential for physical diagnosis. In addition to severity, these characteristics include the temporal pattern of the pain (constant or episodic) and its quality. Episodic or incident pain is much more difficult to control than continuous pain. Other important characteristics of pain are its relationship to physical activity and what seems to alleviate it. The physical examination of the patient includes examination of the painful area as well as neurologic and orthopedic assessment. Since bone metastases are a common cause of pain and since pain can occur with changes in bone density not detectable on x-ray film, bone scans can be helpful. Computed tomographic (CT) scanning is useful in the evaluation of retroperitoneal, paravertebral, and pelvic areas as well as the base of the skull. Myelography may be necessary to determine the cause of pain. Diagnostic nerve blocks can provide information concerning the pain pathway and can determine the potential effectiveness of neuroablative procedures.

When pain is moderate or severe, we can assume that it is damaging the patient's quality of life. That damage, including problems with sleep and depression, must be evaluated. The number of hours the patient is now sleeping compared with the last pain-free interval, difficulties with sleep onset, frequent interruptions of sleep, and/or early morning awakening suggest the need for appropriate pharmacologic intervention, often the addition of a low-dose antidepressant at bedtime. Just as patients hesitate to report severe pain, they may hesitate to report depression. Having the patient report depression or tension on a scale of 0 to 10 may help overcome some of this reluctance. Significant depression should be treated through psychiatric or psychologic consultation, especially if it persists in the face of adequate pain relief.

A very small number of patients in severe psychosocial distress will express many of their losses and concerns as physical pain. It is important to recognize severe somatization and to provide psychiatric referral or counseling to these patients. However, more often physicians misdiagnose true pain as depression or anxiety. Patients who are cognitively impaired, particularly those with agitation, may be extremely difficult to assess. In these patients, the differentiation between agitated delirium and pain may be extremely difficult. Patients in whom pain was well controlled before the development of delirium are unlikely to be agitated due to uncontrolled pain. Frequent discussions between various health care professionals and the patient's family will be required.

Some patients with a history of severe alcoholism or drug addiction may request analgesics for their psychological effects. This is unlikely to occur in patients without a clear history of severe addictive behavior. Although their care is more complex, patients with a history of drug or alcohol addiction should never be denied appropriate pain medications. If this diagnosis is suspected, the patient should be confronted with this behavior and an agreement should be made about the use of opioids for the management of pain as opposed to mood alterations. With this group of patients, long-acting opioids or continuous infusion is preferable to short-acting opioids or patient-controlled analgesia. Prescriptions by a single physician would make the negotiation process with a patient much simpler.

■ TREATMENT

All health care professionals who see cancer patients should be familiar with the Agency for Health Care Policy and Research (AHCPR) guidelines *Management of Cancer Pain.* The prompt relief of pain from cancer frequently involves the use of simultaneously rather than serially administered combinations of drug and nondrug therapies. Identification of a treatable neoplasm as a factor in pain production will call for appropriate radiotherapy (to bone metastases, for example), chemotherapy, or in some instances surgical debulking. Until such treatment can be effective (this may take days to weeks), the patient's pain must be managed with analgesics. In many instances analgesics are the only pain treatment available because of the patient's condition, the physical basis of the pain, or limited treatment options. The principles of pharmacologic management of pain are evolving through studies of analgesic effectiveness and research on the use of combinations of palliative medications.

There is a growing consensus concerning the types of drugs to use, their routes of administration, and how best to schedule them. The first step is the choice of *analgesic* drug to be used (nonopioid, opioid, or a combination). The second step is the choice of *adjuvant* drugs, which can increase the analgesic's effectiveness and can produce other palliative effects to counter the disruptive consequences of pain.

Nonsteroidal Anti-Inflammatory Drugs

Nonsteroidal anti-inflammatory drugs (NSAIDs) constitute the majority of nonopioid analgesics. Their effect on the inflammatory process is a key to their analgesic property. Tumor growth produces inflammatory and mechanical effects in adjacent tissues that can trigger the release of prostaglandins, bradykinin, and serotonin, which in turn may precipitate or exacerbate pain in the surrounding tissues. Prostaglandin-mediated actions on peripheral receptors probably include both direct activation and sensitization to other analgesic substances. Prostaglandins are frequently associated with painful bone metastasis because of their involvement of bone reabsorption. The NSAIDs seem to exert their analgesic, antipyretic, and anti-inflammatory actions by blocking the synthesis of prostaglandins. By virtue of their different mechanisms of action and toxicity profiles, the NSAIDs and opioids are often administered together. Enteric-coated aspirin is one of the first-choice drugs for mild to moderate cancer pain. Other NSAIDs such as ibuprofen, diflunisal, naproxen, and trilisate have established value in the management of clinical pain. These drugs are better tolerated than aspirin but are usually significantly more expensive. Individual differences in response to the various NSAIDs are not yet well understood.

Acetaminophen is a peripherally acting analgesic that does not inhibit peripheral prostaglandin synthesis. Therefore, it does not have anti-inflammatory effects or the side effects associated with the use of NSAIDs. Acetaminophen should be considered for patients who have contraindications to the use of the NSAIDs.

Commercial preparations containing codeine or oxycodone and acetaminophen or aspirin are among the most widely prescribed scheduled analgesics and are frequently administered to cancer patients. This is generally appropriate because of their synergistic effects. Such a combination is reported to be particularly effective for bone pain.

NSAIDs have a number of serious side effects such as gastritis and gastrointestinal hemorrhage, bleeding due to platelet inhibition, and renal failure. Most of these side effects are related to the prostaglandin inhibitory effect of these drugs and are therefore common to all these drugs. Renal failure due to the inhibition of renal medullary prostaglandins can be of particular concern in patients also receiving opioids. Decreased renal elimination of active opioid metabolites can result in somnolence, confusion, hallucinations, or generalized myoclonus. Therefore, kidney function should be monitored in patients receiving a combination of NSAIDs and opioids.

Gastrointestinal complications include gastric pain, nausea, vomiting, hemorrhage, and in extreme cases, perforation. Gastrointestinal damage is mediated by prostaglandin inhibition. The most common form of nephrotoxicity associated with NSAIDs is renal failure related to prostaglandin inhibition and consequent vasodilation. Hepatic injury has been reported with the use of aspirin, benoxaprofen, and phenylbutazone and less commonly with diclofenac, ibuprofen, indomethacin, naproxen, pirbrofen, and sulindac. Sulindac, however, seems to be associated with a higher incidence of cholestasis.

NSAID use is also associated with a variety of hypersensitive reactions involving the skin (rash, eruption, itching), blood vessels (angioneurotic edema, vasomotor disorders), and the respiratory system (rhinitis, asthma). In particular, aspirin may cause anaphylactic crisis, a syndrome characterized by dyspnea, sudden weakness, sweating, and collapse. Undesirable hematologic effects of NSAIDs include platelet

Table 1 Opioid Dosing Equivalence

DRUG	APPROXIMATE EQUIANALGESIC DOSE			
	ORAL		PARENTERAL	
Morphine	30 mg	q3–4hr[a]	10 mg	q3–4hr
Hydromorphone	4–8 mg	q3–4hr	1.5 mg	q3–4hr
Codeine[b]	130 mg	q3–4hr	—	
Propoxyphene[b]	See comment below[c]		—	
Hydrocodone[b]	30 mg	q3–4hr	—	
Oxycodone[b]	30 mg	q3–4hr	—	
Methadone	5–20 mg	q6–8hr[d]	5–10 mg	q6–8hr[d]
Levorphanol	4 mg	q6–8hr[d]	2 mg	q6–8hr[d]
Meperidine[e]	300 mg	q2–3hr	100 mg	q3hr
Transdermal fentanyl	25 µg patch = 8–22 mg/24 hr IV/IM morphine sulfate = 45–134 mg/24 hr PO morphine sulfate			

[a]Slow-release formulations of oral morphine have 8–12 hour duration of analgesic action.
[b]Codeine, propoxyphene, hydrocodone, and oxycodone are often given as combination products with aspirin and/or acetaminophen.
[c]Propoxyphene is a weak analgesic; 65–130 mg is equivalent to about 650 mg of aspirin. It has a duration of action 3–4 hours; however, its duration of action increases with chronic dosing.
[d]The duration of analgesia of methadone and levorphanol may be significantly longer than 6–8 hours in some patients.
[e]Not recommended for chronic use.
From Weissman DE, Burchman SL, Dinndorf PA, Dahl JL. Handbook of cancer pain management. 4th ed. Wisconsin Cancer Pain Initiative, 1993; with permission.

dysfunction, aplastic anemia, and agranulocytosis. Factors often considered in the empirical selection of an NSAID for a given patient include their relative toxicity, cost, dosage schedule, and prior experience. The use of certain aspirin analogues (choline magnesium trisalicylate) has been suggested to be associated with a low incidence of gastropathy and platelet dysfunction. Used as single agents in the management of cancer pain, the effects of NSAIDs are characterized by a ceiling effect, beyond which further increases in dose do not enhance analgesia.

Opioid Analgesics

The choice of an opioid as opposed to nonopioid analgesic follows from an assessment of the severity of pain. The decision is relatively easy when pain is mild (choose nonopioid) or severe (choose opioid, usually in combination with a nonopioid). The choice is more difficult when the patient reports moderate pain, especially when there is reason to suspect that the patient may be under-reporting its severity. Several studies have documented that many cancer patients are inadequately managed because of the physician's reluctance to use opioids in dosages and with schedules known to be sufficient to relieve moderate pain.

Opioid analgesics should be prescribed as soon as there is evidence that pain is not well controlled with nonopioid analgesics. Usually nonopioid analgesics can be continued as a way of maximizing analgesia because their site of action is different from that of the opioids. Except in a minority of patients whose pain is clearly episodic, analgesics should be given around the clock, with the time interval based on the duration of effectiveness of the drug and the patient's report of the duration of effectiveness.

There is evidence that total opioid requirement is lower when opioids are given on a schedule, preventing peaks of pain. Putting patients in the position of having to ask for medication or continually making a judgment about whether their pain is severe enough to take analgesics focuses their attention on pain, reminds them of their need for drugs, and allows pain to reach a severity not readily controlled by a dose that would be effective with scheduled administration. It is important to remember that there may be large individual differences in the required dose of opioid, depending on such factors as the patient's prior opioid history, activity level, and metabolism. The patient's report of severity and relief is the best guideline for opioid titration.

The so-called weak opioids, including codeine and oxycodone, usually formulated in combination with acetaminophen or aspirin, can provide active patients with good pain relief for long periods. As disease advances, oral administration of the more potent opioids provides the majority of patients with pain relief. There is considerable agreement that meperidine should not be used on a chronic basis because it produces the toxic metabolite normeperidine, which is a central nervous system (CNS) stimulant, has a long serum half-life, and has no analgesic properties. Oral administration is preferred, but the physician must remain flexible to changes that are dictated by the patient's ability to take drugs orally. This may include the use of opioid and nonopioid suppositories and other alternate routes of administration (transdermal, sublingual, rectal, subcutaneous).

Oral morphine, either in immediate- or sustained-release preparation, is the analgesic of choice for moderate to severe cancer pain. Long-acting morphine preparations are convenient for both patient and health care staff. Immediate-release morphine is much cheaper and as effective. A typical starting dose of immediate-release oral morphine is 10 to 30 mg every 4 hours in patients not previously taking opioids. When a patient is switching from another opioid (usually codeine or oxycodone) to morphine, it is important to calculate the equianalgesic morphine dose as a basis for determining what morphine-equivalent doses are the threshold for pain control (Table 1). The starting dose may not be sufficient, and relatively rapid upward titration may be needed, especially if pain is severe. When an effective dose of short-acting morphine has been established, the required dose for a long-acting preparation can be calculated. An additional supply of short-acting morphine, given when necessary, will help the patient manage breakthrough pain. Consistent need for this additional morphine will dictate an upward adjustment of the dose of sustained-release drug. Orders for immediate-release morphine should allow for some upward titration of dose by the patient or by the nurse.

While the opioid agonist-antagonist analgesics have established their effectiveness in the control of acute (especially procedurally related) pain, their use in chronic cancer pain is limited by the possibility of precipitous withdrawal in the patient who has been taking morphine-type drugs, by their analgesic ceiling effect (when the drug does not provide more pain relief), and by the lack of an oral form of administration (with the exception of pentazocine, which yields a relatively high proportion of patients reporting disturbing psychotomimetic effects).

Alternate Routes

Approximately 70 percent of patients will benefit from the use of an alternate route of opioid administration sometime before death. The duration for which patients need these routes varies between hours and months. While intermittent injections can be effective for a brief time, this method is painful for the patient, time-consuming for the nursing staff, and difficult to manage at home.

A number of studies have shown that intravenous infusions of narcotics produce stable blood levels of drug and that they are safe and effective for treating both postoperative and cancer pain. The main problem associated with continuous intravenous infusions is the prolonged maintenance of an intravenous line. Patients may have to be subjected to numerous venipunctures when peripheral intravenous lines are used. Totally implantable intravenous catheters are a major improvement, permitting long-term intravenous access. However, these catheters are expensive and must be surgically implanted, and their maintenance requires considerable nursing expertise and patient teaching. If such a catheter is already available in an advanced cancer patient with pain, it certainly can be used for the administration of opioids.

Subcutaneous Route. Subcutaneous injection has been found to be safe and effective for the administration of morphine, hydromorphone, and levorphanol. Subcutaneous opioids can be administered both as a continuous infusion using a portable or nonportable pump or as an intermittent injection. A butterfly needle can be left under the skin approximately 7 days, making both intermittent injections and continuous infusion painless. The needles are commonly inserted in the subclavicular region, anterior chest, or abdominal wall. This allows patients to have free limbs.

Rectal Route. The majority of the experience reported in the literature is with the short-term use of rectal opioids for the management of acute pain. Both solid and liquid solutions have been used. While there is considerable interindividual variation in the bioavailability of rectally administered morphine, there is generalized consensus that this drug is well absorbed following rectal administration. A number of authors have treated terminally ill cancer patients with rectal morphine with good pain control until death. Advantages of the rectal route include no need for the insertion of needles or the use of portable pumps. However, rectal administration can be uncomfortable, absorption may be decreased by the presence of stool in the rectum, diarrhea, or simply by normal bowel movements, and progressive titration may be difficult because of the limited availability of different commercial preparations.

Transdermal Route. The recent development of a transdermal preparation of fentanyl citrate has revitalized interest in this route. Pharmacokinetic data suggest that transdermal fentanyl is well absorbed, although there is considerable delay in reaching steady-state blood levels and a slowly declining plasma concentration after removal of the patch. These characteristics may be obstacles to its regular clinical use, particularly in unstable patients. Although clinical experience is still very limited, treatment appears to be well tolerated. Future research should focus on comparisons among the transdermal route, long-acting morphine preparations, and continuous subcutaneous infusions of opioids.

Adverse Effects

Sedation. Sedation occurs in the majority of patients during the beginning of opioid treatment or after a major increase in dose. Most patients develop rapid tolerance to this side effect, and while the sedation disappears within 3 to 5 days, the analgesic effect persists. When sedation occurs in cancer patients receiving a stable dose of opioid, it is necessary to suspect the accumulation of active opioid metabolites such as morphine-6-glucuronide. This occurs most frequently in patients who are receiving high doses of opioids or who have renal failure. It is also important to suspect other nonopioid causes, since these patients are frequently very ill. Opioid-induced sedation can be managed by opioid rotation (some opioids have a higher ratio of analgesic effects to sedation than others) or by the addition of amphetamine derivatives such as methylphenidate or dextroamphetamine.

Nausea and Vomiting. Most patients have nausea and vomiting after initial administration or a major increase in dose. Some authors propose the use of prophylactic antiemetics on a regular basis during the first days of treatment, since in most patients nausea disappears after that period. The mechanism for the nausea is central. These side effects can be well antagonized by antidopaminergic agents such as metoclopramide. Dexamethasone is also a useful antiemetic that potentiates metoclopramide in these patients. As with sedation, nausea is a multicausal syndrome in cancer patients receiving opioids: severe constipation, cancer-induced autonomic failure, gastritis, increased intercranial pressure, and opioid metabolite accumulation are all possible causes of nausea.

Constipation. This is probably the most common adverse effect of opioids. Opioids act at multiple sites in the gastrointestinal tract and spinal cord. The result is decreased intestinal secretions and peristalsis. While tolerance to both sedation and nausea develops quickly, it develops very slowly to the smooth muscle effects of opioids, so constipation will persist when these drugs are used for chronic pain. When the use of opioid analgesics is initiated, provision for a regular bowel regimen, including stimulants and stool softeners, should be instituted to diminish this adverse effect.

Respiratory Depression. This is the most serious adverse effect of opioid analgesics. Opioids can cause respiratory depression to the point of apnea. In humans, death from overdose of opioids is nearly always due to respiratory arrest. At equinalgesic doses, the morphine-like agonists produce an equivalent degree of respiratory depression. When respiratory depression occurs, it is usually in opioid-naive patients following acute administration of an opioid and is associated with other signs of CNS depression including sedation and mental clouding. Tolerance quickly develops with repeated drug administration, allowing the opioid analgesics to be used without significant risk of respiratory depression. If respiratory depression occurs, it can be reversed by the administration of the specific opioid antagonist naloxone. In patients chronically receiving opioids who develop respiratory depression, naloxone diluted 1:10 should be titrated carefully to prevent the precipitation of severe withdrawal syndromes while reversing the respiratory depression. Long-acting drugs such as methadone, fentanyl patches, and slow-release morphine are likely to cause a higher incidence of respiratory depression. The accumulation of active opioid metabolites and the simultaneous use of other depressants such as benzodiazepines or alcohol are risk factors for respiratory depression. While this is the most feared side effect of opioid analgesics, it occurs very seldom in patients receiving chronic opioid therapy for the treatment of cancer pain.

Allergic Reactions. Allergy to opioids is rare. However, it is very common that patients are described as allergic to a number of opioid analgesics. This commonly is due to a misinterpretation by the patient or clinician of some of the common side effects of opioids such as nausea, sedation, vomiting, and sweating. In most instances a simple discussion with the patient is enough to clarify this issue.

Urinary Retention. The increase in the tone of smooth muscle of the bladder induced by opioids results in an increase in the sphincter tone leading to urinary retention. This is most common in the elderly patient. Attention should be directed to the possibility of this side effect; catheterization may be necessary to manage this transient side effect.

Newer Side Effects. During recent years, as a result of increased education on the assessment and management of cancer pain, patients have been receiving higher doses of opioids for longer periods than ever before.

Cognitive Failure. Patients can experience transient decrease in concentration and psychomotor coordination after starting opioids or after a sudden increase in the opioid dose. In some cases the opioid-induced cognitive failure is permanent. Some of the cognitive effects can be reversed by the administration of amphetamine derivatives such as methylphenidate. Screening tools such as the Mini-Mental State Questionnaire are useful in patients receiving high doses of opioids.

Other Central Effects. Organic hallucinosis, myoclonus, grand mal seizures and even hyperalgesia have been described in patients receiving high doses of opioids for long periods. These effects are likely due to the accumulation of active opioid metabolites. Improvement is frequently seen after a change in the type of opioid.

Severe Sedation and Coma. When coma occurs in patients receiving a stable dose of opioids for a long time, it should be suspected that accumulation of active opioid metabolites has occurred. These patients usually improve quickly after discontinuation of opioids.

Pulmonary Edema. While noncardiogenic pulmonary edema is a well-recognized complication of narcotic overdose in addicts, until recently it was not recognized as a possible complication of cancer pain treatment. Pulmonary edema usually occurs when patients have undergone rapid increases in dose as a result of severe neuropathic pain. While the mortality of the syndrome is very low among patients presenting with acute opioid overdoses, because of the conservative nature of the treatment of terminally ill cancer patients, the mortality of pulmonary edema is much higher within this population.

Adjuvant Drugs

Opioid analgesics are the most important drugs for the treatment of cancer pain. Although these drugs can usually control severe pain when they are used appropriately, they may produce new symptoms or exacerbate pre-existing symptoms, most notably nausea and somnolence. This aspect of treatment with opioid compounds is particularly problematic in patients with advanced cancer. The combination of severe pain, anorexia, chronic nausea, asthenia, and somnolence is a frequent finding in patients with advanced cancer. The term *adjuvant drug* has been used in a variety of ways even in the context of cancer pain management. For the purposes of the following paragraphs, an adjuvant drug meets one or more of the following criteria; (1) it increases the analgesic effect of opioids (adjuvant analgesia); (2) it decreases the toxicity of opioids; (3) it improves other symptoms associated with terminal cancer.

Claims have been made for the adjuvant analgesic effect of many drugs, but unfortunately, most of the evidence for these effects is anecdotal. Controlled clinical trials are needed to clarify the indications and risk-benefit ratios. These agents, some of which have the potential to produce significant toxicity, can aggravate the toxicity of opioids.

Most symptomatic cancer patients receive more than one or two adjuvant drugs. Unfortunately, there is still very limited consensus as to the type and dose of the most appropriate adjuvant drugs.

Tricyclic Antidepressants

In contrast to the frequent use of these agents in British hospices and South American and European cancer centers, the use of tricyclics in North American cancer centers has been infrequent. Tricyclic antidepressants have been found to be useful in a variety of neuropathic pain syndromes, especially when pain has a prominent dysesthetic or burning character. Both amitriptyline and desipramine have been found to be effective in the management of postherpetic neuralgia, diabetic neuropathy, and other neurologic conditions. There is, however, only very limited evidence for significant analgesic effect in cancer pain. Clinical effects suggest that tricyclics could be tried for the management of pain of central, deafferentation, or neuropathic origin. The optimal drug and dosing regimen are unknown. The effects of newer analgesics such as the selective serotonin uptake inhibitors (SSRIs) or specific monoamine oxidase inhibitors (MAOI) on pain control have not been clearly established. Until further evidence is available, the more traditional tricyclics should be used as adjuvant analgesics. The toxic effects of these drugs are mainly autonomic (dry mouth, postural hypotension) and centrally mediated (somnolence, confusion). Because their use may contribute to symptoms already present in debilitated patients, they should be administered cautiously to susceptible patients.

Anticonvulsants

Carbamazepine, phenytoin, valproic acid, and clonazepam, alone or in combination with the tricyclic antidepressants, have been used successfully to treat neuropathic pain. On the basis of well-documented efficacy for the treatment of trigeminal neuralgia, considerable anecdotal experience has accumulated for the use of these agents for neuropathic cancer pain syndromes, including neural invasion by tumor, radiation fibrosis, surgical scarring, herpes zoster, and deafferentation. Based on clinical observations, improvement can be expected in a proportion of patients whose predominant complaint is pain of a lancinating, burning, or hyperesthetic nature. Side effects of therapy can be serious, particularly in patients with advanced cancer, and can include bone marrow depression, hepatic dysfunction, ataxia, diplopia, and lymphadenopathy. Periodic monitoring of complete blood count and liver function tests are recommended.

Corticosteroids

Controlled studies suggest that the administration of corticosteroids to selected patients with advanced cancer results in decreased pain and improved appetite and activity. Unfortunately, the duration of the effects is probably short. The mechanism by which corticosteroids appear to produce beneficial symptom effects in patients with terminal cancer is unclear but may involve their euphoriant effects or the inhibition of prostaglandin metabolism. The optimal drug and dosing regimens have not been established. For the treatment of painful conditions, prednisone and dexamethasone are often administered in doses totaling 30 to 60 mg per day and 8 to 16 mg per day, respectively. As soon as symptomatic relief is obtained, attempts should be made to taper off to the minimally effective dose. Although long-term side effects are not an important consideration in many advanced cancer patients, treatment may produce limiting side effects in these patients, particularly immunosuppression (candidiasis will occur in most patients), proximal myopathy, and psychiatric symptoms. The incidence of psychological disturbances ranges from 3 to 50 percent, with severe symptoms occurring in about 5 percent of affected patients. The spectrum of disturbances ranges from mild to severe affective disorders, psychotic reactions, and global cognitive impairment.

Neuroablative Procedures

The evaluation of the physical basis of the pain may indicate that a neuroablative procedure, wherein the pain pathway is destroyed, would be of benefit for pain control. Such destructive procedures will probably be used more in countries where adequate analgesics are subject to supply constraints or regulatory restrictions. The experience in several countries has been that as opioid analgesia becomes available, the great majority of cancer patients do not require these neuroablative interventions. Destruction of the pain pathway can be accomplished surgically or through destructive nerve blocks using an agent such as phenol. The major barrier to the more widespread application of these techniques is the limited number of experts in their use. The most frequently used neurosurgical procedure is the anterolateral or spinothalamic cordotomy. This is often performed as closed percutaneous cordotomy by stereotaxically placing a radiofrequency needle in the anterolateral quadrant of the cervical cord. Unilateral pain control can unmask significant pain on the opposite side of the body. For pain of head and neck cancer, procedures such as percutaneous radiofrequency coagulation of the glossopharyngeal nerve may be used. Pituitary ablation via injection (hypophysectomy) has been reported to be of benefit for diffuse pain. It is important to remember that performance of such procedures does not eliminate the need to titrate analgesics. Because of afferent regeneration, neurosurgical procedures have had their greatest application to patients whose expected life span is only a few months.

Destructive anesthetic block of the celiac plexus had been used for several decades in the management of pain in the abdominal region. This block, which can be preceded by reversible diagnostic block, is especially useful in the pain syndrome accompanying cancer of the pancreas and may also be helpful for pain from cancer of the liver, gallbladder, or stomach. If success is achieved with the diagnostic block, lasting disruption of the pain pathway can be achieved using alcohol or phenol. Pain from rib metastases or tumors of the chest wall can be relieved with intercostal nerve blocks. Intrathecal and epidural nerve blocks have provided pain relief, but those procedures carry a risk of sensory and motor deficit.

Coping Techniques

Specific skills to manage pain can help most patients, especially those who face pain for months to years. Evaluation and prescription of the specific skills most beneficial to the individual can often be obtained through consultation with a behavioral psychologist, psychiatrist, or pain nurse specialist. Such techniques should never be used as a substitute for appropriate analgesia. The skills include relaxation, self-hypnosis, and other distraction and cognitive control techniques. These measures can affect the sensation of pain by reducing muscle tension on pain-generating lesions, as well as by maximizing the patient's ability to cope with the pain and remain as active as their disease permits.

Suggested Reading

Agency for Health Care Policy and Research. Management of cancer pain. Rockville, MD: U.S. Department of Health and Human Services, 1994.

Bruera E, Ripamonti C. Adjuvants to opioid analgesics. In: Patt R, ed. Cancer pain. Philadelphia: JB Lippincott, 1992:142.

Bruera E, Ripamonti C. Alternate routes of administration of opioids for the management of cancer pain. In: Patt R, ed. Cancer pain. Philadelphia: Lippincott, 1992:161.

Cleeland CS, Gonin R, Hatfield AK, et al. Pain and its treatment in outpatients with metastatic cancer. N Engl J M 1994; 330:592–596.

World Health Organization. Cancer pain relief and palliative care. Geneva: WHO, 1990.

ONCOLOGIC EMERGENCIES

Elizabeth Krecker, M.D.
Franco M. Muggia, M.D.

Knowledge of the natural history and course of disease and the early institution of treatment may prevent oncologic emergencies in any individual instance. Nevertheless, these emergencies may occur at presentation and may be most prevalent in malignancies occurring in areas with potentially life-threatening implications or disseminating in an unpredictable way. For example, lung cancers commonly invade the pericardium or obstruct the superior vena cava and disseminate widely to compromise spinal cord function or involve the central nervous system. In addition, lung cancers are often associated with paraneoplastic syndromes and critical metabolic changes such as hypercalcemia. In describing each oncologic emergency it is important to keep in mind the clinical setting, since it will lead not only to early recognition and definition of the problem but also to the appropriate treatment. A listing of oncologic emergencies appears in Table 1. With the exception of tumor lysis syndrome, emergencies related to treatment are not further described in this chapter. Hypersensitivity reactions are common with the wide range of drugs used. Overhydration may occur with the administration of anticancer drugs. In both these instances pre-existing pulmonary pathology may quickly lead to life-threatening pulmonary edema. Hormones may precipitate hypercalcemia or cord compression as part of disease flares in hormone-dependent cancers.

Myelosuppression, acute abdominal catastrophes, mucosal ulceration and bleeding, and liver and/or renal failure may occur with any number of chemotherapeutic regimens alone or in combination with radiation. Finally, in many of the oncologic emergencies listed, radiation plays a therapeutic role, but often some deterioration is seen prior to the onset of beneficial responses. High doses of steroids are considered to prevent such deterioration.

Table 1 Tumor-Related Oncologic Emergencies

- Metabolic emergencies
  - Hypercalcemia
  - Syndrome of inappropriate ADH secretion
  - Tumor-associated hypoglycemia
- Tumor lysis syndrome (usually treatment related)
- Cerebral herniation syndrome
- Spinal cord compression
- Malignant pericardial effusion*
- Superior vena cava syndrome*

*Most often do not require emergency treatment.

■ SUPERIOR VENA CAVA SYNDROME

Superior vena cava (SVC) syndrome is the clinical result of an obstruction of venous blood flow from the head, neck, upper thoracic region, and upper extremities. The SVC is a large thin-walled vessel with low intravascular pressure that is easily compressed by adjacent expanding masses arising in any of its bounding contiguous structures (trachea, heart, aorta, azygous vein, and paratracheal and bronchial lymph nodes). The SVC arises from the innominate veins, which in turn arise from the internal jugular and subclavian veins. The azygous vein is the last main auxiliary vessel of the SVC draining blood from the chest wall. As a result of this anatomic relationship, if the SVC is obstructed above or at the level of the azygous vein, collateral circulation through the chest wall vessels occurs, rejoining the SVC via the azygous vein. Obstruction at or below the azygous vein causes retrograde blood flow down the azygous and other chest wall veins to reach drainage into the inferior vena cava, producing more prominent symptoms and more significant compromise to the patient. Faster-growing tumors leave less time for collateral vessel growth and lead to more symptomatic presentations.

Primary intrathoracic tumors cause over 80 percent of the cases of SVC syndrome, with 75 percent and 10 percent of these cases secondary to lung cancer (most commonly of the small cell or squamous cell types) and lymphoma (most commonly diffuse large cell non-Hodgkin's lymphoma), respectively. Neoplastic SVC syndrome is also seen in association with mediastinal germ cell tumors, malignant thymoma, and metastases to the mediastinum from carcinoma of the breast (most common), ovary, cervix, thyroid, and larynx. An increasing cause of SVC syndrome in the cancer patient is thrombosis due to central venous catheters used for hyperalimentation and chemotherapy. It is estimated that 100,000 devices are inserted per year with a potential incidence of thrombosis of 30 percent or more. Tuberculosis is the most common non-neoplastic cause of extrinsic obstruction.

Clinical Presentation

The diagnosis of SVC syndrome can usually readily be made by the presence of a mediastinal mass on chest x-ray film along with a classic constellation of signs and symptoms. Because collateral circulation develops as the expanding mass encroaches on the SVC, the syndrome usually has an insidious onset, and the edema may progress slowly. Early presenting signs may include periorbital edema, conjunctival suffusion, and facial swelling, which are most evident in the early morning. Dyspnea is the most common symptom, present in over 60 percent of patients, and may be associated with pleural effusions. Swelling of the face, trunk, and upper extremities is observed in 40 percent of patients. Other presenting complaints are a sensation of fullness in the head and face, cough, chest pain, hoarseness, fatigue, dysphagia, headache, and lethargy. Most of the symptoms worsen when the patient is supine or bending forward. As the impedance to blood flow increases, the full-blown syndrome manifests with thoracic and neck vein distention, facial edema, tachypnea, tightness of the shirt collar (Stoke sign), plethora of the face, edema of the upper extremities, and cyanosis. The life-threatening manifestations of SVC syndrome are airway obstruction from laryngeal edema and central nervous system (CNS) complications of cerebral edema.

Diagnostic Workup

Historically, SVC syndrome has been characterized as a medical emergency with life-threatening potential. This commonly led to empiric treatment with initial high–dose fraction radiotherapy in the absence of a histologic diagnosis. This therapeutic philosophy is no longer valid with refinements in diagnostic approaches. With rare exceptions, treating SVC syndrome without a tissue diagnosis is to be avoided. The more pressing issue in a patient with SVC syndrome is to establish a specific histologic diagnosis so that a potentially curable cancerous lesion can be optimally treated. The goal of accurate tissue diagnosis should be kept in mind as the evaluation of such patients is undertaken.

The most common radiographic abnormalities on chest film are superior mediastinal widening and pleural effusion; only 15 percent of patients with SVC syndrome have normal chest roentgenograms. A computed tomograph (CT) scan will provide more detailed information about the SVC and its tributaries, will provide accurate guidance for percutaneous biopsy, and may identify a thrombus in the SVC. In the absence of a central venous catheter, venography does not add useful diagnostic information. Sputum should be sent for cytologic examination upon presentation, as this establishes the diagnosis in as many as 50 percent of patients. In most cases bronchoscopy provides a histologic diagnosis of small cell lung cancer. A diagnostic thoracentesis should be performed if there is a pleural effusion. Bone marrow aspiration and biopsy may prove rewarding, as small cell lung cancer and lymphoma frequently involve the bone marrow. Biopsy of any palpable supraclavicular lymphadenopathy is diagnostic in two-thirds of patients. If the aforementioned procedures do not yield a diagnosis, mediastinoscopy or thoracotomy should be undertaken. There is minimal evidence to suggest that invasive diagnostic procedures carry excessive risk in patients presenting with SVC syndrome in the absence of tracheal obstruction.

Treatment

The goal of treatment of SVC syndrome is to relieve the symptoms of venous obstruction while optimally treating the underlying disease. The prognosis of SVC syndrome directly relates to that of the underlying disease. Small cell carcinoma of the lung, non-Hodgkin's lymphoma, and germ cell tumors, all curable diseases, afflict a majority of patients presenting with the SVC syndrome. In patients with non–small cell carcinoma radiotherapy is the primary modality of treatment. The fractionation schedule uses initial high daily doses of 400 cGy for 3 days followed by 150 to 200 cGy daily for a total dose of 3,000 to 5,000 cGy. The radiation port should include a 2 cm margin around the tumor with expansion to include mediastinal, hilar, and supraclavicular nodes in the absence of obvious metastatic disease. Chemotherapy, particularly based on platinum compounds, can be given in conjunction with radiotherapy. In patients with limited-stage small cell lung cancer, randomized trials have demonstrated an advantage for combining radiotherapy with chemotherapy. Chemotherapy alone is used if the disease is extensive. The choice of treatment in patients with lymphoma should be based upon the histologic subtype and stage.

Large controlled studies of the use of anticoagulation therapy in patients with SVC syndrome are lacking. In catheter-induced SVC, heparin and warfarin (Coumadin) may reduce thrombus propagation. Streptokinase and urokinase may be used early in formation of the thrombus. The catheter should be removed as the patient is anticoagulated to prevent embolization.

General supportive measures that may help alleviate the symptoms of SVC include bed rest with head elevation, diuresis and salt restriction, steroids (dexamethasone 6 mg IV or orally every 6 hours for 3 days), and supplemental oxygen. These are usually instituted if diagnostic attempts fail, with radiation being justified if malignancy is likely and yet the diagnosis proves elusive.

■ HYPERCALCEMIA

Hypercalcemia is the most common life-threatening metabolic emergency associated with cancer. Although hypercalcemia is a rare presenting sign of neoplastic disease, its prevalence secondary to malignancy is probably about 15:100,000 to 20:100,000. The tumors most commonly associated with hypercalcemia are carcinomas of the breast and lung. Approximately 45 percent and 12 percent of patients with those diseases respectively will manifest hypercalcemia sometime during their course. Hypernephroma, head, neck, esophageal, and thyroid cancer and lymphoma are also commonly associated with hypercalcemia. Neoplastic disease is the leading cause of hypercalcemia in hospitalized patients.

Hypercalcemia occurs when calcium mobilization and resorption from bone exceeds the renal threshold of calcium excretion. Intake of calcium and vitamin D only rarely contribute to hypercalcemia. This occurs by direct osteoclast activity by metastases; indirectly by ectopic humoral osteolytic substances such as osteoclast-activating factors, parathormone (PTH) or related hormones (rPTH), or prostaglandins; or by miscellaneous undefined mechanisms. Diminished renal excretion may result in rapid hypercalcemia in a patient previously compensating with sufficient intake. Thiazide diuretics often contribute to diminished excretion. Some 75 percent of cancer patients with hypercalcemia have metastatic sites of disease; 85 percent of those patients have

Table 2 Clinical Presentation of Hypercalcemia

GENERAL
Somnolence, fatigue, lethargy, weakness, dehydration, anorexia, polydipsia, pruritus
NEUROLOGIC
Muscle weakness, hyporeflexia, behavioral disturbance, confusion, psychosis, seizures, obtundation, coma
GASTROINTESTINAL
Anorexia, nausea, vomiting, abdominal pain, peptic ulcer, pancreatitis, constipation, obstipation, ileus
GENITOURINARY
Polyuria, renal insufficiency, nephrocalcinosis, renal failure
CARDIAC
Bradycardia, prolonged PR interval, shortened QT interval, atrial and ventricular arrhythmias

bone metastases. However, the extent of bone disease does not correlate with the severity of hypercalcemia. Furthermore, 15 to 20 percent of solid tumors associated with hypercalcemia have no evidence of bone disease. Hypercalcemia is almost never seen with small cell cancer and adenocarcinoma, despite the high association of these tumor types with skeletal metastasis. Hypercalcemia occurs often in large cell and squamous cell lung cancer, probably from ectopic secretion of rPTH, as suggested by low immunoreactive PTH with otherwise typical laboratory findings of hyperparathyroidism.

Patients with malignancy-related hypercalcemia can present with a wide range of signs and symptoms (Table 2). The most common presenting symptoms in cancer patients with evolving hypercalcemia are fatigue, lethargy, polyuria, and nausea. The severity of symptoms is related to the rate of increase of ionized serum calcium more than to degree of elevation.

Because serum calcium is approximately 50 percent protein bound and total serum calcium fluctuates with changes in serum protein concentrations, it is necessary to measure the serum protein when initially evaluating a patient with hypercalcemia. Calcium circulates in the blood in bound, complexed, and ionized forms. Only the ionized calcium exerts important biologic effects. It is also occasionally helpful to measure the ionized calcium level, which correlates to the clinical manifestations of hypercalcemia. For instance, a patient with multiple myeloma–associated hyperproteinemia may have an elevated serum calcium secondary to abnormal paraprotein binding with a normal ionized serum calcium. Conversely, a patient with a normal serum calcium and hypoalbuminemia may manifest clinical signs and symptoms of hypercalcemia due to an elevated ionized calcium. An approximation of the severity of hypercalcemia can be determined by using the following formula, which adjusts serum calcium levels for serum concentrations of albumin:

$$\text{corrected } Ca^{++} \text{ (mg/dl)} = \text{measured } Ca^{++} \text{ (mg/dl)} - \text{albumin (g/dl)} + 4$$

Other laboratory studies that should be done in the initial diagnostic workup of the patient with hypercalcemia include serum electrolytes, blood urea nitrogen (BUN), creatinine, phosphorus, and alkaline phosphatase. Hypophosphatemia may occur in ectopic hyperparathyroidism (most commonly

Table 3 Treatment of Hypercalcemia

IV normal saline to achieve euvolemia
IV furosemide after adequate urine output has been established
Mobilization if feasible
Bisphosphonate therapy (pamidronate 60–90 mg IV over 2–4 hours)
Other measures (if serum calcium >14 or patient is symptomatic):
Calcitonin
Glucocorticoids
Gallium nitrate
Treatment of underlying malignancy

seen with carcinomas of the lung, kidney, head, and neck), but low phosphorus also raises the possibility of hypercalcemia due to coexistent hyperparathyroidism. Since PTH suppresses the renal clearance of calcium, patients with cancer tend to have higher urinary calcium values than those with primary hyperparathyroidism. Assays for serum immunoreactive PTH determinations may be clinically useful when evaluated in relation to the concentration of serum calcium. Since hypercalcemia causes a reduction of endogenous PTH, inappropriately elevated PTH levels have been detected in varying proportions of patients with cancer-related hypercalcemia. Studies looking at the PTH-specific mRNA have shown that PTH production cannot be a common cause of cancer-related hypercalcemia and that rPTH proteins are humorally produced by certain tumors implicated in the hypercalcemia of malignancy. Assays for rPTH are becoming available, and its presence may be suspected when PTH is very low with obvious humoral causes.

Treatment

A general approach to the treatment of malignancy-associated hypercalcemia is outlined in Table 3. Treatment directed at the underlying malignancy is the most effective way of achieving long-term eucalcemia. However, hypercalcemia usually accompanies advanced disease in patients who may have failed therapy and who fail to maintain adequate hydration because of other manifestations of progressive disease. Unless the short-term prognosis is known to be poor, hypercalcemic patients should receive vigorous acute intervention. The treatment of cancer-related hypercalcemia is based on augmenting the renal excretion of calcium, decreasing the bone resorption of calcium, and treating the underlying tumor.

General Measures

Before treatment of hypercalcemia in cancer patients is begun, a clinical assessment of the degree of symptoms should be determined. Symptomatic patients or those with a corrected calcium concentration greater than 14 mg/dl should receive prompt and aggressive treatment. Medication that may potentiate hypercalcemia (thiazides, vitamins A and D) should be stopped. Patients with breast cancer who have hypercalcemia precipitated by hormonal therapy can be continued on the drug safely unless they exhibit severe, life-threatening symptoms, in which case the drug should be discontinued. If possible, immobilization should be avoided. Dietary intake of calcium does not significantly contribute to the hypercalcemia of malignancy, and dietary restrictions are impractical and not warranted. Oral phosphates are usually poorly tolerated and may lead to diarrhea, compounding the threat of dehydration.

Intravenous Fluids

Almost all patients with significant hypercalcemia are dehydrated because of polyuria from renal tubule dysfunction, vomiting, and poor oral intake. Intravenous hydration and intravascular volume replacement should be achieved with isotonic normal saline, which promotes calcium excretion by increasing renal blood flow as well as by its natriuretic effect (based on the ionic exchange of calcium for sodium in the distal tubule).

The rate of hydration should be based on the extent of dehydration, the cardiovascular reserve, the renal excretory capacity, and the severity of hypercalcemia. It is common to administer loop diuretics such as furosemide, which in theory should induce natriuresis and enhance urinary excretion. However, this drug increases the risk of worsening hypovolemia, which in turn may decrease glomerular filtration rate further and stimulate renal calcium resorption. Furosemide should be used only after the patient appears to be euvolemic on careful clinical evaluation or if the hydration rate is adjusted to prevent further dehydration. Patients should be closely monitored for clinical volume status (i.e., correction of orthostatic hypotension), evaluation of cardiac status, and measurement of urinary output. The serum electrolytes, creatinine, and calcium should be followed carefully, and potassium and magnesium losses, which frequently occur, should be replaced. In most patients repletion in excess of 2 L of saline during the initial 24 hours decreases serum calcium by 1 to 2 mg/dl. Intravenous (IV) hydration alone may be sufficient treatment in lowering serum calcium concentration levels in patients with mild (less than 12 mg/dl) or asymptomatic hypercalcemia. In hypercalcemic patients with higher serum calcium concentration or those presenting with clinical manifestations of hypercalcemia, it is desirable to implement other measures concomitantly.

Bisphosphonates

Hypercalcemia can easily be treated with intravenous bisphosphonates (i.e., etidronate, pamidronate). These drugs act by inhibiting osteoclast activity, as they adsorb to the surface of crystalline hydroxyapatite and directly inhibit calcium release from the bone. Diphosphonates have rapid and prolonged hypocalcemic effects. Etidronate was the first diphosphonate to be marketed in the United States. Used intravenously, this drug produces normal calcium levels in 75 to 100 percent of patients with malignancy-related hypercalcemia. Etidronate is given in doses of 7.5 mg per kilogram per day IV over 2 to 4 hours (to reduce renal toxicity) for 3 days. Calcium-lowering effects are usually seen within 48 to 72 hours. Oral etidronate has been used to prolong normocalcemia in patients initially treated with the IV form, although controlled studies do not suggest that the oral therapy is beneficial, probably because of limited potency and poor bioavailability. The newer-generation drugs of the bisphosphonate series, such as disodium pamidronate, are more potent than etidronate and have effects that are observed within 1 day. Pamidronate may be given as a single infusion one-time dose of 60 to 90 mg over 2 to 4 hours, to be repeated biweekly, or at greater intervals.

Other Measures

When hypercalcemia is life threatening, other measures may be initiated simultaneously with IV hydration and bisphosphonate therapy as outlined in Table 3. Calcitonin, secreted by the parafollicular cells of the thyroid gland, plays a poorly understood role in calcium homeostasis. In pharmacologic doses, salmon calcitonin can reduce serum calcium by increasing renal calcium excretion and inhibiting bone resorption. Calcitonin is devoid of serious toxicity, but its effect is weak and transient. Glucocorticoids may lower serum calcium by increasing urinary calcium excretion and by inhibiting bone reabsorption induced by lymphokines. Corticosteroids are most beneficial in patients with underlying malignancies that may be responsive to their cytostatic action such as lymphoma, multiple myeloma, leukemia, and breast cancer. In the latter, steroids have a role in counteracting hypercalcemia as part of a flare response to hormone treatment. Also there is some suggestion that glucocorticoids may prevent the escape phenomenon seen with calcitonin by regulating calcitonin receptors. Gallium nitrate was initially developed as an antitumor agent, and hypocalcemia was noted incidentally. In vitro, gallium nitrate produces a concentration-dependent reduction in the osteolytic response to PTH and certain lymphokines that cause hypercalcemia. Thus, this drug directly inhibits bone resorption without causing toxicity to bone cells. Initial studies demonstrated a normalization of calcium in 86 percent of patients treated with 200 mg per square meter per day for 5 consecutive days. The major disadvantage of the drug is a continued parenteral requirement for administration. The drug should not be given until the patient has been rehydrated with a daily urine output of 2 L per day, since nephrotoxicity has been observed. Mithramycin is a cytotoxic antibiotic that inhibits DNA-directed RNA synthesis. It acts as an effective agent for hypercalcemia by directly inhibiting osteoclastic bone resorption. It has a prolonged and potent hypocalcemic effect in the presence or absence of bone metastasis, but its use has been displaced by the bisphosphonates that lack its vesicant, myelosuppressive, and hepatotoxic properties. Most patients can be effectively managed with the measures shown in Table 3. In hypercalcemic patients in whom volume expansion is precluded by renal failure or impaired cardiac function, dialysis with calcium-free dialysate has been used to lower serum calcium. The use of intravenous phosphate has been abandoned because of its excessive toxicity, including renal failure, hypotension, hypocalcemia, extraskeletal calcification, and death.

■ INAPPROPRIATE ANTIDIURETIC HORMONE SECRETION

The diagnostic criteria for the syndrome of inappropriate antidiuretic hormone secretion (SIADH) are listed in Table 4. Cancer is the most common cause of nonpituitary SIADH and constitutes a medical emergency when a patient presents with symptoms due to hyponatremia. Small cell malignancies of the lung are the most common cause, but SIADH occurs with a large list of tumors. Patients may develop anorexia and nausea followed by CNS symptomatology—lethargy, confusion, seizures, and coma.

Table 4 Diagnostic Criteria for SIADH

Hyponatremia (Na^+ <135 mEq/L) with a disproportionately low BUN
Decreased serum osmolarity (<280 mOsm/L)
Urine osmolarity that is not maximally dilute (>75–100 mOsm/L)
Absence of volume contraction
Absence of hypervolemic state (ascites, edema)
Normal renal function
Normal thyroid and adrenal function

Table 5 Treatment of Hyponatremia

1. Fluid restriction to 500–800 ml/day
2. Demeclocycline 150 to 300 mg PO q.i.d.
Severe hyponatremia (Na^+ >115 mEq/L)
1. IV infusion of 3% NaCl at 1 L q6–8h
2. Furosemide 40 mg IV q6–8h

The treatment of SIADH secondary to malignancy (most notably small cell lung cancer and brain metastasis) is aimed at treating the underlying malignancy whenever possible. The first-line therapy for correcting hyponatremia is water restriction to 500 ml per day, which with insensible water loss will result in a negative water balance. Patients who present with acute severe hyponatremia (less than 120 mEq per liter) and severe symptoms (coma, seizures, mental status changes) require intravenous hypertonic saline solution oral (3 percent) to correct hyponatremia slowly (0.5 to 10 mEq per hour). In mild to moderate cases of hyponatremia oral demeclocycline 150 to 300 mg four times a day facilitates free water excretion by producing nephrogenic diabetes insipidus. A general treatment approach is outlined in Table 5.

■ TUMOR-ASSOCIATED HYPOGLYCEMIA

Hypoglycemia is a rare but well-defined presentation of neoplastic disease encountered in association with insulin-secreting pancreatic islet tumors. Rarely, hypoglycemia is a paraneoplastic syndrome observed in association with bulky sarcomas, hepatocellular carcinoma, and tumors of adrenocortical origin, probably due to production of an insulin-like substance, glucose use of the tumor or loss of hormonal regulation of glucose. Presenting symptoms usually occur when serum glucose is less than 40 mg/dl and include diaphoresis, weakness, tremor, lassitude, drowsiness, and coma. For the patient with frank mental status changes due to hypoglycemia, medical stabilization is achieved with serial injections of $D_{50}W$ (glucose solution). After other causes of hypoglycemia have been ruled out, an insulinoma can be distinguished from a non–insulin-secreting tumor by measuring immunoreactive insulin following an overnight fast. Treatment for tumor-associated hypoglycemia includes the following options: IV dextrose, frequent meals, corticosteroid, growth hormones, glucagon, diazoxide, and somatostatin. Definitive treatment requires treatment of the underlying neoplasm, most often with surgery. Nonpancreatic tumors are usually nonresectable, bulky, and slow growing, in which case treatment is palliative and can consist of combined modalities (i.e., surgery, chemotherapy, radiation).

■ TUMOR LYSIS SYNDROME

Acute tumor lysis syndrome is the constellation of life-threatening metabolic abnormalities that result from the release of intracellular contents into the bloodstream following effective chemötherapy for the treatment of tumors with high growth rate fractions and rapid cell turnover. This syndrome is most commonly seen in association with acute leukemia, high-grade lymphomas (i.e., Burkitt's and lymphoblastic lymphomas), and Hodgkin's disease. Cases reported in association with small cell lung cancer and metastatic adenocarcinoma are complicated by concomitant nephrotoxicity possibly due to cisplatin. The hallmarks of tumor lysis syndrome are hyperphosphatemia, hyperkalemia, hypocalcemia, and hyperuricemia. These usually occur within 1 to 2 days of the initiation of chemotherapy but may be seen to some extent before treatment. Risk factors for developing tumor lysis syndrome are elevated lactate dehydrogenase, a rapidly growing bulky tumor, a highly chemosensitive tumor, pretreatment hyperuricemia, and decreased renal function. The major complications of tumor lysis syndrome are renal failure due to hyperuricemia and hyperphosphatemia and malignant cardiac arrythmias due to severe hyperkalemia. Uric acid nephropathy, historically the first manifestation described, is a result of urine urate supersaturation with uric acid crystal formation in the renal tubules and distal collecting system from a combination of heavy urate load and low urine output usually in individuals with pre-existing excellent renal function. In addition, hyperphosphatemia and hyperphosphaturia can further compromise renal tubule function by forming triple phosphate crystals of calcium, magnesium, and ammonium. The precipitation of calcium phosphate salts results in severely low serum calcium levels, which may cause neuromuscular instability with muscle cramps, confusion, tetany, and cardiac arrhythmia characterized by lengthening of the QT interval.

Management of tumor lysis syndrome should begin with awareness and prevention through preserving renal integrity. Patients should receive IV hydration at 200 to 300 ml per hour at least 1 day prior to chemotherapy. Allopurinol 300 mg twice daily is given orally to block uric acid production and reduce serum uric acid levels. Urine alkalinization to maintain a pH above 7 with IV sodium bicarbonate 100 mEq per square meter maximizes uric acid solubility. Urine output should optimally exceed 3 L per day. However, even when renal function appears normal at the initiation of chemotherapy, the rapid lysis of certain tumors may overwhelm the excretory capacity of the kidney, resulting in the aforementioned abnormalities and necessitating additional measures. Electrocardiogram (ECG), serum electrolytes, blood urea nitrogen (BUN), creatinine, calcium, phosphorus, and urate should be monitored every 6 hours after onset of chemotherapy in patients at high risk for developing tumor lysis. If oliguric renal failure ensues despite the institution of proper therapy, diuretics and/or mannitol 12.5 g in 20 percent solution over 3 minutes may be used to maintain urine output. Severe hyperkalemia is the most critical occurrence and should be

Table 6 Indications for Hemodialysis in Patients with Tumor Lysis Syndrome

Serum potassium >6 mEq/L despite Kayexalate (15 g PO q6h)
Serum uric acid >10 mg/dl
Serum creatinine >10 mg/dl
Serum phosphorus >10 mg/dl
Volume-overloaded state
Symptomatic hypocalcemia
Deteriorating renal function
Oliguria

promptly recognized and treated according to standard medical protocol. Severe hyperphosphatemia with renal insufficiency is the next most life-threatening event. ECG monitoring may be useful in recognizing hypocalcemia (prolonged QT interval). Alkalinization of the urine must be discontinued, as this enhances calcium phosphate precipitation. Hypocalcemia can be corrected with IV calcium gluconate. If renal function continues to deteriorate, hemodialysis may be lifesaving and should be instituted early, while renal failure may still be reversible. The indications for hemodialysis are listed in Table 6. The prognosis of tumor lysis syndrome in the absence of renal failure is good. The prognosis is grave in patients requiring hemodialysis for more than 5 days.

■ CEREBRAL HERNIATION SYNDROME

Cerebral herniation is a result of increased intracranial pressure caused by mass lesions in the cerebrum or dural spaces displacing the brain across the hard structures in the skull and shifting the brain parenchyma caudally in the direction of least resistance through the tentorial opening and the foramen magnum. The most common causes of cerebral herniation in cancer patients are primary and metastatic tumor (each accounts for 50 percent of intracranial brain tumors), intracerebral hemorrhage, subdural hematoma, and acute hydrocephalus. Benign origins such as cerebrovascular thrombosis, intracranial hemorrhage, metabolic disturbances, brain abscesses, meningitis, and postradiation brain necrosis must be excluded in a patient presenting with signs and symptoms of cerebral herniation. Given the prolonged survival with chemotherapy and radiotherapy, the incidence of brain metastases has risen in patients with small cell lung and breast cancer. Brain metastases occur in approximately 30 percent of cancer patients, most frequently in association with carcinomas of the lung, breast, kidney, choriocarcinoma of the testis, and less commonly with colon and thyroid cancer. Cancer-related intracerebral hemorrhage is seen in two settings: long-standing thrombocytopenia secondary to hematologic malignancies (multiple myeloma, acute leukemia) and hemorrhagic metastases from melanoma, hypernephroma, choriocarcinoma, and testicular carcinoma. Acute hydrocephalus occasionally occurs secondary to cerebellar metastasis.

Clinical Presentation

Progressive headache, worse in the morning and remitting upon rising, is present in over 50 percent of patients. Cognitive or affective changes, deteriorating mental status, weakness, nausea, vomiting, abnormal pupillary reactions, abnormal posturing, hypertension, bradycardia (except in cerebellar lesions, with which the opposite is found), and seizures are also characteristic of increased intracranial pressure. One-fourth of patients will have engorged retinal veins and/or papilledema on fundoscopic examination. Presenting signs and symptoms vary with the location of the focal lesion, with 90, 8, and 2 percent of metastatic brain lesions occurring in the cerebrum, cerebellum, and brain stem, respectively.

Table 7 Treatment of Cerebral Herniation

Intubation and hyperventilation to a P_{CO_2} of 25 to 30 mm Hg
Dexamethasone 24–100 mg IV followed by 24 mg q6h
Dilantin 1–1.5 g IV (50 mg/min)
Emergent CT scan
Emergent neurosurgical consultation and decompression when feasible
If not improving:
Infuse mannitol 1 g/kg in 20% solution
Monitor serum osmolality and avoid osmolality >320 mosm
Monitor urinary output and osmolality
Replace fluids appropriately

There are three important clinically distinct herniation syndromes: uncal, central, and tonsillar herniation. Uncal herniation is characteristic of a laterally placed supratentorial lesion displacing the temporal lobe (i.e., uncus) medially and caudally, causing compression of the upper brain stem, the third cranial nerve, and the posterior cerebral artery. Clinical features of uncal herniation are a rapid loss of consciousness, an ipsilateral third nerve palsy, contralateral hemiparesis (ipsilateral hemiparesis is also seen when shift of the brain stem compresses the contralateral cerebral peduncle), and decerebrate posturing. Central herniation generally occurs in conjunction with slowly expanding multifocal, supratentorial lesions in the frontal or parietal lobes or acute hydrocephalus. The manifestations are secondary to caudal shift of the diencephalon and upper pons through the tentorium. The typical findings are headache, progressive drowsiness, small reactive pupils, Cheyne-Stokes respirations, and bilateral Babinski responses. In its early stages central herniation mimics metabolic encephalopathy (i.e., hypercalcemia). As central herniation evolves, the patient becomes comatose with fixed, dilated, midpositioned pupils, Cheyne-Stokes respiration, loss of oculocephalic reflexes, and decerebrate posturing. Tonsillar or cerebellar herniation is produced by posterior fossa lesions displacing the cerebellar tonsils through the foramen magnum and compressing the medulla. Occipital headache, meningismus, vomiting, hiccups, rapid deterioration of mental status, hypertension, skew deviation of the eyes, and irregular respiration culminating in respiratory arrest are the hallmarks of cerebellar herniation.

Once cerebral herniation is suspected, emergency management is mandatory before the cause can be established (Table 7). Acutely deteriorating patients require immediate treatment to reduce intracranial pressure. Stuporous and comatose patients require intubation for maintenance of an airway and hyperventilation. Hyperventilation produces cerebral vasoconstriction if the partial pressure of carbon dioxide (P_{CO_2}) is maintained between 25 and 30 torr. Excessive hyperventilation should be avoided because it causes a paradoxical vasodilation. Steroids (dexamethasone 12 to 24 mg IV) are generally administered acutely but do not decrease brain edema for hours. Patients should also receive a loading dose of phenytoin (Dilantin) or another anticonvulsant therapy. Osmotic agents raise the osmotic pressure of the intravascular compartment, rapidly decreasing brain water content and reducing intracranial pressure temporarily, but rebound edema is of concern. A neurosurgeon should be consulted before osmotic diuretics are given.

Once emergency stabilization is under way, a CT of the brain should be obtained. Admission to an intensive care unit is mandatory. After an acutely deteriorating patient has been medically stabilized, prompt neurosurgical intervention may be lifesaving. Such intervention may include ventriculostomy to remove cerebrospinal fluid, decompression with craniotomy, and tumor removal.

SPINAL CORD COMPRESSION

Metastasis to the vertebral body with erosion into the anterior or anterolateral epidural space above the level of the cord termination (L1) is the usual mechanism of spinal cord compression in cancer patients. It is seen most commonly in association with carcinomas of the lung, breast, and prostate and with multiple myeloma. Direct extension of paraspinal tumor through the intervertebral foramina without bony involvement to the lateral epidural space occurs with lymphomas and some retroperitoneal tumors. Spinal cord compression is a medical emergency, as delay in treatment may result in irreversible neurologic damage. The most important factors influencing the neurologic outcome are neurologic status of the patient at the initiation of therapy and the rapidity with which signs become manifest.

Clinical Presentation

Over 95 percent of patients with epidural metastases present with the initial complaint of back pain, which may be either localized or radicular. The thoracic, lumbosacral, and cervical spine are involved approximately 70, 20, and 10 percent of the time, respectively. Back pain precedes other symptoms by weeks to months depending on the particular biology of a given tumor. The pain is usually exacerbated by recumbency, the Valsalva maneuver, cough, and weight bearing. There may be tenderness to palpation over a particular vertebral body due to bone destruction by tumor. The pain may also be radicular, localizing the lesion to one or two vertebral segments. While radicular pain at most sites is lancinating and sharp, thoracic epidural cord involvement presents as a constricting, bandlike feeling around the chest or abdomen. The development of midline neck or back pain in a cancer patient should be considered an ominous symptom warranting prompt investigation. Without treatment the next symptom is usually weakness, which may be accompanied by sensory loss. Sensory disturbances (loss of pinprick and temperature sensation) are most marked distally, ascending to the level of the cord compression. Position and vibratory loss are later findings. Finally, myelopathic signs develop, indicating that the cord is being compromised. These motor signs include increased tone (spasticity and hyper-reflexia), true muscle weakness, abnormal stretch reflexes, and extensor plantar responses. Autonomic dysfunction leading to urinary retention and incontinence strongly suggests the diagnosis. Early diagnosis is crucial to avoid neurologic damage. Patients who are treated while they are ambulatory avoid neurologic compromise in 80 percent of instances, whereas once the patient has lost the ability to walk, permanent invalidism is more common.

Diagnostic Evaluation

Evaluation should include a careful physical examination, complete spinal radiographs and either magnetic resonance imaging (MRI) or complete myelography of the suspected level. Over two-thirds of patients with spinal cord compression will have abnormal bone radiographs of the spine. Diagnostic clues to tumor involvement of vertebrae include erosion and loss of a pedicle (early sign), partial or complete collapse of the vertebral body (late sign), and paraspinous soft tissue masses and/or sclerotic or lytic lesions. Normal spine films do not exclude the diagnosis of epidural metastasis, as there may be tumor invasion through the foramina without bony destruction. Moreover, tumor can be present for 6 months without x-ray changes.

The most definitive and important studies are the myelogram metrizamide CT scan and MRI. MRI has a distinct advantage over myelography in that no uncomfortable positions or contrast injections are required. MRI also avoids the risk of neurologic deterioration after lumbar puncture, which may rarely occur in patients with complete myelographic block. It also has the advantage of distinguishing extradural, intradural, extramedullary, and intramedullary lesions as well as demonstrating multiple sites of epidural metastasis, which may not be obvious on the initial myelogram. One of these diagnostic studies should be performed immediately in all patients to determine the proximal and distal extent of the tumor mass and to determine whether multiple lesions are present.

Treatment

Patients presenting with spinal cord compression should be promptly evaluated by a medical oncologist, a radiation oncologist, and a neurosurgeon. The therapy of patients with spinal cord compression is usually palliative and directed toward the preservation of neurologic function, local tumor control, spinal stability, and pain control. The mainstays of treatment are steroids, radiotherapy, and occasionally systemic anticancer therapies. Glucocorticoids reduce peritumoral edema and may temporarily improve neurologic status and pain. The optimal dose is not known. Dexamethasone is usually given as a 10 mg IV bolus followed by 4 mg orally every 6 hours for 2 days and then tapered. Large doses of dexamethasone (100 mg per day) may be more effective in relieving pain but have not been shown to be statistically superior to conventional doses in overall outcome. Radiotherapy is the primary treatment for most patients with spinal cord compression and should be initiated immediately after the diagnosis is confirmed. When surgical decompression and postoperative radiotherapy were retrospectively compared with radiotherapy alone in a nonrandomized trial, there were no significant differences in the percentages of patients remaining ambulatory at the completion of treatment. The optimum radiation dose and fractionation scheme have not been definitively established. Radiation ports usually extend one or two vertebral segments on either side of the tumor. Most patients will receive 3,000 to 4,000 cGy in 10 to 20 fractions over 2 to 4 weeks. Paravertebral areas and any paraspinous tumor masses are included in the radiation field. These doses of radiation are not associated with increased edema or neurologic decompensation if appropriate doses of steroid are concomitantly administered.

Historically and theoretically laminectomy may provide prompt decompression of the spinal cord and nerve roots. However, a posterior laminectomy frequently produces an unstable spine, and removal of the total tumor is usually impossible. Furthermore, most epidural metastases are anterior to the spinal cord, making it difficult to remove tumor without damaging the spine. Improved results have been reported with an anterior surgical approach with removal of the tumor-laden vertebral body and associated epidural tumor in select patients. Laminectomy is contraindicated in patients with vertebral body collapse because of a higher incidence of neurologic complications. Surgical intervention may be indicated in the following patients: those who have failed radiotherapy and have clinical deterioration; those who have relapsed in an area of prior radiotherapy; and those who appear to have a possibility of complete tumor removal.

Systemic treatment with chemotherapy or hormonal therapy rarely has a role in the management of cancer patients with spinal cord compression. However, if the tumor is responsive (i.e., lymphoma and germ cell tumors) and not refractory to such modalities, treatment should be administered in conjunction with radiotherapy. Another example is women with metastatic breast cancer, who may benefit from systemic chemotherapy and pamidronate to prevent further bone destruction. Hormonal manipulation may also be instituted and is likely to be of benefit in a patient with recently diagnosed metastatic prostate cancer. Treatment decisions must be based on tumor type and prior treatment, the level of the spinal cord compression, and the tempo of progression of neurologic deficits. It is to be reiterated that the appropriate treatment in each case will be most effective when instituted early in the development of signs and symptoms and in the absence of serious neurologic findings.

■ MALIGNANT PERICARDIAL EFFUSION

The development of a malignant pericardial effusion in patients with disseminated malignancy is not uncommon. Incidences range from 5 to 50 percent and vary with histologic diagnosis in autopsy and clinical studies. The most common tumors to involve the pericardium are lung, breast, mesothelioma, gastrointestinal primaries, leukemias and lymphomas, sarcomas, and melanoma. Lung and breast carcinomas predominate. Pericardial disease due to malignancy is clinically apparent in approximately 20 percent of patients found to have pericardial disease postmortem. Because approximately 40 percent of patients presenting with symptomatic pericardial effusion and an underlying malignancy may have nonmalignant pericardial disease, it is of critical importance to define the specific cause. The differential diagnosis in such patients includes radiation pericarditis, drug-induced pericarditis, infection, hypothyroidism, autoimmune disorders, and idiopathic pericarditis. It is easily distinguished from SVC obstruction by the presence of pulsating neck veins.

Clinical Presentation

Malignant pericardial effusion often has an insidious onset encompassing several clinical entities, including asymptomatic chronic pericardial effusion, constrictive pericarditis, effusive constrictive pericarditis, and cardiac tamponade. It may take place in patients who have been in remission, although most often it appears in the presence of disease elsewhere. Symptoms depend on the rate of accumulation of fluid, the volume of fluid, and the underlying cardiac reserve. Symptoms of malignant pericardial effusion include dyspnea, cough, chest pain, orthopnea, palpitations, weakness, fatigue, and dizziness. Cardiac tamponade is characterized by anxiety and severe dyspnea with upright, forward-leaning posture for relief of symptoms, severe tachycardia, narrowing of pulse pressure (falling arterial pressure and rising venous pressure), pulsus paradoxus, and hypotension. These patients may have cardiac enlargement, distant heart sounds, pericardial friction rub, and pulsating neck veins, which easily distinguish pericarditis from SVC obstruction.

Diagnostic Evaluation

A change in the contour of the heart on chest x-ray film classically, (there is an enlargement of the cardiac silhouette described as a water-bottle heart) together with the presenting symptoms mentioned above should raise the possibility of malignancy-related pericarditis. ECG may show sinus tachycardia or changes typically described with pericardial effusion, including low QRS voltage in the limb leads, elevation of the ST segment, T-wave changes, or electrical alternans. Echocardiography is the most precise and least invasive method for diagnosing and measuring a pericardial effusion. Right-heart catheterization and intracardiac pressure tracings may be implemented when the differentiation between pericardial disease and myocardial disease is not clear from information obtained on physical examination and noninvasive studies.

Treatment

After the diagnosis of a malignant pericardial effusion is firmly established, the treatment approach should take into consideration the patient's life expectancy, whether or not the tumor is sensitive to chemotherapy or radiotherapy, and whether or not the patient has cardiac tamponade. The overall treatment plan in cancer patients with pericardial effusions depends on the performance status of the patient, hemodynamic compromise, histology, and the extent of the underlying malignancy. Currently, there are five major methods of treating cancer-related pericardial effusions: pericardiocentesis, pericardial sclerosis, systemic chemotherapy, radiotherapy, and surgery.

Pericardiocentesis should always be performed for therapeutic and diagnostic purposes in a cancer patient with a clinically significant pericardial effusion. When clinical signs and symptoms suggest cardiac tamponade, pericardiocentesis should be performed emergently. The standard methods of pericardiocentesis use a left subxipoid approach, performing the procedure under fluoroscopic, echocardiographic, or electrocardiographic guidance when the clinical situation permits. The complication rates of pericardiocentesis are in the 7 to 15 percent range, with a mean mortality rate of 6 percent in five large series. The causes of morbidity and mortality include induced arrhythmias, perforation of the myocardium, hemopericardium secondary to laceration of the coronary pericardial or internal mammary arteries, and cardiac arrest. The amount of fluid obtained by pericardiocentesis varies from 250 to 2000 ml. The fluid may appear serous or serosanguinous but is most often hemorrhagic. The fluid should be analyzed for cell count, culture, and cytology. Cytologic examination is quite accurate in the diagnosis of malignant pericardial disease, documenting malignant cells in 85 percent of cases. Unless definitive local therapy is initiated, reaccumulation of the fluid and tamponade will occur within 24 to 48 hours following pericardiocentesis. Indwelling catheters are usually left in place to drain reaccumulating fluid and for the administration of intrapericardial sclerosing agents, although the need for sclerosis is far from clear.

The use of cardiac irradiation alone in the management of a malignant pericardial effusion is limited by the time required for response and the fact that non–small cell lung carcinoma, for example, may be relatively radioresistant. However, radiotherapy may be indicated for patients with tumors that either are known to be radiosensitive or are refractory to chemotherapy, such as lymphoma, leukemia, small cell lung cancer, testicular cancer, and breast cancer. Generally, 2,000 to 4,000 cGy is delivered to a port that includes the heart and pericardial structures in daily fractions of 150 to 200 cGy over 3 to 4 weeks. Response, defined as relief of cardiac symptoms, is seen in 70 percent of patients with breast cancer, 25 percent of patients with lung cancer, and 85 percent of patients with hematologic malignancy.

If effective systemic chemotherapy is available, it should be given concurrently with local measures. It is most appropriate in patients with chemosensitive tumors, especially those who have never been treated, such as lymphoma and breast cancer.

Patients with reasonable performance status who have effusive pericarditis and are not candidates for immediate radiation and/or chemotherapy or who have required repeated pericardiocentesis should be considered for surgical intervention. Surgical treatment of malignant pericardial effusion is accomplished with a subxiphoid approach, a left anterior thoracotomy, or a median sternotomy. The subxiphoid approach, which is relatively simple, is the procedure of choice, as it can be done under local anesthesia and has a lower morbidity and mortality than those requiring thoracotomy. A midline incision is done, the xiphoid process is removed to provide maximal access to the substernal space, the pericardium is grasped with clamps, creating a window, and a thoracic catheter is inserted along the inferior aspect of the pericardium. Constrictive pericarditis due to radiation or tumorous thickening of the pericardium may be better treated with an extensive pericardial resection through a median sternotomy. However, debilitated patients with a poor prognosis and active malignancy are best managed with tube drainage. Although the type of procedure performed (pericardiectomy versus pericardial window) does not appear to influence the postoperative survival, patients who have undergone total pericardiectomy do appear to have fewer late failures than those with window pericardiectomy. For this reason, radiation-induced effusions in patients who may be cured of their cancer should not be treated with a pericardial window.

A number of sclerosing agents and radioisotopes have been used to obliterate the pericardial space by inducing an inflammatory response and fibrosis. These agents include nitrogen mustard, 5-fluorouracil, bleomycin, thiotepa, tetracycline, talc, and radioactive gold and phosphorus. Bleomycin has fewer side effects than other agents and may be as effective, but no comparative studies with drainage alone exist. The procedure is considered effective if the pericardial effusion and symptoms thereof disappear for over 30 days and there is no requirement for repeated pericardiocentesis. Patients who are most appropriate for pericardial sclerosis are those who present with cardiac tamponade requiring emergent pericardial drainage, those who do not have radiotherapy- or chemotherapy-sensitive tumors, and those who are poor surgical candidates.

Suggested Reading

DeVita VT Jr, Hellman S, Rosenberg S, eds. Cancer: Principles and practice of oncology. 5th ed. Philadelphia: JB Lippincott, 1997:2461.

Dutcher JP, Wiernik PH. Oncologic emergencies. In: Kelley WN, ed. Textbook of internal medicine. 2nd ed. Philadelphia: JB Lippincott, 1992: 1231.

Wilkes JP, Fidios P, Vaickur L, Perce RP. Malignancy-related pericardial effusion: 127 cases from Roswell Park Cancer Institute. Cancer 1995;76:1377.

EPIDURAL SPINAL CORD COMPRESSION AND NEOPLASTIC MENINGITIS

Mark R. Gilbert, M.D.
Taseer A. Minhas, M.D.

■ EPIDURAL SPINAL CORD COMPRESSION

Epidural spinal cord compression (ESCC), a very common neurologic complication of systemic malignancy, has been estimated to occur in 5 to 12 percent of patients with cancer. The incidence of ESCC is expected to increase as survival from systemic cancer improves. ESCC is often a neurologic emergency, and neurologic expertise can often expedite evaluation and treatment by improving anatomic localization and diagnostic accuracy.

ESCC is defined as spread of tumor into the epidural space. Spinal cord compression develops as the tumor grows in the region adjacent to the spinal cord or cauda equina. Tumor will usually not traverse the dura but grows in a rostral and caudal direction virtually unimpeded by the blood vessels and fat in the epidural space. Contiguous extension of tumor several vertebral levels away from the primary location of the epidural tumor is very common.

There are two routes that tumors use to infiltrate the epidural space. The most common is by direct extension from bone metastases in the vertebral bones. Metastases to the vertebral bodies are most common. Tumor destroys the cortical margin of bone adjacent to the spinal canal, allowing growth into the epidural space. Similarly, extensive destruction of vertebral bones, particularly the vertebral body, can lead to collapse of the bone and extrusion of tumor, along with remnants of the bone, into the spinal canal. The high incidence of vertebral bone metastases in patients with solid tumors has been hypothesized to be secondary to tumor cell drainage from thoracic, abdominal, and pelvic organs into the vertebral venous plexus. The second route of entry into the epidural space is by tumor growth through the intervertebral foramina. This most commonly occurs with retroperitoneal tumors and tumors that spread from paravertebral lymph nodes, such as lymphoma.

Epidural tumor most commonly presents with local or radicular pain. In fact, more than 95 percent of patients with epidural tumors have pain as their initial symptom. Furthermore, in most cases weeks to months may pass from the onset of pain before neurologic dysfunction occurs. In one study, the median time from onset of pain to diagnosis was 7 weeks. Unfortunately, by the time the diagnosis was made, more than 75 percent of the patients had evidence of neurologic dysfunction. The most common neurologic findings are weakness in the extremities, sensory loss (often in a dermatomal distribution, then evolving to a sensory level), and ataxia. Urinary and fecal abnormalities (incontinence and retention) are also frequent complaints. The finding of Brown-Séquard syndrome on examination is highly suggestive of ESCC in a patient with cancer.

Virtually all types of metastatic cancer have been reported to cause ESCC. Breast cancer, lung cancer, prostate cancer, melanoma, gastrointestinal (primarily colon) cancers, renal cell carcinoma, and sarcomas are the most common cancers that cause epidural metastases. The location of the spinal metastases varies with the type of tumor. For example, lung and breast cancer tend to spread to thoracic vertebrae, whereas prostate cancer has a predilection for the lumbar spine. Several factors determine the relative frequency that a specific tumor type causes ESCC: (1) the overall incidence of the tumor; (2) the propensity for the tumor to spread to bone or the periaortic region; and (3) the overall duration of survival of patients with the tumor type. ESCC is often a late complication of cancer; therefore patients with rapidly fatal malignancies, such as pancreatic carcinoma, infrequently develop spinal cord compression.

Diagnosis

Early diagnosis of epidural tumor is essential to successful management. As just described, pain is almost always the initial symptom. Therefore patients with known malignancy and back pain warrant a prompt evaluation for epidural tumor. As outlined in Figure 1, the presence or absence of neurologic findings dictates the initial treatment and evaluation. Patients with neurologic dysfunction warrant immediate treatment with corticosteroids (see following text) followed by a rapid diagnostic evaluation. Patients with back pain and a normal neurologic examination can be evaluated on an urgent basis and often in the outpatient setting. Magnetic resonance imaging (MRI) is currently the diagnostic test of choice. It offers several advantages over computed tomography (CT) myelography: (1) MRI is noninvasive; (2) there is no risk of causing brain herniation if cerebral metastases are present; (3) there is no risk of worsening spinal cord compression by lowering CSF pressure caudal to a complete block, so-called spinal cord herniation; and (4) MRI is superior in distinguishing epidural tumors from intramedullary tumors. The use of gadolinium and recent technical advances in scanning including the use of "fat saturation" algorithms have greatly improved the sensitivity of MRI in detecting epidural tumors. Unfortunately, patient cooperation is essential for a high-quality scan. Often patients with epidural tumors are in severe pain and are unable to lie still for the entire study. This leads to a technically limited study. In my practice I have CT myelograms performed on patients with suspected epidural tumor who have a negative, but technically limited MRI scan. In this situation, the CT myelogram often demonstrates deposits of tumor.

Visualization of the entire extent of tumor is essential for treatment planning. Tumor often extends more than five vertebral bodies away from the primary epidural tumor location. Failure to delineate the full extent of tumor may result in regrowth of tumor at the margins of radiation treatment, preventing further treatment of that area because of concern for overlapping radiation fields and overexposure of the spinal cord. A survey of the entire spine with either

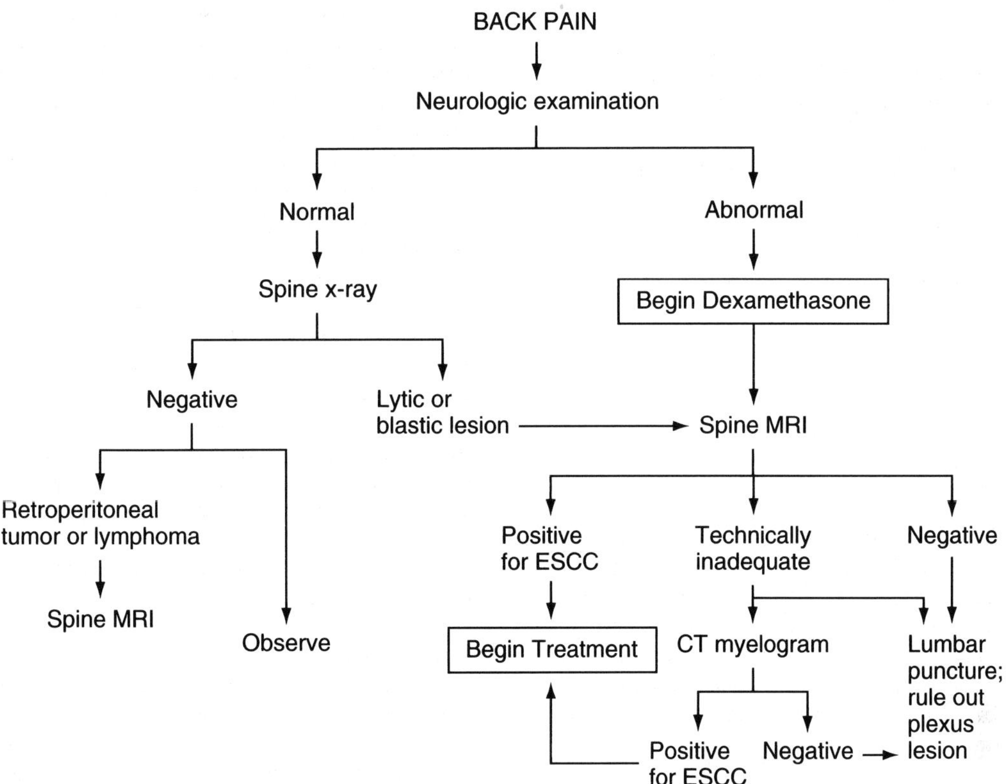

Figure 1
Algorithm for the differential diagnosis of spinal cord dysfunction in patients with cancer. MRI, magnetic resonance imaging; ESCC, epidural spinal cord compression; CT, computed tomography.

sagittal MRI images or myelography should be considered to uncover synchronous epidural tumors, which can then be included in treatment planning.

Differential Diagnosis

The differential diagnosis of spinal cord dysfunction in patients with cancer is outlined in Table 1. Although epidural tumor is the most common cause of spinal cord problems in patients with cancer, the other diagnoses need to be considered. The neurologic examination can be helpful in distinguishing intramedullary from epidural processes. Patients with a suspended sensory level or early loss of fecal or urinary continence are likely to have an intramedullary process. The absence of pain in the setting of progressive neurologic dysfunction is also more commonly seen with intramedullary processes. Rapid progression of neurologic dysfunction with only a short prodrome of pain suggests either epidural abscess or hematoma. The finding of cranial nerve palsies or multilevel radiculopathy suggests neoplastic meningitis either as the primary diagnosis or as a concurrent problem. Additionally, spinal arachnoiditis can present in a similar fashion to ESCC, particularly in the lumbar region.

Chemotherapy-induced myelopathy is a rare complication of repeated intrathecal chemotherapy and is seen only with the lumbar administration of drug. No diagnostic test exists, although MRI scans often reveal local T2 changes and spinal cord enlargement consistent with regional edema. There are reports that CSF myelin basic protein levels are elevated early in the course of the myelopathy. This marker may be useful in making the early diagnosis, stopping treatment, and preventing further progression of neurologic loss. Radiation myelopathy is rare with current radiotherapy techniques and has been reported only when the dose to the spinal cord exceeds 45 Gy. The diagnosis is made by excluding other causes of myelopathy. Similarly, paraneoplastic myelopathy has been reported as a very rare complication of various carcinomas and lymphomas. The diagnosis is made by excluding other causes. MRI scans show regional cord swelling and edema.

Therapy

Corticosteroids

Corticosteroids are the initial treatment of patients with suspected ESCC. Experimental studies have shown that corticosteroid administration is effective in reducing the edema associated with compression of the spinal cord parenchyma. Dexamethasone is the most commonly used corticosteroid, although the dosing is controversial. I recommend that a high-dose regimen be used in patients with progressive neurologic dysfunction. These patients receive an initial bolus of 100 mg intravenously and then receive 96 mg the following day in divided doses. The dose is tapered over the following 2 to 3 weeks depending on stability or improvement in neurologic function. The corticosteroid dose can be modified after imaging studies determine the extent of the spinal cord compression. For example, a patient with neurologic findings with only a partial cord compression can often have the dose of corticosteroid rapidly reduced. Patients with back pain and

Table 1 Causes of Spinal Cord Dysfunction in Patients with Cancer

Epidural cord compression
Tumor
Abscess
Hematoma
Intramedullary processes
Metastases
Abscess
Hematoma
Syrinx
Radiation myelopathy
Chemotherapy myelopathy
Paraneoplastic myelopathy
Neoplastic meningitis
Spinal arachnoiditis

a normal neurologic examination receive 16 mg of decadron each day in divided doses. This dose often provides prompt pain relief while the patient is undergoing diagnostic studies.

Surgery

The role of surgery as a primary treatment of ESCC is evolving. Several studies have clearly shown that the role of laminectomy is limited and that radiation therapy alone is equivalent to radiation therapy following laminectomy. However, recent advances in spine surgery have made anterior or anterolateral resection of tumor more practical, although these are major operations that involve significant morbidity and mortality. Currently a multicenter randomized trial is under way comparing radiotherapy alone with surgical tumor resection plus radiotherapy. I reserve this technique for patients with limited systemic and vertebral disease who have a long life expectancy.

There are several situations in which surgical intervention is either necessary or potentially beneficial:

1. Spine instability caused by destruction of vertebral bones by tumor necessitates a surgical procedure.
2. Patients with ESCC without a known malignancy should undergo a rapid systemic evaluation to find a more accessible lesion. If none is found, then a needle biopsy may be sufficient to make a histologic diagnosis.
3. The possibility of an epidural abscess warrants a biopsy and possibly drainage.
4. Progression of symptoms during radiotherapy may necessitate a surgical decompression before proceeding with the radiation.
5. Tumor recurrence at a previously irradiated region may be temporarily treated with resection, awaiting the effects of another treatment modality, such as systemic chemotherapy. A recent study, however, indicates that retreatment of the spine with radiotherapy can be safely administered providing tumor and pain control in many patients.

Radiation Therapy

Radiation therapy is the primary treatment for spinal cord compression. Effective treatment requires that the extent of the tumor be fully delineated. As discussed previously, tumor can extend several vertebral bodies away from the primary site, and failure to discover this may lead to a lesion at the margin of the radiation port. Likewise, surveying the spine, either with sagittal MRI or myelography, will determine whether there are additional lesions that should be included in treatment planning. A recent report indicates that reirradiation of the spinal cord is possible in patients with recurrent ESCC. In this study, patients maintained ambulatory function and some showed improved neurologic function. The risk of radiation myelopathy was minimal because the overall median survival from the time of re-treatment was short.

Chemotherapy

The role of chemotherapy and immunotherapy in the treatment of ESCC is limited. There are reports of significant improvement in neurologic function after treatment of chemosensitive tumors, such as lymphoma. For the majority of solid tumors, however, response to systemic chemotherapy is slow and a surgical debulking of tumor may be required to allow time for response to chemotherapy to occur.

Outcome

Neurologic function at the time of treatment initiation is the best prognostic factor regarding ultimate outcome, underscoring the need for early diagnosis. Patients who are ambulatory at the time of diagnosis generally remain so at the completion of treatment, whereas patients with paraplegia rarely recover function, particularly if the duration of paraplegia is greater than 48 hours at the time of diagnosis. Laboratory studies suggest that irreversible loss of neurologic function in ESCC is due to vascular compromise, predominantly of the venous plexus adjacent to the spinal cord. There are reports of significant recovery of neurologic function after anterior resection for ESCC, but this technique is usually only used in selected patients with limited vertebral disease and recent onset of neurologic dysfunction.

■ NEOPLASTIC MENINGITIS

Neoplastic meningitis is defined as the infiltration of the pial and arachnoidal membranes of the central nervous system by tumor cells, accompanied by free-floating cells in the CSF. The incidence of neoplastic meningitis, generally a late complication of cancer, is increasing as a consequence of improved survival from systemic malignancies. Neoplastic meningitis has been reported to occur in 0.8 to 8.0 percent of patients with systemic cancer, although the incidence greatly varies by the type of malignancy. Adenocarcinomas, such as breast and lung, have a high incidence, along with other carcinomas such as small cell lung cancer and melanoma. Acute leukemias and high-grade non-Hodgkin's lymphoma spread to the CSF so frequently that in many instances prophylactic treatment of the meninges is indicated.

The pathogenesis of neoplastic meningitis is not known, although it is speculated that tumor cells infiltrate the CSF either by direct extension from metastases within the central nervous system or along nerve sheaths or that hematogenous tumor cells infiltrate via arachnoid vessels, choroid plexus, or via paravertebral or endoneural lymphatics of spinal nerves. Neurologic dysfunction occurs either by infiltration of brain parenchyma via the Virchow-Robin spaces or infiltration of nerve roots. Cortical irritation by tumor can lead to seizures or global neurologic impairment. Furthermore, tumor-related alterations in CSF flow can lead to communicating or noncommunicating hydrocephalus with resulting increased intracranial pressure. Communicating hydrocephalus is due to impaired resorption of CSF at the arachnoid granulations over the cortical convexities. Noncommunicating hydrocephalus is most commonly caused by tumor cells occluding the aqueduct of Sylvius or other narrow CSF pathways.

The most common presentation is with either loss of cognitive function or altered sensorium. Patients with neoplastic meningitis frequently complain of headache, which is secondary to increased intracranial pressure. Cranial nerve and spinal radicular findings are also common. Cranial nerve involvement may present as blindness secondary to optic nerve or chiasm infiltration, diplopia, peripheral facial nerve palsy, loss of gag reflex, and, less frequently, hearing loss, and facial numbness. Spinal radicular symptoms are predominantly lumbosacral, possibly caused by gravity-related settling of tumor cells in the thecal sac. Patients may present with low back pain that has a radicular component, along with lower extremity weakness, incontinence, sensory loss in a dermatomal pattern, and a selected loss of deep tendon reflexes.

Diagnosis

Demonstration of malignant cells in the CSF by cytologic examination of the cerebrospinal fluid is the definitive diagnostic test. This may require multiple lumbar punctures. The diagnostic yield of a single cytologic specimen has been reported to be 50 percent. Three sequential samples improves the yield to 85 percent, and five samples increases the yield of positive cytology to 95 percent. Greater than 95 percent of lumbar punctures are abnormal in patients with neoplastic meningitis. The CSF protein is elevated in 60 to 80 percent, hypoglycorrhia is present in 25 to 40 percent, and an elevated opening pressure is present in 50 percent. Prompt processing for cytologic analysis is critical because neoplastic cells undergo degeneration over time, thereby decreasing the sensitivity of the examination. Various biochemical markers such as carcinoembryonic antigen (CEA), alpha fetoprotein, beta-human chorionic gonadotropin (β-hCG), melanin, glucuronidase, and beta-2-microglobulin can be helpful for diagnosis and monitoring treatment if present in the CSF in excess of serum concentrations. Flow cytometry, particularly for lymphoma, can confirm that there is a clonal population of lymphocytes in the CSF, supporting the diagnosis of lymphomatous meningitis. Monoclonal antibodies for specific tumor antigens may play an important role in diagnosis in the near future. Rarely, a leptomeningeal biopsy is required to make the diagnosis.

Radiologic studies may be helpful in supporting the diagnosis of neoplastic meningitis. MRI scanning particularly with gadolinium administration may reveal enhancement along the walls of the ventricles and over the convexities. MRI of the spine may reveal "sugar coating," a fine line of enhancement over the surface of the cord or thickening of the nerve roots in the cauda equina. Both CT and MRI scanning will reveal either communicating or noncommunicating hydrocephalus. None of the radiographic findings are specific for neoplastic meningitis, and similar changes can be detected in both acute and chronic inflammatory conditions.

Therapy

Radiation Therapy

Cranial radiotherapy is now considered an adjunct to chemotherapy. We generally limit the use of radiotherapy to symptomatic areas. For example, a patient with focal cranial nerve dysfunction or obstructive hydrocephalus secondary to tumor infiltration may benefit by local radiotherapy. Whole-brain radiotherapy is of little long-term therapeutic benefit and is associated with a very high risk of neurotoxicity, particularly when the radiotherapy is followed by intrathecal chemotherapy. Likewise, craniospinal radiation treatment is of limited value in controlling tumor but will markedly reduce bone marrow reserves potentially precluding future chemotherapy administration. The treatment of leptomeningeal leukemia may be the exception because relatively low dose (1,800 cGy) of craniospinal radiotherapy may have significant clinical benefit when administered after intrathecal chemotherapy. Most other leptomeningeal malignancies do not show a significant response to this low dose of radiation.

Newer techniques are being developed to deliver radiation directly to the tumor cells. Radioisotopes such as ^{131}I are coupled directly to monoclonal antibodies that are specific for the tumor cell type. This technique should markedly reduce systemic toxicity while targeting both free-floating and adherent cells in the leptomeninges.

Chemotherapy

Chemotherapy is now considered the mainstay of treatment. Both systemic and intrathecal chemotherapy can be used, although only a small percentage of chemotherapy agents are effective. Systemic administration generally requires that high doses are used and that the drug can cross the blood-brain barrier. Methotrexate, cytosine arabinoside (ara-C), thioTEPA, and procarbazine can achieve therapeutic concentrations in the CSF when administered systematically, but the doses required will often cause myelosuppression and may cause neurotoxicity. Direct administration of chemotherapy into the CSF either via lumbar puncture or ventricular reservoir (i.e., Ommaya reservoir) is the mainstay of treatment of neoplastic meningitis. Three drugs, methotrexate, ara-C, and thioTEPA, are commonly used for direct spinal fluid administration. The usual dosing and use of these agents are listed in Table 2.

These chemotherapeutic agents can be administered either via a ventricular reservoir or by lumbar puncture and administration into the thecal sac. There are advantages and disadvantages to both routes, summarized in Table 3. In general, patients who require many treatments will tolerate treatment better if a ventricular reservoir system is placed. We recommend that the chemotherapeutic agent be mixed in a volume of 10 cc and that a 3 cc nonbacteriostatic saline flush be used. Before administering the treatment, an equal volume of CSF must be removed; then the chemotherapy can be given at a rate of 1 cc per minute. This may reduce immediate side effects such as headache, nausea, and vomiting that may result from the rapid administration of both drug and fluid.

Patients with ventricular reservoirs require a CSF flow study. Most commonly, ^{111}In-labeled albumin is used. The

Table 2 Agents Used for Direct Spinal Fluid Treatment of Neoplastic Meningitis

DRUG	TYPICAL DOSING	FREQUENCY	TUMOR TYPES
Methotrexate	6.25 mg/m^2 or 10–12 mg in adults	1–2/week	Solid tumors, lymphoma, leukemia
Ara-C	50 mg or 30 mg/day × 3 days (adult dosing)	1/week	Leukemia, lymphoma
thioTEPA	10 mg via ventricular reservoir, 15 mg via lumbar puncture	1/week	Solid tumors, primary central nervous system tumors

Table 3 Routes of Administration

ROUTE	ADVANTAGES	DISADVANTAGES
Lumbar	Does not require reservoir placement CSF has better diagnostic value Potentially less neurotoxicity	Drug delivered into CSF only 85%–90% of the time Poor drug delivery into lateral ventricles Possible myelopathy
Lateral ventricle	Easy administration of drug Better drug distribution, particularly lateral ventricles Certainty of drug administration into CSF	Probable increased neurotoxicity compared with lumbar administration Requires neurosurgical placement Requires CSF flow study CSF sampling has lower diagnostic yield

CSF, cerebrospinal fluid.

tracer is injected into the reservoir and scans are performed at 6 hours, 24 hours, and 48 hours. The reasons for this study are several. First, the initial scan confirms that the reservoir and catheter system drain into the lateral ventricle. The subsequent studies will determine whether CSF flow out of the lateral ventricles is normal. Outflow obstruction, such as a noncommunicating hydrocephalus, will result in delayed clearance of drug from the lateral ventricle, markedly accelerating the development of chemotherapy neurotoxicity. Similarly, blockage of the arachnoid granulations over the cortical convexities will prevent CSF resorption and ultimately cause communicating hydrocephalus. This will result in reflux of CSF into the lateral ventricles, again delayed clearance of drug, and potentially accelerating toxicity. Noncommunicating hydrocephalus can often be treated with a short course of radiotherapy to the blocked region, whereas communicating hydrocephalus may require a short course of cranial radiotherapy. After completion of the radiotherapy, the CSF flow study should be repeated to confirm normalization of CSF flow.

Outcome and Prognosis

Neoplastic meningitis is associated with a grim prognosis. For most malignancies, patients have a median survival of 3 to 6 weeks with supportive care alone. The overall prognosis in patients undergoing treatment is based on several factors. Tumor histology and chemotherapy sensitivity are the most important prognostic factors. Some cancers, such as lymphoma and leukemia, can be very responsive, and in certain patients complete remission and long-term control of the meningeal disease can be obtained. This is not the case for most solid tumors; although breast cancer and small cell lung cancer will often respond well to treatment, non–small cell lung cancer will show only a modest response. Other cancers such as malignant melanoma and renal cell carcinoma will rarely respond to chemotherapy. In general, tumor response to systemic chemotherapy will correlate with leptomeningeal response to intrathecal treatment. Other important prognostic factors include the extent of parenchymal infiltration by the leptomeningeal tumor, extent of systemic disease, degree of neurologic dysfunction, and the patient's overall performance status.

Future Directions

There are several areas of active investigation in both diagnosis and treatment of neoplastic meningitis. Polymerase chain reaction (PCR) technology is being applied to assist in the diagnosis of leukemic and lymphomatous meningitis. PCR can often determine that many of the cells are of monoclonal origin by determining that the immunoglobulin-gene rearrangement or T cell receptor gene rearrangement is identical for many of the cells present, distinguishing this population from reactive lymphocytes. Monoclonal antibodies are being increasingly used to stain cytologic preparations and improve the yield of cytology in both solid tumors and lymphoma. Antibodies against specific markers, such as glial fibrillary acidic protein and carcinoembryonic antigen, are undergoing investigation as adjunctive tests.

New therapies are being developed including immunotherapy, gene therapy, and radioimmunoconjugates. Immunotherapy studies have primarily focused on the use of biologic response modifiers (i.e., interferons, interleukins) to stimulate a local host response against the tumor cells. Gene therapy studies are attempting with the use of retroviral vectors, to transduce tumor cells with specific genes such as the herpesvirus thymidine kinase gene, thereby making the tumor cells sensitive to well-tolerated treatment such as ganciclovir. The problems of delivery of retrovirus to tumor cells, a major problem with parenchymal tumor, is markedly reduced with intrathecal administration. Radioimmunoconjugate studies involve generating specific monoclonal antibodies against an antigen on the tumor cell surface and conjugating a radioisotope to the antibody. Administration of the radiolabeled antibody into the CSF should specifically target tumor cells if there is adequate exposure and binding.

The incidence of neoplastic meningitis is increasing, and the impact of this diagnosis on survival and patient's quality of life is obvious. Increased awareness and prompt diagnosis may permit institution of treatment before significant neurologic impairment develops, potentially improving the success of treatment and preventing loss of function. Recognition of potential treatment consequences will reduce the risk of neurotoxicity. Although in most cases the prognosis is poor, future advances in both diagnostic techniques and treatment should markedly alter the outcome for patients with neoplastic meningitis.

Suggested Reading

Byrne TN. Spinal cord compression from epidural metastases. N Engl J Med 1992; 327:614–619.

Chamberlain MC, Corey-Bloom J. Leptomeningeal metastases: ^{111}In-DTPA CSF flow studies. Neurology 1991; 41:1765–1769.

Shiff D, Shaw EG, Cascino TL. Outcome after spinal reirradiation for malignant epidural spinal cord compression. Ann Neurol 1995; 37:583–589.

Wasserstrom WR, Glass JP, Posner JB. Diagnosis and treatment of leptomeningeal metastases from solid tumors: Experience with 90 patients. Cancer 1982; 49:759–772.

Zachariah, B, Zacharial SB, Varghese R, et al. Carcinomatous meningitis: Clinical manifestations and management. Int J Clin Pharm Ther 1995; 33:7–12.

UNKNOWN PRIMARY CANCER

F. Anthony Greco, M.D.
John D. Hainsworth, M.D.

Patients with metastatic cancer and no obvious primary site are relatively common, accounting for about 5 to 10 percent of all cancer patients. Until recently this group of patients attracted little attention, since their prognosis was uniformly poor regardless of treatment. However, effective therapy is now available for many types of advanced cancer, and it is therefore not surprising that some carcinomas of unknown primary site are very sensitive to chemotherapeutic agents. The clinician must approach each patient with carcinoma of unknown primary site with two objectives: (1) to identify patients with treatable malignancies, using both clinical and pathologic criteria, and (2) to avoid superfluous diagnostic procedures and inappropriate treatment for patients with unresponsive neoplasms.

The typical patient with cancer of unknown primary site develops initial symptoms at a metastatic site; routine history, physical examination, chest radiograph, and laboratory studies fail to identify the primary site. In this clinical setting, light microscopic examination of the biopsy specimen usually identifies one of four major categories: (1) poorly differentiated neoplasm, (2) adenocarcinoma, (3) squamous carcinoma, or (4) poorly differentiated carcinoma. These four groups vary with respect to clinical characteristics, recommended diagnostic evaluation, treatment, and prognosis.

■ POORLY DIFFERENTIATED NEOPLASMS OF UNKNOWN PRIMARY SITE

The diagnosis of poorly differentiated neoplasm can describe any of a large number of neoplasms, many of which are highly responsive to systemic therapy. The diagnosis implies the inability of the pathologist to distinguish between carcinoma and other cancers, such as lymphoma, sarcoma, and melanoma. Further evaluation, always necessary in these patients, frequently results in a more precise diagnosis, often with specific therapeutic implications. The most common cause of a nonspecific pathologic diagnosis is an inadequate biopsy. Fine-needle aspiration biopsy usually provides inadequate amounts of tissue for the initial diagnosis of metastatic cancer, since histology is poorly preserved and adequate material is not available for special studies. Often, a specific and more definitive diagnosis can be made by obtaining a larger biopsy. Some pathologic studies require special processing of the biopsy specimen; therefore, close communication with the surgeon and pathologist is important if repeat biopsy is performed.

Occasionally light microscopic examination alone fails to provide a diagnosis more specific than poorly differentiated neoplasm or poorly differentiated carcinoma, even when a large, adequately preserved biopsy specimen is available. Immunoperoxidase staining and electron microscopy are indicated to study the neoplasm further. Immunoperoxidase staining is now widely available, and a number of useful stains have been developed (common leukocyte antigen, epithelial membrane antigen, keratins, vimentin, S-100, prostate specific antigen [PSA], neuron specific enolase, and others). Since these stains are not usually specific, they should not be used alone to make a diagnosis but are frequently useful in conjunction with the light microscopic examination and clinical features. These stains can suggest the diagnosis of lymphoma, melanoma, neuroendocrine carcinoma, sarcoma, or germ cell tumor. However, some neoplasms can only be classified as carcinomas, while in up to 30 percent, immunoperoxidase staining gives inconclusive results.

The examination of cellular ultrastructure by electron microscopy can also provide important information in the differential diagnosis of poorly differentiated neoplasms, and should be considered when immunoperoxidase staining is inconclusive. The important distinction between lymphoma and carcinoma can be made in most instances. Other important ultrastructural findings include neurosecretory granules (neuroendocrine tumors such as small cell lung cancer, carcinoid tumors, neuroblastoma), premelanosomes (melanoma), and intracellular lumina or surface microvilli (adenocarcinoma).

Molecular genetic studies are becoming more feasible and on occasion may help to diagnose poorly differentiated neoplasms. Specific chromosomal abnormalities associated with a few tumors have been identified. A large percentage of germ cell tumors (both testicular and extragonadal) have an isochromosome of the short arm of chromosome 12 (i12p). Peripheral neuroepithelioma and Ewing's tumor share a specific chromosomal translocation (11:22). Many lymphomas and leukemias are characterized by relatively specific chromosomal changes or molecular fingerprints. In the future the recognition of additional specific genetic abnormalities may facilitate the identification of tumor lineage or origin in other patients.

■ ADENOCARCINOMA OF UNKNOWN PRIMARY SITE

Clinical Features and Natural History

About 60 percent of all carcinomas of unknown primary site are well-differentiated adenocarcinomas. The typical patient with this diagnosis is elderly and has metastatic tumor at multiple sites. The most common sites of involvement are the liver, lungs, and bones, but many other sites are also involved.

In most patients, the clinical course is dominated by symptoms related to the sites of metastases. The primary site becomes obvious during the clinical course in only 15 to 20 percent of patients. However, at autopsy, a primary site can be detected in 60 to 80 percent of patients. The most common primary sites are pancreas and lung, accounting for approximately 40 percent of all cases; other gastrointestinal sites (stomach, colon, liver) are also frequent. Adenocarcinomas of the breast and prostate, which occur commonly in the general population, are infrequently identified in this group of patients.

Pathology

The diagnosis of adenocarcinoma is based on the formation of glandular structures by neoplastic cells and is usually made without difficulty using light microscopy. All adenocarcinomas share these histologic features, and therefore the site of origin usually cannot be ascertained. Specialized pathologic evaluation infrequently provides useful additional information; one exception is the immunoperoxidase stain for PSA, which is quite specific for prostate cancer and should be used in men with suggestive clinical findings. Immunoperoxidase stains for estrogen and progesterone receptors should be considered for women with metastatic adenocarcinoma in whom biochemical assays for estrogen and progesterone receptors were not obtained.

The histopathologic diagnosis of *poorly differentiated* adenocarcinoma should be viewed differently, since these patients may vary both with respect to tumor biology and responsiveness to systemic therapy. This diagnosis is made when only minimal glandular formation is seen by light microscopy; sometimes it is based on a positive mucin stain alone in a tumor that would otherwise be called poorly differentiated carcinoma. Additional pathologic study with electron microscopy and immunoperoxidase stains should be performed on these tumors. Evaluation and treatment of these patients is similar to those for patients with poorly differentiated carcinoma, as discussed later.

Diagnostic Evaluation

A summary of the recommended evaluation for this group of patients is outlined in Table 1. All patients with adenocarcinoma of unknown primary should undergo a thorough history and physical examination, including pelvic examination in female patients, standard laboratory screening tests (complete blood count, serum electrolytes, creatinine, glucose, and liver function tests [SMA18], and urinalysis), and chest radiograph. Serum PSA should be measured in male patients, and all women should have mammography, since palliative therapy is available for patients with advanced prostate or breast cancer. Computed tomography of the abdomen can identify the primary site in 20 to 35 percent of patients and should possibly be included in the routine evaluation. Additional radiologic evaluation should evaluate clues and abnormalities identified by history, physical examination, or routine laboratory studies; radiologic evaluation of asymptomatic areas is rarely useful.

Treatment and Prognosis

Therapy for patients with adenocarcinoma of unknown primary site depends on the recognition, based on clinical features, of certain treatable patient subgroups. Women who have adenocarcinoma involving axillary lymph nodes should be suspected of having breast cancer. Documentation of estrogen receptors in the tumor tissue is strong supportive evidence for this diagnosis. Women who have no evidence of other metastatic sites may have stage II breast cancer and therefore may be curable with appropriate therapy. Even when physical examination and mammogram are negative, 50 to 60 percent of women have a small breast primary found following mastectomy. Therapy includes a simple mastectomy and axillary node dissection; radiotherapy to the breast and axilla may be an equally effective alternative. Women with other metastatic sites in addition to axillary lymph nodes may have metastatic breast cancer; treatment with either hormonal therapy or combination chemotherapy is often of major palliative benefit.

Women with peritoneal carcinomatosis sometimes can be treated effectively using the guidelines established for ovarian cancer. Some of these women may have unrecognized ovarian cancer; however, excellent treatment results can also be

Table 1 Cancer of Unknown Primary Site

HISTOPATHOLOGY	CLINICAL EVALUATION (IN ADDITION TO HISTORY, PHYSICAL EXAMINATION, BLOOD COUNTS, SERUM CHEMISTRIES, CHEST X-RAY FILM)	SPECIAL PATHOLOGIC STUDIES	SUBGROUPS WITH TREATABLE TUMORS	PROGNOSIS
Well-differentiated adenocarcinoma	CT scan of abdomen Men: acid phosphatase Women: mammogram Additional radiologic studies to evaluate abnormal symptoms, signs, laboratory values	Men: Prostate specific antigen (immunoperoxidase); Women: Estrogen receptor, progesterone receptor	Women with axillary node metastasis Women with peritoneal carcinomatosis Men with blastic bone metastasis	Poor for entire group (median survival 4 months) Better for treatable subgroups
Poorly differentiated carcinoma and adenocarcinoma	CT abdomen, chest Serum hCG, AFP Additional radiologic studies to evaluate abnormal symptoms, signs, laboratory values	Immunoperoxidase staining Electron microscopy	Atypical germ-cell tumors (identified by chromosomal study only) Neuroendocrine tumors Predominant tumor location in mediastinum, retroperitoneum, lymph nodes	Treatment results similar to extragonadal germ-cell tumors Variable; about 15% curable with cisplatin-based chemotherapy; many others receive useful palliation
Squamous carcinoma (cervical lymph nodes)	Direct laryngoscopy with visualization of nasopharynx Fiberoptic bronchoscopy		Nodes located in high or mid cervical region	30–50% long-term survival with radical surgery and/or radiotherapy

AFP, alpha-fetoprotein; hCG, human chorionic gonadotropin.

achieved in women who have previous oophorectomy or normal ovaries. Therapy should include laparotomy with maximal surgical cytoreduction, followed by combination chemotherapy known to be useful for ovarian carcinoma. With optimal treatment, median survival in this group is about 2 years, with 15 percent achieving long-term disease-free survival.

Men with blastic bone metastases, elevated serum PSA, or tumor staining with PSA should be suspected of having prostate adenocarcinoma. Hormonal therapy may provide effective palliation.

For the remainder of patients with metastatic adenocarcinoma of unknown primary site, treatment is relatively ineffective. This is not surprising, since the majority of these patients have primary sites in either the lung or the gastrointestinal tract, which are relatively unresponsive to systemic therapy. Treatment with a variety of chemotherapeutic agents, used either singly or in combination, produces low response rates (5 to 30 percent) and has little impact on the short median survival, 3 to 6 months. Regimens with partial response rates of 20 to 30 percent include 5-fluorouracil-doxorubicin-mitomycin C and cisplatin-etoposide. Responses with these regimens are usually partial and persist for only a few months. Although a brief trial of such treatment is reasonable, it is also appropriate to treat these patients with symptomatic care alone, particularly if they are elderly or debilitated.

SQUAMOUS CARCINOMA OF UNKNOWN PRIMARY SITE

Squamous carcinoma accounts for approximately 5 percent of cancers of unknown primary site, and usually presents in either cervical or inguinal lymph nodes. Effective treatment is available for some of these patients, and appropriate evaluation is important.

Cervical lymph nodes are the most common metastatic site for squamous carcinoma of unknown primary. Patients are usually middle-aged or elderly and have a history of substantial tobacco use. Patients with squamous carcinoma in upper or mid cervical lymph nodes should be suspected of having a primary tumor in the head and neck region. They should have thorough examination of the oropharynx, nasopharynx, hypopharynx, larynx, and upper esophagus by direct laryngoscopy, with biopsy of any suspicious areas. Patients with squamous carcinoma involving the lower cervical or supraclavicular lymph nodes are more likely to have lung cancer, and fiberoptic bronchoscopy is indicated if the head and neck examination and chest radiograph are unrevealing.

For patients with no identified primary site, treatment should be given to the involved neck. Similar treatment results have been obtained with radical neck dissection, high-dose radiotherapy, or a combination of these modalities. Since occult primaries in the head and neck region became manifest in up to 40 percent of patients treated in the neck dissection colony, radiation therapy (including the hypopharynx and larynx) should be included in the treatment plan. In patients with high or mid cervical adenopathy, 3 year survival after such treatment ranges from 35 to 60 percent. These patients probably have clinically undetectable primaries in the head and neck, which are effectively treated with the local metastatic disease. Long-term survival is poor for patients with lower cervical or supraclavicular adenopathy, probably because most of these patients have lung cancer. However, a small group (10 to 15 percent) achieve long-term survival after local treatment to the cervical area.

Squamous carcinoma appearing in inguinal lymph nodes usually arises from primaries in the genital or anorectal areas. Women should undergo careful examinations of the vulva, vagina, and cervix, with biopsy of any suspicious areas. Men should have careful inspection of the penis. The anorectal area should be examined by digital examination and anoscopy in both sexes, with biopsy of suspicious areas. Finding a primary site in these patients is important, since therapy of carcinomas of the vulva, vagina, cervix, and anus may be curative even after spread to regional lymph nodes.

Metastatic squamous carcinoma in other visceral sites almost always represents metastatic lung cancer. The clinician should be suspicious of the diagnosis of poorly differentiated squamous carcinoma, particularly if other clinical features are unusual for lung cancer (i.e., young patient, nonsmoker, unusual metastatic site). Additional pathologic evaluation with immunoperoxidase studies or electron microscopy should be considered, and a trial of therapy as described later for patients with poorly differentiated carcinoma should be considered. If clinical features suggest the possibility of a lung cancer, computed tomography of the chest and fiberoptic bronchoscopy are appropriate.

■ POORLY DIFFERENTIATED CARCINOMA OF UNKNOWN PRIMARY SITE

Approximately 35 percent of carcinomas of unknown primary site have a poorly differentiated histology. In the past patients with this diagnosis were not considered separately from the larger group with well-differentiated adenocarcinoma of unknown primary site and were assumed to have similar poor response to treatment and short survival. Increasing evidence indicates that these patients form a distinct group with respect to clinical features, tumor biology, and responsiveness to systemic therapy. All patients in this group should be carefully evaluated. Some have extremely responsive neoplasms, and some are curable with appropriate systemic therapy.

Clinical Characteristics

These patients are frequently younger than patients with well-differentiated adenocarcinoma of unknown primary site and often give a history of rapid progression of symptoms and have objective evidence of rapid tumor growth. Tumor in lymph nodes, mediastinum, and retroperitoneum is fairly common in this group, although many sites can be involved with metastases.

Pathology

Patients with a light microscopic diagnosis of poorly differentiated carcinoma should undergo additional pathologic study with immunoperoxidase staining and electron microscopy as described for patients with poorly differentiated neoplasms. These studies can suggest unsuspected diagnoses in up to 25 percent of this patient group, including some for which a specific therapy is available (e.g., lymphoma, neuroendocrine tumors. Ewing's tumor).

Diagnostic Evaluation

The initial diagnostic evaluation of these patients should be similar to that described for patients with adenocarcinoma of unknown primary site (Table 1). Computed tomography of the chest and abdomen should be performed because these tumors frequently involve the mediastinum and retroperitoneum. Measurement of the serum tumor markers human chorionic gonadotropin (hCG) and alpha-fetoprotein (AFP) is essential for all patients, since elevated levels of these substances suggest the diagnosis of a germ-cell tumor.

Treatment

When a specific diagnosis of a treatable neoplasm is made on the basis of specialized pathologic study, patients should be treated appropriately. In addition, patients with elevated levels of hCG or AFP should be treated with combination chemotherapy effective against germ-cell tumors, even if this histologic diagnosis cannot be made definitively.

The majority of patients in this group will have no diagnosis more specific than poorly differentiated carcinoma or poorly differentiated adenocarcinoma, and will have normal serum tumor markers. Some of these patients have highly responsive neoplasms, and up to 30 percent will have complete response to combination chemotherapy with intensive cisplatin-based regimens such as those used in the treatment of germ-cell tumors. Approximately 50 percent of the complete responders (15 percent of the entire group) have prolonged disease-free survival. Clinical features associated with chemotherapy responsiveness include location of tumor in the mediastinum, retroperitoneum, or lymph nodes as opposed to other visceral sites, and younger age. Chemotherapy-responsive tumors cannot always be reliably predicted using clinical and pathologic criteria; therefore, it is reasonable to give all patients in this group a trial of cisplatin-based chemotherapy. A trial of one or two courses should be followed by re-evaluation for response; responders should receive a total of four courses, while nonresponders should be removed from treatment.

A subset of patients have neuroendocrine features identified only by electron microscopy or immunoperoxidase staining. The nature of these tumors is unclear; some patients may have unrecognized small cell lung cancer, but approximately 50 percent of patients in this group are nonsmokers, making the diagnosis of small cell lung cancer unlikely. Although optimal therapy for these patients is undefined, a high response rate can be achieved using cisplatin-based chemotherapy. Some achieve complete response to therapy, and a small percentage are long-term survivors.

Suggested Reading

Greco FA, Vaughn WK, Hainsworth JD. Advanced poorly differentiated carcinoma of unknown primary site: Recognition of a treatable syndrome. Ann Intern Med 1986; 104:547.

Hainsworth JD, Greco FA. Treatment of patients with cancer of an unknown primary site. N Engl J Med 1993; 329:257–263.

Hainsworth JD, Johnson DH, Greco FA. Poorly differentiated neuroendocrine carcinoma of unknown primary site: A newly recognized clinicopathologic entity. Ann Intern Med 1988; 109:364–372.

Hainsworth JD, Johnson DH, Greco FA. Cisplatin-based combination chemotherapy in the treatment of poorly differentiated carcinoma and poorly differentiated adenocarcinoma of unknown primary site: Results of a 12-year experience. J Clin Oncol 1992; 10:912–922.

Patel J, Nemoto T, Rosner D, et al. Axillary lymph node metastasis from an occult breast cancer. Cancer 1981; 47:2923–2930.

HODGKIN'S DISEASE: CHEMOTHERAPY

Gianni Bonadonna, M.D.

Over the past quarter of a century, treatment of Hodgkin's disease has evolved considerably through innovations in the management of various stages. The impact of various treatments on the 5, 10, and 15 year results is being balanced against delayed morbidity, such as organ damage (e.g. heart, lung) and second malignancies, produced by the intensity of therapy or the prolonged delivery of given drugs.

Certain procedures and indications that were routine in the past decade (e.g., staging laparotomy, primary radiotherapy for almost all subsets of patients with nodal disease, a single polydrug regimen such as nitrogen mustard, vincristine, procarbazine, and prednisone, or MOPP) should now find more flexible applications. In fact, multiple trials have produced a variety of treatment options, and most of them appear relatively good. In other words, in many disease stages there is a choice of treatments rather than a treatment of choice. Their merits and demerits will find an important component in the cost-benefit ratio.

Experience confirms that the complexity of clinical evaluation and the modern, sophisticated treatment modalities demand considerable technical resources and qualified personnel. Practicing physicians should therefore carefully and honestly evaluate whether their own experience and the facilities available to them are adequate. If not, referral of patients to specialized centers remains a wise professional response. I cannot foresee a departure from complex treatment programs for the next decade or so. The treatment of Hodgkin's disease is not ready as yet to be relegated to the care of a single physician in his private office or local hospital.

■ DIAGNOSIS AND STAGING

The ideal method of establishing or confirming a pathologic diagnosis of Hodgkin's disease is excision biopsy of one or more enlarged lymph nodes. This procedure also provides sufficient material for immunophenotyping and cytogenetic studies as well as long-term storage. Aspiration cytology and drill biopsies have generally been thought to be unrewarding and unreliable because the amount of tissue obtained is limited and there may be significant cellular trauma and distortion of the architecture. Also, the possibility of sampling error increases in an inverse relationship with the size of the sample. Although in experienced hands the diagnostic accuracy of fine-needle aspiration in diagnosing Hodgkin's disease can be as high as 90 percent, subtype classification can be assigned in only about 60 percent of cases.

The staging of patients with malignancy is a fundamental principle in cancer therapy. The systematic documentation of the extent of disease provides information that physicians use to make appropriate treatment decisions, delineate prognosis, and continue research. The staging of Hodgkin's disease is not new. Over the years, changes have been made along the information provided by given diagnostic methods, namely lymphangiography, laparotomy, bone marrow biopsies, and new imaging techniques. In 1965 the four-stage system was proposed by Peters in 1950. In 1965 the four-stage Rye classification distinguished nodal disease above and below the diaphragm as defined by lymphangiography (stage III) from disease that has extended to involve extranodal tissues (stage IV). The Ann Arbor classification (1971) took into consideration the contribution of staging laparotomy and splenectomy if subsequent management could be influenced by findings from these procedures. Within less than 2 decades from the Ann Arbor classification several changes in the management of Hodgkin's disease have taken place. In particular, important prognostic criteria have been recognized, with bulky lymphoma and multiple sites of disease affecting the outlook adversely, if such patients are treated with radiation alone. Also, computed tomography (CT) and magnetic resonance imaging (MRI) have been introduced. Both have been demonstrated to be accurate and efficient imaging techniques in staging and should be legitimized as staging procedures.

During a meeting organized at Cotswolds, England, in 1986 it was decided to retain the general framework of the Ann Arbor classification, extending it to define bulky lymphoma and subdividing pathologic stage III disease into substages III_1 and III_2. Also the clinical criteria for hepatic and splenic involvement were tightened (Table 1). Furthermore, the Cotswolds meeting addressed the question of post-treatment evaluation and in particular recognized the

Table 1 The Cotswolds Stage Classification

STAGE I:
Involvement of a single lymph node region or lymphoid structure (e.g., spleen, thymus, Waldeyer's ring)
STAGE II:
Involvement of two or more lymph node regions on the same side of the diaphragm (the mediastinum is a single site; hilar lymph nodes are lateralized). The number of anatomic sites should be indicated by a suffix, e.g., II_3
STAGE III:
Involvement of lymph node regions or structures on both sides of the diaphragm
III_1: With or without splenic hilar, celiac, or portal nodes
III_2: With para-aortic, iliac, mesenteric nodes
STAGE IV:
Involvement of extranodal site(s) beyond that designated *E:*
A: No systemic symptoms
B: Fever, drenching sweats, weight loss >10% of body weight
X: Bulky disease: mediastinal mass greater than one-third the widest internal diameter of the thorax, or >10 cm maximum dimension of nodal mass
E: Involvement of a single extranodal site, contiguous or proximal to known nodal site
CS: Clinical stage
PS: Pathologic stage

difficult situation of persisting minor radiologic abnormality in a patient in otherwise normal health and without clinical evidence of lymphoma. In this situation the outcome should be designated as CRU (unconfirmed or uncertain complete remission).

■ CLINICAL EVALUATION

CT scanning is recommended for all new patients. Several studies have demonstrated that 10 to 20 percent of lymphoma cases are upstaged after CT scanning compared with plain chest radiography, and the management is altered in up to 60 percent of patients. In fact, CT has greater accuracy in detecting parenchymal abnormalities, pericardial involvement, chest wall involvement, and retrocardiac nodes. MRI appears superior to CT in the post-treatment evaluation of residual radiologic abnormalities in the mediastinum. Abnormal widening of mediastinum consistent with radiation fibrosis may persist for many years. Although the role of gallium-67 scanning in the staging of Hodgkin's disease has yet to be clearly defined, it is very useful for evaluating mediastinal disease and posttreatment assessment.

Bipedal lymphangiography remains the most accurate method to provide information on retroperitoneal node distribution and architecture. Indeed, the difficult aspect of evaluating Hodgkin's disease is to distinguish the lymphoma neoplastic process from a benign inflammatory process. Distortion of nodal architecture due to replacement is a reliable sign of tumor involvement, but false-positive findings may result from a benign replacement by fat, fibrosis, or reactive hyperplasia and may be as high as 12 percent. The advent of CT has made it easier to detect intra-abdominal disease. This noninvasive procedure is easier to administer and less labor intensive than bipedal lymphangiography. It is also better at defining celiac, retrocrural, splenic, renal, hilar, and porta hepatis nodes. Schematically, it is assumed that lymph nodes of more than 1.5 cm cross-sectional diameter in the abdomen and pelvis are unequivocally abnormal on CT scanning and represent Hodgkin's disease, even though there is a risk of false-positives. For smaller nodes within the abdomen, lymphangiography may clearly be helpful. Today, only a few research institutions continue to do lymphangiograms. Although we are losing information from this decision, it can be expected that CT and MRI will ultimately replace lymphangiography as well as staging laparotomy by the end of this decade.

The CT or MRI scan also provides detailed information about the liver and spleen, which are involved at diagnosis in 4 to 5 percent and 20 to 30 percent, respectively. However, splenic involvement (multiple focal defects) has not been reliably and accurately predicted by CT or MRI, radioisotope, or ultrasound scans. Recent reports suggest that the accuracy of MRI may be significantly enhanced by the use of a new contrast agent, superparamagnetic iron oxide, which causes a change in splenic magnetic resonance signal intensity.

Bone disease at presentation is uncommon but may be present at some time in the course of disease in up to 20 percent of patients. Isotope bone scans using radiolabeled technetium (^{99}Tc) pyrophosphate or ^{99}Tc methylene diphosphonate are very sensitive; specificity can be enhanced by using another imaging technique to support the isotope scan finding.

The laboratory investigations listed in Table 2 may not necessarily contribute directly to staging. However, they may influence treatment modification and guide further investigations to other possible sites of disease.

Most of these studies should be repeated after the initial treatment to assess the status of complete remission properly or restaging in the presence of a single recurrence. Once the patients have been determined to be free of Hodgkin's disease, follow-up examinations are recommended every 2 to 3 months for the first year, with physical examinations, chest radiographs, and abdominal radiographs for patients who have had a prior lymphangiogram. In addition to routine laboratory tests, determining sequential erythrocyte sedimentation rate and serum lactate dehydrogenase levels are helpful in following patients with Hodgkin's disease. A serial increase in either of these two laboratory tests from previously normal values is predictive of recurrent lymphoma. From

Table 2 Recommendations for the Diagnostic Evaluation of Patients with Hodgkin's Disease

I. Mandatory procedures
   A. Biopsy, with interpretation by a qualified pathologist
   B. History, with special attention to the presence and duration of fever, night sweats, and unexplained loss of 10% or more of body weight during previous 6 months
   C. Physical examination
   D. Hematology
      1. Complete blood cell count
      2. Absolute lymphocyte count
      3. Erythrocyte sedimentation rate at 1 hour
      4. Bone marrow biopsy (needle or open)
   E. Biochemistry
      1. Tests of liver and renal function
      2. Serum albumin, lactate dehydrogenase, calcium levels
   F. Radiographic examination
      1. Chest (posteroanterior and lateral)
      2. Computed tomography of the thorax
      3. Computed tomography of the abdomen and pelvis
      4. Lymphangiogram
II. Procedures under certain circumstances
   A. Other surgical procedures
      1. Laparotomy with splenectomy and nodal abdominal biopsies, if decisions regarding management are likely to be influenced
      2. Selective biopsy of any suspicious extranodal lesion(s)
      3. Cytologic examination of any effusion
   B. Other imaging techniques
      1. Ultrasonographic scanning
      2. Magnetic resonance imaging
      3. Isotope scanning (gallium, technetium)

time to time, patients in continuous complete remission should be carefully evaluated to rule out delayed iatrogenic morbidity (e.g., sterility, cardiac and pulmonary damage, second malignancies).

PROGNOSTIC INDICATORS

The results of clinical trials performed during the past 2 decades have allowed us to reconsider the various prognostic variables. The major unfavorable prognostic factor is tumor mass (e.g., bulky mediastinal lymphoma, multiple extranodal involvement, five or more splenic nodules). The biologic implications of large tumor volume have been extensively studied: the greater the tumor cell population, the more likely it is to contain significant numbers of various classes of drug-resistant cells. Modern clinical research should improve the correct assessment and even quantification of tumor volume. Disease progression while on chemotherapy or short-term complete remission despite intensive multiple drug regimens indicates poor prognosis because of primary cell resistance. In general, prognosis is inversely related to age, since children and young adults fare better than older people. In particular, patients older than 60 years often present with advanced disease and other medical problems that cause difficulties in the proper staging and treatment of their disease. Recent observations have confirmed that lymphocyte-depleted Hodgkin's disease is a rare but very aggressive form of lymphoma whose prognosis is still unfavorable because of widespread nodal and extranodal involvement. The presence of systemic (B) symptoms in general carries unfavorable prognostic significance, especially in patients with advanced disease. Patients with stage IIB disease appear to have an adverse prognosis when they manifest all three systemic symptoms; this finding is often associated with bulky mediastinal disease. Male patients almost always have a less favorable prognosis than do female patients.

PRINCIPLES OF MANAGEMENT

Although there is today a variety of treatment options for almost every disease stage, physicians should not forget these points: (1) Total tumor cell burden and optimal drug dose intensity will remain the most critical treatment variables. (2) Primary tumor cell resistance is the major stumbling block to all impeccably delivered chemotherapy regimens. Furthermore, because of the known limitations of radiotherapy alone in stages II and III and the risk that splenectomy could contribute to the incidence of fulminant infections and second malignancies, staging laparotomy is almost completely abandoned. Since also lymphangiography is falling into disuse, the decrease in intensity and accuracy of staging procedures will make combined modality treatment a necessity to ensure optimal results in terms of cure rate with the first treatment approach. However, it remains important to identify patients who would benefit from combined modality therapy. It may well be that in the future the preferred therapy for most patients with nodal Hodgkin's disease will use combined modality programs to avoid staging laparotomy with splenectomy and to reduce the cumulative doses of both irradiation and the most toxic chemotherapeutic agents.

Among the several polydrug regimens available for the treatment of Hodgkin's disease (Table 3), doxorubicin, bleomycin, vinblastine, and dacarbazine (ABVD) have been confirmed in recent years to be superior, alone or with irradiation, to the classical MOPP. The superiority of the ABVD regimen can be summarized as follows: comparatively high incidence and duration of complete remission, less severe myelosuppression allowing a more intensive dose administration of doxorubicin (Adriamycin) and vinblastine than mechlorethamine and procarbazine, and virtual absence of alkylating-induced sterility and acute leukemia. VBM (vinblastine, bleomycin, and methotrexate) combined with irradiation has been shown in a long-term experience at Stanford University to be practically devoid of sterility and leukemogenesis (see Table 3).

GUIDELINES TO PRIMARY TREATMENT

Stages IA and IIA with No Bulky Adenopathy

Treatment guidelines depend on whether physicians use staging laparotomy or not. After this surgical procedure, patients with supradiaphragmatic disease and no bulky mediastinum are treated with subtotal nodal irradiation delivered with high-energy equipment at conventional tumoricidal doses (involved areas, 40 to 44 Gy; uninvolved areas, 35 Gy). In rare cases (4 to 5 percent) with subdiaphragmatic nonbulky

Table 3 Commonly Used Drug Regimens in Hodgkin's Disease

DRUG REGIMEN	CONVENTIONAL DOSE* (MILLIGRAMS PER SQUARE METER OF BODY SURFACE AREA)	ROUTE	CYCLE DAYS*
ABVD			
Doxorubicin	25.0	Intravenous	1 and 15
Bleomycin	10.0	Intravenous	1 and 15
Vinblastine	6.0	Intravenous	1 and 15
Dacarbazine	375.0	Intravenous	1 and 15
MOPP			
Mechlorethamine	6.0	Intravenous	1 and 8
Vincristine	1.4	Intravenous	1 and 8
Procarbazine	100.0	Oral	1–14
Prednisone**	40.0	Oral	1–14
ChlVPP			
Chlorambucil	6.0	Oral	1–14
Vinblastine	6.0	Intravenous	1 and 8
Procarbazine	100.0	Oral	1–14
Prednisone	40.0	Oral	1–14
VBM			
Vinblastine	6.0	Intravenous	1 and 8
Bleomycin	10.0	Intravenous	1 and 8
Methotrexate	30.0	Intravenous	1 and 8
MOPP-ABVD in alternating monthly cycles	As for MOPP and ABVD above		
MOPP-ABV hybrid			
Mechlorethamine	6.0	Intravenous	1
Vincristine	1.4 (maximum, 2)	Intravenous	1
Procarbazine	100.0	Oral	1–7
Prednisone	40.0	Oral	1–14
Doxorubicin	35.0	Intravenous	8
Bleomycin	10.0	Intravenous	8
Vinblastine	6.0	Intravenous	8

*Each cycle lasts 28 days.
**During cycles 1 and 4.

Hodgkin's disease, radiotherapy is administered through an inverted Y field including the splenic pedicle in stage I and through total nodal irradiation (including the mediastinum) in stage II, respectively. With this strategy, if radiotherapy is impeccably delivered, the 20 year relapse-free survival (RFS) is about 65 to 70 percent; total survival following salvage chemotherapy in relapsing patients ranges from 80 to 95 percent. Late relapses, (i.e., 3 years or more after completion of radiotherapy) are 10 to 20 percent and are often related to technique; also, they occur more often in patients with stage I disease and a nodular sclerosis histology.

Treatment guidelines for patients not subjected to staging laparotomy are less well defined. A full course of MOPP chemotherapy was reported by the National Cancer Institute to yield relapse-free survival of 86 percent and a total survival of 92 percent at 10 years. Most clinicians now prefer to use a combined modality approach with radiotherapy limited to the involved nodal regions. The chemotherapy regimen of choice should exclude alkylating agents to reduce the risk of second malignancies and drug-related sterility. These combined programs are very effective and well tolerated, with a freedom from progression in the range of 95 percent whether four courses of primary ABVD (Milan Cancer Institute) or six radiation-adjuvant courses of VBM (Stanford University) are used.

Stages IB and IIB with No Bulky Adenopathy

Only in patients with true (i.e., after staging laparotomy) stage IB or IIB disease with a solitary systemic symptom, subtotal or total nodal radiotherapy can yield a 10 year RFS of about 80 percent. In contrast, in stage IIB patients presenting with all three systemic symptoms, prognosis following extensive radiotherapy alone is extremely poor, since the 5 year freedom from relapse is only about 40 percent. In this subset of patients with one or more systemic symptoms, laparotomy is no longer performed, and combined modality therapy is recommended. Treatment usually begins with 4 to 6 cycles of ABVD alone or alternated with MOPP (see Table 3), following which involved field radiotherapy (36 Gy) is delivered. Alternatively, the primary irradiation program can be followed by 6 courses of VBM chemotherapy.

Stages IIA and IIB with Bulky Adenopathy and Limited Extranodal Extension

All oncologists agree that this stage group should be managed with combined modality therapy. In general, patients present with multiple supradiaphragmatic nodal groups involved and may have extension of tumor into the lung, pericardium, or chest wall. Because effective combination chemotherapy is able to induce prompt tumor shrinkage of compressive symptoms from mediastinal-hilar adenopathy, medical treatment should precede irradiation: radiotherapy can be delivered as mantle or subtotal nodal irradiation including spleen once four to six cycles of the selected combination are completed (i.e., ABVD or MOPP alternated with ABVD). With this strategy most patients begin the radiation program in complete or almost complete clinical remission, thus avoiding cardiac and pulmonary sequelae following high-dose primary irradiation of huge mediastinal-hilar adenopathy. With a combined modality approach, both 5 to 10 year RFS and survival rates are over 75 percent.

Stage IIIA

There is still debate as to how to treat this subset of patients, which includes various prognostic subsets depending on the extent and the bulkiness of disease. If after careful surgical staging patients with Cotswolds stage IA or IIA show histologic involvement limited to the lymphatic structures in the upper abdomen that accompany the celiac-axis group of arteries (substage III_1), subtotal or total nodal irradiation may still be the treatment of choice in the absence of bulky adenopathy and extensive splenic involvement. In fact, the overall survival results, inclusive of salvage chemotherapy for relapsing patients, are comparable with those reported with Peters stage IIA.

The controversy arises when there is involvement of low para-aortic nodes and iliac nodes (substage III_2). The results of numerous trials of systemic drug therapy when the lymphographic patterns appear typical for retroperitoneal node involvement have prompted clinicians to avoid staging laparotomy and to use combination chemotherapy with or without radiotherapy. A once-common approach was total nodal irradiation followed by chemotherapy, usually six cycles of MOPP, but this form of treatment carried a high risk of acute leukemia even if irradiation was limited to involved fields. A more recent approach consists first in the delivery of three to four cycles of ABVD chemotherapy to be followed by total nodal irradiation with 30 to 36 Gy if the patient achieves complete or almost complete remission after drug therapy. This approach is particularly useful in patients with extensive Hodgkin's disease and in the presence of bulky mediastinal or para-aortic nodes. In the experience of the Milan Cancer Institute, three cycles of ABVD delivered before and after radiotherapy yielded superior 10-year results (RFS 97 percent, survival 80 percent) to those of MOPP plus radiotherapy (RFS 64 percent, survival 63 percent) and was devoid of leukemogenesis and irreversible gonadal dysfunction. The frequency of solid tumors was about the same between the two drug combinations. As far as comparative delayed toxicity was concerned, no clinical or laboratory studies detected signs of doxorubicin-related myocardial damage. The ABVD group showed more radiation fibrosis than MOPP group (59 percent versus 30 percent). This finding occurred particularly during the last three cycles of bleomycin-containing chemotherapy.

In light of contemporary concepts about drug-resistant tumor cells, it appears highly questionable whether further chemotherapy with the same drug regimen after completion of the irradiation program is strategically important to influence the duration of complete remission. On the contrary, chemotherapy after extensive irradiation must often be delivered in low-dose regimens because of prolonged myelosuppression and may increase the incidence of treatment-related sequelae. To make combined treatment more tolerable, one should limit the radiation program to involved fields or even to the bulky sites of lymphoma. Also, the radiotherapy dose to the mediastinum should not exceed 36 Gy in complete responders to avoid or limit delayed cardiac complications.

Many investigators have not found that in randomized trials the superior freedom from progression or the RFS achieved with combined treatment over chemotherapy alone translated into a significant advantage in terms of total survival. However, detailed comparative analysis of prognostic subsets prevents today a firm conclusion on the real equivalence between a combined modality approach and impeccably delivered chemotherapy. Because recurrences often occur in previously involved nodal sites, irradiation of the mediastinum, if initially bulky, appears indicated.

Stage IIIB

The treatment options are similar to those for stage $IIIA_2$. Modern chemotherapy regimens often involve ABVD, MOPP alternated with ABVD, or MOPP-ABV (doxorubicin, bleomycin, vinblastine), a hybrid regimen. Six cycles are sufficient to achieve complete remission in about 90 percent of cases. Most clinicians supplement drug therapy with irradiation to the site(s) of initial bulky lymphoma. In the experience of the Milan Cancer Institute with ABVD followed by extensive irradiation, complete remission was documented in 94 percent; the 10 year results yielded an RFS of 78 percent and total survival of 81 percent, respectively.

Stages IVA and IVB

This group is best managed with intensive full-dose combination chemotherapy. However, it is possible that irradiation limited to the site(s) of initial bulky disease can further improve the long-term RFS.

During the past decade, MOPP alternated with ABVD was shown by the Milan Cancer Institute to be superior to MOPP alone in terms of complete remission (89 versus 74 percent), 10 year freedom from progression (61 versus 37 percent), RFS (68 versus 46 percent), and total survival (69 versus 58 percent). In particular, the superiority of alternating chemotherapy was evident in the subsets known to be prognostically unfavorable or less affected by MOPP chemotherapy (i.e. age over 40 years, systemic symptoms, nodular sclerosis, and bulky lymphoma). Comparable results were achieved by the American Intergroup, the Canadian hybrid regimen (MOPP-ABV) and by ABVD alone as tested by Cancer and Acute Leukemia Group B.

It is important to administer chemotherapy through six to eight cycles with the appropriate dose intensity unless peripheral leukocytes are below 3,500 per millimeter cubed and/or platelets below 100,000 per millimeter cubed, respectively, on the planned day of drug administration. In this case physicians can decide whether to delay therapy for a few days or continue chemotherapy, reducing temporarily by 50 percent the dose of myelosuppressive drugs such as mechlorethamine, procarbazine, doxorubicin, and vinblastine. Vomiting and alopecia are more frequent and severe after ABVD than MOPP, and severe neurotoxicity is more often detected after MOPP. To decrease the incidence and degree of vomiting,

Canadian investigators have deleted dacarbazine from their hybrid regimen (MOPP-ABV).

■ SALVAGE CHEMOTHERAPY

Patients who are candidates for salvage chemotherapy can be divided into four groups: those failing on primary radiotherapy, those with advanced disease who have not achieved a complete remission, those with complete remission that lasts less than 12 months, and those who relapse after a remission of 12 months or more.

Relapse from Primary Radiotherapy

After proper restaging, further irradiation can be delivered, if technically feasible, to patients with marginal or true recurrence followed by combination chemotherapy. The response to chemotherapy is as good as that of patients with newly diagnosed lymphoma of the same disease extent. Recent results indicate that doxorubicin-containing regimens (ABVD, MOPP-ABVD) can yield superior results to those of MOPP. Chemotherapy should be administered for a minimum of six cycles or to complete tumor remission plus two consolidation cycles.

Relapse After a Year

If the first complete remission lasts longer than 12 months, re-treatment with the original drug regimen or a program that does not involve cross-resistance remains the standard approach; it can yield a second complete remission in about 80 percent of patients, and in most cases remission is durable.

Relapse in Resistant Patients

Most patients who do not attain complete remission following adequately delivered chemotherapy and those with complete remission lasting less than 12 months are considered resistant to conventional drug programs. Although treatment with non–cross-resistant drugs such as six cycles administered monthly of CEP (lomustine, or CCNU, 80 mg per meter squared orally on day 1, etoposide 100 mg per meter squared orally or intravenously days 1 through 5, prednimustine 60 mg per meter squared orally days 1 through 5 or the equivalent dose of chlorambucil and prednisone) can be tried. However, objective tumor response occurs in only 40 percent of patients, complete durable remissions are rare, and the 5 year survival is about 20 percent. Thus, in these resistant tumors, a program of high-dose chemotherapy with autologous stem cell or bone marrow transplantation is indicated.

Bone Marrow Transplantation

In recent years intensive (myeloablative) chemotherapy followed by the reinfusion of autologous bone marrow and/or circulating progenitor cells has been applied to patients with advanced Hodgkin's disease in relapse or refractory to first or second line chemotherapy. Several drug regimens are being tested in the United States and Europe with the support of hematopoietic growth factors. At present this promising form of salvage therapy, which confirms the importance of the drug dose, remains experimental; patients should be referred to specialized centers for proper evaluation and treatment. The experience of the Milan Cancer Institute in resistant Hodgkin's disease has been favorable without treatment-induced mortality. Schematically, drug treatment includes cyclophosphamide (7 g per meter squared) followed sequentially by vincristine plus high-dose methotrexate, etoposide, total body irradiation (10 Gy) and high-dose melphalan. In patients relapsing within 12 months following complete remission after MOPP, ABVD or MOPP-ABVD, the results at 6 years revealed a RFS of 78 percent. It is quite possible that in the future the indications to use this new intensive approach will be further expanded to other patient subsets and total body irradiation replaced by involved field radiotherapy to minimize the risk of treatment-induced morbidity, including second malignancies.

■ TREATMENT-RELATED MORBIDITY

The most serious consequence of curative therapy for Hodgkin's disease is second malignancies. Most common among these are acute nonlymphocytic leukemia, myelodysplastic syndromes including preleukemia, and diffuse aggressive non-Hodgkin's lymphomas. In patients treated with MOPP or one of its variants, i.e., treatment including alkylating agents, procarbazine, or nitrosourea derivatives (BCNU, CCNU), the risk of leukemia within 10 years is 3 to 4 percent. This risk seems to be increased when patients are subjected to splenectomy or are older than 40 years at the time of systemic treatment and when combined treatment modality is used, especially if salvage MOPP is given after irradiation failure (over 15 percent). The overall risk of non-Hodgkin's lymphomas is about 2 percent. The risk of developing a secondary solid tumor is continuing to increase beyond 10 years (a finding not seen with leukemia), and the risk is highest in older patients; approximately two-thirds of the tumors have occurred so far in the radiotherapy field. Since the selection of agents may be important (ABVD does not appear to be as toxic as MOPP in terms of the development of secondary leukemias), the accrual of more data from patients who receive alternate drug regimens is essential in assessing the relative carcinogenicity of the treatment modalities.

Gonadal dysfunction is another important iatrogenic toxicity that considerably affects the quality of life in patients with Hodgkin's disease. A few cycles of MOPP or MOPP-like combinations induce azoospermia in 90 to 100 percent of patients, and this finding is associated with germinal hyperplasia and increased follicle-stimulating hormone levels, with normal levels of luteinizing hormone and testosterone. In addition, only 10 to 20 percent of patients eventually show recovery of spermatogenesis after long periods, even up to 10 years. Following MOPP alternated with ABVD the incidence of permanent azoospermia is about 50 percent. About half of women become amenorrheic, and premature ovarian failure appears to depend on age (over 30 years, 75 to 85 percent; under 30 years, about 20 percent). This is most probably related to the total dose of drugs and is a progressive rather than an all-or-none phenomenon. The Milan Cancer Institute has reported that the administration of ABVD chemotherapy produces only a limited and transient germ cell toxicity in men and no drug-induced amenorrhea. Thus, to circumvent chemotherapy-induced sterility, the use of drug regimens not containing alkylating agents, procarbazine, or nitrosourea derivatives is highly recommended. An alternative for men undergoing MOPP or MOPP-ABVD is represented by sperm storage prior to chemotherapy; however, both physicians and patients should be aware that about one-third of male patients with Hodgkin's disease have low sperm count or sperm motility before starting cytotoxic treatment. The usefulness of the administration of analogues of gonadotropin-releasing hormone in men or oral contraceptives in premenopausal women remains to be fully confirmed. Libido tends to decrease after both the diagnosis of Hodgkin's disease and treatment with combination chemotherapy. There is no evidence of teratogenicity in patients treated for Hodgkin's disease.

Pericarditis, both acute and chronic, is the most common symptomatic cardiovascular complication of mediastinal irradiation. The incidence of pericarditis is related to the dose, dose rate, and volume irradiated. Clinically evident pericarditis occurs in about 15 percent following anteroposterior fields from a linear accelerator to a mean mediastinal dose of 44 Gy. Pericardial effusions develop in 25 to 30 percent of patients within 2 years of irradiation. Surgical stripping of the pericardium remains the only definitive therapy for chronic constrictive pericarditis. Radiation-induced myocardial fibrosis at the subclinical level occurs in over 50 percent of irradiated patients. Those who receive mediastinal irradiation of 40 to 44 Gy, particularly children and adolescents, run an increased risk of death from coronary artery and other cardiac diseases. Chronic cardiomyopathy may occur after anthracycline administration if the cumulative dose of doxorubicin exceeds 400 to 450 mg per meter squared. Careful cardiac screening of treated patients is now highly recommended, for high-dose mediastinal irradiation can predispose to premature coronary artery disease, and this risk may be further increased by the administration of anthracyclines.

Acute irradiation pneumonitis and chronic restrictive fibrosis are the most important pulmonary complications of mantle irradiation. Both are related to the total dose, dose rate, and volume of lung tissue irradiated. The overall incidence is about 20 percent. Patients with relapsed Hodgkin's disease who receive total body irradiation in preparation for bone marrow transplantation are also at risk for pneumonitis. The drugs with greatest potential for pulmonary toxicity are bleomycin and BCNU. In patients treated with ABVD followed by radiotherapy, overt bleomycin-related lung toxicity is uncommon, and no pulmonary damage was seen in patients given MOPP alternated with ABVD.

Suggested Reading

Bonadonna G. Modern treatment of malignant lymphomas: A multidisciplinary approach? The Kaplan Memorial Lecture. Ann Oncol 1994; 5(Suppl 2):55–S16.

Canellos GP, Anderson JR, Propert KJ, et al. Chemotherapy of Hodgkin's disease with MOPP, ABVD, or MOPP alternating with ABVD. N Engl J Med 1992; 327:1478–1484.

De Vita VT Jr, Hubbard SM. Hodgkin's disease. N Engl J Med 1993; 328: 560–565.

Gianni AM, Siena S, Bregni M, et al. Prolonged disease-free survival after high-dose sequential (HDS) polychemotherapy in poor prognosis Hodgkin's disease: A 6-year update. Ann Oncol 1993;4: 889–891.

Hancock SL, Donaldson SS, Hoppe RT. Cardiac disease following treatment of Hodgkin's disease in children and adolescents. J Clin Oncol 1993; 11:1208–1215.

Lister TA, Crowther D, Sutcliffe SB, et al. Report of a committee convened to discuss the evaluation and staging of patients with Hodgkin's disease: Cotswolds meeting. J Clin Oncol 1989; 7:1630–1636.

LOW-GRADE NON-HODGKIN'S LYMPHOMA: CHEMOTHERAPY

Antonio Ucar, M.D.
Peter A. Cassileth, M.D.

The non-Hodgkin's lymphomas are an extremely heterogeneous group of neoplasms whose clinical course varies by histologic type. Over the past decades several pathologic classifications have been proposed to categorize these entities by their morphologic appearance, lymph node architecture, cell of origin, or immunophenotype. Pathologists and clinicians have had difficulty translating the different subtypes from one classification to another. A working formulation was therefore developed to allow such translation. It generated three major categories that grouped 10 histologic subtypes by differences in survival. The three groupings are low, intermediate, and high grade, which correlate with their respective favorable, intermediate, or unfavorable prognosis for survival. The low-grade lymphomas comprise three histologic subtypes: small lymphocytic (SLL), follicular small cleaved (FSCL), and follicular mixed small and large cell (FML). These correlate with the older Rappaport classification of diffuse lymphocytic well-differentiated (DLWD), nodular lymphocytic poorly differentiated (NLPD), and nodular mixed lymphoma (NML), respectively. This chapter focuses on the chemotherapeutic management of these low-grade or indolent lymphomas. Early studies often included other histologic subtypes under the heading of favorable lymphomas, including follicular large cell (nodular histiocytic lymphoma) and diffuse small cleaved (diffuse lymphocytic poorly differentiated). These latter subtypes, now classed with the intermediate-grade lymphomas, are not discussed here.

The histopathologic diagnosis and classification of lymphoid neoplasms is constantly being re-evaluated. An International Lymphoma Study Group has proposed the REAL (Revised European-American Lymphoma) classification of lymphomas which emphasizes B and T cell immunophenotyping, thereby creating an expanded histologic roster. Within this modified classification, lymphoplasmacytoid lymphomas, mantle zone lymphoma, marginal zone lymphoma, and MALT lymphomas are being considered for inclusion among the low-grade subtypes. Detailed assessment of the chemotherapy of these other lymphomas is not discussed here. Mantle zone lymphoma is often moderately aggressive rather than low-grade in clinical behavior, and extensive clinical studies of the treatment of these relatively recently defined subtypes are not yet available. Moreover, this histopathologic categorization of immunophenotypes requires validation as representing significantly different clinical entities.

The low-grade lymphomas as a group have a median survival of approximately 7 years. This compares favorably with the median survival of the intermediate- and high-grade lymphomas of 2.5 and 1 year, respectively. The plot of relapse-free survival after chemotherapy-induced remission shows other differences between these groups. The relapse curve has an early constant slope in the low-grade lymphomas. The more aggressive subtypes display biphasic curves with a pattern of early relapse associated with short survival followed by a plateau and only rare relapses after 3 to 4 years. In low-grade lymphomas, remissions invariably are followed by relapses, the degree of response to chemotherapy (partial versus complete responses) does not correlate with survival, and cures are rare. In contrast, the intensive treatment of the more aggressive lymphomas leads to durable remissions and cures in a substantial proportion of patients.

■ INCIDENCE AND NATURAL HISTORY

An estimated 43,000 new cases of non-Hodgkin's lymphoma (NHL) were diagnosed in the United States in 1993. Of the low-grade lymphomas, FSCL is the most common, comprising approximately 20 to 25 percent of all NHL. The FML histologic type comprises 10 percent of all NHL and is twice as frequent as SLL. The median age of patients at diagnosis is 50 to 60 years. It is rare for the indolent lymphomas to present within the first 2 decades of life.

Low-grade lymphomas typically present with progressive, nontender lymph node enlargement, usually slowly increasing in size over months to years, at times achieving significant bulk. Some patients exhibit waxing and waning lymph node size. As will be discussed later, more than 75 percent of patients present with disseminated disease, either stage III or IV. Bone marrow and liver are the most commonly involved extralymphatic sites.

An important biologic feature of the low-grade lymphomas is their tendency to become clinically more aggressive with time. This can occur without a change in histologic pattern, but in approximately one-third of patients it is associated with histologic transformation to intermediate or high-grade subtypes. All follicular lymphomas have a tendency to progress from a purely follicular to a follicular and diffuse pattern of growth; more important, they progress to lymphomas of higher histologic grade by an increase in the fraction of tumor cells that are large, with an attendant acceleration in aggressiveness. In one study, 94 percent of the patients with the initial diagnosis of follicular lymphoma who died with lymphoma had only diffuse lymphoma at autopsy; only 6 percent of the patients' lymphomas had maintained the original follicular pattern. Clinical and histologic transformation are marked by decreased responsiveness to chemotherapy, and the median survival from the time of transformation is less than 1 year.

■ DIAGNOSIS

Although subtypes of NHL are classified on the basis of morphologic criteria alone, further characterization of the low-grade lymphomas by surface marker, molecular, or chromosomal analysis is frequently performed. The malignant cells almost invariably originate from B cells. Southern blot analysis with probes for the immunoglobulin genes demonstrates rearrangements consistent with a monoclonal B cell population. Chromosomal analysis of the follicular lymphomas reveals the presence of the t(14;18) translocation in approximately 85 percent of patients. Cloning of the t(14;18) break points (involving the bcl-2 proto-oncogene on chromosome 18 and the immunoglobulin heavy-chain locus on chromosome 14) has made it possible to identify lymphoma cells containing this translocation by oligonucleotide probes and to amplify by the polymerase chain reaction (PCR) the detection of minimal residual disease in bone marrow and peripheral blood.

Staging of the low-grade lymphomas is usually based on clinical evaluation without laparotomy, using the Ann Arbor classification devised for Hodgkin's disease. At presentation more than 50 percent of patients demonstrate advanced stage of disease (III or IV). Of patients with clinical stage I or II who are subjected to staging laparotomy, 40 to 50 percent are found to have disease below the diaphragm. Among the three histologic subtypes of low-grade lymphoma, bone marrow involvement is most common in SLL and least common in FML, occurring in 79 and 30 percent of patients, respectively. Conversely, apparently localized disease occurs more frequently in FML, less often in FSCL, and rarely in SLL. Despite the frequent finding of advanced stage at presentation the low-grade lymphomas are associated with long survival. The extensive involvement at diagnosis appears to reflect the capacity of the small malignant lymphocytes to circulate and readily populate a wide variety of organs.

■ EARLY-STAGE DISEASE

Although this discussion focuses on the chemotherapeutic management of the low-grade lymphomas, it is important to note that primary radiotherapy may be the treatment of choice for stages I and II. Truly limited stage low-grade lymphoma occurs very infrequently. Local radiotherapy in doses of 3,500 to 4,000 cGy causes complete remission in virtually all such patients. With this approach 5 year disease-free survival ranges from 40 to 83 percent, and overall survival is 69 to 100 percent. In two studies with median follow-up greater than 5 years, late relapses are rare and survival curves

Table 1 Results of Therapy with Single Agents

DRUG	NO. OF PATIENTS	CR RATE (%)	PERCENT SURVIVAL (YEARS)	STUDY
CYT or CHL	38	40	50 at (2½‡)	Stanford
CYT	13	47	50 at (2½)	Minnesota
BCNU ± Pred vs CYT ± Pred*	97	47	83 at (2)	Eastern Cooperative Oncology Group
CHL	60	68	—	St. Bart's
CHL	67	65	50 at (3¾)	Capetown
CYT or CHL	17	64	60 at (4)	Stanford
CYT or CHL	20	55	90 at (2½)	Stanford
CHL†	33	33	60 at (5)	Yale
CYT + MED†	22	27	50 at (1¼)	St. Bart's
Weighted Mean		52		

CR, complete remission; CYT, cyclophosphamide; CHL, chlorambucil; MED, methylprednisolone; Pred, prednisone.
*Followed by randomization in CR to maintenance CHL or BCNU, CYT, PRED, and vincristine.
†High-dose pulse therapy.
‡Median survival of patients with FSCL; median survival was 20 months for patients with FML.

flatten, suggesting curability of limited disease after local radiotherapy. Extended-field ports do not provide better survival than generous involved-field irradiation. Younger patients with stage I disease fare better than older patients or patients with stage II disease. Few studies of the combination of chemotherapy and local irradiation in limited-stage low-grade lymphoma have been conducted. Some nonrandomized studies claim improved disease-free survival when systemic therapy is added to local radiotherapy, but they show no improvement in overall survival. A recent prospectively randomized study from the Memorial Sloan-Kettering Cancer Center failed to demonstrate an improvement in disease-free survival or overall survival when adjuvant chemotherapy was added to radiotherapy. The number of patients was small.

■ ADVANCED-STAGE DISEASE

For patients with stage III or IV and most patients with clinical stage II (representing 85 to 90 percent of the low-grade lymphomas), chemotherapy is the treatment of choice. Treatment regimens range from single alklyating agents to aggressive Adriamycin (doxorubicin) combination chemotherapy. An analysis of the literature does not define a clear chemotherapy program of choice for these patients; rather, one selects an optimal individual approach based upon clinical presentation and patient characteristics.

Single-agent alkylator chemotherapy is effective for low-grade lymphomas with minimal toxicity; therefore, it should be considered the standard against which newer approaches are evaluated. Table 1 summarizes the results of studies of single-agent therapy. The overall complete remission (CR) rate is 52 percent. Median survival varies from 20 months to more than 5 years and does not correlate with the frequency of CR induction. The variability in long-term outcome in different studies is due to variations in patient population. Patients with FSCL survive longer than patients with FML, and patients with asymptomatic disease live longer than symptomatic patients. Outcome will necessarily vary with the distribution of these and other characteristics. Because patients with low-grade lymphomas have long survival, lengthy follow-up is required to assess outcome accurately. This is especially problematic at the tail of the survival curve, when it may be possible to demonstrate a plateau (potential cures).

Most of the studies of single-agent therapy used relatively modest doses, usually a daily oral dose. The two studies at the bottom of Table 1 employed intermittent high-dose therapy (chlorambucil 80 mg per square meter over 5 days orally and cyclophosphamide 2.5 to 5 g per square meter over 5 days intravenously). A number of patients in these two trials had poor prognostic features contributing to the low CR rates. Nevertheless, single-agent alkylator therapy by intermittent high doses does not appear to have an advantage over modest daily oral doses. At the same time, the risks of alkylating agent–induced secondary acute leukemia may be lower after pulse therapy than after long-term chronic administration.

Detailed analysis of other single-agent alkylator therapy studies leads to the following conclusions: CR is achieved in more than one-half of treated patients; maximal benefit from low-dose therapy may require 9 to 12 months or more of treatment; and therapy is well tolerated with a minimum of side effects. After partial remission (PR) or CR is achieved and therapy is discontinued, a pattern of continuous relapse emerges. Finally, the response to therapy does not correlate with survival; patients in PR have the same survival as patients in CR.

In an attempt to improve on these results, combination chemotherapy has been extensively evaluated in the management of the low-grade lymphomas. Results from nonrandomized studies using cyclophosphamide, vincristine, and prednisone (CVP) are listed in Table 2. The addition of vincristine and prednisone to the alkylating agent cyclophosphamide in these regimens yields CR rates in the range of 60 to 80 percent, higher than those obtained with single-agent chemotherapy. Several randomized as well as nonrandomized trials comparing a CVP-type of regimen with single-agent alkylator therapy have been performed (Table 3). These studies fail to demonstrate a survival difference between CVP and single-agent therapy despite a higher CR rate and shorter time to CR with CVP therapy. Given the small number of

Table 2 Results of CVP Combination Chemotherapy

NO. OF PATIENTS	CR RATE (%)	PERCENT SURVIVAL (YEARS)
30	40	96 at 2
23	83	65 at 5
41	61	50 at 2½
31	50	73 at 2
37	54	60 at 5
Weighted Mean	57	

CVP, cyclophosphamide, vincristine, and prednisone.

Table 3 Results of Comparative Chemotherapy Trials

THERAPY	NO.	CR RATE (%)	PERCENT SURVIVAL (YEARS)
CHL		68	50 at (9)
vs	104	(P = <.01)	
CVP		89	
C-V-P		47	
vs	29	NS	50 at (2)
CVP		82	
CHL		13	
vs	66	NS	5 at (3)
CVP		37	
CHL		64	
vs	34	NS	72 at (2½)
CVP		88	
Weighted mean		73	

C-V-P, sequential administration of each drug singly after progression.
NS, not significant; CHL, chlorambucil; vs, randomized study.

Table 4 Results of Intensive Chemotherapy Programs

THERAPY	NO. OF PATIENTS	CR RATE (%)	PERCENT SURVIVAL (YEARS)
COP*P	34	50	—
COP*P	13	16	—
COP*P		56	70 at (5)
vs			
CP	128†	54	63 at (5)
vs			
BCVP		53	
COP*P		61	
vs			58 at (5)
CP	52‡	65	
vs			
BCVP		50	
BCVP	42	42	
CHOP-B*	16	62	72 at (2)
B*ACOP	11	82	
COPA		70	54 at (3)
vs			
CVP	41	65	69 at (5)
BCVP Mlp	35	88	90 at (5)
vs			
CHOP	415	64	35 at (10)

C, cyclophosphamide, O; vincristine; P, prednisone; P*, procarbazine; B, BCNU; H or A, doxorubicin; B*, bleomycin; Mlp, melphalan.
†Patients with FSCL in Eastern Cooperative Oncology Group study.
‡Patients with FML in Eastern Cooperative Oncology Group study.

patients in these studies, a modest but meaningful difference in survival may have been missed.

Attempts to improve response rates by means of chemotherapy combinations more intensive than CVP have generally been unsuccessful and have added toxicity. Unfortunately, few studies have been randomized. Table 4 lists the response rates to these regimens. The most common combinations employ CVP in conjunction with BCNU (BCVP), doxorubicin (CHOP), or procarbazine (COPP). The Eastern Cooperative Oncology Group study, randomizing patients to receive CP, COPP, or BCVP, found equivalent pathologically documented complete response rates of 54, 56, and 53 percent, respectively. Overall survival at 5 years was similar among all three groups, but progression-free survival was significantly better for the COPP regimen. Both BCVP and COPP were more toxic than CP and entailed significantly greater leukopenia, nausea, and vomiting. The same study included C2 patients with FML. In these patients, CP, COPP, and BCVP produced similar CR rates and no significant differences in disease-free or overall survival.

Although doxorubicin is an important component in the successful treatment of high-grade lymphomas, its value in the low-grade lymphomas is unclear because it has not been adequately evaluated in randomized trials. In a retrospective review of follicular lymphomas, including some patients with follicular large cell lymphoma who were treated at M.D. Anderson on several combination chemotherapy protocols over an 11 year period, a logistic regression model suggested that doxorubicin-containing regimens were associated with significantly better CR and overall survival. However, another partially randomized study from Paris comparing patients with FSCL treated with CVP with or without doxorubicin demonstrated no difference in response rates or survival. Other trials of intensive regimens adding bleomycin to doxorubicin and CVP have in small numbers of patients with low-grade lymphomas demonstrated that CR rates are in the range of 60 to 80 percent. However, a pattern of continuous relapse is still noted, and toxicity is significantly greater than with either CVP or single-agent therapy.

Increasing the intensity of chemotherapy by use of higher doses of individual agents in combination does speed the time to response and may even prolong the time to relapse. Peculiarly, however, and unlike most other cancers, these responses to treatment of patients with low-grade lymphomas do not translate into increased survival. Relapses still occur after CR, indicating persistence of the malignant clone of lymphocytes. There is no evidence that maintenance therapy after CR has a significant impact on overall survival. Biologically, survival is determined by the ultimate transformation of these lymphomas into clinically aggressive disease. Except perhaps for the FML subtype, which is discussed later, chemotherapy is by definition palliative.

Table 5 Randomized Trials of Chemotherapy Versus Radiation Therapy

TREATMENT	NO. OF PATIENTS	CR RATE (%)	PERCENT SURVIVAL (YEARS)
CHL		65	50 at (4½)
vs	67		
TBI		53	50 at (4½)
CYT or CHL		64	60 at (4)
vs			
CVP	51	88	90 at (4)
vs			
TBI		71	90 at (4)
CVP		67	
vs	44		—
TBI		75	
CVP (FSCL)		62	
or			50 at (>5)
COPP (FML)	75		
vs			
TNI or TBI		85	50 at (>5)

CHL, chlorambucil; TBI, total body irradiation; CYT, cyclophosphamide; CVP, cyclophosphamide, vincristine, and prednisone; COPP, cyclophosphamide, vincristine, procarbazine, and prednisone; TNI, total nodal irradiation.

Radiotherapy, either total body or total nodal, is effective in the management of advanced-stage low-grade lymphomas. Nonrandomized trials reported CR rates of 80 to 100 percent. Most of these studies did not require rebiopsy of involved visceral sites to document CR, as was done in chemotherapy trials. This may contribute to the high CR rate noted in radiotherapy trials. Two studies of central lymphatic radiation for stage III nodular malignant lymphoma have demonstrated an identical life-table actuarial disease-free survival rate of 40 percent at 15 years with median follow-up of 9 to 10 years. Four randomized trials comparing radiotherapy with chemotherapy are listed in Table 5. Response rates and survival are equivalent with the two modalities in these small trials. Upon failure, patients who receive initial total-body radiotherapy are often poorly tolerant of chemotherapy because of impaired marrow reserve.

In patients treated initially with chemotherapy, failures tend to occur in sites of previously documented disease, suggesting that it is more effective in controlling microscopic than bulk disease. Relapse after TNI (total nodal irradiation) usually occurs outside the treatment portals, indicating that local treatment fails to control the disease systemically. The value of combined modality therapy was evaluated at Stanford, randomizing patients to receive chronic oral single-agent alkylator therapy, CVP for 2 years beyond CR, or CVP before and after TNI in a sandwich fashion. Response rates and 30 month survival data were equivalent, with a pattern of continuous late relapse demonstrable for all groups. Combined modality therapy does not appear to be better than chemotherapy alone.

■ OBSERVATION

In the 1970s, Rosenberg at Stanford began to follow a number of asymptomatic or minimally symptomatic patients with newly diagnosed advanced low-grade lymphoma without any initial therapy. Patients received involved-field radiotherapy as needed for locally progressive disease. The institution of chemotherapy was reserved until the patient developed constitutional symptoms or the disease showed rapid progression, threatened a vital organ, or extended beyond a reasonably encompassing radiation therapy port. Patients who were selected for observation gave a history of slowly progressive lymph node enlargement associated with either advanced age or concurrent medical problems that could complicate chemotherapy. In their initial report of 44 patients with stage III or IV low-grade lymphoma, most eventually required systemic therapy, although the median time to treatment was 37 months. When survival of this group of treatment-deferred patients was compared with that of 112 patients treated on protocols during the same years, the overall 4 year survivals (77 percent versus 83 percent, respectively) were similar. The Stanford group later reported on a total of 83 patients whose treatment was deferred. Median follow-up of these patients was 50 months. Spontaneous regression of disease occurred in 23 percent of patients after a median 8 months of observation, and one-third of these were clinical CRs. Therapy was required in 61 percent of the group at a median of 3 years of observation. Median time to initiation of treatment was longer for SLL (6 years) and FSCL (4 years) than for FML (16 months). The overall actuarial median survival was 11 years, but it was significantly greater for patients with FSCL than for FML. The incidence of histologic transformation in these patients was similar to that of a group of comparable patients receiving chemotherapy on protocol during the same period.

In an attempt to confirm Stanford's results, the National Cancer Institute conducted a randomized trial of 84 patients comparing initial observation with an aggressive combined modality approach consisting of ProMACE/MOPP (prednisone, methotrexate, doxorubicin, cyclophosphamide, etoposide plus nitrogen mustard, vincristine, procarbazine, prednisone) chemotherapy and 2,400 cGy of total nodal irradiation. The patients randomized to initial observation were treated palliatively when feasible with involved-field radiotherapy to control local disease manifestations. When these patients later experienced symptomatic or rapidly progressive disease, they were treated with the same combined modality program. Of the 41 patients observed without therapy, 16 required local radiotherapy and 18 crossed over to systemic treatment at a median of 34 months. Approximately one-half of the patients received no therapy at a median 2 years of follow-up. The CR rate was 78 percent for patients randomized to initial treatment, and the median duration of CR is more than 45 months. In contrast, the CR rate was only 43 percent for 18 patients on observation initially who later received therapy. Nevertheless, with short follow-up, overall survival is similar in the two treatment arms—83 percent at 5 years. An update of this trial with extended survival data is needed to determine whether early, aggressive therapy alters the long-term outcome in the low-grade lymphomas. Because of the small number of patients in each arm, survival differences between them will have to be substantial to be significant. As expected, the combined modality regimen was toxic, and to date four patients (10 percent) have developed other malignancies. The cost-benefit analysis of the risk of secondary cancer versus the potential for improved survival must be considered in choosing to treat with combined-modality therapy.

The preceding discussion of the low-grade lymphomas has considered the three subtypes SLL, FSCL, and FML to be equivalent because of their similar natural histories. Because FSCL constitutes 60 to 70 percent of the low-grade lymphomas and few studies involve more than 100 patients, it is difficult to document significant biologic differences between the other subtypes, although they undoubtedly exist.

IS FML CURABLE?

The National Cancer Institute, in a 1977 review of 80 patients with FSCL and FML treated with either CVP or COPP combination chemotherapy, noted better survival in patients with FML than in those with FSCL. Of 24 FML patients treated with COPP, the CR rate was 77 percent and only 4 of 18 CRs relapsed at a median follow-up of 3 years. The survival curve reached a plateau, suggesting possible cures. In contrast, in 49 patients with FSCL, nearly all of whom were treated with CVP, the survival curve demonstrated the typical pattern of continuous late relapse. In a later report of these patients with median follow-up of 7 years, the expected 5 year disease-free survival in FML is 57 percent, with a median CR of more than 7 years. Although late relapses were seen, the survival curve still demonstrates a plateau and is significantly better than that for FSCL treated with CVP. In two other studies of single-agent chemotherapy, FML was noted to have significantly longer CR than FSCL. As noted earlier, a randomized study (see Table 4) by the Eastern Cooperative Oncology Group failed to show any differences in disease-free or overall survival between combinations of varying intensity in either FML or FSCL. Moreover, in a retrospective review of four Eastern Cooperative Oncology Group trials involving the treatment of 80 patients with FML, the 2 year survival was found to be inferior to that of patients with FSCL. However, in FSCL the 2 year survival for patients achieving CR (88 percent) did not differ from that of patients achieving PR (83 percent). In contrast, in FML the 2 year survival was 85 percent for patients achieving CR versus 33 percent for patients achieving PR. The survival curve for patients with FML in a retrospective review of three Southwestern Oncology Group trials suggests a possible plateau of 20 to 25 percent long-term survivors, although late deaths have occurred. Whether FML is curable by chemotherapy remains controversial.

EXPERIMENTAL APPROACHES

Fludarabine phosphate, a fluorinated analogue of adenosine arabinoside that is resistant to deamination, is highly active in chronic lymphocytic leukemia. Several phase II studies have tested the activity of this drug in previously treated patients with low-grade lymphomas. The largest series, from the Eastern Cooperative Oncology Group and the M.D. Anderson Hospital, reported response rates of 45 to 55 percent with complete responses of 13 to 20 percent. 2-Chlorodeoxyadenosine, another purine analogue resistant to deamination, when used in previously treated patients has resulted in similar response rates. It is clear that both drugs are active in low-grade lymphomas, and their efficacy alone and in combination in previously untreated patients is now under study. In addition to the wide range of effective chemotherapeutic drugs in the low-grade lymphomas, a number of biologic response modifiers have demonstrated activity. Recombinant interferon-alpha; given in a variety of doses and schedules, produces response rates of approximately 40 percent, but only 10 percent are complete. The median response duration is usually brief, only 6 to 12 months. Response to IFN does not correlate with histology, stage, symptoms, bulk of disease, or prior therapy. Although the optimal dose and schedule of interferon are unknown, it appears that lower doses are as effective as higher, more toxic doses. Trials in patients with newly diagnosed low-grade lymphoma are in progress in the United Kingdom and Italy. Both trials randomize patients to receive chlorambucil alone or chlorambucil plus interferon-alpha-2b. Responding patients are then randomized to receive either interferon maintenance for up to 12 months or no further treatment. A similar large intergroup study is under way in the United States, using daily oral cyclophosphamide. Preliminary results show that the addition of interferon to an alkylating agent does not improve the early response rate but does cause added toxicity, primarily myelosuppression. With limited follow-up, fewer relapses have occurred in patients receiving maintenance interferon, but so far there is no difference in survival between the two groups. These studies use simultaneous chemotherapy and interferon. A previous study of combination chemotherapy with or without IFN by the Eastern Cooperative Oncology Group in advanced progressive lymphomas showed improved time to treatment failure when IFN was administered at an interval separated from the chemotherapy. It may be that the timing of IFN in combined modality therapy is an important variable.

Monoclonal antibodies are another possible treatment for the low-grade lymphomas. Anti-idiotype antibodies have been custom made for patients and infused in doses ranging from 400 to 15,000 mg. Only a small number of patients have been treated to date; responses approximate 50 percent, but CR is rare. In a murine model the combination of interferon-alpha and monoclonal antibodies was synergistic because interferon seemed to counter the emergence of idiotype-negative clones that appear when antibodies are used alone. Investigators at Stanford used this combination in 11 patients and achieved two CRs and seven PRs. The median duration of response was 7 months (range of 2 to more than 24 months). There was no difference in the emergence of idiotype-negative clones compared with patients treated with antibodies alone. Antibodies to B cell markers, such as CD20, that are linked to toxins or radioisotopes can induce regression of lymphomas and may find increased application in the future.

High-dose chemoradiotherapy with bone marrow rescue has an established role as curative salvage therapy in the management of the intermediate- and high-grade NHLs. Coupled with the sensitivity of low-grade lymphomas to therapy, it forms the rationale for using this therapeutic approach. To date, trials have included patients in second or subsequent complete or partial remission. Studies conducted at the Dana Farber Cancer Institute and St. Bartholomew's

Hospital in London failed to demonstrate a significant difference in disease-free survival when patients are transplanted in complete as opposed to partial remission. Recurrences were seen, but with a lower frequency than expected in comparison with prior experience. The most frequently used conditioning regimen was a combination of cyclophosphamide and total-body irradiation. Due to the high incidence of bone marrow involvement in low-grade lymphoma and the risk of returning occult residual lymphoma cells in the reinfused bone marrow to the patient, investigators have attempted to purge the bone marrow in vitro by exposing it to anti–B cell antibodies or cytotoxic drugs. At the Dana Farber Cancer Institute amplification by PCR was used to detect residual lymphoma cells before and after antibody purging of bone marrow from patients with B cell NHL carrying the translocation t(14;18). After treatment of the marrow with three different anti–B cell antibodies, only one-third of the bone marrows remained positive for lymphoma. Although follow-up is limited, recurrences have been much less common in patients whose reinfused marrow tested PCR negative than in patients with PCR-positive marrow. Although these lymphomas are usually indolent initially, they eventually progress, and conventional chemotherapy does not cure the patient or alter survival. Given these facts and the suggestive data from the NCI chemotherapy-TNI program, bone marrow transplantation is a reasonable option for young patients with these lymphomas. At the same time, the long natural history of low-grade lymphoma requires lengthy follow-up to document whether the early application of bone marrow transplant is of benefit.

Suggested Reading

Gallagher CJ, Gregory WM, Jones AF, et al. Follicular lymphoma: Prognostic factors for response and survival. J Clin Oncol 1986; 4:470–480.

Glick JH, Barnes JM, Ezdinli EZ, et al. Nodular mixed lymphoma: Results of a randomized trial failing to confirm prolonged disease-free survival with COPP chemotherapy. Blood 1981; 58:920–925.

Gribben JG, Freedman AS, Neuberg D, et al. Immunologic purging of marrow assessed by PCR before autologous bone marrow transplantation for B-cell lymphoma. N Engl J Med 1991; 325:526–533.

Hochster HS, Kim K, Green, MD, et al. Activity of fludarabine in previously treated non-Hodgkin's lymphoma: results of an Eastern Cooperative Group study. J Clin Oncol 1992; 10:28–32.

Portlock CS. Management of the low-grade non-Hodgkin's lymphomas. Semin Oncol 1990; 17:51–59.

Rosenberg SA. Classification of lymphoid neoplasms. Blood 1994; 84: 1369–1380.

Smalley RV, Andersen JW, Hawkins MJ, et al. Interferon alfa combined with cytotoxic chemotherapy for patients with non-Hodgkin's lymphoma. N Engl J Med 1992; 327:1336–1341.

Young RC, Johnson RE, Canellos GP, et al. Advanced lymphocytic lymphoma: Randomized comparisons of chemotherapy and radiotherapy, alone or in combination. Cancer Treat Rep 1977; 61:153–159.

Young RC, Longo DL, Glatstein E, et al. The treatment of low-grade lymphomas: Watchful waiting versus aggressive combined modality treatment. Semin Hematol 1988; 25(Suppl 2):11–16.

UNFAVORABLE NON-HODGKIN'S LYMPHOMA

Ellen R. Gaynor, M.D.
Richard I. Fisher, M.D.

The non-Hodgkin's lymphomas (NHL) are a diverse group of diseases with regard to both their natural history and their response to therapy. The Working Formulation groups the lymphomas together according to their natural history as low grade, intermediate grade, and high grade (Table 1). From a clinical standpoint the lymphomas may be conveniently grouped as favorable and unfavorable. Paradoxically, lymphomas in the favorable category are usually not curable, while those in the unfavorable category are commonly curable with aggressive combination chemotherapy.

It is likely that no classification system of the NHL will be permanent. Several new subgroups of aggressive lymphomas do not fit well into the Working Formulation. Examples of newly described aggressive lymphomas include anaplastic large cell lymphoma and adult T cell leukemia/lymphoma.

Anaplastic large cell lymphoma, a subtype of diffuse large cell lymphoma, can be confused histologically with carcinoma because of the anaplastic appearance of the cells. The lymphoma usually originates in the T cells, and the cells usually express the Ki-1 or Hodgkin's-associated antigen CD30. A characteristic chromosomal abnormality, t(2:5), is sometimes seen. This type of lymphoma occurs in adults but is more common in children, who frequently present with extranodal involvement of the skin. Current treatment is the same as for other types of large cell lymphoma.

Adult T cell leukemia/lymphoma is a rare disease associated with infection by the human T cell lymphotropic virus HTLV-1. The disease shows a striking geographic variation, being particularly common in Japan and the Caribbean. Clinically it is commonly associated with skin involvement, lytic bone lesions, and hypercalcemia. While it is responsive to chemotherapy, the patients usually do poorly and follow a rapid downhill course.

In this chapter we discuss briefly the clinical features and management of lymphoblastic lymphoma and Burkitt's lymphoma. We discuss in detail staging, prognostic characteristics, and treatment of diffuse large cell lymphoma, the most common of the unfavorable lymphomas in adults.

Table 1 Working Formulation Nomenclature for the Non-Hodgkin's Malignant Lymphomas

LOW GRADE	
Small lymphocytic	Favorable
Follicular; predominantly small cleaved cell	Favorable
Follicular mixed, small cleaved, and large cell	Favorable
INTERMEDIATE GRADE	
Follicular, predominantly large cell	Unfavorable
Diffuse mixed, small, and large cell	Unfavorable
Diffuse large cell	Unfavorable
HIGH GRADE	
Large cell, immunoblastic	Unfavorable
Lymphoblastic	Unfavorable
Small non-cleaved cell	Unfavorable

BURKITT'S AND LYMPHOBLASTIC LYMPHOMA

Lymphomas of the small non-cleaved cell (Burkitt's type) are endemic in certain parts of Africa. In these areas the disease appears to be causally related to Epstein-Barr virus (EBV). It is also seen in this country, and its incidence is increasing particularly in human immunodeficiency virus (HIV)-infected patients. The relationship of EBV to nonendemic Burkitt's is not clear. Burkitt's lymphoma is seen in children and is frequently associated with bulky disease, primarily involving the jaw or abdomen, with frequent involvement of the bone marrow and meninges. While it is very aggressive in its clinical behavior, it is also exquisitely sensitive to chemotherapy.

Lymphoblastic lymphoma is also aggressive and usually of T cell origin. In many ways it is similar to acute lymphoblastic leukemia, and in some instances distinction between the two diseases may be difficult. Like Burkitt's, lymphoblastic lymphoma is seen primarily in children, although it does occur in adults. Typically it presents with a mediastinal mass in association with peripheral adenopathy. Bone marrow and central nervous system (CNS) involvement are common in this disease.

Because of the systemic nature of both Burkitt's and lymphoblastic lymphoma and because of the extremely rapid growth of these lymphomas, intensive chemotherapy including CNS prophylaxis is standard. For lymphoblastic lymphoma it is not clear whether the disease is best treated as a very aggressive lymphoma or as acute lymphocytic leukemia. It is clear, however, that the regimens used to treat diffuse large cell lymphoma are not adequate for this disease.

DIFFUSE LARGE CELL LYMPHOMA

Treatment approaches to diffuse large cell lymphoma provide the basis for decisions regarding the management of patients with follicular large cell, diffuse small cleaved cell, and diffuse mixed cell lymphoma. The best approach to treatment of the relatively uncommon diffuse small non-cleaved cell (non-Burkitt's) lymphoma has not yet been defined. Many clinicians approach treatment in the same way as with diffuse large cell lymphoma.

Table 2 The Ann Arbor Staging Classification

STAGE I
Involvement of a single lymph node region or of a single extranodal organ or site (I_E)
STAGE II
Involvement of two or more lymph node regions on the same side of the diaphragm or localized involvement of an extranodal site or organ (II_E) and of one or more lymph node regions on the same side of the diaphragm
STAGE III
Involvement of lymph node regions on both sides of the diaphragm, which may also be accompanied by localized involvement of an extranodal organ or site (III_E) or spleen (III_S) or both (III_{SE})
STAGE IV
Diffuse or disseminated involvement of one or more distant extranodal organs with or without associated lymph node involvement

Fever >38° C, night sweats, and/or weight loss >10% of body weight in the 6 months preceding admission are defined as systemic symptoms and denoted by the suffix B. Asymptomatic patients are denoted by the suffix A.

Staging and Prognostic Factors

For many years the most widely used staging system for NHL was the Ann Arbor system (Table 2), originally proposed as a staging system for Hodgkin's disease (HD). The Ann Arbor system is based on the anatomic extent of disease and the presence or absence of B symptoms. Modifications of the system have recently been proposed for the staging of HD; for many years it has been recognized that the system is inadequate for the staging of NHL. Unlike HD, NHL does not commonly spread through contiguous groups of lymph nodes, it is frequently disseminated at the time of diagnosis, and it frequently involves extranodal sites at the time of diagnosis.

Other pretreatment prognostic factors for NHL include patient age, presence or absence of B symptoms, serum lactate dehydrogenase (LDH), performance status, tumor size (specifically bulky disease), the number of nodal and extranodal sites of disease, and the stage of disease at diagnosis. Each of these has been identified in one or more series of patients with unfavorable lymphoma to affect outcome.

Recently the International Non-Hodgkin's Lymphoma Prognostic Factors Project used pretreatment prognostic factors in a sample of several thousand patients with aggressive lymphomas treated with doxorubicin-based combination chemotherapy to develop a predictive model of treatment outcome for aggressive NHL. Pretreatment characteristics found to be independently statistically significant included age above or below 60 years, tumor stage I or II (localized) versus III or IV (advanced), the number of extranodal sites of involvement (none or one versus more than one), patient performance status (0 or 1 versus 2 or higher), and serum LDH (normal or abnormal).

With these five pretreatment risk factors patients could be assigned to one of four risk groups: low risk (0 or 1), low intermediate risk (2), high intermediate risk (3), and high risk (4 or 5). When patients were analyzed according to risk factors, they were found to have very different outcome with respect to complete response (CR) rate, relapse-free survival (RFS), and overall survival (OS). For example, low-risk patients had an 87 percent CR rate and an OS at 5 years of 73 percent. This contrasts with a 44 percent CR rate and a 26 percent 5 year survival in patients identified as being in the high-risk category.

Pretreatment prognostic factors are known to be surrogate markers of the biologic heterogeneity of the lymphomas. Their biologic diversity is only beginning to be understood. Such biologic parameters as the expression of the nuclear Ki-67 antigen, which is an index of cell proliferation, the expression of cell surface adhesion molecules, and the presence of karyotypic abnormalities are being investigated in large numbers of patients with unfavorable lymphomas.

The value of any staging system is its ability to predict the likelihood of response to a proposed therapy. It is hoped that the use of a predictive model such as that proposed by Shipp and associates will allow clinicians to predict prior to therapy the patient's likelihood of responding adequately to the proposed treatment. Those whose outcome is predicted to be favorable with conventional therapy should be spared the added toxicity often associated with more aggressive experimental therapy. On the other hand, those in whom a complete response is unlikely with conventional therapy should be candidates for more aggressive treatment.

Treatment

The unfavorable lymphomas are systemic at the time of diagnosis, and chemotherapy is therefore the mainstay of treatment. A variety of chemotherapeutic regimens have been used over the past 25 years. Those most commonly used today and discussed in this chapter are shown in Table 3.

Localized Disease

Localized disease includes patients with stage I and nonbulky stage II disease. Any tumor mass greater than 10 cm in diameter or any mediastinal mass greater than one-third of the chest diameter is bulky disease. Cure rates for patients with stage I and nonbulky stage II disease are very high, and the variety of treatment approaches includes radiotherapy alone, chemotherapy alone, and chemotherapy (either full course or abbreviated course) followed by tumoricidal doses of RT.

Radiotherapy alone was studied at the University of Chicago. These studies, now very mature, have clearly shown that patients with pathologically staged early disease could be cured with extended field radiotherapy. In the most recent update of this series, Vokes and associates report a 70 percent 10 year survival for patients with pathologic stage I (PSI) diffuse large cell lymphoma. These studies are mainly of historical interest because the morbidity associated with the staging laparotomy required to identify this subset of patients is not acceptable, since many such patients are elderly. More important, the results obtained with radiotherapy alone in pathologically staged patients is not superior to results obtained in clinically staged patients treated with chemotherapy, either alone or in combination with radiotherapy.

One of the earliest studies employing a doxorubicin (Adriamycin)-based chemotherapy regimen in patients with stage I and II large cell lymphoma was reported by Jones and colleagues. In this nonrandomized study most patients received eight cycles of CHOP chemotherapy. In patients in whom tumor was slow to respond to chemotherapy or in whom significant chemotherapy dose modifications were needed, radiotherapy to an involved field was given at 4,000 cGy. A comparison between patients receiving chemotherapy alone and those treated with chemotherapy plus radiotherapy failed to reveal any statistical difference in relapse rate or overall survival.

Short-course chemotherapy followed by involved-field radiotherapy was popularized by Connors and associates, who treated 78 patients with good-prognosis stage I or II large cell lymphoma with three cycles of CHOP chemotherapy followed by involved-field radiotherapy. Some 99 percent of the treated patients achieved a CR, and 85 percent are long-term survivors.

The Southwest Oncology Group (SWOG) is conducting a randomized trial of eight cycles of CHOP alone versus three cycles of CHOP followed by involved-field radiotherapy for patients with clinical stage I and nonbulky stage II disease with aggressive lymphomas. The main objective of this study is to compare these two curative approaches with respect to differences in survival, time to treatment failure, and toxicity.

There are few trials using more aggressive chemotherapy regimens in the treatment of early-stage disease. Longo and associates have employed four cycles of ProMACE-MOPP, with 75 percent of the dose of myelotoxic drugs followed by involved-field radiotherapy, to treat 49 patients with stage I or IE disease. Forty-seven patients achieved a CR, and 94 percent remained alive with a median follow-up of 4 years. This limited experience supports this treatment approach for patients with very early stage disease, although such aggressive therapy as this is probably not necessary.

The issue of the need for radiotherapy in addition to chemotherapy is also being defined by the Eastern Cooperative Oncology Group (ECOG). That group is conducting a study of CHOP for eight cycles versus CHOP for eight cycles plus radiotherapy in a randomized trial. The data from the Connors and Longo groups suggest that radiotherapy adds to chemotherapy by allowing fewer cycles of chemotherapy with equivalent results, by reducing the toxicity of chemotherapy, and by allowing the use of less chemotherapy, which has particular importance in the treatment of the elderly.

The best approach to management of patients with early-stage aggressive lymphoma is participation in a clinical trial. If this is not possible, it is reasonable to treat these patients with either eight cycles of CHOP or three cycles of CHOP followed by involved-field radiotherapy at tumoricidal doses.

Advanced Disease (Stages II, Bulky III, IV)

Investigators at the National Cancer Institute (NCI) were among the first to document the potential curability of these diseases. Using combination chemotherapy regimens, they achieved complete remission in 45 percent and cure in approximately 37 percent of treated patients. In these early trials investigators noted that relapses beyond 2 years were rare and a disease-free survival of 2 years was tantamount to cure. These observations led investigators to reason that treatment approaches which increased the number of pa-

Table 3 Chemotherapeutic Regimens

REGIMENS	DOSE AND ROUTE	DAY	FREQUENCY
CHOP			
C = cyclophosphamide	750 mg/m^2 IV	1	Repeat every 21 days
H = doxorubicin	50 mg/m^2 IV	1	
O = vincristine	1.4 mg/m^2 IV (max 2 mg)	1	
P = prednisone	100 mg PO	1–5	Repeat every 21 days
M-BACOD			
M = methotrexate*	3,000 mg/m^2 IV	15	Repeat every 21 days
B = bleomycin	4 mg/m^2 IV	1	
A = doxorubicin	45 mg/m^2 IV	1	
C = cyclophosphamide	600 mg/m^2 IV	1	
O = vincristine	1 mg/m^2 IV	1	
D = dexamethasone	6 mg/m^2 PO	1–5	
m-BACOD			
m = methotrexate*	200 mg/m^2 IV	8, 15	Repeat every 21 days
B = bleomycin	4 mg/m^2 IV	1	
A = doxorubicin	45 mg/^{2} IV	1	
C = cyclophosphamide	600 mg/m^2 IV	1	
O = vincristine	1.4 mg/m^2 IV	1	
D = dexamethasone	6 mg/m^2 PO	1–5	
ProMACE-MOPP			
Pro = prednisone	60 mg/m^2 IV	1–14	Repeat every 28 days
M = methotrexate*	1,500 mg/m^2 IV	15	
A = doxorubicin	25 mg/m^2 IV	1,8	
C = cyclophosphamide	650 mg/m^2	1,8	
E = etoposide	120 mg/m^2 IV	1,8	
Followed by MOPP after maximal response			
M = mechlorethamine	6 mg/m^2 IV	1,8	Repeat every 28 days
O = vincristine	1.4 mg/m^2 IV	1,8	
P = procarbazine	100 mg/m^2 PO	1–14	
P = prednisone	40 mg/m^2 PO	1–14	
ProMACE-CytaBOM			
Pro = prednisone	60 mg/m^2 IV	1–14	Repeat every 21 days
A = doxorubicin	25 mg/m^2 IV	1	
C = cyclophosphamide	650 mg/m^2 IV	1	
E = etoposide	120 mg/m^2 IV	1	
Cyta = cytarabine	300 mg/m^2 IV	8	
B = bleomycin	5 mg/m^2 IV	8	
O = vincristine	1.4 mg/m^2 IV	8	
M = methotrexate*	120 mg/m^2 IV	8	
MACOP-B			
M = methotrexate*	400 mg/m^2 IV	8,36,64	
A = doxorubicin	50 mg/m^2 IV	1,15,29,43,57,71	
C = cyclophosphamide	350 mg/m^2	1,15,29,43,57,71	
O = vincristine	1.4 mg/m^2 IV (max 2 mg)	8,22,36,50,64,78	
P = prednisone	75 mg/m^2 PO	1–84	
B = bleomycin	10 mg/m^2 IV	22,50,78	

*Leucovorin rescue is given 24 hours after each methotrexate dose.

tients achieving a CR should ultimately translate into improved survival.

CHOP was one of the first combination chemotherapy regimens to employ the drug doxorubicin, one of the most active drugs for lymphoma. This regimen has been studied extensively in cooperative group trials, and it remains the "gold standard" against which newer treatment regimens must be measured. CHOP did result in an increased number of CRs, as had been hoped. Unfortunately, relapses and deaths were not limited to the first 2 years after treatment; in fact, relapses were seen as long as 6 and 7 years after the completion of therapy. Hence, the higher percentage of CRs did not translate into improved survival compared with earlier regimens employed at the NCI.

Recognizing the need to improve on results obtained with CHOP, new and more complex regimens were developed in the 1980s. These are frequently called second- and third-generation regimens to distinguish them from early regimens such as CHOP. The newer regimens continued to rely heavily on the most active drugs, cyclophosphamide and doxorubicin, but in addition they incorporated other drugs with less single-agent activity such as methotrexate, cytarabine, etoposide, and bleomycin. Initial reports appeared very promising, suggesting that the number of patients cured might be double the number seen with regimens such as CHOP.

Two of the more widely used second-generation regimens were M-BACOD, which was developed and piloted at the Dana Farber Cancer Institute and ProMACE-MOPP, which was developed and piloted at the NCI. M-BACOD added high-dose methotrexate to the standard drugs used in the first-generation regimens. Patients participating in this study were relatively young, with a median age of 48. Patients entered on study included both early-stage (I, IE, II, IIE) and advanced (III, IV) disease. Initial results were excellent, with a reported CR rate of 72 percent and a projected 5 year survival of 65 percent. Unfortunately, in a subsequent report the 3 year survival had fallen to 54 percent.

The ProMACE-MOPP regimen used etoposide and high-dose methotrexate as well as standard chemotherapy drugs. The sample included 74 patients with Stage II, III, and IV diffuse mixed, diffuse large cell, and undifferentiated lymphoma. Of these 74 percent achieved a CR, and the projected 4 year survival was 65 percent. In a recent update, however, with 9 years of follow-up, the long-term survival has decreased to 50 percent. The median age of patients treated was 44 years as compared with a median age of 55 years for patients treated in CHOP trials. Furthermore, the study included patients with stage II disease, whereas previous NCI trials of first-generation regimens included only patients with stage III and IV disease.

In an attempt to improve results and possibly decrease cost and toxicity, several single institutions piloted and reported results obtained with the so-called third-generation regimens. These included m-BACOD, which substitutes moderate-dose methotrexate for the high-dose methotrexate of M-BACOD; ProMACE-CytaBOM, which employs cytarabine and bleomycin in addition to the ProMACE drugs; and MACOP-B, an intensive 12 week program employing conventional drugs given on an unconventional dosing schedule. Once again early results were very promising, with CR rates ranging from 68 to 86 percent and projected survival of 58 to 69 percent.

Confirmatory trials of each of these third-generation regimens were conducted by SWOG. Unfortunately, results were considerably poorer than in the initial single-institution results. CR rates ranged from 49 to 65 percent, and survival projections ranged from 50 to 61 percent. In fact, the results were very similar to those obtained with CHOP. Such results are not surprising considering that in the single-institution studies patients tended to be younger and in some of the studies the patients had less advanced disease than in the SWOG trials.

Because the second- and third-generation regimens are more toxic and more costly, it was apparent that they must be compared in a randomized fashion to the older CHOP regimen. Increased cost and toxicity are acceptable if there is a significant improvement in outcome. Results of Intergroup Trial 0067, a phase III comparison of CHOP versus m-BACOD versus ProMACE-CytaBOM versus MACOP-B, have recently been published.

In that study 1,138 previously untreated patients with bulky stage II, stage III, or stage IV disease were randomized between 1986 and 1991 to one of four treatment arms. Each treatment was administered exactly as initially described. There were 239 ineligible patients, most so designated on pathology review. The reported results are those seen in the 899 eligible patients.

The group as a whole had very poor prognostic characteristics. The median age was 56, and one-fourth were older than 64 years. Bulky disease was present in 40 percent, and 46 percent had an elevated pretreatment LDH. The treatment arms were well balanced for these and all other patient characteristics. At the time of publication of results, the median follow-up was 49 months, with a maximum follow-up of 84 mos.

There was no significant difference in CR rate or overall response rate among the four treatment arms. Because persistent abnormalities make it difficult to assess CR on computed tomography scan after treatment, the time to progression, relapse, or death from any cause was analyzed as a more accurate estimate of the fraction of patients who were cured by the initial therapy. Some 43 percent of all eligible patients were estimated to be alive without disease at 3 years. The percentage of patients alive without disease is estimated to be 43 percent on the CHOP arm, 43 percent on the m-BACOD arm, 44 percent on the ProMACE-CytaBOM arm, and 40 percent on the MACOP-B arm. Also, 52 percent of all eligible patients are estimated to be alive at 3 years: 49 percent on MACOP-B, 51 percent on m-BACOD, 53 percent on ProMACE-CytaBOM, and 55 percent on CHOP.

The toxicities observed were similar to those reported in the phase II studies. Most severe toxicities were related to granulocytopenic infections. Fatal toxicities occurred in 1 percent of CHOP-treated patients, 5 percent of m-BACOD–treated patients, 3 percent of ProMACE-CytaBOM–treated patients, and 6 percent of MACOP-B–treated patients.

An attempt was made to identify subsets of patients who might have a better outcome if treated with one of the third-generation regimens as compared with CHOP. The International NHL Prognostic Factors Project's predictive model showed no significant difference in time to treatment failure or overall survival with low, low intermediate, high intermediate, and high-risk groups when analyzed according to treatment arm.

Based on the available data and on the lower cost and lower severe toxicity seen with the CHOP regimen, CHOP remains the standard treatment for patients with advanced-stage aggressive lymphoma. This is not to imply that CHOP is adequate therapy in most cases, and there is clearly a need for better therapies. We strongly advocate participation in a clinical trial; participation in such trials is the best treatment available at present. Outside of a clinical trial, CHOP is the standard treatment for these lymphomas.

There are several possible approaches to improve treatment outcome. These include identification of new active chemotherapeutic agents, the use of standard drugs in escalated doses with colony-stimulating factor support, the use of the predictive prognostic factor model to identify prior to therapy patients who may be candidates for more aggressive experimental therapies, and the use of agents in combination with conventional drugs that may overcome chemotherapy resistance of the lymphoma cells.

Salvage Therapy

As is obvious from the results of the intergroup trial, large numbers of patients with advanced-stage intermediate and high-grade lymphoma either are refractory to initial therapy or relapse after an initial response to first-line therapy. Effective salvage therapy is needed for these patients. For appropriate candidates, bone marrow transplant (usually autologous; ABMT) should be considered, since this approach offers an extended disease-free survival in 20 to 25 percent of patients. Patients who are likely to benefit from this approach are those who had an initial response to therapy and those whose relapsed disease has responded to conventional dose salvage therapy.

Many patients are not candidates for ABMT due to age, bone marrow involvement, performance status, or other medical problems. These patients are usually treated with conventional-dose salvage therapy. Many such regimens have been reported to act on relapsed disease. Comparison of one salvage program with another is difficult or impossible, since many regimens have been used only in small numbers of patients, and selection criteria and patient characteristics have varied widely for the reported salvage regimens.

Despite these limitations, available data allow one to draw tentative conclusions. The DHAP (dexamethasone, high-dose cytarabine, cisplatin) regimen has been used as salvage therapy in several series, with almost 300 patients treated. This regimen has consistently produced response in more than 50 percent and has led to complete response in 15 to 30 percent. DHAP is commonly used prior to ABMT to debulk the lymphoma. The response to this regimen frequently is used to determine whether relapsed disease is sensitive or resistant, since patients with sensitive relapse are most likely to benefit from ABMT.

Other approaches to salvage therapy have been explored. Monoclonal antibody therapy has been used in this situation; there have been two recent promising reports of radiolabeled antibody therapy in this setting. Cytokine therapy with interleukin-2 has minimal activity; perhaps newer cytokines will have greater activity. Finally, approaches aimed at reversing chemotherapy drug resistance offer promise as an approach to salvage therapy.

■ COMMENTS

The unfavorable lymphomas are among the most curable of human malignancies. However, cure is limited in patients presenting with advanced disease. Clearly, better treatment approaches are needed for those identified clinically or biologically as being at risk for treatment failure. The ability to identify such patients depends upon continued basic science and clinical research to further our understanding of these diseases.

Suggested Reading

Armitage JO. Treatment of non-Hodgkin's lymphoma. N Engl J Med 1993; 328:1023–1030.

Connors JM, Klimo P, Fairey RN, Voss N. Brief chemotherapy and involved field radiation therapy for limited stage, histologically aggressive lymphoma. Ann Intern Med 1987; 107:25–30.

Fisher RI, Gaynor ER, Dahlberg S, et al. Comparison of CHOP vs m-BACOD vs ProMACE-CytaBOM vs MACOP-B in patients with intermediate or high-grade non-Hodgkin's lymphoma. N Engl J Med 1993; 328:1002–1006.

Jones SE, Miller TM, Connors JM. Long term follow-up and analysis for prognostic factors for patients with limited stage diffuse large cell lymphoma treated with initial chemotherapy with or without adjuvant radiotherapy. J Clin Oncol 1989; 7:1186–1191.

The International Non-Hodgkin's Lymphoma Prognostic Factors Project. A predictive model for aggressive non-Hodgkin's lymphoma. N Engl J Med 1993; 329:987–994.

T CELL LYMPHOMAS AND LEUKEMIAS IN ADULTS

Timothy M. Kuzel, M.D.
Elaine Lee Wade, M.D.
Steven T. Rosen, M.D., F.A.C.P.

Nowhere in hematology or oncology is the careful clinical evaluation of a patient's history, examination of the presenting lesion or lesions, and review of the histology as important as it is in determining the approach to the adult patient with a T cell lymphoma or leukemia involving the skin. A number of disorders have been included in the spectrum of cutaneous T cell lymphomas (Table 1): mycosis fungoides and the related Sézary syndrome, the adult T cell leukemia/lymphoma (ATLL) associated with human T cell lymphotropic virus (HTLV) 1, peripheral non-Hodgkin's T cell lymphomas, lymphomatoid papulosis, lymphomatoid granulomatosis, angioimmunoblastic lymphadenopathy, and T-gamma lymphoproliferative disorders. Although these diseases all have skin involvement, they have widely disparate causes, histologic appearances, prognoses, and need for and response to treatment. This chapter describes salient clinical and histologic features we use to categorize the lymphoproliferative disorder and suggests various modalities that may have benefit in the treatment of the systemic disorders.

Table 1 Cutaneous T Cell Lymphomas
Mycosis fungoides
Sézary syndrome
Adult T cell leukemia/lymphoma
Peripheral T cell lymphoma
Lymphomatoid papulosis
Lymphomatoid granulomatosis
Angioimmunoblastic lymphadenopathy
T-gamma lymphoproliferative disorders

■ ADULT CELL LEUKEMIA AND LYMPHOMA

Epidemiology and Etiology

HTLV-1 is a human RNA retrovirus of the family Retroviridae, categorized as human type C oncornavirus. HTLV-1 infects both the T and B cells in humans but causes symptomatic processes in only a small percentage of those infected. Routes of infection include venereal transmission, vertical transmission from mother to child, and exchange of blood in shared needles or with unscreened blood transfusions. HTLV-1 is associated with ATLL. An additional spectrum of diseases including myelopathy, tropical spastic paraparesis, and HTLV-1 associated arthropathy are associated with this virus. Approximately 0.5 to 2 percent of HTLV-1 positive individuals develop ATLL. The age of patients ranges from the mid-teens to late 70s, with the mean in the sixth decade of life. There is a slight male predominance, with a ratio of approximately 1.5 : 1.

HTLV-1 infection is endemic in a variety of tropical areas of the world, including the southeastern United States, the Caribbean, Hawaii, southern Japan, South America, and several regions in Africa. Overall, the incidence of ATLL in endemic areas of Japan and the Caribbean for HTLV-1 infection ranges from 1 to 5.5 cases per 100,000 per year. In the United States it is significantly less (0.025 percent). Risk factors for progression to ATLL include living or being raised in an endemic area and early exposure to the virus. No family history is seen. However, increased rates of HTLV-1 seropositivity have been found among spouses and other family members of patients. Overall lifetime risk may be as high as 6 percent for those living their entire life in such an area. The virus can exhibit a long latent period; therefore, symptomatic diseases such as ATLL may not arise for years after an individual has left the endemic area. HTLV-1 is now routinely screened for in blood donors as a result of its increasing incidence. Analysis of ethnic and cultural backgrounds reveals increased incidence of HTLV-1 in African-Americans, Hispanics, intravenous drug abusers, and those being treated in a venereal disease clinic. The rapidity with which the disease process reveals itself depends on the route of transmission and the immune status of the patient.

The HTLV-1 virus itself was isolated in the early 1980s in work done by Poiesz and Gallo. This retrovirus is genetically quite similar to HIV in that it contains GAG, POL, and ENV regions. It behaves as a traditional RNA-based retrovirus, using reverse transcriptase to take over the host DNA network to produce its own genetic material. HTLV-1 does not, however, use the CD4 receptor for cell entry, as does human immunodeficiency virus (HIV). The exact receptor is unknown at present but is believed to be encoded on chromosome 17.

The specific mechanism by which HTLV-1 infection results in leukemogenesis has yet to be determined. A number of theories concerning proliferation and deregulation of T cells via influences by HTLV-1 have been advanced. T cells are normally activated by binding to antigen, which results in cell-surface expression of interleukin (IL) 2R (the IL-2 binding site). Normal resting T and B cells do not express this receptor. However, activated T cells and the neoplastic T cells in ATLL do express this receptor, often at a high level. An interesting proposal by Rosenblatt and associates suggests that the Tax gene, encoded in the 3′ end of the HTLV-1's genetic material, induces generalized, nonspecific proliferation of T cells with increased production of IL-2 and IL-2R. This may be followed by a series of yet-undefined steps that result in the expansion of a monoclonal population of neoplastic T cells. Polymerase chain reaction (PCR) techniques have revealed Tax expression in ATLL cells, suggesting a maintenance role for this gene in this clonal neoplastic disorder.

Histopathology and Cytogenetics

Classically, large atypical lymphoid cells show in the peripheral smear with convoluted or multilobed nuclei. The cells are sometimes called flower cells because of their nuclear appearance. Abnormal lymphocytes in the peripheral smear are seen in approximately 75 percent of patients. Lymph node and extranodal pathology is more difficult to classify. Extranodal sites of involvement include the skin, bone marrow, liver, spleen, lungs, and central nervous system (CNS), particularly the meninges. In tissue sections the lymphoid cells may be medium to large with prominent nuclei and an abundance of nuclear pleomorphism. Cytoplasm may be moderate to abundant without significant granularity. The lymph node architecture is usually effaced by the neoplastic T cells. Numerous chromosomal aberrations, present at high frequency, involving 1p, 6q, 12q, 3q, 9q, and 14q. Trisomy 7 is also seen. Eighty percent of patients with ATLL exhibit DNA aneuploidy. Phenotypically the neoplastic T cells are characterized as mature or post-thymic. They are positive for CD2, CD3, CD4, and CD25. They are TDT and CD8 negative. Thus, the cells appear to be helper T cells, although cells consistent with a reactive suppressor T-cell population are seen occasionally. In contrast to mycosis fungoides, these cells are Leu-8 positive and CD7 negative.

Staging and Prognosis

ATLL typically progresses rapidly. However, its initial clinical presentation encompasses a wide range of characteristics and degrees. Patients with ATLL may be asymptomatic or severely compromised, with acute symptoms including fever, weakness, malaise, lethargy, and pruritus. Weight loss and lymphadenopathy are seen in up to 70 percent of patients. Cutaneous changes including erythema and tumor nodules are frequently seen. Biopsy of those skin lesions reveals lymphocytic infiltrates. Hepatosplenomegaly is seen in approximately 50 percent of cases. Laboratory evaluation often reveals hypercalcemia, increased lactic dehydrogenase (LDH) levels and elevated liver enzymes including aspartate aminotransferase (AST), alanine aminotransferase (ALT), and alkaline phosphatase. Anemia and thrombocytopenia are not common. Increased rates of infection may be seen. These clinical findings may be related to the production of transforming growth factor-beta$_2$ which has been hypothesized to contribute to immunosuppression.

Prominent eosinophilia has occasionally been seen in patients with ATLL, which seems to correlate with the number of ATLL cells and the patient's symptoms. Theories regarding a common growth factor have not been substantiated. A search for endocrine factors that play a role in the hypercalcemia in ATLL has been undertaken by several investigators. In the late 1980s complementary DNA for PTH-related protein was cloned and amino acids sequenced. Comparison with cultured HTLV-1 cell lines reveals a related messenger RNA. Actual secretion of these PTH-like hormones has not yet been documented in ATLL cell studies. Interestingly, the calcium may be used as a marker for measurement of disease activity. If the disease responds to therapy, the calcium level may return to normal as well. The above findings are more common in the acute or relatively aggressive forms of ATLL. In contrast, the smoldering form accompanies underlying rheumatologic or autoimmune disorders. Calcium is frequently normal in these individuals, with few to rare abnormal circulating lymphocytes; however, hypergammaglobulinemia may be present.

The staging of ATLL requires a rigorous evaluation schema. A thorough history and physical examination, routine blood chemistries, complete blood count, and a bone marrow aspirate and biopsy should be obtained. Clusters of lymph nodes or suspicious cutaneous changes should be subjected to biopsy as well. Examination of the peripheral smear may be helpful if flower cells are present. Immunophenotyping and cytogenetics can help significantly, as does serum testing for HTLV-1 antibodies. The distinctive monoclonal population of CD4-positive, CD8-negative mature T cells in the presence of HTLV-1 antibodies is definitive. Rarely a case without antibodies to HTLV-1 has been described. In these instances evidence for increased surface expression of the IL-2R may be helpful but is not diagnostic. ATLL has four stages, acute, lymphomatous, chronic, and smoldering, according to activity of disease. Acute or lymphomatous ATLL is quite evident clinically, with prominent peripheral lymphadenopathy, hepatosplenomegaly, hypercalcemia, increased LDH, and leukocytosis with a significant percentage of ATLL cells evident on peripheral smear. Chronic ATLL is more apparent clinically, manifesting as mild hepatosplenomegaly, moderate lymphadenopathy, and mildly elevated LDH and leukocyte counts, with small percentages (usually less than 5 percent) of ATLL cells. These patients also survive for fairly long periods without therapy, often taking several years to progress to an acute form. Smoldering ATLL, sometimes called pre-ATLL, has few or no symptoms. Mild erythematous cutaneous changes are sometimes evident, with the primary laboratory abnormality consisting of low numbers (0.5 to 3 percent) of ATLL cells in the peripheral smear. Patients in this category appear to have fairly good survival over years.

Management

For purposes of treatment and prognosis it may be wise to view ATLL as a spectrum with two subgroups, acute or lymphomatous and the others, with treatment, though inadequate, reserved for those with acute or lymphomatous ATLL. Observation and close follow-up appear to be more appropriate for both the chronic and smoldering groups. Treatment regimens, while numerous, are for the most part ineffective. Intensive multiagent chemotherapy regimens have been attempted at various institutions without change in the poor survival rates, with median durations of 4 to 6 months.

Deoxycoformycin was tested in various clinical trials initiated by the National Cancer Institute (NCI) in the late 1980s. An antimetabolite that inhibits adenosine deaminase, deoxycoformycin has been shown to have mild to moderate activity but with unacceptable and unpredictable toxicity. A regimen involving therapy directed against the IL-2R has demonstrated some positive response in preliminary studies. Waldmann and associates used monoclonal antibody to the IL-2 receptor, called anti-Tac, to block the growth-stimulating effect of IL-2 on these neoplastic cells, perhaps causing growth inhibition and cell death. Problems with this method include the observation that T cells involved in the aggressive phase of ATLL sometimes no longer require IL-2 for growth, using other autocrine growth factors. Thus other studies using *Pseudomonas* exotoxin and ^{90}Y conjugated to the anti-Tac to deliver a direct cytotoxic effect are now in progress. In vitro studies performed in Japan by Kiyokawa and colleagues revealed an inhibition of protein synthesis in a patient's ATLL cells using a recombinant fusion toxin consisting of IL-2 and portions of the diphtheria toxin protein. Another investigative approach is directed against the surface protein Apo-1, a member of the tumor necrosis factor family in ATLL cells. In vitro studies using a monoclonal antibody to the receptor (anti-Apo-1) caused activation of the cell resulting in subsequent programmed cell death. Clinical trials are anticipated.

Most recently, encouraging results in small numbers of patients have been reported with a combination of interferon alpha and oral zidovudine. Several investigators have observed response rates of approximately 60 percent, with some very durable responses. In a noninvestigational setting, this therapy may be the most appropriate first-line therapy for a patient in need of treatment.

■ PERIPHERAL T CELL LYMPHOMA

Etiology and Epidemiology

Peripheral T cell lymphoma (PTCL) is a heterogenous group of T cell non-Hodgkin's lymphomas (NHL). The term *peripheral* refers to the mature T cell surface phenotype. This heterogenous group of disorders has no working classification system and is categorized according to histologic appearance as large cell, mixed large and small cell, and rarely, small cell lymphocytic lymphoma. Typically, 10 to 15 percent of cases manifest cutaneous disease. According to tabulations from two large series, 40 to 60 percent of cases reveal mixed pathology, 20 to 40 percent are categorized as large cell, and the remaining 20 percent are composed of small cells. Covering a broad spectrum of clinical presentations and outcomes, as a rule they are somewhat aggressive lymphomas that exhibit behavior analogous to that of the spectrum of B-cell NHL. The distinguishing feature of PTCL with primary cutaneous presentation consists of an infiltration of mature or post-thymic T lymphocytes in the dermis associated with lymph node and occasional visceral involvement. Epidermotropism is not seen. The characteristics of the population in which PTCL is found are as diverse as the disease entity itself. It is seen in both sexes, with a slight male predominance. Median age approaches 55; however, cases have been seen in patients as young as 16 and as old as 80 years. Elderly patients commonly present with bulky, advanced disease. Epstein-Barr virus (EBV) has been shown to be present in tumor cells of some patients with PTCL; however, a true causative relationship has not been established at this point. A report of three cases of PTCL in EBV patients with acquired immunodeficiency syndrome (AIDS) does suggest an association.

Histopathology

PTCL are a group of lymphomas that manifest a diffuse growth pattern composed of a mixture of lymphoid cells of varying sizes. Vascularity is commonly increased. Other reactive cells such as eosinophils, histiocytes, and plasma cells are present. Small lymphocytes with a low nuclear to cytoplasmic ratio and large T cell immunoblasts with irregular nuclei and definitive nucleoli are evident. Features of these tumors, including the varying combinations of lymphocytes, presence of benign reactive cells, and wide range of atypia all work against rigidly classifying these lymphomas. An immunohistochemical workup is essential, for morphologically it is frequently quite difficult to distinguish among PTCL, other B-cell NHL, and Hodgkin's disease. CD5 and either CD8 or CD4 antigens can be detected in these cases. Much confusion has been generated by the large, atypical Reed-Sternberg–like cells in some instances. The absence of CD15 in these instances diminishes the likelihood of Hodgkin's disease. On occasion all T cell antigens are negative. In these cases gene rearrangement studies may be necessary for the diagnosis.

Staging and Prognosis

The symptomatic manifestations of these disorders result from the infiltration of T cells into the skin or other organs. Staging should include the routine procedures used in the evaluation of non-Hodgkin's lymphomas. These patients present most commonly with diffuse lymphadenopathy. Skin manifestations, which are frequent, can include a diffuse maculopapular rash, diffuse erythema, pitting edema, erythematous plaques, and desquamative changes. Respiratory symptoms and abdominal discomfort may also be seen. Radiologic abnormalities can include pulmonary processes such as pleural effusions, pulmonary nodules, or mediastinal masses. Concurrent laboratory abnormalities can include anemia, lymphopenia, circulating T-helper lymphocytes, eosinophilia, and hypergammaglobulinemia or hyporgammaglobulinemia. These patients tend to present at an advanced stage and *may* frequently exhibit evidence of B symptoms. Survival statistics reveal an unfavorable outcome in the majority of patients, with survival times ranging from 5 to 30 months and with a median of 9 months. Prognostic features include performance status, age, tumor bulk, stage, and grade of the tumor.

Cytogenetic abnormalities and specific cell surface phenotype may factor into the prognosis. The use of Ki-67, a monoclonal antibody that binds to nuclear antigens present during cellular proliferation (during G1, G2, M, and S) has become more frequent and appears to be a helpful indicator of cell growth. Therefore, a highly Ki-67–positive specimen may reflect a more rapid proliferative rate and therefore a worse prognosis.

Therapy

Treatment is typically aggressive but is based on extent of disease, age, and performance status of the individual. Radiotherapy to localized sites of disease may be quite acceptable and provide significant improvement or even complete remission of the malignancy. More often than not, however, patients present with generalized constitutional symptoms and bulky or systemic disease, implying a need for a combination chemotherapy regimen. Chemotherapeutic trials employing standard combination regimes used to treat non-Hodgkin's lymphoma have been done. Some studies suggest results comparable with those of B cell lymphomas when stratified by stage and grade. Other studies suggest a lower response and cure with PTCL. Collectively, in patients with advanced disease outcomes are poor and survival limited even with the most aggressive treatment regimens.

■ KI-1 LYMPHOMAS

A spectrum of PTCL express the Ki-1 (CD30) antigen. This antigen is also expressed in other tumor cells, including the Reed-Sternberg cell in Hodgkin's. The peripheral cutaneous CD30+ large cell lymphomas most often occur in a population in the mid to late 20s, though a secondary peak is seen at age 50. There is a slight male predominance (3:2). The clinical presentation is characterized by localized cutaneous lesions, consisting of either nodules or tumorlike growths, sometimes with evidence of ulceration. This type of lymphoma is classified as high grade yet often has a better prognosis than other PTCL. They are classically defined by the following criteria: (1) greater than 75 percent predominance or large clusters of CD30+ cells in the initial skin biopsy specimen; (2) clinically no evidence of regression and chronic recurrence, as seen in lymphomatoid papulosis; (3) no pre-existent or concurrent peripheral T cell process such as mycosis fungoides or lymphomatoid papulosis; and (4) no extracutaneous sites of disease at the time of presentation. On biopsy, these CD30+ cutaneous lymphomas reveal dense infiltrates of large tumor cells with abundant cytoplasm, round or irregular nuclei, and one to several nucleoli. High rates of mitosis are evident. The cells cluster together and are often surrounded by inflammatory cells, such as histiocytes or lymphocytes. Occasional multinucleated giant cells are present. Anaplastic changes predominate but frequently are absent. When analyzed with phenotypic studies, these cells most frequently show a T cell phenotype. CD2, CD3, CD5, and CD15 antigens are absent. However, antigens including CD25 (IL-2 receptor antigen), HLA-DR (histocompatibility antigen), and epithelial membrane antigens are present. T cell receptor gene rearrangements have been noted in 50 to 70 percent of cases.

Treatment is tailored to the extent of disease and overall condition of the patient. Truly localized cutaneous disease is usually treated with radiotherapy, though on occasion one may see spontaneous regression. Systemic chemotherapy consisting of a multidrug regimen is often reserved for individuals who have progressed with extracutaneous sites of involvement, such as liver, spleen, or lymph nodes. Response rates are excellent, and with therapy 4 year survival rates of approximately 90 percent have been noted. On occasion cases of CD30+ cutaneous lymphoma have arisen from a preexistent lymphoproliferative disorder such as mycosis fungoides. In these cases response to treatment and overall survival is significantly worse.

LYMPHOMATOID PAPULOSIS

Lymphomatoid papulosis (LyP) is a benign cutaneous eruption that in 20 to 30 percent of patients is associated with the development of non-Hodgkin's and Hodgkin's lymphomas. The classic presentation of LyP includes recurrent episodes of disseminated papules and nodules that typically ulcerate and then heal with scarring. The course is usually indolent, spanning decades. Routine histology demonstrates two morphologic presentations. Type A lesions are more common, are nonepidermotropic, and contain prominent large atypical cells (Reed-Sternberg–like cells) and depending on the age of the lesion, an inflammatory component. Type B lesions are epidermotropic and contain mainly mononuclear cerebriform cells resembling Sézary cells but relatively few inflammatory cells. An erroneous diagnosis of large cell lymphoma is often entertained. LyP has been shown to be clonal process by analysis of T cell receptor gene rearrangements. Immunophenotyping shows a mature T-helper cell profile (CD3+, CD4+) and expression of activation antigens CD30, CD25, and Ia. Therapeutic interventions (PUVA, or psoralen–ultraviolet A, methotrexate, steroids) are reserved for patients with cosmetic consequences of the disease and have a minimal effect on the natural history of this disorder.

LYMPHOMATOID GRANULOMATOSIS

Lymphomatoid granulomatosis is a rare multiorgan disease of the lungs, nasopharynx joints, peripheral and central nervous system, and skin. Cutaneous involvement is seen in 25 to 50 percent of patients. Though cutaneous nodules with pulmonary involvement are most common, some patients have nonspecific macules, papules, or ulcerations. Histologic evaluation usually reveals an angiocentric, polymorphous infiltrate of both atypical lymphocytes and histiocytes surrounding and invading blood vessels. Immunologic studies suggest a mature clonal helper T cell process, but only rare cases have demonstrated clonal T cell receptor rearrangements. Epstein-Barr virus DNA sequences are frequently present. Though the clinical course is variable, the prognosis for patients with diffuse pulmonary involvement or the appearance of high-grade lymphoma is poor, with a median survival of less than 2 years. Treatment, which depends on histologic findings and extent and location of disease, may include corticosteroids, radiotherapy, and/or systemic chemotherapy. Recent reports also suggest a role for interferon-alpha.

ANGIOIMMUNOBLASTIC LYMPHADENOPATHY

Angioimmunoblastic lymphadenopathy is a rare lymphoproliferative disorder frequently accompanied by hepatosplenomegaly, fever, skin rash, and generalized malaise. Common laboratory features include anemia (often Coombs-positive hemolytic), thrombocytopenia, leukocytosis with lymphopenia, and polyclonal hypergammaglobulinemia. Histologic features of lymph node biopsies include complete architectural effacement with replacement by a diffuse polymorphous cellular infiltrate composed of lymphocytes, immunoblasts, and plasma cells, with or without histiocytes and eosinophils. Prominent arborization of postcapillary venules and atrophic germinal centers are seen. Histologic progression to an appearance of a high-grade lymphoma is common. Approximately 50 percent of patients have skin involvement at presentation. Histologic findings are nonspecific; they consist of a perivascular lymphocytic infiltrate in the dermis with a cytologic composition similar to that of the lymph nodes. Molecular and immunologic studies suggest an activated mature clonal T cell phenotype. The median survival is approximately 1.5 years, and only 30 percent of patients survive 2 years. Treatment with corticosteroids and/or chemotherapy has been of modest benefit. An association with Kaposi's sarcoma has been presumed to be a consequence of the patient's immune-depressed state.

T-GAMMA LYMPHOCYTOSIS

T-gamma lymphocytosis is a rare, chronic lymphoproliferative disorder of large granular lymphocytes (LGL). LGL cells are large mononuclear cells with abundant cytoplasm containing eosinophilic granules. There are two predominant phenotypic subsets, T cells and natural killer cells. In both instances a clonal expansion of the malignant population has been demonstrated. T cell LGL express the T cell receptor and are CD2+, CD8+, CD16+, CD56±, and CD57±. Natural killer cell LGL are CD2+, CD11+, CD16+, CD18+, CD45+, CD56+, CD57+, NKR-P^2+, and NKR+. A typical clinical presentation includes a mild to moderate lymphocytosis (4,000 to 30,000 lymphocytes per cubic millimeter) with recurrent infection secondary to neutropenia. In addition, pure red cell aplasia, autoimmune anemia, thrombocytopenia, and rheumatoid arthritis have been associated with this disease. Mild to moderate splenomegaly is common, hepatomegaly is seen less frequently, and lymphadenopathy and cutaneous involvement are unusual. Though T-gamma lymphocytosis usually runs an indolent course, patients may progress to a fulminant leukemic form with high circulating LGL cell counts and generalized organ infiltration. In rare instances, spontaneous resolution of the disease has been witnessed. Treatment in general has been ineffective. Corticosteroids and alkylating agents have modest activity and may increase the neutrophil count. Interferon and purine analogues have been generally disappointing. Splenectomy is rarely useful. Patients at times are most disabled by their chronic neutropenia, thought to be autoimmune in nature, and future therapeutic investigations should address this issue. The use of colony-stimulating factors has not been adequately evaluated in this disorder.

Suggested Reading

Burt RK, Young N. Pathogenesis of T-gamma-lymphocytosis. Contemp Oncol 1992; 2:21–28.

Carlson KC, Gibson LE. Cutaneous signs of lymphomatoid granulomatosis. Arch Dermatol 1991; 127:1693–1698.

Chott A, Augustin I, Wrba F, et al. Peripheral T cell lymphomas: A clinicopathologic study of 75 cases. Hum Pathol 1990; 21:1117–1125.

Gill PS, Horrington W, Jr Kaplan MH, et al. Treatment of adult T-cell leukemia and lymphoma with a combination of interferon alpha and cidovudine. N Engl J Med 1995; 332:1744–1748.

Höllsberg P, Hafler DA. Pathogenesis of diseases induced by human lymphotropic virus type I infection. N Engl J Med 1993; 328:1173–1182.

Kuzel TM, Roenigk HH Jr, Rosen ST. Mycosis fungoides and the Sézary syndrome: A review of pathogenesis, diagnosis, and therapy. J Clin Oncol 1991; 9:1298–1313.

Macaulay WL. Lymphomatoid papulosis update. Arch Dermatol 1989; 125: 1387–1389.

Rosenblatt JD, Danon Y, Block AC. A decade with HTLV-I/HTLV-II; lesions in viral leukemogenesis. Leukemia 1992; 6(Suppl 1):18–23.

Steinberg AD, Seldin MF, Jaffe ES, et al. Angioimmunoblastic lymphadenopathy with dysproteinemia. Ann Intern Med 1988; 108:575–584.

Willemze R. Beljaards RC. Spectrum of primary cutaneous CD30 (Ki-1)-positive lymphoproliferative disorders. J Am Acad Dermatol 1993; 28:973–980.

LUNG CANCER: RADIOTHERAPY

Ritsuko Komaki, M.D., F.A.C.R.
James D. Cox, M.D., F.A.C.R.

Carcinoma of the lung is no longer the most common malignant tumor in the United States, but it is by far the most frequent cause of death from cancer. Estimates from the American Cancer Society for 1997 indicate that lung cancer will be diagnosed in 178,000 Americans, less than cancer of the prostate or breast, but it will kill 160,000 patients, including more than twice as many men as prostatic cancer and fully 25 percent more women than mammary cancer. Radiotherapy is a major component of treatment in most of these patients—as surgical adjuvant therapy, definitive treatment for inoperable patients, and palliation for patients with disseminated disease.

PRESENTATION AND DETECTION

Although the propensity for dissemination is a hallmark of cancer of the lung, patients most frequently present with symptoms resulting from the primary tumor or its intrathoracic regional extensions. Cough, hemoptysis, and pain in the chest, shoulder, or arm are common symptoms; weight loss and bone pain are the first symptoms of systemic disease.

Paraneoplastic phenomena are not rare. A myasthenic syndrome and other peripheral nervous system disorders may be seen, and limbic encephalopathy and other central nervous system (CNS) syndromes may be disclosed by careful testing. Inappropriate secretion of antidiuretic hormone, Cushing's syndrome, hypertrophic pulmonary osteoarthropathy, and hypercalcemia are among the most frequent: all but the last two syndromes are more common with small cell carcinoma.

Although most patients are found to have evidence of the disease by chest roentgenogram, computed tomography (CT) and bronchoscopy are indicated in symptomatic patients if the chest films are unrevealing; even if the chest film is abnormal, these two procedures are appropriate in most patients for diagnosis and staging.

STAGING

Treatment of cancer of the lung in general and the role of radiotherapy in particular are closely related to the stage of the disease, i.e., the anatomic extent of tumors and the histopathologic type of cancer. In addition, the intensity of symptoms as reflected in performance status scores and weight loss are important in determining the goal of therapy.

The staging classification in use is the 1992 version of the American Joint Committee on Cancer (AJCC) (Table 1).

The major histopathologic distinctions are small cell carcinoma, squamous cell carcinoma, adenocarcinoma, and large cell carcinoma, the latter three grouped as non–small cell carcinoma of the lung (NSCCL) because of their very different responses to chemotherapy and their cellular and subcellular characteristics. Small cell carcinoma of the lung (SCCL) is usually classified not by the AJCC criteria, since virtually all are either stage III or IV, but as limited—tumor confined to the thorax and ipsilateral supraclavicular lymph nodes (AJCC stages IIIA and IIIB)—or extensive—evidence of dissemination (AJCC stage IV).

The presence of pleural effusion has been considered by some to be T4 for NSCCL or limited disease for SCCL, whereas others have considered pleural and pericardial effusions to be manifestations of disseminated disease. Although effusions may be transudates secondary to obstruction, they can never be encompassed within the high-dose volume of irradiation, and thus for practical purposes they are best classified with extensive disease.

Minimal studies required to establish extent of disease are CT of the chest and upper abdomen, liver function tests, bone scan, and CT or magnetic resonance imaging (MRI) of the brain for all but squamous cell carcinoma. If none of these

Table 1 AJCC Staging Classification for Lung Cancer

Primary Tumor (T)		
T1	Tumor ≤3 cm surrounded by lung or visceral pleura without invasion more proximal than lobar bronchus	
T2	Tumor >3 cm or involving main bronchus 2 cm or more distal to carina or invading visceral pleura or with atelectasis or obstructive pneumonitis involving less than entire lung	
T3	Tumor that invades the chest wall (including superior sulcus tumors), diaphragm, mediastinal pleura, or parietal pericardium; tumor in main bronchus <2 cm from carina but not invading it; tumor with atelectasis or obstructive pneumonitis of entire lung	
T4	Tumor that invades either mediastinum, heart, great vessels, trachea, esophagus, vertebral body, carina	
Lymph Node (N)		
N0	No regional lymph node metastasis	
N1	Metastasis in ipsilateral peribronchial or hilar lymph nodes	
N2	Metastasis in ipsilateral mediastinal or subcarcinal lymph nodes	
N3	Metastasis in contralateral mediastinal, hilar, or ipsilateral supraclavicular lymph nodes	
Distant Metastasis		
M0	No distant metastasis	
M1	Distant metastasis	
Stage Groupings		
Stage I	T1,T2	N0 M0
Stage II	T1,T2	N1 M0
Stage IIIA	T3	N0 M0
	T1,T2,T3	N2 M0
Stage IIIB	Any T	N3 M0
	T4	Any N M0
Stage IV	Any T	Any N M1

studies indicates extrathoracic dissemination and there is no pleural effusion, treatment can be undertaken with curative intent.

When all pretreatment evaluations are completed, approximately equal proportions of patients have localized disease and disseminated disease (Figure 1). Two other factors identifiable at the time of diagnosis influence the goal of therapy. Performance status scores are strongly related to outcome. We use the Karnofsky scale (KPS), an abbreviated version of which is given in Table 2.

The other major factor in consideration of treatment is weight loss. Although these criteria have been questioned, since they rely entirely on the medical history, they have consistently been very important prognostic factors for survival.

■ MANAGEMENT

Non–Small Cell Carcinoma of the Lung

Stage I

All patients with NSCCL who are candidates for thoracotomy and complete resection should be afforded this option. The vast majority of patients with stage I NSCCL can undergo complete resection, and the prognosis is quite favorable if a formal mediastinal nodal dissection is performed and careful histopathologic assessment reveals no evidence of metastasis to lymph nodes. There is no evidence that adjuvant therapy of any type is indicated. Clinical investigations of systemic therapy are appropriate, and there is considerable interest in chemopreventive studies beyond smoking cessation to reduce the risk of second primary carcinomas arising in the remaining lung, but there is no established value of these measures.

Stage II

Tumors with the demonstrated ability to spread to regional lymph nodes, even to peribronchial nodes, carry a much poorer outlook than stage I tumors, and they justify adjuvant therapy. There is no documented benefit from preoperative adjuvant therapy, although there is interest in this area. Since most of these patients only have documentation of regional lymph node involvement after histopathologic analysis of the resected specimen, postoperative therapy is the standard. Postoperative irradiation has the advantage of reducing the frequency of recurrence in the mediastinum. There are insufficient data to confirm the value of such treatment on survival in patients with squamous cell carcinoma, but a large body of data supports the reduction in local failure, and several studies suggest an improvement in survival 3 and 5 years after therapy. The addition of postoperative systemic chemotherapy to irradiation is under investigation, but its value is not yet established.

Radiotherapy may begin as soon as 2 weeks after resection if there have been no complications. Treatment planning requires postoperative CT of the chest, as the anatomic relationships may be different than indicated on the preoperative studies, and maximum effort to avoid normal lung is imperative. If the tumor was completely resected, the aim of radiotherapy is to deliver a total dose of 50 Gy in fractions of 1.8 or 2 Gy, five fractions per week for 5 to 5½ weeks, to the remaining nodal regions at risk. For tumors that arose in the upper or middle lobes, the ipsilateral supraclavicular fossa is added to a field that encompasses the mediastinum from the thoracic inlet to approximately 5 cm below the carina. Our usual approach is to use parallel opposed anterior and posterior fields with no correction for tissue in homogeneities within the thorax. After 40 Gy has been delivered to the midplane of the chest, oblique or occasionally lateral fields are used and the supraclavicular region is omitted. In this manner the supraclavicular region receives approximately 45 Gy in the first 4 weeks. The entire width of the mediastinum is encompassed, and the hilar regions are included bilaterally with rather narrow margins. There have been suggestions that smaller volumes may be used, but the morbidity of the treatment described is minimal, and no data suggest that there is value in more restricted treatment. Similarly, it has been suggested that the total dose should be higher than 50 Gy, but elimination of local recurrence is nearly complete at this dose unless the margin of resection was positive, in which case an additional 10 Gy in five fractions may be justified.

The only modifications we make for tumors arising in the lower lobes are elimination of the supraclavicular field and extension of the inferior border of the mediastinal field to the diaphragm.

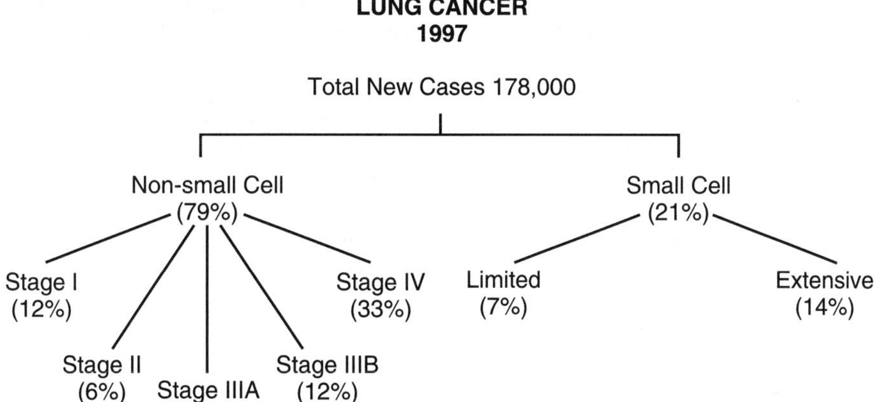

Figure 1
New cases of lung cancer by cell type and stage.

Table 2 Karnofsky Scale for Scoring Performance Status

100	Asymptomatic
90	Minor signs or symptoms; normal activity
80	Normal activity with effort
70	Activity compromised; cares for self
60	Need help to care for self
50	Unable to care for self; not hospitalized
40	Disabled; requires special care
30	Hospitalization necessary
20	Major inpatient support required
10	Near death

Stage IIIA

In principle, patients with stage IIIA NSCCL have resectable tumors. The major reason for dividing stage III into A and B was to distinguish resectable from unresectable tumors. If the tumors are resectable and the resected lymph nodes reveal no evidence of involvement, the treatment plan described for stage II is appropriate.

A large proportion of patients with stage IIIA NSCCL have mediastinal lymph node involvement. There is much interest in induction chemotherapy or combined radiotherapy and chemotherapy for stage IIIA tumors with metastasis to mediastinal lymph nodes, but there is as yet no established benefit of induction therapy before resection. In fact, although thoracotomy and pulmonary resection with mediastinal lymph node dissection for patients with stage IIIA NSCCL who prove to have mediastinal nodal involvement is widely practiced, it is not clear that this approach is superior to combinations of radiotherapy and chemotherapy without resection. This is discussed with clinical stage IIIB.

Stage IIIB

Tumors classified as unresectable by virtue of supraclavicular or contralateral mediastinal lymph node involvement or by virtue of extensions of the primary tumor across midline or to involve major vessels, vertebrae, or other structures not considered resectable except by extraordinary means can still be treated with curative intent. To this group must be added the patients with stage IIIA tumors deemed inoperable due to pulmonary or cardiac compromise and those who refuse surgical intervention. With rare exception, long-term survival has only been described in patients with stages IIIA and IIIB who have KPS scores above 70 and weight loss totaling no more than 5 percent prior to presentation. This represents approximately 40 percent of all patients with inoperable NSCCL.

For many years the standard of therapy for patients with unresectable stage IIIA and IIIB NSCCL was high-dose radiotherapy. Our practice has been to deliver a total dose of 60 Gy at 2 Gy per fraction or occasionally 63 Gy at 1.8 Gy per fraction in 6 or 7 weeks respectively to the primary tumor and all sites of regional involvement. This includes the occasional tumor with metastasis to the supraclavicular fossa. The entire mediastinum and both hilar regions receive a minimum dose of 45 Gy. For upper lobe lesions the lower border of the mediastinal field extends at least 5 cm below the carina; it extends to the diaphragm for primary tumors arising in the lower lobes.

Reports of carefully conducted clinical trials have confirmed the advantage of combining chemotherapy with such irradiation in favorable patients (KPS ≥, weight loss ≤ 5 percent). It is evident that a reduction in distant metastasis results from combinations of cisplatin with vinblastine or etoposide and possibly other agents given before standard radiotherapy. Moreover, concurrent administration of cisplatin with radiotherapy appears to increase local control. This is an area of intense research at present, and any recommendation is likely to be superseded as more data become available. It is our practice to offer every patient the opportunity to participate in prospective clinical trials. If patients are not willing to participate or logistic considerations prohibit one arm of a study, our standard is to use cisplatin 75 mg per square meter IV on days 1, 29, and 50 plus vinblastine 5 mg per square meter IV weekly for 5 weeks. Radiotherapy begins on day 50 after the start of chemotherapy. Daily fractions of 2 Gy are administered. A large field which encompasses sites considered at high risk for extension and metastasis receives a total dose of 42 Gy to 44 Gy; gross disease receives 60 Gy in 6 weeks.

Preliminary results suggest that concurrent use of cisplatin and vinblastine or etoposide with standard or hyperfractionated radiation therapy (1.2 Gy twice daily to 69.6 Gy) may be superior to sequential use of the modalities.

There is little morbidity from standard radiotherapy based on CT treatment planning. Patients usually have odynophagia during the third week of radiotherapy; it decreases in severity during the next weeks due to the cyclic nature of the reactions of the esophageal squamous mucosa, but the discomfort does not disappear completely until after the treatment is over. Pulmonary morbidity is a function of the volume irradiated rather than the total dose, since any portion of the normal lung that receives a total dose above 25 Gy will respond with radiation pneumonitis and subsequent scarring. Therefore, the aim of treatment planning is to keep to a minimum the volume of lung that receives 25 Gy or more.

The addition of chemotherapy increases both the frequency and severity of acute reactions, primarily in the esophagus, especially if the two modalities are given concurrently. Induction chemotherapy is associated with lesser effects on the esophagus, but bone marrow suppression is at least as severe as it is with concurrent chemotherapy and radiotherapy.

Apical Sulcus (Pancoast) Tumors

Tumors that arise in the extreme apex of the lung have a natural history different from other carcinomas of the lung. Patients usually present with shoulder and arm pain and may have Horner's syndrome, extension to the brachial plexus and rib, or vertebral destruction. Although all histopathologic types of carcinoma can be seen in the pulmonary apex, SCCL is least common. The most frequent types are adenocarcinoma and large cell carcinoma. The diagnosis can be made with fine-needle aspiration. CT is useful, but MRI frequently shows much greater extension, especially superiorly, than other imaging procedures.

Tradition has called for preoperative radiotherapy followed by resection, but our experience has shown this less satisfactory than immediate operation. If the tumor is resectable, there is no demonstrated advantage and probably little disadvantage of preoperative irradiation. However, if the tumor proves to be unresectable, such irradiation makes it impossible to deliver the most effective irradiation—which by itself may be curative in a substantial proportion of patients. Our policy is immediate exploration and complete resection if possible. If there is tumor at the margins of resection or regional lymph node involvement, postoperative irradiation is administered. We are investigating the addition of concurrent chemotherapy with cisplatin and oral etoposide. If the tumor is unresectable, we proceed with definitive radiotherapy with concurrent chemotherapy as with stage IIIB tumors.

Small Cell Carcinoma of the Lung

Limited Disease

Chemotherapy is essential in the management of patients with SCCL. As more effective combinations of drugs were developed, some investigators considered radiotherapy to be important only in reducing recurrence in the thorax and of little consequence in determining survival. It is now generally accepted that thoracic irradiation is very important for long-term survival. The best way of combining radiotherapy with chemotherapy is still controversial. We have pursued a number of studies, the results of which have convinced us that concurrent thoracic irradiation with chemotherapy is more effective than giving one modality and then the other. Concurrent therapy produces more side effects during the treatment, but vigorous support of the patients during this time is appropriate, as the reactions subside after the radiotherapy is over, and a higher probability of control within the thorax and long-term survival result.

Studies undergoing analysis will determine whether accelerated fractionation using 1.5 Gy twice daily separated by 6 hours to a total dose of 45 Gy in 3 weeks is superior to 1.8 Gy delivered once daily to a total dose of 45 Gy in 5 weeks. When either of these fractionation schemes is combined with cisplatin 60 mg per square meter IV on day 1 with etoposide 120 mg per square meter days 1 to 3, repeated every 3 weeks for 4 cycles, the survival has been better in our experience than any regimen we have used.

Prophylactic cranial irradiation (PCI) is useful in reducing the very high likelihood of CNS metastasis with SCCL. PCI is more effective when administered early in the course of treatment, and we prefer to use it as soon after completion of chemotherapy as possible. Whole brain irradiation is given with fields that extend inferiorly to encompass the middle cranial fossa; a total dose of 25 Gy given to the midsagittal plane in 10 fractions of 2.5 Gy over a 2 week period is sufficient to control the subclinical metastasis presumed to be present. Late neuropsychologic deficits in patients treated for SCCL raised concerns about PCI, as they were assumed to be sequelae of treatment. Recent studies have shown that specific cognitive deficits are present in patients with SCCL before they receive PCI, and there is no short-term worsening of those deficits.

Extensive Disease

There is no established role for the use of radiotherapy in patients with extensive SCCL. The outlook for such patients is much graver than for those with limited disease, and it is largely determined by the effectiveness of combination chemotherapy. A small proportion will have clinical complete responses documented by chest CT in addition to physical examination and other imaging studies. The single most likely site of recurrence in patients with extensive disease and complete response is in the thorax at the site of the original primary and regional lymph node metastasis. It is reasonable to consider irradiation to the chest for such patients.

■ PALLIATIVE RADIOTHERAPY

At least half the patients who are found to have carcinoma of the lung have distant metastasis at the time of diagnosis. Another large group will have dissemination beyond the thorax after initial treatment. Radiotherapy can be used to relieve symptoms, especially from cerebral and skeletal metastases. A total dose of 30 Gy given in 10 fractions of 3 Gy is usually sufficient to accomplish symptomatic relief. Full benefit is usually seen well after the completion of radiotherapy. It is uncommon to have to repeat a course of such palliative irradiation, but it may be possible if this dose fractionation regimen is used.

Suggested Reading

Komaki R, Cox JD. The lung and thymus. In: Cox JD, ed. Moss' radiation oncology: Rationale, technique, results. 7th Ed. St. Louis: Mosby, 1994:320.

Lee JS, Scott C, Komaki R, et al. Concurrent chemoradiation therapy with oral etoposide and cisplatin for locally advanced inoperable non-small-cell lung cancer: Radiation therapy oncology group protocol 91-06. J Clin Oncol 1996; 14:1055–1064.

Sause WT, Scott C, Taylor S, et al. Radiation Therapy Oncology Group 88-08 and Eastern Cooerative Oncology Group 4588: Preliminary results of a phase III trial in regionally advanced, unresectable non-small cell lung cancer. J Natl Cancer Inst 1995; 87:198–205.

LUNG CANCER: CHEMOTHERAPY

Joan H. Schiller, M.D.

Lung cancer is a major health problem in the United States today. Despite public awareness of the health hazards of smoking, the incidence of lung cancer is increasing because of the increasing incidence of smoking in the late 1960s and 1970s and the long latent period before the appearance of this disease. Thus, knowledge and management of this disease continue to be essential for physicians caring for an adult population.

Lung cancer consists of four general histologic types: adenocarcinoma, squamous cell carcinoma, large cell carcinoma, and small cell carcinoma. Small cell carcinoma of the lung (SCCL) differs from the other three types in its rapid clinical course, propensity to metastasize early, features of neuroendocrine differentiation and association with paraneoplastic syndromes, and unique sensitivity to chemotherapy and radiotherapy. Because of this the other three types are often collectively termed non–small cell carcinoma of the lung (NSCCL).

As with other malignancies, management of NSCCL is based primarily on the stage of the disease at the time of diagnosis. Because of SCCL's unique sensitivity to chemotherapy and propensity for rapid dissemination, chemotherapy forms the backbone of treatment regardless of the extent of disease at diagnosis. This chapter discusses the role of chemotherapy in the management of both localized and advanced SCCL and NSCCL.

■ NON–SMALL CELL LUNG CANCER

Staging

Stage I NSCCL

Stage I NSCCL (T1-T2, N0, M0) is potentially curable with surgical resection, with cure rates of 60 to 80 percent reported. Despite the high cure rates, however, 20 to 40 percent of patients will develop recurrent disease. Prospective studies under way will determine whether prognostic factors (K-ras, p53, blood group antigens) that will help identify patients at high risk for recurrent disease can be identified. At this point, however, no role for postoperative chemotherapy has been identified.

Patients with a history of one lung cancer are at risk of developing a second primary, probably due to the field, or multifocal, effect of the neoplastic process. Based upon encouraging results observed in head and neck cancer patients, an intergroup randomized placebo-controlled study is now under way to determine the role of *cis*-retinoic acid in preventing second primaries in this group of patients.

Locally Advanced NSCCL

The treatment of locally advanced NSCCL is one of the most controversial issues in the management of lung cancer. Treatment options include surgery, chemotherapy, radiotherapy, and any combination thereof. Interpretation of the results of clinical trials involving patients with locally advanced disease has been clouded by a number of issues. Older trials have used older diagnostic techniques and different staging systems, making direct comparisons with current technologies difficult. Although the prognoses for these three stages vary (stage II, 30 to 40 percent 5 year survival; stage IIIA, 10 to 20 percent; stage IIIB, 5 to 10 percent), many trials contain a mix of patients, raising concerns about the heterogeneity of the patient populations studied.

The treatment for stage II NSCCL is surgical resection. Several studies have examined the issue of postoperative adjuvant chemotherapy for stage II and stage IIIA disease. The Lung Cancer Study Group (LCSG) randomized 141 patients with resected stage II and III adenocarcinoma and large cell undifferentiated carcinoma to receive postoperative cyclophosphamide 400 mg per square meter, doxorubicin 40 mg per square meter, and cisplatin (CAP) 40 mg per square meter or bacillus Calmette-Guérin (BCG) and levamisole immunotherapy. Disease-free survival was significantly prolonged in the group receiving chemotherapy, and overall survival bordered on statistical significance. In another study by the LCSG 172 patients with incompletely resected NSCCL were randomized to receive postoperative CAP plus radiotherapy or radiotherapy alone. The chemotherapy arm showed a significantly longer recurrence-free interval. An improvement in the survival rate at 1 year was also observed, although overall survival was not significantly improved.

Despite these results, however, postoperative adjuvant che-

Dr. Schiller is supported in part by the Department of Veterans Affairs.

motherapy for stage II disease cannot be routinely recommended. A randomized intergroup study is under way to define further the role of postoperative chemotherapy in patients with resected stage II or IIIA NSCCL. In that study patients are randomized to receive either radiotherapy plus chemotherapy (cisplatin 60 mg per square meter and etoposide 120 mg per square meter) or radiotherapy alone.

The optimal treatment for stage IIIA and IIIB disease is controversial. Current investigational efforts are directed at identifying the optimal combined modality approach, involving treatments directed at local control of the disease (surgery or radiotherapy) and micrometastatic disease (chemotherapy). Possibilities include preoperative or postoperative chemotherapy and chemotherapy plus radiotherapy.

The use of preoperative chemotherapy with or without radiotherapy is gaining interest. Several nonrandomized studies suggest that such therapy renders unresectable disease resectable and results in prolonged survival. The Memorial Sloan-Kettering Cancer Center has reported response rates of 73 percent in patients with clinical N2, M0 disease following two to three cycles of chemotherapy with cisplatin 120 mg per square meter and vindesine 3 mg per square meter or vinblastine 5 mg per square meter on days 1, 8, 15, 22, and 29. Survival at 3 years was 34 percent for all 41 patients, 40 percent for the 21 who completed the combined treatment (chemotherapy and surgery), and 54 percent for the 8 patients who had a complete resection. Other studies failed to confirm the prolonged median survival, and the role of preoperative chemotherapy is being investigated in a randomized intergroup trial.

The use of chemotherapy plus radiotherapy remains an area of active investigation. The Cancer and Leukemia Group B (CALGB) conducted a randomized trial of induction chemotherapy plus high-dose irradiation versus irradiation alone in stage IIIA and B NSCCL; 155 patients were randomized to receive cisplatin 100 mg per square meter on days 1 and 29 and vinblastine 5 mg per square meter on days 1, 8, 15, 22, 29, followed by radiotherapy on day 50 (60 Gy over 6 weeks) or to receive radiotherapy alone. The median survival was significantly longer in the chemotherapy group (13.8 versus 9.7 months), prompting some clinicians to regard this regimen as the standard treatment for stage IIIA and IIIB NSCCL. However, other randomized trials have failed to confirm the survival advantage of chemotherapy plus radiotherapy over radiotherapy alone. A National Cancer Institute (NCI) high-priority study evaluating the role of chemotherapy plus radiotherapy has recently been completed. In it patients were randomized to standard fractionation radiotherapy, twice daily fractions (hyperfractionation), or chemotherapy plus radiotherapy. Results of this trial, when available, should help define the role of chemotherapy plus radiotherapy for locally advanced disease.

Metastatic Disease

The median survival of patients with metastatic NSCCL is only about 6 months. The effect of chemotherapy treatments on survival is modest at best, with few patients achieving a complete response. Therefore, important questions can be raised regarding the routine use of chemotherapy, whether to treat at all, when to treat, the appropriate patients to treat, and quality of life issues.

Table 1 Chemotherapy Regimens for Metastatic Non–Small Cell Lung Cancer

AGENTS	DOSE
PE	
Cisplatin	60 mg/m^2 IV day 1
Etoposide	120 mg/m^2 IV days 1–3
Cycle to be repeated every 3 weeks	
CAP	
Cyclophosphamide	400 mg/m^2 IV day 1
Doxorubicin (Adriamycin)	40 mg/m^2 IV day 1
Cisplatin	40 mg/m^2 IV day 1
Cycle to be repeated every 4 weeks	
Carbo/VP-16	
Carboplatin	300 mg/m^2 IV day 1
Etoposide	100 mg/m^2 IV days 1–3
Cycle to be repeated every 3 to 4 weeks	

Chemotherapy Regimens

Only a handful of drugs clearly have activity in NSCCL as a single agent. These include cisplatin, ifosfamide, vinblastine, vindesine, mitomycin, and etoposide. No role has been demonstrated for high-dose cisplatin (100 to 120 mg per square meter) compared with more standard doses of cisplatin (50 to 60 mg per square meter).

A variety of cisplatin-based chemotherapy regimens have been used for NSCCL (Table 1). However, in randomized phase III trials no one regimen has been shown to produce a clear survival benefit or higher response rate. Treatment with a brief intensive chemotherapy regimen, CODE (cisplatin, vincristine, doxorubicin, and etoposide plus antibiotic), has yielded promising results that must be confirmed in a randomized trial. Similarly, phase II trials of ifosfamide-based regimens also have demonstrated high response rates. Toxicity can be high, and further studies are needed to determine the ultimate role of these regimens in our chemotherapy armamentarium.

Given the poor response rates and overall survival, it is reasonable to question whether there is any benefit to chemotherapy for metastatic NSCCL patients. At least six randomized trials have compared chemotherapy with best supportive care (i.e., palliative radiotherapy and optimal medical management of other malignancy-related problems). Two of these trials demonstrated an improvement in median survival (8.5 months versus 4 months in an Italian study; 24.7 weeks versus 17 weeks in a trial by the National Cancer Institute of Canada). The other four trials demonstrated a trend toward improved survival that was not statistically significant. The National Cancer Institute of Canada performed a cost-effect analysis of their study and demonstrated that the least expensive treatment was the chemotherapy arm compared with the best supportive care group, due to longer hospital admissions and more radiotherapy in the patients randomized to receive best supportive care. In none of the studies was quality of life studied.

When to Treat

Given these data, it is important to discuss with each patient the possible benefits, goals, chance of response, and quality of life with treatment. Since chemotherapy is rarely curative, goals for treatment should be palliation of symptoms and a modest improvement in survival. Arguments against treatment that should be taken into consideration include the low response rates (15 to 25 percent), side effects of treatment, and marginal improvement in survival. On the other hand, arguments for treatment include the fact that some patients will respond, with palliation of symptoms and presumably improved survival.

Appropriate patient selection is essential. The principal factors predicting response to chemotherapy and survival are performance status and extent of disease. Patients with a poor performance status (Eastern Cooperative Oncology Group [ECOG] performance status of 3 to 4) and bulky disease are unlikely to respond to treatment. Other favorable prognostic factors include no weight loss, female sex, normal serum lactate dehydrogenase (LDH), and no bone or liver metastases. Since one of the major goals of treatment is palliation of symptoms, it may be reasonable to delay chemotherapy in an asymptomatic patient.

If treatment is elected, response and tolerance to treatment can usually be determined within two cycles of therapy. Patients who have not responded within two cycles are unlikely to do so, and treatment should be discontinued.

New Agents

Because of the dismal results with standard chemotherapy regimens, it is imperative to develop new active agents if clear survival benefits are to be achieved. New chemotherapy agents with possible activity include the following:

Camptothecans. Camptothecan, a plant alkaloid derived from *Camptotheca acuminata,* is a potent inhibitor of DNA topoisomerase I. A derivative, CPT-11, has been reported in the Japanese literature to have response rates of 25 to 30 percent as a single agent and response rates over 50 percent when combined with cisplatin. Confirmatory studies are under way in the United States with CPT-11 and another camptothecan derivative, topotecan.

Paclitaxel (Taxol). Taxol, a novel antitubular agent derived from the bark of the Pacific yew tree, has significant antitumor activity in a number of diseases. In two recent studies by ECOG and M.D. Anderson Cancer Center, response rates of 21 to 25 percent and median survival of 24 weeks and 40 weeks respectively were observed. The 1 year survival rate of 41.7 percent observed in the ECOG study was the highest that ECOG has observed in the past 10 years in phase II trials of a single agent in metastatic NSCCL. Studies of taxotere, a semisynthetic paclitaxel derivative prepared from the needles of the yew tree, are also being conducted.

Vinorelbine (Navelbine). Navelbine is a semisynthetic vinca alkaloid that has produced response rates of 12 to 30 percent in phase II trials. In a U.S. trial in which patients were randomized to Navelbine or 5-fluorouracil (5-FU) plus leucovorin, patients treated with Navelbine had a statistically significant prolongation in median survival (29 weeks versus 21 weeks).

Edatrexate. Edatrexate (10-EdaM), a water-soluble methotrexate derivative, has been reported to have response rates of 10 to 30 percent as a single agent in phase II trials. When it is combined with another agent such as vinblastine, mitomycin, cyclophosphamide, or cisplatin, response rates of 27 to 59 percent have been reported.

Gemcitabine. Gemcitabine is a novel deoxycytidine analogue with properties similar to those of cytarabine. Early phase II studies have reported response rates of 20 to 24 percent.

■ SMALL CELL LUNG CANCER

Small cell lung cancer accounts for about 25 percent of all lung malignancies. Compared with the other three forms of bronchogenic carcinomas, it is unique in its rapid clinical course, propensity for rapid dissemination, neuroendocrine features, and association with paraneoplastic syndromes. It is also unique because of its exquisite sensitivity to cytotoxic agents. The responsiveness of this disease to chemotherapy regimens, coupled with the inability of local therapies such as radiotherapy or surgery to control this disease, have made chemotherapy the backbone of treatment.

Staging

Because SCCL usually presents with micrometastases and thus is not curable with surgical resection, staging for SCCL differs from the TNM staging classification of NSCCL. Instead, it is simplified to *limited* (disease combined to one hemithorax and regional lymph nodes and encompassed within one radiation port) and *extensive* (disease outside these boundaries). Patients with limited disease may be candidates for local treatment (i.e., thoracic irradiation) in addition to chemotherapy and—if they have a complete response—prophylactic cranial irradiation (PCI).

Staging workup for SCCL traditionally has encompassed a chest radiograph, computed tomography (CT) scans of the head and abdomen, bone marrow biopsy, and a radionuclide bone scan. However, this information is necessary only if knowledge of the extent of the disease will change treatment, if the prognostic information it yields is important for the patient, or if a patient is being evaluated for study. For example, if a patient is not a candidate for thoracic irradiation or PCI and is not a study candidate, a complete staging workup is probably not necessary.

As in NSCCL, the major pretreatment prognostic factors are stage, performance status, and bulky disease. Hepatic metastases also confer a poorer prognosis. If the patient's initial poor performance status is due to the underlying malignancy, these symptoms can often disappear with treatment, resulting in a net improvement in quality of life. However, major organ dysfunction from nonmalignant

Table 2 Major Active Agents in Small Cell Lung Cancer

Carboplatin	Ifosfamide
Cisplatin	Teniposide
Cyclophosphamide	Vincristine
Doxorubicin	Vindesine
Etoposide	

causes often results in inability of the patient to tolerate chemotherapy.

Single-Agent Chemotherapy

At least 12 agents have been demonstrated to have activity in SCCL (Table 2). An additional 34 agents have been described as having indeterminate activity, and 12 drugs are inactive. Etoposide, one of the most active single agents in SCCL, has a response rate of approximately 45 percent. With the recent availability of an oral preparation, preliminary studies suggest that extended administration of low-dose oral etoposide may be effective and well tolerated as a single agent, particularly in the elderly.

Combination Chemotherapy

With the observations that single agents had activity in this disease, later trials used combinations of drugs. Randomized studies subsequently demonstrated combination chemotherapy to be superior to single-agent chemotherapy. A number of regimens have been studied, with no clear advantage in prolonged survival to any one (Table 3). Cisplatin plus etoposide regimens may have less myelosuppression than regimens containing cyclophosphamide and doxorubicin. As in NSCCL, ifosfamide regimens in phase II trials have yielded promising results that should be confirmed in larger trials. Toxicity considerations must be weighed as well when deciding on a particular regimen.

With these chemotherapy regimens, overall response rates of 75 to 90 percent and complete response rates of 50 percent for localized disease can be anticipated. For extensive disease, overall response rates of about 75 percent with complete response rates of 25 percent are common. Despite these high response rates, however, median survival remains about 14 months for limited disease and between 7 and 9 months for extensive disease. Only 15 to 20 percent of limited-disease patients survive beyond 2 years, and the long-term prognosis for extensive-disease patients is less than 5 percent.

Dose Intensity

Recent trials have explored the use of high-dose, dose-intense regimens, with or without bone marrow transplantation. Despite significant response rates, no major benefit in median survival has been observed. A recent dose-intensity meta-analysis of chemotherapy in SCCL showed no consistent correlation between dose intensity and outcome.

Another method of increasing the intensity of chemotherapy is to intensify the schedule. Promising results of weekly intensive chemotherapy with CODE (cisplatin, vincristine, doxorubicin, and etoposide plus prophylactic antibiotics) have been observed (median survival, 61 weeks; 2 year survival rate, 30 percent) in extensive stage SCCL patients. The mortality rate from toxicity was 4 percent. Current

Table 3 Chemotherapy Regimens for Small Cell Lung Carcinoma

CISPLATIN BASED	
EP	
Etoposide	120 mg/m^2 IV days 1–3
Cisplatin	60 mg/m^2 IV day 1
Repeat cycle every 3 weeks	
or	
Etoposide	240 mg/m^2 PO in two divided doses on days 1–3
Cisplatin	60 mg/m^2 IV day 1
Repeat cycle every 3 weeks	
or	
Cisplatin	25 mg/m^2 IV days 1–3
Etoposide	100 mg/m^2 IV days 1–3
Repeat cycle every 3 weeks	
CARBOPLATIN BASED	
Carboplatin	300 mg/m^2 IV day 1
Etoposide	100 mg/m^2 IV days 1–3
Repeat cycle every 4 weeks	
or	
Carboplatin	100 mg/m^2 IV days 1–3
Etoposide	120 mg/m^2 IV days 1–3
Repeat cycle every 4 weeks	
DOXORUBICIN	
CAV	
Cyclophosphamide	1 g/m^2 IV on day 1
Doxorubicin (Adriamycin)	45 mg/m^2 IV day 1
Vincristine	2 mg IV on day 1
Repeat cycle every 3 weeks	
CAE	
Cyclophosphamide	1 g/m^2 IV on day 1
Doxorubicin (Adriamycin)	45 mg/m^2 IV day 1
Etoposide	50 mg/^{2} IV days 1–5
Repeat cycle every 3 weeks	
CAVE	
Cyclophosphamide	1 g/m^2 IV on day 1
Doxorubicin	50 mg/m^2 IV day 1
Vincristine	1.5 mg/m^2 IV on day 1*
Etoposide	60 mg/^{2} IV days 1–5
Repeat cycle every 3–4 weeks	
COMBINATIONS	
Consolidation	
CAV-EP	
Cyclophosphamide	1 g/m^2 IV on day 1
Doxorubicin	40 mg/m^2 IV day 1
Vincristine	1 mg/m^2 IV on day 1*
Repeat cycle every 3–4 weeks for 6 cycles	
followed by	
Cisplatin	20 mg/m^2 days 1–4
VP-16	100 mg/m^2 days 1–4
Repeat cycle every 4 weeks for 2 cycles	
Alternating	
Cisplatin	100 mg/m^2 IV days 1–3
Etoposide	100 mg/m^2 IV days 1–3
Alternating with the following every 3 weeks for a total of 3 cycles each	
Cyclophosphamide	750 mg/m^2 IV on day 1
Doxorubicin	50 mg/m^2 IV day 1
Vincristine	1 mg/m^2 IV on day 1*

*Maximum dose of vincristine—2 mg

randomized trials will determine the role and toxicities of this regimen in the treatment of SCCL patients.

Alternating Therapy, Consolidation Chemotherapy

Use of alternating non–cross-resistant chemotherapy regimens has been explored because of the mathematical model created by Goldie and Coldman, which predicts improved tumor response when more chemotherapy agents of different mechanisms are used concurrently and early. Despite the mathematical model, randomized trials of alternating chemotherapy regimens versus standard regimens have not consistently yielded significant improvements in survival. The lack of benefit may represent not a failure of the Goldie-Coldman model but lack of two totally non–cross-resistant chemotherapy regimens.

A randomized study by the Southeastern Oncology Group found an improvement in median survival in limited-stage patients who received consolidation cisplatin and etoposide following six cycles of CAV (cyclophosphamide, doxorubicin, and vincristine) compared with patients who received CAV alone (22.8 months versus 15.9 months, respectively). Although these results are promising, it is unclear whether they are due to the consolidation chemotherapy or the introduction of cisplatin and etoposide into a CAV regimen.

A study by the Dana Farber Cancer Institute observed promising results with high-dose chemotherapy with bone marrow transplantation support as consolidation therapy. Patients with limited-stage SCCL who were in near or complete remission from first-line conventional-dose chemotherapy and thoracic irradiation underwent treatment with high-dose cyclophosphamide, cisplatin, and carmustine combined with autologous bone marrow transplantation. A 53 percent 2 year survival was observed in 19 patients.

Duration of Therapy

The optimal duration of treatment for SCCL is 4 to 6 months. A recent study by the European Organization for Research and Treatment of Lung Cancer Cooperative Group treated 687 patients with five cycles of CAE (cyclophosphamide, doxorubicin, and etoposide). Nonprogressing patients were then randomized to either no further therapy or an additional seven cycles. The median survival for patients receiving no further treatment and for those receiving maintenance chemotherapy was 288 days and 275 days, respectively ($p = 0.70$). This study and others suggest that there is no role for prolonged treatment in SCCL.

Chemotherapy Plus Chest Irradiation

The benefit of chest irradiation for limited-stage patients receiving chemotherapy is widely debated. Numerous trials have been conducted with different chemotherapy regimens and different schedules integrating chemotherapy and thoracic irradiation (concurrent, sequential, sandwich), with conflicting reports of the effects on survival. Two meta-analyses have concluded that thoracic irradiation does result in a small but significant improvement in survival and a major control in the chest. However, this improvement is achieved at the cost of a small increase in side effects and occasional mortality. In these analyses, no definite benefit could be ascertained with concurrent versus sequential chemotherapy plus thoracic irradiation treatments, although most of the benefits that have been observed with the combined modality approach have been with concurrent chemotherapy and radiotherapy.

Initial reports using doxorubicin-based regimens with concurrent radiation reported significant toxicities, with enhanced myelosuppression, pneumonitis, and esophagitis. Cisplatin and etoposide, however, are associated with less toxicity when administered concurrently with thoracic irradiation. Preliminary reports suggested that twice-daily (hyperfractionated) radiotherapy, when given concurrently with cisplatin and etoposide, may be more effective than standard fractionation in preventing local recurrence and prolonging survival. Results of a multi-institutional randomized trial comparing hyperfractionated with standard radiotherapy are pending and will answer this important question.

New Agents

Identification of new active agents is clearly crucial if the outcome of this disease is to be improved. However, because of the sensitivity of the disease to standard agents, questions have been raised as to the ethical nature of conducting phase II trials in previously untreated SCCL patients. Recently, phase II trials evaluating new agents have not shown a reduction in survival of patients treated with new drugs who go on to receive salvage chemotherapy. This suggests that within appropriate guidelines, it is safe and ethical to conduct phase II trials with new drugs in this group of patients. Promising agents for SCCL include the following:

Paclitaxel (Taxol). An ECOG phase II trial of 250 mg per square meter of paclitaxel for 4 cycles demonstrated a 34 percent response rate. Studies combining paclitaxel with cisplatin are under way.

Camptothecans. Both CPT-11 and topotecan are undergoing evaluation in phase II and III trials. Response rates of 42 to 47 percent have been reported in early phase II trials.

Epirubicin. The 4′ epimer of doxorubicin had a 50 percent response rate in a phase II study by the National Cancer Institute of Canada, with a median survival of 8.3 months.

Colony-Stimulating Factors

A randomized phase III trial demonstrated that extensive stage SCCL patients treated with granulocyte colony-stimulating factor (G-CSF) and cyclophosphamide, doxorubicin, and etoposide (CAE) had a decreased incidence of neutropenic fevers and a decrease in the median duration of neutropenia, days of hospitalization, and days of treatment with antibiotics, compared with patients who received CAE alone. However, the intensity of chemotherapy was somewhat higher than standard CAE, and the patients were very carefully monitored for any signs of fever. More important, the clinical benefit of maintaining a dose-intense approach in the treatment of SCCL has not been established.

Caution must be exercised when using colony-stimulating factors in patients receiving both chemotherapy and thoracic irradiation. A randomized study by the Southwestern Oncology Group found patients receiving granulocyte-macrophage colony-stimulating factor (GM-CSF) and chemotherapy with concurrent thoracic irradiation had a significant increase in thrombocytopenia over that of patients receiving concurrent chemotherapy and radiotherapy without growth factor.

Recurrent Disease

No effective therapy has been identified for patients with recurrent disease. One study from Vanderbilt University reported a 45 percent response rate for oral etoposide 50 mg per square meter per day for 21 days in 22 patients with recurrent disease, 18 of whom had received previous intravenous etoposide. Responses were most common in patients who had responded to previous chemotherapy and who had not received any treatment in the 90 days before initiation of oral etoposide. Median duration of response was only 4 months.

Suggested Reading

Chang A, Kim K, Glick J, et al. Phase II study of Taxol, merbarone, and piroxantrone in stage IV non-small-cell lung cancer: The Eastern Cooperative Oncology Group results. J Natl Cancer Inst 1993; 85:388–394.

Dillman RO, Seagren SL, Propert KJ, et al. A randomized trial of induction chemotherapy plus high-dose radiation versus radiation alone in stage III non-small cell lung cancer. N Engl J Med 1990; 323:940–945.

Grant S, Gralla R, Kris M, et al. Single-agent chemotherapy trials in small-cell lung cancer, 1970 to 1990: The case for studies in previously treated patients. J Clin Oncol 1992; 10:484–498.

Holmes E, Gail M. Group LCS: Surgical adjuvant therapy for stage II and III adenocarcinoma and large-cell undifferentiated carcinoma. J Clin Oncol 1986; 4:710–715.

Ihde D. Chemotherapy of lung cancer. N Engl J Med 1992; 327:1434–1441.

Johnson D. Chemotherapy for metastatic non-small cell lung cancer: Can that dog hunt? J Natl Cancer Inst 1993; 85:766–767.

Johnson D. Treatment of the elderly with small-cell lung cancer. Chest 1993; 103:72s–74s.

Klasa R, Murray N, Coldman A. Dose-intensity meta-analysis of chemotherapy regimens in small-cell carcinoma of the lung. J Clin Oncol 1991; 9:499–508.

Lad T, Rubinstein L, Sadeghi A. The benefit of adjuvant treatment for resected locally advanced non-small-cell lung cancer. J Clin Oncol 1988; 6:9–17.

Lilenbaum R, Green R. Novel chemotherapeutic agents in the treatment of non-small cell lung cancer. J Clin Oncol 1993; 11:1391–1402.

Martini N, Kris MG, Gralla RJ, et al. The effects of preoperative chemotherapy on the resectability of non-small cell lung carcinoma with mediastinal lymph node metastases. Ann Thorac Surg 1988; 45:370–379.

Murray NOD, Shah A, Page R, et al. Brief intensive chemotherapy for metastatic non-small-cell lung cancer: A phase II study of the weekly CODE regimen. J Natl Cancer Inst 1991; 83:190–194.

Pignon J-P, Arriagada R, Ihde D, et al. A meta-analysis of thoracic radiotherapy for small-cell lung cancer. N Engl J Med 1992; 327:1618–1624.

Strauss GM, Langer MP, Elias AD, et al. Multimodality treatment of stage IIIA non-small-cell lung carcinoma: A critical review of the literature and strategies for future research. J Clin Oncol 1992; 10:829–838.

Warde P, Payne D. Does thoracic irradiation improve survival and local control in limited-stage small-cell carcinoma of the lung? A meta-analysis. J Clin Oncol 1992; 10:890–895.

LUNG CANCER: SURGERY

Steven M. Keller, M.D.

The first reported resection of lung cancer was performed in 1933 by Evarts Graham at the Barnes Hospital in St. Louis. A pneumonectomy was performed on the patient, a 48-year-old physician, who survived 24 years. This chapter will review the role of surgery in both non–small cell carcinoma of the lung (NSCCL) and small cell carcinoma of the lung (SCCL).

■ STAGING

Thorough, uniform staging is crucial for recommending appropriate treatment and to allow comparison of results published from different institutions. The TNM staging system was modified in 1986, when the American Joint Committee on Cancer and the Union Internationale Contre Cancer (UICC) adopted changes designed to create groups that had similar survival rates and therapeutic approaches. The most significant alterations included creation of the T4 and N3 categories and stages IIIA, IIIB, and IV (see Table 1 on p. 978).

Though the ability of the new staging system to predict outcome reliably has been documented in both prospective and retrospective studies (Figs. 1 and 2), not all of the stages are truly homogeneous with regard to either treatment or prognosis. Survival following resection of pathologic stage I NSCCL is generally reported to be in the range of 70 percent. However, the survival of patients with T1 tumors is significantly better than that of patients with T2 neoplasms. This has prompted some authors to propose a subdivision into stages IA and IB. Similarly, stage IIIA includes both patients with N2 lymph node involvement and those with chest wall extension (T3) but no lymph node metastases. Treatment of the latter is radically different from that of the former, as is the long-term survival. These examples demonstrate that the most accurate manner to report results is by the TNM categories themselves rather than overall stage.

The TNM staging system was designed to apply equally to NSCCL and SCCL. More commonly, however, SCCL is described in terms of limited or extensive disease. The former is disease contained within the hemithorax, and the latter is extrathoracic spread. Though these more general terms adequately describe the results of nonoperative treatment, they are insufficient when the role of surgery in SCCL is evaluated.

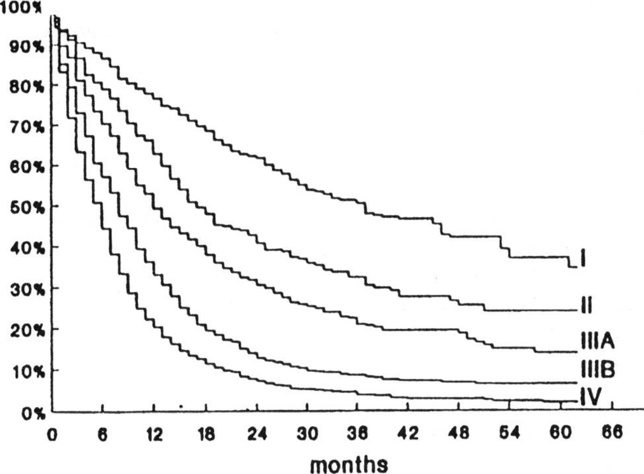

Figure 1
Prognosis based on clinical classification (n = 3,770; stage I = 506; stage II = 373; stage IIIa = 834; stage IIIb = 852; stage IV = 1,205). Stage I versus stage II: p < .001; stage II versus stage IIIa:p < .001; stage IIIa versus IIIb: p < .001; stage IIIb versus stage IV: p < .001. *(From Bulzebrück H, Bopp R, Drings P, et al. New aspects in the staging of lung cancer. Cancer 1992; 70:1102–1110; with permission.)*

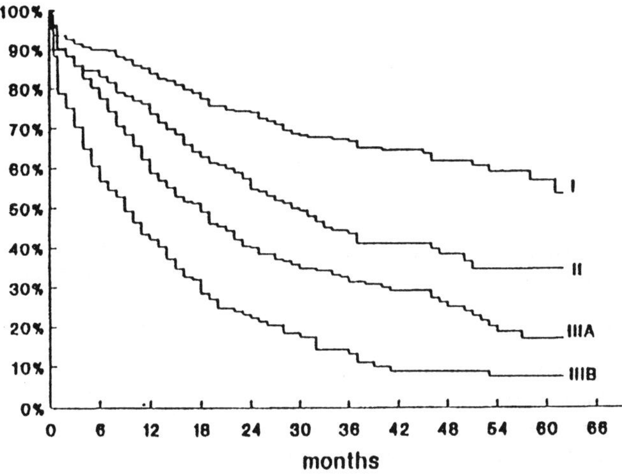

Figure 2
Prognosis based on pathologic classification (n = 1,243; stage I = 439; stage II = 256; stage IIIa = 351; stage IIIb = 197). Stage I versus stage II: p < .001; stage II versus stage IIIa: p < .001; stage IIIa versus stage IIIb: p < .001. *(From Bulzebrück H, Bopp R, Drings P, et al. New aspects in the staging of lung cancer. Cancer 1992; 70:1102–1110; with permission.)*

Preoperative staging is essential. It begins with a thorough history and physical examination. The patient should be questioned about palpable masses, the new onset of bone pain, headache, or change in vision. The supraclavicular fossa and axilla should be carefully evaluated for evidence of metastatic disease. Auscultation and percussion of the thorax may suggest atelectasis or a pleural effusion.

The posteroanterior and lateral chest x-ray films provide a wealth of information regarding not only tumor location but also the appropriate avenue of therapy. The films should be scrutinized for unsuspected pleural effusion, other pulmonary nodules representing either intrapulmonary metastases or a concomitant second primary lung cancer, and osseous metastases. A widened mediastinum is usually indicative of mediastinal metastases (N2 disease). If available, previous x-ray films should be obtained for comparison.

A computed tomography (CT) scan of the chest, including the upper abdomen, is routinely performed to identify any lymphatic or parenchymal metastases. Mediastinal lymph nodes smaller than 1 cm rarely contain tumor. The decision to evaluate lymph nodes of greater size further depends on how the information will be used (see later section). The liver is a frequent site of metastases, and the adrenal gland may harbor tumor in 10 percent of patients with otherwise resectable disease. The chest CT is also useful in planning the technical aspects of the surgery, particularly when the tumor is in a central location.

Serum chemistries are helpful in identifying clinically silent hepatic and osseous metastases. The measurement of tumor-associated antigens in the serum has no role in the management of lung cancer and should be performed only within the context of an approved research project. The utility of routine bone scans and brain CT or magnetic resonance imaging (MRI) remains controversial, though in the absence of symptoms the yield is certainly low.

A histologic diagnosis is not necessary to recommend surgery to a patient with a new operable lung mass that is suspicious for NSCCL and no contraindications to surgery. In such a patient the results of bronchoscopy or percutaneous needle biopsy would not change the therapeutic recommendation and so are unnecessary. SCCL within a solitary nodule is extremely unusual and should not be used as justification for routine preoperative biopsies. However, bronchoscopy and percutaneous needle biopsy are useful when a diagnosis is necessary prior to embarking on palliative therapy.

A thorough preoperative evaluation will show stage IV disease in approximately half of patients with NSCCL and with rare exceptions these patients are treated palliatively. Another 10 percent of patients have inoperable locally advanced disease (stage IIIA or IIIB). Only 40 percent have localized disease amenable to surgical resection (stages I, II, IIIA).

Intraoperative staging is the responsibility of the surgeon and is absolutely crucial for the accurate reporting of results. This must include either a complete mediastinal lymph node dissection or sampling. Mere inspection or digital palpation produces false-negative information. The mediastinal lymph node levels have been meticulously defined by the American Thoracic Society and are described by their relation to constant anatomic structures. Detailed diagrams are available for posting in the operating room to assist the surgeon in the proper identification of each lymph node station. A complete mediastinal lymph node dissection lengthens the operation by only a brief interval and is associated with little morbidity. Appropriately labeled samples should be sent to the pathologist for individual analysis. While there is no evidence of a direct therapeutic effect of complete lymph node dissection, the staging information obtained permits a more detailed knowledge of prognosis and the ability to refer patients for adjuvant therapy.

SURGERY

Both the cardiac and pulmonary systems require careful evaluation prior to surgery. A patient with a normal physical examination and electrocardiogram (ECG) who has no history of coronary disease requires no further evaluation of the heart. Patients with stable, well-controlled cardiac disease can undergo resection with little increase in risk. Previously unrecognized symptoms require further evaluation before surgery, as does unstable or poorly controlled disease. Though atrial arrhythmias may occur in as many as 20 percent of patients and are more common after pneumonectomy, the utility of digitalis prophylaxis remains unproven.

Detailed pulmonary function testing and arterial blood gas readings should be obtained for each patient. An arterial Po_2 below 60 mm Hg or a Pco_2 above 45 mm Hg is associated with increased morbidity. Similarly, DLCO below 60 percent of predicted and MVV below 35 percent predict postoperative complications. Perhaps the single most useful test is the FEV_1. To avoid postoperative respiratory failure the patient must have a postresection FEV_1 above 800 ml, preferably 1 L. If the preoperative FEV_1 is below 2 L, a split-function ventilation perfusion scan should be obtained to document how much function is contributed by the affected lung. This information may be crucial when an unplanned pneumonectomy is necessary to achieve a complete resection.

Intraoperative monitoring includes urinary and indwelling arterial catheters and a pulse oximeter. Right-heart catheterization is performed as necessary. Routine central line placement is not necessary. A double-lumen endotracheal tube is commonly used to permit collapse of the ipsilateral lung and selective ventilation of the contralateral lung. Lower extremity compression boots are employed as deep vein thrombosis prophylaxis. All patients receive perioperative antibiotics.

Most complications following pulmonary resection involve the cardiopulmonary systems. Asymptomatic atelectasis occurs commonly, though clinically significant pneumonia occurs in fewer than 3 percent of patients. Bronchopleural fistulas occur rarely, and wound infections are essentially nonexistent. Approximately 20 percent of patients require blood transfusion. Accepted mortality following pneumonectomy and lobectomy approximate 7 percent and 3 percent, respectively.

Pneumonectomy was the procedure of choice for all stages of NSCCL until the late 1950s, when lobectomy was accepted as equally efficacious. This assertion was never demonstrated in a randomized trial. The claim of some surgeons that wedge resection or formal segmentectomy of stage I NSCCL produced results similar to those of lobectomy has been refuted by a prospective randomized trial conducted by the Lung Cancer Study Group (LCSG). The early results of this study have demonstrated a threefold increase in local recurrence when a more conservative operation was performed. Lobectomy is therefore the procedure of choice when the patient's pulmonary function permits and when negative surgical margins can be obtained. Pneumonectomy is performed only when tumor size or location mandates it. Wedge resection is reserved for patients who will not tolerate removal of greater amounts of pulmonary parenchyma.

The role of video-assisted thoracoscopy in the treatment of NSCCL remains to be determined. The indications for this surgical approach should not be based on unproven claims of decreased duration of hospitalization or postoperative pain. Even the most fervent advocates of this technical advance caution against its use if there may be any compromise in the patient's treatment.

After hospital discharge the patient must be regularly evaluated for evidence of recurrence. Since most tumors that recur will do so within the first 2 years, this interval must be one of careful observation. A careful history and physical examination along with chest x-ray film are sufficient to identify the majority of metastases or local recurrences. Routine chest CT is not indicated.

Most patients do not require narcotic analgesia longer than 8 weeks. Approximately 10 percent of patients develop a postthoracotomy pain syndrome characterized by pain along the incision, in the midback, and beneath the breast. The combination of a nonsteroidal anti-inflammatory agent and a tricyclic antidepressant is frequently successful in ameliorating this vexing problem.

ADJUVANT AND NEOADJUVANT THERAPY OF NSCCL

Survival after complete resection of pathologic stage I NSCCL ranges from 60 and 80 percent (Table 1). Patients with T2N0 tumors do not fare as well as those with T1N0 cancers, and some authors have proposed creating IA and IB categories. The excellent results following surgery have rendered the practical evaluation of additional treatment difficult. However, a number of studies have addressed the potential role of adjuvant therapy.

The LCSG conducted a randomized prospective trial comparing the postoperative intrapleural administration of bacillus Calmette-Guérin (BCG) with placebo and found no survival advantage. The LCSG later compared CAP chemotherapy (cyclophosphamide 400 mg per square meter, doxorubicin 40 mg per square meter, cisplatin 40 mg per square meter) with an untreated control arm in a phase III trial. The majority of patients, 86 percent, were T2N0. The remainder had N1 disease. No survival advantage was found for patients who received chemotherapy.

A phase III trial comparing six cycles of monthly CAP with no treatment demonstrated a significant increase in disease-free survival. This study was flawed by the inclusion of a small

Table 1 Survival After Resection of Stage I NSCCL

STUDY	N	5 YEAR SURVIVAL (%)
Martini (1977)	115	77*
Williams (1981)	331	72
Pairolero (1984)	328	65
LCSG (1990)	907	65†‡

*3 years.
†Approximate.
‡T1N0 only.

number of non–stage I patients. Independent confirmation is required before the routine administration of adjuvant chemotherapy for patients with resected stage I NSCCL can be recommended.

Second primary tumors develop at a rate of 1 percent per year in patients who have undergone resection of stage I NSCCL. A phase III chemoprevention trial (Intergroup 0125) is being conducted by all the cooperative groups in an effort to identify a drug that can prevent formation of a second cancer. Patients will be randomized to receive either oral 13-*cis* retinoic acid 30 mg daily or a placebo. The 1,260 patients necessary for this study will require a 4 year follow-up to prove or disprove the utility of this drug.

Stage II, T1N1 and T2N1, comprises approximately 10 percent of patients with NSCCL. Since the difference between stage II and stage IIIA may depend on the zeal with which the surgeon pursues a lymph node dissection, survival statistics understandably vary widely. Median survival of 54 months has been reported from the Memorial Sloan-Kettering Cancer Center (MSKCC) though other smaller retrospective series have published median survivals of 12 to 14 months (Table 2). Patients with involvement of only a single nodal level have the longest survival.

Three phase III trials that included patients with stage II NSCCL have been reported by the LCSG. CAP chemotherapy administered in six 1 month cycles was compared with a control arm of intrapleural BCG. Patients who received cytotoxic therapy had a median survival 7 months longer than those who received immunotherapy. Patients in another study received either radiotherapy (5,000 cGy, 180 to 200 Gy daily fractions) or no further treatment after complete resection of all stage II disease. Though no survival advantage was demonstrated, there was a decrease in local recurrence. Finally, a small number of patients with pathologic stage II disease were included in a trial comparing the combination of radiotherapy (4,000 cGy in 2,000 cGy split course fractions) and CAP with radiotherapy alone. The median time to recurrence for all participating patients who received the combination therapy was 14 months, significantly longer than the 6 months for patients treated with radiotherapy alone. Due to the relatively few patients with stage II disease, no conclusions regarding therapeutic recommendations could be reached.

Patients with completely resected stage II NSCCL are eligible for participation in Intergroup Trial 0115, a prospective randomized trial comparing concomitant radiotherapy (5,040 cGy in 180 cGy daily fractions) and chemotherapy (cisplatin 60 mg per square meter and etoposide 120 mg per square meter) with radiotherapy alone. The objectives of this study are to investigate the efficacy of combination chemotherapy and radiotherapy in prolonging survival and preventing local recurrence. There is no accepted adjuvant treatment for patients with resected stage II NSCCL. Patients should be carefully observed or offered participation in an approved investigation.

The two major subcategories of stage IIIA are T3N0 and T1-3N2. The treatment and prognosis of these diverse groups of patients differ so substantially that they are best considered separately. Patients with peripheral chest wall invasion (T3) should undergo resection of the involved ribs and underlying lung. The pulmonary resection is the same as that for the absence of rib invasion. Large defects not covered by the chest wall musculature are repaired with a combination of Marlex mesh and methyl methacrylate. Five year survival rates approximate 50 percent (Table 3). The preoperative demonstration of mediastinal lymph node metastases is a contraindication to surgery, as no patient with T3N2 has benefited from operation. Adjuvant therapy has not been shown effective in preventing recurrent disease, which is usually systemic.

Henry K. Pancoast described the tumor that bears his name in 1924. Due to the proximity of the brachial plexus, major thoracic vessels, and vertebral bodies, the tumor was considered inoperable. The first reported resection was not performed until 3 decades later. The tumor is usually found only after a prolonged investigation of shoulder and arm pain that results from rib destruction and/or involvement of the C8 or T1 nerve roots. Frequently the patient has been evaluated by an orthopedist, neurologist, neurosurgeon, and chiropractor. Not uncommonly the cancer is an incidental finding noted on a radiologic investigation of the shoulder or cervical spine. Sometimes Horner's syndrome is the presenting symptom.

A thorough investigation of the surrounding structures is mandatory prior to recommending a course of therapy. The presence of tumor within mediastinal lymph nodes, direct invasion of a vertebral body, and tumor encirclement of the major vessels are contraindications to surgery. Pretreatment symptoms suggesting T1 or C8 nerve root involvement are not contraindications to surgery, as the former nerve root may be removed and the latter may improve with preoperative therapy.

Table 2 Survival After Resection of Stage II NSCCL

STUDY	N	5 YEAR SURVIVAL (%)
Martini (1983)	75	50*
Newman (1983)	20	40
Ferguson (1986)	34	30
Martini (1992)	214	39

*Some patients received adjuvant therapy.

Table 3 Survival After Chest Wall Resection (T3N0)

STUDY	N	5 YEAR SURVIVAL (%)
Piehler (1982)	31	54
Trastek (1984)	29	38
McCaughan (1985)	66	56
Albertucci (1992)	21	41

Table 4 Survival After Resection of Pancoast Tumors (N0)

STUDY	N	5 YEAR SURVIVAL (%)
Paulson (1975)	40	17*
Miller (1978)	25	40
Shahian (1987)	18	56
Wright (1987)	21	27
Sartori (1991)	42	30

*3 years.

Table 5 Subgroups of N2 Disease

MEDIASTINUM CHEST X-RAY		CHEST CT	MEDIASTINOSCOPY	THORACOTOMY
1	Normal	–	–	+
2	Widened	–	–	+
3	–	–	Negative	+
4	–	–	Positive	+
5	–	Positive	–	+

Traditional treatment has been preoperative radiotherapy (2,000 to 3,000 cGy) followed in 2 to 6 weeks by surgery. In addition to the affected lobe, complete removal of the tumor usually involves resection of ribs 1 to 3. The sequela of stellate ganglia resection should be explained to patients prior to surgery. Five year survival ranges from 27 to 56 percent (Table 4). Neoadjuvant chemotherapy may be as effective as radiotherapy and is employed by a number of investigators. The small number of these patients renders a meaningful phase III trial difficult.

The treatment of patients with suspected or documented N2 disease (mediastinal lymph node metastases) remains the most controversial issue in NSCCL. Comparative analysis of the literature is not possible because of the variety of ways in which investigators have reported their results. In fact, five different unintentionally created subgroups of N2 disease were defined by whether the presence or absence of N2 disease was assumed because of a chest x-ray film or CT scan or whether mediastinoscopy was routinely performed (Table 5).

A 30 percent 5 year survival of 151 patients with clinical N0 or N1 disease (subgroup 1) but pathologic N2 disease was reported from the MSKCC. They maintained that since more than 90 percent of these patients were technically resectable and their long-term survival was superior to that of patients who had nonoperative therapy, prethoracotomy mediastinoscopy was unnecessary. However, patients whose chest x-ray film demonstrated bulky mediastinal disease (subgroup 2) were rarely resectable, and even among the few patients who were to have a complete resection, survival was dismal. They concluded that these patients should undergo documentation of N2 disease and then either be treated with palliation or entered in a neoadjuvant therapy protocol.

Other investigators have reported 40 percent 5 year survival in patients who were found to have N2 disease following a false-negative mediastinoscopy (subgroup 3). Five year survival following resection of N2 disease previously demonstrated at mediastinoscopy was only 15 percent (subgroup 4). Presumed N2 disease seen on a preoperative CT scan and later confirmed during a complete resection (subgroup 5) is associated with a similar 20 percent 5 year survival. Regardless of the N2 subgroup, patients who survive 5 years generally have tumor limited to a single mediastinal nodal level.

Patients found to have N2 disease after complete resection are eligible for participation in intergroup adjuvant therapy trial 0115. Ineligible patients or those who refuse randomization are observed closely or treated with mediastinal radiotherapy. The latter is effective in preventing local recurrence but has had no impact on survival.

Patients in whom bulky or multimediastinal nodal level N2 disease is histologically documented prior to surgery may be offered one of three treatment options: observation, palliative radiotherapy, or participation in an approved neoadjuvant therapy protocol. The latter usually consists of chemotherapy with or without radiotherapy. Numerous phase II trials, usually employing a platinum-containing regimen, have demonstrated the ability to convert inoperable bulky mediastinal disease into a technically resectable tumor. Patients who are able to undergo complete resection may have a 5 year survival as high as 26 percent.

Recently, two prospective randomized trials designed to evaluate the efficacy of neoadjuvant therapy in patients with stage III NSCCL that have been completed. Rosell and Roth each reported individual trials containing approximately 60 patients. In both studies those patients who received chemotherapy before surgery had significantly improved disease-free and overall survivals when compared to those patients who went directly to operation. However, the results of these two small studies should not be accepted as definitive. Patients with N2 disease should receive neoadjuvant therapy only within the context of an approved protocol. A randomized stage III trial is now being conducted by the National Cancer Institute–sponsored Cooperative Groups to evaluate the role of surgery in patients with N2 disease.

Direct tumor invasion of mediastinal structures or the presence of metastases in N3 lymph nodes (stage IIIb) is generally considered a contraindication to surgery. However, the Southwest Oncology Group has recently presented the results of a phase II trial in which patients with stage IIIb disease were treated with preoperative concomitant radiochemotherapy. Projected 2 year survival was 40 percent. Other investigators have reported less impressive results, with a median survival approximating 1 year.

Synchronous solitary brain metastases are not an absolute contraindication to surgery. A median survival of 14 months was documented in a cohort of 65 patients from the MSKCC; 2 year survival was 27 percent. Similar results have been obtained by others.

■ SMALL CELL LUNG CANCER

Surgical therapy of SCCL may be beneficial for two patient subgroups: those with early-stage disease and those with a residual lung mass and no evidence of metastatic disease after definitive systemic treatment. Though the vast majority of patients with SCCL have disseminated cancer when their illness is first diagnosed, perhaps 5 to 10 percent have disease limited to the lung parenchyma without mediastinal lymph node metastases. Numerous retrospective reports have demonstrated 5 year survival over 50 percent for patients with pathologic stage I neoplasms (Table 6). Such tumors are frequently undiagnosed preoperatively, and most patients

Table 6 Results of Surgical Resection of SCCL

STUDY	5 YEAR SURVIVAL (%)		
	STAGE I	STAGE II	STAGE III
Karrer* (1990)	61†	35	50
Shepherd* (1991)	51	28	30
Shah‡ (1992)	57	0	55

*All patients received preoperative and/or postoperative systemic therapy.
†4 year survival.
‡No patient received additional treatment.

receive some form of adjuvant therapy. The excellent outcome of this cohort represents another reason for not obtaining a routine preoperative biopsy of all lung nodules suspicious for lung cancer. Some authors have published similar results for stage II and stage IIIA (N0) cancers. In general, the presence of mediastinal lymph node disease places the patient in a group not benefited by surgery. Therefore, when the diagnosis of SCCL is known preoperatively, a thorough evaluation of the mediastinum is required.

When a patient has responded well to the usual systemic therapy for SCCL but is left with residual parenchymal disease, a NSCCL component must be considered. The existence of such mixed SCCL and NSCCL neoplasms is well documented. If a thorough metastatic evaluation is negative, the remaining tumor should be surgically resected.

Suggested Reading

American Thoracic Society. Clinical staging of primary lung cancer. Am Rev Resp Dis 1983; 127:659–670.

Lung Cancer Study Group. The benefit of adjuvant treatment for resected locally advanced non-small-cell lung cancer. J Clin Oncol 1988; 6:9–17.

Martini N, Kris MG, Flehinger BJ, et al. Preoperative chemotherapy for stage IIIa (N2) lung cancer: The Sloan-Kettering experience with 136 patients. Ann Thor Surg 1993; 55:1365–1374.

Pearson FG, DeLarue NC, Ilves R, et al. Significance of positive superior mediastinal nodes identified at mediastinoscopy in patients with resectable cancer of the lung. J Thorac Cardiovasc Surg 1982; 83:1–11.

Roth JA, Fossella F, Komaki R, et. al. A randomized trial comparing perioperative chemotherapy and surgery with surgery alone in resectable stage IIIA non-small cell lung cancer. J Natl Cancer Inst 1994; 86:673–680.

Rusch VW, Albains KS, Crowley JJ, et al. Surgical resection of stage IIIa and stage IIIb non-small-cell lung cancer after concurrent induction chemoradiotherapy. J Thorac Cardiovasc Surg 1993; 105:97–106.

Shepherd FA, Ginsberg RJ, Feld R, et al. Surgical treatment for limited small-cell lung cancer. J Thorac Cardiovasc Surg 1991; 101:385–393.

BREAST CANCER: SURGERY

Monica Morrow, M.D.

Breast cancer is the most common malignancy of American women and the second most common cause of cancer death, accounting for approximately 46,000 deaths in 1995. The modern era of breast cancer surgery began with Halsted's description of the radical mastectomy in 1894, and surgical therapy remained largely unchanged for the next 70 years. Since the 1970s the recognition that radical surgery alone fails to cure most women with breast cancer, coupled with changes in our understanding of the biology of breast cancer, have resulted in great changes in the surgical management of the disease. In June 1990 a National Cancer Institute Consensus Development Conference declared that breast-conserving surgery not only was acceptable but should be considered the preferred treatment for early-stage breast cancer.

The modern approach to breast cancer therapy is a multidisciplinary collaboration among surgeons, radiologists, pathologists, radiation oncologists, and medical oncologists to provide an integrated treatment plan that allows the patient to participate in the decision-making process.

PRESENTATION AND DIAGNOSIS

A palpable mass continues to be the most common clinical indication for breast biopsy and the most common sign of breast cancer. The initial step in the evaluation of a dominant breast mass is fine-needle aspiration (FNA). If the mass is a cyst, the procedure is both diagnostic and therapeutic. If the lesion is solid, material should be obtained for a cytologic examination. Note that aspiration cytology, even in the hands of experienced operators and cytopathologists, has a false-negative rate of 5 to 10 percent. If cytology is used as a diagnostic technique for a solid mass and malignant cells are not obtained, the mass should be excised for definitive diagnosis. False-positive aspirates are uncommon, but until experience is gained at an individual institution, positive aspirates should be confirmed with frozen section at the time of definitive surgery. Aspiration cytology is a rapid and relatively painless office procedure. It is an excellent technique for establishing the diagnosis of breast cancer before incising the breast. With a firm diagnosis a woman can select a treatment option, and only a single operative procedure is needed. When no experienced cytologist is available, core cutting needle biopsy is an alternative office diagnostic technique. Accuracy rates are similar to those reported for aspiration cytology, but more details of tumor histology are available.

Excisional biopsy has been the standard technique for the diagnosis of breast masses. The major advantage of this approach is the ability to evaluate completely the tumor size and histologic characteristics before definitive surgical therapy.

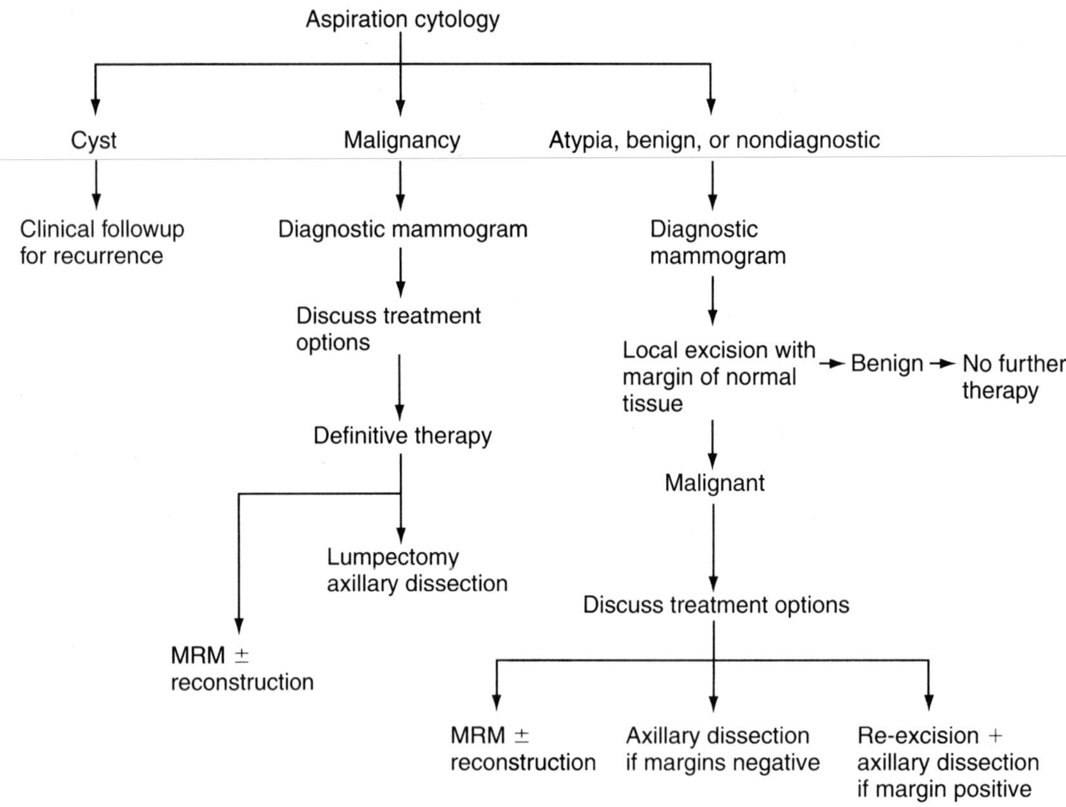

Figure 1
Management of the palpable breast mass. (MRM, Modified radical mastectomy.)

Excisional biopsy should be done as a lumpectomy with the removal of 1 to 2 cm of grossly normal tissue around the mass and inking of the specimen to allow evaluation of the margins. Negative margins are obtained in approximately 95 percent of cases with this approach, which avoids the need for re-excision in women with cancer who opt for breast-conserving therapy. Excisional biopsy is an outpatient procedure that can be done with local anesthesia and supplemental sedation. There is no evidence that a one-step procedure (biopsy under general anesthesia followed by definitive surgery if positive) is associated with any survival benefit compared with biopsy and surgery at a later date. The treatment algorithm for the management of palpable breast masses is shown in Figure 1.

Incisional biopsy is used to establish a diagnosis of breast cancer in masses too large to excise completely. Its main use is in women with locally advanced breast cancer who will receive systemic therapy as an initial treatment and in those with metastatic disease. FNA avoids the problem of occasional poor wound healing and may be preferable for establishing the diagnosis of advanced breast cancer.

Clinically occult breast lesions detected by screening mammography are responsible for an increasing number of breast biopsies each year. The most common indications for biopsy are clustered microcalcifications and nonpalpable masses, each accounting for about 45 percent of biopsies in most series. Asymmetric densities and architectural distortions are the other mammographic indications for biopsy. Mammographic abnormalities have a low positive predictive value for carcinoma, with positive biopsy yields of only 15 to 30 percent. Mammographic abnormalities must be localized prior to excision to ensure removal of the abnormality with a limited amount of normal breast tissue. Localization can be done with straight needles, hook wires, or dye injection along a needle tract. The most important factor in the successful excision of a mammographic abnormality is how close the localizing wire is to the mammographic abnormality. Specimen radiography must be carried out in all biopsies done for microcalcifications to confirm the presence of the calcifications in the biopsy specimen. Although mass lesions may be evident intraoperative specimen radiography documents that the mammographic abnormality has been removed. The specimen should then be marked with orienting sutures and inked to allow evaluation of margins.

Although frozen section is a reliable method for the diagnosis of palpable masses, its role in the management of nonpalpable lesions is limited. Many of the abnormalities being sought by needle localization are very small, representing histologically borderline lesions that are difficult to diagnose on frozen section. Since needle localization is seldom undertaken with a plan to proceed with definitive surgery at the same operation, a careful examination of the entire biopsy specimen with high-quality paraffin sections seems to be the most prudent course. Failure to remove the mammographic abnormality occurs in up to 10 percent of needle localization biopsies. Findings of fibrocystic disease in histologic sections should not be assumed to represent the mammographic abnormality unless the lesion is clearly seen on a specimen radiograph. If a missed lesion is suspected, its presence should

Table 1 TNM Staging System, American Joint Committee on Cancer, 1992

	PRIMARY TUMOR (T)				
TX	Primory tumor cannot be assessed				
T0	No evidence of primary tumor				
Tis	Carcinoma in situ: intraductal carcinoma, lobular carcinoma in situ, or Paget's disease of the nipple with no tumor				
T1	Tumor 2 cm or less in greatest dimension				
T1a	0.5 cm or less in greatest dimension				
T1b	More than 0.5 cm, but not more than 1 cm in greatest dimension				
T1c	More than 1 cm but not more than 2 cm in greatest dimension				
T2	Tumor more than 2 cm but not more than 5 cm in greatest dimension				
T3	Tumor more than 5 cm in greatest dimension				
T4	Tumor of any size with direct extension to chest wall or skin				
T4a	Extension to chest wall				
T4b	Edema (including peau d'orange) or ulceration of the skin of breast or satellite skin nodules to same breast				
T4c	Both T4a and T4b				
T4d	Inflammatory carcinoma				
	REGIONAL LYMPH NODE (N)				
Ipsilateral axillary, interpectoral (Rotter's), and intrammamary nodes are coded as axillary nodes					
NX	Regional lymph nodes cannot be assessed (e.g., previously removed or not removed for pathologic study)	Stage 0	TIS	N0	M0
		Stage I	T1	N0	M0
N0	No regional lymph node metastasis	Stage IIA	T0	N0	M0
N1	Metastasis to movable ipsilateral axillary lymph node(s)		T1	N1	M0
			T2	N0	M0
N1a	Only micrometastasis (none larger than 0.2 cm)				
N1b	Metastasis to lymph node(s), any larger than 0.2 cm	Stage IIB	T2	N1	M0
N1bi	Metastasis in 1 to 3 lymph nodes, any more than 0.2 cm and all less than 2 cm in greatest dimension		T3	N0	M0
N1bii	Metastasis to 4 or more lymph nodes, any more than 0.2 cm and all less than 2 cm in greatest dimension	Stage IIIA	T0	N2	M0
			T1	N2	M0
N1biii	Extension of tumor beyond the capsule of a lymph node metastasis less than 2 cm in greatest dimension		T2	N2	M0
			T3	N1	M0
N1biv	Metastasis to a lymph node 2 cm or more in greatest dimension		T3	N2	M0
N2	Metastasis to ipsilateral axillary lymph nodes that are fixed to one another or to other structures	Stage IIIB	T4	Any N	M0
			Any T	Ne	M0
N3	Metastasis to ipsilateral internal mammary lymph node(s)	Stage IV	Any T	Any T	M1
	DISTANT METASTASIS (M)				
MX	Presence of distant metastasis cannot be assessed				
M0	No distant metastasis				
M1	Distant metastasis (includes metastasis to ipsilateral supraclavicular lymph node(s))				

be confirmed with mammography and a repeat biopsy undertaken.

Recently the nonoperative diagnosis of mammographic abnormalities using a stereotactic device to position a needle for cytologic aspirates or core biopsies has become popular. The final role of this technique in the diagnosis of nonpalpable abnormalities is not yet clear, but it appears to be a reliable method of sampling low-suspicion but not unequivocally benign mammographic abnormalities, avoiding an excessive number of benign biopsies. Further study is required, particularly of the ability of stereotactic biopsy to reliably identify ductal carcinoma in situ and microinvasion before determining whether this technique should be used for the diagnosis of all mammographic abnormalities.

■ STAGING

The initial assessment of stage must be a clinical one used to direct surgical therapy. The major discrepancy between the clinical and the final pathologic stage in breast cancer is the evaluation of axillary lymph node status. About 30 percent of women without palpable axillary adenopathy will have histologic evidence of nodal metastases. Conversely, palpable nodes do not contain tumor in as many as 25 percent of women. Supraclavicular adenopathy is classified as distant metastatic disease in recognition of the poor outcome associated with spread to this site. The current TNM staging definitions are shown in Table 1.

■ PREOPERATIVE WORKUP

The pretreatment evaluation of the breast cancer patient is directed at identifying disease sites in the breast and elsewhere in the body that would alter the treatment plan. In addition to a complete history and physical examination, detailed bilateral mammography is essential. Ideally, mammography should be obtained before excisional breast biopsy to allow adequate evaluation of the index breast for breast-conserving

Table 2 Characteristics of LCIS and DCIS

	LCIS	DCIS
Age	Usually premenopausal	Pre- or postmenopausal
Presentation	Incidental finding	Palpable mass, mammographic mass, microcalcifications, nipple discharge
Cancer risk	Bilateral, throughout breasts	Unilateral, usually at biopsy site
Predictors of invasive cancer risk	None identified	Size, histologic subtype, grade
Treatment options	Observation, prophylactic bilateral mastectomy ± reconstruction	Excision and radiotherapy; total mastectomy ± reconstruction, excision alone

therapy. Magnification views often identify areas of multifocal carcinoma that may preclude the use of a breast-conserving approach. Clinically occult contralateral breast cancer is detected mammographically in approximately 2.4 percent of women.

The likelihood of identifying metastases by the routine use of scans in the asymptomatic patient is greatly influenced by the clinical stage of disease. The incidence of occult bony metastases detected by scanning in asymptomatic women with stage I and II breast cancer is less than 5 percent in most series, and false-positive results are frequent. In contrast, 20 to 25 percent of women with locally advanced breast cancer will have positive bone scans, making this a worthwhile screening test for stage III disease. The yield of screening liver scans is even lower than the yield of bone scans, and false-positive results are more frequent than true positive results. Liver imaging should be reserved for women with abnormal liver chemistries, hepatomegaly, or significant weight loss suggesting hepatic metastases.

Serum tumor markers have not been shown to be useful preoperative tests in women with breast cancer. Carcinoembryonic antigen (CEA) is infrequently elevated in primary breast cancer. Other markers (CA15-3, CA549) are more commonly elevated in primary breast cancer, but elevated levels are also observed in a variety of benign conditions. In summary, for the woman with stage I or II breast carcinoma, bilateral mammography, a chest roentgenogram, complete blood count, and liver chemistries are the only preoperative tests required. For women with ductal carcinoma in situ the only study needed is the mammogram, since the detection of occult metastatic disease is not an issue.

■ NONINVASIVE CARCINOMA

Lobular Carcinoma in Situ

Lobular carcinoma in situ (LCIS) is an incidental microscopic finding that cannot be identified clinically or by gross pathologic examination. Since LCIS lacks clinical or mammographic signs, its true incidence is unknown. LCIS is found in 0.8 to 8 percent of breast biopsies, and the frequency with which it is diagnosed appears to be increasing. LCIS was first described in 1941 as the anatomic precursor of invasive carcinoma. Subsequent information strongly suggests that LCIS is a risk factor for the development of breast cancer rather than a premalignant lesion.

Lobular carcinoma in situ is a disease of premenopausal women. It is usually multicentric and frequently bilateral. The risk of subsequent breast cancer development after a diagnosis of LCIS, approximately 1 percent per year, seems to persist indefinitely. However, subsequent carcinomas are equally distributed between the index and the contralateral breast, even when the LCIS is unilateral. Recognition of this fact has eliminated the use of mirror image biopsies in most centers. The amount of LCIS is not predictive of the risk of development of cancer, and infiltrating ductal carcinomas are the most common tumor type observed. The foregoing information suggests that most women with LCIS will not develop breast cancer and that the risk of breast cancer development is equal in both breasts.

There are two options available for the woman with LCIS. The first is careful observation, as would be carried out for any woman known to be at increased risk for breast cancer on the basis of family history or other risk factors. In women unwilling to accept the risk of breast cancer development associated with this policy, prophylactic bilateral simple mastectomies, usually with immediate breast reconstruction, are another option. Radiotherapy has no role in the management of LCIS. It is unnecessary to obtain negative histologic margins in women who will be followed expectantly, since LCIS is known to be a diffuse lesion. To date efforts to identify features of LCIS associated with a higher likelihood of the development of malignancy have been unsuccessful.

Ductal Carcinoma in Situ

In contrast to LCIS, ductal carcinoma in situ (DCIS) has a variety of both clinical and mammographic presentations. Clinically, DCIS may present as a palpable mass or nipple discharge or be detected mammographically as microcalcifications or a nonpalpable mass. The features of DCIS and LCIS are compared in Table 2. Ductal carcinoma in situ was an infrequent clinical problem prior to the use of screening mammography. The increased use of mammography has resulted in a dramatic increase in the number of cases of DCIS treated annually. In the past, the gross (palpable) form of DCIS was treated exclusively by mastectomy. Axillary node involvement was present in fewer than 5 percent of cases, and both disease-free and overall survival rates exceeded 95 percent.

The increasing use of breast-conserving approaches for the treatment of invasive breast cancer, the increasingly frequent identification of microscopic DCIS by mammography, and the recognition that not all DCIS is an obligate precursor of invasive carcinoma have resulted in attempts to treat DCIS with excision alone or excision and radiotherapy. Retrospective studies indicate that local recurrence rates after excision and breast irradiation are approximately 50 percent lower than local recurrence rates after excision alone. Since approximately half of the local failures in women with DCIS contain invasive tumor, local recurrence in this clinical setting is associated with a small but real risk of breast cancer mortality. Findings from the National Surgical Adjuvant Breast and Bowel Projects (NSABP) randomized trial (protocol B17) comparing excision with negative margins with or without irradiation in the management of DCIS confirms the findings of the retrospective studies. At a mean follow-up of 4 years a significant reduction in the incidence of invasive recurrences was seen in the irradiated group.

The current treatment options for the woman with DCIS are total (simple) mastectomy, which is curative in 99 percent of cases, or excision and radiotherapy, which carries approximately a 10 to 15 percent risk of local recurrence in a 10 year period. Nonrandomized studies suggest that highly selected groups of patients with DCIS can be treated with excision alone with a similar risk of local recurrence. Because of the potential for invasive recurrences, breast conservation in DCIS has a 2 to 3 percent risk of mortality at 10 years. Selection of a treatment option in DCIS depends on whether the small risk associated with breast preservation is acceptable to the patient.

INVASIVE CARCINOMA, STAGES I AND II

The surgical therapy of invasive breast carcinoma has changed dramatically in the past 20 years as our understanding of the biology of breast cancer evolved. Current therapeutic options include modified radical mastectomy, breast-conserving surgery, and modified radical mastectomy with immediate reconstruction.

Modified Radical Mastectomy

Modified radical mastectomy remains the most common surgical treatment for invasive breast cancer, accounting for 60 to 70 percent of procedures performed in the United States in 1990. A modified radical mastectomy includes removal of the entire breast and some or all of the axillary lymph nodes. The pectoralis minor muscle may be removed or transected but is usually preserved. Although the entire breast is removed, the modified radical mastectomy is associated with less arm edema and shoulder dysfunction than the radical mastectomy, and the cosmetic defect is less noticeable in a variety of types of clothing. Breast reconstruction is more easily performed after modified radical mastectomy.

Breast-Conserving Surgery

Breast-conserving surgery involves removal of the primary tumor and a variable margin of surrounding normal breast tissue, usually accompanied by an axillary dissection. A variety of imprecise terms are used to describe this approach to the surgical therapy of breast cancer. They include lumpectomy, tumorectomy, and local excision, which imply the removal of a relatively small amount of normal breast tissue, and partial mastectomy, segmentectomy, and quadrantectomy, which usually imply the excision of a larger amount of breast tissue.

The goal of breast-conserving surgery is to maintain local tumor control in the breast while preserving a good cosmetic appearance. The amount of breast tissue that should be excised is a matter of some debate. The lowest rates of local failure are reported in patients treated with quadrantectomy. A randomized trial comparing quadrantectomy and external beam irradiation with tumor excision with a margin of 1 cm of grossly normal breast tissue followed by an iridium-192 implant and external beam therapy was performed at the National Cancer Institute of Italy in Milan. Local recurrence was decreased from 7.2 percent in the local excision group to 2.5 percent in the quadrantectomy group. However, significantly better cosmesis was obtained in the wide excision group, and no survival differences were noted.

Table 3 Factors Not Predicting Local Failure After Breast Conservation

Tumor size
Tumor histology
Tumor location
Tumor grade
Hormone receptor status
Family history of breast cancer

The amount of breast tissue removed appears to be only one of several factors that may influence the rate of local recurrence after breast-conserving therapy. While gross residual tumor in the breast is associated with increased local failure rates, the value of obtaining histologically negative margins of resection in the prevention of local recurrence is somewhat unclear, since microscopic tumor at resection margins does not clearly correlate with local failure. The lack of a standard definition of a positive margin, variations in sampling techniques, and the presence of additional foci of tumor elsewhere in the breast even if margins are negative limit the utility of margin status as a predictor of local failure. Age less than 35 to 40 years has been associated with an increased risk of local failure in several series, but other reports have failed to substantiate this finding. The microscopic finding of extensive intraductal carcinoma in association with invasive carcinoma has also been a predictor of local recurrence in some studies, but this effect is mitigated if negative margins can be obtained. A number of other factors, many of which are reliable predictors of systemic relapse, do not correlate with local failure rates after breast preservation. These are listed in Table 3. In contrast, the use of adjuvant chemotherapy or hormonal therapy, when combined with breast irradiation, does lower the risk of recurrent tumor in the breast. As larger numbers of women with breast cancer are receiving systemic therapy, a decrease in the overall incidence of local failure has been observed.

Available data suggest that the amount of breast tissue that must be excised should be individualized. For the majority of women, a 1 to 2 cm margin of excision results in good cosmesis and low rate of local recurrence. In patients with positive margins after a conservative excision, an extensive intraductal component associated with the invasive carcinoma, and perhaps very young women, a wider excision may be necessary to maintain local control.

Breast Reconstruction After Mastectomy

Reconstruction may be done at the time of mastectomy or as a secondary procedure, but the possibility should be discussed prior to definitive surgery. The only true contraindication to immediate reconstruction is the presence of significant comorbid conditions that would interfere with the patient's ability to tolerate a longer operative procedure. The patient's age, the need for adjuvant chemotherapy, and poor prognosis are not contraindications to reconstruction. Retrospective studies have shown that breast reconstruction does not impair the detection of local recurrence or increase its incidence. No delay in the time to initiating adjuvant chemotherapy has been noted in several studies of women undergoing immediate reconstruction. The advantages of immediate reconstruction include avoidance of an additional operative procedure, decreased psychological trauma, and improved coordination of the efforts of the oncologic and reconstructive surgeons to produce an optimal cosmetic result without compromising cancer care.

Reconstruction may be accomplished with implants, either saline or silicone gel filled, or with myocutaneous flaps. The availability of adequate skin coverage, the size and shape of the patient's contralateral breast, the patient's cosmetic expectations, and the amount of surgery she is willing to undergo influence the choice of reconstructive technique.

Axillary Dissection

Whether or not mastectomy or breast-conserving surgery is employed, axillary dissection is an important part of the local therapy of breast cancer. The primary purpose of axillary dissection is to provide prognostic information to direct systemic therapy. In addition, axillary dissection is an excellent method of maintaining local control in the axilla. The removal of axillary nodes does not influence survival, and as axillary dissection has come to be regarded as a staging procedure rather than a therapeutic one, dissections limited to the lower levels of the axilla have become more popular. Removal of the nodes below and behind the pectoralis minor (level I and II) provides accurate staging information in 98 percent of women, since isolated disease in the upper axilla (skip metastases) is extremely infrequent. If grossly positive axillary nodes are present or if knowledge of the exact number of positive nodes will alter treatment, a complete dissection should be carried out, since there is a 20 to 30 percent chance that additional positive nodes will be present in the upper axilla if metastases are present in the low axillary nodes.

Major complications of axillary dissection such as injury or thrombosis of the axillary vein and injury to the motor nerves of the axilla are rare. Mild lymphedema is seen in 10 to 15 percent of women, but severe persistent lymphedema occurs in less than 2 percent of patients. Other minor complications include wound infection, persisting seroma, mild shoulder dysfunction, and loss of sensation in the distribution of the intercostobrachial nerve.

The increasingly frequent identification by screening mammography of very small breast cancers with a low risk of axillary node metastases has stimulated interest in avoiding axillary dissection in some patients. Sentinel lymph node biopsy is a technique for identifying the axillary node most likely to contain metastases. Initial reports indicate that the sentinel node accurately predicts the histologic status of the remaining axillary nodes in 95 percent of cases. Additional study is needed before this technique replaces axillary dissection as a routine practice.

■ SELECTION OF LOCAL THERAPY

The ultimate selection of local therapy rests with the patient. The role of the surgeon is to exclude medical contraindications to different forms of local therapy, to educate the patient, and to provide access to multidisciplinary consultation. There is general agreement that first- and second-trimester pregnancy, multiple primary tumors in separate quadrants of the breast or diffuse microcalcifications with an indeterminate appearance, and prior therapeutic irradiation are absolute contraindications to breast preservation. A large tumor to breast ratio is a relative contraindication, but this varies with the patient's cosmetic expectations and the location of the tumor in the breast. Approximately 20 percent of women with Stage 0, I, or II breast carcinoma will have medical contraindications to breast preservation, and an even smaller number have significant comorbidities that preclude immediate reconstruction. For the remainder, factors affecting the decision include access to a radiotherapy facility, the frequency of follow-up exams and mammograms after each procedure, ability to cope with the possibility of recurrent cancer in the preserved breast, and feelings about body image. Consultation with a group of professionals from different disciplines allows a woman to obtain a variety of perspectives when making this difficult decision. In my experience, when offered an informed choice, 80 percent of eligible women will opt for breast preservation.

■ LOCALLY ADVANCED BREAST CANCER

The designation locally advanced breast cancer (LABC) encompasses a heterogeneous group of tumors that corresponds to stage III as defined by the American Joint Cancer Committee (AJCC) staging system. The biologic diversity seen in this group makes the formation of a single treatment recommendation difficult. The goals of therapy for women with LABC are to maintain local control on the chest wall and to prolong survival.

In women with stage IIIA disease on the basis of large primary tumor size alone, modified radical mastectomy followed by systemic adjuvant therapy and irradiation of the chest wall and nodal areas are often the treatments of choice. The use of induction chemotherapy in this group of patients will sometimes allow breast conservation therapy to replace mastectomy. In the presence of skin edema, ulceration, chest wall fixation, skin satellites, inflammatory carcinoma, or fixed axillary nodes, surgical resection as an initial therapeutic step is contraindicated. At most institutions a combined modality approach consisting of induction chemotherapy, mastectomy, radiotherapy, and further chemotherapy is employed. Typically, primary chemotherapy is given at full dose for three to six cycles or to response plateau. No data indicate that either approach is more advantageous, and most women will have achieved maximum response by cycle four. If the local disease has become technically operable and skin changes have resolved, mastectomy is carried out. In cases that remain technically unresectable, high-dose irradiation is used to achieve local control. Mastectomy has the advantage of allowing an accurate pathologic assessment of the extent of residual disease after induction chemotherapy, since physical examination is quite unreliable in this circumstance. Mastectomy following chemotherapy has not been associated with a higher incidence of wound complications than conventional mastectomy. After wound healing is complete, additional chemotherapy is followed by irradiation of the chest wall and lymphatics. This approach has the potential benefits of prompt treatment of presumed systemic disease, reduction of the tumor burden before definitive local therapy, and the use of the response of the primary tumor as an in vivo chemosensitivity assay. Clinical response rates of 70 to 90 percent are reported after induction therapy, and pathologic complete remissions are seen in 5 to 10 percent of cases. In spite of this, high rates of systemic failure are still seen.

Suggested Reading

Donegan WL. Evaluation of a palpable breast mass. N Engl J Med 1992; 327:937–942.

Fisher B, Costantino J, Redmond C, et al. Lumpectomy compared with lumpectomy and radiation therapy for the treatment of intraductal breast cancer. N Engl J Med 1993; 328:1581–1586.

Harris JR, Morrow M. Local management of invasive breast cancer. In: Harris JR, Lippman ME, Morrow M, Hellman S, eds. Diseases of the breast. Philadelphia: Lippincott-Raven, 1996:487.

Harris JR, Morrow M, Norton L. Malignant tumors of the breast. In: DeVita VT, Hellman S, Rosenberg SA, eds. Cancer: Principles and practice of oncology, 5th ed. Philadelphia: Lippincott-Raven, 1997:1557.

Morrow M. When can stereotactic core biopsy replace excisional biopsy?—A clinical perspective. Breast Cancer Res Treat 1995; 36:1-9.

Morrow M. Clinical crossroads: A 47-year-old woman with ductal carcinoma in situ. JAMA 1996; 775:61.

Morrow M, Schnitt S, Harris JR. Ductal carcinoma in situ. In: Harris JR, Lippman NE, Morrow M, Hellman S, eds. Diseases of the Breast. Philadelphia: Lippincott-Raven, 1996:335.

Winchester DP, Cox JD. Standards for breast conservation treatment. Cancer 1992; 42:134-162.

BREAST CANCER: CHEMOTHERAPY

James A. Stewart, M.D., F.A.C.P.

Treatment of breast cancer with systemic medicines is established and useful. Both cytotoxic drug treatment and hormonal strategies can change the natural history of early as well as advanced breast cancer. Nearly all women diagnosed with breast cancer can benefit from a discussion about systemic therapy for either enhancement of survival or improved symptom control. With women for whom systemic treatment is not indicated, such a discussion should result in greater confidence that the chosen treatment plan is sound.

Current incidence estimates for the United States describe 183,000 new diagnoses and 46,000 breast cancer deaths per year. Some 12 percent of U.S. women will be diagnosed with breast cancer, and 3.5 percent of them will die of it. Incidence rates have risen slightly in recent years in part because of increased mammography use but also for other less well understood reasons. Most breast cancer diagnoses occur in women over age 55, yet it is the leading cause of death in U.S. women between the ages of 40 and 55. Considerable anxiety among women of all age groups is generated by the threat of breast cancer. This concern has not been lessened by intense controversy over mammographic screening strategies. Data from controlled trials do not support widespread mammographic screening for populations under age 50 years, the group most vocal about the need for progress in breast cancer detection and treatment. In any case, despite the increase in incidence, the age-adjusted mortality in the United States is stable, perhaps reflecting a benefit from not only earlier detection but also improved systemic treatment.

■ SYSTEMIC APPROACHES

Cytotoxic Chemotherapy

Clinical breast cancer responds to a wide array of cytotoxic and hormonal agents. The choice of treatment for an individual patient depends on many factors (Table 1). Estrogen receptor positivity, metastases to soft tissue or bone rather than liver or lung, and a long interval (several years) from initial diagnosis to metastasis, all predict for response to hormonal therapy. If cytotoxic chemotherapy is used, optimal dosing should be prescribed. Standard regimens with tested doses and schedules have been established for initial treatment in adjuvant or advanced disease. However, the ideal regimen has not been devised for any subset of breast cancer. Whenever possible patients should be encouraged to participate in clinical trials designed to improve standards.

Breast cancer responds to agents from most of the major classes of cytotoxic drugs (see Table 1). Preferred regimens depend in part on the clinician's training, cooperative group affiliation, and geographic location. For example, the anthracycline doxorubicin, the most active single agent, is commonly used in the United States, but in Europe, epirubicin, a stereoisomer of doxorubicin, is more often prescribed. Clinicians affiliated with the Eastern Cooperative Oncology Group (ECOG) are familiar with cyclophosphamide, doxorubicin,

Table 1 Systemic Approaches to Metastatic Breast Cancer

ENDOCRINE THERAPY	DOSE/SCHEDULE	COMMENTS
Tamoxifen	20 mg/day oral	Generally well tolerated
Oophorectomy	Surgical or medical (LH-RH agents)	Laparoscopic procedure possible
Aminoglutethiamide	500–1,000 mg/day oral	Hydrocortisone not needed at lower doses
Megestrol acetate	160 mg/day oral	Weight gain a significant toxicity
Cytotoxic Chemotherapy		
AC	Every 3 weeks	
Doxorubicin	50–60 mg/m^2 q 3 weeks IV	With current antiemetics very well tolerated; also used in many adjuvant programs
Cyclophosphamide	500–600 mg/m^2 q 3 weeks IV	
CMF	Monthly	
Cyclophosphamide	100 mg/m^2/day oral monthly days 1–14	Large clinical experience; oral (C) not well tolerated by some patients
Methotrexate	40 mg/m^2 IV monthly days 1 & 8	
5-Fluorouracil	600 mg/m^2 IV monthly days 1 & 8	
VATH	Every 3 weeks	
Vinblastine	4.5 mg/m^2 IV day 1	Often used in patients with progressive disease after adjuvant CMF
Doxorubicin	45 mg/m^2 IV day 1	
Thiotepa	12 mg/m^2 IV day 1	
Fluoxymesterone	10 mg t.i.d. oral	
Paclitaxel (Taxol)	135–175 mg/m^2 IV q 21 days	Benefit of 3 hour vs. 24 hour infusion under study. Combination with doxorubicin under study.

5-fluorouracil (CAF)-type regimens, while National Surgical Adjuvant Breast Project (NSABP) physicians are experienced with the AC combination. Most first-line chemotherapy treatments involve multiple drugs, but single agents may palliate advanced disease and provide a better toxicity profile.

Although CMF (cyclophosphamide, methotrexate, 5-fluorouracil) and CAF regimens have been the mainstay of cytotoxic breast cancer therapy, new agents and combinations are being evaluated. The most promising drug is paclitaxel (Taxol), a tubulin-binding agent extracted from the bark of the Pacific yew tree *(Taxus brevifolia)*. Expected toxicities with this agent include myelosuppression, alopecia, and cumulative dose-dependent sensory neuropathy. The possibility of hypersensitivity reactions to paclitaxel is markedly lessened with a pretreatment regimen of corticosteroids and antihistamines (H_1 and H_2 blockers). Risk of hypersensitivity is also reduced by prolonging infusion time, although issues of convenience, cost, and efficacy also influence the choice of a 3 hour or 24 hour infusion schedule. One mechanism of paclitaxel resistance involves the increased expression of membrane p-glycoproteins resulting in the multidrug resistant (MDR) phenotype. Phase II studies in breast cancer have demonstrated substantial activity in both previously treated patients (56 percent overall response) and patients with prior adjuvant therapy or no history of chemotherapy (62 percent). Ongoing studies will delineate the role of paclitaxel in combination with other agents such as doxorubicin.

A variety of other drugs, including mitoxantrone, epirubicin, antraphyrazole, platinum compounds, epipodophyllotoxins, vinorelbine, and taxotere, have received phase II testing. To date paclitaxel is the most promising new agent, with the other drugs exhibiting differences in toxicity profiles but no major increase in anticancer effect.

Hormonal Agents

Hormonal therapy benefits many patients with breast cancer. Response rates of 30 percent in unselected patients can result from a variety of endocrine manipulations including tamoxifen or other additive (estrogens) or ablative (oophorectomy) approaches. The nonsteroidal antiestrogen tamoxifen is the agent of first choice for both adjuvant and advanced disease. Tumors that measure positive for hormone receptor exhibit at least a 50 percent response rate. Toxicity is mild, with hot flashes and vaginitis the most common short-term side effects. Tamoxifen is considered cytostatic rather than cytotoxic, and for adjuvant use prolonged administration (2 years plus) is more beneficial than shorter periods. There is evidence that with prolonged use (years) patients have at least a threefold increased risk of uterine endometrial cancer due to the partial estrogen agonist effect of this agent. Surveillance strategies to detect endometrial cancer are necessary for women with an intact uterus when tamoxifen is used long term. The dose of 20 mg per day can be given at one time or in divided doses.

Aminoglutethimide (AG), an aromatase inhibitor, blocks the conversion of androstenedione to estrone in muscle, fat, and liver. The resulting reduction in estrogen production is an effective hormonal treatment for breast cancer in postmenopausal or younger women who have had an oophorectomy. The dose is 1,000 mg per day given orally in divided doses with replacement doses of hydrocortisone (20–40 mg per day) given to suppress adrenocorticotropic hormone (ACTH) and prevent cortisol deficiency. Often lower doses of AG (500 mg per day) are given without supplemental hydrocortisone with successful reduction in estrogen. Toxicities of AG include initial drowsiness and skin rash, which both tend to resolve with continued treatment. Marrow toxicity is rare but does

Table 2 Systemic Treatment of Breast Cancer at the Time of Initial Diagnosis* (Adjuvant Therapy)

	NODE +	NODE – (FAVORABLE)‡	NODE – (UNFAVORABLE)
Premenopausal	ER+ Chemotherapy ± tamoxifen	Observation vs. tamoxifen	Chemotherapy ± tamoxifen
	ER– Chemotherapy	Observation vs. chemotherapy	Chemotherapy
Postmenopausal	ER+ Tamoxifen†	Observation vs. tamoxifen	Tamoxifen ± chemotherapy
	ER– Chemotherapy ± tamoxifen	Observation	Chemotherapy ± tamoxifen

*There is no subset of patients for whom an ideal approach is known. Whenever possible patients should participate in appropriate clinical trials.
†The overview suggests benefit from the addition of chemotherapy. Large individual trials now under way should clarify this issue.
‡Ongoing evaluation of prognostic and predictive factors should improve treatment decision for node-negative patients. Tumor size remains an important factor in node-negative patients.

occur, so it is reasonable to check white blood cell and platelet counts after a period of treatment. New aromatase inhibitors that are more selective and will not require glucocorticoid replacement therapy are in clinical development.

Megestrol acetate is a progestational agent commonly used as second- or third-line endocrine therapy. The standard dose is 40 mg four times a day. The most significant toxicity is weight gain, an effect that has led to the use of high-dose megestrol acetate as a treatment for cancer or acquired immunodeficiency syndrome (AIDS)–related cachexia. Progesterone antagonists are in development as treatments for breast cancer. Drugs such as mifepristone (RU 486) and onapristone block progesterone function at the receptor level.

Just as AG was developed as a medical adrenalectomy, analogues of the naturally occurring luteinizing hormone-releasing hormone (LH-RH) have been developed to provide a medical castration. Leuprolide and goserelin are two such agents; with chronic administration they lead to suppression of pituitary gonadotropins. Depot injection formulations allow for once a month treatment. The high cost of these agents and the need for repeated dosing will have to be weighed against the availability of laparoscopic surgical oophorectomy when this approach is selected in premenopausal women.

■ ADJUVANT THERAPY

Any patient diagnosed with invasive breast cancer is at some risk for distant recurrence regardless of the local therapy (surgical or irradiation) directed at the breast and regional nodes. The current understanding is that breast cancer does indeed begin in the breast, but metastatic spread to bones, liver, lungs, or other sites can occur at any time in the natural history of a breast tumor. Unfortunately, this occurs before diagnosis of the primary breast tumor, and generally the metastases are not detectable by clinical testing. Thus, for every patient with stage I or II breast cancer the reality of metastases is unknown and the risk of such can be estimated only with the prognostic information of anatomic stage, histologic grade, and surrogates for biologic behavior such as tumor hormone receptor measurement.

We do know that the natural history of stage I and II breast cancer can be favorably altered with adjuvant systemic treatment using cytotoxic and hormonal drugs. The result is that disease-free and overall survival for groups of patients given adjuvant treatment is better than that of those not treated. A major difficulty lies in translating the statistical improvement for groups to a treatment decision for an individual. In fact, patients think of themselves as individuals rather than part of a prognostic subset. Unfortunately, it is problematic to describe to an individual patient what her absolute benefit would be with or without adjuvant treatment.

This setting has enough complexity and uncertainty that discussions with patients about the goals of adjuvant treatment, including potential benefits and risks, must be thorough and unhurried. Fortunately, a large body of clinical trials data can support certain approaches. It must be emphasized that there is no subset of breast cancer whose systemic adjuvant treatment is good enough, as judged by efficacy and toxicity, to allow us to be content with the current standards.

The laboratory data that supported early trials of adjuvant therapy for operable breast cancer suggested greater benefit at a time of minimal tumor cell burden, a benefit that was dose dependent, and superior results with combination over single-agent chemotherapy. Issues of treatment timing and optimal dose are still being tested clinically 30 years later.

In terms of adjuvant therapy patients are generally categorized by the presence or absence of lymph node involvement and menopausal status, with further grouping by hormone receptor status of the primary tumor (Table 2). Over 100 randomized trials evaluating systemic adjuvant treatment provide a sizable database from which to estimate reduction of risk of mortality. The so-called overview analysis published early in 1992, an important example of collaboration among many investigators, provides a meta-analysis of data from 133 randomized studies. This effort focuses much of the current discussion regarding clinical recommendations as well as directions for future trials. It is important to remember that there is a continued need for randomized studies in this setting, in which at best new treatments will likely offer only moderate improvements in survival. As stated in the overview, "non-randomised methods . . . . cannot reliably exclude moderate biases." Despite the moderate differences between treated and untreated women, breast cancer is such a common disease that if we apply currently accepted adjuvant therapy to appropriate women, significant delays or reductions in mortality will occur for thousands of women yearly.

Node-Positive Disease

Cytotoxic Chemotherapy

Adjuvant cytotoxic chemotherapy is now considered standard for premenopausal women with node-positive disease regardless of hormone receptor status of the primary tumor. In recent years nearly 50 percent of women diagnosed with breast cancer have metastases in axillary nodes, although this percentage should decrease with increasing mammography and earlier cancer detection. Premenopausal women in the control arms of early studies had a 10 year survival of only 35 to 45 percent, demonstrating the need for improvement. Numerous randomized trials have compared cytotoxic chemotherapy with no systemic therapy. These studies have defined disease-free and overall survival benefits but leave unanswered questions regarding the optimal timing and duration of treatment, the best drug regimen, and the role of dose intensity.

An early clinical trial of the NSABP tested the single agent L-phenylalanine mustard given orally for 5 days every 6 weeks for 2 years against no chemotherapy. A subsequent study of the National Cancer Institute of Milan also evaluated node-positive women but with a combination of drugs (CMF for 1 year) or no chemotherapy. In both trials there was a significant survival benefit at 10 years, with the greatest effect seen in premenopausal women with one to three positive nodes. The 15 year analysis of the Milan study demonstrated that early differences between arms predicted long-term outcome, and the 20 year update confirms the long-term benefit of adjuvant therapy in node-positive women. This suggests that despite the potential long time to recurrence of breast cancer, studies did not have to be followed for many years before initiation of subsequent trials. Also, the number of positive nodes related inversely to outcome, and postmenopausal women accrued less benefit than younger women. How this age difference relates to dose delivery, as older women had more dose reductions, or to a chemotherapy-related oophorectomy effect in younger women is still unclear. The overview analysis reports a reduction in the annual odds of death of 17 percent for women less than 50 years of age and 9 percent for women aged 50 years and older.

Hormonal Treatment

It has long been known that some breast cancer cells are hormone dependent. Oophorectomy was first used in premenopausal women with metastatic disease nearly 100 years ago. Enthusiasm for testing the adjuvant use of hormonal approaches increased in the mid-1970s with the ability to measure hormone receptors and the subsequent evaluation of tamoxifen as a breast cancer treatment. A number of trials evaluating oophorectomy done before this time are limited by the relatively small numbers of patients, the lack of estrogen receptor (ER) data, and inconsistent information regarding node status. In spite of these deficiencies the recent overview analysis emphasizes the importance of ovarian ablation in women under age 50 years. By 15 years the difference in overall survival is approximately 10 percent among the population studied. Since these groups include both hormone receptor-positive and -negative women, the benefit for known receptor-positive women may be greater. New methods of ovarian ablation, including LH-RH agonists and laparoscopic oophorectomy, will aid the necessary continued study of this adjuvant treatment.

The lack of significant acute toxicities for tamoxifen as well as its known activity in metastatic disease led to large trials of this antiestrogen in the adjuvant setting. Over 1,000 node-positive and node-negative women were randomized to tamoxifen or placebo in the Nolvadex Adjuvant Trial Organization study begun in 1977. Again, a 10 percent advantage in favor of treatment was found at 8 years in this mostly postmenopausal population. Surprisingly, there was even a survival advantage in receptor-negative patients. The Scottish Trial also evaluated tamoxifen compared with no adjuvant therapy and demonstrated a significant survival benefit in favor of adjuvant treatment despite the use of tamoxifen in the no-treatment group at recurrence. Current data support the standard of adjuvant tamoxifen for postmenopausal women with positive nodes.

The optimal duration of tamoxifen use is also being evaluated. The long-term use of tamoxifen has been studied at the University of Wisconsin and in ECOG. The potential for beneficial effects on bone mass and cardiovascular risk factors such as serum lipid levels as well as possible induction of endometrial cancer may affect the optimal duration of therapy. Current practice is that adjuvant tamoxifen is given for at least 3 to 5 years. This regimen is in part based on animal studies showing that longer rather than shorter periods are more effective and on the premise that tamoxifen is a cytostatic rather than a cytotoxic agent. Further follow-up of trials with randomization to longer or shorter treatment is necessary to make firm recommendations. As of now there are no clinical trial data to support treatment longer than 5 years.

Node-Negative Disease

There is certainly much controversy among clinicians and anxiety among patients over treatment decisions in the node-negative setting. Following convincing reports that adjuvant chemotherapy or tamoxifen could favorably alter node-positive breast cancer, studies to test adjuvant treatment in node-negative patients also showed positive results. The NSABP B-13 trial for ER-negative cancers showed a benefit in both older and younger women for a nonalkylating agent chemotherapy regimen compared with no adjuvant therapy. The B-14 trial included estrogen receptor-positive breast cancer and tested tamoxifen against placebo, again with benefit shown for the treated group. This study was also instrumental in helping define the toxicity of tamoxifen compared with placebo. ECOG led an intergroup trial of CMF with prednisone chemotherapy versus no adjuvant therapy in cancer that was ER negative or ER positive but with tumor size of at least 3 cm, again in premenopausal and postmenopausal women. This trial also favored the use of adjuvant therapy, with statistically significant improvement in disease-free survival.

It is clear, then, that node-negative breast cancer can be influenced with adjuvant therapy. However, which individual patients will benefit is a difficult question. The discussion with an individual patient regarding the balance among toxicity, cost, and benefit is also difficult. Because of the generally good prognosis of node-negative patients (10 year relapse-free survival in the 70 percent range), the absolute magnitude of benefit is less than for node-positive populations despite similar proportional reduction of recurrence. Rather than treating all patients, most of whom do not need treatment but will experience the toxicity, it would be ideal to treat only those at highest risk.

Non-nodal prognostic factors obviously influence treatment decisions. Tumor size, nuclear grade, and ER status are established risk factors. ER status has the added advantage of predicting for hormonal response. Other potential indicators of invasiveness or metastatic potential include S-phase fraction and DNA ploidy as measured by flow cytometry, and the enzyme cathepsin-D. Unfortunately, the utility of these tests is unclear in the general clinical setting even though they may be ordered routinely along with hormone receptors. Though they may indicate increased aggressiveness, neither these nor other markers predict for treatment effectiveness. What is needed is a single indicator or profile of tests that can not only identify high-risk patients among the node-negative population but also guide treatment that is predictably effective.

The clinician is assisted by several sources of guidance regarding treatment recommendations. In 1990 the NIH Consensus Development Conference Statement on the treatment of early breast cancer summarized recommended approaches for operable breast cancer and the role of adjuvant therapy in node-negative cancer. In addition to encouraging participation in clinical trials the panel recommended adjuvant treatment with chemotherapy or tamoxifen for tumors larger than 1 cm. In 1992 another consensus panel met in St. Gallen, Switzerland, and devised guidelines based on data from individual studies, personal experience, and conclusions from the overview. They divided node-negative patients into minimal to low, good, and high risk. Only for the lowest-risk category (not more than 1 cm, up to 2 cm with very favorable histology, or noninvasive cancer) is an observation-only approach considered. All other categories call for tamoxifen and/or chemotherapy. This group met again in 1995 and underscored the need to determine baseline risk, particularly in the node-negative population. Of note, they specifically did not recommend the measurement of ploidy or S phase to help determine risk.

The overview analysis, the single most influential report on the benefits of adjuvant therapy, is worth close review and deliberation by all physicians. The emphasis on *proportional* effects of adjuvant therapy is worth noting. This requires that the baseline risk of recurrence be estimated prior to applying the derived relative reduction in risk. Patients who start with a relatively small risk (small, node-negative tumors) may benefit, but with less absolute reduction in risk of recurrence or death. Those with a higher natural history risk will gain a larger absolute benefit from adjuvant therapy. It is not clear whether benefit as measured by proportional reduction in annual odds of recurrence and death is accrued to the individual or the group at large. It is also important to weigh the cost (toxicity, dollars) against the absolute benefit expected. This is not easy for many clinicians or most patients, who expect a simpler answer regarding chance for cure and how to optimize the likelihood of cure.

Metastatic Disease

One of the most difficult discussions relates to defining goals of therapy in a patient with evident distant metastatic disease. Many patients who have disease recurrence after earlier adjuvant treatment have been told that cure is a goal at initial diagnosis but not at relapse. Nevertheless, many patients are treated with so-called salvage regimens with good response rates. Patients who recur more than a year after completion of adjuvant therapy can be treated with the same drugs; the resulting response rate is 50 percent. The broad range of treatments, including cytotoxic chemotherapy and hormonal therapy, allow for continued sequential treatment of metastatic breast cancer using multiple regimens. For example, even in heavily pretreated patients certain combinations or single agents such as paclitaxel can induce measurable responses or symptom improvement. Unfortunately, most salvage regimens after the initial postadjuvant treatment are not very useful. Rather than subjecting the patient to third- and fourth-line combination chemotherapy, it is generally wiser to encourage participation in phase I or II clinical trials if systemic treatment is to be used.

The variety of treatment options and the need for repeated assessment of goals raises the issue of optimal duration of treatment. For hormonal therapy of metastatic disease, unless there is clear progression, patients should be treated for at least 3 months even if there is only stable disease before deciding the cancer is not responding. Several chemotherapy studies, some including quality of life evaluation, have randomized patients to arms of different duration. These trials suggest that it may be better to treat for longer continuous periods or until disease progresses, rather than for a defined shorter period followed by observation. Again, the balance between toxicity and therapeutic gain is complex, and repeated reassessment of goals is useful.

Another area of controversy is the combination of endocrine and cytotoxic therapy. The cellular heterogeneity of tumors supports such an approach; that is, a given tumor is composed of both hormone-responsive and nonresponsive cells. Unfortunately, no significant increase in response rate or survival has occurred with this strategy. Another disadvantage of a chemohormonal treatment is assessment of which modality is to be discontinued if there is a tumor response but toxicity is unacceptable.

Another approach is to stimulate breast cancer growth with the appropriate dose of estrogen and then follow with cytotoxic chemotherapy, expecting that the increased cycling induced by the hormone will result in better chemotherapy drug kill. Again, clinical testing of this approach has not increased time to progression or survival. Thus, for metastatic cancer the standard remains the use of either cytotoxic or hormonal therapy at any one time. It is interesting that in the adjuvant setting there is increasing enthusiasm for the use of long-term tamoxifen for premenopausal women who will receive chemotherapy and who have receptor-positive cancer.

■ HIGH-DOSE THERAPY

One of the most emotional debates regarding breast cancer treatment is about high-dose chemotherapy. As in other areas of medicine, the technical ability to administer very high doses of cytotoxic therapy with bone marrow or stem cell support has outpaced our knowledge of how useful this approach may be. Reimbursement battles, sensationalist publicity, and litigation rather than orderly clinical trials have taken center stage.

Alkylating agents tested in laboratory models show a steep dose-response curve. The somatic mutation hypothesis (Goldie-Coldman) predicts decreased likelihood of cure with increased tumor burden because of a greater likelihood of resistant cells. Because of these and other considerations numerous programs are evaluating marrow-ablative doses of chemotherapy with bone marrow or peripheral stem cell support. Unfortunately, the strength of the overview analysis based on data from randomized trials of conventional chemotherapy is lacking in this area of high-dose treatment. Randomized studies designed for both the adjuvant and advanced setting have been slow to accrue. At present, despite the huge effort expended in developing bone marrow transplant type treatments for breast cancer, we do not know even aside from cost issues whether any benefits outweigh the toxicities. The proper trials to test efficacy have not yet been completed.

Dose intensity is also being tested with treatment regimens that are less than marrow ablative. An intergroup trial is evaluating higher than usual doses of doxorubicin and cytoxan with colony-stimulating factor and prophylactic antibiotic support in the adjuvant setting. In this trial women will have a better prognosis than the usual patient treated in marrow-ablative regimens, e.g., those with stage IV or more than 10 positive nodes.

Breast cancer treatment with systemic agents is slowly improving. Better regimens with improved efficacy and less toxicity as well as better selection of women for treatment are possible. Continued and increased emphasis on clinical trials participation is a necessary part of this advancement.

Suggested Reading

Bonadonna G, Valagussa P, Moliterni A, et al. Adjuvant cyclophosphamide, methotrexate, and fluorouracil in node positive breast cancer. N Engl J Med 1995 332:901–906.

Early Breast Cancer Trialists' Collaborative Group. Systemic treatment of early breast cancer by hormonal, cytotoxic, or immune therapy: 133 randomized trials involving 31,000 recurrences and 24,000 deaths among 75,000 women. Lancet 1992; 339:1–5, 71–85.

Fisher B, Redmond C, Dimitrov NV, et al. A randomized clinical trial evaluating sequential methotrexate and fluorouracil in the treatment of patients with node-negative breast cancer who have estrogen-receptor-negative tumors. N Engl J Med 1989; 320:473–478.

Fisher B, Costantino J, Redmond C, et al. A randomized clinical trial evaluating tamoxifen in the treatment of patients with node-negative breast cancer who have estrogen-receptor-positive tumors. N Engl J Med 1989; 320:479–484.

Gasparini G, Pozza F, Harris AL. Evaluating the potential usefulness of new prognostic and predictive indicators in node-negative breast cancer patients. J Natl Cancer Inst 1993; 85:1206–1219.

Glick JH, Gelber RD, Goldhirsch A, Senn H-J. Meeting highlights: Adjuvant therapy for primary breast cancer. J Natl Cancer Inst 1992; 84:1479–1485.

Goldhirsch A, Wood WC, Senn HJ, et al. Meeting Highlights: International Consensus Panel on the Treatment of Primary Breast Cancer. J Natl Cancer Inst 1995; 87:1441–1445.

Mansour EG, Gray R, Shatila AH, et al. Efficacy of adjuvant chemotherapy in high-risk node-negative breast cancer. N Engl J Med 1989; 320:485–490.

Pfeiffer P, Cold S, Rose C. Cytotoxic treatment of metastatic breast cancer. Acta Oncologica 1992; 31:219–224.

Reichman BS, Seidman AD, Crown JPA, et al. Paclitaxel and recombinant human granulocyte colony-stimulating factor as initial chemotherapy for metastatic breast cancer. J Clin Oncol 1993; 11:1943–1951.

Silliman RA, Balducci L, Goodwin JS, et al. Breast cancer care in old age: What we know, don't know, and do. J Natl Cancer Inst 1993; 85:190–199.

Tancini G, Bonadonna G, Valagussa P, et al. Adjuvant CMF in breast cancer: Comparative 5-year results of 12 versus 6 cycles. J Clin Oncol 1983; 1:2–10.

BREAST CANCER: RADIOTHERAPY

Richard A. Steeves, M.D., Ph.D.

Breast-conserving surgery and radiotherapy are now considered an acceptable alternative to mastectomy for patients with stage I or II breast cancer. In 1992 the American College of Surgeons, the American College of Radiology, and the American Cancer Society agreed on the following criteria to identify patients for whom breast-conserving therapy would be appropriate:

1. Early breast cancers (no larger than 1 cm) detected by mammography
2. A single cancer up to 5 cm in diameter if the affected breast is large enough to allow lumpectomy with a good cosmetic result
3. Breast cancer even if the cancer has spread to the ipsilateral axillary lymph nodes

Only a few of these candidates would lose their eligibility for breast-conserving therapy as a result of the following contraindications for breast irradiation:

1. Prior radiotherapy to the same breast
2. Pregnancy
3. Collagen vascular disease
4. High probability of a significant residual tumor volume post lumpectomy, as suggested by gross multicentric breast cancer or extensive in situ carcinoma

Thus, the goals of breast-conserving therapy are as follows:

1. To eradicate microscopic foci of multicentric cancer with moderate doses of radiation
2. To minimize the probability of local recurrence at the primary site
3. To maximize the quality of life benefit with a low risk of complications and an acceptable cosmetic result

Table 1 Comparison of Disease-Free Survival After Breast Conservation Treatment Versus Mastectomy in Prospective, Randomized Trials

	NUMBER OF PATIENTS	DURATION OF FOLLOW-UP IN YEARS	DISEASE-FREE SURVIVAL		
			CONSERVATIVE SURGERY + IRRADIATION (%)	MASTECTOMY (%)	*P* VALUE
National Surgical Adjuvant Breast Project (NSABP)	1,219	8	59	58	.20
National Cancer Institute (Milan)	701	10	77	76	.27
Institut Gustave-Roussy (Paris)	179	10	65*	56*	N.S.
Danish Breast Cancer Group	905	6	70	66	N.S.
National Cancer Intitute (USA)	237	8	66	76	N.S.
Total =	3,241				

*Estimated from curves.
N.S., Not significant.

This chapter summarizes the randomized trials comparing breast-conserving surgery plus irradiation against mastectomy, reviews patient selection and radiotherapeutic technique, and examines locoregional control, complications, and cosmetic results.

RANDOMIZED TRIALS

Overwhelming evidence from over 3,000 randomly assigned patients (Table 1) demonstrates that disease-free survival is the same for 6 to 10 years after treatment whether it was by modified radical mastectomy or by breast-conserving surgery followed by irradiation. All of these studies were conducted on patients with stage I or II infiltrating ductal cancers. The evidence is not so strong for ductal carcinoma in situ (DCIS), however, because random assignment to undergo either mastectomy or lumpectomy for such small cancers would be unacceptable to many women. Instead, the National Surgical Adjuvant Breast Project (NSABP) conducted a randomized trial of lumpectomy alone versus lumpectomy plus breast irradiation (50 Gy) among 790 women with this disease. After a median follow-up of 43 months, the incidence of ipsilateral breast cancer was 16.4 percent in the former group (lumpectomy alone) versus 7 percent in the latter group (lumpectomy and irradiation). Much longer follow-up will be needed before these results can be considered definitive, but the study suggests that radiotherapy decreases the rate of local recurrences in women with ductal carcinoma in situ.

ANALYSIS OF STAGE, SURGICAL MARGINS, AND REGIONS TO BE TREATED

The staging for breast cancer is primarily surgical (see Table 1 in the chapter *Breast Cancer: Surgery*) because clinical judgments of both tumor size and axillary metastases are known to be unreliable. Much emphasis, therefore, is placed on detailed communication with the surgeon and pathologist regarding the size of the primary tumor, the proximity of the margins, and the extent of involvement of the axillary nodes. Since other factors such as the degree of anaplasia and infiltration by lymphocytes are also of prognostic significance, it is ideal to review the slides with the pathologist personally. This is not to lessen the value of a thorough physical examination, for a supraclavicular metastasis drastically alters the prognosis as well as the treatment plan. Careful assessment of the location and the rate of healing of the surgical scar, the volume of induration or hematoma in the remainder of the affected breast, any arm swelling, and a comparison with the opposite breast are needed. A review of the preoperative mammogram, chest x-ray film, and liver function tests usually completes the staging analysis. In the absence of bone pain a bone scan can also be obtained, primarily as a baseline study, for it rarely reflects metastatic disease in patients with early breast cancer.

To aid in treatment planning, it is important to have a thorough understanding between the surgeon and radiation oncologist to ensure that the axilla is meticulously evaluated. Because axillary metastases are known to skip the lower (level 1) nodes 25 percent of the time, an axillary dissection that includes not only level 1 but also level 2 nodes (i.e., those behind the pectoralis minor insertion) is usually performed. Only with this procedure can the axillary and supraclavicular regions be shielded with confidence when cancer cells have not been found in the axillary nodes. Node-positive axillae are irradiated only if four or more nodes contained cancer cells or if lymph nodes were replaced by tumor cells, with a high probability of extranodal spread. If the axillary dissection includes level 3, most radiation oncologists consider the procedure therapeutic as well as diagnostic, and refrain from adding radiation to this region and increasing the risk of arm edema.

Irradiation of the internal mammary nodes (IMN) is becoming increasingly controversial and unpopular. There is a low risk of clinical IMN failure in patients with early-stage breast cancer. Patients with more advanced, medially located lesions may have their IMN included within the tangential breast beams. However, this is done only after precise computed tomography (CT) based treatment planning because it significantly increases the volume of normal tissue treated, and it may compromise subsequent therapy to the opposite breast.

■ RADIOTHERAPEUTIC TECHNIQUE

Treatment planning is generally started 3 to 4 weeks post surgery to allow for wound healing and arm mobility. Individually contoured cradles made of polyurethane foam are formed prior to the CT scan and used during simulation and all treatments to minimize any variation in the patient's supine position. CT scans are obtained to define breast boundaries and underlying normal tissues. At simulation the CT scans are used to determine appropriate field sizes and beam angles. Tangential fields are simulated using visible light and x-ray beams. The films are then used to draw customized blocks that shield heart and lung tissues. The upper portions of the tangential fields and the lower half of the supraclavicular field (if used) are blocked to avoid any divergence into adjacent fields (Fig. 1). This improves the cosmetic result and reduces the risk of a rib fracture.

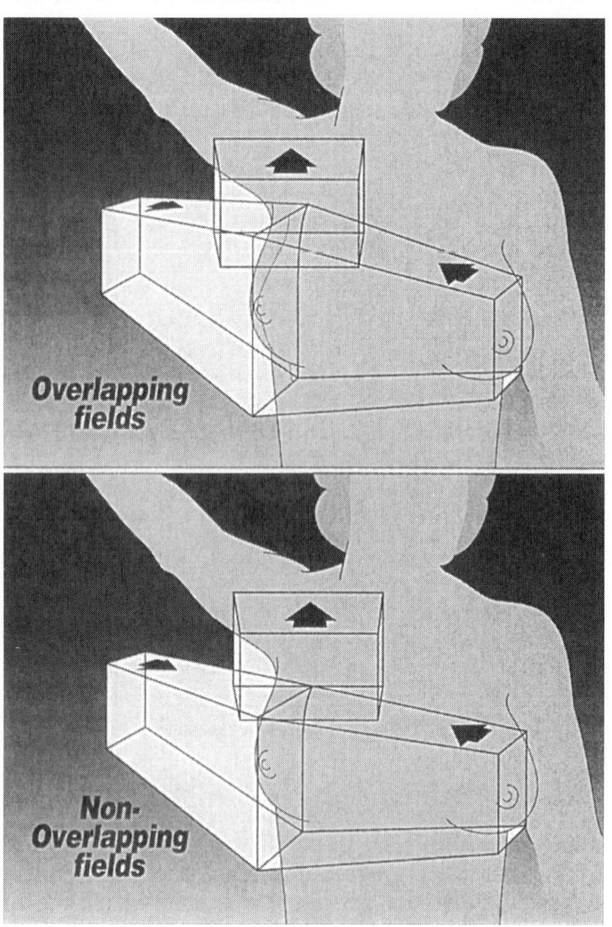

Figure 1
Diagrammatic illustration of the difference between overlapping and nonoverlapping fields when treating the breast and regional lymph nodes.

The doses generally used to treat these regions are 50 Gy in 25 fractions over 5 weeks, although slightly lower doses (46 to 48 Gy) in 1.8 Gy fractions may be used if the patient is obese or has recently completed cytotoxic chemotherapy. The energy of the photon beam can range from 1 to 6 MV. Cobalt γ-rays have become less popular recently because they provide less homogeneity in dose throughout the target region than higher-energy x-ray beams. However, the much sharper penumbra associated with x-rays can lead to greater variations in dose between adjacent fields unless great care is taken with each treatment setup. Application of tissue-equivalent bolus to the skin is not usually needed with cobalt but may be indicated with higher-energy x-rays, especially if there has been invasion of the dermal lymphatic vessels. Treatment of all fields each day is essential for good cosmetic results.

If the margins of resection were negative, the bed from which the tumor was excised is usually boosted to 60 Gy. Deep lesion sites are best treated with photon therapy through coned tangential portals, whereas superficial lesion sites can be encompassed with a minimum volume of normal tissue with shaped electron fields. However, if there is a question about the presence of carcinoma cells near the resected margin, doses of 70 to 75 Gy are preferred. Boost doses of this magnitude cannot be given by external beam with satisfactory cosmetic results, so the dose is delivered with a two- or three-plane interstitial implant that is afterloaded with iridium-192. The dose rate is usually 0.4 to 0.5 Gy per hour, and the entire boost dose is given over a 2 to 3 day period. If care is taken to place the most superficial iridium seeds at least 1 cm deep from the skin, a good cosmetic result is still feasible.

■ LOCOREGIONAL RECURRENCE

Regular physical examinations and mammograms every 6 to 12 months are essential for detecting recurrences as early as

Table 2 Breast Cancer Recurrences 5 Years After Conservative Surgery and Irradiation Related to Tumor Size or Nodal Status

	BREAST CANCER RECURRENCE RATE (%)			
RADIOTHERAPY CENTER	T_1	T_2	N−	N+
NSABP B-06*	7	10	12	6
Curie Institute, Paris	7	11	6	4
Gustav-Roussy Institute, Paris	6	3	4	7
Joint Center, Boston	10	10	12	10
Leuven University, Belgium	5	15	10	15
University of Pennsylvania, Philadelphia	5	8	7	4
University of Wisconsin, Madison	4	7	5	5
Average	6.3	9.1	8.0	7.3

*National Surgical Adjuvant Breast Project, protocol B-06, organized by the University of Pittsburgh.

possible in their evolution. As shown in Table 2, locoregional recurrence rates 5 years after conservative therapy correlate with tumor size but not with nodal status. Other risk factors relate to the probability of residual tumor cells left in the tumor bed after lumpectomy. For example, the presence of gross multicentric carcinoma or extensive intraductal component of the neoplasm should alert the surgical oncologist to resect wide (1.5 to 2 cm) margins of normal tissue around the tumor to reduce the likelihood of local recurrence. Early recurrences are often at or near the tumor bed, whereas late (after 3 years) recurrences occur more often in other quadrants, suggesting a new primary tumor. Prompt treatment with mastectomy provides over 90 percent locoregional control, but carefully selected patients with smaller than 2 cm tumors can be managed successfully with a second lumpectomy followed by localized irradiation to the tumor bed.

Table 3 Criteria for Scoring Cosmetic Results

Score	Criterion
	EFFECTS OF SURGERY
3	Scar unapparent
2	Scar apparent
1	Major tissue loss
	EFFECTS OF IRRADIATION
3	None
2	Slight
1	Moderate
0	Severe
	(Skin changes (diffuse or along match lines); Fibrosis (diffuse or focal); Retraction of the breast)
	PHOTOGRAPHIC ASSESSMENT
4	Excellent: hard to distinguish treated from untreated breast
3	Good: treated breast slightly different from untreated breast
2	Fair: treated breast clearly different from untreated breast
1	Poor: treated breast seriously distorted

Added scores from all three categories range from 10 (excellent) to 7 (good) to 2 (worst case).

■ COMPLICATIONS

Irradiation of the breast is generally well tolerated. Many brochures for patients warn of fatigue, but even this is becoming rarer now that most patients receive irradiation to the breast only. Some redness and edema of the skin are common during the last half of the treatment course, with tenderness persistent for a month or two after treatment. A small percentage of patients may suddenly develop an inflammatory episode

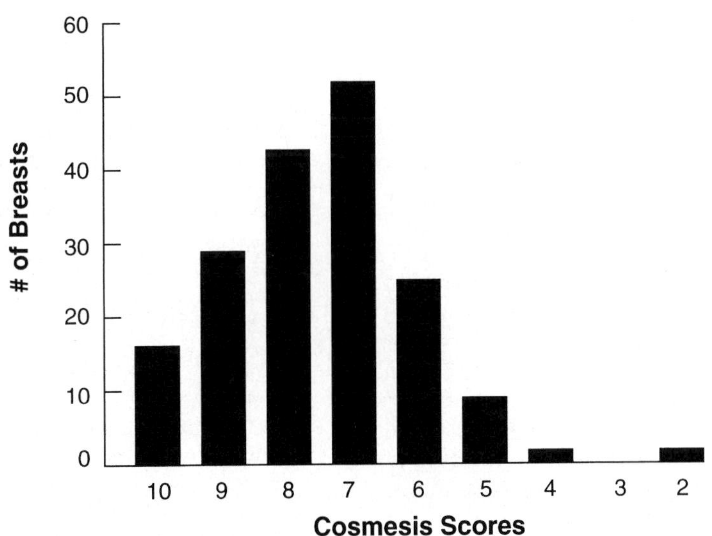

Figure 2
Frequency distribution of cosmesis scores post breast irradiation.

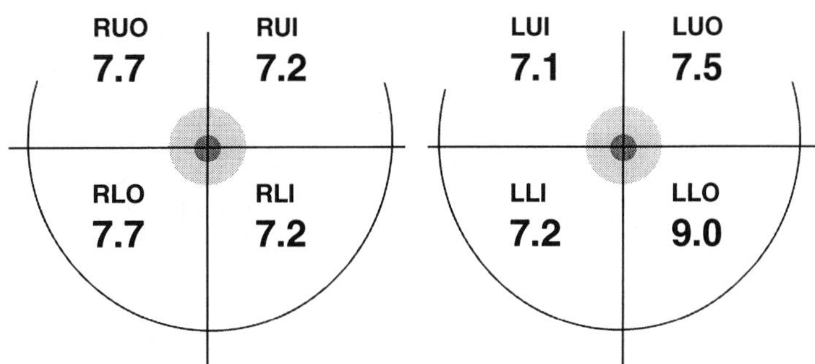

Figure 3
Mean cosmesis scores post irradiation of cancers in different breast quadrants.

Table 4 Mean Cosmesis Scores Post Irradiation Alone or Radiation Coupled with Various Types of Chemotherapy

CHEMOTHERAPY	NUMBER OF PATIENTS	MEAN COSMESIS SCORE
None	101	7.6
CMF-based	10	6.7
CAF-based	38	7.7
Tamoxifen only	26	7.6
Total	175	7.5

6 months or so after radiotherapy. Such patients may notice warmth, tenderness, and limited motion in the treated area, particularly in the pectoral muscles. Not to be confused with recurrence or infection, these symptoms generally last for a few weeks and improve after conservative measures such as aspirin and gentle stretching exercises.

Other complications, such as radiation pneumonitis, pericarditis, or brachial neuropathy, rare in my experience, are reported among published reports in 0.5 to 2 percent of patients. Precise techniques and careful attention to detail are required to maintain a low risk of such complications. Contralateral breast tumors have not been found to be more frequent in irradiated patients than in mastectomy patients in randomized trials.

■ COSMESIS

The overall cosmetic outcome after breast-conserving therapy depends as much on the effects of surgery (tissue loss, nipple distortion, scar appearance) as on the effects of radiation (areolar depigmentation, diffuse fibrosis, breast retraction). Therefore, we have developed a numeric scoring system that assesses the effects of both types of therapy and overall appearance (Table 3). The use of a precise number allows for simpler data analysis than a descriptive qualifier such as good, poor, or fair. This is evident in the frequency distribution of 178 scores after a median of 5 years of follow-up (Fig. 2) and in the cosmetic analysis for cancers that arose in different breast quadrants (Fig. 3). It was also noted that the administration of chemotherapy before breast irradiation did not adversely affect cosmetic outcome (Table 4) once the older age of CMF-treated patients had been taken into account. Other factors that do affect cosmesis include tumor size (smaller is better), daily dose of radiation (less is better), and radiation technique, with improved cosmetic results coming from megavoltage equipment, wedges to reduce dose inhomogeneity, and avoidance of the use of skin bolus.

■ INTEGRATION OF IRRADIATION AND CHEMOTHERAPY

There has been understandable reluctance to delay chemotherapy until after radiotherapy because of the potential for growth of cancer cells at distant metastatic sites. Consequently, several investigators have integrated the two forms of therapy with a modest reduction in the dose of certain drugs and a modest increase in the rate of radiation complications. At the University of Wisconsin it was decided that the surgical margins of resection were wide enough to take the risk of giving all cytotoxic chemotherapy first and then starting the radiotherapy 2 weeks after the last cytotoxic drug. Our 5 year results (Table 2, last line) show no difference in recurrence rate between patients who were axillary node–positive, most of whom received prior cytotoxic chemotherapy, and patients who were node negative and received either tamoxifen or no chemotherapy. Perhaps because of the wide surgical margins, the 5 year recurrence rates at UW were only 5 percent.

Suggested Reading

Fisher B, Redmond C, Poisson R, et al. Eight-year results of a randomized clinical trial comparing total mastectomy and lumpectomy with or without irradiation in the treatment of breast cancer. N Engl J Med 1989; 320:822–828.

Fowble B, Goodman R, Glick J, et al. Breast cancer treatment: A comprehensive guide to management. St. Louis: Mosby–Year Book, 1991.

Rose M, Olivotto I, Cady B, et al. Conservative surgery and radiation therapy for early breast cancer: Long-term cosmetic results. Arch Surg 1989; 124:153–157.

Sarrazin D, Le M, Arrigada R, et al. Ten-year results of a randomized trial comparing a conservative treatment in mastectomy in early breast cancer. Radiother Oncol 1989; 14:177–184.

Steeves RA, Phromratanapongse P, Wolberg WH, et al. Cosmesis and local control after irradiation in women treated conservatively for breast cancer. Arch Surg 1989; 149:1369–1371.

Veronesi U, Banfi A, Salvadori B, et al. Breast conservation is the treatment of choice in small breast cancer: Long-term results of a randomized trial. Eur J Cancer 1990; 26:668–670.

COLORECTAL CANCER: SURGERY

James M. Stone, M.D., F.A.C.S.
John E. Niederhuber, M.D.

EPIDEMIOLOGY AND PATHOLOGY

Colorectal cancer is the second most common visceral malignancy in the United States; approximately 160,000 new cases will occur this year. There is strong evidence that both environmental and genetic factors are involved in the genesis of colorectal cancer. Epidemiologic studies demonstrate a wide variation in the incidence of colorectal cancer in different populations; however, migration studies show that the incidence rates of immigrant populations readily equalize with the host population. Diet is believed to be the dominant environmental factor, and populations that ingest diets high in fat and low in fiber have the highest rates, while Western vegetarians and those in developing nations have the lowest rates.

The genetic predisposition to colorectal cancer is most clearly demonstrated in the familial adenomatous polyposis (FAP) syndrome. In this autosomal dominant, heritable syndrome, essentially 100 percent of affected individuals develop colorectal cancer. The genetic locus linked to FAP has been mapped to a specific chromosome (5q). Colorectal cancer may also be inherited in an autosomal dominant fashion in the hereditary nonpolyposis colon cancer syndrome (HNPCC). This syndrome is characterized by early age of cancer onset, predominance of right-sided lesions, and frequent synchronous and metachronous cancers in the absence of multiple polyps. Approximately 5 percent of patients with colorectal cancer have the HNPCC syndrome while an even larger proportion will have a positive family history for colorectal cancer. Persons with a single first-degree relative with colorectal cancer have a threefold increase in risk of colorectal cancer compared with the general population; two first-degree relatives confers a ninefold increase in risk.

Vogelstein and others have outlined a sequence of genetic abnormalities leading to malignant neoplasia of the colon. Some genetic abnormalities are inherited while others reflect spontaneous somatic mutations or the carcinogenic effect of environmental factors. Eventually, the accumulated activation of oncogenes and inactivation of tumor suppresser genes leads to step-wise transformation of colonic epithelium. The identification of genetic alterations in colon cancer holds great promise in the prevention and early diagnosis of colorectal cancer.

Epidemiologic and pathologic data have long supported the concept that the great majority of colorectal cancers arise from benign polyps. The validity of the polyp to cancer sequence has been supported by recent molecular genetic studies: adenomas usually have one mutation or deletion, in situ carcinomas may have two, invasive cancers may have three or four. Colorectal polyps therefore are an important marker for genetic abnormality and cancer risk.

Ninety-five percent of colorectal cancers are adenocarcinomas. On rare occasions lymphomas, malignant carcinoid, melanoma, leiomyosarcomas, or squamous cancers may also arise from the large bowel. The large bowel is rarely the site of metastatic disease, however, melanoma, lymphoma, and carcinomas of the breast, ovary, lung, and stomach occasionally involve the colon. Usually such metastases occur late in the course of disease. Prostate cancer in rare cases invades the rectum by direct extension.

Colorectal cancers are termed *invasive* when they grow through the muscularis mucosa into the submucosa. Prior to this point, hematogenous or lymphatic metastases are very uncommon. The growing tumor mass may extend circumferentially around the lumen to give the typical "apple-core" appearance seen on barium enema. Intramural spread of the tumor, parallel to the long axis of the bowel, generally does not occur. Recognition of this pattern of tumor growth has enabled surgeons to perform sphincter-sparing, low anterior resection for tumors in the mid to lower rectum.

The pattern of spread of colorectal tumors depends on the anatomy of the involved bowel segment, as well as its lymphatic and vascular supply. The rectum is generally divided into upper, middle, and lower thirds. The tight anatomic confines of the bony pelvis, the diffuse nature of the lymphatic drainage, and the dual blood supply of this area make the pattern of spread from the extraperitoneal rectum different from the intraperitoneal rectum or the colon. Cancers in the lower third of the rectum may spread either via the superior hemorrhoidal veins to the portal system and the liver, or via the middle hemorrhoidal veins to the systemic circulation and the lung. Pulmonary metastases, without intervening liver metastases, are unusual in patients with primary tumors proximal to the lower rectum. Tumor cells of the extraperitoneal rectum may also enter the prevertebral venous plexus and result in thoracic or lumbar spinal metastasis. Tumor cells of the extraperitoneal rectum commonly invade the vagina by direct extension, and on occasion may also directly invade the seminal vesicles, prostate, uterus, urinary bladder, pelvic floor, or sphincter mechanism.

The natural history of tumors arising in the colon and upper rectum are similar. Lymph node metastases generally parallel the arterial supply of the colon, and hematogenous metastases almost always present first in the liver. Tumors that erode through the serosal surface may spread to adjacent or distant peritoneal surfaces. Ovarian metastases occur in approximately 5 percent of women with colon cancer.

Dukes correlated the degree of tumor invasion at the time of resection with survival and proposed the following classification in 1929: tumor confined to the bowel wall (stage A); tumor through the bowel wall, no lymph node metastases, (stage B); lymph node metastases (stage C). Although Dukes' classification was originally derived from patients with rectal cancer, it has been useful in staging patients with colon cancer as well. Numerous modifications of Dukes' classification have been proposed with the intent of increasing its prognostic value. The most popular of these is the Astler-Coller system (Table 1). To provide a uniform and orderly classification for

Table 1 Classification of Colorectal Cancer

DUKES'	ASTLER-COLLER	5 YEAR SURVIVAL
A Limited to bowel wall	A Limited to mucosa	90%–95%
B Through bowel wall	B1 Into muscularis propria	60%
	B2 Through serosa	50%
C Regional node metastasis	C1 Into musc. propria, lymph node metastasis	40%
	C2 Through serosa, lymph node metastasis	25%

Table 2 TNM and Endorectal Ultrasound Classification of Colorectal Cancer

TNM CLASSIFICATION	DESCRIPTION	ERUS CLASSIFICATION
Tis	Carcinoma in situ	uT0
T1	Tumor invades submucosa	uT1
T2	Tumor invades muscularis propria	uT2
T3	Tumor invades subserosa or nonperitonealized pericolic or perirectal tissue	uT3
T4	Tumor perforates visceral peritoneum or directly invades other structure	uT4
N0	No regional node metastases	uN0
N1	1–3 pericolic or perirectal nodes involved	uN1
N2	>4 pericolic or perirectal nodes involved	uN1
N3	Node metastasis along major vascular trunk	—
M0	No distant metastasis	—
M1	Distant metastasis	—

Stage 0: Tis, N0, M0; Stage I: T1–2, N0, M0; Stage II: T3–4, N0, M0; Stage III: T1–4, N1–3; M0; Stage IV: T1–4; N1–3; M1.
ERUS, endoluminal rectal ultrasound

cancer of the colon and rectum, the American Joint Committee on Cancer Staging has proposed a TNM classification (Table 2). Accurate classification is essential for determining prognosis, entering patients into therapeutic trials, and determining the outcome of therapy.

■ PREVENTION AND SCREENING

Primary prevention of colorectal cancer through interventions that reduce or eliminate the genetic changes responsible for malignant transformation is not yet available, but is the goal of much of today's research. Secondary prevention of colon cancer, however, is possible through the elimination of colon polyps. Colonoscopy is the most reliable method for detecting colorectal polyps and it offers the opportunity to remove polyps and subject them to histologic review. However, colonoscopy is impractical as a screening test because it is expensive, time-consuming, and likely to cause complications.

Current screening techniques are primarily designed to detect colorectal cancer while it is in a curable stage, however, an attempt should also be made to eliminate colon polyps when they are found. Recently published data from the University of Minnesota shows that screening a normal-risk population for colon cancer with the fecal occult blood test diminishes the likelihood of dying of colorectal cancer by 33 percent. In 1992 the American Cancer Society revised its recommendations for screening for colon and rectum cancer. Asymptomatic individuals should undergo digital rectal examination starting at age 40 and beginning at age 50, should have yearly fecal occult blood tests and sigmoidoscopy (preferably flexible) repeated at 3 to 5 year intervals. Individuals with one or more first-degree relatives who have colon or rectum cancer before the age of 55 should undergo colonoscopy or barium enema examination at 5 year intervals, starting at 35 to 40 years of age. If occult blood is found or if an adenomatous polyp is present at flexible sigmoidoscopy, colonoscopy or air contrast barium enema (ACBE) should be performed. If a cancer of the distal colon or rectum is found on flexible sigmoidoscopy, colonoscopy or ACBE should be performed in the perioperative period.

Table 3 Patients at Increased Risk for Colorectal Cancer

- Personal history of:
  - Colorectal cancer
  - Adenoma
  - Ureterosigmoidostomy
  - Radiation therapy involving large bowel
  - Ulcerative colitis
- Family history of:
  - Colorectal cancer
  - Polyposis syndrome
  - Hereditary nonpolyposis colon cancer syndrome

As suggested in the American Cancer Society recommendations, patients with higher than normal risk of developing colon cancer (Table 3) should be screened more aggressively, preferably with interval colonoscopy (Tables 4 and 5).

■ DIAGNOSIS AND EVALUATION

The signs and symptoms of colorectal cancer are determined by the location, size, and invasiveness of the primary tumor. Rectal cancers usually present with bright red rectal bleeding.

Table 4 American Cancer Society Recommendations for Early Detection of Colorectal Cancer—Normal Risk

TEST OR PROCEDURE	GENDER	AGE	FREQUENCY
Sigmoidoscopy, preferably flexible	M & F	50 yr and over	Every 3–5 yr
Fecal occult blood testing	M & F	50 yr and over	Every yr
Digital rectal examination	M & F	40 yr and over	Every yr

Table 5 American Cancer Society Recommendations for Early Detection of Colorectal Cancer—Increased Risk

RISK FACTOR	TEST	AGE	FREQUENCY
1st-degree relative with colorectal cancer onset <55 yr old	Colonoscopy or ACBE	35–40 yr	5 yr intervals
Family hx of familial adenomatous polyposis	Proctoscopy	13 yr	Yearly to 45 yr old
Familial adenomatous polyposis trait	Colonoscopy and biopsies	Discovery to time of colectomy	Yearly
Ulcerative pancolitis	Colonoscopy and biopsies	10 yr after onset of disease	Yearly
Ureterosigmoidostomy	Flexible sigmoidoscopy	5 yr after ureterosigmoidostomy	Yearly
Radiation proctosigmoiditis	Flexible sigmoidoscopy	10 yr after radiation	Yearly
Hereditary nonpolyposis cancer syndrome	Colonoscopy or ACBE	5 yr before the onset of earliest cancer	Yearly

ACBE, air contrast barium enema

Adapted from Levin B, Murphy GP. Revision in American Cancer Society recommendations for the early detection of colorectal cancer. CA Cancer J Clin 1992; 42:296–299; with permission.

In later stages, they may cause tenesmus, fecal urgency, a sense of incomplete evacuation, and the need to have frequent small bowel movements. Large tumors may cause symptoms of colonic obstruction. Invasion of adjacent structures may result in fecal incontinence, rectovaginal or rectovesical fistula, or sacral pain.

Tumors in the distal colon tend to cause obstructive symptoms because the lumen is relatively narrow and the stool is more solid. Conversely, tumors of the proximal colon are slower to cause obstruction because of the larger size of the lumen and the more liquid nature of the stool. These tumors are more likely to manifest with the symptoms of anemia or an abdominal mass. An exception is tumors arising at the ileocecal valve, which tend to cause obstruction of the narrow terminal ileum. These patients present with symptoms of distal small bowel obstruction or right lower quadrant pain, and may come to operation with a diagnosis of adhesive band obstruction, inflammatory bowel disease, or acute appendicitis.

When colorectal cancer is suspected because of clinical signs or symptoms the preferred diagnostic test is total colonoscopy. If colonoscopy cannot be performed or is incomplete, sigmoidoscopy followed by ACBE is the required evaluation. Sigmoidoscopy is important to prevent the inadvertent infusion of barium above a distal obstructing lesion and because most of the lesions missed on ACBE are in the rectum or sigmoid colon. The area of rectum posterior and immediately proximal to the sphincter mechanism falls back into the sacral hollow and is not seen well during routine colonoscopy. This area should be palpated by digital examination before inserting the colonoscope. The ACBE is preferred over a full-column barium study because it is more sensitive. Complete colonoscopy should be the goal even if an obvious cancer is identified because the incidence of synchronous cancers is 2 to 4 percent and the incidence of concomitant adenomatous polyps is nearly 50 percent. If colonoscopy cannot be completed preoperatively because of an obstructing lesion, it should be completed after the patient recovers from excision of the obstructing lesion.

After the diagnosis of colon or rectum cancer is established, certain laboratory and radiologic studies may be of use in planning therapy. Measurement of the hematocrit determines the presence of anemia and the ability of the patient to donate autologous blood. The blood carcinoembryonic antigen (CEA) level is determined preoperatively. If the preoperative CEA level is greatly elevated, liver metastasis should be strongly suspected. A rising CEA level in the postoperative period may be an early indication of cancer recurrence. A chest radiograph will reveal lung metastasis. Although the cost effectiveness of routine preoperative computed tomography (CT) remains unproven, several factors support the use of CT as part of the preoperative evaluation. If resectable liver metastases are found, the surgeon should be prepared to resect them at the same time that the primary tumor is resected. Patients with multiple metastases may be candidates for hepatic artery infusion therapy. Preoperative CT scans demonstrating multiple liver metastases prepare the patient and the surgeon for placement of an infusion device at the time of the initial operation. The CT scan may also provide information about invasion of the primary tumor into adjacent structures which is important for planning the operative approach. The scan serves as a baseline for patients with high-risk lesions who will be followed for recurrence by serial CT scans.

Although CT scans are more sensitive than palpation for identifying liver metastases deep within the liver, the most sensitive method of identifying liver metastases is intraoperative hepatic ultrasound combined with palpation to identify small surface lesions. Intraoperative ultrasound is not performed on all patients operated on for colon and rectum cancer because of the time, cost, and need to surgically expose the liver. Intraoperative ultrasound is very useful in patients with planned hepatic resection to identify previously unsuspected lesions, and to more precisely understand the relationship between the tumor(s) and major intrahepatic structures, to better delineate CT findings that are suspicious but inconclusive, and in patients with suspected liver metastases but normal CT scans (CEA > 100 ng per deciliter, or prior to resection of a pulmonary metastasis from colon cancer).

THERAPY

The most effective therapy for primary colon and rectum cancer remains surgical resection. The goals of surgical resection are removal of the primary tumor with an adequate margin of normal proximal and distal colon along with the lymphatics draining the involved bowel. Recently, postoperative adjuvant therapy has been shown to diminish the likelihood of tumor recurrence and to increase survival in patients with certain stages of colon or rectum cancer. Although colon and rectum tumors are histologically indistinguishable, differences in regional anatomy, venous and lymphatic drainage, accessibility, and response to treatment cause them to be managed in very different ways.

Colon Cancer

The blood supply and concomitant lymphatic drainage are the major determinants of the extent of resection performed for colon cancer. Traditional radical lymphadenectomy involves ligation of the appropriate colic vessel(s) as close as possible to their origin off the superior mesenteric artery for the right and transverse colon, or the aorta for the left colon. A further consideration is the ability to bring two healthy bowel ends, with good arterial blood supply, together without tension. Tumors arising in the left colon may require resection back to the transverse colon solely for this purpose. The adequacy of proximal and distal colon margins is rarely a consideration because proper lymphatic resection necessitates a generous resection of normal proximal and distal colon. Although there is no prospectively derived, controlled evidence that radical lymphadenectomy enhances the cure rate in patients with colon cancer, there is good reason to continue the practice. Radical lymphadenectomy is likely to be helpful because (1) the best chance to cure a colon cancer is at the time of the first operation; (2) many patients with excised lymph node metastases will be cured; (3) lymph node metastases are only reliably diagnosed by histologic examination; (4) the presence or absence of lymph node metastases has important prognostic implications and guides effective, but toxic, adjuvant therapy, and traditional radical lymphadenectomy adds little to morbidity.

The anastomosis may be effected by either a sutured or stapled technique. Although it is not difficult to find vigorous proponents of one technique over the other, in the intraperitoneal colon, either technique properly performed will give equivalent results. We prefer to perform intraperitoneal anastomosis by an end-to-end sutured technique. A sutured anastomosis can be performed almost as quickly as a stapled anastomosis and eliminates the cost of the three to four stapler firings used in a typical anastomosis. The anastomosis may be performed via an end-to-end, end-to-side, side-to-end, or stapled "functional" end-to-end technique. The colonoscopist should understand the various techniques, so that they may be recognized at the time of follow-up endoscopy.

Obstruction or perforation of the primary tumor may create special situations which necessitate changes in the operative approach. Ten to 20 percent of colon and rectum cancers present with signs of obstruction. Management is determined by the degree of luminal obstruction, the location of the lesion, and the overall condition of the patient. Most patients with partial obstruction can undergo elective resection, and obstructing cancers in the right colon can usually be managed with a standard right hemicolectomy. The treatment of obstruction distal to the splenic flexure has been associated with higher complication rates so a greater variety of management strategies have been developed. The traditional three-stage approach, proximal colostomy, resection, and anastomosis in three separate operations, is now rarely performed. When there is complete distal colonic obstruction and the patient's condition precludes resection, a loop colostomy should be performed. Unless there is evidence of perforation, the colostomy can be performed through a limited incision under local or general anesthesia. Approximately 1 week later, resection of the tumor—carried back to the colostomy—and primary anastomosis is possible.

If the patient with a distal obstruction can tolerate a laparotomy and the amount of intestinal distention does not preclude a standard lymphadenectomy, resection with anastomosis and a proximal loop colostomy may be performed. The colostomy is closed after healing of the anastomosis has been confirmed by contrast enema. Since the ileocecal valve usually protects the ileum from the effects of distention, one modern approach has been to carry the resection back to the terminal ileum and perform a primary ileorectal or ileosigmoid anastomosis. Although anastomotic leaks are rare with this approach, an extensive operation is required and functional results are often poor. Recently, some surgeons have advocated resection followed by on-table bowel prep and primary anastomosis. This approach has been successful but should only be attempted when two healthy, well-vascularized bowel ends can be brought together without tension.

Perforation occurs most commonly in the cecum, the most easily distended part of the colon, or at the site of the tumor itself. Perforation is a surgical emergency and is managed by prompt resuscitation and resection of the perforated area. Performing proximal colostomy and drainage of the area of perforation does not reliably control sepsis and should only be used in the most desperate situations. If at all possible the area of perforation should be resected. If the peritoneal soilage is localized away from the anastomosis, the bowel may be reconnected in a standard fashion. An unprotected anastomosis should not be performed in a region of established peritonitis.

Laparoscopic colectomy is increasingly popular; however, claims that the extent of lymphadenectomy, morbidity, and ultimate survival are equivalent to conventional techniques remain unsubstantiated. Currently, most "laparoscopic" colectomies are actually performed through a combination of conventional and laparoscopic techniques (laparoscopic-assisted colectomy). A limited incision is necessary to remove the specimen, and to re-establish bowel continuity because intracorporeal anastomotic techniques are cumbersome and unreliable. It is likely that improvements in instrumentation and technique will increase the application of minimal access surgery in colon cancer in the future.

Adjuvant Therapy

An indication that many patients have undetected spread beyond the margins of resection is that 40 to 50 percent of patients who undergo an attempted curative resection eventually die of disseminated disease. The need to eliminate these microscopic metastatic deposits before they can grow into overt metastases has led to an extensive search for effective adjuvant therapy. The success of combined 5-fluorouracil (5-FU) and levamisole in trials from the Mayo Clinic and the North Central Cancer Treatment Group (NCCTG), led to a large multicenter trial of 5-FU and levamisole in stage II and stage III colon cancer in 1985. Over 2 years, 1,296 patients were randomized into groups receiving levamisole alone, levamisole and 5-FU, or no treatment beyond surgery. With a median 3 year follow-up, there was a significant reduction in disease recurrence and a significant improvement in overall survival in the stage III patients who received 5-FU and levamisole. There was no benefit demonstrated in the stage II patients. These results generated a clinical alert from the NIH which recommended the 5-FU-levamisole regimen for "nearly every" patient with colon cancer and lymph node metastases. Although the local recurrence rate for high-risk colon tumors (T3 tumors, especially in the retroperitoneal colon) is almost 40 percent, there has been little role for radiotherapy in colon cancer. This is because colon tumors, which are relatively radioresistant, are surrounded by radiosensitive organs such as the small bowel, kidney and liver which limit radiation dose.

Rectal Cancer

While the surgical treatment of colon cancer has changed little in the past 50 years, the treatment of extraperitoneal cancer of the rectum has been changing rapidly over the past 10 years. As with colon cancer, the time-honored approach to rectal cancer is radical excision which involves removal of the tumor-bearing rectum along with its lymphatic drainage, and an acceptable distal margin. Since the appearance of circular staplers in the early 1980s, the generally accepted paradigm has been: cancer of the upper and middle rectum—perform sphincter-sparing (low anterior) resection; cancer of the lower third of the rectum—perform abdominal-perineal resection (APR) with permanent colostomy. Radical excision was felt to be necessary because there was no way of knowing preoperatively which tumors were confined to the bowel wall (curable with a local excision), and which had metastasized to regional nodes (require radical lymphatic excision for cure). On the other side of the equation, cancer recurred in the operative field in 20 to 40 percent of patients with advanced primary cancers. This suggested that standard radical surgical techniques were insufficient to provide local control in some circumstances.

The advent of effective adjuvant therapy, and the ability to more accurately stage tumors preoperatively, has further modified thinking about the treatment for rectum cancer. The current trend is best categorized as an attempt to match the invasiveness of the therapy to the risk from the tumor. Low-risk cancers are treated with minimal operations such as transanal local resection, while tumors at the highest risk for local or distant failure are treated with radical excision, radiation, and chemotherapy. The challenge posed by this treatment model is that there must be a way to differentiate high-risk from low-risk cancers preoperatively.

Table 6 Rectal Cancer: Depth of Primary Tumor Invasion and Incidence of Lymph Node Metastases

Depth of invasion:	T0	T1	T2	T3
Lymph node metastases:	≥0	5%	20%	35%–55%

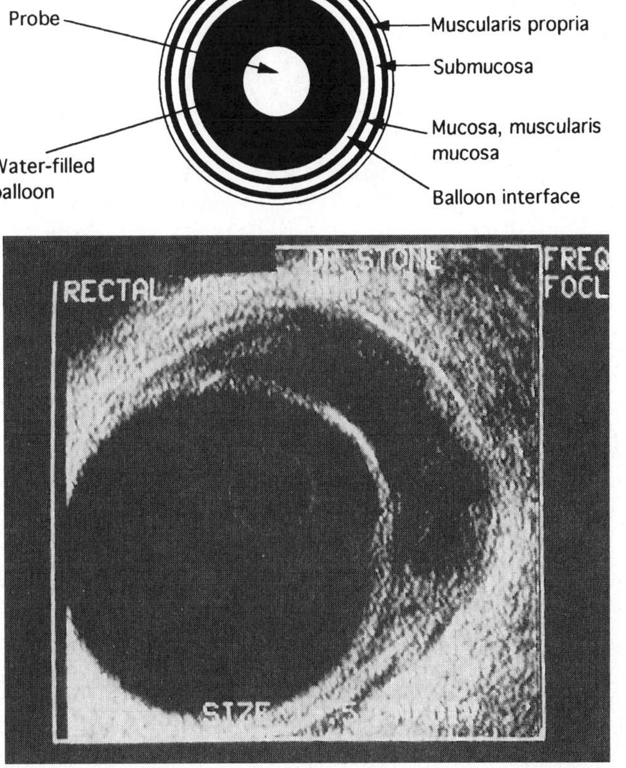

Figure 1
A. Five layer model of the rectal wall. Obliteration of normal interface echoes indicates depth of invasion into the rectal wall. *B.* Lesion—note break in second bright line, thickening of outer dark line, and maintenance of outer bright line, interface between muscularis propria, and perirectal tissue.

Pathology studies, performed on radical excision specimens, have shown a strong correlation between the depth of primary tumor invasion and lymph node metastases (Table 6). Today, depth of invasion of the primary tumor is determined with greater than 90 percent accuracy by ERUS. This technique utilizes a 7 MHz probe which is inserted into the rectum, above the tumor, through a modified proctoscope. A five layer image of the rectal wall is obtained and the probe is pulled down over the tumor (Fig. 1). The depth of tumor invasion is determined by the disruption of the normal tissue interfaces within the rectal wall. Lymph nodes in the perirectal area may also be imaged in this way, however, the accuracy of determining lymph node metastasis with ERUS is only about 66 percent. An ERUS staging system has been devised that parallels the TNM system (Table 2). One of the major advantages of preoperative staging with ERUS is the ability to select good-risk candidates for local excision. Full-

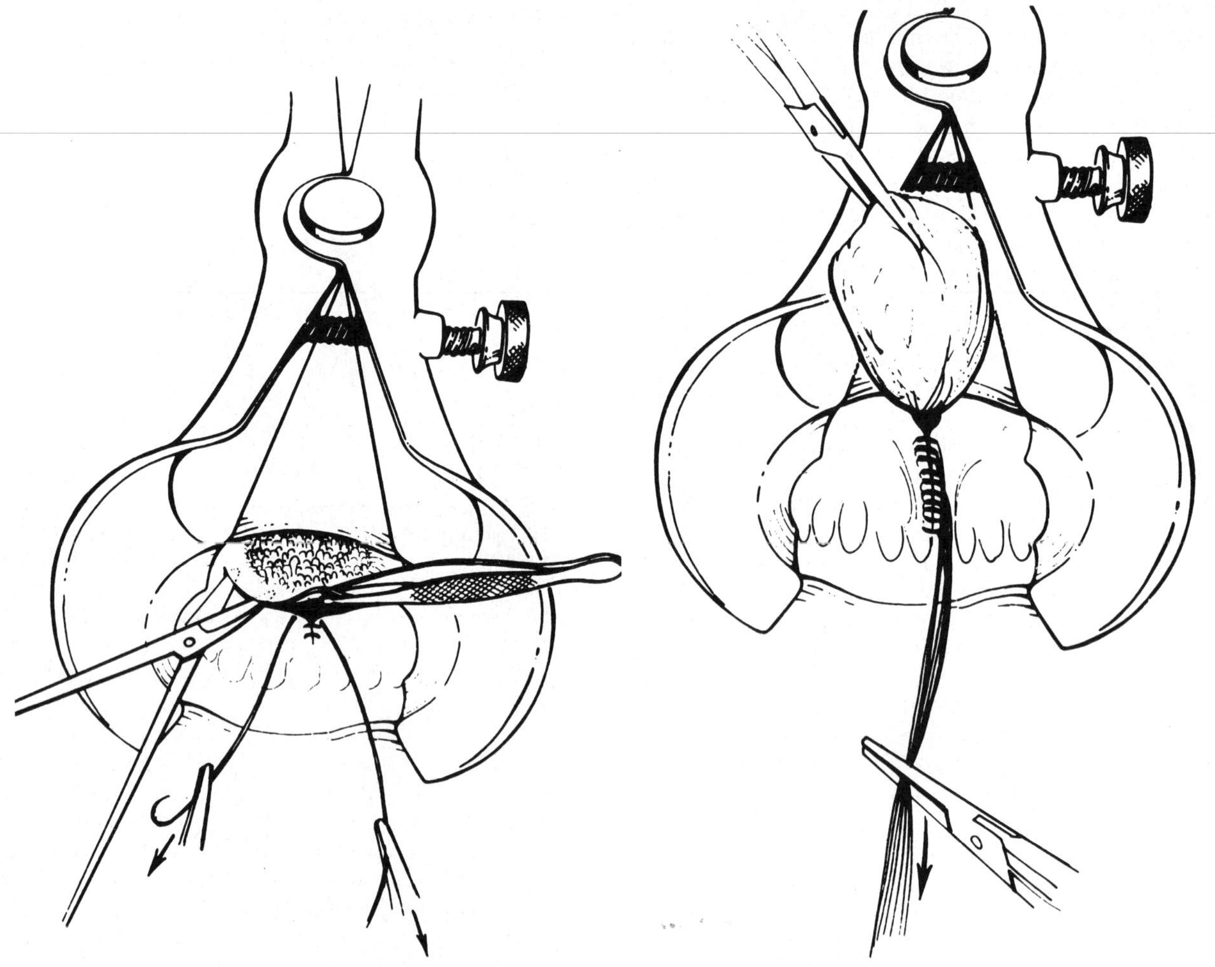

Figure 2
Technique of transanal excision. An anoscope is placed and stay sutures adjacent to the tumor are used to pull the rectal wall distally. An incision is made at the distal end of the tumor. The incision is closed as dissection proceeds into the more proximal rectum. The sutures are left long and are used to place further traction on the rectal wall.

thickness excision of the extraperitoneal rectal wall may be performed with minimal morbidity via the transanal route. In this technique, a retractor is placed in the anus, the rectal wall is pulled down with stay sutures, and a full-thickness disk of the rectal wall encompassing the tumor is removed (Fig. 2). The defect is repaired by suturing. The operation generally requires a general or regional anesthetic and a full bowel prep. Many of the problems with conventional radical surgery such as impotence, small bowel obstruction, incontinence, need for transfusion or colostomy are avoided. Other perineal approaches such as the transsacral or transsphincteric approach give somewhat wider exposure but at the price of higher complication rates. In general, local excision is preferred over nonresectional therapies such as electrofulguration, laser photoablation, or endocavitary radiation because excision allows complete pathologic examination of the tissue.

Tumors that are accessible through one of the perineal approaches should be treated by local excision if they are well or moderately well differentiated, and do not invade beyond the submucosa (uT1). Tumors that invade into, but not through the muscularis propria (uT2), have a local recurrence rate of approximately 20 percent when treated by local excision. These patients typically are treated with radical resection, however, preliminary work suggests that adjuvant therapy improves the success rate of local excision to approximately 90 percent in patients with T2 tumors. Consideration should be given to local excision in patients with uT2 tumors who are poor operative risks. Tumors that invade into the perirectal fat (T3) must be treated by radical excision because the failure rate of local excision is greater than 50 percent.

Radical excision of low rectal tumors traditionally has included excision of the anus, rectum, and distal sigmoid colon along with its mesentery and creation of a permanent end-colostomy (abdominal-perineal resection). The introduction of circular stapling devices, along with the understanding that distal spread along the bowel wall is rare, has greatly diminished the number of APRs performed. Indications for APR now are inability to obtain a 2 cm unstretched distal margin, poorly differentiated tumors of the lower rectum, pre-existing fecal incontinence, or invasion of the sphincters or adjacent organs. If APR is not necessary, an anastomosis from the proximal colon to the rectum is per-

Table 7 Adjuvant Radiation and Chemotherapy Studies for Rectal Cancer

STUDY	INCLUDED	TREATMENT (N)	5 YEAR SURVIVAL
GITSG	B2 or C <12 cm	Observation (58)	45%
		ChemoRx (48)	54%
		Radiation (50)	52%
		Chemo-Rad (46)	67%*
NCCTG	T3 or T4 and N1 or N2	Radiation (100)	48%
		Chemo-Rad (104)	58%
NSABP R-01	B2 or C	Observation (184)	43%
		Radiation (184)	41%
		ChemoRx (187)	53% (p = 0.05 men only)

*$p < 0.05$.

formed. When the anastomosis is below the peritoneal reflection it is termed a *low anterior resection.* Anastomosis to the extraperitoneal rectum is best performed with a circular stapling device. If the anastomosis is not technically perfect or the health of the bowel is questioned, a temporary colostomy or ileostomy may be created. The stoma is closed 6 weeks later after healing has been confirmed by a contrast enema.

Adjuvant Therapy

Although several studies have shown adjuvant radiation therapy to be effective in decreasing the incidence of local failure, it has not been possible to demonstrate that there is a survival benefit from adjuvant radiation alone. An improvement in local control, however, is a worthwhile goal because local recurrence of rectal cancer is a very morbid process (sacral pain, fistulae, obstruction) for which there is no effective therapy.

Combined adjuvant radiation and chemotherapy has been shown to provide a survival benefit in recent studies (Table 7). The Gastrointestinal Tumor Study Group (GITSG) data showed a survival benefit to patients treated with adjuvant combined chemotherapy and radiation over those treated with adjuvant chemotherapy or radiotherapy alone. A multicenter study performed by the NCCTG compared radiation and chemotherapy with radiation alone and again found a survival benefit to the combined regimen. The NSABP R-01 study is significant because it supported the efficacy of chemotherapy by showing a survival benefit over radiation therapy alone (albeit only in men and at the $p = 0.05$ level). Based on these studies, the National Cancer Institute (NCI) issued a clinical announcement in March 1991 recommending combined 5-FU and postoperative radiation therapy for extraperitoneal rectal tumors that penetrated through the full thickness of the rectal wall or had regional lymph node metastases. Semustine (MeCCNU) was used in addition to 5-FU in all three studies, but was omitted from the NCI recommendations because of the risk of leukemia and renal failure, and the finding in subsequent studies (GITSG 7180, NSABP R-02) that it added no benefit to 5-FU. Adjuvant therapy of rectal cancer is also discussed in the next chapter.

■ FUTURE CONSIDERATIONS

At present almost one-half of patients treated for colon and rectum cancer will eventually die of their disease. Epidemiologic studies suggest that in the United States, modest dietary changes including a one-third reduction in dietary fat, would result in a substantial decrease in the incidence of colon and rectum cancer. Improvement in secondary prevention may come from detection of genetic markers in stool. Although the maturation of minimal access techniques will probably diminish the length of hospitalization and allow people to return to work sooner, it is unlikely that changes in surgical technique will have a major impact on survival. Improvements in preoperative staging through the use of intrarectal magnetic resonance imaging, ultrasound, and laparoscopy will allow the extent of surgery to be better matched to the risks presented by the tumor, and thereby improve outcome. The development of new multi agent chemotherapy regimens, optimization of dosage, and delivery regimens for 5-FU, as well as improved modulation of 5-FU with other agents such as leucovorin, will also likely lead to improvement in outcome. Radiolabeled monoclonal antibodies have been developed that can be used in the detection of metastatic lesions from colon and rectum cancer. The new approach of immunotargeted therapy links the same antibodies to cytotoxic agents with the intent of killing metastatic deposits. Attempts to modulate the host immune system via nonspecific immune stimulants or transfer of sensitized lymphocytes may also prove useful. In the future, elucidation of the genetic and protein abnormalities involved in colon carcinogenesis will present new intracellular targets for therapy.

Suggested Reading

Fearon ER, Vogelstein JB. A genetic model for colorectal tumorogenesis. Cell 1990; 61:759–767.

Krook JE, Moertel CG, Gunderson LL, et al. Effective surgical adjuvant therapy for high risk rectal carcinoma. N Engl J Med 1991; 326:709–715.

Levin B, Murphy GP. Revision in American Cancer Society Recommendations for the early detection of colorectal cancer. CA Cancer J Clin 1992; 42:296–299.

Mandel JS, Bond JH, Church TR, et al. Reducing mortality from colorectal cancer by screening for fecal occult blood. N Engl J Med 1993; 328: 1365–1371.

Moertel CG, Fleming TR, MacDonald JS, et al. Levamisole and fluorouracil for adjuvant therapy of resected colon cancer. N Engl J Med 1990; 322: 352–358.

COLORECTAL CANCER: CHEMOTHERAPY

Elaine Lee Wade, M.D.
Al B. Benson III, M.D., F.A.C.P.

Despite efforts at both primary prevention via dietary modifications and secondary prevention via screening maneuvers, colon carcinoma continues to be a common malignancy in the Western world. Metastases are noted primarily within the abdominal cavity, with extra-abdominal disease (e.g., lung metastases) observed less than 20 percent of the time. The likelihood of recurrence has been linked to objective prognostic factors including grade, stage of tumor, depth of invasion, frequency of nodal involvement, number of lymph nodes involved, bowel obstruction secondary to tumor, and tumor perforation. Advances in the treatment of colorectal cancer have resulted from improved surgical staging and resection, improved local control with radiation, and improved disease-free survival and overall survival for patients with Dukes' C colon cancer after adjuvant systemic therapy. Presence of aneuploidy with high proliferative activity (percent cells in S phase), gene amplification, gene deletions, and tumor antigen expression are new prognostic indicators and potential markers to predict treatment response. Treatments for metastatic disease have produced higher response rates than previous regimens, although overall survival benefits have been limited. This chapter focuses on the systemic and regional therapies used in the treatment of colorectal carcinoma, both in the adjuvant and advanced disease settings.

TREATMENT OF ADVANCED COLORECTAL CANCER

After 30 years of investigation, 5-fluorouracil (5-FU) continues to be the most effective chemotherapeutic agent for colorectal cancer. The initial choice of 5-FU was based in part on murine models suggesting survival advantages for animals that received 5-FU with or without methyl CCNU compared with surgical controls. Its mechanism of action depends on two active metabolites, fluorouracil triphosphate (FUTP) and 5-fluodeoxyuridine monophosphate (FdUMP). FUTP inhibits RNA function, while FdUMP acts via formation of a stable ternary complex with the enzyme thymidylate synthase (TS), inhibiting the formation of dTTP and eventually DNA, resulting in cell death. Resistance to 5-FU arises via the absence or deletion of an enzyme involved in 5-FU activation or a relative increase in thymidylate synthase thought to be related to TS gene amplification. Treatment strategies to circumvent resistance or enhance cytotoxicity include 5-FU combinations with other antineoplastics or with levamisole, leucovorin, phosphonacetyl-L-aspartate (PALA), and/or interferon-alpha (IFN-alpha) and continuous infusion regimens of 5-FU alone.

Through the years numerous clinical trials evaluating single-agent bolus 5-FU therapy have demonstrated response rates of 12 to 20 percent in patients with metastatic colorectal cancer. Most of the trials administered 5-FU as a bolus injection on 5 consecutive days repeated monthly or as weekly bolus doses. Within the past 10 years 5-FU has been given a number of ways: as a weekly bolus, at a dose range of 600 to 700 mg per square meter; as a bolus injection 5 days every month; as a continuous infusion for 5 days repeated monthly; as protracted venous infusions given until toxicity is noted. Promising results from the Mid-Atlantic Oncology Group revealed an increase in response with protracted continuous infusion 5-FU (300 mg per square meter) for patients with metastatic disease (30 percent) compared with intravenous bolus dosing (7 percent); however, overall survival was unchanged. During the 1980s, several clinical trials explored the use of single-agent 5-FU given as a continuous infusion after laboratory data revealed improved tumor cell kill after prolonged exposure to the agent. Initially 24 hour infusional studies were undertaken in patients with metastatic disease. The most dose-intensive schedule at a maximally tolerated dose of 2600 mg per square meter per week given as a continuous intravenous infusion over 24 hours produced partial response rates of 25 percent. Trials involving patients with advanced disease exposed to 48 hour and 120 hour infusions resulted in acceptable toxicities at doses of 2,400 mg per square meter per week. Response rates varied widely, from 30 percent in the 48 hour group to 3 percent in the 120 hour group. No survival advantage was seen in either study, and the question of benefit was not clearly answered. Subsequently, in 1987 a dose intensity analysis of 28 clinical trials was completed. This review found a direct correlation between drug intensity and response rate (Table 1). Overall survival advantage is not clear at this point.

Toxicity of 5-FU is primarily gastrointestinal (GI) or hematologic, with varying grades of side effects correlating with the method and timing of drug administration, total dose, and combinations used. While continuous infusion frequently causes GI toxicity such as mucositis and diarrhea or the hand-foot syndrome, bolus dosing may cause significant myelosuppression. Examples of 5-FU combinations with other antineoplastics include the addition of cisplatin, doxorubicin, etoposide, methyl CCNU, ifosfamide, and streptozotocin, often with no substantial increase in response. The Mayo Clinic randomized trial of methyl CCNU, vincristine, and 5-FU (MOF) versus 5-FU alone raised initial optimism, with response rates of 43.5 versus 19.5 percent respectively in 80 patients. This finding was confirmed by several studies. Memorial Sloan-Kettering Cancer Center (MSKCC) followed with a randomized trial comparing 5-FU alone with MOF and streptozotocin, a combination yielding partial response rates above 30 percent in patients with advanced colon carcinoma. Since that time, however, analogous clinical trials, including those performed by the Piedmont Oncology Association, revealed comparable survival and response data in the two groups.

Initial interest in combination therapy with cisplatin and 5-FU arose when synergistic effects were noted in colon carcinoma murine models. Phase II trials of the combination

Table 1 Comparison of 5-FU Infusion Dose Intensity

INVESTIGATOR	5-FU INFUSION* SCHEDULE	5-FU DOSE INTENSITY (MG/M²/WK)	5-FU RESPONSE (%)
Ardalan et al.	2,600 mg/m²/d × 1 q 7 days	2,600	25
Kemeny et al.	1,000 mg/m²/d × 5 q 28 days	1,250	3
Lokich et al.	300 mg/m²/d qd × 70 days	2,100	30
NCI-Canada	350 mg/m²/d × 14 q 28 days	1,225	12
Shah et al.	1,200 mg/m²/d × 2 q 7 days	2,400	30

*24 hour continuous intravenous infusion
Adapted from Anderson N, Lokich J. Controversial issues in 5-fluorouracil infusion use: Dose intensity, treatment duration and cost comparisons. Cancer 1992; 70:998–1002.

involving a total of 323 patients resulted in response rates of 30 percent. These preliminary findings encouraged the design of prospective randomized trials comparing cisplatin plus 5-FU with 5-FU alone (bolus and continuous infusion regimens). The cisplatin was administered on a number of schedules, including weekly, monthly, and three times per week. Neither response nor overall survival was significantly improved with combination cisplatin and 5-FU. For example, the Eastern Cooperative Oncology Group (ECOG) initiated one of the largest randomized trials including 497 patients comparing bolus 5-FU (500 mg per square meter daily for 5 days followed by 600 mg per square meter IV weekly) with low-dose protracted venous infusion 5-FU (300 mg per square meter per day) with or without cisplatin (20 mg per square meter per week). The continuous infusion produced significantly higher response rates than bolus 5-FU ($p = 0.02$); however, the addition of cisplatin did not offer a statistically significant advantage over continuous infusion alone. Combination cisplatin and 5-FU is therefore not recommended for the routine treatment of metastatic colorectal carcinoma.

Incorporation of 5-FU into colon cancer cell DNA and RNA is the key to 5-FU's activity. To augment this effect or overcome inherent or acquired resistance of cells to 5-FU, additional biochemical agents have been employed to modulate or augment 5-FU's cytotoxic effects. Methotrexate has been thought to increase the conversion of 5-FU to its active metabolites via inhibition of purine metabolism. Clinical trials have confirmed the beneficial effect of using methotrexate in conjunction with 5-FU, provided that the timing of the agents is properly sequenced. The most significant response rates have been shown in studies by Marsh and associates in a randomized group of 168 patients with untreated metastatic colon carcinoma. The trial incorporated methotrexate at a dose of 200 mg per square meter followed either 1 hour or 24 hours later by IV 5-FU at 600 mg per square meter. Survival (15.3 versus 11.4 months, $p = 0.003$), response rates (29 versus 14.5 percent, $p = 0.026$) and duration of response (9.9 versus 5.9 percent, $p = 0.009$) were all enhanced when 5-FU was administered 24 hours after methotrexate.

Leucovorin, or folinic acid, has been shown to enhance the cytotoxicity of 5-FU by increasing the intracellular concentration of reduced folate. This in turn enhances stability of the ternary complex, FdUMP-TS, which directly enhances the inhibition of TS. Phase I and II trials of the 5-FU and leucovorin combination were pursued at Roswell Park and the City of Hope using intravenous bolus dosing of 5-FU in conjunction with limited continuous infusions of leucovorin. Toxicities included granulocytopenia, mucositis, and severe diarrhea. Subsequent clinical trials for advanced disease confirmed response rates of 30 to 45 percent, an improvement over 5-FU alone. Compared with various combinations of 5-FU with levamisole or IFN in advanced disease, 5-FU in conjunction with leucovorin has provided the most benefit in terms of response rates and survival, despite lower doses of 5-FU needed to control toxicity. Multiple phase III trials for metastatic colorectal cancer comparing high-dose leucovorin plus 5-FU with 5-FU alone revealed a significant response advantage for the combination. Mayo Clinic and the North Central Cancer Treatment Group (NCCTG) conducted a randomized clinical trial in the late 1980s comparing single-agent 5-FU (500 mg per square meter per day, days 1 to 5) with two combination regimens including high-dose leucovorin, (200 mg per square meter per day with 5-FU 370 mg per square meter per day, days 1 to 5), and low-dose leucovorin at 20 mg per square meter with 5-FU (370 mg per square meter per day, days 1 to 5). Low-dose leucovorin plus 5-FU was the most beneficial regimen, with response rates of 43 percent compared with 10 percent with 5-FU alone and 26 percent with the higher-dose leucovorin. Both high- and low-dose leucovorin improved the time to disease progression over 5-FU alone. Beneficial palliative effects, including improvement in performance status, symptoms, or body weight, were seen more frequently with 5-FU and leucovorin. A meta-analysis of nine randomized trials showed significant improvement in response rate when 5-FU plus leucovorin administered either weekly or monthly was compared with single-agent 5-FU (23 versus 11 percent, respectively) with no improvement in overall survival ($p = 0.57$).

The clinical use of PALA to modulate the cytotoxicity of 5-FU originates from the laboratory investigations using the murine breast carcinoma model CD8F1, which demonstrated increased cytotoxicity with the combination of 5-FU plus PALA compared with 5-FU alone. PALA blocks de novo pyrimidine synthesis pathways by inhibiting aspartate transcarbamylase. Combining PALA with 5-FU enhances tumor cytotoxicity by increasing the incorporation of 5-FU into RNA. O'Dwyer demonstrated that low doses of PALA (250 mg per square meter), given 24 hours prior to high-dose continuous infusion 5-FU (2,600 mg per square meter over 24 hours) in a group of 39 patients resulted in total response rates of 43 percent, similar to another small trial reported by Ardalan. Significant side effects included GI and neurologic toxicity.

IFN-alpha has been shown in preclinical investigations to result in a biochemical modulation of 5-FU, both increasing intracellular levels of 5-FdUMP and binding to thymidylate synthase, 5-dUMP's target enzyme. The combination of IFN-alpha and 5-FU as developed by Wadler and associates has been under clinical investigation since the late 1980s. Initial clinical trials of 5-FU plus IFN-alpha reported response rates of 55 to 65 percent. Subsequent trials have shown increased toxicity and diminished efficacy, with response rates of 25 to 40 percent. In 1993 results of two randomized trials were reported. There was no statistically significant difference in survival when 5-FU was compared with 5-FU (750 mg per square meter daily for 5 days as a continuous infusion followed by weekly bolus 5-FU at a dose of 750 mg per square meter) plus IFN-alpha 2a (9 million units three times weekly), although initial response data favored the combination (31 versus 19 percent). A multicenter phase III randomized trial by the Corfu-A Collaborative Group revealed equivalent response results (21 versus 19 percent) in a group of 496 patients. The study compared 5-FU 750 mg per square meter IV days 1 to 5, then 750 mg per square meter weekly plus IFN-alpha 9 million units three times a week with 5-FU 370 mg per square meter IV bolus plus leucovorin 200 mg per square meter IV bolus days 1 to 5 every 28 days.

The addition of leucovorin to 5-FU and IFN-alpha would theoretically potentiate 5-FU activity. Grem and associates have reported a phase I trial of IFN-alpha 2a 5 million to 10 million units per square meter subcutaneously days 1 to 7, leucovorin 500 mg per square meter per day IV over 30 minutes, days 2 to 6, and 5-FU 370 to 425 mg per square meter per day IV days 2 to 6, 1 hour after leucovorin, for 22 previously untreated patients with advanced GI malignancies. The overall response rate was 45 percent. Pharmacokinetic studies demonstrated that IFN-alpha produced a 30 percent increase in the 5-FU area under the concentration-time curve (AUC) and a dose-dependent decrease in 5-FU clearance.

Subsequently, Grem and associates studied 44 advanced colorectal patients in a phase II trial to evaluate the previously defined best tolerated schedule of IFN (5 million units per square meter per day subcutaneously days 1 to 7) and leucovorin (500 mg per square meter per day IV over 30 minutes) followed 1 hour later by 5-FU (370 mg per square meter per day IV days 2 to 6). Overall response rate was 54 percent with four complete responses. Patients with an ECOG performance status of 2 did not respond to treatment. Median survival was 16.3 months and median time to treatment failure for responding patients was 9.3 months. Grade 3 and 4 toxicities included diarrhea, rash, fatigue, mucositis, vomiting, and neutropenia.

To test 5-FU biochemical modulation concepts more definitively, two large cooperative group trials were designed. The Southwestern Oncology Group (SWOG) recently reported a phase II seven arm study that randomized patients to varying regimens of 5-FU given by bolus with and without high- or low-dose leucovorin, protracted continuous infusion with and without low-dose leucovorin, or 24 hour high-dose 5-FU infusion with and without PALA. The trial, designed to screen the most promising regimens for phase III evaluation, showed a trend favoring survival for the infusion arms.

ECOG, in collaboration with the Cancer and Leukemia Group B (CALGB), has conducted a 1,100 patient randomized phase III trial designed as a definitive investigation of a high-dose 24 hour infusion of 5-FU with or without PALA, 5-FU and IFN-alpha, and 5-FU with high-dose intravenous or oral leucovorin. Preliminary data analysis suggests the following: 5-FU plus high-dose IV leucovorin is not superior to high-dose 24 hour infusional 5-FU; 5-FU plus IV leucovorin is not superior to 5-FU plus oral leucovorin; and 5-FU plus interferon is not superior to 5-FU plus IV leucovorin. Table 2 lists the most commonly used metastatic colorectal regimens.

■ HEPATIC ARTERIAL INFUSION

Colorectal carcinoma commonly metastasizes to the liver and subsequently produces significant morbidity and mortality. Techniques originating in the 1950s were developed to deliver localized chemotherapy through an intra-arterial route as an attempt to administer higher doses of chemotherapy locally for extended periods with less systemic toxicity. Furthermore, the hepatic artery provides most of the blood supply to hepatic metastases, and chemotherapy drugs including 5-FU and fluorodeoxyuridine (FUDR) are extracted nearly completely after the first pass through the liver. Studies revealing response rates of 35 to 75 percent were published based on regimens using 5-FU, FUDR, and mitomycin C in various combinations.

The administration of these drugs required significant intervention by highly skilled physicians, restricting this method of treatment to a few select medical centers. During the 1970s renewed interest in intra-arterial therapy developed after pharmacologic studies revealed significantly increased intrahepatic drug delivery while maintaining low systemic levels of drug. In addition, more practical implantable pumps greatly facilitated the mechanical aspects of treatment. Commencing in the early 1980s, studies evaluated FUDR doses at 0.1 to 0.5 mg per kilogram per day. The pumps were equipped with an additional external port to provide access for infusion of chemotherapy, infusion of nuclear contrast material for angiography to ensure adequate hepatic perfusion, and clearing of the pump if needed. Patients were followed for 13 to 28 weeks at the University of Minnesota on continuous FUDR with mixed results, though some response was noted. Studies at the University of Michigan were then performed on 13 patients who were treated for 6 to 8 week periods determined by patient tolerance. This group showed evidence of a partial response rate of 85 percent assessed by direct measurement on physical exam or via computed tomography (CT) scan. By the end of this period toxicities, consistently present in more than 50 percent of patients, consisted of gastritis and a chemical hepatitis or biliary sclerosis with increased transaminases and bilirubin. Other phase II studies with slightly decreased response rates of 45 to 50 percent were completed. They are difficult to interpret, for all used different criteria for response such as carcinoembryonic antigen (CEA), physical examination, and CT scan findings.

Randomized trials have compared intra-arterial therapy with systemic 5-FU or FUDR demonstrating superior response rates with the intra-arterial therapy (42 to 62 percent) versus the intravenous treatment (10 to 21 percent). Combination intra-arterial FUDR and leucovorin (0.3 mg per kilogram per day and 30 mg per square meter per day, respectively) has been administered for 14 day periods in a small

Table 2 Advanced Disease Colorectal Cancer Chemotherapy Regimens

DRUG	DOSE	SCHEDULE
5-FU	500 mg/m^2	IVP × 5 days q 4–5 wk
5-FU	300 mg/m^2/d	CI days 1–28 q 5 wk
5-FU	2600 mg/m^2	CI over 24 hours, repeat weekly
LV 5-FU	20 mg/m^2 followed by 425 mg/m^2	IVP LV days 1–5 q 4 wk × 2 then q 5 wk
LV 5-FU	500 mg/m^2 600 mg/m^2	LV 2–3 hr IV infusion IVP 5-FU 1 hr after beginning LV days 1, 8, 15, 22, 29, 36 q 8 wk
LV 5-FU	20 mg/m^2 200 mg/m^2/d	IVP days 1, 8, 15, 22 q 5 wk CI days 1–28 q 5 wk
LV 5-FU	125 mg/m^2 600 mg/m^2	PO q hour × 4 IVP 1 hour after LV
LV 5-FU	200 mg/m^2 370 mg/m^2	IVP days 1–5 q 4–5 wks
Methotrexate 5-FU LV	200 mg/m^2 1,100 mg/m^2 14 mg/m^2	CI × 4 hr IVP at hr 7 Begin at 24 hr PO q 6 hr × 8; q 3–4 wk
α IFN 5-FU	9 × 10^6 U SC 750 mg/m^2/d	TIW CI × 5 days then weekly bolus beginning day 15
LV 5-FU αIFN	500 mg/m^2/d 370 mg/m^2/d 5 × 10^6 U/m^2 SC	Days 2–6 IV over 30 min Days 2–6 IV 1 hr after LV Days 1–7 prior to LV q 28 days
PALA 5-FU	250 mg/m^2 2,600 mg/m^2	IV day 1 weekly CI over 24 hr, 24 hr after PALA weekly

CI, Continuous IV infusion; LV, leucovorin; SC, subcutaneous; IVP, intravenous push.

group of patients diagnosed with hepatic metastases. Though response rates were high, toxicities were increased as well, especially hepatotoxicity (increased transminases and sclerosing cholangitis). Most recently the results of a combined intra-arterial plus systemic regimen for metastatic colorectal cancer were published. FUDR was given intrahepatically as a continuous infusion over 14 days, and bolus 5-FU and leucovorin were administered systemically (280 mg per square meter and 200 mg per square meter, days 1 to 5, every 28 days respectively) to 29 patients. The partial response rate of 56 percent is comparable with those of previous intra-arterial trials. Moderate hepatotoxicity was seen. Eight patients received the same therapy after complete resection of hepatic metastases. Toxicities were similar, with disease-free survival to date of approximately 23 months.

Another randomized phase III trial of 100 patients compared hepatic arterial infusion of FUDR with no therapy other than palliative care for previously untreated patients with metastatic colorectal cancer to the liver. This was the first trial to demonstrate a survival advantage with normal quality of life for patients with metastatic colorectal cancer to the liver (median 405 days versus 226 days, $p = 0.03$).

ECOG and SWOG are conducting a randomized phase III trial for patients with surgically resectable liver metastases (1 to 3 metastases) comparing postoperative observation with four 2 week cycles of intra-arterial FUDR (0.1 mg per kilogram per day for 14 days) plus eight 2 week cycles of continuous infusion 5-FU (200 mg per square meter per day for 14 days). CALGB intends to conduct another phase III trial comparing intra-arterial infusion with FUDR (0.18 mg per kilogram), leucovorin (10 mg per square meter), and dexamethasone (20 mg) per day for 14 days, repeated every 28 days versus systemic therapy with leucovorin (20 mg per square meter) and 5-FU (425 mg per square meter) IV daily for 5 days every 28 days for patients with metastatic colorectal cancer.

Present use of intra-arterial therapy is palliative for patients with good to excellent performance status and metastatic disease confined to the liver. Despite high response rates, overall survival is not prolonged.

■ CHEMOEMBOLIZATION

The majority (85 to 90 percent) of patients with documented hepatic metastases are unresectable at diagnosis due to metastatic involvement beyond the liver parenchyma, presence of multiple lesions (more than four) or lesions in more than one lobe of the liver. Brief beneficial results have been shown when patients with hepatic metastases underwent hepatic artery ligation. The technique of chemoembolization incorporates the simultaneous use of liquid or particulate embolic matter with multiple chemotherapeutic agents including mitomycin C, doxorubicin, and cisplatin. Only patients with symptomatic, unresectable, progressive, and localized hepatic disease are routinely eligible. Good performance status and lack of other effective modalities are usual criteria. Patients are treated on a schedule of biweekly to bimonthly administrations over periods extending up to 24 months with a range of one to eight treatments. Much of the experience with (chemo) embolization has been obtained from Southeast Asia and Japan, an endemic area for hepatocellular carcinoma. Overall, comparisons of chemoembolization with surgical resection indicate that surgery is indeed a superior treatment for hepatomas. However, good outcomes have been documented with chemoembolization. One particular series from Japan quoted 3 year survival rates of 40 to 50 percent in patients who had small to moderate tumor burdens (a low number of lesions, each less than 5 cm in size).

In the United States there have been several small series of phase I and II chemoembolization trials, including limited studies of patients with metastatic colorectal carcinoma to the liver. For example, Daniels treated 52 patients with chemoembolization consisting of doxorubicin, cisplatin, and mitomycin C in viscous collagen (Angiostat). This trial demonstrated a greater than 50 percent reduction of CEA in 78 percent of patients, and one-third of patients had more than 50 percent tumor reduction on CT scan. In a series at Northwestern University 30 to 100 patients treated with chemoembolization had metastatic colorectal carcinoma to the liver. In this subgroup of patients, 63 percent displayed radiographic evidence of response, often accompanied by a decrease in tumor markers (e.g., CEA) and tumor-related discomfort after an average of three chemoembolizations, each administered every 4 to 8 weeks. At present, patients with metastatic colorectal cancer (hepatic disease only) are entering a multicenter randomized phase III trial comparing a 3 hour intra-arterial infusion of mitomycin C, doxorubicin, and cisplatin with Angiostat chemoembolization. Toxicities include postoperative right upper quadrant pain, fever, and nausea. Over the 1 to 3 weeks following the procedure, patients may note gastritis and fatigue. The gastritis can be attributed in part to reflux of the chemotherapeutic agents into the gastric circulatory bed. Rarely, renal failure, hepatic failure, hepatic abscess, biliary sclerosis, and tumor hemorrhage are seen. The risk of hepatic failure is greatest when more than 50 to 75 percent of the liver is replaced by tumor. Prophylactic pain medications and antibiotics are administered to diminish or alleviate common complications. At present chemoembolization is a palliative regimen for patients with unresectable hepatic metastases secondary to colorectal carcinoma, carcinoid and islet cell tumors, cholangiocarcinoma, and perhaps sarcoma and melanoma.

■ INTRAPERITONEAL CHEMOTHERAPY

At present intraperitoneal administration of chemotherapeutic agents such as 5-FU is experimental, particularly for patients with carcinomatosis, designed to elevate levels of drug in the hepatic circulatory system. Issues concerning local absorption rates, consistency of drug availability, and local irritation remain.

■ ADJUVANT THERAPY FOR COLON CANCER

Historically, clinical trials for colon cancer were initiated in the late 1950s and involved preoperative and intraoperative regimens of nitrogen mustard or thiotepa. Intravenous and oral routes were attempted without success in terms of survival. The 1960s marked the development of improved chemotherapeutic trial design, and limited treatment effects were noted. Subsequent studies by the VA Surgical Oncology Group in the mid to late 1960s and by the Central Oncology Group (COG) from 1971 to 1976 compared treatment with surgery alone with that of surgery and adjuvant 5-FU. Results suggested an increase in disease-free survival, particularly for patients with positive lymph nodes. Overall, a 10 percent survival advantage was noted. More sophisticated clinical trials in the 1980s accrued large numbers of patients who received newer combinations of agents including immunologic modalities. Specifically, the National Surgical Adjuvant Breast and Bowel Project (NSABP) compared postoperative observation with nonspecific immunotherapy using bacillus Calmette-Guérin (BCG) versus MOF. Patients receiving MOF demonstrated significant increases in both disease-free (67 versus 58 percent) and overall (67 versus 59 percent) survival when compared with control. BCG-treated patients displayed a mild increase in overall survival alone; however, when noncancer deaths were excluded, this difference was no longer statistically significant. Nonetheless, this landmark study demonstrated for the first time the benefits of chemotherapy in terms of disease-free and overall survival.

Levamisole, a synthetic phenylinidazothiazole, has been used for years as an anthelmintic. In the early 1970s this drug was noted to have immunomodulatory effects, the mechanism of which has not been elucidated 25 years later. In vitro analysis of levamisole has revealed increased rates of chemotaxis of monocytes and macrophages, a finding not duplicated in vivo. The promising preliminary animal studies suggesting beneficial effects against tumor metastases in conjunction with its low-toxicity profile made levamisole an ideal agent for clinical investigation. The NCCTG conducted a randomized trial comparing surgery alone with surgery and levamisole plus or minus 5-FU. In patients with stage III disease, the subset receiving 5-FU plus levamisole displayed a statistically significant improvement in disease-free survival over 7 years. Overall survival was unchanged. A confirmatory intergroup trial included NCCTG, ECOG, and SWOG. At 3.5 years, 929 stage III patients enrolled in the 5-FU plus levamisole arm were found to have better overall (71 versus 55 percent) and disease-free (63 versus 47 percent) survival than surgical controls. After more than 5 years the combination of 5-FU and levamisole has resulted in a 39 percent decrease in recurrence rate ($p < 0.0001$) and a 32 percent decrease in cancer-related deaths ($p < 0.004$) for patients with stage III colon cancer. Levamisole alone produced no beneficial effects. The 318 stage II patients were randomized to surgery alone versus 5-FU plus levamisole. There is no survival advantage for stage II patients who received the combined treatment (Table 3).

A University of Wisconsin study showed a survival advantage for patients with advanced colon cancer treated with 5-FU plus levamisole versus 5-FU alone. ECOG subsequently designed the largest randomized study of patients with known minimal residual (nonmeasurable) colorectal cancer (339 patients). There was no survival advantage for 5-FU plus levamisole over 5-FU alone nor over 5-FU plus hepatic radiation (for patients with nonmeasurable hepatic metastases). Both survival and time to progression were shorter for patients with hepatic metastases. The NCCTG also demonstrated neither a response nor a survival advantage using 5-FU plus levamisole versus 5-FU alone in 135 previously untreated patients with metastatic colorectal cancer.

Side effects of levamisole and 5-FU can include mild

Table 3 Adjuvant Studies of Levamisole Plus 5-FU

INVESTIGATIONS	NO. OF PATIENTS	DUKES' STAGE	5-FU*	LEVAMISOLE†	SURVIVAL (%)
Bancewicz et al.	52	B and C	A. None	200 mg/d PO days 1–2 q wk‡ × 1 y	81
			B. 440 mg/m^2/d × 5 d q 4 wk	200 mg/d PO days 1–2 q wk‡ × 1 y	76
			C. None	None	89
Laurie et al.	401	B and C	A. 450 mg/m^2/d × 5 then q wk	†	64
			B. None	†	60
			C. None	None	58
Moertel et al.	929	C§	A. 450 mg/m^2/d × 5 then q wk	†	71
			B. None	†	65
			C. None	None	55
Sertoli et al.	29	C	A. 325 mg/m^2/d × 5 q 5 wk plus methyl CCNU 150 mg/m^2 q 10 wk × 14 cycles	† weeks 2, 4; q 10 wk	60
			B. As above	None	50
Windle et al.	131	B and C	A. 1 g days 1–3 then 1 g PO q wk × 6 mo	†	68
			B. As above	None	48
			C. None	None	56

*Administered by intravenous push except when marked PO.
†50 mg PO t.i.d. d1–3 qow.
‡Levamisole not administered during chemotherapy week.
§Analysis of Dukes' B patients showed no survival advantage with the addition of 5-FU/levamisole.
Adapted from Jaiyesimi I, Pazdur R. Colorectal cancer: Diagnosis and management. In: Medical oncology: A comprehensive review. Huntington, NY: PRR; 148; Grem JL. Oncology 1991; 5(3):63–73.

nausea and leukopenia, the latter reported in 2 to 10 percent of cases. Flulike symptoms such as arthralgias and myalgias are sometimes reported, as is a metallic taste. Elevations in serum alkaline phosphatase, serum aminotransferase, and bilirubin have been reported in nearly 40 percent of patients, with occasional reversible fatty changes of the liver noted by CT scan with a rise in serum CEA. Rarely, patients have been noted to display changes in mood and temperament. Other neurologic toxicities include cerebellar changes and cognitive dysfunction (4.5 percent of cases) occasionally associated with magnetic resonance imaging (MRI) changes. Desquamative dermatitis may be seen as well. As a result of the adjuvant levamisole trials, the National Institutes of Health (NIH) Consensus Development Conference recommended adjuvant 5-FU and levamisole for all Dukes' C patients not enrolled in clinical trials. Beyond these guidelines, specific recommendations for patients diagnosed with stage II and III disease are not yet defined (Table 4). Third-generation colon adjuvant clinical trials have recently reached accrual goals and further explore biochemical modulation concepts. Analysis of these study results may refine treatment recommendations.

Table 4 NIH Consensus 1990

Stage I (colon-rectum)
- No adjuvant treatment

Stage II (colon)
- No recommended adjuvant therapy
- Participation in clinical trials recommended

Stage III (colon)
- Participation in clinical trials
- 5-FU plus levamisole for patients not on trial

Stage II and III (rectum)
- Postoperative high-dose pelvic radiation
- Adjuvant chemotherapy

Additional recent adjuvant protocols include NSABP CO-3 investigating the benefit of MOF versus 5-FU plus leucovorin. Patients treated with 5-FU plus leucovorin had a 32 percent less mortality risk than those treated with MOF (3 year survival, 84 versus 73 percent, $p = 0.003$). More recently the NSABP compared 5-FU plus leucovorin with 5-FU plus levamisole with or without leucovorin; the results are pending. The largest adjuvant chemotherapy trial for patients with colon cancer recently reached accrual, with a total of 3,794 patients. This intergroup project (ECOG, SWOG, CALGB) compares high- or low-dose leucovorin plus 5-FU, 5-FU plus levamisole, and a combination of all three agents. Preliminary results are available for some of these comparisons and suggest that 5-FU plus high-dose leucovorin is not superior to 5-FU plus low-dose leucovorin; 5-FU plus high-dose leucovorin is not superior to 5-FU plus levamisole; and 5-FU plus levamisole plus low-dose leucovorin is not superior to 5-FU plus low-dose leucovorin. Other groups also are performing studies on a smaller scale to investigate the benefits of combination therapy. This includes the NCCTG randomized trial for patients with Dukes' B2 or C colon cancer evaluating 5-FU and levamisole (6 months versus 1 year) with 5-FU, levamisole, and leucovorin (6 months versus 1 year). The National Cancer Institute of Canada trial is comparing surgery with 5-FU plus leucovorin for Dukes' B2 patients. Over the next several years the results of these clinical trials should provide essential information about the benefit of biochemical modulation in the adjuvant setting (Table 5).

Table 5 Current or Recent Colon Cancer Adjuvant Trials

COOPERATIVE GROUP PROTOCOL NUMBER	TREATMENT RANDOMIZATION	STAGE
NCCTG 89-46-51 (closed)	5-FU[a]/Lev[b] × 1 yr 5-FU/Lev × 6 mo 5-FU/Lev/LV[c] × 1 yr 5-FU/Lev/LV × 6 mo	B2, C
NCIC CO.3 (closed)	Obs 5-FU, LV[d]	B2, C
ECOG 5283 (closed)	Obs Vaccine[e]	B2, C
NSABP C-04 (closed)	5-FU/LV[f] (6 cycles) 5-FU/LV[f]/Lev[b] (6 cycles) 5-FU/Lev (one year)	B2, C
INT 0089 (ECOG 2288) (closed)	5-FU/LV-low[g] 5-FU/LV-high[f] 5-FU/Lev 5-FU/LV/Lev[g]	High-risk B2, C
NSABP C-05 (closed)	5-FU/LV 5-FU/LV/IFN[h]	B2, C
ECOG 1290	5-FU/Lev 5-FU/Lev/vaccine[e]	C
INT-0136 (ECOG 1292)	Perioperative 5-FU[i] vs obs (5-FU/Lev for B3, C)	B2, B3, C
INT 0130 (NCCTG 91-46-52)	5-FU/Lev 5-FU[j]/Lev/RT[k]	B3, C2, C3
INT (SWOG 9415)	5-FU/LV/Lev[g] CI 5-FU/Lev[l]	High-risk B2, C

[a]5-FU: 450 mg/m^2 IV d 1–5, then q weekly beginning d 29 × 48 weeks
[b]Lev: 50 mg PO t.i.d. d 1–3, q 2 weeks × 1 year for all levamisole regimens (exceptions are noted)
[c]5-FU: 370 mg/m^2/d d 1–5, d 29, 57 (5 day cycles) then q 5 wk LV: 20 mg/m^2/d d 1–5, d 29, 57 (5 day cycles) then q 5 wk
[d]5-FU: 370 mg/m^2/d × 5 d LV: 200 mg/m^2/d × 5 d q 28 d × 6
[e]Autologus tumor/BCG vaccine administered as intradermal injection weekly × 3
[f]5-FU 500 mg/m^2 LV: 500 mg/m^2 qw × 6, 4 courses
[g]5-FU: 425 mg/m^2 d 1–5 LV: 20 mg/m^2 d 1–5 d 29, 57 (5 day cycles) then q 5 wk × 6
[h]IFNα-2a: 5 × 10^6 u/m^2 s.c. qd d 1–7 LV: 500 mg/m^2.d d 2–6 5-FU: 370 mg/m^2/d d 2–6q 28 d × 6 courses
[i]600 mg/m^2/d CI × 7d
[j]5-FU: cycle 1 5-FU[a]/Levamisole pre-RT during RT, 5-FU d 1–3, 23–25
[k]RT: 45 Gy to tumor-nodal field
[l]5-FU 250 mg/m^2/d × 8 wks, 3 courses; levamisole[b] × 1 year
Obs, observation; LV, leucovorin; Lev, levamisole; IFN, Interfero–alpha; MOF, methyl CCNU, vincristine, 5-FU; CI, continuous IV infusion.

New Colon Adjuvant Trials

The interest in adjuvant therapy given to a localized area was generated by data published by Taylor and associates in Great Britain. Some 250 patients' status post surgical resection without hepatic metastases were randomized to observation versus a perioperative portal vein infusion of 5-FU and heparin at doses of 1 g and 5,000 U, respectively, given for 7 days. Both incidence of hepatic metastases and overall survival were improved for patients with Dukes' B colon cancer and Dukes' C rectal cancer. The NSABP conducted the largest randomized trial of portal vein infusion (1,158 patients). Patients with surgically resected colon cancer were randomized to observation versus an immediate postoperative 7 day continuous infusion of heparin 5,000 U per day and 5-FU 600 mg per square meter per day administered via a portal vein catheter placed at the time of surgery. The trial was based on the theory that tumor emboli are increased during and just after surgical manipulation and that the emboli predominantly retire via the portal circulation and liver. Significant disease-free and overall survival advantages were seen despite no significant decrease in the incidence of hepatic metastases. It has since been postulated that the 5-FU provided a systemic effect resulting in increased survival. A confirmatory study of 400 patients performed in London by Felding and associates demonstrated similar results. Mayo Clinic and the NCCTG investigated portal vein 5-FU infusion therapy but without heparin in 225 patients with Dukes' B2 or C colon cancer. This group, which had a particularly high percentage of Dukes' B2 patients, demonstrated no beneficial effect compared with controls in the incidence of hepatic metastases, disease-free survival, or overall survival. The importance of adding the anticoagulant heparin, given to reduce incidence of portal vein thrombosis, is unclear. Taylor raises the question of an antitumor effect of heparin, suggested by Mooney's studies with warfarin in murine colon cancer models. Antiangiogenesis effects may also play a role, but at present that role is not defined. To investigate the possible systemic advantage of perioperative therapy, the GI intergroup has recently activated a large, randomized phase III trial comparing a control group with patients receiving perioperative IV continuous infusion 5-FU (600 mg per square meter per day) for 7 days. Patients with Dukes' B3 or C disease will receive 5-FU and levamisole 1 month after surgery.

In an attempt to enhance the clinically proven benefit of 5-FU plus levamisole given in the adjuvant setting, an intergroup trial was recently developed to employ adjuvant radiotherapy with 5-FU plus levamisole for completely resected colon cancer patients at high risk for local recurrence. Patients will be randomized to receive 1 year of 5-FU 450 mg per square meter IV push for 5 days, then weekly beginning day 29 for 48 weeks and oral levamisole 50 mg three times a day for 3 days every 2 weeks or 5 days of 5-FU plus levamisole followed by 5-FU IV push 450 mg per square meter days 1 to 3 and days 23 to 25, oral levamisole 50 mg three times a day beginning day 1, 11, and 23 and local radiation (45 to 50 Gy) followed by 43 weeks of 5-FU plus levamisole. Another intergroup adjuvant protocol will compare 5-FU plus leucovorin plus levamisole with protracted intravenous infusion 5-FU plus levamisole.

Immunotherapy has been employed in the treatment of colon carcinoma both in the adjuvant setting and for patients with advanced or metastatic disease. There have been several investigations evaluating the potential benefits of BCG based on the theory that malignant cells express cell surface antigens not present on normal cells. By upregulating the immune surveillance network, BCG may activate the host immune system to recognize and attack cancer cells at an increased frequency. When combined with autologous tumor cells and readministered to an animal host, the BCG vaccine has been observed to increase the host's immune response and diminish or even eliminate the residual tumor burden. In clinical human trials to date, side effects have been minimal, while one small adjuvant colorectal cancer pilot study suggested increases in disease-free survival and overall survival for patients receiving an autologous tumor cell vaccine combined with BCG. ECOG has designed two randomized adjuvant colon trials for further testing of the efficacy of autologous tumor vaccine. The first of these trials was originally designed to compare vaccine with observation for patients with Dukes' B2, B3, and C colon cancer. When the intergroup levamisole and 5-FU results were reported, acrrual of Dukes' C patients was suspended. There is no difference in survival between the two groups (420 patients), although there is a statistically insignificant trend favoring vaccine therapy for Dukes' C patients. ECOG is evaluating 5-FU and levamisole with or without vaccine in patients with Dukes' C (stage III) colon cancer. This combination of vaccine with chemotherapy reproduces the original animal model, which also included autologous tumor vaccine and BCG followed by chemotherapy.

In animals a synergistic effect doubled survival over that of animals receiving immunotherapy alone (Table 5). In Europe, a new randomized phase III trial is planned for patients with Dukes' B colon cancer, comparing autologous tumor vaccine and BCG followed by 6 months of chemotherapy with 5-FU plus low-dose leucovorin followed by a vaccine boost.

Monoclonal antibody therapy also is under investigation for patients with colon cancer. Riethmüller et al., representing six medical centers in Germany, have reported a phase III trial of 189 patients with Dukes' C colon or rectal cancer who were randomly assigned to either observation or to postoperative treatment with 17-1A antibody (500 mg IV 2 weeks post surgery followed by 100 mg IV every 4 weeks for four doses). The 17-1A monoclonal antibody is a murine IgG2a antibody which has been shown to induce antibody-dependent cellular cytotoxicity (ADCC). It is a cell-surface glycoprotein expressed on malignant and normal epithelial cells. After a median follow-up of 5 years, patients who received the antibody treatment had a reduction in overall death rate by 30 percent, with the most pronounced effect in those patients who had distant metastases as the first sign of relapse, compared to those with local relapses. Additional studies are planned to further evaluate the effectiveness of this monoclonal antibody.

■ RECTAL CARCINOMA

Rectal carcinoma occurs in the region of bowel below the peritoneal reflection, including approximately 15 cm of intestine above the anal verge. After surgical resection locoregional recurrence can produce significant morbidity in as many as 50 percent of untreated patients. Clinical trial groups in North America and Europe have clearly demonstrated that either preoperative or postoperative radiotherapy will produce considerable improvement in local disease control. Neither has resulted in an increase in overall survival, nor has the optimal radiation schedule been defined. Compelling data supporting the benefit of combined modality adjuvant therapy for rectal carcinoma have only recently become available. The rationale for postoperative radiotherapy and chemotherapy includes improved patient selection with more accurate operative staging prior to treatment. The Gastrointestinal Tumor Study Group (GITSG) developed the first trial to show a survival advantage with combined modality treatment. Patients were randomized to surgery alone or radiation alone (40 to 48 Gy) or chemotherapy alone including 5-FU 325 mg per square meter days 1 to 5, 375 mg per square meter days 36 to 40, and methyl CCNU 130 mg per square meter day 1 given every 10 weeks over 18 months. The fourth regimen of this trial combined radiation with 5-FU and methyl CCNU. Accrual reached 227 of the 500 patients expected due to early cessation of the trial after significant differences in recurrence became apparent. With a median follow-up of over 8 years, overall survival data are as follows: 28 percent for surgery alone; 44 percent in the radiotherapy or chemotherapy subgroups; and 58 percent in the combination subgroup. The greatest effect is that of combination therapy on local control, with local relapse rates of 11 percent for patients treated with radiation and chemotherapy and 24 percent for those who received surgery alone. The NCCTG–Mayo Clinic confirmed these results in a similar trial of just over 200 patients with Dukes' B2, B3, or C rectal cancer. Patients were randomized to receive postoperative radiotherapy or radiotherapy with methyl CCNU and 5-FU. Combined therapy produced significant improvement in disease-free (58 versus 38 percent, $p = 0.0025$) and overall survival (63 versus 48 percent, $p = 0.04$) compared with radiation alone. Local recurrence was also significantly decreased with combined treatment (13.5 versus 25 percent).

The NSABP completed a study (RO1) of 555 patients with Dukes' B2 or C disease who were randomized to one of three

Table 6 Recent Adjuvant Rectal Trials

STUDY	SCHEMA	ACCRUAL	SURVIVAL
GITSG	RT + MF → MF	210	54% (3 yr DFS)
7180	RT + 5-FU → 5-FU		68% p = 0.20
NCCTG	RT alone	204	48% (7 yr)
79-47-51	MF → RT + 5-FU → MF		63% p = 0.04
NSABP	Control	574	42% (5 yr)[a]
R01	RT		42%
	MOF		52%
Intergroup	↗ 5-FU ↘	664	No advantage with methyl CCNU
NCCTG	MF RT MF		
86-17-51	↘ CI 5-FU ↗		
	↗ 5-FU ↘		CI + RT 4 yr survival advantage vs. bolus
	5-FU RT 5-FU		5-FU (70% vs 60%) p = 0.02
	↘ CI 5-FU ↗		
NSABP	MOF[b]	741	Analysis pending
R02	MOF + RT[b]		
	LV + 5-FU		
	LV + 5-FU + RT		
INT 0114	5-FU[c] → RT + 5-FU[d] → 5-FU[e]	1,792	Analysis pending
	5-FU/LV[f] → RT + 5-FU/LV[g] → 5-FU/LV[h]		
	5-FU[e]/Lev[i] → RT + 5-FU[j] → 5-FU[k]/Lev[m]		
	5-FU/LV[f]/Lev → RT + 5-FU/LV[g] → 5-FU/LV[l]/Lev[m]		

[a]Observed survival advantage of chemotherapy (p = 0.001) was restricted to males
[b]Males only
[c]500 mg/m^2/d, days 1–5, 29–33
[d]d57–59, 85–87
[e]450 mg/m^2/d, days 1–5, 29–33
[f]5-FU 425 mg/m^2/d, LV 20 mg/m^2/d days 1–5, 29–33
[g]5-FU 400 mg/m^2/d + LV days 1–5, 57–60, 85–88[b]
[h]5-FU 380 mg/m^2/d + LV days 1–5, 29–33 (28 days post RT)
[i]50 mg PO t.i.d. × 3 d q 2 weeks
[j]500 mg/m^2/d, days 57–59, 85–87
[k]400 mg/m^2, days 1–5, 29–33
[l]5-FU 300 mg/m^2 days 1–5, 29–33 + LV
[m]Lev = 4 cycles (28 days post RT)
MF, methyl CCNU, 5-FU; MOF, methyl CCNU, vincristine, 5-FU; RT, radiation therapy; CI, continuous IV infusion; LV, leucovorin; Lev, levamisole.

arms: observation, postoperative radiation, or MOF chemotherapy. The study confirmed the benefit of radiation for local disease control, and MOF chemotherapy increased disease-free survival in men only. The first large intergroup postoperative combined modality rectal trial (NCCTG, CALGB, ECOG, SWOG), compared four treatment regimens for patients with B2, B3, and C rectal cancer. Patients received two cycles of preradiation and two cycles of postradiation bolus chemotherapy with 5-FU with or without methyl CCNU. Radiation was administered with either bolus 5-FU or low-dose protracted infusion 5-FU. With a median follow-up of 4 years, decreases in rate of tumor relapse (37 versus 47 percent) and distant metastases (31 versus 40 percent) were seen for patients who received prolonged infusion with radiation. Relapse-free (p = 0.02) and overall survival (p = 0.01) were also significantly improved. Furthermore, the addition of methyl CCNU produced no benefit over 5-FU alone, results which were also confirmed by a previous GITSG trial.

The NSABP completed its second large postoperative combined modality rectal trial (RO2) in 1992. Patients with Dukes' B and C rectal cancer were randomized to receive postoperative leucovorin and 5-FU with and without pelvic radiation versus MOF with and without radiation. In 1993 the second large intergroup project also reached accrual goals (CALGB, ECOG, NCCTG, NCIC, RTOG, SWOG). It further evaluated chemotherapy followed by concomitant chemotherapy and radiation followed by additional chemotherapy. Comparative chemotherapy regimens included 5-FU with or without leucovorin or levamisole versus 5-FU, leucovorin, and levamisole (Table 6).

The third-generation postoperative intergroup trial, opened in 1994, will further explore the utility of low-dose protracted venous infusion 5-FU with radiation (Table 7).

Traditionally, patients diagnosed with resectable rectal carcinoma have been treated with adjuvant postoperative combined modality therapy consisting of chemotherapy and radiotherapy. To date, while benefit in terms of improved overall survival and local control have been observed, toxicity consisting primarily of diarrhea and cytopenias has been very common, often leading to incomplete treatment cycles. Multiple preoperative radiotherapy trials have been completed using relatively low-dose regimens, including the European Organization on Research and Treatment of Cancer, the

Table 7 Current Rectal Adjuvant Trials

COOPERATIVE GROUP PROTOCOL NUMBER	TREATMENT RANDOMIZATION	STAGE
Intergroup (SWOG 9304)	A. 5-FU[a] → PVI 5-FU[b]/RT → 5-FU[c]	B2, C
	B. PVI 5-FU[d] → PVI 5-FU[b]/RT → PVI 5-FU[e]	
	C. 5-FU[f]/LV[g]/Lev[h] → 5-FU[i]/LV[j]/RT → 5-FU[k]/LV[g]/Lev[h]	
Intergroup (RTOG 94-01)	A. Preop 5-FU/LV/RT	B2, C
	5-FU 325 mg/m^2/d days 1–5, 29–33	
	LV 20 mg/m^2/d days 1–5, 29–33	
	RT 50.4 Gy	
	4–6 wks postop:	
	5-FU 425 mg/m^2/d days 1–5, 29–33	
	380 mg/m^2/d days 57–61, 85–89	
	LV 20 mg/m^2/d with the 5-FU	
	B. Postop 5-FU/LV/RT	
	5-FU 425 mg/m^2/d days 1–5, 29–33	
	LV 20 mg/m^2/d days 1–5, 29–33, 57–60	
	5-FU 400 mg/m^2/d days 57–60	
	RT 50.4 Gy	
	28 days post RT begin	
	5-FU 380 mg/m^2/d days 1–5, 29–33	
	LV 20 mg/m^2/d days 1–5, 29–33	
NSABP R03	A. 5-FU/LV[l] → 5-FU[m]/RT → surgery → 5-FU/LV[n]	
	B. Surgery → 5-FU/LV → 5-FU/RT → 5-FU/LV	

[a] 500 mg/m^2/d days 1–5, 29–33
[b] 225 mg/m^2/d + heparin 7,500 U/d begin day 57 protracted venous infusion during RT
[c] 450 mg/m^2/d days 1–5, 29–33 (begin 28 days post RT)
[d] 300 mg/m^2/d + heparin × 42 d
[e] 300 mg/m^2/d + heparin × 56 d (begin 28 days post RT)
[f] 425 mg/m^2/d days 1–5, 29–33
[g] 20 mg/m^2/d days 1–5, 29–33
[h] 50 mg PO t.i.d. × 3 d q 14 d × 4 courses
[i] 400 mg/m^2/d days 57–60, 85–88
[j] 20 mg/m^2/d days 57–60, 85–88
[k] 380 mg/m^2/d days 1–5, 29–33 (begin 28 days post RT)
[l] 5-FU: 500 mg/m^2 qw × 6 LV: 500 mg/m^2 qw × 6
[m] 400 mg/m^2 IV 1st & last 3d of RT
[n] 3 cycles
PVI, protracted venous infusion; RT, radiation therapy; LV, leucovorin; Lev, levamisole.

Stockholm Rectal Cancer Study, and the Veterans Administration Surgical Oncology Group trial II.

Their results reveal improved local recurrence without survival benefit. Those who support this method of treatment stress that sphincter preservation and downstaging of tumors are seen with increased frequency. Combined modality preoperative therapy could provide benefits including the preservation of the anal sphincter and improved tolerance.

Two preoperative versus postoperative combined modality trials, developed by NSABP and the intergroup (RTOG, CALGB, ECOG, SWOG) are presently accruing patients. Both trials include leucovorin plus 5-FU with radiation (see Table 7).

INVESTIGATIONAL AGENTS

Phase II trials of promising drugs are now available for patients with metastatic colorectal cancer. Topoisomerase I inhibitors have been under investigation with some encouraging results.

Topoisomerase is a nuclear enzyme essential for both the unwinding of DNA and creating breaks in single-stranded DNA. The intermediate forms of DNA exist as cleavable and noncleavable complexes. Topotecan, an analogue of camptothecan, is a water-soluble inhibitor of topoisomerase I and is cell cycle specific. Topotecan alters transiently cleavable complexes to disrupt DNA chains permanently. Human tumor xenograft models reveal positive activity of topotecan with minimal toxicity when given at a low dose via subcutaneous infusion. Myelosuppression is the primary toxicity. Topotecan may be given as a continuous infusion at 0.2 mg per square meter per day over 21 days, after which the dose may be increased to 0.7 mg per square meter per day if tolerated. Transient partial responses have been seen thus far in patients with ovarian carcinoma and non–small carcinoma of the lung. Phase II trials for metastatic colorectal cancer are now accruing patients.

Recently a new class of folate-based specific inhibitors of thymidylate synthase has been developed. The agent ZD1694 (Tomudex) is a member of this group of inhibitors that are approximately 100 times more potent than 5-FU in terms of direct activity on the enzyme. Cells resistant to 5-FU due to increased intracellular levels of dihydrofolate reductase remain susceptible to ZD1694. This agent is retained for extended periods within the cell and has displayed evidence of diminished cell growth in lung, ovarian, and colonic cell lines. Phase I trials of ZD1694 suggest a maximum tolerated dose of 4 mg per square meter. Dose-limiting toxicities include nausea, vomiting, diarrhea, and myelosuppression. Transient elevations of liver enzymes, flulike symptoms, and mucositis were also reported. Unlike its predecessors, ZD1694 caused no nephrotoxicity. Colon cancer Phase III trials in the United States will include dosing at 3.0 mg per square meter.

Other camptothecan derivatives under investigation include 9-amino camptothecan and irinotecan (CPT-11). Phase II trials of irinotecan in advanced colorectal cancer, including patients who have progressed following 5-FU treatment, have produced response rates between 14 and 32 percent. The recommended dose is 125 mg per square meter IV weekly for 4 weeks followed by a 2 week rest. Other drugs in development include the combination of uracil and ftorafur (UFT) plus oral leucovorin, which is presently being compared to IV 5-FU plus leucovorin in a randomized phase III trial. Ftorafur was the first 5-FU prodrug to undergo evaluation. In addition, 5-ethynyluracil, a potent, irreversible inhibitor of the enzyme dihydropyrimidine dehydrogenase (DPD) is under investigation in combination with 5-FU.

■ COMMENTS

The evolution of chemotherapy treatment strategies for colorectal cancer has produced both improved survival for patients with surgically resectable disease and enhanced palliation for those with metastatic cancer. The current adjuvant and advanced disease colorectal trials represent a continuum in the strategic effort to build upon past advances. Participation in this next generation of large intergroup clinical trials is essential to determine the benefits of treatment concepts including biochemical modulation, continuous infusion schedules, and combined modality therapy. Critical advances in laboratory science have encouraged the development of translational research projects using tissue from colorectal cancer patients. Molecular biologic observations have improved understanding of the chromosomal and molecular genetic alterations in colorectal cancer. Allelic losses on chromosome arms 1, 5, 8, 17, and 18 are frequently observed in colorectal cancer. Tumor suppressor genes have been identified on chromosomes including the mutated in colorectal cancer (mcc) gene on chromosome 5q, the p53 gene on 17p, and the deleted in colorectal cancer (dcc) gene on chromosome 18q. Such allelic deletions may become important prognostic markers. The current generation of adjuvant colorectal clinical trials are prospectively evaluating the roles of aneuploidy, percent of cells in S-phase, p53, and the dcc gene in the prognosis of colon cancer and are evaluating whether response to chemotherapy can be predicted by molecular genetic alterations and/or flow cytometry. Other trials are now investigating the roles of thymidylate synthase expression, as measured by immunohistochemical techniques, for example, as a prognostic marker and predictor for response to chemotherapy. The goal is careful selection of patients who would most benefit from adjuvant therapy by using the prognostic information from one or more laboratory parameters.

Suggested Reading

Allen-Mersh TG, Earlam S, Fórdy C, et al. Quality of life and survival with continuous hepatic-artery floxuridine infusion for colorectal liver metastases. Lancet 1994; 344:1255–1260.

Anderson N, Lokich J. Controversial issues in 5-fluorouracil infusion use. Dose intensity, treatment duration and cost comparisons. Cancer 1992; 70:998–1002.

Ensminger WD, Rosowsky A, Rasso V, et al. A clinical-pharmacological evaluation of hepatic arterial infusions of 5-fluoro-2′deoxyuridine and 5-fluorouracil. Cancer Res 1978; 38:3784–3792.

Gastrointestinal Tumor Study Group. Prolongation of the disease-free interval in surgically treated rectal carcinoma. N Engl J Med 1985; 312: 1465–1472.

Gastrointestinal Tumor Study Group. The modulation of fluorouracil with leucovorin in metastatic colorectal carcinoma: A prospective randomized phase III trial. J Clin Oncol 1989; 7:1419–1426.

Grem JL, Jordan E, Robson ME, et al. Phase II study of fluorouracil, leucovorin and interferon alfa-2a in metastatic colorectal carcinoma. J Clin Oncol 1993; 11:1737–1745.

Grem JL, King SA, O'Dwyer PJ, et al. Biochemistry and clinical activity of N-(phosphonacetyl)-L-aspartate: A review. Cancer Res 1988; 44:4441–4454.

Hoover HC, Brandhorst JS, Peters LC, et al. Adjuvant active specific immunotherapy for human colorectal cancer: 6.5 year median follow-up of a phase III prospective randomized trial. J Clin Oncol 1993; 11:390–399.

Kemeny N, Lokich JJ, Anderson N, Ahlgren JD. Recent advances in the treatment of advanced colorectal cancer. Cancer 1993; 71:9–18.

Krook JF, Moertel CH, Gunderson LL, et al. Effective surgical adjuvant therapy for high risk rectal carcinoma. N Engl J Med 1991; 324:709–715.

Laurie JA, Moertel CG, Fleming TR, et al. Surgical adjuvant therapy of large-bowel carcinoma: An evaluation of levamisole and the combination of levamisole and fluorouracil: A study of the North Central Cancer Treatment Group (NCCTG) and the Mayo Clinic. J Clin Oncol 1989; 7:1447–1456.

Lyster MT, Benson AB III, Vogelzang R, Talamonti M. Chemoembolization: Alternative for hepatic tumors. Contemp Oncol 1993; 8:17–28.

Marsh JC, Bertino JR, Katz KH, et al. The influence of drug interval on the effect of methotrexate and fluorouracil in the treatment of advanced colorectal cancer. J Clin Oncol 1991; 9:371–380.

Mayer RJ. Systemic therapy for colorectal cancer: an overview. Semin Oncol 1991; 18(Supp 7):62–66.

Mayer RJ. Chemotherapy for metastatic colorectal cancer. Cancer 1992; 70: 1414–1424.

Moertel CG, Fleming TR, Macdonald JS, et al. Levamisole and fluorouracil for adjuvant therapy of resected colon carcinoma. N Engl J Med 1990; 322:352–358.

O'Connell MJ, Martenson JA, Wieand HS, et al. Improving adjuvant therapy for rectal cancer by combining protracted-infusion fluorouracil with radiation therapy after curative surgery. N Engl J Med 331:502–507.

Petrelli N, Herrera L, Rustum Y, et al. A prospective randomized trial of 5-fluorouracil versus 5-fluorouracil and high-dose leucovorin versus 5-fluorouracil and methotrexate in previously untreated patients with advanced colorectal carcinoma. J Clin Oncol 1987; 5:1559–1565.

Poon MA, O'Connell MJ, Moertel CG, et al. Biochemical modulation of fluorouracil: Evidence of significant improvement of survival and quality of life in patients with advanced colorectal carcinoma. J Clin Oncol 1989; 7:1407–1417.

Stagg RJ, Lewis BJ, Friedman MA, et al. Hepatic arterial chemotherapy for colorectal cancer metastatic to liver. Ann Intern Med 1984; 100:736–743.

Advanced Colorectal Cancer Meta-Analysis Project. Modulation of fluorouracil by leucovorin in patients with advanced colorectal cancer: Evidence in terms of response rate. J Clin Oncol 1992; 10:896–903.

Wadler S. Wiernik PH. Clinical update on the role of fluorouracil and recombinant interferon alfa-2a in the treatment of colorectal carcinoma. Semin Oncol 1990; 17(Suppl 1):16–21.

Wolmark N, Fisher B, Rockette H, et al. Postoperative adjuvant chemotherapy of BCG for colon cancer: Results from NSABP protocol C-01. J Natl Cancer Inst 1988; 80:30–36.

Wolmark N, Rockette H, Wickerham DL, et al. Adjuvant therapy of Dukes' A, B and C adenocarcinoma of the colon with portal vein fluorouracil hepatic infusion: Preliminary results of National Surgical Adjuvant Breast and Bowel Project Protocol C-02. J Clin Oncol 1990; 8:1466–1475.

OVARIAN CANCER: COMBINED MODALITY THERAPY AND CHEMOTHERAPY

Robert F. Ozols, M.D., Ph.D.

Ovarian cancer is the most common fatal gynecologic malignancy in women in the United States. Approximately 26,500 new cases are diagnosed yearly and there are nearly 14,500 deaths. The vast majority of ovarian tumors arise in the coelomic epithelium, and the most common histologic type is serous cystadenocarcinoma. Other epithelial tumor histologic types include mucinous cystadenocarcinoma, endometrioid carcinoma, undifferentiated carcinoma, and clear cell carcinoma. Approximately 10 percent of epithelial tumors are classified as germ cell or sex-cord stromal tumors, primarily granulosa cell and Sertoli-Leydig cell tumors.

The incidence of epithelial ovarian carcinoma increases with age, with 80 percent of women being diagnosed after menopause. There are no specific signs or symptoms of ovarian cancer. Among the common symptoms are pelvic pressure, vague abdominal pain, alterations in bowel function, and abdominal distention. Ovarian cancer tends to remain confined to the peritoneal cavity during its entire clinical course, although pleural and liver involvement occurs in 5 to 10 percent of cases.

Screening for ovarian cancer has been hampered by a lack of an identifiable high-risk group of patients and by the absence of sufficiently sensitive and specific diagnostic tests. Hereditary ovarian cancer accounts for less than 5 percent of cases and is due to mutations of the BRCA1 gene, a tumor-suppressor gene which is also responsible for early-onset breast cancer. The pathogenesis of sporadic ovarian cancer is unclear. It has been postulated that incessant ovulation leads to an aberrant repair process in the ovarian surface epithelium, hence to the development of the tumor. In support of this hypothesis is the observation that factors that decrease the number of ovulatory cycles such as pregnancy, lactation, and some oral contraceptives, have a protective effect against ovarian cancer. While serum levels of CA-125, ultrasound examinations including transvaginal sonography, and routine pelvic exams may be useful in monitoring women at high risk for ovarian cancer, it has not been established that these techniques can diagnose women at an earlier stage of disease. It seems prudent that all women over age 40 have yearly pelvic exams and that women in high-risk categories also be evaluated using ultrasonography and serum CA-125 levels.

DIAGNOSIS AND INITIAL EVALUATION

When epithelial ovarian cancer is suspected, the initial staging workup should include chest x-ray film, computed tomography (CT) scan of the pelvis and abdomen; serum CA-125 levels; and radiographic studies of the gastrointestinal system in symptomatic women. Surgery plays a critical role in the initial staging and therapeutic approach to women with ovarian cancer. The staging laparotomy should be exhaustive, including a midline incision that extends above the umbilicus. This enables the surgeon to visualize and examine the peritoneal contents in a systematic fashion. The primary tumor must be carefully examined for presence of capsular integrity, tumor excrescences, and dense adhesions. A bilateral salpingo-oophorectomy, hysterectomy, and partial omentectomy should be performed. All peritoneal surfaces should be closely inspected, with biopsies obtained from suspicious areas. Blind biopsies from the abdominal wall and the right diaphragm may also be useful. The retroperitoneal lymph nodes should be carefully evaluated and biopsies performed. Peritoneal washings should be obtained if there is no ascites present. The Federation Internationale of Gynecology and Obstetrics (FIGO) staging system for epithelial ovarian carcinoma used to select postoperative therapy is detailed in Table 1. Besides accurately staging the patient, the goal of surgery is to remove as much disease as possible, since the volume of residual disease at the time chemotherapy is initiated is a major prognostic factor for achievement of a complete remission. Consequently, cytoreductive surgery should be attempted in all patients with stage III epithelial ovarian cancer. The role of cytoreductive surgery in patients who present with pleural and/or liver metastases (stage IV) is controversial.

For limited-stage ovarian cancer (stages I and II) survival is correlated with the presence of well-defined clinicopathologic factors. Among the factors associated with a favorable

Table 1 Staging of Ovarian Cancer

Stage I	Growth limited to the ovaries.	
	Stage IA	Growth limited to one ovary; no ascites. No tumor on the external surface; capsule intact.
	Stage IB	Growth limited to both ovaries; no ascites. No tumor on the external surface; capsule intact.
	Stage IC*	Tumor either stage IA or IB but with tumor on the surface of one or both ovaries; or with capsule ruptured; or with ascites present containing malignant cells or with positive peritoneal washings.
Stage II	Growth involving one or both ovaries with pelvic extension.	
	Stage IIA	Extension and/or metastases to the uterus and/or tubes.
	Stage IIB	Extension to other pelvic tissues.
	Stage IIC*	Tumor either stage IIA or IIB but with tumor on the surface of one or both ovaries; or with capsule(s) ruptured; or with ascites containing malignant cells or with positive peritoneal washings.
Stage III	Tumor involving one or both ovaries with peritoneal implants outside the pelvis and/or positive retroperitoneal or inguinal nodes. Superficial liver metastasis constitutes stage III. Tumor is limited to the true pelvis but with histologically verified malignant extension to small bowel or omentum.	
	Stage IIIA	Tumor grossly limited to the true pelvis with negative nodes but with histologically confirmed microscopic seeding of abdominal peritoneal surfaces.
	Stage IIIB	Tumor of one or both ovaries with histologically confirmed implants of abdominal peritoneal surfaces, none exceeding 2 cm in diameter. Nodes negative.
	Stage IIIC	Abdominal implants >2 cm in diameter and/or positive retroperitoneal or inguinal nodes.
Stage IV	Growth involving one or both ovaries with distant metastasis. If pleural effusion is present, there must be positive cytologic test results to allot a case to stage IV. Parenchymal liver metastasis constitutes stage IV.	

*To evaluate the effect on prognosis of the different criteria for alloting cases to stage IC or IIC it is helpful to know whether rupture of the capsule was (1) spontaneous or (2) caused by the surgeon and whether the source of malignant cells detected was (1) peritoneal washings or (2) ascites.

prognosis are well differentiated or moderately well differentiated histology, disease confined to the ovaries, no malignant ascites or cytologically positive peritoneal washings, no excrescences on the tumor capsule, and no dense adhesions. Factors associated with a less favorable outcome in limited-stage ovarian cancer include a poorly differentiated tumor, malignant ascites or cytologically positive cells in peritoneal washings, dense adhesions, a ruptured capsule or extracystic excrescences, and clear cell histology. Limited-stage disease afflicts a clinically important minority of patients with ovarian carcinoma. The vast majority (80 to 85 percent) of women will have widespread intra-abdominal disease (FIGO stage III) at the time of diagnosis; however, 2,000 to 3,000 women will have limited-stage disease. Stage IV disease has a distinctly worse prognosis, as does the presence of bulky residual disease (any tumor mass greater than 2 cm in diameter). Other poor prognostic factors include advanced age, high grade, mucinous or clear cell histology, and ascites. In addition, most studies have demonstrated that amplification of the Her-2/neu oncogene also confers an unfavorable prognosis in patients with advanced disease.

With more accurate staging and improved treatments, there has been a modest overall improvement in survival for patients with epithelial ovarian cancer. For limited-stage favorable disease patients, 5 year survivals are approaching 90 percent. In contrast, for women with limited-stage disease and unfavorable clinicopathologic features, 5 year survival is approximately 75 to 80 percent. In patients with advanced ovarian cancer, the overall 5 year survival has increased to 20 to 25 percent. Consequently, while progress has been made with more aggressive surgery and new chemotherapy regimens, most patients with advanced ovarian cancer still die of the disease.

■ TREATMENT OF LIMITED STAGE

The treatment of patients with limited-stage ovarian cancer is based on clinicopathologic parameters determined after the initial careful staging laparotomy. In patients with favorable prognostic characteristics, it has recently been demonstrated that adjuvant therapy is not necessary, since 5 year survival is approximately 90 percent with surgery alone. It has also been demonstrated in a prospective randomized trial that the 5 year survival was identical in patients with unfavorable parameters treated with either intermittent melphalan or intraperitoneal phosphorus-32. The toxicity of melphalan (myelosuppression and gastrointestinal toxicity) was significantly greater than the toxicities observed with intraperitoneal ^{32}P, and consequently the latter treatment has been adopted by the Gynecologic Oncology Group as the standard treatment, against which an intensive combination chemotherapy regimen is being evaluated. Patients with unfavorable prognosis and limited-stage disease are randomized to receive either intraperitoneal ^{32}P or three cycles of cisplatin 100 mg per square meter plus cyclophosphamide 1 g per square meter. Recent trials have demonstrated cisplatin chemotherapy to be superior to irradiation in these patients. Current clinical trials are evaluating the role of paclitaxel-platinum combinations in these patients. Outside of a clinical trial setting, it seems prudent to treat early-stage disease with the same chemotherapy regimens used for advanced disease.

■ TREATMENT OF ADVANCED DISEASE

Ovarian cancer is a highly drug-sensitive tumor. Until recently the most active agents in this disease were the platinum complexes, and their use with bifunctional alkylating agents

Table 2 Combination Chemotherapy in Advanced Ovarian Cancer

DRUG COMBINATION	SCHEDULE	COMMENT
Cisplatin (75 mg/m^2) plus paclitaxel (135 mg/m^2)	Paclitaxel (24 hr infusion) followed by cisplatin	Shown to be superior to cisplatin plus cyclophosphamide
Carboplatin (AUC = 7.5) plus paclitaxel (175 mg/m^2 in 3 hr infusion)	Both drugs on day 1	Outpatient regimen

such as cyclophosphamide constituted the treatment of choice. However, recently paclitaxel has been shown to be a highly active agent in this disease, and paclitaxel plus a platinum compound has become the new standard chemotherapy for patients with advanced ovarian cancer.

A series of clinical trials have evaluated the contribution of cisplatin and Adriamycin (doxorubicin) to the combination chemotherapy of patients with advanced ovarian cancer. The two-drug regimen of cisplatin plus cyclophosphamide has been prospectively compared with the three-drug regimen of cyclophosphamide, Adriamycin, and cisplatin and with the CHAP-5 regimen (cyclophosphamide, hexamethylmelamine, Adriamycin, and cisplatin). Although in some trials Adriamycin-containing combinations have produced higher response rates, there is no significant improvement in survival, and the two-drug combination of cisplatin and cyclophosphamide has been considered the treatment of choice.

Retrospective studies have suggested that the dose intensity (milligrams of drug per square meter per week) of cisplatin is an important factor in achieving optimal results in patients with advanced disease. However, prospective evaluation of high-dose cisplatin regimens has been limited by the toxicity of cisplatin. Cisplatin, particularly at high doses, is associated with nephrotoxicity, severe nausea and vomiting, myelosuppression, and a dose-limiting peripheral neuropathy. Patients receiving cisplatin and cyclophosphamide should be routinely monitored with weekly white blood cell counts and with careful neurologic examinations. Unfortunately, the peripheral neuropathy can be delayed in onset and can progress even after the cessation of cisplatin therapy. The nephrotoxicity can usually be well managed using aggressive hydration techniques and is no longer considered dose limiting.

The second-generation cisplatin analogue carboplatin has essentially replaced cisplatin in the treatment of patients with advanced ovarian cancer. Carboplatin is not nephrotoxic, has less nausea and vomiting, and is essentially devoid of neurotoxicity. However, it does have more myelosuppression, particularly thrombocytopenia, than the parent compound. Carboplatin and cisplatin share the same active intermediate, and consequently there is almost complete cross-resistance between these two agents. Patients who are resistant to cisplatin therapy have less than a 10 percent likelihood of responding to carboplatin treatment.

Carboplatin is excreted extensively in the urine within the first 24 hours of administration. While it is not nephrotoxic, patients with a decreased clearance of carboplatin on the basis of altered renal function will have substantially more hematologic toxicity. Consequently dose adjustments for carboplatin should be made in patients who have severe renal dysfunction or a prior history of chemotherapy or who are elderly.

Some formulas can be used to calculate a dose that will produce a desired degree of thrombocytopenia based on the patient's history of chemotherapy and the creatinine clearance or glomerular filtration rate. In particular, the Calvert formula, total dose in milligrams = target area under the curve (AUC) × (GFR + 25), is useful in calculating an effective dose with acceptable toxicity. However, in most clinical trials, which compared carboplatin combinations with cisplatin combinations, formulas were not routinely used to select dosage. The initial dose of carboplatin was 300 to 350 mg per square meter in these trials, and doses were adjusted on the basis of thrombocytopenia after the first course. On the basis of prospective randomized trials that have demonstrated equal efficacy of carboplatin and cisplatin regimens as well as markedly less toxicity, carboplatin plus cyclophosphamide until recently was considered the treatment of choice for patients with advanced ovarian cancer (Table 2). In previously untreated patients the Calvert formula can be used to select an AUC of approximately 7, and this can be combined with a cyclophosphamide dose of 600 mg per square meter. If a formula is not used to calculate the dosage, the dose should be 300 to 350 mg per square meter with the dosage adjusted after the first course. If the platelet count does not drop below 100,000, the dose of carboplatin on the second cycle can be increased by 25 to 33 percent. If platelet toxicity is severe, the dose of carboplatin can be decreased. For clinical trials evaluating new combinations with carboplatin, it seems imperative that the Calvert formula be used to calculate the dose of carboplatin to provide meaningful comparisons of toxicity.

More recently, paclitaxel has been included as part of initial chemotherapeutic regimens in patients with advanced disease. An important Gynecologic Oncology Group trial randomized suboptimal stage III and stage IV patients to standard therapy with cisplatin 75 mg per square meter plus cyclophosphamide 750 mg per square meter or paclitaxel 135 mg per square meter plus cisplatin 75 mg per square meter. The paclitaxel combination was superior with regard to overall response rate, disease-free survival, and overall survival. Carboplatin plus paclitaxel can also be combined with acceptable toxicity. While long-term survival data are not available from the use of paclitaxel in combination with platinum compounds in previously untreated patients, most investigators in the United States consider standard therapy to be paclitaxel plus a platinum compound (see Table 2).

Induction therapy should be administered on a 3 to 4 week schedule for at least six cycles. There is no evidence that additional therapy will increase the complete remission rate, prevent or delay relapses, or prolong survival.

SECONDARY CYTOREDUCTION

Approximately 25 to 40 percent of patients after their initial surgery will have bulky residual ovarian cancer. Patients who cannot be effectively cytoreduced at the time of diagnosis have approximately a 10 percent chance of achieving a complete remission with chemotherapy. The feasibility and efficacy of secondary or delayed cytoreductive surgery after two or three cycles of induction chemotherapy has been studied. In a randomized trial reported from the EORTC patients who were not able to be debulked received three cycles of chemotherapy and then were randomized to interval debulking followed by three more cycles of chemotherapy on continuation of chemotherapy without interval debulking. The preliminary results suggest that interval debulking may be beneficial with regard to time to progression and survival. A confirmatory trial of interval debulking is in progress in the United States by the Gynecologic Oncology Group.

There appears to be no significant role for cytoreductive surgery in patients after completion of a full six cycles of induction chemotherapy. However, surgery is important after initial chemotherapy for palliation of intestinal obstructions.

COMBINED MODALITY APPROACHES WITH RADIOTHERAPY

In previously untreated patients with small-volume residual disease, pelvic plus abdominal radiotherapy can produce similar survival to what has been observed with combination chemotherapy. Abdominal radiotherapy is not effective in previously untreated patients with bulky residual ovarian cancer. There has not been a prospective randomized trial comparing radiation with chemotherapy in advanced ovarian cancer patients who have been optimally surgically cytoreduced. While abdominal radiation is effective in previously untreated patients with small-volume disease, it appears to have little role in the treatment of patients after induction chemotherapy. Numerous uncontrolled trials have used radiotherapy in patients who have documented residual disease after induction chemotherapy. In these trials only patients with microscopic disease had prolonged survival. Furthermore, abdominal radiotherapy in this situation is usually associated with considerable toxicity, primarily related to effects on the gastrointestinal tract.

It has been suggested that whole abdominal radiotherapy may have a role in patients with microscopic disease at second-look surgery or in patients who have a negative second look but who are at high risk for relapse. The overall relapse rate in patients who achieve a complete remission is approximately 30 to 50 percent. Risk factors for relapse from a negative second-look laparotomy include a high-grade tumor and bulky disease prior to the initiation of chemotherapy. It has been speculated that whole abdominal radiotherapy may decrease the relapse rate in this group of patients, although no prospective trial has demonstrated the efficacy of any form of treatment in decreasing the relapse rate.

INTRAPERITONEAL CHEMOTHERAPY

Ovarian cancer remains confined to the abdominal cavity virtually throughout its clinical course. In an effort to increase the delivery of chemotherapeutic agents directly to the tumor, phase I and pharmacologic studies have evaluated the role of intraperitoneal chemotherapy in patients with ovarian cancer. It has been demonstrated that the intraperitoneal administration of most drugs active in ovarian cancer is associated with a pharmacologic advantage. Administration of drugs directly into the peritoneal cavity leads to higher levels in the fluid bathing of the tumor cells than can be achieved in the systemic circulation. Furthermore, with drugs such as cisplatin, cytotoxic concentrations can also be achieved in the systemic circulation. Consequently, in theory, after intraperitoneal administration a peritoneal tumor is exposed to high levels of drug, which can directly diffuse into the outer layers of the tumor mass; hence, the inner core of the tumor can be effectively treated by cytotoxic drug concentrations via the microcirculation. While clinical studies have demonstrated that intraperitoneal therapy is technically feasible, the role of intraperitoneal therapy in the management of patients with ovarian cancer remains to be established.

In initial trials a Tenckhoff catheter was used for peritoneal access. However, more recently totally implantable Port-a-Cath systems have been used and are associated with a lower complication rate and with increased patient acceptance. However, intraperitoneal catheters are still associated with significant toxicities including bowel perforation, sepsis, and outflow obstruction.

Cisplatin has been the most active single agent when used intraperitoneally in patients with residual ovarian cancer. Approximately 30 percent of patients who have residual disease at second-look laparotomy can be converted to a complete remission by the intraperitoneal administration of cisplatin or cisplatin-based combinations. In uncontrolled trials a 74 percent 5 year survival has been reported in patients with a small volume of residual disease who have received intraperitoneal platinum or platinum-containing combinations. The combination of platinum plus VP-16 appears to be the most active regimen reported for patients with residual ovarian cancer.

The results of a prospective randomized trial comparing intraperitoneal versus intravenous cisplatin in previously untreated patients with small-volume residual disease have recently been reported. Patients were randomized to receive either intraperitoneal or intravenous cisplatin at 100 mg/m^2 and all patients received intravenous cyclophosphamide (600 mg/m^2). Median survival was increased by 20 percent (49 months versus 41 months) in the intraperitoneal group which also experienced less toxicity. Confirmatory studies in which cyclophosphamide is replaced by paclitaxel have been completed and are maturing. Most investigators consider intraperitoneal chemotherapy investigational, pending the results of ongoing trials.

SECOND-LOOK SURGERY

The role of second-look surgery following completion of induction chemotherapy is itself controversial. It is clear that second-look surgery per se has no therapeutic value. The only reason for a second look is if subsequent therapy will depend on findings at the exploratory laparotomy. Patients who have evidence of residual disease after induction chemotherapy, including a persistently elevated CA-125 or radiographic or clinical evidence of residual masses, should not routinely undergo a second-look laparotomy but instead should be treated with salvage regimens. Approximately 25 to 35 percent of patients who are clinically disease free at the completion of induction therapy will be found to have residual disease at a second-look laparotomy.

Clinical trials are in progress to determine whether intraperitoneal therapy can prevent relapses in patients who have a negative second-look laparotomy. While intraperitoneal ^{32}P, whole abdominal radiation, intraperitoneal chemotherapy, and systemic chemotherapy have all been advocated by some investigators to prevent or decrease the relapse rate in patients with a negative second look, no prospective data document that the relapse rate can be decreased by any type of therapy.

Table 3 Second-Line Therapy in Ovarian Cancer

DRUG	COMMENT
Paclitaxel (175 mg/m^2)	30–48% response rate in patients not previously treated with paclitaxel
Carboplatin (AUC = 5)	Response rate dependent upon prior response to platinum
Topotecan (1.5 mg/m^2 qd × 5)	Comparable activity to paclitaxel in patients relapsing after platinum plus cyclophosphamide
Gemcitabine (800–1,000 mg/m^2 q wk × 3)	In vitro synergy with platinum: 15–20% response rate in platinum resistant patients
Oral etoposide (50 mg/m^2 qd × 21 d)	Active in both platinum sensitive (34%) and resistant patients (17%)
Tamoxifen (20 mg PO b.i.d.)	Minimal toxicity

SALVAGE CHEMOTHERAPY

Most patients who do achieve a complete remission with induction chemotherapy unfortunately will recur. Consequently the selection of salvage therapy is an important consideration in the overall management of patients with recurrent disease. However, overall survival remains poor for patients who have recurrent disease, and there is no evidence that any salvage regimen can cure patients once their disease has relapsed.

Several agents have demonstrated activity in previously treated patients with advanced disease. Paclitaxel has been demonstrated by several groups to have an overall response rate of approximately 30 percent in previously treated patients with advanced disease, including a 20 to 25 percent response rate in patients who have been deemed truly platinum refractory. Platinum-refractory patients are those who either progress on platinum therapy or have a response that lasts less than 6 months. The optimum dose and schedule of paclitaxel remain to be defined. Prospective randomized comparisons have demonstrated that a 3 hour infusion at 175 mg per square meter is as effective as a 24 hour infusion at 135 mg per square meter, and consequently the short infusion can be used in previously treated patients with advanced ovarian cancer. If patients recur after initial therapy with paclitaxel plus platinum compound, retreatment with paclitaxel is often associated with a beneficial response if the disease-free interval is greater than 6 months.

Retreatment with platinum compounds also is an effective approach to the management of patients with recurrent ovarian cancer. However, platinum compounds should be used as salvage therapy only in patients who have had prior response to induction chemotherapy with platinum that lasted more than 6 months. Whether to use carboplatin or cisplatin for salvage is based primarily on toxicity considerations. Most patients who have received induction chemotherapy with cisplatin should be retreated with carboplatin, since retreatment with cisplatin will exacerbate any underlying peripheral neuropathy. On the other hand, if the patient had induction chemotherapy with carboplatin and has had substantial hematologic toxicity, cisplatin may produce less toxicity.

Ifosfamide is an alkylating agent whose clinical development was initially limited by severe hemorrhagic cystitis. However, the availability of Mesna, which protects the uroepithelium from the toxic metabolites of ifosfamide, has permitted a more exacting evaluation of ifosfamide in ovarian cancer and other tumors. Ifosfamide as a single agent produces objective responses in approximately 20 percent of previously treated patients, including a response rate of approximately 10 percent in platinum-refractory patients. Hexamethylmelamine has also been shown to have activity in recurrent disease, including platinum-resistant disease. Tamoxifen has also been shown by the Gynecologic Oncology Group to be an effective salvage regimen in previously treated patients with advanced ovarian cancer. An overall response rate of 18 percent was reported for patients treated with tamoxifen 20 mg twice a day.

Several new drugs have recently been shown to be active in recurrent ovarian cancer (Table 3). Topotecan, a topoisomerase I inhibitor, has been approved by the FDA for this indication. Oral etoposide has similar activity in these patients whereas intravenous etoposide is inactive. Other, less studied active agents include gemcitabine, vinorelbine, and encapsulated doxorubicin. Phase II trials remain an appropriate option for all patients with recurrent ovarian cancer.

INVESTIGATIONAL TREATMENTS

High-Dose Chemotherapy

There remains considerable debate regarding the importance of dose intensity in the treatment of patients with advanced ovarian cancer. A prospective randomized trial by the Gynecologic Oncology Group failed to demonstrate any benefit for patients treated with a dose-intense regimen compared with patients treated with a more standard regimen. In this trial patients were randomized to receive either eight cycles of cisplatin 50 mg per square meter plus cyclophosphamide

500 mg per square meter or a double-dose-intense regimen that consisted of cisplatin 100 mg per square meter and cyclophosphamide 1 g per square meter with both drugs administered for only four cycles. Patients randomized to the high-dose regimen had no improvement over patients receiving the standard therapy. It has been speculated that doubling the dose intensity may not be sufficient to produce a clinically significant improvement in survival. Clinical trials in progress with high-dose carboplatin may permit a larger increase in dose than with cisplatin. In these trials peripheral blood stem cell transfusions or cytokines are required to deal with the severe hematologic toxicity. However, there is no evidence that high-dose chemotherapy with peripheral blood stem cell transfusions or autologous bone marrow transplantation is useful in any subset of patients with advanced ovarian cancer. Most clinical trials now are focusing on patients who still have drug-sensitive disease and who have small-volume tumors.

Biologic Agents

Ovarian cancer is well suited for the study of biologic agents and biologic response modifiers. Ovarian cancer cells express antigens including cerbB, and access to the peritoneal cavity permits assessment of the immune response following biologic treatments. Clinical trials examined the toxicity and efficacy of monoclonal antibody–immunotoxin conjugates in patients with refractory ovarian cancer. These studies were based on prior demonstration in preclinical models of human ovarian cancer that immunotoxins have marked antitumor effects. Monoclonal antibodies used in these studies were directed either against tumor-associated antigens or the transferin receptor. The transferin receptor is primarily expressed in dividing cells, and in the abdominal cavity only malignant cells should be expressing this receptor. Toxins used in these studies included recombinant ricin A chain as well as *Pseudomonas* exotoxin. While encouraging clinical activity was observed, these trials have been associated with unacceptable neurotoxicity. Additional studies linking monoclonal antibodies with radioisotopes or with bispecific antibodies are also in progress.

A combination of interleukin-2 and lymphokine activated killer cells (LAK) is effective in a murine model of human ovarian cancer. Based upon these observations, clinical trials have evaluated IL-2 plus LAK in patients with residual ovarian cancer. While activity has been reported, enthusiasm for this approach has been dampened by the severe intraperitoneal toxicity. The intraperitoneal administration of interferon also has been shown to produce responses in patients with small-volume disease. While biologic approaches have activity, improved efficacy and decreased toxicity remain the goals of experimental protocols.

Reversal of Drug Resistance

The biochemical basis for drug resistance in ovarian cancer remains to be completely established. However, it has been demonstrated in preclinical models of ovarian cancer that resistance to cisplatin and alkylating agents is associated with increased glutathione (GSH) levels and in an increased DNA repair capacity. In preclinical systems, it has been demonstrated that inhibition of GSH synthesis with buthionine sulfoximine (BSO), an irreversible inhibitor of the key enzyme in the biosynthesis of GSH, leads to the potentiation of cytotoxicity of alkylating agents and platinum compounds. Furthermore, inhibition of DNA repair with drugs such as aphidicolin, an inhibitor of DNA polymerase alpha, also potentiates the cytotoxicity of cisplatin in drug-resistant tumor cells. Based upon these preclinical observations, clinical trials of agents that can reverse drug resistance such as BSO have recently been initiated.

■ NONEPITHELIAL OVARIAN TUMORS

Ovarian Germ Cell Tumors

Cisplatin-based regimens have led to a dramatic improvement in the prognosis of women with germ cell tumors of the ovary. These tumors occur more frequently in younger patients than epithelial ovarian carcinomas. Patients usually present with symptoms resulting from a pelvic mass such as urinary frequency and lower abdominal pain or pressure. Serum alpha-fetoprotein (AFP) and human chorionic gonadotrophin (hCG) frequently can be detected in patients with germ cell tumors and are useful in the diagnosis and monitoring of patients after surgery.

The most common malignant germ cell tumor of the ovary is a dysgerminoma. Approximately three-quarters of patients are diagnosed with stage I disease, and 10 percent of patients have bilateral tumors. A unilateral salpingo-oophorectomy can be performed if patient desires fertility. Dysgerminoma has long been known to be highly sensitive to radiotherapy, which frequently has been administered when the tumor has metastasized. More recently it has been demonstrated that the combination of cisplatin, vinblastine (Velban), and bleomycin (PVB) is also effective therapy for patients with metastatic germ cell tumors of the ovary. Furthermore, it has been demonstrated that replacement of vinblastine by etoposide in this regimen leads to less toxicity and possibly more efficacy, and consequently the BEP regimen (cisplatin, etoposide, and bleomycin) can be considered the regimen of choice for women with metastatic germ cell tumors of the ovary.

Immature teratomas are the second most common germ cell malignancy. Bilateral ovarian involvement is rare and a unilateral salpingo-oophorectomy can be performed to preserve fertility. Adjuvant chemotherapy has been shown to be successful, and patients with stage IA, grade 2 or 3 should be treated with the BEP regimen with three or four cycles. Patients with stage IA, grade 1 lesions have an excellent prognosis, and adjuvant therapy is not indicated. Similarly, patients with endodermal sinus tumors (EST) are initially treated with unilateral salpingo-oophorectomy. All patients with an EST of the ovary are treated postoperatively with BEP chemotherapy.

Sex-Cord Stromal Tumors

This group of tumors includes granulosa cell tumors and Sertoli-Leydig cell tumors. The granulosa cell tumors are often estrogen secreting and associated with endometrial carcinoma. Most granulosa cell tumors are diagnosed at an early stage, although tumors may recur years after the initial diagnosis. There is no evidence that either radiation or chemotherapy after surgical removal of the tumor prevents recurrences. Similarly, Sertoli-Leydig cell tumors, which frequently present with virilization due to the production of androgens, are also treated with surgery alone in most instances. Chemotherapy has been reserved for patients with persistent or recurrent disease with the BEP combination currently under investigation by the 909.

Borderline Tumors of the Ovary

Borderline tumors are a clearly identifiable subset of epithelial tumors of the ovary that have a markedly superior prognosis to that of invasive carcinoma of the ovary. These tumors, also termed tumors of low malignant potential, are histologically characterized by the absence of invasion into stromal tissues. In contrast to invasive carcinomas of the ovary, most patients with borderline tumors present with stage I disease. The primary treatment for borderline tumors is surgery, a bilateral salpingo-oophorectomy and hysterectomy. In stage I disease there is no demonstrated efficacy for adjuvant therapy. A unilateral salpingo-oophorectomy may be adequate therapy for patients in whom fertility is of concern. It has not been established that postoperative chemotherapy is beneficial for patients who present with advanced stage disease. The primary approach is to remove as much disease as possible. The disease has a long natural history, and even in patients with advanced disease, death from borderline tumor is uncommon in the first 5 years. Consequently, patients with advanced disease have frequently been managed with surgery as needed to deal with symptoms. The current recommendation is to reserve chemotherapy for patients with recurrent disease who cannot undergo successful surgical cytoreduction.

Suggested Reading

Advanced Ovarian Cancer Trialists Group. Chemotherapy in advanced ovarian cancer: An overview of randomised clinical trials. BMJ 1991; 303:884–893.

Alberts DS, Liu PY, Hannigan EV, et al. Intraperitoneal cisplatin plus intravenous cyclophosphamide versus intravenous cisplatin plus intravenous cyclophosphamide for stage III ovarian cancer. N Engl J Med 1996; 335:1950–1955.

Bookman MA, McGuire WP III, Kilpatrick D, et al. Carboplatin and paclitaxel in ovarian carcinoma: A phase I study of the Gynecologic Oncology Group. J Clin Oncol 1996; 14:1895–1902.

Calvert AH, Newell DR, Gumbrell LA, et al. Carboplatin dosage: Prospective evaluation of a simple formula based on renal function. J Clin Oncol 1989; 7:1748–1756.

Chambers JT. Borderline ovarian tumors: A review of treatment. Yale J Biol Med 1989; 62:351–365.

Hatch KD, Beecham JB, Blessing JA, Creasman WT. Responsiveness of patients with advanced ovarian carcinoma to tamoxifen: A Gynecologic Oncology Group study of second-line therapy in 105 patients. Cancer 1991; 68:269–271.

Hoskins WJ, Bundy BN, Thigpen JT, Omura GA. The influence of cytoreductive surgery on recurrence-free interval and survival in small-volume stage III epithelial ovarian cancer: A Gynecologic Oncology Group study. Gynecol Oncol 1992; 47:159–166.

Levin L. Hryniuk WM. Dose intensity analysis of chemotherapy regimens in ovarian carcinoma. J Clin Oncol 1987; 5:756–767.

McGuire WP, Hoskins WJ, Brady MF, et al. Cyclophosphamide and cisplatin compared with paclitaxel and cisplatin in patients with stage III and stage IV ovarian cancer. N Engl J Med 1996; 334:1–6.

Omura GA, Brady MF, Homesley HD, et al. Long-term follow-up and prognostic factor analysis in advanced ovarian carcinoma: The Gynecologic Oncology Group experience. J Clin Oncol 1991; 9:1138–1150.

Ovarian Cancer Meta-Analysis Project. Cyclophosphamide plus cisplatin versus cyclophosphamide, doxorubicin, and cisplatin chemotherapy of ovarian carcinoma: A meta-analysis. J Clin Oncol 1991; 9:1668–1674.

Ozols RF. Ovarian Cancer, Part II: Treatment. Curr Prob Cancer 1992; 63–126.

Ozols RF, Thigpen JT, Dauplat J. et al. Dose intensity. Ann Oncol 1993; 4:S49–S56.

Rowinsky EK, McGuire WP, Donehower RC. The current status of Taxol. Principles and Practice of Gynecologic Oncology Updates. 1993; 1(1): 1–16.

Schilder, RJ. High-dose chemotherapy with autologous hematopoietic cell support in gynecologic malignancies. Principles and Practice of Gynecologic Oncology Updates. 1993; 1(3):1–14.

Williams SD, Blessing JA, Hatch KD, Homesley HD. Chemotherapy of advanced dysgerminoma: Trials of the Gynecologic Oncology Group. J Clin Oncol 1991; 9:1950–1955.

BENIGN PROSTATIC HYPERTROPHY

Jack Geller, M.D.

Benign prostatic hypertrophy (BPH) represents a newly recognized area of endocrine disease that is treatable with medical therapy. Two-thirds of men over the age of 55 have symptoms of BPH. The number of men over age 55 in the United States is approximately 20 million. Therefore, approximately 14 million men have symptoms. Until now surgical transurethral resection (TURP) of the prostate has been the only established therapy for BPH. Because only 400,000 operations a year for BPH are performed in the United States, the vast majority of patients with this disease are receiving no specific therapy presently as surgery is usually reserved for more advanced and serious cases. The following discussion focuses on recently developed medical treatment for BPH that can be introduced at an earlier stage of disease and provide therapy for the vast majority of men for whom no therapy except surgery has been available to date.

BPH does not occur in men who have been castrated prior

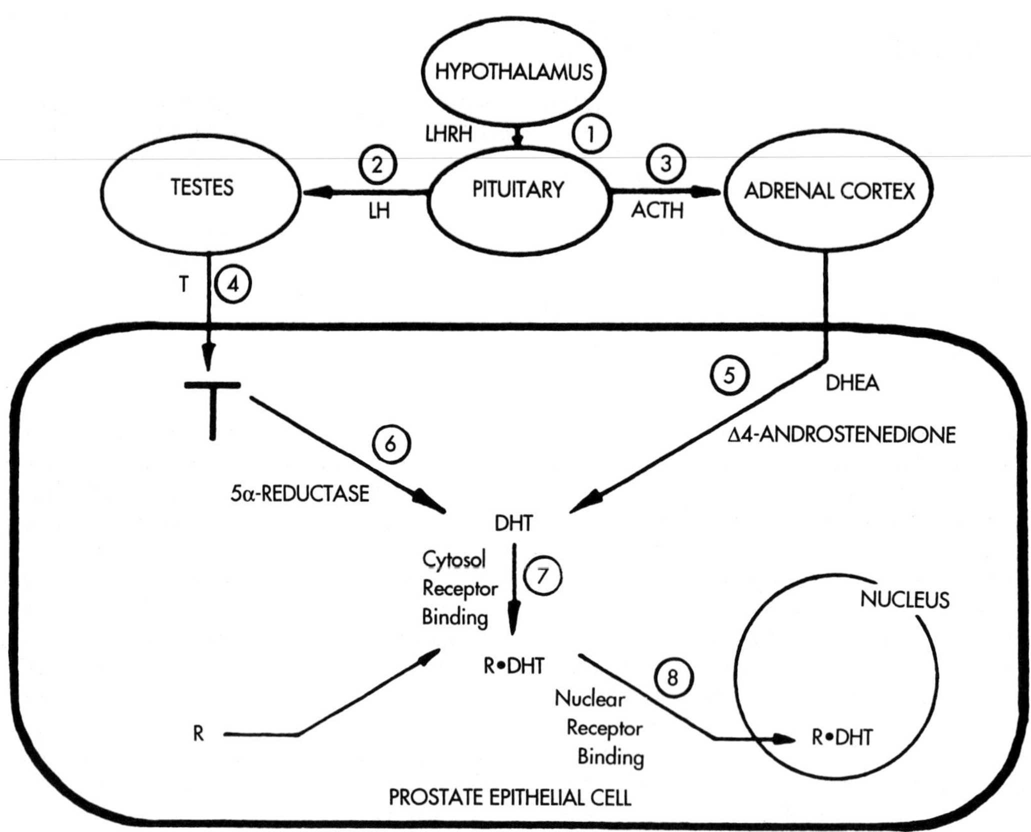

Figure 1
Multiple factors contributing to androgen-mediated action. Pathway for synthesis of dihydrotestosterone is shown; primary loci at which various androgen withdrawal therapies block androgen action are indicated by numbers as follows: surgical castration, 4; medical castration with progestational antiandrogens, 2, 3, 4, 6, 7; androgen blockade with pure antiandrogens, 7; medical castration with gonadotropin-releasing hormone agonist, 1; androgen blockade with 5α-reductase inhibitors, 5 and 6; no therapy, 8. LHRH, Luteinizing hormone–releasing hormone; LH, luteinizing hormone; ACTH, adrenocorticotropic hormone; T, testosterone; DHT, dihydrotestosterone; DHEA, dehydroepiandrosterone; R, androgen receptor; R-DHT, androgen receptor–steroid complex.

to age 40 or in those born with 5α-reductase deficiency or testicular feminization. The major factors in the development of BPH appear to be related to aging, functioning testes, and an intact pathway of androgen-mediated action (Fig. 1). The fact that prostate size decreases following androgen withdrawal has set the stage for the current endocrine therapy of BPH (Table 1).

Symptoms of BPH, referred to as prostatism, include both irritative and obstructive symptoms. The irritative symptoms, which are related to detrusor instability secondary to bladder outlet obstruction, include nocturia, frequency, and urgency of urination. Obstructive symptoms consist of decreased strength of urinary stream, hesitancy, intermittency, and incomplete emptying of the bladder. Outlet obstruction of the bladder causing prostatism is primarily a result of mechanical enlargement of the prostate, which narrows the prostatic urethra. In addition, a dynamic component of outlet obstruction related to $alpha_1$-adrenergic–mediated smooth muscle contraction may exist. The bladder outlet is innervated extensively by $alpha_1$-adrenergic nerves. When these nerves are stimulated, smooth muscle surrounding the inner sphincter at the bladder neck contracts. In addition, prostatic smooth muscle itself is contracted by $alpha_1$-adrenergic stimuli, resulting in increased intraurethral pressure and obstruction.

Medical therapy of BPH must consider treatment of both of these potential causes of outlet obstruction. Mechanical obstruction would appear to be more important than the dynamic factor as a cause of symptoms of bladder outlet obstruction, because surgical removal of the obstructing periurethral adenoma alone by urologists has been demonstrated to be a successful treatment for BPH for over 90 years. Additional evidence for the critical role of prostate volume to bladder outlet obstruction is supported by the urodynamic studies of Tammela et al., who showed a very significant reduction in detrusor pressure at maximal urine flow together with an increase in maximum urinary flow rates following a decrease in prostate size after 6 months of finasteride treatment. Although three-quarters of the decrease in prostate volume that occurs following finasteride therapy occurs in the periurethral adenoma, this decrease is approximately one-fourth that achieved following surgery; therefore, additional

Table 1 Effect of Androgen Withdrawal on Prostate Size

ANDROGEN BLOCKERS	MEAN % DECREASE IN PROSTATE VOLUME (TYPE OF MEASUREMENT)	AVERAGE TIME FOR MAXIMAL DECREASE IN SIZE	LARGE DOUBLE-BLIND STUDIES OF CLINICAL EFFECTS
Surgical castration	30% (TRUS)	3–6 months	No
Progestational antiandrogens (cyproterone acetate)	30% (TRUS)	3–6 months	No
Flutamide	40% (TRUS)	3–6 months	No
Gonadotropin-releasing hormone agonists	25% (TRUS)	3–6 months	No
5α-reductase inhibitors (finasteride)	20% (MRI)	3–6 months	Yes

TRUS, transrectal ultrasound; MRI, magnetic resonance imaging.

medical therapy to decrease the dynamic component of BPH with alpha$_1$-adrenergic blockade may be very useful as an adjunct to the finasteride therapy.

As in any medical disorder, specific therapy for BPH can only be given when the diagnosis has been established and other conditions that may have overlapping symptoms have been excluded. The therapy for BPH is highly specific and should be initiated only after eliminating other conditions (e.g., chronic prostatitis, chronic and acute urinary tract infections, prostate cancer, bladder cancer, neurogenic bladder and urethral stricture) considered in the differential diagnosis. They can be easily excluded by routine urinalysis, comparison of counts of white blood cells and bacteria in urethral and bladder urine with those in postprostatic massage urine, serum prostate-specific antigen (PSA) testing, digital rectal examination, and analysis of postvoid catheterized residual urine to rule out a neurogenic bladder or advanced decompensated BPH.

■ ADMINISTRATION OF FINASTERIDE

Once the diagnosis of BPH has been established by appropriate history, physical examination, and tests, the initial therapy should be based upon the size of the prostate as estimated by rectal exam. This approach represents an important change in the use of medical therapy for the treatment of BPH and is the result of a recently reported VA study that showed finasteride to be ineffective in patients with an average gland size of 36 to 37 g (see Lepor, et al, 1996). In five previously published studies of the effect of finasteride on large numbers of patients with BPH, the average gland size was greater than 40 g in all studies. After the VA study, a retrospective analysis of subsets of patients in each previously published finasteride study, including the VA study, showed than finasteride was consistently effective in significantly decreasing maximal flow rates and AUA symptom score when prostate size was greater than 40 g and ineffective when prostate size was less than 40 g. Most patients with symptomatic BPH will have enlarged prostates greater tham 40 g and initial therapy in this group should, therefore, be directed at the mechanical factor (enlarged prostate) and involves prescribing finasteride, which can decrease prostate size and appears to arrest the disease. Finasteride is a competitive inhibitor of the enzyme 5α-reductase and reduces plasma dihydrotestosterone concentration by approximately 70 percent. Plasma testosterone is statistically increased, but mean values remain in the normal range. No other effects on plasma hormones have been noted. The drug has no effect on plasma lipids or renal, liver, or marrow function. In a dose-response study designed to measure drug effect on prostatic dihydrotestosterone concentrations, daily doses of finasteride ranging from 1 to 80 mg were given. An optimal dose appeared to be 5 mg per day as it maximally decreased both prostate size and tissue dihydrotestosterone concentrations. In a large phase III study, a daily dose of 5 mg finasteride was clinically and significantly effective in reducing symptoms of BPH, decreasing prostate size by 20 percent at 1 year and increasing maximal urinary flow rates in patients with BPH compared with controls. In a follow-up of over 200 of these patients in an open extension study for 3 years, prostate volume decreased by 27 percent from baseline; maximum urinary flow rates increased by 3 ml or more in 40 percent of these patients; and 48 percent of patients experienced a 50 percent or greater improvement in symptom score. In addition, in a recent publication of a 5 year follow-up of a subset of 55 original patients, it was noted that changes in prostate volume, maximum urinary flow rate, and symptom score noted at 1 year all persisted relatively unchanged at the end of 5 years. It is likely that these patients, if continued on therapy, will remain stable indefinitely. Finasteride would appear to have distinct advantages over the other drugs approved for medical therapy, the alpha$_1$-adrenergic blockers, with regard to fewer side effects (Table 2) and a significantly longer track record of proven effectiveness. Therefore, finasteride is the preferred approach to the medical therapy of BPH in patients with moderate or greater sized prostates.

In studies of prostate tissue androgens in patients treated for 7 days with 5 g finasteride daily, dihydrotestosterone levels in the prostate were reduced to 0.6 mg per gram, a value significantly less than the 1.2 mg per gram level noted in prostates from surgical castrates or 4 mg per gram in patients with untreated BPH. Testosterone levels, on the other hand, are increased in prostate tissue by five to seven times above control values following administration of finasteride. Although this rise is impressive, it must be remembered that the affinity of testosterone for the androgen receptor in the prostate is only one-fourth that of dihydrotestosterone, making it a relatively weak prostatic androgen.

Other major support for the rationale of finasteride therapy for BPH is the fact that the prostate in patients born with 5α-reductase deficiency, an experiment of nature, is very

Table 2 Side Effects in Men with Benign Prostatic Hyperplasia Treated with Finasteride or Placebo for 12 Months

SIDE EFFECTS	5 MG FINASTERIDE (N = 297)	PLACEBO (N = 300)
DIGESTIVE SYSTEM		
Abdominal pain	1.0	0.3
Diarrhea	0	0
Flatulence	1.0	0.7
Nausea	0.7	1.0
NERVOUS SYSTEM		
Dizziness	0	0.7
Headache	0.7	0.7
Decreased libido	4.7*	1.3
UROGENITAL SYSTEM		
Breast pain	0.3	0
Dysuria	0.7	0
Ejaculatory disorder	4.4*	1.7
Impotence	3.4	1.7
Orgasm dysfunction	0.7	0.3
Testicular pain	1.0	0.7
Loss of libido	4.3*	1.3
Gynecomastia	rare	0
EYE		
Lens change	0.7	0
Lens opacities	0	0.7
MISCELLANEOUS		
Rash	0.7	0.3
Asthenia	1.0	1.0
Pelvic pain	0.3	0.7

*$p < .05$ versus placebo.

small or vestigial in adults in spite of high prostatic testosterone levels in the presence of very low dihydrotestosterone levels.

There are other drugs that inhibit androgen action and reduce prostate size (see Table 1), but they all have major side effects, particularly loss of libido and impotence. They have been studied mostly in small series of uncontrolled subjects. In addition, large double-blind controlled studies of the effect of these drugs on clinical symptoms and urine flow rates have not been done.

Initiating Treatment and Selection of Patients

Selection of patients for medical therapy of BPH is best accomplished by determining the extent and rate of progression of prostatism with a validated American Urological Association (AUA) symptom score questionnaire filled out by the patient. This AUA symptom score is also very useful for following the progression of BPH and triggering a decision to start medical therapy (for details of symptom score, see Barry et al., 1992, under Suggested Reading). Seven symptoms of prostatism are evaluated to determine the symptom score. Each symptom is given a value of 1 to 5 points, with 5 representing the severest symptom; therefore, the highest score possible is 35. A total of 0 to 8 points represents mild BPH and patients with such a score should be followed yearly but do not usually require treatment; 9 to 19 points signifies moderate disease and scores above 20 represent advanced stage BPH. An ideal time to start therapy for BPH is when there is an increase in the symptom score into the 9 to 19 range. Patients with advanced-stage disease (greater than 20 points) generally respond poorly to finasteride therapy, and such patients should be sent directly to surgery. In untreated mild or moderate BPH the natural history of disease is for symptoms to increase to advanced-stage disease and require surgery in approximately 20 to 40 percent of patients over 5 years.

Finasteride, because of its sustained effectiveness in reducing the size of the prostate and improving clinical symptoms of BPH as previously described, could have a significant effect on decreasing the ultimate need for surgical therapy of BPH. Finasteride should be given once daily in a 5 mg dose; no effect of food on absorption is noted. No modification of dosage for age or renal insufficiency is required. The drug arrests the disease process by shrinking the prostate, which then remains stable at the reduced size for at least 5 years according to the longest follow-up information available. About 40 to 50 percent of patients treated with 5 mg finasteride show significant clinical improvement approximately 6 to 12 months following initiation of therapy. Other patients show lesser degrees of or no clinical improvement, although most prostates shrink in size. In our experience to date, symptoms of prostatism rarely, if ever, progress in patients following initiation of therapy.

Certain patients are unlikely to benefit from therapy. In addition to patients with small glands, these include patients with advanced disease who have either elevated residual urines, bladder stones, repeated gross hematuria, a history of repeated urinary tract infections related to obstruction, or denervation hypersensitivity of the bladder with inability to void more than 100 to 125 ml bladder urine accompanied usually by severe urgency. These patients should be advised to undergo surgery. Patients with elevated PSA levels (greater than 4.0 ng per milliliter with Hybritech method) should be referred to a urologist to rule out prostate cancer.

Monitoring

Patients should be seen at 3 month intervals for re-evaluation of symptoms during the first year of therapy; measurement of maximum urinary flow rate is optional and, if available, should be repeated at 6 month intervals. Digital rectal examination for estimate of prostate size and detection of nodules and plasma PSA determination (a blood test should be done prior to digital examination) should be performed every 6 months for the first year. The same laboratory technique should be utilized for all PSA levels. No quantitative measurement of gland size is recommended. If the baseline PSA level drops by 30 to 50 percent at 1 year (the expected decrease as noted in a large phase III study), the frequency of PSA testing and digital rectal examination should be extended to yearly testing. If the PSA does not drop by at least 30 percent at 12 months, the patient should be rechecked at 18 months. If the PSA level is still unchanged, rises to above upper normal test limits, or shows two consecutive 6 month rises within the normal range, it is advisable to refer the patient for transrectal ultrasound to rule out prostate cancer.

Does finasteride mask prostate cancer? In a large double-blind study to date, prostate cancer was discovered as frequently in patients on finasteride as in those on placebo. However, if an undiagnosable early prostate cancer is present in a patient placed on finasteride therapy, the PSA level may indeed decrease because finasteride, an inhibitor of androgen-mediated action, has been shown to cause a significant decrease in PSA, an androgen-dependent protein, in advanced prostate cancer in a small double-blind study.

Because PSA is a good tumor marker for prostate cancer and predicts tumor mass, a small, undiagnosable early prostate cancer present at initiation of finasteride therapy would not become inoperable if the instructions outlined in this section on monitoring PSA are followed.

Routine monitoring of hormonal steroids or gland size measurements are not required as they do not correlate with clinical response.

Side Effects

As previously stated, no side effects associated with administration of 5 mg finasteride were noted on any organ system, plasma lipids, electrolytes, or chemistries. Other common complaints such as constipation, headache, or fatigue did not differ between finasteride-treated and placebo-treated patients in over 300 patients studied in each group in a phase III double-blind trial (see Table 2). Statistically significant differences between the placebo-treated and 5 mg finasteride-treated groups occurred in the following parameters: decreased libido occurred in 4.7 percent of the patients given finasteride compared with 1.3 percent of the placebo group. Likewise, complaints of decreased ejaculate were noted in 4.4 percent of the finasteride group compared with 1.7 percent of the placebo group. Impotence was also noted in 3.4 percent of the treated patients compared with 1.7 percent of the controls. No other differences of any kind were noted between the placebo and the treated groups in this large phase III trial.

The decrease in volume of ejaculate was anticipated as a side effect as the 5α-reductase inhibitor blocks prostate androgen-dependent function, which is to produce seminal fluid. Patients should be reassured about this; the complaint has no implications with regard to other aspects of sexual function or in regard to their general health.

An uncommon, but recently demonstrated, side effect of finasteride is gynecomastia. Although the drug has not generally been shown to affect serum estrogen levels, rarely it may promote gynecomastia in a patient by either decreasing the conversion of testosterone to dihydrotestosterone in breast tissue or by decreasing total androgen (testosterone plus dihydrotestosterone) because androgens are known to suppress the stimulatory effects of estrogens.

It is difficult in the BPH age group to be certain whether any drug under study is causing a sexual disorder because spontaneous decrease in sexual function occurs in men of this age. We suggest an off-drug trial for 1 to 2 months followed by rechallenge if indicated to determine whether a complaint regarding sexual dysfunction is drug related or coincidental.

Duration of Therapy

Initial therapy should be given to all patients for at least 6 months, the time it takes for a significant decrease in prostate size to occur; improvement in obstructive and irritative symptoms of BPH is seen by several months or more after size reduction. If therapy is effective in improving symptoms, treatment should be continued indefinitely as the gland will regrow if therapy stops.

Drug Interactions

Finasteride had no effect on drug levels or pharmacologic actions of propranolol, digoxin, theophylline, or warfarin. In addition, during large clinical trials finasteride was used concomitantly with a variety of commonly used drugs including angiotensin-converting enzyme inhibitors, analgesics, HMG CoA reductase inhibitors, nonsteroidal anti-inflammatory drugs, benzodiazepine compounds, H2-antagonists, and quinolone antibiotics without any clinically significant adverse actions, although blood levels of these drugs were not studied.

Contraindications

Pregnant women should not be exposed to the drug because the development of external genitalia in the male fetus may be affected. Men interested in reproduction should not be given finasteride because the effects of chronic administration of the drug on fertility are not known. Additionally, the drug is found in semen and theoretically might contaminate pregnant females and cause defects in the male fetus, although drug levels in semen are minuscule.

■ ADVANTAGES AND DISADVANTAGES OF TREATMENT

Anticipated Clinical Response

As previously noted, about 40 to 50 percent of patients in a large phase III double-blind controlled study showed unequivocal improvement in obstructive and irritative symptoms of prostatism. Based on a large phase III trial of approximately 200 patients given the 5 mg dose who have been followed in open extension for 3 years, stability of clinical symptoms and prostate size is maintained following initiation of therapy and thereafter at least for the interval stated. For the 50 to 60 percent of patients who, in spite of reduction in prostate size, have only modest or no clinical improvement following therapy, we suggest the following: If the patient has BPH with annoying but not quality-of-life–threatening symptoms, the outlook is good for stability at whatever level of prostatism exists as long as the patient continues taking the drug. If the patient is not satisfied with the result, he may elect to undergo surgery or to add an alpha$_1$-adrenergic blocker such as terazosin (Hytrin) or doxazosin (Cardura) to the regimen. No data are available regarding the effect of increasing the dosage of finasteride in patients unresponsive to the 5 mg dose.

Alpha$_1$-Adrenergic Blockers as Treatment for BPH

Two alpha$_1$-adrenergic blockers, terazosin and doxazosin, are now approved by the Food and Drug Administration for use in BPH.

Alpha$_1$-adrenergic blockers decrease smooth muscle tension at the bladder neck and in the prostate itself, which relieves the dynamic aspect of outlet obstruction; they have no effect on gland size. This relaxation of smooth muscle may result in easier and more complete emptying of the bladder

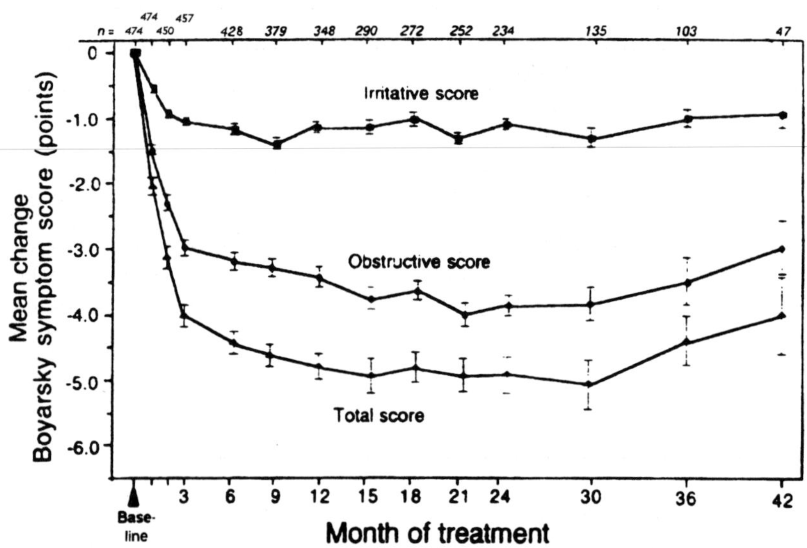

Figure 2
Mean change in Boyarsky symptom scores from baseline to 42 months. Baseline scores were 10.5 for total score, 6.2 for obstructive scores, and 4.3 for irritative scores. The numbers across the top of the graph indicate number of patients available at each time interval. All changes were significant at the $P \leq 0.05$ level. *(From Lepor H. Long-term efficacy and safety of terazosin in patients with benign prostatic hyperplasia. Urology 1995; 45:406–413; with permission.)*

and improvement in symptom score as shown in a large study reported by Lepor in 1995 (Fig. 2).

I do not recommend alpha$_1$-adrenergic blockers as primary medical therapy for BPH except in the case of patients with symptoms of BPH but relatively small prostates. Although the long-term effectiveness of finasteride in controlling prostate size has been well established, alpha$_1$-adrenergic blockers do not affect gland size. Therefore, if the prostate should continue to grow, as occurs in 25 percent of patients, this may be an overriding factor in the progression of prostatism. Although one publication has reported a 42 month follow-up of patients on alpha-blockers, significant patient numbers are available only for 3 years thus far (Lepor, 1995). A recent meta-analysis of alpha-blockers by Eri and Tveter indicated that "tolerance to treatment appeared to develop in a large proportion of patients after six months of therapy." It remains to be seen whether alpha$_1$-adrenergic blockers will be suitable for long-term medical management of BPH.

Alpha-blockers, however, may be very useful as adjunctive therapy in patients being treated medically for BPH, if the finasteride therapy does not adequately control symptoms. In addition, they can be used in conjunction with finasteride to treat patients in whom rapid symptom improvement in 1 to 2 weeks is important. Although alpha-blockers probably do not affect the long-term natural history of BPH as do the 5α-reductase inhibitors, clinical benefits of combining alpha-blockers with a 5α-reductase inhibitor may provide excellent long-term control of BPH.

Doxazosin has the longest half-life of the alpha-blockers available; it can be given once daily. The dose should be titrated by starting at 1 mg at bedtime and increasing the night dose by 1 mg every 4 days until the prostatism improves or postural dizziness secondary to postural hypotension supervenes. Other side effects of alpha-blockers include nasal stuffiness and fatigue.

Additional clinical trials of combined finasteride and alpha-blockers are currently under study.

Morbidity and Mortality Associated with Surgery

TURP is the usual surgery employed to treat BPH (Table 3). Mortality following TURP is 0.2 percent in patients 65 or younger according to a recent large series; however, in patients greater than 85 years of age, a 6.2 percent mortality has been recorded.

Morbidity following TURP has been reported to be 18 percent. This includes postoperative infections, bleeding complications, thromboembolic problems, and incontinence (see Table 3). Late complications of TURP include strictures in 0.6 to 5.0 percent of patients. Another common problem following TURP is retrograde ejaculation as a result of surgical impairment of the internal urethral sphincter.

Recurrence Rate of BPH Following TURP Versus Finasteride Treatment

The recurrence rate of BPH with requirement for repeat TURP is 10 percent at 5 years, 12 percent at 8 years, and 16 percent at 10 years. Finasteride appears to arrest BPH over a 5 year follow-up to date. Patients on open extension with finasteride are still being followed and long-term data on their continued treatment with the drug will be forthcoming. It must be re-emphasized that discontinuation of finasteride is followed by regrowth of the prostate and probable return of prostatism.

Table 3 Comparison of TURP with Finasteride

	TURP	FINASTERIDE
Mortality	Age 65 or less; 0.2% Age 85 or more; 6.2%	—
Morbidity	18% (includes incontinence of 0.4–3.3%)	—
Recurrence	Repeat TURP required in 12% at 8 years, 16% at 10 years	No evidence of tachyphylaxis up to 5 years
Clinical Effectiveness	3 yr following TURP: 75% well 15% unchanged 6% worse	Effect on volume reduction of 24% stable over 5 years; 40% of patients show >3 ml/sec increase in max flow rate over 3 years; symptom score decreased by 50% or more in 50% of patients at 3 years. All of these changes appear to be stable over 5 years in smaller subset of patients.
Impotence	Low	3.4%

Effectiveness of TURP Versus Finasteride

Surgery is usually done for advanced, bothersome symptoms of BPH. Approximately 75 percent of patients were asymptomatic at 5 to 8 years following surgery in one series; 75 percent of patients were improved, and 13 percent of patients were unchanged at follow-up 3 years after surgery in a second series; and 79 percent of patients were improved, 15 percent were unchanged, and 6 percent had worsened following TURP in a third series.

Finasteride treatment alone results in significant clinical improvement in prostatism when compared with a placebo group in a 1 year double-blind study recently completed. Using an identical questionnaire for patients treated with finasteride and patients treated with TURP, improvement in the finasteride group after 1 year of therapy was approximately 50 percent of that noted in the surgical patients at a 1 year follow-up. The groups were not necessarily matched for symptoms because patients treated with surgery may have had more advanced disease than those on finasteride.

In a 3 year open extension of a large phase III trial, 40 percent of patients treated with 5 mg finasteride a day for 3 years showed 3 ml per second or greater increase in maximal urinary flow rate compared to a maximum increase in flow rates of approximately 10 ml per second in 80 percent of patients 1 year following TURP.

Cost of Finasteride Versus Surgery

Finasteride costs approximately $500 per year. Based on the average cost of TURP, 10 years of finasteride therapy approximately equals the cost of prostate surgery.

Finasteride in Combination with Other Therapies

Currently, trials of combinations of finasteride with other drugs are being conducted to see if further clinical benefits can be achieved. As already mentioned, $alpha_1$-adrenergic blockers relieve smooth muscle tension in the bladder neck and prostate itself. A three-armed controlled trial comparing finasteride alone, an alpha-blocker alone, and a combination of both therapies is under way. In addition, aromatase inhibitors are being studied for possible inhibitory effects on prostate stromal growth. Estrogen receptors are found primarily in prostatic stroma; estrogen has been shown by Walsh and collaborators (1976) to increase nuclear androgen receptor concentration in studies in the dog prostate. This may be true in the human as well, although definitive data are lacking. If effective in reducing prostate size by a nonandrogenic mechanism, aromatase inhibitors may be useful in potentiating the clinical effects of finasteride. However, in a recent double-blind, randomized controlled trial, an aromatase inhibitor, Atamestane, did not show any clinical effectiveness or significant change in prostate size compared with controls in an 18 month trial.

This discussion has referred to a single 5α-reductase inhibitor, finasteride, as treatment for BPH. It is likely that several other 5α-reductase inhibitors will be put into clinical trials in the near future.

Suggested Reading

Barry MM, Fowler FJ Jr, O'Leary MP, et al. The American urological association symptom index for benign prostatic hyperplasia. J Urol 1992; 148:1549–1557.

Boyle P, Gould AL, Roehrborn CG. Prostate volume predicts outcome of treatment of benign prostatic hyperplasia with finasteride: Meta-analysis of randomized clinical trials. Urology 1996; 48:398–405.

Eri LM, Tveter KJ. α-Blockade in the treatment of symptomatic benign prostatic hyperplasia. J Urol 1995; 154:923–934.

Geller J. Effect of finasteride, a 5α-reductase inhibitor on prostate tissue androgens and prostate specific antigen. J Clin Endocrinol Metab 1990; 71:1552–1555.

Geller J. Benign prostatic hyperplasia: Pathogenesis and medical therapy. J Am Geriatr Soc 1991; 39:1208–1216.

Geller J. Non-surgical treatment of prostatic hyperplasia. Cancer 1992; 70: 339–345.

Geller J. Five-year followup of patients with benign prostatic hyperplasia treated with finasteride. Eur Urol 1995; 27:267–273.

Horton R. Benign prostatic hypertrophy: A disorder of androgen metabolism. Am J Geriatr 1984; 32:320.

Imperato-McGinley J, Guerrero L, Gautier T, et al. Steroid 5α-reductase deficiency in man: An inherited form of male pseudohermaphroditism. Science 1974; 186:1213–1215.

Isaacs J, Brendler C, Walsh P. Changes in the metabolism of dihydrotestosterone in the hyperplastic human prostate. J Clin Endocrinol Metab 1983; 56:139.

Lepor H. Long-term efficacy and safety of terazosin in patients with benign prostatic hyperplasia. Urology 1995; 45:406–413.

Lepor H. Nonoperative management of benign prostatic hyperplasia. J Urol 1989; 141:1283–1289.

Lepor H, Williford WO, Barry MJ, et al. The efficacy of terazosin, finasteride, or both in benign prostatic hyperplasia. N Engl J Med 1996; 335:533–539.

MK-906 (Finasteride) Study Group. One-year experience in the treatment of benign prostatic hyperplasia with finasteride. J Androl 1991; 12:372–375.

Moore E, Bracken B, Bremner W, et al. Proscar: Five-year experience. Eur Urol 1995; 28:304–309.

Moore RA. Benign hypertrophy and carcinoma of the prostate: Occurrence and experimental production in animals. Surgery 1944; 16:152.

Morimoto I, Edmiston A, Horton R. Alteration in the metabolism of dihydrotestosterone in elderly men with prostatic hyperplasia. J Clin Invest 1980; 66:612.

Siiteri P, Wilson J. DHT in prostatic hypertrophy. J Clin Invest 1970; 49: 1737.

Tunn UW, Kaivers P, Schweikert HU. Conservative treatment for human benign prostatic hyperplasia. In: Bruchovsky N, Chapdelaine A, Newmann F, eds. Regulation of androgen action. West Berlin: Congressdruck R Bruckner, 1985:87.

Walsh PC, Madden JD, Harrod MJ, et al. Familial incomplete male pseudohermaphroditism type 2: Decreased dihydrotestosterone formation in pseudovaginal perineoscrotal hypospadias. N Engl J Med 1974; 291:944–949.

Walsh P, Wilson J. The induction of prostatic hypertrophy in the dog with androstanediol. J Clin Invest 1976; 57:1093.

Wenderoth U, George F, Wilson J. The effect of 5α-reductase inhibitor on androgen mediated growth of dog prostate. Endocrinology 1983; 113:569.

Wilson J. The pathogenesis of benign prostatic hyperplasia. Am J Med 1980; 68:745.

TESTICULAR CANCER

Patrick J. Loehrer Sr., M.D.

Testicular cancer constitutes approximately 1 percent of malignancies, yet it is the most common cancer in young men. Despite the dramatic decrease in mortality over the past 2 decades, the incidence of this disease is increasing for unclear reasons. Improvement in the diagnostic imaging of patients, the advent of the reliable serum markers beta subunit human chorionic gonadotropin (BHCG) and alphafetoprotein (AFP), and most important, the development of effective systemic chemotherapy have been the major factors behind the progress in the treatment of this disease. Over 95 percent of those diagnosed with testicular cancer are curable with proper treatment, including 80 percent of patients who present with disseminated disease. This chapter focuses upon the recent advances and current controversies in the treatment of early- and advanced-stage germ cell neoplasms.

PRESENTATION AND DETECTION

Germ cell neoplasms can be divided into two histologic categories: seminoma and nonseminomatous germ cell tumors (embryonal carcinoma, yolk sac carcinoma, teratoma, choriocarcinoma, or any combination). The distinction between seminomatous and nonseminomatous germ cell tumors (NSGCT) is most important for patients with early-stage disease. Radiotherapy is the treatment of choice for early-stage seminoma. In contrast, early-stage NSGCT is primarily managed by surgery. Germ cell neoplasms most commonly arise within the gonads, but approximately 10 percent arise in extragonadal (usually midline) sites such as the retroperitoneum, mediastinum, and the pineal gland.

The typical presenting complaint of a patient with testicular cancer is an enlarging scrotal mass. Although the malignant testicular masses are usually painless, do not be led to believe that this is universal. The definitive diagnosis of testicular cancer is delayed in many patients with painful masses who are inappropriately treated with antibiotics for presumed epididymitis. Other presenting symptoms include back pain from enlargement of retroperitoneal lymph nodes; gynecomastia, unilateral or bilateral; and in patients with advanced disease, cough; dyspnea; hemoptysis; headache; and seizures.

Physical examination will reveal a mass not separable from testis. In patients with advanced abdominal disease, a palpable mass may be appreciated. With the exception of supraclavicular lymphadenopathy, peripheral adenopathy is not a feature of this disease. Testicular ultrasound is the best available noninvasive tool to detect testicular tumors. Transillumination of the scrotum may help distinguish whether a hydrocele is present but approximately 20 percent of patients with testicular cancer have an associated hydrocele. Patients with mediastinal germ cell tumors present with chest pain or cough. An association with Klinefelter syndrome and acute megakaryocytic leukemia has been well documented in patients with primary mediastinal tumors.

STAGING

The clinical staging of patients with testicular cancer is as follows: stage A, or I, in which cancer appears to be confined to the testis alone; stage B, or II, in which disease has spread to the retroperitoneal lymph nodes; and stage C, or III, which includes any supradiaphragmatic extension and pulmonary or other visceral organ involvement. The approximate frequency of presentation for each of these stages is 40, 40, and 20 percent for stages A, B, and C, respectively.

The initial evaluation is to determine whether a patient has early-stage disease requiring local treatment or more advanced disease, which requires systemic therapy. Patients with early-stage disease are generally treated with primary retroperitoneal lymphadenectomy (or surveillance, as will be discussed later) for NSGCT or radiotherapy for seminoma. For patients with bulky abdominal disease or any stage C disease, primary therapy should consist of cisplatin-based combination chemotherapy.

Evaluation should include a careful history and physical examination, radiographic evaluation including a chest x-ray film and a computed tomographic (CT) scan of the chest if chest x-ray film is normal and abdominal CT scan. About one-third of patients with clinical stage A disease will have retroperitoneal lymph node involvement despite normal serum markers. In addition, AFP and BHCG levels should be obtained. Approximately 90 percent of patients with advanced or recurrent testicular cancer have an elevation in one or both of these serum markers.

PROGNOSIS

Nonseminomatous Germ Cell Tumor

Approximately 10 percent of patients with pathologically proven stage A disease relapse following retroperitoneal lymphadenectomy (RPLND), but with close follow-up with chest x-ray film and markers, recurrences should be discovered in low tumor volume, when chemotherapy is highly effective. Patients who present with clinical stage A disease should have virtually a 100 percent chance for cure with RPLND and follow-up chemotherapy when needed.

The cure rate for patients with pathologic stage B disease is also excellent. Approximately 98 percent of such patients should be curable (50 to 70 percent with surgery alone and the remainder with salvage chemotherapy). Alternatively, two cycles of cisplatin-based adjuvant chemotherapy will virtually eliminate the chance of recurrence following complete resection of disease in a primary RPLND.

For patients with stage C disease, chemotherapy alone or with subsequent resection of residual disease will cure approximately 80 percent of patients. The cure rate for patients with minimal and moderate disease (Indiana staging system; see Table 3) is approximately 90 to 95 percent. For patients with advanced-stage disease, the cure rate is approximately 50 percent.

Seminoma

The primary treatment for clinical stage I seminoma is infradiaphragmatic radiotherapy, which is associated with a cancer-specific survival of 95 to 100 percent. For clinical stage II disease the prognosis with radiotherapy alone is approximately 95 percent for nonpalpable (or less than 5 cm) and 65 to 75 percent for palpable (at least 5 cm) disease treated with radiotherapy alone. The results with chemotherapy parallel those of NSGCT for stage C disease and largely depend on volume and distribution of disease.

MANAGEMENT

Clinical Stage A

The time-honored approach for a patient presenting with clinical stage A testicular cancer is RPLND. Properly performed, RPLND will cure approximately 70 percent of patients with carcinoma involving the lymph nodes with minimal chances of local recurrence. Approximately 10 percent of pathologic stage A patients and 30 percent of resected stage B patients will develop recurrent disease after primary RPLND. When monitored with monthly chest x-ray film and serum markers during the first year and every 2 months during the second year, virtually all patients with recurrent disease will present with minimal metastatic disease, for which the cure rate with cisplatin-based combination chemotherapy is 99 percent or greater.

One of the major drawbacks of a traditional bilateral RPLND as initial treatment of clinical stage A patients is retrograde ejaculation and sterility. In addition, 70 percent of patients will undergo this operation needlessly (i.e., without documentation of retroperitoneal metastases). Modifications of the RPLND have improved the ability to maintain antegrade ejaculation in over 80 percent of patients. Donohue and associates of Indiana University have recently developed a nerve-sparing RPLND in which the sympathetic nerves are carefully dissected, leading to maintenance of normal ejaculatory function and virtually eliminating retrograde ejaculation.

An alternative approach to clinical stage A disease is observation. This practice stems from concerns of surgically induced ejaculatory dysfunction and is supported by the tremendous success seen with chemotherapy for patients with advanced disease. Peckham and colleagues in England introduced surveillance for patients with clinical stage A disease. In similar trials in the United States such patients have been carefully followed with monthly chest x-ray film, markers, and every 2 months CT scans of the abdomen. These series had the anticipated 30 percent recurrence rate. In some series patients also were followed by lymphangiograms. Multivariate analysis has suggested several prognostic factors predicting relapse for clinical stage A patients, including invasion of the venous and lymphatic vessels, absence of yolk sac elements, and presence of undifferentiated (embryonal carcinoma) tumor. Unfortunately, even when all of these factors are present, the positive predictive values remain only 50 percent. In addition, the time of relapse differs from that of patients undergoing RPLND as primary therapy, whose recurrence after 2 years is quite uncommon, as there is a continuous 4 percent per year relapse rate beyond 2 years.

Approximately 5 to 12 percent of patients with recurrent disease following surveillance will not be cured because of greater tumor volume upon recurrence. One explanation is the reliability of patient and supportive service. CT scans must be of excellent quality and interpreted by skilled radiologists. For patients who recur with bulky abdominal disease and pulmonary metastases, a less favorable outcome with subsequent chemotherapy is achieved. Surveillance for patients with stage A disease remains an option *only* for the most highly motivated group of patients and physicians, who maintain a rigorous follow-up schedule including frequent

Table 1 Results of Sequential PVB Studies at Indiana University

YEAR OF STUDY	NO. OF PATIENTS	NO. WITH CR (%)	NED WITH SURGERY (%)	CURRENTLY NED (%)
1974–76	47	33 (70)	5 (11)	25 (57)
1976–78	78	51 (65)	13 (17)	57 (73)
1978–81	147	72 (63)	31 (21)	117 (80)

CR, complete remission; NED, no evidence of disease

CT scans of the abdomen. A modified retroperitoneal lymph node dissection, performed by a skilled urologist, remains the standard for the majority of patients. Efforts to delineate those patients clearly destined to benefit from RPLND are under way.

Stage B Disease

Stage B testicular cancer, which has spread to the retroperitoneal lymph nodes, can be subdivided into B1 (microscopic only), B2 (macroscopic but smaller than 10 cm), or B3 (palpable, or larger than 10 cm). Indications for surgical intervention for patients with stage B disease have been modified in the postcisplatin era. Nonetheless, RPLND alone in such patients is associated with a 50 to 70 percent relapse-free survival, making this one of the few malignancies with such a cure rate in the face of lymphatic involvement.

In light of the effectiveness of chemotherapy in metastatic disease, the issue of adjuvant therapy in patients with resected stage B disease was addressed by the Testicular Cancer Intergroup Study. Following RPLND, 195 patients with completely resected stage B disease were randomized to observation only or to receive two postoperative courses consisting of cisplatin and vinblastine and bleomycin (PVB) or a variation (VAB-6). This study confirmed that patients treated with surgery alone had a relapse rate of approximately 48 percent. All but three patients were subsequently cured with four cycles of systemic chemotherapy upon disease recurrence. In the patients who received two cycles of adjuvant therapy, there have been two recurrences and one cancer death. Thus, the overall survival of 98 to 99 percent was not significantly different between the two arms. This study demonstrated that two cycles of adjuvant chemotherapy would virtually eliminate the chance for disease recurrence; however, similar long-term results were attainable with patients who were carefully followed with monthly chest x-ray film and serum markers alone. It is important to recognize, however, that two cycles of adjuvant therapy does not supplant an inadequate RPLND. Patients who undergo debulking procedure should be treated with more aggressive combination chemotherapy (three or four cycles of therapy) as if they had metastatic disease.

Patients with early stage B disease manifested by elevated markers followed by orchiectomy or minimal abnormalities on CT scans present a mild therapeutic dilemma. Some investigators are exploring the option of giving systemic chemotherapy to such patients, reserving surgery for patients who have persistent residual disease. In general, patients who present with lymph nodes measuring 3 cm or less in greatest diameter should be referred to an experienced urologist for RPLND.

Stage C Disease

Combination chemotherapy is the mainstay of treatment for patients who present with advanced testicular cancer. The dramatic change in therapeutic outcome during the past 15 to 20 years has been outlined in several reviews. The single most important breakthrough came with the discovery of cisplatin and its activity in patients with refractory testicular cancer. Prior to the use of cisplatin, various regimens demonstrated objective remissions, but only rare patients attained durable, complete remissions. In 1974, Einborn at Indiana University combined cisplatin with the active drug combination of vinblastine and bleomycin to produce PVB. The rationale of this combination included single-agent activity, different mechanisms of action, and differing dose-limiting toxicities for each of the three drugs.

In the first 47 patients with disseminated germ cell tumor treated with PVB, 70 percent attained a complete remission, and an additional 11 percent were rendered free of disease with surgical extirpation of residual disease, which revealed teratoma of persistent carcinoma. Two additional cycles of chemotherapy were administered to patients with resected carcinoma. Of these patients, 57 percent remain continuously free of disease. Subsequent trials at Indiana University and the Southeastern Cancer Study Group confirmed this activity (Table 1).

Although 70 percent of patients would be cured of their disease with PVB, a cohort of patients would be candidates for salvage chemotherapy. At that time, for patients progressing on cisplatin, etoposide (VP-16) was the only phase II drug evaluated that demonstrated single-agent activity. Based upon preclinical data demonstrating synergy of cisplatin plus etoposide, this combination was used as salvage therapy in patients failing to be cured with initial PVB therapy. Approximately 25 to 30 percent of such patients were subsequently cured. This formed the basis of a prospective randomized trial that compared cisplatin plus etoposide plus bleomycin (PVP-16B) with PVB (Table 2). Also, 89 of 121 (73.5 percent) patients who were treated with PVB compared with 102 of 123 (83 percent) treated with PVP-16B obtained a complete remission or were rendered disease free following resection of teratoma or carcinoma. Although hematologic toxicity was comparable in the two groups of patients, neuromuscular side effects including paresthesias, myalgias, and abdominal cramps were significantly less in patients receiving PVP-16B. Furthermore, for patients with advanced disease, the PVP-16B regimen was associated with a significantly improved survival. Therefore, PVP-16B has become the preferred induction chemotherapy for metastatic disease.

Evaluation of patients with disseminated germ cell tumors has led to various staging systems to evaluate prognosis. The Indiana University staging system (Table 3) separated patients with good-risk (minimal and moderate) disease (over 90 percent cure rate) from patients with advanced disease with a 50 to 60 percent cure rate. Subsequent research strategies have turned to minimizing toxicity for patients

Table 2 Treatment Arms of Southeastern Cancer Study Group Trial Comparing PVB and PVP-16B

R	Cisplatin 20 mg/m^2 × 5 days every 3 weeks × 4
A	Vinblastine 0.15 mg/kg days 1 and 2 every 3 weeks × 4
N	Bleomycin 30 units weekly × 12
D	
O	
M	
I	Cisplatin 20 mg/m^2 × 5 days every 3 weeks × 4
Z	VP-16 100 mg/m^2 × 5 days every 3 weeks × 4
E	Bleomycin 30 units weekly × 12

Table 3 Indiana University Staging System for Disseminated Testicular Cancer

Minimal Extent
1. Elevated markers only
2. Cervical nodes (± nonpalpable retroperitoneal nodes)
3. Unresectable, nonpalpable retroperitoneal disease
4. Fewer than five pulmonary metastases per lung field and largest <2 cm ± nonpalpable retroperitoneal nodes

Moderate
1. Palpable abdominal mass only (no supradiaphragmatic disease)
2. Moderate pulmonary metastases: 5–10 metastases per lung field and largest <3 cm OR solitary pulmonary metastasis of any size >2 cm ± nonpalpable retroperitoneal disease

Advanced
1. Advanced pulmonary metastases: Any primary mediastinal nonseminomatous germ cell tumor, primary mediastinal seminoma >50% of intrathoracic diameter OR >10 pulmonary metastases per lung field OR multiple pulmonary metastases with largest >3 cm ± nonpalpable retroperitoneal disease
2. Palpable abdominal mass + supradiaphragmatic disease
3. Liver, bone, or CNS metastases

with good-risk disease while looking at more innovative and intense therapy for patients with poor prognosis.

Good-Risk Testicular Cancer

The Southeastern Cancer Study Group subsequently completed a trial to evaluate the optimal duration of therapy with good-risk disease. In 184 patients with minimal or moderate disease, therapy was either the standard four cycles of PVP-16B over 12 weeks or three cycles of the same regimen over 9 weeks. Of 96 patients, 93 (97 percent) randomized to receive four cycles of therapy achieved a disease-free status compared with 86 of 88 (98 percent) patients receiving three cycles. Overall, 91 and 92 percent of the patients, respectively, remain continuously free of disease with three and four cycles, respectively. Thus, therapy in good-risk disease can be shortened to three cycles of therapy in just 9 weeks.

Alternative treatment studies in good-risk disease have looked at the omission of bleomycin. In a trial reported by the Australian Germ Cell Neoplasm Trial Group, 104 patients received either PVB or the same regimen without bleomycin (PV). Although differences in the complete remission rate (89 versus 94 percent), relapse rate (7 versus 5 percent) respectively were not statistically different between PV and PVB, deaths for progressive cancer were (15 versus 5 percent; $p = 0.02$). In another trial performed by investigators at Memorial Sloan-Kettering Cancer Center, 140 good-risk patients randomized to receive VAB-6 or four cycles of cisplatin plus etoposide (EP). No significant differences between these two regimens were noted. Another trial in good-risk disease was conducted by the European Organization for Research on Treatment of Cancer. Patients were randomized to receive cisplatin plus etoposide (120 mg per square meter days 1, 3, 5) alone or with weekly bleomycin. Although initially there was no advantage with the addition of bleomycin, with longer follow-up, an increased recurrence rate is suggested for patients who did not receive bleomycin.

The Eastern Cooperative Oncology Group performed a prospective randomized trial comparing EP alone or with bleomycin (BEP). In 172 patients with minimal or moderate disease entered on this trial, disease-free status was achieved in 82 of 86 (95 percent) with BEP and 78 of 86 (90 percent) with EP. However, the number of patients with unfavorable outcomes (persistent carcinoma, relapse, death) was much greater in the EP group. Only 60 of 86 (70 percent) of patients treated with EP compared with 74 of 86 (86 percent) treated with BEP remain continuously disease free ($p = 0.03$). This cumulative experience underscored the importance of bleomycin when three cycles of cisplatin plus etoposide combination therapy is administered to patients with good-risk disease.

In another attempt to modify cisplatin plus etoposide, Memorial Sloan-Kettering Cancer Center and the Southwest Oncology Group (SWOG) evaluated the substitution of carboplatin for cisplatin. Unfortunately, greater myelosuppression and relapses were noted in the patients treated with carboplatin. In sum, these trials appear to have clarified the minimum threshold of therapy for patients with good-risk disease to be three cycles of BEP or four cycles of EP.

Poor-Risk Patients

In a retrospective review of prospective clinical trial data in germ cell neoplasms, improved survival is associated with patients who receive more intense cisplatin (33 mg per square meter per week versus no more than 25 mg per square meter per week) dosage. This seems to support the concept of dose intensity in this disease. In one prospective randomized trial performed by SWOG patients who received 120 mg per square meter of cisplatin had a significant improvement in response rate and overall survival over those of patients treated with 75 mg per square meter (both groups receiving vinblastine and bleomycin). Whether further escalation of cisplatin dosage can improve the therapeutic outcome was uncertain. Ozols and his colleagues at the National Cancer Institute reported a trial using high dosages of cisplatin (40 mg per square meter daily for 5 days) in combination with etoposide, bleomycin, and vinblastine (PVeBV). Later, in a prospective randomized trial comparing PVeBV with PVB using standard-dose cisplatin, an improvement in response rate and survival was noted in patients treated with the high-dose regimen. However, it was unclear whether the improvement in survival in this latter study was associated with the intense cisplatin or the addition of etoposide.

As a consequence, a prospective randomized trial by the Southeastern Cancer Study Group, Indiana University, and SWOG randomly assigned patients to receive cisplatin at two

Table 4 Consensus Conference Criteria for Good- and Poor-Risk Testicular Cancer Patients

NONSEMINOMA

Good Prognosis

All of the following:

- AFP <1,000 ng/mL, HCG <5,000 IU/L, and LDH <1.5 × upper limit of normal
- Nonmediastinal primary
- No nonpulmonary visceral metastasis

Intermediate Prognosis

All of the following:

- AFP = 1,000–10,000 ng/mL, HCG = 5,000–50,000 IU/L, or LDH = 1.5 to 10 × normal
- Nonmediastinal primary site
- No nonpulmonary visceral metastasis

Poor Prognosis

Any of the following:

- AFP >10,000 ng/mL, HCG >50,000 IU/L, or LDH >10 × normal
- Mediastinal primary site
- Nonpulmonary visceral metastasis present

SEMINOMA

Good Prognosis

- No nonpulmonary visceral metastasis

Intermediate Prognosis

- Nonpulmonary visceral metastasis present

dosages, 20 mg per square meter and 40 mg per square meter daily for 5 days, with the identical dosages of etoposide (100 mg per square meter daily for 5 days) and bleomycin (30 U per week for 12 weeks). From October 1984 through August 1989, 150 patients with advanced germ cell tumors were entered on this protocol. Some 44 of 68 patients treated with the high-dose cisplatin (65 percent) achieved a disease-free status with chemotherapy or resection of teratoma and carcinoma, compared with 51 of 73 (70 percent) treated with standard-dose therapy. There was significantly greater neurologic and hematologic toxicity associated with the more intense regimen. Thus, doubling the dose of cisplatin, the most effective single agent in germ cell malignancies, did not improve the therapeutic outcome of such patients.

Most recently a large progressive intergroup trial evaluated the role of ifosfamide as part of initial induction chemotherapy for patients with advanced disease. Preliminary results from this trial demonstrated a disease-free status in 66 of 130 (51 percent) patients treated with four cycles of BEP compared with 78 of 136 (57 percent) patients treated with four cycles of cisplatin, etoposide, and ifosfamide (VIP). However, the toxicity, primarily hematologic, was greater on the VIP arm, leaving BEP as the standard treatment regimen for advanced disease.

Currently, an intergroup trial is evaluating the role of BEP × four cycles versus BEP × two followed by tandem transplants with high-dose chemotherapy. The trial incorporates the new international staging system (Table 4).

Salvage Therapy

Although virtually all patients respond to initial induction chemotherapy, early recognition of resistance is important. Observation of the decline of serum markers provides some early clues. For instance, at least a 1 log reduction of BHCG should occur with each successful course of therapy (e.g., 10,000 to 1,000 to 100 to 10 . . .). Salvage regimens can be successfully implemented before the overt development of resistance to cisplatin manifested by rising markers on therapy. Furthermore, persistent elevation of markers may occur with cancer within sanctuary sites such as the brain or testis. Occasionally, patients inappropriately were given salvage chemotherapy based on erroneous impressions of tumor progression either with growing benign teratoma on therapy, false elevations of serum markers with BHCG (marijuana, cross-reactivity with luteinizing hormone, antibodies), or AFP (hepatitis). Pseudonodules on chest radiographs may occur with bleomycin and may mimic metastatic disease.

Despite the success of cisplatin combination chemotherapy over the past 20 years, approximately 20 to 30 percent of patients with disseminated germ cell tumors will be candidates for salvage chemotherapy. In such patients phase II trials have demonstrated activity of several drugs, including etoposide and ifosfamide.

Ifosfamide is an oxazaphosphorine (analogue of cyclophosphamide) found to be active in cisplatin-refractory patients by investigators in Europe and in the United States. Yet as with single-agent etoposide in the salvage setting, ifosfamide alone failed to produce durable complete remissions. In a trial at Indiana University, 56 patients who were previously treated with cisplatin, vinblastine, and etoposide were treated with a regimen of cisplatin, ifosfamide, and either vinblastine (VelP) or etoposide (VIP). Overall, 20 (36 percent) patients achieved disease-free status, and 19 patients remain disease free for 16 to 63 months, including nine patients remaining continuously free of disease. As initial salvage therapy for BEP failures, VelP produces durable complete remissions in approximately 30 percent of patients previously treated with BEP chemotherapy.

In a further effort to overcome drug resistance, high-dose chemotherapy with autologous bone marrow rescue was developed. The regimen developed at Indiana University used two courses of high-dosage carboplatin (900 to 2,000 mg per square meter) plus etoposide (1.2 g per square meter), each followed by autologous bone marrow transplant. In 20 highly refractory patients receiving this therapy, durable complete remission was attained in five (25 percent) patients. As part of a trial in second-line therapy, two cycles of conventional chemotherapy followed by one cycle of high-dose chemotherapy with autologous bone marrow transplant was performed. Seven of 18 (39 percent) patients who received therapy achieved a durable complete remission. Further efforts to improve results are under way with one or two cycles of standard induction therapy followed by two courses of high-dose chemotherapy with bone marrow transplant. Desperation surgery for patients with localized disease is another option in refractory disease. Approximately 20 percent of selected patients have achieved durable complete remissions in this setting.

Toxicity of Chemotherapy

The acute toxicity associated with chemotherapy is well recognized. Although nephrotoxicity was a serious problem in early phase II trials with cisplatin, with adequate hydration clinically significant nephrotoxicity is relatively uncommon.

Nonetheless, be cautious with concurrent use of other nephrotoxic agents, including contrast dyes and aminoglycosides.

Nausea and emesis have historically been the major acute toxicity for patients treated with cisplatin combination chemotherapy. However, this toxicity has largely been abrogated with the use of combination antiemetic therapies as well as newer 5 Hydroxytriptomine ($5HT_3$) antagonists, which minimize and frequently eliminate nausea and vomiting associated with cisplatin. Raynaud's phenomenon has been reported with bleomycin and appears to be enhanced with cisplatin. Persistent paresthesias is a dose-related toxicity. Although there is some controversy as to the potential for cardiovascular complications of cisplatin combination chemotherapy, a recent analysis of patients who were treated on a testicular cancer intergroup trial revealed no significant difference in hypertension, coronary artery disease, or cerebral vascular events in patients who were observed versus those receiving two or four cycles of cisplatin-based combination chemotherapy.

Most patients who present with disseminated germ cell tumors are severely oligospermic or azospermic. Following four cycles of PVB, 96 percent of patients are azospermic. However, with time, approximately half of patients will have a normal sperm count and motility. Thus far, no congenital abnormalities have been observed in the children of patients who have undergone this therapy.

In a review of 207 previously treated patients with a minimal follow-up of 5 years, I noted relatively few long-term severe side effects other than sterility and Raynaud's phenomenon. Late recurrences of cancer and leukemia are generally not observed in the absence of the use of more classic alkylating agents other than cisplatin.

Recurrence beyond 2 years is unusual in testicular cancer and has generally been associated with resection of benign teratoma or persistent abdominal disease which implies residual teratoma. Nonetheless, about 2 to 3 percent of recurrences have been beyond 2 years. Virtually none of these patients are cured with chemotherapy alone. As a consequence, surgery is the mainstay of treatment. There is, however, a close association between mediastinal germ cell malignancies and acute megakaryocytic leukemia.

More recently acute leukemia associated with etoposide (generally greater than 400 mg per square meter cumulative dose) has been reported but still represents only 1 percent of treated patients.

Seminoma

As mentioned previously, early-stage seminoma can be treated with radiotherapy in lieu of a RPLND with a 95 percent cure rate. Low levels of BHCG may be observed in some patients with pure seminoma, and in general they are treated as having seminoma without elevation of markers. However, any patient who has nonseminomatous elements or an elevated AFP should be treated as a similarly staged patient with NSGCT.

Some controversy exists regarding the role of observation for clinical stage A patients. Thomas and associates in Canada have reported that a recurrence rate of clinical stage I seminoma patients is much less frequent than previously appreciated (fewer than 10 percent). Yet other investigators are concerned with the surveillance policy for patients with seminoma, who may recur with more advanced disease, as they differ from NSGCT in that they rarely have elevated serum markers on recurrence.

The most appropriate treatment approach for patients with bulky stage B disease is controversial. Approximately 60 percent of patients will be cured with infradiaphragmatic radiotherapy alone. Cisplatin-based chemotherapy should be successful for the vast majority of those who recur following radiotherapy. Prophylactic mediastinal radiotherapy does not appear to improve the cure rate for stage B disease but will significantly impair the ability to give full-dose chemotherapy to patients failing to be cured and is associated with increased risk of a second malignancy and cardiovascular complications. Chemotherapy without radiotherapy should cure over 90 percent of previously untreated patients with bulky stage B seminoma. Therefore, either infradiaphragmatic radiotherapy or cisplatin combination chemotherapy is a reasonable therapeutic option for patients with stage B disease.

Cisplatin-based combination chemotherapy is the treatment of choice for patients with advanced seminoma. These patients have a similar prognosis as those with similarly staged NSGCT. Extensive prior radiotherapy (mediastinal and infradiaphragmatic) and extent of disease (Indiana staging system) seem to indicate relatively poor prognosis. Management of seminoma patients with residual bulky disease following chemotherapy is unclear. Some data suggests that residual masses 3 cm or larger have a greater chance of being persistent carcinoma. In such cases resection may be difficult, and careful observation by serial CT scans is a viable option.

Extragonadal Germ Cell Tumors

Although commonly arising in the testis, germ cell tumors may arise at various midline structures, such as the mediastinum, retroperitoneum, or pineal gland. Historically, patients with extragonadal germ cell tumors present with more advanced disease leading to a poorer outcome with therapy, but in general they have a similar chemosensitive response to that of their testicular cancer counterparts.

Primary mediastinal germ cell tumors appear unique in their propensity to present with more advanced disease as well as their association with chromosomal abnormalities and atypical syndromes. A close association with Klinefelter's syndrome and primary mediastinal tumors has been recently elucidated. Furthermore, the development of non–germ cell malignancies (e.g., sarcomatous elements, adenocarcinoma), acute megakaryocytic leukemia and other myelodysplastic disorders occur much more frequently in patients with mediastinal germ cell tumors than in patients with germ cell neoplasms of testicular origin.

Extragonadal germ cell tumors must be considered in the differential diagnosis of a patient with a carcinoma of unknown primary. The typical profile of such a patient is a young man with mediastinal or retroperitoneal tumor. For such patients serum HCG and AFP should be performed. An empiric trial of PVP-16B should be strongly considered for such patients. Approximately 50 to 60 percent of patients with extragonadal germ cell tumors should be cured with cisplatin combination chemotherapy, with complete excision of residual disease being extremely important.

Table 5 Treatment Recommendations

CLINICAL SETTING	STANDARD THERAPY	INVESTIGATIVE THERAPY
NSGCT		
Stage A	Retroperitoneal lymphadenopathy modified or nerve sparing	Surveillance (including first year) CT scan of abdomen every 2 months; chest x-ray and markers (AFP, BHCG, LDH) q month × 1 year. Second year: Abdominal CT q 4 months with chest x-ray and serum markers every 2 months.
Stage B1 or B2 (S/P RPLND)	Observation with PVP-16B on relapse OR two cycles of PVP-16B as adjuvant	None
Stage B3 or C		
Minimal or moderate	PVP-16B × 3 cycles (or PVP-16 × 4 cycles) plus resection of residual disease	None
Advance	PVP-16B × 4 cycles plus resection of residual disease	Clinical trials ongoing such as PVP-16B plus ABMT
Seminoma		
Stage A	Infradiaphragmatic radiotherapy (2,500 cGy)	Surveillance (including first year) CT scan of abdomen every 2 months, chest x-ray and markers (AFP, BHCG, LDH) q month × 1 year. Second year: Abdominal CT q 4 months with chest x-ray and serum markers every 2 months.
Stage B1 or B2 (<5 cm)	Infradiaphragmatic radiotherapy (2,500 cGy)	
Stage B3 (palpable or ≥5 cm)	Infradiaphragmatic radiotherapy or cisplatin-based combination chemotherapy (PVP-16B or PVP-16 × 4 cycles)	Management of residual mass of ≥3 cm following chemotherapy is controversial (observe or resect)
Stage C	Cisplatin-based combination chemotherapy (PVP-16B × 3 or 4 cycles)	Clinical trials based upon tumor extent

■ COMMENTS

Successful use of combination chemotherapy for metastatic disease has made a major impact on the prognosis of patients with disseminated germ cell tumors. Current therapeutic recommendations are demonstrated in Table 5; the continued direction of clinical research is to evaluate novel approaches for patients with advanced disease.

Acknowledgement

Supported in part by The Walther Cancer Institute, NCI Grant #2 R 35 CA 39844-08, The Cancer Center Planning Grant #P 20 CA 57114-02, The General Clinical Research Center #MO 1 RR 00750-06, and R 10 CA 28171-04 from the Public Health Service.

Suggested Reading

Einborn LH. Treatment of testicular cancer: A new and improved model. J Clin Oncol 1990; 8:1777–1781.

Horwich A, Dearnaley DP. Treatment of seminoma. Semin Oncol 1992; 19: 171–180.

Loehrer PJ, Sledge GW, Einhorn L. Heterogeneity among germ cell tumors of the testis. Semin Oncol 1985; 304–316.

Rorth M. Therapeutic alternatives in clinical stage I nonseminomatous disease. Semin Oncol 1992; 19:190–196.

Williams SD, Birch R, Einhorn LH, et al. Disseminated germ cell tumors: Chemotherapy with cisplatin plus bleomycin plus either vinblastine or etoposide: A trial of the Southeastern Cancer Study Group. N Engl J Med 1987; 316:1435–1440.

SARCOMA: CHEMOTHERAPY

Mark M. Zalupski, M.D.
Laurence H. Baker, D.O.

The treatment of patients with soft-tissue sarcoma presents a significant challenge because of a number of factors associated with this tumor. Soft-tissue sarcoma is uncommon, accounting for approximately 1 percent of all cancers diagnosed annually in the United States. Yet within this group of uncommon cancers there is great heterogeneity in behavior. The intent of therapy in most patients with soft-tissue sarcoma is curative, but the cancer can be fatal, and there is increased morbidity and mortality when it is managed inappropriately. The variety of histologies and sites of presentation in association with its rarity places soft-tissue sarcoma among the least well understood and poorly treated of all cancers.

The use of systemic chemotherapy for soft-tissue sarcoma is evolving. Variables recognized to influence outcome to systemic therapy include histologic grade of the tumor, site of metastasis, and in some instances histologic type of the tumor. With metastatic disease limited to the lung, dose-intensive doxorubicin combinations have been associated with high response rates, and in combination with surgical resection they offer hope for sustained remission. Patients with extrapulmonary metastasis, conversely, rarely benefit from an aggressive surgical approach, and therefore, the likelihood of complete remission is less, which suggests a decreased role for aggressive combination chemotherapy. Patients with low-grade disease may do well with a single drug or sequential administration of active agents, with less toxicity than with combination chemotherapy. In primary disease the risk of metastasis in patients with large, high-grade lesions is significant, prompting continued investigation of adjuvant systemic therapy. In addition to benefits for distant disease control, adjuvant chemotherapy may improve local control. Functional considerations in primary management have led to a re-examination of the role of chemotherapy as an adjunct to surgery, particularly preoperative chemotherapy, in this disease.

■ PATHOLOGY AND PROGNOSTIC FACTORS

The histologic classification of a soft-tissue sarcoma is based on the benign mesenchymal counterpart of the presumed origin of the malignant cell. Inconsistencies in this classification and variation in the reported frequency of sarcoma types are due to interobserver differences in assignment of type and the existence of sarcomas that remain unclassified. While the histologic type of soft-tissue sarcoma is associated with prognosis, it appears the histologic grade of the tumor is of greater significance.

A number of investigators have shown strong correlations with histopathologic grade, disease-free survival, and overall survival for specific histologic types and within mixed series of soft-tissue sarcomas. The importance of histopathologic grade is recognized in the staging system for this disease. Histopathologists assign sarcoma grade based on mitotic rate, extent of necrosis, vascularity, tumor matrix, nuclear pleomorphism, and tumor cellularity. The precision of this grading depends on the experience of the pathologist and is hindered by tumor heterogeneity and the subjectivity of the characteristics that determine grade. For example, Coindre and associates reported only a 75 percent consensus regarding grade between a study and reference group of pathologists. Nevertheless, even with this imprecision, the designation of grade is the most important variable in predicting the subsequent behavior of soft-tissue sarcomas. The grade is reported, depending on the institution, on a two-, three-, or four-grade scale.

Clinical treatment decisions are based primarily on grade, although other factors have also been shown to influence therapy and prognosis. Both site and size of the tumor are important in determining local therapy and have prognostic value independent of histopathologic grade. Similarly, the depth and compartmentalization of the tumor influence the outcome of therapy in this disease. In most instances the histopathologic type is not as important in therapy or prognosis as the other factors just discussed. Exceptions to this statement include histologically uniformly high-grade sarcomas (e.g., rhabdomyosarcoma) and histologic types in which standard therapy approaches have been demonstrated to be ineffective (e.g., gastrointestinal leiomyosarcomas). Recent clinical trials in metastatic disease have also suggested differences in response rate based on assigned histologic type. The clinical utility of these observations of variable response rates between types is undergoing further evaluation.

Biologic parameters being studied as prognostic factors for localized soft-tissue sarcoma include DNA content, cytogenetic aberrations, and protein products of oncogenes and tumor suppressor genes. Sarcomas with abnormal DNA content (DNA aneuploid) have been shown to have a higher risk of metastasis than DNA diploid tumors. In some instances DNA ploidy has also been shown to correlate with response to cytotoxic therapy. Karyotypes of soft-tissue sarcomas are being increasingly reported, and besides being useful for diagnostic purposes, cytogenetic aberrations may soon provide prognostic information as well as identifying areas warranting further molecular study. Activation of oncogenes and loss or mutation of tumor suppressor genes (retinoblastoma and P53) have been described in sarcomas and are likely to relate to clinical behavior of individual tumors. The union of clinical observation and biologic findings will be at the core of improving the outcome in the future for patients afflicted with these diseases.

■ PRIMARY MANAGEMENT

While the treatment of soft-tissue sarcomas must be individualized, a few principles are applicable. Due to the propensity of soft-tissue sarcomas to recur locally and for treatment to result in loss of function, primary therapy must be carefully considered and executed. To obtain local control, radical or wide surgical margins are necessary when surgery is the sole primary therapy. The breadth of the surgical margin is influenced by the grade, size, and site of the primary tumor. Acceptable local control with the combination of radiotherapy and a smaller surgical margin than with surgical therapy alone has led to functional as well as therapeutic considerations when planning primary therapy. Increasing application of preoperative therapies, including radiation and/or chemotherapy, appears to be achieving local control previously seen only with radical operations. In addition to functional considerations, theoretic advantages to preoperative therapies include earlier exposure of any micrometastasis to systemic chemotherapy and in vivo assessment of the effectiveness of therapy through evaluation of histopathologic necrosis and other experimental parameters. The relative value of the different local therapeutic approaches can be assessed only in randomized clinical trials. The details of local therapies are discussed elsewhere in this text.

Sarcomas arising in visceral sites necessitate special consideration regarding primary therapy. Because of their internal location visceral sarcomas are generally advanced when diagnosed, and the surgical principles regarding compartmental resection of sarcomas are often not applicable because of the lack of natural barriers to sarcoma extension. The effective use of adjunctive radiotherapy is made more difficult in this situation because of the radiosensitive organs in the field at risk for recurrence. The use of adjuvant chemotherapy has no demonstrated value in this setting. Alternative approaches to delivering radiotherapy, such as brachytherapy, the use of radiosensitizers, innovative sequencing, and delivery of chemotherapy must be explored as additional therapies to surgery in this setting.

■ ADJUVANT THERAPY

The randomized adjuvant chemotherapy studies conducted to date in soft-tissue sarcoma are inconclusive regarding the value of systemic treatment. Most of the trials show a trend in favor of adjuvant therapy, although in only two trials is a statistically significant improvement in survival observed with such treatment. Combining all trials, a summary overview using published data suggested improvements in survival and disease-free survival of approximately 15 and 30 percent respectively with adjuvant therapy.

Risk factors for the development of metastatic disease following primary management of extremity soft-tissue sarcoma include grade, size, and depth of the primary tumor. Patients with high-grade lesions larger than 5 cm and deep to the superficial fascia have been reported to have approximately a 75 percent risk of developing metastatic disease, half within 18 months of diagnosis. The use of adjuvant chemotherapy in high-grade lesions is considered investigational and optimally should be given in a clinical trial. If an adjuvant study is not available, however, treatment of patients with high-grade nonvisceral lesions larger than 5 cm is probably warranted from the available data. Currently, adjuvant chemotherapy cannot be recommended for low- or intermediate-grade lesions that have received adequate primary treatment.

Table 1 MAID Chemotherapy

Doxorubicin 60 mg/m^2 IV over 96 hr
Dacarbazine (DTIC) 1 g/m^2 IV over 96 hr
Ifosfamide 2 g/m^2 over 24 hr qd for 3 days
Mesna 2 g/m^2 over 24 hr qd for 4 days

Primary or preoperative chemotherapy for high-grade soft-tissue sarcoma is under investigation in a number of centers. Favorable effects on the primary tumor, including the conversion of patients from amputation to limb salvage candidates, have been demonstrated. In addition to a possible benefit for local control, the earlier application of intensive chemotherapy in high-grade soft-tissue sarcoma may result in improved control of micrometastatic disease. Both experimental and clinical data support a relationship between tumor burden and the ability to eradicate tumor with chemotherapy. The Southwest Oncology Group (SWOG) is doing a pilot study of preoperative MAID chemotherapy (doxorubicin, ifosfamide, dacarbazine, and Mesna; see Table 1) in patients with large, high-grade extremity and trunk lesions. Primary tumor regression has been observed in approximately one-third of the cases, and while follow-up is short, local and distant disease control rates have been high with this approach.

■ METASTATIC DISEASE

Metastatic soft-tissue sarcoma can occasionally be cured. Aggressive use of surgery for pulmonary metastasis is reported to result in long-term survival in up to 25 percent of patients treated in this manner. Larger chemotherapy series also report that approximately one-third of patients who achieve complete remission with chemotherapy, albeit a small minority, enjoy long-term disease-free survival. Attempting to increase the number of patients rendered disease free with the use of multimodality therapies in metastatic soft-tissue sarcoma appears warranted.

The majority of patients with metastatic soft-tissue sarcoma develop disease initially restricted to the lungs. A surgical approach to pulmonary metastasis should be considered in such patients. The doubling time of the metastatic nodules, the number of metastases, and the disease-free interval from primary disease to metastasis all influence the likelihood of disease control with surgery in this setting. Patients with bilateral pulmonary disease, synchronous metastatic disease, and extrapulmonary disease should not be considered categorically unresectable. As improvements are made in the systemic therapy of sarcoma, the role of surgery in metastatic disease will likely increase.

Using a surgical approach discussed above, it is unclear what role, if any, chemotherapy has in the patients' postoperative treatment. Patients failing following pulmonary metastatectomy do so because of progression of unrecognized micrometastatic lesions. It has been reported that patients achieving partial response to chemotherapy, subsequently rendered disease free through surgery, have an equivalent survival to patients achieving complete response to chemotherapy alone. We have adopted the approach of treating patients with pulmonary metastasis with two or more cycles of chemotherapy prior to surgical resection. Patients demonstrating a partial or minor response are continued postoperatively with the same combination in an effort to eliminate microscopic foci of disease. Patients without response and those with disease progression need not be treated postoperatively or can be treated with different drugs following surgery in an attempt to consolidate the remission obtained through surgery. The optimal approach to combining surgery and chemotherapy for metastatic disease must be studied further.

The most active chemotherapeutic agent for the treatment of soft-tissue sarcoma is doxorubicin. Its activity in sarcoma was identified soon after its clinical introduction. The response rate to single-agent doxorubicin in soft-tissue sarcoma ranges from 15 to 35 percent. Complete responses, some of long duration, have been observed. A dose-response relationship with doxorubicin is the cornerstone of therapeutic strategy in soft-tissue sarcoma.

The utility of doxorubicin as an anticancer agent is limited by the cumulative cardiotoxicity produced by this drug. It appears that doxorubicin can be given to a greater cumulative dose by an infusional schedule (48 to 96 hours) with a lower risk of cardiotoxicity than comparable doses delivered as a bolus. When used as a single agent in soft-tissue sarcoma, doxorubicin can be administered in doses of 60 to 90 mg per meter squared depending on patient tolerance.

Ifosfamide is an important drug in the treatment of soft-tissue sarcoma. Phase II studies with ifosfamide have demonstrated response rates of 20 to 40 percent. Significantly, responses have been observed in patients who progressed on doxorubicin. Additionally, ifosfamide is the only single agent besides doxorubicin that reliably produces complete responses in this disease.

Ifosfamide has been administered in sarcoma as a single agent in cycles of 1 to 5 days. With daily doses of 3 g per meter squared or greater, neurotoxicity has been reported. To maximize dose and safety, ifosfamide is generally given over 3 to 5 days with a total dose of 7.5 to 10 g per meter squared per cycle. Infusional administration of ifosfamide has been studied and has produced less neurotoxicity. Ifosfamide must be given with attention to hydration and concurrently with the uroprotector Mesna to prevent urothelial toxicity.

More recently, higher doses of ifosfamide, 12 to 16 g per meter squared per course, have been reported to produce responses in patients who progressed on lower doses of ifosfamide. This intensity of therapy is associated with renal toxicity requiring attention to fluids and electrolytes, neurotoxicity, and profound myelosuppression requiring growth factor support. What advantage, if any, high-dose ifosfamide has in soft-tissue sarcoma remains to be determined.

Dacarbazine (DTIC) has a low level of activity in soft-tissue sarcoma, including patients who have progressed on doxorubicin. While response rates to single-agent DTIC are less than 20 percent and complete responses are rarely observed, DTIC is used in combination therapy. It has been suggested that DTIC is active in gastrointestinal leiomyosarcomas, a subtype resistant to doxorubicin, but this has not been well studied.

Other commercially available agents that have been studied primarily in combination therapy include cyclophosphamide, methotrexate, actinomycin D, and vincristine. The true response rates of any of these drugs in adult soft-tissue sarcomas is probably less than 15 percent. Cyclophosphamide, compared with ifosfamide in a European trial, demonstrated an 8 percent response rate. Methotrexate appears to have a low level of activity. Analogues of methotrexate are under evaluation. Actinomycin D and vincristine as single agents have been studied in few adult patients, but when used in combination therapy appear to add little, if anything, to doxorubicin.

Cisplatin, except with uterine sarcomas, does not appear to be active in this group of diseases. A SWOG study that attempted dose intensification of cisplatin did not demonstrate improved response. Etoposide and mitomycin C, despite showing minimal single-agent activity in this disease, are being evaluated in various combinations at some centers. Etoposide is attractive because of demonstrated schedule dependency in other diseases and the availability of an oral formulation. Mitomycin C has been suggested to be synergistic with cisplatin in hypoxic tumor environments, which has led to combination studies. A phase II trial of paclitaxel (Taxol) in untreated soft-tissue sarcoma by SWOG reported a 12 percent response rate.

The initial chemotherapeutic approach to most patients who develop metastatic disease involves combination chemotherapy. While a number of studies of combination chemotherapy in this disease are reported in the literature, the greatest experience is with doxorubicin-based combinations. The highest response rates reported with doxorubicin-based combinations include DTIC, cyclophosphamide, and vincristine (Cy-VADic).

Sequential randomized trials with doxorubicin combinations have been reported by SWOG. The first trial compared doxorubicin, cyclophosphamide, and vincristine plus either DTIC or actinomycin D. The DTIC arm demonstrated improved response and survival. The second randomized trial compared doxorubicin plus DTIC to doxorubicin plus DTIC and either cyclophosphamide or vincristine. There were no significant differences in response or survival among the three arms. As a result of these sequential studies the two-drug combination of doxorubicin and DTIC became the standard SWOG combination in metastatic soft-tissue sarcoma.

More recently the Intergroup Sarcoma Study Group completed a phase III trial evaluating the addition of ifosfamide to the doxorubicin-DTIC combination. While response rates were higher in the ifosfamide regimen (32 versus 17 percent), overall survival favored the two-drug regimen. Analysis of response and survival according to age and tumor grade suggested benefit for the three-drug combination in younger patients with high-grade tumors. Conversely, much of the benefit of the two-drug regimen was seen in older patients with lower-grade tumors. As expected, myelotoxicity in the three-drug arm was higher, with a resultant decrease in doxorubicin dose intensity received.

The introduction of growth factors to ameliorate the myelosuppression associated with chemotherapy has resulted in a number of studies designed to increase dose intensity of doxorubicin in an attempt to improve response and survival. The use of the colony-stimulating factor G-CSF or GM-CSF has decreased leukopenia following combination chemotherapy. However, thrombocytopenia and anemia are increased when colony-stimulating factors are used. Response rates in programs using growth factor have generally been higher than in previous trials, but direct comparisons with and without growth factors have yet to be reported.

More recently, attention has focused on the use of combinations of growth factors including G-CSF, GM-CSF, the interleukins IL-3 and IL-6, and pIXY 321 to circumvent pancytopenia observed following combination chemotherapy. The value of more intensive chemotherapy awaits comparative phase III trials.

CONCLUSIONS AND FUTURE DIRECTIONS

The treatment of patients with metastatic soft-tissue sarcoma depends on the goal of therapy. Patients with good performance status, smaller disease burdens, and high-grade lesions can be approached aggressively with MAID chemotherapy in combination with surgical resection of residual disease. The goal of therapy in this situation is complete response, and a fraction of these patients are likely to have durable remissions. For patients with extrapulmonary metastasis, concurrent medical problems, and/or poor performance status, palliative therapy with single-agent doxorubicin or doxorubicin and DTIC (doxorubicin 60 mg per meter squared and DTIC 1 g per meter squared infused together over 96 hours) is well tolerated. Outpatient therapy is possible for most patients thus treated, and the decreased cardiac toxicity of the infusional schedule permits continued therapy in those responding. Single-agent ifosfamide or experimental therapy is also an option for metastatic disease, either as initial treatment or in patients failing doxorubicin.

The dose-response relationship observed with doxorubicin in the treatment of soft-tissue sarcoma makes intensification of therapy a reasonable approach to improve outcome. Further examination of this relationship with concurrent growth factors and stem cell support is the focus of clinical research. The low incidence of bone marrow metastasis in soft-tissue sarcoma and the relative youth of patients afflicted with this disease suggest the use of alternative high-dose chemotherapy with autologous bone marrow rescue as a possible therapy. The curative potential of autologous transplant in metastatic sarcoma appears promising for some histologies and is under investigation in a number of centers. Until these and other new approaches become available, the use of doxorubicin-based combination chemotherapy, with careful attention to dose intensity and availability of medical support for complications of therapy, remains the optimal approach to patients with metastatic disease.

Understanding the biologic differences among soft-tissue sarcomas, which account for the heterogeneity in clinical behavior, holds the promise of improvement in the therapy of these malignancies. Characterization of tumor phenotypes that predict for micrometastasis would allow more effective targeting of patients for adjuvant treatment. The next generation of adjuvant trials will likely define subgroups of patients based on parameters besides histopathologic grade. In metastatic disease, detection and quantitation of drug resistance could influence choice of therapy or allow modifications in treatment to circumvent or overcome drug resistance. Systemic therapy of sarcomas with agents other than cytotoxic chemotherapy may also be possible once we understand the carcinogenic process.

Suggested Reading

Antman K, Crowley J, Balcerzak S, et al. An intergroup phase III randomized study of doxorubicin and dacarbazine with or without ifosfamide and Mesna in advanced soft tissue and bone sarcomas. J Clin Oncol 1993; 11(7):1276–1285.

Edmonson JH, Ryan LM, Blum RH, et al. Randomized comparison of doxorubicin alone versus ifosfamide plus doxorubicin or mitomycin, doxorubicin, and cisplatin against advanced soft tissue sarcomas. J Clin Oncol 1993; 11(7):1269–1275.

Gaynor JJ, Tan CC, Casper ES, et al. Refinement of clinicopathologic staging for localized soft tissue sarcoma of the extremity: A study of 423 adults. J Clin Oncol 1992; 10:1317–1329.

Steward WP, Verweij J, Somers R, et al. Granulocyte-macrophage colony-stimulating factor allows safe escalation of dose-intensity of chemotherapy in metastatic adult soft tissue sarcomas: A study of the European Organization for Research and Treatment of Cancer soft tissue and bone sarcoma group. J Clin Oncol 1993; 11(1):15–21.

Zalupski MM, Ryan JR. Hussein ME, Baker LH. Systemic adjuvant chemotherapy for soft tissue sarcomas of the extremities. Surg Oncol Clin North Am 1993; 2(4):621–637.

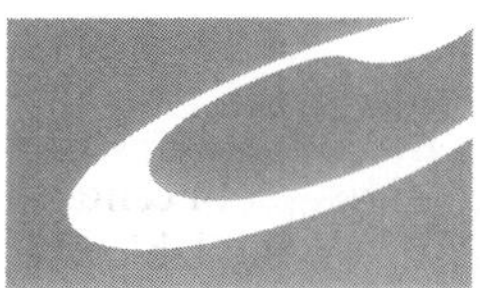

RENAL DISEASES

HYPONATREMIA

John F. Wade III, M.D.
Robert J. Anderson, M.D.

Hyponatremia is a common electrolyte disorder with a prevalence of 2 to 3 percent in hospitalized patients. Central to the understanding of hyponatremia and its therapy is the concept that the plasma sodium concentration reflects the ratio between the amount of sodium and the amount of water in the body. Hyponatremia results from an excess of water relative to sodium. Such an excess of water occurs from continued water intake (oral or intravenous) in the presence of impaired renal water elimination. Decreased renal water excretion is usually caused by the action of antidiuretic hormone causing the kidney to retain water. Occasionally, decreased renal water elimination is caused by renal failure. The rational treatment of hyponatremia depends on whether it is symptomatic or not, whether it is acute or chronic, and on the underlying cause (Table 1).

Table 1 Causes and Treatment of Hyponatremia

CAUSE	TREATMENT
Erroneous and factitious hyponatremia and pseudohyponatremia	No specific therapy needed
Normovolemic hyponatremia (SIADH)	Treat underlying disorder Water restriction Hypertonic saline with or without a loop diuretic Loop diuretics with sodium chloride supplementation Demeclocycline Induce urea diuresis
Primary polydipsia	Water restriction
Hypovolemic hyponatremia	Isotonic saline Rarely, hypertonic saline
Hypervolemic (edematous) hyponatremia	Treat underlying disease Salt and water restriction Loop diuretics Converting enzyme inhibitors for heart failure

■ SYMPTOMATIC HYPONATREMIA

Since body water is in osmotic equilibrium, positive water balance dilutes plasma, decreasing the sodium concentration and osmolality. This leads to a shift of water from extracellular (low osmolality) to intracellular (normal osmolality) spaces. The subsequent cell swelling can produce central nervous system dysfunction since the brain is encased within a rigid skull. The severity of brain edema and dysfunction depends on the rate and magnitude of the decrease in plasma sodium concentration. Acute marked hyponatremia leads to cerebral edema with progressive anorexia, nausea, vomiting, lethargy, headaches, confusion, seizures, and ultimately transtentorial herniation with cardiopulmonary arrest and death. With a more gradual decline in the plasma sodium concentration, brain cells can extrude osmotically active particles such as sodium, potassium, amino acids, and other osmolytes. This decreases cell osmolality and water uptake and mitigates cerebral swelling and dysfunction. The clinical corollary is that acute hyponatremia is often symptomatic while chronic hyponatremia is usually well tolerated.

Acute symptomatic hyponatremia should be considered a medical emergency. Although most symptomatic hyponatremic patients have a plasma sodium concentration of less than 120 mEq per liter, life-threatening hyponatremia can occur with higher concentrations of plasma sodium. The optimal management of acute symptomatic hyponatremia is currently under debate. Untreated symptomatic hyponatremia can lead to seizures and death. Alternatively, an "osmotic demyelination syndrome" with pontine and extrapontine myelinolysis resulting in pseudobulbar palsy, quadriplegia, a "locked-in" state, and other neurologic deficits has occurred after therapy. Risk factors for the development of neurologic sequelae following treatment of symptomatic hyponatremia include chronic hyponatremia (>48 hours), overcorrection, a large magnitude of correction (>15 in 24 hours), rapid correction (>1 to 2 mEq per liter per hour), severe underlying disease such as malnutrition, malignancy, alcoholism, female sex, and an associated hypoxic event.

One approach to the management of acute symptomatic hyponatremia is to administer hypertonic sodium chloride (3 percent or, rarely, 5 percent) at approximately 100 ml per hour until seizures and other symptoms resolve. The endpoint of therapy is either cessation of major symptoms or a 10 to 15 percent increase in plasma sodium concentration. Acutely, 3 percent saline increases the plasma sodium concentration because the concentration of the sodium (513 mEq per liter) exceeds that of the plasma. To produce a sustained, significant increase in the plasma sodium concentration, removal of excess free water from the body is necessary. The administration of hypertonic saline results in negative water balance as long as the osmolality of the administered fluid exceeds that of the urine. In patients with a fixed high urine osmolality, 3 percent sodium chloride (osmolality of 1,026 mOsm per kilogram of H_2O) may result in only a slow correction of hyponatremia. In symptomatic hyponatremic patients with a high urine osmolality, administration of a loop diuretic (i.e., 0.5 to 1 mg per kilogram of furosemide) usually results in a large diuresis of isotonic urine. Repletion of urinary electrolytes lost after the administration of furosemide with a small volume of 3 percent sodium chloride functionally results in the rapid removal of a large amount of free water and in an increase in the plasma sodium concentration. In the treatment of symptomatic hyponatremia of unknown or chronic duration, a reasonable plan is to administer 3 percent sodium chloride (with or without a loop diuretic) to increase the plasma sodium concentration by about 5 percent. In the acute treatment of symptomatic hyponatremia, frequent monitoring of the plasma sodium concentration during therapy (i.e., every 2 to 3 hours) is necessary to ensure a rate of correction of less than 1.5 to 2 mEq per liter per hour and a total magnitude of acute correction of less than 15 mEq per liter over 24 to 48 hours. After the discontinuation of 3 percent sodium chloride, water restriction alone should be undertaken to bring about a slower normalization of plasma sodium.

■ ASYMPTOMATIC HYPONATREMIA

The majority of patients with hyponatremia are asymptomatic. In such asymptomatic patients, the risks of emergent therapy outweigh any potential benefits. The appropriate treatment of asymptomatic hyponatremia depends on the underlying cause of the disorder (see Table 1).

Erroneous Translocation and Factitious Hyponatremia

In approximately 20 percent of patients with hyponatremia, the low plasma sodium concentration can be attributed to laboratory error, blood drawing error (i.e., from a vein proximal to an intravenous infusion of hypotonic fluid), or the presence of high blood concentrations of an osmotically active particle, which is usually glucose but may on rare occasions be mannitol or glycine. Rarely, marked hyperlipidemia or hyperproteinemia can artifactually lower the plasma sodium concentration. In the case of hyperglycemia mannitol and glycine the osmotic effect of glucose results in a shift of water from the intracellular space to the extracellular space, thereby diluting plasma and producing translocation hyponatremia. In these settings, hyponatremia occurs without hypotonicity and therefore requires no specific therapy.

Syndrome of Inappropriate Secretion of Antidiuretic Hormone

Once erroneous and translocation hyponatremia have been excluded, it is useful to categorize patients on the basis of the clinical assessment of their extracellular fluid volume status. Most hyponatremic patients (30 to 40 percent) appear to be euvolemic and meet the criteria for the diagnosis of syndrome of inappropriate secretion of antidiuretic hormone (SIADH). Common clinical settings of SIADH include the postoperative state, the presence of intrathoracic and intracranial disease, selected hormone deficiency states (glucocorticoid and thyroid), psychosis, and cancer, and the use of selected medications such as chlorpropamide. In these disorders, the combination of nonosmotic secretion of antidiuretic hormone plus continued water intake leads to positive water balance and hyponatremia.

The treatment of SIADH varies with the severity of the hyponatremia and the magnitude of the increase in urine osmolality. In all cases, recognition and treatment of the underlying disease is important. Asymptomatic patients with mild to moderate hyponatremia may respond to water restriction sufficient to achieve negative water balance. To achieve negative water balance, the sum of the amount of water intake and of water produced by metabolism must be less than that lost through perspiration, breathing, and urination. Negative water balance with an improvement in the hyponatremic patient's condition can usually be accomplished in patients with urine osmolalities of approximately 300 mOsm per kilogram of H_2O. Successful therapy with water restriction thus requires good patient compliance and a relatively low urine osmolality.

For patients with chronic SIADH in whom urine osmolality is higher and compliance is poor, additional therapy directed toward decreasing urinary osmolality, which increases renal water excretion, is often needed. This therapy may consist of a loop diuretic such as furosemide or bumetanide combined with sodium chloride supplementation (intravenous or oral) to prevent hypovolemia. A second line of therapy used to decrease urine osmolality and increase renal water excretion is the administration of a drug that inhibits the ability of antidiuretic hormone to increase renal collecting tubular water reabsorption. Two such agents are demeclocycline (300 to 600 mg twice daily) and lithium. Because of the potential significant toxicity associated with lithium, demeclocycline is usually preferred, except in children, where this tetracycline can interfere with bone growth. The onset of action of demeclocycline is slow, and it may take several days for an effect to be seen. A final form of therapy for chronic SIADH, infrequently used in the United States, is to decrease urine osmolality by inducing a solute (urea) diuresis by administration of 30 to 60 g of oral urea per day. Oral urea is often successfully used in Europe to treat chronic SIADH with good results.

Occasionally, the clinician encounters a patient with SIADH and moderate to severe hyponatremia in whom it is difficult to determine if any of the symptoms can be attributed to hyponatremia. In such a case, a modest increase of plasma sodium concentration (5 to 10 percent) may be advisable. In this setting, it is tempting to consider normal (0.9 percent) saline therapy. Normal saline (total osmolality of 308 mOsm per kilogram of H_2O; 154 mEq of sodium and 154 mEq chloride) has a higher sodium concentration than plasma and would produce an initial small increase in plasma sodium concentration. If, however, the patient has a fixed high urine osmolality (for example, 616 mOsm per kilogram of H_2O), then worsening of hyponatremia may ultimately occur after administration of normal saline. With a urine osmolality of 616 mOsm per kilogram of H_2O, the 308 mOsm of sodium chloride in the 1 L of normal saline would be excreted in 0.5 L of urine, leaving approximately 0.5 L of free water retained in the body and subsequently causing a slight decrease in the plasma sodium concentration. Thus the key to success in raising a low plasma sodium concentration in disorders associated with high urinary osmolality is either to give the patient a solute (hypertonic saline or urea) with a greater osmolality than the urine or to decrease urinary osmolality (via loop diuretics). Either approach favors renal free water excretion. When used together, hypertonic saline and furosemide allow for rapid increments in the plasma sodium concentration. Furosemide with normal saline (to replace about one-half of the urine output) can result in a modest increase in serum sodium concentration.

Thiazide diuretics are a relatively common cause of hyponatremia, particularly in frail, elderly women. The pathogenesis of hyponatremia in these patients, who usually appear to be euvolemic, is multifactorial. Thiazides may induce polydipsia and also mild volume depletion with enhanced antidiuretic hormone secretion, which results in retention of ingested water. Also, thiazide diuretics exert a renal tubular effect that impairs kidney water elimination. Profound potassium depletion usually accompanies thiazide diuretic–associated hyponatremia. Cessation of the diuretic agent, restoration of any volume deficits through the administration of normal saline, and aggressive potassium repletion constitute the cornerstone of therapy. Repletion of potassium often increases the plasma sodium concentration, presumably because potassium enters cells in exchange for sodium, which is extruded into extracellular fluid.

Normal individuals are capable of excreting large volumes of administered free water. Occasionally, patients with profound psychogenic polydipsia present with euvolemic hyponatremia. In these patients, the rapid ingestion of large volumes of water temporarily exceeds renal excretory capacity. In contrast to patients with SIADH, these patients usually have hypotonic urine (osmolality less than plasma) since the antidiuretic hormone secretion is suppressed. These patients usually need no therapy other than water restriction, as the excess water ingested is rapidly excreted in the urine.

True Volume Depletion

Extracellular fluid volume depletion resulting from gastrointestinal losses (caused by vomiting, diarrhea, blood loss), renal losses (caused by diuretics), skin losses (caused by burns), and other losses or sequestration (caused by pancreatitis, muscle crush injury) is a common clinical setting of hyponatremia. In such cases, the volume depletion leads to antidiuretic hormone release and decreased renal function, which combine to impair renal water excretion. When such patients orally ingest free water or are given hypotonic fluids intravenously, the water is retained, thereby lowering the plasma sodium concentration. Significant weight loss, orthostatic hypotension and tachycardia, decreased skin turgor, dry mucous membranes, and low jugular venous pressure strongly suggest hypovolemia. Often it is difficult to assess extracellular fluid volume status accurately from clinical parameters alone. In circumstances in which volume status remains unclear after clinical evaluation, a spot urinary sodium concentration may be helpful. A urinary sodium concentration of less than 30 to 40 mEq per liter suggests hypovolemia with diminished renal perfusion.

In hyponatremic, volume-depleted patients, the restoration of effective circulating blood volume with appropriate therapy, usually the administration of normal saline, normalizes the plasma sodium concentration. The rate at which the plasma sodium concentration is normalized tends to be slow initially. However, once euvolemia is restored, antidiuretic hormone secretion diminishes and renal function improves, resulting in a water diuresis and a later rapid return of plasma sodium to normal. If hypovolemic patients are symptomatic from hyponatremia, initial administration of 3 percent sodium chloride may rarely be indicated, following the guidelines discussed previously.

■ EDEMATOUS STATES

Hyponatremia occurring in the presence of an edematous disorder (heart failure, cirrhosis, nephrosis) accounts for approximately 30 percent of all cases of hyponatremia. In these settings, a diminished "effective circulating blood volume" leads to decreased renal perfusion with avid renal salt and water retention. If excess free water is ingested or given intravenously, hyponatremia in the context of an increase in both total body water and salt occurs. Thus in hyponatremic edematous disorders, both salt and water restriction are often indicated. Additional therapy in the hyponatremic edematous states should be directed first against the primary disease state. In patients with heart failure, reduction of preload (venodilation, loop diuretics), and afterload (vasodilators and angiotension-converting enzyme inhibitors) and improvement in myocardial contractility (digitalis) may improve effective circulating blood volume sufficiently to suppress antidiuretic hormone secretion and improve renal perfusion, thereby increasing renal water excretion. In patients with congestive heart failure, loop diuretics and converting enzyme inhibitors appear synergistic with regard to enhancing renal water elimination. Converting enzyme inhibitors potentially improve cardiac output and renal perfusion, which enhance renal hemodynamic parameters and thereby increase renal water excretion. Converting enzyme inhibitors also directly inhibit the ability of antidiuretic hormone to increase collecting tubular water reabsorption.

Increasing the effective circulating blood volume is more difficult in patients with severe hepatic cirrhosis and nephrotic syndrome. Loop diuretics may be beneficial in both conditions. In advanced hepatic cirrhosis, effective arterial blood volume can be restored with a peritoneovenous shunt, although this procedure is usually reserved for patients with severe, refractory ascites or the hepatorenal syndrome.

Therapy directed at the primary glomerular pathology may result in amelioration of the nephrotic syndrome. Intravenously administered albumin may temporarily improve renal perfusion and enhance renal water excretion in patients with severe nephrosis. Demeclocycline has also been used in the treatment of chronic hyponatremia of the edematous disorders. Although demeclocycline is efficacious, the drug may accumulate in the body in the presence of liver disease and passive hepatic congestion and lead to severe vomiting and nephrotoxicity. Thus this agent should be used with extreme caution in the setting of cardiac and liver disease.

Hyponatremia associated with edematous states is rarely symptomatic. If it is symptomatic, administration of a loop diuretic with replacement of urinary electrolyte losses through hypertonic saline and peritoneal dialysis and hemodialysis are the preferred modes of therapy.

Suggested Reading

Anderson RJ, Chung HM, Luge R, Schrier RW. Hyponatremia: a prospective analysis of its epidemiology and pathogenetic role of vasopressin. Ann Intern Med 1985; 102:164–168.

Decaux G, Prospert F, Pennincky R, et al. 5-year treatment of the syndrome of inappropriate secretion of ADH with oral urea nephron 1993; 63:468–476.

Oh MS, Kim NJ, Carroll HJ. Recommendations for: treatment of symptomatic hyponatremia. Nephron 1995; 70:143–150.

HYPERNATREMIA

Paul M. Palevsky, M.D.
Irwin Singer, M.D.

Hypernatremia is a common clinical problem, with a prevalence in hospitalized patients of 0.5 to 2 percent. The maintenance of the serum sodium concentration within the normal range of 135 to 145 mEq per liter depends on homeostatic mechanisms that balance water intake and excretion. Hypernatremia is usually the result of impaired water intake in the setting of increased renal or extrarenal water losses (in excess of electrolyte losses, if any).

In the adult population, hypernatremia is most prevalent among the elderly, who are frequently less able to resist dehydration. Several defenses are impaired with aging: body water content, as a percentage of body weight, decreases; maximal urinary concentrating capacity diminishes; and thirst perception declines.

In adults, hypernatremia occurs primarily in the setting of systemic illness, confounding the ability to attribute symptoms precisely and to attribute morbidity and mortality to the hypertonic stress. Although hypernatremia can serve as a marker for the severity of underlying illness, there is little doubt that substantial morbidity and mortality are directly attributable to the hypernatremic state itself. Mortality rates ranging from 40 percent to greater than 70 percent have been reported, depending on the magnitude and duration of the hypernatremia. Survivors of hypernatremia often exhibit significant decreases in functional capacity and the ability to care for themselves.

Hypernatremia can produce clinically important central nervous system (CNS) dysfunction: confusion, lethargy, weakness, and seizures may be presenting symptoms. In acute hypernatremia, the rise in extracellular fluid osmolality results in intracellular dehydration as water redistributes across cell membranes to maintain osmotic equilibrium. Cellular dehydration results in a loss of brain volume, increases the mechanical traction on intracranial vessels, and can result in intracranial bleeding.

The cerebral response to hypernatremia and other hypertonic states is a function of the rapidity of onset and duration of hypertonicity. In animal studies, acute hypernatremia from hypertonic saline infusion produces a rapid decrease in brain water content and an increase in intracellular electrolyte concentration. Intracellular osmolality increases as a result of cellular water loss and electrolyte accumulation. In chronic hypernatremia the increase in intracellular osmolality is the same; however, the relative contributions of intracellular water loss and solute accumulation differ. Brain water content is relatively preserved in chronic hypernatremia; intracellular osmolality increases primarily as the result of the accumulation of "idiogenic osmoles." These solutes, primarily organic metabolites such as polyols, polyamines, and amino acids, accumulate after several hours of hypertonic stress as part of an adaptive mechanism that regulates intracellular brain volume. Although the accumulation of intracellular "idiogenic osmoles" minimizes cerebral shrinkage and the risk of intracranial bleeding, the production of "idiogenic osmoles" increases the risk of developing cerebral edema during rehydration.

■ CAUSES

In the majority of patients, hypernatremia develops as a result of the combination of inadequate water intake and increased electrolyte-free water loss. Occasional patients develop hypernatremia as the result of hypertonic sodium intake in the absence of concomitant water intake. The common denominator of all forms of hypernatremia is an inadequate ingestion or administration of water to maintain a normal serum tonicity.

Although impaired water intake and hypernatremia may result from primary hypodipsia, adult hypernatremia is usually secondary to an intercurrent illness or alteration in mental

Table 1 Causes of Hypernatremia

PATHOPHYSIOLOGIC CONDITIONS	TOTAL BODY SODIUM	TOTAL BODY WATER	TYPICAL ETIOLOGIES
Pure water loss	Near normal	↓	Diabetes insipidus Nephrogenic Hypothalamic Increased insensible losses Fever Mechanical ventilation Hyperventilation
Hypotonic water loss	↓	↓↓	Gastrointestinal losses Vomiting Nasogastric drainage Enterocutaneous fistulae Diarrhea Renal losses Diuretic administration Osmotic diuresis Postobstructive diuresis Nonoliguric ARF
Pure sodium gain	↑	Near normal	Salt ingestion
Hypertonic sodium gain	↑↑	↑	Intravenous hypertonic saline Intravenous sodium bicarbonate

status that has diminished thirst or restricted water intake. The importance of thirst in the regulation of plasma tonicity is exemplified by patients with diabetes insipidus. Despite massive polyuria, patients with diabetes insipidus maintain a serum sodium concentration in the normal range as long as they have adequate thirst perception and unrestricted access to water. In the setting of intercurrent illness or depressed sensorium, their ability to maintain sufficient water intake is diminished, and hypernatremia rapidly develops. Elderly patients with febrile or diarrheal illness, patients with neurologic disease (e.g., stroke or chronic dementia), and patients with acute obtundation or delirium are particularly vulnerable to the development of hypernatremia. In the majority of patients in whom hypernatremia develops during the course of hospitalization the hypernatremia is iatrogenic, resulting from the inadequate or inappropriate prescription of fluids to patients with impaired water ingestion and predictably increased water losses.

Hypernatremia can be divided into four categories on the basis of total body sodium and water content (Table 1). Pure water deficits, with little change in total body sodium, may develop in patients with increased insensible water losses (e.g., water losses secondary to fever, increased ambient temperature, mechanical ventilation without humidification, or hyperventilation), and in patients with hypothalamic or nephrogenic diabetes insipidus. Hypotonic fluid losses from the gastrointestinal tract, skin, or kidneys, may produce hypovolemia and hypernatremia. Large volumes of hypotonic gastrointestinal secretions can be lost during prolonged vomiting or nasogastric suction, through enterocutaneous fistulae, and in cases of severe diarrhea. Hypotonic polyuria may be produced by diuretic administration, osmotic diuresis caused by the excretion of glucose, mannitol, or urea, or nonoliguric acute renal failure, any of which may result in hypernatremia and volume depletion. Hypertonic sodium gain produces hypervolemic hypernatremia; it is usually iatrogenic, developing from the intravenous administration of hypertonic sodium bicarbonate or sodium chloride solutions. Pure sodium gain from voluntary or iatrogenic oral salt ingestion may also produce hypernatremia and sodium overload. Hypernatremia secondary to dialysis against hypertonic or high-sodium baths has also been described.

■ DIAGNOSIS

The diagnosis of hypernatremia is made through laboratory testing. Symptoms and physical signs are nonspecific and may be obscured by underlying medical illnesses. Thirst, the hallmark of dehydration, may not be verbalized or perceived as the result of depressed mental status. Classic physical signs of dehydration, such as poor skin turgor and sunken eyes, are unreliable in the elderly patients most susceptible to the development of hypernatremia.

Clinical hypernatremia is primarily manifest as central nervous system dysfunction. Although a depressed sensorium may precede hypernatremia, hypernatremia may produce CNS depression, which may range from lethargy to coma, in previously alert patients. Myoclonic twitching and generalized seizures may also develop; seizures are uncommon in patients with chronic hypernatremia, but have been described in as many as 40 percent of patients after the initiation of therapy.

■ CALCULATION OF WATER DEFICITS

A hypernatremic patient's water deficit may be estimated from his or her serum sodium concentration and body weight. Assuming that total body sodium has remained unchanged and that the hypernatremia is entirely the result of water loss, one may estimate the water deficit through the following equation:

$$\text{Water Deficit} = (\text{Total Body Water}) \times \frac{\text{Serum } [\text{Na}^+] - 140}{140}$$

The total body water is usually assumed to be 60 percent of body weight.

Although this formula provides a useful first approximation of the water deficit and can be used to guide initial therapy, several important caveats must be recognized.

First, the assumption that total body water is a fixed percentage of body weight is incorrect; total body water is a function of the patient's age, gender, and percentage of body fat. As a general rule, the total body water is a smaller percentage of body weight in women than in men and declines with age. Thus, while a 25-year-old man may have a water content that is 60 percent of his body weight, body water may comprise only 55 percent of body weight in a 25-year-old woman. At 75 years of age, in men, body water may decrease to 50 percent of body weight, and in women, it may decrease to 45 percent of body weight.

Second, the above-mentioned calculation assumes that changes in serum sodium concentration reflect changes in plasma tonicity. This assumption is correct only if there is no elevation in other osmotically active solutes, such as glucose or mannitol. Because these solutes shift water from the intracellular to the extracellular compartments, an elevation in their concentration dilutes other solutes and decreases the serum sodium concentration. In this circumstance, the calculation of the water deficit must be based directly on the change in plasma osmolality, and not just on the serum sodium concentration.

Finally, the above-mentioned formula assumes that total body sodium and other electrolytes have remained constant. In the setting of depletion or overload of sodium or other electrolytes, the calculation must be corrected by the volume of isotonic sodium (or electrolyte) lost or gained.

THERAPY

The treatment of hypernatremia is water repletion. There are a paucity of data regarding the rapidity with which water deficits should be corrected. Although hypernatremia is potentially lethal, overly rapid water repletion may result in the development of cerebral edema or seizures. Because mortality rates may increase with increasing rates of water repletion, therapy should be instituted promptly, but it should also be sufficiently gradual so as to prevent rapid transcellular fluid shifts.

In hypernatremic patients with hypovolemia and evidence of circulatory compromise, the initial therapy is volume replacement. Isotonic saline or colloid should be administered promptly to correct hypotension and restore plasma volume. Severe acidosis (pH <7.15) should also be treated; moderate acidosis, which does not compromise myocardial contractility, does not require rapid bicarbonate supplementation. Undiluted solutions of sodium bicarbonate are hypertonic (a standard 50 ml ampule of 7.5 percent $NaHCO_3$ has a sodium concentration of 892 mEq per liter) and can increase hypernatremia. If bicarbonate must be administered, it can be diluted to isotonicity (e.g., 100 ml of 7.5 percent $NaHCO_3$ added to 1,000 ml of 0.45 percent saline) before infusion.

Once adequate volume replacement has been achieved, the water deficit should be estimated and replacement initiated. Water repletion should be gradual; no more than half of the calculated deficit should be replaced over the first 12 to 24 hours, with the remainder of the deficit corrected during the ensuing 48 to 72 hours. The rate of correction of the serum sodium concentration should not exceed 2 mEq per liter per hour. Throughout the course of therapy, neurologic status should be monitored closely; an abrupt deterioration after initial improvement in mental status may suggest the development of cerebral edema from overly rapid rehydration.

No individual fluid regimen is of documented superiority in the treatment of hypernatremia. Enteral water repletion, administered either orally or by gavage, may be sufficient but is frequently limited by the magnitude of the water deficit or by the patient's underlying medical condition. Intravenous repletion should consist of 5 percent glucose in water or another solution with a low electrolyte content; pure water should not be infused intravenously, as it can cause intravascular hemolysis.

In addition to the repletion of the water deficit, all ongoing fluid and electrolyte losses must be continuously replaced. Plasma electrolytes must be monitored frequently, at a minimum of 6 hour intervals, throughout the course of therapy. Replacement fluid solution should be modified on the basis of response to the prescribed therapy. Insensible water losses may be estimated to be 0.6 ml per kilogram per hour in an afebrile patient, and increase by 20 percent for each 1°C rise in body temperature. Urinary, gastrointestinal, and other fluid losses must be quantitated and their electrolyte content determined. The replacement fluid prescription should be based on these measured and estimated losses so as to achieve and maintain euvolemia.

The reduction of ongoing fluid losses is also of paramount importance. Fever should be reduced by cooling and through the use of antipyretics to minimize insensible water losses. Ongoing osmotic diuresis should be reduced by controlling hyperglycemia and reducing urea synthesis (by treating catabolic states and avoiding protein loads). Osmotic diarrhea from hypertonic enteral nutritional supplements can be reduced by altering the nutritional prescription or with the use of antidiarrheal agents. The polyuria of hypothalamic diabetes insipidus can be minimized by vasopressin administration. Aqueous vasopressin may be used for diagnostic testing, and occasionally for acute therapy; DDAVP, a synthetic analogue of vasopressin with less pressor activity and a longer duration of action, is the preferred therapy and may be administered subcutaneously or intravenously (1 to 2 μg twice daily) during acute illness, or intranasally (10 to 20 μg twice daily) as chronic therapy.

For patients in whom hypernatremia results from the administration of hypertonic saline or bicarbonate or from salt ingestion, treatment requires both water administration and diuresis. Loop-acting diuretics should be used to reduce volume overload. If renal failure prohibits the establishment of diuresis, dialysis may be required.

Since many patients develop hypernatremia as an iatrogenic complication, greater emphasis must be placed on prevention. In patients at high risk for the development of hypernatremia, particularly the elderly and patients with increased fluid losses, fever, or obtundation, more frequent monitoring of the serum sodium concentration is required. Therapy should be initiated early, with prompt treatment of mild hypernatremia, so as to prevent the development of life-threatening water deficits.

Suggested Reading

Alvis R, Geheb M, Cox M. Hypo- and hyperosmolar states: diagnostic approaches. In: Arieff AI, DeFronzo RA, eds. Fluid electrolyte and acid-base disorders. New York: Churchill Livingstone, 1985:185.

Cox M, Geheb M, Singer I. Disorders of thirst and renal water excretion. In: Arieff AI, DeFronzo RA, eds. Fluid electrolyte and acid-base disorders. New York: Churchill Livingstone, 1985:119.

Palevsky P, Bhagrath R, Greenberg A. Hypernatremia in hospitalized patients. Ann Intern Med 1996; 124:197–203.

Robertson GL. Abnormalities of thirst regulation. Kidney Int 1984; 25: 460–469.

Snyder NA, Feigal DW, Arieff AI. Hypernatremia in elderly patients: a heterogeneous, morbid, and iatrogenic unity. Ann Intern Med 1987; 107:309–319.

DYSKALEMIAS: HYPOKALEMIA AND HYPERKALEMIA

Kamel S. Kamel, M.D., F.R.C.P.C.

The dyskalemias are common electrolyte disorders that may have serious sequelae, particularly cardiac arrhythmias. Potassium (K) is the major intracellular cation with only 1.5–2.5 percent (close to 65 mmol) of total body K (approximately 4,000 mmol) residing in the extracellular fluid (ECF) volume of a 70 kg adult. This delicate balance of K concentration on both sides of the cell membrane is strongly influenced by the cell resting membrane potential (RMP). Moreover, this ratio has to be maintained in the face of a daily intake of K in adults that, on average, equals the content of K in the ECF. While the control of the transcellular distribution of K is vital for survival, it is the regulation of K excretion by the kidney that maintains the overall K balance. This discussion begins with a brief synopsis of K physiology because an understanding of the physiology of the internal and external balance of K is central to determine where leverage could be exerted in the management of patients with dyskalemias. The clinical tools that can be used to determine "where is the lesion" in the renal handling of K are then outlined. The approach to therapy in patients with hypokalemia or hyperkalemia emphasizes circumstances in which these disorders represent a life-threatening condition that requires emergency treatment.

■ K PHYSIOLOGY

Internal K Balance

The rapid shift of K between the ICF and ECF acts to limit acute changes in plasma [K]. To induce internal shift of K, either the cell RMP must change or the cell membrane conductance to K ions must be altered. To change the RMP to allow for the shift of K into cells, there must be the net export of positive charges. This occurs when intracellular sodium (Na) ions or those Na ions that have entered the cells in an "electroneutral" fashion are exported from the cell via the "electrogenic" Na-K-ATPase.

Hormones

Two major hormones promote the relocation of K ions into cells: insulin and catecholamines. The effect of insulin to shift K into cells is well recognized and has been utilized clinically in management of patients with hyperkalemia. Insulin promotes the entry of Na ions into cells via the "electroneutral" Na/H exchanger. This increased influx of Na ions stimulates the Na-K-ATPase. For each Na ion that exits the cells, there will be the net export of one-third of a positive charge and therefore, the RMP becomes more electronegative. β_2 agonists lower the plasma K concentration by shifting K ions into cells, probably as the result of stimulating of the Na-K-ATPase via a cyclic-AMP dependent mechanism. The translocation of intracellular Na ions via the Na-K-ATPase exports ⅓ of a positive charge per Na ion that exits. Clinically, hypokalemia due to an acute shift of K may be seen in conditions associated with a surge of catecholamines (e.g., in patients with subarachnoid hemorrhage or myocardial ischemia). β_2 agonists have been used in treatment of patients with acute hyperkalemia.

Acid-Base Disorders

Respiratory acid-base disorders cause only small changes in plasma K concentration. The effect of metabolic acidosis on the distribution of K between ICF and ECF depends on the permeability of the cell membrane to the anion that accompanies the added H^+. Infusion of L-lactic acid or ketoacids in nephrectomized dogs did not cause the shift of K ions out of cells. It appears that the accompanying organic anions entered the cells to the same degree as the H^+ ions, and hence no shift of K out of cells was required for electrical neutrality. A shift of K will occur, however, if the anion that accompanies H^+ is distributed primarily in the ECF as seen experimentally with the infusion of hydrochloric acid. Several clinical implications follow from these observations. First, if hyperkalemia is present in a patient with an organic acidosis, a cause for the hyperkalemia other than the acidosis should be sought (e.g., insulin lack in patients with diabetic ketoacidosis (DKA), ATP depletion in patients with hypoxic lactic acidosis). Second, although inorganic acidosis causes the shift of K from the ICF, patients with chronic hyperchloremic acidosis (e.g., diarrhea, renal tubular acidosis usually present with normal or even low plasma [K] because of the loss of K in the diarrheal fluid or the urine. Therefore, a defect in K excretion is to be suspected if hyperkalemia were to persist in these patients.

Hypokalemia is a common finding in patients with metabolic alkalosis. This, however, reflects the renal K wasting due to the underlying disorder (e.g., vomiting, diuretic use, hyperaldosteronism) rather than the small effect of alkalemia to shift K ions into cells.

Tissue Anabolism–Catabolism

K ions can move into or out of the ICF in response to major changes in the content of intracellular anions such as organic phosphates (anionic charges on the phosphate groups in DNA or RNA counterbalance the bulk of the positive charge of K in the ICF). Severe hyperkalemia is seen in patients with crush injury and also in patients with the tumor-lysis syndrome. In these patients, other factors that compromise the kidney's ability to excrete K are also usually present. In patients with DKA, tissue catabolism with the loss of organic phosphates leads to a parallel loss of K and total body K depletion. Nevertheless, these patients usually present with hyperkalemia, as K ions shift from ICF to ECF because of the lack of insulin.

Hypokalemia may be seen in conditions associated with rapid cell growth and the accumulation of intracellular organic phosphates. Examples include patients treated with total parenteral nutrition (TPN), patients with rapidly growing leukemias and lymphomas, and during the course of treatment in patients with DKA or pernicious anemia.

External K Balance

Long-term K homeostasis is a function of regulation of K excretion by the kidney. Control of K excretion occurs primarily in the late distal tubule and the cortical collecting duct (CCD). The principal cells of these segments are the ones responsible for the net secretion of K. Reabsorption of K may occur by α-intercalated cells in the CCD and medullary collecting duct (MCD) via a H-K-ATPase. This mechanism may play an important role in diminishing renal K losses in K depleted subjects.

The rate of K excretion is determined by the activity of K secretion in the CCD and the rate of flow in that nephron segment. The rate of flow in the distal nephron is influenced by the rate of excretion of osmoles (electrolytes, urea, glucose). Hence in a patient with hyperkalemia, the rate of K excretion could be augmented with the administration of diuretics that inhibit the reabsorption of Na proximal to the CCD. The activity of K secretion in the CCD is modulated by factors that affect the generation of a lumen-negative voltage in the CCD and the conductance of the apical K channels.

The generation of a lumen-negative voltage in the CCD requires that Na ions are reabsorbed at a faster rate than the accompanying anion, usually chloride (Cl), i.e., electrogenic reabsorption of Na. Reabsorption of Na occurs via its channel in the apical membrane of principal cells. Whereas aldosterone is known to activate this channel, the K-sparing diuretic, amiloride, and the antibiotic, trimethoprim, decrease the activity of K secretion by blocking that channel. Glucocorticoids, have both a much higher concentration in blood than aldosterone and an equal affinity for the mineralocorticoid receptor, but they do not directly stimulate K secretion because principal cells have the enzyme 11-β hydroxysteroid dehydrogenase (11-βHSDH). This enzyme converts cortisol to an inactive metabolite (cortisone) that does not bind the mineralocorticoid receptor. Glucocorticoids, however, can exert a mineralocorticoid effect if this enzyme activity is decreased (e.g., in patients with apparent mineralocorticoid excess syndrome), inhibited (e.g., by licorice, carbenoxolyn or chewing tobacco), or if it is overwhelmed by an abundance of cortisol (e.g., in patients with ACTH-producing tumors or severe Cushing's syndrome).

The pathway of reabsorption of Cl in the CCD is not well defined. Nevertheless, changes in the "apparent" permeability for Cl in the CCD have been postulated in some patients with dyskalemia. For example, an increase in Cl reabsorption in the CCD, the so-called "Cl shunt disorder" is thought to be the underlying pathophysiology for hyperkalemia in patients with Gordon's syndrome and in patients treated with cyclosporine.

Under most circumstances, variations in the luminal [Na] do not play a major role in the regulation of K secretion. The delivery of Na without its usual accompanying anion, Cl, however, is an important factor in modulating the rate of secretion of K. The action of anions like sulfate seems to be nonspecific and depends on the presence of a very low luminal [Cl]. Bicarbonate ions (or alkaline luminal pH) activate K secretion even when luminal [Cl] is high; one speculation is that bicarbonate may inhibit the reabsorption of Cl in the CCD. In a patient with hyperkalemia, the rate of excretion of K may be enhanced by the induction of bicarbonaturia (e.g., with the administration of acetazolamide).

■ CLINICAL TOOLS TO ASSESS PATIENTS WITH DYSKALEMIAS

A pathophysiologic classification of the causes of hypokalemia and hyperkalemia is provided in Tables 1 and 2, respectively. Since the kidney plays a major role in long-term K homeostasis, the approach to the diagnosis in patients with chronic dyskalemias focuses on identifying the component of renal excretion of K that is defective in these patients.

K Excretion Rate

In subjects who were rendered hypokalemic with dietary K deprivation, K excretion fell to 10 to 15 mmol/day. On the other hand, with chronic K loading in healthy subjects, rates of excretion of K of 400 mmol/day, that matched their intake, were observed. If a deviation from these "expected" responses in patients with hypokalemia or hyperkalemia is observed, a renal component to the pathophysiology of their disorder must be present.

Components of K Excretion

Two noninvasive tests are used to reflect the components of K excretion in the CCD.

Table 1 Pathophysiologic Classification of the Causes of Hypokalemia

Decreased intake of K
Shift of K into cells
Hormones: Insulin, B_2 sympathomimetics
Gain of anions in the intracellular fluid (recovery phase of ketoacidosis, refeeding after cachexia, treatment of pernicious anemia)
Metabolic alkalosis
Others: Hypokalemic periodic paralysis
Intestinal loss of K
Diarrhea, ileus
Excessive loss of K in urine
High flow CCD, e.g., diuretics, genetic disorders with inhibition of N, K, 2Cl transporter (Bartter's syndrome) or NaCl cotransporter (Gitelman's syndrome)
High $[K]_{CCD}$
Disorders leading to a relatively "Fast Na" in the CCD
High aldosterone, high renin: Low effective circulating volume (diuretics, vomiting, diarrhea), malignant hypertension, renal artery stenosis, renin-secreting tumor
High aldosterone, low renin: Adrenal adenoma or bilateral adrenal hyperplasia, glucocorticoid remediable aldosteronism
Low aldosterone, low renin: Decreased 11-βHSDH activity (apparent mineralocorticoid excess syndrome), inhibition of 11-βHSDH (e.g., licorice, carbenoxolyn, swallowed chewing tobacco), very high levels of glucocorticoids (e.g., ACTH-producing tumor or severe Cushing's disease), increased activity of Na channel (Liddle's syndrome), drugs that increase permeability for Na (e.g., amphotericin B)
Disorders leading to a relatively "Slow Cl" in the CCD
Bicarbonaturia: Vomiting, use of acetazolamide, patients with distal RTA, patients with proximal RTA treated with alkali
?Hypomagnesemia

Table 2 Pathophysiologic Classification of the Causes of Hyperkalemia

Pseudohyperkalemia:
Fist clenching
Thrombocytosis with megakaryocytes
High WBC count with cell lysis
Excess intake of K (in patients with impaired renal excretion of K)
Shift of K from the ICF to the ECF:
Catabolism (rhabdomyolysis, tumor lysis syndrome)
Metabolic acidosis (acute phase of inorganic acidosis)
Drugs (β-blockers, digitalis, depolarizing agents)
Fasting hyperkalemia (dialysis patients)
Hyperkalemic periodic paralysis
Decreased K excretion:
Decreased flow in the CCD:
Low rate of excretion of osmoles (urea, NaCl)
Low $[K]_{CCD}$:
Disorders leading to a relatively "slowNa" in the CCD:
Chronic renal failure (excessive flow per nephron may limit the rate of electrogenic reabsorption of Na)

Low renin:	Damage to, or synthetic defect in, JG apparatus
Low aldosterone:	Hyporeninemia, damage to adrenal glands (autoimmune disorder, granulomatous disease), defect in aldosterone biosynthesis: congenital or acquired (heparin, ketoconazole), decreased aldosterone binding to its receptor (competitive inhibition by spironolactone)
Sodium channel defect:	Type I pseudohypoaldosteronism, drugs that block the Na channel (amiloride, triamterene, trimethoprim, pentamidine)

Disorders leading to a relatively "fast Cl" in the CCD:
Gordon's syndrome
Some patients with hyporeninemic hypoaldosteronism
Cyclosporine A

Flow Rate in the CCD

When antidiuretic hormone (ADH) acts, the major determinant of the rate of flow in the CCD is the number of osmoles to be excreted. A minimum estimate of the rate of flow in terminal CCD could be obtained by dividing the rate of excretion of osmoles by the osmolality at the end of the CCD (equals plasma osmolality when ADH acts).

Transtubular [K] Gradient (TTKG)

The TTKG provides a semiquantitative reflection of the activity of K secretion in terminal CCD.

$$\text{TTKG} = \frac{[\text{K}]\text{urine}/[\text{K}]\text{plasma}}{\text{Uosm}/\text{Posm}}$$

In a patient with hypokalemia, a value for the TTKG that is greater than 2 indicates an inappropriately higher than expected activity of K secretion in the CCD. On the other hand, a TTKG that is less than 10 in a patient with hyperkalemia indicates an inappropriately low activity of K secretion in that nephron segment.

Driving Force for K Secretion

Hypokalemia

A higher than expected TTKG suggests an increased luminal-negative electrical gradient in the CCD. This could be due to either a relatively "faster" rate of reabsorption of Na or a relatively "slower" rate of reabsorption of Cl. Assessment of ECF volume and measurement of blood pressure, plasma renin activity, and plasma aldosterone provide clues to further characterize the patients with a relatively "faster" rate of Na reabsorption (see Table 1). Patients with a "slower" rate of reabsorption of Cl are expected to have a low ECF volume, high plasma renin activity, and an inability to excrete a Na- and Cl-poor urine despite ECF volume contraction.

Hyperkalemia

In these patients, a lower than expected TTKG suggests a lower luminal negativity in the CCD (or decreased activity of luminal K channels, if these are in fact rate-limiting for the secretion of K). A lower luminal negativity could be due to a relatively "slower" rate of reabsorption of Na or a "faster" rate of reabsorption of Cl. Patients with a "slow" Na type of defect are expected to have ECF volume contraction due to renal salt wasting. Measurements of plasma renin activity and plasma aldosterone would help characterize the pathophysiology in these patients (see Table 2). On the other hand, patients with a "Cl shunt disorder" would likely have a normal or expanded ECF volume, low plasma renin activity and should be able to produce a Na- and Cl-poor urine when ECF volume contraction is induced.

Molecular Studies

Recently the molecular basis of a number of the genetic disorders which cause hypokalemia or hyperkalemia have been identified and hence, characterization of the molecular defect can be carried out in the appropriate patients.

For example, mutations in the gene encoding for the 2 Cl, 1 Na, 1 K cotransporter have been characterized in patients with Bartter's syndrome. Patients with Gitelman's syndrome have been found to have mutations in the thiazide-sensitive Na Cl cotransporter in the distal convoluted tubule. The basis for the hypokalemia in patients with Liddle's syndrome is demonstrated to be mutations in the β-subunit of the epithelial Na channel that lead to impaired internalization of these channels and hence increase its "openness". In patients with type 1 pseudohypoaldosteronism, mutations in the α or β subunits of this Na channel resulted in its inhibition and the development of hyperkalemia. The molecular basis of glucocorticoid remediable aldosteronism (GRA), an autosomal dominant form of mineralocorticoid-induced hypertension in which aldosterone biosynthesis is regulated by ACTH rather than the renin-angiotensin system, has also been identified. The defect is one of a chimeric gene in which the regulatory region of $P\text{-}450_{11B}$, the enzyme required for production of cortisol, is linked to the coding sequence of $P\text{-}450_{C18}$, the zona glomerulosa enzyme required for the synthesis of aldosterone. Hence aldosterone secretion in patients with this chimeric gene is regulated exclusively by ACTH. Further, because of an aberrant expression in the zona fasciculata, cortisol, a 17-hydroxylated steroid is also hydroxylated at the C-18 position, with the production of cortisol-aldosterone hybrid steroids. In patients with hypokalemia due to apparent mineralocorticoid excess syndrome a mutation in the gene encoding for the kidney isoform of the enzyme 11-βHSD has been identified.

■ TREATMENT OF HYPOKALEMIA

Emergent Hypokalemia

Hypokalemia is potentially life threatening in three circumstances: in patients with cardiac arrhythmias; if hypokalemia leads to respiratory muscle weakness in a patient with respiratory or metabolic acidosis; and hypokalemia in patients with hepatic encephalopathy.

Under these emergent circumstances, K must be given intravenously. Since a large dose and a high [K] are required, K must be administered via a large central vein. Electrocardiographic (ECG) monitoring is mandatory. The aim of therapy should be to give enough K to get the patient out of danger as fast as is safe. Replacement of the remainder of the K deficit can be done later at a much slower pace.

The following calculation may serve as a guideline in determining how much K to give. Let us consider, for example, a patient with severe hypokalemia that led to cardiac arrhythmias. A reasonable aim in this situation is to raise the plasma [K] by 1 mmol/L in 1 minute. The amount of K that must be given to accomplish this can be calculated by considering that in a typical adult, the blood volume is 5 L, and if the hematocrit is 40 percent, then the plasma volume is 3 L. Assuming a cardiac output of 5 L/min, then 3 mmol of K need to be given to achieve our goal and avoid a high local concentration of K in the heart that may cause serious cardiac disturbances. The rise in plasma [K] will be less than 1 mmol/L, however, as some of the infused K will be distributed to the interstitial space. After this bolus of K, one would infuse K at 1 mmol/min. The plasma [K] should be measured in 5 minutes. If the arrhythmia persists, the procedure should be repeated. One cannot overemphasize, with such a high rate of infusion of K, the requirement for vigilant monitoring of plasma [K].

Another note of caution, the administration of glucose or HCO_3 may lead to the shift of K into cells and thus aggravate an already severe degree of hypokalemia. Therefore one should avoid giving glucose or HCO_3 in the initial management of these patients.

Nonemergent Hypokalemia

Whether mild hypokalemia as might occur in patients treated with diuretics for essential hypertension should be treated or not is debatable. My view is that patients with ischemic heart disease, those with left ventricular hypertrophy and those treated with digitalis may be at risk for arrhythmias and therefore even mild hypokalemia should be avoided in these patients.

Although it is generally stated that a fall in plasma [K] from 4 to 3 mmol/L indicates a total body deficit of 100 to 400 mmol of K, and may be as much as 800 mmol if plasma [K] falls to 2 mmol/L, this is not a useful quantitation in any individual patient. Factors that induce a shift of K into the ICF may also be present, and hence make it difficult to determine the magnitude of the total body deficit of K based on the value of plasma [K]. The bottom line is careful monitoring of plasma [K] as the K deficit is being repleted is required. Two other issues are worth mentioning in this regard. First, during the course of hypokalemia, the CCD may become hyporesponsive to the kaliuretic effect of aldosterone and hence there is a risk for the development of hyperkalemia. Patients who have disorders, or are taking drugs, that may impair their ability to shift K into cells or to excrete K in the urine (e.g., patients with chronic renal failure or diabetes mellitus, patients treated with β-blockers, angiotensin-converting enzyme [ACE] inhibitors or nonsteroidal anti-inflammatory drugs [NSAID's]) may be particularly at risk. Second, in patients in whom the loss of K was accompanied by the loss of intracellular anions (phosphate) (e.g., patients with catabolic disorders such as DKA), restoration of the total body K may require the provision of intracellular constituents (phosphates, amino acids, magnesium, etc.) and the presence of anabolic signals, a process that may take several days to complete.

In the absence of conditions that may limit the ingestion of K or its absorption by the gut (e.g., vomiting, ileus), the oral route is usually preferred. At times also, the urgency of treatment may necessitate using the intravenous (IV) route. If given IV through a peripheral vein, the [K] should preferably not exceed 40 mM as higher concentrations may irritate small veins and cause painful phlebitis. In general, the rate of K administration should not exceed 60 mmol/hr.

Tablets are usually better tolerated than the liquid form. Most tablets are "slow release" preparations, either microencapsulated or in wax matrix, which have occasionally caused ulcerative or stenotic gastrointestinal lesions. "Salt substitutes" may be an inexpensive and generally well tolerated form of K supplementation (Co-salt, for example, provides 14 mmol of K per gram). Contrary to the customary belief, increasing intake of K-rich food (e.g., bananas) is not an effective way to replace a K deficit. Bananas provide little K (about 1 mmol per inch), so one would need to eat 8 inches of bananas to get the same amount of K as in one tablet of Slow K.

In a patient with a K and Cl deficit (e.g., patients with hypokalemia due to diuretics or chronic vomiting), and those in whom the loss of K was accompanied by a gain of Na (e.g., patients with primary hyperaldosteronism), K should be given as its Cl salt. In a patient with hypokalemia and metabolic acidosis (e.g., due to diarrhea or renal tubular acidosis), K is usually given with HCO_3 or other anions that yield HCO_3 on metabolism (e.g., citrate). Nevertheless, since the administration of HCO_3 may induce the shift of K into cells, KCl should be given initially. In patients with rapid anabolism, K will need to be given along with intracellular constituents. In patients on TPN, phosphate is usually added to their therapy. In patients with DKA, K can be given as KCl, while the patient's dietary intake would provide the required phosphate and other intracellular constituents.

Some Specific Disorders of Hypokalemia

Diuretic-Induced Hypokalemia

Since the risk of development of hypokalemia is dose-dependent, and increasing the dose of hydrochlorothiazide beyond 12.5 to 25 mg per day does not usually result in further gain in control of blood pressure, the lowest effective dose of this drug should be used. The degree of renal wasting of K can be minimized by restricting the intake of NaCl to 100 mmol/day. The use of a K-sparing diuretic provides an effective way of reducing the renal loss of K. The Na channel blockers (amiloride, triamterene) are generally better tolerated and lack the gastrointestinal and hormonal side effects (impotence, decreased libido, amenorrhea, gynecomastia) that may occur with the aldosterone competitive inhibitor spironolactone. The availability of combination tablets of hydrochlorothiazide with amiloride or triamterene improves compliance. These drugs, however, blunt the renal response to an increase in plasma K concentration and also have a long half-life. They should therefore only be used cautiously in patients on β-blockers, ACE inhibitors, or NSAIDs and those with underlying renal disease.

Primary Hyperaldosteronism

In a patient with an adrenal adenoma, unilateral adrenalectomy is usually the preferred treatment. In patients with bilateral adrenal hyperplasia, or those with unilateral adenomas who are not suitable surgical candidates, medical therapy with K-sparing diuretics is recommended.

Bartter's and Gitelman's Syndromes

The correction of hypokalemia in patients with these uncommon disorders is usually difficult even with large doses of K supplementation. Hypomagnesemia seems to be an important factor in the enhanced kaliuresis in some, but not all patients with Gitelman's syndrome. Correction of hypomagnesemia with oral magnesium is usually limited by gastrointestinal complaints. K-sparing diuretics may help conserve K, but may exacerbate the renal salt wasting that is present in patients with these disorders. ACE inhibitors have been tried in some patients but with variable results, hypotension is of course a concern. I do not use NSAIDs in the treatment of these patients because of the potential for chronic renal dysfunction.

Other Genetic Disorders

A number of patients with GRA do not have hypokalemia. Administration of glucocorticoids (dexamethasone or prednisone) will correct the overproduction of aldosterone by suppressing the release of ACTH. Control of hypertension and hypokalemia in patients with Liddle's syndrome is achieved with the administration of amiloride or triamterene, drugs which directly inhibit the sodium channel. Since the increase in sodium channel activity is not mediated by aldosterone, its antagonist, spironolactone is not effective in this disorder. In cases of apparent mineralocorticoid excess syndrome, the administration of dexamethasone (which does not bind the mineralocorticoid receptor) helps to correct the hypokalemia by suppressing endogenous cortisol production.

■ TREATMENT OF HYPERKALEMIA

Emergent Hyperkalemia

Regardless of the magnitude of the rise in serum [K], the presence of ECG changes of hyperkalemia warrants emergency treatment. An increase in the amplitude or tenting of the T waves is the earliest ECG change observed in hyperkalemia. As conduction becomes delayed, the P-R intervals become prolonged, and the QRS complexes widen. The P waves become progressively flattened. The wide QRS complexes merge with the T waves, and the ominous sine-wave pattern appears. Ventricular fibrillation or a systole may follow shortly. Because even mild ECG changes may progress rapidly into dangerous cardiac arrhythmias, these patients should be treated aggressively. I also consider severe hyperkalemia ([K] >6.5 mM), even in the absence of ECG changes, a potential medical emergency that requires rapid intervention. The ECG does not always reliably predict the severity of hyperkalemia. Hyperkalemia may be better tolerated if its onset is slow as in patients with chronic renal failure. On the other hand, hyponatremia, hypocalcemia, or hypomagnesemia may potentiate the cardiac toxicity of hyperkalemia.

Emergency measures are aimed at antagonizing the cardiac toxicity of hyperkalemia, inducing a shift of K into the ICF, and removing K rapidly from the body.

Antagonizing Cardiac Toxicity of Hyperkalemia

This can be achieved with the administration of calcium usually as an IV bolus of 10 ml of 10 percent calcium gluconate solution. The onset of action is rapid (1 to 3 minutes) and the effect may last for 30 to 60 minutes. If the ECG changes persist, this dose can be repeated in 5 minutes. As hypercalcemia may precipitate digitalis toxicity, extreme caution should be taken using calcium salts in patients taking digitalis.

Inducing a Shift of K into ICF

Insulin. Recent studies have confirmed the efficacy of insulin (given as a bolus or an infusion) in lowering the plasma [K] in dialysis patients with hyperkalemia. The effect of insulin is evident within 15 minutes, with a mean decrease of plasma [K] of 0.6 to 1 mmol/L after 1 hour. Usually a bolus of 6–10 units of regular insulin is given IV along with 50 g of glucose to avoid hypoglycemia. Delayed hypoglycemia, however, develops in as many as 75 percent of patients receiving this therapy. A continuous infusion of glucose may be needed, and a careful monitoring of blood sugar is required.

$NaHCO_3$. The utility of this time-honored intervention in the acute management of hyperkalemia has recently been challenged. In recent studies in "mildly hyperkalemic" patients on hemodialysis, the administration of $NaHCO_3$ did not result in any significant change in plasma [K] after 1 or 3 hours. With the continuous infusion of $NaHCO_3$ for 6 hours, a drop of approximately 0.5 mmol/L in plasma [K] was only evident after 4 hours of therapy. It is important to note that all of these studies utilized patients with only a mild degree of metabolic acidosis. Perhaps the effect of $NaHCO_3$ is more prominent in patients with a more severe degree of acidosis. Also, all of these studies utilized patients on dialysis; whether $NaHCO_3$ is more effective in patients who are not on dialysis is unclear.

I still recommend that $NaHCO_3$ be given in the acute treatment of hyperkalemia in patients with serum bicarbonate levels <20 mM. It should not be used, however, as the "only" therapy. In fact, the K-lowering effect of insulin/glucose therapy is enhanced when it is given in combination with $NaHCO_3$. Overzealous use of $NaHCO_3$ may result in ECF volume expansion, CO_2 retention and hypernatremia (if not infused as an isotonic solution). In patients with hypocalcemia, administration of alkali may increase the binding of Ca^{2+} to albumin and further lower the serum level of its ionized fraction and provoke an episode of tetany. In these patients, calcium should be administered prior to $NaHCO_3$.

β_2-Adrenergic Agonists. Albuterol or other selective β_2-agonists are available in the United States or Canada only in their nebulized form. In hemodialysis patients with hyperkalemia, the use of nebulized albuterol in a 10 mg dose resulted in a 0.6 mM decrease in plasma [K], while a mean fall of plasma [K] of 1 mmol/L was obtained with the administration of 20 mg. These doses are four- to eightfold higher than what is generally used in treatment of acute asthma. This K-lowering effect is evident in 30 minutes and lasts for 2 hours. It should be noted, however, that the effect of β_2-adrenergics to induce an intracellular shift of K is impaired in some 20 to 40 percent of patients with uremia. Combining these agents with insulin/glucose therapy seems to have an additive effect. In a number of studies, only a modest increase in heart rate was observed when these agents were used in IV or in a nebulized form. Nevertheless, there is the potential risk for tachyarrhythmias. Also, the possibility of inducing myocardial ischemia in a population with a high prevalence of coronary artery disease is of concern. Because of this and the inconsistent responsiveness, these drugs should be tried only cautiously and when other interventions have proved unsuccessful.

Rapid Removal of K

While maneuvers to remove K from the body via the urine or the gastrointestinal tract may be tried (when feasible), rapid removal of K from the body can only be achieved via dialysis. In this regard, hemodialysis is much more effective than peritoneal dialysis. As glucose-stimulated release of insulin may induce the shift of K into the ICF and hence hinder its removal from the body, the use of glucose-free dialysate is preferable. For the same reason, insulin/glucose therapy should be discontinued when dialysis is initiated. In patients susceptible to hypoglycemia, a dialysate with a concentration of glucose of 100 mg/dl should be used.

Nonemergency Hyperkalemia

The focus here is on therapies that will allow for the removal of excess K from the body, measures to avoid the recurrence of hyperkalemia, and interventions that are specific for certain disorders associated with hyperkalemia.

Removal of K from Body

K can be removed from the body via the urine, the gastrointestinal tract or dialysis.

Urinary Excretion of K. The options here are to increase the urine volume and/or the [K] in each liter of urine. The former can be achieved with the administration of a loop diuretic. To avoid unwanted ECF volume contraction, NaCl may need to be administered.

The activity of K secretion in the CCD may be stimulated by the administration of exogenous mineralocorticoids (fludrocortisone 0.1 mg) and/or the induction of bicarbonaturia with the administration of acetazolamide. The bicarbonate lost in the urine may need to be replaced.

Cation Exchange Resins. In these resins an unabsorbable and nonmetabolizable anion, usually sulfonate attached to a polystyrene skeleton, is balanced by an exchangeable and absorbable cation. The one most often used in the treatment of hyperkalemia is Na polystyrene sulfonate (Kayexalate), where Na is exchanged for K. While the resin binds about 3.5 mEq cation per gram, the actual amount of K removed in vivo is close to 0.5 to 1 mmol/g of resin. The resin can be given orally or via a retention enema, resin enemas are less effective than resin given by mouth. When used orally, 25 to 50 g of resin is usually given with 100 ml of 20 percent sorbitol solution to avoid constipation. This may be repeated every 4 to 6 hours as needed. When given as an enema, 50 g of the resin is usually mixed with 50 ml of a 70 percent sorbitol solution and 100 ml of tap water, the enema should be retained for 30 to 60 minutes or even longer. Rectal administration of resin together with sorbitol has been associated with colonic necrosis and perforation in postoperative patients. This is possibly because of decreased colonic motility in the postoperative period, and hence a longer duration of contact between the hypertonic-sorbitol solution and the colonic mucosa. A cleansing enema may be used to remove the resin-sorbitol mixture.

Measures to Avoid Recurrence of Hyperkalemia

The source of increased input of K should be eliminated. A common source is the routine addition of KCl to intravenously administered fluids. Salt substitutes are another source of unrecognized high intake of K. The dietary intake of K should be restricted to 40 mEq/day. Several drugs may predispose to hyperkalemia. This may occur, for example, because of impairing the ability to shift K into cells (e.g., β-blockers), inducing a state of hypoaldosteronism (e.g., ACE inhibitors, NSAIDs, heparin, ketoconazole), competitive inhibition of the binding of aldosterone to its receptor (e.g., spironolactone) or directly blocking the Na channel in the CCD (e.g., amiloride, triamterene, trimethoprim, pentamidine). These drugs should be avoided in patients with a tendency to hyperkalemia.

Therapy for Specific Causes of Hyperkalemia

Syndrome of Hyporeninemic Hypoaldosteronism

Patients with this syndrome represent a heterogeneous group with regard to the pathophysiology of their hyperkalemia. This disorder is commonly seen in patients with diabetes mellitus but also in many other renal diseases. In one group of patients, damage of, or a biosynthetic defect in, the juxtaglomerular apparatus leads to hyporeninemia and hypoaldosteronism. These patients would be expected to manifest ECF volume contraction with renal salt wasting and hyperkalemia. The administration of exogenous mineralocorticoid should lead to stimulation of K secretion and the expected rise in TTKG. These findings, however, are not seen in another group of hyperkalemic patients with hyporeninemia and hypoaldosteronism. These patients tend to have normal or expanded ECF volume; a large rise in TTKG with the induction of bicarbonaturia is observed but not after the administration of mineralocorticoids. This constellation of findings could be explained by the presence of a "Cl-shunt disorder" in the CCD, where the increased electroneutral reabsorption of NaCl could lead to hyperkalemia, ECF volume expansion, and the suppression of renin and aldosterone.

The distinction between these two groups of patients with hyperkalemic hyporeninemic hypoaldosteronism is important because of its therapeutic implications. In the group with a Cl-shunt disorder, the administration of exogenous mineralocorticoids is of no benefit and may further aggravate hypertension. These patients, however, benefit from the administration of diuretics which enhance the rate of K excretion by increasing the rate of flow through the CCD, and may also help blood pressure control. Clearly, the use of diuretics is not suggested for the group of patients with hyperkalemic hyporeninemic hypoaldosteronism with ECF volume contraction and renal salt wasting. Administration of exogenous mineralocorticoids is the appropriate therapy for these patients.

Addison's Disease

Patients with symptomatic primary adrenal insufficiency should receive replacement with both a glucocorticoid and a mineralocorticoid. For the former, 25 mg of hydrocortisone (15 mg in the morning and 10 mg in the afternoon) is usually given; however, the smallest dose that will alleviate the patient's symptoms should be given to avoid weight gain and osteoporosis. For mineralocorticoid replacement, fludrocortisone in a single dose of 50 to 200 μg is usually given. Dose adjustments are made based on the patient's ECF volume status, blood pressure measurement, and plasma [K].

Gordon's Syndrome, Cyclosporine-Induced Hyperkalemia

The pathophysiology of hyperkalemia in patients with these two disorders seems to be one of a Cl-shunt disorder in the CCD. Again, the use of diuretics may enhance kaliuresis and be of benefit for blood pressure control. Since these patients demonstrate a rise in their TTKG with the induction of bicarbonaturia, the use of acetazolamide may be considered, but the loss of bicarbonate may need to be replaced.

Trimethoprim- or Pentamidine-Induced Hyperkalemia

These drugs induce hyperkalemia by blocking the Na channel in the CCD, an effect similar to that of amiloride. In patients treated with these agents who develop hyperkalemia, stopping the offending drug may not always be feasible. It has been suggested that inducing bicarbonaturia may lessen the degree of inhibition of K secretion induced by trimethoprim. The rationale here is that it is the protonated species of trimethoprim that block the Na channel; with increasing urine pH less of the drug will be in its cationic form.

Fasting Hyperkalemia

Recently, hyperkalemia has been described in fasted, hemodialysis patients. The mechanism seems to be related to a relative lack of insulin causing an outward shift of K from the ICF. Hyperkalemia may develop in hemodialysis patients who are kept fasted preoperatively. The rise in plasma [K] in these patients is attenuated with the infusion of glucose (which stimulates endogenous release of insulin), but is completely prevented when exogenous insulin is given with glucose.

Suggested Reading

Allon M. Treatment and prevention of hyperkalemia in end-stage renal disease. Kidney Int 1993; 32:1197–1209.

Kamel K, Halperin ML, Faber MD, et al. Disorders of potassium balance: the dyskalemic syndromes. In: Brenner BM, ed. Brenner & Rector's The Kidney, 5th ed. Philadelphia: WB Saunders 1996:999–1037.

Salem M, Rose R, Battle CD. External potassium tolerance in chronic renal failure: Implications for the treatment of acute hyperkalemia. Am J Kidney Dis 1991; 18:421–444.

HYPERCALCEMIA AND HYPOCALCEMIA

Renee E. Garrick, M.D.
Stanley Goldfarb, M.D., F.A.C.P.

An understanding of the plasma forms of calcium is a critical first step in assessing the clinical significance of serum calcium values. Calcium exists in serum in three forms: a non diffusible protein (primary albumin) bound fraction, constituting approximately 40 percent of the total; a diffusible nonionized fraction chelated with bicarbonate, citrate, and phosphate, constituting about 10 percent of the total; and a free, ionized fraction. Although the ionized fraction represents the physiologically active moiety, most laboratories measure only total calcium. Thus, it is important to recognize that the ionized fraction may vary independently of total calcium. For example, since 85 to 90 percent of the nondiffusible calcium is bound by albumin and only 10 to 15 percent is bound by globulin, hypoalbuminemia will reduce the bound fraction and the total calcium measurement, but will not change the ionized fraction. Therefore, the patient will not exhibit signs or symptoms of hypocalcemia. Conversely, acid-base changes may affect the ionized fraction without changing the total calcium measurement. An alkaline pH will increase the binding of calcium to protein, lowering the ionized fraction, while total calcium is unchanged. Finally, certain forms of hyperglobulinemia may increase total calcium without affecting ionized calcium.

■ FACTORS REGULATING SERUM CALCIUM

Three systems participate in the regulation of serum calcium: intestine, bone, and kidney. Dietary calcium is absorbed in the proximal small bowel primarily under the influence of vitamin D and its metabolites; it is deposited into and released from bone under the influence of parathyroid hormone (PTH), vitamin D, and phosphorus; and it is excreted by the kidney. The renal excretion of calcium is regulated by both the filtered load of calcium (glomerular filtration rate × diffusible calcium) and PTH. High levels of PTH increase the reabsorption of filtered calcium in the distal nephron segments. Most clinical disorders of serum concentration can be traced to abnormalities in either intestinal absorption or bone resorption, with the kidney playing a secondary role.

■ HYPERCALCEMIA

With the advent of the autoanalyzer, the detection of hypercalcemia has become increasingly common. Table 1 lists the major causes of hypercalcemia together with some comments on the associated mechanisms. The most common causes of hypercalcemia are malignancy and hyperparathyroidism. Granulomatous disorders, as a group, are the third most common cause of hypercalcemia.

Table 1 Causes of Hypercalcemia

Hyperparathyroidism
Adenoma
Hyperplasia—familial, multiple endocrine neoplasia syndrome
Malignancy associated
Metastatic resorption of bone
Osteoclast activating factors
PTH-like substances (humoral hypercalcemia of malignancy)
$1,25(OH)_2D$ production by tumor
Prostaglandin-mediated bone resorption
Granulomatous disorders
Tuberculosis, sarcoidosis, histoplasmosis, coccidioidomycosis
Drugs
Hormonal therapy of breast cancer
Lithium
Thiazides
Vitamin D and A intoxication
Isoretinoic acid
Systemic disease
Paget's
Addison's
Thyrotoxicosis
Immobilization
Postrenal transplant; polyuric phase of acute renal failure
Familial hypocalciuric hypercalcemia
Breast implants

Signs and Symptoms

Since hypercalcemia frequently occurs in association with other disorders, many of the signs and symptoms present may reflect the primary disorder, rather than the hypercalcemia per se. The major symptoms directly attributable to hypercalcemia are given in Table 2. These findings are independent of the cause of hypercalcemia, and their severity is influenced by the degree of hypercalcemia and perhaps by the rate at which the calcium level rises. Although many patients with mild hypercalcemia (11 to 12 mg per deciliter) are either asymptomatic or complain of only malaise, patients with severe, acute hypercalcemia (usually 15 mg per deciliter or higher) may present with potentially life-threatening nervous system, cardiac, and renal dysfunction. Within this spectrum, symptomatic hypercalcemia is usually characterized by complaints of anorexia, constipation, polyuria, polydipsia, mild confusion, and memory lapses. Hypercalcemia may be associated with hypertension, which is most frequently seen with the hypercalcemia of parathyroid, granulomatous, and malignant disease.

With the exception of the electrocardiogram (ECG) and urinalysis, the laboratory findings of hypercalcemia are fairly nonspecific. The ECG changes include shortening of the Q-T interval and ST-T segment coving. As hypercalcemia progresses, T wave widening and ventricular arrhythmias as well as heart block may occur. Hypercalcemia potentiates the effects of digitalis and may induce digitalis-associated arrhythmias.

Table 2 Signs and Symptoms of Hypercalcemia

Gastrointestinal
Anorexia, nausea, vomiting, constipation, pancreatitis
Central nervous system
Confusion, memory loss, stupor, coma
Cardiovascular
ECG changes, hypertension, arrhythmias
Renal
Polyuria, polydipsia, acute and chronic renal insufficiency, nephrolithiasis, nephrocalcinosis
Systemic
Hyperchloremic acidosis, metastatic calcification

The most consistent renal defect in hypercalcemia is a reduction in urinary concentrating ability. This occurs with relatively mild (11 to 12 mg per deciliter) hypercalcemia, and although the defect is typically not severe (urine osmolality is usually isotonic or greater), in some cases the urine may be frankly hypotonic and significant polyuria may ensue. The loss of urinary concentrating ability, coupled with hypercalcemia-induced nausea, vomiting, and anorexia, may lead to significant extracellular volume depletion. Extracellular volume depletion will in turn lead to enhanced proximal tubular sodium and calcium reabsorption and may thereby further exacerbate the hypercalcemia. More marked elevations in serum calcium (>13 mg per deciliter) affect both renal blood flow and glomerular permeability and may lead to acute renal insufficiency. This reduction in glomerular filtration rate and the concomitant impairment in renal calcium excretion may be important contributory factors in the genesis of the severe hypercalcemia of certain malignancies—most notably multiple myeloma. With the exceptions of lithium- and thiazide-induced hypercalcemia and familial hypocalciuric hypercalcemia, hypercalciuria is present. Long-standing hypercalcemia, such as that seen with hyperparathyroidism and granulomatous disease, may cause nephrolithiasis and/or nephrocalcinosis, and chronic renal insufficiency may ensue.

Therapeutic Modalities

The basic pharmacologic approaches available for the management of hypercalcemia, together with their possible side effects, are outlined in Table 3. Each of these treatments has certain limitations and some are more likely to be beneficial in certain settings.

Table 3 Therapeutic Modalities for Hypercalcemia

THERAPEUTIC MODALITIES	POTENTIAL SIDE EFFECTS
Increased renal excretion	
Saline	Extracellular volume expansion
Loop diuretics	Hypokalemia, hypomagnesemia, volume depletion
Decreased gastrointestinal absorption	
Glucocorticoids (may inhibit vitamin D metabolism)	Hyperglycemia, immunosupresion
Oral phosphates*	Diarrhea, ? worsening of hyperparathyroid bone disease, extravascular calcification
Decreased bone resorption	
Oral phosphates*	
Calcitonin	Resistance frequently develops
Mithramycin	Renal, hepatic, and bone marrow toxicity
Diphosphonates	Osteomalacia (long-term use)
Prostaglandin inhibitors	Gastrointestinal bleeding, renal toxicity, salt retention
Chelation of ionized calcium	
Intravenous phosphates*	Widespread metastatic calcification
EDTA⁺	Renal toxicity
Removal of calcium	
Dialysis—dialysis plus EDTA	Useful in acute renal failure and chronic renal failure; transient effect

*Also increases calcium movement into bone.
⁺Chelation will lower ionized calcium immediately and chelated calcium will be cleared by renal excretion.

Saline and Loop Diuretics

Most patients with severe, symptomatic hypercalcemia are depleted of extracellular fluid volume. This loss of both the water and sodium results from the renal tubular effects of hypercalcemia. Also, mental obtundation may limit intake of sodium and water. Infusion of isotonic saline solution by expanding the plasma volume with non–calcium-containing solutions will acutely lower the serum calcium level by dilution. Moreover, increasing urinary calcium excretion is an effective and relatively safe method of further lowering the serum calcium level. A brisk saline diuresis alone will substantially increase urinary calcium excretion by minimizing tubular calcium reabsorption at those sites where sodium and calcium transport are linked. Although the addition of a loop diuretic such as furosemide can further potentiate calciuria by inhibiting sodium and calcium reabsorption at sites distal to the proximal tubule, the major aim of furosemide therapy is to maintain the saline diuresis and to reduce the risk of saline-induced extracellular volume overload and congestive failure. Thus, when the diuretic is used, it should *not* be administered until after a saline diuresis has been established, and great care must be taken to avoid diuretic-induced extracellular volume depletion because this will serve to increase proximal tubular sodium and calcium reabsorption and thereby aggravate the hypercalcemia. The approach we prefer is as follows:

1. Begin with 1 to 2 L of isotonic saline over 1 hour to produce the initial volume expansion.
2. Administer furosemide, 20 to 40 mg IV and repeat every 4 to 5 hours.
3. Measure urine volume every hour and urine potassium and sodium concentration every 4 to 6 hours.
4. Replace urine volume with saline and added potassium chloride (20 to 40 mEq of potassium chloride per liter is usually adequate).
5. Measure serum electrolytes and calcium every 4 hours.

A urine volume of 250 to 300 ml per hour is the minimum amount required for adequate calciuria, and effective treatment of severe hypercalcemia (≥15 mg per deciliter) may require urine volumes of 400 to 500 ml per hour. Clearly, close monitoring of urinary sodium and potassium losses and serum electrolytes is imperative. Since optimal management requires infusions of large amounts of saline, central venous pressure determinations should be used as a guide for fluid administration. Elderly patients, patients with cardiovascular disorders, and patients with severe hypercalcemia (>15 mg per deciliter) are best managed in an intensive care unit with central venous pressure or, where appropriate, Swan-Ganz monitoring. Although saline diuresis is effective therapy for most cases of hypercalcemia, the presence of severe renal insufficiency or congestive heart failure will preclude its use. Further, since serum calcium concentration usually falls relatively slowly with this treatment (2 to 3 mg per deciliter per 24 to 36 hours), when severe, symptomatic hypercalcemia is present, modalities capable of inducing a more rapid decline in calcium level must also be employed.

Glucocorticoids

These agents reduce serum calcium concentration by limiting gastrointestinal absorption either directly or via a reduction in 1,25$(OH)_2$D levels. They are very effective agents for the treatment of hypercalcemia due to vitamin D intoxication, sarcoidosis, and perhaps other granulomatous disorders. In the case of vitamin D intoxication, glucocorticoids limit the production of the active vitamin D metabolite, 1,25$(OH)_2$D, and reduce both gut absorption and bone resorption. In sarcoidosis, glucocorticoids reduce the production of 1,25 $(OH)_2$D by the granulomatous tissue and also impair its actions at the level of the gut and the bone. In both vitamin D intoxication and sarcoidosis, very small doses of glucocorticoids may be effective (10 to 15 mg of prednisone or prednisone equivalent per day) and the onset of action is usually between 3 and 5 days. Glucocorticoids may also effectively control the hypercalcemia of certain malignancies—most notably multiple myeloma, breast cancer, and lymphoproliferative disorders. In these settings, glucocorticoids presumably act through a direct tumorlytic effect and by limiting the production of bone resorbing factors such as osteoclast activating factor. Additionally, certain lymphoproliferative disorders (T cell lymphomas) may produce 1,25 $(OH)_2$D, and in these conditions glucocorticoids may also reduce serum calcium concentration via an inhibitory effect on the production and action of 1,25 $(OH)_2$D. When used for malignancy-associated hypercalcemia, doses of 60 mg per day of prednisone or prednisone equivalent are usually required. In this setting, glucocorticoid therapy has the disadvantage of being relatively slow acting: Serum calcium concentration usually falls 5 to 10 days after the start of therapy. In addition, glucocorticoids may (1) lead to increased risk of infection; (2) worsen the catabolic effects of malignancy, chemotherapy, and poor nutrition; and (3) exacerbate skeletal demineralization through a direct effect. Glucocorticoids are generally ineffective in parathyroid-mediated hypercalcemia or in the management of solid-tumor–associated hypercalcemia due to the presence of PTH-like substances (humoral hypercalcemia of malignancy).

Oral Phosphates

In hypercalcemic patients with normal or reduced serum phosphate levels, oral phosphate supplementation is a very reliable, relatively safe treatment. The anticalcemic effects of phosphate are expressed primarily at the level of the bone where there is reduced calcium resorption and enhanced calcium uptake. Phosphates are usually given as 1.5 to 3.0 g of elemental phosphorus per day in divided doses. Neutra-Phos (250 mg phosphorus per capsule) and other phospho-soda preparations are safe, inexpensive preparations. Serum calcium concentration usually declines with 48 hours. Oral phosphate should never be used if renal insufficiency or hyperphosphatemia is present, since the attendant increment in the calcium-phosphate product will greatly increase the risk of extravascular calcification. Serum calcium, phosphorus, and creatinine levels should be closely followed in the hospital until a therapeutic response is seen and the absence of hyperphosphatemia assured. Diarrhea frequently occurs with large doses of oral phosphate and is a major reason for patient noncompliance.

Calcitonin

This agent inhibits osteoclastic bone resorption. Calcitonin acts rapidly (hours) and has a low incidence of toxicity (rash, flushing, rare allergic reactions). These characteristics would suggest that calcitonin is an ideal drug for the treatment of severe hypercalcemia, or the long-term management of malignancy-associated hypercalcemia. Unfortunately, about 20 percent of patients do not respond to calcitonin and the majority of patients who do initially respond become resistant to its effects after several days of therapy. In some patients, concurrent glucocorticoid therapy (30 to 60 mg per day of prednisone) may prevent the development of resistance, but this effect is generally not long lasting. Despite these drawbacks, its safety and rapid onset of action make calcitonin an attractive agent for treatment of hypercalcemia. Although allergic reactions are rare, prior to therapy a 1.0 unit intradermal skin test should be performed. If the skin test is negative then the recommended initial dose of salmon calcitonin is 4 units per kilogram subcutaneously every 12 to 24 hours. The need for dosage increments is guided by the serum calcium level; the maximum recommended dose is 8 units per kilogram every 6 hours.

Mithramycin

Inferential data suggest that this antitumor agent reduces serum calcium levels by inhibiting osteoclastic bone resorption. The usual hypocalcemic dose is 25 µg per kilogram of body weight, although occasionally smaller doses may suffice (10 to 15 µg per kilogram). Its onset of action is less rapid than that of calcitonin; serum calcium usually begins to fall 10 to 20 hours after administration. If an adequate response is not initially obtained, the dose can be repeated daily for 3 to 4 days. The hypocalcemic effect typically lasts from 2 to 6 days. These dosage regimens are only 10 percent of those used to treat malignancy and they are relatively safe and effective even in the presence of renal insufficiency. When several repeated doses are required, however, renal, hepatic, and platelet dysfunction and bone marrow toxicity (thrombocytopenia) may develop. Although weekly administration of mithramycin has been successfully used in the long-term management of malignancy-associated hypercalcemia, the risk of toxicity necessitates close monitoring of renal, hepatic, and platelet function.

Diphosphonates

Normally, the pyrophosphate (P-O-P) bonds of the bone calcium-phosphate crystal hydroxyapatite are cleaved by local pyrophosphatases. The diphosphonates, which contain a pyrophosphatase-resistant P-C-P bond, prevent bone dissolution in part by chemiabsorption to bone calcium-phosphate surfaces and in part by a cellular action on osteoclasts. Additionally, some diphosphonates interfere with bone formation and thus may lead to osteomalacia. Experimental trials have been conducted with three diphosphonate compounds: ethane-hydroxy-diphosphonate (EHDP), dichloromethylene diphosphonate (Cl_2MDP), and amino-hydroxy-propylidine-diphosphonate (APD).

Both EHDP and Cl_2MDP, administered intravenously, have been shown to be effective in the treatment of malignancy-associated hypercalcemia. Cl_2MDP act slightly more rapidly than EHDP, and a reduction in calcium concentration usually occurs within 24 hours, with a maximum effect observed by 5 days. Neither of these compounds is available for parenteral use in the United States.

Oral EHDP has met with only minimal success as a treatment for malignancy-associated hypercalcemia, and in the United States it is currently approved for use only in Paget's disease and heterotopic calcification (myositis ossificans). Since EHDP interferes with bone formation as well as bone resorption, long-term use may be complicated by osteomalacia. In addition, hyperphosphatemia may occur during the initial phases of EHDP therapy. Oral Cl_2MDP effectively reduces serum calcium concentrations, but oral Cl_2MDP is not available in the United States because of purported side effects (possible hematologic malignancies).

Oral APD has also been successfully used to treat the hypercalcemia of malignancy and hyperparathyroidism. A significant fall in calcium level usually occurs within 72 hours of treatment, but in some cases an adequate response may take longer. Unlike EHDP, therapy with APD is not associated with the development of osteomalacia. Although APD appears to be a promising agent for the treatment of hypercalcemia, it is not yet approved for use in the United States.

Prostaglandin Inhibition

Several early reports suggested that inhibitors of prostaglandin synthesis (NSAIDs) could effectively control malignancy-associated hypercalcemia, presumably by blocking prostaglandin-mediated bone resorption. Along these lines, in vitro studies demonstrated that under certain conditions, the bone resorbing activity of cultured human breast cancer cells could be inhibited by the addition of indomethacin to the cell cultures. However, in recent clinical trials, the systemic administration of indomethacin and related agents only rarely resulted in successful control of the serum calcium. Since the vasodilatory prostaglandins may help to counterbalance the vasoconstrictive effects of hypercalcemia, NSAIDs could theoretically worsen renal function. Given these considerations, prostaglandin inhibitors are not recommended for the routine treatment of hypercalcemia.

Intravenous Phosphate

Infusion of 0.70 mmol per kilogram of phosphate over 10 to 12 hours will rapidly lower the ionized calcium by chelation. The dose-dependent fall in serum calcium occurs almost immediately, and it is one of the most potent therapies available. Although a large portion of the calcium-lowering effect may be due to inhibition of bone resorption, the effect also depends on the deposition of complexed calcium and phosphate in bone and extraskeletal sites. Thus deposits may form in the kidney or the heart, and hypotension, acute renal failure, cardiac arrest, and sudden death have been reported. For these reasons, intravenous phosphate is very rarely indicated for the treatment of hypercalcemia, and it should never be used if renal insufficiency is present.

Sodium-EDTA

Sodium disodium-ethylene diamine tetraacetate (sodium-EDTA) can immediately lower ionized calcium by chelation with the serum ionized fraction. Although the total serum calcium level will not fall until after the chelated calcium has been excreted by the kidney, the immediate reduction of the physiologically active ionized fraction provides protection against the toxicities of hypercalcemia. Reports of severe nephrotoxicity have limited its use, but many of those cases involved higher doses than those currently recommended. However, in view of its potential toxicity, we recommend that its use be restricted to the treatment of severe life-threatening hypercalcemia (arrhythmias, seizures, obtundation) where immediate reduction of ionized calcium is critical. The recommended dose is 15 to 50 mg IV over 4 hours. In patients with renal insufficiency and life-threatening hypercalcemia, sodium-EDTA administration can be used in conjunction with dialysis.

Dialysis

Hemodialysis against a low or calcium-free bath can effectively remove calcium and lower the serum calcium level. This treatment is useful if the hypercalcemia is accompanied by oliguria, or if the patient is unable to tolerate saline infusions. The fall in serum calcium concentration is only transient, however, and this therapy usually only serves as a stopgap measure until other agents can begin to exert their effect.

Therapeutic Approach

The first step in the management of hypercalcemia is to determine whether the total serum calcium measurement accurately reflects the ionized calcium level. In view of the calcium-binding properties of serum proteins (as discussed), the serum albumin concentration must always be considered when interpreting the total calcium value. A useful clinical rule of thumb is that the total serum calcium level is decreased by 0.8 mg per deciliter for every 1 g per deciliter decrement in the serum albumin level. Thus, if the serum calcium level is 11.0 mg per deciliter and the albumin is 1 g per deciliter, the corrected serum calcium level would be 13.4 mg per deciliter, and the symptoms consistent with moderate hypercalcemia would be expected. Conversely, an increase in serum albumin concentration, secondary to hemoconcentration, can result in hypercalcemia due to an increase in calcium binding, but the ionized fraction will be normal and the patient will be asymptomatic. Abnormalities of serum globulins are less common; however, as previously noted, in certain cases of multiple myeloma, calcium binding by the paraprotein can result in marked hypercalcemia without an increase in ionized calcium. Proper interpretation of the laboratory values together with careful history and physical examination will help to avoid unnecessary therapeutic maneuvers.

Acute Hypercalcemia

The initial treatment of acute hypercalcemia is guided by the clinical manifestations and the severity of the hypercalcemia. Rarely, a patient with severe hypercalcemia (>15 mg per deciliter) presents with acute oliguric renal failure along with neurologic and cardiovascular complications (hypercalcemic crisis). This constitutes a medical emergency and immediate reduction of the ionized calcium may be lifesaving. An acute saline infusion is the first treatment to use. If potentially fatal cardiac arrhythmias or shock are present, sodium-EDTA infusion and/or short-term hemodialysis should be instituted. Since hemodialysis reduces calcium only transiently, agents such as mithramycin or calcitonin, which work independently of renal function, must also be employed.

A more common presentation is that of moderate to severe hypercalcemia (13 to 15 mg per deciliter) without associated life-threatening neurologic or cardiovascular complications, and here the therapy must be individualized. If the calcium is in the range of 15 mg per deciliter or higher, our initial approach is calcitonin in combination with saline and furosemide. The selection of calcitonin stems from the fact that, although it is less uniformly effective than mithramycin, it has a faster onset of action and fewer side effects. If the serum calcium level does not fall after 8 to 12 hours of treatment, mithramycin can be added.

In symptomatic patients with mild to moderate hypercalcemia, therapy with saline alone or saline and furosemide will usually suffice. If the serum calcium level remains above 12 mg per deciliter after 12 to 24 hours of brisk saline-furosemide diuresis or if a continuous saline infusion is required to maintain the calcium level at less than 12 mg per deciliter, then additional therapy is usually warranted. This is especially true if the glomerular filtration rate fails to normalize after volume expansion, since not only does renal insufficiency blunt the calciuric response to saline and furosemide, but also hypercalcemia per se can worsen renal function. In this setting the choice of therapeutic agents remains somewhat controversial; however, for the reasons enumerated above, we prefer to try first calcitonin and then mithramycin if calcitonin fails. Other potentially useful agents include oral phosphates, which can safely be employed if the serum phosphate concentration is normal or low and if renal and gastrointestinal functions are intact, and glucocorticoids, which may be effective if the underlying cause of the hypercalcemia is myeloma, lymphoma, or breast cancer.

Chronic Hypercalcemia

Therapy for chronic mild hypercalcemia depends to a certain extent on the cause of the hypercalcemia. In the case of malignancy-associated hypercalcemia, specific treatment directed at the underlying tumor is crucial. Glucocorticoid therapy may be useful for the chronic hypercalcemia associated with sarcoidosis, myeloma, lymphoma, and breast cancer. In the setting of glucocorticoid-unresponsive malignancy, oral phosphates may provide effective control. However, if the serum phosphate level is elevated or if the patient is unable to tolerate the associated gastrointestinal discomfort, then mithramycin at 5 to 7 day intervals is a reasonable alternative. This agent may be effective at reduced doses (10 to 15 μg per kilogram) in this setting. If the use of phosphorus or mithramycin is contraindicated, therapy with calcitonin together with glucocorticoids may be attempted. If effective oral diphosphonates become available, this would be an ideal setting for their use.

Surgery is the most appropriate management for symptomatic chronic hypercalcemia of hyperparathyroidism. Medical management is indicated only in patients in whom surgery has repeatedly failed or is contraindicated. When medical management is necessary, oral phosphates can be used to control the serum calcium level, but these may potentially worsen the bone disease, since at least in some patients the reduction in serum calcium concentration will be accompanied by an increase in PTH release. In postmenopausal women, estrogen therapy may be useful in about 50 percent of cases for management of the hypercalcemia of primary hyperparathyroidism. The management of hyperparathyroidism accompanied by mild asymptomatic hypercalcemia detected on routine screening studies remains a difficult issue. We believe that unless adequate follow-up can be ensured, the risk of bone disease, renal stones, and kidney damage usually justifies surgical intervention.

Special Considerations

Mild asymptomatic hypercalcemia is present in familial hypocalciuric hypercalcemia. Associated findings include hypermagnesemia, low fractional excretion of calcium (<1 percent), and hypercalcemia in family members. Although the serum PTH level may be slightly elevated, parathyroidectomy is of no value and this diagnosis must be excluded prior to parathyroid exploration, particularly if the hypercalcemia is asymptomatic.

The hypercalcemia of hyperthyroidism frequently responds to propranolol. This can be administered intravenously (5 to 10 mg per hour) if acute reduction in calcium is necessary. When propranolol is given orally (80 to 100 mg per hour), the serum calcium level usually declines within 5 to 7 days, during which time specific therapy directed at restoration of a euthyroid state should be initiated. Thiazide-induced hypercalcemia can be effectively treated by discontinuation of the drugs and treatment with saline and furosemide. These patients should be evaluated for possible parathyroid abnormalities and should be questioned regarding their use of over-the-counter vitamin D supplements or calcium supplements.

The mild-alkali syndrome, characterized by hypocalciuria, hypercalcemia, hyperphosphatemia, renal insufficiency, and alkalosis, was more common when large amounts of calcium carbonate and milk were prescribed for the treatment of duodenal ulcer disease. The increased calcium intake alone cannot account for the hypercalcemia; since alkalosis reduces urinary calcium excretion, it is likely that this combination of events is responsible for the maintenance of the elevated calcium. The serum calcium can usually be reduced by discontinuation of both the calcium and the alkali. If these measures fail, other causes of hypercalcemia, including hyperparathyroidism, should be considered.

■ HYPOCALCEMIA

Etiologic Agents

As discussed earlier, most laboratories measure only total serum calcium concentration, which is the sum of the free-ionized moiety, the complexed calcium, and the protein-

Table 4 Causes of Hypocalcemia

Disturbances in parathyroid function
Hypoparathyroidism—surgical, infiltrative, idiopathic
Pseudohypoparathyroidism
Pseudoidiopathic hypoparathyroidism
Disturbances in vitamin D
Decreased intake—nutritional deficiency
Decreased absorption—gastrointestinal disorders
Decreased production of 25(OH)D—hepatic disorders
Increased metabolism of 25(OH)D—anticonvulsants, alcohol
Accelerated loss of 25(OH)D—impaired enterohepatic circulation, nephrotic syndrome
Decreased production of $1,25(OH)_2D$
Renal disorders, hyperphosphatemia, hereditary vitamin D–dependent rickets
Resistance to $1,25(OH)_2D$ end-organ effects
Removal of calcium
Hyperphosphatemia
Osteoblastic metastases
Hungry bones
Acute pancreatitis

bound calcium. Approximately 40 percent of the total calcium is bound by albumin and globulin. Hypoalbuminemia lowers the total serum calcium level by reducing the fraction that is bound to protein. The physiologically relevant ionized fraction is not affected by this reduction, and therefore the patient is asymptomatic. When direct measurement of the ionized fraction is not available, the effect of albumin on the serum calcium level can be approximated by assuming that for every 1 g decrement in the serum albumin, the serum calcium level will fall by 0.8 mg per deciliter.

The etiologic factors in reduced ionized calcium are given in Table 4. Since PTH serves to regulate $1,25(OH)_2D$ synthesis, and since $1,25(OH)_2D$ is necessary for the action of PTH at the level of the bone, abnormalities in one system may not be compensated for by the other. Most cases of hypocalcemia can be linked to abnormalities in the production, metabolism, or response to vitamin D and/or PTH. The removal of calcium from the serum and deposition in extravascular sites can also produce hypocalcemia.

Disorders of Vitamin D

Vitamin D deficiency may occur in a variety of ways. An understanding of the normal metabolic pathways of vitamin D allows one to better predict how a given clinical disorder might disrupt vitamin D synthesis and thereby lead to hypocalcemia. Following absorption from the duodenum and jejunum as a fat-soluble vitamin (D_2, D_3), or dermal synthesis under the influence of ultraviolet radiation (D_3), vitamin D_2 and D_3 are hydroxylated to 25(OH)D. 25(OH)D rapidly leaves the liver and a portion of this intermediate compound is further metabolized by the kidney to form $1,25(OH)_2D$—the most active D metabolite. 25(OH)D also participates in an enterohepatic circulation, and after biliary secretion approximately 80 percent of 25(OH)D or its conjugate forms are reabsorbed by the liver. The blood level of 25(OH)D is not directly influenced by primary changes in parathyroid function, calcium balance, or phosphate balance. The synthesis of $1,25(OH)_2D$ is dependent upon adequate renal function and is stimulated by PTH, hypophosphatemia, and hypocalcemia.

Dietary vitamin D deficiency is very uncommon in the United States because milk and other food products are fortified with vitamin D_2. Gastrointestinal disease, primarily gastric surgery, is now the predominant cause of vitamin D deficiency in the United States. Partial gastrectomy, small-bowel disease, steatorrhea, malabsorption, and intestinal resection are all associated with impaired vitamin D absorption or enhanced fecal loss of 25(OH)D due to impaired enterohepatic circulation. Hepatobiliary dysfunction may lead to reduced production or enhanced metabolism of 25(OH)D. Drugs that alter hepatic metabolism, such as phenobarbital and phenytoin, may induce vitamin D deficiency via increased metabolism of 25(OH)D and impairment of vitamin D–dependent calcium absorption. Primary biliary cirrhosis is the hepatic disease most frequently associated with vitamin D deficiency. The deficiency of 25(OH)D may stem from either diminished production or reduced enterohepatic reabsorption. Losses of vitamin D can also occur via the kidney. The nephrotic syndrome can result in the loss of vitamin D binding protein together with 25(OH)D. In each of these disorders, the serum levels of 25(OH)D are low. The levels of $1,25(OH)_2D$ may be normal or low depending on the presence or absence of hypocalemia-induced secondary hyperparathyroidism.

Hyperphosphatemia per se suppresses $1,25(OH)_2D$ synthesis. Defective $1,25(OH)_2D$ production can occur in association with renal parenchymal disease or as a hereditary defect of 1-hydroxylase activity (vitamin D–dependent rickets). Recently a vitamin D deficiency-like syndrome has been reported in association with elevated $1,25(OH)_2D$ levels, and these patients appear to have end-organ resistance to vitamin D metabolites.

Disorders of the Parathyroid System

Hypocalcemia can arise from either reduced production of PTH (hypoparathyroidism) or end-organ resistance to PTH (pseudohypoparathyroidism). Hypoparathyroidism commonly occurs following thyroid, parathyroid, or radical neck surgery. Other causes include infiltrative disorders (amyloidosis, hemochromatosis, malignancy) and idiopathic hypoparathyroidism. The latter disease is often associated with idiopathic adrenal insufficiency, pernicious anemia, hypothyroidism, and diabetes mellitus.

Most patients with pseudohypoparathyroidism have a characteristic short stature, mental retardation, and shortening of the third and fourth metacarpals. Although usually both the kidney and bone demonstrate resistance to the effects of PTH, resistance may rarely exist only at one end organ. Pseudoidiopathic hypoparathyroidism is associated with high PTH levels and a normal renal response to exogenous PTH infusion. Thus, this disorder appears to be due to the secretion of a defective species of PTH. A similar defect may be present in some patients with pseudohypoparathyroidism.

Hypomagnesemia and Hypermagnesemia

With hypomagnesemia of any cause (serum magnesium <1 mg per deciliter), hypocalcemia can occur due to reduced PTH secretion and/or to inhibition of the skeletal effects of PTH. Brisk saline diuresis, loop diuretics, aminoglycosides, and cis-platinum therapy may all increase magnesium excretion. Alcoholism, small-bowel disease, and diarrhea are common causes of impaired magnesium absorption.

Table 5 Signs and Symptoms of Hypocalcemia

Neuromuscular
Paresthesias, tetany, muscle cramps, seizures, anxiety, depression, dementia, movement disorders, proximal myopathy
Cardiovascular
ECG changes, hypotension, congestive heart failure, arrhythmias
Ectodermal
Brittle, dry hair, alopecia, dry skin, cataracts, delayed dentition

Increases in serum magnesium (>5.5 mg per deciliter) may suppress PTH release and reduce renal calcium reabsorption and lead to hypocalcemia. Hypermagnesemia frequently occurs during the acute management of eclampsia and during the inadvertent use of magnesium-containing cathartics in patients with renal insufficiency.

Hyperphosphatemia, Pancreatitis, Osteoblastic Metastases, and "Hungry Bones"

The removal of calcium from the circulation and its deposition elsewhere can produce severe, acute hypocalcemia. Acute hyperphosphatemia from any cause (infusion, ingestion, use of phosphate enemas and laxatives) can lead to hypocalcemia by chelation with ionized calcium. Severe hyperphosphatemia may be seen with rhabdomyolysis and often accompanies the cytotoxic treatment of lymphoma and leukemia. Hyperkalemia, hyperuricemia, and renal failure may occur in these settings. Chronic hyperphosphatemia can lead to hypocalcemia by reducing $1{,}25(OH)_2D$ synthesis and enhancing extravascular deposition. The precipitation of calcium soaps appears to be the major mechanism responsible for the hypocalcemia associated with acute pancreatitis. Additionally, pancreatitis may lead to suppression of PTH release.

The osteoblastic metastases which occasionally accompany carcinoma of the breast, prostate, and lung lead to enhanced deposition of calcium into bone. Enhanced bone formation may also occur following the surgical treatment of hyperparathyroidism. When bone formation is greatly stimulated, the skeletal deposition of calcium, phosphate, and magnesium may result in marked reductions in the serum levels of these minerals. This "hungry bone" syndrome is most likely to occur when radiographic evidence of significant osteitis fibrosa and an elevated alkaline phosphatase level are present preoperatively. It is frequently seen following parathyroidectomy in patients with chronic renal failure and secondary hyperparathyroidism.

Signs and Symptoms

The manifestations of hypocalcemia range from a vague feeling of ill health to life-threatening neuromuscular and cardiovascular dysfunction. The development of symptomatic hypocalcemia probably relates to the rate at which the ionized calcium level falls. A relatively small, acute drop in ionized calcium may produce symptoms, whereas moderate chronic hypocalcemia is often asymptomatic.

The symptoms of hypocalcemia are given in Table 5. The hallmark of hypocalcemia is tetany with markedly enhanced neuromuscular irritability. Latent tetany may be detected in otherwise asymptomatic patients by tapping over the facial nerve to produce a facial twitch (Chvostek's sign) or by inflating a blood pressure cuff over systolic pressure for 3 minutes to produce carpal spasms (Trousseau's sign). Clinically, tetany usually begins with circumoral and facial paresthesias. Motor manifestations include stiffness, muscle cramps, and the characteristic spontaneous carpopedal spasms. Other less common complications of severe hypocalcemia include laryngeal stridor with ventilatory failure, frank seizures, hypotension and congestive heart failure due to decreased myocardial contractility, and ventricular arrhythmias. Resistance to digitalis may occur with hypocalcemia. The electrocardiogram reveals a characteristic lengthening of Q-T interval, which is best detected by measuring the Q-T intervals, since the ST segment is lengthened but the T wave is not affected.

More chronic manifestations of hypocalcemia include mental retardation in children and psychosis and dementia in adults. In children, delayed or defective dentition and extrapyramidal movement disorders may be present. Anterior and posterior subcapsular cataracts, dermatitis, and patchy alopecia may occur. Although skeletal abnormalities (osteomalacia, osteopenia) are often present, their pathogenesis appears to be more closely linked to deficiencies of vitamin D and phosphate rather than to hypocalcemia per se. Similarly, the occurrence of proximal myopathy is most closely related to the presence of secondary hyperparathyroidism, phosphate depletion, or vitamin D deficiency.

Therapeutic Modalities

The preparations of calcium and vitamin D commonly available are given in Table 6. The calcium preparations vary greatly in their elemental calcium content and this must be taken into consideration when prescribing them. Similar care must be taken when recommending over-the-counter calcium preparations, since some of these compounds contain both calcium and vitamin D. We generally prefer to use calcium carbonate, as it is relatively well tolerated and inexpensive. Numerous vitamin D preparations are available and, as will be discussed, some are more likely to be effective in selected situations. Dihydrotachysterol (DHT), $1{,}25(OH)_2D$ (calcitriol), and 1α-hydroxycholecalciferol (1α-OH-D_3, available in Europe) do not require renal metabolism to be effective.

Therapeutic Approach

Acute Hypocalcemia

Acute hypocalcemia accompanied by tetany or cardiovascular or respiratory complications demands emergency therapy. Findings of latent tetany alone do not indicate the need for emergency therapy. However, if these are accompanied by early signs of tetany (circumoral paresthesia) or other symptoms, then therapy is warranted. The treatment of acute hypocalcemia of any cause begins with intravenous infusion of 200 to 300 mg of elemental calcium. We prefer to use calcium gluconate since it is less irritating than calcium chloride. Each 10 ml ampule of 10 percent calcium gluconate provides 93 mg of elemental calcium and two to three ampules can be infused over 10 to 15 minutes. If the symptoms are severe or fail to resolve after the initial therapy, calcium can be administered by continuous intravenous infusion. Fifteen milligrams per kilogram of body weight of elemental calcium

Table 6 Therapeutic Modalities for Treatment of Hypocalcemia

CALCIUM PREPARATIONS	PERCENT ELEMENTAL CALCIUM		
Calcium carbonate	40		
Calcium chloride	36		
Calcium lactate	12		
Calcium gluconate	8		
VITAMIN D PREPARATIONS	**DAILY ANTIRACHITIC DOSE (μg)***	**DAILY DOSE IN HYPOPARATHYROIDISM (μg)***	**TIME REQUIRED TO ACHIEVE EFFECT (WK)**
Vitamin D_2 (erocalciferol)	2–10	700–8,000	4–8
25(OH)D (calcifediol)	1–5	20–100	2–4
Dihydrotachysterol (DHT)	100–500	250–1,000	1–2
1,25 $(OH)_2D$ (calcitriol)	0.25–0.75	0.25–2.0	0.5–1

*These are average doses; individual requirements vary. During dosage titration period serum calcium level should be measured one or two times per week.

(as calcium gluconate) can be administered in D5W every 6 hours. If magnesium depletion is possibly present, blood should be drawn for a magnesium determination, and if renal function is intact, magnesium sulfate should be administered. Several magnesium preparations of varying strengths are available and care must be taken to ensure that the dose of elemental magnesium is appropriate. Each 10 ml ampule of 10 percent magnesium sulfate contains 97 mg of elemental magnesium and one to two ampules can be administered intravenously over a 60 minute period. Every effort should be made to obtain the serum magnesium value as quickly as possible. Until the serum magnesium is available, if magnesium depletion is strongly suspected, intramuscular injections of 2 to 3 ml of a 50 percent magnesium sulfate solution can be given every 4 to 6 hours (2 ml of a 50 percent magnesium sulfate solution contains 97 mg of magnesium). Once significant magnesium depletion is documented, its cause should be evaluated and oral magnesium (as MgO) or intramuscular magnesium should be continued until the serum value returns to normal. Empiric magnesium therapy is absolutely contraindicated in the presence of renal insufficiency.

Acute Hypocalcemia: Specific Clinical Settings

Postsurgical. Transient hypocalcemia frequently occurs after surgery on the parathyroid glands or adjacent structures. If acute symptomatic hypocalcemia occurs, it should be managed as outlined above. More commonly, subacute hypocalcemia is present and this is best managed with slow, continuous intravenous calcium infusion followed by oral calcium supplementation when oral intake is resumed. Postsurgical hypoparathyroidism often persists for 10 to 14 days, and during this interval we recommend continued oral calcium supplements along with a modest restriction in phosphate intake. If the hypocalcemia or hyperphosphatemia persists beyond 14 days, it is likely that the hypoparathyroidism will be permanent and chronic therapy should be instituted. Close follow-up is important, since even patients with protracted postsurgical hypoparathyroidism may recover and become hypercalcemic on therapy.

Subtotal parathyroidectomy for marked secondary hyperparathyroidism is often complicated by the hungry bone syndrome. If preoperative evaluation reveals evidence of significant PTH-related skeletal disease, the patient is more likely to develop this syndrome, and in this setting it is often helpful to increase the serum calcium level to 11 to 12 mg per deciliter a few days before surgery by calcitriol supplementation (0.25 to 0.5 μg per day). Both calcium and calcitriol should be continued postoperatively and the serum calcium, phosphate, and magnesium levels must be closely monitored. Initially, adequate maintenance of serum calcium may require 1.0 to 2.0 μg per day of calcitriol and 3 to 4 g of oral calcium daily, along with phosphate and magnesium. In very severe cases intravenous calcium may be necessary. As bone healing occurs the calcium requirement falls and the therapeutic regimen must be appropriately adjusted. Since serum alkaline phosphatase levels decline as bone healing occurs, to avoid hypercalcemia the calcium and calcitriol dosages should be reduced as soon as these levels begin to fall.

Hypocalcemia with Acute Hyperphosphatemia. As indicated, hyperphosphatemia from any cause can lead to hypocalcemia. Usually, the hypocalcemia is associated with only mild symptoms, and in view of the concomitant hyperphosphatemia, calcium therapy should be avoided. Therapy should be aimed at reducing the serum phosphate concentration and at correcting the underlying cause of the hyperphosphatemia.

Chronic Hypocalcemia

Hypoparathyroidism and Hypocalcemia. In hypoparathyroidism the initial therapy is to provide calcium in the range of 2 to 4 g of elemental calcium per day. In patients with mild hypoparathyroidism calcium alone may be sufficient. However, in most cases therapy with vitamin D is also required. As indicated in Table 6, large doses of either vitamin D_2 or calcifediol can be used effectively. The need for these pharmacologic doses reflects the loss of the stimulating effect of PTH on renal $1,25(OH)_2D$ production. Alternatively, one may use smaller doses of either DHT or calcitriol. We prefer to use these compounds and usually begin therapy with calcitriol. The advantage of calcitriol is that it will quickly improve the hypocalcemia, and if the patient become hypercalcemic with therapy, it will resolve quickly upon discontinuation of the drug. The disadvantages are its expense and the fact that it bypasses the renal hydroxylation feedback mechanism that normally serves to regulate the synthesis of $1,25(OH)_2D$ from 25(OH)D. We believe that usually these disadvantages are outweighed by calcitriol's ability to reliably achieve calcemic control without risking the "overshoot" hypercalcemia that frequently occurs with D_2 and calcifediol therapy, or prolonged periods of hypercalcemia that occur with these agents and DHT. The goal of therapy is to maintain the serum calcium level between 8 and 9.5 mg per deciliter. Values within this range protect against the untoward effects of hypocalcemia, but avoid the occurrence of marked hypercalciuria. The hypercalciuria is due to the loss of the renal action of PTH. In all cases of hypoparathyroidism therapy must be individualized. Some patients may require only calcium or calcitriol, whereas others will require both modalities to maintain the serum calcium concentration in an acceptable range. Additionally, there is always a risk of unexpected hypercalcemia, especially in patients receiving both vitamin D and calcium, and thus routine monitoring of the serum calcium level is mandatory.

Finally, in patients with mild hypoparathyroidism receiving only calcium supplements, the addition of thiazide diuretics may maintain the serum calcium level between 9 and 10 mg per deciliter while simultaneously reducing the hypercalciuria. Unless very close follow-up can be ensured, we do not recommend the use of thiazides in conjunction with vitamin D therapy because potentiation of hypercalcemia may occur unpredictably.

Patients with pseudohypoparathyroidism are best managed with calcitriol. In this disorder the depressed levels of $1,25(OH)_2D$ are due, at least in part, to renal unresponsiveness to PTH. Thus, small doses of this preparation will usually suffice.

Chronic Hypocalcemia: Vitamin D–Deficiency States. Optimal management of hypocalcemia due to vitamin D deficiency is partly dependent upon the underlying cause of the disorder. The rare patient with nutritional deficiency can be managed with small, physiologic doses of vitamin D_2 (2 to 10 μg daily). Disorders associated with malabsorption can be managed with pharmacologic amounts of vitamin D_2 (100 to 300 μg or more daily). In the presence of malabsorption concurrent magnesium depletion should always be considered. If the vitamin D deficiency is secondary to intestinal resection or impaired enterohepatic circulation, calcifediol therapy (50 to 100 μg daily) may be adequate. In all cases of gastrointestinal dysfunction, adequate calcium intake must be maintained. This can usually be achieved by dietary calcium supplementation to ensure daily intake of 2 to 3 g of elemental calcium. Finally, since certain gastrointestinal disorders, such as Crohn's disease, display less marked resistance to vitamin D, it is critical that the optimal regimen be found for each patient, and in some cases, such as celiac sprue, appropriate treatment of the underlying disorder may obviate the need for exogenous supplementation.

Primary biliary cirrhosis can be adequately managed with calcium (1 to 2 g per day) and either vitamin D_2 or calcifediol. Although larger doses of vitamin D_2 are required, it is less expensive than calcifediol. Altered vitamin D metabolism secondary to anticonvulsants can be treated with vitamin D_2 (250 μg daily) and prevented by doses of 125 to 375 μg weekly. Alternatively, physiologic doses of 25(OH)D can be used. These patients usually do not require calcium supplementation. Similarly, if true (ionized) hypocalcemia is present in association with the nephrotic syndrome and vitamin D deficiency, it can be managed with either vitamin D_2 or 25(OH)D.

In general, states of vitamin D deficiency in which 1-hydroxylation is intact should not be treated with compounds such as DHT and calcitriol. These compounds bypass the renal site of feedback control of $1,25(OH)_2D_3$ synthesis and carry a greater risk of inducing hypercalcemia. Periodic measurement of 25(OH)D levels is useful in assessing adequacy of therapy, and since alterations in a variety of factors, such as endogenous estrogens, renal functions, and dietary calcium intake, may occur over time, all patients receiving long-term calcium and vitamin D supplementation must have their serum values routinely monitored.

Chronic Hypocalcemia-Renal Disorders. Vitamin D–dependent rickets, due to defective renal hydroxylation of 25(OH)D, is best managed with small physiologic doses of calcitriol. As long as dietary calcium intake is adequate (1 to 2 g daily), additional calcium supplementation is usually not required. The hypocalcemia of acute renal failure is usually asymptomatic or associated with only minimal symptoms and the initial therapy should be directed at correcting the serum phosphate level by administration of phosphate-binding antacids. During the recovery phase of acute renal failure, especially in the setting of rhabdomyolysis and hyperphosphatemia, hypocalcemia can quickly resolve and frank hypercalcemia may occur. One must anticipate this possibility so that the needed adjustments in the therapeutic regimen can be made. The hypocalcemia of chronic renal insufficiency and end-stage renal disease is usually asymptomatic, and therapy is aimed at preventing or treating the associated secondary hyperparathyroidism and bone disease. Since both hyperphosphatemia and $1,25(OH)_2D$ deficiency contribute to the hypocalcemia, a two-pronged therapeutic approach is useful. The first step is the reduction of hyperphosphatemia with dietary phosphate restriction and phosphate-binding antacids. In early renal insufficiency this alone may be adequate. As renal parenchymal mass decreases, therapy with calcium and then with vitamin D is usually required. An elemental calcium intake of 1 to 2 g per day and vitamin D, as either DHT or calcitriol (0.25 to 1.5 μg daily), are useful, since these compounds do not require renal hydroxylation to be effective. The goal of therapy is to maintain the serum calcium level between 10 and 10.5 mg per deciliter and the serum phosphate level between 4 and 5 mg per deciliter. Calcium therapy should not be instituted if hyperphosphatemia is present, and patients receiving such treatment must have their blood levels of calcium and phosphate routinely monitored.

HYPOPHOSPHATEMIA AND PHOSPHATE DEPLETION

George C.S. Yu, M.D., F.A.C.P., F.C.C.P.
David B.N. Lee, M.D.

Phosphorus is an essential element for all human tissues and is the major intracellular anion. It exists in both organic and inorganic forms. Organic phosphorus comprises the phospholipids, nucleic acids, and phosphoproteins that are needed for cellular integrity and metabolism. Intracellular inorganic phosphorus provides substrate for the synthesis of a large number of life-sustaining phosphorus compounds, including adenosine triphosphate (ATP). Serum phosphorus is mostly in inorganic forms consisting of orthophosphate ions. In an adult, the normal serum phosphorus concentration ranges from 3.0 to 4.5 mg per deciliter. The human body contains about 600 to 700 g of phosphorus, of which 80 to 85 percent is found in bone, 10 to 15 percent in soft tissue, and only about 1 percent in the extracellular fluid (ECF).

Average dietary phosphorus intake varies from 800 to 1,200 mg per day. The percentage of dietary phosphorus absorbed by the intestine remains remarkably constant at 60 to 65 percent over a wide range of phosphorus intake (4 to 30 mg per kilogram per day). Thus, the dietary intake of phosphorus is an important determinant of the amount of phosphorus absorbed. In addition, phosphate absorption is regulated by vitamin D, mainly through the action of its active metabolite 1, 25-dihydroxyvitamin D (1, 25 $(OH)_2D$). Phosphorus is present in most food, especially red meat, dairy products, fish, poultry, and the legumes. The phosphorus, absorbed as phosphate ions from the intestinal lumen into ECF, is handled by two general processes: an intracellular-extracellular phosphate shift mechanism and the renal phosphate excretory mechanism. The absorbed phosphate is first "buffered" by shifting into the soft tissue cells (and probably also the skeleton). Any excess phosphate is ultimately excreted by the kidneys. Shifts of phosphate between extracellular and intracellular compartments cause acute changes in serum phosphorus levels without changes in total phosphorus balance. Renal phosphate excretion is determined by the difference between phosphate filtered at the glomerulus and phosphate absorbed by the tubule. Normally, about 85 percent of the filtered phosphate is reabsorbed by the tubule, and the remaining 15 percent is excreted in the urine. The maximal tubular phosphate reabsorptive capacity (TmP) plays a major role in the maintenance of long-term, steady-state serum phosphorus concentration, i.e., the higher the TmP, the higher the serum phosphorus concentration. The total body phosphorus balance is maintained by urinary excretion of the excess phosphate absorbed by the intestine. In an individual who is in phosphorus balance, urinary phosphate would equal the phosphate absorbed. Factors that may influence renal phosphate reabsorption are listed in Table 1.

Table 1 Factors Influencing Renal Handling of Phosphates

Decreased Renal Phosphate Absorption
Hormonal
Parathyroid hormone
Glucocorticoids
Sex hormones
Calcitonin
Thyroid hormone
Metabolic
High dietary phosphate intake
Metabolic acidosis
Alcoholism
Urinary alkalinization
Diuresis
Diuretics
Osmotic load
Extracellular fluid volume expansion
Increased Renal Phosphate Absorption
Hormonal
Insulin
Vitamin D metabolites
Growth hormone
Metabolic
Dietary phosphate restriction
Hypercalcemia
Hypermagnesemia

It is important to distinguish the terms *hypophosphatemia, phosphorus deprivation,* and *phosphorus depletion.* Hypophosphatemia simply means a serum phosphorus concentration below the range found in the normal population. Sustained hypophosphatemia encountered in clinical practice generally represents conditions with abnormal reduction in TmP, rather than phosphorus deprivation or depletion. Reduction in TmP can be caused by excessive parathyroid hormone secretion or by intrinsic tubular transport defects. Phosphorus deprivation is generally used to mean selective omission of phosphorus from the diet, sometimes accompanied by the administration of intestinal phosphate binders. This should be distinguished from complete starvation, which implies total caloric deprivation. Starvation leads to a catabolic state with loss of water, nitrogen, potassium, phosphorus, and magnesium in the same proportion as in the tissues. The phosphorus content of the remaining tissue would therefore be normal for the reduced body mass. Thus, hypophosphatemia is not a feature of starvation per se. Phosphorus depletion indicates a state in which actual reduction in the body phosphorus store occurs. The distinction between phosphorus deprivation and phosphorus depletion is important because many biochemical changes attributed to phosphorus depletion in fact develop within hours of phosphorus removal from the diet, i.e., long before appreciable net phosphorus loss from the body can occur.

Hypophosphatemia associated with ample phosphate in the urine suggests an abnormally low TmP as the cause of the reduction in serum phosphorus concentration. In such conditions, total body phosphorus balance may still be maintained, and phosphorus depletion may not develop. The laboratory hallmark of phosphorus deprivation and phosphorus depletion is hypophosphatemia associated with the virtual absence of phosphate in the urine. The reappearance

Table 2 Conditions Associated with Hypophosphatemia

CONDITIONS	ALTERED PHOSPHATE METABOLISM		
	INCREASED TRANSCELLULAR SHIFT	DECREASED INTESTINAL ABSORPTION	REDUCED RENAL REABSORPTION
Carbohydrate load	+		
Nutritional recovery syndrome and hyperalimentation*	+		
Respiratory alkalosis	+		
Rapid cell growth*	+		
"Hungry bone" syndrome	+		
Selective dietary phosphorus deprivation*		+	
Administration of phosphate-binding antacids*		+	
Vomiting		+	
Prolonged nasogastric suction		+	
Severe malabsorption disorders		+	
Hyperparathyroidism			+
Primary renal tubular disorders			+
Secondary renal tubular disorders			+
Acidosis	+		
Severe burns*	+		
Gout	+		
Sodium lactate administration	+		
Abnormal vitamin D metabolic states		+	+
Oncogenic hypophosphatemia		+	+
Hemodialysis*		+	+
Diabetic ketoacidosis*	+	+	+
Alcoholism*	+	+	+
Postrenal transplantation	+	+	+

*Conditions that may cause severe hypophosphatemia and phosphorus depletion.

of phosphate in the urine indicates phosphate repletion through either exogenous phosphate administration or endogenous release of phosphate into ECF. The latter condition may be brought about by catabolic states such as starvation or the administration of large doses of glucocorticoids.

■ CAUSES OF HYPOPHOSPHATEMIA AND PHOSPHORUS DEPLETION

Hypophosphatemia may result from three general mechanisms. They are increased phosphate shift into cells and bone, decreased intestinal phosphate absorption or increased intestinal loss of phosphate, and inappropriate urinary phosphate loss through reduction in renal phosphate reabsorptive capacity. Chronic, stable hypophosphatemia of moderate severity (serum phosphorus level 1.5–2.5 mg per deciliter) is generally caused by a reduction in the maximal renal phosphate absorptive capacity and does not manifest characteristics of the phosphorus depletion syndrome. Severe hypophosphatemia (serum phosphorus level <1.5 mg per deciliter), on the other hand, is often associated with phosphorus deprivation or depletion and may be accompanied by clinical manifestations of the phosphorus depletion syndrome. It is obvious, however, that hypophosphatemia does not always indicate phosphorus depletion. Table 2 summarizes the hypophosphatemic disorders encountered in clinical practice.

Hypophosphatemia Associated with Increased Phosphate Shift into Cells and Bone

The most common cause of acute hypophosphatemia in hospitals is the intravenous administration of carbohydrate, usually glucose. The reduction in serum phosphorus concentration is usually modest and transient. Fructose administration, on the other hand, may lead to more prolonged and pronounced decrease in serum phosphorus. This is due to the intracellular trapping of phosphate as fructose-1-phosphate. The lack of negative feedback by the end-product fructose-1-phosphate on the enzyme fructokinase allows for the continual cellular uptake of phosphate. Severe hypophosphatemia may develop especially in those with congenital fructose intolerance.

The nutritional recovery syndrome was first observed during rapid refeeding of severely malnourished prisoners of war. The modern equivalent of this syndrome can be seen in intravenous feeding of patients with severe debilitation or anorexia nervosa, especially if the hyperalimentation solutions are deficient in phosphates. The anabolic state from refeeding promotes an intracellular shift of phosphate and may lead to severe hypophosphatemia, frequently associated with hypokalemia and hypomagnesemia.

Respiratory alkalosis is a common cause of moderate to severe hypophosphatemia. This may be seen in chronic obstructive pulmonary disease patients who undergo mechanical ventilation with reversal of their chronic hypercarbia. Hypophosphatemia is also a common metabolic abnormality during the emergency treatment of asthma. Hyperventilation leads to a reduction of intracellular carbon dioxide and an increase of intracellular pH, which activates phosphofructokinase. This results in accelerated glycolysis, and the enhanced glucose phosphorylation promotes transcellular phosphate influx. Salicylate overdose and gram-negative sepsis are thought to cause hypophosphatemia through respiratory alkalosis. In addition, the massive release of catecholamines with sepsis also promotes cellular uptake of phosphate.

Rapid tumor growth may cause hypophosphatemia by increasing phosphate demand for cell proliferation and growth. An interesting case of recurrent, severe hypophosphatemia has been reported in a patient with T cell lymphoblastic leukemia accompanied by an increase in tumor burden followed by hyperphosphatemia after chemotherapy. The underlying mechanism of hypophosphatemia was thought to be the rapid tumor growth and the high intracellular phosphate content of a lymphoblast compared with a mature lymphocyte.

The "hungry bone" syndrome is a rare disorder in which hypophosphatemia develops as a result of therapy leading to rapid new bone formation in a severely demineralized skeleton. This may follow subtotal parathyroidectomy in a patient with primary or secondary hyperparathyroidism.

Hypophosphatemia Associated with Decreased Absorption or Increased Loss of Phosphate in the Intestine

Because of the universal presence of phosphate in food, selective dietary phosphorus deficiency is generally achieved only under experimental conditions. Certain aluminum- and magnesium-containing antacids avidly bind to intestinal phosphate and render it nonabsorbable. When this condition is superimposed on poor oral intake, vomiting, or prolonged nasogastric suction severe hypophosphatemia may result. Malabsorptive disorders, per se, rarely cause significant net phosphate loss.

Hypophosphatemia Associated with Reduced Maximal Renal Phosphate Reabsorptive Capacity

Hyperparathyroidism is a common cause of moderate hypophosphatemia. Parathyroid hormone reduces renal phosphate reabsorptive capacity and leads to a low serum phosphorus concentration. Primary renal tubular disorders associated with hypophosphatemia include renal tubular acidosis and the Fanconi syndrome. The conditions that lead to secondary renal tubular dysfunction and renal phosphate wasting are listed in Table 1.

Hypophosphatemia Associated with Both Increased Intracellular Phosphate Shift and Decreased Renal Phosphate Reabsorptive Capacity

Acidosis induces decomposition of intracellular organic compounds with release of inorganic phosphate, which is subsequently excreted in the urine. Hypophosphatemia generally develops during the treatment of acidosis from resynthesis of organic compounds and intracellular shift of inorganic phosphate.

Severe burn injury may also induce hypophosphatemia. The lowest serum phosphorus level is commonly seen on the fifth day. Hypophosphatemia may last from 2 to 10 days. Possible mechanisms include respiratory alkalosis, gram-negative sepsis, and pain as well as rapid tissue build-up. These patients also have an inappropriate phosphaturia in the face of severe hypophosphatemia, thus suggesting a defect in renal tubular phosphate reabsorption. In trauma patients, hypophosphatemia with massive urinary phosphate excretion may be observed in the immediate post-traumatic period.

The hypophosphatemia of untreated gout has been attributed to respiratory alkalosis produced by pain-induced hyperventilation and a reduction in renal phosphate reabsorption secondary to tubular damage.

Sodium lactate infusion promotes phosphaturia through volume expansion. The lactate also increases hepatic glucose production and consequent intracellular phosphate shift.

Hypophosphatemia Associated with Reduced Renal Phosphate Reabsorptive Capacity and Decreased Intestinal Absorption of Phosphate

Hypophosphatemia, renal phosphaturia, and impaired intestinal absorption of calcium and phosphate are common features of vitamin D–deficient, –dependent, and –resistant rickets or osteomalacia.

Oncogenic hypophosphatemia is an interesting entity associated with mesenchymal tumors. The underlying mechanism is unclear but may be related to an increased sensitivity to the phosphaturic effect of parathyroid hormone, a reduced level of $1{,}25(OH)_2D$, or the production of an unknown phosphaturic agent.

Severe hypophosphatemia has been described in dialysis patients and attributed to a combination of phosphate loss through dialysis and intensive use of phosphate-binding antacids.

Hypophosphatemia Associated with Increased Intracellular Phosphate Shift and Reduction in Both Renal Phosphate Reabsorptive Capacity and Intestinal Absorption of Phosphate

In clinical practice, severe hypophosphatemia is often encountered in patients recovering from diabetic ketoacidosis and alcohol withdrawal. Patients with diabetic ketoacidosis often have decreased phosphate intake from anorexia, nausea, and vomiting prior to hospitalization. Concomitant metabolic acidosis enhances breakdown of intracellular organic phosphates, and the catabolic effects of insulin deficiency promote a phosphate shift into the ECF, thereby leading to increased phosphaturia. Glycosuria and ketonuria induce further renal phosphate loss. Before treatment, despite normal or even increased serum phosphorus concentrations, these patients have a total body phosphorus deficit. During treatment, insulin administration promotes glycolysis and oxidative phosphorylation with a rapid shift of phosphates into the cells. In addition, vigorous fluid replacement may enhance renal phosphate excretion. Usually, 6 to 12 hours following the initiation of therapy for diabetic ketoacidosis, the serum phosphorus level may fall precipitously.

Another clinical setting in which severe hypophosphatemia often arises is in the hospitalized patient with chronic alcoholism. The patient may have decreased phosphate intake from poor diet or vomiting. Steatorrhea and malabsorption due to chronic pancreatitis and alcoholic cirrhosis may lead to vitamin D deficiency and resultant secondary hyperparathyroidism. Both entities lead to increased renal and intestinal loss of phosphates. In addition, concomitant alcoholic ketosis, hypokalemia, and hypomagnesemia may promote further renal phosphate clearance. During hospitalization, nutritional repletion with intravenous glucose solution leads to increased cellular phosphate uptake. This transcellular phosphate shift is further enhanced by respiratory alkalosis from alcohol withdrawal, hepatic encephalopathy, or concomitant sepsis. The use of phosphate-binding antacids for gastrointestinal bleeding or lactulose further aggravates hypophosphatemia. Typically, severe hypophosphatemia can develop 24 to 72 hours following hospital admission.

Hypophosphatemia may be seen in one-third of renal transplant recipients. Reduced renal phosphate reabsorptive capacity is an important contributing factor. The possible mechanisms for renal phosphate wasting include persistent hyperparathyroidism, subnormal graft function, corticosteroid and diuretic therapy, and chronic volume expansion. The use of phosphate-binding antacids for peptic ulcer prophylaxis leads to decreased intestinal absorption of phosphate. In addition, the resolution of hyperparathyroidism coupled with an increase in circulating $1,25\,(OH)_2D$ may promote healing of renal osteodystrophy with rapid cellular influx of calcium and phosphorus. In some chronically malnourished uremic patients, a post-transplant anabolic state may promote a further intracellular shift of phosphate for cell synthesis.

CLINICAL CONSEQUENCES OF SEVERE HYPOPHOSPHATEMIA AND PHOSPHORUS DEPLETION

Multiple organ dysfunction may occur as a result of severe hypophosphatemia and phosphorus depletion. These disturbances from hypophosphatemia invariably occur in patients with chronic debilitation, often in the setting of pre-existing cellular injury. Increases in mortality rate among hospitalized patients with severe hypophosphatemia have been demonstrated. This metabolic abnormality is often not recognized or inappropriately treated. Acute hypophosphatemia in experimental animals resulting from transcellular phosphate shift is not associated with manifestations of the phosphorus depletion syndrome.

The clinical sequelae of severe hypophosphatemia and phosphorus depletion are the results of three critical biochemical disturbances. First, the level of 2,3-diphosphoglycerate (2,3-DPG) in the erythrocyte is decreased, leading to increased oxygen affinity of the hemoglobin and resultant tissue hypoxia. Second, there is a decrease in the intracellular concentration of ATP, the energy source needed for cell functions. Third, inorganic phosphate is a crucial cofactor in the glyceraldehydephosphate-dehydrogenase step of the Embden-Meyerhof pathway, and a deficiency of intracellular inorganic phosphate may impair glycolysis.

The critical determinants of cellular injury appear to be the level of inorganic phosphate and adenine nucleotide in the cytosol. When cytosolic ATP decreases below a critical level, cellular dysfunction or necrosis may ensue. The cytosolic inorganic phosphate is essential for the formation of ATP from ADP. In addition, intracellular inorganic phosphate has an important role in determining the cellular pool of adenine nucleotides. Normally, ATP, ADP, and adenosine monophosphate (AMP) are related by the following reaction:

$$2\ \text{ADP} \gtrless \text{AMP} + \text{ATP}$$

A major degradation pathway for AMP is the irreversible deamination to inosine monophosphate (IMP) through the action of AMP-deaminase. This enzyme is inhibited by a normal intracellular phosphate concentration. Therefore, a significant reduction in intracellular inorganic phosphate may result in AMP degradation and a decrease of the total adenine nucleotide pool. In addition, a drop in ATP concentration enhances the action of 5′ nucleotidase, which further reduces the amount of nucleotides. Any demand in energy production may place the cell in danger of disintegration from a further decrease in intracellular ATP concentration. The various systemic dysfunctions in severe hypophosphatemia and phosphate depletion are listed in Table 3.

Experimental evidence points to a significant impairment of the cardiovascular system in severe hypophosphatemia. An increased cardiac index was found in critically ill hypophosphatemic patients given phosphorus replacement. Cardiac

Table 3 Clinical Manifestations of Severe Hypophosphatemia and Phosphorus Depletion

Cardiac
Reversible cardiomyopathy
Depressed vascular response to vasopressors
Respiratory
Acute respiratory failure
Hyper- or hypoventilation
Neurologic
Paresthesia
Confusion
Seizures
Coma
Intention tremor
Ataxia
Guillain-Barré–like syndrome
Muscular
Generalized weakness
Proximal myopathy
Rhabdomyolysis
Hematologic
Reduced red cell 2,3-DPG
Hemolytic anemia
Impaired leukocytic chemotaxis, phagocytosis, and bacterial killing
Platelet dysfunction
Skeletal
Osteomalacia with bone pain and pseudofractures
Nonosteomalacic bone disease
Renal
Hypophosphaturia
Hypercalciuria
Hypermagnesuria
Hyperchloremic metabolic acidosis
Endocrine
Functional hypoparathyroidism
Glucose intolerance

arrhythmia can occur in acute hypophosphatemia. Reversible congestive heart failure has been found in patients taking large amounts of phosphate binders. Decreased vascular reactivity to angiotensin II and norepinephrine has been shown in phosphorus-depleted animals. Severe hypophosphatemia may also contribute to the myocardial depression, inadequate peripheral vasodilatation, and acidosis in septic shock.

Acute respiratory failure from respiratory muscle weakness is a serious complication of severe hypophosphatemia. Reversible hypophosphatemia-induced diaphragmatic weakness and pulmonary insufficiency has been demonstrated. Hypophosphatemia may induce hyperventilation, possibly the result of poor tissue oxygenation from decreased erythrocyte 2,3-DPG levels. Hyperventilation leads to respiratory alkalosis and further lowering of the serum phosphorus. The vicious cycle may finally induce hypoventilation due to respiratory muscle fatigue.

Various neurologic manifestations may follow phosphorus depletion. Severe hypophosphatemia can result in a metabolic encephalopathy with paresthesia, tremor, ataxia, weakness, irritability, confusion, seizure, and eventually coma. This has been shown in patients receiving phosphate-deficient hyperalimentation and could be prevented with adequate phosphate supplementation.

Muscle biopsy of hypophosphatemic alcoholics has revealed a decrease in cellular phosphorus and an increase in intracellular sodium, chloride, and water. This may account for the generalized weakness or proximal myopathy seen in some hypophosphatemic patients. Severe hypophosphatemia may induce rhabdomyolysis with elevations of serum creatine phosphokinase levels. This is usually asymptomatic or clinically mild. Occasionally, profound weakness, muscle pain, and acute myoglobinuric renal failure may develop.

A fall in serum phosphorus level leads to a decrease in intracellular inorganic phosphate in the erythrocyte. This in turn leads to impaired glycolysis with a fall in intracellular ATP. The elasticity of the red cell membrane is maintained by a microfilament system dependent on ATP for energy sources. Therefore, insufficient ATP causes erythrocyte rigidity and may lead to fragmentation in the microcirculation. Hemolytic anemia may occur when serum phosphorus concentration falls below 0.5 mg per deciliter. Another important biochemical consequence of hypophosphatemia in erythrocytes is the drop in 2,3-DPG, which leads to a leftward shift in the hemoglobin-oxygen dissociation curve. The increased oxygen binding by the red cell results in decreased peripheral oxygen delivery and tissue hypoxia.

Experimental studies have shown defects of chemotaxis, phagocytosis, and bacterial killing in leukocytes of hypophosphatemic animals. This may be related to impaired microtubular actions from low cellular ATP and abnormal membrane synthesis.

Thrombocytopenia, decreased platelet survival, and impaired clot retraction have been demonstrated in experimental hypophosphatemic animals. These may be due to a reduction of platelet ATP content. However, similar clinical findings have not been observed in humans.

Osteomalacia and pathologic fractures have been described in antacid-induced phosphate depletion. A recent study reported 10 male patients with chronic hypophosphatemia due to renal phosphate wasting and with bone disease other than osteomalacia. These patients have decreased parathyroid hormone, osteopenia, normal osteoid volume, and calcification front. A possible X-linked transmission was proposed.

Phosphorus depletion leads to hypophosphaturia, hypercalciuria, and hypermagnesuria. Measurements of these urinary electrolytes have been proposed as diagnostic criteria for a true phosphorus deficient state.

Metabolic acidosis may also result from severe hypophosphatemia via three mechanisms. First, a decrease in titratable acid excretion follows hypophosphaturia. Second, a fall in renal ammonia excretion secondary to hypophosphatemia leads to decreased acid clearance. Third, reduced renal tubular bicarbonate reabsorption occurs and leads to a hyperchloremic metabolic acidosis. Clinically the degree of acidosis is usually mild as a result of skeletal buffering from mobilization of both phosphorus and bicarbonate. However, severe metabolic acidosis has been observed in hypophosphatemic malnourished children receiving hyperalimentation. This may be related to defective mobilization of skeletal buffers.

Hypophosphatemia has been shown to cause glucose intolerance, probably due to insulin resistance. A state of functional hypoparathyroidism exists in severe hypophosphatemia and phosphorus depletion.

■ DIAGNOSTIC APPROACH

As with most disorders, appropriate therapy rests upon accurate diagnosis. Generally, the cause of hypophosphatemia is apparent from the history or clinical setting in which it occurs. Measurement of urinary phosphorus level is helpful in difficult cases. A fractional phosphate excretion of under 10 percent or 24 hour phosphorus output of less than 100 mg should direct attention to causes other than renal phosphate wasting. Such patients may have transcellular phosphate shift, increased nonrenal loss, or decreased phosphate intake or absorption. Transcellular phosphate shift is the most common cause of hypophosphatemia in the hospitalized patient.

Renal phosphate wasting is suggested by a urinary fractional phosphate excretion of greater than 20 percent or a 24 hour phosphorus output of more than 100 mg in the face of hypophosphatemia. An associated increase in urinary glucose, amino acid, bicarbonate, and uric acid points to Fanconi's syndrome as the underlying disease. Measurement of serum calcium and parathyroid hormone levels distinguishes hyperparathyroidism from the other causes of renal phosphate leak.

■ TREATMENT

At normal body pH (7.40), serum phosphorus exists in two forms, $H_2PO_4^-$ and HPO_4^-. Their relationship can be expressed by the following chemical reaction:

$$H_2PO_4 - \gtreqless H^+ + HPO_4^-$$

The relative proportion of these ions in the serum can be calculated from the Henderson-Hasselbalch equation:

Table 4 Commonly Available Phosphate Preparations

PREPARATIONS	PHOSPHORUS (1 G)	NA (MEQ)*	K (MEQ)*
ORAL			
Skim milk	1,000 ml	28	39
Neutra-Phos	300 ml or 4 caps	28	28
Neutra-Phos-K	300 ml or 4 caps	0	57
Fleet Phospho Soda	6.2 ml	57	0
K-Phos neutral tabs	4 tabs	50	5
K-Phos tabs	7 tabs	0	26
PARENTERAL			
Hyper-Phos-K	15 ml	0	50
In-Phos	40 ml	65	8
Sodium phosphate	11 ml	45	0
Potassium phosphate	11 ml	0	45

Adapted from Lee DBN, et al. Disorders of phosphorus metabolism. In: Bronner F, Coburn J, eds. Disorders of mineral metabolism. Vol III. New York: Academic Press, 1981.
*In 1 g of phosphorus.

$$pH = pK + \log [HPO_4^{=}]/[H_2PO_4^{-}]$$

Since normal serum pH is 7.40 and the physiologic pK is 6.80, we have:

$$7.40 = 6.80 + \log [HPO_4^{=}]/[H_2PO_4^{-}]$$

or

$$0.60 = \log [HPO_4^{=}]/[H_2PO_4^{-}]$$

Antilog 0.60 = 4, therefore:

$$[HPO_4^{=}]/[H_2PO_4^{-}] = 4$$

or

$$[HPO_4^{=}] = 4\,[H_2PO_4^{-}]$$

Since the orthophosphate ions are expressed in molar concentration in the Henderson-Hasselbalch equation, the *molar* ratio of $HPO_4^{=}$ to H_2PO_4- is 4 : 1 under normal serum pH. A solution containing the two orthophosphate ions in this ratio has a pH of 7.40 and is commonly called a "neutral phosphate" solution.

It follows that in normal serum, every 5 mmol of serum phosphate contains 4 mmol of divalent phosphate and 1 mmol of monovalent phosphate, giving a total of nine negative charges per five phosphate ions, or a valence of $9/5 = 1.8$. Therefore, the interconversion of serum phosphate from millimoles to milliequivalents at normal serum pH is: 1 mmol = 1.8 mEq.

It is also apparent that changes in pH affect the ratio of the phosphate ions and thus alter the concentration of the solution expressed in milliequivalents per liter. To avoid confusion, all therapeutic phosphate preparations should be expressed in millimoles per liter and elemental phosphorus in milligrams per deciliter, since these concentrations are independent of pH. Each millimole per liter of phosphate contains 3.1 mg per deciliter of elemental phosphorus. For example, the concentration of elemental phosphorus in 40 mmol per liter of K_2HPO_4 can be calculated as follows: atomic weight of P = 31; 40 mmol per liter K_2HPO_4 contains 40 mmol per liter P, therefore it has 40×3.1 mg per deciliter = 124 mg per deciliter P.

■ MODES OF THERAPY

Asymptomatic moderate hypophosphatemia usually requires attention only to the underlying etiologic agent. For hyperalimentation solutions, the addition of 15 mmol per liter of phosphate normally prevents hypophosphatemia. The judicious use of phosphate-binding antacids in patients with peptic ulcer disease or chronic renal failure avoids hypophosphatemia. For patients with respiratory alkalosis, treatment of the underlying disorder (sepsis, acute gout, or metabolic encephalopathy) reverses the hypophosphatemia.

Treatment of hypophosphatemia in patients with diabetic ketoacidosis remains controversial. Despite normal or elevated levels of serum phosphorus before treatment, these patients become hypophosphatemic and hypophosphaturic when given fluids and insulin. Clinical manifestations of severe hypophosphatemia usually do not develop however, and serum phosphorus normalizes with resumption of oral intake. In addition, several studies have failed to show improvement in insulin requirement, degree of acidosis, glucose metabolism, and red cell abnormalities with phosphate supplementation. Nonetheless, the small proportion of patients who present with hypophosphatemia *prior* to treatment require close monitoring. They have significant phosphorus depletion and are likely to develop severe hypophosphatemia during treatment for diabetic ketoacidosis. These patients may benefit from phosphate administration.

Chronic alcoholics, on the other hand, frequently have phosphorus depletion at the time of hospitalization. Frequent monitoring of their serum phosphorus levels is indicated. Oral phosphate supplementation may be given when an evolving trend toward hypophosphatemia becomes clear, so that a full-blown phosphorus depletion syndrome may be aborted.

For patients with severe hypophosphatemia associated with clinical manifestations of phosphorus depletion, therapy should be instituted without delay. As a general rule, oral therapy is preferred unless the patient cannot tolerate oral feeding or has continual seizures or coma.

Skim milk has about 1 g per liter of both phosphorus and calcium. It is a safe and desirable form of phosphorus supplementation. If the patient cannot tolerate lactose or substantial fluid intake, a commercial phosphate preparation may be used. A total daily amount of 2 to 3 g of elemental phosphorus may be given in two to four divided doses. Mild diarrhea is a frequent side effect. Various commonly available phosphate preparations are listed in Table 4.

In the patient requiring parenteral phosphate, caution must be exercised to prevent hyperphosphatemia. The volume of distribution of the administered phosphate varies widely among individuals and is affected by the serum pH, glucose, and insulin availability. In addition, phosphorus-depleted patients are extremely hypophosphaturic and may remain so for some time despite correction of their hypophosphatemia. Consequently, they are vulnerable to developing hyperphosphatemia when a large quantity of phosphate is given parenterally over a short period of time. We recommend that no more than 1 g of elemental phosphorus be given by steady infusion over 24 hours. In patients with renal failure or oliguria, potassium phosphate preparations should be avoided. An initial phosphate dose of 0.08 mmol per kilogram of body weight (2.5 mg per kilogram of body weight) may be given over 6 hours. The dose may be increased to 0.16 mmol per kilogram (5.0 mg per kilogram) if the patient has serious life-threatening clinical manifestations. Thereafter, serum phosphorus, calcium, potassium, and magnesium should be determined and the rate of phosphate infusion adjusted accordingly. Parenteral phosphate infusion should be discontinued when the serum phosphorus level is higher than 2 mg per deciliter or the serum calcium level is less than 8 mg per deciliter. In a recent report, a rapid intravenous phosphate repletion regimen has been shown to be safe and effective for ICU patients with severe hypophosphatemia. An initial dose of 15 mmol of sodium phosphate was infused over 2 hours. The same dose was repeated to a maximum of 45 mmol in a 24 hour period if the follow-up serum phosphorus level remained less than 2 mg per deciliter.

The hazards of parenteral phosphate therapy include hyperphosphatemia, hypocalcemia, hypomagnesemia, metastatic calcification, hypotension, and renal failure. Diuresis may accompany phosphate administration and lead to dehydration, hypokalemia, and hypernatremia. Patients with renal failure receiving parenteral phosphate therapy are especially susceptible to serious complications.

HYPOMAGNESEMIA AND HYPERMAGNESEMIA

Nachman Brautbar, M.D.

■ BODY MAGNESIUM

Distribution

Body magnesium is distributed in three major compartments—in (1) extracellular fluid, 1.3 percent; in (2) intracellular fluid, 13 percent; and in (3) bone, 67 percent. Thus, magnesium is mainly located in areas that are poorly accessible to study, i.e., the intracellular and the bony compartments. Unfortunately, most of the available data on magnesium metabolism are derived from measurements of the blood concentration of magnesium. The limitations of such information is obvious.

Balance

The role of magnesium has recently been reviewed by Flink and co-workers and by Seelig and co-workers who concluded that at least 6 mg per kilogram per day is required to maintain magnesium balance. The Food and Nutrition Board of the National Academy of Sciences recommend an intake of 300 to 350 mg per day for adults or approximately 5 mg per kilogram per day. The requirement for magnesium may increase in pregnant women or in adolescents. Table 1 shows magnesium requirements for various age groups.

Table 1 Daily Requirements for Magnesium

	AGE IN YEARS	DAILY NEED IN MG (MEQ)
Infants	0.0–0.5	50 (4.2)
	0.5–1.0	70 (5.8)
Children	1–3	150 (12.5)
	4–6	200 (16.6)
	7–10	250 (20.8)
Males	11–14	350 (29.2)
	15–18	400 (33.3)
	>19	350 (29.2)
Females	11–14	300 (25.0)
	>15	300 (25.0)
	Pregnancy	450 (37.5)
	Lactation	450 (37.5)

The magnesium content of food as calculated from tables of food consumption and from chemical analysis shows that, in a mixed general American diet, the intake of magnesium is closely correlated with the number of calories consumed. This is true as long as the calories are not consumed in the form of alcohol or sugar, since both have little or no mineral content and can also cause renal wasting of magnesium. Magnesium is found in great concentration in nuts, green vegetables,

Table 2 Causes of Hypomagnesemia and Magnesium Depletion

Decreased Intake	Excessive Urinary Losses
Protein-calorie malnutrition	Diuretic therapy (especially "loop" agents)
Starvation	Diuretic phase of acute renal failure
Prolonged intravenous therapy	Chronic alcoholism
Decreased Intestinal Absorption	Primary aldosteronism
Malabsorption syndromes, including nontropical sprue	Hypercalcemic states: malignancy, hyperparathyroidism, and vitamin D excess
Massive surgical resection of the small intestine	Renal tubular acidosis
Neonatal hypomagnesemia with selective malabsorption of magnesium	Diabetes, especially during and following treatment of acidosis
Excessive Losses of Body Fluids	Hyperthyroidism
Prolonged nasogastric suction	Idiopathic renal magnesium wasting
Excessive use of purgatives	Chronic renal failure with renal magnesium wasting
Intestinal and biliary fistulas	Gentamicin toxicity
Severe diarrhea as in ulcerative colitis and infantile gastroenteritis	Tobramycin nephrotoxicity
Rarely, prolonged lactation	Cisplatinum nephrotoxicity
	Miscellaneous
	Idiopathic hypomagnesemia
	Acute pancreatitis
	Porphyria with inappropriate secretion of antidiuretic hormone
	Multiple transfusions or exchange transfusions with citrated blood
	Bartter's Syndrome

soybeans, chocolate, and whole cereal grains. In some countries, the drinking water contains some magnesium that depends on the hardness of the water.

■ HYPOMAGNESEMIA AND MAGNESIUM DEPLETION

Definitions

Hypomagnesemia can develop without concomitant magnesium losses, and cellular magnesium depletion can occur in the presence of normomagnesemia. However, low plasma magnesium levels may not always indicate magnesium depletion. Since magnesium is primarily an intracellular cation, in clinical reports and experimental studies that only measure serum magnesium, it is sometimes extremely difficult to judge precisely the status of body magnesium content and with all its limitations, the serum magnesium level remains the prime clinical diagnostic tool. If patients are found to be hypomagnesemic, it is safe to assume that, in most cases, the hypomagnesemia is associated with some degree of magnesium depletion. Special care and a high index of suspicion should be utilized in those patients who may be magnesium depleted, but whose serum magnesium is normal or only very slightly reduced. In these special cases, the clinician may look for other laboratory and clinical findings associated with magnesium depletion.

To aid in the diagnosis of magnesium depletion, several investigative tools are available. The magnesium retention test has been used in the study of magnesium depletion and in the evaluation of magnesium balance. The test is relatively easy to perform and requires the intravenous loading of magnesium and the collection of urine. In a normal subject, 75 to 80 percent of an administered load is excreted in the urine within 24 hours. In a magnesium-deficient individual, less than 75 percent of the administered magnesium is excreted in this period of time, provided no tubular defect in magnesium reabsorption is present. Retention of less than 20 percent indicates that magnesium depletion is unlikely.

Prevalence of Magnesium Depletion in Men

The prevalence of hypomagnesemia (serum magnesium <1.53 mEq per liter) among 5,100 ambulatory and hospitalized patients is approximately 10.2 percent. However, caution should be exercised in the interpretation of these data regarding the presence and/or the severity of magnesium depletion since these studies did not evaluate other definitive parameters of magnesium depletion. However, it is safe to conclude that hypomagnesemia and possibly magnesium depletion are common in the clinical practice of medicine.

Causes of Hypomagnesemia and Magnesium Depletion

The causes and disease entities where magnesium depletion and hypomagnesemia are common are shown in Table 2.

Redistribution of Magnesium in Hypomagnesemia without Net Magnesium Losses

Hypomagnesemia without a net total body magnesium loss occurs from maldistribution of magnesium from the blood to the intracellular, bone, and soft-tissue compartments. Refeeding after starvation is associated with hypomagnesemia without magnesium losses from the body. This hypomagnesemia is attributable to increased trapping of the cation in newly formed tissue. The same mechanism is responsible for the development of hypomagnesemia in patients maintained with intravenous feedings containing glucose, amino acids, and inadequate amounts of magnesium. Potts and Roberts found that hypomagnesemia commonly develops following parathyroidectomy from hyperparathyroidism. This reduction in serum levels was attributed to the fall in circulating parathyroid hormone (PTH) levels and the restoration of normal cellular function. The hypomagnesemia complicating acute pancreatitis is most likely due to deposition of magnesium in injured tissues.

Hypomagnesemia Due to Reduced Dietary Intake Without Losses of Magnesium

Reduced oral intake of magnesium in adults has been associated with hypomagnesemia and evidence of magnesium depletion. During long-term dietary magnesium restriction (>6 weeks), signs of hypomagnesemia such as Trousseau sign, abnormal skeletal muscle electromyograms, and spasticity may develop. Both plasma and red blood cell magnesium levels and urinary magnesium excretion became significantly reduced by 7 days of dietary magnesium restriction. All these clinical findings can be reversed after the administration of magnesium salts. Thus, hypomagnesemia and magnesium depletion can develop when magnesium intake is severely reduced despite the absence of excessive losses of magnesium from the body. Magnesium depletion in these patients is caused by the constant cellular need for magnesium by the turnover of tissue. Relatively reduced magnesium intake in settings in which magnesium requirements are increased (pregnancy and infancy) could also result in magnesium depletion. The formation of new tissue in pregnancy requires that dietary magnesium be higher compared to that of non-pregnant women of the same age.

Protein calorie malnutrition is commonly associated with magnesium depletion. Reduced urinary magnesium excretion, negative magnesium balance, and reduced red blood cell magnesium content have been described. The mechanism is related to both reduced intake and reduced intestinal absorption of magnesium.

Hypomagnesemia with Net Loss of Total Body Magnesium

Gastrointestinal Losses. Increased intestinal loss is a common cause of magnesium depletion and hypomagnesemia, especially in disease entities that produce steatorrhea, such as nontropical sprue, short-bowel syndrome, and malabsorption secondary to inflammation of the intestinal wall or pancreatic insufficiency.

Biliary fistulas and prolonged nasogastric suction with the administration of magnesium-free parental fluids are commonly associated with hypomagnesemia and magnesium depletion. Acute pancreatitis is frequently associated with hypocalcemia and hypomagnesemia. The mechanism is not clear, but is at least partially attributable to the deposition of magnesium within the fatty soaps of injured tissues in and around the pancreas.

Renal Losses. Magnesium depletion, hypomagnesemia, and negative magnesium balance can result from impaired renal reabsorption of the cation. The various disease entities associated with renal magnesium wasting are shown in Table 3.

Table 3 Conditions Associated with Renal Wasting of Magnesium

Primary renal magnesium wasting
Loop diuretics
Diabetic ketoacidosis (osmotic diuresis)
Bartter's syndrome
Hyperaldosteronism
Syndrome of inappropriate ADH secretion
Alcoholism
Hypercalciuria or salt-wasting states
Amphotericin toxicity
Aminoglycosides (gentamicin)
Cisplatin

Several drugs that cause renal wasting have been described. "Loop" diuretics (e.g., furosemide), may be associated with severe hypomagnesemia. This is associated with a marked reduction in muscle potassium content which is not improved by potassium supplementation, but which was reversed after intravenous magnesium administration. Thus, hypomagnesemia is common in patients receiving potent diuretics, and muscle potassium depletion may be a serious complication of this magnesium depletion.

Cisplatin administration is associated with a nephropathy and with hypomagnesemia secondary to increased urinary excretion of magnesium. The pathogenetic factor responsible for the magnesium wasting is not clear. The possible mechanisms to be considered include (1) the direct effect of cisplatin on the renal absorption of magnesium and (2) the interstitial nephritis secondary to cisplatin with damage to the loop of Henle and, in turn, reduced magnesium absorption.

Aminoglycosides may be associated with nephrotoxicity and urinary magnesium wasting. Although the precise mechanism underlying the magnesuria is not known, some indirect information is available. The nephrotoxic effect of aminoglycosides is exerted mainly on the proximal tubule. It is possible that inhibition of proximal magnesium transport leads to increased magnesium delivery to the loop of Henle, thereby exceeding the loop's reabsorptive capacity and thus resulting in magnesuria. A possible direct effect on the loop of Henle cannot be ruled out.

Phosphate depletion is commonly associated with hypomagnesemia and renal magnesium wasting. The magnesuria is correlated with the degree of the hypophosphatemia and the administration of phosphate.

Prevention and Therapy of Magnesium Depletion and Hypomagnesemia

Basic Concepts That Determine the Relationship Between Millimoles, Milligrams, and Milliequivalents

Magnesium has an atomic weight of 24.312 and an atomic number of 12; it carries the valency of 2. Millimoles (mmol) are weight (in mg) divided by the atomic weight, and milliequivalents are mmol times valence. For example, let us take the most commonly used salt of magnesium, $MgSO_4$. The atomic weights of this compound are as follows: Mg, 24; S, 32; and O_4, 64. Therefore, 1 g mol of $MgSO_4$ is 120. That means that for each mol of $MgSO_4$ given to the patient, we deliver 24:120 × 100 percent of elemental magnesium, which means 20 percent of this weight is elemental magnesium. Therefore, 2 ml of 50 percent of a $MgSO_4$ ampule delivers about 4 mmol or 8 mEq per milliliter of Mg.

Prevention. In this category, we can include the following groups of patients: (a) patients on total parenteral nutrition,

(b) patients with chronic diarrheal conditions who waste magnesium, (c) patients with renal wasting of magnesium, and (d) lactating females and growing youngsters. In this group of patients, both oral and intravenous supplementation can be used. In groups (a) to (c), the most appropriate route is the parenteral route, which can be either intramuscular or intravenous. In these patients, 15 to 25 mmol of magnesium should be considered as adequate to prevent depletion. In groups (c) to (d), oral intake is advised. Several preparations are available. Magnesium gluconate tablets, 500 mg, deliver 1.2 mmol of magnesium per tablet. In each 15 g of magnesium sulfate powder there are 12.5 mmol of magnesium. Four hundred mg tablets of $Mg(OH)_2$ deliver 7 mmol. Our own experience has shown that patients readily tolerate magnesium gluconate administered orally. Although $MgSO_4$ powder delivers more magnesium, the side effects of diarrhea and abnormal cramps are disturbing. In all cases, the physician must make sure that renal function is normal. In some patients who require total parenteral nutrition (TPN), intravenously delivered $MgSO_4$ can be used even in the case of renal failure. This procedure needs the monitoring of daily magnesium blood levels. The intravenous dose should not exceed 4 mmol per day.

Treatment

In patients whose clinical and chemical evidence indicate magnesium depletion, such as in the alcoholic patient or in the diabetic with ketoacidosis, administration of intravenous magnesium is indicated. The dose should be considered in relation to renal function. If renal function is normal, the administration of $MgSO_4$, intramuscularly or intravenously, at doses of 16 to 20 mmol per day for several days is recommended. Daily determination of serum magnesium levels should be undertaken.

Maintenance. In patients who have already established a clinical condition that leaves them prone to develop Mg depletion, a daily maintenance oral or intravenous dose should be determined. Again, renal functional assessment is an integral part of the management of these patients.

Emergency Administration. In the patient who develops severe hypomagnesemia and hypocalcemia and who exhibits one or more of the complications of magnesium depletion, administration of high intravenous doses of magnesium supplements are imperative. In these cases, 4 ml of 50 percent $MgSO_4$ diluted in 500 ml of 5 percent glucose and water should be given over a period of 10 to 15 minutes followed by continuous intravenous administration of $MgSO_4$ at a daily dose of 20 mmol per day. To prevent magnesium toxicity and death, renal function measurement is important in any of these cases.

HYPERMAGNESEMIA AND MAGNESIUM TOXICITY

Since large loads of magnesium can easily be eliminated in the urine when renal function is normal, it is unusual to encounter hypermagnesemia unless renal function is impaired. Table 4 lists the various clinical conditions in which hypermagnesemia has been noted. As the glomerular filtration rate declines, absolute magnesium excretion falls, and this may result in hypermagnesemia. As long as the patient remains on a normal diet, the serum levels of magnesium stabilize at around 2.5 mEq per liter. However, when patients with chronic renal failure are treated with magnesium-containing antacids, the plasma level can reach 14 to 16 mEq per liter, thus providing symptoms of toxicity.

Table 4 Conditions Associated with Hypermagnesemia

Acute renal failure
Chronic renal failure
Infants of mothers treated with Mg for eclampsia
Adrenal insufficiency
Administration of pharmacologic doses of Mg and use of oral purgatives or rectal enemas containing Mg, especially in patients with impaired renal function

Many geriatric patients risk the development of magnesium toxicity owing to (1) reduced renal function with age, (2) increased consumption of antacids containing magnesium, and (3) increased intake of vitamins containing mineral salts as magnesium. The sources of magnesium can be classified as magnesium-containing antacids, magnesium-containing laxatives, and urologic lubrication solutions containing magnesium.

Signs and Symptoms

The signs and symptoms of hypermagnesemia are the result of the pharmacologic effects of this ion on the nervous and the cardiovascular systems. Deep tendon reflexes are usually lost when blood magnesium concentration exceeds 6 mEq per liter. Respiratory paralysis, narcosis, hypotension, and abnormal cardiac conduction may occur as blood levels of magnesium approach 10 mEq per liter.

The diagnosis of magnesium toxicity in the elderly patient is of great importance since they are the ones to utilize much of the magnesium-containing medications, and also they commonly have reduction in renal function, at least 50 percent of glomerular filtration rate (GFR). Several reports have suggested a relationship between the blood levels of magnesium and the symptoms. However, there seems to be a great deal of variability from one individual to another; some report drowsiness and altered levels of consciousness at levels of 5 mEq per liter whereas, at the same levels, others report normal mental responses with these blood magnesium levels. The most common clinical signs and symptoms described in patients whose blood magnesium rose to 4 mEq per liter were drowsiness, lethargy, and diaphoresis.

Treatment

Discontinuation of magnesium ingestion or administration and the intravenous injection of calcium compounds are the initial steps in the treatment of symptomatic hypermagnesemia. The administration of 100 to 200 mg of calcium may be adequate to reverse the manifestations of hypermagnesemia, but greater amounts may be required. Peritoneal or hemodialysis may be needed to lower the concentration of blood magnesium in patients with severe hypermagnesemia.

RESPIRATORY ACIDOSIS

Karlman Wasserman, M.D., Ph.D.
Richard Casaburi, M.D., Ph.D.
Darryl Y. Sue, M.D.

Respiratory acidosis is the acid-base state in which the arterial carbon dioxide (CO_2) pressure ($PaCO_2$) is elevated above its normal value (38 to 42 mm Hg at sea level, but less at higher altitudes). The increase in dissolved CO_2 causes a shift in the bicarbonate buffer system so that more carbonic acid is formed, which then dissociates in the body fluid to increase the hydrogen ion (H^+) concentration (and thus decreases the pH). This acidosis is referred to as respiratory acidosis because the mechanism for regulation of $PaCO_2$ is ventilation of the blood perfusing the lungs. Respiratory acidosis occurs when alveolar ventilation decreases relative to metabolic CO_2 production. Clinically, respiratory acidosis is observed in many conditions and may develop rapidly (as acute acidosis) or gradually (as chronic acidosis).

ACUTE RESPIRATORY ACIDOSIS

Acute respiratory acidosis occurs because of an abrupt decrease in alveolar ventilation (the proportion of ventilation that is effective in producing pulmonary gas exchange) relative to the CO_2 produced by metabolic processes. Because of the rapidity with which the $PaCO_2$ increases, there is not sufficient time for compensatory mechanisms (principally renal bicarbonate generation) to respond to prevent a decrease in pH. The primary mechanisms for acute respiratory acidosis are (1) failure of the ventilatory control mechanism to sense the CO_2 stimulus adequately and thereby regulate it; (2) a defect in the respiratory pump resulting from failure of respiratory muscle function; and (3) increased work of breathing and inefficiency in gas exchange resulting from pulmonary pathologic factors.

CHRONIC RESPIRATORY ACIDOSIS

Chronic respiratory acidosis is the state in which the $PaCO_2$ has elevated gradually, allowing sufficient time for a compensatory increase in bicarbonate to occur, with the result being that the arterial pH is usually in the normal range (7.38 to 7.42). In this state, the kidneys have had sufficient time to generate bicarbonate, and metabolic compensation for the respiratory acidosis is usually complete. Respiratory acidosis appears to be the one simple acid-base disturbance that can be completely compensated. Although some authorities maintain that in chronic respiratory acidosis, the pH is low and the degree of acidemia is greater for greater degrees of CO_2 retention, this conclusion is generally based on data collected from experiments with animals. In most mammals, the respiratory system is used to control body heat as well as pH, whereas in humans, it is used primarily to control pH and is not needed for heat elimination. This might account for the more precise pH regulation observed in humans in contrast to that of animals with fur coats.

MECHANISM OF CO_2 REGULATION

CO_2 regulation is accomplished by chemoreceptors that control ventilation. In humans, these receptors include the chemoreceptors in the medulla in close relation to the floor of the fourth ventricle that respond to pH changes of both cerebrospinal fluid and blood, and the carotid bodies that are perfused by a branch of the internal carotid artery near the bifurcation of the common carotid artery. The operative stimulus to the chemoreceptive cells appears to be the H^+ generated by CO_2 and not CO_2 itself. Thus the chemoreceptor stimulation that occurs in association with the high $PaCO_2$ of chronic compensated respiratory acidosis is not substantially different from that which occurs when the $PaCO_2$ and acid-base status are normal. In situations in which the bicarbonate level is low, such as chronic metabolic acidosis, the CO_2 is sensitively regulated because any change in $PaCO_2$ produces a greater H^+ change than occurs when the bicarbonate level is high. Because of the location of the respiratory chemoreceptors, it is the arterial and cerebrospinal fluid pH values that appear to be the set point around which the ventilatory control mechanisms operate.

PATHOPHYSIOLOGY

Mechanisms causing respiratory acidosis include the following: (1) central respiratory depressants (drugs, central nervous system [CNS] infection, brain injury); (2) idiopathic loss of respiratory drive (primary alveolar hypoventilation); (3) impaired chemoreceptor function; (4) muscle or motor endplate dysfunction; (5) chest wall deformity or extreme obesity; and (6) mechanical limitation to pulmonary ventilation or gas exchange. If the pathophysiology is of central origin, breathing appears to be slow and shallow and, if acute, the patient may lapse into coma. If the cause is acute failure of the respiratory pump (respiratory muscle failure) or air flow obstruction, the patient becomes tachypneic and complains of breathlessness.

The most common cause of respiratory acidosis is air flow obstruction such as that associated with one of the obstructive lung diseases (bronchial asthma, bronchitis, emphysema). Chronic respiratory acidosis is commonly associated with obstructive lung disease. It is difficult for patients with these diseases to maintain $PaCO_2$ in the normal range because of the combination of high respiratory work, inefficiency of gas exchange associated with intrapulmonary mismatching of ventilation and perfusion, and lung hyperinflation putting the diaphragm at a mechanical disadvantage. Many of these patients therefore ventilate inadequately, allowing their $PaCO_2$ to increase. Because this generally occurs gradually, the renal generation of bicarbonate is usually sufficient to maintain the arterial pH near the normal range.

Chronic respiratory acidosis also occurs in patients with chest wall deformities such as kyphoscoliosis. Similarly, the morbidly obese patient may retain CO_2 (obesity-hypoventilation or the pickwickian syndrome).

Respiratory acidosis can be a feature of any neuromuscular disorder that sufficiently involves the respiratory muscles (polymyositis, muscular dystrophy), spinal cord (amyotrophic lateral sclerosis, poliomyelitis, spinal cord trauma, transverse myelitis, multiple sclerosis), peripheral nerves (Guillain-Barré syndrome), or motor endplates (botulism, myasthenia gravis). Patients with isolated phrenic nerve or diaphragmatic disease may also present with respiratory acidosis. The respiratory acidosis can be acute or chronic depending on the nature and severity of the neuromuscular disease, or in the presence of other disorders. Rarely, patients with endocrinopathy (hypothyroidism or hyperthyroidism) or electrolyte disturbances (hypokalemia, hypophosphatemia) may have muscle weakness severe enough to cause acute respiratory acidosis.

Central respiratory depression secondary to ingestion or injection of drugs that have respiratory depressant properties is another common cause of CO_2 retention. Central respiratory depression can usually be distinguished from the mechanical causes of respiratory acidosis by observation of the patient's pattern and rate of breathing. Respiratory depression is associated with bradypnea and mechanical limitation to breathing is associated with tachypnea.

■ SYMPTOMS AND SIGNS

Virtually all of the symptoms of respiratory acidosis are secondary to the consequent acidemia. The symptoms and signs of acute respiratory acidosis without associated hypoxia are (1) tachypnea, (2) dyspnea on exertion, (3) asterixis, (4) obtundation, (5) coma, (6) headache, (7) papilledema, (8) heart failure, (9) hypertension, and (10) arrhythmia. Other manifestations may occur if hypercapnia is accompanied by hypoxia; compensated respiratory acidosis in which the pH is normal generally does not cause symptoms. Tachypnea and dyspnea are secondary to the acute decrease in arterial and cerebrospinal fluid pH. The cause of the twitching of muscles held in sustained contraction, best marked by the inability to hold the wrists in extension (asterixis), is uncertain but seems to be related to the effect of pH on the transmembrane potential of the peripheral nerves. Headaches and the papilledema may occur secondary to cerebral vasodilation caused by the low pH. Obtundation and coma may also be precipitated by the acute central nervous system acidosis. Heart failure and arrhythmia may result from the direct effects of acidemia on Ca^{++} and K^{+} flux in the myocardium as well as from the increased pulmonary and peripheral vascular resistance that accompanies systemic acidosis.

A variety of CNS signs can be precipitated by pH disturbances that result from acute changes in $PaCO_2$. When the pH decreases to less than 7.35, asterixis is commonly noted. When the pH decreases to less than 7.30, asterixis tends to disappear but obtundation supervenes. The patient becomes semicomatose and eventually lapses into coma. Generally these effects can be quickly reversed by ventilating the patient and returning the pH to normal.

Neurologic effects can also be induced by an acute decrease in $PaCO_2$ in patients with chronic respiratory acidosis by the creation of alkalemia. When the pH is greater than 7.55, seizures are common, and they are almost inevitable when the pH is increased to more than 7.60. This is especially likely to occur if the blood bicarbonate level is elevated, because a small decrease in $PaCO_2$ results in a greater alkaline swing than that which occurs when the bicarbonate level is normal.

■ TREATMENT

Because respiratory acidosis always results from insufficient ventilation of the blood perfusing the lungs (alveolar ventilation), treatment is directed at increasing the alveolar ventilation. The method of choice depends on the mechanism of disease and the urgency of treatment.

Acute Respiratory Acidosis

The elevation of $PaCO_2$ that occurs with severe acute respiratory acidosis generally necessitates immediate treatment because of the effects of acidosis on the CNS (e.g., lethargy, coma) and the hypoxemia that usually accompanies this elevation. Treatment is directed at restoring a sufficient amount of alveolar ventilation by reversing the condition that led to the hypoventilation and/or by providing artificial ventilation to the patient.

Patients with central depression of ventilation may have CNS injury or disease or may have taken sedatives or narcotics. These patients may need to receive mechanical ventilation until the CNS damage is reversed or the effects of depressant drugs have disappeared. In both cases, maintenance of an effective airway is important. For patients known to have or suspected of having opiate depression of respiration, the specific antagonist naloxone is useful, and other specific pharmacologic antagonists may be available in the future. For depression of respiration caused by the use of other drugs, such as long-acting sedative-hypnotics, supportive care including mechanical ventilation seems to be the most appropriate treatment. Efforts to enhance elimination of such drugs by hemodialysis or other means are not usually beneficial, and nonspecific respiratory stimulants are of little value. Patients in whom central depression of ventilation is the cause of respiratory acidosis may initially have normal lung function, but complications of altered mental status and supportive care may lead to secondary pulmonary problems such as atelectasis and aspiration pneumonia.

Some neuromuscular and chest wall abnormalities that lead to acute respiratory acidosis can be effectively treated, while others are benefited only by supportive care. Correction of hypophosphatemia and hypokalemia may reverse transient muscle weakness in patients with severe abnormalities of these electrolytes. Patients with neuromuscular diseases such as myasthenia gravis, Guillain-Barré syndrome, and muscular dystrophy generally do not develop respiratory acidosis until the vital capacity reaches less than 40 percent of the predicted value or less than approximately 1,200 ml in the typical adult patient. Some investigators believe that, in this setting, the measurement of maximal inspiratory and expiratory pressure generated at the mouth has particular predictive value for the development of respiratory acidosis. These patients should be monitored with frequent vital capacity measurements as well as by neurologic assessment. Treatment should be individualized on the basis of the type of neuromuscular problem. It should also be noted that because patients with respiratory muscle weakness have particularly ineffective coughing and breathe at low lung volume, they are prone to lung infection and atelectasis that further decrease the respiratory ability to ventilate and oxygenate the blood.

The largest group of patients with acute respiratory acidosis are those with chronic obstructive lung disease who have acute decompensation. These patients, some of whom have chronic respiratory acidosis as well, may have mechanical and ventilatory control abnormalities that need to be identified and corrected. First, because the primary problem is airway obstruction, bronchodilators are useful (theophylline, aerosolized and oral beta-adrenergic agonists, and, in most patients with chronic bronchitis, ipratropium bromide, an anticholinergic agent). Corticosteroids should be given to those patients whose obstruction is due to asthma, but these drugs should be used judiciously in patients with chronic obstructive lung disease, the elderly, and those with increased risk of complication from corticosteroids. Airway secretions are an important component of obstruction. Suctioning, coughing, mucolytic agents, and mechanical mobilization of secretions may be of value. Antibiotics that work against usual airway pathogens such as *Haemophilus influenzae* and *Streptococcus pneumoniae* are generally regarded as effective in decreasing the severity of acute exacerbations. Second, it is now recognized that respiratory muscle fatigue is an important aspect of acute respiratory failure in these patients. This should be treated by correction of electrolyte abnormalities such as hypokalemia and hypophosphatemia or by "resting" the respiratory muscles through the use of mechanical ventilation. Improvement of respiratory muscle function after the administration of theophylline has been reported; this may cause the respiratory acidosis to lessen while the underlying mechanical derangement is corrected. On the other hand, respiratory muscle weakness may be induced in a relatively short time by high doses of corticosteroids. Third, because central respiratory depression is often a factor in acute decompensation, the use of sedatives and narcotics should be avoided. Fourth, although it is often anticipated that oxygen administration will worsen acute respiratory acidosis in patients with chronic obstructive lung disease by suppressing the output of the carotid bodies, its benefit in improving central nervous system oxygenation and in relieving pulmonary artery hypertension generally outweighs its adverse effects. Oxygen should be given at a low concentration (24 to 30 percent), and the consequent acid-base status should be carefully monitored. Finally, endotracheal intubation and mechanical ventilation should be considered for those patients who cannot be managed otherwise.

It is important to remember that patients with chronic lung diseases other than chronic bronchitis and emphysema can also have acute respiratory acidosis. These conditions include severe asthma, restrictive lung disease (especially disease caused by chest wall deformity), and adult respiratory distress syndrome. Although the management of acute respiratory acidosis is generally similar in each of these disorders, specific treatment of the underlying problem may be different.

After the patient with acute respiratory acidosis begins receiving mechanical ventilation, adjustments are made to give the appropriate $PaCO_2$ value. This is generally the $PaCO_2$ that results in an acceptable pH value (7.35 to 7.42). This $PaCO_2$ may not necessarily be within the normal range if the plasma bicarbonate value is high (in cases of chronic respiratory acidosis or metabolic alkalosis) or low (in cases of chronic respiratory alkalosis or metabolic acidosis). $PaCO_2$ and alveolar ventilation are inversely related, but the volume of air per minute provided to the patient, the minute ventilation (V_E), is related to alveolar ventilation as the sum of alveolar ventilation plus dead space ventilation.

The adult patient with normal lungs usually has a V_E of 7 L per minute and a dead space ventilation of approximately 2.3 L per minute. For the production of CO_2 at rest, this ventilation is sufficient to maintain a $PaCO_2$ at 40 mm Hg. In patients with abnormal lungs, the dead space ventilation is increased, so that the V_E must increase to maintain a normal $PaCO_2$. Furthermore, if the metabolic rate increases as a result of fever, infection, or physical activity, the V_E must also increase proportionally to maintain a normal $PaCO_2$. Thus the relationship of V_E to $PaCO_2$ and the amount of V_E ordered for the patient undergoing mechanical ventilatory support may vary considerably.

The required ventilation for a desired $PaCO_2$ for given values of the ratio of dead space volume to tidal volume (V_D/V_T) (or, equivalently, the ratio of dead space ventilation to V_E) is shown in Figure 1. This nomogram assumes a constant CO_2 production of 200 ml per minute. The V_D/V_T ratio can be determined at the intersection of the $PaCO_2$ value (measured by arterial blood gas analysis) and the V_E (measured by the mechanical ventilator). Alternatively, from a given $PaCO_2$ and V_E and an assumed constant V_D/V_T ratio, the necessary V_E for any desired $P{CO_2}$ value can be determined.

Recently, a number of studies have demonstrated the beneficial effects of noninvasive positive pressure ventilation delivered by mask in selected patients with acute respiratory failure from chronic obstructive lung disease, congestive heart failure, and a variety of other problems. These patients seem to be helped by temporary unloading of inspiratory respiratory muscles, allowing the muscles to recover function and generate enough pressure subsequently to generate enough minute ventilation to maintain appropriate $P{CO_2}$. This technique may avoid the complications and discomfort associated with endotracheal intubation.

A special problem of acute respiratory acidosis may occur during weaning from mechanical ventilation if the patient cannot provide sufficient spontaneous ventilation to maintain arterial pH and $P{CO_2}$ as mechanical ventilation is withdrawn. This may be caused by insufficient resolution of the underlying lung disease, the increased load imposed on the patient by the endotracheal tube or ventilator circuit, respiratory muscle fatigue, electrolyte abnormalities, corticosteroids contributing to muscle weakness, malnutrition, infection, or patient anxiety. Prolonged muscle weakness has been observed in patients who receive high-dose corticosteroids plus neuromuscular blocking agents such as pancuronium or vecuronium during mechanical ventilation. Correction of these contributing factors is necessary for successful withdrawal of mechanical ventilation.

In some patients with acute respiratory failure, a strategy termed *permissive hypercapnia* has recently been advocated.

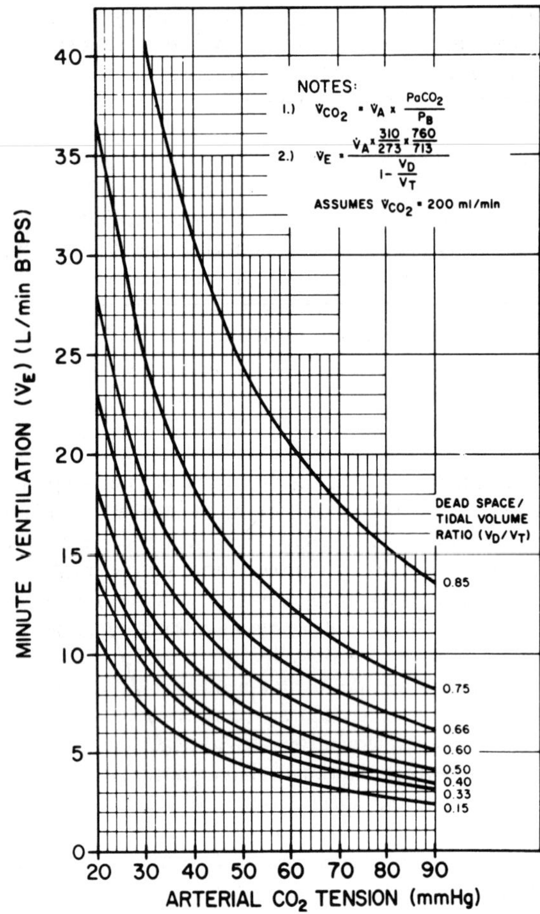

Figure 1
The $\dot{V}_B$ is selected according to the desired $PaCO_2$. These curves have been drawn for an average adult with a CO_2 production ($\dot{V}co_2$) of 200 ml per minute (STPD). However, this nomogram yields good results even when the $\dot{V}co_2$ is not 200 ml per minute, since a $\dot{V}co_2$ differing mildly from this value is compensated for by a false estimate of $\dot{V}_D/\dot{V}_T$, thereby providing a relatively valid $\dot{V}_E$. When the $\dot{V}co_2$ is known to differ from 200 ml per minute, the true $\dot{V}_D/\dot{V}_T$ value can be estimated by multiplying the measured $\dot{V}_E$ value by the measured $\dot{V}co_2$ divided by 200 before determining the intersection of the $\dot{V}_E$ and $PaCO_2$ lines.

Using permissive hypercapnia, patients undergoing mechanical ventilation deliberately receive insufficient minute ventilation to maintain normal $PaCO_2$. This strategy gives priority to preventing injury to the lung by avoiding use of excessively high tidal volume (>6–8 ml/kg) or high respiratory frequency at the cost of acute respiratory acidosis. The first patients for which permissive hypercapnia was used had severe acute asthma, a disorder associated with a high rate of complications such as pneumothorax and hypotension during mechanical ventilation. It has subsequently been recommended for patients with acute respiratory distress syndrome (ARDS) who have very stiff, noncompliant lungs, and who are also subject to an increased risk of pneumothorax and injury to the lung from mechanical ventilation. Permissive hypercapnia usually requires sedating patients heavily or using neuromuscular relaxants so that patients can have their minute ventilation carefully controlled. Then, tidal volumes of 6 to 8 ml/kg ideal weight are given with the goals of keeping peak airway pressure <30 to 40 cm H_2O and avoiding lung hyperinflation. Using this method, arterial Pco_2 would be expected to rise in many, but not all, patients to as high as 50 to 80 mm Hg with subsequent fall in pH to 7.20 to 7.25. Despite severe acute respiratory acidosis, studies have reported that this degree of acidosis is remarkably well tolerated, at least for 24 to 48 hours, and there has been agreement that complications of lung injury from mechanical ventilation have been decreased with this strategy.

Chronic Respiratory Acidosis

Patients with chronic respiratory acidosis have an increased serum bicarbonate concentration that results in a nearly normal pH. Thus the elevated $PaCO_2$ itself does not require treatment. However, the increased CO_2 in the alveolar gas displaces the oxygen resulting in chronic hypoxemia. Because patients with chronic respiratory acidosis almost always have parenchymal lung disease (except those with chest wall deformities such as kyphoscoliosis), the resultant hypoxemia may be severe. The treatment is directed at increasing the PaO_2 directly and/or by indirectly raising the PaO_2 by reducing the $PaCO_2$.

Oxygen

Long-term studies have shown that supplemental oxygen has a beneficial effect in patients with chronic obstructive lung disease. The goal is reduction of pulmonary hypertension that leads to right ventricular failure and its complications. Although there is concern that inhibition of hypoxic drive with the administration of oxygen may cause respiratory acidosis to worsen, it seems that stable patients with chronic respiratory acidosis tolerate oxygen safely. Oxygen is usually administered at low concentrations sufficient to increase the PaO_2 to approximately 60 mm Hg or to increase the oxyhemoglobin saturation to more than 90 percent. In patients with sleep-disordered breathing syndromes, nocturnal hypoxemia associated with apnea may sometimes be treated with oxygen. In some patients, however, the periods of apnea may be prolonged with oxygen administration. It is therefore appropriate to monitor the effect of oxygen in such patients with appropriate studies.

Long-Term Mechanical Ventilation

Long-term mechanical ventilation, either nocturnal or continuous, may be helpful in selected patients. Patients with mild-to-moderate respiratory muscle weakness in particular may require supplemental ventilation from negative-pressure or positive-pressure ventilation during sleeping hours, although they have sufficient muscle strength during the day to support ventilation. Other patients may require longer periods of ventilatory assistance. Patients and their families may require considerable training and orientation to use the mechanical ventilator at home.

Nasal Continuous Positive Airway Pressure

Patients with significant obstruction of the upper airway during sleep (obstructive sleep apnea syndrome) may be helped by the application of nasal continuous positive airway pressure (nasal CPAP). Positive pressure applied over the nose during sleep may reduce the periods of obstructive apnea and decrease the duration of hypoxemia. Patients considered for nasal CPAP should be studied during sleep for the presence of obstructive sleep apnea, and the benefit of nasal CPAP should be tested. Some patients who do not respond to nasal CPAP alone will have a decrease in obstructive apnea during sleep with a combination of CPAP plus increased positive pressure during inspiration (bilevel positive airway pressure). Supplemental oxygen administration is sometimes combined with nasal CPAP. Surgical approaches to obstructive sleep apnea include uvulopalatoplasty and tracheostomy; patients should be carefully selected for these procedures. Finally, in some obese patients with obstructive sleep apnea, reduction of weight by the use of severely restricted diets or by surgical procedures may be indicated.

There is some evidence that the strength and endurance of the inspiratory muscles improves after specific training of these muscles. Some investigators have found that training of the inspiratory muscles achieved by inhalation through a device with a small orifice improves exercise tolerance in patients with chronic obstructive lung disease. The role of respiratory muscle training in the prevention or management of chronic respiratory acidosis is unclear. Similarly, it has been suggested that theophylline and dopamine have a beneficial effect on the strength and endurance of the diaphragm but, again, the precise effect of these drugs on respiratory acidosis is not known.

Drug Therapy

Doxapram Hydrochloride. Doxapram hydrochloride is a reliable respiratory stimulant with a wide range of doses that may be used safely (toxicity is usually manifested by hypertension and seizures). It stimulates both central and peripheral chemoreceptors. At present, in the United States it is available only as an intravenous preparation, so it may be used for short-term therapy only. It has been found useful in the treatment of primary alveolar hypoventilation syndrome. It may also be used in treating hypoventilation secondary to chronic lung diseases, but, as with the use of other respiratory stimulants, dyspnea may be exacerbated. The drug may be administered by constant intravenous infusion, with 3 to 6 mg per minute being an effective dose.

Progesterone. This hormone has been found effective in the treatment of some patients with chronic CO_2 retention secondary to obesity-hypoventilation syndrome. Progesterone seems to act as a central respiratory stimulant, but it does not appear to be an especially potent stimulant. Oral forms are available, and chronic therapy has been accomplished. Medroxyprogesterone in a dose of 20 mg three times per day has been used with success. Potential side effects are thromboembolism and impotence in the male.

Almitrine. Almitrine is a respiratory stimulant currently unavailable in the United States. It has been studied in patients with chronic obstructive pulmonary disease and has been found capable of reducing $PaCO_2$ and increasing PaO_2 when administered chronically by the oral route. Respiratory stimulation takes place by sensitization of the carotid chemoreceptors. A seemingly independent effect is enhancement of hypoxic pulmonary vasoconstriction, which may serve to improve oxygenation by reducing ventilation-perfusion inequality.

Acetazolamide. This drug is not actually a respiratory stimulant, but may be used to "decompensate" a compensated respiratory acidosis. Acting as a carbonic anhydrase inhibitor, it facilitates a bicarbonate diuresis, leading to a mild hyperchloremic metabolic acidosis. The relative acidosis stimulates ventilation to reduce $PaCO_2$. This approach, while useful, is not without hazard; if the patient is unable to increase ventilation in response to the induced acidemia, dyspnea and the consequences of metabolic acidosis will ensue. The drug may be administered orally or intravenously in a single dose of 250 to 500 mg. Subsequent doses depend on the arterial blood gas and pH response.

Theophylline. This agent, given in usual doses as a bronchodilator, appears to be a mild respiratory stimulant acting on the central nervous system. It may be useful in patients with hypoventilation associated with Cheyne-Stokes breathing. There is some evidence that theophylline has beneficial effects on maintaining diaphragmatic strength and endurance during severe loading (i.e., acute exacerbation of chronic obstructive lung disease), but this has not been proven.

Suggested Reading

Aldrich TK. Respiratory muscle fatigue. Clin Chest Med 1988; 9:225–236.

Altose MD, Hudgel DW. The pharmacology of respiratory depressants and stimulants. Clin Chest Med 1986; 7:481–494.

Feihl F, Perret C. Permissive hypercapnia. How permissive should we be? Am J Respir Crit Care Med 1994; 150:1722–1737.

Johanson WG, Peters JL. Respiratory failure: pathophysiology and treatment. In: Murray JF, Nadel JA, eds. Textbook of respiratory medicine. Philadelphia: WB Saunders, 1988:2017.

Weinberger SE, Schwartzstein RM, Weiss JW. Hypercapnia. New Engl J Med 1989; 321:1223–1231.

RESPIRATORY ALKALOSIS

Richard M. Effros, M.D.
Marshall Dunning III, Ph.D.

Respiratory alkalosis occurs when the rate of alveolar ventilation exceeds that needed to keep arterial carbon dioxide partial pressure ($PaCO_2$) below 38 mm Hg and consequently results in an alkalosis. Implicit in this definition is the assumption that alveolar ventilation is increased relative to the rate at which carbon dioxide (CO_2) is produced. Furthermore, it is assumed that the alveolar hyperventilation is not secondary to an underlying metabolic acidosis. It must be emphasized that it is the alveolar ventilation rather than the total ventilation that must increase under these circumstances; ventilation of dead space within the lungs does not contribute to the loss of CO_2. The relationship between arterial carbon dioxide pressure ($PaCO_2$), alveolar ventilation ($\dot{V}_A$), and CO_2 production ($\dot{V}co_2$) can be readily understood in terms of the following alveolar ventilation equation:

$$PaCO_2 = \frac{\dot{V}co_2\,(P_B - PH_2O)}{\dot{V}_A}$$

where P_B is the atmospheric pressure. Not uncommonly, dead space and total ventilation is increased in patients with severe lung disease, but $\dot{V}_A$ is actually reduced and hypercapnia is consequently observed. Diagnosis of respiratory alkalosis must depend on measurements of Pco_2 and pH. Hyperventilation can be quite subtle and is frequently overlooked by clinicians. Furthermore, it is difficult to distinguish between total and alveolar hyperventilation and between primary and secondary disorders without arterial blood data.

After the onset of acute respiratory alkalosis, the level of plasma bicarbonate decreases rapidly by approximately 4 mEq per liter, from 24 to 20 mEq per liter, when the $PaCO_2$ is decreased from 40 to 20 mm Hg. This change in bicarbonate is related in large part to tissue and blood buffering, and to a lesser extent, to lactate accumulation. Under these circumstances, actual pH is 7.6 rather than 7.7, the pH which would have been observed had the level of bicarbonate not decreased. Over the next few days, renal excretion of bicarbonate may result in an additional decrease in bicarbonate to 15 mEq per liter, with a further improvement of arterial pH to 7.49.

■ CAUSES RELATED TO HYPOXIA

High Altitude Exposure

Hypoxia is an inevitable consequence of residence at high altitudes (Table 1). The response of the peripheral chemoreceptors to acute hypoxia is stimulation of the respiratory center, causing the PCO_2 to decrease rapidly. Increased ventilation is helpful because it tends to increase the partial pressure of oxygen (Po_2). Over the next few days, the kidneys respond to the respiratory alkalosis by increasing bicarbonate excretion. This causes the arterial pH to return toward normal and reduces the restraint on ventilation exerted by alkalosis. Ventilation consequently increases further, and there are additional decreases in the Pco_2 and increases in the Po_2 during this period of compensation. In some individuals, the hyperventilatory response to hypoxia appears to be less than optimum, and these patients may complain of dyspnea, malaise, headaches, insomnia, anorexia, nausea, and vomiting after a day or two of residing at high altitudes. These symptoms are referred to as "acute mountain sickness" and are probably related to hypoxia rather than hypocapnia. They can be avoided if a metabolic acidosis with secondary hyperventilation is induced through administration of acetazolamide before ascent into high altitudes. It should be noted that long-term residents of high altitudes seem to lose their sensitivity to hypoxia and typically have less severe hypocapnia and are less hypoxic than visitors. In a small number of natives, decompensation eventually develops with severe hypoxemia, polycythemia, and cor pulmonale. At altitudes over 8,000 feet, acute pulmonary edema, retinal hemorrhage, and cerebral edema may occur. The onset of these events is unpredictable, and pulmonary edema is more commonly seen in healthy young people. It may recur in these individuals and has not been linked to respiratory alkalosis.

Table 1 Causes of Respiratory Alkalosis

- Hypoxia
  - High altitudes
  - Lung disease
    - Pneumonia
    - Pulmonary vascular disease
    - Pulmonary restrictive disease
    - Pulmonary obstruction (early)
  - Anemia
  - Hypotension
- Central nervous system
  - Anxiety and pain
  - Central nervous system injuries
    - Cerebrovascular disorders
    - Tumors
    - Infections
- Other causes
  - Drugs
    - Salicylates
    - Xanthines
    - Catecholamines
    - Nicotine
    - Progestational agents
  - Gram-negative sepsis
  - Liver failure
  - Mechanical ventilation
  - Treatment of metabolic acidosis
  - Atelectasis
  - Carbon monoxide poisoning

Lung Disease

Hypoxia can occur with a wide variety of pulmonary diseases and stimulates ventilation. In restrictive disease associated with decreased lung or chest wall compliance, patients characteristically remain hypocapnic until late stages, when $\dot{V}_A$ becomes compromised. Hypocapnia may also be seen in association with asthma and relatively mild obstructive lung disease, but CO_2 retention eventually occurs as obstruction worsens. Pulmonary vascular and embolic disease are usually associated with respiratory alkalosis. Pneumonias also tend to stimulate ventilation, and hyperventilation may be observed in as many as 10 percent of patients with pulmonary edema. It should be emphasized that the degree of hyperventilation found in patients with these pulmonary disorders is often out of proportion to the amount of hypoxia seen and seems to be related in part to the stimulation of pulmonary parenchymal receptors that respond to stretch or deformation. Thus even if administration of oxygen in these individuals corrects the arterial Po_2, it may fail to eliminate the respiratory alkalosis. Chronic hyperventilation is frequently observed in the presence of intrapulmonary or intracardiac shunting of venous blood into the systemic arteries.

Anemia and Hypotension

If sufficiently severe, either anemia or hypotension may result in tissue hypoxia and hyperventilation. The tendency for anemia to stimulate ventilation is particularly pronounced if an acute loss of blood has occurred.

■ CAUSES RELATED TO THE CENTRAL NERVOUS SYSTEM

Anxiety

Anxiety is probably the most common cause of respiratory alkalosis. This may be a transient problem related to acute stress, or it may recur in individuals who chronically hyperventilate. Episodes of hyperventilation may be initiated by anxiety, anger, or grief, and patients experiencing these emotions are particularly likely to be symptomatic.

Central Nervous System Injury

Any injury involving the brainstem may result in hyperventilation; this sign generally indicates a poor prognosis. Cerebrovascular disorders, tumors, and infections may be responsible for moderate or severe hyperventilation, and CO_2 tensions may decrease dramatically. Respiration may become extremely irregular, having an increased rate and depth of ventilation, and the patient is usually (although not always) unconscious. Alternatively, patients with central nervous system disease may manifest Cheyne-Stokes respiration with episodes of hyperventilation interrupted by apneic spells. The level of the $PaCO_2$ is then dependent on the stage of respiration during which blood is sampled; it is characteristically lower during the apneic phase. This pattern of ventilation is also seen in patients with severe congestive heart failure in whom prolonged circulation times may contribute to this cyclic ventilatory abnormality.

Drug Toxicity

High doses of salicylates stimulate medullary chemoreceptors and cause hyperventilation. The Pco_2 may decrease to 30 mm Hg if the patient is taking a dose of 4 g of aspirin per day and to 10 mm Hg if the dose is 12 g per day. This hyperventilation occurs independent of the metabolic acidosis that follows and persists even if metabolic acidosis is corrected. The metabolic acidosis is in turn related to the uncoupling of oxidative phosphorylation and may be accompanied initially by hyperglycemia, and later by hypoglycemia with ketosis and lactic acidosis. Acutely, patients experience nausea, agitation, confusion, seizures, and coma. Tinnitus is common with chronic salicylate ingestion. Young children are more likely to present at the hospital with metabolic acidosis.

Respiratory alkalosis may also be related to the use of theophyllines, catecholamines, progestational compounds, and nicotine.

■ OTHER CAUSES

Hyperventilation is observed in more than 50 percent of patients with gram-negative sepsis and may precede other manifestations such as fever, hypotension, and metabolic acidosis. Gram-positive sepsis may also cause hyperventilation in some patients.

Not uncommonly, respiratory alkalosis is observed after correction of metabolic acidosis. The delay in slowing of ventilation is presumably related to persistence of acidosis in the cerebrospinal fluid, and care must be taken to avoid correcting the metabolic acidosis too rapidly with bicarbonate infusions. Another common iatrogenic problem is encountered in patients with chronic CO_2 retention who are placed on ventilators. If mechanical ventilation is overly vigorous, the underlying compensatory metabolic alkalosis will become evident, and if this is sufficiently severe, it may result in seizures and death, even when the Pco_2 level remains above normal.

Virtually any kind of severe liver disease with hepatic failure can be associated with moderate or severe respiratory alkalosis, and levels of arterial Pco_2 of less than 25 mm Hg carry a grave prognosis.

By the end of the first trimester of pregnancy, the $PaCO_2$ decreases by approximately 12 mm Hg and stays close to this level throughout the remainder of the pregnancy. During childbirth, the $PaCO_2$ decreases even further and may cause a typical hyperventilation syndrome. It is generally believed that this response to pregnancy is related to the level of progesterone, and ventilation returns to normal as this level declines with the termination of pregnancy. Mild hyperventilation is also common during the progestational stage of the menstrual cycle.

Fever, pain, speech (prolonged conversations), hypotension, delirium tremens, hyperthyroidism, heat stroke, and heat exhaustion have all been reported to cause hyperventilation.

■ SYMPTOMS AND SIGNS

Patients with respiratory alkalosis are usually unaware of the fact that they are hyperventilating. They may complain of difficulty breathing, especially with inhaling ("air hunger") and hyperventilation may actually induce bronchospasm.

Table 2 Symptoms and Signs of Acute Respiratory Alkalosis

Dyspnea
Substernal and epigastric discomfort
Anxiety
Confusion
Diaphoresis
Aerophagia
Paresthesias
Carpopedal spasm
Dizziness
Syncope
Seizures
Arrhythmias in patients with coronary artery disease

Other common complaints are a sense of imminent doom and substernal or epigastric discomfort, which can resemble that of angina, esophageal reflux, or pulmonary embolism. These symptoms may be particularly confusing because respiratory alkalosis can also result in depressions of the ST segments of the electrocardiogram that resemble those of myocardial ischemia. It has been suggested that respiratory alkalosis may aggravate myocardial ischemia in patients with either arteriosclerotic coronary artery disease or Prinzmetal's angina by increasing the affinity of hemoglobin for oxygen or by promoting coronary artery constriction. In the presence of coronary artery disease, hypocapnia can promote both atrial and ventricular arrhythmias that may respond to correction of the arterial P_{CO_2}.

Chest discomfort may also be related to mitral valve prolapse, which appears to be enhanced by hyperventilation. When related to anxiety, hyperventilation is often accompanied by aerophagia, with a sensation of bloating and cramping, and the patient may complain of palpitations. Lightheadedness and confusion may be encountered when the P_{CO_2} level acutely decreases to less than 25 mm Hg. Paresthesias are common. They are usually, but not always, bilateral and are characterized by numbness about the mouth and extremities. If hyperventilation is sufficiently severe, carpopedal spasm, syncope, or seizures may follow. The neuromuscular complications of respiratory alkalosis appear to be related to a decrease in ionized calcium in the serum and perhaps to the alkalosis itself.

Symptoms and signs of acute respiratory alkalosis are summarized in Table 2. They are responsible for many of the symptoms associated with "neurocirculatory asthenia," "panic disorders," and agoraphobia. Because modest increases in ventilation, including occasional sighs, can substantially decrease P_{CO_2}, hyperventilation is often not clinically obvious.

Although arterial blood gas is used to document hypocapnia, measurements of P_{CO_2} in the expired air (capnometry) may provide a convenient, noninvasive method of diagnosing hyperventilation in patients with normal lungs. End-tidal values less than 30 mm Hg either at rest or after mild exercise are suggestive of hyperventilation. Psychogenic hyperventilation subsides during sleep, distinguishing it from organic disorders. Decreased venous HCO_3^- is consistent with chronic hyperventilation, but may be due to a primary metabolic acidosis. An increase in the A-a O_2 difference should alert the clinician to the presence of lung disease.

■ THERAPY

Treatment of respiratory alkalosis is frequently more perplexing than is its detection. Success is much less frequent if hyperventilation is chronic. In patients with primary hyperventilation secondary to anxiety, rebreathing into a relatively noncompliant paper bag about the size of a lunch bag quickly increases the $PaCO_2$ and reverses symptomatology. Rebreathing must continue as long as the patient continues to hyperventilate. Reassurance and other modes of relieving anxiety may be needed. Beta-adrenergic blockade has recently been reported to be helpful, presumably because it reduces adrenergic stimulation of ventilation, but must be avoided if asthma is suspected. Tricyclic antidepressants may be useful in mitigating symptoms associated with panic attacks.

Emergency treatment of hyperventilation is seldom necessary unless arterial pH increases to levels well above 7.5. $PaCO_2$ tensions can be increased by raising inspired CO_2 tensions or, if the patient is mechanically ventilated, by increasing the dead space of the ventilator. These maneuvers stimulate respiration and may promote fatigue. Furthermore, attempts to increase the $PaCO_2$ in patients with respiratory alkalosis associated with serious illness are seldom helpful, although they may reverse arrhythmias in patients with coronary artery disease. In patients with brain injury, increasing the $PaCO_2$ may cause more damage by increasing cerebral perfusion and intracerebral pressure.

Treatment of undiagnosed asthma may relieve episodes of hyperventilation. Reversal of hypoxia by administration of oxygen (or by return to normal altitudes) can reverse respiratory alkalosis secondary to hypoxemia.

Salicylate poisoning can be treated by urinary alkalinization and diuresis, and these measures can increase salicylate excretion by an order of magnitude. Alkaline fluids that contain both potassium and glucose are generally administered, but care must be taken to avoid overhydration since some patients with salicylate poisoning seem predisposed to pulmonary edema. Furthermore, administration of alkaline solutions is contraindicated in patients with severe respiratory alkalosis. Either hemodialysis or hemoperfusion is indicated when blood levels of salicylate are very high or when severe neurologic signs or cardiovascular complications appear. In addition, it may be possible to remove tablets from the stomach by gastric lavage, and the absorption of residual medication from the gut can be enhanced by administering activated charcoal with sorbitol.

Suggested Reading

Ferguson A, Addington W, Gaensler E. Dyspnea and bronchospasm from inappropriate postexercise hyperventilation. Ann Intern Med 1969; 71: 1063–1072.

Gardner WN. The pathophysiology of hyperventilation disorders. Chest 1996; 109:516–534.

Leibowitz MR. Imipramine in the treatment of panic disorder and its complications. Psychiatr Clin North Am 1985; 8:37–47.

McHenry PL, Cogan OJ, Elliott WC, Knoebel SB. False-positive ECG re-

sponse to exercise secondary to hyperventilation: cineangiographic correlation. Am Heart J 1970; 79:683–687.
Okel BB, Hurst JW. Prolonged hyperventilation in man: associated electrolyte changes and subjective symptoms. Arch Intern Med 1961; 108: 757–762.
Rice RL. Symptom patterns of the hyperventilation syndrome. Am J Med 1950; 8:691–700.
Saltzman HA, Heyman A, Sieber HO. Correlation of clinical and physiologic manifestations of hyperventilation. N Engl J Med 1963; 268: 1431–1436.
Tavel ME. Hyperventilation syndrome with unilateral somatic symptoms. JAMA 1964; 187:301–303.
Tavel ME. Hyperventilation syndrome: hiding behind pseudonyms? Chest 1990; 97:1285–1287.

METABOLIC ACIDOSIS

Jaime Uribarri, M.D.
Hugh J. Carroll, M.D.

Normal metabolic processes generate daily approximately 1 mEq of hydrogen ion per kilogram of body weight, leading to the daily consumption of the same amount of buffer, which for practical purposes can be designated as bicarbonate. Reversal of this physiologic tendency toward metabolic acidosis is normally accomplished by two renal mechanisms: (1) complete renal tubular reabsorption of all filtered bicarbonate and (2) generation of new bicarbonate by a mechanism that excretes acid in the urine.

Metabolic acidosis is caused by a diminution in body bicarbonate content. The mechanisms of this process include loss of bicarbonate in stool or urine, failure of the kidney to generate new bicarbonate appropriately, generation of acid by metabolic processes (e.g., ketoacids and lactic acid), and ingestion of acids or their precursors (e.g., methanol, ethylene glycol).

COMPENSATORY MECHANISMS

All of the four primary acid-base disorders are tempered by compensatory alterations in the parameters not primarily involved. In the case of metabolic acidosis, the acidemia caused by the decrease in serum bicarbonate stimulates central and peripheral chemoreceptors, and hyperventilation ensues. This compensatory decline in carbon dioxide partial pressure (Pco_2) raises the blood pH toward (although not to) the normal level. A useful approximation of appropriate respiratory compensation for metabolic acidosis is given by the following formula:

$$\Delta Pco_2 = (\Delta\ HCO_3 \times 1.2) \pm 2$$

Respiratory compensation usually reaches its appropriate level within 12 to 24 hours. If Pco_2 is inappropriately high, two causes should be considered: (1) acidosis of short duration or (2) a complicating primary respiratory acidosis. If Pco_2 is inappropriately low, respiratory alkalosis is also present and its cause must be sought.

Renal compensation for metabolic acidosis relies upon an increase in ammonia excretion and may require more than 24 hours to be fully established.

Although it is not truly a compensatory mechanism, metabolic alkalosis complicating metabolic acidosis ameliorates the acidosis or restores the pH to normal. If the alkalosis is more severe than the acidosis, the pH rises to levels higher than normal.

THE ANION GAP

The concentration of serum cations must equal the concentration of serum anions. For purposes of defining the anion gap, we designate sodium, chloride, and bicarbonate as the "measured ions." Albumin, sulfate, phosphate, and organic anions (a total of 23 mEq per liter) are the "unmeasured anions," and potassium, calcium, and magnesium (a total of 10 mEq per liter) are the "unmeasured cations." Although the anion gap is estimated as $Na- (Cl + HCO_3)$, it is actually determined by the difference between unmeasured cations and unmeasured anions. Thus, in ketoacidosis, an accumulation of 12 mEq per liter of organic acid increases the level of unmeasured anions from 23 to 35 mEq per liter, and thus the anion gap is $35 - 11 = 24$ mEq per liter. In renal tubular acidosis (RTA), the normal anion gap reflects the normal concentrations of unmeasured ions.

CLASSIFICATION OF METABOLIC ACIDOSIS ACCORDING TO THE ANION GAP

The anion gap (normally 12 ± 4 mEq per liter) serves as a useful point of departure for classifying metabolic acidosis (Table 1). However, proper interpretation of the anion gap for the differential diagnosis of metabolic acidosis requires the recognition of conditions that may alter the anion gap independently of acid-base disorders. For example, hyperglobulinemia, as in multiple myeloma, may reduce serum sodium without reducing chloride or bicarbonate and to the same extent reduces the anion gap. Similarly, in hypoalbuminemic states, chloride replaces the anions normally contributed by albumin, and the resulting hyperchloremia decreases the anion gap. Thus, a cirrhotic patient with hypoalbuminemia and hyperchloremia who has suffered rupture of esophageal

Table 1 Classification of Metabolic Acidosis According to the Anion Gap

Increased anion gap (normochloremic acidosis):
Ketoacidosis
Beta-hydroxybutyric acidosis
Lactic acidosis
D-lactic acidosis
Uremic acidosis
Salicylate, methanol, ethylene glycol, and paraldehyde intoxications
Normal anion gap (hyperchloremic acidosis):
Renal tubular acidosis
Early uremic acidosis
Intestinal loss of bicarbonate
Urinary diversion procedures
Acidosis caused by chloride-containing acids (e.g., hydrochloric acid, ammonium chloride, arginine hydrochloride, lysine hydrochloride)
Acidosis caused by the use of anion-exchange resins (e.g., cholestyramine)
Ketoacidosis during recovery phase
Dilutional acidosis
Acidosis following respiratory alkalosis
Acidosis caused by a shift of H^+ from the cell
Acidosis by the use of acetazolamide
Organic acidosis with narrow normal anion gap

varices and shock might develop lactic acidosis and manifest a normal anion gap because the accumulation of lactate in his blood has simply raised an initially low anion gap into the normal range.

The causes of acidosis with increased anion gap are usually apparent from the clinical presentation and, except for uremic acidosis, which is readily identified by assessment of renal function, these disorders tend to develop very rapidly. Ketoacidosis is diagnosed by a positive serum ketone test (Acetest). Lactic acidosis is usually suggested by tissue underperfusion, ethanol intoxication, or severe liver disease and is confirmed by a high serum lactate level. D-Lactic acidosis should be suspected in a patient with short-bowel syndrome and neurologic abnormalities. Acidosis resulting from ingestion of toxins may be suspected on the basis of the history and is confirmed by measurement of the concentration of toxins in the blood; a serum osmolar gap in excess of 10 mOsm per liter in an appropriate clinical setting supports the diagnosis of ethylene glycol or methanol poisoning. The serum osmolar gap is estimated as the difference between the measured osmolality and that estimated from the following formula:

$$\text{serum osmolality} = \text{serum sodium} \times 2 + \text{BUN}/2.8 + \text{glucose}/18$$

Clinically, the most common cause of an increased osmolar gap is ethanol intoxication, which can cause lactic acidosis and ketoacidosis.

In those cases in which bicarbonate is not replaced by an "unmeasured" anion, the chloride is elevated and hyperchloremic acidosis results. Serum chloride must always be interpreted in relation to serum sodium; with states of dehydration, water retention, or salt loss, serum chloride varies with serum sodium. Thus a dehydrated patient with lactic acidosis may present with hyperchloremia, while a patient with fecal loss of bicarbonate may have a hyperchloremic acidosis despite a serum chloride level that is absolutely low. A common error is to mistake compensated respiratory alkalosis (low bicarbonate and high chloride) for hyperchloremic acidosis; the problem is quickly resolved by measurement of blood pH.

The cause of hyperchloremic acidosis is usually apparent from the history and clinical findings. When the cause is not clear, measurement of net acid excretion (titratable acidity + ammonia − bicarbonate) distinguishes renal acidosis (low or normal net acid excretion) from extrarenal acidosis (increased net acid excretion). It has been suggested that the urinary anion gap (urinary sodium + potassium − urinary chloride) is a rough but useful estimate of ammonia excretion. If the urinary anion gap is negative, the ammonia excretion will be greater than normal and the acidosis is extrarenal. A positive urinary anion gap, on the other hand, will indicate low ammonia excretion and suggest acidosis of renal origin. These calculations are useful only when the urine has an acid pH and is not infected. The glomerular filtration rate (GFR) may be frankly below normal in the presence of hyperchloremia, in which case the diagnosis of early uremic acidosis may be made; if the GFR is normal or only minimally impaired, RTA is present.

■ TREATMENT

Attempts should always be made to reverse the underlying disorder. If conditions cannot be re-established in which the patient can maintain his own bicarbonate balance, the patient must be provided in the long-term with bicarbonate or with a bicarbonate precursor such as citrate; in the patient with renal tubular acidosis or uremia who presents with severe acidosis, bicarbonate is a required part of the immediate therapy. The patient with diabetic ketoacidosis, however, usually has two major sources of endogenous bicarbonate: (1) the ketone anions, which produce bicarbonate on their metabolism, and (2) the bicarbonate-generating capacity of the renal tubules. In the great majority of diabetics, these two sources suffice and exogenous bicarbonate is unnecessary, but in some instances of diabetic ketoacidosis or in other varieties of acidosis in which the patient has the capability ultimately to reverse the acidosis, severe acidemia must be directly dealt with and bicarbonate must be given.

The relationship between bicarbonate dosage and the increase in serum bicarbonate is curvilinear, the lower the level of serum bicarbonate, the less is its increase for a given quantity of alkali. As a useful approximation, it may be calculated that 2 mEq of bicarbonate per kilogram of body weight will raise serum bicarbonate by 4 mEq per liter in mild acidosis but only 2 mEq per liter in severe acidosis. The amount actually required to produce a given effect in a given individual is hard to calculate for several reasons—for example, in lactic acidosis, bicarbonate therapy may stimulate the glycolytic pathway to produce more lactic acid, and in diabetic ketoacidosis (DKA) the metabolism of ketones may produce additional alkali. An acceptable approach is to give one or two ampules of bicarbonate (50 to 100 mEq) initially with repetition of the same dosage as indicated by the results of repeated blood gas measurement.

The precise conditions under which bicarbonate should be

given is to some extent a matter of individual experience, but most physicians consider administration of bicarbonate when the pH falls below 7.1. A particular hazard of acidosis is cardiovascular collapse due to arteriolar dilation and decreased myocardial contractility. In general, older patients and patients with diminished myocardial reserve tolerate acidosis very poorly, and therefore bicarbonate therapy should probably begin at a pH of 7.2.

The following reasons have been given for avoiding rapid correction of severe acidosis:

1. "Overshoot alkalosis" caused by the summation of exogenous bicarbonate and that which results from the metabolism of organic anions.
2. Elevation of pH at such a rapid rate that low levels of red blood cell 2,3-diphosphoglycerate cannot increase rapidly enough to avoid tissue hypoxia.
3. Alkalosis caused by persistent hyperventilation in the presence of bicarbonate administration.
4. Paradoxical central nervous system (CNS) acidosis caused by the fact that carbon dioxide can enter the CNS more rapidly than bicarbonate.

It must be pointed out, however, that these arguments have been overemphasized and should not cause the physician to deny the patients the beneficial effect of at least modest amounts of bicarbonate when acidosis is severe. The administration of bicarbonate for specific indications is discussed later in this chapter.

Metabolic Acidosis in Specific Clinical States

Diabetic Ketoacidosis

In the average patient with DKA, the anion gap approximately equals the decrement in serum bicarbonate concentration and the test for ketones in serum and urine is strongly positive. However, neither of these two conditions is mandatory. In some patients, the anion gap exceeds the decrement in bicarbonate because ketone excretion has not been excessive and the retained ketones accumulate preferentially in the extracellular space, whereas in other patients, excretion of large amounts of ketones makes the anion gap somewhat smaller and the serum chloride somewhat higher. The occurrence of frank hyperchloremia, however, is unusual unless the serum sodium is also elevated. The patient may have DKA with a weakly positive or, rarely, a negative Acetest reaction if most or all of the ketoacid is in the reduced form as beta-hydroxybutyric acid. The conditions under which this event occurs are those in which tissue oxygenation is markedly reduced (e.g., septic shock), and in this event, serum lactate is usually higher than the 3 to 4 mEq per liter usually found in DKA.

When the diagnosis of DKA has been confirmed, a flow sheet is prepared in which the patient's clinical and chemical indices and fluid balance are carefully recorded.

Insulin. The patient should receive regular insulin as an intravenous bolus of 10 to 20 U, followed by either an intravenous infusion at a rate of 0.1 U per kilogram per hour or intramuscular injections of 10 U per hour. Insulin administration is continued at this rate until the serum ketone reaction becomes negative. If the blood glucose decreases to less than 300 mg per deciliter before the disappearance of serum ketones, glucose-containing solutions should be substituted and insulin administration continued at the same rate.

Fluids. Water and salt replacement is needed in all patients. Theoretically, the patient should receive hypotonic saline because he has lost water in excess of salt, but the fear of cerebral edema has popularized the practice of starting fluid replacement therapy with 1 L of normal saline and thereafter alternating normal saline with half-normal saline. The actual rate of infusion is determined by the needs of the individual, but the state of dehydration (4 to 5 L of water in adults) is such that 1 L is commonly administered with the first hour; most patients require 4 to 6 L during the first 24 hours. Many pediatric textbooks advise the administration of large amounts of hypotonic solution, but the ubiquity of cerebral edema in DKA and the propensity of children to die of or be disabled as a result of cerebral herniation suggest that avoidance of plasma hypotonicity in children is a prudent measure, and that small volumes of more concentrated salt solutions should be used in children than is currently the practice.

Potassium. Although potassium depletion is a universal phenomenon in DKA, the serum potassium level may range from low to high; usually it is slightly elevated. The effects of several events—e.g., insulin administration, an increase in blood pH, glycogen synthesis—combine to cause a decline in serum potassium, sometimes precipitously, and care must be taken to avoid hypokalemia. If at the start of therapy serum potassium is less than 5 mEq per liter and urine output is normal, potassium administration can be started at a rate of 10 mEq per hour and thereafter modified according to the results of repeated serum potassium levels. Although it is appropriate to be cautious with regard to the rate of potassium administration, no upper limit (e.g., 20 to 30 mEq per hour) can be arbitrarily assigned. If, for example, a patient has life-threatening acidosis and must receive bicarbonate, while the serum potassium is already very low, the intracellular shift of potassium may cause lethal hypokalemia unless potassium is administered at a rate much more rapid than those cited.

Bicarbonate. Treatment with insulin not only stops excessive gluconeogenesis and restores normal glucose metabolism, it also stops mobilization of fatty acids, the precursors of ketoacids, and the blood pH increases as glucose decreases. The blood pH increases primarily because the ketone anions, acetoacetate, and beta-hydroxybutyrate are converted to bicarbonate, but renal generation of bicarbonate also makes a contribution. As noted earlier, insulin alone is usually sufficient to improve serum bicarbonate, and administration of bicarbonate is therefore not necessary. In many patients, when the anion gap returns to normal levels (indicating metabolism of all bicarbonate precursors), only a modest increase in serum bicarbonate occurs, and at this point, the chemical pattern of the blood is that of hyperchloremic (normal anion gap) acidosis. This chemical pattern obtains because a significant portion of the ketone anions are excreted in the urine before the patient's admission to the hospital. Despite this failure of serum bicarbonate to increase promptly to normal levels, blood pH is usually satisfactory because hyperventilation persists for many hours and, eventually, renal generation of bicarbonate normalizes the serum bicarbonate level. Although routine administration of bicarbonate to patients with DKA is not necessary, small amounts should be given to patients with severe acidosis. For example, as was discussed earlier in this chapter, bicarbonate should be given to older patients with poor myocardial reserve when the arterial pH is less than 7.2, and to younger patients when the pH decreases to less than 7.1.

Phosphate. The routine administration of phosphate is probably unnecessary in most patients with DKA, but the serum level should be followed and phosphate supplement should be given if the serum level decreases to less than 2 mg per deciliter. Phosphate can be given as the potassium salt, and the total intravenous dose should not exceed 1 g of phosphorus per day. Excessively rapid administration of phosphate can lead to hypocalcemia.

Indices of Successful Treatment. The endpoint in the treatment of DKA should be the disappearance of ketone anions from the patient's serum. This is best indicated by a negative Acetest reaction and usually coincides with the disappearance of the excess anion gap. Early in the treatment period, despite a decrease in the total ketone concentration, the Acetest reaction may suggest that ketonemia is worsening. This is because the test measures acetoacetate and acetone and not beta-hydroxybutyrate, and with the improvement of the oxidation status of tissues, the ratio of acetoacetate to beta-hydroxybutyrate increases. Normalization of the anion gap is usually a less reliable marker for the disappearance of ketonemia because substantial laboratory errors are often associated with its measurement. Delayed excretion of acetone by lungs and kidneys may sometimes explain a normal anion gap and a positive serum Acetest, since acetone is not a charged moiety.

Alcoholic Ketoacidosis

Alcoholic ketoacidosis typically occurs in chronic alcoholics after a binge during which they have eaten poorly and vomited severely. The possible mechanisms of this acidosis include insulin deficiency caused by hypoglycemia induced by fasting, and an increase in lipolysis. The latter mechanism may be caused by vomiting, which causes an increased secretion of glucocorticoids and catecholamines, and by the ketogenic effect of alcohol or alcohol withdrawal. The Acetest reaction may be only weakly positive in those instances in which most of the ketone anions are in the form of beta-hydroxybutyrate rather than acetoacetate. A modest degree of lactic acidosis may accompany alcoholic ketoacidosis.

The administration of glucose without bicarbonate or insulin terminates alcoholic ketoacidosis easily. An initial dose of 150 ml per hour of any solution containing 5 percent dextrose is reasonable. As in the case of diabetic ketoacidosis, serum levels of potassium and phosphate tend to decrease during treatment, and these ions should be provided according to need. Hyperglycemia is frequently observed during recovery and may reflect the transient inability of the liver to handle a glucose load.

Lactic Acidosis

Lactic acid, the product of glycolysis, is produced by most tissues and carried to the liver and kidney to be oxidized and converted back to glucose. When oxidative processes are interfered with (e.g., with severe liver disease), particularly when the blood supply and therefore the oxygen supply to the liver is reduced, the excess lactic acid titrates the body buffers and metabolic acidosis results. Tissue hypoxia is by far the most common cause of lactic acidosis. Other causes of this disorder are listed in Table 2. Excessive intake of alcohol can induce severe lactic acidosis because the oxidation of alcohol interferes with the mechanism that ordinarily oxidizes lactate to pyruvate. When the alcohol has been metabolized, the lactic acidosis quickly resolves and, curiously, does not recur when the patient drinks again.

Table 2 Causes of Lactic Acidosis

Type A (caused by tissue hypoxia)
Circulatory shock
Severe anemia
Cardiopulmonary arrest
Type B
Drugs and Toxins
Biguanides, alcohol, fructose, sorbitol, xylitol, methanol, epinephrine, ethylene, glycol, streptozotocin, papaverine, isonizid, salicylates
Idiopathic
Diabetes, neoplastic diseases, liver disease, renal failure
Congenital enzymatic defect
Glucose-6-phosphatase deficiency, fructose-1, 6-diphosphatase deficiency, pyruvate carboxylase deficiency, pyruvate dehydrogenase deficiency

Some aspects of the treatment of lactic acidosis are disputed, but the consensus is that the underlying abnormality must be reversed. Lactic acidosis is a metabolic emergency and should be treated in an intensive care unit with appropriate monitoring of metabolic and hemodynamic parameters. Volume replacement is commonly necessary, but care must be taken to prevent fluid overload.

Although bicarbonate does not improve the underlying disorder, it does protect against the harmful effects of extreme acidemia and should be administered when the arterial pH is less than 7.15. A few clinical reports and experimental studies suggest that bicarbonate therapy for the treatment of lactic acidosis may have some detrimental effects (e.g., negative cardiovascular response, reduction of lactate extraction by the liver, and direct stimulation of lactate production), but no significant adverse effects have been clearly documented in humans. Sufficient bicarbonate should be administered to increase the pH to at least 7.2. Because of the potential for volume overload when bicarbonate is being administered, furosemide may be needed, and if the patient has renal failure, dialysis may be indicated. Recovery from lactic acidosis is commonly characterized by "overshoot alkalosis" as the large amounts of lactate are converted to bicarbonate while hyperventilation persists. Dichloroacetate, an experimental drug that enhances the oxidation of lactate, has shown some initial encouraging results, but larger clinical trials are needed.

Chronic lactic acidosis may occur in patients with cancer, and in general it is not advisable to treat this disorder with bicarbonate. The bicarbonate increases glycolysis and more lactate is formed and excreted in the urine. To provide substrate for this process, protein is broken down and converted to glucose. Hence, in the end, such treatment of this form of lactic acidosis may markedly accelerate cachexia.

D-Lactic Acidosis

The lactic acid produced by humans is the L-isomer. In patients with the short bowel syndrome D-lactic acid is produced by the action of colonic bacteria on unabsorbed dietary carbohydrates.

The critical elements in the diagnosis of D-lactic acidosis include (1) rapid development of a high anion gap acidosis; (2) laboratory reports of normal serum lactate levels; (3) a negative Acetest reaction; and (4) the appearance of characteristic neurologic findings (e.g., confusion, disorientation, slurred speech, staggering gait, nystagmus, and delirium). The diagnosis is confirmed by measurement of the serum and urinary D-lactate levels, a procedure identical to the measurement of L-lactate, except for the substitution of D-lactate dehydrogenase (LDH) for L-LDH in the reaction mixture. The development of D-lactic acidosis seems to be caused by a defect in the utilization of as well as by the overproduction of D-lactic acid, since ordinarily humans metabolize D-lactate quite effectively.

For the acute attack, therapy may include administration of intravenous fluids and bicarbonate but relies most on the elimination of the offending colonic bacteria by the administration of oral antibiotics. Subsequent management may include recolonization of the large intestine with Julia flora, a population of bacteria that do not produce D-LDH, and a low-carbohydrate diet.

Salicylate Intoxication

Although salicylate intoxication is generally included in the differential diagnosis of high anion gap metabolic acidosis, the earliest abnormality and the one most commonly found in patients admitted with salicylate intoxication is respiratory alkalosis, which is attributable to the direct effects of salicylate on the respiratory center. When acidosis does occur, it results in part from the compensatory loss of bicarbonate during the phase of hyperventilation and also from interference with metabolic pathways that lead to the accumulation of organic anions (lactate + ketones). The salicylate ion itself may make a small contribution to the anion gap. The toxicity of salicylate depends on its intracellular concentration, and its rate of cellular penetration depends on the concentration of unionized salicylic acid. Thus, acidemia increases the toxicity of salicylate by increasing the rate of its cellular penetration.

The treatment of salicylate intoxication relies primarily on promoting salicylate excretion by alkalinization of urine with administration of bicarbonate. An alkaline blood pH reduces the cell uptake of salicylate, but the blood pH should be monitored hourly, and if it is found to exceed 7.55, acetazolamide should be given to increase bicarbonate excretion. In patients with severe toxicity and worsening neurologic symptoms, hemodialysis should be performed.

Toxic Organic Acidosis Caused by Ethylene Glycol and Methanol

Methanol and ethylene glycol (the latter usually in the form of antifreeze) are sometimes ingested as substitutes for alcohol. Although neither is toxic, both are broken down into toxic organic compounds, most of which are strong acids. Therefore, although patients present with certain individual clinical characteristics, two common features are seen: severe anion gap acidosis and an increased osmolar gap, the latter representing that portion of the ingested substance that has not yet been converted to organic acid. Although fairly typical symptoms may point to the correct diagnosis, confirmation can be rapidly obtained by identification of toxic compounds in the serum. Some hospital laboratories and many commercial laboratories are equipped with constantly available chromatographic apparatus for this type of diagnosis.

Ethylene Glycol Intoxication. Ethylene glycol is metabolized to a series of compounds including glycolic, glyoxalic, and oxalic acids. During the early stages of ethylene glycol intoxication, one finds in addition to profound metabolic acidosis a CNS dysfunction characterized by ataxia, confusion, coma, and seizures. Patients may then develop cardiopulmonary failure and later acute tubular necrosis. The anion that accumulates is predominantly glycolate, but lactate may also accumulate because of the increased production of NADH. In this clinical setting, the appearance of large amounts of urinary oxalate crystals favors the diagnosis of ethylene glycol poisoning.

Therapy is based on the administration of ethanol to prevent ethylene glycol metabolism while simultaneously correcting the severe acidosis and removing ethylene glycol. Unlike ketone anions and lactate, glycolate is not a bicarbonate precursor, and bicarbonate must be administered to treat the acidosis. The loading dose of ethanol is 0.6 g per kilogram of body weight given either intravenously or orally, and the maintenance dose is 0.15 g per kilogram per hour in chronic alcoholics and 0.07 g per kilogram per hour in nonalcoholics. Hemodialysis removes ethylene glycol and glycolate efficiently and should be used in severely intoxicated patients. The ethanol dosage should be increased by 50 percent when hemodialysis is used. Recently, a specific inhibitor of alcohol dehydrogenase—4, methylpyrazole—has been used to treat ethylene glycol poisoning.

Methanol Intoxication. Metabolic acidosis in methanol intoxication results from the metabolism of methanol to formic acid. A prominent complication is optic neuritis, which can cause blurred vision and may progress to blindness. Fundoscopic examination may reveal retinal edema and inflammation of the optic disc. As in the case of ethylene glycol poisoning, excessive production of NADH during the metabolism of methanol leads to an excessive production of lactic acid. A diagnostic clue to severe methanol intoxication can be missed if measurement of the osmolar gap is delayed; because methanol is continuously metabolized, the serum osmolar gap may have returned to normal. However, measurement of serum formate concentration provides confirmation of the diagnosis in the latter case. The treatment of methanol intoxication is the same as that of ethylene glycol poisoning.

Chronic Renal Failure

Advanced renal disease of any cause tends to be associated with some degree of acidosis by the time the GFR decreases to less than 20 ml per minute. The predominant mechanism of the acidosis is diminished ammonia production. The acidosis of advanced renal failure is associated with retention of anions such as sulfate and phosphate, with an elevation in the anion gap. However, with milder degrees of renal insufficiency, the acidosis may be hyperchloremic before significant retention of anions occurs. Predominantly tubulointerstitial renal disease may present with defective excretion of ammonia earlier, and hyperchloremic acidosis that is out of proportion to the decline in the GFR may be found.

In renal disease, the rate of acid production is unchanged and the alkali requirement for neutralizing the daily acid production does not usually greatly exceed 1 mEq per kilogram of body weight per day. For patients who tolerate oral bicarbonate pills poorly, Shohl's solution (sodium citrate with some citric acid for flavoring) may be used. One milliliter of Shohl's solution provides 1 mEq of bicarbonate. The serum bicarbonate level should be kept close to the normal range in order to limit progressive bone disease. In children, the goal should be to maintain a normal serum bicarbonate concentration.

Gastrointestinal Loss of Bicarbonate

Fecal, pancreatic, or biliary loss of bicarbonate causes hyperchloremic metabolic acidosis and hypokalemia. The amount of bicarbonate lost depends on the type of diarrhea. For example, in malabsorption syndrome, some of the organic acids produced by bacteria are titrated by bicarbonate and excreted in the stools as the salts of the organic anions. The alkali loss in the stools can be approximated by measuring the stool anion gap (Na + K − Cl). Alkali, fluid, and potassium are replaced according to the patient's specific needs.

Urinary Diversion Procedures

The association of hyperchloremic metabolic acidosis with urinary diversion procedures is well known. In the past, when ureterosigmoidostomy was the procedure of choice, the incidence of acidosis was nearly 80 percent. Later, with the use of other diversion procedures such as the ileal conduits, the incidence of metabolic acidosis diminished markedly. The mechanism of acidosis seems to be excessive urinary loss of bicarbonate secondary to active chloride absorption in exchange for bicarbonate, which normally takes place in the terminal ileum and ascending colon. Close follow-up of serum bicarbonate is required during the period after surgery to determine whether and how much alkali therapy is needed. Progressive renal insufficiency is common and is caused by obstruction due to ureteral stenosis, stones, and recurrent malignancy. Patients may become salt- and volume-depleted, a condition that markedly worsens the metabolic acidosis and often necessitates hospital admission for water and electrolyte replacement as well as for treatment of acidosis.

Renal Tubular Acidosis

RTA comprises a set of disorders characterized by hyperchloremia associated with hypokalemia of varying severity. In proximal RTA, a low threshold for bicarbonate excretion prevents the maintenance of normal serum bicarbonate, while in distal RTA, the crucial dysfunction is an inability to maintain high concentrations of hydrogen ion in the urine. The diagnosis of distal RTA can be made outright in a patient with hyperchloremic acidosis, frank acidemia, and inappropriately "alkaline" urine (pH > 5.5). In proximal RTA, the urine pH may become fairly acidic and may overlap with the range found with distal RTA. Hence, an acid load is sometimes needed to distinguish proximal from distal RTA. If a documented decrease in plasma bicarbonate of 3 to 5 mEq per liter is not accompanied by a decline in urine pH to less than 5.5, the diagnosis of distal RTA is confirmed. The administration of furosemide can be substituted for an acid load, since furosemide promotes hydrogen ion secretion by increasing the distal delivery of sodium.

Proximal Renal Tubular Acidosis. Defective reabsorption of bicarbonate by the proximal nephron may occur as an isolated event in children, but most commonly it occurs as part of a generalized proximal tubular dysfunction (Fanconi's syndrome). Carbonic anhydrase inhibitors produce the same alteration in acid-base metabolism as proximal RTA.

For acidosis to be corrected, large amounts of bicarbonate must be administered because the low tubular threshold causes the bicarbonate to be wasted. As the excess bicarbonate passes through the collecting tubule, excessive secretion of potassium occurs, and hypokalemia is a common consequence of bicarbonate therapy in the treatment of proximal RTA. Despite this difficulty, even mild acidosis should be treated in children because acidosis severely impairs growth. Volume depletion with thiazide diuretics and a low-salt diet may increase the renal bicarbonate threshold and reduce bicarbonate requirements. Alkali is usually given as sodium bicarbonate or as Shohl's solution with potassium supplements. As an alternative, part of the alkali replacement can be given as oral potassium citrate.

Distal Renal Tubular Acidosis. Acidosis is more severe in distal RTA than in proximal RTA, and the severe chronic acidosis leads to potassium wastage. Hence patients commonly present with weakness caused by profound hypokalemia. Nephrolithiasis, nephrocalcinosis, and pyelonephritis frequently complicate distal RTA and may led to progressive renal insufficiency. The daily dosage of alkali required to correct acidosis is determined by trial; since varying but modest amounts of bicarbonate may be excreted in the urine, the dosage is generally in the range of 1 to 3 mEq per kilogram per day. Although potassium supplementation is necessary for patients with acidosis and hypokalemia, it is not regularly required if the alkali supplements are keeping the blood pH within the normal range. In the acute phase of therapy, when acidosis and hypokalemia are severe, therapy should always be directed first at correction of the serum potassium in order to avoid acutely worsening hypokalemia with respiratory paralysis and potentially lethal cardiac arrhythmias.

Hyperkalemic Hyperchloremic Acidosis (Type IV RTA)

In a variety of clinical circumstances in which the common pathophysiologic feature is a lack of aldosterone or that the collecting tubules apparently fail to respond to aldosterone, hyperchloremic acidosis presents with sustained elevation in serum potassium. A noteworthy feature of the hyperkalemic state is that the electrocardiogram is usually unaffected. The most common cause of sustained hyperkalemia is the syndrome of hyporeninemic hypoaldosteronism (SHH). In this disorder, renin, and consequently aldosterone, are suppressed by volume expansion caused by a primary but unexplained exaggeration in renal salt reabsorption. About half of the patients with this disorder are diabetics, two-thirds have elevated blood pressure, and most have mild-to-moderate renal insufficiency. Interstitial nephropathy, acute glomerulonephritis, and urinary tract obstruction are other common causes of sustained hyperkalemia. The principal cause of the acidosis is suppression of ammonia production due to an excess of body potassium, but the lack of aldosterone, in addition to limiting potassium secretion, also limits hydrogen ion secretion. A liberal salt intake combined with the use of diuretics can diminish the excess total body salt and water and enhance the excretion of potassium, while permitting at least partial return of plasma renin and aldosterone. With this regimen, blood pressure may also decrease. Part of the sodium may be given as bicarbonate or citrate in addition to chloride. Relief of hyperkalemia may ameliorate acidosis. If the suggested program is inadequate, mineralocorticoid replacement can be added (e.g., fluorohydrocortisone 0.1 mg per mouth daily), although mineralocorticoid replacement alone is not appropriate therapy. In many patients, the hyperkalemia is mild and well tolerated. Such individuals may not require therapy. Nevertheless, in these patients, care must be taken to avoid clinical conditions and drugs that may provoke hyperkalemia by reducing distal sodium delivery, reducing aldosterone, or hampering potassium secretion—for example, volume depletion, nonsteroidal anti-inflammatory agents, angiotensin-converting enzyme inhibitors, beta-blockers, heparin, and potassium-sparing diuretics. The underlying cause of type IV RTA should always be sought and, if possible, treated. For example, in patients with obstructive uropathy, relief of obstruction could reverse the defect. Chronic administration of ion-exchange resins (e.g. Kayexalate) is often unsatisfactory because of severe constipation or undesired sodium retention.

Pseudohypoaldosteronism. Pseudohypoaldosteronism type I is a congenital and often transient disorder of infants in which the renal facet of a generalized unresponsiveness to aldosterone is reflected in salt loss, dehydration, hyperkalemia, and hyperchloremic acidosis. A similar disorder may present after infancy as a consequence of chronic renal insufficiency, most often because of tubulointerstitial disease, and is generally described as salt-losing nephropathy. In these disorders, the available evidence shows elevated plasma renin and aldosterone. Treatment consists primarily of supplementation with salt and alkali, sometimes accompanied by thiazide diuretics.

Pseudohypoaldosteronism type II, which is probably identical to Gordon's syndrome, is a variant of hyporeninemic hypoaldosteronism and is treated similarly. In this disorder, primary salt retention is believed to be caused by the inappropriate reabsorption of chloride in the collecting tubule; failure to establish a negative charge in the lumen limits the secretion of both potassium and hydrogen. As in all disorders in which potassium retention leads to hyperkalemia, suppression of ammonia production worsens the acidosis.

Suggested Reading

Batlle DC, Hizon M, et al. The use of the urinary anion gap in the diagnosis of hyperchloremic metabolic acidosis. N Engl J Med 1988; 318:594.

Halperin ML, Hammeke M, et al. Metabolic acidosis in the alcoholic: a pathophysiologic approach. Metabolism 1983; 32:308.

Jacobson D, Bredsen JE, Eidel I, Ostborg J. Anion and osmolal gaps in the diagnosis of methanol and ethylene glycol poisoning. Acta Med Scand 1982; 212:17.

Oh MS, Carroll HJ. The anion gap. N Engl J Med 1979; 197:814.

Oh MS, Carroll HJ, Uribarri J. Mechanism of normochloremic and hyperchloremic acidosis in diabetic ketoacidosis. Nephron 1990; 54:1.

Oh, MS, Uribarri J, Carroll HJ. Electrolyte case vignette: a case of unusual organic acidosis. Am J Kidney Dis 1988; 11:80.

Rocher LL, Tannen RL. The clinical spectrum of renal tubular acidosis. Ann Rev Med 1986; 37:319.

METABOLIC ALKALOSIS

Robert G. Luke, M.D.
John H. Galla, M.D.

DIAGNOSIS

Metabolic alkalosis is the most common acid base disorder in hospitalized patients. Alkalemia is the elevation of arterial blood pH above normal; alkalosis is a tendency toward elevation of arterial blood pH. This difference is important diagnostically because in mixed disturbances, alkalosis may conceal a primary metabolic or respiratory acidosis. Metabolic alkalosis occurs when an acid-base disturbance tends to increase the plasma bicarbonate concentration as a primary event; the usual associated increment in arterial carbon dioxide concentration ($PaCO_2$) is a compensatory secondary phenomenon and never fully corrects arterial pH to normal in the absence of an associated primary respiratory acidosis. Patients with hypochloremia and hyperbicarbonatemia may have either respiratory acidosis or metabolic alkalosis; the anion gap tends to be elevated in metabolic alkalosis but not in respiratory acidosis unless there is associated lactic acidosis caused by severe hypoxia. Thus, to determine an accurate acid-base diagnosis, a determination of arterial pH and $PaCO_2$ is essential before the treatment of hypochloremic hyperbicarbonatemia is instituted. On the average, respiratory compensation for chronic metabolic alkalosis is $PaCO_2$ increase of 0.6 mm Hg for each milliequivalent increase in the plasma bicarbonate concentration above normal. In extreme

Table 1 Causes and Treatment of Maintained Elevation of Plasma Bicarbonate on Chronic Metabolic Alkalosis

MECHANISM	CAUSES OF MAINTAINED ELEVATION OF HCO_3	THERAPEUTIC OPTIONS
Chloride depletion (chronic vomiting)	Chloride depletion	Replace Cl as NaCl, KCl, or HCl
	Continuing H^+ loss	Gastric acid inhibitor
	Ineffective CBV	Improve cardiac output; acetazolamide
	Moderately depressed GFR	NaCl; restore ECF or cardiac output
	Severely depressed GFR (at least temporarily irreversible)	HCl; dialysis against high Cl dialysate
Potassium depletion—mineralocorticoid excess (Bartter's syndrome)	Potassium depletion (depresses GFR and increases tubule reabsorption of bicarbonate)	Discontinue diuretic; KCl; amiloride, triamterene or spironolactone; indomethacin; Mg^{++} repletion
With hypertension (primary aldosteronism)	Excess mineralocorticoid and/or glucocorticoid activity	Low-NaCl diet; remove adenoma; spironolactone (primary aldosteronism); Treat hypertension; KCl; spironolactone (secondary aldosteronism); Pituitary surgery or irradiation; remove tumor—metyrapone or aminoglutethimide (Cushing's syndrome)
Base loading (multiple blood transfusions)	Administration of $NaHCO_3$ or its precursors (e.g., citrate) *plus* bicarbonate-maintaining cause	Stop base; correct underlying cause
With hypercalcemia and hypoparathyroidism (milk-alkali syndrome)	Depression of GFR and enhanced tubular reabsorption of bicarbonate	Stop high intake of base and Ca^{++}; replete Cl and ECF volume deficit

*Example of clinical cause; CBV, circulating blood volume; GFR, glomerular filtration rate; ECF, extracellular fluid.

metabolic alkalosis, the $PaCO_2$ may reach 60 mm Hg or more. It is especially important to recognize that the latter situation is not a primary respiratory disorder, since treatment aimed primarily at reducing $PaCO_2$ produces a life-threatening increase in arterial pH. In primary metabolic alkalosis, specific acid-base therapy is generally indicated when the plasma bicarbonate concentration is greater than 33 mEq per liter or the arterial pH is greater than 7.50.

The clinical manifestations of metabolic alkalosis per se are difficult to separate from those of the commonly associated volume or potassium depletion. However, neuromuscular irritability, cardiovascular instability and arrhythmias, and mental confusion are common when alkalosis is severe. The potential adverse effects of compensatory hypoventilation on other pulmonary functions or on the development of infections of the respiratory tract in the seriously ill patient or the immunocompromised host may be significant. Metabolic alkalosis is clearly not an innocuous condition; in one large series, for patients with an arterial pH of 7.65 or greater the mortality rate was 80 percent. Again, associated conditions may be important, but treatment of the metabolic alkalosis per se in such circumstances is a medical emergency and requires a rapid assessment of the relevant causative mechanisms in order to prescribe corrective therapy, as discussed below.

Metabolic alkalosis can be divided into two phases: generation (loss of hydrogen ion from or gain of bicarbonate by the body) and maintenance. In the absence of the conditions outlined in Table 1, it is difficult to exceed the capacity of the normal kidney to excrete administered bicarbonate or its metabolic precursors such as citrate or carbonate. Iatrogenic acute metabolic alkalosis related to oral or intravenous sodium bicarbonate administration is thus usually transient in the presence of a normal kidney. Especially when sodium bicarbonate has been given intravenously, transient metabolic alkalosis may also occur as the accumulated organic ions of diabetic ketoacidosis or lactic acidosis are metabolized to bicarbonate secondary to insulin administration and/or volume repletion. Since base loading alone rarely produces a sustained elevation of plasma bicarbonate concentration by more than ≈ to 3 mEq per liter in the absence of bicarbonate-retaining mechanisms, the focus of this chapter is on the treatment of chronic metabolic alkalosis in which one of the sustaining causes is virtually always evident. Not included in Table 1 is the recent observation that hypoproteinemia may also be associated with mild alkalosis, which resolves with the restoration of the serum protein concentration to normal. On occasion, the pathogenesis of the generation phase of metabolic alkalosis is obscure and cannot be established by the time the physician is faced with the clinical problem. This, however, need not deter effective therapy. The paramount question to be answered by the physician prior to initiation of appropriately designed therapy is: Why is this patient's kidney not excreting the retained extracellular bicarbonate?

In most patients, the history and physical examination strongly suggest the mechanisms responsible for the maintenance of the elevated plasma bicarbonate concentration. If the cause is not obvious, determination of urinary chloride and potassium concentrations may be helpful. Patients with chloride depletion metabolic alkalosis have a urinary chloride concentration less than 10 mEq per liter except when renal chloride wasting is the cause of chloride depletion, as for example within the period of therapeutic efficacy of administered diuretics or in severe chronic potassium depletion (plasma potassium < 2.4 mEq per liter); in the latter instance, chloride will not be retained until repletion of potassium is initiated. Unless these rather unusual circumstances of renal chloride wasting are present or the patient is ingesting diuret-

Table 2 Differential Diagnosis of Bartter's Syndrome

DIAGNOSIS	COMMENT
Diuretic abuse	Low urine chloride when not ingesting diuretics
Bulimia	Low urine chloride: disequilibrium metabolic alkalosis may occur (see text)
Laxative abuse	Metabolic alkalosis usually not severe
Magnesium depletion	May complicate diuretic abuse or Bartter's syndrome
Bartter's syndrome	High urine chloride

ics surreptitiously a urinary chloride concentration greater than 20 mEq per liter usually suggests that therapy other than chloride repletion is necessary.

Metabolic alkalosis is often also associated with increased urinary potassium excretion, and a urinary potassium concentration of greater than 30 mEq per liter despite hypokalemia would be anticipated unless potassium depletion is profound (i.e., a deficit > 500 mEq in an adult man of average weight). In such circumstances, the urinary potassium concentration may be less than 20 to 30 mEq per liter and yet potassium depletion may be a major contributory cause of the metabolic alkalosis. Primary potassium losses from the bowel, as that which occurs with laxative abuse or villous adenoma of the colon, are also associated with low urinary potassium concentrations.

A urinary sodium concentration of greater than 20 to 30 mEq per liter is unusual in chloride depletion alkalosis, especially when urinary pH is acidic (< 5.5) as is customary when the kidney is conserving bicarbonate. In acute or chronic vomiting, as the plasma bicarbonate concentration is further elevated above its chronic stable high plasma level, transient renal wasting of sodium and bicarbonate may occur. This clinical state is sometimes termed *disequilibrium metabolic alkalosis*. In such patients, urinary sodium concentration may be greater than 20 mEq per liter—even in the presence of overt clinical volume depletion—but the urine is quite alkaline (i.e., the pH is greater than 6.5 and contains significant amounts of bicarbonate), and the urine chloride concentration is less than 15 mEq per liter.

Patients who have alkalosis caused by mineralocorticoid excess with potassium depletion can be subdivided into those with a normal or low blood pressure and plasma volume and those with extracellular fluid (ECF) volume expansion and high blood pressure (see Table 1). In the former case, mineralocorticoid excess is associated with renal wasting of sodium chloride and hence an inability to develop hypertension. In the latter case, an intact kidney responds to mineralocorticoid excess with both sodium chloride retention and potassium loss.

A particularly vexing diagnostic problem is posed by those patients who can best be described as belonging to the group representing the differential diagnosis of Bartter's syndrome (Table 2). Bartter's syndrome is thus important beyond its frequency of occurrence because it illustrates the pathophysiology and treatment of the several much more common conditions listed in Table 1. It further illustrates how several mechanisms may interact with one another to maintain an elevated plasma bicarbonate concentration. The syndrome is characterized by normotension, a tendency to renal sodium, chloride, and potassium wasting, and marked stimulation of the renin-aldosterone system and of renal prostaglandin (Pg) production. Some cases are familial and develop in childhood, although the syndrome may also be diagnosed for the first time in adult life. One plausible explanation for the syndrome is a defect in sodium chloride reabsorption in the thick ascending limb of the loop of Henle (the site of action of loop diuretics) with increased delivery of sodium and fluid to the more distal potassium secretory sites. Potassium loss is accelerated by both macula densa and baroreceptor stimuli for renin release and the resultant hyperaldosteronism. Potassium depletion stimulates renal synthesis of PgE2, which in turn further impairs sodium chloride reabsorption in the thick ascending limb and sets up a vicious circle. A milder variant, Gitelman's syndrome, is consistent with a defect in NaCl transport in the diluting segment (the site of action of thiazides). Diuretic abuse, which may be continually denied by the patient (usually female) mimics these syndromes by impairing sodium chloride transport in the thick ascending limb of the loop of Henle (furosemide) or in the cortical diluting segment (thiazides). Urinary chloride concentration is high in diuretic abuse only during the therapeutic duration of action of the drug. Bulimia may also mimic the syndrome, but the urinary chloride concentration in patients with bulimia is usually low during the metabolic alkalosis. Once the diagnosis is made, the need for therapy is obvious in the case of diuretic abuse or bulimia; expert psychiatric help is usually needed.

■ THERAPEUTIC OPTIONS

The mechanisms listed in the first column of Table 1 are almost always responsible for the inability of the kidney to excrete the retained extracellular bicarbonate. In many patients, two or more mechanisms may contribute and interact. In most, the major mechanism relates to either chloride depletion or mineralocorticoid excess with potassium depletion; associated potassium depletion is also common with chloride metabolic alkalosis. In general, however, the alkalosis *can* be corrected in such patients without concomitant restoration of potassium balance. For the second group, by contrast, repletion of potassium is necessary for correction of metabolic alkalosis. There are, however, cogent clinical reasons to also correct the associated potassium depletion during treatment of metabolic alkalosis even when it is primarily due to chloride depletion.

If the kidney function is severely depressed and the glomerular filtration rate (GFR) cannot be improved by increasing cardiac output or improving effective circulating blood volume, some form of dialysis using a dialysate with a chloride concentration significantly above that in the patient's plasma may be necessary (see Table 1).

■ SPECIFIC THERAPY

For full correction of metabolic alkalosis, the chloride deficit must be replaced, usually intravenously. Judicious selection of

Table 3 Indications for Hydrochloric Acid Administration

Arterial pH >7.55 and NaCl or KCl administration is contraindicated
Need for immediate amelioration of metabolic alkalosis because of:
- Hepatic encephalopathy
- Cardiac arrhythmia
- Digitalis intoxication
- Central nervous system effect of high arterial pH
  - Arterial pH >7.6 when initial renal response to NaCl or KCl or acetazolamide is likely to be sluggish or is in doubt

the accompanying cation—sodium, potassium, or hydrogen ion—depends on careful assessment of (1) ECF volume status and the presence or absence of cardiac failure, (2) the presence and degree of associated potassium depletion, and (3) the degree of impairment and reversibility of the depression of the GFR. If the kidney is capable of excreting sodium and/or potassium, it will excrete bicarbonate with those cations and thus rapidly correct the metabolic alkalosis as chloride is made available. When renal function is too severely depressed by acute or chronic intrinsic renal disease however, or when there is intractable congestive cardiac failure, especially with hyperkalemia, administration of chloride with sodium or potassium may not be feasible. Two therapeutic strategies may be taken in such situations: infusion of chloride as hydrochloric acid (HCl), or providing chloride by dialysis across the peritoneal or hemodialysis membrane so that potassium status, sodium status, and plasma volume can be contemporaneously corrected. An additional indication for HCl is when speed of correction is essential and if there is doubt about the capacity of the kidney to excrete bicarbonate rapidly enough (Table 3).

Administration of isotonic NaCl is the preferred therapy if, as is most commonly the case, there is associated ECF volume depletion. This simultaneously corrects the chloride deficit, the ECF volume deficit, and the associated depression in GFR. Even though repletion of potassium is not essential for the correction of the alkalosis, potassium administration is usually indicated because some degree of potassium depletion is usually present and because kaliuresis may occur as plasma volume, GFR, and urine flow rate are restored to normal. Potassium can be provided conveniently by adding KCl to isotonic NaCl in a concentration of 10 to 20 mEq per liter. In most patients with overt signs of volume contraction such as hypotension (including postural hypotension), tachycardia, and diminished skin turgor, administration of 3 to 5 L of 0.15 M NaCl is necessary to correct volume deficits and metabolic alkalosis. The physician must also include replacement of ongoing losses in the fluid and electrolyte replacement schedule. As the chloride deficit is corrected, a brisk alkaline diuresis should occur with a fall in plasma bicarbonate concentration. This alkaline diuresis may increase urinary potassium losses and reinforces the point of concurrently replacing potassium to avoid the effects of hypokalemia.

When the ECF volume is assessed to be normal, total body chloride deficit in milliequivalents can be estimated by the formula: body weight × 0.2 × the desired increment in the plasma chloride concentration. If there is associated hypokalemia, as is customary, the deficit can be repleted conveniently by either oral or intravenous KCl.

Some recent animal studies in our laboratories suggest that chloride depletion, independent of volume depletion, may contribute not only to maintenance of chronic metabolic alkalosis, but also to a reduction in the GFR and to stimulation of the renin aldosterone system. This may explain the occasional patients we have seen with hypochloremic metabolic alkalosis, hypertension in the recumbent position, and a significant elevation of serum creatinine but without overt sodium or volume depletion. In such patients—although not as yet under study conditions of metabolic balance—administration of KCl alone has been associated with restoration of a normal serum creatinine level, amelioration of hypertension, and correction of both potassium deficits and alkalosis; even when quite severe, potassium depletion by itself is associated with only a slight-to-moderate depression of the GFR. Our studies suggest that chloride depletion leads to depression of the GFR in part via activated tubuloglomerular feedback and to stimulation of renin release from the kidney by a macula densa mechanism.

In the clinical setting of ECF volume overload and/or congestive cardiac failure in association with chloride depletion and metabolic alkalosis, administration of NaCl is clearly inadvisable. As in euvolemic patients, hypokalemia may facilitate repletion of chloride as KCl, but KCl may also be contraindicated either because of concurrent hyperkalemia or concern about the ability to deal with the potassium load in the presence of renal failure. If renal function is still reasonable in this situation (serum creatinine <4 mg per deciliter), the use of acetazolamide in a dosage of 250 mg two or three times daily can be considered. Such an approach could be used for a patient with an acute exacerbation of chronic lung disease and cor pulmonale who develops metabolic alkalosis after therapeutic reduction in $PaCO_2$ in the presence of hyperkalemia. Occasionally, the judicious intermingling of acetazolamide with a loop diuretic in patients with cor pulmonale or in any patient in whom severe metabolic alkalosis is impeding the use of loop diuretics will dampen the magnitude of the chloride depletion. If acetazolamide is used in a patient without hyperkalemia, KCl should be concurrently administered because the risk of development of hypokalemia during the ensuing alkaline diuresis is high. Administration of acetazolamide should be stopped when the plasma bicarbonate concentration approaches baseline levels for that patient, and plasma electrolyte composition should be followed daily during its administration.

When the kidney is incapable of responding to chloride repletion or when dialysis is necessary for the control of renal failure, exchange of bicarbonate for chloride across the semipermeable membrane used during hemodialysis or peritoneal dialysis is an effective mechanism for correcting metabolic alkalosis. Current routine dialysate solutions for both peritoneal dialysis (including continuous ambulatory peritoneal dialysis) and hemodialysis contain concentrations of bicarbonate or its metabolic precursors, such as acetate, equivalent to 35 mEq per liter and therefore must be modified in circumstances of metabolic alkalosis. In an emergency, peritoneal dialysis can be performed against solutions of 0.15 M NaCl with appropriate maintenance of plasma potassium, calcium, and magnesium concentration by intravenous infusion. Most large hospital pharmacies, however, can prepare appropriate special dialysate solutions for both hemodialysis and peritoneal dialysis in these circumstances.

The indications for the use of intravenous HCl administration are given in Table 3. Again, most hospital pharmacies are capable of preparing HCl as 100 mEq per liter (i.e., a 0.1 M solution). The amount of HCl (in milliequivalents) needed to correct alkalosis is calculated by the formula: $0.4 \times$ body weight (kg) $\times$ desired decrement in plasma bicarbonate concentration (mEq per liter). Since the goal of such therapy is to get the patient out of the danger zone in terms of acid-base balance, it is usually prudent to plan initially to restore the plasma bicarbonate concentration halfway toward normal. The HCl must be given through a catheter placed in the vena cava or a large vein draining into it, and placement of the catheter must be confirmed radiographically, since extravasation of HCl can lead to sloughing of the mediastinal tissues. The rate of infusion should not exceed 0.2 mEq per kilogram of body weight per hour. The patient is best managed in an intensive care unit with frequent measurement of arterial blood gases and electrolytes. The above formula does not allow for ongoing loss of hydrogen ion or gain of base by the ECF. An alternative to HCl is ammonium chloride which may be administered via a peripheral vein. The rate of infusion should not provide more than 300 mEq NH_4^+ per 24 hours, and NH_4Cl should be avoided in the presence of renal or hepatic insufficiency. We use HCl only when indicated (see Table 3) and prefer it to NH_4Cl in such circumstances. NH_4Cl is contraindicated in patients with liver or renal failure. The HCl salts of the cationic amino acids lysine or arginine should probably not be used because of the association with dangerous hyperkalemia.

Additional therapeutic approaches are necessary in the following clinical situations associated with chloride depletion metabolic alkalosis. In the presence of pernicious vomiting or the surgical requirement for continual removal of gastric secretions, metabolic alkalosis will continue to be generated and replacement of pre-existing deficits may be complicated by these ongoing losses. In these circumstances, the administration of an H2-receptor blocker, such as cimetidine or ranitidine, will blunt acid production of the stomach and decrease gastric HCl losses. Fairly high doses of cimetidine may be required—e.g., as much as 200 to 600 mg of intravenous cimetidine every 4 hours; omeprazole, an inhibitor of H^+K^+ ATPase, may be more efficacious. Because serious side effects such as acute confusion can complicate these dose levels, it is reasonable to check the pH of the gastric aspirate to determine the lowest effective dose. Even in the presence of achlorhydria, however, gastric secretions contain significant amounts of sodium, potassium, and chloride. In a few gastrocytoplasties usually with high serum gastrin concentrations, the loss of HCl in the urine has resisted treatment with oral chloride replacement as well as histamine and proton-pump inhibitors. Revision of the gastric augmentation may be necessary in these patients.

Although diarrhea is normally associated with metabolic acidosis, in two circumstances metabolic alkalosis can occur in association with increased fecal loss of fluid. About 10 to 15 percent of villous adenomas are associated with alkalosis; these require surgical removal after correction of the sodium chloride, potassium, and volume deficits. The second condition is the rare familial disease of chloridorrhea in which massive amounts of chloride, potassium, and fluid are secreted into the ileum because of a transport defect. This condition has been responsive only to continued repletion of these losses by supplementation of the dietary intake.

Table 4 Estimation of Potassium Deficit

CORRECTED PLASMA POTASSIUM (mEq/L)*	APPROXIMATE TOTAL BODY POTASSIUM DEFICIT %	mEq†
3–3.5	5	100–200
2.5–3.0	5–10	200–400
2–2.5	10–15	300–600
<2.0	15–20+	500–800+

*Increase plasma K by 0.6 mEq per 0.1 increment in arterial pH.
†For the 70 kg subject.

■ POTASSIUM DEPLETION-MINERALOCORTICOID EXCESS

In humans, severe potassium depletion is associated with a mild-to-moderate metabolic alkalosis unless there is complicating chloride depletion or mineralocorticoid excess, in which circumstance severe metabolic alkalosis may occur. In the presence of normotension, the cause of the metabolic alkalosis can usually be determined by the differential diagnosis. Administration of thiazide or loop diuretics should be discontinued. Oral KCl given in the liquid form diluted with fruit juice or in the slow-release form can be given in doses of up to 40 to 60 mEq four or five times per day. If serious effects of potassium depletion and/or metabolic alkalosis are present such as cardiac arrhythmias or muscle paralysis, intravenous HCl may be given at rates as high as 40 mEq per hour in concentrations not to exceed 60 mEq per liter. These are high rates and should be employed only if life-threatening hypokalemia and/or metabolic alkalosis is present; the patient should be monitored by electrocardiogram and frequent determination of plasma potassium concentration (Table 4). It is critical that the solution used to administer potassium or the solution given immediately before the administration of potassium (for example, in the emergency room) not contain glucose, since this will stimulate insulin secretion and cause hypokalemia to worsen. Once potassium repletion is clearly under way, the presence of glucose in the infusion may facilitate cellular potassium repletion, but hypokalemic nephropathy may impair free water excretion and plasma sodium concentration should also be monitored if a free water load is being administered.

Because Bartter's syndrome probably comprises several disorders with different pathophysiologies, the degree to which other solute deficiencies, such as sodium, chloride, magnesium, or calcium deficiencies, occur in or contribute to the disorder varies. Nevertheless, the principal goal of therapy is to prevent the loss of excessive potassium in the urine. Angiotensin-converting enzyme inhibitors—in particular, enalapril in doses of 20 to 40 mg per day—have been shown to correct hypokalemia, hypomagnesemia, and alkalosis; caution is necessary during the first few days of treatment because of possible hypotension. Potassium-sparing diuretics (amiloride, 5 or 10 mg daily: triamterene, 100 mg twice daily: or spironolactone, 25 to 50 mg four times daily) are effective for this purpose, but dietary potassium supplementation is often also needed. Spironolactone may produce tender gynecomastia in men. Renal production of PgE2 is increased and may contribute to sodium, chloride, and potassium wasting; Pg synthetase inhibitors such as indomethacin or ibuprofen may blunt, but usually *do* not completely correct, the hypokalemic alkalosis. Because magnesium depletion may increase urinary potassium wasting, an attempt should be made to correct hypomagnesemia and replete magnesium stores. The degree to which the correction of magnesium depletion blunts the alkalosis is uncertain, however, and magnesium salts usually produce an unacceptable degree of gastrointestinal irritation that may compound the patient's problems. Oral magnesium oxide can be given in doses of 250 to 500 mg four times daily (12.5 to 25 mEq Mg). If severe hypomagnesemia is contributing to seizures or tetany, 4 ml of a 50 percent solution of magnesium sulfate (16 mEq Mg) can be given in 100 ml of 5 percent glucose over 10 to 20 minutes.

In the group of alkaloses characterized by an excess of mineralocorticoid, therapy is directed at either removal of the source of blockade of the mineralocorticoid. Hypertension, often severe, may complicate many of these disorders (specific therapy for this is discussed elsewhere in this text). Since mineralocorticoids directly and indirectly stimulate potassium and hydrogen ion secretion (equivalent to bicarbonate reabsorption) in the distal convoluted tubule and collecting duct (in part in exchange for sodium), the administration of potassium-sparing diuretics will effectively reverse the adverse effects of mineralocorticoid excess on sodium, potassium, and bicarbonate.

The stimulation of net sodium reabsorption and potassium secretion by the effect of excess mineralocorticoid on the kidney may also be ameliorated by adjustments to diet. If hypokalemia and potassium depletion develop, as is common, bicarbonate reabsorption in the proximal tubule of the kidney is stimulated and alkalosis is further intensified. By contrast, the stimulated sodium reabsorption produces volume expansion which tends to diminish fluid and HCO_3 reabsorption in the proximal tubule; however, as noted, distal bicarbonate reabsorption is stimulated by the mineralocorticoid. Thus the restriction of sodium and the addition of potassium to the diet should aid in the control of the alkalosis as well as the hypertension that often accompanies these disorders.

Many primary disorders of mineralocorticoid excess are definitively treated by tumor ablation. Adrenocorticotropic hormone-secreting pituitary tumors may be removed by transsphenoidal resection or ablated by irradiation, With adrenal tumors, adrenalectomy—either unilateral or bilateral as appropriate—is curative. In the ectopic adrenocorticotropic hormone syndrome, the ideal treatment of the secreting tumor can rarely be accomplished. In this instance and in metastatic adrenal tumors, metyrapone, which inhibits the final step in cortisol synthesis, and aminoglutethimide, which inhibits the initial step in steroid biosynthesis, will blunt the myriad manifestations of excess cortisol. In 11-β-hydroxysteroid dehydrogenase deficiency, dexamethasone has been shown to correct the hypokalemic alkalosis. In those disorders in which curative surgery cannot be carried out, mitotane (p,p-DDD), which produces selective destruction of the zona fasciculata and reticularis and leaves aldosterone production intact, has also been used to control effectively many of the manifestations of the disease. To the extent that severe fluid and electrolyte disturbances are due to aldosterone production, this drug may not suffice. Thus, metyrapone, ketoconazole, or aminoglutethimide may be better choices when hypokalemic alkalosis is present. Cisplatin has also recently been used in the treatment of adrenal malignancies: however, a detailed discussion of the use of such drugs is beyond the scope of this review.

Among the alkaloses associated with excess exogenous base administration, the milk-alkali syndrome, characterized by metabolic alkalosis hypercalcemia and renal insufficiency, is now infrequently seen. Cessation of alkali ingestion and the calcium sources (often milk and calcium carbonate) and chloride and volume repletion for the commonly associated vomiting will usually lead to the prompt resolution of all abnormalities. Occasional occult sources of base loading are citrate in blood transfusions or release of base by metastases in bone.

ACUTE HYPERSENSITIVITY INTERSTITIAL NEPHRITIS

Peter S. Heeger, M.D.
Eric G. Neilson, M.D.

Acute tubulointerstitial nephritis, often referred to as simply "acute interstitial nephritis," accounts for nearly 15 percent of cases of acute renal failure. Individuals with acute interstitial nephritis (AIN) typically experience a sudden decrease in renal function, with the hallmarks of acute interstitial injury on renal biopsy manifested by mononuclear cell infiltrates (lymphocytes and plasma cells), occasional eosinophils, tubular destruction, and relatively normal glomeruli. It is also important that as many as 25 percent of patients with chronic renal failure have sustained injury from the concealed, long-term sequelae of what probably began as acute interstitial inflammation. In such patients, biopsy reveals progressive pathologic injury involving interstitial fibrosis, tubular atrophy, and tubular dropout with or without senescent glomerular tufts. Largely because of the work done in experimental systems, there is a growing knowledge of the pathophysiologic mechanisms involved in the production of interstitial injury. Applying this insight to human renal disease has resulted in a reasoned clinical method for evaluating patients suspected of having acute interstitial nephritis and in a firmer groundwork for the discussion of therapeutic options. The approach we use emphasizes the establishment of a diagnosis, the removal of potentially causative agents, and the attempt to treat the destructive lesion with chemotherapy when necessary.

CLINICAL FEATURES

The wide variety of etiologic factors that have been implicated in the development of AIN can be divided into three broad categories: pharmacologic agents, infectious diseases, and autoimmune phenomena (Table 1). Rarely, the presentation of interstitial nephritis is simply idiopathic. A thorough exploration of these potential causes is essential. The initial approach to the treatment of AIN is to remove any inciting agents and to treat any underlying disease.

The diagnosis of interstitial nephritis is relatively straightforward in the classic setting in which a rapidly rising serum creatinine level (0.3 to 0.5 mg per deciliter per day) accompanied by fever, rash, and eosinophilia occurs 10 to 15 days after beginning treatment with a pharmaceutical agent. Unfortunately, this presentation of a hypersensitivity reaction is the exception, not the rule. Skin rash occurs in less than 50 percent of patients, fever in approximately 75 percent, eosinophilia in about 80 percent, and the triad is found in less than 30 percent. Therefore, when AIN is suspected, the physician must first systematically exclude prerenal and obstructive causes of acute renal failure from the differential diagnosis and then proceed to distinguish interstitial nephritis from acute tubular necrosis, glomerulonephritis, or vasculitis. A careful urinalysis is usually helpful in this regard. In interstitial nephritis, the urinalysis reveals mild to moderate proteinuria (although the nephrotic syndrome has been reported, especially with use of alpha-interferon and nonsteroidal anti-inflammatory drugs [NSAIDs]), and microscopic hematuria may be present. Sterile pyuria and/or white blood cell casts are usually encountered, but red blood cell casts are so rare that their presence should suggest the alternative diagnosis of glomerular injury. Additionally, the presence of eosinophiluria, as demonstrated by Hansel's stain, supports the diagnosis of interstitial nephritis. This finding is not entirely sensitive or specific, however, and must be considered in the context of the clinical setting.

Table 1 Etiology of Acute Interstitial Nephritis

Drugs
Antibiotics (e.g., penicillin derivatives, cephalosporins, rifampin, sulfonamides, fluoroquinolones)
Nonsteroidal anti-inflammatory drugs (NSAIDs)
H_2-blockers
Diuretics
Others (phenytoin, allopurinol, alpha-interferon)
Infectious Diseases
Diphtheria
Scarlet fever
Subacute bacterial endocarditis
Leptospirosis
Human immunodeficiency virus
Epstein-Barr virus
Legionella
Syphilis
Autoimmune Diseases
Systemic lupus erythematosus
Sjögren's syndrome
Sarcoidosis
Antitubular basement membrane disease
Tubulointerstitial nephritis-uveitis syndrome
Idiopathic

Often, the available clinical data are insufficient to provide a definitive diagnosis without a renal biopsy. There are many reported cases of clinically unsuspected AIN diagnosed by renal biopsy, as well as multiple reports of biopsy-documented acute tubular necrosis in patients clinically suspected as suffering from AIN. Additionally, renal biopsy can provide important prognostic information based on the extent and character of the renal lesion. The presence of advanced renal insufficiency with significant fibrosis and an extensive mononuclear infiltrate on biopsy, for example, portend a poor renal outcome. In such a situation, it may be best to institute conservative treatment with preparation for renal replacement therapy, and to avoid the potential complications of immunosuppressive therapy. Establishment of a firm diagnosis must be made as quickly as possible because minimizing the time that elapses from the onset of renal injury to the institution of appropriate therapy allows the greatest possibility for return of normal renal function. In experimental interstitial nephritis, substantial irreversible interstitial fibrosis can develop in as little as 10 days. We recommend rapidly obtaining a tissue diagnosis in all cases of suspected interstitial nephritis, provided that the patient is medically stable enough to tolerate a biopsy, and there are no contraindications to immunosuppressive therapy.

■ MECHANISMS OF DISEASE

A general understanding of the underlying pathophysiologic processes leading to interstitial injury is helpful in the selection of appropriate therapy. We believe that virtually all forms of human interstitial nephritis have an immunologic basis, and several reports in the clinical literature are consistent with this view. Most of the detailed information, however, comes from studies in experimental animals. Rodent models of interstitial nephritis implicate humoral and/or cellular arms of the immune system in the expression of the disease. In some experimental models, animals with a genetic predisposition to interstitial nephritis lose their protective immunologic tolerance to self-antigens and subsequently develop an immune response against themselves. In other situations, molecular mimicry from infectious agents and drugs acting as a hapten-bridge with the tubulointerstitium can target an immune response towards previously unrecognized (or unexposed) self-antigens. Other drugs can damage interstitial structures through toxic mechanisms and thereby produce novel antigens that are immunogenic. Obviously, avoidance or removal of exogenous factors that mimic or lead to antigen expression is the first step in the treatment of interstitial nephritis.

Once the target nephritogenic antigen is recognized by the immune system, several immunoregulatory factors, including suppressor T-cell networks, anti-idiotypic networks, and the regulation of major histocompatibility complex (MHC) molecular expression, can modulate the severity of disease. Therapies that make use of these endogenous control mechanisms are at the forefront of immunologic research and are discussed at the end of this chapter.

Actual damage to the kidney can be mediated by several effector mechanisms, including complement activation, and the release of proteases, leukotrienes, superoxides, and peroxides by infiltrating eosinophils, basophils, and mast cells. The hallmark of AIN, however, is the presence of mononuclear cells, particularly T lymphocytes. These T cells cause injury through several discrete mechanisms including: (1) delayed-type hypersensitivity with the release of inflammatory lymphokines, (2) cell-mediated cytotoxicity through protease release, and (3) the production of lymphokines that modulate the biosynthesis of extracellular matrix in epithelial cells and fibroblasts. The majority of therapeutic interventions probably modify some element of this effector response, although the exact mechanisms are not clear.

■ TREATMENT

Once the diagnosis of AIN has been firmly established, the first and most obvious intervention is to identify and discontinue the use of any potential offending drugs or to treat any underlying systemic infection. In some cases, this may constitute definitive therapy. Renal function, as assessed by daily blood urea nitrogen (BUN) and/or creatinine measurements, should improve within several days of removal of the potential inciting immunogenic stimuli.

For those patients whose condition does not improve or in whom the disease process appears to be secondary to an autoimmune disease or to be idiopathic, treatment with corticosteroids should be considered as adjunctive therapy. The decision to treat with corticosteroids must be based on biopsy documentation of histologic AIN without evidence of significant renal fibrosis. We do not recommend steroid therapy without a biopsy, and we feel that immunosuppressive therapy in the presence of significant fibrosis would subject the patient to the risks of treatment without significant potential benefit. The decision to begin corticosteroid treatment should be additionally tempered by the marginal published clinical data to support its widespread use. One often quoted report of 14 patients with methicillin-induced interstitial nephritis suggests that treatment with corticosteroids leads to a faster (9 days versus 54 days) and fuller recovery of renal function (a lower final creatinine level) than with supportive therapy alone. This study is methodologically flawed, however, in that it is retrospective, nonrandomized, and nonblinded. Other similar reports and anecdotes pervade the clinical literature, some suggesting a marked efficacy of corticosteroid treatment, while others showing that the treatment has no effect on outcome. No properly designed study has yet been published. Nevertheless, many physicians have treated patients with AIN whose conditions have improved temporally (and probably causally) with the initiation of steroid therapy. We therefore recommend beginning steroid treatment in a patient with biopsy-proven interstitial nephritis of noninfectious etiology, which does not demonstrate significant fibrosis, and has not immediately responded to withdrawal of potential inciting factors. Since the likelihood of recovery of renal function decreases when azotemia persists for more than 1 to 2 weeks, therapy should be initiated early. We recommended a 4 to 6 week course of prednisone in a dose of 1 mg per kilogram per day (or in a patient incapable of oral intake, an equivalent dose of intravenous prednisolone), followed by a taper over an additional 2 to 3 weeks. Although shorter courses of therapy are endorsed by some authors, occasional patients with AIN will exhibit a clinical exacerbation following 10 days of treatment alone.

It should be noted that steroids themselves improve the glomerular filtration rate by 10 to 25 percent independent of any specific effect they may have on the destructive tubulointerstitial lesion. The mechanism for this is not fully known, but it seems to be related to volume expansion. As a result of this nonspecific effect, one may anticipate aggravated heart failure or pre-existing hypertension. Also, because steroid treatment results in accelerated protein catabolism, the patient with renal failure is at higher risk for developing hyperkalemia, hyperphosphatemia, and hyperuricemia out of proportion to the degree of renal compromise. The diabetic patient will additionally develop a worsening of serum glucose that may require a change in insulin therapy. Despite these potential side effects, we believe that the risk-benefit ratio of a well-defined course of steroid therapy is favorable. Although the risks of long-term steroid treatment are more significant, we are unaware of any cases of AIN in which the maintenance of improved renal function has been dependent on steroids, except in the setting of AIN from sarcoidosis.

The mechanism whereby corticosteroids exert a beneficial influence in the treatment of AIN can only be inferred from their known effects on other immunologic processes. A specific assessment of their action has not been made in either human or experimental interstitial nephritis. Corticosteroids are known to impair cell-mediated immunity and have been shown to abrogate delayed-type hypersensitivity responses in humans. Numerous investigators have noted that pharmacologic doses of steroids inhibit production of interleukin 1, interleukin-2, and gamma-interferon by macrophages and T cells and may impair T-cell responsiveness to these and other lymphokines. There is some evidence that steroids suppress antibody production. In addition, steroids stabilize lysosomal membranes, and thereby suppress the release of proteolytic enzymes. It is therefore reasonable to speculate that the beneficial effects of corticosteroids in interstitial nephritis interrupt the effector phase of the immune response through one or more of the above mechanisms.

In a small number of patients with AIN who do not respond to steroid therapy alone, a more aggressive intervention may be required to produce a remission. In the occasional patient who has little to no fibrosis on renal biopsy and who has not responded to the removal of inciting factors and to 1 to 2 weeks of daily prednisone treatment, cytotoxic treatment may be offered. Under these conditions, it would be reasonable to begin cyclophosphamide at a dosage of 2 mg per kilogram per day in addition to the steroids. If no response is noted within 5 to 6 weeks, the cyclophosphamide should be discontinued and the steroids tapered over several weeks. On the other hand, if an improvement in renal function coincides with the initiation of cyclophosphamide therapy, then, based on anecdotal experience, treatment should be continued for 1 year. As always, with cyclophosphamide, the white blood cell count must be monitored closely and the drug discontinued or decreased in dosage if the total white blood cell count decreases to less than 3,500 per cubic millimeter (2,000 neutrophils). We do not believe that cyclophosphamide poses a serious oncogenic threat within this time frame and there is only a small chance of its limiting fertility. Given that fertility is likely to be decreased with chronic renal failure, we tend to accept these risks with consultation and guidance from the patient. Although there are no controlled clinical data to support the use of cyclophosphamide, there are anecdotal reports in which a response was noted in several patients. In addition cyclophosphamide is extremely effective in preventing irreversible damage in experimental interstitial nephritis, provided that it is given early at an appropriate dosage. Unfortunately, because of the limited numbers of patients, it is not likely that cytotoxic therapy will be systematically evaluated in controlled trials.

The possible beneficial effect of cyclophosphamide seems to be mediated through the functional inhibition of T cells, in that cyclophosphamide has been demonstrated to abrogate the delayed-type hypersensitivity response in experimental animals, without an effect on the humoral immune response.

Finally, one of the most important features of immunosuppressive management is knowing when to stop treatment. With all of the interventions mentioned above, it takes time for the maximum effect to be achieved. Within several weeks, however, one should be able to make a rational decision to provide no further treatment. Protracted treatment in patients with renal failure can lead to metabolic and infectious complications that occasionally prove fatal. The positive renal transplant experience and the consistent improvement in dialytic techniques have demonstrated that patient survival and well-being must always take precedence over attempts to treat hopeless renal failure. It is clearly preferable, at some point, to accept the irreversibility of progressive renal insufficiency and plan for chronic dialysis and/or renal transplantation rather than prolong treatment with powerful immunosuppressive agents. Our overall approach to the treatment of AIN is summarized in Figure 1.

■ EXPERIMENTAL THERAPY

Data from experimental animal studies support the use of cyclosporine A in the therapy of acute interstitial nephritis. This drug has been shown to be an effective prophylactic and therapeutic agent probably by direct inhibition of T-cell activation. With a small but growing experience with this therapy in the treatment of autoimmune diseases in humans, we can anticipate the occasional use of cyclosporine A in the treatment of interstitial nephritis. Nevertheless, since its long-term administration in some transplant settings has raised questions about cyclosporine A's ability to induce fibrogenesis and since the number of steroid-unresponsive cases of AIN are relatively small, it remains unlikely cyclosporine A will be extensively studied as a treatment modality for this disease entity. We believe, however, that further evaluation of the beneficial effects of cyclosporine A is warranted, since it is likely that the drug will be used for only a limited time in any given patient.

The use of plasmapheresis may also be considered in those rare patients who, in addition to meeting the criteria for cyclophosphamide therapy, have antitubular basement membrane antibodies demonstrable by renal immunofluorescence. The rationale for this is parallel to the rationale for treating antiglomerular basement membrane disease with plasmapheresis, cyclophosphamide, and steroids—antitubular basement membrane antibodies are playing a critical role in the disease process and their removal disturbs an immune effector mechanism that contributes to renal injury. Normally we would use 3 to 4 liter exchanges every day for 5 days, and every other day for a second week. Anecdotal reports on its limited use have been mixed.

On the forefront of immunologic research is the use of antigen-specific therapy in the treatment of immune-mediated diseases. The ultimate goal of these approaches is to eliminate or inhibit autoreactive, disease-producing T lymphocytes, while leaving the rest of the immune system intact, thus avoiding the complications of global immunosuppression. Towards this goal, studies in experimental interstitial nephritis have shown that the induction of a specific suppressor T-cell response, or the induction of specific anti-idiotypic antibodies (antibodies directed towards unique gene products of the T-cell receptor region that are in or near the antigen-binding site) can prevent or decrease the severity of

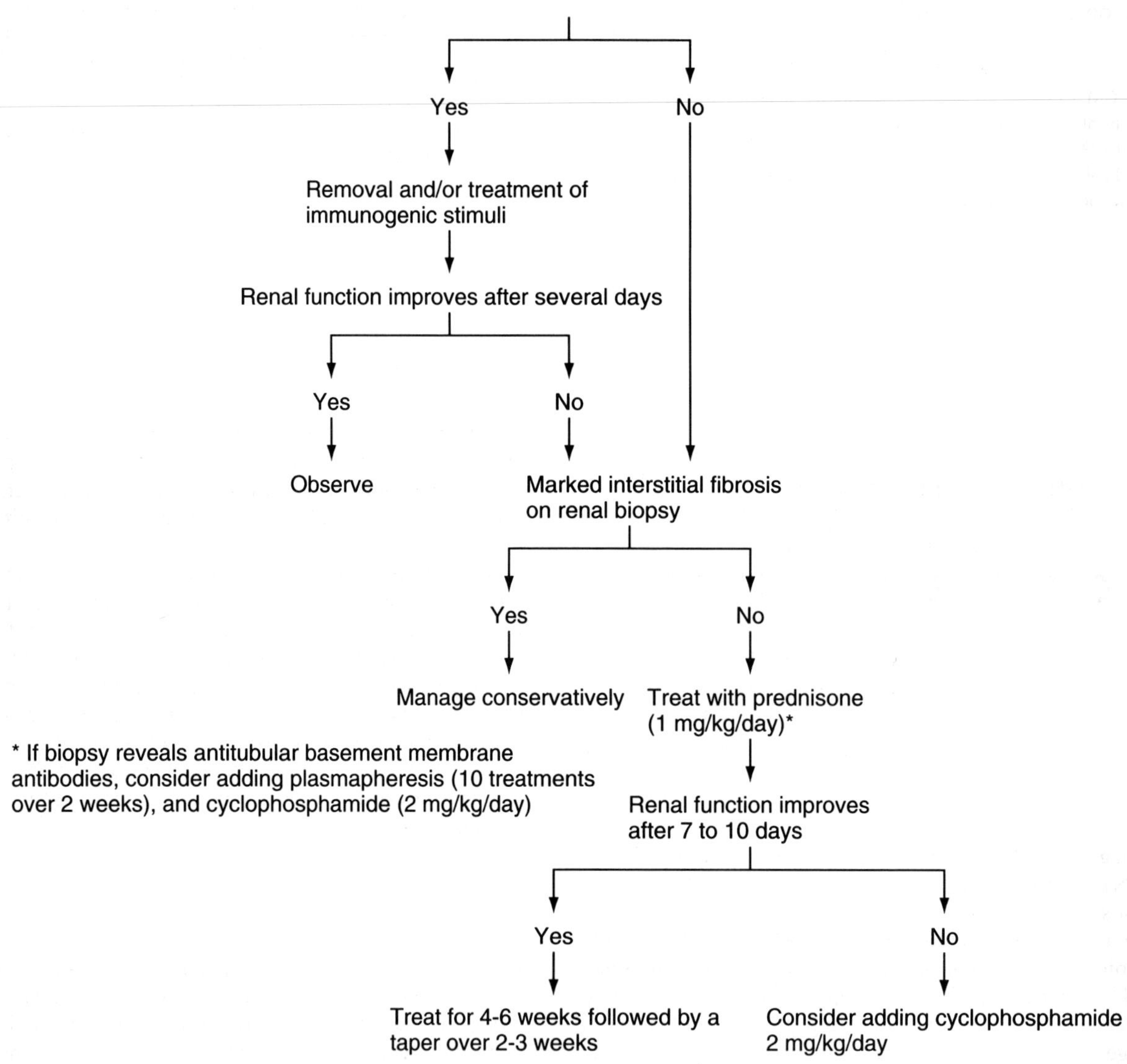
Presence of potential causative factors that can be removed or treated
Yes
No
Removal and/or treatment of immunogenic stimuli
Renal function improves after several days
Yes
No
Observe
Marked interstitial fibrosis on renal biopsy
Yes
No
Manage conservatively
Treat with prednisone (1 mg/kg/day)*
* If biopsy reveals antitubular basement membrane antibodies, consider adding plasmapheresis (10 treatments over 2 weeks), and cyclophosphamide (2 mg/kg/day)
Renal function improves after 7 to 10 days
Yes
No
Treat for 4-6 weeks followed by a taper over 2-3 weeks
Consider adding cyclophosphamide 2 mg/kg/day

Figure 1
Treatment of acute interstitial nephritis.

interstitial injury, even after the disease is well established. The use of T-cell receptor vaccines and the induction of specific T-cell tolerance through antigenic peptide antagonists are additional modalities under evaluation. Although there are many practical obstacles to overcome before such therapy can be used in humans, these novel approaches hold considerable promise for the future.

■ SUPPORTIVE THERAPY

While a variety of specific renal tubular disorders, electrolyte abnormalities, and acid-base disturbances accompany the development of chronic interstitial nephritis, the complications of AIN are, in essence, the general complications of acute renal failure. Thus, the supportive therapy of AIN may involve the treatment of volume overload, hyponatremia, hyperkalemia, hypocalcemia, hyperphosphatemia, and acidosis. (These aspects of patient care are discussed in standard textbooks of nephrology and therefore will not receive further attention here.) Some recent evidence also suggests the potential efficacy of dietary protein restriction in slowing the progression of some forms of chronic renal insufficiency. Interestingly, the cellular lesions of experimental interstitial nephritis can be largely attenuated by dietary protein restriction, probably through a nonspecific inhibition of T-cell function. Bearing in mind that this finding has not been formally investigated in humans, one may consider decreasing protein intake to approximately 0.5 to 0.6 g per kilogram per day in those patients left with chronic renal insufficiency after an episode of acute tubulointerstitial nephropathy. However, considering the overall catabolic and relatively malnourished state of most hospitalized patients with acute renal failure, protein restriction during the acute phase is probably best delayed until ambulatory health is fully established and the patient may be treated on an outpatient basis.

Suggested Reading

Buysen JGM, Houthoff HJ, Krediet RT, Arisz L. Acute interstitial nephritis: A clinical and morphological study in 27 patients. Nephrol Dial Transplant 1990; 5:94–99.

Galpin JE, Shinberger JH, Stanley TM, et al. Acute interstitial nephritis due to methicillin. Am J Med 1978; 65:756–765.

Hannedouche T, Grateau G, Noel LH, et al. Renal granulomatous sarcoidosis: Report of six cases. Nephrol Dial Transplant 1990; 5:18–24.

Koselj M, Kveder R, Bren AF, Rott T. Acute renal failure in patients with drug-induced acute interstitial nephritis. Renal Failure 1993; 15:69–72.

Laberke HG, Bohle A. Acute interstitial nephritis: Correlations between clinical and morphological findings. Clin Nephrol 1980; 14:263–273.

Neilson EG. Pathogenesis and therapy of interstitial nephritis. Kidney Int 1989; 35:1257–1270.

IDIOPATHIC RAPIDLY PROGRESSIVE GLOMERULONEPHRITIS

Peter I. Lobo, M.D.
W. Kline Bolton, M.D.

A diagnosis of rapidly progressive glomerulonephritis (RPGN) is conventionally made in patients presenting with a rapid loss of renal function associated with glomerulonephritis, usually with extensive glomerular crescent formation, on renal biopsy. Deterioration in renal function is considered "rapid" if there is a doubling of serum creatinine or a halving of the creatinine clearance within 3 months or less. Immunopathogenetically, RPGN is divided into three main categories:

1. Immune-complex–induced RPGN, comprising 30 to 40 percent of cases with RPGN. It is frequently associated with postinfectious processes (e.g., poststreptococcal nephritis) or a form of systemic immune complex disease (e.g., lupus nephritis, vasculitis, and cryoglobulinemia). Characteristically, this category is associated with granular immune deposits.
2. Antiglomerular basement membrane (GBM) antibody–induced RPGN, comprising 20 to 30 percent of cases of RPGN.
3. RPGN without glomerular immune deposits (no immune deposits [NID], or "pauci-immune" deposits), comprising approximately 30 to 40 percent of patients with RPGN.

The term *idiopathic* RPGN applies to those types of glomerulonephritis of unknown etiology, regardless of whether crescents are present or not. It includes all three categories described above since its etiologies, except as delineated by specific diseases, are unknown, regardless of the fluorescence or ultrastructural appearance. RPGN associated with immune deposits, as immune complexes or anti-GBM disease, is addressed in other chapters of this text. Therefore this chapter addresses only the NID or "pauci-immune" deposit subtype of idiopathic RPGN associated with crescents.

Most patients with NID-RPGN have a primary renal disease of uncertain etiology and pathogenesis. Some patients with this subtype of RPGN have a form of vasculitis (e.g., polyarteritis nodosa) with inflammation confined to the glomerular capillaries. The presence of antineutrophil cytoplasmic antibodies (ANCA, a marker of vasculitic disease) in some of these patients supports this concept. The therapeutic approaches to each of these categories may differ. This chapter deals with the therapy of the NID subtype of idiopathic RPGN.

■ DIAGNOSIS

Few true emergencies exist in the area of nephrology. One of these, however, is RPGN, especially the crescentic variety. It is critical to make the correct diagnosis to avoid needless and inappropriate therapy for other disease processes, and yet to make the diagnosis that directs therapy at the specific type of RPGN. We routinely perform an emergent renal biopsy in any patient with the de novo clinical presentation of RPGN if no obvious precipitating cause is found (e.g., vasomotor nephropathy, trauma, acute interstitial nephritis with eosinophils in the urine, and an allergic exposure). We perform a biopsy in patients with nosocomial acute renal failure with atypical manifestations such as red blood cell casts, heavy hematuria, and/or proteinuria in the absence of overt causes; with oliguria or anuria in the absence of pressors or obvious causes of severe acute tubular necrosis; and with systemic diseases that have a clinical presentation consistent with the diagnosis of RPGN. Biopsies are also performed in patients with known pre-existing disease who have a sudden change in renal function consistent with RPGN. In our geographic region, one-third of all patients who undergo biopsy are found to have glomerulonephritis. Twenty percent of these have crescents (7 percent of the total number of biopsies). Approximately 12 percent of patients with glomerulonephritis (4 percent of total biopsies) have the clinical course of RPGN. A diagnosis of idiopathic NID-RPGN is made when the biopsy shows greater than or equal to 20 percent cellular crescents in the glomeruli and if immunofluorescence fails to detect anti-GBM antibody or significant immune complex deposits. The idiopathic nature of RPGN is also verified by the absence of antistreptococcal, antinuclear, anti-GBM, and hepatitis B surface antigen antibodies and cryoglobulins. The presence of ANCA does not exclude the diagnosis of idiopathic RPGN, but it becomes necessary to exclude the possibility of systemic necrotizing vasculitis, including Wegener's granulomatosis and polyarteritis.

PROGNOSIS

The prognosis of idiopathic RPGN in general has been poor. Precise figures are difficult to obtain from the existing literature, as most series consist of patients with several types of RPGN. Additionally, follow-up is usually of short duration, and the patients have received variable forms of therapy. However, available data would indicate that 75 percent of such patients become dialysis dependent (or die) within months if they are untreated or treated only with oral steroids and/or immunosuppressive agents.

Recent advances in the therapy of idiopathic RPGN are related to the introduction of intravenous bolus injections of methylprednisolone and plasma exchange. In this chapter, we emphasize our experience with intravenous bolus injections of methylprednisolone (pulse therapy).

TREATMENT REGIMEN

We have used the following regimen at our institution over the past several decades. With pulse methylprednisolone therapy, methylprednisolone is administered intravenously in doses of 30 mg per kilogram of body weight given over a 20 minute period with monitoring of blood pressure. The methylprednisolone is given over a period not greater than 20 minutes and not less than 15 minutes. It is ascertained that patients are volume replete and have not received diuretics within the past 3 hours, and they should not receive any diuretics for 24 hours after therapy. The methylprednisolone should be administered as soon as the patient is stabilized and volume repleted. The maximum dose administered at any single time must not exceed 3 g. This dose of methylprednisolone is repeated every other day for a total of three doses. Forty-eight hours after the last dose of methylprednisolone is administered, treatment with oral alternate-day prednisone is instituted, as detailed in Table 1.

We have a few patients treated with cyclophosphamide or dipyridamole. For such patients, we administer approximately 100 mg per day of cyclophosphamide and 200 mg per day dipyridamole in divided doses. The dose of oral prednisone is adjusted for any patient 60 years of age or older; such patients receive 75 percent of the dose recommended in Table 1. The regimen is accelerated to the next steroid dose (Table 1) if the patient develops and maintains normal renal function for 1 month. Thus the shortest duration of treatment in responding patients is approximately 1 year, and the longest duration is approximately 5 years. Reactivation of disease, documented clinically and with repeat biopsy, is treated as de novo RPGN according to protocol; treatment is repeated as often as three times if the response has previously been good.

Table 1 Protocol for Administering Oral Prednisone Therapy

ALTERNATE-DAY DOSE OF PREDNISONE*	DURATION OF THERAPY (MOS.)
2.00 mg/kg	0.5
1.75 mg/kg	1.0
1.50 mg/kg	3.0
1.25 mg/kg	6.0
1.00 mg/kg	6.0
0.75 mg/kg	6.0
0.50 mg/kg	6.0
0.25 mg/kg	6.0
0.125 mg/kg	12.0
0.0625 mg/kg	12.0

*75 percent of dose for patients 60 years of age or older.

Patients we have excluded from treatment with pulse methylprednisolone therapy include those with an unexplained acute febrile illness, overt psychosis, active peptic ulcer, terminal irreversible illness, and those who have undergone major surgery within the past 2 weeks. We do not permit the use of any steroidal medications, aspirin, phenylbutazone, or other steroid-type drugs while patients are taking methylprednisolone and prednisone.

CRITERIA FOR RESPONSE

Patients are considered to be treated adequately if they survive for 6 weeks or longer, since more than 90 percent of patients respond within the first 6 weeks. Patients' conditions are considered to be stable or improved if the serum creatinine level remains stable or is decreased by 30 percent or more or if the patients were receiving dialytic support and are able to discontinue it.

Table 2 provides the results of treatment with pulse therapy with methylprednisolone in our patients with idiopathic RPGN. Data presented pertain to the average percentage of crescents, whether or not patients were improved, and whether they were receiving dialysis and were able to discontinue it. Twenty-one patients had the histologic diagnosis of idiopathic NID-RPGN. Sixteen of the 21 patients (76 percent) who received pulse therapy showed an improvement. Ten of 15 patients who received pulse therapy and were receiving dialysis were able to discontinue dialysis. An analysis of response relative to the extent of glomerular involvement with crescents showed that 75 percent of patients with 60 percent or more crescents improved with pulse therapy and that 64 percent of patients who received dialysis with 60 percent or more of the glomeruli involved with crescents were able to discontinue dialysis. Ninety percent of patients who were oliguric showed improvement with pulse therapy.

We have also evaluated the effect that associated glomerulosclerotic lesions have on the response to pulse therapy in these patients. Of patients with less than 33 percent glomerular obsolescence, 92 percent demonstrated initial improvement and 85 percent continued to show long-term improvement. The response in those patients exhibiting a glomerular

Table 2 Results of Pulse Methylprednisolone Therapy in the Treatment of Idiopathic NID-RPGN

Total number of patients	21
Mean age	59
Percentage of crescents	69
Percentage of patients whose condition improved	76
Number of patients requiring dialysis	15
Number of patients in whom dialysis was discontinued	10

obsolescence of more than 33 percent was not as promising. Seventy-one percent of these patients had initial improvement, with only 36 percent maintaining improvement over the long term. More importantly, a short duration of disease before the institution of therapy was significantly associated with less chronicity and better response to therapy. This again emphasizes the importance of early biopsy with this disease.

■ COMPLICATIONS

Our treatment regimen has been associated with no major complications. There have been complaints of a metallic taste in the mouth, muscle weakness, "seeing bright lights" and other psychotropic effects, nausea, arthralgia, and discomfort at the site of infusion. Arrhythmia was noted in one patient with a previous cardiac abnormality. No patient has had decreased blood pressure. In patients observed over a long period, we have noted cataracts, cushingoid facies, acne, hirsutism, and occasionally, glaucoma. Our experience over the past 2 decades indicates that a significant steroid-associated side effect such as myocardial infarct, pulmonary embolus, or stroke may be expected once in each 12 patient years of therapy.

■ OTHER TYPES OF THERAPY

A comparison of pulse therapy with methylprednisolone with the other types of therapy for RPGN is difficult to make because of the general lack of discrimination in including patients with different diagnoses in the category of RPGN. Nevertheless, several other general types of treatment have been used successfully. *Conventional therapy* consists of all types of therapy other than pulse therapy, quadruple therapy, and plasma exchange. *Quadruple therapy* consists of prednisone, dipyridamole, cyclophosphamide or azathioprine, and anticoagulation. Regimens of *pulse therapy* other than our own include those consisting variously of 1 g daily administered for up to 11 days or given on an alternate-day schedule or on other schedules. The results of these latter regimens have not necessarily been comparable to our experience. *Plasma exchange therapy* is given in combination with immunosuppressive agents (i.e., prednisone, cyclophosphamide, and azathioprine).

Approximately 25 percent of patients show improvement with a variety of types of therapy (e.g., prednisone alone or combined with azathioprine). This contrasts markedly with the results of quadruple therapy, pulse therapy, and plasma exchange treatment, all of which result in a response in approximately 75 to 80 percent of patients.

We prefer to treat idiopathic RPGN with pulse therapy for several reasons. Quadruple therapy, while apparently effective in non–anti-GBM disease, does require the use of anticoagulants and cytotoxic drugs; and the potential for infection and other complications may therefore be higher. The patient who eventually experiences a relapse, progresses to chronic renal failure, or requires transplantation may already have received enough cytotoxic therapy to increase his or her susceptibility to malignant disease after the institution of immunosuppressive therapy during the transplant period. In addition, a significant number of patients—perhaps half—treated with quadruple therapy eventually progress slowly to chronic renal failure. In our experience, fewer patients treated with pulse therapy alone gradually progress to renal failure. Since the rate of response to pulse therapy in patients with oligoanuria and high degrees of crescent formation is comparable with or better than the rate of response to quadruple therapy and because progression of fibrosis to end-stage disease appears to be less (and the side effects are less), we believe that pulse therapy is indicated over quadruple therapy.

Plasma exchange in combination with prednisone, azathioprine, and cyclophosphamide has been used for a wide variety of types of glomerulonephritis. The complication rate during the initial period of exchange may be higher than that of pulse therapy. Once again, this type of therapy may possibly be associated with the later higher risks of malignant disease because cyclophosphamide is given as part of the regimen. It is also possible that some protective factors that are circulating may be removed as well as harmful factors; we have seen several patients with glomerulonephritis whose conditions actually appeared to deteriorate with the initiation of plasma exchange. In addition, plasma exchange is much more expensive and is inconvenient for the patient. Since the results of therapy with plasma exchange appear to be comparable to those of pulse therapy for idiopathic RPGN, we continue to prefer pulse therapy.

Steroid pulse therapy in idiopathic NID-RPGN has generally not included the use of concomitant cytotoxic agents. Currently there is increasing evidence to implicate a vasculitic process with some patients having idiopathic RPGN. It would therefore seem reasonable to add cyclophosphamide to pulse therapy in those patients with circulating ANCA, as this subgroup may represent a forme fruste of vasculitis. After all, long-term therapy with cyclophosphamide appears to be beneficial for polyarteritis nodosa and Wegener's granulomatosis.

It remains to be determined whether newer approaches (e.g., the use of cyclosporine and normal pooled human gamma globulin) will also be effective for idiopathic RPGN. The latter approach has been used with some success in the therapy of Kawasaki disease and ANCA-positive systemic necrotizing vasculitis.

■ MECHANISM OF DRUG ACTION

The exact mechanism by which pulse therapy with methylprednisolone followed by an alternate-day regimen of prednisone achieves its beneficial effects is not known. The rationale for using pulse therapy was derived from the similarities between crescentic glomerulonephritis and the interstitial reaction that occurs with transplant rejection. Prednisone and large doses of methylprednisolone are known to impair lymphocyte function and to have a dramatic effect on macrophages and monocytes, with depletion of their numbers and impairment of their ability to phagocytose and present antigens. Fibroblast formation is impaired, and lysosomal membranes are stabilized. Arachidonic acid metabolites may also be decreased. It has been our experience that the use of larger doses of methylprednisolone given over 20 minutes is associated with a slightly better response rate than methylprednisolone given in smaller doses over a longer period of time. However, no specific studies on this have been performed.

Suggested Reading

Bolton WK. The role of high-dose steroids in nephritic syndromes: the case for aggressive use. In: Narins RG, ed. Controversies in nephrology and hypertension. New York: Churchill Livingstone, 1984: 421.

Bolton WK, Sturgill BC. Methylprednisolone therapy for acute crescentic rapidly progressive glomerulonephritis. Am J Nephrol 1989; 9:368–375.

Couser WG. Rapidly progressive glomerulonephritis: classification, pathogenetic mechanisms, and therapy. Am J Kidney Dis 1988; 11:449–464.

Jacquot C, Baran D, Vendeville B, et al. Update on immunosuppressive therapy in human and experimental glomerulonephritis. Adv Nephrol 1988; 17:77–99.

POSTSTREPTOCOCCAL GLOMERULONEPHRITIS

Frank G. Boineau, M.D.
John E. Lewy, M.D.

In its typical form poststreptococcal glomerulonephritis has various manifestations, including hematuria, oliguria, proteinuria, reduced glomerular filtration rate, and hypertension. Many patients do not have all of the typical features, and the symptoms and signs may be very mild. This is especially true in family contacts, in whom this disease often goes unrecognized unless the family member is examined and laboratory evidence of the disease is sought.

CLINICAL FEATURES

Epidemiology

Acute poststreptococcal glomerulonephritis (APSGN) is extremely rare before the age of 2 years. Thereafter it may occur at any age, but it is most common in school-aged children. In many studies, the mean age of onset of the sporadic form of APSGN is approximately 7 years. The male-female ratio is 2:1.

Preceding Infection

APSGN has long been known to follow certain types of group A beta-hemolytic streptococcal infections of either the throat and upper respiratory tract or skin. Upper respiratory infections are associated with most cases of APSGN in the northern United States, whereas skin infections are frequently associated with cases in the southern United States. The latent interval is usually 8 to 14 days after a respiratory infection, while the latent interval after skin infection is usually longer (21 to 28 days). Direct culture of streptococcal organisms from the pharynx or skin is not common, but serologic evidence of a preceding group A beta-hemolytic streptococcal infection is usually present. After an upper respiratory tract infection, the antistreptolysin O (ASO) antibody titer is elevated in about 90 percent of the patients with APSGN. After skin infections, the ASO titer is elevated in only about half of the patients, but Streptozyme, antihyaluronidase, or antideoxyribonuclease B antibody titers are usually elevated. If titers of antibodies to these streptococcal antigens are not elevated when APSGN is recognized, serial quantitation of the titers usually reveals a significant rise over 1 to 3 weeks after onset of the clinical illness.

Clinical Manifestations at Onset

Typically the child or adult with APSGN has a history of gross hematuria and edema. He may also have oliguria or anuria, and gastrointestinal, pulmonary, and/or central nervous system manifestations. Because neither gross hematuria nor edema may be present in an individual patient, and the predominant symptoms may be related to the gastrointestinal, central nervous system, cardiovascular, or pulmonary system, APSGN must be considered when these symptoms are present, and the urine carefully examined. The presence of microscopic hematuria or proteinuria or both should alert the physician to pursue the diagnosis of APSGN.

The presenting signs in patients with APSGN mirror the symptoms recorded above. Elevation in blood pressure above 140/90 is present in from 30 to 80 percent of patients. Other evidence of an expanding extracellular fluid volume is often noted. Skin infection may also be present.

Laboratory Data at Onset

Laboratory data at the time APSGN is diagnosed reflect the reduced glomerular filtration rate (GFR), serologic evidence of a preceding streptococcal infection, and consumption of complement. It is well to remember that the degree of hematuria and proteinuria may be very mild and that nephrotic range proteinuria is uncommon. Thus the diagnosis of APSGN must be considered in patients with even mild degrees of hematuria and proteinuria.

■ PREFERRED APPROACH TO MANAGEMENT AND DRUG THERAPY

Hospitalization

Many patients with APSGN can be treated at home. The principal considerations are the severity of the clinical abnormalities and the family's and physician's ability to provide close observation and care at home. Patients with moderate to severe reductions in renal function (creatinine clearance <50 ml per minute per 1.73 m^2, blood urea nitrogen [BUN] >50 mg per deciliter); those with oliguria or anuria; those with any symptoms of hypertensive encephalopathy, including lethargy, vomiting, or ophthalmologic changes; and significant edema or pulmonary congestion should be hospitalized. If hypertension is absent or mild and responds promptly to antihypertensive measures, including bed rest and medication, hospitalization can often be avoided.

Bed rest has been an extremely controversial therapeutic modality. It was once considered appropriate to maintain bed rest until all signs of nephritis were past. However, it appears that ambulation has not been associated with worsening of any variables of renal function once gross hematuria, edema, hypertension, and azotemia have resolved. A reasonable guide is that patients who have gross hematuria, hypertension, edema, evidence of circulatory congestion, or moderate to severe depression of renal function be kept on bed rest as much as possible.

Nutritional Management

Alterations in diet depend on the severity of the edema, renal failure, and hypertension. If the BUN concentration is less than 75 mg per deciliter, dietary protein need not be restricted. If the BUN concentration is above this level, intake should be restricted to 1 g per kilogram of body weight per day of proteins of high biologic value until renal function improves and the BUN concentration spontaneously decreases to below 75 mg per deciliter. Calorie intake should be maintained as near to normal as possible to reduce catabolism. In patients with hypertension or edema, sodium intake should be restricted to 1 to 2 g each day. More severe degrees of sodium restriction are usually not required and lead to poor caloric intake. Fluid balance should be carefully monitored and fluid should be restricted in the presence of severe edema, oliguria, or anuria. In these patients, fluid intake should not exceed the sum of urine output and insensible water loss minus planned weight loss. Measurement of body weight daily, or more often if needed, is an effective way to determine whether fluid intake is appropriate. Fluid and sodium restriction with a decrease in extracellular volume will assist in the management of hypertension. Once edema has resolved, fluid intake should be restricted to insensible water loss plus measured fluid output as long as oliguria persists.

Treatment of Hypertension

Hypertension may be mild or severe. There is considerable disagreement regarding levels of blood pressure in APSGN which require therapeutic intervention. Hypertension often resolves with bed rest alone. If the diastolic blood pressure is below 100 mm Hg and falls further with the patient on bed rest, sodium restriction and continued bed rest are sufficient. If the blood pressure does not decline in 2 to 4 hours, or symptoms of encephalopathy develop (headache, lethargy, nausea, vomiting, seizures), treatment should be instituted promptly. Treatment of acute hypertension in APSGN can often be accomplished by administration of oral nifedipine. In children, nifedipine 0.25 to 0.5 mg per kilogram per dose (maximum 10 mg per dose) may be given orally every 4 to 6 hours to reduce blood pressure. The liquid must be removed from the capsule and administered orally if rapid reduction in blood pressure is needed. Occasionally the blood pressure remains moderately but persistently elevated and treatment with oral nifedipine or propranolol is useful. If oral administration is impossible, parenteral antihypertensive medication must be used. Intravenous nitroprusside or diazoxide has been used successfully to treat severe acute hypertension. Hypertension in APSGN is largely attributable to an expanded extracellular fluid volume. Renin levels at the onset of the disease are characteristically normal or suppressed. Common antihypertensive drugs used in APSGN are listed in Table 1. Diuretics can assist in lowering the blood pressure. Furosemide, 2 mg per kilogram orally or 1 mg per kilogram intravenously, is often effective in producing a diuresis and reducing the extracellular fluid volume. An improvement in encephalopathy has been seen in patients treated with intravenous furosemide even when only minimal or no changes in blood pressure have occurred. These observations imply that edema of the central nervous system plays an important role in hypertensive encephalopathy in APSGN.

Treatment of Edema

If there is fluid overload, diuretics are indicated to reduce edema, to test renal responsiveness, and as an adjunct in the treatment of hypertension. Persistent edema can be treated with oral furosemide, 2 mg per kilogram once to twice daily. Hydrochlorothiazide, 2 mg per kilogram per day, is effective when renal function is normal or nearly normal, but not when there is marked depression of the GFR. Pulmonary congestion in APSGN usually reflects fluid overload and not myocardial failure. It is therefore *not* responsive to administration of digitalis. Vascular congestion can usually be treated effectively with fluid and sodium restriction and the use of diuretics as outlined above.

Antibiotics

Cultures of the throat and skin lesions if present should be obtained in all patients with suspected APSGN and all immediate family members. Those with positive cultures should be treated with appropriate antibiotics. In patients with sus-

Table 1 Common Antihypertensive Drugs Used in Acute Poststreptococcal Glomerulonephritis

DRUG	INITIAL DOSE/ROUTE (MG/KG)	DOSE INTERVAL (HOUR)	MAXIMUM DOSE	COMMON SIDE EFFECTS
DIRECT VASODILATORS				
Hydralazine	0.1–0.5 IV or IM	4–6	25 mg/dose	Tachycardia, palpitations, hypotension
Hydralazine	0.25 PO	4–6	200 mg/day	Tachycardia, palpitations, headaches
Diazoxide	3–10 IV over 30 min	Repeat once in 30 min if needed	10 mg/kg/dose	Dizziness, tachycardia, nausea, rapid fall in BP, hyperglycemia, fluid retention
Nitroprusside	0.5–8 μ/kg/min	Constant infusion		Tachycardia, fluid retention, nausea, headaches, dizziness, cyanide poisoning
CALCIUM CHANNEL BLOCKER				
Nifedipine	0.25–0.5 PO	4–6	10 mg/dose	Flushing, tachycardia, headaches, dizziness, palpitations, syncope
ADRENERGIC INHIBITING DRUGS				
Propranolol	1–2 PO	6–12	10 mg/kg/day	Lethargy, fatigue, bradycardia, depression, insomnia
PLASMIC VOLUME REDUCING DRUGS				
Furosemide	1–4 PO	12–24	8 mg/kg/dose	Hypokalemia, metabolic alkalosis, postural hypotension
Chlorothiazide	5 PO	12	20 mg/kg	Hypokalemia, metabolic alkalosis, postural hypotension

Adapted from Arbus G, Farine M. Management of hypertensive emergencies in children; Boineau FG, Lewy JE. Renal parenchymatous diseases causing hypertension. In: Loggie JMH, ed. Pediatric and adolescent hypertension. Boston: Blackwell Scientific Publications, 1992:374 and 214.

pected APSGN, even if beta-hemolytic streptococcus is not cultured, it is probably safest to treat with a 10 day course of penicillin (or erythromycin in penicillin-sensitive patients). Additional antibiotics are not used unless infectious complications are present. Prophylactic antibiotics are not indicated in this disease, since recurrence of APSGN is very rare.

Subclinical Cases

Subclinical asymptomatic cases of APSGN have been reported by several investigators. When first-degree relatives of an index case were studied, the ratio of subclinical to clinical disease was 4:1 and there was documented evidence of APSGN occurring in about 33 percent of household patient contacts. Thus it seems prudent to recommend evaluation of household family members (throat or skin culture, physical examination, and urinalysis) when an index case of APSGN is identified. If symptoms of acute nephritis develop in family members, serologic and renal function tests should be performed. Serial evaluation of family members is not indicated. The prophylactic treatment of household members with antibiotics is controversial and currently, unless skin or throat cultures are positive, prophylactic treatment is not indicated.

Renal Biopsy

In a typical case of APSGN, a renal biopsy is not required to diagnose the disease. There are, however, times when a renal biopsy should be considered, either because of atypical presentation or because resolution does not follow the expected course. The reasons for considering a renal biopsy are listed in Table 2. None of these is an absolute indication, but should alert the physician that APSGN may not be present and a renal biopsy should be considered for diagnostic reasons. If a renal biopsy is considered, it should be done early, since pathologic changes such as generalized proliferation tend to become focal and subepithelial deposits of immunoglobulin G (IgG) and complement tend to resolve after the first few weeks of the illness, making the diagnosis of APSGN more difficult. It should be emphasized that there are no pathognomonic features of APSGN and the renal biopsy must be interpreted in conjunction with the clinical findings.

Table 2 Relative Indications for Renal Biopsy in Suspected Acute Poststreptococcal Glomerulonephritis

- At onset of illness
  - Absence of reduced serum complement
  - Anuria
  - Nephrotic syndrome
  - Prior history of renal disease
  - Retarded linear growth in children
  - Family history of nephritis
- During period of expected resolution
  - Persistence of oliguria beyond 3 weeks
  - Low C3 or total hemolytic complement beyond 6 weeks
  - Gross hematuria beyond 3 weeks
  - Persistence of hypertension

Immunosuppressive Therapy

Corticosteroids and other immunosuppressive drugs are not indicated in the treatment of APSGN. Mild or moderate cases have an excellent prognosis with supportive therapy, particularly in children. Even in cases of severe APSGN, supportive therapy alone frequently results in complete recovery of renal function. Recent studies that have compared supportive care with immunosuppressive plus anticoagulant therapy in a nonrandomized fashion in crescentic glomerulonephritis of poststreptococcal origin in adults suggest that the renal outcome is equally good in the two groups. Thus the known risks of immunosuppressive medications are not justified in APSGN even when there are diffuse crescents on the biopsy specimen.

■ COURSE AND PROGNOSIS

Resolution of the Acute Phase

The overt manifestations of APSGN, which include gross hematuria, edema, reduced urine output, hypertension, and central nervous system symptoms, usually resolve in the first 1 to 2 weeks of the illness in most patients. Diuresis with loss of edema is usually complete by the end of the second week or sooner. Even those with severe renal failure will begin to show an improvement in the GFR in the first 2 to 3 weeks after the clinical onset of the disease. Hypertension disappears in many patients once they begin bed rest or after a short course of antihypertensive treatment. An improvement in the GFR and renal blood flow results in diuresis with loss of edema and return of plasma volume to normal. This is one of the factors leading to a decrease in blood pressure. The total hemolytic or third component of complement (C3) usually returns to normal within 6 weeks after the clinical onset of APSGN. Failure of complement to return to normal suggests that the patient may have membranoproliferative glomerulonephritis instead of APSGN. Microscopic hematuria will persist after gross hematuria disappears but it too will gradually resolve. Complete disappearance of hematuria may take several months to several years. Occasionally, intermittent or orthostatic proteinuria is noted. Some studies of sporadic APSGN in adults have documented persistence of abnormal proteinuria for 2 years or more. Such persistent proteinuria, especially if associated with hypertension and a reduced GFR, may be a manifestation of a chronic form of glomerulonephritis. If the nephrotic syndrome is present at onset, it tends to be very transient and disappears in the early phase of the illness.

Long-Term Prognosis

The long-term prognosis of APSGN is controversial and depends on the age of the patient at the onset of illness, the severity of the acute disease, and epidemiologic considerations. The prognosis of epidemic APSGN in children seems very favorable, even in those with severe acute disease. Severe oliguria and the presence of diffuse crescents on biopsy suggest a more guarded prognosis.

The long-term prognosis of the sporadic form of APSGN is less favorable in adults than in children. Severe initial disease with a creatinine clearance below 40 ml per minute per 1.73 m^2, persistent heavy proteinuria (above 2 g a day), and older age at the time of onset contribute to a guarded prognosis.

Serial renal biopsies in adult patients with APSGN have demonstrated chronic findings such as glomerulosclerosis, varying degrees of interstitial fibrosis, and arterial changes in one-third to one-half of some series. Whether these changes represent progression of the disease or simply healing of the acute process and static pathologic changes is unknown. The incidence of progression to end-stage renal disease is much less than that of chronic changes found on histopathologic examination of tissue. A review of recent literature with medium to long-range follow-up of adults reveals that chronic renal failure develops in 3 percent of the cases of sporadic symptomatic APSGN. Follow-up studies of longer duration will better answer the question of long-term functional outcome in APSGN.

LUPUS NEPHRITIS

Claudio Ponticelli, M.D., F.R.C.P.
Gabriella Moroni, M.D.

Renal disease is very common in patients with systemic lupus erythematosus (SLE). At presentation, about half of the patients have some clinical signs of kidney involvement, but renal disease may eventually develop in about three-fourths of the patients. Most cases of renal involvement in SLE are caused by glomerulonephritis, which can eventually result in arterial hypertension, nephrotic syndrome, and renal failure with related complications.

■ PRESENTATION AND COURSE OF LUPUS NEPHRITIS

Lupus nephritis, or lupus glomerulonephritis, may present with a nephrotic syndrome (proteinuria more than 3.5 g per day, hypoalbuminemia, hypercholesterolemia, various degrees of edema), a nephritic syndrome (macroscopic or microscopic hematuria, erythrocyte or hemoglobin casts, proteinuria, hypertension, impairment of renal function), or an already established renal insufficiency. In rare but dramatic instances, postpartum or postabortum acute anuric renal failure with or without microangiopathic hemolytic anemia is the first manifestation of kidney involvement or even of SLE. However, many patients may have lupus nephritis without any particular symptoms, and it is diagnosed only by routine analysis. It is possible that underlying, sometimes progressive renal disease may be present in these asymptomatic patients. From a practical point of view it is recommended that blood pressure, serum creatinine, and urinalysis be regularly

Table 1 Clinical Characteristics of the Different Histologic Classes of Lupus Nephritis According to WHO Classification

	I	II	III	IV	V
Histology	Normal glomeruli	Mesangial GN	Focal proliferative GN (50%)	Diffuse proliferative GN	Membranous GN
Frequency	Quite rare	10%–30%	10%–25%	40%–60%	10%–20%
Renal signs and symptoms	No urine abnormalities	Mild proteinuria and urine sediment abnormalities	Proteinuria; hematuria	Heavy proteinuria; telescoped sediment; hypertension; renal failure	Proteinuria; often nephrotic syndrome
Renal prognosis	Excellent	Excellent if no transformation	Good	Severe if untreated	Renal failure 30%–50%; remission 30%
Transformation	To class II or IV 15%–20% To class V, 2%–5%	To class IV 20%–40%	To class V, 2%–5%	To class III or V 5%–10%	Rare

checked, even in patients with minimal or no signs or symptoms of disease-related renal activity. It is also important to study the urinary sediment. The amounts of erythrocytes and leukocytes and the presence of erythrocyte and leukocyte casts are often related to the renal activity of SLE.

The clinical outcome of lupus nephritis is highly variable and may be strongly influenced by therapy. Some patients continue to have minimal urinary abnormalities during follow-up, but others with mild renal disease at presentation may later develop nephrotic proteinuria, hypertension, and renal insufficiency. About half of the patients with nephrotic syndrome at presentation may slowly progress towards uremia, but others maintain stable renal function, with fluctuation of proteinuria and sometimes complete remission.

In patients with nephritic syndrome the extrarenal activity of SLE is often severe. The clinical course of these patients is punctuated by renal flare-ups alternated with periods of clinical quiescence often induced by therapy. If untreated, most nephritic patients will develop end-stage renal disease within a short time. Despite aggressive treatment, a few patients have tumultuous progressive courses with severe hypertension, heart failure, and rapidly progressive renal insufficiency. Black race, severe anemia, and renal insufficiency at presentation are associated with poor prognoses.

Renal failure and infections are the most frequent causes of death in the first few years after diagnosis of lupus nephritis. In the long term, many deaths are related to atherosclerotic disease. Prolonged glucocorticoid therapy, persistent immunologic activity of SLE, hypertension, and nephrotic syndrome may all contribute to the development of cardiovascular disease. Renal failure, infection, and malignancy account for most of the other deaths during long-term follow-up.

RENAL PATHOLOGY AND CLINICOPATHOLOGIC CORRELATIONS

Although some clinicians think that the therapeutic decisions for lupus nephritis can be made even without the help of renal histology, there are few doubts that a kidney biopsy may provide reliable information about the type and the severity of renal involvement. Any form of glomerulonephritis (GN), from the mildest to the most severe, can be seen in SLE patients. Several classifications of renal lesions in SLE have been proposed. Although not universally accepted, the World Health Organization's (WHO) classification remains the most commonly adopted. According to that classification, there are five main patterns of glomerular disease: class I: Normal glomeruli; class II: Mesangial glomerulonephritis; class III: Focal proliferative glomerulonephritis; class IV: Diffuse proliferative glomerulonephritis; class V: Membranous glomerulonephritis. The different types of glomerulonephritis usually have different clinical presentations, natural outcomes, and responses to therapy (Table 1). It must be remembered, however, that the correlation between the findings of the initial biopsy and ultimate survival is weakened by the variable courses of each subtype of glomerulonephritis by transformation from one class to another and by possible overlap of two classes.

The sum of the semiquantitative scores of certain glomerular vascular and tubulointerstitial features provides activity and chronicity indexes (Table 2). An elevated activity index means that there are many lesions that can progress to irreversible damage, and it is a good indication for aggressive treatment. A high chronicity index shows that there are irreversible lesions that are hard to modify by therapy. Unfortunately, there are important differences among pathologists' interpretations that may limit the clinical impact of these important indices.

THERAPY

Treatment of lupus nephritis remains controversial. Therapy can reduce the disease activity, improve proteinuria, and prevent renal insufficiency. On the other hand, therapy can expose patients to disabling and even life-threatening complications. Therefore, the indications for treatment, the choice of drugs, and their dosage are of utmost prognostic importance.

Indications for Therapy

The therapeutic decisions for patients with lupus nephritis present peculiar difficulties that are related not only to the low therapeutic indexes of the available drugs but also to the heterogeneous nature of the disease and to the possible discrepancies between clinical features and histologic patterns. In principle, however, the type of therapy should be

Table 2 Renal Pathology Score System in Lupus Nephritis

ACTIVITY INDEX 0–3*	CHRONICITY INDEX 0–3*
GLOMERULAR CHANGES	
1. Fibrinoid necrosis × 2† Karyorrhexis	1. Glomerular sclerosis
2. Cellular proliferative	2. Fibrous crescents × 2†
3. Cellular crescents	
4. Hyaline thrombi	
5. Leukocyte infiltration	
TUBULOINTERSTITIAL CHANGES	
1. Mononuclear cell infiltration	1. Interstitial fibrosis
	2. Tubular atrophy

From Austin HA III, Muenz LR, Joyce KM, et al. Prognostic factors in lupus nephritis. Am J Med 1983; 75(3):382–391; with permission.

*Each factor is scored from 0 to 3.

†Fibrinoid necrosis and cellular crescents are weighted by a factor of 2 because such lesions are disproportionately more ominous than other active lesions.

dictated by the severity of the clinical and histologic features rather than by the diagnosis of lupus nephritis or by immunologic parameters.

Patients with minor renal abnormalities (proteinuria less than 1 g per day, inactive urine sediment, normal renal function and blood pressure) and with minimal or pure mesangial lesions in a renal biopsy do not require specific treatment. However, because of the possibility of clinicohistologic worsening, periodic clinical surveillance of these patients is mandatory. Therapeutic measures should be aimed at checking the extrarenal activity of SLE when present. Arthralgias, arthritis, myalgias, and fever can often be controlled with salicylates and nonsteroidal anti-inflammatory drugs. Hydroxychloroquine and quinacrine are effective against most dermatologic manifestations. Hemolytic anemia, leukopenia, and thrombocytopenia usually respond to moderate doses of glucocorticoids. Lupus-related inflammations of the lung or heart may be controlled by prednisone, at an initial dose of 1 mg per kilogram per day. Cerebral thromboembolism, often related to the presence of antiphospholipid antibodies, requires anticoagulation. The diffuse central nervous system manifestations caused by primary angiopathy do not always respond to high-dose glucocorticoids, administered either orally or intravenously. Better results have been obtained with a combination of glucocorticoids with intravenous high-dose cyclophosphamide, 1 g per 1.73 square meters.

Whether or not to treat patients with focal proliferative lesions affecting only a minority of glomeruli is optional. If there are neither clinical nor histologic features of lupus activity, we prefer to use symptomatic treatment alone. Others suggest the use of small doses of glucocorticoids (prednisone, 10 to 20 mg per day) and/or immunosuppressive agents (cyclophosphamide, 1 mg per kilogram per day or azathioprine, 1.5 to 2 mg per kilogram per day) to inhibit the immunologic activity of SLE and to prevent potential transformation into more severe forms of lupus nephritis. There is no evidence, however, that such an approach is of any benefit. Patients with focal lesions affecting more than 50 percent of glomeruli and associated with proteinuria more than 2 g per day, elevated serum creatinine, and/or active nephritic sediment should be treated as patients with class IV lupus nephritis.

Patients with membranous glomerulonephritis, nonnephrotic proteinuria, and stable renal function usually have an excellent natural outcome. These patients do not require any specific treatment. Symptomatic therapy may also be useless, since extrarenal activity is usually mild. The indications for glucocorticoid and/or immunosuppressive therapy of patients with membranous nephritis and nephrotic syndrome are still under discussion. Since the natural course of class V nephritis is relatively good, with many patients maintaining normal renal function over time, a number of clinicians use symptomatic therapy alone. However, some patients do progress to renal failure and others are exposed to the potential complications of the nephrotic syndrome, such as intravascular thrombosis, cardiovascular disease, malnutrition, and so on. There are no prognostic clues at presentation to indicate which patients will have a favorable evolution and which will not. Since a 6 month treatment of alternating glucocorticoids and cytotoxic agents may obtain remission of the nephrotic syndrome in about two-thirds of cases and may prevent progression to renal failure in responders, we are in favor of such a treatment. Good results with cyclosporine have also been reported.

Diffuse proliferative nephritis (class IV) is the most severe form of renal disease in SLE, although there are considerable variations in clinical presentation and outcome between one patient and another. Whether or not to treat patients with class IV nephritis as evidenced by a renal biopsy but without clinical signs of renal activity (clinical silent form) is still a matter of controversy. Low-dose prednisone (10 to 20 mg per day) has been advocated to prevent possible evolution to chronic histologic lesions and deterioration of renal function, but there is no proof that such an approach is really useful. These patients should be checked regularly over time and aggressive treatment should be started when there is an increase in serum creatinine or in proteinuria to more than 2 g per day (see following discussion). Most patients with class IV nephritis have a nephritic syndrome, a nephrotic syndrome, or renal insufficiency at presentation or in their early follow-up. These patients need vigorous therapy with high-dose glucocorticoids and/or immunosuppressive agents in order to cure the potentially reversible inflammatory lesions. Careful surveillance is necessary even for cases showing improvement or normalization of renal signs in order to recognize SLE flare-ups early. Ideally, serum complement levels should be normal and anti-DNA antibodies should be negative. However, we prefer to assess the activity of lupus nephritis and to modulate therapy based on the levels of serum creatinine, the amount of daily proteinuria, and the urine sediment, since a relationship between clinical and biologic parameters is often lacking.

Glucocorticoids

There is general agreement that glucocorticoids have improved the survival of patients with lupus nephritis. Although these agents are universally considered for the first-line therapeutic approach, there is no absolute guide in lupus nephritis for the dosage and type of administration. The early experiences clearly showed that low-dose prednisone is unable to interfere with the unfavorable course of severe class IV lupus nephritis. Thus, for patients with severe diffuse proliferative

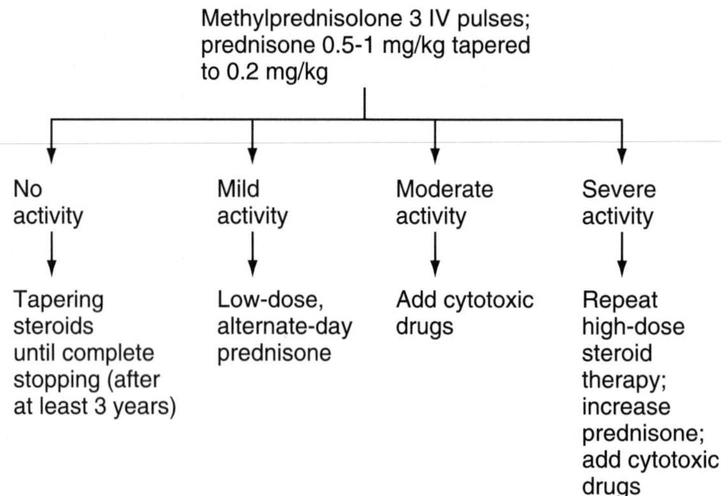

Figure 1
A possible flexible therapeutic strategy for patients with class III and class IV lupus nephritis.

lupus nephritis, many clinicians today start prednisone at doses of 1 to 2 mg per kilogram per day. The doses are tapered off only when renal disease and serologic parameters improve. However, in some patients this may happen only after several months, while progressive renal disease unresponsive to increased dosage of prednisone can develop in another 30 to 40 percent of patients. Moreover, independently of the clinical response, many patients given high-dose prednisone for a long time are prone to the devastating side effects of glucocorticoids, which include hypertension, infection, accelerated atherosclerosis, cushingoid features, obesity, diabetes, aseptic bone necrosis, cataracts, myopathy, and growth retardation in children.

Since low-dose prednisone is ineffective and high-dose prednisone is toxic, an intermediate approach is advisable. For patients with moderate disease, prednisone should be started at dosages not exceeding 1 mg per kilogram per day. It should be taken in a single dose, between 7:00 and 9:00 AM to mimic the circadian rhythm of endogenous cortisol, which is maximal in the morning. If lupus nephritis improves, prednisone may be tapered off to a low-dose maintenance (0.2 to 0.4 mg per kilogram per day). The dose should be reduced gradually and slowly over several months to prevent possible flare-ups. For those patients who tolerate low-dose prednisone without signs of renal and extrarenal activity, a switch to an alternate-day regimen may be tried after some months. Such a therapeutic schedule may control lupus nephritis in many patients, but it is insufficient for more severe cases.

A number of patients may have frequent flare-ups that require repeated administration of high-dose prednisone. Alternative approaches for controlling SLE activity while reducing glucocorticoid toxicity are recommended in these instances. Several reports have shown that a short course of intravenous high-dose methylprednisolone pulses (generally one pulse of 1 g given every 24 hours for 3 consecutive days) can dramatically reverse extrarenal symptoms and can rapidly improve renal function, particularly in patients who have had a recent rise in serum creatinine.

Proteinuria is usually improved more slowly and it may take as long as 6 months. The clinical remission is often maintained with moderate doses of prednisone, thus reducing the iatrogenic risks related to intensive and prolonged glucocorticoid therapy. In some patients rapid injection of high-dose methylprednisolone may induce flushing, tremor, nausea, and altered taste, which spontaneously disappear within a few hours. More severe but very rare complications include seizures, anaphylaxis, and arrhythmia. The risk of these adverse effects can be minimized if methylprednisolone is infused over at least 30 minutes instead of being injected rapidly. Some investigators suggest the regular administration of a single pulse of IV steroid every month for 6 to 12 months or until immunologic improvement occurs.

In view of the large interpatient variability in the severity of the disease and in the responses to therapy, we suggest a more flexible strategy. We start with one methylprednisolone pulse (0.5 to 1 g each according to the size of the patient) for 3 consecutive days and then the patient is given oral prednisone in a single morning dose (0.5 to 1 mg per kilogram per day according to the severity of the disease). The dose is gradually tapered to the minimum amount possible, with conversion to the alternate-day regimen when possible. Whenever a flare-up of SLE occurs (increase in plasma creatinine of at least 30 percent over the basal value and/or increase in proteinuria of at least 2 g per day) a new course of IV methylprednisolone pulses is given and the oral prednisone dose is increased. For patients with persistent activity or with frequent flare-ups, an immunosuppressive agent is added (Fig. 1). With this therapeutic strategy, we have obtained satisfactory long-term clinical results in 58 patients with diffuse proliferative lupus nephritis (Fig. 2).

Immunosuppressive Agents

Immunosuppressive agents can interfere with both the immune and the inflammatory responses and are therefore of potential benefit in treating lupus nephritis. On the other hand, these agents may also have disquieting side effects in either the short term or the long term and should therefore

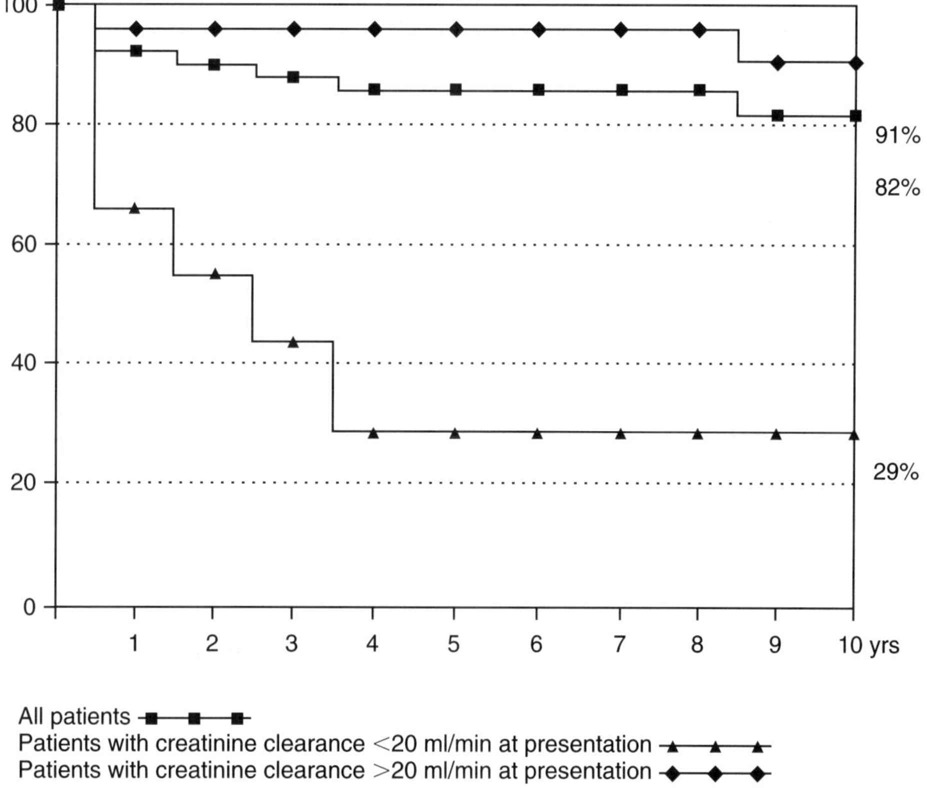

Figure 2
Survival with kidney functioning in 58 patients with diffuse proliferative lupus nephritis.

be used with caution. Several drugs have been tried, including methotrexate, chlorambucil, and vincristine, but the two immunosuppressive agents most widely employed in SLE are cyclophosphamide and azathioprine. Whether or not they have any advantages over glucocorticoids is still disputed. Clinical experience shows, however, that immunosuppressive agents can be useful in the following instances: (1) for treatment of severe phases, (2) when glucocorticoids alone are unable to control the activity of the disease, and (3) for maintenance treatment if one needs to reduce the doses of glucocorticoids because of iatrogenic toxicity.

Since alkylating agents may be oncogenic and since the risk of neoplasia seems to relate to their cumulative doses, it is advisable to limit cyclophosphamide treatment to short periods, reserving longer courses for the more difficult cases. The risk of neoplasia seems to be lower (but not absent!) for azathioprine, which may be preferred for long-term treatment. Although not currently supported by pertinent studies, there is the clinical impression that cyclophosphamide is more effective in obtaining a clinical response, whereas azathioprine is better tolerated, having less bladder, gonadal, and bone marrow toxicity. One possible therapeutic strategy might be to add cyclophosphamide (1.5 to 2 mg per kilogram day) for those patients who show persistent proteinuria, renal insufficiency, and extrarenal activity in spite of adequate glucocorticoid treatment. If a good response is obtained with cyclophosphamide, the drug may be stopped after 2 to 3 months and then may be replaced by azathioprine (2 to 2.5 mg per kilogram per day for 12 to 24 months) for those cases that cannot be controlled with low-dose prednisone alone.

For several years, the National Institutes of Health (NIH) group has been administering cyclophosphamide as intermittent intravenous pulses. A controlled study showed that the 10 year kidney survival of patients with lupus nephritis was significantly better for patients given intravenous cyclophosphamide plus moderate doses of prednisone than for those given prednisone alone. Although there was a trend to a better outcome for patients assigned to intravenous cyclophosphamide than for patients given various types and combinations of oral immunosuppressive drugs, this difference was not significant. Neither malignancy nor bladder toxicity developed in patients given intermittent pulses of cyclophosphamide.

In the first experience of the NIH group, pulses of 0.75 g per square meter were given indefinitely every 3 months. Then the administration was limited to 5 years or until remission was sustained for 2 years. More recent protocols are based on the administration of intravenous cyclophosphamide (0.75 g per square meter) every month for 6 months, followed by one pulse of cyclophosphamide every 3 months for maintenance. Treatment is continued for at least 1 year after remission, asdefined by inactive urinary sediment, reduction of proteinuria to a non-nephrotic range and inactivity of extrarenal lupus.

Several groups from all over the world have confirmed the efficacy of intravenous cyclophosphamide. Forced diuresis and intravenous hydration are recommended to protect from bladder toxicity. Nausea and vomiting are relatively frequent. Alopecia is common. In a few patients the white blood cell count may fall below 1,000 per cubic millimeter, with increased risk of infection. A major problem is represented by ovarian failure. The risk of sterilization may be reduced but not eliminated by administering the cyclophosphamide pulse at the time of menstruation.

Other Treatments

Alternative approaches to glucocorticoids and immunosuppressive agents have been tried for patients with lupus nephritis. Several uncontrolled studies of intensive plasma-exchange therapy in patients with severe disease reported good results. However, an American multicenter controlled study did not show any benefit from plasmapheresis.

The experience with cyclosporine is still preliminary and lacks controlled studies. In view of antiproteinuric properties, this drug might be indicated for patients with nephrotic syndrome refractory to treatment. Cyclosporine might also replace glucocorticoids for maintenance therapy in patients with severe hypercorticism. However, because of its nephrotoxicity, cyclosporine should be used with caution. Patients with renal insufficiency, hypertension, or severe tubulointerstitial lesions in a kidney biopsy are at increased risk for renal toxicity and should not be treated with cyclosporine. The initial doses should not exceed 5 mg per kilogram per day and should be gradually tapered to a maintenance dose of 3 to 4 mg per kilogram per day, if possible. Serum creatinine, blood trough levels of cyclosporine, and blood pressure should be carefully monitored in patients receiving cyclosporine treatment.

Impressive results have been reported for the defibrinogenating agent ancrod. Unfortunately, the studies were not controlled, and the drug has been tested by only one group.

Thromboxane antagonists might potentially have some role, but no clinical experience with these agents in lupus nephritis has been reported.

Fish oil may improve lipid parameters, but it neither improves renal function nor reduces the activity of the disease.

Suggested Reading

Austin HA III, Muenz LR, Joyce KM, et al. Prognostic factors in lupus nephritis. Am J Med 1983; 75:382–391.

Boumpas DT, Austin HA III, Vaughn EM, et al. Controlled trial of pulse methylprednisolone versus two regimens of pulse cyclophosphamide in severe lupus nephritis. Lancet 1992; 340:741–745.

Cameron JS. Lupus nephritis in childhood and adolescence. Pediatr Nephrol 1994; 8:230–249.

Ponticelli C. Current treatment recommendations for lupus nephritis. Drugs 1990; 40(1):19–30.

GOODPASTURE'S SYNDROME

Andrew J. Rees, M.B., Ch.B., M.Sc., F.R.C.P.

The term *Goodpasture's syndrome* was originally applied to all patients with necrotizing glomerulonephritis and pulmonary hemorrhage. Today it is used most frequently to describe only those patients in whom the syndrome is caused by autoantibodies to the glomerular basement membrane (anti-GBM). Nevertheless, it is important to remember that anti-GBM antibodies are responsible for the pulmonary hemorrhage and nephritis in less than half the patients who present with these conditions. Other causes include various types of systemic vasculitis associated with antineutrophil cytoplasmic antibodies (ANCA), systemic lupus erythematosus, and occasionally cryoglobulinemia. This chapter deals exclusively with the management of the anti-GBM antibody-mediated disease except where differences in clinical presentation are contrasted.

Two aspects of antibody-mediated Goodpasture's syndrome have ensured that its importance far exceeds its prevalence, and both have obvious consequences for therapy. First, anti-GBM disease is almost always severe and is frequently life-threatening. It may evolve with great rapidity, sometimes with complete loss of renal function within 24 hours, or the loss of several liters of blood into the lungs within a similar time frame. Thus, treatment is urgent and the disease should be regarded as a medical emergency. Second, anti-GBM disease is the first type of glomerulonephritis in which the pathogenesis (autoimmunity to the GBM) is known and can be quantified by measurement of circulating anti-GBM antibodies. This means that is possible to diagnose the disease noninvasively, to design rational therapies to remove anti-GBM antibodies, and to monitor disease activity. It has also been possible to study the relationship between circulating anti-GBM antibodies and the damage they cause. Such studies have demonstrated the influence of secondary factors such as intercurrent infection and cigarette smoke on the natural history of the disease. Thus, a better understanding of pathogenesis has improved management.

■ CLINICAL ASPECTS

Anti-GBM disease affects people of both sexes and of all ages. It presents most commonly during the third decade of life but there is a second peak in incidence in patients older than 60 years of age. Originally it was suggested that most patients were men, but this greatly exaggerates the sex difference, and most current series record male : female ratios of less than 2 : 1. Some authors have found elderly female patients to be less severely affected than other groups, but this has not been my experience.

The anti-GBM antibodies react with the same antigen in all patients and have highly restricted specificity. The target has been identified as the carboxy-terminal NCI domain of the α_3 chain of type (IV) collagen (α_3[IV]NCI), with very little cross-reactivity with NCI domains from other collagen chains. The gene encoding α_3(IV)NCI has been cloned and expressed in *Escherichia coli* and insect cells, but only the latter has the correct conformation to bind anti-GBM antibodies with similar affinity to the natural antigen. The antibodies are usually IgG with subclasses IgG_1 or IgG_4 predominating. Some patients also have IgA or IgM antibodies and in very rare instances isolated IgA anti-GBM antibodies have been described.

It is not known why tolerance to α_3(IV)NCI is lost, but there is strong evidence of an inherited predisposition. The frequency of the class II major histocompatibility molecules HLA-DR15 (present in 70 percent to 80 percent of patients compared to 25 percent of controls) and HLA-DR4 are increased in patients, and those of DR1 and DR7 are decreased. There is also an association with immunoglobulin allotypes; inheritance also appears to influence the severity of anti-GBM nephritis. Even so, it is unclear what initiates anti-GBM antibody synthesis. Despite repeated claims and a few convincing anecdotes, there is no real evidence to link anti-GBM disease with exposure to hydrocarbon fumes. The evidence that specific viral infections cause anti-GBM disease is equally unconvincing. An association with Hodgkin's disease (or its treatment) has been reported. Perhaps the simplest explanation for these findings is that anti-GBM disease can occur in a genetically susceptible individual when there is local inflammation or injury to the kidney. Recent reports of the development of anti-GBM disease after lithotripsy is perhaps the clearest example of this.

Patients with anti-GBM antibodies usually present with glomerulonephritis, which is associated with hemoptysis or a past history of hemoptysis in one-half to three-quarters of patients. It is uncommon for patients to have signs or symptoms suggestive of generalized disease such as rashes, arthralgia, myalgia, or fever; these are much more characteristic of other types or rapidly progressive nephritis. Typically, the glomerulonephritis is severe and progresses to renal failure in weeks or months if left untreated, but exceptional patients have more indolent disease. However, progression can be much more rapid in the presence of intercurrent infection and renal function can be destroyed within hours or days. At present it is impossible to tell whether an individual who presents with comparatively little renal injury is at risk of sudden deterioration or whether they have truly indolent disease. Evidence from renal biopsies, including those from patients who have already developed renal failure, suggests an explosive final event, in that necrosis and extracapillary proliferation (crescents) in glomeruli all appear to be at a similar stage of evolution. This contrasts with the appearances in biopsies from patients with other forms of rapidly progressive nephritis in whom crescents are found in all phases of evolution from cellular to fibrous, which implies repeated episodes of disease activity.

The severity of pulmonary hemorrhage is highly variable. It is found in 50 to 70 percent of patients and usually precedes evidence of nephritis, sometimes by many years. It is episodic, and varies in severity from mild hemoptysis to severe respiratory failure. It is the most common aspect of the disease in exceptional patients. These differences are not due to the specificity of anti-GBM antibodies, which bind α_3(IV)NCI regardless of clinical presentation. Thus, environmental factors must determine whether the lungs are affected, and exposure to cigarette smoke is the best characterized of these. This is evidenced by the observation that almost all current cigarette smokers who develop Goodpasture's syndrome have pulmonary hemorrhage, but its occurrence is rare in nonsmokers. Cigarette smoke also appears to precipitate acute pulmonary hemorrhage, as can intercurrent infection, fluid overload, and high concentrations of inspired oxygen (at least experimentally in rodents). Cocaine inhalation can also provoke lung hemorrhage. Avoidance of circumstances known to aggravate damage caused by anti-GBM antibodies is as crucial to effective management of antibody-mediated nephritis as are attempts to control antibody levels and to suppress inflammation.

The effectiveness of therapy is greatly influenced by the speed of diagnosis because of the rapidity with which anti-GBM disease can destroy the kidneys. Anti-GBM disease can often be suspected clinically, even in the absence of pulmonary hemorrhage, for example, in patients with deteriorating renal function and a diagnosis of nephritis (evidenced by the urinalysis and microscopy) not accompanied by vasculitis or the signs of generalized illness. Glomerulonephritis should be confirmed by renal biopsy and pulmonary hemorrhage by the presence of hemoptysis, alveolar shadows on chest radiographs, or an increased diffusing capacity for carbon monoxide after correction for lung volumes and for the patient's hemoglobin concentration (κCO). The specific diagnosis is confirmed by demonstrating the presence of anti-GBM antibodies either in the serum by solid phase immunoassays (older tests using indirect immunofluorescence are too insensitive) or in kidney tissue by immunohistochemical demonstration of linear deposition of immunoglobulin along the GBM. The antibodies are most frequently IgG with or without IgM. Occasional patients have been reported with isolated IgA anti-GBM antibodies. Linear staining of the alveolar basement membrane is variable, and its absence on biopsy specimens cannot be used to exclude the diagnosis. This is probably because of variable accessibility of α_3(IV)NCI to circulating anti-GBM antibodies.

Serum and tissue diagnoses are equally effective, but the radioimmunoassay has the advantage of serial measurements that can be used to follow the patient's response to treatment to ensure that anti-GBM antibodies are undetectable before renal transplantation is undertaken. The main conditions that need to be distinguished from anti-GBM disease are other types of rapidly progressive glomerulonephritis (principally those associated with vasculitis), pneumonia complicated by acute tubular necrosis, toxins such as paraquat that damage lungs and kidneys, and finally, any cause of renal failure complicated by pulmonary edema. The principal difficulties usually come either from confusing rapidly progressive glomerular nephritis (RPGN) accompanied by anemia with chronic renal failure, or failing to distinguish anti-GBM disease from systemic vasculitis. The recent demonstration that active systemic vasculitis and idiopathic RPGN are both very strongly associated with antibodies to neutrophil cytoplasmic antigen (ANCA) has greatly facilitated the distinction, even though up to 5 percent of patients may have ANCA as well as anti-GBM antibodies.

APPROACHES TO TREATMENT

The immediate aim of treatment in anti-GBM disease is to control pulmonary hemorrhage and glomerular inflammation as swiftly as possible, thereby providing the best chance of healing and repair. Simultaneously, it may be necessary to treat infection and to support renal and pulmonary function. The longer-term objective is to suppress anti-GBM antibody synthesis permanently. Before discussing our preferred regimen, it is important to recognize the grim prognosis for untreated patients. In their 1973 survey, Wilson and Dixon reported that 25 of their 53 patients died and only seven retained useful renal function. Although the general availability of dialysis and better diagnosis of less severely affected cases have improved prognosis, less than 15 percent of untreated patients in reported series of more than five patients who presented with raised plasma creatinine have retained useful renal function.

Immunosuppressive drugs by themselves appear to have little influence on the course of anti-GBM antibody-mediated nephritis, regardless of whether they are prescribed singly or in combination; this observation is in contrast with their effectiveness in treating other types of rapidly progressive nephritis. It is possible that pulmonary hemorrhage can be controlled by drugs more easily than nephritis, since intravenous boluses of methylprenisolone have been reported to be effective. However, this has not been my experience, and pulmonary hemorrhage tends to be episodic. In the past, bilateral nephrectomy was advocated for treating severe pulmonary hemorrhage in patients with anti-GBM disease. The original rationale for bilateral nephrectomy was that removal of the GBM would minimize the stimulus to further anti-GBM synthesis. However, nephrectomy has no effect on anti-GBM antibody titres. This is not surprising since the autoantigen is found in the lungs as well as the kidneys, and with hindsight, the case reports that originally suggested benefit are unconvincing. This approach is strongly contraindicated and should be abandoned as ineffective and potentially dangerous.

Against this background, it was argued that effective treatment should combine measures to rapidly reduce the concentration of anti-GBM antibodies with those to limit their synthesis and to suppress inflammation. Thus, a treatment regimen was developed that combined repeated large volume plasma exchange with cytotoxic drugs and steroids. Ideally, this regimen should have been assessed by a prospective controlled trial, but unfortunately this has proved impossible because of the rarity of anti-GBM disease and the rapidity with which it progresses. Consequently, the usefulness of the therapy has to be judged by its ability to control anti-GBM antibody titers and to suppress disease activity, and also by the frequency and severity of the complications.

MANAGEMENT

Specific Therapy

Our standard regimen for treating Goodpasture's syndrome is outlined in Table 1. It consists of daily whole volume (4 L for adults) plasma exchanges for albumin, combined with 60 mg of prednisolone daily, and cyclophosphamide, 100 to 150 mg per day administered orally, depending on weight. Originally we used azathioprine as well, but this proved unnecessary and its use has been abandoned. The regimen is modified in patients older than 55 years of age who are rarely given more than 100 mg cyclophosphamide. Plasma exchanges are performed for 14 days or until clinical evidence of continuing injury has subsided. They are restarted if disease activity recurs or if the anti-GBM antibody titer increases rapidly after the first course has been completed; both circumstances are relatively uncommon. Five plasma exchanges are the routine when a second course is required. Other groups have reported on the use of less intensive plasma exchange, and so their results are not directly comparable. It should be emphasized that daily whole volume exchanges combined with immunosuppressive drugs are needed to ensure rapid lowering of anti-GBM antibody concentrations in all patients. Cyclophosphamide is discontinued after 8 to 12 weeks, provided that anti-GBM antibody titers are no longer detectable. The prednisolone dose is also reduced rapidly. Patients receive 60 mg of prednisolone daily for 1 week, and then the dose is reduced at weekly intervals to 45 mg daily, 30 mg daily, 25 mg daily, and 20 mg daily. Thereafter, the dose of prednisolone is reduced by decrements of 5 mg weekly until it is stopped after 8 to 12 weeks. The prolonged use of immunosuppressive drugs is unnecessary in this condition provided that anti-GBM antibodies remain undetectable.

Table 1 Plamsa-Exchange Regimen

Plasma exchange:	Daily 4 L exchanges for albumin for 14 days
Corticosteroids:	Prednisolone 60 mg daily for 7 days; thereafter 45, 30, 25, 20, 15, 10, 5 mg for 1 week each
Cytotoxic drugs:	Cyclophosphamide 100–150 mg/day given for 8–12 weeks
	Cyclophosphamide 100 mg/day in patients over 55 years of age

Plasma Exchange

The development of automatic techniques for plasma separation by centrifugation or filtration opened the way for therapeutic plasma exchange. This is a technique in which whole blood is removed from a patient and separated into its plasma and cellular constituents before the cells are reinfused with fresh albumin instead of the patient's plasma, which is discarded. A single 4 L plasma exchange removes approximately 90 percent of an intravascular marker injected at the start of plasma exchange, and results in a 45 percent decrease in the serum concentration of IgG, and thus is a highly effective way to remove circulating autoantibodies. Unfortunately, anti-GBM antibodies are rapidly resynthesized, and repeated exchanges, as well as the concurrent administration of immunosuppressive drugs, are needed to reliably reduce their concentration in most patients.

Veno-venous circuits are inadequate for plasma exchange of this intensity and central vein catheters are most suitable. All types of cell separators are effective at removing IgG, and so the choice between centrifugation and filtration or the recently developed immunoabsorption columns, which remove IgG specifically, is a personal one and depends on the

Table 2 Practical Considerations to Minimize the Dangers of Plasma Exchange

Proper extracorporeal techniques to prevent air embolism
Accurate volume replacement to maintain blood volume
Sterile techniques to minimize the risk of infection
Use of albumin solutions not contaminated with vasoactive substances
Addition of potassium chloride and calcium glucose to each 400 ml unit of albumin to prevent acute electrolyte disturbances
Diluting replacement albumin solutions given to hypoalbuminemic patients because of the risk of acute hypovolemia
Prevention of chronic fluid overload caused by sodium loading imposed by exchanges

facilities available. Albumin solutions should be used as the plasma substitute and should have potassium and calcium added in sufficient amounts to bring their concentrations into the physiologic range. Plasma exchange removes coagulation factors as well as immunoglobulins. These are returned as 2 U of fresh frozen plasma at the end of exchange in all patients who are at risk from bleeding. Clearly this should include those with fresh pulmonary hemorrhage or who have had recent renal biopsies. The anticoagulation needed to prevent clotting in the extracorporeal circuit also poses a potential danger for these patients, but only a slight one because most of the anticoagulant is discarded with the patient's plasma rather than being returned to the patient.

Plasma exchange shares the complications of all extracorporeal circuits, such as infection of vascular access sites and embolism. In addition, there is a tendency to overload patients with renal failure with sodium because the sodium concentration of most plasma substitutes is greater than that of plasma. Thus, each whole volume exchange is often associated with a sodium load of 100 to 150 mmol. Fluid overload should be anticipated by daily measurement of body weight, and excess fluid should be removed by appropriate use of diuretics or dialysis. Acute hypervolemia associated with severe hypertension can be a problem, especially in children, because of rapid redistribution of fluid, which is caused by the sudden increase of plasma albumin concentration to normal levels in previously hypoalbuminemic patients. Finally, repeated plasma exchange can cause thrombocytopenia because of platelet destruction in the extracorporeal circuit. Table 2 outlines practical steps to minimize the complications.

Cytotoxic Drugs

Anti-GBM antibody titers rapidly return to pre-exchange values without the concomitant use of cytotoxic drugs. The main drug used is the alkylating agent cyclophosphamide. It is rapidly converted by hepatic microsomes to a series of active metabolites, which are incorporated into host DNA at all stages of the cell cycle; cells are killed only during division. In humans, cyclophosphamide suppresses primary antibody responses when given in daily doses of more than 2 mg per kilogram. It has been found to shorten significantly the duration of anti-GBM antibody synthesis in Goodpasture's syndrome when given to patients being treated by plasma exchange. The principal early complication of cyclophosphamide is myelotoxcity. It can occur at any stage of treatment and should be anticipated by daily measurement of the leukocyte count and prevented by appropriate reduction of the dosage. Later complications include hemorrhage cystitis caused by excretion of toxic metabolites, infertility (especially in men), and a small but perceptible risk of malignancy. Eight to 12 week courses in the doses advocated here have minimal short-term and long-term risks.

Prednisolone

Corticosteroids are the most powerful anti-inflammatory drugs available, and they also have some immunosuppressive properties. The pharmacologic aspects of these drugs are discussed extensively in other chapters. In anti-GBM antibody-mediated disease, corticosteroids are used predominantly for their anti-inflammatory properties and are prescribed in short, intensive courses to control the inflammatory response until anti-GBM antibody synthesis has been suppressed. There is no rationale for continuing their use beyond this point.

Supportive Treatment

Renal Failure

Patients with Goodpasture's syndrome may progress to end-stage renal failure within 24 hours and so need to have their renal function assessed daily in the early stages of their disease. Dialysis may be needed either because of azotemia or fluid retention (exacerbated by plasma exchange or blood transfusion), which can cause new life-threatening pulmonary hemorrhage.

Respiratory Failure

The treatment of respiratory failure in patients with anti-GBM disease is also controversial. Although hypoxemia may need to be corrected by increasing the inspired concentration of oxygen, there are sound experimental reasons for being anxious about such therapy. Oxygen toxicity exacerbates anti-GBM antibody-mediated pulmonary injury in rats and rabbits, probably increasing alveolar-capillary-endothelial cell permeability and thus the accessibility of the GBM to circulating antibody. It is impossible to test whether high concentrations of inspired oxygen have similar effects in patients with Goodpasture's syndrome; however, it seems prudent to limit the inspired oxygen concentration to the absolute minimum necessary to maintain safe levels of arterial oxygen concentration. Continuous positive airway pressure should be used as required.

Anemia

Some patients with Goodpasture's syndrome are severely anemic and may present with a hemoglobin concentration of less than 5 g per deciliter. Care must be taken to avoid hypervolemia, which exacerbates pulmonary hemorrhage, when blood transfusions are given.

Infection

Intercurrent infection is the most powerful cause of relapse with anti-GBM disease and appears to produce the effect by enhancing the potency of inflammatory mediators rather than by changing anti-GBM antibody synthesis. Recent experimental evidence has implicated the release of cytokines such as tumor necrosis factor and interleukin-1 in this phenomenon. Meticulous care must be taken to prevent infection during the course of treatment, especially because the risks substantially increase by the presence of indwelling catheters (intravenous, peritoneal, or urinary) and by the use of high doses of steroids.

Other Nonspecific Measures

Cigarette smoking has been identified as an important cause of pulmonary hemorrhage in patients with Goodpasture's syndrome, and resumption of smoking can precipitate relapse. These data provide exceptionally powerful reasons for patients with this disease to stop smoking. Goodpasture's syndrome has frequently been associated with exposure to hydrocarbon fumes. Whether or not the nature of this association and its effects are analogous to those of cigarette smoke is impossible to tell; it seems prudent to limit such exposure as much as possible.

Table 3 Outcome at 2 Months of Patients with Anti-GBM Disease Treated with Plasma Exchange

PRESENTING CREATININE	INDEPENDENT RENAL FUNCTION	DIALYSIS	DEATHS
Dialysis (30)	4 (13%)	19	7
>600 μmols/L (8)	4 (50%)	3	1
<600 μmols/L (2)	18 (86%)	2	1
Total (59)	26 (44%)	24	9

■ RESULTS OF THERAPY

At the Hammersmith Hospital, we have used plasma exchange to treat antibody-mediated Goodpasture's syndrome for the past 15 years and during this time have treated 63 patients. Since 1980, we have also performed serial assays of anti-GBM antibodies and advised on the management of many more patients treated in other units throughout the United Kingdom.

Control of Anti-GBM Antibody Titer

Anti-GBM antibody titers fell immediately after the start of therapy in all patients treated with the combination of plasma exchange and immunosuppressive drugs, and there has been little tendency for anti-GBM antibody titers to increase once the concentrations have been reduced to background values. Long-term, possibly permanent, disappearance of anti-GBM antibodies was achieved within 8 weeks in 29 to 30 patients who received a full course of a plasma-exchange regimen. A full course was defined as at least 12 plasma exchanges and at least 8 weeks of treatment with cyclophosphamide. By contrast, anti-GBM antibodies persisted for much longer in patients who did not receive complete treatment, and only three of 33 patients were cleared of antibodies by 8 weeks; the autoantibodies persisted for more than 1 year in 12 of these patients. Thus, it appears that cyclophosphamide and plasma exchange act synergistically to promote long-term control of anti-GBM antibody synthesis.

Renal Function

Nephrons that have been destroyed cannot regenerate, and so it comes as no surprise that the degree of improvement of renal function depends on the severity of injury at the time that treatment is initiated (Table 3). The plasma exchange regimen has been used on 30 dialysis-dependent patients with anti-GBM disease under our direct supervision, and only four regained useful renal function despite control of autoantibody titers. Similarly, the results in patients whose serum creatinine exceeds 600 μmols per liter (6.8 mg per deciliter) at the start of treatment were only moderately encouraging, with improvement in only four of eight such patients. By contrast, renal function improved in 18 of 21 patients with plasma creatinines that were rapidly increasing, but were less than 600 μmols per liter (6.8 mg per deciliter). Improvement in these patients was evident as soon as the plasma-exchange regimen was started, which argues strongly that it was a direct result of treatment. Seven patients with biopsy-proven nephritis and whose serum creatinine levels were within the normal range were also treated. They all improved as assessed by changes in serum creatinine levels within normal range or by improvement of the urine sediment. Thus, the plasma-exchange regimen is effective treatment for nephritis in Goodpasture's syndrome provided that it is introduced before the kidneys have been severely damaged. Late deterioration of renal function because of progressive fibrosis has occurred in a few patients without recurrence of detectable anti-GBM antibody synthesis. These patients have not been treated by reintroduction of plasma exchange or drug therapy, but have received nonspecific treatment until dialysis or transplantation.

Pulmonary Hemorrhage

Pulmonary hemorrhage in anti-GBM antibody-mediated disease has a much greater tendency to be episodic than does nephritis, and the lungs have a much greater capacity to recover. The patients who died of respiratory failure had pulmonary hemorrhage that was aggravated by intercurrent infection, hypervolemia, or the resumption of cigarette smoking in various patients. None of the surviving patients has developed clinically detectable pulmonary fibrosis, possibly because the lung injury is highly focal even when pulmonary hemorrhage is widespread.

Mortality

The overall mortality rate at 8 weeks in patients treated at Hammersmith Hospital was 15 percent (nine of 59 patients). In three patients, death was unrelated to the treatment regimen, but rather to unsuitability for long-term dialysis in two and an acute myocardial infarct in the third; pulmonary hemorrhage was the cause of death in the remaining five patients.

■ MONITORING THE EFFECTS OF THERAPY

The effects of treatment should be monitored meticulously by repeated assessments of disease activity and fluid balance, and for the possibility of complications. Routine investigations include daily measures of body weight, urine microscopy, serum creatinine, and complete blood count. Chest radiographs and κCO are assessed three times weekly when clinically indicated. Cultures of urine, sputum, and vascular access sites are taken three times weekly, but antibiotics are given only when clinically indicated. Whenever possible, it is helpful to frequently monitor anti-GBM antibody titers. Anti-GBM antibody concentrations are measured daily for the first 2 weeks and three times weekly thereafter. Many clinicians do not repeat assays as frequently as we do; however, it is important to measure antibody titers at presentation to confirm the diagnosis, and also at the end of therapy to assess the need for continued immunosuppression. Titers should also be measured in all patients with deteriorating renal function to distinguish active disease from progressive scarring and before transplantation in patients who develop end-stage renal failure.

■ PATIENT SELECTION

The plasma-exchange regimen described here is arduous and exposes the patient to discomfort as well as some risk. It should not be used indiscriminately, but should be reserved for those patients who are likely to benefit. Presently, we use plasma exchange in all patients with active pulmonary hemorrhage and all those with nephritis and declining renal function. We also treat the majority of patients with nephritis and creatinine levels within the normal range if they have clinical or morphologic evidence of active nephritis. Patients who are anuric but do not have pulmonary hemorrhage are not usually treated unless the renal biopsy contains a surprising number of glomeruli with patent capillary loops; similarly, dialysis-dependent patients who are still passing 500 to 1,000 ml of urine per 24 hours are also sometimes treated. Occasionally, treatment is given to limit the duration of anti-GBM antibody synthesis and to allow earlier renal transplantation.

Although this plasma-exchange regimen appears to be the first consistently effective treatment for anti-GBM disease, it is clearly unsatisfactory because it is cumbersome and lacks specificity. Presently, understanding of autoimmunity and the control of autoantibody responses are advancing rapidly, and it is hoped that the development of more specific ways to suppress anti-GBM antibody synthesis will result. It is also a depressing fact that many patients present after their kidneys have been destroyed, and this clearly indicates the need for earlier diagnosis.

■ ANTI-GBM DISEASE IN ALPORT'S SYNDROME

The development of anti-GBM antibodies after renal transplantation provides a special case. Alport's syndrome is an X-linked disease that results in progressive renal failure usually caused by mutations of the α_5- or α_6-chains of type IV collagen. These chains are present in the same specialized basement membranes that express the α_3- and α_4-chains, and probably form a distinct collagen network with them. Thus, patients with Alport's syndrome do not express α_3(IV)NCI in glomeruli. Transplantation of a normal kidney into patients with Alport's syndrome is sometimes followed by the development of anti-GBM antibodies; in this instance, of course, they are alloantibodies rather than autoantibodies. It was originally thought that anti-GBM antibodies were directed against the α_3(IV)NCI as is the case in the autoimmune form of the disease. However, we have recently developed more specific assays using conformationally correct recombinant α_3(IV)NCI and α_5(IV)NCI and have shown that this is not the case. Anti-GBM antibodies after renal transplantation in patients with Alport's are usually specific for α_5(IV)NCI and have minimal cross-reactivity with α_3-chains. This has serious implications for the diagnosis and the monitoring of anti-GBM antibody responses in this setting. Apparently low antibody titers in conventional anti-GBM assays may conceal very high anti-α_5-activity. It follows that patients with Alport's syndrome need to be very carefully monitored after renal transplantation preferably with an anti-α_5 (NCI) specific assay. Treatment is with plasma exchange and cyclophosphamide in addition to or as partial substitution for conventional antirejection therapy.

Suggested Reading

Herody M, Bobrie G, Gonarin C, et al. Anti-GBM disease: Predictive value of clinical, histological and serological data. Clin Nephrol 1993; 40: 249–255.

Turner AN, Lockwood CM Rees AJ. In: Shrier RW, Gottschalk CW, eds. Diseases of the kidney. 5th ed. Boston: Little, Brown, 1993: 1865.

IgA NEPHROPATHY (BERGER'S DISEASE)

Bruce A. Julian, M.D.
A.W.L. van den Wall Bake, M.D., Ph.D.

IgA NEPHROPATHY (BERGER'S DISEASE)

IgA nephropathy has become recognized worldwide as the most common form of primary glomerulonephritis in the 28 years after its description by Berger and Hinglais. Originally entitled *les depots inter-capillaires d'IgA-d'IgG,* this entity has been also labelled *mesangial IgA disease, IgA-IgG nephropathy,* and *IgA mesangial glomerulonephritis.* Because of the enthusiasm of its champion and the evolving controversies about the pathogenesis of this disorder, the eponym *Berger's disease* has gained increasing favor. The hallmark feature of this kidney disease is the dominant presence of IgA in the mesangium on immunofluorescence examination of the glomeruli. Light microscopy shows variable degrees of mesangial expansion and hypercellularity. Indistinguishable immunohistologic patterns may be found in the kidney biopsy specimens of patients with nephritis due to Henoch-Schönlein purpura. Furthermore, similar pathologic findings have been described in patients with a wide spectrum of diseases, including dermatitis herpetiformis, psoriasis, ankylosing spondylitis, celiac disease, regional enteritis, ulcerative colitis, carcinomas (especially of the colon, oral pharynx, and lung), IgA monoclonal gammopathy, alcoholic cirrhosis, chronic hepatitis, mycosis fungoides, and (rarely) acquired immunodeficiency syndrome. IgA nephropathy in patients with these latter conditions is referred to as secondary in contrast to primary in patients with the idiopathic form (Berger's disease) or Henoch-Schönlein purpura, considered by some investigators to be the 'systemic form' of this process. We will devote our discussion in this chapter to Berger's disease.

DIAGNOSTIC FEATURES

Immunohistologic Features

The diagnosis of IgA nephropathy requires an immunofluorescence examination of kidney tissue. Mesangial deposits of IgA are found in all glomeruli, even in those with a normal histologic appearance or minimal changes. Occasionally the IgA deposits may extend to the peripheral capillary loops. IgG and/or IgM are detected less often. C3 (the third component of complement) is usually found in a similar mesangial distribution. Other components of the alternative complement pathway, including properdin and factor H (β1H), as well as the membrane attack complex (C5b-9) are often detected. The absence or minimal intensity of the staining for C1q is a very useful criterion to distinguish IgA nephropathy from lupus nephritis if IgG is present. The intensity of immunofluorescence staining for lambda usually exceeds that for the kappa light chain isotype. Light microscopy usually shows mild mesangial proliferation and matrix expansion, although the pattern may vary within a biopsy specimen and be segmental (only a portion of a glomerulus affected) or focal (not all glomeruli affected). Segmental sclerosing lesions and cellular crescents are less common. Electron-dense deposits in the mesangial and paramesangial areas are generally found on electron microscopy. Small deposits may be located infrequently in the subendothelial or subepithelial areas.

Clinical Features

IgA nephropathy usually becomes manifest in adolescence and young adulthood, and about three times more often in males than females. The clinical features commonly comprise two syndromes. The more characteristic is an episode of macroscopic hematuria concurrent with infection of the upper respiratory tract or with gastroenteritis. In contrast to the 10 to 14 day delay for the onset of macroscopic hematuria in patients with poststreptococcal glomerulonephritis, urinary blood in patients with IgA nephropathy appears 1 to 2 days after the onset of symptoms and is rarely accompanied by hypertension or edema. Some patients, especially children, experience loin pain. The episode generally lasts only a few days, but may recur with a similar illness months or years later. Strenuous exercise or a nonspecific febrile illness occasionally may induce macroscopic hematuria. Examination of the urinary sediment by phase-contrast microscopy reveals deformed red blood cells, indicating glomerular bleeding rather than bleeding from a site in the urinary tract. Macroscopic hematuria is more common in children and adolescents than in adults and its frequency decreases with increasing age. The second syndrome entails asymptomatic microscopic hematuria with proteinuria of various magnitudes. Such patients are usually discovered upon routine urinalysis testing for insurance, employment, or check-up examinations. Less common clinical presentations include nephrotic syndrome, chronic renal insufficiency, and malignant hypertension. In a few patients, evidence of renal dysfunction is first detected during an episode of macroscopic hematuria; renal biopsies may show two distinctly different patterns: cellular crescents in many glomeruli or tubular necrosis with red blood cell casts.

IgA nephropathy is diagnosed most frequently in the second and third decades of life. The likelihood of documenting the disease depends greatly upon the threshold for performing the requisite renal biopsy. In several geographic regions with a previously low incidence of IgA nephropathy, subsequent screening programs with follow-up evaluation substantially increased the incidence of known disease. In some regions, genetic factors probably influence the prevalence of IgA nephropathy. The disease is rare in a few ethnic groups, especially in blacks. Families with multiple members with IgA nephropathy have been described, including some with relatives with Henoch-Schönlein purpura. Abnormalities of the IgA immune system may be found in patients with biopsy-confirmed disease and unbiopsied first-degree relatives with hematuria. Nonetheless, no HLA antigen, restriction fragment length polymorphism, or other genetic marker has been linked with IgA nephropathy in family studies. In our experience, familial IgA nephropathy is clinically indistinguishable from the sporadic form (individuals without a relative known to be affected by the disease).

Prognosis

For several years after its initial description, IgA nephropathy was assumed to follow an uneventful course and was labelled *benign recurrent hematuria.* However, as many as 20 to 30 percent of patients will reach end-stage renal failure after 20 years of known disease. The clinical markers for an unfavorable long-term prognosis include increased serum creatinine concentration at diagnosis, proteinuria greater than 2 g per day, older age at diagnosis (perhaps indicating a longer duration of disease), male gender, and hypertension. Although IgA nephropathy is uncommon among blacks, the clinical course in this racial group appears to be worse than in whites. Whether this less favorable outcome arises from a higher prevalence of hypertension due to causes independent of IgA nephropathy remains unclarified. Several laboratory findings have been associated with a poor prognosis. Patients homozygous for the deletion (D) allele for the gene encoding the angiotensin-converting enzyme have a worse prognosis than individuals heterozygous or homozygous for the insertion (I) allele. End-stage disease is more common in patients with the HLA-DR1 allele or deficient for the C4A complement protein. Serum IgA concentrations, increased in about 50 percent of patients, have not correlated with the long-term outcome. Some histologic features in the renal biopsy specimen portend a poor outcome, including segmental glomerular sclerosis, interstitial fibrosis, and extension of the IgA immune deposits to the peripheral capillary walls.

Patients may spontaneously enter a prolonged quiescent phase and maintain normal renal function. In our experience, the urinalysis becomes normal for years in about 20 to 30 percent of patients. Nevertheless, some of these patients remain hypertensive. Repeat renal biopsies performed during clinical remission generally show persistent immunohistologic findings diagnostic of IgA nephropathy; resolution of the immune deposits has been described only rarely.

Pregnancy and IgA Nephropathy

Because IgA nephropathy commonly affects young adults, the safety of pregnancy is a concern. Women in whom the creatinine clearance exceeds 70 ml per minute and the blood pressure is normal generally fare well. However, women with renal insufficiency or hypertension frequently experience obstetric complications, including low-birth-weight babies and fetal death and may show an accelerated rate of loss of renal function. Although patients with familial IgA nephropathy comprise a small minority of the total patient population, prospective parents may ask about genetic counseling before pregnancy. At present, neither the genetic basis nor mode of inheritance in this setting is known.

■ PATHOGENESIS

Despite intensive efforts by many investigators in centers throughout the world, the pathogenesis of IgA nephropathy has, at best, been only partially uncovered. As in many diseases, it is probable that a truly effective and safe therapy will be developed only after our insight into the pathogenesis has become more complete. We will briefly review some of the generally accepted concepts, and focus on areas of controversy.

Circulating IgA-Containing Immune Complexes

The mesangial deposits of IgA, often accompanied by other immunoglobulin isotypes and complement, arise from the circulation rather than being synthesized locally in the kidney. This is most clearly shown by the transplant experience whereby mesangial deposits of IgA recur in the allograft of many patients after several years. Conversely, the immune deposits in a kidney with mesangial IgA deposits inadvertently transplanted into a recipient suffering from another type of renal disease disappeared within several months. Other features illustrating the systemic nature of IgA nephropathy include the vascular deposits of IgA in muscle and skin of some patients, and the abnormalities of the circulating IgA reported in many patients. The prevalence of IgA deposits in the skin is controversial, and the predictive value of a skin biopsy is certainly too low to render it a suitable diagnostic alternative to a kidney biopsy.

The appearance of the mesangial IgA, by immunofluorescence and electron microscopy, suggests an immune complex pathogenesis. However, it is not clear whether the mesangial immune complexes are deposited as such from the circulation or, alternatively, formed in the mesangium through an in situ mechanism. Using a variety of techniques, many investigators have found immune complexes in the circulation that contain IgA, complement, and frequently other immunoglobulin isotypes. However, the prevalence of such complexes is lower (25 to 50 percent of patients) than suggested in early reports. Despite occasional descriptions of microbial or alimentary antigens in the mesangial deposits, the identity of antigens inciting formation of the complexes remains unknown.

IgA Subclasses

Of the two subclasses of IgA in man, only the IgA1 subclass appears to be involved in this disease. There is nearly general agreement that the mesangial IgA is exclusively IgA1 in most patients. The IgA in the circulating immune complexes is also restricted to IgA1, and the increased serum concentration of total IgA detectable in 50 percent of patients is due to an increased concentration of this subclass. The percentage of the total IgA produced by lymphocytes from the peripheral blood, bone marrow, and tonsils that is IgA1 is greater than in normal controls. Immunization studies of patients with IgA nephropathy, using both systemic and mucosal immunogens, have yielded conflicting results. Although some studies did not show an increased IgA immune response in patients, others provided evidence of overproduction of IgA antibodies. The IgA hyper-response in patients was limited to the IgA1 subclass, and to polymeric forms of IgA in some of these studies.

IgA Molecular Forms

IgA occurs in two molecular forms in humans: the monomeric form that predominates in the circulation and the polymeric form that is found mainly in mucosal secretions. The pathogenetic role of the polymeric forms of IgA in IgA nephropathy is very controversial. Much recent work has shown no increase in the proportion of the polymeric forms in the serum total IgA, the IgA produced in response to vaccination, the IgA in immune complexes, or the IgA produced by lymphocytes from the blood or bone marrow. Nonetheless, two studies suggested that polymeric IgA, which may be phlogistically more active than monomeric IgA, may comprise a pathogenetically significant fraction of the mesangial IgA. Unfortunately, the deposited IgA is technically difficult to isolate and characterize.

Metabolism of IgA1 and Circulating IgA1-Containing Immune Complexes

The amount of circulating IgA1 and IgA1-containing immune complexes may increase theoretically through either of two mechanisms: decreased catabolism and increased synthesis. Initially, the study of the catabolism of IgA-containing immune complexes was approached by only a very indirect method, using IgG- or complement-coated red blood cells to gauge the function of the mononuclear phagocytic system. In these analyses, a prolonged elimination half-life was found, but the relevance to the disposal of IgA-containing immune complexes is unclear. The rate of removal of altered red blood cells measures predominantly splenic function, and the observed abnormalities may be secondary rather than primary. More recently, two studies using aggregated human IgA have, unfortunately, yielded conflicting results; the role of a postulated disturbed clearance of IgA-containing immune complexes remains uncertain.

Compared to the findings in the catabolism studies, the data supporting an increased synthesis of IgA1 as a mechanism leading to increased circulating levels of IgA are much more solid. Numerous experiments using peripheral blood lymphocytes have shown both increased and normal synthetic rates for IgA. The basis for an increased synthetic rate has been postulated to be an increased function of helper T cells or a decreased function of the suppressor T cell subset. Recent studies have found evidence of an increased production of several cytokines (transforming growth factor beta-1, interleukin-6) that may be involved in the isotype switching to IgA, and the subsequent synthesis of this isotype. Conversely, active disease was associated with decreased production of tumor necrosis factor alpha. The relative contribution of the IgA1 subclass to the total IgA produced by blood mononuclear cells was increased. In interpreting these results, it is important to remember that peripheral blood cells comprise a negligible in vivo source of plasma immunoglobulin, and rather are cells in transit from one lymphoid organ to another. Although IgA1 is produced in both compartments (systemic and mucosal) of the IgA immune system, considerable debate has ensued about which compartment predominates as the origin of the mesangial IgA. An increased production of IgA1 has been shown for the bone marrow and the tonsils of patients with IgA nephropathy. We favor the bone marrow rather than the mucosal compartment as the origin of the mesangial IgA1. In healthy humans the bone marrow is the predominant source of plasma IgA, and the contribution from the mucosal surfaces is very small. Three studies of the small bowel mucosa have shown no increase of IgA or IgA1 plasma cells in patients with IgA nephropathy. In fact, the percentage of IgA plasma cells, and the percentage of IgA plasma cells expressing J chain as a marker for the synthesis of polymers, was recently found to be significantly decreased. Mucosal infections certainly play an important clinical role in IgA nephropathy, as illustrated by the frequent association with episodes of macroscopic hematuria. Perhaps such infections, usually in the upper respiratory tract, lead not only to a local immune response, but also to a circulating antibody response through increased synthesis of IgA in the bone marrow. Indeed, evidence for such a linkage between the two compartments of the IgA system has been observed in experimental animals and humans. The IgA1 hyperresponsiveness would produce elevated plasma levels of IgA1 and IgA1-containing immune complexes after many everyday infections. Possibly an increased permeability of the mucosae permits antigens greater access to the circulation, thereby contributing to the formation of immune complexes. Evidence for such an increased permeability is not firm. Moreover, although the barrier function of the mucosa is often compromized in inflammatory bowel disease, this group of diseases is only rarely complicated by secondary IgA nephropathy.

Other Pathogenetic Considerations

The immune hyper-response described above is probably not the sole pathogenetic factor in IgA nephropathy. Other disease states also characterized by increased plasma levels of IgA1 or IgA1-containing immune complexes (such as IgA myeloma and acquired immunodeficiency syndrome) generally do not manifest mesangial deposits of IgA1. Another, yet unidentified, factor must determine whether or not the elevated plasma level of IgA1 will lead to mesangial deposition and the consequent inflammatory damage. In our opinion, the identification of this factor (or factors) will greatly improve the understanding of this disease. Theoretically, it may entail a biochemical characteristic of the IgA1 unrelated to its antigen specificity or, conversely, involve the capacity of the IgA1 to bind antigen. Examples of the first category include charge, size, and glycosylation of the IgA1 molecule. Glycosylation of the IgA1 molecule in the hinge region has important effects with regard to IgA catabolism in the liver, and possibly also the regulation of IgA synthesis and the interaction of IgA molecules with tissue components. Recent studies have shown that the IgA1 in patients with IgA nephropathy is deficient in galactose residues. With respect to antigenic specificity, autoantigens (native to the glomerulus or not) or exogenous antigens may play a role. In recent years, several studies have described immunoglobulin binding to glomerular structures. One such interaction encompasses the binding of IgA-fibronectin aggregates to collagen; another, the binding of autoantibodies of the IgG isotype to glomerular antigens.

Mesangial Cell Physiology

Very recent data pertaining to mesangial cell physiology may have important implications for the pathogenesis of IgA nephropathy. The emergence of mesangial cell culture techniques has greatly advanced our understanding of the physiology of these cells. The results have changed our previous perception of the mesangial cells as merely innocent bystanders in this disease to one in which they may actively participate. Mesangial cells express surface receptors for IgA, and thereby may play an active role in the accumulation of the mesangial immune deposits. Furthermore, these cells appear capable of synthesizing a large array of inflammatory mediators and expressing receptors for such mediators. Consequently, mesangial cells may mediate the inflammation and sclerosis which characterize the glomerular damage in more advanced disease. Overall, considerable uncertainty persists about the inflammatory mechanisms damaging the glomerulus after the IgA has been deposited. Complement almost certainly plays an important role, as illustrated by the nearly universal finding of mesangial deposits of C3, components of the alternative pathway, and the membrane attack complex. Whether IgA alone is capable of activating the alternative pathway, or whether another co-deposited isotype or perhaps a certain biochemical property of the antigen is necessary remains hotly debated. The wide spectrum of clinical and histologic expression of IgA nephropathy, ranging from almost normal histology to crescentic glomerulonephritis, suggests that various inflammatory mechanisms may be activated, depending on the patient and the phase of the disease.

Thus, many aspects of the pathogenesis of IgA nephropathy unfortunately remain unclear, despite considerable research devoted to the issue. Some of the controversy has arisen because cross-sectional studies frequently did not consider the clinical phase of the patients. We expect that longitudinal studies and basic research about mesangial cell physiology and immune regulation will provide sorely needed insight into the basis of this disease.

■ TREATMENT

No consensus has emerged for a disease-specific approach to treatment of most patients with IgA nephropathy, especially for those with chronic disease. Unfortunately, the beneficial effects of some therapeutic regimens, touted after anecdotal experiences or retrospective reviews, have been disproven in studies with more patients. Few carefully designed, prospective studies have been undertaken. The outcomes of treatment trials will require years of observation because of the generally indolent clinical course. Table 1 summarizes our assessment of the fragmented opinions of various treatment options.

Table 1 Potential Therapeutic Approaches for Patients with IgA Nephropathy

THERAPY	COMMENTS
COINCIDENT MINIMAL CHANGE DISEASE	
Glucocorticoids	Induce remission of nephrotic syndrome
ACUTE RENAL DYSFUNCTION	
Crescentic glomerulonephritis	
Glucocorticoids	Generally beneficial
Cytotoxic agents	Controversial
Plasmapheresis	No proven benefit
Acute tubular necrosis	
Supportive	No immunosuppression warranted
CHRONIC DISEASE	
Immunosuppression	
Glucocorticoids	Beneficial in uncontrolled studies
Immunoglobulin	Beneficial in uncontrolled study
Cytotoxic agents	No proven benefit
Cyclosporine	No benefit
Antiinflammatory agents	
Fish oil	May preserve GFR
Antiplatelet	No proven benefit
Hypertension	
Angiotensin-converting enzyme inhibitor	Preserves GFR, reduces proteinuria
Calcium channel blocker	May reduce glomerular scarring
Dietary restrictions	
Salt restriction	Augments antihypertensive therapy
Protein	May reduce proteinuria
Alcohol	May reduce frequency of macroscopic hematuria
Tonsillectomy	For recurrent tonsillitis
Transplantation	High rate of recurrent disease by immunofluorescence; loss of allograft uncommon Recurrence not greater with living-related donor

GFR, Glomerular filtration rate

Acute Clinical Presentation

Acute renal dysfunction may complicate an episode of macroscopic hematuria. As noted above, renal biopsy specimens occasionally show crescents in more than 50 percent of glomeruli. Many investigators advocate treatment with high-dose glucocorticoids, perhaps including bolus intravenous therapy, as given to patients with other types of immune-complex crescentic glomerulonephritis. Less agreement exists about glucocorticoid treatment of patients with crescents in a small percentage of glomeruli. Some centers have added therapy with plasmapheresis, cytotoxic agents, or anticoagulants. Anecdotal reports of early treatment-associated improvement in renal function often described progressive renal insufficiency after longer observation. Notably, some authors have reported spontaneous resolution of renal dysfunction in patients with crescentic IgA glomerulonephritis. For patients with macroscopic hematuria and tubular necrosis with large casts of red blood cells in the biopsy specimen, supportive therapy with control of blood pressure and dialysis as necessary will suffice; renal function often returns to baseline.

Chronic Disease

General

As with patients with a variety of glomerulopathies, several general approaches to treatment apply to patients with IgA nephropathy. Hypertension often reflects progressive renal damage and, in turn, undoubtedly accelerates the rate of deterioration of renal function. Its control remains vitally important for long-term therapy. In animal models of glomerulonephritis, calcium channel blocker agents and angiotensin-converting enzyme inhibitors decrease glomerular scarring. In this setting, angiotensin-converting enzyme inhibitors blocked the synthesis of several cytokines, including transforming growth factor-β, that may cause fibrosis. Clinical studies have shown that treatment with angiotensin-converting enzyme inhibitors slows the rate of decline in renal function in patients with progressive renal insufficiency due to several kidney disorders, including IgA nephropathy. Whether treatment with this class of agents should include patients with normal blood pressure is unproven. Moderate salt restriction improves the benefits of this pharmacotherapeutic regimen and should be routinely prescribed. Reduction of dietary protein intake to about 0.8 g per kg body weight per day may slow progressive renal insufficiency, although the magnitude of benefit remains controversial despite a large multicenter trial.

Reduction of Synthesis of IgA or IgA-Immune Complexes

Because macroscopic hematuria frequently coincides with an upper respiratory tract infection, eradication of septic foci in the oropharynx has been advocated. While treatment for a year with daily antibiotics, such as tetracycline, may reduce the magnitude of microscopic hematuria in some patients, long-term benefits on renal function have not been proven. Tonsils produce substantial quantities of IgA1 and ultrasonic stimulation of the tissue increases the magnitude of microscopic hematuria in patients with IgA nephropathy. Several centers, initially in Spain and later in Japan, found that tonsillectomy decreased the frequency of the bouts of macroscopic hematuria and the magnitude of microscopic hematuria and proteinuria. In addition, some investigators found that 2 years after surgery the percentage of circulating lymphocytes producing polymeric IgA had significantly decreased. Although tonsillectomy has not yet undergone rigorous testing, the procedure seems reasonable in the setting of recurrent tonsillitis. Other efforts to lower the concentration of circulating IgA have included treatment with phenytoin. The magnitude of hematuria decreased in one study, but no histologic manifestation of disease activity improved during this interval. Investigators in Italy found that a gluten-free diet decreased levels of circulating IgA-containing immune complexes and lessened microscopic hematuria, but the long-term efficacy of this difficult dietary restriction has not been tested. A study in Australia associated bouts of macroscopic hematuria with increased intake of alcoholic beverages, and limiting their regular usage seems prudent.

A different approach has been tried in France where pooled intravenous followed by intramuscular immunoglobulins were given for 9 months. The investigators postulated that immunoglobulin therapy may inhibit B-cell differentiation and immunoglobulin production by acting on B-cell IgG Fc receptors, thereby reducing the levels of the putative nephritogenic IgA molecules. In this uncontrolled study, nine patients with IgA nephropathy showed decreases in the magnitude of proteinuria and rate of decline of creatinine clearance. Repeat renal biopsies after treatment found diminished IgA and C3 deposits and less histologic disease activity. Treatment was well tolerated, but several patients showed clinical relapse within 3 months of stopping therapy.

Immunosuppression

In the absence of a disease-specific therapy, treatment trials have often used agents with broad immunosuppressive effects. Glucocorticoids certainly benefit the few patients with nephrotic-range proteinuria in whom renal biopsy specimens show minimal cellular proliferation or expansion of the matrix and fusion of the epithelial foot processes on electron microscopy. Although some investigators propose that these patients exhibit a coincidental occurrence of minimal change glomerulonephritis and IgA nephropathy, they may comprise a special subset of patients with IgA nephropathy. As in minimal change glomerulonephritis, proteinuria is quite selective whereby small molecules such as albumin account for most of the protein. Treatment with glucocorticoids clears the nephrotic syndrome, but the signs and symptoms may relapse after stopping treatment. The glomerular IgA may clear after a glucocorticoid-induced clinical remission.

Glucocorticoid treatment of patients with nonselective proteinuria or glomerular scarring on biopsy has produced more controversial findings. Short-term courses for less than 6 months have shown no long-term benefit on creatinine clearance. In contrast, more prolonged therapy may preserve renal function. In a nonrandomized study in the United States, 13 children with histologic features associated with progressive disease were treated with alternate-day prednisone for a mean period of 34 months. At the end of a mean observation period of 67 months, 12 had preserved normal renal function and a normal urinalysis. Eleven patients underwent repeat renal biopsy; all showed mesangial IgA deposits of an intensity similar to pretreatment biopsies. The clinical course of these treated children was compared to that of 15 untreated controls, chosen retrospectively, with similar pathologic and clinical findings. After a similar duration of follow-up, only one had a normal urinalysis and seven had progressed to chronic renal insufficiency or end-stage disease. A retrospective study of adults in Japan evaluated treatment with daily prednisone for 18 months. Patients with moderate proteinuria (ranging from 1 to 2 g per day) and a creatinine clearance before treatment greater than 70 ml per minute maintained their renal function during 10 years of observation. Patients treated with nonsteroidal anti-inflammatory or antiplatelet agents showed progressive renal dysfunction after several years. Prednisone treatment failed to preserve renal function in patients with creatinine clearances less than 70 ml per minute. The authors concluded that prednisone therapy may stabilize the clinical course of IgA nephropathy if started in the early stages of disease. In an uncontrolled study, prednisone (an initial daily regimen was tapered to an alternate-day schedule) was combined with azathioprine for a 1 year treatment of 10 children with decreased renal function, proteinuria greater than 1 g per day, and hypertension. The mean serum creatinine concentration did not change after 2 .5 years; proteinuria, magnitude of microscopic hematuria and frequency of macroscopic hematuria all decreased. However, treatment was not risk-free: each patient showed cushingoid features and one developed osteonecrosis of the femoral heads.

Fish Oil

Fish oil, rich in omega-3 fatty acids such as eicosapentanoic acid, has been evaluated for its efficacy to slow deterioration of renal function of patients with IgA nephropathy. The rationale for its use is a postulated effect of omega-3 fatty acids to diminish synthesis or action of cytokines and eicosanoids evoked by an initial immunologic glomerular injury, thereby presumably reducing renal damage. The results of 5 clinical trials have been conflicting. Studies in Hong Kong, Sweden, and Australia have shown no long-term benefit on renal function. In contrast, in a small Japanese study, treatment for 1 year maintained renal function, as measured by the reciprocal of the serum creatinine concentration. More recently in a multicenter, placebo-controlled, randomized study in the United States, supplements of 12 g of fish oil given for 2 years to patients with persistent proteinuria significantly slowed the annual decline in renal function. Proteinuria did not significantly change and blood pressure was similar in the two patient groups. No patient discontinued treatment because of an adverse event. The difference in the effects of fish oil in these 5 studies may reflect differences in the stage of disease, pretreatment rate of progression of disease, composition of the fish oil, and the length of treatment.

Other Approaches

Other immunosuppressive agents have been sporadically evaluated in patients with IgA nephropathy. In two centers, a regimen of cyclophosphamide, dipyridamole, and warfarin reduced the magnitude of proteinuria without altering creatinine clearance. In a study in Hong Kong, cyclosporine for 3 months decreased proteinuria, but at the expense of lower glomerular filtration rates. A controlled trial of antiplatelet therapy with aspirin and dipyridamole showed no clinical benefit. Danazol increased the capacity of patients' sera to remove glomerular immune deposits in kidney biopsy specimens. While treatment with this agent decreased proteinuria, serum creatinine concentrations did not improve. Urokinase, given on the premise that anticoagulation therapy would lessen glomerular damage associated with intraglomerular thrombosis in some biopsy specimens, has not proven beneficial. Neither sodium cromoglycate nor dapsone has shown any clinical effects.

Transplantation

For patients reaching end-stage renal failure, transplantation affords an excellent therapeutic option. Recurrent disease, defined by the characteristic immunohistologic features, has been documented in about 50 percent of patients by 2 years after transplantation. It is difficult to predict which recipients will develop recurrence, but it may be more common in patients with persistently increased circulating levels of IgA-containing immune complexes post transplant. The rate of recurrence has not decreased in the cyclosporine era. Fortunately, loss of the allograft from recurrent disease is uncommon. The milder clinical course may reflect a benefit from immunosuppressive therapy starting at the first exposure of the allograft to the pathogenetic milieu in the recipient. Some investigators have shown better allograft survival in recipients with IgA anti-HLA antibodies; they postulate that these antibodies block the IgG response to the allograft. Kidneys from living-related donors are not at greater risk than cadaveric allografts for recurrent disease and we continue to use relatives as donors after the customary evaluation.

Suggested Reading

Abe S. Pregnancy in IgA nephropathy. Kidney Int 1991; 40:1098–1102.

Chauveau D, Droz D. Follow-up evaluation of the first patients with IgA nephropathy described at Necker Hospital. Contrib Nephrol 1993; 104:6–13.

Clarkson AR, Woodroffe AJ. eds. IgA nephropathy: pathogenesis and treatment. Contrib Nephrol 1995; 111:1–208.

D'Amico G, Imbasciati E, Barbiano di Belgioioso G, et al. Idiopathic IgA mesangial nephropathy. Clinical and histological study of 374 patients. Medicine 1985; 64:49–60.

Galla JH. Perspectives in clinical nephrology: IgA nephropathy. Kidney Int 1995; 47:377–387.

Julian BA, ed. Proceedings from the National Symposium on IgA Nephropathy. Am J Kidney Dis 1988; 12:377–453.

MEMBRANOUS NEPHROPATHY

Wadi N. Suki, M.D.

J. Pedro Frommer, M.D.

Membranous nephropathy (also called idiopathic membranous, epimembranous or extramembranous nephropathy, glomerulonephropathy, or glomerulonephritis) is the most common biopsy diagnosis in adult patients with nephrotic syndrome, accounting for about 25 to 35 percent of cases. Its clinical presentation is proteinuria, with or without the full-blown nephrotic syndrome. Because there are no clinical or laboratory features specific to the disease, its identification depends on performing a renal biopsy.

In mild cases, the biopsy findings on light microscopic examination may appear quite normal and be indistinguishable from minimal-change nephropathy. More commonly, however, hematoxylin, eosin, and periodic acid-Schiff stains show a diffuse and global change consisting of uniform thickening of the glomerular capillary walls. Silver stains, immunofluorescence, and electron microscopic studies demonstrate the abnormalities in greater detail. Electron-dense deposits of varying sizes and shapes are present on the subepithelial surface of the capillary basement membrane.

These appear to correspond to finely granular deposits containing IgG and C3 (and sometimes IgA and IgM), which are seen with immunofluorescence microscopy. As the deposits thicken, the normal basement membrane material appears to grow out between them. This membrane material stained with silver gives the "spiked" appearance characteristic of the disease.

Most patients with this biopsy picture have idiopathic disease, but in most series, 20 to 30 percent of cases are associated with and presumably caused by systemic disease. Systemic lupus erythematosus is the most common association, but tumors, drugs, toxins, sickle cell disease, and particularly infections, including hepatitis and parasitic disease, are also seen. In some cases, cure of the associated disease leads to a remission of the membranous nephropathy; in others, the renal disease persists. Membranous nephropathy occurs in patients of all ages, although its peak incidence is between 35 and 55 years of age. In childhood it is much less common than minimal-change nephrosis and tends to occur in later childhood through young adulthood. There is a male predominance of approximately 2:1. Perhaps as many as 30 to 50 percent of patients with membranous histologic findings have asymptomatic (less than nephrotic) proteinuria.

The cause of membranous nephropathy and the pathogenesis of its accompanying proteinuria are not well understood. Evidence from experimental models suggests that the basement membrane deposits may be the result of in situ formation of immune complexes, the result of a reaction between circulating antibodies with antigens (either endogenous or exogenous) lodged in the glomerular capillary wall.

The course of the disease is variable. After 10 years of observation, perhaps one-third of patients will be in renal failure, another third will have persisting proteinuria with preserved renal function, and one-third will be apparently cured. Patients who have normal renal function and non-nephrotic proteinuria and are normotensive, women, and children appear to have relatively good prognoses.

EVALUATION

When a biopsy specimen in a patient with proteinuria demonstrates membranous nephropathy, the physician should be alert for the possible presence of associated diseases (Table 1). A careful history and physical examination will identify many of these diseases. Laboratory investigations, including determinations of antinuclear antibodies, anti-DNA antibodies, complement, antithyroid antibodies, hepatitis B antigens and antibodies, hepatitis C antibodies, blood glucose, serologic tests for syphilis, and hematocrit, may be useful. The importance of a search for malignancy in a patient presenting with membranous nephropathy is difficult to assess. Some series have found neoplasms in as many as 10 percent of patients with membranous nephropathy, and almost one half of these tumors were unknown at the time of the renal biopsy. The likelihood of tumor increases with the patient's age, and a reasonable search for common tumors (lung, kidney, breast, colon) should be undertaken in individuals 40 years of age or older.

Table 1 Diseases Associated with Membranous Nephropathy

IMMUNOLOGIC ABNORMALITIES
Systemic lupus erythematosus*
Rheumatoid arthritis, Sjögren's syndrome, Hashimoto's thyroiditis, dermatitis herpetiformis, myasthenia gravis, Guillain-Barré syndrome, Weber-Christian panniculitis, dermatomyositis
INFECTIONS
Hepatitis B, especially in childhood*; hepatitis C
Quartan malaria, schistosomiasis, leprosy, congenital and acquired syphilis, hydatid disease, filariasis, and scabies may be significant causes in areas where they are prevalent
NEOPLASMS
Cancers of the lung,* breast,* colon, stomach, kidney, esophagus, carotid body, and melanoma
Lymphoma (more frequent association with minimal-change lesion in Hodgkin's disease) and leukemia
DRUGS AND TOXINS
Gold therapy for rheumatoid arthritis*
Penicillamine*
Captopril*
Nonsteroidal anti-inflammatory drugs
Mercury (in skin-lightening cosmetics), other heavy metals, trimethadione or paramethadione, volatile hydrocarbon solvents
OTHER CONDITIONS
Diabetes mellitus
Sarcoidosis
Sickle cell disease

*Signifies relatively frequent causes.

TREATMENT

General

Patients with membranous nephropathy will of course benefit from salt restriction and appropriate use of diuretics, as do patients with nephrotic syndrome from other causes. Some patients also appear to achieve symptomatic benefits from the combination of nonsteroidal agents such as indomethacin or meclofenamate with diuretics. Diuretics and nonsteroidal agents, however, may compromise renal function and may even result in acute tubular necrosis, and therefore should be used with caution.

Diet

A substantial body of evidence now indicates that lowering protein intake in patients with renal disease in general, and with the nephrotic syndrome in particular, has a beneficial effect. Reducing protein intake to a level of 0.6 to 1 g per kilogram of body weight often results in a reduction in urinary protein excretion without causing protein malnutrition. Also, in those patients whose renal function is declining, curtailing protein intake may also retard or arrest the progression of the disease.

It has been suggested that lipids have a role in the pathogenesis of progressive glomerular disease. Since nephrotic patients are often hyperlipidemic and are at increased risk for atherosclerosis and coronary heart disease, a diet with reduced fat content, and even the use of lipid-lowering drugs, is indicated.

Associated Disease

When an underlying cause or associated disease is present, every effort should be made to treat it successfully. With the removal of an underlying cause, the membranous nephropathy will often, although not always, remit. Furthermore, resolution of hepatitis-associated membranous nephropathy has been reported after alpha-interferon therapy.

Asymptomatic Proteinuria

Although there is evidence that proteinuria in the range of 1 to 2 g per day will remit with prolonged low-dose steroid therapy, there is also evidence that the prognosis for such patients is good without treatment. There would seem to be little need for urgency in treating such patients and no evidence exists that the disease is more harmful than the treatment.

Nephrotic Syndrome with Normal Glomerular Filtration Rate

Corticosteroids

In a large collaborative trial in the United States, prednisone therapy was randomly and prospectively compared with placebo. The patients were adults with idiopathic membranous nephropathy and nephrotic syndrome. The treatment consisted of oral prednisone administered on an alternate-day basis, with the average dose being 125 mg every other day for a period of 2 months, with tapering over an additional 4 to 8 weeks. Patients who received treatment had more frequent remissions of proteinuria, but the occurrence of relapses led to few long-term differences between the groups. Of greater importance was that fewer of the treated patients progressed to renal failure during the period of observation, although more of the untreated patients progressed to renal failure than would have been anticipated during the period of observation. Contrasting with the results of the aforementioned study are the findings of the Toronto Glomerulonephritis Study Group, who also conducted a prospective randomized study in which patients with biopsy-confirmed membranous nephropathy were given a 6 month course of alternate-day prednisone (45 mg per m^2 body surface area) or no specific treatment. No differences could be found between the two groups in terms of remission of proteinuria during the short term (6 months) or the long term (48 months). Unlike the U.S. collaborative study, no differences could be found between the two groups with respect to decline in creatinine clearance, progression to renal failure, or death. Similarly negative findings have been reported by the Medical Research Council of Great Britain. It is therefore safe to conclude that there is no place for the use of alternate-day prednisone therapy in the treatment of nephrotic patients with membranous nephropathy.

Several uncontrolled observations have suggested that daily corticosteroid therapy is helpful in this disease, while others failed to demonstrate that such therapy is of benefit. In our experience, daily therapy with prednisone (1 mg per kilogram) for a period of 2 to 3 weeks, after which the dose is increased by 20 percent and an alternate-day regimen is used, followed by a tapering of the alternate-day dose by 5 mg per week down to a dose of 30 to 40 mg, has resulted in remission in 30 percent of patients when the treatment was maintained for several months (16 months or more). Another 60 percent of patients, who had not responded to prednisone alone, remitted after therapy with cyclophosphamide (see later), accounting for a total remission rate of nearly 90 percent.

Immunosuppressive Therapy

In a randomized, prospective, controlled trial performed in Italy, 6 months of alternating steroids and chlorambucil was compared with no therapy. The initial month began with three 1 g pulses of intravenous methylprednisolone followed by daily oral methylprednisolone (0.4 mg per kilogram per day) or prednisone (0.5 mg per kilogram per day). At the end of the first month, the steroid was discontinued and chlorambucil (0.2 mg per kilogram per day orally) was given for 1 month. This 2 month cycle was repeated three times during a total of 6 months of therapy. At the end of 10 years' follow-up, 26 of 42 of the treated patients (62 percent) were in complete or partial remission, compared with 13 of 39 controls (33 percent), and there was a statistically significant (49 percent) decline in the reciprocal of the serum creatinine in the controls as compared with a 17 percent decline in the treated group. Short-term complications of this therapy were few, and none were serious. The probability of being alive with renal function at 10 years was 0.92 for the treated patients and 0.6 for the untreated controls. Other studies have suggested benefit from cyclophosphamide combined with prednisone or anticoagulants. In our experience, almost all patients who had not responded to prednisone alone went into remission when given cyclophosphamide (2 mg per kilogram) for as long as 12 months or more, giving us a total remission rate of almost 90 percent (see earlier).

It is therefore our belief that cyclophosphamide or chlorambucil is indicated for the treatment of patients who do not respond to prednisone alone. There is no evidence that pulse cyclophosphamide is of any benefit.

Nephrotic Syndrome with Renal Insufficiency

A group from Toronto conducted a controlled trial of cyclophosphamide (maximum of 2 mg per kilogram) in nephrotic patients with membranous nephropathy whose serum creatinine concentration at the time of initiation of therapy exceeded 135 μM (>1.5 mg per deciliter). Most of these patients and all of the controls had received prednisone. After a mean follow-up of 83 months, the serum creatinine in the control group had risen to greater than 500 μM (>5.7 mg per deciliter) in 10 of 17 patients, while in the treated group, it was somewhat lower than the starting value. Complete or partial remission of the nephrotic syndrome was observed in all of the treated patients. Of the control patients five of six developed end-stage renal disease whereas only one of eight treated patients (12.5%) did so. An alternative strategy is to administer cyclosporine in a dose of 3.5 mg per kilogram per day (in two divided 12-hourly doses) with the dose adjusted to maintain a 12-hour trough level of 110 to 170 μg per liter. In a controlled trial using this regimen a significant reduction in proteinuria and an arrest of the progressive loss of proteinuria was achieved. It is evident from these experiences that aggressive therapy is indicated even in patients with renal insufficiency. Up to what degree of renal insufficiency one can intervene and still expect to see a benefit is not clear at present. Considering, however, that patients with more advanced renal insufficiency are otherwise destined to develop renal failure, it would seem that giving the patient the benefit of aggressive therapy is indicated.

In light of the above-mentioned information, it is our practice to be content to follow blood pressure, renal function, and urinary protein excretion in patients with proteinuria less than 2 g per 24 hours. For nephrotic patients, we institute therapy with prednisone in a dose of 1 mg per kilogram of body weight per day for 2 to 3 weeks. The dose of prednisone is then raised by 20 percent and the drug is given on alternate days. The alternate-day dose of prednisone is tapered at the rate of 5 mg every week, reaching a dose of 30 to 40 mg after about 3 months of therapy. Unless protein excretion has decreased by 50 percent or to less than 2 g, the patient is then given cyclophosphamide in a dose of 2 mg per kilogram, and the dose is adjusted to maintain the leucocyte count above 3,000 per cubic millimeter. Patients with renal insufficiency may be candidates for cyclophosphamide therapy right from the outset. Immunosuppression is discontinued when daily protein excretion has decreased to less than 2 g, and the patient is maintained on 20 to 30 mg of prednisone on alternate days thereafter. In our experience, nearly 30 percent of the patients have one or more relapses, and when they occur, these are treated in the same manner as that outlined earlier in this chapter. Subsequent remissions, however, are achieved in about half the time it takes for the first remission.

■ COMPLICATIONS

General

Hypovolemia resulting from hypoproteinemia combined with overvigorous diuretic therapy may impair renal function in membranous nephropathy as it may in other forms of nephrotic syndrome. Allergic interstitial nephritis may result from the use of diuretics, antibiotics, or other drugs and be superimposed on the underlying membranous nephropathy. This should be considered particularly in patients in whom there is a sudden decline in renal function.

Renal Vein Thrombosis

One complication that seems to appear quite frequently in patients with membranous nephropathy is renal vein thrombosis. This complication—which is so common that it was formerly believed to be a major cause of membranous nephropathy—has been reported in up to 50 percent of patients in some series, but probably averages 10 to 15 percent. When this complication leads to thromboembolism, it should be treated with heparin followed by long-term warfarin. Treatment usually leads to the disappearance of the clot on subsequent angiographic studies and to the protection against further embolism. It is not clear when treatment should be discontinued; the propensity to thrombosis probably remains for as long as the nephrotic syndrome persists. The question arises as to whether all nephrotic patients should routinely receive prophylactic oral or parenteral (low molecular weight heparin) anticoagulant therapy. A recent report employing decision analysis provided an affirmative answer. This practice, however, does not appear to have been widely adopted.

When renal vein thrombosis is present without any evidence of acute or chronic embolization, it is unclear whether a serious reduction in renal function or an increase in proteinuria results. Thus, in patients who show no evidence of embolization, it may not be necessary to perform routine renal vein angiography, renal vein Doppler study, or magnetic resonance imaging.

Rapidly Progressive Glomerulonephritis

Clinical signs and symptoms of rapidly progressive glomerulonephritis with the biopsy finding of crescentic glomerulonephritis superimposed on membranous nephropathy are occasionally seen. Antibodies directed against glomerular basement membrane antigens may or may not be present. There is no evidence to recommend any different management from that indicated in the classic form of rapidly progressive glomerulonephritis (described elsewhere in this text).

Transplantation

In patients in whom membranous nephropathy has progressed to end-stage renal failure, transplantation is often performed. Although the membranous lesion may occasionally recur in the transplanted kidney, it frequently does not impair its function.

Suggested Reading

Cameron JS, Healy MJR, Adu D. The Medical Research Council trial of short-term high-dose alternate day prednisolone in idiopathic membranous nephropathy with nephrotic syndrome in adults. Q J Med 1990; NS 74:133–156.

Cattran C, Greenwood C, Ritchie S, et al. A controlled trial of cyclosporine in patients with progressive membranous nephropathy. Kidney Int 1995; 47:1130–1135.

Cattran DC, Delmore T, Roscoe J, et al. A randomized controlled trial of prednisone in patients with idiopathic membranous nephropathy. N Engl J Med 1989; 320:210–215.

Donadio JV Jr, Torres VE, Velosa JA, et al. Idiopathic membranous nephropathy: The natural history of untreated patients. Kidney Int 1988; 33:708–715.

Jindal K, West M, Bear R, Goldstein M. Long-term benefits of therapy with cyclophosphamide and prednisone in patients with membranous glomerulonephritis and impaired renal function. Am J Kidney Dis 1992; 19:61–67.

Ponticelli C, Zucchelli P, Passerini P, et al. A 10-year follow-up of a randomized study with methylprednisolone and chlorambucil in membranous nephropathy. Kidney Int 1995; 48:1600–1604.

MEMBRANOPROLIFERATIVE GLOMERULONEPHRITIS

Daniel C. Cattran, M.D.

Membranoproliferative glomerulonephritis (MPGN) is a chronic nephritis that has had a number of different labels over the past 20 years, including lobular glomerulonephritis, mesangiocapillary glomerulonephritis, and chronic hypocomplementemic glomerulonephritis.

The prevalence of the disease is decreasing worldwide. During the 1970s, it represented approximately 10 percent of the annual total in several renal biopsy surveys, including our own, but during the last 5 years, its incidence has dropped in many reviews to less than 5 percent. It remains an important type of glomerulonephritis, however, since more than 50 percent of the patients eventually progress to end-stage renal failure. The list of secondary causes has increased, and although it is dominated by systemic diseases such as mixed essential cryoglobulinemia and systemic lupus erythematosus, other causes (e.g., malignancies including lymphoma, carcinomas, and infections such as subacute bacterial endocarditis and acquired immunodeficiency syndrome) have also been recognized as etiologic agents. Hepatitis C virus (HCV)–associated MPGN has been found in up to 40 percent of patients previously ascribed to have idiopathic MPGN. Although this has almost always been associated with some degree of liver enzyme elevation, evidence for chronic liver disease may be slight or absent. Most cases (>65 percent) are associated with the findings of a mixed (type 2) cryoglobulin in the serum with the usual associated laboratory and clinical features. The lobular pattern observed on light microscopy represents an accentuation of the segmental nature of the glomerulus and is caused by proliferation of the mesangial cells and their associated matrix. The mesangial expansion extends out and around the capillary loops, and the subsequent laying down of new basement membrane on the surface of this matrix produces the double-layered appearance to the glomerular basement membrane and the classic "tram tracking" noted on periodic acid-Schiff (PAS) staining. The two major variants of MPGN are distinguished by their appearance on electron microscopy. Type I has subendothelial deposits and type II has a ribbonlike continuous "deposit" of electron-dense material within the basement membrane. A less common type III has features of type I combined with subepithelial deposits.

There does appear to be a genetic marker or link of the disorder to a particular major histocompatibility complex—i.e., the extended haplotype HLA-B8, DR3, SCO1, GLO2, with a relative risk score of 15 to 1. The actual pathogenesis of the disorder, however, remains obscure. Discovery of the unique autoantibody C3 nephritic factor (C3NeF) was initially believed to be a major link to disease pathogenesis, but its importance has been reduced by the finding of the antibody in patients without significant renal disease, in patients with no functioning renal mass, in patients who had undergone bilateral nephrectomy, and even in patients with secondary forms of the disorder. The role of cell-mediated immunity also remains poorly defined, and although there is some in vitro evidence to support T-cell malfunction, in vivo these cells appear to perform normally.

It has been recognized for the past decade that platelet survival is significantly reduced in patients with active MPGN. Although this abnormality may not be of primary pathogenetic importance, it has been the rationale for several different treatment protocols.

Eighty percent of patients with MPGN have the type I variant, 10 to 20 percent have type II, and less than 5 percent type III. The mode of presentation of MPGN is extremely variable and includes the acute nephritic syndrome (10 to 20 percent of patients), asymptomatic proteinuria (20 to 30 percent), and the nephrotic syndrome (10 to 20 percent). Other findings at onset include gross hematuria in 5 to 10 percent of patients, hypertension in as many as 20 percent, and asymptomatic but significant elevations of serum creatinine values in a further 10 to 20 percent.

Type I MPGN can be seen in patients of any age, although it is most common in patients between the ages of 5 and 40 years. Type II, on the other hand, is almost always seen in patients 3 to 20 years of age. The third component of complement (C3) may be depressed in type I but is very commonly depressed in type II and can be extremely low. A C3 level of less than 10 percent of normal in a patient with no evidence of systemic disease is almost pathognomonic for idiopathic type II MPGN. In many cases of type II and some type I MPGN, the autoantibody C3NeF is present and is the likely cause of this hypocomplementemia. The precise relationship between the complement abnormalities and immunopathogenesis is poorly defined, but the important clinical point is the lack of correlation between the level of the complement components and disease activity. Sex distribution is the same for all types of MPGN, and although whites are the race most commonly affected, the disease has been reported in both blacks and Asians. Table 1 outlines the common clinical, laboratory, and pathologic features of types I and II MPGN. Type II MPGN is the one associated with partial lipodystrophy (in 5 percent of patients), but otherwise it and type III MPGN, by mode of presentation and survival, are indistinguishable from type I MPGN. The natural history of patients with MPGN has been difficult to determine because many have received drug treatment either because they had an acute, catastrophic presentation or because the physician believed that the process was going to be progressive and wanted to "do something." Most series of untreated patients have indicated that the overall 50 percent actuarial renal survival in types I, II, and III MPGN is reached between the eighth and twelfth year after presentation.

■ MANAGEMENT

Prognosis

There is no proven definitive treatment for MPGN. A major problem in interpreting therapeutic efficacy is the fluctuations that occur in the natural history of many MPGN

Table 1 Pathologic Variates and Their Clinical Features

CLINICAL	TYPE I	TYPE II
Mean age	18 yrs	12 yrs
Age range	5–60 yrs	3–35 yrs
Sex (M/F)	1/1	1/1
Blood pressure	N/↑	N/↑
Urinalysis	Active	Active
24 hour protein	0.1–>5 g	0.1–>5 g
Creatinine clearance	N/↓	N/↓
C3	N/↓	↓↓
Renal survival*		
5 yrs	85%	85%
10 yrs	60%	60%
Pathology		
Light microscopy	Mesangial cell proliferation and increased mesangial matrix, classic double contouring of basement membrane	Mesangial cell proliferation, apparent basement membrane thickening that tends to be segmental
Immunofluorescence	Peripheral C3, ± IgG ± mesangial deposits	C3-interrupted peripheral deposits ± "mesangial rings"
Electron microscopy	Subendothelial ± paramesangial deposits with mesangial matrix interposition and basement membrane splitting	Intramembranous diffuse dense "deposits" in the capillary loops ± mesangium and rarely Bowman's capsule and proximal tubule membrane

*From presentation.

patients. This variability includes periods of acute deterioration and rapid spontaneous improvement in both the glomerular filtration rate and proteinuria in as many as one-third of patients. However, there are certain clinical features associated with a poor prognosis, including a persistent nephrotic-range proteinuria lasting for more than 6 months and/or a progressive decline in creatinine clearance over a similar time frame. Unfavorable histologic features include significant glomerulosclerosis and crescent formation. By contrast, isolated focal and segmental MPGN lesions rather than diffuse involvement carries with it a much more benign prognosis.

Features of no prognostic importance include a nephritic presentation, the initial creatinine and proteinuria values, the age of onset, gender, and the complement profile.

Anticoagulants

The following comments with regard to drug therapy are limited to type I MPGN since there have been no series large enough to permit valid conclusions to be drawn relative to type II or type III. The most intriguing therapeutic trial was the use of a combination of aspirin (975 mg per day) and dipyridamole (325 mg per day). The study was a well-designed, randomized, 1 year trial. The rate of change in renal function was measured not only by the standard creatinine clearance but also by the more precise radioisotope iothalamate method. An additional interesting feature of this study was the monitoring of the patient's platelet survival times. At follow-up there was both better preservation of the glomerular filtration rate and better platelet survival in the drug-treated group compared with the control group. There was no improvement in the urine sediment activity, the complement profile, or the severity of proteinuria. The majority of the treated patients continued to receive the medication, and after an average of 4 years of follow-up, they had a lower percentage of end-stage renal failure than the control group. This drug combination can produce problems, especially in the more advanced renal failure patients, and three of the treated patients (15 percent) had to discontinue the medication because of bleeding complications.

Another trial used a regimen of warfarin combined with dipyridamole and was also shown to have a beneficial effect. These results were much less convincing considering the sample size and complication rate; the trial was designed to be a randomized, crossover, prospective study of 22 patients, but because of problems, only 13 completed the study. Significant side effects included one death due to a cerebrovascular accident, two significant hemorrhagic episodes (in two patients), and a duodenal ulcer (in one patient). I do not use or recommend this regimen.

The introduction of anticoagulant therapy and antiplatelet agents was based on the observation that platelet survival time is reduced in patients with MPGN. These drugs may reduce platelet-derived growth factor release, decrease smooth muscle cell proliferation, and reduce chemotaxis of monocytes and neutrophils to the area, thereby helping to limit the severity of injury. The aspirin and dipyridamole may also act via inhibition of intrarenal prostaglandin synthesis and/or through a change in the balance between platelet thromboxane production and endothelial cell prostacyclin release.

Anticoagulant Plus Cytotoxic Agents

An uncontrolled study done in the early 1970s combined a cytotoxic agent with an oral anticoagulant and dipyridamole and showed this therapy to produce a dramatic improvement in MPGN. A more rigorous, prospective study done by our group using a similar therapy showed it to be of no benefit in the treatment of MPGN, and I therefore believe that this approach should no longer be considered for these patients.

Corticosteroids

An alternate therapeutic approach has been prednisone therapy. Studies of this therapy have been confined to children, and although the studies have been performed over the long term, they have been uncontrolled. The authors' latest results indicate that steroid treatment for patients with type I MPGN results in a significant improvement in both renal survival and severity of proteinuria. It is interesting to note that this beneficial effect was demonstrated only after 3 years of treatment and only if the prednisone was initiated within 12 months of presentation. The dose is substantial; alternate-day prednisone is begun at 2 to 2.5 mg per kilogram and is reduced to 1.5 to 2.5 mg per kilogram after 1 year, to 1 to 1.5 mg per kilogram after 2 years, and to 0.8 to 1.5 mg per kilogram after 3 years. These patients are still receiving significant prednisone in a dose between 0.2 and 1 mg per kilogram at 4 years. The International Study of Kidney Disease in Children (ISKDC) carried out a prospective randomized trial to test this regimen. In MPGN patients with a glomerular filtration rate of greater than 40 ml per minute and significant proteinuria, they compared the effects of prednisone, 40 mg per m^2 given on alternate days, with those of placebo. Patients excluded from the study were those with any evidence of systemic disease and those previously treated with steroids or immunosuppressive drugs. There were 37 patients entered into the study, 23 of whom received treatment and 14 of whom received placebo. There was better preservation of creatinine clearance in the prednisone group; however, survival rates at years 2 through 5 were not different, and significant side effects did occur in the treated patients. These included seizures (in 8 percent of patients), severe hypertension (in 4 percent), growth retardation (in 4 percent), osteoporosis (in 4 percent), glycosuria (in 4 percent), and cushingoid features and obesity (in 8 percent). Taking into account the risks of therapy, they concluded that the marginal improvement in preservation of the glomerular filtration rate did not outweigh the risks. A recently published article has advocated pulse or oral corticosteroids plus cyclophosphamide. They induced a clinical remission in 15 out of 19 patients treated, but the follow-up was only 10 months and toxicity information was difficult to assess.

Other Therapeutic Approaches

Other treatment routines have been advocated. These have included the long-term use of nonsteroidal anti-inflammatory drugs (NSAIDs) and, more recently, the immunosuppressive agent cyclosporine. The former is associated with a significant reduction in the glomerular filtration rate, although uncontrolled trials have shown some evidence to suggest that the improvement in proteinuria is disproportionate to the reduction in the glomerular filtration rate. This reduction in the glomerular filtration rate may be acceptable, especially if the patient is rescued from severe hypoalbuminemia and the associated debilitating edema. Cyclosporine may act through its suppression of T-cell activity or have an effect similar to that of the NSAIDs, with the improvement in proteinuria being related to an overall reduction in the glomerular filtration rate. This drug does have other significant side effects and its use must be considered experimental. Although the HCV-RNA and HCV antibodies are commonly found in the cryoglobulin, they have not yet been found in the immune complexes in the kidney. A response of the proteinuria component of the kidney disease to alpha-interferon treatment is often dramatic when the disease has been associated with HCV, especially if cryoglobulins are found in the circulation. However, the relapse rates are as high as 80 percent once the treatment is discontinued.

My own approach to this disorder is conservative. We are now very familiar with the patients (as many as one-third of those with the disease) who spontaneously improve after an acute nephritic syndrome presentation. If severe proteinuria (>4 g per day) or persistent and increasing creatinine (>1.5 mg per deciliter but less than 4 mg per deciliter) persists for more than 6 months, I initiate therapy using a low dose of aspirin (325 mg per day) combined with dipyridamole (225 mg per day). If the glomerular filtration rate stabilizes and proteinuria does not worsen over 6 months and if the patient is tolerating the medication without problems, I have the patient continue with this regimen indefinitely. If, however, during this period, the patient's condition deteriorates but the glomerular filtration rate is still greater than 50 percent of normal, I may try alternate-day prednisone or other experimental therapy, although only after the risk-benefit ratio has been carefully considered. On the other hand, if the initial biopsy shows only focal segmental lesions and the proteinuria remains at less than 3 g per day (<40 mg per kilogram) with good preservation of serum albumin and a serum creatinine of less than 1.5 mg per deciliter, I limit my treatment to symptomatic therapy—i.e., diuretics for edema, antihypertensive drugs (I use the angiotensin-converting enzyme inhibitors) for blood pressure control, and a modest restriction in dietary protein intake.

■ SPECIAL ASPECTS OF MPGN

As many as 100 percent of patients with type II MPGN have a recurrence in the renal allograft. Despite the presence of the dense "deposits," however, transplant survival seems to be unaffected and is equal to that of other primary types of glomerulonephritis. By contrast, although the recurrence of type I lesions occurs much less frequently (in 20 to 30 percent of patients), long-term preservation of the graft may be adversely affected. If patients with type I MPGN have had a rapid deterioration in native kidney function, a similar pattern is more likely to occur in their transplant allograft. Despite this problem, I still recommend transplantation for all patients with end-stage MPGN renal disease.

Suggested Reading

Cattran DC, Cardella CJ, Roscoe JM, et al. Results of a controlled drug trial in membranoproliferative glomerulonephritis. Kidney Int 1985; 27: 436–441.

Donadio JV, Anderson CF, Mitchell JC, et al. Membranoproliferative glomerulonephritis: A prospective clinical trial of platelet-inhibitor therapy. N Engl J Med 1984; 310:1421–1426.

Donadio JV, Offord KP. Reassessment of treatment results in membranoproliferative glomerulonephritis, with emphasis on life-table analysis. Am J Kidney Dis 1989; 14:445–451.

Faedda R, Satta S, Tanda F, et al. Immunosuppressive therapy of membranoproliferative glomerulonephritis. Nephron 1994; 67:59–65.

Johnson RJ, Willson R, Yamabe H, et al. Renal manifestations of hepatitis C virus infection. Kidney Int 1994; 46:1255–1263.

McEnery PT, McAdams AJ, West CD. The effect of prednisone in a high-dose, alternate-day regimen on the natural history of idiopathic membranoproliferative glomerulonephritis. Medicine 1986; 64:401–424.

Watson AR, Poucell S, Thorner P, et al. Membranoproliferative glomerulonephritis type I in children: Correlation of clinical features with pathologic subtypes. Am J Kidney Dis 1984; 9:141–146.

Zauner I, Bohler J, Braun N, et al. Effects of aspirin and dipyridamole on proteinuria in idiopathic membranoproliferative glomerulonephritis: a multicenter prospective clinical trial. Nephrol Dial Transplant 1994; 619–622.

MESANGIAL PROLIFERATIVE GLOMERULONEPHRITIS

Arthur H. Cohen, M.D.
Sharon G. Adler, M.D.

Glomerular lesions with mesangial IgM deposits (in this chapter to be synonymous with mesangial proliferative or injury glomerulonephritis or "IgM nephropathy") represent a somewhat controversial glomerulopathy. Since the initial emphasis of this immunopathologic "entity" in the mid-1970s, reports have both attested to, and disagreed with, the concept of it as a distinct pathologic or clincopathologic process.

The precise categorization of this "lesion" is difficult. One prevailing view is that in patients with nephrotic syndrome, glomerulonephritis with mesangial IgM deposits is part of a spectrum of injury with a common pathogenesis that includes minimal change disease at the benign end and focal and segmental glomerulosclerosis at the more malignant end. The mesangial "injury" lesion, because of clinical and pathological similarities to each of the others, is in an intermediate position. In support of this concept is the occasional finding of transitions between these three lesions in patients who undergo serial biopsies. A polar view is that it is a distinct entity unto itself. An intermediate consideration is that, regardless of the categorization, the presence of mesangial IgM deposits in glomeruli in a patient with nephrotic syndrome might be a marker for a poor response to corticosteroids and/or progression to renal failure, despite the relatively normal appearance of glomeruli.

This "lesion" is defined by its immunopathologic features: IgM (and often C3) granular deposits in all mesangial regions of all glomeruli. The light microscopic appearance may vary, ranging from normal glomeruli ("mesangial injury") to those with moderate degrees of mesangial hypercellularity. In general, all glomeruli in a biopsy are reasonably similar to one another. Capillary lumina are patent, and capillary walls and basement membranes are thin and single-contoured. Unless complicated, there are no segments of sclerosis. Ultrastructurally, there are small electron-dense deposits in mesangial regions in approximately 50 percent of the cases. When heavy proteinuria is present, the foot processes of visceral epithelial cells are completely effaced. The morphologic features of mesangial proliferative glomerulonephritis may also be associated with diffuse mesangial IgA deposites (Berger's disease), isolated C3 deposits, predominant IgG deposits, or no Ig or complement deposits. Thus "IgM nephropathy" is but one portion of a heterogeneous group of disorders having mesangial proliferation or hypercellularity in common.

There are four common presentations of this form of glomerular injury: asymptomatic proteinuria, heavy proteinuria often in the nephrotic range, isolated microscopic hematuria, or heavy proteinuria with hematuria. Mild hypertension is present in up to one-third of the patients. Laboratory studies are not diagnostically helpful. Serum albumin is low and hyperlipidemia is present in association with the nephrotic syndrome. Mild to moderate azotemia may be present in 25 to 50 percent of patients at the time of diagnosis. Serum complement and immunoglobulin levels are usually normal. Antibodies to nuclear or streptococcal antigens are absent. Genetic determinants have not been identified.

The clinical course is variable and, for the most part, depends upon the initial manifestation. Patients with isolated hematuria usually maintain normal renal function for a considerable period of time, although microscopic hematuria persists, occasionally punctuated by bouts of gross hematuria. Apparently, those with low-grade proteinuria also have a good long-term prognosis. On the other hand, patients with heavy proteinuria may progress to renal insufficiency. This usually occurs within several years of the onset and is heralded by increasing proteinuria and hypertension. It is invariably in patients who are, or have been, steroid-dependent, or, more commonly steroid-resistant and who have persistent heavy proteinuria, often with hematuria. In most instances, repeat renal biopsy discloses either the same lesion or segmental glomerulosclerosis and variable presence of mesangial IgM deposits.

The approach to therapy has not been well defined. The most common indication for treatment is the nephrotic syndrome. The effects of therapy on isolated microhematuria, non–nephrotic-range proteinuria, and progressive azotemia are less well appreciated. Reports from the United Kingdom in the early 1970s suggested that the prevalence of steroid-responsiveness in patients with primary mesangial proliferative glomerulonephritis was low. As a result, few patients were subsequently treated. More recently, however, many investigators have approached therapy in a manner similar to that given patients with minimal change disease. Utilizing high-dose oral prednisone (i.e., 60 mg per day or 120 mg every other day in adults or equivalent in children), the nephrotic syndrome has been reported to respond in up to 65 percent of patients, although frequent relapses, steroid dependence, and partial remissions are common. Nephrotic patients with prominent hematuria are less likely to respond to steroids than those without hematuria.

The use of cytotoxic agents is more controversial than corticosteroids. However, in a few cases, agents such as chlorambucil or cyclophosphamide have been utilized for their steroid-sparing effects in patients with frequently relapsing or steroid-dependent nephrotic syndrome. An occasional report has suggested that cytotoxic agents may be useful in inducing remission in small numbers of steroid-unresponsive patients. Cyclosporine has now been utilized in patients with minimal change disease and focal and segmental glomerulosclerosis who are either steroid-resistant, steroid-dependent, or frequent relapsers. The usefulness of this agent in mesangial proliferative glomerulonephritis remains to be determined. Similarly, the efficacy of nonsteroidal agents, angiotensin-coverting enzyme inhibitors, and low-protein diets in inducing remission or amelioration of nephrotic syndrome has not been specifically studied.

In summary, mesangial proliferative glomerulonephritis with IgM deposits is an uncommon form of renal disease. Its pathogenesis is poorly understood, but some now believe that it may be an intermediate form in a spectrum of disorders including minimal change disease and focal and segmental glomerulosclerosis. The prognosis also appears to be intermediate, with end-stage renal disease developing in a substantial, but not a precisely quantitated, number of patients over the course of many years. Patients most often present with nephrotic syndrome, but less common manifestations include non–nephrotic-range proteinuria and macroscopic or microscopic hematuria. Steroid responsiveness occurs in 25 to 65 percent of patients. In a small number of patients, cytotoxic agents may be useful adjuncts in treating steroid-unresponsive, steroid-dependent, or frequently relapsing nephrotic syndrome. A prospective randomized controlled trial, although difficult to achieve for this group, would be useful to define better the natural history and responsiveness to therapy of this form of glomerular injury.

OBSTRUCTIVE UROPATHY

Saulo Klahr, M.D.

In humans, the effects of urinary tract obstruction on renal function are diverse. Marked reductions in renal blood flow and glomerular filtration rate and significant changes in renal tubular function may occur. Chronic partial obstruction of the urinary tract can lead to progressive atrophy and destruction of nephrons and ultimately chronic renal insufficiency. Unilateral complete obstruction may be well tolerated for several days; however, if the obstruction persists for more than 1 week, some permanent damage ensues. By the end of 3 weeks of complete obstruction, recoverable function is usually nil. On the other hand, complete bilateral obstruction results in acute renal failure. Because obstructive uropathy is generally a remediable cause of kidney failure, early and accurate diagnosis and prompt treatment are vital to the preservation and restoration of renal function.

The clinical manifestations of obstructive uropathy vary. Bilateral complete obstruction of urine flow is manifested as anuria. Partial obstruction can cause fluctuating urine output, alternating from oliguria to polyuria, urinary tract infection that is usually refractory to treatment, abdominal or flank pain, or unexplained acute or chronic renal failure. Obstruction must always be included in the differential diagnosis of acute renal failure, especially when urine output fluctuates or anuria occurs suddenly (Tables 1 and 2).

GENERAL THERAPEUTIC CONSIDERATIONS

Once the diagnosis of obstructive uropathy is established, the next decision is whether or not surgical or instrumental procedures should be performed. High-grade or complete bilateral obstruction presenting as acute renal failure requires intervention as soon as possible. In these patients, the site of obstruction frequently determines the approach. If the obstructive lesion is distal to the bladder, passage of a urethral catheter may suffice, although this may require the aid of a urologist. In some cases, suprapubic cystostomy may be necessary. On the other hand, if the lesion lies proximal to the bladder (upper tract lesion—e.g., a malignant infiltration of the trigone by cervical or prostatic adenocarcinoma), then placement of nephrostomy tubes at the time of ultrasonography or passage of a retrograde ureteral catheter should be undertaken. Tubes should be placed in both obstructed renal calyces, since the potential for recovery of function by either kidney is not easily predicted at the time of the procedure. Such an approach may circumvent the need for dialysis and allows the physician time to determine the specific site and nature of the obstructing lesion. Further, the nephrostomy tube may be used for the local infusion of pharmacologic agents with which to treat infection, malignancy, or calculi. In patients with obstruction complicated by urinary tract infection and generalized sepsis, appropriate antibiotics and other supportive therapy are indicated.

Table 1 Causes of Upper Urinary Tract Obstruction

Urolithiasis	Gartner's duct cysts
Transitional cell cancer of the pelvis/ureter	Tubo-ovarian abscess
Blood clot	Endometriosis
Renal papillae	Uterine prolapse
Fungus ball	Diseases of the gastrointestinal tract
Ureter ligation	Crohn's disease
Primary obstruction of the ureteropelvic junction; intrinsic (congenital) vs. acquired (vessel crossing, postsurgical)	Diverticulitis
	Appendiceal abscess
Ureteral valve	Pancreatic lesions
Ureteral polyp	Diseases of the retroperitoneum
Vascular lesions	Retroperitoneal fibrosis
Abdominal aortic aneurysm	Tuberculosis
Iliac artery aneurysm	Sarcoidosis
Retrocaval ureter	Radiation fibrosis
Puerperal ovarian vein thrombophlebitis	Retroperitoneal hemorrhage
Fibrosis following vascular reconstructive surgery	Primary retroperitoneal tumors (e.g., lymphomas, sarcomas)
Diseases of the female reproductive tract	Secondary retroperitoneal tumors (e.g., cervix, bladder, colon, prostate)
Pregnancy	
Mass lesions of the uterus and ovary	Lymphocele
Ovarian remnants	Pelvic lipomatosis

Table 2 Causes of Lower Urinary Tract Obstruction

Phimosis	Prostatic calculi
Meatal stenosis	Neurogenic bladder
Paraphimosis	Benign prostatic hyperplasia
Urethral stricture	Psychogenic urinary retention
Urethral stone	Bladder calculus
Urethral diverticulum	Bladder cancer
Periurethral abscess	Ureterocele
Posterior urethral valves	Trauma
Anterior urethral valves	Straddle injury
Urethral surgery	Pelvic fracture
Prostatic abscess	

In patients with low-grade acute obstruction or partial chronic obstruction, surgical intervention may be delayed for a few weeks or even months. However, prompt relief of partial obstruction is indicated when: (1) there are multiple repeated episodes of urinary tract infection; (2) the patient has significant symptoms (flank pain, dysuria, voiding dysfunction); (3) there is urinary retention; and (4) there is evidence of recurrent or progressive renal damage. The presence of postvoid residual urine, urinary extravasation, ureterovesical reflux, or dilatation of the collecting system despite sterile urine are not indications for surgical intervention.

MANAGEMENT

Calculi

Stones are the most common cause of ureteral obstruction. The immediate treatment for ureteral stones consists of relief of pain, elimination of obstruction, and control of infection. Relief of pain in this setting is best accomplished by intramuscular injection of adequate doses of a narcotic analgesic. If the stone's diameter is less than 5 mm, urologic instrumentation or surgical intervention is not required, since 80 to 90 percent of these ureteral stones will pass spontaneously. Among ureteral stones in the 5 to 7 mm range, however, only 40 to 50 percent will pass, and stones larger than 7 mm will rarely pass spontaneously. High fluid intake designed to achieve urine volumes of at least 1.5 to 2.5 L daily help pass the stone. The urine must be strained through a gauze sponge to recover the calculi and the stone should be sent for analysis. If a stone completely blocks a ureter and does not move, surgical treatment should commence within a few days. However, if the obstruction is partial, the urine sterile, and the pain manageable, the patient may be observed for weeks or months before surgical therapy is undertaken.

Stone removal is indicated when there is complete obstruction, unremitting colic, urinary tract infection, and urosepsis, or a calculus that is too large to pass (i.e., >7 mm) or that has failed to move despite a trial of time (usually months) and increased fluid intake.

The treatment of urolithiasis has undergone marked changes during the past 10 years. A number of modalities for stone removal are available, including extracorporeal shock wave lithotripsy (ESWL), percutaneous nephrostolithotomy, a combination of these two therapies, ureteroscopic removal, open surgery, laparoscopic surgery, and chemolysis. Treatment selection is based on stone size, position and composition of the stone, anatomy of the collecting system, and the patient's health status and preferences.

The preferred therapeutic modality for patients with stones proximal to or at the level of the iliac vessels is ESWL. This treatment is effective and has a low complication rate. Individuals with stones distal to the iliac vessels that do not pass spontaneously are candidates for ESWL or ureteroscopic removal. The advantages of ureteroscopic removal are the high success rate (approaching 100 percent) of this procedure and its lower cost. New technologies including smaller rigid and flexible ureteroscopes, the development of electrohydraulic probes, the pulse dye laser, and new basket extraction devices have greatly improved ureteroscopic stone removal and decreased substantially the incidence of associated complications.

Patients with renal stones smaller than 2 cm are usually

treated with ESWL. Percutaneous nephrostolithotomy is preferred for larger stones, since the procedure provides a higher rate of stone-free results and fewer interventions are required. The composition of the stone should also be considered; brushite and cystine stones appear to be more resistant to shock-wave energy, and hence ESWL. In both in vitro models and in clinical practice, inferior stone-free intervals have been reported in patients with brushite and cystine stones. Open surgery is utilized in patients with large staghorn calculi having extremely dilated renal collecting systems with or without infundibular stenosis—factors which are known to impair the likelihood of obtaining a stone-free status. Open surgery is used relatively infrequently now because of the advent of ESWL, and ureteroscopic and percutaneous stone removal. The use of open surgery has varied from 0.3 to 4.1 percent of patients requiring stone removal since ESWL became available.

Broad-spectrum antibiotics are useful when infections complicate the presence of renal calculi. The choice of drugs should be based on the sensitivity studies of the organism isolated from the urine. However, antimicrobial therapy without relief of obstruction is not effective in controlling the infection. Therefore, when primary or secondary obstruction accompanies renal calculi, temporary relief of obstruction should be instituted promptly by insertion of a retrograde ureteral catheter. If the attempted retrograde catheter diversion is unsuccessful, a percutaneous nephrostomy tube can be placed. Whenever possible, relief of obstruction and infection should be achieved before stone manipulation and open surgery.

In summary, a stone less than 5 mm in diameter is likely to be passed without the need for surgical intervention. Even when stone removal appears necessary, in 95 percent of patients this can be achieved with ESWL or via a percutaneous nephrostomy alone, regardless of the size or location of the calculus. Surgical therapy is largely reserved for the few patients in whom the aforementioned measures fail. Earlier intervention is certainly indicated for patients whose history, laboratory data, and radiologic studies suggest complete obstruction, patients with infected urine, and patients with partial obstruction whose stone remains in the same position in the ureter for more than a few months.

Obstruction of the ureter by blood clots, a fungus ball, or papillary tissue can be managed by techniques similar to those employed in the treatment of stones. Significant obstruction attributable to neoplastic, inflammatory, and neurologic diseases must be treated aggressively, since it is unlikely to remit spontaneously. A decision as to whether to divert the urine in patients who have metastatic malignant disease must be made on an individual basis.

Patients with sterile hydronephrosis secondary to advanced pelvic malignancy and a short life expectancy are usually not considered for percutaneous nephrostomy, while those with a reasonable prospect for tumor response to chemotherapy and radiotherapy are strong candidates for the procedure.

Intramural Causes of Obstructive Uropathy

Intramural causes of upper urinary tract obstruction are managed by several diverse techniques. Infundibular stenosis is most commonly found following chronic infection of the renal parenchyma. This disorder can be managed either percutaneously through a nephrostomy tube (see later) into the affected infundibulum and subsequent infundibular dilatation or incision or through open exposure of the infundibulum and spatulation. Intramural obstruction due to congenital causes, such as ureteropelvic or ureterovesical junction obstruction or upper ureteral valves, requires open surgery. Ureteropelvic junction obstruction is managed by pyeloplasty. This technique can create a widely patent ureteropelvic junction. Ureterovesical junction obstruction can be corrected by resection of the distal end of the ureter and reimplantation of the remaining ureter into the bladder. Congenital ureteral valves often require surgical excision and ureteroureterostomy. Intrinsic masses in the ureter or renal pelvis should be approached carefully, as if they were carcinomas, so as to avoid seeding and dissemination of the tumor. Treatment for high-grade transitional carcinoma requires nephroureterectomy with an en bloc resection of a 1 cm cuff of bladder around the ureteral orifice. Benign tumors (papillomas, polyps of the ureter), and certain low-grade transitional cell carcinomas may be treated using laser ablation.

Extrinsic Causes of Obstructive Uropathy

Extrinsic obstruction of the ureter usually requires correction of the causative disease process. Ureteral obstruction as a result of an aneurysm of the abdominal aorta is treated by repair of the vascular lesion. Idiopathic retroperitoneal fibrosis is treated by open surgical ureteral lysis and intraperitoneal placement of the ureters. Distal ureteral obstruction from pelvic lipomatosis requires either ureteroneocystostomy into the anterior portion of the bladder or supravesical urinary diversion.

■ ROLE OF NEPHROSTOMY IN MANAGEMENT OF UPPER URETERAL OBSTRUCTION

Nephrostomy refers to the insertion of a tube through the kidney into the renal pelvis to provide immediate urinary drainage. Until the 1950s, all nephrostomy tubes were placed via an open surgical approach. This resulted in significant morbidity and mortality, since patients requiring emergency nephrostomy tube placement were often quite debilitated. In 1955, Goodwin reported the first case of a needle-derived nephrostomy tube placed under fluoroscopic guidance. The technique did not gain popularity until the 1970s, when the advent of ultrasonography and improved methods of fluoroscopy made the percutaneous approach more feasible. Currently, almost all nephrostomy tubules are placed percutaneously by an interventional radiologist or urologist. This is usually done with local anesthesia and takes less than 40 minutes.

The most common indications for placement of a nephrostomy tube are the need to provide a conduit to the kidney for percutaneous stone removal and the need to relieve ureteral obstruction secondary to neoplasia, inflammatory disease, or lower tract extrinsic or intrinsic obstruction in which the patient's condition does not permit a more definitive surgical procedure. Likewise, unmanageable infection in an obstructed system is another common indication. It is not unusual to note dramatic clinical improvement within hours of percutaneous drainage in the patient with urosepsis.

Potential early complications of nephrostomy are perirenal hemorrhage and acute obstruction from clot formation. One of the more serious delayed complications is dislodgement of the nephrostomy tube. This is considered an emergency; the tube should be replaced immediately, otherwise the tract will seal off, usually within 24 hours. Another problem occurring after nephrostomy tube removal is the exsanguinating hemorrhage from a renal pseudoaneurysm. This occurs in 0.5 to 1 percent of patients and is best managed by immediate selective embolization of the affected vessel. Long-term complications, such as infection, calculus formation, and pyelonephritis, are significant and may lead to renal failure.

Except in unusual circumstances, long-term urinary diversion by the nephrostomy tube is not recommended. In many patients, however, several years may pass without the development of serious complications from their nephrostomy tubes. Also, in patients with extrinsic obstruction secondary to metastatic carcinoma, the nephrostomy tract can be used to manipulate a catheter into the bladder. A small tube can be placed through the affected flank and kidney with its pigtail end left in the bladder. The external portion of the stent can be clamped, thereby providing unobstructed flow from the affected kidney to the patient's bladder. This eliminates the need for external drainage bags and also facilitates in the changing of the tube. In essence, all nephrostomy tubes or indwelling stents are changed every 3 months to decrease the build-up of concretions and to preclude breakage of ureteral stents within the collecting system.

For chronically obstructed kidneys, a period of percutaneous drainage may permit significant restoration of renal function. With this knowledge and with periodic determination of split renal function studies, treatment can be planned effectively. A lack of significant improvement in function might suggest, for example, that nephrectomy rather than reparative surgery should be undertaken.

■ LOWER URINARY TRACT OBSTRUCTION

Bladder Neck and Urethra

Bladder neck and urethral obstruction should be surgically repaired in ambulatory patients who have recurrent infections, especially when associated with reflux, evidence of renal parenchymal damage, total urinary retention, repeated bleeding, or other severe symptoms. Difficulties with voiding secondary to benign prostatic hyperplasia do not always follow a progressive course. Therefore, a man with minimal symptoms, no infection, and a normal upper urinary tract may be observed safely until he and his physician agree that surgery is desirable. Urethral stricture in men that is secondary to infection or trauma is frequently treated by simple dilation or direct vision internal urethrotomy. In these patients, radiographic and endoscopic follow-up care is essential to rule out recurrence. The incidence of bladder neck and urethral obstruction in women is low and has been overestimated in the past; hence urethral dilation, internal urethrotomy, meatotomy, and revision of the bladder neck are seldom indicated. In some patients, suprapubic cystostomy may be necessary for bladder drainage. This is especially indicated in patients who are unable to void after sustaining injury to the urethra or who have an impassable urethral stricture.

Again, advances in urologic instrumentation have further decreased the indications for open surgery. Almost all suprapubic cystostomies are performed using a percutaneous approach under fluoroscopic guidance. Open cystostomy is rarely performed. In addition, a closed transurethral approach is used to treat most patients with prostatic hyperplasia (≥60 g of tissue), urethral strictures, bladder neck contractures, bladder calculi, and superficial bladder tumors.

Bladder Dysfunction

When obstructive uropathy is a consequence of neuropathic bladder function, urodynamic studies are essential to establish a treatment regimen. In all cases, the main therapeutic goals are to establish the bladder as a site of urine storage without causing renal parenchymal injury and to provide a mechanism for bladder emptying that is acceptable to the patient. In general, these patients fall into one of two groups: those with bladder atony secondary to lower motor neuron injury and those with unstable bladder function attributable to upper motor neuron disease. In both cases, ureteral reflux and renal parenchymal injury may occur, although it is more common with the hyperactive upper motor neuron bladder. This problem may be potentiated by sphincter-detrusor dyssynergia or by using external compression (Credé maneuver) or increasing abdominal pressure (Valsalva maneuver) to aid voiding.

Neurogenic bladder function caused by diabetes mellitus is a classic example of lower motor neuron disease. Voiding at regular intervals is one method to aid satisfactory bladder emptying in patients with the condition. Occasionally, these individuals respond to cholinergic medications. Publications on the use of bethanechol chloride (Urecholine), 50 mg orally, have seriously questioned its long-term value. Overdistention of the bladder impairs emptying, since detrusor contraction is essential to sphincter relaxation. Thus, bladder outlet obstruction may be a major problem. Alpha-adrenergic blockers such as phenoxybenzamine hydrochloride relax urethral sphincter tone but have only limited success because of side effects. Table 3 summarizes the drugs used in the treatment of lower urinary tract dysfunction and their proposed mechanism of action.

Another alternative for men with a flaccid bladder is external sphincterotomy. This transurethral procedure may be successful in relieving outlet obstruction and promoting bladder emptying, but it has the disadvantage of causing urinary incontinence and requires that the patient wear an external collection device. In men, this problem can be obviated by the use of a penile clamp; however, the clamps often result in significant morbidity owing to urethral erosion and penile edema. In women, the incontinence associated with external sphincterotomy precludes its use. In addition, the implantation of artificial urinary sphincters has been partially successful. Although these devices are useful, problems with their longevity have hindered their widespread acceptance.

The most ideal treatment for patients with significant residual urine and recurrent bouts of urosepsis is clean intermittent catheterization (CIC) performed at regular in-

Table 3 Drugs Used in the Treatment of Lower Urinary Tract Dysfunction

Drugs that facilitate urine storage
1. By increasing urethral tone
   Beta-blockers (propranolol hydrochloride)
   Alpha-adrenergic agonists (imipramine hydrochloride, phenylpropanolamine hydrochloride)
2. By inhibiting bladder (detrusor) contractility
   Anticholinergic agents (propantheline hydrochloride)
   Smooth muscle depressants (imipramine hydrochloride, dicyclomine hydrochloride, oxybutynin chloride)
   Alpha-adrenergic antagonists (prazosin hydrochloride, phenoxybenzamine hydrochloride)

Drugs that facilitate voiding
1. By increasing bladder (detrusor) contractility
   Cholinergic agents (bethanechol chloride)
2. By decreasing sphincter tone
   Alpha-adrenergic antagonists (prazosin hydrochloride, phenoxybenzamine hydrochloride, clonidine hydrochloride)
   Skeletal muscle relaxants (diazepam, dantrolene sodium)

tervals. Ideally catheterization should be performed four to five times per day, so that the amount of urine drained from the bladder does not exceed 300 to 400 ml. This technique has met with considerable success in almost all age groups but requires patient acceptance and careful training.

In patients with unstable urine bladder function attributable to upper motor neuron lesions, the major goal is to improve the storage function of the bladder. Pharmacologic maneuvers include the use of anticholinergic agents such as oxybutynin chloride (Ditropan), 5 mg every 4 to 6 hours. Adjunctive therapy such as CIC is frequently necessary to ensure complete bladder emptying and prevent incontinence.

In all patients with neurogenic bladders, chronic indwelling catheters are to be avoided if possible. In addition to problems of external drainage, bladder stones, urosepsis, and urethral erosion, chronic indwelling catheters are associated with the occurrence of squamous cell carcinoma of the bladder. Patients managed in this fashion for more than 5 years should undergo yearly cystoscopic examinations.

Finally, surgical diversions are indicated for (1) deterioration of renal function despite conservative measures, (2) intractable incontinence, (3) a small contracted bladder, and (4) multiple bladder fistulae. Intermittent bacteriuria is seldom an indication for this treatment, since it is common to all therapeutic approaches to the neurogenic bladder. The ileal conduit is the operation of choice for permanent diversion. Although many individuals do well after this procedure, operative mortality, postoperative intestinal obstruction, and stomal obstruction are complications that make the operation far from ideal. Further, recent studies have indicated that in as many as 80 percent of patients, there will be a progressive decline in renal function. A continent form of ileal diversion has become available: the Koch pouch. With this procedure, an ileal reservoir with a 300 to 500 ml capacity is made. A continent stoma is placed in the right lower quadrant of the abdomen, which the patient must empty by catheterization four times per day. This method of diversion alleviates the need for any external collection devices.

In patients requiring short-term indwelling urethral catheters, good care is necessary to prevent urinary tract infection. Men are instructed to cleanse the glans twice per day with an antimicrobial soap and then to apply an antibiotic ointment. Given specific indications for catheter drainage, proper patient selection, aseptic technique, closed urinary drainage, the judicious use of systemic antimicrobials, and proper catheter care, the indwelling urethral catheter is a satisfactory means of short-term diversion, and in rare instances, of long term urinary diversion. The principles of closed drainage are that the system never be open, that the urine in the drainage tube never come in contact with the urine in the collecting bag, and that, at all times, the bag be in a dependent position. Cultures can be obtained by clamping the catheter for a few minutes and then using a small needle and syringe to aspirate urine from the lumen of the catheter. I prefer not to break the drainage system for catheter irrigation or for the use of antibiotic irrigating solutions to reduce infection, as has been advocated by some. In patients requiring long-term catheter drainage, intermittent irrigation with an acid citrate solution is useful in reducing encrustation.

In the past, there has been some concern and controversy regarding the possible complications of rapid decompression of a severely distended bladder. It has been advised that the grossly distended bladder be drained slowly over a period of hours rather than all at once. It has also been suggested that rapid emptying of the distended bladder may be followed by hypotension and syncope or hemorrhagic cystitis attributable to sudden decompression of stretched mucosal blood vessels. These concerns appear unjustified, since it has been found that the intravesical pressure in patients with acute urinary retention falls precipitously to near-normal values after the first deciliter of urine is withdrawn, indicating that any sudden decompressive effect on blood vessels would be maximal during the removal of the initial volume of urine.

POSTOBSTRUCTIVE DIURESIS

Postobstructive diuresis refers to the marked polyuria that can occur after relief of urinary tract obstruction. This polyuria is usually associated with the excretion of large amounts of sodium, potassium, magnesium, and other solutes. Although self-limited (it may last several days), the losses of salt and water may be of such magnitude as to cause hypokalemia, hyponatremia or hypernatremia, hypomagnesemia and/or marked contraction of the extracellular fluid (ECF) volume, and peripheral vascular collapse. In many patients, however, a brisk diuresis after relief of urinary tract obstruction may be physiologically appropriate rather than caused by an inability of the postobstructed kidney to maintain volume and solute homeostasis. A postobstructive diuresis is appropriate and does not compromise the volume status of the patient when it is caused by excretion of excess salt, water, and urea retained during the period of obstruction. This diuresis is transient and usually subsides within the first day or two after relief of obstruction without causing depletion of the ECF volume. It is often impossible, however, to distinguish patients experiencing benign postobstructive diuresis from those who have a true defect in tubular reabsorption of salt and water on the basis of urine volume and composition alone. Thus, replacement therapy should be guided by clinical and laboratory evidence of the adequacy of the ECF volume and not by the volume of the urine only.

Postobstructive diuresis may be artificially prolonged by overzealous administration of salt and water after relief of obstruction. Replacement of excreted salt and water maintains a state of expansion of the ECF and hence results in the continuous excretion of the excess salt and water administered. Thus, fluid replacement may be justified only when excessive losses of sodium and water occur that are inappropriate for the volume status of the patient and are presumably caused by an intrinsic tubular defect in the reabsorption of sodium and water.

For patients with postobstructive diuresis, the appropriate fluid replacement depends largely on what is excreted. Although intravenous fluid administration may be necessary, urinary losses should be replaced only to the extent necessary to prevent hypovolemia, hypotension, hypokalemia, and/or hypomagnesemia. Excessive fluid administration only prolongs the duration of the postobstructive diuresis. Orthostatic hypotension and tachycardia are perhaps the best indicators of when intravenous fluid administration is needed. To distinguish between inappropriate diuresis and the excretion of fluid retained or excess fluid administration, it may be necessary to decrease the rate of intravenous fluid administration to levels below those of urinary output and observe the patient carefully for signs of volume depletion (hypotension, tachycardia, and stabilization or elevation in the level of blood urea nitrogen, which was previously decreasing). In the case of inappropriate diuresis, appropriate fluid replacement consists of the prompt quantitative replacement of urinary losses of water, sodium, potassium, and magnesium. This is best accomplished by frequent measurements of urine volume and serum and urine electrolytes. With massive diuresis, such measurements may be required every 6 hours. The patient's body weight should be measured daily and occasionally even more often. Fluids administered should be tailored to match the urinary excretion of water and electrolytes.

In most instances, urinary losses of salt and water may be replaced with solutions of 0.45 percent sodium chloride to which sodium bicarbonate and potassium chloride have been added. Replacement of magnesium may be accomplished by adding magnesium sulfate (supplied as 2 ml ampules containing 8 mEq magnesium) to the sodium chloride solution. Sometimes replacement of phosphate losses may be necessary. Either 42 percent sodium phosphate (15 ml ampules containing 45 mmol phosphate and 60 mEq sodium) or 46 percent potassium phosphate (15 ml ampules containing 45 mmol phosphate and 66 mEq potassium) may be added to 5 percent dextrose of 0.45 percent sodium chloride solutions.

Suggested Reading

Coplen DE, Hare JY, Zderic SA, et al. Ten year experience with prenatal intervention for hydronephrosis. J Urol 1996; 156:1142–1145.

Lau MWM, Temperley DE, Mehta S, et al. Urinary tract obstruction and nephrostomy drainage in pelvic malignant disease. Br J Urol 1995; 76: 565–569.

Watkinson AF, A'Hern RP, Jones A, et al. The role of percutaneous nephrostomy in malignant urinary tract obstruction. Clin Radiol 1993; 47:32–35.

Weon AJ. Neuromuscular dysfunction of the lower urinary tract. In: Walsh PC, Retik AB, Stamey TA, Vaughan ED, eds., Campbell's Urology, 6th ed. Philadelphia: WB Saunders, 1992:573–642.

Wilson WT, Preminger GM. Extracorporeal shock wave lithotripsy: an update. Urol Clin North Am 1990; 17:231–242.

NEPHROLITHIASIS

Charles Y.C. Pak, M.D.

Nephrolithiasis is a common disorder affecting 1 to 5 percent of the population, with an annual incidence rate of 0.1 to 0.3 percent in the Western world. It may result in considerable morbidity by causing obstruction, hematuria, or infection.

Although the ultimate symptomatic presentation may be the same, it is clear that nephrolithiasis is heterogeneous with respect to composition and etiologic factors. Renal stones typically contain calcium (calcareous calculi, composed of calcium oxalate and/or calcium phosphate). They are less commonly composed of uric acid, cystine, or struvite (magnesium ammonium phosphate) (noncalcareous calculi). Many patients with stones have been found to suffer from a variety of physiologic or metabolic disturbances, including hypercalciuria, hyperuricosuria, hyperoxaluria, and hypocitraturia. Some of these derangements may be endocrinologic, involving altered metabolism of parathyroid hormone and vitamin D.

The above recognition has led to the refined classification and treatment of nephrolithiasis. Thus, it has been possible to formulate reliable diagnostic criteria on the basis of underlying metabolic derangements in patients with nephrolithiasis. Moreover, treatments could be specifically selected for the ability to "reverse" the particular underlying physiologic disturbances.

This selective approach argues for a thorough diagnostic differentiation of various causes of nephrolithiasis and emphasizes the need for a careful selection of treatment program for each cause of nephrolithiasis. Its feasibility and practicality are considered in detail here.

Table 1 Classification of Nephrolithiasis

CALCAREOUS RENAL CALCULI	NONCALCAREOUS RENAL CALCULI
Hypercalciuria	Uric acid stones
Resorptive	Cystine stones
Absorptive	Cystinuria
Renal	Infection stones
Hyperuricosuria	Infection with urea-splitting organisms
Hyperoxaluria	
Primary	
Secondary	
Hypocitraturia	
No "metabolic" abnormality	

METABOLIC CLASSIFICATION OF NEPHROLITHIASIS

A simple and logical method of diagnostic differentiation of nephrolithiasis is the categorization on the basis of underlying physiologic abnormalities (Table 1). This classification assumes that these physiologic disturbances are pathogenetically important in stone formation. Although complete validation is lacking, it is generally agreed that excessive renal excretion of calcium, oxalate, uric acid, or cystine may contribute to stone formation by rendering the urinary environment supersaturated with respect to stone-forming salts. Hypocitraturia increases urinary saturation and reduces inhibitor activity against the crystallization of calcium salts. This classification is based on major or principal physiologic abnormalities. It is recognized that several disturbances may coexist in a given disorder.

THERAPEUTIC CONSIDERATIONS

Improved elucidation of pathophysiology and formulation of diagnostic criteria for different causes of nephrolithiasis have made feasible the adoption of a selective or an optimum treatment program. Such a program should (1) reverse the underlying physiologic derangements, (2) inhibit new stone formation, (3) overcome nonrenal complications of the disease process, and (4) cause no serious side effects.

The rationale for the selection of a certain treatment program according to its ability to reverse physiologic abnormalities as outlined previously is the assumption that the particular physiologic aberrations identified with the given disorder are etiologically important in the formation of renal stones and that the correction of these disturbances would prevent stone formation. Moreover, it is assumed that such a selective treatment program would be more effective and safe than a "random" treatment. Despite a lack of conclusive experimental verification, these hypotheses appear reasonable and logical.

General Treatment Measures

In patients with calcium stones, moderate oxalate restriction should be imposed by discouraging ingestion of dark greens (such as spinach), rhubarb, brewed tea, and chocolate. Ascorbic acid supplementation should be denied because of potential metabolism of vitamin C to oxalate. A high sodium intake should be discouraged; the avoidance of "salty" foods and using salt shakers should be advised. A moderate dietary calcium restriction is advisable in patients with intestinal hyperabsorption of calcium (by limiting dairy products and dark roughage). In patients with hyperuricosuria and hypocitraturia, there should be an increased intake of fruit juices and an avoidance of excessive animal protein intake. All patients with any form of calculi should be encouraged to drink sufficient fluids to achieve a minimum urine output of 2 L per day.

Selective Treatment Programs

Nephrolithiasis has a high recurrence rate of 50 to 80 percent. The objective of medical treatment is the prevention of further stone formation. Specific treatments should be considered for patients with recurrent nephrolithiasis, especially in those with active disease (for example, stone formation or growth within 3 years of examination). In patients with a single stone episode, selective treatments should also be considered if metabolic derangements (such as hypercalciuria) are disclosed and if patients are in the "high-risk" group in which recurrence is likely (i.e., young adult white men with a family history of stones).

Primary Hyperparathyroidism (Resorptive Hypercalciuria)

Parathyroidectomy is the optimum treatment for nephrolithiasis of primary hyperparathyroidism. Following removal of abnormal parathyroid tissue, the urinary calcium level is restored to normal, commensurate with a decline in serum concentration of calcium and in intestinal calcium absorption. Urinary environment becomes less saturated with respect to calcium oxalate and brushite (calcium phosphate), and its limit of metastability of these calcium salts increases. There is typically a reduced new stone formation rate, unless urinary tract infection is present.

There is no established medical treatment for the nephrolithiasis of primary hyperparathyroidism. Although orthophosphates have been recommended for disease of mild to moderate severity, their safety or efficacy has not yet been proven. They should be used only when parathyroid surgery cannot be undertaken. In postmenopausal women with primary hyperparathyroidism, estrogen (e.g., conjugated estrogen 0.625 mg per day for 25 days each month) may control the hyperparathyroid state and might be useful in those in whom parathyroid surgery is contraindicated or refused.

Absorptive Hypercalciuria

The presumed principal defect of absorptive hypercalciuria is the intestinal hyperabsorption of calcium that accounts for hypercalciuria and calcium nephrolithiasis. This condition may be subdivided into two types. In type I, the intestinal absorption and the renal excretion of calcium are increased during a high as well as during a low calcium diet. In type II, a normal urinary calcium concentration may be restored by dietary calcium restriction alone, although hypercalciuria is present on a high calcium diet. The hyperabsorption of calcium is believed to occur from 1,25-dihydroxyvitamin D_3 excess, hypersensitivity, or an independent process.

Absorptive Hypercalciuria Type I. There is currently no treatment program capable of correcting the basic abnormality of absorptive hypercalciuria, although several drugs are available that have been shown to restore normal urinary calcium excretion.

When sodium cellulose phosphate is given orally, this nonabsorbable ion exchange resin binds calcium and inhibits calcium absorption. However, this inhibition is caused by limiting the amount of intraluminal calcium available for absorption and not by correcting the basic disturbance in calcium transport.

The above mode of action accounts for the two potential complications of sodium cellulose phosphate. First, the treatment may cause magnesium depletion by binding dietary magnesium as well. Second, sodium cellulose phosphate may produce secondary hyperoxaluria by binding divalent cations in the intestinal tract, reducing divalent cation-oxalate complexation, and making more oxalate available for absorption. These complications may be overcome by oral magnesium supplementation (1.0 to 1.5 g magnesium gluconate twice daily, separately from sodium cellulose phosphate) and moderate dietary restriction of calcium (by avoidance of dairy products) and oxalate. Under such circumstances, sodium cellulose phosphate at a dosage of 10 to 15 g per day (given with meals) has been shown to lower urinary calcium without significantly altering urinary oxalate or magnesium, to reduce urinary saturation of calcium salts, and to retard new stone formation. This drug therapy is contraindicated in other forms of hypercalciuria because it may overly stimulate parathyroid function or embarrass skeletal status. It should be used with caution in postmenopausal women, growing children, and patients with low bone density, because of potential dangers of exaggerating bone loss or impairing skeletal growth.

Thiazide exerts the same hypocalciuric action and physicochemical effects in absorptive hypercalciuria as in renal hypercalciuria (see treatment of renal hypercalciuria for action, type, and dosage). Unfortunately, the intestinal hyperabsorption of calcium is not corrected by this treatment in absorptive hypercalciuria, unlike in renal hypercalciuria. Perhaps owing to this reason, some patients with absorptive hypercalciuria type I show an attenuation of hypocalciuric action of thiazide after 2 years of treatment. Moreover, thiazide treatment may cause hypocitraturia (inhibitor deficiency).

Because of the previously mentioned problems with thiazide therapy and difficulties in diagnostic differentiation, the following practical treatment regimen has often been employed. All patients with absorptive hypercalciuria type I may be begun first on a combined therapy with thiazide (e.g., trichlormethiazide, 4 mg per day) and potassium citrate (30 to 60 mEq per day in divided doses) in order to prevent hypocitraturia or raise the urinary citrate level). When thiazide is ineffective in controlling hypercalciuria, treatment with potassium phosphate may be considered.

Absorptive Hypercalciuria Type II. In type II hypercalciuria no specific drug treatment may be necessary. Normal urinary calcium may be obtained by a moderate dietary calcium restriction. Because urinary output is often low in this condition, a high fluid intake sufficient to produce urinary volume of at least 2 L per day should be encouraged.

Renal Hypercalciuria

Renal hypercalciuria is characterized by a "primary" impairment in the renal tubular reabsorption of calcium, secondary hyperparathyroidism, and compensatory intestinal hyperabsorption of calcium from the parathyroid hormone–dependent stimulation of 1,25-dihydroxyvitamin D_3 synthesis.

Thiazide is ideally indicated for the treatment of renal hypercalciuria. This form of diuretic has been shown to correct the renal leak of calcium by augmenting calcium reabsorption in the distal tubule and by causing extracellular volume depletion and stimulating proximal tubular reabsorption of calcium. The ensuing correction of secondary hyperparathyroidism restores normal serum 1,25-dihydroxyvitamin D_3 levels and intestinal calcium absorption. Physicochemically, the urinary environment becomes less saturated with respect to stone-forming salts (calcium oxalate and brushite) during thiazide treatment, largely because of the reduced calcium excretion. Moreover, urinary inhibitor activity is increased by a heretofore undisclosed mechanism.

These effects are shared by hydrochlorothiazide, 25 to 50 mg twice daily, chlorthalidone, 50 mg per day, or trichlormethiazide, 4 mg per day. Excessive sodium intake must be avoided because it could attenuate the hypocalciuric action of thiazide.

Side effects are mostly due to extracellular volume depletion and hypokalemia. Thiazide treatment should be avoided or stopped in the presence of excessive extrarenal loss of fluids and electrolytes. Renal excretion of citrate, an inhibitor of stone formation, may decline due to potassium loss. Thus, potassium citrate (30 to 60 mEq per day in divided doses) should be coadministered whenever thiazide (without potassium-sparing agent) is given.

Concurrent use of triamterene, a potassium-sparing agent, should be undertaken with caution because of reports of triamterene stone formation. Amiloride may potentiate the hypocalciuric action of thiazide or may itself reduce urinary calcium, but it does not alter citrate excretion. In patients with normal citrate excretion, amiloride (5 mg per day) in combination with thiazide (e.g., hydrochlorothiazide, 50 mg per day) without potassium citrate supplementation, may be useful.

Thiazide is contraindicated in primary hyperparathyroidism because of potential aggravation of hypercalcemia.

Hyperuricosuric Calcium Oxalate Nephrolithiasis

In this condition hyperuricosuria develops, usually from dietary "overindulgence" with purine-rich foods and occasionally from uric acid overproduction. The ensuing hyperuricosuria is believed to cause calcium stone formation from urate-induced calcium oxalate crystallization.

Allopurinol (300 mg per day) is the physiologically meaningful drug of choice in hyperuricosuric calcium oxalate nephrolithiasis, if hyperuricosuria is severe (greater than 800 mg per day) or if hyperuricemia coexists. Physicochemical changes ensuing from restoration of normal urinary uric acid by allopurinol include a reduction in urinary saturation of monosodium urate and a commensurate increase in the urinary limit of metastability of calcium oxalate. Thus, the spontaneous nucleation of calcium oxalate is retarded by treatment, probably via inhibition of monosodium urate-induced stimulation of calcium oxalate crystallization.

Side effects of allopurinol are uncommon in patients with stones, although hepatotoxicity, bone marrow depression, and rash have been reported. The complication of xanthine stone formation is rare.

If hyperuricosuria is mild to moderate (less than 800 mg per day) and serum uric acid is normal, potassium citrate alone may be used. The induced hypercitraturia has been shown to prevent urate-induced calcium oxalate crystallization.

In patients with combined disturbances, allopurinol may be given with other agents (e.g., allopurinol and thiazide for patients with hyperuricosuria and hypercalciuria).

Hyperoxaluria

Primary Hyperoxaluria. Primary hyperoxaluria is caused by an accelerated oxalate synthesis. Magnesium gluconate (4 g per day in divided doses) and large doses of pyridoxine may lower urinary oxalate in some patients. Orthophosphate (0.5 g phosphorus three to four times per day orally) may be useful in controlling stone formation, probably by increasing inhibitor activity.

Secondary Hyperoxaluria. In ileal disease (surgical resection, intestinal bypass, inflammatory disease), urinary oxalate may be high secondary to intestinal hyperabsorption of oxalate (enteric hyperoxaluria). Other factors that may contribute to stone formation include low urine volume, low urinary acidity (predisposing to uric acid lithiasis), hypocitraturia, and hypomagnesiuria. Dietary oxalate restriction should be imposed. A high fluid intake should be encouraged. Magnesium gluconate or citrate may be tolerated without aggravating diarrhea. Potassium citrate (40 to 120 mEq in divided doses) may augment citrate excretion and raise urinary pH. If bone disease is also present, 25-hydroxyvitamin D (50 μg per day) may be given with calcium supplements. Should hypercalciuria ensue, thiazide may be added.

Hypocitraturia

Renal Tubular Acidosis. Distal renal tubular acidosis (complete and incomplete) may be found in some patients with calcium nephrolithiasis. Acidosis may cause hypercalciuria by impairing renal tubular resorption of calcium, at least during the early stages of the disease before a significant renal impairment ensues. Because of high urinary pH, more phosphate is dissociated. Thus the urinary environment may become supersaturated with respect to calcium salts, particularly calcium phosphate. There is a defective renal excretion of citrate; this defect may therefore facilitate the crystallization process in urine.

Potassium citrate (40 to 100 mEq per day in divided doses) may correct the acidosis, reduce urinary calcium, augment urinary citrate, and retard the crystallization of calcium salts. This alkali therapy may also improve calcium balance by lowering urinary calcium and increasing intestinal calcium absorption. It should be used with caution in patients with renal insufficiency (glomerular filtration rate less than 40 ml per minute).

Other Causes. Hypocitraturia is present in approximately 50 percent of patients with calcium nephrolithiasis, even in the absence of renal tubular acidosis. Other causes of hypocitraturia include metabolic acidosis of enteric hyperoxaluria and thiazide-induced potassium depletion. Chronic diarrheal states (other than ileal disease) may also cause hypocitraturia. A strenuous physical exercise and ingestion of a high acid-ash diet (animal protein) may contribute to reduced citrate excretion. In some patients, the cause for the hypocitraturia remains unknown (idiopathic).

Potassium citrate (usually 30 to 60 mEq per day in divided doses) sufficient to restore normal urinary citrate is recommended. In chronic diarrheal states with fast intestinal transit or adhesions, a liquid form of potassium citrate may be preferable. In remaining conditions, the tablet form given with meals may be better tolerated and may provide a more consistent rise in citrate excretion.

Uric Acid Stones

The critical determinant in the formation of uric acid stones is the passage of unusually acid urine (pH 5.5) in which uric acid is stable. Uric acid lithiasis is found in gout, secondary causes of purine overproduction (e.g., myeloproliferative states and malignancy), and chronic diarrheal syndromes.

The oral administration of sodium alkali may increase urinary pH and create an environment in which uric acid is unstable. Although this treatment may inhibit the formation of uric acid stones, it may cause complication of calcium stone formation. In contrast, potassium citrate (30 to 60 mEq per day in divided doses) sufficient to raise urinary pH to a range of 6 to 6.5 may be helpful in the prevention of uric acid lithiasis, without producing a significant risk of calcium stone formation.

Allopurinol may be used to control hyperuricosuria (if present); a dose of 300 mg per day is generally sufficient to restore normal urinary uric acid. Dietary purine restriction is seldom practical. Probenecid is contraindicated because of its uricosuric action.

Patients with uric acid lithiasis may also form calcium stones, as manifestations of gouty diathesis. Potassium citrate is the preferred treatment for the prevention of both uric acid and calcium stones.

Cystine Stones

Stone formation is the result of an excessive renal excretion of cystine and the low solubility of this dicarboxylic acid in the normal pH of urine.

The initial treatment program includes a high fluid intake to promote an adequate urine flow (minimum of 2 L per day) and soluble alkali (e.g., potassium citrate 30 to 60 mEq per day in divided doses) to raise urinary pH to 6.5 to 7, in order to lower cystine concentration and raise cystine solubility. If this program is ineffective, α-mercaptopropionylglycine (Thiola) (1 to 2 g per day in divided doses) may be used. This treatment reduces cystine excretion by forming a more soluble mixed disulfide with cysteine. The dose of Thiola should be adjusted in order to maintain cystine concentration in urine below saturation. Potential side effects include nephrotic syndrome, dermatitis, pancytopenia, and arthralgia. These side effects are less common with Thiola than with D-penicillamine.

Infection Stones

Urinary tract infection sometimes accompanies nephrolithiasis. When urea-splitting organisms (*Proteus*, certain species of *Staphylococcus*, *Pseudomonas*, *Klebsiella*) are responsible for infection, stones typically contain struvite (magnesium ammonium phosphate) with varying amounts of apatite.

In some patients, struvite stones may have formed de novo as a consequence solely of infection. In others, specific metabolic disorders associated with the formation of other types of renal stones could be identified; these derangements include hypercalciuria, hyperuricosuria, hyperoxaluria, and cystinuria. Struvite stone formation in the latter group probably results from a metabolic disorder causing formation of nonstruvite stones and resulting in urinary tract infection with urea-splitting organism, eventually leading to formation of struvite stone.

The physicochemical basis for struvite lithiasis is probably the same whether such a stone forms primarily or secondarily. The initial event is the formation of ammonium in urine on enzymatic degradation of urea by bacterial urease. The ammonia undergoes hydrolysis to form ammonium and hydroxyl ions. The resulting alkalinity of urine stimulates the dissociation of phosphate to form more trivalent phosphate ions and lowers the solubility of struvite. The activity product or the state of saturation of urine with respect to struvite is therefore increased. Stone formation ensues when sufficient oversaturation is reached.

If a longstanding effective control of infection with urea-splitting organisms can be achieved, there is some evidence that new stone formation can be averted or some dissolution of existing stone may occur. Unfortunately, such a control is difficult to obtain with antibiotic therapy. If there is an existing struvite stone, it is difficult to clear the infection completely because the stone often harbors the organisms within its interstices. Even if "sterilization" of urine had been achieved by antibiotic therapy, reinfection could occur by a harbored organism. For these reasons it has been customary to recommend surgical removal of struvite stones.

Prevention of new stone formation requires sterilization of urine with an appropriate antibiotic therapy or prevention of the generation of ammonium and hydroxyl ions with urease inhibitors (e.g., acetohydroxamic acid 250 mg three times per day).

Suggested Reading

Pak CYC. Etiology and treatment of urolithiasis. Am J Kid Dis 1991; 18: 624–637.

Pak CYC. Citrate and renal calculi: an update. Min Elect Metab 1994; 20: 371–377.

Pak CYC. Kidney stones. In: Wilson JD, Foster DW, Reed Larsen P, et al., eds. Williams textbook of endocrinology. 9th ed. Philadelphia: WB Saunders, 1996, in press.

CYSTIC DISEASE OF THE KIDNEY

Vicente E. Torres, M.D.

A cyst is a gross cavity lined by epithelium or abnormal tissue usually containing fluid or other material. Renal cysts are usually of tubular origin and are lined by tubular epithelium. Many heterogeneous conditions—whether congenital, developmental, or acquired and with or without a genetic cause—that have in common the presence of renal cysts are classified as "renal cystic diseases." There have been many more or less arbitrary provisional classifications of these diseases. In one such classification, based on pathogenetic considerations, they are divided into (1) those caused by defects of metanephric differentiation (cystic dysplasias), (2) those associated with hereditary interstitial nephritis, (3) those with tubular epithelial hyperplasia without dysplasia, (4) cystic conditions of inflammatory or neoplastic origin, and (5) renal cystic diseases of nontubular origin. Only the most common of these disorders are discussed in this chapter (Table 1).

Table 1 Renal Cystic Disease

Multicystic renal dysplasia
Medullary cystic disease
Simple renal cysts
Medullary sponge kidney
Autosomal recessive polycystic kidney disease
Autosomal dominant polycystic kidney disease
Tuberous sclerosis
von Hippel-Lindau disease
Acquired cystic kidney disease
Multilocular cysts
Cystic disease of the renal sinus

■ MULTICYSTIC RENAL DYSPLASIA

Renal cystic dysplasias comprise a spectrum of renal abnormalities resulting from an interference with the normal metanephric differentiation. Multicystic renal dysplasia is a result of an early inhibition of ampullary activity. The ureter is absent or atretic, and the kidneys consist of a grapelike cluster of cysts. When bilateral, multicystic renal dysplasia is incompatible with life. When unilateral or segmental, it can be diagnosed in the newborn or go undetected and be discovered years later as an abdominal mass or an incidental finding.

Treatment

Because these kidneys tend to decrease in size, most authors recommend a nonsurgical approach when the diagnosis of multicystic renal dysplasia can be firmly established by noninvasive techniques. In the newborn, it is essential that this condition be differentiated from hydronephrosis, since the treatment is markedly different. Excretory urography is frequently unsatisfactory because of decreased renal concentrating ability and glomerular filtration in the newborn, resulting in poor visualization of hydronephrotic kidneys, as well as because of the occasional puttering of contrast material in delayed films in multicystic kidneys. Renal scintigraphy has similar limitations. The most useful diagnostic technique is ultrasonography. The criteria to distinguish multicystic renal dysplasia from congenital hydronephrosis include the presence of interfaces between the cysts, nonmedial location of the larger cysts, absence of identifiable renal sinus, and absence of parenchymal tissue. The diagnosis can be confirmed by retrograde pyelography showing an absent or atretic proximal ureter and by angiography revealing an absent or hypoplastic renal artery.

Clear indications for surgical removal of a multicystic dysplastic kidney are pain, increase in size, infection, and hypertension with lateralizing renal vein renin studies. Some authors, however, recommend nephrectomy of all multicystic dysplastic kidneys because of the risk of hypertension or malignant degeneration. Since most patients with unilateral multicystic kidneys diagnosed during infancy or early childhood have been treated surgically, the natural history of this condition is unclear. Considering the large population at risk, very few cases of proven causally related hypertension have been reported. Similarly, there have been only a few reports of Wilms' tumors and renal cell carcinomas developing in unilateral multicystic kidneys. Several of the reported cases of renal cell carcinoma occurred in women, three of whom were young (25, 26, and 33 years of age). The early development of renal cell carcinoma in these patients may support the concept that a dysplastic kidney has a significantly increased likelihood of malignant degeneration.

■ MEDULLARY CYSTIC DISEASE

Medullary cystic disease and nephronophthisis are synonymous terms that denote a heterogeneous group of diseases characterized by small kidneys with interstitial nephritis and cysts in the cortical medullary junction, clinically characterized by an insidious onset, polydipsia and/or polyuria, benign urinary sediment, mild proteinuria, frequent sodium wasting, and relentless progression to renal failure. The pathogenesis of these disorders is not known, but a primary tubular basement membrane defect and autoimmune mechanisms have been considered likely. Two main forms are recognized on the basis of inheritance and age at diagnosis, a juvenile recessive form and an adult dominant form. Sporadic presentations may represent recessive cases in families with a small offspring or new dominant mutations. The autosomal recessive form is frequently associated with extrarenal abnormalities such as retinitis pigmentosa (renal-retinal syndrome), skeletal abnormalities (cono-renal syndromes including chondroectodermal dysplasia, asphyxiating thoracic dystrophy, Saldino-Mainzer syndrome, and peripheral dysostosis with medullary cystic disease), congenital hepatic fibrosis, and central nervous system abnormalities (cerebro-oculo-hepato-renal syndrome). A renal disease consistent with medullary cystic disease also occurs in two additional autosomal recessive syndromes, the Laurence-Moon-Bardet-Biedl syndrome (obesity, polydactyly, retinitis pigmentosa, mental retardation, and hypogenitalism) and Alström's syndrome (obesity, diabetes mellitus, retinitis pigmentosa, and nerve deafness). The recessive form of nephronophthisis without extrarenal manifestations is genetically heterogeneous, with a gene in chromosome 2q13 being responsible for most, but not all, cases.

Treatment

The treatment of medullary cystic disease is supportive. Hypertension is not a prominent manifestation of the disease but, when present, it should be carefully controlled. Volume contraction and prerenal azotemia, unnecessary sodium restriction, and diuretics should be avoided because of the tendency to sodium wasting. Some patients may require sodium chloride supplementation to maintain sodium balance during a phase of their disease. Administration of sodium bicarbonate may be necessary to correct a renal tubular acidosis. Osteomalacia or secondary hyperparathyroidism should be treated if present. In children with failure to thrive, consideration might be given to treatment with growth hormone. Eventually, dialysis and/or renal transplantation are needed. Precautions should be taken to use only unaffected relatives for living-related kidney transplantation. The living-related donors should undergo meticulous diagnostic evaluation and should be at least 10 years older than the affected child or sibling. The patient and his or her family should be provided with genetic counseling based on the mode of inheritance.

■ SIMPLE RENAL CYSTS

Simple cysts, like most renal cysts of tubuloepithelial origin, are believed to originate from diverticula and localized defects in the tubular wall. The frequency of both tubular diverticula and cysts increases with age. More than 50 percent of people older than 50 years of age have at least one cyst on postmortem examination.

Evaluation and Treatment

Simple cysts most often produce no symptoms and require no specific treatment. Differentiation from more severe conditions, such as renal cell carcinoma and, when multiple, polycystic kidney disease, is therefore essential. Characteristic features on ultrasonography (lack of internal echoes, smooth walls, and enhancement of echoes deep to the lesion) and computed tomography (CT) (density near that of water, thin wall, sharp interface, and no enhancement with contrast material) allow one to distinguish clearly between a benign simple cyst and a renal cell carcinoma in the majority of cases. The presence of a few delicate septa within a cyst is of no clinical significance. When these criteria are not met, percutaneous needle aspiration or, rarely, angiography is necessary. Calcification confined to the cyst wall is not an indication for puncture if all of the CT characteristics for a benign renal cyst are seen. Some findings on ultrasonography or CT, such as a discrete nodule in the wall of the cyst, constitute an indication for surgery regardless of the result of cyst aspiration. Differentiation of multiple simple cysts from mild forms of polycystic kidney disease is difficult and requires a careful family history, search for cysts in other organs, and a careful assessment of clinical correlations.

The incidental discovery of simple renal cysts should not distract one from other more important lesions. They can rarely cause abdominal or flank pain, microscopic or macroscopic hematuria, and renin-dependent hypertension, but other causes of these manifestations should always be sought. For example, simple cysts are often found in the vicinity of a renal cell carcinoma ("sentinel cysts"). Patterns of extrinsic compression and infundibular obstruction caused by cysts on excretory urography are often found to be of no functional significance by furosemide radioactive renal scan.

At present, surgery is indicated only in the rare cases in which there is still doubt regarding the precise diagnosis after using less invasive investigations, in the rare complicated cyst that cannot be adequately treated percutaneously, and in the symptomatic cyst that recurs rapidly after percutaneous drainage. Percutaneous aspiration of a renal cyst is easily accomplished and should be done for diagnostic purposes whenever a cyst might be responsible for pain, obstruction, or hypertension. In some cases, there is no reaccumulation of cyst fluid, and the aspiration is of therapeutic value. Reaccumulation of cyst fluid, however, occurs in 30 to 80 percent of the cases. Several sclerosing agents, including glucose, phenol, bismuth phosphate, iophendylate iodophenylundecanoate (Pantopaque), and ethanol have been used to prevent the reaccumulation of fluid. The best results are obtained with ethanol, but because of the highly sclerosing properties of this substance, introduction of a pigtail catheter into the cyst is required. The technique described by Bean is usually followed: the cyst contents are totally aspirated, and 25 percent of the original cyst volume is replaced with 95 percent ethanol. The patient is then placed in the supine and prone positions and both lateral decubitus positions for 5 minutes to allow adequate contact of the alcohol with all the areas of the cyst wall. The alcohol is then aspirated, and the catheter is removed. It has been shown that after 1 to 3 minutes of contact with the ethanol, the epithelial cells lining the cyst walls become fixed and nonviable, without significant damage to the adjacent normal renal parenchyma. When performed by a radiologist with extensive experience, this procedure is relatively safe, with less than 1 percent of major complications and less than 10 percent of minor complications. The most common major complication is perirenal hemorrhage. The most common minor complication is pain following the procedure, which may persist for several days. Infections of simple renal cysts are very rare, usually occur in female patients, and are caused by *Escherichia coli*. The treatment of infected simple cysts consists of drainage combined with antibiotic therapy. Although surgery used to be required for cyst drainage, percutaneous drainage is equally successful.

■ MEDULLARY SPONGE KIDNEY

Medullary sponge kidney is a common disorder characterized by tubular dilatation of the collecting ducts and cyst formation strictly confined to the medullary pyramids, especially their inner, papillary portions. It is regarded as a nonhereditary disease, but autosomal dominant inheritance has been suggested in several families. It is usually a benign disorder that may remain asymptomatic for life, but mild tubular function abnormalities, such as a concentration defect, a reduced capacity to acidify the urine after ammonium chloride administration, and a reduced maximal excretion of potassium after potassium chloride loading are common. The diagnosis of medullary sponge kidney is usually established during the course of evaluation of episodes of renal colic, hematuria, or urinary tract infections. Nephrolithiasis is the major complication. Patients with medullary sponge kidney have a higher rate of stone formation than other patients with nephrolithiasis. It is uncertain whether hypercalciuria and hyperparathyroidism are more prevalent in these patients than in other patients with nephrolithiasis. Women with medullary sponge kidney and nephrolithiasis are more likely to have cystoscopic examinations and higher rates of urinary tract infections than other women with nephrolithiasis. There is no evidence that medullary sponge kidney per se that is unrelated to the nephrolithiasis predisposes to urinary tract infection. Hypertension does not occur more frequently in these patients than in the general population. The renal function remains normal except in rare patients with complicated nephrolithiasis and chronic pyelonephritis.

Treatment

Patients with medullary sponge kidney should be informed of the benign nature of this disorder, provided that the nephrolithiasis is controlled. Unnecessary repetitious investigations for hematuria should be avoided. As in other patients with nephrolithiasis, metabolic factors contributing to the formation of stones should be identified and treated. Adequate fluid intake to maintain a 24 hour urine volume of more than 2.5 L in men and 2 L in women is essential. Thiazide or orthophosphate may be effective in the patients who continue to form stones. Alkali as potassium citrate may be a more simple alternative to orthophosphate treatment in the patients with medullary sponge kidney and impaired distal acidification with hypocitric aciduria. Because of the blunted kaliuretic response to potassium loading reported to occur in patients with medullary sponge kidney, potassium plasma levels in patients treated with potassium citrate should be rechecked, but hyperkalemia in these patients has not been a problem. As in other patients with nephrolithiasis, urinary tract infections should be aggressively treated, the results of therapy adequately assessed, and chronic suppression or prophylactic therapy instituted if one is unable to eradicate the infection or in patients with frequent recurrences. The treatment of patients with medullary sponge kidney and infected stones with urea-splitting organisms may pose a special problem since complete removal of the stone and adequate acidification of the urine with ammonium chloride may be difficult to achieve in these patients. The roles of surgery and percutaneous or extracorporeal lithotripsy in these patients are not different from those in other patients with nephrolithiasis.

■ AUTOSOMAL RECESSIVE POLYCYSTIC KIDNEY DISEASE

Autosomal recessive polycystic kidney disease (ARPKD) is characterized by various combinations of bilateral renal cystic disease and congenital hepatic fibrosis. It has been mapped recently to chromosome 6p. The cysts in this disorder result from giantism of the collecting tubules. They are elongated, of similar size, and extend from the medulla to the cortex. Congenital hepatic fibrosis is a developmental abnormality that leads to portal hypertension and is characterized by

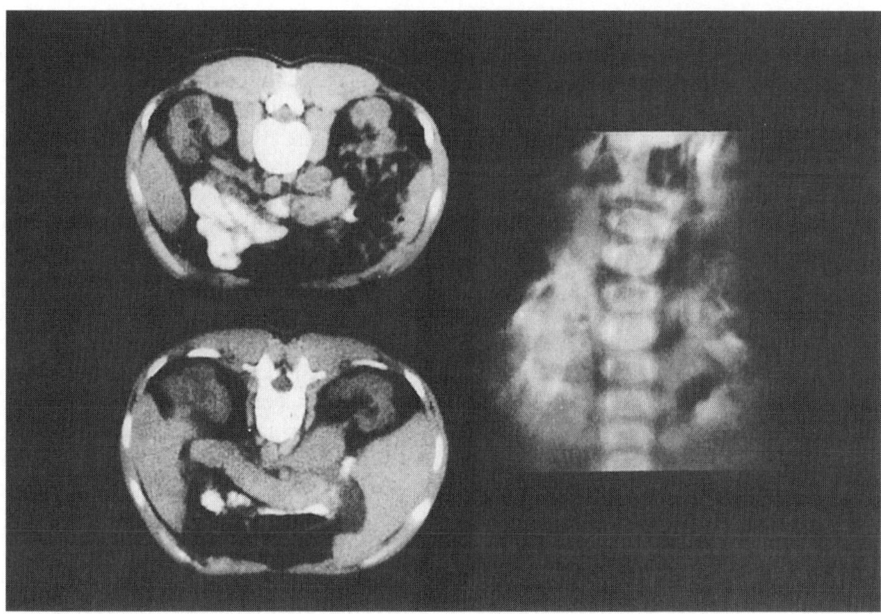

Figure 1
Left, Excretory urography in a 12-month-old male with ADPKD showing large kidneys with a characteristic nephrogram of radiating streaks of contrast. *Right,* CT scan of the abdomen 20 years later showing a relative reduction in the size of the kidneys, multiple renal cysts, and a prominent inferior vena cava consistent with previous portocaval shunting.

enlarged and fibrotic portal areas with an apparent proliferation of bile ducts, absence of central bile ducts, hypoplasia of the portal vein branches, and sometimes, prominent fibrosis around the central veins. It can also occur as an isolated finding or in association with renal dysplasia and hereditary tubulointerstitial nephritis. In newborns and infants, the clinical presentation of ARPKD is dominated by the manifestations of the renal disease, and in older children and adolescents, by the manifestations of portal hypertension. In older children and adolescents, the cystic dilatation of the collecting tubules may be less pronounced and can be confused with medullary sponge kidney. The differential diagnosis of ARPKD and autosomal dominant polycystic kidney diseases in infancy or childhood is usually possible on the basis of the family history and the findings on excretory urography, ultrasonography, and CT. Liver histology is sometimes needed to establish the diagnosis.

Treatment

ARPKD is not always fatal, as was initially believed, and some patients may have a prolonged survival. In fact, the enlarged kidneys may decrease in relative size in patients who survive the neonatal phase of the disease, while the renal function may remain stable for many years or slowly progress to renal failure (Fig. 1). Accurate blood pressure assessment and strict control are essential in these young children. Many require dialysis or renal transplantation at an early age. The surviving patients and those who present during later childhood or adolescence are likely to require treatment for portal hypertension to prevent life-threatening hemorrhages from esophageal varices. The liver function tests are usually normal, although mild elevations of the serum alkaline phosphatase and transaminase can occur. These patients are good candidates for portal systemic shunting procedures, with portocaval shunting being preferred by some. The renal disease may progress to renal failure years after successful shunting. Patients with associated nonobstructive intrahepatic biliary dilatation (Caroli's disease) may have recurrent episodes of cholangitis and may require antimicrobial therapy. Partial hepatectomy can be considered in patients with recurrent episodes of cholangitis and segmental dilatation of the intrahepatic bile ducts.

■ AUTOSOMAL DOMINANT POLYCYSTIC KIDNEY DISEASE

Autosomal dominant polycystic kidney disease (ADPKD) is an autosomal dominant multisystem disease with high penetrance, mainly affecting the kidney, and with a wide range of ages of clinical presentation and a great variation in severity. ADPKD is a genetically heterogeneous disease. The PKD1 gene on chromosome 16p13.3 is responsible for most cases. The PKD2 gene on chromosome 4q13-q23 is responsible for a milder form of the disease. It seems likely that PKD2 accounts for at least 10 to 20 percent of families with ADPKD. In addition there is evidence for at least a third gene (PDK3), as well as for another gene causing polycystic liver disease without renal involvement. Both the PKD1 and the PKD2 gene have been identified and completely sequenced. The PKD1 gene encodes a protein of high molecular weight ("polycystin"), the function of which is not yet known. The PKD2 gene encodes a protein of lower molecular weight (110 KD) which has similarities to a family of voltage-activated calcium and sodium α_1, channel proteins.

Presymptomatic screening for ADPKD should be performed only in individuals who have been properly informed on the advantages and disadvantages of screening and should be followed by appropriate counseling if ADPKD is diagnosed. Presymptomatic screening can be performed by ultrasound, which may not be conclusive before the age of 20 years, or by genetic linkage analysis, which is possible only in families of sufficient size and informativeness. At present, the diagnosis of ADPKD by direct mutation analysis is difficult and not clinically available. Screening by ultrasound is adequate in most cases. The sonographic diagnostic criteria for individuals known to be at 50 percent risk for ADPKD are two cysts either unilateral or bilateral for individuals less than 30 years old, two cysts in each kidney for those 30 to 59 years of age, and at least four cysts in each kidney for those over the age of 60 years. Young adults may benefit from presymptomatic screening. If nonaffected, they will be reassured. If affected, they may benefit from specialized counseling for family planning, from the identification and management of treatable complications such as hypertension, and from avoiding unnecessary evaluations for manifestations of ADPKD. The disadvantages of presymptomatic screening relate to insurability and employability. Recommendations for presymptomatic screening will change when more effective therapies for the disease become available.

Treatment

Despite major advances in the understanding of the process of cystogenesis and some observations that bear hope that the rate of cyst growth may someday be affected by pharmacologic intervention, the therapy of ADPKD at present is still restricted to the treatment of its symptoms and complications. The main renal manifestations of ADPKD are abdominal or flank pain caused by cyst enlargement, bleeding, nephrolithiasis, or infection; hematuria; hypertension; and renal insufficiency. Whether patients with ADPKD are at increased risk for developing gout, especially during diuretic therapy, is uncertain. Renal cell carcinomas in ADPKD patients are rare and possibly not more frequent than in the general population, although they are more frequently bilateral when they occur. The extrarenal manifestations of ADPKD include hepatic cysts, intracranial aneurysms, cardiac valve abnormalities, dilatation of the aortic root, and rarely, aortic aneurysms. It has been suggested that ADPKD patients have an increased incidence of diverticulosis and diverticulitis, but this association needs further confirmation.

Patients with ADPKD often have a sensation of flank or abdominal fullness or heaviness, but this sensation is not painful and requires no analgesics. In a small subset of patients, the renal enlargement and distortion are accompanied by chronic, severe, disabling flank pain. These patients often become analgesic or narcotic dependent. As is the case in other patients with chronic pain, the evaluation and treatment of these patients are difficult. Other renal causes of the pain, such as an infected renal cyst or undetected uric acid calculi, as well as extrarenal processes, need to be ruled out. A psychologic assessment and an understanding and supportive attitude on the physician's part are essential. Reassurance and changes in lifestyle with avoidance of certain activities may provide some relief. In some cases, a pain clinic evaluation and the use of transcutaneous electric nerve stimulation (TENS), celiac plexus, or sympathetic lumbar blocks may be helpful. In other situations, especially when CT reveals considerable distortion and stretching of the kidney by large cysts and conservative measures have been exhausted, cyst decompression should be considered.

The selection of the best option for cyst decompression in a particular patient is a function of the severity of the symptoms, the number, size, and location of the cysts, the level of renal function, and the presence of comorbid conditions. Percutaneous needle aspiration may be of some diagnostic and prognostic value, but it does not usually provide permanent pain relief because of fluid reaccumulation. Ethanol sclerosis may be helpful to treat one or a small number of cysts, but cannot be safely and effectively accomplished in most patients with chronic, severe pain, with many cysts contributing to the pain. These patients may benefit from laparoscopy or from surgical cyst fenestration through a lumbotomy or flank incision. Intraoperative ultrasound is helpful in the localization of unidentified cysts during both laparoscopic and open surgical procedures. Surgical cyst fenestration provides sustained pain relief in approximately 70 percent of patients without an adverse effect on renal function (Fig. 2). The results of laparoscopic surgery (pain relief in 62 percent of the patients at 2 years) approach the results of open surgical treatment.

Episodes of hemorrhage in a polycystic kidney are usually confined inside cysts or lead to gross hematuria. They are self-limited and usually can be treated at home with bed rest, hydration, and analgesics such as acetaminophen with codeine. Rarely, the episodes of bleeding are more severe with extensive subcapsular or retroperitoneal hematomas and significant decreases in hematocrit or hemodynamic instability and require hospitalization and investigations with CT or angiography. Urinary tract obstruction by a hemorrhagic cyst or a clot may also require hospitalization and stent placement. In cases of unusually severe or persistent hemorrhage, segmental arterial embolization or surgery needs to be considered. The episodes of bleeding in a polycystic kidney can sometimes be explained by trauma or unusual physical activity or may be triggered by the use of an anticoagulant medication or by uncontrolled hypertension. Often there is no obvious cause. ADPKD patients should be advised against the practice of contact sports and the use of constrictive belts.

Early detection and strict treatment of hypertension and correction of other cardiovascular risk factors are most important in ADPKD, since cardiovascular complications constitute the main cause of death for patients with this disease. In addition, several studies have shown that ADPKD patients with hypertension are more likely to have a faster deterioration of renal function than those without. The pathogenesis of hypertension in ADPKD is not completely understood, and therefore the best antihypertensive treatment has not been established. Most studies on the pathogenesis of hypertension in ADPKD are consistent with the hypothesis of an increased intrarenal angiotensin effect, with a reduced renal blood flow, increased filtration fraction, and an abnormal renal handling of sodium leading to an absolute or relative expansion of the extracellular fluid volume and hypertension. Given the central role that the renin-angiotensin system is thought to play in this pathogenetic scheme, a converting enzyme inhibitor may be the antihypertensive agent of choice in the presence of normal or near-normal renal function, but this requires further study. It has also been observed that the hypertension

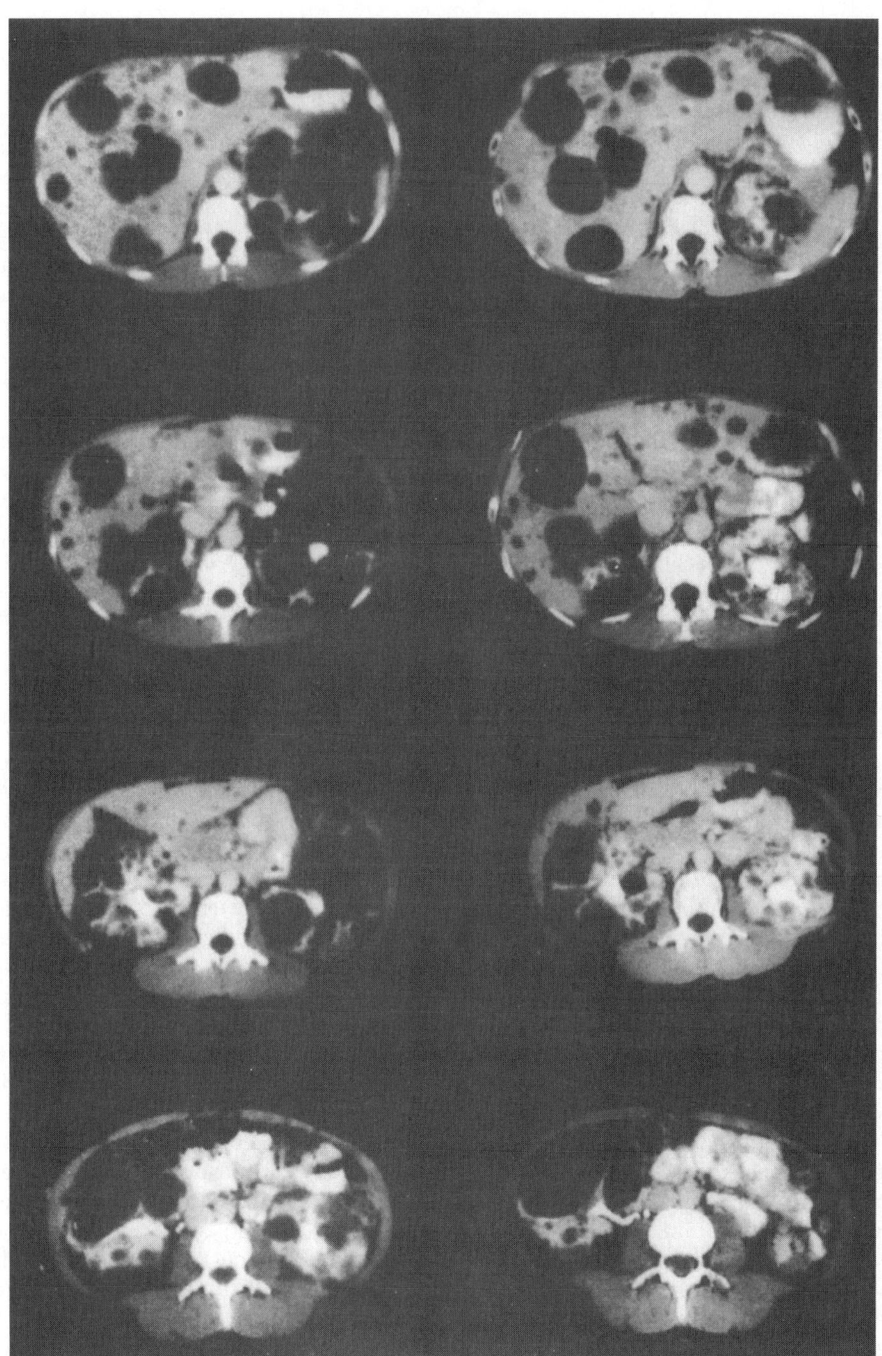

Figure 2
Contrast-enhanced CT scans of the abdomen before *(left)* and after *(right)* surgical decompression of a left polycystic kidney.

in ADPKD becomes less severe with the progression of the renal insufficiency, possibly because of a tendency to sodium wasting. For this reason, diuretics should be administered with caution in these patients to avoid volume contraction and deterioration of renal function. With the currently available antihypertensive medications, the use of diuretics in ADPKD is often unnecessary and contributes to hyperuricemia, hyperlipidemia, hypokalemia, and hyper-reninemia, which may have a negative effect on the course of the disease.

It has been assumed that nephrolithiasis, which occurs in 20 percent of ADPKD patients, is caused mostly by the anatomic obstruction of the collecting system by the cysts. In a recent study, the chemical composition of the stones (mainly uric acid and calcium oxalate) and the frequency of hypocitraturia and low urine pH suggest that both metabolic and mechanical factors are responsible for the frequent occurrence of nephrolithiasis in these patients. Identification and treatment of these metabolic factors should be performed as in other stone-forming patients. Both percutaneous lithotripsy and extracorporeal shock-wave lithotripsy have been performed in patients with ADPKD, but the experience with these procedures is so limited that no conclusions should be reached on their safety with regard to this disease.

Infection of a renal cyst in ADPKD is usually the result of a retrograde infection from the urinary bladder. Unnecessary urinary tract manipulations should therefore be avoided. When absolutely necessary, antimicrobial prophylaxis should be prescribed. The findings on CT or magnetic resonance imaging (MRI) are not specific, and the results of nuclear medicine scans, such as gallium and indium-111 leukocyte scans, are not always positive. The failure of conventional antibiotic therapy, despite favorable in vitro sensitivities, may be the best single diagnostic indicator of renal cyst infection. The treatment of infected renal cysts poses a special problem because of the variable penetration of different antibiotics. Most antibiotics enter the proximal, nongradient cyst to some extent. However, only lipid-soluble antibiotics (e.g., ciprofloxacin, trimethoprim, chloramphenicol, and metronidazole) and not other more conventionally used polar lipid-insoluble antibiotics (e.g., aminoglycosides, penicillins, and cephalosporins) enter the distal, gradient cysts well. The initial treatment of an acutely ill patient with a suspected cyst infection should be an appropriate wide-spectrum antibiotic combination, such as ampicillin and aminoglycoside, because adequate treatment of septicemia takes precedence over the treatment of cyst infections. In addition, it is difficult to separate a cyst from a parenchymal infection in ADPKD, and both may occur simultaneously. Patients with no response to the initial therapy after 5 days of treatment should begin receiving a lipid-soluble agent if the in vitro sensitivities are favorable. In refractory cases, the possibility of an anaerobic or hematogenously disseminated gram-positive infection should be considered.

A decline in renal function eventually occurs in most patients with ADPKD. The relative sparing of the renal parenchyma on ultrasonography or CT at the time of the initial evaluation is helpful in establishing a prognosis. ADPKD patients have a prolonged period of stable renal function followed by a slow decline. Therefore, it is unnecessary to recheck the renal function more than once every 1 to 3 years until significant deterioration of renal function has already occurred. With well-known limitations, a reciprocal plot of plasma creatinine against time is useful in the follow-up of patients with depressed renal function and may alert the physician to the possibility of an intercurrent renal disease or complication if a major diversion from the initial slope occurs. The prevention and treatment of renal insufficiency in ADPKD should include the avoidance of nephrotoxic drugs and the chronic use of analgesics; prevention, early detection, and treatment of complications; strict control of hypertension; and a prudent diet with mild protein (0.8 g per kilogram of ideal body weight) and phosphorus restriction when the renal function starts to deteriorate. Surgical decompression of polycystic kidneys in patients with advanced renal insufficiency and a decline in renal function does not have a beneficial effect. Protection of renal function is not an indication for surgery in patients with ADPKD.

The value of strict blood pressure control and protein restriction have been the subject of a large prospective, multicenter study, the Modification of Diet in Renal Disease (MDRD) trial, which included 200 patients with ADPKD. This trial consisted of two studies. The patients in study A had moderate renal insufficiency with a glomerular filtration rate (GFR) of 38 ml/min/1.73 m^2 at entry. The patients in study B had advanced renal insufficiency with a GFR of 17 ml/min/1.73 m^2 at entry. In both studies, the patients were randomized to usual blood pressure control (mean arterial pressure [MAP] goal ≤107 mmHg for participants ≤60 years old and ≤115 mmHg for participants >60 years) and blood pressure supercontrol (MAP goal ≤92 mmHg for participants ≤60 years old and ≤98 mmHg for participants >60 years). Patients in study A were also randomized to a normal (1.3 g/kg/day) and low (0.58 g/kg/day) protein intake and patients in study B were randomized to low (0.58 g/kg/day) and very low (0.28 g/kg body weight supplemented with ketoacids and essential amino acids) protein diets. In study A, neither the supercontrol of blood pressure nor the low-protein diet had an effect on the yearly rate of decline of GFR. In study B the patients with the low blood pressure goal showed a faster decline of GFR than those with the usual blood pressure goal, but the achieved blood pressure readings at follow-up were not significantly correlated with the rate of GFR decline. The very low-protein diet had a slight beneficial effect of borderline statistical significance. Since the interventions in the MDRD trial were introduced at a late stage in the natural history of ADPKD, the results do not exclude a beneficial effect of these interventions at an earlier stage of the disease, as observed in experimental animal models.

When end-stage renal disease occurs, dialysis and, in the younger patients, renal transplantation are indicated. Patients with ADPKD receiving maintenance hemodialysis do as well as and possibly better than patients with other types of renal disease, probably because they maintain a higher hemoglobin. Bleeding secondary to heparinization during dialysis rarely occurs and can usually be satisfactorily managed by using low or regional heparinization. The evaluation of living-related donors for renal transplantation is not different from that for other diseases, but CT and DNA linkage analysis (in informative families) should be considered in the young patient to rule out ADPKD. The inclusion of CT of the abdomen, MRI of the circle of Willis, and an evaluation of the colon is advisable in the pretransplant evaluation of the recipient. Bilateral nephrectomy before transplantation is indicated in patients with a history of infected cysts or, rarely, in patients with massive organ enlargement with kidneys extending into the pelvis. Most ADPKD patients do not need bilateral nephrectomy before transplantation. There has been some concern that these patients might be at an increased risk for developing a renal cell carcinoma in the native kidneys. So far, this has not been a problem, but more information is needed on long-term renal allograft recipients with ADPKD who have not had a bilateral nephrectomy. After renal transplantation, ADPKD patients may have an increased, although small, risk for some morbidity events related to the extrarenal manifestations of the disease. Overall, however, the long-term outcome of renal transplantation in patients with ADPKD is similar to that of patients with other renal diseases with the exclusion of diabetes mellitus.

Hepatic cysts are frequently associated with ADPKD and usually develop later than the renal cysts. Recent studies indicate that the patient's age, the degree of renal impairment, the female gender, and the number of pregnancies the patient has had correlate with the presence and severity of the cystic liver disease. The latter factors suggest that estrogen has an effect on the development of hepatic cysts in ADPKD. This may have some practical implications when one is advising a patient with significant liver cystic involvement on the safety of future pregnancies or the use of oral contraceptives or postmenopausal estrogens. Preliminary observations that the epithelium lining the hepatic cysts is sensitive to hormones that have an effect on the biliary system, such as secretin, suggest that these cysts might also be influenced pharmacologically. For example, it has been shown in one patient that cimetidine reduces the secretion rate of unroofed hepatic cysts, possibly by inhibiting gastric acidity and secretin secretion. Despite the frequency of their occurrence, hepatic cysts rarely become symptomatic or cause laboratory abnormalities. As in the kidney, intracystic hemorrhage causes acute pain and is most often self-limited. Chronic symptoms usually result from liver enlargement and compression of adjacent structures. Sometimes the enlargement is caused by only a few dominant, very large cysts that can be treated by percutaneous drainage and ethanol sclerosis (Fig. 3). Extended cyst fenestration and segmental hepatic resection should be reserved for those rare patients with massive polycystic liver disease who are disabled by marked abdominal distention and physical disability, early satiety and weight loss, and respiratory compromise, or who have obstructive jaundice or hepatic venous outflow obstruction caused by extrinsic cyst compression. Segmental hepatic resections are often possible without detriment to the liver function because even patients with massive polycystic liver disease frequently have relative sparing of a few hepatic segments (Fig. 4). Rarely, when there is no relative sparing of any hepatic parenchyma or when there is evidence of hepatic insufficiency (which is exceptionally rare in polycystic liver disease), liver transplantation can be considered. Obviously, these surgical options are associated with significant morbidity and mortality rates and should be considered only for highly symptomatic patients in centers with sufficient expertise with these procedures.

A rare complication of polycystic liver disease is hepatic cyst infection. Usually, this occurs in patients who are immunosuppressed, are receiving maintenance hemodialysis, or who have undergone renal transplantation. Enterobacteriaceae in pure culture are the micro-organisms more commonly recovered. The best management is percutaneous drainage combined with antibiotic therapy. Ciprofloxacin is concentrated severalfold in the liver cysts relative to the serum. There is little information on the liver cyst pharmacokinetics of other antibiotics. Surgical drainage or resection and long-term antibiotic suppression may be needed for those patients in whom percutaneous drainage is not possible or successful.

The association of ADPKD and intracranial aneurysms (ICAs) has been well documented. At autopsy ADPKD and ICAs coexist 7.6 times more frequently than would be expected by chance association alone. Subarachnoid hemorrhage (SAH) accounted for 6.9 percent of the mortality in the ADPKD patients of Olmsted County, Minnesota. The incidence of aneurysmal SAH in the ADPKD population of Rochester, Minnesota (1/2,089 persons/yr) is five times higher than in the general population of the same community (1/10,000 persons a year). Aneurysmal rupture in ADPKD occurs at a younger age as compared with sporadic aneurysms. With the development of magnetic resonance angiography, sensitive, noninvasive, presymptomatic screening for ICAs has become possible. With this technique, ICAs were found in 22 percent of patients with a family history of ICA or SAH and in 5 percent of patients without such history. These aneurysms were all small (<6.5 mm in diameter).

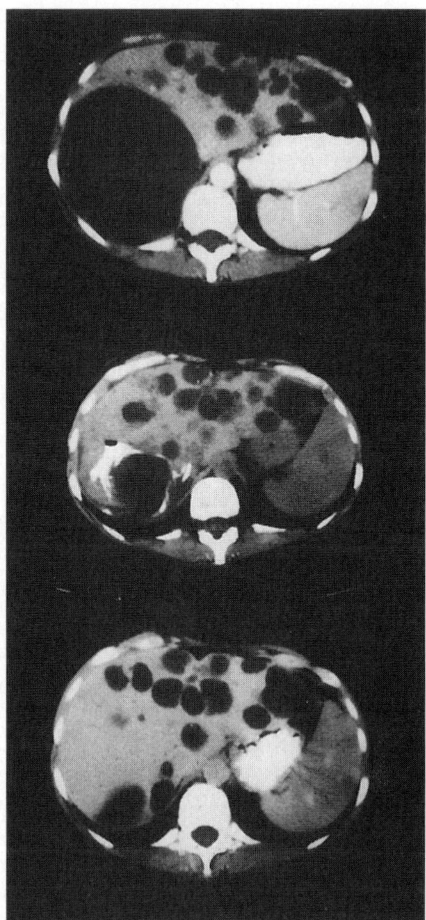

Figure 3
Ethanol sclerosis of a dominant hepatic cyst. *Top,* CT scan showing a large, dominant cyst in the right hepatic lobe. *Middle,* The cyst has been drained and a small amount of contrast material has been injected into the cyst before ethanol sclerosis; a small, adjacent cyst, previously concealed by the dominant cyst, is now seen. *Bottom,* Three months after the ethanol sclerosis, the large dominant cyst is no longer present.

The value of presymptomatic screening for ICAs depends not only on their prevalence and on the yield and risk of the screening procedure but also on the likelihood of benefit from treatment if an aneurysm is found. This, in turn, depends on the risk of rupture, morbidity and mortality from rupture, surgical risk, and rate of formation of de novo aneurysms. The risk of rupture of an asymptomatic aneurysm depends on the size of the aneurysm and on whether there has been an SAH from a different aneurysm in the same patient. Yearly rupture rates range from less than 0.5 percent to 4 percent. Serious morbidity and mortality from aneurysmal rupture ranges

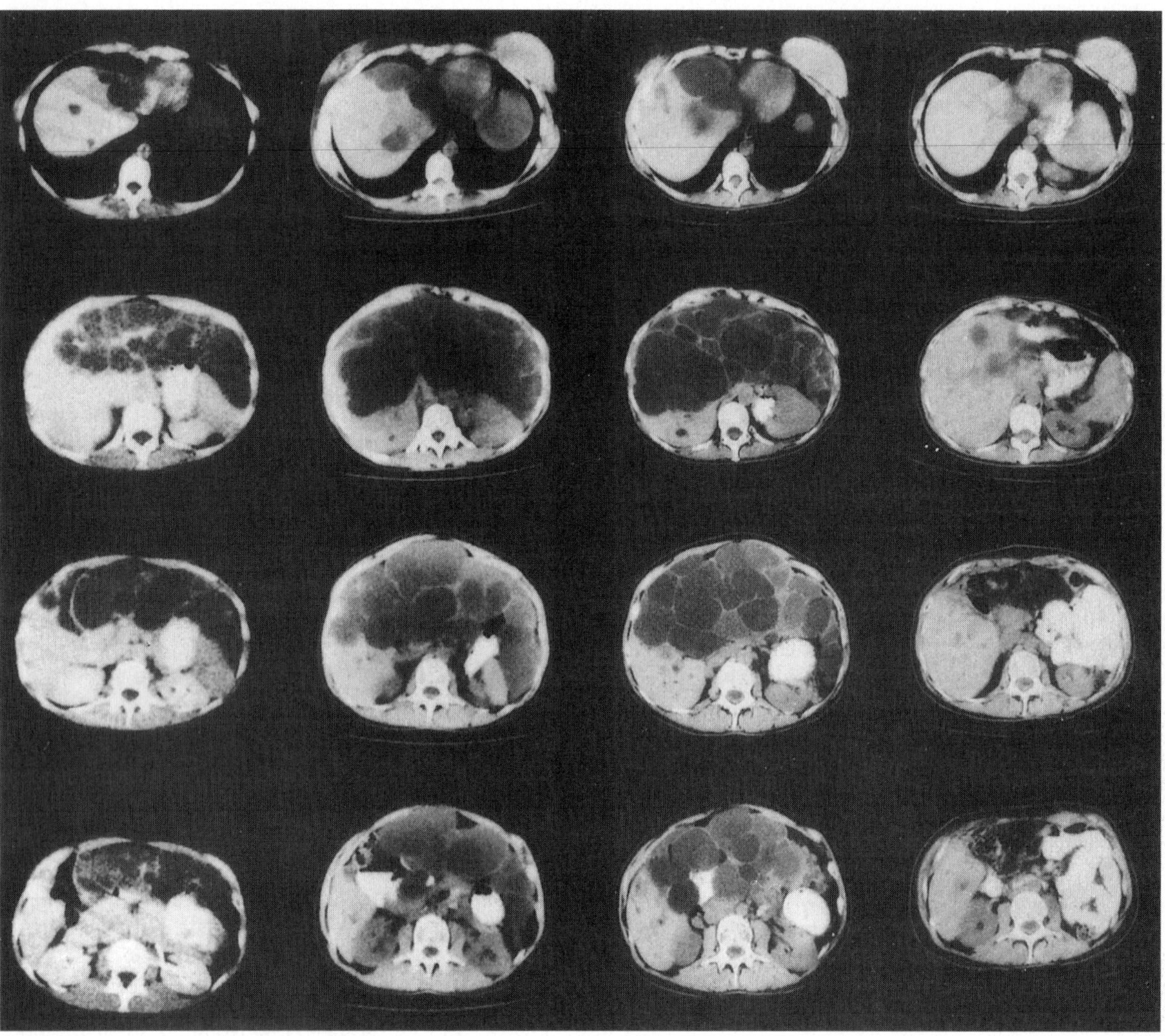

Figure 4
Massive polycystic liver disease. CT scans of the abdomen obtained 10 years before *(left),* 4 years before *(center left),* 1 month before *(center right),* and after *(right)* a combined hepatic resection fenestration procedure.

from 30 to 50 percent with a trend toward lower mortality in recent years. The risk of serious morbidity and mortality from surgery depends on the number, size, and location of the aneurysms and on the presence of comorbid factors, and it ranges from less than 1 percent to 30 percent. Finally, the rate of development of the de novo aneurysms is approximately 2 percent per year. After considering all of these factors and in view of the fact that most incidental asymptomatic ICAs detected in ADPKD patients are small and probably have a low risk of rupture, most investigators have concluded that generalized screening of ADPKD patients is not cost effective or justifiable. It seems reasonable to restrict the screening to patients with good life expectancy and a family history of ICA or SAH and to those with a previous episode of aneurysmal rupture. Other possible indications include preparation for major elective surgery with anticipated hemodynamic instability, indeterminate symptoms that might suggest the presence of an ICA, high-risk occupations, and patients who, having been adequately informed, still want the reassurance that the screening can provide.

Asymptomatic ICAs found concurrently with ruptured aneurysms appear to have a higher risk of rupture and should be surgically treated if technically feasible. An intracranial operation to isolate from the circulation incidental asymptomatic aneurysms measuring 10 mm or more in diameter is clearly indicated in women under 75 years of age and in men under 60 years of age. Reassurance and observation are indicated for asymptomatic aneurysms measuring 5 mm or less in diameter, whereas the treatment of asymptomatic aneurysms measuring 6 to 9 mm in diameter remains controversial. Intravascular occlusion of ICA with detachable platinum coils may be preferable to surgery when the surgical risk is high because of the location or size of the aneurysm or because of the patient's condition.

Physicians caring for patients with ADPKD should be aware of the disease's association with cardiovascular abnormalities, especially mitral valve prolapse, aortic insufficiency, and aortic aneurysms, and with colon diverticula. Patients with associated cardiovascular abnormalities should be informed of the importance of strictblood pressure-control and endocarditis prophylaxis. Because of the possible increased risk for colonic diverticulosis, these patients should be advised to follow a high-fiber diet and to avoid constipation.

■ TUBEROUS SCLEROSIS

Tuberous sclerosis is an autosomal dominant disease with high penetrance, an extremely variable expression, and a high rate of spontaneous mutation. It is genetically heterogeneous with one gene in chromosome 9q34 (TSC1) and another gene in chromosome 16p13.3 (TSC2). It may affect the central nervous system (cortical tubers, subependymal nodules, and giant cell tumors), skin (facial angiofibroma or adenoma sebaceum, fibrous plaques, periungual or subungual fibromas, hypomelanotic macules, and shagreen patches), retina (hamartoma), kidneys (angiomyolipomas, cysts, and, more rarely, renal cell carcinomas), heart (rhabdomyoma), and lungs. Other organs may also be involved, and cysts can occur in the liver. The association of renal cysts and angiomyolipomas is pathognomonic of tuberous sclerosis. In the absence of a family history or angiomyolipomas, the renal cystic disease can be confused with ADPKD.

Treatment

Renal angiomyolipomas require no treatment except in the event of life-threatening bleeding, which may require arterial embolization or segmental nephrectomy or enucleation. Patients with severe, diffuse bilateral cystic involvement often have hypertension and may develop renal failure, usually in the second or third decade of life. The treatment of hypertension and renal failure in these patients is similar to that in ADPKD. Bilateral nephrectomy performed before renal transplantation is indicated in these patients because of the risk of bleeding caused by the angiomyolipomas and because of a likely increased risk for renal cell carcinoma in tuberous sclerosis.

■ VON HIPPEL-LINDAU DISEASE

Von Hippel-Lindau disease is an autosomal dominant disorder with high penetrance and variable expression. It has been mapped to chromosome 3p25-26.

It affects most frequently the cerebellum, medulla oblongata, spinal cord (hemangioblastomas), retina (angiomatosis), kidney (cysts, hemangiomas, adenomas, and carcinomas), pancreas (cysts and, rarely, tumors), and adrenal gland (pheochromocytoma). The renal cysts are usually multiple and limited in number. Occasionally the kidneys may be diffusely cystic, with characteristics resembling those of ADPKD. Some of the patients described in the literature as having renal cell carcinomas and ADPKD probably had von Hippel-Lindau disease.

Treatment

An effort to spare renal tissue in the treatment of renal cell carcinoma in this disease has been recommended, since bilateral and multiple carcinomas are likely to be present or develop subsequently. Early diagnosis of these lesions is essential and CT of the abdomen performed annually is recommended. The renal cysts usually require no treatment. For those patients who have extensive cystic disease and renal failure that require dialysis, nephrectomy should be performed because of the risk of carcinoma.

■ ACQUIRED CYSTIC KIDNEY DISEASE

The term *acquired cystic kidney disease* denotes the cystic degeneration of the renal parenchyma in end-stage kidneys that is probably the result of prolonged uremia. It occurs most often in patients receiving maintenance hemodialysis or peritoneal dialysis, but it has also been described as occurring before the initiation of dialysis after prolonged uremia in native as well as in transplanted kidneys with chronic rejection. The number of patients with cysts, as well as the number and size of the cysts, increases with the duration of uremia and dialysis. The frequency of acquired cystic kidney disease depends on the sensitivity of the diagnostic techniques. Contrast-enhanced CT with thin sections has greater resolution than ultrasonography, and both underestimate the number of cysts observed by direct examination of the kidneys. Using sensitive CT techniques, multiple renal cysts are observed in approximately 80 percent of patients who have been receiving hemodialysis for more than 3 years. It is usually a silent process. Symptoms are related to complications, which include intracystic bleeding, gross hematuria, retroperitoneal hemorrhage, cyst infection, and malignant transformation.

Treatment

As in the treatment of ADPKD, the treatment of a cyst hemorrhage is usually conservative, consisting of bed rest and analgesics. Regional heparinization should be used for dialysis. Occasionally, renal artery embolization or nephrectomy is required. Percutaneous drainage in addition to antibiotic therapy is an alternative to surgical drainage or nephrectomy in the treatment of cyst infection in acquired renal cystic disease (ACRD). It has been estimated that 20 percent of patients with acquired renal cystic disease have tumors, adenomas, or adenocarcinomas. The categorization of these tumors as adenomas or carcinomas is difficult and depends on size and cytologic features. Most tumors less than 3 cm in diameter do not metastasize, but exceptions do occur. It has been estimated that 5 percent of the patients with acquired cystic disease and solid tumors develop metastases. Risk factors for the development of renal cell carcinoma in ARCD include male gender and large renal volume. The diagnosis of ARCD can be made by sonography, but contrast-enhanced MR imaging are the best techniques to detect a solid mass within hyperechoic cystic kidneys. It remains controversial whether patients on dialysis should be screened for the presence of ARCD and renal cell carcinoma. Some investigators have concluded that generalized screening is of little, if any, benefit, and not cost effective. Other investigators recommend annual or biannual screening for patients who have been on dialysis for 3 or more years, with few comobid factors and reasonable life expectancy. Small renal tumors measuring less than 3 cm in diameter should be followed at 6 month intervals. Surgical intervention is indicated for large solid tumors or when there is evidence of progressive tumor enlargement. Because of the frequent multicentricity of these tumors and current availability of erythropoietin, bilateral nephrectomy is recommended. Although acquired renal cystic disease can regress after renal transplantation, there have been some reports of patients with acquired renal cystic disease developing a metastatic renal cell carcinoma years after renal transplantation. A recent report has suggested that 2 percent of deaths occurring among patients who have undergone renal transplantation are secondary to metastatic renal cell carcinoma arising from the native kidneys. It therefore seems prudent to recommend that patients with renal failure, especially those who have been receiving dialysis for more than 1 or 2 years, should have an evaluation of the native kidneys by CT or ultrasonography before transplantation. Patients with solid tumors should undergo bilateral nephrectomy before transplantation.

■ MULTILOCULAR CYST

The multilocular cyst or multilocular cystic nephroma is a well-defined entity consisting of a well-circumscribed, encapsulated renal mass composed of multiple noncommunicating cysts of varying size. The loculi of the cysts are lined with flattened or plump reactive epithelial cells. In some cases, proliferation of these cells has been interpreted as evidence of their neoplastic nature, and occasionally histologic evidence of renal cell adenocarcinoma is found. The biologic course of these tumors is usually benign. Approximately half of the cases occur in children and the other half in adults.

Treatment

The treatment of choice, when technically possible, is partial nephrectomy. At the time of surgery, thorough tissue sampling for histologic studies and frozen sections should be used to rule out the presence of a renal cell carcinoma that would require a total nephrectomy.

■ CYSTIC DISEASE OF THE RENAL SINUS

The cystic disorders of the renal sinus are benign conditions. The most common cysts in this area are of lymphatic origin and are often multiple and bilateral. Despite considerable distortion of the calices and infundibula, the pressure in these lymphatic cysts is usually low, not causing significant functional obstruction. Ultrasonography and CT have facilitated the differential diagnosis of these cysts from other benign conditions such as renal sinus lipomatosis, as well as from serious diseases such as neoplasms of the renal pelvis and kidney or ADPKD.

Treatment

The therapeutic approach to these cysts should be conservative, since the cystic disease of the renal sinus is a benign condition.

Suggested Reading

Fick GM, Gabow PA. Hereditary and acquired cystic disease of the kidney. (Review) Kidney Int 1994; 46:951–964.

Gardner KJ, Bernstein J, eds. The cystic kidney. The Netherlands: Kluwer Academic Publishers, 1990.

Watson ML, Torres VE, eds. Polycystic Kidney Disease. Oxford: Oxford University Press, 1996.

NUTRITIONAL AND NONDIALYTIC MANAGEMENT OF CHRONIC RENAL FAILURE

Joel D. Kopple, M.D.

Nutritional therapy for patients with chronic renal failure has three major goals. These are (1) to retard the rate of progression of renal failure (in the nondialyzed patient), (2) to maintain good nutritional status, and (3) to prevent or improve the uremic syndrome. A reduction in the intake of certain nutrients may retard the progression of renal disease and, in patients with advanced renal failure, reduce uremic toxicity. However, there is much evidence that many patients undergoing maintenance dialysis have wasting and malnutrition. The wasting is usually mild or moderate, but frequently it can be severe. Since in the Western world maintenance dialysis therapy is readily available, it is more advisable to provide a diet for a patient with renal failure that maintains good nutritional status than to prescribe a nutritional therapy that may reduce uremic toxicity at the expense of inducing malnutrition. A proposed recommended intake for adult uremic patients and patients undergoing maintenance hemodialysis or continuous ambulatory peritoneal dialysis (CAPD) is shown in Table 1.

Note: When the recommended nutrient intake is given in terms of kilograms of body weight, this refers to the Metropolitan Life Insurance's desirable body weight, expressed according to the age, height, sex, and frame size of the patient.

Monitoring Nitrogen Intake: Urea Nitrogen Appearance and the Serum Urea Nitrogen to Serum Creatinine Ratio

It is important to ensure that the dietary protein intake in patients with renal failure is neither too low nor too high.

Table 1 Recommended Daily Intakes for Nondialyzed Patients with Chronic Renal Failure and Patients Undergoing Maintenance Hemodialysis or Continuous Ambulatory Peritoneal Dialysis

	CHRONIC RENAL FAILURE*†	HEMODIALYSIS (HD) AND CONTINUOUS AMBULATORY (CAPD) OR CYCLIC PERITONEAL DIALYSIS (CCPD)
Protein‡	0.55–0.60 g/kg/day (about ≥35 g/kg/day high biologic value); maximum intake is 45 g/day Very-low-protein diet (about 0.28 g/kg/day of protein of any biologic value) supplemented with either a ketoacid and amino acid mixture or essential amino acid mixture	HD: 1.0–1.2 g/kg/day; ≥50% high biologic value protein; 1.2 g/kg/day is prescribed unless patient has normal protein status with intakes of 1.0–1.1 g protein/kg/day CAPD: 1.2–1.3 g/kg/day; ≥50% CCPD: High biologic value protein; for malnourished patients, up to 1.5 g/kg/day may be given
Calories§	≥35 Kcal/kg/day unless the patient's relative body weight is >120%	
Fat (% of total calorie intake)**††	40–55	40–55
Polyunsaturated : saturated fatty acid ratio††	1.0 : 1.0	1.0 : 1.0
Carbohydrate‡‡	Rest of nonprotein calories	Rest of nonprotein calories
Total fiber intake††	20–25 g/day	20–25 g/day
Minerals		
Sodium	1,000 to 3,000 mg/day§§	750 to 1,000 mg/day§§
Potassium	40 to 70 mEq/day	40 to 70 mEq/day
Phosphorus	4 to 12 mg/kg/day***	8 to 17 mg/kg/day***
Calcium	1,400 to 1,600 mg/day†††	1,400 to 1,600 mg/day†††
Magnesium	200 to 300 mg/day	200 to 300 mg/day
Iron	10 to 18 mg/day‡‡‡	10 to 18 mg/day‡‡‡
Zinc	15 mg/day	15 mg/day
Water	Up to 3,000 ml/day as tolerated§§	Usually 750 to 1,500 ml/day§§
Vitamin supplements	Diets to be supplemented with these quantities	
Thiamin	1.5 mg/day	1.5 mg/day
Riboflavin	1.8 mg/day	1.8 mg/day
Pantothenic Acid	5 mg/day	5 mg/day
Niacin	20 mg/day	20 mg/day
Pyridoxine HCl	5 mg/day	10 mg/day
Vitamin B_{12}	3 μg/day	3 μg/day
Folic Acid	1 mg/day	1 mg/day
Vitamin A	None	None
Vitamin D	See text	See text
Vitamin E	15 IU/day	15 IU/day
Vitamin K	None§§§	None§§§

*GFR >4–5 ml/min and ≤70 ml/min/1.73 meters squared.
†When recommended intake is expressed per kg body weight, this refers to the patient's desirable weight as determined from the Metropolitan Life Insurance tables.
‡The protein intake is increased by 1.0 g/day of high biologic value protein for each g/day of urinary protein loss.
§This includes energy intake from dialysate in CAPD and CCPD patients.
**Refers to percent of total energy intake (diet plus dialysate).
††These dietary recommendations are considered less crucial than the others.
‡‡Should be primarily complex carbohydrates, if tolerated by the patient.
§§Can be higher in nondialyzed chronic renal failure or maintenance dialysis patients who have greater urinary losses or in CAPD or CCPD patients.
***Phosphorus intake should be 4–9 mg/day for patients ingesting a very low-protein diet supplemented with ketoacids or amino acids; with the 0.55–0.60 g protein/kg/day diet, a phosphorus intake of 8–12 mg/kg/day is more tolerable. Phosphate binders are usually needed as well (see text).
†††Dietary intake must be supplemented to provide these levels.
‡‡‡≥10 mg/day for males and nonmenstruating females; ≥18 mg/day for menstruating females.
§§§Vitamin K supplements may be needed in those who are eating and are receiving antibiotics.

Thus, it is of value to estimate accurately a patient's actual nitrogen intake. Since urea is the major nitrogenous product of protein and amino acid metabolism, the urea nitrogen appearance (UNA, net urea generation) usually correlates closely with, and can be used to estimate, total nitrogen output. UNA is calculated as follows:

$$\text{UNA} = \text{urinary urea nitrogen (UN)} + \text{dialysate UN} + \text{change in body UN}$$

$$\text{Change in body UN} = (\text{SUN}_f - \text{SUN}_i) \times \text{BW}_i \times 0.60 \text{ L per kilogram} + (\text{BW}_f - \text{BW}_i) \times \text{SUN}_f \times 1.0 \text{ L per kilogram}$$

Where UNA and UN are given in grams per day, and final values for the period of measurement, SUN is serum urea nitrogen (g per liter), and BW is body weight (kg). The fraction of body weight that is water is represented by 0.60. Greater or lesser numbers may be used depending on whether the patient is lean, edematous, obese, old, or young. The assumption is made that in a uremic patient any change in BW occurring during a 1 to 3 day interval is attributable to accrual or to loss of water. Therefore, the fraction of weight change that represents gain or loss of water is taken as 1.0.

In our experience, the relationship between UNA and total nitrogen output in chronically uremic patients not undergoing dialysis is as follows:

$$\text{Total nitrogen output (g per day)} = 0.97 \text{ UNA (g per day)} + 1.93 \text{ (g per day)}$$

Since protein contains about 16 percent nitrogen, the relation between UNA and net protein breakdown in these patients can be estimated from the following equation:

$$\text{Net protein breakdown (g per day)} = 6.1 \text{ UNA (g per day)} + 12 \text{ (g per day)}$$

If patients are in neutral balance, this same equation can be used to estimate protein intake; about 3.0 g per day of protein may be added to the value to adjust for unmeasured nitrogen losses.

In nondialyzed patients with chronic renal failure, there is a direct correlation between the ratio of the serum urea nitrogen (SUN) to the serum creatinine and the protein intake. This relationship can be used to estimate daily protein intake or, conversely, to select the optimal quantity of protein to be prescribed for a patient. Although this technique is easy to use and fairly accurate, several factors may reduce its usefulness. A urine flow less than 1,500 ml per day may increase the SUN-serum creatinine ratio for a given protein intake because, in contrast to the creatinine clearance, the urea clearance tends to fall progressively as urine flow decreases below this level.

The SUN-serum creatinine ratio increases with catabolic stress and with reduced muscle mass, as is found in women, children, and very wasted men. Also, with a change in dietary protein, a period of 2 to 3 weeks may be necessary for the SUN to stabilize and the SUN-serum creatinine ratio to reflect the new protein intake. In clinically stable, chronically uremic men with a protein intake of 20, 40, or 60 g per day, the SUN-serum creatinine ratio should be, on an average, 3.4, 6.0, and 8.6, respectively.

Protein Intake

A number of studies in both rats and humans with renal insufficiency indicate that a diet low in protein and phosphorus may retard the rate of progression of renal failure. This effect has been observed not only in patients with advanced renal failure, but also in those with mild to moderate renal failure (serum creatinine values of 2 to 6 mg per deciliter). Although each of the studies carried out in humans suffers from weaknesses in experimental design, almost all reports indicate that in some patients such diets may retard progression of renal failure. The most dramatic effects have been reported with ketoacid- and hydroxyacid-supplemented diets. There are several ketoacid and hydroxyacid formulations currently in use. They usually provide four essential amino acids (histidine, lysine, threonine, and tryptophan) and the ketoacid or hydroxyacid salts of the other five essential amino acids. The ketoacids and hydroxyacids have the same structure as the respective essential amino acids except that the alpha-amino nitrogen is removed and a keto or hydroxy group is substituted.

Chronic Renal Disease with GFR Greater Than 70 ml per Minute per 1.73 Meters Squared

Most studies of the effects of diets low in protein and phosphorus on the rate of progression of renal failure have examined patients with moderately advanced to advanced renal failure (serum creatinine ≥5mg per deciliter). Hence, there is virtually no information concerning the optimal dietary protein (or phosphorus) prescription for patients with chronic renal disease and mild impairment in renal function. Until more information is available, it is recommended that protein (and phosphorus) intake should be restricted for patients with GFR greater than 70 ml per minute per 1.73 meters squared only if there is evidence that renal function is continuing to decline. In this latter case, the patient is treated as indicated in the following paragraph.

Chronic Renal Disease with GFR 5 to 70 ml per Minute per 1.73 Meters Squared

It is the author's policy to discuss with the patient the evidence that low-protein, low-phosphorus diets may retard progression and to indicate that the data, although not conclusive, are strong enough to justify the patient ingesting a restricted protein and phosphorus diet. If the patient agrees to dietary treatment, the patient is prescribed a diet providing about 0.60 to 0.70 g protein per kilogram per day. At least 0.35 g per kilogram per day of the protein should be of high biologic value (eggs, meat, fish, and milk and its products), because these proteins contain a high proportion of essential amino acids that are present roughly in the proportions required by humans. Hence, these proteins are utilized more efficiently than are proteins of lower quality. On the other hand, low-quality proteins, which are prevalent in foods derived from plants (e.g., grains and vegetables), are particularly valuable for increasing the palatability and acceptability of the diet. At least 12 to 16 g per day of low-quality protein seem to be necessary for a palatable diet. An intake of 0.55 to 0.60 g protein per kilogram per day provides about 30 to 35 g per day for women and small men and about 40 g per day for normal sized men. In general, we do not prescribe more than about 45 g per day of protein for any patient with a GFR below 10 ml per minute. In clinically stable patients, the SUN can almost always be maintained below 90 mg per deciliter with these low-protein diets until the GFR falls below 4 to 5 ml per minute. This amount of protein should maintain neutral or positive nitrogen balance and should not be excessively burdensome for most patients.

Amino acid- and ketoacid-supplemented diets may also be offered to the patient. Currently, these diets generally provide about 0.28 g protein per kilogram per day (16 to 20 g protein per day) supplemented with about 10 to 20 g of the essential amino acids or mixtures of essential amino acids and ketoacids. Since the amino acid and ketoacid supplements provide sufficient essential amino acids, the protein derived from food does not have to be of high biologic value, thereby increasing the patient's freedom of food selection. In the author's experience, most, but not all, patients seem to prefer the 0.55 to 0.60 g protein per kilogram per day diet over the essential amino acid-supplemented diet. This former diet is less expensive than is the essential amino acid-supplemented diet.

There are several potential advantages to using amino acid or ketoacid formulations. First, with more advanced renal failure (i.e., GFR <15 to 25 ml per minute per 1.73 meters squared), potentially toxic products of nitrogen metabolism begin to accumulate in increasing quantities. Since the ketoacids and hydroxyacids lack the alpha-amino group, for the same intake of amino acid equivalents less nitrogen is provided and there is less generation of potentially toxic nitrogenous compounds. Second, because the amino acid and ketoacid preparations do not contain phosphorus (or potassium), the content of these elements in the diet can be markedly decreased (see section on recommended phosphorus intake). Third, by modifying the proportions of individual amino acids, ketoacids, or hydroxyacids in the diet, it may be possible to normalize more of the altered plasma and muscle-amino acid concentrations that develop in advanced renal failure—whether this normalization is of value to the patient is not yet established. Finally, as indicated above, these semisynthetic diets may be more effective at retarding the rate of progression of renal failure.

Given the dramatic results described with certain ketoacid formulations, it would seem reasonable that when the GFR decreases to about 25 ml per minute per 1.73 meters squared, patients should be prescribed a diet providing 0.28 g protein per kilogram per day supplemented with a mixture of about 13 to 18 g of ketoacids and amino acids, if the formulation is available. Ketoacid supplements have not yet been approved for clinical use in the United States. Where ketoacids are not available, essential amino acid supplements may be substituted for the ketoacid mixture or patients may be prescribed 0.55 to 0.60 g protein per kilogram per day with at least 0.35 kg per kilogram per day of protein of high biologic value. All three of these diets generally maintain neutral or positive nitrogen balance and generate a low UNA. The protein content of each of the diets prescribed for patients with mild to severe renal failure should be increased by 1.0 g per day of high biologic value protein for each gram of protein excreted in the urine each day. Whether the ketoacid- or essential amino acid-supplemented very-low-protein diets should be prescribed for patients with a GFR above 25 ml per minute per 1.73 meters squared is not known.

When the GFR falls below 5 ml per minute per 1.73 meters squared, there is no conclusive evidence that patients fare as well with low-nitrogen diets as with regular dialysis therapy and higher protein intakes. Since these latter patients may be at high risk for wasting or malnutrition, it is recommended that maintenance dialysis treatment or renal transplantation should be inaugurated at this time. Patients with diabetes mellitus may develop uremic symptoms at a higher GFR; thus, such individuals are often started on maintenance dialysis or undergo renal transplantation when their GFR is between 5 and 10 ml per minute per 1.73 meters squared.

Adherence to low-protein, low-phosphorus diets requires a major change in dietary habits and even in life style. Prior to beginning dietary therapy, the patient and, if possible, close family members or other participants in his or her support network must be informed of the magnitude of this undertaking and must agree to the commitment. Otherwise, there is small likelihood that the patient will adhere successfully to this dietary prescription.

Maintenance Dialysis Therapy

Patients undergoing hemodialysis three times per week should receive a minimum of 1.0 and preferably 1.2 g of protein per kilogram per day (Table 1). Patients undergoing CAPD should receive 1.2 to 1.3 g per kilogram per day of protein. In malnourished CAPD patients, up to 1.5 g protein per kilogram per day can be taken. At least half of their dietary protein should be of high biologic value.

Energy Intake

Studies of energy expenditure in nondialyzed chronically uremic patients and patients undergoing maintenance hemodialysis indicate that energy expenditure is normal during resting and sitting, following ingestion of a standard meal, and with graded exercise. Nitrogen balance studies in nondialyzed chronically uremic patients indicate that the amount of energy necessary to ensure neutral or positive nitrogen balance is approximately 35 Kcal per kilogram per day. However, virtually every survey of energy intake in nondialyzed chronically uremic and hemodialysis patients indicates that, on average, it is lower than this level and usually 30 Kcal per kilogram per day or less.

We currently recommend that nondialyzed chronically uremic patients and patients undergoing maintenance hemodialysis or CAPD should receive about 35 Kcal per kilogram per day. Patients who are obese with an edema-free body weight greater than 120 percent of desirable body weight may be treated with lower calorie intakes. There are many commercially available high-calorie foodstuffs that are low in protein, sodium, and potassium. A nephrology dietitian can recommend these foodstuffs as well as other low-protein high-calorie foods that can be prepared easily at home.

Hyperlipidemia

A large proportion of chronically uremic and dialysis patients have type IV hyperlipoproteinemia with elevated serum triglyceride levels and a low serum HDL cholesterol. Since in uremic patients these alterations in serum lipoproteins may contribute to the high incidence of atherosclerosis and cardiovascular disease, attention has been directed toward reducing serum triglycerides and increasing HDL cholesterol. Elevated serum triglyceride levels in uremia appear to be caused primarily by impaired clearance from blood. Also, since diets in renal failure are usually restricted in protein, sodium, potassium, and water, it is often difficult to provide sufficient energy without resorting to a large intake of purified sugars, which can increase triglyceride production. Serum triglycerides may be lowered by feeding a diet in which the carbohydrate content is reduced to supply 35 percent of calories, the fat content is increased to provide 50 to 55 percent of calories, and the polyunsaturated-saturated fatty acid ratio is raised to 1 : 1.

Although elevated serum triglyceride levels do not appear to be a strong risk factor for arteriosclerotic disease, this dietary treatment should be employed at least for uremic patients with markedly elevated serum triglyceride levels (e.g., greater than 1.5 to 2.0 times the upper limits of normal). L-carnitine, 1.0 g per day orally, may also decrease serum triglyceride concentrations, and patients with this magnitude of hypertriglyceridemia who have low serum carnitine should probably also be given a trial period with this compound. Low serum HDL cholesterol levels are a strong risk factor for cardiovascular disease. Serum concentrations may increase with daily exercise.

Mineral and Water Intake

Sodium and Water

As renal failure progresses, both the glomerular filtration and fractional reabsorption of sodium fall progressively. Thus, sodium balance is usually well maintained in patients with chronic renal failure when they ingest a normal salt intake. However, there is an impaired ability to handle both a sodium load and to conserve sodium normally during intake of a low-sodium diet. Normally, only about 1 to 3 mEq per day of sodium are excreted in the feces, and in the nonsweating individual, only a few mEq per day of sodium are lost through the skin. If sodium intake exceeds the ability of the kidney to excrete sodium, sodium and water retention, hypertension, edema, and congestive heart failure may develop. Certain conditions predispose to sodium retention and may dictate earlier restriction of sodium or water intake or the use of diuretic agents. These conditions include congestive heart failure and advanced liver disease. When the GFR falls below 4 to 10 ml per minute, the ability to handle even a normal sodium intake may fall. In addition, in renal failure, hypertension may be more easily controlled with sodium restriction and may be accentuated with normal or increased sodium intakes. On the other hand, if sodium intake is not sufficient to replace obligatory renal sodium losses, sodium depletion and contraction of extracellular fluid volume may occur and may lead to reduced renal blood flow and further impairment of GFR. Hence, when evaluating patients with renal failure who do not have evidence of fluid overload or hypertension, they should be given a careful trial of sodium loading to assess whether renal function may be improved.

In general, if sodium balance is well controlled, the patient's thirst adequately controls water balance. However, when the GFR falls below 2 to 5 ml per minute, the water intake often must be controlled independently of sodium to prevent overhydration. In diabetics, hyperglycemia may increase thirst and enhance positive water balance. In patients whose total body water is at the desired level, urine excretion may be a good guide to water intake. Daily water intake should equal the urine output plus approximately 500 ml to adjust for insensible losses.

Most nondialyzed chronically uremic patients maintain sodium and water balance with an intake of 1,000 to 3,000 mg of sodium per day and 600 to 3,000 ml of fluid per day. However, the requirement for sodium and water varies markedly, and each patient must be managed individually. Usually, patients undergoing maintenance hemodialysis or peritoneal dialysis are severely oliguric or anuric. For hemodialysis patients, sodium and total fluid intake generally should be restricted to 1,000 to 1,500 mg per day and 700 to 1,500 ml per day, respectively. Patients undergoing CAPD usually tolerate a greater sodium and water intake because salt and water can be easily removed by using hypertonic dialysate. By maintaining a larger dietary sodium and water intake, the quantity of fluid removed from the CAPD patient and, hence, the daily dialysate volume can be increased. This may be advantageous since with CAPD, the daily clearance of small molecules is directly related to the volume of dialysate outflow. With this in mind, some nephrologists have recommended a larger dietary sodium and water intake for CAPD patients in order to increase the hypertonic dialysate and thus increase dialysate outflow. This treatment may be undesirable for obese or hypertriglyceridemic patients because of the greater need for hypertonic glucose exchanges that increase the glucose load. Also, there is the potential disadvantage that some patients may become habituated to high salt and water intakes; if they are changed to hemodialysis therapy, they may have difficulty curtailing ingestion of sodium and water.

One way to monitor sodium requirements in nondialyzed patients is to follow carefully the body weight, blood pressure, and serum sodium. When sodium intake is inadequate, there is often negative water balance, a decrease in body weight, and a fall in blood pressure. Excessive sodium intake is often associated with positive water balance, a rise in body weight, and an increase in blood pressure. Serum sodium concentrations may rise, fall, or not change depending upon the water balance. On the other hand, a decrease in serum sodium in the presence of an unchanging or falling body weight usually indicates that there is a need for more sodium. The dietary sodium requirement may also be determined by decreasing or raising sodium intake for several days and monitoring body weight, blood pressure, appearance of edema, serum creatinine or clearance, serum sodium, and urinary sodium output. The optimal dietary sodium can be assessed by comparing the effects of the sodium intake on excess water gain or loss, the blood pressure, and the creatinine clearance.

In nondialyzed chronically uremic patients or patients undergoing maintenance dialysis who gain excessive sodium or water despite attempts at dietary restriction, furosemide may be used to increase urinary sodium and water excretion.

Potassium

Most patients who have nonoliguric advanced renal failure or who are undergoing maintenance dialysis can tolerate up to

70 mEq of potassium per day without hyperkalemia. Patients with hyporeninemic hypoaldosteronism, however, may be intolerant to this amount of potassium unless they are given a mineralocorticoid, such as 9-alpha-fluorohydrocortisone. In some patients who are given this mineralocorticoid, sodium retention with hypertension or congestive heart failure may occur. In susceptible patients, this usually can be prevented by administering a diuretic simultaneously with the mineralocorticoid.

Phosphorus

It is important to restrict phosphorus intake to prevent or to minimize hyperparathyroidism and possibly to retard the rate of progression of renal failure (as already discussed). The degree to which dietary phosphorus should be reduced is not well established. Clearly, phosphorus restriction should be employed to keep serum phosphorus within normal levels. However, some nephrologists have questioned whether in order to prevent or to ameliorate hyperparathyroidism, the phosphorus intake should be reduced to maintain a normal renal tubular reabsorption of phosphorus; this would require a very low phosphorus intake. The restriction of phosphorus intake that may be necessary to retard the progression of renal failure is not known. The phosphorus intake can be reduced to 300 to 500 mg per day with the essential amino acid- or ketoacid-supplemented very-low-protein diets. One small clinical trial suggests that a prescribed phosphorus intake of 6.5 mg per kilogram per day will slow progression more than an intake of 12 mg per kilogram per day.

Until more information is available, it seems prudent to use a combination of dietary phosphorus restriction and chemical binders of phosphate to maintain the morning serum phosphorus concentrations well within the normal range. Since there is a rough correlation between the protein and phosphorus content of the diet, it is easier to restrict phosphorus if protein intake is reduced. With a 0.55 to 0.60 g per kilogram per day protein diet, phosphorus intake can be decreased to 10 to 12 mg per kilogram per day and sometimes to as low as 8 mg per kilogram per day. This level of dietary phosphorus restriction usually does not maintain serum phosphorus levels within normal limits in patients with a GFR under about 15 ml per minute, and phosphate binders are therefore also employed.

Formerly, the two most commonly used phosphate binders were aluminum carbonate and aluminum hydroxide. Usually, two to four capsules are taken three to four times per day as needed. Greater doses may be used if necessary. Recent evidence that aluminum-induced osteomalacia is causally related to the total lifetime dose of aluminum phosphate binders has made many nephrologists reluctant to use them. However, the hazards of severe uncontrolled hyperparathyroidism would seem to outweigh the potential dangers of aluminum-induced osteomalacia. Thus, if serum phosphorus levels cannot be maintained within normal limits by diet alone, phosphate binders are used.

Several nonaluminum phosphate binders are now being investigated. Calcium carbonate and calcium citrate both appear to bind phosphate effectively. These calcium binders can be given in divided doses with meals and should not be given unless the serum phosphorus level is normal in order to avoid precipitation of calcium phosphate in soft tissues. Thus, hyperphosphatemic patients may be treated with an aluminum binder of phosphate until serum phosphorus falls to normal. At that time, they may be changed to calcium carbonate or calcium citrate. Normally, patients should probably not receive more than about 5 g per day of calcium carbonate or 8.3 g per day of calcium citrate (about 2 g per day of elemental calcium) in order to prevent excessive accumulation of calcium in soft tissues. Calcium carbonate also may counteract the metabolic acidosis frequently found in patients with renal failure. Calcium citrate may be advantageous for the same reason, since the citrate may be metabolized to generate bicarbonate.

As previously indicated, since the essential amino acid and ketoacid supplements do not contain phosphorus, one advantage to diets providing these formulations with about 0.28 g of protein per kilogram per day is the greater degree to which the phosphorus intake can be reduced, often to as low as 4 to 6 mg per kilogram per day. If future studies confirm that these very low phosphorus intakes are both safe and beneficial for patients with mild, moderate, or severe renal insufficiency, this would provide additional justification for the use of these semisynthetic diets.

Calcium

Patients with chronic renal failure have an increased dietary calcium requirement because there is often both vitamin D deficiency and resistance to the actions of vitamin D. These disorders, which lead to impaired intestinal calcium absorption, are compounded by the low calcium content of diets for uremic patients. A 40 g protein diet, for example, provides only about 300 to 400 mg per day of calcium. Dietary calcium intake is low because many foods that are high in calcium are high in phosphorus (e.g., dairy products) and are therefore restricted for uremic patients.

Chronically uremic patients usually require about 1,200 to 1,600 mg per day of calcium for neutral or positive calcium balance, and the diet, therefore, should be supplemented with elemental calcium. Probably, a good target level for total daily calcium intake (food plus supplemental calcium) is 1,400 to 1,600 mg per day. As indicated, up to 2 g of elemental calcium may be given as calcium salts to bind phosphate. Supplemental calcium therapy should not be initiated unless the serum phosphorus concentration is normal (i.e., 3.5 to 4.5 mg per deciliter) to prevent calcium phosphate deposition in soft tissues. Also, frequent monitoring of serum calcium is important since hypercalcemia may develop, particularly if serum phosphorus should fall to low or low-normal levels. Patients undergoing maintenance hemodialysis or peritoneal dialysis may also require 1.0 g per day of supplemental calcium even though there is net calcium uptake from dialysate.

Calcium comprises 40 percent of calcium carbonate, 24 percent of calcium citrate, 18 percent of calcium lactate, and 9 percent of calcium gluconate. Oral calcium chloride should be avoided in uremic patients because of its acidifying properties. As indicated above, calcium carbonate and calcium citrate have both been shown to be effective intestinal phosphate binders. Several proprietary calcium carbonate or calcium citrate tablets have been given a pleasant flavor and are well accepted.

Magnesium

In chronically uremic patients, there is net absorption from the intestinal tract of about 50 percent of ingested magnesium (net absorption is the difference between dietary intake and fecal excretion). The absorbed magnesium is excreted primarily by the kidney, and in renal failure, hypermagnesemia may occur. However, the restricted diets of uremic patients are low in magnesium (usually about 100 to 300 mg per day for a 40 g protein diet), and their serum magnesium levels are usually normal or only slightly elevated. Clinically significant hypermagnesemia usually occurs only when there are additional sources of magnesium intake such as magnesium-containing antacids and laxatives. The nondialyzed chronically uremic patient requires about 200 mg per day of magnesium to maintain neutral magnesium balance. The optimal dietary magnesium allowance for the dialysis patient has not been defined.

Trace Elements

Increased or decreased tissue levels of many trace elements are often observed in patients with chronic renal failure. Adverse clinical effects have not been identified for most of these disorders. Dietary requirements for trace elements have not been defined for uremic patients. Many trace elements are bound avidly to serum proteins, and when present in dialysate, even in small quantities, they may be taken up in the blood. It is therefore recommended that trace elements be removed routinely from the dialysate prior to use.

Since iron deficiency is common and can cause anemia, chronically uremic and dialysis patients may be given oral iron supplements. Ferrous sulfate, 300 mg three times a day after meals, may be used. Patients who do not tolerate this or other oral iron supplements or who have iron deficiency are usually best treated with intramuscular or intravenous iron.

The zinc content of most tissues is normal in renal failure. However, serum and hair zinc may be low, and the red cell zinc is increased. Some reports indicate that dysgeusia and impaired sexual function, which occur commonly in renal failure, may be improved by giving patients zinc supplements. There is not yet sufficient evidence that routine zinc supplementation is beneficial; additional studies are clearly indicated. It is probably of value to ensure that patients ingest the recommended dietary allowance for zinc, 15 mg per day.

Increased body burden of aluminum has been implicated in dialysis patients as a cause of a progressive dementia syndrome, osteomalacia, and anemia. Current data suggest that both contamination of dialysate with aluminum and ingestion of aluminum binders of phosphate may contribute to the excess body burden of aluminum. Recent evidence that bone aluminum levels correlate with total lifetime dosage of aluminum binders of phosphate have led many nephrologists to use aluminum binders more sparingly and to rely more upon low phosphorus diets to control serum phosphorus levels. As indicated above, calcium carbonate and calcium citrate have also been used in place of aluminum hydroxide or carbonate to bind phosphate.

Alkali

Metabolic acidosis is common in nondialyzed patients with chronic renal failure because of the impaired ability of the kidney to excrete acidic metabolites and/or the renal losses of bicarbonate. Acidosis can promote bone reabsorption and many symptoms. Ingestion of low-nitrogen diets may prevent or reduce the severity of the acidosis by decreasing the endogenous generation of acidic products of protein metabolism. Alkali supplements are usually effective for preventing or treating acidosis. Calcium carbonate or calcium citrate, may correct mild acidosis and provide needed calcium. In cases of more severe acidosis, sodium bicarbonate or citrate may be administered orally or intravenously. If the nondialyzed uremic patient is not oliguric and is not particularly likely to develop edema, sodium is usually readily excreted when administered as sodium bicarbonate or citrate. Alkali therapy should probably be initiated if the arterial pH is below 7.35 or the serum bicarbonate is less than 20 mEq per liter. Before implementing alkali therapy, it must be ascertained whether the low serum bicarbonate is not a compensatory response to chronic respiratory alkalosis. If acidosis is severe and not controlled by the foregoing measures, hemodialysis or peritoneal dialysis may be employed.

Fiber Intake

A number of studies suggest that dietary fiber intake may lead to a lower incidence of constipation, irritable bowel syndrome, diverticulitis, neoplasia of the colon, and possibly greater glucose tolerance. Since the patient with renal failure also may benefit from fiber intake, we currently prescribe 20 to 25 g per day of total dietary fiber. There are so many more important nutritional restrictions on the dietary intake of the chronically uremic and dialysis patient, however, that we do not insist vigorously that the patients adhere to a high-fiber diet.

Vitamins

Unless supplements are given, uremic patients have a tendency to develop deficiency of the water-soluble vitamins. Vitamin deficiencies are due to poor intake, altered metabolism (attributable to medicinal intake and, possibly, to uremia per se), or to losses into dialysate. Thus, deficiency of water-soluble vitamins tends to occur more frequently in dialysis patients. Vitamin B_{12} deficiency is uncommon in uremia because this vitamin is protein-bound in plasma.

In renal failure, the daily requirements for most vitamins are not well defined. There is evidence that, in addition to vitamin intake from foods, the following daily supplements of vitamins can prevent or correct vitamin deficiency: pyridoxine hydrochloride, 5 mg in nondialyzed patients and 10 mg in hemodialysis or peritoneal dialysis patients; ascorbic acid, 60 mg; folic acid, 1 mg; and the recommended daily allowance for normal individuals for the other water-soluble vitamins. High serum oxalate levels have been described in chronically uremic patients given large doses of ascorbic acid; therefore, the recommended supplement for vitamin C has been limited to the recommended dietary allowances for healthy adults. Since serum retinol-binding protein and vitamin A are elevated, supplemental vitamin A is not recommended. Additional vitamin E and K are probably not necessary. An exception is the patient who receives antibiotics for extended periods of time and who is not ingesting sufficient quantities of vitamin K; such individuals may need supplements of this vitamin. Treatment with vitamin D analogues is discussed in the chapter on renal osteodystrophy.

Some authors have reported that maintenance hemodialysis patients not receiving vitamin supplements may not develop water-soluble vitamin deficiencies. They have recommended that vitamin supplements should not be prescribed routinely to maintenance dialysis patients. However, these patients were generally followed for less than 1 year and it is possible that with longer periods of time, the incidence of vitamin deficiency may increase. Poor nutrient intake is common in chronically uremic patients, and recent reports continue to show that many renal failure patients have evidence of vitamin deficiencies. Since water-soluble vitamin supplements are safe, it would seem wise to use them routinely until these issues are more completely resolved.

Methods for Attaining Successful Nutritional Therapy

Successful dietary therapy usually requires that the patient make a major change in his lifestyle. The patient must procure special foods, prepare special recipes, usually must forgo or severely limit his intake of many favorite foods, and is often compelled to eat foods that he may not desire. There are demands made on the time, the effort, and the emotional support system of his family or close associates.

In order to ensure successful dietary therapy, patients with renal failure must undergo extensive training concerning the principles of nutritional therapy and the design and preparation of diets. Also, they need continuous encouragement regarding dietary adherence. They must receive repeated retraining regarding their nutritional therapy, and their dietary intake and nutritional status must be closely monitored. Patients who are not monitored carefully usually do not adhere closely to their diets. They may eat too little rather than too much, particularly when undergoing maintenance dialysis therapy.

A team approach to dietary management is often critical. The team should include the physician, dietitian, close family members, the nursing staff, and, when available, psychiatrists or social workers. The diet plans should be designed specifically for each patient and should take into account his or her individual tastes. At each visit, the physician should discuss dietary intake with the patient. The adequacy of energy and protein intake and nutritional status should be frequently assessed. The dietitian is often the best qualified person to perform anthropometric measurements of nutritional status because of her training, interest in nutritional therapy, and access to the patient. The physician must strongly support the efforts of the dietitian. Generally, the spouse or other close relatives or friends should work closely with the patient to provide moral support and to assist with the acquisition and preparation of foods. Nurses, psychiatrists, and social workers can encourage patients and help them work through emotional conflicts that can affect dietary compliance. They are also a valuable source of information concerning the patient's attitude toward dietary therapy, his ability to adhere to the diet, and his actual dietary intake. The important lesson is that if dietary therapy is prescribed to a patient, it requires a major commitment and effort by the patient and the medical staff to attain good results.

The most sensitive, reproducible, and readily available methods for assessing nutritional status in chronically uremic and dialysis patients include the serum albumin and total protein, relative body weight (patient's weight × 100 divided by body weight of a normal person of the same age, height, and sex), patient's weight expressed as a percentage of his weight prior to his illness, triceps and subscapular skinfold thickness, and midarm muscle circumference or cross-sectional area. Serum transferrin may also be helpful; in my experience, values are usually low even in well-nourished patients with chronic renal failure and decrease further when malnutrition is present.

DRUG PRESCRIBING IN RENAL FAILURE

George R. Aronoff, M.D., F.A.C.P.
Michael E. Brier, Ph.D.
Rosemary Ouseph, M.D.

This chapter provides strategies for administering therapeutic agents to patients with renal impairment. Uremia affects every organ system and every aspect of drug disposition. Since the kidney is the major regulator of the internal fluid environment, the physiologic changes associated with renal disease have pronounced effects on the pharmacology of many drugs.

Decreased gastrointestinal absorptive function, impaired motility, the alkalinizing effect of accumulating urea and ammonia formation, and the concurrent administration of cation-containing antacids may reduce oral drug absorption in patients with renal impairment. Edema, dehydration, and impaired protein binding alter drug distribution as renal function decreases. Impaired drug metabolism, frequent drug interactions, and alterations in first-pass hepatic biotransformation may complicate drug dosing. Drugs and their metabolites can accumulate to toxic levels. These changes in drug disposition require clinicians to have a basic understanding of the biochemical and physiologic effects of drugs in patients with renal disease.

APPROACH TO THE PATIENT WITH RENAL IMPAIRMENT

Figure 1 outlines the approach to drug dosing in patients with renal disease. When possible, a specific diagnosis should be established before drug therapy is initiated. The use of fewer drugs and the recognition of potential drug interactions decreases adverse drug effects.

History and Physical Examination

Clinical evaluation always begins with a careful history and physical examination. Particularly important is the history of previous drug allergy or toxicity and the use of concurrent medications or recreational drugs. Physical assessment should include an estimate of the extracellular fluid volume. Edema or ascites increases the distribution volume of many drugs, while dehydration contracts this volume. Measurements of body weight and height can be used to tailor the dosage regimen. Evidence of impaired function of other excretory organs should be sought. Stigmata of liver disease are clues that the drug dose may need to be altered.

Measurement of Renal Function

The rate of elimination of drugs excreted by the kidneys is proportional to the glomerular filtration rate (GFR). The

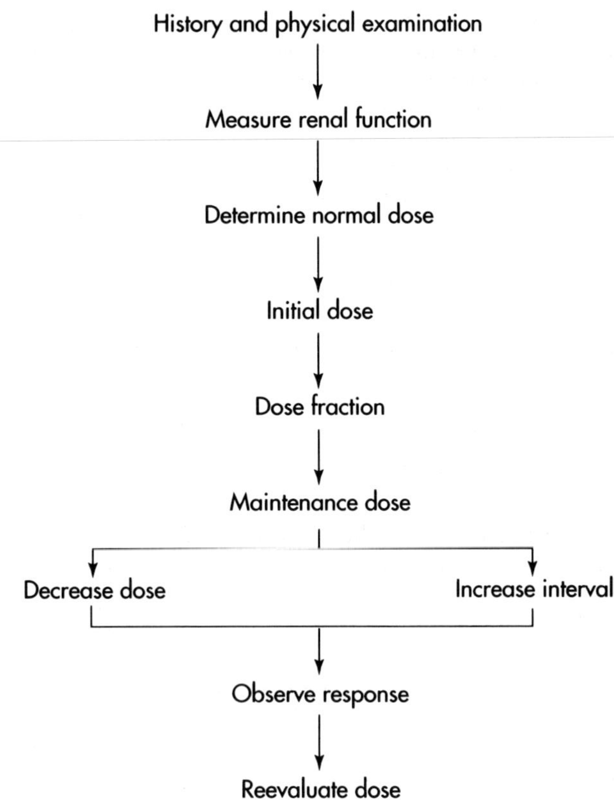

Figure 1
A schema for drug dosing in patients with impaired renal function.

serum creatinine or creatinine clearance is useful in assessing renal function before prescribing any drug. The Cockroft and Gault equation is useful for this purpose:

$$\text{Clcr} = \frac{(140 - \text{age}) \times (\text{Wt})}{72 \times \text{Scr}} \times (0.85 \text{ if female})$$

where Clcr = creatinine clearance (ml/min),
Scr = serum creatinine (mg/dl), and
Wt = body mass (Kg).

In cases of changing renal function, the serum creatinine will no longer reflect the true clearance rate. In these cases, renal function can be estimated by a timed urine collection. The midpoint serum creatinine is used to calculate the creatinine clearance for the collection period. If the patient is oliguric, the creatinine clearance is less than 5 ml per minute.

The serum creatinine reflects muscle mass as well as GFR. Serum creatinine measurements within the "normal" range are frequently used to establish "normal" renal function. This erroneous assumption may cause serious overdose and resultant toxic drug accumulation in elderly or debilitated patients with decreased muscle mass. The Cockroft and Gault equation for estimating the creatinine clearance includes adjustments for the patient's age, body mass, and gender.

Calculation of Initial Dose

The purpose of the initial dose is to achieve therapeutic drug concentrations rapidly. A loading dose should be considered when the half-life of a drug is particularly long in patients with impaired renal function. When the physical examination suggests that the extracellular fluid volume is normal, the loading dose of a drug given to a patient with renal insufficiency is the same as the initial dose given to a patient with normal renal function. If the patient has edema or ascites a larger loading dose may be required. Conversely, dehydrated or debilitated patients should receive smaller initial drug doses.

Calculation of Maintenance Dose

Several methods can be used to decide subsequent doses. Calculate the fraction of the normal dose recommended for a patient with renal insufficiency from the following relationship:

$$\text{Dose fraction} = F\,[(\text{Clcr}/120) - 1)] + 1$$

where F = fraction of the drug excreted unchanged in the urine, and Clcr = creatinine clearance.

When F is not known, the ratio of the drug's half-life in patients with normal renal function ($T_{1/2}$ normal) to that measured in patients with renal failure ($T_{1/2}$ may be substituted as below:

$$\text{Dose fraction} = \frac{T_{1/2}\text{ normal}}{T_{1/2}\text{ renal failure}}\,[(\text{Clcr}/120) - 1] + 1$$

To maintain the same dose interval as for patients with normal renal function, one may decrease the amount of each individual dose given in renal impairment as outlined below:

$$\text{Drug dose in renal impairment} = \text{Normal dose} \times \text{Dose fraction.}$$

This method is effective for drugs with narrow therapeutic ranges and short plasma half-lives in patients with renal insufficiency.

Extension of the dose interval can be calculated by dividing the dose interval for patients with normal renal function by the dose fraction found for the patient with impaired renal function, as below:

$$\text{Dose interval in renal impairment} = \frac{\text{Normal dose interval}}{\text{Dose fraction}}$$

Prolonging the dose interval is often a convenient and cost-effective method for altering the drug dose in patients with renal impairment. This method is particularly useful for drugs with wide therapeutic ranges and long plasma half-lives. Extended parenteral therapy can be completed without prolonged hospitalization, when the dose interval can safely be lengthened to allow for home therapy. If the range between the therapeutic and toxic levels is too narrow, either potentially toxic or subtherapeutic plasma concentrations may result when the dose interval is prolonged.

In practice, a combination of the methods is often effective and convenient. The combination method uses modification of both the dose and dose interval. Multiply the maintenance dose in patients with normal renal function by the dose to decide the total daily dose for a patient with renal insufficiency. For drugs with particularly long half-lives in patients with impaired renal function, give the total daily dose as a single dose each day. Alternatively, divide the total daily dose in half and give twice daily.

The decision to extend the dosing interval beyond a 24 hour period should be based on the need to maintain therapeutic peak or trough drug levels. When the peak level is most important, prolong the dose interval. However, when the minimum trough level must be maintained, modification of the individual dose or a combination of the dose and interval methods may be required.

Drug Dosing in Dialysis Patients

Drug removal by routine hemodialysis is most effective for drugs that weigh less than 500 daltons, those that are less than 90 percent protein bound, and those that have small volumes of distribution. High-flux dialyzers allow for the removal of larger molecules but do not increase the elimination of highly protein-bound drugs or those with a large volume of distribution. For many drugs, the physician must alter the dosage schedule such that the dose can be given at the end of the hemodialysis treatment, thus eliminating the need for a reloading dose.

Although drug removal by continuous ambulatory peritoneal dialysis (CAPD) is minimal, drug absorption following intraperitoneal administration may be substantial. Intraperitoneal antibiotic administration results in therapeutic serum concentrations. Other drugs including insulin have been effective when given in the peritoneal dialysate.

Adverse Drug Reactions

Adverse drug reactions occur more frequently in patients with impaired renal function. Untoward effects may be the result of direct toxicity or additive effects of the drug or its metabolites. The lack of efficacy of the drug in patients with compromised renal function, or increased drug-induced metabolic load also cause adverse drug effects.

Therapeutic Drug Monitoring

Measurement of plasma drug concentrations may be helpful in assessing a particular drug dosing regimen when efficacy or toxicity corresponds to drug levels. These measurements are most important for drugs with a narrow therapeutic range or for drugs whose pharmacologic effects are not easily measured.

Measure serum levels after administration of an appropriate loading dose. If no loading dose is administered, give three or four doses of the drug before measuring serum levels to ensure that steady-state serum concentrations have been established. For some drugs, both maximum and minimum concentrations are relevant. Peak levels are most meaningful when measured after rapid drug distribution has occurred. Trough concentrations are usually measured just before administration of the next scheduled dose. Appropriate pharmacokinetic application of drug level measurements can improve patient care and decrease cost.

Patients with renal disease are heterogeneous and their responses to drug therapy are variable. Dosage nomograms, drug tables, and computer-assisted dosing recommendations should not be taken as a fixed approach to therapy in patients with decreased renal function. They are initial attempts to arrive at an effective dose regimen. Physicians using sound clinical judgment in caring for patients with renal disease evaluate each situation, choose a drug regimen based on all factors, and continually re-evaluate the response to therapy.

Suggested Reading

Aronoff GR, Abel SR. Practical guidelines for drug dosing in renal impairment. In: Schrier RW, ed. Manual of nephrology. 4th ed. Boston: Little, Brown, 1995.

Aronoff GR, Erbeck KR. Drug prescribing for dialysis patients. In: Henrich WL, ed. Principles and practice of dialysis. Baltimore: Williams & Wilkins, 1994:89–97.

Bennett WM, Aronoff GR, Golper TA, et al. Drug prescribing in renal failure: dosing guidelines for adults. 3rd ed. Philadelphia: American College of Physicians, 1994.

Erbeck KM, Aronoff GR. The use of anesthetic drugs in patients with impaired renal function. In: Kaufman L, Taberner PV, eds. Pharmacology in the practice of anaesthesia. Kent, England: Edward Arnold, 1996.

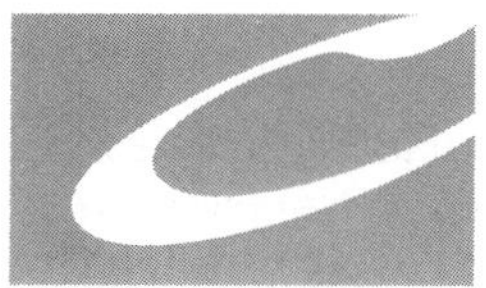

ENDOCRINE DISORDERS

DIABETES INSIPIDUS

Alan G. Robinson, M.D.
Joseph G. Verbalis, M.D.

Diabetes insipidus is literally the excretion of a dilute (tasteless) urine. Once an osmotic diuresis is excluded, hypotonic polyuria can be due to the absence of vasopressin (hypothalamic, or central, diabetes insipidus), lack of renal response to vasopressin (nephrogenic diabetes insipidus), or physiologic suppression of vasopressin in response to ingestion of water (primary polydipsia). We have assumed that appropriate testing to allow an accurate differential diagnosis among these three conditions has been accomplished before beginning therapy. We have also assumed that the cause of the lack of vasopressin (tumor, trauma, infiltrative disease, or idiopathic) has been diagnosed and treated appropriately.

■ GOALS

Maintain a Normal Lifestyle

Most patients with diabetes insipidus have an intact thirst mechanism and are able to drink sufficient water to maintain a relatively normal state of fluid balance. Since lack of vasopressin per se does not cause progressive morbidity nor secondary complications in other vital systems, the major manifestation in many cases is the inconvenience of thirst and frequent urination. Therapeutic agents should therefore be effective in the prevention of polyuria and nocturia, convenient for the patient's lifestyle, and easy for the patient to administer and monitor. The patient should have sufficient knowledge of the mechanism of the therapy to be flexible with dosage and timing depending on daily activities. Finally, because of the benign course of the disorder, the safety of any therapy must be an overriding consideration. Also, even with the use of safe and effective therapy, overtreatment should be avoided because the side effects from this are often more detrimental than from undertreatment.

Control of Potentially Life-Threatening Situations

The benign nature of diabetes insipidus is predicated on the ability of the patient to respond appropriately to signals from an intact thirst center. In any situation in which the patient is either unable to sense thirst or unable to respond by drinking water, the disease is potentially life threatening. If the patient is rendered unconscious (e.g., after an accident), diabetes insipidus may not be apparent when the patient is first seen by a physician because of the sustained effects of therapy. However, as the therapeutic agent reaches its normal duration of pharmacologic effect, polyuria may recur abruptly, and the large volumes of urine may produce severe dehydration and cardiovascular collapse in just a few hours. To avoid this threat, every patient with diabetes insipidus should carry a medical card indicating that diabetes insipidus is present and should wear a medical alert tag identifying the disorder. Diabetes insipidus is rare and in an emergency the patient may be seen by a physician who is unfamiliar with the disorder. The medical alert tag and card should therefore indicate that vasopressin may need to be administered and should also contain the name and telephone number of a physician who is familiar with the disorder, has been involved in the therapy of the patient, and can be contacted.

■ AVAILABLE AGENTS

Water

Water is listed as an agent to treat diabetes insipidus to emphasize that water alone taken in sufficient quantity corrects any metabolic abnormality secondary to diabetes insipidus. All the therapies described below are designed to reduce the amount of water intake necessary to a tolerable level. This level varies from patient to patient and from day to day in a given patient. The physician (and a knowledgeable patient) should not be disturbed that occasional lapses in pharmacologic treatment require temporary increases in water ingestion. In fact, such lapses are at times beneficial to avoid overtreatment and subsequent water intoxication.

Antidiuretic Hormones

L-Arginine Vasopressin

L-Arginine vasopressin is the natural vasopressin of humans and all mammals except the pig.

Aqueous vasopressin is a buffered solution of L-arginine vasopressin that can be given parenterally. It is provided in 1 ml snap-top vials at a concentration of 20 U per milliliter. It is usually given subcutaneously with an onset of action within 1 to 2 hours and duration of effect from 4 to 8 hours. Intravenous bolus administration should be avoided because of an even shorter duration of action and because of potential significant pressor effects (hypertension, angina).

1-(3-Mercaptopropionic Acid)-8-D-Arginine-Vasopressin (Desmopressin)

Desmopressin is a synthetic analogue of L-arginine vasopressin in which the terminal amino group of cystine has been removed and D-arginine has been substituted for L-arginine in position 8. Removal of the terminal amine prolongs the half-life of the drug in plasma, and substitution of D- for L-arginine in position 8 reduces the pressor activity. The agent is approximately 2,000 times more specific for antidiuresis than is natural L-arginine vasopressin. Desmopressin for clinical use is available for administration intranasally, orally, or parenterally. The intranasal preparation is a buffered aqueous solution containing 100 μg per milliliter. It is available in two forms: a nasal spray bottle that delivers a fixed 100 μl volume containing 10 μg desmopressin and a multidose vial that can be used to load varied volumes, 50 to 200 μl (5 to 20 μg DDAVP), into a rhinal catheter and the dose administered by blowing into the nose. The onset of action is rapid and the duration of effect is 6 to 24 hours. Despite this large range of duration of effect between individuals, the effect of similarly administered doses is reproducible in a given patient. Desmopressin for parenteral injection is available in 2 ml vials of 4 μg per milliliter. When administered parenterally, 5 to 20 percent of the agent produces an effect similar to that produced when it is administered intranasally. Desmopressin is also available in 0.1 mg and 0.2 mg tablets for oral administration. Tablets are taken two to four times a day (usually three). Diuresis decreases within 30 to 60 minutes after taking the tablet and reaches a maximum at 1 to 2 hours. The usual duration of effect is about 8 hours. One advantage of the oral preparation of desmopressin is the stability of the tablet at room temperature. The intranasal preparation should be refrigerated.

Lysine Vasopressin

Lysine vasopressin is the naturally occurring vasopressin of the pig. A synthetic form is available in an aqueous buffer of 50 U per milliliter to be used as a nasal spray. The agent comes in a plastic atomizer bottle and can be sprayed directly into each nostril. Absorption of the vasopressin occurs rapidly across the nasal mucosa, but the duration of effect is only 2 to 6 hours.

Orally Administered Pharmacologic Agents

Chlorpropamide

Chlorpropamide (Diabinese) was discovered by serendipity to decrease free water excretion in patients with diabetes insipidus. The major action is to enhance the effect of vasopressin on the renal tubule by increasing the hydro-osmotic action of vasopressin. In experimental studies, vasopressin is necessary for chlorpropamide to exert its antidiuretic effect; therefore, the drug is most often used in patients with partial diabetes insipidus and some residual ability to secrete vasopressin. The usual dose is 100 to 500 mg orally per day; maximal antidiuresis is observed after 4 days of therapy. One must be cautious of the development of hypoglycemia when treating patients with diabetes insipidus, especially in children and in cases of concurrent hypopituitarism.

Carbamazepine

Carbamazepine (Tegretol) has been shown to cause the release of antidiuretic hormone in patients with partial diabetes insipidus. The dosage used is 200 to 600 mg per day. Before prescribing this drug, the physician should be thoroughly familiar with the potential toxicities.

Clofibrate

Clofibrate (Atromid-S) has also been shown to stimulate the release of endogenous arginine vasopressin. Patients with partial diabetes insipidus may respond to 500 mg every 6 hours with a decreased urinary volume. However, because of the possibility of an increased incidence of gallbladder disease and carcinoma in patients taking clofibrate, this agent cannot be recommended for routine treatment of diabetes insipidus.

Thiazide Diuretics

Thiazides are usually thought of as diuretic rather than antidiuretic agents, but they also decrease urinary volumes in patients with both hypothalamic and nephrogenic diabetes insipidus. The mechanism is clearly different from that of the other oral agents and is probably secondary to primary natriuresis with subsequent volume contraction, decreased glomerular ultrafiltrate, and increased proximal tubular reabsorption of salt and water. Hydrochlorothiazide at a dose of 50 to 100 mg per day is usually sufficient. Potassium replacement should be given as necessary to prevent hypokalemia.

Indomethacin (Indocin)

Prostaglandin E in the renal medulla is thought to inhibit the action of vasopressin. Indomethacin, which decreases the concentration of medullary prostaglandin E, results in an increased responsiveness of the distal tubule to vasopressin and enhances the effect of administered antidiuretic hormones. Although this should not be considered primary therapy for diabetes insipidus, it is important to be aware of this action in those patients for whom the drug is prescribed for other reasons.

■ CLINICAL SITUATIONS

Acute Postsurgical Diabetes Insipidus

Acute postsurgical diabetes insipidus occurs frequently after surgery in the suprasellar hypothalamic area. Often the patient is receiving high doses of glucocorticoids, and hyperglycemia with glycosuria may confuse the initial diagnosis of diabetes insipidus. Thus, the blood glucose must first be brought under control to eliminate glycosuria as the cause of the polyuria. Second, it should be noted that excess fluids administered intravenously may be retained during surgery and normally excreted postoperatively. If this large output is matched with continued intravenous input, an incorrect diagnosis of diabetes insipidus may be made. Therefore, if the serum sodium is not elevated concomitantly with the polyuria, the rate of parenterally administered fluid should be slowed with careful monitoring of serum sodium and urinary output to establish the diagnosis. Once the diagnosis is ascertained, the only available pharmacologic therapy is an antidiuretic agent. However, because many neurosurgeons fear water overload and brain edema after this type of surgery, the patient is sometimes treated only with intravenous fluid replacement for a considerable time before the use of an antidiuretic hormone. If the patient is awake and able to respond to thirst, one can treat with an antidiuretic hormone and allow the patient's thirst to be the guide for water replacement. If the patient is unable to respond to thirst, either from a decreased level of consciousness or from hypothalamic damage to the thirst center, fluid balance may need to be maintained by intravenously administered fluid. Urine osmolality and serum sodium *must* be checked every several hours during the initial therapy and then at least daily until stabilization or resolution of the diabetes insipidus. One must also exercise caution with the volume of water replacement administered because excess water during continued administration of vasopressin can create a syndrome of inappropriate antidiuresis and potentially severe hyponatremia.

In some cases, transient postoperative diabetes insipidus is part of a "triphasic" pattern that has been described with stalk section. The initial diabetes insipidus (first phase) is due to axon shock and lack of function of the damaged neurons. This phase lasts from several hours to several days and is followed by an antidiuretic phase (second phase) that is due to the uncontrolled release of vasopressin from the disconnected posterior pituitary or from the remaining severed neurons. Overly aggressive administration of fluids during this second phase does not suppress the vasopressin and leads to hyponatremia. The antidiuresis can last 2 to 14 days, after which the diabetes insipidus (third phase) may return.

Postoperatively, desmopressin for parenteral administration may be given in a dose of 1 to 4 µg subcutaneously, intramuscularly, or intravenously. The intravenous route is preferable because it obviates any concern about absorption, has no significant pressor activity, and has the same total duration of action as other parenteral routes. Prompt reduction in urinary output should occur, and the duration of effect is generally 6 to 24 hours. Usually the patient is hypernatremic with a dilute urine when therapy is started. One should follow the urine osmolality and urine volume to be certain the dose was effective, and check the serum sodium to ensure some improvement of hypernatremia. We allow some return of polyuria before administration of subsequent doses of desmopressin because postoperative diabetes insipidus is often transient, and return of endogenous vasopressin secretion will be apparent by lack of return of polyuria. Some recent publications have reported using a continuous intravenous infusion of a dilute solution of L-arginine vasopressin to control diabetes insipidus postoperatively; an infusion of 1 to 3 mU per kilogram per hour in a dextrose or saline solution decreases the polyuria within 4 hours. Because of the short half-life of vasopressin (10 to 20 minutes), the pharmacologic action can be rapidly terminated in the event of any undesired effects. We have not used such continuous infusion of L-arginine vasopressin, but it may have merit in some clinical situations. As with parenterally administered desmopressin, fluid intake must be monitored and the vasopressin infusion interrupted periodically to check for continued diabetes insipidus. If diabetes insipidus persists, the patient should eventually be switched to maintenance therapy for chronic disease, as described below.

Acute Traumatic Diabetes Insipidus

Acute traumatic diabetes insipidus can occur after an injury to the head, usually an automobile accident. Diabetes insipidus is more common with injuries to the lateral skull that result in a shearing action on the pituitary stalk and/or cause hemorrhagic ischemia of the hypothalamus and posterior pituitary. Like the onset postsurgically, the diabetes insipidus is recognized by hypotonic polyuria in the face of an increased serum osmolality. Management is similar to that of postsurgical diabetes insipidus, except that the possibility of anterior pituitary insufficiency must be considered and the patient given stress doses of hydrocortisone until anterior pituitary function can be definitively evaluated.

Chronic Complete Diabetes Insipidus

Complete diabetes insipidus describes cases in which there is no vasopressin in the circulation and no ability to concentrate urine with a standard dehydration test. These patients require replacement with some form of antidiuretic hormone. The treatment of choice is desmopressin.

Most patients prefer to use an intranasal spray with a metered spray bottle to deliver 10 µg of desmopressin per dose or the recently available desmopressin tablets containing 0.1 or 0.2 mg. When initiating therapy, the duration of action of individual doses should be determined. This is best done in a controlled environment where each voided urine sample can be measured for volume and osmolality. An alternative is to measure volume and specific gravity or, as a last resort, volume alone. In fact, measurement of urinary volume can provide an acceptable index of the duration of drug action. The patient is allowed to escape from the effects of any previous medication, thereby establishing a baseline polyuria. In patients with complete diabetes insipidus, polyuria returns promptly.

When polyuria of approximately 14 ml per minute is established, one dose of desmopressin is administered: either a single spray of 10 µg or half of a 0.1 mg tablet. A decrease in urinary volume occurs within 1 to 2 hours. The duration of effect of the dose can be determined by measuring urine output as described above to determine return of polyuria. The duration of action will range from less than 6 to 24 hours. With the intranasal dose the duration is usually 8 to 12 hours and a schedule can be set for administration two or three times daily. For the orally administered tablets, increasing doses to 0.1 and 0.2 mg can be tried sequentially. Little additional duration of action is achieved by increasing doses above the 0.2 mg tablet. A dose for three times a day can usually be determined. Establishing this duration of action in individual patients is helpful in planning therapy and in assuring the patient (and the physician) that early administration of a second dose of drug (which may be necessary) will not lead to any adverse effect.

For the tablets there is considerable flexibility in the dosage by using whole or split tablets. If more flexibility in dosage is desired, the patient must be taught to use the rhinal catheter and to measure an appropriate dose of desmopressin. A solution of saline can be utilized to fill the tubing for practice administration. Once an appropriately measured dose is in the catheter, the patient should hold it in a U shape with the two ends in a superior position, allowing the measured dose of hormone to roll to the dependent loop of the tube. The patient raises the catheter to the mouth and inserts about 0.5 inch (1.25 cm) into the nostril, being careful to maintain the other end above the bottom of the U. The patient then takes a moderate inspiration and holds the breath while placing the other end of the catheter in the mouth. Blowing through the catheter with a swift puff, as one might imagine doing to blow a ball out of a straw, delivers the hormone high into the nose. A physician or assistant trained in the proper use of the rhinal catheter should train the patient. Inadequate training causes wasted hormone because of dripping out of the end of the catheter, swallowing the hormone, or blowing it into the external nares in a position too low for absorption. It is desirable in each patient to determine the duration of effect of 50, 100, and 200 μl using the measures of urinary volume and osmolality to determine the allowable flexibility.

Once the duration of action of the drug is determined, it is necessary to decide on the dose and time of day for administration. Individualization of this protocol is emphasized. Occasionally, patients maintain satisfactory control of urinary output with a single dose per day, but most require two doses per day intranasally or three doses orally. Two small doses per day (e.g., 50 μl) with the rhinal catheter may be more cost effective than one large dose (e.g., 200 μl) with the rhinal catheter or two sprays with the metered dose.

Similarly, with the orally administered tablets a small dose three times a day may be more cost effective than a larger dose twice a day. Because the biologic half-life of desmopressin is about 4 hours, doubling the dose extends the duration only by that amount of time. Many authors suggest that when a single dose of drug per day is used, the dose be given at bedtime to allow the patient to sleep throughout the night. We find that many patients would rather have the drug administered in the morning to allow a full day of work or other activities without interruption for frequent voiding. A single episode of nocturia may be preferable to multiple interruptions of the workday. When two or three doses of desmopressin are necessary, the time of administration should again be based on the activity of the patient for that day. The first dose should almost always be given in the morning to allow an uninterrupted workday. Timing of the second and third dose (if needed) should be individualized. If the patient is home for the evening, it is usually best to delay administration of the last dose until late in the evening to allow a full night's sleep. If the patient is going out for the evening and by experience knows that polyuria will occur before he or she returns home, it is best to administer the second dose of medication in the late afternoon or early evening to allow an evening free of worry about polyuria. If this dose is insufficient to allow an adequate night of sleep, a third dose of medication may be taken on that particular day just before bedtime. New patients will probably be started on the oral preparation. However, patients who are accustomed to using the intranasal preparation may want to use a flexible program in which intranasal and orally administered drugs are used interchangeably depending on the particular properties of that agent. For example, the intranasal preparation may have a longer duration of action at bedtime and be preferred, whereas tablets of desmopressin may be more convenient to carry and take during the day.

The obvious danger of a flexible program is the possibility that the patient may take repeated doses of desmopressin to always maintain urinary volume at a low output and on occasion may become volume expanded, natriuretic, and hyponatremic. To avoid this complication, the patient should withhold desmopressin, at least once and preferably two to three times a week, until polyuria recurs. This procedure guards against hyponatremia occurring from overzealous use of desmopressin and provides ongoing documentation that diabetes insipidus persists. The latter is especially useful in cases of postsurgical or post-traumatic diabetes insipidus in which renewed ability to secrete vasopressin may occur within the first year after the initial insult.

The only disadvantage of desmopressin is expense: it costs \$50 to \$100 per month whereas chlorpropamide is only \$3 to \$6 per month. Because of the expense, some physicians prescribe a combination of an oral agent with desmopressin to prolong the action of desmopressin and decrease the expense. Both chlorpropamide and indomethacin prolong the effect of an administered dose of desmopressin. However, our feeling is that potential complications from agents that are not otherwise indicated make this attempt to reduce the cost of therapy undesirable. It is also important to recognize that when any of the oral agents described previously are given for routine medical indications, they may augment the effect of desmopressin and predispose the patient to water retention and hyponatremia. Thus, the dose of desmopressin may have to be altered if one such agent is utilized for treatment of another disease.

Chronic Partial Diabetes Insipidus

"Partial" diabetes insipidus refers to patients who have some endogenous secretion of vasopressin but not a sufficient amount to achieve maximal urinary concentration and keep them asymptomatic regarding polyuria and thirst. Most patients do not become hypernatremic but do complain of excessive thirst and polyuria. Probably the safest form of therapy for these patients is also desmopressin. The guidelines for initiating and maintaining therapy in partial diabetes insipidus are essentially identical to those described for the treatment of complete diabetes insipidus, except that these patients often tolerate a somewhat less frequent administration of the agent because the intensity of the polyuria and the thirst is not so severe.

In some of these patients, administration of pharmacologic agents that increase the effectiveness of vasopressin may be preferable. In the rare patient with the unhappy concurrence of diabetes insipidus and either diabetes mellitus or congestive heart failure, treatment of both diseases with a single agent may be appropriate—chlorpropamide for diabetes mellitus and thiazide diuretics for congestive heart failure. One of these agents is prescribed as necessary to treat the primary disease (e.g., diabetes mellitus or congestive heart failure), and the effect on the diabetes insipidus is observed. The need for further therapy with an antidiuretic hormone depends on the initial response.

In a patient with partial diabetes insipidus, chlorpropamide is an acceptable alternative. Therapy can be initiated with 100 mg per day and increased every 4 days until appropriate antidiuresis is obtained. Usually, little further antidiuresis is achieved by doses above 500 mg per day. When an oral agent is begun, the appropriate indices of therapeutic effectiveness are the 24 hour urinary volume and the patient's symptomatic response in terms of thirst. In patients with coexistent panhypopituitarism and lack of adrenocorticotropic hormone and growth hormone, the increased potential for hypoglycemia during treatment with chlorpropamide must be recognized, and frequent feedings given and routine blood glucose levels obtained. In mild cases of partial diabetes insipidus, a trial of thiazide diuretics may be undertaken. Some patients have sufficient reduction of urinary output and decrease of thirst with this agent alone, so that they are satisfactorily controlled. We do not use clofibrate or carbamazepine for the treatment of partial diabetes insipidus. In our opinion, the side effects of each of these agents are too great to justify their use to treat a disease for which other acceptable forms of therapy are available. Furthermore, patients with partial diabetes insipidus who respond to treatment with any oral agents usually respond to either chlorpropamide or thiazides.

Diabetes Insipidus in Pregnancy

Some cases of adult-onset diabetes insipidus have started during pregnancy. The diabetes insipidus has generally not interfered with the progress of parturition and lactation. The agent of choice to treat diabetes insipidus in pregnancy is again desmopressin. This agent has four to 75 times less oxytocic activity than does arginine vasopressin or lysine vasopressin, so that it is possible to obtain potent antidiuresis with minimal uterotonic action.

When diabetes insipidus occurs in pregnancy, it may be especially severe because increased serum oxytocinase activity decreases the effectiveness of endogenously secreted vasopressin. Indeed, rapid destruction of endogenous arginine vasopressin may unmask longstanding partial diabetes insipidus with little secretory reserve. The presence of diabetes insipidus should be confirmed as usual and the pathologic cause determined (e.g., suprasellar tumor) and treated appropriately. The same protocol for initiation of therapy as in complete diabetes insipidus can be undertaken. The physician must be cognizant of the volume expansion and decrease in serum sodium that occurs during normal pregnancy and adjust the desmopressin dose accordingly. Although desmopressin seems to be unaffected by oxytocinase, these patients may nonetheless require a three-times-a-day schedule of administered desmopressin. At parturition, they are usually alert enough to take intermittent doses of desmopressin intranasally. The only caution is that excessive amounts of fluids should not be administered with the desmopressin because this may cause water intoxication and hyponatremia. After parturition, the dosage of desmopressin may have to be adjusted downward. In some cases of partial diabetes insipidus, there is sufficient residual vasopressin secretory capacity to keep the patient asymptomatic when the oxytocinase activity in serum disappears.

Desmopressin does not have specific approval for use in pregnancy but is logically the appropriate agent when some therapy must be given. Any of the oral agents described has the potential for teratotoxicity. Lysine vasopressin gives unacceptable levels of control in most normal subjects, and this effect is magnified in pregnant women. Arginine vasopressin has the potential for inducing uterine cramps and must be given by injection. Since desmopressin is similar to the natural hormone, has no known teratogenic effects, and provides adequate control of antidiuresis, it is the best agent to prescribe in this situation.

Diabetes Insipidus with Inadequate Thirst

Inadequate thirst constitutes the most difficult management problem in patients with diabetes insipidus. Some patients secrete vasopressin when volume depleted but do not respond normally to increased serum osmolality with either thirst or secretion of vasopressin. Because these cases represent a variant of partial diabetes insipidus, there is the potential for an adequate response to oral agents. A trial of chlorpropamide up to 500 mg per day is indicated because in some cases this therapy not only decreases urinary volume, but also increases the recognition of thirst. If chlorpropamide is ineffective, desmopressin is the agent of choice.

To determine the duration of action of desmopressin, it may be necessary to give a water load either orally or intravenously to bring the sodium level into the normal range and ensure a good urinary output. Desmopressin can then be administered, as described previously, but in these patients it is advised that the volume of voided urine be matched with administered fluid until the antidiuresis is terminated. At this point a second dose of desmopressin is administered as described for chronic complete diabetes insipidus. Once the duration of effect of desmopressin is established, a rigid regimen of desmopressin and water intake must be prescribed. It is usually necessary to prescribe an exact volume of fluid to be administered over a given duration of time each day. Even with careful monitoring of desmopressin and water, regular measurement of serum sodium is necessary, because these patients are prone to develop water intoxication with hyponatremia or, alternatively, recurrent dehydration with hypernatremia.

Influence of Diabetes Insipidus on Other Therapeutic Decisions

Routine Surgical Procedures

For most surgical procedures, intranasal desmopressin on the morning of surgery, followed by careful and limited administration of intravenous fluids during the surgery, provide adequate control of fluid balance. For long procedures, serum sodium should be checked during the procedure and in all cases at the end of surgery. If the patient is unable to administer desmopressin intranasally before or after the surgical procedure, parenterally administered desmopressin should be used.

Diabetes Insipidus with Panhypopituitarism

Because diabetes insipidus is frequently caused by a sellar or suprasellar tumor, it is commonly accompanied by panhypopituitarism. In these cases, concurrent hypoadrenalism or hypothyroidism may cause an inability to excrete a water load. In a patient with diabetes insipidus, there may be no polyuria when hypoadrenalism and/or hypothyroidism is present, and consequently the diagnosis of diabetes insipidus may go unsuspected during initial evaluation. As the patient receives thyroid hormone and (more dramatically) hydrocortisone, a prompt increase in urinary output and obvious manifestations of diabetes insipidus are noted. At this time, the patient requires evaluation for complete or partial diabetes insipidus, and initiation of therapy as outlined in the sections on chronic complete diabetes insipidus and chronic partial diabetes insipidus.

In patients taking concurrent maintenance therapy for diabetes insipidus, hypoadrenalism, and hypothyroidism, it is essential to maintain the treatment of all three conditions. Patients who continue treatment for diabetes insipidus but interrupt therapy for adrenal or thyroid deficiency are especially prone to water intoxication and hyponatremia.

Craniopharyngioma

In patients with craniopharyngioma or other suprasellar lesions treated by transfrontal cranial surgery, there is great danger of damaging the neurohypophyseal system and causing permanent diabetes insipidus. This is an almost invariable outcome of attempts at radical, complete removal of a craniopharyngioma. Lifelong diabetes insipidus is sufficiently onerous for this possibility to provide a continuing stimulus to develop safer modes of therapy for craniopharyngioma, as described recently with stereotaxic implantation of radioisotopes into cystic lesions.

Granulomatous Diseases

Diabetes insipidus in these cases may be partial or complete and may require specific therapy, as described previously. In some cases, there has been remission of the diabetes insipidus with appropriate therapy for the underlying condition.

Cardiovascular Disease

A few patients with coronary vascular disease may experience angina pectoris after lysine vasopressin or injected L-arginine vasopressin. This problem has been eliminated by desmopressin because of the markedly reduced pressor activity at the dosages used to produce effective antidiuresis.

Suggested Reading

Bononi PL, Robinson AG. Central diabetes insipidus: Management in the postoperative period. Endocrinologist 1991; 1:180–185.

Czernichow P, Robinson AG, eds. Diabetes insipidus in man. Basel, Switzerland: S. Karger, 1984.

Fjellestad A, Czernichow P. Central diabetes insipidus in children V. Oral treatment with a vasopressin hormone analogue (DDAVP). Acta Paediatr Scand 1986; 75:605–610.

Fjellestad-Paulsen A, Laborde K, Kindermans C, Czernichow P. Water-balance hormones during long-term follow-up of oral dDAVP treatment in diabetes insipidus. Acta Paediatr Scand, 1993; 82:752–757.

Ralston C, Butt W. Continuous vasopressin replacement in diabetes insipidus. Arch Dis Child 1990; 65:896–897.

Reeves WB, Andreoli TE. The posterior pituitary and water metabolism. In: Wilson JD, Foster DW, eds. Williams textbook of endocrinology. 8th ed. Philadelphia: WB Saunders, 1992:311.

Richardson DW, Robinson AG. Desmopressin. Ann Intern Med 1985; 103: 228–239.

Robinson AG. Disorders of antidiuretic hormone secretion. J Clin Endocrinol Metab 1985; 14:55–88.

Robinson AG, Amico JA. "Non-sweet" diabetes in pregnancy. N Engl J Med 1991; 324:445–458.

Robinson AG, DeRubertis FR. Disorders of sodium and water balance associated with adrenal, thyroid and pituitary disease. In: Schrier RW, Gottschalk CW, eds. Diseases of the kidney. Vol 3. Boston: Little, Brown, 1993:2795.

PRIMARY HYPOTHYROIDISM

Eduardo Gaitan, M.D., F.A.C.P.
David S. Cooper, M.D., F.A.C.P.

Primary hypothyroidism is a common medical problem, occurring in approximately 1 to 3 percent of the total population with annual incidence rates of 1 to 2 in 1,000 for females and 2 in 10,000 for males. Overt hypothyroidism is associated with typical symptoms and signs, as well as easily definable functional alterations in many organ systems. The diagnosis is confirmed by an elevated basal serum thyrotropin (TSH) and a depressed total thyroxine (T_4), free-thyroxine estimate (e.g., free-T_4 index: FT_4I), or direct free-thyroxine measurement (FT_4). Subclinical hypothyroidism (SH), with minimal or absent clinical manifestations, is present in about 5 percent of the total population. Subclinical hypothyroidism, the earliest definable stage of primary hypothyroidism, is characterized by normal thyroid hormone concentrations (T_4, FT_4I, FT_4, and triiodothyronine [T_3]) and elevated circulating TSH levels. Primary hypothyroidism occurs at all ages, but postmenopausal women and the elderly, particularly females, are at greatest risk. Elevated TSH levels with normal free-T_4 estimate (or direct free-T_4 measurement) are present in as many as 15 percent of the population older than 65 years. The presence of goiter, positive antithyroid peroxidase antibody (TPO Ab), a history of treatment for hyperthyroidism with surgery, radioactive iodine, or antithyroid drugs, and exposure to lithium or iodine-containing compounds (e.g., amiodarone) are also risk factors for the development of primary hypothyroidism. If left untreated, hypothyroidism is associated with a high degree of morbidity and may ultimately be fatal. Fortunately, the diagnosis is simple and certain, and oral levothyroxine

Table 1 Thyroid Hormone Preparations

SYNTHETIC AGENTS	
Levothyroxine (L-T_4)*	(Levo-T, Levothroid, Levoxyl, Synthroid, and generic)
Liothyronine (L-T_3)	(Cytomel and generic)
Liotrix (L-T_4 + L-T_3)	(Thyrolar)
BIOLOGIC AGENTS	
Desiccated thyroid	(Armour Thyroid, Westthroid, Thyrar, Thyroid Strong, and generic)
Thyroglobulin	(No longer commercially available in the United States)

*Recommended as the only preparation for chronic therapy of hypothyroidism.

replacement, the only therapeutic option recommended, is inexpensive, safe, and curative.

■ THYROID HORMONE PREPARATIONS

The United States Pharmacopoeia (USPDI—1995) lists five thyroid hormone preparations for clinical use: the synthetic preparations, L-T_4, liothyronine (L-T_3), and liotrix (a combination of synthetic T_4 and T_3 in a 4:1 ratio) and the natural or biologic preparations, desiccated thyroid and thyroglobulin (Table 1). Biologic formulations should be of historical interest only as thyroglobulin is no longer commercially available in the United States.

Synthetic Preparations

Levothyroxine sodium is the monosodium salt of the levo isomer of thyroxine. L-T_4 is the thyroid preparation of choice for routine treatment of primary hypothyroidism. L-T_4 is absorbed (about 60 to 80 percent in normal subjects) from the small intestine. Its approximate 6 day half-life permits single daily dosing and produces stable thyroid hormone levels in serum, with only a slight (10 percent) rise a few hours after ingestion and minimal day-to-day variability. Since about 80 percent of extrathyroidal T_3 originates from tissue conversion of T_4, a preparation consisting solely of T_4 provides stable and physiologic quantities of T_3 to the peripheral tissues. Controversy persists on the reliability of stated hormonal content and bioavailability among different brand and generic L-T_4 preparations. Proprietary preparations almost always have reliable hormonal content within 90 to 110 percent of stated values, as assessed by high-pressure liquid chromatography according to the Food and Drug Administration (FDA) specifications. Generic L-T_4 tablets have not consistently met FDA standards for the stated amounts of L-T_4, which may vary depending on the manufacturer and the available lots. Variable hormonal content and differences in particle size, solubility, inert ingredients, and other indeterminate factors that may affect bioavailability could result in substantial changes in circulating thyroid hormone levels, if a different preparation is substituted for the one the patient had previously been taking. This is most likely to occur when a prescription for levothyroxine is refilled and a generic is substituted for a proprietary drug, or vice versa. Therefore, monitoring of the correct thyroid hormone dose (see Monitoring L-Thyroxine Therapy) is necessary under these circumstances. Proprietary preparations are 2 to 10 times more expensive than their generic counterparts. According to the *1995 Red Book of Medical Economics Data*, the average wholesale prices of L-T_4 100 tablets (100 μg) are \$8.25, \$16.31, \$18.56, and \$21.42 for Levoxyl, Levo-T, Levothroid, and Synthroid, respectively, while the cost of the same amount of six generic preparations not Ab coded by the FDA (products will be coded Ab if a study is submitted demonstrating necessary equivalence requirements) ranges from \$2.08 to \$4.28. At present, the cost-benefit advantage of generic over proprietary preparations is minimal, because TSH levels probably should be monitored more frequently with generic drugs.

Liothyronine sodium (sodium L-triiodothyronine, or L-T_3) is the sodium salt of the L-isomer of 3,3′,5 triiodothyronine. Because of the short 1 day half-life of T_3, the use of L-T_3 (Cytomel) in primary hypothyroidism is restricted to short-term therapy of patients with thyroid cancer undergoing L-T_4 withdrawal for radioiodine scanning or therapy. L-T_3, 25 to 75 μg daily, is given for only 4 weeks. L-T_3 is not indicated for the chronic management of patients with hypothyroidism. Like other T_3-containing formulations, L-T_3 itself often results in intermittent supraphysiologic serum T_3 levels after ingestion, and it is typically associated with low serum thyroxine concentrations owing to suppression of endogenous TSH (see Biologic Preparations).

Liotrix (T_3-T_4 liotrix) (Thyrolar) is a mixture of synthetic L-T_4 and L-T_3 in a 4:1 ratio. It was developed because of the uncertainties surrounding the biologic potency of desiccated thyroid, in an era before it was recognized that approximately 80 percent of circulating T_3 is derived from peripheral deiodination of T_4 rather than from direct thyroidal secretion. In addition to all of the same problems inherent in any preparation containing T_4, liotrix preparations are at least twice as expensive as levothyroxine.

Biologic Preparations

Thyroid (desiccated thyroid), the first thyroid hormone preparation to be available on a large scale, is prepared from the dried thyroid glands of slaughterhouse animals, and it contains both T_4 and T_3. The content and relative amounts of T_4 and T_3 in desiccated thyroid may vary according to animal species, season, diet, and geographic region. Thus, desiccated thyroid preparations may have variable potency, either because of metabolically inactive iodothyronines, causing low bioactivity, or a relative increase in T_3 content, causing excessively high bioactivity. Desiccated thyroid also suffers from two problems common to all T_3-containing thyroid hormone preparations. Since T_3 is more rapidly and completely absorbed and has a shorter serum half-life than T_4, serum T_3 levels often transiently rise into hyperthyroid range after ingestion, occasionally causing symptoms, particularly in the elderly or in patients with cardiac disease. Furthermore, patients taking these preparations often have serum T_4 levels in the low-normal range, owing to suppression of endogenous thyroid hormone secretion. Monitoring of hormonal replacement is, therefore, more difficult and may cause inappropriate increases in drug dosage by the physician, resulting in iatrogenic T_3 thyrotoxicosis. Similar problems arise with thyroglobulin, a more highly purified extract of hog thyroid glands, which is no longer commercially available in the United States.

For these reasons, patients taking thyroid hormone preparations other than levothyroxine (L-T_4) should be urged to switch to an equivalent dose of L-T_4. One grain (60 mg) of desiccated thyroid USP or liotrix-1 (containing 60 μg L-T_4 and 15 μg L-T_3) are both roughly equivalent to 100 μg L-T_4. However, prescribing a dose of L-T_4 based on body weight (see Guidelines for Therapy) is preferable to approximating the dose to the metabolic equivalent of desiccated thyroid, and optimal dosing requires individualization on the basis of clinical and laboratory criteria.

GUIDELINES FOR THERAPY

Primary and Secondary Hypothyroidism

In primary hypothyroidism, the correct thyroid hormone dose would be that which normalizes the serum TSH. High-sensitivity TSH assays can accurately determine whether the TSH is normal or below normal, the latter indicating over-replacement. Over-replacement must be avoided because of evidence indicating that doses of L-T_4 sufficient to suppress TSH secretion are associated with subtle hyperthyroidism in certain tissues (i.e., heart, kidney, bone, and liver). Adjustment or replacement therapy to maintain circulating TSH levels in the normal range is associated with normalization of peripheral tissue markers of hyperthyroidism.

In secondary forms of hypothyroidism, i.e., those resulting from pituitary or hypothalamic disease, TSH measurements are not useful in determining levothyroxine dosage; FT_4I or FT_4 levels in the mid-normal to high-normal range are a reasonable end point. For most hypothyroid adults, the replacement dose of levothyroxine is approximately 1.7 μg per kilogram (average 112 μg per day), but some older patients may need less than 1 μg per kilogram body weight. The average daily dose in children is 2 to 4 μg per kilogram body weight and is age dependent, 10 to 15 μg per kilogram body weight in infants for the first 6 months with lower dose thereafter depending on circulating TSH levels. L-T_4 tablets are available in multiple potencies (25 to 300 μg tablets), enabling the physician to individualize therapy with reasonable precision.

Hypothyroid adults in good general health can, from the beginning, use replacement with the optimal calculated dose of L-T_4. Caution should be exercised, however, when treating longstanding hypothyroid patients, particularly the elderly or those with manifestations of ischemic heart disease. Replacement is started with an initial oral dose as small as 12.5 μg to 25 μg per day, with stepwise increases in dosage of 25 μg at 3 to 4 week intervals depending on clinical response. TSH monitoring is conducted 6 to 8 weeks after the therapy has been initiated (see Monitoring L-Thyroxine Therapy). About 40 percent of patients with a combination of hypothyroidism and angina cannot tolerate full replacement therapy, and in rare instances thyroid replacement cannot be given at all. On the other hand, some patients with angina actually improve with thyroid hormone replacement therapy.

Subclinical Hypothyroidism

The treatment of subclinical hypothyroidism (SH), defined by elevated TSH levels but normal serum free-T_4 estimate (or normal free-T_4 measurement) and minimal or no clinical manifestations, is controversial. Most arguments at present are in favor of replacement therapy. First, the use of sensitive TSH assays now permits precise titration of the L-T_4 dosage to bring TSH levels within the normal physiologic range, thus avoiding the previous problem of excessive dosage. Second, there is evidence that thyroid hormone replacement in SH can normalize subtle functional changes in target tissues, particularly the heart. These changes are less pronounced but are similar to those observed in overt hypothyroidism. Recent data also suggest that unfavorable lipoprotein patterns may also be correctable in SH by L-T_4. L-T_4 therapy may also improve symptoms, i.e., cold intolerance and easy fatigue, consistent with mild hypothyroidism, as well as subtle neuropsychiatric changes that are more commonly observed in the elderly. Third, replacement therapy serves prophylactic purposes by preventing progression to overt hypothyroidism. Indeed, in the presence of positive antithyroid antibodies, the rate of conversion of SH to overt hypothyroidism is 5 percent per year and may be as high as 20 percent per year in the elderly. However, in asymptomatic subjects with elevated TSH levels without goiter, TPO Ab, or a history of previous treatment for hyperthyroidism, progression to overt hypothyroidism is unusual, and prophylactic L-T_4 therapy is probably not necessary.

Transient Hypothyroidism

Temporary forms of hypothyroidism lasting from a few weeks to several months are being diagnosed more frequently. Transient hypothyroidism may be observed during the recovery phase of subacute (de Quervain's) and postpartum (silent) thyroiditis; it is also seen in about 15 percent of patients in the first few months after ^{131}I treatment of hyperthyroidism, in patients with excess iodine intake or administration; with lithium therapy; and occasionally in adolescents and young adults with goiter and autoimmune thyroiditis who recover spontaneously. Although replacement therapy is not indicated, in most of these situations the physician is occasionally compelled to initiate L-T_4 therapy because of markedly abnormal thyroid hormone levels and/or clinical manifestations. Replacement therapy under these circumstances is maintained for a 3 to 6 month period, at which time L-T_4 is discontinued. Serum T_4, FT_4I, or FT_4 values are usually low 2 weeks after discontinuing the drug, whereas TSH levels are still within the normal range. Therefore, a final diagnosis and recommendations should be based on TSH measurements made 6 to 8 weeks after the drug has been withdrawn. A normal TSH concentration at that time substantiates a diagnosis of transient hypothyroidism and recovery of normal thyroid function.

Hypothyroidism and Pregnancy

The treatment of hypothyroidism during pregnancy differs in many instances from its treatment in nonpregnant women. Patients who are biochemically euthyroid when first seen in pregnancy usually require subsequent increase in L-T_4 dosage, so evaluation of serum TSH to assess adequacy of replacement therapy should be performed during each trimester of pregnancy. The L-T_4 dose should return immediately after delivery to the same dose before pregnancy, and a serum TSH level complemented with a FT_4 estimate (or direct FT_4 measurement) should be obtained 6 to 8 weeks postpartum.

■ MONITORING L-THYROXINE THERAPY

Given the long half-life of L-T_4, steady-state serum levels of T_4 are achieved after approximately 6 weeks of treatment. In addition, serum TSH levels in hypothyroid patients generally reach their nadir within 6 weeks of initiating treatment. Therefore, the serum TSH and FT_4I or FT_4 at 6 to 8 weeks should enable the clinician to know whether the L-T_4 dose is appropriate. Once the proper dose has been achieved, and its stability confirmed 3 to 6 months later, visits to the physician and thyroid function tests do not need to be repeated more often than once a year, provided the patient's compliance with the prescribed regimen is adequate with maintenance on the same L-T_4 preparation.

The use of TSH levels to judge the adequacy of therapy is not foolproof. For example, suppressed TSH levels may be observed in situations other than thyrotoxicosis or excess thyroid hormone dosage, e.g., with dopamine hydrochloride and glucocorticoid administration, acute psychiatric illness, severe nonthyroidal illness, and occasionally during pregnancy. Under these circumstances, TSH is not a reliable indicator of L-T_4 therapy, and FT_4I or FT_4 values in the mid- to high-normal range become the end point of adequate replacement. None of these situations, except pregnancy, requires adjustment of a previously standardized L-T_4 dose, which should continue to be given to the patient.

It is recognized that some clinically euthyroid L–T_4-treated patients have T_4 levels above the upper limit of normal. Such patients usually have T_3 levels well within the normal range in contrast to iatrogenically thyrotoxic patients who generally have elevated serum T_3 and T_4 values. Euthyroid hyperthyroxinemia is not necessarily an indication to lower the L-T_4 dose. However, a suppressed serum TSH level obtained in a high-sensitivity assay does suggest the possibility of over-replacement, i.e., subclinical thyrotoxicosis. In this situation the dose should be lowered until the serum TSH level is within the normal range.

Failure to respond adequately to an oral L-T_4 dose exceeding 200 to 300 μg daily is rare and should prompt consideration of drug interference with absorption (see Drug Interactions), malabsorption, or patient noncompliance, the latter being the most common cause of treatment failure. Elevated TSH levels with concomitant normal or elevated T_4, FT_4I, or FT_4 values may be seen in noncompliant patients taking large amounts of L-T_4 just before a scheduled visit with their physician. In seriously ill patients, particularly those with gastrointestinal disease or ileus, L-T_4 is preferably administered intravenously to ensure adequate serum levels. Since about 80 percent of a dose is normally absorbed from the gastrointestinal tract, the intravenous dose is proportional to the oral dose.

■ EDUCATION

Hypothyroidism, like any other chronic condition, requires continued surveillance to ensure compliance with long-term therapy in the recommended dose and, preferably, on the same L-T_4 preparation. Therefore, education and recalling (i.e., local or regional computer facilities) are most important. Patients with hypothyroidism may be inclined to discontinue medication once euthyroidism has been attained. Therefore, the physician must stress the following points to the patient and the immediate family: (1) thyroid hormone replacement therapy is lifelong; (2) insidious multiple organ deterioration, e.g., brain and heart, occurs if hypothyroidism remains untreated; and (3) any new physician must be informed of the patient's condition.

■ DRUG INTERACTIONS

By increasing the catabolism of vitamin K–dependent clotting factors, L-T_4 may potentiate the hypoprothrombinemic effect of oral anticoagulant agents. Therefore, when L-T_4 is administered to hypothyroid patients already on anticoagulant therapy, the prothrombin time should be determined regularly and the oral anticoagulant dose adjusted accordingly. The oral anticoagulant dose may be reduced by one-third when L-T_4 is started. Requirements of insulin and oral hypoglycemic agents increase in hypothyroid diabetic patients once L-T_4 replacement therapy is instituted. Similarly, the serum levels of digitalis may be significantly reduced in hypothyroid patients who begin thyroid hormone replacement.

Phenytoin, carbamazepine, phenobarbital, and rifampin may accelerate the metabolism of levothyroxine, resulting in greater demand and increased hormone dosage. The bile acid–binding resins cholestyramine and colestipol, aluminum hydroxide, sucralfate, ferrous sulfate, and ferrous gluconate substantially decrease absorption of L-T_4 from the gastrointestinal (GI) tract. To prevent this interaction, there should be a 4 to 5 hour interval between administration of these medications and L-T_4. Soybean infant formula also decreases GI absorption of L-T_4. The use of androgens in breast cancer treatment may decrease T_4 requirements.

■ ADVERSE REACTIONS

L-T_4 is remarkably free of side effects and allergic reactions. Iatrogenic hyperthyroidism is practically the only side effect of replacement therapy. Over-replacement can be manifested by anxiety, nervousness, tremor, palpitations, headaches, insomnia, sweating, tachycardia, and weight loss. Angina, arrhythmias, and cardiac decompensation and failure are more common in the elderly with previous chronic hypothyroidism and patients with ischemic heart disease. Even subtle over-replacement has been implicated in the development of atrial fibrillation and as the cause of reduced bone density in postmenopausal women on prolonged L-T_4 replacement therapy. The advent of sensitive TSH assays to monitor thyroid hormone replacement has enabled the clinician to avoid excessive L-T_4 dosages, by maintaining the TSH in the normal range.

Finally, when adrenal insufficiency coexists with hypothyroidism, corticosteroids to correct the adrenal insufficiency must be administered before therapy with L-T_4 is initiated. This is because thyroid hormone accelerates the metabolic clearance rate of endogenous glucocorticoids and may cause adrenal crisis.

Suggested Reading

Choe W, Hays MT. Absorption of oral thyroxine. Endocrinologist 1995; 5:222–228.

Mandel SJ, Brent GA, Larsen PR. Levothyroxine therapy in patients with thyroid disease. Ann Intern Med 1993; 119:492–502.

Oppenheimer JH, Braverman LE, Toft A, et al. A therapeutic controversy—Thyroid hormone treatment: When and what? J Clin Endocrinol Metab 1995; 80:2873–2883.

Roti E, Minelli R, Gardini E, Braverman LE. The use and misuse of thyroid hormone. Endocr Rev 1993; 14:401–423.

Singer PA, Cooper DS, Levy EG, et al. Treatment guidelines for patients with hyperthyroidism and hypothyroidism. JAMA 1995; 273:808–812.

Toft AD. Thyroxine therapy. N Engl J Med 1994; 331:174–180.

HYPERTHYROIDISM

Kiyoshi Hashizume, M.D., Ph.D.
Satoru Suzuki, M.D., Ph.D

Graves' disease is the most frequent thyroid disorder that results in thyrotoxicosis. The symptoms of this disease are hyperthyroidism, exophthalmos, and swelling of the thyroid gland. It is well known that hyperthyroidism that is due to Graves' disease is caused by stimulation of thyroid with certain antibodies against the thyroid-stimulating hormone (TSH) receptor. Those anti-TSH receptor antibodies (TRAb) stimulate thyroid cells to produce a high concentration of serum thyroid hormones (3,5,3′-triiodo-L-thyronine [T_3] and L-thyroxine [T_4]). Many of the symptoms of hyperthyroidism resulting from Graves' disease are caused by the increase in the actions of these hormones in target tissues.

It is thus reasonable that reduction of the serum levels of these thyroid hormones is the main goal of the management of Graves' hyperthyroidism. The decrease in the hormone levels, however, is not always accompanied by a decrease in the production of antibodies and the symptoms that are directly related to antibodies rather than T_4 and T_3. For example, these antibodies enlarge the thyroid. Exophthalmos is another symptom of Graves' disease that is thought to be related to the action of these antibodies. In the management of patients with Graves' hyperthyroidism, therefore, we have focused on the following three points: (1) patients should be relieved of clinical symptoms of hyperthyroidism without repetitive hypothyroidism and hyperthyroidism, (2) thyroid hormones should be maintained at their normal serum levels, and (3) the abnormal production of TRAb must be allowed to diminish or be reduced to low levels, if possible.

GENERAL THERAPEUTIC CONSIDERATIONS

Thyroid Hormone Action

Thyroid hormone activates nuclear receptors, which regulate the expression of thyroid hormone-responsive genes. Four different receptors (three thyroid hormone receptor isoforms, alpha-1, beta-1, and beta-2, and a nonreceptor alpha-2 variant) are well documented. Age-dependent, sex-dependent, and target tissue-dependent thyroid hormone actions are present, although it is not certain what kind of receptor is related to each action. In the fetus and neonate, the hormones mainly contribute to the cellular differentiation of each target tissue. In childhood, not only differentiation but also cellular proliferation is induced by thyroid hormones. In the adolescent, especially in the young female, the hormone may play a role in the action of sex steroids. In subjects of all ages, thyroid hormones are important regulators of energy production, functional and structural proteins, and the actions of other hormones, such as glucocorticoids, mineralocorticoids, growth factors (e.g., insulin, insulin-like growth factor-1 [IGF-1]), and biogenic amines (e.g., catecholamines). When possible, the actions of thyroid hormone should be monitored during treatment of patients with Graves' hyperthyroidism.

Measurement of serum TSH concentration is useful in the assessment of thyroid hormone action in patients who have no abnormal function in hypothalamo-hypophyseal axis. Thyroid hormone inhibits pituitary secretion of TSH through the mechanism of negative feedback regulation. The concentration of TSH is a sensitive index of thyroid hormone action. Maintaining the normal serum levels of TSH is an important goal of therapy. Antithyroid drugs (ATDs), radioactive iodide, or surgical removal of thyroid glands sometimes leads to hypothyroidism and to an increase in serum levels of TSH. High serum levels of TSH should be avoided during the course of therapy, especially in pregnant women, neonates, and children.

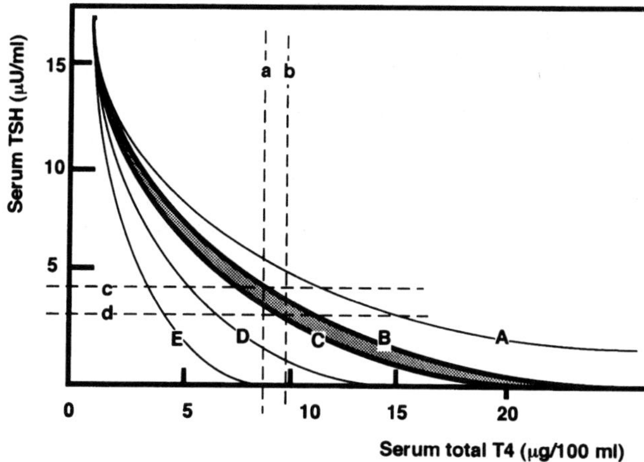

Figure 1
Modification of negative feedback regulation by thyroxine-binding globulin. Thyroid hormone inhibition of TSH secretion is modified by TBG. The relationship between serum T_4 and TSH concentrations is represented between lines B and C. In subjects with high serum TBG, the relation shifts to the right in the figure (from B to A). The relation shifts to the left (from C to D or E) in patients with TBG deficiency. The dashed lines show the normal range for total T_4 (a and b) and TSH (c and d).

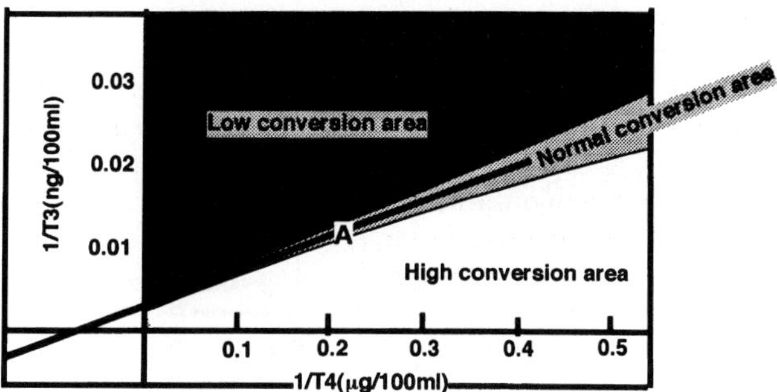

Figure 2
A method for estimating the presence of factors that modify the conversion of T_4 to T_3. The relationship (line A) between serum concentrations of total T_4 and total T_3 is obtained by double reciprocal analysis, using one maximal converting activity and one converting velocity. This line divides two populations; one has low converting activity (area above the line) and the other is high converting activity (area under the line). In the former, undernutrition, chronic liver disease, and acute excess iodide administration are included. In the latter, hypersecretion of growth hormone and PTU administration are included.

Negative Feedback Regulation

As mentioned, evaluation of negative feedback regulation is one of the methods of demonstrating the effectiveness of thyroid hormone action during treatment of hyperthyroidism. Serum thyroid hormones and serum TSH levels are maintained in a certain relationship in normal subjects. The relationship, however, is modified by thyroxine-binding globulin (TBG). In subjects who have high serum levels of TBG, serum thyroid hormone concentration, which maintains the normal serum levels of TSH, is increased. In contrast, serum thyroid hormone concentration is decreased in subjects who have low serum levels of TBG (Fig. 1). Thus, it is important to keep in mind that the serum concentration of TBG influences negative feedback regulation, and that thyroid hormone concentrations which are required to suppress TSH secretion differ depending on the serum concentration of TBG. Measurement of free thyroid hormone levels using radioimmunoassays is not available to evaluate the relationship in those who have extremely high or low serum levels of TBG.

Serum Levels of Thyroid Hormones

Peripheral action of thyroid hormone is mainly governed by T_3, because the affinity for T_3 binding to the receptor is higher than that for T_4 binding. Thus the serum concentration of T_3, but not T_4, strongly reflects the level of thyroid hormone action. T_3, as well as T_4, is released from thyroid glands. The majority of T_3 present in serum, however, is generated from T_4 in the presence of converting enzyme (deiodinase). The conversion is held at target tissues and regulated by intracellular concentration of iodide. There are two different isozymes. One (type I) is widely distributed in many tissues and plays an important role in maintaining the normal serum levels of T_3. Double reciprocal analysis of serum concentrations of T_3 and T_4 reveals the velocity and quantity of peripheral converting activity (Fig. 2). In some patients who suffer from damage in peripheral converting tissues (e.g., liver) the maximal converting activity is decreased, resulting in low serum levels of T_3 despite high levels of serum T_4. In addition, subjects who are undernourished or have low levels of serum GH show decreased conversion of T_4 to T_3. In such cases, differential diagnosis is required before beginning therapy for hyperthyroidism. Also remember that propylthiouracil (PTU), an antithyroid drug, inhibits the enzyme activity.

TBG Metabolism

T_4 is transported to the peripheral converting system by TBG. The presence of excess amounts of TBG in serum reduces the serum concentration of free T_4, which in turn decreases the amount of substrate (T_4) that can be converted to T_3. In patients with high serum concentrations of TBG (liver damage, pregnancy), serum concentrations of TBG and TSH as well as serum thyroid hormone levels should simultaneously be monitored during therapy for hyperthyroidism.

Production of Anti-TSH Receptor Antibodies

Many patients who are treated with any of the antithyroid therapies, including ATDs, radioactive iodide, and the partial surgical removal of the thyroid, experience recurrence of hyperthyroidism. The recurrence is induced by activation of the thyroid with TRAb, which are produced by autoimmune mechanisms. When antibodies are present, recurrence is likely. Glucocorticoids (e.g., prednisolone) are effective in reducing the levels of TRAb. However, long-term administration of steroids should be avoided because of their side effects. ATD is known as one of the agents that diminishes the production of TRAb.

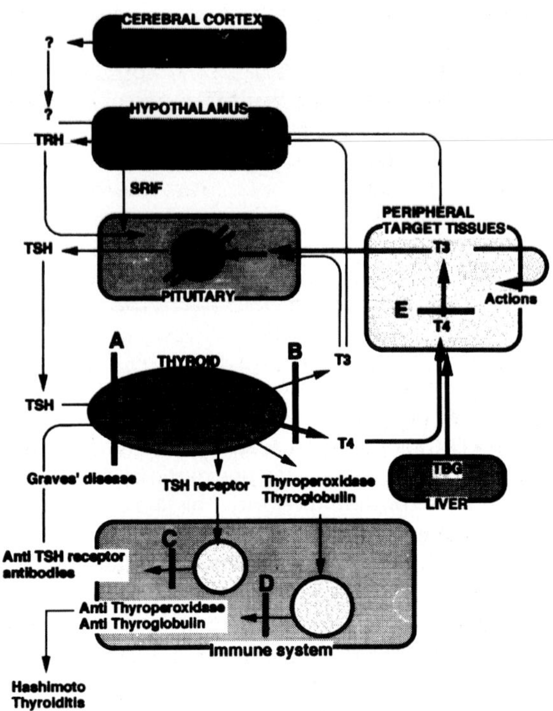

Figure 3
Regulation of thyroid hormone action in normal subjects and patients with Graves' disease. Mechanisms of antithyroid therapies in Graves' disease are shown. *A*, iodide, surgery, and radiation; *B*, Antithyroid drugs (ATD) (MMI and PTU); *C*, Glucocorticoids and ATD; *D*, Glucocorticoids; *E*, PTU and acute excess iodide.

The autoantigens recognized by the immune system are on the TSH receptor itself or fragments of the receptor. Inhibition of exposure of these autoantigens to the immune system is an alternative method to decrease the rate of production of antibodies. The exposure of these autoantigens is enhanced by activation of thyroid glands with TSH or TRAb. Although the initial treatment with ATD decreases the level of TRAb, long-term administration of excess amounts of ATD increases serum levels of TSH, which is induced by decreasing the serum levels of thyroid hormones. The presence of these modifications during ATD therapy for TSH secretion indicates that long-term treatment with these agents easily gives the chance to expose autoantigens (TSH receptor or its fragments) to the immune system. The mechanisms of therapy for Graves' hyperthyroidism are summarized in Figure 3.

■ PREFERRED THERAPEUTIC APPROACH

Initial Therapy

Thyroid hormone facilitates the action of the adrenergic system in the target tissues. Tachycardia, atrial fibrillation, and fine tremor are observed with other manifestations, such as loss of body weight, sweating, autonomic lability, heat intolerance, intestinal hyperactivity, and mental disorder in untreated hyperthyroidism. Usually, administration of ATD and beta-adrenergic blockades (30 to 60 mg per day of d, l-propranolol) is effective in reducing the degree of these symptoms. In addition to these symptoms, dehydration and consciousness disturbance with heart failure are observed in severe cases (thyroid storm or hyperthyroid crisis). Excess stimulation of the beta-adrenergic system increases heart rate, cardiac contractile activity, and cardiac conduction velocity, which requires high cardiac O_2 consumption. This stimulation is adequate to the requirement of high cardiac output for the peripheral demand of high O_2. However, when the stimulation exceeds the upper limit of cardiac function, the output promptly shrinks and results in a sudden drop in circulation volume.

The therapeutic approach to hyperthyroid crisis is divided into two components: (1) preventing overactivity of thyroid hormone in target peripheral tissues including heart, and (2) preventing hypersecretion of thyroid hormones from thyroid glands. In the former, infusion of water and adequate supplementation of electrolytes with intravenous administration of beta-adrenergic blockade is begun under monitoring electrocardiography (ECG). After confirmation of a decrease in the heart rate with normal sinus rhythm, the rate of administration of beta-adrenergic blockade can be reduced. The agent is continued with drip infusion under monitoring ECG thereafter. After the patient regains consciousness, the route of administration of the blockade is changed from intravenous to oral. In the initial treatment, hydrocortisone (200 to 600 mg per day) reduces the peripheral action of thyroid hormone. In the latter, excess amounts of ATD are given by intravenous injection. Oral administration of excess iodide is also effective in acute prevention of hormone secretion. Excess glucocorticoid (hydrocortisone) is also useful in inhibiting the release of excess thyroid hormone by stabilizing the thyroid plasma membranes. Infection (both viral and bacterial) often triggers the storm in patients with Graves' hyperthyroidism. Further, the storm easily occurs in patients receiving inadequate treatment with ATD. ATD may decrease the immune activity and results in the augmentation of inflammatory processes induced by microbial infections. In these cases, antibiotics or antiviral agents are administered.

Antithyroid Drug Therapy

Methimazole (MIM) and PTU inhibit thyroid hormone synthesis in thyroid glands and are used as ATDs in the treatment of thyrotoxicosis of Graves' disease. The mechanisms of inhibition are preventing peroxidation of iodide and blocking iodination of monoiodotyrosine and tyrosine in thyroid. Although the activity is not sufficient, immune suppressive activity is observed in these agents. In addition to the effects on the thyroid gland and on the immune system, PTU inhibits the peripheral deiodination from T_4 to T_3.

Usually, 30 to 60 mg per day of MMI or 300 to 600 mg per day of PTU is administered in the initial treatment of Graves' hyperthyroidism. The initial dosage may be increased depending on the degree of symptoms of thyrotoxicosis, size of goiter, serum levels of thyroid hormones, and the levels of TRAb. Appropriate administration of these agents leads to a decrease in the serum levels of thyroid hormones. This decrease accompanies a decrease in serum levels of TRAb though the effect is not sufficient. Thus, the initial treatment with these agents dramatically improves any symptoms and laboratory data. TSH secretion from pituitary is suppressed during the hyperthyroid state. The low serum levels of TSH continue for several months even after normalization of serum concentrations of thyroid hormones. This phenomenon results from a preceding long-term thyrotoxicosis. The long-term inhibition of TSH synthesis decreases the amount of TSH stored in thyrotrophs of the pituitary; thus TSH secretion does not respond to lowering of serum thyroid hormone concentration during the early stage of therapy.

Whether the initial dose should be continued or decreased cannot be determined when TSH secretion is suppressed. With continued treatment the suppression of the pituitary is reversed and the serum level of TSH increases. The rise in TSH stimulates thyroid growth without increasing thyroid hormone synthesis. Not only thyroid growth but also exposure of thyroid autoantigens (thyroperoxidase, thyroglobulin, and fragments of TSH receptors) to the immune system is accelerated by this stimulation. As expected, the production of autoantibodies (TRAb) is augmented. Thus, the dose of ATD should be reduced depending on the level of serum thyroid hormones and on the degree of improvement of clinical symptoms. The decrease in the dose of ATD leads to an euthyroid state without increasing the serum level of TSH. However, hyperthyroidism frequently recurs after the dose of ATD is reduced or discontinued, because incomplete decrease in TRAb easily induces recurrence even after normalization of serum levels of thyroid hormones. Discontinuation of ATD or reduction of dose is not adequate in patients who have high titers of TRAb even though the thyroid hormone levels are normalized.

Combination Therapy of Methimazole with T_4

Without increasing serum TSH levels, ATD must be continued during the follow-up period of therapy. Administration of T_4 (1.8 μg per kilogram per day or more) with an initial dose of ATD can prevent the progression of ATD-induced hypothyroidism. During the course of this combination, serum levels of TSH could be maintained to 0.05 m IU per milliliter (mild hyperthyroidism or less). The diminished TSH levels do not stimulate thyroid and decrease the chance of exposing autoantigens to immune system, which results in a decrease in the activity of TRAb production. By this combination therapy, both TSH- and TRAb-induced growth of thyroid glands are suppressed. The decrease in the size of thyroid further accelerates the decrease in the activity of TRAb production. PTU, but not MIM, has the ability to inhibit the conversion from T_4 to T_3. Thus, MIM is preferred as an ATD in combination therapy.

The combination of ATD with T_4 has a therapeutic effect on exophthalmos. The occurrence of Graves' ophthalmopathy also is known to be related to the action of TRAb. Long-term administration of ATD alone, which fails to decrease the level of TRAb, accelerates the progression of ophthalmopathy. The prevention of antibody production, therefore, is important in the management of ophthalmopathy. Fully 80 to 90 percent of ophthalmopathy is improved by the combination therapy. In our studies, however, although the progression of exophthalmos was inhibited, it was not normalized by the combination treatment in some cases. The reason for this is uncertain. Long-term exposure of retro-orbital tissues to antibodies probably induces changes that are not reversible.

Once the size of the thyroid gland is normal and serum levels of TRAb are low, the dose of ATD can be reduced. On the other hand, discontinuation of T_4 rapidly increases the serum level of TSH, which results in an increase in TRAb even after normalization of any other monitoring indicators during administration of ATD. In order to prevent TSH-induced reactivation of TRAb production, T_4 alone is continued for 2 to 3 years or more after discontinuation of ATD.

With combination therapy, TRAb levels decrease in 60 to 70 percent of patients with Graves' disease. As is well known, a lifelong memory for recognizing the thyroid autoantigens (TSH receptor) is a main pathogenic cause of Graves' hyperthyroidism. It is important to remember the patient still has a disordered immune system, which can lead to the recurrence of hyperthyroidism. Thus, long-term follow-up is important.

Combination Therapy in Gestational Hyperthyroidism and Postpartum Recurrence of Hyperthyroidism

Fetal growth is dependent on the maternal thyroid hormones, especially after the formation of the placenta. T_4 derived from the maternal thyroid is carried to the placenta as a TBG-bound form. The T_4 transferred to fetal circulation can be converted to T_3 in fetal liver; it then plays a role in the development of fetal peripheral tissues including the central nervous system. Maternal serum total T_4 levels increase after formation of placenta, which is associated with increasing serum levels of TBG. Thus, in normal pregnant women, serum T_4 concentrations of 20 μg per 100 milliliters or more are maintained after placental completion. The high T_4 levels of pregnancy should not be confused with hyperthyroidism. Symptoms of hyperthyroidism may decrease during pregnancy because of decreasing serum levels of TRAb and increasing TBG after placenta formation. Hypothyroidism can occur, which may put the fetus at risk. The hypothyroidism results from the decrease in TRAb and the delayed recovery of TSH secretion. Therefore, ATD which has been administered early in gestation can be discontinued at this time. In some cases, exogenous administration of T_4 is required. Usually 1.8 μg per kilogram per day is recommended to maintain normal fetal growth. Although maternal mild hyperthyroidism is induced, no underlying thyrotoxic manifestations will be observed. Even at the time of delivery, the administration of T_4 does not produce risk for the mother and neonate.

Administration of T_4 to the lactating mother does not alter the pituitary-thyroid axis of the child. Maternal hyperthyroidism may recur 2 to 3 months postpartum. When this happens, administration of ATD should be resumed. The ATD given to the mother accumulates in milk. The breast-feeding infant can obtain ATD from the mother's milk and could become hypothyroid. Since neonatal development requires relatively high levels of serum thyroid hormones, the mother given ATD should avoid breastfeeding. Milk production is easily prevented by 2 days administration of bromocriptine (5.0 to 7.5 mg per day), which inhibits pituitary secretion of prolactin.

Postpartum recurrence of hyperthyroidism is frequently observed in women with Graves' disease. The rate of recurrence is decreased by administration of T_4 1.8 μg per kilogram per day or more during pregnancy. The T_4 is begun from the time of completion of placenta formation. This treatment inhibits TSH secretion during the latter course of pregnancy, which subsequently prevents reactivation of the autoimmune system during the postpartum period.

Combination Therapy in Infantile Hyperthyroidism Resulting from Graves' Disease

Hyperthyroidism caused by Graves' disease is not rare in childhood. The symptoms are similar to those observed in adults except for the presence of marked dehydration. The pathogenesis of the disease is the abnormal production of TRAb. Thus the therapeutic approach is similar to that for adults. However, low levels of serum thyroid hormones must strictly be avoided because normal infant growth and development are entirely dependent on thyroid hormone. The combination of ATD with thyroid hormones is preferred. It is better to administer thyroid hormone (T_4) (2.2 μg per kilogram per day or more) at the beginning of ATD administration. Surgical treatment may also be used. Administration of T_4 is also recommended to prevent thyroidectomy-induced hypothyroidism, which follows even partial thyroidectomy.

In the adolescent, normal maturation depends not only on gonadotropins, IGF-1, and insulin but also on thyroid hormone, which plays a role in the permissive actions with these other hormones. Hypothyroidism induced by antithyroid therapies must be avoided. Radioactive iodide is not recomended in these young patients.

Side Effects of Antithyroid Drugs

Although infrequent, side effects of ATD are observed. One of the most important is leukocytopenia. Pancytopenia is not observed. Pernicious anemia and thrombocytopenia are also associated with Graves' disease per se but the incidences are low. Agranulocytosis is the most dangerous state induced by ATD administration. The mechanism by which this side effect is produced is not thoroughly understood. Although agranulocytosis may be observed during initial treatment with ATD, this hematopoietic disorder is also observed even after long-term administration of ATD. Acute suppurative inflammations, such as acute tonsillitis, acute pneumonia, and acute urinary tract infections, may be the initial symptoms of the agranulocytosis. After discontinuation of ATD the agranulocytosis resolves over several months. The therapy of hyperthyroidism in such cases must be changed from ATD to radioactive iodide or a surgical approach.

Hepatic dysfunction is a common side effect of ATD. An increase in the serum hepatic transaminases and alkaline phosphatase (Alp) is observed. An increase in the bone-derived Alp is common in patients with untreated Graves' hyperthyroidism. Additional increases in serum Alp derived from both bone and liver are frequently observed during initial therapy with ATD.

The skin lesions induced by ATD are caused by a reaction of drug-induced allergy. The lesions sometimes begin as discoid rashes which look like those observed in patients with systemic lupus erythematosus (SLE). Patients with ATD-induced skin rashes sometimes show positive antinuclear antibodies.

Graves' disease frequently is associated with other autoimmune diseases, such as rheumatoid arthritis, SLE, myasthenia gravis, Sjögren's syndrome, and idiopathic thrombocytopenic purpura (ITP). Differential diagnosis of these disorders must be distinguished from the side effects of ATD. These hepatic and dermatologic side effects disappear after discontinuation of ATD or reduction of the dose of ATD.

Complications Induced by Combination Therapy

The combination of ATD and T_4 induces no underlying complications other than those described for ATD alone, even after long-term treatment. Administration of T_4 sometimes induces a mild thyrotoxic state. However, the dose of 1.8 μg per kilogram per day is not sufficient to induce the symptoms of thyrotoxicosis. T_4-induced thyrotoxicosis is only observed in the Graves' patients with TBG deficiency. Serum levels of TBG, therefore, should be monitored during the course of combination therapy.

Recent studies show that osteoporosis is frequently observed in patients who have experienced long-term hyperthyroidism. Bone mineral density, however, is not decreased by the combination therapy. Patients with long-term hyperthyroidism show no decrease in bone strength. No further decrease in bone strength is observed even in the combination therapy–treated patients with low bone density. Further, the frequency of bone fracture is low in these patients.

Limitations of Therapy

As mentioned earlier in this chapter, Graves' disease is caused by abnormal production of autoantibodies against TSH receptor. The mechanism of this abnormal production occurs during fetal development of the immune system. It is, therefore, not possible to make patients free from abnormal production of antibodies. It is important to conduct a long-term follow-up survey. Clinical symptoms, size of goiter, serum levels of thyroid hormones and TSH, and serum levels of TRAb must be carefully monitored.

Other Therapeutic Approaches

Radioactive iodide therapy (not indicated in childhood and young patients) and surgery are classic treatments of Graves' hyperthyroidism. In any therapy, long-term follow-up is important because these therapies fail to introduce permanent remission. TRAb certainly stimulates thyroid tissues, even though its volume is reduced.

■ SPECIAL STATES OF HYPERTHYROIDISM

Hyperthyroidism in Subacute Thyroiditis

Spontaneous hyperthyroidism is sometimes observed during the course of subacute thyroiditis. The structural destruction of thyroid glands is related to the increase in the serum levels of thyroid hormones. In the case of severe thyrotoxic state, beta-adrenergic blockade is useful to remove tachycardia, tremors, and mental irritability. Anti-inflammatory agents are useful against severe thyroid pain. In the case of unresponsiveness to these medications, glucocorticoids (such as prednisolone) are effective. Long-term administration of glucocorticoids, however, delays healing (recurrence is common). Thus, the administration of glucocorticoid is not recommended. In the stage of hypothyroidism, T_4 (1.5 μg per kilogram per day or less) should be given, because the dramatic increase in serum TSH modifies the structure of the thyroid, which increases the chance of recurrent virus-induced inflammation.

Hyperthyroidism Caused by Toxic Adenoma

The constitutive activation of thyroidal adenylate cyclase is caused by the mutation(s) of TSH receptor molecule. The sites of mutation are not uniform. Disordered signal transduction at the coupling between TSH receptor and guanosine triphosphate–binding protein(s) is a major mechanism introducing constitutive activation. There is no way to normalize the coupling. Surgical approach for the tumor mass is preferred to decrease the serum levels of thyroid hormones. Since ATD inhibits thyroid hormone synthesis, these agents are of benefit to induce an euthyroid state before operation.

Hyperthyroidism Induced by TSH-Producing Pituitary Tumor

A TSH hypersecretion may result from a pituitary adenoma or hyperplasia. The transsphenoidal approach to the tumor is indicated. ATD is effective in inhibiting the TSH-induced oversecretion of thyroid hormone. However, the administration of ATD further increases the synthesis of TSH by decreasing the serum levels of thyroid hormones, which accelerates the growth of pituitary tumor. Thus, immediately after obtaining the euthyroid state with ATD, the surgery should be performed.

The diagnosis of a TSH-producing tumor is made as a syndrome of inappropriate TSH secretion (SITSH). The syndrome is observed not only in patients with TSH-producing tumor but also in those with resistance to thyroid hormone. In the latter case, the patients may have symptoms of hypothyroidism.

In elderly subjects, relatively high serum TSH concentration is observed although the serum thyroid hormone levels are normal. Probably the partial (pituitary) resistance to thyroid hormone presents in these subjects. In such cases, clinical symptoms of manifested hyperthyroidism or hypothyroidism (subclinical hypothyroidism may be present) are not observed. Before undertaking a surgical approach to the TSH-producing tumor, differential diagnosis of the tumor from other SITSH must carefully be made.

Suggested Reading

Thyroid gland. In: DeGroot L, et al., eds. Endocrinology. 3rd ed.Vol. 1. Philadelphia: WB Saunders, 1995:507.

DeGroot L, et al., eds. The thyroid and its diseases. 5th ed. New York: John Wiley & Sons, 1984.

Hashizume K, et al. Administration of thyroxine in treated Graves' disease. Effects on the level of antibodies to thyroid hormone-stimulating receptors and on the risk of recurrence of hyperthyroidism. N Engl J Med 1991; 324:947–953.

Hashizume K, et al. Effect of administration of thyroxine on the risk of postpartum recurrence of hyperthyroid Graves' disease. J Clin Endocrinol Metab 1992; 75:6–10.

THYROID STORM

Wolfgang H. Dillmann, M.D.

Thyroid storm, also termed *thyrotoxic crisis,* is a rarely occurring, severe form of hyperthyroidism leading to systemic decompensation and a high mortality (20 to 50 percent in different series). Improving medical care has led to a decreased incidence in recent decades, but the occurrence of thyroid storm may still approach approximately 1 percent of hospitalizations for hyperthyroidism. Thyroid storm occurs more frequently with Graves' disease but is sometimes found in conjunction with toxic nodular goiter and other rarer causes of hyperthyroidism.

The diagnosis of thyroid storm has to be made on clinical grounds. Thyroid hormone values are elevated, but no specific abnormality of free thyroxine (T_4), triiodothyronine (T_3), or thyroid-stimulating hormone can be taken to distinguish severe but compensated hyperthyroidism from thyroid storm. Cardinal clinical signs include a high fever (temperature, 102 to 105° F) with profuse sweating, marked tachycardia (pulse, 120 to 140 beats per minute and higher), atrial fibrillation, and sometimes congestive heart failure; in addition central nervous system signs such as confusion, severe restlessness, and agitation which can cause a lapse into coma. Marked gastrointestinal symptoms with vomiting, profuse diarrhea, and hepatomegaly with jaundice can also occur. These clinical signs are not specific and suspicion that the patient's decompensation could be due to underlying hyperthyroidism is the key to the diagnosis.

The pathophysiologic mechanisms turning severe hyperthyroidism into thyroid storm are not clear, but two general mechanisms are most likely important contributors. One mechanism relates to a sudden increase in the amount of thyroid hormone released from the thyroid gland into the systemic circulation. Examples of this are thyroid surgery in hyperthyroid patients. This accounted frequently for the occurrence of thyroid storm in the past and was termed *surgical storm.* Induction of thyroid storm has also been reported in patients treated with radioactive iodine or in hyperthyroid patients who stopped antithyroid medication. A second mechanism contributing to the development of thyroid storm results from a sudden increase in the amount of free thyroid hormone available to the cells of the body as it

Table 1 Management of Thyroid Storm (To Be Undertaken in Intensive Care Unit)

INTERVENTION AND ITS AIM	AGENT AND DOSE PROCEDURE
INHIBITION OF NEW THYROID HORMONE FUNCTION	
Propylthiouracil	200 mg every 4 hours (orally or nasogastric tube)
Methimazole	20 mg every 4 hours (orally or nasogastric tube)
INHIBITION OF THYROID HORMONE RELEASE	
Iodine	Lugol's solution (10 drops t.i.d.) Potassium iodide (SSKI) (3 drops t.i.d.) Na I IV 1 g 24 hrs
ADRENERGIC BLOCKADE	
Propranolol (Esmolol)	40–80 mg every 4–6 hrs PO; 0.5–1 mg IV every 5–10 mins
SUPPORTIVE THERAPY	
Hydrocortisone	100 mg IV push; repeat 8 hrs for total of 300 mg/day
Treatment of hyperthermia	Cooling blanket; acetaminophen
Fluid replacement	Including 5% dextrose, electrolytes, multivitamins
Treat heart failure	Digoxin
Identify and treat precipitating illness	E.g., infection with appropriate antibiotics

Table 2 Alternative Therapy for Thyroid Storm

Removal of Thyroid Hormone from Blood
Plasmapheresis
Charcoal plasma perfusion
Peritoneal dialysis
Inhibition of Thyroid Hormone Release
Lithium carbonate 300 mg every 6 hours
Inhibition of Peripheral T_4 to T_3 Conversion
Ipodate 1 g PO daily
Alternatives to Adrenergic Blockade
Calcium channel blockers
Diltiazem 30–60 mg every 4–6 hours/day

occurs when the binding capacity of serum proteins for thyroid hormone markedly decreases. An example is thyroid storm that is triggered by an intercurrent illness, for example, an infection like pneumonia or pyelonephritis. In some patients the simultaneous occurrence of a severe illness leading to the nonthyroidal illness syndrome can markedly lower thyroid hormone values like T_4 and T_3 and add further complexity to the diagnosis. Combination of severe hyperthyroidism and diabetic ketoacidosis can result in thyroid storm without significant increases in T_4 and T_3 levels. After treatment of the diabetic ketoacidosis, T_4 and T_3 levels will markedly increase. It is frequently difficult to differentiate between severe thyrotoxicosis complicated by an intercurrent illness and thyroid storm itself. The intercurrent illness may, however, trigger the development of thyroid storm. In some sense the distinction between thyroid storm and hyperthyroidism with intercurrent illness may be artificial and the main question to be decided is whether the patient needs emergency therapy. When in doubt, a diagnosis of an impending storm should be made and the treatment appropriate for thyroid storm initiated as described below.

■ PREFERRED THERAPY

Patients with fully developed or impending thyroid storm should be managed in the intensive care unit by the approach outlined in Table 1. The aims of therapy are (1) inhibit thyroid hormone formation, (2) inhibit release of thyroid hormone from the thyroid gland, (3) provide beta-adrenergic blockade, (4) provide supportive therapy, (5) identify and treat the precipitating illness, and (6) consider long-term therapy to prevent recurrence of thyroid storm. Alternate approaches and other treatment considerations are also discussed and are summarized in Table 2. Treatment has to be frequently initiated on the basis of the clinical diagnosis because laboratory confirmation of elevated thyroid hormone levels cannot be obtained rapidly enough.

Treatment Directed at Inhibition of Thyroid Hormone Formation

Rapid lowering of thyroid hormone synthesis and resultant lowering of thyroid hormone levels is crucial for the successful treatment of thyroid storm. Propylthiouracil (PTU) is administered orally or by nasogastric tube. PTU therapy can be initiated by giving a loading dose of 600 mg and then continued at a dose of 1,200 mg per day administered in 200 mg doses every 4 hours. This dose completely blocks thyroid hormone formation. PTU is currently available in 50 mg tablets. In addition, PTU inhibits the peripheral conversion of T_4 to T_3, which is the biologically active thyroid hormone. In patients who cannot take oral medication, rectal administration of PTU has been successfully used. Currently, no parenteral preparation of antithyroid medication is available in the United States. In patients with prior severe reactions to PTU, like agranulocytosis, this form of therapy is contraindicated. The other antithyroid drug that is available is methimazole. Because methimazole does not inhibit peripheral T_4 to T_3 conversion, it is not the preferred treatment compound. Methimazole is given in a daily dose of 120 mg with 20 mg given every 4 hours. The general side effects of PTU and methimazole, like agranulocytosis and skin rash, also apply to the treatment of thyroid storm. PTU or methimazole only inhibit thyroid hormone synthesis, but not thyroid hormone release from the thyroid gland. Patients with Graves' disease can have significant stores of T_4 and T_3 in their thyroid and inhibition of thyroid hormone release is, therefore, important.

Inhibition of Thyroid Hormone Release

Several hours (2 to 3 hours) after antithyroid medication in the form of PTU has been started, thyroid hormone release should be inhibited by administration of iodine. It is important to first block thyroid hormone formation so that iodine cannot exert a potential stimulating effect on thyroid hormone synthesis. Iodine can be given as Lugol's solution (10 drops, three times a day) or as a saturated solution of potassium iodine (3 drops, three times a day). Intravenous sodium iodine at a dose of 1 to 2 grams every 24 hours can also be used. This preparation is currently not on the market in the United States. Increasing the amount of inorganic iodine in the thyroid results in increased iodination of thyroglobulin, which is more resistant to proteolysis leading to decreased release of T_4 and T_3 from the gland. This effect starts very rapidly and remains for 1 to 3 weeks. In addition, a short-time inhibitory effect on thyroid hormone synthesis (Wolff-Chaikoff effect) occurs. Iodine administration precludes radioactive iodine treatment for hyperthyroidism within several weeks after the thyroid storm has been resolved. The iodine load has to be cleared before a good radioactive iodine uptake can be obtained for successful radioactive iodine treatment. Iodine cannot be used in patients with a history of iodine anaphylaxis. Such patients should be treated with lithium carbonate, which also inhibits thyroid hormone release as described below under Alternatives to the Use of Iodine.

Beta-adrenergic Blockade

Patients in thyroid storm have many signs and symptoms which are compatible with increased beta-adrenergic activity. This includes increased agitation and restlessness, tremor, profuse sweating, and tachycardia. These effects could come about by an increased sensitivity of the beta-sympathetic system to beta-adrenergic stimulation in the hyperthyroid state. An alternate explanation may be that both thyroid hormone and beta-adrenergic agonists stimulate the same parameter, for example leading to an increase in heart rate. Use of beta-adrenergic blockers, like propranolol, in patients with thyroid storm has significant beneficial effects and beta-adrenergic blockade is part of the standard therapy for thyroid storm.

Propranolol is most widely used in an oral dose of 40 to 80 mg every 4 to 6 hours per day for a total dose of 240 to 480 mg per day. Considerable variability in this dose is frequently needed to achieve adequate beta-blockade. Peak effects after oral propranolol administration occur within 2 hours after administration and effects dissipate with a half-life of 3 hours. A mild inhibitory effect on the conversion of T_4 to T_3 is also obtained with propranolol. In patients with acute heart rate related problems, like a rapid ventricular response to atrial fibrillation, propranolol can be administered intravenously at a dose of 1 mg every 5 to 10 minutes until the ventricular rate is controlled. This approach requires careful cardiac monitoring, which is best provided in the setting of an intensive care unit. As a consequence of propranolol therapy, improvement in tachycardia, palpitation, tremors, restlessness, muscle weakness, heat intolerance, and hyperreflexia can be obtained. Despite these beneficial effects, the underlying metabolic disturbance is not influenced and concurrent use of high doses of antithyroid medication and iodine is important in the treatment of thyroid storm. In patients with a history of asthma and bronchial spasms, the use of propranolol is contraindicated. In patients with congestive heart failure, the use of propranolol needs to be considered on an individual basis. If the heart failure is largely caused by a rapid ventricular response, propranolol can be used as described. Because of the overall negative contractile effect of propranolol it may be contraindicated in patients with bradycardia and in patients who are in severe congestive heart failure.

An alternative to propranolol are more recently developed, very short acting beta-blockers, like esmolol. Initially a loading infusion of 250 to 500 µg per kilogram is given over several minutes' time, followed by a maintenance infusion of 50 µg per kilogram per minute. The maintenance dose should be maintained until a decrease of supraventricular tachycardia occurs.

Supportive Therapy

Supportive therapy can be divided into those measures that should be undertaken in every patient with thyroid storm and those measures that require an individual approach according to the underlying symptoms.

Improved survival of patients with thyroid storm who receive adrenal crisis type doses of hydrocortisone have been reported. Hydrocortisone at an initial dose of 300 mg IV followed by 100 mg every 8 hours should, therefore, be administered to every patient with thyroid storm. The pathophysiologic basis for this therapy can be found in the increased cortisol turnover in markedly hyperthyroid patients leading to normal rather than elevated cortisol levels in patients with thyroid storm. In addition, high levels of glucocorticoids inhibit the peripheral conversion of T_4 to T_3. Once the thyroid storm is reversed, the dose can be reduced and subsequently discontinued. Short-term administration of glucocorticoids for several days, but overall for less than a week, does not lead to significant depression of the pituitary-adrenal axis.

High fevers are a hallmark of thyroid storm and need to be controlled. Acetaminophen should be used for pharmacologic antipyretic therapy. Salicylate displaces thyroid hormone from thyroid hormone-binding proteins in the serum and may increase free thyroid hormone concentrations and should, therefore, be avoided. Cooling blankets or ice packs can further help with temperature control. Central thermal regulation, especially shivering, can be inhibited with chlorpromazine (25 to 50 mg IV every 4 to 6 hours), which also has a sedative effect for restlessness, agitation, and tremor.

Profuse sweating, diarrhea, and vomiting can lead to significant fluid loss during thyroid storm and results in intravascular volume depletion and cardiovascular collapse. Dehydration with massive rhabdomyolysis has also been seen. Fluid replacement needs to be individualized in patients, but 100 to 200 ml per hour is sometimes required. In patients with congestive heart failure, fluid replacement needs to be undertaken with caution and is sometimes contraindicated. Inclusion of electrolytes, 5 percent dextrose, and a supply of multiple vitamins in the replacement regimen is advisable in patients with thyroid storm. In a great majority of patients with thyroid storm congestive heart failure results from a too rapid ventricular response resulting in inefficient cardiac contraction. Ventricular rate should be lowered by beta-adrenergic blockade as described in the preceding section. Atrial fibrillation can lead to embolic events and requires anticoagulation. It should be taken into consideration that warfarin anticoagulants have a higher potency in hyperthyroid patients.

The combined use of beta-adrenergic blockers plus digoxin leads to a synergistic effect by increasing atrial ventricular conduction time and prolonging the refectory period of the atrial-ventricular node. The ventricular response of patients with atrial fibrillation is, therefore, diminished. The main benefit of digoxin in thyrotoxic patients is related to its effect on conduction time. Because of the increased distribution space and more rapid metabolism, larger than usual loading dose and maintenance doses of digoxin are sometimes required. The safety margin for digoxin seems to be narrowed in hyperthyroid patients and digoxin toxicity is not infrequent. Rapid changes in the degree of hyperthyroidism may lead to alterations in digoxin metabolism and distribution and it is best to obtain frequent digoxin serum levels.

Patients in thyroid storm and congestive heart failure are best treated in a coronary care unit where monitoring with a Swan-Ganz catheter is possible. The vascular bed is already dilated and frequently volume depletion occurs in patients in thyroid storm. Vasodilators are, therefore, not indicated and diuretics should be used with great caution.

Identification and Treatment of Precipitating Event or Illness

In many patients in thyroid storm, the precipitating event is easily identified. It may relate to discontinuation of PTU treatment in a severely hyperthyroid patient or use of radioactive iodine or a surgical procedure. In other hyperthyroid patients, an interfering illness such as a pneumonia diagnosed on a chest x-ray may present the precipitating event. Vigorous therapy with appropriate antibiotics needs to be undertaken. General antibiotic coverage without identification of a specific infection or organism is, however, not advisable. Some of the more difficult diagnostic dilemmas occur in stuporous or comatose patients with no available history from relatives or friends. In addition, because of an intervening nonthyroidal illness syndrome caused by, for example, diabetic ketoacidosis, T_3 levels may only be modestly elevated. The precipitating illness like the underlying pneumonia or diabetic ketoacidosis needs to be vigorously treated. In about one-third of all patients, thyroid storm is not precipitated by an identifiable event or illness.

Longterm Therapy to Prevent Recurrence of Thyroid Storm

With the treatment regimen outlined above, significant clinical improvement with decreases in T_4 and T_3 levels occurs, in general, within 1 to 2 days; however, full recovery from thyroid storm takes a week or longer. Once the episode of thyroid storm has subsided, iodine therapy should be stopped, glucocorticoids can be rapidly tapered, and, after a normal pulse rate and cardiac action have been obtained, beta-adrenergic blockers can be tapered and then withdrawn. Because of the iodine load received during acute treatment, radioactive iodine treatment for hyperthyroidism is precluded within several weeks after the thyroid storm has resolved. The iodine load has to be cleared before a good radioactive iodine uptake can be obtained for successful radioactive iodine treatment. Once the patient has become euthyroid, surgical therapy using a subtotal thyroidectomy can be performed. In the hands of an experienced thyroid surgeon, this presents a safe procedure with a low rate (about 2 percent) of laryngeal nerve damage or hypoparathyroidism. Surgery in a hyperthyroid patient can induce thyroid storm. Preparation for surgery with propranolol alone does not alleviate the metabolic consequences of hyperthyroidism and thyroid storm and should not be undertaken. The decrease in the occurrence of thyroid storm during the last several decades results most likely from improved therapy of hyperthyroidism using adequate doses of antithyroid medication and beta-blockade and the more adequate preparation of the hyperthyroid patient before thyroid surgery. In addition, the ready use of a thyroid storm regimen in severely hyperthyroid patients with an intercurrent illness probably also markedly contributed to the decreased occurrence of thyroid storm. Continued vigilance for the occurrence of signs of metabolic decompensation in severely hyperthyroid patients and vigorous treatment of the intercurrent illness will probably lead to further decreases in the mortality from thyroid storm.

■ ALTERNATIVE THERAPY FOR THYROID STORM

Alternatives to the Antithyroid Medications

Rarely, one encounters patients in thyroid storm who had a prior severe reaction to PTU or methimazole, such as an episode of agranulocytosis, and these compounds cannot be used. The crossover occurrence of side effects from one compound to the other is probably in the range of 50 percent. Use of radioactive iodine and surgery is also precluded because of the resulting high mortality with these procedures in severely hyperthyroid patients. Direct removal of thyroid hormone from the blood of patients in thyroid storm has been described. The procedures applied include plasmapheresis, charcoal plasma perfusion, and peritoneal dialysis. Plasmapheresis needs to be repeated several times because only one-fifth of the total thyroid hormone pool is removed per session. Plasmapheresis may also decrease the level of thyroid-stimulating immunoglobulin, the causative factor in Graves' disease.

In severely hyperthyroid patients who exhibit signs compatible with thyroid storm, such as a rapid tachycardia, I have used the oral radiographic dye, ipodate. The medication is not a prescription drug, but is available in x-ray departments or from x-ray supply companies and is used as an oral gallbladder dye. Ipodate inhibits peripheral T_4 to T_3 conversion and, because of its large iodine content, also inhibits thyroid hormone release. Ipodate is given as a loading dose of 1.5 g and a daily dose of 0.5 to 1 g subsequently. It should be limited to the acute phase and should not be administered for more than 2 weeks, because the increased iodine exposure can increase thyroid hormone formation. The effect of the drug can be monitored by determining T_3 levels, which should decrease rapidly after the start of the compound. Beta-adrenergic blockade and high doses of glucocorticoids can also be used in such patients.

Alternatives to the Use of Iodine

Iodine cannot be used in patients with a history of iodine anaphylaxis. Such patients should be treated with lithium carbonate, which also inhibits thyroid hormone release. Lithium carbonate is given at a dose of 300 mg every 6 hours. Serum lithium levels should be lower than 1 m per dose equivalent per liter, otherwise the dose needs to be lowered. Too high plasma levels of lithium carbonate can result in nausea, vomiting, cardiac arrhythmias, nephrogenic diabetes insipidus, and muscle hyperactivity. Because of the overall more severe side effects of lithium carbonate in comparison to iodine, the latter is preferred in treatment of patients with severe hyperthyroidism unless contraindicated. Iodine is also not useable in patients with iodine-overload–induced hyperthyroidism or thyroid storm. This has been reported in patients treated with the cardiac antiarrhythmic drug amiodarone, which is highly iodinated and is deiodinated during its metabolism resulting in iodine-induced hyperthyroidism (Jod-Basedow disease), which can lead to thyroid storm. In such patients, antithyroid drugs should be used as described in combination with potassium perchlorate, which blocks the uptake of iodine into the thyroid cells. A dose of 0.5 g potassium per chlorate a day should be used. Higher doses of perchlorate can lead to bone marrow suppression. Perchlorate by itself has been used for the treatment of hyperthyroidism in the past. The use of a dose higher than 1 g per day is repeatedly required and resulted in gastric and bone marrow toxicity and made it a less favored antithyroid drug.

Alternatives to Beta-Adrenergic Blockade

In patients with severe asthma, in whom even more cardioselective agents like esmolol may be too dangerous to use, the hyperdynamic cardiac effects can be inhibited by using reserpine at a dose of 2.5 mg every 4 hours. In addition, guanethidine given orally at 30 mg every 6 hours can be efficient. This drug should not be used in patients with hypertension or congestive heart failure. Calcium channel blockers in patients in thyroid storm with a rapid heart beat and hyperdynamic cardiac action have been employed with good results. Congestive heart failure excludes the use of calcium channel blockers. Diltiazem can be given orally for total doses of 180 to 360 mg a day using 30 to 60 mg tablets in divided doses four to six times a day. Parenteral preparations of diltiazem are also available.

Suggested Reading

Burch HB, Wartofsky L. Life-threatening thyrotoxicosis: Thyroid storm. Endocrinol Metab Clin North Am 1993; 22:263–277.

Burger AG, Philippe J. Thyroid emergencies. Baillieres Clin Endocrinol Metab 1992; 6:77–93.

Candrina R, DiStefano O, Spandrio S, Giustina G. Treatment of thyrotoxic storm by charcoal plasmaperfusion. J Endocrinol Invest 1989; 12:133–134.

Gavin LA. Thyroid crises. Med Clin North Am 1991; 75:179–193.

Lazarus JH, Richards AR, Addission GH, Owen GH. Treatment of thyrotoxicosis with lithium carbonate. Lancet 1974; 2:1160–1163.

Tajiri J, Katsuya H, Kiyokaya T, et al. Successful treatment of thyrotoxic crisis with plasma exchange. Crit Care Med 1984; 12:536–537.

THYROIDITIS

Paul G. Walfish, C.M., M.D., F.R.C.P. C., F.A.C.P., F.R.S.M.

It has been well established that inflammation of the thyroid induced by acute bacterial or viral infections may be accompanied by typical features of pain and fever. However, over the past decades, cytotoxicity secondary to underlying autoimmune thyroiditis has been recognized to result in subacute or chronic thyroiditis without the typical clinical features of inflammation that can lead to either progressive thyroid gland enlargement or atrophy. Additionally, it is now known that patients who are predisposed to episodes of destructive painless autoimmune thyroiditis may be in a latent (subclinical) predisposed stage which is unmasked by disruptions in the immune system or hormonal milieu that can trigger transient cytotoxic episodes. Although the inflammatory process is often associated with a mononuclear cell infiltrate, lymphocytic thyroiditis has been associated with many causes such as chronic autoimmune thyroiditis, spontaneously resolving painless (postpartum or nonpostpartum) thyroiditis, spontaneously resolving subacute (pseudogranulomatous thyroiditis, de Quervain's thyroiditis), localized infection, perineoplastic (hot or cold nodules) thyroiditis, or a "malignant pseudothyroiditis" syndrome.

In my practice the commonest cause of thyroiditis encountered is chronic autoimmune thyroiditis (CT) followed by painless (postpartum or silent) thyroiditis (PT). The next most frequent cause is typical subacute thyroiditis, which often requires differentiation from the less frequently occurring acute suppurative thyroiditis (AT). Other less common but increasingly recognized causes of thyroiditis have been documented from trauma to the thyroid gland after parathyroidectomy and following lymphokine-cytokine therapy or with changes in adrenal gland corticosteroid function that results in a transient destructive injury to the thyroid gland

Supported in part by grants from the Saul A. Silverman Family Foundation and Temmy Latner/Dynacare as well as The Meadowcroft Group and The Mount Sinai Hospital Department of Medicine Research Fund.

simulating either PT or subacute thyroiditis (ST) syndromes. Lymphomas and metastases to the thyroid gland rarely cause a "malignant pseudothyroiditis" syndrome, and inflammatory perineoplastic infiltrates around benign or malignant thyroid nodules can lead to a false suspicion of thyroiditis.

In the management of thyroiditis, the precise cause must first be correctly determined by obtaining a detailed history and physical examination as well as appropriate initial biochemical and radioisotopic laboratory tests followed by serial biochemical studies of thyroid function to monitor the effects of destruction on thyroid gland function. With this information the underlying causes of thyroiditis can usually be assigned to one of the following categories: acute: (pyogenic-bacterial or opportunistic infections); subacute: typical (painful pseudogranulomatous, de Quervain's) or painless (silent, postpartum; postlymphokine-cytokine-adrenocortical dysfunction, postparathyroidectomy and other thyroidal injuries); and chronic: (autoimmune) goitrous (Hashimoto's) or atrophic (idiopathic myxedema) or fibrotic (Riedel's struma).

Once the underlying cause of thyroiditis has been correctly diagnosed, I then prescribe appropriate treatment that is directed toward (1) the control of the disabling symptoms of neck pain dysphagia and systemic complaints (fever, malaise, and myalgia); (2) the amelioration of transient or persistent disturbances in thyroid dysfunction; and when indicated (3) specific therapy for pyogenic-bacterial or opportunistic infections. The remainder of this chapter will deal with my management strategies to ensure that an accurate diagnosis is made and that the appropriate therapy for the various types of thyroiditis is administered.

■ CHRONIC (AUTOIMMUNE) THYROIDITIS

Diagnosis

CT most commonly presents as a diffuse goitrous enlargement of the thyroid gland (Hashimoto's thyroiditis), which is usually relatively asymptomatic and nontender. Alternatively, CT can be associated with an atrophic thyroid gland (idiopathic myxedema). CT reaches a prevalence (as high as 10 to 15 percent) particularly in geographic regions with a high iodine intake. CT is 4 to 10 times more frequent in females than males and often occurs when there is a strong family history of either Hashimoto's thyroiditis or Graves' disease. Circulating antimicromsomal antibody (AMA) and/or antithyroglobulin thyroid antibody (ATA) titers are positive in 90 percent of affected subjects and are often accompanied by varying degrees of hypothyroidism. In euthyroid subjects, the finding of negative AMA and ATA titers will require fine-needle aspiration (FNA) biopsy to differentiate CT from other causes of euthyroid goiter. On regional surveys, approximately 1 percent of the population will develop autoimmune hypothyroidism with subnormal levels of circulating thyroid hormone, whereas other patients may have a compensated phase of subclinical hypothyroidism. However, when there is an elevated serum TSH, positive AMA and/or ATA titers as well as goiter, CT can progress to overt thyroid failure at a rate of approximately 3 to 5 percent per year.

Therapy

Patients who have symptoms consistent with thyroid failure and reduced free thyroxine levels in the presence of an increased serum thyrotropin (TSH) are treated with lifelong thyroid hormone replacement. Maintenance doses of L-thyroxine (L-T_4) usually range from 75 to 200 μg daily. The rapidity with which thyroid function is restored depends on such factors as the duration and severity of the hypothyroidism, the age of patient, and the presence of other clinical problems, particularly cardiovascular disease.

When initiating treatment for patients over 50 years of age or with known cardiovascular disease, I commence L-T_4 therapy using small doses at 12.5 to 25 μg per day and gradually increase the dose by 12.5 to 25 μg per day at 6 week intervals until a maximal daily dose of approximately 100 to 150 μg is reached. L-T_4 is administered at sufficient dosage to restore serum T_4 levels to the mid- to lower levels of normal and maintain the serum TSH at the upper limits of normal or even slightly elevated in patients with active coronary insufficiency and cardiac arrhythmias. Adequate replacement therapy can result in a reduction of thyroid size in most but not all patients with goitrous thyroiditis.

In general, I do not routinely prescribe L-triiodothyronine (L-T_3) for thyroid hormone replacement unless severe symptoms of hypothyroidism are present and there is no risk of underlying cardiovascular disease. L-T_3 is begun at doses of 5 to 12.5 μg administered two to three times daily and increased at weekly intervals to a total dosage of 50 to 75 μg per day. I do not prescribe desiccated thyroid, thyroglobulin, or combined T_4 and T_3 preparations because of their variable content of L-T_3, which induces acute elevations in serum T_3 levels 4 to 8 hours after administration and lowers serum T_4 normal ranges and complicates both clinical and laboratory assessment. Adequacy of L-T_4 replacement therapy requires serial clinical and laboratory test monitoring of a serum T_4 and TSH at 6 to 8 week intervals until a suitable maintenance dosage is established. Failure to check for patient compliance and repeat laboratory testing at less than 6 to 8 week intervals (when stable serum levels have not been reached) can lead to errors in L-T_4 replacement dosage. L-T_4 therapy for CT is not indicated when the only abnormality is a positive antithyroid antibody titer. However, in the presence of an elevated serum TSH and normal serum T_4 and T_3 levels (subclinical hypothyroidism), particularly when accompanied by either goiter and/or other coexistent clinical problems such as elevated lipids, premenstrual tension, menorrhagia, or infertility, I will often recommend a trial of L-T_4 to normalize thyroid functional status and determine whether hypothyroidism was a secondary cause of these concomitant problems.

Surgery is rarely indicated for CT. However, a surgical referral should be considered when despite adequate L-T_4 replacement therapy there is (1) local compression of esophagus, recurrent laryngeal nerve, or trachea; (2) localized hypofunctional nodules on scintiscan that are suspicious for thyroid neoplasia, cancer, or lymphoma; and/or (3) nodules that persist or increase in size despite thyroid hormone therapy and thereby require the exclusion of coexisting malignant neoplasia, i.e., a cellular FNA biopsy aspirate associated with a variable degree of lymphocytic thyroiditis.

Very rarely, a fibrotic type of chronic autoimmune thyroiditis (Riedel's struma) may be encountered which represents a predominantly fibrotic replacement of thyroid glandular tissue. It may be associated with mediastinal or retroperitoneal fibrosis. In this situation the thyroid gland is stony hard and the accompanying sclerosing fibrosis lead to fixation of the thyroid gland with adherence to trachea, esophagus, and recurrent laryngeal nerves. A cutting needle or open surgical biopsy is often required to confirm the diagnosis. Surgical resection is often difficult and of limited efficacy in relieving the compression symptoms resulting from adherence to adjacent structures. Although thyroid hormone replacement therapy is indicated and a trial of corticosteroid therapy often considered, these measures are usually not successful in completely eliminating compressive symptomatology.

■ PAINLESS (SILENT, POSTPARTUM, LYMPHOCYTIC) THYROIDITIS

Diagnosis

PT commonly has an initial spontaneously resolving thyrotoxic phase accompanied by a suppressed radioiodine thyroid uptake that is followed by variable degrees of transient hypothyroidism. In contrast to typical ST, there are no clinical features to suggest a viral etiology such as previous upper respiratory infection, fever, malaise, headache, or myalgia. Also, there is no increase in sedimentation rate, leukocyte count, or viral antibody titers.

Neck examination reveals that the thyroid gland is either normal sized or enlarged to less than twice normal and is nontender to palpation. FNA biopsy usually reveals only lymphocytic infiltration and occasional focal follicular epithelial cell atrophy. Approximately 50 percent of patients with PT will have a positive AMA titer at the onset of the disease and about 85 percent of patients will develop a positive antithyroid antibody titer during the course of their illness. Often there is a threefold rise in AMA titer particularly in the hypothyroid phase. While PT may be observed in either gender and at any age, it has been observed to have a particular predilection for occurring postpartum where it is estimated to occur at a prevalence of between 2 to 6 percent in some geographic regions. Moreover, PT has been increasingly recognized to account for between 5 to 20 percent of all detected causes of hyperthyroidism.

In the hyperthyroid phase, differentiation of PT from Graves' disease can be best achieved by obtaining a radioisotopic thyroid uptake test. For lactating mothers, a ^{99m}Tc or ^{123}I thyroid uptake study can be performed provided that breastfeeding is suspended for 48 hours. When a radioisotopic thyroid uptake study cannot be obtained, spontaneous resolution to a subsequent hypothyroid phase also supports a diagnosis of PT. Current clinical and experimental evidence favors the view that PT is a subclinical variant of autoimmune thyroiditis, which is secondary to a transient destructive (cytotoxic) phase of inflammation that often remits to a latent form of autoimmune thyroiditis.

Therapy

Symptoms resulting from the thyrotoxic phase of PT are treated conservatively with beta-adrenergic blockers such as propranolol 40 to 160 mg per day every 4 to 6 hours in divided doses for relief of tachycardia, tremor, and sweating. For patients with concomitant asthma, propranolol is avoided and instead cardioselective beta-adrenergic blockers such as metoprolol or atenolol are administered. For concomitant nervousness and anxiety, tranquilizers such as diazepam (5 mg) several times daily are occasionally prescribed. Serial clinical and laboratory follow-up assessments are performed at 4 to 6 week intervals to document the spontaneous resolution of thyrotoxic symptoms and to detect the possible development of symptomatic hypothyroidism. Hypothyroidism often requires only short-term treatment with either L-T_3 50 to 75 μg per day in divided dosage or L-T_4 100 to 200 μg daily for 6 to 12 months before attempting withdrawal. After 6 to 12 months of hormone replacement, long-term follow-up at 1 year intervals is indicated. In the presence of a small goiter and low AMA titer, a trial withdrawal of all thyroid hormone replacement is justified to determine whether euthyroidism can be maintained. Although 85 to 90 percent of patients will have no evidence for persistent hypothyroidism, recurrence of symptomatic hypothyroidism in the remaining PT will require reinstitution of thyroid hormone replacement for another 6 to 12 months before considering another withdrawal trial to assess whether long-term thyroid hormone replacement will be necessary.

Because approximately 25 percent of PT patients are at risk for persistent goiter and positive AMA titers, long-term follow-up for many years to detect possible PT recurrences and/or the gradual onset of persistent hypothyroidism is warranted. Female patients with previously documented PT should be observed in the first trimester of pregnancy. If a positive AMA and minimal elevation of serum TSH are present, these abnormalities often remit to euthyroidism by the end of the second trimester and euthyroidism is maintained throughout the third trimester of pregnancy without the need for thyroid hormone replacement. However, such mothers are at risk for an episode of postpartum thyroiditis between 2 and 6 months after delivery. For those mothers who have recurrent episodes of PT, prophylactic steroid therapy beginning 2 to 3 weeks after delivery may be rarely considered. Because most PT have a spontaneously resolving course that can be controlled by symptomatic therapy, thyroidectomy or radioiodine ablation in the recovery phase of PT is seldom justified unless several severe and disabling recurrent episodes have occurred.

■ SUBACUTE (PAINFUL, DE QUERVAIN'S, PSEUDOGRANULOMATOUS) THYROIDITIS

Diagnosis

When there is acute pain localized to the thyroid gland region, which may also be referred to as the ear or angle of jaw and often migrates to the contralateral lobe to produce similar symptoms, a diagnosis of ST should be strongly considered. ST is often accompanied by a fever and leukocytosis and elevated sedimentation rate of greater than 50 mm per hour in association with malaise, myalgia, and headache. Often a preceding upper respiratory infection can be documented. In keeping with its infection etiology, ST frequently occurs as seasonal and geographic epidemics. Although 50 percent of

ST patients have positive antiviral antibody titers to one of several viruses (mumps, measles, echovirus, Coxsackie), I do not routinely test for viral antibodies to these possible pathogenic agents. Affected thyroid lobes are typically exquisitely painful and indurated when palpated. Thyroid gland enlargement is almost always less than twice normal in size. However, unlike AT, there are no inflammatory features of superficial erythema, i.e., overlying redness, heat, and swelling.

Similar to PT but unlike AT, ST is commonly accompanied by a significant release of thyroid hormonal stores which results in transient increases in thyroid function (i.e., elevated levels of total and free T_4 and T_3 with a low thyroidal radioisotopic uptake). Subsequently, the thyrotoxicosis will spontaneously resolve to euthyroidism and varying degrees of hypothyroidism will occur over the next 6 to 12 months (i.e., variable reductions in serum T_4 and a reciprocal increase in serum TSH). Although routine FNA biopsy in the thyrotoxic phase usually demonstrates lymphocytic thyroiditis, it is not diagnostic of ST unless giant cells and pseudogranulomata are also demonstrated. FNA biopsy is also valuable in differentiating ST from AT as well as in excluding other unsuspected pathology such as acute hemorrhage into neoplasm or "malignant pseudothyroiditis" (see the section Malignant Pseudothyroiditis). Also, patients with ST seldom have positive AMA or ATA titers and very rarely have underlying autoimmune thyroid disease. Less common, atypical seasonal syndromes of ST can occur with lesser degrees of biphasic thyroid dysfunction as well as symptoms of inflammation, which will thereby require very little if any medical therapy.

Therapy

For mild to moderate localized neck pain, analgesics such as acetaminophen or nonsteroidal anti-inflammatory agents can be administered several times daily. However, when there is severe and prolonged pain accompanied by disabling systemic symptoms, I prescribe prednisone at an initial divided dosage of 40 to 60 mg per day. This therapy should provide a prompt and dramatic reduction in localized pain, swelling, and dysphagia, as well as systemic complaints of malaise within 3 to 5 days. If this does not occur, the diagnosis of ST is very likely incorrect and an alternative cause should be suspected. For patients who have good responses to prednisone, the daily dose is gradually reduced in 5 mg decrements every 10 to 14 days over a 3 to 4 month interval. A too rapid withdrawal of prednisone risks a relapse of ST symptoms and the necessity to return to a higher dose, i.e., to 30 mg per day prednisone, with a more gradual reduction over another 2- to 3 month interval.

Similar to PT, symptoms in the thyrotoxic phase are treated conservatively with beta-adrenergic blockers such propranolol (40 to 160 mg per day) in divided doses for relief of tachycardia, tremor, and sweating. Concomitant tranquilizers may also be prescribed. Serial clinical and laboratory follow-up visits at 4 week intervals are indicated to monitor the response to prednisone. Upon the resolution of thyrotoxic symptoms, beta-blockers and antianxiety medications are then gradually withdrawn over 1 to 2 weeks. When there is a severe destructive phase of ST accompanied by hyperthyroidism, there is greater risk for the development of symptomatic transient hypothyroidism and the need for short-term thyroid hormone replacement. For the therapy of hypothyroidism, I administer either L-T_3 (in gradually increasing divided doses to a maximum of 50 to 75 µg per day) or L-T_4 (100 to 200 µg per day). Since it is very unlikely that ST will lead to permanent hypothyroidism or recurrences, withdrawal of thyroid hormone therapy should be possible after 6 to 12 months and long-term follow-up will not be indicated.

■ ACUTE (SUPPURATIVE, BACTERIAL, OR OPPORTUNISTIC INFECTIONS) THYROIDITIS

Diagnosis

Most often, patients who present with AT have a rapid onset of a localized neck pain and swelling which may radiate to the angle of the jaw or ear and have accompanying malaise, fever, and increased erythrocyte sedimentation rate. However, in contrast to ST, there is often a localized tender, erythematous, and fluctuant mass palpable over one or both lobes of the thyroid gland which can progress to abscess formation and extend to adjacent structures. Differentiation of this rare cause of thyroiditis from typical subacute thyroiditis or hemorrhage into a neoplasm can be more accurately determined by performing a FNA biopsy to detect the presence of pus and abundant polymorphonuclear leukocytes. Although the most common cause of AT is bacterial, mycobacterial or fungal infection may be rarely encountered. Patients who have been exposed to immunosuppressive therapy for malignancy or are known to have immune response defects to infection (i.e., HIV-positive subjects) are at risk for opportunistic infections such aspergillosis and *pneumocystis carinii.* Pediatric or adolescent patients with recurrent episodes with localized perithyroidal space AT infection should be investigated by a barium swallow study with special views of the hypopharynx to exclude a congenital fistula arising from the apex of the left pyriform sinus which will permit the extension of oral bacterial flora into the perithyroidal space. Also, radiographic studies as well as esophagoscopy and biopsy are indicated in older patients to exclude esophageal perforation into the perithyroidal space due to underlying malignancy.

Therapy

To confirm a diagnosis of AT and exclude other unsuspected underlying pathology, it is essential to perform a FNA biopsy. Whenever a suppurative aspirate is encountered, the needle tip is corked and the contents sent to the lab for aerobic and anaerobic bacterial cultures as well as stains. Subsequently, I commence broad-spectrum antibiotic therapy coverage which can be subsequently revised as indicated when the results of specific bacterial studies become available. Since the most common source of AT infection now encountered is from contiguous extension of oral flora bacteria rather than spread from distant sites, penicillin G is most frequently employed at high doses (preferably intravenously rather than orally) with the addition of metronidazole 500 mg every 8 hours when there is the possibility of severe anaerobic infection. When mixed anaerobes are cultured in severely ill patients, clindamycin at high dosage 300 mg orally or intravenously every 6 hours is recommended. If bacterial spread from distant sites is suspected, broader antibiotic coverage for penicillin-resistant staphylococci as well as *Escherichia coli* are covered with a third generation cephalosporin such as cefotaxime. Opportunistic infections such as aspergillosis and *pneumocystis carinii* will require the selection of specific antibiotic therapy. If repeated needle aspiration continues to yield the presence of pus after 1 week of intensive antibiotic therapy, I recommend surgical incision and drainage which is followed 6 to 8 weeks later with a lobectomy. Since the excision of any residual pyriform sinus or esophageal fistulae is necessary to prevent recurrences of perithyroidal space infections, a detailed barium swallow cine examination of the hypopharynx and esophagus should be obtained prior to scheduled surgery.

■ POST-TRAUMA INDUCED THYROIDITIS

Diagnosis

Episodes of a painless thyroiditis-like syndrome with transient hyperthyroidism followed by hypothyroidism can occur following inadvertent trauma to the thyroid gland during parathyroidectomy as well as from FNA biopsy of a thyroid cyst, accidental electrocution burns to thyroid gland, or hemorrhage into the thyroid while on anticoagulant therapy.

Therapy

Such causes of thyroiditis only require symptomatic management during the transient phase of thyroid dysfunction and often no long-term therapy or follow-up is required.

■ CYTOKINE/LYMPHOKINE AND ADRENOCORTICAL DYSFUNCTION–RELATED PAINLESS THYROIDITIS

Diagnosis

Approximately 30 percent of patients with underlying autoimmune thyroid disease (e.g., goiter and positive antithyroid antibodies as well as strong family history of autoimmune thyroid disease) are at risk for episodes of destructive painless thyroiditis or Graves' hyperthyroidism after cytokine or lymphokine therapy. Also, following the removal of an adrenocortical adenoma or inadequate steroid replacement in patients with coexisting Addison's disease and/or polyglandular insufficiency type 2B syndromes, alterations in immune network regulation from changes in glucocorticoid function can trigger episodes of transient destructive thyroiditis that through the unmasking of underlying autoimmune thyroid disease resembles a PT syndrome.

Therapy

Because over 90 percent of patients revert to a subclinical form of autoimmune thyroiditis once the disturbance in hormone milieu and immune regulation are stabilized, symptomatic therapy during the different phases of thyroid dysfunction is the only therapy required. For most affected patients, symptomatic therapy can be eventually withdrawn as euthyroidism returns. However, longterm followup for risks of recurrent PT or persistent hypothyroidism is warranted particularly if repeat exposure to cytokine or lymphokine therapy is planned.

■ MALIGNANT PSEUDOTHYROIDITIS

A malignant pseudothyroiditis syndrome consisting of hyperthyroxinemia and suppressed thyroidal radioisotopic uptake has been rarely encountered after there is invasion of the thyroid gland by lymphoma or metastatic cancer. However, the degree of thyroid dysfunction is usually mild and the hypothyroidism is not persistent unless there is concurrent autoimmune thyroiditis. Recognition of the underlying malignant pathology by FNA biopsy of any dominant nodules will lead to a correct diagnosis and management as indicated by surgery, external beam irradiation, or chemotherapy.

Suggested Reading

Baudin E, Marcellini P, Pouteau M, et al. Reversibility of thyroid dysfunction induced by recombinant alpha interferon in chronic hepatitis C. Clin Endocrinol 1993; 39:657–661.

Rosen IB, Strawbridge HTG, Walfish PG, Bain J. Malignant pseudothyroiditis: A new clinical entity. Am J Surg 1978; 136:445–448.

Walfish PG. Are silent thyroiditis and post-partum thyroiditis forms of chronic thyroiditis? In: Hamburger JI, Miller JM, eds. Controversies in thyroidology. New York: Springer Verlag, 1981:52.

Walfish PG. Spectrum of thyroiditis. 46th post-graduate assembly syllabus. The Endocrine Society, 1994:333–340.

Walfish PG, Badenhoop K. Postpartum thyroiditis: A variant of Hashimoto's thyroiditis? In: Nagataki S, Mori T, Torizuka K, eds. 80 years of Hashimoto's disease. Amsterdam: Elsevier Science, 1993:171–172.

Walfish PG, Caplan D, Rosen IB. Post-parathyroidectomy transient thyrotoxicosis. J Clin Endocrinol Metab 1992; 75:224–227.

Walfish PG, Chan JYC. Postpartum hyperthyroidism. In: Toft AD, ed. Clinics in endocrinology and metabolism. Philadelphia: WB Saunders, 1985:417.

Walfish PG, Myerson J, Provias PJ, et al. Prevalence and characteristics of post-partum thyroid dysfunction: Results of a survey from Toronto, Canada. J Endocrinol Invest 1992; 15:265–272.

DIFFUSE NONTOXIC AND MULTINODULAR GOITER

Manoochehr Nakhjavani, M.D.
Hossein Gharib, M.D., F.A.C.E.

Nontoxic goiter refers to thyroid gland enlargement, diffuse or nodular, that is not associated with hyperthyroidism or hypothyroidism. It is the most common thyroid problem encountered in clinical practice. This type of glandular enlargement cannot be attributed to autoimmunity or neoplasm. In the United States, nontoxic goiter affects more than 5 percent of the adult population. If in a geographic region, etiologic factors such as iodine deficiency or environmental goitrogens affect more than 10 percent of the local population, the term *endemic goiter* is used. Otherwise, goiter is considered sporadic. Nonendemic goiter may be caused by hereditary defects in biosynthesis of thyroid hormones, exposure to radiation, nutritional factors such as excessive iodine intake in the form of drugs or food, thyroid growth-stimulating immunoglobulins, and unidentified goitrogens in the environment. An inherited predisposition seems to be key in the development of nontoxic goiter. Women are more commonly affected in both iodine-deficient and iodine-sufficient areas, and goiter may run in families. An interaction between genetic and environmental factors may be the cause of goiter in some patients.

Regardless of different possible mechanisms of development, diffuse thyroid enlargement eventually evolves into a nodular stage and for this reason the terms *nontoxic diffuse* and *nodular goiter* are used together.

DIFFERENTIAL DIAGNOSIS

The common conditions that should be considered in the differential diagnosis of nontoxic diffuse or nodular goiters are listed in Table 1. Questions regarding the rate of thyroid growth and recent changes in size, hoarseness, neck pain, odynophagia, dysphagia, and past radiation history are all important in the assessment of thyroid cancer. Although the incidence of clinically significant malignancy in nontoxic goiter is low, the presence of a discrete nodule is always a cause for concern.

Table 1 Major Causes of Diffuse and Nodular Thyroid Enlargement

DIFFUSE ENLARGEMENT
Physiologic goiter in puberty
Chronic lymphocytic thyroiditis
Early stages of Graves' disease
Iodine deficiency (endemic goiter)
Goitrogens (drugs, diet)
NODULAR ENLARGEMENT
Sporadic goiter (colloid goiter)
Chronic lymphocytic thyroiditis
Neoplasms
Inherited disorders of thyroid hormone biosynthesis

Diagnosis

Clinical evaluation of patients with goiter is critical in choosing an appropriate therapeutic approach. Commonly, goiters are asymptomatic and discovered by the physician on routine physical examination or by the patient. Less frequently, patients may be evaluated for recent growth of either a part of or the entire thyroid gland or sudden onset of pain in the thyroid due to hemorrhage into a thyroid nodule.

The physical examination should evaluate not only the thyroid gland but also the eyes, neck, skin, and other major organ systems for evidence of hyperthyroidism or hypothyroidism. Ophthalmopathy or pretibial dermopathy suggests concomitant Graves' disease. Palpation of a firm, rubbery gland suggests Hashimoto's thyroiditis. Neck adenopathy raises the question of local lymph node metastases from papillary thyroid carcinoma, and a fixed or hard nodular thyroid mass is concern for a primary or secondary thyroid malignancy. More often, however, nodular irregularity of the thyroid is due to a benign single nodule or a benign multinodular gland. Few data are available on the growth patterns in patients with nontoxic goiters. Whereas the natural course of nodular goiter is progressive enlargement, clinical observation suggests that most goiters stop growing by the fifth decade of life.

Laboratory testing in patients with nontoxic diffuse or nodular goiters is important in dictating optimal management. By definition, euthyroidism must be present because these goiters are nontoxic. New, highly sensitive TSH assays are more reliable than free or total T_4 measurements in detecting thyroid dysfunction. The concentration of serum TSH is usually normal in nontoxic goiters. In areas of severe iodine deficiency, serum TSH level may be elevated. Approximately 80 percent of patients with multinodular goiters are euthyroid at initial presentation, with hyperthyroidism developing in 10 percent within 10 years. It is important to define the functional state of the gland precisely since a nontoxic goiter may evolve into an autonomous and later into a toxic multinodular gland. The presence of antithyroglobulin antibodies, antithyroid peroxidase antibodies (previously known as antimicrosomal antibodies), and thyroid-stimulating immunoglobulins suggests underlying autoimmune thyroid disease.

Fine-needle aspiration (FNA) biopsy for cytologic examination is recommended for all thyroid nodules, and helps in formulating a treatment plan. The effect of FNA biopsy on the management of thyroid nodules has been dramatic. FNA biopsy is a safe, simple, reliable, and cost effective means of detecting benign nodules. Furthermore, it has substantially increased the yield of malignant tumors found at thyroid operation and has decreased the total number of thyroidectomies. Benign colloid nodules should be observed conservatively, whereas surgical excision is recommended when cytologic results are positive or suspicious for malignancy. If results are nondiagnostic, reaspiration is performed since a second biopsy increases the diagnostic yield by 50 percent. We perform FNA biopsy as the initial procedure in the diagnostic management of a nodular goiter.

Thyroid scanning with either technetium pertechnetate (^{99m}Tc) or radioiodine (^{123}I) is generally not helpful except in patients who have presumed toxic nodules, for evaluation of compressive symptoms, and with neck or upper mediastinal masses suspected to be of thyroid origin.

High-resolution ultrasonography is helpful in documenting the size and structure of the goiter. It is used by some to assess the results of T_4 suppressive therapy since ultrasonography is more precise than palpation in judging the effects of treatment.

A standard chest x-ray should be obtained in any patient with a large goiter. The chest x-ray is helpful to assess tracheal deviation or compression with multinodular goiters.

■ THERAPY

Suppressive Therapy

The rationale for suppressive therapy is based on the observation that thyroid growth is initiated and/or maintained by TSH. Therefore, it seems reasonable to reverse or arrest growth of a nontoxic goiter by inhibiting endogenous TSH secretion. In addition, indirect permissive effects of other growth factors such as epidermal growth factor may be inhibited by thyroid hormones. The goal of therapy is suppression of TSH to a low-normal range, which is different from replacement therapy in primary hypothyroidism. Further TSH suppression is not recommended in order to avoid possible untoward effects of subclinical hyperthyroidism on bone mass in postmenopausal women and on the cardiovascular system in the elderly. The use of second- or third-generation high sensitivity TSH assays has shown that patients with suppressed TSH concentrations have increased nocturnal heart rate, increased urinary sodium excretion, increased muscle and liver serum enzyme levels, decreased serum cholesterol concentrations, and possibly decreased bone mineral density.

Levothyroxine (L-T_4) as well as T_3 may be equally effective in reducing the size of nontoxic nodular goiters. Levothyroxine costs less, has a longer half-life, and can be administered in a single daily dose. A rather moderate daily dose, 100 μg L-T_4, is sufficient to achieve the therapeutic goal, provided it is administered over months. For most patients on T_4 therapy a sensitive TSH assay with a functional sensitivity of 0.1 mIU per liter is sufficient to allow precise titration of the L-T_4 dose without overshooting. Periodic monitoring of serum TSH is necessary to assess the possible development of functional autonomy. This should be kept in mind if serum TSH decreases while the dose of L-T_4 has not changed.

The reported success of L-T_4 suppressive therapy to reduce the size of nontoxic multinodular goiters may be related to iodine intake within the population studied. Failure of L-T_4 to significantly reduce the volume of multinodular goiters is common in countries where iodine supplementation has almost eradicated endemic goiter. However, in a report from the Netherlands, thyroid volume decreased by 25 percent in 58 percent of patients with nontoxic multinodular goiters receiving thyroid hormone therapy after 9 months, with a daily iodine intake of 150 to 300 μg. The possibility exists that a subset of patients may respond to T_4 treatment, although this subgroup has not been clearly identified.

A maximum reduction of thyroid volume by 20 to 30 percent at 3 months has been reported after T_4 treatment of diffuse goiters from iodine-deficient areas. Any factor interfering with normal iodine usage may sensitize the follicular thyroid cells to the effects of TSH, resulting in goiter development despite normal concentrations of TSH. Even in areas where iodine-deficiency goiter is still endemic, half of all goiters may be caused by other factors.

The results of suppressive T_4 therapy to decrease thyroid size in patients with multinodular goiters are unpredictable. Suppressive therapy should be avoided if serum TSH level is borderline low or suppressed; further TSH decline will result in subclinical or overt hyperthyroidism. Furthermore, the extent of decrease in goiter size achieved by T_4 therapy may depend on such factors as the amount of autonomously functioning parenchyma, the presence of connective tissue, and irreversible structural changes. Complete regression of thyroid enlargement is unusual. The outcome of therapy appears not to be related to pretreatment variables such as patient's age, duration of goiter, family history of thyroid disease, thyroid volume, thyroid nodularity, TSH response to TRH, or radioiodine uptake.

The optimal duration of treatment is not clearly defined. An initial success in reducing thyroid volume does not preclude later goiter growth. Recurrence of the goiter after discontinuation of treatment has been reported both from iodine-deficient and iodine-sufficient areas. Regrowth of the goiter raises the important issue that suppression therapy is a long-term commitment which should be discussed thoroughly with the patient. Assessment of failure or success of treatment is recommended after 1 year. One approach is to discontinue T_4 therapy after 1 year of treatment and follow the patient for changes in the thyroid gland.

Shortcomings of L-T_4 therapy include persistence of one or more nodules, requiring long-term treatment and T_4 suppressive therapy inducing subclinical hyperthyroidism with its attendant untoward effects. Subclinical hyperthyroidism due to autonomy of the thyroid is present in up to 20 percent of clinically "euthyroid" patients with multinodular goiters and L-T_4 therapy may further exacerbate the state of subclinical hyperthyroidism in these patients. Postmenopausal women on T_4, in doses that suppress serum TSH levels to less than 0.1 mIU per liter, even with initial normal serum free thyroxine (FT_4) and T_3 levels and/or without thyrotoxic symptoms, have lower bone mineral densities than matched patients with normal serum TSH. In elderly patients, in the absence of recent goiter growth, our approach is observation without treatment and with periodic thyroid testing.

The choice of L-T_4 preparation remains a source of controversy. Levothyroxine is the fifth most commonly dispensed drug in the United States. Since 1984, most studies have suggested therapeutic similarity between brand names Synthroid and Levothroid made in the United States, and Eltroxin made in the United Kingdom, in normalizing serum TSH in patients with hypothyroidism. The required 90 to 110 percent of stated content of levothyroxine is found in the three brand name preparations as demonstrated by high-performance liquid chromatography (HPLC). Generic

Table 2 Commonly Used L-T_4 Preparations

PRODUCT NAME	TABLET STRENGTH AVAILABLE (μg)	COST* PER 100 TABLETS (100 μg) $ U.S.
Synthroid	25, 50, 75, 88, 112, 125, 150, 175, 200, 300	18.00–24.50
Levothroid	As above	16.50–22.50
Levoxyl	As above	8.00–10.50
Generic	100, 150, 175, 200, 300	5.50–8.50

*Obtained from three midwestern pharmacies, January 1996.

preparations have not consistently met Food and Drug Administration standards for L-T_4 content as evaluated by HPLC and are not available in less than 0.1 mg tablet strengths. Although European endocrinologists continue to prescribe generic L-T_4, in the United States brand preparations are more popular but also more expensive (Table 2).

Perhaps more important than the issue of generic versus brand L-T_4 is the recognition that patients must take their L-T_4 tablets regularly and that serum TSH measurements determine the exact dose of L-T_4. Serum TSH concentration should be measured 8 to 12 weeks after initiating therapy and with any change in the type or dosage of L-T_4. Any interchange between generic and brand L-T_4 preparations requires TSH testing, thus adding to the cost of patient care.

Radioiodine Therapy

When ablative therapy for nontoxic multinodular goiter is necessary, thyroidectomy is our first choice. But in some elderly patients with coexistent medical problems in whom the risks of surgery are high, ^{131}I therapy is an attractive alternative. Also, ^{131}I treatment may be recommended in patients with recurrent multinodular nontoxic goiters after thyroid surgery or in patients who refuse surgery. Radioiodine has been used primarily to treat toxic multinodular goiters (Plummer's disease) and, more recently, to treat large, nontoxic multinodular goiters. Results of treatment are unpredictable, however, because cold areas within the gland are not affected by ^{131}I or may even continue growing after treatment. In a recent report, thyroid volume of small multinodular goiters (median volume 73 ml) after ^{131}I treatment decreased 34 percent and 55 percent at 12 and 24 months, respectively, as determined by careful sonography. Furthermore, ^{131}I treatment resulted in a 40 percent reduction of thyroid volume as measured by magnetic resonance imaging, with a significant decrease in tracheal compression and widening of tracheal lumen by more than 10 percent in large, compressive goiters. As with ^{131}I treatment of toxic multinodular goiters, there was no relationship between the initial goiter size and post-treatment thyroid volume reduction. Although it is not uncommon to see an initial increase in thyroid volume at 1 month after ^{131}I therapy, treatment did not aggravate obstructive symptoms.

Surgery

Overall, the enthusiasm for medical treatment of nodular goiters in nonendemic areas is on the wane. Surgery in experienced centers may be considered for the following conditions: documented recent growth of a nodule or goiter, suspicion of malignancy based on FNA cytology, potential or actual encroachment on the trachea, recurrent hemorrhage into cysts or nodules causing pain, large multinodular goiters, or large substernal goiters. For most patients a subtotal thyroidectomy is adequate with removal of most nodules. Prophylactic surgery to avoid cancer development is not justified for nodular goiters.

The most frequent complication of thyroidectomy is recurrent laryngeal nerve damage, followed by hypoparathyroidism. Postoperative bleeding or upper airway obstruction are less frequent. It should be mentioned that surgical complications may be increasing because in most centers fewer thyroid surgeries are performed, resulting in fewer properly trained surgeons. Nevertheless, in centers with available surgical expertise, complications of thyroidectomy remain acceptably low.

The use of postoperative T_4 to prevent nodular recurrence in the thyroid remains controversial. In several recent large retrospective studies with mean follow-up periods ranging from 5 to 10 years, postoperative T_4 therapy did not decrease the frequency of recurrent goiters. Furthermore, in three prospective randomized studies that compared T_4 with no treatment there were no differences between the two groups. Thyroxine replacement is clearly indicated if postoperative TSH is elevated or if near-total thyroidectomy is performed, resulting in a high likelihood of postoperative hypothyroidism. T_4 therapy is also advocated for patients undergoing thyroidectomy with a prior history of radiation exposure.

Suggested Reading

Berghout A, Wiersinga WM, Drexhage HA, et al. Comparison of placebo with L-thyroxine alone or with carbimazole for treatment of sporadic non-toxic goitre. Lancet 1990; 336:193–197.

Cooper DS. Thyroxine suppression therapy for benign nodular disease. J Clin Endocrinol Metab 1994; 80:331–334.

Dworkin HJ, Meier DA, Kaplan M. Advances in the management of patients with thyroid disease. Semin Nuc Med 1995; 25:205–220.

Gharib H. Current evaluation of thyroid nodules. Trends Endocrinol Metab 1994; 5:365–369.

Gharib H, James EM, Charboneau WJ, et al. Suppressive therapy with levothyroxine for solitary thyroid nodules. A double-blind controlled study. N Engl J Med 1987; 317:70–75.

Oppenheimer JH, Braverman LE, Toft A, et al. A therapeutic controversy. Thyroid hormone treatment: When and what? J Clin Endocrinol Metab 1995; 80:2873–2878.

Studer H, Peter HJ, Gerber H. Natural heterogeneity of thyroid cells: The basis for understanding thyroid function and nodular goiter growth. Endocr Rev 1989; 10:125–135.

SINGLE THYROID NODULE

Hossein Gharib, M.D., F.A.C.P.

Thyroid nodules are very common and despite the fact that most are benign, the fear of malignancy is the principal concern of both the physician and the patient. The primary challenge for the physician is to identify and manage medically the benign nodules (majority) and select for surgery the nodules with high risk for malignancy (minority). This chapter describes the clinical importance of thyroid nodules and the changing management of various types of thyroid nodules. My emphasis in discussing assessment and treatment is a strategy that is accurate, efficient, and cost effective.

CLINICAL IMPORTANCE

A thyroid nodule can be described as a single palpable abnormality within an apparently normal gland without reference to pathologic or functional characteristics. The term *nodular thyroid disease* is preferred because it is recognized that at least 50 percent of single, palpable nodules are found to be within a multinodular gland by ultrasonography. The prevalence of thyroid nodules varies according to the methods of evaluation. For example, several autopsy as well as ultrasound studies suggest that 50 percent of the adult population in the United States will have one or more nodules. In the Framingham, Massachusetts, population, there was a 4.2 percent overall incidence of thyroid nodules—6.4 percent in women and 1.6 percent in men (Table 1). In the United States the annual incidence of thyroid nodules becoming clinically recognizable is 0.1 percent, translating into approximately 250,000 new nodules per year. Based on current data, the estimated lifetime risk of developing a thyroid nodule is between 5 percent and 10 percent, with an increased prevalence in women and older subjects.

Although thyroid nodules are common, most are benign. In this country, the annual incidence of thyroid cancer is 0.004 percent in the general population, or 12,000 new cancer cases per year. This would mean that approximately 1 in 20 nodules (5 percent) is likely to be malignant. Therefore, the examining physician must select for surgery the few malignant lesions, identify and follow medically the many benign nodules, and do this without unnecessary testing.

CLINICAL EVALUATION

History and Examination

Thyroid nodules are usually asymptomatic and are discovered by the patient as a "lump" in the neck or by the physician on careful neck palpation. Clinical features that increase the likelihood of thyroid malignancy include a family history of thyroid cancer, young age (less than 20 years), and a past history of head or neck irradiation. Nodules are more common in women but more likely to be malignant in men. Important features on physical examination include the size, consistency, and mobility or fixation of the nodule as well as the presence of lymphadenopathy.

The appearance of a new nodule or increase in size while the patient is on levothyroxine (L-T_4) therapy is always worrisome for malignancy. Symptoms of hyperthyroidism or hypothyroidism are usually associated with a benign process. Local symptoms such as hoarseness, dysphagia, or obstruction suggest malignancy but may also occur in connection with benign goiters. In general, historical features and physical characteristics of the nodule lack specificity and are poor predictors of malignancy.

Table 1 Single Thyroid Nodule

Palpable in 4%–7% of adult population
95% are benign
85% are cold on scan
50% are multiple by sonography

Laboratory Tests

Thyroid function tests including serum thyroxine (T_4), triiodothyronine (T_3), and thyroid-stimulating hormone (TSH) levels are usually normal. The serum TSH determination alone is usually sufficient to screen for hypothyroidism or hyperthyroidism. A subnormal high-sensitivity serum TSH level suggests thyroid autonomy or thyrotoxicosis. Antimicrosomal antibodies and antithyroglobulin antibodies may be seen in patients with autoimmune disease (Hashimoto's thyroiditis). Serum calcitonin determination should be done only if medullary thyroid carcinoma is suspected or there is a family history of this cancer. Contrary to two recent reports, the practice of routine serum calcitonin measurement in all patients with thyroid nodules seems to be neither necessary nor cost effective.

Radionuclide Imaging

Historically, radionuclide scanning was the first diagnostic test in the evaluation of the thyroid nodule. The two most commonly used isotopes are technetium (^{99m}Tc) and radioiodine (^{123}I). Both isotopes are transported into the thyroid follicular cells, but only iodine is organified. A malignant thyroid nodule could therefore appear to function on a technetium scan but be "cold" on an iodine scan.

The radionuclide scan may demonstrate four different patterns of function. A hypofunctioning (cold) nodule means no or subnormal isotope concentration in the nodular tissue. The likelihood of malignancy in cold nodules is less than 15 percent. Because approximately 85 percent of nodules are cold, it is evident that surgical treatment based on radionuclide scan proves to be costly, resulting in removal of many benign nodules (see Table 1). A second scan pattern is the presence of isotopic concentration in the nodule similar to the remainder of the thyroid gland. In this case the nodule is considered functioning (warm) or, more correctly, indeterminate because it is often difficult to properly define the functional status of such a nodule. A third scan pattern is represented by the nodule exhibiting marked increase in isotope concentration with the absence or near absence of isotope in the remainder of the thyroid gland, either labeled as a hyperfunctioning (hot) nodule or an autonomous adenoma. A fourth scan pattern is seen as an irregular or "patchy" appearance with functioning and nonfunctioning areas within the gland, suggestive of a multinodular goiter.

Most centers have abandoned the routine use of thyroid scanning in nodule evaluation because while cold nodules are more likely to be malignant than functioning nodules, most cold nodules are benign. Thyroid scan is useful as the initial test only if a nodule is suspected to be hyperfunctioning.

Ultrasonography

High-resolution (7.5 to 10.0 MHZ) sonography has exceptional ability to measure the volume of the gland as well as the number, the size, and characteristics of nodules within it. High-resolution sonography can identify cystic or solid lesions as small as 2 to 4 mm within the gland. Ultrasound patterns include consistency, echogenicity, and pattern of calcification. On the basis of consistency, thyroid nodules are divided into solid, cystic, and mixed solid-cystic; purely cystic lesions are extremely rare. The benign nodule characteristically has a large cystic component, peripheral calcification, and a hyperechoic texture. The malignant thyroid nodule is typically an irregular, solid mass that is hypoechoic. Microcalcifications are particularly important because they occur in 10 to 15 percent of all nodules, peripheral calcifications being characteristic of benign nodules, whereas internal or punctate calcifications within a nodule are suggestive of papillary carcinoma.

Unfortunately, sonographic features are not sufficiently accurate indicators of malignancy and cannot reliably distinguish benign from malignant nodules. Ultrasonography is expensive and is not essential for routine nodule evaluation. However, in selected cases sonography is helpful to guide a fine-needle aspiration (FNA) biopsy of a nodule with nondiagnostic results or when direct FNA biopsy is technically difficult.

Fine-Needle Aspiration Biopsy

It is no exaggeration to state that FNA biopsy has revolutionized the current management of thyroid nodules. FNA biopsy is now established as an expedient, accurate, inexpensive test, and the most effective method for differentiating benign from malignant thyroid nodules. It is quite safe, and in my experience with more than 15,000 biopsies, I have not encountered serious complications, although minor pain or hematoma is common.

Thyroid fine-needle biopsy, performed with a 25 guage 1.5-inch needle, can be done with or without aspiration. The nonaspiration technique requires no suction, causes less trauma to nodular tissue, and is best suited for vascular lesions that bleed easily. Aspiration biopsy is the technique most commonly used, employing a 10 ml disposable plastic syringe often attached to a syringe pistol. This technique involves inserting the needle directly into the nodule, moving it gently back and forth, and preparing smears from the aspirated material. Usually, two to four aspirations from different sites in each nodule are made, resulting in two to four slides per aspiration. Slides are then immediately placed in 95 percent alcohol and prepared with a modified Papanicolaou stain or, alternatively, are allowed to air dry and are stained by the May-Grünwald technique.

Table 2 Results of FNA Biopsy*

FEATURE	PERCENT
Sensitivity	80–90
Specificity	90–98
Accuracy	95
False negative	1–5
False positive	1–10

*Data from several FNA series 1985–1995.

Accurate cytologic interpretation of aspirated material from the thyroid requires special cytologic training and expertise. Cytologic results are usually sufficient for diagnosis (diagnostic) in 85 percent and insufficient for diagnosis (nondiagnostic) in the remaining 15 percent. The benign category may include normal thyroid, colloid goiter, Hashimoto's thyroiditis, subacute thyroiditis, and so on. The most common benign cytologic picture is a "colloid nodule" that manifests as a macrofollicular process. The malignant category indicates either primary or metastatic cancer with the most common diagnosis being papillary carcinoma. The suspicious or indeterminate category includes cellular neoplasms with atypical features suggestive of, but not definitive for, malignancy. This group includes aspirates suspicious for papillary carcinoma, follicular neoplasms, or Hürthle cell neoplasms. An unsatisfactory or nondiagnostic specimen usually has blood and some colloid or macrophages, but there are insufficient numbers of follicular epithelium for proper diagnosis.

Published FNA results from many centers confirm its utility and accuracy. Although it is a relatively simple procedure, the success of biopsy depends on the experience of the operator and the availability of cytopathologic expertise. In my opinion, the endocrinologist is most qualified to palpate thyroid glands, assess number and size of nodules, and perform FNA biopsies. In experienced centers, the accuracy of FNA biopsy approaches 95 percent, sensitivity 80 to 85 percent, and specificity 90 to 95 percent. False-negative rates vary from 1 to 5 percent, representing missed malignancies, either the result of sampling errors or interpretative mistakes; both improve with experience. False-positive rates vary from 1 to 10 percent, representing benign nodules unnecessarily removed (Table 2). Overall, FNA biopsy is the single best method to identify benign and malignant nodules.

■ MANAGEMENT

Figure 1 summarizes my current approach to thyroid nodules, placing primary reliance for management on FNA and cytology. Whenever necessary, TSH determination, scanning, and ultrasound are used to further direct treatment. The following discusses management of different nodules.

Benign Nodules

Nearly 75 percent of satisfactory aspirates are benign, the majority being from colloid nodules, and require no further

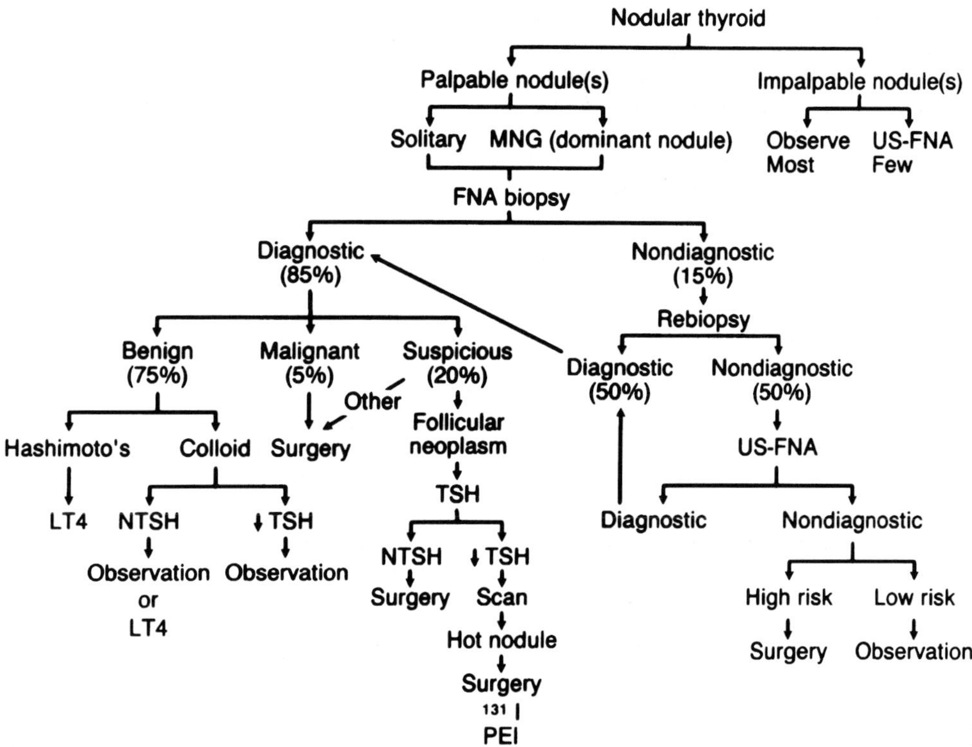

Figure 1
Sequence for diagnostic management of patients with thyroid nodules using FNA biopsy as the routine, initial test, and selecting treatment based on cytologic characteristics. When cytology shows follicular neoplasm and serum TSH is suppressed, a thyroid scan is the next test. For toxic hot nodules, management options include surgery, ^{131}I therapy, and percutaneous ethanol injection (PEI). For nondiagnostic nodules, direct rebiopsy and, later, ultrasound-guided biopsy (US-FNA) seem reasonable. For the vast majority of nonpalpable nodules, observation is sufficient. MNG, multinodular gland.

workup. Biopsy may be repeated if the nodule enlarges or becomes clinically suspicious. In centers with experience in FNA, routine reaspiration is seldom necessary. For clinicians beginning a FNA program, acquisition of adequate experience and good technique requires time and training; it is prudent to rebiopsy nodules in 1 to 2 years for cytologic re-evaluation until adequate confidence and results are achieved.

An important question in patient management is whether TSH suppression with levothyroxine (L-T_4) should be considered for benign nodules. At one time, short-term suppressive therapy was undertaken as a diagnostic tool to separate benign nodules (responders) from malignant nodules (nonresponders); the latter group was then selected for surgical treatment. However, FNA biopsy is far more reliable and practical, and short-term suppression can no longer be justified as a means of separating benign from malignant nodules. The aim of long-term suppressive therapy, on the other hand, is to shrink thyroid nodules or, at least, arrest their further growth. In recent years, several prospective randomized studies have shown little or no benefit from T_4 suppression therapy. Furthermore, additional recent data suggest that suppressive therapy may exacerbate cardiac disease or osteoporosis.

Considering the unproven effectiveness of suppressive therapy and its possible side effects, my personal preference is not to advocate T_4 therapy for cytologically benign nodules. In this regard, I agree with Mazzaferri that "the long-term potential risks outweigh the potential benefits in most patients, especially postmenopausal women." My approach to colloid nodules is observation, periodic palpation, and rebiopsy if nodules grow. I favor treating nodules with T_4 when cytology shows lymphocytic thyroiditis (Hashimoto's thyroiditis), keeping TSH in the low-normal range. Physicians choosing suppressive therapy for colloid nodules should remember a few caveats. Do not suppress postmenopausal women for fear of accelerating bone loss or patients with underlying cardiac disease. Use T_4 doses sufficient to suppress TSH levels to 0.2 to 0.5 mIU per liter. In men and premenopausal women with benign nodules, shrinkage may be more likely if the nodule is solid (not cystic), if pretreatment TSH is greater than 1.0 mIU per liter (not suppressed), and if nodule diameter is less than 3.0 cm. If no shrinkage of the nodule occurs after 1 year, therapy should be stopped.

Malignant and Suspicious Nodules

In general, 5 percent of nodules are cytologically malignant and require surgical excision. Papillary thyroid carcinoma is the most frequent cancer found, and appropriate treatment consists of near-total thyroidectomy with modified neck dissection if lymph node metastasis is detected. The application of FNA biopsy has increased the frequency of carcinoma in excised thyroid nodules from an estimated 15 percent to almost 50 percent.

In most large FNA series, approximately 20 percent of aspirates are labeled *suspicious for malignancy* because it is not possible to separate benign Hürthle cell or follicular cell neoplasms from their malignant counterparts (Fig. 1). Rebiopsy seldom changes diagnosis or management and is not recommended. Approximately 25 percent of nodules with suspicious cytology are malignant at surgery. In general, cytologically suspicious nodules should be surgically removed unless follicular lesions are very small or if Hürthle cell lesions are identified with lymphocytes suggestive of Hashimoto's thyroiditis. When histology is benign, lobectomy-isthmectomy on the side of lesion is almost always adequate treatment, although some advocate a subtotal thyroidectomy even for benign lesions.

Nondiagnostic Nodules

Approximately 15 percent of nodules yield insufficient material for proper cytologic diagnosis, usually because of improper techniques or cystic lesions (see Fig. 1). Reaspiration gives satisfactory results in 50 percent of cases. In cases when repeated aspirations are unsatisfactory, rebiopsy with ultrasound guidance increases the chance of adequate smears. A small group of nodules remains nondiagnostic despite careful, repeated aspirations. In this small subset, high-risk patients (younger than 20 years of age or older than 60 years of age, large recurrent cyst, history of neck irradiation) can be treated surgically and low-risk patients (middle age, small cyst, stable nodule) are managed conservatively (see Fig. 1).

Cystic Nodules

Anywhere from 15 to 25 percent of all nodules are cystic. Commonly, these represent degenerated benign colloid nodules, but neoplasms also undergo cystic degeneration. In most series the incidence of malignancy varies from 5 to 20 percent with an average less than 10 percent. The rate of nondiagnostic aspirates and false-negative rates are higher because of dilution, too few cells, and sampling errors. The presence of malignant cells is diagnostic, but uncommon; the absence of benign follicular cells does not exclude cancer and is considered nondiagnostic.

The aspirated fluid volume varies from 1 to 30 ml, and the color may be clear, watery, yellow, or brownish. A colorless, crystal-clear fluid is likely of parathyroid origin; a frankly hemorrhagic fluid suggests malignancy. In my experience, there is little relationship between the character (volume and color) of cystic fluid, and the incidence of malignancy.

Some cysts collapse after aspiration, and rebiopsy should be attempted on the residual solid mass. It is my practice to surgically excise cysts greater than 4 cm in diameter. T_4 therapy is ineffective in shrinking cysts, and sclerotherapy with tetracycline injection is no longer used. Recently, several studies from Italy reported successful treatment of cysts with percutaneous ethanol injection (PEI).

Hot Nodules

Approximately 5 percent of solitary nodules are hyperfunctioning (hot) on thyroid scintigraphy, concentrating radioisotope greater than the remaining thyroid tissue. These nodules are autonomously functioning and have been referred to as autonomously functioning thyroid adenomas or solitary toxic nodules. Hot nodules are often solitary in otherwise normal glands and are commonly nontoxic. The clinically toxic nodule produces hyperthyroidism with suppressed serum TSH; the nontoxic nodule is associated with a clinically euthyroid state and normal or low-normal TSH levels. Nontoxic hot nodules can be followed, realizing that they are more likely to become toxic if larger than 3 cm in size or in patients older than 60 years of age. Hot nodules are far more common in women.

Table 3 Hot Nodule

Accounts for 5% of all nodules
Toxicity = clinical hyperthyroidism + suppressed TSH
More likely toxic if diameter >3.0 cm or age >60 years
Treat toxic nodules with surgery, ^{131}I, or PEI
Observe nontoxic nodules

PEI, percutaneous ethanol injection.

Treatment is clearly indicated for toxic hot nodules and includes radioiodine ablation, surgery, or percutaneous ethanol injection (Table 3). Surgery is simple, safe, and effective; simple lumpectomy or lobectomy is usually sufficient. The incidence of hypothyroidism postoperatively varies from 10 to 20 percent. Toxic nodules are relatively radioresistant requiring ^{131}I. Doses have varied from 20 to 100 mCi, depending on nodule size and ^{131}I uptake. The incidence of hypothyroidism after radioiodine therapy varies from 5 to 40 percent, depending on whether treated patients are biochemically hyperthyroid and also on the magnitude of the treatment dose of radioiodine.

Several Italian groups have recently used PEI to ablate toxic nodules. With the assistance of ultrasonography, 2 to 4 ml of 95 percent ethanol is injected directly into the hot nodule with a fine needle. Treatment is repeated once or twice per week until ablation is accomplished. Follow-up to 2 years has shown reduction of nodule size in most patients with no recurrence of toxicity. Complications have included pain, fever, and dysphonia. In the United States PEI ablation has not gained acceptance as a routine modality for treating toxic nodules.

Occult Nodules

Nonpalpable thyroid nodules found incidentally by imaging procedures are referred to as "occult" nodules or thyroid "incidentalomas." These are usually found during ultrasonography of the neck for carotid artery disease or parathyroid evaluation. This is not surprising because ultrasound studies have shown that approximately 50 percent of patients beyond the fifth decade of life have one or more small thyroid nodules. These nodules are commonly small, less than 1.5 cm in diameter, and are considered of little clinical importance. My approach to most occult nodules is observation, follow-up neck palpation, and avoiding unnecessary tests or treatment (see Fig. 1). In a rare patient with a history of external neck irradiation, a strong family history for thyroid carcinoma, or sonographic appearance suspicious for malignancy, biopsy under ultrasound guidance would be appropriate. Management depends on cytology; however, ultrasound FNA is seldom necessary.

Table 4 Multinodular Gland

Usually asymptomatic and benign
Only 50% of palpable nodules are truly solitary
Evaluation by TSH and FNA
Mild to moderate goiter: observe
Large or symptomatic goiter: treat with surgery or ^{131}I

Multinodular Glands

A detailed discussion of the multinodular thyroid gland is beyond the scope of this review. Sporadic nontoxic goiters may have solitary or multiple palpable nodules. Recent ultrasound studies suggest that in 50 percent of cases a clinically palpable solitary nodule represents a dominant nodule in a gland with several smaller nonpalpable nodules (Table 4). A recent publication from Spain suggested that the frequency of cancer in patients with solitary nodules is similar to that in patients with multinodular glands (4.7 percent vs. 4.1 percent, respectively). Since the risk of malignancy in a multinodular goiter is not negligible, a dominant nodule in a multinodular thyroid should be carefully evaluated as if it were a solitary nodule.

Appropriate laboratory evaluation at a minimum should include high-sensitivity TSH determination, and serum T_4 and T_3 levels if hyperthyroidism is suspected. FNA biopsy of the dominant nodule as well as other accessible nodules is essential to elucidate the pathologic process. Occasionally, a radionuclide thyroid scan is helpful in defining the size of the goiter. An irregular, patchy uptake pattern is consistent with a multinodular goiter.

For small to moderate, nontoxic multinodular glands with normal serum TSH and benign cytology, observation with medical follow-up is reasonable (see Table 4). If cytology suggests either a suspicious or malignant process, thyroidectomy is the appropriate next step. For patients with growing or symptomatic goiters causing local or systemic symptoms, thyroidectomy is the treatment of choice. The effectiveness of radioiodine therapy in shrinking the size of nontoxic nodular goiters is still controversial. The decision to treat these patients with T_4 is difficult because many are elderly and have large goiters and coexistent cardiac disease. Often, serum TSH level is low or low-normal, suggestive of an autonomous goiter. My approach in these cases is observation without T_4 therapy.

Suggested Reading

Devorkin HJ, Meier DA, Kaplan M. Advances in the management of patients with thyroid disease. Semin Nucl Med 1995; 25:205–220.

Gharib H. Current evaluation of thyroid nodules. Trends Endocrinol Metab 1994; 5:365–369.

Gharib H, Goellner JR. Fine-needle aspiration biopsy of the thyroid. Endocr Pract 1995; 1:410–417.

Giuffrida D, Gharib H. Controversies in the management of cold, hot, and occult thyroid nodules. Am J Med 1995; 99:642–650.

Mazzaferri EC. Management of a solitary thyroid nodule. N Engl J Med 1993; 328:553–565.

Papini E, Panunzi C, Pacella CM, et al. Percutaneous ultrasound-guided ethanol injection: A new treatment for toxic autonomously functioning thyroid nodules. J Clin Endocrinol Metab 1993; 76:411–416.

Tan GH, Gharib H, Reading CC. Solitary thyroid nodule: Comparison between palpation and ultrasonography. Arch Intern Med 1995; 155:2418–2423.

MEDULLARY THYROID CARCINOMA

Douglas B. Evans, M.D.
M. Andrew Burgess, M.D., B.S., F.R.A.C.P.
Helmuth Goepfert, M.D.
Robert F. Gagel, M.D.

Medullary thyroid carcinoma (MTC) originates in the thyroid C cells, which produce both calcitonin (iCT) and carcinoembryonic antigen (CEA). Unlike most other solid tumors, the presence of subclinical microscopic disease within the thyroid, local-regional lymph nodes, or distant metastasis can be detected by elevated serum iCT and CEA levels. MTC occurs either as a sporadic event or secondary to a germline mutation with an autosomal dominant pattern of inheritance. Familial MTC may occur as part of multiple endocrine neoplasia type 2A (MEN 2A) (MTC, pheochromocytoma, and parathyroid hyperplasia) or MEN 2B (MTC, pheochromocytoma, mucosal and alimentary neuromas, and marfanoid habitus) or without other endocrinopathies (familial non–MEN MTC). Until recently, patients who were known members of a familial MTC kindred were screened by measurement of serum levels of pen–tagastrin-stimulated iCT. An abnormal response to pentagastrin would indicate the need for thyroidectomy in an attempt to remove the thyroid prior to the development of invasive carcinoma and metastases to lymph nodes, liver, lung, or bone. Patients with sporadic MTC are diagnosed as a result of the presence of a thyroid nodule. Similar to the prognosis with papillary and follicular thyroid carcinoma, the prognosis with MTC depends on the extent of disease. Surgery remains the most effective therapeutic weapon against thyroid cancer; in general, irradiation and cytotoxic chemotherapy are utilized only as adjuvant or palliative therapies.

Single point mutations within the RET proto-oncogene on chromosome 10 have recently been found responsible for all forms of familial MTC. Each of the identified mutations

Table 1 TNM Staging System

DEFINITION OF TNM			
Primary Tumor (T)			
T0	No evidence of primary tumor		
T1	≤1 cm		
T2	>1 and ≤4 cm		
T3	>4 cm		
T4	Any size, tumor extends beyond the thyroid capsule		
Regional Lymph Nodes (N)			
N0	No lymph node metastases		
N1	Lymph node metastases		
Distant Metastasis (M)			
M0	No distant metastases		
M1	Distant metastases		
STAGE GROUPING			
Stage I	T1	N0	M0
Stage II	T2–4	N0	M0
Stage III	Any T	N1	
Stage IV	Any T	Any N	M1

From Beahrs OH, Henson DE, Hutter RVP, Kennedy BJ, eds. American Joint Committee on Cancer Manual for Staging of Cancer. 4th ed. Philadelphia: JB Lippincott, 1992:53–54; with permission.

changes cysteine to another amino acid at one of five codons. Once the exact base substitution is identified for a given family by DNA sequence analysis, screening of family members can be done through the use of restriction endonuclease digestion now available through several commercial sources. The mutant nucleotide sequence creates a new restriction enzyme cleavage site, giving rise to a different size (length) DNA fragment. The mutant fragment is then easily separated from the normal or wild-type fragment by electrophoresis. The use of DNA testing in at-risk family members has multiple advantages over testing with pentagastrin-stimulated iCT: (1) DNA testing will allow early thyroidectomy prior to the development of invasive MTC; in patients with MEN 2A, thyroidectomy should be performed prior to the age of 6 years; (2) DNA testing will eliminate the need for repeated pentagastrin testing, which is unpleasant, and will prevent the occasional patient from suffering the consequences of failing to return for annual testing; and (3) DNA testing will eliminate the potential for false-positive pentagastrin tests (incidence 3 to 5 percent), which may result in unnecessary thyroidectomy.

Despite the tremendous advances made in the molecular biology of MTC, the opportunity to improve the outcome for the majority of patients who present with sporadic disease still lies in the performance of a safe and comprehensive initial surgical procedure. An understanding of the natural history and patterns of tumor recurrence is important in the development of a surgical strategy.

■ NATURAL HISTORY AND PROGNOSTIC FACTORS

Multiple large institutional and cooperative group studies have demonstrated that stage of disease (Table 1) at diagnosis most accurately predicts length of patient survival. In the absence of metastatic disease or progressive, unresectable local-regional disease, long-term survival (≥10 years) is common (60 to 90 percent). In contrast, patients with metastatic disease (stage IV) have a 5 year survival rate of approximately 50 percent.

Table 2 Cervical Recurrence of MTC Requiring Reoperation

		NO. OF PATIENTS	
FIRST AUTHOR	YEAR	TOTAL	CERVICAL RECURRENCE (%)
Simpson	1982	16	8 (50)
Saad	1984	143	39 (27)
Gharib	1992	52	18 (35)
Dralle	1994	39	23 (59)

Unlike with other solid tumors, very sensitive and specific markers of persistent (and recurrent) disease exist in the form of iCT and CEA. It is possible to detect MTC by measuring iCT or CEA at a stage when there is no detectable disease by any other technique. There is general agreement that individuals with detectable iCT and CEA have residual MTC. However, no consensus has developed on what percentage of patients with detectable iCT or CEA will develop identifiable metastases and what percentage will die of metastatic tumor; it remains impossible to accurately predict the course of the disease in patients with nonmetastatic disease (stages I, II, or III) based on the iCT level following thyroidectomy. This group represents the majority of patients with MTC. While MTC often has an indolent course in patients with no obvious metastatic disease, management is complicated by the frequent progressive rise in iCT (and CEA) levels seen in such patients during outpatient follow-up. The lack of prospective, long-term follow-up data on patients with elevated postoperative iCT levels and no measurable distant organ metastatic disease has contributed to the controversy over appropriate treatment.

Factors associated with an increased rate of tumor recurrence include age greater than 40 years, male gender, extension of cervical disease to the mediastinum, extranodal tumor extension, and incomplete surgical resection of the primary tumor and adjacent lymphatic metastases. In contrast to patients with papillary carcinoma of the thyroid, data are not currently available to translate these prognostic factors into specific treatment recommendations. This is largely because radioactive iodine ablation and thyroid suppression are ineffective therapies in MTC.

MTC is characterized by early spread to regional lymph nodes. It is likely that the majority of patients with invasive MTC have metastasis to regional lymph nodes at the time of diagnosis. This is supported by the frequent finding of persistent elevations in iCT levels following primary tumor resection (thyroidectomy) and the high rates of recurrence in the cervical lymph nodes reported in retrospective studies (Table 2). These data have provided the rationale for surgeons to perform a more extensive lymphadenectomy at the time of initial thyroidectomy and to consider reoperative cervical lymphadenectomy in patients with persistent elevation in iCT level following thyroidectomy.

Distant metastases occur in the liver, lung, bone, and occasionally brain. Similar to metastases from other neuroendocrine tumors, liver metastases are poorly visualized by computed tomography (CT) and best seen with magnetic resonance imaging (MRI) or good-quality sonography. The frequency with which early-stage (stage I, II, or III) MTC spreads to the liver is unknown. Only with long-term patient follow-up in prospective studies will we be able to correlate extent of cervical disease and iCT elevation with a patient's likelihood of having subclinical hepatic metastases. In the absence of significant (moderate to high volume) liver, lung, or bone metastases, therapeutic efforts should focus on obtaining maximal local-regional tumor control to prevent loss of speech or swallowing as a result of tracheal and/or esophageal invasion.

SURGICAL THERAPY

The majority of patients diagnosed with MTC come to medical attention when a dominant thyroid nodule is discovered on physical examination. The diagnosis of MTC is accurately established with fine-needle aspiration cytology; the tumor cell cytoplasm stains positively with iCT antiserum. All patients with a preoperative diagnosis of MTC should be screened for pheochromocytoma with a 24 hour urine collection for metanephrine, vanillylmandelic acid, and free catecholamines. Blood should also be drawn for DNA testing because approximately 7 percent of patients with sporadic MTC have hereditary disease.

Total thyroidectomy is recommended in all patients with biopsy-proven or suspected MTC. Patients with familial MTC have bilateral, multifocal disease, and patients with presumed sporadic disease have a 20 to 30 percent incidence of multifocal disease and may also represent the index case of familial MTC. Because of the frequent finding of lymph node metastases in the central compartment, central neck dissection has been advocated for all patients with palpable primary thyroid tumors even in the absence of grossly evident lymphatic metastases. Central neck dissection is defined as the removal of all fibrofatty lymphatic tissue from the level of the hyoid bone down to the innominate vessels. The upper aspect of the thymus is removed with the paratracheal lymph nodes while preserving the recurrent laryngeal nerve. The lateral limits of the dissection are the internal jugular veins. The inferior parathyroids are often inseparable from the cluster of lymph nodes and thymic horn that extends from the lower pole of the thyroid gland just inferior and anterior to the junction of the inferior thyroid artery and recurrent laryngeal nerve. Therefore, a standard central neck dissection often involves removal of the inferior parathyroid glands. These should be identified when possible, confirmed histologically (so as not to autograft a lymph node metastasis), and autografted into either the sternocleidomastoid muscle in the neck or the brachioradialis muscle in the nondominant forearm.

Total thyroidectomy and central neck dissection are safely performed in a patient who has not had previous cervical surgery. The incidences of permanent hypoparathyroidism and palsy of the recurrent laryngeal nerve should be no greater than 1 or 2 percent. However, when they occur, these complications significantly impact the patient's quality of life and are painfully obvious to both the surgeon and endocrinologist. The potential for such visible complications combined with the known indolent biologic behavior of MTC is likely responsible for the inadequate lymphadenectomy (at least in the central neck compartment) that accompanies many thyroidectomies performed for this disease. It has been clearly demonstrated that compartment-oriented systematic lymphadenectomy decreases local-regional recurrence rates and may improve length of survival in patients with MTC. In contrast, reoperative surgery in the central neck compartment, even when done by experienced surgeons, is associated with a marked increase in the risks of permanent hypoparathyroidism and vocal cord palsy.

The extent of primary surgery performed should also be based on the anticipated plan for postoperative follow-up and management. For example, the vast majority of patients with a palpable (larger than 1 cm) primary tumor will have a persistent postoperative elevation in iCT level if a central compartment lymphadenectomy is not performed at the time of thyroidectomy. Postoperative iCT levels are routinely measured during follow-up and invariably continue to rise slowly. Because of increasing patient and physician anxiety, often prompting multiple radiologic studies, patients are referred for second opinions regarding the potential benefit of reoperative cervical lymphadenectomy. However, patients who have had adequate (compartment-oriented) initial surgery need to be considered for reoperative cervical procedures only in the presence of documented recurrent disease seen on imaging studies (MRI, sonography).

These considerations have led to the following specific surgical recommendations (Table 3).

Table 3 Operative Management of Patients with MTC

	OPERATION PERFORMED	
EXTENT OF DISEASE AT PRESENTATION	**SPORADIC MTC**	**FAMILIAL MTC**
Elevated stimulated iCT	NA	TT
Elevated basal iCT	NA	TT, CND
Palpable thyroid nodule	TT, CND, UMRND	TT, CND, BMRND
Palpable cervical lymphadenopathy	TT, CND, BMRND	TT, CND, BMRND

NA, not applicable; TT, total thyroidectomy; CND, central neck dissection; UMRND, unilateral modified radical neck dissection; BMRND, bilateral modified radical neck dissection.

Patients with MEN 2A or Familial Non-MEN MTC

Patients with a positive RET mutational analysis, a normal basal iCT level, and a normal cervical sonogram undergo total thyroidectomy without lymphadenectomy. Surgery is performed either at the age of 5 years in children known to carry a mutation of the RET proto-oncogene, or when the annual pentagastrin test result becomes positive. In patients with an elevated basal iCT level, total thyroidectomy is combined with a central compartment lymphadenectomy. If a thyroid nodule is visualized by sonography or present on physical examination, we perform total thyroidectomy with central compartment lymphadenectomy and bilateral modified neck dissection.

Patients with MEN 2B

Thyroidectomy should be performed as early as possible in children born with the clinical manifestations of MEN 2B, such as mucosal neuroma syndrome. Analysis for a RET mutation at codon 918 should be performed in all children born to parents with MEN 2B and in all children with ambiguous clinical features suggestive of MEN 2B. Because invasive MTC has been found at birth in children with MEN 2B, thyroidectomy should not be delayed.

Patients with Presumed Sporadic MTC

The majority of patients with MTC (75 percent) have the sporadic form of this disease. As illustrated in Table 3, we advocate an aggressive approach to this disease based on published data demonstrating improved local-regional disease control and suggesting improved survival in patients treated with compartment-oriented lymphadenectomy at the time of total thyroidectomy. Therefore, in patients with a palpable thyroid nodule diagnosed as MTC by fine-needle aspiration cytology, we perform total thyroidectomy with incontinuity clearance of the central neck and standard modified radical neck dissection on the side of the lesion. The inferior parathyroid glands are routinely resected with the paratracheal lymphatic tissue. The operative specimen should be carefully examined for parathyroid glands; when found, they should be confirmed as parathyroid tissue with frozen-section analysis and autografted into either the sternocleidomastoid muscle or the nondominant forearm. In any patient with palpable cervical lymphadenopathy, a bilateral modified radical neck dissection is performed at the time of total thyroidectomy. The goal of this aggressive surgical approach is to maximize local regional tumor control and survival while minimizing the need for reoperation.

Modified radical neck dissection uses as its limits of dissection the posterior belly of the digastric muscles superiorly, the eleventh nerve posterolaterally, and the thoracic inlet inferiorly. The sternocleidomastoid muscle, jugular vein, carotid artery, and vagus nerve are skeletonized and preserved. The only potential morbidity of this procedure is injury to the eleventh nerve. Injury to the phrenic nerve or sympathetic ganglion should be exceedingly uncommon in the absence of advanced, large-volume disease. Therefore, the addition of a lateral or jugular compartment dissection to a standard total thyroidectomy and central neck dissection adds minimal morbidity, simplifies follow-up, and obviates reoperative cervical surgery in the absence of recurrent cervical disease identified on imaging studies.

■ EVALUATION OF THE PATIENT WITH ELEVATED iCT AFTER THYROIDECTOMY

Evaluation of the patient with elevated postoperative iCT levels focuses on sites of expected disease recurrence: cervical and mediastinal lymph nodes, liver, lung, and bone (Fig. 1). Because iCT is such a sensitive marker of recurrent disease, standard radiographic imaging studies are often normal despite significant elevations in basal iCT levels. Therefore,

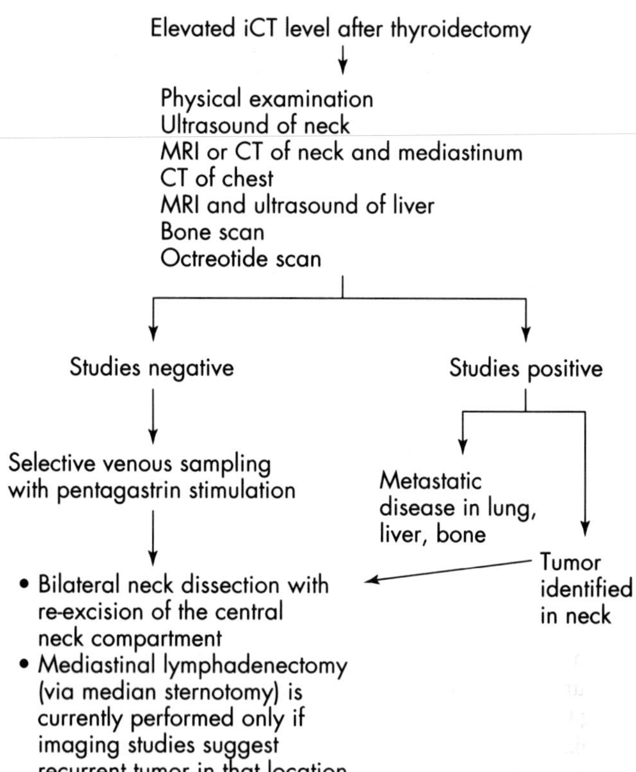

Figure 1
Diagnostic and treatment algorithm for patients with elevated iCT levels following thyroidectomy for MTC. In patients with metastatic disease, reoperative cervical surgery is considered only as a palliative procedure to prevent tracheal or esophageal invasion from resulting in the loss of speech or swallowing.

physicians have searched for an improved method of excluding liver metastases prior to considering reoperative cervical lymphadenectomy. Selective venous sampling after pentagastrin stimulation involves transfemoral catheterization of the superior vena cava, inferior vena cava, and jugular, mediastinal, and hepatic veins. The iCT gradient after pentagastrin stimulation can be expressed as the ratio of the selective sample over the peripheral (forearm) sample. Recent data have suggested that selective venous sampling may be the most sensitive method of detecting occult hepatic metastases. However, the technical aspects of venous sampling have not been standardized, making comparison of data between institutions difficult.

In addition to selective venous sampling, laparoscopy has been advocated for the diagnosis of subclinical hepatic metastases prior to reoperative cervical surgery. Unfortunately, laparoscopy will detect only surface metastases. Laparoscopic hepatic sonography may prove valuable in detecting small lesions within the hepatic parenchyma.

Various scanning techniques have been used to evaluate patients with elevated iCT levels. These techniques involve the use of agents such as iodine-131 metaiodobenzylguanidine (MIBG), iodine-123 MIBG, technetium-99m (V)-dimercaptosuccinic acid (DMSA), thallium-201, thallium/technetium subtraction, technetium-99m Sestamibi, in-

Table 4 Normal Postoperative iCT in Patients Who Underwent Reoperation for MTC

FIRST AUTHOR	YEAR	NO. OF PATIENTS TOTAL	FAMILIAL/ SPORADIC	PG STIMULATION NEGATIVE FOLLOWING REOPERATION (%)
Norton	1980	7	2/5	1/7 (14)
Tisell	1986	11	4/7	4/11 (36)
van Heerden	1990	11	NA	0/11 (0)
Moley	1993	32	17/15	9/32 (28)
Dralle	1994	55	NA	8/55 (15)*
Abdelmoumene	1994	13	4/9	1/13 (8)
Buhr	1995	53	9/44	8/53 (15)
Total				31/182 (17)

PG, pentagastrin; NA, not available.
*Four of 15 (27%) in patients treated with more aggressive compartment-oriented microdissection.

dium 111-labeled anti-CEA monoclonal antibody, and indium-111 pentetreotide (Octreoscan). None of these scanning techniques can reliably exclude the presence of microscopic hepatic metastases and, therefore, have not received widespread use. However, when combined with the intraoperative use of surgical probes, these scanning techniques may prove useful in reoperative cases when mediastinal dissection (via median sternotomy) is being considered.

REOPERATION IN PATIENTS WITH ELEVATED iCT

Despite MTC's propensity for early metastatic spread to regional lymph nodes, controversy persists regarding the merits of elective lymphadenectomy or the removal of clinically normal regional lymph nodes. In oncologic surgery, there are three reasons to remove lymph nodes: (1) staging of disease, (2) local tumor control, and (3) patient cure. The presence of microscopic metastatic MTC in lymph nodes does not, at this time, indicate the need for adjuvant therapy, making staging information of limited value. As mentioned, retrospective data suggest that local disease control is improved with a systematic, compartment-oriented lymphadenectomy. In solid tumor oncology, lymph node metastases are believed to be a marker of systemic disease, and we rarely associate local-regional lymphadenectomy with cure of the disease. However, in contrast to most other solid tumors, MTC may be associated with prolonged periods of apparent tumor latency, during which tumor implantation in distant organs may not have occurred despite the presence of metastases in regional lymph nodes. Proponents of elective lymphadenectomy for asymptomatic elevations in iCT level have as their goal the removal of microscopic metastatic nodal disease to prevent dissemination to distant organs (liver, lung, and bone). However, several investigators have demonstrated that only a minority of patients achieve a biochemical cure (normal pentagastrin-stimulated iCT level) following reoperative regional lymphadenectomy (Table 4). The lack of prospectively acquired data and the relatively short follow-up in available studies have hindered the development of definitive treatment recommendations.

We perform reoperative lymphadenectomy only as part of a standardized diagnostic and treatment algorithm for patients with asymptomatic elevations in iCT level (see Fig. 1). When surgery (elective lymphadenectomy) is to be performed in patients who have elevated iCT levels following previous thyroidectomy but there is no evidence of disease recurrence on CT, MRI, or sonography, we proceed with bilateral modified neck dissection and re-excision of the central neck compartment. The limits of the dissection are the posterior belly of the digastric muscle superiorly, the eleventh nerve posterolaterally, the trachea and esophagus centrally, and the innominate vein inferiorly. The thymic fat pad is removed, and the extent of transcervical mediastinal dissection is based on anatomic considerations related to body habitus and the extent of previous operative procedures. The strap muscles are routinely excised en bloc with the specimen; detachment of their sternal heads greatly increases exposure for the mediastinal dissection. Every attempt is made to preserve (in situ) the superior parathyroid glands, which are usually seen just superior and posterior to the junction of the recurrent laryngeal nerve and inferior thyroid artery. The inferior parathyroid glands are removed with the paratracheal nodal tissue, identified when possible, and autografted.

ADJUVANT EXTERNAL-BEAM RADIATION THERAPY

Adjuvant external-beam radiation therapy (EBRT) should be considered in patients at high risk for local-regional tumor recurrence following maximal surgical therapy. Although prospectively acquired data are lacking, we use postoperative EBRT in patients with positive surgical margins of excision, extranodal soft tissue extension, and extensive mediastinal tumor extension (often requiring median sternotomy). In such patients, tumor recurrence in the central neck compartment or anterior mediastinum would result in invasion of the trachea and/or esophagus, causing loss of speech or swallowing. EBRT should not be used as a replacement for surgical excision in patients who have potentially resectable recurrent or locally advanced cervical disease. The EBRT treatment field extends from the mastoid to approximately the carina based on the individual clinical situation. AP/PA fields are used to deliver approximately 44 Gy (spinal cord tolerance less than 45 Gy) at a rate of 2 Gy per fraction, Monday through Friday. A four-field technique is then used to boost the total dose to 60 Gy in the most high-risk region.

■ TREATMENT OF DISTANT METASTATIC DISEASE

For patients with both the familial and sporadic forms of MTC, chemotherapy is considered only in the presence of either progressive metastatic disease, or advanced regional disease no longer amenable to surgery or EBRT. Initial reports of the use of chemotherapy in patients with MTC included single-agent trials using doxorubicin and other anthracylines, cisplatin, and etoposide. Partial responses of generally short duration were achieved. More recently, combination therapy has been reported to produce more frequent and more durable responses. These combinations have had one drug in common, imidazole carboxamide (DTIC), which is known to be effective against other neuroendocrine tumors. Combinations of DTIC with vincristine and cyclophosphamide with or without doxorubicin have produced significant and durable responses (or stabilization of disease) in more than 50 percent of treated patients. Similarly, DTIC combined with 5-fluorouracil has resulted in regression of metastatic liver, bone, and lung disease, significant reductions in iCT and CEA levels, and the amelioration of symptoms. However, such chemotherapy combinations remain a palliative treatment and their use in patients with elevated iCT levels in the absence of demonstrable metastatic disease cannot be recommended.

Future experimental approaches include the use of radionuclide-labeled monoclonal antibodies against CEA and the potential for gene therapy directed toward inhibiting the effects of RET activation.

Suggested Reading

Abdelmoumene N, Schlumberger M, Gardet P, et al. Br J Cancer 1994; 69: 1141–1144.

Buhr HJ, Kallinowski F, Raue F, et al. Microsurgical neck dissection for metastasizing medullary thyroid carcinoma. Eur J Surg Oncol 1995; 21: 195–197.

Cote GJ, Wohllk N, Evans D, et al. RET proto-oncogene mutations in multiple endocrine neoplasia type 2 and medullary thyroid carcinoma. Baillieres Clin Endocrinol Metab 1995; 9:609–630.

Dralle H, Damm I, Scheumann GFW, et al. Compartment-oriented microdissection of regional lymph nodes in medullary thyroid carcinoma. Jpn J Surg 1994; 14:112–121.

Ellenhorn J, Shah JJP, Brennan MF. Impact of therapeutic regional lymph node dissection for medullary carcinoma of the thyroid gland. Surgery 1993; 114:1078–1082.

Gharib H, McConahey WM, Tiegs RD, et al. Medullary thyroid carcinoma: Clinicopathologic features and long-term follow-up of 65 patients treated during 1946 through 1970. Mayo Clin Proc 1992; 67:934–940.

Moley JF, Wells SA, Dilley WG, Tisell LE. Reoperation for recurrent or persistent medullary thyroid cancer. Surgery 1993; 114:1090–1096.

Saad MF, Ordonez NG, Rashid RK, et al. Medullary carcinoma of the thyroid. Medicine 1984; 63:319–341.

Simpson WJ, Palmer JA, Rosen IB, Mustard RA. Management of medullary carcinoma of the thyroid. Am J Surg 1982; 144:420–422.

Tisell LE, Dilley WG, Wells SA. Progression of postoperative residual medullary thyroid carcinoma as monitored by plasma calcitonin levels. Surgery 1996; 119:34–39.

Tisell LE, Hansson G, Jansson S, Salander H. Reoperation in the treatment of asymptomatic metastasizing medullary thyroid carcinoma. Surgery 1986; 99:60–66.

van Heerden JA, Grant CS, Gharib H, et al. Long-term course of patients with persistent hypercalcitoninemia after apparent curative primary surgery for medullary thyroid carcinoma. Ann Surg 1990; 212:395–401.

INSULIN-DEPENDENT DIABETES MELLITUS IN ADULTS

Lucy A. Levandoski, P.A.-C.
Julio V. Santiago, M.D.

Over 14 million people in the United States have diabetes mellitus, a heterogeneous group of disorders characterized by abnormal insulin secretion and abnormalities in carbohydrate, protein, and fat metabolism. The vast majority of these individuals have non–insulin-dependent diabetes (NIDDM). Insulin-dependent diabetes mellitus (IDDM) accounts for only about 5 to 10 percent of all cases of diabetes. While both NIDDM and IDDM are associated with common tendencies to develop long-term complications, only IDDM is thought to be the result of an immune-related destruction of insulin-producing pancreatic beta cells.

The goals of treating IDDM are twofold. The primary goal is to establish and maintain a state of clinical well-being characterized by the absence of symptoms attributable to hyperglycemia or hypoglycemia, maintenance of normal body weight, and the ability to participate fully in the activities of daily life. The second goal is to provide treatment that reduces the risk for the development and progression of the long-term microvascular, neuropathic, and macrovascular complications of diabetes. The latter goal is by far the more ambitious and clearly requires the greatest effort on the part of the patient and the physician. The Diabetes Control and Complications Trial (DCCT) and the Stockholm Diabetes Intervention Study (SDIS) have demonstrated that many of the long-term microvascular and neuropathic complications of diabetes can be delayed or prevented by treatment strategies that maintain, for 5 years or more, lower mean blood glucose concentrations. However, both studies also indicate that normoglycemia is rarely achieved with any form of treatment of IDDM and that treatment goals and methods must be individually set and adjusted to balance the potential benefits of glucose lowering with patient acceptance and risks for hypoglycemia.

THE DCCT AND SDIS RESULTS

The association of an increased risk for the microvascular and neuropathic complications of diabetes with the severity of hyperglycemia was an old idea supported by a variety of epidemiologic studies conducted prior to the 1990s. Attempts were made during the 1970s and 1980s to extend these observations by demonstrating that lowering mean blood glucose levels could reduce these risks. Most failed to do so, primarily because all of these trials lasted less than 3 years.

The DCCT and SDIS, completed in 1993, demonstrated conclusively that reducing mean blood glucose levels from 230 to 150 mg per deciliter (and mean HbA_{1c} concentrations from 9.0 to 7.2 percent) for 5 to 9 years could substantially reduce the early appearance or progression of retinopathy, neuropathy, and nephropathy in carefully selected and closely supervised adult and adolescent IDDM patients.

The methods used to treat DCCT and SDIS patients have been described as conventional or intensive therapy. In the DCCT, conventional insulin therapy was arbitrarily defined as the type of treatment used by the majority of diabetes experts in the early 1980s to treat most IDDM patients. This treatment consisted of injections of mixtures of regular and NPH insulin, given before breakfast and before the evening meal. Intensive insulin therapy, as defined by the DCCT, involved the use of three or more daily insulin injections or an insulin infusion pump. The key characteristics of these two regimens are shown in Table 1.

Even when intensive therapy was implemented in highly motivated patients by experienced diabetes health care providers using extraordinary resources, most intensively treated DCCT patients were unable to consistently achieve and maintain normoglycemia. For example, approximately 75 percent of the bedtime and prebreakfast blood glucoses were greater than 120 mg per deciliter. The mean hemoglobin A_{1c} for this group was 7.2 percent, and the mean of seven daily blood glucoses was 155 mg per deciliter. These results were accompanied by a threefold increase in the incidence of hypoglycemia with neuroglycopenia severe enough to require assistance when compared with less intensively managed patients whose mean fasting blood glucose level was 200 mg per deciliter and mean HbA_{1c} was 9 percent.

Despite the inability to achieve and maintain normoglycemia and the increased risk for hypoglycemia, some form of intensified therapy is now viewed as the treatment of choice for most IDDM patients. In coming years, with a growing emphasis on preventive measures to reduce the risk of long-

Table 1 DCCT and SDIS Treatment Methods

	CONVENTIONAL THERAPY	INTENSIVE THERAPY
Reduce symptoms of high/low blood glucose	Yes	Yes
Insulin injections	b.i.d.	3–4 or pump
Blood glucose monitoring	1–2/day	4–5/day
Target glucose goals	None*	70–120 mg/dl before meals; >65 mg/dl at 3 AM
Frequent adjustments in treatment to meet goals	Uncommon*	Common, detailed
Feedback on HbA_{1c}	None*	Monthly
Office visits	Quarterly	Monthly

*These components of conventional treatment make this treatment archaic and unwarranted post-DCCT.

Table 2 Available Insulin Preparations

	MANUFACTURER	ONSET (HR)	PEAK (HR)	DURATION (HR)
SHORT-ACTING (REGULAR)				
Human				
Humulin R	Lilly	0.5	2–4	3–6
Novolin R	Novo Nordisk	0.5	2.5–5	8
Novolin BR (Velosulin)	Novo Nordisk	0.5	2.5–5	8
Beef/Pork				
Iletin I	Lilly	0.5	3–4	4–8
Pork				
Iletin II	Lilly	0.5	3–4	4–8
Novo Nordisk R	Novo Nordisk	0.5	2.5–5	8
INTERMEDIATE-ACTING				
Human				
Humulin N	Lilly	2–4	4–10	10–18
Humulin L	Lilly	3–4	4–12	12–20
Novolin N	Novo Nordisk	1.5	4–12	24
Novolin L	Novo Nordisk	2.5	7–15	22
Beef/Pork				
Iletin I NPH	Lilly	4–6	8–14	16–24
Iletin I Lente	Lilly	4–6	8–14	16–24
Pork				
Iletin II NPH	Lilly	4–6	8–14	16–24
Iletin II Lente	Lilly	4–6	8–14	16–24
Novo Nordisk N	Novo Nordisk	1.5	4–12	24
Novo Nordisk L	Novo Nordisk	2.5	7–15	22
LONG-ACTING				
Human				
Humulin U	Lilly	6–10	8–24	18–28
FIXED-RATIO INSULIN				
Human				
Humulin 70/30	Lilly			
Humulin 50/50	Lilly			
Novolin 70/30	Novo Nordisk	0.5	2–12	24

term complications, the treatment of IDDM should be facilitated by more physiologic methods for insulin replacement coupled with a more acceptable, reliable method for continuous or more frequent blood glucose monitoring, and a wider availability of cost effective programs for diabetes education, self-management training, and supervision.

This chapter describes the treatment strategies currently used in our center for the management of adolescent and adult patients with IDDM. The treatment strategies described can be used by nonspecialty physicians in a general practice setting provided that key components of the program are available. Each of these components of IDDM management including insulin preparations, treatment regimens, nutrition, exercise, and patient education are discussed.

COMPONENTS OF DIABETES MANAGEMENT

Insulin

Pancreatic beta cell destruction, the hallmark of IDDM, results in potentially lethal insulin deficiency. Exogenous insulin replacement is the only pharmacologic modality available for the treatment of this disorder. Unfortunately, despite tremendous advances in the treatment of diabetes, insulin replacement regimens remain imperfect and nonphysiologic.

Insulin Preparations

Insulin is classified by source (beef, pork, or biosynthetic human) and by pharmacokinetics (onset, peak, duration of action). Table 2 provides a summary of currently available insulin preparations.

Until the 1980s, all insulins were derived from animal sources. The earliest insulins contained immunogenic impurities that were commonly responsible for lipoatrophy at injection sites, local and systemic insulin allergies, and sometimes with insulin resistance secondary to insulin antibody formation. These problems have been virtually eliminated by the introduction of highly purified animal insulins and human insulin. All currently available animal insulins are either pure pork or a beef and pork combination. It is likely that most animal insulin preparations will be phased out by the end of the century in most countries due to more cost effective production of biosynthetic human insulin.

Biosynthetic human insulin, produced by recombinant DNA technology, has been available since the early 1980s. Biosynthetic human insulin is structurally identical to endogenous insulin, rendering it somewhat less immunogenic than highly purified pork insulin. Human insulin preparations are generally absorbed faster from subcutaneous tissue than pork or beef insulins. This characteristic has two practical consequences, a faster onset of action and peak, and a shorter duration of action.

Human insulin is now used almost exclusively in newly diagnosed IDDMs and in NIDDMs requiring insulin therapy after failure to respond to diet and/or oral hypoglycemic agents. Human insulin should be used in all NIDDMs needing intermittent insulin therapy, such as during surgery, an intercurrent illness, or at times of unusual stress associated with severe hyperglycemia and/or ketosis. Any woman with IDDM who is planning pregnancy or who is already pregnant should be on human insulin.

Patients who are adequately controlled on animal insulin need not be switched routinely to human insulin. On the other hand, patients in less than optimal metabolic control may benefit from switching to human insulin by correcting a physiologic condition, e.g., immune-mediated insulin resistance, or by indirectly addressing a psychological condition, thereby giving the patient the opportunity to "make a fresh start."

Insulin Pharmacokinetics

Insulin preparations can be classified as rapid acting, intermediate acting, or long acting based on onset, peak, and duration of action. It is important to note that insulin absorption varies among patients and in individual patients on a day-to-day basis, depending on anatomic location and blood flow at injection sites. In fact, the coefficient of variation for peak plasma insulin levels, rates of absorption of insulin from the skin, and duration of action can be greater than 30 percent in any one individual. Thus, while these classifications of insulin activity are useful, they should be used only as guidelines. One cannot assume that all insulins within a given category will act similarly in all patients at all times. The choice of insulin preparation and principles of dose adjustments must be made based on the clinical response of individual patients under individual circumstances over several days to weeks.

Short-Acting Insulins

Regular insulin has a rapid onset (½ to 1 hour) and a relatively short duration of action. Its peak glucose-lowering activity occurs 2 to 3 hours following subcutaneous injection and declines gradually between 3 and 6 hours after injection. Large doses of regular insulin (greater than 0.4 U per kilogram body weight) can have glucose-lowering effects of 6 to 8 hours or more. A buffered form of regular insulin is available for use in insulin infusion pumps. Buffered insulin is recommended for use in these devices because it is less likely to precipitate and occlude the infusion tubing.

A new drug application has been submitted to the Food and Drug Administration (FDA) and other regulatory agencies for lispro (Humalog) insulin. This biosynthetic insulin has been chemically modified to yield a formulation that tends to be more rapidly converted to a monomeric form that is more rapidly absorbed than regular insulin. At commonly used doses this form of insulin begins to show glucose lowering effects within 10 to 15 minutes after injection, peak plasma levels at 60 to 90 minutes, and virtually no glycemic effect after 4 hours. Lispro insulin is best injected 5 to 15 minutes before meals and requires supplementation with longer-acting forms of insulin overnight and when meals are spaced more than 4 hours apart. It can be mixed with NPH or Ultralente insulin in the morning and evening and injected alone before lunch. Lispro insulin may also be well suited for use in infusion pumps, although discontinuation or interruption of infusion would result in a rapid tendency for hyperglycemia and ketosis.

Intermediate-Acting Insulins

The onset of action for the intermediate-acting insulins, NPH and Lente, is about 1 to 4 hours with peak plasma activity occurring about 6 to 8 hours after injection for pork insulin and 5 to 7 hours for human insulin. The duration of action of these insulins is generally 8 to 12 hours at doses of 0.2 to 0.5 U per kilogram but can be up to 16 to 20 hours at higher doses (0.8 to 1.2 U per kilogram).

The main difference between NPH and Lente insulins is their compatibility with regular insulin. Premixing regular insulin with NPH has little effect on the absorption of either. However, premixing regular insulin with Lente affects the absorption of both components, diminishing the activity of the regular insulin and rendering it more like an intermediate-acting insulin. As noted, both human NPH and Lente insulins are more rapidly absorbed than animal insulins, resulting in faster onset but shorter duration of action. A major practical consequence of this difference is that human NPH insulin, when given before supper to meet nocturnal needs, is more likely to result in early morning (1:00 to 3:00 AM) hypoglycemia and prebreakfast hyperglycemia than pork NPH insulin.

Long-Acting Insulins

Protamine zinc insulin (PZI) was heralded in the 1940s as a breakthrough in diabetes therapy because, due to its 24 to 36 hour duration of action, it could be given as a once daily injection. This would spare IDDM patients from having to take more frequent injections. Unfortunately, giving PZI insulin once a day did not meet physiologic insulin requirements. The peak activity did not coincide with peak needs after meals and its long duration of action often caused problems with nocturnal hypoglycemia in the predawn period when insulin needs were lowest. PZI insulin is no longer available in North America.

Ultralente insulin has replaced PZI only in North America. Its onset of activity begins between 4 and 6 hours after subcutaneous injection. Technically, Ultralente insulin does not produce a pronounced peak, although it may in some individuals when taken as a single large dose. The duration of action of Ultralente insulin at doses of 0.3 to 0.5 U per kilogram is between 16 and 20 hours.

In recent years there has been renewed interest in long-acting insulin as the basal (i.e., between meal and overnight) component of insulin replacement in intensive insulin therapy using multiple daily injections. The advantage of Ultralente insulin over NPH insulin in multiple injection regimens is its reduced peak activity 4 to 6 hours after injection, allowing for a more physiologic replacement profile that reduces hyperglycemic rebound between meals and hypoglycemic nadirs in the predawn period or when meals are widely spaced, e.g., 6 or more hours. As with NPH and Lente insulins, human Ultralente insulin is more rapidly absorbed than animal preparations. This places it at a relative disadvantage as a once daily basal insulin. As a result, many intensively treated patients using Ultralente take it as twice daily injections approximately 12 hours apart. As a practical matter, titration of Ultralente insulin given in the evening is based on achieving satisfactory blood glucose control before breakfast without inducing hypoglycemia during the early morning predawn period. Titration of the prebreakfast Ultralente dose is based on the avoidance of afternoon hypoglycemia or hyperglycemia when lunch is missed and no regular insulin has been given since the prebreakfast dose.

Premixed Insulins

For convenience, insulin manufacturers have developed premixed insulins. These are most often used by us in NIDDM patients requiring insulin in a fixed ratio or in individuals who have difficulty mixing insulin from two vials. They are not commonly used by us in patients with IDDM because they do not permit independent adjustment of the individual insulin components. However, their relative convenience has led some centers to use them routinely, in a 70 percent NPH, 30 percent regular formulation, as twice daily injections. Premixed insulins are currently available in three different ratios of NPH to regular insulin. The prototype of these preparations is 70/30 insulin (70 percent NPH, 30 percent regular). More recently, 50/50 and 80/20 combinations have been developed. The 50/50 formulation is commonly given before dinner to help reduce nocturnal hypoglycemia that can occur when 70/30 is given at this time. The 80/20 formulation is rarely used.

Prefilled Cartridges

Insulin cartridges are available for pen injectors. These devices make giving away-from-home injections much easier and thus improve patient compliance with prelunch and supplemental insulin doses. As important as their convenience is the fact that pen injectors allow for more precise measurement of doses in less than optimally attentive or visually impaired patients than conventional syringe techniques.

Insulin Analogues

The first of the insulin analogues, lispro (Humalog), became available in the United States in 1996. As reviewed above, these modified insulins have a very rapid onset of action and very short duration of activity. They help reduce optimal timing of premeal injections from 30 to 60 minutes to 20 minutes when compared with regular insulin. These properties make insulin analogues ideally suited for intensive regimens that rely on premeal injections, given 5 to 15 minutes before meals three times daily, to reduce postprandial hyperglycemia and postabsorptive hypoglycemia 3 to 6 hours after injection. Indeed, reduction of hypoglycemia has been an important advantage in lispro use among well-controlled IDDM and NIDDM patients in phase III clinical trials in North America and Europe. When lispro injections are more than 4 hours apart (e.g., breakfast at 6:00 AM, lunch at 1:00 PM) some form of basal insulin (e.g., NPH or Ultralente) will be needed before breakfast.

Frequency and Size of Injections and Daily Doses

It is well known that physiologic insulin delivery consists of normal bursts of secretion after meals and more gradual, glucose-regulated secretion between meals and during the night. During the development of absolute insulin deficiency in the months to years after diagnosis of IDDM, the ability to rapidly release insulin after meals is reduced earlier than the ability to slowly release lesser amounts of insulin during the night. This natural evolution from moderate to severe insulin deficiency is an important component of the "honeymoon phase" of IDDM during which reasonable control of IDDM is achieved with two (and in some cases one) daily injections of relatively reduced amounts of insulin. As insulin deficiency becomes more complete and peak plasma C-peptide levels in the blood fall from above 0.5 nmol per liter to less than 0.2 nmol per liter, IDDM patients require increased amounts of insulin and more frequent insulin injections to maintain optimal blood glucose control. From a practical standpoint, the main consequence of the end of the honeymoon period is that a second insulin injection is needed to maintain acceptable blood glucose levels before breakfast.

Regardless of the type of insulin regimen used, most postpubertal IDDMs require 0.5 to 1.2 U per kilogram per day. Increased adiposity, sedentary lifestyle, and puberty are associated with higher insulin needs. Newly diagnosed IDDM patients will likely need less insulin early in the course of their disease (honeymoon phase), prior to complete or near-complete beta cell destruction. Higher insulin doses are generally needed during febrile illnesses and administration of corticosteroids.

Treatment Implementation

The choice of treatment regimen will be influenced by a number of factors that, in our experience, commonly evolve in specific patients. These factors include (1) the current status of insulin deficiency, (2) the current level of metabolic control, (3) the desired level of metabolic control, (4) extenuating circumstances such as recent history of severe hypoglycemia and concurrent medical problems, (5) the patient's ability and willingness to follow an intensified regimen, (6) financial considerations, and (7) the current resources available to the physician and patient.

Initiating Insulin Therapy

The acutely ill adolescent or adult patient who presents with signs and symptoms of diabetic ketoacidosis (DKA) is usually hospitalized for stabilization and initiation of insulin therapy. Most large hospitals employ diabetes nurses and dietary specialists who provide initial diabetes education and training. For nonacidotic patients this initial treatment is increasingly being provided in an outpatient setting.

Whether a patient is referred to a diabetes specialist immediately after diagnosis will be determined, in large measure, by the resources, time, and experience of the primary care provider. Diabetologists utilize diabetes educators and dietitians to provide education, nutrition counseling, and self-management training needed by IDDMs. These specialists have the requisite staff and time for frequent phone calls and treatment adjustments needed during the first months after diagnosis. Some primary care physicians feel comfortable providing this level of care themselves. Others will see the diabetes specialist as the most efficient way to stabilize and educate a newly diagnosed IDDM patient. Too often, however, there is a reluctance on the part of the diagnosing physician to refer patients to a diabetologist, even for initial management, for fear of losing the patient. Increasingly, "co-management" arrangements are being made whereby the specialist supervises initial management and training and the primary care physician assumes most of the responsibility for day-to-day care and uses the specialist when specific problems emerge or metabolic control is suboptimal.

In the newly diagnosed adolescent or adult patient, the key objective is to stabilize the patient, provide basic survival skills training, and begin the long process of self-management training under professional supervision.

We generally begin subcutaneous insulin treatment with two daily injections based on the patient's weight. Depending on frequently measured (four to seven times per day) blood glucose levels and HbA_{1c} responses, we modify treatment as needed taking into consideration their risk for hypoglycemia, their desired lifestyle, and their ability and willingness to adapt to more rigorous regimens. As an initial dose we give a total of 0.5 to 1.0 U insulin per kilogram body weight, giving two-thirds of the total dose prebreakfast and one-third presupper. The morning insulin dose is distributed as one-third regular insulin and two-thirds NPH insulin. The presupper dose consists of equal parts of regular and NPH insulin. The patient is started on a meal plan calculated by the dietitian to meet nutritional requirements but which includes mid-afternoon and bedtime snacks. The patient is monitored for signs of hypoglycemia and blood glucose levels are measured before each main meal, at bedtime, and at 3:00 AM. The lower total daily insulin doses of 0.5 U per kilogram per day are given to exceptionally lean, nonketotic, and active patients. The higher doses are given to relatively overweight, ketotic, and inactive patients. The average starting dose is 0.6 U per kilogram per day. The four components of insulin treatment are adjusted daily during the first week following diagnosis based on the previous day's experience.

A nonobese, 70 kg person who has average physical activity and is initially started on a dose of 0.6 U per kilogram per day would be given 42 U per day with 28 U given in the morning (9 U regular and 19 U NPH) and 14 U given in the evening (7 U regular and 7 U NPH). Insulin doses are then adjusted daily depending on the patient's ability to achieve blood glucose levels in the initial target range of 70 to 180 mg per deciliter before meals, at bedtime, and during the night. After the end of the first week, insulin dose adjustments are made over the telephone every 2 to 3 days until blood glucose levels are stable. Each insulin component of this initial dose is usually modified only by 10 to 15 percent at a time. For example, hypoglycemia or blood glucose levels below 70 mg per deciliter before breakfast would result in a 10 percent reduction of the evening NPH dose while blood glucose levels above 180 mg per deciliter before supper would result in a 10 percent increase in the morning NPH dose. Generally, these insulin adjustments are made less frequently after the first 2 weeks as the patient regains weight, settles into a consistent eating pattern, and becomes more active.

Sometime after the first 1 to 3 weeks of treatment patients commonly need less insulin as they regain some of their own insulin secretory capacity and insulin requirements decline to 0.2 to 0.5 U per kilogram per day. During this honeymoon phase, which may last weeks or months, blood glucose control is often excellent and the overall blood glucose target range before meals can be reduced to 60 to 160 mg per deciliter. Sometimes it is even possible to temporarily achieve near-optimal control with one daily injection during the honeymoon phase. We rarely discontinue insulin completely in our newly diagnosed IDDM patients.

Patients who maintain, over 2 months, a mean premeal blood glucose level of 120 mg per deciliter generally have HbA_{1c} concentrations below 7 percent. This is considered excellent metabolic control in any IDDM patient. Values approaching the upper limit of normal (6 percent for HbA_{1c}) are sometimes seen but can seldom be maintained safely with two injections of insulin per day after the completion of the honeymoon phase. Excellent metabolic control during the honeymoon phase of IDDM will help preserve insulin secretory capacity in some adolescent and adult patients and should serve as an incentive to maintain exceptional control during this period.

Two alternative treatment strategies are also available during the early honeymoon phase. One is to begin more highly intensified treatment with regular insulin given before each main meal and one or two injections of a longer-acting insulin to meet basal needs during the night and between meals. The second involves use of an insulin infusion pump. We usually do not begin either of these more intensive regimens until the end of the honeymoon period, which is usually heralded by gradually increasing nocturnal insulin requirements to maintain prebreakfast blood glucoses in the 60 to 160 mg per deciliter range and frequent glucose excursions above 240 mg per deciliter after meals. It may be argued, however, that initiation of highly intensive regimens earlier in the course of IDDM will have long-term benefits because it introduces this more physiologic form of insulin replacement sooner when control is more easily achieved and before "bad habits" are fortified with less intensive regimens. The earlier, routine introduction of four daily injections is more common in European centers than in North America, where the majority of IDDM patients treated by diabetes specialists are still being treated with only two or three daily injections.

Post-Honeymoon Treatment

If two daily injections of insulin become inadequate, as evidenced by a HbA_{1c} concentration rising above 7 percent and premeal blood glucose levels becoming more erratic and frequently ranging below 60 mg per deciliter or above 160 mg per deciliter, a more intensive regimen is indicated. The decision to start intensified insulin therapy requires consideration of several factors. These include (1) the patient's willingness to assume a greater role in glucose monitoring and frequent insulin dose adjustments as a routine in his or her diabetes management; (2) the patient's ability, both financially and psychologically, to follow a more demanding treatment regimen; (3) the patient's complication status, i.e., patients with advanced complications are less likely to benefit from intensive therapy and because of the increased risk for severe hypoglycemia, it may not be safe in patients with cardiovascular disease, autonomic neuropathy, and hypoglycemia unawareness; (4) the patient's past history of adherence to the prescribed treatment regimen including blood

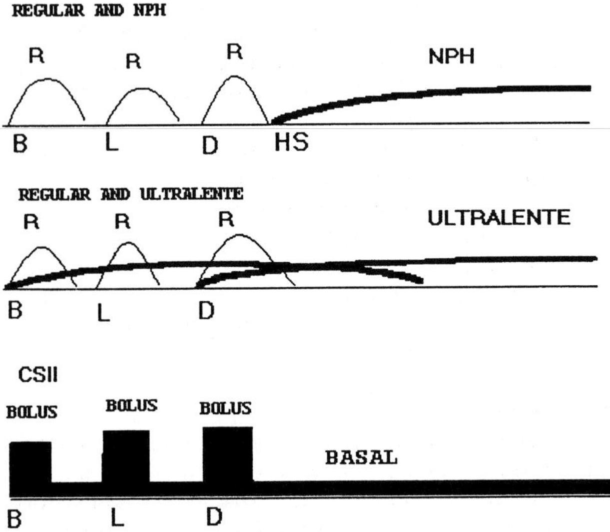

Figure 1
Three intensive insulin regimens used in the DCCT.

glucose monitoring, diet, and insulin injections; and (5) the physician's ability to provide the necessary education, training, and follow-up. All IDDM patients should be informed about the risks and benefits of intensive therapy. Those reluctant to monitor blood glucose four to five times daily, inject insulin before each meal, and follow a predictable meal plan are poor candidates for intensive therapy with the goal of maintaining near normoglycemia.

The cost of intensive therapy regimens needs to be considered. Multiple daily insulin injection regimens are less expensive than continuous subcutaneous insulin infusion (CSII) therapy. Insulin pumps cost about $4,000. The cost of infusion sets, insulin syringes for pump use, and taping preparations is about $600 to $800 per year. This is in addition to the cost of frequent blood glucose monitoring. Some private insurance companies will pay for a portion of the cost of pump therapy. Medicare and some health maintenance organizations will generally not.

Figure 1 illustrates three commonly used intensive insulin regimens that approximate normal pancreatic beta cell function. The first regimen utilizes preprandial regular insulin and bedtime NPH. This regimen is most popular in Europe. The premeal doses are adjusted based on the blood glucose level, the composition of the next meal, the anticipated level of activity, and prior experience. This regimen approximates physiologic insulin replacement fairly well but sacrifices mealtime flexibility insofar as meals cannot be omitted or delayed for 2 or more hours. The regular insulin must be given every 4 to 6 hours to maintain basal insulinemia during the day. Omitting a meal and the premeal insulin dose almost always results in hyperglycemia prior to the next meal. To overcome the lack of "basal" insulin, some physicians prescribe a small dose of NPH (0.15 to 0.20 U per kilogram) along with the prebreakfast regular. This may permit greater flexibility with meal timing but potentially could result in postlunch hypoglycemia because of the overlapping effect of the NPH peak and the prelunch regular.

Using Ultralente insulin as the source of basal insulinemia substantially reduces problems with mealtime flexibility. If the dose of Ultralente is adequate, a meal can be omitted or substituted by a light snack without precipitating hyperglycemia by the next meal. Because human Ultralente has been shown to peak, especially when given in large doses (more than 15 to 20 U), we generally split the Ultralente dose and give about 50 percent of the dose before breakfast and before dinner. Patients who have a marked dawn phenomenon may benefit from giving a higher percentage of the total Ultralente dose in the evening (i.e., 60 to 70 percent of the total dose). These individuals may also benefit from giving the evening Ultralente dose at bedtime. Some patients may require a small amount of regular insulin, taken with their bedtime snack, to prevent fasting hyperglycemia. This must be done judiciously to avoid nocturnal hypoglycemia.

CSII is another option for providing physiologic insulin replacement. With CSII therapy, small amounts of regular insulin are infused hourly based on a preset basal rate. Before each meal, or as needed to correct hyperglycemia, the pump is programmed to give a bolus dose of insulin as determined by the blood glucose level or meal composition. Currently available insulin pumps can be programmed to deliver multiple, different basal rates. This feature allows for customization of the basal rate to compensate for periods of either increased (e.g., 5:00 to 8:00 AM) or decreased (e.g., 1:00 to 3:00 AM) insulin need.

None of these insulin regimens is perfect. All are capable of providing more physiologic insulinemia, but none will produce near-normoglycemia by themselves. Patients must learn, through extensive and ongoing self-management training, how to adjust their insulin, diet, and activity in response to the blood glucose levels obtained several times each day. Without these daily adjustments even the most sophisticated insulin regimen will fail to safely produce optimal control. Near-normoglycemia (i.e., more than 75 percent of blood glucoses between 70 and 120 mg per deciliter before each meal) was rarely maintained long term even in the DCCT. Indeed, less than 25 percent of patients in the DCCT had mean prebreakfast blood glucose levels below 120 mg per deciliter.

Treatment Goals

The DCCT results have prompted a committee of experts to suggest optimal blood glucose values that are slightly less demanding than those used in the DCCT intensive management group. We find these suggested "target values" unrealistic for several reasons. First, post-DCCT glucose values have been higher in the DCCT volunteers seen less than once monthly in nonresearch settings. Second, it is hard for us to recommend that the primary care physician in a nonresearch setting attempt to achieve a degree of blood glucose control not obtained even in the DCCT's average patient. For example, the suggested 80 to 120 mg per deciliter target range for blood glucose levels before breakfast is lower than that achieved by 75 percent of the DCCT intensively treated patients. Third, giving a target value does not tell us what to do when over 50 percent of the values are above the suggested target yet 10 percent or more are below it.

Based on our interpretation of the DCCT data, we believe a more realistic operational goal is to try to have over 50 percent of the premeal blood glucose values between 60 mg per deciliter and 160 mg per deciliter and less than 10 percent below 60

Table 3 Realistic Glycemic Targets

For patients with adequate recognition of hypoglycemia:	
Fasting	60–160 mg/dl
Before meals and bedtime	60–160 mg/dl
3:00 AM	>65 mg/dl
For optimal control, >50% of measured glucose values should be within the above ranges with <10% below or above the target range.	
For patients with hypoglycemia unawareness:	
Fasting	80–180 mg/dl
Before meals and bedtime	80–180 mg/dl
3:00 AM	>80 mg/dl

mg per deciliter. Table 3 lists our target blood glucose goals for a typical IDDM patient who is cooperative and has no history of severe, recurrent hypoglycemia. The lower prebreakfast target value of 60 mg per deciliter that we recommend for optimal patients is driven by the fact that occasional (e.g., 10 percent or 1 to 2 per week) values in the 60 to 80 mg per deciliter range before meals should not necessarily call for an adjustment of treatment while more than 10 percent of blood glucose values over 2 weeks below 60 mg per deciliter should, in our view, prompt a change in treatment to reduce the risk of severe hypoglycemia and iatrogenic hypoglycemia unawareness. The use of the higher target value of 160 mg per deciliter was chosen because more than 75 percent of prebreakfast glucose values among intensively managed DCCT patients were below this value. Overall, our goal is to try to replicate in the post-DCCT "real world" what was actually achieved by the average patient in the DCCT.

In patients with a history of severe hypoglycemia or in patients in whom the potential for severe hypoglycemia is of great concern, higher targets (e.g., 80 to 180 mg per deciliter) can be used. Broad targets of 60 to 180 mg per deciliter or even 60 to 200 mg per deciliter can be used in patients unwilling to pursue a more intensive blood glucose monitoring and dietary regimen. Regardless of the individual target ranges selected, we think that the selected range should be attainable over 50 percent of the time by a given patient doing his or her best and should result in acceptable (i.e., safe, mutually accepted by physician and patient) rates of hypoglycemia. This point is key. A patient who rarely (less than once per month) experiences blood glucose levels below 60 mg per deciliter either does not have true IDDM or is most likely suboptimally controlled with HbA_{1c} values above 8 percent. In the DCCT the average well-controlled patient had two to three self-treated episodes of hypoglycemia per week.

Routine HbA_{1c} assays measured every 1 to 3 months and analyses of patterns of glycemia every 1 to 2 weeks are the mainstays of long-term management. The long-term goal of treatment is to try to maintain mean levels of glycemia that result in HbA_{1c} levels at or below 7 percent with acceptable rates of hypoglycemia. During the DCCT, median blood glucose levels in carefully selected, closely supervised, and highly motivated patients resulted in a median HbA_{1c} of 7 percent, mean blood glucoses of 150 mg per deciliter, and mean prebreakfast blood glucoses of 140 mg per deciliter. Values were higher in the patients entering the study as adolescents and slightly lower in adults. The yearly rate of hypoglycemia severe enough to require assistance was approximately 50 cases per 100 patient years. Over half of the episodes of severe hypoglycemia occurred at night and about one-third of daytime episodes were associated with poor or no recognition of hypoglycemic warning symptoms. The risks of hypoglycemia during highly intensive treatment of IDDM are clearly substantial. However, results similar to those achieved in the DCCT are worth pursuing in the majority of patients early in the course of IDDM because they can reduce the appearance and early progression of most of the microvascular and neuropathic complications of IDDM by 50 to 80 percent or more if a glucose-lowering effect equivalent to 2 percent HbA_{1c} is sustained for 5 to 9 years or more.

Dose Adjustments

Acute adjustments in insulin dose, meal composition, or waiting time between insulin dose and the meal are made when individual premeal blood glucose levels are outside the target range of 60 to 160 mg per deciliter. Premeal insulin dose adjustments are generally dependent on four factors: the premeal blood glucose level, the size and content of the meal, the anticipated level of exercise before the next meal, and prior experience under similar circumstances.

A blood glucose level above 160 mg per deciliter can be corrected in several ways. One option is to increase the usual waiting time between insulin injection and the meal from 15 to 30 minutes to 45 to 60 minutes. The second involves adding small amounts, usually 1 to 4 U, to the premeal regular insulin dose. The third involves using one or both of the above adjustments and reducing the intake of carbohydrates so that blood glucose levels return to their target range by the next meal. For example, decreasing the carbohydrate content of the breakfast meal will likely reduce the prelunch glucose level.

Blood glucose levels below 60 mg per deciliter also warrant an acute adjustment. Most commonly, the premeal regular insulin dose is reduced by 1 to 2 U and it is given immediately before the meal.

If the premeal blood glucose levels are outside the target range for 5 of 7 consecutive days, a long-term change in the appropriate dose is indicated. For example, if the prelunch blood glucose level exceeds 160 mg per deciliter for 5 of the last 7 days, the prebreakfast dose of regular insulin should be increased by about 10 to 15 percent, provided there has been no hypoglycemia on the other days.

The management of nocturnal glycemia poses different problems. When more than one fasting blood glucose measurement per week (or more than 10 percent of fasting values over 2 to 4 weeks) are below 60 mg per deciliter, reductions in the nocturnal insulin dose are initiated and adjusted based on both the following day's 3:00 AM level and fasting blood glucose level. With most modes of insulin replacement, blood glucose levels in well-controlled IDDM patients reach a nadir sometime between 1:00 AM and 4:00 AM and then rise during the dawn period. The rising glucose levels can be the result of both a "rebound" from hypoglycemia and the increased insulin needs at dawn, independent of antecedent hypoglycemia. We do not usually decrease insulin doses when prebreakfast blood glucoses are 60 to 80 mg per deciliter, but we do encourage routine 3:00 AM monitoring in these circumstances, even in the absence of symptomatic hypoglycemia. There are two reasons for this approach. First, 1:00 to 4:00 AM blood glucose nadirs at or below 40 to 50 mg per deciliter often go unnoticed and result in glycemic rebounds into the normoglycemic range of 70 to 120 mg per deciliter before breakfast. Second, recurrent episodes of inadvertent nocturnal hypoglycemia have been shown to impair subsequent awareness of hypoglycemia and blunt normal epinephrine responses that provide counter-regulatory protection against severe hypoglycemia.

The best predictors of nocturnal hypoglycemia are blood glucose levels below 100 mg per deciliter before the bedtime snack and before breakfast. This information has practical consequences because normoglycemic glucose levels before the bedtime snack should prompt a larger bedtime snack and/or the addition of extra protein to this snack. Increased protein intake may help prevent nocturnal hypoglycemia by increasing glucagon levels, which remain responsive to protein ingestion even when hypoglycemia no longer stimulates glucagon release. Glucagon release is the most important normal component of protection against nocturnal hypoglycemia induced by inadvertent hyperinsulinemia. When it is lost, a common event after 5 years' duration of IDDM, epinephrine assumes a predominant role. In situations when both are deficient, intensively managed patients' risk of severe nocturnal hypoglycemia increases more than twentyfold.

HbA_{1c} Measurements

HbA_{1c} measurements are the "gold standard" in assessing long-term glycemic control as well as the long-term risk for complications. In our practice, we use an immunoassay kit that provides results within 10 minutes so that these results can be incorporated into each visit. Previously, because results were not available for several days, patients had to be tracked down after the visit to inform them of the results. HbA_{1c} measurements are made every 1 to 2 months while major changes are being made and every 3 to 4 months in stable IDDM patients in good control (i.e., HbA_{1c} is less than 7.5 to 8 percent). Feedback regarding HbA_{1c} results is considered essential.

Nutrition

Comprehensive nutritional counseling is a necessary component of long-term diabetes management. Three key roles of modern dietary care of IDDM patients are (1) to teach patients to read nutritional labeling on common foods, (2) to provide flexibility in meal planning, and (3) to communicate effectively with other members of the treatment team.

Most people with IDDM are at or near ideal body weight. Unlike NIDDM, where weight loss is the primary goal, the main nutrition goals in IDDM are (1) to provide appropriate calories and nutrients, (2) to provide nutrients that are eaten at desired times and can be matched with insulin replacement patterns, (3) to adjust caloric intake for exercise and hypoglycemia, (4) to encourage eating habits that reduce cardiovascular risks, and (5) to develop meal plans that enhance patient satisfaction and long-term adherence.

In 1995 the American Dietetic Association and the American Diabetes Association revised their nutritional guidelines to reflect a trend toward more flexible meal planning and liberalized food choices. The general recommendation is to provide a balanced diet with 45 to 55 percent of the calories derived from carbohydrate, 15 to 20 percent from protein (0.8 g per kilogram body weight) and less than 30 percent from fat. Total caloric intake should be sufficient to achieve and maintain reasonable body weight (25 to 35 kcal per kilogram ideal body weight, depending on age and activity). The meal plan should take into consideration patient preferences and lifestyle.

Meal timing, composition, and insulin doses are integrated to achieve optimal blood glucose control. More physiologic insulin regimens and the use of blood glucose monitoring permit greater flexibility in meal planning. However, day-to-day consistency with meal times and meal composition is still needed to obtain optimal blood glucose control. One way to increase flexibility with meal composition is to use carbohydrate (bread, fruit, milk) counting to determine premeal regular insulin doses. In general, 1 to 2 U regular insulin is used for each carbohydrate exchange consumed. For example, if a patient wishes to add two extra 15 g carbohydrate exchanges at a given meal, 2 to 4 U regular insulin is added to their usual preprandial dose. Obviously, this works best when patients take regular insulin before a given meal. Using carbohydrate counting is also an effective way to determine the usual premeal insulin dose. For example, if a middle-aged patient usually eats only three carbohydrate exchanges at breakfast, a reasonable starting dose for the prebreakfast regular insulin would be 3 to 6 U.

All patients started on insulin or any intensified regimen that will lower mean blood glucose levels and reduce glycosuria should be warned about potential weight gain. DCCT patients who reduced their HbA_{1c} from 9 to 7 percent gained an average of 10 pounds, usually within the first few months of treatment. To the extent that weight gain is viewed as a disincentive, particularly for women, dietary modifications should start prior to any intensification and should be reviewed regularly by an experienced nutritionist. Usually, a long-term reduction of 300 to 500 kcal per day prevents undesirable weight gain and avoids the need for overtreatment of hypoglycemia.

A more comprehensive guide to nutritional management of IDDM is beyond the scope of this chapter. It is our recommendation that all patients have access to an experienced dietitian on a regular basis. Any preprinted dietary materials should be accompanied by a thorough explanation by a qualified dietitian. Both physicians and nurses should work closely with the dietitian to coordinate insulin dose adjustments in response to permanent or temporary dietary alterations and to reinforce the principles of good nutrition.

Exercise

Exercise, along with insulin and diet, plays a key role in diabetes management. Regular exercise increases insulin sensitivity and reduces insulin requirements. It has a favorable impact on self-esteem, body weight, lipid profiles, and cardiovascular health. Unfortunately, exercise can produce wide fluctuations in blood glucose levels. The most common adverse reaction to exercise is hypoglycemia resulting from increased glucose utilization by exercising tissue and enhanced insulin absorption due to increased subcutaneous blood flow. Conversely, exercising at a time of relative insulin deficiency can lead to hyperglycemia and ketosis due to the

Table 4 Exercise Guidelines for IDDM

1. All patients should undergo a complete evaluation for the detection of diabetes complications including cardiovascular disease, retinopathy, and neuropathy prior to beginning an exercise program.
2. Blood glucose levels should be checked before, during (if activity is >45 minutes), and after exercise.
3. Avoid exercising at the time of peak insulin activity.
4. Exercise 60–90 minutes after a meal to reduce the likelihood of postexercise hypoglycemia and limit postprandial hyperglycemia. Reduce the appropriate pre-exercise insulin dose, as needed, to prevent hypoglycemia during or after exercise.
5. Check blood glucose level before exercise.
   If <100 mg/dl, a snack consisting of 1 carbohydrate exchange should be consumed.
   If >250 mg/dl, check ketones. If present, delay exercise until ketones are gone.
6. For every 30–45 minutes of moderate activity, consume 1–2 carbohydrate exchanges.
7. Avoid giving pre-exercise insulin injections in extremities that will be used during exercise.
8. If exercise has been strenuous and prolonged, hypoglycemia can occur several hours (up to 24 hours) after the exercise is completed.
9. All patients should carry a source of fast-acting carbohydrate with them. They should wear or carry diabetes-specific identification at all times.

release of glucagon and catecholamines with resulting lipolysis, hepatic glucose release, and ketogenesis.

Unlike NIDDM, there is little evidence that routine exercise alone improves metabolic control in IDDM. However, we believe that any patient who wants to participate in an exercise program should be encouraged to do so, providing there is no medical contraindication to exercise. It is the responsibility of the health care team to provide each patient with realistic guidelines for exercise that promote physical and mental well-being without compromising metabolic control. Table 4 summarizes general exercise guidelines.

The metabolic response to exercise depends on a number of factors. These include the time and site of the last injection, the time of the last meal, the blood glucose level at the start of exercise, the amount of glucose stored as glycogen in the liver, and the duration and intensity of the activity. Because of these factors, incorporation of an exercise program into the diabetes treatment plan is not a simple task. Many motivated patients have started an exercise program only to abandon it quickly when they find that it disrupts their previously stable metabolic control.

In order to derive the most benefit, exercise must be done regularly, at predictable times of day. To reduce frustration associated with fluctuating blood glucose levels, patients need to carefully plan for periods of increased physical activity. The use of SMBG before, during, and after exercise helps determine individual response to exercise and for making appropriate compensatory changes in insulin and/or diet to prevent hypoglycemia or hyperglycemia.

Exercise prescriptions should be tailored to the individual patient, taking into consideration overall health, metabolic control, and the presence of complications or other risk factors. Any patient who is over 30 years of age or who has had diabetes for 10 to 15 years should undergo a complete evaluation including screening for cardiovascular disease and complications of diabetes. Patients with advanced sensory neuropathy or severe retinopathy may need to be given very specific recommendations to prevent exacerbation of preexisting complications. For example, patients with advanced, proliferative retinopathy should avoid activities that increase blood pressure, such as weight lifting. Patients with neuropathy need to be instructed about proper footwear, footcare, and the avoidance of lower extremity injuries.

Providing patients with written exercise guidelines is useful but patients will need to take a "trial-and-error" approach to determine their individual response to exercise. Insulin doses, mealtimes, and meal composition may have to be modified to prevent acute and/or delayed hypoglycemia. For short periods (30 to 45 minutes) of moderate exercise all that may be needed is an extra one or two carbohydrate exchanges. For more prolonged exercise, especially if strenuous (e.g., racquetball, biking, hiking, or swimming for 1 to 2 hours), the regular insulin dose before the activity may have to be reduced by 50 percent and one to two carbohydrate exchanges consumed every 30 to 60 minutes. It is especially important that patients realize that exercise, particularly if it has been strenuous and prolonged, can produce hypoglycemia for 12 to 24 hours after exercise. Care should be taken to avoid postexercise and nocturnal hypoglycemia. Extra blood glucose monitoring, including 3:00 AM measurements, may be necessary to detect delayed, postexercise induced hypoglycemia.

Patient Education and Self-Management Training

From the perspective of diabetes care, it is known that certain patient behaviors can reduce acute and long-term complications while others will enhance their risk. Thus, the goal of diabetes education is to promote those behaviors that result in an overall reduction in risk for the development of complications. However, patient education, although essential, is relatively ineffective if it is not accompanied by measures designed to enhance desirable and reduce undesirable behaviors. One of the major advances in diabetes care is that a growing proportion of management responsibilities are being transferred to well-instructed, carefully supervised consumers.

Of necessity, the person with IDDM becomes the most important member of the diabetes treatment team and the primary provider of care. Without adequate self-management training, all but the most motivated and resourceful patients will struggle to manage their disease. A patient's ability and willingness to follow the diabetes treatment regimen is directly related to effective initial and ongoing patient education, guidance, and motivation.

Diabetes education is an ongoing, dynamic process. Every encounter with a patient, e.g., an office visit or a phone call,

Table 5 Basic and Advanced Self-Management Training

BASIC "SURVIVAL SKILLS" TRAINING
1. Pathophysiology of IDDM
2. Insulin dosages and administration
3. Blood glucose monitoring
4. Prevention and treatment of hypoglycemia
5. Sick-day management
6. Basic meal planning

ADVANCED TRAINING
1. Principles of intensive insulin therapy
2. Algorithms for dose adjustments to accommodate changes in routine and to achieve near-normoglycemia
3. Carbohydrate counting and dietary modifications
4. Pathogenesis, detection, and treatment of complications

may provide opportunities to educate. Lifestyle changes (marriage, divorce, going to college) or the development of complications should be viewed as an opportunity to reassess patient knowledge, skills, and goals. Patients need to know the impact these changes will have on their disease.

Many patients with IDDM followed by primary care physicians were initially diagnosed and trained as children or adolescents. As adults, their educational self-management needs may be different or require updating. For example, with longer duration of diabetes comes the potential for the development of complications, a topic that may not have been considered relevant during childhood. An important role of the diabetes nurse specialist and consultant diabetologist is periodic assessment of a patient's current knowledge and treatment behaviors as well as establishment of a program for ongoing training.

A multidisciplinary team approach to diabetes education is ideal. Patients are more likely to assimilate the principles of diabetes management if those principles are reinforced by all members of the team, each providing a different perspective based on their area of expertise. To be effective, all members of the treatment team must have similar treatment goals and provide consistent instructions. When the team management model is employed, the traditional role of the physician as principal care provider is abandoned and more responsibility for diabetes education and management is assumed by nonphysician providers. Flexibility of professional boundaries ("cross-training") is a prerequisite for successful team management. There is no justification for having a physician teach a patient about insulin administration when an experienced diabetes nurse educator can provide this service more efficiently and cost effectively. Conversely, a nutritional consultation may be unnecessary if a knowledgeable, cross-trained physician or nurse can suggest simple dietary modifications.

Essential components of diabetes education and self-management training are listed in Table 5. At the time of diagnosis, all IDDM patients must be instructed on the basic "survival skills." These skills permit patients to incorporate diabetes care into their normal activities. Once these skills have been mastered, patient education training should focus on more advanced topics related to self-management training and the prevention of long-term complications.

Whenever possible, family members and significant others should be included in educational sessions. This serves two purposes. First, occasionally a family member or significant other may be called on to assist in the care of the patient, such as during an intercurrent illness. Second, well-informed family members or significant others can provide support and encouragement to patients with IDDM.

Patients who are beginning an intensive insulin regimen may need extensive self-management training. This includes accurate blood glucose monitoring, adjusting insulin doses, and adjusting diet and activity to achieve target blood glucose goals. Patients should be provided with individualized algorithms for making appropriate dose adjustments. These algorithms must be reviewed regularly in order to insure that treatment goals are achieved.

Patients using subcutaneous insulin infusion via an insulin pump will need instructions specific for CSII therapy including how to operate the pump, how to insert and secure the infusion set, and how to troubleshoot hyperglycemia and hypoglycemia. They must be given instructions on how to manage their diabetes in the event of an insulin pump failure. All intensively treated patients should have 24 hour access to a health care professional experienced in intensive diabetes management.

Because hypoglycemia is the most common acute complication of diabetes treatment, it should be reviewed frequently. To minimize their risk for severe hypoglycemia, patients need to be reminded that their symptoms of hypoglycemia can change over time and that their ability to recover from hypoglycemia can become impaired with longer disease duration. Intensive insulin therapy with resultant near-normoglycemia can lead to a lowering of threshold for the recognition of hypoglycemia. Additionally, the ability to recognize and recover from hypoglycemia may deteriorate with improved blood glucose control.

Follow-Up

The frequency of follow-up visits should, in part, be determined by the patient's HbA_{1c}. Patients in stable, good control with HbA_{1c} of 7.5 percent or less can be seen every 3 to 4 months. Patients making major adjustments or being followed more intensively because of poor control or recurrent hypoglycemia may require return visits every 1 to 2 months. More important than a fixed follow-up schedule is the need to have the patient understand the criteria for routine calls, fax messages, and emergency consultations when glycemic goals are not being met.

Advances in treatment have greatly altered the course of IDDM. Patients with IDDM live longer with fewer complications. But with increased longevity comes an increased incidence in the long-term microvascular, neuropathic, and macrovascular complications of diabetes. We know conclusively that the complications of diabetes that exact a tremendous toll on people with diabetes, their families, and the health care industry can be prevented or delayed. Advances in the treatment of complications, such as laser photocoagulation for retinopathy and the use of ACE inhibitors for persistent proteinuria, as well as the knowledge that early treatment has a more favorable outcome, provides a rationale for early screening for diabetes complications such as retinopathy and neuropathy.

Routine follow-up of patients with IDDM should include careful, periodic assessment for detecting diabetes complications. Blood pressure and weight should be obtained at each follow-up visit. Aggressive treatment of hypertension is crucial to prevent its deleterious effects on the kidney. Assistance should be provided to enhance smoking cessation.

Careful examination of the feet for the detection of lesions and neuropathic disease should be a routine part of follow-up care. Foot-care instructions should be reviewed frequently, especially when the patient begins to lose ankle reflexes or show evidence of decreased sensation to a 10 g filament during periodic examinations for neuropathy. The following should be obtained at least annually in any patient who has had IDDM for more than 5 years: (1) a complete, dilated ophthalmologic examination by an ophthalmologist to detect retinopathy; (2) a timed urine collection for measurement of microalbuminuria and a serum creatinine for all patients with microalbuminuria; and (3) a lipid profile including high-density and low-density lipoprotein levels.

■ LIMITATIONS OF THERAPY

Even though intensive therapy is the treatment of choice for most patients with IDDM, this therapymay not be acceptable or appropriate for all patients. Successful lowering of mean blood glucose levels using an intensive therapy regimen requires extensive selfmanagement skills. Some patients are not willing or able to assume this degree of responsibility for their diabetes care. Others may feel the financial and psychological demands of intensive therapy outweigh any potential long-term benefit. Even highly motivated, closely supervised patients may have difficulty maintaining lower target blood glucose levels for an extended period of time for a variety of reasons, including reduced frequency of blood glucose monitoring, less meticulous attention to insulin dose adjustments and meal planning, and fear of hypoglycemia.

Patients' motivation for selecting intensive therapy will influence ultimate success. Some patients will chose an intensified treatment regimen for the express purpose of increasing their lifestyle flexibility, e.g., delaying or skipping meals. In these patients, achieving better blood glucose control may be a secondary goal. However, to the extent that any lowering of mean blood glucose levels has been shown to impact favorably on the development of long-term complications, all patients with IDDM should be encouraged to achieve the best metabolic control possible without compromising safety or lifestyle choices.

Suggested Reading

American Diabetes Association. Intensive diabetes management. Alexandria, VA: American Diabetes Association, 1995.

American Diabetes Association. Clinical practice recommendations 1996. Diabetes Care 1996; 19(Suppl 1).

The Diabetes Control and Complications Trial Research Group. The effect of intensive treatment of diabetes on the development and progression of long-term complications of insulin-dependent diabetes mellitus. N Engl J Med 1993; 329:977–986.

The Diabetes Control and Complications Trial Research Group. Implementation of the treatment protocols in the Diabetes Control and Complications Trial. Diabetes Care 1995; 18:361–376.

Haire-Joshu D, ed. Management of diabetes mellitus: Perspectives of care across the life span. St. Louis: Mosby–Year Book, 1996.

Reichard P, Nilsson B-Y, Rosenquist U. The effect of long-term intensified insulin treatment on the development of microvascular complications of diabetes mellitus. N Engl J Med 1993; 329:304-309.

NON–INSULIN-DEPENDENT DIABETES MELLITUS

Steven V. Edelman, M.D.
Robert R. Henry, M.D.

It is estimated that there are currently 13 to 16 million Americans with diabetes, more than 90 percent of whom have the adult-onset form termed type II or non–insulin-dependent diabetes mellitus (NIDDM). Of this number, approximately one-half are undiagnosed. Eighty to 90 percent of NIDDM patients are obese. Infrequently, insulin-dependent diabetes mellitus (IDDM) does develop in adults. In NIDDM, both microvascular and macrovascular complications may be present at the time of diagnosis, implying that the diabetic state often develops many years earlier than when it is recognized. At present, the incidence of NIDDM in the United States is stable at 650,000 new cases per year. NIDDM aggregates within families and has a strong genetic component as well as contributing environmental determinants. Factors that are known to influence the development of NIDDM include obesity; sedentary lifestyle; high-fat, low-fiber diets; previous gestational diabetes; impaired glucose tolerance; lipid abnormalities; hypertension; and aging. The risk of developing diabetes is greatly increased in minority populations such as African Americans, Hispanic Americans, Native Americans, and Asian and Pacific Island Americans. In these groups, diabetes is approaching or has reached epidemic proportions and its occurrence is strongly related to cultural changes in lifestyle and economy.

In the United States, diabetes is the seventh leading cause of death and a major contributor to an additional 300,000 deaths. Diabetes is associated with specific long-term microvascular complications that include retinopathy, neuropathy, nephropathy, and a markedly increased risk of premature atherosclerotic vascular disease. In adults, diabetes is the most common cause of end-stage renal disease, new-onset blindness, and lower extremity amputations. Compared with their nondiabetic counterparts, men with NIDDM have a twofold to threefold increased risk and women a fourfold to fivefold increased risk of cardiovascular disease. The economic burden imposed by diabetes is immense, accounting for one-seventh of the total annual U.S. health care expenditure.

■ TREATMENT

The primary objectives of management of NIDDM are to achieve and maintain normal metabolic and biochemical status in order to reduce hyperglycemic symptoms and prevent or delay the development of microvascular and macrovascular complications. Despite a clear understanding of the pathophysiologic mechanisms contributing to the development of hyperglycemia in NIDDM and the availability of therapeutic agents to control this disorder, most patients remain under less than ideal metabolic control. The failure to achieve optimal glycemic regulation is multifactorial in origin but is rooted to some extent in the long-held misconception that NIDDM is a mild disease that is easily treated. In addition, the metabolic nature and ramifications of NIDDM have only recently been fully recognized and appreciated. The hyperglycemia of NIDDM is often associated with numerous other metabolic abnormalities that also favor the development of diabetic complications and premature cardiovascular disease. Furthermore, hyperglycemia itself contributes to perpetuating hyperglycemia through the effects of so-called glucose toxicity. This refers to the ability of glucose to be toxic to multiple organ systems and to further impair the pathophysiologic abnormalities causing NIDDM, such as the insulin-resistant state. Any approach that is used to optimally manage NIDDM must consider all of these aspects and be multifaceted in nature.

In the past, definitive data confirming the benefits of near-normal glucose levels on microvascular complications of diabetes have been lacking. The Diabetes Control and Complications Trial (DCCT) was a long-term study that provided compelling evidence that glycemic control does matter and that near normalization of blood glucose levels can delay the development and progression of retinopathy, nephropathy, and neuropathy in IDDM patients. A major issue derived from these studies is whether the conclusions about the benefits of aggressive glycemic management are equally applicable to those individuals with NIDDM. At present, unequivocal data on this issue are not available. However, there is substantial evidence indicating that the severity and duration of hyperglycemia is a critical factor in the pathogenesis of microvascular complications in both forms of diabetes. This has led to the current recommendation by the American Diabetes Association that even in the absence of confirmatory data, it is warranted to expect that NIDDM patients will also benefit from improved glycemic control. Therefore, they advise that management should be directed at safely achieving the best possible glycemic control in this group as well.

Table 1 Target Levels of Glucose Control

BIOCHEMICAL MEASUREMENT	NORMAL	ACCEPTABLE	POOR
Preprandial glucose (mg/dl)	<115	80–120	>150
Bedtime glucose (mg/dl)	<120	100–140	>200
Glycosylated hemoglobin (%)*	<6	<7	>8

*Normal reference range: 4–6%.

Goals of Therapy

Based on evidence that good glycemic control reduces the risks of complications in diabetes, the goals of therapy have been recently redefined and are shown in Table 1. Although treatment goals should be individualized, the glycemic targets for diabetes reflect the belief that efforts to achieve near normal glucose levels should be attempted, whenever possible. The current glycemic goals to strive for are a fasting and preprandial glucose level of 80 to 120 mg per deciliter, a bedtime or evening glucose of 100 to 140 mg per deciliter and a glycosylated hemoglobin of less than 7 percent or 3 standard deviations from the mean. Normalizing glycemia and glycosylated hemoglobin is not only difficult to attain but also must be done while minimizing weight gain and hypoglycemia and maintaining a reasonable quality of life. Reducing cardiovascular risk factors is important in NIDDM because of the high incidence of macrovascular disease and can be achieved by optimizing diet, body weight, blood pressure, and lipoprotein levels. Patients should also be encouraged and assisted with discontinuing cigarette smoking.

Both glycemic control and cardiovascular risk factors should be managed initially by dietary modification and exercise therapy. Even though these modalities do not usually result in complete normalization of metabolic abnormalities by themselves, they are beneficial. Adherence should be constantly encouraged and reinforced because the response to the subsequent institution of pharmacologic therapy will be enhanced. Not only must every effort be made to optimally control glycemia in NIDDM, major macrovascular risk factors such as hypertension and dyslipidemia must be promptly identified and aggressively treated as well.

Multidisciplinary Approach

The most effective management of diabetes is achieved when a coordinated team approach that involves active participation and encouragement by the physician, diabetes nurse educator, and dietitian. The achievement of normal or near-normal glucose levels requires comprehensive training in self-management and monitoring of blood glucose levels. Continuing education and reinforcement are necessary to ensure that treatment goals are understood and that appropriate attention is given to meal planning, exercise, and therapeutic regimens including the prevention and treatment of hyperglycemia and other acute and chronic complications. Self-glucose monitoring or home glucose monitoring (HGM) of capillary blood glucose is one of the most significant recent developments available to improve glycemic control. This technique enables the patient to be involved in self-management and understand the influence of pharmacologic and nonpharmacologic therapy on blood glucose levels. Because HGM facilitates glycemic control and reinforces adherence to therapy, virtually all diabetic patients should perform HGM with a daily frequency depending on the complexity of the antidiabetic regimen. In patients achieving acceptable control on diet, exercise, and oral hypoglycemic agents, an overnight fasting value alternating with a 2 hour postprandial value may be sufficient. When less than optimal control is achieved or intensive management with oral antidiabetic agents and/or insulin is instituted, four to six daily measurements should be made and recorded. In this situation the recommended times for self-monitoring are before each meal and at bedtime. To assess the glucose response to food intake, intermittent measurements can be made 1 to 2 hours after meals. Measurements should also be made whenever the patient suspects hypoglycemia, including if the patient awakens during the night. The diabetic regimen is adjusted based on HGM results attained on a regular basis. Patients should be educated on how to analyze and respond to HGM data.

Nonpharmacologic Modalities

Nutrition Therapy

Nutrition therapy should be tailored to the individual needs and requirements of the patient. An appropriate diet should account for factors such as age, sex, activity level, degree of obesity, presence of complications, medications, and current nutritional status of the patient. Cultural, ethnic, and socioeconomic status must also be considered when formulating a diet. Following the diagnosis of diabetes, a dietitian or nutritionist should be involved in the management to record a diet history, including lifestyle and eating habits; to review basic principles of diet therapy; and to develop a meal plan. If the fasting glucose level is less than 150 mg per deciliter, diet manipulation alone may be sufficient therapy. When the blood glucose is above this level, patients tend to be symptomatic and diet must usually be combined with pharmacologic therapy. In obese adults with diabetes, caloric restriction and increased physical activity to achieve weight loss, as well as optimal dietary composition, are necessary. Even small amounts of weight loss can have dramatic benefits on metabolic control.

To improve glycemic control, meals should be spaced throughout the day, spreading the calories to allow sufficient time for insulin to be effective. Large caloric loads at any one time tend to produce large glycemic excursions. Considerable controversy continues about the optimal diet composition for adults with diabetes. In the most recent recommendations of the American Diabetes Association, emphasis has been placed on diets that achieve and maintain a reasonable body weight and reduce both blood glucose and cholesterol levels. The basic recommendation is to limit dietary cholesterol to less than 300 mg per day and to restrict saturated fat intake to less than 10 percent of calories and protein to 12 to 20 percent of total daily calories. In contrast with previous recommendations, the absolute intake of carbohydrate and fat in the diet should be based on an individual nutritional assessment and metabolic response to diet. In general, reduction of carbohydrate intake is probably best offset by increasing the content of monounsaturated fat intake such as canola and olive oil.

Exercise

Unless contraindications exist, exercise should be an integral component of the treatment program for adults with diabetes. Exercise increases energy expenditure and enhances the response to dietary and pharmacologic therapy. An exercise program must be individually planned and tailored to meet physical limitations. Many adults with diabetes are sedentary and deconditioned. Therefore, exercise should be started at a low level and gradually increased to limit adverse effects such as physical injury, cardiac problems, or hypoglycemia. Before initiating an exercise program in most adults with diabetes, an exercise stress test should be performed to rule out significant cardiovascular disease or silent ischemia. To avoid hypoglycemia in patients treated with oral antidiabetic agents or insulin, blood glucose should be self-monitored both before and after exercise, with consumption of appropriate snacks, as necessary. A regular exercise routine also minimizes the likelihood of exercise-induced hypoglycemia. Walking, stationary cycling, aerobic water exercises, or lap swimming three to four times per week for 20 to 30 minutes can expend 100 to 200 kcal per session and are safe and effective activities. Any increase in exercise intensity needs to be closely monitored to allow for adjustment of medication. A more intensive program should be managed by a physical therapist knowledgeable in exercise therapy for diabetes.

Pharmacologic Therapies

Oral Antidiabetic Agents: Mechanism of Action

When diet and exercise are unable to maintain plasma glucose levels within the glycemic objectives, oral antidiabetic agents are usually instituted. Oral medication should not be used as a substitute for diet and exercise but as adjunctive therapy. Currently available therapy includes the first-generation and second-generation sulfonylureas and the recently approved biguanide, metformin (Glucophage), and the carbohydrate absorption inhibitor, acarbose (Precose). These three classes of drugs are all effective in the management of glycemia but differ in their mechanism of action. Sulfonylureas work primarily by stimulating pancreatic insulin secretion, whereas the main effect of metformin is to suppress excessive production of glucose by the liver. Acarbose works by delaying the absorption of carbohydrates locally in the gastrointestinal tract and is most effective at reducing the postprandial blood glucose value. Although sulfonylureas tend to cause some weight gain, use of metformin and acarbose in obese adults with NIDDM is reported to result in weight loss or no weight gain. Sulfonylureas are capable of producing severe hypoglycemia, but this side effect is rare with metformin and acarbose when used alone since these agents do not stimulate endogenous insulin secretion. Unlike the previous biguanide, phenformin, which was associated with a substantial incidence of lactic acidosis that led to its withdrawal from clinical use, this complication is uncommon with metformin. The sulfonylureas and metformin should be used with caution when evidence of significant hepatic or renal dysfunction is present. Acarbose is not absorbed systemically and has a better safety profile.

Some of the more commonly used oral antidiabetic agents currently available in the United States are shown in Table 2. There is little difference in the efficacy between first-generation and second-generation sulfonylureas, but the

Table 2 Oral Antidiabetic Agents Commonly Used in NIDDM

AGENT	RECOMMENDED STARTING DOSE (mg)*	RECOMMENDED MAXIMUM DOSE (mg)
Sulfonylureas		
First generation		
Tolazamide	100	1,000
Acetohexamide	250	1,500
Second generation		
Glyburide	2.5	20
Glipizide	5	40
Biguanide		
Metformin	500 b.i.d.†	2,500
Carbohydrate absorption inhibitor		
Acarbose	25 t.i.d.†	300

*Starting dose for elderly and lean adults with diabetes may need to be reduced by up to 50%.
†Dose must be titrated slowly.

first-generation agents are less expensive. The second-generation sulfonylureas are more potent on a per milligram basis and tend to have fewer side effects. These medications should be started at the lowest possible dose and given before breakfast, with progressive increments every 1 to 2 weeks until the desired therapeutic response is achieved. When the daily dose approaches 50 percent or more of the maximum recommended dose, these agents are usually given twice daily, before breakfast and supper. Chlorpropamide (Diabinese) has a very long half-life and can lead to prolonged hypoglycemia especially in the elderly. Chlorpropamide also leads to hyponatremia and can cause the antibuse reaction.

Oral Diabetic Agents: Monotherapy

Now that there are three different classes of oral antidiabetic agents on the U.S. market, initial and combination therapy are not as straightforward as they were when only the sulfonylureas were available. It is important that every patient be evaluated on an individual basis, taking into account many different variables, such as age, body weight, duration of diabetes, presence of dyslipidemia, severity of hyperglycemia, glucose toxicity, and other concomitant conditions. The recommended starting and maximal doses are shown in Table 2.

In patients with newly diagnosed diabetes who are obese and have dyslipidemia, metformin or acarbose therapy would be a good logical choice after failing a 3 month trial of nonpharmacologic maneuvers. Metformin and acarbose both have the advantage of not causing weight gain, a problem often observed with sulfonylurea and insulin therapy. Neither of these agents has an effect on insulin secretion, and hence the risk of hypoglycemia is low. Metformin has the added advantage of lowering the triglyceride and raising the high-density lipoprotein cholesterol levels, in addition to the beneficial effects on the lipoprotein profile that would be expected by improving the glycemic control. When metformin is initiated, it should be titrated up slowly in order to avoid the gastrointestional side effects (500 mg with dinner for 1 week, then twice a day).

If the patient has an elevated serum creatinine (1.5 mg per deciliter or greater in men and 1.4 mg per deciliter in women), metformin should be avoided. Caution should be taken in thin elderly patients with an elevated serum creatinine, but still below the above creatinine limits. In these patients we recommend measuring a creatinine clearance. If the creatinine clearance is below 60 ml per minute, metformin should be avoided or used with extreme caution.

Acarbose may be especially useful in patients with acceptable fasting glucose values, but with elevated glycohemoglobin levels. This scenario would indicate probable excessive postprandial hyperglycemia. HGM 1 to 2 hours after eating would help confirm the need for, and evaluate therapeutic success of, a carbohydrate absorption inhibitor such as acarbose. It is very important to start with a low dose of acarbose and titrate the dose slowly so that the gastrointestinal side effects are avoided (see patient instruction sheet, Table 3).

In nonobese individuals, it is our experience that oral antidiabetic agents have a more variable success rate. It has been reported that as many as 15 percent of these thin individuals may actually have late-onset type 1 IDDM. This would lead to an unsuccessful trial of the different oral agents that commonly is extended over weeks to months. Measuring glutamic acid decarboxylase antibodies may prove to be very useful in identifying these older insulin-dependent diabetics.

In nonobese patients with mild glucose intolerance, a trial with any of the three classes of oral agents would be appropriate. If the patient's glucose values are consistently in the 200 to 300 range, the sulfonylureas or metformin would be indicated because these two agents are more potent than acarbose in lowering the glucose values. These two classes of drugs can also be titrated up more rapidly to the higher dose ranges.

Prolonged severe hyperglycemia or glucose toxicity (prolonged hyperglycemia leading to a worsening of the insulin-resistant state and further impairing beta cell secretory function) is probably the major cause of primary failure of oral antidiabetic agents. Unless the patient concomitantly restricts his or her calorie intake, therapy with oral agents is doomed to fail. Ideally, the patient should be treated with insulin for a few to several weeks before oral agent therapy is attempted. Temporary insulin therapy will reduce glucose toxicity and allow for a better chance of success with oral agents alone. Many clinical trials are now under way to demonstrate that many insulin-requiring NIDDM patients can be weaned off of insulin and be treated with oral agents alone.

Combination Therapy with Oral Antidiabetic Agents

Many patients with type II diabetes will not have adequate glycemic control with monotherapy. The reason a patient fails monotherapy is multifaceted, although one possible explanation is that the patient is undergoing beta cell exhaustion, thus reducing the response to any one agent. Combination therapy with two or more of the oral antidiabetic agents has been used extensively in many countries with excellent results. Each of the different combinations has certain advantages that may be suitable for any given patient. The different combinations

Table 3 Precose (Acarbose) Instruction Sheet

1. You have been given Precose because your blood sugar control needs improvement. Precose is a very safe medication that has been proven to be very effective in improving overall blood sugar control in people with diabetes.
2. Precose works by preventing and delaying the absorption of carbohydrates (sugars) in the gut.
3. Precose works mainly to reduce the rise in blood sugar after eating. Marked elevation in blood sugar after eating is a very common and important problem, which is frequently overlooked.
4. Precose *may* cause you to have flatulence (excess gas), *mild* stomach pain and/or diarrhea. If these side effects occur, it is usually during the first 2 months of starting Precose. For these reasons, it is extremely important to start with a low dose of Precose and increase the dose very slowly.
5. Suggested dosing schedule
   Step 1: Start with 25 mg* with breakfast only for 1 week.
   Step 2: Take 25 mg with breakfast and dinner for 1 week.
   Step 3: Take 25 mg with breakfast, lunch, and dinner for 1 week.
   Step 4: Take 50 mg with breakfast and 25 mg with lunch and dinner for 1 week.
   Step 5: Take 50 mg with breakfast and dinner and 25 mg with lunch for 1 week.
   Step 6: Take 50 mg with breakfast, lunch, and dinner.**
   *Break the 50 mg pill in half or use a pill cutter.
   **Do not increase your dose to 100 mg three times a day until you speak with your caregiver.
6. Do not go to a higher step if you are having bothersome flatulence, stomach pain, or diarrhea. Stay at your current step or go to a lower step until your symptoms improve.
7. It is extremely important to take Precose with the beginning of your meal. Precose will not work to lower your blood sugar if you take it more than 5–10 minutes before you eat.

are discussed below. In general, when monotherapy is failing, addition and not substitution of another oral agent will be necessary to improve metabolic control.

Sulfonylurea and Metformin

Sulfonylureas and metformin have been proven to be a very effective combination. Patients who are failing with maximum doses of either metformin or a sulfonylurea can be given the other medication in combination therapy. No additional benefit is gained by substituting one oral agent for another if the patient is not controlled adequately on a single agent. Some patients may have blood glucose values that are too low (i.e., less than 80 mg per deciliter) during the daytime after beginning combination therapy. In such cases the dose of the sulfonylurea should be lowered to achieve consistent daytime glucose values in a safe range. Metformin will also blunt the weight gain that is seen with the use of sulfonylureas alone. This combination also is the most potent, in terms of lowering the glycosylated hemoglobin, than any other two oral agents used together.

Sulfonylurea and Acarbose

Acarbose and the sulfonylureas also work well together. Acarbose, in a similar fashion as metformin, will blunt the weight gain that is seen with the sulfonylureas when used alone. Acarbose complements the sulfonylureas in this combination because of their unique mechanisms of action to reduce the fasting and postprandial glucose values.

Metformin and Acarbose

Both of these drugs do not cause weight gain or hypoglycemia. Metformin will have a significant effect on the fasting blood glucose whereas acarbose will reduce the postprandial values. These two medications have been used together successfully without excessive gastrointestinal side effects. Clinical trials are currently under way to determine the efficacy and safety of the various combination regimens.

Sulfonylurea, Metformin, and Acarbose

In Europe the combination of all three oral agents is commonly used in clinical practice. All of the oral antidiabetic agents have unique mechanisms of action and potentially can complement the others to improve glycemic control in patients with type II diabetes, thus avoiding insulin therapy. The cost effectiveness of such a regimen has not been determined.

Insulin Therapy

Exogenous insulin therapy should be reserved for patients with NIDDM who have failed other therapeutic modalities such as dietary manipulation, exercise programs, and maximum doses of oral antidiabetic agents. It is apparent from a review of the available literature that there is no one perfect insulin regimen for insulin-requiring type II patients. The success of normalizing the glycosylated hemoglobin with a particular regimen is dependent on numerous variables including the severity of insulin resistance, the extent and type of obesity, endogenous insulin secretory reserves, preceding degree of glucose control, and other complicating medical conditions. Thus, the metabolic success of these different insulin regimens can be quite variable.

The availability of the new oral antidiabetic agents has allowed for the possibility of taking patients with type II diabetes off of insulin. This therapeutic strategy has not been studied, although several trials are under way to try to determine the most effective and safest manner to remove patients with type II diabetes from insulin. In general, if a patient is on less than 40 to 50 U insulin per day, and well controlled, the success of achieving adequate control on oral agents alone is good. Additional clinical characteristics that may indicate success in taking patients off insulin include: (1) duration of diabetes for less than 10 to 15 years; (2) normal or above ideal body weight; (3) glucose toxicity not present, i.e., fasting blood glucose values less than 200 mg per deciliter and/or postprandial blood glucose less than 250 mg per deciliter; and (4) diabetes diagnosed after the age of 35 to

40 years. It is important to emphasize that these characteristics are not written in stone and should be used only as guidelines.

If a patient is on a combination of a daytime oral antidiabetic agent and bedtime insulin, then adding a sulfonylurea, metformin, or acarbose during the day may prove effective. When the new oral agent is started, the patient's insulin dose should be reduced by one-third to one-half depending on the degree of glycemic control at the time of the attempted switch-over. As the dose of the oral agent is increased, usually to the maximum dose, the insulin could be further reduced and eventually discontinued depending on the home glucose readings.

If a patient is on a full insulin regimen, one could attempt to titrate metformin up to 500 mg three times a day while reducing the insulin dose by one-third. The next step would be to increase metformin to 2,500 mg per day while decreasing the insulin dose by another one-third of the total dose. If the glucose control is adequate, the remaining one-third of the insulin dose should be discontinued and the patient's blood glucose values monitored for decompensation. If the home glucose values worsen, or the patient never achieves adequate control on the maximum dose of metformin and one-third of the total insulin dose, add a sulfonylurea, i.e., Glucotrol XL at 2.5 mg per day, and titrate up as necessary. Adding acarbose is also an option if the combination of metformin and a sulfonylurea do not adequately control 24 hour glycemia. One could also start with a sulfonylurea first, then add metformin while titrating the insulin dose downward. To ensure safety, the patient should be reliable, be competent at HGM, and have telephone access to his or her caregiver.

Combination Therapy

Combination therapy usually refers to the use of oral antidiabetic agents together with a single injection of intermediate-acting insulin at bedtime. The underlying tenet for combination therapy assumes that if evening insulin lowers the fasting glucose level to normal by suppressing hepatic glucose output, the daytime sulfonylureas will be more effective at maintaining euglycemia throughout the day.

Patient selection is very important when considering combination therapy. The question of whether a patient is still responding in a satisfactory manner to oral agents is of primary importance. Patients have a higher likelihood of success using daytime sulfonylureas and bedtime insulin if they are obese, have had overt diabetes for less than 10 to 15 years, are diagnosed with NIDDM after the age of 35, and have glucose values less than 250 to 300 mg per deciliter consistently.

Combination therapy can be beneficial for a number of practical reasons. The patient does not need to learn how to mix different types of insulin, hospitalization is not required, and patient compliance and acceptance are better with a single injection of insulin than with multiple injections of insulin. Combination therapy also requires a lower total dose of exogenous insulin than a two- or three-injection-a-day regimen. This usually contributes to less weight gain and peripheral hyperinsulinemia. Calculation of the initial bedtime intermediate-acting insulin dose can be based on clinical judgment or by various formulas based on the fasting

VA Endocrinology Clinic Patient Self-Adjustment of Evening Insulin

1. Begin with a dose of _____ units of NPH insulin administered just before bedtime.
2. If the prebreakfast blood sugar is greater than 140 mg/dl for 3 days in a row, then increase the evening NPH insulin dose by _____ units.
3. If the prebreakfast blood sugar is less than 100 mg/dl for 2 days in a row, then decrease the evening NPH insulin by _____ units.
4. Remember not to increase the insulin dose more frequently than every 3 days.
5. If you have any questions, please call me at
_______________________________ .
6. Provider's name: _______________________

____
Physician/Nurse Practitioner

Figure 1
Patient's self-adjustment form for evening insulin therapy. Reliable patients properly educated in HGM techniques can safely and efficiently adjust insulin doses at home based on HGM results. Patients' self-adjustment can allow for a more rapid time course to achieve normoglycemia and reduce physician and staff workload.

blood glucose level or body weight. For example, one can divide the average fasting blood glucose (mg/dl) by 18 or divide the body weight in kilograms by 10 to calculate the initial dose of NPH or Lente insulin to be started at bedtime (ideally between 10:00 PM and midnight). One can also safely start 5 to 10 U of intermediate-acting insulin for thin patients and 10 to 15 U for obese patients at bedtime as an initial estimated dose. In both cases the dose is increased in 2 to 5 U increments every 3 to 4 days until the morning fasting blood glucose level is consistently in the 70 to 140 mg per deciliter range. Reliable patients can be instructed to make their own adjustments using HGM (Fig. 1). It is recommended that the patient stay on his or her maximal dose of oral antidiabetic agent. However, if the daytime blood glucose levels start to become excessively low, then the dose of oral medication must be adjusted downward. When the fasting blood glucose is brought under control, the success of combination therapy is dependent on the ability of the daytime oral antidiabetic agents to maintain euglycemia. If this cannot be achieved, then the oral hypoglycemic agents should be stopped and conventional insulin regimens employed.

Multiple Injections Regimens

One of the most common insulin regimens utilized in patients with NIDDM is the split-mixed combination, consisting of a prebreakfast and predinner dose of an intermediate-acting and fast-acting insulin. In most cases, single injection therapy with an intermediate-acting or long-acting insulin has been shown to be inadequate to normalize glycosylated hemoglobin and maintain 24 hour euglycemia in patients with NIDDM. The literature also supports the concept that there is no added benefit of a three- or four-dose insulin regimen over

Table 4 Stepwise Approach to Initiate a Split-Mixed Regimen in Type II Diabetes

1. First Goal: Fasting CBG 4.5–6.5 mM
   - Initial dose of NPH insulin 0.2 U/kg before dinner
   - Change dose of evening NPH insulin based on subsequent fasting CBG as follows: >9.5 mM—increase by 0.5 U/kg; 6.5–9.5 mM—increase by 0.05 U/kg; 4.5–6.5 mM—no change in dose; <4.5 mM—decrease by 0.1 U/kg.
2. Second Goal: Presupper CBG 4.5–6.5 mM
   - Initial dose of NPH insulin before breakfast and criteria for adjustment identical to first goal except based on subsequent pre-supper CBG.
   - Proceed to third goal only after first and second goals are achieved.
3. Third Goal: Postprandial (2 h) CBG <9.5 mM (after breakfast and supper)
   - Change each dose of regular insulin based on subsequent postprandial (2 h) CBG as follows: >9.5 mM—increase by 0.025 U/kg; 6.5–9.5 mM—no change in dose; 4.5–6.5 mM—decrease by 0.025 U/kg; <4.5 mM—decrease by 0.05 U/kg.
   - All injections were given subcutaneously in the periumbilical region 30 minutes before breakfast and dinner.

CBG, Capillary blood glucose.
Henry et al. With permission of the American Diabetes Association.

a conventional split-mixed regimen in obese patients with NIDDM failing oral antidiabetic agents.

There are a number of important aspects of insulin therapy in obese patients with NIDDM failing sulfonylurea therapy. First, the average daily dose of insulin needed to control such patients will approximate 1 U per kilogram body weight. Second, the total daily insulin requirement can successfully be split equally between the prebreakfast and predinner injections consisting of 70 percent intermediate-acting and 30 percent fast-acting insulin. Third, the split-mixed regimen in patients with NIDDM is usually devoid of the problems such as overnight hypoglycemia and fasting hyperglycemia that are commonly observed with this regimen in IDDM. Fourth, a regimen of two shots per day is equally effective as a three- or four-shot-per-day regimen. Finally, severe and mild hypoglycemic events are much less frequent in patients with NIDDM undergoing insulin therapy than in patients with IDDM.

There are several acceptable methods to initiate insulin therapy in NIDDM. A conservative yet effective strategy utilizing a stepwise approach to institute a split-mixed regimen begins with NPH prebreakfast and predinner and then later adding regular to control the prelunch and bedtime glucose values (Table 4).

A simple alternative method to initiate a split-mixed regimen in obese patients with NIDDM would be to use a premixed insulin with an initial total daily insulin dose (0.4 to 0.8 U per kilogram) equally split between the prebreakfast and predinner meals. Adjustments are then made on HGM results, which may dictate the need to change the ratio of intermediate-acting to regular-acting insulin either upward or downward. For morbidly obese patients, the insulin requirements rise almost exponentially as the percent ideal body weight increases above 150 percent. In contrast, caution should be used when starting thin patients with NIDDM on insulin, especially premixed insulins with fixed doses of regular insulin (initial total daily dose 0.2 to 0.5 U per kilogram). This group tends to be more sensitive to the glucose lowering effects and thus more prone to severe hypoglycemia. If a multiple insulin injection regimen is to be initiated, Ultralente should be used to provide a steady basal rate of insulin bioavailability. This component should constitute approximately 50 to 60 percent of the total daily insulin requirements. Premeal boluses of regular insulin are also given with adjustments based on the 2 hour postprandial blood glucose measurements.

Insulin Infusion Pumps

Continuous subcutaneous insulin infusion (CSII) pumps have been used primarily for patients with IDDM. At present, there is a paucity of clinical trials using CSII in patients with NIDDM. Although some studies demonstrate metabolic benefits of CSII in patients with NIDDM, they are all limited by their relatively short duration of evaluation and small numbers of heterogeneous subjects. However, an external insulin pump can be benefical in any NIDDM failing exogenous insulin regimens.

Implantable programmable variable rate pumps with intraperitoneal insulin delivery are currently being evaluated in patients with type I and type II diabetes mellitus. The major advantage of implantable over subcutaneous infusion pumps is the more physiologic absorption of the delivered insulin. The implantable insulin pump is surgically placed below the subcutaneous fat just above the rectus sheath in the abdominal area, and only the distal portion of the catheter is placed through the rectus sheath in order to float freely in the peritoneal cavity. The majority of insulin delivered into the peritoneal cavity drains to the liver via the portal vein where hepatic extraction (approximately 50 percent) occurs before the insulin is delivered to the systemic circulation. This results in lower peripheral insulin levels and is more rapidly and predictably absorbed than subcutaneously delivered insulin with direct effects on the liver. Implantable pumps should be available in the near future.

Benefits and Risks of Insulin Therapy

The potential benefits of normoglycemia in NIDDM are numerous. As hyperglycemia is diminished, many acute complications such as excessive thirst, nocturia, sleep disturbances, poor wound healing, and generalized lack of well-being improve. In addition, because the pathophysiologic basis for microvascular complications is due to hyperglycemia, a decline in the incidence and severity of retinopathy, nephropathy, and neuropathy may be expected in patients with NIDDM with improved long-term glycemic control.

Insulin therapy, similar to any form of pharmacologic or

nonpharmacologic modalities that reduce hyperglycemia, improves the dyslipidemia of type II diabetes. These therapies work primarily by reducing free fatty acids and glucose levels, which are substrates for triglyceride production. Despite the development of hyperinsulinemia, insulin therapy has also been shown to induce antiatherogenic changes in the lipoprotein composition of patients with NIDDM. This results not only by improving glycemic control, but also by stimulating lipoprotein lipase activity. Intensive insulin therapy may also reduce the amount of protein-rich or small and dense low-density lipoprotein as well as glycosylation and oxidation of lipoproteins. These changes could have favorable effects on the cardiovascular risk profile.

Weight Gain

A rise in endogenous and exogenous insulin increases the risk of hypoglycemia and leads to marked increases in weight. Not only has hyperinsulinemia been found to occur more frequently in centrally obese individuals but this obese subpopulation is also at increased risk for cardiovascular disease. Several studies have brought attention to the risk factors associated with differences in body fat distribution and the evidence linking central or abdominal obesity with cardiovascular disease. The lowering of blood glucose to normal levels usually requires large doses of exogenous insulin, resulting in hyperinsulinemia and weight gain. Therefore, attention must be focused on the association between hyperinsulinemia and obesity and the potential atherogenicity of both when considering the institution of insulin therapy in NIDDM.

Numerous studies previously cited have demonstrated that treatment of type II diabetes with exogenous insulin resulted in an average increase in pretreatment body weight of between 3 and 9 percent depending on the length of the study and the intensity of glucose control. Development of weight gain during exogenous insulin therapy is a serious clinical problem. The degree of obesity usually dictates the amount of exogenous insulin required to achieve normal glycemia and thus the propensity for weight gain. Excessive weight gain can be minimized by utilizing the lowest dose of insulin possible to achieve the desired glycemic goals and by educating the patient regarding proper diet, exercise, and appropriate caloric response to hypoglycemia.

Hypoglycemia

Intensive insulin therapy brings with it an increased risk of hypoglycemic reactions. Severe hypoglycemia is usually defined as the inability to self-treat with a need for the assistance of others to properly administer therapy. On reviewing the literature, most studies report on the incidence of severe, rather than mild, hypoglycemia, because severe hypoglycemia is a more objective and definitive finding that does not tend to be over-reported. It is also important to recognize that neuroglycopenia can masquerade as a neurologic or cardiovascular event and thus go unrecognized.

The development of severe hypoglycemia is dependent on numerous variables, which makes evaluation of risk factors and comparison of different study results difficult. The duration of diabetes and insulin therapy, the degree of glycemic control, and a history of prior severe hypoglycemic reactions have all been associated with a higher incidence of severe hypoglycemic reactions. Additional recognized causal factors for hypoglycemia include overinsulinization, underfeeding, strenuous unplanned exercise, excessive alcohol intake, and hypoglycemia unawareness.

The risk of severe hypoglycemia in insulin-requiring NIDDM patients has consistently been reported to be significantly reduced compared to insulin-dependent diabetic patients undergoing intensive insulin therapy. Recent studies of intensive insulin therapy confirm that the risk of severe hypoglycemic reactions in NIDDM patients is low and of several orders of magnitude less than in IDDM patients.

The lower incidence of severe hypoglycemia in NIDDM patients may be best explained by the presence of insulin resistance, which is often quite severe. It is interesting to note that an inverse relationship has been reported between body mass index and the incidence of hypoglycemia in NIDDM patients, suggesting that the obese insulin-resistant state may protect against the development of insulin-induced hypoglycemia. Other investigators have hypothesized that NIDDM patients may not be fundamentally different but have less hypoglycemia principally because they tend to receive less aggressive diabetes management and have been treated with insulin for a shorter duration of time than IDDM patients. Regardless of the reasons, it appears that NIDDM patients receiving aggressive insulin therapy are less prone to severe hypoglycemia than are IDDM patients.

DIABETIC KETOACIDOSIS AND HYPERGLYCEMIC HYPEROSMOLAR COMA

Saul M. Genuth, M.D.

Diabetic coma comprises a spectrum of serious and sometimes lethal metabolic decompensation ranging from pure diabetic ketoacidosis (DKA) to nonketotic hyperglycemic hyperosmolar coma (HHC). About one-third of cases can be considered mixed because both a degree of hyperosmolarity sufficient to cause central nervous system dysfunction and significant ketosis are present. The pathogeneses of DKA and HHC have fundamental similarities; the differences largely reflect a functionally lesser degree of insulin deficiency and greater degree of dehydration in HHC. In a modern series of approximately 500 cases of DKA, overall mortality rate was 5 percent, and that ascribable to the metabolic disturbance alone was 0.2 percent. Mortality in HHC is on the order of 20 to 30 percent. Although most deaths are from serious concurrent illness such as sepsis, death from DKA and HHC can occur from therapeutic errors. This danger underscores the continuing importance of basing treatment on a firm understanding of pathophysiology.

■ DIABETIC KETOACIDOSIS

Pathophysiology

Regardless of whether DKA is the presenting mode of new-onset insulin-dependent diabetes mellitus (IDDM) or is a recurrent episode in a previously treated patient, the critical abnormality is insulin deficiency (Fig. 1). This is the case even if the usual insulin doses have been taken and the plasma free insulin level appears to be in the normal fasting range or even elevated. This is because the insulin level is never appropriate for the concurrent degree of hyperglycemia. However, secondary to insulin deficiency itself, to dehydration, and often to precipitating medical stresses are simultaneous elevations in the plasma levels of all the insulin antagonistic hormones. These include glucagon, epinephrine, and norepinephrine; growth hormone; and cortisol. These hormones, along with elevated free fatty acids, acidosis, and hypertonicity, add an important—though not overwhelming—element of insulin resistance. Aldosterone and antidiuretic hormone levels are also elevated in response to dehydration and hyperosmolarity.

The extreme lack of insulin action is manifest by: (1) excessive hepatic glucose production resulting from increased glycogenolysis and gluconeogenesis; (2) decreased glucose clearance by peripheral tissues, both of which lead to hyperglycemia and hyperosmolarity; (3) excessive adipose tissue lipolysis and free fatty acid delivery to the liver, leading to heightened ketogenesis and hyperketonemia (i.e., high plasma levels of beta-hydroxybutyrate and acetoacetate) and often to hypertriglyceridemia, as well; (4) increased muscle proteolysis and diminished protein synthesis, leading to catabolic transfer of amino acids, potassium, phosphate, and magnesium from the intracellular to the extracellular fluid with consequent loss of nitrogen and these electrolytes in the urine.

Hyperglycemia in excess of the renal threshold causes osmotic diuresis with loss of water in excess of sodium, hypovolemia, and decreased glomerular filtration rate. Reduction in the filtered load of glucose by the kidney significantly aggravates the hyperglycemia. Vomiting and increased insensible loss of water because of hyperventilation add to the state of hypotonic dehydration. Hyperketonemia causes an anion gap metabolic acidosis. The resultant ketonuria adds to the osmotic diuresis and causes additional losses of sodium, potassium, calcium, and magnesium as buffering cations for the urinary excretion of the relatively strong ketoacids. Hyperkalemia is common because of insulinopenia and accelerated release of intracellular potassium generated by protein and glycogen breakdown (see Fig. 1). Hyperkalemia is further driven by extracellular acidosis and by the phenomenon of solvent drag as extracellular fluid hyperosmolarity attracts water from the intracellular space.

Diagnosis

The resulting laboratory picture is so characteristic as to make the diagnosis almost always obvious. A urine dipstick will be strongly positive for glucose and ketones. Analysis of blood will reveal the following values (average and typical range): glucose, 600 mg per deciliter (250–2,000); semiquantitative ketones by Acetest tablet or ketosticks, positive 1:16 (1:4–1:64); beta-hydroxy-butyrate plus acetoacetate 12 mM (6–20); pH, 7.15 (6.80–7.30); HCO_3^-, 10 mEq per liter (4–15). PCO_2, 20 mm Hg (14–26). The calculated anion gap $[Na^+-(Cl^-+HCO_3^-)]$ is generally greater than 18 mEq per liter and the excess above the average normal of 12 mEq per liter is approximately equal to the decrement in HCO_3^-. Serum sodium is usually modestly low or low-normal, but when it is corrected for the hyperglycemia it may be normal or even slightly elevated.

Corrected sodium =

$$\frac{\text{measured sodium} + 1.6 \times \text{plasma glucose in mg/dl} - 100}{100}$$

or

$$\frac{\text{measured sodium} + 1.6 \times \text{plasma glucose in mMol/L} - 5.5}{5.5}$$

Serum effective osmolality ($2 \times Na^+ + \frac{\text{glucose in mg/dl}}{18}$) averages 300 (285–340). Serum potassium will usually be normal to modestly elevated, masking the total body potassium depletion. Other causes of ketoacidosis such as total starvation, ethanol, paraldehyde, or isopropyl alcohol intoxication, or glucose-6-phosphatase deficiency, are apparent from history, screening for toxins, and absence of hyperglycemia.

Exceptional circumstances may modify the above findings. In 1 percent of patients, plasma glucose may be normal if prior to presentation insulin has been taken in normal or

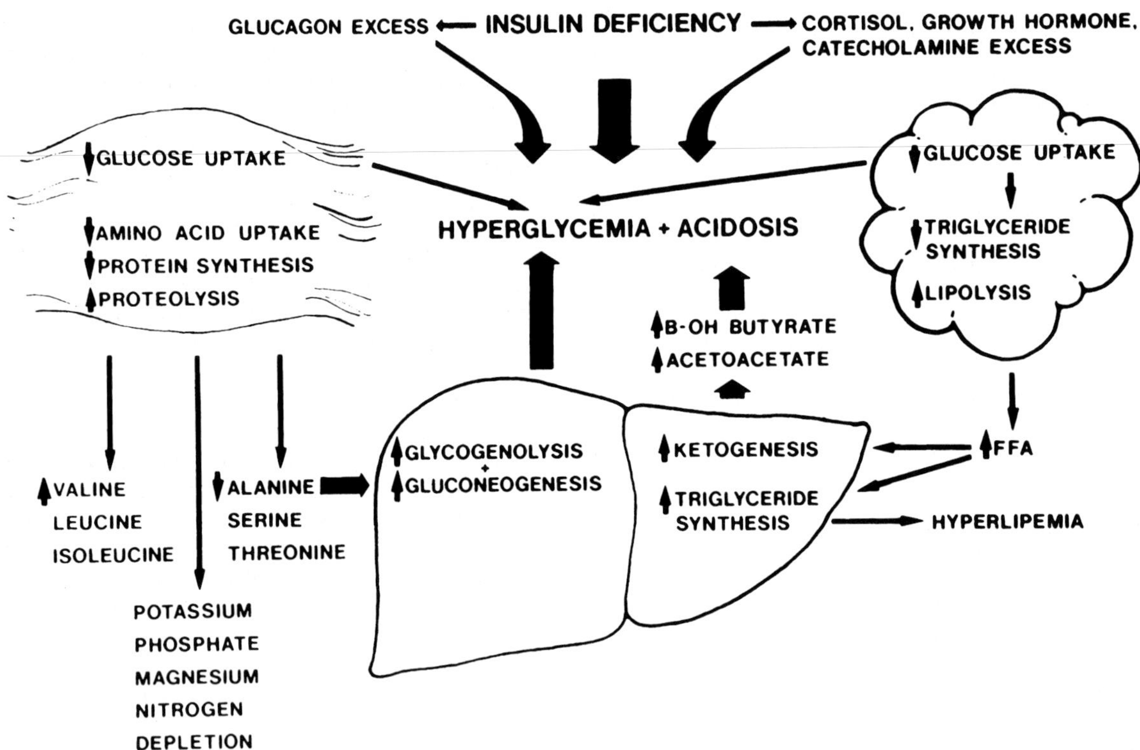

Figure 1
The pathogenesis of diabetic ketoacidosis is depicted. FFA, free fatty acids. *(From Genuth S. Diabetic ketoacidosis. In: Podolsky S, ed. Clinical diabetes: Modern management. New York: Appleton & Lange, 1980:173; with permission.)*

increased amounts without concurrent carbohydrate, or if there is coexisting alcoholism. Ketones that current routine tests detect only as acetoacetate and acetone may be missing from the urine or serum if the redox potential of the patient is very high as in alcohol intoxication or shock. This shifts the equilibrium of the ketoacids far toward the reduced partner beta-hydroxybutyrate. Application of a newly available clinical laboratory measurement of beta-hydroxybutyrate should detect such cases readily, however. HCO_3^- levels may be normal and Pco_2 normal or elevated if there is coexisting respiratory acidosis. The decrement in HCO_3^- may be less than the increase in the anion gap, and the pH may be normal if there is coexistent chronic metabolic alkalosis attributable to diuretic ingestion, pernicious vomiting, or excessive mineralocorticoid action. Occasionally, hyperchloremic acidosis rather than anion gap acidosis (or a mixture of the two) is seen if ketoacids have been cleared by the kidney at a very rapid rate. A Pco_2 lower than predicted from the pH or serum HCO_3^- for a pure metabolic acidosis ($Pco_2 = 1.5 \times HCO_3^- + 8$) suggests a superimposed respiratory alkalosis, possibly caused by sepsis.

Clinical Assessment

The degree of dehydration is most accurately judged by comparing the admission weight, which should always be obtained, with a recent known dry weight. Quantitative estimates of extracellular or total body fluid deficits based on lying or standing blood pressure and pulse, skin turgor, neck veins, and eyeball softness have never been validated in DKA. Supine hypotension probably indicates at least 10 percent dehydration, shock even more. A corrected serum sodium (see the section Diagnosis) that is above normal and a high blood urea nitrogen (BUN) indicate a large volume deficit. Very obvious Kussmaul's breathing suggests an unusually low Pco_2 and pH. Because infection, especially respiratory or urinary, is a frequent precipitant, a thorough history and physical examination with chest x-ray and other appropriate radiologic examinations should always follow the initial rapid emergency assessment. Fever most often indicates infection, but because hypothermia has been described consequent to DKA itself, absence of fever does not rule out infection. On the other hand, leukocytosis up to 20,000 white blood cells per cubic millimeter with neutrophilia is common, may be secondary to the dehydration, and does not itself indicate infection unless the percentage of bands is increased. The somnolent patient should be checked for meningeal signs, and a lumbar puncture, preceded by a computed tomography (CT) scan of the head, should be performed if there is any suspicion of meningitis. The nasal turbinates and palate should be scrutinized for necrotic lesions of mucormycosis. Sinusitis secondary to candidiasis or aspergillosis can also occur. Appendicitis, diverticulitis, cholecystitis, or pelvic inflammatory disease should be considered in the patient with abdominal pain; rectal and pelvic examinations should not be omitted because of the metabolic emergency. Serum amylase and even lipase can be nonspecifically elevated and should not be taken by themselves to prove the presence of pancreatitis. White blood cells in the urine may suggest gram-negative sepsis as well as a urinary tract infection. In older patients, acute myocardial

Table 1 Monitoring the Patient in DKA or HHC

1. Weigh on admission and q6–12 h
2. Record cumulatively intake and output q1–2 h (Foley catheter if incontinent).
3. Check blood pressure, pulse, respiration, mental status q1–2 hr and temperature q8 h.
4. Check blood (fingerstick) or plasma (laboratory) glucose q1–2 hr.
5. Check serum potassium q2–4 h; other electrolytes and serum ketones q4 hr.
6. Check arterial blood pH and gases on admission (in children, venous pH may be substituted; add 0.1 to result). If pH <7.0 on admission, recheck prn until pH exceeds 7.1.
7. Check serum phosphate, magnesium, calcium on admission; if low, repeat q4 hr; otherwise, q8–12 h.
8. Spot check all voidings for ketones and glucose.
9. Perform ECG on admission; repeat if follow-up serum potassium is abnormal or unavailable.
10. Perform complete blood count, blood urea nitrogen, creatinine, urinalysis, appropriate cultures, chest radiography.

All of the above should be carried out until the patient is stable, glucose levels have reached and are maintained at 250 mg per deciliter, and acidosis is largely reversed. An intensive care setting is preferred.

infarction—occasionally without chest pain—is an important precipitant of DKA. In patients using insulin infusion pumps, interruption of delivery can lead to DKA with dangerous hyperkalemia within 12 hours.

Treatment

Whenever possible, treatment of more than mild DKA is best provided in an intensive care unit. There, the desirable clinical observation; vital signs and fluid status monitoring; frequent serum biochemical measurements; and rapid changes in insulin, fluid, and electrolyte administration can be optimally carried out (Table 1). Wherever DKA is treated, however, a written protocol should be available. The use of formal critical care pathways or CareMaps may enhance cost effectiveness.

Insulin

Insulin therapy is now founded on a knowledge of the responsiveness of its target tissues to various doses and on its metabolic clearance rate (approximately 12 ml per kilogram per minute). Lipolysis is inhibited by an insulin concentration of 5 µU per milliliter, proteolysis by 10 µU per milliliter, and hepatic glucose production by 20 µU per milliliter, whereas peripheral glucose utilization is not maximally stimulated by insulin until a concentration of at least 100 µU per milliliter is achieved. All of these insulin actions are desired in treatment of DKA, although inhibition of free fatty acid and glucose release is the most important. To allow for the usual state of moderate insulin resistance, I prefer to maintain a peripheral insulin concentration of 200 µU per milliliter. This is most readily and reliably achieved by an intravenous infusion of regular insulin with a pump at a rate of 10 U per hour (e.g., 200 U per liter at 50 ml per hour). An initial 10 U intravenous bolus, though not strictly necessary, ensures immediate establishment of a therapeutic level while an infusion is being prepared and other measures taken. In adults it is not wise to initiate treatment with less than 5 U per hour. In children a dose of 0.1 U per kilogram per hour gives satisfactory results. If facilities for intravenous insulin infusion are not available, an intravenous bolus of 10 U and doses of 10 U regular insulin IM or SC every hour will eventually achieve the same plateau plasma insulin concentrations. However, this is not advisable for a patient in shock. An average fall in plasma glucose of approximately 75 mg per deciliter per hour is expected, some of which is accounted for by initial rapid rehydration. If no response is evident within 2 hours, one may be dealing with an unusual degree of insulin resistance. Although many authorities recommend doubling the insulin dose every hour or two until response is evident, I prefer increasing the rate of insulin infusion fivefold to tenfold to 50 to 100 U per hour and doubling this every 2 hours thereafter if plasma glucose does not quickly fall. This is to allow for the very rare but endangered patient who has extraordinary insulin resistance and may need thousands of units to recover. So long as serum potassium is carefully monitored, more aggressive insulin doses are safe. Recent experimental reports suggest that administration of insulin-like growth factor as a substitute for insulin or the somatostatin analogue octreotide to decrease secretion of insulin antagonists may be of use in refractory cases.

In a routine case, insulin should be infused at 10 U per hour (or 0.1 U per kilogram) until plasma glucose has decreased to approximately 250 mg per deciliter, and continued until the anion gap has also decreased to near normal (12 to 15 mEq per liter) and serum bicarbonate has increased to at least 15 to 18 mEq per liter. Usually, serum ketones will also have decreased significantly by then, unless acetoacetate and acetone have accumulated to a large extent. If available, blood or plasma beta-hydroxybutyrate measurement should have fallen to less than 2 to 3 mmol per liter by this time. The insulin infusion rate can then be lowered to 2 U per hour (0.02 U per kilogram per hour in children) and individually adjusted along with 5 percent glucose in replacement fluids to maintain plasma glucose around 200 mg per deciliter and to prevent hypoglycemia. This is continued until the patient feels well enough to drink and eat. One to 2 hours before stopping the infusion, it is mandatory to give the adult patient 5 to 10 U (and a weight-adjusted amount for a child) of regular insulin subcutaneously. It is a common mistake not to do so because plasma glucose levels seem satisfactory. However, intravenous insulin has a plasma half-life of only 6 to 8 minutes and a biologic half-life of 30 to 45 minutes, so that failure to give subcutaneous insulin promptly will initiate a recurrence of hyperglycemia and ketosis. Additional 5 to 10 U doses of regular insulin should continue to be given proactively every 4 to 6 hours until it is convenient to either begin or to resume previously prescribed longer-acting insulin as well. The latter can ordinarily be done the morning following recovery from DKA.

Fluids and Electrolytes

Volume repletion is as important as insulin therapy and should be started immediately on suspicion of DKA, even before insulin, while the diagnosis is being ascertained. Indeed, patients without complications can survive for 24 hours and lower their serum glucose levels 200 to 300 mg per deciliter without insulin, if given adequate intravenous fluids and electrolytes. By contrast, if insulin is given without adequate fluids, the fall in extracellular glucose and osmolality causes a shift of fluid from the intravascular space into the intracellular space. This can exacerbate hypotension or even cause vascular collapse.

Repletion of fluids and electrolytes has two goals and two phases. The first goal is restoration of the circulating volume so that in this rapid phase of treatment isotonic fluid is needed. In general, 0.9 percent NaCl is quite adequate for this purpose, though Ringer's lactate can also be used. One liter should be given in the first ½ hour and a second liter in the ensuing ½ to 1 hour, depending on the presenting clinical state of dehydration. For children, 20 ml per kilogram or 500 ml per square meter per hour should be used in this phase. The faster rates are dictated by hypotension; with its persistence, a third or fourth rapid liter of 0.9 percent NaCl may be needed in adults. A colloidal volume expander should be given to patients in shock. At the opposite extreme, in adults with moderate dehydration, 500 ml of 0.9 percent NaCl per hour for 4 hours followed by 500 ml of 0.45 percent NaCl per hour for 4 hours has been reported to be effective.

The second goal is to replace intracellular and total body fluid losses, and this phase is carried out more gradually, usually over about 12 hours in adults. Because the average losses of water and sodium are in one-half isotonic proportions (10 ml per kilogram and 7 mEq Na^+ per kilogram), 0.45 percent NaCl is appropriate for this later phase. In adults the needed rates range from 150 to 500 ml per hour; and this must be individually based on initial estimates of the degree of dehydration, age, and cardiac and renal status. A continuing positive fluid balance should be documented (see Table 1), because urinary losses from the osmotic diuresis will continue until plasma glucose levels have been brought down to the renal threshold of approximately 200 mg per milliliter. The ultimate positive balance in adults *averages* 6 liters. If cardiac function is compromised or renal failure is present, central pressure monitoring with a Swan-Ganz right-heart catheter may be necessary.

In children, the vulnerability to cerebral edema has suggested to some the wisdom of a slower rate of replacement and a slower shift to hypotonic fluids, incomplete replacement of ongoing urine losses, a limitation of 4 L per square meter per 24 hours, and complete replacement—including maintenance estimates—over 48 hours. This subject remains controversial, but a range of rates of 3 to 6 ml per kilogram per hour seems reasonable in children, and, at recovery, average weight gains of 7 to 8 percent can be expected. In children under age 2, higher free water maintenance requirements dictate a lower average sodium concentration in replacement fluids. In small children, very close monitoring and frequent changes of individually tailored fluid rates and compositions are essential to achieving the best outcomes.

Once plasma glucose reaches 250 mg per deciliter, replacement fluids should contain 5 percent glucose. This is given in 0.45 percent NaCl or, in the later phases where more free water may be needed, in 0.2 percent NaCl or in water. The choice of sodium concentration depends on how much sodium was given in the rapid phase and the subsequent serum sodium levels. The higher the corrected serum sodium becomes, the more free water should be given. The use of 10 percent glucose solutions may decrease ketoacid levels slightly faster but has clinical benefit only when plasma glucose falls much more rapidly than ketoacids, e.g., in alcoholics with markedly depleted liver glycogen stores. Ice chips may be given in the later phase for comfort. In circumstances where intravenous fluids cannot be administered and the patient is conscious and not vomiting, World Health Organization oral rehydration salt therapy at 1 L per hour has been reported to be effective.

Potassium

No element of DKA management is more important than potassium replacement, because a major error can lead to death from hypokalemia or, much less commonly, hyperkalemia. Serum potassium is usually normal or increased on admission; higher levels correlate with rapid onset of DKA, lower pH, higher serum osmolality, and higher BUN. The average deficit of potassium is of the order of 5 mEq per kilogram, but this may be much greater if the admission serum potassium is less than 4.0 mEq per liter or if the patient has ben in DKA for more than 24 hours. The goal of intravenous potassium replacement is not total body repletion but to maintain serum potassium above 3.5 mEq per liter, a level that should prevent fatal cardiac arrhythmias or respiratory failure. Total potassium repletion can be completed once DKA is over and oral intake is resumed.

Serum potassium decreases as soon as insulin action begins; hence, potassium administration should begin after the initial liter of 0.9 percent saline has been administered and as soon as serum potassium is known to be less than 6.0 mEq per liter and urine flow is documented. This should not be delayed more than 1 to 2 hours after insulin has been administered. The urgency of administering potassium cannot be overemphasized; life-threatening hypokalemia has been reported within 2 hours of initiating insulin in rare cases. If for any reason a serum potassium determination cannot be obtained promptly, a normal baseline electrocardiogram will give considerable assurance that dangerous hyperkalemia is not present. However, anuria or marked oliguria calls for extreme caution.

The required rate of replacement of potassium usually ranges from 10 to 40 mEq per hour. If the admitting serum potassium is less than 3.5 mEq per liter, the total deficit is enormous and 60 to 80 mEq per hour will be needed initially. In addition, insulin should be temporarily withheld until serum potassium is greater than 4.0 mEq per liter. A concentration of potassium chloride up to 40 mEq per liter in replacement fluids is generally tolerated by peripheral veins. If bicarbonate is administered, extra potassium is indicated (see the section Bicarbonate). Initially, potassium is given as the chloride. Later it may be given as potassium phosphate, remembering that each mmol of phosphate (31 mg phosphorus) provides 1.5 mEq potassium. Reliance should not be placed on oral potassium preparations until DKA is reversed. Serum potassium should be monitored every 2 hours until the insulin infusion rate is lowered (see the section Insulin) and every 4 to 6 hours thereafter until the patient has resumed oral intake. Although serial electrocardiograms (ECGs) can provide some assessment of potassium status (flattened T waves and the presence of U waves indicating hypokalemia), discrepancies and/or misinterpretations are possible, so the ECG can supplement but should not substitute routinely for direct measurement of serum potassium.

Bicarbonate

Insulin treatment alone will gradually eliminate the metabolic acidosis as lipolysis and ketogenesis are inhibited. Although this takes longer than does the reversal of hyperglycemia, blood pH can be expected to normalize over 12 to 24 hours. Furthermore, the routine addition of sodium bicarbonate to replacement fluids has not been shown to accelerate the insulin-induced fall in plasma glucose or ketoacid levels in several randomized studies, even when pH was as low as 6.9. Therefore, bicarbonate is not needed as standard therapy in the vast majority of DKA cases. There are, however, situations where the severity of the metabolic acidosis per se is immediately harmful or dangerous to the patient and where bicarbonate therapy may be advisable.

1. Severe hyperkalemia with characteristic ECG changes (tall, peaked T waves, widened QRS) on admission is an indication for administration of bicarbonate with insulin.
2. Hypotension that does not respond to aggressive infusion of 0.9 percent NaCl or plasma expanders may be caused by an inhibition of vascular responsiveness to catecholamines by acidosis. Such patients may be in "warm shock," and their arteriolar tone and blood pressure may be improved by raising the pH.
3. Left ventricular failure can also result from severe acidosis and may improve with bicarbonate infusion.
4. Deep coma, though largely caused by hyperosmolarity, may be contributed to by a very low pH.
5. A pH less than 7.0 and/or a plasma bicarbonate less than 5.0 mEq per liter indicate a patient with little if any buffering reserve. A slight reduction in compensatory hyperventilation or a small increase in ketoacid or lactic acid production could produce a further catastrophic drop in pH. Bicarbonate should be given to raise pH to 7.1 to 7.2 and/or bring HCO_3^- to 10 to 12 mEq per liter. (The theoretic dose required to increase HCO_3^- from 4 to 10 mEq per liter in a typical 70 kg adult $= 0.4 \times 70 \times (10 - 4) = 168$ mEq.)

If required by any of the above circumstances, sodium bicarbonate should be given promptly. Ampules of 50 to 100 mEq added to 500 to 1,000 ml 0.45 percent saline, respectively, yield slightly hypertonic solutions that can be administered over 30 to 60 minutes in adults. The lower the pH, the larger the bicarbonate dose should be. In left ventricular failure or in hyperkalemia, a 44 mEq dose can be injected directly intravenously over 15 minutes. The arterial pH should then be rechecked, and if less than 7.1 a second dose of bicarbonate should be given. Once undertaken, treatment should be carried through until the pH has risen to at least 7.1 to 7.2. More aggressive therapy may be dangerous. The main risk of bicarbonate therapy is induction of severe hyperkalemia, as potassium enters the cells in exchange for hydrogen ion. Therefore, unless the patient was hyperkalemic at the outset, at least an extra 10 mEq potassium should be administered with each 50 mEq dose of bicarbonate. There are other theoretic disadvantages to bicarbonate treatment. As P_{CO_2} and HCO_3^- rise in blood, central nervous system (CNS) acidosis may worsen from the more rapid diffusion of CO_2 than HCO_3^- into the cerebrospinal fluid (CFS). A decrease in tissue O_2 delivery could result as the rise in pH shifts the oxyhemoglobin dissociation curve to the left. Alkalinization also stimulates ketoacid production. However, none of these potential adverse effects has proven to be of clinical significance.

In the recovery phase of DKA, a state of nonanion gap hyperchloremic acidosis commonly develops. Serum chloride levels of up to 120 mEq per liter are not unusual. This is due to the typical use of physiologically excessive amounts of chloride in replacement fluids as well as to prior urinary losses of sodium and potassium ketoacids that would otherwise have yielded sodium bicarbonate had they been retained and completely oxidized. Subsequent renal compensation generally reverses the hyperchloremic acidosis, but in rare instances it may require temporary bicarbonate treatment.

Phosphate and Magnesium

Crude estimates of phosphate depletion in DKA are at least 1.0 mmol per kilogram. Even if double this amount, such losses of phosphate constitute only 4 percent of soft tissue stores and less than 1 percent of total body stores. On these grounds alone, there is no necessity to administer phosphate acutely. Moreover, prospective randomized studies have shown no significant beneficial effect of routine phosphate administration on the rate of recovery from DKA. Nonetheless, serum phosphate usually plummets in response to insulin treatment, and 6 to 12 hours later values below 1.5 mg per deciliter are not at all unusual. By depleting red blood cells of 2,3-diphosphoglycerate, this theoretically shifts the oxyhemoglobin dissociation curve to the left and decreases tissue O_2 delivery. However, hypophosphatemia is usually clinically silent and eventually reverses with dietary intake, so intravenous phosphate is not essential. If left ventricular dysfunction, rhabdomyolysis, CNS deterioration, respiratory muscle failure, or hemolysis develops with hypophosphatemia (serum phosphate is usually less than 1 mg per deciliter), treatment is indicated. Sixty mmoles of phosphate as the potassium salt (in children 1 mmol per kilogram) should be given over 4 hours and repeated if necessary to normalize serum phosphate. Because this can cause hypocalcemia and even tetany, especially in children, serum calcium should be monitored every 4 hours during phosphate treatment.

Some degree of magnesium depletion is also present in DKA, and hypomagnesemia can develop with insulin treatment. This also does not require routine intravenous replacement. However, if with hypomagnesemia ventricular irritability is observed on the ECG and serum potassium is normal, then 10 to 20 mEq magnesium may be given intravenously as 25 to 50 ml of 5 percent magnesium sulfate over 30 to 60 minutes with ECG monitoring, and the dose may be repeated if necessary.

HYPERGLYCEMIC HYPEROSMOLAR COMA

As previously noted, in many respects the pathophysiology and management of HHC are quite similar to those of DKA. Therefore, the following discussion concentrates on the differences.

Presentation and Pathophysiology

HHC occurs almost exclusively in older patients who have non–insulin-dependent diabetes mellitus (NIDDM) and is rare in IDDM. Typically, a previously undiagnosed elderly person (about half the cases) or an NIDDM patient on diet therapy or oral hypoglycemic drugs becomes progressively hyperglycemic and fails to compensate for polyuria with adequate fluid intake. The fluid that is ingested is often high in carbohydrate content. Gradually, the increasingly hyperosmolar patient lapses into a state of confusion, somnolence, or coma, a seizure occurs, or a strokelike picture appears. The greater propensity to coma in HHC than in DKA is due to the much higher serum osmolarity in the former. In contrast to DKA, generalized or focal convulsions, myoclonic jerking or movement-induced seizures, and even reversible hemiparesis can occur. The seizures do not ordinarily respond well to anticonvulsant medications. The syndrome may be precipitated by a stroke, myocardial infarction, acute pancreatitis, or sepsis. HHC has also occurred from the initiation of treatment with thiazide or loop diuretics, glucocorticoids, phenytoin, diazoxide, cimetidine, loxapine, calcium channel blockers, and immunosuppressive drugs. The key difference from DKA is the absence or minimal nature of ketosis, which prevents the symptoms of DKA—especially vomiting—from alarming the patient. This has been speculatively explained by a higher plasma level of biologically active insulin or by an inhibitory effect of extreme hyperglycemia or hyperosmolarity on adipose tissue lipolysis. The higher plasma glucose levels in HHC than DKA are caused by the greater degree of dehydration and reduction in glomerular filtration that impairs glucose excretion by the kidney. On admission, plasma glucose ranges from 600 to 3,000 mg per deciliter, serum osmolarity from 340 to 440 mOsm per kilogram, with effective serum osmolarity greater than 320. If the measured serum osmolarity exceeds the calculated value ($2 \times Na^+ + \frac{\text{glucose}}{18} + \frac{\text{BUN}}{28}$), ingestion of alcohol or other osmolytes should be suspected. Because serum ketones are usually absent or neglible, pH and HCO_3^- will be near normal unless there is secondary lactic acidosis. Serum creatinine, BUN, and hematocrit are almost always elevated, and to higher levels than in DKA, because the degree of dehydration is greater and often extreme (10 to 20 percent). Unlike in DKA, the serum sodium corrected for hyperglycemia is usually normal or elevated. When even the uncorrected serum sodium is elevated, the degree of free water loss is enormous. Total body sodium and potassium depletion is on an order of magnitude similar to that in DKA, but serum potassium is less often elevated, due to the usual absence of acidosis. Patients with the highest serum levels of sodium, osmolarity, glucose, and BUN have the poorest outcomes.

Management

Insulin therapy is given in similar fashion to that described for DKA, and the expected response rate is similar. Although doses smaller than those advocated for DKA may be effective, it is not worthwhile to do this routinely. Insulin may be withheld briefly in the patient who presents in vascular collapse until isotonic fluid resuscitation is carried out. Potassium therapy may be given less aggressively, and always so in patients who are initially oliguric because of their dehydration. Bicarbonate should not be needed unless severe lactic acidosis is also present.

The crucial element in the management of HHC is the rate and type of fluid administration, over which some controversy exists. The fluid losses are unquestionably hypotonic and much free water is ultimately needed to rehydrate the cells, but the patient is often near or in circulatory collapse. Hence, in the hypotensive patient especially, at least 1 L of 0.9 percent NaCl should be administered within the first 15 to 30 minutes and in some cases, a second liter of 0.9 percent NaCl in the next 30 minutes. Once systolic blood pressure exceeds 110 to 120 mmHg, it is reasonable to give 2 to 3 L of 0.45 percent NaCl at rates of 500 ml per hour for the next 4 to 6 hours. The rate may then be slowed, but ultimately a total of as much as 12 L may be required, at least half of it in the first 18 to 24 hours. In these generally elderly patients, the rates of fluid administration must be guided by blood pressure, urine output, change in body weight, presence or absence of pulmonary congestion, jugular venous pressure or pressures recorded from a Swan-Ganz catheter, and CNS status. In particular, improvement in the latter should slow the rate of fluid replacement. Five percent glucose in 0.2 percent NaCl or in water should be introduced when plasma glucose reaches 250 mg per deciliter.

The optimal rate of fluid replacement or of decrease in plasma glucose or serum osmolarity in HHC has not been established. Concern has been expressed that too rapid correction of extracellular osmolarity will lead to a disequilibrium syndrome within the CNS. The brain has adapted to the hyperglycemic state not only by transferring some water out of its cells but also by increasing intracellular sodium concentration and by taking up diverse osmotically active organic molecules such as myoinositol, taurine, and betaine from the extracellular fluid. Therefore, when hypotonic fluid replacement is carried out along with insulin, which decreases plasma glucose, a strong reverse osmolar gradient drives water back into brain cells, which may become temporarily overhydrated. This may prolong or worsen CNS dysfunction. In practice, some patients take several days to return to their baseline mental status, and this can occur long after plasma glucose has been returned to an acceptable range. Whether this slow recovery is due to a metabolic insult to the brain occurring prior to treatment (analogous to slow CNS recovery sometimes seen after severe prolonged hypoglycemia), or whether it reflects either inappropriately fast or slow cellular rehydration during the active treatment phase, is not clear. Although a slow or delayed rate of clinical recovery always generates great concern, so long as brain function does not deteriorate further and an actual stroke has not occurred, the outcome may still be satisfactory.

As plasma glucose declines with insulin treatment, it is not unusual for measured serum sodium to rise from low normal to levels of 160 to 170 mEq per liter, indicating a continued hyperosmolar state. In some such patients who also have elevated serum creatinine levels, a high plasma antidiuretic hormone level and unresponsiveness to the exogenous hormone suggest a temporary state of nephrogenic diabetes insipidus. This can sustain hypernatremia at levels of 150 to 155 mEq per liter for several days unless there is sufficient administration of 0.45 percent NaCl or 5 percent glucose in water. Care must still be taken, however, not to overload the patient with water in attempts to lower serum sodium to normal.

■ MANAGEMENT OF COMPLICATIONS OF DKA AND HHC

1. For persistent vomiting or gastric dilation (DKA) and in comatose patients, nasogastric suction is advisable. The aspirate may be positive for occult blood because of chemical gastritis in DKA, but overt bleeding is unusual and transfusion is rarely necessary.
2. Any identified focus of infection should be treated with appropriate antibiotics vigorously. Amphotericin B or ketoconazole is indicated for systemic or severe localized fungal infections. Whether to administer broad-spectrum antibiotics immediately to all febrile patients, even without an identified bacterial infection, is arguable and depends on clinical circumstances. Empiric antibiotics are certainly recommended for those who are very ill, hypotensive, elderly, or who have many band neutrophils. After blood and other cultures are obtained, antibiotic coverage should include gram-positive, gram-negative, and anaeraobic bacteria.
3. Prophylactic low-dose heparin is not of proven benefit in uncomplicated DKA. It should, however, be considered in the elderly patient with HHC, particularly if there is a prior history of venous thrombosis or if the patient is likely to remain immobile for days. If a fresh cerebral thrombosis has occurred secondary to HHC, heparin may be considered in the absence of hypertension, but this is controversial and a neurologist should be consulted.
4. Acute respiratory distress syndrome, sometimes induced by overhydration with crystalloid solutions that lower plasma oncotic pressure too much, is manifest by hypoxemia and pulmonary edema in the absence of left ventricular failure. This requires positive pressure oxygen, Swan-Ganz monitoring of fluid replacement, and pulmonary consultation. Pneumomediastinum, which resolves spontaneously, has also been reported.
5. Acute renal failure secondary to extreme volume depletion, papillary necrosis, or overt rhabdomyolysis may require hemodialysis. Rhabdomyolysis in subclinical form, detected by grossly elevated creatine phosphokinase levels, has been reported to occur in 15 percent of cases of DKA and HHC and is associated with an increased mortality rate.
6. Cerebral edema is a rare, often fatal complication seen only in children and young adults with DKA and usually as part of the presentation of their diabetes. The exact cause remains debatable, but it has been suggested that overhydration with hypotonic fluids may play a role. Typically, cerebral edema is manifest—after biochemical recovery has begun—by headache, nausea and vomiting, recurrent somnolence after initial improvement in sensorium, convulsions, diabetes insipidus, and papilledema. The only laboratory clue may be a decrease in measured or calculated serum sodium, rather than the expected increase, as plasma glucose declines. Death from brain herniation often results. If cerebral edema is even suspected clinically, mannitol, 1 to 2 g per kilogram, should be given intravenously over 30 minutes at once, along with 8 mg dexamethasone phosphate. Neither of these therapies is particularly harmful if the diagnosis is not subsequently confirmed by a CT scan of the head, which will show compression of the lateral ventricles. (It should be remembered that elevation of CSF pressure and a clinically inapparent slight degree of cerebral edema probably occur routinely during the rehydration phase of DKA.) Intensive care unit monitoring is mandatory, and neurosurgical consultation is advisable.

■ PREGNANCY

DKA in a pregnant woman deserves special comment. Although the modern incidence in maternal mortality rate is low, the mortality rate for the fetus is still up to 35 percent. DKA can be the presenting event of IDDM during pregnancy, or in a known diabetic patient DKA can be precipitated by hyperemesis; by infection of the urinary tract, sinuses, middle ear, and mastoids; or by the increase of insulin resistance that occurs after 20 to 24 weeks of gestation. The normal physiology of pregnancy entails a state of "accelerated starvation," a lowered renal threshold for glucose, respiratory alkalosis, and a reduced buffering capacity. Thus, DKA in pregnancy can develop unusually rapidly yet plasma glucose levels may be normal on presentation, obscuring the diagnosis. Fluid deficits tend to be 6 to 10 L.

The treatment of the metabolic abnormalities of DKA should be carried out in the same manner as already presented, but if possible with an even greater sense of urgency and in an intensive care unit setting. The earlier the diagnosis and initiation of treatment, the more likely is the fetus to survive. If plasma glucose does not fall 10 percent within the first hour, the insulin infusion rate should be doubled. Other recommendations include continuous fetal monitoring, a left lateral tilt position for the mother, and maintenance of arterial oxygen saturation greater than 95 percent. If preterm labor occurs, magnesium sulfate rather than beta-agonists are employed because the latter can precipitate or aggravate DKA. Surgical intervention for fetal distress should be deferred until the acidosis is reversed, because the fetal mortality rate is high and stabilization of the mother's metabolic status may itself improve the viability of the fetus.

■ PREVENTION OF DKA AND HHC

Many cases of DKA can be prevented by early and continuous contact between the patient and the health care team. Therefore, after the patient recovers from an episode, it is important to address prevention. "Sick day management" should be reviewed, i.e., the necessity to test urine ketones as well as blood glucose when illness or symptoms of decompensation appear, to continue insulin therapy, and to call promptly for advice. In some instances, incipient or already established mild cases of DKA can be managed at home by telephone if oral intake of fluids such as broth and regular soda can be maintained with administration of an antiemetic. Blood glucose and urine ketones must be measured and reported every 2 to 4 hours, and supplemental regular insulin administered by instruction of the diabetes nurse and physician. Alternatively, mild cases without serious concomitant disease can be treated in an emergency room or observation unit and sent home within 6 to 12 hours.

Psychosocial issues that may lead children, particularly adolescents, or even adults to omit insulin should be thoroughly explored. If the cause is interruption of insulin delivery from a pump, the patient's understanding and technique of pump use should be reviewed. Prevention of HHC is dependent on educating the elderly patient with diabetes and his or her family and by maintaining community awareness of the symptoms of hyperglycemia. It is especially important to educate nursing home personnel to this syndrome and to instruct them in blood glucose monitoring techniques, because a sizable portion of patients with HHC develop it in this setting and their mortality rate is unusually high.

■ LACTIC ACIDOSIS

Lactic acid is the major product of anaerobic glucose metabolism. Normal plasma lactate is less than 1.5 mmoles per liter. Significant lactic acidosis is present when the plasma level is greater than 5 mmol per liter and blood pH is less than 7.35.

Lactic acidosis fundamentally results from (1) decreased tissue delivery of oxygen as in cardiovascular collapse or pulmonary failure (type A) or (2) overproduction of lactate as in extreme exercise, status epilepticus, sepsis, or decreased utilization of lactate as in severe liver disease or sepsis (type B). Many cases are of mixed type. Either type A or type B lactic acidosis can occur in association with and as a further complication of DKA (rarely) or HHC (more commonly). In DKA, lactic acidosis is seldom severe unless there is a concomitant cause of cardiovascular collapse (e.g., acute myocardial infarction). In HHC, profound dehydration itself may cause low tissue perfusion and reduced oxygen delivery, but sepsis is also a frequent cause. With the recent introduction of metformin for treatment of NIDDM in the United States, it has again become necessary to be alert for biguanide-induced lactic acidosis. The reported incidence in metformin-treated patients is 3 per 100,000. Because many of these patients also had cardiac or renal insufficiency (contraindications to use of the drug), prevention of metformin-induced lactic acidosis by appropriate patient selection deserves emphasis.

The current prognosis for severe lactic acidosis is poor. With current management, lactic acidosis itself resolves in about one-third of patients. Nonetheless, the overall survival is only 59 percent at 24 hours and 17 percent at 30 days. In all instances—whether associated with diabetes or not—the most effective therapy is restoration of tissue oxygen delivery by volume repletion, augmentation of cardiac function, improvement in ventilation, and administration of appropriate antibiotics. The use of antibodies to endotoxins is being actively investigated. Whether it is truly useful to raise pH with alkali therapy is moot. If to meet basic cellular energy needs, hypoxic peripheral and central nervous system tissues anaerobically glycolized only an extra 45 g glucose per day, this would generate an additional 500 mEq lactate. To the extent that a hypoxic, septic, or otherwise diseased liver cannot metabolize such a load of lactate to glucose and/or CO_2, this would require administration of hundreds of milliequivalents of sodium bicarbonate with the attendant dangers of volume overload in the cardiac compromised patient. Furthermore, raising intracellular pH with alkali may itself stimulate further lactate production, negating the benefit. Raising pH with bicarbonate therapy is rarely decisive if tissue hypoxia or hepatic failure cannot be corrected. However, bicarbonate may improve the prognosis in reversible instances of type B lactic acidosis. A trial of sodium bicarbonate in a quantity sufficient to raise pH to 7.2 may be carried out, but if no clinical benefit is observed, further alkali treatment is likely to be futile. If benefit is observed, diuretics and dialysis with alkaline solutions containing sodium bicarbonate or acetate may be employed to deal with or prevent sodium overload. Dialysis also has the advantage of removing metformin in cases caused by the drug. Dichloroacetate, an experimental drug that activates the enzyme pyruvate dehydrogenase and thereby increases lactate utilization, can lower lactate levels and raise pH, but no survival benefit accrues.

Suggested Reading

Androgue HJ, Barrero J, Eknoyan G. Salutory effects of modest fluid replacement in the treatment of adults with diabetic ketoacidosis. Use in patients without extreme volume deficit. JAMA 1989; 262:2108–2113.

Androgue HJ, Wison H, Boyd AE, et al. Plasma acid-base patterns in diabetic ketoacidosis. N Engl J Med 1982; 307:1603–1610.

Arieff AI. Pathogenesis of lactic acidosis. Diabetes Metab Rev 1989; 5:637–649.

Berger W, Keller U. Treatment of diabetic ketoacidosis and non-ketotic hyperosmolar diabetic coma. Balliere's Clin Endocrinol Metab 1992; 6:1–22.

Chauhan SP, Perry KG Jr. Management of diabetic ketoacidosis in the obstetric patient. Obstet Gynecol Clin North Am 1995; 22:143–155.

Cruz-Caudillo JC, Sabatini S. Diabetic hyperosmolar syndrome. Nephron 1995; 69:201–210.

DeFronzo RA, Matsuda M, Barrett EJ. Diabetic ketoacidosis: A combined metabolic-nephrologic approach to therapy. Diabetes Metab Rev 1994; 2:209–238.

Ellis EN. Concepts of fluid therapy in diabetic ketoacidosis and hyperosmolar hyperglycemic nonketotic coma. Pediatr Clin North Am 1990; 37:313–321.

Fleckman AM. Diabetic ketoacidosis. Endocrinol Metab Clin North Am 1993; 22:181–207.

Foster DW, McGarry JD. The metabolic derangements and treatment of diabetic ketoacidosis. N Engl J Med 1983; 309:159–169.

Gamba G, Oseguera J, Castrejon M, Gomez-Perez FJ. Bicarbonate therapy in severe diabetic ketoacidosis. A double blind, randomized, placebo-controlled trial. Rev Invest Clin 1991; 43:234–238.

Hagay ZJ. Diabetic ketoacidosis in pregnancy: Etiology, pathophysiology, and management. Clin Obstet Gynecol 1994; 37:39–49.

Hamblin PS, Tapliss DJ, Chosich N, et al. Deaths associated with diabetic ketoacidosis and hyperosmolar coma, 1973–1988. Med J Aust 1989; 151:439–444.

Harris GD, Fiordalisi I. Physiologic management of diabetic ketoacidemia: A 5-year prospective pediatric experience in 231 episodes. Arch Pediatr Adolesc Med 1994; 148:1046–1052.

Jenkins D, Close CF, Krentz AJ, et al. Euglycaemic diabetic ketoacidosis: Does it exist? Acta Diabetol 1993; 30:251–253.

Kitabchi AE, Wall BM. Diabetic ketoacidosis. Med Clin North Am 1995; 79:9–37.
Lalau JD, Lacroix C, Compagnon P, et al. Role of metformin accumulation in metformin-associated lactic acidosis. Diabetes Care 1995; 18:779–784.
Lalau JD, Westeel PF, Debussche X, et al. Bicarbonate haemodialysis: An adequate treatment for lactic acidosis in diabetics treated by metformin. Intensive Care Med 1987; 13:383–387.
Lorber D. Nonketotic hypertonicity in diabetes mellitus. Med Clin North Am 1995; 79:39–52.
Matz R. Hyperosmolar nonacidotic uncontrolled diabetes: Not a rare event. Clin Diabetes 1988; 6:25.
May ME, Young C, King J. Resource utilization in treatment of diabetic ketoacidosis in adults. Am J Med Sci 1993; 306:287–294.
McManus ML, Churchwell KB, Strange K. Regulation of cell volume in health and disease. N Engl J Med 1995; 333:1260–1266.
Mel JM, Werther GA. Incidence and outcome of diabetic cerebral oedema in childhood: Are there predictors? J Paediatr Child Health 1995; 31: 17–20.
Piniés JA, Cairo G, Gaztambide S, et al. Course and prognosis of 132 patients with diabetic non-ketotic hyperosmolar state. Diabete Metab 1994; 20:43–48.
Riley L Jr, Cooper M, Narins R. Alkali therapy of diabetic ketoacidosis: Biochemical physiologic and clinical perspectives. Diabetes Metab Rev 1989; 5:627–636.
Rother KI, Schwenk WF. Effect of rehydration fluid with 75 mmol/L of sodium on serum sodium concentration and serum osmolality in young patients with diabetic ketoacidosis. Mayo Clin Proc 1994; 69:1149–1153.
Sauve DO, Kessler CA. Hyperglycemic emergencies. Clin Issues Crit Care Nurs 1992; 3:350–360.
Siperstein MD. Diabetic ketoacidosis and hyperosmolar coma. Endocrinol Metab Clin North Am 1992; 21:415–432.
Stacpoole PW, Wright EC, Baumgartner TG, et al. Natural history and course of acquired lactic acidosis in adults. Am J Med 1994; 97:47–53.
VanBuskirk MC, Vanderbilt D. Evaluating patient care by the use of a diabetic ketoacidosis CareMap in an intensive care unit setting. J Nurs Care Qual 1995; 9:59–68.
Wachtel TJ, Tetu-Mouradjian LM, Goldman DL, et al. Hyperosmolarity and acidosis in diabetes mellitus: A three-year experience in Rhode Island. J Gen Intern Med 1991; 6:495–502.
Walker M, Marshall SM, Alberti KGMM. Clinical aspects of diabetic ketoacidosis. Diabetes Metab Rev 1989; 5:651–663.
Wang L-M, Tsai S-T, Ho L-T, et al. Rhabdomyolysis in diabetic emergencies. Diabetes Res Clin Pract 1994; 26:209–214.

HYPOALDOSTERONISM

Richard Horton, M.D.
Jerry Nadler, M.D.

Aldosterone deficiency is a rare disorder with a considerable but rational differential diagnosis based on knowledge of the renin-aldosterone system. Although aldosterone is one of the mechanisms of sodium conservation, it is critically involved in potassium secretion. Hyperkalemia (greater than 6 mEq per liter) therefore is the key finding. Although the kidney is involved in the secretion of potassium, mild or even moderate renal disease is not usually associated with hyperkalemia because the hormonal mechanisms of secretion (aldosterone and insulin) as well as potassium itself lead to adequate potassium excretion in spite of reduction in glomerular filtration. Acute renal failure, tissue damage, or destruction of blood cells can cause hyperkalemia; however, these causes are usually obvious. In advanced renal disease or acute renal shutdown, hyperkalemia and acidosis would be expected. Salt substitutes, potassium penicillin, or potassium-sparing diuretics, especially in the presence of renal disease, can induce hyperkalemia.

Table 1 Adrenal Causes of Hypoaldosteronism

	ALDOSTERONE	RENIN
Addison's disease (cortisol and aldosterone deficiency)	↓	↑
Adrenogenital syndrome (salt wasting in infants)	↓	↑
Aldosterone biosynthesis defect (types I and II methyl oxidase)	↓	↑
Hyper-reninemic hypoaldosteronism	↓	↑

■ ADRENAL CAUSES OF HYPOALDOSTERONISM

See Table 1 for a list of the four major adrenal disorders. Addison's disease must always be considered in a patient with unexplained hyperkalemia (and hyponatremia). Treatment involves replacement doses of cortisol and a mineralocorticoid. The objectives of mineralocorticoid therapy are to normalize serum electrolyte level and plasma volume.

An additional group of patients with acquired immunodeficiency syndrome (AIDS) has been described; hypoaldosteronism in these patients is the result of infection (tuberculosis, cytomegalovirus) or use of drugs such as ketoconazole to treat fungus infections or rifampin for tuberculosis. In our experience, however, the vast majority of AIDS patients with wasting, hypotension, infection, and hyponatremia (but without hyperkalemia) do not have adrenal insufficiency and their cortisol levels are not abnormally low (less than 10 μg per deciliter in the morning).

The salt-wasting type of adrenogenital syndrome includes a defect in the biosynthesis of both cortisol and aldosterone. The condition affects infants and children but improves with renal maturation and adequate dietary sodium. Early in life this syndrome must be treated with salt supplementation and mineralocorticoid (fludrocortisone [Florinef]; about 1 μg per pound up to 0.1 mg daily orally). Side effects of this synthetic mineralocorticoid are limited to hypokalemia with excessive doses and a tendency to elevated blood pressure when given chronically. Sodium retention occurs only in the presence of cardiac, liver, or renal disease, as discussed later. The rare disorders of aldosterone biosynthesis include either type I (defect in corticosterone conversion to 18-OH corticosterone) or type II (impaired conversion of 18-OH to aldosterone) and can be diagnosed from a positive family history and the presence of elevated precursor steroids (corticosterone or 18-OH corticosterone, respectively). Patients in whom salt wasting occurs are treated with mineralocorticoids (usually fludrocortisone), as they are not deficient in glucocorticoid.

An additional disorder associated with low aldosterone levels has been described recently in critically ill patients. In this syndrome, termed *hyper-reninemic hypoaldosteronism*, the adrenocorticotropic hormone (ACTH)–cortisol axis is normal. Renin secretion is elevated, as most patients are septic and hypotensive. However, there is a marked deficiency of aldosterone in spite of the high renin secretion. Although the adrenal cells synthesizing aldosterone may be partially damaged because of a decreased blood supply, new data suggest that cytokines such as tumor necrosis factor or interleukin-1 stimulate renin and ACTH but inhibit angiotensin effects in the adrenal gland. Treatment of the infection reverses the disorders.

Pseudohypoaldosteronism is a very rare error of peripheral aldosterone receptors. At birth infants with this condition produce large amounts of aldosterone, which lacks biologic activity on renal tubules. This rapidly leads to sodium depletion and hyperkalemia. Emergency treatment with parenteral saline followed by salt supplementation is necessary. Some patients respond to high doses of desoxycorticosterone (10 to 20 mg per square meter) or fludrocortisone. As the kidney further develops after birth, the syndrome may become less severe.

In all these primary adrenal disorders, aldosterone deficiency or resistance is associated with increased renin blood levels (Table 1).

A number of drugs can also suppress aldosterone synthesis, although a second factor such as renal disease is usually also present. Heparin can occasionally interfere with the biosynthesis of aldosterone, but hyperkalemia is seldom observed. Spironolactone can produce hyperkalemia as a result of its competitive antagonism of aldosterone action on the distal renal tubule as well as its impairment of adrenal aldosterone synthesis. Other agents that can impair steroidogenesis, such as mitotane, aminoglutethimide, or ketoconazole, theoretically could produce hypoaldosteronism in a susceptible individual. The hyperkalemia of digitalis is rarely seen and is a direct result of cellular impairment of the Na^+-K^+ adenosine triphosphatase pump.

■ LOW RENIN STATES OR REDUCED RENIN ACTION CAUSING HYPOALDOSTERONISM

Hyporeninemic hypoaldosteronism is the result of an inability of the kidney to process and secrete active renin. A fixed secretion of renin leads to inadequate aldosterone secretion. The syndrome is typically observed in older, insulin-dependent diabetics with varying degrees of diabetic renal vasculopathy. Insulin normally plays a secondary role in the regulation of potassium balance. However, the key disorder is inadequate aldosterone synthesis secondary to renin and angiotensin II deficiency. New studies suggest that there is an imbalance between certain vascular prostaglandins (prostacyclin) and a relative excess in the lipoxygenase pathway product hydroxyeicosatetraenoic acid. The result is a defect in processing prorenin to renin and a tendency to hypertension, low prostacyclin, and reduced aldosterone secretion, in spite of the hyperkalemia. The acidosis is out of proportion to renal function and reflects the aldosterone deficiency and the action of hyperkalemia on renal ammonium formation and hydrogen ion excretion.

Hyponatremia is not usually part of the syndrome, as cortisol secretion is intact and low levels of aldosterone are present; however, other renal mechanisms of sodium conservation at sites along the nephron are active and prevent salt wasting unless there is severe salt restriction. Increased levels of prorenin or an abnormal renin-prorenin ratio are present in diabetic hyporeninemic hypoaldosteronism.

Hyporeninemic hypoaldosteronism has been reported in other types of renal disease, including systemic lupus erythematosus, periarteritis, and glomerulonephritis (Table 2). Although the pathophysiology of this disorder is similar in most patients and includes renin deficiency, the disorder in the conversion of prorenin to active renin is not so apparent. In addition, some patients have resistance to aldosterone, resulting from renal tubular damage or immunologic effects on the nephron.

Hyporeninemic hypoaldosteronism is now recognized as much more common than adrenal insufficiency as a cause of hyperkalemia. It is also becoming clear that all aging patients with chronic diabetes, particularly those who are insulin dependent, have potential microvascular disease of the kidney and tend to have a limited ability to secrete renin.

In full-blown hyporeninemic hypoaldosteronism the diagnosis can be confirmed by demonstrating inadequate levels of renin and aldosterone after administration of furosemide (40 mg), following which the patient remains 1 hour in an upright position.

Beta-adrenergic blockers can, in addition to altering cardiac output and peripheral resistance, lower renin secretion. Their use in diabetics and in patients with renal disease should be accompanied by monitoring of serum potassium concen-

Table 2 Causes of Hyporeninemic Hypoaldosteronism

Diabetes
Other renal disorders (systemic lupus erythematosus, pyelonephritis)
Drug induced

Table 3 Treatment of Hyporeninemic Hypoaldosteronism

ACUTE THERAPY OF HYPERKALEMIA (>6 MEQ/L)
Intravenous salt and water with furosemide
Insulin (5 U) in a liter of 5% glucose
Intravenous sodium bicarbonate (45–90 mEq)
10% calcium gluconate
Hemodialysis
CHRONIC THERAPY OF HYPERKALEMIA
Restrict dietary potassium to 40–50 mEq/day
Fludrocortisone 0.05–0.1 (rarely 0.2) mg/day
Diuretics for sodium retention
Potassium oxalate resins are not well tolerated

trations. Converting enzyme inhibitors are being widely used to reduce afterload in patients who have experienced heart failure and those with a wide spectrum of hypertensive disorders. The logic of these agents is clear; they interfere with the generation of angiotensin II. In otherwise normal patients the body retains some renin-angiotensin activity, because the kidney normally responds to reduced angiotensin II feedback by secreting increased renin. In certain patients with diabetes or those with renal disease, this compensation does not occur and hyperkalemia may ensue. Therefore potassium levels should be monitored in patients with diabetes or those with renal disease taking converting enzyme inhibitor drugs. Cyclosporine also has been reported to alter the renin-angiotensin system and to produce hyperkalemia.

Renal prostaglandins play an important role in maintaining renal blood flow, glomerular function, and renin secretion in all types of renal disease as well as in heart and liver failure. Nonsteroidal anti-inflammatory agents are commonly used for diverse purposes by the physician. In the presence of significant renal, liver, or cardiac disease, nonsteroidal anti-inflammatory agents can reduce renal function, even to the point of producing an oliguric state. An additional and often separate effect of aspirin-like drugs is to interfere with renin secretion, producing hyporeninemic hypoaldosteronism and hyperkalemia by blocking prostaglandin (prostacyclin) formation. We believe that an increased number of cases of drug-induced hypoaldosteronism and hyporeninism will be observed as the result of the widespread use of adrenergic blockers, nonsteroidal anti-inflammatory agents, and the broadened spectrum of use for agents that inhibit the generation of angiotensin or block its actions.

■ TREATMENT OF HYPORENINEMIC HYPOALDOSTERONISM

In a patient with hyperkalemia (potassium greater than 6 mEq per liter), it must first be confirmed that this level reflects true hyperkalemia and not spuriously high levels resulting from hemolysis. A simple procedure is to perform electrocardiography. Progressive electrocardiographic changes seen with hyperkalemia include peaking of T waves progressing to widening of the QRS complex and cardiac standstill at extremely elevated potassium levels. The urgency of treatment depends on the level of serum potassium and electrocardiographic findings. As outlined in Table 3, various therapeutic modalities can be used to correct the hyperkalemia. Any medications that may be precipitating the increase in potassium should be removed, including beta-blockers, nonsteroidal anti-inflammatory agents, converting enzyme inhibitors, and potassium-sparing diuretics.

The most logical approach for chronic therapy is replacement of the mineralocorticoid deficiency. Aldosterone is not effective when administered orally, and desoxycorticosterone acetate must be given by injection. The synthetic mineralocorticoid fludrocortisone (Florinef) is the mainstay of therapy to control potassium retention and acidosis. This steroid is active when taken by mouth and similar by weight in dose effects to aldosterone. Fludrocortisone is usually given as a single daily dose, although some patients with resistant disease should take tablets twice a day. Most adult patients require 0.1 mg daily, which is similar to the dosage used in the treatment of Addison's disease. As noted previously, an occasional case, as a patient with lupus nephritis in which there is a tubular resistance component, requires up to 0.2 mg. Like all mineralocorticoids, fludrocortisone has salt-retaining properties, but uniquely this compound has been shown to have a hypertensive effect independent of its salt-retaining action. Therefore, the dose must be adjusted by balancing the improvement in potassium level with sodium retention and blood pressure elevation.

Patients with diabetes and hyporeninemic hypoaldosteronism are usually elderly and have long standing diabetes. The incidence of cardiac and peripheral vascular disease and advanced diabetic nephropathy in these patients is high. The physician may be faced with a therapeutic dilemma. The hyperkalemia must be improved, but even replacement doses of mineralocorticoid can induce sodium retention with adverse cardiac consequences. A compromise might be to reduce the dose of fludrocortisone (e.g., to 0.05 mg daily or on alternate days) and to place the patient on a strict (but adequate) potassium and protein diet. However, a diet of less than 40 mEq per day of potassium is neither palatable nor well tolerated. We are therefore often forced to utilize a combination of fludrocortisone for kaliuresis and a diuretic such as furosemide for the natriuresis and kaliuresis. This balancing act can be very difficult, and certain patients cannot be treated optimally. Our aim in many of these fragile patients is to control the serum potassium to levels (less than 6 mEq per liter) that do not induce atrioventricular dissociation or other major cardiac arrhythmias.

Suggested Reading

Clive D, Stoff J. Renal syndromes associated with nonsteroidal anti-inflammatory drugs. N Engl J Med 1984; 310:563–572.

De Fronzo R. Hyperkalemia and hyporeninemic hypoaldosteronism. Kidney Int 1980; 17:118–134.

Etzel J, Brocavich J, Torre M. Endocrine complications associated with HIV. Clin Pharm 1992; 11:705–713.

Nadler J, Lee F, Hsueh W, et al. Evidence of prostacyclin deficiency in the syndrome of hyporeninemic hypoaldosteronism. N Engl J Med 1986; 314:1015–1020.

Natrajan R, Ploszaj S, Horton R, et al. Tumor necrosis factor and interleukin-I are potent inhibitors of angiotensin-II induced aldosterone synthesis. Endocrinology 1989; 125:3084–3089.

Schambelan M, Sebastian A. Hyporeninemic hypoaldosteronism. Adv Intern Med 1979; 24:385–405.

Zipser R, Davenport M, Martin K, et al. Hyperreninemic hypoaldosteronism in the critically ill; a new entity. J Clin Endocrinol Metab 1981; 53:867–872.

PRIMARY ALDOSTERONISM

Gail K. Adler, M.D., Ph.D.
Gordon H. Williams, M.D.

Primary aldosteronism, hypersecretion of aldosterone in the absence of definable stimulus, is most commonly associated with a unilateral adrenal adenoma. However, a significant minority of patients have bilateral adrenal hyperplasia. In rare cases, an adrenal carcinoma, an ectopic source of aldosterone, or glucocorticoid-suppressible cortical nodular hyperplasia can cause primary aldosteronism. Primary aldosteronism usually is detected in persons between the ages of 30 and 50 and has an incidence of approximately 1 percent in populations of unselected hypertensive patients. Since aldosterone causes sodium reabsorption and hydrogen and potassium ion excretion, signs and symptoms of primary aldosteronism are attributable to the hypertension (headache and infrequently visual disturbances) or, more commonly, to potassium depletion (fatigue, polyuria, muscle weakness, and cramps). Unfortunately, on the basis of the symptoms alone, patients with primary aldosteronism cannot be readily distinguished from patients with other forms of hypertension.

■ SCREENING

Even though primary aldosteronism occurs relatively infrequently, because it is a potentially curable disease it is important to have a simple, inexpensive screening test. In our opinion, no clinical characteristics distinguish the patient with primary aldosteronism. Studies conducted a number of years ago suggested that a low plasma renin activity may be an effective screen for primary aldosteronism. This was based on the observation that patients with primary aldosteronism are volume expanded and therefore would have suppressed renin levels. Unfortunately, we as well as others have not been particularly enchanted with plasma renin activity as a screening test since it is relatively expensive ($30 to $50) and not very specific (roughly 20 percent of patients with essential hypertension also have low renin levels). We believe that if certain precautions are taken, a more reliable, and certainly cheaper, screening test is a serum potassium level. In our experience, spontaneous hypokalemia in a hypertensive patient is almost invariably a sign of aldosterone excess. Whether it is primary or secondary, aldosteronism can readily be distinguished by measuring plasma renin activity (Fig. 1).

Unfortunately, spontaneous hypokalemia is unusual in hypertensive patients. In most instances a low serum potassium concentration is a result of treatment with potassium-wasting diuretics. Thus, if a patient is hypokalemic and taking potassium-wasting diuretics, the diuretics need to be discontinued for 10 to 14 days and the serum potassium concentration remeasured. If it is still low, this would suggest that the patient has mineralocorticoid excess.

What is the sensitivity of this procedure? Theoretically, all patients with primary aldosteronism should have hypokalemia unless they are on a low-sodium diet (thereby preventing the reabsorption of sodium, a necessary prerequisite for the potassium wastage with aldosterone), are ingesting potassium-sparing diuretics, or have renal failure. Thus, in interpreting a serum potassium level, we take the following precautions to prevent a false-negative result. If patients are on potassium-sparing diuretics, these drugs are discontinued for 10 to 14 days and the serum potassium concentration is remeasured. During this period the patient should be maintained on a normal sodium (100 to 200 mEq) and potassium (60 to 100 mEq) intake. If the serum potassium level is normal while the patient is on a liberal sodium intake, off potassium-sparing diuretics, and free of evidence of renal failure (by blood urea nitrogen and/or creatinine), we believe that primary aldosteronism is effectively excluded.

Several concerns need to be addressed in performing what appears to be a relatively simple procedure. First, discontinuing diuretic therapy for 14 days may produce a rise in blood pressure that could be intolerable for the patient. Under these circumstances, if other antihypertensive agents are not effective and one is concerned about whether a low serum potassium level is secondary to potassium-losing diuretics or excess aldosterone, one could simply obtain a 24 hour urine potassium value after discontinuing the drug. Under most circumstances, if the hypokalemia is drug-induced, urinary potassium excretion declines markedly (less than 30 to 40 mEq per 24 hours). On the other hand, if the hypokalemia is secondary to aldosterone excess, the urinary potassium excretion rate remains elevated (greater than 50 to 60 mEq per 24 hours). Second, care should be taken when increasing a patient's

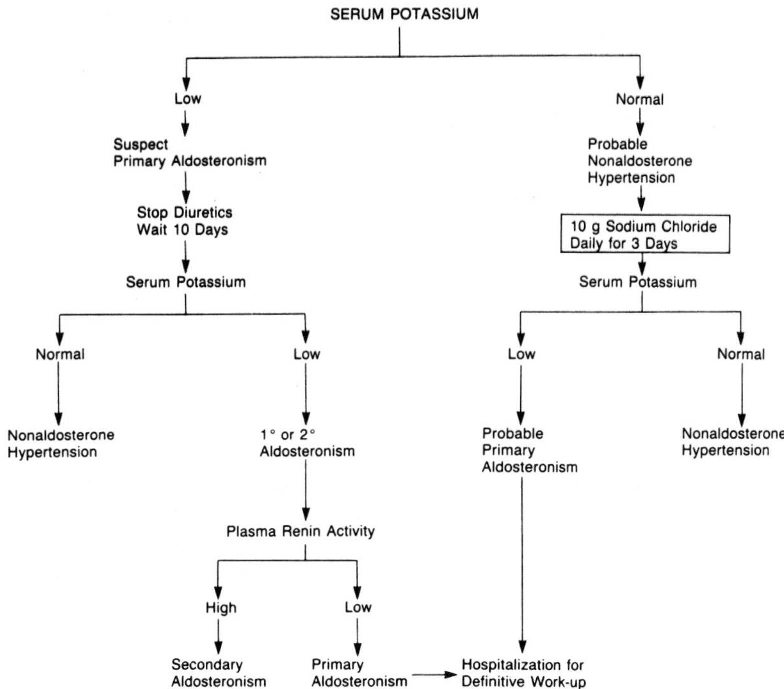

Figure 1
Flowchart for office screening of hypertensive patients for hyperaldosteronism. *(Reprinted with permission from Williams GH, Dluhy RG. How to evaluate and manage hypokalemic high blood pressure. In: Wolf GL, Eliot RS, eds. Contemporary problems in cardiology. Vol 2. Practical management of hypertension. Mt. Kisco, NY: Futura, 1975.)*

dietary sodium intake, particularly in those who may have severe hypertension or incipient congestive heart failure. Finally, sodium should never be administered to a hypokalemic patient in whom you suspect primary aldosteronism. If the suspicion is correct, salt losing will promote further potassium loss, more hypokalemia, and potentially, severe adverse cardiac manifestations of the hypokalemia.

A screening test for primary aldosteronism has been proposed in which patients are given 26 mg of captopril by mouth and their plasma aldosterone and renin levels measured 2 hours later. It is suggested that in patients with primary aldosteronism no change in renin or aldosterone levels will occur, whereas other patients show a rise in renin and a fall in aldosterone. A postcaptopril plasma aldosterone level greater than 15 ng per deciliter and a ratio of plasma aldosterone (ng per deciliter) to plasma renin activity (ng per milliliter per hour) greater than 50 indicate primary aldosteronism. We have had limited experience with this test but are concerned about two potential shortcomings: (1) the cost is probably greater than $100, and (2) the results are highly dependent on the reliability of blood sample collection and the processing of the laboratory samples. Both reasons in all probability exclude this test as a standard screening procedure.

■ DEFINITIVE DIAGNOSIS

If the techniques outlined previously reveal a hypertensive patient with spontaneous hypokalemia and a suppressed plasma renin activity, admission to a metabolic unit for a definitive workup of primary aldosteronism should be arranged. In our experience, the definitive diagnosis of primary aldosteronism should be made on the basis of the following four criteria: (1) plasma or urinary aldosterone levels that do not suppress when salt loaded; (2) plasma renin activity that cannot be stimulated with salt restriction and upright posture; (3) potassium wasting and/or hypokalemia when salt loaded; and (4) normalization of serum potassium with sodium restriction. The easiest way to evaluate a patient suspected of having primary aldosteronism is as follows. The patient is admitted to a metabolic unit and placed on low (10 mEq) sodium and relatively high (100 to 150 mEq) potassium intake. After approximately 5 days when balance is achieved on this diet, supine and upright plasma renin activities are obtained. The patient is then given a saline load—3 L of normal saline intravenously over a 6 hour period. Plasma aldosterone and cortisol levels are obtained before starting the saline infusion and at 6 hours. In our laboratory the normal 6 hour aldosterone value should be less than 5 ng per deciliter. The cortisol level is obtained to rule out a false-positive elevation of aldosterone secondary to stress and adrenocorticotropic hormone (ACTH) stimulation.

The advantages of this approach are as follows:

1. The low-sodium diet prepares the patient for the appropriate renin stimulation test. In our laboratory the upright plasma renin activity has been less than 2 ng angiotensin I per milliliter per hour in every patient with primary aldosteronism whom we have studied on a sodium-restricted diet.
2. Often, by first restricting the patient's salt, both blood

pressure and potassium are normalized. The saline load now can be given with less potential danger to the patient (hypokalemia and/or hypertension).

3. Since approximately 40 percent of patients with essential hypertension have difficulty handling the sodium load and may take longer than 4 hours to suppress their plasma aldosterone levels, we prefer a 6 hour saline infusion and do not recommend a shorter 4 hour infusion. Because the renin levels also fail to suppress normally in these patients, the false-positive elevation of aldosterone usually becomes apparent if one obtains a simultaneous plasma renin activity.

Two other parameters are assessed during the course of the saline infusion: (1) urine potassium excretion (in primary aldosteronism the increment in 24 hour potassium excretion is at least 30 percent over basal), and (2) serum potassium levels. Although serum potassium levels can fall precipitously, we often do not observe a significant change in serum potassium at the conclusion of the 6 hour saline infusion but do observe it the following morning—24 hours after initiating the saline infusion. The reason we fail to see the rapid development of hypokalemia may be in part our preparation of the patients—high potassium, low sodium intake.

We have had an occasional patient in whom we were unable to carry out the foregoing procedures. These patients had concomitant mild to moderate renal failure: thus, the sodium-restricted intake produced a deterioration in renal function and the development of hyperkalemia. In these patients, we elected to perform a 4 hour saline infusion under closely monitored conditions both for blood pressure and potassium shifts. In each case, we observed no change in the plasma aldosterone levels over the 4 hour infusion. Each had an aldosterone-secreting adenoma removed at surgery, with lowering of blood pressure and normalization of the hypokalemia. However, each has required continued medication to normalize the blood pressure. The saline infusion should not be performed in patients with severe hypertension or in patients who have a stroke, myocardial infarction, or congestive heart failure within the past 6 months (Fig. 2).

BILATERAL ADRENAL HYPERPLASIA VERSUS AN ALDOSTERONE-PRODUCING ADENOMA

Once the diagnosis of primary aldosteronism is established, its etiology should be determined since the treatments for an adenoma and for bilateral adrenal hyperplasia differ. Initially, a high-resolution computed tomography (CT) scan should be obtained. The CT scan will detect approximately 90 percent of all adenomas with a less than 1 percent false-positive rate. In our experience, if both adrenal glands are visualized and a unilateral adrenal mass is found, further workup is unnecessary, and the patient can be assumed to have an aldosterone-producing adenoma. Adenomas that are less than 1 cm in diameter are most difficult to detect by CT scan, especially if they are isodense with surrounding tissues and have not changed the contour of the gland. These small adenomas account for most of the 10 percent false-negative rate associated with CT scans.

If by CT scan both adrenals are of equal size, or if one adrenal is not seen, we believe that the patient should undergo adrenal vein sampling. This study should be performed by an experienced radiologist because technical problems can lead to inadequate adrenal vein sampling and significant complications including adrenal vein thrombosis, adrenal infarction, rupture of the adrenal vein, and extravasation of contrast. The sensitivity of adrenal venous sampling is greater than 90 to 95 percent. Bilateral adrenal vein sampling for determination of aldosterone and cortisol concentrations should be obtained to look for lateralization of aldosterone secretion. Lateralization indicates an adenoma, and equal aldosterone levels indicate bilateral hyperplasia. The cortisol levels indicate whether the samples are adequate and should show no lateralization, although differences in levels between the two sides if samples are not obtained concomitantly may result from the normal episodic secretion of this steroid. Adrenal venography has a lower sensitivity of 75 to 90 percent with up to 30 percent false-positives and a slightly higher complication rate than just adrenal venous sampling. Because of the complication rate, the high cost of the procedure, and the relatively little added information obtained with adrenal venography, we no longer obtain this study.

The adrenal iodocholesterol scan is less sensitive (70 to 90 percent sensitivity) and more expensive, and it results in five to ten times more adrenal radiation than a CT scan. In addition, the radioisotopes used are not yet approved by the Food and Drug Administration except for research purposes. For these reasons, we do not perform adrenal iodocholesterol scintigraphy routinely. We have found that other procedures that have been advocated to distinguish an adenoma from hyperplasia are less reliable. They include plasma aldosterone response to upright posture. About 80 percent of patients with an aldosterone-producing adenoma have a decrease in their aldosterone level after 2 hours of upright posture. However, up to 25 percent of patients with bilateral hyperplasia also show this decrease in aldosterone. A second discriminant is an elevated 18-OH corticosterone level in a supine patient on an ad lib sodium intake. In our experience, there are both false negatives and false positives with this test.

Consideration should also be given to the rare causes of primary aldosteronism. An adrenal carcinoma probably would be detected by CT scan since these tumors tend to be inefficient producers of aldosterone and would be large by the time the patient developed symptoms of primary aldosteronism. Overproduction of additional adrenal hormones would also suggest carcinoma. Since our initial treatment for both adrenal adenomas and carcinomas is surgical removal of the affected adrenal, further preoperative testing to distinguish between these possibilities is seldom warranted. Finally, patients with a family history of primary aldosteronism should be evaluated for glucocorticoid-suppressible hyperaldosteronism. Prednisone, 5 mg twice a day for 4 to 6 weeks, will normalize blood pressure, potassium, plasma renin activity, and plasma aldosterone in patients with glucocorticoid-suppressible hyperaldosteronism. A transient decrease in aldosterone production during the

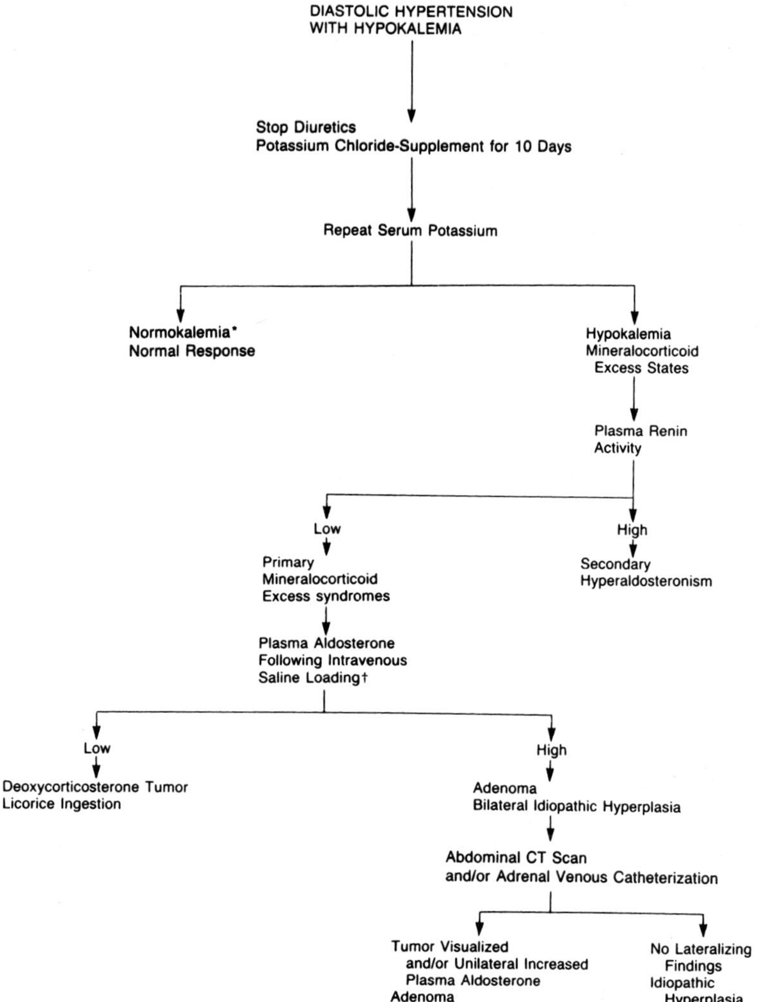

* Serum K^{+} may be normal in some patients with hyperaldosteronism who are taking potassium-sparing diuretics (spironolactone, triamterene) or ingesting low sodium-high potassium intakes.

† This step should not be taken if hypertension is severe (diastolic greater than 115 mm Hg) or if cardiac failure is present. Also, serum potassium levels should be corrected before the infusion of saline.

Figure 2
Diagnostic flowchart for evaluating patients with suspected primary aldosteronism. *(Reprinted with modifications from Williams GH, Dluhy RG. Diseases of the adrenal cortex. In: Petersdorf RG, Adams RD, eds. Harrison's principles of internal medicine. 10th ed. New York: McGraw-Hill, 1983.)*

first few days of prednisone suppression occurs in some patients with primary aldosteronism.

■ APPROACH TO TREATMENT

While waiting for study results, patients with suspected primary aldosteronism should be given a trial of medical therapy. Patients should be placed on less than an 80 mEq sodium diet. With less sodium available for exchange with potassium in the distal renal tubule, patients tend to conserve potassium. In addition, the mild volume depletion that accompanies a low sodium diet may lead to a decrease in the patient's blood pressure. Compliance with a low sodium diet can be monitored by obtaining a 12 hour urine for sodium and creatinine. At the same time, treatment with a potassium-sparing diuretic should be initiated (Table 1).

We usually use spironolactone, a competitive antagonist for the mineralocorticoid receptor. We start at 50 mg twice a day. The dose can be increased in increments of 100 mg at 1 or 2 week intervals up to 300 to 400 mg a day. The patient's blood pressure and serum potassium level should be followed weekly. With spironolactone there is an average increase in serum potassium levels of 1.5 mEq per liter. In addition, the majority of patients with primary aldosteronism become normotensive with spironolactone therapy. Unfortunately,

Table 1 Drug Therapy for Patients with Primary Aldosteronism

MEDICATION	INITIAL DOSE	MAXIMUM DOSE	COST/TABLET*	SIDE EFECTS
Spironolactone	50 mg b.i.d.	200 mg b.i.d.	9¢–17¢ for 25 mg (generic) 29¢–40¢ for 25 mg (Aldactone) 95¢–$1.18 for 100 mg (Aldactone)	Impotence, decreased libido, gynecomastia, lassitude, gastrointestinal complaints
Amiloride	10 mg qd	40 mg qd	24¢–54¢ for 5 mg	Headaches, lassitude, muscle cramps, impotence, gastrointestinal complaints, increased blood urea nitrogen and uric acid levels

*Cost/tablet was obtained from a sampling of pharmacies in the Boston area.

up to 20 percent of patients develop side effects with spironolactone. In males these include decreased libido, impotence, gynecomastia, lassitude, and gastrointestinal disturbances. The gastrointestinal complaints can be minimized, however, if spironolactone is taken with meals.

An alternate potassium-sparing diuretic, amiloride, acts on the distal renal tubules to block sodium channels. Thus, sodium and chloride excretion is increased and potassium excretion decreased. Amiloride does not directly inhibit aldosterone's action. The initial oral dose is 10 mg a day, which may be increased at 10 mg intervals up to 40 mg a day. As with spironolactone therapy, average serum potassium levels rise by roughly 1.5 mEq per liter. Again the majority of patients with an aldosterone-producing adenoma become normotensive. A somewhat smaller decrease in blood pressure is seen in patients with bilateral adrenal hyperplasia. The side effects of amiloride are mild. They include headaches, lassitude, muscle cramps, gastrointestinal complaints, and occasionally impotence. A mild increase in blood urea nitrogen and uric acid levels can occur.

A combination of triamterene and thiazide has been tried, but in our opinion it is less effective than spironolactone or amiloride in reversing potassium depletion. The dose of triamterene-thiazide (50 mg-25 mg) tablets is up to two tablets twice a day. Side effects include blood dyscrasias, liver damage, gastrointestinal disturbances, weakness, headaches, and anaphylaxis.

Rarely, a low sodium diet and maximum therapy with either spironolactone or amiloride does not control a patient's hypokalemia. In these cases, we have begun potassium supplementation. Potassium supplementation and a potassium-sparing diuretic should not be started simultaneously because of the danger of hyperkalemia. Rather than initiating potassium supplementation, there is theoretical support for considering a combination of amiloride and spironolactone to control resistant hypokalemia. Spironolactone and amiloride exert their effects by different mechanisms and could have a synergistic effect on serum potassium. However, we have no practical experience with this approach.

If the patient's blood pressure is not controlled with a low-salt diet and a potassium-sparing diuretic, an aldosteronoma alone is unlikely. The patient has bilateral hyperplasia and/or renal damage secondary to the elevated blood pressure. In these patients, we have found a beta-blocker or a converting enzyme inhibitor (captopril) good first choices. Calcium channel blockers decrease aldosterone levels in isolated glomerulosa cells and have been used with varying success in treating primary aldosteronism. Cyproheptadine, an antiserotoninergic agent, and bromocriptine, a dopamine agonist, have both proved to be ineffective in treating primary aldosteronism. Potential new drugs that exploit the ability of atrial natriuretic factor to inhibit aldosterone secretion may prove useful in the future. These medications were tested because of the hypotheses that aldosterone production is under tonic dopaminergic inhibition and that there exists a pituitary aldosterone-stimulating hormone under serotoninergic stimulation.

If test results indicate bilateral adrenal hyperplasia, patients should be continued on medical therapy. For unknown reasons, bilateral adrenalectomy, despite correcting the biochemical abnormalities in patients with bilateral adrenal hyperplasia, is generally ineffective in reversing hypertension, with only 15 percent of patients becoming normotensive after surgery. In addition, these patients face the problem of adrenal insufficiency. Because of the complications associated with long-term steroid administration, patients with glucocorticoid-suppressible hyperaldosteronism may need to be treated in the same way as patients with bilateral adrenal hyperplasia if a large glucocorticoid dose is required.

The treatment for a patient with an aldosterone-producing adenoma is surgical removal of the adenoma and the affected adrenal gland. Patients who refuse therapy or who are poor surgical candidates because of other medical problems may be treated medically. A posterior rather than a transabdominal surgical approach is preferred. With the posterior approach, patients tend to recover more rapidly and have fewer complications. In our experience, roughly 95 percent of patients who undergo adrenalectomy for an aldosterone-producing adenoma become normotensive and normokalemic in the first 3 to 6 months after surgery. Over the next 2 to 3 years, however, 20 to 25 percent again develop hypertension. When hypertension recurs, it is usually easier to control and is not associated with hypokalemia.

Preoperatively, patients should be treated with a low-sodium diet, potassium-sparing diuretics, and antihypertensive agents as needed to control serum potassium and blood pressure. Intraoperatively, a patient's potassium level should be monitored, and because the remaining adrenal may not produce cortisol adequately, a patient should receive high-dose steroids. The intraoperative steroid dose is 10 mg hydrocortisone per hour by constant intravenous infusion. This dose also prevents rebound mineralocorticoid deficiency. Postoperatively, the patient can be switched to oral steroid supplementation and the dose gradually tapered to zero over a 2 to 6 week period. In the postoperative period, a patient may develop hypoaldosteronism with elevated serum potassium levels owing to inadequate functioning of the remaining adrenal cortex. It may take 3 to 6 months before the adrenal cortex fully recovers from the long-term suppressive effects of high aldosterone levels produced by the tumor. During this time a patient should follow a liberal sodium diet, follow daily weights, and be alert for signs of hypovolemia. Fluorohydrocortisone should be avoided since this can further suppress the adrenal cortex.

Finally, how does one treat a patient with an aldosteronoma who refuses surgery? We have had several such patients. All have been treated with spironolactone with normalization of blood pressure. The longest treatment has been 14 years. We have been successful with this approach only in women: no complications have occurred in them. We have not had any men who have tolerated the side effects, i.e., impotence, associated with long-term spironolactone therapy.

Suggested Reading

Drury PL. Disorders of mineralocorticoid activity. Clin Endocrinol Metab 1985; 14:175–202.

Hsueh WA. New insights into the medical management of primary aldosteronism. Hypertension 1986; 8:76–81.

Lyons DF, Kem DC, Brown RD, Hanson CS, Carollo ML. Single-dose captopril as a diagnostic test for primary aldosteronism. J Clin Endocrinol Metab 1983; 57:892–896.

Melby JC. Diagnosis and treatment of primary aldosteronism and isolated hypoaldosteronism. Clin Endocrinol Metab 1985; 14:977–995.

Young WF, Klee GG. Primary aldosteronism—diagnostic evaluation. Endocrinol Metab Clin North Am 1988; 17:367–395.

CUSHING'S DISEASE: PITUITARY MICROSURGERY

Jules Hardy, O.C., M.D., F.R.C.S.C.

Trans-sphenoidal pituitary microsurgery has reached a general consensus as the primary treatment for Cushing's disease. It has proved the most accurate, rapid, and effective method in the hands of skilled and experienced neurosurgeons. Patients with histologically proven pituitary adenoma may have a 90 percent chance of remission.

Preoperative radiologic investigation is focused on a computed tomographic (CT) scan and magnetic resonance imaging (MRI) of the sella turcica. Most frequently the regular tomogram shows a normal sella turcica contour that gives no clues to the presence of a tumor. CT with contrast infusion of the gland is sensitive enough to detect a pituitary microadenoma in about 60 percent of cases. Tumor may be found to be hyperdense or, most often, hypodense and occasionally isodense (i.e., undetectable). MRI with gadolinium enhancement has increased the accuracy of diagnosis in about 80 percent of cases. Another method is inferior petrosal sinus blood sampling, which allows the source of adrenocorticotropic hormone (ACTH) secretion to be clearly distinguished as coming from the pituitary gland or from ectopic tissue. Furthermore, it may localize the side of predominant ACTH secretion, thus orienting the surgeon to search for the lesion on that side or to perform an ipsilateral hemihypophysectomy. In the absence of a clear differential gradient of ACTH secretion between the right and left side by 50 percent or more, and of radiologic visualization of the pituitary adenoma, it may be difficult to tell whether the origin of Cushing's disease is a diffuse hyperplasia or an isodense adenoma. A recent study suggests that patients with Cushing's disease without pituitary adenoma have high prolactin levels after thyrotropin-releasing hormone–luteinizing hormone-releasing hormone (TRH–LHRH) administration. The TRH–LHRH test appears to be more sensitive than CT in distinguishing the latter condition from pituitary ACTH adenoma.

Optimal results can be achieved when careful preoperative investigation has established the biologic cause of the hypercortisolism and confirmed its pituitary origin. The success rate is further increased when the pituitary adenoma has been delineated by CT or MRI. The alternative surgical procedures may be chosen according to the clinical indication. Cushing's disease in children and young adolescents requires the most careful microsurgical selective adenomectomy with preservation of normal pituitary function in order to avoid growth hormone (GH) and thyroid-stimulating hormone (TSH) deficiencies, or to favor the recovery of GH deficit. Some patients in this group have been in remission without recurrence of disease after more than 10 years. Trans-sphenoidal tumor resection is also recommended and does not interfere with pregnancy.

In adult patients of reproductive age who desire pregnancy, selective removal of the tumor is again mandatory. In patients who are no longer in their reproductive years, the different alternatives can be considered, especially when no tumor is visible at preoperative radiologic examination or at surgical exploration. In such cases, hemihypophysectomy, central core hypophysectomy, or even total hypophysectomy may result in satisfactory remission of the disease despite the inconvenience of partial or total hypopituitarism. In the most recent therapeutic approach, trans-sphenoidal surgery is offered as a staged method. Selective microadenomectomy is attempted in a first stage with 90 percent success when the tumor is well circumscribed and selectively removed. Patients with incomplete tumor removal as verified by intraoperative biopsies may benefit from a second exploration shortly after the first surgery to complete the tumor excision.

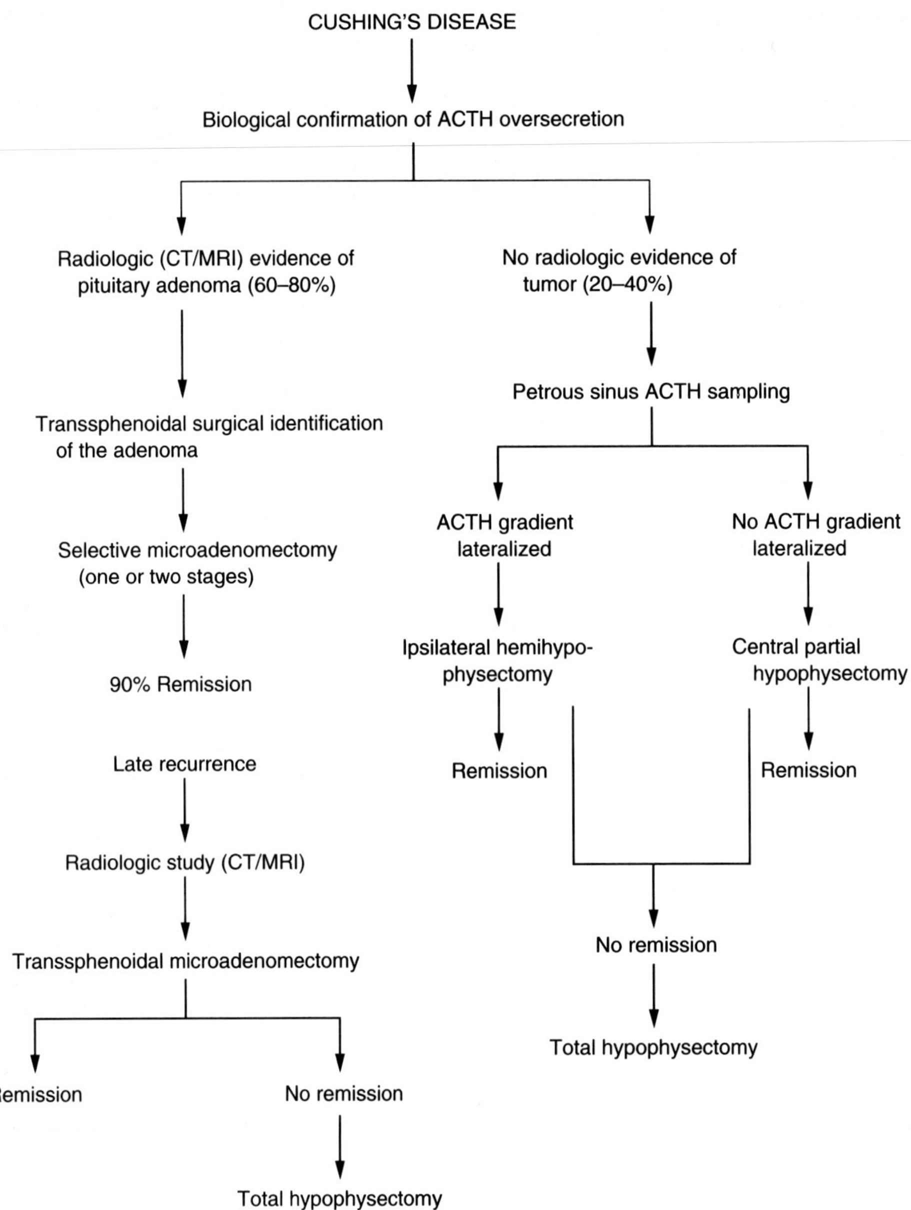

Figure 1
Algorithm used in trans-sphenoidal microsurgery for treatment of Cushing's disease.

Again, a high percentage of cures during this second stage has been obtained while preserving other pituitary functions (Fig. 1).

Patients with late recurrence of a tumor that was visible at the time of the first operation are treated in the same way as a new patient with a first pituitary tumor, i.e., with a selective microadenomectomy. These patients again have a 90 percent chance of remission. When operation on a late recurrence is not satisfactory, total hypophysectomy can be offered as a last resort. If the tumor cannot be totally excised because of invasion of surrounding dural and bony structures, further treatment with radiation and pharmacologic adrenal-blocking agents is possible; however, the final outcome can be determined only after several years. For this reason, radiation therapy should not be used as a first-line treatment for enclosed, noninvasive tumors. More recently, gamma radiation therapy was reported effective in patients with recurrent disease and visible lesion on MRI.

■ SURGICAL TECHNIQUE

The trans-sphenoidal approach to the sella turcica is essentially an extracranial route that encompasses a sublabial gingival incision, elevation of the rhinoseptal mucosa, and opening of the sphenoid sinus to expose the sella turcica. From then on, the operation is carried out with the additional help of magnification with the surgical microscope and an image intensifier to monitor the surgical maneuvers through a fluoroscope on a television screen. The sella turcica is entered with a blunt-ended instrument, and a small window about 8 × 10 mm square is made. The dura is incised in a cruciate fashion. Frequently, a tumor measuring more than 6 mm is readily seen bulging at the surface of the gland; it can be easily shelled out with a microenucleator and removed in one piece, leaving a clear margin cavity within the normal gland. Occasional irregularly shaped tumors require further frozen biopsies of the surrounding margin of the cavity to verify that the remaining tissue is normal adenohypophyseal or neurohypophyseal tissue, thus confirming the total excision of the tumor.

Tumors smaller than 6 mm may not be seen at the surface of the gland and require incision and exploration within the parenchyma. According to the location revealed on the preoperative imaging study, the area is explored until the typical grayish purple or whitish adenomatous tissue that is distinct from the normal gland is seen and selectively removed.

When a pituitary tumor has not been demonstrated preoperatively and is not found during surgical exploration at high-power magnification (×20), alternative surgical techniques can still be offered. When petrous venous blood samples have shown a predominant gradient of ACTH secretion on one side, an ipsilateral hemihypophysectomy is performed. Careful dissection should avoid disrupting the inferior hypophyseal artery, which may result in ischemic damage to the neurohypophysis and infundibulum, producing permanent diabetes insipidus.

When there is no ACTH gradient or when a petrous venous sample has not been obtained, the alternative is partial central core resection of the mucoid zone that contains the majority of ACTH-secreting cells, as demonstrated by immunostaining methods. This procedure is associated with a 82 percent remission of disease.

Finally, in patients with a nondemonstrable adenoma on preoperative radiologic studies or with recurrence of disease after partial resection, total hypophysectomy after pituitary stalk section would ensure complete removal of ACTH and other pituitary secretions, resulting in panhypopituitarism.

The trans-sphenoidal procedure closure is very simple. The sella turcica is packed watertight with lyophilized dura and/or muscle, and then a piece of cartilage from the nasal septum is snapped in the sellar window and covered with tissue adhesive. Antibiotic powder is dusted in the sphenoid sinus, and the nasal mucosae are reapproximated and maintained with endonasal tampons; a few loose catgut sutures are placed on the gingival margin. This relatively nontraumatic procedure allows the patient to resume an oral diet as soon as the anaesthetic agents are dissipated and to be ambulant the night of surgery. Nasal discomfort is relieved when the tampons are removed on the third postoperative day. Numbness of the gum margin prevents postoperative pain, and normal sensation returns within a few weeks.

Perioperative management of patients undergoing trans-sphenoidal surgery requires an intravenous infusion of hydrocortisone, 100 mg every 8 hours, beginning with the start of the operation. After surgery, the medication is tapered by 50 percent each day until a single oral dose is reached. However, careful monitoring of blood pressure and cortisol secretion in the urine allows the detection of early hypoadrenalism. A successful outcome will be followed by low or undetectable plasma values of cortisol and ACTH that will require replacement therapy. In the months after successful surgery the progressive tapering of cortisone may allow the normal cells to resume their own secretion of ACTH. This occurs between the sixth and twelfth months postoperatively in over 80 percent of patients. The incidence of partial insufficiency of TSH requiring replacement therapy is between 5 and 20 percent for patients who have had a microadenomectomy. Because of the susceptibility to infection, patients with Cushing's disease receive prophylactic antibiotic therapy preoperatively and during the first postoperative week.

Possible surgical complications are excessive bleeding, cerebrospinal fluid fistula, and meningitis, which occur in less than 2 percent of cases.

■ COMMENTS

The trans-sphenoidal microsurgical approach, in comparison with other methods (pharmacologic, medical, and radiation therapy) is the most accurate, rapid, and effective treatment for Cushing's disease. It is accurate because it is a direct, open, microsurgical approach that allows the surgeon to visualize the pituitary adenoma and tailor the microsurgical dissection to the form, consistency, and location of the microadenoma within the normal pituitary gland, which in turn can be carefully preserved. It is a rapid procedure that can be performed in less than 2 hours by an experienced surgeon. Within 24 hours of surgery, endocrine tests can confirm remission of the disease by low plasma cortisol secretion. Incomplete remission can be detected early so that reoperation can be offered within a week after the first procedure, obviating the long wait of months and sometimes years before remission due to radiation therapy can be confirmed.

Finally, trans-sphenoidal pituitary microsurgery is an effective treatment that yields immediate results. With this procedure, complete remission is obtained by removing the tumor entirely and thus obliterating the oversecretion of ACTH and cortisol. This is followed by transient hypocortisolism and eventually a restoration of normal pituitary function, thus attaining the goal of ideal therapy for Cushing's disease.

Suggested Reading

Chandler WF, Schteingard DE, Lloyd RV, McKeever PE. Surgical treatment of Cushing's disease. J Neurosurg 1987; 66:204–212.

Comtois R, Beauregard H, Somma M. High prolactin levels in patients with Cushing's disease without pituitary adenoma. Clin Endocrinol 1993; 38:601–607.

Coyne TJ, Atkinson RL, Prins JB. Adrenocorticotropic hormone-secreting pituitary tumor associated with pregnancy: Case report. Neurosurgery 1992; 31:953–955.

Fahlbusch R, Buchfelder M, Muller OA. Transsphenoidal surgery for Cushing's disease. J R Soc Med 1986; 79:262–269.

Hardy J. Transsphenoidal microsurgery of the normal and pathological pituitary. Clin Neurosurg 1969; 16:185–217.

Laws ER. Pituitary tumors—therapeutic considerations: Surgical. In: Barrow DL, Salman W, eds. Concepts in neurosurgery. Neuroendocrinology 1992; 5:395–400.

Ludecke DK, Niedworok G. Results of microsurgery in Cushing's disease and effect of hypertension. Cardiology 1985; 72(Suppl 1):91–94.

Mampalam TJ, Tyrell JB, Wilson CB. Transsphenoidal microsurgery for

Cushing's disease. A report of 216 cases. Ann Intern Med 1988; 109: 487–493.
Marcovitz S, Wee R, Chan J, Hardy J. The diagnostic accuracy of preoperative CT scanning in the evaluation of pituitary ACTH-secreting adenomas. AJNR 1987; 8:641–644.
Melby JC. Therapy of Cushing disease: A consensus for pituitary microsurgery. Ann Intern Med 1988; 109:455–456.
Robert F, Hardy J. Cushing's disease: A correlation of radiological, surgical and pathological findings with therapeutic results. Pathol Res Pract 1991; 187:617–621.
Seo Y, Fukuoka S, Takanashi M, et al. Gamma knife surgery for Cushing disease. Surg Neurol 1995; 43:170–176.
Takashi N, Kuwayama A, Seo H, et al. Endocrinological evaluation of ACTH-secreting pituitary microadenomas: Their location and X-melanocyte stimulating hormone immunoreactivity. J Neurosurg 1992; 76:944–947.
Tindall GT, Herring CJ, Clark RV, et al. Cushing's disease: Results of transsphenoidal microsurgery with emphasis on surgical failures. J Neurosurg 1990; 72:363–369.

POSTMENOPAUSAL OSTEOPOROSIS

Bruce Ettinger, M.D.

A 70-year-old woman is first seen for intense mid-back pain of 2 weeks' duration that began after lifting a suitcase. Spinal X-rays show diffuse osteopenia, moderate wedge deformities of T8-T9, and a crush fracture of L1. The patient has no serious health problems and uses no medications. When menopause occurred 20 years previously, estrogen was prescribed only briefly. Physical examination reveals a thin, slightly kyphotic woman, who measures 4 cm shorter than her height at age 25 years. The patient hesitates to move because of back pain and the upper lumbar spine is tender to percussion.

This patient requires treatment to alleviate the pain of her acute L1 vertebral fracture and to prevent new fractures. The pain of her present fracture will diminish in a few months, although she may have some disability for a year or more. Being healthy, she will probably live to be 85 years old. However, because she experienced one vertebral fracture, she has an annual recurrence risk of 10 to 20 percent; thus over the next 15 years she may experience two or three additional vertebral fractures. Her lifetime risk of hip fracture is about 25 percent, and, should this occur, she would have a 30 percent chance of losing her independence and a 15 percent chance of dying within 6 months.

■ PRETREATMENT EVALUATIONS: NECESSARY AND UNNECESSARY

Measuring Bone Density: Unnecessary

Although bone densitometry facilitates diagnosing osteoporosis and guiding osteoporosis prevention strategies in younger patients, it is unnecessary in older patients. This patient has osteopenia, because a minimum 30 percent reduction in bone density must occur before osteopenia becomes apparent on x-ray films. Because of the patient's advanced age and the multiple vertebral deformities, it is certain that she has osteoporosis, a condition marked by both low bone density and fractures resulting from bone fragility.

Knowing her exact bone density might allow a more accurate prediction of her future risk of osteoporotic fractures but would not alter treatment decisions. If a nonstandard treatment were to be used (see following discussion), it would be necessary to monitor its effects by annually comparing bone density to results obtained before treatment.

Measuring Markers of Bone Turnover: Necessary

Newer biochemical tests, which give indirect evidence of bone turnover rate, may predict bone loss rate and response to therapy. A high bone turnover rate in an untreated postmenopausal woman indicates that bone loss is probably rapid. Nearly all women show high bone turnover for a few years after menopause, but about one-third continue to have high turnover 10 to 20 years later. Many physicians believe such women invariably experience extensive bone loss and therefore should receive aggressive medical therapy, usually with an agent that blocks bone resorption.

Bone turnover occurs by the coupled processes of bone resorption and bone formation. When bone collagen is destroyed, its pyridinium cross-links are released into the circulation and are excreted in urine without being metabolized. The pyridinium cross-links test has replaced measurement of urinary hydroxyproline because it is more specific and sensitive. When bone is formed by osteoblasts, osteocalcin is released into the serum. Both pyridinium cross-links and osteocalcin tests are commercially available through many reference laboratories. Measurement of either bone marker indicates bone turnover rate. Changes in these indicators occur quickly and thus provide a convenient assessment of treatment effects within a few months.

■ TREATMENT OF CHOICE

Correction of Adverse Habits and Lifestyle

With the exception of vertebral fractures, all osteoporotic fractures are preceded by an injury, frequently a fall. Reducing the risk of falling is a positive step toward reducing the risk of fracture. The patient's home can be made safer if handrails are installed in bathrooms and halls and along stairways. Hazards

Table 1 Calcium Preparations

PREPARATION	% CALCIUM	CALCIUM PER TABLET (MG)	YEARLY COST FOR 1,000 MG/ DAY ($)*
Calcium carbonate	40		
Caltrate		600	108
Oyster Shell (generic)		250, 500, 600	40
Os-Cal		250, 500	108
Tums E-X		300	55
Calcium phosphate			
Posture		600	115
Calcium lactate (generic)	13	85	350
Calcium gluconate (generic)	9	90	522
Calcium citrate	8		
Citracal		200, 315	162

*Discount retail price.

from poor lighting, loose rugs, and cluttered furniture should be corrected. Any physical deficiencies of the patient that can increase the propensity to fall, such as poor vision and difficulty in walking, should be corrected. Progress is being made in the development of plastic hip protectors to reduce the force that is transmitted to the femur when patients fall impacting on the buttocks. Once back pain has resolved, suggest an exercise program to improve mobility and neuromuscular coordination. Review the patient's medications and, when possible, stop those that may impair perception or coordination (particularly tranquilizers and hypnotics). Stopping alcohol abuse can limit its adverse effects on bone metabolism and should reduce the risk of drinking-related injuries.

Correction of Deficiencies of Calcium and Vitamin D

Bone loss in the early postmenopausal years is unrelated to any abnormality of calcium metabolism and is not prevented by high calcium intake. However, beginning 5 or more years after menopause, estrogen-dependent bone loss slows and calcium and vitamin D intake may play an increasingly important role in skeletal homeostasis. Several factors may combine to create calcium deficiency in women of advancing age: (1) dietary intakes of calcium and vitamin D may decrease, (2) intestinal calcium absorption becomes less efficient, and (3) 25-hydroxyvitamin D-1α-hydroxylase activity diminishes. Reduced calcium intake is very common among the elderly; 75 to 80 percent of elderly women consume less than the 800 mg daily of the recommended dietary allowance (RDA) of calcium and 80 percent consume less than the 400 U daily of the RDA of vitamin D. Additionally, elderly people who remain indoors have less exposure to ultraviolet light and thus produce less vitamin D in the skin.

The adequacy of calcium and vitamin D intake can be assessed by asking about dairy product intake and by measuring 24 hour urinary calcium excretion. Instead of an elaborate dietary history, use the following formula: the dairy-free diet provides about 300 mg calcium, each full serving of a dairy product (e.g., a cup of milk or slice of cheese) adds about 300 mg, and each serving of a calcium-fortified food adds 160 mg. Add to the dietary intake the milligrams of elemental calcium from supplements (Table 1). Vitamin D intake is 100 U per cup of milk plus any taken in vitamin preparations. Calcium carbonate is the most often used and least expensive calcium supplement. Chewable calcium supplements are preferable because chewing improves dispersion and bioavailability. Bedtime dosage may be especially effective because bone turnover (and loss) is greatest when people are recumbent at night. Absorption is enhanced by taking calcium with a small snack. Avoiding high calcium dosages minimizes the risk of associated constipation.

Make sure that at least 400 U vitamin D are also taken daily. Vitamin D is available combined with calcium, usually 125 to 200 U per tablet. Another convenient vitamin D source is a liquid pediatric preparation, ergocalciferol oral suspension, which provides 200 U per drop and is well absorbed by the elderly. In addition to increasing gastrointestinal calcium absorption, vitamin D may improve osteoblastic function and may have other anabolic effects.

While the patient is ingesting a usual diet (including usual supplements), measurement of 24 hour urinary calcium can be done to show calcium bioavailability. If less than 50 mg a day is excreted, intake and/or absorption are insufficient. In such cases the intake of calcium should be increased to at least 1,200 to 1,500 mg daily, after which a 24 hour urine calcium can be rechecked. If urinary calcium remains low, vitamin D intake should be increased to 800 to 1,200 U daily.

Several studies have shown reduced bone loss among older women who receive calcium or vitamin D supplements, especially if they initially had low dietary calcium or low vitamin D intakes. Vitamin D and calcium correct the biochemical abnormalities indicative of calcium deficiency, reduce bone loss, and appear to reduce the risk of hip fractures.

The goal of this intervention is physiologic correction of dietary and absorptive inadequacy of calcium and not pharmacologic vitamin D effects. There is virtually no risk of toxicity at these low dosages, and close monitoring is unnecessary. The main potential toxicity involves diminished renal function and/or nephrolithiasis. The lifetime risk of calcium stones among women is less than 5 percent, and the disease rarely begins when women are elderly. Studies of the epidemiology of nephrolithiasis indicate urinary calcium has little

Table 2 Equivalent Estrogen Preparations

BRAND NAME	FORMULATION	ROUTE	DOSE (mg)	SCHEDULE	YEARLY COST ($)*
Estrace	17β-estradiol (micronized)	Oral	1.0	Daily	89
Estraderm	17β-estradiol (reservoir)	Transdermal	0.05	Change twice weekly	254
Climara	17β-estradiol (solid matrix)	Transdermal	0.05	Change once weekly	270
Ogen	Piperazine estrone sulfate	Oral	1.25	Daily	237
Premarin	Conjugated equine estrogens	Oral	0.625	Daily	77

*Average retail price.

impact on stone risk until calcium excretion exceeds 350 to 400 mg daily. The prevalence of hypercalciuria among older women is quite low, and there has not been an increase in calcium nephrolithiasis among elderly women in spite of widespread use of calcium supplements in the past 10 to 15 years. Recent epidemiologic studies indicate an inverse relationship between calcium intake and nephrolithiasis. Thus, use of calcium supplement may actually be protective.

Antiresorption Therapy

Estrogen, thyrocalcitonin, and alendronate are Food and Drug Administration (FDA)–approved treatments for osteoporosis; they are more likely to benefit women with mild to moderate bone loss, because neither treatment can restore the aged skeleton to a youthful density. These agents reduce the rate of bone turnover through a reduction in osteoclastic resorption. When treatment is initiated, a temporary imbalance between bone resorption and formation is produced, which may result in increased bone density. The amount of increase is dependent on the rate of bone turnover when therapy is initiated; a high rate of skeletal turnover is associated with numerous, large resorption spaces that fill with new bone. Antiresorption therapy usually increases bone density 5 to 10 percent but only during the first few years of treatment. Thereafter treatment decreases bone turnover, and very slow bone loss is the long-term result. Fracture risk is reduced by about 50 percent in spite of the relatively small gain in bone density. It has been hypothesized that these treatments may improve bone quality, perhaps by increasing its architectural (structural) integrity, enhancing its ability to resist mechanical stress, and increasing its density.

Practitioners should become competent in administering all three drugs because some circumstances favor using one rather than the others; the choice is made on the basis of benefits and risks, but patient acceptability is often a deciding factor. The supporting literature on the role of estrogen in prevention of bone loss and fracture is extensive, but estrogen may cause return of menses, mastalgia, and bloating. Several studies report a possible 30 to 40 percent increase in breast cancer in women taking high-dose estrogens over 10 or more years. However, estrogen therapy may be preferred for the woman who has had a hysterectomy (by age 70, 30 to 35 percent of women). Not only is there no return of menses but in addition the potential adverse symptoms associated with progestogen use can be avoided. In my practice, most elderly women with osteoporosis prefer not to use hormone therapy. Thyrocalcitonin is preferred for the patient who experiences prolonged or severe fracture pain, because studies indicate that endorphin, released from the pituitary by thyrocalcitonin, may reduce pain perception.

Alendronate, the first bisphosphonate approved for treatment of osteoporosis, has been enthusiastically received. Being oral, nonhormonal, and relatively free of side effects has enhanced its acceptance. Some have recommended that it be used by any postmenopausal woman whose bone density is low. However, until more experience is gained with this new drug, I reserve it for older women with overt osteoporosis (low bone density *and* fractures).

Thyrocalcitonin

With experience investigators recognized that administration of thyrocalcitonin at lower dosages and decreased frequency may be as effective as the daily larger dosages initially used. Presently, I give 50 Medical Research Council (MRC) units subcutaneously three times a week and reduce the dose to 30 to 40 MRC units in the 10 to 20 percent of patients who develop flushing or nausea. This treatment schedule costs about $500 annually. Some researchers believe intermittent treatment (e.g., 6 months on, 6 months off) is more effective than continuous therapy because it may avoid development of drug resistance. I prefer a 1 month break at the end of each year of treatment. The drug is available in 2 ml multiple-use vials at a concentration of 200 MRC units per ml for injections of 0.25 ml each. Intranasally administered thyrocalcitonin is now available. Intranasal doses must be about four times the amount needed for subcutaneous route administration to achieve comparable effects. It costs $441 a year. Both subcutaneous and intranasal thyrocalcitonin have been shown to have an analgesic effect that usually becomes evident within 1 to 2 weeks of starting treatment. In my experience, clinically significant analgesia occurs in a minority of patients. I generally use twice the usual dosage for the first few weeks to enhance pain relief.

Estrogen

In treating postmenopausal osteoporosis, standard dosages of estrogen should be used (Table 2). However, to minimize side effects such as mastalgia and bloating, it is prudent to begin using half-strength doses for a few months. When prescribing estrogen for a woman over the age of 65 who still has a uterus, combine estrogen with daily low-dose medroxyprogesterone acetate. Most older women have no menses on this combined hormone regimen. In contrast, the combined continuous hormone regimen causes nearly half of younger women to have irregular bleeding. Other progestin regimens are shown in Table 3.

High calcium intake may allow half the customary estrogen dose to have the same skeletal effects as the standard dosage. For example, 0.3 mg conjugated estrogens combined with a calcium intake of at least 1,500 mg daily for up to 3 years

Table 3 Alternative Medroxyprogesterone Acetate* Regimens

DOSE (mg)	DURATION	SCHEDULE	YEARLY COST ($)†
2.5	Daily	Continuously	123
5.0	12 days	1st–12th of month	70
10.0	14 days	1st–14th of every third month	33

*All dosages are available as generics.
†Average retail price.

appears to have no different effect than 0.6 mg conjugated estrogen given without calcium supplements. When standard doses of estrogen are given, calcium intake does not need to exceed 1,000 mg.

Biphosphonates

Encouraged by recent publications, some physicians have been prescribing etidronate (Didronel) for osteoporosis. Unfortunately, additional follow-up years of patients in a U.S. multicenter trial did not confirm vertebral fracture protection and serious doubts have been raised over detrimental effects to bone health. Currently, a number of newer bisphosphonates are being tested that appear to have less adverse effects on bone mineralization.

Osteoporotic women using alendronate, on average, gain 8 percent in spinal mineral and 4 percent in hip mineral over 2 to 3 years. Nearly all women respond with gains in density. The increased bone mineral produces stronger bone; compared with calcium alone, alendronate reduced new spinal fractures by 48 percent over 3 years. Hip fracture studies of alendronate are ongoing, but early results indicate a similar degree of risk reduction.

Alendronate is usually well tolerated and appears safe. In patients who have taken alendronate up to 3 years, bone biopsies appear normal, but there are no studies of long-term skeletal effects. Alendronate becomes part of the bone and accumulates there. Bone biochemical markers indicate that alendronate suppresses bone turnover about the same amount as estrogen and that this suppression does not increase over 3 years' use. However, I am concerned about cumulative adverse effects on bone and bone marrow from very long-term use. Another drug similar to alendronate was withdrawn from use after possibly increasing the incidence of leukemia. Occasionally alendronate can cause gastritis and esophagitis. These problems appear dose related but are more common in patients with gastric reflux. The drug is very poorly absorbed, so patients must be carefully instructed to take it on an empty stomach with a glass of water and to allow 30 to 60 minutes for absorption before ingesting any food or medications. The annual cost of alendronate treatment, 10 mg once daily, is about $500.

Monitoring Treatment

The ultimate test of osteoporosis treatment is prevention of fractures; thus, annual monitoring for new vertebral fractures should be accomplished by measuring the patient's height and obtaining a single lateral thoracolumbar spine radiograph (instruct the technician to include T6 through L3).

Table 4 Nonstandard Osteoporosis Treatments (Investigational Use Only)

CLASS OF DRUG	PRESUMED MECHANISM OF ACTION	POTENTIAL PROBLEMS WITH USE
Androgen	↑ Formation	Hirsutism, voice deepening, adverse effect on lipoproteins
Coherence therapy (AFDR)	↑ Formation	(Theoretical concept—never implemented)
Fluoride	↑ Formation	Cortical stress fractures, gastrointestinal side effects, poor quality of new bone
Progestin	Unknown	Fails to protect spine, premenstrual syndrome, adverse effect on lipoprotein and vascular tone
Raloxifene	↓ Resorption	Estrogen deficiency symptoms
Tamoxifen	↓ Resorption	Expensive, liver toxicity, estrogen deficiency symptoms
Thiazide diuretic	↓ Urinary calcium	Hypokalemia, orthostatic hypotension
Vitamin D analogue	↑ Formation	Hypercalcemia, hypercalciuria, renal damage, kidney stones

Intermediate end points of treatment success are changes in biochemical measures of bone turnover. These tests are usually high normal or slightly elevated at baseline and should decrease within a few months of treatment to 30 to 50 percent of baseline values.

Bone densitometry is increasingly used for monitoring treatment response. Whereas dual photon absorptiometry lacked sufficient precision to monitor individual patients, newer dual-energy x-ray absorptiometry (DEXA) has excellent precision and monitoring potential. DEXA can show treatment effects at various skeletal sites if careful attention is given to quality assurance and if newer automated techniques are used to minimize repositioning errors. When using agents such as estrogen, thyrocalcitonin, or alendronate that are effective in 90 percent of women, I believe that follow-up densitometry studies are not cost effective.

■ POTENTIAL THERAPIES

A number of new regimens are being actively investigated (Table 4). Until long-term safety and effectiveness are established, these treatments should not be used by practitioners.

Raloxifene, tamoxifen, and progestins appear to inhibit bone resorption; fluoride, 1,25-dihydroxyvitamin D, anabolic steroids, and parathyroid hormone appear to stimulate bone formation; and coherence therapy may do both.

Coherence Therapy

Coherence therapy (or ADFR), first proposed in 1979, involves cyclic administration of a series of agents. The goal is to tip the balance between bone resorption and bone formation toward increased formation. The ADFR acronym stands for the four phases of the regimen: *a*ctivation of new osteoclasts, *d*epression of these same cells before their resorption potential is fully realized, a drug-*f*ree period to allow bone formation at newly activated sites, and *r*epetition of the cycle. A number of activators and depressors are being evaluated, and a number of different timing sequences are being considered. The activators currently in use include inorganic phosphate, parathyroid hormone, and 1,25-dihydroxyvitamin D. Depressors include bisphosphonates and calcitonin. Ideally, this treatment makes all bone metabolic units do the same thing at the same time (coherence), manipulating them by sequential treatments given at critical times in their life cycle. Unfortunately, current ADFR regimens fail to achieve skeletal coherence and without repeated bone biopsies it is not possible to know a person's bone metabolic unit life cycle.

Fluoride

Studies of sodium fluoride have taught an important lesson—increased bone density cannot always be equated with increased bone strength. Sodium fluoride markedly stimulates new bone formation, especially in the spine; it can increase spinal bone density 9 to 10 percent each year. In a 4 year clinical trial sponsored by the National Institutes of Health (NIH), 70 mg sodium fluoride a day increased spinal density 36 percent, on average, but the newly formed bone was not strong; treatment did not reduce the incidence of spinal fractures and appeared to increase severalfold the incidence of peripheral fractures. In addition, many women given sodium fluoride developed troublesome gastrointestinal symptoms and periarticular pains in the lower limbs. After these disastrous results, it appeared that fluoride would never again be used to treat osteoporosis. Recently, enthusiasm for fluoride is again increasing based on studies employing lower dosages. Reanalysis of the NIH clinical trial showed that women who used half the usual dosage of fluoride (because of gastrointestinal intolerance) and whose spinal density increased on average only 4 to 5 percent, showed reductions in spinal fracture rate. Other investigators have since found that 30 to 50 mg sodium fluoride per day may be ideal for increasing bone density and improving bone quality. Development of "slow-release" fluoride has allowed better control of the serum and bone levels of fluoride and has reduced the problem of side effects. Over 2½ years, about one in six women taking slow-release fluoride had a new fracture, compared with about one in three taking calcium alone. A safe serum level of fluoride is 5 to 7 μM per liter (women not taking fluoride will have serum fluoride levels of about 2 μM per liter; toxicity is observed when the serum level reaches 10 μM per liter). Maintaining a therapeutic level of fluoride in the serum should produce a safe increment in spinal bone density, about 4 to 5 percent annually. Slow-release fluoride has recently been recommended by an FDA advisory panel and thus is likely to become available in 1997. The narrow toxic-therapeutic window for fluoride will mandate careful monitoring of serum fluoride levels and annual measurements of spinal and hip bone density. Bone density monitoring will also detect the 30 percent of women who do not respond. Treatment should include 800 to 1,000 mg daily supplemental calcium, and there should be a 2 month break in fluoride administration after each 12 months of use. The expected annual cost of this drug is $350.

Vitamin D Analogues

Vitamin D is converted in the body to 25-hydroxyvitamin D and then to 1,25-dihydroxyvitamin D, the active form of the vitamin that is responsible for physiologic actions on bone and intestine. In some countries, the 25- and 1,25-vitamin D metabolites are the preferred method of treating osteoporosis. A recent, large-scale clinical trial showed 1,25-dihydroxyvitamin D was effective in preventing recurrent vertebral fractures. Having used this drug, I have serious concern about its toxic effects, particularly with respect to hypercalcemia, hypercalciuria, and renal damage. Potent vitamin D analogues have an extremely narrow therapeutic area, and the high risk of toxicity mandates careful monitoring of serum and urine calcium. Thus I do not recommend their general use in treatment of osteoporosis.

Estrogen Analogues

Tamoxifen's antiestrogen effect on breast cell receptors is the rationale for its use in prophylaxis and treatment of breast cancer. However, tamoxifen acts as a weak estrogen on bone and may act as a powerful estrogen on the endometrium. Tamoxifen should not be considered as an alternative to estrogen for osteoporosis because it does not produce comparable skeletal effects, it can worsen estrogen deficiency symptoms, and it can cause endometrial cancer. However, women receiving tamoxifen for breast cancer can be reassured that this drug reduces the rate of postmenopausal bone loss. Experience with tamoxifen has led to the development of other estrogen analogues. Raloxifene and droloxifene have thus far shown promise in limited studies. These drugs appear to act selectively on different estrogen receptors, blocking estrogen's actions on breast and endometrium, but stimulating estrogen's actions on bone and liver. Results of ongoing clinical trials will be available in 1998.

Suggested Reading

Avioli LV. Calcitonin in the prevention and therapy of osteoporotic syndromes. Endocrine Practice 1995; 1:33–38.

Dequeker J, Geusens P. Treatment of established osteoporosis and rehabilitation: Current practice and possibilities. Maturitas 1990; 12:1–36.

Ettinger B, Grady D. Maximizing the benefit of estrogen therapy for prevention of osteoporosis. Menopause 1994; 1:19–24.

Heaney RP. Calcium in the prevention and treatment of osteoporosis. J Intern Med 1992; 231:169-180.

Kanis JA. Treatment of osteoporosis in elderly women. Am J Med 1995; 98(Suppl 2A):60S–66S.

Kanis JA, Gertz BJ, Singer F, Ortolani S. Rationale for the use of alendronate in osteoporosis. Osteoporos Int 1995; 5:1–13.

Kleerekoper M. Extensive personal experience: The clinical evaluation and management of osteoporosis. J Clin Endocrinol Metab 1995; 80:757–763.

Liberman UA, Weiss SR, Bröll J, et al. Effect of alendronate on bone mineral density and the incidence of fractures in postmenopausal osteoporosis. N Engl J Med 1995; 333:1437–1443.

Pak CYC, Sakhaee K, Piziak V, et al. Slow-release sodium fluoride in the management of postmenopausal osteoporosis. Ann Intern Med 1994; 120:625–632.

Riggs BL. Overview of osteoporosis. West J Med 1991; 154:63–77.

Ringe JD, Meunier PJ. What is the future for fluoride in the treatment of osteoporosis? Osteoporos Int 1995; 5:71–74.

Seeman E, Tsalamandris C, Bass S, Pearce G. Present and future of osteoporosis therapy. Bone 1995; 17:23S–29S.

OBESITY

Lawrence J. Cheskin, M.D.

■ THE CLINICAL PROBLEM

Malnutrition is a major health problem worldwide and, as such, is most commonly equated with undernourishment. However, in the developed world, and especially in the United States, malnutrition takes a different form—overnourishment. This type of malnutrition leads to an excess of body fat, also known as obesity, and to its myriad medical complications. Obesity is the most important risk factor in the development of non–insulin-dependent diabetes, and it is a significant risk factor for diseases of virtually every organ system (Table 1), even certain cancers. The risk of most of these complications increases with the degree of obesity, though for some, notably coronary vascular disease and strokes, the risk correlates best with the regional distribution of fat. Abdominal deposition of fat (android or apple-shape pattern), seen commonly in men and less often in women, is associated with a high risk for cardiovascular disease; in contrast, excess fat in the thighs, hips, and buttocks (the gynecoid or pear-shape pattern) is associated with a lower risk of such complications.

Table 1 Health Risks of Obesity

- NIDDM
- Hypertension, CAD
- Hyperlipidemia
- Strokes
- Cancer (endometrial, postmenopausal, breast, colorectal)
- Sleep apnea
- Gallbladder disease
- Gastroesophageal reflux disease
- Fatty liver
- Osteoarthritis
- Gout
- Infertility
- Thromboembolism

NIDDM, non–insulin-dependent diabetes mellitus; CAD, coronary artery disease.

Moderate to severe obesity also elevates overall mortality, carrying a relative risk of death of almost 1.9 for adult men and women at least 40 percent over ideal body weight, according to actuarial tables. Although still controversial, recent epidemiologic evidence suggests that even slight elevations above ideal body weight is associated with excess mortality. In addition to the medical risks, and perhaps more motivating for many of those seeking to lose weight, are the unfortunate psychosocial consequences of obesity. Our society fosters widespread prejudice against obese individuals, detectable in the opinions of children as young as 6 years of age, according to one study. The resulting social and job discrimination contributes to low self-esteem and the high rate of depression among the obese who have sought treatment. Also noteworthy in this vein are the association of childhood sexual abuse with subsequent obesity, the greater social stigma borne by obese women compared with obese men in our society, and the higher prevalence of obesity among those of low socioeconomic status, Anglo-American and Hispanic women, and Native Americans.

What, then, defines this condition, obesity? We all know it when we see it, but a method of standardization is desirable. Obesity is technically defined as an excess of body *fat* (>25 percent of body weight for men and >30 percent for women), rather than an excess of body *weight.* With the exception of patients with marked thyroid overload and very muscular individuals (e.g., certain types of athletes and laborers), relative weight is a reasonable surrogate measure for the less readily obtained measure of adiposity (percent of body weight constituted by fat).

Weight adjusted for height, or body mass index (BMI), defined as weight in kilograms divided by the square of the height in meters, is very useful for defining and grading the severity of obesity (Table 2) and attendant risks. Grade 0 is associated with the lowest mortality risk, as derived from life insurance data. These data are most commonly summarized in tables of "ideal" body weight (IBW) for different heights and frame sizes (Table 3), but some caveats are in order. First, at least one-third of the adult U.S. population is more than

Table 2 Grading Obesity of Body Mass Index (BMI)*

GRADE	DEGREE OF OBESITY	BMI
3	Morbid	>40
2	Moderate to severe	30–40
1	Mild to trivial	25–29.9
0	Not obese	20–24.9

*BMI, weight (kg)/height (m^2).

20 percent over IBW, as are 60 percent of middle-aged black women. The public tends to treat these "ideal" weights as gospel, and much unnecessary deprivation and unhappiness can be attributed to generally unsuccessful attempts to attain and maintain these weights. Second, not only are IBWs unrealistic goals for most obese people, they also apply only to the population from which the data were drawn—middle-class whites in their twenties. This must be considered in light of evidence that the relative weight associated with lowest mortality increases with age (Table 4). Third, although existing evidence is not compelling, it is possible that "yo-yo" dieting may pose greater health risks than staying at a moderately obese level.

Therefore, it is probably best to steer patients away from IBW tables and to strongly encourage weight loss for medical reasons only in those with grade 2 or 3 obesity, especially if they are young, already suffer from complicating medical conditions, or have a strong family history of diabetes, cardiovascular, or cerebrovascular disease. For those with trivial obesity (grade 1) the benefits of successful weight loss are primarily psychosocial rather than medical. These patients should be encouraged to focus on a healthier (low-fat, high-fiber) diet and increased physical fitness (exercise) rather than just the number on the scale.

In the case of abdominal fat deposition, however, even mild excess adiposity may pose a medical problem. A waist-hip ratio of more than 1.0 for men and 0.8 for women suggests abdominal obesity, and can be easily measured with a tape rule around the narrowest point above the umbilicus and the widest point below the hips. Fortunately, this metabolically active abdominal fat is usually first to go with weight loss. The pear shape is both safer and more durable than the apple, as many women who attempt to lose weight have learned. From an evolutionary perspective, lower-body obesity may have conferred a selective advantage by helping to ensure survival through times of food shortage. Lower fat is easily mobilized only under the hormonal influences of pregnancy and breast-feeding.

Despite the inescapable fact that genetic influences exist (witness at least two recently cloned "fat" genes and various adopted-twin studies), genetics does not appear to account for the majority of variability in BMI seen in the population, nor is it an insurmountable barrier in those who were fortunate (or unfortunate) enough to draw the putative genes leading to metabolic efficiency in the lottery of conception.

Table 3 Metropolitan Height-Weight Table, 1983*

	WEIGHT	
HEIGHT	MEN	WOMEN
4′10″		100–131
4′11″		101–134
5′0″		103–137
5′1″	123–145	105–140
5′2″	125–148	108–144
5′3″	127–151	111–148
5′4″	129–155	114–152
5′5″	131–159	117–156
5′6″	133–163	120–160
5′7″	135–167	123–164
5′8″	137–171	126–167
5′9″	139–175	129–170
5′10″	141–179	132–173
5′11″	144–183	135–176
6′0″	147–187	
6′1″	150–192	
6′2″	153–197	
6′3″	157–202	

*For individuals 25 to 59 years old.

Table 4 Desirable Weight by Age

	20–29 YR	30–39 YR	40–49 YR	50–59 YR	60–69 YR
4′10″	84–111	92–119	99–127	107–135	115–142
4′11″	87–115	95–123	103–131	111–139	119–147
5′0″	90–119	98–127	106–135	114–143	123–152
5′1″	93–123	101–131	110–140	118–148	127–157
5′2″	96–127	105–136	113–144	122–153	131–163
5′3″	99–131	108–140	117–149	126–158	135–168
5′4″	102–135	112–145	121–154	130–163	140–173
5′5″	106–140	115–149	125–159	134–168	144–179
5′6″	109–144	119–154	129–164	138–174	148–184
5′7″	112–148	122–159	133–169	143–179	153–190
5′8″	116–153	126–163	137–174	147–184	158–196
5′9″	119–157	130–168	141–179	151–190	162–201
5′10″	122–162	134–173	145–184	156–195	167–207
5′11″	126–167	137–178	149–190	160–201	172–213
6′0″	129–171	141–183	153–195	165–207	177–219
6′1″	133–176	145–188	157–200	169–213	182–225
6′2″	137–181	149–194	162–206	174–219	187–232
6′3″	141–186	153–199	166–212	179–225	192–238
6′4″	144–191	157–205	171–218	184–231	197–244

Adapted from Andres R. Mortality and obesity. In: Hazzard WR, et al, eds. Principles of geriatric medicine and gerontology. 3rd ed. New York: McGraw-Hill, 1994:852.

Both the environment and learned behaviors are supremely important as modifiers of genetic predisposition and are good places to focus treatment.

■ TREATMENT

Perhaps no other field of medicine today is as subject to the fads, hype, and unreasonable expectations as the treatment of obesity. Part of the reason lies in the inherent difficulty of reconciling a society whose main fuels are fat sucrose, and ethanol, with an ideal body form typified by the Barbie doll. Given that our profession is unlikely to have any say in what body form people are striving for, the next best approach is to lobby for reasonable goal weights for our own patients, encourage those who really need to lose weight to do so, and steer them toward safe, comprehensive treatment.

The components of a comprehensive approach to weight loss are listed in Table 5. The omission of any of these items is likely to adversely affect long-term results. The long-term success rate, defined as losing weight and keeping most of it off for 5 years, is quite low, perhaps 5 to 15 percent in the few studies available. Although this rate is clearly poor, it must be viewed in context and compared with our similarly poor success in treating other chronic conditions and addictions, for example, cigarette smoking and drug abuse. In fact, if one views the chronic pleasurable overconsumption of food energy as a kind of addiction, an instructive distinction between food and other reinforcing substances appears. The cigarette smoker need never smoke again; the obese person, however, must learn to coexist with the offending substances in order to live. In this light, the treatment of obesity should be likened not to the cure of an infectious disease but to the control of a chronic condition. As such, we cannot expect many complete cures and will need to be constantly on the alert for relapses in those who appear to be in remission.

Medical Assessment

The first step in treating the obese patient is the medical assessment. The patient may desire weight loss or may be reluctant. By all means encourage the reluctant patient with medical complications of obesity to lose weight but recognize that any attempt at weight loss will be almost certain to fail, even in the short run, if the patient is not self-motivated to change.

Begin as always with a thorough history and physical. The *weight history* may be of value in identifying precipitants of weight gain and suggesting fruitful avenues for treatment. For example, a change in job leading to a reduction in physical activity may be detected. Also of interest is whether the onset of obesity was in childhood or later in life. Although only about a fifth of obese adults were obese children, about four-fifths of obese children become obese adults. Obesity in childhood often results in hyperplasia of fat cells, an actual increase in number of cells, while adult-onset obesity results in only an increase in average cell size, not number. Treatment of the hyperplastic form of obesity is said to be more difficult because weight reduction does not greatly reduce the number of fat cells, only their average size.

Other information that can be gleaned from the weight history includes postpartum weight gain (the average woman weighs about ten pounds more 2 years postpartum compared with prepregnancy, but the amount is extremely variable), weight gain after smoking cessation (average gain of about 6 lb, again highly variable, and the most common excuse women give for not wanting to quit), and evidence of yo-yo dieting and disorders such as binge eating (consuming inordinately large amounts of food within a short period twice a week or more in private for over 1 year with loss of control and negative emotional sequelae) and bulimia nervosa (binge eating plus purging by vomiting and/or laxatives or diuretics). When an eating disorder is suspected, prescribing a diet and exercise program will not be helpful and may even be counterproductive. Instead, referral to a center experienced in the treatment of these problems is recommended. There is a separate chapter on eating disorders.

The history should also include questions to help rule out *endocrinologic* causes of obesity such as hypothyroidism, hyperadrenalism, and neuroendocrine tumors, though in adults even the most common of these, hypothyroidism, is rarely a significant factor in causing obesity. Also inquire about *drugs* that may be associated with weight gain (Table 6) and symptoms suggestive of diseases that often complicate obesity, such as diabetes, coronary artery disease, hypertension, arthritis, and sleep apnea. Symptoms and signs of *depression* should also be sought, as depression is a common accompaniment of severe obesity and may require additional treatment. *Childhood sexual abuse* is also common, and is best brought up late in the interview after a rapport has been established. Individual or group counseling may be helpful when sexual or other abuse is detected. The family history is of interest for endocrinologic diseases, obesity, and its complications.

The physical examination may be somewhat limited when the patient is morbidly obese, but it can yield evidence of endocrinologic causes and detect complicating conditions. It is necessary to obtain not only an accurate weight and height for calculation of the BMI but also the two simple tape measurements for the waist-hip ratio, an important modifier of risk in obesity, as previously noted.

Laboratory evaluations should serve to screen for the complications of obesity. Blood chemistries should include fasting serum glucose, cholesterol, triglycerides, and liver

Table 5 Components of Comprehensive Weight-Loss Programs

Medical assessment
Behavioral modification
Dietary modification
Exercise modification
Long-term follow-up

Table 6 Drug Causes of Weight Gain

Steroids
Progestins
Tricyclics
Phenothiazines
Lithium

function tests. In addition, an electrogram should be taken, as well as a complete blood count and urinalysis to establish a baseline prior to beginning treatment. A measurement of thyroid-stimulating hormone (TSH) should be obtained if there is any suspicion of thyroid dysfunction, and other endocrine and metabolic tests if indicated.

Behavioral Assessment

It is critical to gain a sense of the behavioral as well as the medical aspects of the patient's situation. This can be accomplished by referral to an appropriately skilled psychologist or through your own guided discussions with the patient.

First, it is important to assess not only specific behaviors but also the impact of these behaviors, and the obesity itself, on the patient's level of functioning and quality of life. It may only emerge with inquiry that the patient has withdrawn from all unnecessary social interactions, or is no longer able to enjoy certain activities or interests because of weight gain, or has suffered job discrimination, to name just a few examples.

Also related to quality of life are the patient's expectations about what changes will occur with successful weight control. Although it may be motivating for the patient to believe that life will improve with weight loss, disappointment may follow unless the changes likely to occur have been placed in proper perspective. Medical benefits can certainly be expected with weight loss in the obese suffering from medical complications. For example, type II diabetics can often discontinue insulin or oral agents, antihypertensive medications may become unnecessary, and sleep apnea usually disappears with as little as a 10 to 15 percent loss of initial weight. On another level, however, although self-assurance often increases, the wallflower does not become the life of the party, and the competent worker does not get a promotion upon losing weight. Encourage obese patients toward a balanced view by reminding them that societal prejudices about body weight and character are in no way based on fact, and that they are the same good and worthy people whether they weigh 250 or 125 pounds.

In exploring specific behaviors, it is useful to assist the patient in identifying various *eating cues.* These cues are situations or feelings that lead to eating, often in an inappropriate way. It is axiomatic in our society that physical hunger is rarely a significant part of life, even for the poorest among us. In fact, physical hunger is not an eating cue for most obese people, because we rarely let ourselves get to the point of true hunger. Instead, we eat in response to a whole host of other cues, most of which are inappropriate. The most common eating cues cited are: habit ("It's 12:30 so I guess I'll have lunch" or "I have a jelly doughnut and coffee in the car on the way to work"), stress ("I've got to finish this paper, and eating while I work helps me concentrate"), boredom ("There's nothing else to do" [a subcategory is watching television and eating at the same time]), emotions ("I eat when I'm depressed or upset"), and food as a reward ("After a hard day, I deserve a rich dessert"). Underlying some of these cues is the association of food with love, caring, and comfort, which may have its antecedents in early childhood but persists into adult life and pervades our culture.

The patient should be helped to recognize that using food to deal with stress, boredom, and emotions is, at best, ineffective. The stressful situation, for example, does not resolve with eating. In fact, eating may worsen the problem by distracting one from dealing directly with the situation while adding the stresses of obesity and its sequelae.

Simply telling a patient not to eat when under stress is useless, of course. Instead, try the following three-step approach. First, recommend a period of observation and recording to enable the patient to recognize the cue. For instance, one can ask the patient to wear his or her watch upside-down as a reminder to ask "Why am I reaching for the food at this time?" If the patient is not physically hungry, one of the possibly inappropriate cues is most likely in play, and its nature should be guessed at and recorded. Second, suggest the substitution of other responses for inappropriate eating. For stress, this might be writing down what the stress is, formulating a plan for doing something about it, doing something (besides eating) to relieve the stress on the spot, or, at the very least, substituting a walk around the block or a call to a friend for the bag of potato chips. The third step is repetition, that is, to keep making appropriate responses to the problematic cue and to reap the rewards of the new behavior, which include the positive responses of others to the change in approach, not just to eating, but to life, that the patient makes.

Although some degree of change is necessary and beneficial, not every maladaptive behavior must be completely eliminated nor must every rich food be replaced by celery sticks without dip. While losing a large amount of weight in a reasonable amount of time does require a fairly aggressive diet and exercise program, maintaining a new lower weight does not. If the patient can learn to control even partially a few of the more important inappropriate eating behaviors and to shift to a diet somewhat lower in fat and calories than baseline, that is usually sufficient to maintain weight in the new, lower range. This is easy to see and difficult to do, but impossible if behaviors are not addressed as part of a comprehensive approach to the treatment of obesity.

Another behavior of interest in obesity is restraint. One can simplistically categorize patients as restrained or unrestrained eaters. Restrained eaters believe that they must exercise a good deal of control over their eating—they are always conscious of what they can and cannot eat. Unrestrained eaters do not control their eating to any great extent. Restrained eating may lead to some paradoxical results—once restraint is relaxed, an exaggerated response may ensue in a frenzy of all or nothing behavior. Such patients may be superb dieters, but are equally superb at overeating once the diet has been "broken." The issue is one of too much of a good thing. Although a certain amount of control and monitoring is necessary for maintaining weight loss, high levels of restraint may be more problematic than low ones in the long run. One solution is to couple the teaching of ways to control inappropriate eating cues with dietary changes that emphasize foods lower in fat and calories, so that lower restraint is required to maintain a given intake. This scheme definitely discourages skipping meals when the patient is physically hungry.

Dietary Assessment

Although many aspects of diet are more properly characterized as behaviors, the need remains to understand patients' tastes and the macronutrient composition of their usual array of food choices. This information is a tool for suggesting behavioral changes that will comport with the patient's preferences and lifestyle. Although the physician can and should get some idea of these things in talking with the patient, a formal dietary assessment is best done by a dietitian using either a prospective or retrospective food diary.

The results of such an assessment must be interpreted with caution, as both retrospective under-reporting and prospective restrained eating are common. Despite these shortcomings, the information gathered can be very useful. For example, the macronutrient composition of a patient's diet will often be weighted toward fats, protein, and simple carbohydrates. By cutting fat and increasing the intake of complex carbohydrates, such patients can considerably increase the volume of food they consume as they attempt to reach and maintain a lower weight.

A helpful tool in altering the composition of the patient's diet is the technique of gradual change. For example, a patient reluctant to switch from whole milk to skim milk could first try 2 percent milk (which is actually 37 percent fat), get used to that in a month or two, and then move on to 1 percent for another month. At this point, the patient should notice something interesting—the once-favored whole milk will now taste too oily. At some later date, the final step to skim milk can be made with few or no feelings of deprivation, demonstrating that taste preferences are acquired and eminently changeable even in later life.

Recommend scouring the supermarket aisles (at a time when the patient is not hungry) for tasty, fat-free alternatives to favored foods. Encourage the patient to explore the wide variety of fat-free foods now available and to focus on the good taste of the new choice rather than comparing it to the "real thing." The presentation of nutritional information on foodstuffs was recently improved. The new food labels list not just grams of fat but also the percentage of the daily dietary fat allotment those grams represent. The patient should be taught (usually by the dietitian) how to read both the old and new labels and to stay within a "fat budget."

This is also a good time to be improving the dietary habits of the patient's family, something that is particularly easy to do when the patient is the primary cook and food-shopper. Including the family in this process not only improves their diet but also makes it easier for the patient if at least the house can be a temptation-free zone. Even if other members of the family must have junk food, they can be instructed to partake outside the home or to put only individually packaged items in the cupboard. Small-size purchases of rich desserts and the like are desirable in general—the smaller the dietary indiscretion, the less severe the consequences.

Specific recommendation are given under "Types of Diets."

Exercise Assessment

Exercise alone is, unfortunately, not a terribly effective method of losing weight. It is difficult for the untrained person to do enough of it, and most if not all of the expended energy is compensated by increased caloric intake. Exercise is, however, a superb way to *maintain* a lower weight after weight loss, enabling a person to eat somewhat more than a nonexerciser and maintain the same given weight. Regular aerobic exercise will also improve cardiovascular fitness, trim inches, and promote growth of metabolically more active muscle tissue.

An exercise assessment should include a record of the usual degree of physical activity, any limiting factors such as joint disease or previous injuries, types of activity the patient finds enjoyable, and a measurement by an exercise physiologist of the current fitness level. A formal stress test is not required unless active cardiovascular disease is suspected.

The rule of thumb in devising an exercise regimen is the phased-in approach. Most obese patients have a very limited capacity to exercise. Rather than suggesting a type or level of activity that is unlikely to inspire adherence, make sure that the plan fits into the patient's schedule and lifestyle.

The first phase consists of increasing the amount of everyday physical activity, without introduction of a formal exercise regimen. This includes taking the stairs in gradually increasing increments, parking the car farther away from the mall entrance, walking to the mailbox, and the like. This step alone may double the level of physical activity in a very sedentary person.

The next phase is a walking plan. People are most likely to comply with such a plan if the walk is scheduled during a break or lunchtime at work, and/or when the daily energy level is highest, for example, early morning. Having a companion to walk with and a place to walk indoors are also helpful in increasing compliance.

One-half hour is the minimum amount of time a patient should make available for each session of exercise. The intensity of the exercise is not critical to the burning of calories—walking at a leisurely pace for 1 hour is roughly equal to walking briskly for half an hour. Allow the patient to set the pace. Initially, it may be quite slow, but in the absence of pulmonary or cardiovascular disease, most patients soon find the going easier and faster. This reinforcement can be strengthened by goal setting. Have the patient keep a log of the time spent walking and the distance covered after each session. The patient can then see the progress being made and set the goal a bit higher from time to time.

Next, the types of activities performed should be broadened. Walking or jogging can and should remain an ingredient at this stage, but with the addition of other forms of aerobic exercise. Recommend aerobics classes, stationary or outdoor bicycling, swimming, a cross-country skiing machine, or just about anything else that will burn calories and be enjoyable. Team or racquet sports and golf can be suggested to provide social interaction as well as to increase energy expenditure. Again, the most important criterion for a good exercise plan is that it be one that patients are likely to follow and be comfortable with as a habit for the rest of their lives.

Types of Diets

It is best to start by instilling in your obese patients a degree of skepticism about commercially advertised diets that are not part of a comprehensive approach to weight management. Many are based on very limited menus, the rationale being that monotony helps curb consumption. Others involve diuretic agents. In fact, any reduced-calorie diet will initially cause diuresis, which makes the diet seem efficacious. The diuresis will usually result in an approximately 2 percent to 4 percent loss of body weight during the first 7 to 10 days, but most of this weight will be regained as soon as the period of severe caloric restriction ends.

After the diuretic phase, the amount of weight loss to be expected on any diet obeys a simple formula. Lipolysis of one pound of adipose tissue yields about 3,500 kilocalories; it is therefore necessary to restrict energy intake and/or increase energy expenditure by about 500 kilocalories per day to lose one pound of fat per week. Because some muscle may also be lost and muscle is poorer in energy than fat, the rate of weight loss may be somewhat higher than predicted. However, two countervailing factors are at work. First, with sustained moderate to severe caloric restriction, a modest reduction in metabolic rate occurs. This decrease makes weight loss somewhat more difficult to achieve, but caloric requirement, corrected for the new, lower weight, fortunately appears to return to prediet level within a few months of resuming a balanced diet. Second, because lower weight means reduced caloric need, the same caloric intake will represent less of a deficit as the patient loses weight. A regular program of physical activity can partially compensate for both these factors by helping to blunt the decrease in metabolic rate and by building muscle mass, which is more metabolically active and therefore has a higher caloric requirement than adipose tissue.

How much of a caloric deficit should be recommended, and in what form should the calories be taken? The answer depends on the degree of obesity, the presence or absence of comorbidities, such as diabetes and hypertension, the results of the behavioral assessment, and, to some extent, the patient's preferences. In any case, it is important to remind the patient that the diet is only part of an overall plan and will fail in the long term unless accompanied by changes in behavior.

For patients with grade 1 obesity, it is best to recommend a caloric deficit of at most 500 to 750 calories per day to achieve 1 to 1.5 pounds of weightloss per week. As a very rough guide, daily caloric requirements to maintain a given body weight equals body weight in pounds times 13 for a completely sedentary individual. The dietitian can design a low-calorie, food-based diet that is either balanced-deficit, reducing total number of calories while keeping proportions from carbohydrate, fat, and protein roughly the same as before, or fat-deficit, with most of the caloric reduction resulting from restriction of fat intake. The latter approach is preferable in light of the typical American diet that is too high in fat (37 percent of total calories). Also, a greater volume of food can be eaten on a diet that emphasizes complex carbohydrates and reduces fat to 20 percent of calories consumed. The new labeling regulations help identify dietary fat.

Patients with grade 2 obesity will also benefit from the safety and nutritional soundness of a fat-deficit diet. It is important, however, to recognize that at this level of caloric restriction it will take more than a year to attain a weight-loss of 50 to 70 pounds. Few patients can sustain this degree of restriction for that long; therefore, for a limited period a greater than 500 to 750 calorie daily deficit or even a very low-calorie diet (VLCD) (fewer than 800 total calories per day) may be needed. The VLCD is justified particularly if the patient already suffers from comorbidities that are likely to be alleviated with significant weightloss and/or if the patient is near the upper end of grade 2 obesity.

VLCDs can consist of food, commercially available liquid supplements, or a combination of both. With full compliance, the amount of weight lost on a VLCD ranges from 2.5 to 4 pounds per week, depending on body mass and level of physical activity. The initial diuretic phase may be pronounced and accompanied by (usually transient) lightheadedness, headache, or fatigue. Later symptoms may include constipation and intolerance of cold. Electrolyte abnormalities are rare, but serum must be monitored at least monthly and more often during the first month of the VLCD. Renal insufficiency and severe cardiopulmonary disease are relative contraindications to a VLCD.

Gallstones may arise or become symptomatic, probably due to gallbladder stasis, and a decrease in bile acids, which occurs during or immediately after any severely restricted (especially fat-restricted) diet. To prevent stasis, the patient can add to the diet a tablespoon of a fat such as canola oil taken in *one* daily dose, which will allow the gallbladder to contract.

A VLCD should be administered only under a physician's supervision and with full attention to the behavioral changes necessary to sustain the weightloss that this regimen can produce.

In grade 3 (morbid) obesity, corresponding to twice ideal body weight or more, the only practical diet for most patients is a VLCD or somewhat less restrictive diet with careful medical monitoring and long-term follow-up. It should be noted, however, that even a modest weightloss can yield substantial health benefits for morbidly obese patients. Sleep apnea often disappears with as little as a 10 percent loss in weight, and hypertension, diabetes and gastroesophageal reflux may also improve significantly. Do not view, nor let your patient view, modest weight loss as a failure or a waste of time. The same is true for lower grades of obesity.

Drugs and Surgery

Adjuvant anorectic medications may be useful for the morbidly obese patient, either from the start, to enhance compliance with the diet or later, when compliance begins to waver or hunger becomes an issue. There is little doubt that such medications are generally safe and substantially increase weight loss during the period in which they are used. Currently popular anorectic drugs include phentermine, dex/dl fenfluramine and a combination of the two. These are controlled substances, but though tolerance may develop, the abuse potential is low. One reasonably effective agent, phenylpropanolamine, is available over the counter. The true amphetamines and thyroid medications should not be prescribed for weight loss.

Whether obesity should be considered a chronic disease and treated on a long-term basis with anorectic drugs is in part a philosophic issue. In the present climate of medical treatment, these agents are best used only after attempts at dieting have failed in patients who are seriously obese and/or suffer from comorbid conditions.

The surgical treatment of morbid obesity has improved considerably since the days of the jejunoileal bypass and jaw wiring. Probably the best procedure currently available is the gastric bypass that combines stapling of the stomach to make a small-capacity proximal gastric pouch with a short-segment bypass of the proximal small bowel created by a Roux-en-Y loop. Results are quite good in the short term. Long-term results, as with all methods of weight loss, depend largely on the patient's ability to sustain behavioral changes. Therefore, aside from access to a hospital with adequate experience in this procedure, the best chance of long-term success will come with referring the patient to a center that offers and insists upon extensive preoperative evaluation and maintenance

Table 7 Key Ingredients of a Weightloss Plan

Be ready
Set reasonable goals
Find a reliable support system
Build in maintenance from the outset
Become invested in your goals
Make gradual changes
Keep records (be compulsive)
Make it enjoyable
Be flexible

therapy of long duration consisting of regular sessions in dietary management and behavior modification. Do not make the mistake of viewing surgery as a treatment that does not require the patient's active involvement—an unmotivated or unguided patient can and will defeat the procedure.

■ MAINTENANCE

The physician and the patient should both know that the long-term results of attempts at weight loss are often poor. It is therefore important to expose the patient, at the beginning of treatment, to the attitudes and behaviors that are likely to foster long-term maintenance of weight loss (Table 7). These may be summarized as follows.

- Readiness—Correct timing for change is vital. It is folly for your patient to begin a diet when he or she is not yet convinced of the need to do so or is in the midst of a stressful life event such as divorce.
- Setting reasonable goals—Aiming for an attainable rather than an "ideal" body weight is advisable. A reasonable long-term goal might be the lowest weight the patient has successfully maintained for one year or more during the previous ten years.
- Reliable support systems—Obtaining helpful assistance aids in both weight loss and maintenance. This usually involves seeking out a friend or relative who knows how to listen and not just give advice.
- Building in maintenance—Planning and executing behavioral changes from day 1 is essential.
- Becoming invested in one's goals—Learning how to talk to oneself in a positive way in order to enhance commitment to self-set objectives is a useful technique.
- Making gradual changes—Modifying food choices and level of physical activity reduces the sense of deprivation and may make the process of change easier and the changes themselves more likely to be permanent.
- Keeping records—Recording weight, foods eaten, exercise, and precipitants of inappropriate eating is an excellent way to identify problem areas and to spot a relapse before it gets out of hand, thereby improving the chances of long-term success.
- Making it enjoyable—This is self-explanatory. It is much easier to comply with new behaviors if they can be enjoyed. If your patient cannot stand to exercise, do not tell him or her to do it anyway. Instead, suggest taking a child to the park or walking around the mall to people-watch. The achievement of a positive change in lifestyle is, by itself, very reinforcing and should not be discounted as a source of satisfaction and enjoyment.
- Being flexible—This applies to both the physician and the patient. If an approach that has been given a fair trial is not working, or if the patient's circumstances change (a new job, for example), the weightloss plan may need to change, too.

In closing, it should be obvious that helping patients lose weight and keep it off requires a comprehensive and sustained effort. Although it is true that only the patient can do it, this is one area where the diligent and caring physician can make a real difference.

Suggested Reading

Folsom AR, Kaye SA, Sellers TA, et al. Body fat distribution and risk for death in older women. JAMA 1993; 269:483–487.

Garrow JS. Treatment of obesity. Lancet 1992; 340:409–413.

Kayman S, Bruvold W, Stern JS. Maintenance and relapse after weight loss in women-behavioral aspects. Am J Clin Nutr 1990; 52:800–807.

Must A, Jacques SD, Dallal GE, et al. Long-term morbidity and mortality of overweight adolescents. N Engl J Med 1992; 327:1350–1355.

NIH Technology Assessment Conference. Methods of voluntary weight loss and control. Ann Intern Med 1993; 119:641–770.

Ravussin E, Swinburn BA. Pathophysiology of obesity. Lancet 1992; 340:404–408.

IMMUNE, ALLERGIC, AND RHEUMATOLOGIC DISEASES

ALLERGIC AND NONALLERGIC RHINITIS

Harold S. Nelson, M.D.

Rhinitis is a common affliction that varies in severity, producing nearly disabling symptoms in some patients, whereas in others producing such mild symptoms that they are not easily distinguished from heightened awareness of the normal mucus production of the nose. The types of rhinitis also present a broad spectrum. Seasonal allergic rhinitis is usually clearly distinguishable; perennial rhinitis may be separated less precisely into (1) a group of disorders having an allergic basis, (2) a group that is nonallergic but clearly is associated with other allergic or potentially allergic conditions, and (3) the group formerly called vasomotor rhinitis. The last named could more accurately be called nonallergic, noneosinophilic rhinitis, since little is known of its cause or mechanisms. The importance of distinguishing among these types of rhinitis is that they affect the therapeutic approach. Clearly, allergen avoidance and allergy immunotherapy are indicated only for rhinitis that truly has an allergic basis. Nonallergic rhinitis associated with asthma, eczema, or seasonal allergic rhinitis does not benefit from an allergen-directed therapy but often responds more satisfactorily to pharmacotherapy than does nonallergic rhinitis not sharing these associations.

■ CLASSIFICATION OF RHINITIS

Seasonal allergic rhinitis is characterized by symptoms of nasal and ocular pruritus, repetitive sneezing, watery rhinorrhea, and nasal obstruction occurring during a particular season corresponding to the appearance in the air of an allergen to which the subject can be demonstrated to be sensitive. Significant seasonal allergic rhinitis in the absence of skin test reactivity to the suspected allergen has not been convincingly demonstrated.

Perennial allergic rhinitis, in areas where the occurrence of frost ensures a season without significant outdoor aeroallergens, is primarily due to sensitivity to animal dander and insect allergens, particularly those from the house dust mite but perhaps more often than appreciated those from the cockroach. The importance of indoor molds in the etiology of perennial allergic rhinitis is suspected in some instances when damp areas exist in homes, but few studies have attempted to document their clinical importance. Ingestant allergens have been even less well studied, but the usual opinion is that they are of little importance as a cause of rhinitis beyond infancy and early childhood.

Perennial nonallergic eosinophilic rhinitis is a condition that has only slowly been recognized. It has been known for over 50 years that patients with nonallergic asthma have associated rhinitis and hypertrophic sinusitis with a tendency toward nasal polyps and that their nasal secretions, like their sputum and blood, are characterized by an excess of eosinophils. Nasal biopsies, or examination of tissue removed at the time of sinus surgery, has regularly shown an eosinophilic infiltration of the tissue. It is a reasonable assumption that the same nonallergic rhinitis, characterized by eosinophilic infiltration of the tissues and eosinophilia of the secretions, can occur alone as well as in conjunction with diseases, such as seasonal allergic rhinitis, bronchial asthma, and atopic eczema. Also, just as patients with atopic eczema and bronchial asthma may have positive skin test results that are not clinically relevant to their disease, so, too, may patients with nonallergic eosinophilic rhinitis. Finally, since evidence has been presented that in patients with atopic diseases there may be enhanced mediator release in response to nonimmunologic stimuli, it should not be surprising that patients with nonallergic eosinophilic rhinitis may experience symptoms suggesting the release of histamine, with itchy eyes and nose, sneezing, and rhinorrhea of a degree seen in seasonal allergic rhinitis.

Perennial nonallergic noneosinophilic rhinitis is often termed *vasomotor rhinitis* with the proposal that these patients experienced symptoms as a result of an excessive parasympathetic response to various noxious nonimmunologic stimuli. Although these patients do respond with symptoms to irritating odors and temperature changes, so, too, do virtually all patients with rhinitis. Since there is no convincing evidence that these patients' symptoms are caused by autonomic mechanisms or even that they constitute a single disease entity, a new term is needed that more accurately reflects the state of our knowledge. In general, the response of these patients to pharmacotherapy is not as favorable as it is in patients with the other types of rhinitis. However, there are a few well-categorized conditions that might be separated from this group, such as the rhinitis of pregnancy and hypothyroidism, and rhinitis medicamentosa due to either the topical use of decongestants or systemically administered medications. These conditions offer the prospect of a more successful resolution.

■ THERAPY

The therapies of allergic and nonallergic rhinitis may be justifiably considered together. Measures directed toward allergens—avoidance and immunotherapy—are appropriate only in cases of rhinitis in which a significant allergic component has been demonstrated. Usually the treatment of rhinitis includes a major component of pharmacotherapy, and here the drugs employed are the same, although the response to the drug varies with the type of the rhinitis.

Avoidance

The first consideration in the treatment of allergic rhinitis should be an attempt to avoid completely or decrease the exposure to the offending allergen. Although with the exception of family pets complete elimination is seldom possible, substantial reduction in exposure often can be accomplished. In most pollen seasons the periods of peak counts are of limited duration, and these counts are generally highest during the mid-day or afternoon. Pollen concentrations are considerably reduced indoors, particularly if air conditioning is employed, allowing windows and doors to remain closed. For these reasons patients with pollen-induced seasonal allergic rhinitis often can avoid excessive symptoms by not undertaking outdoor recreational activities during the times of highest pollen counts. Although the season for the dry spore molds, such as *Alternaria* and *Cladosporium,* is more prolonged than it is for most pollens, peak counts are again encountered during dry, windy summer afternoons, allowing for some reduction in exposure by avoiding outdoor activities at these times. The spores that particularly characterize periods of dampness and rain—basidiospores and ascospores—are especially numerous during the early morning hours. If they are suspected of causing allergic problems (a determination more dependent on history than testing because of the general lack of relevant extracts), closing windows at night, through the use of air conditioning if necessary, would be expected to effect a major reduction in exposure.

The most important allergens causing perennial allergy and the major components of "house dust" are animal danders and allergens derived from the house dust mite. The latter is ubiquitous except in the drier portions of the country, such as the Rocky Mountains and the southwest. An additional significant component—cockroach allergen—is encountered in areas where these insects are prevalent, such as the inner city areas of the north and the warmer portions of the country. Since house dust mites tend to accumulate in bedding, upholstered furniture, and adjacent carpeting, some control of allergen exposure is possible. When this has been undertaken in a thorough manner, a significant decrease in symptoms of asthma in both children and adults has been reported. The role of air-cleaning devices in the avoidance of house dust mite allergen is not clear, since the allergen occurs predominantly in relatively large fecal pellets, which would be expected to fall rapidly from the air by gravity. Thus, local reservoirs, such as pillows, mattresses, and bed covers, appear more likely to be an important source than the allergen floating in the air.

Dander from pets, particularly cats and dogs, is a major perennial allergen. Clearly, complete avoidance should be possible, but emotional ties or the presence of pets in the homes of others often frustrates avoidance measures. It should be possible to "animal proof" the bedroom by excluding the pet from this room and keeping the door and heating ducts closed. There are no data that indicate whether under these circumstances the use of a room air-filtering device in the bedroom would be a worthwhile additional measure. However, dander remains airborne longer than mite antigen, and therefore some effect from air cleaner devices is likely. There is evidence that with the continued access of the pet to the bedroom, the concentration of allergen in the furnishings would negate any impact of the use of air filtration on the total allergen load. If only partial elimination of the family pet is possible, the more restricted the area in which the animal is allowed and the less furniture and carpeting to which it has access, the better for the containment of allergens.

The role of indoor mold allergy in producing allergic rhinitis is unclear. Damp areas in the house that cause symptoms should be dehumidified if possible, and if humidifiers are employed, care should be taken that they are cleaned regularly and do not become a source of spore aerosols.

For all patients with rhinitis, nonimmunologic irritants are a problem. Some can be avoided, and tobacco smoking within the home or workplace should be eliminated. It should also be possible, at least within the family, to avoid the use of strongly scented toiletries and cleaning products.

Pharmacotherapy

Antihistamines

Competitive antagonists of the histamine-1 (H_1) receptor have been the traditional basic treatment for allergic and nonallergic rhinitis. The older preparations have been grouped into six classes in part with the expectation that changing from one class to another might evade the tolerance that develops to this group of drugs. However, the tolerance is probably related to the histamine receptor and is not specific for the class of agent that induced it.

In general the alkylamines, represented by chlorpheniramine and brompheniramine, are preferred by the largest number of subjects, while hydroxyzine in the doses commonly employed appears to be slightly more effective than chlorpheniramine but also causes slightly more side effects, making it generally less satisfactory. A limited number of studies suggest that azatadine may also cause relatively few side effects.

The side effects of the traditional antihistamines are primarily of two types. There are direct central nervous system (CNS) effects, which sometimes include stimulation, restlessness, and nervousness but much more often are characterized by drowsiness or incoordination. The second major group of side effects is related to anticholinergic actions of these drugs and includes dryness of the mouth, urinary retention, impotence, and blurring of vision. Tolerance to the CNS side effects develops rapidly, and by 4 to 10 days the incidence of drowsiness in many studies is similar to that with placebo. Tolerance to the desired antihistaminic properties also develops by 3 weeks, but this does not appear to be as profound in degree as the CNS tolerance, effectively improving the therapeutic ratio for these drugs. Antihistamines are now available that are nonsedating because they do not cross the blood-brain barrier. Furthermore, these drugs are free of anticholinergic action, thus avoiding some of the other side effects of the traditional antihistamines. This group includes terfenadine, astemizole, loratadine, and cetirizine.

Antihistamines block some but not all of the symptoms of allergic rhinitis. They effectively relieve pruritus, sneezing, and rhinorrhea, but they are largely ineffective for nasal congestion. This shortcoming is compensated for in part by the addition of a sympathomimetic decongestant. The availability of relatively pure H_1 antagonists, such as astemizole, has demonstrated that histamine is important in the production of symptoms in nonallergic as well as allergic rhinitis. The decision of whether to try antihistamine therapy is best made based on the types of symptoms the patient is experiencing rather than on the perception of whether the symptoms have an allergic basis.

Pharmacokinetic studies in adults have revealed unexpectedly long serum half-lives for a number of antihistamines. Hydroxyzine, chlorpheniramine, and brompheniramine all have serum half-lives of approximately 24 hours, suggesting that once-daily dosing at bedtime with non–sustained-release formulations should be adequate for the relief of symptoms. This dosing schedule has the advantage that maximal serum levels and therefore sedation occur while the patient is asleep. The use of single bedtime dosing, in addition to a gradual build-up of the dosage over 1 to 2 weeks, may allow the use of an inexpensive medication effectively with minimal side effects. In children the serum half-lives of these drugs are about 12 hours, perhaps accounting for the relatively higher doses of antihistamines employed in children but also making single daily dose therapy in children impractical. The new nonsedating antihistamine terfenadine has a half-life somewhat shorter than that of the preparations just listed, and twice-daily dosing appears to be appropriate. Loratadine and cetirizine have longer half-lives consistent with once-daily dosing. Astemizole, on the other hand, possesses pharmacokinetic properties of a different order; with a prolonged half-life for both the drug and its active metabolite, astemizole suppresses skin test reactions for several months after the discontinuation of therapy.

In comparative trials, usually of only 1 or 2 weeks' duration, terfenadine, 60 mg twice daily, has produced control of symptoms equivalent to that with dosages of chlorpheniramine of 6 to 16 mg per day but with a lower incidence of side effects. Loratadine and cetirizine each at a dosage of 10 mg daily have been at least as effective as terfenadine, 60 mg twice a day. Astemizole, 10 mg once daily, on the other hand, has been consistently more effective than terfenadine, 60 mg twice daily, for both seasonal and perennial allergic rhinitis.

Astemizole has been compared in double-blind trials to both cromolyn and nasal beclomethasone dipropionate for the treatment of seasonal allergic rhinitis. It was found to be of equal effectiveness to a combination of nasal cromolyn six times daily and ocular cromolyn four times daily when administered as a once-daily treatment. On the other hand, astemizole was found to be less effective than nasal beclomethasone for control of nasal symptoms although better for eye symptoms.

It is frequently stated that the antihistamines are more effective when administered on a regular basis rather than being taken as needed for the relief of already existing symptoms. Another argument for the regular use of the older preparations is that tolerance develops to the CNS side effects, improving their therapeutic ratio.

Decongestants

The drugs employed as decongestants are nonselective alpha-adrenergic agonists capable of constricting blood vessels elsewhere in the body. For that reason the preferred route of administration would be topical application to the nasal mucosa. Long-acting topical decongestant therapy is recommended for the treatment of nasal congestion associated with viral respiratory infections, to promote drainage during acute infections of the paranasal sinuses and middle ears, and to facilitate penetration during the first few days of topical corticosteroid therapy in patients with marked nasal obstruction. The limitation to their use is the well-recognized development of rebound obstruction, probably due to the induction of down regulation of the alpha-adrenergic receptors.

Orally administered alpha-adrenergic decongestants are also available, both as single drugs and in combination with antihistamines. They produce well-recognized side effects of tremor, restlessness, and agitation and can cause hypertension and urinary retention. Hypertension particularly has been reported with phenylpropanolamine, which appears to have a very narrow therapeutic range. Pseudoephedrine, the other commonly employed drug, has been implicated less frequently. Nevertheless, a recent review concluded that there were inadequate studies to ensure the safety of oral decongestant therapy in patients with hypertension.

There also are few studies that have addressed the effectiveness of these drugs as decongestants during the course of long-term administration when some degree of alpha-adrenergic tolerance may be presumed to have developed. A reduction in nasal airway resistance was demonstrated following a dose of 60 mg of pseudoephedrine, but it persisted for only 2 hours. The sympathomimetics, however, have one advantage—their side effects tend to be directly opposed to those of the older antihistamines, making the combination attractive from the standpoint of reduced side effects. When combined with the nonsedating antihistamines, however, insomnia is a problem in some patients.

Cromolyn Sodium

A nasal solution of 4 percent cromolyn sodium, administered four to six times daily, has been demonstrated to provide moderate relief of the symptoms of seasonal allergic rhinitis. As would be anticipated for a nasal spray, it does not alleviate eye symptoms. Cromolyn nasal solution also has been tested in patients with perennial rhinitis, in whom it produced a modest reduction in symptoms in those with positive skin test results but no better results than placebo in patients with negative skin test results, even in those who had profuse nasal eosinophilia. The topically applied steroid sprays have consistently demonstrated marked superiority over cromolyn in comparative trials and appear to be the preferred treatment except in patients with significant local side effects from the topical use of steroid preparations or those with marked "steroid phobia." Antihistamines have been demonstrated to be as effective as cromolyn and have the advantage of less frequent dosing, control of eye symptoms, and usually lower costs. Therefore, in patients tolerating antihistamines, they would appear to be the preferred initial treatment.

Cromolyn also is available as a 4 percent solution for use in the eyes. Again there is the inconvenience of six time daily use, but this preparation does provide good control of ocular symptoms as well as some effect on nasal symptoms and thus may complement topical nasal steroid therapy in the treatment of seasonal allergic rhinitis in patients whose ocular symptoms are prominent.

Corticosteroids

Several nasal steroids are available, both as a micronized powder in a freon-propelled vehicle and in an aqueous vehicle delivered by a pump spray. The initial dosage is usually two discharges into each nostril once or twice daily, depending on the drug. In recommended dosages the topically applied corticosteroids appear to be of similar efficacy. They have some tendency to cause mucosal bleeding.

Nasal steroids are very effective in seasonal allergic rhinitis, although symptom control is seldom complete. They do not relieve eye symptoms. Furthermore, there is a delay of several days for maximal effect. If marked nasal obstruction is present, they may be ineffective because of lack of access to the nasal mucosa, and initiation of therapy with 3 to 5 days of prednisone, 40 mg per day, or the topical use of a decongestant spray before each dose of corticosteroid for the same period may be necessary. Several studies suggest that antihistamines and topical corticosteroid therapy are complementary; there are no similar data for cromolyn and topical corticosteroid therapy.

It is clear that the topical corticosteroid therapy is more effective in nonallergic eosinophilic rhinitis than in rhinitis that is not related to the atopic diseases. Thus, a positive family history of atopic diseases, positive skin test results, pale swollen mucosa, or the presence of eosinophils in the nasal secretions all were predictors of a likely favorable response to topical corticosteroid therapy. The absence of these markers indicated perhaps a less than 50 percent chance of improvement. Despite this unpromising likelihood of a response, since these are generally patients who have failed to respond to other medications, a 2 week, carefully evaluated trial is indicated.

In patients with recurrent sinusitis or nasal polyps, the treatment of the associated nasal symptoms with topical corticosteroid therapy had been reported to diminish recurrences.

Miscellaneous Treatments

Saline nasal sprays and washes have been reported to diminish symptoms of perennial rhinitis, and in some cases this has been accompanied by an improvement in histopathologic findings.

The anticholinergic properties of the older antihistamines were thought to contribute to their efficacy by exerting a drying effect. Ipratropium bromide, a recently introduced anticholinergic nasal spray, has been reported to decrease rhinorrhea but not other nasal symptoms.

Immunotherapy

Immunotherapy is reserved for last because that is its proper role in the treatment of allergic rhinitis. This is not a reflection of a lack of efficacy. Placebo-controlled studies have clearly demonstrated that injection of extracts of pollens, animal danders, and house dust mite produces not only a decrease in clinical symptoms on natural exposure but also immunologic changes, which include a progressive decline in the levels of IgE specific for the substances being injected. Thus, unlike the other treatment modalities mentioned, allergy immunotherapy offers the promise of actually reversing the sensitized state.

Why then is the use of allergy immunotherapy deferred until other forms of therapy have first been tried and failed? The reason is the rigorous requirements placed upon the physician and the patient if allergy immunotherapy is to succeed. First the physician must determine that the symptoms are truly allergic—that the nature and timing of symptoms, the patient's exposure, and the patient's degree of sensitivity strongly suggest a causal relationship. Next the allergen must be specifically identified; this often is possible with pollens but rarely is possible with molds. Then potent extracts of these substances must be injected, ultimately at high concentrations, which carry the danger of serious or rarely even fatal reactions. The requirement on the patient's part is the investment in time and money over several years if lasting results are to be obtained. Anyone working in the field of allergy has to be concerned about the frequency with which immunotherapy is undertaken without these requisites being satisfied and the number of patients who report no decrease in symptoms after an investment of several years and many hundreds of dollars. Under present circumstances allergy immunotherapy should be reserved for clear-cut allergy to well-defined allergens in patients who have responded poorly to symptomatic therapy and have a prolonged season or perennial symptoms.

Suggested Reading

Corren J, Adinoff AD, Buchmeier AD, Irvin CG. Nasal beclomethasone prevents the seasonal increase in bronchial responsiveness in patients with allergic rhinitis and asthma. J Allergy Clin Immunol 1992; 90:250.

Hillas J, Booth RJ, et al. A comparative trial of intra-nasal beclomethasone dipropionate and sodium cromoglycate in patients with chronic perennial rhinitis. Clin Allergy 1980; 10:253–258.

Howarth PH, Holgate ST. Comparative trial or two non-sedating H_1 antihistamines, terfenadine and astemizole, for hay fever. Thorax 1984; 39: 668–672.

Juniper EF, Kline PA, Hargreave FE, Dolovich J. Comparison of beclomethasone dipropionate aqueous nasal spray, astemizole, and the combination in the prophylactic treatment of ragweed pollen-induced rhinoconjunctivitis. J Allergy Clin Immunol 1989; 83:627.

Nelson HS. Chronic rhinitis: Diagnosis and management. In Stults BM, Dere WH, eds.: Practical care of ambulatory patient. Philadelphia: WB Saunders Co, Philadelphia, 1989.

Turkeitaub PC, Norman PS, et al. Treatment of seasonal and perennial rhinitis with intranasal flunisolide. Allergy 1982; 37:303–311.

Viner AS, Jackman N. Retrospective survey of 1271 patients diagnosed as perennial rhinitis. Clin Allergy 1976; 6:251.

Welsh PW, Stricker WE, Chu C-P, et al. Efficacy of beclomethasone nasal solution, flunisolide, and cromolyn in relieving symptoms of ragweed allergy. Mayo Clin Proc 1987; 62:125.

Wohl J-A, Peterson BN, et al. Effect of the nonsedative H_1 receptor antagonist astemizole in perennial allergic and nonallergic rhinitis. J Allergy Clin Immunol 1985; 75:720–727.

PERENNIAL NONALLERGIC RHINITIS

Valerie J. Lund, M.S., F.R.C.S., F.R.C.S.Ed.

Rhinitis in its broadest sense may be defined as inflammation of the lining of the nose, characterized by one or more of the following symptoms: nasal congestion, rhinorrhea, sneezing, itching, and disturbance of the sense of smell. The relative importance of each symptom depends upon the cause of the inflammation. However, the nose should not be considered in isolation and from a clinical perspective, "rhinosinusitis" better indicates the areas affected. Indeed, the entire respiratory tract should be regarded as a single organ and many forms of rhinitis are paralleled by lower respiratory tract diseases.

A classification of rhinitis is shown in Table 1, which also includes a number of conditions that must be considered in the differential diagnosis and that may coexist or contribute to the inflammation. It has been suggested that the term *nonallergic rhinitis* should be reserved for inflammation of the nasal mucosa that is unrelated to allergy, infection, structural lesions, or other systemic disease; nonallergic rhinitis is variously described as idiopathic, hyper-reactivity, intrinsic, or vasomotor rhinitis. This latter term is the least satisfactory because it implies that the cause is known. Since this is not the case, idiopathic is preferred, encompassing the provocation of watery rhinorrhea, nasal congestion, and sneezing in response to irritants such as tobacco smoke, strong smells, and changes in environmental temperature and humidity, all manifestations of an exaggerated defense response. Cold air-induced rhinitis may occur because of the release of mast cell mediators involving a non–IgE-dependent mechanism. Neurogenic mechanisms may be involved such as the watery rhinorrhea in response to temperature change, eating spicy foods (gustatory rhinorrhea), or the effect of emotion and stress. It should also be remembered that a variety of foods, alcohol, and drugs may produce hypersensitivity (e.g., aspirin), as well as specific allergic reactions. A subgroup, nonallergic rhinitis with eosinophilia syndrome (NARES), is characterized by the symptoms of rhinitis in the presence of nasal eosinophilia but in the absence of positive skin prick tests and raised IgE levels.

The diagnosis of perennial nonallergic rhinitis relies heavily upon a detailed history and a general ear, nose, and throat (ENT) examination, including, whenever possible, endoscopy of the nose. A considerable range of other investigations is available, only a small number of which are routinely employed (Table 2), but they may be applicable to individual cases. The most important thing to consider in the differential diagnosis is the possibility of rarer and more

Table 1 Classification of Rhinitis

CLASSIFICATION

1. Allergic
   - Seasonal
   - Perennial
   - Occupational
2. Infectious
   - Acute
   - Chronic
     - Specific
     - Nonspecific
3. Nonallergic, noninfectious
   - Idiopathic
   - Occupational
   - NARES
   - Hormonal
   - Drug-induced
   - Irritants
   - Food
   - Emotional
   - Atrophic

DIFFERENTIAL DIAGNOSIS

1. Polyps
2. Mechanical factors
   - Deviated septum
   - Hypertrophic turbinates
   - Adenoidal hypertrophy
   - Anatomic variants in the ostiomeatal complex
   - Foreign bodies
   - Choanal atresia
3. Tumors
   - Benign
   - Malignant
4. Granulomas
   - Wegener's granulomatosis
   - Sarcoid
   - Infective
     - Tuberculosis
     - Leprosy
   - Malignant
     - Midline destructive granuloma
5. Cerebrospinal rhinorrhea

From International Rhinitis Management Working Group. International consensus report on diagnosis and management of rhinitis. Eur J Allergy Clin Immunol 1994; 49(Suppl 19):5; with permission.

Table 2 Diagnostic Techniques

History
General ENT examination

In addition where appropriate and/or test is available

Allergy tests
- Skin tests
- Serum specific IgE
- Total serum IgE

Endoscopy
- Rigid
- Flexible

Nasal smear—cytology
Nasal swab—bacteriology
Radiology
- Plain sinus x-rays
- Computed tomography (CT)
- Magnetic resonance imaging (MRI)
- Chest radiograph

Mucociliary function
- Nasomucociliary clearance (NMCC)
- Ciliary beat frequency (CBF)
- Electron microscopy

Nasal airway assessment
- Nasal inspiratory peak flow (NIPF)
- Rhinomanometry (anterior and posterior)
- Acoustic rhinometry

Olfaction
- Quantitative suprathreshold and threshold testing
- Qualitative

Blood tests
- Full blood count and white cell differential
- Erythrocyte sedimentation rate
- Thyroid function tests
- Antineutrophil cytoplasmic antibody (ANCA)
- Immunoglobulins and IgG subclasses
- Antibody response to immunization with protein and carbohydrate antigens

From International Rhinitis Management Working Group. International consensus report on diagnosis and management of rhinitis. Eur J Allergy Clin Immunol 1994; 49(Suppl 19):13–18; with permission.

serious conditions such as malignancy and thereby eliminate them. Unilateral disease should always be regarded with suspicion. It is also important to consider factors that may contribute to the development of chronic inflammation of the nose (Table 3).

Table 3 Contributory Factors in the Development of Chronic Rhinosinusitis

Anatomic Variants
- Concha bullosa
- Enlarged ethmoidal bulla
- Everted uncinate process
- Paradoxical middle turbinate
- Agger nasi pneumatization
- Haller cells
- Septal deflection

Mucociliary Abnormalities
- Congenital
- Acquired

Immune Deficiency
- Congenital
- Acquired

Allergy

PREFERRED APPROACH

Avoidance

In all cases of perennial nonallergic rhinitis, avoidance of irritants and provoking circumstances should be discussed. This can be a counsel of perfection, but requires patient acceptance and compliance to be effective. Recognition of the problem may allow them to reduce exposure to irritants such as cigarette smoke, either active or passive. Patients should be encouraged to stop the excessive long-term use of topical decongestants, which can result in rhinitis medicamentosa, and should be offered alternative therapy such as topical steroids.

Topical Nasal Steroids

Timing of Therapy and Patient Selection

The availability of topical nasal steroids with a high therapeutic ratio attributable to first-pass deactivation in the liver and thus a negligible effect on the hypothalamic-pituitary-adrenal axis has significantly assisted our management of perennial nonallergic rhinitis. Since the introduction of beclomethasone dipropionate (BDP) in 1973, a range of preparations has become available, including budesonide, flunisolide, triamcinalone, and, most recently, fluticasone propionate. In addition, topical formulations of betamethasone sodium phosphate and dexamethasone may be prescribed but may also have systemic effects. As soon as a working diagnosis is established, a topical steroid may be administered, and this applies even in the presence of other forms of rhinitis.

Mechanisms of Action

Some aspects of steroid action are as yet unclear, but it is established that the steroid molecule penetrates the cell membrane and binds to hormone receptors in the cytoplasm. The steroid receptor complex is transferred to the nucleus where it binds to specific sites on the DNA molecule that have a regulatory influence on protein synthesis. The inflammatory cell infiltrate, in particular the number of mast cells and eosinophils, is reduced in the superficial mucosa, diminishing hyper-reactivity, vascular permeability, and release of mediators. Consequently, intranasal steroids are effective against all symptoms of rhinitis, in particular nasal congestion and hyposmia.

Dosage, Routes, and Practical Considerations

Topical steroids are generally administered by freon-driven aerosols, by mechanical pump sprays in aqueous or glycol solutions, or as a dry powder given as two actuations to each side of the nose. Recommended frequency for BDP and flunisolide is twice daily; for budesonide, fluticasone, and triamcinalone, it is once daily. Recommended total daily dosage ranges from 200 to 400 μg.

Method of Instillation

Patients should be instructed to direct the spray superiorly and laterally, avoiding contact with the nasal septum, while breathing in. Betamethasone sodium phosphate, which is available as aqueous drops and also in a form containing neomycin, may be instilled in the head-down and -forward position to enhance penetration into the middle meatus. This is particularly useful in chronic rhinosinusitis where mucopurulent secretion and obstruction of the ostiomeatal region is present.

Side Effects and Complications

Side effects and complications are minor and include dryness, crusting, slight spotting of blood, and occasional discomfort, which may be overcome by a change of delivery system such as to an aqueous form. Rarely, septal perforation has been reported with topical steroid use. However, the modern generation of topical steroids administered at the recommended dosage may be given with confidence to patients of all ages (≥4 years) and during pregnancy. In contrast, because both betamethasone sodium phosphate and dexamethasone are capable of producing minor systemic steroid effects, their use in the very young, during pregnancy, and in the long term is not recommended, but they are useful as the initial therapeutic agent in uncomplicated perennial rhinitis.

Assessment of Therapeutic Response

It is important that patients have an adequate therapeutic trial of daily medication for at least 4 weeks before assessing clinical efficacy. Compliance will be significantly improved if patients understand that the clinical effect is not instantaneous and that it will only continue as long as the medication is administered. Once symptoms are controlled, the daily dosage may be reduced. Depending on the underlying cause of the condition, medication is usually required long term. Patients may be reassured that this poses no safety issues and should be advised to titrate dosages based on individual circumstance. The presence of eosinophils in nasal cytology specimens appears to be a particularly successful predictor of therapeutic efficacy for intranasal steroids.

■ THERAPEUTIC ALTERNATIVES

Systemic Corticosteroids

A short course of oral steroid such as prednisolone or dexamethasone can be useful in severe cases of rhinitis in emergency situations such as prior to an examination or job interview. They allow symptomatic control to be achieved rapidly, after which topical preparations may be used. The regimens for these agents follows: prednisolone 20 mg for 3 days, 15 mg for 3 days, 10 mg for 3 days, and 5 mg for 3 days; dexamethasone: 12 mg for 3 days, 8 mg for 3 days, and 4 mg for 3 days.

There are a number of contraindications to the use of systemic corticosteroids, including herpes keratitis, advanced osteoporosis, severe hypertension, diabetes mellitus, gastric ulceration, and chronic infection. They are not indicated in the treatment of rhinitis in children or in pregnant women.

Depot preparations of steroids (e.g., methylprednisolone) and ACTH analogues (e.g., Synacthen) are also available and although effective, they may produce severe side effects that cannot be reversed and may suppress adrenal cortex function for long periods. Consequently, their use in perennial nonallergic rhinitis is rarely warranted.

Anticholinergics

In some cases of perennial nonallergic rhinitis, watery rhinorrhea is the predominant symptom. Under these circumstances the anticholinergic agent ipratropium bromide can be useful. It acts as an antagonist against the muscarinic receptors of the seromucinous glands. It has been shown to markedly inhibit methacholine-induced and cold air-induced nasal hypersecretion, but it has no effect on congestion, itching, or sneezing. It is administered as a topical spray and works rapidly if it is effective. The side effects are those of any nasal spray—dryness, crusting, irritation, and spotting of blood. In addition, excessive dryness of the throat is sometimes experienced. Ipratropium bromide is not recommended in patients with glaucoma or prostatic hypertrophy.

Saline Douching

Saline douching can be most effective in cases of chronic rhinosinusitis, particularly when mucopurulent discharge is significant before instillation of active medication. Patients are asked to sniff or spray in a solution made of a pinch of table salt and a pinch of bicarbonate of soda dissolved in half a glass of warm water two to three times a day.

Decongestants

Systemic and topical decongestants remain popular with the general public, being readily available without prescription. Systemic decongestants are often sold in combination with antihistamines but evidence is lacking for their efficacy in nonallergic rhinitis. Long-term reliance on topical decongestants should be actively discouraged but the prior use of an agent such as oxymetazoline may facilitate instillation of an intranasal steroid for the first few days of treatment when congestion is severe, without fear of provoking rhinitis medicamentosa.

Antibiotics

Although the treatment of infectious rhinitis is beyond the scope of this chapter, broad-spectrum antibiotics can be helpful in the presence of mucopurulent nasal secretion, which can occur in perennial nonallergic rhinitis. The choice of antibiotics is determined by microbiology, clinical severity, and patient factors. In chronic situations, those agents that inhibit *Haemophilus influenzae*, *Streptococcus pneumoniae*, and anaerobes will be most effective (e.g., amoxicillin clavulanate, cerfuroxime axetil with or without metronidazole).

Surgery

The majority of cases of simple perennial nonallergic noninfectious rhinitis can be managed medically. However, there are a number of contributory elements that may exacerbate the situation and may require surgical intervention, in particular, mechanical factors such as a deviated nasal septum, hypertrophied inferior turbinates, and anatomic variants within the middle meatus causing narrowing of the ostiomeatal complex (see Table 3). When considering surgery the following points should be borne in mind:

1. Surgical correction should be considered when medical treatment fails, but this will not necessarily obviate the need for long-term medication.
2. The sensation of nasal congestion may be due to

Table 4 Methods for Reduction of the Inferior Turbinate

Submucous diathermy
Linear cautery
Submucous resection
Submucous outfracture
Laser cautery/reduction
Cryosurgery
Turbinectomy
Partial
Radical/subtotal

many factors. It is advisable to exclude disease in the middle meatus by endoscopy and/or CT scanning before attacking the nasal septum and inferior turbinates.

3. Anatomic variants in the middle meatus should not be operated on per se as they occur in the normal population. Only do so if they are obstructing sinus outflow with associated infection.

There are many methods of inferior turbinate reduction producing varying periods of symptomatic relief (Table 4). Mucosal preservation is better achieved by submucous diathermy, submucous resection, and submucous outfracture (SMOFIT), but resection of variable amounts of the inferior turbinate remains popular. The effect of a decongestant spray may be helpful in deciding between reduction by shrinkage procedures and excision. When resecting the inferior turbinate, it should be remembered that it is the anterior turbinate that has the greatest effect on resistance to flow in the valve area. Techniques that produce fibrosis may also have an effect on local neuronal control of secretion as well as turbinate mass. However, any surgical interference with the turbinate can produce significant hemorrhage, adhesions, and crusting.

Vidian neurectomy represents a more direct surgical approach to secretion control by aiming to ablate the parasympathetic supply. A variety of routes to the vidian nerve may be chosen, but results, especially in the long term, are disappointing.

Table 4 shows the more common anatomic variants found in the middle meatus. The rationale and details of surgery in this area are beyond the scope of this chapter. Suffice it to say that based on pathophysiologic principles of disrupted mucociliary clearance from the sinuses, there has been a general move away from radical ablative surgery such as the Caldwell Luc approach to a more conservative and precise removal of diseased tissue within the critical drainage areas of the nose (i.e., the ostiomeatal complex). This has been facilitated by improved visualization, both diagnostically and therapeutically, with rigid endoscopy and CT scanning. Nevertheless, patients still receive medication, in particular topical nasal steroids both before and after surgery. Indeed surgery is not generally undertaken unless the patient has had at least 3 months of medical therapy.

Table 5 Complications of Nasal Polypectomy

Death
Intracranial
Meningitis
Hemorrhage
Cerebrovascular accident
Orbital
Blindness
Diplopia
Epiphora
Hematoma
Nasal
Hemorrhage
Adhesions

NASAL POLYPS

The term *nasal polyposis* covers a wide spectrum of disease from the polypoid change often encountered in the middle meatus during chronic infection to the aggressive massive and recurrent polyps of cystic fibrosis or the aspirin-sensitive asthma (ASA) triad. In between lie "ordinary" polyps, the cause of which remains obscure. A condition characterized by obstruction and anosmia, polyps behave like garden weeds, generally defying all medical and surgical efforts to eradicate them. Once diagnosed and differentiated from neoplasia (usually, though not exclusively, by their bilateral occurrence), corticosteroids in their many forms may be tried. Although allergy does not appear to cause polyp formation, mast cell reactions and eosinophil activation with subsequent inflammation appear to be important. For primary treatment betamethasone drops or parenteral steroids can be most useful. Surgery is frequently required and may take the form of conventional nasal polypectomy with snares up to and including total fronto-ethmo-sphenoidectomy. These procedures may be performed using a headlight, microscope, and fiberoptically illuminated speculum, or under endoscopic control. My preference is the latter, but such a procedure is always preceded by 6 to 8 weeks of medical treatment and CT scanning. Following surgery, any of the intranasal steroid sprays may be given ad infinitum. The complications of polypectomy, irrespective of the instrumentation and approach, are shown in Table 5.

Suggested Reading

International Rhinitis Management Working Group. International consensus report on the diagnosis and management of rhinitis. Eur J Allerg Clin Immunol 1994; 49(Suppl 19):1–34.

Mackay IS, ed. Rhinitis: mechanisms and management. London: Royal Society of Medicine Services, 1989.

Mackay IS, Lund VJ. Surgical management of sinusitis. In: Mackay IS, Bull TR, eds. Scott Brown's otolaryngology. 6th ed. Vol 4, Chap 12. London: Butterworths (in press).

Mygind N, Naclerio RM, eds. Allergic and non-allergic rhinitis: clinical aspects. Copenhagen: Munksgaard, 1993.

PENICILLIN ALLERGY

Michael S. Kaplan, M.D.

IMMUNOLOGIC REACTIONS TO PENICILLIN

Penicillins are capable of producing a broad spectrum of immunologic reactions. The scope of these reactions is depicted in Table 1 in approximate order of decreasing frequency. The true incidence of immunologic reactions is unknown but may be as high as 8 percent of all treatment courses in adults and children. The majority of reactions are cutaneous in nature and not serious. A maculopapular or morbilliform nonpruritic eruption occurs in 9 percent of treatment courses with ampicillin. The incidence approaches 100 percent in patients with infectious mononucleosis and is also increased in patients who are receiving allopurinol. This rash and the maculopapular nonpruritic rash associated with penicillin therapy are not IgE mediated, tend to occur late in the course of therapy, are not associated with a risk of anaphylaxis, and can dissipate with continued therapy. The rash can begin even after the penicillin or ampicillin has been discontinued. Reactions encompassing four Gell and Coombs' classes of immunopathic responses have been described with the penicillins and are depicted in Table 2. This chapter is devoted to a discussion of type I hypersensitivity.

Table 1 Hypersensitivity Reactions to Penicillins (in Approximate Decreasing Frequency)

Maculopapular rash
Urticarial rash
Fever
Bronchospasm
Vasculitis
Serum sickness
Exfoliative dermatitis
Stevens-Johnson syndrome
Anaphylaxis
Interstitial nephritis

IgE-MEDIATED REACTIONS

Type I hypersensitivity reactions can occur at any dose and with oral, topical, or parenteral preparations. Reactions may occur without previous known exposure. Hidden exposures are thought to occur in foods of animal origin when animals are treated with penicillin injections; from airborne penicillin particles inhaled by health care or pharmaceutical workers; or from small amounts of penicillin in penicillium mold-contaminated foods.

IgE-mediated reactions to penicillin have been classified according to onset of reaction. *Immediate reactions* occur within minutes to 1 hour after a dose of penicillin and present as urticaria, angioedema, laryngeal edema, bronchospasm, or anaphylaxis. *Accelerated reactions* occur within 1 to 72 hours after starting penicillin, manifesting with urticaria, angioedema, laryngeal edema, or bronchospasm. *Late reactions* occur more than 72 hours after penicillin exposure. Late reaction symptoms include morbilliform rash, interstitial nephritis, hemolytic anemia, neutropenia, thrombocytopenia, serum sickness, drug fever, Stevens-Johnson syndrome, and exfoliative dermatitis. These reactions are not IgE mediated, but represent a heterogeny of immune mechanisms. IgE-mediated reactions to penicillin occur in about 2 percent of adult treatment courses.

Anaphylaxis to penicillin is rare, occurring in 0.04 percent to 0.2 percent of treated individuals. Fatal anaphylaxis occurs in one of every 100,000 treated patients; only one-third of patients who had previously received penicillin had a history of a prior reaction. Anaphylaxis may occur after oral penicillin

Table 2 Classification of Immunopathic Responses to Penicillins

GELL AND COOMBS CLASS	MECHANISM	REACTION	COMMENTS
Type I	IgE immediate hypersensitivity	Urticaria; flushing; laryngeal edema; bronchospasm; abdominal pain; diarrhea; hypovolemic shock	Skin testing with PPL, MDM, Pen G; avoid Pcn or desensitize
Type II	IgG, IgM, C′ cytoxic	Hemolytic anemia; thrombocytopenia; nephritis	Pcn determinants bound to cell surface; Coombs'-positive anemia; skin test and desensitization not applicable
Type III	Soluble immune complexes, C′, and in some patients IgE	Serum sickness	Circulating immune complexes may be positive; ICs plus C′ on biopsy of involved tissue; some patients have intense IgE response; avoid Pcn, desensitization *not* applicable
Type IV	Delayed hypersensitivity	Contact dermatitis	DH skin test or patch test; avoid Pcn contact

MDM, minor determinants; Pcn, penicillin; Pen G, penicillin G; PPL, penicilloyl polylysine.

administration or even during skin testing with penicillin determinants. Atopic predisposition is not a factor contributing to overall risk of a hypersensitivity reaction to penicillin, nor is sensitivity to penicillium mold. However, fatal anaphylactic penicillin reactions tend to occur in atopic individuals, and serum sickness reactions to desensitization may occur more frequently in patients with an IgE-mediated penicillin hypersensitivity.

■ PENICILLIN SKIN TESTING

Who Should Be Tested?

Skin testing all individuals who are to receive penicillin is neither practical nor cost effective. Three to 10 percent of the adult population will have positive skin tests to penicillin irrespective of a positive history. Patients with a history of only skin reactions to penicillin will have less than a 30 percent skin test reaction rate using accurate test reagents. If the history is one of a morbilliform eruption, the skin test reactivity rate is less than 10 percent.

One school of thought recommends that penicillin skin testing be done only in those patients who have a positive history and in whom therapeutic intervention is imminent. The penicillin testing is valid only for the immediate therapeutic course. If skin testing is negative, the subsequent course of penicillin rarely resensitizes the patient. Testing is recommended before each future treatment course, depending on the severity of prior reactions, skin test responses, and subsequent rechallenges. There is a refractory period of skin test unresponsiveness immediately following a treatment course of penicillin, particularly high-dose therapy. Skin reactivity to penicillin determinants returns within 1 to 3 months.

The incidence of positive skin tests in children with a history of penicillin reactions is low (10 percent), yet many children carry a lifelong label of penicillin allergy. One approach to "clear the air" regarding penicillin sensitivity is to skin test history-positive children when penicillin therapy is desirable. If the skin test is negative, then an oral challenge with penicillin is given under observation for 1 hour. The oral challenge is likely to be negative in the face of negative skin tests. Skin test–negative, oral challenge–negative patients can then be given a full therapeutic course of penicillin. Only a few patients will develop a rash under those circumstances, but not a serious systemic reaction. Retesting 4 to 6 weeks after completion of the treatment course will detect patients who have become resensitized or initially sensitized. The incidence of a subsequent positive skin test is low (10 percent). If the skin test is positive, the risk of subsequent reaction is 40 to 73 percent. Approximately one-half of these reactions will be systemic, and one of the 10 systemic reactions is fatal or near fatal.

Unfortunately, there are no clear-cut risk factors for fatal anaphylaxis. Two-thirds of fatal anaphylactic reactions occur in individuals who have had penicillin before, but without a reaction. However, patients with penicillin hypersensitivity have a higher incidence of other drug reactions, and fatal anaphylaxis tends to occur more frequently in atopic individuals and asthmatics with active disease. Using the above information, the best risk profile for fatal anaphylaxis may be those *atopic individuals*, especially *asthmatics* with *other drug sensitivities* who have received penicillins before, regardless of a history for a prior reaction. The use of beta-blockers is an additional risk when combined with the above factors.

Skin test reactivity to penicillin declines with time. Seventy to 100 percent of history-positive patients will have a positive skin test for at least one of the reagents when tested 2 weeks to 3 months after a penicillin reaction. By 5 years after a reaction, 50 percent of history-positive patients are skin-test negative. Skin-test positivity declines to 20 to 30 percent by 10 years. At any given time, the skin tests are 96 percent reliable. Four percent of history-positive, skin-test negative patients will react to penicillin treatment with approximately 1 percent as accelerated reactions and 3 percent as mild, cutaneous reactions. In one large study, anaphylaxis did not occur in skin-test negative patients.

In vitro assays for specific penicilloyl IgE antibodies are less sensitive than skin tests. Radioallergosorbent test (RAST) or enzyme linked immunosorbent assay (ELISA) for penicilloyl-specific IgE antibodies detects only 60 to 95 percent of patients who have a positive skin test to penicilloyl polylysine (PPL).

An in vitro enzyme-linked immune assay for the detection of histamine release from peripheral blood leukocytes (basophils) holds some promise in early trials for detecting penicillin-induced histamine release. Its use as a diagnostic tool is still investigational.

■ SKIN-TEST REAGENTS

Ninety-five percent of benzylpenicillin is metabolized to the penicilloyl moiety (the major determinant). The remainder is metabolized to a variety of minor determinants which include benzylpenicilloate and penilloate. These metabolic products of penicillin combine easily with serum proteins, creating immunogenic complexes. Thus the penicillins are one of the most common drugs to cause adverse immunologic reactions.

The penicilloyl moiety has been combined with polylysine and is commercially available as PrePen. A positive skin test to PPL is thought to reflect a risk for non–life-threatening reactions such as urticaria, whereas a positive skin test to minor determinants indicates a risk for anaphylaxis.

The minor determinants are not commercially available. Alternatively, fresh benzylpenicillin G has been used along with PPL as a skin-test reagent. Skin testing to penicillin G (Pen G) alone would miss approximately 60 percent of allergic individuals. Aging Pen G to generate minor determinants has no advantage over fresh Pen G when minor determinants are unavailable. If there is a history of serious reaction, then epicutaneous testing (scratch or prick) with a 5 unit per milliliter concentration is used. If the history of a reaction is vague or mild in nature or if the initial skin test with 5 units per milliliter is negative, epicutaneous testing is then performed with a 10,000 unit per milliliter solution. Patients with negative or equivocal responses to the above testing are tested intradermally with 0.02 to 0.04 ml of a 10,000 unit per milliliter mix. A net wheal of 2 mm diameter or greater after 15 to 20 minutes compared to a diluent or saline control is considered positive. A positive histamine control is also used: one drop of 1 mg per milliliter histamine phosphate for

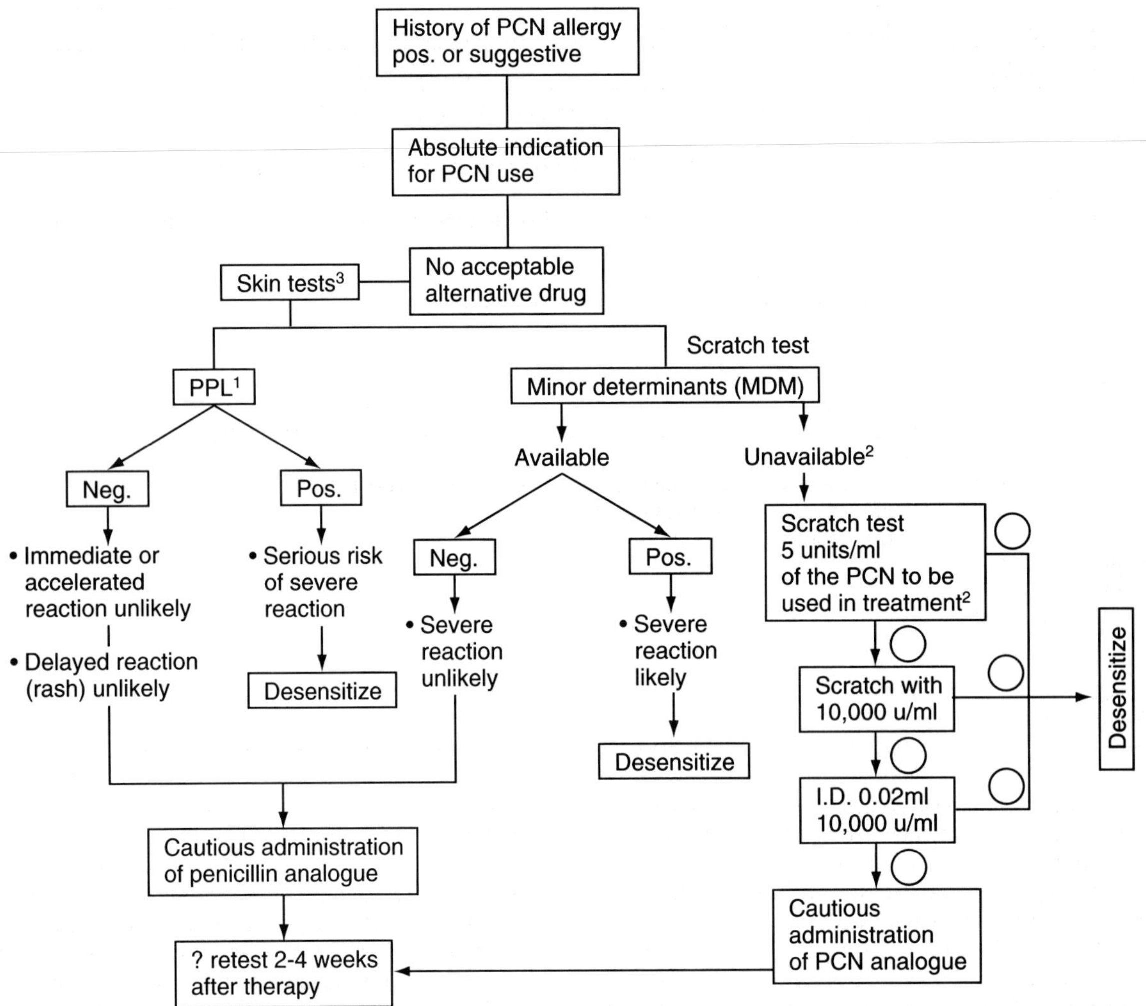

[1] Kremers-Urban Co., Milwaukee, WI.

[2] Fresh Benzyl potassium penicillin 1 million unit vial reconstituted to 100,000 units/ml (stock vial: good for one week). Make 10,000 unit/ml and 5 unit/ml fresh daily; MDM made fresh daily.

[3] Epicutaneous tests are done first; if negative after 20 minutes intradermal tests are done with the same, diluted, reagent as indicated.

Figure 1
Skin testing and treatment.

epicutaneous tests and 0.02 to 0.04 ml of 0.1 mg per milliliter for intradermal tests.

The semisynthetic penicillins contain the same 6 aminopenicillic acid nucleus as benzylpenicillin G. Thus there is a great deal of cross-reactivity with Pen G. Extensive studies indicate that a negative skin test with penicillin G determinants excludes patients at risk for a reaction to semisynthetic penicillins. There may be a small risk for patients to react to antigenic determinants unique to the semisynthetic penicillins. The reagents for these determinants are not commercially available. Serial testing can be done with the specific agent by epicutaneous techniques using concentrations of 0.25 mg per milliliter, 2.5 mg per milliliter, and 25 mg per milliliter. If the epicutaneous tests are negative or equivocal, then intradermal testing can be done serially with concentrations of 2.5 mg per milliliter and 25 mg per milliliter. The testing is interpreted by the same criteria as penicillin G. Skin test reactivity may predict the safe starting level for desensitization. Patients with prick test or low-dose intracutaneous test sensitivity may have to start at one-one thousandth of step 1 doses as listed in the desensitization protocols in Table 5 and 6. An algorithm for skin testing and treatment is presented in Figure 1.

■ DESENSITIZATION

If any of the skin tests are positive and an alternative antibiotic (non–beta-lactam) cannot be used, then a protocol to desensitize to penicillin must be employed. It is unclear whether benzylpenicillin G desensitization will provide protection from a reaction to the semisynthetic penicillins or the cephalosporins. It is probably best to desensitize with the specific agent to be used in therapy, employing a modified protocol

Table 3 Complications During Desensitization (or as a Consequence of Continued Drug Exposure)

COMPLICATION	COMMENTS
Cutaneous (not uncommon)	Do not give higher doses of Pcn when reaction begins to develop
Morbilliform	Treat with oral antihistamine (AH)
Urticarial	For reactions resistant to AH, use Prednisone 20–40 mg per day for 4–7 days (0.5–1 mg/kg/day for children <60 lbs)
Maculopapular	
Angioedema	Continue protocol by resuming at 50% of last tolerated dose (2 steps back from the dose that caused the reaction)
	Can resume while rash is still present
Respiratory (rare)	Stop protocol. Stabilize respiratory function
Asthma	Restart protocol at 1/100 of original step 1
Angioedema	
Anaphylaxis (rare)	Stop protocol. Treat anaphylaxis
	Re-examine risks vs. benefits of continuing desensitization
	May resume "low and slow." Restart protocol at 1/100 or less of original step 1. Proceed in half-steps of the original protocol
Serum Sickness (late response)	Patients with IgE-mediated Pcn reactions may be at more risk
	Prolonged treatment with Prednisone
Nonallergic Serious Reactions	Contraindicated to continue Pcn
Toxic epidermal necrolysis	
Exfoliative dermatitis	
Stevens-Johnson syndrome	
Hepatitis	
Nephritis	
Hemolysis	
Systemic Vasculitis	

based on benzylpenicillin desensitization. The mechanism for desensitization is unknown. The overall incidence of immunologic reactions to penicillin during desensitization and subsequent therapy is 27 percent. Most of these reactions are consistent with an IgE-mediated mechanism, but one must also watch for other immunologic reactions such as serum sickness, hemolytic anemia, and interstitial nephritis. The later reactions occur in 5 percent of desensitized patients. Complications encountered during and after desensitization are listed in Table 3. Most reactions encountered during desensitization are fleeting, mild, cutaneous reactions, rhinitis, or wheeze. These reactions can be treated while desensitization proceeds. Skin tests can revert to negative during desensitization.

A checklist as depicted in Table 4 for patients undergoing desensitization is a useful safeguard. Oral desensitization (Table 5) is associated with fewer anaphylactic reactions than parenteral desensitization. This may be a dose-dependent factor. Parenteral desensitization (Table 6) allows visualization for local reactions to allow adjustments in the protocol. If a reaction begins to occur during parenteral desensitization, a tourniquet can be placed proximal to the injection site and ice applied.

Doses are given 15 to 20 minutes apart. Any dose that provokes a mild systemic reaction should be repeated until the patient tolerates that dose, then resume the protocol. Serious systemic reactions should be treated appropriately. If desensitization is continued, then the dose is withheld until the patient has been stabilized. The dose is then reduced by two, tenfold dilutions and advanced per protocol as tolerated. In general, it is not advisable to pretreat with antihistamines or corticosteroids. This may mask milder reactions that signal a need to alter the desensitization protocol. There is also no firm evidence that such pretreatment is effective for IgE-mediated anaphylaxis. Once therapeutic doses are achieved, the course of therapy should not be interrupted. A lapse of 10 to 12 hours between doses may breach tolerance.

Chronic desensitization is applicable for individuals who are at risk for serious reactions and who frequently encounter beta-lactam antibiotics; examples include nurses or pharmacists who mix penicillin powders and certain patients with frequent bacterial infections. This may be achieved by daily administration of 250 mg tablets of Pen G. As in acute desensitization, treatment must not lapse more than 8 to 12 hours in order to maintain tolerance.

When a rapid desensitization is needed, such as in a pregnant woman with syphilis, a protocol such as in Table 7 can be used. For exquisitely sensitive patients, a lower starting dose may be used.

Carbipenems

The carbipenems have a bicyclic nucleus analogous to penicillin. It is not surprising that studies have demonstrated a high degree of cross-reactivity between penicillin and imipenem skin-test reagents. Penicillin-allergic individuals should also be considered sensitive to carbipenems.

Monobactams

There is no evidence that aztreonam cross-reacts with penicillin. Penicillin-sensitive patients have been treated with aztreonam without adverse sensitivity reactions.

Cephacarbams

Cross-reactivity to penicillin has not been determined.

Cephalosporins

General Considerations

The beta-lactam nucleus of penicillin is attached to a five-member thiazolidine ring. Cephalosporins have a six-member dihydrothiazine ring attached to the beta-lactam

Table 4 Penicillin Desensitization Check List

1. **Document** the absolute need for penicillin
   Life-threatening infection
   No acceptable alternative drug
2. **Informed consent.** Document that risks and benefits were explained to patient or patient's proxy
3. If patient has asthma, **stabilize asthma** first
   Peak flow rate ≥85% of personal best, *or*
   ≥80% of predicted value
4. Perform desensitization **in hospital,** preferably on intensive care unit
   Adequate **personnel** for close observation and monitoring
   Appropriate **equipment and medications** in the immediate area to treat anaphylaxis
   Discontinue beta-blocking agents
5. Start at **lower dose** for patients with stronger skin test responses (i.e., prick vs. intracutaneous response)
6. Ultimately, the **route of administration** by which the drug is to be given should be part of the desensitization protocol
7. Successful desensitization should **proceed immediately into the therapeutic regimen.** Breaks in dosing can result in hypersensitivity reactions
8. **Monitor vital signs frequently** during desensitization and for the first 12 hours on full therapy
9. Ordinarily do not use antihistamines or corticosteroids to premedicate. These agents may mask signs of impending anaphylaxis that allow proper adjustments of the protocol

Table 5 Oral Desensitization Protocol

STEP*	PHENOXYMETHYL† PENICILLIN (U/ml)	AMOUNT (ml)	DOSE (U)	CUMULATIVE DOSAGE (U)	CUMULATIVE TIME COURSE
1	1,000	0.1	100	100	
2	1,000	0.2	200	300	
3	1,000	0.4	400	700	
4	1,000	0.8	800	1,500	
5	1,000	1.6	1,600	3,100	
6	1,000	3.2	3,200	6,300	
7	1,000	6.4	6,400	12,700	
8	10,000	1.2	12,000	24,700	
9	10,000	2.4	24,000	48,700	
10	10,000	4.8	48,000	96,700	
11	80,000	1.0	80,000	176,700	
12	80,000	2.0	160,000	336,700	
13	80,000	4.0	320,000	656,700	
14	80,000	8.0	640,000	1,296,700	260 min
		Observe patient for 30 minutes			
	Change to benzylpenicillin G administered IV				
15	500,000	0.25	125,000		
16	500,000	0.50	250,000		
17	500,000	1.0	500,000		
18	500,000	2.25	1,125,000		350 min
19	Contine with regular therapeutic doses. NOTE: A break in dosing risks a systemic reaction.				

From Sullivan TJ. Penicillin allergy. In: Lichtenstein LM, Fauci AS, eds. Current therapy in allergy, immunology and rheumatology. Toronto: BC Decker, 1985:60.
*Interval between steps: 20 minutes.
†Solution 1: Stock solution prepared fresh 400,000 U/5 ml (80,000 U/ml).
Solution 2: Take 2 cc of solution 1 and add 14 cc sterile water (= 10,000 U/ml).
Solution 3: Take 2 cc of solution 2 and add 18 cc sterile water (= 1,000 U/ml).

nucleus. Cephalosporins are metabolized to the major determinant cephaloyl moiety, which cross-reacts with the penicillin major determinant. Cross-reactivity of penicillin and cephalosporin minor determinants is limited. In a large survey of adverse drug reactions, penicillin accounts for 10.4 percent of all adverse reactions whereas cephalosporins account for 1.3 percent.

The risk of an adverse reaction to cephalosporin in a penicillin-sensitive patient is somewhat controversial. Sullivan reported an overall 51 percent skin test reactivity rate to cephalosporin in 123 penicillin skin test–positive patients. Cephalosporin challenge was not performed in the study; but in another study, 27 history-positive, skin test–positive penicillin-allergic patients were challenged with cephalosporin and none reacted. Cephalosporin skin test was not done. The expected cephalosporin reaction rate in penicillin-allergic

Table 6 Parenteral Desensitization Protocol

STEP*	CONCENTRATION OF β-LACTAM DRUG (mg/ml)	BENZYL-PENICILLIN (UNITS/ml)	AMOUNT (ml SUBCUTANEOUSLY)	CUMULATIVE TIME COURSE
1	0.1	100	0.10	
2	0.1	100	0.20	
3	0.1	100	0.40	
4	0.1	100	0.80	
5	1	1,000	0.15	
6	1	1,000	0.30	
7	1	1,000	0.60	
8	10	10,000	0.10	
9	10	10,000	0.20	
10	10	10,000	0.40	
11	10	10,000	0.80	
12	100	100,000	0.15	
13	100	100,000	0.30	
14	100	100,000	0.60	
15	1,000	1,000,000	0.10	
16	1,000	1,000,000	0.20	
17	1,000	1,000,000	0.40	
18	1,000	1,000,000	0.50	340 min
		Observe patient for 30 minutes		
19	1,000	1,000,000 U/hr continuous	IV (0.5 g)	370 min
20	1,000	Continuous IV	IV (1.5 g)	400 min
		NOTE: A break in dosing risks a systemic reaction.		

From Sullivan TJ. Penicillin allergy. In: Lichtenstein LM, Fauci AS, eds. Current therapy in allergy, immunology and rheumatology. Toronto: BC Decker, 1985:61.
*Interval between steps: 20 minutes.

Table 7 An Example of Rapid Desensitization to Benzathine Penicillin

CONCENTRATION (UNITS/cc)	DOSE (UNITS/0.1 cc)	CUMULATIVE DOSE (UNITS)	ELAPSED TIME
1	0.1 SC	0.1	
10	1.0 SC	1.1	
100	10 SC	11.1	
1,000	100 SC	111.1	
10,000	1,000 SC	1,111.1	
100,000	10,000 SC	11,111.1	
1,000,000	100,000 SC	111,111.1	
	200,000 IM	311,111.1	
	2.1 million IM	2,411,111.1	170 min

patients would be 6 or 7 patients (27 patients × 0.51 cross-reaction rate × 0.5 expected reaction rate to challenge in history-positive–skin test-positive patients). Petz reported an overall reaction rate of 8 percent to cephalosporins in 450 penicillin-sensitive patients. The risk of cross-reaction with penicillin differs among the various cephalosporins; in general, it is more common with the first- and second-generation cephalosporins (Cephaloridin 16.5 percent, Cephalothin 5 percent, Cephalexin 5.4 percent). In Petz's survey only one patient of 9,385 without a history of penicillin sensitivity had an anaphylactic reaction to a cephalosporin (0.1 percent). The risk for anaphylaxis to cephalosporins in penicillin-sensitive patients was 0.4 percent. The rate of urticarial reactions to cephalosporins was 1.3 percent in penicillin-sensitive patients and 0.4 percent in patients without a history of penicillin sensitivity. However, the reaction rate to immunologically unrelated drugs is also of this magnitude in penicillin-allergic patients. Since cephalosporin skin testing was not done in this survey, the precise relationship between cephalosporin and penicillin cross-reactivity is unclear.

The extent of cross-reactivity among the cephalosporins is unknown. It is likely to be low if the clinically relevant antibodies are side-chain specific. Antibodies to the monobactam, aztreonam are side-chain specific and therefore do not cross-react with either penicillin or cephalothin. Ceftazidine, which has an identical aminothiazolyl side-chain, can inhibit aztreonam antibodies in vitro.

Cephalosporin Skin Tests

The predictive value of using native cephalosporins as skin-test reagents is unknown. The nature of the haptenic determinants is also unknown. Native cephalosporins in concentrations of 1 mg per milliliter or greater cause nonspecific skin reactivity. The skin-test reagent for cephalosporin is prepared by making a 10^{-3} mol per liter solution in phosphate-buffered saline. This stock solution is made fresh. Sequential epicutaneous tests are then done with 1:10,000, 1:1,000, and 1:100 dilutions. Negative or equivocal reactions are followed by intradermal testing in the same sequence. The use of penicillin skin-test reagents to predict cephalosporin sensitivity is not completely clear since the studies that suggest cross-reactivity did not challenge patients with cephalosporins, and challenge studies in penicillin-sensitive patients did not look at cephalosporin skin reactivity. On the other hand, the rate of reactions to cephalosporins in penicillin-sensitive patients is low and usually limited to cutaneous reactions and the occurrence of anaphylaxis is very low. At this time a positive skin test to dilute native cephalosporin should be interpreted as reflecting a risk for a hypersensitivity reaction. However, a negative skin test does not rule out this risk and should be taken as "no information."

Before treating with a cephalosporin, patients with a history of penicillin sensitivity should be skin tested with penicillin reagents. Those patients with a negative skin test may be treated with penicillin or cephalosporin. The reaction rate is likely to be very low and limited to cutaneous reactions. Patients who are history-positive and skin-test positive to penicillin should be skin tested with the cephalosporin of choice. Individuals who are also cephalosporin skin-test positive should avoid both drugs. Alternatively, cautious administration of cephalosporin as dictated by the clinical situation should follow the desensitization model used for penicillin.

Suggested Reading

Anderson JA. Cross-sensitivity to cephalosporins in patients allergic to penicillin. Pediatr Infect Dis J 1986; 5:557–561.

Cameron W, Windt M, Borish L, et al. A complicated case of penicillin allergy. Ann Allergy 1984; 53:455.

Green G, Rosenblum A, Sweet L. Evaluation of penicillin hypersensitivity: Value of clinical history and skin testing with penicilloyl-polylysine and penicillin G. J Allergy Clin Immunol 1977; 60:339–345.

Levine BB. Immunologic mechanisms of penicillin allergy. A haptenic model system for the study of allergic disease of man. N Engl J Med 1966; 275:1115–1125.

Lin RY. A perspective on penicillin allergy. Arch Intern Med 1992; 152: 930–937.

Petz LD. Immunologic reactions of humans to cephalosporins. Postgrad Med J 1971; 47(Suppl):64–69.

Saxon A, Beall GN, Rohr AS, Adelman DC. Immediate hypersensitivity reactions to beta-lactam antibiotics. Ann Int Med 1987; 107:204–215.

Sogn DD, Evans R III, Shepherd GM, et al. Results of the NIAID collaborative clinical trial to test the predictive value of skin testing with major and minor penicillin derivatives in hospitalized adults. Arch Intern Med 1992; 152:1025–1032.

Sullivan TJ, Wedner H, Shatz G, et al. Skin testing to detect penicillin allergy. J Allergy Clin Immunol 1981; 68:171–180.

Weiss ME, Adkinson NF. Immediate hypersensitivity reactions to penicillin and related antibiotics. Clin Allergy 1988; 18:515–540.

INSECT STING ALLERGY

David F. Graft, M.D.

Allergic reactions to insect stings are a more serious problem in adults than in children since the reactions tend to be more severe and death occurs much more frequently. Stinging insects (honeybees, yellow jackets, hornets, wasps, and imported fire ants) are members of the order Hymenoptera. Honeybees are small fuzzy insects with alternating tan and black stripes. They are often seen pollinating clover and flowering plants, are relatively nonaggressive, and generally sting only when caught underfoot or if their hive is disturbed. The barbed stinger usually remains at the site of the sting, a feature that can be an important diagnostic clue. Another strain of honeybee ("African" bee or "killer" bee) has been steadily migrating northward from Central and South America and has now reached Texas. They will probably continue to move gradually to the north until their progression is limited by climatic factors. These bees, as compared with the established "European" honeybees, exhibit strong defensive behavior, consider a much wider area to be part of their domain, and sting in large numbers when provoked. Bumblebees are large, slow-moving, noisy bees with hairy bodies of alternating yellow and black stripes. They are nonaggressive and account for only a small fraction of stings.

The vespids include yellow jackets, hornets, and wasps. Yellow jackets have alternating yellow and black body stripes and a characteristic hovering-darting flight pattern. They nest in the ground or in decaying logs and scavenge for food, frequenting garbage cans and picnics where they fly sorties at soda cans and other foodstuffs. They are short tempered and sting upon minor provocation. Closely related are the yellow and white-faced hornets, which build teardrop-shaped nests in trees or shrubs. Not quite as aggressive as the other vespids, the thin-bodied paper wasps build nests in the eaves of buildings in which the hexagonal development cells are not covered by a paper envelope. Imported fire ants are primarily found in the Gulf Coast states. Their dirt mounds of one to two feet in height contain thousands of ants.

■ SPECTRUM OF REACTIONS

A normal reaction to a Hymenopteran sting is transient redness and itching at the sting site. About 10 percent of the population develop large local reactions. These vary in severity from just a few inches of swelling to involvement of an entire extremity and may last for several days. Fire ants usually cause a semicircle of vesicles at the sting sites that results from repetitive stinging as they pivot around, anchored by their mandibles to the victim.

Systemic IgE-mediated reactions occur in 0.4 to 0.8 percent of individuals and by definition involve body sites distant from the sting location. They usually commence within minutes after the sting but occasionally several hours may transpire before symptoms start. Milder reactions may be limited to generalized pruritus or urticaria; more severe manifestations include respiratory or cardiovascular symptoms. Systemic reactions tend to be more severe in adults than children. Furthermore, adults suffer almost all of the 40 to 50 deaths per year in the United States that are attributed to insect sting anaphylaxis.

A toxic reaction may result if a person receives a large number of stings in rapid fashion. These reactions are rare and tend to occur when a nest is disturbed. Over the past 20 years, incidents of 500 or more stings by African honeybees have been reported. Some of these have been fatal, but a healthy adult may tolerate over 5,000 stings without sequelae. Several types of delayed adverse responses have been reported including serum sickness–like reactions, transverse myelitis, and myocarditis. The pathophysiology of delayed reactions remains in doubt; immunologic mechanisms may not be involved.

■ ACUTE MANAGEMENT

Individuals presenting with anaphylaxis require careful observation. A subcutaneous injection of epinephrine (1:1,000) at a dose of 0.3 to 0.5 ml is the cornerstone of management and often is sufficient to terminate a reaction. This may be repeated in 10 to 15 minutes if necessary. An oral antihistamine such as diphenhydramine hydrochloride (Benadryl), 12.5 to 50 mg is also usually given. It may lessen urticaria or other cutaneous symptoms, but in more serious or progressive reactions, its use should not delay the administration of epinephrine. Diphenhydramine (Benadryl) may also be administered parenterally (50 mg; 5 mg per kilogram per 24 hours) for more serious reactions.

Inhaled sympathomimetic agents such as isoproterenol or albuterol may decrease bronchoconstriction but do not address other systemic manifestations such as shock. Aminophylline may be helpful if bronchoconstriction persists following epinephrine. Severe reactions often require treatment with oxygen, H_2-antihistamines such as cimetidine (Tagamet), volume expanders, and pressor agents. Corticosteroids such as prednisone (0.5 to 2 mg per kilogram per 24 hours) are commonly used, but their delayed onset of action (4 to 6 hours) limits their effectiveness in the early stages of treatment. Intubation or tracheostomy is indicated for severe upper airway edema not responding to therapy. Allergic reactions are generally more severe in patients who take beta-blocker drugs. Furthermore, reactions in these patients may be more difficult to treat because beta-blockers impede the response to epinephrine and other sympathomimetic medications. Glucagon, 50 mg per kilogram given over 2 minutes intravenously, may be helpful in this clinical situation.

Systemic reactions commencing more than several hours after a sting usually manifest only mild symptoms. Most are easily managed with oral antihistamines and observation. Occasionally, anaphylaxis may be prolonged or biphasic in nature. Close observation and continued treatment are essential in this situation. The administration of corticosteroids as early in treatment as feasible may help to diminish later symptoms. Overnight hospitalization is indicated for patients who have experienced severe reactions or who have complicated medical problems.

Treatment recommendations for large local reactions include ice, elevation, and antihistamines. A short course of prednisone (0.5 to 2 mg per kilogram per day for 5 days), especially if initiated immediately after the sting, may be the best treatment to prevent symptoms in patients who usually develop massive, large local reactions.

■ DECREASING FUTURE REACTIONS

Preventing Stings

Future stings can be avoided by taking common sense precautions to significantly reduce exposure. Shoes should always be worn outside. Hives and nests around the home should be exterminated. Good sanitation should be practiced since garbage and outdoor food, especially canned drinks, attract yellow jackets. Perfumes and dark and floral-patterned clothing should be avoided.

Emergency Epinephrine

To encourage prompt treatment, epinephrine is available in emergency kits for self-administration. These are used by insect-sting–allergic individuals immediately after the sting to "buy time" to get to a medical facility. The Ana-Kit contains a preloaded syringe that can deliver two 0.3 ml doses of 1:1,000 epinephrine. Incremental doses may also be given. The physician who prescribes this kit must provide thorough instruction and must be confident that the patient can perform the injection procedure. These kits may be confusing to nonmedical personnel and some patients have a petrifying fear of needles. A practice self-injection with saline will help to allay such fears. The Epipen (0.3 mg epinephrine) and EpiPen Jr. (0.15 mg epinephrine) offer a concealed needle and a pressure-sensitive spring-loaded injection device that make them suited for patients and families who are uncomfortable with the injection process. Epinephrine, 1.3 to 3.9 mg by inhalation (6 to 18 puffs of Primatene Mist) may also be used to achieve a therapeutic plasma level and may be especially helpful for laryngeal edema and bronchospasm. Patients who are receiving maintenance injections of venom immunotherapy are advised that emergency self-treatment will probably not be required; however, they should have the kit available if they are distant from medical facilities. A Medic-Alert bracelet is also advised.

Venom Immunotherapy

The clinical history is the key to determining the need for venom immunotherapy (VIT). A careful history discloses the type, degree, and time course of symptoms, and often identifies the culprit insect. An individual who has experienced a sting-induced systemic reaction should be referred to an allergist who will perform skin tests with dilute solutions of

Table 1 Indications for Venom Immunotherapy in Adults

CLASSIFICATION OF STING REACTION BY HISTORY	VENOM SKIN TEST	VENOM IMMUNOTHERAPY
Large local	Positive or negative	No
Systemic (mild)	Positive	Patient-MD decision
	Negative	No
Systemic (moderate-severe)	Positive	Yes
	Negative	No
Toxic	Not indicated	No

Table 2 Typical Dose Schedule for Venom Immunotherapy*

1 μg/ml	10 μg/ml	100 μg/ml
1. 0.05 ml	5. 0.05 ml	9. 0.05 ml
2. 0.10 ml	6. 0.10 ml	10. 0.10 ml
3. 0.20 ml	7. 0.20 ml	11. 0.20 ml
4. 0.40 ml	8. 0.40 ml	12. 0.40 ml
		13. 0.60 ml
		14. 0.80 ml
		15. 1.00 ml

*Mixed vespid venom contains three times the venom per ml shown in this table.

honeybee, yellow jacket, yellow hornet, white-faced hornet, and *Polistes* wasp venoms and, if indicated, imported fire ant whole body extract. Radioallergosorbent testing (RAST) cannot replace venom skin testing but may provide additional information. Whole body extract materials were used before 1979 to diagnose and treat flying Hymenopteran allergy, but they were shown to be ineffective and venoms supplanted their use. To date, fire ant venom has only been available in small research quantities; fortunately, the fire ant whole body extract material seems more potent than those previously available for the other Hymenopteran and has been successfully used for skin testing and treatment. Table 1 lists the indications for VIT in adults. Some clinicians would recommend VIT for an adult who experienced any degree of systemic reaction. However, most individuals have a stereotypic response to a sting with the symptoms on subsequent stings closely resembling the first episode. Therefore, when only a mild reaction has occurred, the physician and patient may jointly decide whether to embark on a course of VIT.

Individuals with large local reactions or negative skin tests are not candidates for venom therapy. Finally, a positive venom skin test or RAST in the absence of a sting-induced systemic reaction is not an indication for therapy. Approximately 25 percent of the general population may have such evidence of sensitization to venom antigens, apparently resulting from past stings. This is usually transient, disappearing in 1 to 3 years.

Other factors may influence the decision concerning the need for VIT. Those with an increased risk of being stung, such as landscapers or other individuals who engage in outdoor activities, especially those that take them far away from available medical care, will dispose the physician towards initiating venom treatment. Part of the morbidity associated with stinging insect allergy includes psychological effects of anxiety in the victim and family because of the threat of a sudden "unpreventable" systemic reaction. This high level of anxiety has frequently been exacerbated by a physician warning that "the next sting may be your last." Actually, most victims exhibit an individual pattern of anaphylaxis that varies only slightly in severity from one sting to another. Some investigators have proposed that a diagnostic sting challenge be used to select patients for VIT. Patients who did not react would not be placed on VIT. However, a recent report described individuals who tolerated one sting challenge, but reacted later to a second challenge. Therefore, further study is needed before definitive recommendations can be made.

The venoms used for immunotherapy are the same as those used for skin testing (honeybee, yellow jacket, yellow hornet, white-faced hornet, and wasp). The regimen begins with an injection of 0.01 μg and advances weekly to 100 μg (Table 2). The maintenance dose of 100 μg (chosen empirically because it is about twice the venom content of a sting) is given every 4 weeks for a year, after which the interval is lengthened to 6 to 8 weeks. A trial of very rapid 1 day rush regimen had some success but caused many systemic reactions and had to be performed in a hospital. More recently, a 2 to 5 hour regimen of VIT in which 10 gradually increasing doses were administered every 10 to 15 minutes to achieve a total dose on day 1 of about 55 μg per venom was described. However, local reactions occurred in over half the patients, and 12 percent experienced mild systemic reactions. A recent report described individuals who had the maintenance interval lengthened to 3 months and then tolerated intentional challenge stings without problem. If these results are verified by further studies, the cost of VIT can be reduced.

Venom immunotherapy is extremely effective. Studies employing intentional stings have demonstrated a 97 to 100 percent protection rate in adults and children after 3 months of treatment. The small percentage of patients who were not protected experienced very mild reactions and perhaps more properly should be considered partial successes instead of failures. In most of the early studies regarding venom efficacy, the majority of the patients demonstrated sensitivity to vespid (usually yellow jacket) venom. The success rate in preventing future systemic reactions may be somewhat less with honeybee venom. Although one group advocates the use of a smaller maintenance venom dose (50 μg), data have been published that demonstrate a superior protective effect with 100 μg doses.

Patients usually receive all the venoms to which they show significant positive skin test results. The venoms are given in separate injections except in cases of multiple vespid sensitivity. In this common clinical situation, a single injection of a mixed-vespid preparation containing full doses of yellow jacket, yellow hornet, and white-faced hornet venom may be employed. Because of the cross-allergenicity of vespid venoms, patients usually have positive skin test results to more than one venom following a single vespid sting. Sometimes the wasp venom skin test is positive, but requires a higher concentration of venom to achieve this than for the other vespid venoms; in this particular situation, RAST inhibition studies can disclose whether patients are sensitive to a cross-reacting allergen or multiple unique allergens.

Venom injections, like other forms of allergen immunotherapy, are administered subcutaneously in the middle third of the outer aspect of the upper arm. The usual care in matching patient and correct allergen extracts and doses, aspirating to be sure no blood is obtained (which, if present, would indicate intravascular placement of the needle and the need to select a different site), and observing the patient in the office for 30 minutes after the injection needs to be followed.

Most patients have short-lived erythema, itching, or swelling at the injection site. Large local reactions, which measure larger than 5 cm in diameter and last longer than 24 hours, occur in about 20 percent of patients. Interestingly, they tend to commence at venom doses between 10 and 30 mg. Generally, unless the local reactions are very large, the schedule of increasing doses is continued since these local reactions usually cease when the venom dose reaches 60 mg. Systemic reactions, including generalized pruritus, urticaria, angioedema, bronchospasm, laryngeal edema, or hypotension, occur in a minority of patients. Treatment with epinephrine is the cornerstone of therapy, which may also include antihistamines, beta$_2$-agonists, glucocorticoids, and fluids. The next dose needs to be decreased before the schedule can be resumed. Sometimes large local reactions may continue to occur. Although some clinicians have recommended using a lower concentration of venom (by increasing the diluent and thus the total volume injected), others have employed the use of a higher concentration (using less diluent) with success.

Venom skin tests are generally repeated every 2 to 5 years. Most patients maintain positive venom skin tests, although many will demonstrate a tenfold or greater decline in venom sensitivity after 5 years. If a patient develops negative skin tests, venom immunotherapy is generally discontinued. A 5 year duration of therapy is sufficient for many venom-sensitive patients since studies have shown that 90 percent of such patients tolerate subsequent stings with impunity. However, patients with initial sting reactions that were graded as severe are more likely to react to post-VIT stings. Patients whose initial sting-induced reactions were of mild to moderate severity usually stop injections after 5 years. However, at this time, we recommend that those patients who have suffered severe reactions continue their injections indefinitely.

Suggested Reading

Golden DBK, Addison BI, Gadde J, et al. Prospective observations on stopping prolonged venom immunotherapy. J Allergy Clin Immunol 1989; 84:162.

Graft DF, Schoenwetter WF. Insect sting allergy: analysis of a cohort of patients who initiated venom immunotherapy from 1978 to 1986. Ann Allergy 1994; 73:481–485.

Keating MU, Kagey-Sobotka A, Hamilton RG, Yunginger JW. Clinical and immunologic follow-up of patients who stop venom immunotherapy. J Allergy Clin Immunol 1991; 88:339–348.

Reisman RE. Natural history of insect sting allergy: Relationship of severity of symptoms of initial sting anaphylaxis to re-sting reactions. J Allergy Clin Immunol 1992; 90:335–339.

Valentine MD. Allergy to stinging insects. Ann Allergy 1994; 70:427–432.

Van der Linden PWG, Struyvenberg A, Kraaijenhagen RJ, et al. Anaphylactic shock after insect-sting challenge in 138 persons with a previous insect-sting reaction. Ann Intern Med 1993; 118:161–168.

SYSTEMIC ANAPHYLAXIS

Alexandra S. Worobec, M.D.
Dean D. Metcalfe, M.D.

Systemic anaphylaxis is an acute allergic reaction involving the release of mediators from mast cells, basophils, and secondarily recruited inflammatory cells, which may occur within a few minutes to a few hours following exposure to a triggering agent. Literally meaning "antiprotection" from the Greek "ana" = no and "phylaxis" = protection, anaphylaxis is potentially life threatening and therefore constitutes a medical emergency that requires prompt recognition and therapy.

Anaphylactic reactions have been classically divided into two categories based on mechanism: (1) anaphylaxis that is traditionally considered to involve IgE, mast cells, and basophils; and (2) anaphylactoid reactions that may be due to other immunologic as well as nonimmunologic mechanisms. Recent murine work using an IgE knockout model is consistent with the hypothesis that non–IgE-mediated signal pathways may also initiate a systemic reaction resembling anaphylaxis. A representative list of etiologic agents involved in anaphylactic syndromes classified according to possible mechanism is included in Table 1. Nonetheless, these distinctions remain a matter of semantics since clinical symptomatology and treatment of all categories is essentially the same.

The signs and symptoms of anaphylaxis may be isolated to one or involve several organ systems. Cutaneous manifestations include erythema, flushing, pruritus, urticaria, and angioedema. Gastrointestinal symptoms include crampy abdominal pain, nausea, vomiting, and diarrhea. Uterine cramping may occur. Life-threatening manifestations most commonly involve respiratory distress secondary to upper airway obstruction from angioedema of the tongue, oropharynx, or larynx, or secondary to lower airway obstruction from bronchospasm. Cardiovascular symptoms are often severe and refractory and include hypotension, arrhythmias, and

Table 1 Classification of Anaphylactic Syndromes

MECHANISM	ETIOLOGIC AGENTS*
I. IgE Mediated Haptens	Most antibiotics: penicillins, cephalosporins, sulfonamides, tetracycline, bacitracin, nitrofurantoin, amphotericin
	Industrial chemicals: ethylene oxide, glue, formaldehyde
Complete Antigens	Allergen extracts: pollens, molds, danders
	Venoms: hymenoptera (including fire ant), snake, deer fly (Chrysops species), kissing bug (Triatoma species)
	Foreign proteins: chymopapain, horse serum
	Foods: peanut, milk, egg, seafood, grains, tree nuts
	Vaccines contaminated with egg protein: influenza
	Human proteins: insulin, vasopressin, serum, and seminal proteins
	Enzymes: streptokinase, trypsin, L-asparaginase
	Protamine
	Latex
	Immunomodulators: cyclosporine
	Ruptured hydatid cyst
II. Direct Mast Cell Activation	Hypertonic solutions: radiocontrast media, mannitol
	Opiates
	Polysaccharides: acacia, dextran, iron-dextran
	Muscle depolarizing agents: curare, d-tubocurarine
	Polymyxin B, vancomycin
	Some chemotherapeutic agents
III. Complement Mediated: C3a, C5a	Human proteins: immunoglobulins, plasma
	Dialysis membranes
IV. Arachidonic Cascade Mediated	Nonsteroidal anti-inflammatory agents, aspirin
V. Mechanism Unknown	
Exercise-induced anaphylaxis	
Idiopathic recurrent anaphylaxis	
Cholinergic urticaria with anaphylaxis	
Cold-induced urticaria with anaphylaxis	
Steroid preparations	Progesterone, hydrocortisone
Mastocytosis	
Sulfites	

*Examples only; list is not complete.

hypovolemic shock. Involvement of the cardiovascular system constitutes the second most common cause of death in anaphylactic syndromes. In general, the magnitude of the anaphylactic response parallels the magnitude of the stimulus, with more severe reactions occurring closer temporally to the time of exposure to the inciting agent.

RECOGNITION AND TREATMENT OF ANAPHYLAXIS

Treatment of anaphylaxis requires early recognition of clinical symptoms associated with the syndrome and a history of possible antigen exposure. Several disorders may present with clinical manifestations not unlike anaphylaxis and hence, comprise the differential diagnostic list for this syndrome (Table 2). The vasovagal reaction is perhaps the most common diagnosis which is confused with anaphylaxis. It presents with symptoms of pallor, profuse sweating, weakness, bradycardia, hypotension, and occassionally syncope. Because bradycardia is an early manifestation of hypovolemic shock, heart rate cannot be used reliably to differentiate a vasovagal reaction from anaphylaxis. Indeed, the heart rate has been

Table 2 Differential Diagnosis of Anaphylaxis

Pulmonary	*Endocrine*
Laryngeal edema	Hypoglycemia
Epiglottitis	Pheochromocytoma
Foreign body aspiration	Carcinoid syndrome
Pulmonary embolus	Catamenial (progesterone-induced) anaphylaxis
Asphyxiation	
Hyperventilation	*Psychiatric*
Cardiovascular	Vocal cord dysfunction syndrome
Myocardial infarction	
Arrhythmia	Munchausen's disease
Hypovolemic shock	Panic attack/Globus hystericus
Cardiac arrest	*Other*
CNS	Hereditary angioedema
Vasovagal reaction	Cold urticaria
Cerebrovascular accident	Idiopathic urticaria
Seizure disorder	Mastocytosis
Drug overdose	Serum sickness
	Idiopathic capillary leak syndrome
	Sulfite exposure
	Scombroid poisoning (tuna, bluefish, mackerel)

Table 3 Stepwise Treatment of Systemic Anaphylaxis: General Measures*

NOTE: To be performed at the time of administration of the first dose(s) of epinephrine SC

1. Removal or discontinuation of inciting agent
   Special case for insect sting or allergen injection:
   Application of a loose tourniquet proximally if an allergen, injection, or sting is on an extremity with further loosening of the tourniquet q15min. The insect stinger should be gently flicked off. 0.1–0.3 ml of aqueous epinephrine may be administered SC at the site of antigen injection to delay its absorption
2. Examination of skin color, upper and lower airway patency. Secure and maintain adequate airway
3. Monitoring of vital signs: BP, pulse, respiratory rate
4. Monitoring of patient's level of consciousness
5. Placement of patient in Trendelenburg position as appropriate
6. High-flow supplemental oxygen (100%) with pulse oximetry monitoring
   Dose: 4–10 L/min via a non-rebreather mask such as the Venturi
   Intubation and mechanical assistance indicated when the Pa_{CO_2} is greater than or equal to 65 mm Hg
7. Insertion of a short, large-bore peripheral IV line as appropriate for age with administration of fluids
   IV fluids: **a. Initial recommendation:**
   Crystalloid solutions:
   1. 0.9% normal saline or
   2. Lactated Ringer's solution
      Monitor vital signs, pulmonary status, and urine output
      Keep SBP greather than or equal to 90 mm Hg
      This may require up to 1 L q15–30min in an adult or 20–30 ml/kg/hr in the pediatric age group for the first several hours

   b. Severe or persistent hypotension:
   Colloid solutions:
   i. Dextran—available in 2 forms:
      1. Dextran 70 (6% solution)
      2. Dextran 40 (10% solution)
   ii. Hetastarch (Hespan)
   iii. Serum Albumin—available in 2 concentrations:
      1. 5% solution: effective plasma expander
      2. 25% solution: more potent elevator of plasma oncotic pressure
8. For severe or refractory hypotension:
   a. Also consider use of antishock trousers to increase afterload. (Note: controversial efficacy in the treatment of peripheral shock)
   b. Lack of efficacy of measures discussed in steps one to seven above, including fluid resuscitation may mandate use of inotropic agents. By this stage, a central line to determine central venous pressure and/or Swan-Ganz catheter insertion is recommended. For unresponsive hypotension due to myocardial depression, an intra-aortic balloon counterpulsation pump may be considered
9. Observation in a monitored setting (i.e., ICU) for at least 24 hours after a moderate-severe anaphylactic reaction; for at least 8–12 hours after a mild reaction

*Exclusion of drug treatment, which is presented in Tables 4 and 5.

reported to be low, normal, or elevated during anaphylaxis. Elevated plasma histamine or tryptase levels, particularly the latter, are retrospective supportive findings in favor of a mast cell–mediated disorder such as anaphylaxis.

The immediate treatment of anaphylaxis begins with a rapid assessment of the patient's level of consciousness, along with the patient's airway, breathing, and circulation (ABCs). A broad outline of measures to be instituted in a patient with probable anaphylaxis is presented in Table 3. The management of anaphylaxis must take into consideration the severity of the reaction.

The first-line drug of choice for treating anaphylaxis is subcutaneous epinephrine. The dose of epinephrine injected subcutaneously is usually 0.3 ml of 1:1,000 aqueous epinephrine in the adult, although the dosage may need to be decreased in the elderly (to say, 0.2 ml) or increased in patients receiving beta-adrenergic blockers (to 0.5 ml). Dosing of epinephrine in children is based on weight, or 0.01 ml per kilogram of a 1:1,000 dilution up to a maximum of 0.3 ml of epinephrine injected subcutaneously. A second epinephrine injection (0.1 to 0.2 ml of 1:1,000 epinephrine) may be given into the site of an insect sting or drug or allergen injection site to delay systemic absorption of the agent if the antigen source is not a digit or other terminal region of the anatomy.

The 1993 report of the Working Group on Asthma in Pregnancy with the National Heart, Lung, and Blood Institute (NIH publication #96-3279) considering the treatment of pregnant women with epinephrine (and likewise diphenhydramine) listed epinephrine as the initial pharmacologic agent of choice in the management of anaphylaxis. A second-line agent of choice for some obstetricians for the treatment of hypotension secondary to anaphylaxis in the pregnant patient is ephedrine, 10 to 15 mg, administered IV push. Although less effective than epinephrine, it is believed that its predominant beta-adrenergic activity may cause less reduction in uterine blood flow than epinephrine.

Along with the administration of epinephrine to increase systemic vascular resistance and elevate diastolic pressure, produce bronchodilation, and increase inotropic and chronotropic cardiac activity, additional measures may be required to stabilize and maintain oxygenation and cardiac output. Other medications may be administered to supplement the effect of epinephrine. Clinical and experimental evidence suggests that treatment with a combination of H_1- and H_2-receptor antagonists such as diphenhydramine and ranitidine may be more effective than treatment with an H_1-antihistamine alone in preventing histamine-induced hypotension. Patients with severe anaphylaxis or those who have received systemic corticosteroid therapy within the previous 6 months should receive pharmacologic doses of parenteral glucocorticoids, given the low but discernible frequency of biphasic and protracted anaphylactic reactions.

For respiratory involvement, patients must be managed aggressively with nebulized and parenteral agents (Table 4). Most commonly, nebulized beta-adrenergic agonists are administered for bronchospasm, with nebulized epinephrine or racemic epinephrine given for upper airway edema. Supplemental oxygen should always be administered in the highest concentration possible, with serial arterial blood gas analyses performed to maintain oxygen saturation greater than or equal to 90 percent ($Po_2 > 60$ mm Hg, $Pco_2 < 65$ mm Hg). In recalcitrant cases, endotracheal intubation, cricothyroid membrane puncture (avoid this procedure in children younger than 10 years of age), or tracheostomy may be necessary to ensure adequate airflow.

Hypotension is generally managed initially via administration of crystalloid solutions (Table 3) such as 0.9 percent normal saline or lactated Ringer's solution through a large-bore intravenous line at a rate depending on the degree of hypovolemia, status of the vital signs, pulmonary exam, and urine output. The goal of treatment is to maintain the systolic blood pressure (SBP) greater than or equal to 90 mm Hg. Because these isotonic solutions contain small molecules that rapidly escape from the vascular space into the interstitium, their volume expansion effects are short-lived. Nonetheless, crystalloids offer the advantage of being nonallergenic and virus free and having no potential to produce a hypotensive reaction.

Refractory hypotension or frank shock in a patient with anaphylaxis warrants a twofold approach to therapy. First, central venous access should be established for monitoring of the central venous pressure and possible need for Swan-Ganz catheter placement and monitoring of cardiac output and the pulmonary capillary wedge pressure. Concomitantly, colloids or solutions containing large macromolecular polymers should be administered intravenously. These solutions allow a greater increase in the plasma oncotic pressure via attraction of water from the interstitium, thereby actually producing intravascular volume expansion in an increment above that which is administered. Example colloid solutions are dextran, hetastarch (Hespan), and serum albumin. Dextran solutions are available in two forms—a high molecular weight form (dextran 70, 6 percent solution) and a low molecular weight form (dextran 40, 10 percent solution)—which have intravascular half-lives of 2 to 3 days and 12 to 18 hours, respectively. Disadvantages of dextran administration include the potential for anaphylaxis and a bleeding diathesis, along with agglutination of red blood cells, thus making subsequent blood cross-matching difficult or impossible. Hetastarch (Hespan), an artificial polymer with a M_r 450 kD, displays a long-lasting volume expansion effect of 24 to 36 hours, is relatively nonallergenic, and does not interfere with blood typing and cross-matching. Disadvantages include alteration of the coagulation function. Serum albumin, available in a 5 percent and 25 percent solution, is the most commonly used plasma expander, but it is expensive and occasionally associated with increased pulmonary interstitial edema.

In addition to fluid resuscitative measures, treatment of refractory hypotension and shock may require pharmacologic intervention. Replacement of serial subcutaneous or intramuscular epinephrine injections with an intravenous bolus, followed by a continuous intravenous 1:10,000 epinephrine drip, is generally recommended as first-line therapy. Lack of response to this measure may warrant addition of an intravenous continuous infusion of dopamine or dobutamine, depending on the patient's underlying cardiovascular status, followed by norepinephrine or amrinone. Patients on maintenance beta-blocker therapy may be relatively resistant to epinephrine; in these patients intravenous glucagon should be considered as a treatment for refractory hypotension, followed by isoproterenol. Established dosages of these vasoactive inotropic medications (Tables 4 and 5) are as provided by the American Heart Association (AHA) guidelines. Patients receiving any of these agents must be monitored for development of anginal symptoms and possible arrhythmias in an intensive care unit setting, with both reactions being treated according to AHA guidelines with the appropriate agent. Hypertension resulting from unopposed beta-adrenergic and alpha-adrenergic activity may require prompt treatment with nitroprusside (initial dose: 10 μg per minute IV, increasing by 10 μg per minute IV every 4 minutes to 10 to 20 mg per minute IV until BP stabilizes) or phentolamine (initial dose: 0.5 mg per minute IV to a maximum of 10 mg IV, maintenance dose: 25 to 50 mg IV every 3 to 6 hours). Even with close cardiac monitoring and titration, myocardial infarction is a known associated sequela of systemic anaphylaxis, either from the initial hypotensive insult to the myocardium or from alpha- and/or beta-adrenergic effects on an already compromised cardiovascular system.

Patients with a mild to moderate anaphylactic reaction should have their vital signs and cardiac and respiratory status monitored for at least an additional 8 to 12 hours after clinical signs and symptoms of anaphylaxis abate. For moderate reactions (i.e., bronchospasm, generalized urticaria) antihistamines and steroids may be continued for several days after the initial reaction, and the patient may be given a self-injectable epinephrine device (EpiPen or Ana-Kit) with a prescription for refills and counseled in its proper use before being discharged. Patients with severe reactions may require monitoring for a minimum of 24 hours after stabilization and warrant close outpatient follow-up and allergy evaluation.

PREVENTION AND PROPHYLAXIS

Basic principles in the prevention of anaphylaxis in high-risk individuals are outlined in Table 5. Identification and avoidance of causative agents, if feasible, remains the most important step in the management of susceptible individuals. Patients should be taught to recognize the clinical signs of impending anaphylaxis (i.e., lump in the throat with difficulty breathing, lightheadedness, feeling of impending

Table 4 Stepwise Treatment of Systemic Anaphylaxis: Pharmacologic Therapy in Adults

MEDICATION	ROUTE	DOSAGE	COMPLICATIONS
A. Indicated for all reactions (urticaria, angioedema, bronchospasm, laryngeal edema, and systemic symptoms)			
1. Epinephrine (drug of first choice)	SC	0.3 ml of a 1:1,000 dilution (usual range 0.2–0.5 ml) q10–15 min × 3 doses, if necessary	Tachycardia, tremor, anxiety, arrhythmias
	IM	0.3 ml of a 1:1,000 dilution q10–15 min (pregnant patient)	
2. Ephedrine	IV push	10–25 mg (only to be considered in the pregnant patient)	
3. Antihistamines			
H_1-Blockers:			
Diphenhydramine	IM or IV	50–75 mg q6h Drip may afford better control of sxs: 5 mg/kg/24h	Large doses: anticholinergic effects, may depress respiration
H_2-Blockers:			
Ranitidine	PO (mild sxs)	150 mg q8–12h	
	IV	50 mg q6–8h	
Cimetidine	PO (mild sxs)	300 mg q6–8h	*Note:* cimetidine is not compatible with IV aminophylline
	IV	300 mg q6–8h	
Famotidine	IV	20 mg q12h	
B. Indicated for laryngeal edema			
1. Epinephrine	Nebulized	1% solution of 1 : 100 epinephrine via hand bulb nebulizer, 1–3 deep inhalations q3h	
2. Racemic epinephrine	Nebulized	2.25% solution of 1 : 100 racemic epinephrine via hand bulb nebulizer, 1–3 deep inhalations q3h	*Note:* racemic epinephrine has approximately half the activity of epinephrine
C. Indicated for bronchospasm			
1. Beta-adrenergic bronchodilators:			Nausea, vomiting, arrhythmias
Albuterol	Nebulized	2.5–5.0 mg (0.5 ml of 0.5% solution diluted to a final volume of 3 ml with 0.9% NS) given over 5–15 min. Each dose, q20min × 6 doses maximum	
Metaproterenol	Nebulized	0.3 ml of 5% solution diluted in 2.5 ml of 0.45% or 0.9% NS, given over 5–15 min each dose, q4h	
Terbutaline	Metered	400 μg or 2 inhalations (200 μg/metered spray), q4–6h	
2. Steroids:			
Methylprednisolone	IV	60–80 mg × 1 dose, followed by prednisone 60 mg PO qd × 2d	*Note:* steroids have no antianaphylactic actions and do not alleviate immediate acute, life-threatening manifestations
Hydrocortisone	IV	100–200 mg q6–8h (up to 5–10 mg/kg q6–8h)	
Prednisone	PO (mild rxns)	20–40 mg qd with quick taper	
3. Aminophylline (second-line therapy)	IV	5–6 mg/kg in 20 ml D_5W over 10–15 min (loading dose), 0.5–1.0 mg/kg/h (maintenance dose)	Nausea, vomiting, seizures, arrhythmias
D. Indicated for cardiovascular collapse (refractory hypotension, shock)			
1. Epinephrine (initial therapy)	Via ETT	1 mg = 10 ml of a 1: 10,000 dilution in 5 ml 0.9% NS, given via a long needle or catheter into an ETT, followed by hyperventilation	*Note:* given when response to SC Epi is too slow or adequate vascular access has not been obtained yet
	IV push	0.1–0.2 ml of 1:1,000 dilution in 10 ml 0.9% NS, given over 5′. This may require follow-up administration of an epinephrine IV drip	
	IV drip	0.1 μg/kg/min, use 1 ml of 1:1,000 dilution in 250 ml D_5W (4 μg/ml) at 1 μg/min, increasing to a maximum of 4–10 μg/min	
2. Dopamine	IV drip	2–20 μg/kg/min (2 amps = 400 mg in 500 ml D_5W)	Arrhythmias
3. Dobutamine	IV drip	2–30 μg/kg/min (2 amps = 500 mg in 500 ml D_5W)	Arrhythmias, esp. tachycardia
4. Norepinephrine	IV drip	0.5–1.0 μg/min (initial dose), followed by 2–12 μg/min	Arrhythmias
5. Amrinone	IV drip	0.75 mg/kg IV bolus over 2–3 min, then 2–15 μg/kg/min (maintenance)	
E. Indicated for patients on beta-blockers with refractory shock			
1. Glucagon (first-line therapy)	IV push	1–5 mg over 2–5 min IV push	Nausea, vomiting
	IV drip	1 mg in 1 L D_5W at 5–15 μg/min	
2. Isoproterenol	IV drip	2–10 μg/min, start with 0.1 μg/kg/min (1 mg in 500 ml D_5W), doubling dose q15′	Tachycardia, arrhythmias

D_5W, 5% glucose in distilled water; ETT, endotracheal tube; NS, normal saline; rxns, reactions; sxs, symptoms.

Table 5 Strategies to Prevent or Lessen the Severity of Anaphylactic Reactions

I. General Principles:
  A. Obtain accurate and complete patient medical history. Skin tests or RAST are valuable in identifying individuals at risk for anaphylaxis from agents such as penicillin and insect venoms
  B. Patient avoidance of allergens known to precipitate anaphylaxis
  C. Medic-Alert bracelet should be worn by at-risk patients at all times
  D. Patients at risk should carry an EpiPen or Ana-Kit at all times and be properly skilled in its correct use
    Adults: 0.3 ml of 1:1,000 dilution of Epinephrine (EpiPen)
    Pediatric: 0.15 ml of 1:1,000 dilution of Epinephrine (EpiPen Jr.)
  E. Desensitization may be recommended for patients with Hymenoptera sensitivity
  F. Require a clear indication for drug use. Consider desensitization by oral route
  G. Desensitize patients to any drug known to have caused anaphylaxis if urgently required to treat a life-threatening disease. Prefer oral desensitization, if feasible
  H. Avoid use of beta-blockers, NSAIDs, or aspirin or replace with reasonable alternatives

II. Prophylaxis of Exercise-Induced Anaphylaxis:
  A. Avoid food ingestion for approximately 6 hours before exercise
  B. Avoid intake of NSAIDs or ASA
  C. In general, prophylactic antihistamines (H_1- and H_2-receptor antagonists) and cromolyn are ineffective

III. Prophylaxis (Desensitization procedures, necessary administration of agent known to cause anaphylaxis):
  A. Pretreatment with an H_1-receptor and possibly H_2-receptor antagonist 12 to 24 hr before administration of agent known to cause anaphylaxis
    1. H_1-blocker: **diphenhydramine IV** 5 mg/kg/24 hr (**adult + pediatric**) in divided doses q6h (25–75 mg IV q6h)
    2. H_2-receptor blocker: **ranitidine IV** 1–2 mg/kg/24 hr (**adult + pediatric**) in divided doses q6–8h or **cimetidine IV** 20–40 mg/kg/24 hr (**adult + pediatric**) in divided doses q6–8h
  B. Pretreatment with steroids. **Hydrocortisone 100 mg PO or IV** qd, q8h (adult)
  C. Avoid use of beta-blockers
  D. Continue above medications for the duration of the administration of the inciting agent

IV. Radiocontrast Allergy Prophylaxis (Adults):
  A. Switch to low osmolar nonionic contrast agents when possible
  B. Administer steroids before scheduled test:
    1. **Prednisone: 30–50 mg PO q6–8h** (i.e. 13, 7, and 1 hour prior to the study)
    2. **Methylprednisolone: 32 mg PO 12 and 2 hr before study**
  C. H_1-receptor antagonists: **Diphenhydramine: 50 mg PO 7 hr and 1 hr, or 50 mg IM 1 hr before study**
  D. H_2-receptor antagonists: **Ranitidine: 150 mg PO 7 hr and 1 hr, or 50 mg IM 1 hr before study**
  E. **Ephedrine: 25 mg PO 1 hr before study**

doom) and feel comfortable and skilled in the technique of self-administration of subcutaneous epinephrine. An epinephrine autoinjector device should be carried by the patient at all times, with several spares in convenient locations (home, work) and these should be renewed on a yearly basis.

Patients with idiopathic anaphylaxis who experience more frequent attacks should be placed on maintenance therapy with oral antihistamines and perhaps steroids (i.e., oral prednisone 20 to 40 mg daily), until the episodes abate, with tapering of steroids thereafter. High-risk patients on beta-blocker therapy, including topical medications used in the treatment of glaucoma, should be continued on these medications only if feasible alternatives are unavailable and the drug is medically indicated.

Short-term desensitization to agents such as penicillin or beta-lactam antibiotics, insulin, antithymocyte globulin, or aspirin should be performed if clearly indicated, and then so in a closely monitored setting such as an intensive care unit. Patients may be considered for premedication with H_1- and H_2-antihistamines and steroids. Because this procedure constitutes a form of "controlled anaphylaxis," patients will likely require repeat desensitization in the event of a future requirement for readministration of the known agent. Immunotherapy is often efficacious and indicated for the prevention of Hymenoptera hypersensitivity.

Radiocontrast allergy, usually due to high osmolar ionic contrast agents, may be significantly decreased via the use of nonionic contrast agents. Pretreatment with oral steroids such as prednisone or methylprednisolone, an H_1-antihistamine such as diphenhydramine, and possibly an H_2-antihistamine such as ranitidine (with or without ephedrine) at least 2 hours before administration of radiocontrast media has been shown to decrease the risk of fatal anaphylaxis.

Suggested Reading

AAAI. Position statement: The use of epinephrine in the treatment of anaphylaxis. J Allergy Clin Immunol 1994; 94:666–668.

Cummins RO. Hypotension/shock/acute pulmonary edema. In: Textbook of advanced cardiac life support. Dallas: American Heart Association 1994:1.40–1.47.

Metcalfe DD. Acute anaphylaxis and urticaria in children and adults. In: Schocket AL, ed. Clinical management of urticaria and anaphylaxis. New York: Marcel Dekker, 1992:1–20.

Schatz M, Zeiger RS. Management of asthma, rhinitis, and anaphylaxis during pregnancy. Curr Obstet Gynecol 1991; 1:65.

HEREDITARY ANGIOEDEMA

Allen P. Kaplan, M.D.

Hereditary angioedema is an autosomal dominant disorder associated with severe episodes of swelling of submucosal and subcutaneous tissues. Attacks may affect virtually any part of the body but most commonly involve the extremities or the face. Occasionally there may be edema of the submucosa of the small bowel that causes episodes of abdominal pain; the most severe of these may resemble an "acute abdomen." Episodes of swelling may also affect the upper respiratory tract to include the tongue, pharynx, and larynx. Laryngeal edema, in particular, can cause acute obstruction, stridor, and asphyxiation and therefore can present as a medical emergency. Attacks are sporadic and often occur in the absence of any precipitating event. However, in some patients there appears to be a preponderance of episodes in association with local trauma, concomitant illness, or emotional stress. The age of onset of episodes of angioedema can vary greatly; it most often occurs during childhood. However, episodes are seldom severe prior to puberty. The duration of attacks is typically 1 to 4 days; they are self-limited and most often require no therapy. However, attacks involving the upper airway or gastrointestinal tract require particular precautions, to be outlined.

Hereditary angioedema is caused by depressed function of the inhibitor of the activated first component of complement (C1 INH). Approximately 85 percent of the cases are attributable to diminished levels of the protein (typically less than 25 percent of normal), and 15 percent of the cases are attributable to synthesis of a dysfunctional protein and plasma levels may be normal or elevated. This protein is the only known physiologic inhibitor of the C1r and C1s components of the first component of complement. It is also the main plasma inhibitor of activated Hageman factor and kallikrein and is therefore the critical protein regulating the formation of the vasoactive peptide bradykinin. The swelling seen in hereditary angioedema is thought to be due to either a kinin-like molecule, which may be derived from one of the complement components, or to bradykinin (or both). Since the disease is transmitted as a dominant gene and patients are heterozygotes, one normal gene is present. The cause of C1 INH levels lower than 25 percent of normal (rather than the expected 50 percent) appears to be excessive catabolism. Similarly when an abnormal C1 INH is synthesized, small amounts of normal C1 INH are also present owing to transcription of the one normal gene.

In a patient presenting with angioedema, the diagnosis of hereditary angioedema is suspected if there is a positive family history. A low C4 level is suggestive regardless of the history, since sporadic cases or a new mutation occasionally may be found. A low C1 INH level is confirmatory. However, if the C1 INH level is normal or elevated in the presence of a low C4 level, a functional determination should be performed. During episodes of swelling the C4 level may approach zero and the C2 level also declines. Acquired angioedema with C1 INH deficiency is to be distinguished from the familial disorder. This is most often associated with B cell lymphomas or connective tissue diseases in which C1 INH levels are low as a result of unusual consumption. In these cases the C1q level is also often depressed; C1q levels are typically normal in hereditary angioedema. Therapy in acquired cases of C1 INH deficiency is directed to the underlying disease, but the modalities used to treat hereditary angioedema also can be utilized to prevent episodes of swelling. A second form of acquired C1 INH deficiency is due to an IgG autoantibody directed to C1 INH. Its effect is to allow C1 INH cleavage by enzymes which bind to it but the enzymes are not inactivated. A lower molecular weight C1 INH circulates which is inactive. It is not familial or associated with systemic diseases. Therapy can utilize plasmapheresis or even immunosuppression in addition to agents used for the hereditary disorder.

Not all patients with hereditary angioedema require therapy. Some may have only mild attacks that do not have a major effect on lifestyle. Others may have an attack frequency of fewer than one or two episodes per month. These do not require therapy unless severe episodes or life-threatening situations are encountered. However, occasional patients such as these may be treated if the death of family members has created such anxiety that they prefer the risk of possible side effects associated with drug therapy. The clinical course of the patient should be the primary guide for therapy rather than the level of C4 or C1 INH.

TREATMENT OF ACUTE ATTACKS

Angioedema affecting the extremities requires no specific therapy, and the episode usually abates within a few days. Swelling affecting the face is more troublesome, and severe attacks can be aborted with repeated subcutaneous doses of epinephrine 1 : 1000. For example, 0.3 cc every 45 minutes for one to three doses would suffice for an otherwise healthy adult with prominent facial, lip, or tongue swelling. Abdominal attacks, although painful, require only supportive therapy. The main symptom is cramping abdominal pain, sometimes associated with nausea, vomiting, or diarrhea. These episodes are similarly self-limited, lasting for 1 to 4 days, but require careful observation if an episode is severe.

We admit patients with severe abdominal attacks, administer fluids intravenously (particularly if dehydration might result from fluid loss), and use mild analgesics. We generally avoid the use of narcotic analgesics; however, a single dose of Demerol administered early in an attack can be helpful. Repeated doses of epinephrine 1:1000 given every 1 to 2 hours sometimes can abort episodes after a few doses. An abdominal examination should be performed periodically with particular attention to the status of bowel sounds and evidence of rigidity. Typically a patient has areas of tenderness to palpation, or rebound may be elicited; bowel sounds are more often hyperactive than hypoactive. The areas of tenderness may vary over time as can rebound (likely the result of stretching of visceral but not parietal peritoneum). However, the abdominal wall remains soft. Fever, leukocytosis, an elevated sedimentation rate, and progressive rigidity of the abdominal wall are signs of an "acute abdomen" and alert one to the uncommon occurrence of another disease for which surgery might really be indicated.

Involvement of the airway is a true medical emergency, which is generally unresponsive to antihistamines or corticosteroids and may or may not respond to epinephrine. Early signs of laryngeal involvement include a change in voice, tone, or pitch or frank hoarseness. Pharyngeal involvement may cause a choking sensation and difficulty in swallowing food. This may not be an emergency, but careful observation is indicated because it can progress to difficulty in swallowing secretions, the risk of aspiration, or laryngeal symptoms. More severe laryngeal involvement can lead to inspiratory stridor and asphyxia. When angioedema of the airway appears likely, an otolaryngologic evaluation to examine the vocal cords and the laryngeal-pharyngeal area should be performed. Epinephrine should be administered (assuming that there are no contraindications)—about 0.3 ml of a 1:1000 dilution given repeatedly. Vital signs should be monitored to be sure that the cardiovascular effects of one dose have passed before another is given. Spacing can vary from every 45 to 120 minutes as indicated. Antihistamines or short-acting corticosteroids may be given, but there is little rationale for their use and they are not likely to help.

The condition in a patient with airway involvement who is seen within hours after onset or during the first day may worsen during the ensuing 1 to 2 days before resolving by day 3 or 4. Such a patient should be observed, and if the attack appears to be progressive, admission to the hospital, the intravenous administration of fluids, and epinephrine are indicated. A patient seen at day 2 or 3 of an episode need not be admitted if the swelling is clearly nonprogressive after observation for many hours. Epsilon-aminocaproic acid can be used in an attempt to ameliorate the severity of edema of the airway. A dose of 8 g is given within the first 4 hours and then 16 g per day for the next 24 to 48 hours until the episode has ended. Thus a combination of subcutaneous doses of epinephrine administered periodically on day 1 with epsilon-aminocaproic acid for a few days is recommended. However, there is no truly reliable modality that one can count on and attacks may nevertheless progress in some patients.

In such a circumstance tracheostomy is indicated. An alternative is nasotracheal intubation in an operating room setting. The staff should be prepared to perform a tracheostomy if intubation is not successful. The tube remains in place until the episode abates.

The use of fresh frozen plasma in such circumstances is controversial. On the one hand C1 INH is being replenished and on the other hand substrate for circulating active enzyme is being given and generation of more permeability factor is possible. Fresh frozen plasma is best utilized as prophylactic therapy (to be discussed) and not administered during acute episodes.

■ SHORT-TERM PROPHYLACTIC THERAPY

Patients with hereditary angioedema may require minor surgical or other invasive procedures, which could precipitate angioedema. Those involving the respiratory tract are of particular concern and include such circumstances as dental procedures (gingivectomy, extraction, root canal work, or even routine local anesthesia) and endoscopy. In such cases the use of fresh frozen plasma in a patient who is receiving no other therapy can prevent attacks. We recommend the infusion of 2 units of fresh frozen plasma the day prior to surgery and 2 units just before the procedure. One must be cautious because there is a finite risk of transmission of hepatitis or even AIDS, and all recommended precautions must be followed. Single donor volunteers who have been screened serologically may be used to allay patient anxiety. If such surgery is elective, the administration of androgens for 5 days prior to the procedure (e.g., 4 mg of stanozolol four times daily) should obviate the need for fresh frozen plasma and is a reasonable alternative. For major surgical procedures the approach is similar. In patients who are already taking maintenance dosages of androgens the dosage should be increased for the aforementioned 5 day period so that C4 and C1 INH levels rise.

■ MAINTENANCE THERAPY

The object of maintenance therapy is to prevent episodes of swelling by utilizing the least quantity of medication that is efficacious to minimize side effects and costs. The most effective drugs are androgens or androgen derivatives, such as methyltestosterone, danazol, and stanozolol. Methyltestosterone was the first androgenic compound shown to be effective in hereditary angioedema; its use is restricted to men but it is otherwise a satisfactory drug. It is efficacious, the cost is low, and the toxicity is minimal. One can start with 10 mg three times daily and, once the disease is quiescent, gradually decrease the dosage. The major danger in its use is cholestatic jaundice, and liver function should be assessed periodically—perhaps monthly at the start and then every few months.

For both women and men one can use attenuated androgens such as danazol or stanozolol. Both these drugs are capable of increasing synthesis of normal C1 INH and thereby correct the underlying biochemical defect. C4 levels also rise with therapy. In women taking birth control pills (estrogenic) there may be an increase in attacks, which can be reversed by discontinuing birth control tablets without further therapy. It has become clear that either drug can be effective for long-term maintenance at dosages that produce little or no change in the plasma C4 or C1 INH level. It is not known whether the drug works by some other mechanism or whether small changes, perhaps within tissues, suffice in terms of protection. The main side effects of danazol use are weight gain (due in part to fluid retention and increased appetite), menometrorrhagia, headaches, muscle cramps, mild androgenic effects (voice deepening, hirsutism, alopecia, acne, altered libido), and a mild increase in the SGOT and SGPT levels.

The starting dosage is 600 mg per day and the dosage is then gradually decreased. As little as 50 mg every other day suffices for some patients, but this is highly variable. My experience with stanozolol is greater than that with danazol, and we utilize this as our first choice for long-term therapy. Its efficacy is essentially the same as for danazol, the cost is less (about 10 to 20 percent), and the side effects, although similar in type, seem less prominent. An increase in SGOT, SGPT, or LDH levels can be seen but not frank jaundice or irreversible changes suggestive of chronic hepatitis or cirrhosis. Lowering the dosage or stopping therapy for a while leads to rapid reversal of the enzyme elevations. Stanozolol is marketed as a 2 mg tablet and most patients are controlled with 2 mg per day. For some, as little as 2 mg every other day is sufficient. One can proceed from 2 mg per day to 4 mg every other day and then to 2 mg every other day.

Epsilon-aminocaproic acid (7 to 8 g per day) also has been shown to control attacks of hereditary angioedema, although it has no effect on C4 or C1 INH levels, its mechanism of action is unclear. It is known to inhibit plasmin, plasminogen activation, and C1 activation even by immune complexes. Its effect is to decrease the severity of attacks of swelling rather than decreasing the frequency. It could be considered in severely ill patients who are unable to take any of the aforementioned androgens. It is clearly a "second-line" drug and particular caution is needed when there is a predisposition to thrombosis because it is antifibrinolytic. Thus it could be dangerous if a patient were to have a myocardial infarction or cerebrovascular accident. Epsilon-aminocaproic acid can also cause severe muscle toxicity, with pain and elevation of the aldolase and creatine phosphokinase levels. Therapy should be discontinued immediately if this occurs.

It is uncommon for therapy to be required in children prior to puberty, although episodes of swelling may occur. However, severe or life-threatening episodes are rare in this age group and avoiding treatment is best. If therapy is needed, the minimal androgenic dosage should be used. This is perhaps less of a problem for males. Therapy of prepubescent girls should be carried out in conjunction with an endocrinologist. Epsilon-aminocaproic acid can be considered in this circumstance, since it does not affect gonadal development. We have successfully treated young females (age 10 to 14) with 2 mg of stanozolol every other day, with a normal onset of puberty, normal menses, and no evident side effects. We assess liver function every 3 months during the first year of therapy and every 6 months thereafter.

Suggested Reading

Frank MM, Sergeant JS, Kane MA, Alling DW. Epsilon aminocaproic acid therapy of hereditary angioneurotic edema: a double blind study. N Engl J Med 1972; 286:808–812.

Gelfand JA, Boss GR, Conley CL, Reinhart R, Frank MM. Acquired C1 esterase deficiency and angioedema: a review. Medicine 1979; 58:321–328.

Gelfand JA, Sherms RJ, Alling DW, Frank MM. Treatment of hereditary angioedema with danazol: reversal of clinical and biochemical abnormalities. N Engl J Med 1976; 295:1444–1448.

Kaplan AP. Urticaria and angioedema. In: Kaplan AP, ed. Allergy, 2nd ed. Philadelphia: WB Saunders, 1997:573–597.

Sheffer AL, Fearon DT, Austen KF. Clinical and biochemical effects of stanazolol therapy for hereditary angioedema. J Allergy Clin Immunol 1981; 68:181–187.

Sheffer AL, Fearon DT, Austen KF. Hereditary angioedema: a decade of management with stanozolol. J Allergy Clin Immunol, 1987; 80:855–867.

SYSTEMIC LUPUS ERYTHEMATOSUS

Michelle Petri, M.D., M.P.H.

Lupus occurs in three major forms: systemic, discoid lupus without systemic involvement, and drug-induced (the most common drugs that induce lupus are phenothiazines, isoniazid, and procainamide). Systemic lupus erythematosus (SLE) is one of the most fascinating and challenging of the autoimmune diseases. Although SLE most often presents with cutaneous, arthritis, or renal manifestations, almost any organ system can be involved, in any combination. It occurs in approximately one of 250 African-American women and one of 400 Caucasian women; the female-male ratio is 9:1. The etiology of SLE is not known, but several inciting or enabling factors have been identified, including female hormones, pregnancy, infections, antibiotics (especially sulfas), and ultraviolet light exposure. Genetic predispositions have been identified as HLA-DR2 and HLA-DR3, and null complement alleles. The diagnosis of SLE requires a thorough history and physical examination with laboratory and, in some cases, radiographic tests to ascertain organ system involvement. Serologic tests such as high-titer ANA, lupus-specific autoantibodies (anti-Sm, anti-dsDNA), other autoantibodies (anti-Ro, anti-La, anti-RNP, antiphospholipid antibodies), and low serum complement (C3, C4) levels can help to confirm the clinical diagnosis.

■ GENERAL MEDICAL MANAGEMENT

Although the 10 and even 20 year survival of SLE patients after diagnosis is better than 90 percent in most centers, one-half of SLE patients are surviving with damage to one or more major organ systems. The challenge in the treatment of SLE is not only to control the inflammatory component of the disease, but also to recognize the toxicity of some of the major treatments, including corticosteroids and immunosuppressive drugs. Even without immunosuppressive treatment, patients with SLE are at increased risk of infection. Opportunistic infections must be considered in any SLE patient treated with immunosuppressive drugs who presents with fever.

The general medical management of a lupus patient includes routine follow-up visits (usually every 3 months if the patient is doing well) to assess and treat disease activity, complications of lupus and/or its treatment, and comorbid factors, such as hypertension, hyperlipidemia, and obesity.

SLE, however, is frequently characterized by unpredictable "flares" or exacerbations that require urgent outpatient visits or even hospitalization. Pneumococcal vaccination and yearly influenza vaccination are recommended.

CUTANEOUS LUPUS

Sun avoidance and the use of sunscreens that block both UV-A and UV-B are the cornerstone of the treatment of cutaneous lupus, whether it be a malar rash, generalized photosensitive cutaneous lupus, subacute cutaneous lupus, or discoid lupus (Table 1). The antimalarial drug hydroxychloroquine is the first line of pharmacologic treatment. Patients who have G6PD deficiency cannot take hydroxychloroquine. A baseline ophthalmology examination is recommended before starting antimalarial therapy. The frequency of retinal toxicity with hydroxychloroquine (the major antimalarial used in the United States) is less than 1 percent. Follow-up ophthalmologic monitoring can be done on a 6 month basis. The usual dose of hydroxychloroquine in an adult is 400 mg a day. Cutaneous lesions may begin to respond in 2 weeks, but full response may take several months. SLE patients with cutaneous vasculitis or severe cutaneous involvement will require corticosteroids, but every attempt is made to quickly taper the daily dose or to add "steroid-sparing agents" (such as methotrexate or azathioprine) to the regimen. A rare form of cutaneous lupus, bullous lupus, responds to dapsone. Both dapsone and retinoids may be helpful in some patients with cutaneous lupus. Potent topical fluorinated steroids cannot be used on the face, because of the risk of cutaneous atrophy, but can be used on the extremities and trunk. Although thalidomide appears to be a very effective drug for discoid lupus, teratogenicity and toxicity limit its use.

MUSCULOSKELETAL LUPUS

Over 90 percent of SLE patients have polyarthralgia or polyarthritis at some point in the evolution of their disease. Nonsteroidal anti-inflammatory drugs (NSAIDs) and antimalarial drugs (hydroxychloroquine) are the mainstay of treatment (Table 2). Some unusual reactions to NSAIDs that have occurred in patients with SLE include aseptic meningitis, most commonly reported with ibuprofen, and salicylate hepatitis, most commonly occurring with aspirin (but occasionally occurring with other NSAIDs). NSAIDs are available from multiple classes; a patient who develops an intolerance to one may usually be given an NSAID from another class. However, a patient with a severe allergic reaction (such as urticaria and/or angioedema or anaphylaxis) should not be rechallenged with any NSAID. The major toxicities of NSAIDs in SLE patients are NSAID gastropathy, renal toxicity, or platelet dysfunction and bleeding. Corticosteroids, usually prednisone in doses of 5 to 20 mg daily, may be required for severe polyarthritis. The addition of an immunosuppressive agent (methotrexate or azathioprine) may allow corticosteroid taper.

The major musculoskeletal damage in SLE patients is due to avascular necrosis of bone and to osteoporotic fractures. Both complications are highly associated with corticosteroid use. Every attempt should be made to keep the maintenance prednisone dose below 20 mg daily, the threshold above which the odds ratio of avascular necrosis of bone rises dramatically. Early avascular necrosis of bone may respond to surgical core decompression. Osteoporosis in SLE is multifactorial, with corticosteroids, disease activity, and other risk factors contributing. Preventive measures, including an exercise regimen, calcium and vitamin D supplementation, and smoking cessation are encouraged. Severe premenopausal osteoporosis can be treated with calcium supplementation, vitamin D, calcitonin, and bisphosphonates. In addition to these measures, the postmenopausal SLE patient is a candidate for

Table 2 Treatment of Lupus Arthritis

Nonsteroidal anti-inflammatory drugs (NSAIDs)
- Once-daily NSAIDs: piroxicam, nabumetone, oxaprozin
- Twice-daily NSAIDs: naproxen, sulindac, diclofenac
- Thrice-daily NSAIDs: tolmetin, indomethacin, flurbiprofen, etodolac, ketoprofen
- Over-the-counter NSAIDs: ibuprofen, naproxen
- Monitor renal function, liver function, hematocrit, and gastrointestinal symptoms

Antimalarial drugs
- Hydroxychloroquine
- Check G6PD status and monitor for toxicity with 6 month ophthalmology examinations

Corticosteroids
- Monitor glucose, electrolytes, lipids, and blood pressure

Methotrexate
- Monitor complete blood counts and liver function tests
  - Methotrexate muse be stopped in a woman planning pregnancy

Table 1 Treatment of Cutaneous Lupus

Sunblock

Antimalarial drugs (usually hydroxychloroquine)
- Check G6PD status. Monitor for retinal toxicity (rare) with a baseline eye examination followed by 6 month follow-ups

Dapsone
- Check G6PD status. Monitor hematocrit and liver function tests, and check for peripheral neuropathy

Etretinate or isotretinoin
- Retinoids should not be prescribed to women at risk of pregnancy. Monitor serum lipids, which may increase

Methotrexate
- Monitor complete blood counts and liver function tests. Methotrexate must be stopped in a woman planning pregnancy

Corticosteroids: topical or oral
- Monitor glucose, electrolytes, lipids, and blood pressure in patients on oral corticosteroids

estrogen replacement therapy (ERT). In established SLE patients, ERT does not appear to increase the risk of disease flare, although this has not been extensively studied.

■ RENAL LUPUS

Approximately 50 percent of SLE patients will have some renal involvement. Active renal lupus will present as hematuria and/or proteinuria, usually in the setting of active serologic tests (low complement and high anti-dsDNA) (Table 3). The goal of treatment is to reduce inflammation, thereby improving or maintaining the glomerular filtration rate (GFR) and decreasing proteinuria (Table 4). Minor renal involvement may respond to a low (<20 mg prednisone daily) to moderate dose (20 to 40 mg prednisone daily) of corticosteroids. Moderate renal involvement may respond to moderate-dose corticosteroid therapy (20 to 40 mg of prednisone daily) and the addition of azathioprine (100 to 150 mg daily). Attention should always be paid to other factors that hasten renal decline, including hypertension and hyperlipidemia. However, severe or rapidly progressive lupus nephritis will usually require an alkylating agent. Based on clinical trails at the National Institutes of Health, the alkylating agent of choice is intravenous "pulse" cyclophosphamide, 750 to 1,000 mg per square meter of body surface area, monthly for 6 months. Adjustments of dose are made on the basis of clinical response and toxicity (such as cytopenias or serious infections). A maintenance schedule of cyclophosphamide treatment every third month for 2 years may be needed to maintain disease control, or it may be possible to maintain the patient on an agent with less toxicity such as azathioprine. Cyclophosphamide has more toxicity (especially in terms of hemorrhagic cystitis and malignancy) when used in a daily oral regimen, but even intravenous pulse cyclophosphamide can have important toxicity, including cytopenias, infection, and premature gonadal failure. SLE patients who develop renal failure do better, in terms of disease activity, with hemodialysis rather than with peritoneal dialysis. SLE patients with renal failure are candidates for renal transplantation.

Table 3 Determining the Activity and Monitoring of Renal Lupus

1. Determine and monitor GFR by a cimetidine-corrected creatinine clearance (because of tubular secretion of creatinine) *or* nuclear medicine GFR, such as technetium-DTPA or iothalamate
2. Quantitate the 24 hour urine protein excretion
3. Look for RBC casts in a morning urinalysis and quantitate urine RBCs per high-power field
4. Determine serum C3 and C4 (or CH50, total hemolytic complement) and anti-dsDNA
5. Consider a renal biopsy if
   a. the diagnosis of SLE is unclear,
   b. it is necessary to differentiate ongoing active renal lupus from inactive, sclerosed kidneys, *or*
   c. it will influence the choice of therapy (i.e., the use of alkylating agents)

■ HEMATOLOGIC LUPUS

Many of the hematologic manifestations of SLE are mild, including leukopenia and mild chronic thrombocytopenia. However, SLE patients can have life-threatening hemolytic anemia and thrombocytopenia, requiring intravenous

Table 4 Treatment of Renal Lupus

Corticosteroids
- May be the sole agent for mild or moderate renal lupus
- In patients with rapidly progressive glomerulonephritis or diffuse proliferative glomerulonephritis, may be initially given as pulse methylprenisolone, 1,000 mg a day for 3 days, followed by a daily maintenance dose of oral prednisone, in the range of 40 to 60 mg a day

Azathioprine
- May be added to corticosteroids in patients who have a partial, but incomplete response to corticosteroids and are not considered candidates for alkylating agents
- May be added as a "steroid-sparing agent" in a patient who has responded to corticosteroids, but who cannot be tapered to an acceptable maintenance prednisone dose (usually ≤20 mg daily)
- Monitor complete blood counts, liver function tests, and amylase

Cyclophosphamide
- May be used initially (with corticosteriods) in patients with rapidly progressive glomerulonephritis or diffuse proliferative glomerulonephritis
- Monthly "pulse" intravenous cyclophosphamide (750 to 1,000 mg/m^2 body surface area) is preferable to daily oral cyclophosphamide, because of lower toxicity (malignancy)
- Monitor complete blood counts. Sodium 2-mercaptoethanesulfonate (MESNA) and hydration are used to prevent hemorrhagic cystitis. Infections must be identified early and treated appropriately. Cyclophosphamide cannot be used during pregnancy because it can cause birth defects. Even IV pulse cyclophosphamide may lead to later malignancy, including leukemia

Plasmapheresis
- Plasmapheresis may be helpful in some patients resistant to corticosteroids and alkylating agents
- Experimental regimens of sequential plasmapheresis followed by cyclophosphamide are currently being tested

Reduce or control comorbid factors that contribute to renal sclerosis
- Hypertension
- Hyperlipidemia
- Diabetes mellitus

"pulse" methylprednisolone therapy, 1,000 mg a day for 3 days. Patients who do not respond may require intravenous gammaglobulin (IVIG). Patients who are IgA deficient should not receive IVIG. Induction therapy consists of 0.4 g IVIG per kilogram body weight for 2 to 5 days. If maintenance therapy on a monthly basis is necessary, 0.4 g per kilogram of body weight can be given as a single infusion. For patients who respond to high-dose corticosteroid therapy but relapse when the dose is tapered, the addition of danocrine or an immunosuppressive agent such as azathioprine may be beneficial. A rare patient may require splenectomy and although this procedure may not result in a cure of the hemolytic anemia or thrombocytopenia, it is usually easier to manage the cytopenia after splenectomy.

■ NEUROLOGIC LUPUS

The neurologic manifestations of lupus are varied and must always be differentiated from infection, thrombotic diathesis secondary to antiphospholipid antibody syndrome, metabolic imbalance, and drug toxicity. Seizures are managed with antiepileptics and control of any underlying active lupus. Psychosis is treated with major tranquilizers and control of the underlying disease. Severe neurologic lupus, whether presenting as organic brain syndrome, coma, transverse myelitis, or other disorder, is treated aggressively with intravenous pulse methylprednisolone. Patients who do not respond may require the addition of cyclophosphamide or plasmapheresis. SLE patients can rarely develop a syndrome resembling thrombotic thrombocytopenic (TTP) purpura, which will respond to plasmapheresis.

Serositis

SLE can cause pericarditis, pleurisy with pleural effusions, or peritonitis. Mild serositis will respond to NSAIDs and/or low doses of daily prednisone. Severe serositis may require intravenous pulse methylprednisolone therapy and the addition of immunosuppressive therapy. Rare patients require surgical intervention for pericardial "window" or chest tube drainage with later sclerosis.

Antiphospholipid Antibody Syndrome

Between 10 and 15 percent of SLE patients will eventually develop the secondary form of antiphospholipid antibody syndrome (APS). This hypercoagulable state is defined by the presence of venous or arterial thrombosis, pregnancy loss (fetal death or recurrent first trimester spontaneous abortions) or thrombocytopenia, in the presence of the lupus anticoagulant or moderate to high titer anticardiolipin (IgG or IgM isotype). SLE patients with the lupus anticoagulant or anticardiolipin antibody, who have not had a clinical criterion for APS, are not currently treated prophylactically (Table 5). It is prudent to remove other factors such as smoking and estrogen-containing oral contraceptives that might further increase the risk of thrombosis. Patients who have had a venous or arterial thrombotic event are preferably anticoagulated with warfarin, aiming for an international normalized ratio (INR) of 3.0. Patients with fetal death or recurrent pregnancy losses can be treated with subcutaneous heparin and low-dose (80 mg) aspirin during a subsequent pregnancy. Warfarin cannot be used during pregnancy because of its teratogenic potential.

Pregnancy

Pregnancy in a woman with SLE is high risk from both the maternal and fetal viewpoint. The woman with SLE is at risk for flare of her disease (occurring in as many as 60 percent of pregnancies) or a renal exacerbation (due to SLE, pre-eclampsia, or both). We have found, however, that flares are severe in only 11 percent of pregnancies. Corticosteroids are metabolized by the placenta and can be used as needed to control SLE disease activity. NSAIDs are stopped in the first trimester because of their potential adverse effect on fetal cardiac involvement. Azathioprine is continued during pregnancy if its use has been shown to be required to control renal, hematologic, or neurologic lupus. Because of its teratogenic potential, cyclophosphamide must be stopped while the woman with SLE is trying to conceive. Chloroquine, one of the antimalarial drugs, has been shown to cross the placenta. Decisions on the use of hydroxychloroquine must be made on an individual basis, weighing risks and benefits in an informed manner.

Risks to the fetus include fetal death secondary to the antiphospholipid antibody syndrome, preterm birth, and neonatal lupus. We have found that 15 percent of pregnancies end in fetal loss. Preterm birth is a significant problem, occurring in over one-third of pregnancies. Preterm birth is multifactorial, with pre-eclampsia and/or toxemia, material HELLP syndrome (hemolysis, elevated liver enzymes, and low platelet count), fetal distress, oligohydramnios, and premature rupture of membranes all contributing. Therefore, we recommend that SLE pregnancies be followed by an obstetrician who specializes in high-risk pregnancies. If the pregnant woman with lupus has anti-Ro antibodies, fetal four-chamber cardiac echocardiograms should be performed, starting at the sixteenth week of gestation, to identify fetal heart block and/or myocarditis early ("neonatal lupus") when it is amenable to treatment with dexamethasone and plasmapheresis.

Patient Education

Immediately after the diagnosis of SLE, the patient is often overwhelmed and frightened. Patients with SLE may benefit from the support groups and educational materials offered by the Lupus Foundation of America (4 Research Place, Suite 180, Rockville, MD 20850-3226; telephone: 1-301-670-9292) and their State Lupus Foundation Chapter. The eventual goal is to have the patient be an equal partner with the physician in her care.

Table 5 Treatment of Antiphospholipid Antibody Syndrome

After a venous or arterial thrombotic event
- *Acute management* with heparin, thrombolytic agent, and/or angioplasty, as appropriate
- *Chronic management* with warfarin (INR 3.0 to 4.0); occasional patients require low-dose aspirin in addition

To prevent fetal death
- Heparin: 8,000–10,000 units subcutaneously twice a day AND low-dose aspirin (80 mg)
- Continue therapy for 6 weeks postpartum; low-dose aspirin may be continued indefinitely

Suggested Reading

Alarcon-Segovia D, Deleze M, Oria CV, et al. Antiphospholipid antibodies and the antiphospholipid syndrome in systemic lupus erythematosus: a prospective analysis of 500 consecutive patients. Medicine 1989; 68:353–374.

Canadian Hydroxychloroquine Study Group: A randomized study of the effect of withdrawing hydroxychloroquine sulfate in systemic lupus erythematosus. N Engl J Med 1991; 324:150–154.

Felson DT, Anderson JA. Treatment of lupus nephritis. N Engl J Med 1986; 315:458.

McCune WJ, Golbus J, Zeldes W, et al. Clinical and immunologic effects of monthly administration of intravenous cyclophosphamide in severe systemic lupus erythematosus. N Engl J Med 1988; 318:1423–1431.

Petri M. Systemic lupus erythematosus and pregnancy. Rheum Dis Clin North Am 1994; 20:87–116.

RHEUMATOID ARTHRITIS

W. Neal Roberts Jr., M.D.
Shaun Ruddy, M.D.

■ PROBLEMS IN PLANNING THERAPY

Rheumatoid arthritis (RA) is a chronic systemic inflammatory disease of unclear etiology, the sine qua non of which is joint inflammation. Other prominent characteristics are symmetry of joint involvement over time (although not necessarily at presentation), variability of presentation, and volatility of clinical course. Spontaneous partial remissions and exacerbations during the disease course are characteristic in three-quarters of patients with RA; in another 10 percent the disease progresses rapidly and relentlessly to debilitating deformity, and 15 percent have monocyclic disease with no recurrence after the first episode (Fig. 1). This extreme variability has suggested to some that patients who initially meet the American College of Rheumatology (ACR) criteria for the diagnosis of RA represent more than one genetically distinct disease. In fact, it is already possible to use HLA-DR subtyping to pick patients at presentation who have a poorer prognosis.

The joints involved during the first year or two tend to be the most troublesome joints throughout the course. Admixtures of inflammatory joint symptoms, secondary mechanical joint symptoms, nonarticular pain (fibrositis, bursitis, ten-

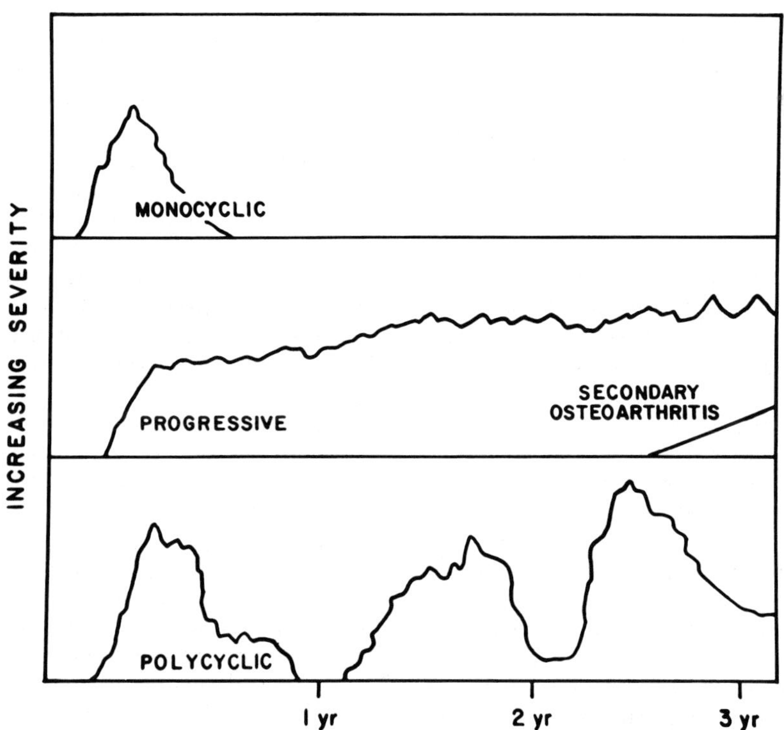

Figure 1
Clinical courses of rheumatoid arthritis. Note secondary osteoarthritis beginning in the second panel.

dinitis), the psychological impact of chronic disease, an increased incidence of septic joints, and extra-articular features (including Sjögren's syndrome, scleritis, vasculitic skin ulcers, and Felty's syndrome) can all contribute to the variability of the clinical course, precluding a linear approach to the therapeutic choices.

There is no cure for or prevention of RA. Early diagnosis and introduction of toxic drugs reduce the probability of irreversible joint damage. Timing is critical. ACR guidelines emphasize that "the initiation of DMARD [disease-modifying antirheumatic drug] therapy should not be delayed beyond three months for any patient with an established diagnosis who, in spite of adequate treatment with NSAIDs (nonsteroidal anti-inflamatory drugs), has ongoing joint pain, significant morning stiffness or fatigue, active synovitis, or persistent elevation of ESR (erythrocyte sedimentation rate) or CRP (C-reactive protein)." Because the goal of treatment is to intervene with the disease before joints are damaged, any patient with persistent synovitis and joint damage already documented by joint examination or radiograph should be started promptly on DMARDs to prevent or slow further damage.

Of the patients who require a DMARD for RA, most will have ceased taking the medication within several years unless the drug is methotrexate. The extensive dropout from this second-line antirheumatic therapy is attributable partially to side effects and partially to a lack of efficacy, but in any case the overall impact of these drugs on the course of the disease probably is not as great as initial responses to therapy would lead one to suspect. There are many treatments for which the efficacy in the usual clinical situation, the benefit-toxicity ratio, or the role relative to other established therapies is as yet poorly defined. Examples include supplemental eicosopentanoic acid and thalidomide. Untraditional remedies, many with little or no apparent efficacy, add complexity.

Finally, surgical replacement of worn-out joints with extensive cartilage loss remarkably improves the function of hips and knees. The threshold for invoking this therapy continues to decrease every few years as technical improvements in joint replacement, particularly at the prosthesis–cement-bone interfaces, lengthen the half-lives of these implants. Therefore, in the face of DMARD toxicity or lack of efficacy, the strategy of last resort for severe rheumatoid arthritis is to abandon DMARD therapy, using only NSAIDs plus monthly intra-articular corticosteroid injections, and replacement of joints as they fail.

■ SPECIFIC THERAPIES AND MANAGEMENT APPROACHES

Physical Measures

The goal of physical management—including formal physiotherapy as well as specific prescriptions for rest, exercise, and splinting of involved joints—is to steer a course between overuse of a joint leading to an increase in inflammatory symptoms and underuse permitting contractures of the surrounding joint capsule with loss of range of motion. The more actively involved a joint, the more immobilization it requires, sometimes requiring splinting accompanied by local steroid injection. With lessening inflammation, range of motion exercise should be intensified in order to recover range lost during the exacerbation.

The most frequent error in general physical management is failure to withdraw a prescription for rest after an exacerbation subsides. After several exacerbations and admonitions to rest, the patient forms the impression that activity should be restricted even when inflammation is minimal. The resulting generalized deconditioning and excessive fatigue may be difficult to distinguish from systemic disease activity.

The most frequent error in physical treatment of specific joints is failure to splint involved wrists in order to prevent excessive flexion while the patient is sleeping. Also important is the liberal use of metatarsal bars, orthotics, or metatarsal pads to decrease the load on the most involved metatarsophalangeal joints.

In two randomized trials comparing inpatient multidisciplinary treatment of flares of RA to vigorous outpatient team treatment with home visits, hospitalization proved to be more expensive and more effective, with benefits lasting for up to 1 year. The low priority accorded patients with RA by health planners and cost-control schemes obviates this approach in most settings. In contrast to acute care hospitals, rehabilitation units are more protected from regulations and may sometimes provide a setting for more prolonged care of patients with RA.

Family and Social Considerations

Support groups of patients with RA as well as other social services serve two important functions. First, they may help the patient define functional thresholds such as the appropriate degree of social activity in adolescents, the ability to remain on a job, and the ability to move around the house and carry out the activities of daily living sufficiently well to remain independent of the extended family. These thresholds should be vigorously defended with a multidisciplinary approach involving social services and toxic drugs for disease control. Even when the patient's course of deterioration has slowed and is not approaching one of these functional thresholds, a social support group can combat the unfavorable psychological aspects of chronic illness.

Second, social services, hospital admissions, and interviews with the family regarding drug toxicity serve to certify the patient in the sick role. Without this certification, the family may see no obvious deformity in the early stages and may conclude that the patient's fatigue and complaints are out of proportion to physical changes.

Monitoring Disease Activity and Treatment

All patients need to be followed indefinitely but monitoring varies with severity and activity of RA. Patients with disease in remission or near remission and not on a toxic drug may be seen semiannually, with frequency of laboratory or other monitoring dictated by their drug program. Patients with early disease, flares, or persistently active disease may require frequent physician visits and rheumatology consultation until disease control is established.

At each visit the physician must assess whether the disease is active. Symptoms of inflammatory (as contrasted to mechanical) joint disease, the duration of morning stiffness, fatigue, and active synovitis on joint examination all indicate active disease and suggest a change in treatment program, particularly changing or adding a DMARD. The joint examination alone may not sensitively reflect disease activity and structural damage and, therefore, periodic ESR or CRP measurements and radiographic examinations of involved joints are also necessary.

NSAIDs

Of all the medications effective for symptoms of RA, aspirin and NSAIDs are the ones with which physicians generally have the most experience. The traditional argument in favor of aspirin as an initial drug was its lower cost. However, if costs of diagnosis and treatment of peptic ulceration and gastrointestinal (GI) hemorrhage are counted, the cost advantage of aspirin over the NSAIDs disappears. The toxic consequences of continuous, full anti-inflammatory dosages of aspirin include one death from GI hemorrhage in every 100 patients every 5 years. Another major advantage of the NSAIDs is their longer pharmacologic half-lives, which lengthen the dosing interval, thereby increasing compliance. For example, piroxicam can be given once a day. Once or twice a day dosing can limit dosage flexibility, however. For example, stiffness may be much worse in the morning, suggesting weighting the major portion of the day's dosage toward the previous night. Indomethacin seems to cause a higher incidence of central nervous system side effects such as headache and dysphoria in older patients. Consequently, the first choice of rheumatologists is an NSAID, avoiding indomethacin in older patients. Sulindac may be particularly valuable in patients with mild renal insufficiency when a minimal effect on renal prostaglandins is desired, and when the patient is taking other medications that are renally excreted and whose toxicity may be augmented by any decrease in glomerular filtration rate. In patients over the age of 60 years in whom clearance is likely to be diminished despite an apparently normal serum creatinine concentration, intrarenal hemodynamic effects secondary to prostaglandin inhibition within the kidney may be more important. Many practitioners check serum creatinine concentration within a few weeks of starting NSAIDs in patients over 60 years old.

How long should therapy with an ineffective NSAID be continued before switching to another medication? The only prospective trial that specifically sought an answer to this question suggested that new responses still occurred 4 weeks into the therapy. The usual recommendation is for 2 weeks of full doses of NSAIDs before concluding that there is a lack of efficacy. When patient noncompliance is factored in, the average trial is probably 7 to 10 days, however. This discrepancy between data and practice probably arises from differences between the patient's and the physician's concerns, the former being more interested in the immediate analgesia and the latter in the slower anti-inflammatory effect. Combinations of NSAIDs with salicylates or other nonsteroidal drugs appear to increase the risk of toxic effects with no increase in efficacy. Most patients decide for themselves to use some additional medication for analgesia. In most cases this is acetaminophen, but sometimes it is an aspirin-containing medication or over-the-counter ibuprofen.

When the first NSAID employed proves ineffective after at least 2 weeks, what drug should replace it? Most rheumatologists pick second and third choice NSAIDs on the basis of the principle of switching from one chemical class to another. There are six or seven chemically distinct groups of NSAIDs, all of which inhibit cyclo-oxygenase activity. The major classes other than salicylates are propionic acids (ibuprofen, naproxen), indole-related compounds (indomethacin, sulindac, tolmetin), which are structurally closest to phenylbutazone, arylacetic acids (diclofenac), and oxicams (piroxicam). Data supporting the switching of classes over random choice of subsequent NSAIDs or their complete omission are lacking.

The main toxic effects of salicylates and NSAIDs are peptic gastritis, erosions, and ulcers. These lesions correlate imperfectly both with symptoms of upper GI upset and with detectable GI blood loss. For example, ulcers can occur, bleed, and heal while the patient continues to take NSAIDs without symptoms. By default most clinicians merely monitor symptoms to detect erosions and ulcers, although a case can be made for periodic monitoring of the hematocrit. Periodic testing of the stool for occult blood is of no value because positive test results occur in most patients taking these drugs for long periods. A strategy for handling GI upset is to discontinue all nonsteroidal and salicylate medications until 5 days after all symptoms have subsided. Therapy with the same or a different drug then can be restarted if there is no practical alternative to maintain joint function. Misoprostil, extra small meals, over-the-counter antacids, H_2 blockers, sodium pump inhibitors, and sucralfate may permit continued NSAID therapy when it is absolutely needed and the risk justified. Misoprostil is probably most effective in preventing ulceration, but also less well tolerated due to cramping and diarrhea. Nonacetylated salicylates (magnesium choline salicylate or salicyl salicylate) have the least effect on the gastric mucosa, but may be less effective in moderate to severe inflammation.

Risk factors for major GI toxicity include advanced age, dose relative to weight, history of peptic ulceration or bleeding, concurrent corticosteroid use, and cardiovascular disease. Reversible renal insufficiency, papillary necrosis, nephrotic syndrome, interstitial nephritis and renal failure can result from any NSAID. Risk factors for renal toxicity include the advancing age, renal vascular disease on diuretics, other forms of renal disease, congestive heart failure, cirrhosis, and atherosclerotic heart disease. Heart disease appears on this list of statistically prominent risk factors, probably because it implies a physiologic state in which renal blood flow is being maintained by prostaglandin-mediated compensatory vasodilation blocked by NSAIDs.

Additional NSAID effects for which there is no agreed-upon detection strategy include drug-induced hepatitis and agranulocytosis. A complete blood count (CBC) including a differential count and a chemistry battery should be carried out within the first few weeks after initiating NSAID treatment.

Often the patient's expectation for relief from a NSAID exceeds what the medication can accomplish. The total effect of these drugs on the pain and inflammation of moderate RA may be in the range of 15 percent on a visual analogue scale, so that the medication may be of benefit, but be seen by the patient as only "taking the edge off." The effect of the NSAID may be evident only when it is discontinued. If pain is due to cartilage loss and secondary osteoarthritis, the patient almost certainly will be disappointed with the effect of the drug.

DMARDs

The therapy of RA with DMARDs is one of the most unusual areas in modern medicine: the doctor gives the drug and then waits for 1 to 6 months for a clinical response. This delay in response makes the clinical effect of the drug difficult to differentiate from the natural history of a variable disease. Clinical parameters to follow are the patient's global assessment, measured grip strength, length of the period of early morning stiffness, and the erythrocyte sedimentation rate. In general, DMARDs have minimal immediate anti-inflammatory effects, but in the long run are severalfold more effective against moderate rheumatoid inflammation than are NSAIDS. True remissions are rare, but approximately two-thirds of the patients who are able to take a full course of a given DMARD improve and about half of these do so to a great degree. The most effective is methotrexate which works well enough to be continued in 50 to 75 percent of patients for five years or longer. In contrast, gold is taken for more than 5 years by less than 25 percent of patients. Adverse drug reactions requiring discontinuation of therapy occur in about one-third of the patients. Long-term benefit from these drugs is reduced because of the continuing occurrence of side effects throughout the period of drug use and the tendency of the disease to relapse when the drugs are withdrawn. It is probable, but not certain, that a patient who initially responds to a slow-acting antirheumatic drug can be "recaptured" with the same medication later. Failure to respond to one such drug does not predict a failure to respond to another; neither does toxicity with one accurately predict a recurrence of similar toxicity with another.

Some side effects of DMARDs, particularly oral ulcers and mild skin rashes from gold, can be circumvented by discontinuing the medication long enough for the side effect to resolve and then reinstituting the same drug, perhaps by a different route of administration (e.g., oral instead of injectable doses of gold), or at a low dosage, and slowly advancing the dosage over a period of weeks to months. Methotrexate oral ulcers often can be prevented with supplemental folic acid, 1 mg per day, or by giving the drug by subcutaneous route. Methotrexate hepatotoxicity can be "treated through" by lowering the dose until the enzyme elevations completely disappear. Toxic effects for which the "treating through" strategy definitely should *not* be tried include methotrexate-induced pulmonary or methotrexate liver disease with biopsy evidence of precirrhotic change, agranulocytosis, hydroxychloroquine retinopathy, proteinuria with a change in renal function from gold (in contrast to mild proteinuria with a normal creatinine level), and gold colitis.

The choice of timing for beginning DMARD therapy is complex (Table 1). The choice of such a drug is influenced by additional factors shown in Table 2. Hydroxychloroquine is clearly the least toxic, but it is also less effective than methotrexate, gold, penicillamine, and cytotoxic drugs. Of all the medications other than NSAIDs and aspirin, methotrexate and steroids in low oral doses act most rapidly. Penicillamine is the slowest. Despite the multiple in vitro mechanisms of action ascribed to each of the DMARDs, it appears likely that gold and hydroxychloroquine operate by affecting monocyte function and that penicillamine interferes with T-lymphocyte function. Methotrexate suppresses interleukin-1 (IL-1), which, along with tumor necrosis factor (TNF), is important in causing erosions, but the actual mechanism of action of methotrexate remains obscure.

Table 1 The Decision to Begin Therapy with Disease-Modifying Antirheumatic Drugs

IN FAVOR

- Early loss of function or progressive deformity; later persistent active inflammation despite nonsteroidal anti-inflammatory drug therapy
- Radiographic evidence of erosions
- Lack of steroid responsiveness
- HLA DR typing suggesting persistent disease
- Positive test for rheumatoid factor

AGAINST

- No evidence of active synovitis on physical examination
- Questionable diagnosis
- Less than 3 months of disease
- Childbearing potential, off birth control therapy
- Lack of compliance or laboratory follow-up

In summary the best initial DMARD for patients with rheumatoid arthritis varies according to severity. Because of safety, convenience, and cost, hydroxychloroquine and sulfasalazine are often selected first for patients with milder disease; methotrexate is most often used first for those with more severe disease. Generally well tolerated, hydroxychloroquine requires no laboratory monitoring, but patients need periodic ophthalmologic examinations for the rare complication of retinal damage. Sulfasalazine requires monitoring for rare myelosuppression. Within 3 to 6 months, the response to these agents may be assessed and the need for other DMARDs determined.

Hydroxychloroquine

Although the beneficial effects of hydroxychloroquine are not marked, this drug is the easiest of the DMARDs to administer. It only rarely leads to GI upset and otherwise causes a vanishingly small incidence of nuisance side effects. Skeletal muscle and myocardial toxic effects have been reported rarely. The abrupt onset of new heart failure in a patient taking hydroxychloroquine is reason to discontinue the drug. Unfortunately, rare instances of pigmentary macular degeneration in the retina occur with hydroxychloroquine. Most reported cases have occurred at high doses; it is recommended that the dosage not exceed 6.5 mg per kilogram per day. Dosage schedules that vary every other day may have to be used because the tablets come in only a 200 mg size and the pill tastes intolerably bitter when split. With this low dosage of one or two tablets per day, the incidence of pigmentary macular degeneration appears to be less than 0.1 percent. Unfortunately, the prospect of visual loss, no matter how small statistically, often frightens patients. Nevertheless, informed consent about visual loss is mandatory.

Appropriate monitoring of hydroxychloroquine includes a full retinal examination initially to exclude senile macular degeneration, which may be difficult to differentiate from pigmentary macular degeneration, along with an ophthalmologic follow-up examination every 6 months. It may take three months for the drug to have a beneficial effect. Patients who are in need of a rapid decrease in inflammatory symptoms are often given a more rapidly acting drug such as

Table 2 Slow-Acting Antirheumatic and Cytotoxic Drugs for the Treatment of Rheumatoid Arthritis

DRUG	HYDROXYCLOROQUINE (HCQ)	METHOTREXATE	AURANOFIN	INJECTABLE GOLD SALTS	PENICILLAMINE	SULFASALAZINE	AZATHIOPRINE
Indications	Mild to moderate synovitis, symptoms unresponsive to nonsteroidal anti-inflammatory drugs, splinting, physiotherapy, local steroid injections	Failure of HCQ & sulfasalazine, need (often social or psychological) for rapid reliable response, early aggressive disease	Persistent or progressive disease despite hydroxychloroquine therapy	Persistent or progressive disease with hydroxychloroquine, diarrhea with auranofin	Failure of gold and methotrexate	Mild to moderate synovitis, symptoms incompletely responsive to nonsteroidal anti-inflammatory drugs	Failure of gold and methotrexate
Relative contraindications	Pre-existing macular disease	Liver disease; alcohol consumption 4 oz/wk; renal disease; trimethoprim sulfa	Proteinuria, renal disease, expected poor compliance with monitoring	Proteinuria, renal disease, history of gold rash, oral lesions	Proteinuria, renal disease, history of drugs rash, oral lesions	Sulfa allergy	Renal disease, liver disease
Usual dosage	200 mg qd or b.i.d.	2.5 or 5.0 mg q 12h × 3 doses weekly	3 mg b.i.d.	10 mg test dose, week 1; 50 mg/week × 20 weeks; taper to 50 mg/mo	125 mg daily, raising dose by 125 mg/mo	500 mg b.i.d. × 1 wk; advance to 1 g b.i.d.	50 mg daily, raising dose by 25 mg over 2 wk, guided by CBC
Maximal dosage	200 mg b.i.d.	20 mg/week	3 mg t.i.d.	50 mg/week	750 mg daily	1,500 mg b.i.d.	200 mg daily
Major toxic effects	Pigmented macular degeneration (1%); gastrointestinal upset (11%)	Hepatic fibrosis; rarely cirrhosis (irreversible), hematologic side effects and mouth ulcers often prevented by addition of 1 mg/day folic acid	Mucocutaneous lesions (23%), rare exfoliation, diarrhea (25%), membranous nephropathy (2%), hematologic complication (7%)	Mucocutaneous lesions (48%), rare exfoliation, membranous nephropathy (6%), hematologic complication (7%)	Mucocutaneous lesions (30%), membranous nephropathy (15–20%), hematologic complications (5%), autoimmune syndromes (1%)	Nausea (not ulcerogenic), rash, bone marrow suppression	Bone marrow suppression, hepatitis (1%)
Recommended monitoring	Baseline and q6mo retinal examination with photographs and Ishikawa dot and Amsler grid tests	CBC, differential and platelet counts, liver chemistries, creatinine q2wk, may lengthen interval to q3wk at 2 mo	CBC, differential and platelet counts, urine dipstick for protein q2wk, may lengthen interval to q3wk at 2 mo	Same as oral gold, but check laboratory test results prior to each injection	CBC, differential and platelet counts, urine dipstick for protein q2wk, may lengthen intervals to monthly at 6 mo	CBC q2wk, adjust dosage monthly thereafter	CBC, differential and platelet counts prior to adjusting dose, liver chemistries monthly
Length of usual trial	3 mo	3 mo (many respond in first month)	6–8 mo	4–6 mo	7–9 mo	2 mo	3 mo

CBC, complete blood cell count.

methotrexate. For those who need therapy in addition to nonsteroidal drugs but who can be expected to maintain function for a number of months, hydroxychloroquine is the DMARD of choice along with sulfasalazine. Sulfasalazine is useful in this role especially when the better tolerated enteric-coated formulation is available.

Methotrexate

For the treatment of moderate to severe RA, methotrexate is both more effective and more rapidly acting than other DMARDs (see Table 2). Responses to methotrexate occur between 2 and 12 weeks of treatment in contrast to the 6 months or more required for the evaluation of gold salt or penicillamine therapy. Methotrexate also compares favorably with the other DMARDs in that patients are more likely to tolerate the drug for longer periods, an important consideration in the treatment of a chronic disease. Although joint disease usually improves, an increase in the size and number of rheumatoid nodules sometimes occurs.

The most common and troublesome toxicity is GI, including anorexia, vomiting, and diarrhea; stomatitis is less frequent. These may respond to adjustments in dosage. Parenteral administration of the drug may decrease the frequency of GI disturbances.

The main clinical complications of methotrexate include hepatic fibrosis, and interstitial pulmonary infiltrates with fibrosis. These occur in 1 to 2 percent of patients, and there is no reliable way to predict when they will occur or to treat them when they do. Methotrexate is contraindicated in patients who consume more than 4 ounces of ethanol per week or who are so obese as to preclude liver biopsy and to have increased risk of hepatic steatosis. Detection of hepatic toxicity is facilitated by measuring liver enzymes at the recommended interval of 4 to 8 weeks; a decrease in the serum albumin concentration may signify the onset of hepatic fibrosis. Routine surveillance liver biopsies should not be performed, but biopsy is indicated when liver blood tests have been persistently abnormal.

Pneumonitis is an uncommon complication of long-term methotrexate therapy with a frequency of 2 to 6 percent; pre-existing pulmonary disease is a contraindication to methotrexate use. A baseline chest radiograph within 1 year prior to starting therapy is recommended, both for future reference and to exclude pre-existing lung disease. Pulmonary toxicity occurs at any time during therapy and is not related to dose. Shortness of breath, a nonproductive cough, and fever are the hallmarks of this disease. A "chest cold" without rhinorrhea should prompt a physician's evaluation for the pulmonary toxicity of methotrexate.

Myelosuppression is not usually a problem with the low doses of methotrexate used to treat rheumatoid arthritis. Risk factors include the use of antifolate agents such as trimethoprim, the presence of folate deficiency, and renal insufficiency; an additional risk factor may also be a mean corpuscular volume of greater than 100. The frequency of macrocytic anemia is reduced by the concomitant administration of folic acid, 1 mg daily, without lessening the efficiency of treatment for the arthritis. Rarely, lymphoproliferative disorders occur in patients taking methotrexate. The relationship to the drug is unclear, but some of the malignancies have regressed after stopping methotrexate.

Gold

Adverse drug reactions to gold include extensive skin eruptions, oral ulcers, and a membranous glomerulopathy, the latter manifested by proteinuria. There may be about a 0.5 percent incidence of mortality from agranulocytosis, aplastic anemia, or uncontrollable secretory diarrhea due to gold-induced colitis. Patients with HLA-DR3 disease may be more susceptible to gold-induced thrombocytopenia. Rarely, intramuscular doses of gold result in a "nitratoid" reaction of acute vasodilation and hypotension when the rapidly absorbed aqueous solution (thiomalate salt) is used.

Most toxic reactions to gold occur during the first 4 months of treatment, but they may occur at any time during treatment, making CBCs with differential counts and urine test for protein every 2 to 4 weeks the standard for monitoring gold therapy, whether given by injection or orally. Hematuria without proteinuria probably is not gold membranous nephropathy and should be studied diagnostically as would any other hematuria.

Laboratory monitoring is the major expense in gold therapy. On the other hand, all the slow-acting antirheumatic drugs (with the exception of hydroxychloroquine) require similar monitoring. Monthly laboratory monitoring can be decreased in frequency to every 2 months in patients who are stable with gold therapy for years. Oral gold therapy may not be the equivalent of injectable therapy; the disease in patients who are stable on injectable gold therapy often flares when they are switched to the oral preparation. Auranofin (oral gold) is associated with lower rates of both renal and hematologic toxicity than parenteral gold compounds. Its minor toxicities include diarrhea (common) and mucocutaneous reactions, but the dose must be adjusted to avoid both of these.

D-Penicillamine

D-Penicillamine is a difficult drug to manage. In addition to the membranous nephropathy and bone marrow toxicity characteristic of gold, penicillamine produces the nuisance side effect of loss of taste in 20 percent of patients and rarely the more serious autoimmune side effects of a myasthenia gravis–like syndrome and pemphigus. If the dosage is accelerated rapidly (e.g., over 2 months rather than 6 months), the incidence of thrombocytopenia, gastrointestinal intolerance, and other adverse reactions increases significantly. On the "go low, go slow" regimen (125 mg as a starting dose with 125 mg monthly increments to a daily dose of 750 mg), it takes 6 months to reach the full dosage and another month to decide that the full dosage has been of no value. Patients not successfully treated with methotrexate, hydroxychloroquine, sulfasalazine, and gold, which are all clearly preferable, may take penicillamine. Patients who seem likely to tolerate the 6 to 9 months with no response to therapy without much functional loss are the best candidates for penicillamine. Penicillamine may be ineffective in seronegative RA.

Cytotoxic Drugs

Anecdotal evidence indicates that azathioprine may be somewhat less effective than methotrexate and more apt to produce GI intolerance in the dosage commonly used. GI intolerance is the most common side effect of azathioprine therapy, requiring discontinuation in approximately 10 percent of treated patients. Rarely pancreatitis may occur with azathioprine. The one controlled comparison between methotrexate and azathioprine showed only a trend toward greater efficacy of methotrexate. Rarely, idiosyncratic hepatotoxicity from azathioprine occurs in the first few weeks of the course. An excess of lymphoreticular malignant disease has been observed among allograft recipients treated with azathioprine but not among patients with rheumatic diseases treated with this drug. Azathioprine is a purine analogue which is capable of inducing myelosuppression at doses used to treat RA (1 to 2mg per kilogram per day). Risk factors for myelosuppression include the use of concomitant allopurinol or ACE inhibitors, or the presence of renal insufficiency. Prevention consists of dose reduction with allopurinol to one-third to one-half the usual dose, avoiding the use of concomitant ACE inhibitors and reducing the dose of azathioprine in patients with renal insufficiency.

Severe effects of rheumatoid vasculitis such as nonhealing lower extremity ulcers may require brief pulse treatment with cyclophosphamide for which there is an established protocol. Despite its efficacy, continuous use of cyclophosphamide for RA without vasculitis is precluded by an increased incidence of the development of neoplasia, particularly lymphoma and bladder cancer.

Combinations of DMARDs

Whether DMARDs should be given in a sequential or additive fashion for patients with persistently active disease remains controversial. Most rheumatologists treat patients who have had a partial response to a DMARD, or have been refractory to different DMARDs, with combinations of DMARDs. The most commonly used combinations are methotrexate-hydroxychloroquine, methotrexate-sulfasalazine, and gold-hydroxychloroquine. Several studies document the efficacy of low dose cyclosporine (2.5 to 5 mg per kilogram per day) in treating RA in combination with methotrexate, but its use is limited by cost and potential long-term renal toxicity.

Corticosteroids

The side effects of systemic glucocorticoids appear increasingly with higher doses and longer duration of treatment. For RA, prednisone should not be given in a dose higher than 10 mg daily. Effort should be made to limit its use to a short course or, if maintenance treatment is necessary, to use the lowest possible dose. There may be some role for low dosage of 5.0 to 7.5 mg a day as a disease-modifying agent.

There is general agreement that the risks of osteoporosis and other adverse effects from pharmacologic doses of prednisone (greater than 5 to 10 mg per day) are great enough to counterbalance their beneficial effect in RA. Using corticosteroids in higher doses for RA is like buying an automobile on time: all the benefits occur in the first 2 years, and payment continues almost indefinitely. Nevertheless, 15 or 20 percent of patients with moderately severe RA take steroids. Every-other-day regimens usually fail owing to an exacerbation of symptoms on the "off" day ("every-other-day arthritis"). The role of steroid therapy hinges on the critical question of how much treatment with low dosages adds to the risk of osteoporosis. The risk-benefit ratio for low-dose prednisone treatment of RA therefore may be affected profoundly by increase in use of estrogen, alendronate, and nasal calcitonin for the prevention of postmenopausal osteoporosis or, in the case of estrogen, coronary artery disease prevention. Prednisone given at a dose of 7.5 mg daily is probably a reasonable addition to DMARD treatment for patients with a lower baseline risk of osteoporosis, including those with high bone density determined by densitometry, large-framed individuals, men and blacks. Postmenopausal women whose bone mass is stable on supplemental calcium and vitamin D may also try low-dose oral prednisone with bone density monitoring.

Injectable Steroids

Steroid injections are most useful when one or a few joints dominate the clinical picture. Almost any joint or surrounding periarticular structure can be injected successfully by an experienced operator. Intra-articular injections should be limited to three or four per joint per year to avoid atrophy of adjacent soft tissues and to one to two total injections per month to avoid systemic corticosteroid side effects. Serious complications from steroid injections are rare, although "postinjection flares" from steroid crystal deposition can occur 2 to 8 hours following the injection. The vitiligo that occurs when some of the injectable steroid infiltrates the dermis in black patients is cosmetically undesirable. Local steroid injection is one of the most effective treatments for geographically limited RA. It does not appear to decrease bone mass or increase the rate of total joint arthroplasty in RA when used according to the above protocol.

Surgery

Secondary osteoarthritis and "bone on bone" pain are indications for joint replacement. Open surgical synovectomy is no longer performed, but arthroscopic synovectomy of the knee may provide relief of symptoms if the knee dominates the clinical picture or is the remaining troublesome joint after successful DMARD or cytotoxic drug therapy. The effects of arthroscopic synovectomy persist for about 2 years. Total joint replacement of the hips and the knees has a 95 percent certainty of affording pain relief, a 1 percent per year chance of resulting in loosening, and a 1 percent chance of resulting in postoperative infection. Prosthetic replacements of other joints are less satisfactory. There is still no widely available prosthesis that withstands the stress put on an ankle. If the ankle joints or joints of the midfoot are destroyed by RA but remain painful, arthrodesis is the best option; the same is generally true of the wrist. Elbow replacement can be successful but is technically difficult. Shoulder replacement eliminates pain as effectively as lower extremity joint replacements but adds little to function because the rotator cuff is usually destroyed and cannot be reconstructed. Silastic joint replacements in the small joints of the hands improve the hands cosmetically but often fracture and fail to increase strength even though they restore mechanical relationships. It is wise not to use hand surgery as a patient's first joint replacement surgery in order to avoid leaving the patient with an unrealistically pessimistic view of the functional value of joint replacement. Dorsal synovectomy to prevent rupture of the extensor tendons of the hands with consequent loss of function is an effective prophylactic surgical measure.

Experimental Treatments

There are a number of apparently effective treatments with major limitations imposed by side effects or inconvenience.

Among these are radiation synovectomy with injected yttrium or dysprosium, which can be performed only in centers adjacent to a cyclotron or linear accelerator capable of creating these short-lived isotopes. Radiation synovectomy is 90 percent effective and may be superior to surgical synovectomy. Total nodal irradiation (2,000 to 3,000 rad) has produced remissions lasting 2 years, but also deaths due to infection. Plasmapheresis is ineffective. Various biologic agents, particularly those aimed at blocking the erosive effect of IL-1 and TNF alpha, appear to offer great promise; their actual clinical role remains uncertain. Pulse methylprednisolone offers no advantage over low-dose steroid therapy. Needed advances include foremost, a clearer definition of the risk-benefit ratio inherent in the strategy of using biologic, immunomodulatory, and disease-modifying antirheumatic drugs earlier in the course of the disease, for example within 6 to 12 weeks after onset.

SPECIAL PROBLEMATIC SITUATIONS

Early Aggressive Disease

The patient who has severe synovitis during the first year of disease with considerable functional loss poses a major question. Does early aggressive treatment as soon as one is certain of the diagnosis have a better chance of succeeding than later treatment? If so, one should use the drug most likely to suppress synovitis before the disease gets a foothold. The contrasting point of view suggests that DMARDs other than methotrexate are rarely continued for many years consecutively and ultimately have little impact on the final outcome. One therefore should withhold these drugs as long as possible in order to avoid unnecessary exposure to toxic drugs in patients in whom spontaneous remission or improvement might occur. Most rheumatologists have become increasingly aggressive in the early use of DMARDs. Previous recommendations centered on the caution that one should avoid such drugs during the first year when the likelihood of spontaneous remission was the greatest. Most rheumatologists now place this window at 3 to 6 months. Toxicity profiles make NSAIDs, methotrexate, hydroxychloroquine, sulfasalazine, and low-dose prednisone the best drugs for early use.

The Discouraged Patient

The patient who adopts a therapeutically nihilistic attitude and gives up trying to maintain joint mobility is in a precarious situation. Flexion contractures may become permanent, and often function lost in this way cannot be regained even surgically. Two approaches greatly encourage the patient at almost no cost. The first is to allow the patient as much control over the therapy as possible. Creating options of more or less equal value and presenting them to the patient as choices generate a sense of control on the part of the patient. Second, steroids can be injected into the two or three most actively inflamed joints. A long-lasting (e.g., 3 month) benefit from injection may occur, and the systemic spillover during the initial week after injection may also help the patient psychologically. The contrast between the response to intra-articular steroid therapy, even if it is shortlived, and the baseline to which the patient returns demonstrates that effective treatment is at least possible and that the situation is not hopeless.

Table 3 Rheumatic Diseases that may Resemble Rheumatoid Arthritis

Consider the following in seronegative rheumatoid arthritis that fails to respond to treatment:
- Erosive interphalangeal osteoarthritis
- Calcium pyrophosphate deposition disease
- Chronic tophaceous gout (especially steroid treated)
- Ankylosing spondylitis (especially if metacarpophalangeal involvement is asymmetric)
- Reiter's syndrome (especially if metacarpophalangeal involvement is asymetric)
- Psoriatic arthritis
- Systemic lupus erythematosus

Night Pain

Pain that awakens the patients at night usually leads to a specific treatment. The three most likely causes of night pain in patients with RA are (1) bursitis-tendinitis in the shoulder, hip, or anserine bursa, which responds to local steroid injections (patients use the medial surface of the knees to push off against the mattress when turning over and may experience patellar and anserine bursa pain from this seemingly innocuous action); (2) compression neuropathy, which can be treated with steroid injection or decompression of the nerve (e.g., carpel tunnel, median nerve release); and (3) structurally diseased joints with bone on bone pain from cartilage loss (these patients may benefit from surgery).

The Patient Who Has Failed to Improve

The diagnosis of the patient who has failed to improve should be reviewed (Table 3). In the patient who has experienced failure with multiple slow-acting antirheumatic drugs as a result of toxicity, a detailed re-examination of the history should be made in order to determine whether the "toxicities" that led to discontinuing such a drug, particularly methotrexate, are toxicities that definitely warrant abandoning the drug. These include methotrexate pulmonary disease, gold nephrotoxicity with rising creatinine levels, cytopenias, and gold colitis. Mild (trace to 1+) gold proteinuria, stomatitis, or a mild skin rash sometimes can be "treated through" by restarting at a lower dosage and advancing the dosage more slowly. The probability of success using this strategy may be augmented by switching the route or form of administration of gold. Thus, if the toxic effect was minor and occurred with aurothioglucose, the patient is switched to gold sodium thiomalate, or auranofin. As an alternative to restarting slow-acting antirheumatic drug therapy, local steroid injections and NSAIDs may be used for the control of symptoms, using surgical replacements for joints as they fail. A patient with advanced widespread disease is sometimes paradoxically a very good candidate for multiple joint replacements, since the level of physical activity is so low that it puts little stress on the bone-cement interface. This conservative strategy of NSAIDs and injection combined with replacement of joints as they fail from cumulative cartilage loss is often superior to repeated excursions into obscure areas of therapeutics such as long-term cyclophosphamide therapy.

The "Burned Out" Patient

There is some debate about whether RA "burns" itself out. Fibrotic pannus may both insulate the examining hand from signs of inflammation in the joint and physically limit the volume of effusion. Some patients appear to have very limited inflammation on examination and yet have malaise and easy fatigability accompanied by laboratory evidence of disease activity, such as decreased albumin and hemoglobin levels with increased ESR. These patients sometimes benefit from aggressive treatment even though they have long-standing RA with little apparent evidence of active synovitis on examination.

Generalized Fatigue and Aching Without Physical Signs

A patient who has had RA for a short time may not have the deformity and scarred pannus of the "burned out" patient but still may not be doing well. Such a person may complain of generalized aching, which may turn out to be secondary fibromyalgia or depression (treatable with amitriptyline, other tricyclics in the case of fibromyalgia) comorbidity such as hypothyroidism is common. When symptoms of aching are disproportionate to physical findings or laboratory test results, special attention to the patient's home, family, or other social situation is indicated.

Single Inflamed Joint or a Dominant Joint

This is the most important special situation in the treatment of patients with RA. A single dominant joint in a patient with RA should be aspirated the first time it is seen to effect symptomatic relief, diagnosis by culture, and drainage of a potentially infected joint space. Shoulders in particular require prompt aspiration. Unlike joints in the lower extremities, shoulders usually can be spared physical stress and are voluntarily and involuntarily splinted by the patient when a small effusion stretches the joint capsule. Therefore, a large palpable effusion makes the shoulder more likely to be infected even if it is not warm. In patients with RA there may be several reasons why there is not so much warmth over a septic joint as in other patients. NSAIDs, steroids, and generalized debility may contribute to decreasing the signs of inflammation. In a particularly stubborn, culture-negative joint, especially one that is as anatomically complex as the shoulder, the failure of one local steroid injection to produce relief should prompt more careful examination of all the tendon and bursal structures around the joint. Injections directed at the structure that seems by physical examination to be most involved are more successful than steroid injections given intra-articularly by the anterior approach regardless of physical findings.

Suggested Reading

Ad Hoc Committee on Clinical Guidelines of the American College of Rheumatology. Guidelines for the management of rheumatoid arthritis. Arthritis Rheum 1996; 39:713–722.

Helewa A, Bombardier C, Goldsmith CH, et al. Cost-effectiveness of inpatient and intensive outpatient treatment of rheumatoid arthritis: A randomized, controlled trial. Arthritis Rheum 1989; 32:1505–1514.

Kremer JM, Alarcon GS, Lightfoot RW Jr, et al. Methotrexate for rheumatoid arthritis: Suggested guidelines for monitoring liver toxicity. Arthritis Rheum 1994; 37:316–328.

Panush RS. Controversial arthritis remedies. Bull Rheum Dis 1985; 34:5.

Scott DGI, Bacon PA. Intravenous cyclophosphamide plus methylprednisolone in the treatment of systemic rheumatoid vasculitis. Am J Med 1984; 76:377–384.

Tugwell P, Pincus T, Yocum D, et al. Combination therapy with Cyclosporine and Methotrexate in severe rheumatoid arthritis. N Engl J Med 1995; 333:555–556.

ANKYLOSING SPONDYLITIS

Joseph H. Korn, M.D.

Ankylosing spondylitis, or Marie-Strümpell arthritis, is the prototype of the group of disorders known as the seronegative spondyloarthropathies. It is both a true arthritis or synovitis of diarthrodial joints and an enthesopathy, an inflammatory and destructive process involving tendinous and ligamentous attachments to bone. It differs from the other polyarthritides such as rheumatoid arthritis in the pattern of joint involvement. Although peripheral joint disease does occur in ankylosing spondylitis, the hallmark of the disease is axial involvement—the spine and the pelvic and shoulder girdles. It is this pattern of involvement that both distinguishes the disease from most inflammatory arthritides and leads to confusion with degenerative and muscular conditions of the lower back. Thus, diagnostic accuracy is important in selecting an appropriate approach to therapy.

In making the correct diagnosis, historical and physical findings are paramount. Clinical studies have shown that the patient's history is reliable in distinguishing inflammatory (e.g., spondylitic) back pain from mechanical back pain. An early age of onset, such as the late teens and early twenties, is found more commonly in ankylosing spondylitis. In addition, the back pain is more diffuse than in mechanical disorders, involving the entire spine and not just the lower back; thus, the symptoms are concordant with the radiographic and pathologic findings. Like other inflammatory arthritides, spondylitic back pain improves with activity, is made worse by prolonged recumbency, and is characterized by stiffness after sitting or lying in a single position (gelliag). Night pain is a common associated feature. Finally, the presence of inflammatory peripheral arthritis, inflammatory enthesopathy, and extra-articular disease manifestations (see later discussion) distinguishes the spondyloarthropathies, including ankylosing spondylitis, from mechanical back pain.

The distinction between ankylosing spondylitis and other spondyloarthropathies is made largely on the basis of associated clinical findings. Extra-articular features of ankylosing spondylitis include uveitis, aortitis, apical pulmonary fibrosis, and enthesopathic findings (e.g., heel pain). Both uveitis and aortitis may be found in Reiter's syndrome, and the distinction between ankylosing spondylitis and Reiter's syndrome is often difficult. Such characteristic features of Reiter's syndrome as balanitis, keratodermia, blennorrhagia, and urethritis, when present, differentiate the disorder from ankylosing spondylitis. Similarly, the presence of inflammatory bowel disease or psoriasis allows the distinction of spondyloarthropathy associated with these disorders from ankylosing spondylitis.

Early in the disease the symptom complex is a result of inflammatory processes in diarthrodial (synovial) joints, in synarthroses (nonsynovial joints), at cartilage-bone junctions, and at ligamentous and tendinous attachments to bone and cartilage. Thus, involvement of apophyseal and costovertebral joints leads to limited motion of the spine (at the intervertebral joints) and rib cage, respectively. Sacroiliac pain, often referred to the buttocks, is a result of involvement of both the true sacroiliac joints (approximately the lower two- thirds of the sacroiliac articulation) and the synarthrosis of the upper articulation. Enthesopathy is common at ligamentous attachments to vertebrae, pelvic bones, ankles (Achilles tendon and plantar fascial attachment), and femurs. At the intervertebral discs, costochondral junctions, and symphysis pubis, inflammatory processes lead to pain, swelling, and erosive changes at the cartilage-bone interfaces. During the course of the disease there is both fusion of diarthrodial and synarthrodial joints and calcification of ligamentous structures leading to loss of mobility and function. These processes obviously are not amenable to medical therapy. The cauda equina syndrome with sphincter dysfunction secondary to root compression has been reported occasionally and may require surgery.

As noted earlier, the diagnosis of ankylosing spondylitis is best made on the basis of a characteristic symptom complex. In early disease both physical and radiographic findings may be normal. With progression, physical examination shows decreased chest expansion and decreased flexion of the lumbar spine. Physical maneuvers to elicit the pain of sacroiliitis, such as sacroiliac compression or hyperextension of the opposite hip, have not been of demonstrated value. With progressive disease there is often forward protrusion of the neck, kyphosis in the upper thoracic spine, and fixed flexion at the hips giving rise to a characteristic posture. Such features as iritis, aortic regurgitation, apical pulmonary fibrosis, and enthesopathic signs and symptoms (e.g., costochondral pain and tenderness) are unusual in mechanical back disease and in inflammatory arthritides other than the spondyloarthropathies, and their presence lends support to a diagnosis of ankylosing spondylitis. Laboratory tests show no consistent abnormalities that are diagnostically useful; the erythrocyte sedimentation rate, which is usually abnormal in other types of inflammatory arthritis, is often normal in ankylosing spondylitis.

Radiographic findings are helpful in the diagnosis. In the spine these include erosions at the vertebral corners and, vertebral squaring, calcification in the outer border of the annulus fibrosus (syndesmophyte) followed by calcification of the anterior longitudinal ligament and other ligamentous structures giving the characteristic bamboo spine appearance, and erosion and fusion at apophyseal and costochondral joints. The sacroiliac joints may show definite erosions, which may be manifested as irregular widening of the joint, areas of narrowing and sclerosis, and, later, fusion. Calcification of ligamentous structures, heel spurs, and costochondral erosion are a few of the other radiographic changes that may be seen.

No discussion of ankylosing spondylitis would be complete without mention of the genetic associations of this disorder. In various studies, 90 to 95 percent of Caucasian patients with ankylosing spondylitis have the histocompatibility antigen HLA-B27; a similar association exists for B27 and Reiter's syndrome. In contrast, HLA-B27 is found in only 6 to 8 percent of the control population. Epidemiologic studies suggest that 1 to 2 percent of the population have symptoms attributable to ankylosing spondylitis; one may then calculate an attack incidence of approximately 20 percent for the B27 positive population. Interestingly, in epidemics of Reiter's syndrome associated with bacterial agents, susceptibility is largely limited to B27 positive individuals, and the attack incidence among these is approximately 20 percent.

Clinically overt ankylosing spondylitis is predominantly a male disease. Subclinical or undiagnosed disease occurs with considerable frequency in women; similarly, there is a reservoir of low- grade disease—under the tip of the iceberg, so to speak—among B27 positive males. This is supported by the demonstration of radiographic evidence of sacroiliitis in B27 positive individuals who have not had symptoms of back pain requiring medical consultation. However, given the fact that approximately one of 14 individuals in the population is B27 positive, and given the high incidence of mechanical back pain in the population, a positive test for HLA-B27 does not sustain a diagnosis of ankylosing spondylitis. Indeed, in most instances testing for B27 is not diagnostically helpful.

Genetic linkage of a disorder raises questions in patients as to genetic transmission. Although half the children of B27 positive patients with ankylosing spondylitis are B27 positive, it is not clear that the risk of ankylosing spondylitis in these children is substantially greater than that in other B27 positive individuals. Although families with several cases of ankylosing spondylitis have been observed, it is clear that the disease is not transmitted in a typical mendelian dominant fashion. A key role for B27 per se, rather than a closely linked gene, is demonstrated by studies in transgenic animals. Introduction as a transgene of the human B27 gene into rats resulted in the development of spondyloarthropathy.

■ THERAPY

In the treatment of the arthritis of ankylosing spondylitis the goals are to provide pain relief and to limit deformity, thus providing maximal function. It is not clear that any therapy, with the possible exception of axial irradiation, halts the erosive, destructive, and ankylosing features of the disease. Nonetheless a program encompassing both anti-inflammatory therapy and physical therapy can prove of long-term benefit to the patient. If ankylosis of the spine or other joints is to occur, these measures can help to insure that joint fusion will occur in the best functional position. The patient in whom the hips are fused in flexion and who has severe dorsal kyphosis and anterior protrusion at the neck represents a failure of medical management.

Physical Measures

Physical measures and physical therapy should be directed at mitigating the deformities just outlined and maintaining maximal mobility of the spine and hips. The physician's role in this regard is educating the patient as to possible long-term consequences of the disease and the important role that the patient can play in treatment. Prolonged periods in any position are harmful, certainly in regard to immediate symptoms and probably long-term outcome as well. Jobs requiring prolonged periods of sitting in one place, particularly while stooping forward, as over a desk or workbench, aggravate forward displacement of the head and dorsal kyphosis. The patient should make a point of arising from a sitting position at least hourly for a short walk. Standing jobs similarly require frequent changes of position and intermittent exercise. When possible, raising the work surface to obviate the need for leaning forward is helpful. Long drives, in the course of either work or leisure, should be interrupted hourly for brief periods of standing, stretching, or walking.

Furniture should be chosen for proper support of the spine rather than for apparent immediate comfort. Chairs should be straight-backed and not deeply cushioned; furthermore, the patient should be instructed to sit with appropriate posture, not curled up or slouched. The patient should sleep on his back and not in a fetal position with hips flexed. Pillows should be thin and compressible, if used at all. Firm back support is essential; because one rarely encounters a patient who admits to anything other than a "firm" mattress, the most prudent course is to use a ¼ inch thickness of plywood even under "firm" mattresses.

"Physical therapy" should combine a generous measure of general physical activity along with specific exercises. Swimming provides excellent range of motion for most joints, including the spine, and at the same time protects joints from weight-bearing stress. In this respect it is perhaps the best form of general exercise for arthritis. Depending on the individual patient, the severity and activity of the disease, and pre-existing deformity, activities ranging from walking to vigorous competitive sports may be appropriate.

Specific exercises should be directed at maximizing the range of motion of the spine and other joints and counteracting the direction in which deformities tend to develop. In the latter regard, instruction should be provided in exercises to counter forward propulsion of the head, to extend the dorsal spine, and to extend the hips. Other exercises should be directed at improving motion of the spine in all planes: rotation, flexion-extension, and lateral flexion. Breathing exercises to maintain the capacity for full chest expansion are often overlooked. A commitment of time for training with a physical therapist who understands the disease and the goals of physical therapy in ankylosing spondylitis is a worthwhile investment for the patient.

Table 1 Nonsteroidal Anti-Inflammatory Drugs for Ankylosing Spondylitis*

DRUG	TOTAL DAILY DOSAGE	FREQUENCY OF ADMINISTRATION
Ibuprofen	2,400–3200 mg†	t.i.d.–q.i.d.
Indomethacin	100–200 mg	b.i.d.–t.i.d.
Diclofenac	150 mg	b.i.d.
Naproxen	750–1,500 mg	b.i.d.
Phenylbutazone	300–400 mg‡	t.i.d.–q.i.d.
Piroxicam	20 mg	t.d.
Sulindac	300–400 mg	b.i.d.
Tolectin	1,200–1,600 mg	t.i.d.–q.i.d.

This is not an all encompassing list but rather those with which the author has had experience.
†Dosages of 3,600 to 4,200 mg daily have been used: 3,200 mg represents upper limit of the officially recommended dosage.
‡400 mg only rarely required, may not be available.

Drug Management

The ability of the patient to function normally in day-to-day activities and to follow an outlined program of physical activity is dependent upon the control of the inflammatory process. To the extent that physical therapy protects from or limits spinal and joint deformity and disability, control of acute symptoms of pain and stiffness permits the execution of a physical program that, we hope, leads to better spine and joint function in the long term. Conversely, there is no evidence to indicate that anti-inflammatory therapy retards the destructive joint disease, and it is unlikely that ankylosis that would otherwise occur can be more than partially ameliorated.

Nonsteroidal anti-inflammatory drugs (NSAIDs) form the basis of therapy. The list of these drugs grows longer each year, and a comprehensive review of the benefits, side effects, and dollar cost of each is both beyond the scope of this article and unnecessary. Several general statements may be made. To varying degrees, all are effective in the management of ankylosing spondylitis. Indomethacin and phenylbutazone, in my experience and that of most others, are considerably more efficacious than other NSAIDs in most patients. Aspirin, for reasons that are unclear, is least effective in this disorder; this is in contrast with rheumatoid arthritis in which aspirin is effective on a par with all the newer NSAIDs. In general, the newer NSAIDs are equivalent to each other in effectiveness, although individual patients appear to respond better to one or another drug. In addition to effectiveness, both side effects and relative costs of the various drugs must be considered.

My preference is to initiate therapy with an NSAID other than indomethacin and phenylbutazone, which, though generally more effective, are associated with greater toxicity. It is important to use these drugs at an adequate dosage (Table 1); too commonly they are prescribed at the lowest recommended dosage and the erroneous conclusion is drawn that they are ineffective. Within the group of available drugs the choice is based on drug half-life and cost. Drugs with short half-lives are less effective in the management of morning stiffness, and the requirement for more frequent daily administration decreases compliance. It is important that patients take the drug around the clock and not only when they hurt. I would thus initiate treatment with a drug that requires no more than a three times daily dosage. It is worth advising the patient to check several pharmacies for relative cost as this may vary considerably in a given geographic area.

In my experience at least half the patients do not achieve sustained relief of symptoms with NSAIDs, even when taken at maximal therapeutic dosages. Most of these respond well to indomethacin. Taken at a dosage of 150 to 200 mg daily initially, indomethacin provides good relief from pain and stiffness. The patient should be cautioned to take the drug with meals to ameliorate headache, light headedness, and other neurologic symptoms. After an initial response the dosage of the drug may be tapered. It is not clear that sustained-release formulations of the drug greatly enhance its effectiveness, but the incidence and severity of side effects may be lower. In patients who do not respond to indomethacin, phenylbutazone is usually effective. Despite the potential for serious side effects (to be outlined), ankylosing spondylitis is one disorder in which use of this drug is clearly indicated.

Side Effects of Therapy

Many of the adverse effects of therapy are shared, to greater or lesser extent, by all the NSAIDs and are a direct result of the pharmacology of drug action. All these drugs inhibit prostaglandin (PG) synthesis, and PGE_2 prevents back-diffusion of hydrogen ion in the gastric mucosa; this effect may be related to the high frequency of gastric irritation and, in some patients, gastrointestinal (GI) ulceration or bleeding. Bleeding is promoted by the inhibitory effects of these drugs on platelet function via inhibition of thromboxane and PGE synthesis. In patients with pre-existent gastric or duodenal ulcers, exacerbation of symptoms, new ulceration, and GI bleeding should be carefully watched for. Some patients cannot tolerate any of the NSAIDs without the concomitant use of antacids, H_2-antagonists, or cytoprotective drugs. These, however, should not be used as a routine adjunct of NSAID therapy in most patients.

Like the GI side effects, renal toxicity may result from pharmacologic effects of the drug. Inhibition of renal prostaglandin synthesis results in decreased renal blood flow, an effect that is most often of clinical consequence in the elderly and those with pre-existent renal disease. The pharmacologic decrease in renal blood flow, however, is reversible, and a mild stable increase in the serum creatinine level should not require drug discontinuation. Sulindac, which is administered as a prodrug and not metabolized efficiently to an active metabolite in the kidney, appears to be associated with a lower incidence of decreased renal function.

More serious is the infrequent development of irreversible and, in rare instances, fatal renal disease. This has been reported with the majority, if not all, of the NSAIDs, is apparently due to an idiosyncratic reaction, and is usually manifested histologically as interstitial nephritis. Elderly patients and those with pre-existent renal disease may be at greater risk for the development of this side effect as well. In addition to the shared side effects already noted, individual drugs have unique but generally not serious side effects.

Indomethacin and phenylbutazone, because of their unique role in the treatment of ankylosing spondylitis and because of their generally greater toxicity, should be discussed separately. As noted, indomethacin causes neurologic side effects that are more pronounced in the elderly but are seen in all age groups, particularly when the drug is taken on an empty stomach. Thrombocytopenia has been reported as a consequence of indomethacin treatment, and platelet counts should be checked every few months, at least initially. Indomethacin is generally more gastric irritative than other NSAIDs, and gastric bleeding may be seen. Despite these side effects, indomethacin is a singularly useful drug in the management of ankylosing spondylitis.

Phenylbutazone is also associated with a greater frequency and severity of gastric intolerance than other NSAIDs and in my experience is associated with a greater frequency of GI bleeding. Phenylbutazone may cause sodium retention to an extent sufficient to precipitate cardiac failure. Most worrying to many are the reported instances of agranulocytosis and general bone marrow depression due to this drug. Estimates suggest that this complication occurs in one of 10,000 treated patients each year and that half the reactions are fatal. For many patients, however, phenylbutazone is the only drug that provides relief from symptoms and allows physical mobility and function; the physician and patient therefore must weigh these benefits against the potential risk. If therapy with phenylbutazone is instituted, hematologic parameters should be followed regularly. Once an initial response is achieved, the patient may be able to be managed with another drug. Unfortunately, efforts to limit the widespread use of phenylbutazone for other conditions have resulted in difficulty in obtaining it for spondylitis.

Corticosteroids and Immunosuppressive Drugs

There is no demonstrated benefit from corticosteroids in the management of spinal disease in ankylosing spondylitis. Occasional patients with peripheral arthritis may benefit from brief courses of steroids in low dosages (5 to 15 mg of prednisone daily) to suppress disease activity. When single peripheral joints are a persistent problem, intra-articular steroid instillation may be beneficial. Immunosuppressive drugs have not been shown to have a place in the treatment of ankylosing spondylitis. One exception may be in the rare patient who has predominant peripheral disease in whom weekly low-dose methotrexate (5 to 15 mg) may be tried. This approach is directed by analogy to Reiter's syndrome and psoriatic arthritis, as there is no published experience with methotrexate in ankylosing spondylitis. Whether axial disease might also respond to methotrexate is unknown, and I have had no experience in this regard.

Evidence from controlled studies suggests that sulfasalazine is beneficial in the treatment of ankylosing spondylitis. It is clear that some patients show significant improvement with sulfasalazine therapy, while others are unresponsive. The mechanism of action of the drug is unknown. Gastrointestinal toxicity may be a limiting factor in therapy.

Irradiation

Irradiation of the axial skeleton can ameliorate spinal arthritis. This modality of treatment has been largely abandoned after reports of leukemia in patients with ankylosing spondylitis who had received irradiation. Nonetheless, in the patient who cannot tolerate any of the NSAIDs (e.g., because of activation of peptic ulcer disease), irradiation may be the only therapeutic intervention that will enable the patient to function. Administration of 400 to 600 rads to the axial skeleton over two sessions may provide good relief while leading to lower risks than previously encountered with higher dosages of radiation.

Surgery

The most common surgical procedure required in patients with ankylosing spondylitis is total hip replacement to correct or prevent hip ankylosis. These patients unfortunately have a tendency to develop periarticular calcium deposition and reankylosis following total hip replacement. The frequency of reankylosis has varied among different series, and the possibility of ankylosis should not preclude total hip replacement which is otherwise indicated. Surgery to correct spinal deformity is of limited utility and should not be attempted unless the deformity markedly limits function and the surgeon has had experience with these patients. There has been some experience with spinal osteotomy to correct severe kyphosis. Finally, it should be noted that many patients with ankylosing spondylitis, owing to a failure of diagnosis, have undergone surgical procedures for low back pain. The clinician should entertain the diagnosis of ankylosing spondylitis in young men with back disease and protect them from surgical procedures that will provide no therapeutic benefit.

Extra-Articular Disease

Most extra-articular disease manifestations are not readily amenable to therapy. Thus, the cardiac abnormalities of conduction disturbances and aortitis have not been treated medically except for control of arrhythmias; aortic valve replacement may be necessary, depending on the hemodynamic consequences of the lesion. There is little published experience about treatment of the pulmonary fibrotic lesion; although occasionally cavitary, it is more commonly a mild fibrosis. Acute iritis requires the use of topical corticosteroid therapy.

■ PATIENT EDUCATION

As with other disorders, taking the time to explain the disease to the patient—what we know about its course and its treatment, what the patient is free to do and what he should avoid, and how even if a disease is incurable, that does not mean that it is untreatable—is critically important. This is often best done over a period of several office visits rather than all at one time during the first encounter. Questions about the hereditary nature of the disease and the risk in offspring should be discussed frankly. Finally, in the course of a chronic disease it is a rare patient who does not seek second, third, or more opinions. This option should be discussed with the patient openly both so that care can be coherent and coordinated and so that the patient may be referred to knowledgeable specialists (lists are usually available from the local Arthritis Foundation). Otherwise many patients will find those who promise cures from diet, vitamins, enemas, or magic drugs, treatments that will have a great impact on the patient's wealth but no beneficial effect on his health.

Suggested Reading

Calin A, Fries JF. Striking prevalance of ankylosing spondylitis in healthy W27 positive males and females. N Engl J Med 1975; 293:835–839.

Calin A, Porta J, Fries JF. The clinical history as a screening test for ankylosing spondylitis. JAMA 1977; 237:2613–2617.

Carette S, Graham D, Little H, Rubenstein J, Rosen P. The natural disease course of ankylosing spondylitis. Arthritis Rheum 1983; 26:186–190.

Clegg DO, Reda DJ, Weisman MH, et al. Comparison of sulfasalazine and placebo in the treatment of ankylosing spondylitis. Arthritis Rheum 1996; 39:2004–2012.

Hammer RE, Maika SD, Richardson JA, et al. Spontaneous inflammatory disease in transgenic rats expressing HLA-B27 and human beta 2m: an animal model of HLA-B27-associated human disorders. Cell 1990; 63:1099–1112.

SJÖGREN'S SYNDROME

Juan-Manuel Anaya, M.D.
Norman Talal, M.D.

Sjögren's syndrome (SS) is a chronic autoimmune disease characterized by a progressive lymphocytic and plasma cell infiltration of the salivary and lachramal glands leading to xerostomia and xerophthalmia (sicca complex). SS is associated with the production of rheumatoid factor and other autoantibodies including anti-Ro/SSA and anti-La/SSB. The spectrum of the disease extends from an organ-specific autoimmune disorder (autoimmune exocrinopathy) to a systemic process. Despite being a "benign" autoimmune process, adult patients with SS are known to have increased risk of developing lymphoma.

SS may occur alone (primary SS) or in association with almost all of the autoimmune diseases (secondary SS). Prevalence of SS in the general population is nearly 2 percent. Although SS can occur in patients of all ages, it affects primarily females during the fourth and fifth decades of life with a female-male ratio of 9:1.

The clinical presentation of SS may be quite variable. Sicca complex is the main clinical presentation in adults, whereas in children swelling of the parotid glands is the most common symptom. Xerostomia, xerophthalmia, and swelling of the

Table 1 Differential Diagnosis of Oral and Ocular Involvement in Sjögren's Syndrome

PAROTID GLAND SWELLING	XEROSTOMIA	XEROPHTHALMIA
Infectious	**Infectious**	**Drugs**
Viral	**Drugs**	**Ocular diseases**
Mumps	Psychotherapeutic	Chronic conjunctivitis
Influenza	Parasympatholytic	Bullous dermatitis
Epstein-Barr	Beta-blockers	Chronic blepharatis
Coxsackie virus	Phenylbutazone	Blink abnormality
Cytomegalovirus	**Psychogenic**	**Senile xerophthalmia**
HIV	**Dehydration**	**Neurologic diseases**
Bacterial*	**Congenital**	V and VII cranial nerve involvement
Streptococcus	**Senile xerostomia**	**Hypovitaminosis A**
Staphylococcus	**Oral breathing**	**Virus**
Salmonella	**Neurologic diseases**	Epstein-Barr
Actinomyces	Multiple sclerosis	HIV
Tuberculosis	Parkinson's disease	HTLV-1
Sarcoidosis	**Irradiation**	**Graft-vs-host disease**
Amyloidosis		**Cystic fibrosis**
Metabolic/endocrine		**Diabetes mellitus**
Hyperlipoproteinemias		
Chronic pancreatitis		
Cystic fibrosis		
Hepatic cirrhosis		
Diabetes mellitus		
Acromegaly		
Malnutrition		
Hypovitaminosis A, B_6, C		
Recurrent parotitis of childhood*		
Tumors*		

*May be unilateral.

parotid glands may be observed in other conditions summarized in Table 1. These conditions must be excluded before a diagnosis of SS is made.

DIAGNOSIS

Many diagnostic tests exist to assess salivary and lachrymal involvement in SS. Although there is no worldwide consensus regarding the diagnostic criteria for SS, we use the validated European diagnostic criteria (Table 2). In addition to subjective symptoms of xerostomia and xerophthalmia, an assessment of oral and ocular involvement is considered essential to the diagnosis of SS. The degree of oral and ocular involvement is measured using several parameters, such as the quantity and quality of secretions and morphologic changes in the glands. A test for autoantibodies (rheumatoid factor, antinuclear antibodies, anti-Ro/SSA, and anti-La/SSB) should be performed on every patient suspected of SS. However, some primary SS patients may lack these autoantibodies.

Secretions can be measured quantitatively by Schirmer's test for the eye and by collecting saliva from the mouth. The Schirmer's test, in which a strip of Whatman No. 41 filter paper is folded and placed in the lower conjunctival sac, is a simple measure of tear production. A positive test is considered when patients moistened less than 5 mm of the test paper after 5 minutes of the test. A more reliable diagnostic sign for xerophthalmia is the rose Bengal score (RBS) performed by placing 25 μl rose Bengal solution in the inferior fornix of each eye and asking the patient to make one to two full blinks. The number of red spots formed are counted and scored: 1+ (sparsely scattered), 2+ (densely scattered), or 3+ (confluent) in lateral and nasal conjunctiva and the cornea. The sum of scores from the three regions of one eye form the RBS of that eye and define the presence of keratoconjunctivitis sicca (KCS). A score greater than or equal to 4 in at least one eye is considered abnormal.

Unstimulated whole saliva collection should be performed in the morning. Patients should not be allowed to eat or drink, brush their teeth, rinse their mouth, or smoke tobacco 1 hour prior to the procedure. Saliva is collected in conical calibrated tubes for 15 minutes. The normal limit is greater than 1.5 ml of saliva. Other tests used to evaluate salivary gland involvement in SS are parotid sialography and salivary gland scintigraphy.

Minor salivary gland biopsy is the test most widely used as a specific diagnostic criterion for the salivary component of SS. Site of biopsy (through histologically normal oral mucosa) and size of biopsy (at least four evaluable salivary gland lobules) are essential for analysis to yield interpretable results. The characteristic histopathologic feature in SS labial salivary glands is the presence of focal lymphocytic sialadenitis in all or most of the glands. Focal lymphocytic sialadenitis (FLS) has been defined as multiple, dense aggregates of 50 or more lymphocytes (one focus) in perivascular or periductal locations. The FLS is graded in focus score, meaning the number of foci per 4 mm^2. A focus score of 10 is generally the highest value that can be counted before foci become confluent. A

Table 2 European Criteria for the Diagnosis of Sjögren's Syndrome

(Patients must meet 4 of 6 criteria in the absence of pre-existing lymphoma, acquired immunodeficiency, sarcoidosis, or graft-versus-host disease)

1. **Ocular symptoms**
   Definition: A positive response to at least one of the following:
   a. Have you had daily, persistent, troublesome dry eyes for more than 3 months?
   b. Do you have a recurrent sensation of sand or gravel in the eyes?
   c. Do you use tear substitutes more than three times a day?
2. **Oral symptoms**
   Definition: A positive response to at least one of the following:
   a. Have you had a daily feeling of dry mouth for more than 3 months?
   b. Have you had recurrent or persistently swollen salivary glands as an adult?
   c. Do you frequently drink liquids to aid in swallowing dry foods?
3. **Ocular signs**
   Definition: A positive result on at least one of the following two tests:
   a. Schirmer test (<5 mm in 5 minutes)
   b. Rose Bengal score (>4)
4. **Histopathologic features**
   Definition: Focus score >1 on minor salivary gland biopsy
5. **Salivary gland involvement**
   Definition: A positive result on at least one of the following three tests:
   a. Salivary scintigraphy
   b. Parotid sialography
   c. Unstimulated salivary flow (<1.5 ml in 15 minutes)
6. **Autoantibodies**
   Definition: Presence of at least one of the following:
   a. Anti-Ro/SSA or anti-La/SSB
   b. Antinuclear antibodies
   c. Rheumatoid factor

value of 12 is assigned to those specimens having two or more glands with confluent lymphocytic infiltration. A focus score greater than one focus per 4 mm^2 has a specificity of 95 percent and a sensitivity of 63 percent in the diagnosis of SS. Inaccurate methods in biopsies and failure to record the focus score are common problems with this technique.

No single test measuring oral or ocular involvement is sufficiently sensitive and specific to form the basis for diagnosis of SS. Tear secretion and saliva production may be physiologically reduced in elderly patients. Also, FSL may be observed in other conditions different from SS. Therefore, only the simultaneous positivity of various tests in conjunction with the presence of subjective symptoms and serologic abnormalities allow sufficient accuracy in the diagnosis of SS.

■ TREATMENT

Sjögren's syndrome is often a neglected disease, adding greatly to the distress of the patient. The physician must remember that there is nothing minor about dryness of the eye and mouth, as well as dryness of other mucosal surfaces. Patients with SS should be seen regularly by a rheumatologist, an ophthalmologist, and a dentist. Patients should also be properly informed about the nature of their illness and the goals of therapy. Patients with SS should be followed closely for significant functional deterioration, significant changes in the course of the disease, or the appearance of symptoms attributable to drug side effects or comorbid conditions (i.e., depression, fibromyalgia).

Treatment of Glandular Disease

Dry Eyes

The patient may notice accumulation of thick ropy secretions along the inner canthus owing to a decreased tear film and an abnormal mucous component. Related complaints include erythema, photosensitivity, eye fatigue, decreased visual acuity, and the sensation of a "film" across the field of vision. Desiccation can cause small superficial erosions of the corneal epithelium. In severe cases, slit lamp examination may reveal filamentary keratitis (filaments of corneal epithelium and debris). Other complications may include conjunctivitis caused by *Staphylococcus aureus.*

Low levels of humidity in air-conditioned environments may worsen symptoms. Similar problems arise in windy or dry climates, in patients who either smoke cigarettes or are exposed to cigarette smoke, and in patients taking drugs with anticholinergic side effects. The most implicated drugs are phenothiazines, tricyclic antidepressants, antispasmodics, antiparkinsonian, and decongestant medications.

The mainstay of treatment for dry eyes is lubrication through the use of artificial tear drops, which may be used as often as necessary (generally once every 1 to 3 hours). Varieties of such drops are available without prescription, differing primarily in viscosity and preservative (Table 3). The thicker, more viscous drops require less frequent application, although they may cause blurring and leave a residue on the lashes. Many patients prefer thinner drops, which require more frequent applications. An apparent failure to respond to artificial tears may be indicative of eye irritation caused by the topical application of preservatives such as benzalkonium chloride, chlorobutanol, or thimerosal. Also available are lubricating ointments that may produce significant blurring and are best used at night to provide protection over a longer period of time (Table 4).

Other steps may be taken to preserve tears if tear substitutes are insufficient to control symptoms. Water tight swimmer's goggles can be very helpful in creating a moisture chamber effect by preventing evaporation. Goggles also protect against wind and dust particles. The same effect can be achieved with ordinary food plastic wrap taped over the eyes. Commercial "bubble" bandages are also available.

Punctual occlusion is another method of conserving the few tears that SS patients produce. This procedure should be considered only in severe cases. Stents have been devised as nonsurgical means of occlusion; this is a good way to predict the success of surgical occlusion.

Sympathomimetics and parasympathomimetics serve to stimulate tear flow. Pilocarpine administered either orally or topically to the eye has been reported to be successful. In patients with a relative excess of mucin production and formation of filaments, a mucolytic agent such as acetylcysteine has been found to be useful. However, other investigators have failed to confirm this. The use of topical steroids for

Table 3 Artifical Tear Preparations (Demulcents)

MAJOR COMPONENTS	TRADE NAME	PRESERVATIVE
Hydroxyethylcellulose	Tear Guard	Sorbic acid + edetate disodium
Hydroxypropylcellulose	Lacrisert (Rx)	Benzalkonium chloride + edetate disodium (water-soluble insert)
Hydroxypropyl methylcellulose	Lacril	Chlorobutanol
	Moisture Drops (0.5%)	Benzalkonium chloride
	Tears Renewed	Benzalkonium + edetate disodium
Carboxymethylcellulose	Cellufresh (0.5%)	Preservative free
	Celluvisc (1%) (unit dose)	Preservative free
	Gum cellulose (Rx) (0.3%, 0.625%, 0.9%)	Unpreserved; refrigerate after opening
Polyvinyl alcohol	Liquifilm Tears	Chlorobutanol
	Liquifilm Forte	Thimersol + edetate disodium
	Dakrina	Potassium sorbate + EDTA
	Dwelle	Potassium sorbate + EDTA
	Nutratear	Benzalkonium 0.004% + 0.08% EDTA
Polyvinyl alcohol and povidone	Refresh (unit dose)	Preservative free
Other Polymeric Systems	Comfort Drops	Benzalkonium chloride + edetate disodium
	Hypotears	Benzalkonium chloride + edetate disodium
	Hypotears P.F. (unit dose)	Preservative free
	Tears Naturale	Benzalkonium chloride + edetate disodium
	Tears Naturale II	Polyquad
	Tears Natural Free (unit dose)	Preservative free
Sterile saline	Unisol	Preservative free
Methylcellulose 1%	Murocel	Methylparaben 0.023% + Propylparaben 0.01%

Table 4 Other Products for Dry Eyes

TRADE NAME	COMPOSITION
OCULAR EMOLLIENTS	
Akwa-Tears Ointment	Petrolatum, liquid lanolin, mineral oil
Duolube	Sterile ointment containing white petrolatum and mineral oil
Duratears	Sterile ointment containing white petrolatum, liquid lanolin, mineral oil, methylparaben, and polyparaben
Hypotears	Sterile ointment containing white petrolatum and light mineral oil
Acri-Lube S.O.P.	Sterile ointment with 42.5% mineral oil, 55% white petrolatum, lanolin, and chlorobutanol
*Refresh P.M.	White petrolatum, mineral oil, lanolin, purified water, sodium chloride
SPECIAL PREPARATIONS AND EQUIPMENT FOR THE EYE	
EV Lid Cleanser II	Mild cleansing formula for eyelid and delicate skin
EV Lid Cleanser Kit	Includes pads and cleaning lotion
EV Lid Cleanser Travel Pak	½ oz cleanser and 10 pads
Clearclenz	Sterile eyelid cleanser
Opticrom (Rx)	Cromolyn sodium solution for allergic manifestations
Vistacrom	Cromolyn sodium solution for allergic manifestations
I-Scrub	Eyelid cleanser
OCuSOFT	Lid scrub lotion and pads
Medicool Medication Protector	Case and holder in which to carry preservative-free eyedrops or other medications that should be kept refrigerated
Moist Eye Moisture Panels	Can be fitted to most configurations of eyewear to create a moisture chamber
Muro-128	Hypertonic sodium chloride 5% and 7% for corneal edema

corneal ulcers of SS was associated with a worsening clinical course and is not recommended.

Dry Mouth

Xerostomia is often the initial symptom of SS. However, it is a common and subjective clinical complaint with a large variety of etiologies (see Table 1). Patients with dry mouths have various complaints. The "cracker sign" describes the difficulties such patients encounter when trying to eat dry foods without sufficient lubrication. Additional features include oral soreness, adherence of food to buccal surfaces, fissuring of the tongue, and dysphagia. Dental caries may also appear, as well as angular cheilitis associated with superimposed candidiasis. Patients may lose their ability to discriminate foods on the basis of taste and smell.

Treatment of xerostomia associated with SS is difficult. Currently, there is no single method that is completely effective. Treatment of oral SS should include (1) methods to

Table 5 Products for the Dry Mouth

TRADE NAME	COMPOSITION
SALIVA SUBSTITUTES	
Mouthkote	Citrus flavor in spray bottle with Mucroprotective Factor
Oral Balance	Moisturing gel
Orex	Squirt bottle; several flavors
Salivart	Pressurized container; can use with one hand
Xero-Lube	Regular 6 oz pump container; some patients recommend diluting slightly with water. Mint flavor available in ½ oz squirt container
Evian mineral water spray	Other mineral waters can be used the same way
SPECIAL TOOTHPASTES AND MOUTHWASHES	
Aquafresh for kids	Contains sodium monofluorophosphate; sugarless (sorbitol main sweetener)
Biotene toothpaste	Contains glucoseoxidase/lactoperoxidase
Biotene mouthwash	Alcohol free
Crest for kids	Contains fluoristat
Saline solution	Mouth rinse; breaks up thick mucus
Alkalol	Mucolytic agent; mouth rinse and nasal douche
PRODUCTS THAT STIMULATE SALIVARY FLOW	
Biotene chewing gum	Contains glucoseoxidase/lactoperoxidase sweetened with xylitol
Extra sugarless gum	Contains Nutrasweet; several flavors, including peppermint, spearmint, winter fresh, bubble gum
Oralbalance	Soothing gel
Pro-Flow	Stimulates saliva; nonacidic
Sialor (Rx) (Anetholtrithion)	Stimulates salivary flow
Sugarless candies	To be sucked
Trident sugarless gum	Contains sorbitol; in Canada, available with xylitol; several flavors
Xylitol mints	To be sucked, not chewed
PRODUCTS TO SOOTHE THE ORAL MUCOSA AND/OR LIPS	
Blistex	
Boric Acid Ointment	Does not contain lanolin
Borofax	Contains boric acid ointment and lanolin; also good inside tips of nostrils
Mouthkote	Citric flavor in spray bottle with Mucoprotective Factor
Phen-oris	Medicated lip care
Smile lip moisturizer	
Vaseline	

increase salivary flow and selective use of saliva substitutes, (2) elimination or replacement of factors contributing to decreased salivary secretions (mouth breathing, heavy smoking, drugs), (3) prevention of dental caries and provision of ongoing dental treatment, and (4) diagnosis and treatment of oral candidiasis (Table 5). Most patients discover that it is helpful to carry water, sugarless lemon drops, or chewing gum. Fluids ad libitum should be utilized for all meals and snacks. The consumption of large amounts of water during the day, though symptomatically helpful, may produce nocturia that interrupts sleep patterns and leads to fatigue.

Artificial saliva substitutes offer some additional palliation. Mucin-containing saliva substitutes seem to be more effective than substitutes based on carboxymethylcellulose or polyethylenoxide. Mucins tend to protect against desiccation, provide for lubrication and cleaning, and have some antimicrobial effects. However, saliva substitutes should be used sparingly with only the minimum volume necessary for oral lubrication. This usually consists of no more than 2 ml before and after meals, at bedtime, and following oral hygiene.

Increased salivary flow rates may be induced by potassium iodide or parasympathomimetic agents such as pilocarpine or neostigmine, systemically or as a mouthwash. Varying degrees of success have been noted. Bromhexine, a synthetic alkaloid originally used as a mucolytic agent in cough syrups, has been tested with limited success. A new battery-powered electronic device for stimulating salivary flow (Salitron System) has been shown to be effective in stimulating increased production of saliva and in reducing the symptoms of xerostomia in SS patients.

Increased moisture to the upper airways by use of normal saline sprays and humidifiers at night may reduce respiratory symptoms and alleviate mouth breathing. During surgery, SS patients are at increased risk for corneal abrasions because of use of anticholinergic agents by the anesthesiologist and low humidity in the operating room. Also, a risk of atelectasis and pneumonia exists because of upper airway dryness and inspired mucous secretions. Therefore, the use of ocular lubricants, humidified oxygen, and respiratory therapy should help to minimize these potential complications.

Approximately one-half of all SS patients have parotid or other major salivary gland enlargement, often painless, recurrent, and bilateral. Salivary gland enlargement may be due to cellular infiltration or ductal obstruction. There is no effective treatment for parotid gland swelling related with SS, which is a mild, and usually self-limited condition. Methods to increase salivary flow (see Table 5) and local moist heat may be helpful in preventing ductal obstruction. Corticosteroids have transient efficacy, may favor infection, and therefore are not recommended. Local radiation treatment and/or cytotoxic drugs have no long-term efficacy and may increase the risk of malignancy. If the gland remains tender or enlarged, lymphoma must be ruled out. Superficial parotidectomy could be considered in these cases. Tenderness, fever, or erythema suggest superimposed infection, in which treatment includes penicillinase-resistant penicillins combined with beta-lactamase inhibitors (i.e., amoxicillin 500 mg, plus clavulanic acid 125 mg, every 8 hours orally for 7 days), local moist heat, and nonsteroidal anti-inflammatory drugs (NSAIDs).

Nose, Skin, and Vaginal Dryness

Dry nose may also be taken into consideration. In addition to the use of nasal solutions (Table 6), lavage of the sinus to remove crusted secretions allows the nasal passages to remain open and the patient to avoid mouth breathing which is a cause of xerostomia.

Dry skin and lips are common complaints in SS patients. Topical treatments with alcohol-free creams and moisturizing lotions are often helpful, as are cosmetics such as lipstick.

Vaginal dryness is often observed in female patients with SS, and may be a cause of dyspareunia. A gynecologic examination is useful to rule out other causes of vaginal dryness. The most frequent cause of vaginal dryness in perimenopausal or postmenopausal women is declining estrogen levels; therefore, vaginal estrogen creams should be advised. Vaginal yeast infection also must be ruled out and treated promptly. When vaginal dryness occurs as a part of SS, sterile lubricants are helpful (Table 7).

Table 6 Products and Devices to Soothe the Dry Nose and Dry Ear

TRADE NAME	COMPOSITION
Nasal irrigator	Attaches to Water-Pik; loosens dried up mucus; use with saline solution
Nasal douche	Loosens dried-up mucus; use with Alkalol or saline solution
Saline solution	Helps prevent nosebleeds
NaSal	Saline solution to prevent nosebleeds
Ocean	Saline solution to prevent nosebleeds
Salinex	Saline solution to prevent nosebleeds
AYR	Saline solution to prevent nosebleeds
Mineral oil	Use with Q-tip for dry ear

Treatment of Extraglandular Disease

In approximately 50 percent of patients with primary SS, an extraglandular manifestation (EGM) may develop during the evolution of the disease (Table 8). In some cases, one EGM may disclose the disease. Systemic manifestations or EGM seen in primary SS patients may lead to confusion regarding its diagnosis. Nevertheless, EGMs in primary SS are usually mild and sometimes subclinical, revealed only by careful examination. Systemic corticosteroids and immunosuppressive drugs are only used to treat potentially life-threatening disease often involving the lung or kidney. They are not recommended for the treatment of dry eyes and dry mouth. No controlled studies have been performed because relatively few patients require immunosuppressive treatment.

Musculoskeletal Manifestations

Arthralgia or arthritis may occur in 60 percent of patients with primary SS. The arthropathy of primary SS is essentially an intermittent polyarticular arthropathy affecting mostly small joints, sometimes asymmetrically. In most cases, sicca symptoms precede arthropathy in which course and prognosis are generally good. Joint deformity and mild erosions are unusual. Although myalgias are frequently observed, inflammatory muscle disease is confirmed in less than 10 percent of patients.

Musculoskeletal symptoms associated with primary SS respond well to NSAIDs. In cases in which NSAIDs fail to control arthritis, either hydroxychloroquine (6 mg per kilogram per day) or sulfasalazine (3 to 4 g daily in evenly divided oral doses) may be useful.

Pulmonary Involvement

Interstitial lung disease (ILD) is probably the most common functional abnormality identified in patients with primary SS and lung involvement, particularly in those with other EGMs. Obstructive disease is more prevalent in secondary SS to rheumatoid arthritis. It has been shown that over 30 percent of unselected primary SS patients have ILD, in which the majority of cases is subclinical. Fibrosing alveolitis is rare in SS. Lung involvement in SS may originate from the exocrine tissue at the bronchi and from bronchus-associated lymphoid tissue. However, its natural history and prognosis are not well known. Once the diagnosis of ILD is established, clinical assessment, radiographic, and pulmonary function tests

Table 7 Products for Vaginal Dryness

TRADE NAME	COMPOSITION
Astroglide	Provides light lubrication
Estrace Vaginal Cream (Rx)	Synthetic human estrogen
H-R lubricating jelly	Lubricating jelly
K-Y lubricating jelly	Lubricating jelly
Lubrin vaginal inserts	Unscented precoital suppositories
Maxilube	Thickest of the vaginal lubricants
Premarin vaginal cream (Rx)	Conjugated estrogens
Replens	Unit dose applicator filled with polycarbophil
Surgilube	Lubricating jelly
Vitamin E oil, cream, or capsules	For topical application to labia (capsules must be pierced, but are the cheapest form)

should be performed and monitored twice per year to determine the extent of functional impairment. High-resolution computed tomography is useful when open-lung or transbronchial biopsy is planned identifying areas of thickened bronchial walls and alveolitis. These sites often yield more useful histologic information than do areas of fibrotic disease. Lung biopsy should be performed before treatment is started. There is a better chance for therapeutic success if a highly cellular infiltrate is found.

The therapy of progressive ILD, regardless of the agent used, requires 3 to 6 months before its effectiveness can be assessed. Treatment is usually initiated with corticosteroids in the range of 1 to 2 mg per kilogram per day. High-dose intravenous corticosteroid treatment (pulse therapy) may be used at the beginning of treatment or in patients with aggressive and severe disease in hopes of arresting progression (usually methylprednisolone, 10 to 15 mg per kilogram per day IV for 3 days). The reasons for varied patient response to corticosteroids is still poorly understood. Determining whether treatment is producing the desired effect may be difficult. A composite clinical, roentgenographic, and physiologic score (CRP score) has been developed allowing a quantification of the clinical course and the impact of therapy in individual patients. As a patient improves, the dose of steroids may be tapered to a maintenance level of 50 percent of the starting dose. If there is no apparent response within 3 to 6 months, azathioprine should be added in addition to low-dose prednisone. The recommended dose of azathioprine is 2 mg per kilogram per day. Cyclophosphamide may succeed when azathioprine has been tried first and failed. Monthly bolus (0.5 to 1 g per square meter), instead of daily oral cyclophosphamide (2 mg per kilogram), may be administered to reduce the risk of side effects. The duration of immunosuppressive therapy has not been established, but conventional use is generally over the course of several months. Thereafter, a low oral maintenance dose should be attempted. Cyclophosphamide bolus may be administered quarterly for a period of 1 year. Although the risk of lymphoma is an important consideration, in our experience it has not appeared in SS patients treated with cyclophosphamide.

Table 8 Extraglandular Manifestations of Primary Sjögren's Syndrome

Musculoskeletal (40%–60%)	**Pulmonary (10%–30%)**
Arthralgias/arthritis	Xerotrachea
Myalgias/myositis	Interstitial lung disease
Vascular/Skin (30%)	Obstructive lung disease
Photosensitivity	Lymphoma
Vasculitis:	**Gastrointestinal (5%–10%)**
Cutaneous	Dysphagia
Systemic	Atrophic gastritis
Raynaud's phenomenon	Pancreatitis
Thyroiditis (30%)	Autoimmune hepatitis
Renal (5%–20%)	**Hematologic (5%–20%)**
Interstitial nephritis	Anemia
Renal tubular acidosis	Leukopenia (lymphopenia)
Glomerulonephritis	Hypergammaglobulinemia
Neurologic (Rare)	Monoclonal gammopathy
Peripheral and central nervous systems involvement	Cryoglobulinemia
	Lymphadenopathy
	Splenomegaly
	Lymphoma

Vascular Involvement

Raynaud's phenomenon may be observed in nearly 30 percent of patients with primary SS generally associated with other EGMs. The course of Raynaud's phenomenon in SS is usually mild. Treatment includes the use of gloves in colder seasons, and either nifedipine or diltiazem.

Vasculitis may be observed in diseases which SS is associated, such as rheumatoid arthritis and systemic lupus erythematosus. In primary SS, vasculitis may occur in two forms: cutaneous vasculitis or systemic necrotizing vasculitis. Vasculitis limited to the skin may occur in about 30 percent of patients with primary SS, and manifest as purpura (palpable or not) or urticaria-like lesions. Leukocytoblastic vasculitis is the most frequent histologic finding. This form of vasculitis requires no specific therapy. Measures avoiding orthostatism may be helpful. In some patients with longstanding cutaneous vasculitis, low-dose steroids, colchicine, or pentoxyfylline have been used empirically with variable success.

Systemic necrotizing vasculitis is rare in primary SS. It is often associated with mixed cryoglobulinemia. It manifests as ulcerative skin lesions, digital gangrene, mononeuritis multiplex, myositis, and glomerulonephritis. Due to the seriousness of such systemic vasculitis, steroids, cyclophosphamide, and plasmapheresis are the recommended treatment.

Renal Involvement

The renal abnormalities in primary SS arise as a result of either lymphocytic infiltration in the renal parenchyma or immune complex deposition in the glomeruli. Interstitial nephritis in SS is usually mild and subclinical. When clinically detectable, the most common presentations are diminished urinary concentrating ability, and distal (type 1) renal tubular acidosis (RTA). Proximal (type 2) RTA can also occur, although less frequently. Hyposthenuria may be treated by hydric restriction (often difficult in SS patients) or low-dose thiazides. Type 1 acidosis is treated with sodium bicarbonate tablets (0.5 to 2.0 mmol per kilogram in 4 to 5 divided doses daily). In addition, low-dose steroids (0.1 mg per kilogram per day) may be useful.

Renal insufficiency resulting from interstitial nephritis is extremely rare in SS. Steroids and cyclophosphamide have been used empirically with good results in almost all cases. However, some patients require prolonged periods of treatment to maintain normal renal function. Glomerulonephritis is rare in primary SS. Its presence should raise the possibility of systemic vasculitis or an associated condition such as systemic lupus erythematosus.

Lymphoma

Benign polyclonal lymphocytic and plasma cell proliferation localized in exocrine glands may progress into monoclonal malignant lymphoma. The term *pseudolymphoma* has been used to describe an intermediate stage between benign to malignant lymphoproliferation. Histologically tumor-like aggregates of lymphoid cells that do not meet the histologic criteria for malignancy characterize pseudolymphoma. Although monoclonality may occur, lymphocytes eluted from pseudolymphoma biopsies are predominantly polyclonal T cells and contain a small percentage of B cells. When pseudolymphoma is suspected, low-grade B-cell lymphoma, including mucosal-associated lymphoid tissue (MALT) lymphoma, should be ruled out.

Clinical aspects relevant to lymphoma evolution include persistent enlargement of parotid glands, spleen, and lymph nodes. In addition, cough, dyspnea on exertion, mediastinal or hilar lymph nodes, unilaterally localized nodules in the lungs, and persistent Raynaud's phenomenon may also indicate malignancy evolution. Laboratory findings of the appearance of monoclonal gammopathy and mixed cryoglobulinemia, lowered IgM, high-serum beta$_2$-microglobulin, and negative rheumatoid factor (having been positive), all suggest the presence of underlying malignancy.

Prevalence of clinically identifiable lymphoma in SS patients is nearly 5 percent. Malignant lymphoproliferation may be present initially or may develop later in the illness. Most lymphomas complicating SS belong to the B-cell lineage, are of either low- or intermediate-grade malignancy, and are localized in extranodal areas (gastrointestinal tract, thyroid, lung, kidney, orbit, salivary glands). Recent studies have suggested good prognosis for SS-associated lymphoma and have also implied a less aggressive approach to therapy than in the past. Patients with low-grade lymphomas affecting exocrine glands should be completely evaluated for the extent of the disease and, if the disease is localized, a "wait-and-watch" policy should be undertaken. In the case of histologically high-grade and clinically aggressive malignancy, then combination chemotherapy is recommended, and patients should be assessed by a cooperative team with an oncologist.

Treatment of Associated Conditions

Although hypothyroidism is frequently associated with SS, most of the cases are subclinical. Nevertheless, hypothyroidism may be one of the causes of common fatigue observed in SS patients. Substitution therapy is advised when hormone deficiency is confirmed.

Fibromyalgia is a frequent comorbid condition observed in patients with SS and in other connective tissue diseases, including systemic lupus erythematosus and rheumatoid arthritis. Why fibromyalgia is becoming the most frequent rheumatologic disease remains poorly understood. Patients with fibromyalgia may also have chronic fatigue syndrome (CFS), irritable bowel syndrome (IBS), sleep disorder, or depression. The presence of fibromyalgia is not associated with the severity nor the activity of SS. On the other hand, some patients with fibromyalgia, IBS, and CFS may present sicca symptoms, Raynaud's phenomenon, and positive antinuclear antibodies. Some of these patients may have hypothyroidism. In the absence of clear evidence of a connective tissue disease, patients must be informed about the absence of "systemic" involvement in "primary" fibromyalgia, IBS, or CFS.

Treatment of fibromyalgia includes patient education, physical therapy, and an appropriate use of analgesic (usually NSAIDs). Ensuring a patient's own responsibility for the treatment may be critical. Possible environmental factors, including occupational, social, economic and psychological and/or psychosomatic factors should be identified. Measures should be taken against poor physiologic fitness and sleep disturbances. Patients should work toward a balance between rest and aerobic activity over several months.

When antidepressant medication is indicated, drugs that have no anticholinergic side effects are recommended (e.g., fluoxetine, trazodone). Interferon-α (INF-α) has been experimentally used in patients with fibromyalgia. Also, because some patients with hepatitis C virus (HCV) infection may present with sicca symptoms, INF-α has been used in SS patients with positive serology for HCV, regardless of the HCV-associated cryoglobulinemia. However, there is no clear evidence that HCV causes SS, and there is no controlled study using INF-α in SS. Further, since INF-α may induce autoimmune conditions, one should be prudent about its use in SS.

Treatment of secondary SS is usually directed at the associated disease. The treatment of rheumatoid arthritis or systemic lupus erythematosus is not altered because of the concomitant presence of SS. The clinical expression of secondary SS is generally milder and managed as already discussed.

Acknowledgments

We would like to thank our colleagues Drs. Hanna Abboud and Randal Otto for helpful suggestions, and George Tye Liu for his help in the preparation of the manuscript. Funded by the RGK Foundation (Austin, TX).

Suggested Reading

Fox PC, Datiles M, Atkinson JC, et al. Prednisone and piroxicam for treatment of primary Sjögren's syndrome. Clin Exp Rheumatol 1993; 11: 149–156.

Fox RI. Treatment of the patient with Sjögren's syndrome. Rheum Dis Clin North Am 1992; 18:699–709.

Kruize AA, Hené RJ, Kallenberg CGM, et al. Hydroxychloroquine treatment for primary Sjögren's syndrome: a two-year double-blind crossover trial. Ann Rheum Dis 1993; 52:360–364.

Moutsopoulos HM, Vlachoyiannopoulos PG. What would I do if I had Sjögren's syndrome. Rheumatol Rev 1993; 2:17.

Talal N. Clinical and pathogenetic aspects of Sjögren's syndrome. Semin Clin Immunol 1993; 6:11–20.

Talal N, Quinn JH, Daniels TE. The clinical effects of electrostimulation on salivary function of Sjögren's syndrome patients. A placebo-controlled study. Rheumatol Int 1992; 12:43–45.

SYSTEMIC NECROTIZING VASCULITIS

Rex M. McCallum, M.D.
Barton F. Haynes, M.D.

Systemic necrotizing vasculitis comprises a group of clinical syndromes characterized by blood vessel inflammation with resultant vessel injury and organ ischemia. Since inflammation may affect any vessel in the body, the clinical manifestations of the systemic vasculitides are varied and frequently confusing. Systemic necrotizing vasculitis also has a broad range of manifestations from isolated mild cutaneous disease to life-threatening multisystem organ failure. Making a diagnosis of systemic necrotizing vasculitis requires a high degree of clinical suspicion and, frequently, invasive procedures such as angiography and/or tissue biopsy. Ideally, such procedures should be performed before instituting immunosuppressive therapy, which may alter histologic and angiographic patterns.

Despite the heterogeneous nature of systemic necrotizing vasculitis syndromes, several well-characterized clinical entities have been described by studying the histologic pattern of the vessel inflammation, size of the involved vessels, pattern of organ system involvement, and associated clinical abnormalities. With the diagnosis of systemic necrotizing vasculitis, attempted classification into a specific vasculitic syndrome should follow. While the nosology of systemic necrotizing vasculitis continues to evolve, the present classification scheme does have prognostic significance, provides information on preferred therapy, suggests therapeutic alternatives, and suggests associated clinical concerns (Table 1). In addition, defining the extent of vasculitic involvement (severity and number of organ systems involved) and understanding the tempo of the illness is important in clarifying the appropriate intensity of therapeutic intervention, defining the timeliness of treatment, and minimizing treatment-associated morbidity.

The primary focus of this chapter is the treatment of the systemic necrotizing vasculitides of the polyarteritis nodosa (PAN) group, Wegener's granulomatosis, and primary (isolated) angiitis of the central nervous system (CNS).

Table 1 Classification of the Major Systemic Necrotizing Vasculitides

Polyarteritis nodosa group
Classic polyarteritis nodosa
Allergic agniitis and granulomatosis (Churg-Strauss disease)
Polyangiitis overlap syndrome
Wegener's granulomatosis
Giant cell arteritis
Temporal arteritis
Takayasu's arteritis
Primary (isolated) agniitis of the central nervous system
Associated with underlying disease process
Collagen vascular disease
Infections
Neoplasms
Behçet's disease
Other autoimmune illnesses
Hypersensitivity vasculitis
Henoch-Schönlein purpura
Serum sickness–like reaction
Cryoglobulinemic vasculitis

PREFERRED THERAPY

Corticosteroids

Corticosteroids are a major component of the primary therapy of the PAN syndromes, Wegener's granulomatosis, and primary angiitis of the CNS. They should be instituted as soon as the diagnosis of systemic necrotizing vasculitis is made and other differential diagnostic considerations such as infection and neoplasm are excluded. Objective signs of systemic necrotizing vasculitis (Table 2) should be identified in order to monitor response to therapy. Corticosteroids should be started at 1 to 2 mg per kilogram body weight per day of prednisone or equivalent therapy in divided dose, administered either intravenously or orally. The absorption of corticosteroids is identical for oral and intravenous dosing; however, intravenous administration is indicated if a question of gastrointestinal malabsorption exists or if the patient is unable to take oral medications.

All patients with PAN group syndromes, Wegener's granulomatosis, and primary angiitis of the CNS require corticosteroid therapy for the control of the vasculitic syndrome. Corticosteroids are used to down regulate proinflammatory effector mechanisms, such as the influx of inflammatory cells into tissues and cytokine production (Table 3). Divided-dose corticosteroids should be continued until manifestations of the disease cease progression and are reduced. The time required to accomplish this varies for each patient and syndrome, with an average range from 5 to 30 days. Pulse methylprednisolone therapy of 0.5 to 1.0 g per day for 3 days can be used initially in patients with rapidly progressive and life-threatening vasculitic syndromes, although there are no controlled trials comparing this regimen to standard corticosteroid dosing. Divided-dose corticosteroid therapy profoundly suppresses the hypothalamic-pituitary-adrenal axis and causes a high incidence of toxic side effects if continued more than a few weeks; therefore, attempts to consolidate treatment to a single morning dose should be undertaken as soon as early clinical response is evident. A single morning dose of corticosteroid coincides with the normal diurnal variation of plasma cortisone levels and is less toxic. If divided-dose therapy is required less than 10 days, then the dose can be consolidated to a single morning dose rapidly, over 1 to 5 days. If divided-dose therapy is required for more than 14 days, then a more gradual taper over 7 to 10 days to a single morning dose is necessary. The consolidated morning dose of corticosteroids is continued until further clinical improvement is evident in the patient's

Table 2 Objective Signs of Systemic Necrotizing Vasculitis

- Eye
  - Episcleritis/scleritis
  - Retinal vasculitis
  - Ischemic optic neuropathy
  - Retro-ocular inflammatory mass lesion
- Nervous system
  - Mononeuritis multiplex
  - Strokes
- Renal
  - Active sediment with proteinuria and hematuria
  - Renal insufficiency
  - Hypertension of recent onset or exacerbation
- Pulmonary
  - Nodules with or without cavitation
  - Infiltrates
  - Pulmonary hemorrhage
  - Cough
  - Hypoxia
- Skin
  - Palpable purpura
  - Subcutaneous nodules
  - Livedo reticularis
- Upper respiratory tract
  - Opacification of sinuses on imaging study
  - Rhinorrhea and nasal congestion
  - Nasal ulceration
  - Saddle nose deformity
  - Serous otitis media
- Associated clinical features
  - Elevated erythrocyte sedimentation rate
  - Anemia of chronic disease
  - Leukocytosis
  - Thrombocytosis
  - Eosinophilia
  - Cryoglobulinemia
- Other
  - Arthritis
  - Intestinal ulceration, perforation, and infarction
  - Myositis
  - Abnormal angiography

Table 3 Mechanisms of Corticosteroid Immunosuppressive and Anti-Inflammatory Effects

- Inhibition of accumulation of monocytic macrophages at inflammatory sites
- Blockage of accumulation of neutrophils at inflammatory sites
- Selective depletion of T lymphocytes more than B lymphocytes
- Suppression of lymphocytic function in
  - Delayed hypersensitivity skin testing by inhibiting monocyte recruitment
  - Lymphocytic proliferation to antigens
  - Mixed lymphocytic proliferation
  - Spontaneous (natural) cytotoxicity
- Suppression of monocytic-macrophage function in
  - Cutaneous delayed hypersensitivity by inhibition of lymphokine effect on macrophages
  - Blockage of Fc-receptor binding and function
  - Bactericidal activity
  - Inhibition of interleukin-1 production
- Decreased reticuloendothelial clearance of antibody-coated cells
- Decreased synthesis of prostaglandin and leukotrienes
- Inhibition of plasminogen activator release
- Antagonism of histamine-induced vasodilation
- Effect on cytokines
  - Decreased production of interleukin-1

Table 4 Example of Corticosteroid Therapy in Systemic Necrotizing Vasculitis

At the time of diagnosis begin prednisone therapy:

DOSE	FREQUENCY	LENGTH OF THERAPY
15 mg	Four times per day	10 days
20 mg	Three times per day	2 days
30 mg	Two times per day	2 days
60 mg	Once a day in the AM	30 days

At this time the taper to alternate-day therapy begins:

"HIGH-DAY" DOSE	"LOW-DAY" DOSE	LENGTH OF THERAPY
60 mg	50 mg	6 days
60 mg	40 mg	6 days
60 mg	30 mg	6 days
60 mg	20 mg	6 days
60 mg	15 mg	6 days
60 mg	10 mg	6 days
60 mg	7.5 mg	6 days
60 mg	5 mg	6 days
60 mg	2.5 mg	6 days
60 mg	0 mg	6 days

The alternate-day dose can be tapered after the patient has been stable for 1 month on alternate-day therapy. The above regimen is only an example of a corticosteroid taper scheme. The design and tempo of a regimen for individual patients must rely on each patient's clinical signs and symptoms and their response to therapy.

subjective symptoms, and the objective signs of disease activity chosen for monitoring resolve, usually within 1 to 3 months (Table 4).

Once a clinical response occurs and clinical signs and symptoms of active disease abate, attempts should be made to taper the corticosteroid dose to alternate-day therapy. The therapeutic principle to be followed is that the patient should be on the lowest, least toxic corticosteroid regimen that will control signs and symptoms of the vasculitic syndrome. Most patients with a systemic necrotizing vasculitis syndrome can be tapered to alternate-day corticosteroid therapy (see Table 4), but an occasional patient may be refractory. In this case, tapering of corticosteroids to the least effective daily dose of corticosteroid must be undertaken. The protocol in Table 4 shows a taper from 60 mg of prednisone each day to 60 mg on alternate days over approximately 8 weeks. The actual tempo of steroid taper must be dictated by patient signs and symptoms. Since corticosteroid therapy in patients with hepatitis B virus–associated PAN may enhance viral replication in the liver, corticosteroid taper to alternate-day therapy should be attempted more rapidly and discontinued, if clinical parameters allow.

Once corticosteroids are administered on alternate days and signs and symptoms of the systemic necrotizing vasculitis remain stable or quiescent for at least 4 weeks, the alternate-

Table 5 Complications of Corticosteroid Therapy

- Central nervous system difficulties
  - Altered morale/personality
  - Steroid psychosis
  - Pseudotumor cerebri
- Cutaneous difficulties
  - Violaceous striae
  - Subcutaneous tissue atrophy
  - Cushingoid habitus
  - Purpura and ecchymosis
  - Acne
  - Hirsutism
  - Facial erythema
- Deposition of fatty tissue
  - Moon facies
  - Buffalo hump
  - Mediastinal lipomatosis
  - Hepatomegaly
- Delayed wound healing (including peptic ulceration)
- Endocrine and metabolic difficulties
  - Hyperglycemia
  - Osteoporosis
  - Suppression of the hypothalamic-pituitary-adrenal axis
  - Hypokalemic alkalosis
  - Fluid retention
  - Hypertension
  - Growth retardation
  - Proximal myopathy
  - Hyperlipoproteinemia
  - Menstrual irregularity
- Immunosuppression
- Ocular difficulties
  - Cataracts
  - Glaucoma
  - Exophthalmos
- Opportunistic infection
- Osteonecrosis
- Pancreatitis
- Weight gain

day therapy can gradually be tapered to the least effective dose or discontinued, at a rate of 10 mg every 2 weeks or slower. The taper should continue as long as signs and symptoms of the systemic necrotizing vasculitis remain stable or quiescent. If signs or symptoms of the vasculitis recur or worsen, the corticosteroid dose should be increased or the taper should be halted or slowed, depending upon the degree and severity of the recurrent or worsening signs and symptoms.

Alternate-day corticosteroid therapy has a significantly lower incidence of side effects compared to daily oral divided-dose therapy. Conversion from daily to alternate-day corticosteroid therapy should routinely be attempted in all patients with forms of systemic necrotizing vasculitis (except temporal arteritis). Corticosteroid dose is clearly a factor in the toxic and infectious complications of corticosteroid therapy, and thus the dose should continually be tapered to achieve the lowest effective dose. Calcium supplementation at a dose of 1,200 to 1,500 mg of elemental calcium daily in divided dose combined with 400 IU of vitamin D per day may delay or attenuate the development of corticosteroid-related osteopenia. Monitoring for the development of glucose intolerance, hypertension, steroid myopathy, and increased intraocular pressure is also recommended in patients receiving corticosteroid therapy for more than 2 weeks (Table 5).

Table 6 Mechanisms of Immunosuppressive Properties of Cyclophosphamide

- Lymphocytopenia of both T and B lymphocytes
- Suppression of in vitro lymphocyte blastogenic response to specific antigens
- Suppression of antibody response and cutaneous delayed hypersensitivity to new antigen
- Selective suppression of in vitro B lymphocytic function with decrease in immunoglobulin production and suppression of mitogen-induced immunoglobulin production
- Reduction in serum immunoglobulin levels

A few patients with a very mild or slowly progressive PAN group disease, Wegener's granulomatosis limited to the upper respiratory tract, or primary angiitis of the CNS without focal CNS difficulties may be treated with corticosteroids alone. Such patients are rare and must be chosen very carefully and monitored for response to therapy and progression of disease. If response is not documented or disease progression is evident, a second drug must then be added to the regimen.

Cyclophosphamide

Many patients with systemic necrotizing vasculitis as well as the majority of patients with PAN group syndromes, Wegener's granulomatosis, and primary angiitis of the CNS require combination therapy with corticosteroid and another immunosuppressive agent. The most commonly recommended and used second drug is the alkylating agent, cyclophosphamide (Table 6). Patients who fail treatment with corticosteroids alone and patients with renal, pulmonary, neurologic, and gastrointestinal manifestations of PAN group syndromes and Wegener's granulomatosis require treatment with cyclophosphamide and corticosteroids, as do patients with primary angiitis of the CNS with focal neurologic findings and/or rapid tempo of progression.

Patients should be started on cyclophosphamide at a dose of 2 mg per kilogram body weight per day given orally or intravenously. The absorption of cyclophosphamide is identical when given orally or intravenously; therefore, the indications to give the drug intravenously are concerns regarding gastrointestinal absorption secondary to gut malabsorption or inability to swallow oral medication. Cyclophosphamide at 2 mg per kilogram body weight per day is maintained for 2 weeks. If evidence of favorable clinical response is noted, this dose is maintained with subsequent dose level adjustments to keep the peripheral white blood cell (WBC) count at greater than 3,000 cells per cubic millimeter. Suppressing the WBC to a level of 3,000 to 4,000 cells per cubic millimeter represents the most aggressive level of immunosuppression, but many patients will achieve clinical remission with WBCs in the absence of leukopenia. If there is no evidence of favorable clinical response in 2 weeks, daily dose should be increased by 25 mg every 2 weeks until a clinical response occurs or until a WBC count of less than 3,000 cells per cubic millimeter is reached. The complete blood count (CBC) should be monitored 2 to 3 times per week for the first 2 weeks of therapy and with any increase in cyclophosphamide dose. Subsequently, the CBC can be monitored weekly. It is important to remember that the dose of cyclophosphamide given has the maximum effect on the WBC count 7 to 10 days after administration. Thus, a rapid change in WBCs over 1 week (e.g., from 10,000 per cubic millimeter to 5,000 per cubic millimeter) is an indication to temporarily discontinue the cyclophosphamide until the WBC count stabilizes.

In patients with fulminant systemic necrotizing vasculitis involving the kidneys, heart, brain, or lungs, the disease is life threatening and can lead to rapid and irreversible organ damage. Such patients include those with CNS vasculitis and multiple rapid strokes, severe pulmonary involvement with hypoxia, rapidly progressive peripheral neuropathy, and/or rapidly progressive renal insufficiency. Renal failure is the most common clinical manifestation of fulminant vasculitis and constitutes a medical emergency. In patients with fulminant vasculitis, cyclophosphamide is begun at 4 mg per kilogram body weight per day orally or intravenously for 3 days with taper over the subsequent 3 days to a dose of 1 to 2 mg per kilogram body weight per day. This dose is maintained with careful attention to the WBC count and its rate of change because waiting until the WBC count is 3,000 cells per cubic millimeter before modifying the dose of cyclophosphamide may result in clinically significant neutropenia when the nadir is finally reached.

Cyclophosphamide should be continued with careful monitoring of disease activity and potential toxicity for 1 year after remission of the systemic necrotizing vasculitis is believed to have been achieved. As the corticosteroid dose is tapered, the cyclophosphamide dose may have to be tapered because corticosteroid protects the patient from some of cyclophosphamide's effect on lowering the WBC count. A taper to alternate-day corticosteroid often requires a 25 to 50 mg decrease in the cyclophosphamide dose. Prolonged cyclophosphamide therapy may be associated with diminished drug tolerance, calling for further reductions in the cyclophosphamide dose. Finally, decreased renal function also requires modification of the cyclophosphamide dose after the initial 5 to 7 days of therapy because active cyclophosphamide metabolites are renally cleared; therefore, peak drug-induced effects on WBCs may be prolonged. In the setting of a persistent creatinine clearance of less than 15 ml per minute, the dose of cyclophosphamide may be less than or equal to 1 mg per kilogram body weight per day after the first week, depending on the WBC count. After 1 year of therapy in remission, the cyclophosphamide should be reduced 25 mg per day every 1 to 2 months until it is discontinued, provided that disease remains quiescent.

Monitoring of primary angiitis of the CNS is much more difficult than PAN group syndromes and Wegener's granulomatosis. Generally, repeat angiography at 3 to 4 months of therapy is necessary to document a response to therapy. If the angiogram is markedly improved or normal and no new symptoms of cerebral ischemia are present, then it may be possible to say that the patient is clinically in remission.

Cyclophosphamide therapy has many potential complications (Table 7). Patients receiving cyclophosphamide should be told to drink adequate fluids to maintain 3 liters urine output per day to decrease drug-induced bladder toxicity. A careful history of bladder function should be obtained and suggestions of bladder-outlet obstruction and neurogenic bladder should be appropriately evaluated and treated. The failure to empty the bladder may increase the risk of developing cyclophosphamide-related bladder toxicity. Patients treated with daily oral cyclophosphamide require lifelong follow-up regarding their increased risk of bladder cancer. All hematuria (gross and microscopic) should be evaluated with cystoscopy to investigate the possibility of bladder cancer. Yearly urine cytologies should also be performed. If hemorrhagic cystitis complicates a course of cyclophosphamide therapy, methotrexate (20 to 25 mg per week) is the first choice to replace the cyclophosphamide. Methotrexate should not be considered unless the serum creatinine is less than 2.5 mg per deciliter. Azathioprine, chlorambucil, and cyclosporine are alternatives to the use of methotrexate in this situation. Azathioprine seems incapable of inducing a remission in most systemic vasculitides, but it seems to work well for maintaining remission in those patients with cyclophosphamide toxicity. The use of cyclic estrogen birth control may decrease immunosuppressive drug–induced toxicity to the ovary. The possibility of sperm banking should be discussed with male patients prior to institution of immunosuppressive therapy.

Table 7 Complications of Cyclophosphamide Therapy

- Alopecia
- Antidiuretic hormone effect at higher doses
- Bladder toxicity
  - Hemorrhagic cystitis
  - Bladder fibrosis
  - Bladder cancer
- Hypogammaglobulinemia
- Lymphoma/leukemia
- Marrow toxicity
  - Neutropenia/leukopenia
  - Thrombocytopenia
  - Anemia, often macrocytic
  - Leukemia
- Nausea and emesis
- Opportunistic infection
- Pulmonary interstitial fibrosis
- Reproductive system
  - Premature ovarian failure
  - Infertility
  - Sterility
  - Teratogenesis

■ THERAPEUTIC ALTERNATIVES

Methotrexate

Given the toxicity of cyclophosphamide in the treatment of systemic necrotizing vasculitides, other immunosuppressive alternatives have been actively sought. Methotrexate may be an effective and less toxic alternative for many patients with systemic necrotizing vasculitis. The mechanism of action of methotrexate in systemic necrotizing vasculitis is not known. The therapeutic effect of methotrexate may be secondary to antifolate activity, immunomodulating effects, immunosuppressive effects, or anti-inflammatory effects on leukocytes. The most reported experience with methotrexate as a second drug has been in the treatment of Wegener's granulomatosis, but anecdotal experience also exists with PAN group syndromes and Takayasu's arteritis.

Methotrexate should be used in combination with corticosteroids to treat patients with PAN group syndromes and Wegener's granulomatosis that do not have rapidly progressive multisystem disease, life-threatening manifestations, or a serum creatinine of greater than 2.5 mg per deciliter. This regimen should be considered in patients with PAN group diseases and Wegener's granulomatosis who have mild to moderate renal disease, mild to moderate pulmonary disease, mild to moderate disease tempo, and the lack of CNS or severe gastrointestinal difficulties. The patient's concerns regarding fertility may also influence the decision to use methotrexate.

Baseline blood counts, liver function tests, and serum creatinine should be obtained prior to methotrexate therapy. If the hemoglobin (Hgb) level is greater than 10 and liver function tests reveal total bilirubin to be less than 1.5 mg per deciliter, alkaline phosphatase less than 50 percent above upper limits of normal, creatinine less than 2.5 mg per deciliter and SGOT/SGPT less than two times normal, methotrexate therapy can be instituted provided that the patient ceases alcohol intake, is not pregnant, and is not breast feeding. Methotrexate is instituted orally as a single weekly dose of 15 mg. If gastrointestinal symptoms occur, the next dose is given in two divided equal doses at 12 hour intervals once a week. If the gastrointestinal symptoms persist with divided-dose oral methotrexate, it should subsequently be given intramuscularly once a week. If well tolerated for 1 to 2 weeks, the dose is increased by 2.5 mg every week until a dose of 20 to 25 mg per week is reached. This dose is maintained unless there are significant side effects or toxicity of the methotrexate. If renal function is not normal, great care should be exercised as higher dose methotrexate is reached because the major route of methotrexate excretion is the kidneys. Complete blood counts, SGOT, SGPT, and albumin should be monitored every 4 to 6 weeks. If WBC is less than 3,000, SGOT or SGPT rise higher than three times normal, platelets fall to less than 100,000, or Hgb falls to less than 10 mg per deciliter, skipping a dose of methotrexate and downward adjustment by 2.5 to 5 mg per week may be necessary. If SGOT is abnormal, five of nine determinations within a given 12 month interval (six of twelve, if performed monthly), then liver biopsy is indicated to make sure that significant methotrexate hepatotoxicity is not occurring.

If significant improvement in vasculitis clinical activity occurs in the first 4 to 6 weeks, prednisone taper should be begun, as previously described. If remission occurs and is sustained for 1 year of methotrexate therapy, methotrexate taper is begun at the rate of 2.5 mg every 2 to 4 weeks until discontinuation or recurrence of vasculitis disease activity is noted. Potential methotrexate side effects are noted in Table 8. Patients who fail to respond to the combination of corticosteroid and methotrexate within 2 to 3 months or have a significant relapse on the regimen should be treated with the combination of corticosteroids and cyclophosphamide.

Table 8 Complications of Methotrexate Therapy

- Alopecia
- Drug-induced pneumonitis
- Hepatic toxicity
  - Abnormal SGOT/SGPT
  - Fatty liver
  - Fibrosis
  - Cirrhosis
- Marrow toxicity
  - Leukopenia
  - Thrombocytopenia
  - Anemia, often macrocytic
- Nausea, emesis, and weight loss
- Oligospermia
- Opportunistic infections
- Skin rash and photosensitivity
- Stomatitis
- Teratogenic effects

Vasculitis Associated with Other Diseases

When vasculitis is associated with other well-defined illnesses, such as collagen vascular diseases or neoplasms, only the underlying disease should be treated unless the vasculitis is multisystem, rapidly progressive, and life threatening. In such cases, the vasculitis should be treated as a PAN group syndrome with corticosteroids and possibly an immunosuppressive agent.

Monitoring

Systemic vasculitides are often serious and life-threatening illnesses that require aggressive diagnostic and therapeutic approaches. Careful monitoring of treatment with regard to side effects and efficacy gives these challenging patients the best chance for remission without significant toxicity. Unfortunately, recent studies have shown that relapses are common in patients with a systemic necrotizing vasculitis. This, combined with the potential complications of present therapies, lead to the requirement of life-long and informed monitoring of these patients.

Suggested Reading

Gross WL. New developments in the treatment of systemic necrotizing vasculitis. Curr Opin Rheumatol 1994; 6:11–19.

Haynes BF, Allen NB, Fauci AS. Diagnostic and therapeutic approach to the patient with vasculitis. Med Clin North Am 1986; 70:355–368.

Hoffman GS, Kerr GS, Leavitt RY, et al. Wegener's granulomatosis: An analysis of 158 patients. Ann Int Med 1992; 116:488–498.

Hoffman GS, Leavitt RY, Kerr GS, Fauci AS. The treatment of Wegener's granulomatosis with glucocorticoids and methotrexate. Arthritis Rheum 1992; 35:1322–1329.

Langford CS, McCallum RM. Idiopathic Vasculitis. In: Belch J, Zurier R, eds. Connective tissue diseases. London: Chapman & Hall, 1995.

BURSITIS

Richard H. Parker, M.D.

Bursal sacs are synovial membrane–lined structures that secrete and absorb liquid throughout the body, providing a lubrication between bones, tendons, ligaments, muscles, and skin. There are over 150 bursal sacs in the human body, and although usually isolated, occasionally they are in communication with a joint space. New bursae may be created whenever there is friction between musculoskeletal structures.

Septic or infectious bursitis is typically seen in a superficial bursa such as the prepatellar or olecranon. It is most commonly seen in middle-aged and older patients after trauma or repetitive activity. However, septic bursitis may be a complication of bacteremia without a history of trauma to the involved area.

Bursitis usually starts abruptly with localized pain and discomfort that are aggravated by movement. Examination reveals swelling with erythema and tenderness to palpation. However, only tenderness and limitation of motion may be found with inflammation of deep bursae.

Fever and surrounding cellulitis demand aspiration of any fluctuant identifiable swelling to differentiate septic from nonseptic bursitis. The olecranon bursa is a particularly common site of septic bursitis as well as bursitis associated with rheumatoid arthritis and gout. Septic bursitis can coexist with bursitis due to other inflammatory disease. The most important tests on the fluid are the white and red blood cell counts, glucose, and culture (Table 1).

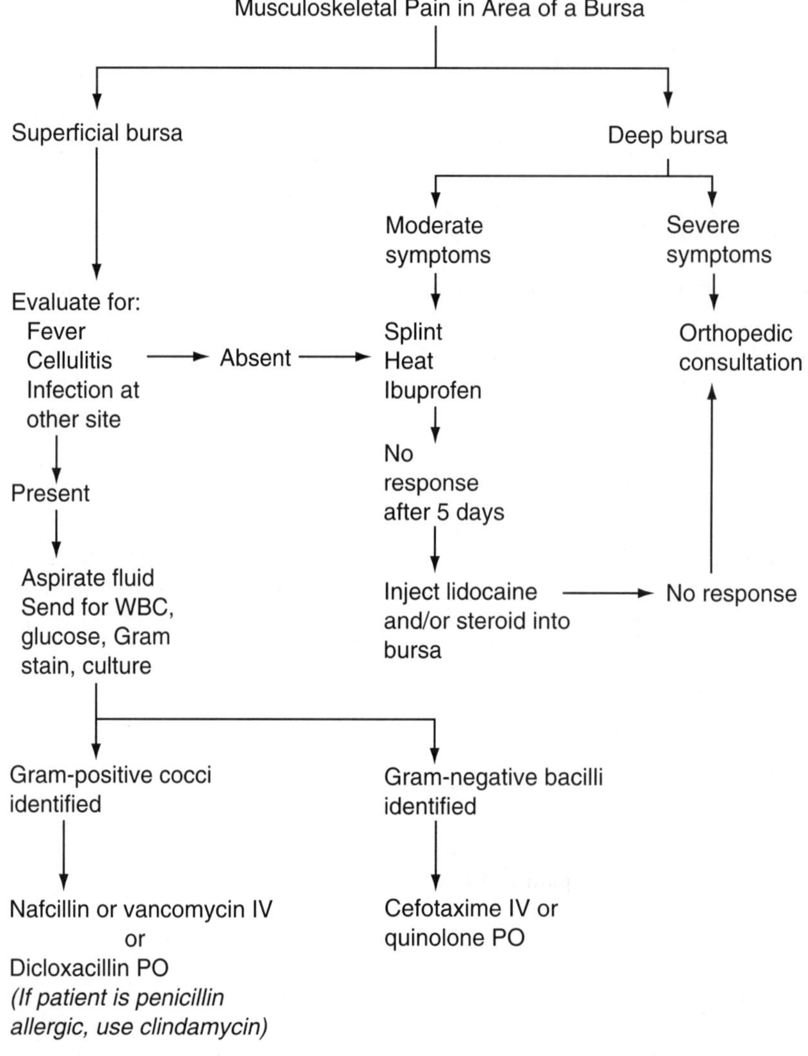

Figure 1
Algorithm for the management of musculoskeletal pain in area of bursa.

Table 1 Findings in Bursal Fluid Related to Causes of Bursitis

FINDING	NORMAL	TRAUMA	SEPSIS	RHEUMATOID INFLAMMATION	MICROCRYSTALLINE INFLAMMATION
Color	Clear yellow	Bloody xanthochromic	Yellow, cloudy	Yellow, cloudy	Yellow, cloudy
WBC	0–200	<5,000	1,000–200,000	1,000–20,000	1,000–20,000
RBC	0	Many	Few	Few	Few
Glucose	Normal*	Normal*	Decreased	Decreased (slight)	Variable
Gram stain, culture	Negative	Negative	Positive	Negative	Negative

*Fluid glucose/blood glucose = 0.6–1.

THERAPY

The first step is deciding whether the inflammation is infectious or noninfectious (Fig. 1). If noninfectious, the therapy is immobilization, heat, and anti-inflammatory agents. If septic bursitis is diagnosed, hospitalization and empiric therapy with intravenous antimicrobial agents should be considered. However, if the patient is not septic, is not an immunocompromised host, and is considered compliant, therapy can be initiated with oral agents and the patient followed closely as an outpatient. Home intravenous infusion therapy is also an option but should be restricted to cases of methicillin-resistant *Staphylococcus aureus* (MRSA), a few other drug-resistant micro-organisms, and for patients who cannot tolerate oral medication.

Most infections are due to *S. aureus;* therefore, initial therapy requires a good antistaphylococcal agent. Where MRSA infections are common, intravenous vancomycin therapy should be initiated. Then, if cultures prove the *S. aureus* is not methicillin-resistant, therapy can be changed to an oral antistaphylococcal drug. Quinolones (ciprofloxacin, ofloxacin) should be avoided as empiric therapy unless streptococcal infection has been ruled out. Also, cefixime (Suprax) should not be used as an oral agent because of its poor antistaphylococcal activity. Gram-negative bacilli and anaerobic microorganisms rarely cause septic bursitis except in complicated cases, such as bursitis in an immunocompromised host. Recurrence of fluid after the initial aspiration and initiation of therapy requires reaspiration. Surgical drainage or bursectomy may be necessary if bursitis has been prolonged prior to initiating therapy, or if there is a history of bursal disease, poor response to medical therapy, or infection with an uncommon micro-organism.

Suggested Reading

Ho G, Tice AD, Kaplan SR. Septic bursitis in the prepatellar and olecranon bursae. Ann Intern Med 1978; 89:21–27.

Ho G, Tice AD. Comparison of nonseptic and septic bursitis. Arch Intern Med 1979; 139:1269–1273.

LaCour EG, Schmid FR. Infections of bursae and tendons. In: Schlossberg D, ed. Orthopedic infections. Springer-Verlag, 1988:92.

LOW BACK PAIN

Don M. Long, M.D., Ph.D.

Low back pain is one of the most common complaints of the American public, equaled only by headache. Population-based studies suggest that 60 to 70 percent of the population will have at least one episode of serious low back pain and that up to 35 percent are complaining at any one time. More than 10 percent of Americans are seeking treatment for low back pain regularly. It is the most common reason for industrial disability and the most common reason to claim disability under Social Security. This is a major public health problem and the cost is enormous. Therefore, it behooves all physicians to understand the appropriate management of the patient with low back pain.

The complaint of low back pain is a relatively nonspecific description of a symptom that may have many causes. There is no good classification system that incorporates physical abnormalities, complaints, and severity or that allows for an accurate prognosis or therapy. Categorization is still descriptive. Our current classification is helpful, but there is great need for a system that differentiates patients according to eventual outcome and therapeutic need.

Even though the existing systems are descriptive only, they do assist in establishing a treatment plan for any individual patient based on what is known today.

CLASSIFICATION OF LOW BACK PAIN

Transient Low Back Pain

The most common occurrences of pain are those that occur briefly. They may be severe, but they rarely last for more than a few hours, and patients usually do not seek medical attention unless the occurrences become repetitive. The causes are unknown, the incidence is almost universal, and it is generally assumed that these transient episodes of pain are muscular or ligamentous in origin. It is better to say the cause is unknown but that these transient episodes do not appear to have any prognostic significance for the development of more serious problems. Unless these episodes become more frequent, they require no evaluation or treatment.

Acute Low Back Pain

Most of what is described under the general rubric of low back pain is termed *acute low back pain.* Acute episodes last from a few days to a few months. They are usually significant, and patients often seek medical help for relief. They may or may not be associated with sciatica, and the issue of disk herniation will be discussed separately. Most patients have back pain and nonsciatic leg pain. The episodes are frequently traumatic in origin but are equally likely to be spontaneous in onset. In order to decide what to do about them, it is important to understand the natural history. There is good evidence that most are self-limited and will disappear within weeks to a few months at most. Nearly all will be gone within 1 month. Treatment used to be prolonged bedrest, but there is evidence that early mobilization is better. Most authorities now restrict patients during only the most severe episodes of pain. There is consensus that plain x-ray examinations are not needed, and other imaging studies should not be done except in unusual circumstances. Treatment is nonspecific and consists of analgesics appropriate to the complaint and findings, rest during the most serious pain, and return to full activity as soon as symptoms allow. That is, the typical patient who presents with the acute onset of low back pain with or without sciatica who does not have any significant neurologic deficit is best treated with pain relievers and a limited period of bedrest, and can return to function as soon as symptoms will allow.

The recently adopted guidelines from the Health Policy Agency include an assessment of physical and manipulation therapies. I disagree with the conclusions of that group concerning the value of therapies for most of these patients for the following reasons. The reports that suggest benefit from either manipulation or passive physical modalities demonstrate only minimal advantage over no therapy, in my opinion. Patients may be made somewhat more comfortable and may return to work a little sooner, but I see no reason to apply these expensive therapies for a benign self-limited process that will disappear without any treatment at all in the majority of patients. Furthermore, the dramatic improvements with manipulation that are much talked about are extremely rare in controlled studies. For these reasons I do not believe the data demonstrate that any form of active or passive therapy at this stage is cost effective.

Who Should Be Evaluated?

The indications for prompt evaluation are not many, and they are reasonably specific. A history of significant trauma that might lead to fracture is an indication for plain x-ray examinations. Unusually severe pain, particularly if unrelieved by narcotics, is another important reason. A history of neoplasm elsewhere, a history of infection, systemic signs of illness, and neurologic deficits are all indications for moving ahead with evaluation promptly.

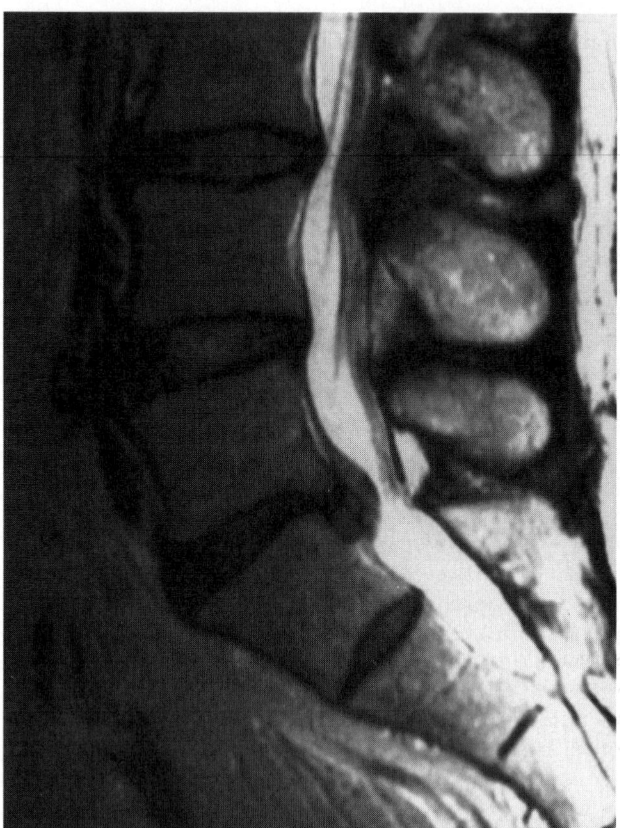

Figure 1
Sagittal magnetic resonance imaging scan. Herniated nucleus pulposus in the canal and L5-S1 with free fragment beneath the ligament.

Low Back Pain with Sciatica and the Acutely Herniated Disk (Fig. 1)

A small number of patients, 1 to 2 percent in most population studies, have a truly herniated disk. Root compression secondary to disk herniation is nearly always accompanied by radiculitis. Since most disk herniations occur at L4-5 or L5-S1, sciatica is the typical manifestation. The signs and symptoms of disk herniation are well known. The predominant pain is sciatica, though back pain may also be important. There is frequently paravertebral muscle spasm with limitation of range of motion; the straight leg raising test is positive; and the crossed straight leg raising test is pathognomonic. There are specific combinations of motor, sensory, and reflex change that indicate the root involved. A diminished knee reflex, weakness in the quadriceps, and anterior thigh and leg numbness suggest an L4 root compression. The L5 root is signaled by weakness of dorsiflexion of the foot and toes and sensory loss on the top of the foot. The medial surface is typically involved more than the lateral. S1 root compression is suspected when the ankle reflex is diminished. There is numbness in the lateral foot, toes, and sole, and plantar flexion is affected. However, in a recent study of more than 500 patients operated on for demonstrated root compression syndromes, these classic triads were present in less than 1 percent, and only 10 percent of patients with disabling pain had even one specific sign. Therefore, it appears that the most important symptom is the severity of the radicular pain.

Even when disk herniation is suspected, there is no reason to move ahead quickly to therapy unless pain is intolerable or significant neurologic deficit occurs. If the patient has weakness that is functionally impairing or any bowel or bladder dysfunction, I believe that urgent evaluation is required. If the pain can be controlled with analgesics and neurologic deficits are not severe, then there is no reason to proceed with therapy immediately. Most patients, even those with classic disk herniations, will recover spontaneously within the first month. Recovery may not be complete in 1 month, but it has clearly begun. Therefore, even when I suspect a typical disk herniation, I do not begin the evaluation or contemplate surgery unless symptoms and signs are severe.

In cases with severe signs and symptoms, the diagnostic study of choice is magnetic resonance imaging (MRI). Many experts still want plain x-ray films. Personally, I believe that the MRI is satisfactory, and I no longer obtain plain x-ray films unless there is an unresolved question apparent on the MRI. Patients with demonstrated disk herniation should proceed to surgery promptly. Our data, derived from a nationwide study of results of surgery for root compression syndromes, indicate that over 90 percent of patients will be satisfactorily relieved and return to full activity and employment.

Persistent Low Back Pain

In a recent multicenter study we have identified a group of patients whose complaints do not improve with time. It had been generally held that all patients with back problems improved and that there was little difference between those operated on and those not operated on after sufficient time had elapsed. Our data indicate that this perception is not true. There are a substantial number of patients whose back pain complaints remain serious and incapacitating. They appear to be stable over years, neither worsening nor improving. These patients are the most important of those complaining of back pain because they seek repeated medical examinations, undergo many treatments, and have substantial vocational disability. Our investigation of this group indicates that the majority suffer from disk herniation or degenerative disk disease with all of the manifestations of lumbar spondylosis. Most suffer from root compression syndromes, but a minority are candidates for surgery given our current criteria. Of this group with persisting pain, some 70 percent had symptoms on the basis of severe lumbar spondylotic disease, 20 percent were thought to have a myofacial syndrome, and only about 10 percent had other unexpected causes.

If a patient's pain has persisted for more than 3 months, investigation may be warranted when pain is severe. If it has been present for 6 months, spontaneous recovery will not occur and the investigation certainly should proceed. Once the physical examination has been done, the imaging studies are the key. Plain x-ray examinations of the spine are still done by most, but MRI will give the most information. If substantial bone pathology is present, computed tomography (CT) scan can be added. CT myelogram is rarely required now. Electrodiagnostic studies are of little value unless peripheral neuropathy and entrapment are issues.

Therapy of Persisting Back Pain with or Without Sciatica

The therapy program that I outline here is controversial. It is in direct opposition to much of what has been done in the past. Traditionally patients with back and leg pain were prescribed physical therapy programs that included many passive modalities such as heat, massage, ultrasound, and traction. Exercises were regularly used, and bracing was commonly employed. There was such faith in conservative care that a trial of physical therapy was obligatory for all patients in whom surgery was contemplated. Chiropractic or osteopathic manipulation was commonly employed, many of these patients sought acupuncture treatment, and a broad spectrum of other therapies have been recommended. The data suggesting that any of these treatments are of value were always marginal.

Recently we conducted a multicenter national study of the effectiveness of these therapies for persistent low back pain, and the results have completely changed my standard practice. In this study we examined a cohort of patients referred to orthopedists and neurosurgeons who had had persisting pain for 6 months or more. One large group of these patients had no treatment during a follow-up period, which was a minimum of 2 years, and 5 years for many. Contrary to expectation, there was no evidence of improvement. Patients worsened slightly, but the numbers did not reach statistical significance. Basically, no patients changed in complaints or incapacitation during the follow-up period. A second, even larger group underwent extensive conservative care. Over 90 percent of the patients had physical therapy, including virtually any known modality. Almost half received manipulation therapy from chiropractors or osteopaths. A significant number were treated with acupuncture, and smaller, though still statistically significant, groups underwent virtually any form of low back pain therapy one might imagine. The results of the follow-up in terms of pain control, functional improvement, and need for further therapy were startling. No conservative program could be differentiated from the no-treatment group. We could not demonstrate any beneficial effect of any of the commonly employed therapies.

Only 14 percent of these patients underwent surgery. Surgery was employed only for root compression syndromes and demonstrated instability. One-half the patients went directly to surgery and one-half had an interposed trial of conservative care. There was no evidence that any patient was improved by the conservative period of waiting and in no case was surgery prevented by either waiting or conservative care. The overall outcome of surgery as done by this group of spinal experts was excellent. Over 90 percent of patients were improved to the point that no further therapy was required, and all returned to presurgery function. For example, all those employed at the time of surgery and not involved in litigation returned to work. Five percent required reoperation during the study period, with almost identical results for a second procedure. Only 2 to 3 percent failed to improve. Fusion was employed in 10 percent and enjoyed an equally good success rate.

My management of these patients has been dramatically altered by these data. If a patient continues to complain of back and leg pain 3 to 6 months after onset, it is virtually certain that spontaneous improvement will not occur. The patient should be examined for a correctable cause of the problem. If one is found, surgery to repair the abnormality should proceed. Of course, it is mandatory that the pain and disability be serious enough to warrant an operation, but when they are, surgery should proceed promptly without interposed conservative care. None of the standard conservative programs, including physical therapy and manipulation, were effective, and I no longer employ any of them.

Intensive Active Physical Therapy for Persistent Low Back Pain

The preceding section pertains to the standard therapies commonly employed by most physicians in the care of these patients. There are strong data suggesting that an intensive therapy program can benefit these patients. That is fortunate, for only a minority of patients are surgical candidates. The best data available suggest that an intensive program of weight control, stretching, muscle strengthening, and reconditioning with attention to focal inflammation, muscle spasm, and impaired range of motion can benefit these patients. I often add a lightweight lumbosacral support for use during periods of greatest activity when the patient can identify those activities that precipitate the pain. Weight control has never been proven to be beneficial, but it is logical that it should be and is a part of my prescribed program.

Thus, when I see a patient with persisting pain of 3 months or more, I look immediately for a remediable cause if the patient has enough symptoms to warrant surgery. If no reparable cause is found, I recommend an intensive program of passive measures to eliminate focal areas of inflammation. Then general reconditioning and back and abdominal muscle strengthening are added. Although no controlled clinical trials exist, the best evidence is that this program must be highly focused and intensive and requires substantial commitments from both therapists and patients.

The Chronic Pain Syndrome

There is a fourth category of patients who are strikingly disabled by pain. From the physical standpoint, it is difficult to differentiate them from those people who complain but are not disabled. This chronic pain group is characterized by extreme disability, fixation upon the pain, a consistent pattern of overuse of medications, reactive depression and anxiety, and a high incidence of premorbid psychological dysfunction. Our examination of these patients over a long period of time suggests that a small number, approximately 30 percent, suffer from severe physical disease and have relatively few comorbidities. About 15 percent seem to have psychiatric disease only with pain being a manifestation of psychiatric symptomatology. The remainder have a lifelong history of personality disorder or dysfunction. Complaints of low back pain account for 80 to 85 percent of chronic pain syndrome patients. My evaluation paradigm for these patients is a thorough medical examination and an equally thorough psychological evaluation with assessment of related comorbidities. These patients require a much more comprehensive program because physical disability is only a part of the overall medical problem. They require the same evaluation for physical causes of low back and leg pain, but psychiatric status, drug utilization, disability, and interpersonal interactions all are disordered and require evaluation. Most of these patients require a multidisciplinary approach or an extremely dedicated personal physician capable of dealing with all of these issues.

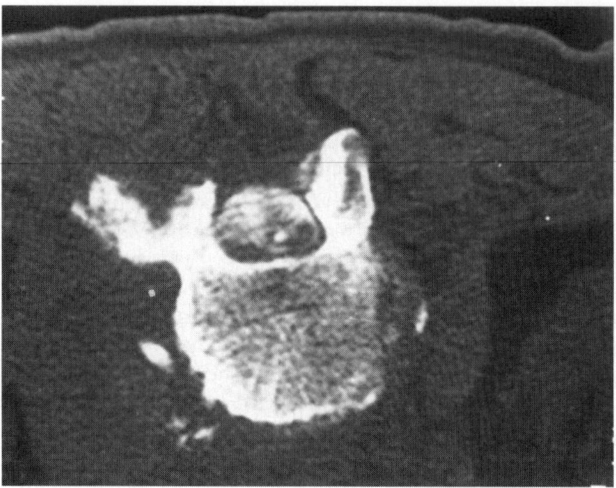

Figure 2
Computed tomographic myelogram L4-5. Decompressive laminectomy for recurrent spinal stenosis. Note square canal and lateral recess decompression. Some patients with failed back syndrome can benefit from reoperation if root compression or instability are demonstrated.

Failed Back Syndrome (Fig. 2)

The so-called failed back or postlaminectomy syndrome is another generic term used to identify a group of patients who may be in the persisting back pain classification or found within the chronic pain syndrome with all of its attendant comorbidities. The designation *failed back* serves little useful purpose and only identifies a group of people who have had one or more operations without benefit. The principles of their evaluation are the same as for any of the serious low back problems. Spontaneous recovery will not occur, so they should be investigated for causes of the pain. This is a business for an expert in spinal surgery and its consequences. Typical conservative care is of no value, but the focused program will benefit a substantial number of these patients by at least improving function. Those with identified abnormalities are candidates for surgical repair. The patients with root compression syndromes who are not candidates for additional surgery are treated by spinal cord stimulation currently.

■ CARE OF THE INTRACTABLE LOW BACK CRIPPLE

These patients fall in two categories in my experience. One group has spinal abnormalities that are beyond any reparative techniques currently available. Pain in the back is intractable. Intrathecal narcotics delivered by implantable pump have been utilized for a small number of these people, but current reports are inadequate to judge efficacy. We are currently testing the hypothesis that these people can be maintained with long-acting narcotic programs that will both relieve pain and allow improved function. The data are insufficient to make a judgment on this point at present, but it is clear from our experience that some patients can be managed successfully in this way. General recommendation for long-term narcotics use would be premature, and these patient evaluations are ongoing.

The second group of these patients have profound psychological dysfunction. Medical management should do two things. Repetitive unnecessary re-evaluation and useless, potentially harmful therapies must be stopped, and the patients should enter an appropriate psychiatric support program. Unfortunately, in my experience the majority refuse to accept either therapy program. I have no solutions for the patient in this category, but at least the physicians involved can withhold unnecessary and potentially harmful evaluations and therapies.

LITIGATION, DISABILITY, AND LOW BACK PAIN

A complaint of intractable low back pain is one of the most common reasons for claimed disability or short-term absence from work. It is my personal view that disability recompense is a worthwhile social program that has been seriously damaged by lack of appropriate controls, biased physicians, and a legal system that have subverted the original goals of the disability program. This is not the place to discuss the issue in detail. However, it is worth remembering that the role of the physician in this equation is to evaluate physical impairments. The American Medical Association guidelines are the standard by which impairment is judged. Disability is a complex issue that takes into account the patient's education, the environment, job opportunities, work history, and many other factors. Few physicians are expert enough to make these judgments alone, and it is not the physician's role in this system to establish disability. Short-term restrictions during a course of therapy are appropriate but should be related to demonstrated abnormalities and a rational treatment program, not simply the patient's complaint of pain and desire not to work.

The issue of litigation is also much discussed. In our recent multicenter study of patients undergoing surgery for spinal problems of all kinds, two very important facts emerged. Every patient who was operated on and not involved in litigation returned to work. No patient operated on who was involved in litigation returned to work during the study. The two groups of patients were indistinguishable in terms of diagnosis, physical impairment, imaging abnormalities, or complaints of pain. In fact, those who were involved in litigation had the same good outcome in terms of pain relief and functional status as those who were not involved in litigation, except for one factor: they did not return to work.

The physician involved in determining impairment and disability for patients with low back pain should be extremely circumspect. Impairment can be established on the basis of known guidelines. Short-term disability related to a treatment program is a reasonable physician decision. An example is the recuperation required after surgery. Long-term disability is a complex issue and not one to be decided by the treating physician alone.

A PARADIGM FOR LOW BACK MANAGEMENT

A major problem with the management of low back pain is that we do not know why the back hurts in the majority of patients. This puts us in the difficult position of having a severe complaint for which the physical examination is of limited value and imaging abnormalities may be very nonspecific. This means that treatments are likely to be nonspecific. It is important to remember that surgery is of proven value for root compression syndromes and demonstrated instability only. To bring some order into what is otherwise a very unsatisfying evaluation and treatment situation, I do the following. For *transient* low back pain that normally lasts less than a day or is trivial in its severity, no evaluation or treatment is required. These patients proceed to evaluation only if the transient episodes become frequent.

The patient suffering from acute back pain that may persist for days to a few months does not need to be evaluated in the early phase of the complaint unless the pain is intractable, there is a neurologic deficit, or systemic signs and symptoms are present. Otherwise, activity should be restricted for as short a time as commensurate with the pain and physical impairment. Early return to activity is desirable. In my view the added benefits of all active and passive therapy modalities and manipulation therapies are insufficient to warrant their cost. I do not employ any of them, and I discourage patients from seeking these kinds of treatments.

Once the patient has recovered, I encourage a program of general physical conditioning; weight control; specific back-, abdominal- and leg-strengthening exercises; and workplace education. Unfortunately, these are available only in a limited number of centers. The majority of treatment programs in my experience wish to focus only on the classic passive modalities repetitively administered by the therapist. I believe our data suggest that these are of no value even for symptomatic relief, and I do not employ them.

Patients with *persistent* low back pain need to be evaluated immediately for the possibility of surgical repair if the symptoms are serious enough. They need to have the implications of their disease seriously discussed. They need to understand that in all likelihood the problem will not disappear spontaneously, but that it is not serious and will not be disabling either. They may need help in adjusting their lifestyle, and they certainly should be involved in the vigorous exercise program described. *Chronic pain syndrome* patients need to be recognized and the comorbidities addressed in addition to the issues with the low back.

Evaluation, including imaging, in the acute back pain problem should begin when it becomes apparent that the pain will not relent spontaneously, that is, usually not before 1 month. The imaging studies will not commonly make a diagnosis, but they will discover the patients with clear-cut disk herniation or other forms of root compression or substantial instability, for whom surgical treatment may be necessary. I rarely proceed to surgery in less than 3 to 6 months after onset unless pain is intractable or there is a substantial neurologic deficit. There is no evidence that conservative care will do anything to change this interval or prevent surgery, but waiting certainly will reduce the number of people who would otherwise be operated on. That is commonly a matter of judgment between patient and physician. Once the problem has been present for 3 to 6 months, there is no reason to wait longer, and no conservative care will prevent an operation.

■ UNPROVEN EVALUATIONS AND THERAPIES

There are a number of omissions in my presentation. These omissions are deliberate because in my view the evaluations or treatments have not been proven by rigorous clinical investigation. These include diskography for determination of a painful disk that is the generator of the patient's symptoms, epidural steroid injection, injection of sclerosants, percutaneous disk surgery, and all surgery based on the diagnostic blocks. These issues are still under investigation, or should be before they are applied generally. When such time-honored treatments as active and passive therapy and manipulation fail to show a benefit in an effectiveness study, it is obvious that new treatments need to be subjected to rigorous evaluation before they are admitted to medical practice.

Suggested Reading

Acute low back problems in adults. Clinical Practice Guideline Number 14. U.S. Department of Health and Human Services, Public Health Service, Agency for Health Care Policy and Research, AHCPR Publication No. 95-0642, December 1994.

Long DM, BenDebba M, Torgerson WS, et al. Persistent back pain and sciatica in the United States: Patient characteristics. J Spinal Disord, in press.

SKIN DISEASES

ACNE

Peter E. Pochi, M.D.

Acne is a prevalent skin disorder, with a peak occurrence in the mid to late teens. However, adults are by no means immune from it, and some dermatologists' practices may actually comprise more adults than teenagers with the disease.

Although research on acne in the past 2 to 3 decades has elucidated a good deal of information about the pathogenic factors involved, two crucial matters about the disease remain elusive, namely, why it comes and why it goes. With time most cases of acne undergo complete or near complete involution, but the reason for it is a mystery. In terms of early development, susceptible pilosebaceous follicles of the face and trunk are affected, with abnormal keratinization occurring in the follicular epithelium. Again the reason for this follicle disturbance has not been adequately explained. Proliferation of anaerobic diphtheroids *(Propionibacterium acnes)* that require sebaceous lipids for subsistence is a central event in the induction of the inflammatory lesions of acne. These bacteria possess chemoattractant properties for neutrophils that initiate a series of events culminating in the expression of inflammation, both immune- and non–immune mediated. Characteristically an inflammatory lesion lasts 2 to 3 weeks, usually healing without a trace but occasionally leaving behind scars, mostly atrophic but occasionally hypertrophic.

■ GENERAL THERAPEUTIC APPROACH AND BASIS OF MANAGEMENT

From the foregoing brief summary of the etiologic events in acne, it is evident that such a multifactorial disorder would require a multifaceted therapeutic regimen. This is often desirable and necessary, although a unitarian approach may prove sufficient to control the disease, particularly mild cases or those early in their onset, or as maintenance therapy. Combination treatment may embrace the topical use of two or even three medications or the use of oral as well as topical therapy.

The decision about specific drugs or measures to use in acne depends on two broad considerations, namely, the severity of the acne and the type of acne present, i.e., whether it is predominantly inflammatory or noninflammatory. Before undertaking or recommending treatment it is important that time be taken to obtain an accurate history from the patient concerning the acne. Too often this aspect is overlooked or glossed over quickly. Important in this regard is the natural evolution of the acne and the response to prior treatments, including over-the-counter preparations. Women should be questioned about menstrual cycles and the presence of other possible manifestations of androgen excess, such as hirsutism or scalp hair recession or thinning. A history of drug ingestion can be important too, since certain medications such as lithium, excessive iodides, and anticonvulsants may aggravate existing acne. Even if little of the history obtained proves helpful for the overall management, the initial visit provides an important basis for a positive interaction between physician and patient. At times the patient, particularly a teenager, may seem indifferent to the physician's inquiry, but the opposite is more often the case.

After examination the disease should be explained to the patient, although the amount of time spent at this point depends on the simplicity or complexity of the problem and the physician's perception of how much of a "didactic" exercise the patient wishes to engage in. However, it is important to mention the general inutility of extrascrupulous cleansing, special diets, and the probable lack of association of the acne with the patient's sexual practices. Once a treatment plan is decided upon, the physician should be sure that the following are explained to the patient: (1) Treatments by and large are suppressive rather than curative, so that therapy must be maintained, or changed if later necessary, until the condition undergoes natural involution, which it does in most cases. (2) Most treatments work by preventing the formation of new lesions rather than by healing more rapidly those lesions already present. Moreover, this preventive effect is not ordinarily observed until 3 to 6 weeks have elapsed. (3) Apropos to this, medications must be applied topically to all the affected areas rather than to individual lesions per se. (4) Trunk acne seems to be less well controlled by topical therapy than facial acne.

Table 1 Tretinoin Preparations

FORM	CONCENTRATION (%)
Cream	0.025
	0.05
	0.1
Gel	0.01
	0.025
	0.1
Liquid	0.05

ANTIKERATINIZING (COMEDOLYTIC) EFFECT

Tretinoin (retinoic acid) is the most effective drug topically because of its capacity to reverse, at least in part, the abnormal follicular hyperkeratosis, the earliest known event in the formation of the acne lesion. By the same token it can help to prevent the transformation of early noninflammatory microcomedones (lesions not clinically visible) into inflammatory sequelae. Salicylic acid also has a keratolytic action, although its benefit in acne via this mechanism appears to be much less than that of tretinoin. Comedolytic assays have shown benzoyl peroxide to have a similar action, but its effect also seems to be comparatively weak.

The commonest objection patients have to the use of tretinoin is the primary irritant reaction it frequently causes. This can be lessened or even prevented by a number of measures that include waiting 20 to 30 minutes after washing before applying it; when using it at bedtime, not retiring until a half-hour has passed; using it every other day at first, rather than the recommended daily application, to allow for accommodation of the skin to its irritant effect; and at first, especially in the winter or dry climates, using the milder cream preparations. Tretinoin is available in creams (0.025, 0.05, and 0.1 percent) gels (0.01, 0.025, and 0.1 percent), and a liquid formulation (0.05 percent) (Table 1).

Another complaint patients may have about tretinoin, which is less frequent but more annoying to the patient, is that there is a flare-up of the acne in the early weeks of treatment. In my experience this occurs to some extent in about 20 percent of the patients and at times can be quite marked. Fortunately the flare-up subsides within a few weeks or sooner, but very uncommonly the worsening may continue unabated and requires discontinuation of medication.

Adapalene, a recently introduced topical antiacne preparation, derived from naphthoic acid and possessing retinoid activity, has shown similar benefit overall compared to tretinoin and with a leser incidence of irritation.

Oral therapy with isotretinoin, the 13-cis isomer of tretinoin, also, as one might expect, has antikeratinizing properties, but it has other antiacne actions as well. Treatment of acne with this drug is described later in this article.

ANTIMICROBIAL THERAPY

The therapy most commonly utilized for acne is antimicrobial therapy, owing in great measure to the availability of a wide variety of preparations for both topical and oral use. Implicit in the widespread use of antibacterial drugs is the recognition,

Table 2 Antibiotics for Acne

TOPICAL THERAPY	ORAL THERAPY
Clindamycin	Tetracycline
Erythromycin	Erythromycin
Meclocycline sulfosalicylate	Minocycline
Tetracycline	Doxycycline
	Trimethoprim-sulfamethoxazole
	Clindamycin

mentioned earlier, that the inflammatory lesions of acne for which most patients seek a physician's attention result from the presence of *P. acnes* within acne susceptible pilosebaceous follicles. One could postulate, with reasonable certainty, that if these follicles could be depleted of these anaerobic diphtheroids, inflammatory acne could be reduced to zero, regardless of whether abnormal keratinization was affected. In actuality suppression of *P. acnes* by antimicrobial therapy, whether topical or oral, is only partially achievable, although sometimes just enough to effect marked or complete amelioration of the inflammatory lesions.

For mild to moderate cases of inflammatory acne, benzoyl peroxide and topical antibiotic therapy have attained prominence in management. Benzoyl peroxide, longest in use for acne, is available in concentrations ranging from 1.0 to 10 percent and in a variety of vehicles—lotions, creams, gels, washes, and soaps. There are at least 30 different marketed preparations that are available with or without a prescription. The majority of nonprescription products are lotions and creams. There is no evidence that prescription products are more efficacious than over-the-counter preparations, although it is possible that gel formulations do possess some superiority.

Benzoyl peroxide may be applied one to two times daily, again being certain that the patient applies it to the entire affected area, although it has been reported that individual lesions may heal more quickly following its use. Benzoyl peroxide possesses two advantages over topical antibiotic therapy. First, it is, in general, more effective. Second, *P. acnes* resistance does not develop, so that if a patient's acne worsens during benzoyl peroxide therapy, it is because the acne has become more active rather than because the benzoyl peroxide somehow has been rendered less effective.

There are, however, disadvantages to the use of benzoyl peroxide compared with antibiotics. First, it is almost invariably more irritating than topically applied antibiotics, even if the lowest concentration, 2.5 percent, is used. Second, sensitization may occur (rare with topical antibiotic therapy), although the precise incidence has not been clearly established. In my experience fewer than one in 100 patients develop allergic contact dermatitis to benzoyl peroxide. Third, the irritant effect of benzoyl peroxide may accentuate the postinflammatory hyperpigmentation seen in dark skinned persons. Last, it may bleach hair and colored fabrics.

An alternative topical antibacterial to benzoyl peroxide is the recently marketed azelaic acid cream, a dicarboxylic acid, that shows significant reduction of *P. acnes* and an antikeratinizing effect as well.

Topical antibiotic therapy has come to occupy a prominent niche in the treatment of minimal to moderately inflamed acne. Such preparations include, in order of their introduction into the clinical practice, tetracycline, clindamycin, erythromycin, and meclocycline sulfosalicylate (Table 2). All have been shown in controlled studies to be more effective in reducing the number of inflammatory lesions than control vehicles, although as a general rule, the percentage difference in inhibition between active drug and control vehicle is less than that between the vehicle and the baseline valves. Tetracycline is the least effective of this group. Most of these antibiotics are in liquid vehicles, although some are available as pledgets, creams, and ointments. The latter two are better tolerated and more useful in patients with sensitive skin. Although, as noted, their effectiveness over a wide range of patients is less than that of benzoyl peroxide, one advantage is that the antibiotics are virtually devoid of allergenicity. A concern in regard to their use has been the potential for the development of resistant bacterial organisms.

The effect of benzoyl peroxide and of topical antibiotic therapy can be enhanced by the concomitant use of tretinoin. Often this combination, i.e., the use of each one daily or more frequently, is not well tolerated. However, if tolerated, a regimen of tretinoin with topical antibacterial therapy remains the most effective way, to date, of suppressing less than severe cases of acne. Benzoyl peroxide has also been combined with erythromycin in a single gel base preparation, and in another with glycolic acid.

Systemic antibiotic therapy has been used for decades in the treatment of acne. The four that are clearly effective in the majority of cases of inflammatory acne are tetracycline, erythromycin, minocycline, and doxycycline (see Table 2). Also effective is clindamycin, although it is infrequently used nowadays because of the risk, albeit very small, of the development of pseudomembranous colitis. The indications for the oral use of antibiotics in acne are as follows: moderately severe to severe inflammatory acne; less severe cases of acne not adequately responsive to topical therapy; still milder cases of acne, in which the individual because of sensitive skin (atopics often) is unable to tolerate topical therapy or in which there is evidence of active scarring; and patients with predominantly truncal acne, which ordinarily does not respond satisfactorily to externally applied medications.

The oral doses of antibiotics used vary with the severity of the disease, although I tend to start with "full" dosages, viz., 1.0 g of tetracycline daily or its equivalent for other antibiotics, even if the acne is only of moderate severity. A more rapid response is achieved and is decidedly preferable if there is any evidence of the development of scarring. An exception to this starting dosage of antibiotic is minocycline, which in dosages of 200 mg per day can cause symptoms of ototoxicity. Only if the disease is severe would I start with this dosage. Tetracycline must be taken on an empty stomach and for logistic reasons can be taken in twice daily doses of 500 mg, although occasionally this amount is not tolerated by the upper gastrointestinal tract. Erythromycin is less affected by the ingestion of food and minocycline, the least.

The advantages and disadvantages of the different antibiotics vary. Gastrointestinal effects occur most frequently with erythromycin. Phototoxicity is moderately severe with doxycycline, moderate with tetracycline, minimal with minocycline, and absent with erythromycin. *Candida* vaginitis is most frequent with tetracycline, occurring in about 15 percent of the patients taking long-term therapy. A special problem with minocycline is the occasional development of pigmentary changes, consisting either of small bluish tattoo-like macules on the face, often in scars, or less commonly a brownish hyperpigmentation elsewhere. These pigmentary changes are reversible on drug discontinuation.

The advantage shared by these three antibiotics is the very low incidence of allergic sensitization with their use. This is in contrast to trimethoprim-sulfamethoxazole, which is also effective for acne but with which allergic reactions are far more common.

Other antibiotics used in acne include ampicillin, amoxicillin, and the cephalosporin group of antibiotics. Controlled studies to assess their effectiveness are lacking. Ampicillin suppresses *P. acnes* weakly.

■ ANTI-INFLAMMATORY DRUGS

The most rapid and most predictable way of reducing the severity of inflammatory acne is the systemic use of corticosteroids in anti-inflammatory dosages, e.g., 30 to 50 mg of prednisone daily. Once the dosage is reduced to 10 to 15 mg per day, the acne begins to flare up. Obviously such treatment is replete with drawbacks, and its use is limited to patients who have periodic severe but infrequent and brief flare-ups.

The principal use of anti-inflammatory steroids is their injection into inflamed lesions to shorten their duration. I use triamcinolone acetonide suspension in a concentration of 2.5 to 10 mg per milliliter. The lower concentration is usually effective. In fact the results of one report have revealed that a concentration of 0.6 mg per milliliter is virtually as effective as higher ones. The risk of a 10 mg per milliliter concentration is the induction of atrophy, even though it almost always reverts with time.

Topical corticosteroid therapy seems to have little effect on acne, although the reason is not certain. The generally held view is that there is inadequate penetration of the steroid into the involved site. Moreover its use is thought to be contraindicated because of the weakening effect of the steroid on the follicular wall, with the possible consequent development of folliculitis ("steroid acne").

Studies with nonsteroidal anti-inflammatory drugs (e.g., naproxen, ibuprofen) have not shown an overwhelming benefit, even when administered in high dosages. However, one study showed unequivocally that the administration of high dosages of ibuprofen (2.4 g per day) enhances the antiacne effect of concomitantly administered tetracycline in a dosage of 1.0 g daily.

■ SEBACEOUS GLAND INHIBITION

Sebum, the secretory product of the sebaceous glands, is an integral factor in the pathogenesis of acne. A substantive reduction in the activity of these androgen-sensitive glands results in a decrease in the intensity of the disease. To date no topical therapy has been discovered that will effectively suppress sebaceous activity. Systemic therapy is required, involving the use of hormonal therapy for androgen suppression.

The drug longest in use for this purpose is estrogen, whose action is to inhibit the pituitary-ovarian axis, with consequent reduction of ovarian androgen production. Some effect on the adrenal gland may occur as well. The drugs are those marketed for oral contraception. Although no controlled studies have clearly delineated the effectiveness of oral estrogen treatment, clinical experience has disclosed that this form of therapy can be beneficial. However, uncomfortably high dosages of estrogen are usually needed, i.e., more than 50 μg of ethinyl estradiol or mestranol daily, to yield a reasonable chance of success. Preparations containing more than 50 μg of estrogen have been withdrawn from the market. The response is slow, requiring 2 to 4 months for clear-cut improvement to become evident. Moreover, as with virtually all other acne treatments, the effect is suppressive rather than curative, so that even if there is a good result, recurrence of the acne is the consequence of treatment discontinuance.

Another disadvantage of estrogen therapy is the problem of the concomitant use or need for oral antibiotic therapy for the acne or other medical conditions. There have been reports that antibiotics may decrease the level of the administered estrogen in the blood. As a consequence, if the estrogen is being taken for the dual purpose of acne treatment and contraception, protection against pregnancy might be reduced. The chance that such an interaction will lead to pregnancy is not known but is likely to be very low.

Another method for androgen suppression is low-dose glucocorticoid administration to decrease adrenal elaboration of androgens, particularly dehydroepiandrosterone. In many studies this androgen, either free or sulfated, has been found to be increased in women with persistent acne, even without collateral signs of androgen excess. Treatment of such patients with dexamethasone, 0.25 to 0.5 mg daily, or with prednisone, 5 to 10 mg daily, has been reported to decrease the acne. However, as with estrogen, controlled studies are still lacking so that the true benefit from low-dose steroid treatment remains unestablished. What has been demonstrated, however, is that combined estrogen-glucocorticoid treatment effects a marked reduction in sebum levels and very significant acne improvement.

Spironolactone in high dosages, i.e., 100 to 200 mg daily, has a peripheral antiandrogen effect. It has been reported to be helpful in women with acne. I have found it to be effective in approximately 50 percent of the patients, the remainder showing only modest to no improvement. Common side effects from spironolactone are menstrual irregularity and fatigue, symptoms that can decrease despite continued administration of the drug.

With any form of hormone therapy I generally try not to exceed 9 months of treatment but occasionally continue the therapy for up to 12 months. The occurrence of side effects in any given patient might curtail the use of whatever regimen has been selected.

■ ISOTRETINOIN

Introduced into clinical practice in 1982, the synthetic retinoid, isotretinoin, has proved to be superior in the treatment of acne and the drug to use in patients with severe nodulocystic acne in whom traditional regimens, including systemic antibiotic therapy, have failed. In fact, it is only in this class of patient that the drug has been approved for use. However, my inclination is to extend its use to the occasional patient who has less severe cystic acne or even noncystic acne but who is developing active scarring and has resisted the standard treatments. The oral dosage of isotretinoin is 0.5 to 2.0 mg per kilogram per day. The dosage that should suffice for most patients is 60 to 80 mg per day, although heavy individuals or those with predominantly truncal acne may require the higher dosages. The drug generally induces a high incidence of remission despite the severity of the disease and its previous recalcitrance to treatment.

Numerous side effects preclude the use of the drug in all forms of acne, although most of the reactions are more of a nuisance than a danger. These changes are chiefly in the skin and mucous membranes and most commonly consist of cheilitis, various types of dry skin rashes, dry eyes, minor degrees of scalp hair loss, and occasional musculoskeletal discomfort. Perhaps the most annoying side effect, insofar as the patient is concerned, is a temporary worsening of the acne, not dissimilar to that seen with tretinoin given topically, but more severe, and observed in about one-third of the patients treated with isotretinoin.

Minimal hyperostoses have been seen in spinal x-ray views in acne patients treated with conventional doses of isotretinoin. They have occurred in 10 percent of the patients, have been asymptomatic, and have not progressed on discontinuation of treatment. Decrease in dark adaptation has been experienced, which reverts to normal when the drug is stopped. The most serious side effect of isotretinoin is its teratogenic potential. One study demonstrates a 25-fold increase in the development of major fetal abnormalities in women who were pregnant or became pregnant while receiving the drug. Prevention of pregnancy while the patient is taking this treatment and for 1 month afterward is an absolute necessity, with the responsibility shared by the physician and the patient.

■ MISCELLANEOUS FORMS OF THERAPY

Cryotherapy

In addition to intralesional injections of steroid to combat inflammation in individual lesions, the use of cryotherapy is a useful alternative, although in my experience not as effective. Liquid nitrogen or dry ice is applied to individual lesions. Even less effective is the application of ice, but this has the advantage that the patient can do it at home. No standard regimen has been developed for lesional "ice cube" treatment, but I suggest to the patient that at the first evidence of a new inflammatory lesion forming, an ice cube be applied for 5 to 10 minutes to the lesion three to four times daily for 1 to 2 days. Some patients claim benefit from this treatment.

Surgical Measures

In active disease both noninflammatory and inflammatory lesions can be decreased by minor surgical procedures. Comedones can be removed with ease and little discomfort. Open comedones can be extracted directly but closed comedones first need to have the small pore opening enlarged by inserting and rotating the opening with a 20 gauge needle.

Inflammatory lesions may be drained if pus is evident, but care must be taken not to incise widely. If the pustular contents cannot be drained easily following simple needle puncture, the lesion is best left alone or instead injected intralesionally with steroid.

A variety of procedures are used to improve the appearance of scars that may form during the healing of inflammatory lesions. If the scars are hypertrophic (usually on the neck, shoulders, upper back, and anterior chest), they can be injected with triamcinolone acetonide suspension in concentrations ranging from 10 to 40 mg per milliliter. Hypertrophic scars, however, have the tendency to decrease slowly in size spontaneously.

Atrophic scars are permanent. A variety of techniques are available for their removal, including dermabrasion, simple excision, excision with punch grafts, and bovine collagen implants, and lasers.

ATOPIC DERMATITIS

Amy S. Paller, M.D.

Atopic dermatitis is a chronic, severely pruritic disorder characterized by dry skin, eczematous patches, lichenification, and a predisposition to staphylococcal pyodermas. The term *atopic* refers to the fact that affected children frequently have elevated IgE levels and a family or personal history of other atopic disorders, especially allergic rhinitis or asthma. The disorder usually begins in infancy but occasionally occurs later in childhood or even in adulthood. The incidence of atopic dermatitis has been rapidly increasing, particularly in urban areas, and the disorder is now thought to occur in 10 percent of 1-year-old infants. The diagnosis is made by the characteristic distribution and clinical features of the rash.

Treatment of atopic dermatitis must be individualized, and based upon several clinical and historical criteria (Table 1). For most patients, atopic dermatitis is a condition that flares readily when therapy is discontinued. Therefore, the regimen must be amenable to long-term patient compliance and safety. For patients with mild atopic dermatitis, the application of emollients and low-strength corticosteroid preparations suffices. For more severely affected patients, the use of stronger corticosteroid preparations and, occasionally, systemic medication may be necessary. Education of patients and parents, including discussions about the chronicity of the disorder and the suppressive, but not curative, effect of medication, is critical for successful therapy. Patients should be reassured, however, that therapy can result in dramatic improvement and that disfiguring pigmentary changes and lichenification can be prevented. Physicians should discuss expected features and complications, exacerbating factors, handling of acute flares, and the choice of reasonable maintenance therapy. The Eczema Association for Science and Education (1221 S.W. Yamhill, Suite 303, Portland, OR 97205, 503-228-4430) provides educational brochures in English and Spanish. In the United Kingdom, the National Eczema Society also has educational materials.

Table 1 Clinical Features That Determine Therapy

Age of patient
Age of onset and course of the dermatitis
Location of involvement, degree of lichenification
Previous response to therapy
Seasonal variation
Occupational history if relevant
Presence of secondary infection
Prior diagnostic studies

■ FACTORS TO CONSIDER IN CHOOSING THERAPY

Initial evaluation should consider the possibility of other diagnostic possibilities, particularly seborrheic dermatitis, juvenile plantar dermatosis, allergic or irritant contact dermatitis, scabies, psoriasis, mycosis fungoides, and rarely, immunodeficiency such as Wiskott-Aldrich syndrome or hyperimmunoglobulinemia E syndrome.

Criteria for the diagnosis of atopic dermatitis have been-well established (Table 2). In addition to the history and examination, the presence of an elevated serum IgE level and eosinophilia may provide further evidence of atopy. Specific tests may be indicated to consider alternative diagnoses, such as mineral oil scrapings to show the scabies mite. Questions regarding the time of onset (usually after the first 2 months of age), degree of pruritus, sensitivity to irritants, and seasonal variations may help to establish the diagnosis. Determining the bathing habits and past experiences with trials of topical corticosteroid preparations and antibiotics will help in management. Attention should be paid to the distribution and character of lesions on physical examination and to the coexistence of secondary infection or other abnormalities that may suggest a systemic abnormality. No routine laboratory testing is necessary.

The rash of atopic dermatitis is aggravated by a number of factors (Table 3). Patients with the disorder have extremely dry skin attributable to increased transepidermal water loss and epidermal hyperproliferation induced by inflammation. The decreased efficiency of the stratum corneum as a protective barrier perpetuates inflammation by increasing the access of allergens and irritants. The dermatitis often becomes aggravated by the low humidity of winter and irritants such as detergents and soaps, wool, and saliva. Dermatitis may be

Table 2 Criteria for Atopic Dermatitis

MAJOR FEATURES (NEED THREE OR MORE)

1. Pruritus
2. Typical appearance and distribution of lesions
   Facial and extensor involvement in infancy and early childhood
   Flexural involvement and lichenification by adolescence
3. Chronic or frequently relapsing dermatitis
4. Personal or family history of atopy (atopic dermatitis, allergic rhinoconjunctivitis, asthma, urticaria)

MINOR, LESS SPECIFIC FEATURES

1. Xerosis
2. IgE reactivity (High serum IgE, prick test or RAST tests positive)
3. Ichthyosis; keratosis pilaris; hyperlinearity of palms
4. Hand/foot dermatitis
5. Periauricular fissures
6. Cheilitis
7. Scalp dermatitis (i.e., cradle cap)
8. Perifollicular accentuation, especially in dark-skinned patients
9. Increased tendency towards cutaneous infections, especially *Staphylococcus aureus* and herpes simplex

Modified from Hanifin JM, Rajka G. Diagnostic features of atopic dermatitis. Acta Dermatol Venereol 1980; 92(suppl):44.

Table 3 Exacerbating Factors in Atopic Dermatitis

Dry skin
Sensitivity to irritants (wool, sweat, saliva)
Sensitivity to allergens (foods, airborne, contact allergens)
Infection (*S. aureus*, molluscum, H. simplex)
Coexisting pruritic disease, such as chickenpox
Emotional stress

exacerbated during summer months because of the irritant reaction to sweat and sweat retention. Soaking in water and frequent handwashing may result in extensive evaporative loss from skin; however, such actions can actually increase the hydration of skin if good emollients are subsequently applied. In general, patients should avoid choosing occupations with frequent handwashing or exposure to irritating chemicals.

The process of rubbing or scratching leads to more rash and more pruritus ("itch-scratch cycle"), so that any cause of pruritus tends to aggravate the dermatitis. Cutaneous infections and superimposed allergic contact dermatitis (see following discussion) may also exacerbate the dermatitis by increasing local inflammation, dryness, and pruritus. Many patients also note a flare of the atopic dermatitis when noncutaneous infections occur such as viral infections or streptococcal pharyngitis.

Emotional stress can impact tremendously on the severity of atopic dermatitis. Familial discord, often triggered by the increased demands of a child with atopic dermatitis, and interpersonal problems with other children at school, including teasing or exclusion of the child, are common problems for the patient with atopic dermatitis. Likewise, major stress such as death of a family member or separation from parents by divorce is also associated with eczematous flares. These psychological problems should be explored and dealt with by the family and personal counseling should be sought, if appropriate.

COMPLICATIONS OF ATOPIC DERMATITIS

The most common complication of atopic dermatitis is secondary bacterial infection of affected areas of skin, especially at excoriated sites. The usual organism is *Staphylococcus aureus*, and the lesions of impetigo usually appear as superficial yellow crusting overlying erythema, although small superficial pustules are sometimes seen. Patients with secondary infection will often not respond to appropriate therapy for the underlying eczema unless the infection is cleared with systemic antibiotics.

Eczema herpeticum (Kaposi's varicelliform eruption) is a complication of atopic dermatitis that is characterized by the abrupt development and rapid spread of the vesicles of herpes simplex. The lesions are usually groups of intact or umbilicated vesicles and pustules overlying erythema. Screening tests, such as Tzanck smear or immunodetection with anti–herpes simplex antibodies should be performed, and viral culture is confirmatory. Children with atopic dermatitis also have an increased risk of the development and spread of molluscum contagiosum, particularly at sites of xerosis and inflammation.

Contact urticaria may manifest as hives or lead to the development of dermatitis such as on the cheeks and perioral area of infants. Older patients may develop contact urticaria from occupational exposure. The reaction usually occurs within 30 minutes at the site of direct contact.

Allergic contact dermatitis may be an important exacerbating factor, and may be difficult to distinguish from the atopic dermatitis itself. Nickel and agents in topical medications are the most important causes in patients with atopic dermatitis. For example, a patch of recalcitrant dermatitis near the umbilical area may be caused by nickel contact from the snap on pants or a belt buckle, rather than the atopic condition.

Neomycin and lanolin frequently cause reactions in patients with atopic dermatitis, since these agents may be present in topical antibiotic preparations and emollients, respectively. Patch testing allows confirmation of the suspected allergen, but false-positive reactions are common in patients with atopic dermatitis.

POSSIBLE ALLERGIC TRIGGERS

The significance of food-induced atopic dermatitis remains controversial. Prick tests and radioallergosorbent test results do not correlate well with response to avoidance and challenge and are most useful if negative. Challenge studies have shown that the ingestion of certain foods, particularly eggs, milk, soy, wheat, and peanuts, can initiate reactions in patients with atopic dermatitis within 2 hours after challenge. However, the unclear relationship between these studies and the occurrence of the dermatitis itself and the fact that removal of these offending allergens does not control the dermatitis suggest that dietary therapy is not of much value for most patients with atopic dermatitis. Furthermore, dietary manipulation may be difficult to implement, particularly in children. Most dermatologists consider food allergies to be of little significance and reserve dietary manipulation for patients with severe eczema who do not respond to more traditional measures.

Airborne allergens have also been implicated as triggers for atopic dermatitis, based largely upon the distribution of lesions at exposed, body areas and supporting evidence by positive patch testing. Airborne allergens, such as dust mites, pets, and molds, are probably more significant for older children and adults, but the allergens are difficult to remove from the environment. Highly motivated patients may take measures to limit dust, such as frequent vacuuming (by another person), encasing mattresses and pillows in occlusive materials, and removing of dust-entrapping curtains, drapes, and stuffed animals.

Table 4 Therapy of Atopic Dermatitis

1. Education and reassurance of patient and family
2. Lubrication: Lukewarm baths or compresses at least once daily, followed by the application of a moisturizing cream or ointment such as petrolatum to the wet skin; moisturizers may be applied more frequently if needed
3. Application twice daily of anti-inflammatory topical corticosteroid preparations, preferably in a moisturizing base. The selection of corticosteroid should be based on the age of the patient, location of lesions, and response to previous therapy
4. Administration of oral antibiotics if eroded, crusted, or pustular lesions are present (e.g., course of cephalexin for 2 weeks)
5. Trial of antihistamines, such as hydroxyzine or combination of H_1- and H_2-blockers. Topical doxepin is now available
6. Alternative agents for more severely involved patients—tar preparations, ultraviolet light therapy, systemic corticosteroids, interferon-gamma, or cyclosporine
7. Avoidance of irritants and specific allergens, such as food or aeroallergens, as appropriate for the individual

■ MANAGEMENT OF ATOPIC DERMATITIS

After the pattern of the dermatitis, aggravating factors, and response to previous therapy are assessed, a therapeutic plan with reasonable goals may be initiated. The regimen usually includes avoidance of exacerbating agents, improved lubrication of skin, and application of anti-inflammatory agents (Table 4).

General Measures

Many patients with atopic dermatitis benefit from a daily bath or shower, which adds water to the outer layer of skin, followed immediately by the application of emollient creams or ointments. Harsh soaps should be substituted with mild or superfatted soaps. The bathwater should be lukewarm since hot water increases skin dryness. Bubble baths are best avoided since they are irritating, but bath oils may be beneficial. Humidifiers are also helpful during dry winter months, but they must be cleaned at least weekly to avoid the dissemination of molds.

Although most patients are troubled by dryness and pruritus in winter, some patients experience more difficulty in the summer, and irritation from sweat may be a major problem. These patients may complain of pruritus with the application of thicker lubricants and benefit from lubricating lotions, which are less occlusive. Such patients are also helped by the use of air conditioners in summer months. Similarly, most patients improve with a regimen of daily baths followed immediately by lubrication. Others cannot tolerate water at all, especially if there are many excoriated or infected sites, and benefit from temporary avoidance of water.

Corticosteroids

Anti-inflammatory topical corticosteroid preparations are usually necessary to clear the inflammatory lesions. The strength and base of the chosen topical preparation depends on the location and severity of the rash and on the age and tolerance of the patient. Fluorinated corticosteroids should never be used for more than a few days on the face or intertriginous areas because of the risk of skin atrophy. Milder eruptions or eruptions on younger children may clear with the use of weak, nonfluorinated agents only such as hydrocortisone or a nonfluorinated medium-strength corticosteroid, whereas patients who are older or with more severe pruritus and inflammation may require a fluorinated moderate- or high-strength corticosteroid. Most patients with dry skin prefer ointment or emollient-based preparations, especially during winter months, while others prefer to use cream-based preparations covered with lubricating agents. Corticosteroid gels and lotions are usually too drying for patients with atopic dermatitis.

Systemic corticosteroids are indicated only for patients with severe involvement who do not respond adequately to topical agents, and short courses are often included for patients who require hospitalization to reverse an acute flare. Exacerbations following discontinuation of systemic corticosteroid therapy are a further disadvantage of this therapeutic approach.

Antipruritics

Oral antihistamine preparations, especially hydroxyzine, doxepin, and diphenhydramine, may be valuable, especially for their sedative effects at night when scratching is most intense. Nonsedating antihistamines usually provide little relief. The addition of the H_2-blocker, cimetidine, has been useful in many patients with atopic dermatitis. The newly released topical doxepin may diminish cutaneous pruritus, but it may also cause sedation if large amounts are applied.

Other Therapy

Weeping dermatitis is often due to secondary infection and requires compresses to dry the areas and to remove crusts and debris. Burow's solution or cool saline compresses should be applied two to three times daily for 20 to 30 minutes using a thin cloth, such as a handkerchief, to allow for evaporative loss. Topical corticosteroid or lubrication may be applied after the compressing.

If bacterial infection is suspected and involves more than a small area, the patient should be treated with systemic antistaphylococcal antibiotics. The choice of systemic therapy should be based upon the local resistance patterns of *S. aureus*, since many staphylococcal organisms are now resistant to erythromycin. Cephalosporins and dicloxacillin are frequently used alternatives. If herpetic infections develop and show a predisposition towards spread, systemic acyclovir therapy is indicated.

Other topical agents that have been helpful for patients with atopic dermatitis include ultraviolet light, mild tar preparations that are applied directly to the skin (e.g., T-derm oil, Estargel, or Psorigel) or added to bathwater (e.g., Balnetar), and keratolytics such as urea or salicylic acid for lichenified plaques. For patients with severe, recalcitrant atopic dermatitis, systemic administration of daily subcutaneous interferon-gamma or oral cyclosporine by a specialist familiar with these medications is an alternative possibility.

Indications for Referral and Admission

Patients who are difficult to manage or who require more than moderate-strength topical corticosteroid preparations should be referred to a dermatologist for management. Patients with severe atopic dermatitis who cannot be managed effectively as outpatients may respond to the intensive topical or systemic management of brief hospitalization. Patients with significant eczema herpeticum or severe secondary bacterial infections may also require observation and treatment in the hospital.

Suggested Reading

Cooper KD. New therapeutic approaches in atopic dermatitis. Clin Rev Allergy 1993; 11:543.

Dahl MV. Atopic dermatitis: the concept of flare factors. South Med J 1977; 70:453.

Hanifin JM, Rajka G. Diagnostic features of atopic dermatitis. Acta Dermatol Venereol 1980; 92(Suppl):44.

Sampson HA. Atopic dermatitis. Ann Allergy 1992; 69:469.

CONTACT DERMATITIS

Vincent A. DeLeo, M.D.

The term *contact dermatitis* is used to describe adverse reactions in the skin that occur secondary to direct contact with chemicals in the environment. The response is one of dermatitis or eczema, which are morphologic responses of the skin, representing inflammation of the epidermis with edema between the keratinocytes. Therefore, the process does not include reactions such as contact urticaria, which result from chemical contact and are not dermatitic. The reaction can be a manifestation of direct damage by the chemical or it can be mediated by immune mechanisms. In the case of the former, the response is referred to as *irritant contact dermatitis,* whereas the immune-mediated response is called *allergic contact dermatitis.* The mechanism of the irritant response is variable and is specific to the chemical structure of the irritant. The mechanism of the allergic reaction is a T-cell mediated, type IV response.

Irritant contact dermatitis is one of the most common of all dermatologic maladies and can be caused by an almost infinite number of naturally occurring and man-made agents. The most common of these are surfactants and solvents. Allergic contact dermatitis, on the other hand, is thought to be related to a finite number of chemicals capable of eliciting the immune response. The number usually quoted is 3,000 different substances (Table 1). Irritant contact dermatitis accounts for approximately 70 to 80 percent of all cases of contact dermatitis, while allergic reactions cause the remainder.

■ DIAGNOSIS

Although the mechanism of the response to the exogenous chemical is different for allergic and irritant contact dermatitis, the response in the clinical setting is very similar. This is probably because the mechanism of both responses ultimately involves many of the same cells, inflammatory mediators, and cytokines. The response is an eczematous dermatitis and can be either *acute* with erythema, edema, and vesicles; *subacute* with erythema, edema, scale, and oozing; or *chronic* with erythema, scale, and lichenification.

The diagnosis of irritant contact dermatitis is based on the appearance of an eczema in a localized distribution combined with a history of exposure to irritating substances. While the diagnosis of allergic contact dermatitis is also suggested by history and physical findings, it is dependent on positive response to patch testing.

The distribution of contact dermatitis is key to the diagnosis of this condition. Most irritant dermatitis involves the hands. This is obviously because the hands are usually the first part of the skin surface to contact the environment, at home and in the workplace. Irritant contact dermatitis of the hands is the most common occupational skin disease. Allergic reactions frequently involve the hands, face, and feet. Other areas can also be involved with specific antigens. Nickel dermatitis, for example, frequently presents in a "jewelry distribution," involving the earlobes, neck, and wrist;

Table 1 The Most Common Agents Causing Allergic Contact Dermatitis

Plants
Toxicodendrum
Poison Ivy, Oak, Sumac
Rubber
Mercaptobenzothiazole
Thiurams
Carbamates
Black Rubber Paraphenylene diamine
Medicaments
Benzocaine
Thimerosal
Neomycin sulfate
Quinolones
Cosmetics
Fragrances
Cinnamic Aldehyde
Balsam of Peru
Vehicles, preservatives and additives
Lanolin alcohol
Imidazolidinyl urea
Quarternium-15
Formaldehyde
Ethylenediamine dihydrocholoride
Cl + Me-isothiazolinone
Parabens
Hair dyes
p-Phenylenediamine
Metals
Nickel sulfate
Potassium dichromate
Cobalt dichloride
Resins
Colophony
Epoxy resin
p-tert-Butylphenol formaldehyde resin

medicament allergy involves those areas where topical medication has been applied, as for example, the lower legs in individuals with stasis dermatitis.

TREATMENT

Treatment of contact dermatitis depends on the morphology of the eczema involved, the distribution and extent of the skin surface involved, the chronicity of the reaction, and the history of chemical exposure. *Treatment consists of identification and avoidance of the offending agent(s) and amelioration of the inflammatory response.*

Reduction of inflammation is based on cool water soaks, which help to dry and cool acute eczema and can be used to help emolliate dry, chronic eczematous skin, and administration of topical or systemic corticosteroids. The strength of the topical steroid used depends on the severity of the dermatitis, the area of the body involved, and the age of the patient (Table 2).

Side effects of topical steroid usage include atrophy, systemic absorption with attendant side effects, and acneform eruptions, especially of the face. Recently even contact allergy has been reported, especially to hydrocortisone. With the exception of contact allergy, the risk of all side effects are increased with increasing potency and when the steroid is used in children, on large surface areas, and in intertriginous areas.

The lowest potency steroids include hydrocortisone and desonide. *Low-potency agents should be the only ones used in children and on the face and in intertriginous areas such as the groin and the axillae in adults. In fact, in very small children and on the face of adults, hydrocortisone is the only agent that can be used with absolute assurance of no significant side effects.*

Medium-range agents include triamcinolone acetonide (<0.1 percent) and betamethasone valerate; the high-potency agents include some products of betamethasone dipropionate and the very highest potency include clobetasol propionate. In addition, the product should be chosen according to the base that will most assist in the therapeutic process—cream, lotion, or ointment.

Systemic antihistamine therapy may be utilized if itching is severe. It should be remembered, however, that the itch of contact dermatitis is not histamine mediated to any great extent and the benefit of antihistamines is based on their sedating qualities. Therefore soporific antihistamines, like diphenhydramine or hydroxyzine, should be used, and the chosen dosage should be sedating. Such agents should be used primarily before bedtime if the patient is to continue to work or drive an automobile.

Contact dermatitis of all types may become secondarily infected with bacteria, usually *Staphylococcus aureus.* When suspected, an antibiotic should be administered. The antibiotic should always be given systemically since topical antibiotics may only complicate the process of contact dermatitis. Erythromycins or cephalosporins are the drugs of choice and the dosage for both drugs, erythromycin and cephalexin, is 250 mg four times per day for 10 days.

With *acute eczema of short duration* (a few days or a week or two) the physician should take a detailed history of exposure of the body part involved. It should include exposure at the workplace, in the home, and in leisure activities. The history should include the topical agents applied by the patient before the visit, since in many cases the initial problem will have been complicated by the application of an irritant or allergen. The patient should be instructed to avoid those agents that may have caused or may be complicating the process. The inflamed skin areas should be soaked in cool water two to four times a day for approximately 10 to 15 minutes. The skin should be gently dried and a topical steroid in a cream base should be applied. In children and for the face, groin, and axillae of adults the mildest group of topical steroids should be used. For other areas of the body the moderate, high, or, less frequently, the most potent classes of agents should be used. The eruption should dry and become subacute within 3 to 4 days. At that point, the soaks can be decreased in frequency or discontinued, and the topical steroid can be maintained. If the skin becomes too dry the topical steroid can be changed to an ointment-based product. The reaction should be completely resolved within 1 to 2 weeks.

If the *acute eczema of short duration* is extensive or involves the face or genital areas with extensive edema, systemic steroids can be used. This usually occurs with allergic disease caused by poison ivy (or oak or sumac) or hair dye. The dosage for an adult is 40 to 60 mg per day of prednisone orally for

Table 2 Topical Adrenocorticoid Strengths

GENERIC NAME	STRENGTH (%)	SOME TRADE NAMES
LOW-POTENCY ADRENOCORTICOIDS		
Alclometasone dipropionate	0.05	Aclovate
Clocortolone pivalate	0.1	Cloderm
Desonide	0.05	Tridesilon
Dexamethasone	0.04–0.1	Decaderm
Dexamethasone sodium phosphate	0.1	Decadron
Flumethasone pivalate	0.03	Locacorten
Flurandrenolide	0.0125	Cordran, Drenison
Hydrocortisone acetate	0.1–1	Cortaid, Cortefete
Methylprednisolone	0.25–1	Medrol
MEDIUM-POTENCY ADRENOCORTICOIDS		
Beclomethasone dipropionate	0.025	Propaderm
Betamethasone benzoate	0.025	Uticort, Beben
Betamethasone valerate	0.05–0.1	Valisone, Betnovate
Clobetasol butyrate	0.05	Eumovate
Desoximetasone	0.05	Topicort
Diflucortolone valerate	0.1	Nerisone
Fluocinolone acetonide	0.01–0.25	Synalar
Flurandrenolide	0.025–0.05	Cordran, Drenison
Hydrocortisone butyrate	0.1	Locoid
Hydrocortisone valerate	0.2	Westcort
Mometasone furoate	0.1	Elocon
Triamcinolone acetonide	0.015–0.1	Aristocort, Kenalog
HIGH-POTENCY ADRENOCORTICOIDS		
Amcinonide	0.1	Cyclocort
Betamethasone dipropionate	0.05	Alphatrex, Diprosone
Desoximetasone	0.05–0.25	Topicort
Diflorasone diacetate	0.05	Florone, Maxiflor
Fluocinonide	0.05	Lidex
Halcinonide	0.025–0.1	Halog
Triamcinolone acetonide	0.5	Halciderm, Aristocort
VERY HIGH-POTENCY ADRENOCORTICOIDS		
Betamethasone dipropionate	0.05	Diprolene, Diprolene AF
Clobetasol propionate	0.05	Dermovate, Temovate
Diflorasone diacetate	0.05	Psorcon

Modified from Maddin S. Dermatologic therapy. In: Moschella S, Hurley H, eds. Dermatology. 3rd edition. Vol 2. Philadelphia: WB Saunders, 1990: 2193.

the first day, with a gradual taper over a period of 14 days. Complications should always be considered before instituting therapy in individuals with other disease processes. The entire dosage should be given in the morning with milk or food and the taper should never be for less than 2 weeks. Shorter courses of steroids frequently result in a rebound flare of the disease. There is no place for systemic steroid therapy in irritant contact dermatitis.

In *subacute eczema of short duration* avoidance of irritants and allergens should be undertaken. Usually soaking of the skin will not be necessary. The patient should be treated with a steroid appropriate for the area of the body and the age of the patient as outlined earlier, but the agent must be in an ointment base.

In *subacute or chronic eczema of long duration,* that is more than 2 or 3 weeks, the same therapeutic maneuvers as just outlined should be undertaken, but patch testing to identify the allergen should be considered. Only such testing can identify the causative agent if allergic disease is present. Once the process has continued, especially in spite of therapy, allergy is more likely.

Only patch testing can identify the causative allergen in allergic contact dermatitis. Identification and instruction of the patient in avoidance of allergen exposure is the only way to "cure" the disease. The physician must keep a high index of suspicion when treating patients thought to have irritant contact dermatitis. If avoidance of irritants and topical steroids do not result in clearing after a few weeks then patch testing must be undertaken. The reader is referred to the references for a discussion of the techniques of patch testing.

In *chronic eczema* topical steroids in ointment bases should be used. Cool water soaks with application of the steroid ointment to moist skin will assist in emolliating the dry, lichenified skin.

In many cases of irritant contact dermatitis of the *subacute or chronic eczematous type of long duration,* irritants cannot be completely avoided. In such cases a strategy of treating chronic disease should be undertaken once contact allergy has been ruled out by adequate patch testing. This most commonly involves treatment of chronic dermatitis of the hand. Such patients should be encouraged to use emolliation, and topical steroids should be saved only for acute flares of disease.

The best agents include petrolatum and hydrophilic ointment, but a multitude of over-the-counter moisturizers are available. Agents with fragrance and, when possible, preservatives should be avoided since these can cause allergy with long-term usage.

Finally, specialized procedures can be used to treat chronic dermatitis, including phototherapy and photochemotherapy, which are available through referral to dermatologists who specialize in those modalities.

The chronic use of systemic corticosteroids in the treatment of dermatitis is to be discouraged and only used with dermatologic consultation and under the direst circumstances. In such cases other diseases like psoriasis should always be considered and appropriate testing, including skin biopsies, may be necessary.

Avoidance Strategy

Instructing patients to avoid irritants or allergens is an essential part of the therapy of contact dermatitis. In the management of most patients this will necessitate an understanding of the patient's job and home environments, including skin care regimens.

As previously stated, if the dermatitis is recurrent or chronic, patch testing must be done to identify the offending allergen or to rule out allergy so that the patient can be treated for chronic dermatitis of the irritant or endogenous type with assurance.

If the patient encounters wet work on the job, such exposure should be minimized. In most cases of suspected occupational contact dermatitis, patch testing should be done initially or shortly after the beginning of therapy if such therapy does not resolve the dermatitis. If no allergy is found, protective gloves may be utilized, depending on the safety of using such protective garments.

In the home environment the patient should be instructed to use rubber gloves whenever wet work is anticipated. Since the hands perspire in such gloves, if the job lasts for more than a few minutes, the patient should be instructed to wear cotton gloves beneath the rubber gloves.

A growing problem is allergy to rubber gloves. The types of reactions caused by such gloves include allergic contact dermatitis of the delayed type, which is due to rubber accelerators and contact urticaria caused by the latex molecule itself, which is an immediate type of sensitivity and can even lead to anaphylaxis. The easiest way to avoid both reactions is to recommend vinyl rather than latex gloves. When such allergy is suspected proper testing (RAST and/or scratch-prick testing) should be carried out since allergy of the immediate type should be known to the patient so as to avoid serious consequences from future exposure.

It should also be remembered that gloves of either latex or vinyl do not prevent the penetration of some allergens. The reader is referred to the reference texts for a discussion of those antigens.

Patients should be instructed to decrease handwashing and to use only cream-based soaps. Antibacterial or deodorant soaps should be avoided and a moisturizer such as petrolatum should be applied immediately after each washing.

Patients with facial dermatitis should be instructed to avoid all cosmetics during acute disease flares. If the reaction recurs the patient should be patch tested. Simply changing from one product or cosmetic line to another is almost always futile since common agents are used in various products. One strategy that may be tried short of patch testing is to switch to fragrance-free cosmetic if fragranced agents were used at the time of the eruption. This may work since the most frequent cosmetic allergen is fragrance.

Frequently, agents used to treat dermatitis induce a secondary allergic contact dermatitis. These agents include topical antibiotics, especially neomycin and bacitracin; topical caines and diphenhydramine; fragrances and preservatives in moisturizers and body lotions; and even topical corticosteroids themselves. The safest agents to use are petrolatum-based ointments that do not contain the agents just listed. Two agents that seem to cause few problems are Synalar ointment and Diprosone ointment.

Suggested Reading

Adams RM. Occupational skin disease. 2nd ed. Philadelphia: WB Saunders, 1990.

Cronin E. Contact Dermatitis. New York: Churchill Livingstone, 1980.

Fisher AA. Contact Dermatitis. Philadelphia: Lea & Febiger, 1986.

Maddin S. Dermatologic Therapy. In: Moschella S, Hurley H, eds. Dermatology. 3rd ed, Vol 2. Philadelphia: WB Saunders, 1990: 2193.

Marks JG, DeLeo VA. Contact and occupational dermatology. 2nd ed. St. Louis: Mosby–Year Book, 1997.

PSORIASIS

Warwick L. Morison, M.B., B.S., M.R.C.P.

We are all familiar with the concept of the "heartbreak" of psoriasis, although it is not clear whether the grief is felt by the physician, the patient, or both. The concept embodies the negative attitude toward treatment of the disease in so many patients and physicians. This negative attitude is unfounded because psoriasis can be successfully treated. However, to achieve this the physician must have a planned approach to the management of the disease. The plan must contain several key elements.

First, the physician must recognize, and explain to the patient, that psoriasis is a chronic disease that usually persists for years, that there is no quick fix or cure, but that there are some very successful treatments that can control the disease in most patients. Second, the initial visit must include a full evaluation of the patient and the disease. Sex, age, occupation, social environment, geographic location, and medical history are important factors in deciding upon the best treatment for the type and extent of disease present. This evaluation takes time, but is essential because the physician must know the patient, the disease, and how the patient feels about the disease. Third, the patient must be educated about the disease and all possible treatments; a handout is an invaluable addition but not a substitute for this explanation. Finally, the treatment program that is agreed upon with the patient must be tailored to the patient and to the disease. The patient must be "sold" on the treatment or it will not be used. The treatment must have a reasonable risk-benefit ratio and be effective for the type of disease being treated.

THERAPEUTIC AGENTS

Treatment modalities with antipsoriatic activity can be broadly divided into three groups: topical, ultraviolet radiation, and systemic. This sequence also roughly defines their risk-benefit ratios: topical agents are usually safest and of benefit only in limited disease, while systemic agents carry greatest risk and should be used only in extensive disease.

Topical Agents

Topically applied corticosteroids are the most frequently prescribed treatment for psoriasis, and this is probably more a tribute to advertising by drug companies rather than their true value as treatment. Only rarely do these agents convert psoriasis to normal skin, and as soon as the treatment is stopped, the psoriasis usually rapidly returns. Tachyphylaxis, permanent atrophy of the skin, and conversion of stable psoriasis to a more aggressive disease, are the chief problems associated with use of these agents. The introduction of clobetasol propionate and betamethasone dipropionate will undoubtedly add new adverse effects. Adrenal suppression and precipitation of generalized pustular psoriasis have been observed frequently in Europe with such potent agents. For all these reasons, corticosteroids should be used in psoriasis only as adjunctive treatment with other more effective agents, in special situations such as the treatment of nails, and in patients who will accept improvement rather than clearance of disease. Systemically administered corticosteroids have no place in the treatment of psoriasis, since rebound spreading disease and serious adverse effects are almost inevitable.

There has been a resurgence of interest in using anthralin in the treatment of psoriasis, mainly because of the introduction of improved formulations and the discovery that its application for 30 minutes yields results as good as those from overnight application. Problems remain: Anthralin stains the skin a grayish color and this persists for several weeks. It also stains porcelain, and because this can be permanent, patients must be warned to wash it off in a fast-flowing shower or to use a rubber basin for washing their hair. Anthralin is also a potent irritant and some patients cannot tolerate the treatment. Reducing the frequency of application and starting with a low strength are the main ways of minimizing the problems. However, despite these disadvantages, it has major advantages over topical corticosteroids: it can clear psoriasis, and remissions often last for months without treatment.

Tar is an effective antipsoriatic agent, but there are several reasons its use should be abandoned. First, it is only weakly effective. Second, it is messy and abhorrent to use. Third, it is carcinogenic in humans, and psoriatic patients are already exposed to enough other carcinogens and immunosuppressive agents. The so-called refined tar preparations appear to have little, if any, therapeutic effect.

Ultraviolet Radiation

The sun has probably been used in the treatment of psoriasis for as long as the disease has existed, since most patients know that they improve during the summer or a winter vacation in the tropics. The latter can be used as an effective and popular treatment in selected patients.

Phototherapy using ultraviolet B (UVB) radiation with prior application of a lubricant is an effective treatment for psoriasis. When erythemogenic doses of UVB radiation are used, about 95 percent of selected patients can be cleared in 20 to 30 treatments. This regimen requires, first, determining the minimal erythema dose, giving 70 percent of that dose as the first exposure dose, and then increasing the exposure dose by 17 percent each treatment. If there is significant disease on the limbs, the same dose is given as an extra exposure while the face and trunk are kept covered. Treatments are given three to five times each week. A lubricant must be applied to each psoriasis plaque that has a surface scale immediately before treatment, since this increases penetration of the radiation. Symptomatic erythema is the main short-term problem. Over the long term this treatment is probably carcinogenic but the risk appears to be low. Photoaging of the skin is another long-term problem. The main disadvantage of the treatment is the lack of a reasonable maintenance regimen. Twice-weekly treatment is usually necessary to maintain a clear state, and most patients find this frequency of treatment economically and socially unacceptable.

Low-dose, nonerythemogenic UVB phototherapy has been used by some people with success. A starting dose well below an erythemal response is selected, and small increments are given with each treatment. A problem with this approach is that patients frequently finish a course of treatment tanned with psoriasis and, not surprisingly, unhappy.

Photochemotherapy, with ingestion of methoxsalen and subsequent exposure to ultraviolet A (UVA) radiation (PUVA therapy), is more effective than UVB phototherapy for both clearance and maintenance treatment. More than 95 percent of the patients with psoriasis can be cleared in 20 to 30 treatments. The treatment is given two to four times each week to clear disease, and the maintenance requirements vary from weekly to monthly treatments; most patients require two treatments each month.

The short-term problems with this therapy are nausea and erythema. Nausea is due to methoxsalen and is dose related; reduction of the dose by 10 mg cures most people. Cataracts, skin cancer, and photoaging are the main long-term concerns. Cataracts should not occur if patients wear ultraviolet-opaque glasses after ingesting methoxsalen. Skin cancer is a risk, especially if a patient has had superficial x-ray or grenz ray treatment, has had skin cancer, or is fair skinned. These risk factors must be evaluated in each patient. In addition, skin cancer is readily amenable to treatment provided the patient is carefully followed and regularly examined. The guidelines for PUVA therapy were published in the *Journal of the American Academy of Dermatology* (1979; 1:106).

Home phototherapy is useful in a few patients. A sunlamp from any drugstore can be used to augment topical treatment for localized psoriasis. Whole body treatment at home is not advisable for several reasons. First, it is not very effective, since patients frequently underdose or overdose themselves. Second, if the treatment is directed by a physician, he or she is taking some responsibility for its safety. Home-built light boxes are unlikely to be electrically safe. Obviously, if the physician supplies plans for the unit, he or she is even more involved. Finally, patients have a tendency to forget to come for follow-up examination until the first skin cancer appears.

The combination of the topical application of tar preparations and exposure to UVB radiation, the Goeckerman regimen, is still used in some centers. This treatment relies on the mild antipsoriatic effect of tar and the much more potent antipsoriatic effect of UVB radiation. On the positive side, the treatment is effective and safe. However, there is a negative side. The treatment is expensive, since it must be done in a hospital or a day care center. Second, because there is no provision for maintenance, the psoriasis gradually returns once the patient has been discharged. Finally, several studies have shown that tar given with UVB radiation is no more effective than a lubricant with UVB radiation; few patients have difficulty in choosing between a lubricant and a messy tar preparation.

Climatotherapy at the Dead Sea, a successful short-term therapy for psoriasis, appears to involve a mixture of UVB phototherapy, psychotherapy, and topical treatment. The main component is phototherapy. Since the Dead Sea is below sea level, sunlight there passes through a greater thickness of atmosphere, which filters out the erythemogenic wavelengths shorter than 300 nm. Consequently, patients can expose themselves to sunlight for long periods each day and receive very high doses of radiation of wavelengths longer than 300 nm, which is more therapeutic for psoriasis. The psychotherapeutic effects of a vacation and association with other people with psoriasis, are also important factors. On the negative side, in many patients the disease does not clear completely, and the duration of a remission appears to be no longer than it is with the Goeckerman treatment. A winter vacation in the Caribbean is probably cheaper, more enjoyable, and equally effective.

Systemic Therapy

Methotrexate is the best systemically administered drug for the treatment of psoriasis. It is an excellent treatment, but it does have serious long-term adverse effects. Therefore, this drug should be held in reserve until other less toxic therapeutic options have been exhausted and the patient has psoriasis of a sufficient severity to warrant taking the risks associated with the treatment. An exception is the short-term use of methotrexate in combination with PUVA therapy or phototherapy.

Depression of the bone marrow is the main short-term problem with methotrexate. The main long-term problem is impairment of liver function, and this occurs in 25 to 40 percent of the patients. Methotrexate is teratogenic, and therefore it should not be used in women of childbearing age without adequate contraception during treatment and for 1 month after cessation of the drug. Another problem is that methotrexate appears to alter the nature of psoriasis, making it a more aggressive disease. Thus, a person may have had the ordinary plaque type of psoriasis but after receiving methotrexate for several years may develop unstable inflammatory psoriasis when an attempt is made to shift to another treatment. The guidelines for methotrexate therapy have been published in the *Journal of the American Academy of Dermatology* (1982; 6:145). Several different regimens are used, but the approach of dividing the weekly dose into three doses given at consecutive 12 hourly intervals appears to be the most effective and safest.

Retinoids have antipsoriatic activity. Etretinate is the preferred drug for the treatment of psoriasis because isotretinoin is much less effective. The main indications for etretinate are the erythrodermic and generalized pustular types of psoriasis, and in a daily dosage of 0.6 to 1 mg per kilogram of body weight this drug is equally as effective as methotrexate in the treatment of these two rare forms of the disease. Etretinate is not very useful in the treatment of the ordinary plaque type of psoriasis; in some patients the disease is partially controlled, but to achieve complete clearance, months of therapy are required. The major disadvantage of etretinate therapy is that it produces side effects in 100 percent of the patients. The most common adverse effects involve the skin and mucous membranes, and these are inconvenient rather than hazardous. However, hyperlipidemia, liver abnormalities, and calcification of tendons occur in 50 to 85 percent of the patients. The long-term significance of some of these side effects is still unknown, and thus use of the drug should be restricted to the rare patient who is unresponsive to other less hazardous therapy. Etretinate is only slowly excreted over 12 to 18 months, and since it is markedly teratogenic, it should not be used in any women of childbearing age as it is impossible to guarantee contraception over such a long period.

Other Treatments

Trauma to the skin is a significant factor in inducing psoriasis, as evidenced by the Koebner phenomenon and localization of the disease to certain areas such as the elbows and knees. Telling patients to reduce the amount of trauma to the skin is good advice, but, except in specific instances, it is not a practical approach to treatment. Use of a condom in a person with psoriasis of the penis and protection of the hands, if they are affected, are two specific instances.

Emotional stress is also a trigger for psoriasis, but, again, telling patients to reduce the amount of stress in their lives is easy rather than practical advice. Perhaps the importance of emotional stress in exacerbating psoriasis is overemphasized. Certainly there are some patients who suffer a flare-up of disease whenever the social milieu becomes stormy. However, there are many other patients who go through deaths, divorces, operations, and other stressful experiences without fluctuation of the disease or requirement for increased treatment to control the disease. Alcohol abuse is an issue that has been raised in psoriatic patients. Anecdotal comments have claimed that alcohol exacerbates psoriasis, but there is no evidence to support this comment. It is possible that patients drink because they have severe psoriasis rather than vice versa, if indeed they do consume more alcohol than other people.

Several medications can induce or exacerbate psoriasis and should be avoided by patients if possible. Lithium and the antimalarial drugs are the main offenders. Beta-blockers can induce a psoriasiform eruption as a rare side effect, and there are a few reports of the exacerbation of existing psoriasis.

Finally, providing information about the National Psoriasis Foundation can be a worthwhile therapeutic measure in some patients. These patients have a desire to "do something" about finding a cause and cure for their disease, and contact with this organization provides an outlet for these feelings. Furthermore, patients feel that they are being kept up to date about psoriasis through information in the foundation's newsletter.

■ THERAPEUTIC REGIMENS

Psoriasis Vulgaris

From a therapeutic standpoint, plaque-form and papular psoriasis of the trunk and limbs can be divided into three categories: minimal psoriasis involving an area less than the surface area of two palms, moderate psoriasis involving an area less than the surface area of one upper limb, and extensive psoriasis involving a surface area greater than one upper limb. Although the extent of disease is usually the main factor dictating a choice of treatment, other characteristics of the disease or the patient may dominate the decision; this applies particularly to patients with moderate disease.

Mild disease localized to a few plaques or papules is best managed by topical therapy. Drithocreme is the linchpin of treatment because it can clear disease and provide a remission for weeks or months. In fair-skinned patients treatment should be started with the 0.25 percent strength, whereas in dark-skinned patients 0.5 percent is a safe preparation as initial therapy. The patient is instructed to apply the preparation daily for 30 minutes and then to wash it off in a shower. Treatment should be reviewed every two weeks, and if the cream is not causing any irritation, a higher strength preparation is prescribed. If the Drithocreme is causing marked irritation, the frequency of application should be reduced until this ceases to be a problem.

A second treatment to be used overnight should always be given in addition to the short-term application of Drithocreme. Keralyt gel under occlusion with Saran Wrap is useful if plaques are thick and hyperkeratotic. Cordran tape, or a medium potency corticosteroid cream under occlusion can be used in other patients and is helpful for the control of irritation from anthralin. Vioform-hydrocortisone cream should be substituted for intertriginous areas. A moisturizing preparation, selected by the preference of the patient for a cream, lotion, or ointment, should be used during the day. Intralesional steroid treatment is sometimes useful in patients with a few small thick lesions, but its use should always be combined with anthralin because otherwise the psoriasis will rapidly return once the effect of the corticosteroid has dissipated.

This regimen for the treatment of minimal psoriasis will be successful only if the physician exhibits enthusiasm and involvement and goals are defined at the initiation of treatment. The patient should be seen at least every 2 weeks, and the aim is to clear the psoriasis in 6 to 8 weeks. Short duration, focused treatment breeds enthusiasm and succeeds, whereas treatment with absence of deadlines and infrequent follow-up is bound to fail.

Psoriasis of moderate extent is a difficult therapeutic problem for two reasons. First, it is an economic and physical logistic problem for the patient to use topical therapy over a moderately extensive area and succeed in clearing the disease. Second, if a more potent therapy is used, such as UVB phototherapy in the office, the patient is frequently unhappy with the end result. The reason for this is simple. Phototherapy usually achieves 95 percent clearance of disease but rarely achieves 100 percent clearance. The patient with moderate disease usually wants 100 percent clearance, whereas a patient with much more extensive disease is usually delighted with 95 percent clearance. Despite these problems, the treatment of choice is topical therapy, as for minimal psoriasis, supplemented in most instances with the use of a small sunlamp at home or a course of UVB phototherapy in the office. The selection of treatment depends on assessment of the disease and the patient. Psoriasis confined mainly to exposed areas and concern about appearance because of employment and social factors are characteristics that weigh in favor of UVB phototherapy. Short-term maintenance UVB treatment for a couple of months is useful in this type of patient to ensure a reasonable remission.

There are a number of therapeutic regimens available for treating psoriasis covering an extensive area. UVB phototherapy in the office is the treatment of choice in the following cases: children, nursing and pregnant women, patients unwilling to use eye protection or take psoralen, patients who have sustained extensive solar damage or who have had significant exposure to grenz rays or superficial x-rays, and patients with psoriasis of recent onset. Whether long-term maintenance treatment is given after clearance of disease is a decision reached after a full discussion with the patient, since usually weekly or more frequent treatment is necessary.

In all other patients the treatment of choice is PUVA

therapy alone or in combination with methotrexate. PUVA therapy is effective in clearing disease in almost all patients and provides convenient maintenance treatment to prevent a recurrence. In the maintenance phase the frequency of treatment is gradually reduced, and if there is no significant flare-up of disease on monthly treatment, the therapy can be suspended. A methotrexate-PUVA combination treatment is useful in patients with very thick plaques, in patients with very active disease, and in those in whom the disease cannot be cleared with PUVA therapy alone. Methotrexate is given for 3 weeks before commencing PUVA therapy and is gradually withdrawn as clearing is achieved.

An alternative combination treatment is UVB phototherapy with PUVA therapy, and this combination is particularly useful in patients in whom methotrexate is contraindicated. Full doses of both treatments are given, exposure to the two wave bands being administered consecutively on the same day. These two combination treatments are very effective, and virtually all patients with psoriasis vulgaris can be cleared of disease using single or multiple treatments.

The main problem with the combination treatments is a high incidence of phototoxicity, but this is a short-term effect that is easily corrected by modifying the exposure dose. Although most patients can be cleared of disease using ultraviolet radiation, a small number cannot be maintained in a clear state using PUVA therapy alone. A combination of low-dose methotrexate and PUVA therapy is often a better treatment for these patients. In addition, there are patients in whom PUVA therapy is contraindicated, and long-term methotrexate treatment must be considered in these cases.

Psoriasis of the Scalp

The scalp requires specific attention when it is involved, except in patients being treated with methotrexate or etretinate. PUVA and UVB therapy are not effective for the treatment of psoriasis on the scalp, but if it is first cleared with topical therapy, UV therapy is often effective in keeping the scalp free of disease without continuation of topical therapy.

The best topical treatment is anthralin as Drithoscalp cream, which is formulated for application to the scalp. The application time is 30 minutes daily or as often as tolerated. A tar shampoo is used, because although the therapeutic effect from this brief exposure to tar is probably minimal, such preparations are labeled for the treatment of psoriasis and thus are favored by patients.

A corticosteroid lotion, such as Lidex solution, is applied overnight for its effect in reducing irritation from the Drithoscalp cream and its antipsoriatic action. If a patient has the thick asbestos type of psoriasis of the scalp. Keralyt gel under occlusion should be used initially to remove all the scale.

Psoriasis of the Palms and Soles

The treatment of choice is oral PUVA therapy. There is the temptation to use topical application of psoralen for this localized disease, but there is a high frequency of blistering burns with that treatment. Between 20 and 30 treatments with oral PUVA therapy are usually required to achieve clearance of disease. The only adjunctive treatment required is application of a keratolytic agent in patients with hyperkeratotic lesions so as to reduce the barrier to radiation. Specialized hand and foot UVA radiators are available and are very efficient, but the door panel of a stand-up unit is almost as effective. Ordinary topical therapy is ineffective in the treatment of psoriasis of the palms and soles. Topical corticosteroid therapy usually produces some improvement, but because it is seldom sustained, the patient is left a virtual cripple in these socially and physically important areas of the body. UVB phototherapy is also without effect because this wavelength cannot penetrate the thick stratum corneum of the palms and soles.

Psoriatic Nail Disease

Involvement of the nail bed or nail matrix by psoriasis is a difficult therapeutic problem. Pitting or a more severe dystrophy can be treated by application of Cordran tape to the skin over the matrix, but the treatment must be continued for months and the incidence of success is low. Onycholysis does not appear to respond to intralesional steroids applied into the nail bed. Nail disease clears in about 50 percent of the patients treated with PUVA therapy, but it usually requires 4 to 6 months of treatment. Local PUVA treatment, with exposure of the dorsa of the hands and feet, is a useful treatment in patients with severe nail disease.

Erythrodermic and Generalized Pustular Psoriasis

These rare forms of psoriasis are usually an indication for hospitalization, since, particularly in the case of the von Zumbusch form of pustular psoriasis, they can be life threatening. If an infection or metabolic disturbance is present, this must be treated. Patients with pustular psoriasis that has been triggered by the abrupt withdrawal of large doses of high-potency corticosteroid preparations must be tested for adrenocortical suppression and given appropriate supplementation. Local care of the skin should be confined to wet dressings and moisturizers. Methotrexate and etretinate are the specific drugs of choice, methotrexate being preferred provided there are no contraindications to its use. When the patient is stabilized, PUVA therapy should be commenced using low doses of UVA radiation and treatment on consecutive days followed by a rest day. Once the lesions have cleared, PUVA therapy usually can be continued as the sole treatment.

Acute Guttate Psoriasis

This variant of psoriasis typically follows an upper respiratory tract infection with a delay of 10 to 14 days. Streptococcal infection used to be the most common cause, but viral infections now seem to be almost as common. A 2 week course of penicillin is indicated if a streptococcal organism grows from a throat swab culture. Many cases of acute guttate psoriasis are said to clear spontaneously, but certainly some do not and the condition can become chronic. Thus, the treatment of choice is a course of UVB phototherapy to ensure that all lesions do clear. Maintenance therapy is usually unnecessary.

Psoriatic Arthritis

There is a form of arthritis that is peculiar to patients with psoriasis and afflicts about 5 percent of the patients. Psoriatic arthritis is rheumatoid factor negative, is usually asymmetric, and affects the distal interphalangeal and sacroiliac joints. A severe form, arthritis mutilans, is fortunately rare. In most instances dermatologists or their patients elect to have an internist or rheumatologist manage the arthritis, but for several reasons the dermatologist should keep in close contact with the progress of therapy for the arthritis. The activities of the skin disease and the arthritis are usually independent of each other, and treatment of the skin seldom affects the arthritis; however, the reverse is not true. Nonsteroidal anti-inflammatory drugs occasionally may exacerbate the skin disease, although this is probably a rare event. Oral doses of corticosteroids should be avoided if at all possible, as has been mentioned. Finally, some internists are not aware that methotrexate is a very effective drug for treating arthritis. Thus, in a patient with significant skin disease and arthritis, methotrexate is often the treatment of choice for both problems. Preliminary reports suggest that etretinate is also effective for psoriatic arthritis, but the toxicity of the treatment may limit its usefulness.

CONCLUSIONS

It is obvious from meeting many patients and from published surveys that many patients with psoriasis are displeased with the management of their disease. There are several common reasons for their displeasure. First, they perceive a lack of interest or a feeling of resignation on the part of many physicians. The "try this; it is new and it might work" attitude is hardly likely to boost morale and engender enthusiasm in a patient with a chronic disease. Second, patients do not like many of the treatments that are frequently used. Tying oneself into a layer of Saran Wrap over a film of grease is not really the nicest way to retire for the evening. Anointing oneself with foul smelling black goop is not a pleasant experience. Third, patients do not like to have psoriasis, any psoriasis, and yet many treatments leave them with a significant level of disease for long periods of time. Topical corticosteroid treatment improves but seldom clears psoriasis. Hospital treatment often flattens psoriasis without clearing it, and then the patient has to endure months of disease until its severity warrants another admission to a hospital or day care center. Finally, many physicians regard psoriasis as being only a cosmetic disturbance. Offering a red, scaly hand for a handshake and leaving a confetti trail of scale behind are more than cosmetic problems; not to mention the soreness and pruritus that can be present.

All these sources of displeasure on the part of the patient must be kept in mind when treating psoriasis. A positive, interested attitude on the part of the physician can work miracles. Selection of a treatment that works, and yet does not totally disrupt the patient's life, is possible with the therapeutic modalities available today. The end result is a happy patient who stays with that physician.

ERYTHEMA MULTIFORME

Marcia G. Tonnesen, M.D.

Erythema multiforme (EM) is an acute, self-limited inflammatory disorder of the skin and mucous membranes, characterized by distinctive skin lesions and histopathologic changes. Currently the classification of EM is evolving as distinct subsets are identified and diagnostic criteria are established. Two clinical forms of EM have been designated EM minor and EM major.

Successful therapeutic intervention in any form of EM is hindered by the fact that specific pathogenic mechanisms of tissue injury have not yet been well defined, and few controlled studies have been performed to evaluate therapeutic effectiveness. A rational approach to therapy should be based on careful consideration of suspected etiologic factors; clinical characteristics, including extent and severity of mucocutaneous lesions and patient discomfort; and potential complications. Elimination of any identified or presumed precipitating factors is of prime importance. Optimal therapy should combine symptomatic and supportive measures with observation for and treatment of associated complications, depending on the severity of the episode (Tables 1 and 2).

ERYTHEMA MULTIFORME MINOR

EM minor is a relatively mild cutaneous illness that is frequently recurrent and usually occurs in young adults. The typical clinical picture is the sudden onset of a symmetric erythematous eruption with a predilection for the extensor aspects of the extremities (hands, elbows, knees). Mucosal involvement, when present, is usually limited to development of a few oral erosions. Skin lesions begin as fixed erythematous papules and may progress to become bullous. At least some of the lesions evolve with concentric zones of color change to form characteristic target lesions, the clinical hallmark of EM minor. Individual lesions, usually symptomless but occasionally associated with burning or itching, appear in successive crops which may coalesce, and then resolve within 2 to 4 weeks, leaving residual postinflammatory hyperpigmentation. Some patients suffer from recurrent episodes, often averaging one every 4 to 5 months. Most, if not all, cases of classic recurrent EM minor are associated with herpes simplex virus (HSV) infection and typically occur 7 to 14 days after the appearance of a recurrent HSV lesion (oral, genital, or other location). Current evidence supports the concepts that HSV is the major precipitating factor of EM minor, and

Table 1 Therapy for EM Minor

Patient Education
- Emphasize:
  - Self-limited course
  - Association with recurrent herpes simplex virus (HSV) infection

Symptomatic Measures
- Antipruritics:
  - Hydroxyzine, 25–50 mg PO q.i.d. *or*
  - Diphenhydramine HCl, 50 mg PO q.i.d.
- Analgesics:
  - Acetaminophen, 650 mg PO q.i.d.

Skin Care for Erosions
- To dry, debride, and cleanse:
  - Open, wet compresses of tepid water *or* aluminum acetate (Burow's solution) for 10 min b.i.d.
- To promote healing:
  - Bacitracin or Polysporin antibacterial ointment
  - Bandage or sterile dressing

Mouth Care for Oral Erosions
- To relieve discomfort:
  - Liquid antacid *or*
  - Topical anesthetic such as:
    - Dyclonine
    - Viscous lidocaine
    - Kaopectate/diphenhydramine 1:1
- To maintain hydration and nutrition:
  - Liquid or soft diet

Preventive Measures for Frequent Recurrences of Herpes-Associated EM Minor
- To prevent or decrease recurrences of herpes simplex infection:
  - Avoid sun
    - Sunscreens (SPF 15 or greater)
    - Sunstick (suncreen in chapstick)
    - Protective clothing
    - No sun exposure 10 AM–3 PM
  - Minimize stress
  - Prophylactic oral antiviral therapy
    - Acyclovir 400 mg PO b.i.d. for 6 months or longer; taper as tolerated
- For continuous or overlapping episodes:
  - Stop treatment with systemic glucocorticosteroids or immunosuppressive drugs
  - Institute oral acyclovir prophylaxis

that recurrent herpes-associated EM minor represents an HSV-specific host immune response in the skin.

Preferred Therapeutic Approach (Table 1)

Patient Education. Patients should be reassured regarding the usual benign, self-limited course and educated regarding the frequent association of EM minor with recurrent herpes simplex viral infection.

Symptomatic Measures. Since most episodes of EM minor are mild, symptomatic care is often sufficient. For pruritic or painful skin lesions, systemic antihistamines (hydroxyzine hydrochloride, 25 to 50 mg taken orally four times a day or diphenhydramine hydrochloride, 50 mg taken orally four times a day) or analgesics (acetaminophen, 650 mg taken orally four times a day) may provide relief.

Skin Care. For crusted erosive skin lesions, mild drying, debridement, and cleansing can be achieved with open, wet compresses of tepid water or aluminum acetate (Burow's solution diluted 1:20, or one Domeboro tablet dissolved in 1 pint of water) applied for 10 minutes twice a day. After cleansing, an antibacterial ointment (Polysporin or Bacitracin) followed by a bandage or sterile dressing should be applied to eroded lesions.

Mouth Care. Liquid antacids or topical anesthetics such as dyclonine, viscous lidocaine, or a 1:1 mixture of Kaopectate and elixir of diphenhydramine used as a mouthwash will provide relief from painful erosions. A liquid or soft diet is usually better tolerated and therefore contributes to the maintenance of hydration and nutrition.

Preventive Measures. Because of the strong etiologic association between recurrent HSV infections and recurrent EM minor, measures that attempt to prevent recurrences of herpes simplex should lessen the frequency of subsequent episodes of EM. Avoidance of sun exposure through the use of sunscreens (SPF 15 or greater), sunsticks (sunscreen-containing chapstick), and protective clothing, and by minimizing sun exposure from 10 AM to 3 PM (the peak period for UVB solar irradiation) may reduce ultraviolet light–induced HSV recurrences on sun-exposed skin. Attempts should be made to minimize stress, a well-known precipitating factor in recurrent HSV.

Thus far, topical antiviral preparations have not been clearly shown to prevent or abort recurrent HSV infections. However, in several uncontrolled studies, prophylactic administration of oral acyclovir has resulted in abolition of recurrent HSV infections and of ensuing episodes of EM minor. Acyclovir does not shorten the duration of an episode of EM once begun, nor does it prevent an EM episode if therapy is started during the antecedent HSV infection. Therefore, in patients with frequently recurrent and debilitating herpes-associated EM minor, the treatment of choice is prophylactic daily oral acyclovir for a period of 6 months or longer. The recommended starting dose is 400 mg orally twice daily, with tapering of the dose after the disease is brought under control. Because of the self-limited nature of EM minor, the known occurrence of acyclovir resistance, and the unknown long-term side effects of chronic acyclovir therapy, the drug should be stopped periodically and the need for its continuance reassessed.

Because systemic glucocorticosteroid or immunosuppressive therapy has been linked to development of continuous or overlapping episodes of EM minor, such therapy is not recommended and should be stopped prior to initiation of a course of prophylactic oral acyclovir. Topical steroid therapy is of little benefit in the treatment of EM.

■ ERYTHEMA MULTIFORME MAJOR

EM major, also known as bullous EM or as Stevens-Johnson syndrome, is a severe, self-limited, variable mucocutaneous illness characterized by an extensive eruption with areas of epidermal detachment, often accompanied by significant involvement of mucosal surfaces, especially the mouth and conjunctivae. A prodrome with constitutional symptoms may herald the onset of the eruption. Skin lesions begin as papules and may evolve to form raised or flat atypical target lesions. Central blister formation may produce areas of epi-

Table 2 Therapy for EM Major

Patient Education
- Emphasize:
  - Self-limited, potentially severe course
  - Association with drugs or infection (*Mycoplasma;* HSV)

Elimination of Etiologic Factors
- Drug:
  - Immediate withdrawal and future avoidance
- *Mycoplasma* infection:
  - Erythromycin, 250–500 mg PO q.i.d. *or*
  - Tetracycline, 250–500 mg PO q.i.d.

Supportive Care
- Hospitalization often necessary
- To maintain hydration and nutrition:
  - Parenteral nutrition, tube feedings, or liquid or soft diet, if tolerated

Symptomatic Measures
- Antipruritics:
  - Hydroxyzine, 25–50 mg PO q.i.d. *or*
  - Diphenhydramine HCl, 50 mg PO q.i.d.
- Analgesics/Antipyretics: Acetaminophen, 650 mg PO q.i.d.

Skin Care for Erosions
- To dry, debride, and cleanse:
  - Open, wet compresses of tepid water *or* aluminum acetate (Burow's solution) for 15 to 20 min b.i.d.
- To soothe and cleanse:
  - Baths in tepid water for 30 min b.i.d.
- To promote healing:
  - Bacitracin antibacterial ointment and sterile dressing or synthetic wound dressing

Mouth Care for Oral Erosions
- To relieve discomfort:
  - Liquid antacid
  - Topical anesthetic such as:
    - Dyclonine
    - Viscous lidocaine
    - Kaopectate/diphenhydramine 1:1
- To treat infection:
  - Erythromycin, 250 mg PO q.i.d. *or*
  - Tetracycline, 250 mg PO q.i.d. for 10 days

Eye Care
- Careful monitoring and early consultation with ophthalmologist

Reduction of Morbidity and Mortality
- For progressive disease:
  - Consider course of Prednisone 1 to 2 mg/kg/day; discontinue when no further disease progression
- For extensive involvement (>10% to 20% total body surface area):
  - Early referral to burn unit
  - Measures to guard against infection:
    - Withdrawal from systemic steroids
    - Limit antibiotic use to culture-proven infections
    - Minimize indwelling lines and catheters
    - Perform daily cultures of skin, blood, and urine
    - Aggressively treat sepsis if it occurs
  - Supportive care:
    - Air-fluidized bed
    - Respiratory and physical therapy
    - Parenteral nutrition or tube feedings
    - Adequate pain relief
    - Avoidance of all unnecessary medications
  - Skin care to facilitate rapid re-epithelialization:
    - Gentle debridement followed by synthetic or biologic dressing

dermal necrosis and detachment. Painful mucosal erosions result in a foul-smelling mouth, typical hemorrhagic crusting of the lips, and decreased oral intake. Ocular involvement may produce red eyes, photophobia, and, if severe, an erosive, exudative conjunctivitis with residual scarring and lash and lacrimal abnormalities. Permanent visual loss may occur.

Certain drugs, particularly sulfonamides, nonsteroidal anti-inflammatory agents, anticonvulsants, penicillins, and allopurinol are important and well-documented etiologic factors in EM major. Infectious agents associated with EM major are *Mycoplasma pneumoniae* and HSV. The duration of erythema multiforme major, reflecting more severe mucocutaneous damage, is typically 4 to 6 weeks. Recurrences are infrequent. EM major is associated with significant morbidity and may be fatal.

Toxic epidermal necrolysis (TEN), characterized by the abrupt, rapid development of extensive mucocutaneous areas of confluent erythema and blistering with sheetlike, full-thickness epidermal necrosis and detachment resembling scalding, is considered by some to be a severe form of EM major, but is viewed by many as a distinct disease entity. Drugs are now believed to be the only documented cause of TEN. TEN can be considered a manifestation of "acute skin failure" with abnormal barrier function resulting in fluid, electrolyte, and protein loss; increased susceptibility to infection; impaired thermoregulation; altered immune status; and increased energy expenditure. Morbidity is significant and the mortality rate is at least 30 percent. The leading cause of death is sepsis.

A new classification for EM major, based on the morphology of skin lesions as well as on the extent of epidermal loss, has recently been formulated in an attempt to standardize diagnosis. Proposed division into five categories and extent of detachment are bullous erythema multiforme (<10 percent), Stevens-Johnson syndrome (<10 percent), overlap Stevens-Johnson–TEN (10 to 30 percent), TEN with discrete lesions (>30 percent), TEN without discrete lesions (>10 percent). Until specific subsets are further identified and defined, the erythema multiforme disease spectrum and its treatment will continue to be controversial.

Preferred Therapeutic Approach (Table 2)

Because of the extensive epidermal and mucosal necrosis that can occur in EM major, careful monitoring is critical, hospitalization is often required, and supportive care is usually necessary.

Patient Education. Patients should be advised that the course is self-limited but potentially severe and educated regarding the frequent association of EM major with drugs or, less commonly, with infection (*Mycoplasma*, HSV).

Elimination of Etiologic Factors. Any suspected or unnecessary drug should be withdrawn and avoided in the future. In particular, no drugs associated with EM major (especially sulfonamides and penicillins) should be used to treat any manifestation of the EM syndrome. If *Mycoplasma pneumoniae* infection is diagnosed or strongly suspected, systemic treatment should be initiated with erythromycin or tetracycline, 1 to 2 g per day. If HSV infection is diagnosed or strongly suspected, measures should be taken to prevent recurrence (see Table 1).

Supportive Care. Hospitalization is often advisable, and intravenous fluid therapy and nasogastric or parenteral feeding may be necessary to maintain hydration and nutrition.

Symptomatic Measures. For pruritic or painful skin lesions, systemic antihistamines (hydroxyzine hydrochloride, 25 to 50 mg taken orally four times a day or diphenhydramine hydrochloride, 50 mg taken orally four times a day) or analgesics (acetaminophen, 650 mg taken orally four times a day) may provide relief.

Skin Care. For bullous or crusted erosive skin lesions, mild drying, debridement, and cleansing can be achieved with open, wet compresses of tepid water or aluminum acetate (Burow's solution diluted 1:20, or a Domeboro tablet dissolved in 1 pint of water) applied for 15 to 20 minutes four times a day. Frequent bathing (30 minutes twice a day) in lukewarm to cool water has a soothing antipruritic effect as well as serving to cleanse the skin lesions and minimize secondary infection. Lesions should be observed for signs of secondary infection, cultured when indicated, and treatment should be initiated with the appropriate systemic antibiotic. Erythromycin, 250 mg taken orally four times a day, is a good first choice, pending culture results. If lesions progress to extensive tissue necrosis with as much as 20 to 30 percent total body surface area involved, surgical intervention and transfer to a burn unit are advisable (see following discussion).

Mouth Care. When extensive painful mouth lesions are present, good oral hygiene is critical to minimize infection and discomfort. Liquid antacids or topical anesthetics such as dyclonine, viscous lidocaine, or a 1:1 mixture of Kaopectate and elixir of diphenhydramine, used as a mouthwash, will provide pain relief. A liquid or soft diet is usually better tolerated and therefore contributes to the maintenance of hydration and nutrition. EM major patients who have extensive oral involvement, however, may be unable to eat or drink despite the use of topical anesthetics, thus necessitating parenteral nutrition or tube feedings. When oral lesions are extensive, purulent, foul smelling, and associated with tender cervical lymphadenopathy, systemic therapy with erythromycin or tetracycline, 1 g per day for 10 days, is appropriate to combat secondary bacterial infection.

Eye Care. Because of the potential for long-term sequelae, resulting in visual loss, careful monitoring of eye involvement is mandatory and early consultation with and continuing care by an ophthalmologist are strongly recommended. Suggested therapeutic measures might include irrigation and compresses to cleanse the eye, lysis of adhesions, and instillation of topical antibiotics when indicated.

Reduction of Morbidity and Mortality. Indication for the use of systemic glucocorticosteroids in EM major is a highly controversial issue, since no controlled studies have been conducted to document efficacy. However, because EM major and TEN can progress to widespread epidermal necrosis with a mortality rate as high as 30 percent, early use of systemic steroids in the progressive phase of the disease process in an attempt to decrease the extent of tissue damage is advocated by some. High-dose therapy (prednisone, 1 to 2 mg per kilogram per day) is administered only during the stage of active extension of lesions. In contrast, systemic steroid use is condemned by others since some retrospective reports have suggested that patients treated with systemic steroids have an increased incidence of complications and death.

If extensive, advanced tissue necrosis occurs or is already

evident (approaching 20 percent total body surface area involvement), immediate transfer of the patient to a burn unit under the care of a surgical burn specialist is strongly advocated. Therapeutic recommendations for care in the burn unit consist of:

1. Measures to guard against iatrogenic infection, including withdrawal from systemic steroids; limitation of antibiotic use to specific culture-proven infections; avoidance of indwelling lines and catheters whenever possible; daily cultures of skin, blood, and urine; and aggressive treatment of sepsis if it occurs;
2. Supportive care consisting of use of an air-fluidized bed, respiratory and physical therapy, parenteral nutrition or tube feedings, adequate pain relief, and continuing care by an ophthalmologist;
3. Avoidance of all unnecessary medications, particularly those which are known etiologic factors of EM-TEN, such as sulfonamides (including sulfa-containing eye preparations, diuretics, and topical dressings); and
4. Skin care with emphasis on early gentle debridement followed by application of a dressing to protect the denuded dermis from desiccation and to facilitate rapid reepithelialization. Reduced mortality has been reported with the use of allografts and porcine xenografts.

THERAPEUTIC OUTCOME

Both EM minor and EM major are self-limited disorders which can be expected to resolve within 4 to 6 weeks. If the disease persists longer than 8 weeks, the diagnosis of EM should be questioned and alternative diagnoses investigated.

Suggested Reading

Halebian PH, Madden MR, Finklestein JL, et al. Improved burn center survival of patients with toxic epidermal necrolysis managed without corticosteroids. Ann Surg 1986; 204:503–512.

Huff JC. Therapy and prevention of erythema multiforme with acyclovir. Semin Dermatol 1988; 7:212–217.

Lemak MA, Duvic M, Bean SF. Oral acyclovir for the prevention of herpes-associated erythema multiforme. J Am Acad Dermatol 1986; 15:50–54.

ERYTHEMA NODOSUM

Mark E. Unis, M.D.

Erythema nodosum is a distinctive clinical entity believed to represent a hypersensitivity reaction to a variety of stimuli and associated diseases. A typical patient presents with the sudden onset of crops of tender, painful, erythematous to purplish subcutaneous, usually pretibial, nodules, biopsy specimens of which show a predominantly septal panniculitis.

Although many cases are idiopathic, several associated diseases listed in Table 1 have been reported frequently. A history, physical examination, and appropriate laboratory evaluation are performed to exclude these associated diseases. If the history and physical findings are unremarkable except for cutaneous findings, a minimal initial evaluation would include a complete blood count, erythrocyte sedimentation rate, and chest x-ray examination. If there is an associated underlying disease, treatment or control of the underlying disease usually improves the erythema nodosum.

Table 1 Erythema Nodosum–Associated Diseases

Sarcoidosis
Inflammatory bowel disease
Crohn's disease
Ulcerative colitis
Collagen vascular diseases
Drugs
Birth control pills
Sulfonamides
Antibiotics
Bromides
Behçet's syndrome
Infections
Streptococcal infection
Atypical mycobacterial infection
Fungal infections
Viral infections
Chlamydial infections
Pregnancy
Lymphoma and leukemia

PREFERRED APPROACH

Evaluation of any particular pharmacologic therapy in patients with erythema nodosum is difficult because of the tendency for spontaneous remission to occur in this disease. Nonetheless, there are several modes of therapy that I have found effective. Nearly all patients with erythema nodosum find relief of symptoms with rest and leg elevation. The preferred approach includes attempts at treatment or control of an underlying disease, if present, bedrest, leg elevation, and pharmacologic therapy, usually potassium iodide or nonsteroidal anti-inflammatory drugs (NSAIDs).

Potassium Iodide

Although there are no established guidelines for the use of potassium iodide in treating erythema nodosum, the medication seems to inhibit mononuclear phagocytes, and this may be the reason for the response of erythema nodosum to therapy with iodides. The reason for their effectiveness is unclear, especially in light of the fact that iodides and bromides have been reported to induce erythema nodosum. I usually prescribe potassium iodide as the 300 mg enteric-coated tablet taken three times daily with meals. Symptomatic improvement usually begins within a few days after starting therapy. If tablets are unavailable, a saturated solution of potassium iodide, 5 to 8 drops orally three times daily in juice or water, may be substituted.

Potassium iodide has a bitter taste. Dyspepsia and heartburn may result from its administration, and small bowel ulcerations have been associated with administration of the enteric-coated potassium iodide preparations.

Potassium iodide is contraindicated during pregnancy because it can induce fetal goiter. Occasional patients display hypersensitivity reactions to iodides, including angioedema, fever, arthralgia, lymphadenopathy, and eosinophilia.

Other effects of iodides are chronic and may include thyroid adenoma, goiter, and myxedema because the drug suppresses thyroid function. Chronic iodism may occur after prolonged treatment, and symptoms may include salivary gland enlargement, increased salivation, coryza, pain in the teeth and gingiva, swelling of the eyelids, headache, and pulmonary edema. Acne may develop or iododerma may occur.

In general, I do not use potassium iodide in chronic or refractory cases of erythema nodosum.

Nonsteroidal Anti-Inflammatory Drugs

I have found several nonsteroidal anti-inflammatory drugs useful in the therapy of erythema nodosum. Their mode of action is not known, but it is believed that inhibition of prostaglandin synthesis by metabolites of NSAIDs may be involved in the anti-inflammatory action of these drugs.

The NSAID I most frequently prescribe is indomethacin in doses ranging from 25 to 75 mg orally three times daily with meals, depending on the age and size of the patient and the severity of the disease. Indomethacin is the most likely of the NSAIDs to cause gastrointestinal disturbance, including dyspepsia, ulceration, perforation, and hemorrhage. Patients should be monitored carefully for development of these problems. Indomethacin can precipitate renal insufficiency, particularly in those with pre-existing renal or hepatic dysfunction. Using the drug for only 2 or 3 weeks of continuous therapy in erythema nodosum usually helps avoid these problems.

Ibuprofen, 400 to 800 mg orally three or four times daily, also may be effective, but I have found it less useful than indomethacin. In general, gastrointestinal side effects are much less frequent with ibuprofen than with other nonsteroidal anti-inflammatory drugs. Its relative safety and efficacy in inflammatory diseases have been well established, as it has been a commonly prescribed medication.

Clinoril 200 mg orally daily or twice daily, might be considered for chronic or recurrent erythema nodosum. Many rheumatologists consider Clinoril to be the most efficacious NSAID with a good safety profile.

All nonsteroidal anti-inflammatory drugs are capable of causing adverse gastrointestinal reactions and platelet dysfunction and are contraindicated in aspirin sensitive patients.

■ MISCELLANEOUS THERAPIES

Aspirin can be effective in treating erythema nodosum, usually in doses of 10 to 15 grains taken orally every 4 hours. Use of enteric-coated preparations again decreases the frequency of side effects, but the efficacy of nonsteroidal anti-inflammatory drugs seems to be greater.

I have had success in one patient with chronic and refractory erythema nodosum by treating with intermittent courses of phenylbutazone. It is usually prescribed in doses of 100 mg three or four times daily with meals. If there is no improvement in the condition within 1 week, the drug should be discontinued. When improvement is obtained, the dosage should be promptly decreased to the minimal effective level necessary to maintain relief, not exceeding 400 mg daily because of the possibility of cumulative toxicity, particularly in terms of bone marrow depression. Aplastic anemia and agranulocytosis have occurred in patients taking phenylbutazone. Like the nonsteroidal anti-inflammatory drugs, phenylbutazone causes gastrointestinal distress and may cause fluid retention. The patient should fail to respond to nonsteroidal anti-inflammatory drugs before one tries phenylbutazone.

I have treated four patients with colchicine, 0.6 mg orally twice daily, and I have had clinical responses in two patients. The most common side effects are nausea, diarrhea, and headache. Long-term use and high doses may be associated with bone marrow depression, among other complications.

I have not found systemic steroid therapy necessary in the treatment of patients with erythema nodosum, but I would not have any reservations about using steroids in patients who are unresponsive to any of the modalities listed, provided the erythema nodosum was not associated with infection. A burst of prednisone, 40 to 60 mg daily tapered over 2 to 3 weeks to avoid chronic side effects would be appropriate.

CHRONIC URTICARIA

Frances Lawlor, M.D., F.R.C.P.I., D.C.H.
Malcolm W. Greaves, M.D., Ph.D., F.R.C.P.

The characteristic skin lesion in urticaria is the wheal, an edematous pale papule, which frequently itches. Since the lesions of urticaria are continually evolving and disappearing, wheals are not invariably seen and when present are associated with a blotchy macular, papular, and annular erythema. In approximately 45 percent of patients with urticaria subcutaneous swelling occurs either at the same time, before, or after the urticarial episode. This frequently affects the mucous membranes and is known as angioedema. Currently when urticaria and angioedema occur together, they are considered part of the same disease. Each urticarial wheal generally lasts less than 24 hours and angioedema swellings less than 72 hours. Both fade to leave normal-appearing skin.

Urticaria can be arbitrarily divided into acute urticaria, which is present less than 12 weeks, and chronic urticaria, which lasts longer than 12 weeks and may last years. In the patients who present with chronic urticaria, a physical urticaria must be considered either as the sole condition or as an associated disease since chronic idiopathic urticaria and the physical urticarias frequently coexist. The diagnosis and treatment of the physical urticarias are considered elsewhere.

Apart from those patients with physical urticaria, the cause of chronic urticaria is unknown, hence its synonym, chronic "idiopathic" urticaria. Allergy or infection do not play a significant role in the pathogenesis of the condition. Thyroid autoantibodies are present more frequently than in the general population but are only occasionally associated with overt thyroid disease. Recently a histamine-releasing IgG autoantibody reacting with the high affinity IgE receptor or with IgE itself has been found in patients' serum, supporting the view that chronic urticaria is an autoimmune disease in some patients. In 75 percent of patients, aspirin worsens the disorder. In a very small number, preservatives, dyes, and colorings can be reproducibly shown to aggravate the condition, possibly through a nonimmunologic mechanism. Drugs such as morphine, codeine, and tubocurarine, which induce mast-cell histamine release, may also augment chronic urticaria.

A careful history (Table 1) taken from a patient suffering from chronic urticaria will generally reveal all the diagnostic information obtainable. A physical examination, including physical urticaria provocation testing where necessary, should confirm the diagnosis.

Table 1 Chronic Urticaria: Taking a History

Lesions on the skin	How long have the symptoms been present? What do they look like? How long do individual lesions last? Is the skin normal after they have gone away? How often do they occur? Are they provoked by exercise, hot baths, emotion, friction, sustained physical pressure, cold, sunlight, or water?
Eyes, lips, face, throat, and tongue	Do they swell? How often does this happen? How long does the swelling last?
Generally	When you have swelling or rash is there any difficulty breathing or swallowing? Any pain in the abdomen or vomiting? Any associated joint pain?

THERAPY OF CHRONIC IDIOPATHIC URTICARIA

The treatment of chronic idiopathic urticaria can be divided into nondrug management and drug treatment for both the urticaria and for the treatment of acute superimposed severe episodes of angioedema, which may have associated systemic symptoms. These are considered separately.

Nondrug Management

Explanation

Chronic idiopathic urticaria is a distressing condition, both because of the itching and the alarming symptoms attributable to involvement of the skin and mucous membranes. It is helpful to explain the nature of the condition with its remissions and exacerbations and to explain that it is unlikely that a direct cause will be found. More than 50 percent of patients remit within 6 months. Although the condition cannot be cured its symptoms can usually be controlled. Treatment is more effective at reducing pruritus and whealing than reducing erythema, and a certain amount of erythema may be expected unless control is complete. Measures to cool the affected skin invariably cause welcome, though temporary, relief. These include wearing light, loose clothes, working and sleeping in a cool room, and frequent showering or bathing with tepid water. Cooling creams or lotion, including calamine lotion, are also useful.

It is important to avoid aspirin and aspirin-containing drugs. Other nonsteroidal anti-inflammatory drugs should be avoided if possible. Paracetamol is safe. Angiotensin-converting enzyme inhibitors should be avoided if a suitable alternative drug is available because these have caused severe angioedema in some people, and their relationship to chronic idiopathic urticaria is unclear.

Avoidance of food additives and antioxidants is controversial, since not all believe that these substances play a part. However, if the patient and the physician wish, a placebo-controlled drug and diet challenge test schedule may be undertaken (Table 2). This can be conducted on an outpatient basis, with the patient keeping a daily diary of the severity of the urticaria. A positive reaction would need to be confirmed by rechallenge before any specific dietary restriction is advised.

Alternatively (and less satisfactorily) the patient could embark (without challenge testing) on a restricted diet avoid-

Table 2 Drug and Diet Challenge Test Schedule Used at St. John's Institute of Dermatology

1. Control
2. Tartrazine 10 mg
3. Control
4. Sodium benzoate 500 mg*
5. Control
6. Hydroxybenzoic acid 200 mg
7. Control
8. Yeast extract 0.6 g
9. Control
10. Penicillin 0.5 mg (not to be given if history of asthma or severe penicillin reaction)
11. Control
12. Aspirin 100 mg (not to be given if history of asthma or severe aspirin reaction)
13. Control
14. New coccine 10 mg*
15. Control
16. Canthaxathine 100 mg*
17. Control
18. Sunset yellow 10 mg*
19. Control
20. Annatto 10 mg
21. Control
22. Butylhydroxytoluene 50 mg
23. Butylhydroxytoluene 50 mg
24. Control
25. Butylhydroxyanisol 50 mg
26. Control
27. Ascorbic acid 600 mg
28. Control
29. Sodium nitrate 100 mg
30. Control
31. Quinoline yellow 10 mg
32. Control
33. Sodium glutamate 200 mg

*One-tenth of the dose is to be given if a patient is under 10 years of age or if there is a history of asthma.

ing the colorings, E102–E180; the benzoate preservatives, E210–219; and the antioxidants, E300–E322. This diet could be continued for 4 to 6 weeks and if there is no major improvement, the diet could be abandoned.

Drug Treatment Using Antihistamine Therapy

The mainstay of drug treatment in chronic idiopathic urticaria is H_1-antihistamine therapy in adequate dosage. The antihistamines block the combination of histamine with its receptors. Generally the half-life of the antihistamines is more prolonged in the elderly than in children. The half-lives of some of the active metabolites are longer than that of the parent compound. There is very little information about the use of antihistamines during pregnancy, although there have been no confirmed reports of teratogenicity. Antihistamine treatment in pregnant women should be avoided if possible, but if it is necessary, the agents of choice are chlorpheniramine and tripelennamine.

The timing of antihistamine ingestion in relation to food is generally not important. Since many patients' urticaria is worse at a particular time of the day, it is wise to take the antihistamine approximately 1 to 2 hours before itching and whealing are maximal. Since each individual responds differently to each antihistamine it is usually necessary to be flexible both in dosage and in the antihistamine used and to be ready to change the antihistamine prescribed until control is optimal and adverse effects are minimal.

The "classic" H_1-antihistamines, apart from hydroxyzine, are generally less effective and cause more unwanted effects than the newer minimally sedating antihistamines. However, the older H_1-antihistamines are useful if night sedation is required. These include chlorpheniramine maleate, diphenhydramine hydrochloride, and hydroxyzine hydrochloride (Table 3). The tricyclic antidepressant doxepin has additional H_2-receptor antagonist properties. It is very useful in depressed and agitated adult patients as a single night-time dose of 25 to 50 mg. It should not be combined with terfenadine or monoamine oxidase inhibitors.

The Newer H_1-Receptor Antagonists

The newer "second-generation" H_1-receptor antagonists seem to have similar efficacy to each other. Their main advantage is that they do not produce atropine-like anticholinergic effects and generally cause little or no drowsiness in the dosage suggested by the manufacturer. However, since it is sometimes necessary to increase the dosage, drowsiness may be a problem at higher dosages (Table 4).

The forerunner of the second-generation antihistamines was terfenadine. All antihistamines have the potential to worsen urticaria for reasons that remain obscure. Occasionally patients taking terfenadine have suffered erythematous rashes, worsening of their urticaria with angioedema, photosensitivity, and peeling of the skin on the hands and feet. The most potentially serious adverse effect of terfenadine is the development of a prolonged QT interval, which may lead to a polymorphic ventricular tachycardia (torsades de pointes). This uncommon problem can be avoided if the adult dosage of terfenadine does not exceed 120 mg per day and if it is not concurrently used with the macrolide antibiotics (e.g., erythromycin), imidazole antifungals (e.g., itraconazole and fluconazole), or the tricyclic antidepressants (e.g., doxepin). Terfenadine should also be avoided in patients with hepatic dysfunction or those with electrolyte imbalance. The exact mechanism of this is not known, although abnormalities in the cytochrome P-450 activity have been postulated.

Astemizole has three properties of note:

1. Its duration of action is prolonged to 4 weeks and its active metabolite is present in the body for 6 weeks.
2. It has been associated with the development of torsades de pointes as described previously, and it should be prescribed using the same precautions as apply to terfenadine. Furthermore, a daily dosage of 10 mg should not be exceeded.
3. Almost all patients who take astemizole gain weight, and if astemizole is used, the patient should be advised to restrict food intake at the same time.

Loratadine has not been associated with adverse cardiac reactions and has been used safely without any reported drowsiness in a dosage of up to 40 mg twice daily. Cetirizine is claimed to have action in addition to its H_1-antihistamine activity, including inhibition of leukocyte activity, especially

Table 3 First-Generation Antihistamines

DRUG	TRADE NAME	FORM/ STRENGTH	USUAL ADULT DOSE	CHILDREN'S DOSAGE	TIME TO PEAK LEVEL AFTER ORAL INTAKE (HOURS)	HALF-LIFE (HOURS)	SIDE EFFECTS COMMON TO ALL	OTHER RARE EFFECTS COMMON TO ALL
Chlorpheniramine maleate	Piriton	Tablets, 4 mg, 8 mg, 12 mg	8 mg–12 mg b.i.d. or t.i.d.	0.35 mg/kg/24 h	2.8 ± 0.8	27.9 ± 8.7	Drowsiness, decreased alertness, GI upset, appetite stimulation, anticholinergic effects, i.e., dry mouth, blurred vision, urinary retention, impotence, abnormalities of liver function	Tachycardia, prolongation of QT interval, heart block, and arrhythmias
Chlorpheniramine maleate	Chlor-Trimeton	Syrup, 2.5 mg/5 ml; Parenteral, 10 mg/ml						
Hydroxyzine hydrochloride	Atarax Ucerax	Capsules, 10 mg, 25 mg, 50 mg, Syrup	10 mg/5 mg 10, 25, 50 mg b.i.d. or t.i.d.	5 mg/kg/24 hr	2.1 ± 0.4	20.0 ± 4.1		
Diphenhydramine hydrochloride	Benadryl	Capsules, 25 mg, 50 mg; Elixir, 12.5 mg/5 ml; Parenteral, 50 mg/ml	25 mg–50 mg t.i.d.	50 mg/kg/24 hr	1.7 ± 1.0	9.2 ± 2.5		
Tripelennamine hydrochloride	PBZ PBZ-SR Pyribenzamine	25 mg, 50 mg; Timed-release, 50 mg, 100 mg	Tablets, 25 mg–50 mg q4–6h	5 mg/kg/24 hr in 4-6 divided doses or if >5 years, 50 mg b.i.d. or t.i.d.				
Doxepin		10 mg, 25 mg	10 mg–25 mg b.i.d. or 50 mg at night					

Table 4 Properties of Second-Generation Antihistamines

DRUG	TRADE NAME	FORM/ STRENGTH	USUAL ADULT DOSAGE	CHILDREN'S DOSAGE	ONSET OF ACTION (HOURS)	DURATION OF ACTION (HOURS)	PRECAUTIONS	DRUG INTERACTIONS	SIDE-EFFECTS	OTHER EFFECTS
Terfenadine	Triludan	60 mg, 120 mg tablets; 30 mg 35 ml suspension	60 mg b.i.d., 120 mg qd; do not exceed	3–6 yr, 15 mg b.i.d.; 7–12 yr, 30 mg b.i.d.	1–2	24	Hepatic impairment, QT prolongation, elecrolyte disturbance	Macrolide antibiotics, imidazole antifungals, neuroleptics, tricyclics, diuretics	Ventricular arrhythmias	
Astemizole	Hismanal	10 mg tablets; 5 mg/1 ml suspension	10 mg qd; do not exceed	6–12 yr, 5 mg qd	Very slow	Up to 4 weeks	Same as for terfenadine; use adequate contraception	Same as for terfenadine	Weight gain, ventricular arrhythmias	
Cetirizine	Zirtek	10 mg tablets, 5 mg/5 ml solution	10 mg qd; increase to 10 mg b.i.d., if necessary	6–12 yr; 10 mg qd	0.5	24	Renal insufficiency		May cause drowsiness in higher dosage	May inhibit mast cell activation; inhibits leukocyte migration; inhibits vascular adhesion molecule expression
Loratadine	Claritin	10 mg q.d.; 5 mg/5 ml syrup	10 mg qd; increase to 10 mg b.i.d., if necessary	2–7 yr, 5 mg qd; 7–12 yr, 10 mg qd	2	12–24			May cause drowsiness in higher dosage	
Acrivastine	Semprex	8 mg capsules	8 mg t.i.d.	None	0.5	<12	Renal failure			

eosinophil adhesion to the endothelium and eosinophil migration. It is excreted unchanged in the urine, and the dosage should be decreased in those with renal impairment.

The antihistamine ketotifen has mast cell stabilizing properties and has been administered in a dose of 1 to 2 mg twice daily. In practice this drug seems to be no more effective than one would expect from its antihistaminic properties. There is evidence that the addition of the H_2-blocker, cimetidine, may confer additional therapeutic benefit but the clinical value of adding H_2- to H_1-antagonists is difficult to demonstrate in clinical practice.

Acrivastine is a short-acting antihistamine that may be most suitable for those who suffer from intermittent symptoms only and is probably best used on demand or possibly added to give extra control in those already taking a longer-acting second-generation antihistamine. It is also excreted unchanged in the urine.

If it proves difficult to achieve control it is often helpful to combine antihistamines (e.g., cetirizine and loratadine) and to take the drugs to coincide with the time of greatest symptoms. Besides antihistamines, other types of drugs have been proposed to suppress the whealing and itching of chronic idiopathic urticaria. These include the calcium channel antagonist, nifedipine, and beta-adrenergic drugs such as terbutaline. These have been disappointing in our experience. Short courses of systemic steroids may rarely have a place in the management of acute crisis during the course of chronic urticaria, but it is unwise to embark on long-term steroid treatment because of development of tolerance and side effects. The recent realization that in some patients with chronic urticaria the disease is attributable to a functional anti–high-affinity IgE receptor on anti-IgE autoantibodies is prompting exploration of nonspecific immunotherapy (cyclosporine, intravenous immunoglobulin), but these are experimental measures at the present time.

Drug Treatment of Nonhereditary Angioedema

Mild to moderate angioedema occurring regularly may often respond to an H_1-antihistamine in adequate dosage taken regularly. Dosages used are similar to those for chronic urticaria. Any of the previously listed drugs that may worsen the condition should be stopped. If the attacks of angioedema are intermittent or unpredictable (i.e., once fortnightly or less frequently) an antihistamine can be taken as soon as symptoms occur and continued until the episode remits.

Table 5 Emergency Treatment of Angioedema

Moderately severe affecting the buccal mucosa:
Medihaler-Epi 4–8 puffs onto the oral mucosa
Severe angioedema:
Adrenaline 1:1,000 (1 mg/ml) subcutaneously to a maximum of 1 ml in divided dosage
IV chlorpheniramine 10–20 mg (max 40 mg/24 hr)
IV hydrocortisone succinate (100-300 mg)
Self-administration of adrenaline:
Adrenaline Min-1-Jet 0.5 ml
Adrenaline EpiPen 0.3 ml (adult) 0.15 ml (pediatric)
In patients with severe oropharyngeal obstruction, with or without anaphylactic symptoms and ventilation, oxygen use may be necessary.

In moderate angioedema affecting the buccal mucosa or throat, other measures are required as necessary in addition to antihistamine treatment (Table 5). Severe oropharyngeal edema with or without anaphylaxis may require introduction of an airway and administration of oxygen. In such patients admission for at least 24 hours for monitoring may be necessary.

In severe angioedema or when systemic symptoms of shortness of breath, wheezing, or difficulty in breathing are present or if there is evidence of systemic anaphylaxis, subcutaneous adrenaline 1:1,000 should be administered. An antihistamine may be administered intravenously in addition to the adrenaline, and intravenous hydrocortisone is usually given at the same time. Patients who experience frequent or severe episodes of angioedema with or without anaphylactic symptoms and those who frequently attend the emergency department can be taught the self-administration of adrenaline. Adrenaline is available for this purpose as the Adrenaline Min-1-Jet or the adrenaline EpiPen and should be administered at the onset of an attack.

Suggested Reading

Simons FER. The therapeutic index of newer H_1-receptor antagonists. Clin Exp Allergy 1994; 24:707.

Simons FER, Simons KS. The pharmacology and use of H_1-receptor-antagonist drugs. N Engl J Med 1994; 330(23):1663.

Sullivan TJ. Pharmacology modulation of the whealing response to histamine in human skin identification of doxepin as a potent in vivo inhibitor. J Allergy Clin Immunol 1982; 69:260.

PEMPHIGUS

José M. Mascaró Jr., M.D.
Luis A. Diaz, M.D.

The term *pemphigus* encompasses a group of chronic autoimmune blistering diseases of the skin characterized by cell-to-cell detachment (acantholysis). This loss of adhesion between keratinocytes induces the formation of intraepidermal blisters. Pressure applied to the edge of a bulla can cause extension of the epidermal separation and, if shearing forces are applied to normal-appearing skin, they produce denudation. These events are both termed *Nikolsky's sign,* a typical finding in pemphigus, although it can be seen in other dermatologic conditions. Pemphigus can be subdivided into four main disease processes: pemphigus foliaceus, pemphigus vulgaris, drug-induced pemphigus, and paraneoplastic pemphigus.

PEMPHIGUS VARIANTS

Pemphigus foliaceus is characterized by blister formation at the level of the stratum granulosum. These are fragile blisters that rupture easily. The disease usually manifests as large areas of desquamated erythematous dermatitis. It can occur all over the body, but it is usually most prominent on the face and trunk. In some cases the lesions can extend, and the disease may present as a generalized exfoliative dermatitis. Mucosal blisters or erosions are rarely observed. Pemphigus foliaceus is usually a benign disease except in older individuals with extensive lesions. In certain areas of Brazil and other South American countries, there is an endemic form of pemphigus foliaceus that is termed Fogo Selvagem (wild fire). The cause of Fogo Selvagem is unknown, but there is substantial epidemiologic evidence indicating that it may be precipitated by an environmental factor (probably an insect). Pemphigus erythematosus (Senear-Usher syndrome) represents a variant of pemphigus foliaceus with features of systemic lupus erythematosus occurring in the same patient.

Pemphigus vulgaris is the most common form of pemphigus on the North American continent and in other parts of the world. Blister formation occurs deeper in the epidermis, just above the basal cell layer. The majority of patients present with oral and/or scalp lesions, and only a few demonstrate glabrous skin lesions initially. In later stages of the disease the skin involvement can be widespread. Cutaneous lesions start as flaccid blisters arising on normal or erythematous skin. They rupture easily, resulting in large, denuded areas that show little tendency to spontaneous healing. Pemphigus vulgaris is a severe disease, and it had a high mortality (60 to 90 percent) before the introduction of glucocorticosteroids in therapy. Pemphigus vegetans, an uncommon variant of pemphigus vulgaris, is characterized by large, fungating lesions occurring predominantly in skin folds (groin and axilla).

Drugs may induce or trigger pemphigus. Penicillamine, captopril, and many other drugs have been implicated in drug-induced pemphigus. These patients usually present with morbilliform or urticarial eruptions, and then skin lesions more typical of pemphigus foliaceus than of pemphigus vulgaris appear. Most cases improve after discontinuation of the causative drug, but some patients will need systemic therapy to control their disease. The mechanism of acantholysis in drug-induced pemphigus is unknown. It is feasible that the drug may have a direct effect in the epidermis where it could unmask antigenic sites that sensitized the patient. The antiepidermal autoantibodies will then cause acantholysis.

Paraneoplastic pemphigus is a recently described autoimmune bullous disease. The clinical features are polymorphous, and the lesions can resemble those of erythema multiforme or lichen planus. Patients usually present with pruritic papulosquamous lesions that evolve to vesicles and blisters. Mucous membrane involvement is a prominent feature of paraneoplastic pemphigus. Patients have persistent painful blisters or erosions of the oral mucosa. There is always an associated neoplasm in paraneoplastic pemphigus. The most frequent neoplasms have been hematologic malignancies (non-Hodgkin's lymphoma, chronic lymphocytic leukemia, Waldenström's macroglobulinemia), but association with thymoma, sarcomas, or squamous cell carcinomas has also been reported.

LABORATORY EVALUATION

Acantholysis is the histologic hallmark of all forms of pemphigus. Histopathologic examination in pemphigus foliaceus reveals the presence of acantholytic intraepidermal blisters located in the subcorneal region of the epidermis. Occasionally the presence of eosinophilic spongiosis can be seen, although this feature is also found in pemphigus vulgaris and bullous pemphigoid. In pemphigus vulgaris, cutaneous biopsies show acantholytic cells and suprabasal intraepidermal blisters. The appearance of basal cells in the floor of the blisters has been described as a "row of tombstones." Histologic findings in the prodromal eruption of drug-induced pemphigus are usually nonspecific. In later lesions the picture can be similar to pemphigus foliaceus or pemphigus vulgaris depending on the clinical appearance. In paraneoplastic pemphigus, light microscopy reveals the presence of suprabasilar acantholysis and intraepidermal clefts. In addition, vacuolar degeneration of the basal cell layer and the presence of necrotic keratinocytes have been described as characteristic findings.

All forms of pemphigus have circulating IgG autoantibodies directed against the cell surface of keratinocytes. Direct immunofluorescence (IF) demonstrates deposition of IgG with or without complement on the cell surfaces of the epidermis from lesional skin of almost all patients. In addition, immunoreactant deposition at the basement membrane zone has also been seen in some patients with paraneoplastic pemphigus. IgG autoantibodies directed against the cell surface of keratinocytes can be demonstrated by indirect IF in the sera of approximately 80 to 85 percent of pemphigus patients tested against stratified squamous epithelia. In general, antibody titers correlate with disease activity, and they can be used to monitor therapy. The antibodies in paraneoplastic pemphigus can also bind with the cell surface of simple, columnar, and transitional epithelia (rodent bladder epithelia), and they are occasionally associated with antibasement membrane zone antibodies.

The serum of pemphigus foliaceus patients recognizes, by immunoprecipitation and immunoblot analyses, a glycoprotein of approximately 160 kD that has subsequently been identified as desmoglein 1 (dsg1). Pemphigus vulgaris antigen is a glycoprotein of approximately 130 kD with significant homologies to dsg1, and it has been designated as dsg3. The serum of paraneoplastic pemphigus patients recognizes by immunoprecipitation a complex of four polypeptides of 250, 230, 210, and 190 kD. The 250 and 210 kD antigens have been identified as desmoplakin I and II, respectively, and the 230 kD corresponds to bullous pemphigoid antigen 1. The 190 kD antigen has not yet been identified.

Pathogenesis

Pemphigus autoantibodies are pathogenic. This was demonstrated by in vitro studies with pemphigus vulgaris IgG in which autoantibodies induced acantholysis of human skin in organ culture model systems. In vivo studies have been performed in pemphigus foliaceus, pemphigus vulgaris, and paraneoplastic pemphigus. The purified IgG from patients infused intraperitoneally into neonatal BALB/c mice has induced the production of acantholysis and intraepidermal vesiculation in the mice. Human IgG is detected by direct IF in the intercellular spaces of lesional skin of these mice. The disease process in mice is dependent on the titers of the infused pemphigus foliaceus or pemphigus vulgaris IgG. Other studies have demonstrated that acantholysis can be induced in the absence of complement or by the injection of $F(ab')_2$ fragments of pemphigus foliaceus IgG. However, the precise mechanism for acantholysis in pemphigus vulgaris and pemphigus foliaceus remains unknown. It has been reported that acantholysis induced by pemphigus autoantibodies may be caused by activation of proteinases such as plasminogen activator.

■ THERAPY

Based on the data outlined in the previous sections the initial goals of therapy are to clear the blistering disease and to allow the healing of previous lesions. Since pemphigus autoantibodies are known to be pathogenic, the aim of the therapy should be to eliminate pemphigus autoantibodies from the patient's serum and skin. Two clinical signs are employed to evaluate therapy in pemphigus patients—the estimated number of new lesions formed per week, and the rate of healing of these new lesions. In addition, pemphigus antibody titers should be performed every 4 to 6 weeks. Combining these clinical and serologic parameters provides the best means for judging the effectiveness of therapy. Therapy with steroids or immunosuppressants must be reduced to the lowest levels required to maintain a clinical remission and lessen side effects.

Currently mortality from pemphigus vulgaris has decreased to about 10 percent over a 5 year period, and approximately 30 to 40 percent of the patients remain in clinical remission off all therapy following successful treatment. Currently, the major cause of death in these patients is secondary to complications of high doses of corticosteroids and/or immunosuppressive therapy. Side effects from steroid therapy are a major, if not the most important, clinical problem in the management of pemphigus patients. Consequently, a history of duodenal ulcers, diabetes, hypertension, osteoporosis, cataracts, or exposure to tuberculosis must be obtained prior to starting therapy. A routine complete blood count (CBC) with differential and urinalysis must also be obtained. Baseline chest radiograph and purified protein derivative (PPD) are recommended prior to initiating steroids and, if positive, isoniazid therapy should be considered. Kidney and liver function should be monitored if immunosuppressive agents are used, since these agents are generally metabolized by these organs. Potential bone marrow toxicity from immunosuppressive agents should also be monitored with a weekly CBC during the first month and every 2 to 4 weeks thereafter.

Corticosteroids

Corticosteroids represent the first-line therapy in pemphigus vulgaris management, but they may need to be combined with an immunosuppressive agent in order to reduce side effects. Patients must initially be treated with enough steroids to suppress the blistering disease. Following the suppression of the disease, the serum is monitored for antibody levels. After they have disappeared the skin is examined by direct IF for the presence of antibody deposition at the cell surfaces of the epidermis. Once the autoantibodies can no longer be detected in the patient's serum or in the skin, steroids should be gradually tapered. Following the complete tapering of steroids patients are observed clinically and serologically, every 3 to 4 months for pemphigus disease activity.

Therapy is usually started at a dose equivalent to 1 to 2 mg per kilogram of prednisone daily in divided doses, depending on disease severity. If blister formation diminishes, prednisone can be consolidated into a single morning dose and rapidly reduced at first (approximately 5 to 10 mg per week) and then more slowly when nearing a dose of 40 mg per day. If the disease remains under control at 40 mg daily, then an attempt to change to an alternate-day therapy should be made by gradually tapering the dose given every other day to zero. The 40 mg every other day should then be tapered as tolerated. However, if after 6 to 8 weeks the patient continues to demonstrate new blister formation, the prednisone dose should be increased by 50 percent of the dose that the patient was receiving, and 50 percent increases of the dose should be done every week until the disease is controlled. Then, the usual tapering rate of prednisone is lower (5 to 2.5 mg per week). Once this dose has been tapered to a level of 80 mg per day, alternate-day tapering is recommended.

Immunosuppressive Agents

If high maintenance doses are required or if the patient is not tolerating prednisone, then addition of an immunosuppressive agent should be considered. The combination of immunosuppressive drugs with low doses of steroids not only controls the disease, but also has a pronounced steroid-sparing effect, resulting in the decreased occurrence of steroid side effects. Cytotoxic agents that have been used in various combinations to treat pemphigus include azathioprine, cyclophosphamide, and methotrexate. These agents take several weeks to take effect and are not drugs of first choice for treating the acute phase of pemphigus vulgaris. They are usually not started until the prednisone has been tapered to about 40 mg daily. When steroids have been discontinued, the immunosuppressive agent should be tapered over a 1- to 2 month period. Cyclophosphamide (Cytoxan) is usually the drug of choice. It is given in doses of 75 to 150 mg per day. Significant adverse effects include bone marrow suppression, hemorrhagic cystitis, bladder fibrosis, sterility, and increased risk of developing malignancies. The risk of cystitis can be reduced by encouraging patients to maintain a high fluid intake. Azathioprine (Imuran) is given in doses of 100 to 200 mg per day. Its major side effects are bone marrow suppression, an increased risk of developing malignancies, and hepatotoxicity. When methotrexate is used, 25 to 50 mg per week are given either intramuscularly (single dose) or orally (divided in three doses given 12 hours apart). Hepatotoxicity is the main side effect of methotrexate. Routine liver function tests as well as liver biopsies (both pretreatment and during therapy) are recommended if long-term treatment is anticipated.

Other Treatments

Intravenous pulse glucocorticosteroid therapy, using supraphysiologic doses of corticosteroids (1 g per day given for 3 days), offers an alternative approach to uncontrollable pemphigus patients. Although there are generally fewer side effects, serious complications also exist, including psychological disturbances, seizures, hypertension, sinus bradycardia, increased blood glucose, and severe arthralgia. After the pulse has been administered, oral glucocorticosteroids in tapering doses are usually required and sometimes, several pulses are necessary to control the disease.

Plasmapheresis, a technique in which antibody-containing plasma is removed from the circulation and replaced with a plasma substitute, has been a useful alternative in patients poorly controlled on high-dose prednisone and/or immunosuppressive agents. It is currently considered an experimental therapy, but it may be contemplated in patients with severe, refractory disease. It should be undertaken while the patient is receiving concomitant treatment with steroids and immunosuppressants. Complications include immunosuppression caused by removal of immunoglobulins and depletive coagulopathy.

Gold therapy has been shown to be effective in the treatment of patients with pemphigus vulgaris. Weekly doses of gold (25 to 50 mg) must be given to reach a cumulative dose of 1,500 mg or higher before any therapeutic effect can usually be detected. After the disease is controlled, the weekly doses of gold can be reduced to once a month and then discontinued. Patients treated with gold can achieve clinical and serologic remissions. Oral gold is now the preferred form of therapy. Complications of this therapy include thrombocytopenia, bone marrow suppression, glomerulonephritis, pneumonitis, and mucocutaneous eruptions.

Dapsone has been used in older individuals in which the concomitant use of steroids and immunosuppressants may be difficult. The standard dose is 50 to 100 mg per day.

Cyclosporine has also been used in the treatment of pemphigus vulgaris, and although there have been several favorable uncontrolled studies, it appears that cyclosporine is ineffective as a single therapy and is associated with a high rate of renal toxicity.

A few patients with drug-resistant pemphigus vulgaris have been successfully treated with extracorporeal photopheresis. However, this procedure is an experimental form of treatment, and therefore more experience is needed before it can be used on a routine basis.

Topical care for crusted lesions and erosions includes wet aluminum subacetate compresses and silver sulfadiazine three to four times daily, which removes crusts, decreases discomfort, and reduces the risk of infection. Patients with oral involvement may benefit from a soft diet and viscous lidocaine before meals; topical steroids in an adherent base may also be of some help.

Treatment of Other Pemphigus Variants

Pemphigus foliaceus is usually a relatively benign and self-limited disorder. The cutaneous eruption of the majority of patients will respond to treatment with systemic corticosteroids alone at 40 to 60 mg of prednisone per day. The disease can usually be controlled in a few weeks, and steroids may be rapidly tapered to every other day and maintained until autoantibodies are not detected. In some patients, however, the disease runs a chronic course and verrucous plaques develop on the trunk that are extremely resistant to therapy. Local fluorinated steroids may be used as an adjuvant to systemic therapy. Immunosuppressive drugs and gold compounds have also been used successfully. In drug-induced pemphigus it is extremely important to discontinue the suspected agent. Most cases will then resolve rapidly and need no further therapy. However, some patients may follow a chronic course similar to idiopathic pemphigus foliaceus or pemphigus vulgaris and will require analogous therapy. Most patients with paraneoplastic pemphigus follow a progressive course that is refractory to all treatments. Although a few patients may improve with therapies used to treat pemphigus vulgaris, most will only have improvement in their cutaneous disease if the malignancy is in remission or cured.

Suggested Reading

Becker BA, Gaspari AA. Pemphigus vulgaris and vegetans. Dermatol Clin 1993; 11(3):429–452.

Crosby DL, Diaz LA. Endemic pemphigus foliaceus. Dermatol Clin 1993; 11(3):453–462.

Pye RJ. Bullous eruptions. In: Champion RH, Burton JL, Ebling FGJ, eds. Rook/Wilkinson/Ebling textbook of dermatology. 5th ed. Oxford: Blackwell Scientific Publications, 1992: 1623–1673.

Stanley JR. Pemphigus. In: Fitzpatrick TB. Eisen AZ, Wolff K, et al, eds. Dermatology in general medicine. 4th ed. New York: McGraw-Hill, 1993: 606–615.

PEMPHIGOID: BULLOUS AND CICATRICIAL

Lawrence S. Chan, M.D.
David T. Woodley, M.D.

■ BULLOUS PEMPHIGOID

Bullous pemphigoid (BP) is an immune-mediated blistering disease of the skin, manifested as tense bullae (either generally or locally) on inflammed or urticarial skin. The mean age of onset of the disease is the late 1960s. In the case of generalized involvement, the lesions preferentially occur in the intertriginous areas. In rare cases, the disease is manifested as pruritic urticarial plaques without clinically visible blisters or even as generalized pruritus without skin lesions. Classically, the histology of bullous pemphigoid is characterized by subepidermal blister formation accompanied by an eosinophilic dermal infiltrate. Direct immunofluorescence microscopy of a perilesional skin biopsy typically reveals the linear deposition of immunoglobulin G and complement at the dermal-epidermal junction. In the majority of cases, circulating antibasement membrane antibodies of the immunoglobulin G class are detected by indirect immunofluorescence microscopy. These autoantibodies bind to hemidesmosomal components of the basal keratinocyte apposed to the cutaneous basement membrane zone. These autoantibodies are targeted to a 230,000 Daltons and/or a 180,000 Daltons glycoprotein associated with hemidesmosomes. If salt-split skin substrate is used, these autoantibodies bind to the epidermal roof. After proper therapy, the disease usually heals without scarring.

Therapy

The treatment plan for bullous pemphigoid should be tailored to suit the individual patient, depending on the severity of the disease and the patient's clinical response. For generalized bullous pemphigoid, systemic corticosteroids are the mainstay of treatment and should be started as soon as the clinical diagnosis is confirmed by lesional histology and perilesional direct immunofluorescence microscopy. Most patients with generalized bullous pemphigoid respond well to a single daily dose of oral prednisone in the range of 0.5 to 1 mg per kilogram body weight. Prednisone taken after breakfast is better tolerated than afternoon or evening administration. The mechanism of action of prednisone on bullous pemphigoid is most likely due to its anti-inflammatory effects.

Oral azathioprine (100 to 250 mg per day) often is used as an adjunct treatment. It was thought that the addition of azathioprine would allow lower total doses of prednisone. However, there is no documentation in the literature that this occurs, and this notion is being challenged. Since azathioprine is a slow-acting drug, it should be initiated early in the treatment regimen. The mechanism of action of azathioprine on bullous pemphigoid is unknown. It may act by decreasing the number of leukocytes through bone marrow suppression. Accordingly, the patient's leukocyte and platelet counts should be monitored monthly. The duration and magnitude of the azathioprine clinical effects correlate with tissue level, but not plasma level, of the metabolite thiopurine nucleotide. Therefore, blood levels of the drug have little predictive value for therapy. Unlike pemphigus vulgaris, the circulating anti-basement membrane antibody titers in patients with BP do not correlate with disease severity. Therefore, indirect immunofluorescence has little value in assessing disease activity or adjusting the dosages of medications. The adjustment of medication should be dependent primarily upon the clinical response of the patient. In general, one expects a decrease in new blisters approximately 1 week after the initiation of therapy of oral prednisone. Healing of the blisters occurs in the subsequent weeks.

Adjunctive topical corticosteroid (mid to high potency) may be added to selected areas in some BP patients. The application of a topical corticosteroid may reduce the need for high doses of oral prednisone. Since blistered skin may increase the chance of systemic absorption, the possible sparing of systemic steroids by the use of topical steroids may not be significant.

The timing for tapering oral prednisone is important, since tapering too early may result in flare of the disease and tapering too late may increase the chance of unnecessary corticosteroid side effects. Two weeks after the cessation of new blister formation and the initiation of healing, tapering of the oral prednisone may begin. In most cases, tapering the prednisone by 5 mg per day every 2 to 3 weeks can be achieved. Some physicians taper oral prednisone using an alternate-day schedule to further reduce potential complications. Our usual approach is to taper the daily prednisone to 20 to 40 mg and then initiate an alternate-day regimen. There are several schedules for converting daily prednisone to an alternate-day regimen. Our preference is to simply double the current daily dose of prednisone but to give it every other day. The patient is then on the same total weekly dose of prednisone. After a week or two on this regimen, we again begin to taper the alternate day prednisone by 5 mg each week.

If oral azathioprine is part of the therapeutic regimen, it should be kept constant while the prednisone is tapered. After the patient is completely off prednisone and remains disease free for several months, azathioprine can then be decreased, usually by 50 mg every week until it is completely discontinued.

When the patient has widespread blisters, erosions, and crusts, topical or systemic antibiotics should be administered to prevent secondary infection or sepsis resulting from denudation of the skin. Systemic antibiotics are usually dicloxacillin, erythromycin, or cephalexin at 1 g per day in divided doses. If the patient becomes febrile, blood cultures should be obtained to monitor for the possibility of sepsis.

Although most patients with generalized bullous pemphigoid respond well to low to medium doses of oral prednisone (with or without adjunctive agents such as azathioprine or topical corticosteroid), some patients respond poorly and may require higher doses of prednisone, longer duration of treatment, and/or more potent immunosuppressants. When dealing with poorly responsive cases, it is recommended that the diagnosis be thoroughly re-evaluated. Indirect immunofluorescence on salt-split skin and immunoblotting should be performed to rule out other more difficult to treat diseases such as epidermolysis bullosa acquisita. Cyclophosphamide (daily dose of 1 to 2 mg per kilogram is a good alternative to azathioprine. We have had severe bullous pemphigoid patients who failed on azathioprine, but then rapidly responded to cyclophosphamide. Nevertheless, one must closely monitor the potential side effects of cyclophosphamide such as bone marrow suppression and hemorrhagic cystitis. A complete blood count and urinalysis should be performed on at least a semiweekly schedule.

For those patients who require long-term oral prednisone, one should consider using therapeutic measures to impede for steroid-induced bone loss. The use of a "triple therapy" (calcium 1 g per day, vitamin D 1,000 IU, diphosphonate EHDP 7.5 mg per kilogram) has been reported recently to impede bone loss in patients on systemic steroids.

Other medications have been used in generalized bullous pemphigoid with the hope of being able to use lower doses of systemic steroids to curtail the disease. Chlorambucil, an alkylating antineoplastic medication, has been used (0.1 mg per kilogram body weight) successfully to treat bullous pemphigoid in combination with low doses of systemic corticosteroid. The potentially serious side effects of chlorambucil include bone marrow suppression, especially thrombocytopenia, and leukemia.

Methotrexate, an antimetabolite, also has been reported to be a good adjunctive medication (weekly single dose of less than 20 mg) for bullous pemphigoid in combination with oral prednisone. The potential hepatotoxicity of methotrexate must be closely monitored by following liver enzymes on a biweekly basis.

A minority of patients respond well to sulfa-containing medications such as dapsone. These agents possess antineutrophil motility effects and may be anti-inflammatory in nature. Since potentially fatal hemolysis may occur in patients with a genetic G6PD deficiency, all patients should be checked for G6PD prior to dapsone treatment (100 to 400 mg per day).

Some patients with bullous pemphigoid respond to oral niacinamide (1.5 to 2.5 g per day in three divided doses) in combination with oral antibiotics such as tetracycline or erythromycin (both given at 2 g per day in four divided doses). Topical steroid creams or ointments may be added to this regimen. This therapy is particularly worth trying in elderly patients with milder disease who can be observed closely and are compliant. Like dapsone, tetracycline and erythromycin are anti-inflammatory in nature because of their inhibitory effects on inflammatory cells such as the neutrophils. Anti-inflammatory effects may be responsible for the clinical response. The treatment of bullous pemphigoid with cyclosporine, an antilymphocyte medication, has been tried but appears to give variable results.

For localized bullous pemphigoid, the potential morbidity and mortality are low. It can be treated with mid to high potency topical corticosteroids alone. In some cases, a low dose of oral prednisone may be added for a short duration to stop the development of new blister formation.

CICATRICIAL PEMPHIGOID

Cicatricial pemphigoid, as currently defined, is not a homogeneous, but rather a heterogeneous group of diseases. In general, cicatricial pemphigoid is characterized clinically by inflammation and blister formation on mucosal surfaces and histologically by a full subepithelial blister and linear immune deposits at basement membrane zone when mucosal biopsy specimens are examined by direct immunofluorescence microscopy. Circulating antibasement membrane antibodies are detected in only a small percent of patients. Scarring may result from the inflammatory process, mostly involving ocular mucosae.

The heterogeneity of the currently defined cicatricial pemphigoid is illustrated by several recent findings. On one hand, a subset of patients who have predominantly mucosal disease and minor skin involvement has been found to have autoantibodies directed against a lower lamina lucida component laminin-5 (also known as kalinin/nicein/BM600/epiligrin). On the other hand, another subset of patients have pure ocular disease and are distinguished from bullous pemphigoid and other mucosal pemphigoid by the high frequency of fibrin deposition at the basement-membrane zone and a virtual absence of circulating antibodies against the basement-membrane zone. Yet another subgroup of patients has only oral mucosal disease without much cicatrization. This appears to be another unique disease entity. In addition, HLA-DQBI* 0301, a specific allele in the class II major histocompatibility complex gene region, was found to be significantly increased in patients with pure ocular cicatricial pemphigoid. Thus at least three distinct subsets of cicatricial pemphigoid can currently be defined—anti–laminin-5 mucosal pemphigoid, pure ocular cicatricial pemphigoid, and oral mucosal pemphigoid.

Therapy

As for bullous pemphigoid, the treatment for cicatricial pemphigoid as a group should be tailored to suit each patient, according to the particular organ involved. For patients who have ocular disease, the physician will face great difficulties in managing the disease. On one hand, untreated or insufficiently treated ocular disease will result in ocular mucosal scarring and potentially lead to blindness. On the other hand, proper treatment of ocular disease requires aggressive usage of potent immunosuppressives. Our initial treatment is oral prednisone (1 mg per kilogram body weight) plus azathioprine (100 to 300 mg per day). If no response occurs in 2 weeks, we add dapsone (100 to 300 mg per day). If no significant response is observed in 2 months with this combination therapy, we then use cyclophosphamide (1 to 2 mg per kilogram body weight) as a replacement for azathioprine. For those patients who cannot tolerate cyclophosphamide because of cystitis or other complications, the alternate therapy is chlorambucil. Patients who require long-term strong immunosuppressives should be properly informed about the potential side effects, such as bone marrow suppression, leukemia and other malignancies, and severe infection. Immunization for influenza and common bacterial infections are recommended. It should be noted that medical treatments do not reverse the formed scar, although they may stop further scar formation. Surgical correction of ocular scarring is not recommended because of the high rate of rescarring. Patients with ocular disease should be managed and monitored by both dermatologists and ophthalmologists.

For patients who do not have ocular disease, treatment should be less aggressive. Usually, a mid to high potency topical corticosteroid should be used as the initial treatment. Since secondary candidiasis may occur as a complication to steroid treatment, a compound medication containing both anticandida and corticosteroid such as Lotrisone cream may be used. In patients with severe oral disease, we give a short course (1 to 2 months) of low dose oral prednisone (20 to 40 mg per day) in conjunction with a topical steroid (Kenalog in orabase or Temovate gel) and/or topical cyclosporine A. Topical cyclosporin A used as a "swish-and-spit" agent is too expensive. We recommend that a small amount of full-strength cyclosporine A solution be poured into a small cup and the patient should then use a cotton applicator to soak the solution and press against the mucosal lesions for 5 minutes, repeated three times a day.

Suggested Reading

Foster CS, Wilson LA, Ekins MB. Immunosuppressive therapy for progressive ocular cicatricial pemphigoid. Ophthalmology 1982; 89:340–353.

Krain LS, Landau JW, Newcomer VD. Cyclophosphamide in the treatment of pemphigus vulgaris and bullous pemphigoid. Arch Dermatol 1972; 106:657–661.

Milligan A, Hutchinson PE. The use of chlorambucil in the treatment of bullous pemphigoid. J Am Acad Dermatol 1990; 22:796–801.

Paul MA, Jorizzo JL, Fleischer AB, White WL. Low-dose methotrexate treatment in elderly patients with bullous pemphigoid. J Am Acad Dermatol 1994; 31:620–625.

Rogers RS, Sheridan PJ, Nightingale SH. Desquamative gingivitis: Clinical, histopathologic, immunopathologic, and therapeutic observations. J Am Acad Dermatol 1982; 77:729–735.

Thivolet J, Barthelemy H, Rigot-Muller G, et al. Effects of cyclosporin on bullous pemphigoid and pemphigus. Lancet 1985; 1:334–335.

DERMATITIS HERPETIFORMIS

Jens Gille, M.D.
Robert A. Swerlick, M.D.

Dermatitis herpetiformis (DH) is a chronic, intensely pruritic, papulovesicular skin eruption typically distributed in a symmetrical fashion on extensor surfaces. DH may present at any age; however, it usually starts in the second or third decade. Characteristically, patients feel localized burning, stinging, or itching about 12 to 24 hours before the appearance of the lesions. Essentially all patients with DH have a gluten-sensitive enteropathy (GSE) that most commonly is asymptomatic. If gastrointestinal symptoms do occur, they clinically resemble celiac sprue. In addition to GSE, DH can be associated with a number of other internal abnormalities (Table 1).

The ability of DH patients to both normalize the morphologic changes of the intestine and to improve their skin lesions by strictly adhering to a gluten-free diet has provided strong evidence that associated GSE plays a fundamental role in the pathogenesis of DH. The high occurrence of certain major histocompatibility complex antigens such as HLA-B8, HLA-DRw17, HLA-DQw2 in DH patients is viewed as a major immunogenic factor contributing to a relative immune susceptibility. Granular deposits of polyclonal IgA found in both involved and uninvolved dermal skin are a universal phenomen in DH patients; however, their role in the pathophysiology of DH is still unknown.

Table 1 Selected Disorders Associated with Dermatitis Herpetiformis
Gluten-sensitive enteropathy (GSE)
Gastric abnormalities (atrophy, hypochlorhydria)
Thyroid abnormalities (autoimmune thyroiditis, hypothyroidism, hyperthyroidism, thyroid nodules, and malignancy)
Gastrointestinal lymphoma
Autoimmune diseases (systemic lupus erythematosus, dermatomyositis, Sjögren's syndrome, rheumatoid arthritis, myasthenia gravis, and others)

Even if the clinical presentation is not classic and straightforward, DH can usually be diagnosed by direct immunofluorescence of perilesional skin. Typically, in vivo–bound granular IgA deposits are found in the papillary dermis, which by definition distinguish the entity DH from other subepidermal blistering eruptions.

■ THERAPY

There are two therapeutic strategies to treat patients with DH—pharmacologic therapy and a gluten-free diet. The choice of therapy depends on a variety of factors, including the knowledge of the benefits and the risks that accompany both drug and dietary treatment. Sulfones are the pharmacologic agents of choice in the therapy of DH. Three drugs within this class, diaminodiphenylsulfone (dapsone, DDS), sulfapyridine, and sulfamethoxypyridazine, are used to treat DH, although only dapsone is freely available in the United States. Drug therapy typically results in rapid relief of severe itching and burning, and the appearance of new lesions ceases within 24 to 48 hours. Sulfones are usually well tolerated, yet

Table 2 Selected Side Effects of Dapsone Therapy

Hemolytic anemia
Methemoglobinemia
Headache
Nausea
Fatigue
Cyanosis
Gastrointestinal irritation
Psychosis
Skin eruption
Hepatitis, infectious mononucleosis-like with lymphadenopathy
Hypalbuminemia
Peripheral neuropathy
Leukopenia-agranulocytosis

Table 3 Absolute and Relative Contraindications of Dapsone Therapy

Sulfa allergy
History of adverse reactions to sulfones
G-6-PD deficiency
Anemia
History of hemoglobulin abnormalities
Ischemic heart disease
Peripheral vascular insufficiency
Liver, lung, and kidney disorders

they do not improve the associated GSE and have a small risk of severe side effects. In contrast, a gluten-free diet treats both bowel and skin disease and is essentially devoid of significant risks. However, a gluten-free diet is difficult for the patient to manage, and effective control of the skin eruption with strict dietary treatment may take many months to years. Therefore, sulfones are generally the initial treatment of choice in order to rapidly control the rash, while a gluten-free diet should be offered to patients with associated symptomatic GSE or those desiring a drug-free treatment.

Dapsone

Diaminodiphenylsulfone (dapsone) is a remarkably effective agent for DH treatment. The responsiveness to dapsone has almost become an additional criterion for the diagnosis of DH. A variety of other skin disorders that are characterized histologically by infiltration with polymorphonuclear leukocytes may also respond to dapsone, but a presumptive diagnosis of DH in patients who fail to respond to dapsone should suggest an alternative diagnosis.

The initial dose for an average adult patient is usually 50 to 100 mg daily, depending on the severity of the disease and the expected risks of dapsone therapy. Approximately two-thirds of all DH patients will sufficiently respond to 100 mg per day of dapsone. Since many side effects (Table 2) are dose dependent, it is critical to establish the minimum dose that is required to suppress symptoms for each patient. However, few patients without other medical problems will experience side effects at daily doses of 100 mg or lower.

If the skin rash is adequately controlled, the daily dose should be reduced every 2 to 4 weeks by 25 to 50 mg until the daily dose is 25 to 50 mg. Subsequently, the dosage should be administered every second day, reviewed in 2 to 4 weeks, and then every third day until skin lesions reappear. In DH patients, who have not responded to 100 mg daily after 2 to 4 weeks, the dose can be increased in 25 to 50 mg increments every 2 to 4 weeks. Patients generally tolerate dosages up to 150 or 200 mg daily. Occasionally, initial dosage of 300 to 400 mg per day may be required, though side effects usually do not allow dapsone treatment at such high doses.

The use of dapsone in the treatment of DH is limited by its side effects and contraindications (see Tables 2 and 3). Two categories of toxicity are appreciated: dose-dependent and idiosyncratic reactions. Dose-dependent side effects include the well-documented hematologic effects of dapsone therapy, such as hemolysis and methemoglobinemia. A dose of 100 mg daily will transiently decrease hemoglobin levels by 1 to 2 g per deciliter. In particular, this will affect the elderly population and patients with ischemic heart disease, peripheral vascular disease, or cerebrovascular insufficiency. Concomitant administration of vitamin E can effectively blunt dose-dependent decreases in hemoglobin levels at daily doses of 800 U.

Methemoglobinemia is regularly seen in patients treated with dapsone, although it is uncommonly symptomatic at doses below 150 mg per day. If methemoglobin concentrations reach critical levels, related symptoms, such as headache, nausea, fatigue, and cyanosis, can occur. Both methylene blue (Urolene blue, Star Pharmaceuticals) and cimetidine (400 mg three times daily) can reduce dose-dependent methemoglobinemia. Levels of methemoglobin can be measured, yet the dose of dapsone and concomitant methylene blue or cimetidine treatment can usually be adjusted on a clinical basis. Although the initial dose of methylene blue is 65 mg twice daily, it can be escalated up to as much as 130 mg four times daily. Methylene blue is well tolerated except for occasional bladder irritation, particularly if it is not administered in divided doses. Patients need to know that this therapy will turn their urine blue.

Dapsone may also cause a variety of other adverse reactions on an idiosyncratic or allergic basis. These reactions include agranulocytosis, infectious mononucleosis-like hepatitis, various cutaneous eruptions, psychosis, and peripheral neuropathy (see Table 2). The severe cases of agranulocytosis almost invariably occur within the first 8 to 12 weeks of therapy. The risk has been estimated to be as high as 1:240 to as rare as 1:20,000.

Because of its potential and pharmacologic side effects, dapsone therapy requires close laboratory monitoring before and during treatment. Complete blood cell counts, differential white blood cell counts, hemoglobin, and renal and liver parameters should be obtained before starting dapsone therapy. Since hemolysis may be life threatening in patients with glucose-6-phosphate dehydrogenase (G-6-PD) deficiency, this condition represents a rigid contraindication for dapsone therapy. Although the incidence of G-6-PD deficiency is considered low in northern European populations who are at greatest risk for DH, we routinely screen all patients prior to treatment. Complete blood counts with differential are checked weekly during the first 2 weeks of therapy and then twice monthly during the next 3 months of therapy to monitor for leukocytopenia or agranulocytosis. Thereafter, complete blood parameters and liver and renal function are periodically determined at 2 to 3 month intervals. Thyroid abnormalities are frequently associated with DH and may affect dapsone metabolism. It may be prudent to obtain functional thyroid parameters if clinical hyperthyroidism or hypothyroidism is suspected.

Sulfapyridine and Sulfamethoxypyridazine

Sulfapyridine and sulfamethoxypyridazine are almost exclusively used as alternative drugs in DH patients who do not tolerate dapsone or in whom its hemolytic potential makes it unsuitable, such as in patients with cardiopulmonary problems. In part, their limited use is also caused by their unavailability in many countries. Sulfapyridine appears to be less effective in controlling DH symptoms than dapsone. The initial dose is 500 mg twice daily, but it may require up to 2 to 3 g daily in order to completely alleviate cutaneous lesions. Sulfamethoxypyridazine, however, is a very effective drug in patients who are at risk under dapsone treatment or who have been unable to tolerate dapsone. An adequate response is seen in most patients at daily doses of 0.5 to 1.0 g.

As with dapsone management, the initial dose of both drugs should be reviewed after 2 to 4 weeks and adjusted to the minimum dose necessary to prevent symptoms. Side effects include morbilliform skin rashes, nausea, depression, and severe bone marrow suppression that requires close monitoring of complete blood counts.

Gluten-Free Diet

Since it has been demonstrated that both skin eruption and associated GSE improve and normalize with strict avoidance of dietary gluten in DH patients, it is commonly accepted that gluten is central to the pathophysiology and development of DH. Strict adherence to a gluten-free diet can substantially reduce the dose of sulfone therapy or even enable the patient to discontinue drug treatment completely. In addition, since sulfone therapy does not affect the enteropathy in DH patients, there are compelling reasons to encourage patients with DH to try the gluten-free diet, particularly those individuals with symptomatic GSE.

Although dietary treatment appears to be an attractive alternative to medication for many patients, it is very difficult to maintain. The gluten-free diet requires a lifelong avoidance of gluten, specifically, the gliadin fraction of gluten found in common grains (wheat, rye, oats, barley, and in some patients also soy, millet, and buckwheat). Even the intake of trivial amounts of gluten may prevent improvement of clinical symptoms. In addition, dietary treatment may need several months to years in order to alleviate cutaneous lesions in DH patients. This is particularly true in patients who have been treated with sulfones for an extended period of time. Nevertheless, a gluten-free diet should be offered as an appropriate and sufficient therapeutic approach for motivated patients who wish to avoid lifelong drug therapy. Additional candidates for a gluten-free diet are patients with any of the disorders listed in Table 3. The patients should be supervised by experienced dietitians who are well versed in a gluten-free diet. Additional information and support are provided by the Celiac Sprue Association, U.S.A. (2313 Rocklyn Drive #1, Des Moines, IA 50322) and by the Gluten Intolerance Group of North America (P.O. Box 23063, Seattle, WA 98102-0353).

Topical Therapy of DH Skin Lesions

Topical treatment of cutaneous lesions may not only decrease the duration of healing and the subjective discomfort caused by severe itching and burning, but it can also aid the patient to better tolerate skin symptoms under a given dose of sulfone therapy or dietary treatment. The occasional development of new lesions in DH patients can usually be managed by topical application of a medium-strength (e.g., triamcinolone 0.1 percent) or high-potency (e.g., betamethasone 0.05 percent) glucocorticoid cream or ointment. Since most patients can predict the sites of newly developing skin lesions because of the localized burning and itching that occurs 12 to 24 hours in advance, the eruption can be repressed by immediate use of topical steroids. DH patients need to be advised on the considerable side effects of topically applied corticosteroids. Their use should be restricted to the minimum possible and has to be avoided in critical areas such as facial and intertriginous skin.

AVOIDANCE OF EXACERBATING FACTORS

Halogens may provoke and exacerbate DH lesions in selected patients. Both the external application through patch testing (10 to 25 percent potassium iodide in petrolatum) and the internal administration (e.g., iodine or potassium periodide) can produce DH symptoms or may result in exacerbation of pre-existing skin lesions. The influence of both medical and dietary treatment on the susceptibility to halogens in DH patients has not been intensively studied. Therefore, it is difficult to precisely determine the dose of exposure required for inducing DH symptoms in a given individual. Our impression is that dietary iodides usually do not affect the clinical course of DH. Nonetheless, patients with DH should be counseled on the exacerbating potential of halogens, especially with regard to diagnostic procedures involving high quantities of iodides.

Furthermore, a subgroup of DH patients is susceptible to induction of DH symptoms by nonsteroidal anti-inflammatory drugs (e.g., indomethacin, ibuprofen). The susceptibility appears to be increased in patients with dapsone therapy. Clinically, the exacerbation can present as a rapid development of new skin lesions that may mimic drug-induced skin eruptions. Since similar reactions have not been reported after administration of acetaminophen, this antianalgesic drug can serve as an alternative medication for temporary relief of minor pains.

Suggested Reading

Coleman MD. Dapsone: Modes of action, toxicity and possible strategies for increasing patient tolerance. Br J Dermatol 1993; 129:507.

Hall RP III. Dermatitis herpetiformis. J Invest Dermatol 1992; 99:873.

Katz SI. Dapsone. In: Fitzpatrick TB, et al. eds. Dermatology in general medicine. 4th ed. New York: McGraw-Hill, 1993: 2865.

Leonard JN, Fry L. Treatment and management of dermatitis herpetiformis. Clin Dermatol 1992; 9:403.

McFadden JP, Leonard JN, Powles AV, et al. Sulfamethoxypyridazine for dermatitis herpetiformis, linear IgA disease and cicatricial pemphigoid. Br J Dermatol 1989; 121:759.

EXFOLIATIVE DERMATITIS

Herman S. Mogavero Jr., M.D.

This entity, also known as erythroderma, is a cutaneous inflammation characterized by an initial erythema with the subsequent development of pronounced scaling or exfoliation. Although it is often initially localized, the process typically has spread to the majority of the cutaneous surfaces at the time of presentation.

There are multiple etiologies for this disorder, recognizing both a primary de novo clinical presentation and secondary underlying causes. These can be conveniently compartmentalized into the following classification:

1. Idiopathic.
2. Generalized or widespread cutaneous disease states such as atopic, contact, or seborrheic dermatitis, psoriasis, lichen planus, pemphigus foliaceus, or pityriasis rubra pilaris.
3. Systemic diseases with cutaneous manifestations such as leukemias, lymphomas (of both the T- and B-cell types), and some solid tumors (e.g., of the lung or rectum).
4. Adverse cutaneous reactions to drugs. This reaction can involve many classes of drugs, including but not limited to antibiotics, antiinflammatory drugs, anticonvulsants, and metallic compounds.

The diagnosis of a pre-existing dermatologic condition in the erythrodermic patient relies on a detailed examination of the whole integument. Dermatologic consultation should be requested to assist in looking for distinct areas of "typical" morphology isolated from the surrounding "sea of erythema." It is in these areas that there is the highest yield of diagnostic skin biopsy findings in specific dermatologic entities. In addition, skin biopsy can be helpful in the diagnosis of underlying leukemia or lymphomas and is indicated in the evaluation of all cases of erythroderma.

The objective cutaneous manifestations of exfoliative dermatitis can extend beyond the obvious erythema and scaling. There can be complete or partial alopecia, onychodystrophy, deep painful fissuring of the skin, and desquamation of the palms and soles in broad thick sheets. Mucous membrane involvement is distinctly unusual in erythroderma.

There are major systemic components of exfoliative dermatitis, and in most cases these features warrant hospitalization for appropriate diagnostic evaluation and therapeutic intervention. Typically there are complaints referable to the inability to maintain thermostability. In spite of multiple layers of clothing, the patient is unable to keep warm at ambient temperatures that are uncomfortably hot for others. The patient reports chills and shaking sensations. On examination there may be either fever or hypothermia. In the latter instance it is important to be sure that the device measuring the temperature can register below 96°F (36°C). The remainder of the physical examination must be complete, with special attention paid to assessing lymphadenopathy, hepatomegaly, and splenomegaly. The distinction of lymphoma from dermatopathic lymphadenopathy often requires lymph node biopsy as well. Other signs of secondary infection, hypervolemia, tachycardia, edema, and high-output cardiac failure must be sought. The laboratory evaluation can parallel that used in a severe burn with prominent fluid and electrolyte abnormalities, including hypoalbuminemia and hypernatremia if increased transepidermal water loss is not corrected. Accurate weight measurements and daily monitoring of fluid intake and output are also required.

■ TREATMENT

The treatment of exfoliative dermatitis is focused on the diagnostic entity responsible. Elimination of an offending drug usually initiates resolution of the dermatitis. Treatment of the underlying systemic disease is necessary to control erythroderma secondary to neoplastic processes. In this setting a consultation with a hematologist or oncologist is appropriate for therapeutic intervention.

The approach in cases of erythroderma related to widespread cutaneous disease or idiopathic exfoliative erythroderma is initially conservative. The patient is often best served by hospitalization in order to allow for the aforementioned diagnostic studies and systemic monitoring and also to remove him or her from any negative environmental factors (e.g., in cases of atopic dermatitis).

The mainstay of therapy is frequent lubrication of the skin with colloidal baths and bland ointments such as Aquaphor or petrolatum. If pruritus is a component of the eruption, antihistamines are given. I routinely employ hydroxyzine as an H_1 blocker and increase the dosage to maximal tolerance (up to 100 mg orally every 6 hours) before adding additional H_1 blockers (cyproheptadine, 4 mg orally every 8 hours, or terfenadine, 60 mg orally every 12 hours) or H_2 blockers (cimetidine, 300 mg orally three or four times daily).

The topical use of corticosteroid ointments is tempered by the realization that the widespread cutaneous inflammation and defective vasoconstriction allow for enhanced absorption percutaneously. I typically begin with 1 percent hydrocortisone ointment applied three times daily. If no response is noted after a brief period of time (while diagnostic studies are pending), one can advance to 0.1 percent triamcinolone ointment or its equivalents (class III or IV) three times daily. The topical use of more potent steroids (class I or II) is modulated by the extent of the cutaneous eruption because widespread disease allows for pituitary-adrenal axis suppression. If the diagnosis of psoriasis has been excluded and the risk-benefit of systemic treatment of severe seborrheic or atopic dermatitis is considered, a course of systemic corticosteroid therapy is warranted, with initial doses of prednisone in the range of 1 to 1.5 mg per kilogram per day. Once control has been achieved the objective of therapy is to consolidate to a single daily dose and then taper to alternate day, low-dose steroid therapy to minimize the well-known complications of daily systemic steroid therapy.

The introduction of retinoids has added greatly to the therapeutic tools available to the dermatologist. In cases of erythrodermic psoriasis, etretinate has proved very effective.

In contrast to pustular psoriasis, the approach in erythrodermic psoriasis is to use a low dose of etretinate (25 mg orally each day) and to increase gradually the amount if necessary. In a similar fashion, generalized or refractory cases of pityriasis rubra pilaris have been responsive to etretinate at doses of 0.5 to 1 mg per kilogram or to isotretinoin in the 1 to 2 mg per kilogram daily dosage range. The use of these retinoids requires a detailed knowledge of their biologic half-life and the associated risks of teratogenicity, skeletal abnormalities, and the signs and symptoms of hypervitaminosis A.

To some extent the use of cytotoxic drugs has been displaced by the retinoids. Methotrexate in the usual dosage of 2.5 to 5 mg every 12 hours for three consecutive doses per week remains an alternative for cases of idiopathic exfoliative dermatitis that are refractory to the foregoing approach.

Mortality from exfoliative dermatitis has been a prominent feature in a number of retrospective studies. The metabolic complications of exfoliative dermatitis have been discussed. There must also be constant vigilance for complications of systemic infections (sepsis, pneumonia, cellulitis), venous thrombosis or embolism, and complications caused by the underlying disease process or its treatment.

PHOTOALLERGIC CONTACT DERMATITIS

Richard D. Granstein, M.D.
Ernesto Gonzalez, M.D.

Photoallergic contact dermatitis (PCD) is an immune response to an offending exogenous chemical, in which participation of the immune system is necessary for the response to occur and in which photons are required with the chemical for immunologic activation. An epidemic of PCD occurred in the 1960s as a result of the use of the potent photoallergen tetrachlorsalicylanilide as an antimicrobial agent in soaps. Other halogenated salicylanilides and related compounds are still used in some toiletries, although their photosensitizing potential seems to be low. More recently musk ambrette and 6-methylcoumarin, contained in perfumes and other fragrance containing toiletries, have been implicated as a cause of PCD; this has required the U.S. Food and Drug Administration to remove 6-methylcoumarin from the market.

PCD is to be distinguished from phototoxic chemical photosensitivity states in which photosensitized damage occurs directly and does not involve the immune system. There is considerable controversy over this distinction in the clinical literature. Numerous drugs and chemicals have been reported in the past to be photoallergens, despite little or no evidence for immunologic involvement in the induced photosensitivity. Phototoxic reactions are characterized by occurrence on the first exposure to the offending agent, with a high incidence among those exposed (theoretically 100 percent if the dose of the chemical and radiation is sufficient) and with subsequent exposures at untreated sites mimicking the time course and intensity of the first exposure. By contrast, photoallergic reactions require previous exposure for sensitization to occur, with subsequent exposures resulting in more severe reactions than the initial exposure. The incidence of photoallergic reactions among those exposed is low, and the dose of chemical required to elicit the reaction in sensitive individuals is usually quite low. Table 1 summarizes these differences. In addition, many, if not most photoallergic agents are also phototoxic, yielding some confusion. Table 2 lists the major agents commonly implicated in PCD.

Table 1 Characteristics of Photocontact Dermatitis

CHARACTERISTIC	PHOTOALLERGIC	PHOTOTOXIC
Occurs on first exposure	No	Yes
Requires previous sensitization	Yes	No
Incidence	Low	High
Dose of agent needed to elicit	Low	High
Flare at nonexposed, previously involved site	Possible	No
Skin changes	Eczematous	Similar to sunburn

In recent years several animal models have been developed to study mechanisms involved in PCD. These models, utilizing guinea pigs or mice, have shown that PCD is a cell-mediated immune response that can be induced in a naive animal by the adoptive transfer to T-lymphocytes from sensitive animals. Indeed PCD appears to be immunologically identical to ordinary allergic contact dermatitis except for the requirement for photons for initiation or elicitation of the response. In animal models it has been demonstrated that irradiation of chlorpromazine or sulfanilamide in vitro results in the production of a photoproduct that is capable of inducing or eliciting ordinary allergic contact dermatitis and that is cross reactive with induced PCD to these agents. Thus, in PCD the mechanism of antigen formation to these agents appears to be the generation of a hapten photoproduct.

Two other mechanisms have been proposed to account for the generation of the antigen in PCD. A photon could be necessary for the binding of a hapten to a carrier protein, or the photon with the chemical may alter a host protein, which becomes antigenic. There are no current experimental data to support these mechanisms.

Table 2 Agents Reported to Induce Photoallergic Contact Dermatitis*

Halogenated phenols	Sunscreens
Tetrachlorosalicylanilide	Para-aminobenzoic acid (PABA)
Tribromosalicylanilide	Glyceryl PABA
Dibromosalicylanilide	Digalloyl trioleate
Multifungin	Mexenone
Trichlorocarbanilide	Cinnamate
Bithionol	Various chemicals
Fentichlor	Moquizone
Hexachlorophene	Quindoxine
Buclosamide (Jadit)	Thiourea
Chloro-2-phenylphenol	Musk ambrette
Drugs	6-Methylcoumarin
Promethazine hydrochloride	Stilbenes
Sulfonamides	Sandalwood oil
Diphenhydramine	
Quinine	
Benzocaine	

*Inclusion of some of these agents is based on a single or very few reports.

Table 3 Photopatch Testing Agents

Benzocaine	5% in petrolatum
Chlorpromazine	0.1% in petrolatum
Diphenhydramine	2% in petrolatum
Hydrochlorathiazide	1% in petrolatum
Musk ambrette	5% in petrolatum and 5% in alcohol
6-Methylcoumarin	10% in alcohol
Sandalwood oil	1% in petrolatum
Sulfanilamide	5% in petrolatum
Tribromosalicylanilide	1% in petrolatum
Bithionol	1% in petrolatum
Buclosamide (Jadit)	10% in water
Fentichlor	1% in petrolatum
Hexachlorophene	1% in petrolatum
Tetrachlorosalicylanilide	1% in petrolatum
Trichlorocarbanilide	1% in petrolatum
Quinine	1% in petrolatum
Para-aminobenzoic acid	1% in petrolatum
Cinnamate	1% in petrolatum
Benzophenone (Piz Buin sunscreen)	Commercial preparation as is

CLINICAL DESCRIPTION

The majority of photoallergic reactions are eczematous. Early changes are acute eczema with vesiculation, which may progress to bullae, with scaling, crusting, and excoriations as variable features. In the chronic stage thick lichenified plaques are present. Urticarial papular and lichenoid eruptions have also been reported as photoallergic reactions, but these are unusual responses described in isolated case reports. The histology of the eruption is that of a spongiotic dermatitis with intercellular edema in the epidermis with or without vesicle formation, depending on the clinical pattern. A dense perivascular dermal lymphohistiocytic infiltrate is present, identical to that found in allergic contact dermatitis. Some authors believe that a biopsy in some cases may make it possible to distinguish a photoallergic reaction from a phototoxic one. The differences observed are those that distinguish allergic contact dermatitis from a primary irritant contact dermatitis.

PCD can occur at any age and in either sex. Males are more commonly affected than females, although it has been postulated that this may reflect differences in exposure to photoallergens. As in other diseases, the history and physical examination should begin the evaluation of the patient. The patient usually presents with a rash, restricted to exposed sites, which he attributes to sunlight exposure. The initial eruption frequently occurs a few days after long exposure to sunlight, but subsequent eruptions may occur within hours after exposure. The face, V of the neck, and dorsum of the hands and arms are usually involved. The areas behind the ears (Wilkinson's triangle), under the chin, between the fingers, and in the skin folds are usually spared. Facial involvement is sometimes surprisingly patchy. The actual distribution of the eruption and the time course are determined, of course, by the dose and site of exposure to the chemical and radiation. When a localized area is exposed to the offending agent as well as the relevant wavelengths of radiation and PCD ensues, a distant, previously involved area may demonstrate a flare of activity.

The differential diagnosis includes phototoxic reactions, contact dermatitis (especially airborne contact dermatitis), photosensitive eczema, and the eczematous form of polymorphous light eruption. Photoallergic reactions also may be a consequence of drugs administered systemically.

In addition to the physical findings and history, photopatch testing can be useful in making a diagnosis. There is no standard procedure, but the approach to testing is uniform. A battery of known photosensitizers is applied in duplicate to small areas of the back, and all sites are covered by an opaque material. Table 3 lists standard photoallergy testing materials. Substances to be tested are prepared in petrolatum at the concentrations listed in Table 3.

After 24 hours one set of the applied substances is exposed to UVA (320 to 400 nm) radiation, because the action spectrum for most photoallergens is thought to be in this range. We use a bank of PUVA fluorescent bulbs filtered through mylar (to remove wavelengths below 320 nm) as the source of radiation in our clinic. The exposure dose is usually 10 J per square centimeter, a dose empirically selected because it is below the minimal erythema dose for most individuals and is presumed to be sufficient to elicit a photoallergic response. However, if the patient's minimal erythema dose for UVA is at or below this level, a lower exposure dose is used. We believe that it is mandatory to do phototesting prior to photopatch testing to ensure that a proper dose of UVA radiation is selected (see later discussion). The sites are then re-covered. Twenty-four and 48 hours later the sites are examined for a reaction. Erythema, edema, and vesiculation are considered positive responses that are graded on a 1+ to 4+ scale of severity. Positive responses of equal intensity at both the nonirradiated and the irradiated sites are interpreted as ordinary allergic contact dermatitis. A positive response at an irradiated site, or in the presence of allergic contact dermatitis, an enhanced response at the irradiated site are interpreted as being consistent with photocontact allergy.

Phototesting in which the minimal erythema dose to UVA and UVB radiation is determined may be helpful in differen-

Table 4 Interpretation of Phototesting

CONDITION	MED TO UVA	MED TO UVB	PHOTOPATCH TEST
PCD	Normal	Normal	Positive
Photosensitive eczema	Normal or decreased	Usually decreased	Negative
Persistent light reaction	Normal or decreased	Decreased	Positive
Actinic reticuloid	Usually decreased	Normal or decreased	Positive or negative

tiating idiopathic photosensitivity states from PCD (Table 4) and is necessary for determining the dose of radiation to use in photopatch testing, as already mentioned. All patients referred for photopatch testing undergo phototesting prior to photopatch testing. This is performed by exposing small areas of non–sun-exposed (buttock) skin to graded doses of radiation, shielding these sites from light exposure, and examining these areas 24 hours later. In our experience the skin type of the patient is not a reliable indicator of the "normal" minimal erythema dose. Generally a minimal erythema dose below 20 mJ per square centimeter for UVB or 20 J per square centimeter for UVA radiation is considered abnormal, depending on the circumstances and characteristics of the patient. We also examine sensitivity to visible radiation by exposing non–sun-exposed skin to graded doses of radiation from a tungsten lamp, shielding these areas from light exposure, and examining them 24 hours later. Any reaction is considered abnormal.

There are limitations to the use and interpretation of the photopatch test. Radiation sources used vary, but most investigators use a source with a main emission spectrum in the UVA range because, as already mentioned, the action spectra of photoallergic reactions to most chemicals are included in this waveband. However, the action spectra of some reactions probably involve UVB (280 to 320 nm) radiation. Therefore, a solar simulator that emits both UVA and UVB radiation is sometimes used. However, because UVB radiation is much more erythemogenic than UVA radiation, problems of dosimetry occur when using a solar simulator source for photopatch testing.

A suberythemal dose of radiation, chosen by testing the patient, is administered when the solar simulator is employed. To increase the probability of detecting a response, a dose of radiation just below the minimal erythema dose could be employed at each of several suspected wavelengths. This could clearly result in very large and impractical amounts of testing.

Other problems of phototesting include determining the amount of photosensitizer to apply and differentiating allergic contact dermatitis from photoallergic contact dermatitis when both occur. In addition, allergic contact dermatitis to some agents could be increased by exposure to ultraviolet radiation. Another problem relates to the possibility that photoallergic contact dermatitis to some chemicals might result from exposure to visible radiation. Finally, the differentiation of phototoxic responses from photoallergic responses can be difficult, although biopsy of test sites can sometimes distinguish these reactions, as already mentioned. Risks and complications of photopatch testing include inadvertent photosensitization to test agents, discomfort at positive test sites, occasional flares of disease activity at sites of previous involvement, and false-positive or false-negative results due to incorrect amounts of chemical or radiation. Despite these caveats, in many circumstances photopatch testing can be very helpful in identifying the offending agent in a patient with PCD.

■ THERAPY

Avoidance of the offending agent is, of course, the single most important therapeutic maneuver. Thus, it is important to identify the offending agent if at all possible. This often can be done by means of the history, but when the history is ambiguous, photopatch testing can be useful. If more than one chemical is implicated by the history, photopatch testing can determine which among them is responsible for the eruption. It also can be used as a confirmatory test when the history suggests only one offending chemical, and occasionally it is useful in diagnosing photosensitivity states when the history does not clearly implicate any substance. Once an offending agent is identified, it is crucial to tell the patient what substances in his environment may contain that chemical or a cross reactive substance. In our clinic we provide the patient with a written list of common materials containing the agent to which he is sensitive.

The avoidance of sunlight can be important in the treatment of acute photoallergic contact dermatitis. This often must be extended beyond the period of acute dermatitis because the offending chemical may persist in the skin for some time. In severe cases confinement to a darkened room for several days may speed recovery. Since most offending agents are activated by exposure to wavelengths above 320 nm, sunlight penetrating window glass can aggravate the dermatitis. When the offending chemical cannot be identified, avoidance of sunlight may become a mainstay of treatment.

The utility of sunscreens is limited by the fact that most transparent sunscreens do not protect against photons of wavelengths in the UVA range. Although some of these agents, especially those that contain benzophenones, afford some protection above 320 nm, the most useful sunscreens are those that form an opaque barrier to all photons of solar radiation. These agents contain opaque powders, such as titanium oxide, kaolin, zinc oxide, or talc. Unfortunately, these are usually not as cosmetically acceptable as sunscreens that are invisible. It should also be pointed out that some sunscreens, notably those that contain para-aminobenzoic acid and its esters, can produce allergic contact dermatitis and sometimes, although rarely, photoallergic contact dermatitis. In addition, various inactive components of these preparations, such as preservatives and fragrances, may produce ACD or PCD.

Symptomatic Therapy

The acute treatment of photoallergic contact dermatitis is similar to that of ordinary allergic contact dermatitis. For vesicular and weeping areas, astringent soaks are appropriate as is topical steroid therapy. It is crucial to keep open areas clean to prevent superinfection. We often prescribe astringent soaks, such as Domeboro's solution, three or four times a day. If large areas are weeping, we also may advise the patient to clean these areas with an antimicrobial cleansing agent, such as Hibiclens antimicrobial cleanser, twice a day. Antihistamines may be helpful for pruritus. In severe cases a short course of systemic steroid therapy can be given. As already implied, removal of the offending photosensitizer and related compounds eliminates the problem once the acute eruption has resolved.

Persistent Light Reaction

A small number of patients with PCD display photosensitivity without apparent continuing exposure to a chemical or a cross-reacting agent to which they are demonstrably sensitive. This condition, termed *persistent light reaction,* was first recognized as a consequence of tetrachlorosalicylanilide exposure. Since that time it has been observed as a consequence of other photosensitizers. The eruption is a chronic eczematous dermatitis initially restricted to light-exposed sites. Patients display marked photosensitivity with a lowered minimal erythema dose to UVB radiation, often to UVA radiation, and sometimes to visible light. Photopatch testing reveals a strongly positive response to a photoallergen. This disorder can be disabling, and severe depression and suicide have been reported among patients with photosensitivity states.

Various hypotheses have been presented to account for this condition. One is that patients continue to encounter the photoallergen or a cross-reacting substance. Another is that an induced photoantigen persists in the skin, and a third is that a normal skin constituent has undergone an alteration and has become antigenic, with subsequent exposure to ultraviolet radiation producing the same or a similar photoproduct without further exposure to an offending chemical. This last possible mechanism is perhaps, supported by the observation that tetrachlorosalicylanilide can photo-oxidize proteins. None of these hypotheses completely explains the broad spectrum of photosensitivity observed in some patients or the abnormal sensitivity of uninvolved skin on phototesting.

The treatment consists of using sunscreens, avoiding sun exposure and, when necessary, fluorescent light exposure. Topical and systemic steroid therapy is useful, especially for acute eruptions. Suppression of persistent light reaction (PLR) by 8-methoxypsoralen and sunlight has been reported. We find this interesting, because a patient with actinic reticuloid was treated in our clinic with PUVA and did very well for a prolonged period.

Patients with actinic reticuloid, photosensitive eczema, and PLR generally share a number of characteristics. They are usually male, middle-aged or older, and the eruption is usually eczematous. The relationship among these three disorders is not clear. For this reason it has been proposed by some authors that the present nomenclature be abandoned and that the term *chronic actinic dermatitis* with appropriate subdivisions be used to classify these diseases.

LEG ULCERS

Donald P. Lookingbill, M.D.

Leg ulcers can be due to a wide variety of etiologies, but the most common is stasis. This section deals primarily with the therapy of venous (stasis) ulcers, although some of the therapeutic measures can be applied to other types of leg ulcers as well.

■ PATIENT EVALUATION

Stasis ulcers result from sustained elevations in venous pressure in the lower extremities. Frequently there is a history of thrombophlebitis. The ulcers typically occur above the malleolus, usually on the medial side of the leg. Venous ulcers are often accompanied by petechiae and a brownish discoloration ("stasis changes") of the surrounding skin. Dermatitis may be present as well and is due either to the stasis itself or to secondary contact dermatitis. Dermatitis, if present, is sometimes confused with cellulitis in that both are manifested by erythematous skin; but dermatitis is often vesicular and almost always pruritic, whereas cellulitis is warm and tender and sometimes is accompanied by fever.

In patients with venous ulcers, leg and pedal edema is usually present and is a critical factor that must be addressed if treatment is to succeed. In the general evaluation of the patient, consideration should be given to other possible causes of edema, including congestive heart failure and kidney disease. The blood pressure should also be obtained and pedal pulses examined to screen for other vascular causes or factors contributing to the leg ulcer. If pedal pulses are absent, a vascular surgery consultation is recommended. In chronic nonhealing ulcers, a biopsy specimen should be taken from the edge of the ulcer to rule out other etiologies, particularly malignant disease.

■ MEDICAL THERAPY

The preferred therapy for venous ulcers is medical. Surgical treatment may be needed if medical management fails or becomes unduly prolonged. The foremost consideration in medical management is to control edema. If this is not achieved, other measures will be of little value. The other measures include treatment of infection (if present), debridement, and wound dressings.

Edema Reduction

Edema control is more easily said than achieved, especially in an outpatient. For patients with severe disease, hospitalization may be necessary. In the hospital setting the patient is put at strict bedrest with the foot of the bed slightly elevated. Pneumatic compression devices such as the Jobst extremity pump can also be used to reduce edema and lymphedema more quickly. In our hospital this is done once or twice daily in the physical therapy department.

For most outpatients, strict bedrest is impossible to achieve, but patients are encouraged to maximize the amount of time they spend lying flat with their legs slightly elevated and minimize time spent sitting in a chair. We have found that in patients who comply with bedrest instructions the ulcers are much more likely to heal than those in patients who are noncompliant.

The judicious use of diuretics may help reduce edema in some patients, but this is not a mainstay of therapy. Unna boots and elastic stockings are also helpful for edema control (to be discussed).

Treatment of Infection

Most ulcers contain potentially pathogenic bacteria, which can be recovered on routine culture. However, cultures are not usually performed, and antibiotic treatment is not instituted, unless there is evidence of cellulitis around the ulcer. If cellulitis is present, a culture is taken and empiric antibiotic therapy is begun to cover gram-positive organisms. If there is no clinical response, the culture results may be of help in selecting alternative antibiotic therapy. When the cellulitis subsides, antibiotics are discontinued. Sterilization of the ulcer is an unrealistic goal; long-term antibiotic therapy only selects out resistant organisms.

Debridement

Necrotic debris enhances bacterial growth and impairs ulcer healing. Physical debridement can be done with a curette or scissors and forceps. Viscous lidocaine may be helpful for local anesthesia. We have not found the topical application of enzymatic preparations to be very useful and they can cause irritation.

Medical measures for debridement include wet-to-dry dressings. Occlusive dressings also provide for debridement and are discussed separately.

Wet Dressings

Wet dressings are most useful in the initial stages of treating ulcers that have abundant debris. Wet dressings are most conveniently used in patients who are at bed rest. For the "wetness" we use saline or quarter-strength Burow's solution (aluminum acetate). Full-strength Burow's solution is not used because evaporation can result in an ultimate concentration that will cause irritation. Since patients with venous ulcers have a predilection for developing contact dermatitis in the area of involvement, the use of potentially sensitizing chemicals should be avoided. This includes antiseptics such as povidone-iodine (Betadine) and topically applied antibiotics such as neomycin.

Wet dressings are applied as follows: Several layers of wet gauze are placed over the ulcer and held in place with tubular gauze. Since evaporation is desired, the dressing should not be occluded. Depending upon the amount of wetness to begin with, it takes 30 minutes to several hours for the dressings to dry. The dressings should be changed every 4 hours. At the time of removal, some of the debris will have stuck to the dressing and hence will have been removed. The ulcer base is then gently cleaned and another dressing applied. Wet-to-dry dressings are used mainly in the initial stages of ulcer therapy or in preparation for grafting.

Occlusive Dressings

Occlusive dressings exploit the theory of "moist wound healing." A number of these dressings are now on the market, including Biocclusive, Duoderm, Op-Site, Synthaderm, Tegaderm, and Vigilon. Most are made of polyurethane, and all but Tegaderm and Vigilon are self-adhesive. All have in common the property of occlusion, which causes an accumulation of exudate (which aids debridement) and accelerates wound healing. We have mainly used Duoderm. The dressing is applied to the ulcer and surrounding skin. With Duoderm, tape is used to further secure the edges. The dressing should not be removed until it loosens naturally or drainage leaks out from under the edges. Most dressings stay in place for at least several days (up to 1 week), but in ulcers with copious exudate, more frequent dressing changes may be necessary. Patients need to be advised that fluid will accumulate under the dressing and that the drainage may have a foul odor. Patient instruction booklets are available for some occlusive dressings (for example, Duoderm). The dressings are moderately expensive, and some patients need help in applying them. Development of cellulitic infection under the occlusive dressing is a theoretical concern, but surprisingly rarely occurs. A major advantage of occlusive dressings is that they usually provide excellent pain relief. Elastic stockings can be used over Duoderm dressings. The use of occlusive dressings can be continued until complete healing occurs.

Unna Boot

The time-tested Unna boot still has a place in the treatment of leg ulcers. It is best used after debridement and edema reduction. It protects the ulcers, provides partial occlusion, and helps to prevent edema. We use a Dome-Paste dressing, which is applied in accordance with the directions on the package. With the foot in a flexed position, the leg is wrapped from the forefoot to just below the knee, including the heel. Wrinkles and reverse turns should be avoided. The dressing should be applied in a "pressure gradient" fashion with more pressure at the ankle than at the knee, but care must be taken not to make the dressing too tight. The entire dressing is used and covers the leg in about three layers. It is then wrapped with a Kling bandage, which is held in place with tape applied to the top, bottom, and sides. Removal is accomplished by carefully cutting the dressing with bandage scissors on the side of the leg opposite the ulcer. At dressing changes, the ulcer and leg are gently cleaned, but no medications are applied except for the fresh dressing.

The Unna boot dressing is changed weekly until healing occurs (often months) or until no further progress is made. The Unna boot method has the advantage of requiring infrequent dressing changes with relatively inexpensive materials, but it is somewhat bulky and requires weekly office (or home) visits and a nurse skilled in its application.

■ SURGICAL THERAPY

With medical therapy many ulcers heal, albeit slowly. At each office visit the ulcer should be measured or traced so that progress can be monitored. The surrounding skin should be checked for edema, and if it is present, the aforementioned measures should be readdressed. If, in the absence of edema, the ulcer is enlarging or not improving over time, surgery should be considered. This is a time to also re-evaluate the original diagnosis. For example, if a biopsy had not been done initially, it might now be considered to rule out malignant disease.

In our hospital ulcer surgery is done by either plastic surgeons or vascular surgeons. An accurate assessment of the patient's vascular status is important prior to leg surgery. Some venous ulcerations occur over incompetent perforating veins in the lower legs, and sclerosing one or several of these vessels may be helpful. The arterial blood supply of course must also be adequate for successful grafting.

If the ulcer bed is clean, the ulcer may be covered directly with a split-thickness skin graft. For necrotic ulcers with poor granulation tissue, excision is needed before grafting.

Properly performed and cared for, skin grafting can result in excellent coverage of long-standing venous ulcers.

■ POSTULCER TREATMENT: ELASTIC SUPPORT STOCKINGS

The successful management of venous ulcers does not end with ulcer healing. Prevention is important. For this, the use of elastic stockings is strongly recommended. Several types are manufactured, and kits are now available for measuring patients in the office. We use knee-length stockings and fit patients for either Jobst Fast-Fit or T.E.D. stockings. The Jobst Fast-Fit stockings are more expensive, but are flesh colored and provide venous pressure gradient support. Measurements are made at the calf and ankle, and the patient is fitted with one of six sizes. The T.E.D. stockings are white and are available in two lengths, each in small, medium, large, and extra large sizes. They are fitted on the basis of calf circumference and leg length measurements. Fitting measurements are preferably made when the patient has no or minimal edema; once fitted, patients are instructed to put the stockings on each morning before getting out of bed.

SUPERFICIAL FUNGAL INFECTION OF SKIN AND NAILS

Arnold W. Gurevitch, M.D.

■ DERMATOPHYTE INFECTIONS

Tineas are infections caused by the group of fungi called dermatophytes. These organisms can infect structures containing keratin, including the skin, hair, and nails. The tineas are clinically classified by the part of the body infected: tinea corporis, tinea cruris, tinea pedis, tinea manuum, tinea faciei, tinea barbae, tinea capitis, and tinea unguium (onychomycosis). The dermatophyte group consists of three fungal genera, *Trichophyton, Microsporum,* and *Epidermophyton.* A given species may cause a variety of skin lesions on different sites.

Specific Infections

Tinea Corporis

Dermatophyte infections of the glabrous (hairless) skin produce the classic ringworm picture. Although seen in any age group, tinea corporis is most common in children. Infection can be acquired from pets, humans, or the soil and may be caused by any species of dermatophytes. The most common fungi are *Microsporum canis, Trichophyton rubrum,* and *Trichophyton mentagrophytes.* The eruption begins as a small erythematous scaling patch. As the infection spreads outward, it tends to clear partially or completely in the center, producing an annular or ringlike lesion. The characteristic lesions are roughly circular, with a well-defined elevated erythematous scaling border. Differential diagnoses include nummular dermatitis, psoriasis, pityriasis rosea, seborrheic dermatitis, impetigo, erythema annulare centrifugum, and granuloma annulare.

Tinea Cruris

Tinea cruris is a fungal infection of the groin and inner thighs with extension to the perineum and buttocks. It is most common in warm, humid climates, and it affects men more often than women. In most cases the patient has coexisting tinea pedis, probably the source of the infection. There is usually a sharply marginated serpiginous scaling border on the inner thighs. Central clearing is common. The scrotum and penis are usually uninvolved, and when they are infected, they have minimal scaling and erythema. Candidiasis is more common in women. It does not have a well-defined raised border, but it does have satellite papules and pustules and intense erythema. In men candidiasis often affects the scrotum and penis. Intertrigo, a dermatitis due to local heat, moisture, and friction, is also common in this area. Other diagnostic considerations are contact dermatitis, psoriasis, seborrheic dermatitis, and erythrasma.

Tinea Pedis

Tinea pedis is the most common dermatophyte infection, affecting 4 percent of the population. Asymptomatic infections are found in up to 20 percent of those surveyed. *Trichophyton rubrum, Trichophyton interdigitale,* and *Epidermophyton floccosum* are responsible for almost all cases. The wearing of shoes, with accompanying sweating and maceration in the toe webs, is considered a major pathogenetic factor. Of the three clinical forms the most common is intertriginous (interdigital). In this type whitish macerated scale in the web spaces between the toes is often accompanied by a foul odor. Fissuring can lead to secondary bacterial infection. An increase in bacterial flora, especially coryneforms, may play a pathogenic role as well. A second highly inflammatory form, vesiculopustular, presents with marked erythema, vesicles, pustules, erosions, fissures, and scaling. The arch of the foot is involved most often, as well as the undersurface of the toes. This variety may resolve spontaneously, only to recur. The most common form of tinea pedis is the dry chronic scaling type caused by *T. rubrum.* The soles are involved with extension to the sides of the feet (moccasin distribution). The nails are often involved as well. This type may be asymptomatic to pruritic. Maceration between the toes due simply to hyperhidrosis, without infection, must be distinguished from interdigital tinea pedis. Interdigital gram-negative bacterial infections can also mimic tinea. Patients with dyshidrotic eczema and pustular psoriasis may develop plantar vesicles and pustules, respectively. Contact dermatitis and dry skin are other diagnostic considerations.

Tinea Manuum

Ringworm of the hands alone is quite uncommon. Tinea manuum most often accompanies tinea pedis. Scaling of the palms and fingers, especially in the creases, is the usual presentation. Much less common are vesicular lesions and involvement of the dorsal surface. In half of cases one hand and both feet (two foot, 1 hand syndrome) are involved. Differential diagnoses are much the same as with tinea pedis.

Tinea Faciei

Tinea faciei is tinea corporis of the face. It is rare, and the diagnosis is often missed. Erythema with or without scale is the usual presentation. A few small vesicles or pustules may be found. The classic ringworm appearance is not usual. Tinea faciei is often misdiagnosed as seborrheic dermatitis, photosensitivity, or rosacea.

Tinea Barbae

Tinea barbae, in contrast to tinea faciei, is a dermatophyte infection of the bearded area of the face and neck with invasion of fungi into the hairs. It occurs in men, most commonly farm workers. The two main causative species are *T. verrucosum* and *T. mentagrophytes.* The clinical picture can range from dry red scaling patches to a deep pustular folliculitis with alopecia. The involved hairs are brittle, lusterless, and easily pulled out. Tinea barbae must be distinguished from bacterial folliculitis, acne, rosacea, and pseudofolliculitis barbae (ingrown hairs).

Tinea Capitis

The vast majority of cases of ringworm of the scalp and hair in the United States are caused by *Trichophyton tonsurans.* This organism does not produce the characteristic green fluorescence under Wood's light. Children are affected almost exclusively and spread is primarily from human to human. African-American children are affected much more commonly than white. In a recent study almost 50 percent of families of an infected child had at least one other member with a positive culture.

Varying combinations of erythema, scaling, and bald patches are seen. One or many infected patches may be found. In some cases erythema and alopecia may be minimal or even absent, with severe scaling the predominant feature. Other children may show severe inflammation. *T. tonsurans* can also cause a black dot alopecia, in which black dots are produced by swollen infected hair shafts which break off at the surface of the scalp.

Occasionally a kerion develops at the infected sites. The kerion is a boggy nodular mass with severe follicular inflammation. The involved hairs are lost, and frequently pustules and crusting appear. Secondary bacterial infection may occur, but the primary pustule is a hypersensitivity reaction to the fungus. Kerions often heal with scarring and some degree of permanent alopecia.

Tinea capitis may mimic psoriasis, seborrheic dermatitis, atopic dermatitis, and lupus erythematosus. However, the primary diagnostic consideration in a child with scalp scaling and no other cutaneous involvement is tinea capitis. The kerion can be confused with a bacterial folliculitis or even a carbuncle.

Tinea Unguium

Tinea unguium, nail plate invasion by a dermatophyte, is one type of onychomycosis. Onychomycosis can also be produced by other types of fungi, including *Candida albicans* and nondermatophyte molds. Only 50 percent of dystrophic nails are actually caused by fungi, and dermatophytes account for 90 percent of these cases. Some 20 percent of adults in the United States have onychomycosis, usually associated with chronic tinea pedis. Toenail infection is four times as frequent as fingernail. Of the several clinical patterns of onychomycosis the most common is the distal subungual form. The fungus first causes hyperkeratosis of the nailbed under the distal aspect of the nail. This is followed by onycholysis (separation of the distal nail from the underlying bed) and thickening and distortion of the nail plate. A second clinical form, proximal white subungual, affects the cuticle and proximal nailbed with a white discoloration of the intact nail plate. This form is common in human immunodeficiency virus (HIV)-infected and other immunocompromised patients. In white superficial onychomycosis, the third type, fungal organisms in the nail plate produce a crumbled white surface. All three clinical patterns can ultimately lead to total nail destruction. Psoriasis in the nails may closely mimic onychomycosis, although fine pitting suggests psoriasis. Chronic eczematous eruptions and lichen planus may also produce nail dystrophy. Candidal nail infection usually begins with a paronychia, seen as erythema and swelling of the nail fold, followed by lateral onycholysis. Chronic trauma may also result in onycholysis and nail alterations that simulate onychomycosis.

Diagnosis

Definitive diagnosis of a dermatophyte infection rests with either a potassium hydroxide (KOH) preparation or a fungus culture. Scales for either technique should be taken from the active border of skin infections. Infected hairs from tinea capitis and tinea barbae can be plucked and used. Another technique in the diagnosis of tinea capitis is to rub a dry toothbrush over the area of alopecia or scale and then place the material on a slide or in a fungal medium. In tinea unguium material should be taken from the infected nailbed (subungual debris) and the involved plate. Nail clippings can be used, especially for culture.

In a KOH preparation the scrapings or hairs are placed on a microscopic slide and covered with a coverslip. One or two drops of 10 to 20 percent KOH are applied to the edges of the coverslip and allowed to run under it. The slide should be gently heated with a low flame, and then the coverslip is lightly pressed to thin the preparation. Initial examination of the field may be performed under the 10 × objective. Lowering the condenser will increase the contrast and make hyphae easier to see. Hyphae will often be visible as translucent, slightly greenish rod-shaped filaments, often with branching. Areas suspicious for hyphae should be examined under the 40 × objective for confirmation. It is often necessary to examine the entire specimen carefully since hyphae may be found in only one small fragment of scale. In tinea capitis and tinea barbae chains of spores will be seen either within or surrounding the hair shaft. Interpretation of the KOH preparation does require a great deal of experience. Often there are very few hyphae and they are difficult to see. Artifacts are common and misleading. Lipid droplets and crystallized KOH may confuse the inexperienced observer, as will a mosaic artifact that resembles true hyphae.

Fungal culture in Sabouraud's glucose agar is the diagnostic method of choice for nail infections, since hyphae are more difficult to find in KOH preparations from that site. One can also examine a nail histologically for evidence of fungi with a periodic acid-Schiff (PAS) or methenamine silver stain. A culture is often necessary in tinea capitis as well. Sabouraud's agar may be supplemented with an antibiotic (e.g., chloramphenicol) to inhibit the growth of bacteria or cycloheximide to suppress the growth of molds. Another medium, DTM, contains a color indicator that turns red in the presence of a dermatophyte. One disadvantage of the culture is the 2 to 4 weeks required to obtain growth.

Therapy

Most dermatophyte infections of limited areas of skin can be managed with topical agents. Several topical antifungals are available over the counter, others are available only by prescription. Most topical antifungal products fall into two classes, the imidazole derivatives and the allylamines. In addition, there are three other products, ciclopirox, haloprogin, and tolnaftate. The imidazoles include clotrimazole, econazole, ketoconazole, miconazole, oxiconazole, and sulconazole. Efficacy rates of these fungistatic agents are generally over 80 percent. Two allylamines, naftifine and terbinafine, are available. These fungicidal products are effective in 90 to 100 percent of cases. In a recent cost analysis of topical drug regimens for dermatophyte infections it was recommended that an inexpensive generic imidazole, such as miconazole or clotrimazole, be used first. Only patients with unresponsive infections should be treated with the higher-priced prescription drugs. In the latter situation the best choice may be an allylamine. The antifungal cream or solution is rubbed in well twice daily for 2 to 4 weeks, at least 1 week beyond clinical clearing. For tinea pedis and tinea cruris I recommend use of an antifungal powder containing miconazole after each application of the cream. The dry chronic type of tinea pedis invariably recurs, and tinea cruris often recurs as well. To prevent recurrence I suggest the regular and continued use of an antifungal powder after the course of a topical antifungal agent has been completed. Persons with recurring tinea cruris should also be advised against wearing tight undergarments. Careful drying between the toes, avoidance of occlusive footwear, and wearing cotton socks help prevent reinfection or recurrence of tinea pedis.

Extensive or resistant cases of cutaneous dermatophyte infections require systemic therapy. The four available systemic agents are griseofulvin, ketoconazole, fluconazole, and itraconazole. The latter two drugs are not approved to treat dermatophyte infections. I use ultramicrosize griseofulvin (Fulvicin P/G, Gris-PEG) 250 mg twice daily for 3 to 4 weeks for the average adult. Griseofulvin is highly effective against dermatophytes and has relatively few significant side effects.

Hair and nail infections require systemic therapy for effective control. For tinea capitis my choice is ultramicrosize griseofulvin 7.5 to 10 mg per kilogram per day or griseofulvin microsize suspension 15 to 20 mg per kilogram per day in two divided doses for 2 weeks beyond clinical clearing of the erythema or scaling. This may require 1 to 3 months of treatment. A complete blood count and liver function tests should be ordered prior to treatment of children with risk factors for liver disease and when treatment extends beyond 3 months. In addition to griseofulvin, kerion is treated with prednisone 1 mg per kilogram per day for the first 2 to 3 weeks of therapy. A topical antifungal shampoo such as selenium sulfide or ketoconazole may help to prevent spread to other children, but they are not effective for definitive therapy.

The treatment of tinea unguium remains difficult. Most of these patients seem to have an underlying inherited immune defect predisposing them to this infection. Therefore, recurrences are common, certainly greater than 50 percent with toenail disease. Whether or not to treat and what form of therapy to use should be individualized. Factors to consider are the age and general health of the patient, compliance, cost of therapy, drug interactions, and side effects. However, it is vital to establish the diagnosis by KOH preparation, culture, or fungal stain before instituting systemic therapy.

For many years griseofulvin was the drug of choice for fungal nail infections. Unfortunately, it has many drawbacks. It must be taken daily for 6 to 9 months for fingernails and 12 to 18 months for toenails. Even with this duration of treatment, only 25 percent of patients with nail disease and

70 percent with fingernail infection are permanently cured. Most patients require 750 mg to 1 g daily to clear the infection. At that dose headaches and gastrointestinal disturbances are the most common side effects. A baseline complete blood count (CBC) and liver panel should be obtained before beginning treatment and every 2 months thereafter. Ketoconazole has limited use in the treatment of nail infections because of the risk of hepatotoxicity. However, two newer oral imidazoles, fluconazole and itraconazole, although not yet approved for this purpose, appear to be quite effective. They have only rarely been associated with hepatotoxicity. Dosage regimens are still being evaluated, but fluconazole 150 mg each week for 6 to 9 months appears to be safe and effective. Itraconazole 200 mg twice daily for 1 week of each month has been used. Duration of treatment is 3 months for fingernail infections and 4 months for toenail infections. Baseline CBC and liver profiles, followed by periodic monitoring every month, are recommended.

For patients unwilling or unable to take systemic medication, topical therapy may inhibit progression of nail disease. Chemical nail avulsion using a 40 percent urea preparation and surgical avulsion are further options. Avulsion works best in combination with either topical or systemic antifungal therapy. Additionally, after control of the nail infection has been achieved, daily to weekly application of a topical antifungal agent may help prevent recurrence.

■ TINEA VERSICOLOR

Tinea versicolor (TV) is a superficial fungal infection of the skin caused by *Pityrosporum ovale (Malassezia furfur)*. This yeast organism is found on the oily areas of the head and upper trunk in 95 percent of normal adults. An overgrowth of its hyphal form produces tinea versicolor. Since the organism is part of normal flora, it is not truly a communicable disease. Factors that promote the development of TV include high humidity and temperature, hereditary predisposition, systemic steroids, and defective cell-mediated immunity. TV is most common in tropical and subtropical climates and tends to appear during the summer, chiefly in persons with high sebum production (puberty through age 50). Recurrences are common.

The most commonly affected sites are the neck, upper trunk, and proximal extremities. However, the entire trunk, distal extremities, and face may be involved. TV begins as small, well-demarcated, finely scaling macules. The scaling can be extremely mild and subtle. Lesions are usually hypopigmented on dark or tanned skin and light pink or tan on pale skin. Some of the small macules usually coalesce into larger patches. Symptoms are often absent, and the patient seeks medical care because of the discoloration. Occasionally mild itching occurs, especially when the patient has been sweating.

Differential diagnosis includes vitiligo, pityriasis alba, pityriasis rosea, and seborrheic dermatitis. Vitiligo is characterized by depigmentation and a lack of scaling, whereas TV is hypopigmented and finely scaling. Pityriasis alba consists of ill-defined hypopigmented dry scaling patches, often seen on the face or upper trunk of atopic children. Seborrheic dermatitis of the chest may resemble TV. Pityriasis rosea does not have coalescent large patches, and it has a distinctive Christmas tree arrangement of lesions.

Diagnosis

KOH examination of scales is the best diagnostic procedure. Clusters of round yeast cells with short rod-shaped hyphae (bats and balls or spaghetti and meatballs) are characteristic. The organism does not grow on routine fungal culture media. Examination with a Wood's light may give a yellow to yellow-green fluorescence. However, this procedure is often negative, especially if the patient has recently showered.

Therapy

Tinea versicolor can usually be managed with topical therapy unless it is very extensive or recalcitrant. I use either 2.5 percent selenium sulfide (Selsun, Exsel) or 2 percent zinc pyrithione (DHS Zinc, Sebulon) shampoo. Ketoconazole (Nizoral) shampoo has also been reported to be effective. Although many regimens have been advocated, I instruct the patient to apply the shampoo as a lotion to the trunk, neck, upper arms, or other involved areas, leaving it on for 10 minutes before showering. This procedure is repeated nightly for 1 or 2 weeks, then weekly for 1 month. I inform the patients that they may prevent recurrences by repeating the procedure monthly. Topical imidazole antifungals are also effective, but they are too expensive if the involvement is widespread. The patient should be informed that repigmentation takes place gradually over several months.

Systemic therapy may be required for widespread disease and in patients unresponsive to topical modalities. Oral ketoconazole has been most commonly used. The proposed treatment schedules vary from a single 400 mg dose to 200 mg a day for 1 to 2 weeks. I usually recommend 400 mg a day for 3 days. Fluconazole 400 mg repeated in 1 week and itraconazole 200 mg for 5 days are also reported to be effective but are not approved for this use in the United States. Although recurrences are less frequent after systemic therapy, I suggest that the topical prophylactic regimen be followed every 1 to 3 months.

Suggested Reading

Borelli D, Jacobs PH, Nall L. Tinea versicolor: Epidemiologic, clinical, and therapeutic aspects. J Am Acad Dermatol 1991; 25:300–305.

Chren M-M, Landefeld CS. A cost analysis of topical drug regimens for dermatophyte infections. JAMA 1994; 272:1922–1925.

Elewski BE. Onychomycosis. Fitzpatrick's J Clin Dermatol 1994; 2:48–54.

Hay RJ. Risk/benefit ratio of modern antifungal therapy: Focus on hepatic reactions. J Am Acad Dermatol 1993; 29:S50–S54.

Macura AB. Dermatophyte infections. Int J Dermatol 1993; 32:313–322.

Roseeuw D, DeDoncker P. New approaches to the treatment of onychomycosis. J Am Acad Dermatol 1993; 29:S45–S50.

Vargo K, Cohen BA. Prevalence of undetected tinea capitis in household members of children with disease. Pediatrics 1993; 92:155–157.

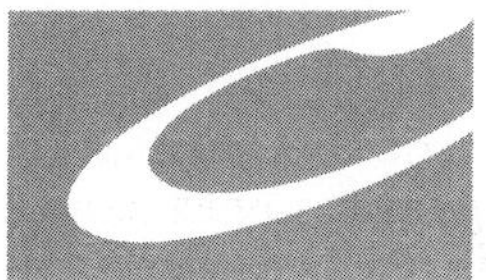

NEUROLOGIC DISEASES

THE COMATOSE PATIENT

Kyra J. Becker, M.D.
John A. Ulatowski, M.D., Ph.D.

Coma is a state of unresponsiveness or unconsciousness characterized by lack of self-awareness and environmental awareness. The term *consciousness* can be modified to refer to a continuum of states ranging from that of awake and alert to that of completely unresponsive (comatose). Intermediate states, variably referred to as sleepy but arousable (lethargic), stuporous, and obtunded, are also included within the spectrum of levels of consciousness. An accurate description of the patient's level of arousal, however, is far more meaningful than an arbitrary categorization, as it conveys more information and eliminates the possibility of semantic differences between individuals. It is important to differentiate those patients with disordered *levels of consciousness* from those with disordered *contents of consciousness,* or delirium, since the diagnostic and therapeutic strategies differ. A change in the level of consciousness can be symptomatic of many different diseases and does not represent a unique illness in itself. Adequate management of the comatose patient depends on identification of the underlying disease process and execution of disease-appropriate treatment. There are, however, certain immutable principles of therapy that are applicable to all comatose patients irrespective of the mechanism of injury. Since many forms of coma are fully reversible, two major goals should guide the clinician rendering therapy. First, prompt institution of basic critical care can prevent ongoing neurologic injury, and second, rapid recognition and treatment of remediable causes of coma can restore neurologic function.

■ IMMEDIATE INITIAL THERAPY

Upon first encounter with an unresponsive patient, the immediate concern should be that of the ABCs (airway, breathing, circulation). The airway must be secured and adequate ventilation, oxygenation, and perfusion established. Failure to do so swiftly may result in hypoxic ischemic injury in addition to the injury produced by the underlying disease process. A *secure airway* implies that the airway is free of obstruction and that the patient is not at risk for aspiration. Thus, depending on the patient's condition, the airway can be secured with placement of an oral obturator, a nasal trumpet, or an endotracheal tube. The need to assist ventilation generally requires endotracheal intubation. The neck needs to be immobilized in any unconscious patient with potential traumatic spine injury to decrease the risk of cervical cord damage and quadriplegia. This should be done before attempts at intubation. Oxygenation can be readily assessed with the use of pulse oximetry. A timeline for therapy is presented in Figure 1. As hypoglycemia can produce coma and cause permanent neurologic dysfunction, unless a dexi stick glucose can be obtained immediately, all unresponsive patients should be given intravenous glucose, an ampule of D_{50} IV and thiamine 100 mg IV to prevent Wernicke's encephalopathy. The risks of prolonged hypoglycemia far outweigh the risks of transient hyperglycemia, but there is now mounting evidence that hyperglycemia can be detrimental to the injured brain. If the etiology of the coma is not readily apparent, initial evaluation must include a blood electrolyte and chemistry profile as well as blood and urine toxicology screens. Blood specimens should be obtained at the time intravenous access is established for glucose administration. Despite noninvasive pulse oximetry and capnography, arterial blood gas determination is important not only for documentation of adequate ventilation and oxygenation, but because the arterial pH may yield clues to the etiology of the unresponsiveness. All of the major causes of anion gap acidoses, lactic acidosis, ketoacidosis, and poisonings (salicylates, ethanol, methanol, and ethylene glycol) can cause coma. Naloxone (Narcan), 0.4 to 2 mg IV, should be given to any patient in whom narcotic use is suspected. The drug should be administered in increments of 40 to 80 μg to avoid the side effects of acute narcotic withdrawal. Flumazenil (Romazicon) should be administered with the same precautions as it can precipitate seizures in normal subjects as well as in patients with benzodiazepine overdose.

■ INITIAL DIAGNOSTIC EVALUATION AND EXAMINATION

Once the patient is rendered stable, diagnostic evaluation should ensue. As the unresponsive patient is incapable of

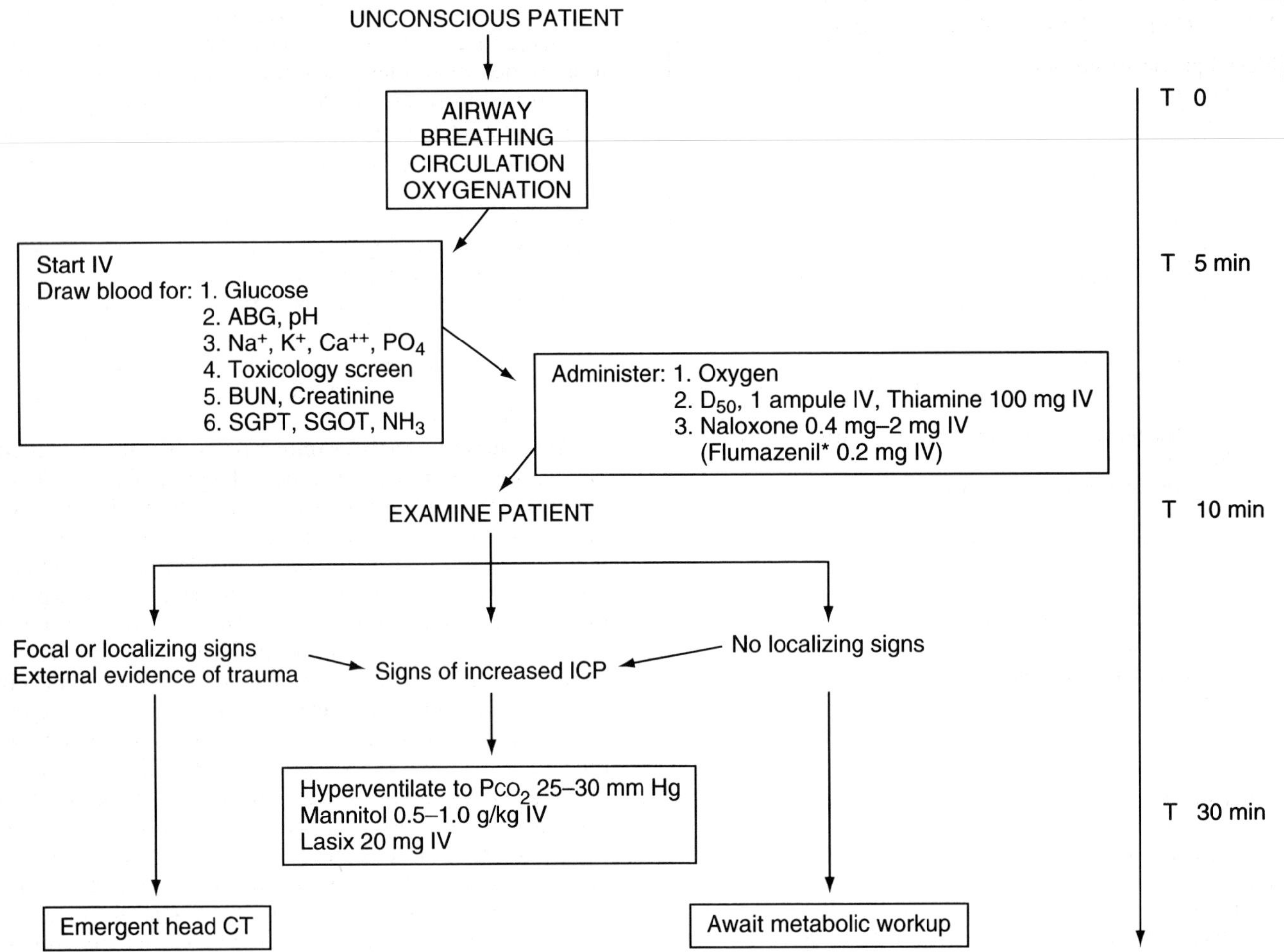

Figure 1
Approach to the unconscious patient. (Use of flumazenil should not be considered routine as it can precipitate seizures in certain subsets of patients.) ABG, arterial blood gas; BUN, blood urea nitrogen; SGPT, serum glutamic pyruvic transaminase; SGOT, serum glutamic oxaloacetic transaminase; ICP, intracranial pressure; CT, computed tomography.

offering a history, and friends and family are often unavailable or unable to provide an adequate history, the clinician must be able to perform a rapid and goal-directed examination that focuses on the diagnostic aspects of the most plausible of the possible treatable etiologies of coma (Table 1). A fundamental knowledge of the neuroanatomic correlates of consciousness allows one to develop a diagnostic approach that significantly abridges the examination and evaluation of the comatose patient. Requisites for consciousness include the reticular activating system (RAS), which ascends through the center of the brainstem, and at least one functional cerebral hemisphere. Coma therefore results from bihemispheric dysfunction, brainstem dysfunction, or both. The dysfunction can be caused by toxic metabolic insults or by structural lesions. *Structural lesions* are those that can be visualized on neuroimaging studies such as magnetic resonance imaging (MRI). These include infarcts and space-occupying lesions such as hemorrhages, tumors, and abscesses. Strategically placed lesions within the brainstem or cerebral cortices, if bihemispheric, can produce coma in the absence of significant mass effect. More commonly, however, lesions in noneloquent cortex or brainstem produce coma by virtue of associated cerebral edema and brainstem compression or midline shift. If midline shift is substantial, dysfunction of the contralateral hemisphere can result. Toxic metabolic insults generally result in global cortical dysfunction with preservation of the brainstem examination, although some toxic substances (such as barbiturates) will eventually paralyze all brainstem reflexes if present at high enough levels. Focal neurologic deficits are characteristically absent. The presence of a focal neurologic deficit should alert one to the existence of a structural lesion and dictates urgent neuroimaging.

While waiting for laboratory results to return, examine the patient in detail for important clues to the etiology of coma. A careful neurologic examination is essential as it will help to differentiate between cerebral dysfunction resulting from structural lesions and cerebral dysfunction mediated by drug or metabolic intoxications. The most important aspects of the brainstem examination are the pupillary responses and extraocular movements. It is essential that the oculocephalic reflex be examined in all comatose patients. If oculocephalic testing reveals no response or if testing is impossible because of cervical spine instability, cold water calorics must be done. The absence of brainstem reflexes (such as oculocephalics, calorics, and corneals) in the presence of reactive pupils

Table 1 Common Differential Diagnosis of Coma

Bihemispheric dysfunction
Functional
Metabolic
Hypoxia*
Hypoglycemia*
Hepatic dysfunction (hyperammonemia)
Uremia
Hyponatremia, hypernatremia
Hyperglycemic hyperosmolar nonketotic coma
Hypothyroidism (myxedema coma)
Toxic
Drug overdose
Drugs of abuse: narcotics, barbiturates, benzodiazepines, etc.
Therapeutic drugs: anticholinergics, tricyclics, etc.
Infectious
Meningitis/meningoencephalitis
Others
Nonconvulsive status epilepticus
Structural
Infarction
Bilateral hemispheric infarcts
Mass lesions
Bilateral hemispheric
Unilateral or bilateral hemispheric with elevated intracranial pressure* or local mass effect
Brainstem dysfunction
Functional
Structural
Infarction
Mass lesion
Mimics
Organic
Bilateral pontine infarcts ("locked-in" syndrome)
Neuromuscular weakness
Acute inflammatory demyelinating polyneuropathy (AIDP)
Myasthenia gravis
Botulism
Drug-induced neuromuscular blockade
Psychiatric
Malignant catatonia
Psychogenic unresponsiveness

*These possibilities need to be treated immediately.

suggests a toxic metabolic insult. Asymmetry of the brainstem examination suggests a structural lesion.

The neurologic examination also allows for the diagnosis of increased intracranial pressure (ICP), which requires immediate attention. Although bilaterally fixed and dilated pupils may result from drug intoxications (atropine, phencyclidine) and brain death, they can also be manifestations of increased ICP. The presence of papilledema, although not always seen acutely, can be helpful. The presence of unilateral mydriasis in a comatose patient, however, is indicative of herniation and requires institution of ICP-reducing therapy without delay. This includes intubation and hyperventilation to a P_{CO_2} of 25 to 30 mm Hg and intravenous mannitol, 0.5 g per kilogram to 1 g per kilogram. Diuresis may be facilitated with furosemide (Lasix) 20 to 40 mg given intravenously. Patients with signs of increased ICP must undergo computed tomography (CT) as soon as it is feasible since the identification of a surgically remediable lesion (such as an epidural, subdural, or lobar hematoma), subarachnoid hemorrhage, or hydrocephalus may be lifesaving. The presence of an asymmetric neurologic examination in the absence of signs of increased intracranial pressure also dictates urgent neuroimaging since early detection and treatment of a mass lesion may avert impending herniation. Evidence of external trauma implies intracranial injury as the etiology of coma and, again, surgically remediable lesions need to be identified as quickly as possible. CT scanning remains the imaging study of choice for preoperative evaluation as it is rapid and extremely sensitive to the presence of acute blood. If CT scanning is unrevealing in the comatose head-injured patient, MRI may reveal the presence of diffuse axonal injury (DAI). MRI is best delayed until the patient is stable, however, since the diagnosis of DAI will not alter therapy.

The general physical examination is also important in determining the etiology of coma and is particularly useful in the patient with bilateral cerebral dysfunction. The presence of an arteriovenous fistula or a peritoneal dialysis catheter should suggest renal disease and uremia. Jaundice, ascites, or gastrointestinal bleeding suggests the presence of hepatic disease and hyperammonemia. Knowledge of the core body temperature is extremely important because hypothermic patients can appear brain dead and yet recover completely with appropriate therapy. Fever and nuchal rigidity suggest meningitis or meningoencephalitis. Broad-spectrum antibiotic therapy should be started immediately if meningitis is suspected. Delay of antibiotics until the lumbar puncture is performed is not necessary as cerebrospinal fluid cultures will remain positive up to 4 hours after the institution of antibiotics and the Gram stain and counterimmune electrophoreses (CIE) will reveal diagnostic information despite antibiotic therapy. CT scanning is necessary prior to lumbar puncture if there are focal neurologic signs.

The possibility of nonconvulsive status epilepticus must also be considered in comatose patients. The diagnosis is easy to make if it is suspected but difficult to make if it is not. Whereas in a young patient with a history of seizures the index of suspicion is usually high, the frequency of nonconvulsive status among elderly patients admitted to the hospital with a change in the level of consciousness is usually underestimated. Urgent electroencephalogram (EEG) can confirm the clinical diagnosis. If the suspicion is great enough, a therapeutic trial of lorazepam (Ativan) 0.5 to 2 mg IV in the adult can be given while awaiting the EEG if the airway is secured and ventilation is adequate. In patients where the diagnosis is less clear, administration of benzodiazepines should be avoided until there is EEG confirmation of seizures, as they will only serve to further depress the level of consciousness.

■ THE UNRESPONSIVE NONCOMATOSE PATIENT

There are important disease entities that mimic coma and must be eliminated from the differential diagnosis. These include those states in which the patient is awake and alert but is unable to respond to the environment. The classic example is the patient with bilateral pontine infarcts, or the "locked-in" patient. Other examples include patients with profound neuromuscular weakness such as acute inflammatory demyelinating polyneuropathy (AIDP), or Guillian-Barré syndrome, severe myasthenia gravis, and drug-induced or toxin-induced (botulism) neuromuscular blockade. The pupils are spared in AIDP and myasthenia gravis, and administration of acetylcholinesterase inhibitors such as neostigmine (1 to 2 mg IV) will reverse the effects of nondepolarizing muscle blockade and may improve the examination of the myasthenic. There are also psychiatric conditions that may mimic coma, such as psychogenic unresponsiveness and malignant catatonia. Clues to the psychiatric nature of unresponsiveness include forced eye closure and the presence of visual tracking responses. The latter is best tested by attempting to get the patient to track the reflection of his or her own eyes in a moving mirror, a reflex that cannot be suppressed by a conscious patient.

■ RECOMMENDATIONS

Detailing specific therapy for each of the diseases that can produce coma is beyond the scope of this chapter. When the patient has been stabilized and (1) immediately remediable forms of coma have been treated (hypoglycemia, hypoxia, and drug overdose), (2) elevated ICP, if present, has been treated, and, when appropriate, (3) surgical intervention has been obtained, the clinician has some leisure of time to embark upon further diagnostic evaluation and therapy of the medically remediable causes of coma. If one adheres to the basic principles of critical care, the comatose patient can be prevented from experiencing further neurologic injury. And if the etiology of the coma is determined, which relies on an accurate neuroanatomic diagnosis, delivery of the appropriate therapy can frequently restore consciousness.

Suggested Reading

Levy DE, Bates D, Caronna JJ, et al. Prognosis in nontraumatic coma. Ann Intern Med 1981; 94:293–301.

Plum F, Posner JB. The diagnosis of stupor and coma. 3rd ed. Philadelphia: FA Davis, 1980.

VERTIGO AND DYSEQUILIBRIUM

Timothy C. Hain, M.D.

Vertigo is the sensation of rotational motion and *dysequilibrium* denotes a disturbance of balance. Together they form the symptom complex that we discuss here. In neurologic practice, the vertigo-dysequilibrium symptom complex is caused mainly by four categories of disorders, with roughly equal numbers in each group. *Otologic disturbances* include disorders of the inner ear such as benign paroxysmal vertigo, vestibular neuritis, and bilateral vestibular loss. *Central nervous system disturbances* include stroke, migraine, and numerous miscellaneous causes. *Psychogenic vertigo* denotes vertigo or dysequilibrium associated with an independently diagnosable psychiatric disturbance. *Vertigo of uncertain origin* denotes the lack of a diagnosis or a situation in which the diagnosis is conjectural because it is based purely on exclusion. In this chapter we review diagnosis and treatment of conditions in these categories.

■ OTOLOGIC VERTIGO

Table 1 lists commonly encountered causes of vertigo associated with *otologic disturbances (inner ear disease)*. There are four subcategories that we discuss in order of their importance.

Benign Paroxysmal Positional Vertigo

Benign paroxysmal positional vertigo (BPPV) is the most common type of otologic vertigo and accounts for approximately half of all cases of otologic vertigo. BPPV is diagnosed by combining a history of positional vertigo with a typical nystagmus pattern (a burst of upbeating and/or torsional nystagmus) that appears on positional testing. It is currently thought that BPPV is caused by free otoconia within in the semicircular canals, dislodged from the otolith organs by trauma, infection, or degeneration. When the head is repositioned, the debris relocates and provokes vertigo. Thus, BPPV is not actually caused by vestibular damage but rather by an abnormal source of stimulation to a normal vestibular system. Patients may be told that they have "ear rocks." BPPV prevalence increases linearly with age.

The most effective treatments for BPPV are the Epley maneuver and the Brandt-Daroff exercises. These are physical maneuvers that reposition the debris to an insensitive location, the vestibule of the inner ear. I perform the Epley maneuver on patients who have positional nystagmus that I can demonstrate on my examination and the Brandt-Daroff exercises on patients in whom I am uncertain as to the side of lesion or who have failed the Epley maneuver. These maneuvers are very effective, and after a visit or two 95 percent of patients are cured. In the remainder, if symptoms have been present for less than a year and are mainly an annoyance, I recommend watchful waiting. If, however, symptoms have been present for a year or longer, or if the patient's livelihood is being adversely affected by positional vertigo, a surgical procedure (posterior canal plugging) is offered. Because most patients improve spontaneously and because the physical treatments of BPPV work so well, only about 1 percent of BPPV patients are referred for surgery. Although drug treatment is not nearly as effective as the physical treatments just described, I use meclizine (12.5 or 25 mg at bedtime) in patients with BPPV whose vertiginous spells are followed by nausea or who are unable to sleep because of positional vertigo.

Vestibular Neuritis and Other Unilateral Vestibulopathies

Vestibular neuritis is a self-limited condition attributed to a viral infection of the vestibular portion of the eighth nerve. Clinically it presents with vertigo, nausea, ataxia, and nystagmus. Hearing is not impaired; when there are similar symptoms with hearing affected, the syndrome is termed *labyrinthitis.* Severe distress associated with constant vertigo, nausea, and malaise usually lasts 2 or 3 days and less intense symptoms ordinarily persist for 1 or 2 weeks. Vestibular neuritis and labyrinthitis occur with fairly equal distribution across all ages. In uncomplicated cases I order no laboratory tests.

Management is ambulatory except when emesis is severe and prolonged. In the first few days of the illness I use vestibular suppressants and antiemetics (Tables 2 and 3), prescribed as suppositories if necessary. By the third day I reduce the dosage of vestibular suppressants and encourage the patient to increase activity. Follow-up visits should be scheduled at 2 weeks, 1 month, and 2 months if symptoms persist.

Roughly 10 percent of patients are still functionally disabled 2 months after onset of symptoms. In this situation I usually obtain a magnetic resonance imaging (MRI) or computed tomography (CT) scan of the head, formally check hearing with an audiogram, and obtain an electronystagmogram (ENG). The scan serves to exclude a central lesion, and the audiogram is obtained mainly to look for signs of Ménière's disease (see the next paragraph). If the audiogram is abnormal, I obtain a serum fluorescent treponemal antibody test (FTA). The ENG helps determine whether there is a good reason for the slow recovery (e.g. a severe vestibular imbalance). If a significant vestibular paresis is not found on ENG, alternative explanations for symptoms (e.g. central or psychogenic cause) are considered. In patients with significant vestibular lesions who are simply slow to recover, I prescribe visual-vestibular exercises provided as a handout or 4 weeks of weekly participation in a specialized vestibular physical therapy program. Alternatively, avocational activities often serve as well to promote vestibular compensation and recovery, and depending on the abilities and interests of my patients, I might prescribe golf, bowling, racquetball, bicycling, or even T'ai Chi.

Table 1 Common Causes of Otologic Vertigo and Dysequilibrium

Benign paroxysmal positional vertigo
Unilateral vestibular paresis or disturbance
Labyrinthitis
Vestibular neuritis
Mass lesions (e.g., acoustic neuroma)
Ménière's disease
Neurovascular compression
Bilateral vestibular paresis
Middle ear dysfunction
Cerumen impaction
Eustachian tube malfunction
Otitis media
Perilymph fistula
Otosclerosis

Ménière's disease is another cause of unilateral vestibular paresis. It is typified by four cardinal symptoms: episodic vertigo, roaring tinnitus, monaural fullness, and fluctuating hearing. Ménière's disease is usually diagnosed by combining the historical elements just noted with a fluctuating low-frequency sensorineural hearing impairment documented with serial audiometry. Treatment involves a combination of prophylactic measures and acute management of vertigo. For acute management I use vestibular suppressants and antiemetics in a way similar to that described for vestibular neuritis. For prevention of attacks, I begin with a 2 g or no-added salt diet. If this is not effective, I will add a diuretic such as Dyazide (given every morning). In patients who have not responded adequately to this regime, I will add verapamil in a sustained-release form (120 to 240 mg SR every morning) combined with daily use of a vestibular suppressant such as meclizine or lorazepam (0.5 mg twice daily). Patients who have unacceptable symptoms after several months of treatment are referred for surgical consideration. An MRI is not needed in the evaluation of most patients with Ménière's, but I usually obtain FTA, thyroid-stimulating hormone (TSH), and antinuclear antibody (ANA) blood tests to exclude treatable medical causes.

Other than vestibular neuritis, labyrinthitis, and Ménière's, there are numerous other potential causes of unilateral vestibular disturbance, but practically they are encountered extremely rarely. *Acoustic neuromas* and other

Table 2 Vestibular Suppressants, Arranged in Order of Preference

DRUG	DOSE	ADVERSE REACTIONS AND PRECAUTIONS	PHARMACOLOGIC CLASS
Meclizine (Antivert, Bonine)	25–50 mg q4–6h	Sedating; precautions in prostatic enlargement	Antihistamine; anticholinergic
Lorazepam (Ativan)	0.5 mg b.i.d.	Mildly sedating; drug dependency	Benzodiazepine
Clonazepam (Klonopin)	0.5 mg b.i.d.	Mildly sedating; drug dependency	Benzodiazepine
Amitriptyline (Elavil)	10–50 mg h.s.	Sedating; anticholinergic	Tricyclic with anticholinergic and antihistamine actions

All doses are those used routinely for adults and will generally not be appropriate for children. This list is not exhaustive, but other available agents are similar in action and have no greater advantage.

Table 3 Antiemetics (in Alphabetical Order)

DRUG	USUAL DOSE (ADULTS)	ADVERSE REACTIONS	PHARMACOLOGIC CLASS
Droperidol (Inapsine)	2.5 mg or 5 mg SL	Sedating; hypotension	Neuroleptic
Granisetron (Kytril)	1 mg PO or IV	Headache	5HT3 antagonist
Meclizine (Antivert, Bonine)	12.5–25 mg q4–6h PO	Sedating; precautions in glaucoma, prostate enlargement	Antihistamine and anticholinergic
Metoclopramide (Reglan)	10 mg PO t.i.d. or 10 mg IM	Restlessness or drowsiness; extrapyramidal	Dopamine antagonist, prokinetic
Ondansetron (Zofran)	4 mg PO or IV	Headache, diarhhea, fever	5HTC antagonist
Prochlorperazine (Compazine)	5 mg or 10 mg IM or PO q6–8h	Sedating, extrapyramidal	Phenothiazine
Promethazine (Phenergan)	25 mg PO q6–8 h or 25 mg PR q12h or 12.5 mg IM q6–8h	Sedating, extrapyramidal	Phenothiazine
Triethylperazine (Torecan)	10 mg PO up to t.i.d. or 2 ml IM up to t.i.d.	Sedating; extrapyramidal	Phenothiazine
Trimethobenzamide (Tigan)	250 mg PO t.i.d. or 200 mg IM t.i.d. or 200 mg rectal t.i.d.	Sedating; extrapyramidal	Similar to phenothiazine

All doses are those used routinely for adults and will generally not be appropriate for children. This list is not exhaustive, but other available agents have similar mechanisms of action.

cerebello-pontine angle tumors are infrequent sources of vertigo—because acoustics grow very slowly, hearing impairment rather than vertigo is ordinarily the presenting symptom. *Neurovascular compression* is discussed under the heading of central vertigo.

Bilateral Vestibular Paresis

Bilateral vestibular paresis is nearly always a consequence of a prolonged exposure to an ototoxic drug. Most commonly the patient has received a 3 week or longer course of gentamicin, although other "mycin" antibiotics, loop diuretics, chemotherapy, and industrial solvents can also produce this picture. Many of these patients have had ambulatory peritoneal dialysis where gentamicin was used to treat a peritonitis. Patients present clinically with dysequilibrium and oscillopsia—an illusory movement of the visual world provoked by head movement. The diagnosis is confirmed by rotatory chair testing. Audiometry is generally normal. Bilateral vestibular paresis is easily separated from the more prosaic "sensory ataxia," actually somatosensory ataxia, by oscillopsia and vestibular testing.

I treat these patients by withdrawing all vestibular suppressants. Patients are given a list of ototoxic drugs and drugs that suppress vestibular function to avoid in the future. I have them undergo 4 or more weeks of specialized physical therapy and expect them to continue to perform these exercises indefinitely.

Middle Ear Disturbances

Middle ear disease is an infrequent cause of vertigo, but there are several conditions that one should be aware of. *Cerumen impaction* responds to wax disimpaction, which should be done in any case, to visualize the tympanic membrane of the vertiginous patient. *Eustachian tube malfunction* causes complaints of a mild and vague dizziness, which fluctuates with aural fullness. I routinely prescribe decongestants, antihistamines, and intranasal steroids, although they generally have little effect. Although ventilation tubes eliminate symptoms, it is generally thought that this is unduly aggressive. I refer patients with *temporomandibular joint (TMJ) dysfunction* to their dentist for a "night guard," a plastic insert worn at night, to reduce bruxism. Amitriptyline (10 to 50 mg at bedtime) is also sometimes helpful. *Otosclerosis* is an uncommon hereditary disorder characterized by a progressive conductive hearing loss and occasionally some vertigo. The vertigo is treated with vestibular suppressants as needed.

Perilymph fistula is another uncommon source of otologic vertigo. The diagnosis is usually made by noting the combination of barotrauma, such as a scuba diving accident or airplane-related ear injury, and dizziness elicited by blowing of the nose or similar activities where middle ear pressure is altered. Fistula is also a common consequence of otologic (stapes) surgery. Initially I get a baseline audiogram and instruct the patient to avoid further barotrauma for 6 months. I also prescribe vestibular suppressants (e.g., lorazepam 0.5 twice daily as needed). Hearing is rechecked if the patient notices a drop. Roughly 90 percent of patients improve spontaneously. If patients do not improve after 6 months of waiting, or hearing deteriorates, these cases are referred to an otologist for surgical exploration and patching of the fistula.

■ CENTRAL VERTIGO

Table 4 lists common causes of "central vertigo." Stroke and transient ischemic attack account for one-third of cases and vertebrobasilar migraine another 15 percent. A large number of individual miscellaneous neurologic disorders such as seizures, multiple sclerosis, and the Arnold-Chiari malformation make up the remainder. Much of central vertigo is basic neurology, which would be inappropriate to review here, but there are several less obvious presentations.

Headache and Vertigo

This symptom complex is usually encountered in females in the 30 to 40 years of age group, where the incidence of migraine peaks in the general population. It is also a common symptom complex after head injury. When vertebrobasilar migraine is suspected, I try a prophylactic drug such as a sustained-release preparation of verapamil (Calan SR, Isoptin SR, Verelan), 120 to 240 mg every morning. A trial of amitriptyline (10 to 50 mg at bedtime) can be made if the

Table 4 Common Causes of Central Vertigo

Stroke and TIA
Cerebellar
AICA distribution
PICA distribution
Vertebrobasilar migraine
Adult form
Childhood variant (benign paroxysmal vertigo of childhood)
Seizure (temporal lobe)
Multiple sclerosis, postinfectious demyelination
Arnold-Chiari malformation, basilar impression
Tumors of eighth nerve, brainstem, or cerebellum
Paraneoplastic cerebellar degeneration

TIA, transient ischemic attack; AICA, anterior inferior cerebellar artery; PICA, posterior inferior cerebellar artery.

patient does not tolerate verapamil because of constipation, palpitations, or ankle edema. I favor amitriptyline over newer antidepressant medications such as the selective serotonin reuptake inhibitor (SSRI) family because the anticholinergic activity of amitriptyline helps suppress vertigo. Beta-blockers form a third line of treatment.

Quick Spins

Patients relate a history of brief episodes of vertigo consisting of one or two spins in a second. Such spells may occur 20 or more times per day. Frequently these patients have a history of head trauma and have sharp waves on their electroencephalogram (EEG). Carbamazepine (Tegretol), in therapeutic doses for epilepsy (100 to 200 mg three times per day), is tried in such cases, especially if symptoms have been persistent over months and have not responded to vestibular suppressant medication. Gabapentin (Neurontia) can also be effective in this situation. If the EEG is normal, in head trauma cases I initially prescribe the Brandt-Daroff exercises because of the high prevalence of BPPV. A variant of "quick spins" is "episodic tilts." Again, these patients often respond to carbamazepine, although the EEG is nearly always normal. Many of these patients have ectatic vertebral and basilar arteries on imaging studies, which may be causing symptoms by compression of the vestibular nerve or the root entry zone of the eighth nerve in the medulla (neurovascular compression).

Structural Lesion of the Brainstem or Cerebellum

I am frequently referred central patients who are not a diagnostic problem but rather need treatment for vertigo. The treatment approach is empiric. Meclizine (12.5 to 25 mg twice daily) is occasionally successful. Benzodiazepines such as lorazepam and clonazepam are frequently helpful (see Table 2 for doses), but one must be wary of psychological addiction and physical dependance. Amitriptyline (25 mg at bedtime) may also be tried. Physical therapy, roughly once per week, and ongoing if possible, can also be very helpful.

■ PSYCHOGENIC VERTIGO

Psychogenic vertigo denotes vertigo accompanying a psychiatric problem (Table 5). Although there is considerable imprecision in diagnosing psychogenic vertigo in the neurologic

Table 5 Types of Psychogenic Vertigo

Anxiety and panic
Agoraphobia
Depression
Malingering
Somatization disorder

Table 6 Diagnoses Made in Patients with Vertigo Without Objective Findings

Vertigo of "unknown cause" or "vertigo, not otherwise specified"
Post-traumatic vertigo and labyrinthine concussion
Hyperventilation syndrome
Dysequilibrium of the elderly.

and otologic community, it seems likely that these patients do account for a substantial number of dizzy patients. The psychogenic diagnosis should not be used as a substitute for "unknown" (see the following section), but rather it requires positive evidence for a psychiatric disturbance. Most frequently this diagnosis is arrived at by psychometric testing or psychiatric evaluation obtained after one has failed to discover an objective cause for vertigo or dysequilibrium. Note that there is a basic chicken-egg problem, because although anxiety may engender vertigo, the reverse is also true. Patients understand this very well.

Agoraphobia, anxiety, and panic are recognized by their situational dependence. These patients respond well to benzodiazepines. Patients with depression or somatization disorder may manifest vague and unquantifiable symptoms such as vertigo, headache, or dysequilibrium. I try an SSRI-type antidepressant such as sertraline (Zoloft, 50 mg at bedtime) in patients with depression and refer to psychiatry for other situations. Malingerers, usually attempting to obtain compensation after an accident, may also choose to manifest vertigo. I request psychometric testing (MMPI) and posturography in cases where there is litigation to document potential symptom amplification and inconsistency.

■ VERTIGO OF UNKNOWN CAUSE

Table 6 enumerates conditions that share the unifying feature of a lack of an objective abnormality. In the vertigo literature, these patients are usually allocated somewhat inconsistently between the "unknown" category, psychogenic category, and the remaining categories in Table 6, presumably reflecting the degree to which the diagnosing physician and/or the patient population being studied are able to tolerate a lack of a definite diagnosis.

The terms listed in Table 6 denote the following clinical situations. *Post-traumatic vertigo* is a vertigo of unknown origin which follows a head injury. *Labyrinthine concussion* is a post-traumatic vertigo in which a new hearing impairment is present. *Hyperventilation syndrome* denotes vertigo of unknown origin that is provoked by rapid breathing. *Dysequilibrium of the elderly* is imbalance of unknown origin in a person aged 75 years or more.

If after a thorough history and neurologic and otologic

examination I am unable to reasonably postulate an otologic, central, or psychiatric disturbance, I obtain audiometric testing. Patients with audiometric abnormalities are tentatively assigned as having otologic vertigo. Patients with positional symptoms are given a trial of the Brandt-Daroff exercises for BPPV. If there are no positional symptoms or the exercises are ineffective, an ENG and an MRI study of the head are recommended. When all results are normal, I gently advise the patient to consult a psychiatrist.

Because it is best that the patient does not conclude that "the doctor thinks this is all in my head," it helps to empirically try several drug manipulations. In patients already taking medication, I withdraw drugs that could affect the vestibular system. This strategy may identify persons with ataxia caused by medication. Several drugs are then tried. Meclizine (12.5 to 50 mg, three times daily), may be prescribed on an as-needed basis. If meclizine is already being used and is ineffective, it may be replaced by a small dose of lorazepam (0.5 mg twice daily). Clonazepam (0.5 mg twice daily) can be used in a similar fashion. It is generally difficult to exclude mild Ménière's disease, and salt restriction (no added salt) and a diuretic such as Dyazide (1 taken every morning) may be tried. Amitriptyline (10 to 25 mg at bedtime) is tried for 4 weeks. If patients do not respond to these regimens, they are followed at 3 to 6 month intervals and undergo yearly audiometric screenings.

Suggested Reading

Brandt T, Daroff RB. Physical therapy for benign paroxysmal positional vertigo. Arch Otolaryngol 1980; 106:484–485.

Epley JM. The canalith repositioning procedure: For treatment of benign paroxysmal positional vertigo. Otol Head Neck Surg 1992; 107:399–404.

Hain TC. Treatment of vertigo. Neurologist 1995; 1:125–133.

Hain TC. Episodic vertigo. In: Rakel R, ed. Conn's current therapy. Philadelphia: WB Saunders. 1996:869.

SLEEP DISORDERS

David W. Buchholz, M.D.

Sleep disorders take three basic forms: insomnia, excessive wake-time sleepiness, and abnormal behaviors associated with sleep.

■ INSOMNIA

There are three patterns of insomnia, each of which has diagnostic implications. Difficulty initiating sleep implies a psychological problem such as anxiety or learned insomnia, although physical disorders, especially restless legs syndrome (RLS), can present in this way. Difficulty maintaining sleep suggests that a physical problem is disrupting sleep. The third pattern of insomnia, early morning awakening, usually indicates depression.

Insomnia can be treated in two ways. The best way is to identify and treat its underlying cause(s). The other way to treat insomnia is symptomatically, using either behavioral therapy or hypnotic medication. Identifying treatable causes of insomnia depends mainly on history-taking and to a lesser extent on physical examination and blood studies. Sleep laboratory testing is generally not indicated in the evaluation of insomnia except for suspected sleep apnea and some cases of periodic limb movements in sleep.

Table 1 Treatable Causes of Insomnia

Medications
Caffeine, nicotine, alcohol, and other drugs of abuse
Medical problems
Painful disorders
Gastroesophageal reflux
Congestive heart failure
Nocturia
Hyperthyroidism
Restless legs syndrome and periodic limb movements in sleep
Sleep apnea
Sleep-wake schedule disorders
Delayed sleep phase syndrome
Problems of the elderly
Time zone changes
Rotating work shifts
Depression
Other psychological and psychiatric disorders
Learned insomnia

Treatable Causes (Table 1)

Medications That Cause Insomnia

The role of medications in causing insomnia is substantial but underappreciated. The offending medications may be either prescription drugs or over-the-counter remedies (Table 2). No step is more important in the treatment of insomnia than identifying and discontinuing, if possible, over-the-counter and prescription medications that contribute to the problem.

Caffeine, Nicotine, Alcohol, and Other Drugs of Abuse

The three most prevalent drugs of abuse—caffeine, nicotine, and alcohol—all contribute to insomnia. Caffeine is a more

Table 2 Medications That Cause Insomnia

OVER-THE-COUNTER MEDICATIONS
Caffeine-containing headache relievers
"Sinus" medications with decongestant ingredients
Diet aids such as phenylpropanolamine
Stimulants (including herbal remedies) containing caffeine, ephedrine, and other sympathomimetics
PRESCRIPTION MEDICATIONS
Stimulants including methylphenidate, pemoline, and methamphetamine
Appetite suppressants including phentermine and fenfluramine
Adrenergic agonists for treatment of asthma
Caffeine-containing headache relievers
Nasal decongestants
Corticosteroids
Selective serotonin reuptake inhibitors
Deprenyl (selegiline)
Beta-blockers, especially propranolol
Diuretics resulting in nocturia
Insulin and oral hypoglycemic agents coupled with inadequate glucose intake before bedtime
Excessive thyroid hormone replacement
Withdrawal from central nervous system depressants, including hypnotic medications

Table 3 Treatment of Restless Legs Syndrome and Periodic Limb Movements in Sleep

Use carbidopa-levodopa ½ of a 25/100 mg tablet ½ hour before bedtime. Increase the dosage by half-tablet increments every several days or more as needed or tolerated up to a maximum of 3 or 4 tablets total. If the patient reawakens with symptoms during the night, divide the dosage between bedtime and later in the night and/or convert some or all of the carbidopa-levodopa dosage to the controlled-release preparation.
Beware of augmentation of RLS due to rebound from carbidopa-levodopa. Avoid using carbidopa-levodopa during the day.
A second option is pergolide starting at 0.05 mg in the evening and repeated at bedtime. The dosage may be gradually increased as needed or tolerated by 0.05 mg added to each of the two doses every several days up to a total daily dosage of 0.5 mg or more as needed or tolerated. The two doses may be consolidated into one if pergolide is well tolerated.
A third option is an opioid such as propoxyphene 100–300 mg or oxycodone 5–15 mg at bedtime. An opioid can be used in combination with carbidopa-levodopa or pergolide.
A fourth option is a benzodiazepine such as triazolam 0.125–0.5 mg or temazepam 15–30 mg at bedtime.
Gabapentin may also be an option, although experience is limited.

potent and prolonged stimulant than most people realize; drinking coffee, tea, or cola in the afternoon or evening may substantially interfere with falling asleep at night. Alcohol is the most widely self-prescribed "sleeping pill," but it yields disturbed and unrefreshing sleep. Surreptitious use of illicit stimulants such as cocaine and speed may further cloud the picture of insomnia, and in some cases the essential problem may be revealed only by drug and alcohol testing.

Medical Problems

Painful disorders such as arthritis, spinal degenerative changes, and carpal tunnel syndrome may produce enough discomfort to awaken your patient and make it difficult for him or her to return to sleep. The patient complaining of difficulty maintaining sleep is waving a red flag indicating that a physical problem is probably disrupting sleep, and making the diagnosis may be as simple as asking the patient what wakes him or her up.

Gastroesophageal reflux is naturally exacerbated in the position of sleep. Patients may awaken with heartburn, other chest pain, or laryngospasm (as a result of reflux into the pharynx and aspiration into the larynx). Patients with *congestive heart failure* (CHF) may have insomnia related to orthopnea, paroxysmal nocturnal dyspnea, and/or nocturia. In older men frequent *awakening to urinate* is usually due to prostatic hypertrophy, but other considerations include diuretic therapy, excessive alcohol or caffeine intake, CHF, urinary tract infection, and diabetes. Patients with *hyperthyroidism* causing insomnia almost always have other easily detected symptoms and signs of hyperthyroidism.

Restless Legs Syndrome and Periodic Limb Movements in Sleep

Restless legs syndrome (RLS) is a common but often overlooked cause of insomnia. In part it is overlooked because it is confused with anxiety, since patients report being fidgety as they try to fall asleep. The diagnosis of RLS is also missed because there is great variability in how patients describe the problem. Most do not use the term *restless* to communicate the discomfort that they experience mainly in their legs as they try to lie still and fall asleep. Some of the terms used to describe RLS include *tension, drawing, tightness, numbness, tingling, burning, cramping, aching,* and *pain.* The hallmarks of RLS are worsening of discomfort in the evening, exacerbation of discomfort at rest, and momentary relief of discomfort with activity of the legs.

Periodic limb movements in sleep (PLMS) are rhythmic triple-flexion movements of one or both legs approximately every 20 to 30 seconds during sleep. These movements may cause difficulty maintaining sleep for the patient and/or the bed partner, although the condition is often relatively asymptomatic. Many individuals with PLMS do not have RLS, but almost everyone with RLS has PLMS. The cause of RLS/PLMS is unknown, but many patients have a positive family history (pointing to genetic influences), and in other cases the problem appears secondary to factors such as uremia, antidepressant medication, neurologic disorders (including polyneuropathy, radiculopathy, and myelopathy), or iron deficiency.

Treatment of RLS/PLMS is usually a rewarding although imperfect experience. The best treatments are carbidopa-levodopa, pergolide, or an opioid (Table 3). The biggest problem with carbidopa-levodopa for RLS/PLMS is the development of rebound augmentation of RLS symptoms earlier in the day in approximately one-half of patients. It is inadvisable to deal with this by having the patient take more carbidopa-levodopa earlier in the day; this is a classic example of chasing one's tail. If augmentation of RLS secondary to carbidopa-levodopa therapy is a substantial problem, I switch to alternative treatment such as pergolide or an opioid. Tolerance and addiction have not been problems in appropriately selected patients with RLS/PLMS who are treated with opioids. Opioid and dopaminergic treatment can be combined.

Benzodiazepines are another option for RLS/PLMS, although in my opinion they are a distant third behind dopamine and opioid therapy. The most conventional benzodiazepine treatment for RLS/PLMS is clonazepam, but it is a long-acting drug, and it seems more rational to use a shorter-acting benzodiazepine such as triazolam 0.125 to 0.5 mg or temazepam 15 to 30 mg, since patients tend to be most symptomatic during the first third of the night and because shorter-acting benzodiazepines are less likely to cause daytime sedation. Gabapentin is another potential option, but experience is limited.

Sleep Apnea

Sleep apnea is discussed later as a cause of excessive waketime sleepiness because that is its usual presentation, but occasionally sleep apnea causes insomnia. Most patients with sleep apnea have subconscious arousals, not awakenings, that terminate their hundreds of apneic episodes during sleep. Occasionally patients with sleep apnea complain of difficulty maintaining sleep because of conscious awakenings rather than subconscious arousals. You might expect that these patients would describe awakening with an awareness of difficulty breathing, but that is rarely the case. The complaint of awakening with difficulty breathing is more suggestive of a problem such as gastropharyngeal reflux, asthma, CHF, or panic attacks.

Sleep-Wake Schedule Disorders

Every person struggles daily to adjust his or her sleep-wake schedule to the 24 hour solar day, since our internal clocks have a natural daily cycle length of approximately 25 hours.

Delayed Sleep Phase Syndrome. Some individuals have even longer than 25-hour natural daily sleep-wake cycle lengths, and these "night owls" habitually find it difficult to stay in sync with the rest of society because of their tendency to both go to bed and get up too late. A combination of bright light exposure (phototherapy) for 1 hour early in the morning (which encourages earlier sleep onset) and strictly enforced early arising may be useful in regulating the sleep-wake schedules of these individuals.

Problems of the Elderly. As we grow older our daily sleep-wake cycle tends to shorten. Consequently, we tend to both fall asleep and wake up earlier. Elderly individuals who are disturbed by awakening before sunrise should postpone bedtime and avoid napping during the day. Many inactive elderly people (especially those who are institutionalized or demented) develop fragmented sleep-wake schedules as a result of napping during the day, and the best strategy is to force them to remain awake during the day and thereby consolidate their need to sleep at night-time.

Time-Zone Changes. Jet lag increases with the number of time zones that are crossed, and it takes approximately 1 day to fully adjust to each hour of time-zone change. Eastward travel is more difficult, because the direction of sleep-wake schedule change is opposite our natural tendency to fall asleep later and wake up later every day (related to our 25 hour daily sleep-wake cycle length). It is advisable to avoid the temptation to use alcohol as a hypnotic agent and caffeine as a stimulant in an effort to help adjust to timezone changes; these measures usually backfire. A short-acting hypnotic medication such as zolpidem or triazolam may be helpful when traveling from the west coast to the east coast of the United States, since it may be used to induce sleep in advance of one's internal clock's schedule. Hypnotic medication may also aid in obtaining sleep during eastward transoceanic flights at night.

Rotating Work Shifts. Approximately 20 percent of the working population is asked to do the impossible: namely, to change their sleep-wake schedule by 8 hours or more as often as weekly. Workers who must rotate shifts are best advised to do so as infrequently as possible and in a forward direction (i.e., from the morning shift to the afternoon shift to the night shift).

Depression

Although depression classically presents as the pattern of insomnia known as early morning awakening, it can cause any type of insomnia. Depression is widely prevalent and is more often than not associated with insomnia. Most cases of depression are readily treatable, and a sedating tricyclic antidepressant (e.g., amitriptyline or imipramine) or trazodone are apt choices when insomnia is a prominent symptom of depression.

Other Psychological and Psychiatric Disorders

Anxiety disorders cause insomnia, and panic attacks may present as abrupt awakenings with difficulty breathing, palpitations, tremors, and a sense of dread. Psychiatric or psychological evaluation and treatment are indicated when these diagnostic considerations arise.

Learned Insomnia

Almost every case of chronic insomnia, regardless of its contributing causes, becomes complicated by a multifactorial phenomenon known as learned insomnia. Part of learned insomnia is one's emotional reaction to the presence of insomnia. A few nights of poor sleep lead to frustration and anticipation of poor sleep, which becomes a self-fulfilling prophecy by virtue of the anxiety and other disquieting emotions that accompany anticipation of poor sleep.

Learned insomnia also has behavioral aspects related to scheduling of sleep. Individuals who sleep poorly at night may attempt to catch up by sleeping late in the morning or napping during the day. Not surprisingly, sleeping at night becomes more and more difficult as a result of sleeping at other times. The treatment of learned insomnia is behavioral treatment including sleep hygiene and sleep restriction (see the following sections).

Symptomatic Treatment

Insomnia can be treated symptomatically whether or not there are identifiable underlying causes of insomnia that can be treated directly.

Table 4 Sleep Hygiene

Maintain a regular sleep-wake schedule. Get out of bed early in the morning whether or not you have slept well.
Avoid naps. Exercise when you might otherwise nap.
Preserve your bed as a haven for sleep and sex. Avoid other activities in bed (e.g., reading, watching television).
Minimize alcohol consumption and avoid caffeine in the afternoon and evening. Don't eat heavily shortly before bed.
Make sure your bedroom environment is conducive to sleep. It should be cool, quiet, and dark.
If your mind is preoccupied by something such that you can't fall asleep, put the problem to rest by writing it down in a sentence or two and set it aside until morning.
Don't try too hard to fall asleep; it will only make things worse. If you can't fall asleep after 20 to 30 minutes, get out of bed, do something relaxing, and go back to bed when you feel sleepy.

Behavioral Treatment

Sleep Hygiene. Table 4 lists advice, collectively known as sleep hygiene, regarding behavioral management of insomnia. This approach often works best when you emphasize a few particular items on the list for each individual patient, based on the details of that patient's history.

Sleep Restriction. This simple but effective approach works best for people with difficulty initiating sleep due to anxiety or learned insomnia. For example, such a person may go to bed at 11:00 PM but be unable to sleep soundly until 2:00 AM. First, you instruct the person to stay out of bed and remain awake until 2:00 AM. It is very likely that the patient will fall asleep quickly when he or she goes to bed that late. Then, after 1 week, you tell the patient that he or she may now get into bed at 1:30 AM. The person will probably still fall asleep promptly at that hour. This process of gradually shifting bedtime is continued until your patient is able to achieve reasonable sleep onset (that is, within one-half hour of turning out the lights) at his or her desired bedtime (for example, 11:00 PM). In order for sleep restriction to work, your patient must be reminded to get up early in the morning, (and not sleep late in response to a delayed bedtime).

Hypnotic Medication

Hypnotic medication is an adjunct to behavioral treatment of insomnia. Hypnotic medication should not be used long-term on a regular basis, but it may be very helpful for intervals of days to weeks in appropriate circumstances. These circumstances especially include transient situational insomnia (e.g., related to transient anxiety or illness) or adjustment to time-zone changes.

I recommend zolpidem 10 mg at bedtime (5 mg in the elderly or for those with hepatic insufficiency). The best alternative is a short-acting benzodiazepine such as triazolam 0.125 to 0.25 mg or temazepam 15 to 30 mg at bedtime. Longer-acting benzodiazepines should be avoided because of their tendency to cause daytime sedation. There is as yet insufficient evidence to support the use of melatonin as a hypnotic agent. Antihistamines have limited efficacy as hypnotics and have a relatively high incidence of side effects, especially in the elderly, including delirium, urinary retention, and constipation.

Table 5 Treatable Causes of Excessive Wake-Time Sleepiness

Sleep deprivation
Medications, alcohol, and other drugs
Medical problems
Sleep apnea
Restless legs syndrome and periodic limb movements in sleep
Narcolepsy and related disorders

■ EXCESSIVE WAKE-TIME SLEEPINESS

It is important to differentiate between excessive wake-time sleepiness (EWS) and fatigue. EWS refers to the inability to stay awake during normal wake-time activities. Fatigue, on the other hand, refers to tiredness and lack of energy but not actually falling asleep inappropriately. Fatigue has many causes, including depression, but it is the issue of EWS to be considered here.

Often the patient with EWS does not appreciate the extent of the problem, and you may need to question family or friends to establish the existence and degree of EWS. In other words, you need to be on the alert for EWS and pay attention to clues, such as the patient who falls asleep in your office or has a history of motor vehicle mishaps.

You have a responsibility to your patient with EWS and society in general to discuss with him or her the issue of potential impairment of the ability to operate motor vehicles and machinery. This concern should be addressed and documented as you would with any other disorder capable of causing episodic disturbance of consciousness, such as epilepsy.

Treatable Causes (Table 5)

Sleep Deprivation

We tend to grossly underestimate our true sleep needs. We need a bare minimum of 7 to 8 hours of solid sleep daily in order to be maximally alert. Far and away the most common cause of EWS is chronic sleep deprivation. If your patient with EWS sleeps less than 7 or 8 hours per day, the first thing to do, if possible, is extend sleep duration to 8 hours per day for at least 2 weeks as a therapeutic trial.

Medications, Alcohol, and Other Drugs

The list of medications that cause EWS is long and includes hypnotics (especially long-acting benzodiazepines), anxiolytics, antidepressants, anticonvulsants, narcotics, antihistamines, and some antihypertensives. Alcohol and sedating illicit drugs not only directly cause EWS but also potentiate EWS from any other cause.

Medical Problems

Patients with EWS should undergo general medical evaluation for considerations including hypothyroidism, anemia, kidney failure, liver disease, pulmonary insufficiency, and diabetes.

In cases where EWS remains unexplained despite adequate consideration of sleep deprivation, medications, alcohol, other drugs, and medical problems, it is likely that a primary sleep disorder (i.e., sleep apnea, RLS/PLMS, or narcolepsy) is present, and evaluation at an accredited sleep disorders center, including sleep laboratory testing, is indicated.

Sleep Apnea

Most sleep apnea is obstructive and occurs as a result of collapse of the upper airway during sleep in the setting of relaxation of the muscles that normally maintain upper airway patency during respiration. Less commonly patients have central sleep apnea in which the primary problem is a failure of respiratory drive. Apneic episodes may occur hundreds of times per night, yet the typical patient with sleep apnea is unaware that this is happening. A bed partner may notice loud snoring and breathing pauses. The cardinal symptom of sleep apnea is EWS, yet many patients underestimate or deny the presence of EWS, a fact that underscores the importance of taking a history from family or friends in cases of suspected sleep apnea.

The consequences of sleep apnea are not only EWS but also globally impaired well-being, motor vehicle and industrial accidents due to falling asleep, hypertension, heart failure, and fatal cardiac arrhythmias. Given these complications and its prevalence of several percent in the general population, the diagnosis of sleep apnea should be diligently sought. If an adult male or postmenopausal female has EWS that is otherwise unexplained, and especially if that person snores loudly or is overweight, he or she should be referred to an accredited sleep disorders center for evaluation of sleep apnea. At this time, optimal evaluation of sleep apnea remains in-laboratory testing; home monitoring or other abbreviated approaches to the diagnosis cannot be recommended.

The treatment of sleep apnea is best left to those with special training and expertise. Weight loss can be curative in those who are overweight. Patients with sleep apnea should be counseled to avoid alcohol and central nervous system (CNS) depressant medications before sleep. Anatomic problems that may contribute to upper airway narrowing may be surgically correctable in some cases. Uvulopalatopharyngoplasty (UPPP) is a surgical procedure designed to create a more capacious oropharynx, which is thereby theoretically less likely to occlude during sleep, but it has been difficult to select patients with a high likelihood of benefiting from this procedure.

The mainstay of treatment for obstructive sleep apnea is continuous positive airway pressure (CPAP). A small, quiet pump sitting at the bedside delivers pressurized air to a tight-fitting mask worn over the nose and mouth. This acts as a "pneumatic splint" of the upper airway, preventing collapse of the pharynx. It is extremely effective, but some patients have difficulty tolerating the discomfort of the mask or the dryness and congestion associated with the pressurized air.

Restless Legs Syndrome and Periodic Limb Movements in Sleep

These conditions, discussed earlier as a cause of insomnia, may also result in EWS as a consequence of difficulty initiating sleep (due to RLS), difficulty maintaining sleep (due to RLS and PLMS), and/or sleep fragmentation (due to PLMS).

Table 6 Treatment of Narcolepsy

Use brief preventive naps throughout the day to restore alertness, especially before driving.
Start with pemoline 18.75 mg on awakening, and gradually increase as needed or tolerated to as much as 150 mg qd in divided doses.
If pemoline fails, try methylphenidate 5 mg b.i.d., gradually increasing as needed or tolerated to as much as 20 mg q.i.d.
If pemoline and methylphenidate fail, other drug options such as amphetamines are best advised by someone with special expertise in treating narcolepsy.
If cataplexy or other accessory symptoms are problematic, try protriptyline 5–30 mg qd in divided doses, imipramine 25–200 mg qd, or fluoxetine 10–60 mg qd

PLMS is a relatively common finding during sleep laboratory testing, and the finding is often irrelevant unless the frequency of PLMS and the percentage of associated arousals are high.

Narcolepsy and Related Disorders

Narcolepsy is probably often undiagnosed, and the reason is that most physicians have the mistaken notion that patients with narcolepsy present dramatically by falling asleep in the middle of wake-time activities. To the contrary, patients with EWS due to narcolepsy behave similarly to patients with EWS from any other cause: they tend to fall asleep too easily in permissive situations. Less than one-half of patients with narcolepsy have cataplexy, which is sudden, transient muscle weakness often triggered by emotional stimulation. Even fewer have other accessory symptoms of narcolepsy such as hypnagogic or hypnopompic hallucinations or sleep paralysis. Symptoms typically begin during teenage or early adult years. The cause of narcolepsy is unknown.

The diagnosis of narcolepsy depends on sleep laboratory testing, and the characteristic sleep study findings include relatively normal nocturnal sleep but abnormally rapid onset of sleep and occurrence of REM sleep during daytime nap testing. Some patients otherwise appear to have narcolepsy but lack the finding of REM sleep onset during naps, and these patients are sometimes labeled as having idiopathic hypersomnolence. As a lumper, I tend to treat them as though they have narcolepsy.

I believe it is a mistake to diagnose or treat narcolepsy based on history alone. Confirmatory sleep laboratory testing is needed. If a patient comes to you with the diagnosis of narcolepsy but has never had confirmatory sleep laboratory testing, and if that patient is requiring high doses of stimulants or is not doing well with treatment, I recommend that you withdraw the patient from stimulant medication for 2 weeks or more and then have the patient undergo nocturnal polysomnography and daytime nap testing at an accredited sleep disorders center.

The treatment of narcolepsy (Table 6) begins with common sense, including avoidance of CNS depressants and the use of one or more brief daytime naps, which are often refreshing for a number of hours. Most patients with narcolepsy require stimulant medication. Cataplexy and the other accessory symptoms of narcolepsy do not usually require treatment, but if they do, certain antidepressants work best.

■ ABNORMAL BEHAVIORS ASSOCIATED WITH SLEEP

The differential diagnosis of abnormal behaviors associated with sleep includes seizures, but primary sleep disorders presenting in this fashion can be divided into non-REM and REM types.

Non-REM Behaviors (Parasomnias)

Sleepwalking, night terrors, and enuresis tend to occur in the transition from the deeper stages of non-REM sleep (slow-wave sleep) to its lighter stages. These behaviors usually occur in childhood and generally resolve with maturation. Persistence or late re-emergence of these conditions may reflect psychological problems. Because slow-wave sleep tends to occur in the first hour or two of sleep, these behaviors typically occur during that early interval. The affected individual has no recall of the event. In the case of night terrors, these historical features (early occurrence and lack of recall) help distinguish night terrors from nightmares, which are REM-related episodes and are therefore later in sleep (when most REM sleep takes place) and more likely to be recalled.

Treatment of non-REM parasomnias begins with reassurance if the patient is a child, because he or she will likely grow out of the problem. Protecting the individual from dangerous situations is the most important consideration with sleepwalking. Behavioral training with an alarm device can be useful for persistent enuresis. Sleep deprivation should be avoided, because the rebound increase in slow-wave sleep that occurs when one catches up after sleep deprivation is more likely to be associated with the occurrence of non-REM parasomnias. Benzodiazepines can be used to suppress both slow-wave sleep and arousals (the situations that foster non-REM parasomnias), but these drugs are rarely appropriate for children.

REM Behavior Disorder

Other than the muscles of respiration, muscles are generally paralyzed during REM sleep. Some individuals lack normal inhibition of muscle activity during REM sleep, and they thus have abnormal REM-related motor activity, which can be relatively complex (such as attempting to strangle one's bed partner while dreaming of an intruder). REM behavior disorder can be treated with a benzodiazepine such as alprazolam or clonazepam.

Suggested Reading

Gillin JC, Byerley WF. The diagnosis and management of insomnia. N Engl J Med 1990; 322:239–248.

Kryger MH, Roth T, Dement WC. Principles and practice of sleep medicine. Philadelphia: WB Saunders, 1994.

RECURRENT GENERALIZED AND PARTIAL SEIZURES

John F. Kerrigan, M.D.
Robert S. Fisher, M.D., Ph.D.

Proper treatment for epilepsy begins with an understanding of the type of seizure (or seizures) and, if possible, the epilepsy syndrome expressed by the patient. This information usually suggests the drug of first choice, as well as therapeutic options if the initial choice fails. The treating physician also needs to appreciate the unique features of the individual patient in order to obtain the best balance between seizure control and medication side effects.

The number of medications available to treat epilepsy has suddenly increased. Since the introduction of valproic acid in 1978, no truly new anticonvulsant medications were available until the release of felbamate in 1993, followed quickly by gabapentin and lamotrigine. A number of other medications are under active study and may expect approval by the U.S. Food and Drug Administration (FDA) over the next several years, including vigabatrin, tiagabine, topiramate, and oxcarbazepine. Increasing diversity of medications for epilepsy will allow us to tailor better treatment for individual patients.

■ THE PROBLEM: RECURRENT SEIZURES

Epilepsy is a condition of recurrent, unprovoked seizures. Approximately 0.5 to 1 percent of the population in the United States has epilepsy, whereas approximately 5 percent may experience a seizure sometime during their life. Seizures that are provoked or precipitated by particular circumstances probably do not require chronic treatment with antiseizure medications. Febrile seizures and alcohol withdrawal seizures are common examples of such situational events. Even patients who have experienced a single unexplained and unprovoked seizure are often better evaluated and observed for a period of time, rather than immediately initiating anticonvulsant treatment.

Even with a diagnosis of epilepsy, not all patients require treatment. The need to treat should take the full risk-benefit analysis into consideration, weighing the consequences of seizure activity against the possible adverse effects of medication treatment. A decision to withhold treatment may be made, for example, in children with benign epilepsy with centro-temporal spikes (benign rolandic epilepsy), where simple partial seizures may occur with an exclusively nocturnal pattern, representing very little threat to the patient's medical and social well-being. For other patients, any uncontrolled seizure activity may be devastating, prompting early and aggressive treatment. For high-functioning adult patients, even one daytime seizure can have adverse consequences with regard to work or driving, or carry the possibility of physical injury.

This chapter focuses on those patients who require ongoing maintenance therapy. The good news is that 50 to 75 percent of these patients will be well controlled with one or two of the conventional medications. The goal for all patients is to achieve complete seizure control with the least amount of medication possible. Patients in whom this goal cannot be readily attained (due to poorly controlled seizures or to excessive medication side effects, or both) have "intractable" epilepsy. Such patients often have complex and interrelated medical, psychological, and social problems and can benefit from the multidisciplinary care available at comprehensive epilepsy centers. They may also be suitable candidates for surgical treatment.

■ EVALUATION OF THE PATIENT WITH EPILEPSY

Patients with epilepsy should be treated by primary care practitioners. However, the initial evaluation of patients with seizures, stabilization at times of seizure breakthrough, and treatment of the patient with intractable epilepsy is best performed by neurologists with an interest in epilepsy and neurophysiology.

After determining that the patient has epilepsy (rather than one of its imitators) and classifying the type of seizure, we next look for the cause for the seizure disorder. The underlying etiology can be established in 25 to 50 percent of patients by consideration of the history, physical examination, family history, and selected neurodiagnostic tests. The tests to be selected vary with the individual case, as the patient's age and history usually suggest the most likely causes.

Sophisticated magnetic resonance imaging (MRI) techniques have increased our ability to identify such lesions as focal cortical dysplasia and hippocampal atrophy, previously missed with older imaging tools. MRI is the initial imaging modality of choice for patients with partial epilepsy, except in selected circumstances, such as a search for calcification or fresh blood with computed tomography (CT). Special MRI sequences may be used to further increase the sensitivity for selected conditions (such as hippocampal atrophy), if relevant.

Most patients with generalized seizures should also undergo brain MRI, particularly in the presence of any associated neurologic problems. Many patients have generalized seizure activity due to either diffuse or multifocal brain disease. In addition, patients with seizures that appear to be generalized may indeed demonstrate focal pathology. Patients with well-defined primary generalized epilepsy (childhood absence epilepsy representing the most common example) do not require MRI or CT.

The underlying etiology itself may require treatment, such as with vascular malformation or tumor. Genetic syndromes require family counseling. Even if no specific treatment is possible, identifying the etiology may provide a more certain prognosis.

■ CLASSIFICATION OF SEIZURES

The now widely accepted International Classification for seizures divides seizure events into focal and generalized categories (Table 1). Partial seizures (also known as *focal* or *localization related*) are those events that result from a seizure discharge within a particular brain region or focus. Simple partial seizures do not induce any loss or alteration of consciousness as part of the clinical symptoms. Complex partial seizures result in some alteration of consciousness or awareness. The aura experienced by many seizure patients represents a simple partial seizure preceding its spread to the complex partial stage. Partial seizures can secondarily generalize to tonic or tonic-clonic activity. Many seizures reported to be generalized (or grand mal) may in fact have partial onset, with rapid secondary spread.

Generalized seizures are those events that demonstrate electroencephalographic seizure activity over widespread and bilateral scalp regions simultaneously. Further classification of generalized seizures (such as atonic, myoclonic, absence, and others) is based on the clinical and electrographic pattern. Seizure recording with video-electroencephalographic techniques may be required for definitive evaluation in difficult cases.

■ CLASSIFICATION OF EPILEPTIC SYNDROMES

The classification of epileptic syndromes incorporates the type (or types) of individual seizures with additional patient information such as age of onset, associated neurologic or developmental problems, and natural history. Both localization-related and generalized epilepsies are designated

Table 1 Seizure Classification

- Partial seizures
  - Simple partial seizures
    - Simple partial seizures with motor symptoms
    - Simple partial seizures with sensory symptoms
    - Simple partial seizures with psychic or autonomic symptoms
  - Complex partial seizures
  - Complex partial seizures beginning as simple partial seizures
  - Complex partial seizures beginning with impairment of consciousness
  - Complex partial seizures with secondary generalization
- Generalized seizures
  - Absence
  - Atonic
  - Tonic
  - Clonic
  - Tonic-clonic
  - Myoclonic
- Unclassified seizures

symptomatic if the seizures result from an identified underlying cerebral insult or disease state, and are considered *cryptogenic* if an underlying disease is suspected but not identified. *Idiopathic epilepsy* indicates (or implies) a genetic predisposition for seizures in patients who are otherwise normal. Seizure classification attempts to describe individual seizures, whereas epilepsy syndrome classification attempts to describe the overall disorder affecting individuals with seizures. A detailed review of the many epilepsy syndromes is beyond the scope of this chapter and may be found in standard references on the subject. For an abbreviated classification of epilepsy syndromes, see Table 2.

Table 2 Classification of Epilepsy Syndromes (Abbreviated)

Localization-related epilepsies
- Idiopathic epilepsies
  - Benign epilepsy with centro-temporal spikes (benign rolandic epilepsy)
  - Childhood epilepsy with occcipital paroxysms
- Cryptogenic or symptomatic epilepsies
  - Simple partial with symptoms suggestive of onset in:
    - Frontal lobe
    - Parietal lobe
    - Temporal lobe
    - Occipital lobe
  - Complex partial with symptoms suggestive of onset in:
    - Frontal lobe
    - Parietal lobe
    - Temporal lobe
    - Occipital lobe
  - Secondarily generalized with initial symptoms suggestive of onset in:
    - Frontal lobe
    - Parietal lobe
    - Temporal lobe
    - Occipital lobe

Generalized epilepsies
- Idiopathic epilepsies (ordered for age of presentation)
  - Benign neonatal convulsion
  - Benign myoclonic epilepsy in infancy
  - Childhood absence epilepsy
  - Juvenile absence epilepsy
  - Juvenile myoclonic epilepsy
  - Generalized tonic-clonic seizures upon awakening

Cryptogenic or symptomatic epilepsies
- Infantile spasms
- Lennox-Gastaut syndrome

The identity of the epilepsy syndrome may allow further refinement or modification of the therapeutic approach, based on prior experience in that particular subgroup of patients. For example, children with infantile spasms (a generalized epilepsy syndrome) are best treated initially with a course of intramuscular adenocorticotropic hormone (ACTH) gel, whereas valproic acid is usually considered to be the drug of first choice for generalized seizures.

■ THERAPY

Selection of Antiepilepsy Drugs

In addition to efficacy against a particular seizure type, we select an antiepilepsy drug (AED) on the basis of recognizing a number of other factors. These include potentially problematic side effects, ease of administration, safety, and cost. These issues affect patient compliance and medication tolerability.

Very few large, controlled studies have been performed with head-to-head comparison between one medication and another in the treatment of specific patient groups. The first Veterans Administration (VA) cooperative study found approximately similar efficacy against partial seizures for carbamazepine, phenytoin, phenobarbital, and primidone. Full seizure control was more often achieved with carbamazepine. Excessive sleepiness early in treatment was more of a problem for those on primidone. In the second VA cooperative study carbamazepine and valproic acid were each shown to be effective against partial seizures, though again with greater efficacy for carbamazepine. The VA studies were conducted with adult patients. In many other instances, "standards" have been established by virtue of collective experience and studies that lack direct comparison of one AED to another.

The pharmacokinetic and dosing features (including formulations) of the commonly used AEDs are shown in Tables 3 and 4. The common idiosyncratic and dose-related side effects of these drugs are shown in Table 5. Additional comments concerning the individual drugs are included in the sections that follow.

Table 3 Pharmacokinetic Aspects of the Anticonvulsant Medications

MEDICATION	HALF-LIFE	METABOLISM/ ELIMINATION	PROTEIN BINDING (% BOUND)	ADULT DOSE
Phenytoin	18 hours (nonlinear kinetics)	Hepatic	85%–90%	200–500 mg/day, qd to t.i.d.
Carbamazepine	14 hours (autoinduction)	Hepatic	60%–70%	600–1600 mg/day, b.i.d. to q.i.d.
Phenobarbital	96 hours (varies with age)	Hepatic	45%–50%	30–120 mg/day, qd to b.i.d.
Primidone	Primidone 12 hours Phenobarbital 96 hours (phenobarbital active metabolite)	Hepatic	<30% (phenobarbital 45%–50%)	300–1,500 mg/day t.i.d.
Valproic acid	10 hours	Hepatic	70%–90%	375–3,000 mg/day, b.i.d. to t.i.d.
Gabapentin	8 hours	Renal	None	600–4,800 mg/day, t.i.d.
Lamotrigine	24 hours (altered by drug interactions)	Hepatic	<55%	200–700 mg/day, qd to t.i.d.
Felbamate	20 hours	Hepatic	25%	1,800–4,800 mg/day, b.i.d. to q.i.d.
Ethosuximide	36 hours	Hepatic	<10%	250–1,000 mg/day, b.i.d. to t.i.d.

Table 4 Applied Pharmacology of the Anticonvulsant Medications

MEDICATION	ROUTE	FORMULATIONS	THERAPEUTIC RANGE (SERUM)
Phenytoin (Dilantin)	IV, PO	Parenteral 50 mg/cc Suspension 125 mg/5 cc Extended-release capsules 100 mg and 30 mg Infatabs 50 mg	10–20 μg/ml
Carbamazepine (Tegretol)	PO	Suspension 100 mg/5 cc Tablet 200 mg Chewable tablet 100 mg	4–12 μg/ml
Phenobarbital	PO	Parenteral 60 mg/cc (and others) Suspension 20 mg/5 cc Tablets 15 mg, 30 mg, 60 mg, 100 mg	10–40 μg/ml
Primidone (Mysoline)	PO	Suspension 250 mg/5 cc Tablets 50 mg, 250 mg	Primidone 5-13 μg/ml; phenobarb 10–40 μg/ml
Valproic acid (Depakene, Depakote)	PO	Suspension 250 m/5 cc Tablets 125 mg, 250 mg, 500 mg Sprinkle capsules 125 mg Capsules 250 mg	50–100 μg/ml (5-150 μg/ml in clinical usage)
Gabapentin (Neurontin)	PO	Capsules 100 mg, 300 mg, 400 mg	Not established
Lamotrigine (Lamictal)	PO	Tablets 25 mg, 100 mg, 150 mg, 200 mg	Not established
Felbamate (Felbatol)	PO	Suspension 600 mg/5 cc Tablets 400 mg, 600 mg	40–100 μg/ml
Ethosuximide (Zarontin)	PO	Suspension 250 mg/5 cc Gelatin capsules 250 mg	40–100 μg/ml

IV, intravenous; PO, *per os* (oral administration).

Table 5 Adverse Effects of Anticonvulsant Medications

MEDICATION	COMMON SIDE EFFECTS (USUALLY DOSE RELATED)	UNCOMMON BUT SERIOUS SIDE EFFECTS (USUALLY IDIOSYNCRATIC)
Phenytoin	Nystagmus, lethargy, ataxia	Rash, hepatitis, gingival hypertrophy, coarsening of facial features (in children), hirsutism, lymphadenopathy
Carbamazepine	Nausea, lethargy, ataxia, diplopia, leukopenia	Rash, hyponatremia, aplastic anemia, hepatitis, pancreatitis
Phenobarbital	Hyperactivity (in children), lethargy, cognitive slowing, ataxia	Rash, Stevens-Johnson syndrome, serum sickness, depression, changes in personality
Primidone	As for phenobarbital	As for phenobarbital
Valproic acid	Nausea, tremor, thrombocytopenia, weight loss or weight gain	Hair loss, hepatitis, pancreatitis
Gabapentin	Lethargy, fatigue, dizziness, nausea	None recognized
Lamotrigine	Rash (up to 10%), lethargy, diplopia, nausea	None recognized
Felbamate	Insomnia, nausea, weight loss, decreased appetite, headache	Aplastic anemia, hepatitis
Ethosuximide	Nausea, abdominal discomfort, lethargy, headache	Rash, lupus-like reaction

Treatment of Partial Seizures

Monotherapy

We consider carbamazepine to be the drug of first choice when treating partial (localization-related) epileptic seizures because of its efficacy and lack of cosmetic side effects. Carbamazepine generally requires three times daily dosing. Phenytoin is useful in those cases in which compliance, cost, or risk of hematologic depression makes carbamazepine less desirable. Valproic acid is an attractive alternative to those failing control with carbamazepine or phenytoin. Although also effective, barbiturate medications, such as phenobarbital or primidone, have a significant likelihood of neurobehavioral side effects (such as sedation in adults and hyperactivity in children) and are more likely to require discontinuation for this reason. Recommendations for monotherapy of partial seizures are shown in Table 6.

In adolescents and adults we initiate carbamazepine in doses of 100 mg (half of a scored 200 mg tablet) three times daily. A written schedule details increases in the daily dose by 100 mg every 3 to 7 days depending on clinical response. Typical side effects include nausea, lethargy or confusion, diplopia, and ataxia. The target dose for initial therapy is 400 mg three times per day, to generate serum drug levels in most laboratories of 6 to 12 μg per milliliter. We will attempt

Table 6 Anticonvulsant Medications for Partial Seizures: Monotherapy

PARTIAL SEIZURE	FIRST-CHOICE OPTIONS	SECOND-CHOICE OPTIONS
All types	Carbamazepine Phenytoin Valproic acid	Phenobarbital Primidone Gabapentin Lamotrigine Felbamate

to use a twice-daily dosing regimen in patients with likely compliance problems.

Phenytoin does not usually require a taper-up schedule and can be started at the initial maintenance dose of 300 mg per day. Steady-state serum levels will be achieved in 5 to 7 days. Patients with difficult to control seizures, or those taking generic phenytoin (which tends to have lower bioavailability), should divide their medication into two or three daily doses. If rapid loading is desired to obtain more rapid seizure control, we give adult patients 1,000 mg divided into three doses on the first day, then 300 mg daily thereafter. Ataxia, somnolence, and cognitive problems are common after a loading dose. Uncommonly, chronic use of phenytoin may cause megaloblastic anemia or osteomalacia. Target serum levels for phenytoin are 10 to 20 μg per milliliter. Phenytoin exhibits zero-order kinetics at higher serum levels, and so small increases in dose may lead to large increases in serum level.

We start valproic acid in the form of divalproex sodium (Depakote) since our experience indicates that it is better tolerated than valproic acid. The starting dose for adults is 125 mg three times daily, with an increase of 125 mg daily every 3 to 7 days for an initial target dose of 500 mg three times daily. Many patients may tolerate twice-daily dosing. Typical side effects of stomach upset, thinning of the hair, tremor, and weight gain or weight loss should be discussed. Valproic acid can depress platelet function or, at higher serum levels, lead to thrombocytopenia, and therefore should be used cautiously prior to surgical procedures. Target serum levels are 50 to 100 μg per milliliter, although many patients require and tolerate higher levels up to 150 μg per milliliter.

Felbamate is effective in treating partial and secondarily generalized seizures in adults, both as monotherapy and as add-on treatment in combination with other medications. Since its introduction in the United States in 1993, this medication has been associated with uncommon but serious adverse events, specifically aplastic anemia and liver injury. A subsequent FDA advisory has effectively restricted the use of this drug. Currently we recommend the use of felbamate only for those patients who have failed adequate seizure control with other medications, and in whom the potential benefits of improved seizure control outweigh the potential of risk. Close follow-up and monitoring of these selected patients is mandatory.

Further study and experience are required before recommending gabapentin or lamotrigine as monotherapy for partial or secondarily generalized seizures. However, the effectiveness of these medications as add-on therapy and the preliminary results as monotherapy look promising.

Table 7 Options for Polytherapy for Partial Seizures

Carbamazepine plus valproic acid
Carbamazepine plus phenobarbital
Carbamazepine plus gabapentin
Carbamazepine plus lamotrigine
Carbamazepine plus clorazepate
Phenytoin plus valproic acid
Phenytoin plus phenobarbital
Phenytoin plus gabapentin
Phenytoin plus lamotrigine
Valproic acid plus gabapentin
Valproic acid plus lamotrigine
Phenobarbital (or primidone) plus gabapentin
Phenobarbital (or primidone) plus lamotrigine

"Rational Polypharmacy"

If possible, we treat seizures with monotherapy. A single medication used optimally often provides seizure control with reduced potential for side effects, drug interactions, and high cost. "Rational polypharmacy" arises from the recognition that approximately 5 to 20 percent of patients can be better controlled with combinations of AEDs, usually two medications. Rarely, three medications may be required. Controlled studies demonstrating the superiority of one regimen over another have not been performed. We therefore employ medications with complementary features: different mechanisms of action, different profiles of side effects, and low potential for drug-drug interaction. Recommendations for polytherapy of partial seizures are shown in Table 7.

The combination of carbamazepine and phenytoin is *not* recommended; these drugs overlap in their mechanism of action and in their side effect profiles. Carbamazepine or phenytoin do combine well with valproic acid or (low-dose) phenobarbital.

The newer anticonvulsants have been best studied in combination with traditional drugs, since the pivotal studies proving their efficacy have consisted of placebo-controlled add-on trials in patients with intractable epilepsy, usually taking one or two other AEDs.

Gabapentin is particularly appealing as an add-on medication for patients with partial seizures because it is generally well tolerated. It binds negligibly to serum proteins, is excreted by the kidneys, does not induce hepatic enzymes, and interacts little with other AEDs. The relatively modest efficacy of this medication when used in combination (approximately 30 percent of subjects demonstrated 50 percent improvement in the frequency of partial onset seizures) has been tempered by the recognition that patients may have improved seizure control at doses higher than those used in the clinical trials. Although the upper end of the dose-response curve has yet to be defined, doses of up to 4,800 mg per day may be recommended in adults, with monitoring for clinical side effects, most typically sedation and ataxia. Gabapentin is initiated with 300 mg per day on the first day of therapy, with 300 mg twice daily on the second day and 300 mg three times daily on the third day. Dosing can be increased by 300 mg per day to initial total daily doses of 1,800 to 3,600 mg.

The combination of traditional medications with lamotrigine can also be advocated. We begin lamotrigine with 25 mg tablets twice daily and increase by 25 mg once every week to

Table 8 Anticonvulsant Medications for Generalized Seizures: Monotherapy

GENERALIZED SEIZURE	FIRST-CHOICE OPTIONS	SECOND-CHOICE OPTIONS
Tonic-clonic	Valproic acid, phenytoin	Carbamazepine, phenobarbital, primidone, lamotrigine, felbamate
Tonic, clonic, atonic	Valproic acid	Phenobarbital, lamotrigine, felbamate
Absence	Ethosuximide, valproic acid	Acetazolamide, lamotrigine, felbamate
Myoclonic	Valproic acid, clonazepam	Lamotrigine, phenobarbital, felbamate

achieve target doses of 200 mg twice daily. As with gabapentin, the upper end of the dose-response curve has not yet been defined, and more aggressive dosing of this medication may prove effective. The hepatic metabolism of lamotrigine is highly influenced by other medications. Enzyme-inducing drugs such as carbamazepine, phenytoin, and phenobarbital decrease the half-life of lamotrigine and increase its dosing requirements. Conversely, valproic acid significantly increases the half-life of lamotrigine, and more cautious dosing is necessary. The risk of skin rash (seen in approximately 10 percent of patients) appears to be increased with rapid titration to the target dose or in combination with valproic acid.

Benzodiazepines, such as diazepam, lorazepam, clonazepam, and clorazepate, are most useful for short-term treatment or for interrupting seizure clusters. Long-term use of benzodiazepines tends to result in tachyphylaxis and sedation.

Our personal strategy for treating seizures of partial origin is as follows: we begin with either carbamazepine or phenytoin. If the initial drug fails, we then attempt monotherapy with the other. If this fails, we then try valproic acid, initially in combination, and as monotherapy if successful. Gabapentin is also an add-on drug of choice, used either before or after valproic acid. With continued seizures or unacceptable side effects, we next try add-on lamotrigine or phenobarbital, or (after obtaining informed consent) monotherapy with felbamate.

Treatment of Generalized Seizures

Monotherapy

Patients with generalized epilepsy syndromes frequently have more than one seizure type and therefore require the use of broad-spectrum medications or, for some, a combination of medications. For instance, patients with juvenile myoclonic epilepsy (a prototypical primary generalized epilepsy) usually have myoclonic and generalized epilepsy) usually have myoclonic and generalized tonic-clonic seizures and may have absence seizures as well. Recommendations for monotherapy of generalized seizures are shown in Table 8.

We consider valproic acid to be the drug of choice in treating most patients with generalized epilepsy over 2 years of age. This drug has a broad spectrum of activity for the different seizures of generalized onset, including generalized tonic-clonic, myoclonic, absence, and the so-called minor motor seizure events (tonic, atonic, and so on). We will increase the dose to achieve blood levels in the 130 to 150 μg per milliliter range if patients continue to have seizures and are tolerating the medication well from a clinical point of view. (Most laboratories report a "therapeutic" range of 50 to 100 μg per milliliter.) Dose-related side effects that may ultimately limit further increases in dosage include lethargy, nausea, tremor, or thrombocytopenia. This medication is usually well tolerated with little or no effect on cognition.

Ethosuximide occupies an important niche for treating children with childhood or juvenile absence epilepsy. Ethosuximide is effective for absence seizures and has low toxicity, and therefore is most often used as monotherapy for this group of patients. However, it is a "narrow-spectrum" drug and may not be satisfactory for those patients who also have generalized tonic-clonic seizures. These patients are better treated with valproic acid, with or without ethosuximide in combination.

Myoclonic seizures are notoriously difficult to treat. Valproic acid is our recommended treatment of choice. Benzodiazepines, such as clonazepam, may also be useful, as either the primary or adjunctive drug, although their sedative character and tendency to pharmacologic habituation limit their attractiveness.

Felbamate is a broad-spectrum anticonvulsant that deserves continued consideration for patients with refractory generalized epilepsy. It is of particular use in children with Lennox-Gastaut syndrome, where the benefits of seizure control in this devastating condition may outweigh the potential risks. Lamotrigine is a broad-spectrum drug that may eventually find a role in monotherapy for generalized seizures, pending further study and clinical experience.

Phenobarbital may be useful as a second-tier medication, or adjunct, though once again it is limited by its potential for neurobehavioral side effects. Phenytoin and carbamazepine are effective for generalized tonic-clonic seizures but have poor efficacy against the other generalized-onset seizure types described previously. Carbamazepine may exacerbate seizures in children with generalized epilepsy.

"Rational Polypharmacy"

Valproic acid may be effective in combination with ethosuximide for absence seizures, with clonazepam for myoclonic seizures, and with phenytoin for tonic-clonic seizures. Additional recommendations are shown in Table 9.

Valproic acid and lamotrigine combines two relatively broad-spectrum drugs that have proven useful for some patients, particularly those with symptomatic epilepsy with mixed seizure types. This combination invokes significant drug-drug interactions that require careful dosing and increased monitoring, specifically due to the tendency for valproic acid to increase the half-life of lamotrigine from 24 hours to approximately 70 hours. Consequently, dosing of lamotrigine in combination with valproic acid should be started at 25 mg every other day and increased cautiously by 25 mg increments.

Table 9 Options for Polytherapy for Generalized Seizures

GENERALIZED TONIC-CLONIC SEIZURES
Valproic acid plus phenytoin
Valproic acid plus lamotrigine
Valproic acid plus felbamate
Valproic acid plus phenobarbital
Phenytoin plus lamotrigine
Phenytoin plus felbamate
Felbamate plus lamotrigine
ABSENCE SEIZURES
Valproic acid plus ethosuximide
Valproic acid plus acetazolamide
Valproic acid plus lamotrigine
Valproic acid plus clonazepam
Valproic acid plus felbamate
MYOCLONIC SEIZURES
Valproic acid plus clonazepam
Valproic acid plus phenobarbital
Valproic acid plus felbamate
Valproic acid plus lamotrigine

SPECIAL POPULATIONS

The Elderly

Along with the very young, older patients have an increased incidence of seizures and epilepsy. Seizures in the elderly are more likely to be symptomatic in cause and partial in type, with seizure activity secondary to acquired pathologies such as stroke.

Aging and coexisting medical conditions may alter the distribution and clearance of AEDs, particularly in the setting of hepatic or renal difficulties. The ranges for "therapeutic" blood levels have not been validated in this age group. The elderly are frequently taking large numbers of other medications, raising the potential for complex and myriad drug-drug interactions and additive side effects, especially affecting cognition. Older patients may prove to be more vulnerable to the cognitive side effects of AEDs, with barbiturates and benzodiazepines being particularly problematic.

Phenytoin is the most commonly used anticonvulsant in elderly patients. In the absence of more definitive studies in this population, the recommendations just discussed for the treatment of partial and generalized seizures may be applied, but increased caution in dosing and compulsive clinical follow-up is advised.

Women

Women need to be aware that many of the widely used antiseizure medications may reduce the effectiveness of oral contraceptive agents. An oral contraceptive dose equivalent of 50 μg per day or more of ethinyl estradiol may reduce, but not eliminate, the risk of oral contraceptive failure.

Currently there is no drug of first choice for pregnant women. Recommendations for antiseizure medication management during pregnancy stresses the trade-off between poorly controlled convulsive seizures and the potential teratogenic effects of the drugs themselves. If at all possible, plan prior to conception. Appropriate management includes the following:

1. Reduce the number of antiseizure medications to monotherapy, if possible. The medication or medications chosen should be the most effective for the patient's individual seizure type and epileptic condition. If possible, it is best to avoid the use of valproic acid, as the risk of neural tube defects is 1 to 2 percent. This malformation occurs during the first month of gestation and can be monitored by measurement of maternal or amniotic alpha-fetoprotein or by ultrasonography after the eighteenth week of the pregnancy.
2. Supplement with folate 0.4 to 1 mg per day prior to conception, reducing the risk of major malformations (including neural tube defects) that occur early in gestation. Consider giving 1 mg of folate daily to women of childbearing potential.
3. Carefully monitor anticonvulsant dose and blood levels, particularly during the third trimester, when significant changes in the volume of drug distribution and clearance kinetics can be seen.
4. Administer vitamin K (phytonadione 10 mg daily) during the last month of gestation as prophylaxis against hemorrhagic disease of the newborn. The increased risk of neonatal bleeding is due to inhibition of vitamin K transfer across the placenta by the mother's AEDs and subsequent deficiency of vitamin K–dependent clotting factors.

SERUM DRUG LEVELS

The ability to routinely monitor anticonvulsant serum levels represents a major practical advance in the treatment of patients with epilepsy. Blood levels (and, by extrapolation, brain levels) do not always show a predictable relationship to drug dosing.

Levels should be obtained when clinically indicated and not on a "routine" basis. Serum levels are indicated (1) to establish compliance with the anticonvulsant regimen, (2) to establish the current level in patients with uncontrolled seizures where an increase in dose is contemplated, or (3) to correlate blood level with clinical signs of toxicity, where a decrease in dose may be needed.

Serum levels must be individualized to the patient's needs. A "low" value may be perfectly effective and appropriate for one patient, whereas another patient may enjoy seizure control (and a lack of side effects) at a serum level that is considered to be in the "toxic" range. We are careful to explain this to patients so that the dosage is not inadvertently lowered at the time of an emergency room or clinic visit.

CHANGING MEDICATIONS

The first-choice medication may require change because of inadequate seizure control or unacceptable side effects. From an actuarial perspective, the second- or third-choice medications are either less likely to work or perhaps more likely to cause adverse side effects. These considerations, which are based on experience with a population of patients, may not apply to the individual patient, and therefore a trial of the alternative medication is justified when the initial choice fails to work. Each medication used should be given an adequate trial and not be discarded prematurely. Failure to maximize the dosing regimen is a frequent cause of medication failure and may necessitate backtracking at a later date for a second, more aggressive trial. Alternatively, a medication may appear to be toxic if introduced too rapidly or if used in combination.

Failure of the initial medication to control seizures should always prompt reconsideration of the original seizure type or, indeed, of the diagnosis of epilepsy itself. Conditions that mimic epileptic seizures, such as psychogenic spells, may need to be considered. Such issues can usually be clarified, if necessary, by video-electroencephalographic monitoring.

We usually perform medication switches over 1 to 2 months, unless serious side effects mandate more rapid changes. If the patient is on monotherapy, we add a second drug to the first and achieve a therapeutic level of the second drug before tapering the first. This minimizes the potential for breakthrough seizures. For patients taking a two-drug regimen, switch of the second drug can usually be made by simultaneous reduction of the original second drug and substitution with the new drug.

■ DISCONTINUING THERAPY

The prognosis for seizure remission can often be predicted based on knowledge of the underlying etiology or identification of the epilepsy syndrome. Decision making at the margins is usually straightforward: patients with progressive neurologic disease will tend to have a continuing seizure risk, and patients with benign self-limited epilepsy syndromes of childhood can be predicted to remit with a high degree of confidence. Patients with known structural pathology or with coexisting neurologic or development problems should be considered as higher-risk patients in comparison to those without such findings.

The role of the routine electroencephalogram (EEG) in predicting risk of relapse following discontinuation of anticonvulsants has been controversial. We believe that the findings on routine EEG offer value in the decision-making process, but only within the context of the entire clinical picture. That is, all other factors being equal, the presence of epileptiform abnormalities indicates increased risk of seizure relapse. However, the power of this finding is relatively modest, as some patients with epileptiform findings may be successfully tapered off medication, and many patients without such EEG abnormalities may subsequently experience seizures.

The decision to taper and discontinue a medication is made with the patient and family. The consequences of a relapse in seizure activity can vary with age. Adults often contend with greater social disability with loss of seizure control in comparison to children, including such issues as restrictions on driving or occupational problems.

There is no firm rule as to how long a patient must be seizure free before considering the discontinuation of treatment. We feel that patients who have been seizure free for 2 years are potential candidates for medication taper and discontinuation. A shorter period of time may be advocated in younger ages. As a general rule, medications should be tapered over a period of 1 to 2 months. Primidone, in particular, may result in breakthrough seizures as a "withdrawal" phenomenon if tapered too rapidly. We ask patients not to drive for 3 months after the end of the taper.

Suggested Reading

Levy RH, Mattson RH, Meldrum BS. Antiepileptic drugs. 4th ed. New York: Raven Press, 1995.

Mattson RH, Cramer JA, Collins JF, et al. Comparison of carbamazepine, phenobarbital, phenytoin, and primidone in partial and secondarily generalized tonic-clonic seizures. N Engl J Med 1985; 313:145–151.

Mattson RH, Cramer JA, Collins JF, et al. A comparison of valproate with carbamazepine for the treatment of complex partial and secondarily generalized tonic-clonic seizures in adults. N Engl Med 1992; 327:765–771.

Wilder BJ, ed. Rational polypharmacy in the treatment of epilepsy. Neurology 1995; 45 (3 Suppl 2):S1–S38.

Wyllie E. The treatment of epilepsy: Principles and practice. Philadelphia: Lea & Febiger, 1993.

Wyllie E, ed. New developments in antiepileptic drug therapy. Epilepsia 1995; 36 (Suppl 2):S1–S118.

COMPLEX PARTIAL SEIZURES

Barbara E. Swartz, M.D., Ph.D.

DIAGNOSIS

Complex partial seizures are one of the most challenging forms of seizures to treat. By definition, they are not generalized but do involve an alteration or loss of consciousness. The first step in diagnosis of complex partial seizures is to elicit a thorough description of the patient's and significant others' perception of the way the seizures begin and the sequential manifestations of the subsequent behavioral changes. If clear, complex, stereotyped automatisms are described in conjunction with clouding of consciousness, it is reasonable to assume that the patient is having complex partial seizures, and therapy can be started while further evaluation is in progress (Fig. 1). Attention needs to be paid to the presence of auras and their symptoms, to the character of the seizures themselves, to the presence of dysphasia occurring before or after the seizure, and to any other postictal neurologic deficits. This information helps to localize or lateralize the seizures. Further discussion of diagnosis can be found in the Suggested Reading list.

INITIAL ADVICE TO PATIENTS

Patients never present with or have a single complex partial seizure (CPS). This somewhat simplifies the initial discussion. The patient needs to understand that he or she has a chronic condition, which is called epilepsy. This condition is not contagious, not inherently lethal, and, with one possible rare exception, not genetic (if CPS exists). It should also be emphasized that it is usually possible to achieve control of seizures with medication. This is the good news. The bad news is that medication will have to be taken the rest of his or her life, again with rare exceptions; all medications have side effects; it often takes some time to find the right medication or combination; and the medications must be taken only as prescribed. I also warn that frequent CPSs over several years may cause memory impairment. The worst news is that driving must be suspended until seizures are controlled, (the exact duration varies from state to state); the current recommendation of the Epilepsy Foundation of America (EFA) is at least 6 months. The physician must be informed about the particular laws of the state he or she practices in, and in particular must explain the reporting guidelines to the patient. It must be clear to the patient and significant others that his or her odd behaviors are not under the patient's control and are not insanity. The patient should be informed about the ADA guidelines or referred to the local EFA chapter for information on this and other advocacy issues that may arise.

This first discussion must also include an interview about the patient's lifestyle and relationship of seizures to external events such as sleep, alcohol, menses, work, stress, and meals. The importance of regular eating and sleeping habits and avoidance of excess alcohol cannot be overemphasized and will probably need repeating more than once. If the patient is a woman who desires pregnancy, the risks of anticonvulsants should also be discussed early rather than late, with a plan for how pregnancy can be approached. However, no study has shown that simple or complex partial seizures without generalization and in the absence of status are dangerous to a fetus.

THERAPY

Pharmacology

I recommend initiation of pharmacologic treatment even if seizures are very brief and nondebilitating or are purely nocturnal, because one can never predict when a tonic-clonic seizure or even status will occur. There is also some experimental and clinical evidence that complex partial seizures can destroy hippocampal neurons. Nevertheless, the advisability of all treatment modalities should be judged in relationship to acute and chronic side effects, and to the lifestyle of the patient, as well as to pharmacologic efficacy. Given the large number of anticonvulsants available today, it is ideal to make a diagnosis of the seizure type or epilepsy syndrome prior to initiating therapy, but that is rarely possible in today's medical environment. Therefore, I start with an interictal electroencephalogram (EEG), with sleep and nasopharyngeal, or true temporal leads as my first diagnostic test. This is done before therapy when the diagnosis of CPS cannot be made on the basis of the history. Seizure types that may be confused with CPS are atypical absence and absence with simple automatisms. If the EEG supports atypical absence, I obtain a magnetic resonance image (MRI) and treat with valproic acid if it does not show a focal lesion. An EEG consistent with primary generalized epilepsy (covered elsewhere), or one in which almost all the spike-wave complexes show secondary bilateral synchrony, also leads to initiation of valproic acid. I know of no published data to support my choice in the latter group; it is simply my personal preference.

Table 1 gives my suggestions for the initial and maintenance doses for the five anticonvulsants I would consider in my major armamentarium. Some have common or particularly bothersome side effects, and my recommendation for serum chemistries monitoring is also given. As just mentioned, for typical complex partial seizures I begin with carbamazepine. I also obtain an MRI and interictal EEG in this group as part of my initial evaluation. The reason is that some patients with potentially malignant lesions can be controlled for some time on anticonvulsants, but the appropriate therapy in this group is surgery *before* neurologic deficits occur.

In Figure 1, I also segregate out a group in whom the EEG shows frequent repetitive focal spike-wave discharges. For this group I recommend surface video-EEG ictal monitoring, because they are at risk for subclinical seizures. If these are demonstrated, and carbamazepine therapy has been maximized, additional or other anticonvulsants should be initiated. I also suggest monitoring with video-EEG if the patient

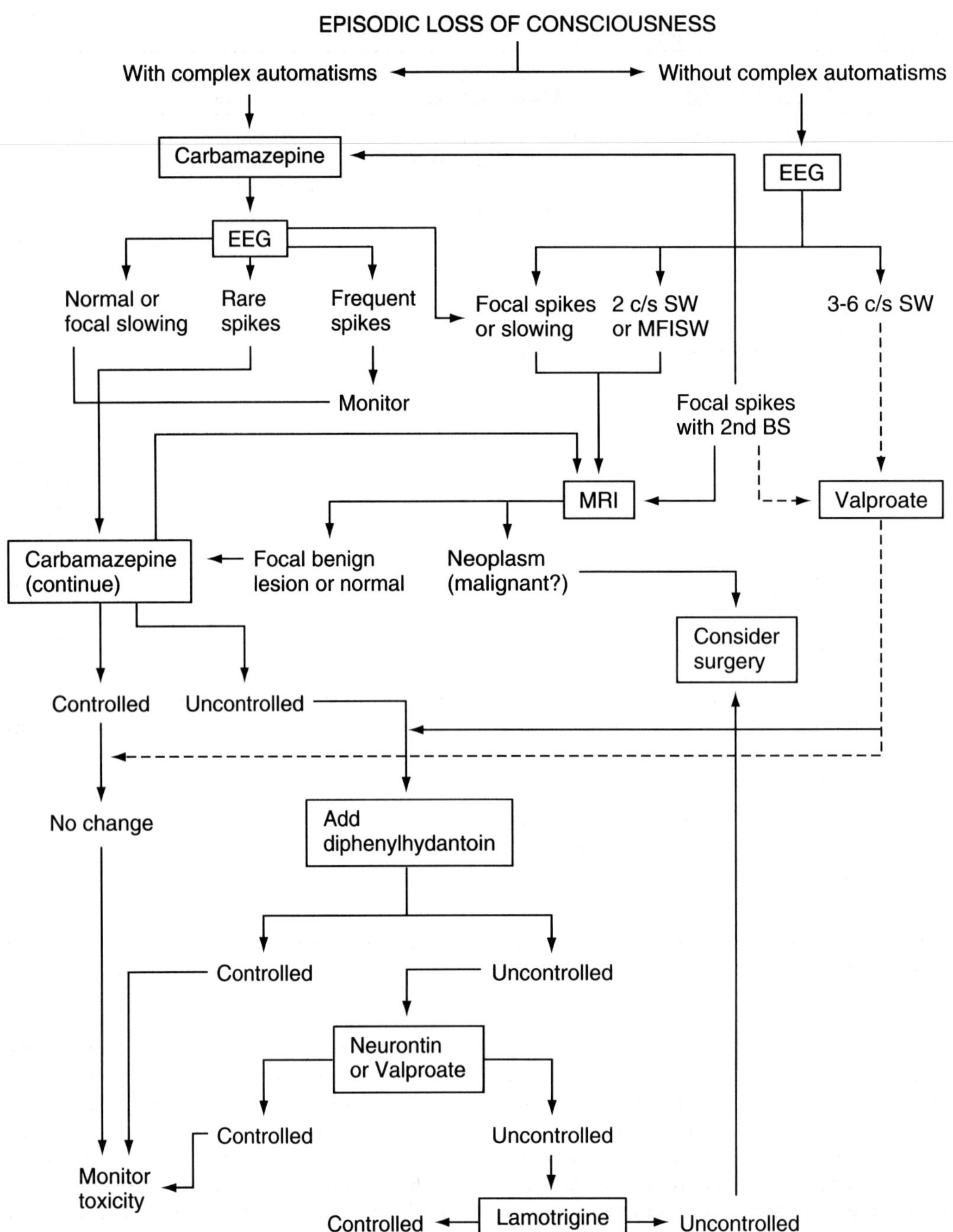

Figure 1
Approach to management of complex partial seizures. The decision tree moves downward except when otherwise indicated by arrows. Dotted line indicates probable primary generalized epilepsy. EEG, electroencephalogram; MRI, magnetic resonance imaging; BS, benign seizure; SW, spike wave; MFISW, multifocal independent spike wave.

reports frequent fluctuations in behavior and cognitive functioning, again suggesting seizures.

My second line drug is diphenylhydantoin, which I usually add to the first drug and, if control is achieved, attempt to taper off the first drug. Many drugs give a "honeymoon" period of 1 to 3 months, so I do not begin the taper before 4 months have passed. If control has not been achieved, I never try to taper off the first drug with the hope that the second alone will be more efficacious than were the two together. I do taper people off multiple drugs when side effects are intolerable, whether or not seizures are controlled. My general rule for tapering is a one tablet reduction each three half-lives. "Rational polytherapy" would dictate that drugs such as carbamazepine and diphenylhydantoin not be used together because they have similar mechanisms of action. Nevertheless, clinical experience shows this combination to be quite effective in many individuals.

As a substitute for diphenylhydantoin (see the following),

Table 1 Anticonvulsants Used to Treat Complex Partial Seizures

DRUG	STARTING DOSE	SERUM MONITORING*	MAINTENANCE DOSE	SIDE EFFECTS
Carbamazepine	100 mg b.i.d. × 3 da. 100 mg q.i.d. × 3 da. 200 mg t.i.d. × 1 wk, check level and titrate.	CBC with diff., liver functions, electrolytes. Repeat q mo. × 3, then 6 mo, 12 mo.	200 mg t.i.d. to 600 mg q.i.d., depending on patient, cost, etc.	Diplopia, ataxia, rash on sun-exposed areas (benign), SIADH, liver and marrow toxicity, ↓ HR, granulocytopenia (dose-dependent)
Valproic acid	125 mg b.i.d. × 3 da. 250 mg b.i.d. × 4 da. 250 mg q.i.d. × 1 wk, check levels, titrate.	CBC with diff., liver functions, amylase, electrolytes, ammonia. Repeat q mo. × 3, then 6 mo, 12 mo.	250 mg t.i.d. to 1,000 mg q.i.d.	Nausea—try sprinkles, ↓ platelets—use L-carnitine; 300 mg t.i.d., hair loss—Zn^{++}, Mg^{++} supplements; tremor—no treatment unless severe; weight gain—diet, exercise; polyuria at high doses—avoid dehydration
Diphenylhydantoin	100 mg t.i.d. × 1 wk. 300 mg q.h.s. × 1 wk., check trough level. Repeat 1 mo, 3 mo, 6 mo, 1 yr.	CBC with diff, liver function	200 mg qd to 300 mg b.i.d.	Ataxia, gum hypertrophy, nystagmus, peripheral neuropathy, sedation, depression
Gabapentin	300 mg qd × 1 da. 300 mg b.i.d. × 1 da. 300 mg t.i.d. × 1 da. 400 mg t.i.d.	CBC with diff, liver function electrolytes. Repeat 1 mo, 3 mo, 6 mo, 1 yr.	400 mg t.i.d. to 1,200 mg t.i.d.	Euphoria, irritability, sedation, headache
Lamotrigine	25 mg qd × 3 da. 50 mg qd × 4 da. 50 mg b.i.d. × 1 wk. 100 mg b.i.d. × 1 wk., 100 mg t.i.d.	CBC with diff, liver functions. Repeat at 1 mo, 3 mo, 6 mo, 1 yr.	100 mg t.i.d. to 500 mg qd in divided doses	Rash, ataxia, sedation

*Serum monitoring may be reduced in less litigious environments and as we gain more experience with the newer anticonvulsants.
CBC, complete blood chemistry; diff, differential; SIADH, syndrome of inappropriate antidiuretic hormone; HR, heart rate.

or if seizures are uncontrolled, I try gabapentin or valproic acid added to the other anticonvulsants and taper off the diphenylhydantoin. Valproic acid is difficult to use with carbamazepine because each induces the other's metabolism, but the combination is often effective when therapeutic levels are achieved. The physician must be aware that toxicity can exist when levels of either drug are normal or even low due to metabolites. Other anticonvulsants can also lower valproate levels, but less so. I particularly like valproic acid when frequent tonic-clonic seizures coexist with CPS. Gabapentin will become a popular drug whether or not it is highly efficacious, because it is very easy to titrate the dose. It has no interference with other anticonvulsants or liver-metabolized drugs and has a very high therapeutic-toxic ratio. The dose may need to reach 3,600 mg per day before significant seizure control is achieved. Finally, lamotrigine, the most recently released anticonvulsant, should be mentioned. Although the package insert makes it appear hard to use, I have not found it so. With a conservative approach it is well tolerated and has decreased, although not eliminated, CPS in some of my patients.

There are other medications available that are not mentioned in Figure 1. I use either phenobarbital or primidone occasionally, in spite of the cognitive and behavioral depression, usually in combination with carbamazepine, and some patients tolerate it well. I almost never use benzodiazepines for chronic therapy of CPS because of the tachyphylaxis and risk of serious withdrawal seizures and pulmonary edema. However, I often prescribe 2 mg lorazepam orally or sublingually to take after the first aura or seizure in patients whose seizures typically come in flurries. I use methylphenytoin when other medications fail. Its side effect profile is like that of diphenylhydantoin but with a much lower therapeutic-toxic ratio. It almost always controls seizures for several months, which is useful to stabilize patients prior to the intracarotid amytal test and surgery. Vigabatrin is expected to be released soon. I have no personal experience with it, but reports from Europe and studies under way in the United States are encouraging, as it appears to have a broad spectrum of action with a high therapeutic index. Information on other, infrequently used anticonvulsants can be found in the Suggested Reading list.

Advice to Patients Taking Anticonvulsants

Carbamazepine. I advise patients that the typical trilogy of side effects for all anticonvulsants, namely sedation, nausea, and ataxia, may be encountered but are usually either transient or occur only at high doses. The most frequent side effect I have seen with carbamazepine is diplopia, which is more common in individuals with pre-existing strabismus. I warn that frequent blood tests to look for marrow and liver toxicity will be done over the first 3 months but less frequently after that, and that anyone can experience an "idiosyncratic" reaction to a drug that may not occur when it is first started. I advise that a drop in the white blood cell count is common and usually of no clinical significance, and so I ask that I be contacted before the patient follows the advice of another physician to discontinue the drug. With this and all other anticonvulsants I warn that patients should never voluntarily discontinue or involuntarily run out of medicine because of the risk of life-threatening status epilepticus. A benign macular rash in sun-exposed areas is not uncommon and is best managed with protective clothing and sunscreen.

Diphenylhydantoin. Diphenylhydantoin is a highly effective agent that is easy to use, but every medical student has had to memorize its multiple acute and chronic, dose-dependent, and idiopathic side effects. As a rule, I give everyone to whom I prescribe diphenylhydantoin 1 mg of folic acid per day and increase this to 3 mg if the patient has any pre-existing peripheral neuropathy or gum hypertrophy, or is a woman of childbearing age. I hesitate to start this drug in children or young adults who may not want to suffer from hirsutism, coarsening of features, and acne, although these are not universal effects. I monitor for liver toxicity early in the course of treatment, and I warn about ataxia, sedation, nausea, and possible depression. I emphasize the importance of dental hygiene and a good calcium intake, as I have had a number of patients on diphenylhydantoin who suffered from easily induced or pathologic fractures. I also inquire about distal burning or paresthesias and examine for peripheral neuropathy at each visit.

Valproic Acid. In addition to the risk of bone marrow toxicity, especially affecting platelet production, the patient should be warned of the symptoms of pancreatitis. Minor symptoms of valproate toxicity that are commonly seen are tremor, weight gain, and hair loss, which is more pronounced in male pattern baldness. Other hair changes may occur, such as straight to curly or color change (red to brown). I give L-carnitine 330 mg daily for signs of decreased platelets, increased serum ammonia, or weight gain and recommend heavy metal supplements (especially zinc) for hair changes, although I warn that there is no proof that these approaches can prevent the side effect from worsening. One can argue that everyone could be treated with L-carnitine for mitochondrial toxicity, but it is not clear that everyone needs it, and, unlike folic acid, carnitine is not inexpensive. At high doses (>2 daily) valproate may evoke polyuria and even enuresis, because the high salt load requires a large amount of urine to excrete. Patients should be advised about this and warned against dehydration. Ataxia does not occur, but nausea is frequent, and although food significantly decreases the rate of absorption of this drug, one may have to resort to sprinkles, which are well tolerated and give good serum levels. Sedation is reported but is rare in my experience.

Gabapentin. This agent is newly released and, as mentioned, is very easy to use. The side effects are the usual trilogy, but in general it is well tolerated. I have had to stop several patients' therapy with this agent due to irritability and dysphoric mood swings, although this is not discussed much in the literature, so I don't bias the patient to expect this until more information is accumulated. Euphoria may occur; I have seen it only once. No significant toxicity is reported or expected because of its renal excretion. However, given my general discomfort with using anticonvulsants without monitoring, and the medical-legal environment of California, I have elected to monitor for liver, electrolyte, and marrow toxicity as I do the other drugs.

Lamotrigine. This is another new agent with a broader spectrum than gabapentin, but it is described as more difficult to use. I have not found its initiation too onerous. The package insert explains the dosing clearly; you must go slower if the patient is on valproate and can go faster if they are on anything else. Patients should be warned that they will be at subtherapeutic levels for some time. The main side effect, other than the usual trilogy, is a rash. Tell your patients to call if one appears and then inquire if it is tender or pruritic (tender is bad), flat or raised (raised is bad), and sparing or including mucous membranes (including is bad). The patient must be seen for any of the bad signs or if fever is present to decide whether hospitalization is necessary, and the drug should be stopped. For benign rash, decrease the dose and rate of increase and monitor more closely. I have initiated therapy more slowly than recommended by the package insert and have seen no rash in a handful of patients. Doses of 300 to 500 mg daily are recommended; above that, there appears to be a plateau effect.

Surgery

Since entire texts are devoted to this topic, it is no small task to provide a brief summary. The first question, that of who should have surgery, is not trivial. I am a strong advocate of surgery given some studies that suggest that the natural history of CPS is gradual deterioration, with ever-worsening seizures and memory over the years. However, I have some patients who stubbornly refuse to consider surgery and gradually have come under complete control, even without a clear relationship to medication changes. It is not obvious what distinguishes this relatively small group from the more typical one, so I do not rush to recommend surgery before I have accumulated significant personal experience with each subject. A good mnemonic is the rule of "fours." A patient who has had seizures for more than 4 years that have never been controlled on therapeutic levels of four major anticonvulsants, and who has four or more seizures per month, should be referred for a surgical evaluation. Some people cannot tolerate two seizures per month; some may be controlled on the fifth drug tried. Nevertheless, these are reasonable guidelines.

Figure 2 is an algorithm for a surgical approach to intractable seizures. There is likely to be little or no disagreement with the left-hand side of the algorithm, and little disagreement about the need to implant nonlesional cases that appear to have extratemporal foci based on electroclinical, neurologic, and neuropsychological tests. Some would not ap-

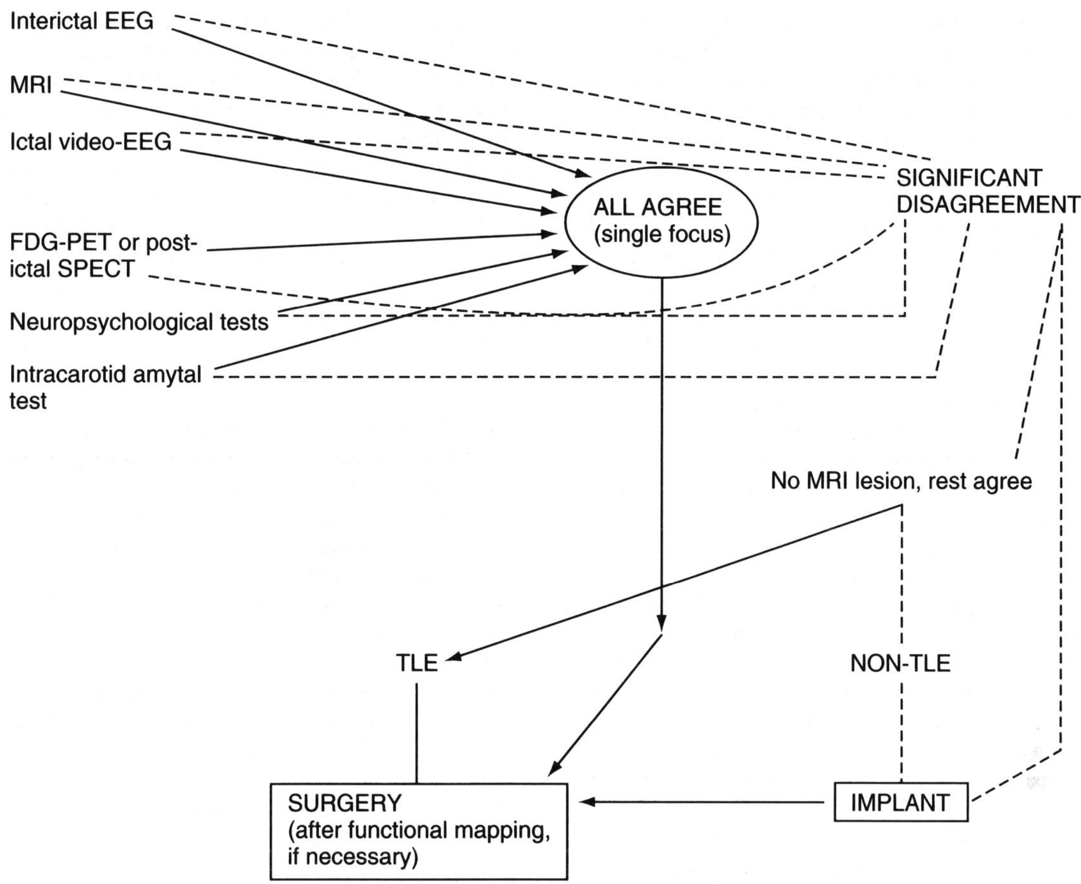

Figure 2
An algorithm for presurgical evaluation of intractable complex partial seizures. Decision tree goes down except for dashed lines, which indicate more testing needed, and where arrows indicate otherwise. EEG, electroencephalogram; MRI, magnetic resonance imaging; FDG-PET, fluorodeoxyglucose positron emission tomography; SPECT, single photon emission computed tomography; TLE, thin-layer electrophoresis.

proach this group at all, which is appropriate if either the neurologist or neurosurgeon is uncomfortable with such cases. Some of the other decision pathways may be more controversial, and all cases must be individualized.

Temporal Lobe Epilepsy

In our group (California Comprehensive Epilepsy Program) we implant subjects who have a high probability of temporal lobe epilepsy but in whom it is unclear whether the focus is medial, lateral, or combined, because the prognosis is worse in the lateral group (70 percent seizure free), and it is best to be able to give the patient accurate information about his or her chance of seizure control. If a patient has medical temporal seizures as determined by intracranial ictal recordings, or by surface recordings with a sphenoid onset and simple seizures consisting of an arrest and oral alimentary automatisms, with or without later dystonic postures and reactive automatisms, he may be a candidate for the so-called Spencer procedure. Naturally the neuroimaging studies have either to agree with or not contradict the diagnosis. This procedure is a limited lateral tip resection (2 to 3 cm) followed by complete amygdalohippocampectomy. This group has an excellent response to surgery—90 percent can be seizure free on medication. Approximately 25 percent will be able to discontinue medication. The medial-lateral group (ictal onsets simultaneously in lateral neocortex and hippocampus) will be more likely to rapidly generalize. Such patients will generally require larger lateral resections (5 to 6 cm) in addition to amygdalohippocampectomy. The chances of being seizure free with this type of seizure focus are intermediate between the medial and lateral types. The lateral temporal type is most difficult to diagnose in the absence of a structural lesion, although auditory hallucinations and conscious dysphasia are strong clues. We have generally also approached these with lateral plus medial resections given the extreme susceptibility of the hippocampus to epileptogenesis. However, if there is no sign of medial temporal dysfunction on neuropsychological tests, intracarotid sodium amytal test, and neuroimaging studies, we may recommend trying focal lateral resection. In our experience this is a palliative, not curative, procedure unless a short-lived lateral temporal lesion is present. For all types of epilepsy surgery we use intraoperative electrocorticography (ECC), relying on interictal spiking, absence of fast frequencies, and presence of polymorphic delta slowing, to guide the extent of the cortical resection. We do not "chase spikes" or perform postoperative corticography.

Extratemporal, Focal Seizures

There is argument about whether implantation is needed when a structural lesion is present. I still require all noninvasive data to agree, for although the epileptogenic zones are more likely to be in the vicinity of a lesion (rather than at the lesion itself), it may be impossible to discern how close or even how remote it is from the lesion. I have seen many patients with intractable seizures who had previous removal of a lesion. I have seen many patients with intractable seizures who had previous removal of a lesion "to control my seizures." If the lesion is located near eloquent or sensory-motor cortex, functional mapping should be used. My preference is to do this with an implantation of a grid of electrodes over and surrounding the lesion, with ictal recordings and functional mapping made in the more readily controlled environment of the patient's room. When this is not possible, and when all data point to a focus near the lesion, intraoperative mapping and ECC are performed.

When no structural lesion is present, even with newer techniques, such as postictal single photon emission computed tomography (SPECT), most groups would implant using large subdural grids. I find this objectionable because if a recording procedure is used to screen for epileptogenic zones it should be as minimally invasive as possible. Thus, when surface recordings and the nature of the seizures themselves do not give enough information to locate a focus, we generally use subdural strips, which are much easier to tolerate. Only 25 percent of the time have I had to go to a second implant with large grids to fine-tune the focus localization or do functional mapping. Another reasonable approach started by the Cleveland Clinic group involves putting spaced epidural pegs in the skull prior to implant.

Even in the absence of a structural lesion I would consider bypassing electrode implantation if the electroclinical manifestations and other noninvasive data pointed to one focus. For instance, I have evaluated a patient whose aura consisted of feeling as if his left hand were not his, followed by left hand and arm paresthesias and posturing. Sometimes a secondarily generalized seizure followed. His interictal EEG showed an occasional P4 spike wave; his ictal recordings started with rhythmic slowing in that region as well. Since there was no structural lesion on MRI and fluorodeoxyglucose positron emission tomography was normal, the surgical group concluded that he should be implanted. The electroclinical manifestations coupled with the neurologic examination, which showed left upper extremity neglect, could not have come from anywhere but the right parietal lobe, but there is an enormous lack of faith in classical neurodiagnostics that is sometimes unwarranted.

Suggested Reading

Broglin D, Delgado-Escueta AV, Walsh GO, et al. Clinical approach to the patient with seizures. In: Chauvel P, Delgado-Escueta AV, et al., eds. Frontal lobe seizures and epilepsies: Adv in Neurology, Vol. 57, New York: Raven Press, 1992; 59–88.

Engel J Jr, ed. Surgical treatment of the epilepsies. New York: Raven Press, 1993.

Levy RH, Mattson RH, Meldrum BS, eds. Antiepileptic drugs. 4th ed. New York: Raven Press, 1995.

Lüders HO, ed. Epilepsy surgery. New York: Raven Press, 1995.

Swartz BE. Unusual seizure types. Semin Neurol 1995; 15:151–157.

FIRST TONIC-CLONIC SEIZURE IN AN ADULT: TREATMENT AND PROPHYLAXIS

Nathan Watemberg, M.D.
John M. Pellock, M.D.

Tonic-clonic convulsions are common. Up to 6 percent of the population will experience at least one nonfebrile seizure during their lives. Therefore the physician is often faced with deciding whether or not to start the patient on antiepileptic drugs (AEDs) after a first event. The etiology, if known, plays a major role in the decision-making process, but the social and economic implications of the convulsion, as well as the patient's and his or her relatives' perception of the significance of the seizure may affect the physician's course of action. The patient's probability of developing more seizures should be assessed, always balancing the potential benefits versus the risks of implementing long-term pharmacologic therapy. Finally, some patients may require treatment during the initial seizure if it is prolonged (status epilepticus), although this does not necessarily imply the need for chronic therapy thereafter.

■ WAS THE EVENT REALLY A SEIZURE?

Previously known as *grand mal* seizures, generalized tonic-clonic (GTC) seizures are among the most impressive happenings in clinical medicine. They may be primarily generalized, involving simultaneous paroxysmal neuronal activity arising from both cerebral hemispheres, or they may have a partial (focal) onset followed by secondary generalization. Frequently the focal onset prior to generalization is too brief to be noticed or may not be clinically apparent. For this reason many instances of secondarily generalized tonic-clonic events are misinterpreted as primary generalized convulsions.

Table 1 Acute Diagnostic Workup After a First Tonic-Clonic Seizure in an Adult

HISTORY AND NEUROLOGIC FINDINGS	SEIZURE TYPE	EEG	LUMBAR PUNCTURE	CT OR MRI
Normal	Provoked	Yes	Yes, if febrile	Yes
Normal	Unprovoked	Yes	No	Yes
Abnormal	Provoked	Yes	Yes	Yes
Abnormal	Unprovoked	Yes	No	Yes

EEG, electroencephalography.

The first step in the decision-making process is to establish whether the described event was really a GTC seizure. Patients experiencing GTC convulsions have no recollection of the event and may show evidence of trauma sustained upon falling to the ground, such as skin lacerations or abrasions. During the tonic phase the tongue can be bitten by clenching teeth, and urinary incontinence can occur. Postictal drowsiness is common. These clues support the diagnosis of GTC seizures. Patients may have GTC without any of these features, but when there is no clinical, electroencephalographic (EEG), or radiologic evidence of an organic cause, their absence suggests nonepileptic paroxysmal events, such as conversion reactions or pseudoseizures.

Next, a detailed description of the event is obtained. The patient's relatives and the witnesses to the seizure should be interviewed in an effort to establish the type of seizure (generalized, partial, complex partial, or partial with secondary generalization). Seizure features such as preictal behavior (confusion or abrupt onset), the initial body parts involved (partial or generalized), and the pattern of muscle activity (tonic, clonic, or tonic-clonic) assist in classifying the seizure and in deciding on further diagnostic workup. The duration of the event should be assessed to avoid overlooking episodes of status epilepticus.

Sometimes the event is described vaguely or is not witnessed, precluding a diagnosis by clinical features. Even after ancillary tests have been performed, whether or not the described first event was a seizure may be uncertain.

■ INITIAL DIAGNOSTIC EVALUATION

The management of the patient with a first GTC seizure is based on a careful search for the etiology of the convulsion and assessment of the prognosis for the specific condition, the chances for recurrence, and the potential benefits versus side effects of AEDs (Table 1).

Etiology of Seizure and Risk of Recurrence

A description of the different etiologies for a GTC convulsion is beyond the scope of this chapter. However, certain common causes are worth reviewing.

Febrile Seizures

GTC seizures may occur with fever during bacterial meningitis and viral encephalitis. In these cases the patients are usually very ill, and the diagnosis of severe infection can be promptly made by lumbar puncture.

Nonfebrile Convulsions

Primary or secondary GTC seizures are the most common clinical type of seizures in the general population. They occur as part of an epileptic syndrome; in neurologically impaired patients; as a generalization of partial seizure; in an idiopathic (genetic) fashion; or as a symptom of brain injury, toxicity, metabolic derangements, neoplasms, and malformations.

A detailed clinical history and neurologic examination will assist in identifying possible epileptic syndromes. If the patient is mentally retarded, has a major neurologic deficit, or has EEG abnormalities (focal or generalized), the chances of the witnessed seizure being the first of a symptomatic epilepsy syndrome are high. Furthermore, if the convulsion clearly commenced as a partial seizure and then generalized, the possibility of a structural or neoplastic lesion is increased, particularly in adolescents and adults. In these situations long-term pharmacologic therapy usually is indicated. When a convulsion occurs immediately after head trauma, in toxic states, or during metabolic impairment, AED treatment may be brief, and may be discontinued after the abnormality is reversed.

In contrast to pediatric patients, in adults a GTC seizure is more likely to be symptomatic (secondary to a previous or an acute cerebral injury). New or old strokes, traumatic lesions, alcohol and substance abuse, tumors, and metabolic impairments are among the causes. Idiopathic GTC seizures are less likely to occur as age increases. New GTC seizures in adults warrant EEG and neuroimaging studies. If brain lesions are detected, AEDs are initiated after only one seizure. The pharmacologic agents chosen for long-term therapy may be different from those used acutely.

Alcohol-related seizures are common enough to be considered separately. The most frequent presentation is withdrawal seizures, occurring 7 to 48 hours after cessation of drinking. This form of GTC seizure, frequent in busy emergency rooms, in our opinion warrants immediate short-term prophylaxis with AEDs. A short course of oral phenobarbital (90 mg followed by 60 mg 24 hours later and 30 mg the next day) probably provides some protection, especially in individuals with previous episodes of withdrawal seizures. The EEG reveals no paroxysmal activity between seizures. Alcohol abuse can also lower the threshold for GTC seizures in patients with epileptic syndromes, head trauma, strokes, and other brain injuries.

Status Epilepticus

Twelve to 15 percent of cases of first GTC present as status epilepticus. This presentation is more common in adults than

Table 2 Risk of Recurrence After a First Tonic-Clonic Seizure in an Adult

HIGH	LOW
Abnormal neurologic finding	Transient metabolic and toxic states
Mental retardation	Benign rolandic seizures
Abnormal EEG findings	Impact seizures in early non-severe head trauma
Myoclonic jerks, absences, or atonic seizures	
Structural brain lesions	
Family history of epilepsy	
Elderly individuals	

EEG, electroencephalogram.

in children and can occur in patients without previous history of seizures.

Factors That Influence Seizure Recurrence

It is impossible to predict exactly which patients will have more convulsions in the future, but several factors can help the physician decide whether AEDs are indicated after a first episode. Abnormal neurologic findings (such as mental retardation or focal features), structural brain lesions in radiologic studies, or an abnormal EEG indicate that the patient has a higher risk for recurrent seizures. This risk also exists in healthy individuals exposed to an acute severe injury to the brain; those who abuse drugs and alcohol or suffer from a severe acute metabolic derangement, intoxication, or central nervous system infection; and in the elderly. A history of epilepsy in first-degree relatives increases the chances of seizure recurrence. A lower risk exists in patients who sustain a convulsion as the result of such transient insults as mild head trauma, readily corrected hypoglycemia, or hypocalcemia. Because a seizure represents a symptom of neurologic dysfunction that can be transient or have more long-lasting consequences, the etiology, length of seizure, and setting truly help define the likelihood of recurrence (Table 2).

Electroencephalography

Electroencephalography is to epilepsy what electrocardiography is to the study of cardiac arrhythmias, an extremely useful ancillary test. Its clinical usefulness may be affected by several factors. First, the routine EEG records brain electrical activity for a short period of time, usually 30 to 45 minutes. Seizure activity and interictal epileptiform discharges may not appear during a specific recording even though the patient has epilepsy. Second, epileptiform activity may not be evident during wakefulness. EEG during sleep or following sleep deprivation may be necessary. Finally, the EEG requires specialized technicians and expert interpreters, often so that early access to adequate testing is sometimes difficult.

Nevertheless, the EEG is an invaluable diagnostic aid in patients with seizures. It provides reliable information on the degree and type of cerebral paroxysmal activity, enabling the neurologist to determine the presence of encephalopathy, toxic states, subclinical seizures, and severe brain impairment. It also provides useful information in delineating those with primary generalized epilepsy syndromes to help establish proper treatment from those with secondarily generalized epilepsy where additional testing should be pursued.

The chance of a second seizure is markedly increased when spikes are present after the first event. Fifty to 90 percent of these patients will have a second seizure, compared with 12 percent to 25 percent of patients who do not have paroxysmal spikes or spike wave on EEG. Conversely, not infrequently even clearly neurologically affected patients may have a normal record. Although in most individuals with epilepsy the EEG will eventually show epileptiform activity (>90 percent by the fourth recording), the initial decision whether to treat the patient must be based on assessment of the patient's overall risk for further seizures.

Neuroimaging Studies

Head computed tomography (CT) and magnetic resonance imaging (MRI) are helpful in ruling out structural brain lesions that could cause seizures, with MRI now being preferred. These tests have a definite role in the evaluation of a first GTC seizure when there is a history of trauma, previous stroke, asphyxia, or an abnormal neurologic examination, especially with focal findings. They are of little value in patients with a syndrome of benign partial or primary generalized epilepsy who are neurologically normal.

■ THERAPY

Is Pharmacologic Therapy Indicated?

Because of the numerous clinical situations that can produce a first GTC seizure, every case should be considered individually. Several general guidelines are helpful in the decision making. Overall the recurrence risk following a first unprovoked seizure is 14 percent within 1 year and 34 percent within 5 years in the general population. The elderly have a higher risk of recurrence because most of their seizures will prove to be symptomatic.

Although the chances of recurrence are lower in adults than in children, seizures in adults are more frequently associated with structural lesions or other chronic insults to the brain. In these almost always symptomatic cases, we initiate treatment. Seizures due to transient metabolic derangement and substance abuse in an otherwise healthy patient may be managed with short-term AED until the pathologic process has resolved. If no cause or associated neurologic abnormality is found, the case is carefully discussed with the patient and treatment is frequently withheld. Patients should be warned not to drive for 3 to 6 months or longer (depending on state laws) whether or not treatment is initiated.

The need for and duration of therapy for patients with head trauma who have experienced seizures remain controversial. In general we provide prophylactic treatment in the settings of penetrating injury and intraparenchymal hemorrhage. A GTC seizure immediately after head trauma is in most cases a benign event. If no other neurologic complications occur, prolonged treatment is not indicated. Figure 1 summarizes the decisions for a first tonic-clonic seizure in an adult.

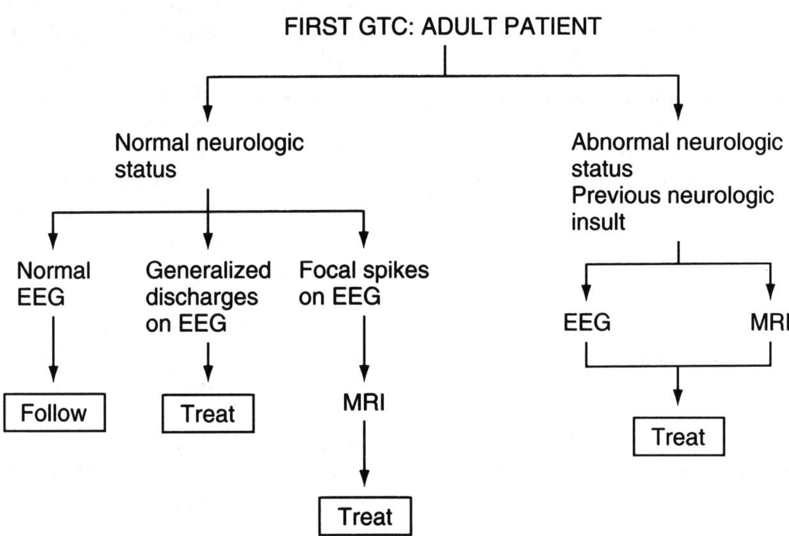

Figure 1
Decision tree for a first tonic-clonic seizure in an adult. EEG, electroencephalogram; MRI, magnetic resonance imaging.

Table 3 Current Antiepileptic Drugs (AEDs)

	MAINTENANCE DOSE (MG/KG/DAY)	INDICATIONS	SERUM LEVELS (MG/L)	HALF-LIFE HOURS (RANGE)	TIME TO STEADY STATE	SIDE EFFECTS
Valproic acid	10–70	GTC, CPSz, absence, myoclonic, atonic	50–120	10 (5–18)	3–4 days	Drowsiness, tremors, gastrointestinal discomfort, hepatitis, pancreatitis, thrombocytopenia, liver failure, weight gain
Carbamazepine	10–40	SPSz, secondary generalized, CPSz	4–12	14 (8–36)	28–42 days	Sleepiness, diplopia, headache, rash, liver toxicity, blood dyscrasia, arrhythmia
Phenytoin	4–12	SPSz, CPSz, secondary generalized	10–20	24 adult, 18 child (5–100)	14–28 days	Ataxia, drowsiness, nystagmus, rash, hirsutism, gum hyperplasia
Phenobarbital	1–5	GTC, CPSz, SPSz	15–40	60–120	14–21 days	Drowsiness, rash, cognitive and behavioral deficits
Ethosuximide	10–75	Absence	40–100	36 (15–68)	14 days	Abdominal discomfort, rash, dizziness, blood dyscrasia, lupus
Gabapentin	30–90	CPSz, SPSz	>5	5–7	1–2 days on full dose	Somnolence, ataxia
Lamotrigine	(>16 years)	CPSz, GTC, SPSz, myoclonic	2–5	1–59*	3–5 days	Rash, dizziness, somnolence
Felbamate	15–45	CPSz, SPSz, GTC	32–137	20–23	5–10 days	Anorexia, insomnia, abdominal discomfort, aplastic anemia, hepatic failure

CPSz, complex partial seizures; GTC, generalized tonic-clonic; SPSz, simple partial seizures.
*Half-life affected by other AEDs.

Choosing the Appropriate Antiepileptic Drug

Not all AEDs offer protection against tonic-clonic seizures. Some rules of thumb are helpful in choosing the "right" drug: patients who also have myoclonic or absence seizures and generalized or bilateral multifocal discharges in their EEG most likely have primarily generalized epilepsy and may benefit from valproate (Depakote, Depakene) or from lamotrigine (Lamictal). Carbamazepine (Tegretol), phenytoin (Dilantin), and gabapentin (Neurontin) along with valproic acid and lamotrigine are effective in partial and complex partial seizures. Phenobarbital and primidone are effective in GTC and complex and simple partial seizures (Table 3).

Three new medications are available in the United States. Felbamate (Felbatol), gabapentin (Neurontin), and lamotrigine (Lamictal) have been licensed for management of simple and complex partial seizure therapy. Felbamate and lamotrigine are effective in GTC seizures. The use of felbamate is currently limited because of the associated idiopathic aplastic anemia and fulminant hepatic failure. Gabapentin seems useful for the treatment of secondarily generalized seizures.

Suggested Reading

DeLorenzo RJ, Towne AR, Pellock JM, Ko D. Status epilepticus in children, adults and the elderly. Epilepsia 1992; 33:S4–S25.

Incidence and prevalence of epilepsy. In: Hauser WA, Hesdorfer DC. Epilepsy: Causes and consequences. Epilepsy Foundation of America. New York: Demos, 1990: 1–52.

Pellegrino TR. An emergency department approach to first-time seizures. Emerg Clin North Am 1994; 4:925–939.

MIGRAINE AND CLUSTER HEADACHES

Stephen D. Silberstein, M.D., F.A.C.P.
William B. Young, M.D.
Richard B. Lipton, M.D.

■ MIGRAINE

Migraine is an episodic headache disorder characterized by various combinations of neurologic, gastrointestinal, and autonomic changes. It affects more than 17 percent of women and 6 percent of men in the United States. The diagnosis of migraine is largely based on the headache's characteristics and associated symptoms. The medical and neurologic examinations as well as laboratory studies are usually normal and, as such, serve to exclude other, more ominous causes of headache.

Since 1988 the International Headache Society (IHS) criteria have been used to classify headache disorders. These criteria identify seven varieties of migraine. The two major varieties are migraine without aura, known formerly as common migraine, and migraine with aura, known formerly as classic migraine. Auras are focal neurologic symptoms typified by the scintillating scotoma that usually precede headache onset. Prodromes are characterized by changes in mood or behavior (i.e., irritability, food cravings), which may occur in migraine with or without aura.

The pain of migraine is invariably accompanied by other features. Anorexia is a common feature, although food cravings also occur. Nausea occurs in up to 90 percent of patients, and vomiting occurs in up to one-third. Many patients experience sensory hyperexcitability, manifest by photophobia, phonophobia, and osmophobia, and seek a dark, quiet room. Other symptoms include blurry vision, nasal stuffiness, cramps, and increased urination (followed by decreased urinary output after the attack). The diagnosis of migraine without aura requires the presence of nausea or vomiting or photophobia and phonophobia. Identifying these features is crucial for the accurate diagnosis of migraine, particularly in the absence of aura. Treatment must address not only the headache of migraine, but also the associated features. Remember that organic headaches sometimes respond to treatments for migraine diagnosis should never be based solely on response to treatment.

Table 1 Behavioral Modifications

MAY HELP	LESS LIKELY TO HELP
Regulate sleep	Avoid milk products
Regular exercise	Avoid citrus products
Regular meals	Avoid chocolate
Avoid tyramine-containing food	
Avoid monosodium glutamate	
Avoid alcoholic beverages	
Limit caffeine	
Limit medications	
Biofeedback or stress management	

Therapy

The goals of treatment are to relieve or prevent the pain and associated symptoms of migraine and to optimize the patient's ability to function normally. The first step in treatment is to tell the patient that he or she has migraine. The benign nature of the disorder, the mechanisms of migraine, and the patient's role as a partner in treatment should be explained. We design a treatment plan that attempts to reduce the impact of the symptoms that are most disturbing to the patient. Our patients are given a headache calendar and told to record the duration and severity of their headaches as well as their response to treatment. Behavioral interventions are an important part of treatment; potential interventions are summarized in Table 1. Biofeedback is a useful treatment and also

Table 2 Abortive Medications: Efficacy, Side Effects, Relative Contraindications, and Indications

			COMORBID CONDITION	
DRUG	EFFICACY*	SIDE EFFECTS*	RELATIVE CONTRAINDICATIONS	RELATIVE INDICATION
Acetaminophen	1+	1+	Liver disease	Pregnancy
Aspirin	1+	1+	Kidney disease, ulcer disease, PUD, gastritis (age <15)	CAD, TIA
Butalbital, caffeine, and analgesics	2+	2+	Use of other sedative; history of medication overuse	
Caffeine adjuvant	2+	1+	Sensitivity to caffeine	
Isometheptene	2+	1+	Uncontrolled HTN, CAD, PVD	
Narcotics	3+	3+	Drug or substance abuse	Pregnancy; rescue medication
NSAIDs	2+	1+	Kidney disease, PUD, gastritis	
Dihydroergotamine				
Injections	4+	2+	CAD, PVD, uncontrolled HTN	Orthostatic hypotension, prominent nausea or vomiting
Intranasal	3+	1+		
Ergotamine				
Tablets	2+	2+	Prominent nausea or vomiting, CAD, PVD, uncontrolled HTN	
Suppositories	3+	3+		
Sumatriptan				
Subcutaneous injection	4+	1+	CAD, PVD, uncontrolled HTN	Prominent nausea or vomiting
Tablets	3+	1+	CAD, PVD, uncontrolled HTN	

*Ratings are on a scale from 1+ (lowest) to 4+ (highest) on response rates and consistency of response in double-blind placebo-controlled trials and our clinical experience.
PUD, peptic ulcer disease; PVD, perhipheral vascular disease; CAD, coronary artery disease; TIA, transient ischemic attack; HTN, hypertension; NSAIDs, nonsteroidal anti-inflammatory drugs.

serves to engage patients in cognitive behavioral therapy. It is especially useful in children, pregnant women, and patients who report stress as a trigger. Although behavioral interventions are important, drugs are the mainstay of treatment for most patients.

Pharmacotherapy of migraine may be acute (abortive, symptomatic) or preventive (prophylactic). Patients with frequent, severe headaches often require both. Symptomatic treatment attempts to abort (stop the progression of) or reverse a headache (and the associated symptoms) once it has started. Preventive therapy is given daily, even in the absence of a headache, to reduce the frequency and severity of anticipated attacks. Acute treatment is almost always indicated, whereas preventive treatment should be used more selectively. We consider using preventive pharmacotherapy when attacks occur 3 or 4 days per month. Specific criteria for preventive treatment are presented in that section.

Medications used for acute headache treatment include analgesics, antiemetics, anxiolytics, nonsteroidal anti-inflammatory drugs (NSAIDs), ergots, steroids, major tranquilizers, narcotics, and selective 5-HT_1 (serotonin) agonists (Table 2). We use various combinations of these medications for headaches of differing severities. Patients should take acute medications at the first reliable indication of a migraine attack (except for sumatriptan, which must be taken after the aura ends and the headache begins). Preventive treatments include a broad range of medications, most notably beta-blockers, calcium channel blockers, antidepressants, serotonin antagonists, and anticonvulsants. Treatment choice should be based on the presence of comorbid and coexistent conditions. Concurrent illnesses should be treated with a single agent when possible, and migraine drugs that might aggravate these disorders should be avoided.

Optimizing therapy requires knowledge about treatment alternatives and the patient's own preferences. Some patients who want to minimize attack frequency are willing to accept significant side effects to achieve this goal. Some patients are eager to try new therapies, whereas others are afraid to change an established regimen even if its benefits are incomplete. Some patients accept parenteral routes of administration readily, but others are horrified by the idea of injections or suppositories. Effective management requires ongoing communication with the patient regarding these issues.

Symptomatic Treatment

Many acute treatments are available for migraine. The choice depends on the severity and frequency of the headaches, the pattern of the associated symptoms, the presence of comorbid illnesses, and the patient's treatment response profile (Table 3). We start with oral medications, such as analgesics, NSAIDs, or a caffeine adjuvant compound, for patients with mild to moderate headache. If treatment fails we move on to dihydroergotamine (DHE) or sumatriptan. If prominent nausea or vomiting is present, we recommend an antiemetic and more readily recommend nonoral treatment. If oral medication is ineffective or cannot be used due to gastrointestinal symptoms, we recommend suppositories, nasal sprays, or injections based on the patient's preferred route of administration. Suppositories include ergotamine, indomethacin, and prochlorperazine. Nasal sprays include transnasal butorphanol and, soon, DHE. Injections include sumatriptan SC and DHE IM, among others. We often prescribe more than

Table 3 Choice of Preventive Treatment in Migraine: Influence on Comorbid Conditions

			COMORBID CONDITION	
DRUG (EXAMPLE)	EFFICACY*	SIDE EFFECTS*	RELATIVE CONTRAINDICATIONS	RELATIVE INDICATION
Anticonvulsants (Divalproex)	4+	2+	Liver disease, bleeding disorders	Mania, epilepsy, anxiety disorders
Antidepressants (Amitriptyline)	4+	3+	Urinary retention, heart block	Other pain disorders, depression, anxiety disorders, insomnia
Antiserotonin (Methysergide)	4+	4+	Angina, PVD	Orthostatic hypotension
Beta-blockers (Propranolol, Nadolol)	4+	2+	Asthma, depression, CHF, Raynaud's disease, diabetes	HTN, angina
Calcium channel blockers (Verapamil)	2+	1+	Constipation, hypotension	Migraine with aura, HTN, angina, asthma
NSAIDs (Naproxen)	2+	2+	Ulcer disease, gastritis	Arthritis, other pain disorders

*Ratings are on a scale from 1+ (lowest) to 4+ (highest) on response rates and consistency of response in double-blind placebo-controlled trials and our clinical experience.
PVD, perhipheral vascular disease; CHF, congestive heart failure; HTN, hypertension; NSAIDs, nonsteroidal anti-inflammatory drugs.

one acute treatment at the time of the initial visit. For example, we may advise patients to use naproxen sodium for mild to moderate headaches and sumatriptan for more severe headaches (Fig. 1).

Simple and Combination Analgesics and NSAIDs. We often begin with simple analgesics for patients with mild to moderate headaches. Many individuals find headache relief with a simple analgesic such as aspirin or acetaminophen, either alone or in combination with caffeine. Butalbital is another effective analgesic adjuvant. We also use the combination of acetaminophen, isometheptene (a sympathomimetic), and dichloralphenazone (a chloral hydrate derivative). For patients who are nauseated we use the antiemetic metoclopramide. We often try naproxen sodium first, but we use all the NSAIDs, often in combination with metoclopramide. Indomethacin, available as a 50 mg rectal suppository, and IM ketorolac are useful in patients with severe nausea and vomiting.

Ergotamine and DHE. We use ergotamine and its derivative, DHE, to treat moderate to severe migraine if analgesics do not provide satisfactory headache relief or if they produce significant side effects. Since rectal absorption is more reliable than oral, we prefer to use ergotamine by suppository. Patients who cannot tolerate ergotamine because of nausea are pretreated with metoclopramide, prochlorperazine, promethazine, or a mixture of a barbiturate and a belladonna alkaloid. Metoclopramide may enhance the absorption of oral ergotamine.

DHE has fewer side effects than ergotamine and can be administered IM, SC, or IV. DHE is given in doses of up to 1 mg IM or IV per treatment with a maximum of 3 mg per day. We typically limit monthly use to 18 ampules or 12 events. DHE is a mainstay of treatment because it is effective in most patients, it is associated with a low headache recurrence rate (less than 20 percent), and it is less likely than ergotamine to exacerbate nausea or produce rebound headache.

We avoid ergotamine and DHE in women who are attempting to become pregnant and in patients with uncontrolled hypertension; sepsis; renal or hepatic failure; and coronary, cerebral, or peripheral vascular disease. Although nausea is a common side effect with ergotamine, it is less common with DHE (unless it is given intravenously). Other side effects include dizziness, paresthesias, abdominal cramps, and chest tightness; rare idiosyncratic arterial and coronary vasospasm can occur. We recommend an electrocardiograph (ECG) on all patients before their first dose of DHE, particularly if there are any cardiac risk factors (including age greater than 40).

Sumatriptan. Sumatriptan, a selective 5-HT$_1$-receptor agonist, is available both as an injection (6 mg SC) and as tablets (25 and 50 mg oral tablets). Sumatriptan SC has a more rapid onset of action than oral sumatriptan. Sumatriptan relieves headache pain, nausea, photophobia, and phonophobia and restores the patient's ability to function normally. We often prescribe sumatriptan at the initial consultation as a first-line drug for severe attacks and as an escape medication for less severe attacks that do not adequately respond to simple or combination analgesics. We prefer the SC injection for patients who need rapid relief or have severe nausea or vomiting. Although 80 percent of patients experience pain relief from an initial dose of sumatriptan, headache recurrence occurs in about 40 percent of patients. Recurrences are most likely in patients with long-duration headaches. Recurrences respond well to a second dose of sumatriptan or to simple and combination analgesics.

Sumatriptan should not be used in patients with clinical or subclinical ischemic heart disease, Prinzmetal's angina, or vertebrobasilar migraine. Common side effects include pain at the injection site, tingling, flushing, burning, and warm or hot sensations. Dizziness, heaviness, neck pain, and dysphoria also can occur. These side effects generally abate within 45 minutes. Sumatriptan causes noncardiac chest pressure in approximately 4 percent of patients. We obtain an ECG on patients over the age of 40 and with risk factors for heart disease before using sumatriptan. We often give the

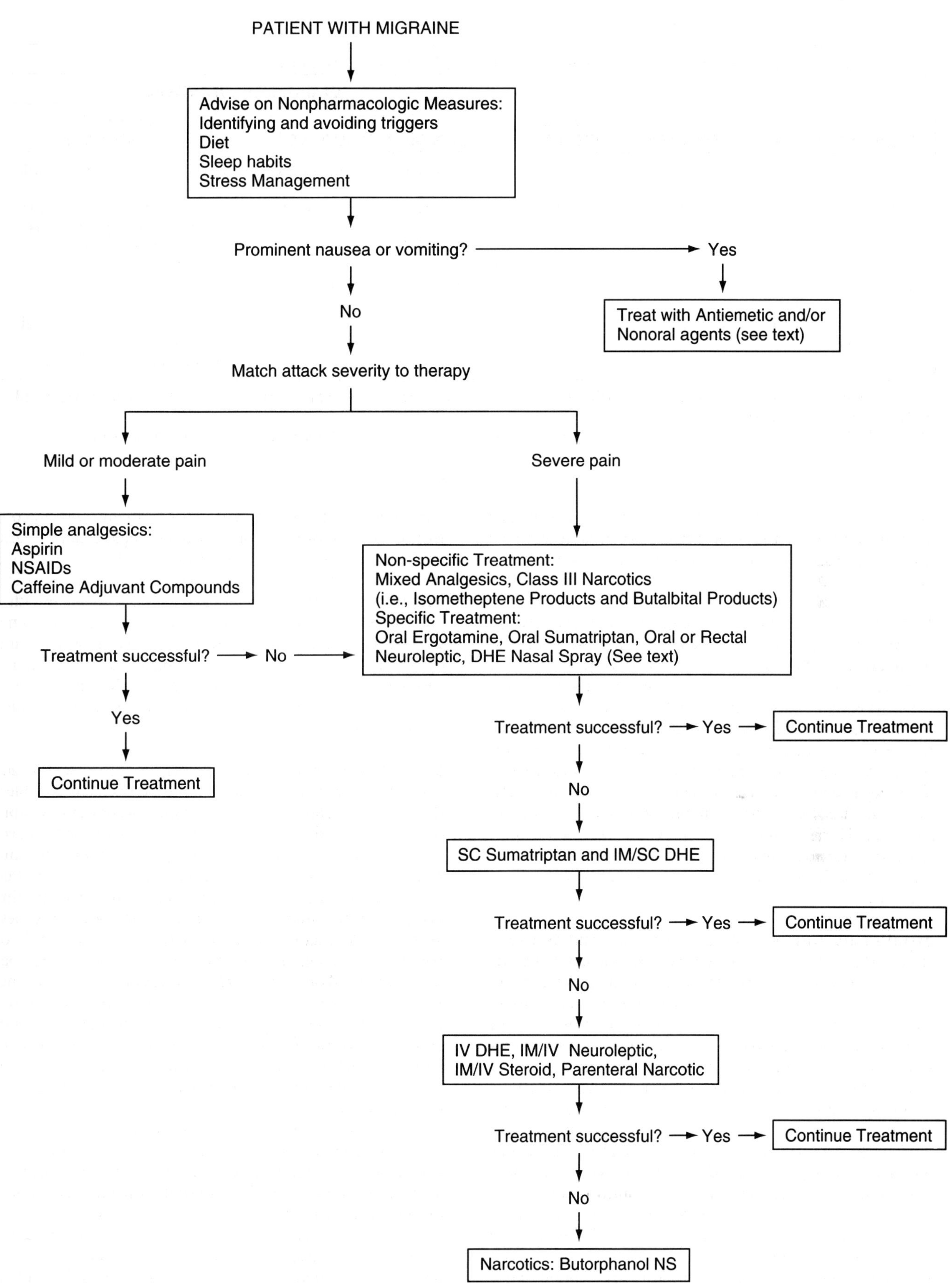

Figure 1
Algorithm for the treatment of migraine. NSAIDs, nonsteroidal anti-inflammatory drugs; DHE, dihydroergotamine; NS, normal saline.

first dose of sumatriptan in the office at a time the patient does not have a headache.

Narcotics. If nonopioid medications do not provide adequate pain relief, we use codeine in combination with simple analgesics and sometimes with butalbital or caffeine. We also use more potent narcotic analgesics such as propoxyphene, butorphanol, meperidine, morphine, hydromorphone, and oxycodone, alone and in combination with simple analgesics. Because medication overuse and rebound headache pose a threat, these agents are most appropriate for patients whose severe headaches are relatively infrequent. The potential for drug abuse is reduced for opiates that are mixed agonist-antagonists, such as butorphanol, although it is not clear whether these agents offer any protection from rebound headache. Transnasal butorphanol tartrate (1 mg followed by 1 mg 1 hour later) is an effective acute outpatient migraine treatment that circumvents problems with oral absorption. Opiates should not be used more than 2 days per week on average.

In specific groups of patients, such as women with intractable menstrual migraine, we use narcotics on a more regular basis. These drugs are also especially helpful to patients who do not respond to simple analgesics and who cannot take ergots or sumatriptan. Pregnant women can use codeine or meperidine with caution. Narcotics are also useful for patients who awaken in the middle of the night with a headache. Sedation, which is at times an undesirable side effect, may help the patient go back to sleep and awaken headache free in the morning.

Adjunctive Therapy

Nausea and vomiting can be as disabling as the headache itself. Gastric stasis and delayed gastric emptying decrease the effectiveness of oral medication. We use metoclopramide as an antiemetic and a prokinetic to enhance the absorption of oral medications. Promethazine and ondansetron (a selective 5-HT_3-receptor antagonist) IV (0.15 mg per kilogram diluted in 50 ml of 5 percent dextrose or normal saline) or orally (8 mg tablet) can be used by patients who cannot tolerate metoclopramide because of side effects. We use the neuroleptics, chlorpromazine and prochlorperazine, IV, IM, and by suppository for nausea, vomiting, and pain. Prochlorperazine suppositories (25 mg) are used as a primary treatment for headache and nausea and also as a rescue medication.

Preventive Therapy

General Principles. We consider preventive medication when (1) two or more attacks per month produce disability lasting 3 or more days per month; (2) symptomatic medications are contraindicated or ineffective; (3) abortive medication is required more than twice per week; or (4) less frequent headache attacks produce profound disruption, as in migraine with prolonged aura or migrainous infarction.

We choose a drug from one of the first-line categories (beta-adrenergic blockers, antidepressants, calcium channel antagonists, and anticonvulsants) based on the drug's side effect profile and the patient's comorbid condition(s). Start the drug at a low dose and increase it slowly until therapeutic effects or side effects develop, or until the maximum dose is reached. (A full therapeutic trial may take as long as 6 months.) To obtain maximal benefit, the patient should not overuse analgesics or ergot derivatives. Migraine may improve with time independent of treatment; if the headaches are well controlled, a drug holiday can be undertaken following a slow taper program.

Beta-Blockers. Since the relative efficacy of the different beta-blockers (propranolol, metoprolol, timolol, nadolol, and atenolol) has not been clearly established, we choose a beta-blocker based on beta selectivity, convenience of drug formulation, side effects, and the patient's individual reaction. We prefer nadolol and atenolol because of their long half-life and favorable side effect profile. Since beta-blockers can produce behavioral side effects, such as drowsiness, fatigue, lethargy, sleep disorders, nightmares, depression, memory disturbance, and hallucinations, we avoid them in patients with depression or low energy. Decreased exercise tolerance limits their use by athletes. Less common side effects include impotence, orthostatic hypotension, significant bradycardia, and aggravation of intrinsic muscle disease. We find beta-blockers especially useful in patients with comorbid angina or hypertension. They are relatively contraindicated in patients with congestive heart failure, asthma, Raynaud's disease, and insulin-dependent diabetes.

Antidepressants. We use both tricyclic antidepressants (TCAs) and selective serotonin reuptake inhibitors (SSRIs). The TCAs we use most commonly are nortriptyline and doxepin, although only amitriptyline has demonstrated benefits in placebo-controlled double-blind studies. We often use TCAs for the patient with a sleep disturbance. We frequently use SSRIs such as fluoxetine, paroxetine, and sertraline, based on their favorable side effect profiles, not their established efficacy. Fluoxetine is of proven value in chronic daily headache. We believe that venlafaxine, the first specific serotonin and norepinephrine reuptake inhibitor, is effective, but no studies have been performed.

Side effects of TCAs are common. Most involve antimuscarinic effects, such as dry mouth and sedation. The drugs also cause increased appetite and weight gain; cardiac toxicity and orthostatic hypotension occur occasionally. Sexual dysfunction is not uncommon with SSRIs and can be treated with amantadine. Antidepressants are especially useful in patients with comorbid depression and anxiety disorders.

Calcium Channel Blockers. Of the calcium channel blockers available in the United States, verapamil is the most effective. It is especially useful in patients with comorbid hypertension or with contraindications to beta-blockers such as asthma and Raynaud's disease. We use verapamil in patients with migraine with prolonged aura or migrainous infarction. Because the drug has an especially favorable side effect profile, we use it preferentially on patients unlikely to tolerate cognitive side effects. Constipation is verapamil's most common side effect.

Anticonvulsant Medications. The most effective anticonvulsant is valproic acid; we use it in the form of divalproex. Divalproex is a very effective preventive medication for migraine, as has been demonstrated by four placebo-controlled

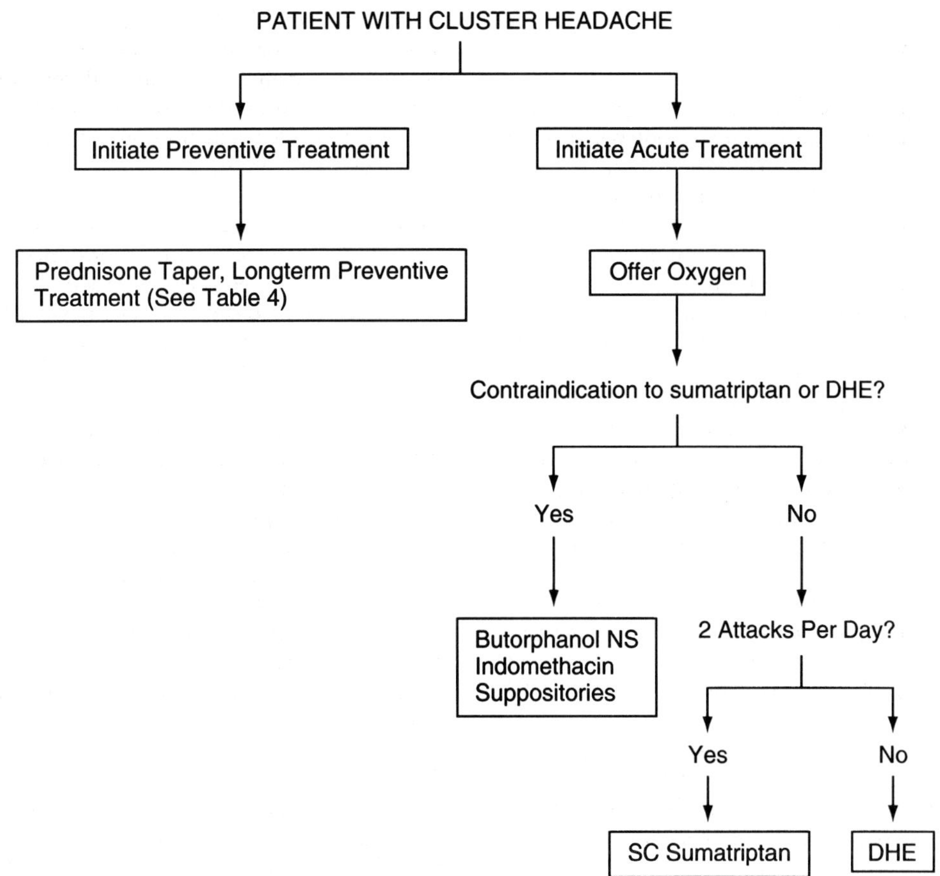

Figure 2
Algorithm for the treatment of cluster headache. DHE, dihydroergotamine; NS, normal saline.

studies. It is effective in many patients at a low dose of 500 to 750 mg per day. In patients who do not respond to lower doses we push the dose of divalproex to a trough level of 120 μg per milliliter.

Side effects include sedation, hair loss, tremor, and changes in cognitive performance. Nausea, vomiting, and indigestion can occur but are self-limited. Hepatotoxicity is the most serious side effect, but irreversible hepatic dysfunction is extremely rare in adults. Baseline liver function studies should be obtained, but routine follow-up studies are probably not routinely needed in adults on monotherapy. Follow-up is necessary to adjust the dose and monitor side effects.

Divalproex is especially useful when migraine occurs in patients with comorbid epilepsy, anxiety disorders, or manic-depressive illness. It can be safely administered to patients with depression, Raynaud's disease, asthma, and diabetes, circumventing the contraindications to beta-blockers.

Serotonin Antagonists. Methysergide is an effective migraine prophylactic drug. Side effects include transient muscle aching, claudication, abdominal distress, nausea, weight gain, and hallucinations. Frightening hallucinations after the first dose are not uncommon. The major complication of methysergide is the rare (1 in 2,500) development of retroperitoneal, pulmonary, or endocardial fibrosis, the unreasonable fear of which prevents its more widespread use. To prevent this complication, a medication-free interval of 4 weeks following each 6 month course of continuous treatment is recommended. We find methysergide to be a very effective drug with minimal side effects, but we reserve its use because of the need for a drug holiday.

Status Migrainosus

Status migrainosus is a condition characterized by severe, persistent headache often associated with intractable nausea and vomiting. We start treatment by rehydrating the patient with IV fluids and giving compazine 10 mg IV followed by DHE 1 mg. If the headache is not relieved we repeat these drugs in 1 to 2 hours or give supplemental corticosteroids (Decadron 4 mg). If the patient cannot tolerate DHE or neuroleptics, we use narcotics, corticosteroids, or ketorolac alone. If the headache cannot be broken, we admit the patient for repetitive IV DHE (Fig. 2).

■ CLUSTER HEADACHE

Although once classified as a vascular headache along with migraine, cluster headache is a distinct clinical and epidemiologic entity. Bouts consist of attacks of severe unilateral, orbital, supraorbital, and/or temporal pain that last 15 to 180 minutes and typically occur once or twice per day. The

Table 4 Agents Used for the Prophylaxis of Cluster Headache

AGENT	DOSAGE	ADVERSE EFFECTS
EPISODIC CLUSTER HEADACHE*		
Divalproex	600–2,000 mg/day in divided doses to maintain fasting blood concentration of 50–120 mg/L	Nausea, lethargy, tremor, weight gain, hair loss; rarely abnormal liver function, pancreatitis
Ergotamine	Up to 4 mg/day (in divided doses)	Nausea, paresthesia, intermittent claudication, ergotism
Lithium	300 mg b.i.d or t.i.d./blood concentration of 0.4–0.8 mmol/L)	Weakness, nausea, thirst, tremor, lethargy, slurred speech, blurred vision
Methysergide	2–8 mg/day	Muscle cramps, nausea, diarrhea, abdominal discomfort
Prednisone	40–100 mg/day initially, taper over 1–2 weeks	Insomnia, restlessness, personality changes, hyponatremia, edema, hyperglycemia, osteoporosis, myopathy, gastric ulcers, hip necrosis
Verapamil	120–640 mg/day	Constipation, edema, dizziness, nausea, hypotension, fatigue
CHRONIC CLUSTER HEADACHE†		
Divalproex	Dosage as for episodic headache	Adverse effects as for episodic headache
Lithium	Dosage as for episodic headache	Long-term use may lead to hypothyroidism and polyuria
Methysergide	Dosage as for episodic headache	Prolonged use may cause fibrotic reactions
Verapamil	Dosage as for episodic headache	Adverse effects as for episodic headache

*Administration of agents should begin early in the cluster period and continue until the patient has been headache free for at least 2 weeks. Subsequently, the dosage should be tapered and then restarted at the beginning of the next cluster period.
†Combinations of agents are often required.

frequency ranges from one attack every other day to eight attacks per day. The pain is associated with at least one autonomic sign ipsilateral to the pain. These most frequently include conjunctival injection, eye tearing, nasal congestion, runny nose, forehead and facial sweating, miosis, ptosis, or eyelid edema. The periods of frequent attacks are referred to as cluster periods. Based on the duration of the cluster period, cluster headache is divided into two clinical entities: episodic cluster, which occurs in periods lasting 7 days to 1 year separated by remission of at least 14 days, and chronic cluster, in which attacks occur for more than 1 year without remission or with remission lasting less than 14 days.

Therapy

Treatment for cluster can be abortive, prophylactic (preventive), or both. An acute attack is relieved most quickly by oxygen inhalation, SC sumatriptan, or DHE. Our cluster headache treatment approach is outlined in Table 4.

Acute Therapy

Oxygen given by face mask (7 to 10 L per minute for 15 minutes) is effective in approximately 70 percent of patients, usually within 10 minutes. We use oxygen as a first-line therapy in our offices and in the emergency department. One limitation of oxygen is that it is not very portable or convenient, although we often prescribe home oxygen. Sumatriptan (SC) is another highly effective acute treatment for cluster headache, with a response in 10 minutes. It is most useful in patients with two or fewer attacks per day. DHE (IM or SC) is also effective. In our experience intranasal lidocaine is occasionally effective. Analgesics and opioids do not play a large role in the treatment of cluster because (1) the multiplicity of attacks necessitates repeated use and so creates the risk of addiction; and (2) these agents are nonspecific medications and are not usually as effective as specific medications for cluster headache.

Preventive Therapy

Cluster headache patients usually require preventive therapy. The goal is to produce a rapid remission and maintain it with minimal adverse effects until the cluster period is over. Effective medications include ergotamine, methysergide, corticosteroids, verapamil, lithium, and valproic acid (divalproex). Indomethacin is occasionally effective.

We start treatment early in the cluster period and continue it until the patient is headache free for at least 2 weeks, and then gradually taper the drug until the next cluster period, at which time we restart it. Treatment must be individualized. We often initiate preventive treatment with a combination of prednisone (60 to 80 mg daily) and verapamil (240 mg per day). Prednisone often produces a rapid remission, but it also produces side effects, which are cumulative. Accordingly, we give 1 week of high-dose prednisone and taper it during the second week. Verapamil has a favorable side effect profile but a delayed onset of action. By the time the prednisone taper is complete, the verapamil usually becomes effective. The verapamil dose may need to be escalated; some patients require daily doses that exceed the 480 mg upper limit recommended on the package insert.

If verapamil fails, methysergide (2 mg three to four times a day) is an effective alternative, especially in younger patients. Because episodic cluster and its treatment are self-limited, fibrotic complications are of less concern. Methysergide should not be combined with daily ergotamine, as it may enhance vasospasm. If methysergide is ineffective, lithium or divalproex can be used alone or in combination with verapamil. While waiting for the other drugs to start working, we use corticosteroids and IM DHE daily to break the headache cycle or to treat severe exacerbations. In patients with exclusively nocturnal attacks we use ergotamine alone at bedtime.

Chronic cluster can be treated with verapamil or lithium, alone or in combination. Divalproex used alone or in combination with verapamil is often very effective. An occasional patient responds to the intranasal application of capsaicin five to six times per day. Occipital nerve blocks may relieve cluster attacks for days or weeks, but it has been our experience that subsequent injections become less effective.

Patients with episodic cluster headache may become resistant to a previously successful prophylactic medication. These patients may require polypharmacy and eventually inpatient treatment. We use DHE given IV every 8 hours (in an inpatient setting) for the rare patient with intractable cluster headache. All our patients become headache free during treatment. The remission is often sustained after discharge from the hospital. If hospitalization and all efforts at prevention fail, some patients require neuroablative procedures.

Surgical procedures include sphenopalatine ganglionectomy and radio frequency thermocoagulation of the trigeminal ganglion and section of the trigeminal nerve. The corneal anesthesia that results from these procedures puts the ipsilateral eye at risk. Recently glycerol injection into the trigeminal cistern has been used as a treatment of intractable cluster headache with significant pain relief and corneal safety.

Suggested Reading

Saper JR, Silberstein SD, Gordon CD, Hamel RL. Handbook of headache management. Baltimore: Williams & Wilkins, 1993.

Silberstein SD. Pharmacologic management of cluster headache. CNS Drugs 1994; 2(3):199–207.

Silberstein SD, Lipton RB. Overview of diagnosis and treatment of migraine. Neurology 1994; 44(7):S6–S16.

Solomon SD, Lipton RB, Newman LC. Prophylactic therapy of cluster headaches. Clin Neuropharmacol 1991; 14:116–130.

PARKINSON'S DISEASE

Garrett E. Alexander, M.D., Ph.D.

Idiopathic Parkinson's disease (PD) is a progressive, age-related neurodegenerative disorder with characteristic neuropathologic changes that include the formation of Lewy bodies and the loss of neuromelanin-containing central neurons, including the dopaminergic neurons of the substantia nigra pars compacta (SNc). The clinical hallmarks of this disorder include tremor at rest, muscular stiffness (rigidity), reduction of facial expressiveness (masking), paucity of spontaneous movements and postural adjustments (akinesia), slowing of voluntary movements (bradykinesia), and postural instability. Although the etiology remains unknown, much has been learned in recent years about the pathophysiology and effective treatment of PD. The loss of dopaminergic innervation of the neostriatum (especially the putamen), which results in excessive and disordered inhibitory outflow from the basal ganglia to the ventrolateral thalamus, is believed to underlie most of the predominantly motor symptomatology of this disorder. Accordingly, some of the most effective therapeutic measures available for treating PD patients are designed to restore dopaminergic tone within the neostriatum or to interrupt disordered outflow from the basal ganglia. The diagnosis of PD continues to be based principally on clinical signs and symptoms, coupled with the active exclusion of other conditions that may mimic PD. As yet there are no laboratory or imaging studies that provide reliable, positive evidence that someone has PD.

■ DIAGNOSIS

There are no formal criteria for making the diagnosis of PD. As indicated in Figure 1, a presumptive diagnosis may be made in the patient who has a strongly lateralized resting tremor with or without accompanying signs of parkinsonism (rigidity, bradykinesia, or akinesia), provided the symptoms began after the age of 50 years. The presence of cogwheeling is supportive but not diagnostic. Although the presence of tremor at rest favors a diagnosis of PD, other conditions such as benign essential tremor or cerebellar disease should be considered when the tremor is much more pronounced during active movements. If the onset of symptoms was before the age of 50, or if signs of akinesia, bradykinesia, or rigidity are not accompanied by an asymmetric resting tremor, it is essential, before making a presumptive diagnosis of PD, to exclude other conditions that may also present with signs of parkinsonism. Most of the conditions listed in Table 1 can be excluded during an initial evaluation, based on a careful history and neurologic examination and appropriate laboratory and imaging studies. Nevertheless, the possibility remains that one may be dealing with a condition other than PD itself. These include the multiple system atrophies (especially striatonigral degeneration), atypical presentations of progressive supranuclear palsy or cortical-basal ganglionic degeneration, and Pick's and Alzheimer's diseases—in those cases when signs of parkinsonism are accompanied by significant dementia. For this reason one can only make a presumptive—rather than definitive—diagnosis of PD until a positive clinical response to dopamine replacement therapy has been documented. Even so, unless or until the patient's parkinsonian symptoms have become sufficiently troublesome to warrant the *therapeutic* introduction of levodopa, it is usually advisable (for reasons discussed later) to delay the use of this drug for as long as possible.

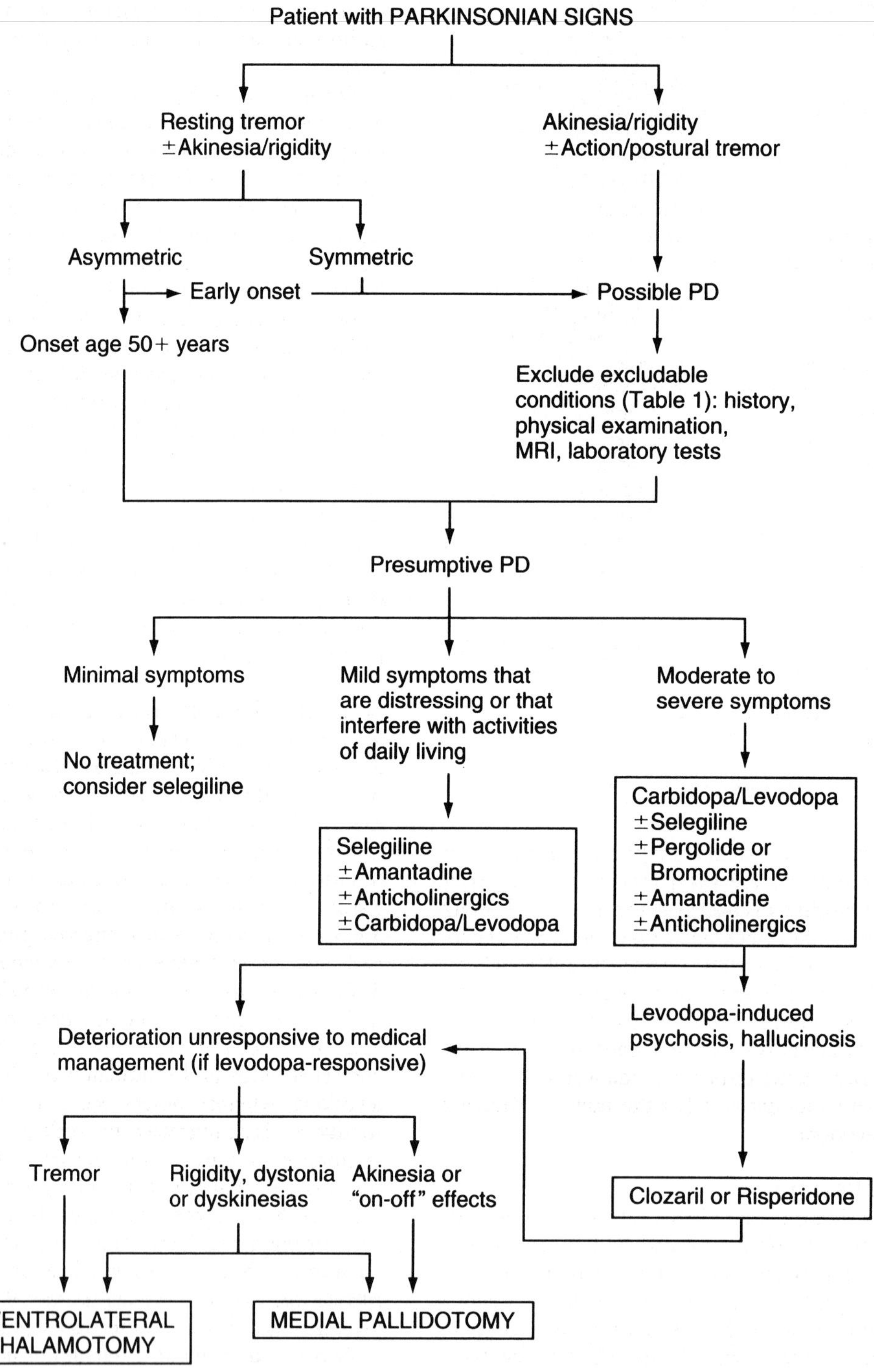

Figure 1
Algorithm for the management of the patient with Parkinson's disease (PD). MRI, magnetic resonance imaging.

Table 1 Other Conditions Associated with Parkinsonian Signs

Multiple system atrophies
  Striatonigral degeneration
  Shy-Drager syndrome
  Olivopontocerebellar degeneration
Progressive supranuclear palsy
Huntington's disease, juvenile form
Wilson's disease
Cortical-basal ganglionic degeneration with neuronal acromasia
Familial basal ganglia calcification
Hallervorden-Spatz disease
Multiple infarct state
Symptomatic hemidystonia (lesions of putamen or posterolateral thalamus)
Creutzfeldt-Jakob disease (if course is prolonged)
Pick's disease
Alzheimer's disease
Amyotrophic lateral sclerosis (ALS)
Corticostriatospinal degeneration (dementia, parkinsonian, and ALS)
	Normal pressure hydrocephalus
	Dementia pugilistica (repeated head injury)
	Anoxic or hypoperfusion encephalopathy
	Metabolic abnormalities
	  Parathyroid abnormalities
	  Hypothyroidism
	  Hepatocerebral degeneration
	Toxin-induced
	  N-Methyl-4-phenyl-1,2,3,6-tetrahydropyridine, manganese, mercury, cyanide, carbon monoxide, carbon disulfide, methanol
	Drug induced
	  Postsynaptic dopamine antagonists (neuroleptics, antiemetics)
	  Presynaptic dopamine antagonists (reserpine, tetrabenazine)
	  Calcium channel blockers (flunarizine, cinnarizine)
	  Alpha-methyldopa

THERAPY: GENERAL APPROACH

As indicated in Figure 1, the patient with presumptive PD who has minimal symptoms that are not in themselves distressing (such as a slight resting or postural tremor that is only troublesome during times of stress) does not require any medical treatment initially, and he or she should merely be reassured that effective therapy will be available when the need arises. However, even at this earliest stage of symptomatic PD, it is useful to discuss with the patient two important, but as yet unresolved, issues of patient management: (1) the issue of antioxidant therapy and (2) the issue of delaying treatment with levodopa.

Antioxidant Therapy

There is indirect evidence that oxidative stress and free radical formation could be responsible for the neuronal injury that is seen in PD. The effects of MPTP (1-methyl-4-phenyl-1,2,3,6-tetrahydropyridine), a neurotoxic agent that destroys SNc neurons and leads to clinical signs of parkinsonism in humans and experimental animals, appear to be medicated primarily by oxidative mechanisms. These observations led to the introduction of selegiline (Eldepryl), a monoamine oxidase (MAO)-B inhibitor, as a potential prophylactic agent in PD. This drug provides a protective effect if given prior to experimental treatment with MPTP. Early clinical trials indicated that the use of selegiline could delay the need for introducing levodopa in patients with PD, and this was interpreted as evidence for a neuroprotective effect that forestalled the natural progression of the disease. However, as a dopaminergic agent selegiline also has positive symptomatic effects in many PD patients. This symptomatic benefit may have been responsible for much of the purported prophylactic effect that was observed in the early studies, and additional studies are under way to address this important issue.

For now, however, the issue is unresolved. As the risks of using selegiline are minimal, as it may provide some minor symptomatic improvement and may delay the need for beginning levodopa therapy, and as the early claims for a prophylactic benefit have yet to be disproven, it seems reasonable to give new PD patients who have minimal, nondistressing symptoms the option of beginning selegiline even before they actually require symptomatic treatment. The principal negative factor is cost, which may easily exceed $1,200 per year. Fortunately, selegiline is relatively low in potential side effects, provided it is used at the recommended dose of 5 mg twice daily, with the last dose being administered by 12 noon. At higher doses, selegiline is no longer a selective inhibitor of MAO-B (which occurs mainly in the central nervous system), so nonspecific inhibition of peripheral MAO-A may result in hypertensive crises should the patient be exposed to a tyramine load, such as may occur with the ingestion of red wine or aged cheese. At the recommended dose, however, dietary restrictions are not necessary. Insomnia may be a problem if selegiline is administered later than noon.

Delaying Treatment with Levodopa

The second issue is whether it is ultimately more beneficial to delay symptomatic treatment with levodopa for as long as possible, and to minimize the cumulative dose of this agent, due to the possibility that it may have a toxic effect on dopamine receptors, may promote neuronal damage through the formation of free radicals, and may hasten the eventual onset of troublesome motor fluctuations. Although levodopa is unquestionably the most effective pharmacologic agent for symptomatic treatment of PD, its effectiveness over time is limited. Eventually, its efficacy diminishes, and progressively higher doses are required to maintain comparable symptomatic relief. Motor fluctuations may ensue, some of which are correlated with and modulated by the dosing schedule of levodopa, whereas others occur at random intervals. Although PD is a progressive neurodegenerative disorder, there is some evidence to suggest that levodopa itself may be responsible for some of these long-term complications. On the other hand, some have argued that early use of levodopa may prolong life span. The issue has yet to be resolved conclusively, but for now it would appear prudent to delay the introduction of levodopa at least until the level of disability becomes distressing to the patient or interferes with the activities of daily living (ADLs). It is also advisable to minimize the total daily dose of levodopa by the judicious use of adjunctive therapies.

Symptomatic Therapy (Table 2)

It is important for the patient with PD to recognize that the most realistic goal of therapy is to control disability, not to eliminate all symptoms of the disorder. Another key principle in PD management is the recognition, by physician and

Table 2 Drugs Useful in the Treatment of Parkinson's Disease

CATEGORY	GENERIC NAME	BRAND NAME	PREPARATION (MG)	DOSING SCHEDULE (MG)	MECHANISM OF ACTION
Dopaminergic agents	Carbidopa/ levodopa	Sinemet	Tabs (25/100, 25/250)	25/100 t.i.d. to 25/250 q4h	DOPA decarboxylase inhibitor; dopamine precursor
	Carbidopa/ levodopa	Sinemet CR	Tabs (25/100, 50/200)	25/100 t.i.d. to 75/300 q4h	DOPA decarboxylase inhibitor; dopamine precursor
	Selegiline	Eldepryl	Tabs (5.0)	5 b.i.d. (before noon)	MAO-B inhibitor
	Amantadine	Symmetrel	Caps (100)	100 b.i.d.	Release of dopamine
	Pergolide	Permax	Tabs (0.05, 0.25, 1.0)	0.05 b.i.d. to 1.0 q4h	Dopamine agonist
	Bromocriptine	Parlodel	Tabs (2.5), caps (5.0)	1.25 b.i.d. to 5 q4h	Dopamine agonist
Anticholinergic agents	Trihexyphenidyl	Artane	Tabs (2.0, 5.0)	1 t.i.d. to 2.5 t.i.d.	Muscarinic antagonist
	Benztropine	Cogentin	Tabs (0.5, 1.0, 2.0)	0.5 qd to 2 b.i.d.	Muscarinic antagonist
Antipsychotic agents	Clozapine	Clozaril	Tabs (25, 100)	12.5 q.h.s to 50 b.i.d.	Dopamine antagonist
	Risperidone	Risperdal	Tabs (1.0, 2.0, 3.0, 4.0)	0.5 q.h.s. to 2.0 b.i.d.	Dopamine and serotonin antagonist

DOPA, 3,4-dihydroxyphenylalanine; MAO, monoamine oxidase.

patient alike, that changes in drug therapy should seldom be made at intervals of less than 2 weeks. This is because of the fluctuating natural history of PD (with "good" and "bad" periods lasting from days to weeks), and the often-delayed effects of the antiparkinson medications themselves. Once the patient with PD has passed from the stage of minimal, nondistressing symptoms to that of mild disability, there are several options available before beginning levodopa therapy. The issue of selegiline should be revisited. Amantadine (Symmetrel), an antiviral agent with dopaminergic and anticholinergic properties, may be beneficial at this stage. The standard dosage is 100 mg twice daily. Common side effects include confusion and hallucinations. Anticholinergic agents, such as trihexyphenidyl (Artane) or benztropine (Cogentin), may also be useful at this early stage, but their efficacy is frequently limited by side effects. Complaints of blurred vision, lethargy, urinary retention, confusion, and memory loss are not uncommon, even among younger patients. In elderly patients, the frequency of cognitive side effects dictates special caution in using either amantadine or one of the anticholinergics.

When it becomes necessary to introduce levodopa, a combined preparation that includes carbidopa, a peripheral decarboxylase inhibitor, should be used in order to minimize the peripheral conversion of levodopa to dopamine. Unless the patient is elderly or extremely frail, an initial dose of regular Sinemet (carbidopa/levodopa) 25/100 three times per day is usually well tolerated. Otherwise, a trial dose of half a tablet three times per day may be necessary, followed by careful titration over 2 to 4 weeks to a target dose of one full tablet three times per day. If there is no clinical response at that level, further titration to a maximum initial dose of 1.5 tablets three times per day may be warranted, because failure to show symptomatic improvement after the latter dose has been maintained for 3 weeks can be taken as an indication of failure to respond to levodopa. This would suggest that the presumptive diagnosis of PD should be reconsidered. Sinemet also comes in strengths of 10/100 and 25/250, but these are of limited usefulness for most patients. The 10/100 tablets contain too little carbidopa and may be poorly tolerated in comparison to comparable amounts of the 25/100 preparation. The 25/250 preparation is too strong for most patients until late in the course of the disease.

In beginning treatment with Sinemet, it is advisable initially for the drug to be taken with meals to minimize the possibility of attendant nausea. However, for many patients there is significant interference with the absorption and blood-to-brain transport of levodopa by dietary neutral amino acids, leading to a sometimes profound loss of efficacy when regular Sinemet is ingested within 90 minutes or less of the nearest meal, especially if the meal is high in protein. Thus, if nausea is not encountered after an initial trial, patients may be advised to try to space their Sinemet away from mealtimes if possible. The optimal spacing of doses is 4 to 5 hours, and the last dose should be administered well before bedtime so that its clinical effect will not be wasted while the patient is asleep. Besides nausea, the principal, dose-dependent side effects of Sinement are confusion, hallucinations, and hypotension.

Sinemet CR, a sustained-release form of carbidopa-levodopa, is also available. This provides a smoother delivery of levodopa, with lower peaks and higher troughs in blood levels. Nevertheless, most patients require a three times per-day dosing schedule as with regular Sinemet, though the spacing can be extended to 5 to 6 hours. Because of this smoothing effect, the clinical response is usually more subtle than with the regular preparation, and for this reason I generally prefer to begin with regular Sinemet unless the presumptive diagnosis of PD is beyond doubt. An initial dose of Sinemet CR 25/100 three times per day is appropriate, but because the effective delivery of levodopa to the bloodstream is less efficient with this preparation, somewhat higher nominal doses of Sinemet CR are required to match a given amount of regular Sinemet (roughly 1.2 to 1.4:1). Thus most patients will require some upward titration from the recommended starting dose. The CR tablets are scored and may be broken, but not crushed, without loss of the sustained-release property.

As the disease progresses, higher doses of Sinemet or Sinemet CR will be required. It is advisable, however, to maintain the total daily dose of levodopa as low as possible. Once the dose of levodopa has reached 400 mg per day (500 mg when using Sinemet CR), direct-acting dopamine agonists may be added for their anti-parkinson and levodopa-sparing effects. The ergot alkaloids pergolide (Permax) and bromocriptine (Parlodel) are often quite useful in this respect. Pergolide, which has roughly 10 times the clinical potency of bromocriptine, is an agonist at D_2 receptors and a mild antagonist at D_1 receptors. Bromocriptine is an agonist at both D_2 and D_1 receptors. Although neither of these agents has very profound antiparkinson properties when taken alone, either drug may provide significant therapeutic benefit when used in combination with Sinemet. As with Sinement, the principal side effects are nausea, hypotension, confusion, and hallucinations.

Eventually, after some 3 to 5 years of Sinemet therapy, some of the major complications of PD are likely to be encountered. From this point on, management of the patient with PD becomes increasingly difficult, as most of the available therapies involve significant trade-offs between antiparkinson effect and amelioration of the complicating condition. The major complications of PD are considered in the following sections.

■ MANAGEMENT OF MOTOR FLUCTUATIONS

Sporadic or periodic motor fluctuations become increasingly more common and problematic as the disease progresses. Some are correlated in time with the dosing schedule of dopaminergic agents; others appear at random. Usually the first to be encountered is a typical "wearing-off" effect at the end of one or more dosing intervals. This is characterized by a recrudescence of the patient's parkinsonian symptoms and may readily respond to an upward titration in the dose of Sinemet or a shortening of the dosing interval. Off-period dystonia is also associated with trough levels of levodopa. This is especially common in the morning, before the first dose of Sinemet, when there is usually selective involvement of the feet.

Peak-dose dyskinesias are another common problem. These occur from 30 minutes to 2 hours after a dose of regular Sinemet and may last for as few as 15 minutes or up to the time of the next scheduled dose. Patients themselves may be relatively unconcerned by these involuntary movements, and they almost universally prefer the dyskinesias associated with excess dopaminergic stimulation to the hypokinesia associated with off periods. However, family members are frequently distressed by these movements, and to the clinician their emergence usually indicates that the therapeutic window is narrowing and further problems may lie ahead. Levodopa-induced dyskinesias may be controlled initially by the discontinuance of selegiline or reduction of dopamine agonist therapy. Otherwise, it may be necessary to lower the dose of Sinemet. If dopamine agonists had not already been in use, the reduction in Sinemet may be offset by the careful addition of pergolide or bromocriptine. Soon after their initial appearance, levodopa-induced dyskinesias associated with regular Sinemet may respond to a conversion to Sinemet CR, but this is usually a transient effect.

As the therapeutic window continues to narrow, some patients may eventually deteriorate to the point where they alternate between sustained periods of dyskinesias preceded or followed by end-of-dose akinesia, with only brief interludes of relative normalcy lasting but a few minutes. Another late and potentially quite troublesome complication is that of random "on-off" effects, comprising sudden and unpredictable motor fluctuations that range from severe dyskinesias to profound akinesia with freezing. Either of these late complications may respond to the rather extreme measure of using an oral liquid preparation of Sinemet. Four tablets of regular Sinemet 25/250 can be dissolved by the patient in 1 L of tap water to which 2 g of ascorbic acid has been added. The patient is instructed to begin by taking the liquid form (1 mg of levodopa per 1 ml of liquid) at the same dose and schedule as was previously prescribed. From this starting point, the dose and dosing interval may be adjusted until a relatively even clinical effect is achieved.

■ DRUG-INDUCED PSYCHOSIS AND HALLUCINOSIS

Cognitive side effects of dopaminergic agents are common among elderly patients with PD but may also occur among younger patients. These usually take the form of confusion, visual or auditory hallucinations, or paranoia. Discontinuation of selegiline, amantadine, and/or direct-acting dopamine agonists may permit Sinemet to be continued, although the dose may need to be reduced. Conversion from regular Sinement to Sinemet CR may be helpful on occasion, especially if this is accompanied by an overall reduction in the total effective dose of levodopa. If psychosis or hallucinosis persist after these measures have been taken, and further reductions of Sinemet are accompanied by unacceptable degrees of parkinsonism, an antipsychotic medication may be necessary.

The most effective antipsychotic agent for most PD patients is clozapine (Clozaril) because of its relative specificity for blocking D_4 dopamine receptors, which are concentrated in the mesolimbic system and are believed to be largely responsible for the psychotogenic effects of dopaminergic drugs. Most of the other neuroleptics have more pronounced effects on D_2 receptors, which are abundant within the basal ganglia motor circuitry and the antagonism of which may be associated with various degrees of parkinsonism. Unfortunately, the use of clozapine is encumbered by the necessity of weekly white blood cell counts for the duration of treatment, due to a 1 percent incidence of drug-induced agranulocytosis. For this reason, it is often worthwhile initially to try another antipsychotic that, though less selective than clozapine, may still permit control of psychotic symptoms with a minimum of parkinsonian side effects. Presently, a reasonable choice is risperidone (Risperdal), which blocks dopamine (mainly D_2) as well as serotonin (mainly 5HT-2) receptors. However, it is important that patients and their families be warned of the distinct possibility that their parkinsonian symptoms may be exacerbated by this drug, so that it can be discontinued quickly if necessary. Despite the need for weekly WBCs, the threshold for introducing clozapine should not be too high, as it can often mean the difference between moderate functionality and total disability. Lethargy and hypotension are common side effects of clozaril and frequently impose limits on its effectiveness.

■ HYPOTENSION

Some degree of orthostatic hypotension is common in PD. When moderate to severe, and disproportionate to the level of parkinsonian disability, hypotension may be an indication of progressive autonomic failure and should raise considerations of multiple system atrophy, specifically, the Shy-Drager syndrome. Most dopaminergic agents, particularly Sinemet and the ergot alkaloids, are also quite commonly associated with hypotensive side effects. Many PD patients are especially sensitive to this complication, even in the absence of preexisting hypotension. When severe parkinsonian symptoms prevent further reductions in dopaminergic agents, salt repletion, pressure stockings, and mineralocorticoid therapy with fludrocortisone 0.1 to 0.5 mg three times per day may be indicated. In severe cases of orthostatic hypotension unresponsive to the preceding measures, inhibitors of prostaglandin synthesis (e.g., indomethacin 25 to 50 mg three times per day), low-dose beta-adrenergic blockade (e.g., propranolol 20 to 40 mg twice per day), or a trial of the alpha-2-adrenergic agonist clonidine (0.1 to 0.3 mg twice per day) may be indicated.

■ DEMENTIA

Dementia may occur in up to 20 percent of patients with PD. Treatable causes should be actively excluded. Because of the cognitive side effects associated with all antiparkinson agents (including dopaminergics and anticholinergics), the management of PD patients with associated dementia may present special challenges. If patients develop disruptive behavior that cannot be controlled by nonsedating doses of benzodiazepines, and if side effects preclude effective treatment with clozaril, it may be necessary to trade some worsening of parkinsonian symptomatology for the potent calming effect of other neuroleptics, such as thioridazine or haloperidol.

■ DEPRESSION

Depression requiring medical therapy may be expected in up to 50 percent of PD patients, and in many of these the depression may have antedated the parkinsonian symptoms. This suggests that in some cases, at least, the depression associated with PD may not be simply a reaction to chronic disability, though in other instances that seems clearly to be the case. There is little correlation between the incidence of depression and the severity or chronicity of motor impairment in PD. Nor is there any predictability in the response to levodopa therapy, with some patients showing improvement in depressive symptoms when Sinemet is introduced and others not.

Depression in PD patients usually responds well to treatment either with tricyclics, such as nortriptyline or amitriptyline, or with serotonin reuptake inhibitors, such as sertraline or fluoxetine. The tricyclics have the slight advantage of an anticholinergic effect, which may provide some added benefit with respect to parkinsonian symptoms, but the disadvantages of requiring more delicate titration of dosing and the monitoring of blood levels at higher doses. Recently, the manufacturer of selegiline announced that this drug, as an MAO inhibitor, should not be used in combination with any other antidepressant medication. At the relatively low dose recommended for prophylactic therapy in PD, selegiline itself does not have any significant antidepressant effect.

Should PD patients suffer from severe depression unresponsive to medical therapy, electroconvulsive therapy (ECT) may be indicated. For reasons as yet unexplained, ECT often results in remarkable improvement in the motoric impairments of PD, and these effects may last for 6 months or more.

■ SURGICAL THERAPY

For patients whose progressive motor dysfunction can no longer be managed adequately with medical therapy alone, ablative stereotactic surgery may provide an effective therapeutic option. Two different procedures, each with its own unique indications, expected outcomes, and potential complications, are now available at a number of institutions.

Ventrolateral thalamotomy was devised in the late 1950s and has been used by numerous neurosurgeons over the past 4 decades. The primary indication is severe appendicular tremor unresponsive to medical therapy. The optimal lesion is directed at the nucleus VIM (ventralis intermedius), which is actually the recipient of cerebellar rather than basal ganglia input. Midline tremors (including head tremor) are less responsive to this approach. Ventrolateral thalamotomy can also be used to treat contralateral rigidity, dystonia, or levodopa-induced dyskinesias, provided that the lesion is extended anteriorly to include the basal ganglia-recipient zone that lies just rostral to nucleus VIM. If the lesion is well targeted, patients may receive moderate or even complete relief of contralateral motor symptoms that may last for many years. Neither bradykinesia nor akinesia is improved by the thalamotomy procedure. PD patients must continue to take antiparkinson medications, although the dosage may occasionally be reduced. Successful surgical control of drug-induced dyskinesias may permit even higher doses of Sinemet to be used postoperatively, for more effective control of akinesia. The most common complication of either form of ventrolateral thalamotomy is mild contralateral facial weakness, which is usually transient. Bilateral procedures are considered more hazardous because of the significant risk of hypophonia, which may be permanent.

Over the past 4 years, medial pallidotomy for PD has come into widespread use. Originally introduced a few years before the thalamotomy procedure, the early experiences of most neurosurgeons were not encouraging due to unacceptably high morbidity. However, over the past 35 years the procedure was steadily refined in Sweden, and eagerly embraced in the United States and Europe after the Swedish results were first publicized in 1991. The optimal lesion targets the caudoventral portion of the medial pallidal segment, which represents the major source of motor influences emanating from the basal ganglia. The enthusiasm for the medial pallidotomy procedure is due to the fact that virtually all of the motor symptoms of PD (with the exception of postural instability) are alleviated in the contralateral extremities when the lesion is well placed. Not only are tremor, rigidity, dystonia, and drug-induced dyskinesias improved, but akinesia and bradykinesia as well. In fact, in some cases there may even be some degree of ipsilateral improvement. Contralateral hemianopsia is a potential complication due to the proximity of the optic tract, but with careful placement of the lesion under microelectrode guidance the risk is relatively small. Despite the remarkable improvements in motor function experienced by many patients, levodopa therapy must be continued postoperatively in nearly all cases, but often at reduced dosage. As with the ventral thalamotomy procedure, the success rate for medial pallidotomy depends critically on the skill and experience of the surgical team.

The development of techniques for the eventual transplantation of dopamine-producing cells into the striatum of patients with PD remains an area of active research. Considerable progress has been made in various animal models, but the use of these approaches in human subjects is still experimental.

Suggested Reading

Fahn S, ed. Therapy of Parkinson's disease: Four critical issues. Neurology 1994; 44 (Supp. 1):S3–S20.

Golbe LI, Sage JI. Medical treatment of Parkinson's disease. In: Kurlan R, ed. Treatment of movement disorders. Philadelphia: JB Lippincott, 1995:1.

Jankovic J, Marsden CD. Therapeutic strategies in Parkinson's disease. In: Jankovic J and Tolosa E, eds. Parkinson's disease and movement disorders. 2nd ed. Baltimore: Williams & Wilkins, 1993:115.

Laitinen LV, Bergenheim AT, Hariz MI. Leksell's posteroventral pallidotomy in the treatment of Parkinson's disease. J Neurosurg 1992; 76:53–62.

Tasker RR, Yamashiro K, Lenz F, et al. Thalamotomy in Parkinson's disease. In: Lundsford D, ed. Modern stereotactic surgery. Norwell, Mass: Academic Press, 1988:297.

ACUTE VIRAL ENCEPHALITIS

Roger T. Inouye, M.D.
Scott M. Hammer, M.D.

Encephalitis is inflammation of the brain parenchyma. In contrast, meningitis is an inflammatory process limited to the leptomeninges and the subarachnoid space, but it can often coincide with encephalitis; hence the overlap term *meningoencephalitis.* Encephalitis or meningoencephalitis is suggested by signs and symptoms of brain parenchymal invasion such as mental status and behavioral changes, seizures, and focal neurologic findings. Possible causes of encephalitis include a wide range of infectious, parainfectious, and noninfectious entities. Among the first group are various viruses, which in the United States cause hundreds to thousands of cases per year as reported to the Centers for Disease Control and Prevention (CDC).

With the introduction over the past decade of sensitive molecular biologic techniques such as the polymerase chain reaction (PCR), which provide relatively specific detection of minute quantities of infectious agents, the ability to identify the causative agents of encephalitis has improved substantially. Early detection makes possible prompt, specific antimicrobial intervention.

■ ETIOLOGY

Viral encephalitis can be subdivided into several clinical and pathogenic categories. These include acute viral encephalitis, slow virus infections, postinfectious encephalitis, and cryptogenic central nervous system (CNS) processes with probable direct or indirect viral associations such as Reye's syndrome. Several viral families are associated with acute encephalitis, the most common of which are Herpesviridae, Picornaviridae, Retroviridae, Paramyxoviridae, assorted respiratory and zoonotic viruses, and the group of RNA viruses formerly called arboviruses, now designated as the families Togaviridae, Flaviviridae, Bunyaviridae, and Reoviridae (Table 1). The acquired immunodeficiency syndrome (AIDS) epidemic and therapeutic immunosuppression in transplant recipients and chemotherapy patients have redefined the differential of infectious disease processes that can cause symptoms and signs consistent with encephalitis. These changes have made the clinician's diagnostic task when confronted with an encephalitic patient all the more complex and challenging. Even before these developments, the list of viral and nonviral causes of encephalitis was extensive (Table 2).

■ EPIDEMIOLOGY

The many virus types that can cause encephalitis vary significantly in their epidemiologic profiles. Therefore, the identification of a particular virus can be aided by clues derived from a careful review of the patient's epidemiologic background, including sexual behavior, intravenous drug use,

Table 1 Significant Causes of Viral Encephalitis in the United States

- *Herpesviridae*
  - Herpes simplex viruses
  - Varicella-zoster
  - Cytomegalovirus
  - Epstein-Barr virus
  - Human herpesvirus 6
- *Bunyaviridae*
  - California encephalitis serogroup
  - LaCrosse virus
  - Jamestown virus
  - Snowshoe hare virus
- *Togaviridae*
  - Alphavirus
  - Eastern equine encephalitis virus
  - Western equine encephalitis virus
  - Venezuelan equine encephalitis virus
- *Flaviviridae*
  - St. Louis encephalitis virus
  - Powassan virus
- *Reoviridae*
  - Colorado tick fever virus
- *Picornaviridae*
  - Echovirus
  - Coxsackievirus
  - Poliovirus
  - Enterovirus
- *Retroviridae*
  - HIV-1
- *Orthomyxoviridae*
  - Influenza virus
- *Paramyxoviridae*
  - Measles virus
  - Mumps virus
- *Miscellaneous viruses*
  - Adenovirus
  - Rubella virus (nonarthropod member of Togaviridae)
  - Lymphocytic choriomeningitis virus
  - Rabies virus

Table 2 Nonviral Causes of Encephalitis-like Presentations

INFECTIOUS

- Bacterial
  - Parameningeal infections
  - CNS infections
  - Subdural empyema
  - Venous sinus thrombophlebitis
  - *Neisseria meningitidis*
  - *Streptococcus pneumoniae*
  - *Haemophilus* spp.
  - *Listeria monocytogenes*
  - *Mycoplasma* spp.
  - *Rickettsia* spp.
  - *Borrelia burgdorferi*
  - *Treponema pallidum*
  - *Legionella* spp.
  - *Mycobacterium* spp.
  - *Brucella* spp.
  - *Leptospira* spp.
  - *Actinomyces* spp.
  - *Nocardia* spp.
  - *Bartonella henselae*
  - *Tropheryma whippeli*
  - Bacterial toxin-mediated processes
- Fungal
  - Zygomycetes
  - *Aspergillus* spp.
  - *Cryptococcus neoformans*
  - *Coccidioides immitis*
  - *Histoplasma capsalatum*
- Parasitic
  - *Toxoplasma gondii*
  - *Plasmodium* spp.
  - *Trypanosoma* spp.
  - *Naegleria fowleri*
  - *Acanthamoeba* spp.
  - *Strongyloides stercoralis*

NONINFECTIOUS

- Parainfectious
  - Reye's syndrome
  - Viral postinfectious syndromes
  - Postvaccination syndromes
- Primary central nervous system or metastatic neoplastic disease
- Cerebrovascular disease
- Subdural hematoma
- Endocrine disorders
- Toxic metabolic encephalopathy
- Connective tissue disease (e.g., systemic lupus erythematosus, Behçet's disease)
- Paraneoplastic syndromes
- Seizures/postictal state

travel, occupation, arthropod or animal contacts, vaccine history, and exposures to ill persons. A summary of representative associations with specific viral and nonviral entities is outlined in Table 3.

■ PATHOGENESIS

Depending on the specific pathogen, viruses gain entry into the CNS mainly through hematogenous or neural spread and cause either direct cytopathic effects or indirect pathology via immune-mediated processes. Bunyaviridae, Flaviviridae, and Togaviridae hematogenously seed the CNS following replication in local tissues after subcutaneous inoculation by the insect vector. In addition to the integument, the initial portal of entry by neurotropic viruses can be the respiratory tract (e.g., adenovirus, measles, influenza) or the gastrointestinal tract (e.g., enteroviruses), or the placenta (e.g., cytomegalovirus [CMV]). Rabies virus is a neurotropic virus that reaches the CNS via intra-axonal transport. In the case of adult herpes simplex virus (HSV) encephalitis, either primary or reactivated, the pathogenesis remains unfully characterized, but virus passage along the olfactory and trigeminal tracts, respectively, would explain the classic temporal lobe localization.

Once the CNS parenchyma has been seeded, predominantly mononuclear cell perivascular infiltrates, glial nodules, and neuronophagia characterize histopathologic changes commonly seen in acute viral encephalitis. Inclusion bodies, such as Negri and Cowdry bodies caused by rabies and herpesviruses, respectively, can reflect infections with specific viruses. The type of CNS parenchymal cell predominantly affected during encephalitis can vary among neurotropic viruses. The role of cytokines in the pathogenesis of encephalitis remains to be defined. Likewise, the possible role of infectious copathogens as in the case of CMV with human immunodeficiency virus (HIV) continues to be elucidated.

In postinfectious encephalitis, pathogenesis occurs via immune-mediated mechanisms rather than through direct cytopathic effects, and manifests as multifocal perivascular demyelination. Viruses implicated in this type of encephalitis include measles, mumps, rubella, varicella-zoster virus (VZV), and Epstein-Barr virus (EBV).

Host factors clearly play a role in the susceptibility to and severity of viral encephalitis. For example, chronic enteroviral meningoencephalitis is seen most commonly in patients with agammaglobulinemia; acute measles encephalitis usually occurs in immunosuppressed patients.

■ CLINICAL MANIFESTATIONS

Usually the clinical features of a particular neurotropic virus alone are not pathognomonic. The clinical presentation of viral infections of the CNS can vary from no symptoms to a fulminantly fatal disease. Although the literature is replete

Table 3 Clinical and Epidemiologic Characteristics of Major Causes of Viral Encephalitis in the United States

VIRUS	MOST AFFECTED HOST	PEAK SEASON	GEOGRAPHIC DISTRIBUTION	CLUES IN PRESENTATION	EPIDEMIOLOGIC CLUES
HERPESVIRIDAE					
Herpes simplex type 1	All ages	Year-round	Ubiquitous	Focal neurologic findings such as hemiparesis, ataxia, visual field loss, dysphasia, seizures	
Varicella-zoster	Healthy and immuno-compromised adults; infants	Year-round	Ubiquitous	Cerebellar ataxia	Primary varicella rash or herpes zoster dermatomal rash possible; onset usually within 2 weeks of rash
Cytomegalovirus (CMV)	Immunocompromised, e.g., person with AIDS; transplant recipients; neonates	Year-round	Ubiquitous	Cranial nerve palsies; radiographic findings of ventriculomegaly or periventricular enhancement	In known HIV+ individuals, CD4 count <100, prior CMV disease; post-transplant individuals: donor and recipient CMV serologic status, most cases occur 3 weeks to 4 months post-transplant; in patients with unknown immune status must elicit HIV risk factors
RETROVIRIDAE					
Human immuno-deficiency virus	All ages	Year-round	Ubiquitous	Subacute onset of cognitive, motor deficits in an HIV+ individual; focal findings rare	HIV risk factor history: sexual practices, intravenous drug use, transfusions
TOGAVIRIDAE					
Eastern equine	Young and elderly	Summer, fall	East, Gulf Coast	High morbidity and mortality, especially in the elderly and young	Contact with Culiseta mosquito; outdoor occupation or activities
Western equine	Young and elderly	Summer, fall	Western North America, Central and South America	Nonfocal presentation common	Contact with Culex mosquito; outdoor occupation or activities; travel or habitation in rural areas
Venezuelan equine	Adults	Summer, fall	South	Nonfocal presentation common	Contact with Culex or Aedes mosquito; outdoor occupation or activities
St. Louis encephalitis	Elderly	Summer, fall	Nationwide	Nonfocal presentation common	Contact with Culex mosquito; in the West, endemic in rural areas; in the East, sporadic urban outbreaks
Powassan	Young	Summer, fall	Nationwide	Nonfocal presentation common	Contact with ticks; possible transmission through unpasteurized dairy products
BUNYAVIRIDAE					
LaCrosse	Young	Summer, fall	Midwest, East	Usually asymptomatic	Contact with Aedes mosquito; outdoor activities
PICORNAVIRIDAE					
Echo Coxsackie Polio Enterovirus	Young, especially agammaglobulinemic children	Summer, fall	Nationwide	Accompanying viral exanthem, conjunctivitis, myopericarditis, herpangina, hand-foot-and-mouth disease	Known community epidemic of picornavirus
RHABDOVIRIDAE					
Rabies	All ages		Nationwide except Hawaii	Animal bite or scratch	Animal contact

with case reports of unique neurologic manifestations of viral encephalitis, the clinical presentation of acute viral encephalitis is generally characterized by a rapidly progressive constellation of symptoms. These typically include fever, altered mental status, headache, nausea, and vomiting. Nuchal rigidity and seizures, either partial or generalized, can also be prominent. Cranial nerve abnormalities are commonly seen in certain encephalitic processes such as HIV-related CMV ventriculoencephalitis. Certain viral pathogens are associated with focal CNS predilections and can cause corresponding deficits. Archetypical of such viruses are HSV with the temporal and fronto-orbital lobes, CMV with the periventricular areas, rabies with the limbic system, and VZV with the cerebellum. Associated extraneural complications of viral encephalitis include inappropriate antidiuretic hormone (ADH) secretion and diabetes insipidus.

Furthermore, any extraneural manifestations of a particular neurotropic virus, such as parotitis with mumps, pharyngitis and lympadenopathy with EBV, and a dermatomal rash with VZV, may aid in the diagnostic workup (see Table 3). However, significant numbers of patients may present without the classic constellation of extraneural signs and symptoms; their absence does not exclude specific pathogens.

DIAGNOSIS

Clues to the cause can be derived from both a patient's epidemiologic background and the clinical manifestations. Several diagnostic tests also have varying utility in the diagnosis of viral encephalitis. Basic laboratory studies such as general chemistries and cell counts have relatively limited value, but occasionally clues can be derived from them. For example, a peripheral blood examination showing atypical lymphocytes or a positive Monospot may suggest EBV infection; hyperamylasemia may suggest mumps virus. Rectal and throat swabs may provide evidence of neurotropic viruses such as enteroviruses. Immunocytochemical analysis of corneal smears occasionally aids in the diagnosis of rabies. However, the absence of such findings does not exclude a particular virus.

Examination of the cerebrospinal fluid (CSF) can show abnormal nonspecific cell counts and chemistries. For example, with HSV encephalitis, except in the initial stages, most patients have a mononuclear pleocytosis typically less than 1,000 cells per cubic millimeter with a median of approximately 130 cells per cubic millimeter. Significant numbers of polymorphonuclear cells (at least 40 percent) can be seen in as many as 10 to 15 percent of patients if the lumbar puncture is done early. Red blood cells (RBCs) are usually present in the CSF, but in a series conducted by the National Institute of Allergy and Infectious Diseases (NIAID) Collaborative Antiviral Study Group, 16 percent of brain biopsy–proven HSV encephalitis cases lacked RBCs in their CSF, and 18 percent of these patients had RBC counts above 500 per cubic millimeter. Although in half of the patients the total protein may be normal in the first week, CSF protein levels are usually elevated, with a range of 7 to 755 and a mean value of 80 mg/dl. In HSV encephalitis, hypoglycorrhachia is relatively uncommon.

The yield (and consequently the utility) of CSF viral culture in adults with encephalitis is low. Because CSF results are relatively nonspecific and may even be normal in early disease, several other diagnostic modalities have been used to obtain clinically useful results and to guide initial therapy.

Radiologic and Electroencephalographic Evidence

The electroencephalogram (EEG) may assist in the diagnosis of acute focal encephalitis such as HSV. Periodic lateralized epileptiform discharges in the temporal lobe classically can be seen within the first days after onset. Although having low specificity, the EEG is reported to have a sensitivity on the order of 81 percent versus 59 percent for computed tomography (CT) and 50 percent for nuclear scans. Encephalitis-induced EEG abnormalities can precede CT changes, which may not be seen until 4 to 5 days after the onset of symptoms. CT abnormalities in HSV are typically characterized by low-density lesions in one or both of the inferomedial temporal lobes. T2-weighted magnetic resonance imaging (MRI) allows for earlier radiographic evidence of encephalitis and more precise imaging of the temporobasal lobes than CT. MRI, therefore, is the radiographic imaging study of choice in patients with suspected encephalitis.

Pathogen-Specific CSF and Serologic Assays

Serum and CSF immunoglobulin assays are available for most neurotropic viruses, including the Herpesviridae, Bunyaviridae, Togaviridae, Picornaviridae, and Rhabdoviridae. Unfortunately, viral-specific antibodies are difficult to detect early in the disease process. For example, HSV-specific antibodies are rarely detected in the first week of illness and so are not very helpful with selection of a specific therapeutic intervention. Furthermore, CSF antibodies may be elevated because of nonencephalitic processes such as viremia without CNS involvement; therefore, serum to CSF antibody ratios may be used to help distinguish between CNS and non-CNS viral processes. Acute and convalescent serum titers alone can retrospectively suggest acute infection, but again, they are not useful when initial therapeutic decisions are made.

PCR has been used to detect a number of neurotropic viruses in CSF, biopsy, and autopsy specimens, including HSV, VZV, CMV, EBV, human herpesvirus (HHV) 6, HIV, measles virus, JC virus, and enteroviruses. This diagnostic technique, applied to CSF, is an attractive alternative to brain biopsy, given its relative noninvasiveness combined with the limitations of the aforementioned modalities in terms of early onset sensitivity and specificity. Again, with HSV, the sensitivity and specificity of PCR of CSF-extracted DNA from patients with presumed HSV encephalitis is reported to be as high as 95 to 100 percent. Positive results are reported as early as a day after onset of symptoms. In comparison, in the same study, HSV antigen detection had a sensitivity of 33 percent, and HSV-specific intrathecal antibody assay by indirect Enzyme-linked immunosorbent assay (ELISA) had a sensitivity of 23 percent.

Brain Biopsy

The role of a diagnostic brain biopsy in the management of HSV encephalitis remains controversial, especially in light of the ability to institute effective empiric antiviral drugs for viruses such as HSV and the rivaling sensitivity and specificity

Table 4 Treatment Regimens for Herpes Viral Encephalitis

VIRUS	DRUG OF CHOICE	MAJOR TOXICITIES	ALTERNATIVE REGIMENS	MAJOR TOXICITIES
Herpes simplex virus	Acyclovir 10 mg/kg IV q8h for 10 to 14 days	Nephrotoxicity, vomiting, diarrhea, mental status changes	Foscarnet 60 mg/kg IV q8h or 90 mg/kg IV q12h for 10 to 14 days	Nephrotoxicity, electrolyte disturbances, nausea, fever
			Vidarabine 15 mg/kg IV qd for 10 to 14 days	Nausea, confusion, hematologic abnormalities
Cytomegalovirus	Foscarnet induction 60 mg/kg IV q8h or 90 mg/kg q12h for 21 days; consider maintenance therapy in HIV+ patients	Nephrotoxicity, electrolyte disturbances, nausea, fever	Foscarnet can be combined with ganciclovir	
	Ganciclovir induction 5 mg/kg IV q12h for 21 days; consider maintenance therapy in HIV+ patients	Bone marrow suppression, rash, fevers		
Varicella-zoster virus	Acyclovir 10 mg/kg IV q8h	As for acyclovir		
Epstein-Barr virus	Acyclovir 10 mg/kg IV q8h	As for acyclovir		

of relatively noninvasive PCR-based assays. Until PCR techniques become more widely available and accepted, brain biopsy remains the gold standard of diagnosis.

■ THERAPY

General Supportive Care

No effective treatment is yet available for many neurotropic viruses such as the Bunyaviridae, Togaviridae, and Picornaviridae. Therefore, it is important to pay particular attention to preventing and treating complications that can arise in any patient with a depressed sensorium, who may require an extended intensive care unit stay with ventilatory support. These include nosocomial infectious diseases such as pneumonias with potentially resistant, gram-negative organisms; device-related infections such as those involving intracranial pressure monitoring bolts, line infections, and indwelling urinary catheters; and antibiotic-related colitis. CNS complications of encephalitis, such as seizures and intracranial hypertension, may necessitate anticonvulsants and intracranial pressure–lowering techniques such as hyperventilation, osmotic agents, and barbiturates. The possibility of noninfectious complications such as deep vein thrombosis, pulmonary embolism, gastrointestinal stress ulcers, decubitus ulcers, musculoskeletal contractures, and malnutrition requires appropriate attention as well.

Antiviral Therapy

While numerous viruses are associated with encephalitis, there remain relatively few effective regimens. Nevertheless, some drugs have activity against several of the more commonly encountered viral pathogens (Table 4).

Herpesviridae

Herpes Simplex Virus. In the United States, HSV is the most common cause of sporadic encephalitis. In the mid-1980s two studies showed acyclovir to work better than vidarabine in adult patients. In one of these studies, recipients of vidarabine had a mortality of 54 percent compared with 28 percent for those who received acyclovir. Additionally, at a 6 month morbidity assessment, 38 percent of acyclovir recipients versus 14 percent of vidarabine-treated patients had normal functional status. The age of the patient (over 30 years), level of consciousness at presentation (Glasgow coma score over 10), and duration of disease (under 4 days) before acyclovir therapy were significant determinants of improved survival. In contrast to these findings in adults, controlled trials comparing acyclovir with vidarabine in neonatal HSV encephalitis failed to show significant differences in outcome.

Relapses have occurred after the administration of standard regimens of both acyclovir and vidarabine and are thought to occur in up to 5 percent of cases. Treatment failures have been attributed to cryptogenic postinfectious mechanisms, failure of the standard 10 day regimen to eradicate the virus, and possibly drug resistance. Acyclovir resistance is most commonly associated with HSV thymidine kinase alteration or deficiency (TK–). Resistant strains have been described as causing acyclovir-refractory HSV meningoencephalitis in HIV-infected individuals.

Cytomegalovirus. With the advent of the AIDS epidemic, CMV infections including encephalitis have unfortunately become more common. Ganciclovir, one of the mainstays in the treatment of CMV retinitis, has yielded inconsistent results in the treatment of CMV encephalitis and ventriculitis. Foscarnet crosses the blood-brain barrier, attaining virustatic concentrations in CSF, and therefore is a reasonable alternative to ganciclovir.

Varicella-Zoster and Epstein-Barr Viruses. High-dose parenteral acyclovir has been used in the treatment of VZV encephalitis, although the use of antiviral drugs in this disease

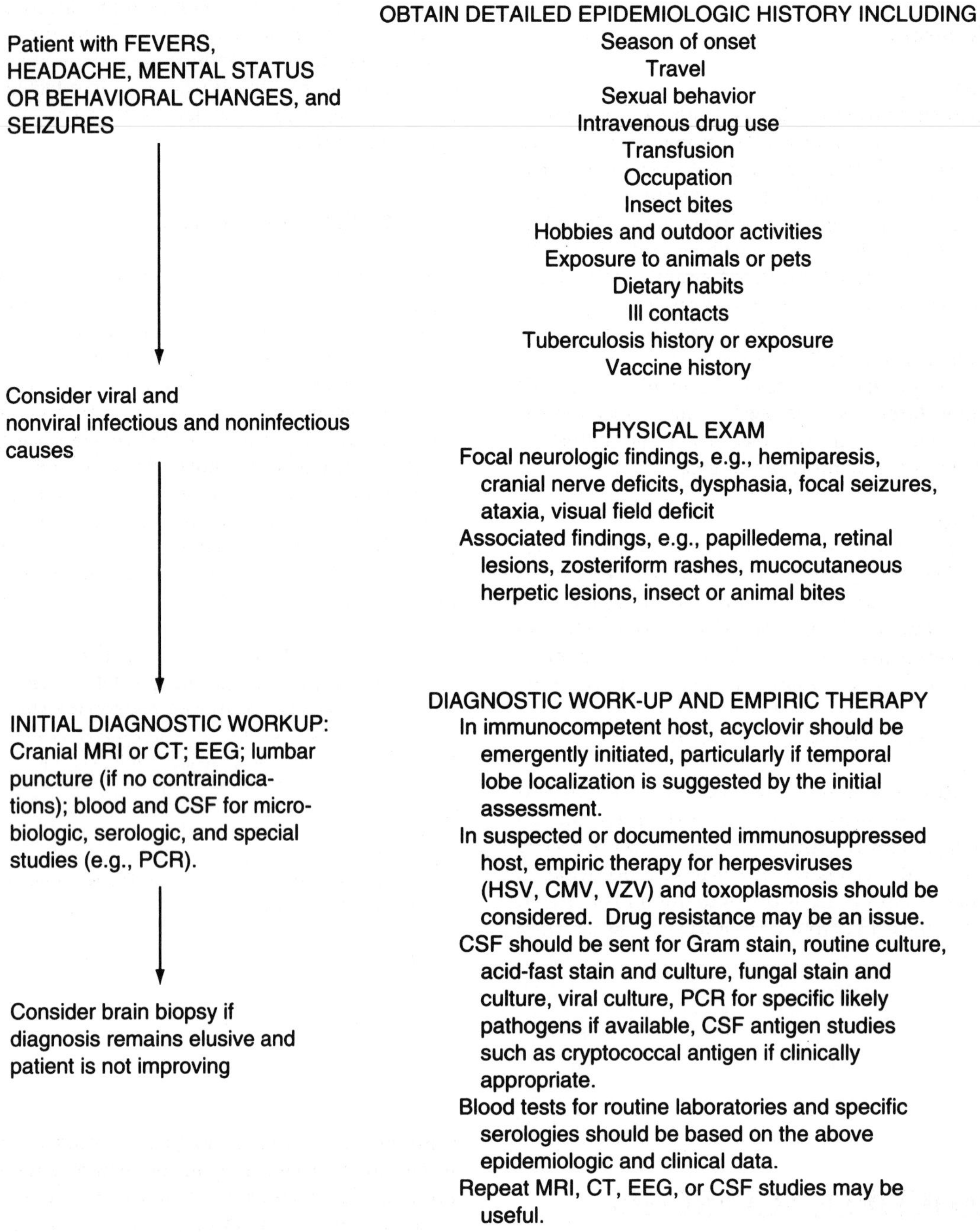

Patient with FEVERS, HEADACHE, MENTAL STATUS OR BEHAVIORAL CHANGES, and SEIZURES

↓

Consider viral and nonviral infectious and noninfectious causes

↓

INITIAL DIAGNOSTIC WORKUP: Cranial MRI or CT; EEG; lumbar puncture (if no contraindications); blood and CSF for microbiologic, serologic, and special studies (e.g., PCR).

↓

Consider brain biopsy if diagnosis remains elusive and patient is not improving

OBTAIN DETAILED EPIDEMIOLOGIC HISTORY INCLUDING
Season of onset
Travel
Sexual behavior
Intravenous drug use
Transfusion
Occupation
Insect bites
Hobbies and outdoor activities
Exposure to animals or pets
Dietary habits
Ill contacts
Tuberculosis history or exposure
Vaccine history

PHYSICAL EXAM
Focal neurologic findings, e.g., hemiparesis, cranial nerve deficits, dysphasia, focal seizures, ataxia, visual field deficit
Associated findings, e.g., papilledema, retinal lesions, zosteriform rashes, mucocutaneous herpetic lesions, insect or animal bites

DIAGNOSTIC WORK-UP AND EMPIRIC THERAPY
In immunocompetent host, acyclovir should be emergently initiated, particularly if temporal lobe localization is suggested by the initial assessment.
In suspected or documented immunosuppressed host, empiric therapy for herpesviruses (HSV, CMV, VZV) and toxoplasmosis should be considered. Drug resistance may be an issue.
CSF should be sent for Gram stain, routine culture, acid-fast stain and culture, fungal stain and culture, viral culture, PCR for specific likely pathogens if available, CSF antigen studies such as cryptococcal antigen if clinically appropriate.
Blood tests for routine laboratories and specific serologies should be based on the above epidemiologic and clinical data.
Repeat MRI, CT, EEG, or CSF studies may be useful.

Figure 1
Diagnostic and therapeutic considerations in acute encephalitis.

has yet to be proved to have clinical benefit. Encephalitis is a rare complication of EBV. The therapeutic effects of acyclovir in EBV encephalitis remain unproven as well but should be strongly considered, given the lack of alternative regimens and the relatively low toxicity of acyclovir.

Paramyxoviridae

Invasion of the CNS by measles virus is associated with several distinct syndromes, including two forms of acute encephalitis. One is characterized by direct cytopathic effects, the other by immunologically mediated mechanisms. The former usually occurs in immunocompromised hosts. Early ribavirin administration in PCR-diagnosed measle encephalitis of this variety has been reported effective in young immunocompromised hosts. The role of steroids in postinfectious immune-mediated measles and other parainfectious encephalitides related to other viruses has yet to be clearly established.

Rhabdoviridae

Because of the lack of effective therapies, the approach to rabies must concentrate on pre-exposure vaccination of high-risk individuals such as veterinarians and postexposure prophylaxis, as there are only extremely rare survivors with symptomatic disease.

Retroviridae

Human Immunodeficiency Virus. With varying degrees of supporting data, a number of compounds have been reported to have an effect on primary HIV-related encephalopathy. The most studied and best proved of these agents are the reverse transcriptase inhibitors, most notably zidovudine (ZDV). After other possible causes have been addressed, ZDV 1 to 2 g per day can be administered empirically to HIV-positive patients with a subacute course of nonfocal cognitive-motor deficits characteristic of HIV encephalopathy. Although having a lower CSF to plasma ratio than ZDV, didanosine also appears to decrease the incidence of HIV encephalopathy. Attempts have been made to increase the CNS concentration of anti-HIV drugs by coupling them to carrier molecules such as dihydropyridine.

Picornaviridae

The mainstay of picornaviral encephalitis treatment is supportive care. Several experimental agents, the WIN compounds, which interfere with the picornaviral capsid, hold promise for treatment. The intraventricular administration of gamma globulin may be beneficial in the treatment of picornaviral encephalitis in agammaglobulinemic children.

Bunyaviridae, Flaviviridae, Togaviridae, and Reoviridae

Treatment of arthropod-transmitted encephalitis is also generally supportive. Adjunctive use of high-dose dexamethasone was tested to reduce intracranial hypertension–related deaths in Japanese B encephalitis (JE) virus infections, but no statistically significant benefit was noted. Immunization has potential to be a means by which selected arboviral encephalitides may be prevented. For example, inactivated JE virus vaccine given in three doses has been shown to induce significant neutralizing antibody titers and should be strongly considered for individuals who plan on traveling to endemic areas, especially for extended periods or during the peak summer months.

■ CLINICAL APPROACH

Several factors should be taken into account when approaching a patient with an encephalitic presentation (Fig. 1). Host factors such as immune status and age should be noted and combined with a full review of epidemiologic clues. Next, associated physical exam findings and general laboratory values should be assessed. Given the significant morbidity and mortality associated with untreated HSV encephalitis, for which effective therapies now exist, combined with the relatively common prevalence of this entity, empiric anti-HSV therapy should be initiated on an urgent basis in the appropriate clinical setting. Concurrently, alternative viral, nonviral, and noninfectious causes should be diagnostically and therapeutically addressed.

Suggested Reading

Fishbein DB, Robinson LE. Rabies. N Engl J Med 1993; 329(22):1632–1638.

Kalayjian RC, Cohen ML, Bonomo RA, Flanigan TP. Cytomegalovirus ventriculoencephalitis in AIDS. Medicine 1993; 72(2):67–77.

Koskiniemi M, Vaheri A, Taskinen E. Cerebrospinal fluid alterations in herpes simplex virus encephalitis. Rev Infect Dis 1984; 6(5):608–618.

Tsai TF. Arboviral infections in the United States. Infect Dis Clin North Am 1991; 5(1):73–102.

Whitley RJ, Lakeman F. Herpes simplex virus infections of the central nervous system: Therapeutic and diagnostic considerations. Clin Infect Dis 1995; 20:414–420.

MULTIPLE SCLEROSIS

J. William Lindsey, M.D.
Staley A. Brod, M.D.
Jerry S. Wolinsky, M.D.

Multiple sclerosis (MS) is a recurrent or chronic disease characterized by damage to central nervous system myelin. MS is quite variable in its clinical presentation and course, and patients may have acute relapses followed by remission, relapses followed by partial remission, chronic progression of symptoms, or any combination of these. The neurologic status of the patient may fluctuate dramatically from month to month, especially early in the disease. Although there is minimal effect on life span, patients often develop significant disability. The long-term prognosis for development of disability is variable; some patients have only minimal disability after years of disease, and others may become rapidly and severely disabled. There are no reliable characteristics that identify the patients destined to do well or those destined to do poorly. Because of the short-term and long-term variability, treatment must be individually tailored for each patient, and the decision to use any medical therapy must balance the risks and benefits of the therapy with the anticipated natural history of the disease.

■ DIAGNOSIS

In spite of the recent advances in imaging technology, the diagnosis of MS is still made on clinical criteria. Accurate diagnosis is essential since other disease processes can produce symptoms and magnetic resonance imaging (MRI) findings similar to those seen in MS. We make the diagnosis of MS only when the patient has experienced two distinct episodes of neurologic symptoms affecting two distinct areas of the central nervous system, and the alternative diagnoses relevant to the individual case have been excluded by appropriate laboratory tests. Recent studies suggest that patients presenting with a monosymptomatic syndrome (optic neuritis, transverse myelitis, or a brainstem syndrome) and typical white matter lesions on brain MRI are at a high risk of progressing to clinically definite MS over the next few years. We discuss this possibility with those patients, but we do not diagnose MS until the clinical criteria are unequivocally satisfied because of the implications of the diagnosis for employment and eligibility for health insurance. We are also careful in diagnosing MS because once the diagnosis is made, it is frequently accepted by subsequent physicians without critical re-evaluation, and all subsequent neurologic symptoms are attributed to MS with little further investigation.

■ NONPHARMACOLOGIC THERAPY

Once the diagnosis of MS is made, our earliest intervention is usually counseling the patient. We inform them directly of the diagnosis and discuss the variable prognosis for development of disability, the typical clinical course, the moderate risk of MS in first-degree relatives, the effect of pregnancy on MS, and the available treatments. Since many patients with the early symptoms of MS will have a relatively benign course, we encourage an optimistic outlook. A statistically better prognosis is associated with younger age at onset, female sex, relapsing rather than progressive symptoms, and visual or sensory symptoms at onset, but none of these factors is useful in predicting individual prognosis. Most patients ask about the effects of stress, diet, lifestyle, exercise, smoking, and alcohol use on the course of MS. We encourage them to pursue a generally healthy lifestyle, but we inform them that there is no special diet or nutritional supplement that affects the course of MS and that exercise neither worsens nor alleviates the symptoms of MS. We advise patients against provoking heat-sensitive symptoms but otherwise suggest no limitations on activity. We refer patients wishing more detailed information to the local chapter of the MS Society or to the excellent text by Kalb and Scheinberg, *Multiple Sclerosis and the Family.* Patients are often interested in whatever alternative therapy is popular in the local MS community at the time. We remind them of the difficulties in assessing the effect of therapies in a relapsing-remitting disease and give them any information available in medical literature. In the interest of preserving the physician-patient relationship, we do not discourage alternative therapies unless they are dangerous or expensive or interfere with other effective treatment.

■ PHARMACOLOGIC THERAPY

Pharmacologic therapy in MS is directed at ameliorating acute exacerbations, modifying the long-term course of disease, or alleviating the various symptoms caused by damaged myelin.

Treatment of Acute Relapses

High-Dose Intravenous Methylprednisolone

Early in disease, patients usually have well-defined exacerbations and remissions. We treat exacerbations that significantly affect function with a 5 day course of intravenous methylprednisolone at a dose of 1,000 mg per day (an alternative dose is 15 mg per kilogram per day). This regimen has been demonstrated in controlled trials to hasten and improve recovery from the acute attack. It may also prolong the time to the next exacerbation. New or recurring symptoms should be present for at least 24 hours before an exacerbation is diagnosed, and treatment should ideally begin early in the course of the exacerbation. Patients should be advised of the symptoms that may occur during an exacerbation and instructed to call if they think they are having an exacerbation. We generally do not treat exacerbations that have only sensory symptoms, those that have no definite signs on examination, or those that are already resolving. We also do not treat symptoms appearing during the course of an acute infection unless they persist after the infection has resolved. We usually give a rapid oral taper of steroids, starting with a dose of 1.5 mg per kilogram of prednisone and decreasing by 20 mg every 2 to 3 days. We feel that the taper reduces the emotional effects of steroid withdrawal and may reduce the possibility of early relapse, but there is no controlled clinical evidence to support this practice. Patients should be re-evaluated within 3 to 4 weeks following the taper of steroids in order to define their new neurologic baseline.

We make sure that any intercurrent infection is recognized and adequately treated before starting high-dose steroids, and we treat patients with an H_2 blocker such as famotidine while they are on steroids. We observe only minimal adverse effects with this brief regimen. Many patients experience mood changes and fluid retention, but these symptoms resolve after the course is finished. We prefer to admit patients to the hospital for treatment if it is their first course of such therapy because of the potentially serious side effects, including psychosis, anaphylaxis, hypertension, and hyperglycemia. Severe attacks that seriously compromise the patient's or caregiver's ability to provide supportive care require acute hospitalization, often with a course of inpatient rehabilitation after methylprednisolone treatment. With this regimen, the total time on corticosteroids should be 14 days or less, so we usually avoid the more serious side effects of long-term steroid therapy.

Alternative Corticosteroid Regimens

A variety of other regimens using different corticosteroids or adrenocorticotropic hormone (ACTH) at different doses by different routes of administration have been used. Studies in small numbers of patients suggest that high-dose intravenous methylprednisolone is equivalent to or better than ACTH, better than lower doses of intravenous methylprednisolone, and similar to equivalent doses of oral methylprednisolone. Until more definitive studies are available, we avoid deviating from the protocol just described. We advise against the use of medium-dose regimens of oral steroids, such as 1 mg per kilogram of prednisone per day for 1 or 2 weeks. These regimens are easy and inexpensive; but there is suggestive evidence that they accelerate the occurrence of future relapses.

Therapies Affecting the Long-Term Course of the Disease

Although treatment of acute exacerbations with corticosteroids hastens recovery, there is no evidence that it affects the long-term accumulation of disability. The most exciting developments in MS therapy over the last few years have been the reports of therapies that either reduce the frequency of relapses or slow the progression of disability. One of these therapies is currently available, and others may be available soon.

Prevention of Relapses

For patients with frequent relapses early in disease, we consider treatment with interferon-beta-1b (Betaseron). This drug reduced the relapse rate by 31 percent when given at a dose of 0.25 mg on alternate days by subcutaneous injection in a 3 year clinical trial. Interferon-beta-1b also reduced disease activity on serial MRI scans, and there was a trend to a decrease in the progression of disability as measured by the Kurtzke Expanded Disability Status Scale (EDSS). The only patient population studied was selected for mild disability, relapsing-remitting disease, and frequent relapses, so efficacy in more severe disease or progressive disease is unknown. Before beginning therapy, patients should understand that interferon-beta-1b reduces the frequency of exacerbations but does not prevent them entirely. We continue to treat acute exacerbations with our standard regimen of corticosteroids while patients are on interferon-beta-1b.

The drawbacks of interferon-beta-1b are the route and frequency of administration, the side effects, and the significant cost. The patients must be trained to give themselves the subcutaneous injections. The most common side effects observed in our practice are injection site reactions and a flulike syndrome of fatigue, malaise, and myalgia on the day following injections. More severe side effects include neutropenia, leukopenia, and elevation of hepatic transaminases, which require every 3 month monitoring; skin necrosis; and depression, which can be severe enough to lead to suicide attempts. Many patients have impressive side effects at the initiation of therapy that become more tolerable with time. About 20 percent of our patients have discontinued the drug because of intolerable side effects.

There are no clear guidelines for discontinuing treatment. There is evidence that some patients develop an antibody response that blocks the effect of the drug. We discontinue treatment in patients who have several severe relapses in 1 year or who develop progressive symptoms.

Two other forms of therapy aimed at preventing relapses and slowing the course of disease have been approved. These are copolymer-1 and a second interferon, interferon-beta-1a. Both have recently been shown in controlled trials to reduce the frequency of relapses in early MS by about 30 percent and to alter the accumulation of disability as measured on the EDSS. Both have to be given by injection, but they are reported to have fewer side effects than Betaseron. Both of these therapies were shown to be effective in patients with relapsing-remitting disease and minimal or moderate disability. The usefulness of the interferon for progressive symptoms or later disease has not been tested. Copolymer-1 appears to be more effective early in disease and has a more impressive effect in relapsing-remitting patients than in chronic-progressive patients.

Progressive Disease or MS with Severe Disability

Unlike the treatment of acute exacerbations and the prevention of exacerbations in early disease, there are no therapies that have been definitively demonstrated to be useful in more severe MS. We often see patients who are rapidly accumulating disability, either following relapses with incomplete recovery or in a chronic progressive course. The need for effective intervention is pressing, but there are no clear guidelines supported by adequate studies.

Our recommendations for treating these patients are extrapolated from the experience in early relapsing-remitting MS just discussed. We often attempt steroid therapy, especially when patients are approaching a major change in function, such as requiring a wheelchair instead of a cane, or becoming unable to transfer without assistance. The results are variable, but sometimes progression is arrested or improvement occurs. We also sometimes try monthly treatments with a single dose of 1,000 mg of methylprednisolone for patients with frequent relapses requiring repeated courses of steroid treatment. It is currently not known whether interferon-beta-1b will be effective in patients with progressive symptoms or with severe disability. A clinical trial to test the efficacy of interferon-beta-1b in progressive MS is currently planned.

If steroids are not effective, we occasionally utilize one of the many other immunosuppressive agents that have been used in MS, but these agents are of limited efficacy. Azathioprine and methotrexate are both well tolerated but probably have at best a modest effect on slowing progression. Cyclosporine also has a modest effect on slowing progression, but its use is limited by the significant side effects of hypertension and renal toxicity and by its high cost. Cyclophosphamide is claimed to be useful for treatment of progressive MS but was never shown to be superior to placebo in a controlled trial. Nevertheless, monthly bolus treatments with cyclophosphamide may be useful in highly selected cases.

The need for effective therapy for this group of patients is obvious, and several clinical trials of various therapies for progressive MS are either planned or under way. Whenever possible, such patients should be encouraged to participate in these controlled trials.

Symptomatic Therapies

Even when we are unable to affect the primary disease process in MS, treatment of the symptoms may significantly improve the quality of life of the patient.

Fatigue

Fatigue is a frequent symptom in MS and may occur either in patients with severe weakness or in patients with minimal findings on examination. We treat fatigue with amantadine 100 mg twice per day. We have patients take the drug for 2 to 3 weeks before deciding whether it is effective and whether to continue therapy. About half of patients will have a beneficial response, although the mechanism of action is unknown. The main side effects are nausea, lightheadedness, and insomnia.

The development of livedo reticularis limits the long-term use of amantidine in some patients. Fatigue in MS is often cyclical, so patients should be encouraged to cycle off the drug periodically. If amantadine is not effective, second-line therapies include pemoline and fluoxetine. Pemoline is given as 18.75 mg tablets, starting with two per day and titrating the daily dose upward at weekly intervals to a maximum of six tablets per day. Fluoxetine is prescribed at 20 to 40 mg per day. We do not use methylphenidate as it is rarely effective if the other drugs fail, and its use creates significant regulatory problems.

Pain

Although generally under-rated as a symptom in MS, pain is a frequent complaint. Some of the pain encountered is paroxysmal in character, whether seen as classic trigeminal neuralgia or as radicular pain, and is presumably related to lesions in sensory pathways. This type of pain usually responds to near-homeopathic doses of carbamazepine. It has recently been suggested that misoprostol, a long-acting prostaglandin E analogue, may be quite effective in this setting. Other effective therapies, listed in the approximate order of benefit, include tricyclic antidepressants, phenytoin, baclofen, or valproate. The lowest effective dose of a given drug should be used. These syndromes are often self-limited, so the need for continued therapy should be re-evaluated at intervals.

More problematic are the more continuous dysesthetic sensations. The drugs just listed should be tried in turn, each pushed to clinical tolerance or benefit, until the list is exhausted. Only then should narcotic or intrathecal administration of narcotics or baclofen be considered on a trial basis.

Musculoskeletal pain related to pyramidal imbalance is common in more severely affected patients. Directed exercise programs with the guidance of a physical therapist are sometimes useful. Hydrotherapy can be particularly helpful, especially in patients whose pyramidal weakness precludes standing or walking on land. More often nonsteroidal anti-inflammatory drugs or non-narcotic analgesics are necessary. Occasionally this type of pain is a manifestation of depression.

Depression

Depression is frequent in MS and several studies document a markedly increased risk of suicide in the MS patient population. Most instances of depression can be managed with supportive treatment and involvement in MS support groups. A list of these can be provided by the local chapter of the National Multiple Sclerosis Society. Some patients may require treatment with antidepressant medication or referral to a psychiatrist. Medications causing depression as a side effect, such as Betaseron, must be used carefully, if at all, in depressed patients.

Bowel and Bladder Symptoms

Complaints of difficulty with bowel and bladder control are common in patients with advanced disease. Patients with MS may have either a small-capacity spastic bladder with urinary urgency, frequency, and incontinence or a large, flaccid bladder with overflow incontinence. Delineation of bladder function often necessitates referral to a urologist for evaluation and urodynamic studies. We treat complaints of urinary urgency with oxybutynin 5 mg two to three times per day, propantheline bromide 15 mg two to three times per day, or hyoscyamine 0.25 mg up to four times per day. Patients with frequent urinary tract infections may have urinary retention and require intermittent catheterization. Constipation is the most frequent bowel complaint and may require stool softeners, laxatives, or suppositories.

Spasticity

Spasticity may limit the activities of patients with moderate to severe paraparesis. Leg stiffness may interfere with walking or with transferring from the wheelchair. Severely affected patients may have extensor or flexor spasms either with attempted movement of the limb or spontaneously. These spasms may prevent movement, can be painful, and often interfere with sleep. Conversely, some degree of spasticity is helpful for patients with paraparesis since the lower extremity extensor tone enables them to bear weight for assisted ambulation or transfers.

We use baclofen for treating patients whose function is limited by spasticity. We explain the necessity for careful titration of the dose so that their disability from spasticity is relieved, but they still have enough remaining extensor tone to maintain their usual level of function. We begin with a dose of 10 mg twice per day and allow patients to titrate this dose upward or downward within set limits every few days until they determine the point of maximum benefit. The usual effective dose is between 30 and 80 mg per day but can be substantially higher. The main side effect is drowsiness, and the manufacturer recommends tapering the medication gradually instead of suddenly discontinuing it. Second-line medications for spasticity include diazepam, clonazepam, and dantrolene, but these are rarely useful when baclofen has failed. For patients with severe spasticity that limits their function, implantation of a pump for intrathecal baclofen administration may be useful.

Tremor

Intention tremor is a not uncommon symptom of MS and can cause severe disability. This tremor is usually refractory to therapy. We start with a trial of clonazepam 0.5 mg two to three times per day and increase gradually until benefit is obtained or intolerable side effects occur. Propanolol, isoniazid, and trihexyphenidyl are other options, but they are rarely effective.

Ancillary Services

Referral to a physician specializing in rehabilitation or to physical or occupational therapists is frequently helpful, particularly just following an exacerbation with development of a new deficit. The appropriate use of canes, walkers, motorized scooters, and other assistive devices may make a considerable difference in the patient's quality of life. Proper cushions and training of caregivers can prevent decubiti. A therapist experienced with MS patients can evaluate the need for such devices and provide instruction in their use.

Disability

Patients who become disabled from MS frequently require the assistance of their physician to obtain benefits. Depending on the institution providing benefits, several attempts may be necessary before disabled MS patients are able to receive the assistance they deserve.

Suggested Reading

The IFNB Multiple Sclerosis Study Group and the University of British Columbia MS/MRI Analysis Group. Interferon beta-1b in the treatment of multiple sclerosis: Final outcome of the randomized controlled trial. Neurology 1995; 45:1277–1285.

Johnson KP, Brooks BR, Cohen JA, et al. Copolymer 1 reduces relapse rate and improves disability in relapsing-remitting multiple sclerosis: Results of a phase III multicenter, double-blind, placebo-controlled trial. Neurology 1995; 45:1268–1276.

Kalb RC, Scheinberg L. Multiple sclerosis and the family. New York: Demos, 1992.

Matthews WB, Compston A, Allen IV, et al. McAlpine's multiple sclerosis. 2nd ed. Edinburgh: Churchill Livingstone, 1991.

Rudick RA, Goodkin DE, eds. Treatment of multiple sclerosis: Trial design, results, and future perspectives. London: Springer-Verlag, 1992.

Wolinsky JS. Multiple sclerosis. In: Appel SH, ed. Current neurology, Vol. 13. St. Louis: Mosby, 1993.

MYASTHENIA GRAVIS AND MYASTHENIC SYNDROME

Andrea M. Corse, M.D.
Ralph W. Kuncl, M.D., Ph.D.

■ MYASTHENIA GRAVIS

Myasthenia gravis (MG) is an autoimmune disorder with an antibody-mediated pathogenesis. Antibodies directed against the nicotinic acetylcholine receptor (AChR) on skeletal muscle are responsible for impaired transmission at the neuromuscular junction, resulting in muscle fatigability and weakness. The prevalence of MG is approximately 5 in 100,000 population. Autoimmune MG affects all ages. Peak incidence occurs in young women and older men. Neonatal MG affects approximately 15 percent of babies born to myasthenic mothers. It is a transient, potentially life-threatening condition resulting from the passive transfer of immunoglobulin from the mother to the baby. By contrast, congenital myasthenic syndromes are nonautoimmune gene defects, usually affecting AChR ion channels or acetylcholinesterase.

Pathogenesis

The defect in MG is a reduction in the number of available AChRs at the neuromuscular junction. Anti-AChR antibodies reduce the number of available receptors via three mechanisms: increased receptor degradation by accelerated receptor endocytosis, receptor blockade, and complement-mediated receptor damage. Additional morphologic alterations of the neuromuscular junction also occur, including simplification of the postsynaptic membrane folds and increased distance between the pre- and postsynaptic membranes.

In MG the amount of acetylcholine released from the presynaptic terminal both at rest and after sustained activity is normal. However, due to the reduced number of AChRs available, the amplitude of motor endplate potentials triggered by the acetylcholine is reduced. Normally, the amplitude of the endplate potentials is more than large enough to trigger an action potential. This excess amplitude termed the *safety margin,* is estimated to be 3 to 4 times greater than the threshold needed to generate a muscle action potential. However, because of insufficient AChRs in MG the endplate potential amplitudes at some neuromuscular junctions may be too low to trigger an action potential, and if transmission is sufficiently impaired at enough neuromuscular junctions, the muscle will be weak.

Normally, with sustained muscle activity the amount of acetylcholine released from the presynaptic nerve terminal is reduced with each successive impulse. Due to the large safety factor, transmission is not affected and strength is sustained. However, in MG the reduced acetylcholine results in further impaired impulse transmission at even more neuromuscular junctions. This is the basis of muscle fatigability and electrophysiologic decrement in MG.

Anti-AChR antibodies are detectable in about 85 percent of patients with MG using the most sensitive radioimmunoassay detection. The antibody titer does not correlate well overall with disease severity, though for an individual patient a significant reduction in serum antibody titer (≥50 percent) is often associated with clinical improvement. Evidence indicates that antibody-negative MG is, nonetheless, autoimmune because it responds to immunotherapy and pheresis and can be passively transferred. Therefore anti-AChR antibodies appear to be present that are not detectable by conventional radioimmunoassay methods.

The thymus gland appears to play a role in the origin and perpetuation of MG. The high incidence of pathologic abnormalities of the thymus gland in patients with MG and the favorable response to thymectomy initially suggested a pathogenetic role for the thymus. The anti-AChR antibody response is T-cell dependent. T cells obtained from thymus glands of myasthenic patients are more responsive to acetylcholine receptors than T cells derived from peripheral blood. Furthermore, the thymus contains myoid cells, which are striated, multinucleate "muscle-like" cells bearing AChRs on their surface. Due to their proximity to the immunocompetent cells of the thymus, the myoid cells may be particularly vulnerable to immune attack and might serve as an antigenic stimulus in MG.

Diagnosis

Every attempt should be made to establish the diagnosis of MG *unequivocally* prior to the initiation of chronic therapies.

Clinical Features

The hallmark clinical features of MG are weakness and muscle fatigability. The latter must be differentiated from tiredness or depression. Symptoms may include diplopia, ptosis, difficulty chewing and swallowing, dysarthria, proximal limb weakness, and shortness of breath. The most common muscles involved, in descending frequency, are the extraocular muscles and levators of the eyelids; proximal limb muscles (especially deltoid, iliopsoas, and triceps); muscles of facial expression, mastication, and speech; and neck extensors. Weakness is often worsened by repetitive or prolonged activity and improved with rest. Rarely, MG can present with respiratory insufficiency.

Diagnostic Tests

Confirmatory laboratory tests are generally performed in this order: edrophonium (Tensilon) test, determination of anti-AChR antibody titers, repetitive nerve stimulation, and single fiber electromyography (EMG).

Tensilon is a short-acting inhibitor of acetylcholinesterase. Acetylcholinesterase inhibitors potentiate the effects of acetylcholine at the neuromuscular junction by inhibiting its degradation. An initial 2 mg test dose of Tensilon is followed by 8 mg, using a double-blind control if possible. If a patient has demonstrable weakness due to MG, intravenous injection of Tensilon should result in transient improvement in strength lasting 1 to 3 minutes. Quantitative measures of endpoints should be used. As an alternative, 1 mg of neostigmine can be given by intramuscular injection, which allows for approximately 30 minutes of observation.

Repetitive nerve stimulation can identify abnormalities in neuromuscular transmission in approximately 80 percent of patients when clinically affected muscles are tested. The typical electrodiagnostic features on repetitive nerve stimulation in MG are decremental responses greater than 10 percent comparing the amplitude or area of the fourth to the initial compound motor unit potential; postactivation facilitation; and later postactivation exhaustion.

Single fiber EMG provides the highest sensitivity in the detection of neuromuscular junction defects, detecting abnormalities in 88 to 99 percent of patients with MG. The hallmark feature of a neuromuscular junction defect by this technique is increased jitter, where jitter is the varying time interval between the triggered muscle action potentials in two muscle fibers belonging to the same motor unit. In patients undergoing evaluation for MG who are antibody negative and in whom repetitive nerve stimulation is normal or equivocal, single fiber EMG is routinely performed.

Chest computed tomography (CT) or magnetic resonance imaging (MRI) to investigate the thymus should be performed in all patients diagnosed with MG. Thymic abnormalities occur in nearly 75 percent of patients with MG and include thymic hyperplasia in 85 percent and thymomas, benign tumors of the thymus gland, in 15 percent.

Screening for other autoimmune diseases often linked with MG, such as hyper- or hypothyroidism, systemic lupus erythematosus, rheumatoid arthritis, or polymyositis, should be performed; these disorders may add to the diagnostic picture of immune dysregulation and may complicate therapy.

Therapy

Cholinesterase Inhibitors

Anticholinesterase agents are the first-line therapy for MG. These drugs prolong the action of acetylcholine by slowing its degradation at the neuromuscular junction, thereby enhancing neuromuscular transmission. Although most patients experience some benefit from anticholinesterase agents, the response is often incomplete, necessitating the addition of immunotherapy.

Pyridostigmine bromide (Mestinon) is the most widely used anticholinesterase. The onset of action occurs within 30 minutes and peaks at 1 to 2 hours. The usual starting dose is one tablet (60 mg) orally every 3 to 4 hours while awake. Doses higher than 120 mg five to six times daily are not often useful. A sustained-release anticholinesterase preparation, Timespan 180 mg, is available; however, because of its irregular absorption, it should be used only for night-time dosing in patients who have weakness during the night or upon awakening.

Anticholinesterases are safe, well-tolerated drugs, though they should be used with caution in patients with asthma or cardiac conduction defects. The most common side effect is diarrhea, which is dose related and which can be controlled with diphenoxylate (Lomotil) or loperamide (Imodium) once or twice a day. Other symptoms of cholinergic excess are tearing, sialorrhea, and fasciculations. Excessive amounts of anticholinesterases may cause increased weakness that is reversible after decreasing or discontinuing the drug.

Thymectomy

Thymectomy is recommended for patients with MG in two instances. First, patients between puberty and age 50 who are inadequately controlled with Mestinon monotherapy may benefit (because of involution, no significant thymic tissue remains beyond middle age). Thymectomy results in clinical improvement in probably 85 percent of patients, with drug-free remission in up to 35 percent and reduced medication requirements in up to 50 percent. The benefit from thymectomy is delayed, rarely occurring within 6 months and requiring up to 2 to 5 years for demonstrated efficacy. Second, at any age thymomas should be removed, because these tumors may spread locally and become invasive, though they rarely metastasize.

Thymectomy is an elective procedure and should be performed when the control of myasthenia is optimal. Patients with significant weakness often benefit from a course of plasmapheresis during the weeks to days prior to thymectomy. Postoperative plasmapheresis may also be necessary if patients have significant weakness. We prefer thymectomy *before* other immunosuppressive therapy. This avoids poor wound healing related to steroids and the potential risk of infections postoperatively because of immunosuppression. If immunosuppressive therapy after thymectomy is indicated, it is generally begun 2 to 6 weeks postoperatively for prednisone or 1 to 2 weeks postoperatively for Imuran.

Median sternotomy and limited transcervical or transcer-

Table 1 Standard Immunotherapy in Myasthenia Gravis

DRUG	USUAL ADULT DOSE	TIME TO ONSET OF IMPROVEMENT	TIME TO MAXIMAL IMPROVEMENT	TOXICITY/EFFICACY MONITORING
Prednisone	Gradually ascending to 60 mg qd orally followed by q.o.d. regimen	2–3 weeks	3–6 months	Weight Blood pressure Fasting blood glucose Electrolytes Ophthalmic examination Bone density 24 h urine calcium 25-OH vitamin D (especially in post-menopausal women)
Cyclosporine (Sandimmune)	5 mg/kg/day orally, divided b.i.d. (125–200 mg b.i.d.)	2–12 weeks	3–6 months	Blood pressure Serum creatinine Blood urea nitrogen Cyclosporine level, 12 h trough by RIA Amylase Cholesterol
Azathioprine (Imuran)	2–3 mg/kg/day orally (100–250 mg daily)	3–12 months	1–2 years	WBC (maintain >3,500) Differential (goal, <1,000 lymphocytes) MCV (goal, >100 fl) Platelets Liver function tests Amylase

RIA, radioimmunoassay; WBC, white blood cell count; MCV, mean corpuscular volume.

vical endoscopic approaches for thymectomy have been used. Despite a cosmetic disadvantage, we advocate a "maximal" transsternal dissection of all thymus, because thymic tissue can extend throughout the mediastinum from the diaphragm to the neck. This is particularly true in cases of thymoma, which can spread throughout the thoracic cavity. If thymomatous tissue cannot be completely excised, nonferromagnetic clips should be placed at the site of the remaining tumor and postoperative radiotherapy administered.

The risks of surgery include injury to the phrenic or recurrent laryngeal nerves, atelectasis, pleural effusion, pneumonia, myasthenic crisis, intercurrent pulmonary embolism, impaired wound healing, and later sternal instability. Therefore, thymectomy should always be performed in an institution where this procedure is performed expertly and regularly, and where the staff is experienced in the anesthetic care and pre- and postoperative management of MG.

Immunosuppressive Drugs

The prognosis for myasthenic patients has improved strikingly as a result of advances in immunotherapy; most myasthenic patients can return to full productive lives with proper therapy. Three agents can now be considered as first-line drugs for chronic immunosuppressive therapy in MG—prednisone, azathioprine, and cyclosporine. The choice among them is made by considering two facts: (1) how the toxicity profile fits the patient and (2) how fast the patient has to improve. Factors by which to compare their use are outlined in Table 1.

We see patients who are not immunosuppressed potently enough, not treated long enough, or are treated without adequate management of side effects or infections. The predictably poor outcomes may end up souring both the patient and doctor on a particular drug, or convincing both that it is ineffective when it could be effective.

Before immunosuppression is begun, the patient's history of tuberculosis (TB) exposure and tuberculin skin testing must be obtained. If the patient has a significantly positive skin reaction, alternative immunomodulatory therapies, such as maintenance plasmapheresis or human immune globulin therapy, should be reconsidered. Alternatively, empiric TB prophylaxis should be given concurrently with immunosuppressive treatment.

Corticosteroids

Indications. Corticosteroids have been the mainstay of MG therapy for over 20 years. Corticosteroids are indicated when MG symptoms are insufficiently controlled by anticholinesterase agents and are sufficiently disabling to the patient that the frequent side effects of these drugs are worth risking. *Sufficient control* is best defined functionally by each individual patient: for example, some patients are willing to live with moderate generalized weakness, whereas for others even mild ptosis or diplopia is intolerable. Corticosteroids can produce improvement in patients with all degrees of weakness, from diplopia to severe respiratory involvement. Diplopia, which is rarely corrected by anticholinesterase agents alone, usually responds well to steroid treatment. Older men with MG seem to respond particularly well to steroid therapy. Steroids may improve overall results following removal of a thymoma because of their lympholytic effects.

More than 80 percent of myasthenic patients can be expected to improve with steroid treatment alone; the clinical effect usually begins within 2 to 3 weeks, and occasionally longer, though maximal benefit may not be realized for up to 6 months or more.

Contraindications. There are no absolute contraindications to the use of corticosteroids. Relative contraindications include severe obesity, diabetes mellitus, uncontrolled hypertension, ulcer disease, osteoporosis, or ongoing infections. These problems can usually be circumvented by appropriate medical measures. Long-term treatment with steroids requires medical attention by an experienced physician; patients who are unable or unwilling to be followed closely should *never* be treated with steroids. Nursing mothers should be warned that steroids may pass into breast milk.

Many of the immunosuppressive effects of corticosteroids may last far longer than the maximal suppression of adrenocorticotropic hormone (ACTH) secretion by the pituitary. This allows effective alternate-day therapy in MG. If the drug is administered as a single dose in the morning at a time when the normal endogenous cortisol level would peak, by evening the administered dose is no longer present in the circulation, and the hypothalamus-pituitary-adrenal axis should secrete ACTH. This, in turn, will stimulate secretion of endogenous cortisol the next morning. The longer immunopharmacologic effect maintains disease control, and the single alternate-morning dose schedule mimics the normal diurnal cortisol cycle, reduces side effects, and facilitates eventual tapering of total dose.

Induction. Patients with moderate to severe generalized weakness or significant respiratory insufficiency or bulbar weakness are at risk of a transient steroid-induced exacerbation and should be admitted to the hospital for initiation of steroid therapy and observation. Nearly 50 percent of such patients have an exacerbation, which lasts days and occurs most commonly during the second 5 days of induction. The cause of this initial steroid-induced deterioration is not clear.

We prefer a gradually increasing schedule, since larger doses may exacerbate weakness. Prednisone is begun at a dosage of 15 to 20 mg per day and increased gradually by about 5 mg every 2 or 3 days, until the patient reaches a satisfactory clinical response or reaches the level of 60 mg daily. Only if the patient is already on a ventilator do we begin with a high dose. Prednisolone is chosen only if a problem in the hepatic metabolism of prednisone to prednisolone is known or suspected. The rate of increase must not be preprogrammed but should be guided by the patient's response. Increasing weakness is a signal to backtrack or proceed more slowly in raising the dose of prednisone.

If a patient has mild MG or purely ocular involvement and can be reliably monitored at about weekly intervals, outpatient initiation of prednisone may be done as follows: begin with 5 to 10 mg per day and increase every week by 5 mg until a response is seen. This usually occurs at a dose of 35 to 60 mg per day.

Maintenance. High-dose prednisone is maintained until clinical improvement levels off, or 3 months, whichever comes first. Then the same total dose is maintained but the dosage schedule is gradually tapered to an alternate-day regimen. The amount on the "on" day is increased by 5 mg, and the amount taken on the "off" day is decreased by the same amount. Eventually an alternate-day regimen is established in most patients; occasionally a small dose of prednisone must be given on the "off" day to prevent fluctuations in strength. Although corticosteroids are effective in lowering the AChR antibody levels, one should avoid treating the antibody level. What is important is the patient's index symptoms and quantitatively measured signs, which served as the original indication for immunotherapy.

Finally, when the patient reaches a plateau of improvement on an alternate-day regimen, the total dose is tapered gradually to seek the smallest effective dose. The goal is not to eliminate all medication, because steroid treatment must be continued indefinitely in nearly all patients (>90 percent), though the dose may be substantially reduced. We recommend reducing the dose at a rate no faster than 10 mg every 2 months, until a dose of about 50 mg every other day is reached, after which the reduction should be at a rate of about 5 mg every 2 months. It usually takes more than a year to determine the minimum requirement for a given patient. It is extremely important to taper the drug very gradually, as the disease may exacerbate with too rapid a taper. The consequences of lowering the dose too far may not be apparent for several months, and higher doses may be needed to achieve the same effect as before the exacerbation. As an alternative to the above scheme, when the patient has responded rapidly to steroids, the dose may be decreased on the "off" day and maintained on the "on" day, a gradual process that usually takes 3 to 6 months or longer, depending on the clinical course.

Corticosteroids should not be used in divided daily doses—this need arises mainly in painful, inflammatory, arthritic or vasculitic diseases, never in MG.

Follow-up visits are usually required every 6 to 12 weeks. Muscle strength should be measured quantitatively by the physician at interval visits. The most useful measurements include forced vital capacity (FVC), forward arm abduction time (arms sustained forward, extended, palms down, parallel to the floor), ptosis time (sustained upgaze until lid fatigues down to predetermined level, e.g., top or middle of the pupil), and measurements of individual muscle strength using a dynamometer.

The following patients should be considered candidates for other forms of immunotherapy, such as azathioprine, cyclosporine, or thymectomy if not already performed: those who have an exacerbation when prednisone is slowly tapered; those who fail to respond; those requiring more than 40 to 50 mg every other day; and those in whom toxicity exceeds benefit.

Toxicity. Physicians must make their patients familiar with the unfortunately long list of side effects of chronic steroid therapy and of their potential seriousness. Of course, not every patient will develop every symptom, but most patients will have some side effects. Almost every patient will gain weight and develop part of the Cushingoid habitus.

In handling toxicity, cooperation and communication between the patient's internist and neurologist is essential. Fortunately, many of the side effects can be minimized with alternate-day dosing and scrupulous attention to follow-up. We routinely monitor weight, blood pressure, the lens, fasting blood glucose, and electrolytes. Much of the toxicity can be prevented. We suggest the following:

Osteoporosis. Preventive treatment, especially in postmenopausal women, includes exercise, calcium supplements (1,500 mg per day, monitoring 24 hour urinary calcium), vitamin D (50,000 units twice weekly, or equivalent, monitoring serum 25-OH vitamin D levels), and replacement of gonadal hormones. Use of calcitonin or etidronate should be considered in patients who develop steroid osteopenia (detected by monitoring baseline and follow-up quantitative bone mineral densitometry) or fractures.

Obesity, hypertension, and diabetes. Monitor caloric intake to prevent weight gain. Restrict sodium intake. Supplement potassium as needed. Monitor fasting serum glucose.

Ulcer and dyspepsia. Give antacids (Tums and Rolaids double as a calcium supplement), H_2 receptor antagonists, or both in susceptible individuals.

Adrenal insufficiency. Double any low-maintenance steroid doses during acute periods of stress.

General. Use the least effective dose—no more than once-daily therapy—and gradually switch to alternate-day dosing when possible.

Azathioprine

Pharmacology. Since a completely intact immune response requires antigen processing and presentation (dependent in part on RNA synthesis) as well as proliferation and differentiation of immunocompetent cells (dependent on DNA and RNA synthesis), purine analogues such as azathioprine can interrupt the immune response potently at multiple sites. A tight relationship exists between azathioprine dose and biologic effects on dividing cells such as lymphoid and erythroid cells. Leukopenia and macrocytosis occur predictably and are monitored as guides to azathioprine dosage. The drug is extensively oxidized and methylated in liver and red blood cells. Concurrent administration of allopurinol (for treatment of gout) can increase the toxicity of azathioprine by interfering with its metabolism by xanthine oxidase, an important degradative pathway. Therefore, azathioprine dosage must be reduced by as much as 75 percent in patients who take allopurinol.

Indications. Azathioprine can be used effectively as initial therapy in MG. The manner in which azathioprine is most often used derives from its chief disadvantage—beneficial effects may take 6 months or more to appear. It therefore tends to be used as additional therapy in patients whose myasthenia has not been adequately controlled by thymectomy and corticosteroids. The combination affords the relatively rapid onset of immunosuppression produced by the steroids and allows tapering of corticosteroids once the azathioprine has had time to take effect. Finally, the addition of azathioprine allows a reduction of steroid dosage in otherwise well-controlled patients with excessive toxic effects of prednisone, or those who require a chronic maintenance dose of prednisone of more than about 50 mg on alternate days.

Contraindications. Patients who are unable or unwilling to be followed medically should *never* be treated with azathioprine. Only approximately 10 percent of patients are unable to tolerate azathioprine because of abnormal liver function, bone marrow depression, or an idiosyncratic reaction consisting of flulike symptoms of fever and myalgia. The question of a small increased risk of malignancy in azathioprine-treated patients has not been resolved; experience with azathioprine in organ transplantation suggests an increased risk of malignancy. However, patients with myasthenia or rheumatoid arthritis have been treated for years with the drug, and no increase in the incidence of malignancies has been found.

Induction. The usual target dose of azathioprine is 2 to 3 mg per kilogram per day. It is important to realize that in obese patients, the optimum dose depends on the *total body weight,* not on lean body weight. A test dose of approximately 50 mg per day should be given for the first week. If this is well tolerated, the dose should be gradually raised by 50 mg each week, while the white blood cell count (WBC), differential count, platelets, and liver function tests are monitored closely. To establish the optimum dose, several endpoints may be used. A total WBC of 3,000 to 4,000 per cubic millimeter is a safe endpoint. Azathioprine should be briefly discontinued if the WBC falls below 2,500 per cubic millimeter or the absolute neutrophil count is less than 1,000 per cubic millimeter, then reintroduced at a lower dose. This measure cannot be used in patients receiving prednisone, because of the steroid-induced leukocytosis. In that situation, an absolute lymphocyte count of 5 to 10 percent is the appropriate target. A rise in the RBC mean corpuscular volume to greater than 100 fl also provides a useful gauge of biologic activity, and in MG usually correlates with clinical improvement, but macrocytosis does not require discontinuation of therapy.

Maintenance. An adequate therapeutic trial of azathioprine as sole therapy must last at least 1 to 2 years, since the lag to onset of effect may range from 3 to 12 months, and the point of maximum benefit may be delayed until 1 to 3 years. Although azathioprine is decidedly slow to act, it is well tolerated by most patients. Close monitoring for toxicity should continue indefinitely, and patients should be seen at a minimum of every 3 months after a stable, nontoxic dose is reached. Although most myasthenic patients require lifelong immunosuppression, it is worthwhile to attempt to taper azathioprine to establish a minimal effective dose. A doubling of the anti-AChR antibody titer (optimally, in sera from two different dates measured in simultaneous assay) may predict clinical relapse. Based on European experience with the drug as sole therapy, only a minority of myasthenic patients remain in remission after discontinuation of azathioprine, so continued close follow-up is necessary after therapy is stopped.

Toxicity. As with other immunosuppressive agents, azathioprine increases susceptibility to opportunistic infections, which should be treated promptly and vigorously. The hematologic toxicity discussed earlier—leukopenia, anemia, and thrombocytopenia—are all reversible upon reduction of the dose of azathioprine. Hepatic toxicity, with mild elevation of transaminases is common, and responds to lowering the dose. A rise in transaminase levels up to twofold is usually well tolerated by patients. Gastrointestinal discomfort, with nausea and anorexia, is usually mild and responds to the use of divided doses taken after meals.

Cyclosporine

Mechanisms. Cyclosporine inhibits the activation of helper inducer ($CD4^+$) T cells and their production of IL-2, while relatively sparing suppressor ($CD8^+$) T cells. Its therapeutic effect in MG is thus explained, because the activation of B cells and production of anti-AChR antibodies are T-cell dependent. This relatively selective immunomodulatory action contrasts with the broad-spectrum effects of corticosteroids, azathioprine, and cyclophosphamide. Unlike cytotoxic immunosuppressants, cyclosporine does not cause generalized myelosuppression, thereby limiting the risk of opportunistic infections.

Pharmacokinetics and Drug Interactions. Cyclosporine reaches peak plasma concentrations within 3 to 4 hours after ingestion. The drug has a large volume of distribution and is sequestered in tissues. It is cleared from blood with a half-life of about 19 hours. Most of the drug is metabolized in the liver and excreted in the bile. This accounts for its ability to potentiate greatly the risk of necrotizing myopathy or myoglobinuria due to lovastatin, which also depends on biliary excretion. Because cytochrome P_{450}-mediated oxidation of the drug is extensive, hepatic dysfunction or concomitant administration of agents that affect the cytochrome P_{450} system can cause dramatic changes in the elimination of cyclosporine. Cyclosporine's independent mechanism of action produces an effect that is additive to that of corticosteroids. Because of evidence that the combination of cyclosporine with azathioprine and prednisone for suppression of organ rejection causes an increased risk of malignancies and infectious complications, most centers prefer to use only prednisone in combination with cyclosporine. It should be noted that corticosteroids increase plasma cyclosporine levels.

Indications. Cyclosporine is the only drug that has been shown to be effective primary immunotherapy for the treatment of MG in a prospective double-blinded, randomized, placebo-controlled trial. Improvement began at about 2 weeks, with maximal improvement by 4 months, correlating with a reduction in anti-AChR antibody levels. Although that original trial was small and limited, reported experience with the drug in open trials for MG has also been generally positive, and a large multicenter controlled trial has been completed and awaits publication. The efficacy of cyclosporine is similar to that of azathioprine, but it has the advantage of a more prompt effect, usually occurring within weeks.

It is becoming more and more justified to use cyclosporine as a first-line drug because of its more targeted immunomodulatory effects. It is also indicated in patients in whom corticosteroids or azathioprine treatment has either failed or been excessively toxic. The general indications for use of the drug in MG are the same as for any immunosuppressant—the severity of the MG must not be functionally trivial, the expected benefit must outweigh the risks of toxicity, and the patient must be reliable.

Induction. The efficacy of cyclosporine relates to the lowest ("trough") plasma levels, whereas toxicity depends on peak concentrations. Therefore the drug is given in a divided-dosage schedule, twice a day. Because it is lipid soluble and variably absorbed, cyclosporine should be taken with a fat-containing meal or snack. The initial dose is 2.5 mg per kilogram twice per day. With this dose and schedule, nephrotoxicity and hypertension occur in less than 8 percent of patients.

Maintenance. Although the dose is eventually guided by clinical efficacy, it is initially adjusted by monitoring (1) plasma cyclosporine levels and (2) side effects. Plasma levels should be measured every 2 weeks until stable, and then approximately monthly. Trough levels are measured in the morning, 12 to 14 hours after the last dose. The reported levels depend on the method of assay; using the radioimmunoassay with a specific monoclonal antibody, the trough level should be maintained between 100 and 200 ng per milliliter. The blood pressure, serum creatinine, and blood urea nitrogen are monitored, and the dose of cyclosporine is decreased if the creatinine level rises above 1.4 times the baseline level.

Toxicity. Compared with corticosteroids, cyclosporine has less frequent serious chronic toxicity. The most worrisome side effects are nephrotoxicity and hypertension. It should therefore be used only with great caution in patients with pre-existing uncontrolled hypertension or significant renal disease. There is an increased risk of nephrotoxicity in elderly patients. Nonsteroidal anti-inflammatory drugs that inhibit prostaglandin generation will potentiate cyclosporine nephrotoxicity. Other side effects include facial hirsutism, gastrointestinal disturbance, headache, tremor, convulsions, and, rarely, hepatotoxicity. These are related to drug level and are reversible with dose reduction. Hypertension usually responds either to dose reduction or, if levels are appropriate, to institution of weight reduction, salt restriction, and/or an antihypertensive drug. Calcium channel blockers are preferred. As with other immunosuppressive agents, there is a theoretically possible increase in the long-term risk of malignancy.

With close attention to management, cyclosporine can be used safely in nearly 90 percent of patients.

Short-Term Immunotherapies

Plasma Exchange. Plasma exchange, which depletes circulating antibodies, can produce short-term improvement in ongoing MG. Several uncontrolled trials as well as long experience have proven its effectiveness. Plasma exchange is now used primarily to stabilize patients in myasthenic crisis or for short-term management of patients undergoing thymectomy, in order to avoid corticosteroids and immunosuppressants. Less commonly it is used as adjuvant therapy in severely ill patients who are slow to respond to immunosuppressants. Repeated plasma exchange as a *chronic* form of therapy, either because the patient is intolerant or unresponsive to conventional immunosuppressant treatment, is rarely indicated.

Plasma exchange works rapidly, with objective improvement measurable within days of treatment. Improvement (in the individual patient) correlates roughly with reduction in anti-AChR antibody titers. The beneficial effects of plasma exchange are temporary, lasting only days to weeks, unless concomitant immunosuppressive agents are used. Even "antibody-negative" patients may improve after plasma exchange.

Many protocols for plasma exchange have been advocated. Five exchange treatments of 3 to 4 liters each over a 2 week period is a typical program at our institution. In centers with adequate experience, plasma exchange is safe. The vital signs and the serum concentrations of potassium, calcium, and magnesium should be monitored. The major risks are due to problems of vascular access. Blood flow from peripheral veins is frequently insufficient for processing by modern high-volume hemapheresis machines. Therefore, indwelling catheters in large veins are used and can cause infection, thrombosis, perforation, and even pneumothorax. Sepsis, arrhythmia, anaphylactic shock, pulmonary embolism, and systemic hemorrhage from disseminated intravascular coagulation, among other hazards, have also been reported. The benefit of plasma exchange must be weighed against problems of vascular access, the risks of pheresis, and the high cost of the procedure.

Intravenous Human Immune Globulin. The indications for use of intravenous human immune globulin (HIG) are the same as those for plasma exchange, i.e., to produce rapid improvement in order to get the patient through a difficult period of myasthenic weakness. The largest review of the efficacy of HIG summarized eight independent studies of 60 patients and reported overall improvement in 73 percent, but this figure is likely to be biased by the selective reporting of positive uncontrolled trials. The usual dose is 400 mg per kilogram per day on each of 5 consecutive days. When patients respond, the onset is within 4 to 5 days and the maximal response occurs within 1 to 2 weeks of initiation of HIG. The effect is transient but may be sustained for weeks to months, allowing intermittent chronic therapy. The mechanism of action of HIG in MG is not known, but it has no consistent effect on the measurable amount of AChR antibody in vivo or in vitro. Possible mechanisms that have been suggested to explain the immunomodulatory action of HIG include (1) block of Fc receptors on macrophages and other cells and (2) inhibition of the immune response to AChR by specific anti-idiotypic antibodies in the HIG pool.

Adverse reactions occur in fewer than 10 percent of patients and are generally mild, including allergy, headache, fluid overload, and various GI symptoms. The process of preparation of HIG has been shown to inactivate HIV and hepatitis B. HIG is very expensive, and this factor as well as the possible risks should be carefully weighed against the potential of rapid benefit.

Comparisons

Each of the available treatment options has its own advantages and disadvantages. Prednisone generally acts rapidly, is tried and true, but is beset by the problems of prevention and treatment of side effects. Azathioprine is safe and moderately effective, but slow. Cyclosporine is about equal to azathioprine in effectiveness; it is rapid in onset but expensive to use. Cyclophosphamide is potent but highly toxic and is therefore reserved for special cases. Plasmapheresis or HIG are often useful for the short-term management of acute problems or as pre- or postoperative therapy. However, the effects of both are transient, and their costs are extremely high. The therapeutic armamentarium now available provides a broad spectrum of effective treatment modalities. However, more specific and long-lasting treatments are still needed.

Myasthenic Crisis

A patient with MG is said to be in myasthenic crisis when significant respiratory insufficiency or dysphagia results. Any patient with MG who reports dyspnea or dysphagia should be evaluated promptly. The two most helpful measurements of respiratory function in myasthenic patients are FVC and negative inspiratory force. Arterial blood gas measurements are not a good determinant as they may be normal despite imminent respiratory failure. If the FVC is reduced to approximately 25 percent of normal or about 1 liter, the patient should be admitted to an intensive care unit for continuous monitoring and intubation if necessary. If the FVC is greater than 1 L, the patient should be hospitalized for close observation of respiratory parameters and pharyngeal function. Anticholinesterase dose and route are optimized. For intravenous or intramuscular administration, neostigmine (Prostigmin) is available. Neostigmine 1 mg is equivalent to 60 mg of pyridostigmine. Neostigmine is given as a continuous IV infusion. Acute immunotherapeutic intervention begins usually with plasmapheresis or, less commonly, HIG in patients known to be HIG-responsive. In patients already on steroids, the dose can be increased abruptly concurrent with the start of pheresis. The beneficial effect of pheresis typically lasts only weeks, by which time the increased steroid dose should be effective. Ventilated patients who have not previously been on steroids can be started on high doses of prednisone (60 mg daily). Steroid dose must be accelerated slowly as previously described in patients not on steroids at the onset of the crisis. Steroids must be used with caution, however, in the setting of infection.

One should have a high suspicion of infection as a potential precipitating cause of myasthenic crisis. These patients are frequently immunosuppressed; furthermore, reduced respiratory function increases their vulnerability to pneumonia. MG patients with respiratory insufficiency (or post-thymectomy) can benefit from periodic inflation of the lungs with intermittent positive pressure therapy three times per day to reduce atelectasis and the risk of pneumonia. Incentive spirometry is discouraged, as it is probably ineffective and may contribute to respiratory muscle fatigue.

Neonatal Myasthenia Gravis

Preparations for the contingency of neonatal myasthenia should be made in the delivery room for all myasthenic mothers, because it is not possible to predict from the severity or laboratory features of the mother's myasthenia (even antibody positivity) whether an infant will be affected. Affected infants have weak suck and cry and may have generalized weakness or impaired swallowing and breathing. The clinical diagnosis is confirmed by repetitive nerve stimulation. The disorder may be recognized anytime in the first 72 hours and abates spontaneously after 2 to 3 weeks. Treatment requires only anticholinesterase agents and support of vital functions. Neostigmine (Prostigmin), 0.005 to 0.020 mg per kilogram per hour, is given by continuous intravenous infusion. Alternatively, 4 to 10 mg pyridostigmine (Mestinon) syrup may be used orally or by nasogastric tube every 4 hours. Cholinergic symptoms should be monitored to prevent overmedication.

LAMBERT-EATON MYASTHENIC SYNDROME

Clinical Features and Pathogenesis

Lambert-Eaton myasthenic syndrome (LEMS) is characterized primarily by weakness but also by fatigability, hyporeflexia, and autonomic dysfunction. Weakness is proximal, more prominent in legs and truncal muscles than in arms. Ocular and bulbar muscles are sometimes affected, but mildly so, in contrast to their prominent involvement in MG. Weakness is more disabling than life-threatening, because the disorder rarely produces respiratory failure. Therefore LEMS is really part of the differential diagnosis of acquired myopathy in adults. It is not often confused with MG, although the two autoimmune disorders may coexist. Reflexes are reduced or absent. Autonomic symptoms and signs include dry mouth, decreased sweating, erectile impotence, and loss of pupillary light reflex. LEMS is autoimmune and is associated commonly with carcinoma (especially small cell lung cancer) or other autoimmune disorders. Paraneoplastic LEMS often presents before (even 2 or 3 years before) the discovery of the neoplasm. As in MG, sex and age affect case incidence. Two-thirds of all are paraneoplastic, mostly men, and one-third are primarily autoimmune, mostly women, accounting for the overall male predominance (M-F, 4:1) in the disorder. In general, LEMS responds to therapy less well than does MG.

The neuromuscular transmission defect in LEMS is presynaptic due to impaired release of acetylcholine at motor nerve terminals. This is caused by antibodies directed against voltage-gated calcium channels in the nerve terminal (and cholinergic autonomic nerve terminals), which reduce calcium uptake, decreasing the probability of synaptosomal acetylcholine release at active sites. As a result, muscle fatigue and evoked compound muscle action potentials are low in amplitude, despite infrequent muscle wasting. The normal increased mobilization of calcium in the nerve terminal and increased release of acetylcholine immediately following exercise or electrical activation of motor nerves transiently increases muscle strength. This facilitation is the basis for the electrophysiologic diagnosis but is only occasionally evident on physical examination. Repetitive nerve stimulation reveals decrement at 2 Hz but marked (40 to 1,000 percent) facilitation of the compound muscle action potential after brief exercise or 50 Hz stimulation. Small cell carcinomas enriched in voltage-gated calcium channels provide the shared antigenic stimulus in paraneoplastic LEMS.

Therapy Prior to Immunosuppressant Drugs

A combined approach to therapy includes treatment of any underlying cancer, pharmacotherapy of the neuromuscular transmission defect, and immunosuppression. There should be a high suspicion of underlying malignancy, especially in smokers. Because the syndrome may precede the discovery of a tumor by years, the evaluation should include not only an initial extensive search for underlying malignancy, including chest CT or MRI, but also frequent surveillance if the initial evaluation is negative. Partial, and occasionally complete, remission may be achieved by removal or control of the underlying small cell cancer with surgery, radiation therapy, or chemotherapy.

3,4-Diaminopyridine

Because the main defect in LEMS is impaired release of acetylcholine from the nerve terminal, neuromuscular transmission is most rationally treated by drugs that enhance release. The family of aminopyridine drugs are potassium channel blockers, which by prolonging the duration of an action potential increase nerve terminal calcium uptake by enhancing the activation of voltage-gated calcium channels. As a result, acetylcholine release (and release of other neurotransmitters at other synapses) is greatly increased. 3,4-diaminopyridine (3,4-DAP) is available under treatment IND protocols for therapeutic use in LEMS. It has been shown to repair the neuromuscular transmission defect, to improve muscle strength quantitatively, to ameliorate autonomic symptoms, and to improve functional measures of strength and well-being significantly. The usual dose range is 20 to 80 mg per day, divided every 4 to 6 hours, tapering upward from a starting dose of 5 mg three times per day. Although 3,4-DAP penetrates the blood-brain barrier less than other aminopyridines do, the risk of seizure toxicity increases over 80 to 100 mg per day. Other toxicity includes paresthesias, gastric upset, and insomnia.

Guanidine was the first effective release agent used in LEMS but is limited by its toxicity and is now supplanted by 3,4-DAP. The analogue, 4-aminopyridine, is also effective but crosses the blood-brain barrier. Because these agents are not very selective for particular ion channels or synapses, they are epileptogenic and rather toxic. Newer potassium channel blockers (linopirdine and analogues) are under development.

Anticholinesterase Agents

As in MG, anticholinesterases can partially repair the neuromuscular transmission defect in LEMS by preventing breakdown of acetylcholine in the synaptic cleft and prolonging the effect of acetylcholine at receptors, even though the primary defect is presynaptic. The effect in LEMS is modest, so anticholinesterases usually supplement other forms of therapy.

Immunotherapy

Immunotherapy is indicated when treatment of the underlying malignancy and treatment with pyridostigmine and 3,4-DAP are insufficiently beneficial and when the potential benefits of immunosuppressants outweigh the risks. Because LEMS rarely remits spontaneously, treatment needs to be continued indefinitely. Immunosuppressants by themselves do not often produce complete symptomatic remission, so that pyridostigmine and/or, 3,4-DAP are usually also required.

Corticosteroids. Corticosteroids are effective in LEMS and may be initiated at a dose of approximately 60 mg per day without upward tapering. Effects begin within weeks, and usually by 2 to 3 months the dose schedule may be converted gradually to 120 mg on alternate days. Once a benefit is consolidated, the dose is tapered slowly downward to the patient's individual "trough" level based on measured efficacy and side effects.

Azathioprine. A steroid-sparing agent is often used in conjunction with corticosteroids, and azathioprine is the usual choice. Azathioprine by itself is often effective, but the extraordinarily slow onset of effect (6 to 12 months) limits its usefulness. The combination of azathioprine and corticosteroids is thought to be more effective than either agent alone. The practical aspects of management with azathioprine are no different in LEMS than in MG (as mentioned earlier).

Plasma Exchange and Human Immune Globulin. Plasmapheresis is effective in LEMS, but as in MG the effect lasts only days to weeks after a series of exchanges. Therefore, maintenance plasma exchange is rational only in exceptional cases refractory to other combined therapies, especially in view of its expense and catheter-related risks. Use of HIG is anecdotal but reportedly effective. The several caveats about its use mentioned for MG apply also to LEMS.

Acknowledgment

The authors wish to acknowledge their support from the Jay Slotkin Fund for Neuromuscular Research. We thank D.B. Drachman for critical review portions of the manuscript.

Suggested Reading

Arsura E. Experience with intravenous immunoglobulins in myasthenia gravis. Clin Immunol Immunopathol 1989; 53:S170.

Drachman DB. Myasthenia gravis. N Engl J Med 1994; 330:1797–1810.

Drachman DB, Kuncl RW. Myasthenia gravis. In: Hohlfeld R, ed. Immunology of neuromuscular disease. Immunology and Medicine Series. Dordrecht, The Netherlands: Kluwer Academic Publishers, 1994:165.

Lisak R. Handbook of myasthenia gravis and myasthenic syndromes. New York: Marcel Dekker, 1994.

Matell G. Immunosuppressive drugs: Azathioprine in the treatment of myasthenia gravis. Ann NY Acad Sci 1987; 505:588–594.

McEvoy KM. Treatment for Lambert-Eaton myasthenic syndrome. In: Lisak RP, ed. Handbook of myasthenia and myasthenic syndromes. New York: Marcel Dekker, 1994.

Penn AS, Richman DP, Ruff RL, et al., eds. Myasthenia gravis and related disorders: Experimental and clinical aspects. Ann NY Acad Sci 1993; 681:1–622

Tindall RSA, Rollins JA, Phillips JT, et al. Preliminary results of a double-blind, randomized, placebo-controlled trial of cyclosporine in myasthenia gravis. N Engl J Med 1987; 316:719–724.

Younger DS, Jaretzki A III, Penn AS, et al. Maximum thymectomy for myasthenia gravis. Ann NY Acad Sci 1987; 505:832–835.

ALZHEIMER'S DISEASE

Claudia Kawas, M.D.
Ann Morrison, M.S., R.N., C.S.

More than 4 million people in the United States have Alzheimer's disease (AD), the most common cause of dementia in the elderly. As our population ages, the number of AD patients may triple by the year 2020. The physician has a particularly important role in providing care for dementia patients and their families. If nursing home placement could be delayed for 1 month for each patient, it would result in an estimated savings of $5 billion, a major consideration in attempts to contain costs of health care. Appropriate management and utilization of services during the course of this disease can maximize patient and caregiver functioning as well as minimize behavioral difficulties and caregiver strain. This chapter provides specific recommendations for achieving this goal.

■ DIAGNOSIS

The first step in the treatment of patients with Alzheimer's disease and other dementias is to make a diagnosis. The routine workup for the evaluation of dementia is shown in Table 1.

Differential diagnosis depends primarily on the history, neurologic and physical examinations, and patterns of cognitive loss rather than on specific laboratory or radiologic tests since no biologic markers are available for the majority of primary dementing illnesses, including AD. Alzheimer's disease, however, is not a diagnosis of exclusion. The diagnosis is made when there is a dementia with a typical course of insidious onset; gradual progression; and absence of focal findings, significant extrapyramidal signs, or other illnesses that could account for the disorder. See the article by McKhann and co-workers in Suggested Reading list for more detail. Procedures such as lumbar punctures are necessary if the course is atypical, if there is an abrupt decline, or if systemic diseases including syphilis and malignancies are present. If depression or seizures are being considered as the

Table 1 Workup for the Differential Diagnosis of Dementia

BY THE EXAMINER
History, physical examination, hearing, vision
Mental status testing
Neurologic examination
SPECIAL TESTS
Blood for:
CBC, metabolic screen, thyroid
B_{12}, serology, HIV, if indicated
EEG
ECG
Brain imaging—CT or MRI
LP, if indicated
Psychometric testing, if indicated

CBC, complete blood cell count; HIV, human immunodeficiency virus; EEG, electroencephalography; ECG, electrocardiography; CT, computed tomography; MRI, magnetic resonance imaging; LP, lumbar puncture.

etiology of the observed cognitive changes, an electroencephalogram may be helpful. Apolipoprotein E genotype is a susceptibility factor for AD, not a diagnostic test, and genotyping is not indicated for the clinical care of most patients.

Making a diagnosis within the best abilities of the clinician is crucial to permit the patient and family to frame appropriate short-term and long-term plans. Even if the physician is not certain of the specific category of primary dementing illness, use of terminology such as *dementia* and *similar to Alzheimer's disease* will support the individual's own quests for information from patient associations, reading materials, and the media. Families who hear that it is due to "getting old" or "hardening of the arteries" are unequipped to take advantage of available materials and support services as they await their next visit.

Should the patient be told of the diagnosis? Although many family members, as well as some physicians, may be uncomfortable with disclosure to the patient, the ethical principle of autonomy requires in most circumstances that the patient be aware of the diagnosis to the extent he or she is capable. Discussion of the diagnosis is best conducted in a multidisciplinary patient and family conference, allowing the patients' relatives to witness the patient's reaction (almost inevitably less catastrophic than anticipated) and the physician's management of questions that arise. Patients' insight and ability to comprehend the illness will vary considerably and must be handled on an individual basis. Even if the patient does not understand the specifics of the discussion, an approach that does not exclude the patient will encourage a sense of unity with his or her family and the health care team.

Frequency of Visits

The frequency of visits undoubtedly will vary depending on the needs of each patient and family. Most will benefit from a visit to the clinic every 3 to 4 months. More frequent evaluations are indicated when patients require medication adjustments or suffer severe affective or behavioral disturbances, and when caregivers are unduly stressed. Conversely, biannual visits may suffice for the most stable patients provided that safety and education issues have been addressed. Telephone support is often required throughout the course of this illness.

Clinical Deterioration

Although patients with dementia gradually deteriorate, precipitous changes in clinical course require investigation, particularly for infections (urinary and pulmonary), subdural hematomas, and seizures. Additional factors that may contribute to abrupt alterations in mental status are new medications and dosage changes, crisis in the home environment, or new surroundings.

■ THERAPY

Treatment of Cognitive Loss

Currently, there is one FDA-approved compound for the treatment of the primary symptoms of Alzheimer's disease. Tacrine (Cognex) is an acetylcholinesterase inhibitor, that can improve cognitive abilities in 30 to 40 percent of AD patients. Indeed, 5 to 10 percent of patients on tacrine show substantial improvement, although they never return to normal levels of cognition. The remaining subjects who respond to treatment have more modest clinical benefits including mild memory enhancement, increased social interaction, or heightened attention.

Tacrine dosage is titrated every 6 weeks (to a maximum of 160 mg per day) until satisfactory clinical improvement is noted or toxicity develops. Asymptomatic elevation of liver transaminases is the most frequent significant side effect, requiring monitoring of liver function tests (aspartate aminotransferase and alanine aminotransferase) every 2 weeks for several months. The *Physicians' Desk Reference* and package insert provide detailed management instructions for adjusting dosage depending on transaminase elevations. When patients do not have observable clinical benefit from tacrine therapy, administration should be stopped.

Treatment of Associated Symptoms

Although in demented patients the focus is often on memory and cognitive loss, the syndrome also includes behavioral and affective disorders that disrupt the life of the patient and caregivers. Treating these symptoms with medications or behavioral management is generally more important for improving the lives of patient and family than attempts to improve the memory disorder. The clinician must help the caregiver generate strategies with the goal of limiting the problem behavior. Identifying unrealistic expectations on the part of the caregiver or family is essential.

Clinical research is sparse on the most effective strategies for managing the behavioral and affective symptoms of dementia and AD. Small doses of familiar medications can produce good results, but it may be very difficult to predict response in individual patients. The general clinical strategy is often reduced to successive medication attempts until there is an adequate clinical response. Behavioral problems change over time. The family (and physician) can generally be assured that today's problems are likely to give way to new issues. Dementia is a dynamic disorder.

Depression

More than one-third of all AD patients have significant depressive symptoms that may respond to antidepressant medications or counseling or both. Depression is particularly

Table 2 Medications for Symptoms of Alzheimer's Disease

SYMPTOM	DRUG	STARTING DOSE AND RANGE
Hallucinations or delusions	Neuroleptics:	
	Haloperidol (Haldol)	1 mg (0.5–2 mg)
	Fluphenazine (Prolixin)	1 mg (1–5 mg)
	Resperidone	1 mg (0.5–6 mg)
Agitation or anxiety	Non-neuroleptics:	
	Buspirone	15 mg (15–30 mg)
	Lorazepam	1 mg (0.5–6 mg)
	Trazodone	100 mg (100–400 mg)
Depression	Nortriptyline (Pamelor)	30 mg (30–100 mg)
	Sertraline (Zoloft)	50 mg (50–200 mg)
	Paroxetine (Paxil)	20 mg (20–50 mg)
Insomnia	Zolpidem (Ambien)	5mg (5–10 mg)
	Chloral hydrate	500 mg (500–1,000 mg)
	Lorazepam (Ativan)	1 mg (1–6 mg)

likely in the earlier stages of the illness and treatment can often improve cognitive and functional abilities. Some commonly used medications and dosages are shown in Table 2. Choice of drugs should be determined by individual patient profile and medical history. For example, the patient with sleep difficulties and agitation might benefit from a mildly sedating tricyclic antidepressant such as nortriptyline, whereas the depressed AD patient who is hypersomnolent may do better with a selective serotonergic reuptake inhibitor.

Delusions and Hallucinations

Paranoid delusions and visual or auditory hallucinations, which occur in more than one-third of AD patients, can be extremely disruptive for both the patient and family. However, management of these distressing symptoms can be very rewarding for the clinician. We primarily use low doses of neuroleptic medications, such as haloperidol, with careful monitoring for anticholinergic and extrapyramidal side effects. A subgroup of AD patients who also have diffuse cortical Lewy bodies (Lewy body variant of Alzheimer's disease) may have a higher rate of delusions and hallucinations but are also likely to be hypersensitive to the extrapyramidal side effects of neuroleptic compounds and have unexplained falls.

Agitation and Sleep-Wake Cycle Disturbances

These frequent symptoms can be difficult to manage and generally require a combination of medical and behavioral strategies. If a patient also has depressive or psychotic symptoms, sedating compounds for treatment are likely to be useful for diminishing agitation. For the patient whose primary symptom is mild to moderate agitation, we generally try buspirone or benzodiazepine-related compounds such as lorazepam (Ativan). Sleep medications such as chloral hydrate or zolpidem (Ambien) may be helpful for some patients.

Table 3 Experimental Compounds for the Treatment of Alzheimer's Disease

- Cholinergic enhancers
  - Cholinesterase inhibitors
  - Muscarinic agonists
  - Cholinergic release enhancers
- Additional agents
  - Serotonin receptor agonists
  - Cholinergic/adrenergic receptor activity
  - Anti-inflammatory compounds
  - Antioxidants
  - Estrogens

Behavioral Strategies

The most successful management of the associated symptoms of dementia combines behavioral and pharmacologic interventions. Behavioral difficulties are often triggered or exacerbated by environmental stimuli. For example, agitation or combativeness may be linked to caregiving strategies. Attempting to force patients usually results in resistance. Activities such as bathing and changing clothes are commonly cited by caregivers as circumstances that trigger agitation. Caregivers need help in identifying alternative approaches. Strategies as simple as changing the time of day of the activity, preceding the task with a favorite activity, limiting choices, or distraction during the task may solve the problem.

Sleep difficulties may be exacerbated by excessive daytime sleeping, presence of pain, or frequent bathroom visits. Limiting alcohol, caffeine, and fluids several hours before bedtime may improve nocturnal restlessness. Early bedtime promotes early awakening, especially in the elderly. It is imperative that caregivers and patients design synchronous sleep schedules to reduce night-time wandering and potential safety hazards.

Experimental Trials

A variety of compounds are under investigation for treatment of Alzheimer's disease. Table 3 lists the categories of investigational treatments by suggested mechanism of action. The design, length, and subject requirements for the research protocol will be influenced by the nature of the compound as well as the phase of the drug approval process. Drug trials may be financially supported by private industry or federal grant programs.

Patients may express interest in participating in experimental trials for the treatment of Alzheimer's disease. Trials can be located through the local Alzheimer's Association or closest teaching university. Study subjects, in general, should have no major medical illnesses or behavioral disturbances, be amenable to cognitive testing, and have scores on the Mini-Mental State Exam that fall in the midrange (10 to 27).

■ COUNSELING

Education, Safety, and Referrals

A number of education and safety concerns need to be addressed with patients and families. Table 4 provides a checklist that can be utilized by the practitioner to document these discussions. Difficult issues such as revoking driving

Table 4 Safety and Education Issues by Stage of Illness

EARLY/MID STAGES
Understanding diagnosis
Safety issues:
MedAlert bracelet
Driving
Smoking
Operating dangerous equipment
Wandering/supervision needs
Legal and financial planning
Advance directives
Day care
LATE STAGES
Nursing home placement
Autopsy

privileges and nursing home placement are made easier when the patient and family are given advance notice that these issues will be discussed at the next visit.

Assistance for families can be obtained through the national and local Alzheimer's Associations. These associations provide reading materials, telephone helplines, educational seminars, support groups, and financial assistance for day care. Available support services include home health aides, respite care, home-delivered meals, and transportation to and from doctor's appointments. Services may be provided free or have a sliding-scale fee. Families should also be referred to the Department of Aging as well as community and local religious organizations to inquire about services available in the area.

A case manager can assist families by providing a range of supportive services such as paying monthly bills or arranging for medication supervision. The plan of care will be tailored to the patient's medical, social, legal, and financial needs. This type of assistance is generally not covered by insurance. This service is particularly useful for family members who care for a patient at a distance or for patients who have no caregiver. Social workers may have much to offer when burdensome family circumstances, poor caregiver adaptation, or the need for extensive one-on-one counseling has been identified. Similarly, referral to psychiatry is helpful when fundamental approaches to managing psychiatric symptoms are not successful.

Genetics

Genetic counseling in AD is a complex issue that the clinician must address, particularly in families with more than one affected relative. Rarely, the clinician will encounter patients from large kindreds with multiple affected members in the same generation. Members of these families are likely to have a 50 percent risk of developing AD, often at an early age (presumed autosomal dominant inheritance). Examination of the pedigree for one of the known genetic mutations on chromosomes 21, 14, or 1 may be considered. These families are not common. Indeed, about 60 percent of all AD patients report no family history of dementia.

In general, a family history of dementia (one or more affected first-degree relatives) appears to increase the lifetime risk of developing dementia, but quantifying the excess risk is difficult. Estimates from the Eurodem meta-analyses report an estimated relative risk of 2.6 (CI 2.0 to 3.5) with one affected family member and 7.5 (CI 3.3 to 16.7) when two or more family members are affected.

Our general clinical approach is to acknowledge the increased genetic risk for the children of our patients, but also to reinforce that we cannot predict individual risk of developing AD even with additional procedures such as apolipoprotein E genotyping or positron emission tomography scanning. In the future, additional genetic and biologic markers are likely to be available for more adequate genetic counseling. More important, interventions to prevent or delay onset of disease are likely to be identified in the next decade.

Suggested Reading

Folstein MF, Folstein SE, McHugh PR. Mini-mental state: A practical method for grading the cognitive state of patients for the clinician. J Psychiatr Res 1975; 12:189–198.

McKhann G, Drachman D, Folstein M, et al. Clinical diagnosis of Alzheimer's disease: Report of the NINCDS-ADRDA Work Group under the auspices of Department of Health and Human Services Task Force on Alzheimer's Disease. Neurology 1984; 49:1253–1258.

Patient Readings

Barusch AS. Elder care: Family training and support. Newbery Park, CA: Sage, 1991.

Hamdy RC. Alzheimer's disease: A handbook for caregivers. 2nd ed. St. Louis: Mosby–Year Book, 1994.

Mace NL, Rabins PV. The 36-hour day: A family guide to caring for persons with Alzheimer's disease, related dementing illnesses, and memory loss in later life. Baltimore: Johns Hopkins University Press, 1981.

Zarit SH, Pearlin KW, Schaie KW. Caregiving systems: Informal and formal helpers. Hillsdale, NJ: Erlbaum, 1993.

THE OTHER DEMENTIAS

Richard K.T. Chan, M.B.B.S., M.R.C.P. (UK)
Vladimir C. Hachinski, M.D., F.R.C.P.C., M.Sc. (DME), D.Sc. (Med)

The management of a demented patient depends on the etiology (Fig. 1). The dementias can be divided into the primary degenerative and the secondary dementias. Primary degenerative dementia is the most common form of dementia in the elderly population, with Alzheimer's disease accounting for the majority of the caseload in a typical neurology clinic. The management of Alzheimer's disease has been discussed elsewhere in this book.

It is traditional to classify dementias into reversible and irreversible forms. The names are misleading. With few exceptions, it is doubtful if the cognitive impairment of the reversible dementias reverts to normal after treatment. In the case of some irreversible dementias, although no treatment is available to reverse the cognitive deficit, there are interventions available to prevent or retard the progression of disease. Clinically, it is more useful to divide the dementias into those in which specific treatments are available versus those without (Table 1).

■ DIFFERENTIAL DIAGNOSIS

Depressed patients may manifest symptoms of cognitive decline. The symptoms usually resolve with appropriate antidepressants. Depression is common among those with dementia, and it may be difficult to isolate the effect of both. In such cases, a therapeutic trial of antidepressant is helpful.

Clinicians should also differentiate the amnestic syndrome from the dementias. Especially noted is Korsakoff's syndrome. There is no treatment available to reverse the memory deficit, but attention to nutrition, especially the B-complex vitamins, helps to prevent further damage to the brain.

■ REVERSIBLE DEMENTIAS

A recommended screening panel is shown in Table 2 to detect the dementias in which specific treatments are available. Once recognized, treatment should be offered to the patient. It is

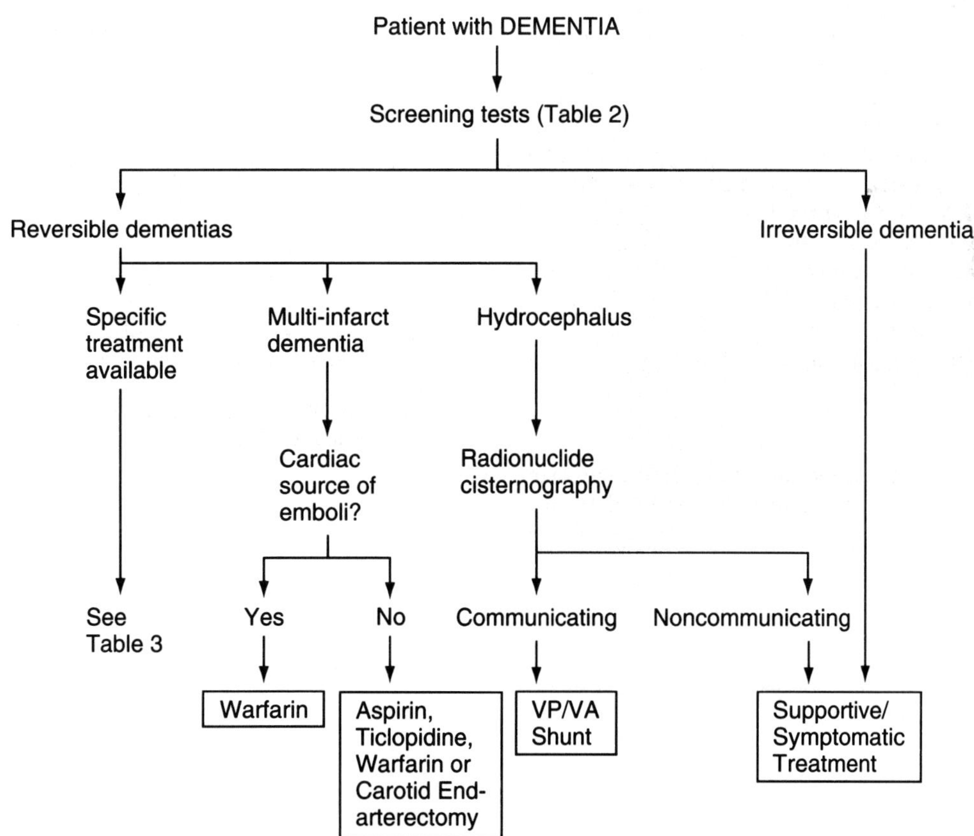

Figure 1
Algorithm for the management of dementia. VP, ventriculoperitoneal; VA, ventriculoatrial.

Table 1 Causes of Dementia

	SPECIFIC TREATMENT AVAILABLE	NO SPECIFIC TREATMENT
Primary degenerative		Alzheimer's disease Huntington's disease Lewy body disease Parkinson's disease Pick's disease
Vascular	Multi-infarct dementia	CADASIL Amyloid leukoencephalopathy Icelandic hereditary leukoencephalopathy
Infectious/parainfectious	Neurosyphilis Chronic meningoencephalitis	HIV encephalopathy AIDS-related dementia Creutzfeldt-Jakob disease
Metabolic/endocrine	Hypothyroidism Cushing's disease/syndrome Vitamin B_{12} deficiency Pellagra Wilson's disease Chronic liver/renal failures	
Toxic	Chronic lung ingestion Solvent abuse	
Others	Normal pressure hydrocephalus	Multiple sclerosis
Differential diagnosis	Depression (pseudodementia)	Korsakoff's syndrome

CADASIL, cerebral autosomal-dominant arteriopathy with subcortical infarcts and leukoencephalopathy.

Table 2 Screening Test for Diagnosis of Dementia

TEST	RATIONALE	REMARKS
Blood test		
Complete blood count	Assess general nutritional status	
Serum B_{12} level	Exclude vitamin B_{12} deficiency	Schilling's test if B_{12} level is low
TSH + Free T_4 *or* TSH + FTI	Exclude primary and secondary hypothyroidism	
HIV serology	Exclude HIV infection	Perform only if indicated; consent from patient required
Cerebrospinal fluid		
Cell count/protein level	Exclude chronic meningitis	Perform only if indicated
Cytology	Exclude carcinomatous meningitis	Perform only if indicated
VDRL	Exclude neurosyphilis	Perform only if indicated; check serum TPHA and HIV serology if CSF VDRL is positive
CT scan/MRI of the brain	Identify infarcts and white matter changes; exclude presence of neoplasm, demyelinating disease, and hydrocephalus; location of atrophy may suggest the diagnosis (e.g., parahippocampal atrophy in Alzheimer's disease, frontotemporal atrophy in Pick's disease)	
Electroencephalogram	Exclude metabolic encephalopathies; useful if Creutzfeldt-Jakob disease or status epilepticus is suspected	Perform only if indicated
Neuropsychological evaluation	Help to characterize pattern of cognitive impairment, which may aid in the classification of dementia; rule out pseudodementia from depression	

TSH, thyroid-stimulating hormone; FTI, free thyroxine index; HIV, human immunodeficiency virus; VDRL, Venereal Disease Research Laboratory test; TPHA, *Treponema pallidum* hemagglutination assay; CSF, cerebrospinal fluid; CT, computed tomography; MRI, magnetic resonance imaging.

Table 3 Specific Therapy for the Common Treatable Form of Dementias

ETIOLOGY	TREATMENT
Multi-infarct dementia	Aspirin, ticlopidine, warfarin, or carotid endarterectomy when indicated (see text)
Neurosyphilis	IV crystalline penicillin 18–24 million units daily × 14 days *or* IM procaine penicillin G 2.4 million units daily, with oral probenecid 500 mg q6h × 10–14 days; this is followed by IM benzathine penicillin G 2.4 million units weekly × 3 weeks *or* Oral erythromycin 500 mg q6h × 30 days *or* oral tetracycline 500 mg q6h × 30 days Repeat treatment every 6 months if CSF protein/cell count remains elevated 6 months after treatment
Vitamin B_{12} deficiency	IM cyanocobalamine 1,000 μg daily × 1 week, then 1,000 μg weekly × 4 weeks then 1,000 μg monthly (lifelong)
Hypothyroidism	Oral L-thyroxine, starting at a dose of 50 μg daily; increase dose slowly by monitoring thyroid function test
Chronic drug ingestion/solvent abuse	Remove offending agents
Chronic subdural hematoma/hygroma	Surgical drainage if mass effect is present
Normal pressure hydrocephalus	Ventriculoperitoneal/ventriculoatrial shunt if indicated
Intracranial neoplasm/obstructive hydrocephalus	Surgical intervention if not contraindicated
Depression	Antidepressant; e.g., amitriptyline, starting at 10 to 25 mg before sleep, increase dose by 25 mg weekly, up to 150 mg before sleep

CSF, cerebrospinal fluid.

important to emphasize the goal of treatment: to halt or retard the progression of disease; normalization of cognitive function may not occur. The treatments of these dementias are summarized in Table 3. Two special categories deserve further discussion here.

Multi-Infarct Dementia

Multi-infarct dementia is the second most common cause of dementia in the elderly. The condition is due to multiple ischemic insults, either embolic or thrombotic or hemorrhagic, in the cerebral hemispheres. Computed tomographic (CT) scans of the brain may be normal; magnetic resonance imaging (MRI) is more sensitive in detecting the ischemic lesions. In severe cases, there are extensive changes involving the deep white matter, a condition called leukoariosis. There are no clinical research data to compare various treatments in preventing deterioration of cognitive function. However, based on studies of primary and secondary ischemic stroke prevention, there is rationale for using antiplatelet agents (aspirin or ticlopidine) or anticoagulant (warfarin), or carotid endarterectomy, in the hope of preventing further cerebral ischemic events. When there is evidence to suspect cardiac emboli causing the recurrent infarctions (e.g., cardiac mural thrombi, chronic valvular atrial fibrillation), warfarin should be prescribed, maintaining the international normalized ratio at 2.0 to 3.0. If the patient has few vascular risk factors and no definite clinical episodes of cerebral ischemia (cerebral infarcts or transient ischemic attacks), we start treatment with low-dose aspirin (325 mg daily). When the rate of deterioration seems rapid, the dose of aspirin can be increased to 1,300 mg daily, or the patient can be put on ticlopidine 250 mg twice daily. Patients taking ticlopidine should have regular blood counts at the initial stage to detect the rare (1 to 2 percent), reversible, but potentially fatal, agranulocytosis associated with the use of this drug. In those with stenosis of the internal carotid artery, endarterectomy should be considered if the appropriate indications are present, i.e., symptomatic patients with stenosis of 70 to 99 percent.

Normal Pressure Hydrocephalus

Normal pressure hydrocephalus manifests itself by the clinical triad of cognitive impairment, sphincteric incontinence, and apraxic gait. However, when the patient has all these signs, the disease is probably in the advanced stage, and little is gained by ventricular shunting procedure at this stage. At the early stage of disease, when cognitive impairment is mild, the only helpful sign is the enlarged ventricles on CT scan or MRI of the brain.

It is difficult to distinguish normal pressure hydrocephalus from hydrocephalus associated with cerebral atrophy (hydrocephalus ex vacuo). The postsurgical result is often poor if the decision to insert a shunt is based on the radiologic appearance alone. If the patient has gait disturbances, a "diagnostic" lumbar puncture can be attempted. In this test, the time required to walk a fixed distance (usually 20 to 50 m) is taken at baseline. Twenty to 50 ml of cerebrospinal fluid (CSF) is then removed via a lumbar puncture needle. The patient is asked to walk the same distance 1 hour and 24 hours after the tap. If there is substantial improvement in performance, a beneficial postsurgical result is more likely. In patients without significant gait disturbance, a radionuclide cisternography can be helpful. In this technique, a radioactive isotope is introduced into the subarachnoid space via a lumbar puncture. If there is reflux of the isotope into the ventricles and decreased pericerebral perfusion, the result of shunting tends to be better. The use of continuous CSF pressure monitoring, with or without intrathecal saline infusion, requires special equipment, and the experience is still quite limited.

In carefully selected patients, shunting of the ventricular system improves the clinical symptoms or, at least, retards the rate of progression. Results tend to be best if there is a prior history of meningitis or subarachnoid hemorrhage.

■ IRREVERSIBLE DEMENTIAS

The management of patients with Alzheimer's disease has been discussed in the previous chapter. For the remaining nontreatable dementias, no pharmacologic or surgical intervention has been shown to be effective in preventing progression. Management of these patients is supportive and symptomatic in nature.

Creutzfeldt-Jakob disease is a rapidly progressive form of dementia, often associated with myoclonic jerks. The patients invariably die within a year from the onset of disease, and most within 6 months. Institutional care is often needed. Family and health care personnel caring for the patient should be warned of the potentially infectious nature of the disease. Body fluid must be handled with caution.

The other dementias in this group are often slowly progressive. The most important aspect of management is to make the patient aware of his or her condition. An honest discussion, with hopeful tone, is appropriate. Introduce family, social, or institutional intervention as and when necessary.

On the individual level, patients should be encouraged to remain active, depending on their level of well-being. Supervision may or may not be required. Discourage any activity that carries some amount of risk of harm to the patient or the other individuals. In a patient with moderately severe cognitive impairment, or when judgment skill is impaired, he or she should not be allowed to drive or operate heavy, fast-moving machines. Patients with dementia are prone to malnutrition. The patient who stays alone should have a visiting person checking on him or her regularly. At this stage, the patient should be encouraged to make up living directives and financial arrangement. This usually proves to be helpful at the later stages of the disease.

When the cognitive impairment is such that the patient is constantly forgetting things, or when there is significant risk of exposure to hazardous situations, he or she should not live alone. Ideally, the patient can still live in his or her own house with other family members or a live-in housesitter. Sometimes this may not be possible, and placement in an independent living facility or nursing home is necessary.

Depression is a common condition associated with the dementing process, further aggravating the cognitive problem. This may be due to structural changes in the brain, although it is commonly reactive in nature. Low-dose antidepressant, such as amitriptyline, is often helpful in elevating the mood. High doses of antidepressant may cause worsening of cognition and must be avoided.

Another common condition is caregiver burnout. It is important for the physician to understand that the caregiver is often under tremendous stress to cope with the ever-changing situation. Family support should be solicited when necessary, and referral to a support group or social agencies can also be helpful.

Suggested Reading

Arnold SE, Kumar A. Reversible dementias. Med Clin North Am 1993; 77: 215–230.

Diaz F, Hachinski V, Merskey H, et al. Leuko-araiosis and cognitive impairment in Alzheimer's disease. In: Iqbal K, McLachian DRC, Winblad B, Wisniewski HM, eds. Alzheimer's disease: Basic mechanisms, diagnosis and therapeutic strategies. New York: Wiley, 1991.

Kramer SI, Reifler BV. Depression, dementia, and reversible dementia. Clin Geriatr Med 1992; 8:289–297.

Stewart JT. Managing the care of patients with dementia. How to maximize level of functioning and minimize behaviour problems. Postgrad Med 1991; 90(4):45–49.

ASEPTIC MENINGITIS SYNDROME

Burt R. Meyers, M.D.
Alejandra C. Gurtman, M.D.

Aseptic meningitis syndrome is associated with symptoms, signs, and laboratory evidence of meningeal inflammation. Clinically, patients usually appear nontoxic but may have changes in mental status, including irritability. Classically, some or all of the following are noted: headache, nausea, vomiting, meningismus, and photophobia. A stiff neck with or without a Brudzinski or Kernig sign may be observed. Other signs of viral infection may include pharyngitis, adenopathy, morbilliform rash, and evidence of systemic viral infection, including myalgia, fatigue, and anorexia. There are usually no signs of vascular instability.

Various causes of this syndrome have been described (Table 1) including infections from bacteria and higher-order organisms such as mycobacteria, fungi, rickettsia, viruses, and parasites. Noninfectious causes include collagen vascular diseases (i.e., lupus erythematosus), granulomatous arteritis, sarcoidosis, cerebral vascular lesions, epidermal cysts, meningeal carcinomatosis, serum sickness, drug reactions, and nonfocal lesions of the central nervous system (CNS). Specific syndromes (i.e., Mollaret's meningitis) may produce a similar clinical picture.

■ PATHOPHYSIOLOGY

Viruses passively enter through skin or respiratory, gastrointestinal, or urogenital tract and may cause initial infection at the entrance site. Growth in extraneural tissue relates to the ability to infect susceptible cells with receptors for the virus and then to replicate viral particles intracellularly. Viruses spread through nerve endings by retrograde trans-

Table 1 Differential Diagnosis of Aseptic Meningitis

INFECTIOUS	
Bacteria	Partially treated bacterial meningitis
	Listeria monocytogenes
	Brucella sp.
	Nocardia
	Streptococcus pneumoniae (uncommon)
	Neisseria meningitidis (uncommon)
	Haemophilus influenzae (uncommon)
Fungi	*Histoplasma capsulatum*
	Cryptococcus neoformans
	Coccidioides immitis
	Candida spp.
	Aspergillus spp., *Phycomyces*
Mycobacteria	*Mycobacterium tuberculosis*
Rickettsia	*Rickettsia rickettsii*
	Ehrlichia spp.
Mycoplasma	*Mycoplasma pneumoniae*
Spirochetes	*Treponema pallidum*
	Borrelia burgdorferi
	Leptospira sp.
Parasites	Angiostrongylus
	Cysticercosis
	Amoebae
Viruses	
Enterovirus	Poliovirus
	Echovirus
	Coxsackievirus
	New enteroviruses
Herpesvirus	Herpesvirus 1 and 2
	Varicella-zoster virus
	Epstein-Barr virus
	Cytomegalovirus
Paramyxovirus	Mumps virus
	Measles virus
Togavirus	Rubivirus, rubella virus
Alphavirus	Eastern equine encephalitis virus
	Western encephalitis virus
	Venezuelan encephalitis virus
Flavivirus	Japanese encephalitis virus
	Murray Valley encephalitis virus
	St. Louis encephalitis virus
Bunyavirus	California encephalitis virus
	LaCrosse encephalitis virus
Reovirus	Colorado tick fever virus
Arenavirus	Lymphocytic choriomeningitis virus
Rhabdovirus	Rabies virus
Retrovirus	Human immunodeficiency virus
NON-INFECTIOUS	
Drug reactions	Nonsteroidal anti-inflammatory agents
	Antineoplastic agents
	Antibiotics (trimethoprim-sulfamethoxazole)
	Immunosuppressants (orthoclone)
	Immunoglobulin
Chemicals	Contrast agents
	Disinfectants, glove powder
Neurologic disorders	Cerebral vascular lesions
	Epidermal cysts
	Brain tumors
	Epidural, subdural abscess
Miscellaneous	Sarcoidosis
	Serum sickness
	Mollaret's meningitis
	Subacute bacterial endocarditis
	Meningeal carcinomatosis
	Vaccination
	Postinfectious viral syndromes

mission via neuronal axons (i.e., poliovirus). Viruses may multiply within an axon as well as within interstitial and lymphatic tissue between nerve fibers. Some viruses enter via the nose, cause infection of the submucosa, and then enter the subarachnoid space. In experimental models, herpes simplex virus (HSV) has been shown to enter by this route. Most viruses probably enter the CNS following viremia; they are either growing in the choroid plexus or pass directly through it into the CNS.

Enteroviruses, lymphocytic choriomeningitis (LCM) virus, mumps, and arthropod-born viruses replicate initially in muscle cells or mesodermal cells. Other agents, such as bacteria, mycobacteria and fungi, enter the body through the respiratory tract, including the pharynx, sinuses, or lung, and travel to the CNS via the blood stream. In the lungs an antecedent pneumonitis may be followed by fungemia or bacteremia. *Treponema pallidum* and *Borrelia burgdorferi* enter the CNS after blood stream invasion. Mechanisms whereby meningeal carcinomatosis, collagen vascular disease, brain tumors, and epidural or subdural abscess cause changes in the cerebrospinal fluid (CSF) have not been described. Antineoplastic agents, immunosuppressants, including orthoclone (OKT-3), trimethoprim-sulfamethoxazole, and nonsteroidal anti-inflammatory drugs (NSAIDs) may produce aseptic meningitis syndrome; the pathophysiology is not known.

■ DIAGNOSTIC WORKUP

The approach to patients with this syndrome should be careful elucidation of the history and then complete physical and CSF examination (Table 2). Time of the year may be an important clue, since many viral infections are seasonal, occurring during late summer and early fall. Examples of this are the enteroviruses, including echovirus and coxsackievirus. Furthermore, a history of exposure to patients with known viral illness often suggests infection. Exposure to mice and rodents suggests infection with LCM, less commonly *Leptospira* sp., or the recently described hantavirus, which may cause a severe pulmonary syndrome.

A history of sexual contacts should be elicited, since HSV and, in appropriate risk groups, human immunodeficiency virus (HIV) may present initially with this syndrome. All patients, including the elderly, should be questioned about risk factors for HIV infection, including sexual promiscuity, intravenous drug use, sexual preference, and history of transfusions with blood or blood products.

Geographic location, in terms of domicile and travel history, should be known. *Histoplasma capsulatum, Coccidioides immitis,* and *B. burgdorferi* occur mainly in certain sections of the United States. Those who have recently been in contact with a pet or been camping may risk infection with *Rickettsia* or *Borrelia* related to a tick bite. Rabies, though rare, should be considered if there was contact with or a bite from a sick animal, including skunk, raccoon, dog, fox, and bat. Drinking local water on backpacking trips may be associated with *Leptospira;* ingestion of unpasteurized milk and cheeses suggests brucellosis.

Physical examination may reveal a typical malar rash or other stigmata of collagen vascular disease. Vasculitides found

Table 2 Diagnositc Workup for Aseptic Meningitis Syndrome

CLINICAL EVALUATION
History
Season (summer, enteroviruses, Rocky Mountain spotted fever)
Geographic area (Colorado tick fever, babesia, Lyme disease)
Exposure to other patients (mumps, varicella)
Tick, mosquito bites (malaria, Lyme disease)
Exposure to animals (rabies, hantavirus)
Sexual history (HIV, herpes simplex virus)
Intravenous drug use (endocarditis)
Drug reactions (immunoglobulin, OKT-3, NSAIDs)
Physical Examination
SPINAL FLUID
Opening pressure low
Leukocyte count predominance
Neutrophils (initially echo [especially 9], polio, TB)
Lymphocytes (coxsackie, enterovirus)
Eosinophils (cystricercosis, angiostrongylus)
Abnormal cells (Mollaret's, lymphoma)
Protein <40 mg/dl
Glucose <40 mg/dl or <50% serum
Gram stain, AFB smear
Cryptotoccal antigen, India ink
Immunoelectrophoresis
VDRL
Wet mount (toxoplasmosis, amoebae)
Bacterial, viral, mycobacterial, fungal cultures
Lactate, C-reactive protein, adenosine deaminase
SEROLOGIC TESTING
Cryptococcal antigen
Histoplasma capsulatum, Coccidioides immitis antibody titer
Mycoplasma complement fixation
Lyme disease, ELISA, Western blot
Rocky Mountain spotted fever complement fixation
Antinuclear antibody (ANA)
HIV-1, HIV-2
OTHER
Chest x-ray film
Computed tomography, magnetic resonance imaging
Echocardiogram

HIV, human immunodeficiency virus; OKT-3, orthoclone; NSAID, nonsteroidal anti-inflammatory drug; AFB, acid-fast bacilli; VDRL, Venereal Drug Research Laboratory; ELISA, enzyme-linked immunosorbent assay.

in patients of Mediterranean origin include Behçet's syndrome and familial Mediterranean fever. Certain drugs, including NSAIDs and immunosuppressants, the latter especially in the transplant patient, have been associated with aseptic meningitis syndrome. Intracranial infections may present with headache and fever. Brain abscess and epidural or subdural abscesses should be considered in patients with a history of upper respiratory tract infection (i.e., otitis media, sinusitis) or infection of the teeth or gums.

Computed tomography (CT) scan or magnetic resonance imaging may aid in this diagnosis. Subacute bacterial endocarditis has been associated with aseptic meningitis syndrome; physical stigmata, including conjunctival petechiae, cardiac murmurs, retinal lesions, and evidence of embolic phenomenon, may be found. Infection with either mycobacteria or fungi or a history of malignancy must be considered.

Equine-associated meningoencephalitis outbreaks occur from late summer to early fall; there is usually an association with infections reported in horses. Avian or equine sources with spread via mosquitoes is the assumed route of infection to humans.

Though it is untreatable at this time, consider enteroviral infection in patients with aseptic meningitis. These viruses are responsible for up to 90 percent of cases of aseptic meningitis. Included in this group are the three polioviruses, group A coxsackievirus (24 types), group B coxsackievirus (6 types), echovirus (33 or 34 types) and enterovirus types 68 through 71. Enteroviruses are most commonly isolated in summer and fall, and they decrease through December.

Enteroviruses, while most commonly causing aseptic meningitis, may also cause encephalitis, ataxia, peripheral neuritis, and even paralysis. The incubation period is 1 to 5 days. Meningeal involvement usually occurs within 7 to 10 days. Most cases occur in children 5 years of age or less, with male predominance of 1.5:1. Children most commonly have fever, rash, and/or other signs of viral infection of the respiratory or gastrointestinal tract accompanied by irritability and lethargy. In adults, headache is a more prominent finding.

Recurrent bouts of meningitis with a benign clinical picture and unknown cause suggest Mollaret's meningitis.

■ PHYSICAL EXAMINATION

The patient is usually febrile and nontoxic appearing, with or without evidence of meningismus. Low-grade fever may be present, the pulse and respiration are usually within normal limits. Examination of the skin may reveal a morbilliform or vesicular rash or evidence of a tick bite. The scalp should be carefully examined along with the area behind the ears. Petechial lesions of the hands and feet usually suggest rickettsial infection. Examination of the eyes for conjunctival petechiae and funduscopic examination are important because they may reveal typical lesions of infectious endocarditis. Other lesions usually diagnosed by funduscopic examination include cytomegalovirus (CMV) retinitis or toxoplasmosis, especially if there is suspicion of HIV. Examination of the oral cavity may show a mild pharyngitis or even vesiculopapular lesions on the buccal mucosa gum margin with or without cervical adenopathy. The chest examination is usually normal, but a murmur in this setting suggests endocarditis; a pericardial rub suggests a collagen or vascular syndrome. Hepatomegaly, splenomegaly, or adenopathy suggests a systemic disease, including disseminated viral or fungal infection. Examination of the genital area may reveal vesicular or ulcerative lesions. Ulcerative lesions in the vagina have been noted in vascular syndromes such as lupus erythematosus. Joint inflammation, particularly monoarthritis, suggests mycobacterial infection. Examination of the neck may reveal evidence of stiffness on flexion and a positive Brudzinski and/or Kernig sign. Focal or multiple cranial nerve involvement suggests central lesions such as a brain, subdural, or epidural abscess; embolic phenomena may also produce these lesions.

■ LABORATORY DATA

The CSF should be examined and opening pressure recorded. Microscopic examination usually reveals a predominance of *lymphocytes.* (Initially, echovirus, polio, mumps, and HSV may have a predominance of polymorphonuclear leukocytes). The cell count is usually less than 100 lymphocytes per milliliter. Pleocytosis has been reported in 25 percent of patients with enteroviral infection. Meningeal carcinomatosis is suggested when abnormal cells are seen; large endothelial cells with indistinct cytoplasm suggest Mollaret's meningitis. Fat droplets have been seen following epidermoid cyst rupture. A wet prep of CSF should be examined on suspicion of *Toxoplasma gondii* or amoebae. Gram stain should be performed, since partially treated bacterial infection or infection with *Listeria monocytogenes* may cause a predominance of lymphocytes. Acid-fast smears to rule out mycobacterial infections and India ink stain for cryptococcal infection should be performed. CSF should be sent for routine fungal, viral, and mycobacterial cultures. If indicated, simultaneous viral cultures should be obtained from throat washings and stool specimens. Eosinophils in the CSF suggest parasitic disease such as angiostrongylus or cysticercosis.

Spinal fluid glucose may be compared with a simultaneously drawn blood glucose. Normal levels of CSF glucose (40 mg per deciliter or more than 50 to 66 percent of the blood levels) suggest viral meningitis. However, viruses like herpes, mumps, LCM, and polio can cause hypoglycorrhachia. The protein is usually elevated in this syndrome; levels above 800 mg suggest CSF block with infection or tumor, though it has been described in chemical meningitis.

Examination of the peripheral blood reveals a white count that is usually normal or may be less than 5,000 per cubic millimeter. The differential is also normal, though occasionally a left shift of polymorphonuclear leukocytes has been observed. Eosinophilia has been described with drug and serum sickness reactions. Sedimentation rate may be normal or elevated. Blood cultures should be performed, since *L. monocytogenes, Brucella,* and some typical pathogens, including *Streptococcus pneumoniae, Neisseria meningitidis,* and *Haemophilus influenzae,* may present initially with a predominance of polymorphonuclear leukocytes in the CSF. Infectious endocarditis from either bacteria or fungi can be considered in the appropriate clinical setting when a patient has positive blood cultures.

If fungal disease is suspected, serologic studies should be performed for cryptococcal antigen, *H. capsulatum,* and *C. immitis.* Complement fixation for *Mycoplasma pneumoniae* is also warranted. Venereal Disease Research Laboratory (VDRL) test should be performed on CSF. When rickettsial diseases are suspected, (i.e., Rocky Mountain spotted fever or Lyme disease), appropriate serologic tests should be performed. If rabies is suspected, an immunofluorescence test on conjunctival scrapings is the best method for establishing the diagnosis.

A chest x-ray film specifically looking for diffuse infiltrates, cavitation, and pleural or pericardial involvement may suggest mycoplasmal, mycobacterial, or fungal infection. Evidence of a mass lesion in this setting suggests carcinoma and possibly meningeal carcinomatosis. Other serologic tests include antinuclear antibody (ANA) to rule out systemic lupus erythematosus. Given the appropriate clinical setting, HIV testing may be warranted. Patients with genital HSV-2 infection and meningitis should have serologic tests performed over 3 to 4 weeks looking for fourfold rise of antibody titer. The virus may be isolated from CSF as well.

With physical findings of focal involvement, a CT scan should be performed to look for evidence of an intracranial infection or malignancy. Epidermoid tumors have often presented with recurrent meningitis mimicking Mollaret's meningitis; macrophages can be seen in the CSF.

If vesicular lesions are present, immunofluorescent staining for HSV-1, HSV-2, and varicella-zoster virus (VZV) should be performed, as should viral culture. If other than vesicular lesions are found, careful examination by dark field may reveal evidence of *T. pallidum.* Petechial lesions should be stained and cultured for bacteria and stained with immunofluorescence antibody for *R. rickettsii.*

Throat and stool cultures should be obtained for confirmation of enteroviral infection. The use of polymerase chain reaction for the diagnosis of aseptic meningitis has resulted in increased identification of the enterovirus, which allows the discontinuation of antimicrobial therapy, decreases hospital length of stay and costs, and enables patients to return to their usual environments.

■ THERAPY

The diagnosis and treatment of the aseptic meningitis syndrome is a challenge; differentiating between infectious and aseptic meningitis can be difficult (see Table 1). While there is no specific treatment for most patients with aseptic meningitis, the management of those with a syndrome of viral origin includes supportive care in most cases, though therapy exists for specific viral pathogens. Acyclovir, ganciclovir, and zidovudine (AZT) may be used to treat meningitis due to HSV, VZV, CMV, and meningitis secondary to HIV infection. Specifically, acyclovir 10 to 12 mg per kilogram every 8 hours is used for HSV and VZV; ganciclovir 5 mg per kilogram twice a day for CMV; and AZT 1,200 mg per day for the treatment of HIV. Still experimental is ribavirin for the treatment of hantavirus. Treatment with doxycycline or chloramphenicol may be indicated for patients suspected of having *Brucella* or Rocky Mountain spotted fever.

Most viral meningitides are benign and require no therapy. For bacterial, fungal, and spirochetal disease antimicrobial therapy directed against the offending agent is required (see specific chapters). However, since *L. monocytogenes* may present rarely with this picture, especially in immunocompromised hosts, specific therapy with ampicillin plus gentamicin is suggested when this organism is a consideration. Other causes of aseptic meningitis syndrome, i.e., measles, mumps and polio, are preventable by vaccination.

Although no specific antiviral therapy exists for enteroviral infection, the administration of gamma globulin has led to improvement in patients with agammaglobulinemia who have chronic enteroviral meningitis as well as in neonates with enteroviral sepsis and meningitis.

Since the differential diagnosis of aseptic meningitis syndrome is so broad, the initial evaluation of the patient in conjunction with the results of CSF studies will determine whether the patient needs empiric antimicrobial therapy to treat bacterial meningitis pending culture results from blood and CSF. Patients who are toxic appearing, in the extremes of life, or with serious underlying disease should be admitted to the hospital and treated empirically until a clear diagnosis is made. Isolation precautions for contagious diseases should be instituted.

Suggested Reading

Connolly KJ, Hammer SM. The acute aseptic meningitis syndrome. Infect Dis Clin North Am 1990; 4:599–622.

Fishman RA. Cerebrospinal fluid in diseases of the central nervous system. 2nd ed. Philadelphia: WB Saunders, 1992.

Greenlee JE. Cerebrospinal fluid in central nervous system infections. In: Scheld WM, Whitley RJ, Durack DT, eds. Infections of the central nervous system. New York: Raven Press, 1991:861–85.

Johnson RT. The pathogenesis of acute viral encephalitis and postinfectious encephalomyelitis. J Infect Dis 1987; 155:359–364.

Melnick JL. Enteroviruses: polioviruses, coxsackieviruses, echoviruses, and newer enteroviruses. In: Fields BM, Knipe DM, eds. Virology. New York: Raven Press, 1990:549.

GUILLAIN-BARRÉ SYNDROMES

John W. Griffin, M.D.
Tony W. Ho, M.D.

The Guillain-Barré syndrome (GBS) is one of the most gratifying neurologic disorders to treat. The mortality has been reduced by nearly tenfold by the employment of modern critical care. Two adjunctive therapies—plasmapheresis and infusion of human immunoglobulin (HIG)—have been proved beneficial in hastening recovery of function. In addition, we believe that the initial diagnosis of GBS is being made more rapidly and efficiently, in part as a result of the dissemination of modern electrodiagnostic testing and in part by widespread postgraduate education about the disease. Yet former patients often recall clearly the distress produced by fear, loss of control, and loss of ability to communicate. This chapter emphasizes patient education, communication tools, and the importance of realistic prognosis in the early stages of the disease.

■ DIAGNOSIS

All other aspects of GBS management stem from prompt initial diagnosis. GBS should be regarded as a true neurologic emergency. In the most dramatic examples, patients can go from being ambulatory but weak to being respirator dependent within a day. The initial symptoms may be dominated by sensory complaints, such as the abrupt onset of paresthesias in the feet or in all extremities, or the appearance of poorly localized back pain. Even at this stage, some weakness is usually detected on examination. The possibility of GBS is often suggested by the finding of hyporeflexia or areflexia in a previously healthy individual. In at least 30 percent of individuals there is no history of antecedent infection, surgery, or other precipitating factors. At this stage, examination of the cerebrospinal fluid (CSF) may exclude other possibilities, such as meningeal infiltration with neoplasm, but it is usually normal in early GBS. The characteristic elevations of spinal fluid protein occur after the first 1 to 2 weeks of illness. Careful electrodiagnostic studies may reveal prolonged distal latencies, abnormalities of F waves, slowing of conduction velocity, or reductions in compound motor action potential (CMAP) amplitudes.

In most patients, it is important to exclude the possibility of spinal cord compression. The absence of cranial nerve palsies and the presence of sensory or bowel and bladder involvement usually make this easy to diagnose. Acute intermittent porphyria should be excluded in patients with predominantly axonal physiology. Periodic paralysis should be considered in patients without sensory symptoms and should be pursued by a detailed family history, a potassium level, and electrodiagnostic studies.

Diagnostic Difficulties

There are several categories of adult patients in whom the initial diagnosis can be difficult.

Previously Ill Individuals

Very confusing pictures can be seen in individuals with a severe pre-existing disease who develop neuromuscular weakness in the hospital. A particularly vexing problem is a patient who fails to be weaned from respiratory support begun for a pulmonary indication. The differential that often arises is whether the patient has GBS or a "critical care" neuropathy. The latter problem presents as a predominantly motor axonal polyneuropathy, usually following sepsis and severe illness. There is no evidence that it is inflammatory or immune mediated, or that it responds to therapies such as plasmapheresis.

HIV Infection

Patients with HIV infection are at greater risk for GBS. Although it can occur during frank acquired immunodeficiency syndrome (AIDS), GBS is more frequently seen in the early phases of human immunodeficiency virus (HIV) infection. In the patient with AIDS, GBS must be differentiated from cytomegalovirus (CMV) polyradiculoneuropathy, another neurologic emergency. The CSF examination is critical

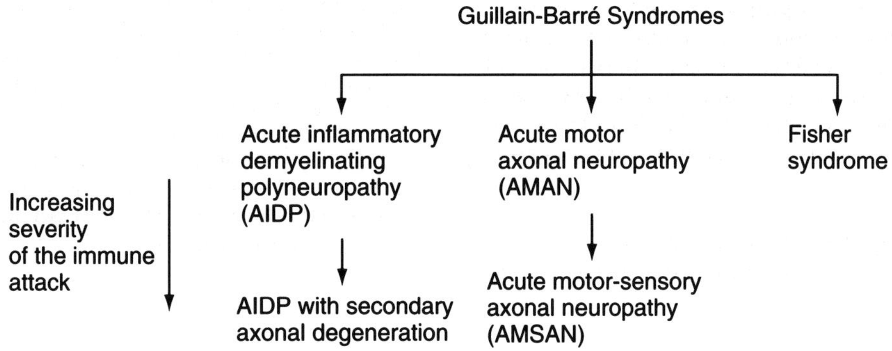

Figure 1
Proposed interrelationship among the forms of Guillain-Barré syndrome.

Table 1 Features of the Guillain-Barré Syndromes

	AIDP	AMAN	AMSAN	FISHER
Motor	Predominant	Predominat	Severe	Rare
Sensory	Frequent	Rare	Usually severe	Some
Reflexes	Absent	Absent	Absent	Absent
Other features				Ophthalmoplegia, ataxia
Electrophysiology				
Distal latency	Increased	Normal	Normal if elicitable	Normal
F wave latency	Increased	Normal	Normal if elicitable	Normal
Conduction velocity	Reduced	Not less than 10% of lower limit of normal	Normal if measurable	Normal
Compound muscle action potential amplitude	Reduced	Reduced	Rapidly and severely reduced	Normal
Sensory nerve action potential amplitude	Often reduced	Normal	Reduced/absent	Normal
Sensory nerve action potential conduction velocity	Often reduced	Normal	Normal if measurable	Normal by standard measures

AIDP, acute inflammatory demyelinating polyneuropathy; AMAN, acute motor axonal neuropathy; AMSAN, acute motor-sensory axonal neuropathy.

to the diagnosis of CMV infection: the CSF typically contains polymorphonuclear leukocytes, and evidence of the virus can be obtained by polymerase chain reaction (PCR) of the spinal fluid or by cytology of a cytospin sample. Because of its responsiveness to ganciclovir and foscarnet, prompt recognition of CMV polyradiculoneuropathy is critical. Other potential causes of neuromuscular weakness in HIV infection include drug-induced neuromuscular diseases and myositis.

Heterogeneity of the Guillain-Barré Syndromes

Guillain, Barré, and Strohl described a clinically defined syndrome of weakness, areflexia, and elevated spinal fluid protein. In 1916, they had no information on the physiology or pathology of their cases. With demonstration of lymphocytic inflammation and demyelination in autopsied cases, and the recognition that the physiologic criteria for demyelination are present in most cases of GBS, the syndrome came to be considered as synonymous with acute inflammatory demyelinating polyneuropathy (AIDP). This view is made explicit in the criteria for diagnosis of GBS promulgated by the National Institutes of Neurologic Diseases and Stroke, in which the presence of demyelination as inferred from electrodiagnosis is included in the criteria for GBS.

It is increasingly clear that, although all forms of GBS presumably represent autoimmune attack on the peripheral nervous system, in some forms the attack is directed primarily against constituents of the Schwann cell and in others against components of the axon. It appears likely that the major antigens are glycoconjugates on cell membranes. However, at the present time there are no clinically useful serologic tests that aid in the diagnosis of the various Guillain-Barré Syndromes (GBSs).

A clinically useful classification of the GBSs is given in Figure 1, and their distinctive features are described in Table 1. Using a combination of clinical and electrodiagnostic criteria, it is usually straightforward to distinguish among AIDP, AMAN (acute motor axonal neuropathy), and the Fisher syndrome. As indicated in Table 1, AMAN is distinguished by the presence of normal sensory nerve action potentials and conduction velocities, in the presence of reduced compound motor action potentials and the absence of features consistent with demyelination. The Fisher syndrome is readily diagnosed by its distinctive clinical picture of ataxia, ophthalmoparesis, and areflexia, with relatively preserved or normal strength. It is often not possible to distinguish between acute motor-sensory axonal neuropathy (AMSAN) and severe AIDP, and yet there are important prognostic differences. Most cases of AMSAN progress rapidly to severe motor and sensory involvement, and recovery is slow and often incomplete, reflecting the degeneration of nerve fibers and the requirement for regeneration for recovery. At the onset, features of demyelination may be demonstrable, but once compound muscle action potentials and sensory nerve action potentials are severely reduced or absent, the distinction between AIDP with nerve terminal demyelination, AIDP with severe secondary axonal degeneration, and AMSAN with primary immune attack on the axon is not possible. For this reason, in severe cases of GBS the early electrodiagnostic studies are often particularly helpful.

■ IMMUNOTHERAPIES

The immunotherapies are discussed first, but it is important to emphasize that the tenfold fall in mortality of GBS in the past 40 years stems not from immunotherapy but from modern means of critical care. In a similar vein, patient satisfaction is not dictated by the choice of the better immunotherapy but by attention to issues of education and communication.

Plasmapheresis was the first treatment shown to hasten recovery. Subsequently, infusion of high-dose intravenous HIG has been proven effective. Comparison studies indicate that there is little difference between the agents. Because infusion of intravenous immunoglobulin does not entail the difficulties in line placement sometimes encountered with plasmapheresis, and because it can be easily arranged on any day and at any hour, it is now the first choice of therapy for most patients.

For both infusions of HIG and plasmapheresis, it is important to check serum immunoglobulin levels. Patients with very low IgA levels (due to congenital abnormalities of IgA) are likely to develop anti-IgA antibodies and are at potential risk for anaphylaxis. Although this may be more true of HIG therapy, there is sufficient IgA in the salt-poor albumin used in plasmapheresis that patients with anti-IgA antibodies are at risk with this procedure as well.

Use of Human Immunoglobulin

All commercial products appear to be equally effective, and all are expensive. The record of safety is excellent, although concern about possible transmission of hepatitis C with one product occurred in 1994. Changes in processing are said to have minimized the possibility of transmission of blood-borne viruses with this product. In particular, HIV is inactivated during the processing, and both the donor pools and the products are tested for evidence of HIV antibody and virus. The two main complications of infusion of HIG are headache and acute renal failure. Headaches may occur more often in migraineurs, but they are associated with a CSF pleocytosis and evidence of aseptic meningitis in many individuals. They are self-limited. More dangerous is the development of acute tubular necrosis and acute renal failure. Pre-existing renal disease is unquestionably a predisposing factor. We have seen acute renal failure develop in patients with vasculitis and with diabetic nephrosclerosis. The renal involvement is always reversible, but a period of dialysis may be required. Finally, patients with high levels of immunoglobulin, as encountered occasionally in patients with HIV infections and in patients with monoclonal gammopathies, may develop hyperviscosity syndromes. Infusion of 1 g per kilogram of HIG can raise the immunoglobulin level to over 3 g per deciliter.

The usual recommendation is for infusion of 0.4 g per kilogram per day for 5 days (total dose, 2 g per kilogram). In the absence of contraindications, we often infuse 1 g per kilogram per day for 2 days. The treatment for GBS is always done in the hospital because of the possibility of idiosyncratic or anaphylactic reactions. On the first day an initial dose of 0.2 g per kilogram is infused. If this is well tolerated, on that same night the remaining 0.8 g per kilogram is infused. The next day, 1 g per kilogram is infused in divided doses.

Use of Plasmapheresis

In patients with relative contraindications to the use of HIG, plasmapheresis is an equally effective alternative, and is also an extremely safe procedure. The biggest risk is the necessity to obtain and maintain venous access in patients with inadequate veins. This often requires placement of a Shiley catheter. The continuous-flow plasmapheresis machines appear to be preferable. The replacement fluid is a 5 percent salt-poor albumin. Four or five exchanges over a period of 8 to 10 days, to a total of 250 cc per kilogram of body weight, are the standard approach. Daily plasmapheresis is disadvantageous, both because the procedure is removing in large part the replacement fluid from the day before, and because the shorter total pheresis time appears to predispose the patient to relapses.

It is not known whether the responsiveness to either immunotherapy is different among the different GBSs. At present the evidence for an antibody- and complement-mediated injury is greatest for the AMAN and AMSAN patterns. For this reason, we treat these disorders as vigorously and promptly as severe AIDP. A further unresolved question is whether there are some instances of GBS too mild to require therapy. As the evidence mounts that early immunotherapy can forestall or prevent progression to more advanced forms, a higher proportion of patients are receiving therapy. The only patients who we are not treating at the present time are those with mild involvement, who are walking without support, and who are stable and improving. A final question is whether re-treatment is advisable in a patient who had one form of immunotherapy early after onset but who continues to progress. There are at present no data to support such an approach, and assessment of the results of a multicenter trial in which plasmapheresis was followed by HIG suggests that there is no or only minimal benefit.

A frequently asked question regards the use of corticosteroids. There has never been convincing evidence for benefit from corticosteroids alone, and a recent multicenter trial has confirmed the lack of efficacy. However, ongoing studies are assessing the possibility that corticosteroids used in conjunction with HIG may provide benefit beyond that of immunoglobulin alone. At present this issue is unresolved.

■ CRITICAL CARE OF GBS PATIENTS

The modern intensive care unit (ICU) is responsible for the dramatic fall in mortality of GBSs. The mortality rate is now 2 to 3 percent, and intercurrent disease such as myocardial infarction contributes heavily to that figure. A major worry is that the ease of HIG therapy will result in patients remaining in hospitals without specialized ICUs that are experienced in GBS. If this occurs, improved immunotherapy might lead indirectly to a higher mortality rate. Ironically, the ICU experience is often that recalled least favorably by the patient. The problem lies in issues of education and communication, as discussed in the following sections.

The Decision to Place a Patient in the ICU

The decision to place a patient in the ICU must be individualized and depends on vital capacity and the rate of change of vital capacity, the presence of associated medical illnesses, and bulbar function. The sequence to be avoided can be summarized as follows: a patient with marginal respiratory function and a degree of bulbar involvement becomes acutely fatigued, often as a result of modest aspiration while eating or drinking, and is unable to cough effectively. The autonomic abnormalities characteristic of GBS result in swings in blood pressure and heart rate, compounding respiratory fatigue. Suddenly, an apparently stable patient undergoes emergency intubation at the bedside. Often the procedure is accompanied by further heart rate and blood pressure swings. Frequent monitoring of vital capacity, early transfer to the ICU, elective intubation, and careful monitoring of fluid volume can prevent such emergencies. We generally consider elective intubation when a patient's forced vital capacity falls below 12 to 15 cc per kilogram or, in patients with bulbar symptoms, 15 to 18 cc per kilogram.

Within the ICU the most important issues are prevention and treatment of respiratory tract infections, prophylaxis of venous thrombosis and pulmonary embolism with subcutaneous heparin (5,000 units every 12 hours), monitoring for inappropriate antidiuretic hormone secretion (an occasional complication of GBS), and protection against urinary tract infection, fecal impaction, and stress ulcers. Prevention of keratitis by using artificial tears and monitoring for loss of lid closure and/or tearing is essential.

The autonomic system is affected in up to 50 percent of GBS patients and is the major cause of mortality. Autonomic involvement can be manifest by systemic hypertension, orthostatic hypotension, altered sweating, or tachy- or bradyarrhythmia. In general, no treatment is necessary for systemic hypertension; antihypertensive drugs must be used with extreme caution because of the risk of sudden drops in blood pressure. An enhanced vagal response may cause bradyarrhythmia during suctioning.

Back pain and dysesthesia in the extremities may be major sources of discomfort; low-dose tricyclics or narcotics are often helpful with these.

Education and Communication

From the earliest diagnosis of GBS, it is important to discuss with a patient in detail the prognosis and the possibilities for progression. We emphasize the possibility of a progression to respirator dependency and outline the likelihood, based on the prognostic information in the electrodiagnostic studies, as well as the patient's age, general medical status, and presence or absence of *Campylobacter jejuni* as an antecedent infection (patients with *Campylobacter* tend to have more severe GBS and a poorer prognosis). We emphasize that GBS is a disease of the peripheral nervous system only and does not produce damage to the brain, with attendant dementia, blindness, and so on, or to the spinal cord. Some patients benefit from visiting the ICU while they are "upright." In addition, patients and family members are encouraged to learn a communication system for use in the event that ventilation is required. An easily learned system that can be used with great efficiency is the clear Lucite letterboard: as long as the patient is able to move the eyes, communication can be achieved by looking from letter to letter to spell out the message, with the letterboard placed between the patient and the reader. Finally, a visit by a former patient can be very useful.

As recovery is commencing, attainable goals are set for physical therapy and rehabilitation and a realistic timetable is outlined. The prognostic information available in follow-up electrodiagnostic studies is often of considerable importance—and usually reassuring—to patients.

Suggested Reading

Feasby TE, Hahn AF, Brown WF, et al. Severe axonal degeneration in acute Guillain-Barré syndrome: Evidence of two different mechanisms? J Neurol Sci 1993; 116:185–192.

Hughes RAC. Guillain-Barré syndrome. New York: Springer-Verlag, 1990.

Nobile-Orazio E, Meucci N, Barbieri S, et al. High-dose intravenous immunoglobulin therapy in multifocal motor neuropathy. Neurology 1993; 43:537–544.

Ropper AH, Wijdicks EFM, Trauax BT. Guillain-Barré syndrome. Philadelphia: FA Davis, 1991.

SPINAL CORD INJURY

Bruce H. Dobkin, M.D.
Eric I. Hassid, M.D.

Traumatic spinal cord injury (SCI) is a leading cause of morbidity in the United States primarily among males at a mean age of 30, with about 60 percent of patients ages 16 to 30 at onset. The prevalence is 200,000 with an annual incidence of 10,000. With exemplary acute and chronic care, survival rates are over 90 percent and most young victims have a near-normal life span. The causes of SCI include motor vehicle accidents (48 percent); falls (21 percent); acts of violence (14 percent), which are increasing as vehicular accidents decline; and sports injuries (14 percent). Management issues can be considered across the phases of acute hospital care, subacute care with inpatient rehabilitation, and chronic care over the lifetime of the disabled person. A neurosurgeon or orthopedist most often provides initial acute care. A neurologist, physiatrist, or internist tends to manage subsequent care, in concert with a team of rehabilitation therapists, an orthotist, a urologist, and others as needed. Chronic medical and rehabilitative management is similar to what may be provided for patients with myelopathies of any etiology, such as cervical spondylosis in older persons and spastic paraparesis due to demyelinating disease.

■ ACUTE MANAGEMENT

The goal of immediate management of SCI is quick recognition of the extent of spine and other injuries, safe stabilization of the spinal column, and rapid management of life-threatening conditions such as respiratory failure and hypotension. Urinary retention commonly follows spinal shock. A Foley catheter should be placed during acute care unless urethral trauma is suspected. Intermittent bladder catheterization should start as soon as it is feasible to reduce the incidence of urinary tract infection. The acute administration of intravenous methylprednisolone at a rate of 30 mg per kilogram over 1 hour followed by 5.4 mg per kilogram per hour for the next 23 hours has been recommended based on the results of a multicenter randomized, placebo-controlled clinical trial. Methylprednisolone-treated patients had a modest gain in strength at 6 weeks and 1 year if the drug was administered within 8 hours of the injury. Other acute neuroprotective trials are in progress.

Once vital signs have been stabilized, a careful examination should include the American Spinal Injury Association (ASIA) Standard Neurological Classification to define the level of injury, motor and sensory scores (Fig. 1), and completeness of the deficit using the impairment scale (Fig. 2). Palpation that produces tenderness can point to vertebral fractures. A variety of fracture patterns and subluxations are found in SCI, related to the summation of directional forces at the time of injury. Radiographic studies may need to include the head, spine, abdomen, chest, lung, pelvis, and long bones. A combination of plain x-ray films and computed tomographic scans provides the best yield for detecting vertebral fractures. Magnetic resonance imaging best detects disk herniations, root compressions, and cord edema. Traction and spine stabilization with external devices such as a thermoplastic jacket may be adequate, but about 60 percent of patients will require surgical decompression or an internal fixation.

Other medical complications that can be prevented during the acute phase include pneumonia, urinary tract infections, deep venous thrombosis (DVT), and skin and gastric ulcers. For DVT prophylaxis, subcutaneous heparin, 5,000 units twice per day, can be continued until lower-extremity hypotonia gives way to hypertonia or the patient is ambulating. In an intubated patient, hypotension and bradycardia can result from vagal stimulation during endotrachial suctioning. Histamine H_2 blockers can prevent gastric ulcer formation due to the stress of the injury.

■ SUBACUTE PHASE

The subacute stage may start toward the end of an acute hospital stay and continue through inpatient rehabilitation. Although they vary widely, mean acute hospital stays are about 30 days and inpatient rehabilitation stays are about 45 days for SCI. Additional medical problems that can develop include pressure sores; bladder storage and emptying dysfunction, often with detrusor-sphincter dyssynergia; bowel incontinence and obstipation; flexor spasms and other sequelae of spasticity; autonomic hyperreflexia; and heterotopic ossification. The effects of a traumatic brain injury, a post-traumatic stress disorder, and premorbid substance abuse may become apparent and will require cognitive and psychosocial interventions.

Pressure sores have been found in 5 percent to 15 percent of SCI patients, and the yearly rate can be considerably higher over the lifetime of patients who are the most immobilized or are not attentive to preventive measures. During rehabilitation, patients are taught to inspect their skin on their own with mirrors or with the help of a caregiver, paying attention to the bony prominences of the sacrum, heel, scapula, foot, and trochanter. Prevention requires daily skin examinations, wheelchair weight shifting, pressure-relieving cushions and pads, and repositioning every 3 hours during sleep.

Detrusor-sphincter dyssynergia results from disruption of motor, sympathetic, and parasympathetic activity. If bladder contractions occur against a closed urethral sphincter, the detrusor muscle can hypertrophy, intravesicular pressure becomes chronically elevated, and ureteral reflux can lead to hydronephrosis and renal insufficiency. Intermittent bladder catheterization with the administration of anticholinergics such as oxybutynin, from 2.5 mg at bedtime to 5 mg four times per day can create a more flaccid bladder, facilitate storage, and decrease reflux. Alpha-1 blockers such as prazosin, 1 to 2 mg twice daily, can decrease urethral sphincter tone and facilitate emptying in the presence of outlet obstruction. When the detrusor does not contract well, bethanechol, 25 mg twice per day to 50 mg four times per day, can facilitate emptying. Imipramine, 25 to 100 mg at bedtime, can facilitate

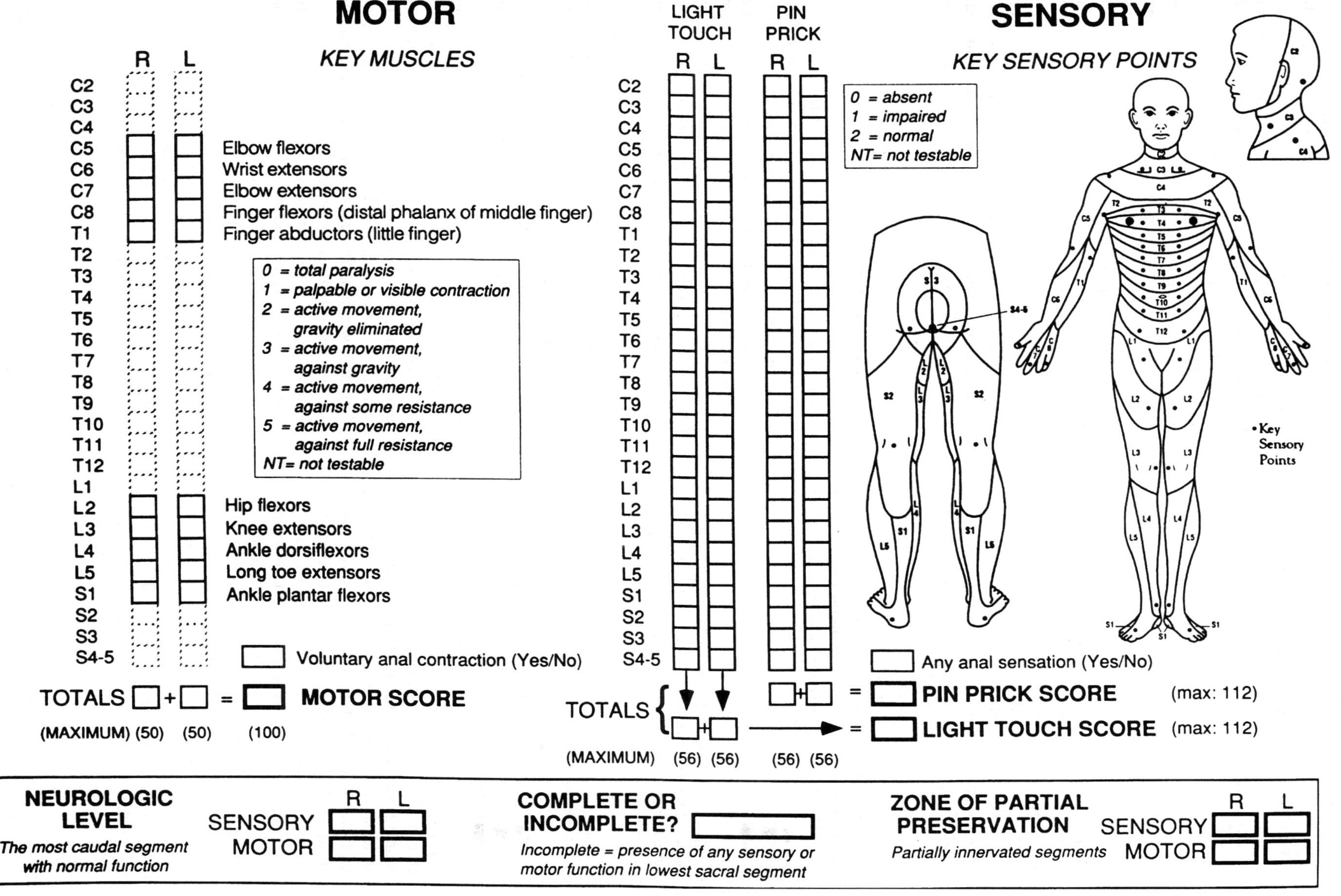

STANDARD NEUROLOGIC CLASSIFICATION OF SPINAL CORD INJURY

MOTOR

KEY MUSCLES

R L

C2
C3
C4
C5 Elbow flexors
C6 Wrist extensors
C7 Elbow extensors
C8 Finger flexors (distal phalanx of middle finger)
T1 Finger abductors (little finger)
T2
T3
T4
T5
T6
T7
T8
T9
T10
T11
T12
L1
L2 Hip flexors
L3 Knee extensors
L4 Ankle dorsiflexors
L5 Long toe extensors
S1 Ankle plantar flexors
S2
S3
S4-5

0 = total paralysis
1 = palpable or visible contraction
2 = active movement, gravity eliminated
3 = active movement, against gravity
4 = active movement, against some resistance
5 = active movement, against full resistance
NT= not testable

☐ Voluntary anal contraction (Yes/No)

TOTALS ☐ + ☐ = ☐ **MOTOR SCORE**

(MAXIMUM) (50) (50) (100)

SENSORY

KEY SENSORY POINTS

LIGHT TOUCH R L — PIN PRICK R L

C2, C3, C4, C5, C6, C7, C8, T1, T2, T3, T4, T5, T6, T7, T8, T9, T10, T11, T12, L1, L2, L3, L4, L5, S1, S2, S3, S4-5

0 = absent
1 = impaired
2 = normal
NT= not testable

• Key Sensory Points

☐ Any anal sensation (Yes/No)

TOTALS ☐ + ☐ = ☐ **PIN PRICK SCORE** (max: 112)

☐ + ☐ = ☐ **LIGHT TOUCH SCORE** (max: 112)

(MAXIMUM) (56) (56) (56) (56)

NEUROLOGIC LEVEL
The most caudal segment with normal function
SENSORY R ☐ L ☐
MOTOR R ☐ L ☐

COMPLETE OR INCOMPLETE? ☐
Incomplete = presence of any sensory or motor function in lowest sacral segment

ZONE OF PARTIAL PRESERVATION
Partially innervated segments
SENSORY R ☐ L ☐
MOTOR R ☐ L ☐

Figure 1
American Spinal Injury Association motor and sensory scales.

ASIA IMPAIRMENT SCALE

☐ A = **Complete:** No motor or sensory function is preserved below the neurologic level or in the sacral segments S4–S5.

☐ B = **Incomplete:** Sensory but not motor function is preserved below the neurologic level and extends through the sacral segments S4–S5.

☐ C = **Incomplete:** Motor function is preserved below the neurologic level, and the majority of key muscles below the neurologic level have a muscle grade less than 3.

☐ D = **Incomplete:** Motor function is preserved below the neurologic level, and the majority of key muscles below the neurologic level have a muscle grade greater than or equal to 3.

☐ E = **Normal:** Motor and sensory function is normal.

Figure 2
American Spinal Injury Association impairment scale.

storage by increasing internal sphincter tone and decreasing detrusor contractions. In addition, most antispasticity agents will facilitate emptying, which can be an unwanted side effect. Measurements of residual urine by catheterization or, better, by ultrasound and a urologic evaluation with a cystometrogram best identify the type of dysfunction and the most appropriate pharmacologic or surgical approach. Electrical stimulation with electrodes implanted over the bladder wall, sphincter, pudendal nerve, and sacral roots has aided continence and emptying in selected SCI patients.

Constipation is common. Enemas or laxatives on a routine basis are not an acceptable means of bowel care. Docusate sodium, 100 mg one to two times daily, and digital stimulation are the best initial approaches for scheduled bowel movements, augmented by bisacodyl or glycerin suppositories. Gastrointestinal hypomotility can be alleviated with cisapride.

Range of motion of all paralyzed extremities at least a few times across all joints performed twice a day is extremely important to prevent contractures. Spinal shock can take weeks to months to resolve. Spasticity and flexor or extensor spasms frequently follow. Spasms and clonus tend to be most apparent in patients with severe but incomplete cervicothoracic injuries. They are often induced by muscle stretch, particularly of the iliopsoas when moving from sitting to supine, or local pain. Many patients use their inducible hypertonicity to increase antigravity muscle tone for pivot transfers or stepping. Management of unwanted spasms includes careful inspection for inciting noxious stimuli such as pressure sores, bladder distention, rectal fissures, ingrown toenails, heterotopic ossification, and DVT. Spasticity should be treated pharmacologically when it causes significant pain or interferes with everyday functioning such as with leg positioning and wheelchair transfers. The most useful drugs are listed in Table 1. The alpha-2 adrenergic drugs such as clonidine and tizanidine can be especially valuable in eliminating noxious stimuli-induced spasms, perhaps by suppressing dorsal horn sensory inputs. Dantrolene tends to cause

Table 1 Pharmacologic Treatments of Spasticity

MEDICATION	DOSAGE RANGE	SIDE EFFECTS
Baclofen	5–40 mg t.i.d.	Confusion, sedation, weakness
Diazepam	2–30 mg t.i.d.	Confusion, sedation, weakness
Dantrolene	25 mg qd–100 mg q.i.d.	Hepatotoxicity, diarrhea, generalized weakness
Clonidine	0.1 mg qd–0.2 mg b.i.d.	Sedation, hypotension
Cyproheptadine	4–12 mg b.i.d.	Sedation, dry mouth

more generalized paresis, even in unaffected muscles. Oral baclofen must be tapered over about 2 weeks if it had been used chronically to avoid withdrawal seizures and delirium. Intrathecal baclofen can eliminate spasms with few side effects in patients who fail other therapies. Any of these drugs, alone or in combination, can occasionally improve stepping in patients who have some ability to walk with assistive devices and bracing. However, a brief drug trial must be monitored closely with an evaluation of the safety of the gait pattern and the speed of locomotion to help determine that the agent is worth continuing. Intramuscular injections of botulinum toxin can lessen unwanted co-contractions of a muscle during walking or allow for easier care when, for example, hip adductor spasticity interferes with perineal skin care. The effect may only last several months. Phenol nerve or motor point blocks, surgical tendon lengthenings, and tendon transplants can improve joint range and occasionally allow better control of a joint movement.

Autonomic hyperreflexia from loss of supraspinal control over autonomic reflexes requires treatment in about 15 percent of SCI patients with lesions above T6 in the first 6 months and in at least that number of ASIA A and B tetraplegic patients on a more chronic basis. It presents as headache, flushing, palpitations, a feeling of doom, and paroxysmal hypertension. Common precipitants include a distended bladder or rectum and noxious stimuli such as an ingrown toenail, DVT, or an acute abdomen without localizing pain. A step-by-step approach to treatment of hyperreflexia is outlined in Table 2.

Heterotopic ossification is a condition in which ossification of subcutaneous and periarticular tissues occurs especially in the hips, knees, and shoulders. Swelling, erythema, pain, and decreasing range of motion are among the first clinical signs. A three-phase bone scan reveals focal uptake prior to radiographic visualization of bone. Range of motion and nonsteroidal anti-inflammatory drugs such as indomethacin, 25 mg three times per day, can help. Etidronate sodium, 20 mg per kilogram per day divided into two daily doses given for up to 6 months, retards the progression of the condition. Persistent pain or immobility can require surgical resection.

Inpatient rehabilitation includes education about how to maintain the SCI patient's health over a lifetime. The rehabilitation team also provides sexual, drug, and vocational

Table 2 Treatment Regimen for Autonomic Hyperreflexia
Sit patient up to 90 degrees.
Monitor blood pressure every 3 minutes.
Catheterize bladder using lidocaine gel.
Disimpact bowel using lidoacine gel.
Look for source of noxious stimuli (ingrown toenail, acute abdomen, DVT).
Give 10 mg nifedipine SL if systolic blood pressure >170; repeat in 10 minutes as needed. Monitor for hypotension.
Give hydralazine 5–10 mg IV if hypertension persists.
Check blood pressure often.
Give prazosin 5 mg up to three times per day for prophylaxis.

counseling and begins the lengthy process of acclimating the patient to the changes in body image and level of independence that so often follow a serious SCI. The physician plays an important role in providing hopeful but realistic information about recovery and about the physical and psychosocial adaptations that may be necessary. For the first several months after an SCI, we do not offer a specific prognosis about the amount of recovery that is likely. No young SCI patient is ready to accept less than near full recovery, and a detailed prognosis is still uncertain in all but the patient who has a complete transection. We ask the patient and family to work with the nurses and therapists on specific goals that will allow the patient to be more functional over the short run so that he or she can return home. However, a few relative prognostic findings from clinical studies give the physician an idea about what is most likely to happen.

The physical therapist assists the patient in attaining the maximum strength possible in functioning muscle groups and tries to bring out activity elsewhere, especially just below the level of impairment. In a quadriplegic, early emphasis is placed on achieving head and trunk control to allow for swallowing, better respiratory function, and sitting balance. The paraplegic and the incomplete or C6 level and below quadriplegic patient are trained to become independent in transfers and wheelchair mobility over a variety of surfaces. If residual strength of the arms and legs is adequate, step training with bracing and assistive devices begins. Ambulation is one of the most sought goals of patients after SCI. The strength of the lower extremities determines the amount of work performed by the upper extremities for support, which in turn determines the rate of oxygen consumption and the practicality of ambulation. Many patients may achieve short-distance walking in the home, but fewer will have the strength and stamina to walk over 500 feet within a reasonable time in the community. The patient who is a complete paraplegic at 1 month postinjury has no more than a 5 percent chance of regaining minimal motor function or in becoming a community ambulator by 1 year post-SCI. However, about 85 percent of muscles in the incomplete paraplegic who has $1/5$ to $2/5$ strength at 1 month will recover to at least $3/5$ strength by 1 year, and 75 percent of these persons will be capable of community ambulation with aids. About 45 percent of incomplete quadriplegic patients become community ambulators.

The occupational therapist works especially with the patient's residual upper extremity motor function. About 75 percent of muscles of the incomplete quadriplegic patient that are graded $1/5$ at 1 month and nearly all muscles that have $2/5$ strength at 1 month will improve to greater than $3/5$ strength by 1 year. This strength is adequate for most self-care tasks. However, only 20 percent of muscles graded $0/5$ at 1 month will recover to at least $3/5$ strength. The therapist and patient are restricted in what can be done manually depending on the motor level and residual strength. Supplemented by assistive devices and physical changes in the home and work environment, most persons with even a C5 level can achieve some independence, and with a level below C6 they will reach considerable independence in self-care and community activities.

■ CHRONIC PHASE

This period extends from the start of outpatient rehabilitation through the lifetime of the disabled person. Rehabilitation efforts often continue for at least 1 year in patients who continue to improve in strength with selective muscle exercises and work on conditioning. A gain of functionally useful strength at one level below the injury can make a dramatic difference in the life of a quadriplegic. Tendon transfers and joint-stabilization procedures can provide greater function if the patient has plateaued at 1 year. For example, a C6 level patient can gain elbow extension and a functional reach by surgically implanting the posterior deltoid tendon over the triceps insertion. Gait training strategies can include treadmill training while some of the patient's body weight is supported by a harness attached to an overhead lift. Functional electrical stimulation of nerve-muscle and a variety of bracing systems have been used to try to increase hand and finger grip and, in the patient with persistently profound lower extremity weakness, to permit stepping over short distances. Few such measures are yet standardized, all require considerable time in therapy and cost $15,000 to $50,000, and most follow-up studies show that patients tend not to use the gait systems over the long run. Wheelchair use is more efficient. Over the years postinjury, many patients will benefit from a brief burst of therapy to deal with overuse of a muscle group and to deal with evolving changes in function.

In addition to continued management of the potential medical complications of immobility, the clinician must monitor urinary function. This includes a urinalysis every 4 months or when the patient recognizes symptoms of infection (greater spasticity, spasms, dysautonomia, cloudy urine, fever), a blood urea nitrogen and creatinine and a renal scan yearly, and urodynamic studies for problems of storage or emptying. Central pain near the site of spinal injury can develop in many patients. Tricyclics, carbamazepine, baclofen, nonsteroidal anti-inflammatory drugs, and transcutaneous electrical stimulation can help. Radiologic studies might pinpoint a contributing cause due to spinal column instability or an enlarging syrinx. A syrinx that produces pain, autonomic hyperreflexia, or severe spasms or leads to a decline in motor and sensory function should be shunted and ablated if possible. In the quadriplegic patient, sleep apnea can impair daytime alertness and may require the use of continuous positive airway pressure.

To be able to handle the searching questions of their patients, clinicians will want to keep abreast of research in spinal cord neuroprotection, central myelin and axonal regeneration, and the efficacy of spinal implants of tissues and bridging materials across an injury. Animal models of neuroplasticity continue to reveal the potential for biologic approaches to one day enhance the outcome of patients with SCI. In the interim, attention to the details of health maintenance and problem solving will enhance a patient's quality of life.

Suggested Reading

Bracken MB, Shepard M, Collins W, et al. A randomized controlled trial of methylprednisolone or naloxone in the treatment of acute spinal cord injury. N Engl J Med 1990; 332:1405–1411.

Ditunnno JF, Formal CS. Chronic spinal cord injury. N Engl J Med 1994; 33:550–556.

Dobkin BH. Neurologic rehabilitation. Philadelphia: FA Davis, 1996: chap. 8.

Johnston RA. The management of acute spinal cord injury. J Neurol Neurosurg Psychiatry 1993; 1046–1054.

Waters RL. Motor and sensory recovery following incomplete paraplegia. Arch Phys Med Rehabil 1994; 75:67–72.

POLYMYOSITIS, DERMATOMYOSITIS, AND INCLUSION-BODY MYOSITIS

Marinos C. Dalakas, M.D.

Inflammatory myopathies are acquired muscle diseases characterized by myopathic muscle weakness, endomysial inflammation, and elevation of serum muscle enzymes. A simple and practical classification of the inflammatory myopathies is into three major groups: polymyositis (PM), dermatomyositis (DM), and inclusion-body myositis (IBM).

DM affects both children and adults. In contrast, PM is seen after the second decade of life and IBM after the age of 40. DM remains a distinct clinical entity because of the characteristic rash that accompanies or, more often, precedes the manifestation of proximal muscle weakness. The earliest lesion in DM is the deposition of complement, C5b-9 membranolytic attack complex (MAC), on the intramuscular capillaries. This is followed by necrosis and marked reduction in the number of capillaries per each muscle fiber, resulting in ischemia, muscle fiber destruction often resembling microinfarcts, and inflammation.

In contrast with DM, PM has no unique clinical features. It is best defined as an inflammatory myopathy with a rather slow onset (weeks to months) and steady progression that occurs mainly in adults and rarely in children who do not have any of the following: a rash, involvement of eye and facial muscles, family history of neuromuscular disease, history of exposure to myotoxic drugs or toxins, endocrinopathy, neurogenic disease, dystrophy, biochemical muscle disease, or IBM.

IBM is often suspected when a patient with presumed PM does not respond to therapy. IBM has now evolved into a distinct clinical entity. It is the most common acquired myopathy above the age of 50 years and remains therapy resistant and predictably disabling. It presents with an often-asymmetric weakness and atrophy and selective involvement of the quadriceps, iliopsoas, triceps, biceps, foot extensors, and finger flexors. Involvement of the flexor digitorum profundus IV and V and the flexor pollicis are early clues to the clinical diagnosis.

In PM there is evidence of an antigen-directed cytotoxicity mediated by $CD8^+$ cytotoxic T cells, which surround healthy and MHC-1 class-expressing non-necrotic muscle fibers that eventually invade and destroy. In IBM, in spite of the same immunopathologic abnormalities as those seen in PM, degenerative causes may coexist because of the presence of amyloid deposition within the vacuolated muscle fibers and the relative resistance of the disease to immunotherapies.

■ GENERAL THERAPEUTIC GUIDELINES

The goal of therapy in PM, DM, and IBM is to improve function in the activities of daily living as the result of improving muscle strength. Creatine kinase (CK) level is a useful marker of disease activity and when the strength improves it falls concurrently. However, the reverse is not always true because most of the immunosuppressive therapies can result in a decrease of serum muscle enzymes without necessarily improving muscle strength. For example, plasmapheresis reduces CK without improving strength. Unfortunately, this has been misinterpreted as "chemical improvement" and has formed the basis for the common habit of "chasing" or "treating" the CK level instead of the muscle weakness, a practice that has led to prolonged treatment with unnecessary immunosuppressive drugs and erroneous assessment of their efficacy.

Most of the treatment trials in inflammatory myopathies have been empiric, and large-scale control therapeutic studies against the immunologically specific forms of childhood DM and adult PM or DM have not been conducted. As the specific target antigens are also unknown, these therapies are not selectively targeting the autoreactive T cells or the complement-mediated process on the intramuscular blood vessels. Instead, they are inducing a nonselective immunosuppression or immunomodulation. Other pitfalls in the therapy of these diseases include lack of objective means of measuring muscle strength; consideration of PM/DM as a homogeneous disease in spite of distinct differences in the clinical, immunologic, and prognostic parameters; reliance on serologic markers, i.e., autoantibodies, with unproven significance in taxonomy, prognosis, and pathogenesis; and lack of data on natural history.

■ THERAPEUTIC STRATEGIES

The therapeutic strategies that I follow in the management of patients with PM and DM are, sequentially, the following:

Corticosteroids

In spite of lack of control trials, steroids remain the first therapeutic option. Because the effectiveness and relative safety of prednisone therapy will determine the future need for stronger immunosuppressive drugs, I prefer an aggressive approach of high-dose prednisone early in the disease. A high dose, 80 to 100 mg per day (or 1 mg per kilogram per day), as a single daily morning dose for an initial period of 3 to 4 weeks is preferable. Prednisone is then tapered over a 10 week period to 80 to 100 mg *single dose, alternate-day,* by gradually reducing an alternate "off day" dose by 10 mg per week, or faster if necessitated by side effects, although this carries a greater risk of breakthrough of disease (Table 1). If there is evidence of efficacy and no serious side effects, the dosage is reduced gradually by 5 to 10 mg every 3 to 4 weeks until the lowest possible dose that controls the disease is reached. In a patient responding to prednisone, a "maintenance" dose of 10 to 25 mg every other day may be needed to secure continuous improvement and stability. On the other hand, if by the time the dosage has been reduced to 80 to 100 mg every other day (approximately 14 weeks after initiating therapy) there is no objective benefit (defined as increased muscle strength and not as lowering of the CK or a subjective feeling of increased energy), the patient may be considered unresponsive to prednisone and tapering can be accelerated while the next-in-line immunosuppressive drug is started.

The single-dose, alternate-day program minimizes side effects (Cushingoid appearance, diabetes, obesity, high blood pressure, osteoporosis, avascular necrosis of the hip, retarded growth in children) and can adequately control the underlying disease. I prefer not to start therapy with alternate-day prednisone without a preceding high daily-dose schedule because, empirically, the response appears to be suboptimal. I

Table 1 Conservative Method of Reducing High Single-Dose Daily Prednisone to Low Alternate-Day Doses in the Treatment of Polymyositis and Dermatomyositis

HIGH-DOSE DAY	LOW-DOSE/ OFF DAY	DURATION	TAPER METHOD
100	100	3–4 wk (100 mg/day)	
100	100–10	9 wk	After 3rd or 4th week, start tapering an alternative (off-day) dose by 10 mg every week; i.e., 100 mg one day, 90 mg the other; a week later, 100 mg one day, 80 mg the other day, etc.
100	10–0	2 wk	By 5 mg every week, i.e., 100 mg one day, 5 mg the other, until 100 mg one day, 0 the other.
100	0	2–4 wk	If no benefit by this time, patient is probably not responding to prednisone; accelerate tapering and start an immunosuppressive drug.
100–70	0	18–22 wk	If there is benefit, start tapering high-day dose by 5 mg every 3 to 4 weeks until 70 mg on alternate days.
70–40	0	36–48 wk	Continue tapering by 2.5 mg every 3 to 4 weeks until 40 mg on alternate days.
40–20	0	8–16 mo	Continue tapering by 2.5 mg every 1 to 2 months until 20 mg on alternate days.
20–10	0	Maintenance dose	Continue tapering by 2.5 mg every 3 to 4 months until 15 mg on alternate days.

Reduction can be slower or faster if dictated by disease status or drug side effects.

also prefer to give the prednisone as a single dose in the morning because the higher morning natural cortisol concentration results in a competitive decrease in the metabolism of the administered prednisone, resulting in a decreased clearance of the unbound (active) prednisolone and, theoretically, a greater beneficial effect. Further, the morning exogenous prednisone dose is less likely to suppress the evening secretion of adrenocorticotropic hormone and, consequently, the endogenous cortisol secretion is anticipated to be unaffected the next morning.

Intravenous methylprednisolone, up to 1 g per square meter per day, over 60 minutes for 3 days is also used by some clinicians, especially in sick patients with gastrointestinal problems who cannot tolerate oral corticosteroids. The value of IV steroids, the recommended dose, the frequency of the administration, and the long-term side effects have not been studied. My own preference in such patients is to switch to oral prednisone as soon as it is felt to be clinically safe.

Collateral Corticosteroid Program

Every patient is requested from the beginning of steroid therapy to start a strict diet of low-carbohydrate, low-salt, high-protein intake. Self-discipline to avoid gaining weight is also emphasized, and the patient's compliance is monitored by checking body weight during each visit. This dietetic regimen decreases the chance for excess weight gain and for developing hypertension, especially in predisposed individuals. For individuals with gastrointestinal discomfort, we use antacids, preferably a calcium-containing one such as Tums, between meals, or Cimetidine, 300 mg three times per day, or Ranidine once daily. Coadministration of calcium supplement (1 g per day) and vitamin D (50,000 units once per week) are considered in postmenopausal female patients when long-term therapy is required. An effort is made to reassure the patients that certain symptoms such as "flushing," or redness in the face, insomnia, and mild action tremor of the hands, which are common with the high doses, will disappear upon lowering the steroid dosage. Patients at high risk of exposure to tuberculosis, those with a recently documented positive purified protein derivative test, or those with a previous history of tuberculosis are given isoniazid (INH) prophylaxis. If INH is used, pyridoxine 100 mg per day is administered concurrently to prevent INH-induced neuropathy.

Steroid-Myopathy Versus Disease Activity

The long-term use of prednisone may cause worsening of muscle strength associated with a normal or unchanged CK level, referred to as *steroid myopathy.* Steroids do not in fact cause histologic signs of myopathy but rather selective atrophy of type II muscle fibers and loss of thick filaments documented by electronmicroscopy. In practice, steroid-induced weakness is not often a major factor because the increasing weakness is usually caused by the underlying disease. In certain circumstances, however, steroid-induced weakness raises diagnostic concerns because it may be difficult to separate it from increased weakness related to disease activity since the two can coexist. Further, the increased weakness may be caused by other factors, such as decreased mobility, infection, or an associated systemic illness. The decision to adjust the prednisone dosage in a patient who has previously responded to treatment may be influenced by reviewing the past 1 to 2 months' history of the muscle strength, mobility, serum CK, medication changes, and associated medical conditions. For example, in a patient who for the past 1 to 2 months has increased CK levels, no new overt signs of steroid toxicity with reduced or unchanged dosage of steroids, and no evidence of a systemic illness or infection, an increasing muscle weakness is most likely due to exacerbation of the disease, which may either require more prednisone or has become steroid resistant. When these signs are not clear, I arbitrarily raise the prednisone dosage and wait for the answer, which can be evident in about 2 to 8 weeks, according to the change in the patient's strength. A new muscle biopsy may not reveal the cause of increased weakness because active inflammatory disease can be present, even when steroid intoxication was the cause of increasing weakness, while type II muscle fiber atrophy can coexist with active inflammation even in a patient who has never received steroids. Electromyography may occasionally be of some help if it shows active myopathic changes with fibrillations and positive sharp waves in many sites of proximal muscle groups. A clinical sign that I have found to be of some help in a few patients is the strength of neck flexor muscles, which usually worsens with exacerbation of the disease but may remain unchanged with steroid-induced muscle intoxication.

Nonsteroidal Immunosuppressive Therapies and "Prednisone Failures"

Although the majority of the patients with bona fide PM or DM respond to steroids to some degree and for some period of time, a number of them fail to respond or become steroid resistant. The decision to start an immunosuppressive drug in PM or DM patients is based on the following factors: (1) need for its "steroid-sparing" effect, when in spite of steroid responsiveness the patient has developed significant complications; (2) attempts to lower a high-steroid dosage have repeatedly resulted in a new relapse; (3) adequate dose of prednisone for at least a 2 to 3 month period has been ineffective; and (4) rapidly progressive disease is present with evolving severe weakness and respiratory failure. The preference for selecting the next-in-line immunosuppressive therapy remains empiric because controlled studies have not been conducted. The choice is usually based on our own prejudices, our personal experience with each drug, and our own assessment of the relative efficacy-safety ratio. In this phase of therapy, my preference is, sequentially, (1) azathioprine or methotrexate, (2) intravenous immunoglobulin (IVIg), and (3) other immunosuppressants.

Azathioprine or Methotrexate

Among the two, my preference is azathioprine, a derivative of 6-mercaptopurine. Although lower doses (1.5 to 2 mg per kilogram) are commonly used, I prefer higher doses up to 3 mg per kilogram for effective immunosuppression. Among immunosuppressants, this drug is my first choice because it is well tolerated, has fewer side effects, and, empirically, appears to be as effective for long-term therapy as the other drugs. Compared to cyclosporine, however, which may work rather fast, the beneficial effect of azathioprine is usually seen after 3 to 6 months of treatment. Patience is therefore required before it is concluded that the drug is ineffective. The major toxicity of azathioprine includes thrombocytopenia, anemia, leukopenia, pancytopenia, drug fever, nausea, and liver toxicity. An elevation of liver enzymes, if slight, needs only observation. Azathioprine, which is metabolized by xanthine oxidase, if given concurrently with allopurinol, can be severely toxic to the liver or bone marrow, and their combined use is not recommended.

Methotrexate, an antagonist of folate metabolism, is a drug with documented efficacy in rheumatoid arthritis. Although in my experience, methotrexate is not more effective than azathioprine, it has the advantage of working faster (if it is going to work at all). It can be given intravenously over 20 to 60 minutes at weekly doses of 0.4 mg per kilogram up to 0.8 mg per kilogram with sufficient fluids, or orally starting at 7.5 mg weekly for the first 3 weeks (given in a total of 3 doses, 2.5 mg every 12 hours), increasing it gradually by 2.5 mg per week up to a total of 25 mg weekly. A relevant side effect is methotrexate-pneumonitis, which can be difficult to distinguish from the interstitial lung disease of the primary myopathy. Other side effects include stomatitis, gastrointestinal symptoms, leukopenia, thrombocytopenia, renal toxicity, hepatotoxicity, and malignancies.

Intravenous Immunoglobulin

IVIg is a promising, although expensive, therapy. In a double-blind study in patients with refractory DM, IVIg was shown to be an effective therapy. Not only did strength improve and skin rash resolve or improve but the underlying immunopathology also improved or resolved. The improvement begins after the first IVIg infusion, but it is more evident by the second monthly infusion. If there is no benefit after the third infusion, it probably does not work. The benefit is short lived (not more than 8 weeks), requiring repeated infusions every 6 to 8 weeks to maintain improvement. In uncontrolled studies, IVIg has been also shown to be effective in PM. Because of its relative safety compared to other immunosuppressants, IVIg is my second choice of immunomodulating drugs following an initial trial with azathioprine or methotrexate. Whether IVIg should be used early or late in the disease, alone or in conjunction with other drugs, or immediately after steroids have failed or are not fully effective is uncertain but the decision may be based on practical issues and clinical judgment. In children or the elderly with DM, IVIg may be considered as a first-line therapy because of fear that long-term steroid therapy in these age groups may result in serious side effects. Although this may be a reasonable consideration, it may not be practical because of the prohibitive expense of IVIg.

All commercial IVIg products appear equally effective and almost equal in safety and cost. The dose of IVIg has been, empirically, 2 g per kilogram. Although this was initially given in five divided doses of 400 mg per kilogram per day, there seems to be no basic reason to spread it in 5 days because the side effects are not different, provided the infusion rate is slow, as noted later. Further, there is experimental evidence suggesting that high serum concentration of IgG (achieved with the 2 day infusion) enhances the immunomodulating action of IVIg. In all our trials, I divide the dose in 2 days (1 g per kilogram per day). The rate of infusion should not exceed 200 cc per hour or 0.08 ml per kilogram per minute. Before using IVIg, we check the following:

1. *Serum IgA.* If IgA is *very low,* presumably due to anti-IgA antibodies, there is a risk of developing severe anaphylactic reactions from the small quantities of IgA present in the infused IVIg. Although this is a very rare condition, I screen all our patients for IgA level.
2. *Serum viscosity.* IVIg can increase serum viscosity by a mean of 0.6 cp (normal serum viscosity is 1.2 to 1.8 cp). Patients with cryoglobulinemias, hypercholesterolemias, or high IgM may already have high, or borderline high-normal, serum viscosity. In these patients, IVIg may cross the symptomatic viscosity threshold. In patients with cerebrovascular or cardiovascular disease, raising the viscosity above 2.5 cp may be a risk for thromboembolic events. The rise in serum viscosity may be the main reason for the few reported incidents of strokes or pulmonary embolisms, especially in the elderly.
3. *Renal function.* Acute tubular necrosis—mostly reversible—has been reported rarely in patients, especially those with pre-existing renal disease. Elderly patients with diabetes may be those to monitor.

Although IVIg is relatively safe, minor adverse reactions occur in up to 10 percent of patients. They include (1) headaches—mild to severe—that respond to nonsteroidal anti-inflammatory medications; (2) chills, myalgia, or chest discomfort, which usually develop the first hour of the infusion and respond to lowering the rate; (3) fatigue, exhaustion, fever, and nausea, which usually develop after completion of the infusion and last about 24 hours; (4) skin reactions, which vary from urticaria to peculiar anamnestic skin lesions thought to be due to reactivation by the IVIg of previous skin antigens (the latter develop usually 2 to 5 days after completion of the infusions and may last up to 30 days); (5) aseptic meningitis, which can occur in up to 10 percent of patients, especially migraine sufferers, and is unrelated to the company's product, the rate of infusion or the type of the underlying disease; (6) severe anaphylactic reaction in those few patients with absent or severely deficient IgA due to IgA antibodies (in such patients, the IVIg preparation Gammagard, which is low in IgA, should be used); (7) renal tubular necrosis, which occurs, rarely, in patients with pre-existing kidney disease, and is linked to one company's product that contains high sucrose as a stabilizing agent; and (8) thromboembolic events, in patients at risk or with high serum viscosity.

Other Immunosuppressants

Many times we are faced with patients who either have not responded or have stopped responding adequately to the measures just described. Our options are limited, but one of the following drugs, although the efficacy has not been established, may be considered according to the clinician's experience, patient's age, or coexistence of other systemic diseases:

Chlorambucil is an alkylating agent of the nitrogen mustard type that has now been rediscovered in the treatment of PM and DM. It has been recently reported that patients with recalcitrant DM treated with 4 mg per day chlorambucil have improved within 4 to 6 weeks, with insignificant side effects (only leukopenia).

Cyclophosphamide, an alkylating agent, is given intravenously or orally at doses of 2 to 2.5 mg per kilogram, usually 50 mg orally three times per day. Cyclophosphamide has been ineffective in our hands in spite of occasional promising results reported by others. The drug may be helpful in a subset of patients who also have interstitial lung disease.

Cyclosporine has been used with limited success. Although the toxicity of the drug can now be monitored by measuring optimal trough serum levels (which vary between 100 to 250 μg per milliliter), its effectiveness is uncertain. Reports that low doses of cyclosporine could be of benefit in children with DM or as a first-line therapy in adults with DM need confirmation. Based on the patients referred to us, the drug has been disappointing.

Plasmapheresis and lymphocytopheresis, without concomitant immunosuppression, was ineffective in a double-blind, placebo-controlled study. This procedure may still have merit, however, in occasional patients with active DM, if combined with immunosuppressive drugs.

Total body or lymphoid irradiation is an extreme remedy for extreme situations. Although it has been helpful for some patients, the long-term side effects may be considerable.

■ TREATMENT OF INCLUSION-BODY MYOSITIS

IBM has become a frequent disease that is desperately disabling, slowly progressive, and resistant to all immunosuppressive therapies, including total body irradiation. Prednisone, together with azathioprine or methotrexate, are not helpful, although most of us try these agents in newly diagnosed patients. Sometimes, occasional patients receiving these drugs may feel subjectively weaker after they discontinue therapy and have the impression that the drugs were halting disease progression. With this rationale in mind, several clinicians maintain these patients on prednisone or azathioprine and methotrexate with the only goal to slow disease progression. Unfortunately, there is no objective evidence to support this practice. To the contrary, exposing the patients to the long-term side effects of these drugs may prove to be more harmful, especially in a disease such as IBM, which is slowly progressive, and its natural history is unknown. My approach is to try prednisone for 3 months and, if not of benefit (as seen in the majority of the patients), try IVIg with guarded optimism. We have been encouraged with the preliminary results from our controlled study that showed a mild, although nonsustained, improvement in the least weak muscles, in up to 25 percent of the IBM patients we have treated.

■ PRACTICAL THERAPEUTIC CONSIDERATIONS

Based on the information just given regarding the efficacy of these therapies and our experience with more than 300 patients, the following observations and practical tips may be useful:

1. Patients with bona fide PM and DM should almost always respond to prednisone to a certain degree and for some period of time.
2. Patients with DM, as a group, respond better than patients with PM.
3. A patient with presumed PM who has not responded to any form of immunotherapy most likely has IBM or another disease. In these cases, a repeat muscle biopsy and a more vigorous search for the "other disease" are recommended.
4. Calcinosis, a manifestation of DM, does not resolve with immunotherapies. New calcium deposits, however, may be prevented if the primary disease responds to the available therapies. Diphosphonates, aluminum hydroxide, probenecid, colchicine, low doses of warfarin, and surgical incision have all been tried without success.
5. If prednisone or the other immunosuppressive therapies have not helped or have become ineffective in improving the patient's strength, they should be discontinued to avoid severe irreversible side effects; contrary to common belief, their continuation does not appear to "maintain stability" or prevent further disease progression.
6. Patients with acute, fulminant course associated with rhabdomyolysis should be treated aggressively with combination therapy, although many times they fail to respond to immunotherapies.
7. Patients with interstitial lung disease may have a high mortality, requiring aggressive treatment especially with cyclophosphamide. In such patients, avoid methotrexate because it can increase the severity of pneumonitis.
8. When the treatment of PM is unsuccessful, the patient should be re-evaluated and the muscle biopsy re-examined. A new biopsy might be considered to make sure that the diagnosis is correct or the disease has not been misdiagnosed as IBM.

■ SUPPORTIVE THERAPY

I recommend physical therapy early in the disease to preserve existing muscle function and avoid disuse atrophy of the weak muscles or joint contractures. Evaluation of swallowing function is also recommended because dysphagia is common, especially in IBM, where it occurs in up to 60 percent of the patients. Speech therapy provides practical tips on how to prevent choking episodes and diminish the anxiety of an impending aspiration.

Occupational and rehabilitation therapists help the patients with their ambulation by providing canes, braces, or wheelchairs, according to the stage of their disease, or by teaching them how to walk without falling and how to perform easier fine motor tasks. The patients should be given the proper emotional support to accept these aids, as in the long run they will help mobility, transportation, and socialization. Falls due to "buckling" of the knees are frequent in IBM patients because of early atrophy and weakness of the quadriceps muscles. Teaching the patients to walk by "locking" on their knees or by using light braces on the knees and ankles (when there is a foot drop) is highly advisable from the outset.

Suggested Reading

Dalakas MC. Polymyositis, dermatomyositis, and inclusion-body myositis. N Engl J Med 1991; 325:1487–1498.

Dalakas MC. How to diagnose and treat the inflammatory myopathies. Semin Neurol 1994; 14:137–145.

Dalakas MC, Illa I, Dambrosia JM, et al. A controlled trial of high-dose intravenous immunoglobulin infusions as treatment for dermatomyositis. N Engl J Med 1993; 329:1993–2000.

Engel AG, Hohlfeld R, Banker. BQ. The polymyositis and dermatomyositis syndromes. In Engel AG, Franzini-Armstrong C, eds. Myology. 2nd ed. New York: McGraw-Hill, 1994: 1335.

Mastaglia F. Treatment of inflammatory myopathies. In: Bailliere's Clinical Neurology. London: WB Saunders, 1993.

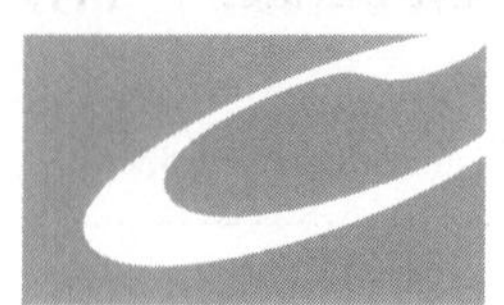

EYE DISEASES

CONJUNCTIVITIS

Robert A. Hyndiuk, M.D.
Bhavna P. Sheth, M.D.

Infection of the conjunctiva is a common cause of red eyes. Although most cases resolve without sequelae, infections such as *Neisseria gonorrhoeae,* herpes simplex virus, keratoconjunctivitis, and trachoma can result in significant loss of vision.

Common symptoms of conjunctivitis, depending on the causative agent, include redness, discharge, tearing, foreign body sensation, and transient blurring of vision with blinking. Symptoms such as vision loss, marked pain, and photophobia suggest a more severe disease process such as glaucoma, iritis, or keratitis (Table 1). Clinical findings may include conjunctival follicles, papillae, and/or preauricular adenopathy.

Gram stain and culture aid in identifying the causative agent and its susceptibility to antibiotics but are not essential in most cases of mild conjunctivitis. They are mandatory in hyperacute conjunctivitis and neonatal conjunctivitis to evaluate for *N. gonorrhoeae.*

Even though most cases of conjunctivitis are self-limited, antibiotic therapy for bacterial conjunctivitis is suggested to reduce the risk of complications, recurrence, and transmission to other individuals.

■ BACTERIAL CONJUNCTIVITIS

Bacterial conjunctivitis may be subdivided into hyperacute, acute, and chronic cases.

Hyperacute Bacterial Conjunctivitis

Hyperacute purulent conjunctivitis is usually caused by the *Neisseria* sp. *N. gonorrhoeae* most commonly occurs in sexually active young adults. The usual mode of transmission is by autoinoculation from infected genitalia. Signs include unilateral or bilateral marked conjunctival redness, chemosis, purulent discharge, and preauricular adenopathy. *N. gonorrhoeae* is one of the few bacteria that cause preauricular adenopathy. This infection is rapidly progressive, with potential for severe ocular destruction due to the bacteria's capability of invading intact conjunctival and corneal epithelium and causing severe corneal ulcers and vision loss. Gram stain to identify intracellular gram-negative diplococci and a culture are necessary in all suspected cases. Systemic treatment with adjunctive topical treatment is required for gonococcal conjunctivitis (Table 2). Also, frequent topical irrigation with saline is recommended. Affected patients are commonly coinfected with chlamydia and require treatment with oral tetracycline, erythromycin, or doxycycline for a week.

Neisseria meningitidis is a rare cause of hyperacute conjunctivitis. Clinical features are similar to those described for gonococcal conjunctivitis, except *N. meningitidis* tends to affect younger individuals. Though primary meningococcal infection of the conjunctiva can occur, the conjunctivitis is more commonly seen secondary to meningococcal septicemia. Systemic treatment, as outlined for gonococcal conjunctivitis, is required to prevent dissemination.

Acute Bacterial Conjunctivitis

Acute bacterial conjunctivitis is characterized by an abrupt onset of conjunctival hyperemia, mild to moderate mucopurulent discharge, and mild foreign body sensation. The disease lasts less than 3 to 4 weeks. Common causative agents include *Streptococcus pneumoniae, Haemophilus* sp., and *Staphylococcus aureus.*

Str. pneumoniae causes a bilateral, self-limited conjunctivitis with small petechial subconjunctival hemorrhages. Infections tend to occur in epidemics in temperate climates. *Haemophilus influenzae* produces a similar acute catarrhal conjunctivitis and is a common cause of infection in children. Systemic symptoms, including fever, otitis media, and upper respiratory infection may also be present. The Koch-Weeks bacillus, a subtype (aegyptius) of *H. influenzae,* also causes an acute mucopurulent conjunctivitis. In contrast to *Str. pneumoniae,* the Koch-Weeks bacillus produces epidemics in warm climates. *S. aureus* is the predominant pathogen implicated in both acute and chronic conjunctivitis in adults.

Treatment of routine acute bacterial conjunctivitis with topical antibiotics, such as bacitracin, erythromycin, combi-

Table 1 Red Eye: Differential Features

	CONJUCTIVITIS			KERATITIS			
	BACTERIAL	VIRAL	ALLERGIC	BACTERIAL	VIRAL	IRITIS	GLAUCOMA (ACUTE)
Blurred vision	0	0	0	+++	0 to ++	+ to ++	++ to +++
Pain	0	0	0	++	0 to +	++	++ to +++
Photophobia	0	0	0	++	++	+++	+ to ++
Discharge	Purulent + to +++	Watery + to ++	White, ropy +	Purulent +++	Watery +	0	0
Injection	+++	++	+	+++	+	0 to + (limbal)	+ to ++ (limbal)
Corneal haze	0	0	0	+++	+ to ++	0	+ to +++
Ciliary flush	0	0	0	+++	+	+++ to +++	+ to ++
Pupil	Normal	Normal	Normal	Normal or miotic (iritis)	Normal	Miotic	Mid-dilated Nonreactive
Pressure	Normal	Normal	Normal	Normal	Normal	Normal, low or high	High
Preauricular nodes	Rare	Usual	0	0	0	0	0
Smear	Bacteria PMNs	Lymphs	Eosinophil	Bacteria PMNs	0	0	0
Therapy	Antibiotics	Nonspecific	Nonspecific	Antibiotics	Antivirals (if herpes)	Cycloplegia Topical steroids	Medical or surgical

+, mild; ++, moderate; +++, severe; PMNs, polymorphonuclear leukocytes.

Table 2 Treatment of Gonococcal Conjunctivitis in Adults

A. Without septicemia
   Ceftriaxone 1g IM × 1 dose
   Frequent topical saline irrigation
   Bacitracin ointment q2h × 2 days, then 5 times a day until resolution
B. With septicemia
   Ceftriaxone 1 g IM or IV q12–24h for at least 3 days
   Frequent topical saline irrigation
   Bacitracin ointment q2h × 2 days then 5 times a day until resolution
C. With corneal ulcer
   Ceftriaxone 1 g IM or IV q12–24h for at least 3 days
   Frequent topical saline irrigation
   Ciprofloxacin or ofloxacin drops every 5 min for 30 min (load); then every 15 min for 6 hours; then every 30 min around the clock for 1–2 days; then hourly with AM and PM load until resolved (5–7 days)

nations of neomycin and polymyxin, or trimethoprim-polymyxin four times a day for 7 days is appropriate. Trimethoprim-polymyxin should never be used if a neisserial infection is suspected, even with aggressive dosing, since Neisseriae are totally resistant to the combination. With *H. influenzae* infections, systemic antibiotics should be added if systemic symptoms or otitis media are present. The topical fluoroquinolones ciprofloxacin and ofloxacin have recently been approved and are very potent and effective against most pathogens, including staphylococcus and even streptococcus. The fluoroquinolones are so well tolerated topically, especially ciprofloxacin, that they may be used more frequently the first 2 to 3 days, i.e., eight times daily. In severe infections ciprofloxacin is so well tolerated that it may be used 16 times daily, i.e., every hour while awake. Ofloxacin more frequently causes a symptomatic toxic epithelial keratitis when used topically more than four times daily.

Chronic Bacterial Conjunctivitis

Chronic bacterial conjunctivitis is often associated with adjacent lid disease and lasts longer than 3 to 4 weeks. Chronic *S. aureus* conjunctivitis can accompany simultaneous lid infection (blepharitis). Symptoms include conjunctival injection and papillae, mild foreign body sensation, mild mucoid discharge, and eyelid crusting. *Moraxella lacunata* can also produce chronic conjunctivitis in association with angular blepharitis involving the lateral canthal region of the eyelid. Treatment of these chronic infections consists of nightly application of bacitracin, erythromycin, or trimethoprim-polymyxin ointment as well as lid hygiene.

■ CHLAMYDIAL CONJUNCTIVITIS

Trachoma

Chlamydia trachomatis (serotype A to C) is the most common cause of infectious blindness in the world. Sporadic cases are seen in various parts of the United States. It is characterized by conjunctival follicles of the superior tarsus that cicatrize to produce a thickened and scarred superior tarsus. The scarring may cause the eyelashes to turn inward and rub against the eye (trichiasis). Corneal involvement with vascularization and opacification may occur later in the course of the disease. Treatment consists of either topical erythromycin or tetracycline ointment or oral tetracycline (Table 3).

Adult Chlamydial Conjunctivitis

Adult chlamydial conjunctivitis is a sexually transmitted disease caused by *C. trachomatis* serotype D to K. Affected individuals usually have concurrent genital infection, which can be asymptomatic. Ocular infection usually results from autoinoculation with genital secretions; rarely, transmission may occur from unchlorinated swimming pools. Symptoms include tearing, foreign body sensation, photophobia, and lid

Table 3 Treatment of Chlamydial Conjunctivitis

TRACHOMA
Erythromycin or tetracycline ointment b.i.d. for 5 days each month for 6 months, or
Tetracycline 1.5 g PO qd for 5 days each month for 6 months
ADULT INCLUSION CONJUNCTIVITIS
Tetracycline 500 mg PO t.i.d. for 3 weeks, or
Doxycycline 100 mg PO b.i.d. for 3 weeks, or
Erythromycin 250 mg PO q.i.d. for 3 weeks

edema. Conjunctival follicles of the lower lid with a preauricular node are present. Corneal involvement may also occur. Treatment of adult infection is with oral tetracycline, doxycycline, or erythromycin for 3 weeks (see Table 3). Affected patients may need further evaluation and treatment of concurrent genital infection.

■ VIRAL CONJUNCTIVITIS

The adenovirus is a common cause of sporadic or epidemic follicular conjunctivitis. It is characterized by unilateral or bilateral conjunctival hyperemia, tearing, irritation, follicles, and tender preauricular nodes. Pharyngoconjunctivitis due to adenovirus types 3 and 7 is a self-limited conjunctivitis associated with fever and pharyngitis. Epidemic keratoconjunctivitis, caused by adenovirus types 8 and 19, is extremely contagious and is transmitted via direct contact, hand-to-eye contact or contaminated water (e.g., swimming pools). Affected patients may also have corneal epithelial or subepithelial infiltrates, which are usually self-limited but may persist for months to years, impairing the vision. Patients are infectious for up to 2 weeks after the start of symptoms. Treatment is supportive, with cool compresses and artificial tears for comfort.

Molluscum contagiosum produces a chronic, toxic follicular conjunctivitis due to release of viral particles from an eyelid lesion. The lesion typically appears as a pearly white raised nodule with an umbilicated center. Treatment consists of removal of the nodule's central core, incision of the nodule to produce bleeding, or complete excision of the nodule.

Primary infection with type 1 herpes simplex virus (HSV) occurs in children and young adults and typically produces a unilateral follicular conjunctivitis with eyelid vesicles and a tender preauricular node. A severe keratitis may also be present. Recurrent HSV infection usually manifests with corneal disease, which may threaten the vision. Treatment of HSV requires antiviral agents.

Enterovirus 70 and coxsackievirus A24 can produce a highly contagious, acute hemorrhagic conjunctivitis. Clinical signs include follicular conjunctivitis with subconjunctival hemorrhages, transient epithelial keratitis, and a preauricular node. The condition is usually self-limited, and treatment is supportive.

■ CONJUNCTIVITIS MEDICAMENTOSA

Conjunctivitis medicamentosa is associated with the overuse of vasoconstricting drops. It is analogous to rhinitis medicamentosa, the well-recognized condition of chronic nasal congestion associated with the overuse of vasoconstricting nose drops. Vasoconstricting eye drops, available over the counter, increase conjunctival injection and often a rebound hyperemia that persists despite discontinuation of eye drops. Vasoconstrictor eye drops should be discontinued in favor of more appropriate treatment of the underlying condition.

Suggested Reading

Hyndiuk R, Ogawa GSH. The fluoroquinolones. In Zimmerman TJ; et al, eds. Textbook of ocular pharmacology. Philadelphia: Lippincott-Raven, 1997.

Jackson WB. Differentiating conjunctivitis of diverse origins. Surv Ophthalmol 1993; 38(Suppl):91–104.

Spector SL, Raizman MB. Conjunctivitis medicamentosa. J Allergy Clin Immunol 1994; 94:134–136.

Tabbara KF, Hyndiuk RA, eds. Infections of the eye. 2nd ed. Boston: Little, Brown. 1996.

World Health Organization. Conjunctivitis of the newborn: Prevention and treatment at the primary health care level, World Health Organization. 1986.

IRITIS

D. Geraint James, M.D., F.R.C.P., F.A.C.P. (Hon.)

The uveal tract is a continuous vascular structure consisting of the iris, ciliary body, and choroid. It is convenient, if somewhat artificial, to subdivide inflammation of the uveal tract into anterior uveitis (iritis, iridocyclitis) and posterior uveitis (choroiditis and choroidoretinitis). Exogenous uveitis may follow injury or surgery to the eye or may have a local intraocular cause, which is usually obvious from history or examination. Endogenous uveitis may be regarded as a symptom of some widespread infection or multisystem disorder.

PRESENTATION

Iritis may have an acute explosive or a chronic insidious onset.

Acute iritis is characterized by pain, photophobia, and blurring of vision. There is circumcorneal injection, which should not be confused with conjunctivitis. There is a ciliary flush, but the pupil is not stuck down. Inflammatory cells (keratic precipitates) are seen on the back of the cornea, or they may settle into a sterile abscess, or hypopyon, in the anterior chamber.

Chronic iritis has an insidious onset. The pupil is small and sluggish, and it may be irregular because of adhesions between the iris and lens (posterior synechiae). The patient may have had previous attacks and be able to anticipate a recurrence. The cause is rarely evident by examination of the eye alone. General examination of the patient is essential, as is slit-lamp examination of the eye (Fig. 1). From this multisystem approach emerge several patterns of uveitis.

PATTERNS OF UVEITIS

Distinctive patterns of multisystem iritis permit more efficient investigation and treatment (Table 1).

Sarcoid Uveitis

Sarcoid uveitis is most common in women of childbearing age. The clinical diagnosis becomes obvious if there are associated skin lesions and an abnormal chest radiograph. The diagnosis is clinched by histology of skin, lung, or liver. Transbronchial biopsy by fiberoptic bronchoscopy is a fruitful source of sarcoid tissue. The course may be acute or chronic.

Behçet's Disease

Behçet's disease is diagnosed at the bedside. There are no definitive laboratory tests. The diagnosis is evident when iritis is associated with orogenital mucocutaneous ulceration, dermatographia, polyarthritis, erythema nodosum, thrombophlebitis, and neurologic and cardiac abnormalities; the pathology is that of a vasculitis.

HLA-B27 Anterior Uveitis

This variant is usually severe, unilateral, and recurrent in young adults. It is often due to ankylosing spondylitis,

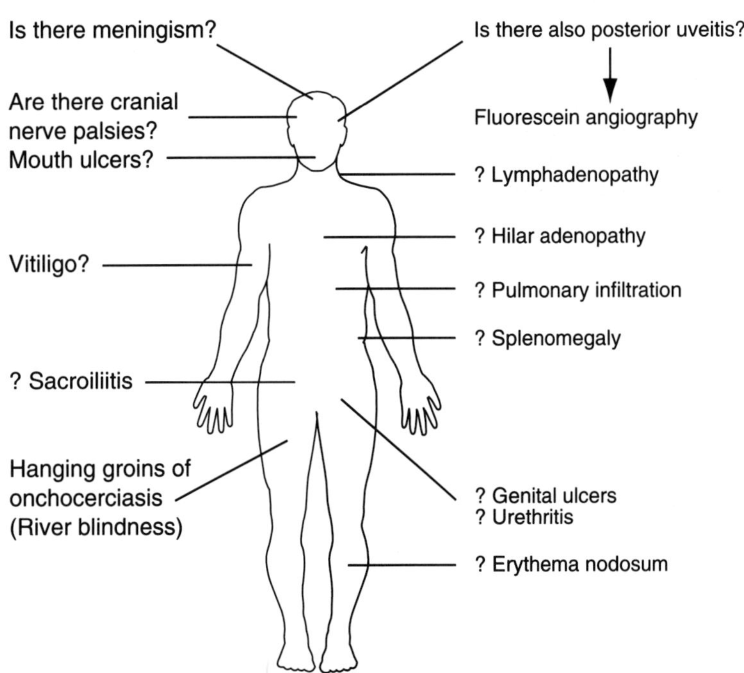

Figure 1
Clinical examination of a patient with uveitis.

Table 1 Patterns of Multisystem Iritis

SYSTEM	DISORDER	OTHER FEATURES	USEFUL INVESTIGATION
Pulmonary	Sarcoidosis	Lacrimals, skin	Chest x-ray
	Tuberculosis	Fever, lassitude	Chest x-ray, tuberculin test
	Churg-Strauss syndrome	Asthma	Eosinophilia
Renal	Wegener's granulomatosis	Scleritis, nasopharyngeal and renal involvement	ANCA, chest x-rays, kidney biopsy
	Interstitial nephritis	Pars planitis	Kidney biopsy
Autoimmune and rheumatic	Behçet's disease	Orogenital ulceration, erythema nodosum	Bedside clinical diagnosis
	Stevens-Johnson syndrome	Erythema multiforme, mucosal ulceration	Cold agglutinins, mycoplasma serology
	Ankylosing spondylitis	Apical fibrosis of lungs	X-rays, HLA-B27
	Reiter's syndrome	Urethritis, aortitis, arthritis	X-rays, HLA-B27
	Polychondritis	Floppy Pinna, aortic aneurysm	Biopsy of cartilage
Infections	Leprosy	Thickened nerves, anesthetic plaques	Biopsy of skin, nose
	Onchocerca	Posterior uveitis	Skin biopsy
	Syphilis	Secondary stage rash; lymph nodes	Treponema antibody
	AIDS	Multisystem involvement	Specific antibody
	Herpes	Vesicles at tip of nose	Virus isolation, cell inclusions
	Lyme Borreliosis	Facial nerve palsy, Erythema migrains	Specific antibody
Intestine	Chronic inflammatory bowel disease	Colitis	Sigmoidoscopy and biopsy
Vascular	Fuchs' Heterochromic Cyclitis	Moth-eaten depigmented iris	Slit lamp

ANCA, antineutrophil cytoplasmic antibody.

particularly in men. These patients or their families may also be identified because of accompanying peripheral arthritis, chronic inflammatory bowel disease, or psoriasis. Infection with *Yersinia enterocolitica, Salmonella* or *Mycoplasma* may trigger iritis, seronegative arthropathy, or erythema nodosum. A careful family history may be most rewarding.

Herpes

Herpes zoster ophthalmicus is due to involvement of the ophthalmic branch of the trigeminal nerve. Jonathan Hutchinson suggested that vesicles on the tip of the nose indicated involvement of the nasociliary branch and therefore ocular inflammation due to the ciliary branch. The earlier the diagnosis is made, the more useful is intravenous acyclovir or famcyclovir. The classical lesion of herpes simplex is dendritic keratitis, but the iris may also be involved.

Table 2 Treatment of Iritis in Addition to Steroid Therapy

IRITIS	TREATMENT
Sarcoidosis	Nonsteroidal anti-inflammatory agents, hydroxychloroquine, methotrexate
Tuberculosis	Isoniazid, rifampicin, pyrazinamide
Behçet's disease	Cyclosporine, azathioprine, colchicine, interferon
Wegener's granulomatosis	Cyclophosphamide, staphylococcal nasal carriage
Leprosy	BCG, ofloxin, rifampicin, dapsone, clofazimine, interferon
Onchocerciasis (river blindness)	Thiabendazole, diethylcarbamazine, suramin
Syphilis	Penicillin
Herpes	Acyclovir, famcyclovir
Inflammatory bowel disease	Sulfasalazine, metronidazole, azathioprine, cyclosporine

BCG, Bacille Calmette-Guérin

■ THERAPY

The immediate treatment is to reduce the inflammation and prevent adhesions within the eye. The pupil is dilated to prevent adhesions between the iris and lens. Inflammatory cells may block the trabecular meshwork and cause a rise of the intraocular pressure, so antiglaucoma treatment must also be considered. Thus, the mainstays of treatment are topical and possibly oral corticosteroids together with local cyclopentolate (mydriatic) eye drops. Steroid eye drops are applied frequently throughout the day and reinforced with a steroid eye ointment at night. If there is no substantial and continuing improvement after a week, the concentration of corticosteroid in the anterior segment of the eye may be increased by a local subconjunctival injection of cortisone or by oral steroid therapy. If ophthalmoscopy reveals posterior uveitis in addition to the anterior uveitis, oral steroids are indicated.

Local steroid therapy must be monitored carefully by intraocular pressure levels, for topical steroids may provoke rises or even precipitate secondary glaucoma. This is not a particular hazard of oral steroids. High intraocular pressure necessitates a switch from topical to oral steroids, and giving timolol eye drops to reduce the pressure to normal. In addition to steroid therapy, there may be specific therapy for the various associated disorders (Table 2).

Suggested Reading

James DG, Friedmann AI, Graham E. Uveitis: A series of 368 patients. Trans Ophthalm Soc UK 1976; 96:108–112.

James DG, Jones Williams W. Sarcoidosis and other granulomatous disorders. Philadelphia: WB Saunders, 1985.

James DG, Studdy PR. Colour atlas of respiratory disorders. 2nd ed. London: Wolfe, 1993.

Wechsler B, Godeau P. Behçet's disease. In: Proceedings of the Sixth International Conference. London and New York: Excerpta Medica, 1993.

ANTIMICROBIAL AGENT TABLES

Rosalie Pepe, M.D.
David Schlossberg, M.D.

Table 1 Antibacterial Agents

NAME		USUAL DOSE		COST (PER DAY)*	CHANGE IN ABSORPTION WITH FOOD	PREGNANCY CLASS†
GENERIC	BRAND	ADULT	PEDIATRIC			
Amikacin‖	Amikin	15 mg/kg/day; divide q8–12h IV	15 mg/kg/day; divide q8–12h	$116.00		D
Amoxicillin	Amoxil	0.25–0.5 g q8h PO	6.6–13.3 mg/kg PO q8h	$0.66	Decreased	B
Amoxicillin-clavulanate	Augmentin	0.25–0.5 g q8h PO	6.6–13.3 mg/kg q8h PO	$5.60	Decreased	B
Ampicillin	Ampen, Omnipen	0.5–1 g q8h PO; 1–2 g q4–6h IV	12.5–25 mg/kg q8h PO 6.25–25 mg/kg q8h IV	$0.53 PO $12.40 IV	Decreased	B
Ampicillin-sulbactam	Unasyn	1.5–3 g q6h IV	25–50 mg/kg q6h IV	$22.90 1.5 g $40.70 3.0 g		B
Azithromycin	Zithromax	5 g day 1; 0.25 g days 2–5 PO	§	$6.03 $36.18/5 day course	Decreased	B
Azlocillin	Azlin	2–4 g q4–6h IV	75 mg/kg q6h IV	Not available		B
Aztreonam	Azactam	1–2 g q6–8h IV	30–50 mg/kg q6–12h (N.A.)	$43.05		B
Bacampicillin	Spectrobid	0.4–0.8 g q12h PO	12.5–25 mg/kg q12h PO	$4.36		B
Carbenicillin indanyl sodium	Geocillin	1–2 0.382 g tabs q6h PO	7.5–12.5 mg/kg q6h PO	$7.20	Decreased	B
Carbenicillin	Geopen	5–6.5 g q4–6h IV	25–100 mg/kg q4–6h IV	Not available		B
Cefaclor	Ceclor	0.25–0.5 g q8h PO	20–40 mg/kg/day; divide q8h PO	$6.34	Decreased	B
Cefadroxil	Duricef	0.5–1 g q12–24h PO	30 mg/kg/day; divide q12h PO	$6.12	Decreased	B
Cefamandole	Mandol	0.5–2 g q4–8h IV	50–150 mg/kg/day; divide q4–8h IV	$36.25 (1 g q6h)		B

*Average wholesale price according to the 1995 Red Book.
†FDA pregnancy categories: A, adequate studies in pregnant women, no risk; B, animal studies no risk, human studies inadequate, or animal toxicity, human studies no risk; C, animal studies show toxicity, human studies inadequate but benefit may exceed risk; D, evidence of human risk, benefit may outweight risk; X, fetal abnormalities in humans, risk exceeds benefit.
‡Use in breastfeeding: limited data are available. Since all drugs are probably excreted in small amounts into breast milk, the potential for adverse reactions in the infant must be considered, although few have been reported. "Probably safe" indicates that breastfeeding can be continued during treatment based on information available at present. "Avoid if possible" indicates that an alternate drug should be chosen or consideration given to discontinuing breastfeeding.
§Insufficient information available to make a recommendation.
‖Aminoglycoside dosing may be modified after obtaining serum levels. The generally desired peak and trough concentrations are: for gentamicin and tobramycin, peak 6–12 μg/ml and trough <2 μg/ml; for netilmicin, peak 6–10 μg/ml, trough <2 μg/ml; for amikacin and kanamycin, peak 15–30 μg/ml, trough <5–10 μl/ml. "Once-daily" administration of aminoglycosides is gaining acceptance. The usual regimen is 5–7 mg/kg q 24h for gentamicin and tobramycin, 15 mg/kg q 24h for amikacin. The dose is infused over 60 minutes to avoid neuromuscular blockade. Dosage may be modified according to creatinine clearance or by following serum levels (see Nicolau et al. in "Suggested Reading").
CRCl, creatinine clearance ml/min; HD, hemodialysis; PD, peritoneal dialysis; CNS, central nervous system; GI, gastrointestinal; pHD, posthemodialysis; N.A., not approved; AST, aspartate aminotransferase; ALT, alanine aminotransferase; NR, not recommended.

USE IN BREASTFEEDING‡	DOSE INTERVAL ADJUSTMENT FOR REDUCED CRCL			SUPPLEMENTAL DOSE IN DIALYSIS		MAJOR TOXICITY
	>50	10–50	<10	HD	PD	
Avoid if possible	q8–12h	q12–48h	>48h	2.5–3.75 mg/kg pHD	2.5 mg/kg/day IV or 3–4 mg/2 L dialysate removed	Renal toxicity, vestibular or auditory toxicity, CNS reactions, neuromuscular blockade (rare)
Probably safe	q8h	q8–12h	q16–24h	0.25–0.5 g	0.25 g q12h	Allergic reactions (rare: anaphylactic), rash, diarrhea, nausea, vomiting
Probably safe	q8h	q12h	q12–24h	0.25 g PO	§	Allergic reactions (rare: anaphylactic), diarrhea, nausea, vomiting, cholestatic hepatitis
Probably safe	q4–6h	q8h	q12–24h	0.5–2 g	0.25 g q12h PO or 1–4 g q24h IV	Allergic reactions (rare: anaphylactic), diarrhea, nausea, vomiting
Probably safe	q6–8h	q8–12h	q24h	2 g ampicillin pHD	§	Allergic reactions (rare: anaphylactic), diarrhea, nausea, vomiting
Probably safe	Usual	Usual	Usual	§	§	GI disturbance, headache
Probably safe	q4–6h	q8h	q12h	3 g pHD	§	Allergic reactions (rare: anaphylactic), diarrhea, nausea, vomiting
Probably safe	q6–8h	q12–18h	q24h	1/8 first dose (60–250 mg) pHD	Usual dose (1–2 g) then 1/4 usual dose at usual intervals	Rash, diarrhea, nausea, vomiting, elevated AST/ALT
Probably safe	q12h	q12h	§	§	§	Allergic reactions (rare: anaphylactic), diarrhea, nausea, vomiting
Probably safe	§	§	§	§	§	Allergic reactions (rare: anaphylactic), diarrhea, nausea, vomiting
Probably safe	q4h	2–3g q6h	N.R.	0.75–2 g pHD	2 g q6–12h	Allergic reactions (rare: anaphylactic), diarrhea, nausea, vomiting
Probably safe	q8h	q8h	q8h	0.25–0.5 g	§	Allergic reactions, GI disturbance, arthritis, serum sickness
Probably safe	q12–24h	0.5 g q12–24h	0.5 g q36h	0.5–1 g	§	Allergic reactions, GI disturbance
Probably safe	q4–8h	q8h	0.5–1 g q12h	0.5–1 g	§	Thrombophlebitis with IV infusion, allergic reactions, GI disturbance

Continued.

Table 1 Antibacterial Agents—cont'd

NAME		USUAL DOSE		COST (PER DAY)*	CHANGE IN ABSORPTION WITH FOOD	PREGNANCY CLASS†
GENERIC	BRAND	ADULT	PEDIATRIC			
Cefazolin	Ancef, Kefzol	0.5–2 g q8h IV	25–100 mg/kg/day; divide q6–8h IV	$9.00 (1g q8h)		B
Cefepime	Maxipime	0.5–2 g q12h IV	50 mg/kg q8h IV (N.A.)	$63.76		B
Cefixime	Suprax	0.4 g q24h PO	8 mg/kg/day; divide q24h PO	$6.40	Decreased	B
Cefmetazole	Zefazone	2 g q6–12h IV	§	$42.99		B
Cefonicid	Monocid	0.5–2 g q24h IV	§	$26.10		B
Cefoperazone	Cefobid	1–2 g q6–12h IV	25–100 mg/kg q12h IV (N.A.)	$35.10		B
Cefotaxime	Claforan	0.5–2 g q8–12h IV 3 g q6h for CNS	50–200 mg/kg/day; divide q4–8h IV	$83.98 2 g q6h		B
Cefotetan	Cefotan	1–2 g q12h IV	40–60 mg/kg/day; divide q12h IV (N.A.)	$46.04		B
Cefoxitin	Mefoxin	1–2 g IV q6–8h IV	80–160 mg/kg/day; divide q4–8h IV	$80.34		B
Cefpodoxime	Vantin	0.1–0.4 g q12h PO	5 mg/kg q12h PO	$3.30	Increased	B
Cefprozil	Cefzil	0.25–0.5 g q12–24h PO	15 mg/kg q12h PO	$6.10		B
Ceftazidime	Fortaz, Tazicef, Tazidime	1–2 g q8–12h IV	25–50 mg/kg q8h IV	$86.40 2g q8h		B
Ceftizoxime	Cefizox	1–3 g q6–8h IV	33–50 mg/kg q6–8h IV	$45.56		B
Cetriaxone	Rocephin	0.5–2 g q12–24h IV	50–100 mg/kg/day; divide q12–24h IV	$66.70 2 g q24h		B
Cefuroxime	Zinacef, Kefurox	0.75–1.5 g q8h IV	50–100 mg/kg/day divide q6–8h IV	$28.30		B
Cefuroxime axetil	Ceftin	0.125–0.5 g q12h PO	0.125–0.25 g q12h PO	$6.32	Decreased	B
Cephlalexin	Keflex, Biocef, Keftab	0.25–1 g q6h PO	25–100 mg/kg/day; divide q6h PO	$2.51 generic $5.32 trade	Unchanged	B
Cephalothin	Keflin	0.5–2 g q4–6h IV	80–160 mg/kg/day; divide q6h IV	$15.90		B
Cephapirin	Cefadyl	0.5–2 g q4–6h IV	40–80 mg/kg/day divide q6h IV	$9.40		B

*Average wholesale price according to the 1995 Red Book.
†FDA pregnancy categories: A, adequate studies in pregnant women, no risk; B, animal studies no risk, human studies inadequate, or animal toxicity, human studies no risk; C, animal studies show toxicity, human studies inadequate but benefit may exceed risk; D, evidence of human risk, benefit may outweight risk; X, fetal abnormalities in humans, risk exceeds benefit.
‡Use in breastfeeding: limited data are available. Since all drugs are probably excreted in small amounts into breast milk, the potential for adverse reactions in the infant must be considered, although few have been reported. "Probably safe" indicates that breastfeeding can be continued during treatment based on information available at present. "Avoid if possible" indicates that an alternate drug should be chosen or consideration given to discontinuing breastfeeding.
§Insufficient information available to make a recommendation.
||Aminoglycoside dosing may be modified after obtaining serum levels. The generally desired peak and trough concentrations are: for gentamicin and tobramycin, peak 6–12 μg/ml and trough <2 μg/ml; for netilmicin, peak 6–10 μg/ml, trough <2 μg/ml; for amikacin and kanamycin, peak 15–30 μg/ml, trough <5–10 μl/ml. "Once-daily" administration of aminoglycosides is gaining acceptance. The usual regimen is 5–7 mg/kg q 24h for gentamicin and tobramycin, 15 mg/kg q 24h for amikacin. The dose is infused over 60 minutes to avoid neuromuscular blockade. Dosage may be modified according to creatinine clearance or by following serum levels (see Nicolau et al. in "Suggested Reading"). CrCl, creatinine clearance ml/min; HD, hemodialysis; PD, peritoneal dialysis; CNS, central nervous system; GI, gastrointestinal; pHD, posthemodialysis; N.A., not approved; AST, aspartate aminotransferase; ALT, alanine aminotransferase; NR, not recommended.

USE IN BREASTFEEDING‡	DOSE INTERVAL ADJUSTMENT FOR REDUCED CRCL			SUPPLEMENTAL DOSE IN DIALYSIS		MAJOR TOXICITY
	>50	10–50	<10	HD	PD	
Probably safe	q8h	0.5–1 g q8–12h	0.5–1 g q24h	0.25–0.5 g	§	Allergic reactions, GI disturbance, diarrhea
Probably safe	0.5–2 g q12h IV	q24h	0.25–0.5 g q24h	dose pHD	0.5–2 g q48h	Nausea, diarrhea, vomiting, rash, phlebitis
Probably safe	q24h	0.3 g q24h	q48h	None	§	Thrombophlebitis, allergic reactions, GI disturbance
Probably safe	q6–12h	q16–24h	q48h	§	§	Thrombophlebitis, allergic reactions, GI disturbance
Probably safe	q24h	4–15 mg/kg q24–48h	4–15	None	§	Allergic reactions, GI disturbance, hypoprothrombinemia or hemorrhage
Probably safe	q6–12h	q6–12h	q6–12h	Dose after HD	§	Thrombophlebitis, allergic reactions, GI disturbance
Probably safe	q8–12h	q12–24h	0.5 g q24–48h	0.5–2 g	§	Thrombophlebitis, allergic reactions, GI disturbance
Probably safe	q12h	q24h	q48h	25% dose nonHD days, 50% HD	§	Thrombophlebitis, allergic reactions, GI disturbance, hypoprothrombinemia, hemorrhage
Probably safe	q6–8h	q12–24h	0.5–1 g q12–24h	1–2 g	§	Thrombophlebitis, allergic reactions, GI disturbance
Probably safe	q12h	q24h	q24h	Dose 3 × wk	§	Allergic reactions, GI disturbance
Probably safe	q12–24h	50% dose q12–24h	50% dose q12–24h	§	§	Allergic reactions, GI disturbance
Probably safe	q8–12h	q12–24h	q24–48h	1 g load then 1 g pHD	0.5 g q24h IV or 250 mg/2 L dialysate	Thrombophlebitis, allergic reactions, GI disturbance
Probably safe	q6–8h	0.25–1 g q12h	0.5 g q24h	Dose pHD	3 g q48h	Thrombophlebitis, allergic reactions, GI disturbance
Probably safe	q12–24h	q12–24h	q12–24h	None	§	Thrombophlebitis, allergic reactions, GI disturbance, cholelithiasis
Probably safe	q8h	q8–12h	0.75 g q24h	0.75 g	15 mg/kg aftr dialysis	Thrombophlebitis, allergic reactions, GI disturbance
Probably safe	q12h	q12h	0.25 g q24h	§	§	Allergic reactions, GI disturbance
Probably safe	q6h	q8–12h	q24–48h	0.25–1 g	§	Allergic reactions, GI disturbance
Probably saffe	q4–6h	1–1.5 g q6h	0.5 g q8h	0.5–2 g	Add up to 6 mg/kg to dialysate	Thrombophlebitis with IV infusion, allergic reactions, GI disturbance
Probably safe	q4–6h	q8h	q12h	7.5–15 mg/kg pHD then q12h	§	Thrombophlebitis, allergic reactions, GI disturbance

Continued.

Table 1 Antibacterial Agents–cont'd

NAME		USUAL DOSE		COST (PER DAY)*	CHANGE IN ABSORPTION WITH FOOD	PREGNANCY CLASS†
GENERIC	BRAND	ADULT	PEDIATRIC			
Cephradine	Velosef	0.25–1 g q6h PO 0.5–2 g q4–6h IV	25–100 mg/kg/day; divide q6–12h PO 50–100 mg/kg divide q6h IV	$3.30 PO	Decreased	B
Chloramphenicol	Chloromycetin	0.25–0.75 g q6h PO 0.25–1 g q6h IV	50–100 mg/kg/day; divide q6h PO, IV	$5.01 PO $16.59 IV	No data	C
Cinoxacin	Cinobac	0.25 g q6h, 0.5 g q12h PO	N.R.	$3.81	No data	C
Ciprofloxacin	Cipro	0.25–0.75 g q12h PO 0.2–0.4 g q12h IV	N.R.	$6.26 PO $60.02 IV	Decreased	C
Clarithromycin	Biaxin	0.25–0.5 g q12h PO	7.5 mg/kg q12h (N.A.)	$6.29	Increased or unchanged	B
Clindamycin	Cleocin	0.15–0.3 g q6h PO 0.3–0.9 g q6–8h IV	8–25 mg/kg/day; divide q6–8h PO 15–40 mg/kg/day; divide q6–8h IV	$8.80 PO $23.32 IV	Unchanged	B
Cloxacillin	Tegopen	0.5–1 g q6h PO	12.5–25 mg/kg q6h PO	$3.18	Decreased	B
Colistin		5–15 mg/kg/day q8h PO 2.5–5 mg/kg/day q6–12h IV	5–15 mg/kg/day; divide q8h PO 2.5–5 mg/kg/day; divide q6–12h IV	$62.02 IV		Not established
Dapsone		0.05–0.1 g q24h PO	1–2 mg/kg/day; divide q24h	$0.34		C
Dicloxacillin	Dynapen	0.25–0.5 g q6h PO	3.125–6.25 mg/kg q6h PO	$1.60	Decreased	Not established
Doxycycline	Vibramycin	0.1 g q12h PO, IV	2.2 mg/kg q12–24h PO, IV	$0.99 PO generic $7.09 PO trade $42.13 IV	Decreased with milk, antacids	D
Enoxacin	Penetrex	0.4 g q12h PO, IV	N.R.	$5.46	Decreased	C
Erythromycin base	EryC, PCE, Emycin, Erytab	0.25–0.5 g q6h PO	30–50 mg/kg/day; divide q6h	$1.00 PO	Decreased	B

*Average wholesale price according to the 1995 Red Book.

†FDA pregnancy categories: A, adequate studies in pregnant women, no risk; B, animal studies no risk, human studies inadequate, or animal toxicity, human studies no risk; C, animal studies show toxicity, human studies inadequate but benefit may exceed risk; D, evidence of human risk, benefit may outweight risk; X, fetal abnormalities in humans, risk exceeds benefit.

‡Use in breastfeeding: limited data are available. Since all drugs are probably excreted in small amounts into breast milk, the potential for adverse reactions in the infant must be considered, although few have been reported. "Probably safe" indicates that breastfeeding can be continued during treatment based on information available at present. "Avoid if possible" indicates that an alternate drug should be chosen or consideration given to discontinuing breastfeeding.

§Insufficient information available to make a recommendation.

||Aminoglycoside dosing may be modified after obtaining serum levels. The generally desired peak and trough concentrations are: for gentamicin and tobramycin, peak 6–12 μg/ml and trough <2 μg/ml; for netilmicin, peak 6–10 μg/ml, trough <2 μg/ml; for amikacin and kanamycin, peak 15–30 μg/ml, trough <5–10 μl/ml. "Once-daily" administration of aminoglycosides is gaining acceptance. The usual regimen is 5–7 mg/kg q 24h for gentamicin and tobramycin, 15 mg/kg q 24h for amikacin. The dose is infused over 60 minutes to avoid neuromuscular blockade. Dosage may be modified according to creatinine clearance or by following serum levels (see Nicolau et al. in "Suggested Reading").

CRCl, creatinine clearance ml/min; HD, hemodialysis; PD, peritoneal dialysis; CNS, central nervous system; GI, gastrointestinal; pHD, posthemodialysis; N.A., not approved; AST, aspartate aminotransferase; ALT, alanine aminotransferase; NR, not recommended.

USE IN BREASTFEEDING‡	DOSE INTERVAL ADJUSTMENT FOR REDUCED CRCL			SUPPLEMENTAL DOSE IN DIALYSIS		MAJOR TOXICITY
	>50	10–50	<10	HD	PD	
Probably safe	q6h	0.5 g q6h	0.25 g q12h	0.25 g before HD, then 12, 36, and 48h pHD	0.5 g q6h	Allergic reactions, GI disturbance
Avoid if possible	Usual	Usual	Usual	Dose pHD	Usual	Blood dyscrasias, gray baby syndrome, GI disturbance
Avoid if possible	q6h	0.25 g q12–24h	N.R.	§	§	Nausea, vomiting, dizziness, headache, tremors, confusion
Avoid if possible	q12h	0.25–0.5 g q12h PO, q12–24h IV	0.25–0.5 g q18h PO, q18–24h IV	0.25–0.5 g q24h, pHD on HD days	0.25–0.5 g q24h	Nausea, vomiting, dizziness, headache, tremors, confusion
Probably safe	q12h	q12–24h	q24h	§	§	GI disturbance, abnormal taste, headache
Avoid if possible	Usual	Usual	Usual	Usual	Usual	Diarrhea, including pseudomembranous colitis, allergic reactions
Probably safe	q6h	q6h	q6h	Usual	Usual	Allergic reactions (rare: anaphylactic), diarrhea, nausea, vomiting
§	q6–12h	2.5 mg/kg/day q12–24h	1.5 mg/kg q36h	§	§	Nephrotoxicity, CNS side effects including confusion, coma, seizures
Avoid if possible	q24h	q24h	q24h	§	§	Rash, headache, GI irritation, infectious mono-like syndrome
Probably safe	q6h	q6h	q6h	Usual	Usual	Allergic reactions (rare: anaphylactic), diarrhea, nausea, vomiting
Avoid if possible	q12h	q12h	q12h	Usual	Usual	GI disturbance, photosensitivity reactions, hepatic toxicity, esophageal ulcers
Avoid if possible	q12h	0.1–0.2 g q12h	0.1–0.2 g q12h	§	§	Nausea, vomiting, dizziness, headache, tremors, confusion
Probably safe	q6h	q6h	q6h	Usual	Usual	GI disturbance; rare: allergic reactions, hepatic dysfunction, hearing loss

Continued.

Table 1 Antibacterial Agents–cont'd

NAME		USUAL DOSE		COST (PER DAY)*	CHANGE IN ABSORPTION WITH FOOD	PREGNANCY CLASS†
GENERIC	BRAND	ADULT	PEDIATRIC			
Erythromycin estolate	Ilosone	0.25–0.5 g q6h PO	3–50 mg/kg/day; divide q6h	$3.05	Decreased	B
Erythromycin ethyl succinate	EES, eryPed	0.4 g q8h PO	30–50 mg/kg/day divide q8h PO	$0.98		B
Erythromycin lactobionate	Erythrocin	0.5–1 g q6h IV	15–20 mg/kg/day; divide q6h IV	$41.20 IV		B
Gentamicin‖	Garamycin	3–5 mg/kg/day; divide q8h IV	3–7.5 mg/kg/day; divide q8h IV	$12.35		C
Imipenem	Primaxin	0.5–1 g q6h IV	15–25 mg/kg q6h IV (N.A.)	$101.65		C
Kanamycin‖	Kantrex	15 mg/kg/day; divide q8–12h IV	15 mg/kg/day; divide q8–12h IV	$13.56		D
Lincomycin	Lincocin	0.5 g q6–8h PO 0.6–1 g q8–12 IV	30–60 mg/kg/day; divide q6–8h PO 10–20 mg/kg/day; divide q6h IV	$5.29 PO $32.16 IV		Not established
Lomefloxacin	Maxaquin	0.4 g q24h PO	N.R.	$6.10	No data	C
Loracarbef	Lorabid	0.2–0.4 g q12–24h PO	15–30 mg/kg/day; q12h	$6.30	Decreased	B
Meropenem	Merrem	0.5–1 g q8h IV	20–40 mg/kg q8h IV	$155.52		B
Metronidazole	Flagyl	0.25–0.5 g q6–12h PO 0.5 g q6–8h IV	15 mg/kg/day; divide t.i.d. (N.A.)	$0.65 PO generic $3.91 PO trade $50.27 IV	Unchanged	B
Mezlocillin	Mezlin	3–4 g q4–6h IV	50 mg/kg q4–6h IV	$62.20 4 g q6h		B
Minocycline	Minocin, Dynacin	0.1 g q12h PO, IV	2 mg/kg q12h PO, IV	$3.11 PO $62.46 IV	Decreased with milk, antacids	D

*Average wholesale price according to the 1995 Red Book.

†FDA pregnancy categories: A, adequate studies in pregnant women, no risk; B, animal studies no risk, human studies inadequate, or animal toxicity, human studies no risk; C, animal studies show toxicity, human studies inadequate but benefit may exceed risk; D, evidence of human risk, benefit may outweight risk; X, fetal abnormalities in humans, risk exceeds benefit.

‡Use in breastfeeding: limited data are available. Since all drugs are probably excreted in small amounts into breast milk, the potential for adverse reactions in the infant must be considered, although few have been reported. "Probably safe" indicates that breastfeeding can be continued during treatment based on information available at present. "Avoid if possible" indicates that an alternate drug should be chosen or consideration given to discontinuing breastfeeding.

§Insufficient information available to make a recommendation.

‖Aminoglycoside dosing may be modified after obtaining serum levels. The generally desired peak and trough concentrations are: for gentamicin and tobramycin, peak 6–12 μg/ml and trough <2 μg/ml; for netilmicin, peak 6–10 μg/ml, trough <2 μg/ml; for amikacin and kanamycin, peak 15–30 μg/ml, trough <5–10 μl/ml. "Once-daily" administration of aminoglycosides is gaining acceptance. The usual regimen is 5–7 mg/kg q 24h for gentamicin and tobramycin, 15 mg/kg q 24h for amikacin. The dose is infused over 60 minutes to avoid neuromuscular blockade. Dosage may be modified according to creatinine clearance or by following serum levels (see Nicolau et al. in "Suggested Reading").
CRCl, creatinine clearance ml/min; HD, hemodialysis; PD, peritoneal dialysis; CNS, central nervous system; GI, gastrointestinal; pHD, posthemodialysis; N.A., not approved; AST, aspartate aminotransferase; ALT, alanine aminotransferase; NR, not recommended.

USE IN BREASTFEEDING‡	DOSE INTERVAL ADJUSTMENT FOR REDUCED CRCL			SUPPLEMENTAL DOSE IN DIALYSIS		MAJOR TOXICITY
	>50	10–50	<10	HD	PD	
Probably safe	Usual	Usual	Usual	No change	No change	Cholestatic hepatitis, hearing loss or tinnitus, GI disturbance, hypersensitivity reactions
Probably safe	Usual	Usual	Usual	Usual	Usual	GI disturbance; rare: allergic reactions, hepatic dysfunction
Probably safe	Usual	Usual	Usual	Usual	Usual	GI disturbance; rare: allergic reactions, hepatic dysfunction, hearing loss
Avoid if possible	q8–12h	q12–48h	>48h	1–1.7 mg/kg pHD	1 mg/2 L dialysate removed	Renal toxicity, vestibular and auditory toxicity, CNS reactions, neuromuscular blockade (rare)
Probably safe	q6h	0.5 q8–12h	0.25–0.5 g q12h	0.25–0.5 pHD then q12h	§	Fever, rash, nausea, vomiting, diarrhea, seizures (rare)
Avoid if possible	q8–12h	q12–48h	>48h	4–5 mg/kg pHD	3.75 mg/kg/day	Cranial nerve VIII and renal damage
Avoid if possible	Usual	Usual	Usual	§	§	Diarrhea, including pseudomembranous colitis, allergic reactions
Avoid if possible	q24h	0.2 g q24h	0.2 g q24h	0.4 g load, then 0.2 g q24h	§	Nausea, vomiting, dizziness, headache, tremors, confusion, photosensivity
Probably safe	q12–24h	q24–48h	q3–5d	Dose after HD	§	Allergic reactions, GI disturbance
Probably safe	0.5–1 g q8h IV	q12h	0.25–0.5 q24h	§	§	Nausea, diarrhea, vomiting, rash
Avoid if possible	Usual	Usual	Usual	Usual	Usual	Nausea, headache, metallic taste
Probably safe	q4–6h	q8h	q8h	2–3 g then 3–4 g q12h	3 g q12h	Allergic reactions (rare: anaphylactic), diarrhea, nausea, vomiting
Avoid if possible	q12h	q12h	q12h	Usual	Usual	GI disturbance, photosensitivity, hepatic toxicity, esophageal ulcers, vestibular toxicity; tooth discoloration

Continued.

Table 1 Antibacterial Agents–cont'd

NAME		USUAL DOSE		COST (PER DAY)*	CHANGE IN ABSORPTION WITH FOOD	PREGNANCY CLASS†
GENERIC	BRAND	ADULT	PEDIATRIC			
Nafcillin	Nallpen, Unipen	0.5–2 g q4–6h IV	150 mg/kg/day; divide q4–6h IV	$22.40 2 g q6h		B
Neomycin	Neo-tabs	50 mg/kg/day; divide q6h PO	§	$1.47	Not established	Not established
Netilmycin‖	Netromycin	4–6.5 mg/kg/day; divide q8–12h IV	3–7.5 mg/kg/day; divide q8–12h IV	$24.16		D
Norfloxacin	Noroxin	0.4 g q12h PO	N.R.	$5.08	Decreased	C
Ofloxacin	Floxin	0.2–0.4g q12h PO, IV	N.R.	$5.60 PO $55.20 IV	Decreased	C
Oxacillin	Bactocil	0.5–1 g q4–6h IV	37.5–50 mg/kg q6h IV	$2.10 PO $17.40 IV	Decreased	B
Penicillin V	Pen-VeeK, Pen-V	0.25–0.5 g q6h PO	6.25–12.5 mg/kg q6h PO	$0.49	Decreased	B
Penicillin G benzathine	Bicillin	600,000–2,400,000 units IM × 1	600,000 units IM × 1	$25.60		B
Penicillin G		0.5–1 g q6h PO 1–4 million units q4–6h IV	25,000–90,000 units/kg/day; divide q4–8h PO 25,000–400,000 units/kg/day; divide q4–6h IV	$0.77 PO $10.16 IV	Decreased	B
Piperacillin	Pipracil	3–4g q4–6h IV	50 mg/kg q4–6h IV (N.A.)	$90.49 4 g q6h		B
Piperacillin-tazobactam	Zosyn	3.375 g q6–8h IV		$44.42		B
Polymyxin B	Aerosporin, Neosporin	15,000–25,000 units/kg/day q12h IV	15,000–25,000 units/kg/day q12h IV	$75.49		Not established
Procaine penicillin G	Wycillin	0.6–1.2 million units q12h IM	25,000–50,000 units/kg q12–24h IM	$5.79		B

*Average wholesale price according to the 1995 Red Book.
†FDA pregnancy categories: A, adequate studies in pregnant women, no risk; B, animal studies no risk, human studies inadequate, or animal toxicity, human studies no risk; C, animal studies show toxicity, human studies inadequate but benefit may exceed risk; D, evidence of human risk, benefit may outweight risk; X, fetal abnormalities in humans, risk exceeds benefit.
‡Use in breastfeeding: limited data are available. Since all drugs are probably excreted in small amounts into breast milk, the potential for adverse reactions in the infant must be considered, although few have been reported. "Probably safe" indicates that breastfeeding can be continued during treatment based on information available at present. "Avoid if possible" indicates that an alternate drug should be chosen or consideration given to discontinuing breastfeeding.
§Insufficient information available to make a recommendation.
‖Aminoglycoside dosing may be modified after obtaining serum levels. The generally desired peak and trough concentrations are: for gentamicin and tobramycin, peak 6–12 μg/ml and trough <2 μg/ml; for netilmicin, peak 6–10 μg/ml, trough <2 μg/ml; for amikacin and kanamycin, peak 15–30 μg/ml, trough <5–10 μl/ml. "Once-daily" administration of aminoglycosides is gaining acceptance. The usual regimen is 5–7 mg/kg q 24h for gentamicin and tobramycin, 15 mg/kg q 24h for amikacin. The dose is infused over 60 minutes to avoid neuromuscular blockade. Dosage may be modified according to creatinine clearance or by following serum levels (see Nicolau et al. in "Suggested Reading"). CRCl, creatinine clearance ml/min; HD, hemodialysis; PD, peritoneal dialysis; CNS, central nervous system; GI, gastrointestinal; pHD, posthemodialysis; N.A., not approved; AST, aspartate aminotransferase; ALT, alanine aminotransferase; NR, not recommended.

USE IN BREASTFEEDING‡	DOSE INTERVAL ADJUSTMENT FOR REDUCED CRCL			SUPPLEMENTAL DOSE IN DIALYSIS		MAJOR TOXICITY
	>50	10–50	<10	HD	PD	
Probably safe	q4–6h	q4–6h	q4–6h	Usual	Usual	Allergic reactions (rare: anaphylactic), diarrhea, nausea, vomiting; platelet dysfunction with high doses
Probably safe	§	§	§	§	§	Cranial nerve VIII and renal damage
Avoid if possible	q8–12h	q12–48h	>48h	2 mg/kg pHD	§	Renal toxicity, vestibular and auditory toxicity, CNS reactions, neuromuscular blockade (rare)
Avoid if possible	q12h	q24h	q24h	§	§	Nausea, vomiting, dizziness, headache, tremors, confusion
Avoid if possible	q12h	q24h	0.1–0.2 g q24h	0.2 g load; then 0.1 g q24h	§	Nausea, vomiting, dizziness, headache, tremors, confusion
Probably safe	q4–6h	q4–6h	q4–6h	Usual	Usual	Allergic reactions (rare: anaphylactic), diarrhea, nausea, vomiting
Probably safe	q6h	q6h	q6h	250 mg	§	Allergic reactions (rare: anaphylactic), diarrhea, nausea, vomiting
Probably safe	Usual	Usual	Usual	Usual	Usual	Allergic reactions (rare: anaphylactic), diarrhea, nausea, vomiting
Probably safe	q4–6h	q4–6h	25–50% of standard dose q4–6h	500,000 U	§	Allergic reactions (rare: anaphylactic), diarrhea, nausea, vomiting
Probably safe	q4–6h	q6–8h	q8–12h	1 g pHD, then 2 g q8h IV	§	Allergic reactions (rare: anaphylactic), diarrhea, nausea, vomiting; platelet dysfunction with high doses
Probably safe	q6–8h	2.25 g q6h	2.25 g q8h	§	§	Allergic reactions (rare: anaphylactic), diarrhea, nausea, vomiting
§	q12h	q12h	2,250–3,750 U/kg/day; divide q12h	§	§	Nephrotoxicity, flushing; CNS effects: confusion, seizures; allergic reactions
Probably safe	q12h	q12h	q12h	§	§	Allergic reactions (rare: anaphylactic), diarrhea, nausea, vomiting

Continued.

Table 1 Antibacterial Agents–cont'd

NAME		USUAL DOSE		COST (PER DAY)*	CHANGE IN ABSORPTION WITH FOOD	PREGNANCY CLASS†
GENERIC	BRAND	ADULT	PEDIATRIC			
Spectinomycin	Trobicin	2 g qd IM	§	$16.13		B
Streptomycin		0.5–1 g q12h IV or IM	20–40 mg/kg/day; divide q6–12h IV or IM	Free from manufacturer		D
Sulfadiazine	Microsulfon	2–4 g/day; q4–8h PO	120–150 mg/kg/ day; divide q4–6h PO	$1.58	Decreased	C
Sulfamethox- azole	Gantanol, Urobac	1 g q8–12h PO	50–60 mg/kg/day; divide q12h PO	Not available	Decreased	C
Sulfisoxazole	Gantrisin	0.5–1 g q6h PO 25 mg/kg/q6h IV	120–150 mg/kg/ day; divide q4–6h PO	$0.90	Decreased	C
Teichoplanin		0.2–0.4 g q24h IV	10 mg/kg q24h IV	Not available		Not established
Tetracycline	Achromycin	0.25–0.5 g q6h PO	25–50 mg/kg/day; divide q6–12h	$0.25	Decreased with milk, antacids	D
Ticarcillin	Ticar	3 g q4–6h	50 mg/kg q4–6h	$59.70		B
Ticarcillin- clavulanate	Timentin	3.1 g q4–8h IV	50 mg/kg q4–6h IV	$42.76		B
Tobramycin‖	Nebcin	3–5 mg/kg/day; divide q8h IV	3–6 mg/kg/day; divide q8h IV	$23.29		D
Trimethoprim- sulfamethox- azole	Bactrim, Septra	0.16–0.8 g q12–24h PO 3–5 mg/kg q6–8h IV trimethoprim	6–12 mg/kg/day; divide q6–12h PO IV	$2.38 PO $14.47 IV	Decreased	C
Trimethoprim	Proloprim	0.1 g q12h PO	4 mg/kg/day; divide q12h PO	$0.40	No data	C
Vancomycin	Vancocin	0.5–2 g q6–8h PO 1 g q12h IV	40 mg/kg/day; di- vide q6–8h PO 40 mg/kg/day; di- vide q6–12h IV	$44.02 IV $8.40 oral solu- tion $14.17 pulvules	Not absorbed	B

*Average wholesale price according to the 1995 Red Book.
†FDA pregnancy categories: A, adequate studies in pregnant women, no risk; B, animal studies no risk, human studies inadequate, or animal toxicity, human studies no risk; C, animal studies show toxicity, human studies inadequate but benefit may exceed risk; D, evidence of human risk, benefit may outweight risk; X, fetal abnormalities in humans, risk exceeds benefit.
‡Use in breastfeeding: limited data are available. Since all drugs are probably excreted in small amounts into breast milk, the potential for adverse reactions in the infant must be considered, although few have been reported. "Probably safe" indicates that breastfeeding can be continued during treatment based on information available at present. "Avoid if possible" indicates that an alternate drug should be chosen or consideration given to discontinuing breastfeeding.
§Insufficient information available to make a recommendation.
‖Aminoglycoside dosing may be modified after obtaining serum levels. The generally desired peak and trough concentrations are: for gentamicin and tobramycin, peak 6–12 μg/ml and trough <2 μg/ml; for netilmicin, peak 6–10 μg/ml, trough <2 μg/ml; for amikacin and kanamycin, peak 15–30 μg/ml, trough <5–10 μl/ml. "Once-daily" administration of aminoglycosides is gaining acceptance. The usual regimen is 5–7 mg/kg q 24h for gentamicin and tobramycin, 15 mg/kg q 24h for amikacin. The dose is infused over 60 minutes to avoid neuromuscular blockade. Dosage may be modified according to creatinine clearance or by following serum levels (see Nicolau et al. in "Suggested Reading").
CRCl, creatinine clearance ml/min; HD, hemodialysis; PD, peritoneal dialysis; CNS, central nervous system; GI, gastrointestinal; pHD, posthemodialysis; N.A., not approved; AST, aspartate aminotransferase; ALT, alanine aminotransferase; NR, not recommended.

USE IN BREASTFEEDING‡	DOSE INTERVAL ADJUSTMENT FOR REDUCED CRCL			SUPPLEMENTAL DOSE IN DIALYSIS		MAJOR TOXICITY
	>50	10–50	<10	HD	PD	
§	q24h	q24h	q24h	§	§	Pain at injection site, nausea, allergic reactions
Avoid if possible	q12h	7.5 mg/kg q24h	7.5 mg/kg q72–96h	0.5 g pHD	§	Cranial nerve VIII damage, paresthesias, rash, fever, renal toxicity, neuromuscular blockade, optic neuritis
Avoid if possible	§	§	§	§	§	Rash, photosensitivity, drug fever
Avoid if possible	§	§	§	§	§	Rash, photosensitivity, drug fever
Avoid if possible	q6h	q8–12h	q12–24h	§	§	Rash, photosensitivity, drug fever
§	q24h	q48h	q72h	§	§	Ototoxicity
Avoid if possible	q6h	Use doxycycline	Use doxycycline	500 mg pHD	§	GI disturbance, photosensitivity, hepatic toxicity, esophageal ulcers
Probably safe	q4–6h	q6–8h	2 g q12h	3 g pHD; then 2 g q12h	3 g q12h	Allergic reactions (rare: anaphylactic), diarrhea, nausea, vomiting
Probably safe	q4–6h	q6–8h	2 g q12h IV	3.1 g	3.1 g q12h	Allergic reactions (rare: anaphylactic), diarrhea, nausea, vomiting
Avoid if possible	q8–12h	q12–48h	>48h	1 mg/kg pHD	1 mg/2 L dialysate removed	Renal toxicity, vestibular and auditory toxicity, CNS reactions, neuromuscular blockade (rare)
Avoid if possible	q6–12h	q24h	Avoid	4–5 mg/kg pHD	0.16–0.8 g q48h	Rash, nausea, vomiting
Probably safe	q12h	q18–24h	Avoid	§	§	Nausea, vomiting
Probably safe	Levels vary; use serum assays and manufacturer's nomogram to guide dosage	Levels vary; use serum assays and manufacturer's nomogram to guide dosage	Levels vary; use serum assays and manufacturer's nomogram to guide dosage	None needed	None needed	Thrombophlebitis, fever, chills, rash, cranial nerve VIII toxicity

Continued.

Table 2 Antimycobacterial Agents

NAME		USUAL DOSE		COST (PER DAY)*	CHANGE IN ABSORPTION WITH FOOD	PREGNANCY CLASS†
GENERIC	BRAND	ADULT	PEDIATRIC			
Capreomycin	Capastat	1 g IM q24h	10–20 mg/kg q24h (N.A.)	$20.86		C
Clofazimine	Lamprene	0.1 g q24h PO	§	$0.26	Increased	C
Cycloserine	Seromycin	0.25–0.5 g q12h PO	10–20 mg/kg q12h (N.A.)	$6.56	No data	C
Ethambutol	Myambutol	15–25 mg/kg q24h PO	10–15 mg/kg q24h (N.R.)	$4.62	Unchanged	B
Ethionamide	Trecator	0.25–0.5 g q12h PO	15–20 mg/kg q24h (N.A.)	$3.40	No data	C
Isoniazid		0.3 g q24h PO, IM	10–20 mg/kg/day; divide q12–24h PO, IM	$0.08	Decreased	C
Para-amino-salicylic acid	PAS	150 mg/kg q6–12h	150–360 mg/kg/day; divide q6–8h	Not available	Decreased but advised	C
Pyrazinamide		15–30 mg/kg q24h PO	30 mg/kg/day; divide q12–24h (N.A.)	$2.62	No data	C
Rifabutin (ansamycin)	Mycobutin	0.3 g q24h PO	§	$6.82	Unchanged	C
Rifampin	Rifadin, Rimactane	.6 g q24h PO, IV	10–20 mg/kg/day; divide q12–24h PO, IV	$3.21 PO $79.38 IV	Decreased	B
Streptomycin		1 g q24h IM	20–40 mg/kg q24h IM	Free		D

*Average wholesale price according to the 1995 Red Book.
†FDA pregnancy categories: A, adequate studies in pregnant women, no risk; B, animal studies no risk, human studies inadequate, or animal toxicity, human studies no risk; C, animal studies show toxicity, human studies inadequate but benefit may exceed risk; D, evidence of human risk, benefit may outweight risk; X, fetal abnormalities in humans, risk exceeds benefit.
‡Use in breastfeeding: limited data are available. Since all drugs are probably excreted in small amounts into breast milk, the potential for adverse reactions in the infant must be considered, although few have been reported. "Probably safe" indicates that breastfeeding can be continued during treatment based on information available at present. "Avoid if possible" indicates that an alternate drug should be chosen or consideration given to discontinuing breastfeeding.
§Insufficient information available to make a recommendation.
CRCl, creatinine clearance ml/min; HD, hemodialysis; PD, peritoneal dialysis; N.A., not approved; GI, gastrointestinal; N.R., not recommended; pHD, posthemodialysis; pPD, postperitoneal dialysis; CNS, central nervous system.

USE IN BREASTFEEDING‡	DOSE INTERVAL ADJUSTMENT FOR REDUCED CRCL			SUPPLEMENTAL DOSE IN DIALYSIS		MAJOR TOXICITY
	>50	10–50	<10	HD	PD	
Probably safe	q24h	7.5 mg/kg q24–48h	7.5 mg/kg 2 × /wk	§	§	Renal and cranial nerve VIII toxicity, hypokalemia, sterile abscesses at injection site
Avoid if possible	q24h	q24h	q24h	§	§	Hyperpigmentation, ichthyosis, dry eyes, GI disturbance
Avoid if possible	q12h	q24h	0.25g q24h	§	§	Anxiety, depression, confusion, hallucinations, headache, peripheral neuropathy
§	q24h	q24–36h	q48h	15 mg/kg/day pHD	15 mg/kg/day	Optic neuritis, allergic reactions, GI disturbance, acute gout
§	q12h	q12h	5 mg/kg q24h	§	§	GI disturbance, liver toxicity, CNS disturbance
Probably safe	q24h	q24h	½ dose in slow acetylators	5 mg/kg pHD	Daily dose pPd	Peripheral neuropathy, liver toxicity (possibly fatal), glossitis, GI disturbance, fever
§	§	§	§	§	§	GI disturbance
Avoid if possible	q24h	q24h	12–20 mg/kg q24h	§	§	Arthralgia, hyperuricemia, liver toxicity, GI disturbance, rash
Avoid if possible	§	§	§	§	§	Uveitis, orange discoloration of urine, sweat, tears; liver toxicity, GI disturbance
Avoid if possible	q24h	q24h	q24h	§	§	Orange discoloration of urine, sweat, tears; liver toxicity, GI disturbance, flulike syndrome
Avoid if possible	q24h	q24–72h	q72–96h	0.5 g pHD	§	Vestibular nerve damage, paresthesias, rash, fever, pruritus, renal toxicity

Table 3 Antifungal Agents

NAME		USUAL DOSE		COST (PER DAY)*	CHANGE IN ABSORPTION WITH FOOD	PREGNANCY CLASS†
GENERIC	BRAND	ADULT	PEDIATRIC			
Amphotericin B	Fungizone	0.25–1 mg/kg q24h IV	0.25–1 mg/kg q24–48h IV	$29.64		B
Clotrimazole	Mycelex	10 mg PO 5 × /day	§	$3.75	Not absorbed	C
Fluconazole	Diflucan	0.05–0.4 g q24h PO, IV	3–6 mg/kg qd (N.A.)	$6.80 PO $81.25 IV	Unchanged	C
Flucytosine	Ancobon	50–150 mg/kg/day; divide q6h PO	50–150 mg/kg/day; divide q6h PO	$15.50	Decreased	C
Griseofulvin	Grisactin, Grifulvin, Fulvicin	0.5–1 g q24h PO	15 mg/kg/day; q24h PO	$1.06	Increased	C
Itraconazole	Sporanox	0.2–0.4 g q24h PO	§	$10.78	Increased	C
Ketoconazole	Nizoral	0.2–0.4 g q12–24h PO	5–10 mg/kg/day; divide q12–24h PO	$5.41	Increased	C
Miconazole	Monostat	0.4–1.2 g q8h IV	20–40 mg/kg/day; divide q8h IV	$230.82		C
Nystatin	Mycostatin	400,000–1,000,000 U q8h PO	400,000–600,000 U q6h PO	$3.89 (20 ml)	Not absorbed	C

*Average wholesale price according to the 1995 Red Book.
†FDA pregnancy categories: A, adequate studies in pregnant women, no risk; B, animal studies no risk, human studies inadequate, or animal toxicity, human studies no risk; C, animal studies show toxicity, human studies inadequate but benefit may exceed risk; D, evidence of human risk, benefit may outweight risk; X, fetal abnormalities in humans, risk exceeds benefit.
‡Use in breastfeeding: limited data are available. Since all drugs are probably excreted in small amounts into breast milk, the potential for adverse reactions in the infant must be considered, although few have been reported. "Probably safe" indicates that breastfeeding can be continued during treatment based on information available at present. "Avoid if possible" indicates that an alternate drug should be chosen or consideration given to discontinuing breastfeeding.
§Insufficient information available to make a recommendation.
CRCl, creatinine clearance ml/min; HD, hemodialysis; PD, peritoneal dialysis; N.A., not approved; GI, gastrointestinal; N.R., not recommended; pHD, posthemodialysis; pPD, postperitoneal dialysis; CNS, central nervous system.

USE IN BREASTFEEDING‡	DOSE INTERVAL ADJUSTMENT FOR REDUCED CRCL			SUPPLEMENTAL DOSE IN DIALYSIS		MAJOR TOXICITY
	>50	10–50	<10	HD	PD	
Avoid if possible	q24h	q24h	q24h	Usual	Usual	Fever, chills, nausea with infusion; renal insufficiency, anemia
Probably safe	§	§	§	§	§	
Avoid if possible	q24h	50% dose q24h	25% dose q24h	§	§	Nausea, vomiting, rash, elevated liver enzymes
Avoid if possible	q6h	q12–24h	15–25 mg/kg q24h	20–37.5 mg/kg pHD	§	Leukopenia
§	q24h	q24h	q24h	§	§	GI disturbance, allergic and photosensitivity reactions, blood dyscrasias, liver toxicity, exacerbation of SLE and leprosy
Avoid if possible	q12–24h	§	§	§	§	Nausea, rash, headache, edema, hypokalemia, hepatotoxicity
Avoid if possible	q12–24h	Usual	Usual	Usual	Usual	Nausea, vomiting, gynecomastia, decreased testosterone synthesis, rash, hepatotoxicity, adrenal insufficiency
§	q8h	q8h	q8h	§	§	Phlebitis, thrombocytosis, pruritus, rash, blurred vision, anaphylaxis (rare)
Probably safe	q8h	q8h	q8h	§	§	GI disturbance, allergic reactions

Table 4 Antiviral Agents

NAME		USUAL DOSE		COST (PER DAY)*	CHANGE IN ABSORPTION WITH FOOD	PREGNANCY CLASS†
GENERIC	BRAND	ADULT	PEDIATRIC			
Acyclovir	Zovirax	0.2–0.8 g 2–5 × / day PO 5–12 mg/kg q8h IV	0.2 g 5 × /day (HSV) PO 20 mg/kg q6h PO, max 800 mg q6h (VZV) 25–50 mg/ kg/day q8h IV	$4.88 PO (200 mg) $18.40 (800 mg) $229.00 IV (10 mg/kg dose)	Unchanged	C
Amantadine	Symmetrel	0.1 g q12h PO	2.2–4.4 mg/kg q12h PO	$0.84	No data	C
Cidofovir	Vistide	5 mg/kg IV q wk × 2 wks, then 5 mg/kg q2wks	§	$100.97		C
Didanosine	Videx	0.167–0.2 g q12h PO	0.143–0.248 mg/m² divided q12h PO	$5.76	Decreased	B
Famciclovir	Famvir	0.125 g q12h PO (HSV) 0.5 g q8h PO (VZV)	§	$18.45	Unchanged	B
Foscarnet	Foscavir	60 mg/kg q8h IV × 14–21 days; then 90 mg/kg/day	§	$145.92		C
Ganciclovir	Cytovene	5 mg/kg q12h IV × 14–21 days; then 5 mg/kg/day or 1 g t.i.d. PO	5 mg/kg q12h IV	$52.20		C
Indinavir	Crixivan	800 mg po q8h	§	$12.00	Decreased	C
Lamivudine	Epivir	150 mg po q12h	4 mg/kg po q12h	$7.46	Unchanged	C
Nevirapine	Ciramune	200 mg po q24h × 14d, then 200 mg po q12h	§	$8.25	Unchanged	C
Ribavirin	Virazole	12–18 hr qd × 3 days via aerosol, PO, IV investiga- tional	12–22 hr qd × 6 days via aerosol	Not available		X
Rimantadine	Flumadine	0.1 g q12h PO	§	$2.55	Unchanged	C
Ritonavir	Norvir	600 mg po q12h	§	$22.26	Unchanged	B
Saquinavir	Invirase	600 mg po q8h	§	$19.00	Increased	B
Stavudine	Zerit	0.04 g q12h PO	§	$7.50	Unchanged	C
Valacyclovir	Valtrex	1 g po tid (V2V) 0.5 g po bic (HSV)	Unchanged	B		
Vidarabine	Vira-A	10–15 mg/kg/day over 12h IV	10–15 mg/kg/day over 12h IV	Not available		Not established
Zalcitabine	Hivid	0.375–0.75 g q8h PO	0.75 g q8h PO (children >13 years)	$5.34	Decreased	C
Zidovudine	Retrovir	0.1 g q4h PO or 0.2 g q8h PO 1–2 mg/kg q4h IV	180 mg/m² q6h PO	$7.74	Decreased	C

*Average wholesale price according to the 1995 Red Book.

†FDA pregnancy categories: A, adequate studies in pregnant women, no risk; B, animal studies no risk, human studies inadequate, or animal toxicity, human studies no risk; C, animal studies show toxicity, human studies inadequate but benefit may exceed risk; D, evidence of human risk, benefit may outweight risk; X, fetal abnormalities in humans, risk exceeds benefit.

‡Use in breastfeeding: limited data are available. Since all drugs are probably excreted in small amounts into breast milk, the potential for adverse reactions in the infant must be considered, although few have been reported. "Probably safe" indicates that breastfeeding can be

USE IN BREASTFEEDING‡	DOSE INTERVAL ADJUSTMENT FOR REDUCED CRCL			SUPPLEMENTAL DOSE IN DIALYSIS		MAJOR TOXICITY
	>50	10–50	<10	HD	PD	
Probably safe	2–5 × /day PO q8h IV	2–5 × /day PO q12–24h IV	0.2–0.8 g q24h PO 2.5–6 mg/kg q24h IV	0.5 g PO pHD	2–5 mg/kg/day	Headache, rash, renal toxicity, CNS symptoms (rare)
Avoid if possible	q12h	0.1–0.2 g 2–3 × /wk	0.1–0.2 g qwk	§	§	Livedo reticularis, edema, insomnia, dizziness, lethargy
Avoid if possible	Check prescribing information	Check prescribing information	Check prescribing information	§	§	Proteinuria, renal insufficiency, neutropenia
Avoid if possible	q12h	q12–24h	100 mg q24h PO	Dose pHD	§	Diarrhea, nausea, vomiting, pancreatitis, peripheral neuropathy
Avoid if possible	0.5g q8h 0.125 g q12h	0.5 g q12–24h 0.125 g q12–24h	0.25 g q48h 0.125 g q48h		ND	Headache, nausea
Probably safe	63–90 mg/kg/day maintenance	78–63 mg/kg/day maintenance	§	§	§	Renal dysfunction, anemia, nausea, disturbances of calcium, magnesium, phosphorus, potassium metabolism
Avoid if possible	q12h	2.5 mg/kg q24h	1.25 mg/kg q24h	1.25 mg/kg pHD	§	Neutropenia, thrombocytopenia
Avoid if possible	§	§	§	§	§	Nephrolithiasis, nausea, headache
Avoid if possible	150 mg po q12h	100–150 g po q D	25–50 mg po q D	§	§	Headache, nausea, neutropenia, increased AST, ALT.
Avoid if possible	§	§	§	§	§	Rash, including Stevens-Johnsons Syndrome; hepatotoxicity
Avoid if possible	§	§	§	§	§	Anemia, headache, hyperbilirubinemia, bronchospasm
Avoid if possible	q12h	q12h	q12h	§	§	Fewer CNS side effects than amantadine
Avoid if possible	Usual	Usual	Usual	Usual	Usual	Nausea, vomiting, diarrhea.
Avoid if possible	§	§	§	§	§	Diarrhea
Avoid if possible	§	§	§	§	§	Peripheral neuropathy, liver toxicity
Probably safe	Usual	112–24h	0.5 g q24h	0.5 g q24h	0.5 g q24h	Nausea, headache; thrombotic thrombocytopenic purpura in immunocompromised pts.
§	Usual	Usual	10 mg/kg/day over 12h	Usual dose pHD	§	GI disturbance, nausea, vomiting, thrombophlebitis
Avoid if possible	q8h	q12h	q24h	§	§	Peripheral neuropathy, stomatitis, esophageal ulcers, pancreatitis
Avoid if possible	q4h	q6h	q6–12h	100 mg pHD	100 mg q6–12h	Anemia, granulocytopenia, headache, nausea, insomnia, nail pigment changes

continued during treatment based on information available at present. "Avoid if possible" indicates that an alternate drug should be chosen or consideration given to discontinuing breastfeeding.

§Insufficient information available to make a recommendation.

CRCl, creatinine clearance ml/min; HD, hemodialysis; PD, peritoneal dialysis; N.A., not approved; GI, gastrointestinal; N.R., not recommended; pHD, posthemodialysis; pPD, postperitoneal dialysis; CNS, central nervous system.

Table 5 Antiparasitic Agents

NAME		USUAL DOSE		COST (PER DAY)*	CHANGE IN ABSORPTION WITH FOOD	PREGNANCY CLASS†
GENERIC	BRAND	ADULT	PEDIATRIC			
Albendazole‖	Zentel	15 mg/kg qd PO	§	Not listed		Not established
Artemisinin#		10 mg/kg qd × 5 days	Same as adult	Not listed		Not established
Atovoquone	Mepron	750 mg t.i.d. PO	§	$24.92	Increased	C
Benznidazole#		5 mg/kg b.i.d. PO 1–4 mo	§	Not listed		Not established
Bithionol¶	Bitin	30–50 mg/kg on alternate days × 10–15 days.	Same as adult	Not listed		Not established
Chloroquine HCL	Aralen HCL	200 mg q6h IM 300 mg qwk PO (prophylaxis) 600 mg PO, then 300 mg after 6, 24, 48 h (treatment)	5 mg/kg qwk PO (for prophylaxis) 10 mg/kg, then 5 mg/kg, same intervals as adult (treatment) IM treatment not recommended	$230.98 IM	Increased	C
Chloroquine phosphate	Aralen phosphate	500 mg qwk PO (prophylaxis) 1 g, then 500 mg after 6, 24, 48 h (treatment)	8.3 mg/kg qwk PO (prophylaxis)	$18.32 (2 day treatment course)	Increased	C
Dehydroemetine†		1–1.5 mg/kg/day IM (maximum dose 90 mg)	1–1.5 mg/kg IM qd, divided in 2 doses	Not listed		Not established
Diethyl carbamazine‖	Hetrazan	Day 1: 50 mg × 1 PO 2: 50 mg t.i.d. 3: 50 mg t.i.d. 4–21: 6 mg/kg/day divided t.i.d.	Day 1: 1 mg/kg × 1 PO 2: 1 mg/kg t.i.d. 3: 1–2 mg/kg t.i.d. 4–21: 6 mg/kg/day divided t.i.d.	Not listed		Not established

*Average wholesale price according to the 1995 Red Book.
†FDA pregnancy categories: A, adequate studies in pregnant women, no risk; B, animal studies no risk, human studies inadequate, or animal toxicity, human studies no risk; C, animal studies show toxicity, human studies inadequate but benefit may exceed risk; D, evidence of human risk, benefit may outweight risk; X, fetal abnormalities in humans, risk exceeds benefit.
‡Use in breastfeeding: limited data are available. Since all drugs are probably excreted in small amounts into breast milk, the potential for adverse reactions in the infant must be considered, although few have been reported. "Probably safe" indicates that breastfeeding can be continued during treatment based on information available at present. "Avoid if possible" indicates that an alternate drug should be chosen or consideration given to discontinuing breastfeeding.
§Insufficient information available to make a recommendation.
‖Available in the United States only from the manufacturer.
¶Available from the Centers for Disease Control and Prevention drug service.
#Not available in the United States.
CRCl, creatinine clearance ml/min; HD, hemodialysis; PD, peritoneal dialysis; AST, aspartate aminotransaminase; ALT, alanine aminotransferase; GI, gastrointestinal; G6PD, glucose-6 phosphate dehydrogenase; AIDS, acquired immunodeficiency syndrome; N.R., not recommended; p.c., after meals; CSF, cerebrospinal fluid.

USE IN BREASTFEEDING‡	DOSE INTERVAL ADJUSTMENT FOR REDUCED CRCL			SUPPLEMENTAL DOSE IN DIALYSIS		MAJOR TOXICITY
	>50	10–50	<10	HD	PD	
§	§	§	§	§	§	Diarrhea, abdominal discomfort, elevated AST, ALT, bone marrow suppression, alopecia with high dose
§	§	§	§	§	§	Transient heart block, elevated AST, ALT, neutropenia, decreased reticulocyte count, abdominal pain, diarrhea, fever
Probably safe	§	§	§	§	§	Rash, GI disturbance, fever, headache
§	§	§	§	§	§	Peripheral neuropathy, rash, bone marrow suppression
§	§	§	§	§	§	
Avoid if possible	§	§	§	§	§	Blurred vision (retinopathy with prolonged use), GI effects, pruritus, hemolysis in patients with G6PD deficiency
Avoid if possible	§	§	§	§	§	Blurred vision (retinopathy with prolonged use), GI effects, pruritus, hemolysis in patients with G6PD deficiency
§	§	§	§	§	§	Diarrhea, nausea, vomiting, cardiac arrhythmias, tachycardia
§	§	§	§	§	§	Headache, malaise, arthralgia, nausea, vomiting, anorexia, pruritus, fever, hypotension, lymphadenitis, encephalopathy

Continued.

Table 5 Antiparasitic Agents–cont'd

NAME		USUAL DOSE		COST (PER DAY)*	CHANGE IN ABSORPTION WITH FOOD	PREGNANCY CLASS†
GENERIC	BRAND	ADULT	PEDIATRIC			
Diloxanide furoate¶	Furamide	500 mg t.i.d. × 10 days	20 mg/kg/day divided t.i.d. × 10 days	Not listed		Not established
Eflornithine‖		400 mg/kg/day IV divided q.i.d. × 14 days then 300 mg/kg/day × 3–4 wk PO	§	Not listed		Not established
Furazolidone	Furoxone	100 mg q6h PO	25–50 mg q6h PO	$7.91		Not established
Halofantrine	Halfan	500 mg q6h PO × 3, repeat in 1 wk	8 mg/kg q6h PO × 3 (pt <40 kg), repeat in 1 wk	Not listed		Not established
Hydroxychloroquine	Plaquenil	400 mg qwk PO (prophylaxis) 800 mg, then 400 mg after 6, 24, 48 h (treatment)	5 mg/kg/qwk PO (prophylaxis) 10 mg/kg, then 5 mg/kg at same intervals as adult (treatment)	$11.59 (2 day treatment course)		C
Iodoquinol	Yodoxin, Diquinol	650 mg t.i.d. PO	30–40 mg/kg/day; divide t.i.d. PO	$1.21	Minimally absorbed	Not established
Ivermectin¶	Mectizan	200 units/kg/day 0.15 mg/kg/day PO	§	Not listed		Not established
Mebendazole	Vermox	100–400 mg q8–24h PO depending on infection being treated	Same as adults	$4.83	Minimally absorbed	B
Mefloquine	Lariam	1,250 mg qwk PO	25 mg/kg qwk PO	$22.24		C
Meglumine antimonate	Glucantine	20 mg/kg IV × 2 days (850 mg/day limit)	§	Not listed		Not established
Melarsoprol B¶	Mel B, Arsobal	1.2 mg/kg t.i.d. IV × 3 days; repeat qwk × 2	§	Not listed		Not established

*Average wholesale price according to the 1995 Red Book.
†FDA pregnancy categories: A, adequate studies in pregnant women, no risk; B, animal studies no risk, human studies inadequate, or animal toxicity, human studies no risk; C, animal studies show toxicity, human studies inadequate but benefit may exceed risk; D, evidence of human risk, benefit may outweight risk; X, fetal abnormalities in humans, risk exceeds benefit.
‡Use in breastfeeding: limited data are available. Since all drugs are probably excreted in small amounts into breast milk, the potential for adverse reactions in the infant must be considered, although few have been reported. "Probably safe" indicates that breastfeeding can be continued during treatment based on information available at present. "Avoid if possible" indicates that an alternate drug should be chosen or consideration given to discontinuing breastfeeding.
§Insufficient information available to make a recommendation.
‖Available in the United States only from the manufacturer.
¶Available from the Centers for Disease Control and Prevention drug service.
#Not available in the United States.
CRCl, creatinine clearance ml/min; HD, hemodialysis; PD, peritoneal dialysis; AST, aspartate aminotransaminase; ALT, alanine aminotransferase; GI, gastrointestinal; G6PD, glucose-6 phosphate dehydrogenase; AIDS, acquired immunodeficiency syndrome; N.R., not recommended; p.c., after meals; CSF, cerebrospinal fluid.

USE IN BREASTFEEDING‡	DOSE INTERVAL ADJUSTMENT FOR REDUCED CRCL			SUPPLEMENTAL DOSE IN DIALYSIS		MAJOR TOXICITY
	>50	10–50	<10	HD	PD	
§	§	§	§	§	§	Flatulence
§	§	§	§	§	§	Anemia, thrombocytopenia, leukopenia, nausea, vomiting, diarrhea, transient hearing loss
§	§	§	§	§	§	Nausea, vomiting, rash, fever, headache, hemolysis in patients with G6PD deficiency
§	§	§	§	§	§	Abdominal pain, vomiting, diarrhea, headache, pruritus, rash
Avoid if possible	§	§	§	§	§	Blurred vision, GI effects, pruritus; rare: cardiomyopathy
§	§	§	§	§	§	Optic neuritis, peripheral neuropathy, anorexia, nausea, vomiting, diarrhea, skin reactions
§	§	§	§	§	§	Fever, pruritus, headache, edema
Probably safe	§	§	§	§	§	Diarrhea, nausea, vomiting, abdominal pain, fever, headache, neutropenia, thrombocytopenia
§	§	§	§	§	§	Nausea, dizziness, seizures, bradycardia, rash
§	§	§	§	§	§	
§	§	§	§	§	§	Fever, hypertension, abdominal pain, vomiting, arthralgia, encephalopathy, rash, hemolysis in patients with G6PD deficiency

Continued.

Table 5 Antiparasitic Agents–cont'd

NAME		USUAL DOSE		COST (PER DAY)*	CHANGE IN ABSORPTION WITH FOOD	PREGNANCY CLASS†
GENERIC	BRAND	ADULT	PEDIATRIC			
Niclosamide	Niclocide	2 g qd PO	0.5–1.5 g qd PO	$11.07	Not absorbed	B
Nifurtimox¶	Lampit	3 mg/kg t.i.d. PO × 3 mos	§	Not listed		Not established
Niridazole	Ambilhar	§	§	Not listed		Not established
Oxamniquine	Vansil	12–60 mg/kg qd or divide b.i.d.	20–60 mg/kg divided b.i.d.	$15.30	Decreased	Not established
Paromomycin	Humatin	25–35 mg/kg PO divided t.i.d. 2–3 g qd divided q.i.d. in AIDS	§	$15.08	Not absorbed	Not established
Pentamidine	Pentam, Nebupent	3–4 mg/kg/qd IV 300 mg aerosolized qmo	3–4 mg/kg qd IV	$98.75 IV $98.75 aer		C
Piperazine citrate	Antepar	2–3.5g qd PO	65–75 mg/kg qd PO	$0.26		Not established
Praziquantel	Bitricide	5–25 mg/kg × 1 (intestinal cestodiasis) 50–75 mg/kg qd, divided t.i.d. other infections	Not shown to be safe for children under 4	$30.94		B

*Average wholesale price according to the 1995 Red Book.
†FDA pregnancy categories: A, adequate studies in pregnant women, no risk; B, animal studies no risk, human studies inadequate, or animal toxicity, human studies no risk; C, animal studies show toxicity, human studies inadequate but benefit may exceed risk; D, evidence of human risk, benefit may outweight risk; X, fetal abnormalities in humans, risk exceeds benefit.
‡Use in breastfeeding: limited data are available. Since all drugs are probably excreted in small amounts into breast milk, the potential for adverse reactions in the infant must be considered, although few have been reported. "Probably safe" indicates that breastfeeding can be continued during treatment based on information available at present. "Avoid if possible" indicates that an alternate drug should be chosen or consideration given to discontinuing breastfeeding.
§Insufficient information available to make a recommendation.
||Available in the United States only from the manufacturer.
¶Available from the Centers for Disease Control and Prevention drug service.
#Not available in the United States.
CRCl, creatinine clearance ml/min; HD, hemodialysis; PD, peritoneal dialysis; AST, aspartate aminotransaminase; ALT, alanine aminotransferase; GI, gastrointestinal; G6PD, glucose-6 phosphate dehydrogenase; AIDS, acquired immunodeficiency syndrome; N.R., not recommended; p.c., after meals; CSF, cerebrospinal fluid.

USE IN BREASTFEEDING‡	DOSE INTERVAL ADJUSTMENT FOR REDUCED CRCL			SUPPLEMENTAL DOSE IN DIALYSIS		MAJOR TOXICITY
	>50	10–50	<10	HD	PD	
Probably safe	§	§	§	§	§	Nausea, abdominal discomfort, diarrhea, drowsiness, dizziness, headache
§	§	§	§	§	§	Nausea, vomiting, abdominal pain, anorexia, weight loss, restlessness, insomnia, paresthesias, seizures, rash, neutropenia
§	§	§	§	§	§	
	§	§	§	§	§	Dizziness, drowsiness, headache, nausea, vomiting, abdominal pain, orange-red discoloration of urine
Probably safe	§	§	§	§	§	Anorexia, nausea, vomiting, abdominal pain, diarrhea, malabsorption
Probably safe	§	§	§	§	§	Nephrotoxicity, hypotension, sterile abscess with IM injection, hypoglycemia or hyperglycemia, nausea, vomiting, abdominal pain, pancreatitis, hypocalcemia, cough and bronchospasm with inhalation
Probably safe	§	§	§	§	§	Nausea, vomiting, diarrhea, abdominal cramps, headache, dizziness, rash, hemolytic anemia, ataxia
Avoid if possible	Usual dose	N.R.	N.R.	§	§	Transient dizziness, headache, drowiness, fatigue, seizures, CSF reaction syndrome with treatment of neurocysticercosis, abdominal pain, nausea, rash

Continued.

Table 5 Antiparasitic Agents–cont'd

NAME		USUAL DOSE		COST (PER DAY)*	CHANGE IN ABSORPTION WITH FOOD	PREGNANCY CLASS†
GENERIC	BRAND	ADULT	PEDIATRIC			
Primaquine phosphate		26.3 mg qd PO × 14 days 29 mg qwk PO × 8 wk	0.5 mg/kg qd PO 1.5 mg/kg qwk PO	$0.64		Not established
Proguanil#	Paludrine	200 mg qd PO	<2 yr 50 mg qd PO 2–6 yr 100 mg PO 7–10 yr 150 mg PO >10 yr 200 mg PO	Not listed		Not established
Pyrantel pamoate	Antiminth	11 mg/kg (max 1 g) qd PO	11 mg/kg qd PO; not recommended for children <2yr	Not listed		Not established
Pyrimethamine	Daraprim	25–75 mg qd PO	0.5–2 mg/kg PO, divide b.i.d. Contraindicated for children <2 yr	$0.75		C
Pyrimethamine + sulfadiazine	Fansidar	1 tab qwk PO (prophylaxis) 3 tabs PO × 1 (treatment)	½ tab PO 5–10 kg 1 tab 10–20 kg 1½ tab 21–30 kg 2 tabs 31–40 kg For children >2 yr	$3.23/wk (prophylaxis) $9.71 (treatment course)		C
Quinacrine HCl	Atabrine	100 mg t.i.d. p.c. × 5 days	6 mg/kg t.i.d. p.c. × 5 days (<50 kg)	Not listed		C
Quinidine		10 mg/kg load over 1–2 hr, then 0.02 mg/kg/min × 72 hr	Same as adult	$55.08		C
Quinine	Legatrin Quinamm	325–650 g PO b.i.d.–t.i.d.	25–30 mg/kg/day PO; divide t.i.d.	$5.40		X

*Average wholesale price according to the 1995 Red Book.
†FDA pregnancy categories: A, adequate studies in pregnant women, no risk; B, animal studies no risk, human studies inadequate, or animal toxicity, human studies no risk; C, animal studies show toxicity, human studies inadequate but benefit may exceed risk; D, evidence of human risk, benefit may outweight risk; X, fetal abnormalities in humans, risk exceeds benefit.
‡Use in breastfeeding: limited data are available. Since all drugs are probably excreted in small amounts into breast milk, the potential for adverse reactions in the infant must be considered, although few have been reported. "Probably safe" indicates that breastfeeding can be continued during treatment based on information available at present. "Avoid if possible" indicates that an alternate drug should be chosen or consideration given to discontinuing breastfeeding.
§Insufficient information available to make a recommendation.
||Available in the United States only from the manufacturer.
¶Available from the Centers for Disease Control and Prevention drug service.
#Not available in the United States.
CRCl, creatinine clearance ml/min; HD, hemodialysis; PD, peritoneal dialysis; AST, aspartate aminotransaminase; ALT, alanine aminotransferase; GI, gastrointestinal; G6PD, glucose-6 phosphate dehydrogenase; AIDS, acquired immunodeficiency syndrome; N.R., not recommended; p.c., after meals; CSF, cerebrospinal fluid.

USE IN BREASTFEEDING‡	DOSE INTERVAL ADJUSTMENT FOR REDUCED CRCL			SUPPLEMENTAL DOSE IN DIALYSIS		MAJOR TOXICITY
	>50	10–50	<10	HD	PD	
Avoid if possible	§	§	§	§	§	Hemolytic anemia in patients with G6PD deficiency, nausea, vomiting, abdominal cramps, headache, pruritus
§	§	§	§	§	§	Rare hematologic toxicity
Probably safe	§	§	§	§	§	Nausea, vomiting, cramps, dizziness, drowsiness, headache
Probably safe	§	§	§	§	§	Bone marrow suppression with high doses, pulmonary eosinophilia, photosensitivity
Probably safe	§	§	§	§	§	Leukopenia, hemolysis in patients with G6PD deficiency, rash and hypersensitivity reactions including Stevens-Johnson syndrome, hepatitis, pulmonary hypersensitivity reactions
§	§	§	§	§	§	Nausea, vomiting, headache, dizziness, yellow discoloration of skin and urine, rash, fever, psychosis
	§	§	§	§	§	Diarrhea, abdominal pain, hypersensitivity reactions, systemic lupus erythematosus like syndrome, elevated AST, elevated alkaline phosphatase, jaundice, cardiac arrhythmias
	§	§	§	§	§	Flushing, pruritus, rash, fever, tinnitus, headache, nausea, thrombocytopenia, hemolysis in patients with G6PD deficiency, hypoglycemia

Continued.

Table 5 Antiparasitic Agents–cont'd

NAME		USUAL DOSE		COST (PER DAY)*	CHANGE IN ABSORPTION WITH FOOD	PREGNANCY CLASS†
GENERIC	BRAND	ADULT	PEDIATRIC			
Spiramycin#		3 g qd PO	§	Not listed		
Stibogluconate¶	Pentostam	20 mg/kg IV qd × 20 days (not to exceed 850 mg)	§	Not listed		Not established
Suramin¶	Germanin	1 g IV qwk × 5 wks (100 mg test dose)	§	Not listed		Not established
Thiabendazole	Mintizol	25 mg/kg PO b.i.d. (max 3 g qd)	22 mg/kg b.i.d. PO	$5.86		Not established
Trimetrexate	Neutrexin	45 mg/m^2 qd with leucovorin 20 mg/m^2 q6h; continue leucovorin at least 72 hr after last dose	§	$150.00 + $66.00 leucovorin		Not established

*Average wholesale price according to the 1995 Red Book.

†FDA pregnancy categories: A, adequate studies in pregnant women, no risk; B, animal studies no risk, human studies inadequate, or animal toxicity, human studies no risk; C, animal studies show toxicity, human studies inadequate but benefit may exceed risk; D, evidence of human risk, benefit may outweight risk; X, fetal abnormalities in humans, risk exceeds benefit.

‡Use in breastfeeding: limited data are available. Since all drugs are probably excreted in small amounts into breast milk, the potential for adverse reactions in the infant must be considered, although few have been reported. "Probably safe" indicates that breastfeeding can be continued during treatment based on information available at present. "Avoid if possible" indicates that an alternate drug should be chosen or consideration given to discontinuing breastfeeding.

§Insufficient information available to make a recommendation.

||Available in the United States only from the manufacturer.

¶Available from the Centers for Disease Control and Prevention drug service.

#Not available in the United States.

CRCl, creatinine clearance ml/min; HD, hemodialysis; PD, peritoneal dialysis; AST, aspartate aminotransaminase; ALT, alanine aminotransferase; GI, gastrointestinal; G6PD, glucose-6 phosphate dehydrogenase; AIDS, acquired immunodeficiency syndrome; N.R., not recommended; p.c., after meals; CSF, cerebrospinal fluid.

USE IN BREASTFEEDING‡	DOSE INTERVAL ADJUSTMENT FOR REDUCED CRCL			SUPPLEMENTAL DOSE IN DIALYSIS		MAJOR TOXICITY
	>50	10–50	<10	HD	PD	
	§	§	§	§	§	
§	§	§	§	§	§	Abdominal pain; nausea; vomiting; malaise; headache; elevated AST, ALT; nephrotoxicity; myalgia; arthralgia; fever; rash; cough
§	§	§	§	§	§	Nausea, vomiting, shock, loss of consciousness, death during administration; fever, rash, exfoliative dermatis, paresthesia, photophobia, renal insufficiency, diarrhea
§	§	§	§	§	§	Anorexia, nausea, vomiting, dizziness
§	§	§	§	§	§	Neutropenia (must be given with leucovorin); rash; elevated AST, ALT; reversible peripheral neuropathy

Suggested Reading

American Academy of Pediatrics Committee on Drugs. Transfer of drugs and other chemicals into human milk. *Pediatrics* 1989; 84:924-931.

Drug Topics Red Book. Montvale, NJ: Medical Economics, 1995.

Fulton B, Moore L. The galactopharmacopedia antiinfectives in breastmilk. I: Penicillins and cephalosporins. Journal of Human Lactation 1992; 8:157-158.

Fulton B, Moore L. The galactopharmacopedia antiinfectives in breastmilk. II: Sulfonamides, tetracyclines, macrolides, aminoglycosides and antimalarials. Journal of Human Lactation 1992; 8:221-223.

Fulton B, Moore L. The galactopharmacopedia antiinfectives in breastmilk. III: Antituberculars, quinolones and urinary germicides. Journal of Human Lactation 1993; 9:43-46.

Mandell GL, Douglas RG Jr, Dolin R, et al., eds., Mandell, Douglas, and Bennett's principles and practice of infectious diseases. 4th ed. New York: Churchill Livingstone, 1995.

McEvoy GK. American hospital formulary service drug information 95. Bethesda, MD: American Society of Hospital Pharmacists, 1995.

Nicolau D, Freeman C, Beliveau P, et al. Experience with a once daily aminolgycoside program administered to 2,184 adult patients. Antimicrob Agents Chemother 1995; 650-655.

INDEX

Pages numbers followed by "*f*" indicate figures; page numbers followed by "*t*" indicate tables.

D

O

W

X

Z